evolve
learning system

To access your Student Resources, visit:

http://evolve.elsevier.com/Lowdermilk/MWHC

- Anatomy Reviews
- Animations
- Answers to Clinical Reasoning Exercises
- Assessment Videos
- Audio Glossary
- Audio Key Points
- Care Plan Constructor
- Case Studies
- Childbirth Videos
- Critical Thinking Exercises
- Nursing Skills
- Resources
- Review Questions
- Spanish Guidelines

ELSEVIER
MOSBY

ELSEVIER
MOSBY

3251 Riverport Lane
St. Louis, MO 63043

MATERNITY & WOMEN'S HEALTH CARE, 10th ed

ISBN: 978-0-323-07429-2

Notice

Knowledge and best practice in this field are constantly changing. As new research and experience broaden our understanding, changes in research methods, professional practices, or medical treatment may become necessary. Practitioners and researchers must always rely on their own experience and knowledge in evaluating and using any information, methods, compounds, or experiments described herein. In using such information or methods they should be mindful of their own safety and the safety of others, including parties for whom they have a professional responsibility.

With respect to any drug or pharmaceutical products identified, readers are advised to check the most current information provided (i) on procedures featured or (ii) by the manufacturer of each product to be administered, to verify the recommended dose or formula, the method and duration of administration, and contraindications. It is the responsibility of practitioners, relying on their own experience and knowledge of their patients, to make diagnoses, to determine dosages and the best treatment for each individual patient, and to take all appropriate safety precautions.

To the fullest extent of the law, neither the Publisher nor the authors, contributors, or editors, assume any liability for any injury and/or damage to persons or property as a matter of products liability, negligence or otherwise, or from any use or operation of any methods, products, instructions, or ideas contained in the material herein.

The Publisher

ISBN: 978-0-323-07429-2

Executive Editor: Robin Carter
Managing Editor: Laurie K. Gower
Publishing Services Manager: Jeff Patterson
Design Direction: Karen Pauls
Cover Illustration: Sally Wern Comport

Printed in the United States of America

Last digit is the print number: 9 8 7 6 5 4 3

ABOUT THE AUTHORS

DEITRA LEONARD LOWDERMILK

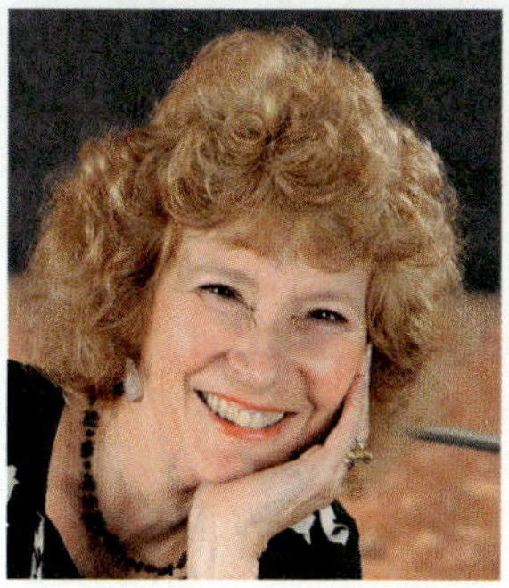

Deitra Leonard Lowdermilk is Clinical Professor Emerita, School of Nursing, University of North Carolina at Chapel Hill. She received her BSN from East Carolina University and her MEd and PhD in Education from UNC-CH. She is certified in In-Patient Obstetrics by the National Certification Corporation. She is a Fellow in the American Academy of Nursing. In addition to being a nurse educator for more than 34 years, Dr. Lowdermilk has clinical experience as a public health nurse and as a staff nurse in labor and delivery, postpartum, and newborn units, and has worked in gynecologic surgery and cancer care units.

Dr. Lowdermilk has been recognized for her expertise in nursing education. She has repeatedly been selected as Classroom and Clinical Teacher of the Year by graduating seniors. She was a recipient of the Educator of the Year Award from both the District IV Association of Women's Health, Obstetric and Neonatal Nurses (AWHONN) and the North Carolina Nurses Association. She also received the 2005 AWHONN Excellence in Education Award.

She is active in AWHONN, having served as Chair of the North Carolina Section of AWHONN and has served as chair and member of various committees in AWHONN at the national, district, state, and local levels. She has served as guest editor for the *Journal of Obstetric, Gynecologic and Neonatal Nursing* and served on editorial boards for other publications.

Dr. Lowdermilk's most significant contribution to nursing has been to promote excellence in nursing practice and education in women's health through integration of knowledge into practice. In 2005 she received the first Distinguished Alumni Award from East Carolina University School of Nursing for her exemplary contributions to the nursing profession in the area of maternal-child care and the community. She was also Alumna of the Year for East Carolina University in 2005, and was selected as one of the 100 Incredible ECU Women in 2007 for Outstanding Leadership Among Women in the first 100 years of the University's founding.

In Fall 2010, the East Carolina University College of Nursing named the Neonatal Intensive Care and Midwifery Laboratory in honor of Dr. Lowdermilk.

SHANNON E. PERRY

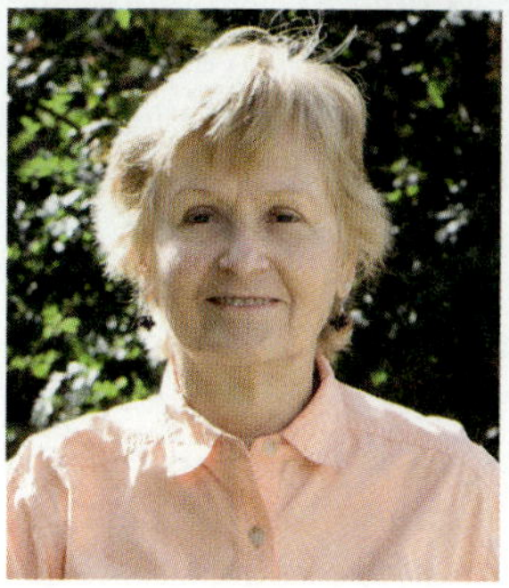

Shannon E. Perry is Professor Emerita, School of Nursing, San Francisco State University. She received her diploma in nursing from St. Joseph Hospital School of Nursing, Bloomington, Illinois; a Baccalaureate in Nursing from Marquette University, an MSN from the University of Colorado Medical Center, and a PhD in Educational Psychology from Arizona State University. She completed a 2-year postdoctoral fellowship in perinatal nursing at the University of California, San Francisco, as a Robert Wood Johnson Clinical Nurse Scholar.

Dr. Perry has had clinical experience as a staff nurse, head nurse, and supervisor in surgical nursing, obstetrics, pediatrics, gynecology, and neonatal nursing. She has served as an expert witness and legal consultant. She has taught in schools of nursing in several states and was interim director and director of the School of Nursing and director of a Child and Adolescent Development baccalaureate program at SFSU. She was Marquette University College of Nursing Alumna of the Year in 1999, was the University of Colorado School of Nursing Distinguished Alumna of the Year in 2000, and received the San Francisco State University Alumni Association Emeritus Faculty Award in 2005.

She is a Fellow in the American Academy of Nursing, a nursing consultant to the International Education Research Foundation, and co-chair of INESA, the International Nursing Education Services and Accreditation, a joint global task force of the National League for Nursing and the National League for Nursing Accreditative Commission.

Dr. Perry's experience in international nursing includes teaching international nursing courses in the United Kingdom, Ireland, Italy, Thailand, Ghana, and China and participating in health missions in Ghana, Kenya, and Honduras. For her "exemplary contributions to nursing, public service, and selfless commitment and passion in shaping the future of international health," she received the President's Award from the Global Caring Nurses Foundation, Inc., in 2008.

KITTY CASHION

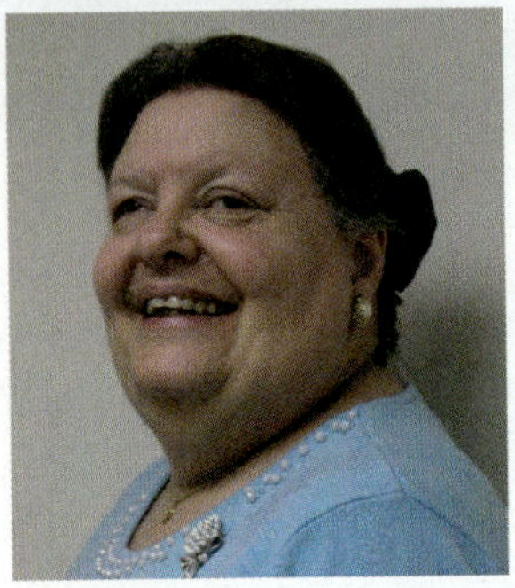

Kitty Cashion is a Clinical Nurse Specialist in the Maternal-Fetal Medicine Division, College of Medicine, Department of Obstetrics and Gynecology at The University of Tennessee Health Science Center in Memphis. She received her BSN from the University of Tennessee College of Nursing in Memphis and her MSN in Parent-Child Nursing from Vanderbilt University School of Nursing in Nashville, Tennessee. Ms. Cashion is certified as a High Risk Perinatal Nurse through the American Nurses Credentialing Center (ANCC).

Ms. Cashion's job responsibilities at the University of Tennessee include providing education regarding low and high risk obstetrics to staff nurses in West Tennessee community hospitals. In addition, she works part-time as a staff nurse in Labor and Delivery at The Regional Medical Center at Memphis (The MED). For more than 15 years, Ms. Cashion has taught Labor and Delivery clinicals for students at Northwest Mississippi Community College in Senatobia, Mississippi, and Union University in Germantown, Tennessee.

Ms. Cashion has been an active AWHONN member, holding office at both the local and state levels. She has also served as an officer and board member of the Tennessee Perinatal Association and as an active volunteer for the Tennessee chapter, March of Dimes Birth Defects Foundation.

Ms. Cashion has contributed many chapters to maternity nursing textbooks over the years. She also coauthored a series of Virtual Clinical Excursions workbooks to accompany six obstetric nursing textbooks published by Elsevier. More recently she served as one of the authors for *Maternity Nursing,* 8th edition and *Clinical Companion for Maternity & Newborn Nursing,* 2nd edition.

KATHRYN RHODES ALDEN

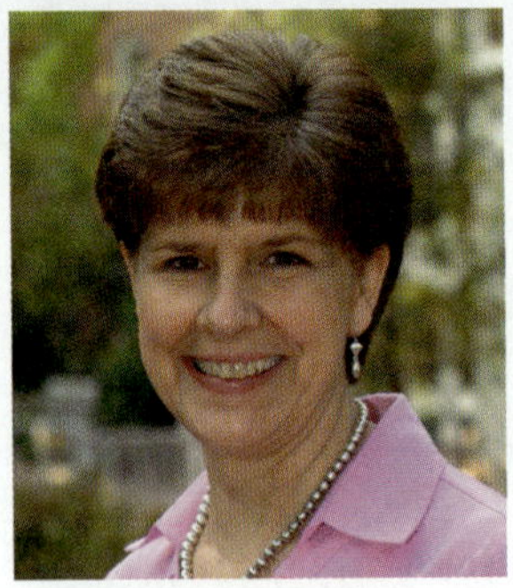

Kathryn Rhodes Alden is Clinical Associate Professor, University of North Carolina at Chapel Hill School of Nursing. She received a BSN from the University of North Carolina at Charlotte, an MSN from the University of North Carolina at Chapel Hill, and a doctorate in adult education from North Carolina State University.

Dr. Alden has extensive experience as a nursing educator. She has more than 25 years experience as an educator for baccalaureate nursing students in maternal-newborn nursing courses. For the past 21 years, Dr. Alden has served on the faculty at the University of North Carolina at Chapel Hill School of Nursing, where she coordinates the maternal-newborn nursing course in the undergraduate program and serves as lead academic counselor for the nursing school. She has been recognized and awarded for her clinical teaching expertise. Dr. Alden has been instrumental in the use of human patient simulation at UNC-Chapel Hill; she has written numerous simulation scenarios and recently developed two obstetric simulation cases for Elsevier. She coauthored a chapter titled "Enhancing Patient Safety in Nursing Education through Patient Simulation" in *Patient Safety and Quality: An Evidence-Based Handbook for Nursing,* published by the Agency for Healthcare Research and Quality (AHRQ).

Dr. Alden is an international board certified lactation consultant and works part-time as a lactation consultant for Rex Healthcare in Raleigh, North Carolina. She teaches prenatal breastfeeding classes to expectant parents and has provided continuing education programs on breastfeeding throughout the state of North Carolina.

She has authored a variety of chapters in maternity texts for Elsevier on endocrine and metabolic disorders of pregnancy; newborn nutrition, assessment, and nursing care; and postpartum care. Her research interests focus on predictors of academic success and retention in baccalaureate nursing students.

CONTRIBUTORS

Dusty Dix, RN, MSN
Clinical Assistant Professor, School of Nursing
University of North Carolina at Chapel Hill
Chapel Hill, North Carolina

Karen F. Dorman, RN, MS
Research Instructor, Obstetrics and Gynecology
University of North Carolina at Chapel Hill
Chapel Hill, North Carolina

Susan M. Ellerbee, PhD, RNC, IBCLC
Associate Professor/BSN Coordinator
University of Oklahoma College of Nursing
Oklahoma City, Oklahoma

Noreen Esposito, EdD, WHNP-BC, FNP-BC
Clinical Associate Professor, School of Nursing
MSN Coordinator, Women's Health Nurse Practitioner Program
University of North Carolina at Chapel Hill
Chapel Hill, North Carolina

Makeba B. Felton, RN, MSN, FNPC, WHNP
Clinical Assistant Professor, College of Nursing and Health Innovation
Arizona State University
Phoenix, Arizona

Anne Hopkins Fishel, PhD, PMH, CNS
Professor Emerita, School of Nursing
University of North Carolina at Chapel Hill
Chapel Hill, North Carolina

Debbie Fraser, MN, RNC-NIC
Associate Professor, Centre for Nursing and Health Studies
St. Boniface General Hospital
Winnipeg, Manitoba, Canada

Pat Mahaffee Gingrich, MSN, WHNP-BC
Clinical Assistant Professor, School of Nursing
University of North Carolina at Chapel Hill
Chapel Hill, North Carolina

Carole Kenner, DNS, BSN, MSN, RNC, FAAN
Dean and Professor, College of Nursing
University of Oklahoma
Oklahoma City, Oklahoma

Denise G. Link, PhD, WHCNP-BC, CNE
Associate Dean, Clinical Practice and Community Partnerships, College of Nursing & Health Innovation
Arizona State University
Phoenix, Arizona

Sharon E. Lock, PhD, ARNP
Associate Professor, College of Nursing
University of Kentucky
Lexington, Kentucky

Jane McAteer, MN, RN
Director of Nursing
College of San Mateo
San Mateo, California

Margaret Shandor Miles, PhD, RN, FAAN
Professor, School of Nursing
University of North Carolina at Chapel Hill
Chapel Hill, North Carolina

Mary Courtney Moore, MSN, PhD, RD
Research Associate Professor, Molecular Physiology and Biophysics
Vanderbilt University School of Medicine
Nashville, Tennessee

Karen A. Piotrowski, RNC, BSN, MSN
Associate Professor, School of Nursing
D'Youville College
Buffalo, New York

Linda Fowler Shahzad, BSN, MSN, RNC
Clinical Nurse II, Women's Services
University of North Carolina at Chapel Hill
Chapel Hill, North Carolina

Lillie D. Shockney, RN, BS, MAS
Administrative Director
University Distinguished Service Associate Professor of Breast Cancer
Associate Professor, Johns Hopkins University School of Medicine
Departments of Surgery/Gynecology and Obstetrics
Associate Professor, School of Nursing
Johns Hopkins Medical Institution
Baltimore, Maryland

Julie Smith Taylor, PhD, RN, WHNP-BC
Assistant Professor/Graduate Coordinator, School of Nursing
University of North Carolina at Wilmington
Wilmington, North Carolina

Marcia Van Riper, PhD, RN
Associate Professor, School of Nursing
Chair, Family Health Division
Carolina Center for Genome Sciences
University of North Carolina at Chapel Hill
Chapel Hill, North Carolina

M. Terese Verklan, PhD, CCNS, RNC, FAAN
Associate Professor, Neonatal Clinical Nurse Specialist
University of Texas Health Science Center at Houston
Staff Nurse, Neonatal Intensive Care Unit
Children's Memorial Hermann Hospital
Houston, Texas

Jan Lamarche Zdanuk, DNP, APRN, FNP-BC, CNS, CWS, FACCWS, FAANP
Clinical Assistant Professor, College of Nursing
University of Texas at Arlington
Arlington, Texas
Family Nurse Practitioner—Board Certified
Clinica Mi Doctor
Fort Worth, Texas

INSTRUCTOR AND STUDENT ANCILLARIES

Case Studies

Stephanie C. Butkus, RN, MSN, CPNP, CLC
Assistant Professor, Division of Nursing
Kettering College of Medical Arts
Kettering, Ohio

Audience Response Questions, Curriculum Guides, PowerPoint Slides, Review Questions, Test Bank

Barbara Pascoe, RN, BA, MA
Director, The Family Place
Concord Hospital
Concord, New Hampshire

Instructor's Manual, Study Guide

Karen A. Piotrowski, RNC, BSN, MSN
Associate Professor, School of Nursing
D'Youville College
Buffalo, New York

REVIEWERS

Sharon Armstrong, MSN, WHNP
Professor of Nursing
St. Clair County Community College
Port Huron, Michigan

Patricia Davidson, MSN, RNC
Assistant Professor/Clinical; Department of Family Nursing Care
University of Texas Health Science Center at San Antonio
San Antonio, Texas

Kathleen K. Furniss, MSN, RNC, DMH
Mountainside Hospital
Montclair, New Jersey

Robin S. Goodrich, EdD (C), MS, RNC-NIC
Assistant Professor, Department of Nursing
Western Connecticut State University
Danbury, Connecticut

Jennifer M. Guay, CNM, MS, BSN
Assistant Professor, School of Nursing
D'Youville College
Kaleida Health, Millard Fillmore Suburban Hospital
Buffalo, New York

Olga Libova, MS, CNM, RN
Nursing Faculty
DeAnza Community College
Cupertino, California

Beryl Stetson, RN, BC, MSN
Assistant Professor, School of Nursing
Raritan Valley Community College
Somerville, New Jersey
Nursing Education Specialist
Robert Wood Johnson University Hospital
New Brunswick, New Jersey

Mary Charles Sutphin MSN, CNM
Clinical Instructor, School of Nursing
University of North Carolina at Chapel Hill
Chapel Hill, North Carolina

PREFACE

WOMEN'S health care encompasses reproductive health care and the unique physical, psychologic, and social needs of women throughout their life span. The specialties of women's health and maternity nursing offer both challenges and opportunities. Nurses are challenged to assimilate knowledge and develop the technical and critical thinking skills needed to provide reflective practice. Each woman, with her individual needs that must be identified and met, presents a challenge. However, the opportunities are sufficiently extraordinary to make this one of the most fulfilling specialties of nursing practice.

The goal of nursing education is to prepare today's students to meet the challenges of tomorrow. This preparation must extend beyond mastery of facts and skills. Nurses must be able to provide safe, quality, client-centered care through the combination of clinical reasoning skills, technical competence, and compassionate caring. They must address the physiologic as well as the psychosocial needs of their clients. They must look beyond the condition and see the woman as an individual with distinctive needs. Yet they must consider her needs in the context of family-centered care, realizing and acknowledging the influence and involvement of family members and significant others. Above all, nurses must strive to improve practice on the basis of sound evidence-based information. In a time of dwindling financial resources for health care, nurses can use evidence-based practice to produce measurable outcomes that can validate their unique and necessary role in the health care delivery system.

Maternity & Women's Health Care was designed to provide students with accurate and up-to-date information so that they can develop the knowledge and skills needed to become clinically competent, to think critically, and to attain the necessary sensitivity to become caring nurses. *Maternity & Women's Health Care* has been a leading maternity nursing text since it was first published in 1977, more than 30 years ago. We are proud of the continued support this text has received. With this tenth edition we have a responsibility to continue this leading tradition.

This tenth edition has been revised and refined in response to comments and suggestions from educators, clinicians, and students. It includes the most accurate, current, and clinically relevant information available. We have had the assistance of expert faculty, nurse clinicians, and specialists from other health disciplines who authored, reviewed, and revised the text. Many exciting updates and new additions will be noted throughout the book; they demonstrate the various dimensions of women's health care and areas of rapid and complex changes such as genetics, fetal assessment, and alternative therapies. However, we have retained the underlying philosophy that has been the strength of previous editions: our belief that pregnancy and childbirth and developmental changes in a woman's life are natural processes. We have also retained a base in physiology and a strong, integrated focus on the family and on evidence-based practice.

The text is also used as a reference for the practicing nurse. The most recent recommendations based on evidence from research and clinical experts have been included from professional organizations such as the Association of Women's Health, Obstetric and Neonatal Nurses; the National Association of Neonatal Nurses; the American College of Obstetricians and Gynecologists; the American Academy of Pediatrics; the American Diabetes Association; the Centers for Disease Control and Prevention; and the U.S. Preventive Health Services Task Force.

Approach

Professional nursing practice continues to evolve and adapt to society's changing health priorities. The ever-changing health care delivery system offers new opportunities for nurses to alter the practice of maternity and women's health nursing and to improve the way care is given. Consumers of maternity and women's health care vary in age, ethnicity, culture, language, social status, marital status, and sexual preference. They seek care with obstetricians, gynecologists, family practice physicians, nurse-midwives, nurse practitioners, nurses, and other health care providers in a variety of health care settings, including the home. Increasingly, many are self-treating, using a variety of alternative and complementary therapies.

Nursing education must reflect these changes. Clinical education must be planned to offer students a variety of maternity and women's health care experiences in settings that include hospitals and birth centers, the home health setting, clinics and private physician offices, shelters for the homeless or women in need of protection, in prisons, and in other community-based settings. Advances in nursing education include the increased use of simulation learning activities. Simulation laboratories have emerged in schools of nursing and in health care institutions to provide students and staff with opportunities to engage in care of clients in focused, challenging situations while in the safety of a controlled environment. Simulation experiences offer students in maternity and women's health courses opportunities that are otherwise unavailable due to shrinking opportunities for clinical placements, decreased clinical time, and increased numbers of students in clinical rotations.

Today's nursing students are challenged to learn more than ever and often in less time than their predecessors. Students are diverse. They may be new high school graduates, college students, or older adults with families. They may be male or female. They may have college degrees in other fields and be interested in changing careers. They may represent various cultures; English may not be their primary language. Students may be enrolled in associate degree or diploma programs, in baccalaureate or accelerated baccalaureate nursing programs, or in entry level master's programs. The tenth edition, with its accompanying teaching and learning package, has been revised to meet these changing needs. Each chapter has been reviewed by a specialist to improve readability and comprehension, especially by a diverse student population. Focused content is presented in a clearly written and easily read manner while retaining the comprehensiveness of previous editions. The text can be used by all levels of nursing education, and in courses of varying lengths.

This tenth edition is also aimed at meeting the learning needs of practicing nurses who work with women and their families in women's health and childbearing. The text can be used to prepare for certification courses and for review in graduate programs of study. The text and its electronic resources would be an excellent reference on the nursing unit.

Health care today emphasizes *wellness and health promotion.* This focus is an integral part of our philosophy. Likewise the developmental changes a woman experiences throughout her life are considered natural and normal. In women's health care, the goal is promotion of wellness for the woman through knowledge of her body and its normal functioning throughout her life span, while developing an awareness of conditions that require professional intervention. The unit on women's health care emphasizes the wellness aspect of care but also includes information about common gynecologic problems as well as breast and gynecologic cancers. This unit has been placed before the units on pregnancy because many of the aspects of assessment and care can be applied to later chapters.

Pregnancy and childbirth are also part of a natural developmental process. We believe that students need to thoroughly understand and recognize the normal processes before they can identify complications and comprehend their implications for care. We present the entire normal childbearing cycle before discussing potential complications.

In this edition of *Maternity & Women's Health Care,* there is expanded and enhanced content related to the risks associated with obesity as it relates to women's health, pregnancy, and neonatal outcomes. In relevant chapters throughout the book, this content is addressed, based on the most current evidence-based information from the medical and nursing literature.

Readers will note that throughout the text, the authors use different terms to describe various racial and ethnic groups. Whenever statistical data are described, the terms in the reference are used, for instance, non-Hispanic black, non-Hispanic white, and Hispanic. When discussing individual clients or population groups and their health beliefs, the more commonly used terms are used, for instance, Latina or Hispanic, Caucasian, African-American, and Asian.

Features

The tenth edition features a contemporary design and spacious presentation. Students will find that the logical, easy-to-follow headings and attractive full-color design highlight important content and increase visual appeal. More than 750 color photographs (many of them new) and drawings throughout the text illustrate important concepts and techniques to further enhance comprehension. Each chapter begins with a list of *Learning Objectives* designed to focus students' attention on the important content to be mastered. *Electronic Resources* that can be found on the companion website and/or the interactive companion CD are listed at the beginning of each chapter to provide the student with additional information. *Key Terms* that alert students to new vocabulary are in blue, defined within the chapter, and included in a glossary at the end of the book. Each chapter consistently ends with *Key Points,* which summarize important content. **NEW *Community Activity*** exercises are included in most chapters to provide opportunities for students to increase their knowledge of community resources. **NEW *Clinical Reasoning*** exercises are integrated to guide students in applying their knowledge and increasing their ability to think critically about maternity and women's health care issues. ***References*** have been updated significantly, with most citations being less than 5 years old and all chapters having citations within 1 year of publication. An expanded Table of Contents and Index make it easier for readers to locate exactly the information they are seeking. More of the additional outstanding features follow:

- ***Care Management*** is used as the consistent framework throughout to discuss collaborative care and more specifically, the nursing care related to each topic.
- ***Nursing Process*** boxes are included as a **NEW** feature in this edition. These boxes provide key points related to assessment, potential nursing diagnoses, goals/expected outcomes, interventions, and evaluation.
- ***Nursing Care Plans*** help students apply the nursing process in the clinical setting and use NANDA-approved nursing diagnoses, describe expected outcomes for client care, provide rationales for interventions, and include evaluation of care.
- ***Protocols*** and ***Procedure*** boxes provide students with examples of various approaches to implementation of care.
- ***Teaching for Self-Management*** boxes emphasize guidelines for the client to practice self-care and provide information to help students transfer learning from the hospital to the home setting.
- ***Emergency*** boxes alert students to the signs and symptoms of various emergency situations and provide interventions for immediate implementation.
- ***Signs of Potential Complications*** boxes alert students to signs and symptoms of potential problems and are included in chapters that cover uncomplicated pregnancy and childbirth.
- ***Nursing Alert*** and ***Safety Alert*** boxes highlight critical information.
- ***Evidence-Based Practice*** is incorporated throughout in **NEW** boxes that integrate findings from several studies on selected clinical practices and changing practice. In addition, research findings summarized in *The Cochrane Pregnancy and Childbirth Database* and other resources for evidence-based practices that confirm effective practices or identify practices that have unknown, ineffective, or harmful effects are integrated throughout the text and identified by this icon in the margin.
- ***Alternative and Complementary Therapies*** are discussed for many women's health and pregnancy-related problems and are identified in the text by this icon in the margin.
- ***Cultural Considerations*** boxes describe beliefs and practices about pregnancy, childbirth, parenting, and women's health concerns and the importance of understanding cultural variations when providing care.
- ***Legal Tips*** are integrated throughout to provide students with relevant information to deal with these important areas in the context of maternity and women's health nursing.
- ***Medication Guide*** boxes include key information about medications used in maternity and women's health care, including their indications, adverse effects, and nursing considerations.

Organization

The tenth edition of *Maternity & Women's Heath Care* comprises eight units organized to enhance understanding and learning and to facilitate easy retrieval of information.

Unit One, Introduction to Maternity & Women's Health Care, begins with an overview of contemporary issues in maternity and women's health nursing practice. Chapter 1 includes a section on historic milestones in maternity care and provides an overview of important therapies that can be used instead of or in addition to traditional techniques used in maternity and women's health care. Chapter 2 addresses the community as a unit of care, incorporating family theory, cultural aspects of care, and home care in relation to maternity and women's health nursing. Chapter 3 provides essential discussion about genetics in relation to maternity and women's health care.

Unit Two, Women's Health, is a thoroughly revised unit on women's health. Eight chapters discuss health promotion, screening, and physical assessment, and then present common reproductive concerns. The chapter on assessment and health promotion incorporates normal anatomy and physiology of the female reproductive system and integrates health promotion for common women's health problems. There are separate chapters on reproductive problems and concerns, sexually transmitted infections and other infections, contraception and abortion, infertility, violence, problems of the breast, and structural disorders and neoplasms of the female reproductive system.

Unit Three, Pregnancy, describes nursing care of the woman and her family from conception through preparation for childbirth. Nursing care during pregnancy includes both physiologic and psychologic aspects of care, as well as information on preparation for childbirth. A separate chapter on maternal and fetal nutrition emphasizes the important aspects of care, highlights cultural variations in diet, and stresses the importance of early recognition and management of nutritional problems.

Unit Four, Childbirth, focuses on collaborative care among physicians, nurse-midwives, nurses, and women and their families during the processes of labor and birth. Separate chapters deal with the nurse's role in management of discomfort during labor and childbirth, and fetal monitoring, both of which have been updated significantly. All four chapters familiarize students with current childbirth practices and focus on evidence-based interventions to support and educate the woman and her family.

Unit Five, Postpartum, deals with a time of profound change for the entire family. Physiologic changes and nursing care based on the changes are addressed. The mother requires both physical and emotional support as she adjusts to her new role. The chapter on transition to parenthood discusses family dynamics in response to the birth of a child and describes ways nurses can facilitate parent-infant adjustment. Anticipatory guidance for the first few weeks at home and home follow-up care is addressed.

Unit Six, The Newborn, has been updated and addresses physiologic adaptations of the newborn and assessment and care of the newborn. Information on the nutritional needs of the newborn and nursing care associated with breastfeeding and formula feeding are highlighted in a separate chapter.

Unit Seven, Complications of Pregnancy, discusses the conditions that place the woman, fetus, infant, and family at risk. This unit has been revised and updated and includes a chapter on assessment of the high risk pregnancy and eight other chapters covering specific pregnancy complications including hypertensive disorders, antepartal hemorrhagic disorders, endocrine and metabolic problems, medical-surgical problems, obstetric critical care, mental health problems and substance abuse, labor and birth complications, and postpartum complications. Care management focuses on achieving the best possible outcomes, as well as supporting the woman and family when expectations are not met.

Unit Eight, Newborn Complications, addresses the most common acquired conditions of the neonate as well as hematologic disorders and congenital anomalies. It then describes the nursing care for high risk newborns, emphasizing the care of the preterm infant. There is enhanced content on care of late preterm infants in this edition. All chapters have been revised and updated. A separate chapter on loss and grief discusses care management of the family experiencing a fetal or neonatal loss.

Teaching/Learning Package

Several ancillaries to this text have been developed for instructors and students to use in classroom and clinical settings.

- ***Evolve.*** Evolve is an innovative website that provides a wealth of content, resources, and state-of-the-art information on maternity nursing. Evolve's wide array of information includes course resources for instructors (Instructor's Manual, Test Bank, Image Collection, PowerPoint slides, Audience Response Questions) and learning resources for students (Case Studies, NCLEX©-style Review Questions, Nursing Skills, Assessment Videos, Animations, Critical Thinking Exercises, Nursing Care Plans, downloadable Audio Key Points, and more).
- ***Instructor's Electronic Resource.*** The innovative electronic resources for the instructor (available online) contain the following components:
    - *Instructor's Manual* contains learning objectives, chapter outlines and accompanying teaching strategies, learning activities, and curriculum guides for courses of varying lengths.
    - *Electronic Test Bank in ExamView format* contains approximately 1,125 NCLEX-style test items, including alternate format questions. An answer key with page references to the text, rationales, and NCLEX-style coding is included.
    - *Electronic Image Collection,* containing more than 500 full-color illustrations and photographs from the text, helps instructors develop presentations and explain key concepts. All images can be printed as acetates for overhead projection, as well as used in Power Point slides.
    - *PowerPoint Slides,* with lecture outlines for each chapter of the text, assist in presenting materials in the classroom.
    - *Audience Response Questions* for i-clicker and other systems provide additional review of content in the classroom.
    - A *Curriculum Guide* that includes a proposed class schedule and reading assignments for courses of varying lengths is provided. This gives educators suggestions for using the text in the most essential manner or in a more comprehensive way. Also, answers are provided for the Clinical Reasoning exercises found in the text.

- ***Study Guide.*** This comprehensive and challenging study aid presents a variety of questions to enhance learning of key concepts and content from the text. Multiple-choice and matching questions are included, as well as Critical Thinking Case Studies. Answers for all questions are included at the back of the Study Guide.
- ***Clinical Companion.*** This handy, portable book provides students with an accessible, quick reference to the information needed in the clinical setting.
- ***Virtual Clinical Excursions: CD and Workbook Companion.*** A CD and workbook have been developed as a virtual clinical experience to expand student opportunities for critical thinking. This package guides the student through a computer-generated virtual clinical environment and helps the user apply textbook content to virtual clients in that environment. Case studies are presented that allow students to use this textbook as a reference to assess, diagnose, plan, implement, and evaluate "real" clients using clinical scenarios. The state-of-the-art technologies reflected on this CD demonstrate cutting-edge learning opportunities for students and facilitate knowledge retention of the information found in the textbook. The clinical simulations and workbook represent the next generation of research-based learning tools that promote critical thinking and meaningful learning.
- ***Simulation Learning System.*** The Simulation Learning System (SLS) is an online toolkit that effectively incorporates medium- to high-fidelity simulation into nursing curricula with scenarios that promote and enhance the clinical decision-making skills of students at all levels. The SLS offers a comprehensive package of resources including leveled patient scenarios, detailed instructions for preparation and implementation of the simulation experience, debriefing questions that encourage critical thinking, and learning resources to reinforce student comprehension.

Acknowledgments

The tenth edition of *Maternity & Women's Health Care* would not have been possible without the contributions of many people. First, we want to thank the many nurse educators, clinicians, and nursing students in the United States, Canada, Australia, and Taiwan whose comments and suggestions about the manuscript led to this collaborative effort by an outstanding group of contributors. A special thanks goes to these contributors, many of whom are new to this edition, whose names appear in the list of Contributors. Their expertise and knowledge of current clinical practice and research have added to the relevancy and accuracy of the materials presented. We also thank Pat Gingrich for contributing to the Evidence-Based Practice boxes; Ed Lowdermilk for his assistance with Medication Guides and verification of other medication information; Julie Taylor for her contributions to the content on obesity as it affects the health of women throughout their life span; and Dusty Dix for her contribution to the development of the new Community Activity boxes.

We are also appreciative of the critiques given by the reviewers, especially their attention to validating the accuracy of content and their challenge to present content differently and to include new ideas. These combined efforts have resulted in a revision that incorporates the most recent research and current information about the practice of maternity and women's health care.

We offer thanks for shared expertise and photographs to the staff of University of North Carolina Women's Hospital; University of North Carolina School of Nursing; Nurses Certificate program in Interactive Imagery; Jane Stansbury, SRS Medical Systems, Inc.; Phil Wilson, Momentum, Inc.; Leonard Nihan, Sea-Band International; Gayle Kipnis, RNC, CHTP, HNC; Tina Whitehorn; Polly Perez, Cutting Edge Press; and Barbara Harper, Global Maternal/Child Health Association.

We also would like to thank the following photographers: Cheryl Briggs, RNC, Annapolis, MD; Michael S. Clement, MD, Mesa, AZ; Julie Perry Nelson, Loveland, CO; and Marjorie Pyle, RNC, Lifecircle, Costa Mesa, CA.

Thanks to the following individuals who allowed us to use their beautiful photos: Freida Belding, Bird City, KS; Jodi Brackett, Phoenix, AZ; David A. Clarke, Philadelphia, PA; Thomas and Christie Coghill, Clayton, NC; Eugene Doerr, Litchfield, KY; Kara and Casey George, Peoria, AZ; Sue George, Hays, KS; Patricia Hess, San Francisco, CA; Sharon Johnson, Petaluma, CA; Sara Kossuth, Los Angeles, CA; Mahesh Kotwal, MD, Phoenix, AZ; Paul Vincent Kuntz, Houston, TX; Nicole Larson, Eden Prairie, MN; Wendy and Marwood Larson-Harris, Roanoke, VA; Lauren and Brian LiVecchi, Raleigh, NC; Ed Lowdermilk, Chapel Hill, NC; Kim Molloy, Knoxville, IA; Chris Rozales, San Francisco, CA; H. Gil Rushton, MD, Washington, DC; Brian and Mayannyn Sallee, Anchorage, AK; Shari Rivera Sharpe, Chapel Hill, NC; Kody Skaggs, Morrison, CO; Margaret Spann, New Johnsonville, TN; Edward S. Tank, MD, Portland, OR; Amy and Ken Turner, Cary, NC; Rebekah Vogel, Fort Collins, CO; Roni Wernik, Palo Alto, CA; and Randi and Jacob Wills, Clayton, NC.

Special words of gratitude are extended to Robin Carter, Executive Editor; Laurie Gower, Managing Editor; Jeff Patterson, Publishing Services Manager; Jeanne Genz, Project Manager; and Karen Pauls, Designer, for their encouragement, inspiration, and assistance in the preparation and production of this text. These talented and hardworking people helped change our manuscript into a beautiful book by editing the manuscript, designing an attractive format for our special features, and overseeing the production of the book from start to finish. We are especially thankful to Laurie Gower, who always had time to answer our questions, kept track of innumerable details, found just the right photo or resource, obtained that elusive permission, and always reassured us that we were doing a great job.

Deitra Leonard Lowdermilk
Shannon E. Perry
Kitty Cashion
Kathryn Rhodes Alden

CONTENTS

UNIT ONE INTRODUCTION TO MATERNITY & WOMEN'S HEALTH CARE

1. 21st Century Maternity and Women's Health Nursing, 1
    - Contemporary Issues and Trends, 2
        - *Healthy People 2020 Goals, 2*
        - *Millennium Development Goals, 2*
        - *Integrative Health Care, 3*
        - *Problems with the U.S. Health Care System, 3*
        - *Health Literacy, 5*
        - *Trends in Fertility and Birth Rate, 5*
        - *Increase in High Risk Pregnancies, 6*
        - *High-Technology Care, 7*
        - *Community-Based Care, 7*
        - *Childbirth Practices, 7*
        - *Involving Consumers and Promoting Self-Management, 8*
        - *Health of Women, 9*
    - Trends in Nursing Practice, 9
        - *Nursing Interventions Classification, 9*
        - *Evidence-Based Practice, 9*
    - Standards of Practice and Legal Issues in Delivery of Care, 11
        - *Risk Management, 12*
        - *Sentinel Events, 12*
        - *Failure to Rescue, 13*
        - *Quality and Safety Education for Nurses, 13*
        - *Teamwork and Communication, 13*
    - Ethical Issues in Perinatal Nursing and Women's Health Care, 14
    - Research in Perinatal Nursing and Women's Health Care, 14

2. Community Care: The Family and Culture, 17
    - Introduction to Family, Culture, Community, and Home Care, 17
    - The Family in Cultural and Community Context, 18
        - *Defining Family, 18*
        - *Family Organization and Structure, 18*
        - *The Family in Society, 19*
    - Theoretic Approaches to Understanding Families, 19
        - *Family Nursing, 19*
        - *Family Assessment, 19*
        - *Family Theories, 19*
        - *Graphic Representations of Families, 21*
    - The Family in a Cultural Context, 21
        - *Cultural Factors Related to Family Health, 21*
        - *Implications for Nursing, 21*
        - *Childbearing Beliefs and Practices, 24*
        - *Personal Space, 25*
        - *Time Orientation, 25*
        - *Family Roles, 25*
    - Developing Cultural Competence, 27
    - Community Health Promotion, 28
        - *Levels of Preventive Care, 28*
        - *Promoting Family Health, 28*
    - Assessing the Community, 29
        - *Data Collection and Sources of Community Health Data, 29*
        - *Vulnerable Populations in the Community, 31*
        - *Implications for Nursing, 33*
    - Home Care in the Community, 34
        - *Communication and Technology Applications, 34*
        - *Guidelines for Nursing Practice, 35*
        - *Perinatal Services, 35*
        - *Client Selection and Referral, 35*
        - *Preparing for the Home Visit, 36*
        - *First Home Care Visit, 36*
        - *Nursing Considerations, 37*
    - Safety Issues for the Home Care Nurse, 38
        - *Personal Safety, 39*
        - *Woman's Home, 40*
        - *Infection Control, 40*

3. Clinical Genetics, 43
    - Nursing Expertise in Genetics and Genomics, 44
        - *Essential Competencies in Genetics and Genomics for All Nurses, 44*
        - *Expanded Roles for Maternity and Women's Health Nurses, 44*
    - Human Genome Project and Implications for Clinical Practice, 44
        - *Importance of Family History, 45*
        - *Gene Identification and Testing, 45*
        - *Pharmacogenomics, 46*
        - *Gene Therapy, 46*
        - *Ethical, Legal, and Social Implications, 46*
        - *Factors Influencing the Decision to Undergo Genetic Testing, 47*
    - Clinical Genetics, 47
        - *Genetic Transmission, 47*
        - *Genes and Chromosomes, 47*

Chromosomal Abnormalities, 48
Patterns of Genetic Transmission, 52
Cancer Genomics, 54
Gene Mutations That Can Lead to Cancer, 54
Hereditary Breast and Ovarian Cancer, 54
Colon Cancer, 55
Genetic Counseling, 55
Definition of Genetic Counseling, 55
Access and Referral to Genetic Counseling, 56
Estimation of Risk, 56
Interpretation of Risk, 57
Multiple Roles for Nurses in Genetics, 57
Future Promise of Genetics, 57

UNIT TWO WOMEN'S HEALTH

4. Assessment and Health Promotion, 60
Female Reproductive System, 60
External Structures, 61
Internal Structures, 61
The Bony Pelvis, 63
Breasts, 64
Menstruation and Menopause, 67
Menarche and Puberty, 67
Menstrual Cycle, 67
Prostaglandins, 69
Climacteric and Menopause, 69
Sexual Response, 69
Reasons for Entering the Health Care System, 69
Preconception Counseling and Care, 70
Pregnancy, 70
Well-Woman Care, 70
Fertility Control and Infertility, 71
Menstrual Problems, 72
Perimenopause, 72
Barriers to Seeking Health Care, 72
Financial Issues, 72
Cultural Issues, 72
Gender Issues, 72
Health Risks in the Childbearing Years, 73
Age, 73
Socioeconomic Status, 74
Substance Use and Abuse, 74
Nutrition, 75
Physical Fitness and Exercise, 76
Stress, 76
Sexual Practices, 77
Medical Conditions, 77
Gynecologic Conditions, 77
Environmental and Workplace Hazards, 78
Violence Against Women, 78
Health Assessment, 78
Interview, 78
Women with Special Needs, 79
History, 82
Physical Examination, 82
Laboratory and Diagnostic Procedures, 88
Anticipatory Guidance for Health Promotion and Illness Prevention, 88
Nutrition, 88
Exercise, 90
Stress Management, 91
Substance Use Cessation, 92
Sexual Practices That Reduce Risk, 92
Health Screening Schedule, 92
Health Risk Prevention, 93
Health Protection, 93

5. Violence Against Women, 95
Historical Perspective, 96
Conceptual and Theoretic Perspectives, 97
Biologic Factors, 97
Psychologic Perspective, 97
Sociologic Perspective, 98
Feminist Perspective, 98
Ecological Model, 99
Women Experiencing Intimate Partner Violence, 100
Characteristics of Women in Abusive Relationships, 100
Cultural Considerations, 101
Intimate Partner Violence During Pregnancy, 103
Nursing Interventions, 105
Sexual Violence, 109
Why Do Some Men Rape? 109
Mental Health Consequences of Sexual Assault, 110
Rape-Trauma, 110
Collaborative Care, 111

6. Reproductive System Concerns, 119
Common Menstrual Disorders, 120
Amenorrhea, 120
Cyclic Perimenstrual Pain and Discomfort, 121
Dysmenorrhea, 121
Premenstrual Syndrome and Premenstrual Dysphoric Disorder, 123
Endometriosis, 125
Alterations in Cyclic Bleeding, 126
Menopause, 130
Physiologic Characteristics, 131
Physical Changes During the Perimenopausal Period, 131
Health Risks of Perimenopausal Women, 133
Menopausal Hormonal Therapy, 134
Sexual Counseling, 137

7. Sexually Transmitted and Other Infections, 143
Prevention, 143
Risk Reduction Measures, 144
Sexually Transmitted Bacterial Infections, 146
Chlamydia, 146
Gonorrhea, 147
Syphilis, 149
Pelvic Inflammatory Disease, 150
Sexually Transmitted Viral Infections, 152
Human Papillomavirus, 152
Genital Herpes Simplex Virus, 153
Viral Hepatitis, 155
Human Immunodeficiency Virus, 156
Vaginal Infections, 159
Bacterial Vaginosis, 159
Candidiasis, 160
Trichomoniasis, 161
Group B Streptococci, 162
Effects of Sexually Transmitted Infections on Pregnancy and the Fetus, 162
TORCH Infections, 162
Infection Control, 165

8. Contraception and Abortion, 169
Contraception, 169
Methods of Contraception, 171
Coitus Interruptus, 171
Fertility Awareness Methods, 171
Spermicides and Barrier Methods, 175
Hormonal Methods, 181
Emergency Contraception, 184
Intrauterine Devices, 185
Sterilization, 186
Breastfeeding: Lactational Amenorrhea Method, 189
Induced Abortion, 189
Incidence, 189
The Decision to Have an Abortion, 190
First-Trimester Abortion, 190
Second-Trimester Abortion, 191
Nursing Considerations, 192

9. Infertility, 194
Incidence, 194
Factors Associated with Infertility, 195
Female Infertility, 195
Male Infertility, 197
Interventions, 202

10. Problems of the Breast, 211
Benign Conditions of the Breast, 211
Fibrocystic Changes, 211
Fibroadenomas, 212
Nipple Discharge, 212
Mammary Duct Ectasia, 213
Intraductal Papilloma, 213
Macromastia and Micromastia, 213
Collaborative Care, 213
Malignant Conditions of the Breast, 214
Incidence, 214
Etiologic Factors, 214
Determining a Woman's Risk of Genetically Related Breast Cancer, 216
Chemoprevention, 217
Pathophysiology, 217
Clinical Manifestations and Diagnosis, 217
Prognosis, 220
Nursing Considerations, 228

11. Structural Disorders and Neoplasms of the Reproductive System, 234
Structural Disorders of the Uterus and Vagina, 234
Alterations in Pelvic Support, 234
Benign Neoplasms, 238
Ovarian Cysts, 238
Uterine Polyps, 240
Leiomyomas, 240
Vulvar Problems, 244
Malignant Neoplasms, 245
Cancer of the Endometrium, 246
Cancer of the Ovary, 248
Cancer of the Cervix, 251
Cancer of the Vulva, 260
Cancer of the Vagina, 262
Cancer of the Uterine Tubes, 262
Cancer and Pregnancy, 263

UNIT THREE PREGNANCY

12. Conception and Fetal Development, 270
Conception, 270
Cell Division, 270
Gametogenesis, 271
Fertilization, 273
Implantation, 273
Embryo and Fetus, 273
Primary Germ Layers, 274
Development of the Embryo, 274
Membranes, 274
Amniotic Fluid, 275
Yolk Sac, 276
Umbilical Cord, 276
Placenta, 277
Fetal Maturation, 279
Multifetal Pregnancy, 286
Nongenetic Factors Influencing Development, 287

13. Anatomy and Physiology of Pregnancy, 289
Gravidity and Parity, 289
Pregnancy Tests, 290
Adaptations to Pregnancy, 291
Signs of Pregnancy, 292
Reproductive System and Breasts, 292
General Body Systems, 296

14. Maternal and Fetal Nutrition, 307
Nutrient Needs Before Conception, 307
Nutrient Needs During Pregnancy, 308
Energy Needs, 308
Protein, 313
Fluids, 314
Minerals and Vitamins, 314
Other Nutritional Issues During Pregnancy, 318
Pica and Food Cravings, 318
Adolescent Pregnancy Needs, 319
Preeclampsia, 319
Physical Activity During Pregnancy, 319
Nutrient Needs During Lactation, 319
Diet History, 320
Physical Examination, 321
Laboratory Testing, 321
Client Education, 321

15. Nursing Care of the Family During Pregnancy, 329
Diagnosis of Pregnancy, 330
Signs and Symptoms, 330
Estimating Date of Birth, 330
Adaptation to Pregnancy, 330
Maternal Adaptation, 331
Paternal Adaptation, 333
Sibling Adaptation, 335
Grandparent Adaptation, 335
Initial Visit, 337
Follow-up Visits, 340
Collaborative Care, 344
Variations in Prenatal Care, 358
Cultural Influences, 358
Age Differences, 360
Childbirth and Perinatal Education, 363
Childbirth Education Programs, 363
Perinatal Care Choices, 364
Birth Plans, 365
Birth Setting Choices, 365

UNIT FOUR CHILDBIRTH

16. Labor and Birth Processes, 369
Factors Affecting Labor, 369
Passenger, 369
Passageway, 371
Powers, 374
Position of the Laboring Woman, 378
Process of Labor, 378
Signs Preceding Labor, 378
Onset of Labor, 379
Stages of Labor, 380
Mechanism of Labor, 380
Physiologic Adaptation to Labor, 382
Fetal Adaptation, 382
Maternal Adaptation, 383

17. Pain Management, 386
Pain During Labor and Birth, 386
Neurologic Origins, 386
Perception of Pain, 387
Expression of Pain, 387
Factors Influencing Pain Response, 387
Nonpharmacologic Pain Management, 389
Childbirth Preparation Methods, 391
Relaxation and Breathing Techniques, 391
Effleurage and Counterpressure, 393
Music, 393
Water Therapy (Hydrotherapy), 394
Transcutaneous Electrical Nerve Stimulation, 395
Acupressure and Acupuncture, 395
Application of Heat and Cold, 396
Touch and Massage, 396
Hypnosis, 396
Biofeedback, 396
Aromatherapy, 396
Intradermal Water Block, 397
Pharmacologic Pain Management, 397
Sedatives, 397
Analgesia and Anesthesia, 397
Systemic Analgesia, 398
Nerve Block Analgesia and Anesthesia, 400
General Anesthesia, 407
Nonpharmacologic Interventions, 408
Pharmacologic Interventions, 408

18. Fetal Assessment During Labor, 415
Basis for Monitoring, 415
Fetal Response, 415
Uterine Activity, 416
Fetal Compromise, 416
Monitoring Techniques, 416
Intermittent Auscultation, 417
Electronic Fetal Monitoring, 418
Fetal Heart Rate Patterns, 420
Baseline Fetal Heart Rate, 421
Periodic and Episodic Changes in Fetal Heart Rate, 422
Electronic Fetal Monitoring Pattern Recognition and Interpretation, 426

Other Methods of Assessment and Intervention, 428
Client and Family Teaching, 430
Documentation, 430

19. Nursing Care of the Family During Labor and Birth, 433
First Stage of Labor, 434
Nursing Care, 448
Second Stage of Labor, 457
Preparing for Birth, 460
Third Stage of Labor, 471
Placental Separation and Expulsion, 471
Fourth Stage of Labor, 472
Care of the New Mother, 474
Care of the Family, 474

UNIT FIVE POSTPARTUM

20. Postpartum Physiology, 478
Reproductive System and Associated Structures, 478
Uterus, 478
Cervix, 480
Vagina and Perineum, 480
Endocrine System, 481
Placental Hormones, 481
Pituitary Hormones and Ovarian Function, 481
Abdomen, 481
Urinary System, 481
Urine Components, 482
Postpartal Diuresis, 482
Urethra and Bladder, 482
Gastrointestinal System, 482
Appetite, 482
Bowel Evacuation, 482
Breasts, 482
Breastfeeding Mothers, 482
Nonbreastfeeding Mothers, 482
Cardiovascular System, 483
Blood Volume, 483
Cardiac Output, 483
Vital Signs, 483
Blood Components, 483
Neurologic System, 484
Musculoskeletal System, 484
Integumentary System, 484
Immune System, 484

21. Nursing Care of the Family During the Postpartum Period, 486
Transfer from the Recovery Area, 486
Planning for Discharge, 487
Laws Relating to Discharge, 487
Criteria for Discharge, 488
Nursing Interventions, 490
Effect of the Birth Experience, 500
Maternal Self-Image, 501
Adaptation to Parenthood and Parent-Infant Interactions, 501
Family Structure and Functioning, 501
Effect of Cultural Diversity, 502
Discharge Teaching, 502
Self-Management and Signs of Complications, 502
Sexual Activity and Contraception, 503
Prescribed Medications, 503
Follow-up After Discharge, 504
Routine Mother and Baby Follow-up Care, 504
Home Visits, 504
Telephone Follow-up, 505
Support Groups, 505
Referral to Community Resources, 505

22. Transition to Parenthood, 507
Parental Attachment, Bonding, and Acquaintance, 507
Assessment of Attachment Behaviors, 510
Parent-Infant Contact, 510
Early Contact, 510
Extended Contact, 510
Communication Between Parent and Infant, 511
The Senses, 511
Entrainment, 511
Biorhythmicity, 512
Reciprocity and Synchrony, 512
Parental Role After Birth, 512
Transition to Parenthood, 512
Parental Tasks and Responsibilities, 512
Becoming a Mother, 514
Becoming a Father, 515
Adjustment for the Couple, 516
Diversity in Transitions to Parenthood, 519
Age, 519
Parenting in the Lesbian Couple, 521
Social Support, 521
Culture, 521
Socioeconomic Conditions, 522
Personal Aspirations, 522
Parental Sensory Impairment, 522
Visually Impaired Parent, 523
Hearing-Impaired Parent, 523
Sibling Adaptation, 523
Grandparent Adaptation, 525

UNIT SIX THE NEWBORN

23. Physiologic and Behavioral Adaptations of the Newborn, 528
Transition to Extrauterine Life, 528
Physiologic Adaptations, 529
Respiratory System, 529
Cardiovascular System, 530
Hematopoietic System, 532
Thermogenic System, 533
Renal System, 534
Gastrointestinal System, 535
Hepatic System, 536
Immune System, 539
Integumentary System, 539
Reproductive System, 541
Skeletal System, 542
Neuromuscular System, 545
Behavioral Characteristics, 545
Sleep-Wake States, 549
Other Factors Influencing Newborn Behavior, 550
Sensory Behaviors, 550
Response to Environmental Stimuli, 551

24. Nursing Care of the Newborn and Family, 553
Care Management: Birth Through the First 2 Hours, 553
Initial Assessment and Apgar Scoring, 554
Physical Assessment, 555
Neurologic Assessment, 565
Gestational Age Assessment, 566
Airway Maintenance, 570
Maintaining an Adequate Oxygen Supply, 571
Maintaining Body Temperature, 571
Immediate Interventions, 572
Care Management: From 2 Hours After Birth Until Discharge, 574
Common Newborn Problems, 574
Physiologic Problems, 575
Laboratory and Diagnostic Tests, 577
Discharge Planning and Teaching, 591

25. Newborn Nutrition and Feeding, 606
Recommended Infant Nutrition, 607
Breastfeeding Rates, 607
Benefits of Breastfeeding, 607
Choosing an Infant Feeding Method, 607
Supporting Breastfeeding Mothers, 608
Cultural Influences on Infant Feeding, 609
Nutrient Needs, 610
Fluids, 610
Energy, 610
Carbohydrate, 610
Fat, 610
Protein, 611
Vitamins, 611
Minerals, 611
Anatomy and Physiology of Lactation, 611
Anatomy of the Lactating Breast, 611
Lactogenesis, 612
Uniqueness of Human Milk, 613
Care Management: The Breastfeeding Mother and Infant, 613
Positioning, 614
Latch, 615
Milk Ejection or Let-Down, 616
Frequency of Feedings, 616
Duration of Feedings, 617
Indicators of Effective Breastfeeding, 617
Supplements, Bottles, and Pacifiers, 617
Special Considerations, 619
Formula Feeding, 629
Parent Education, 629
Readiness for Feeding, 630
Feeding Patterns, 630
Feeding Technique, 630
Common Concerns, 630
Bottles and Nipples, 630
Infant Formulas, 631
Vitamin and Mineral Supplementation, 632
Weaning, 632
Complementary Feeding: Introducing Solid Foods, 632

UNIT SEVEN COMPLICATIONS OF PREGNANCY

26. Assessment for Risk Factors in Pregnancy, 637
Psychologic Considerations Related to High Risk Pregnancy, 639
Antepartum Testing, 639
Biophysical Assessment, 640
Daily Fetal Movement Count, 640
Ultrasonography, 640
Magnetic Resonance Imaging, 645
Biochemical Assessment, 645
Amniocentesis, 645
Chorionic Villus Sampling, 647
Percutaneous Umbilical Blood Sampling, 648
Maternal Assays, 648
Antepartal Assessment Using Electronic Fetal Monitoring, 649
Indications, 649
Nonstress Test, 649
Vibroacoustic Stimulation, 651
Contraction Stress Test, 651
Nurses' Role in Assessment of the High Risk Pregnancy, 652

27. Hypertensive Disorders in Pregnancy, 654
Significance and Incidence, 654
Morbidity and Mortality, 654
Classification, 655
Gestational Hypertension, 655
Preeclampsia, 656
Eclampsia, 656
Chronic Hypertension, 656
Chronic Hypertension with Superimposed Preeclampsia, 656
Preeclampsia, 656
Etiology, 656
Pathophysiology, 657
HELLP Syndrome, 658
Eclampsia, 667
Immediate Care, 667
Chronic Hypertension, 668

28. Antepartum Hemorrhagic Disorders, 670
Early Pregnancy Bleeding, 670
Miscarriage (Spontaneous Abortion), 670
Recurrent Premature Dilation of the Cervix (Incompetent Cervix), 675
Ectopic Pregnancy, 676
Hydatidiform Mole (Molar Pregnancy), 678
Late Pregnancy Bleeding, 680
Placenta Previa, 680
Premature Separation of Placenta (Abruptio Placentae [Placental Abruption]), 683
Cord Insertion and Placental Variations, 685
Clotting Disorders in Pregnancy, 685

29. Endocrine and Metabolic Disorders in Pregnancy, 688
Diabetes Mellitus, 688
Pathogenesis, 689
Classification, 689
Metabolic Changes Associated with Pregnancy, 689
Pregestational Diabetes Mellitus, 691
Preconception Counseling, 691
Maternal Risks and Complications, 691
Fetal and Neonatal Risks and Complications, 693
Gestational Diabetes Mellitus, 701
Fetal Risks, 701
Screening for Gestational Diabetes Mellitus, 701
Hyperemesis Gravidarum, 704
Etiology, 705
Clinical Manifestations, 705
Thyroid Disorders, 706
Hyperthyroidism, 706
Hypothyroidism, 707
Nursing Care, 707
Maternal Phenylketonuria, 707

30. Medical-Surgical Problems in Pregnancy, 709
Cardiovascular Disorders, 709
Congenital Cardiac Disease, 710
Acquired Cardiac Disease, 711
Ischemic Heart Disease, 712
Other Cardiac Diseases and Conditions, 712
Heart Transplantation, 714
Other Medical Disorders in Pregnancy, 720
Anemia, 720
Pulmonary Disorders, 722
Integumentary Disorders, 726
Neurologic Disorders, 727
Autoimmune Disorders, 728
Gastrointestinal Disorders, 729
Inflammatory Bowel Disease, 730
Urinary Tract Infections, 730
Surgery During Pregnancy, 732
Appendicitis, 732

31. Obstetric Critical Care, 735
Obstetric Intensive Care Unit, 735
Equipment and Expertise, 736
Physiologic Changes in Pregnancy, 737
Cardiovascular Changes, 737
Colloid Osmotic Pressure, 738
Respiratory Changes, 738
Hematologic Changes, 738
Systemic Vascular Resistance, 738
Hemodynamic Monitoring, 739
Anatomic and Physiologic Characteristics of Circulation, 739
Cardiac Output, 739
Invasive Hemodynamic Monitoring, 741
Data Collection, 745
Trauma During Pregnancy, 749
Significance, 749
Maternal Physiologic Characteristics, 749
Fetal Physiologic Characteristics, 750
Mechanisms of Trauma, 751
Immediate Stabilization, 751
Electronic Fetal Monitoring, 754
Fetal-Maternal Hemorrhage, 754
Ultrasound, 754
Radiation Exposure, 754
Perimortem Cesarean Birth, 754
Family-Centered Obstetric Critical Care, 754
Maternal Death, 755

32. Mental Health Disorders and Substance Abuse in Pregnancy, 757
Mental Health Disorders During Pregnancy, 757
Mood Disorders, 757
Anxiety Disorders, 759
Substance Abuse During Pregnancy, 761
Prevalence, 761

Risk Factors, 761
Barriers to Treatment, 761
Legal Considerations, 762
Commonly Abused Drugs, 762
Postpartum Psychologic Complications, 767
Mood Disorders, 768
Postpartum Onset of Anxiety Disorders, 775

33. Labor and Birth Complications, 779
Preterm Labor and Birth, 779
Preterm Birth Versus Low Birth Weight, 780
Predicting Spontaneous Preterm Labor and Birth, 780
Causes of Preterm Labor and Birth, 781
Premature Rupture of Membranes, 791
Chorioamnionitis, 791
Dysfunctional Labor (Dystocia), 792
Abnormal Uterine Activity, 792
Secondary Powers, 793
Abnormal Labor Patterns, 793
Precipitous Labor, 794
Alterations in Pelvic Structure, 794
Fetal Causes, 794
Position of the Woman, 797
Psychologic Responses, 797
Obesity, 797
Obstetric Procedures, 799
Version, 799
Induction of Labor, 799
Augmentation of Labor, 805
Operative Vaginal Birth, 806
Cesarean Birth, 807
Trial of Labor, 814
Vaginal Birth After Cesarean, 815
Postterm Pregnancy, Labor, and Birth, 815
Maternal and Fetal Risks, 816
Obstetric Emergencies, 817
Meconium-stained Amniotic Fluid, 817
Shoulder Dystocia, 817
Prolapsed Umbilical Cord, 818
Rupture of the Uterus, 819
Anaphylactoid Syndrome of Pregnancy, 820

34. Postpartum Complications, 824
Postpartum Hemorrhage, 824
Definition and Incidence, 824
Etiology and Risk Factors, 824
Uterine Atony, 825
Lacerations of the Genital Tract, 825
Retained Placenta, 826
Inversion of the Uterus, 826
Subinvolution of the Uterus, 826
Hemorrhagic (Hypovolemic) Shock, 830
Medical Management, 831
Nursing Interventions, 831
Fluid or Blood Replacement Therapy, 831
Coagulopathies, 832
Idiopathic Thrombocytopenic Purpura, 832
von Willebrand Disease, 832
Thromboembolic Disease, 832
Incidence and Etiology, 832
Clinical Manifestations, 832
Medical Management, 833
Nursing Interventions, 833
Postpartum Infections, 833
Endometritis, 834
Wound Infections, 834
Urinary Tract Infections, 834
Mastitis, 834

UNIT EIGHT NEWBORN COMPLICATIONS

35. Acquired Problems of the Newborn, 837
Birth Trauma, 837
Soft-Tissue Injuries, 838
Skeletal Injuries, 839
Peripheral Nervous System Injuries, 840
Central Nervous System Injuries, 841
Infants of Mothers with Diabetes, 841
Pathophysiology, 841
Congenital Anomalies, 842
Macrosomia, 843
Birth Trauma and Perinatal Hypoxia, 843
Respiratory Distress Syndrome, 843
Hypoglycemia, 843
Hypocalcemia and Hypomagnesemia, 843
Cardiomyopathy, 844
Hyperbilirubinemia and Polycythemia, 844
Nursing Care, 844
Neonatal Infections, 844
Sepsis, 844
Transplacental Infections, 848
Bacterial Infections, 853
Fungal Infections, 855
Substance Abuse, 856
Tobacco, 856
Alcohol, 857
Heroin, 858
Methadone, 859
Marijuana, 860
Cocaine, 860
Methamphetamine, 860
MDMA/Ecstasy, 860
Other Drugs of Concern, 861

36. Hemolytic Disorders and Congenital Anomalies, 867
Hyperbilirubinemia, 867
Physiologic Jaundice, 867
Pathologic Jaundice, 868
Hemolytic Disease of the Newborn, 868
Rh Incompatibility, 869
ABO Incompatibility, 869
Other Causes of Hemolytic Jaundice, 870
Acute Bilirubin Encephalopathy, 870
Congenital Anomalies, 873
Cardiovascular System Anomalies, 873
Central Nervous System Anomalies, 876
Encephalocele and Anencephaly, 877
Spina Bifida, 877
Hydrocephalus, 878
Microcephaly, 879
Respiratory System Anomalies, 879
Laryngeal Web and Choanal Atresia, 879
Congenital Diaphragmatic Hernia, 879
Gastrointestinal System Anomalies, 880
Cleft Lip and Palate, 880
Esophageal Atresia and Tracheoesophageal Fistula, 881
Omphalocele and Gastroschisis, 883
Gastrointestinal Obstruction, 883
Imperforate Anus, 884
Musculoskeletal System Anomalies, 884
Developmental Dysplasia of the Hip, 884
Clubfoot, 886
Polydactyly, 886
Genitourinary System Anomalies, 886
Hypospadias and Epispadias, 886
Exstrophy of the Bladder, 887
Ambiguous Genitalia, 887
Prenatal Diagnosis, 888
Perinatal Diagnosis, 888
Postnatal Diagnosis, 888
Genetic Diagnosis, 888
Cytogenetic Studies, 889
Dermatoglyphics, 890
Newborn Care, 890
Parents and Family Support, 891

37. Nursing Care of the High Risk Newborn, 894
Preterm Infants, 894
Late Preterm Infants, 895
Physiologic Functions, 896
Physical Care, 899
Complications in High Risk Infants, 915
Infant Pain Responses, 919
Late Preterm Infants, 922
Postmature Infants, 923
Other Problems Related to Gestation, 924
Discharge Planning, 926
Transport to and from a Regional Center, 926
Anticipatory Grief, 927

38. Perinatal Loss and Grief, 931
Perinatal Loss, 931
Grief Responses, 932
Acute Distress, 932
Intense Grief, 933
Reorganization, 934
Family Aspects of Grief, 934
Grandparents and Siblings, 934
Help the Mother, the Father, and Other Family Members Actualize the Loss, 937
Help the Parents with Decision Making, 940
Help the Bereaved Parents Acknowledge and Express Their Feelings, 942
Normalize the Grief Process and Facilitate Positive Coping, 943
Meet the Physical Needs of the Postpartum Bereaved Mother, 944
Assist the Bereaved in Communicating with, Supporting, and Getting Support from Family, 944
Create Memories for Parents to Take Home, 944
Communicate Using a Caring Framework, 944
Be Concerned About Cultural and Spiritual Needs of Parents, 945
Provide Sensitive Care At and After Discharge, 945
Provide Postmortem Care, 946
Special Losses, 946
Prenatal Diagnoses with Negative Outcome, 946
Loss of One in a Multiple Birth, 947
Adolescent Grief, 947
Complicated Grief, 948

Glossary, 951

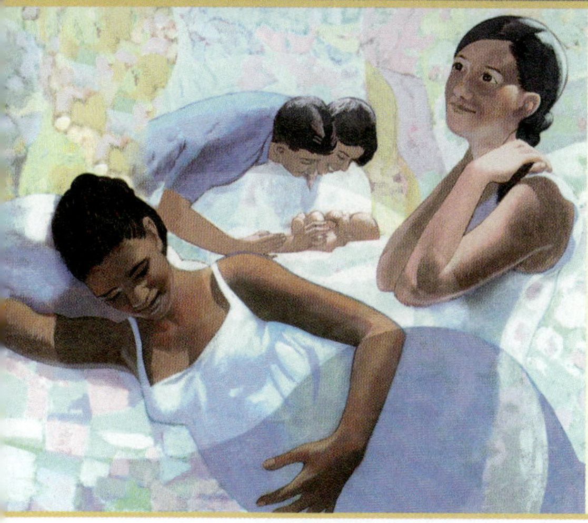

CHAPTER

1

21st Century Maternity and Women's Health Nursing

Shannon E. Perry

evolve WEBSITE

http://evolve.elsevier.com/Lowdermilk/MWHC/
Audio Glossary
Audio Key Points
NCLEX Review Questions

LEARNING OBJECTIVES

- Describe the scope of maternity and women's health nursing.
- Evaluate contemporary issues and trends in maternity and women's health care.
- Examine social concerns in maternity nursing and women's health care.
- Differentiate between standard (allopathic or Western) and holistic health care.
- Describe the scope of perinatal education in the community.
- Explain risk management and standards of practice in the delivery of nursing care.
- Discuss legal and ethical issues in perinatal nursing.
- Examine *Healthy People 2020* goals.

Maternity nursing encompasses care of childbearing women and their families through all stages of pregnancy and childbirth, as well as the first 4 weeks after birth. Throughout the prenatal period, nurses, nurse practitioners, and nurse-midwives provide care for women in clinics and physicians' offices and teach classes to help families prepare for childbirth. Nurses care for childbearing families during labor and birth in hospitals, in birthing centers, and in the home. Nurses with special training may provide intensive care for high risk neonates in special care units and for high risk mothers in antepartum units, in critical care obstetric units, or in the home. Maternity nurses teach about pregnancy; the process of labor, birth, and recovery; and parenting skills. They provide continuity of care throughout the childbearing cycle.

Women's health care focuses on the physical, psychologic, and social needs of women throughout their lives. In the care of women, their overall experience is emphasized: general physical and psychologic well-being, childbearing functions, and diseases. Women's health nurses specialize in and investigate conditions unique to women (such as reproductive malignancies and menopause) and sociocultural and occupational factors that are related to women's health problems (such as poverty, rape, incest, and family violence). They also provide care for women and their families during the childbearing cycle.

Nurses caring for women have helped make the health care system more responsive to women's needs. Nurses have been critically important in developing strategies to improve the well-being of women and their infants and have led the efforts to implement clinical practice guidelines and to practice using an evidence-based approach. Through professional associations, nurses can have a voice in setting standards and in influencing health policy by actively participating in the education of the public and of state and federal legislators. Some nurses hold elective office and influence policy directly. For example, in 2008 the American Nurses Association (ANA) published *ANA's Health System Reform Agenda*, and in 2009 a nurse was appointed Administrator of the Health Resources and Services Administration, the agency that oversees approximately 7000 community clinics that serve low-income and uninsured people (Obama Chooses UND's Mary Wakefield as Health Resources and Services Administration Leader, February 20, 2009).

Although tremendous advances have taken place in the care of mothers and their infants during the past 150 years (Box 1-1), serious problems exist in the United States related to the health and health care of mothers and infants. Lack of access to prepregnancy and pregnancy-related care for all women and the lack of reproductive health services for adolescents are major

BOX 1-1 HISTORIC OVERVIEW OF MILESTONES IN THE CARE OF MOTHERS AND INFANTS

1847—James Young Simpson in Edinburgh, Scotland, used ether for an internal podalic version and birth; the first reported use of obstetric anesthesia
1861—Ignaz Semmelweis wrote *The Cause, Concept and Prophylaxis of Childbed Fever*
1906—First U.S. program for prenatal nursing care established
1908—Childbirth classes started by the American Red Cross
1909—First White House Conference on Children convened
1911—First milk bank in the United States established in Boston
1912—U.S. Children's Bureau established
1916—Margaret Sanger established first American birth control clinic in Brooklyn, New York
1923—First U.S. hospital center for premature infant care established at Sarah Morris Hospital in Chicago, Illinois
1933—*Natural Childbirth* published by Grantly Dick-Read
1941—Penicillin used as a treatment for infection
1953—Virginia Apgar, an anesthesiologist, published Apgar scoring system of neonatal assessment
1958—Edward Hon reported on the recording of the fetal electrocardiogram (ECG) from the maternal abdomen (first commercial electronic fetal monitor produced in the late 1960s)
1958—Ian Donald, a Glasgow physician, was the first to report clinical use of ultrasound to examine the fetus
1959—*Thank You, Dr. Lamaze* published by Marjorie Karmel
1960—American Society for Psychoprophylaxis in Obstetrics (ASPO/Lamaze) formed
1960—International Childbirth Education Association founded
1960—Birth control pill introduced in the United States
1962—Thalidomide found to cause birth defects
1963—Title V of the Social Security Act amended to include comprehensive maternity and infant care for women who were low income and high risk
1965—Supreme Court ruled that married people have the right to use birth control
1967—Rh_o(D) immune globulin produced
1967—Reva Rubin published article on maternal role attainment
1968—Rubella vaccine became available
1969—Nurses Association of the American College of Obstetricians and Gynecologists (NAACOG) founded; renamed AWHONN (Association of Women's Health, Obstetric and Neonatal Nurses) and incorporated as a 501(c)3 organization in 1993
1972—WIC (Special Supplemental Food Program for Women, Infants, and Children) started
1973—Abortion legalized in the United States
1974—First standards for obstetric, gynecologic, and neonatal nursing published by NAACOG
1975—The Pregnant Patient's Bill of Rights published by the International Childbirth Education Association
1978—Louise Brown, first test-tube baby, born
1991—Society for Advancement of Women's Health Research founded
1992—Office of Research on Women's Health authorized by U.S. Congress
1993—Human embryos cloned at George Washington University
1993—Family and Medical Leave Act enacted
1998—Newborns' and Mothers' Health Act went into effect
2000—Working draft of sequence and analysis of human genome completed
2010—Centenary of the death of Florence Nightingale
2010—The Patient Protection and Affordable Care Act signed into law by President Obama

concerns. Sexually transmitted infections, including acquired immunodeficiency syndrome (AIDS), continue to affect reproduction adversely.

Racial and ethnic diversity is increasing within North America. It is estimated that by the year 2050, 50% of the population will be European-American, 15% will be African-American, 24% will be Hispanic, and 8% will be Asian-American (U.S. Census Bureau, 2009). Significant disparity exists in health outcomes among people of various racial and ethnic groups despite the great strides in public health made by the United States.

In addition, people may have lifestyles, health needs, and health care preferences related to their ethnic or cultural backgrounds. They may have dietary preferences and health practices that are not understood by caregivers. This presents a challenge for health care providers to provide culturally sensitive care. To meet the health care needs of a culturally diverse society, there must be increasing diversity of the nursing workforce.

This chapter presents a general overview of issues and trends related to the health and health care of women and infants.

CONTEMPORARY ISSUES AND TRENDS

Healthy People 2020 Goals

Healthy People provides science-based 10-year national objectives for improving health and preventing disease in the United States (www.healthypeople.gov/hp2020). In *Healthy People 2010* the 467 objectives to improve health were organized into 28 specific focus areas, including one related to maternal, infant, and child health.

Healthy People 2020 has four recommended overarching goals: (1) eliminate preventable disease, disability, injury, and premature death; (2) achieve health equity, eliminate disparities, and improve the health of all groups; (3) create social and physical environments that promote good health for all; and (4) promote healthy development and healthy behaviors across every stage of life. The goals of *Healthy People 2020* are based on assessments of major risks to health and wellness, changes in public health priorities, and issues related to the health preparedness and prevention of our nation. Objectives of *Healthy People 2010* have been retained or revised and some new ones included (Box 1-2).

Millennium Development Goals

The United Nations Millennium Development Goals (MDGs) are eight goals to be achieved by 2015 that respond to the world's main development challenges. The MDGs are drawn from the actions and targets contained in the Millennium Declaration that was adopted by 189 nations and signed by 147 heads of state and governments during the United Nations Millennium Summit in September 2000 (www.un.org/millenniumgoals/goals.html). Goals three through five of the MDGs relate specifically to women and children (Box 1-3).

BOX 1-2 *HEALTHY PEOPLE 2020* PERINATAL PROPOSED OBJECTIVES

OBJECTIVES RETAINED FROM *HEALTHY PEOPLE 2010*
- Reduce maternal deaths.
- Reduce maternal illness and complications due to pregnancy (complications during hospitalized labor and delivery).
- Increase the proportion of pregnant women who receive early and adequate prenatal care.
- Reduce cesarean births among low risk (full-term, singleton, vertex presentation) women.
- Reduce low-birth-weight (LBW) and very low-birth-weight (VLBW).
- Reduce preterm births.
- Increase the percentage of healthy full-term infants who are put down to sleep on their backs.
- Increase abstinence from alcohol, cigarettes, and illicit drugs among pregnant women.
- Reduce the occurrence of fetal alcohol syndrome (FAS).
- Increase the proportion of mothers who breastfeed their babies.

OBJECTIVES RETAINED BUT MODIFIED FROM *HEALTHY PEOPLE 2010*
- Reduce fetal and infant deaths.
- Increase the proportion of pregnant women who attend a series of prepared childbirth classes.
- Increase the proportion of mothers who achieve a recommended weight gain during their pregnancies.
- Reduce the proportion of children diagnosed with a metabolic disorder through newborn screening who experience developmental delay requiring special education services.
- Decrease the proportion of children with cerebral palsy born as LBW infants (<2500 grams).
- Reduce the occurrence of neural tube defects.
- Increase the proportion of pregnancies begun with the recommended folic acid level.
- Ensure appropriate newborn blood-spot screening and follow-up.

OBJECTIVES NEW TO *HEALTHY PEOPLE 2020*
- Decrease postpartum relapse of smoking among women who quit smoking during pregnancy.
- Increase the percentage of women giving birth who attend a postpartum care visit with a health care worker.
- Among women delivering a live birth, increase the percentage that receive preconception care services and practice key recommended preconception health behaviors.
- Increase the percentage of employers who have worksite lactation programs.
- Decrease the percentage of breast-fed newborns who receive formula supplementation within the first 2 days of life.
- Increase the percentage of live births that occur in facilities that provide recommended care for lactating mothers and their babies.
- Increase the 1-year survival rates for infants with Down syndrome.
- Reduce the proportion of persons ages 18 to 44 years who have impaired fecundity (i.e., a physical barrier preventing pregnancy or carrying a pregnancy to term).

Source: http://healthypeople.gov/hp2020/Objectives/TopicArea.aspx?id=32&TopicArea=Maternal%2c+Infant+and+Child+Health. Accessed July 27, 2010.

BOX 1-3 UNITED NATIONS MILLENNIUM DEVELOPMENT GOALS

1. Eradicate extreme poverty and hunger
2. Achieve universal primary education
3. Promote gender equality and empower women
4. Reduce child mortality
5. Improve maternal health
6. Combat HIV/AIDS, malaria, and other diseases
7. Ensure environmental sustainability
8. Develop a global partnership for development.

AIDS, Acquired immunodeficiency syndrome; *HIV,* human immunodeficiency virus.

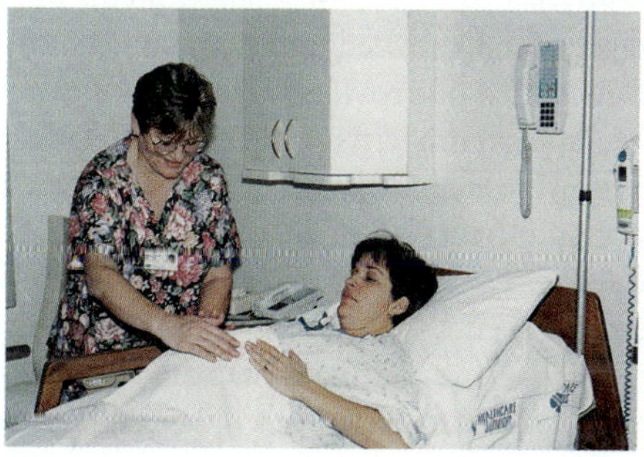

FIG. 1-1 Healing touch with pregnant woman. (Courtesy Wendy Wetzel, Flagstaff, AZ.)

Integrative Health Care

Integrative health care encompasses complementary and alternative therapies in combination with conventional Western modalities of treatment. Many popular alternative healing modalities offer human-centered care based on philosophies that recognize the value of the client's input and honor the individual's beliefs, values, and desires. The focus of these modalities is on the whole person, not just on a disease complex. Clients often find that alternative modalities are more consistent with their own belief systems and also allow for more client autonomy in health care decisions (Fig. 1-1). Examples of alternative modalities include acupuncture, macrobiotics, herbal medicines, massage therapy, biofeedback, meditation, yoga, and chelation therapy. Complementary and alternative therapies are included throughout the text and will be identified with an icon ( ).

The Office of Alternative Medicine (OAM) in the United States supports research and evaluation of various alternative and complementary modalities and provides information to health care consumers about such modalities. The National Center for Complementary and Alternative Medicine (NCCAM) incorporates the work of the OAM in its mission and function.

Problems with the U.S. Health Care System

Structure of the Health Care Delivery System

The health care delivery system offers opportunities for nurses to alter nursing practice and improve the way care is delivered through managed care, integrated delivery systems, and redefined roles. Consumer participation in health care decisions is increasing, information is available on the Internet, and care is provided in a technology-intensive environment (Tiedje, Price, & You, 2008).

BOX 1-4 NATIONAL QUALITY FORUM "NEVER EVENTS" PERTAINING TO MATERNAL AND CHILD HEALTH

- Infant discharged to the wrong person
- Maternal death or serious disability associated with labor or birth in a low risk pregnancy while being cared for in a health care facility
- Death or serious disability (kernicterus) associated with failure to identify and treat hyperbilirubinemia in neonates
- Artificial insemination with the wrong donor sperm or donor egg

Source: The National Quality Forum: *National Quality Forum updates endorsement of serious reportable events in healthcare.* Available at www.qualityforum.org. Accessed May 12, 2010.

Reducing Medical Errors

Medical errors are a leading cause of death in the United States and result in as many as 98,000 deaths per year (Gauthier & Serber, 2005). An investigation by the Hearst media corporation concluded that about 200,000 deaths per year occurred because of preventable medical errors and infections (Harmon, 2009). In Canada adverse events are implicated in up to 23,750 deaths per year (French, 2006). Since the Institute of Medicine released its 1999 report, *To Err Is Human: Building a Safer Health System,* a concerted effort has been under way to analyze causes of errors and develop strategies to prevent them. Recognizing the multifaceted causes of medical errors, the Agency for Healthcare Research and Quality (2000) prepared a fact sheet, *20 Tips to Help Prevent Medical Errors,* for clients and the public. Clients are encouraged to be knowledgeable consumers of health care and to ask questions of providers, including physicians, midwives, nurses, and pharmacists.

In 2002 the National Quality Forum published a list of 27 events that should never occur in a health care facility (Shalo, 2007). The list was updated in 2006 with the addition of one event. Of these 28 events, 4 pertain directly to maternity and newborn care (Box 1-4). The National Quality Forum also published *Safe Practices for Better Healthcare* (www.qualityforum.org). The 30 safe practices included should be used in all applicable health care settings to reduce the risk of harm that results from processes, systems, and environments of care. Box 1-5 contains a selection of practices from that document.

In August 2007 the Centers for Medicare & Medicaid Services (CMS) issued a rule that denies payment for eight hospital-acquired conditions that became effective October 2008 (O'Reilly, 2008). Five of the conditions are also on the National Quality Forum list. Conditions that might pertain to maternity nursing include a foreign object retained after surgery, air embolism, blood incompatibility, falls and trauma, and catheter-associated urinary tract infection. Almost 1300 U.S. hospitals waive (do not bill for) costs associated with "never events" (O'Reilly).

High Cost of Health Care

Health care is one of the fastest-growing sectors of the U.S. economy. Currently, 16% of the gross domestic product is spent on health care, with an expectation that the proportion will rise to 20% by 2016 (Roehr, 2008). A shift in demographics, an emphasis on high-cost technology, and the liability costs of a litigious society contribute to the high cost of care. Most researchers agree that caring for the increased number of low-birth-weight (LBW) infants in neonatal intensive care units contributes significantly to the overall health care costs. Midwifery care has helped contain some health care costs. However, not all insurance carriers reimburse nurse practitioners and clinical nurse specialists as direct care providers. Nor do they reimburse for all services provided by nurse-midwives, a situation that continues to be a problem. Nurses must become involved in the politics of cost containment because they, as knowledgeable experts, can provide solutions to many health care problems at a relatively low cost.

BOX 1-5 SELECTED SAFE PRACTICES FOR BETTER HEALTH CARE

- Create and sustain a health care culture of safety.
- Ask each client or legal surrogate to "teach back" in his or her own words key information about the proposed treatments or procedures for which he or she is being asked to provide informed consent.
- Ensure that care information is transmitted and appropriately documented in a timely manner and in a clearly understandable form to clients and to all of the clients' health care providers or professionals, within and among care settings, who need that information in order to provide continued care.
- Standardize methods for the labeling and packaging of medications.
- Comply with current Centers for Disease Control and Prevention (CDC) hand hygiene guidelines.

Source: National Quality Forum. (2006). *Safe practices for better healthcare—2006 update.* Available at www.qualityforum.org. Accessed May 12, 2010.

Limited Access to Care

Barriers to access must be removed so pregnancy outcomes can be improved. The most significant barrier to access is the inability to pay. The number of uninsured people in the United States in 2006 was 47 million or 15.8% of the population (DeNavas-Walt, Proctor, & Smith, 2007). A more recent study reports that 86.7 million Americans were uninsured at one point during 2007-2008 (Pifer-Bixler, 2009). Lack of transportation and dependent child care are other barriers. In addition to a lack of insurance and high costs, a lack of providers for low-income women exists because many physicians either refuse to take Medicaid clients or take only a few such clients. This presents a serious problem because a significant proportion of births is to mothers who receive Medicaid.

Health Care Reform

In early 2010, President Obama signed into law the Patient Protection and Affordable Care Act. The Act aims to make insurance affordable, contain costs, strengthen and improve Medicare and Medicaid, and reform the insurance market. There are provisions to promote prevention and improve public health, improve the quality of care for all Americans, reduce waste, fraud, and abuse, and reform the health delivery system. There are some immediate benefits but implementation of the Act will occur over the next several years.

Efforts to Reduce Health Disparities

Significant disparities in morbidity and mortality rates are experienced by African-Americans, Native Americans, Hispanics, Alaska Natives, and Asian/Pacific Islanders in comparison with Caucasians. Shorter life expectancy, higher infant and maternal mortality rates, more birth defects, and more sexually transmitted infections are found among these ethnic and racial minority groups. The disparities are thought to result from a complex interaction among biologic factors, environment, and health behaviors. Disparities in education and income are associated with differences in morbidity and mortality.

The Health Resources and Services Administration (HRSA) Health Disparities Collaboratives are part of a national effort with the goal of eliminating disparities and improving delivery systems of health care for all people in the United States who are cared for in HRSA-supported health centers (Calvo, 2006). The National Institutes of Health has a commitment to improve the health of minorities and provides funding for research and training of minority researchers (www.nih.gov). The National Institute of Nursing Research has included the goal of reducing disparities in its strategic plan and supports research for this purpose. A broad public health perspective is needed to reduce these disparities (Satcher & Higginbotham, 2008).

Health Literacy

Health literacy involves a spectrum of abilities, ranging from reading an appointment slip to interpreting medication instructions. These skills must be assessed routinely to recognize a problem and accommodate clients with limited literacy skills. Most client education materials are written at too high a level for the average adult (Wilson, 2009).

As a result of the increasingly multicultural U.S. population, there is a more urgent need to address health literacy as a component of culturally and linguistically competent care. Health care providers contribute to health literacy by using simple, common words, avoiding jargon, and assessing whether the client understands the discussion. Speaking slowly and clearly and focusing on what is important will increase understanding.

Trends in Fertility and Birth Rate

Fertility trends and birth rates reflect women's needs for health care. Box 1-6 defines biostatistical terminology useful in analyzing maternity health care. In 2008 the **fertility rate,** births per 1000 women from 15 to 44 years of age, was 68.7 (Hamilton, Martin, & Ventura, 2010). The highest birth rates occurred among women between 20 and 29 years of age. The **birth rate,** number of live births in 1 year per 1000 population, was 14.3 in 2008; the teen birth rate was 41.5. In 2008 the proportion of births by unmarried women varied widely among racial groups in the United States: African-American, 72.3%; Hispanic, 52.5%; and non-Hispanic white, 28.6% (Hamilton et al.).

Low Birth Weight and Preterm Birth

The risks of morbidity and mortality increase for newborns weighing less than 2500 g (5 lb, 8 oz)—**low birth weight (LBW)** infants. Multiple births contribute to the incidence of LBW. The twin birth rate was 32.1 per 1000 in 2006. The downward trend in the birthrate of higher-order multiples (triplet, quadruplet, and greater) continued in 2006, with a rate of 153.3 per 100,000. In 2003, 58% of all multiple births were LBW. In 2008 the incidence of LBW infants was 8.2% (Hamilton et al., 2010). African-American infants are more than twice as likely as non-Hispanic white infants to be of LBW and to die in the first year of life. For African-American births, the incidence of LBW was 13.7%, whereas the rate was 7.2% for non-Hispanic white births and 6.9% for Hispanic births (Hamilton et al.). Cigarette smoking is associated with LBW, prematurity, and intrauterine growth restriction. In 2007, 13.2% of pregnant women smoked including 18.1% of non-Hispanic white women, 10.6% non-Hispanic black women, and 2.8% of Hispanic women (Heron, Sutton, Xu, Ventura, Strobino, & Guyer, 2010).

The percentage of infants born preterm (i.e., born before 38 weeks of gestation) was 12.3% in 2008. There was variation in the percentage according to race and Hispanic origin: 17.5% for non-Hispanic black births, 12.1% for Hispanic births, and 11.1% for non-Hispanic white births (Hamilton et al., 2010). Multiple births accounted for 3.4% of births in 2006, with most of the increase associated with increased use of fertility drugs and older age at childbearing (Martin, Kung, Mathews, Hoyert, Strobino, Guyer, et al., 2008).

BOX 1-6 MATERNAL-INFANT BIOSTATISTICAL TERMINOLOGY

Abortus: An embryo or fetus that is removed or expelled from the uterus at 20 weeks of gestation or less, weighs 500 g or less, or measures 25 cm or less

Birth rate: Number of live births in 1 year per 1000 population

Fertility rate: Number of births per 1000 women between the ages of 15 and 44 years (inclusive), calculated on a yearly basis

Infant mortality rate: Number of deaths of infants younger than 1 year of age per 1000 live births

Maternal mortality rate: Number of maternal deaths from births and complications of pregnancy, childbirth, and puerperium (the first 42 days after termination of the pregnancy) per 100,000 live births

Neonatal mortality rate: Number of deaths of infants younger than 28 days of age per 1000 live births

Perinatal mortality rate: Number of stillbirths and the number of neonatal deaths per 1000 live births

Stillbirth: An infant who, at birth, demonstrates no signs of life, such as breathing, heartbeat, or voluntary muscle movements

Infant Mortality in the United States

A common indicator of the adequacy of prenatal care and the health of a nation as a whole is the **infant mortality rate,** the number of deaths of infants younger than 1 year of age per 1000 live births. The neonatal mortality rate is the number of deaths of infants younger than 28 days of age per 1000 live births. The perinatal mortality rate is the number of stillbirths plus the number of neonatal deaths per 1000 live births. The U.S. infant mortality rate for 2007 was 6.77 (Heron et al., 2010). The disparity in infant mortality rate between African-American infants and Caucasian infants has increased over time. The infant mortality rate continues to be higher for non-Hispanic black babies (13.63 per 1000) than for non-Hispanic whites (5.76 per 1000) and Hispanic (5.62 per 1000) babies (Heron et al.). Limited maternal education, young maternal age, unmarried status, poverty, lack of prenatal care, and smoking appear to be associated with higher infant mortality rates. Poor nutrition, alcohol use, and maternal conditions such as poor health or hypertension also are important contributors to infant mortality. To address the factors associated with infant mortality, a shift from the current emphasis on high-technology medical interventions to a focus on improving access to preventive care for low-income families must occur.

The leading cause of death in the neonatal period is congenital anomalies. Other causes of neonatal death include disorders related to short gestation and LBW, sudden infant death, respiratory distress syndrome, and the effects of maternal complications. Racial differences in the infant mortality rates continue to challenge public health experts. Increased rates of survival during the neonatal period have resulted largely from high-quality prenatal care and the improvement in perinatal services, including technologic advances in neonatal intensive care and obstetrics.

Commitment at national, state, and local levels is required to reduce the infant mortality rate. More research is needed to identify the extent to which financial, educational, sociocultural, and behavioral factors individually and collectively affect perinatal morbidity and mortality. Barriers to care must be removed and perinatal services modified to meet contemporary health care needs.

International Infant Mortality Trends

In 2005, the infant mortality rate of Canada (5.4/1000) ranked twenty-fifth, and that of the United States (6.9/1000) ranked twenty-ninth, when compared with those of other industrialized nations (Heron et al., 2010). Decreases in the infant mortality rate in the United States do not keep pace with the rates of other industrialized countries. One reason for this is the high rate of LBW infants in the United States in contrast with the rates in other countries.

Maternal Mortality Trends

Worldwide, approximately 1600 women die each day of problems related to pregnancy or childbirth; many of these deaths are preventable. In the United States in 2006, the annual **maternal mortality rate** (number of maternal deaths per 100,000 live births) was 13.3 (Heron, Hoyert, Murphy, Xu, Kochanek, & Tejada-Vera, 2009). The Centers for Disease Control and Prevention (CDC) began working with national and international groups in 2001 to develop and implement programs to promote safe motherhood (Jones, 2008). Although the overall number of maternal deaths is small, maternal mortality remains a significant problem because a high proportion of deaths are preventable, primarily through improving the access to and use of prenatal care services. In the United States, there is significant racial disparity in the rates of maternal death: black women (32.7), Hispanic women (10.2), and Caucasian women (9.5) (Heron et al.). The leading causes of maternal death attributable to pregnancy differ over the world. In general, three major causes have persisted for the last 50 years: hypertensive disorders, infection, and hemorrhage. The three leading causes of maternal mortality in the United States today are gestational hypertension, pulmonary embolism, and hemorrhage. Factors that are strongly related to maternal death include age (younger than 20 years and 35 years or older), lack of prenatal care, low educational attainment, unmarried status, and non-Caucasian race. The *Healthy People 2010* goal of 3.3 maternal deaths per 100,000 posed a significant challenge and was not achieved. Worldwide strategies to reduce maternal mortality rates include improving access to skilled attendants at birth, providing postabortion care, improving family planning services, and providing adolescents with better reproductive health services (Millennium Development Goals, 2008).

Increase in High Risk Pregnancies

Approximately 500,000 of the 4 million births that occur in the United States each year are categorized as high risk because of maternal or fetal complications. The diagnosis of high risk imposes a situational crisis on the family (e.g., loss of pregnancy before the anticipated date, development of gestational diabetes mellitus with its potential complications, or birth of a neonate who does not meet cultural, societal, or familial norms and expectations).

Identification of the risks, together with appropriate and timely intervention during the perinatal period, can prevent morbidity and mortality among mothers and infants. With the changing demographics in the United States, more women and families can be identified as at risk because of factors other than biophysical criteria. The increasing numbers of homeless, single, or uninsured pregnant women who have no access to prenatal care during any stage of pregnancy and the behaviors and lifestyles that pose a risk to the health of the mother and fetus contribute to the problem.

Over 90% of pregnant women take prescription or nonprescription drugs, social drugs (e.g., alcohol, tobacco), or illicit drugs sometime during pregnancy (The Merck Manual Online Medical Library, 2007). Drug use in pregnancy has contributed to higher incidences of prematurity, LBW, congenital defects, learning disabilities, and withdrawal symptoms in infants. Alcohol use in pregnancy has been associated with miscarriages, mental retardation, LBW, and alcohol-related birth defects.

More than one third (35.2%) of women in the United States are obese (body mass index of 30 or greater), with adults ages 45 to 64 having the highest prevalence. Obesity in women demonstrates significant racial disparities: 53.2% of non-Hispanic black women, 41.8% of Mexican-American women, and 31.6% of non-Hispanic white women ages 20 years and older are obese (National Center for Health Statistics, 2009). Almost 20% of women who give birth in the United States are obese. The two most frequently reported maternal medical risk factors are hypertension associated with pregnancy and diabetes, both of which are associated with obesity. Obesity in pregnancy is associated with the use of increased health care services and hospital stays that are longer (Chu, Bachman, Callaghan, Whitlock, Dietz, Berg, et al., 2008).

High risk pregnancy is a critical problem for modern medical and nursing care. The new social emphasis on the quality of life and the wanted child has resulted in a reduction of family size and the number of unwanted pregnancies. At the same time, technologic advances have facilitated pregnancies in previously infertile couples. As a consequence, emphasis is on the safe birth of normal infants who can develop to their potential. Scientific and technologic advances have allowed perinatal health care to reach a level far beyond that previously available.

Early and ongoing risk assessment is a crucial component of perinatal care. Conditions associated with perinatal morbidity and mortality can be prevented, treated, or referred to more skilled health care providers. Factors to consider when determining a woman's risk status include resources available locally to treat the condition, availability of appropriate facilities for transport if needed, and determination of the best match for the woman's needs. In the past, risk factors were evaluated only from a medical viewpoint; therefore, only adverse medical, obstetric, or physiologic conditions were considered to place the woman at risk. Today a more comprehensive approach to high risk pregnancy is used, and the factors associated with high risk childbearing are grouped into broad categories based on threats to health and pregnancy outcome.

Regionalization of Perinatal Health Care Services

Not all facilities develop and maintain the full spectrum of services required for high risk perinatal clients. As a consequence, regionalization of hospital-based perinatal health care services occurred and facilities within a geographic region were organized to provide different levels of care. This system of coordinated care was also applied to preconception and ambulatory prenatal care services.

Guidelines have been established regarding the level of care that can be expected at any given facility. In ambulatory settings, providers must distinguish themselves by the level of care they provide. *Basic care* is provided by obstetricians, family physicians, certified nurse-midwives, and other advanced practice clinicians approved by local governance. Routine risk-oriented prenatal care, education, and support are provided. Providers offering *specialty care* are obstetricians who must provide fetal diagnostic testing and management of obstetric and medical complications in addition to basic care. *Subspecialty care* is provided by maternal-fetal medicine specialists and includes the aforementioned in addition to genetic testing, advanced fetal therapies, and management of severe maternal and fetal complications (American Academy of Pediatrics [AAP] & American College of Obstetricians and Gynecologists [ACOG], 2007).

Specialty hospital care includes these personnel requirements in addition to providing care of high risk mothers and fetuses, stabilization of ill neonates before transfer, and care of preterm infants with a birth weight of 1500 g or more. Women in preterm labor or those with impending births at 32 weeks of gestation or less should be transferred for subspecialty care. Additional criteria for subspecialty care include provision of comprehensive perinatal care for women and infants of all risk categories, evaluation and use of new high risk technologies and therapies, and data collection and retrieval. Collaboration among providers to meet the woman's needs is the key to reducing perinatal morbidity and mortality (AAP & ACOG, 2007).

High-Technology Care

Advances in scientific knowledge and the large number of high risk pregnancies have contributed to a health care system that emphasizes high-technology care. Maternity care has extended to preconception counseling, more and better scientific techniques to monitor the mother and fetus, more definitive tests for hypoxia and acidosis, and neonatal intensive care units. The labors of virtually all women who give birth in hospitals are monitored electronically despite the lack of evidence of efficacy of such monitoring. The numbers of assisted labors and births are increasing. Internet-based information is available to the public that enhances interactions among health care providers, families, and community providers. Point-of-care testing is available. Personal data assistants are used to enhance comprehensive care; the medical record is increasingly in electronic form.

Telehealth is an umbrella term for the use of communication technologies and electronic information to provide or support health care when the participants are separated by distance. Telehealth permits specialists, including nurses, to provide health care and consultation when distance separates them from those needing care. This technology has the potential to save billions of dollars annually for health care, but these technologic advances have also contributed to higher health care costs.

Strides are being made in identifying genetic codes, and genetic engineering is taking place. Women's health has expanded to emphasize care of older women, new cancer-screening techniques, advances in the diagnosis and treatment of breast cancer, and work on an AIDS vaccine. In general, high-technology care has flourished, whereas "health" care has become relatively neglected. Nurses must use caution and prospective planning and assess the effect of the emerging technology.

Community-Based Care

A shift in settings, from acute care institutions to ambulatory settings including the home, has occurred (see Chapter 2). Even childbearing women at high risk are cared for on an outpatient basis or in the home. Technology previously available only in the hospital is now found in the home. This has affected the organizational structure of care, the skills required in providing such care, and the costs to consumers.

Home health care also has a community focus. Nurses are involved in providing care for women and infants in homeless shelters, in caring for adolescents in school-based clinics, and in promoting health at community sites, churches, and shopping malls. Nursing education curricula are increasingly community based.

Childbirth Practices

Prenatal care can promote better pregnancy outcomes by providing early risk assessment and promoting healthy behaviors such as improved nutrition and smoking cessation. Prenatal care ideally begins before pregnancy because early decisions lay the foundation for the entire perinatal year. If at all possible, education continues in each trimester of pregnancy, and extends through the early postpartum weeks. Some health care providers today promote preconception care as an important component of perinatal services. Preconception or early pregnancy classes also emphasize health-promoting behavior as well as choices of care.

In 2006, 69% of all women received care in the first trimester. There is disparity in receiving prenatal care by race and ethnicity: 12.2% of Hispanic women, 11.8% of non-Hispanic blacks, and 5.2% of non-Hispanic whites received late or no prenatal care (Heron et al., 2010). In spite of these statistics, substantial

CLINICAL REASONING

Safety and Efficacy of Midwifery Care

A group of nurse-midwives is setting up practice in your hometown. They are to collaborate with one of the groups of obstetricians in the same city. A letter to the editor appeared in the local newspaper stating that the presence of midwives will jeopardize care of pregnant women in the community because midwives usually care for the poor and indigent, deliver babies at home, and therefore do not have the skills to work in hospitals and care for middle-class women who have insurance. The letter-writer urged the community to boycott the midwives to ensure safe childbirth for women in the community.

1. Evidence—Is there sufficient evidence to document the qualifications of nurse-midwives and their safety record to write a response to this letter?
2. Assumptions—What assumptions can be made about midwifery care and the knowledge base of the public regarding that care?
3. What implications and priorities for nursing can be made at this time?
4. Does the evidence objectively support your conclusion?
5. Are there alternative perspectives to your conclusion?

gains have been made in the use of prenatal care since the early 1990s, which is attributed to the expansion in the 1980s of Medicaid coverage for pregnant women.

Women can choose physicians or nurse-midwives as primary care providers. In 2006, physicians attended 92% of all births and certified nurse-midwives attended 7.4% (Heron et al., 2010). Women who choose nurse-midwives as their primary providers participate more actively in childbirth decisions and receive fewer interventions during labor. The rate of vaginal births after cesarean (VBACs) declined, whereas cesarean births increased to 31.8% of live births in the United States in 2007. The *Healthy People 2010* goal of 15% was not met.

Certified nurse-midwives (CNMs) are registered nurses with education in the two disciplines of nursing and midwifery. **Certified midwives** (direct-entry midwives) are educated only in the discipline of midwifery. In the United States, certification of midwives is through the American College of Nurse-Midwives (ACNM), the professional association for midwives. The Royal College of Midwives is the professional association for midwives in the United Kingdom. In Canada, the Association of Ontario Midwives is the professional association, and the College of Midwives of Ontario is the regulatory body for midwives in Ontario; the other provinces of Canada have similar regulatory bodies (e.g., College of Midwives of British Columbia). Many national associations belong to the International Confederation of Midwives, which comprises 97 member associations from 86 countries in the Americas and Europe, Africa, and the Asia-Pacific region.

With family-centered care, fathers, partners, grandparents, siblings, and friends may be present for labor and birth. Fathers or partners may be present for cesarean births. Fathers or partners may participate in vaginal births by "catching the baby" or cutting the umbilical cord or both (Fig. 1-2). Doulas—trained and experienced female labor attendants—may be present to provide a continuous, one-on-one caring presence throughout the labor and birth. Ideally, newborns are placed skin-to-skin with the mother immediately after birth and are encouraged to breastfeed as soon as possible. Nonseparation is common; neonates often remain in the room with their parents and may never transfer to a newborn nursery. Parents actively participate in newborn care on mother/baby units, in nurseries, and in neonatal intensive care units.

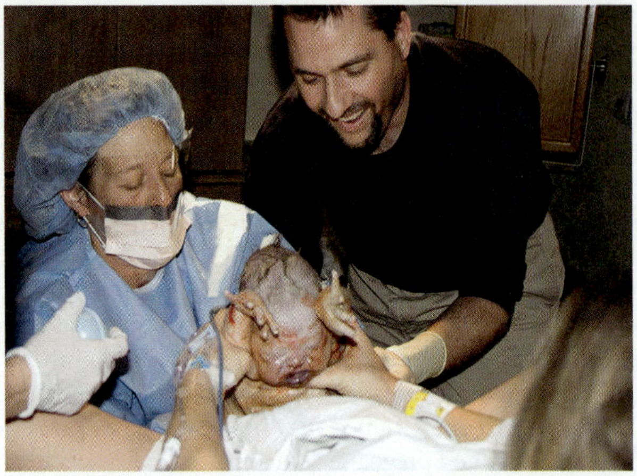

FIG. 1-2 Father "catching" newborn son. Mother is reaching down to help birth the baby. (Courtesy Darren and Julie Nelson, Loveland, CO.)

Neonatal security in the hospital setting is of concern. A significant number of cases of "baby-napping" and of sending parents home with the wrong baby have been reported. Security systems have been placed in nurseries, and nurses are required to wear photo identification or some other security badge.

Discharge of a mother and baby within 24 hours of birth has created a growing need for follow-up or home care. In some settings, discharge may occur as early as 6 hours after birth. Legislation has been enacted to ensure that mothers and babies are permitted to stay in the hospital for at least 48 hours after vaginal birth and 96 hours after cesarean birth although they may choose to leave earlier. Focused and efficient teaching is necessary to enable the parents and infant to make the transition safely from the hospital to the home.

Involving Consumers and Promoting Self-Management

Self-management is appealing to both clients and the health care system because of its potential to reduce health care costs. Maternity care is especially suited to self-management because childbearing is primarily health focused, women are usually well when they enter the system, and visits to health care providers can present the opportunity for health and illness interventions. Measures to improve health and reduce risks associated with poor pregnancy outcomes and illness can be addressed. Topics such as nutrition education, stress management, smoking cessation, alcohol and drug treatment, prevention of violence, improvement of social supports, and parenting education are appropriate for such encounters.

International Concerns

Female genital mutilation, infibulation (surgical closure of the labia majora), and circumcision are terms used to describe procedures in which part or all of the female external genitalia are removed for cultural or nontherapeutic reasons (WHO, 2006). Worldwide, many women undergo such procedures. With the growing number of immigrants from Africa and other countries where female genital mutilation is practiced, nurses in the United States and Canada will increasingly encounter women who have undergone the procedure. Women who have undergone the procedure are significantly more likely to have adverse obstetric outcomes resulting in one or two additional perinatal deaths per 100 births (WHO, 2006). Ethical dilemmas arise when the woman requests that after birth the perineum be repaired as it was after infibulation and the health care provider believes that such repair is unethical. The International Council of Nurses and other health professionals have spoken out against the procedures that result in mutilation as harmful to women's health.

Health of Women

Various factors and conditions affect women's health. Race is a major factor: Caucasian women have a life expectancy at birth of 80.7 years, in contrast with 77.0 years for African-American women (Miniño, Xu, Kochanek, & Tejada-Vera, 2009). In 2010, there were an estimated 207,090 new cases of invasive breast cancer in women in the United States, and 39,840 women were expected to die of the disease (American Cancer Society, 2010). Early detection of breast cancer through mammography can reduce the mortality rate resulting from this type of cancer. However, because of lack of information or lack of insurance and access, many women never have mammograms. Wide disparity exists between Caucasian women and women of other races and between older and younger women in their rates of mammography, detection, and treatment of breast cancer, and in their survival rates (see Chapter 10).

The population has grown older: approximately 50 million women are older than 50 years of age; 51 is the median age for menopause. Hormone replacement therapy for menopausal women has been used for many years and has both benefits and risks (see Chapter 6).

Violence is a major factor affecting women (see Chapter 5). Violence includes battery, rape or other sexual assaults, and attacks with various weapons. Rates of reported intimate partner violence have increased, possibly because of better assessment and reporting mechanisms. Approximately 4% to 8% of pregnant women are battered; the incidence of battering increases during pregnancy. Violence is associated with complications of pregnancy such as bleeding. Alcoholism and substance abuse by the woman and her abuser are associated with violence and homelessness, which affect a growing number of women and children and place them at risk for a variety of health problems.

The rates of pregnancy and elective abortion among adolescents declined from 1991 through 2005 but the pregnancy rate increased between 2005 and 2007; rates are higher in the United States than in any other industrialized country. Single mothers gave birth to 39.7% of the babies born in the United States in 2007 (Heron et al., 2010). Births to unmarried women are frequently related to less favorable outcomes, such as LBW infants or preterm birth.

TRENDS IN NURSING PRACTICE

The increasing complexity of care for maternity and women's health clients has contributed to specialization of nurses working with these clients. This specialized knowledge is gained through experience, advanced degrees, and certification programs. Nurses in advanced practice (e.g., nurse practitioners and nurse-midwives) may provide primary care throughout a woman's life, including during the pregnancy cycle. In some settings, the clinical nurse specialist and nurse practitioner roles are blended, and nurses deliver high-quality, comprehensive, and cost-effective care in a variety of settings. Lactation consultants provide services in the hospital setting, in clinics and physician offices, and during home visits.

Nursing Interventions Classification

When the National Institute of Medicine proposed that all client records be computerized by the year 2000, a need for a common language to describe the contributions of nurses to client care became evident. Nurses from the University of Iowa developed a comprehensive standardized language that describes interventions that are performed by generalist or specialist nurses. This language is included in the Nursing Interventions Classification (NIC) (Dochterman & Bulechek, 2004). Interventions commonly used by maternal-child nurses include those in Box 1-7.

Evidence-Based Practice

Evidence-based practice—providing care based on evidence gained through research and clinical trials—is increasingly emphasized. Although not all practice can be evidence based, practitioners must use the best available information on which to base their interventions. The Association of Women's Health, Obstetric and Neonatal Nurses (AWHONN) *Standards and Guidelines for Professional Nursing Practice in the Care of Women and Newborns* (AWHONN, 2009) and the *Standards for Professional Perinatal Nursing Practice and Certification in Canada* (AWHONN, 2002) include an evidence-based approach to practice. Discussion of nursing care and evidence-based practice boxes throughout this text provide examples of evidence-based practice in perinatal and women's health nursing (see Evidence-Based Practice box).

Cochrane Pregnancy and Childbirth Database

The Cochrane Pregnancy and Childbirth Database was first planned in 1976 with a small grant from the World Health Organization to Dr. Iain Chalmers and colleagues at Oxford. In 1993, the Cochrane Collaboration was formed, and the Oxford Database of Perinatal Trials became known as the Cochrane Pregnancy and Childbirth Database. The Cochrane Collaboration oversees up-to-date, systematic reviews of randomized controlled trials of health care and disseminates these reviews. The premise of the project is that these types of studies provide the most reliable evidence about the effects of care.

The evidence from these studies should encourage practitioners to implement useful measures and to abandon those that are useless or harmless. Studies are ranked in six categories:

1. Beneficial forms of care
2. Forms of care that are likely to be beneficial
3. Forms of care with a trade-off between beneficial and adverse effects
4. Forms of care with unknown effectiveness
5. Forms of care that are unlikely to be beneficial
6. Forms of care that are likely to be ineffective or harmful

BOX 1-7 CHILDBEARING CARE INTERVENTIONS

LEVEL 1 DOMAIN: FAMILY
- Care that supports the family

LEVEL 2 CLASS: CHILDBEARING CARE
- Interventions to assist in the preparation for childbirth and management of the psychologic and physiologic changes before, during, and immediately after childbirth

LEVEL 3: INTERVENTIONS
- Amnioinfusion
- Birthing
- Bleeding reduction: antepartum uterus
- Bleeding reduction: postpartum uterus
- Breastfeeding assistance
- Cesarean section care
- Childbirth preparation
- Circumcision care
- Electronic fetal monitoring: antepartum
- Electronic fetal monitoring: intrapartum
- Environmental management: attachment process
- Family integrity promotion: childbearing family
- Family planning: contraception
- Family planning: infertility
- Family planning: unplanned pregnancy
- Fertility preservation
- Genetic counseling
- Grief work facilitation: perinatal death
- High risk pregnancy care
- Intrapartal care
- Intrapartal care: high risk delivery
- Kangaroo care
- Labor induction
- Labor suppression
- Lactation suppression
- Newborn care
- Newborn monitoring
- Nonnutritive sucking
- Phototherapy: neonate
- Postpartal care
- Preconception counseling
- Pregnancy termination care
- Prenatal care
- Reproductive technology management
- Resuscitation: fetus
- Resuscitation: neonate
- Risk identification: childbearing family
- Surveillance: late pregnancy
- Tube care: umbilical line
- Ultrasonography: limited obstetric

From Dochterman, J., & Bulechek, G. (2004). *Nursing interventions classification (NIC)* (4th ed.). St. Louis: Mosby.

EVIDENCE-BASED PRACTICE *Pat Gingrich*

Searching for and Evaluating the Evidence

Throughout this text you will see Evidence-Based Practice boxes. These boxes provide examples of how a nurse might conduct an inquiry into an identified practice question. Curiosity and access to a virtual or real library are all the nurse needs to be confident that his or her practice has a sound foundation of evidence.

A literature search may reveal up to three levels of evidence. The first level consists of primary studies. The strongest of these are randomized controlled trials. Well-designed studies, even small ones, each add another piece to the puzzle.

These primary studies may be combined into the second level of evidence. In systematic analyses such as those in the Cochrane Database, the researcher uses methods to identify all studies relevant to a particular question. If the data are similar enough, they can be pooled into a metaanalysis. If the evidence is strong, some analyses will form the basis for recommendations for practice and to guide further inquiry.

At the tertiary level, professional organizations such as the Agency for Healthcare Research and Quality (AHRQ) (www.ahrq.gov) or the Academy of Breastfeeding Medicine (ABM) (www.bfmed.org) may decide to address a broad practice question by sorting through all the available primary and secondary evidence in addition to consulting experienced clinicians. After thoughtful review the committee of experts in the organization then crafts its consensus statement. These recommendations for best practice stand on the shoulders of the systematic analysts, who stand on the many shoulders of the primary researchers.

Provided the professional organization is well respected and the process is rigorous, these guidelines in the consensus statement carry enormous authority. Individuals and institutions may choose to adopt these guidelines with confidence. An example of this process is the Association of Women's Health, Obstetric and Neonatal Nurses (AWHONN) (www.awhonn.org) Late Preterm Infant Initiative. This initiative began in 2005 in response to the confusion that surrounded the care of infants who do not qualify for neonatal intensive care admission yet require extra vigilance. Nurseries can adapt these recommendations to their specific institutions, enabling nurses to become more effective at caring for the unique problems of this population of neonates. As is the case with AWHONN, most professional organizations make their guidelines available free of charge on their websites.

Practices that have been reviewed by the Cochrane Collaboration as well as other evidence for practice are identified with a symbol ( ) throughout this text.

Joanna Briggs Institute

Established in 1996 as an initiative of the Royal Adelaide Hospital and the University of Adelaide in Australia, the Joanna Briggs Institute (JBI) uses a collaborative approach for evaluating evidence from a range of sources (www.joannabriggs.edu.au). The JBI has formed collaborations with a variety of universities and hospitals around the world including in the United States and Canada. In 2007, the JBI adopted the following grades of recommendation for evidence of feasibility, appropriateness, meaningfulness, and effectiveness: *A*, strong support that merits application; *B*, moderate support that warrants consideration of application; and *C*, not supported (The Joanna Briggs Institute, 2008). The JBI provides another source for perinatal nurses to access information to support evidence-based practice.

TABLE 1-1 NURSING OUTCOMES CLASSIFICATION

Breastfeeding Establishment: Infant (1000)
Domain—Physiologic health (II)
Class—Nutrition (K)
Scale—Not adequate to Totally adequate (f)
Definition: Infant attachment to and sucking from the mother's breast for nourishment during the first 3 weeks of breastfeeding

BREASTFEEDING ESTABLISHMENT: INFANT	NOT ADEQUATE 1	SLIGHTLY ADEQUATE 2	MODERATELY ADEQUATE 3	SUBSTANTIALLY ADEQUATE 4	TOTALLY ADEQUATE 5
Indicators					
100001. Proper alignment and latch-on	1	2	3	4	5
100002. Proper areolar grasp	1	2	3	4	5
100003. Proper areolar compression	1	2	3	4	5
100004. Correct suck and tongue placement	1	2	3	4	5
100005. Audible swallow	1	2	3	4	5
100006. Swallowing a minimum of 5 to 10 minutes per breast	1	2	3	4	5
100007. Minimum 8 feedings per day	1	2	3	4	5
100008. Urinations per day appropriate for age	1	2	3	4	5
100009. Loose, yellow, seedy stools per day appropriate for age	1	2	3	4	5
100010. Appropriate weight gain for age	1	2	3	4	5
100011. Infant contentment after feeding	1	2	3	4	5

Outcome content references:
Biancuzzo, M. (2003). *Breastfeeding the newborn: Clinical strategies for nurses* (2nd ed.). St. Louis: Mosby.
Henderson, A., Pincombe, J., & Stamp, G. (2000). Assisting women to establish breastfeeding: Exploring midwives practices. *Breastfeeding Review, 8*(3), 11-17.
Lang, S. (2002). *Breastfeeding special care babies* (2nd ed.). London: Bailliere Tindall.
Lawrence, R.A., & Lawrence, R.M. (1999). *Breastfeeding: A guide for the medical professional* (5th ed.). St. Louis: Mosby.
Minchin, M. (1989). Positioning for breastfeeding. *Birth: Issues in Perinatal Care and Education, 16*(2), 67-80.
Mulford, C. (1992). The mother-baby assessment (MBA): An "Apgar Score" for breastfeeding. *Journal of Human Lactation, 8*(2), 79-82.
Neifert, M., & Seacat, J. (1986). A guide to successful breastfeeding. *Contemporary Pediatrics, 3,* 1-14.
Page-Goertz, S. (1989). Discharge planning for the breastfeeding dyad. *Pediatric Nursing, 15*(5), 543-544.
Righard, L., & Alade, M. (1992). Sucking technique and its effect on success of breastfeeding. *Birth: Issues in Perinatal Care and Education, 19*(4), 185-189.
Riordan, J., & Auerbach, K. (1999). *Breastfeeding and human lactation* (2nd ed.). Boston: Jones and Bartlett.
Shrago, L., & Bocar, D. (1990). The infant's contribution to breastfeeding. *Journal of Obstetric, Gynecologic and Neonatal Nursing, 19*(3), 209-215.
Walker, M. (1989). Functional assessment of infant breastfeeding patterns. *Birth: Issues in Perinatal Care and Education, 16*(3), 140-147.
Moorhead, S., Johnson, M., & Maas, M. (Eds.). (2000). *Nursing outcomes classification (NOC)* (3rd ed.). St. Louis: Mosby.

Outcomes-Oriented Practice. Outcomes of care (that is, the effectiveness of interventions and quality of care) are receiving increased emphasis. **Outcomes-oriented care** measures effectiveness of care against benchmarks or standards. It is a measure of the value of nursing using quality indicators and answers the question, "Did the client benefit or not benefit from the care provided?" (Moorhead, Johnson, & Maas, 2004). The Outcome and Assessment Information Set (OASIS) is an example of an outcome system important for nursing. Its use is required by the CMS in all home health organizations that are Medicare accredited. The Nursing Outcomes Classification (NOC) is an effort to identify outcomes and related measures that can be used for evaluation of care of individuals, families, and communities across the care continuum (Moorhead et al.). An example of outcomes classification is provided in Table 1-1.

A Global Perspective. Advances in medicine and nursing have resulted in increased knowledge and understanding in the care of mothers and infants and reduced perinatal morbidity and mortality rates. However, these advances have affected predominantly the industrialized nations. For example, the majority of the 3.2 million children living with human immunodeficiency virus (HIV) or AIDS acquired the infection through perinatal transmission and live in sub-Saharan Africa.

As the world becomes smaller because of travel and communication technologies, nurses and other health care providers are gaining a global perspective and participating in activities to improve the health and health care of people worldwide. Nurses participate in medical outreach, providing obstetric, surgical, ophthalmologic, orthopedic, or other services (Fig. 1-3); attend international meetings; conduct research; and provide international consultation. International student and faculty exchanges occur. More articles about health and health care in various countries are appearing in nursing journals. Several schools of nursing in the United States are World Health Organization Collaborating Centers.

STANDARDS OF PRACTICE AND LEGAL ISSUES IN DELIVERY OF CARE

Nursing standards of practice in perinatal and women's health nursing have been described by several organizations, including the ANA, which publishes standards for maternal-child health nursing; AWHONN, which publishes standards of practice and education for perinatal nurses (Box 1-8); ACNM, which publishes standards of practice for midwives; and the National Association of Neonatal Nurses (NANN), which publishes standards of practice for neonatal nurses. These

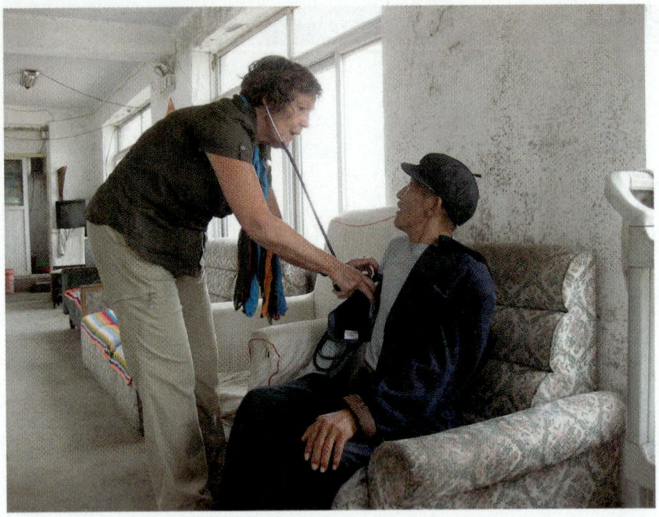

FIG. 1-3 Nurse examining client on a medical mission in China. (Courtesy Sue George, Hays, KS.)

standards reflect current knowledge, represent levels of practice agreed on by leaders in the specialty, and can be used for clinical benchmarking.

In addition to these more formalized standards, agencies have their own policy and procedure books that outline standards to be followed in that setting. In legal terms, the **standard of care** is that level of practice that a reasonably prudent nurse would provide in the same or similar circumstances. In determining legal negligence, the care given is compared with the standard of care. If the standard was not met and harm resulted, negligence occurred. The number of legal suits in the perinatal area has typically been high. As a consequence, malpractice insurance costs are high for physicians, nurse-midwives, and nurses who work in labor and birth settings.

> **LEGAL TIP: Standard of Care**
> When you are uncertain about how to perform a procedure, consult the agency procedure book and follow the guidelines printed therein. These guidelines are the standard of care for that agency.

Risk Management

Risk management is an evolving process that identifies risks, establishes preventive practices, develops reporting mechanisms, and delineates procedures for managing lawsuits. Nurses should be familiar with concepts of risk management and their implications for nursing practice. These concepts can be viewed as systems of checks and balances that ensure high-quality client care from preconception until after birth. Effective risk management minimizes the risk of injury to clients and the number of lawsuits against nurses, doctors, and hospitals. Each facility or site develops site-specific risk management procedures based on accepted standards and guidelines. The procedures and guidelines must be reviewed periodically.

To decrease risk of errors in the administration of medications, The Joint Commission (TJC) (2009) developed a list of abbreviations, acronyms, and symbols *not* to use (Table 1-2). In addition, each agency must develop its own list.

BOX 1-8 STANDARDS OF CARE FOR WOMEN AND NEWBORNS

STANDARDS THAT DEFINE THE NURSE'S RESPONSIBILITY TO THE CLIENT

Assessment
- Collection of health data of the woman or newborn

Diagnosis
- Analysis of data to determine nursing diagnosis

Outcome Identification
- Identification of expected outcomes that are individualized

Planning
- Development of a plan of care

Implementation
- Performance of interventions for the plan of care

Evaluation
- Evaluation of the effectiveness of interventions in relation to expected outcomes

STANDARDS OF PROFESSIONAL PERFORMANCE THAT DELINEATE ROLES AND BEHAVIORS FOR WHICH THE PROFESSIONAL NURSE IS ACCOUNTABLE

Quality of Care
- Systemic evaluation of nursing practice

Performance Appraisal
- Self-evaluation in relation to professional practice standards and other regulations

Education
- Participation in ongoing educational activities to maintain knowledge for practice

Collegiality
- Contribution to the development of peers, students, and others

Ethics
- Use of ANA Code of Ethics for Nurses with Interpretive Statements (ANA, 2001) to guide practice

Collaboration
- Involvement of client, significant others, and other health care providers in the provision of client care

Research
- Use of research findings in practice

Resource Utilization
- Consideration of factors related to safety, effectiveness, and costs in planning and delivering client care

Practice Environment
- Contribution to the environment of care delivery

Accountability
- Legal and professional responsibility for practice

Source: Association of Women's Health, Obstetric and Neonatal Nurses (AWHONN). (2009). *Standards and guidelines for professional nursing practice in the care of women and newborns* (7th ed.). Washington, DC: Author.

Sentinel Events

TJC describes a sentinel event as "an unexpected occurrence involving death or serious physical or psychological injury, or the risk thereof. Serious injury specifically includes loss of limb or function." These events are called *sentinel* because they signal a need for an immediate investigation and response (TJC, 2010). Reportable sentinel events in perinatal nursing include

TABLE 1-2 THE JOINT COMMISSION "DO NOT USE" LIST

DO NOT USE	POTENTIAL PROBLEM	USE INSTEAD
U (unit)	Mistaken for "0" (zero), the number "4" (four), or "cc"	Write "unit"
IU (International Unit)	Mistaken for IV (intravenous) or the number 10 (ten)	Write "International Unit"
Q.D., QD, q.d., qd (daily)	Mistaken for each other	Write "daily"
Q.O.D., QOD, q.o.d., qod (every other day)	Period after the Q mistaken for an "I" and the "O" for "I"	Write "every other day"
Trailing zero (X.0 mg)	Decimal point is missed	Write X mg
Lack of leading zero (.X mg)	Decimal point is missed	Write 0.X mg
MS	Can mean morphine sulfate or magnesium sulfate	Write "morphine sulfate"
MSO_4 and $MgSO_4$	Confused for one another	Write "magnesium sulfate"
Additional Abbreviations, Acronyms, and Symbols*		
> (greater than) < (less than)	Misinterpreted as the number "7" (seven) or the letter "L" Confused for one another	Write "greater than" Write "less than"
Abbreviations for drug names	Misinterpreted due to similar abbreviations for multiple drugs	Write drug names in full
Apothecary units	Unfamiliar to many practitioners Confused with metric units	Use metric units
@	Mistaken for the number "2" (two)	Write "at"
cc	Mistaken for U (units) when poorly written	Write "mL" or "ml" or "milliliters" ("mL" is preferred)
µg	Mistaken for mg (milligrams) resulting in one thousand–fold overdose	Write "mcg" or "micrograms"

*(For possible future inclusion in the Official "Do Not Use" List)

Source: Official "Do Not Use" list. Available at www.jointcommission.org/PatientSafety/DoNotUseList. Updated March 5, 2009. Accessed February 9, 2010.

any maternal death related to the process of birth, any perinatal death unrelated to a congenital condition in an infant having a birth weight greater than 2500 g, severe neonatal hyperbilirubinemia (bilirubin greater than 30 mg/dL), and infant discharge to the wrong family (TJC). Other sentinel events that may occur in perinatal nursing include hemolytic transfusion reaction involving major blood group incompatibilities, leaving a foreign body (e.g., sponge or forceps) in a client after surgery, and falls that result in death or major permanent loss of function that is a direct result of the injuries caused by the fall. When a sentinel event occurs, there must be a root cause analysis and an action plan formulated that identifies strategies to reduce the risk of future similar events.

Failure to Rescue

Failure to rescue is used to "evaluate the quality and quantity of nursing care by comparing the number of surgical clients who develop common complications who survive versus those who do not" (Simpson, 2005). As mothers and babies are generally healthy, complications leading to death in obstetrics are comparatively rare. Simpson proposes evaluating the perinatal team's ability to decrease risk of adverse outcomes by measuring processes involved in common complications and emergencies in obstetrics. Key components of failure to rescue are (1) careful surveillance and identification of complications, and (2) acting quickly to initiate appropriate interventions and activating a team response. For the perinatal nurse, this involves timely identification of complications, appropriate interventions, and efforts of the team to minimize client harm. Maternal complications that are appropriate for process measurement are placental abruption, postpartum hemorrhage, uterine rupture, eclampsia, and amniotic fluid embolism (Simpson). Fetal complications include nonreassuring fetal heart rate and pattern, prolapsed umbilical cord, shoulder dystocia, and uterine hyperstimulation (Simpson). Perinatal nurses can use these complications to develop a list of expectations for monitoring, timely identification, interventions, and roles of team members. The list can be used to evaluate the perinatal team's response.

Quality and Safety Education for Nurses

Quality and Safety Education for Nurses (QSEN) is an effort to provide nurses with the competencies to improve the quality and safety of the systems of health care in which they practice (Cronenwett, Sherwood, Barnsteiner, Disch, Johnson, Mitchell, et al., 2007). The competencies for nursing delineated by the Institute of Medicine (2003) (Box 1-9) were adapted by QSEN faculty members and defined describing essential features of a competent and respected nurse. They then developed knowledge, skills, and attitudes (KSAs) for each competency. Incorporation of these KSAs into prelicensure education for nurses would assist faculty to plan learning experiences to prepare respected and qualified nurses.

Teamwork and Communication

Situation, Background, Assessment, Recommendation

The situation background assessment recommendation (SBAR) technique gives a specific framework for communication among health care providers. SBAR is an easy to remember, useful, concrete mechanism for communicating important information that requires a clinician's immediate attention (Kaiser Permanente of Colorado, n.d.) (Box 1-10). Failure to communicate is one of the major reasons for errors in health care. The SBAR technique has the potential to serve as a means to reduce errors.

TeamSTEPPS

TeamSTEPPS was developed by the Department of Defense's Patient Safety Program in collaboration with the Agency for Healthcare Research and Quality as a teamwork system for health professionals to provide higher quality, safer client care (http://teamstepps.ahrq.gov/about-2cl_3.htm). It provides an evidence-base to improve communication and teamwork skills. Through this system medical teams use information, people,

BOX 1-9 INSTITUTE OF MEDICINE COMPETENCIES FOR NURSING

Client-centered care
Teamwork
Collaboration
Evidence-based practice
Quality improvement
Safety
Informatics

Source: Institute of Medicine. (2003). *Health professions education: A bridge to quality.* Washington, DC: National Academies Press.

and resources to achieve the best possible clinical outcomes, increase team awareness and clarify roles and responsibilities of team members, resolve conflicts and improve sharing of information, and eliminate barriers to quality and safety.

ETHICAL ISSUES IN PERINATAL NURSING AND WOMEN'S HEALTH CARE

Ethical concerns and debates have multiplied with the increased use of technology and with scientific advances. For example, with reproductive technology, pregnancy is now possible in women who thought they would never bear children, including some who are menopausal or postmenopausal. Should scarce resources be devoted to achieving pregnancies in older women? Is giving birth to a child at an older age worth the risks involved? Should older parents be encouraged to conceive a baby when they may not live to see the child reach adulthood? Should a woman who is HIV positive have access to assisted reproduction services? Should third-party payers assume the costs of reproductive technology such as the use of induced ovulation and in vitro fertilizations? With induced ovulation and in vitro fertilization, multiple pregnancies occur, and multifetal pregnancy reduction (selectively terminating one or more fetuses) may be considered. Questions about informed consent and allocation of resources must be addressed with innovations such as intrauterine fetal surgery, fetoscopy, therapeutic insemination, genetic engineering, stem cell research, surrogate childbearing, surgery for infertility, "test tube" babies, fetal research, and treatment of very LBW (VLBW) babies. The introduction of long-acting contraceptives has created moral choices and policy dilemmas for health care providers and legislators; that is, should some women (substance abusers, women with low incomes, or women who are HIV positive) be required to take the contraceptives? With the potential for great good that can come from fetal tissue transplantation, what research is ethical? What are the rights of the embryo? Should cloning of humans be permitted? Discussion and debate about these issues will continue for many years. Nurses and clients, as well as scientists, physicians, attorneys, lawmakers, ethicists, and clergy, must be involved in the discussions.

RESEARCH IN PERINATAL NURSING AND WOMEN'S HEALTH CARE

Research plays a vital role in the establishment of maternity and women's health science. Research can validate that nursing care makes a difference. For example, although prenatal care is clearly associated with healthier infants, no one knows exactly which nursing interventions produce this outcome. The research into women's health must increase. In the past, medical researchers rarely included women in their studies, so more research in this area is crucial. Many possible areas of research exist in maternity and women's health care. The clinician can identify problems in the health and health care of women and infants. Through research, nurses can make a difference for these clients. Nurses should promote research funding and conduct research on maternity and women's health, especially concerning the effectiveness of nursing strategies for these clients.

BOX 1-10 SAMPLE SBAR REPORT TO PHYSICIAN OR MIDWIFE ABOUT A CRITICAL SITUATION

S Situation
I am calling about Mary Smith.
I have just assessed her and she saturated a peripad in the last hour. Her blood pressure is 112/62, pulse 86, and respirations 18.
I think she is bleeding excessively.

B Background
Mrs. Smith is 12 hours postpartum after giving birth vaginally to a 9 lb, 12 oz term infant after an uncomplicated pregnancy. She had a rapid labor, just over 4 hours, and had no analgesia. She plans to bottle-feed this baby. She had an IV with 10 units of pitocin but it was completed and discontinued about 2 hours ago.
This is her sixth birth. All were uncomplicated and she had an uneventful recovery from them.

A Assessment
Her fundus becomes firm after massage but relaxes again. She has voided and her bladder feels empty.
I think she might have retained placenta and she needs to be examined.

R Recommendation
I would like you to come and examine her immediately.
Do you want her IV restarted?
Do you want her to have a Hb and HCT?

Hb, Hemoglobin; *HCT,* hematocrit.
The SBAR tool was developed by Kaiser Permanente. This example was prepared by Shannon Perry.

Ethical Guidelines for Nursing Research. Research with perinatal clients may create ethical dilemmas for the nurse. For example, participating in research may cause additional stress to a woman concerned about outcomes of genetic testing or one who is waiting for an invasive procedure. Obtaining amniotic fluid samples or performing cordocentesis poses risks to the fetus. Nurses must protect the rights of human subjects (i.e., clients) in all of their research. For example, nurses can collect data on or care for clients who are participating in clinical trials. The nurse ensures that the participants are fully informed and aware of their rights as subjects. The nurse may be involved in determining whether the benefits of research outweigh the risks to the mother and the fetus. Following the ANA ethical guidelines in the conduct, dissemination, and implementation of nursing research helps nurses ensure that research is conducted ethically (Silva, 1995).

KEY POINTS

- Maternity nursing focuses on women and their infants and families during the childbearing cycle.
- Women's health nursing focuses on the special physical, psychologic, and social needs of women throughout their life spans.
- Nurses caring for women can play an active role in shaping health care systems to be responsive to the needs of contemporary women.
- Childbirth practices have changed to become more focused on the family and to allow alternatives in care.
- A variety of factors, including race, age, and violence, affect women's health.
- Canada ranks twenty-fifth and the United States ranks twenty-ninth among industrialized nations in infant mortality rates.
- Integrative medicine combines modern technology with ancient healing practices and encompasses the whole of body, mind, and spirit.
- Evidence-based practice and outcomes orientation are emphasized in current practice.
- Risk management and learning from sentinel events can improve quality of care.
- *Healthy People 2020* provides an update on goals for maternal and infant health.
- Research plays a vital role in establishing a scientific base for the care of women and infants.
- Ethical concerns have multiplied with the increasing use of technology and scientific advances.

Audio Chapter Summaries Access an audio summary of these Key Points on evolve

REFERENCES

Agency for Healthcare Research and Quality.(2000). *20 Tips to help prevent medical errors. Patient fact sheet.* Available at www.ahqr.gov/consumer/20tips.htm. Accessed February 9, 2010.

American Academy of Pediatrics & American College of Obstetricians and Gynecologists. (2007). *Guidelines for perinatal care* (6th ed.). Washington, DC: AAP/ACOG.

American Cancer Society. (2010). *Cancer facts & figures 2010.* Atlanta: American Cancer Society. Available at www.cancer.org. Accessed July 27, 2010.

American Nurses Association (2001). Code of Ethics for nurses with interpretive statements. Silver Spring, MD: Author.

Association of Women's Health, Obstetric and Neonatal Nurses (AWHONN). (2002). *Standards for professional perinatal nursing practice and certification in Canada.* Washington, DC: Author.

Association of Women's Health, Obstetric and Neonatal Nurses (AWHONN). (2009). *Standards and guidelines for professional nursing practice in the care of women and newborns* (7th ed.). Washington, DC: Author.

Calvo, A. (2006). *HRSA health disparities collaborative: Executive summary—September, 2006.* Available at www.healthdisparities.net/hdc/html/home.aspx. Accessed February 9, 2010.

Chu, S., Bachman, D., Callaghan, W., Whitlock, E., Dietz, P., Berg, C., et al. (2008). Association between obesity during pregnancy and increased use of health care. *New England Journal of Medicine, 358*(14), 1444–1453.

Cronenwett, L., Sherwood, G., Barnsteiner, J., Disch, J., Johnson, J., Mitchell, P., et al. (2007). Quality and safety education for nurses. *Nursing Outlook, 55*(3), 122–131.

DeNavas-Walt, C., Proctor, B., & Smith, J. (2007). *U.S. Census Bureau, Current Population Reports, P60-233, income poverty, and health insurance coverage in the United States: 2006.* Washington, DC: US Government Printing Office.

Dochterman, J., & Bulechek, G. (2004). *Nursing interventions classification (NIC)* (4th ed.). St. Louis: Mosby.

Drug use in pregnancy. (2007). *The Merck Manuals Online Medical Library.* Available at www.merck.com/mmhe/sec22/ch259a.html. Accessed May 10, 2010.

French, J. (2006). Medical errors and patient safety in health care. *Canadian Journal of Medical Radiation Technology, 37*(4), 9–13.

Gauthier, M., & Serber, M. (2005). *A need to transform the U.S. health care system: Improving access, quality, and efficiency.* The Commonwealth Fund. Available at www.cmwf.org/publications/publications_show.htm?doc_id=302833. Accessed February 9, 2010.

Hamilton, B., Martin, J., & Ventura S. (2010). Births: Preliminary date for 2008. National Vital Statistics Report, *58*(16), 1-18.

Harmon, K. (2009). *Deaths from avoidable medical error more than double in past decade, investigation shows.* Scientific American News Blog, August 10, 2009. Available at www.scientificamerican.com/-blog/post.cfm?id+deaths-from-avoidable-medical-error-2009-08-10. Accessed May 12, 2010.

Heron, M., Hoyert, D., Murphy, S., Xu, J., Kochanek, K., & Tejada-Vera, B. (2009). Deaths: Final data for 2006. *National Vital Statistics Reports, 57*(14), 1–135.

Heron, M., Sutton, P., Xu, J., Ventura, S., Strobino, D., & Guyer, B. (2010). Annual summary of vital statistics: 2007. *Pediatrics, 125*(1), 4–15.

Institute of Medicine. (2003). *Health professions education: A bridge to quality.* Washington, DC: National Academies Press.

The Joanna Briggs Institute. (2008). *JBI grading of recommendations.* (2008). Available at www.joannabriggs.edu.au/pubs/approach.php. Accessed May 12, 2010.

The Joint Commission. (2009). *Official "do not use" list.* Available at www.jointcommission.org/NR/rdonlyres/2329F8F5-6EC5-4E21-B932-54B2B7D53F00/0/dnu_list.pdf. Accessed February 9, 2010.

The Joint Commission. (2010). *Sentinel events.* Available at www.jointcommission.org/SentinelEvents. Accessed February 8, 2010.

Jones, W. (2008). *At a glance. Safe motherhood. Promoting health for women before, during, and after pregnancy.* Atlanta: USDHHS, CDC. Available at www.cdc.gov/nccdphp/publications/aag/pdf/drh.pdf. Accessed February 8, 2010.

Kaiser Permanente of Colorado. (n.d.). *SBAR technique for communication: A situational briefing model.* Available at www.ihi.org/IHI/Topics/PatientSafety/SafetyGeneral/Tools/SBARTechniqueforCommunicationASituationalBriefingModel.htm. Accessed February 8, 2010.

Martin, J., Kung, H., Mathews, T., Hoyert, D., Strobino, D., Guyer, B., et al. (2008). Annual summary of vital statistics: 2006. *Pediatrics, 121*(4), 788–801.

Millennium Development Goals (January 2008). Available from http://siteresources.worldbank.org/DATASTATISTICS/Resources/MDGsOfficialList2008.pdf. Accessed February 9, 2010.

Miniño, A., Xu, J., Kochanek, K., & Tejada-Vera, B. (2009). Death in the United States, 2007. *NCHS Data Brief, 26*(December), 1–20.

Moorhead, S., Johnson, M., & Maas, M. (2004). *Nursing outcomes classification (NOC)* (3rd ed.). St. Louis: Mosby.

National Center for Health Statistics (2009). Health, United States, 2008, Hyattsville, MD: Author.

National Center for Health Statistics. (2009). *Health, United States, 2009: With Special Feature on Medical Technology.* Hyattsville, MD: Author.

Obama Chooses UND's Mary Wakefield as Health Resources and Services Administration Leader. (Feburary 20, 2009). Available at www.GrandForksHerald.com/event/article/id/107444. Accessed February 8, 2010.

O'Reilly, K. (2008). *No pay for "never event" errors becoming standard.* Available at www.ama-assn.org/amednews/2008/01/07/prsc0107.htm. Accessed February 9, 2010.

Pifer-Bixler, J. (2009). *Study: 86.7 million Americans uninsured over last two years*. Available at www.cnn.com/2009/HEALTH/03/04/uninsured.epidemic.obama/. Accessed May 12, 2010.

Roehr, B. (2008). Pressure mounts to cut US spending on health care. *BMJ, 336*(7638), 236–237.

Satcher, D., & Higginbotham, E. (2008). The public health approach to eliminating disparities in health. *American Journal of Public Health, 98*(3), S8–S11.

Shalo, S. (2007). In the news. The price of committing error. *American Journal of Nursing, 107*(8), 20.

Silva, M. (1995). *Ethical guidelines in the conduct, dissemination, and implementation of nursing research*. Washington, DC: American Nurses Association.

Simpson, K. (2005). Failure to rescue in obstetrics. *MCN American Journal of Maternal/Child Nursing, 30*(1), 76.

Tiedje, L., Price, E., & You, M. (2008). Childbirth is changing. What now? *MCN American Journal of Maternal/Child Nursing, 33*(3), 144–150.

U.S. Census Bureau. (2009). *U.S. interim projections by age, sex, race, and Hispanic origin*. Available at www.census.gov/ipc/www/usinterimproj. Accessed February 8, 2010.

U.S. Department of Health and Human Services. (2000). *Healthy People 2010 (conference edition, in two volumes)*. Washington, DC: Author.

Wilson, M. (2009). Readability and patient education materials used for low-income populations. *Clinical Nurse Specialist, 23*(1), 33–40.

World Health Organization study group on female genital mutilation and obstetric outcome, & Banks, E., Meirik, O., Farley, T., Akande, O., Bathija, H., & Ali, M. (2006). Female genital mutilation and obstetric outcome: WHO collaborative prospective study in six African countries. *Lancet, 367*(9525), 1835–1841.

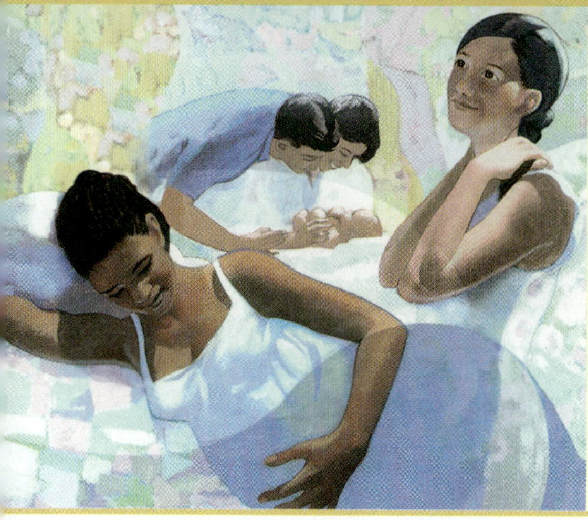

CHAPTER

2

Community Care: The Family and Culture

Makeba Felton

evolve WEBSITE

http://evolve.elsevier.com/Lowdermilk/MWHC/

Audio Glossary
Audio Key Points
Critical Thinking Exercises
- Community Resources for Families
- Cultural Health and the Family

NCLEX Review Questions
Nursing Care Plans
- Community and Home Care
- The Family Newly Immigrated from a Non-English-speaking Country
- Incorporating the Infant into the Family

LEARNING OBJECTIVES

- Describe the main characteristics of contemporary family forms.
- Identify key factors influencing family health.
- Compare theoretic approaches for working with childbearing families.
- Discuss cultural competence in relation to one's own nursing practice.
- Identify key components of the community assessment process.
- List indicators of community health status and their relevance to perinatal health.
- Describe data sources and methods for obtaining information about community health status.
- Identify predisposing factors and characteristics of vulnerable populations.
- List the potential advantages and disadvantages of home visits.
- Explore telephonic nursing care options in perinatal nursing.
- Describe how home care fits into the maternity continuum of care.
- Discuss safety and infection control principles as they apply to the care of clients in their homes.
- Describe the nurse's role in perinatal home care.

INTRODUCTION TO FAMILY, CULTURE, COMMUNITY, AND HOME CARE

The composition, structure, and function of the American family have changed dramatically in recent years, largely in response to economic, demographic, sociocultural, and technologic trends that influence family life and health. Despite current challenges in improving the overall health of the nation, there is widespread concern about family health and well-being as a reflection of individual, community, and national health status. Recent economic changes in society have prompted individuals and families to go without health insurance, thus providing yet another barrier to health care. In addition to facing significant barriers in accessing needed services women and families are faced with the challenge of overcoming discrimination in health care practices. As cultural diversity increases and demographics change, it is essential that nurses become culturally competent in order to provide sensitive and individualized care to women and their families (Cooper, Grywalski, Lamp, Newhouse, & Studlien, 2007).

Trends in maternal and infant health in the United States reveal that progress has been made in relation to reduced infant and fetal deaths, and use of prenatal care (see Chapter 1), but notable gaps remain as the rates of low birth weight, preterm birth, and infant mortality have fallen short of *Healthy People 2010* target goals, with persistent disparities between non-Hispanic whites and African-Americans (March of Dimes, 2009). Because many of these outcomes are preventable through access to prenatal care, the use of preventive health practices clearly demonstrates the need for comprehensive community-based care for mothers, infants, and families. As perinatal health trends emerge, nurses are assuming greater roles in assessing family health status and providing care across the perinatal continuum. This continuum begins with family planning and

COMMUNITY ACTIVITY

- Visit the Health Resources and Services Administration website at www.communityhealth.hrsa.gov. What is the definition of a health center by the HRSA? What populations do they serve? What are the different types of health centers?
- Locate a health center in your community at the HRSA website. What types of services do they provide? Do they provide primary and preventative health services? Is care provided regardless of the client's ability to pay?
- Visit your State Center for Health Statistics (SCHS) website. Evaluate the health status of women and infants in your county. Vital statistics include: live births, physician versus midwife attended, out of wedlock births, cesarean births, low birth weight, maternal smoking, and fetal/infant mortality. Review the BABY BOOK, which according to the website "is comprised of multiple cross-tabulations of various maternal and infant variables such as age, race, birth order, birth weight, and number of prenatal visits as well as medical conditions of the mother, the labor/birth, and the newborn."

continues with the following categories of care: preconception, prenatal, intrapartum, postpartum, newborn, interconception (between pregnancies), and the child from infancy to 1 year of age. In the community, health care ranges from individual care to group and community services, and from primary prevention to tertiary care experiences and home visiting. Depending on the needs of the individual family unit, independent self-management, ambulatory care, home care, low risk hospitalization, or specialized intensive care may be appropriate at different points along this continuum.

In community-based health care, both the aggregate (group of people who have shared characteristics) and the population become the focus of intervention. Health professionals are required not only to determine health priorities but also to develop successful plans of care to be delivered in the health clinic, the community health center, or the client's home (Community Activity). This home and community-based delivery system presents unique challenges for perinatal and maternity nurses.

THE FAMILY IN CULTURAL AND COMMUNITY CONTEXT

The family and its cultural context play an important role in defining the work of maternity nurses. It is therefore essential that nurses become culturally competent in order to provide the most efficient care possible. Despite modern stresses and strains, the family forms a social network that acts as a potent support system for its members. Family care-seeking behavior and relationships with providers are all influenced by culturally related health beliefs and values. Ultimately all of these factors have the power to affect maternal and child health outcomes. The current emphasis in working with families is on wellness and empowerment for families to achieve control over their lives.

Defining Family

The family has traditionally been viewed as the primary unit of socialization, the basic structural unit within a community. The family plays a pivotal role in health care, representing the primary target of health care delivery for maternal and newborn nurses. As one of society's most important institutions, the family represents a primary social group that influences and is influenced by other people and institutions. There are a variety of family configurations.

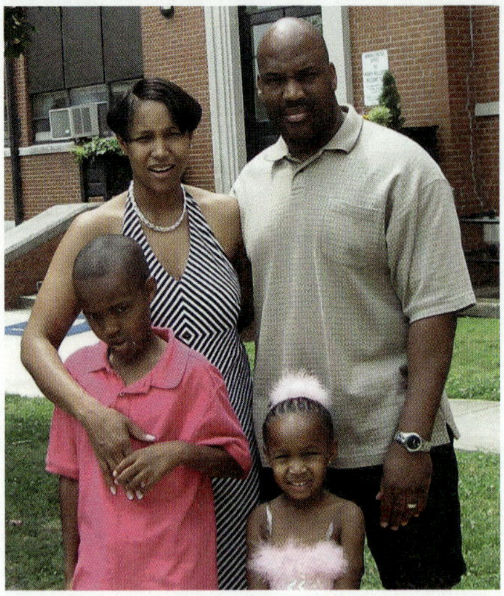

FIG. 2-1 Nuclear family. (Courtesy Makeba Felton, Gilbert, AZ.)

Family Organization and Structure

The **nuclear family** has long represented the traditional American family in which male and female partners and their children live as an independent unit, sharing roles, responsibilities, and economic resources (Fig. 2-1). In contemporary society, this "idealized" family structure actually represents only a relatively small number of families, which is steadily decreasing in number.

Married-parent families (biologic or adoptive parents) account for approximately 64% of American families, representing 69% of Caucasian, 55% of Hispanic, and 26.6% of African-American families (Wherry & Finegold, 2004).

Many nuclear families have other relatives living in the same household.

Extended family members include grandparents, aunts, uncles, or other people related by blood (McEwen & Pullis, 2008) (Fig. 2-2). For some groups, such as African-American and Latin-American, extended family is an important resource in terms of preventive health behavior. Mexican Americans account for the fastest growing minority population in the United States, and they rely on their family to make almost all decisions, including health care (Eggenberger, Grassley, & Restrepo, 2006). The extended family is becoming more common as American society ages. It is therefore important for nurses to recognize the desire for people of many cultures to include their family in making important decisions, and to do everything possible to make this happen.

Married-blended families, those formed as a result of divorce and remarriage, consist of unrelated family members (stepparents, stepchildren, and stepsiblings) who join to create a new household. These family groups frequently involve a biologic or adoptive parent whose spouse may or may not have adopted the child.

Cohabiting-parent families are those in which children live with two unmarried biologic parents or two adoptive parents.

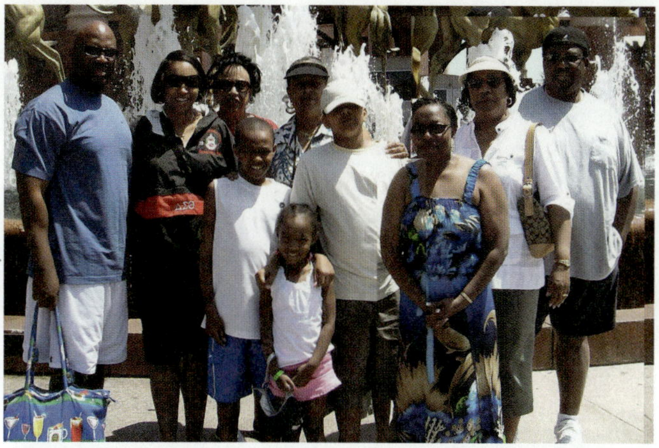

FIG. 2-2 Extended family. (Courtesy Makeba Felton, Gilbert, AZ.)

Hispanic children are more than twice as likely as African-American children to live in cohabiting-parent families and about four times as likely as Caucasian children to live in this kind of family arrangement (Wherry & Finegold, 2004).

Single-parent families comprise an unmarried biologic or adoptive parent who may or may not be living with other adults. The single-parent family may result from the loss of a spouse by death, divorce, separation, or desertion; from either an unplanned or planned pregnancy; or from the adoption of a child by an unmarried woman or man. This family structure is continually on the rise. In 2007 according to the U.S. Census Bureau, 13.6 million single parents lived in the United States. These 13.6 million single parents are raising 26% of the children in the United States younger than age 18 (Wolf, 2008). The single-parent family tends to be vulnerable economically and socially, creating an unstable and deprived environment for the growth of children. Research demonstrates the effect of single parenthood not only in economic instability but also in relation to health status, school achievement, and high risk behaviors for these children. Single mothers are more likely to live in poverty and have poor perinatal outcomes (Schor, 2003; Spencer, 2005; Weitoft, Hjern, Haglund, & Rosen, 2003).

Another family configuration that is less well documented is the increasing number of homosexual families (lesbian and gay), who may live together with or without children. It is estimated that between 800,000 and 7 million homosexual parents are raising between 1 and 9 million children (Cameron, 2004). Although there is no consensus as to what constitutes a gay and lesbian family, these families are rich and diverse in their form and composition. Usually formed by same-sex couples, they can also consist of single gay or lesbian parents or multiple parenting figures.

Children in lesbian and gay families may be the offspring of previous heterosexual unions, conceived by one member of a lesbian couple through therapeutic insemination, or adopted. These trends reflect the increased opportunities for alternative forms of parenthood within our society, owing both to more liberal social mores and to technologic and medical advances that offer the possibility of parenthood to single men and women (Greenfeld, 2005).

No-parent families are those in which children live independently in foster or kinship care such as living with a grandparent. An estimated 6.6 million children in the U.S. have grandparents living in their home. Of these grandparents, 23% are primary caretakers for their grandchildren; nearly half of these have assumed this responsibility for more than 5 years (U.S. Census Bureau, 2009a).

The Family in Society

The social context for the family can be viewed in relation to social and demographic trends that define the population as a whole. U.S. census data indicate that the racial and ethnic diversity of the population has grown dramatically in the past three decades; 30% of all U.S. citizens belong to racial or ethnic minority groups (USDHHS, 2010). Statistics reflect a population that is 79.8% Caucasian, 15.4% Hispanic, 12.8% African-American, 4.5% Asian-American, and Native American or Pacific Islander (U.S. Census Bureau, 2009b). According to these statistics, the Hispanic population continues to comprise the largest minority group in the United States.

THEORETIC APPROACHES TO UNDERSTANDING FAMILIES

Family Nursing

Family plays a pivotal role in health care, representing the primary target of health care delivery for maternal and newborn nurses. It is crucial that nurses assist families as they incorporate new additions to their family (see Nursing Care Plan). The core concepts of woman- and family-centered care are dignity and respect, information sharing, participation, and collaboration (Johnson, Abraham, Conway, Simmons, Edgman-Levitan, Sodomka, et al., 2008). When treating the woman and family with respect and dignity, health care providers listen to and honor perspectives and choices of the woman and family. They share information with families in ways that are positive, useful, timely, complete, and accurate. The family is supported in participating in the care and decision making at the level of their choice.

Family Assessment

When selecting a family assessment framework, an appropriate model for a perinatal nurse is one that is a health-promoting rather than an illness-care model. The low risk family can be assisted in promoting a healthy pregnancy, childbirth, and integration of the newborn into the family. The high risk perinatal family has illness-care needs, and the nurse can help to meet those needs while also promoting the health of the childbearing family.

Family Theories

A family theory can be used to describe families and how the family unit responds to events both within and outside the family. Each family theory makes certain assumptions about the family and has inherent strengths and limitations. Most nurses use a combination of theories in their work with families. A brief synopsis of several theories useful in working with families is included in Table 2-1. Application of these concepts can guide assessment and interventions for the family.

Because so many variables affect ways of relating, the nurse must be aware that most family members will interact and communicate with each other in ways that are very different from

NURSING CARE PLAN

Incorporating the Infant into the Family

NURSING DIAGNOSIS

Readiness for enhanced family coping related to adaptation of family to new infant

Expected Outcome

Family members will verbalize that individual and family goals are met during a smooth transition of new family member into the home.

Nursing Interventions/*Rationales*

- Assess type and amount of support available to family on a daily basis during the postpartum period *to facilitate adaptation of the family to situation of a new member.*
- Encourage family to use past successful coping mechanisms *to enhance ability to cope with new situation and promote self-esteem.*
- Encourage mother to use family and other support or services *to carry out daily household tasks to permit her to focus on herself and infant.*
- Suggest that woman take time to rest when infant sleeps *to conserve energy for healing and limit responsibility to herself and infant.*
- Assess family structure and relationships, including culture, *to evaluate if longer period of adjustment may be expected.*
- Teach family about sensory needs and capabilities of infant *to motivate family to meet infant's needs and set realistic expectations for infant's capabilities.*
- Refer to parent support group or community agencies, as needed, *to facilitate and validate ongoing positive adjustment of family to new family member.*

NURSING DIAGNOSIS

Ineffective role performance related to developmental challenge of addition of new family member

Expected Outcome

Each family member will verbalize realistic expectations regarding his or her role in the family and formulate a plan to incorporate role into overall family goals.

Nursing Interventions/*Rationales*

- Assess family structure, roles, and each member's perception of his or her role in the family *to evaluate the impact of the new member on the structure and roles of the family as perceived by the members.*
- Evaluate individual's perception of goals and new roles during this transition *to promote early intervention and correct any misinterpretation.*
- Encourage discussion of family members' thoughts and feelings regarding this transition *to promote open communication and trust.*
- Provide positive reinforcement for family members' actions that promote a positive environment for the infant *to increase self-esteem and provide encouragement.*
- Refer to community support groups *to provide group reinforcement and further assistance.*
- Give information about sibling and grandparent classes and support groups as available *to promote empowerment and self-esteem for significant others in the family.*

TABLE 2-1 THEORIES AND MODELS RELEVANT TO FAMILY NURSING PRACTICE

THEORY	SYNOPSIS OF THEORY
Family Systems Theory (Wright & Leahy, 2005)	The family is viewed as a unit, and interactions among family members are studied rather than studying individuals. A family system is part of a larger suprasystem and is composed of many subsystems. The family as a whole is greater than the sum of its individual members. A change in one family member affects all family members. The family is able to create a balance between change and stability. Family members' behaviors are best understood from a view of circular rather than linear causality.
Family Life Cycle (Developmental) Theory (Carter & McGoldrick, 1999)	Families move through stages. The family life cycle is the context in which to examine the identity and development of the individual. Relationships among family members go through transitions. Although families have roles and functions, a family's main value is in relationships that are irreplaceable. The family involves different structures and cultures organized in various ways. Developmental stresses may disrupt the life cycle process.
Family Stress Theory (Boss, 1996)	How families react to stressful events is the focus. Family stress can be studied within the internal and external contexts in which the family is living. The internal context involves elements that a family can change or control, such as family structure, psychologic defenses, and philosophic values and beliefs. The external context consists of the time and place in which a particular family finds itself and over which the family has no control, such as the culture of the larger society, the time in history, the economic state of society, maturity of the individuals involved, success of the family in coping with stressors, and genetic inheritance.
McGill Model of Nursing (Allen, 1997)	Strength-based approach in clinical practice with families, as opposed to a deficit approach, is the focus. Identification of family strengths and resources; provision of feedback about strengths; assistance given to family to develop and elicit strengths and use resources are key interventions.
Health Belief Model (Becker, 1974; Janz & Becker, 1984)	The goal of the model is to reduce cultural and environmental barriers that interfere with access to health care. Key elements of the Health Belief Model include the following: perceived susceptibility, perceived severity, perceived benefits, perceived barriers, cues to action, and confidence.
Human Developmental Ecology (Bronfenbrenner, 1979; 1989)	Behavior is a function of interaction of traits and abilities with the environment. Major concepts include ecosystem, niches (social roles), adaptive range, and ontogenetic development. Individuals are "embedded in a microsystem [role and relations], a mesosystem [interrelations between two or more settings], an exosystem [external settings that do not include the person], and a macrosystem [culture]" (Klein & White, 1996). Change over time is incorporated in the chronosystem.

those of the nurse's own family of origin. Most families will hold at least some beliefs about health that are very different from those of the nurse. Their beliefs can conflict with principles of health care management predominant in the Western health care system.

A family assessment tool such as the one outlined by Friedman (1998) (Fig. 2-3) can be used as a guide for assessing aspects of the family.

Graphic Representations of Families

A family genogram (family tree format depicting relationships of family members over at least three generations) (Fig. 2-4) provides valuable information about a family and can be placed in the nursing care plan for easy access by care providers. An ecomap, a graphic portrayal of social relationships of the women and family, may also help the nurse understand the social environment of the family and identify support systems available to them (Fig. 2-5) (Rempel, Neufeld, & Kushner, 2007). Software is available to generate genograms and ecomaps (www.interpersonaluniverse.net).

THE FAMILY IN A CULTURAL CONTEXT

Cultural Factors Related to Family Health

Cultural knowledge includes beliefs and values about each facet of life and is passed from one generation to the next. Cultural beliefs and traditions relate to food, language, religion, art, health and healing practices, kinship relationships, and all other aspects of community, family, and individual life. Culture has also been shown to have a direct effect on health behaviors. Values, attitudes, and beliefs that are culturally acquired may influence perceptions of illness, as well as health care–seeking behavior and response to treatment. The political, social, and economic context of people's lives is also part of the cultural experience.

Culture, shared beliefs and values of a group, plays a powerful role in an individual's behavior, particularly when the individual is sick. Understanding a culture can provide insight into how a person reacts to illness, pain, and invasive medical procedures, as well as patterns of human interaction and expressions of emotion. The effect of these influences must be assessed by health professionals in providing health care and developing effective intervention strategies. Culture is not static; it is an ongoing process that influences a woman throughout her entire life, from birth to death. Culture is an essential element of what defines us as people.

Many subcultures may be found within each culture. **Subculture** refers to a group existing within a larger cultural system that retains its own characteristics. A subculture may be an ethnic group or a group organized in other ways. For example, in the United States and Canada, many ethnic subcultures such as African-Americans, Asian-Americans, Hispanic-Americans, and Native Americans exist. It is important to note that subcultures also exist within these groups. In addition, the Caucasian population in America has multiple subcultures of its own. Because every identified cultural group has subcultures and because it is impossible to study every subculture in depth, greater differences may exist among and between groups than is generally acknowledged. It is important to be familiar with common cultural practices within these subgroups. However, it is also important to avoid the generalization that every person practices every cultural belief within a group.

In a multicultural society, many groups can influence traditions and practices. As cultural groups come into contact with each other, acculturation and assimilation may occur.

Acculturation refers to the changes in one's cultural pattern to those of the host society (Spector, 2008). These changes take place within one group or among several groups when people from different cultures come into contact with one another. People may retain parts of their own culture while adopting cultural practices of the dominant society. This familiarization among cultural groups results in overt behavioral similarity, especially in mannerisms and dress. Language patterns, food choices, and health practices are often much slower to adapt to the influence of acculturation. Furthermore, during times of family transitions such as childbearing, or during crisis or illness, a person may rely on old cultural patterns even after becoming acculturated in many ways. This is consistent with the family developmental theory that states that during times of stress, people revert to practices and behaviors that are most comfortable and familiar.

Assimilation means becoming in all ways like the members of the dominant culture (Spector, 2008). This process involves the complete loss of cultural identity while acquiring a new cultural identity. Assimilation is the process by which groups "melt" into the mainstream, thus accounting for the notion of a "melting pot," a phenomenon that has been said to occur in the United States. This is illustrated by individuals who identify themselves as being of Irish or German descent, without having any remaining cultural practices or values linked specifically to that culture such as food preparation techniques, style of dress, or proficiency in the language associated with their reported cultural heritage. Spector asserts that in the United States the melting pot, with its dream of a common culture, is a myth. Instead, a mosaic phenomenon exists in which we must accept and appreciate the differences among people.

Implications for Nursing

As our society becomes more multiculturally diverse, it is essential that nurses become culturally competent. It is crucial for nurses to be familiar with their own beliefs so that they have a better appreciation and understanding of the beliefs of their clients (see Clinical Reasoning box). Understanding the concepts of ethnocentrism and cultural relativism may help nurses care for families in a multicultural society.

Ethnocentrism refers to the view that one's own culture's way of doing things is best (Giger & Davidhizar, 2009). Although the United States is a culturally diverse nation, the prevailing practice of health care is based on the beliefs and practices held by members of the dominant culture, primarily Caucasians of European descent. This practice is based on the biomedical model that focuses on curing disease states. From this biomedical perspective, pregnancy and childbirth are viewed as processes with inherent risks that are most appropriately managed by using scientific knowledge and advanced technology.

The medical perspective stands in direct contrast with the belief systems of many cultures. Among many women, birth is

The Friedman Family Assessment Model (Short Form)

Identifying Data
1. Family name
2. Address and phone
3. Family composition
4. Type of family form
5. Cultural (ethnic) background
6. Religious identification
7. Social class status
8. Family's recreational or leisure-time activities

Developmental Stage and History of Family
9. Family's present developmental stage
10. Extent of family developmental tasks fulfillment
11. Nuclear family history
12. History of family of origin of both parents

Environmental Data
13. Characteristics of home
14. Characteristics of neighborhood and larger community
15. Family's geographic mobility
16. Family's associations and transactions with community
17. Family's social support system or network

Family Structure
18. Communication patterns
    - Extent of functional and dysfunctional communication (types of recurring patterns)
    - Extent of emotional (affective) messages and how expressed
    - Characteristics of communication within family subsystems
    - Extent of congruent and incongruent messages
    - Types of dysfunctional communication processes seen in family
    - Areas of open and closed communication
    - Familial and contextual variables affecting communication
19. Power structure
    - Power outcomes
    - Decision-making process
    - Power bases
    - Variables affecting family power
    - Overall family system and subsystem power (Family power continuum placement)
20. Role structure
    - Formal role structure
    - Informal role structure
    - Analysis of role models (optional)
    - Variables affecting role structure
21. Family values
    - Compare the family to American or family's reference group values and/or identify important family values and their importance (priority) in family.
    - Congruence between the family's values and the family's reference group or wider community
    - Congruence between the family's values and family member's values
    - Variables influencing family values
    - Values consciously or unconsciously held
    - Presence of value conflicts in family
    - Effect of the above values and value conflicts on health status of family

Family Functions
22. Affective function
    - Family's need–response patterns
    - Mutual nurturance, closeness, and identification
    - Separateness and connectedness
23. Socialization function
    - Family child-rearing practices
    - Adaptability of child-rearing practices for family form and family's situation
    - Who is (are) socializing agent(s) for child(ren)?
    - Value of children in family
    - Cultural beliefs that influence family's child-rearing patterns
    - Social class influence on child-rearing patterns
    - Estimation about whether family is at risk for child-rearing problems and if so, indication of high risk factors
    - Adequacy of home environment for children's need to play
24. Health care function
    - Family's health beliefs, values, and behavior
    - Family's definitions of health–illness and their level of knowledge
    - Family's perceived health status and illness susceptibility
    - Family's dietary practices
    - Adequacy of family diet (recommended 3-day food history record)
    - Function of mealtimes and attitudes toward food and mealtimes
    - Shopping (and its planning) practices
    - Person(s) responsible for planning, shopping, and preparation of meals
    - Sleep and rest habits
    - Physical activity and recreation practices (not covered earlier)
    - Family's drug habits
    - Family's role in self-care practices
    - Medically based preventive measures (physicals, eye and hearing tests, and immunizations)
    - Dental health practices
    - Family health history (both general and specific diseases—environmentally and genetically related)
    - Health care services received
    - Feelings and perceptions regarding health services
    - Emergency health services
    - Source of payments for health and other services
    - Logistics of receiving care

Family Stress and Coping
25. Short- and long-term familial stressors and strengths
26. Extent of family's ability to respond, based on objective appraisal of stress-producing situations
27. Coping strategies utilized (present/past)
    - Differences in family members' ways of coping
    - Family's inner coping strategies
    - Family's external coping strategies
28. Dysfunctional adaptive strategies utilized (present/past; extent of usage)

Family Composition Form

Name (last, first)	Gender	Relationship	Date/place of birth	Occupation	Education
1. (Father)					
2. (Mother)					
3. (Oldest child)					
4.					
5.					
6.					
7.					
8.					

FIG. 2-3 The Friedman Family Assessment Model (short form). (From Friedman, M. [1998]. *Family nursing theory and assessment* [4th ed.]. New York: Appleton & Lange.)

traditionally viewed as a completely normal process that can be managed with a minimum of involvement from health practitioners. When encountering behavior in women unfamiliar with the biomedical model, the nurse may become frustrated and impatient. The nurse may label the women's behavior inappropriate and believe that it conflicts with "good" health practices. If the Western health care system provides the nurse's only standard for judgment, the behavior of the nurse is called ethnocentric.

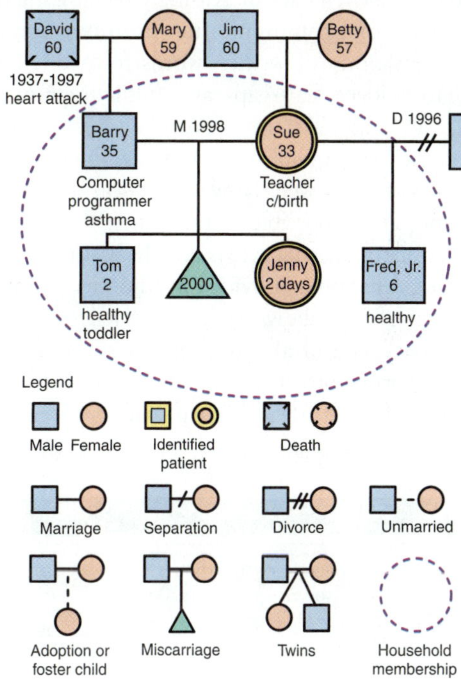

FIG. 2-4 Example of a family genogram.

Cultural relativism is the opposite of ethnocentrism. It refers to learning about and applying the standards of another's culture to activities within that culture. The nurse recognizes that people from different cultural backgrounds comprehend the same objects and situations differently. In other words, culture determines viewpoint.

CLINICAL REASONING

Providing Culturally Appropriate Care

You will be caring for Elisabeth, a 22-year-old first-generation Mexican-American who comes into your office for her initial prenatal visit. You are concerned because Elisabeth's fundal height is consistent with 32 weeks of gestation and she has just begun prenatal care. Elisabeth, who lives with her husband, four children (ages 6, 4, 3, and 15 months), her mother, her aunt, and her uncle, states that she has been doing well this pregnancy and did not start prenatal care in her previous pregnancies until she was almost ready to give birth. She also comments that all the babies were full term with uneventful labors and births. In obtaining the history you note the presence of a safety pin in Elisabeth's shirt, and wonder what this is for. You want to provide culturally competent care to this woman and her family.

1. Evidence—Is there sufficient evidence to support what culturally competent care should consist of for Elisabeth?
2. Assumptions—What assumptions can be made about culturally competent care for Elisabeth?
   a. How is pregnancy viewed in Elisabeth's culture?
   b. What is the role of family in Elisabeth's culture?
   c. How acceptable is it for women Elisabeth's age to begin having children at such young ages?
   d. What religious beliefs may Elisabeth have that may affect contraception?
3. What implications and priorities for nursing care can be made at this time?
4. Does the evidence objectively support your conclusion?
5. Are there alternative perspectives to your conclusion?

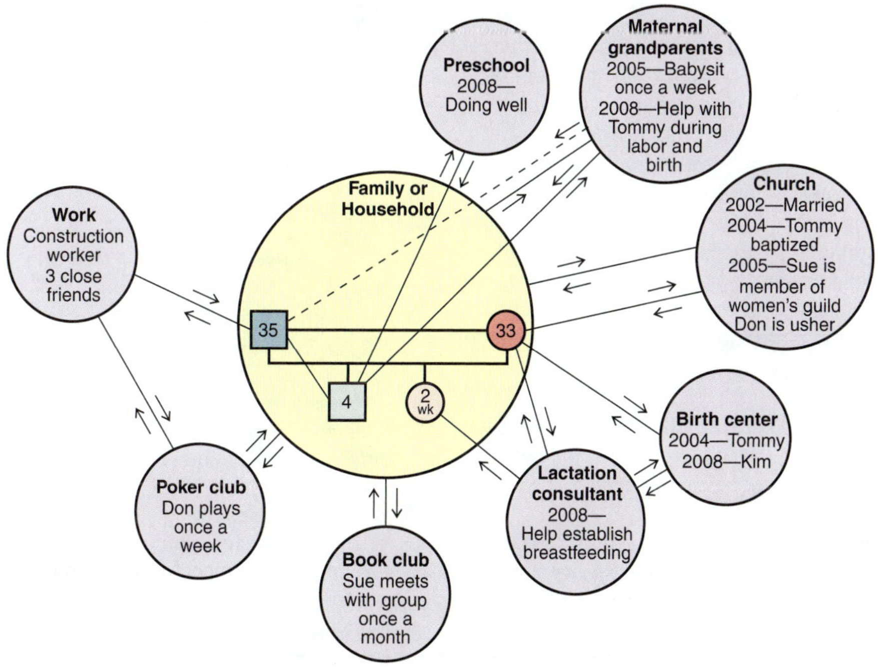

FIG. 2-5 Example of an ecomap. An ecomap describes social relationships and depicts available supports.

Cultural relativism does not require nurses to accept the beliefs and values of another culture. Instead, they recognize that the behavior of others may be based on a system of logic different from their own. Cultural relativism affirms the uniqueness and value of every culture.

Childbearing Beliefs and Practices

Nurses working with childbearing families care for families from many different cultures and ethnic groups. To provide culturally competent care, the nurse should be aware of the spectrum of cultural beliefs and practices important to individual families. When working with childbearing families, a nurse should consider all aspects of culture including communication, space, time orientation, and family roles.

Communication often creates the most challenging obstacle for nurses working with clients from diverse cultural groups. This is because communication is not merely the exchange of words. Instead it involves (1) understanding the individual's language, including subtle variations in meaning and distinctive dialects; (2) appreciation of individual differences in interpersonal style; and (3) accurate interpretation of the volume of speech as well as the meanings of touch and gestures. For example, members of some cultural groups tend to speak more loudly when they are excited, with great emotion and with vigorous and animated gestures; this is true whether their excitement is related to positive or negative events or emotions. It is important, therefore, for the nurse to avoid rushing to judgment regarding a client's intent when the client is speaking, especially in a language not understood by the nurse. Instead, the nurse should withhold an interpretation of what has been expressed until it is possible to clarify the client's intent. The nurse must quickly enlist the assistance of a person who can help, and seek to verify with the client the true intent and meaning of the communication.

Inconsistencies between the language of clients and the language of providers present a significant barrier to effective health care. For example, there are many dialects of Spanish that vary by geographic location. Because of the diversity of cultures and languages within the U.S. and Canadian populations, health care agencies are increasingly seeking the services of interpreters (of oral communication from one language to another) or translators (of written words from one language to another) to bridge these gaps and fulfill their obligation for culturally and linguistically appropriate health care (Box 2-1). Finding the best possible interpreter in the circumstance is critically important as well. However, ideal interpretive services sometimes are impossible to find when they are needed because the nature of nursing care is not always predictable and because nursing care that is provided in a home or community setting does not always allow expert, experienced, or mature adult interpreters. The ideal interpreter has had training in health care interpretation so that she or he can help promote effective communication. Health care providers are encouraged

BOX 2-1 WORKING WITH AN INTERPRETER

Step 1: Before the interview

A. Outline your statements and questions. List the key pieces of information you want/need to know.

B. Learn something about the culture so that you can converse informally with the interpreter.

Step 2: Meeting with the interpreter

A. Introduce yourself to the interpreter and converse informally. This is the time to find out how well he or she speaks English. No matter how proficient or what age the interpreter is, be respectful. Some ways to show respect are to ask a cultural question to acknowledge that you can learn from the interpreter, or you could learn one word or phrase from the interpreter.

B. Emphasize that you do want the client to ask questions, because some cultures consider this inappropriate behavior.

C. Make sure the interpreter is comfortable with the technical terms you need to use. If not, take some time to explain them.

Step 3: During the interview

A. Ask your questions and explain your statements (see Step 1).

B. Make sure that the interpreter understands which parts of the interview are most important. You usually have limited time with the interpreter, and you want to have adequate time at the end for client questions.

C. Try to get a "feel" for how much is "getting through." No matter what the language is, if in relating information to the client, the interpreter uses far fewer or far more words than you do, something else is going on.

D. Stop every now and then and ask the interpreter, "How is it going?" You may not get a totally accurate answer, but you will have emphasized to the interpreter your strong desire to focus on the task at hand. If there are language problems (1) speak slowly; (2) use gestures (e.g., fingers to count or point to body parts); and (3) use pictures.

E. Ask the interpreter to elicit questions. This may be difficult, but it is worth the effort.

F. Identify cultural issues that may conflict with your requests or instructions.

G. Use the interpreter to help problem solve or at least give insight into possibilities for solutions.

Step 4: After the interview

A. Speak to the interpreter and try to get an idea of what went well and what could be improved. This will help you to be more effective in the future with this or another interpreter.

B. Make notes on what you learned for your future reference or to help a colleague.

Remember

Your interview is a *collaboration* between you and the interpreter. *Listen* as well as speak.

NOTES:

1. The interpreter may be a child, grandchild, or sibling of the client. Be sensitive to the fact that the child is playing an adult role.
2. Be sensitive to cultural and situational differences (e.g., an interview with someone from urban Germany will likely be different from an interview with someone from a transitional refugee camp).
3. Younger females telling older males what to do may be a problem for both a female nurse and a female interpreter. This is not the time to pioneer new gender relations. Be aware that in some cultures it is difficult for a woman to talk about some topics with a husband or a father present.

Courtesy Elizabeth Whalley, PhD, San Francisco State University.

Nursing Care Plan—The Family Newly Immigrated from a Non-English-Speaking Country

to use these individuals when communicating with non–English-speaking clients in order to effectively communicate and to prevent possible liability from misinterpretation. However, in crisis or emergency situations, or when family members are having extreme stress or emotional upset, it may be necessary to use relatives, neighbors, or children as interpreters. If this occurs, the nurse must ensure that the client is in agreement and comfortable with using the available interpreter to assist.

When using an interpreter, the nurse respects the family by creating an atmosphere of consideration and privacy. Questions should be addressed to the woman and not to the interpreter. Even though an interpreter will of necessity be exposed to sensitive and privileged information about the family, the nurse should take care to ensure that confidentiality is maintained. A quiet location free from interruptions is ideal for interpretive services to take place. It is also appropriate to use written literature, videos, or other material to help with the woman's understanding of information that is presented. It is important to ensure that the material has been translated by someone who is trained appropriately, to avoid liability issues.

Personal Space

Cultural traditions define the appropriate personal space for various social interactions. Although the need for personal space varies from person to person and with the situation, the actual physical dimensions of comfort zones differ from culture to culture. Actions such as touching, placing the woman in proximity to others, taking away personal possessions, and making decisions for the woman can decrease personal security and heighten anxiety. Conversely, if nurses respect the need for distance, they allow the woman to maintain control over personal space and support the woman's autonomy, thereby increasing her sense of security. For example, many Asian groups have reserved attitudes about physical contact, and this may at times create anxiety when health care is delivered.

Nurses often use touch, and frequently do so without any awareness of the emotional distress they may be causing to clients. In the home care setting, a nurse who must provide physical care to a woman with a disease may cause the woman great anxiety because she fears that her disease will be spread to the nurse. Fears about spreading the disease also may interfere with her acceptance of physical comfort and care from family members.

Time Orientation

Time orientation also is a fundamental way in which culture affects health behaviors. People in cultural groups may be relatively more oriented to past, present, or future. Those who focus on the past strive to maintain tradition or the status quo and have little motivation for formulating future goals. In contrast, individuals who focus primarily on the present neither plan for the future nor consider the experiences of the past. These individuals do not necessarily adhere to strict schedules and are often described as "living for the moment," or "marching to their own drummer." Individuals oriented to the future maintain a focus on achieving long-term goals.

The time orientation of the childbearing family may affect nursing care. For example, talking to a family about bringing the infant to the clinic for follow-up examinations (events in the future) may be difficult for the family that is focused on the present concerns of day-to-day survival. Because a family with a future-oriented sense of time plans far in advance, thinking about the long-term consequences of present actions, they may be more likely to return as scheduled for follow-up visits. Despite the differences in time orientation, each family can be equally concerned for the well-being of its newborn.

Family Roles

Family roles involve the expectations and behaviors associated with a member's position in the larger family system (e.g., mother, father, or grandparent). Social class and cultural norms also affect these roles, with distinct expectations for men and women clearly determined by social norms. For example, culture may influence whether a man actively participates in the pregnancy and childbirth, yet maternity care practitioners working in the Western health care system expect fathers to be involved. This can create a significant conflict between the nurse and the role expectations of very traditional Mexican or Arab families, who usually view the birthing experience as a female affair (see Cultural Considerations box). The way that health care practitioners manage such a family's care molds its experience and perception of the Western health care system.

In maternity nursing and women's health care, the nurse supports and nurtures the beliefs that promote physical or emotional adaptation to childbearing. However, if certain beliefs might be harmful, the nurse should carefully explore them with the woman and use them in the reeducation and modification process. Strategies for care delivery and providing appropriate care are presented in Box 2-2.

Few families are exclusively "Asian" or "Caucasian." Instead they are often blended composites, with one partner bringing to the relationship the traditions of one culture or family of origin and the other partner bringing a slightly differing perspective. Even when partners are both of Asian ancestry, for example, their families of origin may come from different regions of the same country and follow completely different health practices. Table 2-2 provides examples of cultural beliefs and childbearing practices frequently encountered by the nurse who works

BOX 2-2 STRATEGIES FOR CARE DELIVERY AND PROVIDING CULTURALLY APPROPRIATE CARE

STRATEGIES FOR CARE DELIVERY

- Break down the language barriers.
- Explain your rationale and reasons for suggestions.
- Integrate folk and Western treatments.
- Enlist the family caretaker and others.
- Get consent from the right person.
- Provide language-appropriate materials.

PROVIDING APPROPRIATE CARE

- Ask about traditional beliefs, such as the role of hot and cold.
- Be sensitive regarding interpreters and language barriers.
- Ask about important dietary practices, particularly those related to events such as childbirth.
- Ask about group practices and beliefs.
- Ask about a woman's fears, and those of her family, regarding an unfamiliar care setting.

From Mattson, S. (2000). Providing culturally competent care: Strategies and approaches for perinatal clients, *AWHONN Lifelines, 4*(5), 37-39.

TABLE 2-2 TRADITIONAL* CULTURAL BELIEFS AND PRACTICES: CHILDBEARING AND PARENTING

PREGNANCY	CHILDBIRTH	PARENTING
Hispanic (Based primarily on knowledge of Mexican-Americans; members of the Hispanic community have their origins in Spain, Cuba, Central and South America, Mexico, Puerto Rico, and other Spanish-speaking countries.)		
Pregnancy Pregnancy desired soon after marriage Late prenatal care Expectant mother influenced strongly by mother or mother-in-law Cool air in motion considered dangerous during pregnancy Unsatisfied food cravings thought to cause a birthmark Some pica observed in the eating of ashes or dirt (not common) Milk avoided because it causes large babies and difficult births Many predictions about sex of baby May be unacceptable and frightening to have pelvic examination by male health care provider Use of herbs to treat common complaints of pregnancy Drinking chamomile tea thought to ensure effective labor May wear ribbon or band around pregnant belly in belief that baby will be born healthy	***Labor*** Use of *partera* or lay midwife preferred in some places; may prefer presence of mother rather than husband After birth of baby, mother's legs brought together to prevent air from entering uterus Loud behavior in labor ***Postpartum*** Diet may be restricted after birth; for first 2 days only boiled milk and toasted tortillas permitted (special foods to restore warmth to body) Bed rest for 3 days after birth Keep warm Delay bathing Mother's head and feet protected from cold air; bathing permitted after 14 days Mother often cared for by her own mother Forty-day restriction on sexual intercourse Mother may want baby's first wet diaper to wipe her face in belief that it aids in making "mask of pregnancy" go away	***Newborn*** Breastfeeding begun after third day; colostrum may be considered "filthy" or "spoiled" or just not enough nourishment Olive oil or castor oil given to stimulate passage of meconium Male infant not circumcised Female infant's ears pierced Belly band used to prevent umbilical hernia Religious medal worn by mother during pregnancy; placed around infant's neck Infant protected from *mal ojo* ("evil eye") Various remedies used to treat *mal ojo* and fallen fontanel (depressed fontanel)
African-American (Members of the African-American community, many of whom are descendants of slaves, have different origins. Today a number of black Americans have emigrated from Africa, the West Indies, the Dominican Republic, Haiti, and Jamaica.)		
Pregnancy Acceptance of pregnancy depends on economic status Pregnancy thought to be state of "wellness," which is often the reason for delay in seeking prenatal care, especially by lower-income African-Americans Old-wives' tales include beliefs that having a picture taken during pregnancy will cause stillbirth and reaching up will cause cord to strangle baby Craving for certain foods, including chicken, greens, clay, starch, and dirt Pregnancy may be viewed by African-American men as a sign of their virility Self-treatment for various discomforts of pregnancy, including constipation, nausea, vomiting, headache, and heartburn	***Labor*** Use of "Granny midwife" in certain parts of United States Varied emotional responses: some cry out, some display stoic behavior to avoid calling attention to selves Woman may arrive at hospital in far-advanced labor Emotional support often provided by other women, especially the woman's own mother ***Postpartum*** Vaginal bleeding seen as sign of sickness; tub baths and shampooing of hair prohibited Sassafras tea thought to have healing power Eating liver thought to cause heavier vaginal bleeding because of its high "blood" content	***Newborn*** Feeding very important: "good" baby thought to eat well Early introduction of solid foods May breastfeed or bottle-feed; breastfeeding may be considered embarrassing Parents fearful of spoiling baby Commonly call baby by nicknames May use excessive clothing to keep baby warm Belly band used to prevent umbilical hernia Abundant use of oil on baby's scalp and skin Strong feeling of family, community, and religion
Asian-American (Typically refers to groups from China, Korea, the Philippines, Japan, Southeast Asia [particularly Thailand], Indochina, and Vietnam.)		
Pregnancy Pregnancy considered time when mother "has happiness in her body" Pregnancy seen as natural process Strong preference for female health care provider Belief in theory of hot and cold May omit soy sauce in diet to prevent dark-skinned baby Prefer soup made with ginseng root as general strength tonic Milk usually excluded from diet because it causes stomach distress Inactivity or sleeping late may cause difficult birth	***Labor*** Mother attended by other women, especially her own mother Father does not actively participate Labor in silence Cesarean birth not desired ***Postpartum*** Must protect self from *yin* (cold forces) for 30 days Ambulation limited Shower and bathing prohibited Warm room Diet: Warm fluids Some women are vegetarians Korean mother served seaweed soup with rice Chinese diet high in hot foods Chinese mother avoids fruits and vegetables	***Newborn*** Concept of family important and valued Father is head of household; wife plays a subordinate role Birth of boy preferred May delay naming child Some groups (e.g., Vietnamese) believe colostrum is dirty; therefore, they may delay breastfeeding until milk comes in

TABLE 2-2 TRADITIONAL* CULTURAL BELIEFS AND PRACTICES: CHILDBEARING AND PARENTING—cont'd

PREGNANCY	CHILDBIRTH	PARENTING
European-American (Members of the European-American [Caucasian] community have their origins in countries such as Ireland, Great Britain, Germany, Italy, and France.)		
Pregnancy Pregnancy viewed as a condition that requires medical attention to ensure health Emphasis on early prenatal care Variety of childbirth education programs available, and participation encouraged Technology driven Emphasis on nutritional science Involvement of the father valued Written sources of information valued	***Labor*** Birth is a public concern Technology dominated Birthing process in institutional setting valued Involvement of father expected Physician seen as head of team ***Postpartum*** Emphasis or focus on early bonding Medical interventions for dealing with discomfort Early ambulation and activity emphasized Self-management valued	***Newborn*** Increased popularity of breastfeeding Breastfeeding begins as soon as possible after childbirth Parenting Motherhood and transition to parenting seen as stressful time Nuclear family valued, although single-parenting and other forms of parenting more acceptable than in the past Women often deal with multiple roles Early return to prenatal activities
Native American (Many different tribes exist within the Native American culture; viewpoints vary according to tribal customs and beliefs.)		
Pregnancy Pregnancy considered a normal, natural process Late prenatal care Avoid heavy lifting Herb teas encouraged	***Labor*** Prefers female attendant, although husband, mother, or father may assist with birth Birth may be attended by whole family Herbs may be used to promote uterine activity Birth may occur in squatting position ***Postpartum*** Herbal teas to stop bleeding	***Newborn*** Infant not fed colostrum Use of herbs to increase flow of milk Use of cradle boards for infant Babies not handled often

NOTE: Most of these cultural beliefs and customs reflect the traditional culture and are not universally practiced. These lists are not intended to stereotype clients but rather to serve as guidelines while discussing meaningful cultural beliefs with a woman and her family. Examples of other cultural beliefs and practices are found throughout this text.
*Variations in some beliefs and practices exist within subcultures of each group.
Data from Amaro, H. (1994). Women in the Mexican-American community: Religion, culture, and reproductive attitudes and experiences. *Journal of Comparative Psychology, 16*(1), 6-19; Bar-Yam, N. (1994). Learning about culture: A guide for birth practitioners. *International Journal of Childbirth Education, 9*(2), 8-10; Galanti, G. (1997). *Caring for patients from different cultures: Case studies from American hospitals* (2nd ed.). Philadelphia: University of Pennsylvania Press; D'Avanzo, C. (2008). *Mosby's pocket guide to cultural health assessment* (4th ed.). St. Louis: Mosby; Mattson, S. (1995). Culturally sensitive prenatal care for Southeastern Asians. *Journal of Obstetric, Gynecologic and Neonatal Nursing, 24*(4), 335-341; Spector, R. (2008). *Cultural diversity in health and illness* (7th ed.). Upper Saddle River, NJ: Prentice-Hall; Williams, R. (1989). Issues in women's health care. In B. Johnson (Ed.). *Psychiatric mental health nursing: Adaptation and growth.* Philadelphia: JB Lippincott.

CULTURAL CONSIDERATIONS

Questions to Ask to Elicit Cultural Expectations About Childbearing

1. What do you and your family think you should do to remain healthy during pregnancy?
2. What can you do to improve your health and the health of your baby?
3. Who do you want with you during your labor?
4. What can your labor support person do to help you be most comfortable during labor?
5. What actions are important for you and your family after the baby's birth?
6. What do you and your family expect from the nurse(s) caring for you?
7. How will family members participate in your pregnancy, childbirth, and parenting?

with women who identify themselves as European-American (Caucasian), Hispanic-American, Asian-American, African-American (black), or Native American. The cultural beliefs and customs in Table 2-2 are categorized based on distinct cultural traditions and are not practiced by all members of the cultural group in every part of the country. Women from these cultural and ethnic groups may adhere to a few, all, or none of the practices listed. In using this table as a guide, the nurse should use caution to avoid making stereotypic assumptions about any person based on sociocultural-spiritual affiliations. Nurses should exercise sensitivity in working with every family, being careful to assess the ways in which they apply their own mixture of cultural traditions.

DEVELOPING CULTURAL COMPETENCE

In today's society, with its ever-expanding diversity, it is of critical importance that nurses develop more than technical skills. They need to develop cultural competence. There are as many varying definitions of cultural competence as there are for culture. According to Purnell and Paulanka (2008), cultural competence involves respecting the differences in others, including ethnicity, ethnoculture, and religious beliefs.

Key components of culturally competent care include:

- Recognizing that there is disparity between one's own culture and that of the client
- Educating and promoting healthy behaviors in a cultural context that has meaning for clients
- Taking abstract knowledge about other cultures and applying it in a practical way, so that the quality of service improves and policies are enacted that meet the needs of all clients

- Communicating respectfulness for a wide range of differences, including client use of nontraditional healing practices and alternative therapies
- Recognizing the importance of culturally different communication styles, problem-solving techniques, concepts of space and time, and desires to be involved with care decisions
- Anticipating the need to address varying degrees of language ability and literacy, as well as barriers to care and compliance with treatment

Cultural competence affirms the uniqueness and value of every culture in nursing practice (www.bphc.hrsa.gov/cultural competence). For almost two decades, the American Academy of Nursing (1992) has pledged to promote transcultural nursing and to foster nursing expertise in culturally competent care, defined as a complex integration of knowledge, attitudes, and skills that enhance cross-cultural communications and lead to appropriate and effective interaction with others. It has always been vital that nurses develop the ability to relate to others, but the challenges of meeting the broad scope of these needs have never been greater.

Nurses must be continually involved in the development of cultural competence because it is of equal importance in terms of health outcomes as preserving and promoting human dignity. Nurses who relate effectively with clients are able to motivate them in the direction of health-promoting behaviors. Provider competence to address language barriers facilitates appropriate tailoring of health messages and preventive health teaching. Cross-cultural experiences also present an opportunity for the health care professional to expand cultural sensitivity, awareness, and skills.

COMMUNITY HEALTH PROMOTION

Best practices in community-based health initiatives involve understanding of community relationships and resources as well as participation of community leaders. The emphasis on community-based health promotion has grown in recent years, with recognition that many health issues require the collaborative efforts of a diverse community network to achieve public health goals (Cottrell, Girvan, & McKenzie, 2006). These efforts are particularly relevant in relation to maternal-newborn health, which is affected by multiple public health issues: lack of health insurance, recent economic challenges that include job loss, teen pregnancy, substance abuse, and the consequences of no or inadequate prenatal care.

Levels of Preventive Care

In community-based health promotion, there are three levels of prevention of disease. Primary prevention involves promoting healthy lifestyles through immunizations, encouraging exercise, and healthy nutrition. Secondary prevention involves targeting populations at risk for certain diseases. For example, women are encouraged to have mammograms; men are encouraged to have prostate screening. Tertiary prevention focuses on rehabilitation of an individual who already has a disease back to as optimal health as possible. For example, a person who has experienced a stroke has an optimal expectation of being able to function at his or her fullest potential. As nurses, we do what we can to ensure that this occurs.

During pregnancy, primarily primary and secondary prevention are relevant. The goal is to maintain a healthy pregnancy by preventing illness and screening those at risk for potential illnesses or complications that could arise during pregnancy. In pregnancy, primary prevention might involve providing the influenza vaccine to women, whereas secondary prevention might involve performing an amniocentesis for a woman older than age 35.

Promoting Family Health

Functioning within the social, cultural, environmental, and economic context of the community, the family becomes an integral component of community health promotion efforts (Friedman, Bowden, & Jones, 2003). For childbearing families, health promotion is primarily focused on early intervention through prenatal care and prevention of complications during the perinatal period. Often this early exposure to health information sets the stage for a successful birth and positive outcomes for mother and baby. Family systems and developmental theories provide a framework for the appropriate timing and content of health promotion activities. The nurse's role in this process is focused on collaboration with the family, identifying risk factors, and providing health information to facilitate positive health behaviors. Involving expectant mothers and fathers in identification of their learning needs is an essential first step to securing their participation in the health promotion process.

A wide variety of strategies have been used to engage families and groups in health-promoting activities or community health programs. Some are more successful than others. Generally, participant engagement in the planning process and empowerment to create internal solutions are considered key factors in effective interventions. Many communities have organized coalitions to address specific health promotion agendas related to sharing information, educating community members, or advocating for health policies around maternal and child health issues. An example of this is the National Friendly Access Program (2003), a community-based initiative to improve access to maternal and child care by changing provider behaviors. The benefits of partnership with faith-based organizations for community health improvement have been demonstrated in health promotion efforts aimed at lifestyle choices, health education, and maternal-child health outcomes. Another community-based partnership demonstrated the potential for policy and practice improvements in maternal-child health systems around the issues of provider access, transportation, and discrimination in health care practices (Pincus, Thomas, Keyser, Castle, Dembosky, Firth, et al., 2003).

Prepared childbirth classes are a well-established mechanism for increasing awareness of healthy behaviors during pregnancy and preparing parents for the care of themselves and their newborn during the postpartum period. Mass media efforts such as those presented by the March of Dimes "Baby Your Baby" advertisements are clear consumer-friendly messages designed to reach a large target audience. Other venues include public health education in newspapers and magazines, and health department programs such as the Special Supplemental Program for Women, Infants, and Children (WIC), which offers a variety of health education and written information to mothers.

ASSESSING THE COMMUNITY

A community assessment is a tool that is used to assess the health and well-being of a community. One can define "community" either geographically or as having a common characteristic. For example, one can do a community assessment of clients who live in a particular neighborhood or of women who have developed preterm labor. In doing the community assessment, risk factors for certain diseases, patterns of illness, cultural beliefs, religious beliefs, transportation systems, and support systems are just a few factors that are assessed in order to determine how these components relate to certain patterns of illness.

In a community health assessment data are collected, analyzed, and used to educate and mobilize communities, develop priorities, garner resources, and plan actions to improve public health. Many models and frameworks of community assessment are available, but the actual process often depends on the extent and nature of the assessment to be performed, the time and resources available, and the way the information is to be used (www.assessnow.info/resources/models-of-community-health-assessment).

Data Collection and Sources of Community Health Data

Important measures of community health include, for example, access to care, level of provider services available, availability of transportation, and family support. Consideration of a variety of these factors helps one to assess areas that may affect care so that nurses can introduce alternatives to meet the needs of clients. For example, if a client has to work Monday through Friday, from 8 AM to 5 PM, the nurse can facilitate an after-hours appointment. A community assessment model (Fig. 2-6) can be used to provide a comprehensive guide to data collection.

The most critical community indicators of perinatal health relate to access to care; maternal mortality; infant mortality; low birth weight; first trimester prenatal care; and rates for mammography, Papanicolaou smears, and other similar screening tests (Agency for Healthcare Research and Quality [AHRQ], 2005). Nurses can use these indicators as a reflection of access, quality, and continuity of health care in a community. For women and infants, access to a consistent source of care is critical. Those with a regular source of care are more likely to use preventive services and have more positive pregnancy outcomes, but current statistics indicate that many women lack access to a usual source of care or rely primarily on emergency services.

Access to health care relates not only to the *availability* of health department services, hospitals, public clinics, clinic hours, or other sources of care, but also to *accessibility* of care. In many areas where facilities and providers are available, geographic and transportation barriers render the care inaccessible for certain populations. This is particularly true in rural areas or other remote locations that lack such resources as public health departments, public transportation, and other necessary prenatal services. Other barriers to care should also be evaluated including cultural and language barriers, and lack of providers or specialty care.

Some local health departments, due to lack of funding, are not able to provide all services to meet the needs of the communities they serve. For example, health departments may not offer prenatal clinics for pregnant clients, and primary care and adult health clinics are unavailable. Although this can be a result of a lack of financial resources, other contributing factors include a lack of health care providers to staff clinics. Although one growing trend to help provide increased access to care is retail health clinics in pharmacies and retail stores, they often do not provide care to pregnant women.

Health departments at the city, county, and state level are a valuable resource for annual reports of births and deaths. Local health departments also compile extensive statistics about the birth complications, causes of death, and leading causes of morbidity and mortality for each age-group. Local and state health data are compiled and reported through the Centers for Disease Control and Prevention (CDC) (www.cdc.gov) to the National Center for Health Statistics (NCHS). The National Health Survey published annually from this source describes national health trends. However, national data are only as accurate and reliable as the local data on which they are based, so caution is needed in interpreting the data and applying it to specific population groups.

The U.S. census provides data on population size, age ranges, sex, racial and ethnic distribution, socioeconomic status, educational level, employment, and housing characteristics. Summary data are available for most large metropolitan areas, arranged by zip code and census tract, which usually corresponds to a neighborhood comprising approximately 3000 to 6000 people. Looking at individual census tracts within a community helps to identify subpopulations or aggregates whose needs may differ from those of the larger community. For example, women at high risk for inadequate prenatal care according to age, race, and ethnic or cultural group can be readily identified, and outreach activities can be appropriately targeted.

Other sources of useful information are hospitals and voluntary health agencies. The March of Dimes Foundation, for example, has supported perinatal needs assessments in many communities across the United States (www.modimes.org). Other community health resources include health care providers or administrators, government officials, religious leaders, and representatives of voluntary health agencies. Community or county health councils exist in many areas, with oversight of specific health initiatives or programs for that region. These **key informants** often provide a unique perspective that may not be accessible through other sources. Community gatekeepers who address the social and health care needs of the population are also critical links to population-specific health information.

The perinatal health nurse can explore existing community health program reports, records of preventive health screenings, and other informal data. Established programs often provide good indicators of the health promotion and disease prevention characteristics of the population.

Professional publications are a rich and readily accessible source of information for all nurses. In addition to nursing and public health journals, behavioral and social science literature offers diverse perspectives on community health status for specific populations and subgroups. The Internet has increased the availability and accessibility of national, state, and local health data as well. However, the use of Internet-based resources for

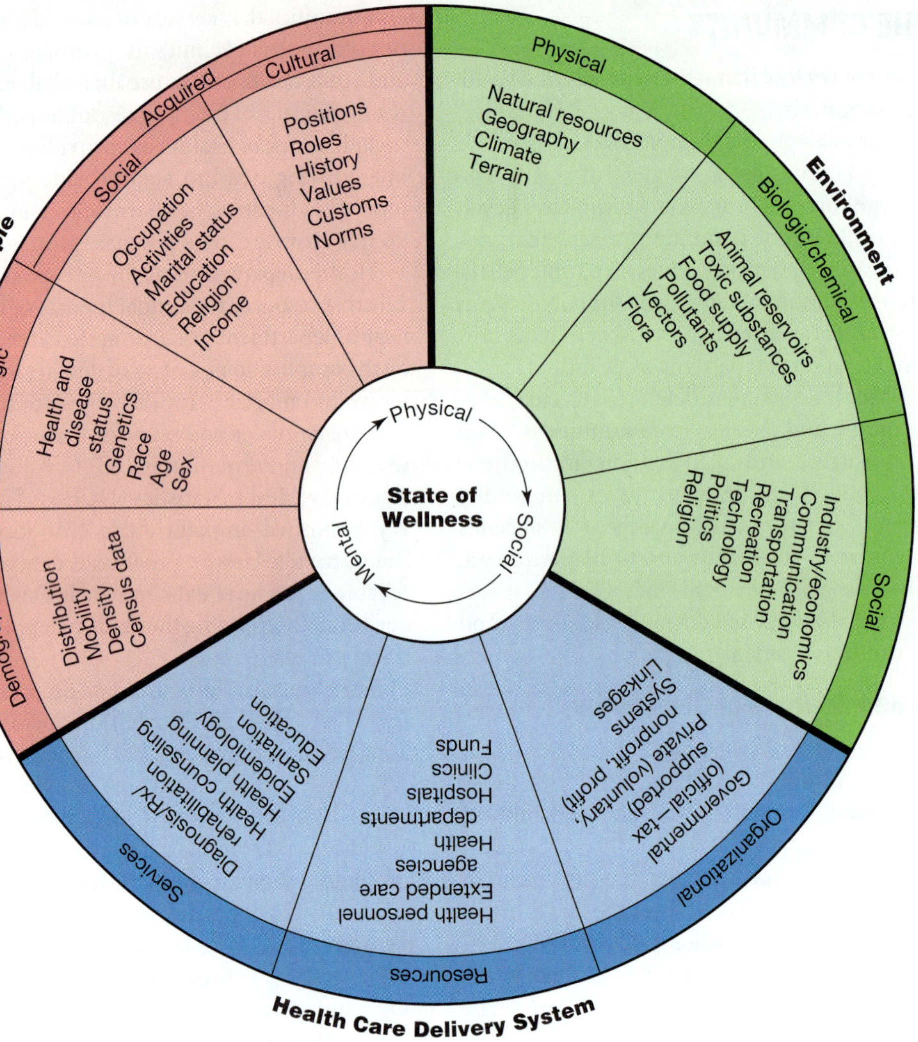

FIG. 2-6 Community health assessment wheel. (From Clemen-Stone, S. (2002). In S. Clemen-Stone, S. McGuire, & D. Eigsti. [2002]. *Comprehensive community health nursing: Family, aggregate, & community practice* [6th ed.]. St. Louis: Mosby.

health information requires caution because data reliability and validity are difficult to verify. (Guidelines for evaluation of Internet health resources can be found on the Health on the Net website, www.hon.ch).

Data collection methods may be either qualitative or quantitative and may include visual surveys that can be completed by walking through a community, participant observation, interviews, focus groups, and analysis of existing data. Potential clients and health care consumers may be asked to participate in focus groups or community forums to present their views on needed community services and programs. Formal surveys, conducted by mail, telephone, or face-to-face interviews, can be a valuable source of information not available from national databases or other secondary sources. Several drawbacks exist with this method: surveys are generally expensive to develop and time-consuming to administer. In addition to the cost of such surveys, poor response rates often preclude a sufficiently representative response on which to base nursing interventions.

A **walking survey** is generally conducted by a walk-through observation of the community (Box 2-3), taking note of specific characteristics of the population, economic and social environment, transportation, health care services, and other resources. With this type of data collection, information is gathered based on what the data collector observes, and is clearly objective data. **Participant observation** is another useful assessment method in which the nurse actively participates in the community to understand the community more fully and to validate observations (Stanhope & Lancaster, 2008).

Finally, as part of the assessment process, nurses working in multiethnic and multicultural groups need an in-depth assessment of culturally based health behaviors.

Analysis and synthesis of data obtained during the assessment process help to generate a comprehensive picture of the community's health status, needs, and problem areas, as well as its strengths and resources for addressing these concerns. The goal of this process is to assign priorities to community health needs and to develop a plan of action for correcting them. A comparison of community health data with state and national statistics can be useful in identification of appropriate target populations as well as interventions to improve health outcomes.

BOX 2-3 COMMUNITY WALK-THROUGH

As you observe the community, take note of the following:

- **Physical environment**—Older neighborhood or newer subdivision? Sidewalks, streets, and buildings in good or poor repair? Billboards and signs? What are they advertising? Are lawns kept up? Is there trash in the streets? Parks or playgrounds? Parking lots? Empty lots? Industries?
- **People in the area**—Old, young, homeless, children; predominant ethnicity, language? Is the population homogeneous? What signs do you see of different cultural groups?
- **Stores and services available**—Restaurants: chain, local, ethnic? Grocery stores: neighborhood or chain? Department stores, gas stations, real estate or insurance offices, travel agencies, pawn shops, liquor stores, discount or thrift stores, newspaper stands?
- **Social**—Clubs, bars, fraternal organizations (e.g., Elks, American Legion), museums?
- **Religious**—Churches, synagogues, mosques? What denominations? Do you see evidence of their use other than on religious/holy days?
- **Health services**—Drugstores, doctors' offices, clinics, dentists, mental health services, veterinarians, urgent care facilities, hospitals, shelters, nursing homes, home health agencies, public health services, traditional healers (e.g., herbalists, palmists)?
- **Transportation**—Cars, buses, taxis, light rail, sidewalks, bicycle paths, access for disabled persons?
- **Education**—Schools, before- and after-school programs, child care, libraries, bookstores? What is the reputation of the schools?
- **Government**—What is the governance structure? Is there a mayor? City council? Are meetings open to the public? Are there signs of political activity (e.g., posters, campaign signs)?
- **Safety**—How safe is the community? What is the crime rate? What types of crimes are committed? Are police visible? Is there a fire station?
- **Evaluation of the community based on your observations**—What is your impression of the community? Is the environment pleasing? Are services and transportation adequate? How difficult is it for residents to obtain needed services—i.e., how far do they have to travel? Would you want to live in this community? Why or why not?

Vulnerable Populations in the Community

Assessment of population health includes indicators related to diverse groups and cultures, particularly disenfranchised or "vulnerable" community members (www.crosshealth.com). Vulnerability in terms of health status and health outcomes may take many forms—including sociocultural, economic, and environmental risk factors that contribute to disparities in health. Health disparities are conditions that disproportionately affect certain racial, ethnic, or other groups. African-Americans, Hispanic-Americans, Native Americans, Pacific Islanders, and Asian-Americans are all considered vulnerable populations because they are more likely to have poor health and die prematurely (CDC, 2007).

The Institute of Medicine report, *Unequal Treatment: Confronting Racial and Ethnic Disparities in Health Care* (2002), provides evidence of racial and ethnic disparities for a number of health conditions and services. According to the National Healthcare Disparities Report (AHRQ, 2008), disparities are pervasive and improvement is possible, but there are still gaps in information for many groups. Although health disparities have been evident across all domains of health care for several decades, the etiology of these differences is still unclear (Jacobs, Karavolos, Rathouz, Ferris, & Powell, 2005). Poverty, poor access to care, lack of preventive services, and inadequate health knowledge and skills all contribute to excess disease burden.

Women

Women comprise 51% of the U.S. population, representing a very diverse, and largely at risk, group in relation to health (USDHHS, 2009c). Although women assume leadership for health care decision making in most families, they also face significant challenges in accessing the health care system and meeting their own health needs and those of family members (Kaiser Family Foundation, 2009). What is the source of women's vulnerability? Although there is no single contributing factor, the primary sources of health disparities for women fall into the areas of gender, socioeconomic status, and race or ethnicity. Significant gaps exist in the quality of care for women when compared with men.

The *National Report Card on Women's Health* describes significant deficiencies in women's health (National Women's Law Center [NWLC], 2007). States' performance in relation to 27 key areas was assessed; most were rated as *unsatisfactory* in relation to women's health status and policies influencing women's health. Key indicators focused on access to services, use of preventive health care and health promotion activities, the occurrence of certain health conditions, and an assessment of the community's effect on women's health. This report suggested that one of the primary factors compromising women's health is lack of access to acceptable-quality health care, which may manifest itself in many forms: lack of health insurance, living in a medically underserved area, or an inability to obtain needed services, particularly basic services such as prenatal care. Federal and state policies and programs also fail to safeguard women's interests in relation to reproductive health and health care coverage (NWLC).

Although many women report that they are in good to excellent health, statistics reveal significant disparities in health status of women from all age-groups and racial and ethnic backgrounds (USDHHS, 2009c). Low levels of educational attainment (high school or lower) are also associated with lack of resources, and difficulty navigating the health care system. This is particularly true of women of ethnic and racial minorities, whose limited English proficiency may compromise provider access and quality of care (Kaiser Family Foundation, 2009). According to recent statistics, 7 out of 10 working women lack health insurance coverage, which equates to 64 million American women (United Press International, 2009). Within this large group of women are those who are in the perinatal period, in which care, or the lack thereof, affects at least two individuals.

Racial and Ethnic Minorities

In addition to social, economic, and cultural barriers to optimal health, women who are in racial and ethnic minorities (29.3% of all U.S. women), experience a disproportionate burden of disease, disability, and premature death. Whereas 63% of non-Hispanic white females reported that they are in excellent or good health, only 53% of Hispanic and 51% of non-Hispanic black women reported this level of health (CDC, 2009a).

Significant health disparities continue to exist in adult women's health and the health of their infants. Although positive trends are evident, there are persistent disparities among racial and ethnic groups in early prenatal care, an important factor in achieving healthy pregnancy outcomes (CDC, 2009a). The goals of *Healthy People 2020* are reflective of the health disparities that exist among various populations, with emphasis on reduction of fetal and infant deaths, reduction of preterm births, reduction of maternal deaths, among others (USDHHS, 2009d) (see Box 1-2).

Minority women, many of whom live in poverty, also have higher rates of chronic disease including heart disease, cancer, hepatitis, and acquired immunodeficiency syndrome (AIDS), and mental health issues (USDHHS, 2009c). Women with underlying health conditions are at especially high risk for poor obstetric outcomes for themselves and their infants. They have high rates of preterm labor and gestational hypertension, and often have intrauterine growth restriction resulting in the birth of infants who are small for gestational age. These are the women for whom the community-based perinatal nurse will be providing care, and their needs are complex, demanding high levels of expertise and skill.

Adolescent Girls

The adolescent population in the United States is generally considered healthy. However, the adolescent population participates in riskier behaviors and their health is often compromised as a result. In 2006 13,739 deaths were reported among teenagers between the ages of 15 and 19, with unintentional injuries being the main cause of death, followed by homicide and suicide (USDHHS, 2009b).

Although adolescents are concerned about becoming pregnant, they still engage in unprotected sex. Adolescents also use a variety of sources for health information—the media, friends, and sex education—yet they are very misinformed, particularly about STIs and human immunodeficiency virus (HIV) transmission. These findings have significant implications for perinatal outcomes and emphasize the importance of aggressive prevention programs and community outreach related to sexuality, teen pregnancy, and substance abuse.

As the rate of adolescent pregnancy continues to rise and as STIs become more prevalent, it is crucial that nurses engage adolescents in health education programs that will encourage them to make informed decisions about their sexual health. It is also vital that nurses be a resource to these women.

Older Women

It is estimated that in the United States in 2008, 22.4 million women were older than age 65 (U.S. Census Bureau, 2009b). Although women have a greater life expectancy than men, they are more likely to have chronic illnesses, less likely to use preventive services, and ultimately spend more on health care (CDC). As nurses, it is important that we engage this population at all levels of prevention, from primary to tertiary.

Incarcerated Women

The number of incarcerated women in the United States has continued to climb in recent years, increasing at a significantly greater rate than for men. In 2008, approximately 207,700 were in prison or jail, with the highest number of these being non-Hispanic black women (Department of Justice, 2009). Many of these women report a history of sexual and physical abuse.

Because their relationship histories are often unstable, and because they often lack the support of family, incarcerated women or those with a history of repeated incarceration frequently have difficulty providing emotional stability, secure housing, and health promotion role modeling for their children.

The lifestyle choices of this group, including risky sexual relationships, illicit drug use, and smoking, place them at high risk for STIs, HIV and AIDS, other chronic and communicable diseases, and complicated pregnancies.

Refugee and Migrant Women

As of 2006, one in every eight residents in the United States was foreign born, the highest number since 1920 (Martin, 2007). This accounts for a rapidly growing diverse population for which nurses will be providing care. California, Texas, New York, Florida, and Illinois are among the states with the highest growing immigrant population, respectively (Martin). An immigrant is an individual who moves from one country to another in an effort to take up legal residency, whereas a refugee is an individual who is forced to leave his or her home country, often in search of a safer and more stable living environment.

Both populations are often challenged with not being able to easily access health care because they are not U.S. citizens. These women often do not seek medical care for fear of deportation. Access to care is further limited by health care policies that restrict Medicaid eligibility for these groups (Kaiser Commission, 2003a). Mohanty and colleagues (2005) compared the health care costs of immigrants to those of U.S. citizens. Refuting the assumption that immigrants place an extra burden on the health care system, the study revealed that total health care expenditures for immigrant adults and children were significantly lower than those of U.S.-born citizens.

Migrant laborers and their families face many problems, including financial instability, child labor, poor housing, lack of education, language and cultural barriers, and limited access to health and social services. Poor dental health, diabetes, hypertension, malnutrition, tuberculosis, skin diseases, and parasitic infections are common health issues among migrant populations (Feldman, Vallejos, Quandt, Fleischer, Schulz, Verma, et al., 2009; Henning, Graybill, & George, 2008). Primary health care services are largely provided by a number of migrant health centers, of which there are more than 400 throughout the United States. In 2008, more than 834,000 seasonal and migrant farm workers and their families were served (USDHHS, n.d.). Routine prenatal care, as well as screening and treatment for hypertension and diabetes, are provided. Community health nurses frequently encounter the challenges of providing culturally and linguistically appropriate care while facing numerous health issues.

Numerous reproductive health issues exist for migrant women, including less consistent use of contraception and increased rates of STIs. Migrants are less likely to receive early prenatal care and have a greater incidence of inadequate weight gain during pregnancy than do other poor women.

Along with their profound resilience and determination, refugees and immigrants have brought rich diversity to the United

States in several important dimensions including cultural heritage and customs, economic productivity, and enhanced national vitality. In general, refugees are more likely to live in poverty than are immigrants. Over time, measures of health and well-being actually decline for the immigrant population as they become part of American society. Many of the conditions or illnesses that they acquire contribute to the persistence of disparities in maternal and neonatal health outcomes for both immigrants and refugees.

Rural Versus Urban Community Settings

Approximately 17% of the U.S. population lives in a rural area, with 80% of the land area considered to be rural (USDA, 2009). Characteristically, rural residents are older, less educated, and generally in poorer health than their urban counterparts. Rural communities are disproportionately affected by poverty and poor access to health care services. Lack of insurance presents an additional factor for poor health in rural areas. Of the 41 million uninsured residents of the United States, 1 in 5 lives in rural communities. In some states, up to 70% of rural residents lack insurance or rely on Medicaid.

Rural women are especially vulnerable to financial and transportation barriers to health care. Although women in rural counties report only *fair* to *poor* health, they pay considerably more for their health care. In rural communities, women have less access to prenatal care, which contributes to higher rates of adverse pregnancy outcomes including higher rates of preterm birth, low birth weight, and infant mortality. The disproportionate distribution of poverty and of variations in race/ethnicity, age, education, and availability and access to medical resources may be the link to infant mortality in rural areas.

Homeless Women

Homelessness among women is an increasing social and health issue in the United States. Although exact numbers are unknown because of the difficulty in tracking individuals without a permanent address, it is estimated that more than 744,000 people were homeless in 2005. Women make up 65% of the homeless population and are increasingly affected by poverty, making homelessness more prevalent for families and children, particularly among rural populations (National Coalition for the Homeless [NCFH], 2009).

Health issues among the homeless are numerous and result primarily from a lack of preventive care and a lack of resources in general. Health problems including chronic illness, asthma, circulatory problems, and diabetes are rampant. Homeless women face many health issues, related to lifestyle factors and the vulnerability resulting from being homeless. In addition to extreme poverty, women are at increased risk for illness and injury; many have been victims of domestic abuse, assault, and rape (American College of Obstetricians and Gynecologists [ACOG], 2005).

Although little is known about pregnancy in this population, about 20% of women do become pregnant while homeless. Conversely, pregnancy and recent birth are highly correlated with becoming homeless (ACOG, 2005). In addition to risk factors related to inadequate nutrition, inadequate weight gain, anemia, bleeding problems, and preterm birth, homeless women face multiple barriers to prenatal care: transportation, distance, and wait times. Most women also underutilize available prenatal services (Bloom, Bednarzyk, Devitt, Renault, Teaman, & VanLoock, 2004). The unsafe environment and high risk lifestyles often result in adverse perinatal outcomes.

Low Literacy

Individuals and groups for whom English is a second language often lack the skills necessary to seek medical care and function adequately in the health care setting. Communication barriers may affect access to care, particularly in such areas as making appointments, applying for services, and obtaining transportation.

Health literacy involves a spectrum of abilities, ranging from reading an appointment slip to interpreting medication instructions. There is growing evidence of the effects of low health literacy on adult health status (Rosal, Goins, Carbone, & Cortes, 2004; www.hsph.harvard.edu/healthliteracy). Low health literacy may also be an independent contributor to a disproportionate disease burden among disadvantaged populations. Disparities in preventive care, early screening for cancer, and utilization of health care services, particularly among minority women, have also been linked to language barriers (Jacobs et al., 2005; www.prenataled.com/healthlit).

As the United States becomes increasingly multicultural, nurses will be required to interact with non–English-speaking groups or those with limited health literacy. Consequently, health literacy must be viewed as a component of culturally and linguistically competent care. These skills must be assessed routinely to recognize a problem and accommodate clients with limited literacy skills.

Implications for Nursing

Although the long-term consequences of contemporary immigration for American society are unclear, the successful incorporation of immigrant families depends on the resources, benefits, and policies that ensure their healthy development and successful social adjustment. Culturally competent health care and involvement of the immigrant community in health care programs are recommended strategies for improving the access to and effectiveness of health care for this population.

The use of camp volunteers has been effective in assisting families living in migrant worker camps to obtain prenatal, postpartum, and infant care. Working in partnership with health professionals such as nurses, lay camp aides have been used effectively for outreach and health education; however, more strategies are needed to link traditional practices with the formal health care system. Guidance and information about other health resources are available to health care providers through the National Migrant Resource Program and the Migrant Clinicians Network.

Nurses working with homeless women and families are challenged to treat them with dignity and respect to establish a therapeutic relationship. Case management is recommended to coordinate the services and disciplines that may be involved in meeting the complex needs of these families. Whenever possible, general screening and preventive health services must be provided when the woman seeks treatment because this may be the only opportunity to provide health information and intervention. Building on existing coping strategies and strengths, the health care provider helps the woman and her family to reconnect with a social support system. Nurses also have an important role in advocating for funding to support health services to the homeless and to improve access to preventive care for all homeless populations.

HOME CARE IN THE COMMUNITY

Modern home care nursing has its foundation in public health nursing, which provided comprehensive care to sick and well clients in their own homes. Specialized maternity home care nursing services began in the 1980s when public health maternity nursing services were limited and services had not kept pace with the changing practices of high risk obstetrics and emerging technology. Lengthy antepartum hospitalizations for such conditions as preterm labor and gestational hypertension created nursing care challenges for staff members of inpatient units.

Many women expressed their concern for the negative effect of antepartum hospitalizations on the family. Although clinical indications showed that a new nursing care approach was needed, home health care did not become a viable alternative until third-party payers (i.e., public or private organizations or employer groups that pay for health care) pushed for cost containment in maternity services.

In the current health care system, home care is an important component of health care delivery along the perinatal continuum of care (Fig. 2-7). The growing demand for home care is based on several factors:

- Interest in family birthing alternatives
- Shortened hospital stays
- New technologies that facilitate home-based assessments and treatments
- Reimbursement by third-party payers

As health care costs continue to rise, and because millions of American families lack health insurance, there is greater demand for innovative, cost-effective methods of health care delivery in the community. Large health care systems are developing clinically integrated health care delivery networks whose goals are: (1) improved coordination of care and care outcomes; (2) better communication among health care providers; (3) increased client, payer, and provider satisfaction; and (4) reduced cost. The integration of clinical services changes the focus of care to a continuum of services that are increasingly community based.

Communication and Technology Applications

As maternity care continues to consist of frequent and brief contacts with health care providers throughout the prenatal and postpartum periods, services that link maternity clients throughout the perinatal continuum of care have assumed increasing importance. These services include critical pathways, telephonic nursing assessments, discharge planning, specialized education programs, parent support groups, home visiting programs, nurse advice lines, and perinatal home care. Hospitals may provide cross-training for hospital-based nurses to make postpartum home visits or to staff outpatient centers for postpartum follow-up.

Telephonic nursing care through services such as warm lines, nurse advice lines, and telephonic nursing assessments is a valuable means of managing health care problems and bridging the gaps among acute, outpatient, and home care services. Providers are using the Internet to communicate with clients who have an Internet service provider (ISP). Nursing care that occurs by telephone is interactive and responsive to immediate health care questions about particular health care needs. **Warm lines** are telephone lines that are offered as a community service to provide new parents with support, encouragement, and basic parenting education. Nurse advice lines, or toll-free nurse consultation services, often are supported by third-party payers or health management organization/managed care organization (HMO/MCO) and are designed to provide answers to medical questions. Nurse care managers are prepared to guide callers through urgent health care situations, suggest treatment options, and provide health education. Telephonic nursing assessments, or nurse consultation, assessment, and health education that take place during a telephone conversation, can be added to the plan of care in conjunction with skilled nursing visits, or they may comprise a separate nursing contact for the woman. Telephonic nursing assessments are commonly used after a postpartum home care visit to reassess a woman's knowledge about the signs and symptoms of adequate hydration in

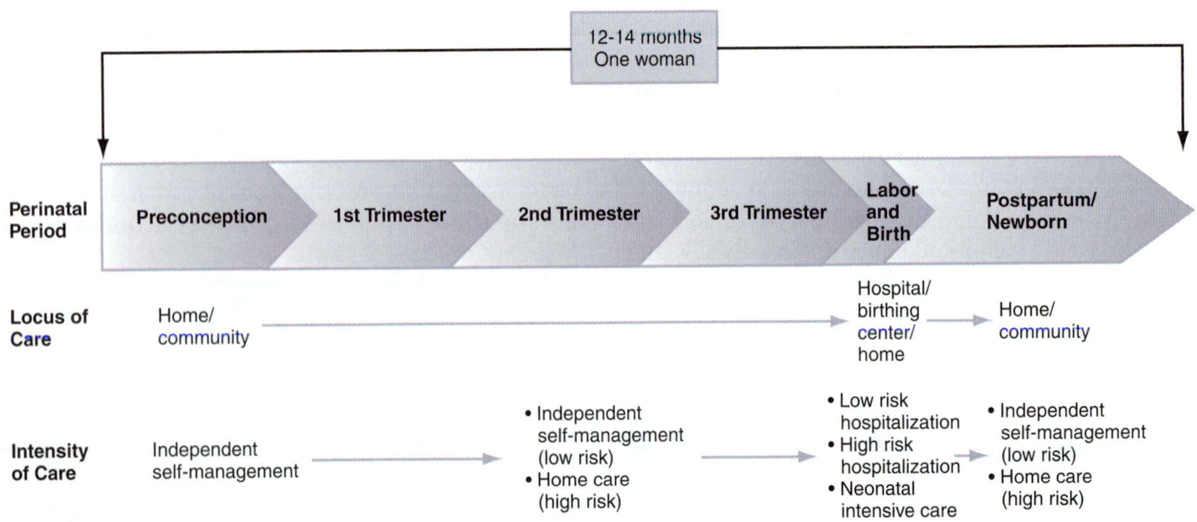

FIG. 2-7 Perinatal continuum of care.

breastfeeding, or, after initiating home phototherapy, to assess the caregiver's knowledge regarding problems with equipment.

Guidelines for Nursing Practice

The Association of Women's Health, Obstetric, and Neonatal Nurses (AWHONN, 2009) defines home care as the provision of technical, psychologic, and other therapeutic support in the woman's home rather than in an institution. The scope of nursing care delivered in the home is necessarily limited to practices deemed safe and appropriate to be carried out in an environment that is physically separated from a health care institution and its resources. Nursing practice at home is consistent with federal and state regulations that direct home care practice. The nurse demonstrates practice competence through formalized orientation and ongoing clinical education and performance evaluation in the respective home care agency. Standards for practice from key specialty organizations such as AWHONN, the ACOG, the American Academy of Pediatrics (AAP), and the Intravenous Nursing Society (INS) provide the basis for clinical protocols and pathways and organizational programs in home care practice. The Joint Commission (www.jointcommission.org) provides criteria for home care operations based on Centers for Medicare & Medicaid Services (CMS) regulations (cms.hhs.gov).

A wide range of professional health care services and products can be delivered or used in the home by means of technology and telecommunication. For example, telehealth and telemedicine make it possible for clients in the home to be interviewed and assessed by a specialist located hundreds of miles away. Home health care can be viewed as an extension of in-hospital care. Essentially, the primary difference between health care in a hospital and home care is the absence of the continuous presence of professional health care providers in a client's home. Generally, but not always, home health care entails intermittent care by a professional who visits the client's home for a particular reason and/or provides care onsite for fewer than 4 hours at a time. The home health care agency maintains on-call professional staff to assist home care clients who have questions about their care and for emergencies, such as equipment failure.

Perinatal Services

Home care perinatal services may be provided by hospital-based programs, independent proprietary (for-profit) agencies, or nonprofit home care agencies, and official or tax-supported agencies. Innovative programs may be supported by research grants for a period of years, but ultimately they must be sponsored by an agency with long-term funding. Home visits have advantages and disadvantages. The pregnant woman is able to maintain bed rest if indicated, and vulnerable neonates are not exposed to the weather or external sources of infection. The nurse can observe and interact with family members in their most natural and secure environment. Adequacy of resources and safety factors can be assessed. Teaching can be tailored to the actual home conditions, and other family members can be included. A home visit is less expensive than a day's hospitalization, but a 60- to 90-minute visit requires 2.5 to 3 hours of nursing time, including travel and documentation. Areas of challenge include limited availability of nurses with expertise in maternity care and concerns about the nurse's physical safety in the community. One alternative that is less expensive is contacting women via telephone.

Visits for outreach and health promotion are an integral part of community (or public) health nursing. In countries with national health systems, a nurse or midwife may see all women during pregnancy and after birth. In the United States, visits of this sort have been provided mainly to low-income families without health insurance and Medicaid recipients who use the clinics provided by local health departments. Until recently, private insurers did not reimburse for health promotion visits. MCOs now recognize that anticipatory guidance can be cost-effective, but home visitation programs for the most part still target specific, high risk populations, such as adolescents and women at risk for preterm labor.

Home care agencies are subject to regulation by governmental and professional organizations and provide interdisciplinary services including social work, nutrition, and occupational and physical therapy. Increasingly, their case loads are made up of women who require high-technology care, such as infusions or home monitoring. Although the home health nurse develops the care plan, all care must be ordered by a physician. In addition, interventions must meet the insurer's criteria for reimbursement, and services are limited to registered clients. Preconception care and low risk antepartum care can usually be provided more efficiently in offices and are not currently reimbursable. High risk antepartum care can be provided by home care agencies; for example, women with hyperemesis gravidarum who require parenteral nutrition may be treated at home. Conditions requiring bed rest, such as preterm labor and hypertension, are other common indications for home care. Other conditions often managed with home care may include cardiac disease, substance abuse, and diabetes in pregnancy.

Insurers may reimburse for at least one postpartum visit to families after early discharge or in the presence of high risk factors. Home phototherapy is used for treatment of neonatal hyperbilirubinemia and to avoid separation of mother and infant. Many other neonates who require long-term high-technology care are also managed with home care.

Client Selection and Referral

The office or hospital-based nurse is often the key person in making effective referrals to home care. When considering a referral to home care, the following factors are evaluated:

- Health status of mother and fetus or infant: Is the condition serious enough to warrant home care, and is it stable enough for intermittent observation to be sufficient?
- Availability of professionals to provide the needed services within the woman's community
- Family resources, including psychosocial, social, and economic resources: Will the family be able to provide care between nursing visits? Are relationships supportive? Is third-party reimbursement available, or can it be negotiated with the insurer? Could a voluntary or tax-supported community agency provide needed care without payment?
- Cost-effectiveness: Is it more reasonable for the woman to receive these services at home or to go to a local outpatient facility to receive them?

Community referrals should not be limited to women with physiologic complications of pregnancy that require medical treatment. Women at risk (e.g., young adolescents, families with a history of abuse, members of vulnerable population groups, developmentally disabled individuals) may need follow-up care at home. As we move more and more into an interdisciplinary health care society, it is crucial that nurses communicate with social workers to tap into valuable community resources that women can use once in their community.

Standardized forms simplify the referral process and ensure that all needed information will be forwarded to the home health agency. The nursing assessment should include the woman's physical and psychologic status, her level of knowledge about self-management activities, her willingness to learn, the availability of caregivers and social support in the home, and her level of comfort with home care. If the referral is for a mother-and-infant home care visit, the nursing assessment should include newborn data.

High-technology home care requires additional information to be collected from the chart, and consultation with the referring physician and other members of the health care team, before a home care referral is made. These additional data include the medical diagnosis, medical prognosis, prescribed therapies, medication history, drug-dosing information, potential ancillary supplies, type of infusion and access device, and the available systems of social support for the woman and family. The nursing assessment and therapy data provide baseline information for the home care nurse and other health care providers involved in the care plan.

Whenever a referral is called in to a home health care agency, a member of the nursing or admissions staff determines the agency's ability to accept the woman for service. The use of telecommunication modalities such as fax machines, cellular phones, electronic files and the Internet to transmit information has eliminated delays in initiating home care services, even in more remote rural areas.

CARE MANAGEMENT

Preparing for the Home Visit

The home care nurse reviews the available clinical data, demographic information, and completed care plan form and consults with the home care pharmacist or other health care team members who have previously contacted the woman to determine the goals of the visit. At this point, the nurse uses the medical diagnosis and the location of the case on the perinatal continuum as a starting point to organize the woman's care. The nurse reviews agency policies and procedures, professional literature about diagnosis, and community resources as part of the previsit preparation work (Box 2-4).

Before going on a home visit, the nurse schedules a time for the visit with the woman. It is essential that the nurse obtain clear driving directions at this time as well.

The nurse identifies himself or herself by name, title, and agency. He or she then explains who referred the woman to the agency for home care and the purpose of the home care visits. The nurse briefly explains what will occur during the visit and approximately how long the visit will last. The woman should be asked to restrain any pets during the visit. Last, the nurse asks about health supplies that may be needed for the woman's care.

First Home Care Visit

Making the first home care visit can be stressful for the nurse and the woman. The home care nurse is faced with an unknown environment controlled by the woman and her family. The woman and her family also experience feelings about the unknown, such as anxiety about the way the nurse will treat them or what the nurse will do during the visit. The challenge for the home care nurse is to establish a positive nurse-client relationship and provide the prescribed home care services within the time provided for the initial home visit.

Implementing the following will generally make the home visit more comfortable for both the nurse and the woman: the nurse wears identification, and introduces herself upon entering the home, clearly states the purpose of the visit, obtains written consent for the visit, provides privacy, as desired by the woman, provides culturally sensitive care, and encourages the woman and family to become actively involved in the care provided. One of the most important roles of the home care nurse is modeling health-related behaviors for the woman and others who are in the home during the visit.

ASSESSMENT AND NURSING DIAGNOSES

The primary goals of the assessment phase are to develop a trusting relationship and collect data by various methods to obtain a comprehensive client profile. It may not be feasible or appropriate to collect in-depth information about all areas of assessment during the first visit. However, in many instances, the nurse may be limited to one visit and must obtain information pertinent to the current situation in that hour.

The major areas of the assessment are demographics, medical history, general health history, medication history, sociocultural assessment (Box 2-5), home and community environment, and physical assessment. Information can be obtained from client records sent to the home care agency at the time of referral or from the previsit interview. These data will be used to develop the nursing care plan and complete the plan of care, which is required for many licensed home health care agencies.

Each plan of care has a different emphasis in the home environment. For example, women receiving infusion therapy for hyperemesis gravidarum need a safe place to store medications and infusion supplies that is out of reach of small children living in the home. The home care nurse should incorporate the agency policies and procedures for the storage and handling of infusion supplies into her walk-through inspection. During the walk-through, the home care nurse looks at the potential storage areas that are dry and clean, and where the temperature can be maintained. The home care nurse should include an inspection of the work areas such as countertops, tabletops, sinks, and trash areas that the woman or caregiver may use for mixing medications, changing infusion tubing, handling supplies, or disposing of used equipment and supplies.

The homes of women using electronic home health care equipment, such as phototherapy equipment or infusion pumps, require physical inspection of any electrical outlets,

BOX 2-4 PROTOCOL FOR PERINATAL HOME VISITS

PREVISIT INTERVENTIONS

1. Contact the family to arrange details for home visit.
   a. Identify self, credentials, and agency role.
   b. Review purpose of home visit follow-up.
   c. Schedule convenient time for visit.
   d. Confirm address and route to family home.
2. Review and clarify appropriate data.
   a. Review all available assessment data for mother and fetus or infant (i.e., referral forms, hospital discharge summaries, identified learning needs of the family).
   b. Review records of any previous nursing contacts.
   c. Contact other professional caregivers as necessary to clarify data (i.e., obstetrician, nurse-midwife, pediatrician, referring nurse).
3. Identify community resources and teaching materials appropriate to meet those needs already identified.
4. Plan the visit, and prepare a bag with equipment, supplies, and materials necessary for assessments of mother and fetus or infant, actual care anticipated, and teaching.

IN-HOME INTERVENTIONS: ESTABLISHING A RELATIONSHIP

1. Reintroduce yourself and establish the purpose of the visit for mother, infant, and family; offer the family the opportunity to clarify their expectations of the contact.
2. Spend a brief time socially interacting with the family to become acquainted and establish a trusting relationship.

IN-HOME INTERVENTIONS: WORKING WITH THE FAMILY

1. Conduct a systematic assessment of the mother and the fetus or newborn to determine their physiologic adjustment and any existing complications (Fig. 2-8).
2. Throughout visit, collect data to assess the emotional adjustment of individual family members to the pregnancy or birth and lifestyle changes. Note any evidence of family-newborn bonding and sibling rivalry; note relationships among mother, father, children, and grandparents.
3. Determine the adequacy of support system.
   a. To what extent does someone help with cooking, cleaning, and other home management tasks?
   b. To what extent is help being provided in caring for the newborn and any other children?
   c. Are support persons encouraging the new mother to care for herself and get adequate rest?
   d. Who is providing helpful information? Emotional support?
4. Throughout the visit observe the home environment for adequacy of resources.
   a. Space: privacy, safe play of children, sleeping
   b. Overall cleanliness and state of repair
   c. Number of steps pregnant woman/new mother must climb
   d. Adequacy of cooking arrangements
   e. Adequacy of refrigeration and other food storage areas
   f. Adequacy of bathing, toilet, and laundry facilities
   g. Arrangements in home for newborn: sleeping, bathing, formula preparation (if needed), layette items, and diapers
5. Throughout the visit, observe the home environment for overall state of repair and existence of safety hazards.
   a. Storage of medications, household cleaners, and other substances hazardous to children
   b. Presence of peeling paint on furniture, walls, or pipes
   c. Factors that contribute to falls, such as dim lighting, broken steps, scatter rugs
   d. Presence of vermin
   e. Use of crib or playpen that fails to meet safety guidelines
   f. Existence of emergency plan in case of fire; fire alarm or extinguisher
6. Provide care to the mother, the newborn, or both as prescribed by their respective primary care provider or in accord with agency protocol.
7. Provide teaching on the basis of previously identified needs.
8. Refer the family to appropriate community agencies or resources, such as warm lines and support groups.
9. Ascertain that the woman knows potential problems to watch for and who to call if they occur.
10. Ensure that used disposable items have been handled appropriately and that reusable items are cleaned and repacked appropriately in the nurse's bag.

IN-HOME INTERVENTIONS: ENDING THE VISIT

1. Summarize the activities and main points of the visit.
2. Clarify future expectations, including the schedule of the next visit.
3. Review the teaching plan and provide major points in writing.
4. Provide information about reaching the nurse or agency if needed before the next scheduled visit.

POSTVISIT INTERVENTIONS

1. Document the visit thoroughly, using the necessary agency forms to serve as a legal record of the visit and to allow third-party reimbursement, as possible.
2. Initiate the plan of care on which the next encounter with the woman and/or family will be based.
3. Communicate appropriately (by telephone, letter, progress notes, or referral form) with the primary care provider, other health professionals, or referral agencies on behalf of the woman and family.

electrical cords, and extension cords that will be used. Homes with faulty electrical wiring may place the woman at risk for being involved in an electrical fire; faulty wiring may require inspection and repair by a professional electrician before electronic devices are used. Findings from the assessment are incorporated into the plan of care.

The nursing plan of care is developed in collaboration with the woman, based on the health care needs of the individual. Home care nurses working in home health care agencies regulated by the CMS use a plan of care that includes client demographics, the health care provider's orders, home care goals, and the woman's level of functioning. This document is initiated at the time of referral to the home care agency and must be updated every 60 days or as specified by state regulations. The frequency of the skilled nursing visit may vary with the individual plan of care and reimbursement criteria established by the third-party payers.

Nursing Considerations

There are several areas of concern when caring for a woman in the home. In home care, the woman or family members are responsible for administration of medications in the absence of the nurse. A careful medication history should be obtained to see if the woman is taking her medications correctly and understands their desired action and potential side effects. It is important that women and caretakers have a clear understanding of

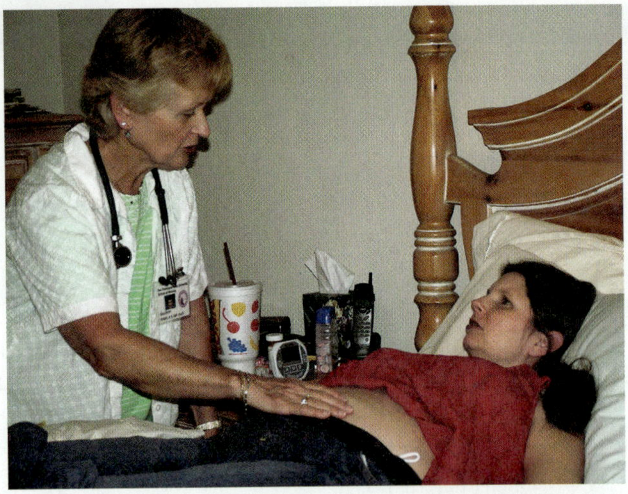

FIG. 2-8 Home care nurse visits with a woman in preterm labor at home on bed rest. (Courtesy Shannon Perry, Phoenix, AZ.)

medication regimens and are notified when medications change in any way. Even more important is ensuring that the woman and her caregivers fully understand the information that they are provided by health care providers.

It is also important that nurses are aware of how to use and educate women on the use of all home care equipment such as infusion pumps and phototherapy lights, for example. Nurses also have to be skilled at performing various procedures such as venipuncture and administration of intravenous medications or fluids. In addition to teaching about medications and equipment, nurses must be sure that women know how to respond in emergency situations. Women need to be able to have 24-hour access to resources in the community in emergency situations. Women and family members are also encouraged to learn how to perform cardiopulmonary resuscitation (CPR), especially for infants.

Additional client and family education in home care includes information about the specific high risk condition(s) involved, implications for pregnancy outcome, and measures for self-monitoring. Verbal explanations should be supplemented with clearly written instructions. General information to promote well-being, such as about nutrition and common discomforts of pregnancy, should also be included. The need for preparation for childbirth can be addressed by using books or videos and supplemented by individual teaching at home. Coping with bed rest or other limitation of activity is a problem for many women with high risk pregnancies. The nurse may share strategies that others have used, help with time management, and provide information about support services. Teaching about infant care or the special needs of the preterm infant may be appropriate during the prenatal period.

Clear documentation of assessments, problems identified, treatments and interventions performed, and the woman's response is essential. Third-party payers base reimbursement on the nurse's written record of providing skilled nursing care and assessments that support the woman's continuing need for those services. The nurse must promptly inform the health care provider by telephone, facsimile, or electronic file of any significant changes. When new orders are transmitted by telephone, a written copy must be sent for the physician's signature.

BOX 2-5 PSYCHOSOCIAL ASSESSMENT

LANGUAGE
- Identify the primary language spoken in the home.
- Assess whether there are any language barriers to receiving support.

COMMUNITY RESOURCES/ACCESS TO CARE
- Identify primary and secondary means of transportation.
- Identify community agencies family uses for health care and support.
- Assess cultural and psychosocial barriers to receiving care.

SOCIAL SUPPORT
- Determine the people living with the pregnant woman.
- Identify who assists with household chores.
- Identify who assists with child care and parenting activities.
- Identify who the pregnant woman turns to for problems or during a crisis.

INTERPERSONAL RELATIONSHIPS
- Identify the way decisions are made in the family.
- Identify the family's perception of the need for home care.
- Identify roles of adults in caring for family members.

CAREGIVER
- Identify the primary caregiver for home care treatments.
- Identify other caregivers and their roles.
- Assess the caregiver's knowledge of treatments and the care process.
- Identify potential strain from the caregiver role.
- Identify the level of satisfaction with the caregiver role.

STRESS AND COPING
- Identify what the woman perceives as lifestyle changes and their effect on her and her family.
- Identify the changes she and her family have made to adjust to her health condition and home health care treatments.

Finally, as soon as home care has been provided, it is essential that the nurse document assessment findings, care provided, recommendations for change, and any client or family teaching. Detailed documentation is necessary to justify the need for the home visit, and is often crucial in attaining reimbursement from insurance companies. The nursing care plan summarizes details to be included in caring for a woman in the home (see Nursing Care Plan).

SAFETY ISSUES FOR THE HOME CARE NURSE

Nurse safety and infection control are two important components of home care. The nurse should be fully aware of the home environment and the neighborhood in which the home care is being provided. Unlike hospitals, in which the environment is more predictable and controlled, the woman's neighborhood and home have the potential for uncertainty. Home care nurses should take necessary safety precautions and avoid dangerous areas.

Agencies that serve clients in high-crime areas may conduct an assessment of the potential for violence by telephone before the visit and enlist the client's cooperation in minimizing risk. Others have hired full-time security personnel to accompany nurses on their visits. Personal strategies recommended for nurses visiting families with a history of violence or substance abuse include: (1) self-awareness; (2) environmental

NURSING CARE PLAN

Community and Home Care

NURSING DIAGNOSIS

Readiness for enhanced family coping related to family growth and development in new community

Expected Outcome

Family will identify at least three community groups that can serve as appropriate resources for an expectant family with small children.

Nursing Interventions/*Rationales*

- Assess family structure and availability of significant others, friends, or family members to assist family with new baby and siblings *to provide database for further interventions.*
- Encourage family to enlist assistance of individuals who are available to help family at birth of new baby *to provide physical and emotional support.*
- Using therapeutic communication, assist the family to assess coping strategies used in the past for new situations *to provide clarification and promote empowerment of family in new situations.*
- Suggest strategies to find resources available in the community *to assist family during pregnancy, with new baby, and with small siblings.*
- Give information regarding community workshops, classes, or support groups *to promote networking, community bonding, and support.*

NURSING DIAGNOSIS

Ineffective community management of therapeutic regimen related to resettlement of refugees in the community

Expected Outcome

The community will develop programs to meet the needs of new members of the community.

Nursing Interventions/*Rationales*

- Conduct a needs assessment of the community *to identify priority needs for new members of the community.*
- Initiate health education programs based on topics identified in the needs assessment *to meet the needs of members of the community.*
- Prepare client education materials in a variety of languages *to enhance understanding of community members.*
- Identify risks in the community (e.g., environmental hazards, drug sales) *to provide a target for community improvement.*
- With community leaders, develop a plan to cope with and reduce environmental hazards *to improve public health and safety.*
- Develop a monitoring or surveillance system *to ensure that progress will continue and new problems will be identified.*

NURSING DIAGNOSIS

Ineffective community coping related to presence of gangs and lack of community programs to redirect activities of youth

Expected Outcome

Health status of the community will improve.

Nursing Interventions/*Rationales*

- Initiate health screening programs for community members *to identify effects of environmental hazards in the community.*
- Work with politicians and policy makers to develop the community *to provide a safe environment with means of economic survival for community members.*
- Initiate programs such as Block Watch, Safe Houses, and Neighborhood Watch *to enhance the safety of the environment.*
- Work with community leaders to develop or clean up playgrounds *to provide a safe place for children to play.*
- With community leaders, develop community grass roots initiatives *to enable community members to take ownership in the community.*
- Identify sites of lead exposure *to decrease the potential for lead poisoning in children.*
- Participate in immunization or vaccination clinics *to reduce the risk in the community of infectious diseases.*
- Develop community education programs on drugs, alcohol, and tobacco *to reduce exposure of young people to these products.*

assessment; (3) using listening and observation skills with clients to be aware of behavioral changes indicating aggression or lack of impulse control; (4) planning for dealing with aggressive behavior (i.e., allowing personal space and taking a nonaggressive stance); (5) making visits in pairs; and (6) having access to a cell phone at all times.

Personal Safety

The home care nurse must be aware of personal safety behaviors before going on a home visit. Dress should be casual but professional in appearance, with a name identification tag. Limited jewelry should be worn. Valuable personal items, such as an expensive purse or coat, should not be worn on a visit. Carrying an extra set of car keys in the nursing home care bag saves time and frustration if the nurse becomes locked out of the automobile. Automobile keys spread between the fingers with sharp ends outward can be used as a weapon if necessary. The same commonsense behaviors and precautions that guide a person's behavior when alone in any setting should be followed by home care nurses.

The agency should have a copy of the nurse's home care itinerary, including contact telephone numbers if a client does not have a telephone and information on the nurse's car (make, model, color, and license plate number). Many home care nurses carry agency-provided pagers or cell phones that allow the agency to contact the nurse throughout the day to give information about client updates, changes in orders or services, schedule changes, and new clients who require an initial visit. The telephone also is useful to notify clients when the nurse is delayed.

The automobile used for the home care visits, whether a personal or an agency-owned vehicle, should have regular preventive maintenance checks, an adequate fuel level, and road safety items stored in the trunk. Items to carry in the vehicle include change for parking fees and tolls, maps, emergency telephone numbers, a flashlight, a first aid kit, flares, a blanket, and equipment for inclement weather conditions. When making a visit to a woman in a more remote rural setting, other travel considerations may be needed, as well as taking additional supplies or medication to the client.

Home care nurses should park and lock their cars in a safe place that is visible from the street and the woman's home and away from hidden alleys. While driving to the woman's home, the nurse should assess the neighborhood for safety, especially if the neighborhood is unfamiliar. All valuable items should be stored out of sight before leaving the office. While walking to the woman's home, nurses should not walk near groups of strangers hanging out in doorways or alleys, enter into vacant buildings, or enter a yard that has an unrestrained dog. The home or building should not be entered if the nurse has any safety concerns. All home care agencies should have policies to follow for such situations.

Woman's Home

Once inside the woman's home, the nurse may encounter unsafe situations such as the presence of weapons, abusive behavior, or health hazards. Each potentially hazardous situation must be dealt with according to agency policies and procedures. If abuse or neglect is reasonably suspected, the home care nurse should follow home care agency and state and federal regulations for reporting and documenting the situation. Nurses should maintain their own safety first and act accordingly throughout the visit.

Infection Control

The nurse carries the necessary supplies and equipment to provide nursing care to the woman. Home care bags should contain infection control supplies, such as personal protection equipment; disposable nonsterile, sterile, and utility gloves; disinfectants; disposable CPR masks; gowns; shoe covers; caps; leak-proof and puncture-resistant specimen containers; sharps container; dry hand disinfectants; and leak-proof barriers. Proper infection control techniques should be used in stocking, storing, handling, and transporting this bag. When a procedure is to be performed, the nurse should set up a clean area for necessary supplies. A "dirty" area is designated with a trash bag for the collection of soiled equipment and supplies. Hands are washed before all supplies and equipment for the visit are removed from the bag and placed in a clean area.

The importance of infection control does not diminish because nursing care is provided in the woman's home rather than in a hospital. Women are not likely to become infected because of their home environment, but the nurse may become exposed to an infectious disease.

The CDC has recommended Standard Precautions guidelines for the protection of health care workers from bloodborne pathogens. These guidelines recommend that Standard Precautions be used whenever a treatment is performed because it is difficult to determine which clients have a communicable disease.

Handwashing remains the single most important infection-control procedure, and the caregiver is in a position to educate about the importance of this practice in preventing disease. Hands should be washed before and after each client contact. Wearing gloves does not eliminate the necessity of handwashing. If running water or clean facilities are unavailable, the hands can be cleaned with a self-drying antiseptic solution.

Using gloves reduces the incidence of exposure to bloodborne pathogens. Gloves should be selected according to the nursing activity to be performed. Nonsterile latex or vinyl gloves should be worn with each procedure that incurs potential contact with bodily substances (e.g., performing venipunctures, heel sticks on the newborn, and perineal care). Sterile gloves should be worn for clinical procedures requiring sterile technique, such as insertion of peripherally inserted central lines and certain dressing changes. General-purpose utility gloves should be used for housekeeping activities, such as cleaning equipment or spills. Nonsterile and sterile gloves should be discarded after each use in a leak-resistant waste receptacle. Utility gloves can be disinfected and reused.

Disposable personal protection equipment should be removed after each use and discarded in a plastic trash container. Safety glasses and goggles can be cleaned with soap and water after each use.

Whenever specimens are collected, Standard Precautions should be used. Any specimen of bodily fluids should be placed in a leak-proof bag and secured in a puncture-proof container. The outside of the container must be washed off, if it was soiled, before transporting it. Specimens should be labeled with the woman's name and additional identifying information according to the home health care agency or laboratory policies. If specimens are being transported, they should be placed in a container on a flat surface in the vehicle. An insulated container may be used to keep specimens cool in transit. The nurse should be aware of the time sensitivity for certain types of specimens and laboratory procedures.

Sharps containers are puncture-proof and leak-proof containers labeled with a biohazard sign on the outside and should be used to collect needles and sharp objects. Women are instructed to fill containers between two thirds and three fourths full to prevent spillage of their contents. As part of the client teaching process, information about storage and handling is covered by the home care nurse. When the container reaches its maximal capacity, it should be returned to the home health care agency and replaced. Medical waste such as urine and secretions can be discarded through the sewer or septic system.

Contaminated dressings and disposable supplies should be placed in a leak-proof plastic bag and securely fastened for disposal at the woman's home. The woman should be instructed regarding the proper disposal of medical waste in the home. Agency policies and procedures and local waste management ordinances should be consulted before the woman is instructed.

SAFETY ALERT

In caring for the home care client, Occupational Safety and Health Administration (OSHA) guidelines should be followed. The use of strict handwashing techniques, personal protective equipment (PPE), and proper equipment is essential in preventing the spread of disease to the care provider, the woman, and her family.

KEY POINTS

- Contemporary American society recognizes and accepts a variety of family forms.
- The family is a social network that acts as an important support system for its members.
- Family theories provide nurses with useful guidelines for understanding family function.
- Family socioeconomics, response to stress, and culture are key factors influencing family health.
- The reproductive beliefs and practices of a culture are embedded in its economic, religious, kinship, and political structures.
- To provide quality care to women in their childbearing years and beyond, nurses should be aware of the cultural beliefs and practices important to both themselves and individual families.
- Most changes aimed at improving community health involve partnerships among community residents and health workers.
- Methods of collecting data useful to the nurse working in the community include walking surveys, analysis of existing data, informant interviews, and participant observation.
- Vulnerable populations are groups who are at higher risk for developing physical, mental, or social health problems.
- Perinatal home care is a unique nursing practice that incorporates knowledge from community health nursing, acute care nursing, family therapy, health promotion, and client education.
- Perinatal home care can be provided for women and infants throughout the perinatal period, beginning before conception and ending in the postpartum period.
- Telephonic nurse advice lines, telephonic nursing assessments, and warm lines are low-cost health care services that facilitate continuous client education, support, and health care decision making, even though health care is delivered in multiple sites.
- Communication protocols among members of the home health care team are critical to diminish fragmentation and duplication of health care services.

Audio Chapter Summaries Access an audio summary of these Key Points on evolve

REFERENCES

Agency for Healthcare Research and Quality (AHRQ). (2008). *National Healthcare Disparities Report, 2008.* Available at www.qualitytools.ahrq.gov/disparitiesreport/browse/browse.aspx?id=32232009. Accessed December 6, 2009.

Agency for Healthcare Research and Quality (AHRQ). (May, 2005). *Women's health care in the United States: Selected findings from the 2004 National Healthcare Quality and Disparities Reports.* Fact sheet. AHRQ Publication No. 05-P021. Rockville, MD. Available from www.ahrq.gov/qual/nhqrwomen/nhqrwomen.htm. Accessed July 29, 2010.

Allen, F. (1997). Comparative theories of the expanded role in nursing and implications for nursing practice. *Nursing Papers, 9*(2), 38–45.

American Academy of Nursing. (1992). AAN expert panel report: Culturally competent health care. *Nursing Outlook, 40*(6), 277–283.

American College of Obstetricians and Gynecologists (ACOG). (2005). Health care for homeless women. ACOG Committee Opinion No. 312. *Obstetrics and Gynecology, 106*(2), 429–434.

Association of Women's Health, Obstetric, and Neonatal Nurses (AWHONN). (2009). *Standards for professional nursing practice in the care of women and newborns* (7th ed.). Washington, DC: Author.

Becker, M. (1974). The health belief model and sick role behavior. *Health Education Monographs, 2,* 409–419.

Bloom, K., Bednarzyk, M., Devitt, D., Renault, R., Teaman, V., & VanLoock, D. (2004). Barriers to prenatal care for homeless pregnant women. *Journal of Obstetric, Gynecologic and Neonatal Nursing, 33*(4), 428–435.

Boss, P. (1996). *Family stress management* (2nd ed.). Newbury Park, CA: Sage.

Bronfenbrenner, U. (1979). *The ecology of human development.* Cambridge, MA: Harvard University Press.

Bronfenbrenner, U. (1989). Ecological systems theory. In R. Vasta (Ed.), *Annals of child development* (vol. 6). Greenwich, CT: JAI.

Cameron, P. (2004). Number of homosexual parents living with their children. *Psychological Reports, 94*(1), 179–188.

Carter, B., & McGoldrick, M. (1999). *The expanded family life cycle: Individual, family, and social perspectives* (3rd ed.). Boston: Allyn & Bacon.

Centers for Disease Control and Prevention (CDC). 2007. Office of Minority Health & Health Disparities (OMHD). Disease burden and risk factors. Available at www.cdc.gov/omhd/AMH/dbrf.htm. Accessed July 28, 2010.

Centers for Disease Control and Prevention (CDC). (2009a). National Center for Health Statistics. *Faststats.* Available at www.cdc.gov/nchs/fastats/prenatal.htm. Accessed May 13, 2010.

Centers for Disease Control and Prevention (CDC). (2009b). National Center for Health Statistics. *Quickstats.* Available at www.cdc.gov/mmwr/preview/mmwrhtml/mm5842a7.htm. Accessed May 13, 2010.

Clemen-Stone, S. (2002). Community assessment and diagnosis. In S. Clemen-Stone, S. McGuire, & D. Eigsti (Eds.), *Comprehensive community health nursing: Family, aggregate, and community practice* (6th ed.). St. Louis: Mosby.

Cooper, M., Grywalski, M., Lamp, J., Newhouse, L., & Studlien, R. (2007). Enhancing cultural competence: A model for nurses. *Nursing for Women's Health, 11*(2), 148–159.

Cottrell, R., Girvan, J., & McKenzie, J. (2006). *Health promotion and education* (3rd ed.). San Francisco: Pearson Benjamin Cummings.

Eggenberger, S., Grassley, J., & Restrepo, E. (July 19, 2006). Culturally competent nursing care for families: Listening to the voices of Mexican-American women. *The Online Journal of Issues in Nursing, 11*(3), 7.

Feldman, S., Vallejos, Q., Quandt, S., Fleischer, A., Schulz, M., Verma, A., et al. (2009). Health care utilization among migrant Latino farmworkers: The case of skin disease. *Journal of Rural Health, 25*(1), 98–103.

Friedman, M. (1998). *Family nursing theory and assessment* (4th ed.). New York: Appleton & Lange.

Friedman, M., Bowden, V., & Jones, E. (2003). *Family nursing: Research, theory, and practice.* Upper Saddle River, NJ: Prentice-Hall.

Giger, J., & Davidhizar, R. (2009). *Transcultural nursing: Assessment and intervention* (5th ed.). St. Louis: Mosby.

Greenfeld, D. (2005). Reproduction in same sex couples: Quality of parenting and child development. *Current Opinion in Obstetrics and Gynecology, 17*(3), 309–312.

Henning, G., Graybill, M., & George, J. (2008). Reason for visit: Is migrant health care that different? *Journal of Rural Health, 24*(2), 219–220.

Institute of Medicine (IOM). (2002). *Unequal treatment: Confronting racial and ethnic disparities in health care.* Washington, DC: National Academies Press.

Jacobs, E., Karavolos, K., Rathouz, P., Ferris, T., & Powell, L. (2005). Limited English proficiency and breast and cervical cancer screening in a multiethnic population. *American Journal of Public Health, 95*(8), 1410–1416.

Janz, N., & Becker, M. (1984). The health belief model: A decade later. *Health Education Quarterly, 11*(1), 1–47.

Johnson, B., Abraham, M., Conway, J., Simmons, L., Edgman-Levitan, S., Sodomka, P., et al. (2008). Partnering with patients and families to design a patient- and family-centered health care system: Recommendations and promising practices. *American Journal of Medical Quality, 23*(4), 279–286.

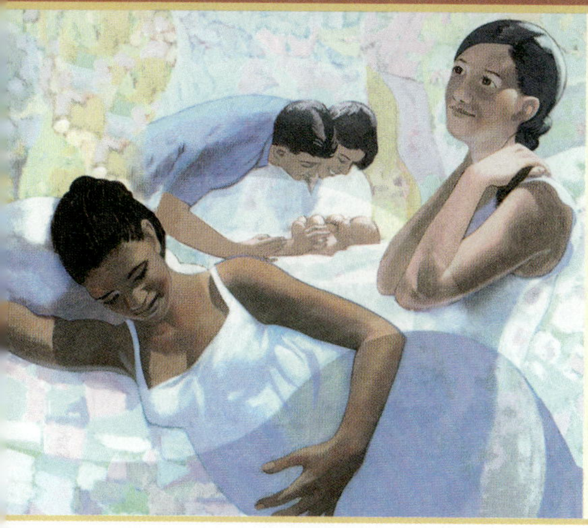

CHAPTER

3

Clinical Genetics

Marcia Van Riper

evolve WEBSITE

http://evolve.elsevier.com/Lowdermilk/MWHC/

Audio Glossary
Audio Key Points
Critical Thinking Exercise
  Genetic Counseling
NCLEX Review Questions
Nursing Care Plan
  The Family Living with a Child with Down Syndrome

LEARNING OBJECTIVES

- Explore how recent advances in genetics have changed the field of health care.
- Discuss the essential competencies in genetics and genomics for all nurses.
- Describe expanded roles for nurses in genetics and genetic counseling.
- Discuss key findings of the Human Genome Project.
- Describe the different types of genetic testing.
- Identify genetic disorders commonly tested for in maternity and women's health nursing.
- Explore the possible benefits and risks of pharmacogenomics.
- Discuss the current status of gene therapy.
- Examine the ethical, legal, and social implications of the Human Genome Project.
- Explain the key concepts of basic human genetics.
- Discuss the education and counseling needs of individuals and families who undergo genetic testing.
- Explore the availability of genetic testing for individuals and families from diverse backgrounds.
- Describe the role of genomics in cancer.
- Identify genetics resources for nurses and other health care professionals.

Recent advances in molecular biology and genomics have revolutionized the field of health care by providing the tools needed to determine the hereditary component of many diseases, as well as improve our ability to predict susceptibility to disease, onset and progression of disease, and response to medications (Feero, Guttmacher, & Collins, 2008; Ginsburg & Willard, 2009, Guttmacher, McGuire, Ponder, & Stefansson, 2010). This increase in genetic knowledge has resulted in a gradual shift from genetics to genomics. **Genetics** is the study of individual genes and their effect on relatively rare single gene disorders, whereas **genomics** is the study of all the genes in the human genome together, including their interactions with each other, the environment, and the influence of other psychosocial factors and cultural factors. **Genes** are basic physical units of inheritance that are passed from parents to offspring and contain the information needed to specify traits. The **genome** is the entire set of genetic instructions found in each cell. For these and other definitions of genetic terms, visit the *Talking Glossary of Genetic Terms* (www.genome.gov/Glossary).

With growing public interest in personalized genomic information (information about much or all of a person's genome), increasing development of practice guidelines, mounting commercial pressures, and ever-increasing opportunities for individuals, families, and communities to participate in the direction and design of their genomic health care, genetic services are rapidly becoming an integral part of routine health care (Guttmacher et al., 2010). Moreover, many individuals and families have participated in direct-to-consumer genetic testing (testing marketed directly to consumers through television, print advertisements, and websites for companies such as DNA Direct [www.dnadirect.com/web], 23 and Me [www.23andme.com], and DeCODEme [www.decodeme.com]). Although much of the information provided by direct-to-consumer testing companies is recreational (ancestry information, information about type of ear wax, and bitter taste perception), some of it is health related and could be interpreted as diagnosis (Evans & Green, 2009). Because of this, direct-to-consumer testing that is provided without the involvement of competent health care professionals may be not only unhelpful but also harmful (Guttmacher et al.; McGuire & Burke, 2010).

Due to their frontline position in the health care system and their long-standing history of providing holistic family-centered care, nurses are likely to be among the first health care professionals to whom individuals and families turn with questions about genetic risk and susceptibility and to seek guidance regarding the complexities of genetic testing and interpretation. Nowhere is this more apparent than in the area of maternity and women's health care (Dolan, Biermann, & Damus, 2007). A growing number of maternity and women's health nurses are offering and interpreting genetic tests. Although most of these tests are being used to determine a client's risk of having a child affected by a genetic condition such as Down syndrome, cystic fibrosis (CF), or sickle cell disease, the number of tests being used to determine the presence of, or susceptibility to, adult-onset disorders (e.g., hereditary colorectal cancer, hereditary breast and ovarian cancer, and Huntington's disease [HD]) continues to rise. Additionally, nurses working in maternity and women's health are caring for an increasing number of individuals and families who are dealing with complex ethical, legal, and social issues associated with genetic testing and the experience of living with someone who has a genetic condition (Hamilton, 2009; Sparbel & Williams, 2009; Van Riper, 2007; Van Riper & Gallo, 2006).

NURSING EXPERTISE IN GENETICS AND GENOMICS

Essential Competencies in Genetics and Genomics for All Nurses

Nearly 50 organizations, including the Association of Women's Health, Obstetric and Neonatal Nurses and the National Association of Neonatal Nurses, have endorsed the Essential Nursing Competencies and Curriculum Guidelines for Genetics and Genomics. The guidelines were developed by an independent panel of nurse leaders from clinical, research, and academic settings and published by the American Nurses Association and the National Human Genome Research Institute (NHGRI) of the National Institutes of Health (Jenkins & Calzone, 2007). According to the guidelines, all nurses need to have minimal competencies in genetics and genomics regardless of their academic preparation, practice setting, or specialty. Some of the competencies most relevant to nurses in the area of maternity and woman's health include:

- Constructs a pedigree from collected family history information using standardized symbols and terminology.
- Develops a nursing care plan that incorporates genetic and genomic assessment information.
- Recognizes when one's own attitudes and values related to genetics and genomic science may affect care provided to clients.
- Provides clients with credible, accurate, appropriate, and current genetic and genomic information, resources, services, and/or technologies that facilitate decision making.
- Demonstrates in practice the importance of tailoring genetic and genomic information and services to clients based on their culture, religion, knowledge level, literacy, and preferred language.
- Assesses client's knowledge, perceptions, and responses to genetic and genomic information.
- Facilitates referrals for specialized genetic and genomic services for clients as needed.

Expanded Roles for Maternity and Women's Health Nurses

- Expanded roles for nurses with expertise in genetics and genomics are developing in many areas of maternity and women's health nursing. These areas include but are not limited to:
  - Prenatal screening and testing (Dolan et al., 2007; Hamilton, 2009; Sparbel & Williams, 2009)
  - Neonatal genetic screening and testing (Kenner, Lewis, Pressler, & Little, 2008)
  - Palliative care for infants with life-threatening genetic conditions and their families (Shaw, 2008; Wirth, 2009)
  - The identification and care of individuals with genetic conditions and their families (Gallo, Knafl, & Angst, 2009; Lynch, Snyder, & Lynch, 2009; Ranweiler, 2009; Schiefelbein & Cheeseman, 2009; Snyder, Lynch, & Lynch, 2009; Van Riper, 2007)
  - The care of women with genetic conditions who require specialized care during pregnancy, such as women with congenital heart disease (Khairy, Ouyang, Fernandes, Lee-Parritz, Economy, & Landzberg, 2006), cystic fibrosis (McMullen, Pasta, Frederick, Konstan, Morgan, Schechter, et al., 2006), and Factor V Leiden (Horne & McCloskey, 2006; Weinstein, 2009)

The Oncology Nursing Society (ONS) (www.ons.org) has taken an active role in providing oncology nurses with the education and resources they need to integrate genetics and genomics into all phases of care for individuals and families affected by chance. ONS offers online updates, regional classes, and position statements related to genetics and genomics (Hamilton, 2009).

HUMAN GENOME PROJECT AND IMPLICATIONS FOR CLINICAL PRACTICE

Two key findings from the Human Genome Project were that (1) all human beings are 99.9% identical at the deoxyribonucleic acid (DNA) level, and (2) there are probably about 20,500 genes in the human genome. The finding that human beings are 99.9% identical at the DNA level should help discourage the use of science as a justification for drawing biologically precise racial boundaries around certain groups of people (Collins, 2004). Originally scientists had estimated that there were 50,000 to 140,000 genes in the human genome. It had been assumed that the main reason that humans are more evolved and more highly sophisticated than other species is that they have more genes. A new explanation for human complexity, given the relatively small number of genes, is that humans are more efficient with their genes. Humans are able to do much more with their genes than are other species. Instead of producing only one protein per gene, most human genes produce at least three proteins.

Importance of Family History

Completion of the Human Genome Project and the resultant identification of the inherited causes for many diseases has created a renewed interest in family history (Clarke, 2009; De Sevo, 2009; Dolan et al., 2007; Dolan & Moore, 2007; Feero et al., 2008; Ginsburg & Willard, 2009; Hinton, 2008; Soloman, Jack, & Feero, 2008; Wattendorf & Hadley, 2005). Although it is easy to be impressed by the almost 1900 genetic tests currently available, family history will most likely continue to be the single most cost-effective piece of genetic information. Rich and colleagues (2004) described family history as the most important tool for diagnosis and risk assessment in health care genetics and a critical tool in the use of predictive testing in primary care. Solomon and colleagues argued that a complete three-generation family history that includes ethnicity information concerning both sides of family is the best genetic "test" applicable to preconception care. When nurses and other clinicians conduct a family history, they can gain not only valuable information about the structure of the family and diseases that affect various individuals in the family, but also a rich understanding of family relationships, social context, occupations, lifestyle, and health habits. In addition, the process of collecting this information often facilitates the development of a relationship between the client/family and the clinician. In 2004, the U.S. Department of Health and Human Services launched the Family History Initiative by designating Thanksgiving Day as National Family History Day. The U.S. Surgeon General encouraged families to use their family gatherings as a time to talk about and collect important family health history. A number of family history tools are available free of charge online. One of the most widely used is the *My Family Health Portrait* (https://familyhistory.hhs.gov). Another recently developed tool is the family health history tool, *Does it run in the family?* that was developed by the Genetic Alliance (www.doesitruninthefamily.org).

Gene Identification and Testing

Initial efforts to sequence and analyze the human genome have proven invaluable in the identification of genes involved in disease and in the development of genetic tests. Hundreds of genes involved in diseases such as breast cancer, colorectal cancer, Alzheimer's disease, and CF have been identified. The number of commercially available genetic tests continues to increase and can be found on GeneTests, a publicly funded genetics information resource for clinicians (www.ncbi.nlm.nih.gov/sites/GeneTests/?db=GeneTests).

Genetic testing involves the analysis of human DNA, **ribonucleic acid (RNA), chromosomes** (threadlike packages of genes and other DNA in the nucleus of a cell), or proteins to detect abnormalities related to an inherited condition. Genetic tests can be used to examine directly the DNA and RNA that make up a gene (direct or molecular testing), look at markers that are coinherited with a gene that causes a genetic condition (linkage analysis), examine the protein products of genes (biochemical testing), or examine chromosomes (cytogenetic testing). Cytogenetic analysis of malignant tissue has become a mainstay of oncology.

Most of the genetic tests now offered in clinical practice are tests for single-gene disorders in clients with clinical symptoms or who have a family history of a genetic disease. Some of these genetic tests are prenatal tests or tests used to identify the genetic status of a pregnancy at risk for a genetic condition. Current prenatal testing options include maternal serum screening (a blood test used to see if a pregnant woman is at increased risk for carrying a fetus with a neural tube defect or chromosomal abnormalities such as Down syndrome, trisomy 18 and trisomy 13), **fetal ultrasound** or **sonogram** (an imaging technique using high-frequency sound waves to produce images of the fetus inside the uterus), and invasive procedures (chorionic villus sampling and amniocentesis) (see Chapter 26 for discussion of these tests). Other tests are carrier screening tests used to identify individuals who have a gene mutation for a genetic condition but do not show symptoms of the condition because it is an autosomal recessive condition (e.g., CF, sickle cell disease, and Tay-Sachs disease). Another type of genetic testing is **predictive testing,** which is used to clarify the genetic status of asymptomatic family members. The two types of predictive testing are presymptomatic and predispositional. Mutation analysis for HD, a neurodegenerative disorder, is an example of **presymptomatic testing.** If the gene mutation for HD is present, symptoms of HD are certain to appear if the individual lives long enough. Testing for a BRCA1 gene mutation to determine breast cancer susceptibility is an example of predispositional testing. **Predispositional testing** differs from presymptomatic testing in that a positive result (indicating that a BRCA1 mutation is present) does not indicate a 100% risk of developing the condition (breast cancer).

In addition to using genetic tests to test for single-gene disorders in clients with clinical symptoms or who have a family history of a genetic disease, genetic tests are being used for population-based screening. For example, newborn screening for phenylketonuria (PKU) and other inborn errors of metabolism (IEMs) has been going on in the United States and many other countries for decades (Guttmacher et al., 2010; Kenner et al., 2008). Initially, state-mandated newborn screening in the United States was concerned with only a few conditions. With the advent of tandem mass spectrometry, the number of conditions tested for during newborn screening grew rapidly. Currently, most states use blood spots collected from newborns to test for at least 30 different metabolic and genetic diseases. The four conditions most commonly tested for are PKU, congenital hypothyroidism, galactosemia, and sickle cell disease. A complete list of conditions tested for in each state is available on the National Newborn Screening and Genetics Resource website.

Another type of population-based screening is carrier screening for single-gene disorders such as CF, sickle cell disease, and Tay-Sachs disease either preconceptually or prenatally. In 2001, the American College of Obstetricians and Gynecologists and the American College of Medical Genetics (ACOG & ACMG) began recommending that clinicians offer carrier screening for CF to individuals with a family history of CF, reproductive partners of individuals who have CF, and couples in whom one or both partners are Caucasian and are planning a pregnancy or seeking prenatal care (ACOG & ACMG, 2001). One outcome of this broader CF carrier screening is that more and more individuals are being informed they have a CF mutation. Unfortunately, the correlation between **genotype** (an individual's collection of genes) and **phenotype** (an individual's observable traits) is poor for many of the more than 1400 CF mutations identified to date. That is, whereas some CF mutations are associated with significant health problems (poor growth, greasy stools, and chronic respiratory problems) others are not. Because of this, the significance of many CF mutations is uncertain. As a result, nurses and other health care professionals are increasingly being asked to communicate results with uncertain significance to individuals and families during the preconception and prenatal period (Dolan et al., 2007). In 2008, the NHGRI held a workshop to discuss lessons learned and new opportunities for population-based carrier screening (www.genome.gov/27026048). One of the main conclusions from this workshop was that a more coherent and systematic approach is needed for the introduction of new tests into population-based screening programs.

Pharmacogenomics

One of the most promising clinical applications of the Human Genome Project has been pharmacogenomic testing (the use of genetic information to guide a client's drug therapy) (Ginsburg & Willard, 2009). Associations between genetic variation and drug effect have been observed for a number of commonly used drugs, including warfarin, an anticoagulant commonly used to reduce the risk of thromboembolic events in clients with a history of deep vein thrombosis, pulmonary embolism, myocardial infarction, or atrial fibrillation (Lanfear & McCleod, 2007; Meckley, Gudgeon, Anderson, Williams, & Veenstra, 2010). Warfarin is a drug with a narrow therapeutic index; it can result in serious bleeding with supratherapeutic doses and thromboembolic events with subtherapeutic doses). Because of this and the fact that there is a great deal of inter- and intraclient dose variation, warfarin is one of the most common causes of serious adverse drug reactions. Fortunately there is mounting evidence that genotype-guided warfarin dosing may not only help reduce the serious adverse drug reactions commonly associated with warfarin, but increase dosing accuracy, shorten the time to dose stabilization, and help identify individuals who may require more frequent monitoring. In August 2007, the U.S. Food and Drug Administration (FDA) approved updated labeling for warfarin. The updated labeling acknowledges that individuals with variations in their CYP2C9 and VKORC1 genes may require a lower initial dose of warfarin. However, there are not enough clinical data yet to recommend that this type of testing be mandatory.

Pharmacogenomic testing can also be used to target therapies. Trastuzumab (Herceptin), a monoclonal antibody that specifically targets HER2/neu overexpressing breast tumors, is an example of a drug for which an obligatory genetic test has been developed (Ginsburg & Willard, 2009). The purpose of this obligatory genetic test is to identify the subset of women with breast cancer who overexpress HER2/neu. Women who overexpress HER2/neu are most likely the only breast cancer clients who will benefit from taking trastuzumab (www.herceptin.com/index.jsp).

Gene Therapy

In the early 1990s, a great deal of optimism was felt about the possibility of using **gene therapy** to correct a long list of inherited diseases. Generally, gene therapy involves inserting a healthy copy of the defective gene into the **somatic cells** (any cell of the body except sperm and egg cells) of the affected individual. Although the early optimism about gene therapy was probably never fully justified, gene therapy has now moved from preclinical to clinical studies for many diseases ranging from hemophilia and other single gene disorders to complex disorders such as cancer, human immunodeficiency virus, and cardiovascular disorders (Gillet, Macadangdang, Fathke, Gottesman, & Kimchi-Sarfaty, 2009). Early hype, failures, and tragic events, such as the death of Jessie Gelsinger (an 18-year-old male with an X-linked genetic liver disease who was the first person publicly identified as having died in a gene therapy clinical trial) have now largely been replaced by stepwise progress in carefully developed, scientifically precise clinical trails (Gillet et al.; Kohn & Candotti, 2009). Major challenges to gene therapy include figuring out how to target the right gene to the right location in the right cells, expressing the transferred gene at the right time, and minimizing adverse reactions.

Ethical, Legal, and Social Implications

Before the beginning of the Human Genome Project, widespread concern about misuse of the information gained through genetics research resulted in 5% of the Human Genome Project budget being designated for the study of the **ethical, legal, and social implications (ELSIs)** of human genome research. Two large ELSI programs were created to identify, analyze, and address the ELSIs of human genome research at the same time that the basic science issues were being studied. During the past decade, issues of high priority for these programs have been privacy and fairness in the use and interpretation of genetic information; clinical integration of new genetics technologies; issues surrounding genetics research, such as possible discrimination and stigmatization; and education for professionals and the general public about genetics, genetics health care, and ELSI of human genome research. Both ELSI programs have excellent websites that include large amounts of educational information, as well as links to other informative sites (www.genome.gov/10001618; www.ornl.gov/sci/techresources/Human_Genome/elsi/elsi.shtml).

The major risk associated with genetic testing concerns what happens with the information gained through testing: it may result in increased anxiety and altered family relationships; it may be difficult to keep confidential; and it may result in discrimination and stigmatization. More important, there is still a large gap between the ability to test for a genetic condition and the ability to treat the same condition. In addition, informed consent is difficult to ensure when some of the outcomes, benefits, and risks of genetic testing remain unknown. Also many of the tests being used are as yet imperfect—few have a 100% detection rate. Individuals and families who receive false-positive results (the test results falsely indicate that a person or fetus is affected by a genetic condition) may terminate an unaffected pregnancy or undergo unwarranted extreme measures such as bilateral prophylactic mastectomy. Individuals and families who receive false-negative results (the test results indicate that a person or fetus is not affected by a genetic condition when in fact the person or fetus is affected) may fail to follow surveillance strategies designed to improve their health outcomes because they have been falsely reassured that they are not at increased risk for a specific condition.

Factors Influencing the Decision to Undergo Genetic Testing

The decision to undergo genetic testing is seldom autonomous and based solely on the needs and preferences of the individual being tested. Instead, it is often a decision based on feelings of responsibility and commitment to others (Van Riper, 2005; Van Riper & McKinnon, 2004). For example, a woman who is receiving treatment for breast cancer may undergo BRCA1/BRCA2 mutation testing not because she wants to find out if she carries a BRCA1 or BRCA2 mutation, but because her two unaffected sisters have asked her to be tested, and she feels a sense of responsibility and commitment to them. A female airline pilot with a family history of HD, who has no desire to find out if she has the gene mutation associated with HD, may undergo mutation analysis for HD because she feels she has an obligation to her family, her employer, and the people who fly with her.

Decisions about genetic testing are shaped, and in many instances constrained, by factors such as social norms, where care is received, and socioeconomic status. Most pregnant women in the United States now have at least one ultrasound examination, many undergo some type of multiple-marker screening, and a growing number undergo other types of prenatal testing. The range of prenatal testing options available to a pregnant woman and her family may vary significantly, based on where the woman receives prenatal care and her socioeconomic status. Certain types of prenatal testing may not be available in smaller communities and rural settings (e.g., chorionic villus sampling and fluorescent in situ hybridization [FISH] analysis). In addition, certain types of genetic testing may not be offered in conservative medical communities (e.g., preimplantation diagnosis). Some types of genetic testing are expensive and typically not covered by health insurance. Because of this, these tests may be available only to a relatively small number of individuals and families: those who can afford to pay for them.

Cultural and ethnic differences also have a significant effect on decisions about genetic testing. When prenatal diagnosis was first introduced, the principal constituency was a self-selected group of Caucasian, well-informed, middle- to upper-class women. Today the widespread use of genetic testing has introduced prenatal testing to new groups of women, women who had not previously considered genetics services. The fact that many of the women undergoing prenatal testing may not share mainstream U.S. views about the role of medicine and prenatal care, the meaning of disability, or how to respond to scientific risks and uncertainties further amplifies the complexity of ethical issues associated with prenatal testing.

The genetic testing experience raises fundamental questions about the mutual obligations of kin. Are individuals morally obligated to alert extended family members about inherited health risks? Conversely, do extended family members have a moral obligation to participate in research designed to determine genetic risk when unwanted information about them may be generated in the process? Another important question that must be considered is "Whose gene is it?" This question is likely to stimulate a great deal of debate, especially in the area of preimplantation genetic testing.

CLINICAL GENETICS

Genetic Transmission

Human development is a complicated process that depends on the systematic unraveling of instructions found in the genetic material of the egg and the sperm. Development from conception to birth of a normal, healthy baby occurs without incident in most cases; occasionally, however, some anomaly in the genetic code of the embryo creates a birth defect or disorder.

Genes and Chromosomes

The hereditary material carried in the nucleus of each of the somatic cells determines an individual's characteristics. This material, called **deoxyribonucleic acid (DNA),** forms threadlike strands known as chromosomes. Each chromosome is composed of the many smaller segments of DNA referred to as genes. Genes, or combinations of genes, contain coded information that determines an individual's unique characteristics. The code is found in the specific linear order of the molecules that combine to form the strands of DNA. Genes control both the types of proteins that are made and the rate at which they are produced. Genes never act in isolation; they always interact with other genes and the environment.

All normal human somatic cells contain 46 chromosomes arranged as 23 pairs of homologous (matched) chromosomes; one chromosome of each pair is inherited from each parent. There are 22 pairs of **autosomes** that control most traits in the body, and one pair of **sex chromosomes.** Whereas the Y chromosome is primarily concerned with sex determination, the X chromosome contains genes that are involved in much more than sex determination. The larger female chromosome is called the X; the smaller male chromosome is the Y. Generally the presence of a Y chromosome causes an embryo to develop as a male; in the absence of a Y chromosome, the individual develops as a female. Thus in a normal female, the homologous pair of sex chromosomes are XX, and in a normal male, the homologous pair are XY.

Homologous chromosomes (except the X and Y chromosomes in males) have the same number and arrangement of genes. In other words, if one chromosome has a gene for hair color, its partner chromosome also will have a gene for hair color, and these hair-color genes will have the same **loci** or be located in the same place on the two chromosomes. Although both genes code for hair color, they may not code for the *same* hair color. Genes at corresponding loci on homologous chromosomes that code for different forms or variations of the same trait are called **alleles.** An individual having two copies of the same allele for a given trait is said to be **homozygous** for that trait; with two different alleles, the person is **heterozygous** for the trait.

The term **genotype** typically is used to refer to the genetic makeup of an individual when discussing a specific gene pair, but at times genotype is used to refer to an individual's entire genetic makeup or all the genes that the individual can pass on to future generations. **Phenotype** refers to the observable expression of an individual's genotype, such as physical features, a biochemical or molecular trait, and even a psychologic trait. A trait or disorder is considered **dominant** if it is expressed or phenotypically apparent when only one copy of an

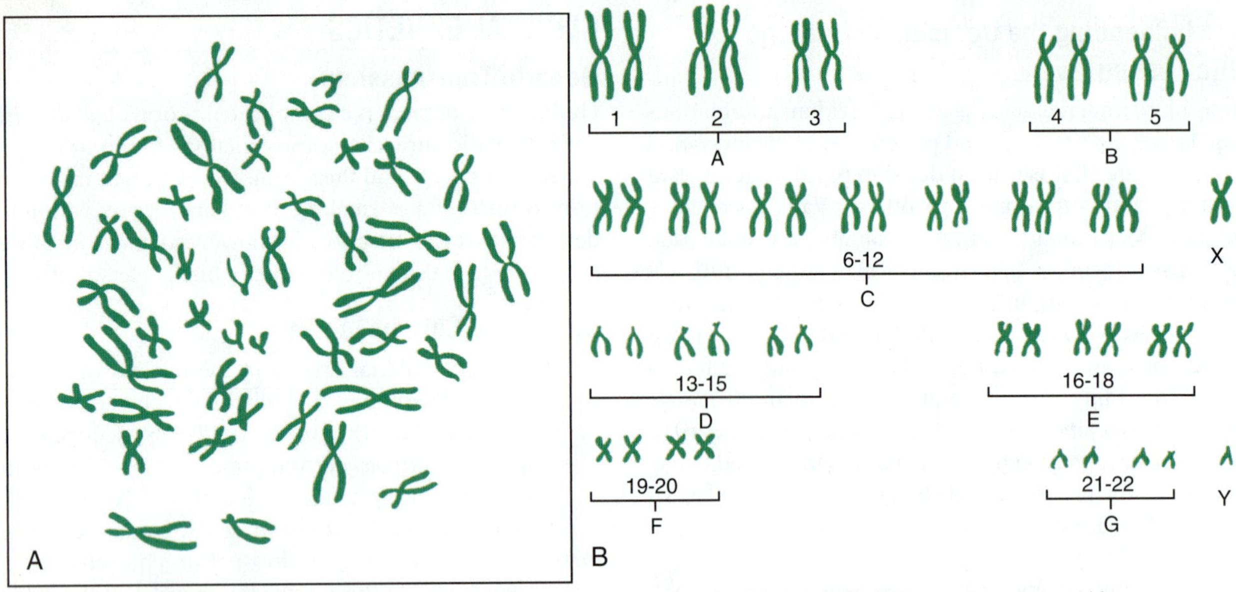

FIG. 3-1 Chromosomes during cell division. **A,** Example of photomicrograph. **B,** Chromosomes arranged in karyotype; female and male sex-determining chromosomes.

allele associated with the trait is present. It is considered recessive if it is expressed only when two copies of the alleles associated with the trait are present.

As more is learned about genetics and genomics, the concepts of dominance and recessivity have become more complex, especially in X-linked disorders. For example, traits considered to be recessive may be expressed even when only one copy of a gene located on the X chromosome is present. This occurs frequently in males because males have only one X chromosome; thus they have only one copy of the gene located on the X chromosome. Whichever gene is present on the one X chromosome determines which trait is expressed. Females, conversely, have two X chromosomes, so they have two copies of the genes located on the X chromosome. However, in any female somatic cell, only one X chromosome is functioning (otherwise, there would be inequality in gene dosage between males and females). This process, known as X-inactivation or the Lyon hypothesis, is generally a random occurrence. That is, there is a fifty-fifty chance as to whether the maternal X or the paternal X is inactivated. Occasionally the percentage of cells that have the X with an abnormal or mutant gene is very high. This helps explain why hemophilia, an X-linked recessive disorder, can clinically manifest itself in a female known to be a heterozygous carrier (a female who has only one copy of the gene mutation). It also helps explain why traditional methods of carrier detection are less effective for X-linked recessive disorders; the possible range for enzyme activity values can vary greatly, depending on which X chromosome is inactivated.

Chromosomal Abnormalities

Chromosomal abnormalities are a major cause of reproductive loss, congenital problems, and gynecologic disorders; the incidence is approximately 0.6% in newborns, 6% in stillbirths, and 60% in spontaneous abortions (Martin, 2008). Errors resulting in chromosomal abnormalities can occur during mitosis (cell division occurring in somatic cells that results in two identical daughter cells containing a diploid number of chromosomes) or meiosis (division of a sex cell into two and four haploid cells). These errors can occur in either the autosomes or the sex chromosomes. Even without the presence of obvious structural malformations, small deviations in chromosomes can cause problems in fetal development.

The pictorial analysis of the number, form, and size of an individual's chromosomes is known as a karyotype. Cells from any nucleated, replicating body tissue (not red blood cells, nerves, or muscles) can be used. The most commonly used tissues are white blood cells and fetal cells in amniotic fluid. The cells are grown in a culture and arrested when they are in metaphase (during metaphase, the chromosomes are condensed and visible with a light microscope), and then the cells are dropped onto a slide. This breaks the cell membranes and spreads the chromosomes, making them easier to visualize. Next the cells are stained with special stains (e.g., Giemsa stain) that create striping or "banding" patterns. These patterns aid in the analysis because they are consistent from person to person. Once the chromosome spreads are photographed or scanned by a computer, they are cut out and arranged in a specific numeric order according to their length and shape. The chromosomes are numbered from largest to smallest, 1 to 22, and the sex chromosomes are designated by the letter X or Y. Each chromosome is divided into two "arms" designated by p (short arm) and q (long arm). A female karyotype is designated as 46, XX and a male karyotype is designated as 46, XY. Figure 3-1 illustrates the chromosomes in a body cell.

Autosomal Abnormalities

Autosomal abnormalities involve differences in the number or structure of autosome chromosomes (pairs 1 through 22). They result from unequal distribution of genetic material during gamete (egg and sperm) formation.

Abnormalities of Chromosome Number. A euploid cell is a cell with the correct or normal number of chromosomes within the cell. Since most gametes are haploid (1N, 23 chromosomes) and most somatic cells are diploid (2N, 46 chromosomes), they are both considered euploid cells. Deviations from the correct number of chromosomes per cell can be one of two types: (1) **polyploidy,** in which the deviation is an exact multiple of the **haploid** number of chromosomes or one chromosome set (23 chromosomes); or (2) **aneuploidy,** in which the numerical deviation is not an exact multiple of the haploid set. A **triploid** (3N) cell is an example of a polyploidy. It has 69 chromosomes. A **tetraploid** (4N) cell, also an example of a polyploidy, has 92 chromosomes.

Aneuploidy is the most commonly identified chromosome abnormality in humans and the leading genetic cause of mental retardation. A **monosomy** is the product of the union between a normal gamete and a gamete that is missing a chromosome. Monosomic individuals only have 45 chromosomes in each of their cells. The product of the union of a normal gamete with a gamete containing an extra chromosome is a **trisomy.** The most common autosomal aneuploid conditions involve trisomies. Trisomic individuals have 47 chromosomes in most or all their cells.

The vast majority of trisomies occur during oogenesis (the process by which a premeiotic female germ cell divides into a mature egg) and the incidence of these types of chromosomal errors increases exponentially with advancing maternal age (Hassold & Hunt, 2009; Hunt & Hassold, 2008). Although variation exists among trisomies with regard to the parent and stage of origin of the extra chromosome, most trisomies are maternal meiosis I (MI) errors. This means that most trisomies are caused by **nondisjunction** during the first meiotic division. The first meiotic division involves the segregation of homologous or similar chromosomes. One pair of chromosomes fails to separate. One resulting cell contains both chromosomes, and the other contains none. The fact that most trisomies are maternal MI errors is not that surprising, because maternal MI occurs over a long time span. It is initiated in precursor cells during fetal development, but it is not completed until the time those cells undergo ovulation after menarche.

The most common trisomal abnormality is **Down syndrome (DS).** Approximately one in every 733 newborns has DS and it is estimated that there are more than 400,000 individuals with DS living in the United States (Canfield, Honein, Yuskiv, Xing, Mai, Collins, et al., 2006). Ninety-five percent of individuals with DS have trisomy 21 or an extra chromosome 21 (47, XX +21, female with DS; or 47, XY +21, male with DS). Another type of DS, translocation, occurs when extra chromosome 21 material is present in every cell of the individual but it is attached to another chromosome. In the third type of DS, mosaicism, extra chromosome 21 material is found in some but not all of the cells.

Although the clinical presentation of DS is complex and variable (Ranweiler, 2009), all individuals with DS have some level of mental retardation. Common characteristics seen in individuals with Down syndrome are as follows:

- Oblique palpebral fissures or an upward slant to the eyes
- Epicanthal folds or small skin folds on the inner corners of the eyes
- Small, white, crescent-shaped spots on the irises called Brushfield spots
- A flat facial profile that usually includes a somewhat depressed nasal bridge and a small nose
- Enlargement of the tongue in relationship to size of the mouth

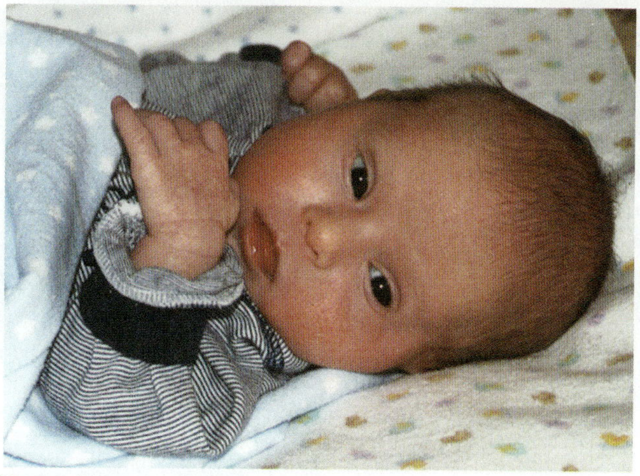

FIG. 3-2 Infant with Down syndrome. Note upward slant to eyes, flat nasal bridge, slightly protruding tongue, and mottled skin. (Courtesy Thomas and Christie Coghill, Clayton, NC.)

- Small ears, which may be abnormally shaped or abnormally rotated
- Short, broad hands with a fifth finger that has one flexion crease instead of two
- A single deep crease across the center of the palm, often referred to as a simian crease
- Excessive space between large and second toe
- Hyperflexibility, an excessive ability to extend the joints
- Muscle hypotonia or low muscle tone

Some individuals with DS have all of these characteristics, but others have only a few. Figure 3-2 is a picture of an infant with DS who has some of the characteristics commonly associated with that syndrome (see Nursing Care Plan).

Congenital abnormalities and diseases found in individuals with DS are the same as those that occur in the general population, but individuals with DS are affected more often and more severely by specific abnormalities and diseases than are typically developing individuals. For example, congenital heart disease occurs in 40% to 50% of individuals with DS, whereas the overall incidence of congenital heart disease in the general populations is around 0.8%. Leukemia occurs in 1 of every 150 children with DS. This is 20 times higher than in the general population. Other health problems commonly seen in individuals with DS include vision and hearing defects, sleep apnea, thyroid disease, atlantoaxial instability, and gastrointestinal abnormalities. Individuals with DS have a higher mortality rate from infectious disease than do individuals who do not have DS (see Chapter 36).

Although the risk of having a child with DS increases with maternal age (incidence is approximately 1 in 1200 for a 25-year-old woman; 1 in 350 for a 35-year-old woman; and 1 in 30 for a 45-year-old woman), children with Down syndrome can be born to mothers of any age (National Down Syndrome Society, 2010). Eighty percent of children with Down syndrome are born to mothers younger than 35 years. The risk of a mother having a second child with Down syndrome is about 1% when the cause of the Down syndrome is trisomy 21.

During the past 30 years fundamental changes have occurred in the care of individuals with DS. These changes, which underscore the importance of the family and emphasize the need for health promotion and health protection activities, have resulted in individuals with DS living longer and enjoying an improved

NURSING CARE PLAN

The Family Living with a Child with Down Syndrome

NURSING DIAGNOSIS

Interrupted family processes related to birth of a neonate with Down syndrome

Expected Outcome

The parents will verbalize accurate information about Down syndrome, including implications for future pregnancies.

Nursing Interventions/*Rationales*

- Assess knowledge base of parents regarding the clinical signs and symptoms of Down syndrome *to correct any misconceptions and establish basis for teaching plan.*
- Provide information throughout the genetic evaluation regarding risk status and clinical signs and symptoms of Down syndrome *to give parents a realistic picture of neonate's defects and assist with decision making for future pregnancies.*
- Use therapeutic communication during discussions with the parents *to provide opportunity for expression of concern.*
- Refer to support groups, social services, or counseling *to assist family with cohesive actions and decision making.*
- Refer to child development specialist *to provide family with realistic expectations regarding cognitive and behavioral differences of child with Down syndrome.*

NURSING DIAGNOSIS

Situational low self-esteem related to diagnosis of Down syndrome as evidenced by parents' statements of guilt and shame

Expected Outcome

The parents will express an increased number of positive statements regarding their neonate with Down syndrome.

Nursing Interventions/*Rationales*

- Assist parents to list strengths and coping strategies that have been helpful in past situations *to use appropriate strategies during this situational crisis.*
- Encourage expression of feelings using therapeutic communication *to provide clarification and emotional support.*
- Clarify and provide information regarding Down syndrome *to decrease feelings of guilt and gradually increase feelings of positive self-esteem.*
- Refer for further counseling as needed *to provide more in-depth and ongoing support.*

NURSING DIAGNOSIS

Risk for impaired parenting related to birth of neonate with Down syndrome

Expected Outcomes

Parents will bond with and provide appropriate care for the infant.

Nursing Interventions/*Rationales*

- *Assist parents to see and describe normal aspects of infant to promote bonding.*
- Encourage and assist with breastfeeding if that is parents' choice of feeding method *to facilitate closeness with infant and provide benefits of breast milk.*
- Assure parents that information regarding the neonate will remain confidential *to assist the parents to maintain some situational control and allow for time to work through their feelings.*
- Discuss and role-play with parents ways of informing family and friends of infant's diagnosis and prognosis *to promote positive aspects of infant and decrease potential isolation from social interactions.*
- Provide anticipatory guidance about what to expect as infant develops *to assist family to facilitate optimum development of their infant.*

NURSING DIAGNOSIS

Spiritual distress related to situational crisis of child born with Down syndrome

Expected Outcome

Parents will seek appropriate support persons (family members, priest, minister, rabbi) for assistance.

Nursing Interventions/*Rationales*

- Listen for cues indicative of parents' feelings ("Why did God do this to us?") *to identify messages indicating spiritual distress.*
- Acknowledge parents' spiritual concerns and encourage expression of feelings *to help build a therapeutic relationship.*
- Facilitate visits from clergy and provide privacy during visits *to demonstrate respect for parents' relationship with clergy.*
- Encourage parents to discuss concerns with clergy *to use expert spiritual care resources to help the parents.*
- Facilitate interaction with family members and other support persons *to encourage expressions of concern and seek comfort.*

NURSING DIAGNOSIS

Social isolation related to full-time caretaking responsibilities for a neonate with Down syndrome

Expected Outcome

Parents will describe a plan to utilize resources to prevent social isolation.

Nursing Interventions/*Rationales*

- Provide opportunity for parents to express feelings about caring for a neonate with Down syndrome *to facilitate effective communication and trust.*
- Discuss with parents their expectations about caring for the neonate *to identify potential areas of concern.*
- Assist parents to identify potential caregiving resources *to permit parents to return to a routine at home.*
- Identify appropriate referrals for home care *to provide continuity of care.*

quality of life. The life expectancy for individuals with DS has increased from 9 years in 1929 to at least 50 to 60 years. For decades it was assumed that living in a family that includes an individual with DS was a negative experience. Findings from more recent studies do not provide support for this notion (Cuskelly, Hauser-Cram, & Van Riper, 2009; Van Riper, 2007). Many families living with DS have described the experience as positive and growth producing (see also Chapter 36).

Other autosomal trisomies that maternity nurses may see in practice are trisomy 18 and trisomy 13. Trisomy 18 (Edward syndrome) is more common than trisomy 13 (Patau syndrome); it occurs in about 1 out of every 3000 live births versus 1 out of every 10,000 live births for trisomy 13. Infants with trisomy 18 may exhibit more than 130 different anomalies, but some of the major phenotypic features and medical complications are small for gestational age or low birth weight; craniofacial abnormalities including cleft lip and/or palate, small mouth, and small jaw; weak cry; feeding difficulties; cardiac malformations; central nervous system manifestations including hypertonia, seizures, and apnea; and extremity malformations such as small fingernails and toenails, clenched fist with index finger overlapping the third finger, and rocker-bottom feet (Shaw, 2008).

As with trisomy 18, infants with trisomy 13 have numerous abnormalities, the most common of which are central nervous system anomalies, visual abnormalities, microcephaly (small head), absent nasal bridge, cleft lip and palate, holoprosencephaly (one large eyelike structure in the center of the face due to fusion of the developing eyes), capillary hemangiomas, cardiac defects, extremity deformities including polydactyly (extra fingers or toes), renal abnormalities, and genital abnormalities (Wirth, 2009).

Infants with trisomy 18 and trisomy 13 are usually severely to profoundly retarded. Although both conditions have a poor prognosis, with the vast majority of affected infants dying before they reach their first birthday, a growing number of infants with these trisomies are living longer and a small number are actually living into their 20s and 30s.

Nondisjunction also can occur during mitosis. If this occurs early in development when cell lines are forming, the individual has a mixture of cells, some with a normal number of chromosomes and others either missing a chromosome or containing an extra chromosome. This condition is known as **mosaicism.** The most common form of mosaicism in autosomes is mosaic Down syndrome.

Depending on when the nondisjunction occurs during development, different body tissues will have different numbers of chromosomes. The clinical characteristics of DS may be mild or with varying degrees of severity, depending on the number and location of the abnormal cells. An individual with mosaic DS may have normal intelligence. Mosaicism of both trisomy 18 and trisomy 13 has been reported. Both situations usually lead to a partial clinical expression of the phenotype. Infants who have mosaic trisomy 18 or trisomy 13 usually have a longer life span than infants with these disorders who are not mosaic.

Abnormalities of Chromosome Structure

Structural abnormalities can occur in any chromosome. Types of structural abnormalities include translocation, duplication, deletion, microdeletion, and inversion. **Translocation** results when there is an exchange of chromosomal material between two chromosomes. Exposure to certain drugs, viruses, and radiation can cause translocations, but often they arise for no apparent reason. The two major types of translocation are reciprocal and robertsonian. Reciprocal translocations are the most common. In a *reciprocal translocation,* either the parts of the two chromosomes are exchanged equally **(balanced translocation)** or a part of a chromosome is transferred to a different chromosome, creating an **unbalanced translocation** because there is extra chromosomal material—extra of one chromosome but correct amount or deficient amount of the other chromosome. In a balanced translocation, the individual is phenotypically normal because there is no extra chromosome material; it is just rearranged. In an unbalanced translocation, the individual will be both genotypically and phenotypically abnormal.

In a *robertsonian translocation,* the short arms (p arms) of two different acrocentric chromosomes (chromosomes with very short p arms) break, leaving sticky ends that then cause the two long arms (q arms) to stick together. This forms a new, large chromosome that is made of the two long arms. The individual with a balanced robertsonian translocation has 45 chromosomes. Because the short arm of acrocentric chromosomes contains genes for ribosomal RNA and these genes are represented elsewhere, the individual usually does not show any symptoms.

Deletions result in the loss of chromosomal material and partial monosomy for the chromosome involved. Loss of chromosomal material at the end of a chromosome is referred to as a **terminal deletion.** In contrast, loss of chromosomal material anywhere else in the chromosome is called an **interstitial deletion.** The resulting clinical phenotype of either a terminal or an interstitial deletion depends on how much of the chromosome has been lost and the number and function of the genes contained in the missing segment. **Microdeletions** are deletions too small to be detected by standard cytogenetic techniques. These deletions can be identified with FISH analysis. FISH technology uses a single-stranded piece of DNA with a fluorescent label that adheres to its complementary piece of DNA in the chromosome being investigated.

Whenever a portion of a chromosome is deleted from one chromosome and added to another, the gamete produced can have either extra copies of genes or too few copies. The clinical effects produced can be mild or severe, depending on the amount of genetic material involved. Two of the more common conditions are the deletion of the short arm of chromosome 5 (cri du chat syndrome) and the deletion of the long arm of chromosome 18. Cri du chat syndrome, so named after the typical mewing cry of the affected infant, causes severe mental retardation with microcephaly and unusual facial appearance. Deletion of the long arm of chromosome 18 causes severe psychomotor retardation with multiple organ malformations. *Velocardiofacial syndrome,* characterized by cardiac and craniofacial abnormalities, is an example of a microdeletion. In this syndrome, a very small piece of the long arm of chromosome 22 is missing. Microdeletions in the Y chromosome have been found in men with infertility problems.

Inversions are deviations in which a portion of the chromosome has been rearranged in reverse order. Few birth defects have been attributed to the presence of inversions, but it is suspected that inversions may be responsible for problems with infertility and miscarriages. Some inversions can be detected prenatally. Inversions do not appear to occur randomly; more than 40% of all inversions involve chromosome 9 (Lashley, 2005).

Sex Chromosome Abnormalities

Several sex chromosome abnormalities are caused by nondisjunction during gametogenesis in either parent. The most common deviation in females is *Turner syndrome* or monosomy X (45, X). The affected female is missing an X chromosome. She usually exhibits juvenile external genitalia with undeveloped ovaries. She is short and often has webbing of the neck, a low hairline in the back, low-set ears, and lymphedema of her hands and feet. Intelligence may be impaired. Most affected embryos miscarry spontaneously. In most cases of Turner syndrome, it is the paternal X or Y that is lost.

The most common deviation in males is *Klinefelter syndrome,* or trisomy XXY. The affected male has an extra X chromosome

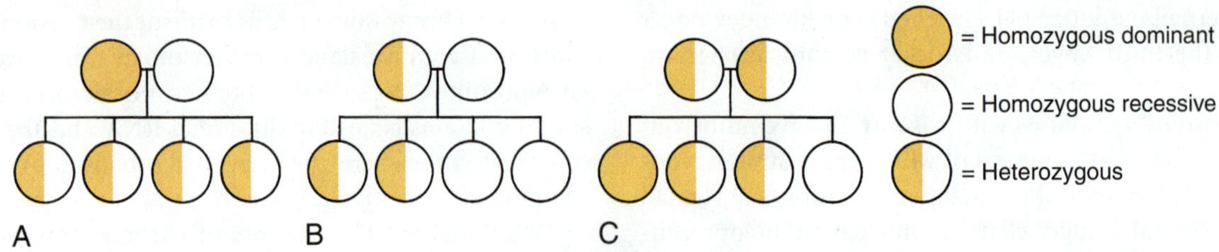

FIG. 3-3 Possible offspring in three types of matings. **A,** Homozygous-dominant parent and homozygous-recessive parent: children all heterozygous, displaying dominant trait. **B,** Heterozygous parent and homozygous recessive parent: children 50% heterozygous, displaying dominant trait; 50% homozygous, displaying recessive trait. **C,** Both parents heterozygous: children 25% homozygous, displaying dominant trait; 25% homozygous, displaying recessive trait; 50% heterozygous, displaying dominant trait.

and exhibits poorly developed secondary sexual characteristics and small testes. He is infertile, usually tall, and may be slow to learn (www.genetic.org). Males who have mosaic Klinefelter syndrome may be fertile.

Patterns of Genetic Transmission

Heritable characteristics are those that can be passed on to offspring. The patterns by which genetic material is transmitted to the next generation are affected by the number of genes involved in the expression of the trait. Many phenotypic characteristics result from two or more genes on different chromosomes acting together (referred to as multifactorial inheritance); others are controlled by a single gene (referred to as unifactorial inheritance). Specialists in genetics (e.g., geneticists, genetic counselors, and nurses with advanced expertise in genetics and genomics) predict the probability of the presence of an abnormal gene from the known occurrence of the trait in the individual's family and the known patterns by which the trait is inherited.

Multifactorial Inheritance

Most common congenital malformations result from multifactorial inheritance, a combination of genetic and environmental factors. Examples are cleft lip, cleft palate, congenital heart disease, neural tube defects, and pyloric stenosis. Each malformation can range from mild to severe, depending on the number of genes for the defect present or the amount of environmental influence. A neural tube defect can range from spina bifida, a bony defect in the lumbar region of the vertebrae with little or no neurologic impairment, to anencephaly, absence of brain development, which is always fatal. Some malformations occur more often in one sex. For example, pyloric stenosis and cleft lip are more common in males, and cleft palate is more common in females.

Unifactorial Inheritance

If a single gene controls a particular trait or disorder, its pattern of inheritance is referred to as *unifactorial mendelian,* or single-gene inheritance. The number of single-gene disorders far exceeds the number of chromosomal abnormalities. Potential patterns of inheritance for single-gene disorders include autosomal dominant, autosomal recessive, and X-linked dominant and recessive modes of inheritance.

Autosomal Dominant Inheritance. Autosomal dominant inheritance disorders are those in which only one copy of a variant allele is needed for phenotypic expression. The variant allele may be a result of a mutation, a spontaneous and permanent change in the normal gene structure, in which case the disorder occurs for the first time in the family. Usually an affected individual comes from multiple generations having the disorder. An affected parent who is heterozygous for the trait has a 50% chance of passing the variant allele to each offspring (Fig. 3-3, *B* and *C*). There is a vertical pattern of inheritance (there is no skipping of generations; if an individual has an autosomal dominant disorder such as HD, so must one of the parents). Males and females are equally affected.

Autosomal dominant disorders are not always expressed with the same severity of symptoms. For example, a woman who has an autosomal dominant disorder may show few symptoms and may not become aware of her diagnosis until after she gives birth to a severely affected child. Predicting whether an offspring will have a minor or severe abnormality is not possible. Examples of autosomal dominant disorders are HD, Marfan syndrome, neurofibromatosis, myotonic dystrophy, Stickler syndrome, Treacher Collins syndrome, and achondroplasia (dwarfism).

Neurofibromatosis (NF) is a progressive disorder of the nervous system that causes tumors to form on nerves anywhere in the body. NF affects all races, all ethnic groups, and both sexes equally. Half of the cases of NF result from a spontaneous genetic mutation, whereas the other half of cases are inherited in an autosomal dominant manner. Individuals with NF due to a spontaneous mutation have a 50% chance of transmitting the variant allele to the next generation with each pregnancy. Two genetically distinct forms of NF include NF1, the most common type, with an incidence of 1 in 4000 and NF2, with an incidence of 1 in 40,000 (Clarke, 2009). The most distinctive features of NF1 are multiple neurofibromas (benign, soft tumors), freckles in the axilla or groin, and patches of skin pigmentation called café-au-lait spots. Generally, symptoms of NF1 are mild and affected individuals are able to live healthy, productive lives. Individuals with NF2 typically develop bilateral vestibular schwannomas (tumors on the eighth cranial nerves, the hearing and balance nerves) that often cause pressure damage to nearby nerves, which may result in headaches, facial pain, and facial numbness. Other symptoms typically experienced by individuals with NF2 include tinnitus (ringing noise in the ear) and poor balance. Some individuals with NF2 experience hearing loss in their teen years.

No treatment for NF is available, other than the surgical removal of the tumors. Once removed, the tumors may grow back.

Factor V Leiden (FVL) is the most common inherited risk factor for primary and recurrent venous thromboembolisms

(Moll, 2006). It is an autosomal dominant disorder that markedly increases an individual's risk for deep vein thrombosis (blood clots in the large veins of the legs) and pulmonary emboli (blood clots that travel through the bloodstream and become embedded in the lungs), especially if the individual is a woman who (1) uses oral contraceptives, (2) is pregnant, or (3) is on hormone replacement therapy during menopause. FVL is due to a mutation in the Factor V gene, which leads to activated protein C (APC) resistance. If a woman is heterozygous (has inherited one copy of the FVL mutation), she has a four- to eightfold increase in her chance of developing venous blood clots, but her risk increases by a factor as high as 75 to 80 if she is homozygous (has inherited two copies of the FVL mutation) (National Institutes of Health, 2010). Women who carry the FVL mutation should not take oral contraceptives. In addition, if they become pregnant and they have a history of blood clots, it is recommended that they receive prophylactic anticoagulation (with low-molecular-weight heparin) during their pregnancy and for 6 weeks postpartum (Marik & Plante, 2008).

FVL can be accurately detected with genetic testing, but the most cost-effective way to screen for FVL is taking a careful individual and family history. Women with a personal or close family history of venous blood clots, pulmonary emboli, early onset and recurrent preeclampsia, recurrent fetal growth restriction, recurrent pregnancy loss and stillbirth, or placental abruption should be screened for FVL.

Autosomal Recessive Inheritance. **Autosomal recessive inheritance disorders** are those in which both genes of a pair are forms associated with the disorder to be expressed. Heterozygous individuals have only one variant allele and are unaffected clinically because their normal gene (wild-type allele) overshadows the variant allele. They are known as **carriers** of the recessive trait. Because these recessive traits are inherited by generations of the same family, an increased incidence of the disorder occurs in consanguineous matings (closely related parents). For the trait to be expressed, two carriers must each contribute a variant allele to the offspring (see Fig. 3-3, *C*). The chance of the trait occurring in each child is 25%. A clinically normal offspring may be a carrier of the gene. Autosomal recessive disorders have a horizontal pattern of inheritance, rather than the vertical pattern seen with autosomal dominant disorders. That is, autosomal recessive disorders are usually observed in one or more siblings, but not in earlier generations. Males and females are equally affected. Most recessive disorders tend to have severe clinical manifestations, and affected offspring may not reproduce. If they do, all their offspring will at least be carriers for the disorder. Most inborns errors of metabolism (IEMs), such as PKU, galactosemia, maple syrup urine disease, Tay-Sachs disease, sickle cell anemia, and CF, are autosomal recessive inherited disorders.

Inborn Errors of Metabolism. More than 350 **inborn errors of metabolism** have been recognized (Jorde, Carey, & Bamshad, 2010). Individually, IEMs are relatively rare, but collectively, they are common (1 in 5000 live births). Archibald Garrod first used the term "inborn errors of metabolism" in 1908 when he described variants of metabolism. Garrod recognized that IEMs illustrate our "chemical individualities." As noted previously, most IEMs are inherited in an autosomal recessive pattern. IEMs occur when a gene mutation reduces the efficiency of encoded enzymes to a level at which normal metabolism cannot occur. Defective enzyme action interrupts the normal series of chemical reactions from the affected point onward. The result may be an accumulation of a damaging product, such as phenylalanine in PKU, or the absence of a necessary product, such as the lack of melanin in albinism caused by lack of tyrosinase. Diagnostic and carrier testing is available for a growing number of IEMs. In addition, many states have started screening for specific IEMs as part of their expanded newborn screening programs using tandem mass spectrometry. However, many of the deaths caused by IEMs are due to enzyme variants not currently screened for in many of the newborn screening programs (Jorde et al.).

Phenylketonuria is a relatively uncommon autosomal recessive disorder. A deficiency in the liver enzyme phenylalanine hydroxylase results in failure to metabolize the amino acid phenylalanine, allowing its metabolites to accumulate in the blood. The incidence of this disorder is 1 in every 10,000 to 20,000 births. The highest incidence is found in Caucasians (from northern Europe and the United States). It is rarely seen in Jewish, African, or Japanese populations. Screening for PKU is routinely performed as part of state-mandated newborn screening in the United States.

Tay-Sachs disease is a lipid-storage disease that occurs more commonly in Ashkenazi Jews and French-Canadians from Quebec (Lashley, 2005). It results from a deficiency in hexosaminidase. Until age 4 to 6 months, infants with Tay-Sachs disease appear normal; their facial features are considered very beautiful. Then the clinical symptoms appear: apathy and regression in motor and social development and decreased vision. Death occurs between ages 3 and 4 years. No treatment exists for Tay-Sachs disease.

Infantile Krabbe's disease or *globoid-cell leukodystrophy* is a lysosomal storage disorder characterized by failure of the process of myelination in the central and peripheral nervous systems, rapidly progressive neurologic deterioration, and death (often before the age of 2 years). Findings from a study by Escolar and colleagues (2005) suggest that transplantation of umbilical-cord blood from unrelated donors in newborns with infantile Krabbe's disease favorably altered the natural history of this disease. Infants who underwent transplantation before the development of symptoms demonstrated continued gains in developmental skills and progressive central myelination, and most had age-appropriate cognitive function and receptive language skills. However, if transplantation occurred after the onset of symptoms, there was minimal neurologic improvement. These findings have implications for decisions regarding the addition of screening for lysosomal storage disorders to existing newborn screening programs.

X-linked Dominant Inheritance. **X-linked dominant inheritance** mimics autosomal dominant inheritance, except that male-to-male transmission cannot occur unless the father has Klinefelter syndrome due to XY disomy (Simpson & Elias, 2003). X-linked dominant inheritance disorders occur in males and heterozygous females, but because of X inactivation, affected females are usually less severely affected than affected males and they are more likely to transmit the abnormal gene (variant allele) to their offspring (Lashley, 2005). Heterozygous females (females who have one wild-type allele and one variant allele) have a 50% chance of transmitting the abnormal gene (variant allele) to each offspring. The variant allele is often lethal in affected males because, unlike affected females, they have no normal gene (wild-type allele). Mating of an affected male and an unaffected female is uncommon as a result of the tendency for the variant allele to be lethal in affected males. Relatively few X-linked dominant disorders have been identified. Two examples are vitamin D–resistant rickets and Rett syndrome.

X-linked Recessive Inheritance. Abnormal genes for X-linked recessive inheritance disorders are carried on the X chromosome. Females may be heterozygous or homozygous for traits carried on the X chromosome because they have two X chromosomes. Males are hemizygous because they have only one X chromosome, which carries genes with no alleles on the Y chromosome. Therefore X-linked recessive disorders are most commonly manifested in the male, with the abnormal gene on his single X chromosome. Hemophilia, color blindness, and Duchenne muscular dystrophy are X-linked recessive disorders.

A man with an X-linked recessive disorder receives the disease-associated allele from his carrier mother on her affected X chromosome. Female carriers (those heterozygous for the trait) have a 50% probability of transmitting the disease-associated allele to each offspring. An affected man can pass the disease-associated allele to his daughters, but not to his sons. The daughters will be carriers of the trait if they receive a normal gene on the X chromosome from their mother. They will be affected only if they receive a disease-associated allele on the X chromosome from both their mother and their father.

Fragile X syndrome (FXS), the most common inherited form of cognitive impairment, is an X-linked disorder that has a complex pattern of inheritance. FXS is caused by a trinucleotide repeat expansion (CGG) at a "fragile site" on the long arm of the X chromosome. Most people have 5 to 40 CGG repeats. Individuals with FXS have more than 200 CGG repeats. The abnormally expanded CGG segment inactivates or silences the FMR1 (fragile X mental retardation) gene, which prevents the gene from producing a protein called fragile X mental retardation protein. Loss of this protein leads to the characteristic physical features (large ears, long face, prominent forehead, protruding ears, hypermobile joints, and macroorchidism or increased testicular volume in postpubertal males) and behavior problems (poor eye contact, hyperactivity, social avoidance, repetitive speech, and self-injurious behavior) associated with FXS (Jorde et al., 2010; Schneider, Hagerman, & Hessl, 2009). Males and females can be affected by FXS, but because males have only one X chromosome, a CGG repeat expansion on one X is likely to affect males more severely than females. Also, the degree of cognitive impairment tends to be milder and more variable in females than in males. Unlike DS, FXS is not generally detectable through a physical examination at birth. Delays and behavioral abnormalities gradually become apparent during the first 2 years of life, but ultimately the diagnosis of FXS can be verified only through DNA testing (Sherman, Pletcher, & Driscoll, 2005).

Individuals with more than 55 but fewer than 200 CGG repeats are said to be permutation carriers. These individuals were originally thought to be unaffected, but recent research has shown that about 20% of adult carrier females may develop premature ovarian failure (cessation of menses before 40 years of age). Elderly male permutation carriers may manifest fragile X-associated tremor/ataxia syndrome (FXTAS), which consists of parkinsonism, intention tremors, autonomic dysfunction, peripheral neuropathy, weakness in the legs, cognitive decline, and cerebellar ataxia (www.nfx.org).

CANCER GENOMICS

Gene Mutations That Can Lead to Cancer

There are three main ways that people acquire gene mutations that can lead to cancer. The first is from the environment. Known factors in the environment that cause cancer are ultraviolet (UV) light (skin cancer) and tobacco smoke (lung cancer). The second way that people acquire mutations is by chance. Normal metabolic processes can generate chemicals that damage DNA. Third, people inherit mutations from their parents; hereditary mutations are thought to be a major factor in about 5% to 10% of all cancers.

The two main types of genes that have been recognized as playing a critical role in the development of cancer are *oncogenes* and *tumor suppressor genes* (American Cancer Society, 2010). Oncogenes are mutated forms of proto-oncogenes. The main functions of proto-oncogenes are to encourage and promote normal growth and development. When proto-oncogenes mutate to become carcinogenic oncogenes, the result is excessive cell multiplication. The activation of oncogenes has been compared to a jammed accelerator in a car. Most mutations of proto-oncogenes are acquired mutations, such as mutations in the KIT gene which are thought to cause most cases of gastrointestinal stromal tumor (GIST). This type of cancer can be treated with drugs that target the KIT gene, such as imatinib (Gleevec). Two examples of inherited mutations of proto-oncogenes are ERBB2, located on chromosome 13, and KRAS2, located on chromosome 12. ERBB2 is involved in breast, ovarian, lung, gastric, and salivary gland cancers. KRAS2 is involved in breast, pancreatic, thyroid, colorectal, bladder, and lung cancers, as well as acute myeloid leukemia.

Tumor suppressor genes normally function to inhibit or "put the brakes on" the cell growth and division cycle. They function to prevent the development of tumors. Mutations in tumor suppressor genes cause the cell to ignore one or more of the components of the network of inhibitory signals, removing the brakes from the cell cycle. This results in a higher rate of uncontrolled growth: cancer. Acquired mutations of the TP53 gene appear in a wide range of cancers, including lung, colorectal, and breast cancer. Examples of inherited tumor suppressor genes include APC, located on chromosome 5 and involved with familial adenomatous polyposis of the colon (FAP); BRCA1, located on chromosome 17 and associated with hereditary breast cancer and ovarian cancer; and RB1, found on chromosome 13 and involved with familial retinoblastoma.

Hereditary Breast and Ovarian Cancer

Breast cancer is a common disease and a central concern in women's health. In the United States, breast cancer is the most common form of cancer for women and the second most common cause of death. Hereditary mutations are considered to be a key factor in approximately 5% to 10% of all breast and ovarian cancers. Another 15% to 20% of female breast cancers occur in women who have a family history of breast and ovarian cancer but do not carry a mutation in one of the genes that are known to be strongly associated with breast and ovarian cancer susceptibility.

BRCA1 and BRCA2 mutations account for approximately 70% to 85% of hereditary breast and ovarian cancer (HBOC). These mutations are inherited in an autosomal dominant pattern; thus each offspring of an individual found to carry a BRCA mutation has a 50% chance of inheriting the same mutation. Ashkenazi Jews are 10 times more likely to have BRCA1 and/or BRCA2 mutations than are the general population. According to estimates of lifetime risk, approximately 12% of women in the general population will develop breast cancer sometime during their lifetime, compared to about 60% of women who have inherited a deleterious mutation in their BRAC1 or BRCA2 gene (National Cancer Institute, 2010). Another way of saying this is that a woman with a deleterious BRCA1 or BRCA2 mutation is about five times more likely to develop breast cancer than a woman who does not carry a deleterious BRCA1 or BRCA2 mutation. Even though only about 6% of the men who carry a BRCA mutation develop breast cancer, men who carry a BRCA mutation have a 50% chance of passing the mutation on to their offspring. As far as lifetime risk estimates for ovarian cancer, about 1.4% of women in the general population will be diagnosed with ovarian cancer during their lifetime, compared with 15% to 40% of women who have a deleterious BRCA 1 or BRCA2 mutation. Carriers of BRCA1 mutations may also be at increased risk for colon cancer, though this has been disputed. Carriers of BRCA2 mutations may be at increased risk for pancreatic, prostate, gallbladder and bile duct, and stomach cancers, hematologic malignancies, and malignant melanoma.

Genetic testing for HBOC has been commercially available in the United States since 1995. The cost for testing (current in 2010) is approximately $3,000 for full-sequence BRCA1 and BRCA2 testing, and $350 for an analysis of relatives of an individual with an identified mutation. Women newly diagnosed with breast cancer are increasingly being asked to consider undergoing BRCA1 and BRCA2 testing before they make decisions about their treatment options. This request for testing is occurring because a number of studies have shown that a woman's short-term risk of developing a second breast cancer is substantially affected by whether she carries a BRCA1 or BRCA2 mutation, and prophylactic surgery has been found to decrease the risk of breast and ovarian cancer by more than 90% (Hartmann, Degnim, & Schaid, 2004; McDonnell, Schaid, Myers, Grant, Donohue, Woods, et al., 2001; Rebbeck, Friebel, Lynch, Neuhausen, van't Veer, Garber, et al., 2004). The main advantage to offering BRCA1 and BRCA2 testing before the onset of treatment is that it gives women who are found to carry a deleterious mutation the option of choosing risk-reduction surgery concurrent with therapeutic surgical treatment.

Colon Cancer

Colon cancer is the third leading cause of cancer-related death in women. According to estimates from the American Cancer Society (2010), 102,900 new cases of colon cancer and 39,670 new cases of rectal cancer were diagnosed in 2009 and there were 51,370 deaths due to colorectal cancer. Only 10% of colon cancer cases are likely to involve a mutation in one of several predisposing genes. Two examples of predisposing genes are mutations in the APC tumor suppressor gene and mutations in a mismatch repair gene. Mutations in the APC tumor suppressor gene have been associated with FAP, a rare, autosomal dominant syndrome that accounts for about 1% of all colon cancer. It is typically diagnosed clinically. Affected individuals have 100 to 1000 polyps in their colon by the time they are 20 to 30 years old. Genetic testing is greater than 80% sensitive. Identification of high risk individuals guides surveillance strategies and the timing of a prophylactic colectomy. Low risk individuals can stop the increased surveillance.

Hereditary nonpolyposis colon cancer (HNPCC) results from mutations in one of many mismatch repair (MMR) genes. Mutations in MSH2 and MLH1 account for 50% to 60% of HNPCC. Families at high risk for HNPCC often have three or more relatives with colorectal cancer; colorectal cancer present in at least two generations; and a diagnosis of colorectal cancer before age 50 years in at least one case. HNPCC is characterized by an increased risk of colon cancer and other cancers that include cancers of the ovary, endometrium, stomach, small intestine, upper urinary tract, hepatobiliary tract, brain, and skin. The lifetime risk of colon cancer for individuals with HNPCC is approximately 80%. The majority of these cancers occur in the proximal colon. Genetic tests are available to test for MSH2 and MLH1. Testing should be done first on the affected family member. At-risk clients should be offered a prophylactic colectomy. Women may be offered a total abdominal hysterectomy with a salpingo-oophorectomy to decrease cancer risk. If colon cancer develops, a total colectomy is recommended.

GENETIC COUNSELING

Genetic counseling is a service that grew out of a need for professionals who could provide genetics information, education, and support to individuals and families with ongoing or potential genetic health concerns. In 2010 there were 31 accredited genetic counseling programs in the United States and international genetic counseling programs in 15 different countries. At the same time, there were 2448 American Board of Genetic Counseling (ABGC)–certified genetic counselors. The National Society of Genetic Counselors was formed in 1979 and the International Society of Nurses in Genetics (ISONG) was formed in 1988. The number of nursing programs offering courses in genetics and genomics is growing rapidly. A small number of graduate nursing programs offer advanced practice courses and/or specialty options in genetics and genomics. Examples of these are the University of California San Francisco School of Nursing, the University of Pittsburgh School of Nursing, and the University of Iowa College of Nursing.

Definition of Genetic Counseling

In 1975 an ad hoc committee of the American Society of Human Genetics developed a formal definition of genetic counseling. According to this definition:

> Genetic counseling is a communication process that deals with the human problems associated with the occurrence or risk of occurrence of a genetic disorder in a family. This process involves an attempt by one or more appropriately trained person to help the individual or family to (1) comprehend the medical facts including the diagnosis, probable course of the disorder, and the available management; (2) appreciate the way

heredity contributes to the disorder and the risk of recurrence in specified relatives; (3) understand the alternatives for dealing with the risk of recurrence; (4) choose a course of action that seems to them appropriate in view of their risk, their family goals, and their ethical and religious standards and act in accordance with that decision; and (5) make the best possible adjustment to the disorder in an affected family member and/or to the risk of recurrence of that disorder.

Access and Referral to Genetic Counseling

Genetic counseling is typically provided by a team of genetics specialists that includes clinical geneticists (physicians with an MD or DO), medical geneticists with a PhD, genetics fellows, genetics counselors, and, in a growing number of cases, advanced practice genetics nurse specialists. Cytogeneticists, biochemical geneticists, and molecular geneticists support the clinical genetics team by providing laboratory expertise that helps with the diagnosis and management of individuals and families affected by genetic conditions.

Until recently, most individuals and families interested in receiving genetic counseling went to regional genetics centers or major medical centers. Genetic counseling also was provided in outreach or satellite genetics clinics, public health clinics, and some community hospitals. Now that genetics is entering the mainstream of health care, genetic counseling is being offered in a wide variety of other settings. These include, but are not limited to, managed health care organizations, commercial facilities, and private practices. A number of specialized groups provide genetics education and counseling for individuals and families affected by specific genetic disorders, such as DS, CF, diabetes, muscular dystrophy, HD, and cancer. Genetic counseling also is offered over the Internet.

Individuals and families seek out, or are referred for, genetic counseling for a wide variety of reasons and at all stages of their lives. Some seek preconception or prenatal information; others are referred after the birth of a child with a birth defect or a suspected genetic condition; still others seek information because they have a family history of a genetic condition. Regardless of the setting or the individual and family's stage of life, genetic counseling should be offered and available to all individuals and families who have questions about genetics and their health. However, there is currently a shortage of appropriately trained genetics professionals who can provide genetic counseling. This means that many individuals and families will not be offered genetic counseling when they undergo genetic testing. Moreover, some of the genetics education and counseling that is provided will be inadequate.

It may take years before a sufficient number of health care professionals feel comfortable and are proficient in providing genetic counseling (Burke & Kirk, 2006; Cashion, 2009). Until then it is imperative that all health care professionals become familiar with existing genetics resources, such as the Centers for Disease Control and Prevention, the Genetic Alliance, the National Coalition for Health Professional Education in Genetics, Genetics Education Program for Nurses at Cincinnati Children's Hospital Medical Center, NHGRI Education, and others. Some of these resources may be in health care professionals' own communities, but others are regional, national, and international.

Critical Thinking Exercise—Genetic Counseling

Estimation of Risk

Most families with a history of genetic disease want an answer to the following question: What is the chance that our future children will have this disease? Because the answer to this question may have profound implications for individual family members and the family as a whole, health care professionals must be able to answer this question as accurately as they can in a timely manner. In some cases, estimation of risk is rather straightforward; in other cases, it is complicated. Because of this, health care professionals should be prepared to refer families with a history of genetic disease to genetics professionals if they are at all unsure. Again, the answer to this question can have profound implications for individual family members and the family as a whole, so health care professionals must do their best to ensure that the question is answered accurately.

If a couple has not yet had children, but they are known to be at risk for having children with a genetic disease, they will be given an **occurrence risk.** Once the mating of a couple has produced one or more children with a genetic disease, the couple will be given a **recurrence risk.** Both occurrence and recurrence risks are determined by the mode of inheritance for the genetic disease in question. For genetic diseases caused by a factor that segregates during cell division (genes and chromosomes), risk can be estimated with a high degree of accuracy by application of mendelian principles.

In an autosomal dominant disorder, both the occurrence and recurrence risk is 50%, or one in two, when one parent is affected and the other is not. The recurrence risk for autosomal recessive disorders is 25%, or one in four, if both parents are carriers (they each have one recessive disease gene and one normal gene). Occasionally an individual homozygous for a recessive disease gene mates with an individual who is a carrier of the same recessive gene. In this case, the recurrence risk is 50%, or one in two. If two individuals affected by an autosomal recessive disorder mate, all of their children will be affected (See Fig. 3-3). For X-linked disorders, recurrence risk is related to the sex of the child. Translocation disorders have a high risk of recurrence.

A number of autosomal disorders display fairly complex patterns of inheritance, making estimation of risk somewhat difficult. For example, if a child is born with a genetic disease and there has been no history of the disease in the family, the disease may have been caused by a new mutation (this is more likely if the disease in question is an autosomal dominant disorder, such as achondroplasia). If the child's genetic disease has been caused by a new mutation, the recurrence risk for the parents' subsequent children is low (1% to 2%), but it is not as low as that for the general population. Offspring of the affected child may have a substantially elevated occurrence risk.

The risk of recurrence for multifactorial conditions can be estimated empirically. An empiric risk is based not on genetics theory but rather on experience and observation of the disorder in other families. Recurrence risks are determined by applying the frequency of a similar disorder in other families to the case under consideration.

An important concept to be emphasized to individuals and families during a genetic counseling session is that *each pregnancy is an independent event.* For example, in monogenic disorders in which the risk factor is one in four that the child will be affected, the risk remains the same no matter how many affected children are already in the family. Families may maintain the erroneous assumption that the presence of one affected child ensures that the next three will be free of the disorder. However, "chance has no memory." The risk is one in four for each pregnancy. Conversely, in a family with a child who has a disorder with multifactorial causes, the risk increases with each subsequent child born with the disorder.

Interpretation of Risk

The guiding principle for genetics counselors has traditionally been **nondirectiveness.** According to the principle of nondirectiveness, the individual who is providing genetic counseling respects the right of the individual or family being counseled to make autonomous decisions. Counselors using a nondirective approach avoid making recommendations and try to communicate genetics information in an unbiased manner. The first step in providing nondirective counseling is becoming aware of one's own values and beliefs. Another important step is recognizing how those values and beliefs can influence or interfere with the communication of genetics information.

If the individual who is providing genetic counseling has difficulty being nonjudgmental and objective, he or she may either intentionally or unintentionally influence the decision-making process. Individuals and families also may pressure the counselor to make decisions for them with questions such as, "What would you do if you were me?" Families and individuals need education, guidance, and support throughout the counseling process. They should be given the facts and possible consequences, as well as all of the assistance they need in problem solving, but the final decision regarding a course of action must be their own.

Multiple Roles for Nurses in Genetics

Nurses play many roles in genetics. Some nurses play a key role in the identification of families in need of genetic counseling, and they collaborate with other health care professionals to make referrals to specialists in genetics. Other nurses take a more active role in genetic counseling. For example, these nurses might provide appropriate genetics information before, during, and after the initial genetic counseling session; construct family pedigrees of three or more generations; clarify the genetics information that family members receive during counseling sessions or from other sources such as the public library, the Internet, or support groups; help families manage the ongoing challenges associated with living with a genetic disorder; make referrals to support groups and national organizations; and provide long-term follow-up of families affected by genetic conditions.

Probably the most important of all nursing functions is to provide emotional support during all aspects of the counseling process. Feelings that are generated under the real or imagined threat posed by a genetic disorder are as varied as the people being counseled. Responses may include a variety of stress reactions, such as apathy, denial, anger, hostility, fear, embarrassment, grief, and loss of self-esteem. Guilt and self-blame are universal reactions. Many look on the disorder as a stigma, especially if the disorder is visible to others. Old wives' tales, superstitions, and long-held misconceptions may influence a family's reaction to a genetic disorder (Clinical Reasoning).

CLINICAL REASONING

Counseling About Genetic Risk

Sylvia confides in you that several infants have been born into her family with serious anomalies. From previous conversations you know that she is opposed to abortion and would never consider having one. Sylvia is currently 6 weeks pregnant, and her physician has urged her to have chorionic villus sampling (CVS). Sylvia asks you for information about CVS and the implications of a finding that her fetus has serious anomalies.

1. Evidence—Is there sufficient evidence to provide Sylvia with answers to her questions about CVS?
2. Assumptions—What assumptions can be made about CVS and what can be discovered using this technology?
   a. The risks of this technology
   b. The benefits of this technology
   c. The fit between Sylvia's beliefs and the implications of a positive diagnosis
   d. Sylvia's acceptance of the birth of a child with an anomaly
3. What implications and priorities for nursing can be made at this time?
4. Does the evidence objectively support your conclusion?
5. Are there alternative perspectives to your conclusion?

FUTURE PROMISE OF GENETICS

Overall, the Human Genome Project and other sequencing efforts have been a huge success. Our understanding of the human genome, as well as other genomes, has grown exponentially during the past decade. The increased availability of genetic testing and other genetics services gives individuals and families unprecedented opportunities to learn whether they have heightened risk for certain diseases or the potential to transmit gene mutations to their offspring. Awareness of genetic risk also can facilitate informed health care decisions and, in some cases, can promote risk reduction behaviors that have the potential to reduce morbidity and mortality. Ultimately it is hoped that advances in molecular biology and genomics will make it possible to offer diagnostic, preventive, and treatment options not only for genetic diseases but also for common diseases such as cancer, atherosclerosis, diabetes, and Alzheimer's disease.

Recent advances made possible through the Human Genome Project have been remarkable, but our ability to offer treatment options, even for single-gene disorders, remains limited. Progress in the acquisition of genetics information and the development of genetics technology continues to outpace the development of therapeutic interventions. For most genetic conditions, therapeutic interventions are nonexistent or disappointingly limited. Consequently the most useful means of reducing the incidence of genetic disorders now is preventing transmission. Only three reproductive options exist for individuals at risk for transmitting a genetic disorder: the avoidance of pregnancy; genetic diagnosis during an ongoing pregnancy; and prevention of transmission of an altered gene or genes through preimplantation genetics. For many families, none of these options is viewed as acceptable.

Dialogue among pregnant women, expectant families, health care professionals, and disability advocates concerning prenatal testing for DS and other genetic disorders is urgently needed. Clinical and technical information must be complemented by social understanding of the experience of disability in contemporary society. The picture of life with a disability should be more balanced than that currently portrayed. It is critical that the voices of individuals and families living with disabilities be heard.

Nurses are in an ideal position to help individuals and families maximize the benefits of the genetics revolution, but first, nurses need (1) a working knowledge of human genetics, (2) an awareness of recent advances in genetics and genomics, and (3) an understanding of the potential effects of genomic discoveries on individual and family well-being. More research is needed concerning the family experience of genetic testing. Nurses must understand why individuals and families decide to undergo genetic testing. Nurses also need to be aware of how individuals and families define and manage ethical, legal, and social issues that emerge during the genetic testing experience.

COMMUNITY ACTIVITY

- Select a hereditary disorder such as cystic fibrosis, muscular dystrophy, hemophilia, Tay-Sachs disease, or sickle cell anemia. Visit the website of the national organization. Locate accredited care centers that are in your community. Do the centers offer preconception counseling?
- Visit the Genetic Alliance website at www.geneticalliance.org. Select a disorder and go to the disease information search link. Review the client information sections about clinical description, insurance issues, research and treatment.
- Share your findings with your classmates in a clinical conference.

KEY POINTS

- Recent advances in molecular biology and genomics have revolutionized the field of health care by providing the tools needed to determine the hereditary component of many diseases.
- Increasingly, nurses from all specialty areas, as well as all practice settings, are expected to have competencies in genetics and genomics.
- The major force behind the genetics revolution has been the Human Genome Project.
- All humans are 99.9% identical at the DNA level.
- Approximately 20,000 to 25,000 genes are found in the human genome.
- Most of the genetic tests being offered in clinical practice are tests for single-gene disorders.
- Pharmacogenomics will probably be the most immediate clinical application of the Human Genome Project.
- The decision to undergo genetic testing is often based on feelings of responsibility and commitment to others.
- Genes are the basic units of heredity responsible for all human characteristics. They comprise 23 pairs of chromosomes: 22 pairs of autosomes and 1 pair of sex chromosomes.
- Chromosomal abnormalities occur in autosomes and sex chromosomes.
- Multifactorial inheritance includes genetic and environmental contributions.
- Advances in genetics have complex ethical, legal, and social implications.
- Cancer genetics is an important emerging field.

Audio Chapter Summaries Access an audio summary of these Key Points on evolve

REFERENCES

American Cancer Society. (2010). *Cancer facts & figures, 2010.* Atlanta: American Cancer Society. Available at www.cancer.org/docroot/STT/stt_0.asp. Accessed February 1, 2010.

American Cancer Society. (2010). *Oncogenes and tumor suppressor genes.* Available at www.cancer.org/docroot/ETO/content/ETO_1_4x_oncogenes_and_tumor_suppressor_genes.asp. Accessed February 1, 2010.

American College of Obstetricians and Gynecologists & American College of Medical Genetics. (2001). *Preconception and prenatal carrier screening for cystic fibrosis; clinical and laboratory guidelines.* Washington DC: Author.

Burke, S., & Kirk, M. (2006). Genetics education in the nursing profession: Literature review. *Advances in Nursing Science, 54*(2), 228–237.

Canfield, M., Honein, M., Yuskiv, N., Xing, J., Mai, C., Colins, J., et al. (2006). National estimates and race/ethnic-specific variation of selected birth defects in the United States, 1999-2001. *Birth Defects Research Part A: Clinical and Molecular Teratology, 76*(11), 747–756.

Cashion, A. (2009). Importance of genetics education for undergraduate and graduate nursing programs. *Journal of Nursing Education, 47*(10), 535–536.

Clarke, L. (2009). Neurofibromatosis 2: A family's journey. *Canadian Journal of Neuroscience Nursing, 31*(4), 7–14.

Collins, F. (2004). What we do and don't know about 'race,' 'ethnicity,' genetics and health at the dawn of the genome era. *Nature Genetics Supplement, 36*(Suppl. 11), S11–S15.

Cuskelly, M., Hauser-Cram, P., & Van Riper, M. (2009). Families of children with Down syndrome: What we know and what we need to know. *Down Syndrome Research and Practice, 12,* 202–210. Available at www.down-syndrome.org/reviews/2079. Accessed February 7, 2010.

De Sevo, M. (2009). Unlocking the clues of family history: The importance of creating a pedigree. *Nursing for Women's Health, 13*(2), 122–131.

Dolan, S., Biermann, J., & Damus, K. (2007). Genomics for health in preconception and prenatal periods. *Journal of Nursing Scholarship, 39*(1), 4–9.

Dolan, S., & Moore, C. (2007). Linking family history in obstetric and pediatric care: Assessing risk for genetic disease and birth defects. *Pediatrics, 120*(Suppl. 2), S66–S70.

Escolar, M., Poe, M., Provenzale, J., Richards, K., Allison, J., Wood, S., et al. (2005). Transplantation of umbilical-cord blood in babies with infantile Krabbe's disease. *New England Journal of Medicine, 352*(20), 2069–2081.

Evans, J., & Green, R. (2009). Direct to consumer genetic testing: Avoiding a culture war. *Genetics in Medicine, 11*(8), 568–569.

Feero, W., Guttmacher, A., & Collins, F. (2008). The genome gets personal—almost. *Journal of the Americal Medical Association, 299*(11), 1351–1352.

Gallo, A., Knafl, K., & Angst, D. (2009). Information management in families who have a child with a genetic condition. *Journal of Pediatric Nursing, 24*(3), 194–204.

Gillet, J., Macadangdang, B., Fathke, R., Gottesman, M., & Kimchi-Sarfaty, C. (2009). The development of gene therapy: From monogenic recessive disorders to complex diseases such as cancer. *Methods in Molecular Biology, 542,* 5–54.

Ginsburg, G., & Willard, H. (2009). Genomic and personalized medicine: Foundations and applications. *Translational Research, 154*(6), 277–287.

Guttmacher, A., McGuire, A., Ponder, B., & Stefansson, K. (2010). Personalized genomic information: Preparing for the future of genetic medicine. *Nature Reviews Genetics, 11*(2), 161–165.

Hamilton, R. (2009). Nursing advocacy in a post-genomic age. *Nursing Clinics of North America, 44*(4), 435–446.

Hartmann, L., Degnim, A., & Schaid, D. (2004). Prophylactic mastectomy for BRCA 1/2 carriers: Progress and more questions. *Journal of Clinical Oncology, 22*(6), 981–983.

Hassold, T., & Hunt, P. (2009). Maternal age and chromosomally abnormal pregnancies: What we know and what we wish we knew. *Current Opinion in Pediatrics, 21*(6), 703–708.

Hinton, R. (2008). The family history: Reemergence of an established tool. *Critical Care Nursing Clinics of North America, 20*(2), 149–158.

Horne, M., & McCloskey, D. (2006). Factor V Leiden as a common genetic risk factor for venous thromboembolism. *Journal of Nursing Scholarship, 38*(1), 19–25.

Hunt, P., & Hassold, T. (2008). Human female meiosis: What makes a good egg go bad. *Trends in Genetics, 24*(2), 86–93.

Jenkins, J., & Calzone, K. (2007). Establishing the essential nursing competencies for genetics and genomics. *Journal of Nursing Scholarship, 39*(1), 10–16.

Jorde, L., Carey, J., & Bamshad, M. (2010). *Medical genetics* (4th ed.). St. Louis: Mosby.

Kenner, C., Lewis, J., Pressler, J., & Little, C. (2008). Neonatal genetic testing is more than screening. *Critical Care Nursing Clinics of North America, 20*(2), 233–237.

Khairy, P., Ouyang, D., Fernandes, S., Lee-Parritz, A., Economy, K., & Landzberg, M. (2006). Pregnancy outcomes in women with congenital heart disease. *Circulation, 113*(4), 517–524.

Kohn, D., & Candotti, F. (2009). Gene therapy fulfilling its promise. *New England Journal of Medicine, 360*(5), 518–521.

Lanfear, D., & McLeod, H. (2007). Pharmacogenetics—Using DNA to optimize drug therapy. *American Family Physician, 76*(8), 1179–1182.

Lashley, F. (2005). *Clinical genetics in nursing practice* (3rd ed.). New York: Springer.

Lynch, H., Snyder, C., & Lynch, J. (2009). Genetic counseling and the advanced practice oncology nursing role in hereditary cancer prevention clinic: Hereditary breast cancer focus. *The Breast Journal, 15*(Suppl. 1), 11–19.

Marik, P., & Plante, L. (2008). Venous thromboembolic disease. *New England Journal of Medicine, 359*(19), 2025–2033.

Martin, R. (2008). Meiotic errors in human oogenesis and spermatogenesis. *Reproductive BioMedicine Online, 16*(4), 523–531.

McDonnell, S., Schaid, D., Myers, J., Grant, C., Donohue, J., Woods, J., et al. (2001). Efficacy of contralateral prophylactic mastectomy in women with a personal and family history of breast cancer. *Journal of Clinical Oncology, 19*(19), 3938–3943.

McGuire, A., & Burke, W. (2010). An unwelcome side effect of direct-to-consumer personal genome testing. *Journal of the American Medical Association, 300*(22), 2669–2671.

McMullen, A., Pasta, D., Frederick, P., Konstan, M., Morgan, W., Schechter, M., et al. (2006). Impact of pregnancy on women with cystic fibrosis. *Chest, 129*(3), 706–711.

Meckley, L., Gudgeon, J., Anderson, J., Williams, M., & Veenstra, D. (2010). A policy model to evaluate the benefits, risks, and costs of warfarin pharmacogenetic testing. *Pharmacogenomics, 28*(1), 61–74.

Moll, S. (2006). Thrombophilias—Practical implications and testing caveats. *Journal of Thrombosis and Thrombolysis, 21*(1), 7–15.

National Cancer Institute. (2010). *BRCA1 and BRCA2; cancer risk and genetic testing.* Available at www.cancer.gov/cancertopics/factsheet/Risk/BRCA. Accessed February 1, 2010.

National Down Syndrome Society. (2010). *Down syndrome fact sheet.* Available at www.ndss.org/index.php?option=com_content&;view=article&id=54&Itemid=74. Accessed February 1, 2010.

National Institutes of Health. (2010). *Learning about Factor V Leiden thrombophilia.* Available at www.genome.gov/15015167. Accessed February 1, 2010.

Ranweiler, R. (2009). Assessment and care of the newborn with Down syndrome. *Advances in Neonatal Care, 9*(1), 17–24.

Rebbeck, T., Friebel, T., Lynch, H., Neuhausen, S., van't Veer, L., Garber, J., et al. (2004). Bilateral prophylactic mastectomy reduces breast cancer risk in BRCA1 and BRCA2 mutation carriers: The PROSE study group. *Journal of Clinical Oncology, 22*(6), 1055–1062.

Rich, E., Burke, W., Heaton, C., Haga, S., Pinsky, L., Short, M., et al. (2004). Reconsidering the family history in primary care. *Journal of General Internal Medicine, 19*(3), 273–280.

Schiefelbein, J., & Cheeseman, S. (2009). Principles of genetics and their clinical application in the neonatal intensive care unit. *Critical Care Nursing Clinics of North America, 21*(1), 67–85.

Schneider, A., Hagerman, R., & Hessl, D. (2009). Fragile X syndrome—From genes to cognition. *Developmental Disabilities Research Reviews, 15*(4), 333–342.

Shaw, J. (2008). Trisomy 18: A case study. *Neonatal Network, 27*(1), 33–41.

Sherman, S., Pletcher, B., & Driscoll, D. (2005). Fragile X syndrome: Diagnostic and carrier testing. *Genetics in Medicine, 7*(8), 584–587.

Simpson, J., & Elias, S. (2003). *Genetics in obstetrics and gynecology*. Philadelphia: Saunders.

Snyder, C., Lynch, J., & Lynch, H. (2009). Genetic counseling and the advanced practice oncology nursing role in hereditary cancer prevention clinic: Hereditary breast cancer focus (part 1). *The Breast Journal, 15*(Suppl. 1), 2–10.

Soloman, B., Jack, B., & Feero, W. (2008). The clinical content of preconception care: Genetics and genomics. *American Journal of Obstetrics and Gynecology, 199*(6 Suppl. 2), S340–S344.

Sparbel, K., & Williams, J. (2009). Pregnancy as foreground in cystic fibrosis carrier testing decisions in primary care. *Genetic Testing and Molecular Biomarkers, 13*(1), 133–142.

Van Riper, M. (2005). Genetic testing and the family. *Journal of Midwifery & Women's Health, 50*(3), 227–233.

Van Riper, M. (2007). Families of children with Down syndrome: Responding to a "change of plans" with resilience. *Journal of Pediatric Nursing, 22*(2), 116–128.

Van Riper, M., & Gallo, A. (2006). Family, health, and genomics. In D. Crane, & E. Marshall (Eds.), *Handbook of families and health: Interdisciplinary perspectives.* Thousand Oaks, CA: Sage.

Van Riper, M., & McKinnon, W. (2004). Genetic testing for breast and ovarian cancer susceptibility: A family experience. *Journal of Midwifery & Women's Health, 43*(3), 210–219.

Wattendorf, D., & Hadley, D. (2005). Family history: A three-generation pedigree. *American Family Physician, 72*(3), 441–448.

Weinstein, S. (2009). Factor V Leiden: Impact on infusion nursing practice. *Journal of Infusion Nursing, 32*(4), 219–223.

Wirth, J. (2009). Case study: Trisomy 13, a palliative care case. *Neonatal Network, 28*(4), 263–266.

CHAPTER

4

Assessment and Health Promotion

Jan Lamarche Zdanuk

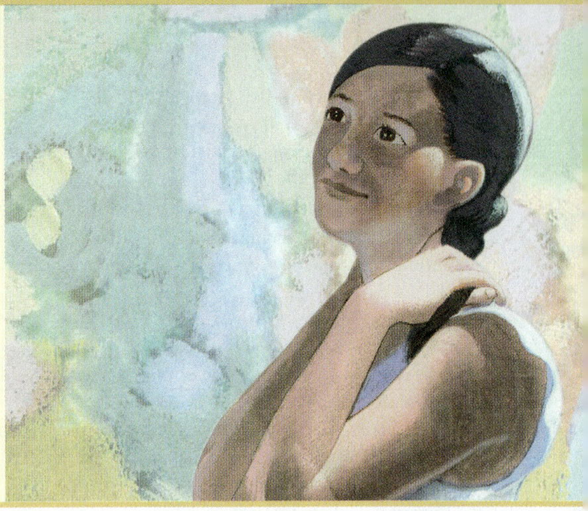

evolve WEBSITE

http://evolve.elsevier.com/Lowdermilk/MWHC/

- Anatomy Review
  - Adult Female Pelvis
  - Female Breast
  - Female External Genitalia
  - Female Pelvic Organs
- Animations
  - Breasts
  - Female Accessory Sex Organs
  - Female External Genitalia
  - Female Reproductive Ducts
  - Menstrual Cycle: Ovarian
  - Ovaries
  - Ovulation
- Audio Glossary
- Audio Key Points
- Case Study
  - Health Assessment
  - Women's Health and Conception Counseling
- NCLEX Review Questions
- Nursing Skill
  - Breast Self-Examination
- Spanish Guidelines
  - Menstruation
  - Physical Examination
- Video—Nursing Skills
  - Assisting with a Pelvic Examination
  - Teaching Breast Self-Examination

LEARNING OBJECTIVES

- Identify the structures and functions of the female reproductive system.
- Describe the menstrual cycle in relation to hormonal, ovarian, and endometrial response.
- Review the four phases of the sexual response cycle.
- Analyze barriers that may affect a woman's decision to seek health care.
- Investigate adaptation of the history and physical examination for women with special needs.
- Examine signs of abuse, screening, and referral to community agencies.
- Describe the history and physical examination.
- Identify the steps for assisting with and collecting specimens for Papanicolaou (Pap) testing.
- Review client teaching of breast self-examination.
- Analyze conditions that increase health risks for women across the life span.
- Describe anticipatory guidance that prevents disease, promotes health and self-management.
- Outline health-screening and immunization recommendations for women across the life span.

Most females initially enter the health care system because of a woman's health-related concern such as the need for a Pap test, vaginal infection, irregular menses, contraceptive needs, or pregnancy. It is important for health care providers to recognize the need for health promotion, health maintenance, and disease prevention and to offer these services across the life span of women.

This chapter reviews female anatomy and physiology including the menstrual cycle. Physical assessment and screening for disease prevention for women are presented. Barriers to seeking health care and an overview of conditions that increase health risks across the life span such as cardiovascular disease, obesity, and nutritional deficiencies are described. Anticipatory guidance suggestions including nutrition, exercise, and health screenings for women across the life span are discussed.

FEMALE REPRODUCTIVE SYSTEM

The female reproductive system consists of external structures visible from the pubis to the perineum and internal structures located in the pelvic cavity. The external and internal female reproductive structures develop and mature in response to estrogen and progesterone, starting in fetal life and continuing through puberty and the childbearing years. Reproductive

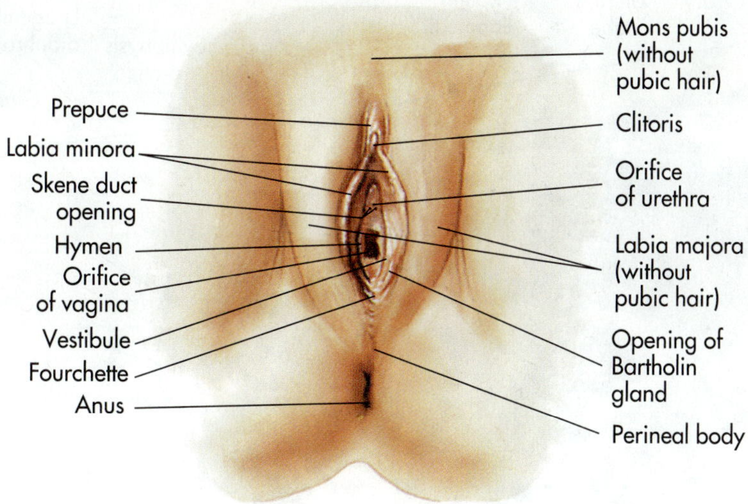

FIG. 4-1 External female genitalia.

Anatomy Review—Female External Genitalia

structures atrophy with age or in response to a decrease in ovarian hormone production. A complex nerve and blood supply supports the functions of these structures. The appearance of the external genitals varies greatly among women. Heredity, age, race, and the number of children a woman has borne influence the size, shape, and color of her external organs.

External Structures

The external genital organs, or *vulva,* include all structures visible externally from the pubis to the perineum: the mons pubis, the labia majora, the labia minora, the clitoris, the vestibular glands, the vaginal vestibule, the vaginal orifice, and the urethral opening. The external genital organs are illustrated in Figure 4-1. The *mons pubis* is a fatty pad that lies over the anterior surface of the symphysis pubis. In the postpubertal female, the mons is covered with coarse, curly hair. The *labia majora* are two rounded folds of fatty tissue covered with skin that extend downward and backward from the mons pubis. The labia are highly vascular structures whose outer surfaces develop hair after puberty. They protect the inner vulvar structures. The *labia minora* are two flat reddish folds of tissue visible when the labia majora are separated. No hair follicles are in the labia minora, but many sebaceous follicles and a few sweat glands are present. The interior of the labia minora is composed of connective tissue and smooth muscle and supplied with extremely sensitive nerve endings. Anteriorly, the labia minora fuse to form the *prepuce* (hoodlike covering of the clitoris) and the *frenulum* (fold of tissue under the clitoris). The labia minora join to form a thin flat tissue called the *fourchette* underneath the vaginal opening at midline. The *clitoris* is located underneath the prepuce. It is a small structure composed of erectile tissue with numerous sensory nerve endings. During sexual arousal the clitoris increases in size.

The vaginal *vestibule* is an almond-shaped area enclosed by the labia minora that contains openings to the urethra, Skene glands, vagina, and Bartholin glands. The urethra is not a reproductive organ but is considered here because of its location. It usually is found about 2.5 cm below the clitoris. Skene glands are located on each side of the urethra and produce mucus, which aids in lubrication of the vagina. The vaginal opening is in the lower portion of the vestibule and varies in shape and size. The hymen, a connective tissue membrane, surrounds the vaginal opening. It can be perforated during strenuous exercise, insertion of tampons, masturbation, and vaginal intercourse. Bartholin glands (see Fig. 4-1) lie under the constrictor muscles of the vagina and are located posteriorly on the sides of the vaginal opening, although the ductal openings are usually not visible. During sexual arousal, the glands secrete a clear mucus to lubricate the vaginal introitus.

The area between the fourchette and the anus is the **perineum,** a skin-covered muscular area that covers the pelvic structures. The perineum forms the base of the perineal body, a wedge-shaped mass that serves as an anchor for the muscles, fascia, and ligaments of the pelvis. The pelvic organs are supported by muscles and ligaments that form a sling.

Internal Structures

Animation—Female External Genitalia

The internal structures include the vagina, the uterus, the uterine tubes, and the ovaries. The vagina is a fibromuscular, collapsible tubular structure that extends from the vulva to the uterus and lies between the bladder and rectum. During the reproductive years the mucosal lining is arranged in transverse folds called rugae. These rugae allow the vagina to expand during childbirth. Estrogen deprivation that occurs after childbirth, during lactation, and at menopause causes dryness and thinning of the vaginal walls and smoothing of the rugae. The vagina, particularly the lower segment, has few sensory nerve endings. Vaginal secretions are slightly acidic (pH 4 to 5) so that vaginal susceptibility to infections is reduced. The vagina serves as a passageway for menstrual flow, as a female organ of copulation, and as a part of the birth canal for vaginal childbirth. The uterine cervix projects into a blind vault at the upper end of the vagina. There are anterior, posterior, and lateral pockets called fornices (singular, fornix) that surround the cervix. The internal pelvic organs can be palpated through the thin walls of these fornices.

The *uterus* is a muscular organ shaped like an upside-down pear that sits midline in the pelvic cavity between the bladder

Animation—Female Reproductive Ducts

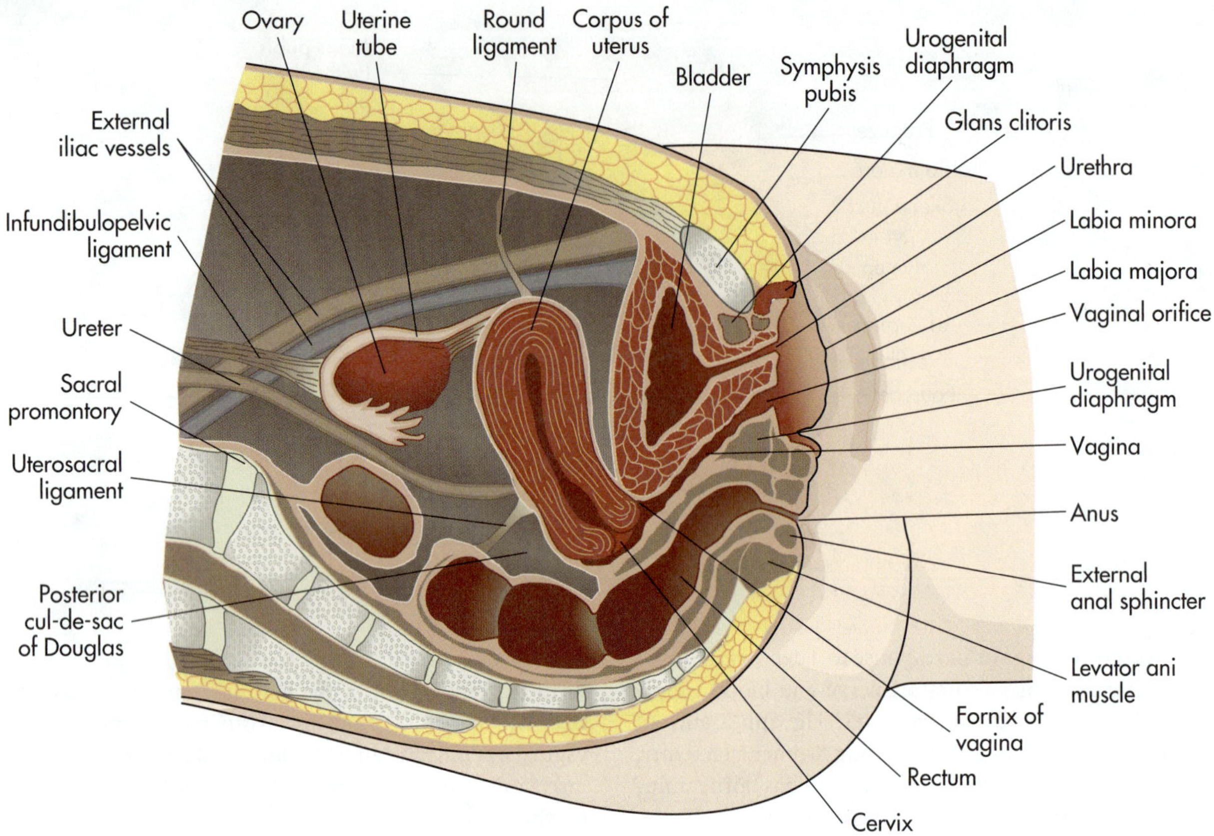

FIG. 4-2 Midsagittal view of female pelvic organs with woman lying supine.

and rectum and above the vagina. Four pairs of ligaments support the uterus: the cardinal, the uterosacral, the round, and the broad. Single anterior and posterior ligaments also support the uterus. The cul-de-sac of Douglas is a deep pouch, or recess, posterior to the cervix formed by the posterior ligament.

The uterus is divided into two major parts, an upper triangular portion called the corpus and a lower cylindric portion called the *cervix* (Fig. 4-2). The *fundus* is the dome-shaped top of the uterus and is the site at which the uterine tubes enter the uterus. The isthmus (lower uterine segment) is a short, constricted portion that separates the corpus from the cervix.

The uterus serves for reception, implantation, retention, and nutrition of the fertilized ovum and later of the fetus during pregnancy, and for expulsion of the fetus during childbirth. It also is responsible for cyclic menstruation.

Anatomy Review—Female Pelvic Organs

The uterine wall comprises three layers: the endometrium, the myometrium, and part of the peritoneum (membrane that covers the abdominal wall). The endometrium is a highly vascular lining made up of three layers, the outer two of which are shed during menstruation. The myometrium is made up of layers of smooth muscles that extend in three different directions (longitudinal, transverse, and oblique) (Fig. 4-3). Longitudinal fibers of the outer myometrial layer are found mostly in the fundus, and this arrangement assists in expelling the fetus during the birth process. The middle layer contains fibers from all three directions, which form a figure-eight pattern encircling large blood vessels. These fibers assist in ligating blood vessels after childbirth and control blood loss. Most of the circular fibers of the inner myometrial layer are around the site where the uterine tubes enter the uterus and around the internal cervical os (opening). These fibers help keep the cervix closed during pregnancy and prevent menstrual blood from flowing back into the uterine tubes during menstruation.

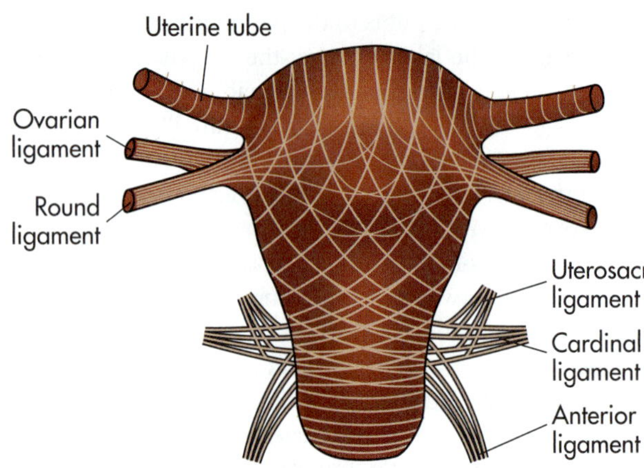

FIG. 4-3 Schematic arrangement of directions of muscle fibers. Note that uterine muscle fibers are continuous with supportive ligaments of uterus.

The cervix is made up of mostly fibrous connective tissues and elastic tissue, making it possible for the cervix to stretch during vaginal childbirth. The opening between the uterine cavity and the canal that connects the uterine cavity to the vagina (endocervical canal) is the internal os. The narrowed opening between the endocervix and the vagina is the external os, a small circular opening in women who have never been pregnant. The cervix feels firm (like the end of a nose) with a dimple in the center, which marks the external os.

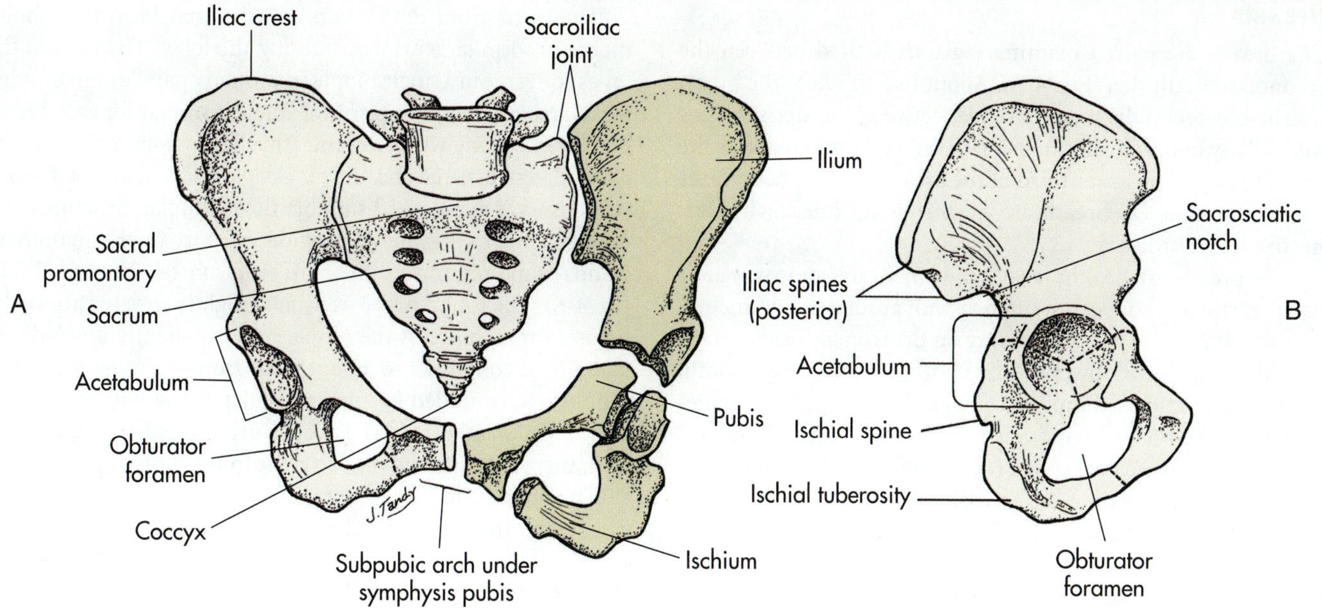

FIG. 4-4 Adult female pelvis. **A,** Anterior view. **B,** External view of innominate bone (fused).

The outer cervix is covered with a layer of squamous epithelium. The mucosa of the cervical canal is covered with columnar epithelium and contains numerous glands that secrete mucus in response to ovarian hormones. The **squamocolumnar junction,** where the two types of cells meet, is usually located just inside the cervical os. This junction also is called the *transformation zone,* the most common site for neoplastic changes (see Fig. 11-12); cells from this site are scraped for the Pap test (see later discussion).

The *uterine tubes* (fallopian tubes) attach to the uterine fundus. The tubes are supported by the broad ligaments and range from 8 to 14 cm in length. The tubes are divided into four sections: the interstitial portion is closest to the uterus; the isthmus and the ampulla are the middle portions; and the infundibulum is closest to the ovary. The uterine tubes form passages between the ovaries and the uterus for the passage of the ovum. The infundibulum has fimbriated ends, which pull the ovum into the tube. The ovum is pushed along the tubes to the uterus by rhythmic contractions of the muscles of the tubes and by the current that is produced by the movement of the cilia that line the tubes. The ovum is usually fertilized by the sperm in the ampulla portion of one of the tubes.

The *ovaries* are almond-shaped organs located on each side of the uterus below and behind the uterine tubes. During the reproductive years they are approximately 3 cm long, 2 cm wide, and 1 cm thick; they diminish in size after menopause. Before menarche each ovary has a smooth surface; after menarche they become nodular because of repeated ruptures of follicles at ovulation. The two functions of the ovaries are ovulation and hormone production. **Ovulation** is the release of a mature ovum from the ovary at intervals (usually monthly). Estrogen, progesterone, and androgen are the hormones produced by the ovaries.

The Bony Pelvis

The bony pelvis serves three primary purposes: protection of the pelvic structures, accommodation of the growing fetus during pregnancy, and anchorage of the pelvic support structures.

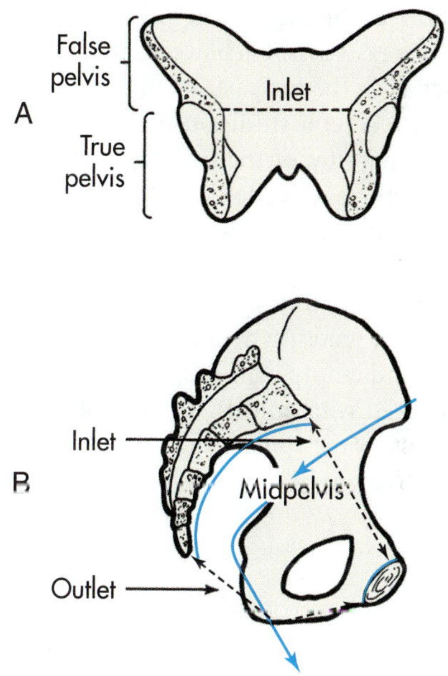

FIG. 4-5 Female pelvis. **A,** Cavity of false pelvis is shallow. **B,** Cavity of true pelvis is an irregularly curved canal *(arrows).*

Two innominate (hip) bones (consisting of ilium, ischium, and pubis), the sacrum, and the coccyx make up the four bones of the pelvis (Fig. 4-4). Cartilage and ligaments form the symphysis pubis, the sacrococcygeal joint, and two sacroiliac joints that separate the pelvic bones. The pelvis is divided into two parts: the false pelvis and the true pelvis (Fig. 4-5). The false pelvis is the upper portion above the pelvic brim or inlet. The true pelvis is the lower, curved bony canal, which includes the inlet, the cavity, and the outlet through which the fetus passes during vaginal birth. The upper portion of the outlet is at the level of the ischial spines, and the lower portion is at the level of the ischial tuberosities and the pubic arch (see Fig. 4-4). Variations that occur in the size and shape of the pelvis are usually due to age, race, and sex. Pelvic ossification is complete at about age 20 years.

Breasts

The breasts are paired mammary glands located between the second and sixth ribs (Fig. 4-6). About two thirds of the breast overlie the pectoralis major muscle, between the sternum and midaxillary line, with an extension to the axilla referred to as the tail of Spence. The lower third of the breast overlies the serratus anterior muscle. The breasts are attached to the muscles by connective tissue or fascia.

The breasts of healthy mature women are approximately equal in size and shape, but often are not absolutely symmetric. The size and shape vary depending on the woman's age, heredity, and nutrition. However, the contour should be smooth, with no retractions, dimpling, or masses. Estrogen stimulates growth of the breast by inducing fat deposition in the breasts, development of stromal tissue (i.e., increase in its amount and elasticity), and growth of the extensive ductile system. Estrogen also increases the vascularity of breast tissue.

Animation—Breasts

Once ovulation begins in puberty, progesterone levels increase. The increase in progesterone causes maturation of mammary gland tissue, specifically the lobules and acinar structures. During adolescence, fat deposition and growth of fibrous tissue contribute to the increase in the gland's size. Full development of the breasts is not achieved until after the end of the first pregnancy or in the early period of lactation.

Findings from several studies using ultrasound imaging to investigate the anatomy of the breast found differences from previous descriptions (Geddes, 2007; Love & Barsky, 2004; Ramsay, Kent, Hartmann, & Hartmann, 2005). The following description incorporates these findings. Each mammary gland is made of a number of lobes that are divided into lobules. Lobules are clusters of acini. An acinus is a saclike terminal part of a compound gland emptying through a narrow lumen or duct. The acini are lined with epithelial cells that secrete colostrum and milk. Just below the epithelium is the myoepithelium (*myo*, or muscle), which contracts to expel milk from the acini.

The ducts from the clusters of acini that form the lobules merge to form larger ducts draining the lobes. Ducts from the lobes converge in a single nipple (mammary papilla) surrounded by an areola. The anatomy of the ducts is similar for each breast but varies among women. Protective fatty tissue surrounds the glandular structures and ducts. *Cooper's ligaments*, or fibrous suspensory, separate and support the glandular structures and ducts. Cooper's ligaments provide support to the mammary glands while permitting their mobility on the chest wall (see Fig. 4-6). The round nipple is usually slightly elevated above the breast. On each breast the nipple projects slightly upward and laterally. It contains 4 to 20 openings from the milk ducts. The nipple is surrounded by fibromuscular tissue and covered by wrinkled skin (the areola). Except during pregnancy and lactation, there is usually no discharge from the nipple.

The nipple and surrounding areola are usually more deeply pigmented than the skin of the breast. The rough appearance of the areola is caused by sebaceous glands directly beneath the skin called *Montgomery tubercles*. These glands secrete a fatty substance, thought to lubricate the nipple. Smooth muscle fibers in the areola contract to stiffen the nipple to make it easier for the breastfeeding infant to grasp.

Besides their function of lactation, breasts function as organs for sexual arousal in the mature adult.

The vascular supply to the mammary gland is abundant. In the nonpregnant state, the skin has no obvious vascular pattern. The normal skin is smooth without tightness or shininess. The skin covering the breasts contains an extensive superficial lymphatic network that serves the entire chest wall and is continuous with the superficial lymphatics of the neck and abdomen. In the deeper portions of the breasts, the lymphatics form a rich network as well. The primary deep lymphatic pathway drains laterally toward the axillae.

The breasts change in size and nodularity in response to cyclic ovarian changes throughout reproductive life. Increasing

Anatomy Review—Female Breast

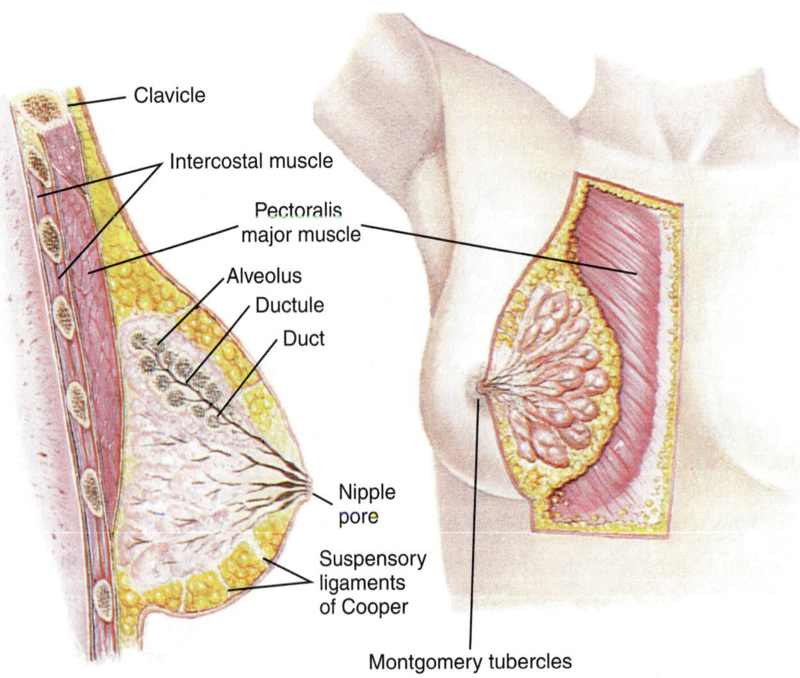

FIG. 4-6 Anatomy of the breast, showing position and major structures. (Adapted from Seidel, H., et al. [2011]. *Mosby's guide to physical examination* [7th ed.]. St. Louis: Mosby.)

levels of both estrogen and progesterone in the 3 to 4 days before menstruation increase the vascularity of the breasts, induce growth of the ducts and acini, and promote water retention. The epithelial cells lining the ducts proliferate in number, the ducts dilate, and the lobules distend. The acini become enlarged and secretory, and lipid (fat) is deposited within their epithelial cell lining. As a result, breast swelling, tenderness, and discomfort are common symptoms just before the onset of menstruation. After menstruation, cellular proliferation begins to regress; the acini begin to decrease in size; and retained water is lost. After breasts have undergone changes numerous times in response to the ovarian cycle, the proliferation and involution (regression) are not uniform throughout the breast. In time, after repeated hormonal stimulation, small persistent areas of nodulations may develop. This normal physiologic change must be remembered when breast tissue is examined. Nodules may develop just before and during menstruation, when the breast is most active. The physiologic alterations in breast size and activity reach their minimal level about 5 to 7 days after menstruation stops.

The best time for a woman who wishes to perform a **breast self-examination (BSE)** (palpation of breasts to detect changes in breast tissue) is during this phase of the menstrual cycle or whenever the breasts are not tender or swollen (see Teaching for Self-Management box: Breast Self-Examination).

Table 4-1 compares the variations in physical assessment related to age differences in women.

Nursing Skill—Breast Self-Examination

TEACHING FOR SELF-MANAGEMENT

Breast Self-Examination

If you choose to perform a breast self-examination, the best time is when breasts are not tender or swollen.

How to examine your breasts:

1. Lie down and put a pillow under your right shoulder. Place your right arm behind your head (Fig. 1).
2. Use the finger pads of your three middle fingers on your left hand to feel for lumps or thickening. Your finger pads are the top third of each finger. Use circular motions of the finger pads to feel the breast tissue.
3. Press firmly enough to know how your breast feels. Use light pressure to feel the tissue just under the skin, medium pressure for a little deeper, and firm pressure to feel the breast tissue close to the chest and ribs. A firm ridge in the lower curve of the breast is normal.
4. Move around the breast in a set way, such as using an up and down or vertical line pattern (Fig. 2). Go up to the collar bone and down to the ribs and from your underarm on the side to the middle of your chest. Use the same technique every time. It will help you to make sure that you have gone over the entire breast area and to remember how your breast feels.
5. Now examine your left breast using the finger pads of your right hand.
6. You may want to check your breasts while standing in front of a mirror. See if there are any changes in the way your breasts look: dimpling of the skin, changes in the nipple, or redness or swelling.
7. You may also want to perform an extra breast self-examination while you are in the shower (Fig. 3). Your soapy hands will glide over the wet skin, making it easy to check how your breasts feel.
8. Checking the area between the breast and the underarm and the underarm itself is important. Examine the area above the breast to the collarbone and to the shoulder while you are standing or sitting up with your arms lightly raised.
9. If you find any changes, see your health care provider right away.

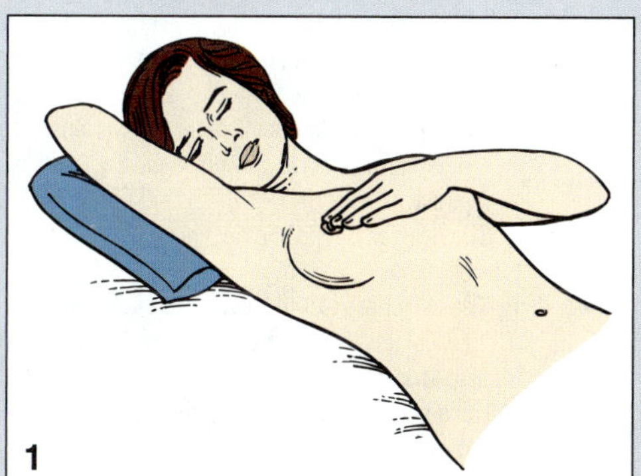
1

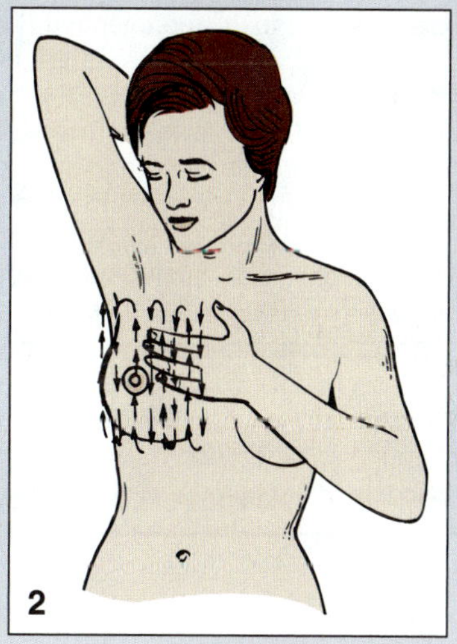
2

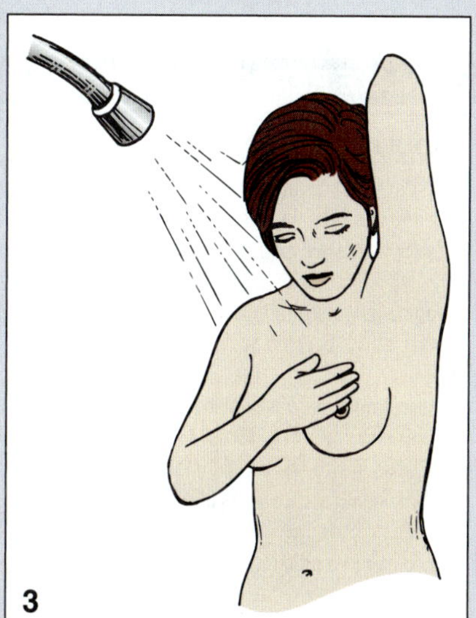
3

Source: American Cancer Society. (2008). *How to perform a breast self-exam.* Available at www.cancer.org. Accessed January 20, 2010.

Video—Nursing Skill: Teaching Breast Self-Examination

EVIDENCE-BASED PRACTICE

Pat Gingrich

Teaching Women Breast Self-Examination: Is It Worthwhile?

ASK THE QUESTION

Does teaching women breast self-examination actually result in fewer deaths from breast cancer?

SEARCH FOR EVIDENCE

Search Strategies

Professional organization guidelines, meta-analyses, systematic reviews, randomized controlled trials, nonrandomized prospective studies and retrospective studies since 2006.

Databases Searched

CINAHL, Cochrane, Medline, National Guideline Clearinghouse, and websites for the Association for Women's Health, Obstetric and Neonatal Nurses, American Cancer Society, and National Cancer Institute.

CRITICALLY ANALYZE THE DATA

The ideal screening test for breast cancer would have a high sensitivity for breast cancer in an early, curable stage, thus decreasing mortality. Moreover, it would have a high specificity, meaning few false positives and thus few unnecessary diagnostic tests. Screening for breast cancer has conventionally consisted of breast self-examination monthly, clinical breast examination (CBE) yearly, and screening mammogram every one to two years after 40 years of age. Of these, screening mammogram has been the gold standard, responsible for a 15% decrease in mortality in a meta-analysis of seven trials, representing 600,000 women (Gotzsche & Nielsen, 2009). Mammograms are limited by their cost, discomfort, geographical availability, skilled interpretation, exposure to radiation, and high false-positive rates and in the meta-analysis led to 30% overdiagnosis and overtreatment.

Mammograms are usually accompanied by a clinical breast examination by a trained examiner. Since the 1970s, women were also routinely taught to do breast self-examination (BSE). The assumption was that BSE was a low-tech screening tool for women to detect tumors in the early, more treatable stages. This theory was challenged by a classic meta-analysis of two randomized controlled trials involving 388,535 women in Russia and Shanghai, which found no difference in cancer mortality between groups taught BSE and control groups without the BSE education (Kosters & Gotzsche, 2003, updated 2007). In fact, the BSE group was twice as likely to undergo unnecessary biopsy with benign results as the control group. The authors noted poor compliance with BSE, but note that it was possible that BSE may have decreased mortality in some countries.

Breast cancer screening recommendations from the National Cancer Institute include CBE and screening mammogram (NCI, 2009). The NCI organization guidelines note that BSE alone has not been shown to reduce mortality, but do encourage women to be alert to any changes in their breasts and report them to their health care provider.

IMPLICATIONS FOR PRACTICE

Breast self-examination is a low-tech, low-cost technique that can empower some women to discover breast changes earlier. It is not clear that this will decrease mortality. BSE and CBE may also result in unnecessary testing. A Breast Health Global Initiative panel recommends "breast health awareness," a combination of education and BSE that may provide the greatest value by promoting breast awareness in low-resource areas (Smith et al. 2006). Nurses should offer to teach the technique to women who wish to learn. However, some women are not comfortable examining their breasts, or find it frightening. All women should be taught to follow the recommended guidelines for clinical breast examination yearly and mammograms based on age and personal history.

References

Gotzsche, P., & Nielsen, M. (2009). Screening for breast cancer with mammography. In *The Cochrane Database of Systematic Reviews 2010*, 4, Chichester, UK: John Wiley & Sons.

Kosters, J., & Gotzsche, P. (2003). Regular self-examination or clinical examination for early detection of breast cancer. *The Cochrane Database of Systematic Reviews 2010*, 4, Chichester, UK: John Wiley & Sons.

National Cancer Institute. (2009). *What you need to know about breast cancer.* Available at www.gov/cancertopics/wyntk/breast. Accessed May 11, 2010.

Smith, R., Caleffi, M., Albert, U., Chen, T., Duffy, S., Franceschi, D., & Nystrom, L. (2006). Breast cancer in limited-resource countries: Early detection and access to care. *Breast J, 12*(Suppl 1), S16–S26, 2006.

TABLE 4-1 FEMALE REPRODUCTIVE PHYSICAL ASSESSMENT ACROSS THE LIFE CYCLE

	ADOLESCENT	ADULT	POSTMENOPAUSAL
Breasts	Tender when developing; buds appear; small, firm; one side may grow faster; areola diameter increases; nipples more erect	Grow to full shape in early adulthood; nipples and areola become pinker and darker	Become stringy, irregular, pendulous, and nodular; borders less well delineated; may shrink, become flatter, elongated, and less elastic; ligaments weaken; nipples are positioned lower
Vagina	Vagina lengthens; epithelial layers thicken; secretions become acidic	Growth complete by age 20	Introitus constricts; vagina narrows, shortens, loses rugation; mucosa is pale, thin, and dry; walls may lose structural integrity
Uterus	Musculature and vasculature increase; lining thickens	Growth complete by age 20	Size decreases; endometrial lining thins
Ovaries	Increase in size and weight; menarche occurs between 8 and 16 years of age; ovulation occurs monthly	Growth complete by age 20	Size decreases to 1 to 2 cm; follicles disappear; surface convolutes; ovarian function ceases between 40 and 55 years of age
Labia majora	Become more prominent; hair develops	Growth complete by age 20	Labia become smaller and flatter; pubic hair sparse and gray
Labia minora	Become more vascular	Growth complete by age 20	Become shinier and drier
Uterine tubes	Increase in size	Growth complete by age 20	Decrease in size

MENSTRUATION AND MENOPAUSE

Nurses should be knowledgeable about menarche, the hypothalamic-pituitary cycle, the ovarian cycle, the endometrial cycle, other cyclic changes, and the climacteric because they provide care for women across the life span.

Menarche and Puberty

Although young girls secrete small, rather constant amounts of estrogen, a marked increase occurs between ages 8 and 11 years. The term **menarche** denotes first menstruation. **Puberty** is a broader term that denotes the entire transitional stage between childhood and sexual maturity. Increasing amounts and variations in gonadotropin and estrogen secretion develop into a cyclic pattern at least a year before menarche. In North America this occurs in most girls at about age 13 years.

Initially, for most women, periods are irregular, unpredictable, painless, and *anovulatory* (no ovum released from the ovary). After 1 or more years, a hypothalamic-pituitary rhythm develops, and the ovary produces adequate cyclic estrogen to make a mature ovum. *Ovulatory* (ovum released from ovary) periods tend to be regular, monitored by progesterone.

Although pregnancy can occur in exceptional cases of true precocious puberty, most pregnancies in young girls occur after the normally timed menarche. All young adolescents of both sexes would benefit from knowing that pregnancy can occur at any time after the onset of menses.

Menstrual Cycle

Menstruation is the periodic uterine bleeding that begins approximately 14 days after ovulation. It is controlled by a feedback system of three cycles: hypothalamic-pituitary, ovarian, and endometrial. The average length of a menstrual cycle is 28 days, but variations are normal. The first day of bleeding is designated day 1 of the menstrual cycle, or menses (Fig. 4-7). The average duration of menstrual flow is 5 days (range, 3 to 6 days), and the average blood loss is 50 ml (range, 20 to 80 ml), but these vary greatly.

For about 50% of women, menstrual blood does not appear to clot. The menstrual blood clots within the uterus, but the clot usually liquefies before being discharged from the uterus. Uterine discharge includes mucus and epithelial cells in addition to blood.

The menstrual cycle is a complex interplay of events that occur simultaneously in the endometrium, the hypothalamus, the pituitary glands, and the ovaries. The menstrual cycle prepares the uterus for pregnancy. When pregnancy does not occur, menstruation follows. The woman's age, physical and emotional status, and environment influence the regularity of her menstrual cycles.

Hypothalamic-Pituitary Cycle

Toward the end of the normal menstrual cycle, blood levels of estrogen and progesterone decrease. Low blood levels of these ovarian hormones stimulate the hypothalamus to secrete gonadotropin-releasing hormone (GnRH). In turn, GnRH stimulates anterior pituitary secretion of follicle-stimulating hormone (FSH). FSH stimulates development of ovarian graafian follicles and their production of estrogen. Estrogen levels begin to decrease, and hypothalamic GnRH triggers the anterior pituitary to release luteinizing hormone (LH). A marked surge of LH and a smaller peak of estrogen (day 12; see Fig. 4-7) precede the expulsion of the ovum from the graafian follicle by about 24 to 36 hours. LH peaks at about day 13 or 14 of a 28-day cycle. If fertilization and implantation of the ovum have not occurred by this time, regression of the corpus luteum follows. Levels of progesterone and estrogen decline, menstruation occurs, and the hypothalamus is once again stimulated to secrete GnRH. This process is called the hypothalamic-pituitary cycle.

Ovarian Cycle

The primitive graafian follicles contain immature oocytes (primordial ova). Before ovulation from 1 to 30 follicles begin to mature in each ovary under the influence of FSH and estrogen. The preovulatory surge of LH affects a selected follicle. The oocyte matures, ovulation occurs, and the empty follicle begins its transformation to the corpus luteum. This follicular phase (preovulatory phase; see Fig. 4-7) of the ovarian cycle varies in length from woman to woman. Almost all variations in ovarian cycle length are the result of variations in the length of the follicular phase (Fehring, Schneider, & Raviele, 2006). On rare occasions (i.e., 1 in 100 menstrual cycles), more than one follicle is selected, and more than one oocyte matures and undergoes ovulation.

After ovulation, estrogen levels decrease. For 90% of women only a small amount of withdrawal bleeding occurs, so it goes unnoticed. In 10% of women there is sufficient bleeding for it to be visible, resulting in what is termed *midcycle bleeding.*

The luteal phase begins immediately after ovulation and ends with the start of menstruation. This postovulatory phase of the ovarian cycle usually requires 14 days (range, 13 to 15 days). The corpus luteum reaches its peak of functional activity 8 days after ovulation, secreting the steroids estrogen and progesterone. Simultaneously with peak luteal functioning, the fertilized ovum is implanted in the endometrium.

If implantation does not occur, the corpus luteum regresses, steroid levels decrease, and the functional layer of the uterine endometrium is shed through menstruation.

Endometrial Cycle

The four phases of the endometrial cycle are (1) the menstrual phase, (2) the proliferative phase, (3) the secretory phase, and (4) the ischemic phase (see Fig. 4-7). During the menstrual phase shedding of the functional two thirds of the endometrium (the compact and spongy layers) is initiated by periodic vasoconstriction in the upper layers of the endometrium. The basal layer is always retained, and regeneration begins near the end of the cycle from cells derived from the remaining glandular remnants or stromal cells in this layer.

The proliferative phase is a period of rapid growth lasting from about the fifth day to the time of ovulation. The endometrial surface is completely restored in approximately 4 days, or slightly before bleeding ceases. From this point on, an eight- to tenfold thickening occurs, with a leveling off of growth at ovulation. The proliferative phase depends on estrogen stimulation derived from ovarian follicles.

The secretory phase extends from the day of ovulation to about 3 days before the next menstrual period. After ovulation

Spanish Guidelines—Menstruation

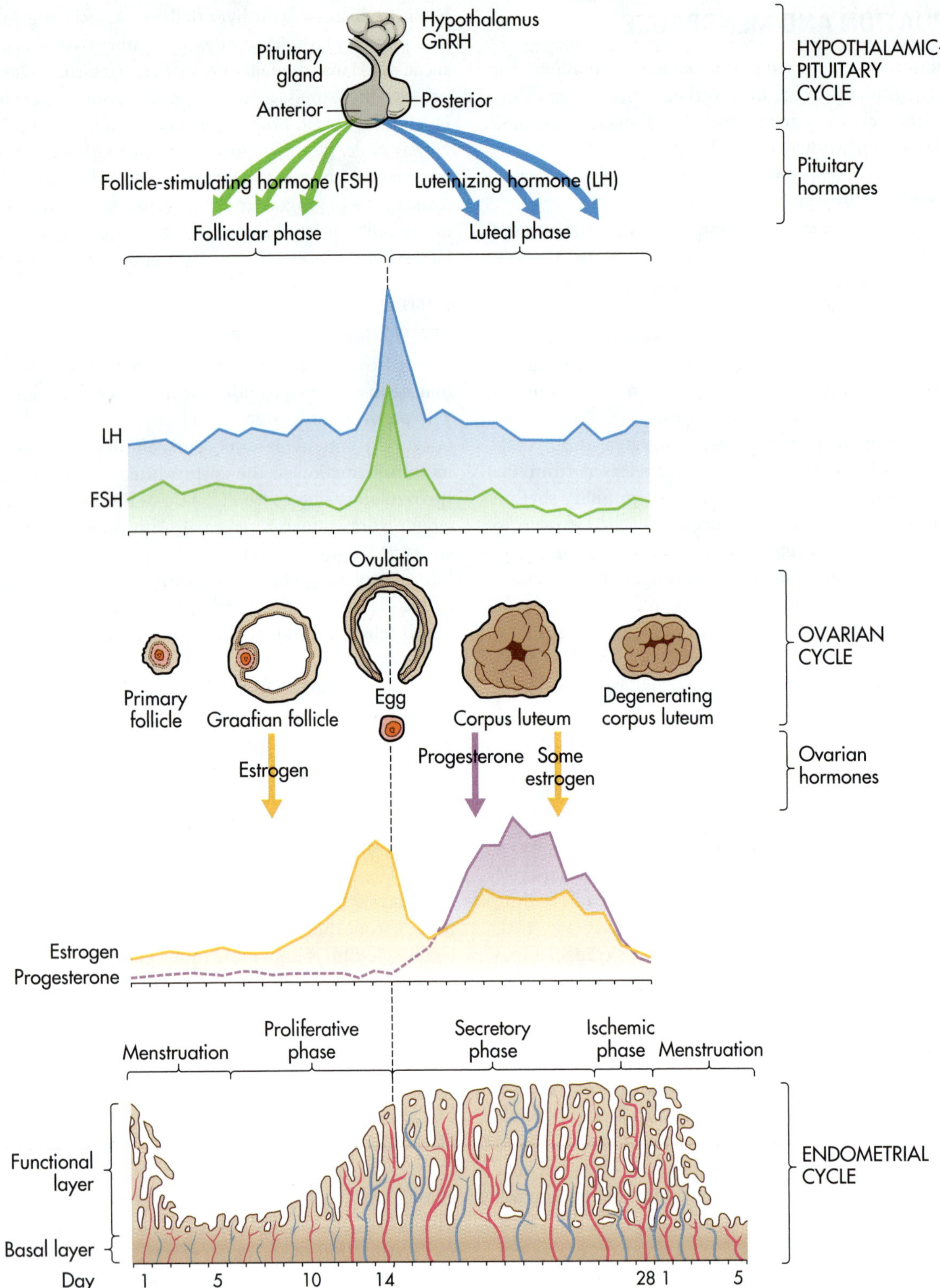

FIG. 4-7 Menstrual cycle: hypothalamic-pituitary, ovarian, and endometrial.

larger amounts of progesterone are produced. An edematous, vascular, functional endometrium becomes apparent. At the end of the secretory phase the fully matured secretory endometrium reaches the thickness of heavy, soft velvet. It becomes luxuriant with blood and glandular secretions, a suitable protective and nutritive bed for a fertilized ovum.

Implantation of the fertilized ovum generally occurs about 7 to 10 days after ovulation. If fertilization and implantation do not occur, the corpus luteum, which secretes estrogen and progesterone, regresses. With the rapid decrease in progesterone and estrogen levels, the spiral arteries go into spasm. During the ischemic phase the blood supply to the functional endometrium is blocked, and necrosis develops. The functional layer separates from the basal layer, and menstrual bleeding begins, marking day 1 of the next cycle (see Fig. 4-7).

Other Cyclic Changes

When the hypothalamic-pituitary-ovarian axis functions properly, other tissues undergo predictable responses. Before ovulation, the woman's basal body temperature (BBT) is often less than 37° C; after ovulation, with increasing progesterone levels, her BBT increases. Changes in the cervix and cervical mucus follow a generally predictable pattern. Preovulatory and postovulatory mucus is viscous (thick), so that sperm penetration is discouraged. At the time of ovulation, cervical mucus is thin and clear. It looks, feels, and stretches like egg white. This stretchable quality is termed *spinnbarkeit* (see Chapter 8). Some women have localized lower abdominal pain called *mittelschmerz* that coincides with ovulation. Some spotting may occur.

Prostaglandins

Prostaglandins (PGs) are oxygenated fatty acids classified as hormones. The different kinds of PGs are distinguished by letters (PGE, PGF), numbers (PGE_2), and letters of the Greek alphabet ($PGF_{2\alpha}$).

Prostaglandins are produced in most organs of the body, including the uterus. Menstrual blood is a potent prostaglandin source. PGs are metabolized quickly by most tissues. They are biologically active in minute amounts in the cardiovascular, gastrointestinal, respiratory, urogenital, and nervous systems. They also exert a marked effect on metabolism, particularly on glycolysis. Prostaglandins play an important role in many physiologic, pathologic, and pharmacologic reactions. $PGF_{2\alpha}$, PGE_4, and PGE_2 are most commonly used in reproductive medicine.

Prostaglandins affect smooth muscle contractility and modulation of hormonal activity. Indirect evidence suggests that PGs have an effect on ovulation, fertility, changes in the cervix, and cervical mucus that affect receptivity to sperm, tubal and uterine motility, sloughing of endometrium (menstruation), onset of abortion (spontaneous and induced), and onset of labor (term and preterm).

After exerting their biologic actions, newly synthesized PGs are rapidly metabolized by tissues in such organs as the lungs, the kidneys, and the liver.

Prostaglandins may play a key role in ovulation. If PG levels do not increase along with the surge of LH, the ovum remains trapped within the graafian follicle. After ovulation, PGs may influence production of estrogen and progesterone by the corpus luteum.

The introduction of PGs into the vagina or into the uterine cavity (from ejaculated semen) increases the motility of uterine musculature, which can assist the transport of sperm through the uterus and into the oviduct.

Prostaglandins produced by the woman cause regression of the corpus luteum, regression of the endometrium, and sloughing of the endometrium, resulting in menstruation. PGs increase myometrial response to oxytocic stimulation, enhance uterine contractions, and cause cervical dilation. They may be a factor in the initiation of labor, the maintenance of labor, or both. They also may be involved in dysmenorrhea (see Chapter 6) and preeclampsia-eclampsia (see Chapter 27).

Climacteric and Menopause

The **climacteric** is a transitional phase during which ovarian function and hormone production decline. This phase spans the years from the onset of premenopausal ovarian decline to the postmenopausal time when symptoms stop. **Menopause** (from the Latin *mensis,* month, and Greek *pausis,* to cease) refers only to the last menstrual period. Unlike menarche, however, menopause can be dated with certainty only 1 year after menstruation ceases. The average age at natural menopause is 51.4 years, with an age range of 35 to 60 years. **Perimenopause** is a period preceding menopause that lasts about 4 years. During this time, ovarian function declines. Ova slowly diminish, and menstrual cycles may be anovulatory, resulting in irregular bleeding. The ovary stops producing estrogen, and eventually menses no longer occur.

Animation—Female Accessory Sex Organs

SEXUAL RESPONSE

The hypothalamus and anterior pituitary gland in females regulate the production of FSH and LH. The target tissue for these hormones is the ovary, which produces ova and secretes estrogen and progesterone. A feedback mechanism between hormone secretion from the ovaries, the hypothalamus, and the anterior pituitary aids in the control of the production of sex cells and steroid sex hormone secretion.

Although the first outward appearance of maturing sexual development occurs at an earlier age in females, both females and males achieve physical maturity at approximately age 17 years; however, individual development varies greatly. Anatomic and reproductive differences notwithstanding, women and men are more alike than different in their physiologic response to sexual excitement and orgasm. For example, the glans clitoris and the glans penis are embryonic homologues. Little difference exists between female and male sexual response; the physical response is essentially the same whether stimulated by coitus, fantasy, or masturbation. Physiologically, according to Masters (1992), sexual response can be analyzed in terms of two processes: vasocongestion and myotonia.

Sexual stimulation results in an increase in circulation to circumvaginal blood vessels (lubrication in the female), causing engorgement and distention of the genitals. Venous congestion is localized primarily in the genitals, but it also occurs to a lesser degree in the breasts and other parts of the body. Arousal is characterized by myotonia (increased muscular tension), resulting in voluntary and involuntary rhythmic contractions. Examples of sexually stimulated myotonia are pelvic thrusting, facial grimacing, and spasms of the hands and feet (carpopedal spasms).

The **sexual response cycle** is divided into four phases: excitement phase, plateau phase, orgasmic phase, and resolution phase. The four phases occur progressively, with no sharp dividing line between any two phases. Specific body changes take place in sequence. The time, intensity, and duration for cyclic completion also vary for individuals and situations. Table 4-2 compares male and female body changes during each of the four phases of the sexual response cycle.

REASONS FOR ENTERING THE HEALTH CARE SYSTEM

Women's health assessment and screening focus on a systems evaluation, beginning with a careful history and physical examination. During the assessment and evaluation, the

TABLE 4-2 FOUR PHASES OF SEXUAL RESPONSE

REACTIONS COMMON TO BOTH SEXES	FEMALE REACTIONS	MALE REACTIONS
Excitement Phase		
Heart rate and blood pressure increase. Nipples become erect. Myotonia begins.	Clitoris increases in diameter and swells. External genitals become congested and darken. Vaginal lubrication occurs; upper two thirds of vagina lengthen and extend. Cervix and uterus pull upward. Breast size increases.	Erection of the penis begins; penis increases in length and diameter. Scrotal skin becomes congested and thickens. Testes begin to increase in size and elevate toward the body.
Plateau Phase		
Heart rate and blood pressure continue to increase. Respirations increase. Myotonia becomes pronounced; grimacing occurs.	Clitoral head retracts under the clitoral hood. Lower one third of vagina becomes engorged. Skin color changes occur—red flush may be observed across breasts, abdomen, or other surfaces.	Head of penis may enlarge slightly. Scrotum continues to grow tense and thicken. Testes continue to elevate and enlarge. Preorgasmic emission of two or three drops of fluid appears on the head of the penis.
Orgasmic Phase		
Heart rate, blood pressure, and respirations increase to maximum levels. Involuntary muscle spasms occur. External rectal sphincter contracts.	Strong rhythmic contractions are felt in the clitoris, vagina, and uterus. Sensations of warmth spread through the pelvic area.	Testes elevate to maximum level. Point of "inevitability" occurs just before ejaculation and an awareness of fluid in the urethra. Rhythmic contractions occur in the penis. Ejaculation of semen occurs.
Resolution Phase		
Heart rate, blood pressure, and respirations return to normal. Nipple erection subsides. Myotonia subsides	Engorgement in external genitalia and vagina resolves. Uterus descends to normal position. Cervix dips into seminal pool. Breast size decreases. Skin flush disappears.	Fifty percent of erection is lost immediately with ejaculation; penis gradually returns to normal size. Testes and scrotum return to normal size. Refractory period (time needed for erection to occur again) varies according to age and general physical condition.

responsibilities for self-management, health promotion, and enhancement of wellness are emphasized. Nursing care includes assessment, planning, education, counseling, and referral as needed, as well as commendations for good self-care that the woman has practiced. This enables women to make informed decisions about their own health care.

Preconception Counseling and Care

Preconception health promotion provides women and their partners with information that is needed to make decisions about their reproductive future. Preconception counseling guides couples on how to prevent unintended pregnancies and to achieve pregnancy when desired, stresses risk management, and identifies healthy behaviors that promote the well-being of the woman and her potential fetus (Moos, 2006).

All providers who treat women for well-woman care or other routine care should incorporate preconception health screening as part of the routine care for women of reproductive age (Johnson, Posner, Biermann, Cordero, Atrash, Parker, et al., 2006). The initiation of activities that promote healthy mothers and babies must occur before the period of critical fetal organ development, which is between 17 and 56 days after fertilization. By the end of the eighth week after conception and certainly by the end of the first trimester, any major structural anomalies in the fetus are already present. Because many women do not realize that they are pregnant and do not seek prenatal care until well into the first trimester, the rapidly growing fetus may be exposed to many types of intrauterine environmental hazards during this most vulnerable developmental phase.

Case Study—Women's Health and Conception Counseling

Preconception care is important for women who have had a problem with a previous pregnancy (e.g., miscarriage, preterm birth). Although causes are not always identifiable, in many cases, problems can be identified and treated and may not recur in subsequent pregnancies. Preconception care is also important to minimize fetal malformations. For example, the woman may be exposed to teratogenic agents such as drugs, viruses, and chemicals, or she may have a genetically inherited disease. Preconception counseling can educate the woman about the effects of these agents and diseases, which can help prevent harm to the fetus or allow the woman to make an informed decision about her willingness to accept potential hazards should a pregnancy occur (Atrash, Johnson, Adams, Cordero, & Howse, 2006).

A model for preconception care of women of reproductive age targets all women from menarche to menopause at every encounter, not just in maternity and women's health. Providing optimal health care for women whether or not they desire to conceive can result in a high level of preconception wellness (Moos, 2006). Suggested components of preconception care, such as health promotion, risk assessment, and interventions, are outlined in Box 4-1.

Pregnancy

A woman's entry into health care is often associated with pregnancy, either for diagnosis or for actual care. The possibility of pregnancy is realized most commonly when a woman is late with her menses. If she is pregnant, it is desirable for a woman to enter prenatal care within the first 12 weeks. This allows early pregnancy counseling, especially for the woman who has had no preconception care. Major goals of prenatal care are found in Box 4-2 and should be initiated at the first visit. Extensive discussion of pregnancy is found in Chapter 15.

Well-Woman Care

Current trends in the health care of women have expanded beyond a reproductive focus. A holistic approach to women's health care includes a woman's health needs throughout her lifetime. This view goes beyond simply her reproductive needs. This restructuring places women's health within the primary

BOX 4-1 COMPONENTS OF PRECONCEPTION CARE

HEALTH PROMOTION: GENERAL TEACHING

- Nutrition
  - Healthy diet, including folic acid
  - Optimal weight
- Exercise and rest
- Avoidance of substance abuse (tobacco, alcohol, "recreational" drugs)
- Use of risk-reducing sex practices
- Attending to family and social needs

RISK FACTOR ASSESSMENT

- Chronic diseases
  - Diabetes, heart disease, hypertension, asthma, thyroid disease, kidney disease, anemia, mental illness
- Infectious diseases
  - HIV/AIDS, other sexually transmitted infections, vaccine-preventable diseases (e.g., rubella, hepatitis B)
- Reproductive history
  - Contraception
  - Pregnancies—unplanned pregnancy, pregnancy outcomes
  - Infertility
- Genetic or inherited conditions (e.g., sickle cell anemia, Down syndrome, cystic fibrosis)
- Medications and medical treatment
  - Prescription medications (especially those contraindicated in pregnancy), over-the-counter medication use, radiation exposure
- Personal behaviors and exposures
  - Smoking, alcohol consumption, illicit drug use
  - Overweight or underweight; eating disorders
  - Folic acid supplement use
  - Spouse or partner and family situation, including intimate partner violence
  - Availability of family or other support systems
  - Readiness for pregnancy (e.g., age, life goals, stress)
  - Environmental (home, workplace) conditions
  - Safety hazards
  - Toxic chemicals
  - Radiation

INTERVENTIONS

- Anticipatory guidance or teaching
  - Treatment of medical conditions and results
  - Medications
  - Cessation or reduction in substance use and abuse
  - Immunizations (e.g., rubella, hepatitis)
- Nutrition, diet, weight management
- Exercise
- Referral for genetic counseling
- Referral to and use of:
  - Family planning services
  - Family and social needs management

AIDS, Acquired immunodeficiency syndrome; *HIV*, human immunodeficiency virus.

BOX 4-2 MAJOR GOALS OF PRENATAL CARE

- Define health status of mother and fetus.
- Determine the gestational age of the fetus, and monitor fetal development.
- Identify the woman at risk for complications, and minimize the risk whenever possible.
- Provide appropriate education and counseling.

health care delivery system. Women's health assessment and screening focus on a multisystem evaluation emphasizing the maintenance and enhancement of wellness.

Many women first enter the health care delivery system for a Pap test or contraception. Visits to the nurse may be their only contact with the system unless they become ill. Some women postpone examination until a specific need arises, such as pregnancy, pain, abnormal bleeding, or vaginal discharge.

Health care needs vary with culture, religion, age, and personal differences. The changing responsibilities and roles of women, their socioeconomic status, and their personal lifestyles also contribute to differences in the health and behavior of women. Employment outside of the home, physical disability, inadequate or no health insurance, divorce, single parenthood, and sexual orientation also can affect women's ability to seek and receive health care in clinical settings. As women age, many continue to address their primary health care needs within their established gynecologic care setting; therefore, well-women's health care should include a complete history, physical examination, age-appropriate screening, and health promotion.

Fertility Control and Infertility

As women become more informed about themselves and their health care, they are more willing to seek counseling and contraception appropriate to their varied and specific needs. Some women first enter the health care system to obtain such advice. More than half of the pregnancies in the United States each year are unintended, many even with contraception use (Trussell, 2007). Education is the key to encouraging women to make family planning choices based on preference and actual benefit-to-risk ratios. Providers can influence the user's motivation and ability to use the method correctly (see Chapter 8 for further discussion of contraception).

The concept of health promotion applies to contraception, as can be seen in Box 4-3. The nurse can influence women positively regarding the need for child spacing, methods of family planning that are consistent with religious and personal preferences, noncontraceptive benefits of certain methods, the appropriate use of methods selected, and the protection of future fertility when so desired.

Women also enter the health care system because of their desire to achieve a pregnancy. Approximately 15% of couples in the United States have some degree of infertility. Many couples have delayed starting their families until they are in their 30s or 40s, which allows more time to be exposed to situations negatively affecting fertility (including age-related infertility for the woman). In addition, sexually transmitted infections (STIs), which can predispose to decreased fertility, are becoming more common, and many women and men are in workplaces and home settings where they may be exposed to reproductive environmental hazards.

BOX 4-3 CONTRACEPTIVE HEALTH PROMOTION

- Child spacing and quality maternity care improve perinatal outcomes and health in general of mother and children.
- Achieving desired family size enables a better sharing of all resources, with attendant increases in education, health care, and other positive societal parameters.
- Contraceptives themselves may positively affect future health. For example, use of condoms may prevent acquisition of HIV infection; combined OCs may provide some protection against later development of cancer of ovary and endometrium; barrier methods decrease transmission of STIs, which can develop into pelvic inflammatory disease with resultant infertility or sterility and thus affect future childbearing capacity.

HIV, Human immunodeficiency virus; *OCs,* oral contraceptives; *STIs,* sexually transmitted infections.

Steps toward prevention of infertility should be undertaken as part of ongoing routine health care, and such information is especially appropriate in preconception counseling. Primary care providers can undertake initial evaluation and counseling before couples are referred to specialists. For additional information about infertility, see Chapter 9.

Menstrual Problems

Irregularities or problems with the menstrual period are among the most common concerns of women and often cause them to seek help from the health care system. Common menstrual disorders include amenorrhea, dysmenorrhea, premenstrual syndrome, endometriosis, and menorrhagia or metrorrhagia. Simple explanation and counseling may handle the concern; however, history and examination must be completed, as well as laboratory or diagnostic tests, if indicated. Questions should never be considered inconsequential. Age-specific reading materials are recommended, especially for teenagers. Information should also consider cultural relevance and be available in languages appropriate for the population with whom the nurse is working. See Chapter 6 for an in-depth discussion of menstrual problems.

Perimenopause

The body responds to this natural transition in a number of ways, most of which are due to the decrease in estrogen. Most women seeking health care during the perimenopausal period do so because of irregular bleeding. Others are concerned about vasomotor symptoms (hot flashes and flushes). Although fertility is greatly reduced during this period, women are urged to maintain some method of contraception because pregnancies still can occur. All women need to have factual information, the dispelling of myths, a thorough examination, and periodic health screenings thereafter. See Chapter 6 for discussion of perimenopause and menopause.

BARRIERS TO SEEKING HEALTH CARE

Financial Issues

Parts of the health care delivery system remain in a state of flux. Great variation occurs depending on type and size of the system, source of payment for services, private versus public programs, availability of and accessibility to providers, individual preferences, and insurance coverage or ability to pay. The existing system continues to be oriented to treatment of acute or episodic conditions rather than the promotion of health and comprehensive care (see discussion in Chapter 1).

A health care reform bill was signed by President Obama on March 23, 2010. However, the impact of this legislation on the American people will not be known for years because not all benefits will be immediate (Gaulin, 2010).

Cultural Issues

As our nation becomes more racially, ethnically and culturally diverse, the health of minority groups becomes a major issue. A variety of reasons are given to explain some of the differences in accessing care when financial barriers are adjusted. Unfair treatment was described by women who experienced racial discrimination or disrespectful, disillusioning, or discouraging encounters with community service providers such as social services and health care providers. A lack of training in cross-cultural communication may present problems. Desired health outcomes are best achieved when the health care providers have a knowledge and understanding about the culture, language, values, priorities, and health beliefs of minority groups. Conversely, members of the group should understand the health goals to be achieved and the methods proposed to do so. Language differences can produce profound barriers between women and health care providers. Even with an interpreter, information may be skewed in either direction.

Providers must consider culturally based differences that could affect the treatment of diverse groups of women, and the women themselves should share their practices and beliefs that could influence their management, responses, or willingness to comply (see Cultural Considerations box: Female Genital Mutilation). For example, women in some cultures value privacy to such an extent that they are reluctant to disrobe and, as a result, avoid physical examination unless absolutely necessary. Other women rely on their husbands to make major decisions, including those affecting the woman's health. Religious beliefs may dictate a specified plan of care, such as limiting assisted reproductive technology, contraception measures, blood transfusions, cardiopulmonary resuscitation, or assisted ventilation. Some cultural groups prefer folk medicine, homeopathy, or prayer to traditional Western medicine, and others attempt combinations of various practices.

Gender Issues

Gender influences provider-client communication and may influence access to health care in general. The most obvious gender consideration is that between men and women. Researchers have reported significant male-female differences in receipt of major diagnostic and therapeutic interventions, especially with cardiac and kidney problems. Women tend to use primary care services more often than men and, some believe, more effectively. The sex of the provider plays a role; studies have shown that female clients have Pap tests and mammograms more consistently if they are seen by female providers.

Sexual orientation may produce another barrier. Lesbian women have primary erotic attractions and relations with other women. Some lesbians may not disclose their orientation to

CULTURAL CONSIDERATIONS

Female Genital Mutilation

Defined by the World Health Organization (WHO), female genital mutilation (FGM) is "all procedures that involve partial or total removal of the external female genitalia, or other injury to the female genital organs for non-medical reasons" (2008). This includes female circumcision and is an attempt to control women through controlling their sexuality. FGM is supposed to remove sexual desire so that the girl will not become sexually active until married (McGargill, 2009).

Female circumcision occurs in women of many different ethnic, cultural, and religious backgrounds. Although circumcision is usually performed during childhood, some communities circumcise infants or older females. The procedure involves the removal of a portion of the clitoris but may extend to the removal of the entire clitoris and labia minora. Additionally, the labia majora, which are often stitched together over the urethral and vaginal openings, may be affected.

The extent of the circumcision site affects the seriousness of complications. Common complications include bleeding, pain, local scarring, keloid or cyst formation, and infection. Impaired drainage of urine and menstrual blood may lead to chronic pelvic infections, pelvic and back pain, and chronic urinary tract infections. Some women may require surgery before vaginal examination, intercourse, or childbirth if the vaginal opening is obstructed.

FGM is illegal in the United States and punishable by fines, prison, and deportation. An obstetrician may incise the closed labia in order to deliver a baby, or remove cysts, but may not sew the labia back to its previous state of reinfibulation. If performed on a minor, FGM is considered child abuse in the United States. "The practice also violates the rights to health, security and physical integrity of the person, the right to be free from torture and cruel, inhuman or degrading treatment, and the right to life when the procedure results in death" (WHO, 2008).

Nurses are providing care to a growing number of women who have emigrated from the Middle East, Asia, and Africa, where female circumcision is more common. Nurses must be sensitive to the unique needs of these clients, especially if these women have concerns about maintaining or restoring the intactness of the circumcision after childbirth.

Sources: McGargill, P. (2009). Female genital mutilation. *On the Edge, 15*(2 Summer). Available at www.cinahl.com/cgi–bin/refsvc?jid=29638accno-2010331425. Accessed August 5, 2010; World Health Organization (WHO). (2008, May). *Female genital mutilation.* Available at www.who.int/mediacentre/factsheets/fs241/en/print.html. Accessed January 20, 2010.

health care providers because they feel they may be at risk for hostility, inadequate health care, or breach of confidentiality. In many health care settings, heterosexuality is assumed, and the setting may be one in which the woman does not feel welcome (magazines, brochures, and environment reflect heterosexual couples, or the health care provider shows discomfort interacting with the woman). Another problem is that lesbians themselves may hold beliefs that are incorrect, such as that they have immunity to human immunodeficiency virus (HIV), STIs, and certain cancers (e.g., cervical). The perceived lack of risk can result in lesbians avoiding medical care as well as in health care providers giving incorrect advice or not doing appropriate cancer screening for these women. Not all gynecologic cancers are related to sexual activity; lesbians who have never had children may be more at risk for breast, ovarian, and endometrial cancer. Their risk for heart disease, cancer of the lung, and colon cancer is the same as that of the heterosexual woman. To offset stereotypes, it is necessary for providers to develop an approach that does not assume that all women are heterosexual. Revising forms to be inclusive of sexual diversity and providing an environment that promotes acceptance and inclusiveness are two strategies suggested by researchers (Goldberg, 2005-2006; Roberts, 2006).

HEALTH RISKS IN THE CHILDBEARING YEARS

Maintaining optimal health is a goal for all women. Essential components of health maintenance are identification of unrecognized problems and potential risks and the education and the health promotion needed to reduce them. This is especially important for women in their childbearing years, because conditions that increase a woman's health risks are not only of concern for her well-being but also are potentially associated with negative outcomes for both mother and baby in the event of a pregnancy. Prenatal care is an example of prevention that is practiced after conception; however, prevention and health maintenance are needed before pregnancy because many of the mother's risks can be identified and then eliminated or at least modified. An overview of conditions and circumstances that increase health risks in the childbearing years follows.

Age

Adolescence

As a girl progresses through development, she may be at risk for conditions that are age related. All teens undergo progressive growth of sexual characteristics and undertake developmental tasks of adolescence, such as establishing identity, developing sexual preference, emancipating from family, and establishing career goals. Some of these situations can produce great stress for the adolescent, and the health care provider should treat her carefully. Female teenagers who enter the health care system usually do so for screening (Pap tests start at age 21 or 3 years after the girl becomes sexually active) or because of a problem such as episodic illness or accidents. Gynecologic problems are often associated with menses (either bleeding irregularities or dysmenorrhea), vaginitis or leukorrhea, STIs, contraception, or pregnancy. The adolescent also is at risk for depression (Huff, Abuzz, & Omar, 2007).

Teenage Pregnancy. Pregnancy in the teenager who is 16 years old or younger often introduces additional stress into an already stressful developmental period. The emotional level of such teens is commonly characterized by impulsiveness and self-centered behavior, and they often place primary importance on the beliefs and actions of their peers. In attempts to establish a personal and independent identity, many teens do not realize the consequences of their behavior, and planning for the future is not part of their thinking processes.

Teenagers usually lack the financial resources to support a pregnancy and may not have the maturity to avoid teratogens or to have prenatal care and instruction or follow-up care. Children of teen mothers can be at risk for abuse or neglect because of the teen's inadequate knowledge of growth, development, and parenting. Implementation of specialized adolescent programs in schools, communities, and health care systems is demonstrating continued success in reducing the birth rate in teens.

Young and Middle Adulthood

Because women ages 20 to 40 years have need for contraception, pelvic and breast screening, and pregnancy care, they can prefer to use their gynecologic or obstetric provider as their primary care provider also. During these years the woman may be "juggling" family, home, and career responsibilities, with resulting increases in stress-related conditions. Health maintenance includes not only pelvic and breast screening but also promotion of a healthy lifestyle, that is, good nutrition, regular exercise, no smoking, little or no alcohol consumption, sufficient rest, stress reduction, and referral for medical conditions and other specific problems. Common conditions requiring well-woman care include vaginitis, urinary tract infections, menstrual variations, obesity, sexual and relationship issues, and pregnancy.

Parenthood After Age 35. A woman older than 35 years does not have a different physical response to a pregnancy, per se, but rather has had health status changes as a result of time and the aging process. These changes may be responsible for age-related pregnancy conditions. For example, a woman with type 2 diabetes may not have had expression of her diabetes at age 22, but may have full-blown disease at age 38. Other chronic or debilitating diseases or conditions increase in severity with time, and these in turn may predispose to increased risks during pregnancy (National Women's Health Resource Center [NWHRC], 2008). Of significance to women in this age-group is the risk of giving birth to a child with certain genetic anomalies (e.g., Down syndrome), and the opportunity for genetic counseling should be available to all (March of Dimes, 2010).

Late Reproductive Age

Women of later reproductive age are often experiencing change and reordering of their personal priorities. Generally the goals of education, career, marriage, and family have been achieved, and now the woman has increased time and opportunity for new interests and activities. Conversely, divorce rates are high at this age, and children leaving home may produce an "empty nest syndrome," resulting in increased levels of depression. Chronic diseases also become more apparent. Most problems for the well woman are associated with perimenopause (e.g., bleeding irregularities and vasomotor symptoms). Health maintenance screening continues to be of importance because some conditions such as breast disease or ovarian cancer occur more often during this stage.

Socioeconomic Status

Differences exist among people from different socioeconomic levels and ethnic groups with respect to risk for illness and distribution of disease and death. Some diseases are more common among people of selected ethnicity, for example, sickle cell anemia in African-Americans, Tay-Sachs disease in Ashkenazi Jews, adult lactase deficiency in Chinese, beta thalassemia in Mediterranean peoples, and cystic fibrosis in northern Europeans. Cultural and religious influences also increase health risks because the woman and her family may have life and societal values and a view of health and illness that dictate practices different from those expected in the Judeo-Christian Western model. These practices may include food taboos or frequencies, methods of hygiene, effects of climate, care-seeking behaviors, willingness to undergo screening and diagnostic procedures, and value conflicts.

Socioeconomic status affects birth outcomes. Social consequences for poor women as single parents are great because many mothers with few skills are caught in the bind of having income that is insufficient to afford child care. These families generate fewer and fewer resources and increase their risks for health problems. Multiple roles for women in general produce overload, conflict, and stress, resulting in higher risks for psychologic illness.

Substance Use and Abuse

Use of illicit drugs and inappropriate use of prescription drugs continue to increase and are found in all ages, races, ethnic groups, and socioeconomic strata. Addiction to substances is seen as a biopsychosocial disease, with several factors contributing to risk. These include biogenetic predisposition, lack of resilience to stressful life experiences, and poor social support. Women are less likely than men to abuse drugs, but the rate in women is increasing significantly. Substance-abusing pregnant women create severe problems for themselves and their offspring, including interference with optimal growth and development and addiction. In many instances, the use of substances is identified through screening programs in prenatal clinics and obstetric units (see Chapter 32).

Smoking

Cigarette smoking is a major preventable cause of death and illness. Smoking is linked to cardiovascular heart disease, various types of cancers (especially lung and cervical), chronic lung disease, and negative pregnancy outcomes. Tobacco contains nicotine, which is an addictive substance that creates a physical and a psychologic dependence. There is little difference in the rate of smoking between men and women, although rates for women are slightly less (American Cancer Society [ACS], 2010a). Cigarette smoking impairs fertility in women and men, may reduce the age for menopause, and increases the risk for osteoporosis after menopause. Smoking during pregnancy is known to cause a decrease in placental perfusion and is a cause of low birth weight (Kliegman, 2006).

COMMUNITY ACTIVITY

- Visit the National Women's Health Resource Center website at www.healthy women.org. Go to the conditions and treatments link and select a condition. Review the client information sections about diagnosis, treatment, prevention, facts to know, questions to ask and lifestyle tips.
- Visit the smokefree.gov website to learn about smoking in your state. What percentage of adults smoke? How does your state rank compared to other states?
- Visit the women.smokefree.gov website. Go to the link about smoking and pregnancy. Review client information regarding the benefits of quitting smoking for the woman, fetus, and newborn. What resources are available to help women quit smoking?

Alcohol

Women ages 35 to 49 years have the highest rates of chronic alcoholism, but women ages 21 to 34 have the highest rates of specific alcohol-related problems. About one third of alcoholics are women, and many relate onset of their drinking problem to stressful events. Women who are problem drinkers are often depressed, have more motor vehicle injuries, and have a higher incidence of attempted suicide than women in the general population. They also are at risk for alcohol-related liver damage. Early case finding and treatment are important in alcoholism for both the ill individual and for family members. See Chapter 32 for further discussion about alcohol use in women.

Prescription Drugs

Psychotherapeutic medications such as stimulants, sleeping pills, tranquilizers, and pain relievers are used by an estimated 2% of American women. Such medications can bring relief from undesirable conditions such as insomnia, anxiety, and pain, but because the medications have mind-altering capacity, misuse can produce psychologic and physical dependency in the same manner as illicit drugs. Risk-to-benefit ratios should be considered when such medications are used for more than short periods.

Depression is the most common mental health problem in women. Many kinds of medications are used to treat depression. All of these psychotherapeutic drugs can have some effect on the fetus when taken during pregnancy and must be very carefully monitored (see Chapter 32).

Illicit Drugs

Illicit drugs are taken for unlawful purposes. When they are unprescribed, they are usually obtained on the street for the purpose of getting high or for their body-mind–altering characteristics. Almost any drug can be abused or even illegal if taken in excess, including alcohol and prescription medication (see Chapter 32 for further discussion of substance abuse).

Nutrition

Good nutrition is essential for optimal health. A well-balanced diet helps prevent illness and treat certain health problems. Conversely, poor eating habits, eating disorders, and obesity are linked to disease and debility.

Dietary Guidelines for Americans 2010 provides evidenced-based recommendations to promote health and reduce risks for chronic diseases through diet (U.S. Department of Health and Human Services [USDHHS] & U.S. Department of Agriculture [USDA], 2010) (www.cnpp.usda.gov/Dietaryguidelines/htm).

Nutritional Deficiencies

Overt disease caused by lack of certain nutrients is rarely seen in the United States; however, insufficient amounts or imbalances of nutrients do pose problems for individuals and families. Overweight or underweight status, malabsorption, listlessness, fatigue, frequent colds and other minor infections, constipation, dull hair and thin nails, and dental caries are examples of problems that can be related to nutrition and indicate the need for further nutritional assessment. Poor nutrition, especially related to obesity and high fat and cholesterol intake, may lead to more serious conditions and is said to contribute to four of the six leading causes of death in the United States: heart disease, malignant neoplasms, cerebrovascular disease, and diabetes (Kung, Hoyert, Xu, & Murphy, 2008).

Obesity

During the last 20 years, obesity in the United States has increased dramatically. Estimates indicate that one third of women older than 20 years are obese (body mass index [BMI] 30 or higher) (NWHRC, 2006). In the United States the prevalence of obesity is highest among non-Hispanic black women, followed by Hispanic women and non-Hispanic white women (CDC, 2009). The BMI is defined as a measure of an adult's weight in relation to his or her height, specifically the adult's weight in kilograms divided by the square of his or her height in meters (see Table 14-2).

Overweight and obesity are known risk factors for premature death, diabetes, heart disease, dyslipidemia, stroke, hypertension, gallbladder disease, diverticular disease, some anemias, oral disease, constipation, osteoarthritis, gout, osteoporosis, respiratory dysfunction and sleep apnea, and some types of cancer (uterine, breast, colorectal, kidney, and gallbladder) (ACS, 2010b). In addition, obesity is associated with high cholesterol, menstrual irregularities, hirsutism (excess body/facial hair), stress incontinence, depression, complications of pregnancy, increased surgical risk, and shortened life span (USDHHS & USDA, 2010). Obesity-related pregnancy complications include macrosomia, gestational diabetes, hypertensive disorders, preterm birth, and cesarean birth. Pregnant women who are morbidly obese are at increased risk for intrauterine growth restriction and intrauterine fetal demise (Smith, Hulsey, & Goodnight, 2008).

Other Considerations

Other dietary extremes also can produce risk. For example, insufficient amounts of calcium can lead to osteoporosis, too much sodium can aggravate hypertension, and megadoses of vitamins can cause adverse effects in several body systems. Fad weight-loss programs and yo-yo dieting (repeated weight gain and weight loss) result in nutritional imbalances and, in some instances, medical problems. Such diets and programs are not appropriate for weight maintenance. Adolescent pregnancy produces special nutritional requirements because the metabolic needs of pregnancy are superimposed on the teen's own needs for growth and maturation at a time when eating habits are less than ideal.

Anorexia Nervosa. Some women have a distorted view of their bodies and, no matter what their weight, perceive themselves to be much too heavy. As a result, they undertake strict and severe diets and rigorous extreme exercise. This chronic eating disorder is known as anorexia nervosa. Women can carry this condition to the point of starvation, with resulting endocrine and metabolic abnormalities. If not corrected, significant complications of arrhythmias, amenorrhea, cardiomyopathy, and congestive heart failure occur and, in the extreme, can lead to death. The condition commonly begins during adolescence in young women who have some degree of personality disorder. They gradually lose weight over several months, have amenorrhea, and are abnormally concerned with body image. Diagnosis can be difficult, especially if the person tries to hide the problem. Denial of a problem and secrecy around eating are common features of anorexia. Depression usually accompanies anorexia. There are no specific tests to diagnose anorexia nervosa. A medical history, physical examination, and screening tests help identify women at risk for eating disorders. Several tools are available to use in primary care settings. The SCOFF questionnaire is easy to administer and can help the nurse decide whether an eating disorder is likely and if the woman needs further assessment and possibly psychiatric and medical intervention (Parker, Lyons, & Bonner, 2005; Wolfe, 2005) (Box 4-4).

Bulimia Nervosa. Bulimia refers to secret, uncontrolled binge eating alternating with methods to prevent weight gain: self-induced vomiting, use of laxatives or diuretics, strict diets, fasting, and rigorous exercise. During a binge episode, large numbers of calories are consumed, usually consisting of sweets and "junk foods." Binges occur at least twice per week. Bulimia usually begins in early adulthood (ages 18 to 25 years) and is found primarily in women. Complications can include dehydration and electrolyte imbalance, gastrointestinal abnormalities, and cardiac arrhythmias (Wolfe, 2005). Bulimia is somewhat similar to anorexia in that it is an eating disorder and usually involves some degree of depression. Unlike those with anorexia, individuals with bulimia may feel shame or disgust about their disorder and tend to seek help earlier. The SCOFF assessment also can be used to screen for bulimia (see Box 4-4).

Binge Eating Disorder. The hallmark of binge eating disorder is eating large amounts of food in a short period (a couple of hours) and not being able to stop eating. The woman may eat when she's not hungry or until uncomfortably full. She may choose to eat alone because she is embarrassed about how much she eats. Binge eating disorder involves bingeing that alternates with a restricted dietary intake. An associated syndrome called night eating syndrome is when limited food is eaten early in the day and most of the day's food intake is consumed after the evening meal. Over time, obesity and related complications of being overweight can develop. Common personality traits found in those with binge eating disorder include excessive concern about body size and shape and low self-esteem. Depression and anxiety commonly occur along with binge eating, which makes treatment and recovery more difficult. Binge eating is not associated with anorexia nervosa or bulimia nervosa.

BOX 4-4 SCREENING FOR EATING DISORDERS

SCOFF QUESTIONS

Each question scores 1 point. A score of 2 or more indicates the person may have anorexia nervosa or bulimia.

1. Do you make yourself **S**ick (i.e., induce vomiting) because you feel too full?
2. Do you worry about loss of **C**ontrol over the amount you eat?
3. Have you recently lost more than **O**ne stone (6.4 kg [14 lb]) in a 3-month period?
4. Do you think you are too **F**at even if others think you are too thin?
5. Does **F**ood dominate your life?

Reference: Morgan, J., Reid, F., & Lacey, J. (1999). The SCOFF questionnaire: Assessment of a new screening tool for eating disorders. *BMJ, 319* (7223), 1467-1468.

Physical Fitness and Exercise

Physical activity promotes health, psychological well-being, and ideal body weight for height. It enhances independence, and improves quality of living across the life span. Women should engage in 2½ hours per week of moderate intensity or 1¼ hours per week of vigorous intensity aerobic physical activity or a combination of both according to the current Physical Activity Guidelines for Americans (USDHHS, 2008).

Exercise can reduce risks for a variety of conditions that are influenced by obesity and a sedentary lifestyle such as cardiovascular disease, cerebrovascular disease, and diabetes. Exercise plays an important role in the management of chronic conditions such as hypertension, arthritis, respiratory disorders, and osteoporosis. Exercise contributes to stress reduction and improving the quality of sleep. Women report that engaging in regular exercise improves their body image and self-esteem and acts as a mood enhancer.

Aerobic exercise contributes to cardiovascular fitness while increasing oxygen levels to working muscles. Anaerobic exercise, such as weight training, improves individual muscle mass without stress on the cardiovascular system. Because women are concerned about both cardiovascular and bone health, weight-bearing aerobic exercises such as walking, running, racket sports, and dancing may be preferred. Sustained excessive exercise can lead to hormonal imbalances, such as amenorrhea, which can usually be reversed when the body returns to normal levels of activity.

SAFETY ALERT

Before beginning any planned physical activity program, a woman should see her primary care nurse practitioner (NP) or physician for a thorough medical evaluation to prevent potential injuries or harm.

Stress

The modern woman faces increasing levels of stress and as a result is prone to a variety of stress-induced complaints and illnesses. Stress often occurs because of multiple roles, such as when coping with job and financial responsibilities conflicts with parenting and duties at home. To add to this burden, women are socialized to be caretakers, which is an emotionally draining role in itself. They also may find themselves in positions of minimal power that do not allow them to have control over their everyday environments. Some stress is normal and contributes to positive outcomes. Many women thrive in busy surroundings. However, excessive or high levels of ongoing stress trigger physical reactions in the body, such as rapid heart rate, elevated blood pressure, slowed digestion, release of additional neurotransmitters and hormones, muscle tenseness, and a weakened immune system. Consequently, constant stress can contribute to clinical illnesses such as flare-ups of arthritis or asthma, frequent colds or infections, gastrointestinal upsets, cardiovascular problems, and infertility. Box 4-5 lists symptoms that may be related to chronic or extreme stress. Psychologic signs such as anxiety, irritability, eating disorders, depression, insomnia, and substance abuse are associated with stress.

BOX 4-5 STRESS SYMPTOMS

PHYSICAL
- Perspiration/sweaty hands
- Increased heart rate
- Trembling
- Nervous tics
- Dryness of throat and mouth
- Tiring easily
- Urinating frequently
- Sleeping problems
- Diarrhea, indigestion, vomiting
- Butterflies in stomach
- Headaches
- Premenstrual tension
- Pain in the neck and lower back
- Loss of appetite or overeating
- Susceptibility to illness

BEHAVIOR
- Stuttering and other speech difficulties
- Crying for no apparent reason
- Acting impulsively
- Startling easily
- Laughing in a high-pitched and nervous tone of voice
- Grinding teeth
- Increased smoking
- Increased use of drugs and alcohol
- Being accident-prone
- Losing appetite or overeating

PSYCHOLOGIC
- Feeling anxious
- Feeling scared
- Feeling irritable
- Feeling moody
- Low self-esteem
- Fear of failure
- Inability to concentrate
- Embarrassed easily
- Worrying about the future
- Preoccupation with thoughts or tasks
- Forgetfulness

Modified from The State University of New York Counseling Center. (2002). *Stress management.* Buffalo: University of Buffalo, The State University of New York.

Sexual Practices

Potential risks related to sexual activity are undesired pregnancy and STIs. The risks are particularly high for adolescents and young adults who engage in sexual intercourse at earlier and earlier ages. Adolescents report many reasons for wanting to be sexually active, among which are peer pressure, desire to love and be loved, experimentation, enhancing self-esteem, and having fun. However, many teens do not have the decision-making or values-clarification skills needed to take this important step at a young age, and they lack the knowledge base regarding contraception and STIs. They also do not believe that becoming pregnant or getting an STI will happen to them.

Although some STIs can be cured with antibiotics, many can cause significant problems. Possible sequelae include infertility, ectopic pregnancy, neonatal morbidity and mortality, genital cancers, acquired immunodeficiency syndrome (AIDS), and even death (CDC, Workowski, & Berman, 2006). The incidence of STIs is increasing rapidly and reaching epidemic proportions. Choice of contraception has an effect on the risk of contracting an STI; however, no method of contraception offers complete protection. (See Chapter 7 for discussion of STIs and Chapter 8 for contraception.)

! NURSING ALERT

A comprehensive sexual assessment should be integrated into all health histories.

Medical Conditions

Most women of reproductive age are relatively healthy. Heart disease; lung, breast, colon, and gynecologic cancers; stroke; chronic lung disease; and diabetes are among the leading causes of death in adult women (Heron & Tejada-Vera, 2008) (Box 4-6). Certain medical conditions present during pregnancy can have deleterious effects on both the woman and the fetus. Of particular concern are risks from all forms of diabetes, urinary tract disorders, thyroid disease, hypertensive disorders of pregnancy, cardiac disease, and seizure disorders. Effects on the fetus vary and include intrauterine growth restriction, macrosomia, anemia, prematurity, immaturity, and stillbirth. Effects on the woman also can be severe. These conditions are discussed in later chapters.

Gynecologic Conditions

Women are at risk throughout their reproductive years for pelvic inflammatory disease, endometriosis, STIs and other vaginal infections, uterine fibroids, uterine deformities such as bicornuate uterus, ovarian cysts, interstitial cystitis, and urinary incontinence related to pelvic relaxation. These gynecologic conditions may contribute negatively to pregnancy by causing infertility, miscarriage, preterm labor, and fetal and neonatal problems. Gynecologic cancers also affect women's health, although the risk for most cancers is low in pregnancy. Risk factors depend on the type of cancer. The effect of developing a gynecologic problem or cancer in women and their families is shaped by a number of factors including the specific type of problem or cancer, the implications of the diagnosis for the woman and her family, and the timing of the occurrence in the

BOX 4-6 TOP 10 LEADING CAUSES OF DEATH IN WOMEN IN THE UNITED STATES

1. Heart disease
2. Malignant neoplasm (cancer)
3. Cardiovascular disease (stroke)
4. Chronic lower respiratory disease
5. Alzheimer's disease
6. Unintentional injury
7. Diabetes mellitus
8. Influenza and pneumonia
9. Nephritis
10. Septicemia

Source: U.S. Department of Health and Human Services, Health Resources and Services Administration. (2009). Maternal and Child Health Bureau. *Women's Health USA 2009.* Rockville, MD: U.S. Department of Health and Human Services, 2009. Available at mchb.hrsa.gov/whusa09/hstat/hi/pages/2081cd.html. Accessed January 20, 2010.

woman's and family's lives. These conditions are discussed in Chapters 6, 7, and 11.

Environmental and Workplace Hazards

Environmental hazards in the home, the workplace, and the community can contribute to poor health at all ages. Categories and examples of health-damaging hazards include the following: (1) pathogenic agents (viruses, bacteria, fungi, parasites); (2) natural and synthetic chemicals (natural toxins from animals, insects, and plants; consumer and industrial products such as pesticides and hydrocarbon gases; medical and diagnostic devices; tobacco; fuels; and drug and alcohol abuse); (3) radiation (radon, heat waves, sound waves); (4) food substances (added components that are not necessary for nutrition); and (5) physical objects (moving vehicles, machinery, weapons, water, and building materials).

Environmental hazards can affect fertility, fetal development, live birth, and the child's future mental and physical development. Environmental hazards are discussed throughout other chapters as they are identified as specific risks to women's and infants' health.

Violence Against Women

Violence against women is a major health care problem in the United States, affecting millions of women each year and costing millions of dollars in annual medical costs. Women of all races and of all ethnic, educational, religious, and socioeconomic backgrounds are affected. Pregnancy is often a time when violence begins or escalates. The magnitude of the problem is far greater than the statistics indicate because violent crimes against women are the most underreported data as a result of fear, lack of understanding, and stigma surrounding violent situations. Maternity and women's health nurses, by the very nature of their practice, are in a unique position to conduct case finding, provide sensitive care to women experiencing abusive situations, engage in prevention activities, and influence health care and public policy toward decreasing the violence. For further discussion of violence against women, see Chapter 5.

HEALTH ASSESSMENT

Case Study—Health Assessment

Women's health trends have expanded beyond a reproductive focus to include a holistic approach to health care across the life span and places women's health within the scope of primary care. Women's health assessment and screening focus on a systems evaluation beginning with a careful history and physical examination. During the assessment and evaluation, the responsibility for self-care, health promotion, and wellness enhancement is emphasized.

In a market-driven system such as managed care, specific guidelines may be provided for health screening by the insurer or the managed care organization. A nurse often takes the history, orders diagnostic tests, interprets test results, makes referrals, coordinates care, and directs attention to problems requiring medical intervention. Advanced practice nurses who have specialized in women's health, such as nurse practitioners, clinical nurse specialists, and nurse-midwives, perform complete physical examinations, including gynecologic examinations.

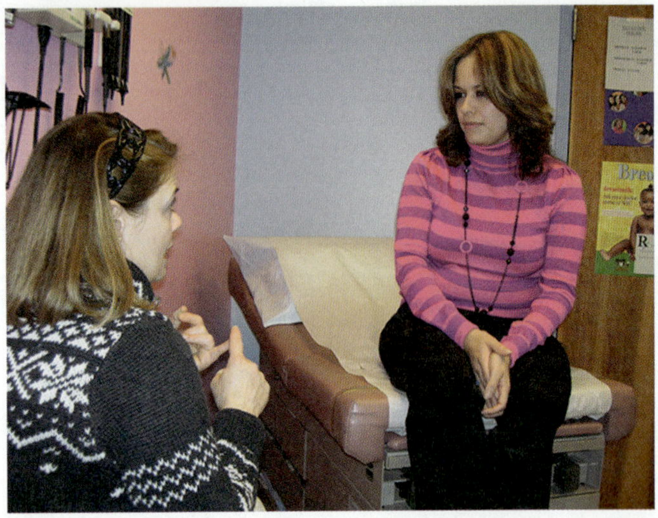

FIG. 4-8 Nurse interviews woman as part of history taking prior to physical examination. (Courtesy Ed Lowdermilk, Chapel Hill, NC.)

Interview

The contact with the woman usually begins with an interview. This interview should be conducted in a private, comfortable, and relaxed setting (Fig. 4-8). The woman is addressed by her title and name (e.g., Mrs. Gonzalez), and the nurse introduces herself or himself by using name and title. It is important to phrase questions in a sensitive and nonjudgmental manner. Body language should match verbal communication. The nurse is cognizant of a woman's vulnerability and assures her of strict confidentiality. For many women, fear, anxiety, and modesty make the examination a dreaded and stressful experience. Many women are uninformed, misguided by myths, or afraid they will appear ignorant by asking questions about sexual or reproductive functioning. The woman is assured that no question is irrelevant. The history begins with an open-ended question such as, "What brings you in to the office/clinic/hospital today? Anything else? Tell me about it."

Additional ways to get women to share information include the following:

- **Facilitation:** Using a word or posture that communicates interest; leaning forward; making eye contact; or saying "Mm-hmmm" or "Go on"
- **Reflection:** Repeating a word or phrase that a woman has used
- **Clarification:** Asking the woman what is meant by a word or phrase
- **Empathic responses:** Acknowledging the feelings of a woman by statements such as "That must have been frightening"
- **Confrontation:** Identifying something about the woman's behavior or feelings not expressed verbally or apparently inconsistent with her history
- **Interpretation:** Putting into words what you infer about the woman's feelings or about the meaning of her symptoms, events, or other matters

Direct questions may be necessary to elicit specific details. These should be worded in language that is understandable to the woman and expressed neutrally, so that the woman will not be led into a specific response. The nurse asks about one item at a time and proceeds from the general to the specific (Seidel, Ball, Dains, Flynn, Soloman, & Stewart, 2011).

CULTURAL CONSIDERATIONS

Communication Variations

- Conversational style and pacing: Silence may show respect or acknowledgment that the listener has heard. In cultures in which a direct "no" is considered rude, silence may mean no. Repetition or loudness may mean emphasis or anger.
- Personal space: Cultural conceptions of personal space differ. Based on one's culture, for example, someone may be perceived as distant for backing off when approached, or aggressive for standing too close.
- Eye contact: Eye contact varies among cultures from intense to fleeting. Consistent with the effort to refrain from invading personal space, avoiding direct eye contact may be a sign of respect.
- Touch: The norms about how people should touch each other vary among cultures. In some cultures, physical contact with the same sex (embracing, walking hand in hand) is more appropriate than that with an unrelated person of the opposite sex.
- Time orientation: In some cultures, involvement with people is more valued than being "on time." In other cultures, life is scheduled and paced according to clock time, which is valued over personal time.

Sources: Galanti, G. (2008). *Caring for patients from different cultures* (4th ed.). Philadelphia: University of Pennsylvania Press; Mattson, S. (2000). Striving for cultural competence: Providing care for the changing face of the U.S. *AWHONN Lifelines, 4*(3), 48-52.

Cultural Considerations

Recognizing signs and symptoms of disease and deciding when to seek treatment are influenced by cultural perceptions. It is essential that a nurse have respect for the rich and unique qualities that cultural diversity brings to individuals. In recognizing the value of these differences, the nurse can modify the plan of care to meet the needs of each woman.

To understand the woman's point of view, it is important to ask the right questions. Galanti (2008) suggests the use of the 4 C's of Cultural Competence. These include:

1. Call—What do you call your problem?
2. Cause—What do you think caused your problem?
3. Cope—How do you cope with your condition?
4. Concerns—What are your concerns regarding your condition?

Using the 4 C's of Cultural Competence along with cultural proficiency, biomedical values and evidence-based practice allows the nurse to individualize care with a client-focused approach. Trust that the woman is the expert on her life, culture, and experiences. If the nurse asks with respect and a genuine desire to learn, the woman will tell the nurse how to care for her. Modifications may be necessary for the physical examination. In some cultures, it may be considered inappropriate for the woman to disrobe completely for the physical examination. In many cultures, a female examiner is preferred. Communication may be hindered by different beliefs even when the nurse and woman speak the same language (see Box 2-1, p. 25, and Cultural Considerations box above).

Women with Special Needs

Women with Disabilities

Women with emotional or physical disorders have special needs. Women who have vision, hearing, emotional, or physical disabilities should be respected and involved in the assessment and physical examination to the full extent of their abilities. The nurse should communicate openly and directly with sensitivity. It is often helpful to learn about the disability directly from the woman while maintaining eye contact (if eye contact is culturally appropriate). Family and significant others should be relied on only when absolutely necessary. The assessment and physical examination can be adapted to each woman's individual needs.

Communication with a woman who is hearing impaired can be accomplished without difficulty. Most of these women read lips, write, or both; thus an interviewer who speaks and enunciates each word slowly and in full view may be easily understood. If a woman is not comfortable with lip reading, she may use an interpreter. In this case, it is important to continue to address the woman directly, avoiding the temptation to speak directly with the interpreter.

The visually impaired woman needs to be oriented to the examination room and may have her guide dog with her. As with all women, the visually impaired woman needs a full explanation of what the examination entails before proceeding. Before touching her, the nurse explains, "Now I am going to take your blood pressure. I am going to place the cuff on your right arm." The woman can be asked if she would like to touch each of the items that will be used in the examination.

Many women with physical disabilities cannot comfortably lie in the lithotomy position for the pelvic examination. Several alternative positions may be used, including a lateral (side-lying) position, a V-shaped position, a diamond-shaped position, and an M-shaped position (Piotrowski & Snell, 2007) (Fig. 4-9). The woman can be asked what has worked best for her previously. If she has never had a pelvic examination, or has never had a comfortable pelvic examination, the nurse proceeds by showing her a picture of various positions and asking her which one she prefers. The nurse's support and reassurance can help the woman to relax, which will make the examination go more smoothly.

Abused Women

Nurses should screen all women entering the health care system for potential abuse. Help for the woman may depend on the sensitivity with which the nurse screens for abuse, the discovery of abuse, and subsequent intervention. The nurse must be familiar with the laws governing abuse in the state in which she or he practices.

Pocket cards listing emergency numbers (abuse counseling, legal protection, and emergency shelter) may be available from the local police department, a women's shelter, or an emergency department. It is helpful to have these on hand in the setting where screening is done. An abuse-assessment screen (Fig. 4-10) can be used as part of the interview or written history. If a male partner is present, he should be asked to leave the room because the woman may not disclose experiences of abuse in his presence, or he may try to answer questions for her to protect himself. The same procedure would apply for partners of lesbians, parents of teens, or adult children of older women.

Fear, guilt, and embarrassment may keep many women from giving information about family violence. Clues in the history and evidence of injuries on physical examination should give a high index of suspicion. The areas most commonly injured in women are the head, the neck, the chest, the abdomen, the breasts, and the upper extremities. Burns and bruises in patterns

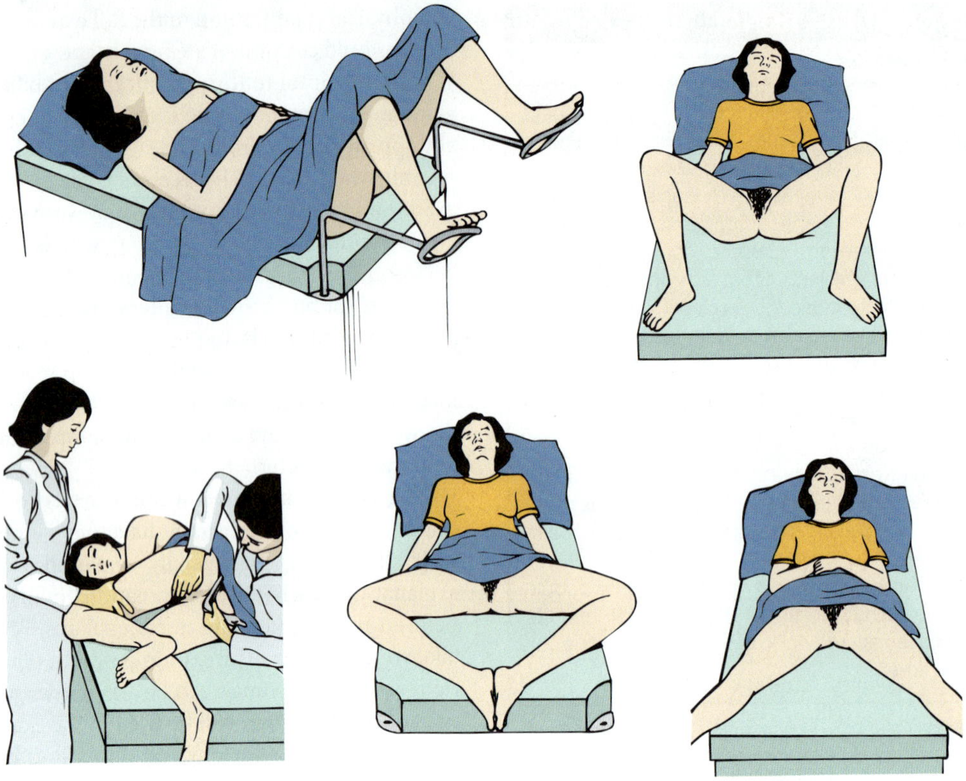

FIG. 4-9 Lithotomy and variable positions for women who have a disability.

ABUSE ASSESSMENT SCREEN

1. Have you ever been emotionally or physically abused by your partner or someone important to you?

YES ☐ NO ☐

2. Within the last year, have you been hit, slapped, kicked, or otherwise physically hurt by someone?

YES ☐ NO ☐

If YES, by whom ____________________

Number of times ____________________

Mark the area of injury on body map.

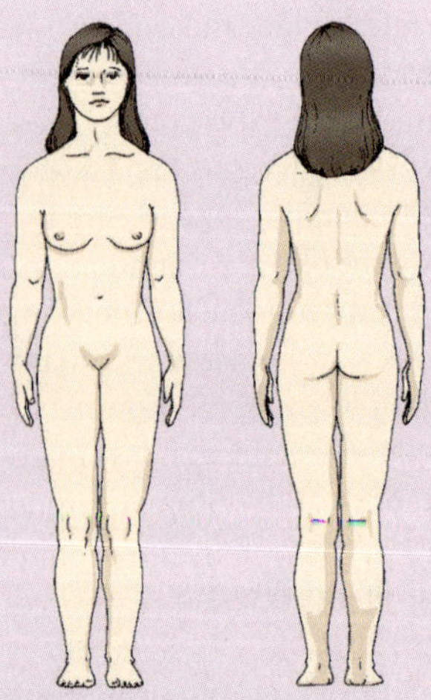

3. Within the last year, has anyone forced you to have sexual activities?

YES ☐ NO ☐

If YES, by whom ____________________

Number of times ____________________

4. Are you afraid of your partner or anyone you listed above?

YES ☐ NO ☐

FIG. 4-10 Abuse assessment screen. (Modified from the Nursing Research Consortium on Violence and Abuse. [1991].)

resembling hands, belts, cords, or other weapons may be seen as well as multiple traumatic injuries. Attention should be given to women who repeatedly seek treatment for somatic complaints such as headaches, insomnia, choking sensation, hyperventilation, gastrointestinal symptoms, and pain in the chest, back, and pelvis. During pregnancy the nurse should assess for injuries to the breasts, the abdomen, and the genitals. See Chapter 5 for further discussion of violence.

Adolescents (Ages 13 to 19 Years)

As a young woman matures, she should be asked the same questions that are included in any history. Particular attention should be paid to hints about risky behaviors, eating disorders, and depression. Do not assume that a teenager is not sexually active. After rapport has been established, it is best to talk to a teen with the parent (partner or friend) out of the room. Questions should be asked with sensitivity and in a gentle and nonjudgmental manner (Seidel et al., 2011).

A teen's first speculum examination is the most important because she will develop perceptions that will remain with her for future examinations. What the examination entails should be discussed with the teen while she is dressed. Models or illustrations can be used to show exactly what will happen. All of the necessary equipment should be assembled so that there are no interruptions. Pediatric speculums that are 1 to 1.5 cm wide can be inserted with minimal discomfort. If the teen is sexually active, a small adult speculum may be used.

Injury prevention should be a part of the counseling at routine health examinations, with special attention to seat belts, helmets, firearms, recreational hazards, and sports involvement. The use of drugs and alcohol and the nonuse of seat belts contribute to motor vehicle injuries, accounting for the greatest proportion of accidental deaths in women. Contraceptive use and STI prevention information may be needed for teens who are sexually active.

To provide developmentally appropriate care, it is important to review the major tasks for women in this stage of life. Major tasks for teens include values assessment; education and work goal setting; formation of peer relationships that focus on love, commitment, and becoming comfortable with sexuality; and separation from parents. Individuality may be reflected in areas such as sexuality, politics, and career choices. Conflict exists between making and keeping commitments to keep options open. The teen is egocentric as she progresses rapidly through emotional and physical change. Her feelings of invulnerability may lead to serious misconceptions, such as that unprotected sexual intercourse will not lead to pregnancy.

Midlife and Older Women (Ages 50 Years and Older)

The assessment of women ages 50 and older presents unique challenges. Women may be experiencing major lifestyle changes, such as children leaving home, care for their aging parents, job change, retirement, separation, divorce or death of a partner, and aging-related changes and health problems. The nurse uses reflection and empathy to communicate in an open and caring manner. It may be necessary to schedule a longer appointment time because older women have longer histories or have a need to talk. Some women may fail to report symptoms because they fear their complaints will be attributed to old age, or they feel that they have lived with a chronic condition (e.g., incontinence, dyspareunia, interstitial cystitis, decreased libido, depression) for so long that nothing can be done. Women may choose to ignore a problem if they have symptoms that are life threatening (e.g., chest pain or a breast lump) because they traditionally put the needs of others first. As a result, the nurse should encourage the woman to express her concerns and fears and reassure her that her problems are important and will be addressed. Exercise, hormone therapy, diet, vitamins, calcium with vitamin D supplementation, daily aspirin, breast self-examination, Pap and mammogram recommendations, colonoscopy, immunization updates, and sun protection should be discussed.

Functional assessment is included as part of the history in women older than 70 years and those with disabilities. In the review of systems, the nurse should ask about self-management activities such as walking, getting to the bathroom, bathing, hair combing, dressing, and eating. Questions about driving, using public transportation, using the telephone or the Internet, hanging up clothes, buying groceries, taking medications, and meal preparation should be included.

Sexual assessment continues to be important in women 50 and older. Unless directly asked, women may omit mention of sexual concerns. Questions asked with sensitivity may invite responses regarding changes in sexual desire or response or physical issues that challenge her sexual enjoyment. Open and reflective questions also affirm a woman's right to sexual enjoyment throughout the life span.

Women older than 50 years commonly experience menopause and have physical changes associated with decreased estrogen. A decrease in estrogen causes numerous cytologic and structural changes of the vagina, vulva, and lower urinary tract. Estrogen deficiency leads to a narrowing and shortening of the vagina and thinning of the vaginal walls. This can result in vaginal dryness, itching, burning, and dyspareunia. Estrogen loss also causes reduced smooth muscle relaxation, decreased vaginal blood flow and decreased vaginal secretions (North American Menopause Society [NAMS], 2007).

Estrogen plays a role in the formation of bone matrix, and a decrease may lead to osteoporosis. The risk for heart disease increases because of changes in lipid metabolism related to declining estrogen levels. Decreases in estrogen can cause a relaxation of ligaments and connective tissue, which affects the support of the bladder and uterus. Decreases in estrogen affect the hypothalamus, causing hot flashes, which are disturbing to most women (see Chapter 6).

Physical changes can result in increased discomfort during the pelvic examination. It is important to be both gentle and thorough during the examination. A small adult speculum may be used to view the cervix. The uterus in a menopausal woman is small and firm, and the ovaries are nonpalpable. In postmenopausal women the specimen from the vaginal pool may be useful to detect endometrial cells. A woman with palpable adnexal masses or vaginal bleeding after menopause needs immediate gynecologic referral.

A respectful and reassuring approach toward caring for women ages 50 and older will ensure their continued participation in seeking health care. Because the risk of breast, ovarian, uterine, cervical, colon, and skin cancers increases with age, the nurse has the opportunity to educate women about the importance of preventive screening. It is the nurse's responsibility to ensure a positive health care experience that encourages future visits for prevention and chronic and acute care.

Advance directives can be introduced on any entry into a health care system. It is a good idea to have a formal statement in the medical record regarding a woman's wishes in the event of accident or illness regarding life-maintaining measures or organ donation. Most states have laws formalizing such statements in writing. The durable power of attorney for health care can be used by a woman to delegate decision-making authority to a trusted relative or friend.

Many studies done on religion and health suggest that religious people are healthier and generally live longer than nonreligious people. Religious people have lower rates of uterine, cervical, and intestinal cancer; ulcer disease; coronary artery disease; and high blood pressure. Those who attend church once a week are less likely to become ill than those who do not. The studies did not control for rates of smoking and drinking, so no inference can be made as to whether the improved health status was from better health habits or religion. In general, it is known that religious people do tend to have healthier lifestyles overall than people who are not religious (Condon, 2004). Spiritual wellness can be estimated by answering questions such as those suggested in Box 4-7.

Healthy Aging. Women in the United States can expect on average to live to be 80 years old and may spend one third of their lives as postmenopausal women. With a healthy lifestyle, many women are living to be 100 years old or older. Proper nutrition, exercise, and mental and social stimulation are critical to keeping the body healthy and the mind active and alert into old age. Menopause is a time to evaluate, take stock, and prepare for many healthy years to come (Minikin & Wright, 2005).

BOX 4-7 SPIRITUAL WELLNESS SELF-ASSESSMENT

The more questions for which you have an answer other than "I don't know," the higher the level of spiritual wellness.

1. What is your purpose in life?
2. What activities do you do regularly that bring you joy?
3. Do you believe in a higher power?
4. Who can you count on for encouragement and/or support?
5. To whom do you give encouragement and/or support?
6. Who loves you?
7. Whom do you love or care about?
8. In what areas are you growing?
9. What activities nurture you?
10. Is there something that you do just for yourself every day?
11. How do you go about forgiving yourself?
12. How do you go about forgiving others?
13. To whom do you confide your hopes, dreams, and pain?
14. What do you hope for in the future?
15. What do you do regularly just for fun?
16. When do you reach out to people?
17. What goals do you have for 6 months from now?
18. What goals do you have for 2 years from now?
19. Do you look forward to getting up in the morning?
20. Would you like to live to be 100?

Source: Condon, M. (2004). *Women's health: Body, mind, spirit: An integrated approach to wellness and illness.* Upper Saddle River, NJ: Prentice-Hall.

Spanish Guidelines—Physical Examination

History

At a woman's first visit, she is often expected to fill out a form with biographic and historic data before meeting with the examiner. This form aids the health care provider in completing the history during the interview. Most forms include information about the following categories:

- Biographic data
- Reason for seeking care
- Present health or history of present illness
- Past health
- Family history
- Review of systems
- Functional assessment (activities of daily living)

Box 4-8 describes a complete health history and review of systems based on the above categories.

Physical Examination

In preparation for the physical examination, the woman is instructed on undressing and given a gown to wear during the examination. She is usually given the opportunity to undress privately. Objective data are recorded by system or location. A general statement of overall health status is a good way to start. Findings are described in detail.

- General appearance: age, race, sex, state of health, posture, height, weight, development, dress, hygiene, affect, alertness, orientation, cooperativeness, and communication skills
- Vital signs: temperature, pulse, respiration, blood pressure
- Skin: color; integrity; texture; hydration; temperature; edema; excessive perspiration; unusual odor; presence and description of lesions; hair texture and distribution; nail configuration, color, texture, condition, or presence of nail clubbing
- Head: size, shape, trauma, masses, scars, rashes, or scaling; facial symmetry; presence of edema or puffiness
- Eyes: pupil size, shape, reactivity, conjunctival injection, scleral icterus, fundal papilledema, hemorrhage, lids, extraocular movements, visual fields and acuity
- Ears: shape and symmetry, tenderness, discharge, external canal, and tympanic membranes; hearing—Weber should be midline (loudness of sound equal in both ears) and Rinne negative (no conductive or sensorineural hearing loss); should be able to hear whisper at 3 feet
- Nose: symmetry, tenderness, discharge, mucosa, turbinate inflammation, frontal or maxillary sinus tenderness; discrimination of odors
- Mouth and throat: hygiene, condition of teeth, dentures, appearance of lips, tongue, buccal and oral mucosa, erythema, edema, exudate, tonsillar enlargement, palate, uvula, gag reflex, ulcers
- Neck: mobility, masses, range of motion, trachea deviation, thyroid size, carotid bruits
- Lymphatic: cervical, intraclavicular, axillary, trochlear, or inguinal adenopathy; size, shape, tenderness, and consistency
- Breasts: skin changes, dimpling, symmetry, scars, tenderness, discharge or masses; characteristics of nipples and areolae
- Heart: rate, rhythm, murmurs, rubs, gallops, clicks, heaves, or precordial movements
- Peripheral vascular: jugular vein distention, bruits, edema, swelling, vein distention, positive Homans sign, or tenderness of extremities

BOX 4-8 HEALTH HISTORY AND REVIEW OF SYSTEMS

Identifying data: Name, age, race, sex, marital status, occupation, religion, and ethnicity

Reason for seeking care: A response to the question, "What problem or symptom brought you here today?" If the woman lists more than one reason, focus on the one she thinks is most important.

Present health: Current health status is described with attention to the following:

- *Use of safety measures:* seat belts, bicycle helmets, designated driver
- *Exercise and leisure activities:* regularity
- *Sleep patterns:* length and quality
- *Sexuality:* Is she sexually active? With men, women, or both? Risk-reducing sex practices?
- *Diet, including beverages:* 24-hour dietary recall; caffeine: coffee, tea, cola, or chocolate intake
- *Nicotine, alcohol, illicit or recreational drug use:* type, amount, frequency, duration, and reactions
- *Environmental and chemical hazards:* home, school, work, and leisure setting; exposure to extreme heat or cold, noise, industrial toxins such as asbestos or lead, pesticides, diethylstilbestrol (DES), radiation, cat feces, or cigarette smoke

History of present illness: A chronologic narrative that includes the onset of the problem, the setting in which it developed, its manifestations, and any treatments received are noted. The woman's state of health before the onset of the present problem is determined. If the problem is long standing, the reason for seeking attention at this time is elicited. The principal symptoms should be described with respect to the following:

- Location
- Quality or character
- Quantity or severity
- Timing (onset, duration, frequency)
- Setting
- Factors that aggravate or relieve
- Associated factors
- Woman's perception of the meaning of the symptom

Past health:

- *Infectious diseases:* measles, mumps, rubella, whooping cough, chickenpox, rheumatic fever, scarlet fever, diphtheria, polio, tuberculosis (TB), hepatitis
- *Chronic disease and system disorders:* arthritis, cancer, diabetes, heart, lung, kidney, seizures, thyroid, stroke, ulcers, sickle cell anemia
- *Adult injuries, accidents*
- *Hospitalizations, operations, blood transfusions*
- *Obstetric history*
- *Allergies:* medications, previous transfusion reactions, environmental allergies
- *Immunizations:* diphtheria, pertussis, tetanus, polio, measles, mumps, rubella (MMR), hepatitis B, varicella, influenza, pneumococcal vaccine, last TB skin test
- *Last date of screening tests:* Pap test, mammogram, stool for occult blood, sigmoidoscopy or colonoscopy, hematocrit, hemoglobin, rubella titer, urinalysis, cholesterol test; electrocardiogram; last vision, dental, hearing examination
- *Current medications:* name, dose, frequency, duration, reason for taking, and compliance with prescription medications; home remedies, over-the-counter drugs, vitamin and mineral or herbal supplements used over a 24-hour period

Family history: Information about the ages and health of family members may be presented in narrative form or as a family tree or genogram: age, health or death of parents, siblings, spouse, children. Check for history of diabetes; heart disease; hypertension; stroke; respiratory, renal, or thyroid problems; cancer; bleeding disorders; hepatitis; allergies; asthma; arthritis; TB; epilepsy; mental illness; human immunodeficiency virus infection; or other disorders.

Screen for abuse: Has she ever been hit, kicked, slapped, or forced to have sex against her wishes? Has she been verbally or emotionally abused? Does she have a history of childhood sexual abuse? If yes, has she received counseling or does she need referral?

Review of systems: It is probable that all questions in each system will not be included every time a history is taken. Some questions regarding each system should be included in every history. The essential areas to be explored are listed in the following head-to-toe sequence. If a woman gives a positive response to a question about an essential area, more detailed questions should be asked.

- *General:* weight change, fatigue, weakness, fever, chills, or night sweats
- *Skin:* skin, hair, and nail changes; itching, bruising, bleeding, rashes, sores, lumps, or moles
- *Lymph nodes:* enlargement, inflammation, pain, suppuration (pus), or drainage
- *Head:* trauma, vertigo (dizziness), convulsive disorder, syncope (fainting); headache: location, frequency, pain type, nausea and vomiting, or visual symptoms present
- *Eyes:* glasses, contact lenses, blurriness, tearing, itching, photophobia, diplopia, inflammation, trauma, cataracts, glaucoma, or acute visual loss
- *Ears:* hearing loss, tinnitus (ringing), vertigo, discharge, pain, fullness, recurrent infections, or mastoiditis
- *Nose and sinuses:* trauma, rhinitis, nasal discharge, epistaxis, obstruction, sneezing, itching, allergy, or smelling impairment
- *Mouth, throat, and neck:* hoarseness, voice changes, soreness, ulcers, bleeding gums, goiter, swelling, or enlarged nodes
- *Breasts:* masses, pain, lumps, dimpling, nipple discharge, fibrocystic changes, or implants; breast self-examination practice
- *Respiratory:* shortness of breath, wheezing, cough, sputum, hemoptysis, pneumonia, pleurisy, asthma, bronchitis, emphysema, or TB; date of last chest x-ray
- *Cardiovascular:* hypertension, rheumatic fever, murmurs, angina, palpitations, dyspnea, tachycardia, orthopnea, edema, chest pain, cough, cyanosis, cold extremities, ascites, intermittent claudication (leg pain caused by poor circulation to the leg muscles), phlebitis, or skin color changes
- *Gastrointestinal:* appetite, nausea, vomiting, indigestion, dysphagia, abdominal pain, ulcers, hematochezia (bleeding with stools), melena (black, tarry stools), bowel-habit changes, diarrhea, constipation, bowel movement frequency, food intolerance, hemorrhoids, jaundice, or hepatitis; sigmoidoscopy, colonoscopy, barium enema, ultrasound
- *Genitourinary:* frequency, hesitancy, urgency, polyuria, dysuria, hematuria, nocturia, incontinence, stones, infection, or urethral discharge; menstrual history (e.g., age at menarche, length and flow of menses, last menstrual period [LMP], dysmenorrhea, intermenstrual bleeding, age at menopause or signs of menopause), dyspareunia, discharge, sores, itching
- *Sexual health and sexual activity:* with men, women, or both; contraceptive use; sexually transmitted infections
- *Peripheral vascular:* coldness, numbness and tingling, leg edema, claudication, varicose veins, thromboses, or emboli

Continued

BOX 4-8 HEALTH HISTORY AND REVIEW OF SYSTEMS—cont'd

- *Endocrine:* heat and cold intolerance, dry skin, excessive sweating, polyuria, polydipsia, polyphagia, thyroid problems, diabetes, or secondary sex characteristic changes
- *Hematologic:* anemia, easy bruising, bleeding, petechiae, purpura, or transfusions
- *Musculoskeletal:* muscle weakness, pain, joint stiffness, scoliosis, lordosis, kyphosis, range-of-motion instability, redness, swelling, arthritis, or gout
- *Neurologic:* loss of sensation, numbness, tingling, tremors, weakness, vertigo, paralysis, fainting, twitching, blackouts, seizures, convulsions, loss of consciousness or memory
- *Mental status:* moodiness, depression, anxiety, obsessions, delusions, illusions, or hallucinations
- *Functional assessment:* ability to care for self

- Lungs: chest symmetry with respirations, wheezes, crackles, rhonchi, vocal fremitus, whispered pectoriloquy, percussion, and diaphragmatic excursion; breath sounds equal and clear bilaterally
- Abdomen: shape, scars, bowel sounds, consistency, tenderness, rebound, masses, guarding, organomegaly, liver span, percussion (tympany, shifting, dullness), costovertebral angle tenderness
- Extremities: edema, ulceration, tenderness, varicosities, erythema, tremor, or deformity
- Genitourinary: external genitalia, perineum, vaginal mucosa, cervix, inflammation, tenderness, discharge, bleeding, ulcers, nodules, masses, internal vaginal support; bimanual and rectovaginal palpation of cervix, uterus, and adnexae
- Rectal: sphincter tone, masses, hemorrhoids, rectal wall contour, tenderness, and stool for occult blood
- Musculoskeletal: posture, symmetry of muscle mass, muscle atrophy, weakness, appearance of joints, tenderness or crepitus, joint range of motion, instability, redness, swelling, or spine deviation
- Neurologic: mental status, orientation, memory, mood, speech clarity and comprehension, cranial nerves II to XII, sensation, strength, deep tendon and superficial reflexes, gait, balance, and coordination with rapid alternating motions

Pelvic Examination

Many women are intimidated by the gynecologic portion of the physical examination. The nurse in this instance can take an advocacy approach that supports a partnership relationship between the woman and the care provider.

The woman is assisted into the lithotomy position (see Fig. 4-9) for the pelvic examination. When she is in the lithotomy position, the woman's hips and knees are flexed, with the buttocks at the edge of the table, and her feet are supported by heel or knee stirrups.

Some women prefer to keep their shoes or socks on, especially if the stirrups are not padded. Many women express feelings of vulnerability and strangeness when in the lithotomy position. During the procedure, the nurse assists the woman with relaxation techniques such as taking slow deep breaths. Distraction is another technique that can be used effectively (e.g., placement of interesting pictures on the ceiling over the head of the table).

Many women find it distressing to attempt to converse in the lithotomy position. Most women appreciate an explanation of the procedure as it unfolds, as well as coaching for the types of sensations they may expect. Generally, however, women prefer not to have to respond to questions until they are again upright and at eye level with the examiner. Questioning during the procedure, especially if they cannot see their questioner's eyes, may make women tense.

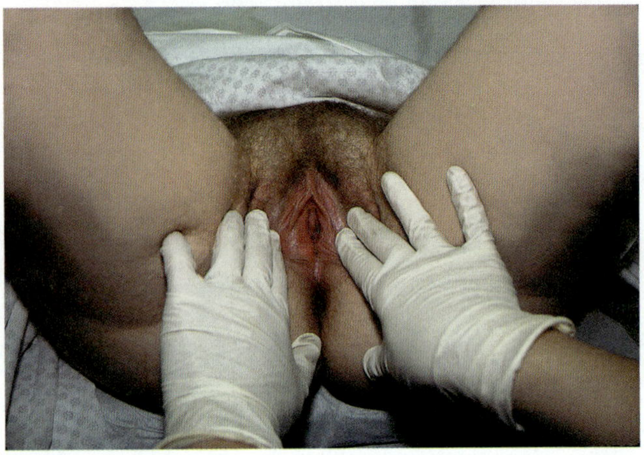

FIG. 4-11 External examination. Separation of the labia. (From Wilson, S., & Giddens, J. [2009]. *Health assessment for nursing practice* [4th ed.]. St. Louis: Mosby.)

External Inspection. The examiner sits at the foot of the table for the inspection of the external genitals and for the speculum examination. In good lighting, external genitals are inspected for sexual maturity: clitoris, labia, and perineum. After childbirth or other trauma, there may be healed scars.

External Palpation. The examiner proceeds with the examination by using palpation and inspection. The examiner wears gloves for this portion of the assessment. Before touching the woman, the examiner explains what is going to be done and what the woman should expect to feel (e.g., pressure). The examiner may touch the woman in a less sensitive area such as the inner thigh to alert her that the genital examination is beginning. This gesture may put the woman more at ease. The labia are spread apart to expose the structures in the vestibule: urinary meatus, Skene glands, vaginal orifice, and Bartholin glands (Fig. 4-11). To assess the Skene glands, the examiner inserts one finger into the vagina and "milks" the area of the urethra. Any exudate from the urethra or the Skene glands is cultured. Masses and erythema of either structure are assessed further. Ordinarily the openings to the Skene glands are not visible; prominent openings may be seen if the glands are infected (e.g., with gonorrhea). During the examination, the examiner keeps in mind the data from the review of systems, such as history of burning on urination.

The vaginal orifice is examined. Hymenal tags are normal findings. With one finger still in the vagina, the examiner repositions the index finger near the posterior part of the orifice. With the thumb outside the posterior part of the labia majora,

Video—Nursing Skill: Assisting with a Pelvic Examination

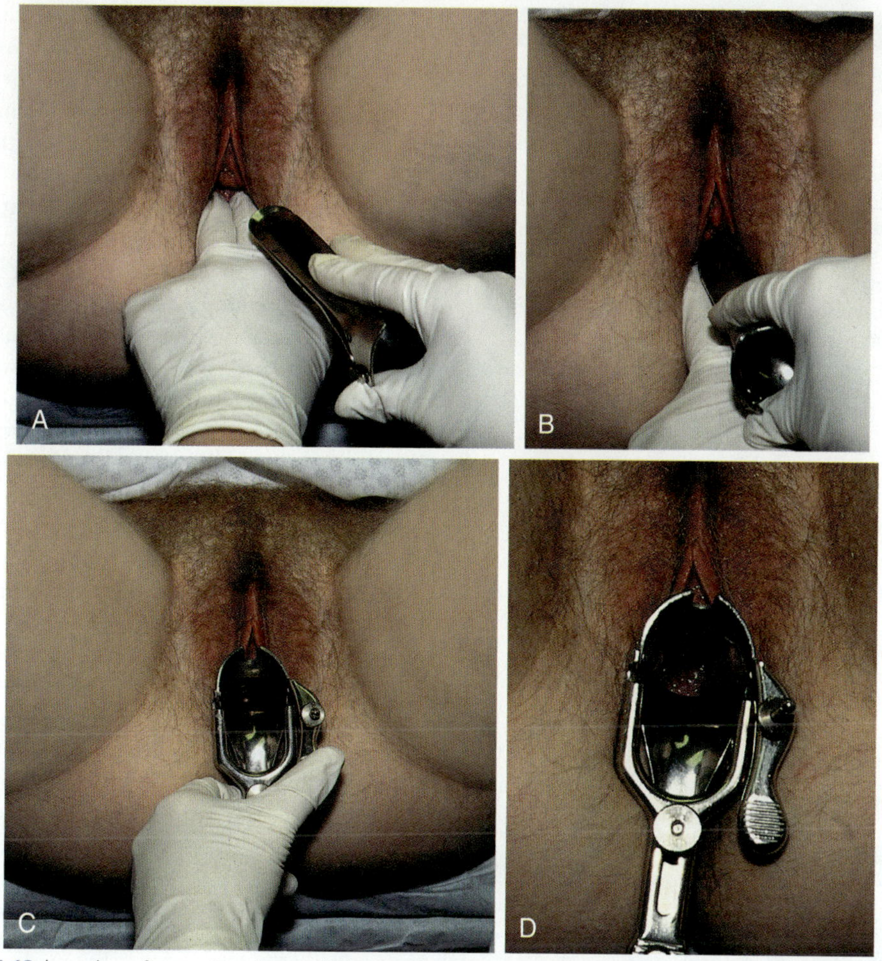

FIG. 4-12 Insertion of speculum for vaginal examination. **A,** Opening of the introitus. **B,** Oblique insertion of the speculum. **C,** Final insertion of the speculum. **D,** Opening of the speculum blades. (From Wilson, S., & Giddens, J. [2009]. *Health assessment for nursing practice* [4th ed.]. St. Louis: Mosby.)

the examiner compresses the area of Bartholin glands located at the 8 o'clock and 4 o'clock positions and looks for swelling, discharge, and pain.

The support of the anterior and posterior vaginal wall is assessed. The examiner spreads the labia with the index and middle fingers and asks the woman to strain down. Any bulge from the anterior wall (urethrocele or cystocele) or posterior wall (rectocele) is noted and compared with the history, such as difficulty to start the stream of urine or constipation.

The perineum (area between the vagina and anus) is assessed for scars from old lacerations or episiotomies, thinning, fistulas, masses, lesions, and inflammation. The anus is assessed for hemorrhoids, hemorrhoidal tags, and integrity of the anal sphincter. The anal area also is assessed for lesions, masses, abscesses, and tumors. If there is a history of STI, the examiner may want to obtain a culture specimen from the anal canal at this time. Throughout the genital examination, the examiner notes the odor. Odor may indicate infection or poor hygiene.

Vulvar Self-Examination. The pelvic examination provides a good opportunity for the practitioner to emphasize the need for regular **vulvar self-examination (VSE) or genital self-examination (GSE)** and to teach this procedure. Because there has been a dramatic increase in cancerous and precancerous conditions of the vulva in recent years, a VSE should be performed as an integral part of preventive health care by all women who are sexually active or ages 18 years or older. Most lesions, including malignancy, condyloma acuminatum (wartlike growth), and Bartholin cysts, can be seen or palpated and are easily treated if diagnosed early.

The VSE can be performed by the practitioner and woman together, by using a mirror. A simple diagram of the anatomy of the vulva can be given to the woman, with instructions to perform the examination herself that evening to reinforce what she has learned. She does the examination in a sitting position with adequate lighting, holding a mirror in one hand and using the other hand to expose the tissues surrounding the vaginal introitus. She then systematically examines the mons pubis, the clitoris, the urethra, the labia majora, the perineum, and the perianal area and palpates the vulva, noting any changes in appearance or abnormalities, such as ulcers, lumps, warts, and changes in pigmentation.

Internal Examination. A vaginal speculum consists of two blades and a handle. Speculums come in a variety of types and styles. A vaginal speculum is used to view the vaginal vault and cervix (see Procedure box: Assisting with Pelvic Examination). The speculum is gently placed into the vagina and inserted to the back of the vaginal vault. The blades are opened to reveal the cervix and are locked into the open position. The cervix is inspected for position and appearance of the os: color, lesions, bleeding, and discharge (Fig. 4-12). Cervical findings that are not within normal limits include ulcerations, masses, inflammation, and excessive protrusion into the vaginal vault. Anomalies,

PROCEDURE

Assisting with Pelvic Examination

- Wash hands. Assemble equipment (see below).
- Ask woman to empty her bladder before the examination (obtain clean-catch urine specimen as needed).
- Assist with relaxation techniques. Have the woman place her hands on her chest at about the level of the diaphragm, breathe deeply and slowly.
- Encourage the woman to become involved with the examination if she shows interest. For example, a mirror can be placed so that she can see the area being examined.
- Assess for and treat signs of problems such as supine hypotension.
- Warm the speculum in warm water if a prewarmed one is not available.
- Instruct the woman to bear down when the speculum is being inserted.
- Apply gloves and assist the examiner with collection of specimens for cytologic examination, such as a Pap test. After handling specimens, remove gloves and wash hands.
- Lubricate the examiner's fingers with water or water-soluble lubricant before bimanual examination.
- Assist the woman at completion of the examination to a sitting position and then a standing position.
- Provide tissues to wipe lubricant from perineum.
- Provide privacy for the woman while she is dressing.

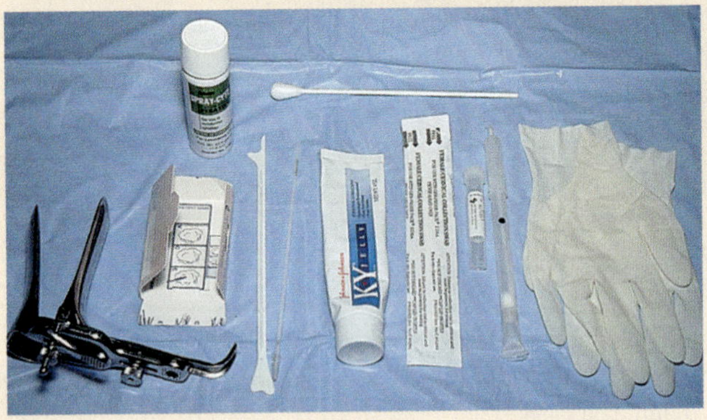

Equipment used for pelvic examination. (Courtesy Michael S. Clement, MD, Mesa, AZ.)

such as a cockscomb (a protrusion over the cervix that looks like a rooster's comb), a hooded or collared cervix (seen in diethylstilbestrol [DES] daughters), or polyps, are noted.

Collection of Specimens. The collection of specimens for cytologic examination is an important part of the gynecologic examination. Infection can be diagnosed through examination of specimens collected during the pelvic examination. These infections include candidiasis, trichomoniasis, bacterial vaginosis, group B streptococci, gonorrhea, chlamydia, and herpes simplex virus (see Chapter 7). Once the diagnoses have been made, treatment can be instituted.

Papanicolaou (Pap) Test. Carcinogenic conditions, potential or actual, can be determined by examination of cells from the cervix collected during the pelvic examination (see Procedure box: Papanicolaou Test). This is termed a Pap test.

Vaginal Examination. After the specimens are obtained, the vagina is viewed when the speculum is rotated. The speculum blades are unlocked and partially closed. As the speculum is withdrawn, it is rotated, and the vaginal walls are inspected for color, lesions, rugae, fistulas, and bulging.

Bimanual Palpation. The examiner stands for this part of the examination. A small amount of lubricant is placed on the first and second fingers of the gloved hand for the internal examination. To avoid tissue trauma and contamination, the thumb is abducted and the ring and little fingers are flexed into the palm (Fig. 4-13).

The vagina is palpated for distensibility, lesions, and tenderness. The cervix is examined for position, shape, consistency, motility, and lesions. The fornix around the cervix is palpated.

The other hand is placed on the abdomen halfway between the umbilicus and the symphysis pubis and exerts pressure downward toward the pelvic hand. Upward pressure from the pelvic hand traps reproductive structures for assessment by palpation. The uterus is assessed for position, size, shape, consistency, regularity, motility, masses, and tenderness.

With the abdominal hand moving to the right lower quadrant and the fingers of the pelvic hand in the right lateral fornix, the adnexa is assessed for position, size, tenderness, and masses. The examination is repeated on the woman's left side.

Just before the intravaginal fingers are withdrawn, the woman is asked to tighten her vagina around the fingers as much as she can. If the muscle response is weak, the woman is assessed for her knowledge about Kegel exercises.

Rectovaginal Palpation. To prevent contamination of the rectum from organisms in the vagina (such as *Neisseria gonorrhoeae*), it is necessary to change gloves, add fresh lubricant, and then reinsert the index finger into the vagina and the middle finger into the rectum (Fig. 4-14). Insertion is facilitated if the woman strains down. The maneuvers of the abdominovaginal examination are repeated. The rectovaginal examination permits assessment of the rectovaginal septum, the posterior surface of the uterus, and the region behind the cervix and the adnexa. The vaginal finger is removed and folded into the palm, leaving the middle finger free to rotate 360 degrees. The rectum is palpated for rectal tenderness and masses.

After the rectal examination, the woman is assisted into a sitting position, given tissues or wipes to cleanse herself, and given privacy to dress. The examiner returns after the woman is dressed to discuss findings and the plan of care.

Pelvic Examination During Pregnancy

The pelvic examination is done in the same way as it is during a routine examination on a nonpregnant woman. Pelvic measurements are completed, and uterine size is estimated. A Pap test may be done initially, as well as collection of cytologic specimens to test for gonorrhea, chlamydia, human papillomavirus, herpes simplex virus, and group B streptococci. As the pregnancy progresses, the nurse will inspect the woman's abdomen, palpate fetal size and position, auscultate fetal heart tones, and measure fundal height at each visit.

While the pregnant woman is in lithotomy position, the nurse must watch for supine hypotension, caused by the weight of the abdomen pressing on the vena cava and aorta and triggering a decrease in blood pressure (see Fig. 19-5). Symptoms of supine hypotension include pallor, dizziness, faintness, breathlessness, tachycardia, nausea, clammy skin, and sweating. The woman should be positioned on her side until symptoms resolve and vital signs stabilize. The vaginal examination can be done with the woman in the lateral position.

PROCEDURE

Papanicolaou Test

- In preparation, make sure the woman has not douched, used vaginal medications, or had sexual intercourse for 24 to 48 hours before the procedure. Reschedule the test if the woman is menstruating. Midcycle is the best time for the test.
- Explain to the woman the purpose of the test and what sensations she will feel as the specimen is obtained (e.g., pressure but not pain).
- The woman is assisted into a lithotomy position. A speculum is inserted into the vagina.
- The cytologic specimen is obtained before any digital examination of the vagina is made or endocervical bacteriologic specimens are taken. A cotton swab may be used to remove excess cervical discharge before the specimen is collected.
- The specimen is obtained by using an endocervical sampling device (Cytobrush, Cervex-brush, spatula, or broom) (see Figs. *A* and *B*). If the two-sample method of obtaining cells is used, the Cytobrush is inserted into the canal and rotated 90 to 180 degrees, followed by a gentle smear of the entire transformation zone by using a spatula. Broom devices are inserted and rotated 360 degrees five times. They obtain endocervical and ectocervical samples at the same time. If the woman has had a hysterectomy, the vaginal cuff is sampled. Areas that appear abnormal on visualization will require colposcopy and biopsy. If using a one-slide technique, the spatula sample is smeared first. This is followed by applying the Cytobrush sample (rolling the brush in the opposite direction from which it was obtained), which is less subject to drying artifact; then the slide is sprayed with preservative within 5 seconds.
- The ThinPrep or Sure Path Pap Test is a liquid-based method of preserving cells that reduces blood, mucus, and inflammation. The Pap specimen is obtained in the manner described above except that the cervix is not swabbed before collection of the sample. The collection device (brush, spatula, or broom) is rinsed in a vial of preserving solution that is provided by the laboratory. The sealed vial with solution is sent off to the appropriate laboratory. A special processing device filters the contents, and a thin layer of cervical cells is deposited on a slide, which is then examined microscopically. The AutoPap and Papnet tests are similar to the ThinPrep test. If cytology is abnormal, liquid-based methods allow follow-up testing for human papillomavirus (HPV) DNA with the same sample.
- Label the slides or vial with the woman's name and site. Include on the form to accompany the specimens the woman's name, age, parity, and chief complaint or reason for taking the cytologic specimens.
- Send specimens to the pathology laboratory promptly for staining, evaluation, and a written report, with special reference to abnormal elements, including cancer cells.
- Advise the woman that repeated tests may be necessary if the specimen is not adequate.
- Instruct the woman concerning routine checkups for cervical and vaginal cancer. Women vaccinated against HPV should follow the same screening guidelines as unvaccinated women. According to revised evidence-based guidelines issued by the American College of Obstetricians and Gynecologists (ACOG) (2009), women should have their first cervical cancer screening at age 21 and be screened less frequently than previously recommended. Women younger than age 30 should undergo cervical screening once every 2 years instead of annually. Women ages 30 and older who have had three consecutive negative cervical cytology test results may be screened once every 3 years. Women with high risk factors such as exposure to diethylstilbestrol (DES) in utero, those treated for cervical intraepithelial neoplasia (CIN) 2, CIN 3, cervical cancer, or human immunodeficiency virus (HIV) may need more frequent screening.

  Young women who have been treated with excisional procedures for dysplasia have an increase in premature births. A large majority of the cervical dysplasias in adolescents caused by HPV resolve on their own without treatment. It is important to avoid unnecessary instrumentation and procedures that negatively affect the cervix. Women who have had a complete hysterectomy for noncancerous reasons that have no history of high-grade CIN, may have routine cervical cytology testing discontinued. Women ages 65 to 70 who have had three or more negative cytology results in a row and no abnormal test results in the past 10 years may discontinue cervical cancer screening (ACOG, 2009). The American Cancer Society 2010 guidelines for cervical cancer screening are slightly different (Table 4-3).

  Record the examination date on the woman's record.

  Communicate findings to the woman per agency protocol.

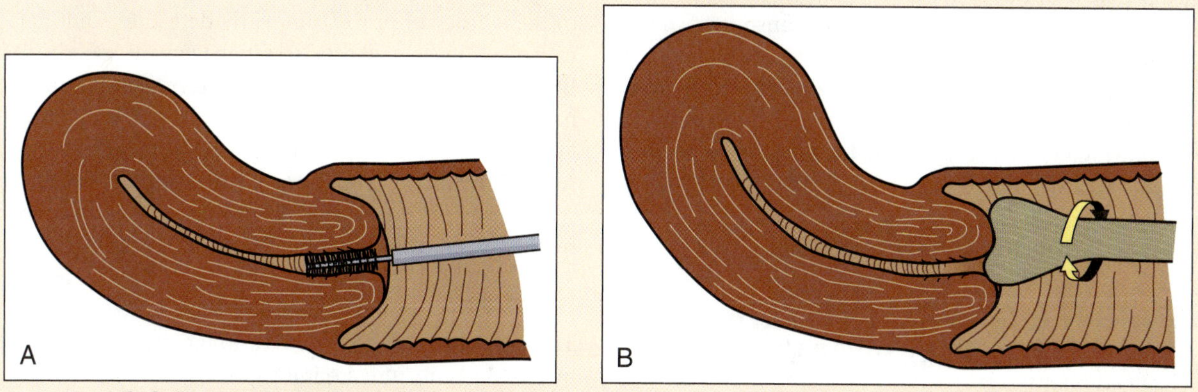

A, Collecting cells from endocervix using a Cytobrush. **B,** Obtaining cells from the transformation zone using a wooden spatula. (From Stenchever, M., Drogemueller, W., Herbst, A., & Mishell, D. [2001]. *Comprehensive gynecology* [4th ed.]. St. Louis: Mosby.)

Source: ACOG. (2009). Cervical cytology screening practice bulletin #109. Accessed January 20, 2010, from www.acog.org.

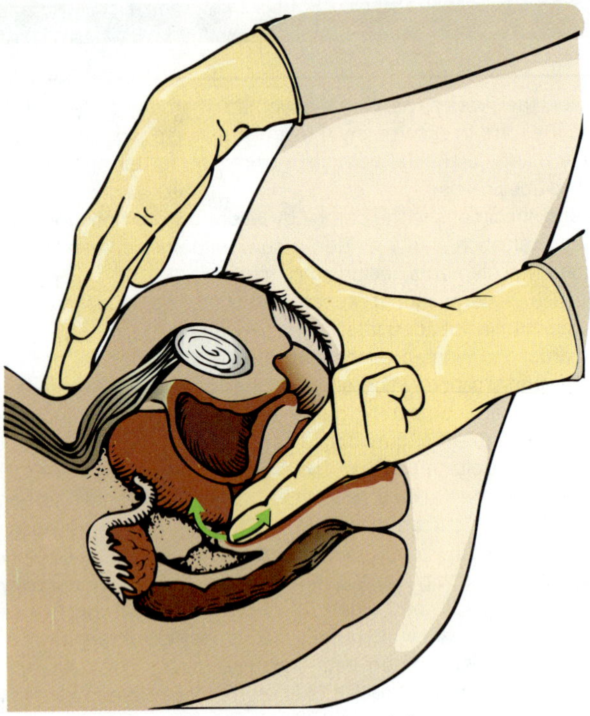

FIG. 4-13 Bimanual palpation of the uterus.

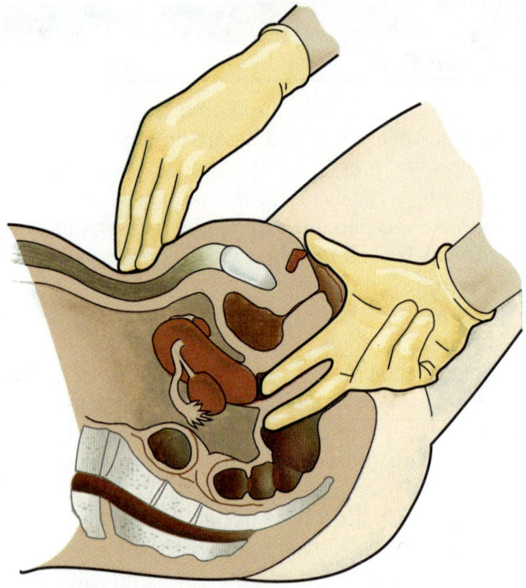

FIG. 4-14 Rectovaginal examination. (From Seidel, H., et al. [2011]. *Mosby's guide to physical examination* [7th ed.]. St. Louis: Mosby.)

Pelvic Examination After Hysterectomy

The pelvic examination is done much as it is done on a woman with a uterus. Vaginal screening using the Pap test is not recommended in women who have had a hysterectomy for benign disease. Because of the epidemic of human papillomavirus, which causes vaginal intraepithelial neoplasia, sampling of the vaginal cuff and vaginal walls after hysterectomy may still be practiced (see Table 4-3).

Laboratory and Diagnostic Procedures

The following laboratory and diagnostic procedures are ordered at the discretion of the clinician, considering the woman and her family history: hemoglobin, fasting plasma glucose, total blood cholesterol, lipid profile, urinalysis, syphilis serology (Venereal Disease Research Laboratory [VDRL] or rapid plasma reagin [RPR]) and other screening tests for sexually transmitted infections, mammogram, tuberculosis skin testing, hearing, visual acuity, electrocardiogram, chest X-ray, pulmonary function, fecal occult blood, flexible sigmoidoscopy, and bone mineral density scan. Results of these tests may be reported in person, by phone call, or by letter. Tests for HIV and drug screening may be offered with informed consent in high risk populations. These test results usually are reported in person.

ANTICIPATORY GUIDANCE FOR HEALTH PROMOTION AND ILLNESS PREVENTION

Over the past several decades women have made tremendous strides in education, careers, policy making, and overall participation in today's complex society. There have been costs for these advances, and although women are living longer, they may not be living better.

As a result, the health care system must pay greater attention to the health consequences for women. In addition, women must be active participants in their own health promotion and illness prevention. **Health promotion** is the motivation to increase well being and actualize health potential. **Illness prevention** is the desire to avoid illness, detect it early, or maintain optimal functioning when illness is present.

Nurses have a major opportunity and responsibility to help women understand risk factors and to motivate them to adopt healthy lifestyles that prevent disease. Lifestyle factors that affect health over which the woman has some control include diet; tobacco, alcohol, and substance use; exercise; sunlight exposure; stress management; and sexual practices. Other influences, such as genetic and environmental factors, may be beyond the woman's control, although some opportunities for prevention exist (e.g., through environmental legislation activism or genetic counseling services).

Knowledge alone is not enough to bring about healthy behaviors. The woman must be convinced that she has some control over her life and that healthy life habits, including periodic health examinations, are a sound investment. She must believe in the efficacy of prevention, early detection, and therapy and in her ability to perform self-management practices, such as BSE. Many people believe that they have little control over their health, or they become immobilized by fear and anxiety in the face of life-threatening illnesses, such as cancer, so they delay seeking treatment. The nurse must explore the reality of each woman's perceptions about health behaviors and individualize teaching if it is to be effective.

Nutrition

To maintain good nutrition, women should be counseled to include recommended servings from the major food categories of MyPyramid. Recommended servings from the food groups also provide adequate vitamins, minerals, iron, and fiber. Fluid intake is not included in the food pyramid, but individuals should be encouraged to drink at least six to eight glasses of water every day in addition to other fluids such as juices. Coffee, tea, soft drinks, and alcoholic beverages should be used in moderation.

TABLE 4-3 HEALTH SCREENING GUIDELINES AND IMMUNIZATION RECOMMENDATIONS FOR WOMEN AGES 18 YEARS AND OLDER

INTERVENTION	RECOMMENDATION*
Physical Examination	
Blood pressure	Every visit, but at least every 2 years
Height and weight	Every visit, but at least every 2 years
Pelvic examination	Annually until age 70; recommended for any woman who has ever been sexually active
Breast Examination	
Clinical examination†	Every 3 years, ages 20 to 39; annually after age 40
High risk	Annually after age 18 with history of premenopausal breast cancer in first-degree relative
Risk Groups	
Skin examination	Family history of skin cancer or increased exposure to sunlight every 3 years between ages 20 to 40; annually after age 40; monthly mole self-examinations also recommended
Oral cavity examination	History of mouth lesions or exposure to tobacco or excessive alcohol at least annually
Laboratory and Diagnostic Tests	
Blood cholesterol (fasting lipoprotein analysis)	At least once between ages 20 and 45; if level is within normal limits, every 5 years; more often if abnormal levels or have risk factors for coronary artery disease
Papanicolaou test†	Initially, 3 years after becoming sexually active but no later than age 21; yearly with conventional Pap test or every 2 years with liquid-based Pap tests. After age 30 and after three normal test results in a row, every 2 to 3 years; after age 70 and no abnormal test results in 10 years or after total hysterectomy, women may choose to stop screening
Mammography‡	Every 1 to 2 years between ages 40 and 49 or earlier if at high risk Annually after age 40 Annually after age 50 Biennially, ages 50 to 74 After age 75 discuss with your health care provider
Colon cancer screening	Use 1 of these 3 methods: -Fecal occult blood test annually ages 50 to 74 -Flexible sigmoidoscopy every 5 years ages 50-74 -Colonoscopy every 10 years ages 50 to 74 Screen more often if family history of colon cancer or polyps After age 75, discuss with your health care provider
Hearing screen	Starting at age 18 then every 10 years until 49 Every 3 years after age 50 Annually with exposure to excessive noise or when loss is suspected
Vision screen	At least once between ages 20 and 29; at least twice between ages 30 and 39 Every 2 to 4 years between ages 40 and 64; every 1 to 2 years after age 65
Risk Groups	
Fasting blood sugar	Annually with family history of diabetes or gestational diabetes or if significantly obese; every 3 to 5 years for all women older than 45 years of age
Thyroid-stimulating hormone (TSH) test	As determined by the health care provider
Sexually transmitted infection test (e.g., gonorrhea, syphilis, herpes)	As needed if sexually active with multiple partners and engaging in risky sexual behaviors
Chlamydia test	If sexually active, yearly until age 25; after age 25, test as needed when sexually active with new or multiple partners
Human Immunodeficiency Virus (HIV) test	At least once between ages 18 to 64 to determine HIV status; test if there is a high risk of HIV infection
Tuberculin skin test	Annually with exposure to persons with tuberculosis or in risk categories for close contact with the disease
Endometrial biopsy	At menopause for women at risk for endometrial cancer; repeat as needed
Bone mineral density testing	All women age 65 and older at least once; repeat testing as needed; younger women with risk for osteoporosis may need periodic screenings
Immunizations	
Tetanus-diphtheria	Booster is given every 10 years after primary series
Measles, mumps, rubella	Once if born after 1956 and no evidence of immunity
Hepatitis A	Primary series of two injections for all who are in risk categories
Hepatitis B	Primary series of three injections for all who are in risk categories
Influenza	Annually after age 65 or in risk categories, such as chronic diseases, immunosuppression, renal dysfunction
Human papillomavirus (HPV) vaccine	Primary series of three injections for girls ages 9 to women 26 years old. Intended for those not previously exposed to HPV.

*The information in this table is only a guide; health care providers will individualize the timing of tests and immunizations for each woman.

†American Cancer Society (ACS). (2010a). *Cancer facts and figures, 2010.* New York: ACS.

‡Note: No consensus has been reached regarding mammograms for women between 40 and 49 years of age; therefore, various recommendations are listed. Women are urged to discuss circumstances with their health care providers.

Sources: American Cancer Society (ACS). (2010a). *Cancer facts and figures, 2010.* New York: ACS; American College of Obstetricians and Gynecologists (ACOG). (2009). *Response of the American College of Obstetricians and Gynecologists to new breast cancer screening recommendations from the U.S. Preventive Services Task Force.* Available at www.acog.org. Accessed January 8, 2010; Centers for Disease Control and Prevention (CDC) Advisory Committee on Immunization Practices. (2009). *Recommended adult immunization schedule, United States, 2009.* Available at www.cdc.gov/vaccines/pubs/ACIP-list.htm. Accessed May 4, 2010; CDC, Workowski, K., & Berman, S. (2006). Sexually transmitted diseases treatment guidelines, 2006. *Morbidity and Mortality Weekly Report. Recommendations and Reports, 55*(RR11), 1-94; Expert Panel on Detection, Evaluation, and Treatment of High Blood Cholesterol in Adults. (2001). Executive summary of the third report of the national education program (NCEP) expert panel on detection, evaluation, and treatment of high blood cholesterol in adults (Adult Treatment Panel III). *Journal of the American Medical Association, 285*(19), 2486-2497; National Women's Health Resource Center. (2007). Women and health screenings. *National Women's Health Report, 29*(5), 1-7; National Women's Health Information Center. (2009). *General screenings and immunizations for women.* Available at www.4woman.gov. Accessed January 20, 2010; U.S. Preventive Services Task Force (USPSTF). (2009). *Guide to clinical preventive services.* Agency for Healthcare Research and Quality (AHRQ) Pub. No. 09-1P006, Rockville MD: AHRQ.

CLINICAL REASONING

Cardiovascular Disease—the Leading Cause of Death in Women

Selena is a 56-year-old Hispanic menopausal female who presents for her annual well-woman exam. She is a nonsmoker and nondrinker who lives a sedentary lifestyle. She does not exercise. Her mother died of a heart attack at age 60.

Body mass index (BMI) at today's visit is 33, BP 150/100, high-density lipoprotein (HDL) 25.

She says she knows that she is overweight and should probably exercise and lose weight. How would you respond to her statement?

1. Evidence—Is there evidence that supports how the nurse should respond?
2. Assumptions—What assumptions can be made about the following issues?
   a. Effects of primary and secondary cardiovascular risk factors
   b. Elevated blood pressure
   c. Low HDL
3. What implications and priorities for nursing care can be made at this time?
4. Does the evidence objectively support your conclusion?
5. Are there alternative perspectives to your conclusion?

Folic acid helps reduce high levels of homocysteine, an amino acid that damages the heart and blood vessels and increases the risk of heart disease, stroke, and dementia. Folic acid is present in citrus fruits, broccoli, spinach, asparagus, peas, lettuce, beans, whole grains, and orange juice. It is in many fortified grains and pasta or can be taken as a daily vitamin supplement (USDHHS & USDA, 2010).

Antioxidants are thought to be effective in helping to prevent oxidative damage in the body such as cancer, heart disease, and stroke; however, more research is needed in this area. Vitamins C and E; selenium (a mineral); and a group known as beta-carotenes (carotenoids) can be found in a diet containing fruits, vegetables, and whole grains.

Most women do not recognize the importance of calcium to health, and their diets are insufficient in calcium. Women who are unlikely to have enough calcium in the diet may need calcium supplements in the form of calcium carbonate with vitamin D, which contains more elemental calcium than do other preparations.

Vitamin D is essential for strong bones and a healthy immune system. Recent epidemiologic studies have shown a relationship between low vitamin D levels and multiple disease states such as increased cardiovascular mortality, cancer incidence, diabetes, osteoporosis, chronic pain and autoimmune diseases such as multiple sclerosis (Kulie, Groff, Redmer, Hounshell, & Schrager, 2009). Women can fulfill their vitamin D requirements by ingesting vitamin D and vitamin D–enhanced foods or being exposed to the sun for enough time to produce adequate amounts. It has been postulated that exposure of the arms and legs for 5 to 30 minutes between the hours of 10 AM and 3 PM twice a week can be adequate to prevent vitamin D deficiency (Holick, 2007). With concerns about skin cancer, most women are cautious about sun exposure. Sources of natural vitamin D include egg yolks, shitake mushrooms, tuna, mackerel, sardines, salmon, and cod liver oil. Vitamin D–enhanced foods include milk, orange juice, infant formulas, yogurt, butter, margarine, cheese, and breakfast cereals. Researchers continue to investigate the optimum levels of vitamin D needed by healthy adults; most experts agree that less than 20 ng/ml represents deficiency (Kulie et al.).

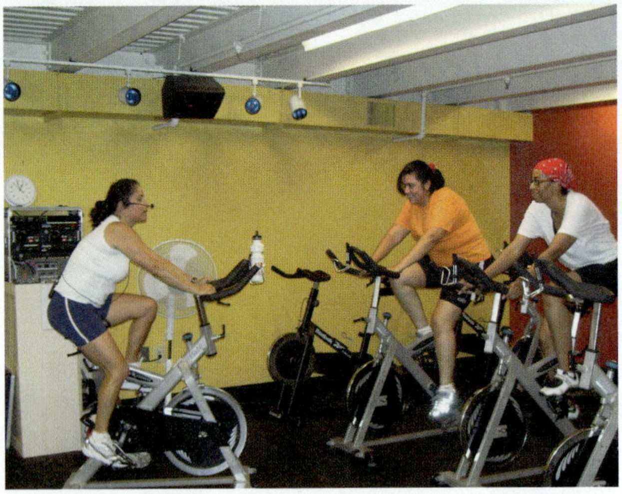

FIG. 4-15 Exercise should be a part of one's regular health routine. A cycle class is fun and provides moderate to vigorous exercise. (Courtesy Shari Rivera Sharpe, Chapel Hill, NC.)

The diet can be assessed by using a standard assessment form—a 24-hour recall is adequate and quick—and then food likes and dislikes, including cultural variations and typical food portions and dietary habits should be discussed and incorporated into counseling (see Chapter 14).

Exercise

Physical activity and exercise counseling for women of all ages should be undertaken at schools, worksites, and primary care settings. American Heart Association (AHA) (2010) recommendations include 30 to 60 minutes of moderate to vigorous activity on most days of the week. Activities do not need to be strenuous to bring health benefits. What is important is to include activities as part of a regular health routine. Activities that are especially beneficial when performed regularly include brisk walking, hiking, stair climbing, aerobic exercise, jogging, running, bicycling, rowing, swimming, soccer, and basketball. Few Americans exercise as often as they should, and physical activity is known to decrease with age, especially during adolescence and early adulthood.

The nurse should stress the importance of daily exercise throughout life for weight management and health promotion, suggesting exercises that are enjoyable to the individual (Fig. 4-15). Physical activity builds healthy bones, muscles, and joints and reduces the risk of colon and breast cancer. It also reduces feelings of depression and anxiety and improves mood and promotes a feeling of well-being. Many women who are sedentary during leisure time can benefit from gradually increasing their physical activity. They may be encouraged to exercise with their children or in groups with friends. Programs such as Curves for women, worksite fitness programs, or community-based programs such as the AHA's Choose To Move are increasingly available. Young women can be involved in fitness centers, cheerleading, gymnastics, sports teams, or individual competitive sports.

For women who are sedentary or are not able to exercise vigorously, even moderate- and low-intensity activities, when performed daily, can have long-term health benefits such as lowering the risk of cardiovascular disease. Regular physical activity can reduce or eliminate some of these risk factors by lowering blood pressure, maintaining a reasonable weight or facilitating weight loss, and lowering cholesterol levels to less than 200 mg/dl.

Home maintenance, yard work, and gardening are other activities that promote health and a sense of well-being, especially for older adults. Attention to safety factors and wearing clothing and shoes appropriate to each activity are advised. Care should be taken not to aggravate existing conditions or create muscle and joint discomfort by an overly aggressive approach to exercise.

Kegel Exercises

Kegel exercises, or pelvic muscle exercises, were developed to strengthen the supportive pelvic floor muscles to control or reduce incontinent urine loss. These exercises also are beneficial during pregnancy and postpartum. They strengthen the muscles of the pelvic floor, providing support for the pelvic organs and control of the muscles surrounding the vagina and urethra. Educational strategies for teaching women how to perform Kegel exercises were compiled by nurse researchers who conducted a research utilization project for the Association of Women's Health, Obstetric and Neonatal Nurses (AWHONN) are described in the Teaching for Self-Management box: Kegel Exercises.

Stress Management

Because it is neither possible nor desirable to avoid all stress, women must learn how to manage stress. The nurse should assess each woman for signs of stress by using therapeutic communication skills to determine risk factors and the woman's ability to function. See Box 4-5 for identifying symptoms of stress.

Women are twice as likely as men to have depression, anxiety, or panic attacks (NWHRC, 2009). Nurses must be alert to the symptoms of serious mental disorders, such as depression and anxiety. Women having major life changes such as divorce and separation, bereavement, serious illness, and unemployment need special attention.

For many women, the nurse is able to provide comfort, reassurance, and advice concerning helping resources, such as support groups. Many centers offer support groups to help women prevent or manage stress. The nurse can help women become more aware of the relationship between good nutrition, rest, relaxation, and exercise, and diversion, and their ability to deal with stress. In the case of role overload, determining what needs immediate attention and what can wait is important. Practical advice includes having regular breaks, taking time for friends, developing interests outside of work or the home, setting realistic goals, and learning self-acceptance. Discussing how women can maintain meaningful relationships is important. Social support and good coping skills can improve a woman's self-esteem and give her a sense of mastery. Anticipatory guidance for developmental or expected situational crises can help her plan strategies for dealing with potentially stressful events.

TEACHING FOR SELF-MANAGEMENT

Kegel Exercises

DESCRIPTION AND RATIONALE

Kegel exercises, or pelvic muscle exercise, is a technique used to strengthen the muscles that support the pelvic floor. This exercise involves regularly tightening (contracting) and relaxing the muscles that support the bladder and urethra. By strengthening these pelvic muscles, a woman can prevent or reduce accidental urine loss.

TECHNIQUE

The woman needs to learn how to target the muscles for training and how to contract them correctly. One suggestion for teaching is to have the woman pretend she is trying to prevent the passage of intestinal gas. Have her use this tightening motion on the muscles around her vagina and the upper pelvis. She should feel these muscles drawing inward and upward. Other suggested techniques are to have the woman pretend she is trying to stop the flow of urine in midstream or to have her think about how her vagina is able to contract around and move up the length of the penis during intercourse.

The woman should avoid straining or bearing-down motions while performing the exercise. She should be taught how bearing down feels by having her take a breath, hold it, and push down with her abdominal muscles as though she were trying to have a bowel movement. Then the woman can be taught how to avoid straining down by exhaling gently and keeping her mouth open each time she contracts her pelvic muscles.

SPECIFIC INSTRUCTIONS

1. Each contraction should be as intense as possible without contracting the abdomen, thighs, or buttocks.
2. Contractions should be held for at least 10 seconds. The woman may have to start with as little as 2 seconds per contraction until her muscles get stronger.
3. The woman should rest for 10 seconds or more between contractions, so that the muscles have time to recover and each contraction can be as strong as the woman can make it.
4. The woman should feel the pulling up over the three muscle layers so that the contraction reaches the highest level of her pelvis.

OTHER SUGGESTIONS FOR IMPLEMENTATION

1. At first the woman should set aside about 15 minutes a day to do the Kegel exercises.
2. The woman may want to put up reminders to do the exercises, such as notes on her bathroom mirror, her refrigerator, her television, or her calendar.
3. Guidelines for practicing Kegel exercises suggest performing between 24 and 100 contractions a day; however, positive results can be achieved with only 24 to 45 a day.
4. The best position for learning how to do Kegel exercises is to lie supine with the knees bent. Another position to use is on the hands and knees. Once the woman learns the proper technique, she can perform the exercises in other positions such as standing or sitting.

Sources: Sampselle, C. (2003). Behavior interventions in young and middle-aged women: Simple interventions to combat a complex problem. *American Journal of Nursing, 103*(Suppl), 9-19; Sampselle, C. (2000). Behavioral interventions for urinary incontinence in women: Evidence for practice. *Journal of Midwifery & Women's Health, 45*(2), 94-103; Sampselle, C., Wyman, J., Thomas, K., Newman, D., Gray, M., Dougherty, M., et al. (2000). Continence for women: A test of AWHONN's evidence-based protocol. *Journal of Obstetric, Gynecologic and Neonatal Nursing, 29*(1), 312-317.

The abundant literature on stress management interventions includes role-playing, relaxation techniques, biofeedback, meditation, desensitization, imagery, assertiveness training, yoga, diet, exercise, and weight control, techniques nurses can include in their repertoire of helping skills. Insufficient time prevents one-on-one assistance in many situations, but the more nurses know about these interventions, the better able they are to intervene, counsel, and direct women to appropriate resources.

Some women must be referred for counseling or other mental health therapy. Careful follow-up of all women experiencing difficulty in dealing with stress is important.

Substance Use Cessation

All women of all ages will receive substantial and immediate benefits from smoking cessation. However, this task is not easy, and most people stop several times before they accomplish their goal (Box 4-9). Many are never able to do so. Those who wish to stop smoking can be referred to a smoking-cessation program where individualized methods can be implemented. At the very least, individuals should be guided to self-help materials available from the March of Dimes, the American Lung Association, and the ACS. During pregnancy, women seem to be highly motivated to stop or at least to limit smoking. Insult to the fetus can be reduced or even prevented if cessation is accomplished by the end of the first trimester (Bernstein, Mongeon, Badger, Solomon, Heil, & Higgins, 2005).

New approaches to increase cessation among smokers and to discourage smoking among young women—especially in adolescence and during pregnancy—are needed. Health care providers can have a positive effect on smoking behavior and should attempt to motivate smokers to stop.

Counseling women who appear to be drinking alcohol excessively or using drugs may include promoting strategies to increase self-esteem and teaching new coping skills to resist and maintain resistance to alcohol abuse and drug use. Appropriate referrals should be made, with the health care provider arranging the contact and then following up to be sure that appointments are kept. General referral to sources of support also should be provided. National groups that provide information and support for those who are chemically dependent have local branches or contacts that are listed in the local telephone book.

Anticipatory guidance includes teaching about the health and safety risks of alcohol and mind-altering substances and discouraging drug experimentation among preteen and high school students, because the use of drugs at an early age tends to be a predictor of greater involvement later.

Sexual Practices That Reduce Risk

Prevention of STIs is predicated on the reduction of high risk behaviors by educating toward a behavioral change. Behaviors of concern include multiple and casual sexual partners and unsafe sexual practices. The abuse of alcohol and drugs also is a high risk behavior and results in impaired judgment and thoughtless acts. Specific self-management measures to reduce risk are described in Chapter 7.

In addition to the prevention of STIs, women of childbearing years need information regarding contraception and family planning (see Chapter 8).

Health Screening Schedule

Periodic health screening includes history, physical examination, education, counseling, immunizations, and selected diagnostic and laboratory tests. This regimen provides the basis for overall health promotion, prevention of illness, early diagnosis of problems, and referral for appropriate management. Such screening should be customized according to a woman's age and risk factors. In most instances it is completed in health care offices, clinics, or hospitals; however, portions of the screening are now being carried out at events such as community health fairs. An overview of health screening recommendations and immunizations for women 18 years and older is provided in Table 4-3.

BOX 4-9 INTERVENTIONS FOR SMOKING CESSATION: THE FIVE A'S

ASK

- What was her age when she started smoking?
- How many cigarettes does she smoke a day? When was her last cigarette?
- Has she tried to quit?
- Does she want to quit?

ASSESS

- What were her reasons for not being able to quit before, or what made her start again?
- Does she have anyone who can help her?
- Does anyone else smoke at home?
- Does she have friends or family who have quit successfully?

ADVISE

- Give her information about the effects of smoking on pregnancy and her fetus, on her own future health, and on the members of her household.

ASSIST

- Provide support; give self-help materials.
- Encourage her to set a quit date.
- Refer to a smoking cessation program, or provide information about nicotine replacement products (not recommended during pregnancy) if she is interested.
- Teach and encourage use of stress-reduction activities.
- Provide for follow-up with a phone call, letter, or clinic visit.

ARRANGE FOLLOW-UP

- Arrange to follow the woman to find out about smoking-cessation status.
- Make a phone call around the time of her quit date. Assess her status at every prenatal visit.
- Congratulate her on her success, or provide support for her if she relapses.
- Referral to intensive treatment may be necessary.

Source: American College of Obstetricians and Gynecologists Committee on Health Care for Underserved Women; ACOG Committee on Obstetric Practice. (2005). ACOG committee opinion No. 316, October, 2005. Smoking cessation during pregnancy. *Obstetrics and Gynecology, 106*(4), 883-888.

Health Risk Prevention

Simple safety factors often are forgotten or perceived not to be important, yet injuries continue to have a major effect on the health status of all age-groups. Being aware of hazards and implementing safety guidelines will reduce risks. The nurse should frequently reinforce the following common-sense concepts that will protect the individual:

- Wear seat belts at all times in a moving vehicle.
- Wear safety helmets when riding a motorcycle, bicycle, or inline skates.
- Follow driving "rules of the road."
- Place smoke alarms throughout the home and workplace. Avoid secondhand smoke.
- Lock doors and windows to ensure personal safety.
- Reduce noise pollution or safeguard against hearing loss.
- Protect skin and eyes from ultraviolet light with the use of sunscreen, protective clothing, sunglasses, and hats.
- Practice water safety.
- Never walk or run alone, especially at night.
- Consider storing personal health information (PHI) in a digital database that can be accessed from anywhere you travel.
- Never share computer passwords with strangers to safeguard financial, personal, and health data.
- Take precautions and avoid dangerous situations.

Health Protection

Nurses can make a difference in stopping violence against women and preventing further injury. Educating women that abuse is a violation of their rights and facilitating their access to protective and legal services constitutes a first step. Encouraging health care institutions to implement appropriate domestic violence screening programs also is of great value (see Chapter 5). Other helpful measures for women to discourage their entry into abusive relationships include promoting assertiveness and self-defense courses; suggesting support and self-help groups that encourage positive self-regard, confidence, and empowerment; and recommending educational and skills development classes that will enhance independence and self-care.

Numerous national and local organizations provide information and assistance for women in abusive situations. All nurses who work in women's health care should become familiar with local services and legal options.

KEY POINTS

- Culture, religion, socioeconomic status, personal circumstances, individual preference, and stage of development are among the factors that influence a woman's desire for care and her response to the health care system.
- The changing status and roles of women affect their health, needs, and ability to cope with problems.
- Anticipatory guidance is enhanced in a private, safe environment in which the interaction is culturally competent, nonjudgmental, and confidential.
- Preconception counseling allows identification and possible remediation of potentially harmful personal and social conditions, medical and psychologic conditions, environmental conditions, and barriers to care before conception.
- Conditions that increase a woman's health risks also increase risks for her offspring.
- Periodic health screening, including history, physical examination, immunizations, and diagnostic and lab tests, provide the basis for overall health promotion, prevention of illness, early diagnosis of problems, and referral for management.
- Physical Activity Guidelines for Americans include 2½ hours a week of moderate intensity or 1¼ hours per week of vigorous-intensity exercise, or a combination of both (USDHHS, 2008).
- Health promotion and prevention of illness assists women in actualizing health potential by increasing motivation, providing information, and incorporating recommendations for accessing specific resources.

Audio Chapter Summaries Access an audio summary of these Key Points on evolve

REFERENCES

American Cancer Society (ACS). (2010). *Women and smoking: An epidemic of smoking-related cancer and disease in women*. New York: ACS.

American Cancer Society (ACS). (2009). *Cancer facts and figures 2010*. New York: ACS.

American College of Obstetricians and Gynecologists (ACOG). (2007). Cervical cytology screening practice bulletin No. 109. *Obstetrics & Gynecology, 114*(6), 1409–1420.

American Heart Association. (2010). *Physical activity and cardiovascular health: Questions and answers*. Available at www.americanheart.org. Accessed May 9, 2010.

Atrash, H., Johnson, K., Adams, M., Cordero, J., & Howse, J. (2006). Preconception care for improving perinatal outcomes: The time to act. *Maternal and Child Health Journal, 10*(Suppl. 5), S3–S11.

Bernstein, I., Mongeon, J., Badger, G., Solomon, L., Heil, S., & Higgins, S. (2005). Maternal smoking and its association with birth weight. *Obstetrics and Gynecology, 106*(5 Part 1), 986–991.

Centers for Disease Control and Prevention (CDC). (2009). Quickstats: Prevalence of obesity among adults aged ≥20 years by race/ethnicity and sex, United States, 2003-2006. *MMWR Morbidity and Mortality Weekly Report, 58*(38), 1075.

Centers for Disease Control and Prevention (CDC), Workowski, K., & Berman, S. (2006). Sexually transmitted diseases treatment guidelines 2006. *MMWR Morbidity and Mortality Weekly Report, 55*(RR11), 1–94.

Condon, M. (2004). *Women's health: Body, mind, spirit: An integrated approach to wellness and illness*. Upper Saddle River, New Jersey: Prentice-Hall.

Fehring, R., Schneider, M., & Raviele, K. (2006). Variability in the phases of the menstrual cycle. *Journal of Obstetric, Gynecologic and Neonatal Nursing, 35*(3), 376–384.

Galanti, G. (2008). *Caring for patients from different cultures* (4th ed.). Philadelphia: University of Pennsylvania Press.

Gaulin, P. (2010). *Health care bill summary and timetable of changes 2010-2018*. Available at www.associatedcontent.com/article/2824522/health_care_bill_summary_and_timeline.html?car=5. Accessed May 9, 2010.

Geddes, D. (2007). Inside the lactating breast: The latest anatomy research. *Journal of Midwifery & Women's Health, 52*(6), 556–563.

Goldberg, L. (2005-2006). Understanding the lesbian experience: What perinatal nurses should know to promote women's health. *AWHONN Lifelines, 9*(6), 463–467.

Heron, M., & Tejada-Vera, B. (2008). Deaths: Leading causes for 2005. *National Vital Statistics Reports, 58*(8), 1–98.

Holick, M. (2007). Vitamin D deficiency. *New England Journal of Medicine, 357*(3), 266–281.

Huff, M., Abuzz, G., & Omar, H. (2007). Detecting and treating depression among adolescents presenting for reproductive care: Realizing opportunities. *Journal of Pediatric and Adolescent Gynecology, 20*(6), 371–376.

Johnson, K., Posner, S., Biermann, J., Cordero, J., Atrash, H., Parker, C., et al. (2006). Recommendations to improve preconception health and health care—United States. A report of the CDC/ATSDR preconception care work group and the select panel on preconception care. *MMWR Morbidity and Mortality Weekly Report. Recommendations and Reports, 55*(RR06), 1–23.

Kliegman, R. (2006). Intrauterine growth restriction. In R. Martin, A. Fanaroff, & M. Walsh (Eds.), *Fanaroff and Martins's neonatal-perinatal medicine: Diseases of the fetus and infant* (8th ed.). Philadelphia: Mosby.

Kulie, T., Groff, A., Redmer, J., Hounshell, J., & Schrager, S. (2009). Vitamin D: An evidence-based review. *Journal of the American Board of Family Medicine, 22*(6), 698–706.

Kung, H., Hoyert, D., Xu, J., & Murphy, S. (2008). Deaths: Final data for 2005. *National Vital Statistics Reports, 56*(10), 1–120.

Love, S., & Barsky, S. (2004). Anatomy of the nipple and breast ducts revisited. *Cancer, 101*(9), 1947–1957.

March of Dimes Foundation. (2010). *Pregnancy after 35*. Available at www.marchofdimes.com. Accessed May 9, 2010.

Masters, W. (1992). *Human sexuality* (4th ed.). New York: HarperCollins.

Minikin, M., & Wright, C. (2005). *A woman's guide to menopause and perimenopause*. New Haven, CT: Yale University Press.

Moos, M. (2006). Preconception care: Every woman, every time. *AWHONN Lifelines, 10*(4), 332–334.

National Women's Health Resource Center (NWHRC). (2006). Women and obesity. *National Women's Health Report, 28*(4), 1–7.

National Women's Health Resource Center (NWHRC). (2008). Pregnancy & women age 35+. *National Women's Health Report, 30*(2), 1–4.

National Women's Health Resource Center (NWHRC). (2009). *Depression*. Available at www.healthywomen.org/condition/depression. Accessed May 9, 2010.

North American Menopause Society (NAMS). (2007). The role of local vaginal estrogen for treatment of vaginal atrophy in postmenopausal women: 2007 position statement of the North American Menopause Society. *Menopause, 14*(3 Part 1), 335–369.

Parker, S., Lyons, J., & Bonner, J. (2005). Eating disorders in graduate students: Exploring the SCOFF questionnaire as a simple screening tool. *Journal of American College Health, 52*(2), 103–107.

Piotrowski, K., & Snell, L. (2007). Health needs of women with disabilities across the life span. *Journal of Obstetric, Gynecologic and Neonatal Nursing, 36*(1), 79–87.

Ramsay, D., Kent, J., Hartmann, R., & Hartmann, P. (2005). Anatomy of the lactating breast redefined with ultrasound imaging. *Journal of Anatomy, 206*(6), 525–534.

Roberts, S. (2006). Health care recommendations for lesbian women. *Journal of Obstetric, Gynecologic and Neonatal Nursing, 35*(5), 583–591.

Seidel, H., Ball, J., Dains, J., Flynn, J., Solomon, B., & Stewart, R. (2011). *Mosby's guide to physical examination* (7th ed.). St. Louis: Mosby.

Smith, S., Hulsey, T., & Goodnight, W. (2008). Effects of obesity on pregnancy. *Journal of Obstetric, Gynecologic and Neonatal Nursing, 37*(2), 176–184.

Trussell, J. (2007). The cost of unintended pregnancies in the United States. *Contraception, 75*(3), 168–170.

U.S. Department of Health and Human Services (USDHHS), & U.S. Department of Agriculture (USDA). (2010). *Dietary guidelines for Americans*. Hyattsville, MD: USDA.

U.S. Department of Health and Human Services (USDHHS). (2008). *Physical activity guidelines for Americans*. Available from www.health.gov/paguidelines. Accessed May 5, 2010.

Wolfe, B. (2005). Reproductive health in women with eating disorders. *Journal of Obstetric, Gynecologic and Neonatal Nursing, 34*(2), 255–263.

CHAPTER

5

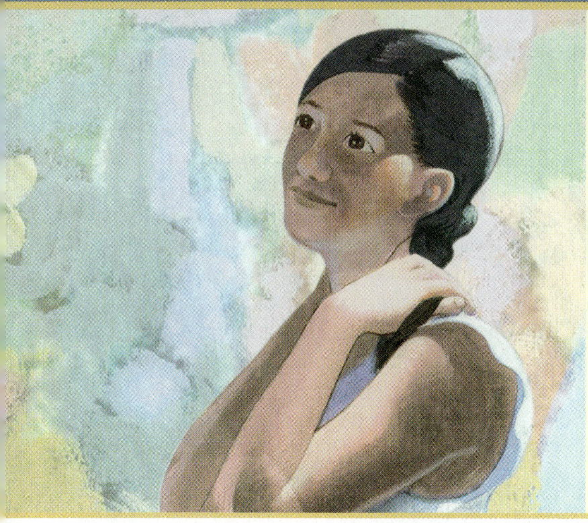

Violence Against Women

Noreen Esposito

evolve WEBSITE

http://evolve.elsevier.com/Lowdermilk/MWHC/

Audio Glossary
Audio Key Points
Critical Thinking Exercise
  Women's Health and Safety
NCLEX Review Questions
Nursing Care Plan
  The Woman Experiencing Intimate Partner Violence
Spanish Guidelines
  Recognizing Violence in a Relationship

LEARNING OBJECTIVES

- Describe the beliefs and practices that historically have perpetuated violence against women.
- Examine the prevalence and effects of intimate partner violence.
- Contrast the theoretic premises underlying the victimization of women.
- Discuss theories of violence and how they can be used in assessment and intervention for women who are abused.
- Develop a plan of care for a woman who is experiencing intimate partner violence.
- Review the dynamics of sexual assault.
- Describe the rape-trauma syndrome.
- Develop a nursing plan of care for a woman in the acute phase of rape-trauma syndrome.
- Evaluate resources available to women experiencing abuse.

Violence against women (VAW) is a worldwide public health problem. The United Nations defines it as "any act of gender-based violence that results in or is likely to result in physical, sexual or mental harm or suffering to women including threats of such acts, coercion, or arbitrary deprivation of liberty whether occurring in public or private" (Blanchfield, 2008; United Nations, 1993). Around the globe VAW takes many different forms including but not limited to intimate partner violence, sexual assault, marital-rape, dowry-related violence, sexual trafficking and exploitation, and female genital mutilation. This chapter focuses on intimate partner violence and sexual assault.

Intimate partner violence (IPV) is the most common form of VAW, with a reported lifetime incidence of one out of every six women (World Health Organization [WHO], 2010). The National Violence Against Women Survey (NVAWS) defines IPV as "the actual or threatened physical, sexual, psychologic, or emotional abuse by a spouse, ex-spouse, boyfriend, girlfriend, ex-boyfriend, ex-girlfriend, date, or cohabiting partner" (Tjaden & Thoennes, 2006). The term generally implies female victims and male perpetrators, but an estimated 7.4% of IPV is committed against men (Tjaden & Thoennes). IPV can be thought of as "a continuum ranging from one hit that may or may not impact the victim to chronic, severe battering" (Centers for Disease Control and Prevention [CDC], 2008). Other terms such as partner abuse and domestic or family violence are common. Older terms such as wife battering or spouse battering are generally not used. Battery has been used in the past to refer to physical contact with another with the intent of harm. IPV is the preferred term in that it encompasses not only physical contact but also emotional and other forms of violence previously ignored (Saltzman, Fanslow, McMahon, & Shelley, 2002).

IPV is a complex, stigmatized problem involving issues of emotional distress, personal safety, and social isolation. In many places in the United States and abroad IPV has been socially tolerated or ignored. Lack of reporting and inconsistent definitions have made it difficult to get an accurate count of the number of victims with wide ranges of estimates. Existing data tell us that IPV is pervasive.

The World Health Organization (WHO) found that the incidence of IPV ranged from 15% to 71% in a sample of 24,097 women from 10 countries not including the United States (Garcia-Moreno, Jansen, Ellsberg, Heise, & Watts, 2006). In an IPV study of 3568 female members of a nonprofit health maintenance organization (HMO), 44% of the predominantly Caucasian college-educated women reported abuse of any kind, 34% reported physical forced sex and/or sexual contact; 35% reported nonphysical abuse (threats and anger, controlling behavior) at some time in their adult lives, and 14% experienced abuse within the last 5 years and 8% in the last year (Thompson, Bonomi, Anderson, Reid, Dimer, Carrell, et al., 2006). In a prospective survey of 2737 urban public hospital emergency department (ED) clients, 548 (20%) identified themselves as victims of IPV. Greater victim-perceived danger was associated with lower physical and mental health functioning in the 216 of those who returned for follow-up (Straus, Cerulli, McNutt, Rhodes, Conner, Kemball, et al., 2009). The National Violent Death Reporting System (NVDRS) indicates that 1 in 5 murders in 2005 were IPV related. IPV was involved in 8 out of every 10 homicides, and 90% of the persons who did the killing were men (CDC, 2008). Although overall U.S. violence rates, including IPV rates, declined between 1998 and 2008 the percentage of women killed by an intimate partner rose from 40% to 45% (Catalano, Smith, Snyder, & Rand, 2009).

Abusive relationships happen to couples who are dating, living together, or married. They can continue after the relationship ends. The abuse may be physical, sexual, psychologic, or financial. One partner behaves in a way that injures, intimidates, humiliates, frightens, or terrorizes the other partner. These behaviors can be insidious, slowly happening over time. Emotional abuse may include name calling, acting in a jealous or possessive manner, trying to isolate the woman from her family or friends, putting her down in front of others, threatening her children or alienating her children from her, not wanting her to go out or go to work, or insisting that she account for every minute she is away from home. Physical violence may never be used, or used rarely, but threats can be as effective as actual violence. Once physical violence happens, the threat of recurrence always exists.

IPV may begin in pregnancy. If it already exists, IPV may increase, decrease, or stay the same during the pregnancy (Macy, Martin, Kupper, Casanueva, & Guo, 2007; Taylor & Nabors, 2009). (See later discussion on p. 103.)

The consequences of IPV are profound. In a study comparing abused women with never abused women, abused women had a higher incidence of social and family problems, substance abuse, menstrual and other reproductive disorders, sexually transmitted infections (STIs), musculoskeletal and gastrointestinal (GI) disorders, chest pain, abdominal pain, urinary tract infections (UTIs), and headaches (Bonomi, Anderson, Reid, Rivara, Carrell, & Thompson, 2009). In another study, women who had experienced abuse had a 50% to 70% increase in central nervous system (CNS), gynecologic, and anxiety-related problems (Campbell, J., Jones, Dienemann, Kub, Schollenberger, O'Campo, et al., 2002). In a study of 82 women diagnosed with depression, the researchers found that 61% of them had experienced IPV in their lifetimes and that the severity of violence was significantly correlated with the severity of depression (Dienemann, Boyle, Baker, Resnick, Wiederhorn, & Campbell, 2000).

Medical costs alone for interpersonal violence are estimated to be $2.7 to $7 billion for the first 12 months after victimization, and annual medical costs for any past intimate partner victimization, not just the last year range from $25 to $59 billion (Brown, Finkelstein, & Mercy, 2008). These figures do not include the cost of police and court costs, shelters, foster care, sick leave, and nonproductivity. Reducing the rate of intimate partner violence was a *Healthy People 2010* objective and a modified version is included in *Healthy People 2020* (U.S. Department of Health and Human Services [USDHHS], 2009).

CLINICAL REASONING

Intimate Partner Violence

Mariana, 21 years old, is in the clinic to discuss birth control options. She missed her last appointment. She is accompanied by her boyfriend, with whom she lives. The nurse suggests that he wait outside while she asks intake questions about Mariana's health. Mariana looks down and says quietly, "It's fine if he stays, really it is." The nurse notices that he is very attentive to Mariana, is very nice to the nurse, and answers for Mariana most of the time she is asked a question. You explain that the clinic has a policy that the interviews are done in private. He reluctantly leaves the room. After some routine questions about her general health the nurse asks her about intimate partner violence and safety. "Have you been hit, slapped, kicked, or in other ways physically hurt by someone?" Mariana shakes her head and says, "No" in a quiet voice. The nurse notices Mariana glance at a small bruise on the inner part of her arm. The nurse asks Mariana if she is being physically hurt or threatened in her relationship. She gets teary but says, "No." What is the nurse's responsibility in this instance regarding confidentiality, questioning Mariana about domestic violence, and risks to Mariana if she admits that she has been hurt by her boyfriend? What is the nurse's responsibility to report the incident to the police?

1. Evidence—Is there sufficient evidence to draw conclusions about Mariana as an abused woman?
2. Assumptions—What assumptions can be made about the following?
   a. Characteristic behaviors of abused woman
   b. Gender equality
   c. Blame and self-doubt
   d. Relationship expectations
3. What implications and priorities for nursing care can be made at this time?
4. Does the evidence objectively support your conclusion?
5. Are there alternative perspectives to your conclusion?

HISTORICAL PERSPECTIVE

Women have been treated inhumanely throughout history. In ancient Rome, wives were divorced or killed by husbands for adultery, public drunkenness, or attending public games, whereas men could engage in these activities daily. In the 1700s, under English common law, the "rule of thumb" gave men permission to chastise their wives physically as long as the implement they used was no wider than their thumbs. In the late 1600s, Pilgrims and Puritans directed male heads of the family to use force when needed to maintain conduct of their wives. Although American law prohibited beating wives, the Puritans supported physical force by husbands as legitimate. In the 1800s men gradually lost the right to beat their wives. Slow progress was made in the early 20th century. There was little awareness from both health care professionals and the legal and justice systems to the plight of women in intimate relationships. As late as the 1960s, it was believed that violence in the family was rare and committed only by the mentally ill.

The first shelter for women opened in London in 1971, and books and articles on domestic violence began to appear in the 1970s. Battered woman syndrome was described by Lenore Walker in 1979 and battered women programs begin to emerge in the 1980s. In the 1990s the American Nurses Association issued a position statement against VAW, the American Medical Association declared that physicians were liable if they did not recognize IPV, and The Joint Commission issued standards to identify and manage IPV patients. The National Domestic Violence Hotline was established in 1996. The CDC issued guidelines promoting the phrase intimate partner violence over domestic violence (Mitchell & Anglin, 2009). Health care providers, law enforcement, the legal system, and the general public are slowly acknowledging IPV, but power imbalances, persistent beliefs that family problems are private matters, and fear continue to keep women from disclosing abuse.

CONCEPTUAL AND THEORETIC PERSPECTIVES

In the late 1970s little was known about IPV. Lenore Walker, a pioneer in the field, interviewed 120 victims. From those interviews with a select group she described the "battered woman syndrome," which identified victim characteristics such as learned helplessness and abuser characteristics such as mental health problems. At the time Walker proposed a model of how IPV might appear in some families. The model, referred to as the *cycle of violence* described three phases in an IPV relationship: tension building, acute battering, and the honeymoon phase. In her proposed model, violence was neither random nor constant but occurred in repeated cycles. Her continued research led to modifications in her early interpretations. Ongoing research from different disciplines has expanded today's understanding of IPV. Current thought does not support the general applicability of the cycle of violence.

IPV is heterogeneous. Not all batterers are alike, not all victims are alike, and not all relationships and patterns of abuse are alike. In some relationships physical and psychologic abuse happen on a regular basis. In other relationships, physical abuse or the threat of abuse may happen rarely, but emotional abuse is more persistent. In some relationships abuse happens after stressful events or pregnancy. Walker's work was an important first step and helped raise awareness and interest. Because the cycle of violence was the only available explanation for IPV, the model became a core part of IPV training for health professionals, social workers, law enforcement officers, and judges. Despite limited evidence of its usefulness many professionals still believe that the cycle of violence explains IPV (Dutton, 2009).

The past 30 to 40 years have seen a growing body of literature about the characteristics and dynamics of IPV. Along with feminist ideologies that play a critical role in gender-based violence, theories from biology, psychology, and sociology all help to partially explain various aspects of violence against women. No single theory can completely explain this complex problem. Following is a brief discussion of some of these theoretic perspectives.

Biologic Factors

A complete explanation of the biologic perspective is beyond the scope of this chapter, but evidence indicates that neurobiologic and hormonal factors influence aggression in men. Areas in the brain believed to play a role in aggressive behavior are the limbic system, the frontal lobes, and the hypothalamus. Changes in structural functioning of the limbic system, such as occur with brain lesions, substance use, epilepsy, and head injuries, affect the emotional experience and behavior of the individual and thus can increase or decrease the potential for aggressive behavior (Stuart & Hamolia, 2009).

Neurochemical factors also can play a role in aggressive behavior so that dysfunction or disregulation of certain neurotransmitters can result in aggression. Increased levels of norepinephrine and L-dopa foster aggressive behavior. Reducing the levels of serotonin in animals causes aggressive behavior. The amino acid gamma-aminobutyric acid (GABA) inhibits aggressive behavior. The occurrence of violence in neurologic disorders also is reported, especially when violent reactions are out of proportion to the provoking events (Stuart & Hamolia, 2009).

In studies of animals, aggression is associated with abnormally high levels of testosterone. Soler, Vinayak, and Quadagno (2000) reported higher testosterone levels in abusive male subjects and suggested that heritability is an issue that warrants the inclusion of this variable in future studies of violent behavior. There is no conclusive evidence in biologic theory, except perhaps in instances of neurologic damage, that it is impossible to control aggressive behavior.

Psychologic Perspective

Psychology, the study of emotion and behavior, places responsibility for behaviors such as aggression on the individual. Early psychoanalytic theory suggested that aggression is a basic instinctual drive leading to mastery and accomplishment. In men aggression was seen as a positive force that connoted boldness, forcefulness, energy, and enterprise. Thus early psychologic theory saw aggression in men as normal. Early psychoanalytic theory promoted gender-stereotypic expectations for women to be caring and nurturing; aggression in women was and still is viewed negatively and aggressive women are often labeled as hostile and belligerent.

The myth that abuse is committed by people who have some type of mental illness perpetuates the notion that violence occurs among people who are not "normal." Mental illness accounts for a very small percentage of IPV. Men who batter range from having modest personality dysfunction to significant personality pathology such as borderline and antisocial personality disorders (Capaldi & Kim, 2007). Although a mental health diagnosis of alcohol abuse is frequently found in abusers, it should not be misconstrued as the cause of violence. There is some evidence that alcohol may increase the risk of violent behavior because survivors of violence often report abuser substance abuse (Torres & Han, 2003). There is no diagnostic profile of an abuser, but Box 5-1 provides some characteristics of men who batter that nurses may consider when assessing clients' relationships.

Women with severe and persistent mental illness are likely to be more vulnerable to being involved in controlling and violent relationships. However, numerous mental health problems (such as depression, psychophysiologic illnesses, substance abuse, eating disorders, posttraumatic stress disorder [PTSD], and anxiety reactions) experienced by women with abusive

BOX 5-1 CHARACTERISTICS OF A POTENTIAL MALE BATTERER

- Low self-esteem
- Problems with abandonment, loss, helplessness, dependency, insecurity, and intimacy
- Inadequate verbal skills, especially difficulty expressing feelings
- Deficits in assertiveness
- Personality disorders frequently diagnosed
- Low frustration tolerance (loses temper easily)
- Higher incidence of growing up in an abusive or violent home
- Denies, minimizes, blames, and lies about own actions
- Violence is consistent with his view of himself and the world; it is an acceptable way of dealing with everyday life
- Inability to empathize with others
- Rigidity in male and female behaviors (sex-role stereotypes)
- Perception of self as "special" and deserving special attention for being the provider, protector
- Substance abuse problems are common
- Display of an unusual amount of jealousy (e.g., expects partner to spend all of her time with him or to keep him informed of her whereabouts)

partners are more likely to be consequences of long-term abuse rather than causes (Moracco, Brown, Martin, Chang, Dulli, Loucks-Sorrell, et al., 2004). Relationship violence differs by the severity and frequency of violence, if the violence is confined to the family or occurs outside the family and by the individual's characteristics. Not all victims see their violence experiences in the same way; different women experience violence differently. Women with dependent personality traits as well as independent women have been victims of IPV. Although there may be shared characteristics, each person's experience and response is individual (Nurius & Macy, 2008).

Newer studies in psychology are exploring the unique differences among individuals who are in violent relationships. We know that men who are involved in relationship violence are not all alike. Heterogeneity is seen in the characteristics of the men, in their partners, and in the relationship dynamics. When trying to understand some types of violence, there is growing interest in considering both members of a relationship. In one conceptual model Capaldi and Kim (2007) explore the typologies of couples experiencing violence. They offer a dynamic systems model that considers what each person brings to a relationship. For example, personal characteristics such as depression or antisocial behavior might be combined with a person's emotional development to create a unique individual. Individuals come together to create a pattern of interactions and these interactions occur in the context of various social stresses such as substance use, financial stress, or separation. The dynamics can lead to some type of incident. Viewed this way, this dynamic model provides many potential areas for intervention. Research is needed to further explore the possibilities of this approach.

Sociologic Perspective

The social structure and conditions in Western society provide the basis for many of the prevailing attitudes toward violent behavior. U.S. history is filled with examples of violence, such as war as a means of social control. Social acceptance and promotion of violence in men are double standards because women are expected to be nonviolent. Thus psychologic theories of gender-based behaviors can influence social beliefs and responses to particular behaviors. Because men are socially expected to be aggressive, their violence is sometimes treated with more leniency and less stigma than women who are violent, particularly in the justice system. The more a culture uses physical force for socially approved ends, the more the violence becomes generalized to other areas of social life (Fishwick, Parker, & Campbell, 2005).

The structure and dynamics of the family—ascribed roles of family members, the amount of time spent together, the private nature of the family, the intensity of emotional involvement, and stress and conflict inherent in families—often set the stage for violent behaviors (Fishwick et al., 2005). Power and violence, or even the threat of physical force, serve to maintain the patriarchal view of woman's place in the home and in the rest of society. Gender inequality, in both economic opportunities and physical strength, serves to perpetuate the power imbalance in relationships.

Another family issue is the multigenerational transmission of violence; some perpetrators of violence and some victims learn about violence in families of origin by either witnessing or experiencing violence while growing up (Cannon, Bonomi, Anderson, & Rivara, 2009; Fishwick et al., 2005). In families in which violence occurs, both the lack of emotional support experienced by children and the awareness that people who love each other can be violent are important factors. Children in these environments do not have role models to help them develop mental models of healthy family dynamics. Abuse as a child does not consistently determine later violent behavior because many children who were abused grow up to avoid violent behavior.

Feminist Perspective

One contemporary view of violence is derived from feminist theory. This view, with the primary theme of male dominance and coercive control, enhances our understanding of all forms of violence against women, including IPV, stranger and acquaintance rape, incest, and sexual harassment in the workplace. This gender and power perspective evolved from women's descriptions of their abusive experiences and from activists attempting to understand the victimization that occurred. In numerous cases, power and control tactics were central events leading to the violence (Renzetti, Edleson, & Bergen, 2001). The power and control wheel developed by the Duluth, Minnesota, Domestic Abuse Intervention Project identified ways that men may exercise the power and control that underlie many types of IPV and has been used to help women, men, and care providers understand violence (Fig. 5-1).

As our understanding of the complexity of violence against women has evolved over time so has the need for an evolving feminist viewpoint. Using frontline workers' perspectives of current feminist thought, one study proposes an integrative feminist model. Keeping gender and other forms of oppression as the roots of IPV, an integrative model offers flexibility in exploring multiple other models emerging in violence research (McPhail, Busch, Kulkarni, & Rice, 2007).

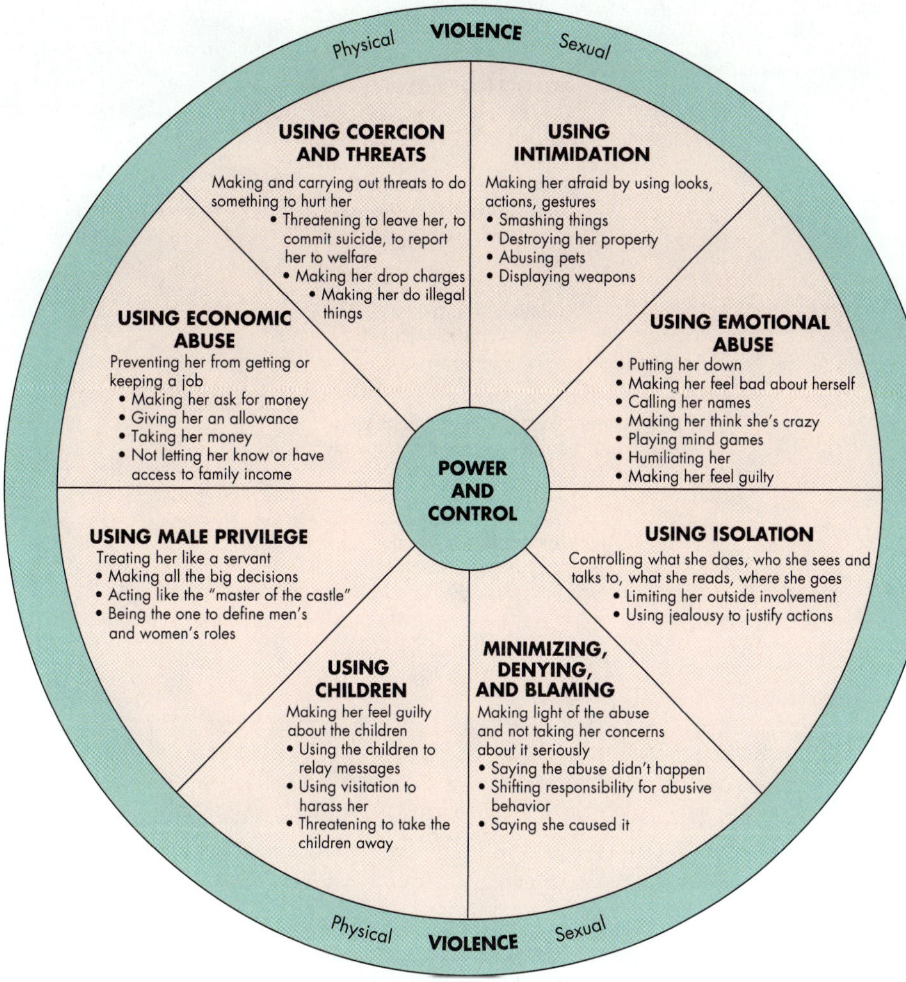

FIG. 5-1 Model of how power and control issues perpetuate battering. (Developed by the Duluth Domestic Abuse Intervention Project, Duluth, MN.)

Ecological Model

An ecological model is a useful tool when trying to understand a complex social issue like IPV. Ecological models help to make apparent the dynamic relationship between the individual and the environment. Bronfenbrenner (1979, 2005) explained how an ecological model might explain child development. An ecological model is sometimes drawn as nested circles that represent characteristics of the individual and the things in that person's immediate and larger environment that influence the phenomenon of concern. The model has been adapted and used to understand a variety of health behaviors and social issues. The WHO uses an ecological model to look at communities. Heise (1998) adapted one for IPV and Campbell and colleagues (2009) developed a similar model for sexual assault.

Figure 5-2 is an ecological model of IPV. The individual woman is at the center of the model. Her unique characteristics, such as age, life experience, race/ethnicity, social class, education, personality, emotional well-being, finances, and so on influence who she is and how she is in the world. In her immediate environment is her intimate partner, his characteristics, and the characteristics of their relationship. At the next level *(microsystem)* are her children, family, friends, and the people and activities in her daily life that are important such as her neighbors, employer, or coworkers. Surrounding the social network are community resources such as women's groups, violence prevention programs, and local resources *(mesosystem)*. The *exosystem* refers to organizations and formal agencies, health care systems, and providers such as nurses, the police, and the legal system. All of these are influenced by the larger sociocultural beliefs, myths, and media *(macrosystem)*. Finally, the *chronosystem* represents the influence of events over time.

For example, a woman (individual) experiencing IPV over time may develop chronic depression and hopelessness, finding it more difficult to mount the energy needed to change or leave the relationship. Her partner interactions may have pushed away her friends, and her emotional state makes it difficult to rebuild relationships. Perhaps her family or friends are influenced by social or cultural expectations not to interfere in someone else's marriage. The woman is socially isolated. She may hear about IPV issues from a local women's group, helping to destigmatize her perception of the issue. If she risks disclosing her experience to a nurse and receives validation and support, she may be more likely to seek help again in the future, perhaps with the health care system, or with another social agency. The nurse who interacted with the woman is also influenced by that experience in providing support to a victim of IPV. All parts of the model are influenced by other parts, and those influences change over time.

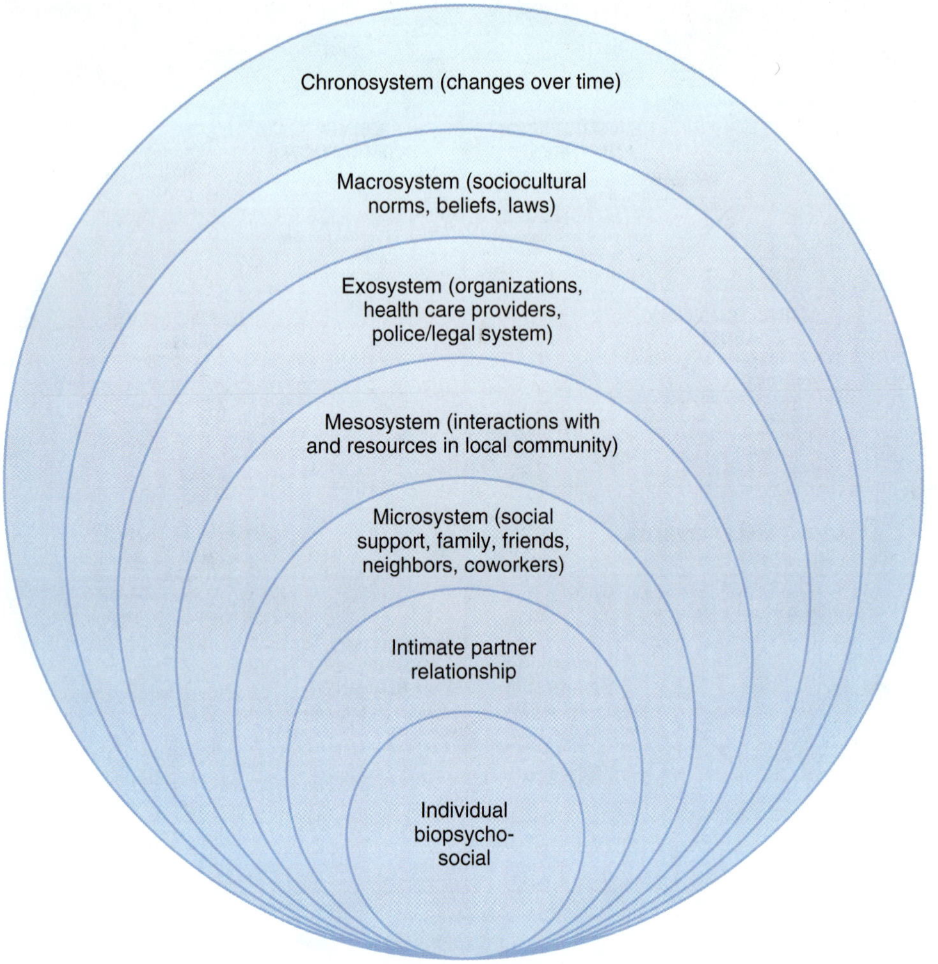

FIG. 5-2 Ecological framework for intimate partner violence. (Adapted from Bronfenbrenner, U. [1979]. *The ecology of human development: Experiments by nature and design.* Cambridge, MA: Harvard University Press; Bronfenbrenner, U. [2005]. *Making human beings human: Bioecological perspectives on human development.* Thousand Oaks, CA: Sage; Heise, L. [1998]. Violence against women: An integrated, ecological framework. *Violence Against Women, 4*[3], 262-290; Campbell, R., Dworkin, E., & Cabral, G. [2009]. An ecological model of the impact of sexual assault on women's mental health. *Trauma Violence and Abuse, 10*[3], 225-246.)

WOMEN EXPERIENCING INTIMATE PARTNER VIOLENCE

Characteristics of Women in Abusive Relationships

Spanish Guidelines—Recognizing Violence in a Relationship

Every segment of society is represented among people experiencing abuse. Race, religion, social background, age, and educational level do not differentiate women at risk. Poor and uneducated women tend to be disproportionately represented because they are seen in EDs, they are financially more dependent, they have fewer resources and support systems, and they may have fewer problem-solving skills. Women with educational or financial resources have been hidden from public awareness but can just as easily be victims (Thompson et al., 2006). They may be disadvantaged in other ways in that they do not fit the stereotype of an abused woman and find it difficult to come to terms with the idea that they are in an abusive relationship (Steiner, 2009).

The value women place on their social roles may have some influence in intimate partner violence. Traditional feminine characteristics such as compassion, sympathy, and yielding often result in greater tolerance of male dominance and more acceptance of partner violence. In contrast the traits of assertiveness, independence, and willingness to take a stand have been viewed as more characteristic in women who are in nonviolent relationships (Faramarzi, Esmailzadeh, & Mosavi, 2005.) There is little research that tells us how these characteristics might change if independent, assertive women found themselves in abusive relationships. Although women who are in abusive relationships may appear passive or even helpless to an outside observer, their behaviors may be active efforts to reduce the risk of violence as they survive day to day (Dutton, 2009).

Survivors of IPV may believe they are to blame for their situations because they are "not good enough, not efficient enough, not pretty enough." The woman may blame herself for bringing on the violent behavior in her relationship because she believes she must try harder to please the abuser. In many cases, a traumatic bonding with the man hinges on loyalty, fear, and terror. Some women have low self-esteem. Some may have histories of domestic violence in their families of origin. Often abused women are socially isolated. This may be the result of stigma, fear, restrictions placed on them by their partners or partner behaviors that discourage others from being involved.

Based on the self-appraisal of 448 victims who filed a police report, Nurius and Macy (2008) identified five subgroups of

TABLE 5-1 COMPARISON OF CHARACTERISTICS OF POSTTRAUMATIC STRESS SYNDROME, BATTERED WOMAN SYNDROME, AND RAPE-TRAUMA SYNDROME

POSTTRAUMATIC STRESS SYNDROME*	BATTERED WOMAN SYNDROME	RAPE-TRAUMA SYNDROME
The person experienced an event that involved or threatened death, a serious injury, or a threat to physical integrity of self or others.	Deliberate and repeated physical or sexual assault experienced by a woman at the hands of an intimate partner.	A violent, aggressive sexual assault on a woman without her consent from a stranger or someone she knows.
The person's response involved intense fear, helplessness, or horror.	The woman responds with terror, entrapment, and helplessness.	The woman responds with shock, terror, and humiliation.
The traumatic event is persistently reexperienced, such as through distressing recollections or dreams.	If the woman remains in the relationship, the repeated experience may be real rather than recalled.	The woman relives the scene and considers what she "should have done"; she experiences a range of emotions and may feel guilty.
Psychologic reactivity occurs on exposure to internal or external cues symbolic of the traumatic event.	The woman feels anxious and isolated (or alone) and reacts to any expression of anger or threat by cowering or attempting to placate the abuser.	Physical symptoms such as muscle tension, hyperventilation, and flushing may occur in response to reexperiencing the rape or when approached by men, especially strangers.
The person persistently avoids stimuli associated with the trauma; responses are numbed.	The woman attempts to avoid arousing the anger of the abuser and tries to please him; she exerts effort to control situations to avoid abuse.	The woman avoids situations in which she feels vulnerable; if in an intimate relationship, she may avoid intercourse.
The person has persistent symptoms of increased arousal, such as difficulty sleeping, hypervigilance, and exaggerated startle response.	The woman is alert to signs of increasing tension in the abuser during the tension-building stages; she withdraws from interaction.	The woman is afraid of being alone or in a crowd and of being attacked from behind; she takes extra precautions when going out and is suspicious.

*Modified from American Psychiatric Association. (2000). *Diagnostic and statistical manual of mental disorders* (4th ed. rev.). Washington, DC: American Psychiatric Association.

victims. Each group varied in their feelings of vulnerability, sense of power, symptoms of depression, social relationships with others, type and duration of exposure to violence, and physical health. The largest group was composed of women who felt vulnerable to continued abuse and had high depression scores. The second group included women struggling with depression but with a low sense of vulnerability. A third group felt vulnerable to violence or abuse but were otherwise healthy with low rates of depression and strong social relationships. One group included women with multiple resources including good health, low depression scores, lower sense of being vulnerable, and high social support. The last group included women with high rates of vulnerability, physical injury, depression, and negative social relationships.

Some survivors of IPV may be formally diagnosed as having PTSD, provided that the symptoms meet the criteria in the *Diagnostic and Statistical Manual of Mental Disorders* (American Psychiatric Association [APA], 2000). Table 5-1 compares the characteristics of PTSD sufferers with characteristics of women survivors of violence and those of rape-trauma victims (discussed later).

Leaving an abusive relationship is extremely difficult and the most dangerous time because most homicides occur shortly after separation (Campbell, 2004b). Health professionals can become frustrated by women they see repeatedly who have numerous signs of abuse but seem unable to liberate themselves from the battering relationships. As with other human dynamics that are not easily explained, health professionals and others may rationalize the woman's behaviors to justify their own uninvolvement. A number of misconceptions are used to account for the woman's perceived self-destructive behavior. If nurses and other professionals believe these misconceptions, they may become judgmental (such as blaming the victim) or respond in unhelpful ways, rather than being empathic and empowering women to take control over their lives (Westbrook, 2009). Empowerment is built on respect for the woman. Providing supportive empathy, validation, and information that can be lifesaving are empowering behaviors. Table 5-2 lists some myths and facts about IPV.

Cultural Considerations

IPV is seen in all races, ethnicities, religions, and socioeconomic backgrounds (Breiding, Ziembroski, & Black, 2009; Mitchell & Anglin, 2009). In the United States, Caucasian women report less IPV than do non-Caucasians. Native American and Alaska Native women report significantly more instances of IPV than do women of any other racial background; Asian women report significantly less IPV than do other racial groups (Montalvo-Liendo, 2009; Tjaden & Thoennes, 2006). Reporting rates may not reflect the magnitude of the problem because many women do not disclose violence because of fear, embarrassment, or not having been asked by those from whom they seek help.

There is a growing official acknowledgment of IPV across the globe. In 1994 the United States enacted the Violence Against Women Act (VAWA) followed by Guatemala and El Salvador in 1996, China in 1997, Colombia in 2000 and Japan in 2001. Mexico passed its first law in 2007 (Montalvo-Liendo, 2009). Women from almost all cultures—Asian women, Mexican immigrants, and Vietnamese—identify fear as a common factor in IPV. An important cultural consideration relates to refugees and immigrants. Immigrant women face unique challenges related to their non-citizen status as well as unfamiliarity with the health care and legal systems. The objectification of women and power inequalities in human social arrangements support the abuse of women. These are especially apparent in any social or cultural system of oppression. The cross-cultural meaning of violence is difficult to ascertain because cultures also differ in their perceptions and definitions of abuse. Accurate data about the incidence and prevalence of violence in ethnic groups are challenging because they are infrequently represented in research studies; violence may be underreported as a result

TABLE 5-2 MYTHS AND FACTS ABOUT INTIMATE PARTNER VIOLENCE

MYTHS	FACTS
Intimate partner violence (IPV) occurs in a small percentage of the population.	One fourth of all women experience IPV.
Being pregnant protects the woman from IPV.	From 4% to 8% of all women who experience violence experience it during pregnancy. IPV frequently begins or escalates in frequency and intensity during pregnancy. Pregnancy may be the result of forced sex or of the man's control of contraception.
IPV occurs only in "problem" or lower-class families.	IPV can occur in any family. Although lower class families have a higher reported incidence of IPV, it also occurs in middle- and upper-income families. Incidence is not really known because of the tendency of middle- and upper-income families to hide their IPV.
IPV women like to be beaten and deliberately provoke the attack. They are masochistic.	Women are terrified of their assailants and go to great lengths to avoid a confrontation. In some cases, the woman may provoke her partner to release tension that if left unchecked might lead to a more severe beating and possible death.
Only men with psychologic problems abuse women.	Many batterers are successful professionals, including politicians, ministers, physicians, and lawyers. Research indicates that only a small number of abusers have psychologic problems.
Only people who come from abusive families end up in abusive relationships.	Most abused women report that their partners were the first person to abuse them.
Alcohol and drug abuse cause IPV.	Although alcohol may be involved in abusive incidents, it is not the cause. Many batterers use alcohol as an excuse to be violent, and shift the blame to the alcohol.
Women would leave the relationship if the abuse were really that bad.	Those women who stay in the relationship do so out of fear and financial dependence. Shelters have long waiting lists.
Victims and perpetrators of IPV cannot change.	Counseling may effectively help both victims and abusers of women.

Sources: Gelles, R. (1997). *Intimate violence in families* (3rd ed.). Thousand Oaks, CA: Sage; National Institute on Alcohol Abuse and Alcoholism. (1997). Alcohol, violence, and aggression. *Alcohol Alert, 38,* 1-6; National Women's Health Information Center. (2002). *Violence against women.* Available at www.4woman.gov/violence/index.cfm. Accessed January 24, 2010.

of cultural norms. For example, groups that distrust police or immigration officials may not report abuse because they fear the repercussions.

The nurse must be sensitive to immigrant women and their intimate partners because acculturation is gradual, and cultural expectations from their birth countries may heavily influence beliefs and behaviors (Shiu-Thornton, Senturia, & Sullivan, 2005). Nurses must consider all forces that shape the woman's identity—ethnicity, race, class, language, citizenship, religion, and culture—while recognizing that abuse is against the law and injurious to the health and well-being of women and children (and men). More than basic awareness of cultural influences on violence toward women is helpful to the nurse who seeks to be more sensitive to the needs of women whose cultural experiences differ from the nurse's own. Becoming familiar with the client's cultural influences and increasing the numbers of nurses from various ethnic groups will increase the opportunity to provide culturally appropriate care.

African-American Culture

The African-American culture supports unity among humans, nature, and the spiritual world, and social connectedness and relatedness as important norms. African-American men are more likely to be psychologically, socially, and economically oppressed and discriminated against. Violence may occur more frequently as a result of anger generated by environmental stresses and limited resources (Campbell, D., Sharps, Gary, Campbell, & Lopez, 2002). No valid evidence of greater violence seems to exist in this population although African-American women tend to report violence at a slightly higher rate than do Caucasian women (McFarlane, Groff, O'Brien, & Watson, 2005). The devalued status of the female survivor, racial stereotype and fear of putting another African-American man in jail, may be barriers to African-American women seeking and receiving help (Morrison, Luchok, Richter, & Parra-Medina, 2006).

Hispanic (and Latino) Cultures

Hispanic (or Latino) describes someone whose country of origin is Mexico, the largest group at 65%, followed by Puerto Rico, Cuba, Spanish-speaking Central and South American countries, or other Spanish cultures (U.S. Census Bureau, 2006). When data are collected, Americans who are of Hispanic descent may be grouped with those born in other countries. Thus Hispanics range from newly immigrated and strongly influenced by their native culture to second-generation Americans steeped in U.S. popular culture. It is difficult to generalize on culture among these groups.

Hispanics as a group are described as family oriented with a strong family network in which unity, cooperation, respect, and loyalty are important. Traditional families, as with most immigrant groups, are very hierarchic, with authority often given to older adults, parents, and men. Sex roles are clearly delineated. Hispanics in the United States have been found to have the same rate of IPV as non-Hispanic women; and in one study, researchers found that they had significantly more mental health issues than non-Hispanic women who experienced IPV (Bonomi, Anderson, Cannon, Slesnick, & Rodriguez, 2009). Another difference is in the characteristics of the abusive relationship. In one study the partners of Hispanic women were more likely to have alcohol problems and to force sex but less likely to own a gun, use illegal drugs, or threaten suicide than non-Hispanics in abusive relationships (Glass, Perrin, Hanson, Mankowski, Bloom, & Campbell, 2009).

Native American Culture

Empiric evidence about abuse in the Native American culture is limited (Duran, Oetzel, Parker, Malcoe, Lucero, & Jiang, 2009). Research indicates the IPV occurs within the context of complex racial and unique sociocultural factors. Native American and Alaska-Native women report the highest rates of IPV in the United States; however, research is needed to determine whether the rate is higher in these women, or the rate of reporting is higher (Tjaden & Thoennes, 2006). Oetzel and Duran (2004) proposed an ecological framework to guide health care providers in understanding the causes and possible areas for intervention with Native American and Alaska Natives.

Asian Women

Asian women are often artificially grouped into one homogeneous group despite their vast and varied cultures.

Reasons for not disclosing IPV vary across cultures. Women from South Asia, including Afghanistan, Bangladesh, Bhutan, Sri Lanka, India, the Maldives, Nepal, and Pakistan, were worried about immigrant laws, were concerned about family honor, and believed that men had the right to abuse. Urban women from Bangladesh were fearful of being killed, felt helpless, and were worried about community retaliation and judgment (Naved, Azim, Bhuiya, & Persson, 2006). Jordanian women expressed fear, shame, religious beliefs, and lack of social support as reasons for not disclosing. The majority of Jordanian men and women deny the problem of wife abuse and oppose discussions of it in society, a reflection of this patriarchal society (Btoush & Haj-Yahia, 2008). Chinese women worried they would be criticized and were fearful of not saving face and disappointing relatives. Japanese women felt shame, were fearful of escalating violence, and victim blaming (Yoshihama, 2002). Vietnamese women put the needs of the family before their individual needs and kept the woman's role subordinate to men to maintain harmony in the family (Shiu-Thornton et al., 2005).

INTIMATE PARTNER VIOLENCE DURING PREGNANCY

IPV has serious consequences for the health of the mother and fetus. The prevalence of IPV during pregnancy is estimated at 4% to 8% (Martin, Mackie, Kupper, Buescher, & Moracco, 2001). It is more common than preeclampsia, gestational diabetes, or an abnormal Papanicolaou (Pap) test in pregnancy (Chambliss, 2008). Women who are abused before pregnancy may continue to be abused during the pregnancy.

Some clinicians believe that abuse may begin or escalate with pregnancy, but some studies suggest that both lethal and nonlethal abuse may actually decrease during pregnancy in some couples (Taylor & Nabors, 2009). In a small longitudinal study Macy, Martin, Kupper, Casanueva, & Guo (2007) found that rates of physical abuse among women with a history of recent abuse peaked during the first 3 months of pregnancy, then declined while women without a recent history of abuse had low rates of abuse during pregnancy. Thus, pregnancy may be protective for some women. In the same study, rates of psychologic abuse were highest in the first month after the birth, as was sexual abuse.

It is clear that IPV has negative effects on pregnancy. Maternal complications of depression, suicide, low weight gain, infections, and substance abuse have been related to being in an abusive relationship (Campbell, J. et al., 2002; Plichta, 2004). Gastrointestinal symptoms may occur from chronic stress, as may hypertension and chest pain. Other conditions are gynecologic problems such as STIs, bleeding, urinary tract infections, chronic pelvic pain, and genital trauma. A history of abuse prior to the pregnancy is associated with a higher risk of postpartum depression (Records & Rice, 2009).

Homicide is the leading cause of trauma death in pregnancy and postpartum (Chang, Berg, Saltzman, & Herndon, 2005; Horon & Cheng, 2005). Estimates are that 16% to 66% of pregnancy-related murders are by intimate partners (Martin, Macy, Sullivan, & Magee, 2007). IPV may be a risk factor for suicide attempts in pregnancy (Martin et al.).

Not only is physical abuse harmful to the mother, the risk of fetal injury also is very high. Trauma may result in low birth weight, preterm birth, fetal demise, premature separation of placenta, hemorrhage, infections, and other trauma-related injuries (Chambliss, 2008; Morland, Leskin, Block, Campbell, & Friedman, 2008). Pregnant adolescents may be abused at higher rates than are adult women, so they should be considered at high risk. There is a greater likelihood of unintended pregnancy in adolescents who often delay prenatal care (Plichta, 2004). Physical abuse and pregnancy in teenagers constitute a particularly difficult situation. Adolescents may be more trapped in the abusive relationship than adult women because of their inexperience. They may ignore the violence because the jealous and controlling behavior is interpreted as love and devotion. Because pregnancy in adolescent girls is frequently the result of sexual abuse, feelings about the pregnancy should be assessed. Teens report abuse from partners, former partners, and family members (Renker, 2002). Many who had been abused through the pregnancy also were abused afterward, and others who were not abused during pregnancy reported initial abuse after giving birth (Harrykissoon, Rickert, & Wiemann, 2002). Adolescents have been found to be at very high risk for abuse in the postpartum period. Quinlivan and Evans (2005) found that IPV and drug abuse in adolescents affected maternal attachment and infant temperament.

CARE MANAGEMENT

Care of the woman experiencing IPV must begin with the nurse's self-assessment. An exploration of attitudes toward women in abusive situations, awareness of feelings that may result in judgmental communication, and knowledge about the many aspects of IPV are preparations for care. Dienemann, Glass, and Hyman (2005) found that women desired health care providers to take an active role, that is, to provide documentation, protection, immediate response, to give options, and to be there for the survivor later. They also wanted to be treated with respect and concern.

Exactly what drives a woman to seek assistance is not clear. Women who belong to any of the following three groups are more likely to seek assistance: (1) women who are beaten frequently and severely; (2) those who have not experienced or witnessed family violence in their family of origin; and (3) those who see an alternative to life in an abusive relationship, specifically women with jobs. Sometimes women seek help after their children have been hurt or when their children start imitating the abuser's behavior.

Women experiencing IPV may be reluctant to seek help for various reasons, including the need to avoid the stigma associated with the nature of the family violence; the fear that they will not be believed; the fear of reprisal from their husbands or partners; and in some states in which battering is a reportable crime, the desire to avoid involvement with police (see Legal Tip: Mandatory Reporting of Domestic Violence).

LEGAL TIP: Mandatory Reporting of Domestic Violence
Domestic violence is considered a crime in all states, but it varies between being categorized a misdemeanor and a felony, the majority calling it a misdemeanor. Mandatory reporting of domestic violence is controversial. Mandatory reporting is appropriate in child abuse because a minor is unable to make an informed decision about his or her own safety. In domestic violence situations involving adults, mandatory reporting takes away a woman's right to make informed decisions and may put her in danger. The Association of Women's Health, Obstetric and Neonatal Nurses (AWHONN) opposes mandatory reporting (AWHONN Board of Directors, 2007). Few states have mandatory reporting for domestic violence of any kind. Forty states and the District of Columbia have laws that mandate reporting by health care providers in situations in which the woman has an injury that may be caused by a deadly weapon. Some states also require reports when there is a reason to believe that the woman's injury may have resulted from an illegal act or an act of violence. California has the strongest reporting law. Colorado, New Mexico, and Kentucky mandate health provider reporting of injuries resulting from IPV to law enforcement or public welfare. Ohio mandates that IPV be documented in the medical record. Rhode Island requires that domestic violence injuries be reported for statistical purposes only. Texas mandates that IPV be documented and that clients be informed that IPV is against the law and be offered shelter referral.

Because of the wide variation from state to state in mandatory reporting, nurses must be knowledgeable about the reporting requirements of the state in which they practice (Family Violence Prevention Fund [FVPF], 2004). Nurses can check the FVPF website—www.endabuse.org—for a listing and evaluation of reporting laws.

Clients in any women's health care setting may be at risk for abuse and nurses are encouraged to assess for abuse in all women entering the health care system (McFarlane et al., 2002) (see Nursing Process box). Health care providers may be the first and only contact that a socially isolated woman makes with someone outside the relationship. Failure to identify IPV and to recognize the risk of serious injury or even death further endangers the lives of women and their children.

A woman suspected of being emotionally abused or physically threatened or abused should be examined and interviewed in private, and, if her partner is male, she may feel safer and more comfortable with a female health care provider. Nurses should *never* ask about abuse with a partner present because this may place the woman in danger. When one is taking a psychosocial history, the following information provides clues to violence or potential for violence: does the woman feel safe at home with her partner, how does the woman and her partner resolve conflict, what happens when the woman's partner becomes angry, does fighting occur during disagreements, and if fighting occurs, does it ever escalate to restraining or physical means. It may help the woman to disclose information if these events are normalized by the nurse stating, "Many people [families] have difficulty in expressing anger or dealing with conflict. What is that like for you and your partner?" The nurse listens for any evidence of power and control in the relationship. While inquiring about past trauma or injuries, the nurse also should ask directly if the woman has been injured by her husband or intimate partner. At least the following questions should be asked:

- Are you with a spouse or partner who threatens or physically hurts you?
- Within the past year or in this pregnancy has anyone hit, slapped, kicked, or otherwise hurt you?
- Has anyone forced you to have sexual activities that made you uncomfortable? (American Congress of Obstetricians and Gynecologists [ACOG], 2010). These questions give a woman permission to disclose sensitive information.

Assessment tools can be a part of the interview that give the nurse useful information. Patterns of violence change over time in some relationships, and reports show an increase in the identification of victims of domestic violence when the nurse inquires at each visit whether a woman has been hit or threatened since her last visit (Macy et al., 2007; Walton-Moss & Campbell, 2002). Cues to abuse are delay in seeking medical assistance (hours or days), missed appointments, vague explanation of injuries, nonspecific somatic complaints, social isolation, lack of eye contact, a husband or partner who does not want to leave the woman alone with the primary health care provider, and substance abuse.

In the United States a pregnant woman is often accompanied by her husband to the antepartum appointment. This is especially true if the woman does not speak English and the husband does. The use of an interpreter is preferred; the interpreter needs to be a woman who can communicate the nurse's sensitivity and concern accurately. All women should be seen for some part of the visit without the partner present.

For some abused women, day-to-day survival is exhausting. They may cope by denying to the nurse the probabilities of impending abuse, severity of injury, future recurrence, and death. Women may be embarrassed about their abusive relationships and believe the abuse is caused by their inadequacies. Other abused women may cope by denying to themselves that their partner's violent behavior will happen again. By asking a woman directly about abuse, telling her that similar injuries are common in women who have been abused, and pointing out that she is not responsible for another's violent behavior, the nurse may help her disclose the violence she is experiencing. During pregnancy the nurse should assess for abuse at each prenatal visit and on admission to labor, although it is not appropriate to ask questions during active labor. Assessment for abuse continues after birth because abuse may begin or escalate then; well-baby clinics may be important settings for screening women for abuse (Martin et al., 2001).

Assessment techniques are straightforward but do require the nurse to be comfortable asking about this socially stigmatized issue. Of utmost importance for women who disclose that they experience IPV (or sexual assault, another hidden trauma) is to validate that you have heard her. Assure her that it is not her fault. The nurse might say something like, "What you have just told me is very important, I'm glad you have shared this with me; no one has the right to hurt you this way." It can be demoralizing when, despite taking the risk to disclose, the health care provider does not acknowledge the import of what has just been said. The next important step is to establish the woman's safety at the moment and in the future. Psychosocial assessment findings may include anxiety, insomnia, self-directed abuse, depression,

Critical Thinking Exercise—Women's Health and Safety

EVIDENCE-BASED PRACTICE

Pat Gingrich

Interventions for Intimate Partner Violence

ASK THE QUESTION

What nursing interventions for women who experience intimate partner violence (IPV) result in increased safety behaviors and decreased violence?

SEARCH FOR EVIDENCE

Search Strategies

Professional organization guidelines, meta-analyses, systematic reviews, randomized controlled trials, nonrandomized prospective studies and retrospective reviews since 2009.

Databases Searched

CINAHL, Cochrane, Medline, PUBMED, NICE, and the professional sites for Guttmacher and AWHONN.

CRITICALLY ANALYZE THE DATA

Macy, Ferron, and Crosby (2009) conducted a systematic review of 28 articles (qualitative and quantitative) involving 3500 diverse women who experience IPV. Women with IPV presented with chronic mental health issues, including depression and anxiety. They sought medical care for vague gastrointestinal issues, headaches, heart disease, and hearing loss. Abuse of illegal substances was strongly correlated with IPV, while alcohol had a much weaker association. A Guttmacher longitudinal study interviewed 526 females interviewed in middle school and again in their mid-twenties. Adult IPV experience was associated with aggressive behavior in middle school, earlier onset of sexual activity, increased number of sexual partners, unintended pregnancy, and living together with the aggressor (O'Donnell, Agronick, Duran, Myint-U, & Stueve, 2009).

A Cochrane Review assessed ten randomized, controlled trials regarding IPV involving 1527 participants (Ramsay, Carter, Davidson, Dunne, Eldridge, Hegarty, et al., 2009). The trials varied greatly in their measures of interventions (counseling lasting from 30 minutes to 80 hours) and outcomes (depression, quality of life, distress, safety behaviors, return to violence). However, the authors were able to conclude that intensive advocacy for women already in shelters did lead to decreased physical abuse one to two years later, and even brief counseling is associated with safer behaviors. The review showed equivocal results regarding the effect of counseling on depression, quality of life, and distress. The authors caution that not enough is known to conclude anything about the benefits of counseling for women still living with their abuser.

Clinic-based counseling was the intervention studied by a randomized controlled trial of 850 pregnant African-American women who were identified as high risk for poor pregnancy outcomes based on smoking, depression, and IPV (Joseph, El-Mohandes, Kiely, El-Khorazaty, Gantz, Johnson, et al., 2009). The authors concluded that the clinic-based counseling significantly reduced psychosocial and behavioral risk factors for IPV.

IMPLICATIONS FOR PRACTICE

All disciplines that potentially interact with women experiencing IPV should be alert to the characteristic signs and symptoms. Macy, et al. (2009) noted that the various professional disciplines tend to compartmentalize people living with IPV according to that discipline's own framework, leaving women underserved in other areas and thus trapped by unsolved problems. For example, a counselor may see only the mental health issues, or the health care provider focuses only on the health problems. Victims of IPV were found to be greatly in need of comprehensive care from a collaborative team of physical, mental health, health education, social work, substance abuse, and legal professionals. The reviewers recommended interagency meetings, and cross training (for example, nurse practitioners can work one day a month at a shelter), as well as collaborative policy changes. In addition, screening for early risk factors for IPV, such as adolescent aggression and early onset of sexual activity, may lead to counseling and education interventions than can prevent the circumstances that foster IPV.

References

Joseph, J., El-Mohandes, A., Kiely, M., El-Khorazaty, M., Gantz, M., Johnson, A., Katz, K., et al. (2009). Reducing psychosocial and behavioral pregnancy risk factors: Results of a randomized clinical trial among high risk pregnant African American women. *American Journal of Public Health, 99*(6), 1053–1061.

Macy, R., Ferron, J., & Crosby, C. (2009). Partner violence and survivors' chronic health problems: informing social work practice. *Social Work, 54*(1), 29–43.

O'Donnell, L., Agronick, G., Duran, R., Myint-U, A., & Stueve, A. (2009). Intimate partner violence among economically disadvantaged young adult women: associations with adolescent risk-taking and pregnancy experiences. *Prospectives on Sexual and Reproductive Health, 41*(2), 84–91.

Ramsay, J., Carter, Y., Davidson, L., Dunne, D., Eldridge, S., Hegarty, K., et al. (2009). Advocacy interventions to reduce or eliminate violence and promote physical and psychosocial well-being of women who experience intimate partner abuse. *The Cochrane Database of Systematic Reviews 2009*, 3, Chichester, UK: John Wiley & Sons.

smoking, and drug or alcohol abuse (Downs & Rindels, 2004; Gerber, Gantz, Lichter, Williams, & McCloskey, 2005). During the physical examination, the woman should be observed for injuries to the face, breasts, abdomen, and buttocks. These injuries may be old or new and may range from minor bruising to serious. Other physical signs include fractures that required significant force or that would rarely occur by accident; multiple injuries at various stages of healing; and patterns left by whatever might inflict injury, such as teeth, utensils, fists, or hot objects.

NURSING INTERVENTIONS

A therapeutic relationship and skillful interviewing help women disclose and describe their abuse. Language is important when talking with women. A major factor in addressing abuse is to identify the woman as a survivor, not a victim. Victim connotes someone who is harmed, is made to suffer, and may have little or no control. Survivor is an empowering term that connotes coping and decision making in relation to taking control of one's life. The nurse might ask the woman how she sees herself. Women who have identified their abuse may appear passive, hostile, anxious, depressed, or hysterical because they may think they are at the mercy of the man's temper. In addition, they may be embarrassed, afraid, angry, sad, and shocked. Transitioning to a different self-image takes time, persistence, and support. A tool that provides a framework for sensitive nursing interventions is the *ABCDES* of caring for the abused woman (Campbell & Furniss, 2002).

- *A* is reassuring the woman that she is not *alone.* The isolation and denigration by the abuser keep her from knowing that others are in the same situation and that health care providers can help.
- *B* is expressing the *belief* that violence against the woman is not acceptable in any situation and that it is not her fault; no one deserves to be hurt or mistreated. This may be the first step in empowering her to think about self-protection and acceptable boundaries.

NURSING PROCESS

Intimate Partner Violence

ASSESSMENT

- Interview the woman in private. Use of assessment tools may be helpful (see text).
  - Take a psychosocial history to elicit information about potential problems such as anxiety, insomnia, drug or alchohol abuse
  - Ask questions about whether the woman has been injured or threatened by her husband or partner, or been forced to have sexual activities that made her uncomfortable
- Physical examination
  - Observe for evidence of injuries–old or new.

NURSING DIAGNOSES

Examples of nursing diagnoses for women experiencing IPV include:

***Hopelessness* related to:**
- prolonged exposure to physical, mental, psychologic, and sexual abuse

***Powerlessness* related to:**
- phenomenon of being abused and isolated

***Fear* related to:**
- potential or real threats to safety

***Risk for Post-trauma Syndrome* related to:**
- experience of interpersonal abuse

***Social Isolation* related to:**
- the stigma of being abused

***Ineffective Family Coping* related to:**
- persistence of victim-abuser relationship

***Injury* related to:**
- physical abuse

***Situational Low Self-esteem* related to:**
- continuing victim-abuser relationship

***Deficient Knowledge* related to:**
- available resources

EXPECTED OUTCOMES OF CARE

Expected outcomes are that the woman will do the following:
- Identify her areas of strength and develop goals for herself.
- State her knowledge of alternatives, options, and choices; community resources (shelters, financial aid, child care, education, job or financial assistance); counseling for the partner
- Express a feeling of empowerment and control as a survivor.
- Perceive herself as deserving of respect and not as "deserving" to be victimized.
- Express measures to protect her children or, if she is pregnant, the fetus from abuse.
- Formulate a plan for safety.

PLAN OF CARE AND INTERVENTIONS

- Use a tool such as the ABCDES of caring for the abuse woman to provide sensitive nursing care (see p. 106 and Nursing Care Plan).
  - Reassure the woman she is not alone.
  - Express the belief that violence against the woman is not acceptable and not her fault.
  - Maintain confidentiality of the information the woman has shared.
  - Document descriptively and objectively the woman's statements of abuse and with her consent, include evidence or photographs of the abuse.
  - Educate about IPV and community resources.
  - Help the woman develop a safety plan.

EVALUATION

Evaluation of the care of the abused woman is based on expected outcomes and must be in harmony with the choices the woman has made.

Nursing Care Plan—Intimate Partner Violence

- *C* is *confidentiality* of the information being shared, particularly because the woman may believe that if the abuse is reported, the perpetrator will retaliate (and in reality, this may happen). Explain the mandatory reporting laws, where applicable.
- *D* is for descriptive *documentation* and includes the following: (1) the woman's quoted statement, "My husband punched me," a clear statement by the woman about the abuse. It should not include her subjective opinion, such as "I provoked the abusive behavior"; (2) accurate descriptions of injuries and a history of the first, worst, and most recent incident of violence may be included; and (3) with the woman's consent, evidence, or photographs (Box 5-2).
- *E* is for *education,* especially that violence is likely to recur and escalate. Education about options including community resources such as where a woman can be referred for help and information about local shelters; for example, National Domestic Violence/Abuse Hotline—800-799-SAFE. Ask if she knows how to obtain a restraining order.
- *S* is for *safety,* the most significant part of the intervention because one of the most dangerous times for a woman is when she decides to leave. Tell the woman to call 911 if she is in imminent danger, and to consider alerting neighbors to call the police if they hear or see signs of conflict. A safety plan should be developed. The safety plan will be adapted based on whether the woman chooses to stay in the relationship or leave. The woman may be conflicted and need support as she goes through a decision-making process (Glass, Eden, Bloom, & Perrin, 2009). The woman can be offered a telephone to call the shelter if this is an option she chooses. If she chooses to go back to the abuser, a safety plan includes necessities for a quick escape: a bag packed with personal items for an overnight stay (can be hidden or left with a neighbor), money or a checkbook, an extra set of car keys, and any legal documents to use for identification. Legal options, such as those for restraining orders or arrest of the perpetrator, also are important aspects of the safety plan. A restraining order can be obtained 24 hours a day from the county court or police department. Many communities have battered women's hotlines where they can get counseling. Pennell and Francis (2005) discuss safety conferencing as a means of building the individual and collective strength to assist women to reshape connections, make sound choices, and promote their safety (see Nursing Care Plan).

One part of safety planning is trying to sort out the potential danger in a relationship. A validated danger assessment tool (Fig. 5-3) was designed to assess the level of violence in a relationship and to identify abused women who are at risk of

BOX 5-2 DOCUMENTING ABUSE

Documentation can be useful to women later in court should they choose to press charges or obtain child support, custody, or alimony. Medical records are most helpful if the examiner:

- Takes photographs of the injuries known or believed to have been caused by domestic violence.
- Writes clearly.
- Sets off the woman's words in quotation marks and use such phrases as "client states" to indicate the information recorded reflected the woman's words. Describes the offender and the event in the words of the woman, for example, the client said, "My husband kicked me in the stomach."
- Avoids such legalistic phrases as "woman claims" or "woman alleges" that cast doubt about the truth of the statements. Avoids terms such as "alleged perpetrator." If the health care provider's observations differ from the woman's account of the victimization, states the reason for the difference.
- Does not summarize a client's report in conclusive terms that lack the supporting factual information, for example, "the client is a battered woman," because it will render the report inadmissible. In the same theme, does not place the term "domestic violence" in the diagnosis section of the medical record, because it does not convey factual information and is not medical terminology.
- Describes the woman's demeanor, whether she is crying, shaking, angry, calm, laughing, or sad, even if it belies the evidence of abuse.
- Records the time of day of the examination and indicates whenever possible how much time has passed since the abuse.

NURSING CARE PLAN

The Woman Experiencing Intimate Partner Violence

NURSING DIAGNOSIS

Risk for self-directed violence related to history of battering by partner as evidenced by physical injuries

Expected Outcomes

Woman will identify dynamics of violence in their unique relationship and develop plan for safety.

Nursing Interventions/*Rationales*

- Provide opportunity to verbalize feelings in a nonthreatening atmosphere *to give emotional support.*
- Be alert for cues indicative of abuse *to provide database for interventions.*
- Provide information on options available to women experiencing intimate partner violence (IPV) (e.g., counseling, shelters, legal assistance) *to provide information in developing a plan for safety for herself and any children.*
- Refer to social services and support groups *to give further information and share experiences.*

NURSING DIAGNOSIS

Social isolation related to stigma of battering as evidenced by behaviors of withdrawal

Expected Outcome

Woman will demonstrate an increase in social contacts.

Nursing Interventions/*Rationales*

- Provide private opportunity to express feelings of aloneness *to initiate and maintain a therapeutic relationship.*
- Support opportunities for social interaction *to increase feelings of self-worth and self-confidence.*
- Encourage interaction with groups for socialization and support *to increase number of social contacts.*

NURSING DIAGNOSIS

Ineffective family coping related to situational crisis

Expected Outcomes

Family will identify feelings and the need for support during this situational crisis.

Nursing Interventions/*Rationales*

- Provide appropriate time and place for therapeutic communication *to promote trust and allow expression of feelings.*
- Identify effective coping mechanisms *to provide the family with a foundation of familiar interventions.*
- List support systems available *to assist the family to use outside resources.*
- Refer the woman and family to counseling and social services *to provide ongoing support.*

being murdered (Campbell, 2004a; Campbell, Webster, & Glass, 2009). The nurse and the abused woman can go through the tool collaboratively. Online training and permission to use the tool are available at www.dangerassessment.org/WebApplication1/pages/product.aspx.

If the woman is pregnant, collaboration with maternity nurses who will be involved in her care during the pregnancy may be helpful. Each nurse can plan care that will point out the woman's strengths and increase her self-esteem. The husband or partner may attend prenatal visits and classes and is included in other ways if the woman chooses to stay with him. The first days after birth are particularly crucial because the mother is physically and emotionally vulnerable and usually tired, and the baby's crying may be intolerable to both the father and the mother. The danger of abuse to mother and child is acute during this time. Facilitating the woman's establishment of a support network of maternity and pediatric staff, community health nurses, and shelter and parental crisis center personnel is important during this crucial period. Referral to resources and provision for follow-up examination by health care providers also should be part of the nursing intervention.

Many nurses become frustrated when a woman returns to a previously abusive situation (Davis, Park, Kaups, Bennink, & Bilello, 2003). It is important to remember that many victims have been abused for a long time, which may make it

DANGER ASSESSMENT

Jacquelyn C. Campbell, Ph.D., R.N.

Several risk factors have been associated with increased risk of homicides (murders) of women and men in violent relationships. We cannot predict what will happen in your case, but we would like you to be aware of the danger of homicide in situations of abuse and for you to see how many of the risk factors apply to your situation.

Using a calendar, please mark the approximate dates during the past year when you were abused by your partner or ex-partner. Write on that date how bad the incident was according to the following scale:

1. Slapping, pushing; no injuries and/or lasting pain
2. Punching, kicking; bruises, cuts, and/or continuing pain
3. "Beating up"; severe contusions, burns, broken bones
4. Threat to use weapon; head injury, internal injury, permanent injury
5. Use of weapon; wounds from weapon

(If **any** of the descriptions for the higher number apply, use the higher number.)

Mark **Yes** or **No** for each of the following. ("He" refers to your husband, partner, ex-husband, ex-partner, or whoever is currently physically hurting you.)

________ 1. Has the physical violence increased in severity or frequency over the past year?
________ 2. Does he own a gun?
________ 3. Have you left him after living together during the past year?
3a. (If have never lived with him, check here ________)
________ 4. Is he unemployed?
________ 5. Has he ever used a weapon against you or threatened you with a lethal weapon?
(If yes, was the weapon a gun?________)
________ 6. Does he threaten to kill you?
________ 7. Has he avoided being arrested for domestic violence?
________ 8. Do you have a child that is not his?
________ 9. Has he ever forced you to have sex when you did not wish to do so?
________ 10. Does he ever try to choke you?
________ 11. Does he use illegal drugs? By drugs, I mean "uppers" or amphetamines, "meth", speed, angel dust, cocaine, "crack", street drugs or mixtures.
________ 12. Is he an alcoholic or problem drinker?
________ 13. Does he control most or all of your daily activities? For instance: does he tell you who you can be friends with, when you can see your family, how much money you can use, or when you can take the car? (If he tries, but you do not let him, check here: ________)
________ 14. Is he violently and constantly jealous of you? (For instance, does he say "If I can't have you, no one can.")
________ 15. Have you ever been beaten by him while you were pregnant? (If you have never been pregnant by him, check here: ________)
________ 16. Has he ever threatened or tried to commit suicide?
________ 17. Does he threaten to harm your children?
________ 18. Do you believe he is capable of killing you?
________ 19. Does he follow or spy on you, leave threatening notes or messages on answering machine, destroy your property, or call you when you don't want him to?
________ 20. Have you ever threatened or tried to commit suicide?

________ Total "Yes" Answers

Thank you. Please talk to your nurse, advocate or counselor about what the Danger Assessment means in terms of your situation.

FIG. 5-3 Danger assessment tool. (From Campbell, J. [2004]. *Danger assessment.* Available at www.dangerassessment.org. Accessed January 5, 2010; Campbell, J., Webster, D., & Glass, N. [2009]. The danger assessment: Validation of a lethality risk assessment instrument for intimate partner femicide. *Journal of Interpersonal Violence, 24*(4), 653-674.)

difficult for them to seek and accept help. Women in repeatedly abusive situations may have lost their ability to perceive the possibility of success and may have become very passive. In addition to understanding the many reasons women stay in abusive relationships, recognizing that the most dangerous period for a woman is when she is in the process of leaving may help nurses to be less judgmental about the woman's dilemma.

A woman may indicate her readiness to leave the relationship when she believes that she is capable of planning for herself, investing in herself, and recognizing that the abuse is part of a continuing pattern. She also needs to believe that she will have economic and other resources to "make it" on her own. Going to a shelter may be an option; however, shelter stays are typically limited to 30 to 90 days, and therefore a long-term plan must be in place. Also, her being in a shelter may make the husband or partner angrier. Nurses can be helpful in directing women to sources of information, continuing to be expert listeners, and offering encouragement as women struggle in their decision-making process toward freedom and control in their lives.

Prevention

Screening is a common approach to preventing the progression of health problems. Currently there is insufficient evidence to say that universal screening prevents further incidents of IPV in asymptomatic women (MacMillan, Wathen, Jamieson, Boyle, Shannon, Ford-Gilboe, et al., 2009; U.S. Preventive Services Task Force, 2004). Nevertheless, because the research is limited, and because screening studies were not paired with interventions, major health care organizations including ACOG continue to recommend universal screening of all women. Screening alone is not helpful but assessment with adequate intervention may be useful in improving outcomes (Klevens & Saltzman, 2009). Because IPV has been linked to many other health problems such as headaches, GI problems, chronic pain, arthritis, STIs, pelvic pain, substance abuse, depression, PTSD and suicide, women with any of these symptoms should be carefully assessed.

Nurses can make a difference in stopping the violence and preventing further injury. Educating women that abuse is a violation of their rights and facilitating their access to protective and legal services constitute a first step. Other measures that may help women to discourage the risk of abusive relationships are promoting assertiveness and self-defense courses; suggesting support and self-help groups that encourage positive self-regard, confidence, and empowerment; and recommending educational and skills-development classes that will enhance independence or at least the ability to take care of oneself (Pennell & Francis, 2005). Classes for learning English may be particularly helpful to immigrant women. Nurses can offer information on local classes.

Preventive education with children encourages and teaches them androgynous gender roles: men and women are equal; both can be nurturing; and neither needs to dominate the other or to engage in violent behavior to have needs met. Helping children to gain problem-solving and conflict management skills may eliminate the need for violent solutions to life stresses. Encouraging schoolchildren to form and participate in Students Against Violence Everywhere (SAVE) groups, which is a nationwide pro-peace effort that promotes justice, respect, and love, gives them an appreciation for these qualities in all facets of life. Adolescents benefit from discussion about sex roles, their relationships, and the consequences of the "macho" concept. School nurses can be instrumental in developing and implementing informational activities for adolescents (Walton-Moss & Campbell, 2002). Other means of prevention are to advocate against violence in all arenas and to participate actively in promoting legislation and policies toward stopping violent acts.

SEXUAL VIOLENCE

Sexual violence is a broad term that encompasses a wide range of sexual victimization including sexual harassment, sexual assault, and rape. *Sexual harassment* includes unwelcome degrading sexual remarks, contact, or behavior such as exhibitionism that makes the work or other environment uncomfortable or difficult. **Sexual assault** refers to intentional unwanted completed or attempted touching of the victim's genitals, anus, groin, or breasts, directly or through clothing as well as by voyeurism (Basile, Chen, Black, & Saltzman, 2007). It also includes exhibitionism, exposing someone to pornography or displays of images taken of the victim in a private context (National Institute of Justice, 2007). **Rape** is a legal term that is defined differently by each state. It usually refers to forced sexual intercourse or penetration of the mouth, anus, or vagina by a body part or object without consent; it may or may not include the use of a weapon. It involves the use of force, threats, or a victim who is incapable of giving consent. The term is a legal and not a medical one. *Molestation* consists of noncoital sexual activity between a child and an adolescent or adult. *Statutory rape* involves penetration as described above by a person who is 18 years or older of a person under the age of consent, and the specifics vary from state to state.

The National Survey on Crime reported 260,940 incidents of sexual assault and attempted or completed rapes (Violence Against Women Online Resources, 2010). Based on another national survey of 5000 women, researchers estimate that more than 1 million women from diverse ethnic and social backgrounds are raped each year in the United States (Kilpatrick, Resnick, Ruggiero, Conoscenti, & McCauley, 2007). Almost one third of all sexual assault victims report that the assault occurred during adolescence (McCauley, Amstadter, Danielson, Ruggiero, Kilpatrick, & Resnick, 2009). Rape may occur within intimate, casual, or work relationships. Rapists may be intimate partners or spouses. They may be family members or acquaintances such as friends, neighbors, or dates. Or they may be strangers, police, prison guards, or soldiers. Rape occurs in the general population, in institutional settings such as colleges, in the military, and in prisons.

Why Do Some Men Rape?

Multiple theories exist on the causes of sexual violence from the perspective of the perpetrator (Stinson, Sales, Becker, & American Psychological Association, 2008). Some risk factors for perpetrators include having themselves been sexually abused in childhood; seeing women as sex objects and viewing them negatively, with hostility, or as dangerous; supporting beliefs that justify rape such as male entitlement to sex or that a woman is asking or deserving to be raped because she dresses provocatively. Some perpetrators are conditioned to become aroused to forced sexual violence. Using violent pornography may normalize preexisting sexually aggressive impulses (Casey & Lindhorst, 2009).

Acquaintance rape involves persons who know one another such as friend, neighbor, family member, classmate, date, or acquaintance. If there is a relationship, then trust is violated. Victims may fear retaliation from the assailant or harassment from family or friends who know the person (Rape, Abuse, and Incest National Network [RAINN], 2009).

Stranger rape is the least common type of rape. The assailant may be a total stranger who suddenly attacks the victim in a public place or in the home. Other stranger rapes occur when the assailant has brief contact with the victim prior to the assault, for example engaging the victim in conversation to earn trust at a bar or party. Women are more likely to report stranger rape than acquaintance rape (Jones, Wynn, Kroeze, Dunnuck, & Rossman, 2004).

Sexual assault and rape are considered forcible when there is threat or actual use of force on an unwilling victim. An incapacitated sexual assault or rape occurs when the victim is under the influence of alcohol or drugs, rendering the person unconscious or otherwise unable to give consent. Estimates are that as many as half of rapes are either drug facilitated or the result of self-induced intoxication. Alcohol is the most common drug associated with sexual assault (Hindmarch, ElSohly, Gambles, & Salamone, 2001). Alcohol makes it more difficult for women to identify potentially dangerous situations and to resist unwanted sexual advances. A drug-facilitated sexual assault occurs when alcohol and/or drugs are taken unwillingly or unknowingly. The use of date rape drugs such as flunitrazepam (Rohypnol, or "roofies"), gamma-hydroxybutyrate (GHB), ketamine, and carisoprodol (Soma) incapacitate the victim and may produce amnesia. These drugs are potentiated by alcohol, and the combination can be lethal. The frequency that these drugs are used may be underestimated because they are rapidly excreted, and lab testing has to be done within a few hours of ingestion (Crawford, Wright, & Birchmeier, 2008). Signs indicating that a woman may have been drugged include having no recall after taking a drink laced with the drug, feeling as if sex has occurred but not having any memory of the incident, feeling more intoxicated than what would be a usual response to the amount of alcohol consumed, or feeling fuzzy on awakening.

Kilpatrick and coworkers (2007) found that only 16% of victims reported the assault to police. Many factors deter a woman from reporting the crime, so data regarding sexual assaults may underestimate the magnitude of the problem. Women do not report rape because of the associated stigma; embarrassment; guilt that in some way they provoked the assault; fear of retribution from the rapist or his friends; dread of being humiliated and figuratively "raped" again by the criminal justice system publicity; distrust of law enforcement; involvement in illegal substance use; and discouragement generated by the dismally small number of convictions. Rape survivors often fear the reactions of husbands, lovers, friends, family, and children and prefer to suffer alone.

Mental Health Consequences of Sexual Assault

Rape produces long-term mental health consequences similar to those experienced by combat veterans. Most sexual assaults result in minor physical injuries; genital trauma may or may not be apparent. However, the psychologic effect can be severe. Sexual assault and rape are associated with depression, rape-trauma syndrome (RTS) and PTSD, substance abuse, suicidality, and a host of physical disorders including chronic pelvic pain and sexual dysfunction. One third of women seek counseling as a direct result of their sexual assault (Tjaden & Thoennes, 2006).

Why is rape so traumatic? Victims may have been threatened by a weapon, pushed, shoved, overpowered, or coerced. The assailant may have threatened to return and kill the victim if the incident is reported to anyone. In the aftermath victims may be frightened, angry, embarrassed, or ashamed. They may feel betrayed if there was a preexisting relationship with the assailant. Some may withdraw, feeling socially isolated, unable to tell the people closest to them, fearful of being judged or rejected. Some victims are afraid to return to their homes, workplace, or wherever the assault happened. The emotional suffering can take over women's lives and whereas some seek support from family, friends, health care professionals, or police, others may carry this experience silently, never telling anyone (Esposito, 2005).

Rape-Trauma

When humans experience fear, horror, or helplessness after a life-threatening traumatic event such as rape or combat there is an intense initial stress response. In the first few hours and days an initial neurobiologic dysregulation in the brain interferes with learning new information, making memories, responding to stress, and regulating the level of arousal. In some survivors this dysregulation and other neurobiologic changes persist (Heim & Nemeroff, 2009). For example, in most trauma survivors cortisol levels in the brain rise in response to stress. It appears from emerging research that in people who then develop PTSD, brain cortisol levels, rather than being elevated during stressful events, are low. Some theories suggest that the brain may become oversensitive to cortisol, and minor stress events may cause the person to overreact and major traumas may produce an underreaction (Wheeler, 2008). Variations in brain function and structure are important in understanding the trauma-related symptoms seen in some but not all rape victims. Why do some victims not recover? Suggested possibilities include genetic differences, neuroanatomic differences, sex differences, personality styles, past exposures to stress, and the characteristics and context of the specific trauma and subsequent experiences. Researchers are working on finding specific neurobiopsychologic strategies such as medications and/or therapies that can prevent and treat trauma sequelae like PTSD.

The neurobiologic changes that occur produce an array of symptoms. In the 1970s RTS was identified as a cluster of characteristic symptoms and related behaviors seen in the weeks and months after a rape (Burgess & Holmstrom, 2000). These researchers described three phases (see following). RTS is consistent with acute and chronic phases of PTSD (APA, 2000). Understanding the pattern of responses that victims may experience is crucial in helping the nurse provide woman-centered supportive and responsive care.

Acute Phase: Disorganization

According to Burgess and Holmstrom (2000) the assault itself marks the beginning of the acute phase of RTS, which can last for several days or up to 3 weeks. Reactions such as shock, denial, and disbelief are common. The rape survivor feels embarrassed, degraded, fearful, angry, and vengeful, and she may blame herself. The victim may feel unclean and want to bathe and douche, although this may destroy evidence. Fear is the primary feeling. Observable reactions may be controlled, expressed, or disoriented. In *controlled emotions* the survivor hides her emotions; has a subdued, calm demeanor; and seems to act as if nothing happened. She may answer questions and interact in a matter-of-fact way. Her affect seems incongruent with what she has just experienced. The second type of acute phase reaction is *expressed emotions*. Here the survivor may appear agitated, pacing, hysterical. She may be restless, crying, tense, or anxiously smiling. Her affect may change rapidly from crying to being calm and controlled. She relives the scene over and over in her mind and considers things she "should have done." *Shocked disbelief* or *disorientation* marks the third type of reaction. The victim may feel disoriented, have difficulty concentrating or making decisions, and may have poor recall of the event. Physiologically she may be uncomfortable, experiencing skeletal muscle pain or tension, gastrointestinal irritability, sighing, hyperventilation, and flushing.

Outward Adjustment Phase

During the adjustment phase the survivor may appear to have resolved her crisis. She may return to a job or to maintaining a household, or both, but she is denying and suppressing her thoughts and feelings. She needs this time to regain some control in her life. She may move, change jobs, buy a weapon to protect herself, or install an alarm system in her home. She may not be able to stop talking about the assault, letting it dominate her life or she may minimize or suppress the event, refusing to discuss it, acting as if it did not happen. She may try to analyze the details of how it happened, trying to explain how it happened and what the rapist was thinking. She may seek safety by fleeing her job, her home, or making other radical changes. She may experience fear, anxiety, phobias, mood swings, anger and rage, depression, insomnia, hypervigilance, and continued flashbacks. She may withdraw from support systems and be afraid to leave her home or go to certain places. She may develop sexual problems.

Long-Term Process: Reorganization Phase

The third phase is reorganization. Denial and suppression are difficult to maintain. Disclosing personal thoughts and feelings has a profound effect on improving health and reducing stress. As a rape survivor's suppression of feelings and emotions starts to deteriorate, she becomes depressed and anxious. Her own healthy spirit pressures her to discuss the rape with someone. Because she is losing her control of denial, her fears start to surface; she may be afraid to be alone or in a crowd or may fear being attacked from behind. Nightmares and eating disorders are common in these last two phases.

The recovery process may take years and can be difficult and painful. The victim has progressed through recovery when the physical distress and the constant memories of the rape have diminished. She no longer blames herself for what happened and can truly call herself a survivor. These phases are not necessarily linear and survivors may move back and forth between the phases. RTS may meet the criteria for PTSD and be formally diagnosed (see Table 5-1).

Collaborative Care

Nurses in women's health care and EDs are most likely to see rape victims in the acute phase. However, all women who manifest any of the signs of other phases should be assessed for posttraumatic experiences (Esposito, 2006). It is important to remember that sexual assault acute care has a dual purpose. First and foremost is to address the health care needs of the woman. The second purpose is to facilitate the collection of evidence and documentation of findings for use by the justice system. Health care is the nurse's first priority.

Facilities that provide initial treatment for rape victims vary in protocols and resources. In its 1992 guidelines, The Joint Commission (TJC) required EDs and ambulatory care departments to have protocols on physical assault; rape or sexual assault; and domestic abuse of older adults, spouses, partners, and children. These protocols must address client consent, examination, and treatment guidelines and the health care facility's responsibility for collecting evidence, photographing injuries, and releasing evidence to law enforcement officials. In addition, the EDs and ambulatory care departments must provide to victims a referral list of community-based and private service agencies dealing with family violence. The nurse interacting with the sexual assault client should be guided by the particular treatment center's protocol (Box 5-3). The first *National Protocol for Sexual Assault Medical Forensic Exams*, although failing to adequately address STIs and pregnancy prevention was important in identifying the unique roles of nurses including sexual assault nurse examiners (SANEs), physicians, police, forensic specialists, prosecutors, and counseling advocacy in the aftercare of a sexual trauma victim (Lewis-O'Connor, Franz, & Zuniga, 2005; U.S. Department of Justice & Office of Violence Against Women, 2004). Agency or state recommendations for care are continually evolving as new research and forensic techniques emerge.

Many treatment centers have initiated the use of SANEs as described in the above protocols. A SANE is educated in the specialty of forensic nursing and is prepared to examine clients; recognize, collect, and preserve evidence; counsel the client; link the client with vital community resources; follow up cases; and, if necessary, testify in court. When cared for by a SANE, victims receive better quality care, appropriate prophylaxis for infection and pregnancy and are more satisfied than when cared for in settings without SANEs (Campbell, 2008). Information on becoming a SANE, which currently requires a 40-hour course, is available at www.iafn.org. If a SANE is not available in a particular facility, TJC member organizations must implement a plan for educating an appropriate staff member about identifying, treating, and referring abuse victims. Additional resources may include a social worker who is called when a woman who has been raped is admitted. A local rape crisis center may have volunteers on call who may provide emotional support; provide transportation; help the woman interact with her family, friends, and various authorities; inform her of RTS; and find other resources for her as needed. Male volunteers may counsel male members of the victim's family and her male friends.

Psychologic First Aid

When victims seek help from people in their social network, from the police or from health care settings, the response they get is critical to their healing process. The goal of supportive

BOX 5-3 ADULT SEXUAL ASSAULT PROTOCOL: EMERGENCY DEPARTMENT

PURPOSE

To outline nursing care of sexual assault (rape and/or sexual offense) clients, which includes participation in the collection of forensic evidence and in the referral of clients for follow-up treatment.

Whenever possible, the sexual assault client will be cared for by an RN who is a sexual assault nurse examiner (SANE). These nurses have successfully completed a continuing education course in forensic and sexual assault evidence collection. This course provides those nurses with the information and skills to care properly for clients after sexual assault by recognizing, collecting, and preserving evidence; interviewing the client; and linking the client to vital community resources for follow-up.

ASSESSMENT

- Assess the client for any life-threatening injuries.
- Assess the client's level of coping, coherence, and ability to control behavior.
- Assess the client's priorities
  - Is client seeking care for prevention of pregnancy or disease only?
  - Is client seeking forensic evidence collection?
  - Does the client want both?

NOTE: Notify a SANE to perform the examination if the client is seeking evidence collection for filing of police charges either at this time or in the future.

- Assess the client's entire body for bruises, lacerations, and/or other skeletal or soft tissue injuries.
- Initiate the collection of evidence using the sexual assault collection kit if client consents.

If SANE is available:

- Complete collection.
- Examine the vagina and rectum to include the speculum examination.

NOTE: Toluidine blue dye, a Wood's lamp and a colposcope may be used to collect evidence.

- Physician performs the bimanual examination.

If SANE is not available:

- Primary nurse initiates collection with the exception of vaginal, rectal, and bimanual examinations.
- Physician performs vaginal, rectal, and bimanual examinations.
- Ask client whether those who are with the client know that the client has been sexually assaulted.

NOTE: This information cannot be given to secondary victims without the client's permission.

SAFETY

- Notify hospital police when a sexual assault client enters the emergency department (ED).

NOTE: Hospital police will complete a risk assessment of client safety.

CARE

- Provide care for any physical injuries.
- Provide for client privacy and nonjudgmental support.
- Protect client confidentiality by identifying the client as "7273" rather than by name or chief complaint.
- Assign one nurse to the client for the duration of his or her stay and disposition of evidence collection.
- Notify the sexual assault advocate office.

NOTE: The client has the right to refuse an advocate. It is the policy of the ED to allow the advocate to offer services directly to the client unless the client expressly forbids it. Notify the advocate of any secondary victims who may have accompanied the client and if the secondary victim is aware that the client has been sexually assaulted.

- Reassure the client that he or she is safe.
- Reassure the client that the incident is not his or her fault.
- Prepare the client for the possibility that some questions asked may be embarrassing.
- Obtain informed consent for the physical examination, to include photographs of injuries.

NOTE: If the client permits the release of information to law enforcement agencies, explain to the victim that the evidence will be turned over to the appropriate jurisdiction for processing. If the client is unwilling to have law enforcement notified at this time, the client should mark "do not (notify)" on the release form. The client may later change this if he or she chooses to file charges or have law enforcement involved.

- Collect the evidence as directed and in accordance with client consent.

NOTE: All evidence should be marked with the client's identification. Any photographs taken should be labeled with the client's information and described in the nursing notes. These photographs should then be sealed in an envelope and secured per ED policy. The evidence *must* remain in the possession of *one nurse* throughout the entire assessment procedure and treatment period, until it is released to a police agency.

- Perform a urine test for pregnancy; the urine can also be tested for drugs if the client suspects that he or she was drugged.
- Provide the opportunity for bathing and clean clothing after the examination.
- Discuss and provide emergency contraception and prophylaxis against sexually transmitted infections (STIs), including human immunodeficiency virus (HIV) if desired.
- Arrange for follow-up care per client preference for any medical and/or psychologic problems and/or injury.

CLIENT/SIGNIFICANT OTHER (SO) TEACHING

- Explain to the client/SO:
  - All procedures and their rationales
  - That feelings of anger, anxiety, and fear are normal
  - That options for medical, legal, and emotional counseling are available to both primary and secondary victims

NOTE: Do not assume that a friend or SO is aware of the assault.

- Inform client/SO of resources available:
  - Judicial system options (e.g., official police report, "blind" report)
  - Financial assistance
  - Local rape crisis center
  - Mental health agency
  - Sites and phone numbers for HIV counseling and testing
  - Resource list of phone numbers (e.g., law enforcement)

DOCUMENTATION

- Complete the forms for sexual assault evidence collection.
- Attach forms to appropriate documents.
- Seal the evidence kit as directed, and deliver it to a sworn law enforcement officer.
- Seal all photographs in an envelope marked with client identification, and secure per ED policy.
- Document care rendered, teaching done, and client response and level of understanding on ED nursing record.

care is to help victims feel less threatened, safer and have lower levels of anxiety. We do not know which victims will go on to develop PTSD but we do know that negative experiences in the health care system are associated with an increase in PTSD. Negative feedback has a powerful impact on survivors, and can be experienced as secondary victimization (Campbell, 2008).

The nurse may be one of the first persons to talk with a victim of sexual trauma. Initial distress is not abnormal and most sexual assault victims are able to recover. Even though there is limited evidence for specific treatments to prevent PTSD in sexual assault victims, trauma experts suggest that one promising approach is Psychological First Aid (Litz, 2008). Psychological First Aid has eight core goals that are consistent with and can be easily adapted to nursing practice. They are to (1) respond when a survivor reaches out to you or when you initiate contact with the survivor, in a nonintrusive, compassionate, and helpful manner; (2) enhance the survivor's safety and provide physical and emotional comfort; (3) stabilize by calming and orienting the survivor if she is emotionally overwhelmed; (4) identify immediate needs and concerns and gather information; (5) offer practical help in addressing needs; (6) offer to help establish contact with personal supports; (7) provide information about stress and coping responses to sexual assault; and (8) link the survivor with community and other services (National Child Traumatic Stress Network and National Center for PTSD, 2005; Ruzek, Brymer, Jacobs, Layne, Vernberg, & Watson, 2007). Nurses who understand postassault experiences can influence the responses of their nursing units, hospital, or institution and community.

The Sexual Assault Examination

Because sexual assault is a crime, the first nurse to see the sexually assaulted client must consider the need to preserve evidence (see Legal Tip: Collector of Evidence). However, the preservation of evidence should not overshadow a survivor's rights to be treated as a human being with respect, courtesy, and dignity. Client-centered care takes into consideration the psychologic needs of the victim, and the nurse adapts the examination accordingly.

> **LEGAL TIP: Collector of Evidence**
> Consent forms must be signed before evidence can be collected and released to the police and before photographs can be taken. If the victim is a minor (see individual state laws for age cutoff) a pediatric SANE, or a child sexual assault pediatrician is notified. Child sexual assault is beyond the scope of this chapter. A parent or guardian is required to sign the consent forms. A children's protective service may need to be called to facilitate consent.

Any health care and/or evidence collection is done only with the permission of the woman. She should be informed of all the steps involved in the sexual assault examination, treatment, and follow-up care. Written, informed consent for medical care and human immunodeficiency virus (HIV) testing must be obtained. In addition, consent must be obtained for collection and storage of sexual offense evidence, including forensic photography. A signed consent for release of evidence must be obtained. The woman may choose to stop her care or the evidence examination at any time. Informed consent includes information on what will happen during the examination, what tests will be done, what treatments can be offered, what risks occur without treatment, and what evidence collection may provide. It is important for the nurse to remember that the examination cannot determine if an assault (nonconsensual sexual encounter) has happened. That is a legal determination that happens in court. The examination provides information that may or may not be consistent with sexual contact. Not all sexual assaults produce trauma, and not all sexual trauma is nonconsensual.

History. History taking is an important step in early care. History includes a statement of the traumatic event whether or not evidence will be collected (Box 5-3). The woman needs privacy but should not be left alone. It is important to tell the woman that she is safe, that the incident is not her fault, and that she is not alone in what she has experienced. She also needs assurance of confidentiality and may need a great deal of support and patience in verbalizing the offender's acts. For example, giving the woman permission to describe the situation however she chooses and restating what the client has said (without minimizing) tells the woman she has been heard and ensures that what the nurse documents accurately reflects what she said. It also is important to obtain sexual, gynecologic, and obstetric histories (see Chapter 4).

The medicolegal record in a sexual assault case is likely to be used in court. A key feature used in court to establish rape is the absence of consent. The victim who is developmentally delayed, who is unconscious or otherwise physically unable to move, who has been drugged without her knowledge, or who is a minor (statutory rape) is not capable of giving consent. Bribery, threat, or coercion implies the lack of consent. The nurse's documentation is an important part of the medicolegal record. The wording of the history should reflect the woman's report, and her exact words should be used as often as possible (New York State Department of Health, 2008). When documenting, it is important for the nurse to remember that care is provided to the woman without judgment. Thus nurses should avoid using legal terms or words that suggest value judgments when documenting or referring to the woman. For example use of the term "alleged" or "claims" suggests that the nurse questions the woman's report. It is not the role of the nurse to determine whether a sexual assault occurred but to treat the woman patient as any other trauma victim. The court must prove absence of consent.

> **LEGAL TIP: Documentation**
> Clear, legible, accurate documentation is imperative. The woman's name should be on each page, and date, times, and signatures should be legible. Document an interpreter's name if one was used.

Physical Examination and Laboratory Tests. The nurse may assist with or, if trained, may perform the physical examination, which is conducted after the procedure is explained to the woman and consent is obtained. Some victims may view the examination as a second traumatic event. Preservation of the woman's dignity is of utmost importance during the examination. The woman may choose a female attendant, rape counselor, or other person to remain with her during the examination. The physician, nurse practitioner, or SANE informs her of every step of the procedure. The content of the examination is based on the history. For example, if there was oral penetration but no removal of clothing and genital contact, a speculum exam may not be appropriate. However many victims do not recall what happened during parts or all of the assault, and examination of all orifices is suggested. A standardized sexual assault evidence collection kit is used to obtain and package specimens. The kit gives detailed instructions on how to collect and package specimens and other evidence.

If the woman needs to urinate or defecate prior to the examination, the nurse should ask her to avoid wiping away vaginal or other secretions until after evidence is collected. Collect the first voided specimen for possible drug-facilitated sexual assault testing and document the time it was collected. If the woman has a tampon, panty liner, or contraceptive devices in the vagina, she should not remove or discard them. The woman remains clothed while her vital signs and blood pressure are determined, and her clothing is inspected for stains, tears, and foreign material. Clothing is handled only by the woman and may be collected, allowed to air dry, then sealed in a bag to be checked for evidence. She is assisted to undress and is draped for the physical examination. Her body is inspected for bruises, swelling, scratches, lacerations, or other wounds. A head-to-toe examination is performed as indicated. Victims may have injuries to other parts of their body including the head, face, and neck. An ultraviolet light (Wood's lamp) is used to find dried secretions on the victim's skin. External genitals, thighs, buttocks, and lower abdomen are assessed, and if there are injuries, bruises, or marks, photographs may be taken or drawings made. Pubic and scalp hair is combed for collection. Perianal, oral, and vaginal swabs are collected. If the victim scratched her attacker, her nails are scraped to obtain material that may aid in identification.

A speculum examination, often using magnification, is performed gently to detect tears or bruises and to collect appropriate specimens. Many victims have some type of genital injury, even if it is asymptomatic. A bimanual pelvic examination is not usually performed for evidence collection if a SANE is doing the examination. Internal pelvic assessment may be done by the nurse practitioner or physician if internal injury is suspected.

Laboratory tests may include oral swabs for the victim's DNA, a urine or blood pregnancy test, blood tests for hepatitis B virus, and oral or blood tests for HIV (CDC, Workowski, & Berman, 2006). A preexisting pregnancy will affect treatment decisions for possible HIV prophylaxis. Cultures for gonorrhea, chlamydia, and syphilis are not recommended because women are treated prophylactically, lab results will not change treatment, and testing may have negative consequences in court (Lewis-O'Connor et al., 2005; New York State Department of Health, 2008). Wet-mount slides may be obtained if symptoms indicate (CDC et al., 2006).

During the examination, the woman's emotional status is assessed, and findings are recorded: what reactions she exhibits to the assault; her orientation to time and place; and her attention span, affect, and verbal description and feelings about the assault. The availability of family or peer-support systems is assessed. She is asked about her plans to report the crime to the police. After the examination, the woman should be allowed to shower and offered fresh clothes or a gown. She may be given time to rest and to talk with the nurse, rape crisis counselor, family, or friends.

It is important that the chain of custody be maintained. *Chain of custody* is a legal term that refers to the continual guarding of evidence and describes evidence from the moment that it is first collected until it appears in court. All items of evidence are individually labeled with the name of examiner, client, date, and source. The evidence is never left unattended or with family, woman, or support person such as an advocate. During the examination chain of custody is the responsibility of the examiner. When evidence is turned over to the next custodian, each person signs. Signing indicates that no one touched or tampered with the evidence during that person's watch. This ensures that the evidence can be used in court.

Immediate Care

Nursing diagnoses for the rape victim during the immediate and later posttrauma period are listed in Box 5-4. Medical management includes (1) treating the physical injuries, including tetanus toxoid booster if indicated; (2) providing prophylactic antibiotic therapy for STIs (e.g., chlamydia, gonorrhea); and (3) providing prophylaxis for pregnancy if the woman is not pregnant. If physical trauma is life threatening, appropriate intervention takes precedence over collecting evidence. If the woman is at risk for pregnancy, emergency contraception should be discussed with her. Emergency contraception with progestin-only such as Plan B One-Step (one pill taken once) or combined

BOX 5-4 NURSING DIAGNOSES FOR THE RAPE VICTIM DURING THE IMMEDIATE AND LATER POSTTRAUMA PERIODS

IMMEDIATE POSTTRAUMA PERIOD

- *Anxiety/fear* related to:
  - rape-trauma experience
  - interactions with police and caregivers
  - physical examination to assess injury and collect evidence
- *Acute pain* related to:
  - physical injury from rape
  - examination
- *Disturbed body image* related to:
  - the rape
- *Rape-trauma* related to:
  - aftermath of being sexually assaulted
  - feelings of being unclean and humiliated
  - silent reaction of being unable to discuss the rape
- *Decisional conflict* related to:
  - discussing rape with family
  - possible pregnancy

LATER POSTTRAUMA PERIOD

- *Risk for infection* related to:
  - sexually transmitted infections
  - sexual assault by an assailant of unknown sexual history
- *Impaired social interaction* related to:
  - the rape
  - strained relationships with family, friends, intimate partners

estrogen and progestin pills can be used up to 120 hours after intercourse (see Table 8-2). The manufacturer recommends taking the medication within 96 hours. But research indicates that Plan B One-Step is effective up to 120 hours (5 days) after intercourse (U.S. Department of Health and Human Services & Office of Women's Health, 2009). The earlier it is taken, the more effective. The woman should be advised that emergency contraception does not guarantee pregnancy prevention, and that she should repeat the pregnancy test if she has not had a menstrual period within 3 to 4 weeks. She is apprised of the availability of abortion or menstrual extraction as a backup measure. If the woman is pregnant at the time of the assault, she should be observed for several hours for uterine contractility.

The woman may be provided with prophylactic antibiotic therapy to prevent STIs, hepatitis B immunization if needed, and HIV postexposure prophylaxis (PEP) (CDC et al., 2006).

Discharge

The woman is discharged with medications and printed instructions about their use, printed instructions for self-care, and names and telephone numbers of resource people if she requires assistance. Money and transportation to wherever she is staying (an alternative place may be found for her) add to the woman's comfort and perception of being in control. A medical follow-up examination in the gynecology or pediatric clinic is scheduled in 1 to 2 weeks for cultures for gonorrhea and other STIs; at 6 weeks for assessment of healing injuries; and at 6, 12, and 24 weeks for repeated serology tests for syphilis and HIV infection if initial test results were negative. The woman and her counselor determine whether there is a need for an additional medical or psychologic follow-up examination between the scheduled visits. The woman has a choice of site for follow-up testing. Some women choose to continue with the health care provider who first performed the examination, some prefer their primary health care provider, and others need referral to a clinic in the area (city, state) in which they live.

Nurses must be aware that responses to sexual assault are variable. Self-blame and humiliation may alternate with anger and fear. The woman needs to be reassured again before she leaves that her feelings are normal and that she is not alone. The initial care of a woman will affect her recovery and her decision to return for follow-up care. Nurses can assist women through an examination that is as nontraumatic as possible, with kindness, skill, and empathy.

After Discharge

Because of the phases of recovery, telephone contact by the health care provider to whomever the woman is referred is continued until the woman has no further need for such help. Education in prevention strategies is often offered by community agencies or rape-awareness groups. The focus of the classes is usually on increasing women's awareness of situations that put them at high risk for rape or sexual assault. Other courses may teach self-defense methods or how to change personal behaviors to reduce the risk of being victimized, such as avoiding being alone in isolated places and being alert to unusual activities or persons in one's environment. Still other courses may focus on changing societal attitudes about rape. Nurses can play a role in preventive education by offering courses or participating in courses offered by community or health care groups. Nurses must be knowledgeable about the epidemiology of sexual assault, reporting requirements, and services available in their community for victims, and should screen all women for a history of assault and any sequelae.

COMMUNITY ACTIVITY

- Research the laws regarding domestic violence in your state. Is it considered a misdemeanor or felony crime? Go to the website www.endabuse.org. Is mandatory reporting of domestic violence by health care providers required in your state? What is the definition of statutory rape in your state?
- What are the resources for victims of domestic violence in your community? Visit the website of a shelter for women and their children who are escaping violent relationships

KEY POINTS

- Violence against women is a major social and health care problem in the United States, costing thousands of lives and billions of dollars in direct and indirect health care costs.
- IPV includes physical, sexual, emotional, psychologic, and economic abuse.
- To provide effective care, nurses must increase awareness of their own beliefs and values regarding victimization of women.
- Theoretic frameworks—psychologic, sociologic, biologic, and feminist perspectives—provide the foundation for understanding the complexity of the victimization of women.
- Cultural influences regarding violent behaviors and relationships sensitize the nurse to the special needs of women from various ethnic groups.
- IPV affects young, middle-aged, and older women of all races; all socioeconomic, educational, and religious groups; and pregnant women.
- All states have mandatory reporting of the abuse of children and older adults; some states have initiated mandatory reporting of wife abuse. Mandatory reporting is controversial and takes away the right for women to choose.
- Rape is a legal term defined by each state differently but usually refers to penetration of an orifice against someone's will.
- Nurses in all professional areas should respond with sensitivity and caring to women who experience abuse and victimization.
- Follow-up and collaborative care are important in all instances of abuse.
- Nurses should be knowledgeable about reporting requirements and available community services for women who have been sexually assaulted.

Audio Chapter Summaries Access an audio summary of the Key Points on evolve

REFERENCES

American College of Obstetricians and Gynecologists. (2010). *Are you being abused? Screening tool for domestic violence.* Available at www.acog.org/departments/dept_notice.cfm?recno=17&bulletin=585. Accessed May 30, 2010.

American Psychiatric Association. (2000). *Diagnostic criteria from DSM-IV-TR.* Washington, DC: American Psychiatric Association.

Association of Women's Health, Obstetric and Neonatal Nurses (AWHONN) Board of Directors. (2007). *Mandatory reporting of intimate partner violence.* Available at www.awhonn.org/awhonn/content.do?name=05_HealthPolicyLegislation%2F5H_PositionStatements.htm. Accessed May 30, 2010.

Basile, K., Chen, J., Black, M., & Saltzman, L. (2007). Prevalence and characteristics of sexual violence victimization among U.S. adults, 2001-2003. *Violence and Victims, 22*(4), 437–448.

Blanchfield, L. (2008). *United Nations system efforts to address violence against women.* Available at http:fpc.state.gov/documents/organization/109495.pdf. Accessed August 8, 2010.

Bonomi, A., Anderson, M., Cannon, E., Slesnick, N., & Rodriguez, M. (2009). Intimate partner violence in Latina and non-Latina women. *American Journal of Preventive Medicine, 36*(1), 43–48.

Bonomi, A., Anderson, M., Reid, R., Rivara, F., Carrell, D., & Thompson, R. (2009). Medical and psychosocial diagnoses in women with a history of intimate partner violence. *Archives of Internal Medicine, 169*(18), 1692–1697.

Breiding, M., Ziembroski, J., & Black, M. (2009). Prevalence of rural intimate partner violence in 16 US states, 2005. *Journal of Rural Health, 25*(3), 240–246.

Bronfenbrenner, U. (1979). *The ecology of human development: Experiments by nature and design.* Cambridge, MA: Harvard University Press.

Bronfenbrenner, U. (2005). *Making human beings human: Bioecological perspectives on human development.* Thousand Oaks, CA: Sage Publications.

Brown, D., Finkelstein, E., & Mercy, J. (2008). Methods for estimating medical expenditures attributable to intimate partner violence. *Journal of Interpersonal Violence, 23*(12), 1747–1766.

Btoush, R., & Haj-Yahia, M. (2008). Attitudes of Jordanian society toward wife abuse. *Journal of Interpersonal Violence, 23*(11), 1531–1554.

Burgess, A., & Holmstrom, L. (2000). Rape trauma syndrome. In A. Burgess (Ed.), *Violence through a forensic lens.* King of Prussia, PA: Nursing Spectrum.

Campbell, D., Sharps, P., Gary, F., Campbell, J., & Lopez, L. (2002). Intimate partner violence in African-American women. *Online Journal of Issues in Nursing, 7*(1), 5.

Campbell, J. (2004a). *Danger assessment.* Available at www.dangerassessment.org. Accessed May 30, 2010.

Campbell, J. (2004b). Helping women understand their risk in situations of intimate partner violence. *Journal of Interpersonal Violence, 19*(12), 1464–1477.

Campbell, J., & Furniss, K. (2002). *Violence against women: Identification, screening and management of intimate partner violence.* Washington, DC: Association of Women's Health, Obstetric and Neonatal Nurses.

Campbell, J., Jones, A., Dienemann, J., Kub, J., Schollenberger, J., O'Campo, P., et al. (2002). Intimate partner violence and physical health consequences. *Archives of Internal Medicine, 162*(10), 1157–1163.

Campbell, J., Webster, D., & Glass, N. (2009). The danger assessment: Validation of a lethality risk assessment instrument for intimate partner femicide. *Journal of Interpersonal Violence, 24*(4), 653–674.

Campbell, R. (2008). The psychological impact of rape victims. *American Psychologist, 63*(8), 702–717.

Campbell, R., Dworkin, E., & Cabral, G. (2009). An ecological model of the impact of sexual assault on women's mental health. *Trauma Violence and Abuse, 10*(3), 225–246.

Cannon, E., Bonomi, A., Anderson, M., & Rivara, F. (2009). The intergenerational transmission of witnessing intimate partner violence. *Archives of Pediatric and Adolescent Medicine, 163*(8), 706–708.

Capaldi, D., & Kim, H. (2007). Typological approaches to violence in couples: A critique and alternative conceptual approach. *Clinical Psychology Review, 27*(3), 253–265.

Casey, E., & Lindhorst, T. (2009). Toward a multi-level, ecological approach to the primary prevention of sexual assault: Prevention in peer and community contexts. *Trauma Violence and Abuse, 10*(2), 91–114.

Catalano, S., Smith, E., Snyder, H., & Rand, M. (2009). *Female victims of violence.* Available at www.ojp.usdoj.gov/bjs/abstract/fvv.htm. Accessed May 30, 2010.

Centers for Disease Control and Prevention (CDC), Workowski, K., & Berman, S. (2006). Sexually transmitted diseases treatment guidelines 2006. *MMWR Morbidity and Mortality Weekly Report, 55*(RR11), 1–94.

Centers for Disease Control and Prevention. (2008). *Intimate partner violence definitions.* Available at www.cdc.gov/ViolencePrevention/intimatepartnerviolence/definitions.html. Accessed January 25, 2010.

Centers for Disease Control and Prevention & National Center for Injury Prevention and Control. (2008). *National violent death reporting system: Monitoring and tracking the causes of violent deaths in 2008.* Available at www.cdc.gov/ncipc/dvp/NVDRS/at_a_glance.htm. Accessed January 25, 2010.

Chambliss, L. (2008). Intimate partner violence and its implication for pregnancy. *Clinics in Obstetrics and Gynecology, 51*(2), 385–397.

Chang, J., Berg, C., Saltzman, L., & Herndon, J. (2005). Homicide: A leading cause of injury deaths among pregnant and postpartum women in the United States, 1991-1999. *American Journal of Public Health, 95*(3), 471–477.

Crawford, E., Wright, M., & Birchmeier, Z. (2008). Drug-facilitated sexual assault: College women's risk perception and behavioral choices. *Journal of American College Health, 57*(3), 261–272.

Davis, J., Park, S., Kaups, K., Bennink, L., & Bilello, J. (2003). Victims of domestic violence on the trauma service: Unrecognized and underreported. *Journal of Trauma, 54*(2), 352–355.

Dienemann, J., Boyle, E., Baker, D., Resnick, W., Wiederhorn, N., & Campbell, J. (2000). Intimate partner abuse among women diagnosed with depression. *Issues in Mental Health Nursing, 21*(5), 499–513.

Dienemann, J., Glass, N., & Hyman, R. (2005). Survivor preferences for response to IPV disclosure. *Clinical Nursing Research, 14*(3), 215–233.

Downs, W., & Rindels, B. (2004). Adulthood depression, anxiety, and trauma symptoms: A comparison of women with nonabusive, abusive, and absent father figures in childhood. *Violence and Victims, 19*(6), 659–671.

Duran, B., Oetzel, J., Parker, T., Malcoe, L., Lucero, J., & Jiang, Y. (2009). Intimate partner violence and alcohol, drug, and mental disorders among American Indian women in primary care. *American Indian Alaskan Native Mental Health Research, 16*(2), 11–27.

Dutton, M. (2009). *Update of the "battered woman syndrome" critique.* Available at http://new.vawnet.org. Accessed August 8, 2010.

Esposito, N. (2005). Manifestations of enduring during interviews with sexual assault victims. *Qualitative Health Research, 15*(7), 912–927.

Esposito, N. (2006). Women with a history of sexual assault. Health care visits can be reminders of a sexual assault. *American Journal of Nursing, 106*(3), 69–71, 73.

Family Violence Prevention Fund (FVPF). (2004). *Mandatory reporting of domestic violence by health care providers.* Available at www.endabuse.org/health/mandatoryreporting. Accessed January 25, 2010.

Faramarzi, M., Esmailzadeh, S., & Mosavi, S. (2005). A comparison of abused and non-abused women's definitions of domestic violence and attitudes to acceptance of male dominance. *European Journal of Obstetrics, Gynecology, and Reproductive Biology, 122*(2), 225–231.

Fishwick, N., Parker, B., & Campbell, J. (2005). Care of survivors of abuse and violence. In G. Stuart & M. Laraia (Eds.), *Principles and practice of psychiatric nursing* (8th ed.). St. Louis: Mosby.

Garcia-Moreno, C., Jansen, H., Ellsberg, M., Heise, L., & Watts, C. (2006). Prevalence of intimate partner violence: Findings from the WHO multi-country study on women's health and domestic violence. *Lancet, 368*(9543), 1260–1269.

Gerber, M., Gantz, M., Lichter, E., Williams, C., & McCloskey, K. (2005). Adverse health behaviors and the detection of partner violence by clinicians. *Archives of Internal Medicine, 165*(9), 1016–1021.

Glass, N., Eden, K., Bloom, T., & Perrin, N. (2009). Computerized aid improves safety decision process for survivors of intimate partner violence. *Journal of Interpersonal Violence*. Available at www.ncbi.nlm.nih.gov/entrez/query.fcgi?cmd=Retrieve&db=PubMed&dopt=Citation&list_uids=20040709. Accessed May 30, 2010.

Glass, N., Perrin, N., Hanson, G., Mankowski, E., Bloom, T., & Campbell, J. (2009). Patterns of partners' abusive behaviors as reported by Latina and non-Latina survivors. *Journal of Community Psychology, 37*(2), 156–170.

Harrykissoon, S., Rickert, V., & Wiemann, C. (2002). Prevalence and patterns of intimate partner violence among adolescent mothers during the postpartum period. *Archives of Pediatric and Adolescent Medicine, 156*(4), 325–330.

Heim, C., & Nemeroff, C. (2009). Neurobiology of posttraumatic stress disorder. *CNS Spectrums, 14*(1 Suppl. 1), 13–24.

Heise, L. (1998). Violence against women: An integrated, ecological framework. *Violence Against Women, 4*(3), 262–290.

Hindmarch, I., ElSohly, M., Gambles, J., & Salamone, S. (2001). Forensic urinalysis of drug use in cases of alleged sexual assault. *Journal of Clinical Forensic Medicine, 8*(4), 197–205.

Horon, I., & Cheng, D. (2005). Underreporting of pregnancy-associated deaths. *American Journal of Public Health, 95*(11), 1879, author reply 1879–1880.

Jones, J., Wynn, B., Kroeze, B., Dunnuck, C., & Rossman, L. (2004). Comparison of sexual assaults by strangers versus known assailants in a community-based population. *American Journal of Emergency Medicine, 22*(6), 454–459.

Kilpatrick, D., Resnick, H., Ruggiero, K., Conoscenti, L., & McCauley, J. (2007). *Drug-facilitated, incapacitated and forcible rape: A national study (No. 219181)*. Charleston, SC: Medical University of South Carolina, National Crime Victims Research and Treatment Center.

Klevens, J., & Saltzman, L. E. (2009). The controversy on screening for intimate partner violence: A question of semantics? *Journal of Women's Health (Larchmont), 18*(2), 143–145.

Lewis-O'Connor, A., Franz, H., & Zuniga, L. (2005). Limitations of the national protocol for sexual assault medical forensic examinations. *Journal of Emergency Nursing, 31*(3), 267–270.

Litz, B. (2008). Early intervention for trauma: Where are we and where do we need to go? A commentary. *Journal of Traumatic Stress, 21*(6), 503–506.

MacMillan, H., Wathen, C., Jamieson, E., Boyle, M., Shannon, H., Ford-Gilboe, M., et al. (2009). Screening for intimate partner violence in health care settings: A randomized trial. *Journal of the American Medical Association, 302*(5), 493–501.

Macy, R., Martin, S., Kupper, L., Casanueva, C., & Guo, S. (2007). Partner violence among women before, during, and after pregnancy: Multiple opportunities for intervention. *Women's Health Issues, 17*(5), 290–299.

Martin, S., Mackie, L., Kupper, L., Buescher, P., & Moracco, K. (2001). Physical abuse of women before, during, and after pregnancy. *Journal of the American Medical Association, 285*(12), 1581–1584.

Martin, S., Macy, R., Sullivan, K., & Magee, M. (2007). Pregnancy-associated violent deaths: The role of intimate partner violence. *Trauma, Violence, & Abuse, 8*(2), 135–148.

McCauley, J., Amstadter, A., Danielson, C., Ruggiero, K., Kilpatrick, D., & Resnick, H. (2009). Mental health and rape history in relation to non-medical use of prescription drugs in a national sample of women. *Addictive Behaviors, 34*(8), 641–648.

McFarlane, L., Campbell, J., Sharps, P., & Watson, K. (2002). Abuse during pregnancy and femicide: Urgent implications for women's health. *Obstetrics and Gynecology, 100*(1), 27–35.

McFarlane, J., Groff, J., O'Brien, A., & Watson, K. (2005). Populations at risk: Empirical studies of prevalence of partner violence against 7,443 African American, white, and Hispanic women receiving care at urban public primary care clinics. *Public Health Nursing, 22*(2), 98–107.

McPhail, B., Busch, N., Kulkarni, S., & Rice, G. (2007). An integrative feminist model: The evolving feminist perspective on intimate partner violence. *Violence Against Women, 13*(8), 817–841.

Mitchell, C., & Anglin, D. (2009). *Intimate partner violence: A health-based perspective.* New York, NY: Oxford University Press.

Montalvo-Liendo, N. (2009). Cross-cultural factors in disclosure of intimate partner violence: An integrated review. *Journal of Advanced Nursing, 65*(1), 20–34.

Moracco, K., Brown, C., Martin, S., Chang, J., Dulli, L., Loucks-Sorrell, M., et al. (2004). Mental health issues among female clients of domestic violence programs in North Carolina. *Psychiatric Services, 55*(9), 1036–1040.

Morland, L., Leskin, G., Block, C., Campbell, J., & Friedman, M. (2008). Intimate partner violence and miscarriage: Examination of the role of physical and psychological abuse and posttraumatic stress disorder. *Journal of Interpersonal Violence, 23*(5), 652–669.

Morrison, K., Luchok, K., Richter, D., & Parra-Medina, D. (2006). Factors influencing help-seeking from informal networks among African American victims of intimate partner violence. *Journal of Interpersonal Violence, 21*(11), 1493–1511.

National Child Traumatic Stress Network and National Center for PTSD. (2005). *Psychological first aid: Field operations guide, 47.* Available at www.vdh.virginia.gov/EPR/pdf/PFA9-6-05Final.pdf. Accessed May 30, 2010.

National Institute of Justice. (2007). *Measuring intimate partner violence.* Available at www.ojp.usdoj.gov/nij/topics/crime/intimate-partner-violence/measuring.htm. Accessed May 30, 2010.

Naved, R., Azim, S., Bhuiya, A., & Persson, L. (2006). Physical violence by husbands: Magnitude, disclosure and help-seeking behavior of women in Bangladesh. *Social Science Medicine, 62*(12), 2917–2929.

New York State Department of Health. (2008). *State of New York protocol for the acute care of the adult patient reporting sexual assault. October 2008.* Available at www.nyhealth.gov/professionals/protocols. Accesed January 25, 2010.

Nurius, P., & Macy, R. (2008). Heterogeneity among violence-exposed women: Applying person-oriented research methods. *Journal of Interpersonal Violence, 23*(3), 389–415.

Oetzel, J., & Duran, B. (2004). Intimate partner violence in American Indian and/or Alaska Native communities: A social ecological framework of determinants and interventions. *American Indian Alaskan Native Mental Health Research, 11*(3), 49–68.

Pennell, J., & Francis, S. (2005). Safety conferencing: toward a coordinated and inclusive response to safeguard women and children. *Violence Against Women, 11*(5), 666–692.

Plichta, S. (2004). Intimate partner violence and physical health consequences. *Journal of Interpersonal Violence, 19*(11), 1296–1323.

Quinlivan, J., & Evans, S. (2005). Impact of domestic violence and drug abuse in pregnancy on maternal attachment and infant temperament in teenage mothers in the setting of best clinical practice. *Archives of Women's Mental Health, 8*(3), 191–199.

Rape, Abuse, and Incest National Network (RAINN). (2009). *Acquaintance rape.* Available at http://rainn.org/get-information/types-of-sexual-assault. Accessed May 30, 2010.

Records, K., & Rice, M. J. (2009). Lifetime physical and sexual abuse and the risk for depression symptom in the first 8 months after birth. *Journal of Psychosomatic Obstetrics and Gynaecology, 30*(3), 181–190.

Renker, P. (2002). "Keep a blank face. I need to tell you what has been happening to me." Teens' stories of abuse and violence before and during pregnancy. *MCN American Journal of Maternal/Child Nursing, 27*(2), 109–116.

Renzetti, C., Edleson, J., & Bergen, R. (2001). *The sourcebook on violence against women.* Thousand Oaks, CA: Sage.

Ruzek, J., Brymer, J., Jacobs, A., Layne, C., Vernberg, E., & Watson, P. (2007). Psychological first aid. *Journal of Mental Health Counseling, 29*(1), 17–49.

Saltzman, L., Fanslow, J., McMahon, P., & Shelley, G. (2002). *Intimate partner violence surveillance: Uniform definitions and recommended data elements.* Available at www.cdc.gov/ncipc/pub-res/ipv_surveillance/intimate.htm. Accessed May 30, 2010.

Shiu-Thornton, S., Senturia, K., & Sullivan, M. (2005). "Like a bird in a cage": Vietnamese women survivors talk about domestic violence. *Journal of Interpersonal Violence, 20*(8), 959–976.

Soler, H., Vinayak, P., & Quadagno, D. (2000). Biosocial aspects of domestic violence. *Psychoneuroendocrinology, 25*(7), 721–739.

Steiner, L. (2009). *Crazy love: A memoir.* New York: St. Martin's Press.

Stinson, J., Sales, B., Becker, J., & American Psychological Association. (2008). *Sex offending: Causal theories to inform research, prevention, and treatment.* Washington, DC: American Psychological Association.

Straus, H., Cerulli, C., McNutt, L., Rhodes, K., Conner, K., Kemball, R., et al. (2009). Intimate partner violence and functional health status: Associations with severity, danger, and self-advocacy behaviors. *Journal of Women's Health (Larchmont), 18*(5), 625–631.

Stuart, G., & Hamolia, C. (2009). Preventing and managing aggressive behavior. In G. Stuart (Ed.), *Principles and practice of psychiatric nursing* (9th ed.). St. Louis: Mosby.

Taylor, R., & Nabors, E. (2009). Pink or blue... black and blue? Examining pregnancy as a predictor of intimate partner violence and femicide. *Violence Against Women, 15*(11), 1273–1293.

Thompson, R., Bonomi, A., Anderson, M., Reid, R., Dimer, J., Carrell, D., et al. (2006). Intimate partner violence: Prevalence, types, and chronicity in adult women. *American Journal of Preventive Medicine, 30*(6), 447–457.

Tjaden, P., & Thoennes, N. (2006). *Extent, nature and consequences of rape victimization: Findings from the National Violence Against Women Survey*. Available at www.ojp.usdoj.gov/nij/pubs-sum/210346.htm. Accessed May 30, 2010.

Torres, S., & Han, H. (2003). Women's perceptions of their male batterers' characteristics and level of violence. *Issues in Mental Health Nursing, 24*(6), 667–673.

U.S. Census Bureau. (2006). *Hispanics in the U.S. 2006*. Available at www.census.gov/population/www/socdemo/hispanic/files/Internet_Hispanic_in_US_2006.pdf. Accessed May 30, 2010.

U.S. Department of Health and Human Services, & Office of Women's Health. (2009). *Emergency contraception*. Available at www.womenshealth.gov/faq/emergency-contraception.pdf. Accessed August 8, 2010.

U.S. Department of Health and Human Services. (2009). *Proposed Healthy People 2020 objectives*. Available at http://healthypeople.gov/HP2020/default.asp. Accessed August 8, 2010.

U.S. Department of Justice, & Office of Violence Against Women. (2004). *A national protocol for sexual assault medical forensic examinations*. Available at www.ncjrs.gov/pdffiles1/ovw/206554.pdf. Accessed May 30, 2010.

U.S. Preventive Services Task Force. (2004). Screening for family and intimate partner violence: Recommendation statement. *Annals of Internal Medicine, 140*(5), 382–386.

United Nations. (December 20, 1993). *Declaration of the elimination of violence against women*. Available at www2.ohchr.org/english/law/eliminationvaw.htm. Accessed May 30, 2010.

Violence Against Women Online Resources. (2010). The facts about sexual violence. *Research in brief*. Available at www.vaw.umn.edu/documents/inbriefs/sexualviolence/sexualviolence-bw.pdf. Accessed May 30, 2010.

Walton-Moss, B., & Campbell, J. (2002). Intimate partner violence: Implications for nursing. *Online Journal of Issues in Nursing, 7*(1), 6.

Westbrook, L. (2009). Information myths and intimate partner violence: Sources, contexts, and consequences. *Journal of the American Society for Information Science and Technology, 60*(4), 826–836.

Wheeler, K. (2008). *Psychotherapy for the advanced practice psychiatric nurse*. St. Louis: Mosby.

World Health Organization. (2010). *The ecological framework*. Available at www.who.int/violenceprevention/approach/ecology/en/index.html. Accessed January 7, 2010.

Yoshihama, M. (2002). Breaking the web of abuse and silence: Voices of battered women in Japan. *Social Work, 47*(4), 389–400.

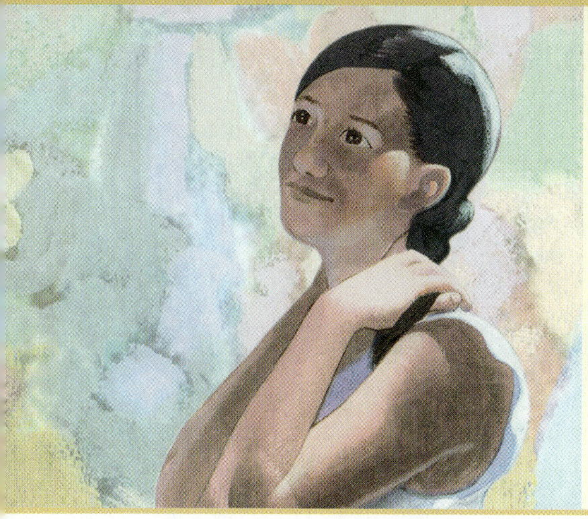

CHAPTER

6

Reproductive System Concerns

Deitra Leonard Lowdermilk

evolve WEBSITE

http://evolve.elsevier.com/Lowdermilk/MWHC/
Audio Glossary
Audio Key Points
NCLEX Review Questions
Nursing Care Plans
  Endometriosis
  Premenstrual Syndrome

LEARNING OBJECTIVES

- Differentiate signs and symptoms of common menstrual disorders.
- Develop a nursing care plan for a woman with primary dysmenorrhea.
- Outline client teaching about premenstrual syndrome (PMS).
- Relate the symptoms of endometriosis to the associated pathophysiology.
- Differentiate the various causes of abnormal uterine bleeding.
- Identify health risks of perimenopausal women.
- Develop an assessment guide for perimenopausal women.
- Develop a nursing plan of care for a postmenopausal woman.
- Examine the risks and benefits of menopausal hormone therapy.
- Summarize client teaching strategies for prevention of osteoporosis.
- Evaluate the use of alternative therapies for menstrual disorders and menopausal symptoms.

Problems may occur at any point in the menstrual cycle. In addition, many factors, including anatomic abnormalities, physiologic imbalances, and lifestyle, can affect the menstrual cycle. Many women seek out nurses as advisers, counselors, and health care providers for information about menstrual cycle experiences, concerns, or disorders. If they are to meet their clients' needs, nurses must have accurate, up-to-date information. This chapter provides information on menstrual cycle experiences, including menarche and menopause; common menstrual disorders; abnormal bleeding problems; and problems associated with menopause.

Knowledge of the normal parameters of menstruation is essential to the assessment of menstrual cycle experiences and disorders. The menstrual cycle is a result of a complex interplay among the reproductive, neurologic, and endocrine systems. The hypothalamus produces gonadotropin-releasing hormone (GnRH), which stimulates the pituitary gland to produce follicle-stimulating hormone (FSH) and luteinizing hormone (LH). In turn, FSH and LH stimulate the ovaries to produce first estrogen and then progesterone. In response to the hormones, the endometrium, or lining of the uterus, proliferates and then sheds. Chapter 4 provides additional information on the menstrual cycle and endocrine physiology.

Normal menstrual patterns are averages based on observations and reports from large groups of healthy women. When counseling an individual woman, remember that these values are averages only. Generally a woman's menstrual frequency stabilizes at 28 days within 1 to 2 years after puberty, with a range from 26 to 34 days (Blackburn, 2007). Although no woman's cycle is exactly the same length every month, the typical month-to-month variation in an individual's cycle is usually plus or minus 2 days. However, greater but still normal variations are noted frequently.

During her reproductive years a woman may have more than one physiologic variation in her menstrual cycle. An understanding of the physiologic variations that occur in several age-groups is essential for nurses. Menstrual cycle length is most irregular at the extremes of the reproductive years including the 2 years after menarche and the 5 years before menopause, when anovulatory cycles are most common. Irregular bleeding, both in length of cycle and amount, is the rule rather than the exception in early adolescence. It takes approximately 15 months for completion of the first 10 cycles and an average of 20 cycles before ovulation occurs regularly. Cycle lengths of 15 to 45 days are not unusual, and during the first 2 years after menarche, intervals of 3 to 6 months between menses can be normal.

Women's knowledge and understanding of the menstrual cycle may be limited and is often influenced by myths and misunderstandings. Women typically have menstrual cycles for about 40 years. Once the irregular nature of menses in the first 1 to 2 years after menarche subsides and a cyclic, predictable pattern of monthly bleeding is established, women may worry about any deviation from that pattern, or from what they have been told is normal for all menstruating women. A woman may be concerned about her ability to conceive and bear children or she may believe that she is not really a woman without monthly evidence. A sign such as amenorrhea or excess menstrual bleeding can be a source of severe distress and concern for women.

COMMON MENSTRUAL DISORDERS

Amenorrhea

Amenorrhea, the absence of menstrual flow, is a clinical symptom of a variety of disorders. Although these criteria for a clinical problem of amenorrhea are not universal, these circumstances should generally be evaluated: (1) the absence of both menarche and secondary sexual characteristics by age 14 years; (2) absence of menses by age 16 years, regardless of presence of normal growth and development (primary amenorrhea); or (3) a 3- to 6-month absence of menses after a period of menstruation (secondary amenorrhea) (Speroff & Fritz, 2005).

Although amenorrhea is not a disease, it is often the sign of one. Still, most commonly and most benignly, amenorrhea is a result of pregnancy. It also may result from anatomic abnormalities such as outflow tract obstruction, anterior pituitary disorders, other endocrine disorders such as polycystic ovary syndrome, hypothyroidism or hyperthyroidism, chronic diseases such as type 1 diabetes, medications such as phenytoin (Dilantin), drug abuse (alcohol, tranquilizers, opiates, marijuana, cocaine), or oral contraceptive use.

Hypogonadotropic amenorrhea reflects a problem in the central hypothalamic-pituitary axis. In rare instances a pituitary lesion or genetic inability to produce FSH and LH is at fault. More commonly it results from hypothalamic suppression as a result of two principal influences: stress (in the home, school, or workplace) or a body fat-to-lean ratio that is inappropriate for an individual woman, especially during a normal growth period (Lobo, 2007d). Research has demonstrated a biologic basis for the relationship of stress to physiologic processes. Amenorrhea is one of the classic signs of anorexia nervosa, and the interrelatedness of disordered eating, amenorrhea, and altered bone mineral density has been described as the female athlete triad (Lebrun, 2007). Calcium loss from bone, comparable to that seen in postmenopausal women, may occur with this type of amenorrhea.

Exercise-associated amenorrhea can occur in women undergoing vigorous physical and athletic training. The pathophysiology is complex and is thought to be associated with many factors, including body composition (height, weight, and percentage of body fat); type, intensity, and frequency of exercise; nutritional status; and the presence of emotional or physical stressors (Lobo, 2007d). In addition, it is probably due to diminished secretion of GnRH. Women who participate in sports emphasizing low body weight are at greatest risk, including the following (Bonci, Bonci, Granger, Johnson, Malina, Milné, et al., 2008):

- Sports in which performance is subjectively scored (e.g., dance, gymnastics)
- Endurance sports favoring participants with low body weight (e.g., distance running, cycling)
- Sports in which body contour–revealing clothing is worn for competition (e.g., swimming, diving, volleyball)
- Sports with weight categories for participation (e.g., rowing, martial arts)
- Sports in which prepubertal body shape favors success (e.g., gymnastics, figure skating)

Assessment of amenorrhea begins with a thorough history and physical examination. An important initial step, often overlooked, is to be sure that the woman is not pregnant. Specific components of the assessment process depend on a client's age—adolescent, young adult, or perimenopausal—and whether she has previously menstruated.

Once pregnancy has been ruled out by a β-human chorionic gonadotropin (β-hCG) pregnancy test, diagnostic tests may include FSH level, thyroid-stimulating hormone (TSH) and prolactin levels, radiographic or computed tomography scan of the sella turcica, and a progestational challenge (Lobo, 2007d).

Management

When amenorrhea is a result of hypothalamic disturbances, the nurse is an ideal health professional to assist women because many of the causes are potentially reversible (e.g., stress, weight loss for nonorganic reasons). Counseling and education are primary interventions and appropriate nursing roles. When a stressor known to predispose a client to hypothalamic amenorrhea is identified, initial management involves addressing the stressor. Together the woman and the nurse plan how the woman can decrease or discontinue medications known to affect menstruation, correct weight loss, deal more effectively with psychologic stress, address emotional distress, and alter her exercise routine.

The nurse works with the woman to help her identify, cope with, and possibly resolve sources of stress in her life. Deep-breathing exercises and relaxation techniques are simple yet effective stress reduction measures. Referral for biofeedback or massage therapy also may be useful. In some instances, referrals for psychotherapy may be indicated.

If a woman's exercise program is thought to contribute to her amenorrhea, several options exist for management. The American College of Sports Medicine (ACSM) recommends increasing nutritional intake to increase energy availability and reducing exercise energy expenditure as the first line of treatment (Nattiv, Loucks, Manore, Sandborn, Sundgot-Borgen, Warren, & ACSM, 2007). Therefore, the woman may decide to decrease the intensity or duration of her training if possible or to gain 2% to 3% in body weight. Coming to accept this alternative may be difficult for one who is committed to a strenuous exercise regimen, and the nurse and the client may have several sessions before the woman elects to try exercise reduction. Many young female athletes may not understand the consequences of low bone density or osteoporosis; nurses can point out the connection between low bone density and stress fractures. The nurse and the woman also should investigate other factors that may be contributing to the amenorrhea and develop plans for altering lifestyle and decreasing stress.

A daily calcium intake of 1000 to 1500 mg and vitamin D 400 to 600 International Units is recommended for women with amenorrhea associated with the female athlete triad (Bonci et al., 2008). Some researchers have found that low-dose oral contraceptives have a positive effect on bone density in premenopausal women with exercise-associated amenorrhea (Liu & Lebrun, 2006; Vescovi, VanHeest, & De Souza, 2008).

Cyclic Perimenstrual Pain and Discomfort

Cyclic perimenstrual pain and discomfort (CPPD) is a concept developed by a nurse science team for a research project for the Association of Women's Health, Obstetric and Neonatal Nurses (AWHONN) (Collins Sharp, Taylor, Thomas, Killeen, & Dawood, 2002). This concept includes dysmenorrhea, premenstrual syndrome (PMS), and premenstrual dysphoric disorder (PMDD) as well as symptom clusters that occur before and after the menstrual flow starts. Symptoms occur cyclically and can include mood swings as well as pelvic pain and physical discomforts. These symptoms can range from mild to severe and can last a day or two or up to 2 weeks (Taylor, Berg, & Fogel, 2008). CPPD is a health problem that can have a significant effect on a woman's quality of life. The following discussion focuses on the three main conditions of CPPD.

Dysmenorrhea

Dysmenorrhea, pain during or shortly before menstruation, is one of the most common gynecologic problems in women of all ages. Many adolescents have dysmenorrhea in the first 3 years after menarche. Young adult women ages 17 to 24 years are most likely to report painful menses. Approximately 75% of women report some level of discomfort associated with menses, and approximately 15% report severe dysmenorrhea (Lentz, 2007b); however, the amount of disruption in women's lives is difficult to determine. Researchers have estimated that up to 10% of women with dysmenorrhea have severe enough pain to interfere with their functioning for 1 to 3 days a month. Severe dysmenorrhea is also associated with early menarche, nulliparity, and stress (Lentz, 2007b). Traditionally dysmenorrhea is differentiated as primary or secondary. Symptoms usually begin with menstruation, although some women have discomfort several hours before onset of flow. The range and severity of symptoms are different from woman to woman and from cycle to cycle in the same woman. Symptoms of dysmenorrhea may last several hours to several days.

Pain is usually located in the suprapubic area or lower abdomen. Women describe the pain as sharp, cramping, or gripping or as a steady dull ache; pain may radiate to the lower back or upper thighs.

Primary Dysmenorrhea

Primary dysmenorrhea, a condition associated with abnormally increased uterine activity, is due to myometrial contractions induced by prostaglandins in the second half of the menstrual cycle. During the luteal phase and subsequent menstrual flow, prostaglandin $F_2\alpha$ ($PGF_2\alpha$) is secreted. The uterine muscle of both normal and dysmenorrheic women is sensitive to prostaglandins; however, the amount of prostaglandin produced is the major differentiating factor. Excessive release of $PGF_2\alpha$ increases the amplitude and frequency of uterine contractions and causes vasospasm of the uterine arterioles, resulting in ischemia and cyclic lower abdominal cramps. Systemic responses to $PGF_2\alpha$ include backache, weakness, sweating, gastrointestinal symptoms (anorexia, nausea, vomiting, and diarrhea), and central nervous system symptoms (dizziness, syncope, headache, and poor concentration). Pain begins at the onset of menstrual flow and lasts from 8 to 48 hours (Lentz, 2007b).

Primary dysmenorrhea is not caused by underlying pathology; rather it is the occurrence of a physiologic alteration in some women. Primary dysmenorrhea usually appears within 6 to 12 months after menarche when ovulation is established. Anovulatory bleeding, common in the few months or years after menarche, is painless. Because both estrogen and progesterone are necessary for primary dysmenorrhea to occur, it is experienced only with ovulatory cycles. This problem is most common in women in their late teens and early 20s; the incidence declines with age. Psychogenic factors may influence symptoms, but symptoms are definitely related to ovulation and do not occur when ovulation is suppressed.

Management. Management of primary dysmenorrhea depends on the severity of the problem and an individual woman's response to various treatments. Important components of nursing care are information and support. Because menstruation is so closely linked to reproduction and sexuality, menstrual problems such as dysmenorrhea can have a negative influence on sexuality and self-worth. Nurses can correct myths and misinformation about menstruation and dysmenorrhea by providing facts about what is normal. Nurses must support their clients' feelings of positive sexuality and self-worth.

Often more than one alternative for alleviating menstrual discomfort and dysmenorrhea can be offered. Women can then try options and decide which ones work best for them. Heat (heating pad or hot bath) minimizes cramping by increasing vasodilation and muscle relaxation and minimizing uterine ischemia. Massaging the lower back can reduce pain by relaxing paravertebral muscles and increasing pelvic blood supply. Soft rhythmic rubbing of the abdomen (effleurage) may be useful because it provides distraction and an alternative focal point. Biofeedback, transcutaneous electrical nerve stimulation (TENS), progressive relaxation, Hatha yoga, acupuncture, and meditation are also used to decrease menstrual discomfort, although evidence is insufficient to determine their effectiveness (Lentz, 2007b).

Exercise has been found to help in relieving menstrual discomfort through increased vasodilation and subsequently decreased ischemia; release of endogenous opiates, specifically beta-endorphins; suppression of prostaglandins; and shunting of blood flow away from the viscera, resulting in less pelvic congestion. A specific exercise that nurses can suggest is pelvic rocking.

In addition to maintaining good nutrition at all times, specific dietary changes may be helpful in decreasing some of the systemic symptoms associated with dysmenorrhea. Decreased salt and refined sugar intake 7 to 10 days before expected menses may reduce fluid retention. Increasing water intake may serve as a natural diuretic. Including natural diuretics such as asparagus, cranberry juice, peaches, parsley, and watermelon in the diet may help reduce edema and related discomforts. Decreasing red meat intake also may help minimize dysmenorrheal symptoms.

CLINICAL REASONING

Relief for Menstrual Discomfort

Kelli, 20, has come to the student health clinic for a checkup. She reports that she has "really bad cramps" for the first 2 days of her period. She has been taking acetaminophen 1000 mg every 6 hours but says it does not help "a lot." She wants to know if there is anything else she can do for her pain. How should the nurse respond?

1. Evidence—Is there sufficient evidence to draw conclusions about what advice the nurse should give?
2. Assumptions—Describe underlying assumptions about the following issues:
   a. Etiology and symptoms of primary dysmenorrhea
   b. Cyclic perimenstrual pain and discomfort
   c. Self-help strategies (e.g., comfort measures, medications)
3. What implications and priorities for nursing care can be drawn at this time?
4. Does the evidence objectively support your conclusion?
5. Are there alternative perspectives to your conclusion?

Medications used to treat primary dysmenorrhea in women not desiring contraception include prostaglandin synthesis inhibitors, primarily nonsteroidal antiinflammatory drugs (NSAIDs) (Lentz, 2007b) (Table 6-1). NSAIDs are effective if begun 2 to 3 days before menses or with the sign of first bleeding; this regimen decreases the possibility of a woman taking these drugs early in pregnancy (Speroff & Fritz, 2005). All NSAIDs have potential gastrointestinal side effects, including nausea, vomiting, and indigestion. All women taking NSAIDs should be warned to report dark-colored stools, because this may be an indication of gastrointestinal bleeding.

! NURSING ALERT

If one NSAID is ineffective, a different one may often be effective. If the second drug is unsuccessful after a 6-month trial, combined oral contraceptive pills (OCPs) may be used. Women with a history of aspirin sensitivity or allergy should avoid all NSAIDs.

TABLE 6-1 NONSTEROIDAL ANTIINFLAMMATORY AGENTS USED TO TREAT DYSMENORRHEA

DRUG	BRAND NAME AND STATUS	RECOMMENDED DOSAGE (ORAL)*	COMMON SIDE EFFECTS†	COMMENTS	CONTRAINDICATIONS
Diclofenac	Cataflam Rx	50 mg tid or 100 mg initially, then 50 mg tid up to 150 mg/day	Nausea, diarrhea, constipation, abdominal distress, dyspepsia, heartburn, flatulence, dizziness, tinnitus, itching, rash	Enteric coated; immediate release	For all NSAIDs: Do not give if woman has hemophilia or bleeding ulcers; do not give if woman has had an allergic or anaphylactic reaction to aspirin or another NSAID; do not give if woman is taking anticoagulant medication
Ibuprofen	Motrin Rx Advil OTC, Nuprin OTC, Motrin IB OTC	400 mg q 6-8 hr 200 mg q 4-6 hr up to 1200 mg/day	See diclofenac	If GI upset occurs, take with food, milk, or antacids; avoid alcoholic beverages; do not take with aspirin; stop taking and call care provider if rash occurs	
Ketoprofen	Orudis Rx Orudis KT OTC, Actron OTC	25-50 mg q 6-8 hr up to 300 mg/day 12.5 mg q 6-8 hr up to 75 mg/day	See diclofenac	See ibuprofen	
Meclofenamate	Meclomen Rx	100 mg tid up to 300 mg	See diclofenac	See ibuprofen	
Mefenamic acid	Ponstel Rx	500 mg initially, then 250 mg q 6 hr up to 1000 mg/day	See diclofenac	Very potent and effective prostaglandin-synthesis inhibitor; antagonizes already formed prostaglandins; increased incidence of adverse GI side effects	
Naproxen	Naprosyn Rx	500 mg initially, then 250 mg q 6-8 hr up to 1250 mg/day	See diclofenac	See ibuprofen	
Naproxen sodium	Anaprox Rx Aleve OTC	550 mg initially, then 275 mg q 6-8 hr or 550 mg q 12 hr up to 1375 mg/day 440 mg initially, then 220 mg q 6-8 hr up to 660 mg/day	See diclofenac	See ibuprofen	
Celecoxib	Celebrex	400 mg initially, then 200 mg bid	See diclofenac	See ibuprofen	

*Dosages are current recommendations and should be verified before use. Recommended doses for over-the-counter preparations are generally less than recommendations for therapeutic doses. As-needed dosing is recommended by manufacturer; scheduled dosing may be more effective.

†Risk with all NSAIDs is gastrointestinal ulceration, possible bleeding, and prolonged bleeding time. Incidence of side effects is dose related. Reported incidence, 1% to 10%.

bid, Twice a day; *GI,* gastrointestinal; *NSAIDs,* nonsteroidal antiinflammatory drugs; *OTC,* over the counter; *q,* every; *Rx,* prescription; *tid,* three times a day.

Sources: Facts and Comparisons (2009). *Nonsteroidal antiinflammatory drugs.* Available at www.factsandcomparisons.com. Accessed February 15, 2010; Lentz, G. (2007b). Primary and secondary dysmenorrhea, premenstrual syndrome, and premenstrual dysphoric disorder: Etiology, diagnosis, and management. In V. Katz, G. Lentz, R. Lobo, & D. Gershenson (Eds.), *Comprehensive gynecology* (5th ed.). Philadelphia: Mosby; U.S. Department of Health and Human Services, U.S. Food and Drug Administration. (2008). *Medication guide for non-steroidal anti-inflammatory drugs (NSAIDs).* Available at www.fda.gov/CDER/drug/infopage/COX2/NSAIDmedguide.htm. Accessed February 15, 2010.

OCPs prevent ovulation and can decrease the amount of menstrual flow, which can decrease the amount of prostaglandin, thus decreasing dysmenorrhea. There is evidence that combined OCPs can effectively treat dysmenorrhea (Lentz, 2007b). OCPs may be used in place of NSAIDs if the woman wants oral contraception and has primary dysmenorrhea. OCPs have side effects, and women who do not need or want them for contraception may not wish to use them for dysmenorrhea. OCPs also may be contraindicated for some women (see Chapter 8 for a complete discussion of OCPs).

Over-the-counter (OTC) preparations that are indicated for primary dysmenorrhea include the same active ingredients (e.g., ibuprofen, naproxen sodium) as prescription preparations; however, the labeled recommended dose may be subtherapeutic. Preparations containing acetaminophen are less effective because acetaminophen does not have the antiprostaglandin properties of NSAIDs.

If dysmenorrhea is not relieved by one of the NSAIDs, further investigation into the cause of the symptoms is necessary. Conditions associated with dysmenorrhea include müllerian duct anomalies, endometriosis, and pelvic inflammatory disease.

Alternative and complementary therapies are increasingly popular and used in developed countries. Therapies such as acupuncture, acupressure, biofeedback, desensitization, hypnosis, massage, Reiki, relaxation exercises, and therapeutic touch have been used to treat pelvic pain (Dehlin & Schuiling, 2006; Taylor et al., 2008). Herbal preparations have long been used for management of menstrual problems including dysmenorrhea (Table 6-2). Herbal medicines may be valuable in treating dysmenorrhea; however, it is essential that women understand that these therapies are not without potential toxicity and may cause drug interactions. It is also important for women to know that research is limited about the effectiveness of use (Dehlin & Schuiling, 2006).

! NURSING ALERT

Nurses must routinely ask women about use of herbal and other alternative therapies, and document their use.

Secondary Dysmenorrhea

Secondary dysmenorrhea is acquired menstrual pain that develops later in life than primary dysmenorrhea, typically after age 25 years. This condition is associated with pelvic pathology, such as adenomyosis, endometriosis, pelvic inflammatory disease, endometrial polyps, or submucous or interstitial myomas (fibroids). Women with secondary dysmenorrhea often have other symptoms that may suggest an underlying cause. For example, heavy menstrual flow with dysmenorrhea suggests a diagnosis of leiomyomata, adenomyosis, or endometrial polyps. Pain associated with endometriosis often begins a few days before menses, but can be present at ovulation and continue through the first days of menses or start after menstrual flow has begun. In contrast to primary dysmenorrhea, the pain of secondary dysmenorrhea is often characterized by dull, lower abdominal aching radiating to the back or thighs. Often women experience feelings of bloating or pelvic fullness. In addition to a physical examination with a careful pelvic examination, diagnosis may be assisted by ultrasound examination, dilation and curettage, endometrial biopsy, or laparoscopy. Treatment is directed toward removal of the underlying pathology. Many of the measures described for pain relief of primary dysmenorrhea also are helpful for women with secondary dysmenorrhea.

Premenstrual Syndrome and Premenstrual Dysphoric Disorder

Approximately 30% to 80% of women experience mood or somatic symptoms (or both) that occur with their menstrual cycles (Lentz, 2007b). Establishing a universal definition of **premenstrual syndrome (PMS)** is difficult, given that so many symptoms have been associated with the condition, and at least two different syndromes have been recognized: PMS and **premenstrual dysphoric disorder (PMDD).**

PMS is a complex, poorly understood condition that includes one or more of a large number (more than 100) of physical and psychologic symptoms beginning in the luteal phase of the menstrual cycle, occurring to such a degree that lifestyle or work is affected, and followed by a symptom-free period. Symptoms include fluid retention (abdominal bloating, pelvic fullness, edema of the lower extremities, breast tenderness, and weight gain); behavioral or emotional changes (depression, crying spells, irritability, panic attacks, and impaired ability to concentrate); premenstrual cravings (sweets, salt, increased appetite, and food binges); and headache, fatigue, and backache.

TABLE 6-2 HERBAL THERAPIES FOR MENSTRUAL DISORDERS

SYMPTOMS OR INDICATIONS	HERBAL THERAPY*	ACTION
Menstrual cramping, dysmenorrhea	Black haw	Uterine antispasmodic
	Catnip	Uterine antispasmodic
	Dong quai	Uterotonic; antiinflammatory
	Ginger	Antiinflammatory
	Motherwort	Uterotonic
	Wild yam	Uterine antispasmodic
	Valerian	Uterine antispasmodic
Premenstrual discomfort, tension	Black cohosh root	Estrogen-like luteinizing hormone suppressant; binds to estrogen receptors
	Chamomile	Antispasmodic
Breast pain	Chaste tree fruit	Decreases prolactin levels
	Bugleweed	Antigonadotropic; decreases prolactin levels
Menorrhea, metrorrhagia	Lady's mantle	Uterotonic
	Raspberry	Uterotonic
	Shepherd's purse	Uterotonic

*Many women's herbs do not have rigorous scientific studies backing their use; most uses and properties of herbs have not been validated by the U.S. Food and Drug Administration.

Sources: Annie's Remedy. (2008). *Herbal remedies for dysmenorrhea.* Available at www.anniesremedy.com. Accessed March 1, 2010; Bascom, A. (2002). *Incorporating herbal medicine into clinical practice.* Philadelphia: F.A. Davis; Fugh-Berman, A., & Awang, D. (2001). Black cohosh. *Alternative Therapies in Women's Health, 39*(11), 81-85; Low Dog, T. (2001). Conventional and alternative treatments for endometriosis. *Alternative Therapies, 7*(6), 50-56; National Center for Complementary and Alternative Medicine. (2009). *Herbs at a glance.* Available at www.nccam.nih.gov. Accessed March 1, 2010; Stevinson, C., & Ernst, E. (2001). Complementary/alternative therapies for premenstrual syndrome: A systemic review of randomized controlled trials. *American Journal of Obstetrics and Gynecology, 185*(1), 227-235.

All age-groups are affected, with women in their 20s and 30s most frequently reporting symptoms. Ovarian function is necessary for the condition to occur because it does not occur before puberty, after menopause, or during pregnancy. The condition is not dependent on the presence of monthly menses: women who have had a hysterectomy without bilateral salpingo-oophorectomy (BSO) still can have cyclic symptoms.

PMDD is a more severe variant of PMS in which 3% to 8% of women have marked irritability, dysphoria, mood lability, anxiety, fatigue, appetite changes, and a sense of feeling overwhelmed (Lentz, 2007b). The most common symptoms are those associated with mood disturbances.

A diagnosis of PMS is made when the following criteria are met (American College of Obstetricians and Gynecologists [ACOG], 2000; AWHONN, 2003):

- Symptoms consistent with PMS occur in the luteal phase and resolve within a few days of menses onset.
- Symptom-free period occurs in the follicular phase.
- Symptoms are recurrent.
- Symptoms have a negative effect on some aspect of a woman's life.
- Other diagnoses that better explain the symptoms have been excluded.

For a diagnosis of PMDD, the following criteria must be met (American Psychiatric Association [APA], 2000):

- Five or more affective and physical symptoms are present in the week before menses and are absent in the follicular phase of the menstrual cycle.
- At least one of the symptoms is irritability, depressed mood, anxiety, or emotional lability.
- Symptoms interfere markedly with work or interpersonal relationships.
- Symptoms are not caused by an exacerbation of another condition or disorder.

These criteria must be confirmed by prospective daily ratings for at least two menstrual cycles.

The causes of PMS and PMDD are not known, but there is general agreement that they are distinct psychiatric and medical syndromes rather than an exacerbation of an underlying psychiatric disorder. They do not occur if there is no ovarian function. A number of biologic and neuroendocrine etiologies have been suggested; however, none have been conclusively substantiated as the causative factor. It is likely that biologic, psychosocial, and sociocultural factors contribute to PMS and PMDD (Lentz, 2007b; Taylor, Schuiling, & Sharp, 2006). Readers are encouraged to explore current feminist, medical, and social science literature for more information on PMS.

Management

There is little agreement on management. A careful, detailed history and daily log of symptoms and mood fluctuations spanning several cycles may give direction to a plan of management. Any changes that assist a woman with PMS to exert control over her life have a positive effect. For this reason, lifestyle changes are often effective in the treatment of PMS.

Education is an important component of the management of PMS. Nurses can advise women that self-help modalities often result in significant symptom improvement. Women have found a number of complementary and alternative therapies to be useful in managing the symptoms of PMS. Nurses can suggest that women:

- Not smoke and limit their consumption of refined sugar (less than 5 tablespoons/day), salt (less than 3 g/day), red meat (up to 3 ounces/day), alcohol (less than 1 ounce/day), and caffeinated beverages.
- Include whole grains, legumes, seeds, nuts, vegetables, fruits, and vegetable oils in their diet.
- Eat three small to moderate-sized meals and three small snacks a day that are rich in complex carbohydrates and fiber (Lentz, 2007b).
- Use natural diuretics (see section on dysmenorrhea management on p. 121) to help reduce fluid retention.

Nutritional supplements can assist in symptom relief. Calcium (1000 to 1200 mg daily), magnesium (300 to 400 mg daily), and vitamin B_6 (100 to 150 mg daily) have been shown to be moderately effective in relieving symptoms, to have few side effects, and to be safe. Daily supplements of evening primrose oil are reportedly useful in relieving breast symptoms with minimal side effects, but research reports are conflicting (Taylor et al., 2008). Other herbal therapies have long been used to treat PMS; see Table 6-2 for specific suggestions.

Regular exercise (aerobic exercise three or four times a week), especially in the luteal phase, is widely recommended for relief of PMS symptoms (Lentz, 2007b). A monthly program that varies in intensity and type of exercise according to PMS symptoms is best. Women who exercise regularly seem to have less premenstrual anxiety than do nonathletic women. Researchers believe aerobic exercise increases beta-endorphin levels to offset symptoms of depression and elevate mood.

Yoga, acupuncture, hypnosis, light therapy, chiropractic therapy, and massage therapy have all been reported to have a beneficial effect on PMS. Further research is needed for all of these suggested therapies.

Nurses can explain the relation between cyclic estrogen fluctuation and changes in serotonin levels, that serotonin is one of the brain chemicals that assist in coping with normal life stresses, and the ways in which the different management strategies recommended help maintain serotonin levels. Support groups or individual or couples counseling may be helpful. Stress reduction techniques also may assist with symptom management (Lentz, 2007b; Taylor et al., 2008).

If these strategies do not provide significant symptom relief in 1 to 2 months, medication is often begun. Many medications have been used in treatment of PMS, but no single medication alleviates all PMS symptoms. Medications often used in the treatment of PMS include diuretics, prostaglandin inhibitors (NSAIDs), progesterone, and OCPs. Selective serotonin reuptake inhibitors (SSRIs) such as fluoxetine (Prozac or Sarafem), sertraline (Zoloft), and paroxetine (Paxil CR) are approved by the U.S. Food and Drug Administration (FDA) as agents for PMS. Use of these medications results in a decrease in emotional premenstrual symptoms, especially depression (Lentz, 2007b). Common side effects are headaches, sleep disturbances, dizziness, weight gain, dry mouth, and decreased libido (see Nursing Care Plan: Premenstrual Syndrome).

NURSING CARE PLAN

Premenstrual Syndrome

NURSING DIAGNOSIS

Acute pain related to cyclic breast changes as evidenced by woman's report

Expected Outcome

Woman will report a decrease in the intensity of pain or discomfort after interventions.

Nursing Interventions/*Rationales*

- Assess timing and intensity of pain or discomfort *to validate relation to cyclic changes.*
- Counsel woman to take medications if prescribed *to minimize breast tenderness.*
- Suggest that woman wear a supportive bra *to minimize breast tenderness.*

NURSING DIAGNOSIS

Situational low self-esteem related to cyclic hormonal changes as evidenced by woman's verbal report

Expected Outcome

Woman will report increased number of feelings of self-worth.

Nursing Interventions/*Rationales*

- Provide therapeutic communication *to validate feelings of depression and mood swings.*
- Encourage woman to limit caffeine and eat small, frequent meals *to lessen irritability aggravated by caffeine and hypoglycemia.*
- Refer woman to support groups *to encourage the sharing of experiences, feelings, and self-help tips.*

NURSING DIAGNOSIS

Excess fluid volume related to cyclic hormonal influences as evidenced by weight gain before start of menstrual period

Expected Outcome

Woman will report no significant changes in body weight before start of menstrual period.

Nursing Interventions/*Rationales*

- Encourage woman to limit intake of salt and sodium-containing foods *to decrease fluid retention.*
- Counsel woman to take diuretics as prescribed *to facilitate fluid excretion.*
- Encourage consumption of natural diuretic foods *to encourage fluid excretion.*

NURSING DIAGNOSIS

Anxiety related to anticipation of cyclic pain

Expected Outcome

Woman will report a decrease in anxiety level.

Nursing Interventions/*Rationales*

- Teach woman to recognize anxiety *to prompt early preventive interventions.*
- Identify relaxation techniques *to decrease anxiety.*
- Encourage woman to attend support groups *to encourage expression of feelings and self-help interventions.*

Endometriosis

Endometriosis is characterized by the presence and growth of endometrial glands and stroma outside of the uterus. The tissue may be implanted on the ovaries; the anterior and posterior cul-de-sac; the broad, uterosacral, and round ligaments; the uterine tubes; the rectovaginal septum; the sigmoid colon; the appendix; the pelvic peritoneum; the cervix; and the inguinal area (Fig. 6-1). Endometrial lesions have been found in the vagina and on surgical scars, as well as on the vulva, the perineum, and the bladder, and sites far from the pelvic area such as the thoracic cavity, the gallbladder, and the heart. A chocolate cyst is a cystic area of endometriosis in the ovary. Old blood causes the dark coloring of the cyst's contents.

Endometrial tissue contains glands and stoma and responds to cyclic hormonal stimulation in the same way that the uterine endometrium does. During the proliferative and secretory phases of the cycle, the endometrial tissue grows. During or immediately after menstruation, the tissue bleeds, resulting in an inflammatory response with subsequent fibrosis and adhesion to adjacent organs.

Endometriosis is a common gynecologic problem, affecting from 6% to 10% of women of reproductive age (Lobo, 2007b). Although the condition usually develops in the third or fourth decade of life, endometriosis is being diagnosed more frequently in adolescents with disabling pelvic pain or abnormal vaginal bleeding (Templeman, 2009). The condition is found equally in Caucasian and African-American women, is slightly more prevalent in Asian women, and may have a familial tendency for development (Lobo). Endometriosis may worsen with repeated cycles, or it may remain asymptomatic and undiagnosed, eventually disappearing after menopause.

Several theories have been offered to account for the cause of endometriosis, yet the causes and pathologic features of this condition are poorly understood. One of the most widely accepted, long-debated theories is transtubal migration or retrograde menstruation. According to this theory, endometrial tissue is regurgitated or mechanically transported from the uterus during menstruation to the uterine tubes and into the peritoneal cavity, where it implants on the ovaries and other organs.

Symptoms vary among women, from nonexistent to incapacitating. Severity of symptoms can change over time and may be disproportionate to the extent of the disease. The major symptoms of endometriosis are pelvic pain, dysmenorrhea, dyspareunia (painful intercourse), abnormal menstrual bleeding, and infertility. Women also may experience chronic noncyclic pelvic pain, pelvic heaviness, or pain radiating to the thighs. Many women report bowel symptoms such as diarrhea, pain with defecation, and constipation caused by avoiding defecation because of the pain. Less common symptoms include abnormal bleeding (hypermenorrhea, menorrhagia, or premenstrual staining) and pain during exercise as a result of adhesions (Lobo, 2007b).

Women who have endometriosis can have fibromyalgia, chronic fatigue syndrome, endocrine disorders, and autoimmune disorders (Tietjen, Bushnell, Herial, Utley, White, & Hafeez, 2007).

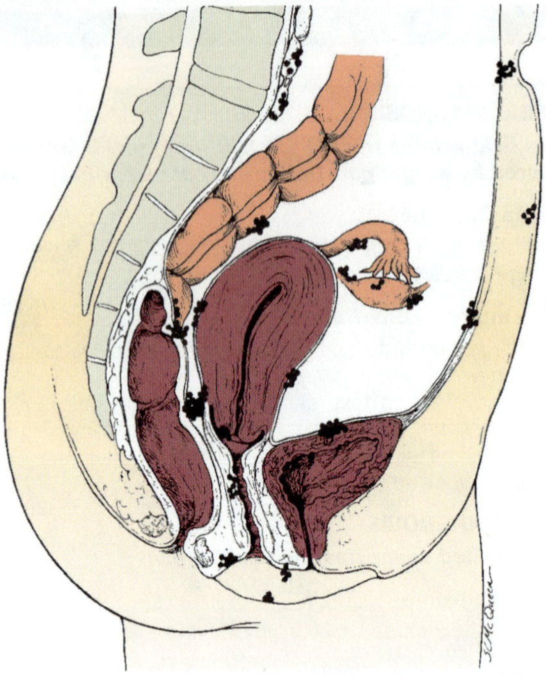

FIG. 6-1 Common sites of endometriosis. (Lobo, R. [2007b]. Endometriosis. In V. Katz, G. Lentz, R. Lobo, & D. Gershenson [Eds.], *Comprehensive gynecology* [5th ed.]. Philadelphia: Mosby.)

Impaired fertility may result from adhesions around the uterus that pull the uterus into a fixed, retroverted position. Adhesions around the uterine tubes may block the fimbriated ends or prevent the spontaneous movement that carries the ovum to the uterus.

Management

Treatment is based on the severity of symptoms and the goals of the woman or couple. Women without pain who do not want to become pregnant need no treatment. Women with mild pain who may desire a future pregnancy may use NSAIDs for pain relief. Women who have severe pain and can postpone pregnancy may be treated with continual OCPs that have a low estrogen-to-progestin ratio to shrink endometrial tissue. However, when this therapy stops, women often experience high rates of pain recurrence and other symptoms.

Hormonal antagonists that suppress ovulation and reduce endogenous estrogen production and subsequent endometrial lesion growth are used to treat mild to severe endometriosis in women who wish to become pregnant at a future time. GnRH agonist therapy (leuprolide, nafarelin [Synarel], goserelin acetate [Zoladex]) acts by suppressing pituitary gonadotropin secretion. FSH and LH stimulation to the ovary declines noticeably, and ovarian function decreases significantly. The hypoestrogenism results in hot flashes in almost all women. In addition, minor bone loss sometimes occurs, most of which is reversible within 12 to 18 months after the medication is stopped. Leuprolide (3.75-mg intramuscular injection given once a month) or nafarelin (200 mcg administered twice daily by nasal spray) are effective and well tolerated. Both medications reduce endometrial lesions and pelvic pain associated with endometriosis and have posttreatment pregnancy rates similar to that of danazol therapy (Lobo, 2007b). Common side effects of these drugs are similar to those of natural menopause—hot flashes and vaginal dryness. Some women report headaches and muscle aches.

Danazol (Danocrine), a mildly androgenic synthetic steroid, suppresses FSH and LH secretion, thus producing anovulation with resulting decreased secretion of estrogen and progesterone and regression of endometrial tissue. Bothersome side effects include masculinizing traits in the woman—weight gain, edema, decreased breast size, oily skin, hirsutism, and deepening of the voice—all of which often disappear when treatment is discontinued. Other side effects are amenorrhea, hot flashes, vaginal dryness, insomnia, and decreased libido. Some women report migraine headaches, dizziness, fatigue, and depression. In addition, some women experience decreases in bone density that are only partially reversible. Danazol should never be prescribed when pregnancy is suspected, and contraception should be used with it because ovulation may not be suppressed. Danazol can produce pseudohermaphroditism in female fetuses. The drug is contraindicated in women with liver disease and should be used with caution in women with cardiac and renal disease (Lobo, 2007b).

Administration of NSAIDs and continuous combined hormonal therapy (oral contraceptive pills, estrogen/progestin patch, estrogen/progestin vaginal ring) for menstrual suppression are the usual treatment of adolescents younger than the age of 16 who have endometriosis. GnRH agonists are not usually used because the resultant hypoestrogenic state can affect bone mineralization (ACOG Committee on Adolescent Health Care, 2005).

Surgical intervention is often needed for severe, acute, or incapacitating symptoms. A woman's age, desire for children, and location of the disease influence decisions regarding the extent and type of surgery. For women who do not want to preserve their ability to have children, the only definite cure is hysterectomy and BSO (total abdominal hysterectomy [TAH] with BSO). In women who are in their childbearing years and who want children if the disease does not prevent pregnancy, surgery or laser therapy is used to carefully remove as much endometrial tissue as possible to maintain reproductive function (Lobo, 2007b).

Short of TAH with BSO, endometriosis recurs in approximately 40% to 50% of women, regardless of the form of treatment. Therefore, for many women, endometriosis is a chronic disease with conditions such as chronic pain or infertility. Counseling and education are critical components of nursing care of women with endometriosis. Women need an honest discussion of treatment options with potential risks and benefits of each option reviewed. Because pelvic pain is a subjective, personal experience that can be frightening, support is important. Sexual dysfunction resulting from dyspareunia may be present and may necessitate referral for counseling. Some locations have support groups for women with endometriosis; Resolve (www.resolve.org), an organization for infertile couples, or the Endometriosis Association (www.ivf.com/endohtml.html) also may be helpful. The nursing care measures discussed in the section on dysmenorrhea are appropriate for managing chronic pelvic pain associated with endometriosis (see Nursing Care Plan: Endometriosis).

Alterations in Cyclic Bleeding

Women often experience changes in amount, duration, interval, or regularity of menstrual cycle bleeding. Commonly, women worry about menstruation that is infrequent or scanty, is excessive, or occurs between periods.

NURSING CARE PLAN

Endometriosis

NURSING DIAGNOSIS

Acute pain related to menstruation secondary to endometriosis

Expected Outcome

Woman will verbalize a decrease in intensity and frequency of pain during each menstrual cycle.

Nursing Interventions/*Rationales*

- Assess location, type, and duration of pain and history of discomfort *to determine severity of dysmenorrhea.*
- Administer analgesics *to assist with pain relief.*
- Administer hormone-altering medications if ordered *to suppress ovulation.*
- Provide nonpharmacologic methods such as heat *to increase blood flow to the pelvic region.*

NURSING DIAGNOSIS

Deficient knowledge related to unfamiliarity with treatment, as evidenced by woman's statements

Expected Outcome

Woman will verbalize correct understanding of the use of self-care methods and prescribed therapies.

Nursing Interventions/*Rationales*

- Assess woman's current understanding of the disorder and related therapies *to validate the accuracy of knowledge base.*
- Give information to woman regarding the disorder and treatment regimen *to empower the client to become a partner in her own care.*

NURSING DIAGNOSIS

Situational low self-esteem related to infertility as evidenced by woman's statements of decreased self-worth

Expected Outcome

Woman will verbalize positive feelings of self-worth.

Nursing Interventions/*Rationales*

- Provide therapeutic communication *to validate feelings and provide support.*
- Refer to support group *to enhance feelings of self-worth through group communication.*

NURSING DIAGNOSIS

Anxiety related to possible invasive surgical procedure as evidenced by woman's verbal report

Expected Outcome

Woman will report a decreased number of anxious feelings.

Nursing Interventions/*Rationales*

- Provide opportunity to discuss feelings *to identify source of anxiety.*
- Reinforce information provided *to keep expectations realistic and dispel myths or inaccuracies.*
- Provide emotional support *to encourage verbalization of feelings.*

NURSING DIAGNOSIS

Risk for injury related to disease progression

Expected Outcome

Woman will report any changes in health status to health care provider.

Nursing Interventions/*Rationales*

- Teach woman to report any changes in health status *to initiate prompt treatment.*
- Review side effects of medications *to recognize possible causes for changes in health status.*
- Encourage ongoing communication with health care provider *to promote trust and comfort.*

Oligomenorrhea/Hypomenorrhea

The term **oligomenorrhea** often is used to describe decreased menstruation, either in amount, time, or both. However, oligomenorrhea more correctly refers to infrequent menstrual periods characterized by intervals of 40 to 45 days or longer, and **hypomenorrhea** to scanty bleeding at normal intervals. The causes of oligomenorrhea are often abnormalities of hypothalamic, pituitary, or ovarian function. Oligomenorrhea also can be physiologic, or part of a woman's normal pattern for the first few years after menarche or for several years before menopause.

Treatment is aimed at reversing the underlying cause, if possible. Hormonal therapy using progestins, with or without estrogens, also may be used to prevent complications of unopposed estrogen production (endometrial hyperplasia or carcinoma) or of absent estrogen (vaginal dryness, hot flashes or flushes, or osteoporosis).

Women with menstruation characterized by prolonged intervals between cycles need education and counseling. The cause of the condition and the rationale for a specific treatment should be discussed, as should advantages and disadvantages of hormonal therapy. If a woman chooses medical intervention, she should be provided with written instructions, taught how to take the medications, and made aware of side effects of any medications. Teaching and counseling should emphasize the importance of the woman keeping careful records of her vaginal bleeding.

One of the most common causes of scanty menstrual flow is OCPs. If a woman is considering OCPs for contraception, it is important to explain in advance that the use of OCPs can decrease menstrual flow by as much as two thirds. This effect is caused by the continuous action of the progestin component, which produces a decidualized endometrium with atrophic glands.

Hypomenorrhea also may be caused by structural abnormalities of the endometrium or the uterus that result in partial destruction of the endometrium. These conditions include Asherman syndrome, in which adhesions resulting from curettage or infection obliterate the endometrial cavity, and congenital partial obstruction of the vagina.

Metrorrhagia

Metrorrhagia, or intermenstrual bleeding, refers to any episode of bleeding, whether spotting, menses, or hemorrhage, that occurs at a time other than the normal menses. *Mittlestaining,* a small amount of bleeding or spotting that occurs at the time of ovulation (14 days before onset of the next menses), is considered normal. The cause of mittlestaining is not known;

EVIDENCE-BASED PRACTICE

Pat Gingrich

Heavy Menstrual Bleeding: Treatments to Improve Quality of Life

ASK THE QUESTION

What treatments are available for women experiencing heavy menstrual bleeding? Is surgery or medicine the better treatment?

SEARCH FOR EVIDENCE

Search Strategies

Professional organization guidelines, meta-analyses, systematic reviews, randomized controlled trials, nonrandomized prospective studies, retrospective studies, and systematic reviews of qualitative research since 2009.

Databases Searched

CINAHL, Cochrane, Medline, National Guideline Clearinghouse, TRIPP Database, and NICE.

CRITICALLY ANALYZE THE DATA

Heavy menstrual bleeding (HMB) is usually defined as anything more than 80 ml lost. A systematic review of qualitative research reported that women experiencing HMB find it to be physically, socially, and emotionally challenging to their quality of life (Garside, Britten & Stein, 2008). The authors reported that uncertainty, embarrassment, feeling that concerns were minimized, difficulty with menstrual etiquette, and fears of anemia and cancer can cause women to experience stress and anxiety.

The range of treatments for HMB includes medication and surgical interventions. Danazol, a modified testosterone, has anti-estrogen and anti-progesterone properties. A meta-analysis of research control trials revealed that danazol was more effective than progesterone, non-steroidal anti-inflammatory medication (NSAIDs), oral contraceptives (Beaumont et al., 2007) or tranexamic acid (Lethaby, Irvine & Cameron, 2008). However, danazol may produce intolerable side effects of masculinization, menopause-like symptoms, weight gain or acne. The recommendation statement of the National Institute for Clinical Excellence (NICE) (2007) lists the first line drug as the levonorgestrel-releasing intrauterine system (an IUD that releases progesterone, preventing endometrial proliferation). Their second line treatments include tranexamic acid, NSAIDs, and combined oral contraceptives. Third line includes oral and injected progesterones.

Surgically, HMB can be treated according to the severity of the symptoms and the woman's desire to preserve fertility. Hysterectomy is successful at stopping the bleeding, but carries the most surgical risk. Endometrial ablation can use several mechanical and thermal techniques to destroy the uterine lining. This more conservative surgery can be done on an outpatient basis, and has less risk of post-operative complications. Kaunitz, Meredith, Inki, Kubba, and Sanchez-Ramos (2009) reported that endometrial ablation had similar therapeutic effects as the levonorgestrel-releasing intrauterine system in managing heavy bleeding. Both hysterectomy and endometrial ablation eliminate future pregnancies. If the bleeding is caused by a fibroid and the woman desires future pregnancies, the blood supply to the fibroid can be blocked using a uterine artery embolization, or the tumor can be removed using a myomectomy. The NICE recommendation guidelines (2007) state that dilation and curettage for HMB is not recommended.

IMPLICATIONS FOR PRACTICE

Women experiencing HMB may delay getting medical care, due to embarrassment or uncertainty. Nurses should regularly ask their female clients about their menstrual cycle amount and duration, including clots. Evaluate for anemia. Concerns about bleeding should trigger a detailed focused menstrual history and pregnancy history, including desire for future pregnancies. The nurse can explain normal parameters for duration and flow. Clots are usually an indicator of heavy flow. Once identified, nurses should ask women experiencing HMB about their concerns and fears. As the health care provider and woman work through the various options, the woman and her partner may need a sounding board and resource for answers to questions. In the event of loss of fertility, counseling and referral to a group such as Resolve (www.resolve.org) may provide support.

References

Beaumont, H., Augood, C., Duckitt, K., & Lethaby, A. (2007). Danazol for heavy menstrual bleeding. *The Cochrane Database of Systematic Reviews 2010, 5*, Chichester, UK: John Wiley & Sons.

Garside, R., Britten, N., & Stein, K. (2008). The experience of heavy menstrual bleeding: A systematic review and meta-ethnography of qualitative studies. *Journal of Advanced Nursing, 63*(6), 550–562.

Kaunitz, A., Meredith, S., Inki, P., Kubba, A., & Sanchez-Ramos, L. (2009). Levonorgestrel-releasing intrauterine system and endometrial ablation in heavy menstrual bleeding: A systematic review and meta-analysis. *Obstetrics and Gynecology, 113*(5), 1104–1116.

Lethaby, A., Irvine, G., & Cameron, I. (2008). Cyclical progesterones for heavy menstrual bleeding. *The Cochrane Database of Systematic Reviews 2010, 5*, Chichester, UK: John Wiley & Sons.

National Institute for Health and Clinical Excellence. (2007). *Heavy menstrual bleeding. NICE Clinical Guideline, 44*, London, 2008, NICE. Available at http://www.nice.org.uk/Guidance/CG44, Accessed May 28, 2010.

however, its common occurrence can be documented by its repetition in the menstrual cycle.

Women taking OCPs may have midcycle bleeding or spotting. (See Chapter 8 for a discussion of the side effects of OCPs.) If the OCP does not maintain a sufficiently hypoplastic endometrium, the endometrium will begin to shed, usually in small amounts at a time, a process termed *breakthrough bleeding*. Breakthrough bleeding is most common in the first three cycles of OCPs. The reduced potency of OCPs (resulting in increased safety) has decreased the amount of available hormones, making it more important that blood levels be kept constant. Taking the pill at exactly the same time each day may alleviate the woman's problem. If the spotting continues, a different formulation of the OCP that increases either the estrogen or progestin component of the pill can be tried.

Progestin-only contraceptive methods (oral and injectable) also may cause midcycle bleeding, especially in the first several cycles. Women should be advised of this and counseled to report continuation of breakthrough bleeding after the first three to six cycles to their health care provider.

Women with an intrauterine device (IUD) may have spotting between their periods and possibly heavier menstrual flow.

The causes of intermenstrual bleeding are varied (Table 6-3). It is important that the nurse always consider the possibility that any woman who has not undergone menopause and who seeks care for intermenstrual bleeding is or recently has been pregnant.

Treatment of intermenstrual bleeding depends on the cause and may include reassurance and education concerning mittlestaining, observation of three menstrual cycles for suspected functional ovarian cyst, adjustment of an OCP, removal of

TABLE 6-3 **CAUSES OF INTERMENSTRUAL BLEEDING**

REPRODUCTIVE DISORDER	PREGNANCY PROBLEMS	INFECTIONS
Functional ovarian cyst	Pregnancy: implantation	Endometritis
Cervical erosion infection	Miscarriage	Sexually transmitted infections
Leiomyoma	Ectopic pregnancy	
Polyps, uterine or endocervical	Molar pregnancy	
Trauma	Retained placenta, miscarriage or induced abortion	
Foreign body	Retained placenta, birth	
Malignancy of reproductive tract		

foreign bodies, and treatment for vaginal infections. More complex treatment may consist of removal of polyps; evaluation and treatment of an abnormal Papanicolaou (Pap) test, including colposcopy, biopsy, cautery, cryosurgery, or conization; and surgery, chemotherapy, or radiation treatment for malignancy. Important nursing roles include reassurance, counseling, education, and support.

Menorrhagia

Menorrhagia (hypermenorrhea) is defined as excessive menstrual bleeding, in either duration or amount. The causes of heavy menstrual bleeding are many, including hormonal disturbances, systemic disease, benign and malignant neoplasms, infection, and contraception (IUDs). A single episode of heavy bleeding may occur, or a woman may have regular flooding as a pattern in which she changes tampons or pads every few hours for several days.

> **! NURSING ALERT**
>
> If the woman herself considers the amount or duration of bleeding to be excessive, the problem should be investigated.

Hemoglobin and hematocrit provide objective indicators to actual blood loss and should always be assessed.

A single episode of heavy bleeding may signal an early pregnancy loss. This type of bleeding is often thought to be a period that is heavier than usual, perhaps delayed, and is associated with abdominal pain or pelvic discomfort. When early pregnancy loss is suspected, a hematocrit and serum β-hCG pregnancy test should be done.

Infectious and inflammatory processes such as acute or chronic endometritis and salpingitis may cause heavy menstrual bleeding. Although rare, systemic diseases of nonreproductive origin such as blood dyscrasias, hypothyroidism, and lupus erythematosus also can cause hypermenorrhea. In obese women anovulation caused by increased peripheral conversion of androstenedione to estrogen may develop and manifest as menorrhagia. Medications also may cause abnormal bleeding. Chemotherapy, anticoagulants, neuroleptics, and steroid hormone therapy all have been associated with excessive flow.

Uterine *leiomyomata* (fibroids or myomas) are a common cause of menorrhagia. Fibroids are benign tumors of the smooth muscle of the uterus, the etiology of which is unknown. Fibroids are estrogen sensitive and commonly develop during the reproductive years and shrink after menopause. Other uterine growths ranging from endometrial polyps to adenocarcinoma and endometrial cancer are other common causes of heavy menstrual bleeding, as well as of intermenstrual bleeding.

Treatment for menorrhagia depends on the cause of the bleeding. If the bleeding is related to the contraceptive method, the nurse provides factual information and reassurance and discusses other contraceptive options. If bleeding is related to the presence of fibroids, the degree of disability and discomfort associated with the fibroids and the woman's plans for childbearing will influence treatment decisions. Treatment options include medical and surgical management. Most fibroids can be monitored by frequent examinations to judge growth, if any, and correction of anemia, if present. Women with menorrhagia should be warned not to use aspirin because of its tendency to increase bleeding. Medical treatment is directed toward temporarily reducing symptoms, shrinking the myoma, and reducing its blood supply (Katz, 2007). This reduction is often accomplished with the use of a GnRH agonist. If the woman wishes to retain childbearing potential, a myomectomy may be done. Myomectomy, or removal of the tumors only, is particularly difficult if multiple myomas must be removed. If the woman does not want to preserve her childbearing function, or if she has severe symptoms (severe anemia, severe pain, considerable disruption of lifestyle), hysterectomy or endometrial ablation (laser surgery or electrocoagulation) may be done (see Chapter 11). Uterine artery embolization, based on the assumption that control of arterial blood flow to the fibroid will control symptoms, has been reported to result in reduced menorrhagia, less dysmenorrhea, and reduced pelvic pressure and urinary symptoms. This method of treatment is used for women who have completed their childbearing since there is a risk for loss of fertility (see Chapter 11).

Dysfunctional Uterine Bleeding

Abnormal uterine bleeding (AUB) is any form of uterine bleeding that is irregular in amount, duration, or timing and not related to regular menstrual bleeding. Box 6-1 lists possible causes of AUB. Although often used interchangeably, the terms AUB and dysfunctional uterine bleeding (DUB) are not synonymous. **Dysfunctional uterine bleeding** is a subset of AUB defined as "excessive uterine bleeding with no demonstrable organic cause, genital or extragenital" (Lobo, 2007*a*). DUB is most frequently caused by anovulation. When there is no surge of LH, or if insufficient progesterone is produced by the corpus luteum to support the endometrium, it will begin to involute and shed. This process most often occurs at the extremes of a woman's reproductive years—when the menstrual cycle is just becoming established at menarche or when it draws to a close at menopause. DUB also can be found with any condition that gives rise to chronic anovulation associated with continuous estrogen production. Such conditions include obesity, hyperthyroidism and hypothyroidism, polycystic ovary syndrome, and any of the endocrine conditions discussed in the sections on amenorrhea and oligomenorrhea. A diagnosis of DUB is made only after all other causes of abnormal menstrual bleeding have been ruled out (Lentz, 2007*a*).

BOX 6-1 POSSIBLE CAUSES OF ABNORMAL UTERINE BLEEDING

ANOVULATION
- Hypothalamic dysfunction
- Polycystic ovary syndrome

PREGNANCY-RELATED CONDITIONS
- Threatened or spontaneous miscarriage
- Retained products of conception after elective abortion
- Ectopic pregnancy

LOWER REPRODUCTIVE TRACT INFECTIONS
- Chlamydial cervicitis
- Pelvic inflammatory disease

NEOPLASMS
- Endometrial hyperplasia
- Cancer of cervix and endometrium
- Endometrial polyps
- Hormonally active tumors (rare)
- Leiomyomata
- Vaginal tumors (rare)

TRAUMA
- Genital injury (accidental, coital trauma, sexual abuse)
- Foreign body
- Primary coagulation disorders

SYSTEMIC DISEASES
- Diabetes mellitus
- Thyroid dysfunction (hypothyroidism, hyperthyroidism)
- Severe organ disease (renal or liver failure)

IATROGENIC CAUSES
- Exogenous hormone use (oral contraceptives, menopausal hormone therapy)
- Medications with estrogenic activity
- Herbal preparation (ginseng)

Sources: American College of Nurse-Midwives (ACNM). (2002). Abnormal and dysfunctional uterine bleeding. ACNM Clinical Bulletin No. 6. *Journal of Midwifery and Women's Health, 47*(3), 207-213; Katz, V. (2007). Benign gynecologic lesions: Vulva, vagina, cervix, uterus, oviducts and ovary. In V. Katz, G. Lentz, R. Lobo, & D. Gershenson (Eds.), *Comprehensive gynecology* (5th ed.). Philadelphia: Mosby.

When uterine bleeding is profuse and a woman's hemoglobin level is less than 8 g/dl (hematocrit of 23% or 24%), the woman may be hospitalized and given conjugated estrogens (e.g., Premarin), 25 mg intravenously. The dose may be repeated until bleeding stops or slows significantly (usually within 1 to 5 hours) (Behera & Price, 2009). If the bleeding has not stopped in 12 to 24 hours, dilation and curettage (D&C) may be done to control severe bleeding and hemorrhage. An endometrial biopsy may be collected at the same time to evaluate endometrial tissue or rule out endometrial cancer. After this treatment, oral conjugated estrogen, 2.5 mg, is given daily followed by the addition of progesterone (e.g., medroxyprogesterone [Provera], 10 mg by mouth), given in the final 10 days of therapy to initiate withdrawal bleeding. Alternatively, a combined OCP is given for 21 days after intravenous therapy. Once the acute phase has passed, the woman is maintained on cyclic low-dose OCPs for 3 to 6 months. Such long-term treatment will help prevent recurrence of the pattern of dysfunctional uterine bleeding and hemorrhage. If the woman wants contraception, she should continue to take OCPs. If the woman has no need for contraception, the treatment may be stopped to assess her bleeding pattern. If menstruation does not resume, a progestin regimen (e.g., medroxyprogesterone, 10 mg/day for 10 days before the expected date of her menstrual period) may be prescribed after ruling out pregnancy. This is done to prevent persistent anovulation with chronic unopposed endogenous estrogen hyperstimulation of the endometrium, which can result in eventual atypical tissue changes (Lobo, 2007a).

If the recurrent, heavy bleeding is not controlled by hormonal therapy or D&C, ablation of the endometrium through laser treatment may be performed. Nursing roles include counseling and educating women about their options as needed and referring women to the appropriate specialists and health care services.

CARE MANAGEMENT

Medical and nursing management have been discussed with each menstrual problem. Specific aspects of the nursing process are listed in the Nursing Process box: Menstrual Disorders.

MENOPAUSE

With the increasing life span of American women, most women can expect to live one third of their lives after their reproductive years. As women age many experience transitions that present challenges and require adaptation such as changing health, work, or marital status. Nowhere is this more true than with the changes associated with menopause. In the United States, most women have menopause during their late 40s and early 50s, with the median age being 51 to 52 years (Lobo, 2007*c*). The average age for the onset of the perimenopausal transition is 46 years; 95% of women experience the onset between ages 39 and 51. The average duration of the perimenopause period is 4 to 5 years, with 95% of women postmenopausal by age 58 (Lobo). Cigarette smoking and a history of short intermenstrual intervals seem to decrease the age at onset of menopause. African-American and Hispanic women in the United States experience menopause earlier than Caucasian women. However, heredity is the major determinant of age at menopause; genetics may explain most of the variation in menopause age (Lobo).

Perimenopause is the period that encompasses the transition from normal ovulatory cycles to cessation of menses and is marked by irregular menstrual cycles. Another term used to signal the period when a woman moves from the reproductive stage of life through the perimenopausal transition and menopause to the postmenopausal years is the **climacteric. Menopause** refers to the complete cessation of menses and is a single physiologic event said to occur when women have not had menstrual flow or spotting for 1 year, and it can be identified only in retrospect. **Surgical menopause** occurs with hysterectomy and bilateral oophorectomy. **Postmenopause** is the time after menopause.

Although all women have similar hormonal changes with menopause, the experience of each woman is influenced by her age, cultural background, health, type of menopause (spontaneous or surgical), childbearing desires, and relationships. Women may view menopause as a major change in their lives—either positive, such as freedom from troublesome dysmenorrhea or the need for contraception, or negative, such as feeling "old" or losing childbearing possibilities.

NURSING PROCESS

Menstrual Disorders

ASSESSMENT

- Take a thorough menstrual, obstetric, sexual, and contraceptive history.
- Explore the woman's perceptions of her condition, cultural or ethnic influences, lifestyle, and patterns of coping.
- Evaluate the amount of pain or bleeding experienced and its effect on daily activities.
- Note any home remedies and prescriptions to relieve discomfort. A symptom diary, in which the woman records emotions, behaviors, physical symptoms, diet, and exercise and rest patterns, is a useful diagnostic tool.

NURSING DIAGNOSES

Nursing diagnoses include:

Risk for Ineffective Individual Coping **related to:**

- insufficient knowledge of the cause of the disorder
- emotional and physiologic effects of the disorder

Deficient Knowledge **related to:**

- self-management
- available therapy for the disorder

Risk for Disturbed Body Image **related to:**

- menstrual disorder
- sexual dysfunction

Risk for Situational Low Self-Esteem **related to:**

- others' perception of her discomfort
- inability to conceive

Acute or Chronic Pain **related to:**

- menstrual disorder

EXPECTED OUTCOMES OF CARE

Expected outcomes for the woman are that she will:

- Verbalize understanding of reproductive anatomy, cause of her disorder, medication regimen, and diary use.
- Verbalize understanding and accept the emotional and physical responses to her menstrual cycle.
- Develop personal goals that benefit her emotionally and physically.
- Choose appropriate therapeutic measures for her menstrual problems.
- Adapt successfully to the condition, if cure is not possible.

PLAN OF CARE AND INTERVENTIONS

- Accept the woman's symptoms as valid.
- Correlate data from the daily diary of emotional status, subjective feelings, and physical state with physiologic changes.
- Encourage the woman to express her feelings about her symptoms.
- Provide information about therapeutic options (pharmacologic and nonpharmacologic) so that the woman (couple) makes choices considered best for her (them).
- Provide information about local support groups.

EVALUATION

Care has been effective when the woman reports improvement in the quality of her life, skill in self-management, and a positive self-concept and body image.

Physiologic Characteristics

Knowledge of the normal changes that occur during the perimenopause is essential to the assessment of menopausal experiences and problems. Natural menopause is a gradual process with progressive increases in anovulatory cycles and eventual cessation of menses. In the 2 to 8 years preceding menopause, subtle hormonal changes eventually lead to altered menstrual function and later to amenorrhea. When women are in their 40s, anovulation occurs more often, menstrual cycles increase in length, and ovarian follicles become less sensitive to hormonal stimulation from FSH and LH. Because of these changes, a follicle is stimulated to the point that an ovum grows to maturity and is released in some months, whereas in other months, no ovulation takes place. Without ovulation and release of an ovum, progesterone is not produced by the corpus luteum. The lining continues to grow until it lacks a sufficient blood supply, at which point it will bleed. During this time a woman's cycle will become more irregular. She may skip or miss periods; have shorter or lighter periods or longer, heavier periods; and have clotting. FSH levels become elevated, reflecting an attempt to stimulate a follicle to produce estrogen.

Physical Changes During the Perimenopausal Period

Bleeding

During the perimenopausal years, women may have longer menstrual periods that differ in the type of bleeding. They may have 2 to 3 days of spotting followed by 1 to 2 days of heavy bleeding, or they may have regular menses followed by 2 to 3 days of spotting. Such symptoms are characteristic of degenerating corpus luteum function. After menopause women continue to have small amounts of circulating estrogen. Although the ovaries do not produce estrogen, androgens (androstenedione and testosterone) are produced for some time after menopause. Androgens produced by the adrenal glands are converted to estrone, a form of estrogen, in the liver and fat cells. With advanced age the ovaries stop producing androstenedione, which further limits the amount of estrone in the body. Obese women are more likely to have dysfunctional uterine bleeding and endometrial hyperplasia because women with more body fat have higher circulating levels of estrone. This occurs because the estrogen that is stored in the fat cells of the body is converted into a form of estrogen (estrone) that is available to the estrogen receptors within the endometrium.

Genital Changes

The vagina and urethra are estrogen-sensitive tissues, and low levels of estrogen can cause atrophy of both. Age-related vaginal changes not affected by estrogen also occur. Through both processes the vaginal membranes thin, hold less moisture, and lubricate more slowly. However, not all women have symptoms of genital atrophy. Women who are sexually active have less vaginal atrophy and fewer problems related to intercourse. Thin women are more likely to have more symptoms related to reduced estrogen levels such as vaginal dryness because of lack of adipose tissue and thus stored estrogen. Additionally, vaginal pH increases, lactobacillus growth can be depressed, and other bacteria tend to multiply. This combination of factors can lead to vaginitis.

Dyspareunia (painful intercourse) can occur because the vagina becomes smaller, the vaginal walls become thinner and drier, and lubrication during sexual stimulation takes longer. Intercourse becomes painful and may result in postcoital bleeding. Some women may decide to forgo intercourse altogether.

In some women the shrinking of the uterus, the vulva, and the distal portion of the urethra associated with aging leads to disturbing symptoms, including urinary frequency, dysuria, uterine prolapse, and stress incontinence. Vaginal relaxation with cystocele, rectocele, and uterine prolapse is not caused by reduced estrogen levels but may be a delayed result of childbearing or other cause of weakness of pelvic support structures. Urinary frequency sometimes occurs after menopause because the distal portion of the urethra, which has the same embryologic origin as the reproductive organs, shortens and shrinks. Irritants have easier access to the urinary tract with its shorter urethra and may cause frequency and urinary tract infections.

Urinary incontinence and uterine displacement are two other common age-related rather than menopause-related findings in the postmenopausal period. These conditions are discussed in Chapter 11.

Vasomotor Instability

During the past three decades investigators have devoted significant attention to identifying ovarian, hypothalamic, and pituitary hormonal mechanisms that produce symptoms related to menopause. Two symptoms appear to increase in incidence as women progress through menopause: hot flashes and night sweats. Many of the other changes commonly associated with menopause, such as decrease in size of genital structures, skin changes, and changes in breast size, are more correctly attributed to aging.

Vasomotor instability in the form of hot flashes or flushes is a result of fluctuating estrogen levels and is the most common disturbance of the perimenopausal years, occurring in up to 75% of women having natural menopause and 90% of women who have a surgical menopause. In the United States, Hispanic and African-American women report a higher incidence of these symptoms than Caucasian women; Asian women have the lowest incidence (Lobo, 2007c). Vasomotor instability occurs most frequently in the first 2 postmenopausal years; the number of episodes decreases over time. However, some women have hot flashes before menopause and continue to have them for 10 or more years afterward. During this time women experience changeable vasodilation and vasoconstriction as a **hot flush** (visible red flush of skin and perspiration) or **hot flash** (sudden warm sensation in neck, head, and chest) and night sweats. These disturbances vary widely in severity, and only about 40% of women seek health care for them (Nedrow, Miller, Walker, Nygren, Huffman, & Nelson, 2006). For some women hot flashes may be an infrequent, possibly pleasant, sensation of warmth; for others, they may be an intensely unpleasant sensation of heat or warmth that may occur 20 to 50 times a day, create intense anxiety, and significantly decrease quality of life. Several factors can precipitate or aggravate an episode, including crowded or warm rooms, alcohol, hot drinks, spicy foods, proximity to a heat source, and stress.

Night sweats, characterized by profuse perspiration and heat radiating from the body during the night, are another form of vasomotor instability experienced by many women. Sleep may be interrupted nightly because nightclothes and bed linens may be soaked. Women may find that they are not able to go back to sleep. Sleep deprivation is a primary complaint of women experiencing hot flashes (Lobo, 2007c). Other problems that may be associated with perimenopausal fluctuations of vasoconstriction or vascular spasms include dizziness, numbness and tingling in fingers and toes, and headaches.

Mood and Behavioral Responses

The tendency to associate hormonal changes with psychologic symptoms in midlife that has been prevalent in medical literature for decades and continues today was fueled by a belief that postmenopausal women have "estrogen deficiency." Contrary to this common belief, there is no concrete evidence that menopause has a deleterious effect on mental health of midlife women. Reviews of epidemiologic studies on menopause and depression found no causal association between menopause and depression (Lobo, 2007c). Women with hot flashes and night sweats do report insomnia, fatigue from loss of sleep, and depressed mood. Women complain of feeling more emotionally labile, nervous, or agitated, with less control of their emotions. However, the interaction of psychologic, biologic, and sociocultural factors is so complex that it is difficult to determine whether a woman's reported mood shifts are the result of hormonal changes, normal aging, or cultural conditioning. Most likely a woman's psychologic makeup, cultural background, intercurrent stresses, and changing life roles and circumstances are more important than estrogen levels. Dealing with teenage children; having teenagers leave home; helping aging parents; becoming widowed or divorced; the onset of a major illness or disability (even death) in a spouse, relative, or friend; grieving for friends and family who are ill or dying; retirement; and financial insecurity are among the many stresses of women in their 40s and 50s.

Cultural messages also influence a woman's perception of menopause. Women's experiences with menopause are not universal and vary among cultural groups. Most North American women do not believe that menopause interferes with their quality of life (National Institutes of Health [NIH], 2005). Women do not find symptoms to be a cause for concern; however, they do report that symptoms are bothersome. Many women have accepted childbearing and child rearing as their major role in life, and the inability to bear children is a significant loss. Others see menopause as the first step to old age and associate it with a loss of attractiveness, physical ability, and energy. Western culture values youth and physical attractiveness; the wisdom gained from life experience is not valued, and older adults have a loss of status, function, and role. No rituals give older women a special place and function. In cultures where postmenopausal women gain status, such as India, the Far East, and the South Pacific islands, depression among menopausal women is not observed. Western women, however, may have little to compensate for their losses.

For other women, menopause is not a loss or a symbol of losses, but a relief. For some, menopause is a relief from the fear of pregnancy, the discomfort and bother of menstruation, and the inconveniences of contraception.

The ability to cope with any stress involves three factors: the person's perception or understanding of the event, the support system, and coping mechanisms. Nurses counseling women in their perimenopausal years must therefore assess their understanding of perimenopausal changes, their perceptions of stressful experiences, their support systems, and their repertoire of coping skills.

Health Risks of Perimenopausal Women

Osteoporosis and coronary heart disease are the major health risks of perimenopausal women and the focus of the following discussion.

Osteoporosis

Aging is associated with a progressive decrease in bone density in men and women. **Osteoporosis** is a generalized, metabolic disease characterized by decreased bone mass and increased incidence of bone fractures. Normally there is a dynamic balance between bone formation (osteoblastic activity) and bone resorption (osteoclastic activity). Because one of the functions of estrogen is to stimulate the osteoblasts, the postmenopausal decrease in estrogen levels causes an imbalance between bone formation and resorption. Old bone deteriorates faster than new bone is formed, resulting in a slow thinning of the bones. Estrogen also is required for the conversion of vitamin D into calcitonin, which is essential in the absorption of calcium by the intestine. Reduced calcium absorption from the gut, in addition to the thinning of the bones, places postmenopausal women at risk for problems associated with osteoporosis.

Osteoporosis is a major health problem in the United States, affecting more than 8 million women older than 45 years (National Osteoporosis Foundation [NOF], 2010). Approximately 50% of U.S. women have some degree of osteoporosis. One in two Caucasian women will have changes severe enough to predispose them to fractures. In the United States, the incidence of osteoporosis-related fractures has increased in the past 20 years. Postmenopausal women with a hip or symptomatic vertebral fracture have a 25% increased risk of death in the year following their fracture. After a hip fracture 25% of women will need long-term care and 50% will have long-term loss of mobility (North American Menopause Society [NAMS], 2010b). During the first 5 to 6 years after menopause, women lose bone six times more rapidly than men. By age 65, one third of women have had a vertebral fracture; by age 81, one third have had a hip fracture. By the time women reach age 80, they have lost 47% of their trabecular bone, concentrated in the vertebrae, the pelvis and other flat bones, and the epiphyses. The most well-defined risk factor for osteoporosis is the loss of the protective effect of estrogen associated with cessation of ovarian function, particularly at menopause. Women at risk are likely to be Caucasian or Asian, small boned, and thin. Obese women have higher estrogen levels resulting from the conversion of androgens in adipose tissue; mechanical stress from extra weight also helps preserve bone mass. A family history of the disease is common. The influences of heredity, race, and sex may result in differences in peak bone mass (NOF, 2010).

Inadequate calcium intake is a risk factor, particularly during adolescence and into the third and fourth decades, when peak bone mass is attained. An excessive caffeine intake increases calcium excretion, causing a systemic acidosis that stimulates bone resorption. Vitamin D deficiency can affect the physiologic regulation and stimulation of intestinal absorption of calcium (NOF, 2010). Smoking is associated with earlier and greater bone loss and decreases estrogen production. Excessive alcohol intake interferes with calcium absorption and depresses bone formation. A greater phosphorus than calcium intake, which occurs with soft drink consumption, may be a risk factor. Other risk factors include steroid therapy and disorders such as hypogonadism, hyperthyroidism, and diabetes mellitus (NOF).

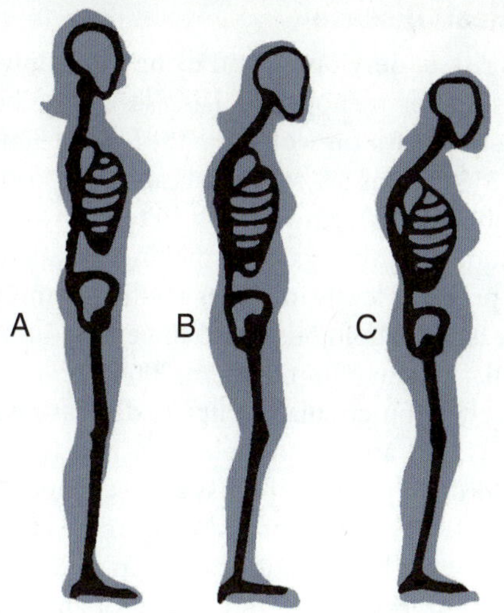

FIG. 6-2 Skeletal changes secondary to osteoporosis assessed by height and body shape at **A,** age 55 years; **B,** age 65 years; and **C,** age 75 years.

The first sign of osteoporosis is often loss of height resulting from vertebral fracture and collapse (Fig. 6-2). Back pain, especially in the lower back, may or may not be present. Later signs include "dowager's hump," in which the vertebrae can no longer support the upper body in an upright position, and fractured hip, in which the fracture often precedes a fall. Damage to the vertebrae usually precedes bone loss in the hip by an average of 10 years. Osteoporosis cannot be detected by radiographic examination until 30% to 50% of the bone mass has been lost; thus routine screening is not warranted in women younger than age 65. However, bone density testing is recommended for women at high risk for osteoporosis at age 60 and for all women older than 65 to assess fracture risk (NOF, 2010; U.S. Public Health Services Task Force, 2002). Medicare will pay for tests for high risk women once every 2 years (NOF, 2008). Insurance reimbursement for the tests varies among insurance carriers and from state to state.

COMMUNITY ACTIVITY

- Visit the National Women's Health Information Center website at www.4women.gov. Select a menstrual disorder and review the client information about diagnosis, treatment, prevention, facts to know, questions to ask and life style tips.
- Visit the National Osteoporosis Foundation website at www.nof.org. Review the client information regarding osteoporosis, prevention, management, and finding a doctor. What are the resources for women with osteoporosis in your community?

Coronary Heart Disease

A woman's risk of developing and dying of cardiovascular disease increases after menopause. Diseases of the heart are the leading cause of death for women in the United States. The lifetime risk is 31% versus 3% for breast cancer in postmenopausal women (Lobo, 2007c). Known risk factors for coronary heart disease include obesity, cigarette smoking, elevated cholesterol and blood pressure levels, diabetes mellitus, family history of cardiac disease, alcohol abuse, and the effects of aging on the cardiovascular system (Cunningham, 2008; Lobo). Estrogen has a favorable effect on circulating lipids, decreasing low-density lipoprotein (LDL) and total cholesterol and increasing high-density lipoprotein (HDL), and has a direct antiatherosclerotic effect on arteries. Postmenopausal women are at risk for coronary artery disease because of changes in lipid metabolism: a decline in serum levels of HDL cholesterol and an increase in LDL levels (Lobo). These changes can be favorably reduced by diet and exercise.

Menopausal Hormonal Therapy

Until 2002 **menopausal hormonal therapy (MHT)**—either as *estrogen replacement therapy (ERT)* or *estrogen therapy (ET)*, in which a woman takes only estrogen, or *hormonal replacement therapy (HRT)* or *hormonal therapy (HT)*, in which she takes both estrogen and progestins—was widely prescribed for discomforts associated with the perimenopausal years, including hot flashes and vaginal and urinary tract atrophy. Further, MHT was aggressively used for therapeutic and preventive management. At the same time its use remained highly controversial in women's health. Some authorities recommended HT or ET for all women; these proponents viewed the perimenopause as a disease or deficiency state. Others insisted that the use of hormones was never indicated for menopausal symptoms. The middle-ground approach advocated the use of MRT for women who have specific discomforts (therapeutic management) and for women in certain high risk groups (preventive management). Research studies challenged these beliefs in the preventive and beneficial effects of HT. Findings from the Women's Health Initiative, a study by the National Institutes of Health, documented increased risks for blood clots, heart attack, stroke, and invasive breast cancer in older women with a uterus (mean age 63, range 50 to 79 years) with long-term use of continuous combined estrogen plus progestin (Kaunitz, 2002; Rossouw, Anderson, Prentice, LaCroix, Kooperberg, Stefanick, et al., 2002).

These findings changed the way MHT is used. Many women stopped taking MHT and sought alternative therapies to treat their menopausal symptoms. Others chose to continue with the MHT but had questions about the available regimens and associated risks. Although the absolute risk for these adverse outcomes in an individual woman is very low, menopausal women should be aware of the most current research to make an informed decision regarding if, when, and for how long they use MHT.

Decision to Use Hormone Therapy

All women considering ET or HT must understand that studies on MHT are ongoing, and there is still much to be learned. Nurses can provide information and counseling to assist women to make decisions regarding MHT use. Important teaching points include the following (National Women's Health Information Center, 2006 [www.4women.gov]; NAMS, 2010a [www.menopause.org]; Santoro & Steunkel, 2009):

- For women taking MHT for short-term (1 to 3 years) relief of menopausal discomforts and who do not have increased risks for cardiovascular disease, the benefits may outweigh the risks. The decision to use MRT should be made between a woman and her health care provider.
- If used, MHT should be taken at the lowest effective dose for the shortest possible duration.
- When a woman decides to stop MHT, a recurrence of symptoms will occur whether the medication is tapered or discontinued abruptly. NAMS makes no recommendation on how to discontinue the medication, although some clinicians recommend a gradual withdrawal.
- Older women who are taking or considering MHT only for the prevention of cardiovascular disease should be counseled on other methods to reduce their risks of cardiovascular disease.
- Alternatively there may be beneficial cardiovascular effects associated with MHT for younger, more recently menopausal women, but research is needed.
- Women who are taking MHT only for prevention of osteoporosis should be counseled regarding their personal risks and benefits for continuing the therapy and reassured that there are effective alternatives for long-term prevention. Bone density studies also may be indicated to determine the degree of risk in an individual woman.
- Women with a high risk for breast cancer or who have had breast cancer should be counseled against using MHT.
- Conjugated estrogens are associated with an increased incidence of gallbladder disease, and women with a known history of gallbladder disease should not use MHT.

Nurses are encouraged to stay current with ongoing MHT research findings. As other Women's Health Initiative (WHI) data on MHT are analyzed, further clarification of the issues will be published.

Side Effects

Side effects associated with estrogen use include headaches, nausea and vomiting, bloating, ankle and feet swelling, weight gain, breast soreness, brown spots on the skin, eye irritation with contact lenses, and depression. The type of estrogen used for postmenopausal hormonal therapy is much less potent than ethinyl estradiol used in OCPs and has fewer serious side effects. Side effects that occur with MHT may disappear with a change in estrogen preparation or a decrease in the dose prescribed.

Treatment Guidelines

Research in MHT continues; however, nurses who counsel women about MHT must understand what is available and teach women who choose to continue MHT how to take the medications correctly. Thus the following discussion about the different regimens of MHT is included.

Many different estrogen preparations, natural and synthetic, and ways of administering them—oral tablets, topical creams, transdermal preparations, suppositories, and vaginal rings—exist (Table 6-4). However, most women today in the United States use tablets (Carroll, 2010).

TABLE 6-4 **HORMONE MEDICATIONS FOR MENOPAUSAL SYMPTOMS**

MEDICATION NAME	COMPOSITION	AVAILABLE DOSES
Oral Estrogens		
Premarin	Conjugated estrogens	0.3 mg; 0.45 mg; 0.625 mg; 0.9 mg; 1.25 mg
Estrace, various generics	Micronized estradiol	0.5 mg; 1 mg; 2 mg
Menest	Esterified estrogens	0.3 mg; 0.625 mg; 1.25 mg; 2.5 mg
Femtrace	Estradiol acetate	0.45 mg, 0.9 mg, 1.8 mg
Ortho-Est	Estropipate	0.625 mg; 1.25 mg; 2.5 mg
Transdermal		
Estraderm	Estradiol reservoir patch	0.05 mg; 0.1 mg twice weekly
Climera, Esclim, Estradot	Estradiol matrix patch	0.025 mg; 0.0375 mg; 0.05 mg; 0.075 mg; 0.1 mg once weekly
Vivelle	Estradiol matrix patch	0.05 mg; 0.1 mg twice weekly
Vivelle-Dot	Estradiol matrix patch	0.025 mg; 0.0375 mg; 0.05 mg; 0.1 mg twice weekly
Menostar	Estradiol matrix patch	0.014 mg once weekly
Alora	Estradiol matrix patch	0.0025 mg; 0.05 mg; 0.075 mg; 0.1 mg twice weekly
Divigel	Estradiol gel 0.1%	0.003 mg; 0.009 mg; 0.027 mg daily
EstroGel	Estradiol gel 0.06%	0.035 mg daily
Elestrin	Estradiol gel 0.06%	0.0125 mg daily
Evamist	Estradiol spray	0.021 mg per spray daily; may increase to 2 or 3 sprays daily
Estrasorb	Estradiol emulsion	0.05 mg/2 packets daily
Vaginal		
Premarin cream	Conjugated estrogens	0.5 g to 2 g/day (0.0625 mg/g)
Estrace cream	Estradiol	1 g/day (0.1 mg/g)
Femring vaginal ring	Estradiol acetate	12.4 mg or 24.8 mg; releases 0.05 mg/day or 0.10 mg/day for 90 days
Estring vaginal ring	Estradiol	2 mg; releases 7.5 mcg daily for 90 days
Vagifem vaginal tablet	Estradiol hemihydrate	25-mcg tablet twice a week
Oral Progestogens		
Provera	Medroxyprogesterone acetate	2.5 mg; 5 mg; 10 mg
Aygestin	Norethindrone acetate	5 mg
Micronor	Norethindrone	0.35 mg
Norgestrel	Ovrette	0.075 mg
Progesterone capsule (in peanut oil)	Prometrium	100 mg; 200 mg
Intrauterine		
Levonorgestrel	Mirena	Approximately 20 mcg/day
Vaginal		
Progesterone gel	Prochieve 4%	45 mg/applicator
Oral Combination Estrogen-Progestin		
Premphase	Conjugated estrogens (E)	0.625 mg E daily for 28 days
	Medroxyprogesterone acetate (P)	5 mg P on day 14 through day 28
Prempro	Conjugated estrogens (E)	0.0625 mg E plus 2.5 or 5 P daily
	Medroxyprogesterone acetate (P)	0.3 mg or 0.45 mg E plus 1.5 P daily
Activella	Estradiol (E) and norethindrone acetate (NETA)	1 mg E plus 0.5 mg NETA daily
Femhrt	Ethinyl estradiol and norethindrone acetate (NETA)	2.5 mcg E plus 0.5mg NETA daily
Transdermal		
CombiPatch	Estradiol/norethindrone acetate (NETA)	0.05 mg estradiol/0.14 mg NETA or 0.05 mg estradiol/0.25 mg NETA twice weekly
Climera Pro	Estradiol and levonorgestrel	0.045 mg/0.015 mg weekly

Source: North American Menopause Society. (2009). *Hormone products for postmenopausal use in the United States and Canada.* Available at www.menopause.org. Accessed March 1, 2010.

There are multiple dosing regimen options for combining progesterone with estrogen for women who have a uterus. According to NAMS (2010a), there is insufficient research to recommend one regimen over another; however, there is evidence to recommend keeping exposure to progesterone at a minimum. An oral continual-cyclic regimen that is most commonly prescribed is estrogen on days 1 to 28 and a progestogen (e.g., medroxyprogesterone) on days 14 to 28. Women usually do not have cyclic bleeding with this regimen and are less likely to have progestin side effects. There are also multiple regimen options for ET for women who have had a hysterectomy.

The transdermal estrogen patch is applied once or twice a week to a hairless area of skin. Transdermal gels and sprays are applied daily. Any site on the trunk or upper arms provides adequate absorption. Sites should be rotated. The patches should not be placed on the breasts because of their sensitivity. Some women report minor skin irritation and reddening at the patch site. Generally transdermal estrogen offers the same relief of menopausal symptoms as the oral preparation. The transdermal method of delivery of estrogen does not have the same side effects such as breast tenderness and fluid retention. Oral progestin therapy can be used with transdermal ET.

Combined estrogen-progestin transdermal patches also are available.

Vaginal creams and tablets are inserted daily or twice a week. Usually these local administrations of low-dose estrogen are used for vaginal symptoms of dryness and atrophy. Vaginal rings are inserted and left in place for 90 days. Although minimal systemic absorption is possible, there are no reports of adverse effects when a low dose is used (NAMS, 2010a).

Bioidentical and Custom-Compounded Hormones

Bioidentical hormones, sometimes referred to as natural hormones, are structurally identical to those produced by the ovary. Bioidentical hormone preparations are available as government approved well-tested brand-name prescription medications. Others are made at compounding pharmacies. Custom-compounded hormones are custom mixes of one or more hormones in varying amounts. These mixes can provide individualized doses and mixtures of hormones that are not available commercially. They also include ingredients that are nonhormonal (e.g., dyes, preservatives). The risks are that these mixtures have not been studied to confirm whether appropriate absorption occurs or if predictable levels can be detected in blood and tissue (NAMS, 2006). Preparations may vary from one pharmacy to another, meaning that a woman may not get consistent amounts of medication. These preparations are not approved by any regulatory agency (NAMS, 2010a). Although these hormones may relieve menopausal symptoms, more research is needed to determine their effects on the body. Women who choose to take these hormones need to understand and accept the potential risks. Expense is also an issue because these drugs often are more expensive and are not covered by third-party payers.

Alternative Therapies

Many complementary and alternative therapies are useful for relieving some of the changes associated with altered estrogen levels. Homeopathy, acupuncture, and herbs have been used with varying degrees of success for menopausal problems such as heavy bleeding, hot flashes, irritability, and headaches.

Homeopathy views menopausal symptoms as the body's efforts to heal itself from the hormonal changes it is experiencing. Examples of remedies commonly prescribed during menopause by homeopaths are sepia, made from the inky juice of the cuttlefish, to relieve symptoms such as dry mouth, eyes, and vagina; nux vomica, derived from the poison nut, to relieve backaches, constipation, and frequent awakenings; and pulsatilla, made from the windflower, to relieve severe menstrual symptoms and hot flashes. Homeopathic remedies are subject to regulation by the U.S. Food and Drug Administration (FDA), although the FDA does not require proof of effectiveness. Most studies have not proven homeopathy to be any more effective than a placebo for relieving menopausal symptoms (Martin, Pinkerton, & Santen, 2009).

Acupuncturists also treat hot flashes, but it is important that women evaluate their acupuncturists carefully. The American Association of Acupuncturists and Oriental Medicine will supply a list of acupuncturists in a given state. Questions to ask are: Is the acupuncturist certified by the National Commission for the Certification of Acupuncture? Is the acupuncturist certified in the state in which he or she practices? Does the acupuncturist carry malpractice insurance? Some clinical trials have shown some improvement in mood and decreased frequency of hot flashes but others have not found hot flashes to be improved (Nedrow et al, 2006).

Herbal therapy also has been used to treat menopausal discomforts (see Table 6-2). Herbs can be ingested as teas or tinctures. Many herbal preparations also are available in capsule form. It is important that women understand mechanisms of action, contraindications, and potential side effects of each herb.

SAFETY ALERT

Most herbal preparations have not undergone long-term testing for safety and efficacy. Benefits and risks are not completely known. Women should always consult with their health care provider before beginning herbal therapy. Questions regarding the use of herbal therapy and other supplements must be a component of a client history.

In addition to resolving physical symptoms, herbs also are used to combat mood swings and depression. Ginseng has been claimed to be helpful in alleviating hot flashes, although research studies have not supported this assertion. Women should be advised against prolonged use of ginseng in high doses because it can increase blood pressure. Oriental herbal teas composed of licorice, ginseng, coptis, red raspberry leaf, and Chinese rhubarb may be of some help in relieving hot flashes.

Dong quai and black cohosh have been used to treat menopausal discomforts; both have been investigated for effectiveness, with varying results (Martin et al., 2009; Palacio, Masri, & Mooradian, 2009; Shams, Setia, Hemmings, McCusker, Sewitch, & Ciampi, 2010).

Some plant foods contain **phytoestrogens** (isoflavones) and are capable of interacting with estrogen receptors in the body. These foods include red clover, wild yams, dandelion greens, cherries, alfalfa sprouts, black beans, and soybeans. Use of soy-rich foods as an alternative to traditional hormonal therapy for menopause has been studied, and beneficial effects on menopausal symptoms and on reducing cholesterol have been reported although results for relief of hot flashes have been inconsistent (Albertazzi, 2005; Martin et al., 2009; Nedrow et al., 2006). More research is needed to better understand the potential effects of soy intake on prevention of osteoporosis and reducing risks of coronary heart disease (Alekel, Van loan, Loehler, Hanson, Stewart, & Hanson 2010; NAMS, 2010a).

For women who want to add soy to their diets, tofu, roasted soy nuts, and soy milk are good sources. Foods should be added gradually because some women have gastrointestinal discomfort from the high fiber content of these foods. Spreading out the daily intake over several meals may be the best way to include soy products in the diet.

Vitamin E is a popular alternative among women who do not take MHT. Women who take vitamin E report relief from hot flushes, leg cramps, and loss of energy; however, research has not supported this clinical finding (Martin et al., 2009; Nedrow et al., 2006). Vitamin E is found in a variety of foods, including spinach, peanuts, wheat germ, vegetable oils, and soybeans, or may be taken as a supplement. Dosage varies widely, from 400 to 800 International Units/day.

TEACHING FOR SELF-MANAGEMENT

Comfort Measures for Menopausal Symptoms

HOT FLASHES/FLUSHES

During the Day

- Wear layered clothing so you can take things off if you get warm.
- Avoid "triggers" that bring on a flash/flush; these include vigorous exercise on hot days, eating spicy foods, caffeine, hot beverages, and alcohol.
- Splash your face with cool water, drink ice water, or take a cool shower if you get warm.
- Try slow, deep breathing.

At Night

- Sleep in cotton clothes, use cotton sheets, and keep room cool.
- Avoid heavy blankets that make you too warm at night.
- Keep a thermos of water by the bed.

INSOMNIA

- Avoid caffeine, alcohol, or tobacco in the evening.
- Avoid liquids after dinner.
- Exercise regularly but limit exercise to the daytime and early evening.
- Develop a bedtime routine.
- Establish a regular time to go to bed.
- Try drinking warm milk or having a hot bath.
- Use your bed only for sleeping or sexual activity; don't watch TV, read, etc.
- Encourage your body's circadian rhythm.
- If you can't sleep, get up and do something until you feel tired.
- Avoid naps during the day.
- Sprinkle lavender oil on the pillow.
- Drink chamomile tea (do not use if allergic to ragweed or chrysanthemums).

HEADACHES

- Try to avoid stress and get plenty of rest.
- Eat or drink foods that contain natural diuretics (parsley).

UROGENITAL SYMPTOMS

- Drink lots of water (i.e., at least 8 glasses a day), and empty bladder frequently.
- Practice Kegel exercises daily.
- Wear cotton underwear and avoid wearing wet bathing suits for a prolonged time.
- Use water-soluble lubricants for vaginal dryness.

NERVOUSNESS, IRRITABILITY

- Practice yoga or other meditation.
- Do relaxation or deep-breathing exercises.
- Practice guided imagery.

Source: Woods, N., & Mitchell, E. (2008). Mid-life women's health. In C. Fogel & N. Woods (Eds.), *Women's health care in advanced practice nursing.* New York: Springer.

Layered clothing, ice packs, ice water, and fans may offer symptomatic relief from hot flashes (see Teaching for Self-Management box: Comfort Measures for Menopausal Symptoms). Women can be counseled to avoid hot curries and other spicy foods. Reassurance that hot flashes will not last forever may be of comfort even if duration of the problem cannot be predicted accurately. Many women find that hot flashes lessen in frequency and intensity or disappear within 4 to 6 years after menopause.

Nurses should be aware of the availability of natural remedies for menopausal symptoms and be knowledgeable about the indications for complementary and alternative therapies so clients can be counseled appropriately.

CARE MANAGEMENT

Most women know little about menopause, and old wives' tales and misinformation can cause anxiety. They need to know what to expect, why it happens, and what measures will help make them more comfortable. Women appreciate the opportunity to discuss what they are experiencing. They need to know that their discomforts have a normal physiologic basis and that other women experience similar discomforts.

Planning for nursing care requires knowledge of the perimenopausal period and great sensitivity. Treatment must be individualized for the specific woman (see Nursing Process box: The Perimenopausal Woman). Informed consent regarding MHT, weight-bearing exercise, and calcium supplements is a major concern because treatment may involve expense, inconvenience, and side effects. Menopause clinics are needed where research on the effects of various treatments can be developed and evaluated and where care by the various specialty groups involved, such as endocrinology, radiology, psychosocial resources, exercise physiology, and nutrition, can be effectively coordinated. Women's support groups also are needed. Sexual counseling, nutrition, exercise, and support are topics that are included for further discussion.

Sexual Counseling

Sexuality is a lifelong behavior, and contrary to common stereotypes, sex does not end with menopause. Many women remain sexually active throughout their entire lives. However, women and their partners may change their expression of sexuality during and after menopause, depending on physical changes, changes in the partner, and cultural myths and messages. Some women report decreases in interest and desire. These decreases in sexuality with aging are influenced more by culture and attitudes than by nature and physiology (hormones). Although some women report that it takes longer to reach orgasm and that the orgasm is not so intense, the capacity for orgasm is not decreased. There is no way to prevent the inevitable aging process that the body undergoes. For people who see aging as loss, sexuality may become difficult to incorporate into what they perceive to be a less attractive identity. The fear of rejection may be present.

Changes in a male partner may influence whether he continues to want to engage in sexual activity. As men age, they, too, take longer to reach orgasm; erections take longer to occur and are less firm. Men may believe they are becoming impotent or ill and give up sexual activity, viewing it as too frustrating. Women may believe their partners are losing interest in them. Couples may need counseling to understand these changes.

NURSING PROCESS

The Perimenopausal Woman

ASSESSMENT

- A thorough health history, physical examination, and laboratory tests are essential to distinguish pathologic conditions from the normal perimenopausal experiences. These assessments include:
  - Personal or family history of breast or uterine cancer, hypertension, thrombophlebitis, liver or gallbladder disease, undiagnosed uterine bleeding, and other acute or chronic diseases are noted, as are hysterectomy and bilateral oophorectomy.
  - Recent changes in menstrual history help identify the phase of the perimenopausal period the woman is experiencing.
  - Risk factors for osteoporosis are identified.
  - The woman's perception of this stage of life, ethnic and cultural factors, and knowledge and concerns about sexuality and care available are all recorded.
  - The practices and remedies the woman has used for menopausal symptoms are assessed, including pharmacologic and alternative therapies.
  - A physical and pelvic examination are performed to note age-related changes.
  - Laboratory tests: Serum FSH level may be done to confirm menopause (12 consecutive months of amenorrhea).

NURSING DIAGNOSES

Nursing diagnoses for perimenopausal women may include:

Deficient Knowledge **related to:**
- menopause and its management

Readiness for Enhanced Family Coping **related to:**
- receiving information about the condition, its management, and prognosis
- emotional support

Risk for Injury **related to:**
- osteoporosis
- heart disease

Sexual Dysfunction **related to:**
- changes associated with decreasing estrogen levels

Risk for Situational Low Self-Esteem **related to:**
- physical and emotional changes during the perimenopausal period

EXPECTED OUTCOMES OF CARE

Expected outcomes are stated in terms of client behaviors. The woman will:
- Explain the physical changes associated with menopause.
- View the perimenopausal period as a normal developmental phase instead of a deficiency disease.
- Have no discomforts that interfere with daily activities.
- Develop no symptoms or signs of osteoporosis or experience only minimal effect.
- Experience a healthy perimenopausal transition.
- Report concerns about changes associated with menopause and treatment.

PLAN OF CARE AND INTERVENTIONS

Interventions are individualized and include information and teaching in the following areas (see text for discussion, specifically Box 6-2 and Teaching for Self-Management box):
- Hormonal therapy and alternative therapies for menopausal symptoms
- Comfort measures for self management of symptoms
- Sexuality
- Nutrition
- Exercise
- Midlife support groups

EVALUATION

The nurse can be reasonably assured that care was effective to the degree that the expected outcomes of care have been met.

The two most important influences on older women's sexual activity are the strength of a relationship and the physical condition of each partner. The lack of available male partners can have a negative effect on sexual expression for many midlife and older women. Women outlive men, and older widowed and divorced women frequently have fewer opportunities to develop relationships because they are less sought after. In counseling older women who do engage in intercourse, the nurse cannot assume that new or nonmonogamous partners are free of sexually transmitted infections (STIs) and should inform women of their risk for human immunodeficiency virus infection (HIV) and other STIs and the need to use condoms.

As long as women are able to bear children, some accept intercourse as part of their responsibility as wives. When menopause frees them from this duty, they may choose to forgo intercourse. For other women, libido may increase without the fuss of contraception, fear of pregnancy, or interruption from menses.

Older lesbian women largely have been a silent group whose sexual needs and special social circumstances have not been acknowledged or recognized. Although lesbian women in midlife and in later years do not face the problem of a lack of available male partners, they are faced with negative attitudes accompanying being old, female, and lesbian—all of which can adversely affect sexuality and sexual expression.

Nurses must give accurate information on matters such as appropriate contraception, sexuality, and the physiology of menopause and should offer support and nonjudgmental guidance. Women need advice about contraception because ovulation may not cease for a year after the last menstrual cycle, and menopausal women can still become pregnant. The nurse's attitude toward sex and the older woman is important. Negative attitudes can reinforce the woman's misgivings about maintaining an active and satisfying sex life. The nurse can reassure the woman grieving over lost youth and attractiveness that the desire for sex into old age is a natural one and that the body has the capacity for sexual satisfaction. Only minor adjustments may be required.

Muscle tone around the reproductive organs decreases after menopause. Kegel exercises (see p. 91) strengthen these muscles, improve tone, and, if practiced regularly, help prevent prolapsed uterus and stress incontinence. This is a low-cost, effective, noninvasive intervention to control symptoms. However, symptoms return if exercises are discontinued.

Lubricating jelly (e.g., K-Y, Femglide, Aqualube) is a water-soluble lubricant that provides relief from painful intercourse. It may be applied directly to the vulva and the penis. Vaginal moisturizers may be water based but also contain other products such as vitamin E and aloe (e.g., K-Y Longlasting, Replens, Astroglide). They are inserted into the vagina using a prefilled applicator. Oil-based lubricants such as petroleum jelly (Vaseline) should not be used because they clog vaginal glands, which can then be sites for bacterial infection.

Prolonged hospitalization of an older adult partner may have a significant effect on the couple's sexual relationship. They may have difficulty renewing sexual activity when the separation is over and may need counseling or referral. In the event that a couple is admitted to a nursing home, the nurse should encourage placement of the couple together. With the aging of the American population and changing attitudes about the appropriateness of lifelong sexual expression, long-term care, extended care, and full-time care facilities are more receptive to providing opportunities for sexual activity between marital partners.

The nurse can refer couples to a counselor or physician for problems beyond the scope of nursing practice.

Nutrition

Obesity and osteoporosis are common health problems of midlife and older women. As women move out of their childbearing years, they may need to change their diets. Because metabolic rates decrease with age and many women exercise less, fewer calories are needed for weight maintenance as women age. In general, foods chosen should be high in nutrients, fiber, and calcium but moderate in calories and low in fat to allow adequate nutritional intake while maintaining body weight. Nurses can suggest that women substitute skim for whole milk or chicken without skin for steak. Excessive protein should be avoided. Fat-free milk and yogurt are good sources of calcium and vitamin D. Women should avoid excessive intake of alcohol, soft drinks, and caffeinated coffee.

Calcium is an essential part of any therapeutic regimen for women with osteoporosis and those who want to prevent osteoporosis. The best source of calcium is food; however, it is difficult to eat other foods that contain calcium (sesame seeds, spinach, greens, broccoli, and seaweed) in quantities sufficient to meet daily requirements. Calcium supplements are recommended when a woman's diet does not supply recommended amounts of calcium. Although calcium cannot reverse loss of bone mass or prevent fractures, calcium supplementation may retard the development of osteoporosis after menopause. Menopausal women without contraindications to calcium supplementation (history of kidney stones, kidney failure, hypercalcemia) should be encouraged to consume a diet that has 1200 to 1500 mg of calcium a day or to add an amount of calcium supplementation that will increase their daily intake to this level. Calcium supplements are best taken in divided doses and with meals because of the increase in acid secretions and extended time in the stomach. At least 8 ounces of water to increase solubility is recommended. Calcium supplements should not be taken with caffeinated beverages. Calcium is most commonly available as calcium carbonate, calcium lactate, and calcium phosphate.

The NOF (2010) recommends that women older than age 50 take vitamin D 800 to 1000 International Units daily. Sources of vitamin D include sunlight, food (e.g., fortified dairy products, fatty fish, liver, egg yolks), and supplements. Usually a supplement is needed to get the required daily dose. A combination of vitamin D and calcium is available, and most multivitamins contain some vitamin D.

Exercise

All too often midlife women are sedentary—the demands of family and work constraints increase, and energy levels decrease. Unfortunately little or no exercise predisposes women to weight gain and does not help prevent cardiac disease or osteoporosis. Exercise alone cannot prevent or reverse osteoporosis, but data indicate that weight-bearing exercise, such as walking and stair climbing, may delay bone loss and increase bone mass at any age. Muscle strengthening exercises combined with weight-bearing exercises also help improve agility, balance, and strength and may reduce the risk of falls and fractures (NOF, 2010). A study by Vallance, Murray, Johnson, and Elavsky (2010) found that women who engage in moderate intensity physical exercise for a minimum of 30 minutes for 5 days a week or vigorous intensity activity for 20 minutes 3 days a week reported higher scores in quality of life and psychosocial health than women who exercised less than the American Heart Association physical activity recommendations.

Water aerobics is excellent for cardiovascular fitness and is a good choice for older women who may be unable to engage in weight-bearing exercises. The nurse can help women plan an exercise program. Examples of exercises are available from the NOF (Fig. 6-3).

Medications for Osteoporosis

In addition to calcium and exercise, there are a number of FDA-approved medications for the prevention and treatment of osteoporosis (Box 6-2). The medications assist in delaying bone loss, increasing bone mass, and preventing fractures. These include salmon calcitonin (Miacalcin); bisphosphonates (alendronate sodium [Fosamax], risedronate sodium [Actonel]), ibandronate [Boniva], zoledronic acid [Reclast]); estrogen agonist/antagonists such as raloxifene (Evista), parathyroid hormone (teriparatide [Fortéo]), and estrogen or hormone therapy (NOF, 2010).

Calcitonin reduces the rate of bone turnover and stabilizes bone mass in women with osteoporosis and may have some analgesic effects. Although calcitonin can reduce the incidence of spinal fractures, no data are available about the use of calcitonin to protect against hip fractures. Calcitonin may be used with women who are at least 5 years postmenopausal and in whom estrogen is contraindicated or not tolerated. The drug usually is administered intranasally on a daily basis; subcutaneous administration is also available. The medication is considered safe; however, side effects of nausea, vomiting, anorexia, and rhinitis (if used intranasally) have been reported (NOF, 2010).

Bisphosphonates are approved for prevention and treatment of osteoporosis, especially in reducing the incidence of spinal fractures. Side effects include gastrointestinal problems such as difficulty swallowing, inflammation of the esophagus, and gastric ulcer. Depending on the medication used, the oral drugs may be taken daily or monthly. Some formulations contain vitamin D (NOF, 2010). Alendronate is available in the United States in a generic preparation. Ibandronate is available as an intravenous injection every 3 months; zoledronic acid is given intravenously yearly for treatment of osteoporosis and every 2 years for prevention (NOF).

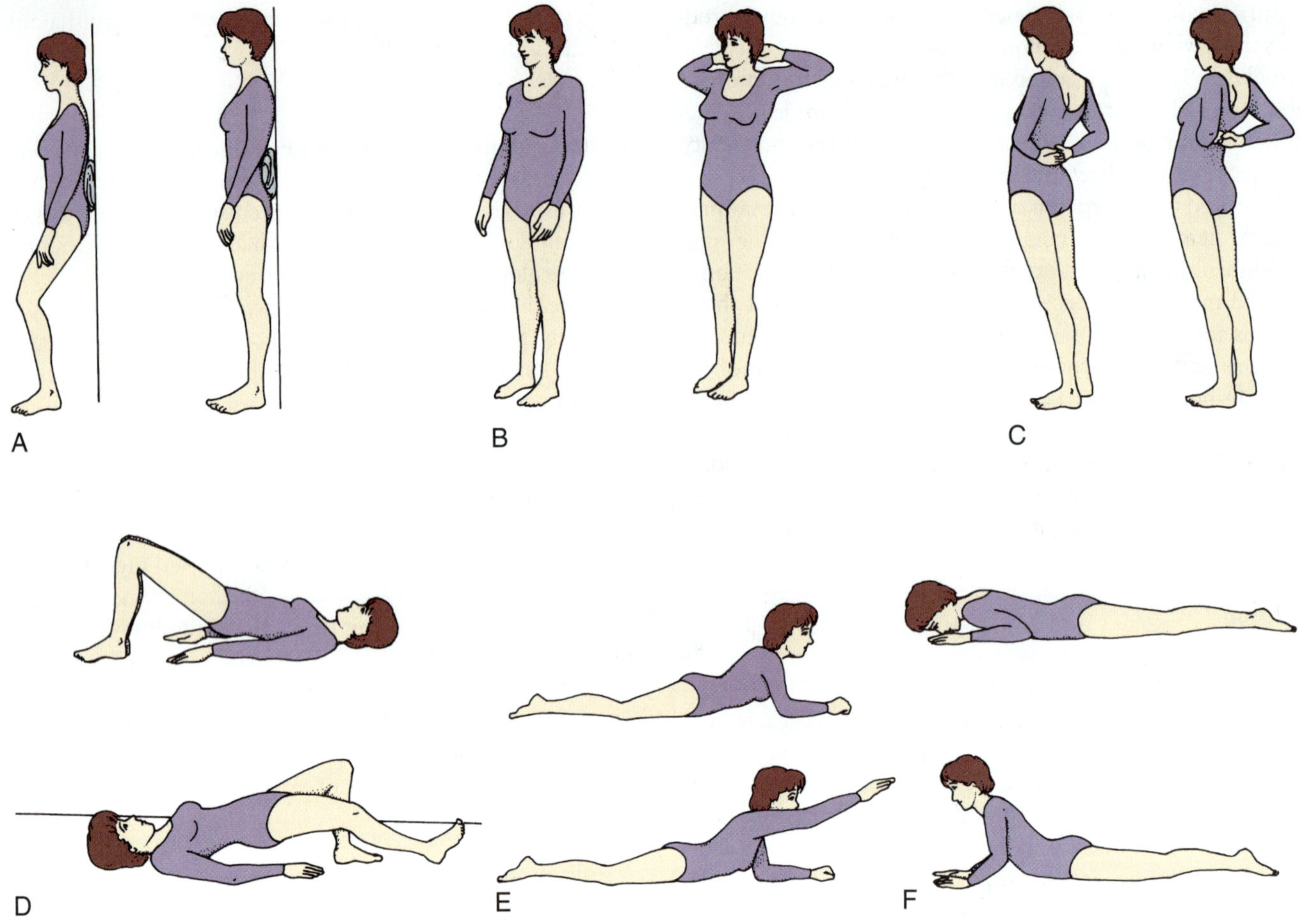

FIG. 6-3 Posture exercises. **A,** Wall standing and pelvic tilt. **B,** Isometric posture correction. **C,** Standing back bend. **D,** The bridge. **E,** The elbow prop. **F,** Prone press-ups with deep breathing. (From *Boning Up on Osteoporosis.* Courtesy the National Osteoporosis Foundation.)

BOX 6-2 PREVENTION OF OSTEOPOROSIS

- All postmenopausal women should be evaluated clinically for risk for osteoporosis and to determine the need for bone mineral density (BMD) testing.
- A BMD test is the only way to diagnose osteoporosis and determine risk for future fracture. The U.S. Preventive Services Task Force and the National Osteoporosis Foundation recommend testing for postmenopausal women and all women ages 65 and older.
- To protect bone health it is important that all individuals have a nutritionally balanced diet, which includes calcium-rich foods and vitamin D. Adults 50 and older need 1200 mg of calcium and 800 to 1000 International Units of vitamin D daily. Adults younger than 50 need 1000 mg of calcium and 400 to 800 International Units of vitamin D daily.
- A program of regular weight-bearing and muscle strengthening exercises further helps promote bone health. Weight-bearing exercises may increase bone density and weight-bearing exercise and muscle strengthening can increase balance and agility and reduce the risk of falls and fractures. Eliminating environmental hazards in the home can decrease the risk of falls.
- Avoidance of excessive alcohol intake and tobacco smoking is advised.
- U.S. FDA-approved medications for the prevention and/or treatment of osteoporosis include:
  - Bisphosphonates: alendronate, alendronate plus D; risedronate, risedronate with 500 mg calcium; ibandronate; zoledronic acid (prevention and treatment)
  - Calcitonin (treatment)
  - Estrogens (estrogen or hormone therapy) (prevention)
  - Estrogen agonist-antagonist (prevention and treatment)
  - Parathyroid hormone (treatment)

! NURSING ALERT

Because food and certain minerals reduce the absorption of bisphosphonates, women must take alendronate sodium and risedronate sodium on an empty stomach with 6 to 8 ounces of plain water only, at least 30 minutes before eating or drinking to improve absorption; remaining upright for these 30 minutes also is recommended (NOF, 2010).

Raloxifene is approved by the FDA for osteoporosis prevention and treatment in postmenopausal women only. This medication seemingly preserves the beneficial effects of estrogen, including protection against cardiovascular diseases and osteoporosis, without stimulating breast and uterine tissues. However, the effects of raloxifene and the risks of breast cancer and heart disease are still under study (NOF, 2006). The medication modestly increases bone density. Calcium supplements up to 1500 mg should be taken if dietary intake is inadequate.

Parathyroid hormone is approved for the treatment of osteoporosis in postmenopausal women at high risk for fractures. It is administered by daily subcutaneous injection. It can be used for a maximum of 2 years. The drug is well tolerated although some women report dizziness and leg cramps (NOF, 2010).

Estrogen/hormone therapy is approved for the prevention of osteoporosis. It should be used in the lowest effective doses for the shortest treatment time. The FDA recommends that it should not be used solely for the prevention of osteoporosis until after approved non-estrogen treatments are tried (NOF, 2010).

Midlife Support Groups

Nurses should be familiar with local resources and direct women to classes that supply appropriate information and support. They can encourage women to develop a supportive network with other women with whom they can share their concerns (Fig. 6-4).

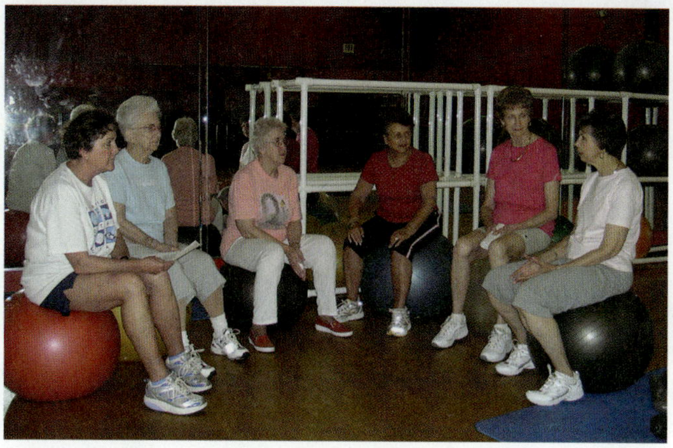

FIG. 6-4 Midlife women can develop a supportive network. (Courtesy Dee Lowdermilk, Chapel Hill, NC.)

Women's centers and clinics may have support groups and classes for women who want to discuss menopause and other midlife events. If no group or class is available in the community, nurses should consider starting one.

KEY POINTS

- Menstrual disorders diminish the quality of life for affected women and their families.
- Amenorrhea is most commonly a result of pregnancy.
- Dysmenorrhea is one of the most common gynecologic problems in women.
- PMS is a disorder with symptoms that begin in the luteal phase of the menstrual cycle and end with the onset of menses.
- Endometriosis is characterized by secondary amenorrhea, dyspareunia, abnormal uterine bleeding, and infertility.
- The perimenopause is a normal developmental phase during which a woman passes from the reproductive to the nonreproductive stage.
- During the perimenopause women seek care for symptoms that arise from bleeding irregularities, vasomotor instability, fatigue, genital changes, and changes related to sexuality.
- Menopausal hormonal therapy, if used, should be taken at the lowest effective dose for the shortest possible time.
- Alternative therapies are beneficial in relieving discomforts associated with menstrual disorders and menopause.
- Osteoporosis, a progressive loss of bone mass that results from decreasing levels of estrogen after menopause, can be prevented or minimized with lifestyle changes and medication.
- Postmenopausal women are at increased risk for coronary artery disease because of changes in lipid metabolism.
- Sexuality and the capacity for sexual expression continue after menopause.

Audio Chapter Summaries Access an audio summary of these Key Points on evolve

REFERENCES

Albertazzi, P. (2005). Alternatives to estrogen to manage hot flushes. *Gynecological Endocrinology, 20*(1), 13–21.

Alekel, D., Van loan, M., Loehler, K., Hanson, L., Stewart, J., Hanson., K., et al. (2010). The soy isoflavones for reducing bone loss (SIRBI) study: A 3-y randomized controlled trial in postmenopausal women. *American Journal of Clinical Nutrition, 91*(1), 218–230.

American College of Obstetricians and Gynecologists. (2000). *Premenstrual syndrome.* ACOG Practice Bulletin, No. 15. Washington, DC: Author.

American College of Obstetricians and Gynecologists Committee on Adolescent Health Care. (2005). Endometriosis in adolescents. ACOG Committee Opinion No. 310. *Obstetrics and Gynecology, 105*(4), 921–927.

American Psychiatric Association (APA). (2000). *Diagnostic and statistical manual of mental disorders* (4th ed., text rev). Washington, DC: American Psychiatric Association Press.

Association of Women's Health, Obstetric and Neonatal Nurses (AWHONN). (2003). *Evidence-based clinical practice guideline: Nursing management for cyclic perimenstrual pain and discomfort.* Washington, DC: Author.

Behera, M., & Price, T. (2009). *Dysfunctional uterine bleeding.* Available at www.emedicine.com. Accessed February 16, 2010.

Blackburn, S. (2007). *Maternal, fetal, & neonatal physiology: A clinical perspective* (3rd ed.). St. Louis: Saunders.

Bonci, C., Bonci, L., Granger, L., Johnson, C., Malina, R., Milne, L., et al. (2008). National Athletic Trainers' Association position statement: Preventing, detecting, and managing disordered eating in athletes. *Journal of Athletic Training, 43*(1), 808-820.

Carroll, N. (2010). A review of transdermal nonpatch estrogen therapy for the management of menopausal symptoms. *Journal of Women's Health, 19*(1), 47–55.

Collins Sharp, B., Taylor, D., Thomas, K., Killeen, M., & Dawood, M. (2002). Cyclic perimenstrual pain and discomfort: The scientific basis for practice. *Journal of Obstetric, Gynecologic and Neonatal Nursing, 31*(6), 637–649.

Cunningham, S. (2008). Cardiovascular disease in women. In C. Fogel, & N. Woods (Eds.), *Women's health care in advanced practice nursing*. New York: Springer.

Dehlin, L., & Schuiling, K. (2006). Chronic pelvic pain. In K. Schuiling, & F. Lokis (Eds.), *Women's gynecologic health*. Boston: Jones and Bartlett.

Katz, V. (2007). Benign gynecologic lesions: Vulva, vagina, cervix, uterus, oviducts and ovary. In V. Katz, G. Lentz, R. Lobo, & D. Gershenson (Eds.), *Comprehensive gynecology* (5th ed.). Philadelphia: Mosby.

Kaunitz, A. (2002). Menopausal hormone therapy: Where do we go now? *Breast Journal, 8*(6), 329–337.

Klaiber, E., Vogel, W., & Rako, S. (2005). A critique of the WHI hormone therapy study. *Fertility and Sterility, 84*(6), 1589–1601.

Lebrun, C. (2007). The female athlete triad: What's a doctor to do? *Current Sports Medicine Reports, 6*(6), 397–404.

Lentz, G. (2007a). Differential diagnosis of major gynecologic problems by age group: Vaginal bleeding, pelvic pain, and pelvic mass. In V. Katz, G. Lentz, R. Lobo, & D. Gershenson (Eds.), *Comprehensive gynecology* (5th ed.). Philadelphia: Mosby.

Lentz, G. (2007b). Primary and secondary dysmenorrhea, premenstrual syndrome, and premenstrual dysphoric disorder: Etiology, diagnosis, and management. In V. Katz, G. Lentz, R. Lobo, & D. Gershenson (Eds.), *Comprehensive gynecology* (5th ed.). Philadelphia: Mosby.

Lewiecki, E. (2009). Current and emerging pharmacologic therapies for the management of postmenopausal osteoporosis. *Journal of Women's Health, 18*(10), 1615–1626.

Liu, S., & Lebrun, C. (2006). Effect of oral contraceptives and hormone replacement therapy on bone mineral density in premenopausal and perimenopausal women: A systematic review. *British Journal of Sports Medicine, 40*(1), 11–24.

Lobo, R. (2007a). Abnormal uterine bleeding: Ovulatory and anovulatory dysfunctional uterine bleeding: Management of acute and chronic excessive bleeding. In V. Katz, G. Lentz, R. Lobo, & D. Gershenson (Eds.), *Comprehensive gynecology* (5th ed.). Philadelphia: Mosby.

Lobo, R. (2007b). Endometriosis: Etiology, pathology, diagnosis, management. In V. Katz, G. Lentz, R. Lobo, & D. Gershenson (Eds.), *Comprehensive gynecology* (5th ed.). Philadelphia: Mosby.

Lobo, R. (2007c). Menopause: Endocrinology, consequences of estrogen deficiency, effects of hormone replacement therapy, treatment regimens. In V. Katz, G. Lentz, R. Lobo, & D. Gershenson (Eds.), *Comprehensive gynecology* (5th ed.). Philadelphia: Mosby.

Lobo, R. (2007d). Primary and secondary amenorrhea and precocious puberty. In V. Katz, G. Lentz, R. Lobo, & D. Gershenson (Eds.). *Comprehensive gynecology* (5th ed.). Philadelphia: Mosby.

Martin, K., Pinkerton, J., & Santen, R. (2009). *Complementary and alternative medicine (CAM) for menopausal symptoms*. Available at www.hormone.org. Accessed February 26, 2010.

National Institutes of Health (NIH). (2005). National Institutes of Health state-of-the-science conference statement: Management of menopause-related symptoms. *Annals of Medicine, 142*(12 Part 1), 1003–1013.

National Osteoporosis Foundation (NOF). (2008). *Frequently asked questions regarding bone density testing for Medicare reimbursement*. Available at www.nof.org. Accessed February 25, 2010.

National Osteoporosis Foundation (NOF). (2010). *Clinician's guide to the prevention and treatment of osteoporosis*. Washington, DC: Author.

National Women's Health Information Center. (2006). *Menopause and hormone therapy*. Available at www.4women.gov/menopause. Accessed February 25, 2010.

Nattiv, A., Loucks, A., Manore, M., Sandborn, C., Sundgot-Borgen, J., & Warren, M., American College of Sports Medicine (2007). American College of Sports Medicine position stand. The female athlete triad. *Medicine and Science in Sports and Exercise, 39*(10), 1867–1882.

Nedrow, A., Miller, J., Walker, M., Nygren, P., Huffman, l., & Nelson, H. (2006). Complementary and alternative therapies for the management for menopause-related symptoms. *Archives of Internal Medicine, 166*(14), 1453–1465.

North American Menopause Society. (2006). *Menopause guidebook* (6th ed.). Available at www.menopause.org. Accessed February 26, 2010.

North American Menopause Society. (2009). *Hormone products for postmenopausal use in the United states and Canada*. Available at www.menopause.org. Accessed February 26, 2010.

North American Menopause Society. (2010a). Estrogen and progestogen use in postmenopausal women: 2010 position statement of the North American Menopause Society. *Menopause, 17*(2), 242–255.

North American Menopause Society. (2010b). Management of osteoporosis in postmenopausal women: 2010 position statement of the North American Menopause Society. *Menopause, 17*(1), 25–54.

Palacio, C., Masri, G., & Mooradian, A. (2009). Black cohosh for the management of menopausal symptoms: A systematic review of clinical trials. *Drugs and Aging, 26*(1), 23–36.

Rossouw, J., Anderson, G., Prentice, R., LaCroix, A., Kooperberg, C., Stefanick, M., et al. (2002). Risks and benefits of estrogen plus progestin in healthy postmenopausal women: Principal results from the Women's Health Initiative randomized control trial. *Journal of the American Medical Association, 288*(3), 321–333.

Santoro, S., & Steunkel, L. (2009). *Get the facts: Risks and benefits of hormone therapy for menopausal women*. Chevy Chase, MD: The Hormone Foundation.

Shams, T., Setia, M., Hemmings, R., McCusker, J., Sewitch, M., & Ciampi, A. (2010). Efficacy of black cohosh–containig preparations on menopausal symptom: A meta-analysis. *Alternative Therapies in Health and Medicine, 16*(1), 36–44.

Speroff, L., & Fritz, M. (2005). *Clinical gynecologic endocrinology and infertility* (7th ed.). Philadelphia: Lippincott Williams & Wilkins.

Taylor, D., Berg, J., & Fogel, C. (2008). Perimenstrual symptoms and syndromes. In C. Fogel, & N. Woods (Eds.), *Women's health care in advanced practice nursing*. New York: Springer.

Taylor, D., Schuiling, K., & Sharp, B. (2006). Menstrual cycle pain and discomforts. In K. Schuiling, & F. Lokis (Eds.), *Women's gynecologic health*. Boston: Jones and Bartlett.

Templeman., C. (2009). Adolescent endometriosis. *Obstetric & Gynecologic Clinics of North America, 36*(1), 177–185.

Tietjen, G., Bushnell, C., Herial, N., Utley, C., White, L., & Hafeez, F. (2007). Endometriosis is associated with prevalence of comorbid conditions in migraine. *Headache, 47*(7), 1069–1078.

U.S. Public Health Services Task Force. (2002). Screening for osteoporosis in postmenopausal women. In *Guide to Clinical Preventive Health Services, 2009. Recommendations of the U.S. Public Health Services Task Force*. Rockville, MD: Agency for Healthcare Research and Quality.

Vallance, J., Murray, T., Johnson, S., & Elavsky, S. (2010). Quality of life and psychosocial health in postmenopausal women achieving public health guidelines for physical activity. *Menopause, 17*(1), 64–71.

Vescovi, J., VanHeest, J., & De Souza, M. (2008). Short-term response of bone turnover to low-dose oral contraceptives in exercising women with hypothalamic amenorrhea. *Contraception, 77*(2), 97–104.

Woods, N., & Mitchell, E. (2008). Mid-life women's health. In C. Fogel, & N. Woods (Eds.), *Women's health care in advanced practice nursing*. New York: Springer.

CHAPTER

7

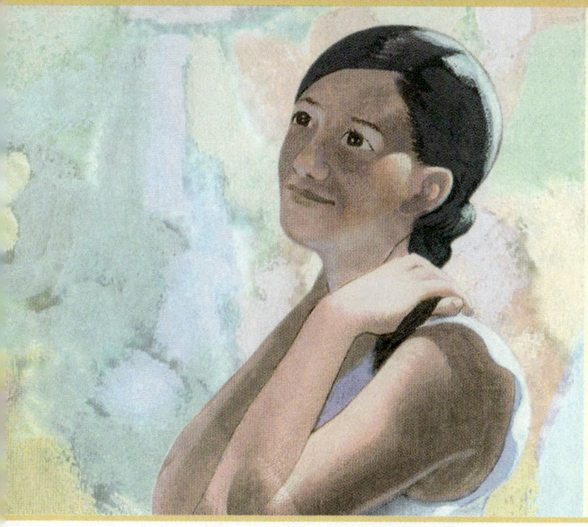

Sexually Transmitted and Other Infections

Deitra Leonard Lowdermilk

evolve WEBSITE

http://evolve.elsevier.com/Lowdermilk/MWHC/

Animation
  Pelvic Inflammatory Disease
Audio Glossary
Audio Key Points
NCLEX Review Questions
Nursing Care Plan
  The Woman with a Sexually Transmitted Infection

LEARNING OBJECTIVES

- Describe prevention of sexually transmitted infections in women, including risk reduction measures.
- Differentiate signs, symptoms, diagnosis, and management of nonpregnant and pregnant women with sexually transmitted bacterial infections.
- Examine the care of nonpregnant and pregnant women with selected sexually transmitted viral infections (human immunodeficiency virus [HIV]; hepatitis A, B, and C; human papillomavirus).
- Compare and contrast signs, symptoms, and management of selected vaginal infections in nonpregnant and pregnant women.
- Discuss the effect of group B streptococci (GBS) on pregnancy and management of pregnant clients with GBS.
- Identify the effects of TORCH infections on pregnancy and the fetus.
- Describe the health consequences (e.g., ectopic pregnancy, infertility) for women who are infected with reproductive tract infections.
- Review principles of infection control for HIV and blood-borne pathogens.

Reproductive tract infection is a term that encompasses both sexually transmitted infections and other common genital tract infections (Marrazzo, Guest, & Cates, 2007). *Sexually transmitted diseases (STDs),* or **sexually transmitted infections (STIs),** include more than 25 organisms that cause infections or infectious disease syndromes primarily transmitted by close, intimate contact (Box 7-1). These terms, used interchangeably in this text, have replaced the older designation, *venereal disease,* which described primarily gonorrhea and syphilis. Caused by a wide spectrum of bacteria, viruses, protozoa, and ectoparasites (organisms that live on the outside of the body, such as a louse), STIs are a direct cause of tremendous human suffering, place heavy demands on health care services, and cost society hundreds of millions of dollars to treat. Despite the U.S. Surgeon General's targeting STIs as a priority for prevention and control efforts, STIs are among the most common health problems in the United States, especially for young people. The Centers for Disease Control and Prevention (CDC) estimate that more than 19 million Americans are infected with STIs every year; almost half of these are between the ages of 15 and 24 (CDC, 2009b). The most common STDs or STIs in women are chlamydia, gonorrhea, human papillomavirus, herpes simplex virus type 2, syphilis, and HIV infection; these are discussed in this chapter. Common vaginal infections are also discussed. Neonatal effects of STIs are discussed in Chapter 35.

PREVENTION

Preventing infection (primary prevention) is the most effective way of reducing the adverse consequences of STIs for women and for society. With the advent of serious and potentially lethal STIs that are not readily cured or are incurable, primary prevention becomes critical. Prompt diagnosis and treatment of

BOX 7-1 SEXUALLY TRANSMITTED INFECTIONS

BACTERIA
- Chlamydia
- Gonorrhea
- Syphilis
- Chancroid
- Lymphogranuloma venereum
- Genital mycoplasmas
- Group B streptococci

VIRUSES
- Human immunodeficiency virus
- Herpes simplex virus, types 1 and 2
- Cytomegalovirus
- Viral hepatitis, types A and B
- Human papillomavirus

PROTOZOA
- Trichomoniasis

PARASITES
- Pediculosis (may or may not be sexually transmitted)
- Scabies (may or may not be sexually transmitted)

current infections (secondary prevention) also can prevent personal complications and transmission to others.

Preventing the spread of STIs requires that women at risk for transmitting or acquiring infections change their behavior. A critical first step is for the nurse to include questions about a woman's sexual history, risky sexual behaviors, and drug-related risky behaviors as a part of her assessment (Box 7-2). Techniques that are effective in providing prevention counseling include using open-ended questions, using understandable language, and reassuring the woman that treatment will be provided regardless of consideration such as ability to pay, language spoken, or lifestyle (Marrazzo et al., 2007; Ravin, 2007). Prevention messages should include descriptions of specific actions to be taken to avoid acquiring or transmitting STIs (e.g., refraining from sexual activity when STI-related symptoms are present) and should be individualized for each woman, giving attention to her specific risk factors.

To be motivated to take preventive actions, a woman must believe that acquiring a disease will be serious for her and that she is at risk for infection. However, most individuals tend to underestimate their personal risk of infection in a given situation; thus many women may not perceive themselves as being at risk for contracting an STI. Telling them that they should carry condoms may not be well received. Although levels of awareness of STIs are generally high, widespread misconceptions or specific gaps in knowledge also exist. Therefore nurses have a responsibility to ensure that their clients have accurate, complete knowledge about transmission and symptoms of STIs and behaviors that place them at risk for contracting an infection.

Primary preventive measures are individual activities aimed at deterring infection. Risk-free options include complete abstinence from sexual activities that transmit semen, blood, or other body fluids or that allow skin-to-skin contact (Marrazzo et al., 2007). Alternatively, involvement in a mutually monogamous relationship with an uninfected partner also eliminates risk of contracting STIs. When neither of these options is realistic for a woman, however, the nurse must focus on other, more feasible measures.

BOX 7-2 ASSESSING STI AND HIV RISK BEHAVIORS

SEXUAL RISK
- Are you sexually active now?
- If no, have you had sex in the past?
- Ever had an oral, vaginal, or anal sexual experience with another person?
- With how many different people? 1? 2 or 3? 4 to 10? More than 10?
- Have your partners been men, women, both?
- Ever thought that a sex partner put you at risk for AIDS or an STI (IV drug user, bisexual)?
- Ever had an STI (herpes, gonorrhea, genital warts, chlamydia)?
- Ever had sex against your will?
- What do you do to protect yourself from HIV and STIs?
- Do you use male condoms? Female condoms? Other barriers?

DRUG USE—RELATED RISK
- Ever injected drugs using shared equipment, including street drugs, steroids?
- Ever had sex with a person who uses and shares?
- Ever had sex while stoned, high, or drunk, so that you can't remember the details?
- Ever exchanged sex for drugs, money, shelter?

BLOOD-RELATED RISKS
- Ever had a blood transfusion?
- Ever had sex with a person who had a blood transfusion?
- Ever had sex with a person with hemophilia?
- Ever received donor semen, egg, transplanted organ or tissue?
- Ever shared equipment for tattoo, body piercing?

OTHER
- Ever had a test for HIV?
- Ever worried about AIDS and would like to talk with someone about it?

AIDS, Acquired immunodeficiency syndrome; *HIV*, human immunodeficiency virus; *IV*, intravenous; *STI*, sexually transmitted infection.
Source: Marrazzo, J., Guest, F., & Cates, W. (2007). Reproductive tract infections, including HIV and sexually transmitted infections. In R. Hatcher, J. Trussell, A. Nelson, W. Cates, F. Guest, & D. Kowal (Eds.), *Contraceptive technology* (19th ed.). New York: Ardent Media.

Risk Reduction Measures

An essential component of primary prevention is counseling women regarding risk reduction practices, including knowledge of her partner, reduction of the number of partners, low risk sex, avoiding the exchange of body fluids, and vaccination (CDC, Workowski, & Berman, 2006).

No aspect of prevention is more important than knowing one's partner. Reducing the number of partners and avoiding partners who have had many sexual partners decreases a woman's chance of contracting an STI. Deciding not to have sexual contact with casual acquaintances also may be helpful. Discussing each new partner's previous sexual history and exposure to STIs are augment other efforts to reduce risk; however, sexual partners may not always be truthful about their sexual history. Women must be cautioned that practicing risk reduction measures is always advisable, even when partners insist otherwise. Critically important is whether male partners resist or accept wearing condoms. This is crucial when women are not sure about their partners' history. Women should be cautioned against making decisions about a partner's sexual and other behaviors based on appearances and unfounded assumptions such as the following (Marrazzo et al., 2007):

- Single people have many partners and risky practices.
- Older people have few partners and infrequent sexual encounters.
- Sexually experienced people know how to use risk reduction measures.
- Married people are heterosexual, low risk, and monogamous.
- People who look healthy are healthy.
- People with good jobs do not use drugs.

Sexually active persons also may benefit from carefully examining a partner for lesions, sores, ulcerations, rashes, redness, discharge, swelling, and odor before initiating sexual activity. Teach women about low risk sexual practices and which sexual practices to avoid (Table 7-1).

The physical barrier promoted for the prevention of sexual transmission of HIV and other STIs is the condom (male and female). Nurses can help motivate clients to use condoms by initiating a discussion of the subject with them. This gives women permission to discuss any concerns, misconceptions, or hesitations they may have about using condoms. Information to be discussed includes the importance of using latex or plastic male condoms rather than natural skin condoms for STI protection. The nurse should remind women to use a condom with every sexual encounter, to use each one only once, to use a condom with a current expiration date, and to handle it carefully to avoid damaging it with fingernails, teeth, or other sharp objects. Condoms should be stored away from high heat. Although it is not ideal, women may choose to safely carry condoms in wallets, shoes, or inside a bra. Women can be taught the differences among condoms: price ranges, sizes, and where they can be purchased. Explicit instructions for how to apply a male condom are included in Box 8-3.

The female condom—a lubricated polyurethane sheath with a ring on each end, one end that is inserted into the vagina and the other end covering the labia (see Figure 8-7, *A*)—has been shown in laboratory studies to be an effective mechanical barrier to viruses, including HIV. Although no clinical studies have been completed to evaluate the efficacy of female condoms in protecting against STIs, laboratory studies have demonstrated that polyurethane can block smaller viruses such as the herpesvirus and HIV (Murphy, Morgan, & Likis, 2006). Further, studies suggest that the female condom is at least as effective as male condoms in preventing transmission of STIs. The CDC, Workowski, and Berman (2006) state that when used correctly and consistently, the female condom may substantially reduce STI risk and recommends its use when a male condom cannot be used properly. What is important and should be stressed by nurses is the consistent use of condoms for every act of sexual intimacy when there is the possibility of transmission of disease.

Despite concern about the potential for cervicovaginal epithelial disruption with nonoxynol-9 (N-9)–based spermicides, interest in vaginally applied chemical barriers that provide dual contraceptive and protection against bacterial STIs remains. Evidence has shown that vaginal spermicides do not protect against certain STIs, although more than 60 potential microbicides are in development and 18 are in clinical trials (Murphy et al., 2006). Condoms lubricated with N-9 are not recommended (American College of Obstetricians and Gynecologists [ACOG], 2008; CDC et al., 2006).

TABLE 7-1 RISK-REDUCTION PRACTICES

SAFEST	LOW BUT POTENTIAL RISK	HIGH RISK (UNSAFE)
Abstinence Self-masturbation Monogamous (both partners and no high risk activities) and tested negative for HIV and other STIs Hugging, massage, touching (assuming no break in skin) Dry kissing Mutual masturbation without contact with semen or vaginal secretions and no broken skin Drug abstinence Sexual fantasy Erotic conversation, books, movies Erotic bathing, showering Eroticizing feet, fingers, buttocks, abdomen, ears	Wet kissing* Vaginal intercourse with condom; anal intercourse with condom Monogamous (both partners and no high risk activities) but not tested for HIV or other STIs Oral sex with woman wearing female condom Oral sex with man wearing condom Mutual masturbation without contact with semen or vaginal secretions; healthy intact skin or use of latex or plastic barrier Urine contact with intact skin	Unprotected anal intercourse; unprotected vaginal intercourse Oral-anal contact Multiple sexual partners, no HIV or STI testing Any sex (fisting, rough vaginal or anal intercourse, rape) that causes tissue damage or bleeding Oral sex on man or woman without a latex or plastic barrier Sharing sex toys, douche equipment Sharing needles Blood contact, including menstrual blood

*Assumes no breaks in skin.

HIV, Human immunodeficiency virus; *STI,* sexually transmitted infection.

Sources: Centers for Disease Control and Prevention, Workowski, K., & Berman, S. (2006). Sexually transmitted diseases treatment guidelines, 2006. *MMMR Morbidity and Mortality Weekly Report, 55*(RR-11), 1-94; Marrazzo, J., Guest, F., & Cates, W. (2007). Reproductive tract infections, including HIV and sexually transmitted infections. In R. Hatcher, J. Trussell, A. Nelson, W. Cates, F. Guest, & D. Kowal (Eds.), *Contraceptive technology* (19th ed.). New York: Ardent Media.

A key issue in condom use as a preventive strategy is to stress to women that in sexual encounters men must comply with a woman's suggestion or request that they use a condom. Moreover, condom use must be renegotiated with every sexual contact, and women must address the issue of control of sexual decision making every time they request a male partner to use a condom. Women may fear that their partner would be offended if a condom were introduced. Some women may fear rejection and abandonment, conflict, potential violence, or loss of economic support if they suggest the use of condoms to prevent STI transmission. For many individuals, condoms are symbols of extrarelationship activity. Introduction of a condom into a long-term relationship in which one has not been used previously threatens the trust assumed in most long-term relationships.

Nurses must suggest strategies to enhance a woman's condom negotiation and communication skills. It can be suggested that she talk with her partner about condom use at a time removed from sexual activity, which may make it easier to bring up the subject. Role playing possible partner reactions with a woman and her alternative responses can be helpful. Asking a woman who appears particularly uncomfortable to rehearse how she might approach the topic is useful, particularly when a woman fears her partner may be resistant. The nurse might suggest the woman begin by saying, "I need to talk with you about something that is important to both of us. It's hard for me, and I feel embarrassed, but I think we need to talk about reducing risk during sex." If women are able to sort out their feelings and fears before talking with their partners, they may feel more comfortable and in control of the situation. Women can be reassured that it is natural to be uncomfortable and that the hardest part is getting started. Nurses should help their clients clarify what they will and will not do sexually because it will be easier to discuss their concerns with their partners if they have thought about what to say. Women can be reminded that their partner may need time to think about what they have said and that they must pay attention to their partner's response.

Many women do not anticipate or prepare for sexual activity in advance; embarrassment or discomfort in purchasing condoms may prevent some women from using them. Cultural barriers also may impede the use of condoms; for example, Hispanic gender roles make it difficult for Hispanic women to suggest using condoms to a partner. In general, suggesting condom use implies that a woman is sexually active, that she is "available" for sex, and that she is "seeking" sex; these are messages that many women are uncomfortable conveying, given the prevailing mores of our country. In a society that commonly views a woman who carries a condom as overprepared, possibly oversexed, and willing to have sex with any man, expecting her to insist on the use of condoms in a sexual encounter is somewhat optimistic at best and unrealistic at worst.

Finally, women should be counseled to watch out for situations that make it hard to talk about and to practice safer sex. These include romantic times when condoms are not available and when alcohol or drugs make it impossible to make wise decisions about safer sex.

Vaccination is an effective method for the prevention of some STIs such as hepatitis B and human papillomavirus (HPV). Hepatitis B vaccine is recommended for women at high risk for STIs (CDC, 2008b, 2008c). A vaccine is available for HPV types 6, 11, 16, and 18 for girls and women. It is recommended for girls 11 and 12, but can be given to girls as early as 9 years of age; catch-up vaccinations for girls and young women ages 13 to 26 may also be given (CDC, 2010b).

SEXUALLY TRANSMITTED BACTERIAL INFECTIONS

Chlamydia

Chlamydia trachomatis is the most commonly reported STI in American women. In 2008 there were 1.2 million cases reported and estimates of more than 2 million cases unreported (CDC, 2009b). These infections are often silent and highly destructive; their sequelae and complications can be very serious. In women, chlamydial infections are difficult to diagnose; the symptoms, if present, are nonspecific, and the organism is expensive to culture.

Early identification of *C. trachomatis* is important because untreated infection often leads to acute salpingitis or pelvic inflammatory disease. Pelvic inflammatory disease is the most serious complication of chlamydial infections, and past chlamydial infections are associated with an increased risk of ectopic pregnancy and tubal factor infertility. Furthermore, chlamydial infection of the cervix causes inflammation, resulting in microscopic cervical ulcerations, and thus may increase the risk of acquiring HIV infection. More than half of infants born to mothers with chlamydia will develop conjunctivitis or pneumonia after perinatal exposure to the mother's infected cervix. *C. trachomatis* is the most common infectious cause of ophthalmia neonatorum. Neonatal ocular prophylaxis with silver nitrate solution or antibiotic ointment does not prevent perinatal transmission from mother to infant, nor does it adequately treat chlamydial infection (see Chapter 35). Sexually active women ages 15 to 19 have the highest rates of infection (CDC, 2009b). Women older than 30 years have the lowest rate of infection. Risky behaviors, including multiple partners and nonuse of barrier methods of birth control, increase a woman's risk of chlamydial infection. Lower socioeconomic status may be a risk factor, especially with respect to treatment-seeking behaviors.

Screening and Diagnosis

In addition to obtaining information regarding the presence of risk factors, the nurse should inquire about the presence of any symptoms. The CDC, Workowski, and Berman (2006) and U.S. Preventive Services Task Force (USPSTF, 2007a) strongly recommend screening of asymptomatic women at high risk in whom infection would otherwise go undetected (see www.cdc.org, and www.ahrq.gov). CDC guidelines recommend yearly screening of all sexually active adolescents, women between ages 20 and 25 years, and women older than 25 years who are at high risk (e.g., those with new or multiple partners). In addition, whenever possible, all women with two or more of the risk factors for chlamydia should be cultured. All pregnant women should have cervical cultures for chlamydia at the first prenatal visit. Screening late in the third trimester (36 weeks) may be carried out if the woman was positive previously, or if she is younger than 25 years, has a new sex partner, or has multiple sex partners.

CLINICAL REASONING

STI Counseling in Pregnancy

Meera is a 19-year-old African-American woman, gravida 1 para 0, who has come to the prenatal clinic for her first visit. She has a history of drug use (marijuana and alcohol). She says her current boyfriend is her support person but he is not the father of the baby. Meera is currently unemployed and living with her mother. She has been given an explanation of the prenatal laboratory tests that will be done during her examination. She says that she does not see why she has to have the tests for sexually transmitted infections (STIs) because she has not had these infections.

1. Evidence—Is there sufficient evidence to draw conclusions about what advice the nurse should give?
2. Assumptions—Describe underlying assumptions about the following issues:
   a. STI effects on pregnancy and the fetus
   b. STI risk factors
   c. Prevention of maternal-fetal transmission of human immunodeficiency virus (HIV)
3. What implications and priorities for nursing care can be drawn at this time?
4. Does the evidence objectively support your conclusion?
5. Are there alternative perspectives to your conclusion?

Although chlamydial infections are usually asymptomatic, some women may experience spotting or postcoital bleeding, mucoid or purulent cervical discharge, or dysuria. Bleeding results from inflammation and erosion of the cervical columnar epithelium. Women taking oral contraceptives may have breakthrough bleeding.

Laboratory diagnosis of chlamydia is by culture (expensive and labor intensive), deoxyribonucleic acid (DNA) probe (relatively less expensive but less sensitive), enzyme immunoassay (also relatively less expensive but less sensitive), and nucleic acid amplification tests (expensive but has relatively higher sensitivity) (CDC et al., 2006). Special culture media and proper handling of specimens are important, so the nurse should always know what is required in his or her individual practice site. Chlamydial culture testing is not always available, primarily because of expense.

Management

The CDC recommendations for treatment of urethral, cervical, and rectal chlamydial infections, which are summarized in Table 7-2, are doxycycline and azithromycin (CDC et al., 2006). Azithromycin is often prescribed when compliance may be a problem, because only one dose is needed; however, expense is a concern with this medication. If the woman is pregnant, erythromycin or amoxicillin is used. Women who have a chlamydial infection and also are infected with HIV should be treated with the same regimen as those who are not infected with HIV.

Because chlamydia is often asymptomatic, the woman should be cautioned to take all medication prescribed. All exposed sexual partners should be treated. Women, especially pregnant women, should be encouraged to be retested 3 to 4 months after treatment, especially if their partners did not seek treatment (CDC, 2007).

Gonorrhea

Gonorrhea is probably the oldest communicable disease in the United States and second to chlamydia in reported cases. The CDC estimates about 700,000 cases of gonorrhea a year will occur in the United States (CDC, 2009b). The incidence of drug-resistant cases of gonorrhea, in particular, penicillinase-producing *Neisseria gonorrhoeae* (PPNG), is increasing dramatically in the United States.

Gonorrhea is caused by the aerobic, gram-negative diplococcus, *N. gonorrhoeae.* Gonorrhea is almost exclusively transmitted by sexual contact. The principal means of communication is genital-to-genital contact; however, it also is spread by oral-to-genital and anal-to-genital contact. There also is evidence that infection may spread in females from vagina to rectum. Age is probably the most important risk factor associated with gonorrhea. In the United States the highest reported rates of infection are among sexually active teenagers, young adults, and African-Americans. In 2008, 70% of cases of gonorrhea were reported by African-Americans, and mostly in young girls ages 15 to 19 (CDC, 2009b).

Women are often asymptomatic, with one third of infections in adolescent women going unnoticed. When symptoms are present they are often less specific than are the symptoms in men. Women may have a purulent endocervical discharge, but discharge is usually minimal or absent. Menstrual irregularities may be the presenting symptom, or women may complain of pain—chronic or acute severe pelvic or lower abdominal pain or longer, more painful menses. Infrequently, dysuria, vague abdominal pain, or low backache prompts a woman to seek care. Gonococcal rectal infection may occur in women after anal intercourse, with 10% to 30% of urogenital infections accompanied by rectal infection. Individuals with rectal gonorrhea may be completely asymptomatic or, conversely, have severe symptoms with profuse purulent anal discharge, rectal pain, and blood in the stool. Rectal itching, fullness, pressure, and pain also are common symptoms, as is diarrhea. A diffuse vaginitis with vulvitis is the most common form of gonococcal infection in prepubertal girls. There may be few signs of infection, or vaginal discharge, dysuria, and swollen, reddened labia may be present.

Gonococcal infections in pregnancy can affect both mother and fetus. In women with cervical gonorrhea, salpingitis may develop in the first trimester. Perinatal complications of gonococcal infection include premature rupture of membranes, preterm birth, chorioamnionitis, neonatal sepsis, intrauterine growth restriction, and maternal postpartum sepsis. Amniotic infection syndrome manifested by placental, fetal, and umbilical cord inflammation after premature rupture of the membranes may result from gonorrheal infections during pregnancy. Ophthalmia neonatorum, the most common manifestation of neonatal gonococcal infections, is highly contagious and, if untreated, may lead to blindness of the newborn (see Chapter 35).

Screening and Diagnosis

Because gonococcal infections in women often are asymptomatic, the CDC recommends screening all women at risk for gonorrhea (CDC et al., 2006). All pregnant women should be screened at the first prenatal visit, and infected women and those identified with risky behaviors rescreened at 36 weeks of gestation. Gonococcal infection cannot be diagnosed reliably by clinical signs and symptoms alone. Individuals may have "classic" symptoms, vague symptoms that may be attributed to a number of conditions, or no symptoms at all. Cultures with selective media are considered the gold standard for diagnosis of gonorrhea. Cultures should be obtained from the endocervix, the rectum, and when indicated, the pharynx. Thayer-Martin cultures are recommended to diagnose gonorrhea in women. Any woman suspected of having gonorrhea should have a chlamydial culture and serologic test for syphilis if one has not been done in the past 2 months, because coinfection is common.

Management

Management of gonorrhea is straightforward, and the cure is usually rapid with appropriate antibiotic therapy (see Table 7-1). Single-dose efficacy is a major consideration in selecting an antibiotic regimen for women with gonorrhea. Another important consideration is the high percentage (45%) of women with coexisting chlamydial infections. The treatment of choice for uncomplicated urethral, endocervical, and rectal infections in pregnant and nonpregnant women is cefixime or ceftriaxone. The CDC recommends concomitant treatment for chlamydia (CDC, 2007). All women with both gonorrhea and syphilis

TABLE 7-2 **SEXUALLY TRANSMITTED INFECTIONS AND DRUG THERAPIES FOR WOMEN***

DISEASE	NONPREGNANT WOMEN (13-17 YR)	NONPREGNANT WOMEN (>18 YR)	PREGNANT WOMEN	LACTATING WOMEN†
Chlamydia	*Recommended:* Azithromycin, 1 g orally once *or* Doxycycline, 100 mg orally bid for 7 days	*Recommended:* Azithromycin, 1 g orally once *or* Doxycycline, 100 mg orally bid for 7 days	*Recommended:* Azithromycin, 1 g orally once *or* Amoxicillin, 500 mg orally tid for 7 days	*Recommended:* Azithromycin, 1 g orally once *or* Amoxicillin, 500 mg orally tid for 7 days
Gonorrhea	*Recommended:* Ceftriaxone, 125 mg IM once (adolescents who weigh >45 kg can be treated with any regimen recommended for adults) Treatment for chlamydia if infection not ruled out	*Recommended:* Ceftriaxone, 125 mg IM once *or* Cefixime 400 mg orally once Treatment for chlamydia if infection not ruled out	*Recommended:* Ceftriaxone, 125 mg IM once Treatment for chlamydia if infection not ruled out	*Recommended:* Ceftriaxone, 125 mg IM once Treatment for chlamydia if infection not ruled out
Syphilis	Primary, secondary, early latent disease: *Recommended:* Benzathine penicillin G, 2.4 million units IM once Late latent or unknown duration disease: *Recommended:* Benzathine penicillin G, 7.2 million units total, administered as three doses, 2.4 million units each, at 1-wk intervals *Penicillin allergy:* Doxycycline, 100 mg orally qid for 14 days *or* Tetracycline, 500 mg orally qid for 14 days	Primary, secondary, early latent disease: *Recommended:* Benzathine penicillin G, 2.4 million units IM once Late latent or unknown duration disease: *Recommended:* Benzathine penicillin G, 7.2 million units total, administered as three doses, 2.4 million units each, at 1-wk intervals *Penicillin allergy:* Doxycycline, 100 mg orally qid for 14 days *or* Tetracycline, 500 mg orally qid for 14 days	Primary, secondary, early latent disease: *Recommended:* Benzathine penicillin G, 2.4 million units IM once (some experts recommend a second dose of benzathine penicillin, 2.4 million units, 1 wk later) Late latent or unknown duration disease: *Recommended:* Benzathine penicillin G, 7.2 million units total, administered as three doses, 2.4 million units each, at 1-wk intervals *Penicillin allergy:* No proven alternatives to penicillin in pregnancy. Pregnant women who have a history of allergy to penicillin should be desensitized and treated with penicillin	Primary, secondary, early latent disease: *Recommended:* Benzathine penicillin G, 2.4 million units IM once Late latent or unknown duration disease: *Recommended:* Benzathine penicillin G, 7.2 million units total, administered as three doses, 2.4 million units each, at 1-wk intervals
Human papillomavirus	*Recommended for external genital warts:* Client-applied: Podofilox, 0.5% solution, or gel to wart bid for 3 days followed by 4-day rest for ≤4 cycles *or* Imiquimod, 5% cream, at hs 3 times a week for ≤16 wk Provider-applied: Cryotherapy with liquid nitrogen or cryoprobe *or* Podophyllin resin, 10%-25% in tincture of benzoin compound weekly (wash off in 1-4 hr). Repeat weekly as necessary *or* Trichloracetic acid (TCA) or bichloracetic acid (BCA) 80%-90% weekly	*Recommended for external genital warts:* Client-applied: Podofilox, 0.5% solution, or gel to wart bid for 3 days followed by 4-day rest for ≤4 cycles *or* Imiquimod, 5% cream, at hs 3 times a week for ≤16 wk Provider-applied: Cryotherapy with liquid nitrogen or cryoprobe *or* Podophyllin resin, 10%-25% in tincture of benzoin compound weekly (wash off in 1-4 hr). Repeat weekly as necessary *or* TCA or BCA 80%-90% weekly	*Recommended for external genital warts:* Provider applied: Cryotherapy with liquid nitrogen or cryoprobe *or* TCA or BCA 80%-90% weekly Imiquimod, podophyllin, and podofilox should not be used in pregnancy—unless benefits outweigh risks, other therapies pose fewer risks	*Recommended for external genital warts:* Provider applied: Cryotherapy with liquid nitrogen or cryoprobe *or* TCA or BCA 80%-90% weekly Imiquimod, podophyllin, and podofilox should not be used during lactation—unless benefits outweigh risks, other therapies pose fewer risks

*List is not inclusive of all drugs that may be used as alternatives.

†These medications are usually compatible with breastfeeding.

bid, Twice daily; *hs,* bedtime; *IM,* intramuscularly; *IV,* intravenous; *qid,* four times daily; *tid,* three times daily.

Sources: American Academy of Pediatrics Committee on Drugs. (2002). The transfer of drugs and other chemicals into human milk. *Pediatrics, 108*(3), 776-789; Centers for Disease Control and Prevention, Workowski, K., & Berman, S. (2006). Sexually transmitted diseases treatment guidelines 2006. *MMWR Morbidity and Mortality Weekly Report, 55*(RR-11), 1-94; Centers for Disease Control and Prevention (CDC). (2007). *Updated recommended treatment regimens for gonococcal infections and associated conditions, United States, April, 2007.* Available at www.cdc.gov/std/ treatment/2006/updated-regimens.htm. Accessed June 2, 2010.

TABLE 7-2 SEXUALLY TRANSMITTED INFECTIONS AND DRUG THERAPIES FOR WOMEN*—cont'd

DISEASE	NONPREGNANT WOMEN (13-17 YR)	NONPREGNANT WOMEN (>18 YR)	PREGNANT WOMEN	LACTATING WOMEN[†]
Genital herpes simplex virus (HSV type 1 or 2)	*Primary infection:* Acyclovir, 400 mg orally tid for 7-10 days *or* Acyclovir, 200 mg orally 5 times a day for 7-10 days *or* Famciclovir, 250 mg orally tid for 7-10 days *or* Valacyclovir, 1 g orally bid for 7-10 days *Recurrent infection:* Acyclovir, 400 mg orally tid for 5 days *or* Acyclovir, 800 mg orally bid for 5 days *or* Acyclovir, 800 mg orally tid for 2 days *or* Famciclovir, 125 mg orally bid for 5 days or 1000 mg orally bid for 1 day *or* Valacyclovir, 500 mg orally bid for 5 days or 1 g orally once a day for 5 days *Suppression therapy:* Daily for 1 year or more Acyclovir, 400 mg orally bid *or* Famciclovir, 250 mg orally bid *or* Valacyclovir, 500 mg orally once a day *or* Valacyclovir, 1 g orally once a day	*Primary infection:* Acyclovir, 400 mg orally tid for 7-10 days *or* Acyclovir, 200 mg orally 5 times a day for 7-10 days *or* Famciclovir, 250 mg orally tid for 7-10 days *or* Valacyclovir, 1 g orally bid for 7-10 days *Recurrent infection:* Acyclovir, 400 mg orally tid for 5 days *or* Acyclovir, 800 mg orally bid for 5 days *or* Acyclovir, 800 mg orally tid for 2 days *or* Famciclovir, 125 mg orally bid for 5 days *or* Valacyclovir, 500 mg orally bid for 5 days *Suppression therapy:* Daily for 1 year or more Acyclovir, 400 mg orally bid *or* Famciclovir, 250 mg orally bid *or* Valacyclovir, 500 mg orally once a day *or* Valacyclovir, 1 g orally once a day	No increase in birth defects beyond the general population has been found with acyclovir use in pregnancy. Acyclovir, 400 mg orally tid for 7 days for first episode or severe recurrent infection. May be given IV if infection is severe. Daily suppression therapy 4 weeks before the birth for women with recurrent infections can reduce the need for a cesarean birth.	Acyclovir usually is considered compatible with breastfeeding Acyclovir, 400 mg tid for 7 days Suppressive therapy: Same as non-pregnant women (>18 yr)

should be treated for syphilis according to CDC guidelines (see discussion of syphilis in this chapter).

Gonorrhea is a highly communicable disease. Recent (past 30 days) sexual partners should be examined, cultured, and treated with appropriate regimens. Most treatment failures result from reinfection. The client must be informed of this, as well as of the consequences of reinfection in terms of chronicity, complications, and potential infertility. Women are counseled to use condoms. All clients with gonorrhea should be offered confidential counseling and testing for HIV infection.

> **LEGAL TIP: Reporting Communicable Diseases**
>
> Gonorrhea is a reportable communicable disease. Health care providers are legally responsible for reporting all cases to the health authorities, usually the local health department in the client's county of residence. Women should be informed that the case will be reported, told why, and informed of the possibility of being contacted by a health department epidemiologist.

Syphilis

Syphilis, one of the earliest described STIs, is caused by *Treponema pallidum*, a motile spirochete. Transmission is thought to be by entry in the subcutaneous tissue through microscopic abrasions that can occur during sexual intercourse. The disease also can be transmitted through kissing, biting, or oral-genital sex. Transplacental transmission may occur at any time during pregnancy; the degree of risk is related to the quantity of spirochetes in the maternal bloodstream.

Rates of syphilis in the United States among women, especially African-Americans have continued to rise since 2004.

Syphilis is a complex disease that can lead to serious systemic disease and even death when untreated. Infection manifests itself in distinct stages with different symptoms and clinical manifestations. *Primary* syphilis is characterized by a primary lesion, the chancre, that appears 5 to 90 days after infection. This lesion often begins as a painless papule at the site of inoculation and then erodes to form a nontender, shallow, indurated, clean ulcer several millimeters to centimeters in size (Fig. 7-1, *A*). *Secondary* syphilis

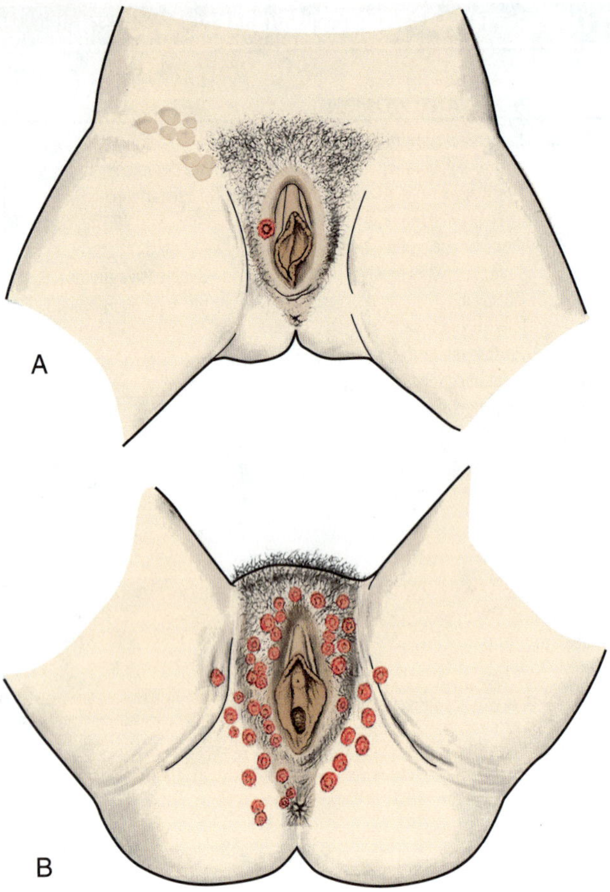

FIG. 7-1 Syphilis. **A,** Primary stage: chancre with inguinal adenopathy. **B,** Secondary stage: condylomata lata.

occurs 6 weeks to 6 months after the appearance of the chancre and is characterized by a widespread, symmetric maculopapular rash on the palms and soles and generalized lymphadenopathy. The infected individual also may experience fever, headache, and malaise. Condylomata lata (broad, painless, pink-gray, wartlike infectious lesions) may develop on the vulva, the perineum, or the anus (see Fig. 7-1, *B*). If the woman is untreated, she enters a latent phase that is asymptomatic for the majority of individuals. Latent infections are those that lack clinical manifestations but are detected by serologic testing. If the infection was acquired in the preceding year, the infection is termed an *early latent* infection. If it is left untreated, tertiary syphilis will develop in about one third of these women. Neurologic, cardiovascular, musculoskeletal, or multiorgan system complications can develop in the third stage.

Animation—Pelvic Inflammatory Disease

Screening and Diagnosis

All women who are diagnosed with another STI or with HIV should be screened for syphilis. All pregnant women should be screened for syphilis at the first prenatal visit and again in early third trimester and at the time of giving birth if high risk (CDC et al., 2006; USPSTF, 2009b). Diagnosis is dependent on microscopic examination of primary and secondary lesion tissue and serology during latency and late infection. A test for antibodies may not be reactive in the presence of active infection because it takes time for the body's immune system to develop antibodies to any antigens. Up to one third of people in early primary syphilis may have nonreactive serologic tests. Two types of serologic tests are used: nontreponemal and treponemal. Nontreponemal antibody tests such as the Venereal Disease Research Laboratories (VDRL) or rapid plasma reagin (RPR) are used as screening tests. False-positive results are not unusual, particularly when conditions such as acute infection, autoimmune disorders, malignancy, pregnancy, and drug addiction exist and after immunization or vaccination. The treponemal tests, fluorescent treponemal antibody absorbed (FTA-ABS), and microhemagglutination assays for antibody to *T. pallidum* (MHA-TP), are used to confirm positive results. Test results in clients with early primary or incubating syphilis may be negative. Seroconversion usually takes place 6 to 8 weeks after exposure, so testing should be repeated in 1 to 2 months when a suggestive genital lesion exists. Tests for concomitant STIs (e.g., chlamydia and gonorrhea) should be done (e.g., wet preps and cultures) and HIV testing offered if indicated.

Management

Penicillin is the preferred drug for treating clients with syphilis (see Table 7-2). It is the only proven therapy that has been widely used for clients with neurosyphilis, congenital syphilis, or syphilis during pregnancy. Intramuscular benzathine penicillin G is used to treat primary, secondary, and early latent syphilis. Although doxycycline, tetracycline, and erythromycin are alternative treatments for penicillin-allergic clients, both tetracycline and doxycycline are contraindicated in pregnancy, and erythromycin is unlikely to cure a fetal infection. Therefore, pregnant women should, if necessary, receive skin testing and be treated with penicillin or be desensitized (CDC, et al., 2006). Specific protocols are recommended by the CDC.

> **! NURSING ALERT**
>
> Clients treated for syphilis may experience a Jarisch-Herxheimer reaction. This acute febrile reaction is often accompanied by headache, myalgias, and arthralgias that develop within the first 24 hours of treatment. The reaction may be treated symptomatically with analgesics and antipyretics. If the treatment precipitates this reaction in the second half of pregnancy, women are at risk for preterm labor and birth. They should be advised to contact their health care provider if they notice any change in fetal movement or have any contractions.

Monthly follow-up is mandatory so that repeated treatment may be given if needed. The nurse should emphasize the necessity of long-term serologic testing even in the absence of symptoms. The woman should be advised to practice sexual abstinence until treatment is completed, all evidence of primary and secondary syphilis is gone, and serologic evidence of a cure is demonstrated. Women should be told to notify all partners who may have been exposed. They should be informed that the disease is reportable. Preventive measures should be discussed.

Pelvic Inflammatory Disease

Pelvic inflammatory disease (PID) is an infectious process that most commonly involves the uterine (fallopian) tubes (salpingitis), uterus (endometritis), and more rarely, the ovaries and peritoneal surfaces. Multiple organisms have been found to cause PID, and most cases are associated with more than one organism. In the past, the most common causative agent was thought to be *N. gonorrhoeae;* however, *C. trachomatis* is now estimated to cause half of all cases of PID. In addition to gonorrhea and chlamydia, a wide variety of anaerobic and aerobic bacteria are recognized to cause PID. PID encompasses a wide variety of pathologic processes; the infection can either be acute, subacute, or chronic and can have a wide range of symptoms.

Most PID results from ascending spread of microorganisms from the vagina and endocervix to the upper genital tract. This spread most frequently happens at the end of or just after menses following reception of an infectious agent. During the menstrual period, several factors facilitate the development of an infection: the cervical os is slightly open, the cervical mucus barrier is absent, and menstrual blood is an excellent medium for growth. PID also may develop after a miscarriage or an induced abortion, pelvic surgery, or childbirth.

Risk factors for acquiring PID are those associated with the risk of contracting an STI, including young age (most cases of acute PID are in women younger than age 25), nulliparity, multiple partners, high rate of new partners, and a history of STIs and PID. Women who use intrauterine devices (IUDs) may be at increased risk for PID up to 3 weeks after insertion (Eckert & Lentz, 2007b).

Women who have had PID are at increased risk for ectopic pregnancy, infertility, and chronic pelvic pain. After a single episode of PID, a woman's risk for ectopic pregnancy increases sevenfold compared with the risk for women who have never had PID. Other problems associated with PID include dyspareunia (painful intercourse), pyosalpinx (pus in the uterine tubes), tuboovarian abscess, and pelvic adhesions.

The symptoms of PID vary, depending on whether the infection is acute, subacute, or chronic; however, pain is common to all types of infection. It may be dull, cramping, and intermittent (subacute) or severe, persistent, and incapacitating (acute). Women may also report one or more of the following: fever, chills, nausea and vomiting, increased vaginal discharge, symptoms of a urinary tract infection, and irregular bleeding. Abdominal pain is usually present (Eckert & Lentz, 2007b).

Screening and Diagnosis

PID is difficult to diagnose because of the accompanying wide variety of symptoms. The CDC recommends treatment for PID in all sexually active young women and others at risk for STIs if the following criteria are present and no other cause or causes of the illness are found: lower abdominal tenderness, bilateral adnexal tenderness, and cervical motion tenderness. Other criteria for diagnosing PID include an oral temperature of 38.3° C or above, abnormal cervical or vaginal discharge, elevated erythrocyte sedimentation rate, elevated C-reactive protein, and laboratory documentation of cervical infection with *N. gonorrhoeae* or *C. trachomatis* (CDC et al., 2006).

Management

Perhaps the most important nursing intervention is prevention. Primary prevention includes education in preventing the acquisition of STIs, and secondary prevention involves preventing a lower genital tract infection from ascending to the upper genital tract. Instructing women in self-protective behaviors such as practicing risk reduction measures and using barrier methods is critical. Also important is the detection of asymptomatic gonorrheal and chlamydial infections through routine screening of women with risky behaviors or specific risk factors such as age.

TABLE 7-3 TREATMENT OF PELVIC INFLAMMATORY DISEASE

PARENTERAL TREATMENT	ORAL TREATMENT
Regimen A—Preferred Treatment Cefotetan, 2 g IV every 12 hr *or* Cefoxitin, 2 g IV every 6 hr *PLUS* Doxycycline, 100 mg IV or orally every 12 hr **Regimen B—Alternative Treatment** Clindamycin, 900 mg IV every 8 hr *PLUS* Gentamycin, loading dose IV or IM (2 mg/kg of body weight), followed by maintenance dose (1.5 mg/kg) every 8 hr. Single daily dosing may be substituted.	Ceftriaxone, 250 mg IM in a single dose *or* Cefoxitin, 2 g IM AND probenecid, 1 g orally in a single dose, concurrently *or* Other parenteral third-generation cephalosporin *PLUS* Doxycycline, 100 mg orally twice a day for 14 days *WITH OR WITHOUT* Metronidazole, 500 mg orally twice a day for 14 days

bid, Twice daily; *IM*, intramuscularly; *IV*, intravenously.
Sources: Centers for Disease Control and Prevention, Workowski, K., & Berman, S. (2006). Sexually transmitted diseases treatment guidelines 2006. *MMWR Morbidity and Mortality Weekly Report, 55*(RR-11), 1-94; Centers for Disease Control and Prevention (CDC). (2007a). *Updated recommended treatment regimens for gonococcal infections and associated conditions, United States, April, 2007.* Available at www.cdc.gov/std/ treatment/2006/updated-regimens.htm. Accessed June 2, 2010.

Although treatment regimens vary with the infecting organism, a broad-spectrum antibiotic is generally used (Table 7-3). Treatment for mild to moderately severe PID may be oral, or a combination of oral and parenteral, and regimens can be administered in inpatient or outpatient settings (CDC, 2007). The woman with acute PID should be on bed rest in a semi-Fowler position. Comfort measures include analgesics for pain and all other nursing measures applicable to a woman confined to bed. The woman should have as few pelvic examinations as possible during the acute phase of the disease. During the recovery phase the woman should restrict her activity and make every effort to get adequate rest and a nutritionally sound diet. Follow-up laboratory work after treatment should include endocervical cultures for a test of cure.

Health education is central to effective management of PID. Explain to women the nature of their disease, and encourage them to comply with all therapy and prevention recommendations, emphasizing the necessity of taking all medication, even if symptoms disappear. Counsel women to refrain from sexual intercourse until their treatment is completed. Provide contraceptive counseling. Suggest that the woman select a barrier method such as condoms or a diaphragm. A woman with a history of PID should not choose an IUD as her contraceptive method (Mishell, 2007).

The potential or actual loss of reproductive capabilities can be devastating and can adversely affect a woman's self-concept. Because PID is so closely tied to sexuality, body image, and self-concept, the woman diagnosed with it will need supportive care. Referral to a support group or for counseling may be appropriate.

SEXUALLY TRANSMITTED VIRAL INFECTIONS

Human Papillomavirus

Human papillomavirus (HPV) infections, also known as *condylomata acuminata,* or *genital warts,* is the most common viral STI seen in ambulatory health care settings. An estimated 20 million Americans are infected with HPV, and about 6.2 million new infections occur every year (CDC, 2009b). HPV, a double-stranded DNA virus, has more than 30 serotypes that can be sexually transmitted, 5 of which are known to cause genital wart formation, and 8 of which are currently thought to have oncogenic potential (CDC et al., 2006). HPV is the primary cause of cervical neoplasia (American Cancer Society [ACS], 2010).

HPV lesions in women are most commonly seen in the posterior part of the introitus; however, lesions also are found on the buttocks, the vulva, the vagina, the anus, and the cervix (Fig. 7-2). Typically the lesions are small—2 to 3 mm in diameter and 10 to 15 mm in height—soft, papillary swellings occurring singly or in clusters on the genital and anorectal region. Infections of long duration may appear as a cauliflower-like mass. In moist areas such as the vaginal introitus, the lesions may appear to have multiple, fine, fingerlike projections. Vaginal lesions are often multiple. Flat-topped papules, 1 to 4 mm in diameter, are seen most often on the cervix and often are visualized only under magnification. Warts are usually flesh colored or slightly darker on Caucasian women, black on African-American women, and brownish on Asian women. The lesions are often painless but may be uncomfortable, particularly when very large, inflamed, or ulcerated. Chronic vaginal discharge, pruritus, or dyspareunia can occur.

HPV infections are thought to be more frequent in pregnant than in nonpregnant women, with an increase in incidence from the first trimester to the third. Furthermore, a significant proportion of preexisting HPV lesions enlarge greatly during pregnancy, a proliferation presumably resulting from the relative state of immunosuppression present during pregnancy. Lesions may become so large during pregnancy that they affect urination, defecation, mobility, and fetal descent, although birth by cesarean is rarely necessary (Duff, 2007). HPV infection may be acquired by the neonate during birth; the frequency of such transmission is unknown. The preventive value of cesarean birth is unknown, and it is not recommended solely to prevent transmission of HPV infection to newborns (Duff).

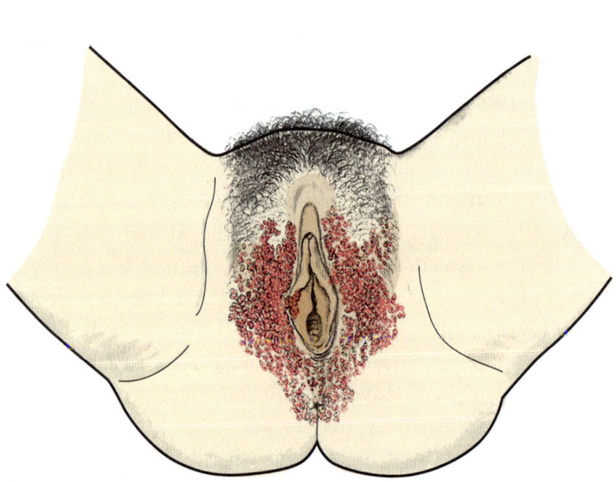

FIG. 7-2 Human papillomavirus infection. Genital warts or condylomata acuminata.

Screening and Diagnosis

A woman with HPV lesions may complain of symptoms such as a profuse, irritating vaginal discharge, itching, dyspareunia, or postcoital bleeding. She also may report "bumps" on her vulva or labia. History of a known exposure is important; however, because of the potentially long latency period and the possibility of subclinical infections in men, the lack of a history of known exposure cannot be used to exclude a diagnosis of HPV infection.

Physical inspection of the vulva, the perineum, the anus, the vagina, and the cervix is essential whenever HPV lesions are suspected or seen in one area. Because speculum examination of the vagina may block some lesions, it is important to rotate the speculum blades until all areas are visualized. When lesions are visible, the characteristic appearance previously described is considered diagnostic. However, in many instances, cervical lesions are not visible, and some vaginal or vulvar lesions also may be unobservable to the naked eye. Because of the potential spread of vulvar or vaginal lesions to the anus, gloves should be changed between vaginal and rectal examinations.

Viral screening and typing for HPV are available but not standard practice. History, evaluation of signs and symptoms, Papanicolaou (Pap) test, and physical examination are used in making a diagnosis. The HPV-DNA test can be used in women older than the age of 30 in combination with the Pap test to screen for types of HPV that are likely to cause cancer or in women with abnormal Pap test results (ACS, 2010). The only definitive diagnostic test for presence of HPV is histologic evaluation of a biopsy specimen.

HPV lesions must be differentiated from molluscum contagiosum and condylomata lata. Molluscum contagiosum lesions are half-domed, smooth, flesh-colored to pearly white papules with depressed centers. Condylomata lata are a form of secondary syphilis and generally flatter and wider than genital warts. A serologic test for syphilis would confirm the diagnosis of secondary syphilis.

Management

Untreated warts may resolve on their own in young women since their immune systems may be strong enough to fight the HPV infection. Treatment of genital warts, if needed, is often difficult. No therapy has been shown to eradicate HPV. The goal of treatment therefore is removal of warts and relief of signs and symptoms. The woman often must make multiple office visits; frequently, many different treatment modalities will be used.

Treatment of genital warts should be guided by preference of the woman, available resources, and experience of the health care provider. None of the treatments is superior to all other treatments, and no one treatment is ideal for all warts (CDC et al., 2006). Available treatments are outlined in Table 7-2. Imiquimod, podophyllin, and podofilox should not be used during pregnancy. Because the lesions can proliferate and become friable during pregnancy, many experts recommend their removal by using cryotherapy or various surgical techniques during pregnancy (CDC et al.).

Women with discomfort associated with genital warts may find that bathing with an oatmeal solution and drying the area with a cool hair dryer will provide some relief. Keeping the area clean and dry will also decrease growth of the warts. Cotton underwear and loose-fitting clothes that decrease friction and irritation also may decrease discomfort. Women should be advised to maintain a healthy lifestyle to aid the immune system; women can be counseled regarding diet, rest, stress reduction, and exercise.

Client counseling is essential. Women must understand how the virus is transmitted, that no immunity is conferred with infection, and that reacquisition of the infection is likely with repeated contact. Women should know that their partners should be checked even if they are asymptomatic. Because HPV is highly contagious, the majority of women's partners will be infected and should be treated. All sexually active women with multiple partners or a history of HPV should be encouraged to use latex condoms for intercourse to decrease acquisition or transmission of condylomata.

Instructions for all medications and treatments must be detailed. Women should be informed before treatment of the possibility of posttreatment pain associated with specific therapies. The importance of thorough treatment of concurrent vaginitis or STI should be emphasized. The link between cervical cancer and HPV infections and the need for close follow-up should be discussed. Annual health examinations are recommended to assess disease recurrence and screening for cervical cancer. Women should be counseled to have regular Pap screening, as recommended for women without genital warts (CDC et al., 2006).

Prevention

Preventive strategies that have been suggested include abstinence from all sexual activity, staying in a long-term monogamous relationship, and prophylactic vaccination (CDC, 2009a, 2010b). Two vaccines, Cervarix and Gardisil, are available and other vaccines continue to be investigated. The vaccines are most effective if given before the woman has her first sexual contact (CDC, 2009a). Practitioners should stay current with results of these clinical trials and make recommendations about vaccination based on the outcomes of the research.

Genital Herpes Simplex Virus

Unknown until the middle of the 20th century, genital herpes simplex virus (HSV) infection is now widespread in the United States. Genital HSV is more common in women: approximately 1 in 5 women ages 14 to 49 are infected (CDC, 2010a). HSV infection results in painful recurrent genital ulcers and is caused by two different antigen subtypes of herpes simplex virus: herpes simplex virus 1 (HSV-1) and herpes simplex virus 2 (HSV-2). HSV-2 is usually transmitted sexually, and HSV-1, nonsexually. Although HSV-1 is more commonly associated with gingivostomatitis and oral labial ulcers (fever blisters; cold sores) and HSV-2 with genital lesions, neither type is exclusively associated with the respective sites.

Although HSV infection is not a reportable disease, it is estimated that about 50 million people in the United States are infected with genital herpes (CDC et al., 2006). Women between the ages of 15 and 34 are most likely to become infected, especially if they have multiple sex partners. Many persons infected with HSV-2 are asymptomatic and therefore undiagnosed. They can transmit the infection unaware that they are infected.

An initial HSV genital infection is characterized by multiple painful lesions, fever, chills, malaise, and severe dysuria and may last 2 to 3 weeks. Women generally have a more severe clinical course than men. Women with primary genital herpes have many lesions that progress from macules to papules, then forming vesicles, pustules, and ulcers that crust and heal without scarring (Fig. 7-3). These ulcers are extremely tender, and primary infections may be bilateral. Women also may have itching, inguinal tenderness, and lymphadenopathy. Severe vulvar edema may develop, and women may have difficulty sitting. HSV cervicitis also is common with initial HSV-2 infections. The cervix may appear normal or be friable, reddened, ulcerated, or necrotic. A heavy, watery-to-purulent vaginal discharge is common. Extragenital lesions may be present because of autoinoculation. Urinary retention and dysuria may occur secondary to autonomic involvement of the sacral nerve root.

Women with recurrent episodes of HSV infections commonly have only local symptoms that are usually less severe than those associated with the initial infection. Systemic symptoms are usually absent, although the characteristic prodromal genital tingling is common. Recurrent lesions are unilateral, are less severe, and usually last 5 to 7 days. Lesions begin as vesicles and progress rapidly to ulcers. Few women with recurrent disease have cervicitis.

During pregnancy, maternal infection with HSV-2 can have adverse effects on both the mother and fetus. Viremia occurs during the primary infection, and congenital infection is possible, though rare. Primary infections during the first trimester have been associated with increased miscarriage rates. The most severe complication of HSV infection is neonatal herpes, a potentially fatal or severely disabling disease occurring in 1 in 2000 to 1 in 10,000 live births. Most mothers of infants who contract neonatal herpes lack histories of clinically evident genital herpes. Risk of neonatal infection is highest among women with primary herpes infection who are near term and is low among women with recurrent herpes (CDC et al., 2006).

Screening and Diagnosis

A history provides much information when making a diagnosis of herpes. A history of exposure to an infected person is important, although infection from an asymptomatic individual is possible. A history of having viral symptoms such as malaise,

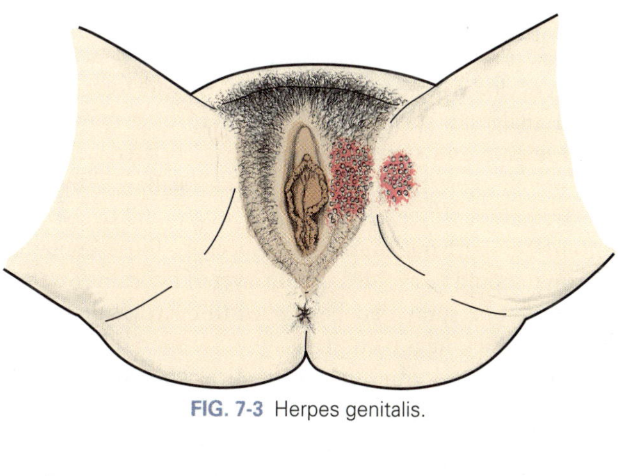

FIG. 7-3 Herpes genitalis.

headache, fever, or myalgia is suggestive. Local symptoms such as vulvar pain, dysuria, itching or burning at the site of infection, and painful genital lesions that heal spontaneously also are highly suggestive of HSV infections. The nurse should ask about a history of a primary infection, prodromal symptoms, vaginal discharge, and dyspareunia. Pregnant women should be asked whether they or their partner(s) have had genital lesions.

During the physical examination, the nurse should assess for inguinal and generalized lymphadenopathy and elevated temperature. The entire vulvar, perineal, vaginal, and cervical areas should be carefully inspected for vesicles or ulcerated or crusted areas. A speculum examination may be very difficult for the woman because of the extreme tenderness often associated with herpes infections. Any suggestive or recurrent lesions found during pregnancy should be cultured to verify HSV. Although a diagnosis of herpes infection may be suspected from the history and physical, it is confirmed by laboratory studies. A viral culture is obtained by swabbing exudate during the vesicular stage of the disease.

Management

Genital herpes is a chronic and recurring disease for which there is no known cure. Management is directed toward specific treatment during primary and recurrent infections, prevention, self-help measures, and psychologic support.

Systemic antiviral medications partially control the symptoms and signs of HSV infections when used for the primary or recurrent episodes or when used as daily suppressive therapy. However, these medications do not eradicate the infection nor do they alter subsequent risk or frequency of recurrences after the medication is stopped. Three antiviral medications provide clinical benefit: acyclovir, valacyclovir, and famciclovir. Treatment recommendations are given in Table 7-2. The safety of acyclovir, valacyclovir, and famciclovir therapy during pregnancy has not been established; however, acyclovir may be used to reduce the symptoms of HSV if the benefits to the woman outweigh the potential harm to the fetus (CDC et al., 2006). Continued investigation of HSV therapy with these medications in pregnancy is needed.

Cleaning lesions twice a day with saline will help prevent secondary infection. Bacterial infection must be treated with appropriate antibiotics. Measures that may increase comfort for women when lesions are active include warm sitz baths with baking soda; keeping lesions dry by blowing the area dry with a hair dryer set on cool or patting dry with a soft towel; wearing cotton underwear and loose clothing; using drying aids such as hydrogen peroxide, Burow's solution, or oatmeal baths; applying cool, wet, black tea bags to lesions; and applying compresses with an infusion of cloves or peppermint oil and clove oil to lesions.

Oral analgesics such as aspirin or ibuprofen may be used to relieve pain and systemic symptoms associated with initial infections. Because the mucous membranes affected by herpes are extremely sensitive, any topical agents should be used with caution. Nonantiviral ointments, especially those containing cortisone, should be avoided. A thin layer of lidocaine ointment or an antiseptic spray may be applied to decrease discomfort, especially if walking is painful.

Counseling and education are critical components of the nursing care of women with herpes infections. Information regarding the etiology, signs and symptoms, transmission, and treatment should be provided. The nurse should explain that each woman is unique in her response to herpes and emphasize the variability of symptoms. Women should be helped to understand when viral shedding and thus transmission to a partner is most likely, and that they should refrain from sexual contact from the onset of prodromal symptoms until complete healing of lesions. Some authorities recommend consistent use of condoms for all persons with genital herpes. Condoms may not prevent transmission, particularly male-to-female transmission; however, this does not mean that the partners should avoid all intimacy. Women can be encouraged to maintain close contact with their partners while avoiding contact with lesions. Women should be taught how to look for herpetic lesions with a mirror and good light source and a wet cloth or finger covered with a finger cot to rub lightly over the labia. The nurse should ensure that women understand that when lesions are active, sharing intimate articles (e.g., washcloths, wet towel) that come into contact with the lesions should be avoided. Plain soap and water is all that is needed to clean hands that have come into contact with herpetic lesions.

Stress, menstruation, trauma, febrile illnesses, chronic illnesses, and ultraviolet light have all been found to trigger genital herpes. Women may wish to keep a diary to identify stressors that seem to be associated with recurrent herpes attacks so that they can then avoid these stressors when possible. The role of exercise in reducing stress can be discussed. Referral for stress-reduction therapy, yoga, or meditation classes may be indicated. Avoiding excessive heat and sun and hot baths and using a lubricant during sexual intercourse to reduce friction also may be helpful. Women in their childbearing years should be counseled regarding the risk of herpes infection during pregnancy. They should be instructed to use condoms if there is any risk of contracting an STI from a sexual partner. If they become pregnant while taking acyclovir, the risk of birth defects does not appear to be higher than for the general population; however continued use should be based on whether the benefits for the woman outweigh the possible risks to the fetus. Acyclovir does enter breast milk but the amount of medication ingested during breastfeeding is very low and is usually not a health concern (Weiner & Buhimschi, 2009).

Because neonatal HSV infection is such a devastating disease, prevention is critical. Current recommendations include carefully examining and questioning all women about symptoms at onset of labor (CDC et al., 2006). If visible lesions are not present at onset of labor, vaginal birth is acceptable. Cesarean birth within 4 hours after labor begins or membranes rupture is recommended if visible lesions are present. Infants who are born through an infected vagina should be carefully observed and cultured (see Chapter 35).

The emotional effect of contracting an incurable STI such as herpes is considerable. At diagnosis, many emotions may surface—helplessness, anger, denial, guilt, anxiety, shame, or inadequacy. Women need the opportunity to discuss their feelings and help in learning to live with the disease. Herpes can affect a woman's sexuality, her sexual practices, and her current and future relationships. She may need help in raising the issue with her partner or with future partners.

Viral Hepatitis

Five different viruses (hepatitis viruses A, B, C, D, and E) account for almost all cases of viral hepatitis in humans. Hepatitis viruses A, B, and C are discussed. Hepatitis D and E viruses, common among users of intravenous drugs and recipients of multiple blood transfusions, are not included in this discussion.

Hepatitis A

Hepatitis A virus (HAV) infection is acquired primarily through a fecal-oral route by ingestion of contaminated food, particularly milk, shellfish, or polluted water, or person-to-person contact. Women living in the western United States, Native Americans, Alaska Natives, and children and employees in day-care centers are at high risk. Hepatitis A, like other enteric infections, can be transmitted during sexual activity.

HAV infection is characterized by flulike symptoms with malaise, fatigue, anorexia, nausea, pruritus, fever, and right upper quadrant pain. Serologic testing to detect the immunoglobulin M (IgM) antibody is done to confirm acute infections. The IgM antibody is detectable 5 to 10 days after exposure and can remain positive for up to 6 months. Because HAV infection is self-limited and does not result in chronic infection or chronic liver disease, treatment is usually supportive. Women who become dehydrated from nausea and vomiting or who have fulminating hepatitis A may need to be hospitalized. Medications and other ingested substances that might cause liver damage or that are metabolized in the liver (e.g., acetaminophen, ethyl alcohol) should be avoided. A well-balanced diet is recommended. Hepatitis A vaccine is recommended for women at high risk for being exposed to HAV infection. The safety of the vaccine has not been established in pregnancy; therefore, immune globulin (gamma globulin) or immune-specific globulin is indicated for a pregnant woman exposed to HAV. All household contacts of the woman also should receive gamma globulin (CDC et al., 2006).

Hepatitis B

Hepatitis B virus (HBV) is the virus most threatening to the fetus and neonate. It is caused by a large DNA virus and is associated with three antigens and their antibodies: hepatitis B surface antigen (HBsAg), HBV antigen (HBeAg), HBV core antigen (HBcAg), antibody to HBsAg (anti-HBs), antibody to HBeAg (anti-HBe), and antibody to HBcAg (anti-HBc). Screening for active or chronic disease or disease immunity is based on testing for these antigens and their antibodies.

Populations at risk include women of Asian, Pacific Island (Polynesian, Micronesian, Melanesian), or Alaskan-Inuit descent and women born in Haiti or sub-Saharan Africa. Women who have a history of acute or chronic liver disease, who work or receive treatment in a dialysis unit, or who have household or sexual contact with a hemodialysis client are at greater risk. Women who work or live in institutions for the mentally challenged are considered to be at risk, as are women with a history of multiple blood transfusions. Health care workers and public safety workers exposed to blood in the workplace are at risk. Behaviors such as having multiple sexual partners and a history of intravenous drug use increase the risk of contracting HBV infections.

HBsAg has been found in blood, saliva, sweat, tears, vaginal secretions, and semen. Drug abusers who share needles are at risk, as are health care workers who are exposed to blood and needlesticks. Perinatal transmission most often occurs in infants of mothers who have acute hepatitis infection late in the third trimester or during the intrapartum or postpartum period from exposure to HBsAg-positive vaginal secretions, blood, amniotic fluid, saliva, and breast milk. HBV has also been transmitted by artificial insemination. Although HBV can be transmitted via blood transfusion, the incidence of such infections has decreased significantly since testing of blood for HBsAg became routine.

HBV infection is a disease of the liver and is often a silent infection. In an adult the course of the infection can be fulminating, and the outcome, fatal. Symptoms of HBV infection are similar to those of hepatitis A: arthralgias, arthritis, lassitude, anorexia, nausea, vomiting, headache, fever, and mild abdominal pain. Later the woman may have clay-colored stools, dark urine, increased abdominal pain, and jaundice. Between 5% and 10% of individuals with HBV have persistence of HBsAg and become chronic hepatitis B carriers.

Screening and Diagnosis. All women at high risk for contracting HBV should be screened on a regular basis. However, screening only individuals at high risk may not identify up to 50% of HBsAg-positive women. Screening for the presence of HBsAg is recommended on allw pregnant women at the first prenatal visit, regardless of whether they have been tested previously; screening should be done on admission for labor and birth for women at high risk for infection during pregnancy or if prenatal test results are not available (CDC, 2008b; USPSTF, 2009a).

The HBsAg screening test is usually performed, given that a rise in HBsAg occurs at the onset of clinical symptoms and usually indicates an active infection. If HBsAg persists in the blood, the woman is identified as a carrier. If the HBsAg test result is positive, further laboratory studies may be ordered: anti-HBe, anti-HBc, serum glutamic-oxaloacetic transaminase (SGOT), alkaline phosphatase, and liver panel.

Management. There is no specific treatment for hepatitis B. Recovery is usually spontaneous in 3 to 16 weeks. Pregnancies complicated by acute viral hepatitis are managed on an outpatient basis. Women should be advised to increase rest periods, eat a high-protein, low-fat diet; and increase their fluid intake. They should avoid medications metabolized in the liver, and alcohol. Pregnant women with a definite exposure to HBV should be given hepatitis B immune globulin and should begin the hepatitis B vaccine series within 14 days of the most recent contact to prevent infection (CDC et al., 2006). Vaccination during pregnancy is not thought to pose risks to the fetus.

All nonimmune women at high or moderate risk of hepatitis should be informed of the availability of hepatitis B vaccine. Vaccination is recommended for all individuals who have had multiple sex partners within the past 6 months (CDC et al., 2006). In addition, intravenous drug users, residents of correctional or long-term care facilities, persons seeking care for an STI, prostitutes, women whose partners are intravenous drug users or bisexual, and women whose occupation exposes them to high risk should be vaccinated. The vaccine is given in a series of three (four if rapid protection is needed) doses over a 6-month period, with the first two doses given at least 1 month apart. The vaccine is given in the deltoid muscle (CDC et al.).

Client education includes explaining the meaning of hepatitis B infection, including transmission, state of infectivity, and sequelae. The nurse also should explain the need for immunoprophylaxis for household members and sexual contacts. To decrease transmission of the virus, women with hepatitis B or who test positive for HBV should be advised to maintain a high level of personal hygiene (e.g., wash hands after using the toilet; carefully dispose of tampons, pads, and bandages in plastic bags; do not share razor blades, toothbrushes, needles, or manicure implements; have male partner use a condom if unvaccinated and without hepatitis; avoid sharing saliva through kissing, or sharing of silverware or dishes; and wipe up blood spills immediately with soap and water). They should inform all health care providers of their carrier state. Postpartum women should be reassured that breastfeeding is not contraindicated if their infants received prophylaxis at birth and are currently on the immunization schedule.

Hepatitis C

Hepatitis C virus (HCV) infection has become an important health problem as increasing numbers of persons acquire the disease. Hepatitis C is responsible for nearly 50% of the cases of chronic viral hepatitis. Risk factors include having STIs such as hepatitis B and HIV, multiple sexual partners, history of blood transmissions, and history of intravenous drug use. HCV is readily transmitted through exposure to blood and much less efficiently via semen, saliva, or urine.

Most clients with hepatitis C are asymptomatic or have general influenza-like symptoms similar to those of hepatitis A. HCV infection is confirmed by the presence of anti-C antibody during laboratory testing. Interferon-alfa alone or with ribavirin for 6 to 12 months is the main therapy for chronic HCV-related liver disease, although effectiveness of this treatment varies. Currently, no vaccine is available for hepatitis C. Transmission of HCV through breastfeeding has not been reported.

Human Immunodeficiency Virus

Approximately 37,000 new HIV infections occur in the United States each year. An estimated 26% of these new infections occur in women. African-American women are estimated to have 64% of these infections, Caucasian women are estimated to have 19%, Hispanic women, 15%, and Native American women less than 1% (CDC, 2008d).

Severe depression of the cellular immune system associated with HIV infection characterizes acquired immunodeficiency syndrome (AIDS). Although behaviors that place women at risk have been well documented, you should assess all women for the possibility of HIV exposure. The most commonly reported opportunistic diseases are *Pneumocystis (jiroveci)* pneumonia (PCP), *Candida* esophagitis, and wasting syndrome. Other viral infections such as HSV and cytomegalovirus infections seem to be more prevalent in women than men (CDC et al., 2006). PID is often more severe in HIV-infected women than in the general population, and rates of HPV and cervical dysplasia are sometimes higher in non–HIV-infected women (Eckert & Lentz, 2007a). The clinical course of HPV infection in women with HIV infection is accelerated while recurrence is more frequent in non–HIV-infected women.

Once HIV enters the body, seroconversion to HIV positivity usually occurs within 6 to 12 weeks. Although HIV seroconversion may be totally asymptomatic, it usually is accompanied by a viremic, influenza-like response. Symptoms include fever, headache, night sweats, malaise, generalized lymphadenopathy, myalgias, nausea, diarrhea, weight loss, sore throat, and rash.

Laboratory studies may reveal leukopenia, thrombocytopenia, anemia, and an elevated erythrocyte sedimentation rate. HIV has a strong affinity for surface-marker proteins on T lymphocytes. This affinity leads to significant T-cell destruction. Both clinical and epidemiologic studies have shown that declining CD_4 levels are strongly associated with increased incidence of AIDS-related diseases and death in many different groups of HIV-infected persons.

Transmission of the virus from mother to child can occur throughout the perinatal period. Exposure may occur to the fetus through the maternal circulation as early as the first trimester of pregnancy, to the infant during labor and birth by inoculation or ingestion of maternal blood and other infected fluids, or to the infant through breast milk (Marrazzo et al., 2007).

Screening and Diagnosis

Screening, teaching, and counseling regarding HIV risk factors, indications for being tested, and testing are major roles for nurses caring for women today. A number of behaviors place women at risk for HIV infection, including intravenous drug use, high risk sexual partners, multiple sex partners, and a previous history of multiple STIs. HIV infection is usually diagnosed by using HIV-1 and HIV-2 antibody tests. Antibody testing is first done with a sensitive screening test such as the enzyme immunoassay (EIA). Reactive screening tests must be confirmed by an additional test, such as the Western blot or an immunofluorescence assay. If a positive antibody test is confirmed by a supplemental test, it means that a woman is infected with HIV and is capable of infecting others. HIV antibodies are detectable in at least 95% of individuals within 3 months after infection. Although a negative antibody test usually indicates that a person is not infected, antibody tests cannot exclude recent infection. Because HIV antibody crosses the placenta, definite diagnosis of HIV in children younger than 18 months is based on laboratory evidence of HIV in blood or tissues by culture, nucleic acid, or antigen detection (CDC et al., 2006).

The U.S. Food and Drug Administration (FDA) (2008) has approved six rapid HIV antibody screening tests. These tests use a blood sample obtained by fingerstick or venipuncture, an oral fluid sample, or a urine sample to provide test results within 20 minutes, with sensitivity and specificity rates of more than 99%. If the results are reactive, further testing is necessary (CDC, Divisions of HIV/AIDS Prevention, 2008). Quicker results mean that clients do not have to make extra visits for follow-up standard tests, and the oral test provides an option for clients who do not want to have a blood test.

The CDC, Workowski, and Berman (2006) and the USPSTF (2007b) recommend offering HIV testing to all women whose behavior places them at risk for HIV infection. It may be useful to allow women to self-select for HIV testing. On entry to the health care system, a woman can be handed written information about the risk factors for the AIDS virus and asked to inform the nurse if she believes she is at risk. She should be told that she does not have to say why she may be at risk, only that she thinks she might be.

Counseling for HIV Testing. Counseling before and after HIV testing is standard nursing practice today. It is a nursing responsibility to assess a woman's understanding of the information such a test would provide and to be sure the woman thoroughly understands the emotional, legal, and medical implications of a positive or negative test before she is ready to take an HIV test.

! NURSING ALERT

Counseling associated with HIV testing has two components: pretest and posttest counseling. During pretest counseling, a personalized risk assessment is conducted, the meaning of positive and negative test results is explained, informed consent for HIV testing is obtained, and women are helped to develop a realistic plan for reducing risk and preventing infection. Posttest counseling includes informing the woman of the test results, reviewing the meaning of the results, and reinforcing prevention messages. Document all pretest and posttest counseling.

Given the strong social stigma attached to HIV infection, nurses must consider the issue of confidentiality and documentation before providing counseling and offering HIV testing to clients.

LEGAL TIP: HIV Testing

If HIV test results are placed in the client's chart—the appropriate place for all health information—they are available to all who have access to the chart. Inform the woman of this availability before testing. Informed consent must be obtained before an HIV test is performed. In some states, written consent is mandated. In many sites, HIV testing is performed unless women decline (i.e., opt-out testing). Nurses must know what procedures are being used for informed consent in their facility.

Unless rapid testing is done, there is generally a 1- to 3-week waiting period after testing for HIV, which can be a very anxious time for the woman. It is helpful if the nurse informs her that this time period between blood drawing and test results is routine. Test results, whatever they are, always must be communicated in person, and women need to be informed in advance that such is the procedure. Whenever possible, the person who provided the pretest counseling also should tell the woman her test results. Some women, when informed of negative results, may escalate their risk behaviors because of an equating of negativity with immunity. Others may believe that negative means "bad" and positive means "good." Women's reactions to a negative test should be explored, such as by asking, "How do you feel?" HIV-negative result counseling sessions are another opportunity to provide education. Emphasis can be placed on ways in which a woman can remain HIV free. She should be reminded that if she has been exposed to HIV in the past 6 months, she should be retested, and that if she continues high risk behaviors, she should have ongoing testing.

In posttest counseling to an HIV-positive woman, privacy with no interruptions is essential. Adequate time for the counseling sessions also should be provided. The nurse should make sure that the woman understands what a positive test means and review the reliability of the test results. Risk reduction practices should be reemphasized. Referral for appropriate medical evaluation and follow-up should be made, and the need or desire for psychosocial or psychiatric referrals should be assessed.

The importance of early medical evaluation so that a baseline assessment can be made and prophylactic medication begun should be stressed. If possible, the nurse should make a referral or appointment for the woman at the posttest counseling session.

Management

During the initial contact with an HIV-infected woman, the nurse should establish what the woman knows about HIV infection and that she is being cared for by a medical practitioner or facility with expertise in caring for persons with HIV infections, including AIDS. Psychologic referral also may be indicated. Resources such as counseling for financial assistance, legal advocacy, suicide prevention, and death and dying may be appropriate. All women who are drug users should be referred to a substance-abuse program. A major focus of counseling is prevention of transmission of HIV to partners.

Nurses counseling seropositive women wishing contraceptive information can recommend oral contraceptives and latex condoms or tubal sterilization or vasectomy and latex condoms. For women who are HIV infected, the diaphragm is classified as having more risks than advantages; the IUD appears safe for selected women (World Health Organization [WHO], 2004). Suggest female condoms or abstinence to women whose male partners refuse to use condoms.

No cure is available for HIV infections at this time. Rare and unusual diseases are characteristic of HIV infections. Opportunistic infections and concurrent diseases are managed vigorously with treatment specific to the infection or disease. Routine gynecologic care for HIV-positive women should include a pelvic examination every 6 months. Thorough Pap screening is essential because of the greatly increased incidence of abnormal findings on examination (CDC et al., 2006). In addition, HIV-positive women should be screened for syphilis, gonorrhea, chlamydia, and other vaginal infections and treated if infections are present. General prevention strategies are an important part of care (e.g., smoking cessation, sound nutrition) as is antiretroviral therapy. Discussion of the medical care of HIV-positive women or women with AIDS is beyond the scope of this chapter because of the rapidly changing recommendations. The reader is referred to the CDC (www.cdc.gov), AIDS hotline (800-342-2437), and Internet websites such as HIV/AIDS Treatment Information Service (www.hivatis.org) for the current information and recommendations.

HIV and Pregnancy

HIV counseling and testing should be offered to all women at their initial entry into prenatal care as part of routine prenatal testing unless the woman opts out of the screening (Branson, Handsfield, Lampe, Janssen, Taylor, Lyss, et al., 2006; USPSTF, 2007b.) Universal testing is recommended versus selective testing for maternal HIV because it results in a greater number of

EVIDENCE-BASED PRACTICE

Pat Gingrich

Venus and Mars and HIV/STD Prevention Interventions

ASK THE QUESTION

Are abstinence-only programs effective at preventing the spread of HIV? Can tailoring HIV and STD prevention counseling interventions to specific populations result in better outcomes?

SEARCH FOR EVIDENCE

Search Strategies

Professional organization guidelines, meta-analyses, systematic reviews, randomized controlled trials, nonrandomized prospective studies and retrospective reviews since 2007.

Databases Searched

CINAHL, Cochrane, Medline, PUBMED.

CRITICALLY ANALYZE THE DATA

Abstinence-only programs emphasize refraining from intercourse, without further information about safe sex practices. In a Cochrane meta-analysis of 13 studies involving 15,940 youth in high-income countries, abstinence-only programs neither increased nor decreased HIV risk. HIV risk behavior included unprotected vaginal sex, number of sexual partners, and/or condom use (Underhill, Operario, & Montgomery, 2007).

Another Cochrane Review meta-analyzed studies of the effectiveness of intervention among men who have sex with men (MSM), the group at greatest risk for HIV infection. Forty-four studies, involving 18,585 men, examined intervention that included individual counseling, group education, and behavioral support such as peer and relational support, as well as leadership training for community leaders and community-building activities. All educational interventions led to reduced self-reported unprotected anal sex (the riskiest for HIV transmission). The effect was most marked for men who did not self-identify as gay. One possible reason suggested was that self-identified non-gay men had not been previously exposed to as many repeated prevention messages as the gay identifiers (Wayne, Rafael, Flanders, Goodman, Hill, Holtgrave, et al., 2008).

African-American women who live in the inner city experience a cumulative incidence of HIV that is more than 20 times higher than the incidence in white women. In a randomized controlled trial of 564 African-American women in New Jersey, nurses led a specific intervention entitled "Sister to Sister-Respect Yourself! Protect Yourself! Because You Are Worth It!" as individual or group counseling. The intervention started with an assessment of risk factors, so as to tailor the session to the individual client. Goals included increasing knowledge and condom self-efficacy, using role-playing, videos, and hands-on condom demonstrations. Each participant was given a condom keychain, an outward sign that this woman intends to protect herself. In addition, the counseling session length varied, from 20 minutes to $3\frac{1}{3}$ hours. The women who received the 20-minute individualized counseling showed sustained decreased exposure to STDs and HIV, even 12 months later. Results suggest that this intervention is a cost-effective and effective prevention measure that can be duplicated by nurses trained in the technique, regardless of the nurse's race (Jemmott, Jemmott, Hutchinson, Cedarbaum, & O'Leary, 2008).

IMPLICATIONS FOR PRACTICE

Clearly, comprehensive educational interventions are effective preventive measures against HIV and STDs. Initial assessment allows tailoring the session to the individual. Interventions include oral and written instructions, and a variety of activities such as role-playing and condom practice that develop the skills needed to negotiate and use abstinence or safe-sex techniques. The nurse needs to be informed and non-judgmental about the wide variety of sexual practices, and negotiate the contradiction between behavior (such as MSM) and the client's perception (self-identified non-gay).

In particular, the "Sister to Sister" intervention uses three themes: (1) helping family and community by HIV prevention, (2) caring about self, future and community, and (3) increasing the feeling of self-worth in a population of women that struggle with self-esteem and self-efficacy (Jemmott, et al., 2008). While further research is needed to see if it can be adapted to other populations, this seems to be a promising evidence-based nurse-led intervention that benefits a very vulnerable population.

References

Jemmott, L., Jemmott, J., Hutchinson, M., Cedarbaum, J., & O'Leary, A. (2008). Sexually transmitted infection/HIV risk reduction interventions in clinical practice settings. *Journal of Obstetric, Gynecologic and Neonatal Nursing, 37*(2), 137–145.

Underhill, K., Operario, D., & Montgomery, P. (2007). Abstinence-only programs for HIV infection prevention in high-income countries. *The Cochrane Database of Systematic Reviews 2007, 4,* Chichester, UK: John Wiley & Sons.

Wayne, W., Rafael, M., Flanders, W., Goodman, M., Hill, A., Holtgrave, D., et al. (2008). Behavioral intervention to reduce risk for sexual transmission of HIV among men who have sex with men. *The Cochrane Database of Systematic Reviews 2008, 3,* Chichester, UK: John Wiley & Sons.

women being screened and treated and can reduce the likelihood of perinatal transmission and maintain the health of the woman (American Academy of Pediatrics Committee on Pediatric AIDS, 2008). The CDC also recommends retesting in the third trimester for women known to be at high risk for HIV and rapid HIV testing in labor for women with unknown HIV status (Branson et al.).

Perinatal transmission of HIV has decreased significantly in the past decade because of the administration of antiretroviral prophylaxis (e.g., zidovudine) to pregnant women in the prenatal and the perinatal periods. Treatment of HIV-infected women with the triple-drug antiviral therapy or highly active antiretroviral therapy (HAART) during pregnancy has been reported to decrease the mother-to-child transmission to 1% to 2% (Volmink, Siegfried, van der Merwe, & Brocklehurst, 2007). All HIV-infected women should be treated with a combination of antiretroviral drugs (e.g., HAART) during pregnancy, regardless of their CD_4 cell counts (Panel on Treatment of HIV-Infected Pregnant Women and Prevention of Perinatal Transmission, 2010). Data are insufficient to support or refute the teratogenic risk of antiretroviral medications given for prophylaxis in the first 10 weeks or pregnancy. Current research does not support major teratogenic effects for most of the antiretroviral agents (Panel on Treatment of HIV-Infected Pregnant Women and Prevention of Perinatal Transmission, 2010). Pregnant women already receiving antiretroviral treatment should continue their regimen, except the use of efavirenz should be avoided. Women who are HIV-infected and need treatment for their own health should start the therapy as soon as possible, even in the first trimester. Women who are taking the therapy as prophylaxis usually start therapy after the first trimester (Panel on Treatment of HIV-Infected Pregnant Women and Prevention of Perinatal Transmission, 2010).

Antiviral therapy is administered orally and is continued throughout pregnancy. The major side effect of this therapy is bone marrow suppression. Periodic hematocrit, white blood cell count, and platelet count assessments should be performed (Panel on Treatment of HIV-Infected Pregnant Women and Prevention of Perinatal Transmission, 2010). Women who are HIV positive should also be vaccinated against hepatitis B, pneumococcal infection, Haemophilus influenzae type B, and viral influenza. To support any pregnant woman's immune system, appropriate counseling is provided about optimal nutrition, sleep, rest, exercise, and stress reduction. Use of condoms is encouraged to minimize further exposure to HIV if her partner is the source.

In the intrapartum period, antiretroviral therapy and cesarean birth are recommended to prevent vertical transmission of HIV (Panel on Treatment of HIV-Infected Pregnant Women and Prevention of Perinatal Transmission, 2010). The Panel recommends a scheduled cesarean birth at 38 weeks of gestation for women with a viral load of more than 1000 copies/ml. A vaginal birth may be an option for HIV-infected women who have a viral load of less than 1000 copies/ml at 36 weeks, if a woman has ruptured membranes and labor is progressing rapidly, or if she declines a cesarean birth. Intravenous zidovudine is recommended for all HIV-infected pregnant women during the intrapartum period. The drug is administered 3 hours before a scheduled cesarean birth and is continued until the baby is born. It should be given during labor if the woman is having a vaginal birth (Panel on Treatment of HIV-Infected Pregnant Women and Prevention of Perinatal Transmission, 2010). Fetal scalp electrode and scalp pH sampling should be avoided because these procedures may result in inoculation of the virus into the fetus. Similarly, the use of forceps or vacuum extractor should be avoided when possible. Infants should receive oral zidovudine for 6 weeks after birth. Avoidance of breastfeeding is recommended in the United States and most developed countries (American Academy of Pediatrics Committee on Pediatric AIDS, 2008).

Women who have HIV but who are without symptoms may have an unremarkable postpartum course. Immunosuppressed women with symptoms may be at increased risk for postpartum urinary tract infections (UTIs), vaginitis, postpartum endometritis, and poor wound healing. Good perineal hygiene should be stressed. Women who are HIV positive but who were not on antiretroviral drugs before pregnancy should be tested in the postpartum period to determine whether therapy that was initiated in pregnancy should be continued (Panel on Treatment of HIV-Infected Pregnant Women and Prevention of Perinatal Transmission, 2010). After the initial bath the newborn can be with the mother. In planning for discharge, comprehensive care and support services will need to be arranged. After discharge the woman and her infant are referred to physicians who are experienced in the treatment of HIV and AIDS and associated conditions for intensive monitoring and follow-up (Panel on Treatment of HIV-Infected Pregnant Women and Prevention of Perinatal Transmission, 2010).

COMMUNITY ACTIVITY

Visit the Centers for Disease Control and Prevention website at www.cdc.gov. Select a sexually transmitted infection. What is the prevalence of the disease in your state? Evaluate the rank, number of cases, rate per 100,000 population and cumulative percent. Review the client information about facts, treatment and other resources. Go to the Life Stages & Specific Populations link and review the information about pregnancy.

VAGINAL INFECTIONS

Vaginal discharge and itching of the vulva and vagina are among the most frequent reasons a woman seeks help from a health care provider. More women complain of vaginal discharge than of any other gynecologic symptom. Vaginal discharge resulting from infection must be distinguished from normal secretions. Women who have adequate endogenous or exogenous estrogen will have vaginal secretions. Normal vaginal secretions, or leukorrhea, are clear to cloudy in appearance and may turn yellow after drying; the discharge is slightly slimy, is nonirritating, and has a mild, inoffensive odor. Normal vaginal secretions are acidic, with a pH range of 4 to 5. Normal vaginal secretions contain lactobacilli and epithelial cells. The amount of leukorrhea differs with phases of the menstrual cycle, with greater amounts occurring at ovulation and just before menses. Leukorrhea also is increased during pregnancy.

The most common vaginal infections are bacterial vaginosis (BV), candidiasis, and trichomoniasis. Vulvovaginitis, or inflammation of the vulva and vagina, may be caused by vaginal infection or copious amounts of leukorrhea, which can cause maceration of tissues. Chemical irritants, allergens, and foreign bodies that produce inflammatory reactions can also cause vulvovaginitis.

Bacterial Vaginosis

Bacterial vaginosis (BV), formerly called nonspecific vaginitis, *Haemophilus vaginitis*, or *Gardnerella*, is the most common type of vaginitis today (Eckert & Lentz, 2007a). BV is associated with preterm labor and birth. The exact etiology of BV is unknown. It is a syndrome in which normal H_2O_2-producing lactobacilli are replaced with high concentrations of anaerobic bacteria (*Gardnerella* and *Mobiluncus*). With the proliferation of anaerobes, the level of vaginal amines is increased, and the normal acidic pH of the vagina is altered. Epithelial cells slough, and numerous bacteria attach to their surfaces (clue cells). When the amines are volatilized, the characteristic odor of BV occurs.

Many women with BV complain of the characteristic "fishy odor." The odor may be noticed by the woman or her partner after heterosexual intercourse because semen releases the vaginal amines. When present, the BV discharge is usually profuse, thin, and white or gray, or milky in appearance. Some women also may experience mild irritation or pruritus.

Screening and Diagnosis

A focused history may help distinguish BV from other vaginal infections if the woman is symptomatic. Reports of fishy odor and increased thin vaginal discharge are most significant, and a report of increased odor after intercourse is also suggestive of BV.

Microscopic examination of vaginal secretions is always performed (Table 7-4). Both normal saline and 10% potassium hydroxide (KOH) smears are made. The presence of clue cells (vaginal epithelial cells coated with bacteria) on wet saline smear is highly diagnostic because the phenomenon is specific to BV. Test vaginal secretions for pH and amine odor. Nitrazine paper is sensitive enough to detect a pH of 4.5 or greater. The fishy odor of BV will be released when KOH is added to vaginal secretions on the lip of the withdrawn speculum.

TABLE 7-4 **WET SMEAR TESTS FOR VAGINAL INFECTIONS**

INFECTION	TEST	POSITIVE FINDINGS
Trichomoniasis	Saline wet smear (vaginal secretions mixed with normal saline on a glass slide)	Presence of many white blood cell protozoa
Candidiasis	Potassium hydroxide (KOH) prep (vaginal secretions mixed with KOH on a glass slide)	Presence of hyphae and pseudohyphae (buds and branches of yeast cells)
Bacterial vaginosis	Normal saline smear	Presence of clue cells (vaginal epithelial cells coated with bacteria)
	Whiff test (vaginal secretions mixed with KOH)	Release of fishy odor

Management

Treatment of bacterial vaginosis with oral metronidazole (Flagyl) is most effective (CDC et al., 2006). Table 7-5 outlines treatment guidelines. Side effects of metronidazole are numerous, including sharp, unpleasant metallic taste in the mouth; furry tongue; central nervous system reactions; and urinary tract disturbances. When oral metronidazole is taken, the woman is advised not to drink alcoholic beverages, or she will experience the severe side effects of abdominal distress, nausea, vomiting, and headache. Gastrointestinal symptoms are common whether alcohol is consumed or not. Treatment of sexual partners is not routinely recommended (CDC et al.).

Metronidazole crosses the placenta but does not pose a major teratogenic risk if used for short durations. Metronidazole is excreted into breast milk; however, limited studies have demonstrated that the risk of adverse effects on the infant is remote (Weiner & Buhimschi, 2009).

Candidiasis

Vulvovaginal candidiasis (VVC), or yeast infection, is the second most common type of vaginal infection in the United States. Although vaginal candidiasis infections are common in healthy women, those seen in women with HIV infection are often more severe and persistent. Genital candidiasis lesions may be painful coalescing ulcerations necessitating continuous prophylactic therapy.

TABLE 7-5 **VAGINAL INFECTIONS AND DRUG THERAPIES FOR WOMEN**

DISEASE	NONPREGNANT WOMEN (13-17 YR)	NONPREGNANT WOMEN (>18 YR)	PREGNANT WOMEN	LACTATING WOMEN
Bacterial vaginosis	*Recommended:* Metronidazole, 500 mg bid for 7 days (no alcohol) *or* Metronidazole gel 0.75%, 5 g intravaginally bid for 7 days *or* Clindamycin cream 2%, 5 g intravaginally at bedtime for 7 days (less effective)	*Recommended:* Metronidazole, 500 mg bid for 7 days (no alcohol) *or* Metronidazole gel 0.75%, 5 g intravaginally bid for 7 days *or* Clindamycin cream 2%, 5 g intravaginally at bedtime for 7 days (less effective)	High risk asymptomatic or symptomatic women *Recommended:* Metronidazole, 500 mg orally bid for 7 days *or* Metronidazole, 250 mg orally tid for 7 days *or* Clindamycin, 300 mg orally bid for 7 days	*Recommended:* Clindamycin cream or ovules
Trichomoniasis	*Recommended:* Metronidazole, 2 g orally once Tinidazole, 2 g orally once	*Recommended:* Metronidazole, 2 g orally once	*Recommended:* Metronidazole, 2 g orally once	Metronidazole not recommended during lactation; stop lactation, treat, resume breastfeeding in 12-24 hr after drug completed Tinidazoles: Stop breastfeeding and resume 3 days after treatment Pump and discard milk to maintain supply
Candidiasis	Numerous OTC intravaginal agents: Butoconazole, clotrimazole, miconazole, tioconazole, terconazole; treatment with "azole" drugs more effective than nystatin Dose varies by agent from one dose a day to one dose for 3 to 7 days *Oral agent:* Fluconazole 150-mg oral tablet once	Numerous OTC intravaginal agents: Butoconazole, clotrimazole, miconazole, tioconazole, terconazole; treatment with "azole" drugs more effective than nystatin Dose varies by agent from one dose a day to one dose for 3 to 7 days *Oral agent:* Fluconazole 150-mg oral tablet once	OTC "azole" intravaginal agents: Butoconazole, clotrimazole, miconazole, terconazole Use for 3 to 7 days Oral agents not recommended	OTC "azole" intravaginal agents: Butoconazole, clotrimazole, miconazole, terconazole Use for 3 to 7 days

bid, Twice daily; *OTC,* over-the-counter; *tid,* three times daily.
Source: Centers for Disease Control and Prevention, Workowski, K., & Berman, S. (2006). Sexually transmitted diseases treatment guidelines 2006. *Morbidity and Mortality Weekly Report, 55*(RR-11), 1-94.

The most common organism is *Candida albicans;* estimates indicate that more than 90% of the yeast infections in women are caused by this organism. However, in the past 10 years, the incidence of non–*C. albicans* infections has risen steadily. Women with chronic or recurrent infections often are infected with these organisms (Eckert & Lentz, 2007a).

Numerous factors have been identified as predisposing a woman to yeast infections, including antibiotic therapy, particularly broad-spectrum antibiotics such as ampicillin, tetracycline, cephalosporins, and metronidazole; diabetes, especially when uncontrolled; pregnancy; obesity; diets high in refined sugars or artificial sweeteners; use of corticosteroids and exogenous hormones; and immunosuppressed states. Clinical observations and research have suggested that tight-fitting clothing and underwear or pantyhose made of nonabsorbent materials create an environment in which a vaginal fungus can grow.

The most common symptom of yeast infections is vulvar and possibly vaginal pruritus. The itching can be mild or intense, interfere with rest and activities, and may occur during or after intercourse. Some women report a feeling of dryness. Others may experience painful urination as the urine flows over the vulva, which usually occurs in women who have excoriations resulting from scratching. Most often the discharge has a thick, white, lumpy, and cottage cheese–like consistency. The discharge may be found in patches on the vaginal walls, cervix, and labia. Commonly, the vulva is red and swollen, as are the labial folds, vagina, and cervix. Although there is not a characteristic odor with yeast infections, sometimes a yeasty or musty smell can be detected.

Screening and Diagnosis

In addition to a complete history of the woman's symptoms, their onset, and course, the history is a valuable screening tool for identifying predisposing risk factors. Physical examination should include a thorough inspection of the vulva and vagina. A speculum examination is always done. Commonly health care practitioners will obtain saline and KOH wet smears and check vaginal pH (see Table 7-4). Vaginal pH is normal with a yeast infection; if the pH is greater than 4.5, trichomoniasis or BV should be suspected. The characteristic pseudohyphae (bud or branching of a fungus) may be seen on a wet smear done with normal saline; however, they may be confused with other cells and artifacts (CDC et al., 2006).

Management

A sizable number of antifungal preparations are available for the treatment of *C. albicans* infection. Intravaginal agents include miconazole, clotrimazole, butoconazole, tioconazole, terconazole, and nystatin; fluconazole is an effective oral agent (CDC et al., 2006). Many of these vaginal medications (e.g., Monistat, Gyne-Lotrimin) are available over the counter (OTC). Exogenous lactobacillus (in the form of dairy products [yogurt] or powder, tablet, capsule, or suppository supplements) and garlic have been suggested for prevention and treatment of vulvovaginal candidiasis, but research is inconclusive, and no recommendations have been developed for use in practice (Eckert & Lentz, 2007a). The first time a woman suspects that she may have a yeast infection, she should see a health care provider for confirmation of the diagnosis and treatment recommendation. If she experiences another infection, she may wish to purchase an OTC preparation and self-treat; if she chooses to do so, she should always be counseled regarding seeking care for numerous recurrent or chronic yeast infections. If vaginal discharge is extremely thick and copious, vaginal debridement with a cotton swab followed by application of vaginal medication is useful.

Women who have extensive irritation, swelling, and discomfort of the labia and vulva may find sitz baths helpful in decreasing inflammation and increasing comfort. Adding colloidal oatmeal powder to the bath may also increase the woman's comfort. Not wearing underpants to bed may help decrease symptoms and prevent recurrences. Completing the full course of treatment prescribed is essential to removing the pathogen. Instruct women to continue the medication even during menstruation. Explain that they should avoid using tampons during menses because the tampon will readily absorb the medication. If possible, women should avoid intercourse during treatment; if abstinence is not feasible, the woman's partner should use a condom to prevent the introduction of more organisms (see Teaching for Self-Management box: Prevention of Genital Tract Infections).

TEACHING FOR SELF-MANAGEMENT

Prevention of Genital Tract Infections

- Practice genital hygiene.
- Choose underwear or hosiery with a cotton crotch.
- Avoid tight-fitting clothing (especially tight jeans).
- Select cloth car seat covers instead of vinyl.
- Limit time spent in damp exercise clothes (especially swimsuits, leotards, and tights).
- Limit exposure to bath salts or bubble bath.
- Avoid colored or scented toilet tissue.
- If sensitive, discontinue use of feminine hygiene deodorant sprays.
- Use condoms.
- Void before and after intercourse.
- Decrease dietary sugar.
- Drink yeast-active milk and eat yogurt (with lactobacilli).
- Do not douche.

Trichomoniasis

Trichomonas vaginalis is almost always an STI and is also a common cause of vaginal infection (5% to 50% of all vaginitis) and discharge (Eckert & Lentz, 2007a).

Trichomoniasis is caused by *T. vaginalis,* an anaerobic one-celled protozoan with characteristic flagellae. Although trichomoniasis may be asymptomatic, commonly women have characteristically yellowish to greenish, frothy, mucopurulent, copious, malodorous discharge. Inflammation of the vulva, the vagina, or both may be present, and the woman may complain of irritation and pruritus. Dysuria and dyspareunia are often present. Typically the discharge worsens during and after menstruation. Often the cervix and the vaginal walls will demonstrate the characteristic "strawberry spots" or tiny petechiae, and the cervix may bleed on contact. In severe infections, the vaginal walls, the cervix, and occasionally the vulva may be acutely inflamed.

Screening and Diagnosis

In addition to obtaining a history of current symptoms, a careful sexual history should be obtained. Any history of similar symptoms in the past and treatment used should be noted. The nurse should determine whether the woman's partner(s) was treated and if she has had subsequent relations with new partners.

A speculum examination is always done, even though it may be very uncomfortable for the woman; relaxation techniques and breathing exercises may help the woman with the procedure. Any of the classic signs may be present on physical examination. The typical one-celled flagellate trichomonads are easily distinguished on a normal saline wet prep. Trichomoniasis also may be identified on Pap tests. Because trichomoniasis is an STI, once diagnosis is confirmed, appropriate laboratory studies for other STIs should be carried out.

Management

The recommended treatment is metronidazole or tinidazole (CDC et al., 2006) (see Table 7-5). Although the male partner is usually asymptomatic, it is recommended that he receive treatment also because he often harbors the trichomonads in the urethra or prostate. It is important that nurses discuss the importance of partner treatment with their clients because if they are not treated, it is likely that the infection will recur.

Women with trichomoniasis need to understand the sexual transmission of this disease. The woman must know that the organism may be present without symptoms being present, perhaps for several months, and that it is not possible to determine when she became infected. Women should be informed of the necessity for treating all sexual partners and helped with ways to raise the issue with their partner(s).

Group B Streptococci

Group B streptococci (GBS) may be considered a part of the normal vaginal flora in a woman who is not pregnant, and it is present in 20% to 30% of healthy pregnant women. GBS infection has been associated with poor pregnancy outcomes. Furthermore, GBS infections are an important factor in neonatal morbidity and mortality, usually resulting from vertical transmission from the birth canal of the infected mother to the infant during birth (Cunningham, Leveno, Bloom, Hauth, Rouse, & Sprong, 2010).

Risk factors for neonatal GBS infection include positive prenatal culture for GBS in the current pregnancy; preterm birth of less than 37 weeks of gestation; premature rupture of membranes for a duration of 18 hours or more; intrapartum maternal fever higher than 38° C; and a positive history for early-onset neonatal GBS (Cunningham et al., 2010).

To decrease the risk of neonatal GBS infection, it is recommended that all women be screened at 36 to 37 weeks of gestation for GBS using a rectovaginal culture, and that intravenous antibiotic prophylaxis (IAP) be offered during labor to all who test positive. If a culture is not available at onset of labor or if a risk factor is present, IAP is also offered. IAP is not recommended before a cesarean birth if labor or rupture of membranes has not occurred. The recommended treatment is penicillin G, 5 million units intravenous (IV) loading dose, and then 2.5 million units IV every 4 hours during labor. Ampicillin, 2 g IV loading dose, followed by 1 g IV every 4 hours, is an alternative therapy (CDC, 2008a).

EFFECTS OF SEXUALLY TRANSMITTED INFECTIONS ON PREGNANCY AND THE FETUS

Sexually transmitted infections in pregnancy are responsible for significant morbidity and mortality. Some consequences of maternal infection, such as infertility and sterility, last a lifetime. Congenitally acquired infection may affect a child's length and quality of life. Table 7-6 describes the effects of several common STIs on pregnancy and the fetus. It is difficult to predict these effects with certainty. Factors such as coinfection with other STIs and, when in pregnancy, the infection was acquired and treated can affect outcomes.

TORCH Infections

*T*oxoplasmosis, *o*ther infections (e.g., hepatitis), *r*ubella virus, *c*ytomegalovirus (CMV), and *h*erpes simplex virus, known collectively as TORCH infections, form a group of organisms capable of crossing the placenta. **TORCH infections** can affect a pregnant woman and her fetus. Generally, all TORCH infections produce influenza-like symptoms in the mother, but fetal and neonatal effects are more serious. TORCH infections and their maternal and fetal effects are shown in Table 7-7. Neonatal effects are discussed in Chapter 35. The following discussion focuses on infections not previously discussed.

TABLE 7-6 PREGNANCY AND FETAL EFFECTS OF COMMON SEXUALLY TRANSMITTED INFECTIONS

INFECTION	MATERNAL EFFECTS	FETAL EFFECTS
Chlamydia	Premature rupture of membranes Preterm labor Postpartum endometritis	Low birth weight
Gonorrhea	Miscarriage Preterm labor Premature rupture of membranes Amniotic infection syndrome Chorioamnionitis Postpartum endometritis Postpartum sepsis	Preterm birth IUGR
Group B streptococci	Urinary tract infection Chorioamnionitis Postpartum endometritis Sepsis Meningitis (rare)	Preterm birth
Herpes simplex virus	Intrauterine infection (rare)	Congenital infection (rare)
Human papillomavirus (HPV)	Dystocia from large lesions Excessive bleeding from lesions after birth trauma	None known
Syphilis	Miscarriage Preterm labor	IUGR Preterm birth Stillbirth Congenital infection

IUGR, Intrauterine growth restriction.

Source: Gilbert, E. (2011). *Manual of high risk pregnancy & delivery* (5th ed.). St. Louis: Mosby; Duff, P., Sweet, R., & Edwards, R. (2009). Maternal and fetal infections. In R. Creasy, R. Resnik, J. Iams, C. Lockwood, & T. Moore (Eds.), *Creasy and Resnik's maternal-fetal medicine: Principles and practice* (6th ed.). Philadelphia: Saunders.

Toxoplasmosis

Toxoplasmosis is a protozoal infection associated with the consumption of infested raw or undercooked meat and with poor handwashing after handling infected cat litter. Pregnant women with HIV antibodies are at higher risk because toxoplasmosis is a common accompanying opportunistic infection. The presence of toxoplasmosis can be determined through blood studies, although laboratory diagnosis is difficult. Women at risk for infection should have toxoplasmosis titers evaluated. Acute infection in pregnancy produces influenza-like symptoms and lymphadenopathy in some women but no symptoms in others. Miscarriage may occur.

TABLE 7-7 TORCH INFECTION: MATERNAL AND FETAL

INFECTION	MATERNAL EFFECTS	FETAL EFFECTS	COUNSELING: PREVENTION, IDENTIFICATION, AND MANAGEMENT
*T*oxoplasmosis (protozoa)	Most infections asymptomatic Acute infection similar to mononucleosis Woman immune after first episode (except in immunocompromised patients)	Congenital infection is most likely to occur when maternal infection develops during the third trimester. The risk of fetal injury, however, is greatest when maternal infection occurs during the first trimester.	Good handwashing technique should be used. Eating raw or rare meat and exposure to litter used by infected cats should be avoided; toxoplasma titer should be checked if there are cats in the house. If titer is rising during early pregnancy, abortion may be considered an option.
*O*ther infections			
Hepatitis A (infectious hepatitis) (virus)	Liver failure (extremely rare) Low-grade fever, malaise, poor appetite, right upper quadrant pain and tenderness, jaundice, and light-colored stools	Perinatal transmission virtually never occurs.	Spread by fecal-oral contact especially by culinary workers; gamma globulin can be given as prophylaxis for hepatitis A. Hepatitis A vaccine is available.
Hepatitis B (serum hepatitis) (virus)	May be transmitted sexually. Approximately 10% of patients become chronic carriers. Some people with chronic hepatitis B eventually develop severe chronic liver disease, such as cirrhosis or hepatocellular carcinoma.	Infection occurs during birth. Maternal vaccination during pregnancy should present no risk for fetus (however, data are not available).	Generally passed by contaminated needles, syringes, or blood transfusions; also can be transmitted orally or by coitus (but incubation period is longer); hepatitis B immune globulin can be given prophylactically after exposure. Hepatitis B vaccine recommended for populations at risk.
*R*ubella (3-day or German measles) (virus)	Rash, fever, mild symptoms such as headache, malaise, myalgias, and arthralgias; postauricular lymph nodes may be swollen; mild conjunctivitis	Approximately 50%-80% of fetuses exposed to the virus within 12 weeks after conception will show signs of congenital infection. Very few fetuses are affected if infection occurs after 18 weeks of gestation. The most common fetal anomalies associated with congenital rubella syndrome are deafness, eye defects (e.g., cataracts or retinopathy), central nervous system defects, and cardiac defects.	Vaccination of pregnant women is contraindicated; pregnancy should be prevented for 1 month after vaccination. Women may breastfeed after vaccination and the vaccine can be administered along with immunoglobulin preparations such as Rh immune globulin.
*C*ytomegalovirus (CMV) (a herpesvirus)	Most adults are asymptomatic or have only mild influenza-like symptoms. The presence of CMV antibodies does not totally prevent reinfection.	The fetus can be infected transplacentally. Infection is much more likely with a primary maternal infection. The most common indications of congenital infection include hepatosplenomegaly, intracranial calcifications, jaundice, growth restriction, microcephaly, chorioretinitis, hearing loss, thrombocytopenia, hyperbilirubinemia, and hepatitis.	The virus is transmitted by transplantation of an infected organ, transfusion of infected blood, sexual contact, or contact with contaminated saliva or urine. Virus may be reactivated and cause disease in utero or during birth in subsequent pregnancies; fetal infection may occur during passage through infected birth canal. Prevention includes use of CMV-negative blood products if transfusion of pregnant women is necessary and teaching all women to wash hands carefully after handling infant diapers and toys.
*H*erpes genitalis (herpes simplex virus, type 1 or type 2 [HSV-1 or HSV-2])	Primary infection with painful blisters, tender inguinal lymph nodes, fever, viral meningitis (rare) Recurrent infections are much milder and shorter.	Transplacental infection resulting in congenital infection is rare and usually occurs with primary maternal infection. The risk mainly exists with infection late in pregnancy.	As many as two-thirds of women with HSV-2 antibodies acquired the infection asymptomatically; however, asymptomatic women can give birth to seriously infected neonates. Risk of transmission is greatest during vaginal birth if woman has active lesions; thus cesarean birth is recommended. Acyclovir can be used to treat recurrent outbreaks during pregnancy or as suppressive therapy late in pregnancy to prevent an outbreak during labor and birth.

Source: Duff, P., Sweet, R., & Edwards, R. (2009). Maternal and fetal infections. In R. Creasy, R. Resnik, J. Iams, C. Lockwood, & T. Moore (Eds.), *Creasy and Resnik's maternal-fetal medicine: Principles and practice* (6th ed.). Philadelphia: Saunders.

The treatment of choice for toxoplasmosis is spiramycin, sulfadine, or a combination of pyrimethamine and sulfadiazine. Treatment of the pregnant woman may reduce the risk of congenital toxoplasmosis (Cunningham et al., 2010).

Other Infections

The primary infection included in the category of other infections is hepatitis, which was discussed previously. Infections other than hepatitis also may be identified as "other" TORCH infections. These include GBS, varicella, and HIV.

Rubella

Rubella, also called German measles or 3-day measles, is a viral infection transmitted by droplets (such as from an infected person's sneeze). Rash, muscle aches, joint pain, and mild lymphedema are usually seen in the infected mother. Consequences for the fetus are much more serious and include miscarriage, congenital anomalies (referred to as congenital rubella syndrome), and death. Vaccination of pregnant women is contraindicated because a rubella infection may develop after the live vaccine is administered. Rubella vaccine is given to women who are not immune as part of preconception counseling or in the postpartum period prior to discharge, with instructions to use contraception for at least 1 month after vaccination (ACOG, 2002).

Cytomegalovirus

Maternal infection with CMV may begin as a mononucleosis-like syndrome. In most adults the onset of CMV infection is uncertain and asymptomatic; however, the disease may become a chronic persistent infection. Approximately 60% of the adult population has antibodies to CMV. This virus is primarily transmitted by close contact but also has been isolated from semen, cervical and vaginal secretions, breast milk, placental tissue, urine, feces, and banked blood. Maternal CMV infection may be diagnosed by presence of CMV in urine or in serum, because many women have evidence of CMV infection. Women who show CMV infection in pregnancy (by positive viral titers) usually have chronic or recurrent infections (Yudkin & Gonik, 2006).

Women at risk for infection include those who work in or have children in daycare centers and women with compromised immune systems.

! NURSING ALERT

Contact with the saliva or urine of young children is a major cause of CMV infection among pregnant women. Women should wash their hands often with soap and water for 15-20 seconds, especially after changing diapers or touching saliva or nasal secretions from a young child.

In the United States, 1% to 2% of infants have congenital CMV infection. Fetal infection can cause microcephaly; eye, ear, and dental defects; and mental retardation. No treatment is available during pregnancy.

Herpes Simplex Virus

The potential pregnancy effects of primary genital herpes infection include miscarriage, preterm labor, and intrauterine growth restriction. The main route of HSV transmission from mother to neonate is through an infected birth canal (see previous discussion on p. 153).

CARE MANAGEMENT

Women may delay seeking care for STIs and other infections because they fear social stigma, have little accessibility to health care services, are asymptomatic, or are unaware that they have an infection. A comprehensive assessment focuses on lifestyle issues that are often personal or sensitive. A culturally sensitive, nonjudgmental approach is essential to facilitate accurate data collection (see Nursing Process box: Woman with a Sexually Transmitted Infection).

The woman with an STI will need encouragement to seek care at the earliest stage of symptoms. Counseling women about STIs is essential for (1) preventing new infections or reinfection; (2) increasing compliance with treatment and follow-up; (3) providing support during treatment; and (4) assisting women in discussions with their partner(s). Women must be made aware of the serious potential consequences of STIs and the behaviors that increase or decrease the likelihood of infection.

The nurse must make sure that the woman understands what infection she has, how it is transmitted, and why it must be treated (see Teaching for Self-Management box: Sexually Transmitted Infections).

TEACHING FOR SELF-MANAGEMENT

Sexually Transmitted Infections

- Take your medication as directed.
- Use comfort measures for symptom relief as suggested by your health care provider.
- Keep your appointment for repeat cultures or checkups after your treatment to make sure your infection is cured.
- Inform your sexual partner(s) of the need to be tested and treated, if necessary.
- Abstain from sexual intercourse until your treatment is completed or for as long as you are advised by your health care provider.
- Use sex practices that decrease risk when sexual intercourse is resumed.
- Call your health care provider immediately if you notice bumps, sores, rashes, or discharges.
- Keep all future appointments with your health care provider, even if things appear normal.

Addressing the psychosocial component of STIs is essential. A woman may be afraid or embarrassed to tell her partner or to ask her partner to seek treatment. She may be embarrassed to admit her sexual practices, or she may be concerned about confidentiality. The nurse may need to help the woman deal with the effect of a diagnosis of an STI on a committed relationship, because the woman is now faced with the necessity of dealing with "uncertain monogamy."

In many instances sexual partners should be treated; thus the infected woman is asked to identify and notify all partners who might have been exposed. Often she will find this difficult to do. Empathizing with the woman's feelings and suggesting specific ways of talking with partners will help decrease anxiety and assist in efforts to control infection. For example, the nurse

NURSING PROCESS

The Woman with a Sexually Transmitted Infection

ASSESSMENT

- A complete history is essential in identifying possible STIs. Factors that may influence the development and management of STIs in women include present symptoms, a history of STI or PID, the number of past or current sexual partners, and types of sexual activity. Women should be queried for specific lifestyle behaviors that place them at risk for STIs. Among these are intravenous drug use or partner intravenous drug use, smoking, alcohol use, inadequate or poor nutrition, and high levels of stress or fatigue.
- A comprehensive physical examination is essential to diagnosing STIs. Because the speculum usually is not lubricated before insertion into the vagina (cultures of vaginal secretions may have to be obtained), insertion may be more uncomfortable than usual.
- Appropriate laboratory studies will be suggested, in part, by the history and physical examination results.
  - Bacterial STIs are easily determined from genital tract, urine, and blood studies.
  - Viral agents also can be cultured.
  - Additional laboratory studies may be done, including Pap smear, wet mounts, gonococcal culture, VDRL or RPR test for syphilis, cultures for HSV.
  - The woman should be offered the HIV-antibody test.

NURSING DIAGNOSES

The following nursing diagnoses are representative of those used in a plan of care for a woman with an STI and/or other vaginal infection:

***Anxiety/Situational Low Self-Esteem/Disturbed Body Image* related to:**
- perceived effects on sexual relationships and family processes
- possible effects on pregnancy or fetus
- long-term sequelae of infection

***Deficient Knowledge* related to:**
- transmission/prevention of infection/reinfection
- behaviors that reduce risk for STIs
- management of infection

***Acute Pain/Impaired Tissue Integrity* related to:**
- effects of infection process
- scratching (excoriation) of pruritic areas
- hygiene practices

***Sexual Dysfunction* related to:**
- effects of infection process

***Social Isolation and Impaired Social Interaction* related to:**
- perceived effects on relationships with others if STI status is unknown

EXPECTED OUTCOMES OF CARE

Outcomes for the woman include that she will:
- Be free of infection or, in the case of viral infection, have remission or stabilization of the infection.
- Identify and be able to discuss the etiology, management, and expected course of the infection and its prevention.
- Be able to identify her risky behaviors and discuss plans for decreasing her risk for infection.

PLAN OF CARE AND INTERVENTIONS

- Provide a brief description of the infection in language that they can understand, including modes of transmission, incubation period, symptoms, infectious period, and potential complications.
- Provide thorough, careful instructions about medications, both verbally and in writing; include side effects, benefits, and risks of the medication.
- Suggest comfort measures to decrease symptoms such as pain, itching, or nausea.
- Advise the woman to refrain from intercourse until all treatment is finished and a repeat culture, if appropriate, is done.
- Teach risk reducing practices, if this has not been done already.

EVALUATION

Evaluation is based on client-centered outcomes identified during the planning stage of nursing care. The nurse can be reasonably assured that care was effective to the extent that expected outcomes have been met.

might suggest that the woman say, "I care about you and I'm concerned about you. That's why I'm calling to tell you that I have a sexually transmitted infection. My clinician will be happy to talk with you if you would like." Offering literature and role-playing situations with the client also may be of assistance. It is often helpful to remind the woman that although this is an embarrassing situation, most persons would rather know than not know that they have been exposed. Health professionals who take time to counsel their clients on how to talk with their partner(s) can improve compliance and case findings.

Interrupting the transmission of infection is crucial to STI control. For treatable and vaccine-preventable STIs, further transmission and reinfection can be prevented with referral of sex partners. Many STIs are reportable; all states require that the five traditional STIs—gonorrhea, syphilis, chancroid, lymphogranuloma venereum, and granuloma inguinale—be reported to public health officials. Many other states require that other STIs such as chlamydial infections, genital herpes, and genital warts be reported. In addition, all states require that AIDS cases be reported; 35 states require that HIV infection be reported.

LEGAL TIP: STI Reporting

A nurse is legally responsible for reporting all cases of those diseases identified as reportable and should know what the requirements are in the state in which she or he practices. The woman must be informed when a case will be reported and be told why. Failure to inform the woman that the case will be reported is a serious breach of professional ethics.

INFECTION CONTROL

Infection-control measures are essential to protect care providers and to prevent health personnel–related infection of clients, regardless of the infectious agent. The risk for occupational transmission varies with the disease. Even when the risk is low, as with HIV, the existence of any risk warrants reasonable precautions. Precautions against airborne disease transmission are available in all health care agencies. Standard Precautions (precautions to use in care of all persons for infection control) and additional precautions for labor and birth settings are listed in Box 7-3.

BOX 7-3 STANDARD PRECAUTIONS

Medical history and examination cannot reliably identify all persons infected with human immunodeficiency virus (HIV) or other blood-borne pathogens. Standard Precautions should therefore be used consistently in the care of all persons. These precautions apply to blood, body fluids, and all secretions and excretions, except sweat, nonintact skin, and mucous membranes. The following infection-control practices should be applied during the delivery of health care to reduce the risk of transmission of microorganisms from known and unknown sources of infection (Seigel, Rhinehart, Jackson, Chiarello, & the Healthcare Infection Control Practices Advisory Committee, 2007):

1. *Hand hygiene.* During the delivery of health care, avoid unnecessary touching of surfaces in close proximity to the client to prevent both contamination of clean hands from environmental surfaces and transmission of pathogens from contaminated hands to surfaces. Wash dirty or contaminated hands with either a nonantimicrobial or an antimicrobial soap and water. If hands are not visibly soiled, decontaminate hands with an alcohol-based hand rub, or hands may be washed with an antimicrobial soap and water. Perform hand hygiene (1) before having direct contact with clients; (2) after contact with blood, body fluids, or excretions, mucous membranes, nonintact skin, or wound dressings; (3) after contact with a client's intact skin (e.g., when taking a pulse or blood pressure or lifting a client); (4) if hands will be moving from a contaminated body site to a clean body site during client care; (5) after contact with inanimate objects (including medical equipment) in the immediate vicinity of the client; and (6) after removing gloves. Wash hands with nonantimicrobial soap and water or with antimicrobial soap and water if contact with spores (e.g., *Clostridium difficile* or *Bacillus anthracis*) is likely to have occurred. The physical action of washing and rinsing hands under such circumstances is recommended because alcohols, chlorhexidine, iodophors, and other antiseptic agents have poor activity against spores. Do not wear artificial fingernails or extenders if duties include direct contact with clients at high risk for infection and associated adverse outcomes.
2. *Personal protective equipment (PPE).* Observe the following principles of use:
   - *Gloves.* Wear gloves when a reasonably anticipated possibility exists that contact with blood or other potentially infectious materials, mucous membranes, nonintact skin, or potentially contaminated intact skin (e.g., of a client incontinent of stool or urine) might occur. Gloves should be worn during infant eye prophylaxis, care of the umbilical cord, circumcision site, parenteral procedures, diaper changes, contact with colostrum, and postpartum assessments. Wear gloves with fit and durability appropriate to the task. Remove gloves after contact with a client or the surrounding environment (including medical equipment) using proper technique to prevent hand contamination. Do not wear the same pair of gloves for the care of more than one client. Change gloves during patient care if the hands will move from a contaminated body site (e.g., perineal area) to a clean body site (e.g., face).
   - *Gowns.* Wear a gown that is appropriate to the task to protect the skin and prevent soiling or contamination of clothing during procedures and client-care activities when contact with blood, body fluids, secretions, or excretions is anticipated. Remove the gown and perform hand hygiene before leaving the client's environment. Do not reuse gowns, even for repeated contacts with the same client. Routine donning of gowns on entrance into a high risk unit (e.g., intensive care unit [ICU], neonatal intensive care unit [NICU]) is not indicated.
   - *Mouth, nose, eye protection.* Use PPE to protect the mucous membranes of the eyes, nose, and mouth during procedures and client-care activities that are likely to generate splashes or sprays of blood, body fluids, secretions, and excretions. Select masks, goggles, face shields, and combinations of each according to the need anticipated by the task performed.
3. *Respiratory hygiene and cough etiquette.* Post signs at entrances and in strategic places (e.g., elevators, cafeterias) within ambulatory and inpatient settings with instructions to clients and other persons with symptoms of a respiratory infection to cover their mouth and nose when coughing or sneezing, use and dispose of tissues, and perform hand hygiene after hands have been in contact with respiratory secretions. Provide tissues and no-touch receptacles (e.g., foot pedal—operated lid or open, plastic-lined wastebasket) for disposal of tissues. Provide resources and instructions for performing hand hygiene in or near waiting areas in ambulatory and inpatient settings; provide conveniently located dispensers of alcohol-based hand rubs and, where sinks are available, supplies for handwashing. During periods of increased prevalence of respiratory infections in the community, offer masks to coughing clients and other symptomatic persons (e.g., persons who accompany ill clients) on entry into the facility, and encourage them to maintain special separation, ideally a distance of at least 3 feet, from others in common waiting areas.
4. *Safe injection practices.* The following recommendations apply to the use of needles, cannulas that replace needles, and, where applicable, intravenous delivery systems:
   - Use aseptic technique to prevent contamination of sterile injection equipment. Needles, cannulas, and syringes are sterile, single-use items; they should not be reused for another client. Use fluid infusion and administration sets (i.e., intravenous bags, tubing, and connectors) for one client only, and dispose appropriately after use. Use single-dose vials for parenteral medications whenever possible. If multidose vials must be used, both the needle (or cannula) and the syringe used to access the multidose vial must be sterile. Do not keep multidose vials in the immediate client treatment area, and store in accordance with the manufacturer's recommendations; discard if sterility is compromised or questionable.

Source: Seigel, J., Rhinehart, E., Jackson, M., Chiarello, L., & The Healthcare Infection Control Practices Advisory Committee. (2007). *2007 Guidelines for isolation precaution and preventing transmission of infectious agents in healthcare settings.* Available at www.cdc.gov/ncidod/dhqp/gl_isolation.html. Accessed March 8, 2010.

KEY POINTS

- Reproductive tract infections include STIs and common genital tract infections.
- Risk-reduction sexual practices are key STI-prevention strategies.
- HIV is transmitted through body fluids, primarily blood, semen, and vaginal secretions.
- Prevention of mother-to-newborn HIV transmission is most effective when the woman receives antiretroviral drugs during pregnancy and labor and birth, and the infant receives the drugs after birth.
- HPV is the most common viral STI.
- Syphilis has reemerged as a common STI, affecting African-American women more than any other ethnic or racial group.
- Chlamydia is the most common STI in women in the United States and the most common cause of PID.
- Viral hepatitis has several forms of transmission; HBV infections carry the greatest risk.
- Young, sexually active women who do not practice risk-reducing sexual behaviors and have multiple partners are at greatest risk for STIs and HIV.
- STIs are responsible for substantial mortality and morbidity, great personal suffering, and heavy economic burden in the United States.
- STIs and vaginitis are biologic events for which all individuals have a right to expect objective, compassionate, and effective health care.
- Pregnancy confers no immunity against infection, and both mother and fetus must be considered when the pregnant woman contracts an infection.
- Because history and examination cannot reliably identify everyone with HIV or other blood-borne pathogens, blood and body-fluid precautions should be used consistently for everyone all the time.

Audio Chapter Summaries Access an audio summary of the Key Points on evolve

REFERENCES

American Academy of Pediatrics Committee on Pediatric AIDS. (2008). HIV testing and prophylaxis to prevent mother-to-child transmission in the United States. *Pediatrics, 122*(5), 1127–1134.

American Cancer Society (ACS). (2010). *Cancer facts and figures 2010*. New York: Author.

American College of Obstetricians and Gynecologists (ACOG). (2008). *ACOG patient education: How to prevent STDs*. Washington, DC: ACOG.

American College of Obstetricians and Gynecologists (ACOG). (2002). ACOG Committee Opinion. No. 281, December, 2002. Rubella vaccination. *Obstetrics and Gynecology, 100*(6), 1417.

Branson, B., Handsfield, H., Lampe, M., Janssen, R., Taylor, A., Lyss, S., et al. (2006). Revised recommendations for HIV testing of adults, adolescents, and pregnant women in health-care settings. *MMWR Morbidity and Mortality Weekly Report, 55*(RR-14), 1–17.

Centers for Disease Control and Prevention (CDC). (2007). *Updated recommended treatment regimens for gonococcal infections and associated conditions, United States, April, 2007*. Available at www.cdc.gov/std/treatment/2006/updated-regimens.htm. Accessed March 3, 2010.

Centers for Disease Control and Prevention. (2008a). *Guidelines for GBS screening*. Available at www.cdc.gov/groupbstrep. Accessed June 2, 2010.

Centers for Disease Control and Prevention (CDC). (2008b). *Hepatitis B information for health professionals—Perinatal transmission*. Available at www.cdc.gov/hepatitis. Accessed June 2, 2010.

Centers for Disease Control and Prevention (CDC). (2008c). *Hepatitis B vaccine*. Available at www.cdc.gov/hepatitis. Accessed June 2, 2010.

Centers for Disease Control and Prevention (CDC). (2008d). *HIV/AIDS among women*. Available at www.cdc.gov/hiv/topics/women/resources/factsheets/women.htm. Accessed June 2, 2010.

Centers for Disease Control and Prevention (CDC). (2009a). *Genital HPV infection—CDC fact sheet*. Available at www.cdc.gov/std/HPV/STDfact-HPV.htm. Accessed June 2, 2010.

Centers for Disease Control and Prevention (CDC). (2009b). *Sexually transmitted diseases in the United States, 2008*. Available at www.cdc.gov/std/stats08/trends.htm. Accessed June 2, 2010.

Centers for Disease Control and Prevention (CDC). (2010a). *Genital herpes—CDC fact sheet*. Available at www.cdc.gov/std/Herpes. Accessed June 2, 2010.

Centers for Disease Control and Prevention (CDC). (2010b). *Human papillomavirus vaccine*. Available at www.cdc.gov/hpv. Accessed June 2, 2010.

Centers for Disease Control and Prevention (CDC), Workowski, K., & Berman, S. (2006). Sexually transmitted diseases treatment guidelines 2006. *MMWR Morbidity and Mortality Weekly Report, 55*(RR-11), 1–94.

Centers for Disease Control and Prevention Division of HIV/AIDS Prevention. (2008). (*FDA-approved rapid HIV antibody screening tests*. Available at www.cdc.gov/hiv/topics/testing/rapid/rt-comparison.htm. Accessed June 2, 2010.

Cunningham, F., Leveno, K., Bloom, S., Hauth, J., Rouse, D., & Sprong, C. (2010). *Williams obstetrics* (23rd ed.). New York: McGraw-Hill.

Duff, P. (2007). Maternal and perinatal infection. In S. Gabbe, J. Niebyl, & J. Simpson (Eds.), *Obstetrics: Normal and problem pregnancies* (5th ed.). New York: Churchill Livingstone.

Eckert, L., & Lentz, G. (2007a). Infections of the lower genital tract. In V. Katz, G. Lentz, R. Lobo, & D. Gershenson (Eds.), *Comprehensive gynecology* (5th ed.). Philadelphia: Mosby.

Eckert, L., & Lentz, G. (2007b). Infections of the upper genital tract. In V. Katz, G. Lentz, R. Lobo, & D. Gershenson (Eds.), *Comprehensive gynecology* (5th ed.). Philadelphia: Mosby.

Marrazzo, J., Guest, F., & Cates, W. (2007). Reproductive tract infections, including HIV and sexually transmitted infections. In R. Hatcher, J. Trussell, A. Nelson, W. Cates, F. Guest, & D. Kowal (Eds.), *Contraceptive technology* (19th ed.). New York: Ardent Media.

Mishell, D. (2007). Family planning: Contraception, sterilization, and abortion. In V. Katz, G. Lentz, R. Lobo, & D. Gershenson (Eds.), *Comprehensive gynecology* (5th ed.). Philadelphia: Mosby.

Murphy, P., Morgan, K., & Likis, F. (2006). Contraception. In K. Schuiling, & F. Likis (Eds.), *Women's gynecological health* Sudbury, MA: Jones and Bartlett.

Panel on Treatment of HIV-Infected Pregnant Women and Prevention of Perinatal Transmission. (2010). *Recommendations for Use of Antiretroviral Drugs in Pregnant HIV-1-Infected Women for Maternal Health and Interventions to Reduce Perinatal HIV Transmission in the United States. May 24, 2010;* pp 1–117. Available at http://aidsinfo.nih.gov/ContentFiles/PerinatalGL.pdf. Accessed June 2, 2010.

Ravin, C. (2007). Preventing STIs: Ask the questions. *Nursing for Women's Health, 11*(1), 88–91.

U.S. Food and Drug Administration (FDA). (2008). *HIV testing*. Available at www.fda.gov/oashi/aidstest.html. Accessed March 8, 2010.

U.S. Preventive Services Task Force (USPSTF). (2009a). *Screening for hepatitis B virus infection in pregnancy. Guide to clinical preventive services, 2009. Recommendations of the U.S. Preventive Services Task Force.* Rockville, MD: Agency for Healthcare Research and Quality.

U.S. Preventive Services Task Force (USPSTF). (2009b). *Screening for syphilis infection. Guide to clinical preventive services, 2009. Recommendations of the U.S. Preventive Services Task Force.* Rockville, MD: Agency for Healthcare Research and Quality.

U.S. Preventive Services Task Force (USPSTF). (2007a). *Screening for chlamydial infection. Guide to clinical preventive services, 2009. Recommendations of the U.S. Preventive Services Task Force.* Rockville, MD: Agency for Healthcare Research and Quality.

U.S. Preventive Services Task Force (USPSTF). (2007b). *Screening for HIV. Guide to clinical preventive services, 2009. Recommendations of the U.S. Preventive Services Task Force.* Rockville, MD: Agency for Healthcare Research and Quality.

Volmink, J., Siegfried, N., van der Merwe, L., & Brocklehurst, P. (2007). Antiretrovirals for reducing the risk of mother-to-child transmission of HIV infection. *Cochrane Database of Systematic Reviews, 2007*, Issue 1, Art. No. CD003510.

Weiner, C., & Buhimschi, C. (2009). *Drugs for pregnant and lactating women* (2nd ed.). Philadelphia: Saunders.

World Health Organization (WHO). (2004). *Medical eligibility criteria for contraceptive use* (3rd ed.). Geneva: WHO.

Yudkin, M., & Gonik, B. (2006). Perinatal infections. In R. Martin, A. Fanaroff, & M. Walsh (Eds.), *Fanaroff & Martin's neonatal-perinatal medicine: Diseases of the fetus and infant* (8th ed.). Philadelphia: Mosby.

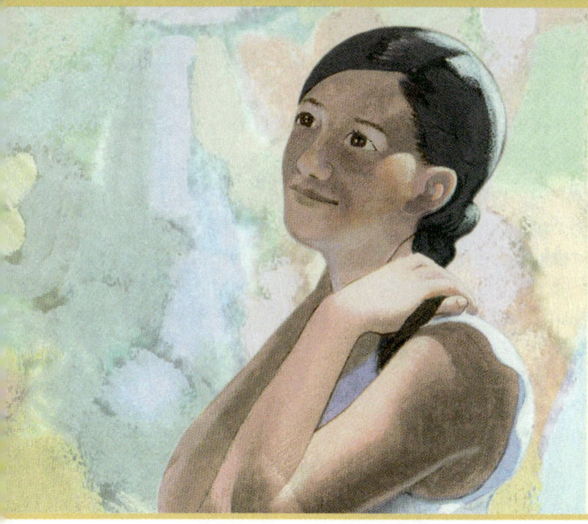

CHAPTER

8

Contraception and Abortion

Sharon E. Lock

evolve WEBSITE

http://evolve.elsevier.com/Lowdermilk/MWHC/

Audio Glossary
Audio Key Points
Critical Thinking Exercise
  Client Teaching – Contraception
NCLEX Review Questions
Nursing Care Plan
  Sexual Activity and Contraception
Spanish Guidelines
  Contraception
Video—Nursing Skills
  Teaching Birth Control Methods

LEARNING OBJECTIVES

- Compare various methods of contraception.
- Identify the advantages and disadvantages of commonly used methods of contraception.
- Explain the common nursing interventions that facilitate contraceptive use.
- Examine the various ethical, legal, cultural, and religious considerations of contraception.
- Describe the techniques used for medical and surgical interruption of pregnancy.
- Discuss the various ethical and legal considerations of elective abortion.

CONTRACEPTION

Contraception is the intentional prevention of pregnancy during sexual intercourse. *Birth control* is the device and/or practice to decrease the risk of conceiving, or bearing, offspring. *Family planning* is the conscious decision on when to conceive, or to avoid pregnancy, throughout the reproductive years. With the wide assortment of birth control options available, it is possible for a woman to use several different contraceptive methods at various stages throughout her fertile years. Nurses interact with the woman to compare and contrast available options, reliability, relative cost, protection from sexually transmitted infections (STIs), the individual's comfort level, and the partner's willingness to use a particular birth control method. Those who practice contraception may still be at risk for pregnancy simply because their choice of birth control method is not perfect or is used inconsistently or incorrectly. Providing adequate instruction about how to use a contraceptive method, when to use a backup method, and when to use emergency contraception can decrease the chance of unintended pregnancy (Stewart, Trussell, & Van Look, 2007).

CARE MANAGEMENT

A multidisciplinary approach may assist a woman in choosing and correctly using an appropriate contraceptive method. Nurses, nurse-midwives, nurse practitioners, and other advanced practice nurses as well as physicians have the knowledge and expertise to assist a woman in making decisions about contraception that will satisfy the woman's personal, social, cultural, and interpersonal needs.

Family, friends, media, partner or partners, religious affiliation, and health care professionals influence a woman's perception of contraceptive choices. These external influences form a woman's unique view. The nurse assists in supporting the woman's decision based on the individual's situation (see Nursing Process box).

Informed consent is a vital component in the education of the client concerning contraception or sterilization. The nurse often has the responsibility of documenting information provided and the understanding of that information by the client. The acronym BRAIDED may be useful (see Legal Tip).

NURSING PROCESS

Contraception

ASSESSMENT

- Determine the woman's knowledge about contraception and her sexual partner's commitment to any particular method.
- Collect data about the frequency of coitus, the number of sexual partners, the level of contraceptive involvement, and her or her partner's objections to any methods.
- Assess the woman's level of comfort and willingness to touch her genitals and cervical mucus.
- Identify any misconceptions, as well as religious and cultural factors. Pay close attention to the woman's verbal and nonverbal responses to hearing about the various available methods.
- Consider the woman's reproductive life plan.
- Complete a history (including menstrual, contraceptive, and obstetric), physical examination (including pelvic examination), and laboratory tests (as needed for identifying presence of STIs).

NURSING DIAGNOSES

Examples of nursing diagnoses include:

***Decisional Conflict* related to:**
- contraceptive alternatives
- partner's willingness to agree on contraceptive method

***Fear* related to:**
- contraceptive method side effects

***Risk for Infection* related to:**
- unprotected sexual intercourse
- use of contraceptive method
- broken skin or mucous membrane after surgery or intrauterine device (IUD) insertion

***Ineffective Sexuality Patterns* related to:**
- fear of pregnancy

***Acute Pain* related to:**
- postoperative recovery after sterilization

***Risk for Spiritual Distress* related to:**
- discrepancy between religious or cultural beliefs and choice of contraceptive method

EXPECTED OUTCOMES OF CARE

The expected outcomes include that the woman or couple will:
- Verbalize understanding about contraceptive methods.
- Verbalize understanding of all information necessary to give informed consent.
- State comfort and satisfaction with the chosen method.
- Use the contraceptive method correctly and consistently.
- Experience no adverse sequelae as a result of the chosen method of contraception.
- Prevent unplanned pregnancy or plan a pregnancy.

PLAN OF CARE AND INTERVENTIONS

- Implement the appropriate teaching for the specific contraceptive used.
- Have the woman perform a return demonstration to assess her understanding.
- Give written instructions and telephone numbers for questions.
- If the woman has difficulty understanding written instructions, offer her (and her partner, if available) graphic material and a telephone number to call as necessary.
- Offer the woman an opportunity to return for further instruction. See text for discussion of methods of contraception.
- Provide information about back up methods of birth control and emergency contraception.

EVALUATION

- Care is effective when the expected outcomes have been achieved: the woman and her partner learn about the various methods of contraception, the couple achieves pregnancy only when planned, and they have no complications as a result of the chosen method of contraception.

Critical Thinking Exercise—Client Teaching: Contraception

LEGAL TIP: Informed Consent

B—Benefits: information about advantages and success rates
R—Risks: information about disadvantages and failure rates
A—Alternatives: information about other available methods
I—Inquiries: opportunity to ask questions
D—Decisions: opportunity to decide or to change her mind
E—Explanations: information about method and how it is used
D—Documentation: information given and client's understanding

To foster a safe environment for consultation, a private setting should be provided in which the client can feel free to be open. Distractions should be minimized, and samples of birth control devices for interactive teaching should be available. The nurse counters myths with facts, clarifies misinformation, and fills in gaps of knowledge. The ideal contraceptive should be safe, easily available, economical, acceptable, simple to use, and promptly reversible. Although no method may ever achieve all these objectives, new contraceptive technologies are being developed (Blithe, 2008; Practice Committee of the American Society for Reproductive Medicine, 2008; Yranski & Gamache, 2008).

Contraceptive effectiveness varies from couple to couple (Box 8-1) and depends on the properties of the method and the characteristics of the user (Kost, Singh, Vaughan, Trussell, & Bankole, 2008). *Contraceptive failure* rate refers to the percentage of contraceptive users expected to have an unplanned pregnancy during the first year, even when they use a method consistently and correctly. Failure rates decrease over time, either because a user gains experience and uses a method more appropriately or because the less effective users stop using the method.

! NURSING ALERT

Make sure the woman has a backup method of birth control and emergency contraceptive pills (ECPs) readily available during the initial learning phase when she uses a new method of contraception to help prevent an unintentional conception.

Safety of a method depends on the woman's medical history. Barrier methods offer some protection from STIs, and oral contraceptives may reduce the incidence of breast, ovarian, and endometrial cancer but increase the risk of thromboembolic problems.

Methods of Contraception

The following discussion of contraceptive methods provides the nurse with information needed for client teaching. After implementing the appropriate teaching for contraceptive use, the nurse supervises return demonstrations and practice to assess client understanding (Fig. 8-1). The woman is given written instructions; if she has difficulty understanding the written instructions, she (and her partner, if available) is offered graphic material and a telephone number to call as necessary, or is offered an opportunity to return for further instruction (see Nursing Care Plan).

BOX 8-1 FACTORS AFFECTING METHOD CONTRACEPTIVE EFFECTIVENESS

- Frequency of intercourse
- Motivation to prevent pregnancy
- Understanding of how to use the method
- Adherence to method
- Provision of short-term or long-term protection
- Likelihood of pregnancy for the individual woman
- Consistent use of method

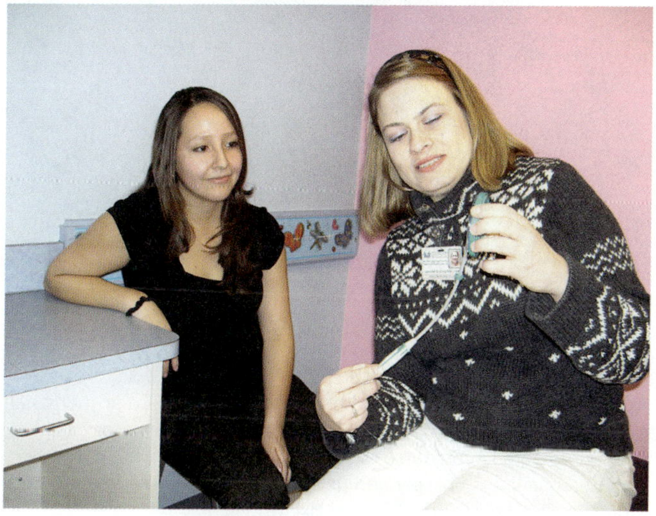

FIG. 8-1 Nurse counseling woman about contraceptive methods. (Courtesy Dee Lowdermilk, Chapel Hill, NC.)

Coitus Interruptus

Coitus interruptus (withdrawal) involves the male partner withdrawing the penis from the woman's vagina before he ejaculates. Although coitus interruptus is one of the least effective methods of contraception, it is a good choice for couples who do not have another contraceptive available (Kowal, 2007). Effectiveness is similar to barrier methods and depends on the man's ability to withdraw his penis before ejaculation. The percentage of women who will experience an unintended pregnancy within the first year of typical use (failure rate) of withdrawal is about 27% (Trussell, 2007). Coitus interruptus does not protect against STIs or human immunodeficiency virus (HIV) infection.

Fertility Awareness Methods (Natural Family Planning)

Fertility awareness methods (FAMs) of contraception, also known as periodic abstinence or natural family planning, depend on identifying the beginning and end of the fertile period of the menstrual cycle. These methods provide contraception by relying on avoidance of intercourse during fertile periods. Natural family planning methods are the only contraceptive practices acceptable to the Roman Catholic Church. When women who want to use FAMs are educated about the menstrual cycle, three phases are identified:

1. Infertile phase: before ovulation
2. Fertile phase: about 5 to 7 days around the middle of the cycle, including several days before and during ovulation and the day afterward
3. Infertile phase: after ovulation

NURSING CARE PLAN

Sexual Activity and Contraception

NURSING DIAGNOSIS

Decisional conflict related to contraceptive alternatives

Expected Outcome

Woman and partner will verbalize understanding of different methods of contraception and will choose the method best suited for their needs.

Nursing Interventions/*Rationales*

- Provide information regarding reliability, use, indications, contraindications, and side effects of different methods of contraception *to facilitate the decision-making process.*
- Use privacy and therapeutic communication during discussion of sexual activity and methods of contraception *to provide clarification of information and client trust of caregiver.*

NURSING DIAGNOSIS

Risk for infection related to ongoing sexual activity as evidenced by client history

Expected Outcome

Woman and her partner will remain free of sexually transmitted infections.

Nursing Interventions/*Rationales*

- Provide information regarding sex practices to reduce risk of STIs and use of barrier methods *to raise client awareness of methods to prevent infection.*

NURSING DIAGNOSIS

Ineffective health maintenance related to unfamiliarity with contraceptive method

Expected Outcome

Woman and partner will verbalize intent to utilize chosen contraception correctly.

Nursing Interventions/*Rationales*

- Review information given regarding use, reliability, and side effects of chosen contraceptive method *to ensure woman's and partner's understanding.*
- Provide list of informational resources *to promote consistency of use of chosen method.*
- Encourage ongoing effective communication with health care provider *to promote trust.*

The human ovum can be fertilized no later than 12 to 24 hours after ovulation (Cunningham, Leveno, Bloom, Hauth, Rouse, & Spong, 2010; Hatcher, 2007). Motile sperm have been recovered from the uterus and the oviducts as long as 60 hours after coitus, but their ability to fertilize the ovum probably lasts no longer than 24 to 48 hours. One problem with FAMs is that the exact time of ovulation cannot be predicted accurately, and couples may find it difficult to exercise restraint for several days before and after ovulation. In addition, women with irregular menstrual periods have the greatest risk of failure with FAMs.

Although ovulation can be unpredictable in many women, teaching the woman about how she can directly observe her fertility patterns is an empowering tool. There are nearly a dozen categories of FAMs. To prevent pregnancy, each one uses a combination of charts, records, calculations, tools, observations, and either abstinence or barrier methods of birth control during the fertile period in the menstrual cycle (Jennings & Arevalo, 2007). The charts and calculations associated with these methods can also be used to increase the likelihood of detecting the optimal timing of intercourse to achieve conception. Signs and symptoms of fertility awareness most commonly used with abstinence are menstrual bleeding, cervical mucus, and basal body temperature (see later discussions) (Jennings & Arevalo).

Advantages of these methods include low to no cost, absence of chemicals and hormones, and lack of alteration in the menstrual flow pattern. Disadvantages of FAMs include adherence to strict record-keeping, unintentional interference from external influences that may alter the woman's core body temperature and vaginal secretions, decreased effectiveness in women with irregular cycles (particularly adolescents who have not established regular ovulatory patterns), decreased spontaneity of coitus, and attending possibly time-consuming training sessions by qualified instructors (Jennings & Arevalo, 2007) (Box 8-2). The typical failure rate for most FAMs is 25% during the first year of use (Trussell, 2007). FAMs do not protect against STIs or HIV infection.

FAMs involve several techniques to identify fertile days. The following discussion includes the most common techniques as well as some promising techniques for the future.

Calendar-Based Methods

Calendar Rhythm Method. Practice of the calendar rhythm method is based on the number of days in each cycle, counting from the first day of menses. With this method the fertile period is determined after accurately recording the lengths of menstrual cycles for at least 6 months. The beginning of the fertile period is estimated by subtracting 18 days from the length of the shortest cycle. The end of the fertile period is determined by subtracting 11 days from the length of the longest cycle (Jennings & Arevalo, 2007). If the shortest cycle is 24 days and the longest is 30 days, application of the formula to calculate the fertile period is as follows:

Shortest cycle : 24 − 18 = sixth day
Longest cycle : 30 − 11 = nineteenth day

To avoid conception the couple would abstain during the fertile period— days 6 through 19. If the woman has very regular cycles of 28 days each, the formula indicates the fertile days to be as follows:

Shortest cycle : 28 − 18 = tenth day
Longest cycle : 28 − 11 = seventeenth day

To avoid pregnancy the couple abstains from day 10 through 17 because ovulation occurs on day 14 plus or minus 2 days. A major drawback of the calendar method is that one is trying to predict future events with past data. The unpredictability of the menstrual cycle also is not taken into consideration. The calendar rhythm method is most useful as an adjunct to the basal body temperature or the cervical mucus method.

Standard Days Method. The Standard Days Method (SDM) is essentially a modified form of the calendar rhythm method that has a "fixed" number of days of fertility for each cycle—that is, days 8 to 19 (Germano & Jennings, 2006). A CycleBeads necklace—a color-coded string of beads—can be purchased as a concrete tool to track fertility (Fig. 8-2). Day 1 of the menstrual flow is counted as the first day to begin the counting. Women who use this device are taught to avoid unprotected intercourse on days 8 to 19 (white beads on CycleBeads necklace). Although this method is useful to women whose cycles are 26 to 32 days long, it is unreliable for those who have longer or shorter cycles. The typical failure rate for the SDM is 12% during the first year of use (Jennings & Arevalo, 2007).

BOX 8-2 POTENTIAL PITFALLS OF USING FERTILITY AWARENESS METHODS OF CONTRACEPTION

Potential pitfalls of using fertility awareness methods include the five *Rs*:

- **R**estriction on sexual spontaneity
- **R**igorous daily monitoring
- **R**equired training
- **R**isk of pregnancy during prolonged training period
- **R**isk of pregnancy high on unsafe days

Source: Zieman, M., Hatcher, R. A., Cwiak, C., Darney, P. D., Creinin, M., & Stosur, H. (2007). *A pocket guide to managing contraception.* Tiger, GA: Bridging the Gap Foundation.

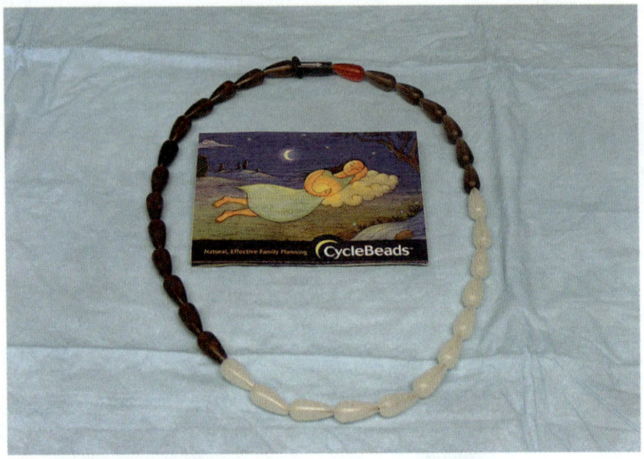

FIG. 8-2 CycleBeads. Red bead marks the first day of the menstrual cycle. White beads mark days that are likely to be fertile days; therefore, unprotected intercourse should be avoided. Brown beads are days when pregnancy is unlikely and unprotected intercourse is permitted. (Courtesy Dee Lowdermilk, Chapel Hill, NC.)

TEACHING FOR SELF-MANAGEMENT

Cervical Mucus Characteristics

SETTING THE STAGE

- Show charts of menstrual cycle along with changes in the cervical mucus.
- Have the woman practice with raw egg white.
- Supply her with a basal body temperature log and graph if she does not already have one.
- Explain that assessment of cervical mucus characteristics is best when mucus is not mixed with semen, contraceptive jellies or foams, or discharge from infections. Tell her to refrain from douching before the assessment.

CONTENT RELATED TO CERVICAL MUCUS

- Explain to the woman (couple) how cervical mucus changes throughout the menstrual cycle.
  - Postmenstrual mucus: scant
  - Preovulation mucus: cloudy, yellow or white, sticky
  - Ovulation mucus: clear, wet, sticky, slippery
  - Postovulation fertile mucus: thick, cloudy, sticky
  - Postovulation, postfertile mucus: scant
- Right before ovulation, the watery, thin, clear mucus becomes more abundant and thick (Fig. A). It feels similar to a lubricant and can be stretched 5+ cm between the thumb and forefinger; this quality of mucus is called spinnbarkeit (Fig. B), and its presence indicates the period of maximal fertility. Sperm deposited in this type of mucus can survive until ovulation occurs.

ASSESSMENT TECHNIQUE

- Stress that good handwashing is imperative to begin and end all self-assessment.
- Start observation from last day of menstrual flow.
- Assess cervical mucus several times a day for several cycles. Mucus can be obtained from vaginal opening; reaching into the vagina to the cervix is unnecessary.
- Record the findings on the same record on which the basal body temperature is entered.

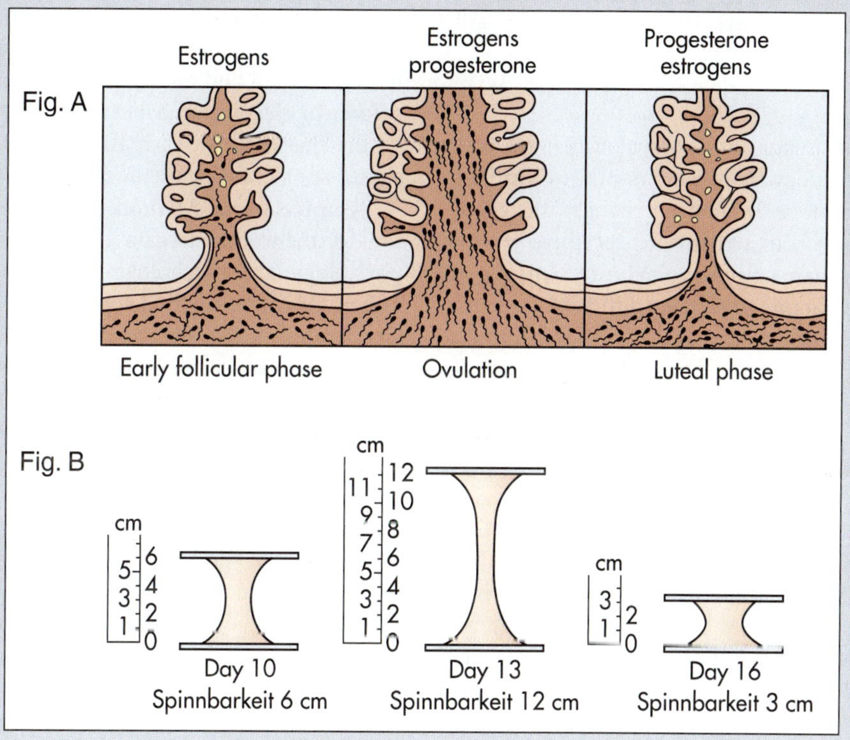

Symptoms-Based Methods

TwoDay Method. The TwoDay Method is based on the monitoring and recording of cervical secretions (Germano & Jennings, 2006). Each day the woman asks herself, (1) "Did I note secretions today?" and (2) "Did I note secretions yesterday?" If the answer to either is yes, she should avoid coitus or use a backup method of birth control. If the answer to both questions is no, her probability of getting pregnant is very low. After 2 days without secretions, the woman may resume unprotected intercourse. The TwoDay Method appears to be simpler to teach, learn, and use than other natural methods. Results suggest that the method can be an effective alternative for low literacy populations or for programs that find current natural family planning methods too time consuming or otherwise not feasible to incorporate into their services. Early studies have found the typical failure rate of the TwoDay Method to be 14% (Germano & Jennings).

Ovulation Method. The cervical mucus ovulation-detection method (also called the Billings method and the Creighton model ovulation method) requires that the woman recognize and interpret the cyclic changes in the amount and consistency of cervical mucus that characterize her own unique pattern of changes (see Teaching for Self-Management box: Cervical Mucus Characteristics). The cervical mucus that accompanies ovulation is necessary for viability and motility of sperm. It alters the pH environment, neutralizing the acidity, to be more compatible for sperm survival. Without adequate cervical mucus, coitus does not result in conception. Women check

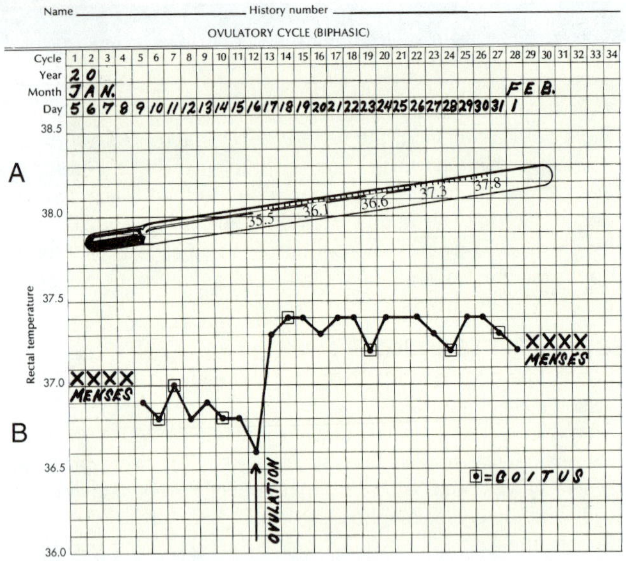

FIG. 8-3 **A,** Special thermometer for recording basal body temperature, marked in tenths to enable person to read more easily. **B,** Basal temperature record shows drop and sharp rise at time of ovulation. Biphasic curve indicates ovulatory cycle.

quantity and character of mucus on the vulva or introitus with fingers or tissue paper each day for several months to learn the cycle. To ensure an accurate assessment of changes, the cervical mucus should be free from semen, contraceptive gels or foams, and blood or discharge from vaginal infections for at least one full cycle. Other factors that create difficulty in identifying mucus changes include douches and vaginal deodorants, being in the sexually aroused state (which thins the mucus), and taking medications such as antihistamines (which dry up the mucus). Intercourse is considered safe without restriction beginning the fourth day after the last day of wet, clear, slippery mucus (postovulation) (Jennings & Arevalo, 2007).

Some women may find this method unacceptable if they are uncomfortable touching their genitals. Whether or not the individual wants to use this method for contraception, it is to the woman's advantage to learn to recognize mucus characteristics at ovulation. Self-evaluation of cervical mucus can be highly accurate and can be useful diagnostically for any of the following purposes:

- To alert the couple to the reestablishment of ovulation while breastfeeding and after discontinuation of oral contraception
- To note anovulatory cycles at any time and at the commencement of menopause
- To assist couples in planning a pregnancy

Basal Body Temperature Method. The basal body temperature (BBT) is the lowest body temperature of a healthy person, taken immediately after waking and before getting out of bed. The BBT usually varies from 36.2° to 36.3° C during menses and for about 5 to 7 days afterward (Fig. 8-3). At about the time of ovulation, a slight decrease in temperature (approximately 0.5° C) may occur in some women, but others may have no decrease at all. After ovulation, in concert with the increasing progesterone levels of the early luteal phase of the cycle, the BBT increases slightly (approximately 0.2° to 0.5° C) (World Health Organization Department of Reproductive Health & Research [WHO/RHR] and Johns Hopkins Bloomberg School of Public Health/Center for Communication Programs [CCP], 2007). The temperature remains on an elevated plateau until 2 to 4 days before menstruation, and then it decreases to the low levels recorded during the previous cycle, unless pregnancy has occurred and the temperature remains elevated. If ovulation fails to occur, the pattern of lower body temperature continues throughout the cycle.

To use this method, the fertile period is defined as the day of first temperature drop, or first elevation through 3 consecutive days of elevated temperature. Abstinence begins the first day of menstrual bleeding and lasts through 3 consecutive days of sustained temperature rise (at least 0.2° C) (Jennings & Arevalo, 2007; WHO/RHR & CCP, 2007). The decrease and subsequent increase in temperature are referred to as the *thermal shift*. When the entire month's temperatures are recorded on a graph, the pattern described is more apparent. It is more difficult to perceive day-to-day variations without the entire picture. Infection, fatigue, less than 3 hours sleep per night, awakening late, and anxiety may cause temperature fluctuations, altering the expected pattern. If a new BBT thermometer is purchased, this fact is noted on the chart because the readings may vary slightly. Jet lag, alcohol and antipyretic medications taken the evening before, or sleeping in a heated waterbed also must be noted on the chart because each affects the BBT. Therefore, the BBT alone is not a reliable method of predicting ovulation.

Symptothermal Method. The symptothermal method is a tool for the woman to gain fertility awareness as she tracks the physiologic and psychologic symptoms that mark the phases of her cycle. This method combines at least two methods, usually cervical mucus changes with BBT, in addition to heightened awareness of secondary, cycle phase–related symptoms (Pallone & Bergus, 2009). Secondary symptoms may include increased libido, midcycle spotting, mittelschmerz, pelvic fullness or tenderness, and vulvar fullness. The woman is taught to palpate her cervix to assess for changes in texture, position, and dilation that indicate ovulation. During the preovulatory and ovulatory periods, the cervix softens, opens, rises in the vagina, and is more moist. During the postovulatory period the cervix drops, becomes firm, and closes. The woman notes days on which coitus, changes in routine, and illness have occurred (Fig. 8-4). Calendar calculations and cervical mucus changes are used to estimate the onset of the fertile period; changes in cervical mucus or the BBT are used to estimate its end.

Biologic Marker Methods

Home Predictor Test Kits for Ovulation. All of the preceding methods discussed are indicative of but do not prove the occurrence and exact timing of ovulation. The urine predictor test for ovulation is a major addition to the NFP and fertility-awareness methods to help women who want to plan the time of their pregnancies and those who are trying to conceive (Fig. 8-5). The urine predictor test for ovulation detects the sudden surge of luteinizing hormone (LH) that occurs approximately 12 to 24 hours before ovulation. Unlike BBT, the test is not affected by illness, emotional upset, or physical activity. For home use, a test kit contains sufficient material for several days of testing during each cycle. A positive response indicative of an LH surge is noted by an easy-to-read color change. Directions for use of urine predictor test kits vary with the manufacturer. Saliva predictor tests for ovulation use dried, nonfoamy saliva

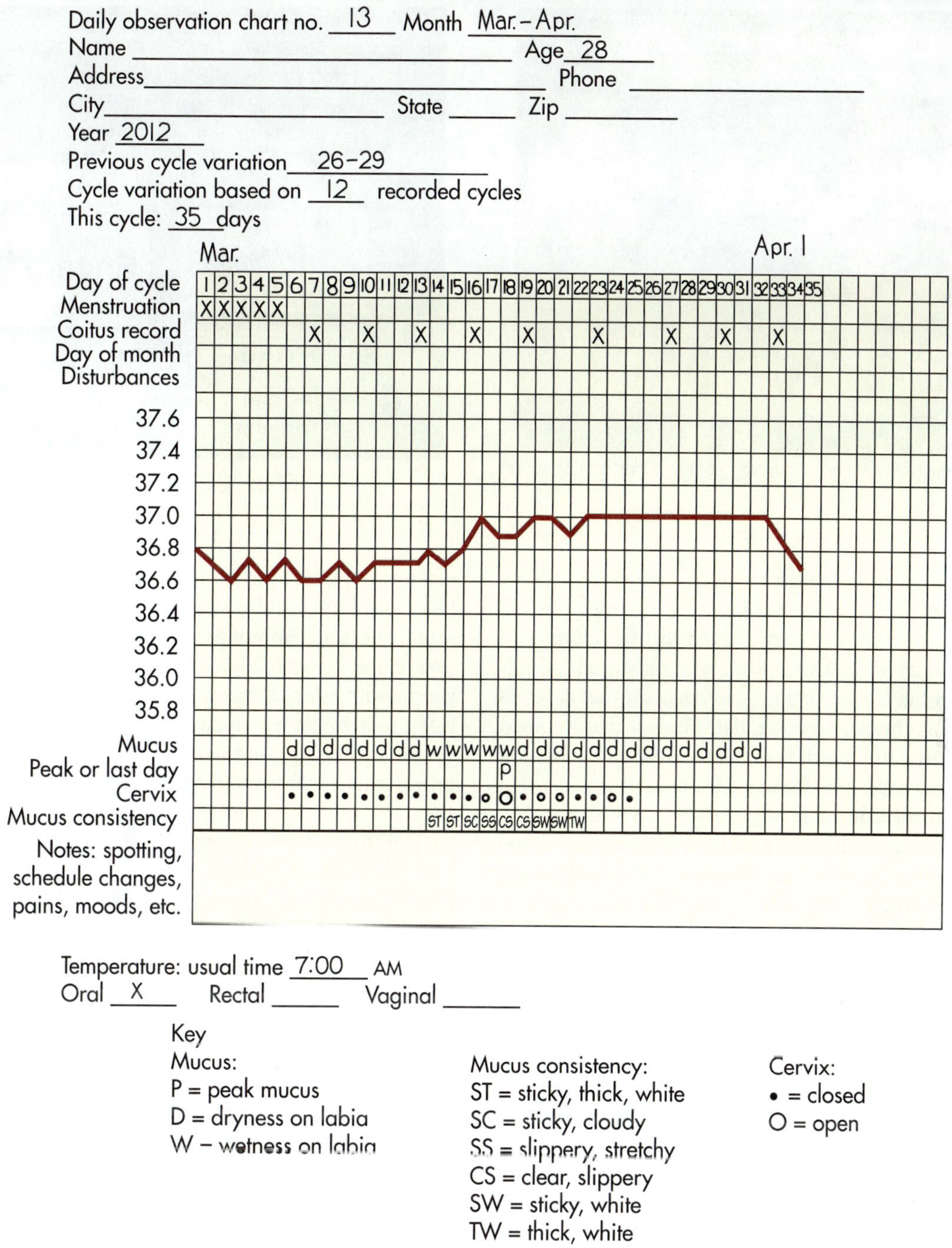

FIG. 8-4 Example of a completed symptothermal chart.

as a tool to show fertility patterns. More research is needed to determine the efficacy of use of these tests for pregnancy prevention.

The Marquette Model. The Marquette Model (MM) is a natural family planning method that was developed through the Marquette University College of Nursing Institute for Natural Family Planning (Fehring, Schneider, & Barron, 2008). The MM uses cervical monitoring along with the ClearPlan Easy Fertility Monitor. The ClearPlan monitor is a handheld device that uses test strips to measure urinary metabolites of estrogen and LH. The monitor provides the user with "low," "high," and "peak" fertility readings. The MM incorporates the use of the monitor as an aid to learning NFP and fertility awareness. The MM is currently being tested at different sites in the United States for its effectiveness in helping couples avoid pregnancy. One study has shown a typical use failure rate of 10.6% (Fehring et al.).

Spermicides and Barrier Methods

Barrier contraceptives have gained in popularity, not only as a contraceptive method but also as a protective measure against the spread of STIs, such as human papillomavirus (HPV) and herpes simplex virus (HSV). Some male condoms and female vaginal methods provide a physical barrier to several STIs, and some male condoms provide protection against HIV (Cates & Raymond, 2007; Warner & Steiner, 2007). Spermicides serve as chemical barriers against the sperm.

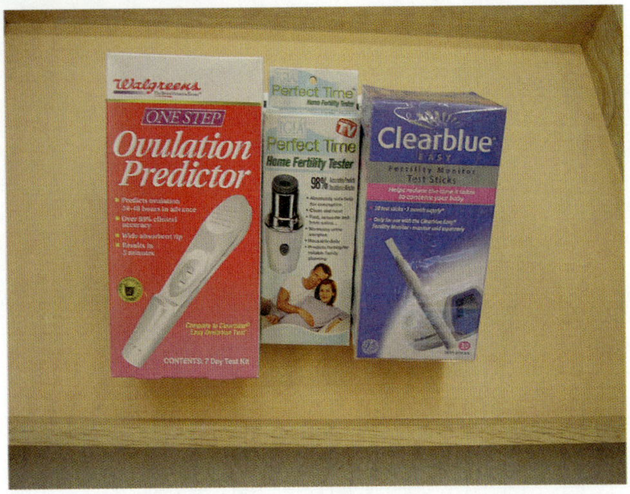

FIG. 8-5 Examples of ovulation prediction tests. (Courtesy Shannon Perry, Phoenix, AZ.)

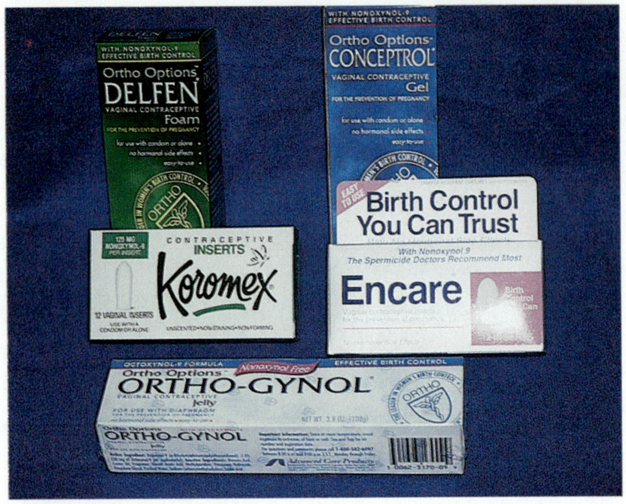

FIG. 8-6 Spermicides. (Courtesy Marjorie Pyle, RNC, Lifecircle, Costa Mesa, CA.)

Spermicides. Spermicides, such as nonoxynol-9 (N-9), work by reducing the sperm's mobility; the chemicals attack the sperm flagella and body, thereby preventing the sperm from reaching the cervical os. N-9, the most commonly used spermicidal chemical in the United States, is a surfactant that destroys the sperm cell membrane; however, data suggest that frequent use (more than two times a day) of N-9, or use as a lubricant during anal intercourse, can disrupt the mucosa, which could increase the transmission of HIV (Cates & Raymond, 2007). Women with high risk behaviors that increase their likelihood of contracting HIV and other STIs are advised to avoid the use of spermicidal products containing N-9, including those lubricated condoms, diaphragms, and cervical caps to which N-9 is added (Centers for Disease Control and Prevention [CDC], Workowski, & Berman, 2006).

Intravaginal spermicides are marketed and sold without a prescription as foams, tablets, suppositories, creams, films, and gels (Fig. 8-6). Preloaded single-dose applicators small enough to be carried in a small purse are available. Effectiveness of spermicides depends on consistent and accurate use. Clients should be cautioned against misunderstanding terms: contraceptive gel differs from fruit jelly, and cosmetics or hair products containing the nonspermicidal forms of nonoxynol are not adequate substitutes. The spermicide should be inserted high into the vagina so that it makes contact with the cervix. Some spermicide should be inserted at least 15 minutes before, and no longer than 1 hour before, sexual intercourse. Spermicide must be reapplied before each additional act of intercourse, even if a barrier method is used. Studies have shown varying effectiveness rates for spermicidal use alone. Typical failure rate for spermicide use alone is about 29% (Trussell, 2007).

Condoms. The male condom is a thin, stretchable sheath that covers the penis before genital, oral, or anal contact and is removed when the penis is withdrawn from the partner's orifice after ejaculation (Fig. 8-7, *A*). Condoms are made of latex rubber, polyurethane (strong, thin plastic), or natural membranes (animal tissue). In addition to providing a physical barrier for sperm, nonspermicidal latex condoms also provide a barrier for STIs (particularly gonorrhea, chlamydia, and trichomoniasis) and HIV transmission. Condoms lubricated with N-9 are not recommended for preventing STIs or HIV (CDC et al., 2006). Latex condoms will break down with oil-based lubricants and should be used only with water-based or silicone lubricants (Warner & Steiner, 2007). Because of the growing number of people with latex allergies, condom manufacturers have begun using polyurethane, which is thinner and stronger than latex. Research is being conducted to determine the effectiveness of polyurethane condoms to protect against STIs and HIV.

! NURSING ALERT

All individuals should be questioned about the potential for latex allergy. Latex condom use is contraindicated for people with latex sensitivity.

A small percentage of condoms are made from lamb cecum (natural skin). Natural skin condoms do not provide the same protection against STIs and HIV infection as latex condoms. Natural skin condoms contain small pores that could allow passage of viruses such as hepatitis B, HSV, and HIV.

A functional difference in condom shape is the presence or absence of a sperm-reservoir tip. To enhance vaginal stimulation, some condoms are contoured and rippled or have ribbed or roughened surfaces. Thinner construction increases heat transmission and sensitivity; a variety of colors and flavors increase condoms' acceptability and attractiveness (Warner & Steiner, 2007). A wet jelly or dry powder lubricates some condoms. Condoms must be discarded after each single use. They are available without a prescription. The typical failure rate in the first year of male condom use is 15% (Trussell, 2007). To prevent unintended pregnancy and the spread of STIs, it is essential that condoms be used consistently and correctly. Instructions, such as those listed in Box 8-3, can be used for client teaching.

The female condom is a lubricated vaginal sheath made of polyurethane and has flexible rings at both ends (see Fig. 8-7, *A*). The closed end of the pouch is inserted into the vagina and is anchored around the cervix, and the open ring covers the labia. Women whose partner will not wear a male condom can use this as a protective mechanical barrier. Rewetting drops or oil or water-based lubricants can be used to help decrease

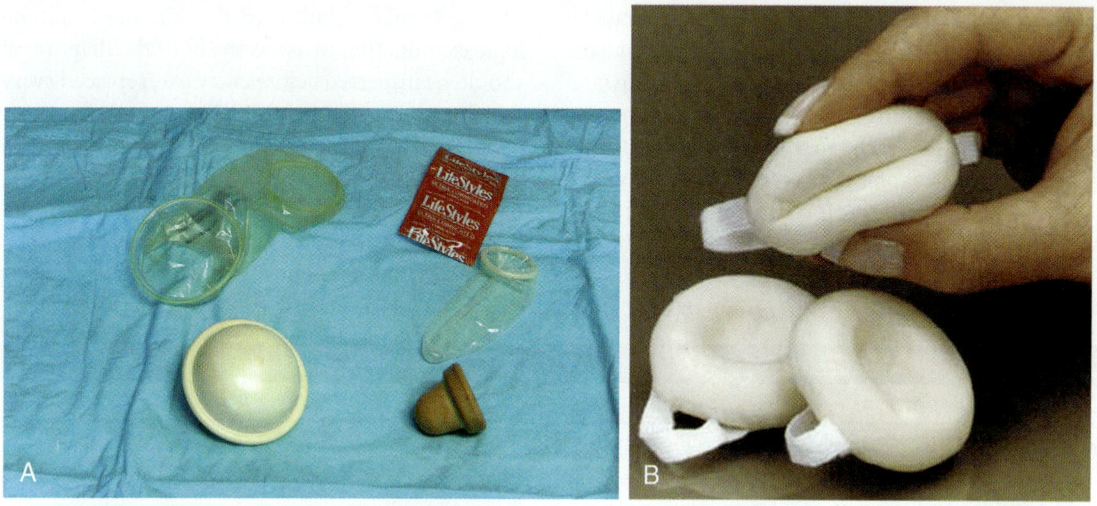

FIG. 8-7 **A,** Mechanical barriers. From the top left corner, clockwise: female condom, male condom, cervical cap, diaphragm. **B,** Contraceptive sponge. (**A,** Courtesy Dee Lowdermilk, Chapel Hill, NC; **B,** courtesy Allendale Pharmaceuticals, Inc., Allendale, NJ.)

BOX 8-3 MALE CONDOMS

MECHANISM OF ACTION
- Sheath is applied over the erect penis before insertion or loss of preejaculatory drops of semen. Used correctly, condoms prevent sperm from entering the cervix. Spermicide-coated condoms cause ejaculated sperm to be immobilized rapidly, thus increasing contraceptive effectiveness.

FAILURE RATE
- Typical users: 15%
- Correct and consistent users: 2%

ADVANTAGES
- Safe
- No side effects
- Readily available
- Premalignant changes in cervix can be prevented or ameliorated in women whose partners use condoms
- Method of male nonsurgical contraception

DISADVANTAGES
- Must interrupt lovemaking to apply sheath
- Sensation may be altered
- If used improperly, spillage of sperm can result in pregnancy
- Condoms occasionally may tear during intercourse

STI PROTECTION
- If a condom is used throughout the act of intercourse and there is no unprotected contact with female genitals, a latex rubber condom, which is impermeable to viruses, can act as a protective measure against STIs.

NURSING CONSIDERATIONS
Teaching should include the following instructions:
- Use a new condom (check expiration date) for each act of sexual intercourse or other acts between partners that involve contact with the penis.
- Place condom after penis is erect and before intimate contact.
- Place condom on head of penis (Fig. A) and unroll it all the way to the base (Fig. B).
- Leave an empty space at the tip (Fig. A); remove any air remaining in the tip by gently pressing air out toward the base of the penis.
- If a lubricant is desired, use water-based products such as K-Y lubricating jelly. Do *not* use petroleum-based products because they can cause the condom to break.
- After ejaculation, carefully withdraw the still-erect penis from the vagina, holding on to condom rim; remove and discard the condom.
- Store unused condoms in cool, dry place.
- Do not use condoms that are sticky, brittle, or obviously damaged.

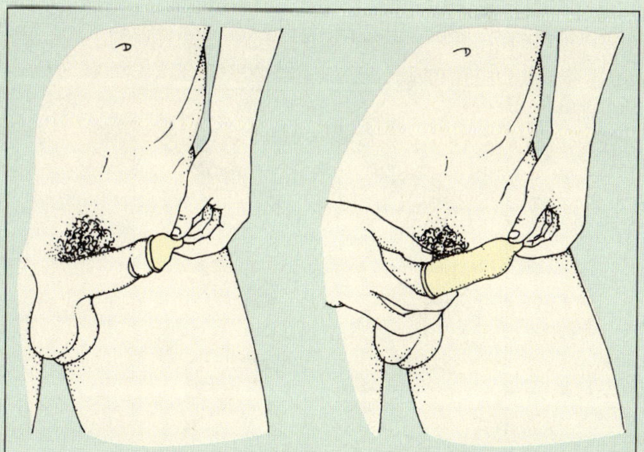

Fig. A　Fig. B

STI, Sexually transmitted infection.

the distracting noise that is produced while penile thrusting occurs. The female condom is available in one size, is intended for single use only, and is sold over the counter. Male condoms should not be used concurrently because the friction from both sheaths can increase the likelihood of either or both tearing (Cates & Raymond, 2007). The typical failure rate in the first year of female condom use is 21% (Trussell, 2007).

Diaphragms. The contraceptive diaphragm is a shallow dome-shaped latex or silicone device with a flexible rim that covers the cervix (see Fig. 8-7, *A*). There are four types of diaphragms: coil spring, arcing spring, flat spring, and wide seal rim. Available in many sizes, the diaphragm should be the largest size the woman can wear without her being aware of its presence. The typical failure rate of the diaphragm combined with spermicide is 16% in the first year of use (Trussell, 2007). Effectiveness of the diaphragm is less when used without spermicide. Women at high risk for HIV should avoid use of N-9 spermicides with the diaphragm (Cates & Raymond, 2007).

The woman is informed that she needs an annual gynecologic examination to assess the fit of the diaphragm. The device should be inspected before every use, replaced every 2 years, and may have to be refitted for a 20% weight fluctuation, after any abdominal or pelvic surgery, and after every pregnancy (WHO/RHR & CCP, 2007). Because various types of diaphragms are on the market, the nurse should use the package insert for teaching a woman how to use and care for the diaphragm (see Teaching for Self-Management box: Use and Care of the Diaphragm).

TEACHING FOR SELF-MANAGEMENT

Use and Care of the Diaphragm

INSPECTION OF THE DIAPHRAGM

You must inspect your diaphragm carefully before each use. The best way to perform this inspection is as follows:

- Hold the diaphragm up to a light source. Carefully stretch the diaphragm at the area of the rim, on all sides, making sure there are no holes. Remember, sharp fingernails can puncture the diaphragm.
- Another way to check for pinholes is to fill the diaphragm with water carefully. If any problem develops, you will see it immediately.
- A diaphragm that is puckered, especially near the rim, could mean thin spots.
- If you see any of these problems, do not use the diaphragm, avoid sexual intercourse or use another method of birth control; consult your health care provider about replacing the diaphragm.

PREPARATION OF THE DIAPHRAGM

Rinse off the cornstarch. Your diaphragm must always be used with a spermicidal lubricant to be effective. Pregnancy cannot be prevented effectively by the diaphragm alone.

Always empty your bladder before inserting the diaphragm. Place approximately 2 teaspoons of contraceptive jelly or contraceptive cream on the side of the diaphragm that will rest against the cervix (or whichever way you have been instructed). Spread it around to coat the surface and the rim. This measure aids in insertion and offers a more complete seal. Many women also spread some jelly or cream on the other side of the diaphragm (Fig. A).

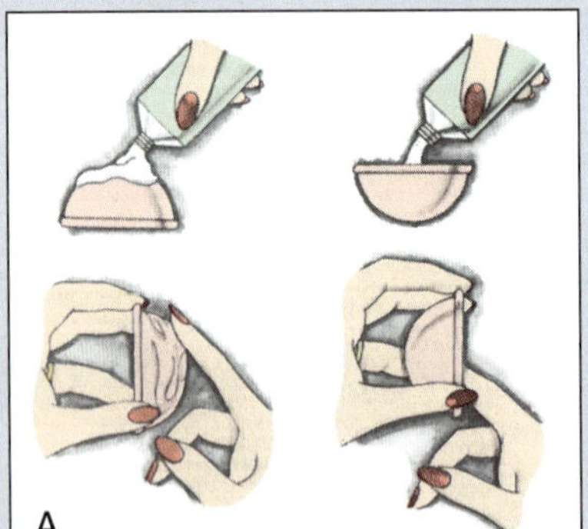

A

POSITIONS FOR INSERTION OF THE DIAPHRAGM

Squatting: Squatting is the most commonly used position, and most women find it satisfactory.

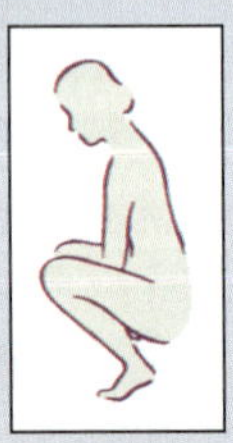

Leg-up method: Another position is to raise the left foot (if right hand is used for insertion) on a low stool, and, while in a bending position, insert the diaphragm.

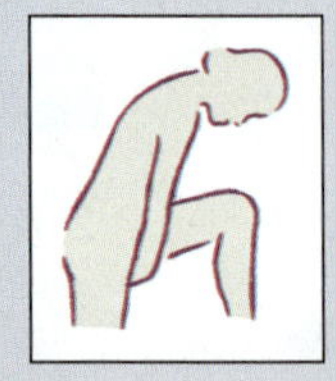

Chair method: Another practical method for diaphragm insertion is to sit far forward on the edge of a chair.

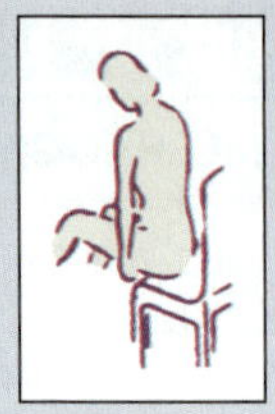

Reclining: You may prefer to insert the diaphragm while in a semireclining position in bed.

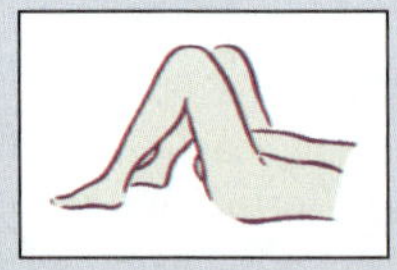

INSERTION OF THE DIAPHRAGM

The diaphragm can be inserted up to 6 hours before intercourse. Hold the diaphragm between your thumb and fingers. The dome can be either up or down, as directed by your health care provider. Place your index finger on the outer rim of the compressed diaphragm (Fig. B).

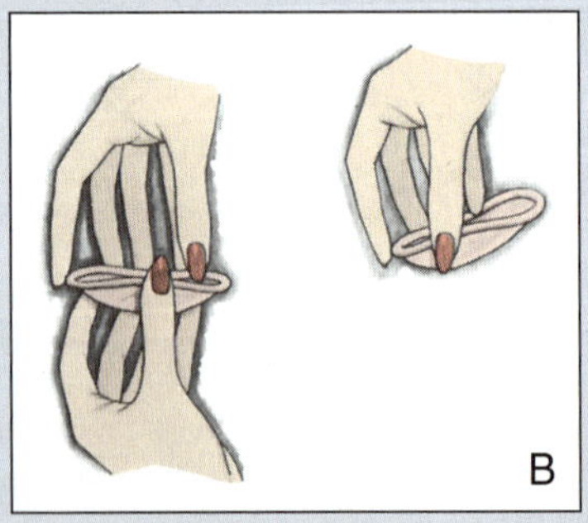

B

Use the fingers of the other hand to spread the labia (lips of the vagina). This action will assist in guiding the diaphragm into place.

TEACHING FOR SELF-MANAGEMENT

Use and Care of the Diaphragm—cont'd

Insert the diaphragm into the vagina. Direct it inward and downward as far as it will go to the space behind and below the cervix (Fig. C).

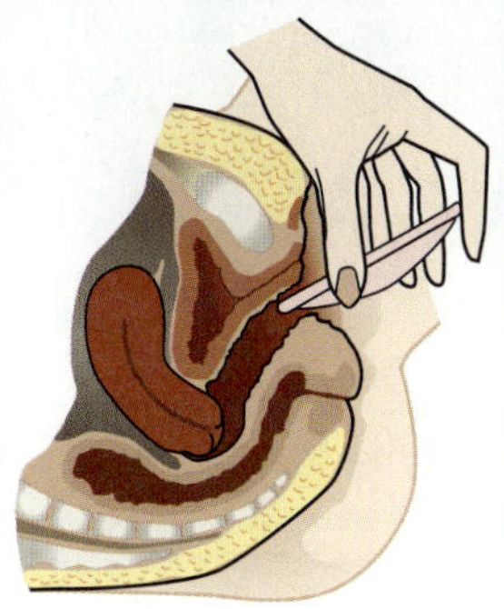

C

Tuck the front of the rim of the diaphragm behind the pubic bone so that the rubber hugs the front wall of the vagina (Fig. D).

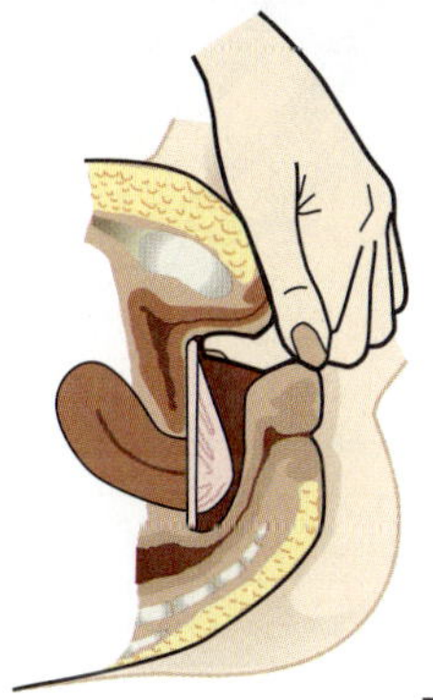

D

Feel for your cervix through the diaphragm to be certain it is properly placed and securely covered by the rubber dome (Fig. E).

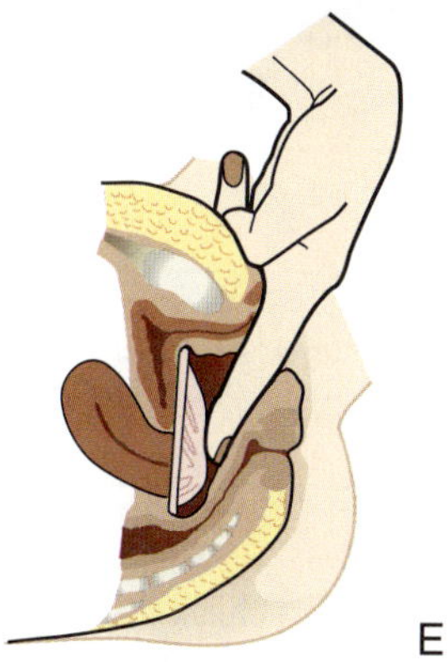

E

GENERAL INFORMATION

Regardless of the time of the month, you must use your diaphragm every time intercourse takes place. Your diaphragm must be left in place for at least 6 hours after the last intercourse. If you remove your diaphragm before the 6-hour period, you will greatly increase your chance of becoming pregnant. If you have repeated intercourse, you must add more spermicide for each act of intercourse.

REMOVAL OF THE DIAPHRAGM

The only proper way to remove the diaphragm is to insert your forefinger up and over the top side of the diaphragm and slightly to the side.

Next, turn the palm of your hand downward and backward, hooking the forefinger firmly on top of the inside of the upper rim of the diaphragm, breaking the suction. Pull the diaphragm down and out. This technique prevents tearing the diaphragm with the fingernails. You should not remove the diaphragm by trying to catch the rim from below the dome (Fig. F).

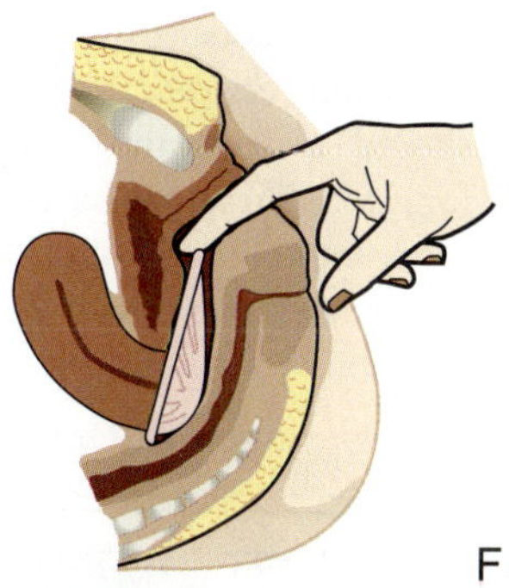

F

CARE OF THE DIAPHRAGM

When using a vaginal diaphragm, avoid using oil-based products, such as certain body lubricants, mineral oil, baby oil, vaginal lubricants, or vaginitis preparations. These products can weaken the rubber.

A little care means longer wear for your diaphragm. After each use, wash the diaphragm in warm water and mild soap. Do not use detergent soaps, cold-cream soaps, deodorant soaps, and soaps containing oil products because they can weaken the rubber.

After washing, dry the diaphragm thoroughly. Remove all water and moisture with a towel. Then dust the diaphragm with cornstarch. Do not use scented talc, body powder, baby powder, or similar products because they can weaken the rubber.

To clean the introducer (if one is used), wash with mild soap and warm water, rinse, and dry thoroughly.

Place the diaphragm back in the plastic case for storage. Do not store it near a radiator or heat source or in a location that is exposed to light for an extended period.

Disadvantages of diaphragm use include the reluctance of some women to insert and remove the diaphragm. Although it can be inserted up to 6 hours before intercourse, a cold diaphragm and a cold gel temporarily reduce vaginal response to sexual stimulation if insertion of the diaphragm occurs immediately before intercourse. Some women or couples object to the messiness of the spermicide. These annoyances of diaphragm use, along with failure to insert the device once foreplay has begun, are the most common reasons for failures of this method. Side effects may include irritation of tissues related to contact with spermicides. The diaphragm is not a good option for women with poor vaginal muscle tone or recurrent urinary tract infections. For proper placement the diaphragm must rest behind the pubic symphysis and completely cover the cervix. To decrease the chance of exerting urethral pressure, the woman should be reminded to empty her bladder before diaphragm insertion and immediately after intercourse. Diaphragms are contraindicated for women with pelvic relaxation (uterine prolapse) or a large cystocele. Women with a latex allergy should not use latex diaphragms.

Toxic shock syndrome (TSS), although reported in very small numbers, can occur in association with the use of the contraceptive diaphragm and cervical caps (Cates & Raymond, 2007). The nurse should instruct the woman about ways to reduce her risk for TSS. These measures include prompt removal 6 to 8 hours after intercourse, not using the diaphragm or cervical caps during menses, and learning and watching for danger signs of TSS.

! NURSING ALERT

The nurse should inform the woman who uses a diaphragm or cervical cap as a contraceptive method to be alert for signs of TSS. The most common signs include a sunburn type of rash, diarrhea, dizziness, faintness, weakness, sore throat, aching muscles and joints, sudden high fever, and vomiting (WHO/RHR & CCP, 2007).

Cervical Caps. Three types of cervical caps are available; two come in varying sizes and one is one-size-fits-all. They are made of rubber or latex-free silicone and have soft domes and firm brims (see Fig. 8-7, *A*). The cap fits snugly around the base of the cervix close to the junction of the cervix and vaginal fornices. It is recommended that the cap remain in place no less than 6 hours and not more than 48 hours at a time. It is left in place at least 6 hours after the last act of intercourse. The seal provides a physical barrier to sperm: spermicide inside the cap adds a chemical barrier. The extended period of wear may be an added convenience for women.

Instructions for the actual insertion and use of the cervical cap closely resemble the instructions for the use of the contraceptive diaphragm. Some of the differences are that the cervical cap can be inserted hours before sexual intercourse without a need for additional spermicide later, no additional spermicide is required for repeated acts of intercourse when the cap is used, and the cervical cap requires less spermicide than the diaphragm when initially inserted. The angle of the uterus, the vaginal muscle tone, and the shape of the cervix may interfere with the cervical cap's ease of fitting and use. Correct fitting requires time, effort, and skill from both the woman and the clinician. The woman must check the cap's position before and after each act of intercourse (see Teaching for Self-Management box).

Because of the potential risk of TSS associated with the use of the cervical cap, another form of birth control is recommended for use during menstrual bleeding and up to at least 6 weeks postpartum. The cap should be refitted after any gynecologic surgery or birth and after major weight losses or gains. Otherwise the size should be checked at least once a year.

TEACHING FOR SELF-MANAGEMENT

Insertion and Removal of the Cervical Cap

- Push the cap (filled with contraceptive cream or jelly) up into the vagina until it covers the cervix.

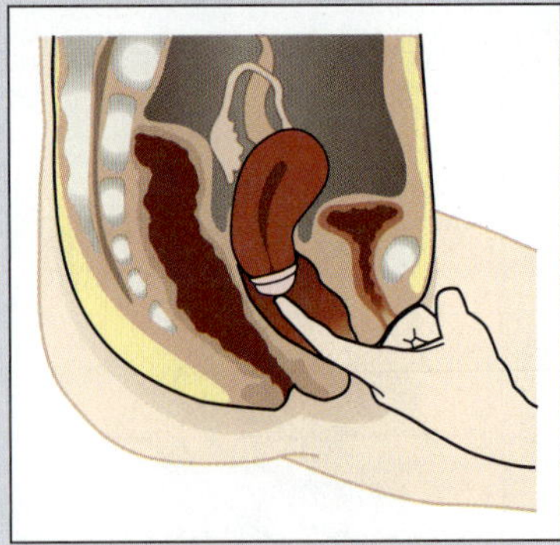

- Press the rim against the cervix to create a seal.

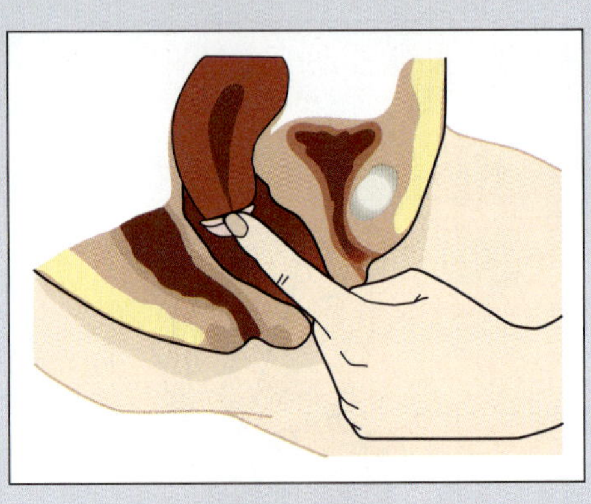

- To remove, push the rim toward the right or left hip to loosen from the cervix, and then withdraw.

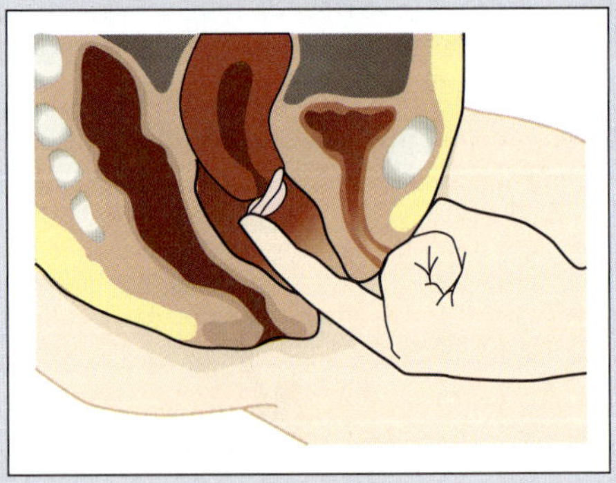

- The woman can assume several positions to insert the cervical cap. See the four positions shown for inserting the diaphragm.

TABLE 8-1 **HORMONAL CONTRACEPTION**

COMPOSITION	ROUTE OF ADMINISTRATION	DURATION OF EFFECT
Combination estrogen and progestin (synthetic estrogens and progestins in varying doses and formulations)	Oral	24 hours; extended cycle—12 weeks
	Transdermal	7 days
	Vaginal ring insertion	3 weeks
Progestin only:		
Norethindrone, norgestrel	Oral	24 hours
Medroxyprogesterone acetate	Intramuscular injection; subcutaneous injection	3 months
Progestin, etonogestrel	Subdermal implant	Up to 3 years
Levonorgestrel	Intrauterine device	Up to 5 years

Women who are not good candidates for wearing the cervical cap include those with abnormal Papanicolaou (Pap) test results, those who cannot be fitted properly with the existing cap sizes, those who find the insertion and removal of the device too difficult, those with a history of TSS, those with vaginal or cervical infections, and those who experience allergic responses to the latex cap or spermicide. Failure rates the first year of use are 16% in nulliparous and 32% in multiparous women (WHO/RHR & CCP, 2007).

Contraceptive Sponge. The vaginal sponge is a small, round polyurethane sponge that contains N-9 spermicide (see previous discussion of N-9) (see Fig. 8-7, *B*). It is designed to fit over the cervix (one size fits all). The side that is placed next to the cervix is concave for better fit. The opposite side has a woven polyester loop to be used for removal of the sponge.

The sponge must be moistened with water before it is inserted. It provides protection for up to 24 hours and for repeated instances of sexual intercourse. The sponge should be left in place for at least 6 hours after the last act of intercourse. Wearing it longer than 24 to 30 hours may put the woman at risk for TSS (Cates & Raymond, 2007). The typical failure rate in the first year of use is 32% for parous women and 16% for nulliparous women (Trussell, 2007).

Hormonal Methods

More than 30 different hormonal contraceptive formulations are available in the United States today. General classes are described in Table 8-1. Because of the wide variety of preparations available, the woman and the nurse must read the package insert for information about specific products prescribed. Formulations include combined estrogen-progestin medications and progestational agents. The formulations are administered orally, transdermally, vaginally, by implantation, by injection, or by intrauterine insertion.

Combined Estrogen-Progestin Contraceptives

Oral Contraceptives. The normal menstrual cycle is maintained by a feedback mechanism. Follicle-stimulating hormone (FSH) and LH are secreted in response to fluctuating levels of ovarian estrogen and progesterone. Regular ingestion of combined oral contraceptive pills (COCs) suppresses the action of the hypothalamus and anterior pituitary, leading to insufficient secretion of FSH and LH; therefore, follicles do not mature, and ovulation is inhibited.

Other contraceptive effects are induced by the combined steroids. Maturation of the endometrium is altered, making it a less favorable site for implantation. COCs also have a direct effect on the endometrium, so that from 1 to 4 days after the last COC is taken, the endometrium sloughs and bleeds as a result of hormone withdrawal. The withdrawal bleeding is usually less profuse than that of normal menstruation and may last only 2 to 3 days. Some women have no bleeding at all. The cervical mucus remains thick from the effect of the progestin (Nelson, 2007).

Cervical mucus under the effect of progesterone does not provide as suitable an environment for sperm penetration as does the thin, watery mucus at ovulation. The possible effect, if any, of altered tubal and uterine motility induced by COCs is not clear.

Monophasic pills provide fixed dosages of estrogen and progestin. Multiphasic pills (e.g., biphasic and triphasic oral contraceptives) alter the amount of progestin and sometimes the amount of estrogen within each cycle. These preparations reduce the total dosage of hormones in a single cycle without sacrificing contraceptive efficacy (Nelson, 2007). To maintain adequate hormonal levels for contraception and enhance compliance, COCs should be taken at the same time each day.

Advantages. Because taking the pill does not relate directly to the sexual act, its acceptability may be increased. Improvement in sexual response may occur once the possibility of pregnancy is not an issue. For some women it is convenient to know when to expect the next menstrual flow.

Evidence of noncontraceptive benefits of oral contraceptives is based on studies of high-dose pills (50 mg estrogen). Few data exist on noncontraceptive benefits of low-dose oral contraceptives (less than 35 mg estrogen) (Nelson, 2007). The noncontraceptive health benefits of COCs include decreased menstrual blood loss and decreased iron deficiency anemia, regulation of menorrhagia and irregular cycles, and reduced incidence of dysmenorrhea and premenstrual syndrome (PMS). Oral contraceptives also offer protection against endometrial cancer and ovarian cancer, reduce the incidence of benign breast disease, improve acne, protect against the development of functional ovarian cysts and salpingitis, and decrease the risk of ectopic pregnancy. Oral contraceptives are considered a safe option for nonsmoking women until menopause. Perimenopausal women can benefit from regular bleeding cycles, a regular hormonal pattern, and the noncontraceptive health benefits of oral contraceptives (Nelson).

A pelvic examination and Pap smear are not necessary before initiating COCs (WHO/RHR & CCP, 2007). If STI screening is indicated, a urine-based test can be used for some infections (e.g. chlamydia, gonorrhea); others will require a pelvic examination and cultures of vaginal or cervical secretions or blood tests (Planned Parenthood, 2010). Most health care providers assess the woman 3 months after beginning COCs to detect any complications.

Use of oral hormonal contraceptives is initiated on one of the first days of the menstrual cycle (day 1 of the cycle is the first day of menses) or after childbirth or abortion. With a "Sunday start," women begin taking pills on the first Sunday after the start of their menstrual period. If contraceptives are to be started at any time other than during normal menses, or within 3 weeks after birth, miscarriage, or induced abortion, another

Video Nursing Skill—Teaching Birth Control Methods

method of contraception should be used throughout the first week to avoid the risk of pregnancy (Nelson, 2007). Taken exactly as directed, oral contraceptives prevent ovulation, and pregnancy cannot occur; the overall effectiveness rate is almost 100%. Almost all failures (i.e., pregnancy occurs) are caused by omission of one or more pills during the regimen. The typical failure rate of COCs due to omission is 8% (Trussell, 2007).

Disadvantages and Side Effects. Since hormonal contraceptives have come into use, the amount of estrogen and progestational agent contained in each tablet has been reduced considerably. This is important because adverse effects are, to a degree, dose related.

Women must be screened for conditions that present absolute or relative contraindications to oral contraceptive use. Contraindications for COC use include a history of thromboembolic disorders, cerebrovascular or coronary artery disease, breast cancer, gallbladder disease, estrogen-dependent tumors, pregnancy, impaired liver function, liver tumor, lactation less than 6 weeks postpartum, smoking if older than 35 years, headaches with focal neurologic symptoms, surgery with prolonged immobilization or any surgery on the legs, hypertension (140/90 mm Hg), and diabetes mellitus (of more than 20 years' duration) with vascular disease (Nelson, 2007; WHO/RHR & CCP, 2007).

Certain side effects of COCs are attributable to estrogen, progestin, or both. Serious adverse effects documented with high doses of estrogen and progesterone include stroke, myocardial infarction, thromboembolism, hypertension, gallbladder disease, and liver tumors (Nelson, 2007). Common side effects of estrogen excess include nausea, breast tenderness, fluid retention, and chloasma. Side effects of estrogen deficiency include early spotting (days 1 to 14), hypomenorrhea, nervousness, and atrophic vaginitis leading to painful intercourse (dyspareunia). Side effects of progestin excess include increased appetite, tiredness, depression, breast tenderness, vaginal yeast infection, oily skin and scalp, hirsutism, and postpill amenorrhea. Side effects of progestin deficiency include late spotting and breakthrough bleeding (days 15 to 21), heavy flow with clots, and decreased breast size. One of the most common side effects of combined COCs is bleeding irregularities (Nelson).

In the presence of side effects, especially those that are bothersome to a woman, a different product, a different drug content, or another method of contraception may be required. The "right" product for a woman contains the lowest dose of hormones that prevents ovulation and that has the fewest and least harmful side effects. There is no way to predict the right dosage for any particular woman. Issues to consider in prescribing oral contraceptives include history of oral contraceptive use, side effects during past use, menstrual history, and drug interactions (Nelson, 2007).

Large prospective studies have not shown a relationship between use of oral contraceptives available and diabetes or glucose intolerance (Nelson, 2007). The risks and benefits should be assessed before prescribing oral contraceptives for women who have diabetes with vascular problems.

The effectiveness of oral contraceptives can be negatively influenced when the following medications are taken simultaneously (Nelson, 2007; WHO/RHR & CCP, 2007):

- *Anticonvulsants:* barbiturates, oxcarbazepine, phenytoin, phenobarbital, felbamate, carbamazepine, primidone, and topiramate
- *Systemic antifungals:* griseofulvin
- *Antituberculosis drugs:* rifampicin and rifabutin
- *Anti-HIV protease inhibitors:* nelfinavir, amprenavir

! NURSING ALERT

Over-the-counter medications, as well as some herbal supplements (such as St John's wort) can alter the effectiveness of COCs. Women should be asked about their use when COCs are being considered for contraception.

No strong pharmacokinetic evidence exists that shows a relation between broad-spectrum antibiotic use and altered hormonal levels among oral contraceptive users, although potential antibiotic interaction can occur. Studies on the incidence of breast cancer in COC users have not found a significant increase of breast cancer in women who use COCs (Nelson, 2007).

After discontinuing oral contraception, return to fertility usually happens quickly, but fertility rates are slightly lower the first 3 to 12 months after discontinuation (Nelson, 2007). Many women ovulate the next month after stopping oral contraceptives. Women who discontinue oral contraception for a planned pregnancy commonly ask whether they should wait before attempting to conceive. Studies indicate that these infants have no greater chance of being born with any type of birth defect than do infants born to women in the general population, even if conception occurred in the first month after the medication was discontinued. Little evidence suggests that oral contraceptives cause postpill amenorrhea. Amenorrhea after oral contraceptive use is probably related to the woman's menstrual cycle before taking the pill (Nelson).

Nursing Considerations. Many different preparations of oral hormonal contraceptives are available. The nurse reviews the prescribing information in the package insert with the woman. Because of the wide variations, each woman must be clear about the unique dosage regimen for the preparation prescribed for her. Directions for care after missing one or two tablets also vary (Fig. 8-8).

Withdrawal bleeding tends to be short and scanty when some combination pills are taken. A woman may see no fresh blood at all. A drop of blood or a brown smudge on a tampon or the underwear counts as a menstrual period.

Only about 68% of women who start taking oral contraceptives are still taking them after 1 year (Trussell, 2007). All women choosing to use oral contraceptives should be provided with a second method of birth control and be instructed in and comfortable with this backup method. Most women stop taking oral contraceptives for nonmedical reasons.

The nurse also reviews the signs of potential complications associated with the use of oral contraceptives (see Signs of Potential Complications box: Oral Contraceptives). Oral contraceptives do not protect a woman against STIs or HIV. A barrier method such as condoms and spermicide should be used for protection.

Oral Contraceptive 91-Day Regimen. Some women prefer to take COCs in 3-month cycles and have fewer menstrual periods. Levonorgestrel/ethinyl estradiol (Seasonale), U.S. Food and Drug Administration (FDA)– approved for extended cycle use, contains both estrogen and progestin and is taken in

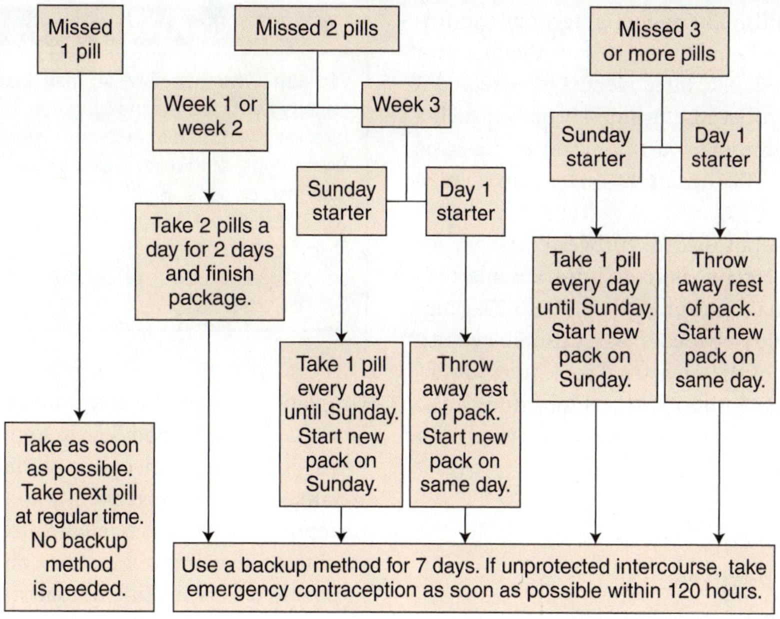

FIG. 8-8 Flowchart for missed active contraceptive pills, 2010. (Courtesy Patsy Huff, PharmD, Chapel Hill, NC.)

SIGNS OF POTENTIAL COMPLICATIONS

ORAL CONTRACEPTIVES

Before oral contraceptives are prescribed and periodically throughout hormone therapy, alert the woman to stop taking the pill and to report any of the following symptoms to the health care provider immediately. The mnemonic ACHES helps in retention of this list:

A—Abdominal pain may indicate a problem with the liver or gallbladder.

C—Chest pain or shortness of breath may indicate possible clot problem within the lungs or heart.

H—Headaches (sudden or persistent) may be caused by cardiovascular accident or hypertension.

E—Eye problems may indicate vascular accident or hypertension.

S—Severe leg pain may indicate a thromboembolic process.

3-month cycles of 12 weeks of active pills followed by 1 week of inactive pills. Menstrual periods occur during the thirteenth week of the cycle. There is no protection from sexually transmitted infections, and risks are similar to COCs. Other monophasic COCs may be prescribed for extended cycle use and must be taken on a daily schedule, regardless of the frequency of intercourse. Because users will have fewer menstrual flows, they should consider the possibility of pregnancy if they do not experience their thirteenth-week flows (Nelson, 2007; WHO/RHR & CCP, 2007).

Transdermal Contraceptive System. Available by prescription only, the contraceptive transdermal patch delivers continuous levels of norelgestromin (progesterone) and ethinyl estradiol. The patch can be applied to intact skin of the upper outer arm, the upper torso (front and back, excluding the breasts), the lower abdomen, or the buttocks (Fig. 8-9). Application is on the same day once a week for 3 weeks, followed by a week without the patch. Withdrawal bleeding occurs during the "no-patch" week. Mechanism of action, efficacy, contraindications, skin reactions, and side effects are similar to those of COCs. The typical failure rate during the first year of use is less than 8% in women weighing less than 198 pounds (Trussell, 2007).

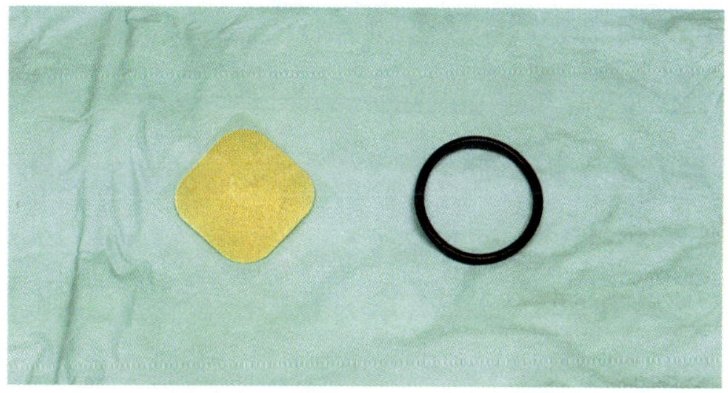

FIG. 8-9 Hormonal contraceptive transdermal patch and vaginal ring. (Courtesy Dee Lowdermilk, Chapel Hill, NC.)

Vaginal Contraceptive Ring. Available only with a prescription, the vaginal contraceptive ring is a flexible ring (made of ethylene vinyl acetate copolymer) worn in the vagina to deliver continuous levels of etonorgestrel (progesterone) and ethinyl estradiol (see Fig. 8-9). One vaginal ring is worn for 3 weeks, followed by a week without the ring. The ring is inserted by the woman and does not have to be fitted. Some wearers may experience vaginitis, leukorrhea, and vaginal discomfort (Nanda, 2007). Withdrawal bleeding occurs during the "no-ring" week. If the woman or partner notices discomfort during coitus, the ring can be removed from the vagina, but only up to 3 hours to still be effective when reinserted. Mechanism of action, efficacy, contraindications, and side effects are similar to those of COCs. The typical failure rate of the vaginal contraceptive ring is reportedly less than 8% during the first year of use (Trussell, 2007).

Progestin-Only Contraceptives. Progestin-only methods impair fertility by inhibiting ovulation, thickening and decreasing the amount of cervical mucus, thinning the endometrium, and altering cilia in the uterine tubes (Raymond, 2007b).

Oral Progestins (Minipill). The failure rate of progestin-only pills for typical users is about 1% to 10% in the first year of use (WHO/RHR & CCP, 2007). Effectiveness is increased if minipills are taken correctly. Because minipills contain such a low dose of progestin, the minipill must be taken at the same time every day (Raymond, 2007b). Users often complain of irregular vaginal bleeding.

Injectable Progestins. Depot medroxyprogesterone acetate (DMPA or Depo-Provera), 150 mg, is given intramuscularly in the deltoid or the gluteus maximus muscle. A 21- to 23-gauge needle, 2.5 to 4 cm long, should be used. DMPA should be initiated during the first 5 days of the menstrual cycle and administered every 11 to 13 weeks. A subcutaneous injection is also available (Practice Committee of the American Society for Reproductive Medicine, 2008).

CLINICAL REASONING

Vaginal Bleeding on Depo-Provera

Julie is a 32-year-old African-American woman who had been using Depo-Provera as a contraceptive for 15 years, but stopped the injections 1 year ago because she thought she had been on it too long. After talking to her primary care provider, she decided to restart the injections and received her first injection 6 weeks ago. When she was on Depo-Provera before, she did not have menstrual periods. Now she is complaining of vaginal spotting for the past 2 weeks.

1. Is there evidence to draw conclusions about how the nurse should respond?
2. Assumptions
   a. Effects of long-term use of Depo-Provera
   b. Effects of Depo-Provera on the menstrual cycle
   c. Side effects of Depo-Provera
3. What implications and priorities for nursing care can be drawn at this time?
4. Does the evidence objectively support your conclusion?
5. Are there alternative perspectives to your conclusion?

NURSING ALERT

When administering an intramuscular injection of progestin (e.g., Depo-Provera), do *not* massage the site after the injection because this action can hasten the absorption and shorten the period of effectiveness.

Advantages of DMPA include a contraceptive effectiveness comparable to that of perfect use of COCs, long-lasting effects, requirement of injections only four times a year, and the improbability of lactation being impaired. Side effects at the end of a year include decreased bone mineral density, weight gain, lipid changes, increased risk of venous thrombosis and thromboembolism, irregular vaginal spotting, decreased libido, and breast changes (Goldberg & Grimes, 2007). Other disadvantages include no protection against STIs (including HIV). Return to fertility may be delayed as long as up to 18 months after discontinuing DMPA. The typical failure rate is 3% in the first year of use (Trussell, 2007).

Implantable Progestins. Contraceptive implants are one or more thin rods that contain progestin. The implants are inserted under the skin of the woman's arm. A single-rod implant (Implanon) that is effective for up to 3 years is the only implant available in the United States. Implants will prevent some, but not all, ovulatory cycles and will thicken cervical mucus. Other advantages include reversibility and long-term continuous contraception that is not related to frequency of coitus. Irregular menstrual bleeding is the most common side effect. Less common side effects include headaches, nervousness, nausea, skin changes, and vertigo. No STI protection is provided with the implant method, so condoms should be used for protection (Raymond, 2007a).

NURSING ALERT

Women who use DMPA may lose significant bone mineral density with increasing duration of use. A systematic literature review found that bone loss is reversible (Kaunitz, Arias, & McClung, 2008). It is unknown if use of DMPA during adolescence or early adulthood, a critical period of bone accretion, will reduce peak bone mass and increase the risk of osteoporotic fracture in later life. Women who receive DMPA should be counseled about calcium intake and exercise (Goldberg & Grimes, 2007).

Emergency Contraception

Emergency contraception (EC) is available in more than 100 countries, and in about one third of these countries it is available without a prescription. In the United States, Plan B has been the only EC method available without a prescription and only in limited pharmacies and clinics in pharmacy access states (states where legislation has been passed to allow this practice)—Alaska, California, Hawaii, Maine, Massachusetts, New Hampshire, New Mexico, Vermont, and Washington. In 2009, the FDA approved Plan B for over-the-counter sale to women ages 17 and older without a prescription (FDA, 2009).

Plan B (levonorgestrel-only) is available in 1 or two dose regimens. Other options that the FDA has determined to be safe for emergency contraception include high doses of oral estrogen or COCs (ECPs) and insertion of a copper IUD (Stewart, Trussell & Van Look, 2007). These options will continue to be available by prescription only.

Emergency contraception should be taken by a woman as soon as possible but within 120 hours of unprotected intercourse, or birth control mishap (broken condom, dislodged ring or cervical cap, missed oral contraceptive pills, late for injection, and so on) to prevent unintended pregnancy (Stewart et al., 2007; WHO/RHR & CCP, 2007). If taken before ovulation, emergency contraception prevents ovulation by inhibiting follicular development. If taken after ovulation occurs, there is little effect on ovarian hormone production or the endometrium. Recommended oral medication regimens with ECPs are presented in Table 8-2. To minimize the side effect of nausea that occurs with high doses of estrogen and progestin, the woman can be advised to take an over-the-counter antiemetic 1 hour before each dose. Women with contraindications for estrogen use should use progestin-only emergency contraception. No medical contraindications for emergency contraception exist, except pregnancy and undiagnosed abnormal vaginal bleeding. If the woman does not begin menstruation within 21 days after taking the pills, she should be evaluated for pregnancy. Emergency

TABLE 8-2 **ORAL EMERGENCY CONTRACEPTIVES**

BRAND NAMES	FIRST DOSE (WITHIN 120 hr)	SECOND DOSE (12 hr LATER)
Progestin only		
Plan B		
Single-dose regimen (1.5 mg levonorgestrel) tablet	1 white tablet	
Two-dose regimen (0.75 mg levonorgestrel tablet)	1 white tablet	1 white tablet
Combined Oral Contraceptives* 100-120 mcg ethinyl estradiol and 0.5-0.6 mg levonorgestrel/tablet		
Ogestrel	2 white tablets	2 white tablets
Cryselle	4 white tablets	4 white tablets
Jolessa	4 pink tablets	4 pink tablets
Portia	4 pink tablets	4 pink tablets
Seasonale	4 pink tablets	4 pink tablets
Lo/Ovral	4 white tablets	4 white tablets
Low-Ogestrel	4 white tablets	4 white tablets
Enpresse	4 orange tablets	4 orange tablets
Nordette	4 light orange tablets	4 light orange tablets
Levora	4 white tablets	4 white tablets
Quasense	4 white tablets	4 white tablets
Trivora	4 yellow tablets	4 yellow tablets
Seasonique	4 light blue-green tablets	4 light blue-green tablets
Lessina	5 pink tablets	5 pink tablets
Aviane	5 orange tablets	5 orange tablets
LoSeasonique	5 orange tablets	5 orange tablets
Syronx	5 white tablets	5 white tablets
Lutera	5 white tablets	5 white tablets
Lybel	6 yellow tablets	6 yellow tablets

Sources: American College of Obstetricians and Gynecologists. (2010). Emergency contraception: ACOG Practice Bulletin No. 112. *Obstetrics and Gynecology, 115*(5), 1100-1109; Emergency Contraception. (2010). *Types of emergency contraception.* Available at http://ec.princeton.edu/questions/dose/html#dose. Accessed June 3, 2010. Stewart, F., Trussell, J., & Van Look, P. (2007). Emergency contraception. In R. Hatcher, J. Trussell, A. Nelson, W. Cates, F. Stewart, & D. Kowal (Eds.), *Contraceptive technology* (19th rev. ed.). New York: Ardent Media.
*Antinausea medications needed for any of the combined oral contraceptives.

contraception is ineffective if the woman is pregnant because the pills do not disturb an implanted pregnancy. Risk of pregnancy is reduced by as much as 75% (estrogen-progestin) and 89% (progestin only) if the woman takes ECPs (Stewart et al., 2007).

! NURSING ALERT

Emergency contraception will not protect a woman against pregnancy if she engages in unprotected intercourse in the days or weeks that follow treatment. Because ingestion of emergency contraceptive pills may delay ovulation, caution the woman that she needs to establish a reliable form of birth control in order to prevent unintended pregnancy (Stewart et al., 2007). Information about emergency contraception method options and access to providers is available at www.NOT-2-LATE.com or by calling 1-888-NOT-2-LATE.

IUDs containing copper (see later discussion) provide another emergency contraception option. The IUD should be inserted within 5 days of unprotected intercourse (Stewart et al., 2007). This method is suggested only for women who wish to have the benefit of long-term contraception. The risk of pregnancy is reduced by as much as 99% with emergency insertion of the copper-releasing IUD.

Contraceptive counseling should be provided to all women requesting emergency contraception, including a discussion of modification of risky sexual behaviors to prevent STIs and unwanted pregnancy.

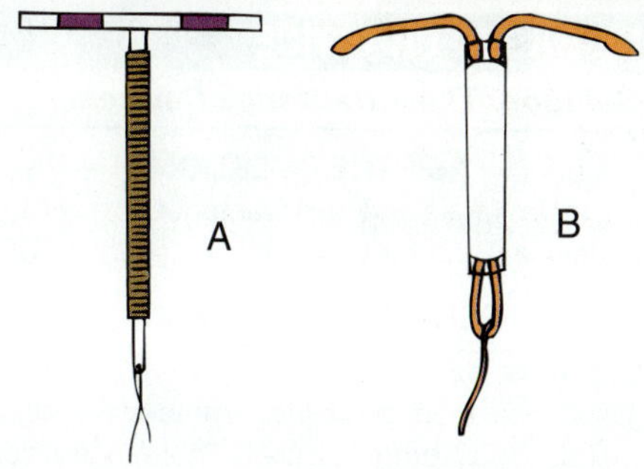

FIG. 8-10 Intrauterine devices (IUDs). **A,** Copper T 380A. **B,** Levonorgestrel-releasing IUD.

Intrauterine Devices

An IUD is a small T-shaped device with bendable arms for insertion through the cervix (Fig. 8-10). Once the trained health care provider inserts the IUD against the uterine fundus, the arms open near the fallopian tubes to maintain position of the device and to adversely affect the sperm motility and irritate the lining of the uterus. Two strings hang from the base of the stem through the cervix and protrude into the vagina for the woman to feel for assurance that the device has not been dislodged (Grimes, 2007). The woman should have had a negative pregnancy test, treatment for dysplasia if present, cervical cultures to rule out STIs, and a consent form signed before IUD insertion. Advantages to choosing this method of contraception include long-term protection from pregnancy and immediate return to fertility when removed. Disadvantages include increased risk of pelvic inflammatory disease (PID) shortly after placement, unintentional expulsion of the device, infection, and possible uterine perforation. IUDs offer no protection against HIV or other STIs. Therefore, women who are in mutually monogamous relationships are the best candidates for this device (see Evidence-Based Practice box).

There are two FDA-approved IUDs, the ParaGard Copper T 380A and the hormonal intrauterine system (Mirena). The ParaGard Copper T 380A is made of radiopaque polyethylene and fine solid copper and is approved for 10 years of use. The copper primarily serves as a spermicide and inflames the endometrium, preventing fertilization (Grimes, 2007). Sometimes women experience more bleeding and cramping within the first year after insertion, but nonsteroidal antiinflammatory drugs (NSAIDs) can be taken for pain relief. The typical failure rate in the first year of use of the copper IUD is less than 1% (Trussell, 2007).

The hormonal intrauterine system (Mirena) releases levonorgestrel from its vertical reservoir. Effective for up to 5 years, it impairs sperm motility, thickens cervical mucus, decreases the lining of the uterus, and has some anovulatory effects (Grimes, 2007). Uterine cramping and bleeding are usually decreased with this device, although irregular spotting are common in the first few months following insertion. The typical failure rate in the first year of use is less than 1% (Trussell, 2007).

EVIDENCE-BASED PRACTICE

Pat Gingrich

An Ideal Solution: The Intrauterine Device

ASK THE QUESTION

What are the advantages and disadvantages for women using the intrauterine device (IUD) for contraception? Which IUD is best?

SEARCH FOR EVIDENCE

Search Strategies

Professional organization guidelines, meta-analyses, systematic reviews, randomized controlled trials, nonrandomized prospective studies and retrospective studies since 2007.

Databases Searched

CINAHL, Cochrane, Medline, National Guideline Clearinghouse, TRIP Database and websites for the Association of Women's Health, Obstetric, and Neonatal Nurses and Royal College of Obstetrics & Gynaecology.

CRITICALLY ANALYZE THE DATA

The IUD is a safe, cost-effective, highly reliable and reversible method of contraception. It may be an ideal option for many women, but remains underused. Forthofer (2009) examined perspectives and knowledge of health care providers and found inaccuracies and bias in medical texts and lack of knowledge and mistaken beliefs among providers. Copper-covered IUDs have been the gold standard for decades, with the longest duration of action (approved for 10 years) and the most effectiveness (Kulier, O'Brien, Helmerhorst, Usher-Patel, & d'Arcangues, 2007). Although several designs are offered in Europe, the copper IUD approved for use in the US is the T 380A. Its mechanism of action is primarily by the prevention of fertilization. More recently, the levonorgestrel intrauterine system (LNG-IUS), which delivers low levels of progestin, has become very popular both as a contraceptive and a treatment for heavy menstrual bleeding or severe dysmenorrhea (RCOGFSRH, 2007). The action of the LNG-IUS is primarily through hormonally affecting the endometrium, preventing implantation. The LNG-IUS is approved for five years of use before it must be replaced. Both the copper and hormonal IUD have pregnancy rates at 5 years of 0.3% to 0.6% (Thonneau & Almont, 2008).

The IUD can be recommended to women regardless of parity, age, or past history of ectopic pregnancy or pelvic inflammatory disease. It can be placed in the immediate postpartum period although expulsion rates are higher than with interval insertions (unrelated to pregnancy) (Grimes,Lopez, Schulz, Van Vliet, & Stanwood, 2010). According to the guidelines of the Royal College of Obstetricians and Gynaecologists (2007), the copper IUD is the first choice for women with diabetes, breast cancer, cardiovascular disease or risk for thrombophlebitis. The LNG-IUS is the best choice for women with anemia, thalassemia, sickle cell, or heavy bleeding. Insertion can occur anytime, as long as there is no pre-existing pregnancy.

The copper IUD is also recommended as an effective form of emergency contraception. Inserted shortly after unprotected intercourse, it works by preventing implantation. It can then be left in place to provide ongoing contraception (Cheng Gülmezoglu, Piaggo, Ezcurra, & Van Look, 2008).

IMPLICATIONS FOR PRACTICE

For many women, the IUD would be the ideal method of contraception throughout their childbearing years, but many don't know much about it. Any doubts about its safety have been long dispelled. The IUD could benefit teens, who have a notoriously difficult time with contraception. Either type of IUD can be inserted immediately after childbirth and can provide reversible spacing between children. At 40 years of age, a woman can get a copper IUD, or at 45 she can get a LNG-IUS, which will then provide contraception for her through menopause. The nurse should counsel the woman about its mode of action, and take a thorough health history. Women should know that there is a very small (2 out of 1000) risk of perforation upon insertion. By giving accurate, evidence-based information, women can make the best choice of contraception for themselves and their families.

References

Cheng, L., Gülmezoglu, A., Piaggo, G., Ezcurra, E., & Van Look, P. (2008). Interventions for emergency contraception. *The Cochrane Database of Systematic Reviews 2008*, 1, CD001324.

Forthofer, L. (2009). A clinical review of the intrauterine device as an effective method of contraception. *Journal of Obstetric, Gynecologic and Neonatal Nursing, 38*(6), 693–698.

Grimes, D, Lopez, L., Schulz, K., Van Vliet, H., & Stanwood, N. (2010). Immediate post-partum insertion of intrauterine devices. *The Cochrane Database of Systematic Reviews, 2010,* 5, CD003036.

Kulier, R., O'Brian, P., Helmerhorst, F., Usher-Patel, M. & d'Arcangues, C. (2007). Copper containing, framed intra-uterine devices for contraception. *The Cochrane Database of Systematic Reviews 2007*, 3, CD005347.

Royal College of Obstetrics & Gynaecology Faculty of Sexual and Reproductive Healthcare (RCOGFSRH). (2007). *Clinical guidance: Intrauterine contraception.* Available at www.fsrh.org/admin/uploads/CEUGuidanceIntrauterineContraceptionNov07.pdf. Accessed June 3, 2010.

Thonneau, P., & Almont,T. (2008). Contraceptive efficacy of intrauterine devices. *American Journal of Obstetrics and Gynecology, 198*(4), 248-253.

Nursing Considerations. The woman should be taught to check for the presence of the IUD strings after menstruation to rule out expulsion of the device. If pregnancy occurs with the IUD in place, an ultrasound should confirm that it is not ectopic. Early removal of the IUD helps decrease the risk of spontaneous miscarriage or preterm labor. The woman should report any signs of flulike illness because this may indicate a septic miscarriage (Grimes, 2007). In some women who are allergic to copper, a rash develops, necessitating the removal of the copper-bearing IUD. Signs of potential complications to be taught to the woman are listed in the Signs of Potential Complications box.

SIGNS OF POTENTIAL COMPLICATIONS

INTRAUTERINE DEVICES (IUDs)

Signs of potential complications related to IUDs can be remembered in the following manner (Zieman, Hatcher, Cwiak, Darney, Creinin, & Stosur, 2007):

P—Period late, abnormal spotting or bleeding
A—Abdominal pain, pain with intercourse
I—Infection exposure, abnormal vaginal discharge
N—Not feeling well, fever, or chills
S—String missing; shorter or longer

Sterilization

Sterilization refers to surgical procedures intended to render a person infertile. Most procedures involve the occlusion of the passageways for the ova and sperm (Fig. 8-11). For the woman, the oviducts (uterine tubes) are occluded; for the man, the sperm ducts (vas deferens) are occluded. Only surgical removal of the ovaries (oophorectomy) or uterus (hysterectomy) or both will result in absolute sterility for the woman. All other sterilization procedures have a small but definite failure rate; that is, pregnancy may result.

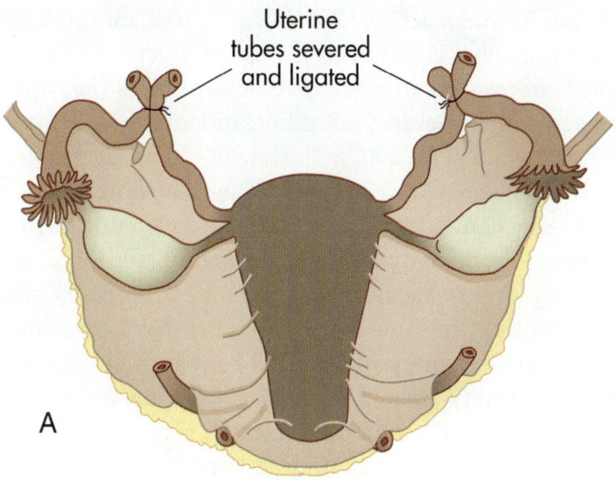

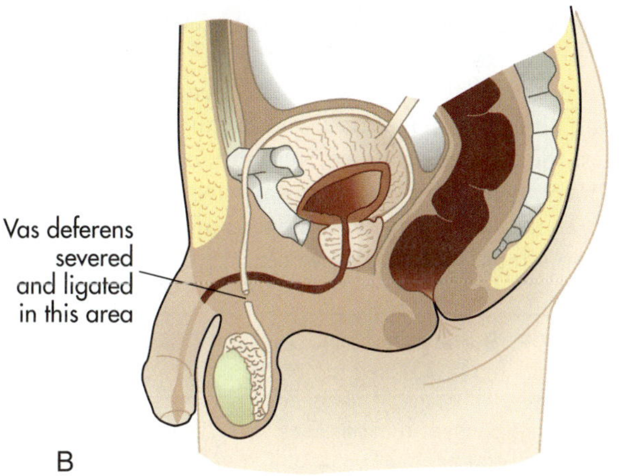

FIG. 8-11 Sterilization. **A,** Uterine tubes severed and ligated (tubal ligation). **B,** Sperm duct severed and ligated (vasectomy).

Female Sterilization. Female sterilization (bilateral tubal ligation [BTL]) may be done immediately after childbirth (within 24 to 48 hours), concomitant with induced abortion, or as an interval procedure (during any phase of the menstrual cycle). If sterilization is performed as an interval procedure, the health care provider must be certain that the woman is not pregnant. Half of all female sterilization procedures are performed immediately after a pregnancy (Pollack, Thomas, & Barone, 2007). Sterilization procedures can be safely done on an outpatient basis.

Tubal Occlusion. A laparoscopic approach or a minilaparotomy can be used for tubal ligation (Fig. 8-12), tubal electrocoagulation, or the application of bands or clips. Electrocoagulation and ligation are considered to be permanent methods. Use of the bands or clips has the theoretic advantage of possible removal and return of tubal patency.

For the minilaparotomy, the woman is admitted the morning of surgery, having received nothing by mouth since midnight. Preoperative sedation is given. The procedure can be carried out with a local anesthetic, but a regional or general anesthetic also can be used. A small incision is made in the abdominal wall below the umbilicus. The woman may experience sensations of tugging, but no pain, and the operation is completed within 20 minutes. She may be discharged several hours later if she has recovered from anesthesia, or next day if done postpartum.

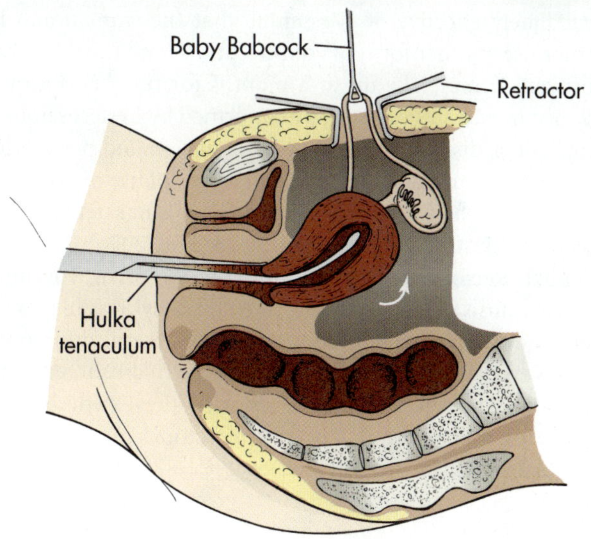

FIG. 8-12 Use of minilaparotomy to gain access to uterine tubes for occlusion procedures. Tenaculum is used to lift uterus *(arrow)* toward incision.

Any abdominal discomfort usually can be controlled with a mild analgesic (e.g., acetaminophen). Within days the scar is almost invisible (see Teaching for Self-Management box: What to Expect After Tubal Ligation). As with any surgery, there is always a possibility of complications of anesthesia, infection, hemorrhage, and trauma to other organs.

TEACHING FOR SELF-MANAGEMENT

What to Expect After Tubal Ligation

- You should expect no change in hormones and their influence.
- Your menstrual period will be about the same as before the sterilization.
- You may feel pain at ovulation.
- The ovum disintegrates within the abdominal cavity.
- It is highly unlikely that you will become pregnant.
- You should not have a change in sexual functioning; you may enjoy sexual relations more because you will not be concerned about becoming pregnant.
- Sterilization offers no protection against STIs; therefore, you may need to use condoms.

Transcervical Sterilization. Still considered experimental, hysteroscopic techniques can be used to inject occlusion agents into the uterine tubes. One FDA-approved device is the Essure system, an interval sterilization method (not intended for the postpartum period). A trained health care professional inserts a small catheter holding the polyester fibers through the vagina and cervix and places the small metallic implants into each uterine tube. The device works by stimulating the woman's own scar tissue formation to occlude the uterine tubes and prevent conception (Abbott, 2007). An advantage is that the nonhormonal form of contraception can be inserted during an office procedure without anesthesia. Analgesia is recommended to decrease mild to moderate discomfort associated with tubal spasm. Particularly convenient for obese women, or those with abdominal adhesions, the transcervical approach eliminates the need for abdominal surgery. Because the procedure is not immediately effective, it is essential that the woman and her partner use another form of contraception until tubal blockage is proven. It may take up to 3 months for tubal occlusion to fully occur, and success must be confirmed by hysterosalpingogram. Other disadvantages include expulsion and perforation. The typical failure rate during the first year of use of the Essure system is less than 1%. Long-term efficacy and safety rates are unknown (Hastings-Tolsma, Nodine, & Teal, 2006).

Tubal Reconstruction. Restoration of tubal continuity (reanastomosis) and function is technically feasible except after laparoscopic tubal electrocoagulation. Sterilization reversal, however, is costly, difficult (requiring microsurgery), and uncertain. The success rate varies with the extent of tubal destruction and removal. The risk of ectopic pregnancy after tubal reanastomosis is increased by 1% to 7% (Pollack et al., 2007).

Male Sterilization. *Vasectomy* is the sealing, tying, or cutting of a man's vas deferens so that the sperm cannot travel from the testes to the penis (Pollack et al., 2007). It is considered the easiest and most commonly used operation for male sterilization. Vasectomy can be carried out with local anesthesia on an outpatient basis. Pain, bleeding, infection, and other postsurgical complications are considered the disadvantages to the surgical procedure. It is considered a permanent method of sterilization because reversal is generally unsuccessful.

Two methods are used for scrotal entry: conventional (scalpel incision) and no-scalpel (small puncture) vasectomy. The surgeon identifies and immobilizes the vas deferens through the scrotum. Then the vas is ligated or cauterized (see Fig. 8-11, *B*). Surgeons vary in their techniques to occlude the vas deferens: ligation with sutures, division, cautery, application of clips, excision of a segment of the vas, fascial interposition, or some combination of these methods (Pollack et al., 2007).

The man is instructed in self-care to promote a safe return to routine activities. To reduce swelling and relieve discomfort, ice packs are applied to the scrotum intermittently for a few hours after surgery. A scrotal support may be applied to decrease discomfort. Moderate inactivity for about 2 days is advisable because of local scrotal tenderness. The skin suture can be removed 5 to 7 days after surgery. Sexual intercourse may be resumed as desired; however, sterility is not immediate. Some sperm will remain in the proximal portions of the sperm ducts after vasectomy. One week to several months are required to clear the ducts of sperm; therefore, some form of contraception is needed until the sperm count in the ejaculate on two consecutive tests is down to zero (Pollack et al., 2007).

Vasectomy has no effect on potency (ability to achieve and maintain erection) or volume of ejaculate. Endocrine production of testosterone continues, so secondary sex characteristics are not affected. Sperm production continues, but sperm are unable to leave the epididymis and are lysed by the immune system. Men occasionally may develop a hematoma, infection, or epididymitis (Pollack et al., 2007). Less common are painful granulomas from accumulation of sperm.

Complications after bilateral vasectomy are uncommon and usually not serious. They include bleeding (usually external), suture reaction, and reaction to anesthetic agent. The failure rate for male sterilization is 0.15% (Trussell, 2007).

Tubal Reconstruction. Microsurgery to reanastomose (restoration of tubal continuity) the sperm ducts can be accomplished successfully in more than 90% of cases (i.e., sperm in the ejaculate); however, the fertility rate varies widely from 38% to 89% (Pollack et al., 2007). The rate of success decreases as the time since the procedure increases. The vasectomy may result in permanent changes in the testes that leave men unable to father children. The changes are those ordinarily seen only in older adults (e.g., interstitial fibrosis [scar tissue between the seminiferous tubules]). In some men, antibodies develop against their own sperm (autoimmunization). The role of antisperm antibodies in fertility after vasectomy reversal has not been completely determined. Additional research is needed to explore a possible link between vasectomy and prostate cancer.

Laws and Regulations. All states have strict regulations for informed consent. Many states permit voluntary sterilization of any mature, rational woman without reference to her marital or pregnancy status. Although the partner's consent is not required by law, the man or woman is encouraged to discuss the situation with the partner, and health care providers may request the partner's consent. Sterilization of minors or mentally incompetent individuals is restricted by most states and often requires the approval of a board of eugenicists or other court-appointed individuals (see Legal Tip).

LEGAL TIP: Sterilization

- If federal funds are used for female or male sterilization, the person must be age 21 years or older.
- Informed consent must include an explanation of the risks, benefits, and alternatives; a statement that describes sterilization as a permanent, irreversible method of birth control; and a statement that mandates a 30-day waiting period between giving consent and the sterilization.
- Informed consent must be in the man's or woman's native language, or an interpreter must be provided to read the consent form to the man or woman.

Nursing Considerations. The nurse plays an important role in assisting people with decision making so all requirements for informed consent are met. The nurse also provides information about alternatives to sterilization, such as contraception. The nurse acts as a "sounding board" for people who are exploring the possibility of choosing sterilization and their feelings about and motivation for this choice. The nurse records this information, which may be the basis for referral to a family-planning clinic, a psychiatric social worker, or another professional health care provider.

Information must be given about what is entailed in various procedures, how much discomfort or pain can be expected, and what type of care is needed. Many individuals fear sterilization procedures because of the imagined effect on their sex life. They need reassurance concerning the hormonal and psychologic basis for sexual function and that uterine tube occlusion or vasectomy has no biologic sequelae in terms of sexual adequacy (Pollack et al., 2007). Preoperative care includes health assessment, which includes a psychologic assessment, physical examination, and laboratory tests. The nurse assists with the health assessment, answers questions, and confirms the client's understanding of printed instructions (e.g., nothing by mouth after midnight). Ambivalence and extreme fear of the procedure are reported to the physician.

Postoperative care depends on the procedure performed (e.g., laparoscopy, laparotomy for tubal occlusion, or vasectomy). General care includes recovery after anesthesia, monitoring of vital signs and fluid and electrolyte balance (intake and output, laboratory values), prevention of or early identification and treatment for infection or hemorrhage, control of discomfort, and assessment of emotional response to the procedure and recovery.

Discharge planning depends on the type of procedure performed. In general, the client is given written instructions about observing for and reporting symptoms and signs of complications, the type of recovery to be expected, and the date and time for a follow-up appointment.

Breastfeeding: Lactational Amenorrhea Method

The *lactational amenorrhea method (LAM)* can be a highly effective, *temporary* method of birth control. It is more popular in underdeveloped countries and traditional societies, where breastfeeding is used to prolong birth intervals. The method has seen limited use in the United States since most American women do not establish breastfeeding patterns that provide maximum protection against pregnancy (Kennedy & Trussell, 2007).

When the infant suckles at the mother's breast, a surge of prolactin hormone is released, which inhibits estrogen production and suppresses ovulation and the return of menses. LAM works best if the mother is exclusively or almost exclusively breastfeeding, if the woman has not had a menstrual flow since giving birth, and if the infant is younger than 6 months of age. Effectiveness is enhanced by frequent feedings at intervals of less than 4 hours during the day and no more than 6 hours during the night, long duration of each feeding, and no bottle supplementation or limited supplementation by spoon or cup. The woman should be counseled that disruption of the breastfeeding pattern or supplementation can increase the risk of pregnancy. The typical failure rate is 2% (Kennedy & Trussell, 2007; King, 2007).

Future Trends

Contraceptive options are more limited in the United States and Canada than in some other industrialized countries. Lack of funding for research, governmental regulations, conflicting values about contraception, and high costs of liability coverage for contraception have been cited as blocks to new and improved methods. Existing methods of contraception are being improved, however, and a variety of new methods are being developed.

Lower-dose COCs (15 mcg of ethinyl estradiol) are available in Europe. Female barrier methods (new female condoms, client-fitted diaphragms, and new vaginal sponges) are being tested. Vaginal delivery systems including progestin-only vaginal rings and progesterone daily suppositories are under investigation. Two new IUDs and spermicidal microbicides are being evaluated. Male hormonal methods are also being investigated, including hormonal injections (testosterone), gonadotropin-releasing hormone antagonists, antisperm compounds, immunologic methods, and contraceptive vaccines (Blithe, 2008; Gabelnick, Schwartz, & Darroch, 2007).

INDUCED ABORTION

Induced abortion is the purposeful interruption of a pregnancy before 20 weeks of gestation. (Spontaneous abortion [miscarriage] is discussed in Chapter 28.) If the abortion is performed at the woman's request, the term *elective abortion* is used; if performed for reasons of maternal or fetal health or disease, the term *therapeutic abortion* applies. Many factors contribute to a woman's decision to have an abortion. Indications include (1) preservation of the life or health of the mother, (2) genetic disorders of the fetus, (3) rape or incest, and (4) the pregnant woman's request. The control of birth, dealing as it does with human sexuality and the question of life and death, is one of the most emotional components of health care and has been the most controversial social issue in the last half of the 20th century and continues to be so today. Regulations exist to protect the mother from the complications of abortion.

Abortion is regulated in most countries, including the United States. Before 1970, legal abortion was not widely available in the United States. However, in January 1973, the U.S. Supreme Court set aside previous antiabortion laws and legalized abortion. This decision established a trimester approach to abortion. In the first trimester, abortion is permissible, the decision is between the woman and her health care provider, and a state has little right to interfere (Paul & Stewart, 2007). In the second trimester, abortion is left to the discretion of the individual states to regulate procedures as long as they are reasonably related to the woman's health. In the third trimester, abortions may be limited or even prohibited by state regulation unless the restriction interferes with the life or health of the pregnant woman (Paul & Stewart).

In 1992, the U.S. Supreme Court made another landmark ruling, this time allowing states to restrict early abortion services as long as the restrictions did not place an "undue burden" on the woman's ability to choose abortion. Since then many bills have been introduced to limit access and funds for women seeking abortion. In 2006, several states introduced bills to ban most abortions; the U.S. Supreme Court will again play a major role in deciding the future of abortions. Hospitals maintained by Roman Catholics and some of those maintained by strict fundamentalists forbid abortion (and often sterilization) despite legal challenges.

> **LEGAL TIP: Induced Abortion**
> It is important for nurses to know the laws regarding abortion in their country or state of practice before they offer abortion counseling or nursing care to a woman choosing an abortion. Many states enforce a mandatory delay or state-directed counseling before a woman may legally obtain an abortion.

Incidence

The number of abortions performed in the United States in 2006 was 846,181 (Pazol, Gamble,, Parker, Cook, Zane, & Hamdan, 2009). Most abortions are performed in the first trimester, with about 62% in the first 8 weeks after the last menstrual period. Only about 5% of abortions are performed after 16 weeks of gestation. Most women who are having an elective abortion are Caucasian, between the ages of 20 to 29 years, and unmarried (Pazol et al.). In 2006, an estimated 91,377 abortions were performed in Canada (Statistics Canada, 2010).

The Decision to Have an Abortion

A woman who is deciding whether to have an abortion is often ambivalent. She needs information and an opportunity to discuss her feelings about pregnancy, abortion, and the effect of either choice on her future. She needs to make her decision without feeling coerced (Levi, Simmonds, & Taylor, 2009).

Nurses and other health care providers often struggle with the same values and moral convictions as those of the pregnant woman. The conflicts and doubts of the nurse can be readily communicated to women who are already anxious and overly sensitive. Regardless of personal views on abortion, nurses who provide care to women seeking abortion have an ethical responsibility to counsel women about their options and to make appropriate referrals (Levi et al., 2009).

The Association of Women's Health, Obstetric and Neonatal Nurses (AWHONN, 2009) continues to support a nurse's right to choose to participate or not in abortion procedures in keeping with his or her "personal, moral, ethical, or religious beliefs." AWHONN also advocates that "nurses have a professional obligation to inform their employers, at the time of employment, of any attitudes and beliefs that may interfere with essential job functions."

LEGAL TIP: Institutional Policies for Nurses' Rights and Responsibilities Related to Abortion

Nurses' rights and responsibilities related to caring for abortion clients should be protected through policies that describe how the institution will accommodate the nurse's ethical or moral beliefs and what the nurse should do to avoid client abandonment in such situations. Nurses should know what policies are in place in their institutions and encourage such policies to be written if there are none (The Joint Commission, 2009).

CARE MANAGEMENT

A thorough assessment is conducted through history, physical examination, and laboratory tests. The length of pregnancy and the condition of the woman must be determined to select the appropriate type of abortion procedure. An ultrasound examination should be performed before a second-trimester abortion is done. If the woman is Rh negative, she is a candidate for prophylaxis against Rh isoimmunization. She should receive Rh_o(D) immune globulin within 72 hours after the abortion if she is D negative and if Coombs' test results are negative (if the woman is unsensitized or isoimmunization has not developed).

The woman's understanding of alternatives, the types of abortions, and expected recovery are assessed. Misinformation and gaps in knowledge are identified and corrected. The record is reviewed for the signed informed consent, and the woman's understanding is verified. General preoperative, operative, and postoperative assessments are performed.

Analysis of data leads to identification of the appropriate nursing diagnoses for the woman undergoing elective abortion. Potential nursing diagnoses are listed in Box 8-4.

Counseling about abortion includes help for the woman in identifying how she perceives the pregnancy, information about the choices available (i.e., having an abortion or carrying the pregnancy to term and then either keeping the infant or placing the baby for adoption), and information about the types of abortion procedures.

BOX 8-4 SELECTED NURSING DIAGNOSES FOR WOMEN HAVING ELECTIVE ABORTION

- *Decisional conflict* related to
  - value system
- *Fear* related to
  - abortion procedure
  - potential complications
  - implications for future pregnancies
  - what others might think
- *Anticipatory grieving* related to
  - distress at loss or feelings of guilt
- *Risk for infection* related to
  - effects of the procedure
  - lack of understanding of preoperative and postoperative self-care
- *Acute pain* related to
  - effects of the procedure or postoperative events

CLINICAL REASONING

Abortion

Caroline is a 19-year-old college student who engaged in unprotected intercourse with her date after attending a party. She has missed a period and at the clinic today learns that she is approximately 9 weeks pregnant. She has requested an appointment for an abortion. She has many questions about the choices she has and what she can expect during the procedure and afterward. How should the nurse respond?

1. Evidence—Is there sufficient evidence to draw conclusions about what response the nurse should give?
2. Assumptions—Describe underlying assumptions about the following issues:
   a. Physical response related to termination of pregnancy with vacuum aspiration
   b. Psychologic and emotional response
   c. Future childbearing
3. What implications and priorities for nursing care can be drawn at this time?
4. Does the evidence objectively support your conclusion?
5. Are there alternative perspectives to your conclusion?

First-Trimester Abortion

Methods for performing early abortion (less than 9 weeks of gestation) include surgical (aspiration) and medical methods (mifepristone with misoprostol, and methotrexate with misoprostol).

Aspiration

Aspiration (vacuum or suction curettage) is the most common procedure in the first trimester, with almost 88% of all procedures being performed by this method (Pazol et al., 2009). Aspiration abortion is usually performed under local anesthesia in the physician's office, the clinic, or the hospital. The suction procedure for performing an early elective abortion (ideal time is 8 to 12 weeks since the last menstrual period) usually requires less than 5 minutes.

A bimanual examination is done before the procedure to assess uterine size and position. A speculum is inserted and the cervix is anesthetized with a local anesthetic agent. The cervix is dilated if necessary and a cannula connected to suction is inserted into the uterine cavity. The products of conception are evacuated from the uterus.

During the procedure the nurse or physician keeps the woman informed about what to expect next (e.g., menstrual-like cramping, sounds of the suction machine). The nurse assesses the woman's vital signs. The aspirated uterine contents must be carefully inspected to ascertain whether all fetal parts and adequate placental tissue have been evacuated. After the abortion the woman rests on the table until she is ready to stand. She remains in the recovery area or waiting room for 1 to 3 hours for detection of excessive cramping or bleeding; then she is discharged.

Bleeding after the operation is normally about the equivalent of a heavy menstrual period, and cramps are rarely severe. Excessive vaginal bleeding and infection, such as endometritis or salpingitis, are the most common complications of elective abortion. Retained products of conception are the primary cause of vaginal bleeding. Evacuation of the uterus, uterine massage, and administration of oxytocin or methylergonovine (Methergine) or both may be necessary. Prophylactic antibiotics to decrease the risk of infection are commonly prescribed (Paul & Stewart, 2007). Postabortion pain may be relieved with NSAIDs such as ibuprofen.

Postabortion instructions differ among health care providers (e.g., tampons should not be used for at least 3 days or should be avoided for up to 3 weeks, and resumption of sexual intercourse may be permitted within 1 week or discouraged for 2 weeks). The woman may shower daily. Instruction is given to watch for excessive bleeding and other signs of complications and to avoid douches of any type.

SAFETY ALERT

The woman who has an induced abortion should be given clear instructions to return immediately to the health care facility or emergency department for any of the following symptoms:

- Fever greater than 38° C (100.4° F)
- Chills
- Bleeding greater than two saturated pads in 2 hours or heavy bleeding lasting a few days
- Foul-smelling vaginal discharge
- Severe abdominal pain, cramping, or backache
- Abdominal tenderness (when pressure applied)

The woman may expect her menstrual period to resume 4 to 6 weeks from the day of the procedure. Information about the birth control method the woman prefers is offered, if this has not been done previously during the counseling interview that usually precedes the decision to have an abortion. Some methods can be initiated immediately such as an IUD insertion. Hormonal methods may be started immediately or within a week (Paul & Stewart, 2007). The woman must be strongly encouraged to return for her follow-up visit so complications can be detected. A pregnancy test may also be performed at that time to determine whether the pregnancy was successfully terminated.

Medical Abortion

Early medical abortion has been popular in Canada and Europe for more than 15 years, but it is a relatively new procedure in the United States. Medical abortions are available for use in the United States for up to 9 weeks after the last menstrual period. Methotrexate, misoprostol, and mifepristone are the drugs used in the current regimens to induce early abortion. About 11% of all reported abortion procedures in 2006 were medical procedures (Pazol et al., 2009).

Methotrexate is a cytotoxic drug that causes early abortion by blocking folic acid in fetal cells so that they cannot divide. Misoprostol (Cytotec) is a prostaglandin analog that acts directly on the cervix to soften and dilate and on the uterine muscle to stimulate contractions. Mifepristone, formerly known as RU 486, was approved by the FDA in 2000. It works by binding to progesterone receptors and blocking the action of progesterone, which is necessary for maintaining pregnancy (Paul & Stewart, 2007).

Methotrexate and Misoprostol. There is no standard protocol, but methotrexate is given intramuscularly or orally (usually mixed with orange juice). Vaginal placement of misoprostol follows in 3 to 7 days. The woman returns for a follow-up visit in 1 week to confirm the abortion is complete. If not, the woman is offered an additional dose of misoprostol, or vacuum aspiration is performed (Paul & Stewart, 2007).

Mifepristone and Misoprostol. Mifepristone can be taken up to 7 weeks after the last menstrual period. The FDA-approved regimen is that the woman takes 600 mg of mifepristone orally; 48 hours later she returns to the office and takes 400 mcg of misoprostol orally (unless abortion has already occurred and been confirmed). Two weeks after the administration of mifepristone, the woman must return to the office for a clinical examination or ultrasound to confirm that the pregnancy has been terminated. In 1% to 5% of cases, the drugs do not work, and surgical abortion (aspiration) is needed (Paul & Stewart, 2007).

Research has demonstrated a more effective regimen that has fewer side effects. This regimen can be given up to 9 weeks after the last menstrual period and includes administration of 200 mg mifepristone orally followed by misoprostol 800 mcg vaginally in 24 to 48 hours. This vaginal insertion can be done at home by the woman. A follow-up visit is in 4 to 8 days (Paul & Stewart, 2007).

With any medical abortion regimen, the woman usually will experience bleeding and cramping. Side effects of the medications include nausea, vomiting, diarrhea, headache, dizziness, fever, and chills. These are attributed to misoprostol and usually subside in a few hours after administration (Paul & Stewart, 2007).

Second-Trimester Abortion

Second-trimester abortion is associated with more complications and costs than first-trimester abortions. Dilation and evacuation (D&E) accounts for almost all procedures performed in the United States. Induction of uterine contractions with hypertonic solutions (e.g., saline, urea) injected directly into the uterus and uterotonic agents (e.g., misoprostol, dinoprostone) account for only about 0.5% of all abortions (Pazol et al., 2009).

Dilation and Evacuation

D&E can be performed at any point up to 20 weeks of gestation although it is most commonly performed between 13 and 16 weeks of gestation (Paul & Stewart, 2007). The cervix requires more dilation because the products of conception are larger. Often, osmotic dilators (e.g., laminaria) are inserted several hours or several days before the procedure, or misoprostol can be applied to the cervix. The procedure is similar to vaginal aspiration except a larger cannula is used and other instruments may be needed to remove the fetus and placenta. Nursing care includes monitoring vital signs, providing emotional support, administering analgesics, and postoperative monitoring. Disadvantages of D&E may include possible long-term harmful effects to the cervix.

Nursing Considerations

The woman will need help exploring the meaning of the various alternatives and consequences to herself and her significant others. It is often difficult for a woman to express her true feelings (e.g., what having an abortion means to her now and how she may feel about her decision in the future and what support or regret her friends and peers may demonstrate). A calm, matter-of-fact approach on the part of the nurse can be helpful (e.g., "Yes, I know you are pregnant. I am here to help. Let's talk about alternatives."). Listening to what the woman has to say and encouraging her to speak are essential. Neutral responses such as "Oh," "Uh-huh," and "Umm," and nonverbal encouragement such as nodding, maintaining eye contact, and use of touch are helpful in setting an open, accepting environment. Clarifying, restating, and reflecting statements, open-ended questions, and feedback are communication techniques that can be used to maintain a realistic focus on the situation and bring the woman's problems into the open.

Information about alternatives to abortion such as referral to adoption agencies or to support services if the woman chooses to keep her baby should be provided. If a decision is made to have an abortion, the woman must be assured of continued support. Information about what is entailed in various procedures, how much discomfort or pain can be expected, and what type of care is needed must be given. A discussion of the various feelings including depression, guilt, regret, and relief that the woman might experience after the abortion is needed. Information about community resources for postabortion counseling may be needed (Paul & Stewart, 2007). If family or friends cannot be involved, scheduling time for nursing personnel to give the necessary support is an essential component of the care plan.

After an abortion, studies have indicated that most women report relief, but some have temporary distress or mixed emotions. A systematic review of the literature found no difference in the long-term mental health outcomes of women who had abortions and women who did not have abortions (Charles, Polis, Sridhara, & Blum, 2008). Because symptoms can vary among women who have had abortions, nurses must assess women for grief reactions and facilitate the grieving process through active listening and nonjudgmental support and care.

COMMUNITY ACTIVITY

- Visit the Planned Parenthood Federation of America website at www.plannedparenthood.org. Locate a Planned Parenthood clinic in your community. Visit the website of the clinic. What types of services are offered for walk-in clients versus clients that need to make an appointment? Does the clinic offer any specialty services? What forms of payment does the clinic accept?
- Visit the Emergency Contraception hotline website at www.not-2-late.com. Research whether emergency contraception is available without a prescription in your state. Are there any pharmacies or clinics that dispense emergency contraception in your community?

Audio Chapter Summaries Access an audio summary of the Key Points on evolve

KEY POINTS

- A variety of contraceptive methods are available with various effectiveness rates, advantages, and disadvantages.
- Women and their partners should choose the contraceptive method or methods best suited to them.
- Effective contraceptives are available through prescription and nonprescription sources.
- A variety of techniques are available to enhance the effectiveness of periodic abstinence in motivated couples who prefer this natural method.
- Hormonal contraception includes both precoital and postcoital prevention through various modalities and requires thorough client education.
- The barrier methods of diaphragm and cervical cap provide safe and effective contraception for women or couples motivated to use them consistently and correctly.
- Intrauterine devices can provide long-term (5 to 10 years) protection.
- Emergency contraception should be taken as soon as possible after unprotected intercourse, but no later than 120 hours.
- Proper, concurrent use of spermicides and latex condoms provides protection against STIs.
- Tubal ligations and vasectomies are permanent sterilization methods used by increasing numbers of women and men.
- Induced abortion performed in the first trimester is safer than an abortion performed in the second trimester.
- The most common complications of induced abortion include infection, retained products of conception, and excessive vaginal bleeding.
- Major psychologic sequelae of induced abortion are rare.

REFERENCES

Abbott, J. (2007). Transcervical sterilization. *Current Opinion in Obstetrics and Gynecology, 19*(4), 325–330.

Association of Women's Health, Obstetric and Neonatal Nurses (AWHONN). (2009). *Ethical decision making in the clinical setting: Nurses' rights and responsibilities.* Available at www.awhonn.org/awhonn/content.do?name=05_HealthPolicyLegislation/5H_PositionStatements.htm. Accessed June 3, 2010.

Blithe, D. (2008). Male contraception: What is on the horizon? *Contraception, 78*(4 Suppl. 1), S23–S27.

Cates, W., & Raymond, E. (2007). Vaginal barriers and spermicides. In R. Hatcher, J. Trussell, A. Nelson, W. Cates, F. Stewart, & D. Kowal (Eds.), *Contraceptive technology* (19th rev. ed.). New York: Ardent Media.

Centers for Disease Control and Prevention (CDC), Workowski, K., & Berman, S. (2006). Sexually transmitted diseases treatment guidelines, 2006. *MMWR Morbidity and Mortality Weekly Report, 55*(RR-11), 1–94.

Charles, V., Polis, C., Sridhara, S., & Blum, R. (2008). Abortion and long-term mental health outcomes: A systematic review of the evidence. *Contraception, 78*, 436–450.

Cunningham, F., Leveno, K., Bloom, S., Hauth, J., Rouse, D., & Spong, C. (2010). *Williams obstetrics* (23rd ed.). New York: McGraw-Hill.

Fehring, R., Schneider, M., & Barron, M. (2008). Efficacy of the Marquette method of natural family planning. *MCN The American Journal of Maternal/Child Nursing, 33*(6), 348–354.

Gabelnick, H., Schwartz, J., & Darroch, J. (2007). Contraceptive research and development. In R. Hatcher, J. Trussell, A. Nelson, W. Cates, F. Stewart & D. Kowal (Eds.), *Contraceptive Technology* (19th rev. ed.). New York: Ardent Media.

Germano, E., & Jennings, V. (2006). New approaches to fertility awareness-based methods: Incorporating the Standard Days and TwoDay methods into practice. *Journal of Midwifery & Women's Health, 51*(6), 471–477.

Goldberg, A., & Grimes, D. (2007). Injectable contraceptives. In R. Hatcher, J. Trussell, A. Nelson, W. Cates, F. Stewart, & D. Kowal (Eds.), *Contraceptive technology* (19th rev. ed.). New York: Ardent Media.

Grimes, D. (2007). Intrauterine devices. In R. Hatcher, J. Trussell, A. Nelson, W. Cates, F. Stewart, & D. Kowal (Eds.), *Contraceptive technology* (19th rev. ed.). New York: Ardent Media.

Hastings-Tolsma, M., Nodine, P., & Teal, S. (2006). Essure: Hysteroscopic sterilization. *Journal of Midwifery & Women's Health, 51*(6), 510–514.

Hatcher, R. (2007). The menstrual cycle. In R. Hatcher, J. Trussell, A. Nelson, W. Cates, F. Stewart, & D. Kowal (Eds.), *Contraceptive Technology* (19th rev. ed). New York: Ardent Media.

Jennings, V., & Arevalo, M. (2007). Fertility awareness-based methods. In R. Hatcher, J. Trussell, A. Nelson, W. Cates, F. Stewart, & D. Kowal (Eds.), *Contraceptive technology* (19th rev. ed.). New York: Ardent Media.

The Joint Commission. (2009). *Standards, intents, and examples for managing staff requests. Comprehensive accreditation manual for hospitals: The official handbook.* Oakbrook Terrace, IL: The Commission.

Kaunitz, A., Arias, R., & McClung, M. (2008). Bone density recovery after depot medroxyprogesterone acetate injectable contraception use. *Contraception, 77*(2), 67–76.

Kennedy, K., & Trussell, J. (2007). Postpartum contraception and lactation. In R. Hatcher, J. Trussell, A. Nelson, W. Cates, F. Stewart, & D. Kowal (Eds.), *Contraceptive technology* (19th rev. ed.). New York: Ardent Media.

King, J. (2007). Contraception and lactation. *Journal of Midwifery & Women's Health, 52*(6), 614–620.

Kost, K., Singh, S., Vaughan, B., Trussell, J., & Bankole, A. (2008). Estimates of contraceptive failure from the 2002 National Survey of Family Growth. *Contraception, 77*(1), 10–21.

Kowal, D. (2007). Coitus interruptus (withdrawal). In R. Hatcher, J. Trussell, A. Nelson, W. Cates, F. Stewart, & D. Kowal (Eds.), *Contraceptive technology* (19th rev. ed.). New York: Ardent Media.

Levi, A., Simmonds, K., & Taylor, D. (2009). The role of nursing in the management of unintended pregnancy. *Nursing Clinics of North America, 44*(3), 1–14.

Nanda, K. (2007). Contraceptive patch and vaginal contraceptive ring. In R. Hatcher, J. Trussell, A. Nelson, W. Cates, F. Stewart, & D. Kowal (Eds.), *Contraceptive technology* (19th rev. ed.). New York: Ardent Media.

Nelson, A. (2007). Combined oral contraceptives. In R. Hatcher, J. Trussell, A. Nelson, W. Cates, F. Stewart, & D. Kowal (Eds.), *Contraceptive technology* (19th rev. ed.). New York: Ardent Media.

Pallone, S., & Bergus, G. R. (2009). Fertility awareness-based methods: Another option for family planning. *Journal of the American Board of Family Medicine, 22*(2), 147–157.

Paul, M., & Stewart, F. (2007). Abortion. In R. Hatcher, J. Trussell, A. Nelson, W. Cates, F. Stewart, & D. Kowal (Eds.), *Contraceptive technology* (19th rev. ed.). New York: Ardent Media.

Pazol, K., Gamble, S., Parker, W., Cook, D., Zane, S., & Hamdan, S. (2009). Abortion surveillance, United States, 2006. *MMWR Morbidity and Mortality Weekly Report, 58*(SS 08), 1–35.

Planned Parenthood. (2010). *STD testing quick reference guide.* Available at www.plannedparenthood.org/health-topics/stds. Accessed June 3, 2010.

Pollack, A., Thomas, L., & Barone, M. (2007). Female and male sterilization. In R. Hatcher, J. Trussell, A. Nelson, W. Cates, F. Stewart, & D. Kowal (Eds.), *Contraceptive technology* (19th rev. ed.). New York: Ardent Media.

Practice Committee of the American Society for Reproductive Medicine. (2008). Hormonal contraception: Recent advances and controversies. *Fertility and Sterility, 90*(Suppl. 3), S103–S113.

Raymond, E. (2007a). Contraceptive implants. In R. Hatcher, J. Trussell, A. Nelson, W. Cates, F. Stewart, & D. Kowal (Eds.), *Contraceptive technology* (19th rev. ed.). New York: Ardent Media.

Raymond, E. (2007b). Progestin-only pills. In R. Hatcher, J. Trussell, A. Nelson, W. Cates, F. Stewart, & D. Kowal (Eds.), *Contraceptive technology* (19th rev. ed.). New York: Ardent Media.

Statistics Canada. (2010). *Induced abortions,* 2006. Available at www.statcan.gc.ca/daily-quotidien/090824/dq090824e-eng.htm. Accessed June 3, 2010.

Stewart, F., Trussell, J., & Van Look, P. (2007). Emergency contraception. In R. Hatcher, J. Trussell, A. Nelson, W. Cates, F. Stewart, & D. Kowal (Eds.), *Contraceptive technology* (19th rev. ed.). New York: Ardent Media.

Trussell, J. (2007). Contraceptive efficacy. In R. Hatcher, J. Trussell, A. Nelson, W. Cates, F. Stewart, & D. Kowal (Eds.), *Contraceptive technology* (19th rev. ed.). New York: Ardent Media.

U.S. Food and Drug Administration. (2009). *FDA approves Plan B One-Step emergency contraceptive; lowers age for obtaining Two Dose Plan B emergency contraceptive without a prescription.* Available at www.fda.gov/Drugs/DrugSafety/PostmarketDrugSafetyInformationforPatientsandProviders/ucm109775.htm. Accessed June 3, 2010.

Warner, L., & Steiner, M. (2007). Male condoms. In R. Hatcher, J. Trussell, A. Nelson, W. Cates, F. Stewart, & D. Kowal (Eds.), *Contraceptive technology* (19th rev. ed.). New York: Ardent Media.

World Health Organization Department of Reproductive Health & Research (WHO/RHR) and Johns Hopkins Bloomberg School of Public Health/Center for Communication Programs (CCP). (2007). *Family planning: A global handbook for providers.* Baltimore & Geneva: WHO & CCP.

Yranski, P., & Gamache, M. (2008). New options for barrier contraception. *Journal of Obstetric, Gynecologic and Neonatal Nursing, 37*(3), 384–389.

Zieman, M., Hatcher, R., Cwiak, C., Darney, P., Creinin, M., & Stosur, H. (2007). *A pocket guide to managing contraception.* Tiger, GA: Bridging the Gap Foundation.

CHAPTER 9

Infertility

Pat Mahaffee Gingrich

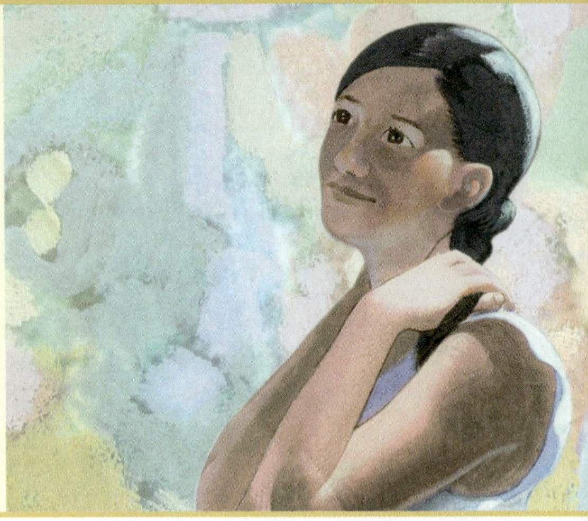

evolve WEBSITE

http://evolve.elsevier.com/Lowdermilk/MWHC/
Audio Glossary
Audio Key Points
NCLEX Review Questions
Nursing Care Plan
Infertility

LEARNING OBJECTIVES

- List common causes of infertility.
- Discuss the psychosocial impact of infertility.
- Identify common diagnoses and treatments for infertility.
- Identify reproductive alternatives for infertile couples.
- Examine the various ethical and legal considerations of assisted reproductive therapies for infertility.

This chapter addresses infertility, associated tests, and common therapies. The available alternatives and the psychosocial implications of infertility are discussed.

INCIDENCE

Infertility is a serious medical concern that affects quality of life and is a problem for 10% to 15% of reproductive-age couples (American Society for Reproductive Medicine [ASRM], 2010a; Nelson, Marshall, Trussell, Stewart, Nelson, Cates, et al., 2007). The term *infertility* implies subfertility, a prolonged time to conceive, as opposed to *sterility*, which means inability to conceive. Normally a fertile couple has approximately a 20% chance of conception in each ovulatory cycle. Primary infertility applies to a woman who has never been pregnant; secondary infertility applies to a woman who has been pregnant.

The prevalence of infertility is relatively stable among the overall population but increases with the age of the woman, particularly in those older than 40 years (Lobo, 2007). Probable causes include the trend toward delaying pregnancy until later in life, when fertility decreases naturally due to ovulatory dysfunction and the accumulated damage from diseases such as endometriosis and tubal infection (ASRM, 2010a). There is some controversy regarding whether there has been an increase in male infertility, or whether male infertility is being more readily identified because of improvements in diagnosis.

Diagnosis and treatment of infertility require considerable physical, emotional, and financial investment over an extended period. Men as well as women can experience emotional vulnerability (Burns, 2007). However, women have more stress from tests and treatments, and place greater importance on having children. In contrast, men express distress in their partner's suffering and the resulting changes in their partnership and sexual relationship (Wischmann, Scherg, Strowitzki, & Verres, 2009).

Same-sex couples desire pregnancy and parenthood for the same reasons as do heterosexual couples, but may feel unaccepted and marginalized in health care settings. Lesbian women are at risk for higher general stress, which can be compounded by the invasive nature of fertility treatments (Weisz, 2009).

In the United States, feelings connected with infertility are many and complex. The origins of some of these feelings are myths, superstitions, misinformation, or magical thinking about the causes of infertility. Other feelings arise from the medicalization of reproduction and from a perception of being "different" from others. The attitude, sensitivity, and caring nature of those who are involved in the assessment of infertility lay the foundation for the clients' ability to cope with the subsequent therapy and management. Couples seeking infertility treatments can benefit from instruction in stress management and coping skills (Cousineau & Domar, 2007). Health team members also must respect affected individuals' and couples' desires in choosing to stop treatment and to select other alternatives, such as adoption (see Clinical Reasoning box).

CLINICAL REASONING

Infertility Counseling

Shauna, age 37, is a CEO of her own company. She has been married for 4 years to Jason, 39, a high school teacher and coach. They have not used contraception for the past 3 years. Shauna had amenorrhea as an adolescent due to an eating disorder, but her weight is normal and her menstrual cycles are monthly now. They arrive together at the assisted reproductive care clinic, seeking advice. They have heard about in vitro fertilization (IVF) and wonder what the costs and treatments involve. What response by the nurse would be appropriate?

1. Evidence—Is there sufficient evidence to draw conclusions about what response the nurse should give?
2. Assumptions—Describe underlying assumptions about the following issues:
   a. Age and fertility
   b. Infertility as a major life stressor
   c. Success rates for IVF—pregnancy and birth
3. What implications and priorities for nursing care can be drawn at this time?
4. Does the evidence objectively support your conclusion?
5. Are there alternative perspectives to your conclusion?

FACTORS ASSOCIATED WITH INFERTILITY

Many factors, both male and female, contribute to normal fertility. A normally developed reproductive tract in both the male and female partner is essential. Normal functioning of an intact hypothalamic-pituitary-gonadal axis supports gametogenesis—the formation of sperm and ova. The life spans of the sperm and the ovum are short. Although sperm remain viable in the female's reproductive tract for 48 hours or more, probably only a few retain fertilization potential for more than 24 hours. Ova remain viable for about 24 hours, but the optimal time for fertilization may be no more than a few hours (Cunningham, Leveno, Bloom, Hauth, Rouse, & Spong, 2010); thus timing of intercourse becomes critical.

An alteration in one or more of these structures, functions, or processes results in some degree of impaired fertility. Causes of impaired fertility are sometimes difficult to assign to either the male or female. In general, about 20% of couples will have unexplained or idiopathic causes of infertility. Among the 80% of couples who have an identifiable cause of infertility, about 40% are related to factors in the female partner, 40% are related to factors in the male partner, and 20% are related to factors in both partners (Lobo, 2007; Nelson et al., 2007). Boxes 9-1 and 9-2 list factors affecting female and male infertility.

Infertility also may be caused by something as simple as poor timing or inadequate frequency of intercourse. The couple should be taught about the menstrual cycle and the ways to detect ovulation (see Chapters 4 and 8).

Female Infertility

Congenital or Developmental Factors

Congenital factors rarely cause impaired fertility. If the woman has abnormal external genitals, surgical reconstruction of abnormal tissue and construction of a functional vagina may permit normal intercourse. Vaginal and uterine anomalies and their surgical repair vary from individual to individual. If a functional uterus can be reconstructed, pregnancy may be possible.

Hormonal and Ovulatory Factors

Anovulation may be primary or secondary (see Chapter 6). Primary anovulation may be caused by a pituitary or hypothalamic hormone disorder or an adrenal gland disorder, such as congenital

BOX 9-1 FACTORS AFFECTING FEMALE FERTILITY

OVARIAN FACTORS
Developmental anomalies
Anovulation, primary
Pituitary or hypothalamic hormone disorder
Adrenal gland disorder
Congenital adrenal hyperplasia
Anovulation, secondary
Disruption of hypothalamic-pituitary-ovarian axis
Amenorrhea after discontinuing oral contraceptive pills
Premature ovarian failure
Increased prolactin levels

UTERINE, TUBAL, AND PERITONEAL FACTORS
Developmental anomalies
Tubal motility reduced
Inflammation within the tube
Tubal adhesions
Endometrial and myometrial tumors
Asherman syndrome (uterine adhesions or scar tissue)
Endometriosis
Chronic cervicitis
Hostile or inadequate cervical mucus

OTHER FACTORS
Nutritional deficiencies (e.g., anemia)
Obesity
Thyroid dysfunction
Idiopathic condition

BOX 9-2 FACTORS AFFECTING MALE FERTILITY

STRUCTURAL OR HORMONAL DISORDERS
Undescended testes
Hypospadias
Varicocele
Obstructive lesions of the vas deferens or epididymis
Low testosterone levels
Hypopituitarism
Endocrine disorders
Testicular damage caused by mumps
Retrograde ejaculation

OTHER FACTORS
Sexually transmitted infections
Exposure to workplace hazards such as radiation or toxic substances
Exposure of scrotum to high temperatures
Nutritional deficiencies
Obesity
Antisperm antibodies
Substance abuse
Changes in sperm—cigarette smoking, heroin, marijuana, amyl nitrate, butyl nitrate, ethyl chloride, methaqualone
Decrease in libido—heroin, methadone, selective serotonin reuptake inhibitors (SSRIs), and barbiturates
Impotence—alcohol, antihypertensive medications
Idiopathic condition

adrenal hyperplasia. It is usually seen in adolescents. Secondary anovulation, usually seen in young to midlife women, is relatively common and is caused by the disruption of the hypothalamic-pituitary-ovarian axis. In amenorrheic states and instances of anovulatory cycles, hormone studies usually reveal the problem.

Although relatively rare, amenorrhea after the discontinuation of oral contraceptives is seen more frequently in women with histories of menstrual dysfunction before initiation of contraceptive use. Because most women resume menstruating within 6 months, the workup should be delayed until that time in the absence of other symptoms.

Occasionally women experience menopause before they are 40 years old. In a vast majority of cases of early menopause, the ovaries do not respond to ovulation-inducing drugs. Obesity and related metabolic disorders, such as polycystic ovary syndrome (PCOS), and eating disorders also contribute to anovulation (Balen & Anderson, 2007; Leddy, Jones, Morgan & Schulkin, 2009; Malik, 2009).

An increased prolactin level may cause anovulation and amenorrhea, in the same way it does during lactation. Hyperprolactinemia can be a side effect of drugs, such as phenothiazine, opiates, diazepam, reserpine, methyldopa, and tricyclic antidepressants. Prolactin may also be elevated as a result of physical stressors such as surgery, cranial lesions, or injury, or severe emotional stress. Benign pituitary adenoma, which is diagnosed through sophisticated radiographic techniques or computed tomography (CT) scan, may also cause hyperprolactinemia.

Cancer treatments involving radiation and chemotherapy can decrease or halt ovarian function (Pauli, Berga, Shang, & Session, 2009).

Age-Related Infertility. The rate of fertility declines dramatically after the age of 35. By 40, the total number of ovarian follicles diminishes and the quality of remaining eggs is poor. Abnormalities of oocytes are thought to be the primary reason for age-associated infertility, followed by cumulative factors such as endometriosis, infection, metabolic disease, and smoking (ASRM, 2008).

Tubal/Peritoneal Factors

The motility of the tube and its fimbriated end may be reduced or absent as a result of infections, adhesions, scarring, or tumors. Chlamydial infection impairs tubal function and impedes fertility. In rare instances one tube may be congenitally absent. One tube may be relatively shorter than the other, which is often associated with an abnormally developed uterus.

Inflammation within the tube or involving the exterior of the tube or the fimbriated ends represents a major cause of impaired fertility. Tubal adhesions resulting from pelvic infections (e.g., ruptured appendix, sexually transmitted infections [STIs]) may impair fertility. When infection with purulent discharge heals, scar tissue adhesions form. In the process, the tube can be blocked anywhere along its length. It can be closed off at the fimbriated end, or it can be distorted and kinked by adhesions. Adhesions may permit the tiny sperm to pass through

EVIDENCE-BASED PRACTICE

Pat Gingrich

Endometriosis Treatments for Infertility

ASK THE QUESTION

What treatments are beneficial for endometriosis? Does treatment for endometriosis improve fertility?

SEARCH FOR EVIDENCE

Search Strategies

Professional organization guidelines, meta-analyses, systematic reviews, randomized controlled trials, nonrandomized prospective studies and retrospective reviews since 2008.

Databases Searched

CINAHL, Cochrane, Medline, PUBMED, ZYNX, NICE, and the professional sites for ACOG and SGOC.

CRITICALLY ANALYZE THE DATA

The monthly proliferation and sloughing cycle of endometrial cells outside the uterine cavity irritate surrounding tissue. The resulting inflammation and scarring contribute to infertility, dysmenorrhea (painful menses) and dyspareunia (painful intercourse). Hormonal treatment suppresses the cyclic changes, but may produce side effects, and are not appropriate for women attempting pregnancy. A Cochrane meta-analysis found that laparoscopic (small incision) surgery to remove visible lesions improves fertility for women with mild to moderate endometriosis (Jacobson, Duffy, Barlow, Farquhar, Koninckx, & Olive, 2010). Pain, subfertility, and recurrence of endometriosis are diminished with laparoscopic excision of endometrial lesions, especially with pre- and/or post-treatment with hormone suppression or insertion of levonorgestrel intrauterine system (LNG-IUS, or progestin IUD) (Yeung, Shwayder, & Pasic, 2009). The use of the LNG-IUS reduces cell proliferation and increases markers for cell apoptosis, thus decreasing the ectopic endometrial lesions, allowing the surrounding tissue to heal (Gomes, Rosa-e-Silva, Garcia, de Sa Rosa-e-Silva, Turatti, Vieira, et al., 2009).

IMPLICATIONS FOR PRACTICE

Sensitive assessment may reveal that women with endometriosis have suffered for years with decreased quality of life from dysmenorrhea and dyspareunia. Careful history-taking can reveal risk factors for peritoneal causes of subfertility, such as pelvic inflammatory disease, complicated appendicitis, pelvic surgery, ectopic pregnancy and endometriosis (Luttjeboer, Verhoeve, van Dussell, van der Veen, Mol & Coppus, 2009). Women undergoing procedures for fertility need good information about the purpose, risks and benefits, as well as anticipatory guidance. Treatments for endometriosis that are not conducive to pregnancy, such as hormone suppression or LNG-IUS, may be discontinued after the endometriosis is diminished.

References

Gomes, M., Rosa-e-Silva, J., Garcia, S., de Sa Rosa-e-Silva, A., Turatti, A., Vieira, C,. et al. (2009). Effects of the levonorgestrel-releasing intrauterine system on cell proliferation, Fas expression, and steroid receptors in endometriosis lesions and normal endometrium. *Human Reproduction, 24*(11), 2736–2745.

Jacobson, T., Duffy, J., Barlow, D., Farquhar, C., Koninckx, P., & Olive, D. (2010). Laparoscopic surgery for subfertility associated with endometriosis. *The Cochrane Database of Systematic Reviews 2010,* 1, CD001398.

Luttjeboer, F., Verhoeve, H., van Dussell, H., vanm der Veen, F., Mol, B., & Coppus, S. F. (2009). The value of medical history taking as risk indicator for tuboperitoneal pathology: A systematic review. *British Journal of Obstetrics and Gynaecology, 116*(5), 612–625.

Yeung, P., Shwayder, J., & Pasic, R. (2009). Laparoscopic management of endometriosis: Comprehensive review of best evidence. *Journal of Minimally Invasive Gynecology, 16*(3), 269–281.

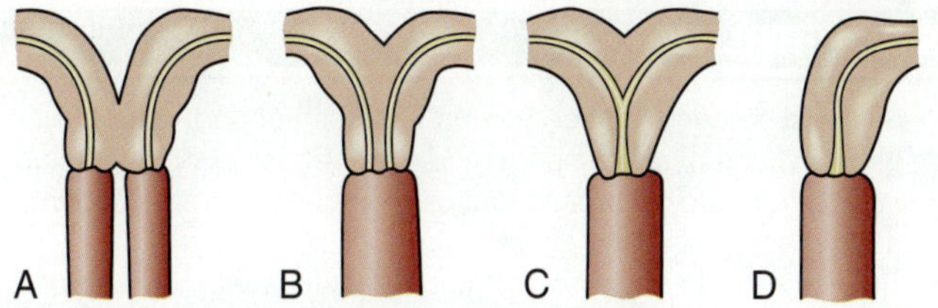

FIG. 9-1 Abnormal uterus. **A,** Complete bicornuate uterus with vagina divided by a septum. **B,** Complete bicornuate uterus with normal vagina. **C,** Partial bicornuate uterus with normal vagina. **D,** Unicornuate uterus.

the tube but may prevent a fertilized egg from completing the journey into the intrauterine cavity. This results in an ectopic pregnancy that can completely destroy the tube and be life threatening. In other cases, adhesion of the tubes to the ovary or the bowel can be caused by endometriosis (see Chapter 6). Endometriosis is more commonly seen in women who delay childbearing until they are older than 30 years. Women who have a first-degree relative with a history of endometriosis also have a slightly higher risk.

Uterine Factors

Abnormalities of the uterus are more common than might be expected. Minor developmental anomalies of the uterus are fairly common; major anomalies occur rarely. Hysterosalpingography may reveal müllerian malformations of the uterine cavity, such as bicornuate or septate uterus (Fig. 9-1) (Chalazonitis, Tzovara, Laspas, Porfyrdis, Ptohis, & Tsimitselis, 2009). Endometrial and myometrial tumors (e.g., polyps or myomas) may also be revealed by x-ray studies of infertile women. These anomalies can affect implantation and the maintenance of a pregnancy.

Asherman syndrome (uterine adhesions or scar tissue) is characterized by hypomenorrhea. The adhesions prevent normal cyclic endometrial proliferation necessary for implantation. This can result from surgical interventions such as too vigorous curettage (scraping) after an elective abortion or miscarriage.

Endometritis (inflammation of the endometrium) may result from any of the causes of infection of the cervix or uterine tubes (e.g., *Chlamydia*). Women who have numerous sexual partners are more susceptible to endometrial infection than are women in monogamous relationships.

Vaginal-Cervical Factors

Vaginal fluid is acidic (pH of 4 to 5), whereas cervical mucus is normally alkaline (pH of 7 or more). Ejaculation should place the sperm at or near the cervical os. The alkalinity of cervical mucus helps support sperm and permits the ascending transportation of sperm around the time of ovulation.

Endocervical mucus normally obstructs or plugs the cervix, acting as a barrier against infection, until increasing estrogen levels cause the mucus to become clear, thin, and nutritionally supportive of sperm. This change occurs around the time of ovulation and lasts approximately 48 to 72 hours. The amount of cervical mucus and its characteristics are influenced by the hormone estrogen (see Teaching for Self-Management box, p. 173 in Chapter 8).

Vaginal-cervical infections (e.g., bacterial vaginosis) cause an increased pH (decreased acidity) of the vaginal fluid, plus the presence of white blood cells. Inflammation from vaginal infection often destroys or drastically reduces the number of viable motile sperm before they enter the cervical canal (Mania-Pramanik, Kerkar, & Salvi, 2009). The amount of mucus and its physical changes are influenced by the presence of blood, pathogenic bacteria, and irritants such as an intrauterine contraceptive device (IUD) or a polyp. Severe emotional stress, antibiotic therapy, and diseases such as diabetes mellitus alter the acidity of mucus.

Some infertile women develop sperm antibodies. The production of antibodies by one member of a species against something that is commonly found within that species is termed **isoimmunization.** Sperm may be immobilized or agglutinated within the cervical mucus, rendering them incapable of migration into the uterus (see Postcoital Test later in this chapter).

Male Infertility

Male infertility can be caused by structural and hormonal disorders such as undescended testes, hypospadias, varicocele (varicose veins of the scrotum), low testosterone levels, or previous vasectomy, all of which can cause azoospermia (no sperm cells produced) or oligospermia (few sperm cells produced). Mumps, especially after adolescence, can result in permanent damage to the testes.

Male infertility also may be caused by some of the same health issues that affect women, such as nutrition, endocrine disorders, genetic disorders, psychologic disorders, and STIs (ASRM, 2010a). Male obesity can lead to decreased semen quality (Shayeb & Bhattacharya, 2009). Exposure to hazards in the workplace such as radiation also can affect sperm production; exposure of the scrotum to high temperatures can both decrease and cause abnormal sperm production. Cancer treatments can decrease production or quality of sperm (Pauli et al., 2009).

Substance abuse can be a major factor in male infertility. Alcohol consumption can cause erectile problems (impotence). In addition, cigarette smoking has been associated with abnormal sperm, a decreased number of sperm, and chromosome damage. Heroin and marijuana use may depress the number and motility of sperm and increase the percentage of abnormally formed sperm. Amyl nitrate, butyl nitrate, ethyl chloride, and methaqualone (used to prolong orgasm) cause changes in spermatogenesis. Heroin, methadone, selective serotonin reuptake inhibitors (SSRIs), and barbiturates decrease libido. Monoamine oxidase inhibitors (MAOIs), a class of antidepressants, adversely affect spermatogenesis. In addition, some antihypertensives may cause impotence.

Male fertility declines slowly after age 40 years; however, no cessation of sperm production occurs analogous to menopause in women.

CARE MANAGEMENT

The nurse assists in the assessment by obtaining data relevant to fertility through interview and physical examination. The database must include information to identify whether infertility is primary or secondary. Religious, cultural, and ethnic data are noted (Box 9-3).

Much of the data needed to investigate impaired fertility are of a sensitive, personal nature. Obtaining these data may be viewed as an invasion of privacy. The tests and examinations are occasionally painful and intrusive and can take the romance out

BOX 9-3 RELIGIOUS AND CULTURAL CONSIDERATIONS OF FERTILITY

RELIGIOUS CONSIDERATIONS

- Civil laws and religious proscriptions about sex must always be kept in mind by the health care provider.
- Conservative and reform Jewish couples are accepting of most infertility treatment; however, the Orthodox Jewish husband and wife may face problems with infertility investigation and management because of religious laws that govern marital relations. For example, according to Jewish law, the Orthodox couple may not engage in marital relations during menstruation and through the following 7 "preparatory days." The wife then is immersed in a ritual bath *(mikvah)* before relations can resume. Fertility problems can arise when the woman has a short cycle (i.e., a cycle of 24 days or fewer; when ovulation would occur on day 10 or earlier).
- The Roman Catholic Church regards the embryo as a human being from the first moment of existence and regards as unacceptable technical procedures such as in vitro fertilization (IVF), masturbation to collect semen for husband/partner or therapeutic donor insemination, and freezing of embryos.
- Other religious groups may have ethical concerns about infertility tests and treatments. For example, most Protestant denominations and Muslims usually support infertility management as long as IVF is done with the husband's sperm, there is no reduction of fetuses, and insemination is done with the husband's sperm. These groups are less supportive of surrogacy and use of donor sperm and eggs. Christian Scientists do not permit surgical procedures or IVF but do permit insemination with husband and donor sperm.
- Care providers should seek to understand the woman's spirituality and how it affects her perception of health care, especially in relation to infertility. Women may wish to seek infertility treatment but have questions about proposed diagnostic and therapeutic procedures because of religious proscriptions. These women are encouraged to consult their minister, rabbi, priest, or other spiritual leader for advice.

CULTURAL CONSIDERATIONS

- Worldwide cultures continue to use symbols and rites that celebrate fertility. One fertility rite that persists today is the custom of throwing rice at the bride and groom. Other fertility symbols and rites include passing out congratulatory cigars, candy, or pencils by a new father and baby showers held in anticipation of a child's birth.
- In many cultures, the responsibility for infertility is usually attributed to the woman. A woman's inability to conceive may be a result of her sins, of evil spirits, or of the fact that she is an inadequate person. The virility of a man in some cultures remains in question until he demonstrates his ability to reproduce by having at least one child.

Source: D'Avanzo, C. (2008). *Mosby's pocket guide to cultural health assessment* (4th ed.). St Louis: Mosby.

of lovemaking. A high level of motivation is needed to endure the investigation.

Many couples have already visited various physicians and have read extensively on the subject. Their previous infertility experiences and knowledge should be explored and recorded.

Because multiple factors involving both partners are common, the investigation of impaired fertility is conducted systematically and simultaneously for male and female partners. Both partners must be interested in the solution to the problem. The medical investigation requires time (3 to 4 months) and considerable financial expense (Box 9-4), and it causes emotional distress and strain on the couple's interpersonal relationship (ASRM, 2010b). Preparatory and concurrent counseling support is recommended (Burns, 2007) (see Nursing Process box).

Investigation of impaired fertility begins for the woman and the man with a complete history and physical examination. A complete general physical examination is followed by a specific assessment of the reproductive tract. Laboratory data are assembled. Data from routine urine and blood tests are obtained along with other diagnostic tests.

ASSESSMENT OF FEMALE INFERTILITY

Diagnostic Tests for Female Infertility. Several examinations and tests for impaired fertility in the woman include the basic infertility survey, which involves evaluation of the cervix, uterus, tubes, and peritoneum; detection of ovulation; assessment of immunologic compatibility; and evaluation of psychogenic factors (Nelson et al., 2007). The nurse can alleviate some of the anxiety associated with diagnostic testing by explaining to clients the timing and rationale for each test (Table 9-1). Test findings that are favorable to fertility are summarized in Box 9-5.

BOX 9-4 INSURANCE COVERAGE FOR INFERTILITY

In 2010 only 15 states had mandated some form of insurance coverage for infertility. These mandates included in vitro fertilization in some states, whereas others only covered some diagnostic tests. Some states require health maintenance organizations (HMOs) to cover some costs, whereas in others, HMOs are exempt. Clients need specific information about what they can expect from their insurers. The websites for the American Society for Reproductive Medicine (www.asrm.org) and RESOLVE (www.resolve.org) have more complete information. For laws in a specific state, the state insurance commissioner's office may be contacted.

Sources: American Society for Reproductive Medicine (ASRM). (2009). *Frequently asked questions about infertility.* Available at www.asrm.org. Accessed June 7, 2010; Resolve. (2010). *Insurance coverage.* Available at www.resolve.org/family-building-options/insurance_coverage.html. Accessed June 7, 2010.

Couples should be cautioned that everything can be normal and conception still may not occur. In addition, pregnancy may still occur even with poor test results.

Detection of Ovulation. All infertile women should have ovulatory function assessed, because a history of monthly menstruation is inadequate to conclude that ovulation is occurring and is optimal for conception.

Documentation of time of ovulation is important in the investigation of impaired fertility. Direct proof of ovulation is pregnancy or the retrieval of an ovum from the uterine tube. Several indirect or presumptive methods for detection of ovulation include assessment of basal body temperature (BBT) and cervical mucus characteristics, as well as endometrial biopsy and pelvic ultrasound examination. A serum progesterone level may be obtained in the latter half of the menstrual cycle to determine

NURSING PROCESS

Infertility

ASSESSMENT

Assessment of female infertility

- Complete a history that includes duration of infertility, past obstetric events, a detailed menstrual and sexual history, medical and surgical conditions, exposure to reproductive hazards in the home and workplace, use of alcohol and other drugs, and emotional stresses.
- Complete a specific assessment of the reproductive tract following a complete general physical examination.
- Obtain data from routine urine and blood tests along with results of other diagnostic tests, e.g., tests to detect ovulation, hormone analyses, ultrasound examination, hysterosalpingogram, endometrial biopsy, hysteroscopic examination, laparoscopic examination, sperm antibody agglutination test, chromosomal studies (see discussion in text).

Assessment of male infertility

- Complete a thorough history that includes nutritional deficiency; debilitating or chronic disease; trauma; exposure to environmental hazards such as radiation, heat, and toxic substances; use of tobacco, alcohol, and marijuana.
- Complete a physical examination.
- Obtain data from noninvasive tests such as the semen analysis and ultrasound examination and additional studies as indicated-e.g., basic endocrine studies (serum FSH, LH, and testosterone levels, triiodothyronine [T_3]; thyroxine [T_4], TSH levels), test for sperm antibodies (autoimmunization), chromosomal studies
  - Testicular biopsy where correct interpretation is available (may give a more accurate diagnosis and prognosis in cases of azoospermia and severe oligospermia)
  - Vasography if indicated and available

NURSING DIAGNOSES

Examples of nursing diagnoses related to impaired fertility include:

***Anxiety* related to:**
- unknown outcome of diagnostic workup

***Disturbed Body Image or Situational Low Self-esteem* related to:**
- impaired fertility

***Risk for Ineffective Individual Coping* related to:**
- methods used in the investigation of impaired fertility
- alternatives to therapy: child-free living or adoption

***Interrupted Family Processes* related to:**
- unmet expectations for pregnancy

***Acute Pain* related to:**
- effects of diagnostic tests (or surgery)

***Ineffective Sexuality Patterns* related to:**
- loss of libido secondary to medically imposed restrictions

***Deficient Knowledge* related to:**
- preconception risk factors
- factors surrounding ovulation
- factors surrounding fertility

EXPECTED OUTCOMES OF CARE

Expected outcomes include that the couple will:

- Verbalize understanding of the anatomy and physiology of the reproductive system.
- Verbalize understanding of treatment for any abnormalities identified through various tests and examinations (e.g., infections, blocked uterine tubes, sperm allergy, varicocele) and be able to make an informed decision about treatment.
- Verbalize understanding of their potential to conceive.
- Resolve guilt feelings and not need to focus blame.
- Conceive or, failing to conceive, decide on an alternative acceptable to both of them (e.g., child-free living, adoption).

PLAN OF CARE AND INTERVENTIONS

- Assist couples to express feelings about their infertility.
- Provide explanations or reinforcement or both about diagnostic tests and results of tests.
- Provide supportive care during diagnostic and treatment phases.
- Implement treatment interventions as ordered.
- Teach and encourage use of stress reducing activities.
- Provide information about available community resources
- Refer for counseling or follow-up as needed.

EVALUATION

Evaluation of the effectiveness of care of the couple experiencing impaired fertility is based on the previously stated outcomes

TABLE 9-1 TESTS FOR IMPAIRED FERTILITY

TEST OR EXAMINATION	TIMING (MENSTRUAL CYCLE DAYS)	RATIONALE
Hysterosalpingogram	7-10	Late follicular, early proliferative phase; will not disrupt a fertilized ovum; may open uterine tubes before time of ovulation
Sonohysterogram	7-10	Same as hysterosalpingogram
Postcoital test	1-2 days before ovulation	Ovulatory late proliferative phase; look for normal motile sperm in cervical mucus
Sperm immobilization antigen-antibody reaction	Variable, ovulation	Immunologic test to determine sperm and cervical mucus interaction
Assessment of cervical mucus	Variable, ovulation	Cervical mucus should have low viscosity, high spinnbarkeit
Ultrasound diagnosis of follicular collapse	Ovulation	Collapsed follicle is seen after ovulation
Serum assay of plasma progesterone	20-25	Midluteal midsecretory phase; check adequacy of corpus luteal production of progesterone
Basal body temperature	Chart entire cycle	Elevation occurs in response to progesterone, documents ovulation
Endometrial biopsy	21-27	Late luteal, late secretory phase; check endometrial response to progesterone and adequacy of luteal phase
Sperm penetration assay	After 2 days but no more than 1 week of abstinence	Evaluation of ability of sperm to penetrate an egg
Hysteroscopy	Variable	Direct visualization of inside of uterus, via cervix
Laparoscopy	Variable	Direct visualization of outside of uterus, ovaries, and tubes, via abdomen

BOX 9-5 SUMMARY OF FINDINGS FAVORABLE TO FERTILITY

1. Follicular development, ovulation, and luteal development are supportive of pregnancy:
   a. Basal body temperature (BBT) (presumptive evidence of ovulatory cycles) is biphasic, with temperature elevation that persists for 12 to 14 days before menstruation.
   b. Cervical mucus characteristics change appropriately during phases of menstrual cycle.
   c. Laparoscopic visualization of pelvic organs verifies follicular and luteal development.
2. The luteal phase is supportive of pregnancy:
   a. Levels of plasma progesterone are adequate.
   b. Findings from endometrial biopsy samples are consistent with day of cycle.
3. Cervical factors are receptive to sperm during expected time of ovulation:
   a. Cervical os is open.
   b. Cervical mucus is clear, watery, abundant, and slippery and demonstrates good spinnbarkeit and arborization (fern pattern).
   c. Cervical examination reveals no lesions or infections.
   d. Postcoital test findings are satisfactory (adequate number of live, motile, normal sperm present in cervical mucus).
   e. No immunity to sperm demonstrated.
4. The uterus and uterine tubes are supportive of pregnancy:
   a. Uterine and tubal patency are documented by hysterosalpingogram.
      (1) Spillage of dye into peritoneal cavity.
      (2) Outlines of uterine and tubal cavities of adequate size and shape, with no abnormalities.
   b. Laparoscopic examination verifies normal development of internal genitals and absence of adhesions, infections, endometriosis, and other lesions.
5. Body mass index less than 30 (or less than 35 in woman older than age 37, with no other risk factor).
6. The male partner's reproductive structures are normal:
   a. No evidence of developmental anomalies of penis, testicular atrophy, or varicocele (varicose veins on the spermatic vein in the groin).
   b. No evidence of infection in prostate, seminal vesicles, or urethra.
   c. Testes are more than 4 cm in largest diameter.
7. Semen is supportive of pregnancy:
   a. Sperm (number per milliliter) are adequate in ejaculate.
   b. Most sperm show normal morphology.
   c. Most sperm are motile, forward moving.
   d. No autoimmunity exists.
   e. Seminal fluid is normal.

the presence of sufficient amounts to accommodate implantation and maintain pregnancy. Occurrence of mittelschmerz and midcycle spotting provides unreliable presumptive evidence of ovulation.

Hormone Analysis. Hormone analysis is performed to assess endocrine function of the hypothalamic-pituitary-ovarian axis when menstrual cycles are absent or irregular, or to assess the woman's ovarian reserve. Determination of blood levels of prolactin, follicle-stimulating hormone (FSH), luteinizing hormone (LH), estradiol (E_2), progesterone, and the thyroid hormones may be necessary to diagnose the cause of irregular or absent menstrual cycles. The clomiphene citrate challenge test (CCCT) may be performed to determine ovarian reserves: fewer eggs means less responsiveness to FSH.

Ultrasonography. Abdominal or transvaginal ultrasound is used to assess pelvic structures (Fig. 9-2). This procedure is used to visualize pelvic tissues for a variety of reasons (e.g., to identify abnormalities such as fibroid tumors and ovarian cysts, to verify follicular development and maturity, and to assess thickness of the endometrium around the time of ovulation). Sonohysterography uses fluid infused into the uterus via the cervix to help define the uterine cavity and the depth of the uterine lining, using vaginal ultrasound.

Hysterosalpingography. Radiographic (x-ray) film examination allows visualization of the uterine cavity and tubes after the instillation of radiopaque contrast material through the cervix (Fig. 9-3). It is possible to see abnormalities of the uterus such as congenital defects or defects produced by submucous myomas and endometrial polyps. Distortions of the uterine cavity or uterine tubes can be a result of current or past pelvic inflammatory disease (PID). Scar tissue and adhesions from inflammatory processes can immobilize the uterus and tubes, kink the tubes, and surround the ovaries.

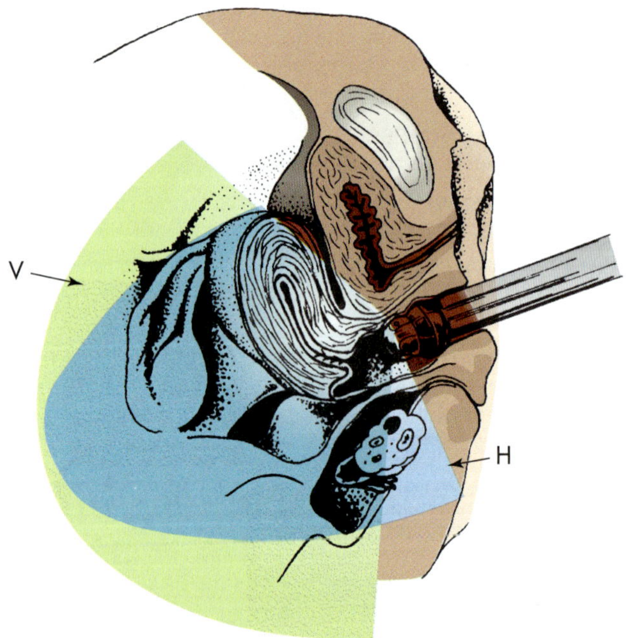

FIG. 9-2 Vaginal ultrasonography. Major scanning planes of transducer. *H*, Horizontal; *V*, vertical.

Hysterosalpingography is scheduled 2 to 5 days after menstruation to avoid flushing a potential fertilized ovum out through a uterine tube into the peritoneal cavity. Endometrial blood vessels are closed at this time, and all menstrual debris has been discharged. This decreases the risk of embolism or of forcing menstrual debris into the peritoneal cavity.

Referred shoulder pain may occur during this procedure. The referred pain is indicative of subphrenic irritation from the contrast media if it is spilled out of the patent uterine tubes.

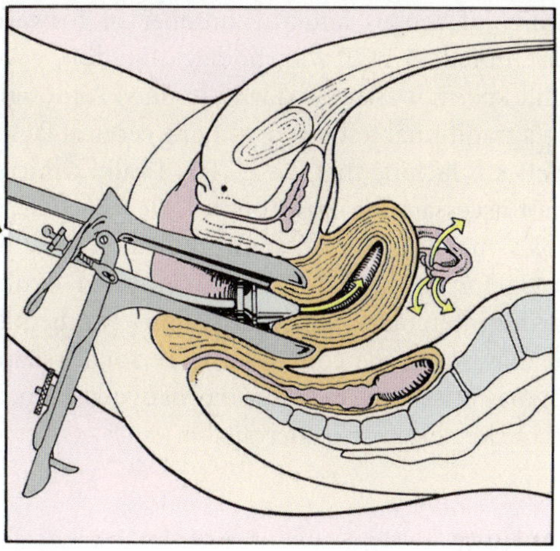

FIG. 9-3 Hysterosalpingography. Note that contrast medium flows through intrauterine cannula and out through the uterine tubes.

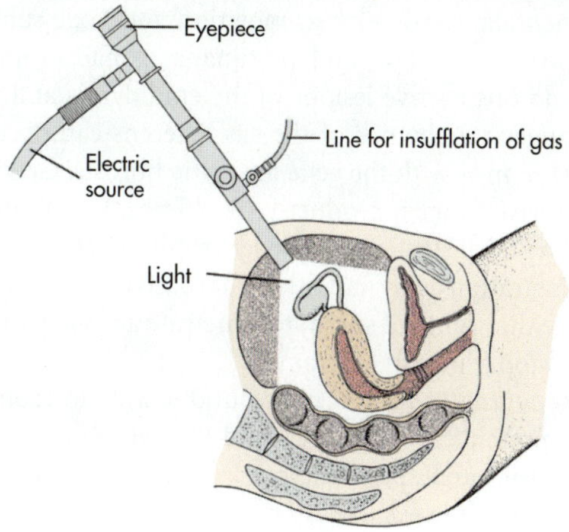

FIG. 9-4 Laparoscopy.

The discomfort can be managed with position change and mild analgesics. Pain usually subsides within 12 to 14 hours. Women with blocked tubes may have cramping for up to 48 hours.

Hysteroscopy. Hysteroscopy uses a flexible scope threaded through the cervix to directly view the uterine cavity. This is the gold standard for evaluation of leiomyomas (fibroids) and adhesions that might impair implantation (Thomson, Abbott, Deans, Kingston, & Vancaillie, 2009).

Timed Endometrial Biopsy. Endometrial biopsy is scheduled after ovulation, during the luteal phase of the menstrual cycle. Late in the menstrual cycle, 2 to 3 days before expected menses, a small cannula is introduced into the uterus, and a small portion of the endometrium is removed for histologic evaluation. To assess the response of the endometrium to progesterone production, the tissue is dated with respect to expected normal menstrual development. Tissue that is "out of phase" with expected development signifies either abnormal function of the corpus luteum or abnormal response of the endometrium.

Findings favorable to fertility include endometrial tissue that shows no signs of tuberculosis, polyps, or inflammatory conditions and that reflects secretory changes normally seen in the presence of adequate luteal (progesterone) phase.

Laparoscopy. Laparoscopy is useful to view the pelvic structures intraperitoneally, outside the uterus, which may reveal endometriosis, pelvic adhesions, tubal occlusion, leiomyomas (fibroids), or polycystic ovaries. Performed early in the menstrual cycle, under either general or local anesthesia, a small endoscope is inserted through a small incision in the anterior abdominal wall. Cold fiberoptic light sources allow superior visualization of the internal pelvic structures (Fig. 9-4). A needle is inserted, and carbon dioxide gas is pumped into the peritoneum to elevate the abdominal wall from the organs, thereby creating an empty space that permits visualization and exploration with the laparoscope. If tubal patency is being assessed, a cannula is used to instill a dye contrast medium through the cervix.

After surgery deflation of most gas is done by direct expression. Trocar and needle sites are closed with a single subcuticular absorbable suture or skin clip, and an adhesive bandage is applied. Referred shoulder pain or subcostal discomfort usually lasts only 24 hours and is relieved with a mild analgesic.

BOX 9-6 SEMEN ANALYSIS

- Semen volume 1.5 to 5 ml
- Semen pH 7.2 or higher
- Viscosity greater than 3 (scale of 0 to 4)
- Sperm density greater than 20 million/ml
- Total sperm count greater than 40 million per ejaculate
- Normal morphologic features greater than 30% (normal oval)
- Motility (important consideration in sperm evaluation)—percentage of forward-moving sperm estimated with respect to abnormally motile and nonmotile sperm, 50%
- Sperm agglutination less than 2 (scale 0 to 3)

Note: These values are not absolute but are only relative to final evaluation of the couple as a single reproductive unit. Values also differ according to source used as a reference.

Source: World Health Organization (WHO). (1999). *Laboratory manual for the examination of semen and sperm-cervical mucus interaction* (4th ed.). Geneva: WHO.

ASSESSMENT OF MALE INFERTILITY

Semen Analysis. The basic test for male infertility is the semen analysis. A complete semen analysis, study of the effects of cervical mucus on sperm forward motility and survival, and evaluation of the sperm's ability to penetrate an ovum provide basic information. Semen is collected by ejaculation into a clean container or a plastic sheath that does not contain a spermicidal agent. The specimen is usually collected by masturbation after 2 to 5 days of abstinence from ejaculation. The semen is taken to the laboratory in a sealed container within 2 hours of ejaculation. Avoid exposure to excessive heat or cold. Commonly accepted values based on the World Health Organization (WHO) criteria for semen characteristics are given in Box 9-6. If results are in the fertile range, no further sperm evaluation is necessary. If results are not within this range, the test is repeated. If subsequent results are still in the subfertile range, further evaluation is needed to identify the problem (Nelson et al., 2007).

Seminal deficiency can be attributable to one or more of a variety of factors. The male is assessed for these factors: hypopituitarism; nutritional deficiency; debilitating or chronic disease, including obesity and metabolic disease (Hammoud, Gibson, Peterson, Meikle, & Carrell, 2008); trauma; exposure to environmental hazards such as radiation and toxic substances; use of tobacco, alcohol, and marijuana; gonadotropic inadequacy; and obstructive lesions of the epididymis and vas deferens. Congenital absence of the vas deferens can occur more frequently in men with the gene for cystic fibrosis. Genetic testing may reveal other reproductive problems. Hormone analyses are done for testosterone, gonadotropin, FSH, and LH. The sperm penetration assay and other alternative tests may be used to evaluate the ability of sperm to penetrate an egg. In addition, testicular biopsy may be warranted.

Ultrasonography. Scrotal ultrasound is used to examine the testes for presence of varicocele and to identify abnormalities in the scrotum and spermatic cord. Transrectal ultrasound is used to evaluate the ejaculatory ducts, seminal vesicles, and the vas deferens.

ASSESSMENT OF THE COUPLE

Postcoital Test. The postcoital test (PCT) is one method used to test for adequacy of coital technique, cervical mucus, antisperm antibodies, sperm, number and quality, and degree of sperm penetration through cervical mucus. Intercourse is synchronized with the expected time of ovulation (as determined from evaluation of BBT, cervical mucus changes, and usual length of menstrual cycle or use of LH detection kit to determine LH surge). It is performed only in the absence of vaginal infection. The test is performed within several hours after ejaculation of semen into the vagina. A specimen of cervical mucus obtained from the cervical os is examined under a microscope. The quality of mucus and the number of forward-moving sperm are noted. A PCT with no agglutination, good mucus, and motile sperm is associated with fertility. Although the PCT has been a traditional test for identifying cervical factor infertility, evidence is lacking that the PCT is a valid clinical tool and thus is not necessary for most couples (Nelson et al., 2007).

Couples may experience some difficulty abstaining from intercourse for 2 to 4 days before expected ovulation and then having intercourse with ejaculation on schedule. Sex on demand may strain the couple's interpersonal relationship. A problem may arise if the expected day of ovulation occurs when facilities or the physician is unavailable (such as over a weekend or holiday).

Interventions

The management of clients with infertility problems includes psychosocial, nonmedical, medical, and surgical interventions. Assisted reproductive therapies may be indicated. Nursing interventions are an important aspect of care (see Nursing Care Plan).

Psychosocial

Infertility is recognized as a major life stressor that can affect self-esteem; relations with the spouse, family, and friends; and careers. Individuals experiencing infertility are at risk for distress, anxiety, anger, lowered self-esteem, isolation, marital dysfunction, and grief. The distress of infertility and its treatment can exacerbate preexisting mental conditions (Burns, 2007). Couples often need assistance in separating their concepts of success and failure related to treatment for infertility

NURSING CARE PLAN

Infertility

NURSING DIAGNOSIS

Deficient knowledge related to lack of understanding of the reproductive process with regard to conception as evidenced by client questions

Expected Outcome

Woman and partner will verbalize understanding of the components of the reproductive process, common problems leading to infertility, usual infertility testing, and the importance of completing testing in a timely manner.

Nursing Interventions/*Rationales*

- Assess woman's current level of understanding of the factors promoting conception *to identify gaps or misconceptions in knowledge base.*
- Provide information in a supportive manner regarding factors promoting conception including common factors leading to infertility of either partner *to raise woman's awareness and promote trust in caregiver.*
- Identify and describe the basic infertility tests and the rationale for precise scheduling *to enhance completion of the diagnostic phase of the infertility workup.*

NURSING DIAGNOSIS

Ineffective individual coping related to inability to conceive as evidenced by woman and partner statements

Expected Outcome

Woman and partner will identify situational stressors and positive coping methods to deal with testing and unknown outcomes.

Nursing Interventions/*Rationales*

- Provide opportunities through therapeutic communication to discuss feelings and concerns *to identify common feelings and perceived stressors.*
- Evaluate couple's support system, including support of each other during this process *to identify any barriers to effective coping.*
- Identify support groups and refer as needed *to enhance coping by sharing experiences with other couples experiencing similar problems.*

NURSING DIAGNOSIS

Hopelessness related to inability to conceive as evidenced by woman's and partner's statements

Expected Outcome

Woman and partner will verbalize a realistic plan to decrease feelings of hopelessness.

Nursing Interventions/*Rationales*

- Provide support for couple while grieving for loss of fertility *to allow couple to work through feelings.*
- Assess for behaviors indicating possible depression, anger, and frustration *to prevent impending crisis.*
- Refer to support groups *to promote a common bond with other couples during expression of feelings and concerns.*

TABLE 9-2 NURSING ACTIONS IN RESPONSE TO BEHAVIOR ASSOCIATED WITH IMPAIRED FERTILITY

BEHAVIORAL CHARACTERISTIC	NURSING ACTIONS
Surprise: Each person assumes she or he is fertile and that pregnancy is an option	Point out resemblance to grieving process—a normal, expected reaction to loss. Refer to support group such as RESOLVE (www.resolve.org).
	Prepare clients for length of time it may take to grieve and for types of feelings (psychologic, somatic) to expect.
	Encourage and allow time to talk of past and present feelings of sexuality, self-image, and self-esteem.
Denial: "It can't happen to me!"	Allow time for denial because it gives the body and mind time to adjust a little at a time.
	Do not feed into the client's denial; instead say, "It must be hard to believe such a devastating report."
Anger: Toward others (perhaps even the nurse) or themselves	Explain that the reaction to loss of control and to a feeling of helplessness is often anger, which can easily be projected onto another person. Anger is a natural feeling.
	Allow time to express anger at losing a sense of control over bodies and destinies.
	A helpful approach may be, "It's okay to be angry…at those who are pregnant, at people who want abortions, at self, at mate, at caregivers" and so forth.
Bargaining: "If I get pregnant, I'll dedicate the child to God."	Accept bargaining statements without comment.
Depression:	
Isolation: Personal	Allow time for both woman and man to talk about how it feels whenever a sight, event, or word serves as a reminder of his or her own state of impaired fertility.
	Develop role-playing situations to practice interactions with others under various circumstances to increase the couple's ability to cope and to solve problems (increases their self-confidence).
	The nurse may say, "You must feel so terribly alone sometimes."
Guilt or unworthiness	Allow time to identify feelings that may be related to earlier behaviors (such as abortion, premarital sex, contact with sexually transmitted infections [STIs]).
Acceptance (resolution)	Couple or person comes to the realization that "unworthiness" and impaired fertility are unrelated.
	Clients need to know that grief feelings are never laid away forever; they may be activated by special reminders (such as anniversaries).

Sources: American Society for Reproductive Medicine (ASRM). (2010b). *Frequently asked questions: The psychological component of infertility.* Available at www.asrm.org. Accessed June 7, 2010; Resolve. (2010). *Emotional aspects of infertility.* Available at www.resolve.org/support-and-services/managing-infertility-stress/emotional-aspects.html. Accessed June 7, 2010.

from personal success and failure. Recognizing the significance of infertility as a loss and resolving these feelings are crucial to putting infertility into perspective, even if treatment is successful (ASRM, 2010b; Nelson et al., 2007; Paterno, 2008).

Nurses can help couples express and discuss their feelings as honestly as possible. Ventilation may help couples to unburden themselves of negative feelings. A meta-analysis found that psychologic interventions alone can improve some couples' chances of becoming pregnant (Hammerli, Znoj, & Barth, 2009).

Psychologic responses to a diagnosis of infertility may tax a couple's giving and receiving of physical and sexual closeness. Sexual dysfunction may manifest as dyspareunia, decreased libido, unrealistic or rigid routines, decreased body image, depression, and ambivalence (Burns, 2007). Couples sometimes report orgasmic dysfunction or midcycle erectile disorders.

To be able to deal comfortably with a couple's sexuality, nurses must be comfortable with their own sexuality so that they can better help couples understand why the private act of lovemaking must be shared with health care professionals. Nurses need up-to-date factual knowledge about human sexual practices and must be accepting and nonjudgmental of the preferences and activities of others (including same-sex couples). They need skills in interviewing and in therapeutic use of self, sensitivity to the nonverbal cues of others, and knowledge regarding each couple's sociocultural and religious beliefs. Gender-neutral and inclusive language, as well as pictures and brochures depicting all types of families, including same-sex couples, establishes a tone of respect and safety in the health care setting (Gay and Lesbian Medical Association [GLMA], 2006).

The woman or couple facing infertility exhibits behaviors of the grieving process that are associated with other types of loss (Table 9-2). The loss of one's genetic continuity with the generations to come leads to a loss of self-esteem, to a sense of inadequacy as a woman or a man, to a loss of control over one's destiny, and to a reduced sense of self. The investigative process leads to a loss of spontaneity and control over the couple's marital relationship and sometimes to a loss of control over progress toward career and life goals. All people do not have all the reactions described, nor can it be predicted how long any reaction will last for an individual.

The support systems of the couple with impaired fertility must be explored. This exploration should include persons available to assist, their relationship to the couple, their ages, their availability, and the available cultural or religious support (ASRM, 2010b). Individuals undergoing infertility evaluation and treatment should be encouraged to share this information with all providers of health care, including mental health practitioners (Burns, 2007).

If the couple conceives, nurses must be aware that the concerns and problems of the previously infertile couple may not be over. Many couples are overjoyed with the pregnancy; however, some are not. Some couples rearrange their lives, sense of selves, and personal goals within their acceptance of their infertile state. The couple may feel that those who worked with them to identify and treat impaired fertility expect them to be happy with the pregnancy. Some couples may be shocked to find that they feel resentment because the pregnancy, once a cherished dream, now necessitates another change in goals, aspirations, and identities. The normal ambivalence toward pregnancy may seem to be a retreat from the original choice to become parents. Reactions of couples range from dealing with the feelings of being overwhelmed to worrying about miscarriage to thinking about choosing to abort the pregnancy. If the couple chooses

with antimicrobials. FSH, hMG, and clomiphene may be used to stimulate spermatogenesis in men with hypogonadism (Attia & Al-Inany, 2007).

The primary care provider is responsible for informing clients fully about the prescribed medications. However, the nurse must be ready to answer clients' questions and to confirm their understanding of the drug, its administration, potential side effects, and expected outcomes. Because information varies with each drug, the nurse must consult the medication package inserts, pharmacology references, the physician, and the pharmacist as necessary.

Surgical

A number of surgical procedures can be used for problems causing female infertility. Ovarian tumors must be excised. Whenever possible, functional ovarian tissue is left intact. Scar tissue adhesions caused by chronic infections may cover the ovary. These adhesions usually necessitate surgery to free and expose the ovary so that ovulation can occur.

Hysterosalpingography, using an oil-soluble contrast medium to flush the tubes, is useful for identification and treatment of tubal obstruction (Johnson, Vanderchove, Lilford, Harada, Hughes, Luttjeboer, et al., 2007). The passage of contrast medium may clear tubes of mucous plugs, straighten kinked tubes, or break up adhesions within the tubes (caused by salpingitis). The procedure may stimulate cilia in the lining of the tubes to facilitate transport of the ovum. It also may aid healing as a result of the bacteriostatic effect of the iodine within the contrast medium.

During laparoscopy, delicate adhesions may be divided and removed, and endometrial implants may be destroyed by electrocoagulation or laser (Zarei, Al-Ghafri, & Tulandi, 2009). Laparotomy and even microsurgery may be required to do extensive repair of the damaged tube. Prognosis is dependent on the degree to which tubal patency and function can be restored.

Reconstructive surgery (e.g., the unification operation for bicornuate uterus) often improves a woman's ability to conceive and carry the fetus to term. Laparoscopic or hysteroscopic surgical removal of tumors or fibroids involving the endometrium or uterus often improves the woman's chance of conceiving and maintaining the pregnancy to viability (Luciano, 2009). Surgical treatment of uterine tumors or maldevelopment that results in successful pregnancy usually requires birth by cesarean surgery near term gestation because the uterus may rupture as a result of weakness of the area of reconstructive surgery.

Chemocautery (destruction of tissue with chemicals) or thermocautery (destruction of tissue with heat, usually electrical) of the cervix, cryosurgery (destruction of tissue by application of extreme cold, usually liquid nitrogen), or conization (excision of a cone-shaped piece of tissue from the endocervix) is effective in eliminating chronic inflammation and infection. However, when the cervix has been deeply cauterized or frozen, or when extensive conization has been performed, extreme limitation of mucus production by the cervix may result. Sperm migration may be difficult or impossible because of the absence of a mucus bridge from the vagina to the uterus. Therapeutic intrauterine insemination may be necessary to carry the sperm directly through the internal os of the cervix.

BOX 9-7 ISSUES TO BE ADDRESSED BY INFERTILE COUPLES BEFORE TREATMENT

- Risks of multiple gestation
- Possible need for multifetal reduction
- Possible need for donor oocytes, sperm, or embryos, or for gestational carrier (surrogate mother)
- Whether to or how to disclose facts of conception to offspring
- Freezing embryos for later use
- Possible risks of long-term effects of medications and treatment on women, children, and families
- Stress management techniques and recommendation for ongoing psychologic and couples counseling

Surgical procedures also may be used for problems causing male infertility. Surgical repair of varicocele has been relatively successful in increasing sperm count but not fertility rates. Microsurgery to reanastomose (restore tubal continuity) the sperm ducts after vasectomy can restore fertility.

Assisted Reproductive Therapies

Although remarkable developments have occurred in reproductive medicine, **assisted reproductive therapies (ARTs)** account for less than 1% of all U.S. births (Wright, Chang, Jeng, Macaluso, & CDC, 2008) and less than 3% of infertility treatment (ASRM, 2010a). They are associated with many ethical and legal issues (Box 9-7). The lack of information or misleading information about success rates and the risks and benefits of treatment alternatives prevents couples from making informed decisions. Nurses can provide information so that couples have an accurate understanding of their chances for a successful pregnancy and live birth. In 2005, the success rate for pregnancy with ART transfer procedures was 42%, whereas the success rate for live births was 35% (Wright, et al.). Nurses also can provide anticipatory guidance about the moral and ethical dilemmas regarding the use of ARTs.

Table 9-3 summarizes the following ART procedures and their possible indications.

In Vitro Fertilization–Embryo Transfer. **In vitro fertilization–embryo transfer (IVF-ET)** is a common approach for women with blocked or absent uterine tubes or with unexplained infertility and for men with very low sperm counts. About 99% of all ARTs use this procedure (Van Voorhis, 2006). Ovarian stimulation using pharmacologic therapy results in multiple mature ova, which are collected at midcycle via intravaginal needle aspiration. The ova are fertilized with sperm in vitro (in a dish) for up to 6 days, then transferred to the uterus using ultrasound guidance (AHRQ, 2008). If sperm are not available via ejaculation, they can be retrieved via needle from the testes or the epididymis (Proctor, Johnson, van Peperstraten, & Phillipson, 2008).

Intracytoplasmic sperm injection (ICSI) is a micromanipulation technique that makes it possible to achieve fertilization even with few or poor-quality sperm by introducing sperm beneath the zona pellucida directly into the egg. ICSI offers the opportunity to enhance the chances of fertilization in cases of a severe male factor (i.e., poor sperm quality) (Pauli et al., 2009; Van Voorhis, 2006). Another micromanipulation option is assisted hatching. In some instances, the zona pellucida is

TABLE 9-3 **ASSISTED REPRODUCTIVE THERAPIES**

PROCEDURE	DEFINITION	INDICATIONS
In vitro fertilization–embryo transfer (IVF-ET)	A woman's eggs are collected from her ovaries, fertilized in the laboratory with sperm, and transferred to her uterus after normal embryo development has occurred.	Tubal disease or blockage; severe male infertility; endometriosis; unexplained infertility; cervical factor; immunologic infertility
Intracytoplasmic sperm injection	Selection of one sperm cell that is injected directly into the egg to achieve fertilization. Used with IVF.	Male partner is azoospermic or has a very low sperm count; couple has a genetic defect; male partner has antisperm antibodies
Assisted hatching	The zona pellucida is penetrated chemically or manually to create an opening for the dividing embryo to hatch and implant into uterine wall.	Recurrent miscarriages; to improve implantation rate in women with previously unsuccessful IVF attempts; advanced age
Gamete intrafallopian transfer (GIFT)	Oocytes are retrieved from the ovary, placed in a catheter with washed motile sperm, and immediately transferred into the fimbriated end of the uterine tube. Fertilization occurs in the uterine tube.	Same as for IVF-ET, except there must be normal tubal anatomy, patency, and absence of previous tubal disease in at least one uterine tube
IVF-ET and GIFT with donor sperm	This process is the same as described above except in cases in which the male partner's fertility is severely compromised and donor sperm can be used; if donor sperm are used, the woman must have indications for IVF-ET or GIFT.	Severe male infertility; azoospermia; indications for IVF-ET or GIFT
Zygote intrafallopian transfer (ZIFT)	This process is similar to IVF-ET; after in vitro fertilization the ova are placed in one uterine tube during the zygote stage.	Same as for GIFT
Donor oocyte	Eggs are donated by an IVF procedure, and the donated eggs are inseminated. The embryos are transferred into the recipient's uterus, which is hormonally prepared with estrogen/progesterone therapy.	Early menopause; surgical removal of ovaries; congenitally absent ovaries; autosomal or sex-linked disorders; lack of fertilization in repeated IVF attempts because of subtle oocyte abnormalities or defects in oocyte-spermatozoa interaction
Donor embryo (embryo adoption)	A donated embryo is transferred to the uterus of an infertile woman at the appropriate time (normal or induced) of the menstrual cycle.	Infertility not resolved by less aggressive forms of therapy; absence of ovaries; male partner is azoospermic or is severely compromised
Gestational carrier (embryo host); surrogate mother	A couple undertakes an IVF cycle, and the embryo(s) is transferred to the uterus of another woman (the carrier) who has contracted with the couple to carry the baby to term. The carrier has no genetic investment in the child. Surrogate motherhood is a process by which a woman is inseminated with semen from the infertile woman's partner and then carries the fetus until birth.	Congenital absence or surgical removal of uterus; a reproductively impaired uterus, myomas, uterine adhesions, or other congenital abnormalities; a medical condition that might be life threatening during pregnancy, such as diabetes, immunologic problems, or severe heart, kidney, or liver disease
Therapeutic donor insemination (TDI)	Donor sperm are used to inseminate the female partner.	Male partner is azoospermic or has a very low sperm count; couple has a genetic defect; male partner has antisperm antibodies; lesbian couple

Data from American Society for Reproductive Medicine (ASRM). (2010a). *Frequently asked questions about infertility.* Available at www.asrm.org. Accessed June 7, 2010; Van Voorhis, B. (2006). Outcomes from assisted reproductive technology. *Obstetrics and Gynecology, 107*(1), 183-200; Pauli, S., Berga, S., Shang, W., & Session, D. (2009). Current status of the approach to assisted reproduction. *Pediatric Clinics of North America, 56*(3), 467-488.

thick or tough and the embryo cannot break through or "hatch" through this coating in the blastocystic phase of development. An infrared laser is used to create a hole in the zona pellucida so that the embryo can break through and implant. This procedure is recommended for couples that have had previous IVF failures (AHRQ, 2008).

Preimplantation genetic diagnosis (PGD) is a form of early genetic testing designed to eliminate embryos with serious genetic defects before implantation through one of the ARTs and to avoid future termination of the pregnancy for genetic reasons. Micromanipulation allows removal of a single cell from a multicellular embryo for genetic study (i.e., embryo biopsy). Couples must be counseled about their options and choices, as well as the implications of their choices, when genetic analysis is considered. For example, the transfer of only embryos that are free from abnormalities can increase the implantation rate and decrease the miscarriage rate and may increase the likelihood of the birth of a healthy infant (Kulieve & Verlinsky, 2008; Pauli et al., 2009).

To minimize the risks of multiple pregnancies, guidelines recommend only two embryos be transferred into women, unless they are older than 37 (Practice Committees of ASRM and the Society for Assisted Reproductive Technology, 2009). Ovarian tissue, oocytes, or embryos can be cryopreserved for later use (Wallberg, Keros, & Hovatta, 2009).

LEGAL TIP: Cryopreservation of Human Embryos

Couples who have excess embryos frozen for later transfer must be fully informed before consenting to the procedure, to make decisions regarding the disposal of embryos in the event of (1) death, (2) divorce, or (3) the decision that the couple no longer wants the embryos.

Success rates for pregnancy and for live births vary widely from center to center. Each couple's physical status and age factor into their individual chances for pregnancy as well as whether the embryos are fresh or frozen and are from eggs of the woman or a donor (Van Voorhis, 2006). Costs vary by treatment and by region of the country: one cycle of IVF-ET averages $12,400 (ASRM, 2010a).

Gamete Intrafallopian Transfer. **Gamete intrafallopian transfer (GIFT)** is similar to IVF-ET. GIFT requires women to have at least one normal uterine tube. Ovulation is induced as in IVF-ET, and the oocytes are aspirated from follicles via

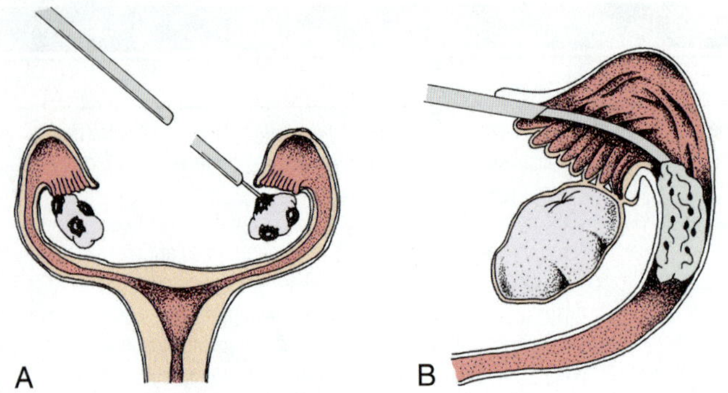

FIG. 9-5 Gamete intrafallopian transfer. **A,** Through laparoscopy, a ripe follicle is located and fluid containing the egg is removed. **B,** The sperm and egg are placed separately in the uterine tube, where fertilization occurs.

laparoscopy (Fig. 9-5, *A*). Semen is collected before laparoscopy, and sperm are capacitated by the same technique used for IVF-ET. The ova and sperm are then transferred to one uterine tube (Fig. 9-5, *B*), permitting natural fertilization and cleavage. Less than 1% of all ARTs use this technique (ASRM, 2010a).

Zygote Intrafallopian Transfer. **Zygote intrafallopian transfer (ZIFT)** is similar to GIFT except that in ZIFT, after in vitro fertilization the ova are placed in the uterine tube during the zygote stage. ZIFT accounts for less than 1% of all ART procedures (ASRM, 2010a).

Complications. Other than the established risks associated with ovarian stimulation, invasive procedures and general anesthesia, few risks are associated with IVF-ET, GIFT, and ZIFT. The more common transvaginal needle aspiration requires only local or intravenous analgesia. Evidence of increased risk of congenital malformations associated with ART is mixed: the anomalies may be related to the underlying cause of infertility (Pauli et al., 2009). In addition, the underlying cause of infertility, such as severe male infertility factor, may be passed on to the offspring. Infertility treatment increases the risk of placental problems (AHRQ, 2008). Multiple gestations are more likely and are associated with increased risks for both the mother and fetuses (Wright et al., 2008). Ectopic pregnancies occur more often, and these carry a significant maternal risk. In addition, psychologic, financial, and emotional stresses are common.

Oocyte Donation. Women who have ovarian failure or oophorectomy, who have a genetic defect, or who fail to achieve pregnancy with their own oocytes may be eligible for the use of donor oocytes. Oocyte donation is usually done by women who are younger than 35 years and healthy, and who are recruited and paid to undergo ovarian stimulation and oocyte retrieval. The donor eggs are then fertilized in the laboratory with the male partner's sperm. The recipient woman undergoes hormonal stimulation to allow development of the uterine lining. Embryos are then transferred. The psychosocial issues are similar to those in therapeutic donor insemination. Historically the courts have upheld the gestational mother as the legal mother. It is expected that the egg donor will have no rights or responsibilities in relation to the offspring.

Embryo Donation. On occasion a couple decides that they do not want their frozen embryos, and they release these for "adoption" by other infertile couples. Infertility centers are struggling to develop guidelines and protocols to address the various legal and ethical issues associated with these procedures. Extensive medical testing of both partners who wish to release the embryos is required as well.

Surrogate Mothers/Embryo Hosts. Surrogate motherhood can be achieved by two methods. The first is for the surrogate mother to be inseminated with semen from the infertile woman's partner and to carry the baby until the birth. The baby is then formally adopted by the infertile couple. A less common method is to retrieve an ovum from the infertile woman, fertilize it with her partner's sperm, and place it into the uterus of a surrogate, who becomes an embryo host or gestational carrier. These interventions raise considerable legal and ethical issues that require extensive counseling of couples and the women who choose to become surrogates.

Therapeutic Donor Insemination. **Therapeutic donor insemination (TDI),** previously referred to as artificial insemination by donor, is used when the male partner has no sperm or a very low sperm count (less than 20 million motile sperm per milliliter), the couple has a genetic defect, or the male partner has antisperm antibodies. Couples need to be counseled extensively regarding the mutuality of their decision, their ability (particularly of the male partner) to grieve the loss of a biologic child, and long-term issues relating to parenting the child conceived through TDI (Van Voorhis, 2006). Couples also must be aware of the legal status of TDI in their state.

In TDI, donor semen is subjected to laboratory testing to reduce the possibility of life-threatening illnesses for the recipient and her fetus, as well as for factors that could jeopardize the woman's future fertility or compromise the chance of the success of the procedure. No increase in maternal or perinatal complications occurs with TDI; the same frequencies of anomalies (about 5%) and obstetric complications (between 5% and 10%) that accompany natural insemination (through sexual intercourse) apply also to TDI.

The intrauterine insemination procedure is done in the physician's office or clinic, usually the day after the woman has an LH surge. The sperm are injected via catheter through the cervix, and placed high in the uterine cavity. The woman lies flat for a few minutes and then can get up and resume her usual activities.

Assuming normal female fertility, intrauterine TDI at or about the time of ovulation has resulted in pregnancy in as many as 70% of cases. If pregnancy has not occurred within six cycles of well-timed insemination, further investigation of the female partner is warranted. The couple must know that there is no guarantee of pregnancy and that the miscarriage rate is approximately the same as in a control population.

Adoption

Couples may choose to build their family through adoption of children who are not their own biologically. With increased availability of birth control and abortion and increasing numbers of single mothers keeping their babies, however, the adoption of Caucasian infants is extremely limited. Minority infants and infants with special needs, older children, and foreign adoptions are other options.

COMMUNITY ACTIVITY

- Visit the Resolve National Infertility Association website at www.resolve.org. Review the client information regarding overview of infertility, diagnosis and management, family building options, support and resources. Research the availability of a Resolve support group in your community. Contact the facilitator and try to attend a meeting.
- Visit the National Adoption Information Clearinghouse website at www.calib.com/naic. Go to the adoption link and review the client information about the steps to adoption, costs and types, issues to consider, alternatives, legal considerations, support, tools and resources. Locate an adoption agency in your community and visit the website. What is the mission of the agency? Are the adoptions domestic or international?

Most adults assume that they will be able to have children of their own. The discovery that they are unable to do so is often accompanied by feelings of inferiority, doubts about masculinity or femininity, and feelings of guilt or blame in relation to the partner. These feelings and frustrations, combined with the anxiety of waiting for pregnancies, feelings of loss, and the multiple medical procedures to investigate infertility, plus the legal uncertainties and potential financial considerations surrounding adoption, create many challenges for the adoptive couple preparing for parenthood.

Couples who decide to adopt a child have decided that being a parent and having a child is more important than the actual process of birthing the baby. The birth process is a very small aspect of becoming a parent. Prospective parents can become so focused on attempting to become pregnant with their own genetic child that they don't see alternate ways of creating a family and parenting a child. The question couples who are considering adoption need to answer is, "What is important to you—that you become parents or that you go through the experience of pregnancy and birth?" Nurses should have information on options for adoption available for couples or refer them to community resources for further assistance (ASRM, 2010b).

KEY POINTS

- Infertility is the inability to conceive and carry a child to term gestation when the couple has chosen to do so.
- Infertility affects between 10% and 15% of otherwise healthy adults. Infertility increases as the woman ages, especially after age 40 years.
- In the United States, about 20% of infertility causes are unexplained; of that 80% in which causative factors are known, about 40% are related to female causes, 40% are related to male causes, and 20% are attributable to both male and female causes.
- Common etiologic factors of infertility include decreased sperm production, ovulation disorders, tubal occlusion, and endometriosis. Obesity in either partner is receiving increasing attention as a cause of infertility.
- The investigation of infertility is conducted systematically and simultaneously for male and female partners.
- The couple's relationship dynamics, sexuality, and ability to cope with the psychologic and emotional effects caused by diagnostic procedures and treatment of infertility must be considered in the plan of care. Ongoing support is recommended.
- Most infertility cases are treated with conventional medical and surgical therapies; less than 3% are treated with in vitro fertilization.
- Reproductive alternatives for family building include IVF-ET, GIFT, ZIFT, oocyte donation, embryo donation, TDI, surrogate motherhood, and adoption.

Audio Chapter Summaries Access an audio summary of the Key Points on evolve

REFERENCES

Agency for Healthcare Research and Quality (AHRQ). (2008). *Effectiveness of assisted reproductive technology.* Rockville, Maryland, Available at www.ahrq.gov/clinic/tp/infertiltp.htm. Accessed June 7, 2010.

American Society for Reproductive Medicine (ASRM). (2008). The Committee on Gynecologic Practice of the American College of Obstetricians and Gynecologists and the Practice Committee of the ASRM. Age-related fertility decline. A committee opinion. *Fertility & Sterility, 90*(Suppl. 3), S154–S155. Available at www.asrm.org. Accessed June 7, 2010.

American Society for Reproductive Medicine (ASRM). (2010a). *Frequently asked questions about infertility.* Available at www.asrm.org. Accessed June 7, 2010.

American Society for Reproductive Medicine (ASRM). (2010b). *Frequently asked questions: The psychological component of infertility.* Available at www.asrm.org. Accessed June 7, 2010.

Anderson, B., Haimovici, F., Ginsburg, E., Schust, D., & Wayne, P. (2007). In vitro fertilization and acupuncture: Clinical efficacy and mechanistic basis. *Alternative Therapies in Health & Medicine, 13*(3), 38–48.

Attia, A., & Al-Inany, H. (2007). Gonadotropins for idiopathic male factor subfertility. (Cochrane Review). *The Cochrane Database of Systematic Reviews, 2007*, 4, CD005071.

Badawy, A., State, O., & Abdelgawad, S. (2007). N-acetylcysteine and clomiphene citrate for induction of ovulation in polycystic ovarian syndrome: A crossover trial. *Acta Obstetrica et Gynecologica Scandinavica, 80*(3), 265–269.

Balen, A., & Anderson, R. (2007). Impact of obesity on female reproductive health: British Fertility Society, policy and practice guidelines. *Human Fertility, 10*(4), 195–206.

Bensdorp, A., Cohlen, B., Heineman, M., & Vanderchove, P. (2007). Intra-uterine insemination for male subfertility (Cochrane Review). *The Cochrane Database of Systematic Reviews, 2007*, 4, CD000360.

Brown, J., Farquhar, C., Beck, J., Boothroyd, C., & Hughes, E. (2009). Clomiphene and anti-oestrogens for ovulation induction in PCOS (Cochrane Review). *The Cochrane Database of Systematic Reviews, 2009*, 4, CD002249.

Burns, L. (2007). Psychiatric aspects of infertility and infertility treatments. *Psychiatric Clinics of North America, 30*(4), 689–716.

Cantineau, A., & Cohlen, B. (2007). Ovarian hyperstimulation protocols (anti-oestrogens, gonadotropins with and without GnRH agonists/antagonists) for intrauterine insemination (IUI) for women with subfertility (Cochrane Review). *The Cochrane Database of Systematic Reviews, 2007*, 2, CD005356.

Chalazonitis, A., Tzovara, I., Laspas, F., Porfyrdis, P., Ptohis, N., & Tsimitselis, G. (2009). Hysterosalpinography: Technique and application. *Current Problems in Diagnostic Radiology, 38*(5), 199–205.

Cheong, Y., Ng, E., & Ledger, W. (2008). Acupuncture and assisted conception (Cochrane Review). *The Cochrane Database of Systematic Reviews, 2008*, 4, CD006920.

Cousineau, T., & Domar, A. (2007). Psychological impact of infertility. *Best Practice & Research Clinical Obstetrics & Gynaecology, 21*(2), 293–308.

Cunningham, F., Leveno, K., Bloom, S., Hauth, J., Rouse, D., & Spong, C. (2010). *Williams obstetrics* (23rd ed.). New York: McGraw-Hill.

Dennehy, C. (2006). The use of herbs and dietary supplements in gynecology: An evidence-based review. *Journal of Midwifery & Women's Health, 51*(6), 402–409.

Gay and Lesbian Medical Association (GLMA). (2006). Guidelines for care of lesbian, gay, bisexual, and transgender patients. Available at www.glma.org. Accessed June 7, 2010.

Hammarberg, K., Fisher, J., & Wynter, K. (2008). Psychological and social aspects of pregnancy, childbirth and early parenting after assisted conception: A systematic review. *Human Reproduction Update, 14*(5), 395–414.

Hammerli, K., Znoj, H., & Barth, J. (2009). The efficacy of psychological interventions for infertile patients: A meta-analysis examining mental health and pregnancy rate. *Human Reproduction Update, 15*(3), 279–295.

Hammoud, A., Gibson, M., Peterson, C., Meikle, A., & Carrell, D. (2008). Impact of male obesity on fertility: A critical review of the current literature. *Fertility & Sterility, 90*(4), 897–904.

Hughes, E., Brown, J., & Tiffin, G. (2007). Danazol for unexplained infertility (Cochrane Review). *The Cochrane Database of Systematic Reviews, 2007*, 1, CD000069.

Johnson, N., Vanderchove, P., Lilford, R., Harada, T., Hughes, E., Luttjeboer, F., et al. (2007). Tubal flushing for subfertility (Cochrane Review). *The Cochrane Database of Systematic Reviews, 2007*, 13, CD003718.

Kulieve, A., & Verlinsky, Y. (2008). Preimplantation genetic diagnosis: Technological advances to improve accuracy and range of applications. *Reproductive Biomedicine Online, 16*(4), 532–538.

Leddy, M., Jones, C., Morgan, M., & Schulkin, J. (2009). Eating disorders and obstetric-gynecologic care. *Journal of Women's Health Care, 18*(9), 1395–1401.

Lobo, R. (2007). Infertility: Etiology, diagnostic evaluation, management, prognosis. In V. Katz, G. Lentz, R. Lobo, & D. Gershenson (Eds.), *Comprehensive gynecology* (5th ed.). Philadelphia: Mosby.

Luciano, A. (2009). Myomectomy. *Clinical Obstetrics and Gynecology, 52*(3), 362–371.

Malik, S. (2009). Impact of obesity on female fertility and fertility treatment. *British Journal of Midwifery, 17*(7), 452–454.

Mania-Pramanik, J., Kerkar, J., & Salvi, V. (2009). Bacterial vaginosis: A cause of infertility? *International Journal of Sexually Transmitted Diseases and Human Immunodeficiency Virus, 20*(11), 778–781.

Masheshwari, A., Stofberg, L., & Bhattacharya, S. (2007). Effects of overweight and obesity on assisted reproductive technology—a systematic review. *Human Reproduction Update, 13*(5), 433–444.

Monti, F., Agostini, F., Fagandini, P., Paterlini, M., La Sala, G., & Blickstein, I. (2008). Anxiety symptoms during late pregnancy and early parenthood following assisted reproductive technology. *Journal of Perinatal Medicine, 36*(5), 425–432.

Nelson, A., Marshall, J., Trussell, J., Stewart, F., Nelson, S., Cates, W., Guest, F., et al. (2007). Impaired fertility. In R. Hatcher, J. Trussell, A. Nelson, W. Cates, F. Stewart, & D. Kowal (Eds.), *Contraceptive technology* (19th rev. ed.). New York: Ardent Media.

Paterno, M. (2008). Families of two: Meeting the needs of couples experiencing male infertility. *Nursing for Women's Health, 12*(4), 300–306.

Pauli, S., Berga, S., Shang, W., & Session, D. (2009). Current status of the approach to assisted reproduction. *Pediatric Clinics of North America, 56*(3), 467–488.

Practice Committees of the American Society of Reproductive Medicine and the Society of Assisted Reproductive Technology. (2009). Guidelines on number of embryos transferred. *Fertility & Sterility, 92*(5), 1518–1519.

Proctor, M., Johnson, N., van Peperstraten, A., & Phillipson, G. (2008). Techniques for surgical retrieval of sperm prior to intra-cytoplasmic sperm injection (ICSI) for azoospermia (Cochrane Review). *The Cochrane Database of Systematic Reviews, 2008*, 2, CD002807.

Sampey, A., Bourque, J., & Wren, K. (2004). Learning scope: Herbal medicines. *Advance for Nurses, 6*(25), 13–19.

Shayeb, A., & Bhattacharya, S. (2009). Male obesity and reproductive potential. *British Journal of Diabetes & Vascular Disease, 9*(1), 7–12.

Sheweita, S., Tilmisany, A., & Al-Sawaf, H. (2005). Mechanisms of male infertility: Role of antioxidants. *Current Drug Metabolism, 6*(5), 495–501.

Thomson, A., Abbott, J., Deans, R., Kingston, A., & Vancaillie, T. (2009). The management of uterine synechiae. *Current Opinions in Obstetrics and Gynecology, 21*(4), 335–341.

Van Voorhis, B. (2006). Outcomes from assisted reproductive technology. *Obstetrics and Gynecology, 107*(1), 183–200.

Wallberg, K., Keros, V., & Hovatta, O. (2009). Clinical aspects of fertility preservation in female patients. *Pediatric Blood Cancer, 53*(2), 254–260.

Wang, J., Davies, M., & Norman, R. (2002). Obesity increases the risk of spontaneous abortion during infertility treatment. *Obesity Research, 10*(6), 551–554.

Weed, S. (1986). *Wise woman herbal for the childbearing years*, Woodstock, NY: Ash Tree.

Weisz, V. (2009). Social justice considerations for lesbian and bisexual women's health care. *Journal of Obstetric, Gynecologic & Neonatal Nursing, 38*, 81–87.

Wischmann, T., Scherg, H., Strowitzki, T., & Verres, R. (2009). Psychological characteristics of women and men attending infertility counseling. *Human Reproduction, 24*(2), 378–385.

Wright, V., Chang, J., Jeng, G., Macaluso, M., & CDC. (2008). Assisted reproductive technology surveillance—United States, 2005. *MMWR Morbidity and Mortality Weekly Report Surveillance Summaries, 57*(5), 1–230.

Zarei, A., Al-Ghafri, W., & Tulandi, T. (2009). Tubal surgery. *Clinical Obstetrics and Gynecology, 52*(3), 344–350.

CHAPTER

10

Problems of the Breast

Lillie D. Shockney

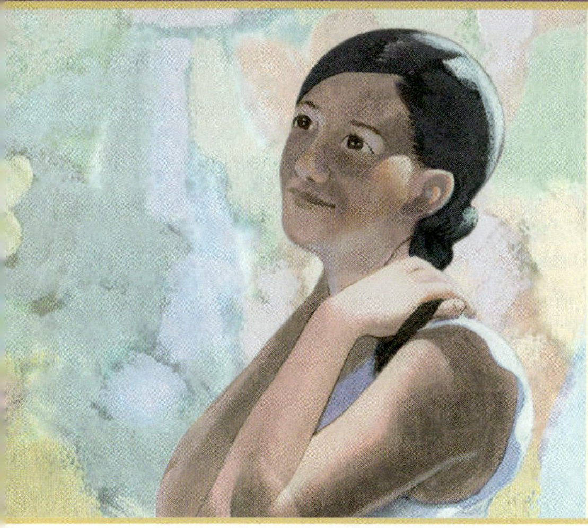

evolve WEBSITE

http://evolve.elsevier.com/Lowdermilk/MWHC/

Audio Glossary
Audio Key Points
Case Study
    Breast Cancer
NCLEX Review Questions
Nursing Care Plans
    Breast Cancer
    The Woman Having Breast-Conserving Surgery and Axillary Node Dissection

LEARNING OBJECTIVES

- Discuss the pathophysiology of selected benign and malignant breast disorders found in women.
- Explain the emotional effects of benign and malignant neoplasms.
- Design a nursing care plan for the woman with a breast disorder.
- Evaluate treatment alternatives for women with breast cancer.
- Integrate critical elements for teaching women who have undergone medical-surgical management of benign or malignant neoplasms of the breast.

Approximately 50% of women have a breast problem at some point in their adult lives. The most common sign of a breast problem is a palpable mass. Most of these lumps are benign, although finding them may produce anxiety for the woman, who may fear she has cancer. The development of breast cancer can have a far-reaching effect on the woman and her family. Beyond the obvious physiologic alterations, she also may experience threats to her self-image and ability to cope. The condition and its treatments can affect a woman's concept of herself as a sexual being. Cancer also presents a challenge for a woman's family. When breast cancer occurs during or after pregnancy, it adds to the complexity of both physical and emotional responses to childbearing.

Nurses have important roles in teaching women about early detection and treatment and in providing supportive care to clients and their families. This chapter presents information that will assist nurses in providing care for women with benign breast conditions or breast cancer. The ongoing investigations of new drug therapies to prevent breast cancer are also introduced.

BENIGN CONDITIONS OF THE BREAST

A benign breast condition often causes a lump or thickened area noted on breast self-examination (BSE) or clinical breast examination. It may or may not feel tender. The most common causes of a single lump are fibroadenoma, fibrocystic changes, cysts, or atypical hyperplasia. The younger a woman is the more likely a single lump will be found to be benign.

Fibrocystic Changes

The most common benign breast problem is fibrocystic change found in varying degrees in healthy women's breasts. Fibrocystic changes are characterized by lumpiness, with or without tenderness, in both breasts (Valea & Katz, 2007). Fibrocystic breast condition involves the glandular breast tissue.

Etiology

Fibrocystic changes tend to appear most commonly in women in their second and third decades of life. The most significant contributing factor to fibrocystic breast condition is a woman's normal hormonal variation during her monthly cycle. Many hormonal changes occur as a woman's body prepares each month for a possible pregnancy. The most important of these hormones are estrogen and progesterone. These two hormones directly affect the breast tissues by causing cells to proliferate. Other hormones also play an important role, however, causing fibrocystic changes. Prolactin, growth factor, insulin, and thyroid hormones are some of the other major hormones that can also affect cell growth within the breast tissue. Except for proliferative change known as hyperplasia, which is associated with a slightly elevated risk of breast cancer, or atypical hyperplasia, which is associated with a moderately increased risk of breast cancer, the histologic findings associated with fibrocystic changes are part of the spectrum of normal involutional patterns of the breast (Valea & Katz).

Clinical Manifestations and Diagnosis

The usual clinical presentation of fibrocystic change is lumpiness in both breasts; however, single simple cysts also can occur. Women in their 20s report the most severe pain. Women in their 30s have premenstrual pain and tenderness; small multiple nodules are usually present. Women in their 40s usually do not report severe pain, but cysts will be tender and often regress in size. Symptoms usually develop about a week before menstruation begins and subside about a week after menstruation ends. They include dull, heavy pain and a sense of fullness and tenderness often in the upper outer quadrant of the breasts that increases in the premenstrual period. The woman with fibrocystic change may form cysts that manifest as painful enlarging lumps in her breasts. Cysts are common in premenopausal women who are not receiving estrogen therapy. Physical examination may reveal excessive nodularity. The cysts are soft on palpation, well differentiated, and movable. Deeper cysts, especially aggregations of cysts, are indistinguishable by palpation from carcinomas, which are malignant growths that infiltrate surrounding tissue.

A first assessment of a breast lump is ultrasonography to determine if it is fluid filled or solid. Fluid-filled cysts are aspirated, and the woman is monitored on a routine basis for development of other cysts. If the lump is solid and the woman is older than 35 years, mammography is obtained. A fine-needle aspiration (FNA) is performed, regardless of the woman's age, to determine the nature of the lump (see Fig 10-4). In some cases, a core biopsy may be necessary after FNA to harvest adequate amounts of tissue for pathologic examination (Lin, Hsu, Yu, Yu, Lee, Hsu, et al., 2009; Valea & Katz, 2007).

Therapeutic Management

Treatment for fibrocystic changes is usually conservative. Management can depend on the severity of the symptoms. Dietary changes and vitamin supplements are one management approach. Although research findings are contradictory, some practitioners advocate reducing consumption or eliminating methylxanthines (i.e., colas, coffee, tea, chocolate) and tobacco (Valea & Katz, 2007). Some symptom relief may be achieved by avoiding smoking and the consumption of alcohol. Recommended pain-relief measures include taking analgesics or nonsteroidal antiinflammatory drugs (NSAIDs) such as ibuprofen, wearing a supportive bra, and applying heat to the breasts.

Vitamin E supplements and decreasing sodium intake or taking mild diuretics before menses have also been reported to reduce some women's symptoms. Some women report relief while taking oral contraceptives, but others report worsening of symptoms. Danazol, bromocriptine, and tamoxifen also have been used with varying degrees of success (Valea & Katz, 2007). Evening primrose oil may be effective for some women, although evidence is lacking. It is important to stress that women may need to try several approaches for a number of months before improvement is noted (Valea & Katz).

Surgical removal of nodules is attempted only in rare cases. In the presence of multiple nodules, the surgical approach involves multiple incisions and tissue manipulation and may not prevent the development of more nodules.

Fibroadenomas

The next most common benign condition of the breast is a **fibroadenoma**. It is the single most common type of tumor seen in the adolescent population, although it can also occur in women in their 20s and 30s. Fibroadenomas are discrete, usually solitary lumps less than 3 cm in diameter (Valea & Katz, 2007). Occasionally the woman with a fibroadenoma will experience tenderness in the tumor during the menstrual cycle. Fibroadenomas do not increase in size in response to the menstrual cycle (in contrast to fibrocystic cysts). The mass tends to remain the same size or increase in size slowly over time. Fibroadenomas increase in size during pregnancy and decrease in size as the woman ages. Diagnosis is made by a review of the client history and physical examination. Mammography, ultrasonography, or magnetic resonance imaging (MRI) may be used to determine the type of lesion, and FNA may be used to determine the underlying disorder. Surgical excision may be necessary if the lump is suspicious or if the symptoms are severe. Fibroadenomas do not respond to either dietary changes or hormonal therapy. Periodic observation of masses by professional physical examination or mammography may be all that is necessary for those masses not requiring surgical intervention (Shockney & Tsangaris, 2007).

Nipple Discharge

Nipple discharge is a common occurrence that concerns many women. Though most nipple discharge is physiologic, each woman who presents with this problem must be evaluated carefully because in a small percentage, nipple discharge may be related to a serious endocrine disorder or malignancy. Bilateral serous discharge expressed during nipple stimulation can be considered a normal finding (Shockney & Tsangaris, 2007).

Another form of nipple discharge not related to malignancy is **galactorrhea**—a bilaterally spontaneous, milky, sticky discharge. It is a normal finding in pregnancy. Galactorrhea can also occur as the result of elevated prolactin levels. Increased prolactin levels may be a result of a thyroid disorder, pituitary tumor, coitus, eating, stress, trauma, or chest wall surgery. Obtaining a complete medical history on each woman is essential. Certain medications may precipitate galactorrhea. Tricyclic antidepressants, phenothiazines, narcotics, antiemetics, and antihypertensive medications, as well as oral contraceptives, can precipitate galactorrhea in some women (Lobo, 2007). Diagnostic tests that may be indicated include a prolactin level, a microscopic analysis of the discharge from each breast, a thyroid profile, a pregnancy test, and a mammogram. The optimal time to draw blood to assess a prolactin level is between 8 AM and 10 AM. Ideally, prolactin levels should not be drawn directly after a breast examination, sexual activity, or exercise session (Lobo, 2007).

Mammary Duct Ectasia

Mammary duct ectasia is an inflammation of the ducts behind the nipple. The cause of mammary duct ectasia is unknown, although chronic inflammation and dilation of the lactiferous ducts has been suggested. This condition occurs most often in perimenopausal women and is characterized by a thick, sticky nipple discharge that is white, brown, green, or purple. Frequently the woman will experience a burning pain, itching, or a palpable mass behind the nipple.

The diagnostic workup consists of a mammogram, aspiration of fluid, and culture of fluid. Duct ectasia is usually self-limiting, requiring only reassurance of the woman. An infection in the inflamed area can occur and requires antibiotic therapy. If an abscess develops, an incision and drainage may be necessary along with a prescription for oral antibiotics. Treatment may also include a local excision of the affected duct or ducts if the woman has no future plans to breastfeed (Mayo Foundation for Medical Education and Research, 2008).

Intraductal Papilloma

Intraductal papilloma is a relatively rare, benign condition that develops in the terminal nipple ducts. The cause is unknown. It usually occurs in women between ages 30 and 50 years. Papillomas are usually too small to be palpated (less than 0.5 cm), and present with the characteristic sign of serous, serosanguineous, or bloody nipple discharge. The discharge is unilateral and spontaneous. A ductogram is a common way of making the diagnosis, along with mammography and core biopsy. After the possibility of malignancy is eliminated, treatment for papillomas includes excision of the affected segments of the ducts and breasts (Shockney & Tsangaris, 2007; Valea & Katz, 2007). Table 10-1 compares common manifestations of benign breast masses.

Macromastia and Micromastia

Macromastia or breast hyperplasia, is a condition in which the woman has very large breasts. The size and weight of the breasts can cause chronic pain in the breast, back, neck, and shoulders, as well as significant disruption in psychosocial functioning and body image. Macromastia also can cause thoracic kyphosis, headache, paresthesia of the upper extremities, and shoulder grooving from brassiere straps. Macromastia is treated by reduction mammoplasty, in which the plastic surgeon removes breast tissue to reduce the size and weight of the breasts. Women who have had breast reduction surgery have significant improvement of preoperative signs and symptoms and their quality of life (Brown, Holton, Chung, & Slezak, 2008). However, risks associated with the surgery include the potential to affect the woman's ability to breastfeed in the future, infection, decreased nipple sensation, and scarring (Rahman, Adigunt, Yusif, & Bamigbade, 2007). Breast reduction surgery is considered reconstructive surgery when done to relieve symptoms of macromastia and may be covered by health insurance policies. Women considering reduction mammoplasty should review their policies to determine exact coverage.

Although it is not a breast disorder, **micromastia,** or having very small breasts, may negatively influence a woman's body image. Augmentation mammoplasty may be done to increase breast size. The plastic surgeon inserts implants filled with normal saline between the breast tissue and the chest wall. Silicone gel–filled implants are not available for breast augmentation done for cosmetic reasons (Rahman et al., 2007) (see later discussion on breast reconstruction). Breast augmentation surgery is considered cosmetic surgery and is usually not covered by health insurance policies. Saline breast implants do not last indefinitely; most must be replaced in 10 to 15 years or sooner (Shockney & Tsangaris, 2007).

Collaborative Care

Assessment should include a thorough client history and physical examination. The history should focus on risk factors for breast diseases, events related to the breast mass, and health maintenance practices. Risk factors for breast cancer are discussed later in this chapter. Information related to the breast mass should include how, when, and by whom the mass was discovered. The interval between discovery and seeking care is crucial. The following client information is documented: presence of pain, whether symptoms increase with menses, dietary habits, smoking habits, use of oral contraceptives or hormone replacement therapy, personal history of breast cancer, family history of breast cancer, use of BSE, and the examination technique if used. The woman's emotional status, including her stress level, fears, and concerns, and her ability to cope also should be assessed.

Physical examination may include assessment of the breasts for symmetry, masses (size, number, consistency, mobility), and nipple discharge.

Nursing actions might include the following:

- Discuss the intervals for and facets of breast screening, including professional examination and mammography (see Table 10-3). Women with breast implants may need special views (called push-backs) of the breast, and precautions might have to be taken not to rupture the implant during mammography.
- Provide written educational materials.

TABLE 10-1 COMPARISON OF COMMON MANIFESTATIONS OF BENIGN BREAST MASSES

FIBROCYSTIC CHANGES	FIBROADENOMA	LIPOMA	INTRADUCTAL PAPILLOMA	MAMMARY DUCT ECTASIA
Multiple lumps	Single lump	Single lump	Nonpalpable	Mass behind nipple
Nodular	Well delineated	Well delineated	Not well delineated	Not well delineated
Palpable	Palpable	Palpable	Nonpalpable	Palpable
Movable	Movable	Movable	Nonmobile	Nonmobile
Round, smooth	Round, lobular	Round, lobular	None	Irregular
Firm or soft	Firm	Soft	Firm or soft	Firm
Tenderness influenced by menstrual cycle	Usually asymptomatic	Nontender	Usually nontender	Painful, burning, itching
Bilateral	Unilateral	Unilateral	Unilateral	Unilateral
May or may not have nipple discharge	No nipple discharge	No nipple discharge	Serous or bloody nipple discharge	Thick, sticky nipple discharge

- Encourage the verbalization of fears and concerns about treatment and prognosis.
- Provide specific information regarding the woman's condition and treatment, including dietary changes, drug therapy, comfort measures, stress management, and surgery.
- Demonstrate correct BSE technique if woman desires to practice it (see p. 91).
- Describe pain-relieving strategies in detail, and collaborate with the primary health care provider to ensure effective pain control.
- Encourage discussion of feelings about body image.
- Refer to a stress management resource if needed to cope with long-term consequences of benign breast conditions.

MALIGNANT CONDITIONS OF THE BREAST

Incidence

The United States has one of the highest rates of breast carcinoma in the world. One in eight American women will develop invasive breast cancer in her lifetime. The American Cancer Society's (ACS) most recent estimates for breast cancer in the United States are for 2010 (ACS, 2010):

- 207,090 new female cases of invasive breast cancer
- 54,010 new female cases of cancer in situ; about 85% will be ductal carcinoma in situ (DCIS)
- 40,230 female deaths from breast cancer

Statistics reported by the ACS indicated that breast cancer incidence increased during the 1990s. This increase may be related to better detection of early-stage breast cancer, increasing rates of obesity, improvements in the quality of mammography (digital), and use of postmenopausal hormonal therapy (ACS, 2010). There has been a decrease in incidence from 1999 to 2006, as many women discontinued hormonal therapy for menopausal symptoms.

It is also important to note that in the United States, the number of women over the age of 55 is larger than ever, which will increase the number of women diagnosed. Breast cancer is the most common cancer among women in the United States, other than skin cancer. It is the second leading cause of cancer death in women, after lung cancer. The chance of dying from breast cancer is about 1 in 35—death rates have declined since 1990. This decline is probably the result of finding the cancer earlier and improved treatment (ACS).

Etiologic Factors

Although the exact cause of breast cancer continues to elude investigators, there are certain factors that increase a woman's risk for developing a malignancy.

Some risk factors are unchangeable; others, associated with lifestyle choices, are changeable. Therefore, being familiar with the entire list is important when a nurse is assessing and counseling a woman about ways to reduce her risk.

Unchangeable risk factors include (ACS, 2009, 2010, Valea & Katz, 2007):

- **Gender:** Simply being a woman is the main risk for breast cancer. Although men also have the disease, it is about 100 times more common in women than in men.
- **Age:** The chance of having breast cancer goes up as a woman gets older. About two out of three women with invasive breast cancer are age 55 or older when the cancer is found.
- **Genetic risk factors:** About 5% to 10% of breast cancers are thought to be linked to inherited changes (mutations) in certain genes. The most common gene changes are those of the BRCA1 and BRCA2 genes. Women with these gene changes have up to an 80% chance of having breast cancer during their lifetimes. Other gene changes, such as Li-Fraumeni syndrome, Cowden syndrome, or Bannayan-Riley-Ruvalcaba syndrome, will raise breast cancer risk as well.
- **Family history:** Breast cancer risk is higher among women whose close blood relatives have this disease. The relatives can be from either the mother's or father's side of the family. Having a mother, sister, or daughter with breast cancer about doubles a woman's risk. (It's important to note that 70% to 80% of women who have breast cancer do not have a family history of this disease.) For a family member who carries a breast cancer gene, however, the risk for other family members is higher than for those whose history does not include a genetic link.
- **Personal history of breast cancer:** A woman with cancer in one breast has a greater chance of having a new cancer in the opposite breast or in another part of the same breast.
- **Race:** Caucasian women are slightly more likely to get breast cancer than are African-American women. But African-American women are more likely to die of this cancer. At least part of the reason seems to be because African-American women have faster-growing tumors. Asian, Hispanic, and Native American women have a lower risk of getting breast cancer (Fig. 10-1).
- **Dense breast tissue:** Women with denser breast tissue have a higher risk of breast cancer. Dense breast tissue can also make it more difficult for a radiologist to see an abnormality on mammograms (Martin, Minkin, & Boyd, 2009).
- **Menstrual periods:** Women who began having periods early (before age 12) or who went through menopause after the age of 55 have a slightly increased risk of breast cancer. They have had more menstrual periods and as a result have been exposed to more of the hormones estrogen and progesterone.
- **Earlier breast radiation:** Women who have had radiation treatment to the chest area (as treatment for another cancer) earlier in life have a greatly increased risk of breast cancer.
- **Treatment with diethylstilbestrol (DES):** In the past, some pregnant women were given DES because it was thought to lower their chances of losing the baby (miscarriage). Studies have shown that these women (and their daughters who were exposed to DES while in the womb), have a slightly increased risk of having breast cancer.

Lifestyle choices increase the risk of breast cancer. These include: (ACS, 2009, 2010)

- **Not having children or having them later in life:** Women who have not had children, or who have their first child after age 30, have a slightly higher risk of breast cancer. Being pregnant more than once and at an early age reduces breast cancer risk. Pregnancy reduces a woman's total number of lifetime menstrual cycles, which may be the reason for this effect.
- **Recent use of birth control pills:** Studies have found that women who are using birth control pills have a slightly greater risk of breast cancer than women who have never used them. Women who stopped using the pill more than 10 years ago do not seem to have any increased risk.

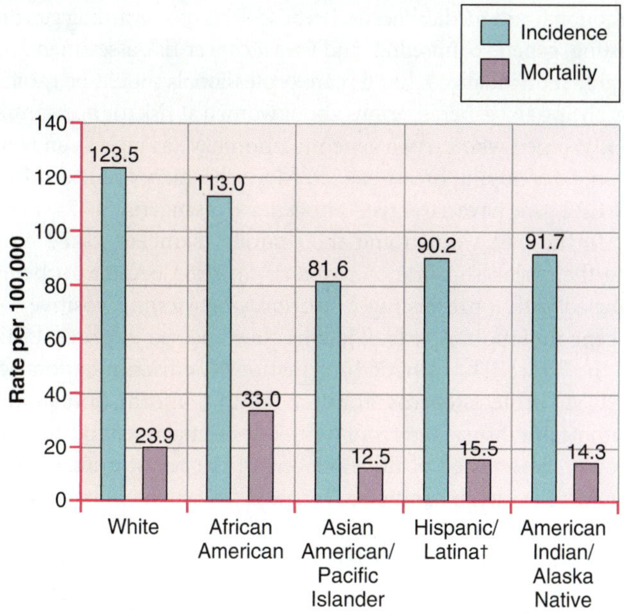

*Rates are age-adjusted to the 2000 US standard population.
†Persons of Hispanic origin may be any race.

Data sources: Incidence – North American Association of Central Cancer Registries, 2009. Incidence data for American Indian/Alaska Natives only includes individuals from Contract Health Service Delivery Areas (CHSDA). Mortality – National Center for Health Statistics, Centers for Disease Control and Prevention, 2009. For Hispanics, information is included for all states except Minnesota, New Hampshire, North Dakota, and the District of Columbia.

American Cancer Society, Surveillance Research, 2009

FIG. 10-1 Female breast cancer incidence and mortality rates by race and ethnicity, U.S. 2002-2006 (From American Cancer Society. [2009]. *Breast cancer facts and figures, 2009-2010.* Atlanta, GA: Author.)

- **Menopausal hormone therapy (MHT):** Either as estrogen replacement therapy (ERT) or hormonal replacement therapy (HRT), MHT has been used for many years to help relieve symptoms of menopause and to help prevent thinning of the bones (osteoporosis).
  - **Combined MHT:** It has become clear that long-term use (several years or more) of combined MHT (estrogen and progestin) (usually prescribed for women who have a uterus) increases the risk of breast cancer. Five years after stopping combined MHT, the risk seems to drop back to normal.
  - **ERT:** The use of estrogen alone (usually prescribed for women without a uterus), does not seem to increase the risk of developing breast cancer. When used long-term (for more than 10 years), some studies have found that ERT increases the risk of ovarian and breast cancer.
- **Not breastfeeding:** Some studies have shown that breastfeeding slightly lowers breast cancer risk, especially if the breastfeeding lasts 1½ to 2 years. This could be because breastfeeding lowers a woman's total number of menstrual periods, as does pregnancy.
- **Alcohol:** Use of alcohol is clearly linked to an increased risk of having breast cancer. Women who have one drink a day have a very small increased risk. Those who have two to five drinks daily have about 1½ times the risk of women who drink no alcohol. The ACS (2010) suggests limiting the amount to one drink per day.
- **Being overweight or obese:** Being overweight or obese is linked to a higher risk of breast cancer, especially for post-menopausal women and if the weight gain took place during adulthood. Central obesity appears to increase this risk even further especially in the post-menopausal woman. The link between weight and breast cancer risk is complex, and studies of fat in the diet as it relates to breast cancer risk have often given conflicting results (ACS, 2009, 2010).
- **Lack of exercise:** Studies show that exercise reduces breast cancer risk. The only question is how much exercise is needed. One study found that as little as 1 hour and 15 minutes to 2½ hours of brisk walking per week reduced the risk by 18%. Walking 10 hours a week reduced the risk a little more (ACS, 2009, 2010).

In addition uncertain risk factors may increase the risk of breast cancer but more research is needed. These factors include:

- **High-fat diets:** Studies of fat in the diet have not clearly shown that this is a breast cancer risk factor. Most studies found that breast cancer is less common in countries where the typical diet is low in fat. On the other hand, many studies of women in the United States have not found the cancer risk to be linked to how much fat they ate. Researchers are still not sure how to explain this difference. More research is needed to better understand the effect of the types of fat eaten and body weight on breast cancer risk.
- **Antiperspirants and bras:** Internet e-mail rumors have suggested that underarm antiperspirants can cause breast cancer. There is very little evidence to support this idea. Also there is no evidence to support the idea that underwire bras cause breast cancer.
- **Abortions:** There is a myth that abortions cause breast cancer. Several studies show that induced abortions do not increase the risk of breast cancer. There is no evidence to show a direct link between miscarriages and breast cancer.
- **Breast implants:** Silicone breast implants can cause scar tissue to form in the breast. But several studies have found that this does not increase breast cancer risk. If a woman has breast implants, she might need special x-ray views during mammograms.
- **Pollution:** Research has been undertaken to learn how the environment might affect breast cancer risk. At this time research does not show a clear link between breast cancer risk and environmental pollutants such as pesticides and polychlorinated biphenyls (PCBs).
- **Tobacco smoke:** Most studies have found no link between active cigarette smoking and breast cancer. An issue that continues to be a focus of research is whether secondhand smoke (smoke from another person's cigarette) may increase the risk of breast cancer. The evidence about secondhand smoke and breast cancer risk in human studies is not entirely clear but is thought to contribute to breast cancer occurrences. A possible link to breast cancer is yet another reason to avoid being around secondhand smoke (Fentiman, Allen, & Hamed, 2005).
- **Night work:** A few studies have suggested that women who work at night (nurses on the night shift, for example) have a higher risk of breast cancer. This is a fairly recent finding, and more studies are being done to look at this issue (Breast Cancer on the night shift, 2007; Stevens, 2009).

Determining a Woman's Risk of Genetically Related Breast Cancer

Although knowing whether one is hereditarily predisposed to breast cancer may have benefits, the extent to which an individual can benefit remains unclear. Confirming one's mutation status may provide a sense of control in life plans, yet may alternatively create high levels of anxiety and distress. Genetic testing can alter decisions regarding family and intimate relationships, childbearing, body image, and quality of life. Regardless of whether results are positive or negative in testing for BRCA1 and BRCA2 mutations, they can have a highly negative effect on women's lives.

Genetic counseling may not be an adequate measure for relieving the ensuing psychologic distress. Women at increased risk for breast cancer need comprehensive information about the benefits and limitations of genetic testing, in addition to alternatives, to ensure that informed decisions can be made about genetic testing. Nurses and other health care professionals should tailor care to women who have undergone genetic testing for hereditary breast cancer or those who plan to undergo testing, and they should impart current information related to these women's specific emotional and medical needs. Because decisions regarding genetic testing, genetic counseling, and breast cancer risk assessment are highly individualized, health care professionals should be careful regarding any generalizations about women at risk for breast cancer. Women who carry a gene mutation have as high as an 80% risk of developing breast cancer. Men who carry the BRCA1 or BRCA2 gene have a 6% risk (Shockney & Tsangaris, 2007).

In the past women and their family members risked having their health insurance coverage canceled because of being labeled with a preexisting condition when testing positive for a gene mutation. A federal law has been passed to prevent this in the future. The Genetic Information Nondiscrimination Act (GINA) protects clients from having that information shared with health insurers or employers. Before enactment of the law, women who tested positive for one of the breast cancer genes could be denied insurance coverage or employment based on a predisposition to developing breast cancer years later. This law (a) prohibits the use of genetic information to deny employment or insurance coverage; (b) ensures that genetic test results are kept private; and (c) prevents an insurer from basing eligibility or premiums on genetic information (Kotz, 2008).

EVIDENCE-BASED PRACTICE

Pat Gingrich

Genetic Risk Assessment for Breast Cancer

ASK THE QUESTION

Is genetic risk assessment for breast cancer beneficial for women? Now that women are able to determine if they have the BRCA1 or BRCA2 mutations, what can they do with that information?

SEARCH FOR EVIDENCE

Search Strategies

Professional organization guidelines, meta-analyses, systematic reviews, randomized controlled trials, nonrandomized prospective studies and retrospective studies since 2007.

Databases Searched

CINAHL, Cochrane, Medline, National Guideline Clearinghouse, Agency for Healthcare Research and Quality, Database and websites for Association of Women's Health, Obstetric and Neonatal Nurses and American Cancer Association.

CRITICALLY ANALYZE THE DATA

Women seeking a risk assessment for breast cancer now have a new and powerful tool: genetic testing. The BRCA1 mutation can greatly predispose a woman to breast cancer, while the BRCA2 can greatly increase the risk for breast and/or ovarian cancer. An accurate reflection of risks could lead to greater psychological well-being and less worry. In a meta-analysis reported in the Cochrane database, women who received genetic risk assessment reported less distress, a more accurate perception of risk, and increased knowledge about breast cancer and genetics (Sivell, Iredale, Gray, & Coles, 2007).

Women with a high risk of breast or ovarian cancer have the choice of risk-reducing surgery or more frequent screening. A study of 517 women, cancer-free but positive for BRCA1 or BRCA2, found that women were more likely to have prophylactic mastectomy and oophorectomy if they have a close family history with breast or ovarian cancer (Metcalfe, Foulkes, Kim-Sing, Ainsworth, Rosen, Armel, et al., 2008). A smaller study of 272 female carriers of the gene noted that predictors for prophylactic surgery were age less than 60 years and previous history of breast or ovarian cancer, and that most made their decision within a median of 4 months (Beattie, Crawford, Lin, Vittinghoff, & Ziegler, 2009).

Women who have already had breast cancer can now assess their risk for recurrence. In a study by the Hereditary Breast Cancer Clinical Study Group, an international cohort of 927 women with hereditary breast cancer were much more likely to undergo prophylactic mastectomy in North America than in Europe (Metcalfe, Lubinski, Ghadirian, Lynch, Kim-Sing, Friedman, et al., 2008). Likewise, the same study revealed that older women and women who chose mastectomy over breast-conserving surgery at the time of original diagnosis were more likely to choose the prophylactic contralateral mastectomy.

IMPLICATIONS FOR PRACTICE

Women at risk for breast and ovarian cancer can have genetic risk assessments that can aid their decision-making and improve their psychological well-being. The regional differences in the decision for prophylactic mastectomy and oophorectomy may indicate a difference in medical opinion, cultural preference, or available medical care and expense. It was not clear what role age plays in the decision-making process. Perhaps young women at high genetic risk might choose to screen frequently, nurse their children, and then undergo the risk-reducing surgery. Much more evidence and ethical guidance is needed to assist women in deciding if and when to have their children tested for the gene.

References

Beattie, M. S., Crawford, B., Lin, F., Vittinghoff, E., & Ziegler, J. (2009). Uptake, time course, and predictors of risk-reducing surgeries in BRCA carriers. *Genetic Testing and Molecular Biomarkers, 13*(1), 51–56.

Metcalfe, K., Foulkes, W., Kim-Sing, C., Ainsworth, P., Rosen, B., Armel, S., et al. (2008). Family history as a predictor of uptake of cancer preventive procedures by women with a BRCA1 or BRCA2 mutation. *Clinical Genetics, 73*(5), 474–479.

Metcalfe, K. A., Lubinski, J., Ghadirian, P., Lynch, H., Kim-Sing, C., Friedman, E., et al. (2008). Predictors of contralateral prophylactic mastectomy in women with a BRCA1 or BRCA2 mutation: The Hereditary Breast Cancer Clinical Group Study Group. *Journal of Clinical Oncology, 26*(7), 1093–1097.

Sivell, S., Iredale, R., Gray, J., & Coles, B. (2007). Cancer genetic risk assessment for individuals at risk of familial cancer. *The Cochrane Database of Systematic Reviews 2007,* 2, CD003721.

Information about breast cancer risks can be confusing, and women can overestimate or underestimate their risks. Women and health professionals can use the Breast Cancer Risk Assessment Tool to calculate risk. This tool was developed and verified by the National Cancer Institute (NCI) to predict the risk of breast cancer in 5 years and over the lifetime (to age 90 years) of a woman. (The risk factors used are in Box 10-1; the tool is available at www.nci.nih.gov/bcrisktool/.)

An accurate estimation of risk for breast cancer is needed in order that women may be given rational management recommendations. During breast cancer risk counseling, facts should be presented to women in a supportive, nondirective way, without personal opinions or preferences. Discussion should also include treatment options and prognosis of breast cancer, as well as risks and benefits of alternative methods of prevention and early diagnosis. A woman's recognition of having increased breast cancer risk can carry psychologic consequences such as anxiety, guilt, depression, and reduced self-esteem. High risk women who pass specific genetic mutations on to their children can experience enormous guilt. Psychologic intervention should be considered to assist these individuals in coping with these significant adverse sequelae (Shockney & Tsangaris, 2007).

Chemoprevention

Ongoing studies by the NCI and other groups are investigating the role of tamoxifen, raloxifene, and anastrozole in the prevention of breast cancer (NCI, 2009). Raloxifene, in postmenopausal women, prevents osteoporosis without the possible increased cancer risks of estrogen therapy. This medication may be an ideal choice for the woman at high risk for both osteoporosis and breast cancer. Tamoxifen has already reduced the recurrence of breast cancer in women with prior breast malignancies. Prevention studies are attempting to identify which women would most benefit from administration of these chemopreventive drugs. Although many women may want to start chemopreventive drugs for breast cancer prevention, the risk of occasional serious side effects demands careful consideration before prescribing these drugs (see later discussion) (Shockney & Tsangaris, 2007).

Pathophysiology

Breast cancer occurs when there are genetic alterations in the deoxyribonucleic acid (DNA) of breast epithelial cells. Many types of breast cancer exist. Genetic alterations, either inherited or spontaneous, are found in the epithelial cells, compromising ductal or lobular tissue. Researchers are investigating which oncogenes (potentially cancer-inducing genes) may cause breast cancer or change its growth pattern and how the process can be stopped.

BOX 10-1 RISK FACTORS INCLUDED IN THE BREAST CANCER RISK ASSESSMENT TOOL

- Woman's age
- Number of first-degree relatives affected
- Age of woman at menarche
- Age of woman at first live birth
- Number of breast biopsies
- History of atypical hyperplasia in biopsy specimens

Breast cancer begins in the epithelial cells lining the mammary ducts of the breast. The rate of breast cancer growth depends on the effect of estrogen and progesterone and other prognostic factors such as its grade, Ki67 score, human epidermal growth factor receptor 2 (HER2)/neu receptor status, and other variables. These cancers can be either invasive (infiltrating) or noninvasive (in situ). Invasive or infiltrating breast cancers can grow into the wall of the mammary duct and into the surrounding tissues.

By far the most frequently occurring cancer of the breast is invasive ductal carcinoma. Ductal carcinoma originates in the lactiferous ducts and invades surrounding breast structures. The tumor is usually unilateral, not well delineated, solid, nonmobile, and nontender.

Lobular carcinoma originates in the lobules of the breasts. This type of breast cancer can be nonpalpable and appear smaller on imaging studies than it actually is.

Nipple carcinoma (Paget's disease) originates in the nipple. It usually occurs with invasive ductal carcinoma and can cause bleeding, oozing, and crusting of the nipple.

A more rare form of breast cancer is known as inflammatory breast cancer. This type of cancer is diagnosed by the appearance of a rash or reddish skin of the breast. It can be misdiagnosed as mastitis. A skin punch biopsy is performed to diagnose it, and the pathology report will state that there are breast cancer cells in the dermal lymphatic channels. It is usually aggressive and is classified as stage II breast cancer from its onset. There are also other types of less common forms of breast cancer such as mucinous and malignant phyllodes tumors.

Breast cancer can invade surrounding tissues in such a way that the primary tumor can have tentacle-like projections (referred to as being a "spiculated mass"). This invasive growth pattern can result in the irregular tumor border felt on palpation. As the tumor grows, fibrosis develops around it and can shorten Cooper's ligaments, which result in the characteristic peau d'orange (orange peel–like skin) changes and edema associated with some breast cancers. If the breast cancer invades the lymphatic channels, tumors can develop in the regional lymph nodes, often occupying the axillary lymph nodes. The tumor may invade the outer layers of skin, creating ulcerations.

Metastasis results from seeding of the breast cancer cells into the blood and lymph systems, leading to tumor development in the bones, the lungs, the brain, and the liver (Table 10-2).

Clinical Manifestations and Diagnosis

Breast cancer in its earliest form can be detected on a mammogram before it can be felt by the woman or her health care provider. It is estimated, however, that women detect 90% of all breast lumps. Of this 90%, only 20% to 25% are malignant. More than half of all lumps are discovered in the upper, outer quadrant of the breast (Fig. 10-2). The most common initial symptom is a lump or thickening of the breast. The lump may feel hard and fixed or soft and spongy. It may have well-defined or irregular borders. It may be fixed to the skin, causing dimpling to occur. A bloody or clear nipple discharge also may be present. Pain may be present in approximately 10% of women.

Unilateral and spontaneous discharge (without nipple manipulation) is associated with mastitis, intraductal papilloma, and cancer. The discharge is usually intermittent and

TABLE 10-2 **STAGING FOR BREAST CANCER***

STAGE	DEFINITION
Stage 0	Carcinoma in situ (intraductal carcinoma, lobular carcinoma, Paget disease) (Tis-N0-M0)
Stage I	Tumor <2 cm with negative nodes (T1-N0-M0) (includes microinvasive T1, <0.1 cm)
Stage IIA	Tumor 0 to 2 cm with positive nodes (including micrometastasis N1, or <0.2 cm), or 2 to 5 cm with negative nodes (T0-N1, T1-N1, T2-N0, all M0)
Stage IIB	Tumor 2 to 5 cm with positive nodes or >5 cm with negative nodes (T2-N1, T3-N0, all M0)
Stage IIIA	No evidence of primary tumor or tumor <2 cm with involved fixed lymph nodes, or tumor >5 cm with involved movable or nonmovable nodes (T0-N2, T1-N2, T2-N2, T3-N1, T3-N2, all M0)
Stage IIIB	Tumor of any size with direct extension to chest wall or skin, with or without involved lymph nodes, or any size tumor with involved internal mammary lymph nodes (T4–any N, any T–N3, all M0)
Stage IV	Any distant metastasis (includes ipsilateral supraclavicular nodes) (any T, any N) (all M1)

*Breast cancer is most frequently staged according to the TNM classification system, which evaluates the tumor size (T), involvement of regional lymph nodes (N), and distant spread of the disease or metastases (M).
Source: From National Cancer Institute. (2010). *Staging information for breast cancer.* Available at www.cancer/gov/cancertopics/pdq/treatment/breast/healthprofessional/pge4#section_30. www.nccn.org. Accessed June 9, 2010.

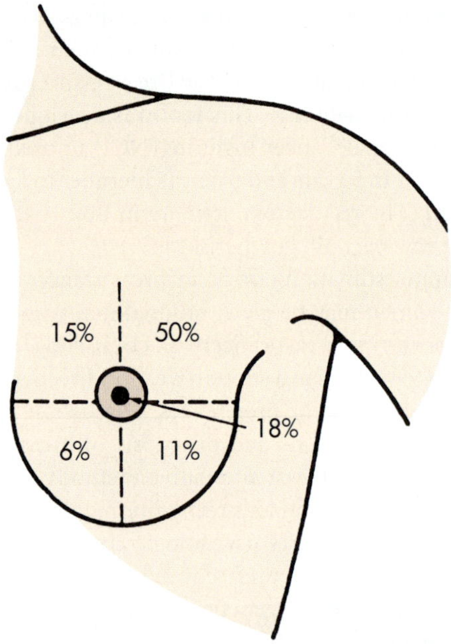

FIG. 10-2 Relative location of malignant lesions of the breast. (Modified from DiSaia, P., & Creasman, W. [2007]. *Clinical gynecologic oncology* [8th ed.]. St. Louis: Mosby.)

persistent and may be clear, serous, green-gray, purulent, serosanguineous, or sanguineous. Women with these findings need a complete diagnostic workup to determine the actual cause of their symptoms.

As a general principle, any unilateral breast symptom (i.e., mass, discharge, pain, or itching) is a more ominous finding than a bilateral symptom. However, all findings must be carefully followed up to avoid missing a serious diagnosis such as cancer. A delay in treatment may adversely affect the woman's subsequent prognosis and treatment options.

Early detection and diagnosis reduce the mortality rate because the cancer is found when it is smaller, lesions are more localized, and there tends to be a lower percentage of positive nodes. Therefore it is imperative that protocols for assessment and diagnosis be established. The use of clinical examination by a qualified health care provider and screening **mammography** (x-ray filming of the breast) (Fig. 10-3) may aid in the early detection of breast cancers. BSE may be beneficial and can lead to a woman reporting new breast symptoms promptly to her health care provider (see Chapter 4). Table 10-3 lists the recommendations of the ACS for breast cancer screening (ACS, 2010). These recommendations stand despite a 2009 recommendation from the U.S. Preventive Services Task Force (USPSTF, 2009) to make changes. Box 10-2 provides the USPSTF recommendations and selected responses from professional organizations.

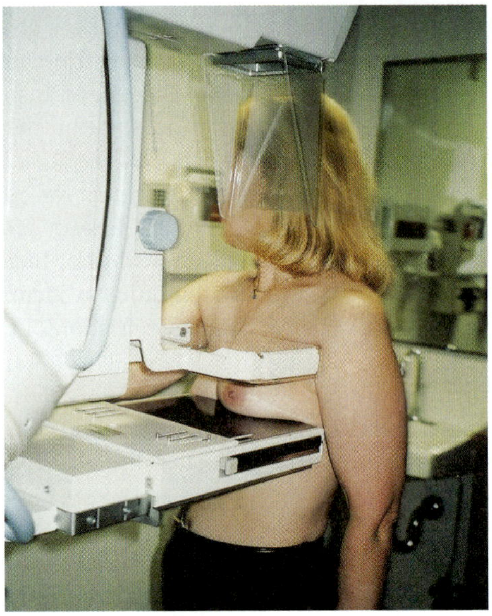

FIG. 10-3 Mammography. (Courtesy Shannon Perry, Phoenix, AZ.)

Research has suggested that the major obstacles to breast cancer screening include older age; fiscal barriers (e.g., expense, lack of health insurance); knowledge, attitudinal and behavioral barriers (e.g., fear, ignorance, lack of motivation); and organizational barriers (e.g., scheduling problems, lack of availability of mammography services, lack of physician referral) (Shockney & Tsangaris, 2007). Strategies that may be helpful to health care providers in improving screening for breast cancer include education and encouragement of older women, continuing education of providers, provision of information about new and affordable screening options, use of reminder systems in office practice, use of client-directed literature, and interventions that will reward, support, and prompt desired screening behaviors (Shockney & Tsangaris). In addition, it is important for a practitioner to assess the technique of a woman who is practicing BSE.

Cultural factors may influence a woman's decision to participate in breast cancer screening. Knowledge of these factors and use of culturally sensitive, tailored messages and materials that appeal to the unique concerns, beliefs, and reading abilities of target groups of underutilizers may assist the nurse in helping women overcome barriers to seeking care (see Cultural Considerations box).

CULTURAL CONSIDERATIONS

Breast Screening Practices

Certain minority women tend to have low compliance rates in the use of early screening methods for breast cancer. Many factors play a role in influencing the screening practices of these women. African-American women reported not participating in early breast cancer screening because of discomfort with impersonal care from providers, lack of health care insurance, lack of funds to pay for mammograms, lack of awareness of community assistance within the health care system, lack of access to transportation, and feelings of fatalism, fear, helplessness, and powerlessness. Hispanic women cited lack of a regular physician, lack of health insurance coverage, inaccessibility of screening facilities, lack of access to transportation, and being unable to obtain time off from work. Asian women cited unawareness of mammography tests, gender and modesty concerns unique to their cultural beliefs, and fear resulting from a sense of vulnerability to breast cancer.

Interventions that will encourage minority women to participate in early breast cancer screening practices begin with the development of culturally sensitive community education programs designed to help women overcome barriers to reaching optimal levels of health. Programs should be designed to educate small groups of women about risk factors of breast cancer, prevention strategies, and early detection methods. Recruitment of women may be communicated through fliers in neighborhoods, women's groups, churches, clubs, and organizations. Use of incentives to reward participation may be helpful. Nurses and guest speakers of similar ethnicity as the attending group who are breast cancer survivors would be valuable in providing meaningful information and support, and providing past, present, and future perspective to the educational content.

Sources: Ansell, D., Grabler, P., Whitman, S., Ferrans, C., Burgess-Bishop, J., Murray, L., et al. (2009). A community effort to reduce the black/white breast cancer mortality disparity in Chicago. *Cancer Causes & Control, 20*(9), 1681-1688; Han, H., Lee, J., Kim, J., Headen, H., Song, H., & Kim, A. (2009). A meta-analysis of interventions to promote mammography among ethnic minority women. *Nursing Research, 58*(4), 246-254; Sim, H., Seah, M., & Tan, M. (2009). Breast cancer knowledge and screening practices: A survey of 1,000 Asian women. *Singapore Medical Journal, 50*(2), 132-138.

Mammography today remains the gold standard for breast cancer screening and early detection. New technologies that are considered for breast cancer screening must equal or exceed the performance of screen-film mammography to be accepted as screening tools for breast cancer. In other words, these technologies must demonstrate identification of more breast cancers that are missed by mammography, such as a higher fraction of early stage cancers (stages 0 and I), and be cost-effective, noninvasive, and available and acceptable to clients. Full field digital mammography (FFDM) is much like standard film mammography in that x-rays are used to produce an image of the breast. Film mammography is captured on x-ray film, however, and digital mammography is recorded using a computer. Digital mammography has proven to be more accurate in identifying subtle abnormalities within the breast architecture and as a result of research studies has proven to be 28% more accurate in identifying cancer than traditional film mammography (Pisano, Acharyya, Cole, Marques, Yaffe, Blevins, et al., 2009). These images enable the radiologist to enlarge the image as well as lighten and darken the background contrast, finding abnormalities that may go undetected with film mammography. It is also critically important that the radiologist reading the mammograms be expert in doing so. Studies have verified that general radiologists reviewing mammograms can miss the presence of breast cancer on imaging 41% of the time compared to dedicated breast imaging radiologists who specialize in breast imaging and read a large volume of mammograms weekly (Ciatto, Ambroghetti, Morrone, & Del Turco, 2006). An additional method to assist radiologists with reading mammograms, which can be important for facilities who do not have dedicated breast imaging radiologists, is computer-aided detection and diagnosis (CAD). For nearly two decades this device has been in use to help radiologists find suspicious changes on mammography studies. This can be especially important for film mammography evaluation. CAD electronically scans the mammogram first. It can detect tumors or other breast abnormalities and flag them for the radiologist to further investigate (ACS, 2010).

TABLE 10-3 SCREENING GUIDELINES FOR EARLY BREAST CANCER DETECTION

AGE (YR)	EXAMINATION	FREQUENCY
Average Risk for Asymptomatic Women		
20-39	Breast self-examination (BSE)	Not specified; inform women about the benefits and limitations of BSE, offer instructions; women may choose to perform regularly, irregularly, or not at all
	Clinical breast examination	At least every 3 years
40 and older	BSE	Not specified; inform women about the benefits and limitations of BSE, offer instructions; women may choose to perform regularly, irregularly, or not at all
	Clinical breast examination	Yearly
	Mammography	Yearly
High Risk Women (>20% Lifetime Risk)		
30 and older*	MRI and mammogram	Yearly
Moderate Risk Women (15% to 20% Lifetime Risk)		
30 and older*	MRI and mammogram	Decision about frequency made between physician and woman after discussing benefits and limitations of MRI screening

*The best age to start should be decided between physician and woman after looking at her individual status.

Source: American Cancer Society. (2010). *Cancer facts and figures, 2010.* Atlanta: Author.

A screening mammogram is performed on women who do not have any signs or symptoms of a breast abnormality. Diagnostic mammograms are performed when a screening mammogram identifies something warranting further inspection or if the woman or her physician or nurse finds a symptom such as a lump, nipple discharge, or other breast symptom that is new.

One of the most valuable uses of mammography is the identification of calcifications within the breast. Though most are benign, some can be an early sign of breast cancer. There are two types of calcifications:

- Macrocalcifications are mineral deposits that are most likely changes in the breast caused by aging of the breast arteries, old injuries, or inflammation. They appear as large white dots or dashes. These deposits are related to noncancerous conditions and do not require a biopsy. These types of

BOX 10-2 SCREENING FOR BREAST CANCER

In a 2009 Clinical Guidelines update, the U.S. Preventive Services Task Force made the following recommendations about screening for breast cancer:

- Recommended against routine screening mammography in women ages 40 to 49
- Recommended biennial screening mammography for women between ages 50 and 70
- Concluded there was insufficient evidence to assess the benefits and harms of screening mammography for women older than the age of 75
- Recommended against teaching breast self-examination (BSE)
- Concluded there was insufficient evidence to assess benefits and harms of clinical breast examination as a supplement to mammography in women older than age 40
- Concluded there was insufficient evidence to assess benefits and harms of digital mammography or magnetic resonance imaging (MRI) as screening tools for breast cancer

In response to these guidelines, several professional organizations issued the following statements:

- The American Cancer Society stated the organization would continue to recommend annual screening with mammography and clinical breast examinations for women ages 40 and older.
- The American College of Obstetricians and Gynecologists (ACOG) would continue to recommend screening mammography every 1 to 2 years for women ages 40 to 49 and yearly screening for women ages 50 and older. ACOG also will continue to recommend BSE.
- The American College of Radiology (ACR) and the Society of Breast Imaging recommend breast cancer screening with mammography to begin by age 40 and earlier for women at high risk for breast cancer.

These professional organizations and others that provide care for women will continue to be committed to finding better screening tests for breast cancer and will update their guidelines and recommendations as new evidence is found through research. Nurses must support their clients who have concerns about the changing recommendations and the effect on their health care. They must also keep themselves informed of the changes in recommendations so they can be better advocates for women.

Source: American Cancer Society (ACS). (2009). Press release. *American Cancer Society responds to changes to USPSTF mammography guidelines 11/16/09.* Available at www.cancer.org. Accessed June 9, 2010; American College of Obstetricians and Gynecologists (ACOG). (2009). *Response of the American College of Obstetricians and Gynecologists to new breast cancer screening recommendations from the U.S. Preventive Services Task Force 11/16/09.* Available at www.acog.org. Accessed June 9, 2010; Lee, C., Dershaw, D., Kopans, D., Evans, P., Monsees, B., Monticciolo, D., et al. (2010). Breast cancer screening with imaging: Recommendations from the Society of Breast Imaging and the ACR on the use of mammography, breast MRI, breast ultrasound, and other technologies for the detection of clinically occult breast cancer. *Journal of the American College of Radiology, 7*(1), 18-27; U.S. Preventive Services Task Force. (2009). Clinical guidelines: Screening for breast cancer: U.S. Preventive Services Task Force recommendation statement. *Annals of Internal Medicine, 151*(10), 716-726.

calcifications are found in about half of women older than age 50 and in 1 in 10 women younger than 50.

- Microcalcifications are fine white specks of calcium in the breast. They may be alone or in clusters and resemble grains of sand or salt. These can be more concerning depending on their pattern and shape. Those that are tightly clustered together and have irregular edges can be a sign of ductal carcinoma in situ (DCIS) or early stage I breast cancer, and warrant biopsy.

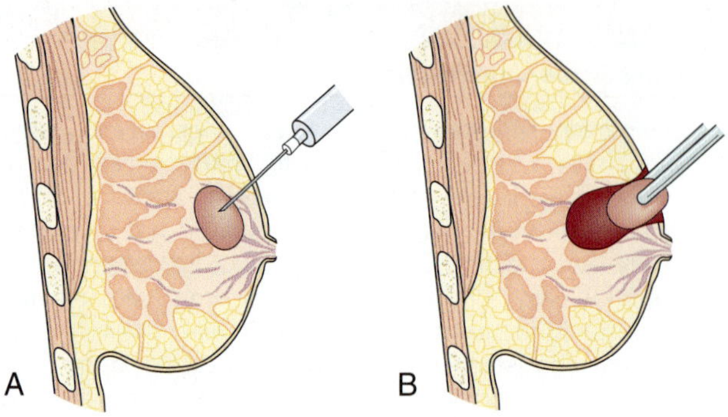

FIG. 10-4 Diagnosis. **A,** Needle aspiration. **B,** Open biopsy.

Mammography does have its limitations. It has not proven helpful in screening younger women due to the high breast density associated with youth. Roughly 80% of breast cancer can be identified through the application of mammography when combined with clinical breast examination; however, 20% may be missed (Shockney & Tsangaris, 2007). Ultrasound has become a valuable screening adjunct to mammography, especially for women with significant breast density. It is cost-effective, noninvasive, and widely available. Ultrasound has been helpful in distinguishing between fluid-filled masses (cysts) and solid masses (benign and malignant). It uses high-frequency sound waves to assess the breast tissue and axillae. The test is painless and noninvasive and requires no exposure to radiation. It has also been useful in performing image-guided biopsies (ACS, 2010).

MRI has also become a valuable screening adjunct to mammography and ultrasound. MRI of the breast has shown an overall sensitivity to breast cancer of 96%. However, factors such as cost, lack of standardized examination technique and interpretation criteria, insensitivity to microcalcifications, and higher rate of false-positive results than mammography have caused concern regarding the potential of breast MRI as a screening method (Shockney & Tsangaris, 2007). There is growing popularity to use it for women diagnosed with breast cancer to rule out the presence of multicentric disease and determine the size of tumors (such as invasive lobular carcinomas), and it has been used increasingly for women who are identified as high risk (such as those who carry a BRCA gene mutution).

When a suspicious finding on a mammogram is noted or a lump is detected, diagnosis is confirmed by core needle biopsy (stereotactically or ultrasound-guided core), or by needle localization biopsy (Fig. 10-4). The latter procedure requires the collaborative efforts of both the radiologist and the surgeon. This often requires that the procedure take place in two different environments (radiology and surgery), so women need specific information regarding procedures, duration, and outcomes. In most facilities, core biopsies can be performed and the pathology results known the following day, providing the woman with rapid results. Recognizing the woman's high anxiety level is important, and the sooner the outcome of the biopsy can be provided the sooner she can have her fears allayed or confirmed.

Prognosis

Major advances have been made in the understanding of the biology of cancer. Breast cancer is thought to be a systemic disease, which means that micrometastasis could be present at the initial

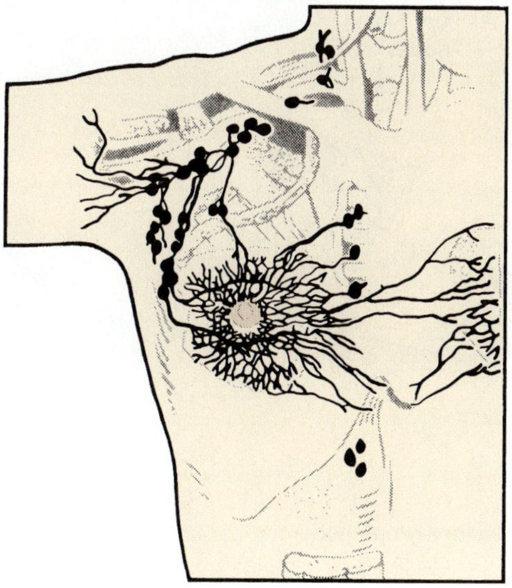

FIG. 10-5 Lymphatic spread of breast cancer.

presentation with or without nodal involvement. The area in which affected lymph nodes are located also is prognostic. The involvement of axillary lymph nodes worsens the prognosis of breast cancer. Nodal involvement and tumor size remain the most significant prognostic criteria for long-term survival (Fig. 10-5).

Other biologic factors have been shown to be helpful in predicting response to therapy or survival. These factors include estrogen receptor assay, progesterone receptor assay, tumor *ploidy* (the amount of DNA in a tumor cell compared with that in a normal cell), S-phase index or growth rate (the percentage of cells in the S phase of cellular division done by flow cytometric determinations of the S-phase fraction), Ki67 (another proliferation marker), and histologic or nuclear grade (Shockney & Tsangaris, 2007). Estrogen and progesterone receptors are proteins in the cell cytoplasm and surface of some breast cancer cells. When these receptors are present, they bind to estrogen or progesterone, and binding promotes growth of the cancer cell. A breast cancer can have estrogen or progesterone receptors (ERs, PRs) or both types. It is valuable to know the ER status of the cancer to predict which women will respond to hormone therapy (Nelson, Fu, Griffin, Nygren, Smith, & Humphrey, 2009). Molecular and biologic factors are valuable indicators for prognosis and treatment of breast cancer. HER2, which is associated with cell growth, is overexpressed in 30% of all breast cancers and is associated with loss of cell regulation and uncontrolled cell proliferation. Thus a positive HER2 status is associated with aggressive tumors, poor prognosis, and resistance to certain chemotherapeutic drugs (ACS, 2010).

CARE MANAGEMENT

Controversy continues regarding the best treatment of breast cancer. Nodal involvement, tumor size, receptor status, and aggressiveness are important variables for treatment selection. Medical management of breast cancer includes surgery, breast reconstruction, radiation therapy, adjuvant hormone therapy, biologic targeted therapy, and chemotherapy. Many women face difficult decisions about the various treatment options. Box 10-3 lists questions that must be addressed in decision making.

BOX 10-3 DECISION-MAKING QUESTIONS TO ASK

1. What kind of breast cancer is it (invasive or noninvasive)?
2. What is the stage of the cancer (i.e., how extensive is the spread)?
3. Did the cancer test positive for hormone (estrogen)? (May be slower growing)
4. What further tests are recommended?
5. What are the treatment options? (Pros and cons of each, including side effects)
6. If surgery is recommended, what will the scar look like?
7. If a mastectomy is done, can breast reconstruction be done (at the time of surgery or later)?
8. How long will the woman be in the hospital? What kind of postoperative care will she need?
9. How long will treatment last if radiation or chemotherapy is recommended? What effects can the woman expect from these treatments?
10. What community resources are available for support?

Source: American Cancer Society. (2009). *Detailed Guide: Breast cancer. What should you ask your doctor about breast cancer?* Available at www.cancer.org/docroot/cri/content/cri_2_4_5x_what_you_should_ask_your_physician_about_breast_cancer_5.asp?sitearea=. Accessed June 9, 2010.

CLINICAL REASONING

Breast Cancer Treatment Options

Beth is a 34-year-old with stage I breast cancer. Her family history includes her mother being diagnosed with breast cancer at age 50 and her maternal aunt being diagnosed with ovarian cancer at age 44. Both succumbed to their diseases. Her menstrual periods started at age 10. She has one sibling, a sister, aged 39, who has had no breast health issues. Beth is divorced, has two young children, one in elementary school and one in daycare, and is employed full-time as a real estate agent. She states that she is scared and doesn't want to have a mastectomy but thinks she should because she has heard that is the best treatment for long-term survival. How would you respond to this statement?

1. Evidence—Is there sufficient evidence to draw conclusions about what the nurse should say?
2. Assumptions—What assumptions can be made about the following issues?
   a. Differences between breast-conserving surgery and mastectomy for stage I cancer
   b. Genetic and family risk factors
   c. Psychosocial and socioeconomic needs of single parent facing breast cancer treatment
3. What implications and priorities for nursing care can be made at this time?
4. Does the evidence objectively support your conclusion?
5. Are there alternative perspectives to your conclusion?

Surgery

After a diagnosis of breast cancer is made, surgical treatment options are offered to the woman. The most frequently recommended surgical approaches for the treatment of breast cancer are lumpectomy and total simple mastectomy. A **lumpectomy** (Fig. 10-6) involves the removal of the breast tumor and a small amount of surrounding healthy tissue to ensure there are clean margins. **Partial mastectomy** (see Fig 10-6, *B*) includes *tylectomy, wide excision,* and *quadrantectomy* or *segmental mastectomy*

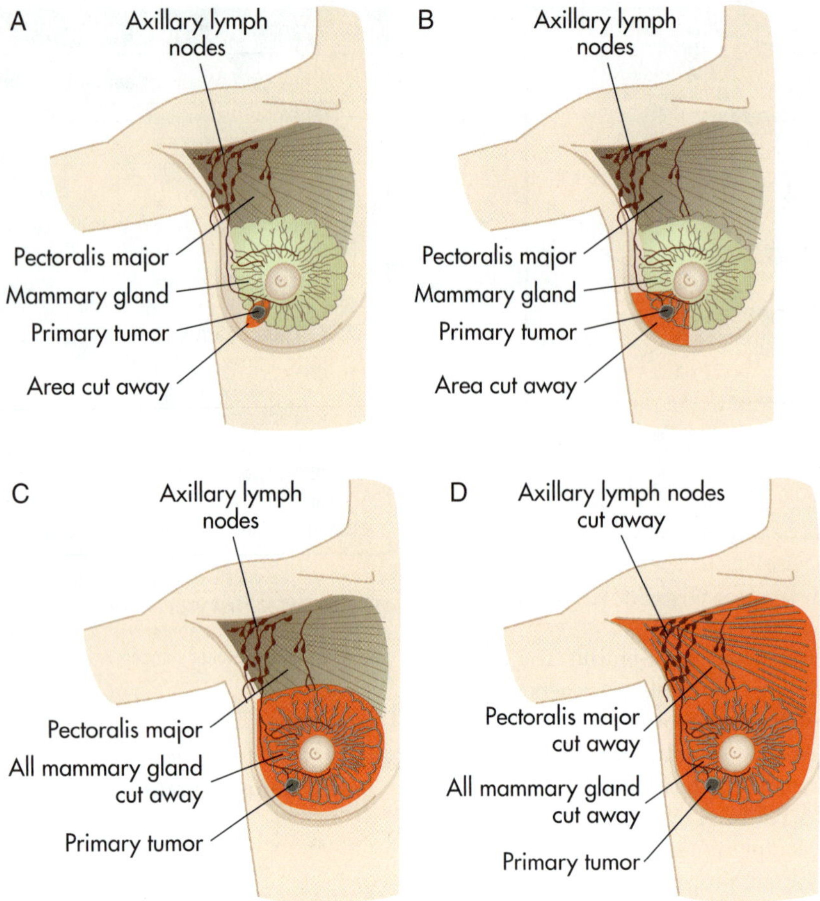

FIG. 10-6 Surgical alternatives for breast cancer. **A,** Lumpectomy. **B,** Partial mastectomy. **C,** Total (simple) mastectomy. **D,** Radical mastectomy.

and involves removal of the tumor, which may be larger, along with a rim of healthy tissue around it, again to ensure clear margins. For women whose breast cancer is invasive, a sentinel node biopsy will be performed. The sentinel node is the first node that receives lymphatic drainage from the tumor, and is identified by injecting vital blue dye or radioactive dye in the area surrounding the tumor. A small incision in the axilla allows for identification of the blue-stained lymphatic channel leading to the blue sentinel node, either visually or by gamma probe. This node then can be removed and examined for the presence of tumor cells, as opposed to an entire axillary dissection.

It is helpful in determining the need for adjunctive systemic treatment by indicating whether nodes are positive for metastatic cells. Lymphatic mapping and sentinel node biopsy are minimally invasive techniques that identify women with axillary node involvement.

Clinical trials have reported identification of the sentinel node in more than 95% of cases, with false-negative rates for predicting axillary nodal metastases of less than 5% (Krag, Ashikaga, Harlow, Skelly, Julian, Brown, et al., 2009; Quan, Wells, McCready, Wright, Fraser, & Gagliardi, 2010).

Identification of the sentinel node is usually done through a separate incision at the time of these procedures, and surgery is usually followed by radiation therapy to the remaining breast tissue (DiSaia & Creasman, 2007). These procedures are used for the primary treatment of women with early stage (I or II) breast cancer. Lumpectomy offers survival equivalent to that of having a total simple mastectomy (DiSaia & Creasman).

Additional criteria for recommending lumpectomy/partial mastectomy are as follows: a tumor that is relatively small compared to breast volume; no previous breast radiation; no previous mantle field radiation (area includes neck, chest, and underarm lymph nodes) as a youth; and no evidence of multicentric disease.

Mastectomy is the removal of the breast, including the nipple and areola. Women who are advised to have mastectomy instead of lumpectomy are women who have:

- Had radiation to the breast
- Multiple tumors in the breast occupying several quadrants of the breast
- Extensive DCIS that occupies a large area of the breast tissue
- A large tumor compared to breast volume

Deciding which mastectomy to have will be guided by the breast surgeon, but as always the woman should have an active part in any decisions that directly affect her treatment. There are several different types of mastectomies. These include:

- **Total simple mastectomy:** This is removal of the breast, nipple and areola. No lymph nodes from the axillae are taken. Recovery from this procedure, if no reconstruction is done at the same time, is usually 1 to 2 weeks. Hospitalization varies; for some it may be an outpatient procedure, whereas other women may require an overnight stay (see Fig 10-6, *C*).
- **Modified radical mastectomy:** This procedure is removal of the breast, nipple and areola as well as axillary node dissection. Recovery, when surgery is done without reconstruction, is usually 2 to 3 weeks.

- **Skin-sparing mastectomy:** This is the removal of the breast, nipple and areola, keeping the outer skin of the breast intact. It is a special method of performing a mastectomy that allows for a good cosmetic outcome when combined with a reconstruction done at the same time. A tissue expander may also be placed as a space holder for later reconstruction.
- **Nipple-sparing mastectomy:** This kind of mastectomy is reserved for a smaller number of women with tumors that are not near the nipple areola area. The surgeon makes an incision on the outer side of the breast or around the edge of the areola and hollows out the breast, removing the areola and keeping the nipple intact. Sometimes the completed reconstruction is performed at the same time and in other cases, a tissue expander is inserted as a space holder for later reconstruction.
- **Nipple- and areola-sparing mastectomy:** In this procedure, the surgeon makes an incision on the side of the breast or in some cases, around the edge of the areola. The breast is hollowed out and reconstruction is performed at the same time. In some cases, a tissue expander may be placed as a space holder for later reconstruction.
- **Scar-sparing mastectomy:** In this procedure, the affected breast is hollowed out. Whether done as skin sparing, nipple sparing, areola sparing or a combination, one goal of this surgery is to minimize visible surgical incisions. It is not uncommon for an entire mastectomy procedure to be performed through an opening that is less than 2 inches in length.
- **Preventive/prophylactic mastectomy:** Prophylactic mastectomy is designed to remove one or both breasts in order to dramatically reduce the risk of developing breast cancer. Women who test positive for certain genetic mutations like BRCA1 and BRCA2, or who have a strong family history of breast cancer, may elect this kind of surgery. They may also elect to have their ovaries removed at the same time. Genetic counseling may help to confirm or eliminate any nagging suspicion about family history. When this type of mastectomy is performed, no lymph nodes need to be removed because there is no evidence of cancer present. It is necessary to have a mammogram performed within 90 days of the procedure to ensure that it is healthy breast tissue being removed for preventive purposes.

Breast Reconstruction

The goals of surgical breast reconstruction are achievement of symmetry and preservation of body image. Surgical reconstruction can be done immediately or at a later date. Immediate reconstruction at the time of mastectomy does not change survival rates or interfere with therapy or the treatment of recurrent disease. It is important that women be aware of this. Women choosing surgical reconstruction offer the following rationale for reconstructive surgery: the need to feel complete again, to avoid using an external prosthesis, to achieve symmetry, to decrease self-consciousness about appearance, and to enhance femininity.

In the past 10 years major achievements have been made in breast reconstruction following mastectomy surgery. No longer do women need to face long, jagged scars that affect their self-image. Instead, advanced techniques have given plastic surgeons the tools to rebuild a woman's breast in such a way that her silhouette is once again whole.

Women with breast cancer have two main considerations when considering reconstructive surgery—when to have surgery and what type of surgery to have. The options for when to have reconstruction are:

- **Simultaneous reconstruction:** Women have the option to have immediate reconstruction of their breast(s) at the same time as their mastectomy. This is a reasonable option for women who do not need breast irradiation.
- **"Staged" reconstruction:** Many women who require radiation therapy are advised to have staged reconstruction. If radiation is done on a newly reconstructed breast, over time it can alter its cosmetic appearance, making an implant hard, painful, deformed, contracted, or even exposed. It may also cause severe fibrosis or shrinkage of the fatty tissue that may have been used in rebuilding the breast.
- **Delayed reconstruction:** A woman may opt for delayed reconstruction if, after her mastectomy, a plastic surgeon was not involved. Many women who did not know their options at the time of mastectomy fall into this category. More and more these women are discovering that surgically re-creating their breasts is possible and is required to be covered by insurance as a result of a federal law passed in 1998.

The types of surgical option for breast reconstruction include implants and flap procedures. Implants are made out of silicone or saline or a combination of both, and can be inserted at the same time as a mastectomy or later. They are placed underneath the chest muscle versus on top of it, as in the case of breast augmentation. Silicone implants have been deemed safe and are an option for women having breast reconstruction following mastectomy.

Flap procedures are done by plastic and reconstructive surgeons who specialize in microsurgery. During flap reconstruction, a breast is created using tissue taken from other parts of the body, such as the abdomen, back, buttocks, or thighs, which is then transplanted to the chest by reconnecting the blood vessels to new ones in the chest region. Due to the high level of skill required for microsurgery, as well as the equipment and staff needed, these techniques are available only at specialized centers. Most breast centers are still performing flap surgery the "old fashioned" way if they do not have surgeons with these skills. These older procedures (transverse rectus abdominis myocutaneous [TRAM] flaps and latissimus dorsi flaps) result in the woman sacrificing either her abdominal muscles or her upper back muscles. Although these procedures were the best options decades ago, there is a higher risk of hernia, weakness, abdominal bulging, and limits on physical activity when these older procedures are performed. There are no physical limitations when today's more sophisticated procedures are performed (Hedén, Bronz, Elberg, Deraemaecker, Murphy, Slicton, et al., 2009). Table 10-4 compares the advantages and disadvantages of the various reconstruction options.

After a woman has recovered from initial reconstructive surgery, she may choose to have nipple and areolar reconstruction. Nipple reconstruction is achieved by using an autologous skin graft to construct a nipple, either from tissue from

TABLE 10-4 **RECONSTRUCTIVE BREAST SURGERY OPTIONS**

NAME OF OPTION	BRIEF DESCRIPTION	ADVANTAGES	DISADVANTAGES
Simultaneous reconstruction	Reconstruction of the breasts done at the same time as surgery to remove the cancer	• The woman wakes up with a breast mound already in place, having been spared the experience of seeing herself with no breast at all. • The process is done in the shortest time possible and is not a series of complex surgeries over a length of time.	• If there is a recurrence of the cancer, the reconstruction may need to be modified. • If there are postsurgery complications, the woman may need to have more surgeries. • Small revision surgeries or matching procedures on the opposing breast may be required. • Rarely it is determined that a woman will need radiation, which can compromise reconstructed breast tissue.
Staged reconstruction	This reconstruction involves placement of a temporary tissue expander at time of mastectomy. The expander gradually stretches the muscle and skin in preparation for either an implant or flap reconstruction.	• The surgeon creates a natural "pocket" in which a permanent implant or a tissue flap may be placed. • The overall result is more symmetric, natural, and aesthetically pleasing. • It allows a woman to complete radiation treatment while having a "placeholder" implanted. • It allows enough time to make sure all of the cancer has been treated.	• It takes longer to "complete" the breast cancer process. • During the time of temporary tissue expansion, the breasts do not look natural. • Small revision surgeries or matching procedures on the opposing breast may be required.
Delayed reconstruction	This reconstruction happens after all of the recommended treatment is completed.	• Some women aren't comfortable weighing all the options at once when they are struggling with a diagnosis of cancer. • Some women need time to come to terms with losing their breast(s). • Some women who are overweight, smokers, or who have high blood pressure may be advised to wait. • It allows enough time to make sure all of the cancer has been treated.	• It takes longer to "complete" the breast cancer process. • Women may not feel whole without their breast(s).
Implant	A breast implant is a silicone shell filled with either silicone gel or a saltwater solution known as saline.	• The recovery from the initial expander placement surgery and from the permanent implant placement surgery is usually quicker than flap surgery. • It may be easier to control the final size of the reconstructed breast with implant reconstruction. • There are no additional scars on the woman's body other than those on the breasts. • For women without excess fatty tissue and who do not require radiation treatment, implants are a good choice, one with good final results.	• Because most women require placement of an expander first followed by secondary replacement of the expander with an implant, this type of reconstruction almost always requires at least two surgical stages and multiple visits to the plastic surgeon's office between these stages for tissue expansion. • It is important to realize that for women who are having a unilateral (one-sided) mastectomy, matching the other natural breast with an implant can be difficult. The shape and feel of an implant are not exactly like that of a natural breast. • In the short term, implants can become infected or malpositioned and require surgery to correct these problems. • Implant-based reconstruction is not generally recommended if women require radiation, due to the risk of complications. In the longer term, implants can develop capsular contracture (tightening of the soft tissues around the implant), implant malposition, and implant rupture. • In the case of complications secondary procedures may be required.
Deep inferior epigastic perforator (DIEP) flap, Superficial inferior epigastric artery (SIEA) flap, Bilateral simultaneous superior gluteal artery perforator (SGAP) flaps	The DIEP flap is the technique in which skin and tissue (no muscle) is taken from the abdomen in order to re-create the breast. Other flap techniques, called the SIEA flap and the SGAP flap take tissue from the lower abdomen or lateral buttock regions.	• Because the reconstruction involves using the woman's own tissues, the risks of implant reconstruction are avoided, particularly in the case of radiation. • Most women have less postoperative pain than after a TRAM flap and are therefore able to leave the hospital sooner and return to normal activities quicker than after a TRAM flap. • Because the abdominal muscle is not removed as in the TRAM flap, women have much less risk of developing hernias, bulges, and core weakness at the site where the flap is removed. This advantage is much greater in bilateral (both sides) reconstruction. • It is typically easier to match the contralateral natural breast with the woman's own tissue when compared with implant reconstruction. • Women essentially end up with a "tummy tuck," "bottom lift," or other cosmetic benefits at the same time as the breast reconstruction.	• DIEP/SIEA/SGAP flap reconstruction generally requires a longer and more challenging surgery at the first stage when compared with implants or TRAM flaps. • Women will have a scar across the lower abdomen or the upper part of the buttock where the flap is obtained. However, this does not differ from the TRAM flap as the abdominal scars are equivalent. • Small revision surgeries or matching procedures on the opposing breast or donor site may be required. • Women who smoke, are obese, or who have diabetes are not ideal candidates for this type of surgery.

TABLE 10-4 **RECONSTRUCTIVE BREAST SURGERY OPTIONS—cont'd**

NAME OF OPTION	BRIEF DESCRIPTION	ADVANTAGES	DISADVANTAGES
Transverse rectus abdominis myocutaneous (TRAM) flap	In a pedicle TRAM flap, the tissue remains attached to its original site, retaining its blood supply. The flap, consisting of the skin, fat, and muscle with its blood supply, is tunneled beneath the skin to the chest, creating a pocket for an implant or, in some cases, creating the breast mound itself, without need for an implant. The free TRAM flap involves less muscle.	• Shorter and less complex surgery than the other flaps	• This was state of the art decades ago and has since been replaced by other, more advanced procedures. • The woman may have more postoperative pain and longer hospital stays. • There is a risk of abdominal bulge or hernias, and as a result there might be a limit to how much weight the woman can lift. • Other newer procedures may offer more natural results.

Source: Shockney, L., & Tsangaris, T. (2008). *Johns Hopkins breast cancer handbook for health care professionals.* Sudbury, MA: Jones and Bartlett.

the remaining nipple or from a donor site. Tiny flaps from the new breast itself also may be used. This outpatient procedure requires local anesthesia, intravenous sedation, or a combination of both, depending on how much sensation has returned to the breast. The procedure lasts about an hour and, 4 weeks later, tattooing may be used to create an areola and match the color of the natural nipple (Valea & Katz, 2007).

Radiation

As mentioned, the conservative approach to treatment involves lumpectomy followed by radiation therapy as standard therapy for early stage breast cancer. Radiation to the breast destroys tumor cells remaining after manipulation and handling of the tumor during surgery. The total recommended radiation dose is 4500 to 5000 cGy over a 6- to 8-week period. A booster dose of up to 1000 cGy may be prescribed with the use of either implants or external beam irradiation (Shockney & Tsangaris, 2007). The risk of local recurrence depends on several treatment factors such as extent of breast resection, tumor margins, technical details of radiation therapy, and the use of adjuvant systemic therapy. Although radiation after lumpectomy surgery is standard protocol, some large breast tumors (due to the disease being locally advanced) may be irradiated before surgery to facilitate easier surgical removal. Side effects of radiation therapy include swelling and heaviness in the breast, sunburn-like skin changes in the treated area, and fatigue. Changes to the breast tissue and skin usually resolve in 6 to 12 months. The breast may become smaller and firmer after radiation therapy. Radiation therapy in the area of the axilla can cause lymphedema of the ipsilateral arm. Close medical follow-up is important after conservative surgery and radiation. Recommended guidelines include a breast physical examination every 4 to 6 months for 5 years, and then yearly. A mammogram is recommended 6 months after radiation and then annually (National Comprehensive Cancer Network [NCCN], 2009).

A variety of radiation methods are widely used. These include accelerated therapy and brachytherapy.

- **Accelerated breast radiation.** External beam radiation for 6 weeks, 5 days a week, can be very inconvenient for a woman. Research has been conducted to develop ways to shorten this time frame and still deliver the therapy needed to prevent recurrence of this disease. Accelerated radiation was created with this goal in mind and delivers a slightly larger dose of radiation over a 3-week period. Skin changes (resembling sunburn) can be slightly more prevalent because of the more intense period of time and corresponding dosage.
- **Brachytherapy.** Initially created for other types of cancer, like prostate, this form of radiation enables the client to complete her radiation in an even shorter time and is not delivered via external beam. Instead a deflated balloon is inserted into the space left by the lumpectomy and is filled with saline. The balloon is left in place until the margins are confirmed as clear. The balloon is removed and replaced with another balloon specifically created to allow radiation to be inserted within it. Radiation rods or seeds are inserted into the balloon device each day for 5 days, and the radiation is completed, at which time the balloon is then removed. This enables partial breast radiation to be delivered, recognizing that most local recurrences happen at or near the location of the original cancer.

Adjuvant Systemic Therapy

Chemotherapy administered soon after surgical removal of the tumor is referred to as adjuvant chemotherapy. The role of adjuvant chemotherapy in the treatment of breast cancer (chemotherapy and endocrine therapy) is either to eradicate or impede the growth of micrometastatic (microscopic cell metastasis) disease. Often it is not possible to detect the presence of micrometastasis at the time of initial treatment, and when it is present, mutations can occur in the tumor cells. These mutations make tumor cells resistant to the effects of chemotherapeutic agents despite tumor sensitivity to drug therapy being greatest when the tumor burden is small. Consequently the prediction cannot be made with confidence that all tumors of 1 cm or less can be cured with initial local and regional treatment. The early introduction of systemic adjuvant therapy, as determined by the estimated risk of tumor recurrence in certain subsets of women with node-negative disease, is a prudent course of treatment. Research findings suggest that adjuvant chemotherapy significantly reduces the risks for recurrence and mortality in women with node-positive disease (Valea & Katz, 2007). For women diagnosed with early stage breast cancer and favorable prognostic factors (hormone receptor positive and HER2/neu negative), a special pathology test may be performed to help determine the woman's risk of recurrence. This test, called Oncotype DX, provides a score that represents the likelihood of her specific cancer recurring. Such information can be useful for women whose known benefit for receiving chemotherapy may be minimal based on her prognostic factors from the tumor itself. For women with a low score, commonly only hormonal therapy is recommended, and for those with a high score usually chemotherapy is strongly considered.

Hormonal therapy. To determine whether a woman is a candidate for hormonal therapy, a receptor assay is done. After the entire tumor or a portion is removed by biopsy or excision, a pathologist examines the cancer cells for ERs and PRs.

The presence of a receptor on the cell wall indicates that the woman is positive for that type of hormone receptor. If these receptors are present, the growth of the woman's breast cancer can be influenced by estrogen, progesterone, or both. It is unknown exactly how these hormones affect breast cancer growth. Bilateral oophorectomy has been noted to benefit women diagnosed with their first breast cancer before age 50 by reducing exposure to endogenous estrogen. Oophorectomy reduces the risk of breast cancer by approximately 50% in BRCA1 carriers (Shockney & Tsangaris, 2007). Thus oophorectomy may be an option that helps decrease the odds of recurrence and improve length of survival. In addition to or instead of oophorectomy, medications may be given to stop tumor growth that is influenced by hormones. Ovarian suppression may also be recommended by a medical oncologist as part of the hormonal therapy treatment.

There are several hormonal therapy drugs. Tamoxifen, the oldest one and the one used the longest, is an oral antiestrogen medication that mimics progesterone and estrogen. Tamoxifen attaches to the hormone receptors on cancer cells and prevents natural hormones from attaching to the receptors. When tamoxifen fits into the receptors, the cell is unable to grow. Research has demonstrated a clear benefit for use of tamoxifen in all age-groups (Brauch, Mürdter, Eichelbaum, & Schwab, 2009). Adjuvant hormonal therapy with tamoxifen is recommended for most premenopausal women with breast cancer whose tumors are hormone receptor positive. In this age-group, adjuvant tamoxifen therapy improves disease-free survival and, in some cases, length of survival. Use of hormonal therapy for 5 years in premenopausal women with breast cancer significantly reduces recurrence and mortality rates.

The NCCN guidelines (2009) recommend giving adjuvant hormonal therapy to women with hormone receptor–positive breast cancer regardless of menopause status, age, or HER2/neu status, with the exception of women with lymph node–negative cancers less than or equal to 0.5 cm, or 0.6 to 1 cm in diameter with favorable prognostic features. Women treated with hormonal therapy should receive therapy for at least 5 years. Use beyond 5 years in node-positive women results in a reduction in beneficial effects with an increase in toxicity, although the optimal duration of tamoxifen administration is under investigation (Brauch et al.) (see Medication Guide: Tamoxifen).

MEDICATION GUIDE

Tamoxifen (Nolvadex)

ACTION

Antiestrogenic effects; attaches to hormone receptors on cancer cells and prevents natural hormones from attaching to the receptors.

INDICATION

For treatment of advanced stage or metastatic breast cancer; treatment of early stage breast cancer after breast cancer surgery and radiation therapy; to reduce the incidence of breast cancer in women at high risk.

DOSAGE AND ROUTE

20 mg orally, daily

ADVERSE REACTIONS

Common side effects include hot flashes, night sweats, nausea, vaginal discharge, and mood swings. Hair loss is an uncommon effect. Serious side effects include deep vein thrombosis, increased risk of endometrial cancer, and stroke. Symptoms include abnormal vaginal bleeding, leg swelling or tenderness, chest pain, shortness of breath, weakness or numbness of extremities, sudden severe headache.

NURSING CONSIDERATIONS

The medication may be taken on an empty stomach or with food. Missed doses should be taken as soon as possible, but taking two doses at once is not recommended. A barrier or nonhormonal form of contraception is recommended in premenopausal women because tamoxifen may be harmful to the fetus if pregnancy should occur.

Raloxifene is an oral selective ER modulator. It is used to prevent osteoporosis in menopausal women. It works as well as tamoxifen in decreasing invasive breast cancer risk in postmenopausal women with a high risk for breast cancer with fewer thromboembolic events and lower risk of uterine cancer (see Medication Guide: Raloxifene Hydrochloride).

Aromatase inhibitors (AIs) is a classification of hormonal therapy in use. It markedly suppresses plasma estrogen levels in postmenopausal women by inhibiting or inactivating aromatase, the enzyme responsible for synthesizing estrogens from androgenic substrates (Brauch et al., 2009). AIs such as anastrozole, letrozole, and exemestane are effective agents in hormonal therapy for breast cancer. Clinical trials indicate that letrozole is convincingly better than tamoxifen in treating advanced disease in postmenopausal women, and anastrozole is at least as good. In early stage breast cancer, adjuvant therapy with anastrozole appears to be superior to adjuvant therapy with tamoxifen in reducing recurrence in postmenopausal women. AIs appear to be well tolerated with lower incidence of adverse effects as compared to tamoxifen. AIs are more commonly given to postmenopausal women whose tumors are hormone receptor positive (Shockney & Tsangaris, 2007) (see Medication Guide: Letrozole).

Chemotherapy. Chemotherapy drugs are most often given in combination regimens, which have been shown to improve or increase the disease-free survival time after therapy. The

MEDICATION GUIDE

Raloxifene Hydrochloride (Evista)

ACTION

A selective estrogen receptor modulator, serving as an agonist and antagonist to estrogen receptor sites.

INDICATIONS

Treatment and prevention of osteoporosis; reduction in the risk of invasive breast cancer in postmenopausal women with osteoporosis; and reduction of risk of invasive breast cancer in postmenopausal women at high risk for invasive breast cancer.

DOSAGE

60 mg orally, daily

ADVERSE REACTIONS

Common side effects include hot flashes, nausea, peripheral edema, joint pain, leg cramps, flu-like symptoms, sweating. Serious and life-threatening side effects can occur from existing condition. Women who have had a heart attack or at risk for a heart attack have increased risk of dying from a stroke. There is an increased risk of blood clots in the legs and lungs: Raloxifene is contraindicated in women with an active or past history of venous thromboembolism.

NURSING CONSIDERATIONS

The medication may be taken on an empty stomach or with food. Missed doses should be taken as soon as possible, but taking two doses at once is not recommended. Counsel woman to contact physician if leg pain or feeling of warmth in lower legs, swelling of hands and feet, sudden chest pain or shortness of breath, or sudden changes in vision occur. Calcium 1500 mg plus vitamin D 400 to 800 International Units daily is recommended.

MEDICATION GUIDE

Letrozole (Femara)

ACTION

An aromatase inhibitor; inhibits the conversion of androgens to estrogen.

INDICATION

For adjuvant treatment of early breast cancer in postmenopausal women who have received 5 years of tamoxifen therapy; first-line treatment of postmenopausal women with hormone receptor–positive or hormone receptor–unknown locally advanced or metastatic cancer; adjuvant treatment of postmenopausal women with hormone receptor–positive early breast cancer

DOSAGE AND ROUTE

2.5 mg once a day by mouth

ADVERSE REACTIONS

Common side effects include hot flashes, nausea, increased sweating, joint or muscle pain, fluid retention, vaginal dryness, constipation, dizziness, fatigue, headache; severe side effects include severe allergic reactions (e.g., rash, hives, difficulty breathing), vomiting, chest pain, severe bone pain, calf pain or tenderness

NURSING CONSIDERATIONS

The medication may be taken on an empty stomach or with food. Missed doses should be taken as soon as possible, but taking two doses at once is not recommended. The woman should use caution if driving or using machinery because this medication may cause drowsiness or dizziness. Women who are not postmenopausal should not take letrozole.

BOX 10-4 COMMON CHEMOTHERAPY REGIMENS FOR ADJUVANT TREATMENT OF BREAST CANCER

- CMF: cyclophosphamide, methotrexate, fluorouracil
- CAF: cyclophosphamide, doxorubicin (Adriamycin), fluorouracil
- AC: doxorubicin, cyclophosphamide
- EC: epirubicin, cyclophosphamide
- A → CMF: doxorubicin followed by CMF
- TAC: docetaxel, doxorubicin, and cyclophosphamide
- AC → T: doxorubicin and cyclophosphamide followed by paclitaxel or docetaxel (Herceptin may be given with the paclitaxel or docetaxel for HER2/neu-positive tumors.)
- CEF: cyclophosphamide, epirubicin, and fluorouracil (this may be followed by docetaxel)
- TC: docetaxel and cyclophosphamide
- TCH: docetaxel, carboplatin, and Herceptin for HER2/neu-positive tumors

Source: American Cancer Society. (2009). *Detailed guide: Breast cancer: Chemotherapy*. Available at www.cancer.org. Accessed June 9, 2010.

most common chemotherapy regimens used for adjuvant treatment of node-positive and node-negative tumors are listed in Box 10-4.

Adjuvant chemotherapy has been most useful in premenopausal women who have breast cancer with positive nodes, regardless of hormone receptor status. It is postulated that younger women often have tumors with a higher S-phase fraction and proliferative rate, which makes the tumors more sensitive to chemotherapy. Although adjuvant chemotherapy effectively decreases the risks for recurrence and mortality in premenopausal women with node-positive disease, postmenopausal women can also be offered chemotherapy, depending on the cancer size, nodal involvement, and morphologic and biologic factors or markers of the particular cancer (Shockney & Tsangaris, 2007).

Chemotherapy with multiple drug combinations is used in the treatment of recurrent and advanced breast cancer with positive results. First-line single agents for women with locally advanced or metastatic breast cancer include paclitaxel, docetaxel, epirubicin, doxorubicin, pegylated liposomal doxorubicin, capecitabine, vinorelbine, and gemcitabine. Combination regimens and sequential single agents may be used (NCCN, 2009). Because chemotherapy drugs kill rapidly reproducing cells, treatment also affects normal body cells that rapidly reproduce (red and white blood cells, gastric mucosa, and hair). Thus chemotherapy can cause leukopenia, neutropenia, thrombocytopenia, anemia, gastrointestinal side effects (nausea, vomiting, anorexia, mucositis), and partial or full hair loss.

Chemotherapy treatments are usually administered in ambulatory care settings once or twice per month. During the informed consent process, before the treatment is selected, the woman and her family members should be educated about the names of the medications, routes of administration, treatment schedule, timing and ordering of medications, length of time of administration, reimbursed and unreimbursed costs of therapy, potential side effects, management of side effects, possible changes in body image (e.g., full or partial hair loss), recovery time after treatment (necessitating lost work time), and need for a caregiver to transport the woman to treatment and care for her afterward. Depending on the medications used, the treatments may include intravenous, subcutaneous, and oral administration. Often a long-term central venous catheter is inserted when the women will be receiving chemotherapy for an extended period or when she will receive medications that may damage the vein. Presence of a central venous catheter, hair loss, loss of part or all of her breast, menopause, and possible infertility all have the potential to cause a change in body image and increase emotional distress for the woman with breast cancer.

Breast cancer treatment with chemotherapy, hormonal therapy, or a combination of the two often causes changes in reproductive function. The premenopausal woman may experience these changes along with symptoms of menopause and possible infertility. It is not known whether hormonal therapy to ease the effects of menopause is safe for women with breast cancer; therefore, it is not recommended. For this reason the nurse must use other measures to help the woman cope with menopause (see Chapter 6). A young woman with breast cancer may become devastated by early and abrupt menopausal symptoms and the possibility of jeopardized reproductive function. A postmenopausal woman must cope with unpleasant side effects from chemotherapy and loss of part or all of her breast, and frequently, with treatment side effects superimposed on the presence of comorbidities that develop with aging.

Women receiving chemotherapy and their partners must understand that chemotherapy can be teratogenic, that is, chemotherapy agents can cause congenital birth defects. Any woman who is of childbearing age and receiving chemotherapy, even though no longer menstruating, must use birth control. Birth control pills are not recommended because they contain hormones that may assist in the growth of cancer. A birth control method must be chosen with the assistance of a gynecologist and a medical oncologist, and it must be used before chemotherapy begins and continue to be used until the medical oncologist and gynecologist believe it is safe to discontinue. Although a woman may not be menstruating, she may still be able to get pregnant.

CARE MANAGEMENT

Nursing Considerations

Nursing care of a woman with breast cancer will depend on the treatment option that has been chosen. Data that will guide the care include a client history, a physical examination, laboratory and diagnostic test results, and psychosocial assessment (see Nursing Process box).

Emotional Support After Diagnosis

When a woman is confronted with a diagnosis of cancer, she faces not only possible major changes in appearance but also the possibility of death. The emotional reaction to the diagnosis of cancer is always intense, and the many disruptions caused by the disease challenge the woman's and family's ability to cope. Disruptions may be caused by costs of treatment, loss of role function, lack of stress-relieving activities, spouse's or child's reaction to the diagnosis, change in body image and sexual function, disability, and pain. The woman may feel despair, fear, and shame. Sexuality issues related to breast cancer include a change in body image, changes in sexual function (such as decreased vaginal lubrication caused by hormonal therapy), and relational distress. Health care providers are responsible for discussing the influence of breast cancer on the woman's life and in assisting the woman and her family in coping effectively with these changes. Nurses need to be especially aware of the individual quality of life needs of their clients and deliver interventions that improve quality of life outcomes within the context of the breast cancer survivor's personal history, life cycle concerns, and psychosocial life stage.

Nursing Care Plan—Breast Cancer

Women and their families often undergo a period of distress after the diagnosis of cancer. It is difficult to accept the diagnosis of cancer when the woman may feel and look well. This period is characterized by anguish and shock followed by disbelief and denial. During this time absorbing information and education can be difficult, and the nurse should be sensitive as to how this may affect decision-making abilities. Flexibility is the key to sensitive nursing care. As the woman and family begin to accept the diagnosis of breast cancer, more and more information can be shared, and care planning with full client participation can take place, including the following:

- Validate and reinforce accurate information processing by the woman and her family.
- Assist in client decision making and arrange for the woman to speak with breast cancer survivors who have chosen a variety of treatment options (see Box 10-3).
- Suggest approaches the woman might take to deal with the sexual concerns of her significant other.
- Discuss the application of alternative therapies to alleviate stress and promote healing, such as exercise, guided imagery, meditation, and progressive muscle relaxation.
- Refer the woman to the ACS's Reach to Recovery program or other resources that provide trained survivor volunteers for one-on-one support.
- Refer the woman to a cancer rehabilitation program, such as ENCORE, an exercise program run by the YWCA.

The NCCN (www.nccn.org) and the ACS (www.cancer.org) provide specific, up-to-date recommendations on breast cancer treatments on the Internet. These are invaluable resources for women to learn about scientifically tested treatment protocols for each stage of breast cancer.

After assisting the woman with accepting the diagnosis and obtaining support, consider nursing care in the preoperative, postoperative, and convalescent periods. The discussion that follows is pertinent to the care required by a woman who is having a modified radical mastectomy (see Nursing Care Plan).

Preoperative Care

General preoperative teaching and care are given, including expectations regarding physical appearance, pain management, equipment to be used (e.g., intravenous therapy, drains), and emotional support. Some emotional support may be obtained by arranging for a visit from a member of an organization such as Reach to Recovery. The woman is reminded that when she awakens after surgery, her arm on the affected side will feel tight.

Immediate Postoperative Care

After recovery from anesthesia, the woman is returned to her room. Special precautions must be observed to prevent or to minimize lymphedema of the affected arm.

NURSING PROCESS

The Woman with Breast Cancer

ASSESSMENT

- Take a thorough history of symptoms, including timing of detection of lump, size, changes, location, nipple discharge, and breast symmetry and risk factors.
- Palpate the breast lump and describe the mass in terms of location (by using the clock-dial method), shape, size, consistency, and fixation to the surrounding tissues. Observe breasts for skin changes, such as dimpling, peau d'orange, increased vascularity, nipple retraction, or ulceration; these may indicate advanced disease.
- Palpate the infraclavicular, supraclavicular, and axillary lymph nodes.
- Evaluate pain and soreness in the affected breast and arm.
- Assess the woman's present emotional state and the reaction of her family and significant others and history of handling crises.

NURSING DIAGNOSES

Nursing diagnoses for women with a diagnosis of breast cancer might include:

***Fear/Anxiety* related to:**
- diagnosis of breast cancer
- treatment choices
- choice of reconstructive procedure

***Decisional Conflict* related to:**
- choices of and controversies about treatment options

***Sexual Dysfunction* related to:**
- altered body image
- side effects of therapy

***Compromised/Disabled Family Coping* related to:**
- diagnosis and prognosis

***Anticipatory Grieving* related to:**
- loss of breast or diagnosis of advanced cancer

***Fatigue* related to:**
- cancer treatments

***Acute Pain* related to:**
- incision or metastatic cancer or side effects of systemic treatment

***Impaired Skin Integrity* related to:**
- surgery or radiation

***Disturbed Body Image* related to:**
- loss of breast
- hair loss (chemotherapy)

EXPECTED OUTCOMES OF CARE

Outcomes might include that the woman will:
- Experience a reasonable level of anxiety related to diagnosis that does not interfere with use of healthy coping mechanisms.
- Elicit appropriate support from significant others.
- Choose among alternative treatment options and verbalize satisfaction with the decision-making process.
- Report satisfactory sexual functioning after surgery.
- Demonstrate necessary self-care techniques correctly.
- Accept a change in body image and demonstrate a positive self-concept.

Other expected outcomes include the following:
- The family will adapt to the diagnosis and provide appropriate support through all stages of treatment.
- The woman's skin will remain intact and will heal without complications.
- The woman will continue usual activities as tolerated during treatment.

PLAN OF CARE AND INTERVENTIONS

Nursing actions that will best assist the woman in achieving her expected outcomes include:
- Provide time to discuss the diagnosis, answer questions, and listen to concerns.
- Provide teaching for the specific treatment.
- Provide nursing interventions for the specific treatment.
- Encourage ventilation of feelings by the woman and family in a nonjudgmental atmosphere.
- Offer information about support groups or individual therapy for the woman and the family members, including children.

EVALUATION

Evaluation is based on the client-centered expected outcomes. The nurse can be assured that care was effective to the extent that the goals for care have been achieved.

! NURSING ALERT

When vital signs are taken, never apply the blood pressure cuff to the affected arm.

The affected arm is elevated with pillows above the level of the right atrium. Blood is not drawn from this arm, and this arm is not used for intravenous therapy or any injections. Early arm movement is encouraged. Any increase in the circumference of that arm is reported immediately.

Nursing care of the wound involves observation for signs of hemorrhage (dressing, drainage tubes, and Hemovac or Jackson-Pratt drainage reservoirs are emptied at least every 8 hours and more frequently as needed), shock, and infection. Dressings are reinforced as necessary. The woman is asked to turn (alternating between unaffected side and back), cough (while the nurse or the woman applies support to the chest), and deep breathe every 2 hours. Breath sounds are auscultated every 4 hours. Active range of motion (ROM) exercise of legs is encouraged. Parenteral fluids are given until adequate oral intake is possible. Emotional support is continued.

Care given during the immediate postoperative period is continued as necessary. Most women who undergo lumpectomy have surgery as ambulatory clients and return home a few hours after surgery. Women are discharged 24 hours or less after mastectomy without reconstruction. Women having a mastectomy with tissue expander placement will be in the hospital for 24 hours. Those having flap reconstruction at the same time will be hospitalized for 3 to 5 days. Because of the generally short time spent in the hospital, thorough teaching is important. It is best to do as much teaching as possible before surgery if the outcome is known. If this is not possible, discharge teaching should be done with the woman's caregiver present. This is to acknowledge the possibility that emotional stress or recovery from anesthesia may cause the woman to forget some of the discharge instructions. Printed information also should be provided for the woman and family to refer to at home. She will also need information about being fitted for a permanent

NURSING CARE PLAN

The Woman Having Breast-Conserving Surgery and Axillary Node Dissection

NURSING DIAGNOSIS

Acute pain related to surgical incision and surgical drains, as evidenced by client verbalizations

Expected Outcome

Woman will report minimal intensity and decreased number of painful episodes.

Nursing Interventions/*Rationales*

- Use pain scale to assess type and intensity of pain *to provide accurate database.*
- Administer analgesics as ordered *to decrease perception of pain.*
- Teach and reinforce use of relaxation techniques *to reduce anxiety and provide distraction that may decrease the perception of pain.*
- Reposition woman with affected arm elevated *to promote comfort and lymphatic channel return.*

NURSING DIAGNOSIS

Risk for infection related to disruption of skin integrity and removal of lymph nodes

Expected Outcome

Woman will experience no clinical manifestations of infection.

Nursing Interventions/*Rationales*

- Assess clinical manifestations of infection at the incision and drain sites that may include redness, swelling, localized heat, fever, increasing pain, and foul-smelling drainage *to facilitate prompt treatment.*
- Demonstrate the procedure for emptying and recording the amount of drainage from the Jackson-Pratt drain(s) *to provide information to the surgeon as to the appropriate removal time of drains.* Drains are usually removed when drainage is less than 30 ml of fluid in 24 hours.
- Explain the need to avoid trauma or irritation to the affected arm *to reinforce to the woman that alterations in sensation and removal of some lymph nodes may affect ability to sense irritation or prevent infection.*
- Reinforce to the woman the need to protect arm from injury and to avoid blood drawing or blood pressures to be taken on the affected arm *to avoid trauma and infection because decreased sensation may be present as well as decreased lymphatic return.*
- Explain the importance of reporting any clinical manifestations of infection to the caregiver as soon as possible *to provide identification and treatment of problem.*

NURSING DIAGNOSIS

Disturbed body image related to loss of all or part of a breast as evidenced by client statements

Expected Outcome

Woman will report acceptance of herself as she is and regain a positive body image.

Nursing Interventions/*Rationales*

- Provide opportunity through therapeutic communication to express feelings about body image changes *to clarify and validate feelings.*
- Refer to support groups to *facilitate verbalization of feelings with women who have similar concerns.*

NURSING DIAGNOSIS

Impaired physical mobility related to pain and tissue trauma

Expected Outcome

Woman will return to her preoperative level of mobility.

Nursing Interventions/*Rationales*

- Encourage woman to do hand, arm, and wrist exercises that can be performed in the immediate postoperative period *to enhance fluid return and prevent muscle atrophy.*
- Encourage woman to perform activities of daily living as much as possible *to encourage woman to focus on her strengths rather than her limitations.*
- Teach woman exercises to be performed after the drains are removed *to promote range of motion in the arm that had the axillary nodes dissected.*
- Teach woman to do exercises slowly and gently *to prevent injury and pain.*
- Caution woman not to lift anything heavier than 10 pounds for 4 to 6 weeks *to avoid exerting strain on affected arm.*

breast prosthesis 6 to 7 weeks after surgery; this fitting should be done by a certified prosthesis fitter. A prescription will be needed specifying the anatomic side and to include mastectomy bras as part of the fitting process.

Women who have had breast cancer surgery are usually seen by their surgeon within 5 to 7 days of surgery. This follow-up visit is important because it allows the physician to assess the outcome of surgical treatment as well as provide reinforcement of education and emotional support. A woman having simultaneous reconstruction will also be seen by her plastic surgeon within a week postoperatively.

Mobility is a key subject to be addressed with women having breast surgery. Early ambulation is encouraged to improve circulation and ventilation and to prevent loss of calcium from bone. The psychologic benefits of early mobility include resumption of self-care and activities of daily living that serve to reinforce the woman's control over her life and help her move from a sick role to the role of breast cancer survivor.

Arm exercises are encouraged at least four times daily (Box 10-5). Exercise is increased as tolerated and is stopped at the point of pain. Initially the woman alternately clenches and extends her fingers and then progresses to wrist and elbow exercises, gradually abducting her arm and raising it to and over her head. She is encouraged to exercise by assisting with her care—washing her face, brushing her teeth, and eating with her hand and arm on the affected side. Physical therapy may be prescribed to improve strength and mobility of the affected arm. Women having a sentinel node biopsy only should have full ROM back within a few days. A woman having axillary dissections will need to work more vigorously at restoring ROM. She should have returned to her baseline range of motion by the end of the third week postoperatively.

It is important to discuss the appearance of the woman's breast if dressings have not been removed before discharge. Some women may not want to view their surgical site, but it is important to give them the opportunity to do so and to provide emotional support at that time. The woman should be encouraged to express her emotions and verbalize her feelings. The woman needs to know that it will take time to become accustomed to her change of appearance. A woman who has

BOX 10-5 ARM EXERCISES AFTER LYMPH NODE DISSECTION

Exercises After Breast Surgery

It is important to talk to your physician before starting any exercises. A physical therapist or occupational therapist can help design an exercise program for you.

Exercises in Lying Position

These exercises should be performed on a bed or the floor while lying on your back with your knees and hips bent, feet flat.

Wand Exercise

This exercise helps increase the forward motion of the shoulders. You will need a broom handle, yardstick, or other similar object to perform this exercise.

- Hold the wand in both hands with palms facing up.
- Lift the wand up over your head (as far as you can) using your unaffected arm to help lift the wand, until you feel a stretch in your affected arm.
- Hold for 5 seconds.
- Lower arms and repeat 5 to 7 times.

Elbow Winging

This exercise helps increase the mobility of the front of your chest and shoulder. It may take several weeks of regular exercise before your elbows will get close to the bed (or floor).

- Clasp your hands behind your neck with your elbows pointing toward the ceiling.
- Move your elbows apart and down toward the bed (or floor).
- Repeat 5 to 7 times

Exercises in Sitting Position

Shoulder Blade Stretch

This exercise helps increase the mobility of the shoulder blades.

- Sit in a chair very close to a table with your back against the chair back.
- Place the unaffected arm on the table with your elbow bent and palm down. Do not move this arm during the exercise.
- Place the affected arm on the table, palm down with your elbow straight.
- Without moving your trunk, slide the affected arm toward the opposite side of the table. You should feel your shoulder blade move as you do this.
- Relax your arm and repeat 5 to 7 times.

Shoulder Blade Squeeze

This exercise also helps increase the mobility of the shoulder blade.

- Facing straight ahead, sit in a chair in front of a mirror without resting on the back of the chair.
- Arms should be at your sides with elbows bent.
- Squeeze shoulder blades together, bringing your elbows behind you. Keep your shoulders level as you do this exercise. Do not lift your shoulders up toward your ears.
- Return to the starting position and repeat 5 to 7 times.

Side Bending

This exercise helps increase the mobility of the trunk/body.

- Clasp your hands together in front of you and lift your arms slowly over your head, straightening your arms.
- When your arms are over your head, bend your trunk to the right while bending at the waist and keeping your arms overhead.
- Return to the starting position and bend to the left.
- Repeat 5 to 7 times.

Exercises in Standing Position

Chest Wall Stretch

This exercise helps stretch the chest wall.

- Stand facing a corner with toes approximately 8 to 10 inches from the corner.
- Bend your elbows and place forearms on the wall, one on each side of the corner. Your elbows should be as close to shoulder height as possible.
- Keep your arms and feet in position and move your chest toward the corner. You will feel a stretch across your chest and shoulders.
- Return to starting position and repeat 5 to 7 times.

Shoulder Stretch

This exercise helps increase the mobility in the shoulder.

- Stand facing the wall with your toes approximately 8 to 10 inches from the wall.
- Place your hands on the wall. Use your fingers to "climb the wall," reaching as high as you can until you feel a stretch.
- Return to starting position and repeat 5 to 7 times.

Source: American Cancer Society. (2009). *Exercises after breast surgery*. Available at www.cancer.org/docroot/CRI/content/CRI_2_6x_Exercises_After_Breast_Surgery.asp?sitearea=CRI&viewmode=print&. Accessed June 9, 2010.

undergone reconstruction at the same time should be encouraged to look at herself as a work in progress—swelling, positioning of tissue expanders, appearance of flaps and presence of multiple drains initially can be difficult to accept. Over time, when drains are out and swelling is subsiding, she will begin to see her new silhouette take shape.

An option for restoration of body image is choosing an external prosthesis to replace the lost breast or portion of breast tissue for women having mastectomy without reconstruction. The external prosthesis is inserted into a mastectomy bra. Women who choose to use a partial external prosthesis after lumpectomy or full external prosthesis after mastectomy need information about where to obtain prostheses and an appropriate bra. Women need to be advised on how to submit the cost of the prosthesis to their insurance company. Volunteers of the Reach to Recovery program are able to provide this information, as well as a list of sources for prostheses, bathing suits, and lingerie. They can offer helpful hints and suggestions for coping with prostheses and wearing apparel. Some women find that an external prosthesis does not restore body image and seek surgical reconstruction of the missing or disfigured breast (see earlier discussion).

Discharge Planning and Follow-up Care

Before discharge, considerable time should be spent counseling the woman and her family about the aspects of self-management. These instructions are summarized in the Teaching for Self-Management box. Printed instructions should be given to the woman and her family. A referral for home nursing care may be made if the woman needs assistance caring for her incision.

Teaching Needs for the Client and Family Undergoing Adjuvant Therapies

It is important that the woman and her family be given thorough instructions regarding side effects and avoidance of possible complications of adjuvant treatment. A common side effect of radiation therapy is skin irritation and breakdown. The woman should avoid using lotions, powders, or ointments on the skin at the radiation site unless instructed by the radiologist. The skin should be cleansed gently with mild soap and water, rinsed thoroughly, and patted dry. Skin markings that direct the placement of the radiation beam should not be removed. Soft, nonirritating clothing should be worn over the site, and the skin should be protected from exposure to sun and heat.

Common side effects of chemotherapy include alopecia, fatigue, nausea, vomiting, mouth sores, and immunosuppression. The woman planning to receive chemotherapy that produces hair loss should be encouraged to obtain a wig matching her own hair color and style before beginning treatments so that she is prepared when hair loss begins. The local ACS can assist in obtaining a wig and head coverings designed for women experiencing hair loss from chemotherapy. The woman should be taught the importance of rest periods when fatigue occurs. She and her family will need to know that work and family schedules may need adjustment to accommodate needed rest. Exercise such as power walking has proven to combat fatigue (Mock, Atkinson, Barsevid, Berger, Cimprich, Eisenberger, et al., 2007). Nausea and vomiting should be reported to the physician and are treated with antiemetics. Mouth sores may be very painful, and the woman should be instructed to maintain good oral hygiene and avoid trauma to the oral mucosa. The mouth should be rinsed frequently with water or saline, and mouthwashes containing alcohol or glycerin should be avoided as well as spicy or irritating foods. Topical anesthetic medications may be prescribed by the physician. The woman with immunosuppression should be instructed to use frequent handwashing and avoid crowds and other large gatherings of people, especially during cold and flu season. She should be taught to avoid eating raw fruits and vegetables (low-bacteria diet) and maintain strict personal hygiene. The woman should be taught the signs and symptoms of infection and to report them to the physician immediately.

COMMUNITY ACTIVITY

- Visit the National Comprehensive Cancer Network website for families, caregivers and their families at www. NCCN.org. Review the client information regarding treatment summaries for each stage of breast cancer, making treatment decisions, living with cancer, paying for treatment and life beyond cancer. Locate a Cancer Center in your state, which is a member of the NCCN. Visit the website of the Cancer Center. How many cancer clients does the Center treat each year? Are there any clinical trials open for breast cancer patients?
- Research the availability of rehabilitation programs for breast cancer survivors in your community such as the American Cancer Society's Reach to Recovery program, or the ENCORE exercise program run by the YWCA.

TEACHING FOR SELF-MANAGEMENT

After a Mastectomy Without Reconstruction

- Wash hands well before and after touching incision area or drains.
- Empty surgical drains twice a day and as needed, recording the date, time, drain sites (if more than one drain is present), and amount of drainage in milliliters in the diary you will take to each surgical checkup until your drains are removed. (Before discharge, you may receive a graduated container for emptying drains and measuring drainage.)
- Avoid driving, lifting more than 10 pounds, or reaching above your head until given permission by the surgeon.
- Take medications for pain as soon as pain begins.
- Perform arm exercises as directed.
- Call physician if inflammation of incision or swelling of the incision or the arm occurs.
- Avoid tight clothing, tight jewelry, and other causes of decreased circulation in the affected arm.
- Until drains are removed, wear loose-fitting underwear (camisole or half-slip) and clothes, pinning surgical drains inside of clothing. (You will be taught how to do this safely.)

You will be provided a surgical bra with pockets on the inside that will hold a temporary breast form for you to wear until you can be fitted for a mastectomy bra and breast prosthesis.

- After drains are removed and surgical sites are healing and still tender, wear a mastectomy bra or camisole with a cotton-filled, muslin temporary prosthesis. Temporary prostheses of this type are often available from Reach to Recovery.
- Avoid depilatory creams, strong deodorants, and shaving of affected chest area, axilla, and arm.
- Sponge bathe for the first 48 hours, then you may shower. Thoroughly dry yourself afterward and reapply fresh dressings.
- Return to the surgeon's office for incision check, drain inspection, and possible drain removal as directed.
- Contact Reach to Recovery or a breast center nursing staff member for assistance in obtaining external prosthesis and lingerie when dressings, drains, and staples are removed and wound is healing and nontender.
- Contact insurance company for information about coverage of prosthesis and wig if needed. Obtain prescriptions for prosthesis and wig to submit with receipts of purchase for these items to the insurance company. If insurance does not pay for these items, contact hospital or agency social worker or local American Cancer Society for assistance.
- Practice BSE of unaffected side and affected surgical site and axilla.
- Keep follow-up visits for professional examination, mammography, and testing to detect recurrent breast cancer.
- Expect decreased sensation and tingling at incision sites and in the affected arm for weeks to months after surgery.
- Resume sexual activities as desired.
- Participate in breast cancer survivor support group if desired.
- Encourage mother, sisters, and daughters (if applicable) to learn and practice BSE and to have annual professional breast examinations and mammography (if appropriate).

ADDITIONAL NURSING CARE FOR WOMEN UNDERGOING MASTECTOMY WITH RECONSTRUCTION

No tight compression of the reconstructed breasts until approved by her plastic surgeon.

Wear loosely fitting garments for first 3 to 4 weeks.

Emphasize to the woman that her surgery is still a work in progress and that final cosmetic result of reconstruction takes many weeks.

Assess skin for potential of poor peripheral circulation that may cause skin necrosis and report any skin changes immediately.

See drain care instructions under axillary dissection section.

KEY POINTS

- The most common benign breast problems are fibrocystic changes and fibroadenomas.
- The development of breast neoplasms, whether benign or malignant, can have a significant physical and emotional effect on the woman and her family.
- The risk of American women developing cancer of the breast is one in eight.
- An estimated 90% of all breast lumps are detected by the woman.
- Clinical breast examinations by a health care provider (starting in one's 20s), and routine screening mammograms (after age 40) are recommended by the ACS for early detection of breast cancer.
- The primary therapy for most women with stage I or stage II breast cancer is breast-conserving surgery followed by radiation therapy.
- Adjuvant chemotherapy is most helpful to premenopausal women with breast cancer that has spread to the lymph nodes.
- Tamoxifen, along with raloxifene and anastrozole, provides the first real hope for the prevention of breast cancer.
- The emotional diagnosis of breast cancer is always intense, and the many disruptions caused by the disease challenge the woman's and her family's ability to cope.
- There are more reconstruction options today than ever before.
- Digital mammography is superior to traditional analog mammography.
- 85% of women diagnosed today with breast cancer will be long-term survivors.

Audio Chapter Summaries Access an audio summary of the Key Points on evolve

REFERENCES

American Cancer Society (ACS). (2009). *Breast cancer facts and figures 2009-2010*. Atlanta: Author.

American Cancer Society (ACS). (2010). *Cancer facts and figures 2010*. Atlanta: Author.

Brauch, H., Mürdter, T., Eichelbaum, M., & Schwab, M. (2009). Pharmacogenomics of tamoxifen therapy. *Clinical Chemistry, 55*(10), 1770–1782.

Breast cancer on the night shift. (2007). *Lancet, 373*(9669), 1054.

Brown, J., Holton, L., Chung, T., & Slezak, S. (2008). Breast feeding, self exam and exercise practices before and after reduction mammoplasty. *Annals of Plastic Surgery, 61*(4), 375–379.

Ciatto, S., Ambroghetti, D., Morrone, D., & Del Turco, M. (2006). Analysis of the results of a proficiency test in screening mammography at the CSPO of Florence: Review of 705 tests. *Radiologica Medica, 111*(6), 797–803.

DiSaia, P., & Creasman, W. (2007). *Clinical gynecologic oncology* (7th ed.). Philadelphia: Mosby.

Fentiman, I., Allen, D., & Hamed, H. (2005). Smoking and prognosis in women with breast cancer. *International Journal of Clinical Practice, 59*(9), 1051–1054.

Fentiman, I., Hamby, A., Allen, D., Key, T., & Meilahn, E. (2006). Hormone dependency of breast tumours developing in the Guernsey Cohort study. *Breast Cancer Research Treatment, 97*(2), 205–208.

Hedén, P., Bronz, G., Elberg, J., Deraemaecker, R., Murphy, D., Slicton, A., et al. (2009). Long-term safety and effectiveness of style 410 highly cohesive silicone breast implants. *Aesthetic Plastic Surgery, 33*(3), 430–436.

Kotz, D. (2008). *New "GINA" law would stop genetic discrimination*. Available at http://health.usnews.com/blogs/on-women/2008/04/25/new-gina-law-would-stop-genetic-discrimination.html. Accessed June 9, 2010.

Krag, D., Ashikaga, T., Harlow, S., Skelly, J., Julian, T., Brown, A., et al. (2009). Surgeon training, protocol compliance, and technical outcomes from breast cancer sentinel lymph node randomized trial. *Journal of the National Cancer Institute, 101*(19), 1356–1362.

Lin, W., Hsu, G., Yu, C., Yu, J., Lee, H., Hsu, H., et al. (2009). Value of sonographically guided needle sampling of cystic versus solid components in the diagnosis of complex cystic breast masses. *Acta Radiologica, 50*(6), 595–601.

Lobo, R. (2007). Hyperprolactinemia, galactorrhea, and pituitary adenomas: Etiology, differential diagnosis, natural history, management. In V. Katz, G. Lentz, R. Lobo, & D. Gershenson (Eds.), *Comprehensive gynecology* (5th ed.). Philadelphia: Mosby.

Martin, L., Minkin, S., & Boyd, N. (2009). Hormone therapy, mammographic density, and breast cancer risk. *Maturitas, 64*(1), 20–26.

Mayo Foundation for Medical Education and Research. (2008). *Mammary duct ectasia*. Available at www.mayoclinic.com/health/mammary-duct-ectasia/DS00751. Accessed June 9, 2010.

Mock, V., Atkinson, A., Barsevid, A., Berger, A., Cimprich, B., Eisenberger, M., et al. (2007). Cancer-related fatigue. Clinical practice guidelines in oncology. *Journal of the National Comprehensive Cancer Network, 5*(10), 1054–1078.

National Cancer Institute (NCI). (2009). *Breast cancer clinical trial results*. Available at www.cancer.org/clinicaltrials/results/breast. Accessed June 9, 2010.

National Comprehensive Cancer Network (NCCN). (2009). *Breast cancer treatment guidelines for patients* (online). Available at www.nccn.org/treatment-summaries.aspx. Accessed June 9, 2010.

Nelson, H., Fu, R., Griffin, J., Nygren, P., Smith, M., & Humphrey, L. (2009). Systematic review: Comparative effectiveness of medications to reduce risk for primary breast cancer. *Annals of Internal Medicine, 17*(10), 703–715.

Pisano, E., Acharyya, S., Cole, E., Marques, H., Yaffe, M., Blevins, M., et al. (2009). Cancer cases from ACRIN digital mammographic imaging screening trial: Radiologist analysis with use of a logistic regression model. *Radiology, 252*(2), 348–357.

Quan, M., Wells, B., McCready, D., Wright, F., Fraser, N., & Gagliardi, A. (2010). Beyond the false negative rate: Development of quality indicators for sentinel lymph node biopsy in breast cancer. *Annals of Surgical Oncology, 17*(2), 579–591.

Rahman, G., Adigunt, I., Yusif, I., & Bamigbade, D. (2007). Macromastia and bilateral axillary breast hypertrophy: A case report. *West Africa Journal of Medicine, 26*(3), 250–252.

Shockney, L., & Tsangaris, T. (2008). *Johns Hopkins breast cancer handbook for health care professionals*. Sudbury, MA: Jones and Bartlett.

Stevens, R. (2009). Light at night, circadian disruption and breast cancer: Assessment of existing evidence. *International Journal of Epidemiology, 38*(4), 963–970.

U.S. Preventive Services Task Force. (2009). Clinical guidelines: Screening for breast cancer: U.S. Preventive Services Task Force recommendation statement. *Annals of Internal Medicine, 151*(10), 716–726.

Valea, F., & Katz, V. (2007). Breast disease: Diagnosis and treatment of benign and malignant disease. In V. Katz, G. Lentz, R. Lobo, & D. Gershenson (Eds.), *Comprehensive gynecology* (5th ed.). Philadelphia: Mosby.

CHAPTER 11

Structural Disorders and Neoplasms of the Reproductive System

Deitra Leonard Lowdermilk

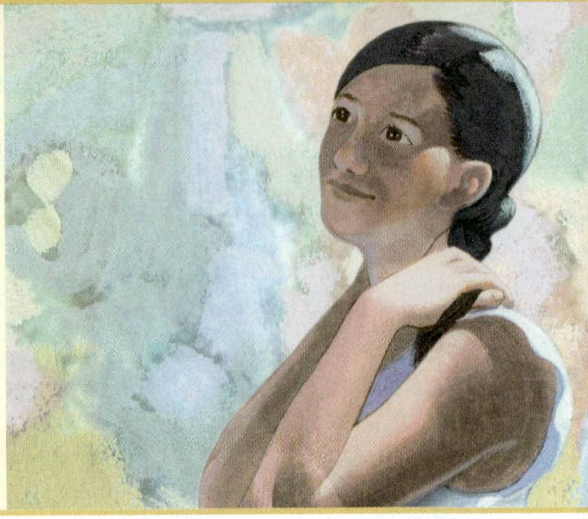

evolve WEBSITE

http://evolve.elsevier.com/Lowdermilk/MWHC/
Audio Glossary
Audio Key Points
NCLEX Review Questions
Nursing Care Plan
Hysterectomy for Endometrial Cancer

LEARNING OBJECTIVES

- Describe the various structural disorders of the uterus and vagina.
- Discuss the pathophysiology of selected benign and malignant neoplasms of the female reproductive tract.
- Compare the common medical and surgical therapies for selected benign gynecologic conditions.
- Explain diagnostic procedures in client-centered terms.
- Examine the emotional effects of benign and malignant neoplasms.
- Develop a nursing care plan for a woman with endometrial cancer who has had a hysterectomy.
- Differentiate treatments for preinvasive and invasive conditions.
- Identify critical elements for teaching clients with selected benign or malignant neoplasms.
- Investigate health-promoting behaviors that reduce cancer risk.
- Assess the effects of and treatments for malignant neoplasms during pregnancy.
- Discuss the development and sequelae of gestational trophoblastic neoplasia.

Women are at risk for structural disorders and neoplastic diseases of the reproductive system from the age of menarche through menopause and the older years. Problems may include structural disorders of the uterus and vagina related to pelvic relaxation and urinary incontinence and chronic pain related to vulvodynia. Benign neoplasms of the reproductive organs, such as fibroids and cysts, and malignant neoplasms of the reproductive system also may occur. Benign tumors usually do not endanger life, tend to grow slowly, and are not invasive. Malignant tumors (cancers) grow rapidly in a disorganized manner and invade surrounding tissues. The development of structural disorders and benign or malignant neoplasms can have far-reaching effects for the woman and her family. Beyond the obvious physiologic alterations, the woman also experiences threats to her self-concept and her ability to cope. A woman's concept of herself as a sexual being can be affected by the condition and its treatments. A woman's family also is challenged in the way it responds to her diagnosis. When cancer occurs with pregnancy, it adds to the complexity of physical and emotional responses to childbearing.

Nurses have important roles in teaching women about early detection and treatment and in providing supportive care to women and their families. This chapter presents information that will assist the nurse in assessing and identifying problems associated with structural problems or benign or malignant reproductive neoplasms. Nursing care concepts related to early detection, treatment methods, and education are included.

STRUCTURAL DISORDERS OF THE UTERUS AND VAGINA

Alterations in Pelvic Support

Alterations in pelvic support include uterine displacement and prolapse, cystoceles and rectoceles, urinary incontinence, and genital fistulas. Research by Wu and colleagues (2009) suggests that the prevalence of these disorders will increase by as much as 55% in the United States between the years 2010 and 2050 as the numbers of older women increase.

Uterine Displacement and Prolapse

The round ligaments normally hold the uterus in anteversion, and the uterosacral ligaments pull the cervix backward and upward (see Fig. 4-3). **Uterine displacement** is a variation of this normal placement. The most common type of displacement is posterior displacement, or retroversion, in which the uterus is tilted posteriorly, and the cervix rotates

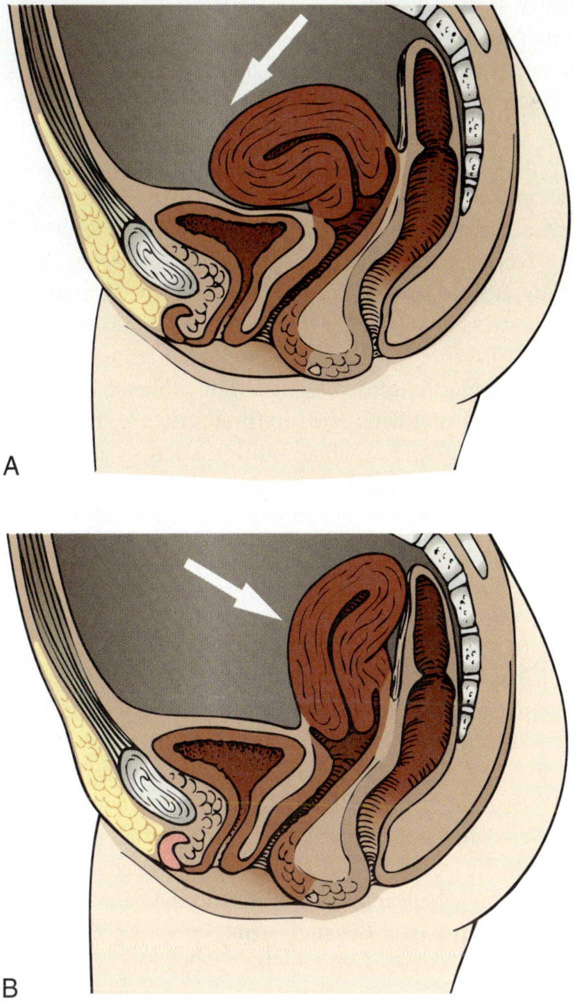

FIG. 11-1 Types of uterine displacement. **A**, Anterior displacement. **B**, Retroversion (backward displacement of the uterus).

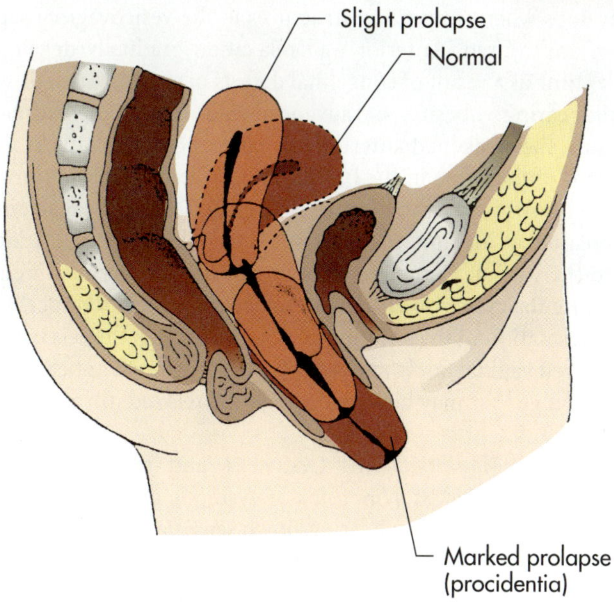

FIG. 11-2 Prolapse of uterus.

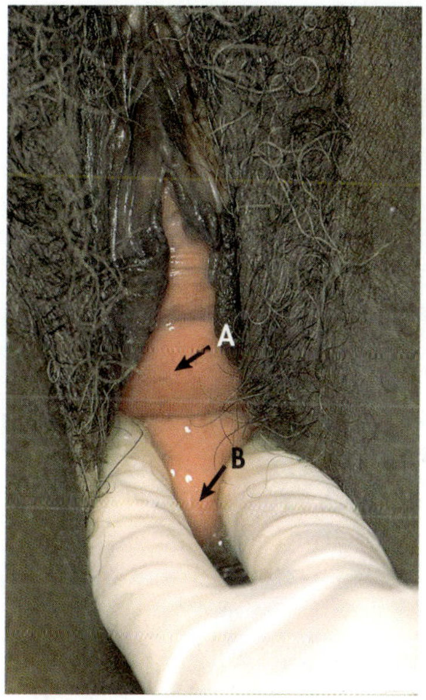

FIG. 11-3 *A*, Cystocele. *B*, Rectocele. (From Seidel, H., Ball, J., Dains, J., Flynn, J., Solomon, B., & Stewart, R. [2011]. *Mosby's guide to physical examination* [7th ed.]. St. Louis: Mosby.)

anteriorly. Other variations include retroflexion and anteflexion (Fig. 11-1).

By 2 months postpartum, the ligaments should return to normal length, but in about one third of women, the uterus remains retroverted. This condition is rarely symptomatic, but conception may be difficult because the cervix points toward the anterior vaginal wall and away from the posterior fornix, where seminal fluid pools after coitus. If symptoms occur, they may include pelvic and low back pain, dyspareunia, and exaggeration of premenstrual symptoms.

Uterine prolapse is a more serious type of displacement. The degree of prolapse can vary from mild to complete. In complete prolapse, the cervix and body of the uterus protrude through the vagina, and the vagina is inverted (Fig. 11-2).

Uterine displacement and prolapse can be caused by congenital or acquired weakness of the pelvic support structures (often called **pelvic relaxation**). In many cases, problems can be a delayed but direct result of childbearing. Although extensive damage may be noted and repaired shortly after birth, symptoms related to pelvic relaxation most often appear during the perimenopausal period, when the effects of ovarian hormones on pelvic tissues are lost, and atrophic changes begin. Pelvic trauma, stress and strain, and the aging process also are contributing factors. Other causes of pelvic relaxation include reproductive surgery and pelvic radiation.

Clinical Manifestations. Symptoms of pelvic relaxation generally relate to the structure involved: urethra, bladder, uterus, vagina, cul-de-sac, or rectum. The most common complaints are pulling and dragging sensations, pressure, protrusions, fatigue, and low backache. Symptoms may be worse after prolonged standing or deep penile penetration during intercourse. Urinary incontinence can be present.

Cystocele and Rectocele

Cystocele and rectocele almost always accompany uterine prolapse, causing the uterus to sag even farther backward and downward into the vagina. **Cystocele** (Fig. 11-3, *A*) is the protrusion of the bladder downward into the vagina that develops when supporting structures in the vesicovaginal septum are injured. Anterior wall relaxation gradually develops over time as a result of congenital defects of support structures, childbearing, obesity, or advanced age. When the woman stands, the weakened anterior vaginal wall cannot support the weight of the urine in the bladder; the vesicovaginal septum is forced downward, the bladder is stretched, and its capacity is increased. With time the cystocele enlarges until it protrudes into the vagina. Complete emptying of the bladder is difficult because the cystocele sags below the bladder neck. **Rectocele** is the herniation of the anterior rectal wall through the relaxed or ruptured vaginal fascia and rectovaginal septum; it appears as a large bulge that may be seen through the relaxed introitus (see Fig. 11-3, *B*).

Clinical Manifestations. Cystoceles and rectoceles often are asymptomatic. If symptoms of cystocele are present, they include complaints of a bearing-down sensation or that "something is in my vagina." Other symptoms include urinary frequency, retention, and/or incontinence, and possible recurrent cystitis and urinary tract infections (UTIs). Pelvic examination will reveal a bulging of the anterior wall of the vagina when the woman is asked to bear down. Unless the bladder neck and urethra are damaged, urinary continence is unaffected. Women with large cystoceles complain of having to push upward on the sagging anterior vaginal wall to be able to void.

Rectoceles may be small and produce few symptoms, but some are so large that they protrude outside of the vagina when the woman stands. Symptoms are absent when the woman is lying down. A rectocele causes a disturbance in bowel function, the sensation of bearing down, or the sensation that the pelvic organs are falling out. With a very large rectocele it may be difficult to have a bowel movement. Each time the woman strains during bowel evacuation, the feces are forced against the thinned rectovaginal wall, stretching it more. Some women facilitate evacuation by applying digital pressure vaginally to hold up the rectal pouch.

Urinary Incontinence

Urinary incontinence (UI) affects young and middle-aged women, with the prevalence increasing as the woman ages. Although nulliparous women can have UI, the incidence is higher in women who have given birth and increases with parity. Women who are overweight and those who have had a hysterectomy are also at increased risk (Sung & Hampton, 2009). There are conflicting data about ethnicity and race as contributing factors (Waetjen, Laio, Johnson, Sampselle, Sternfield, Harlow, & Gold, 2007). Conditions that disturb urinary control include stress incontinence due to sudden increases in intraabdominal pressure (such as that due to sneezing or coughing); urge incontinence, caused by disorders of the bladder and urethra, such as urethritis and urethral stricture, trigonitis, and cystitis; neuropathies, such as multiple sclerosis, diabetic neuritis, and pathologic conditions of the spinal cord; and congenital and acquired urinary tract abnormalities. Research also suggests that a significant number of women have undiagnosed urinary incontinence (Wallner, Porten, Meenan, O'Keefe Rosetti, Calhoun, Sarma, & Clemens, 2009).

Stress incontinence may follow injury to bladder neck structures. A sphincter mechanism at the bladder neck compresses the upper urethra, pulls it upward behind the symphysis, and forms an acute angle at the junction of the posterior urethral wall and the base of the bladder (urethrovesical angle) (Fig. 11-4). To empty the bladder, the sphincter complex relaxes, and the trigone contracts to open the internal urethral orifice and pull the contracting bladder wall upward, forcing urine out. The angle between the urethra and the base of the bladder is lost or increased if the supporting pubococcygeus muscle is injured; this change, coupled with urethrocele, causes incontinence. Urine spurts out when the woman is asked to bear down or cough in the lithotomy position.

Clinical Manifestations. Involuntary leaking of urine is the main sign. Episodes of leaking are common during coughing, laughing, and exercise.

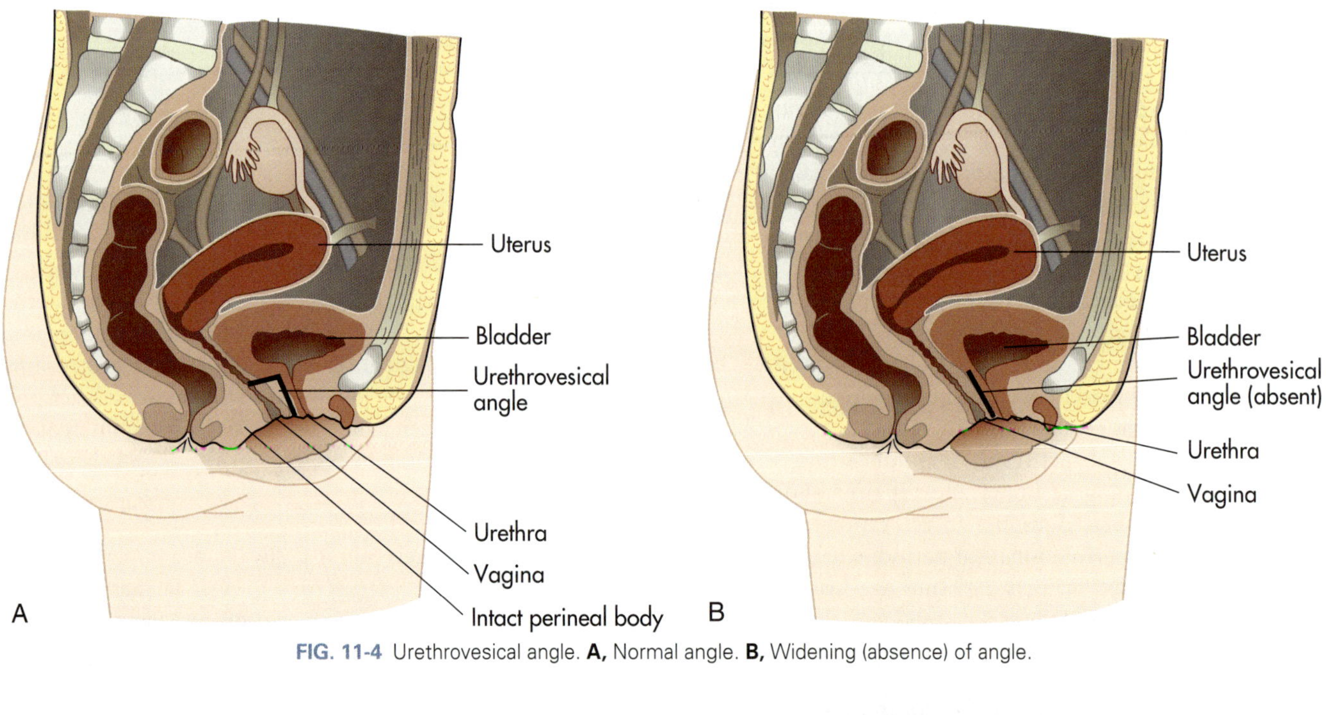

FIG. 11-4 Urethrovesical angle. **A,** Normal angle. **B,** Widening (absence) of angle.

Genital Fistulas

Genital **fistulas** are perforations between genital tract organs. Most occur between the bladder and the genital tract (e.g., vesicovaginal); between the urethra and the vagina (urethrovaginal); and between the rectum or sigmoid colon and the vagina (rectovaginal) (Fig. 11-5). Genital fistulas also may be a result of a congenital anomaly, gynecologic surgery, obstetric trauma, cancer, radiation therapy, gynecologic trauma, or infection (e.g., in the episiotomy).

Clinical Manifestations. Signs and symptoms of vaginal fistulas depend on the site but can include presence of urine, flatus, or feces in the vagina; odors of urine or feces in the vagina; and irritation of vaginal tissues.

Collaborative Care

Assessment for problems related to structural disorders of the uterus and vagina focuses primarily on the genitourinary tract, the reproductive organs, bowel elimination, and psychosocial and sexual factors. A complete health history, a physical examination, and laboratory tests are done to support the appropriate medical diagnosis. The nurse must assess the woman's knowledge of the disorder, its management, and possible prognosis. Possible nursing diagnoses for structural problems of the uterus and vagina include the following:

- *Deficient knowledge* related to:
  - causes of structural disorders and treatment options
- *Constipation or diarrhea* related to:
  - anatomic changes
- *Acute pain* related to:
  - relaxation of pelvic support or elimination difficulties
- *Ineffective coping* related to:
  - changes in body image
- *Interrupted family processes* related to:
  - the woman's anatomic and functional changes
- *Risk for injury* related to:
  - lack of skill in self-care procedures
  - lack of understanding of the reasons for the need to comply with therapy
- *Social isolation, spiritual distress, disturbed body image,* or *chronic low self-*esteem related to:
  - changes in anatomy and function
- *Anxiety* related to:
  - surgical procedure
  - prognosis

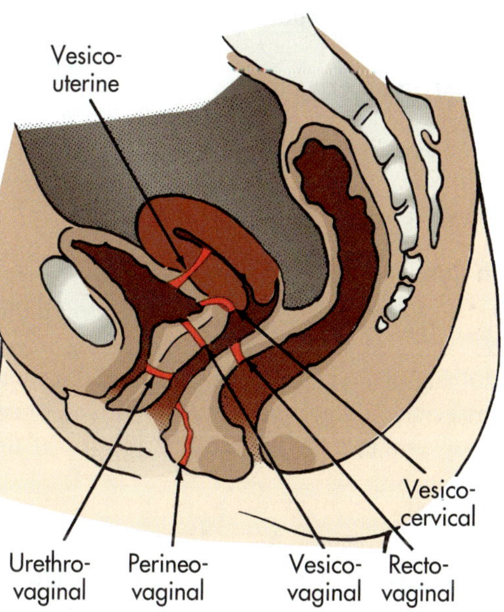

FIG. 11-5 Types of fistulas that may develop in the vagina, uterus, or rectum. (From Monahan F., Sands, J. K., Neighbors, M., Marek, J., & Green, C. (2007). *Phipps' medical-surgical nursing: Health and illness perspectives* (8th ed.). St. Louis: Mosby.

The health care team works together to treat the disorders related to alterations in pelvic support and to assist the woman in management of her symptoms. In general, nurses working with these women can provide information and self-care education to prevent problems before they occur, to manage or reduce symptoms and promote comfort and hygiene if symptoms are already present, and to recognize when further intervention is needed. This information can be part of all postpartum discharge teaching or can be provided at postpartum follow-up visits in clinics or physician/nurse-midwife offices, during postpartum home visits, or during gynecologic health examinations. In addition, information on how to prevent or recognize problems can be a topic for workshops for women or health fairs in community settings.

Besides providing information about prevention, nurses participate in a team effort to prepare the woman for surgery and self-care after discharge. Preoperative teaching involves the primary nurse, operating room nurse, surgeon, and anesthesia provider. Postoperatively, a nurse in the health promotion setting may be most aware of the woman's living circumstances, physical limitations, and social problems and therefore may be best suited to coordinate continuity of care after discharge.

Interventions for specific problems depend on the problem and the severity of the symptoms. If discomfort related to uterine displacement is a problem, several interventions can be implemented. Kegel exercises (see p. 91) can be performed several times daily to increase muscle strength. A knee-chest position performed for a few minutes several times a day can correct a mildly retroverted uterus. A fitted **pessary** to support the uterus and hold it in the correct position (Fig. 11-6) may be inserted in the vagina. Usually a pessary is used only for a short time because it can lead to pressure necrosis and vaginitis. Good hygiene is important; some women can be taught to remove the pessary at night, cleanse it, and replace it in the morning. If the pessary is always left in place, regular douching with commercially prepared solutions or weak white vinegar solutions (1 tablespoon to 1 quart [liter] of water) to remove increased secretions and keep the vaginal pH at 4 to 4.5 is suggested. After a period of treatment, most women are free of symptoms and do not require the pessary. Surgical correction is rarely indicated.

Treatment for uterine prolapse depends on the degree of prolapse. Pessaries may be useful in mild prolapse. Estrogen therapy also may be used in the older woman to improve tissue tone. If these conservative treatments do not correct the problem, or if there is a significant degree of prolapse, abdominal or vaginal hysterectomy (see later discussion) is usually recommended (Lentz, 2007).

Mild to moderate urinary infections can be significantly decreased or relieved in many women by bladder training and pelvic muscle (Kegel) exercises (Bersuk, 2007; Dumoulin & Hay-Smith, 2010). Other management strategies include pelvic flow support devices (i.e., pessaries), vaginal estrogen therapy,

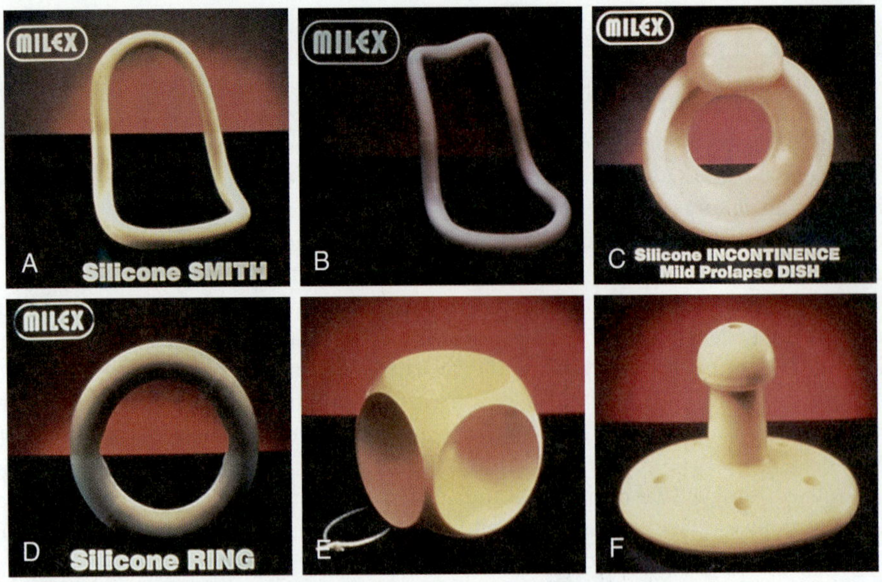

FIG. 11-6 Examples of pessaries. **A,** Smith. **B,** Hodge without support. **C,** Incontinence dish without support. **D,** Ring without support. **E,** Cube. **F,** Gellhorn. (Courtesy Milex Products, Inc., a division of CooperSurgical, Trumbull, CT.)

serotonin-norepinephrine reuptake inhibitors, electrical stimulation, insertion of an artificial urethral sphincter, and surgery (e.g., anterior repair) (Tarnay & Bhatia, 2010).

Nursing care for women with urinary incontinence includes assessment for depression that can result from decreased quality of life and functional status. Women also may need guidance about changes in lifestyle (e.g., losing weight) and education about pelvic muscle exercises (Peterson, 2008; Sung, West, Hernandez, Wheeler, Myers, Subak, et al., 2009).

Treatment for a cystocele includes use of a vaginal pessary or surgical repair. Pessaries may not be effective. *Anterior repair (colporrhaphy)* is the usual surgical procedure and is commonly performed for large, symptomatic cystoceles. This involves a surgical shortening of pelvic muscles to provide better support for the bladder. An anterior repair is often combined with a vaginal hysterectomy. Kegel exercises may be beneficial for symptoms of urinary and fecal incontinence (Lentz, 2007).

Small rectoceles may not require treatment. The woman with mild symptoms may derive relief from a high-fiber diet and adequate fluid intake, stool softeners, or mild laxatives. Vaginal pessaries usually are not effective. Large rectoceles that are causing significant symptoms are usually repaired surgically. A *posterior repair (colporrhaphy)* is the usual procedure. This surgery is performed vaginally and involves shortening the pelvic muscles to provide better support for the rectum (Lentz, 2007). Anterior and posterior repairs may be performed at the same time and with a vaginal hysterectomy.

Management of genital fistulas depends on the location. Surgical repair is the usual treatment; however, it may not be successful.

Nursing care of the woman with a cystocele, rectocele, or fistula requires great sensitivity, because the woman's reactions are often intense. She may become withdrawn or hostile because of embarrassment caused by odors and soiling of her clothing that are beyond her control. She may have concerns about engaging in sexual activities because her partner is repelled by these problems. The nurse can tactfully suggest hygiene practices that reduce odor. Commercial deodorizing douches are available, or noncommercial solutions, such as chlorine solution (1 teaspoon of household chlorine bleach to 1 quart of water) may be used. The chlorine solution also is useful for external perineal irrigation. Sitz baths and thorough washing of the genitals with unscented, mild soap and warm water help. Sparse dusting with deodorizing powders can be useful. If a rectovaginal fistula is present, enemas given before leaving the house may provide temporary relief from oozing of fecal material until corrective surgery is performed. Irritated skin and tissues may benefit from use of the heat lamp or application of an emollient ointment. Hygienic care is time consuming and may need to be repeated frequently throughout the day; protective pads or pants may have to be worn. All of these activities can be demoralizing to the woman and frustrating to her and her family. If surgical repair is performed, nursing care focuses on preventing infection and helping the woman avoid putting stress on the surgical site.

BENIGN NEOPLASMS

Benign neoplasms include a variety of nonmalignant cysts and tumors of the ovaries, the uterus, the vulva, and other organs of the reproductive system.

Ovarian Cysts

Functional ovarian cysts (Fig. 11-7) are dependent on hormonal influences associated with the menstrual cycle. These cysts may be classified as follicular cysts, corpus luteum cysts, theca-lutein cysts, endometrial cysts, and polycystic ovary syndrome. Other benign ovarian neoplasms include dermoid cysts and ovarian fibromas.

Follicular Cysts

Follicular cysts develop most commonly in normal ovaries of young women as a result of the mature graafian follicle failing to rupture, or when an immature follicle does not resorb fluid after ovulation. A cyst is usually asymptomatic unless it ruptures, in which case it causes severe pelvic pain. If the cyst does not rupture, it usually shrinks after two or three menstrual cycles.

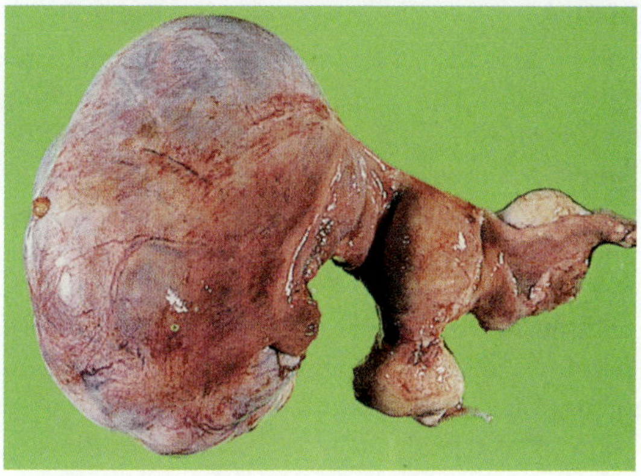

FIG. 11-7 Ovarian cyst. (From Seidel, H., Ball, J., Dains, J., Flynn, J., Solomon, B., & Stewart, R. [2011]. *Mosby's guide to physical examination* [7th ed.]. St. Louis: Mosby.)

Corpus Luteum Cysts

Corpus luteum cysts occur after ovulation and are possibly caused by an increased secretion of progesterone that results in an increase of fluid in the corpus luteum. Clinical manifestations associated with a corpus luteum cyst include pain, tenderness over the ovary, delayed menses, and irregular or prolonged menstrual flow. A rupture can cause intraperitoneal hemorrhage. Corpus luteum cysts usually disappear without treatment within one or two menstrual cycles.

Theca-Lutein Cysts

Theca-lutein cysts are uncommon and in up to 50% of cases are associated with hydatidiform mole (see Chapter 28). **Theca-lutein cysts** develop as a result of prolonged stimulation of the ovaries by human chorionic gonadotropin (hCG). They also may occur if the woman has taken ovulation induction drugs; if she is pregnant and a large placenta is present, such as in the presence of a multiple gestation; or if the woman has diabetes (Katz, 2007). The cysts are almost always bilateral. A feeling of pelvic fullness may be noted by the woman if the ovary is enlarged, but most women are asymptomatic.

Polycystic Ovary Syndrome

Polycystic ovary syndrome (PCOS) occurs when an endocrine imbalance results in high levels of estrogen, testosterone, and luteinizing hormone (LH) and decreased secretion of follicle-stimulating hormone. This syndrome is associated with a variety of problems in the hypothalamic-pituitary-ovarian axis and with androgen-producing tumors. The condition can be transmitted as an X-linked dominant or autosomal dominant trait (Stein-Leventhal syndrome). Multiple follicular cysts develop on one or both ovaries and produce excess estrogen. The ovaries often double in size. Clinical manifestations include obesity, hirsutism (excessive hair growth), irregular menses or amenorrhea, and infertility. Impaired glucose tolerance and hyperinsulinemia occur in about 40% of women with PCOS (Lobo, 2007). Affected women are at high risk for developing type 2 diabetes mellitus and possibly cardiovascular diseases (Benson, Hahn, Tan, Janssen, Schedlowski, & Elsenbruch, 2010). PCOS is often diagnosed in adolescence when menstrual irregularities and other symptoms appear (Lobo).

Collaborative Care

A variety of interventions may be implemented for the woman with a functional cyst. If expectant management is the treatment, the woman is advised to keep appointments for pelvic examinations to monitor the changes in size of the cyst (enlarging or shrinking). Pharmacologic interventions such as analgesics may be prescribed for pain management. Oral contraceptives may be ordered for several months to suppress ovulation for functional cysts. Large cysts (greater than 8 cm) or cysts that do not shrink may be removed surgically (cystectomy). Corpus luteum cysts are treated similarly. Theca-lutein cysts are usually managed conservatively (they usually regress) or by removal of the hydatidiform mole (Katz, 2007).

Nursing care focuses on educating the woman regarding treatment options as well as pain management with analgesics or comfort measures such as heat to the abdomen or relaxation techniques. If surgery is performed, the nurse provides preoperative and postoperative care. Discharge teaching includes signs of infection, postoperative incision care, the possibility of recurrence, and advice regarding follow-up appointments.

The treatment for PCOS depends on what symptoms are of greatest concern to the woman. Lifestyle modifications (e.g., losing weight) and management of presenting symptoms such as infertility, irregular menses, and hirsutism are the focus. Oral contraceptives (OCs) are the usual treatment for irregular menses, if pregnancy is not desired, because they inhibit LH and decrease testosterone levels. OCs can also lessen acne to some degree. Gonadotropin-releasing hormone (GnRH) analogs may be used to treat hirsutism if oral contraceptives do not improve this condition. If pregnancy is desired, ovulation-inducing medications are given (Lobo, 2007). Metformin and other insulin medications for type 2 diabetes also are used to lower insulin, testosterone, and glucose levels, which in turn can reduce acne, hirsutism, abdominal obesity, amenorrhea, and other symptoms in women with PCOS (Lobo).

Nurses can provide information and counseling for women with PCOS. Information may be needed about the syndrome or about its long-term effects on the woman's health. Research has shown that women report symptoms of psychologic distress including depression, anxiety, and social fears (Benson et al., 2010). Women may need to discuss their feelings about the physical manifestations of PCOS and may need emotional support if they have self-image problems related to the symptoms. Teaching about lifestyle modifications such as exercise and diet may be needed as well as education about the medications that are prescribed. Information about finding a support group or information on the Internet may be useful.

Other Benign Ovarian Cysts and Neoplasms

Two other ovarian neoplasms are dermoid cysts and ovarian fibromas. **Dermoid cysts** are germ cell tumors, usually occurring in childhood. These cysts contain substances such as hair, teeth, sebaceous secretions, and bones. Unless the cyst is large enough to put pressure on other organs, it is usually asymptomatic. Dermoid cysts may develop bilaterally and are often attached to the ovary. Treatment is usually surgical removal.

Ovarian fibromas are solid ovarian neoplasms developing from connective tissue and most often occurring after

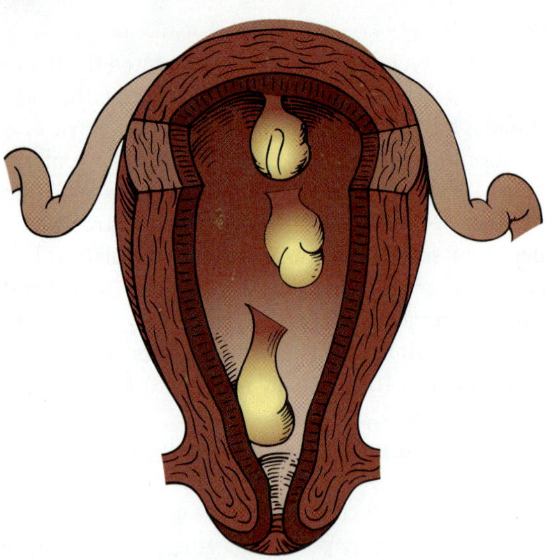

FIG. 11-8 Endometrial polyps.

menopause. Fibromas range in size from small nodules to large masses weighing more than 23 kg. Most fibromas are unilateral. They are usually asymptomatic, but if large enough, they may cause ascites, feelings of pelvic pressure, or abdominal enlargement. Treatment is usually surgical removal.

Nursing care of women who have surgery for the removal of dermoid cysts and ovarian fibromas is similar to that described for functional ovarian cysts.

Uterine Polyps

Uterine polyps may be endometrial or cervical in origin. They are tumors that are on pedicles (stalks) arising from the mucosa (Fig. 11-8). The etiology is unknown, although they may develop in response to hormonal stimulus or be the result of inflammation. Polyps are the most common benign lesions of the cervix and endometrium that occur during the reproductive years. These polyps may be single or multiple. Endocervical polyps are most common in multiparous women older than 40 years. The woman may be asymptomatic or she may have premenstrual or postmenstrual bleeding or postcoital bleeding (Nelson & Gambone, 2010).

Collaborative Care

Clinical management of endometrial polyps is by surgical removal. Cervical polyps are usually removed in an office or clinic procedure without anesthesia. The polyp is grasped with a clamp and twisted or cut off. All polyps should be sent for pathologic examination. Endometrial sampling (which may require local anesthesia) should be done to determine if other pathologic conditions are present (Katz, 2007).

Nursing care includes preparing the woman for what to expect during the removal procedure and encouraging relaxation and breathing exercises and providing support during the procedure. After the procedure the woman is advised to avoid using tampons, sexual intercourse, and douching for up to 1 week or until the site is healed. She is taught how to identify signs of infection and to notify her health care provider if she experiences heavy bleeding (more than one pad in 1 hour).

Leiomyomas

Leiomyomas, also known as fibroid tumors, fibromas, myomas, or fibromyomas, are slow-growing benign tumors arising from the muscle tissue of the uterus (Nelson & Gambone, 2010). They are the most common benign tumors of the reproductive system, occurring most often after age 50 years. They tend to occur more often in African-American women and women who have never been pregnant (Nelson & Gambone). Fibroids also occur more often in women who are overweight (Katz, 2007). They rarely become malignant. Because their growth is influenced by ovarian hormones, these benign tumors can become quite large when the woman is pregnant or taking hormone therapy. They often spontaneously shrink after menopause when circulating ovarian hormones are diminished (Katz; Nelson & Gambone).

CLINICAL REASONING

Informed Decision Making for Treatment of Leiomyoma

Yolanda, a 43-year-old married Hispanic woman, has just been diagnosed with a uterine leiomyoma. She has expressed concern about the treatment because she does not want to have a hysterectomy and her friends have told her that she will probably have to have one. What response by the nurse would be appropriate?

1. Evidence—Is there sufficient evidence to draw conclusions about what the nurse should say?
2. Assumptions—What assumptions can be made about the following issues?
   a. Medical therapy and observation for leiomyomas
   b. Differences between myomectomy and hysterectomy for leiomyoma treatment
   c. Uterine artery embolization as a treatment option for leiomyomas
3. What implications and priorities for nursing care can be made at this time?
4. Does the evidence objectively support your conclusion?
5. Are there alternative perspectives to your conclusion?

Clinical Manifestations and Diagnosis

The cause of leiomyomas remains unknown, although genetic factors may be involved in their development. Most of the tumors are found in the body of the uterus. Leiomyomas are classified according to the location in the uterine wall. *Subserous* leiomyomas develop beneath the peritoneal surface of the uterus and appear as small or large masses that protrude from the outer uterine surface (Fig. 11-9, *A*). *Intramural* leiomyomas are tumors that develop within the wall of the uterus (see Fig. 11-9, *B*). *Submucosal* leiomyomas are the least common tumors, but often cause the most symptoms. These tumors develop in the endometrium and protrude into the uterine cavity (see Fig. 11-9, *C*). Leiomyomas can develop in the cervix and on the broad ligaments (see Fig. 11-9, *D*). They can grow on pedicles or stalks (see Fig. 11-9, *E*). Occasionally these break off the pedicle and attach to other tissues (become parasitic).

Most women are asymptomatic; abnormal uterine bleeding is the most common symptom of fibroids. If the tumor is very large, pelvic circulation may be compromised, and surrounding viscera may be displaced. A woman may complain of backache, low abdominal pressure, constipation, urinary incontinence, or

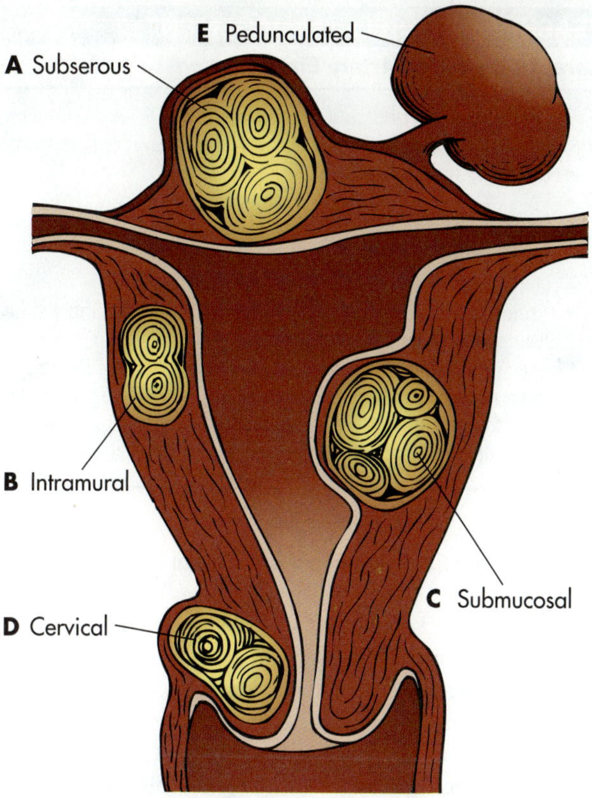

FIG. 11-9 Types of leiomyomas. *A*, Subserous. *B*, Intramural. *C*, Submucosal. *D*, Cervical. *E*, Pedunculated.

dysmenorrhea (painful menstruation). Nausea and vomiting may occur if the tumor is obstructing the intestines. The woman also may notice an abdominal mass if the tumor is large. Anemia can occur if the woman has excessive bleeding. Pedunculated tumors can twist and become necrotic, causing pain.

The tumors appear to be influenced by the presence of estrogen. Fibroids can affect implantation and maintenance of pregnancy. During pregnancy, the tumors may produce complications such as preterm labor, miscarriage, or dystocia (difficult labor). The severity of the symptoms seems to be directly related to the size and location of the tumors.

CARE MANAGEMENT

Knowledge of the medical-surgical management of leiomyomas is essential in planning nursing care. The knowledge enables the nurse to work collaboratively with other health care providers and to meet the woman's informational and emotional needs. Clinical management for benign tumors of the uterus depends on the severity of the symptoms, the age of the woman, and her desire to preserve childbearing potential (see Nursing Process box: Woman with a Leiomyoma).

Medical Management

Medications. If symptoms are mild, regular checkups may suffice to observe for growth or changes in size. Nonsteroidal anti-inflammatory drugs (NSAIDs) may be prescribed for pain; oral contraceptives inhibit ovulation and may relieve symptoms; and GnRH agonists such as leuprolide acetate (Lupron, Synarel) may be prescribed to reduce the size of the leiomyoma. Other medications used include medroxyprogesterone acetate (Depo-Provera), danazol (Danocrine), mifepristone (Mifeprex), and selective estrogen receptor modulators (SERMs) (e.g., raloxifene) (Katz, 2007; Nelson & Gambone, 2010; Wu, Chen, & Xie, 2007). The ideal medical therapy for treating fibroids has not been found, and research in this area continues (Sankaran & Manyonda, 2008).

The woman who prefers medical treatment will need information about the various medications, their actions and side

NURSING PROCESS

The Woman with a Leiomyoma

ASSESSMENT

Assessments include:

- History of symptoms (which might include abnormal bleeding, abdominal pain, dysmenorrhea, pelvic fullness or heaviness, or problems with elimination)
- Pelvic examination that usually identifies the presence of uterine enlargement.
- Pregnancy test—a negative test will rule out pregnancy as the cause of the symptoms.
- Laparoscopy may be used to differentiate ovarian masses from uterine masses.
- Ultrasound examination can differentiate between inflammatory masses or endometriosis and subserous fibroids.

NURSING DIAGNOSES

Possible nursing diagnoses for a woman with a leiomyoma include:

Anxiety **related to:**

- uncertain diagnosis
- fear of malignancy
- potential surgical treatment

Acute or Chronic Pain **related to:**

- leiomyomas

Sexual Dysfunction **related to:**

- dyspareunia

EXPECTED OUTCOMES OF CARE

Expected outcomes for the woman with a leiomyoma might include that the woman will:

- Verbalize a decrease in anxiety related to the diagnosis and therapeutic regimen.
- Verbalize understanding of treatment options to make an informed decision.
- Report no compromise in sexual functioning as a result of the therapeutic intervention.

PLAN OF CARE AND INTERVENTIONS

Nursing interventions will be based on the treatment of leiomyomas (see text and Teaching for Self-Management boxes on pp. 242 and 244) and include:

- Providing information about medications
- Providing teaching about preparation for uterine artery embolization (UAE) or surgical procedure
- Providing postprocedure care and discharge teaching
- Using therapeutic communication skills with the woman to help her express her feelings and concerns
- Referring to a community support group or counseling as needed

EVALUATION

The nurse evaluates the care of the woman who has had treatment of uterine leiomyomas by using the outcome criteria.

effects, and routes of administration. A woman who is receiving GnRH agonists to decrease the size of the fibroid must understand that regrowth will occur after the treatment is stopped. She also must know that a small loss in bone mass and changes in lipid levels can occur; therefore, long-term use is not recommended. Adding raloxifene to GnRH administration has been effective in preventing these effects in some premenopausal women (Nelson & Gambone, 2010; Sankaran & Manyonda, 2008). Amenorrhea may occur; however, women who wish to avoid pregnancy should use a nonhormonal or barrier method of contraception. A discussion of administration methods for GnRH agonists, including subcutaneous and intramuscular injections, intranasal administration, and subcutaneous implantation, will assist the woman in making a decision about her preferred method of administration (see Medication Guide, p. 205).

Uterine Artery Embolization. **Uterine artery embolization (UAE)** is a treatment during which polyvinyl alcohol (PVA) pellets are injected into selected blood vessels to block the blood supply to the fibroid and cause shrinkage and resolution of symptoms (Katz, 2007). The procedure is done under local anesthesia and conscious sedation and can be done as an outpatient procedure, although some women will have the procedure in the hospital setting and remain overnight or be discharged within 4 to 6 hours (Katz; Pisco, Bilhim, Duarte, & Santos, 2009). An incision is made into the groin, and a catheter is threaded into the femoral artery to the uterine artery. An arteriogram identifies the vessels supplying the fibroid. Most fibroids are reduced in size by 50% within 3 months. Temporary amenorrhea or early menopause can occur in some women. Although symptom improvement occurs for most women, data are lacking about the effects on future fertility and pregnancy outcomes. Long-term effects of the procedure are unknown (Katz).

Preoperative teaching includes advising the woman not to drink alcohol or smoke and not to take aspirin or anticoagulant medications 24 hours before the procedure. If the procedure is done on an outpatient basis, the woman will usually need to take acid-suppressing medications, NSAIDs, and antihistaminic drugs as well as laxatives beginning the day before the procedure (Pisco et al., 2009). The woman is told to expect cramping during injection of the PVA pellets. Explanations about what to expect postoperatively include pelvic pain, fever, malaise, and nausea and vomiting that may be caused by acute fibroid degeneration. Pain can be controlled with NSAIDs or narcotic analgesics if needed. Postoperative nursing assessments include checking for bleeding in the groin, taking vital signs, assessing pain level, and checking the pedal pulse and neurovascular condition of the affected leg (Hiller, Miller, & Stavas, 2005). Discharge teaching includes signs of possible complications and when to notify the physician, self-care instructions, and follow-up advice (see Teaching for Self-Management box: Care after Uterine Artery Embolization).

TEACHING FOR SELF-MANAGEMENT

Care After Uterine Artery Embolization

- Take prescribed medications as ordered.
- Call your physician if you have any of the following symptoms:
  - Bleeding
  - Pain
  - Swelling or hematoma at the puncture site
  - Fever of 39° C
  - Urinary retention
  - Abnormal vaginal drainage (foul odor, brown color, tissue)
- Eat a normal diet including fluids and fiber.
- Do not use tampons, douche, or have vaginal intercourse for at least 4 weeks.
- Avoid straining during bowel movements.
- Keep your follow-up appointment.

Surgical Management

In addition to the surgical options of hysterectomy and myomectomy, other techniques have been developed to treat leiomyomas. These include laparoscopic techniques; hysteroscopic techniques; myolysis by heat, cold, and laser; and magnetic resonance–guided focused ultrasound surgery. Not all of these techniques are suitable for every woman nor are all of them universally available to women (Istre, 2008).

Laser Surgery. Laser surgery or electrocauterization can be used to destroy small fibroids through a laparoscopic (abdominal) or hysteroscopic (vaginal) approach. Hysteroscopic uterine *ablation* (vaporization of tissues) can be performed under local or general anesthesia, usually as an outpatient procedure. Medical therapy using GnRH agonists to control bleeding temporarily and to suppress endometrial tissue may be given for 8 to 12 weeks before surgery. Although the uterus remains in place, the vaporization process can cause scarring and adhesions in the uterine cavity, affecting future fertility. Thus this procedure is for women who wish to retain their uterus but no longer desire childbearing potential (Nelson & Gambone, 2010). Risks of the procedure include uterine perforation, cervical injury, and fluid overload (caused by the leaking into blood vessels of fluid used to expand the uterus during surgery). The woman may experience postoperative cramping and a slight vaginal discharge for a few days. Before discharge the following information is given:

- Analgesics or NSAIDs can be used for pain relief as needed.
- Normal activities can be resumed within several days.
- Vaginal discharge is to be expected for 4 to 6 weeks.
- Use of tampons or vaginal intercourse should be avoided for 2 weeks.
- The next menstrual period may be irregular.
- The woman should be reminded about the effects of ablation on her fertility, if appropriate.
- The physician should be called if the woman has heavy bleeding or signs of infection.

Myomectomy. If the tumor is near the outer wall of the uterus, the uterine size is no larger than at 12 to 14 weeks of gestation, and symptoms are significant, **myomectomy** (removal of the tumor) may be performed (Katz, 2007). Myomectomy can be performed through a laparoscopic or abdominal incision approach or a vaginal (hysteroscopic) approach. Myomectomy leaves the uterine muscle walls relatively intact, thereby preserving the uterus and allowing the possibility of future pregnancies (Agdi & Tulandi, 2008). It is usually performed in the proliferative phase of the menstrual cycle to avoid interrupting a possible pregnancy. GnRH therapy may be given before surgery to reduce the size of the fibroid. Fibroids can recur after myomectomy; further treatment may be needed (Nelson & Gambone, 2010).

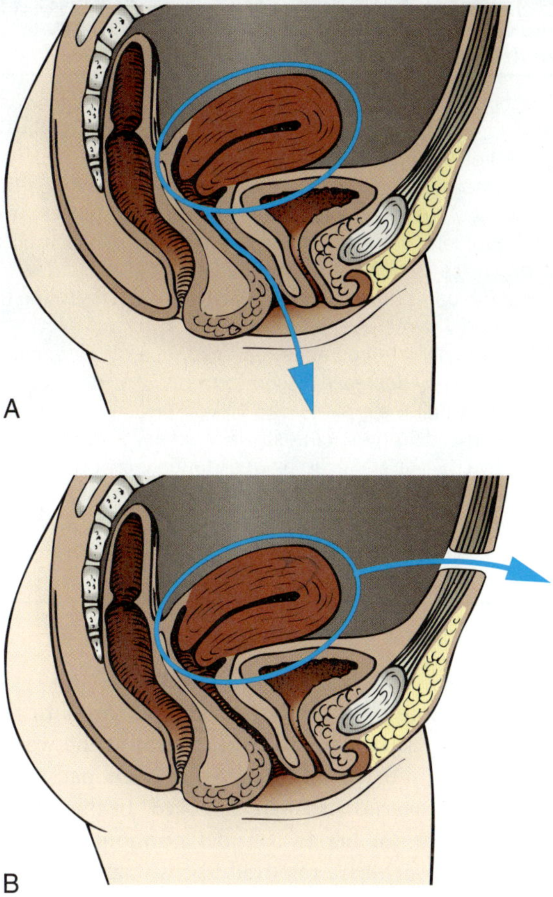

FIG. 11-10 Hysterectomy. **A,** Vaginal. **B,** Abdominal.

BOX 11-1 QUESTIONS FOR A WOMAN TO ASK TO ENSURE INFORMED CONSENT

- Why is this procedure proposed for my condition/problem?
- What are the risks/benefits of the proposed surgery?
- Are there alternatives to this surgery? If so, what are the risks and benefits of these alternatives?
- How many times have you performed this surgery?
- How long will I be hospitalized? Can the procedure be done in an outpatient setting? How long will it take to recover?
- What types of anesthesia can be used?
- What hospital and surgical procedures can I expect?
- How will the surgery affect me (e.g., any changes in physical function, sexual function, or childbearing ability)?

Source: Wade, J., Pletsch, P., Morgan, S., & Menting, S. (2000). Hysterectomy: What do women need and want to know? *Journal of Obstetric, Gynecologic & Neonatal Nursing, 29*(1), 33-42.

BOX 11-2 PREOPERATIVE PROCEDURES FOR HYSTERECTOMY

- Vaginal examination or physical examination
- Laboratory tests
  - Complete blood count, type, and crossmatch
  - Urinalysis
- Chest radiograph
- Electrocardiogram
- Teaching for postoperative routines
  - Turning, coughing, deep breathing
  - Passive and active leg exercises
  - Need for early ambulation
  - Pain relief options
- Nothing by mouth after midnight or as ordered
- Enema if ordered
- Douche if ordered
- Abdominal: mons or perineal shave if ordered
- Removal of makeup, nail polish
- Removal of glasses, contact lenses, dentures, etc.
- Identification band in place
- Signed consent form in chart
- Have woman empty bladder immediately before surgery

Hysterectomy. Hysterectomy (removal of the entire uterus) is the treatment of choice if bleeding is severe or if the fibroid is obstructing normal function of other organs. An abdominal or vaginal surgical approach depends on the size and location of the tumors. For example, abdominal hysterectomy is usually performed for leiomyomas larger than a uterus would be at 12 to 14 weeks of gestation or for multiple leiomyomas. The uterus is removed through either a vertical or transverse incision. In some circumstances the cervix is not removed. Vaginal approaches can be used for smaller tumors. In both abdominal and vaginal approaches, the uterus is removed from the supporting ligaments (broad, round, and uterosacral). These ligaments are then attached to the vaginal cuff, allowing maintenance of normal depth of the vagina (Fig. 11-10). Alternatives to these procedures are the *laparoscopic assisted vaginal hysterectomy (LAVH)* and the *laparoscopic assisted supracervical hysterectomy (LASH)*. LAVH converts an abdominal procedure to a vaginal one by using a laparoscope in the abdomen to assist with removal of the uterus. LASH allows the cervix to remain. Both are associated with a quicker recovery and fewer postoperative complications (Mueller, Renner, Haeberle, Lermann, Oppelt, Beckemann, & Thiel, 2009; Nieboer, Johnson, Lethaby, Tavender, Curr, Garry, et al., 2009).

Preoperative Care. Assessments needed before surgery include the woman's knowledge of treatment options, her desire for future fertility if she is premenopausal, the benefits and risks of each procedure, preoperative and postoperative procedures (Boxes 11-1 and 11-2), and the recovery process (Askew, 2009). If the woman demonstrates understanding of this information, she can make an informed decision about treatment and feel a sense of control over the surgical experience. Resources on helping women to make decisions about treatment can be found at the website for the Fibroid Treatment Collective at www.fibroid.org.

Psychologic assessment is essential, particularly for a woman who is scheduled for a hysterectomy. Areas to be explored include the significance of the loss of the uterus for the woman, misconceptions about effects of surgery, and adequacy of her support system. Women who have not completed their childbearing, who believe that their self-concept is related to having a uterus (to be a complete woman), who feel that sexual functioning is related to having a uterus, or who have too little or too much anxiety about the surgery may be at risk for postoperative emotional reactions (Leppert, Legro, & Kjerulff, 2007). Yen and associates (2008) found that postoperatively most women reported positive feelings about femininity and their body image, less anxiety and depression, but still reported a worsening of sexual functioning.

BOX 11-3 POSTOPERATIVE CARE AFTER HYSTERECTOMY

- Monitor vital signs every 15 minutes until stable; then every 4 hours for 48 hours
- Maintain unobstructed airway
- Turn, cough, deep breathe every 2 hours for 24 hours
  - Assist woman to splint incision with hands or pillow
- Incentive spirometry if ordered
- Leg exercises every 2 to 4 hours until ambulatory
- Assess Homans sign
- Assess bleeding
  - Abdominal: assess dressing or incision
  - Vaginal: perineal pad count (one saturated pad in less than 1 hour is excessive; vaginal bleeding is usually minimal)
- Check laboratory values, especially hematocrit
- Assess lungs
- Assess bowel sounds and monitor bowel function
- Monitor intake and output
  - Foley catheter may be in place for 24 hours after abdominal surgery
  - After vaginal hysterectomy, urinary retention may be a problem because of manipulation of the urethra during surgery
- Assess abdominal incision or vagina for signs of infection
- Observe for signs of complications
  - Abdominal hysterectomy: assess for signs of wound evisceration, pulmonary embolism, thrombophlebitis, pneumonia, bowel obstruction, bleeding (incisional or vaginal)
  - Vaginal hysterectomy: assess for signs of urinary tract infection, urinary retention, wound infection, vaginal bleeding
- Pain relief
  - Pharmacologic measures: patient-controlled analgesia (PCA) or epidural narcotics may be ordered for the first 24 hours, followed by oral analgesics and nonsteroidal anti-inflammatory drugs
  - Nonpharmacologic measures: breathing and relaxation exercises, position changes, guided imagery, application of heat to the abdomen, and sitz baths or ice packs for the perineum; ambulation may relieve gas pains
- Psychologic assessments
  - Assess for depression or other emotional reactions
  - Assess support systems
  - Assess sexual concerns

Postoperative Care. Postoperative assessments and care after myomectomy and abdominal hysterectomy are similar to those for other abdominal surgery (Box 11-3). Assessments specific to abdominal and vaginal hysterectomy include assessment for vaginal bleeding (one perineal pad saturated in less than 1 hour is excessive), urinary retention (especially after vaginal hysterectomy), perineal pain after vaginal hysterectomy, and psychologic assessments (e.g, depression) (Leppert et al., 2007; Yen, Chen, Long, Chang, Yen, & Ko, 2008).

Discharge Planning and Teaching. Discharge planning and teaching are similar for myomectomy and hysterectomy (see Teaching for Self-Management box: Care After Myomectomy or Hysterectomy). Myomectomy and vaginal hysterectomy may be performed in an ambulatory setting, and women may be discharged the evening of the surgery. Women who have an abdominal hysterectomy may have a 1- to 2-day stay in the hospital before being discharged.

TEACHING FOR SELF-MANAGEMENT

Care After Myomectomy or Hysterectomy

- Eat foods high in protein, iron, and vitamin C to aid in tissue healing; include foods with high fiber content; and drink six to eight 8-ounce glasses of water daily.
- Rest when tired; resume activities as comfort level permits. Avoid vigorous exercise and heavy lifting for 6 weeks. Avoid sitting for long periods. Resume driving when comfort allows or on advice from health care provider.
- Avoid tub baths, intercourse (vaginal rest), and douching until after the follow-up examination.
- When vaginal intercourse is resumed, use of water-soluble lubricants may decrease discomfort.
- Report the following symptoms to your health care provider: vaginal bleeding, gastrointestinal changes, persistent postoperative symptoms (cramping, distention, change in bowel habits), and signs of wound infection (redness, swelling, heat, or pain at incision site).
- Keep your follow-up appointment with your health care provider.

If a hysterectomy was performed, the woman is reminded that she will experience cessation of menses. If the woman is premenopausal, she will not experience menopause at this time unless her ovaries also were removed. In this case there will be no reason for her to consider hormone replacement therapy. If the ovaries are removed, the woman will need the most current information on the risks and benefits of hormone replacement therapy (see Chapter 6). Other symptoms she may experience include pain, sleep disturbance, fatigue, anxiety, and depression.

Vaginal intercourse may be uncomfortable at first, especially after vaginal procedures. Use of water-soluble lubricants, relaxation exercises, and positions that control penile penetration may be beneficial (Katz, 2007). Women can be assured that this discomfort will decrease over time.

The schedule for follow-up care depends on the procedure performed, but usually a postoperative visit is scheduled within a week. Vaginal screening with cytology/Papanicolaou (Pap) test after total hysterectomy for a nonmalignant reason is not recommended (American Cancer Society [ACS], 2010a); however, vaginal cancer can occur after hysterectomy and health care providers may continue to recommend Pap screening to assess for vaginal cancer (Slomovitz & Coleman, 2007).

Vulvar Problems

Bartholin Cysts

Bartholin cysts are the most common benign lesions of the vulva. They arise from obstruction of the Bartholin duct, which causes it to enlarge. Small cysts often are asymptomatic; however, large cysts or infected cysts cause symptoms such as vulvar pain, dyspareunia (painful intercourse), and a feeling of a mass in the vulvar area (Eckert & Lentz, 2007).

Collaborative Care. If the woman is asymptomatic no treatment is necessary. If the cyst is symptomatic or infected, surgical incision and drainage may provide temporary relief. Cysts tend to recur; therefore, a permanent opening for drainage may be recommended. This procedure is called *marsupialization* and is the formation of a new duct opening for drainage (Eckert & Lentz, 2007).

Nursing care after surgery includes teaching the woman about pain-relief measures such as sitz baths, heat lamps to the perineum, and use of analgesics. The woman is taught to assess the incision site for signs of healing and infection and to take antibiotics, if prescribed, for prevention of infection.

Vulvodynia

Vulvar pain is a common gynecologic problem. **Vulvodynia,** also called vulvar pain syndrome or vulvovestibulitis, is reportedly experienced by 4% to 27% of women. The incidence is thought to be the same for women of all races and ethnicities (Kingdon, 2009).

Vulvodynia is a complex condition thought to be a chronic pain disorder of the vulvar area. The term vulvodynia is used if pain is present with no visible abnormality or no identified neurologic diagnosis (Katz, 2007). Pain can be described as provoked (e.g., by inserting a tampon or having vaginal intercourse) or unprovoked and localized to the vestibule or generalized over the vulvar area (Kingdon, 2009).

Etiology has not been established although psychologic and biologic theories have been proposed. The most common theory is that vulvodynia is caused by a chronic neuropathic pain syndrome. Inflammation may also be a causative factor and continues to be investigated. (Zolnoun, Hartmann, Lamvu, As-Saine, Maixner, & Steege, 2006). Past sexual and emotional experiences and personality traits are being investigated as causes because they can influence the perception and interpretation of nerve impulses (Kingdon, 2009).

A feature of neuropathic pain is *allodynia,* which is a painful sensation that is from something not supposed to be painful. It commonly occurs in women with vulvodynia. Several triggers that reportedly cause allodynia in the vulvar area include use of oral contraceptives; presence of candidiasis or human papillomavirus; wearing tight-fitting underwear and pants, especially synthetic materials; being a victim of childhood sexual abuse; and using chemical irritants such as scented detergents, soaps, and bubble baths (Arnold, Bachmann, Rosen, & Rhoads, 2007, Goldstein & Burrows, 2008; Harlow, Vitonis, & Stewart, 2008). However, with all these triggers, research evidence is conflicting and the need for scientific evidence is ongoing.

Collaborative Care. Assessment of a woman with possible vulvodynia includes a health history including a mental health history, specifically inquiring about anxiety or depression. A thorough pain assessment is essential. Questions about provoking and palliative factors, the quality of pain, radiation of the pain, strength of the pain and the timing of pain occurrence are included. A history may elicit complaints about burning, stinging or irritation in the vulvar area, and reports of how the woman feels her symptoms affect her physical activities and ability for sexual intimacy.

A thorough pelvic examination is recommended to rule out other causes of pain such as infection or trauma. The vulva should be inspected for erythema, ulcerations, and hyperpigmentation (Goldstein & Burrows, 2008; Katz, 2007). A cotton swab is used to identify areas of pain on pressure to confirm presence of allodynia. A systematic assessment (e.g., using positions of the face of a clock) is suggested, and ratings of pain should be rated as mild, moderate, or severe. Reed (2006) suggests the indentation of the swab be about 5 cm. A speculum examination (a pediatric size is recommended) is used to examine the vagina for redness, erosions, and dryness. A swab of vaginal secretions is obtained and can be tested for yeast, increased white blood cells, and pH. Cultures for *Candida* and bacteria can be obtained. A bimanual examination may be performed (Katz; Reed).

Management strategies are individualized to the woman. Often a series of therapies or a combination of therapies will be implemented to find the best treatment. Currently there is little evidence to support one therapy over another. Oral medications include gabapentin and tricyclic antidepressants (Harris, Horowitz, & Bordiga, 2007; Katz, 2007; Reed, Caron, Gorenflo, & Haefner, 2006). Topical therapies include the use of lidocaine 5% ointment that can be applied nightly or prophylactically (i.e., before sexual intercourse) (Katz, 2007).

Other therapeutic measures that have been tried and are reportedly helpful for symptoms include pelvic floor exercises, biofeedback, vaginal dilator training, hypnosis, and cognitive-behavioral therapy (Hartmann, Strauhal, & Nelson, 2007; Munday, Buchan, Ravenhill, Wiggs, & Brooks, 2007; Katz, 2007; Pukall, Kandyba, Amsel, Khalifé, & Binik, 2007).

Hygienic measures suggested for women with vulvodynia include wearing white cotton underwear, using 100% cotton menstrual pads, using soaps and detergents for sensitive skin, avoiding wearing tight clothing over the vulvar area, avoiding lubricants that contain propylene glycol, and using natural oils such as olive oil for lubricants (Kingdon, 2009).

Surgery is usually not recommended until other measures have proven to be ineffective. The surgical procedure is a vestibulectomy, a difficult procedure that removes the vestibule and hymen and has a high rate of complications (Katz, 2007). Research by Bergeron, Khalife, Glazer, & Binik (2008) found this procedure to be no more effective than less invasive measure such as biofeedback.

Client information about vulvodynia including how to locate support groups is available on various websites including:

- International Society for the Study of Vulvovaginal Disease: www.issvd.org
- National Vulvodynia Association: www.nva.org
- Vulvar Pain Society: www.vulvarpainsociety.org

Nurses can recommend these websites to women who want more information about vulvodynia. Nurses also need to keep current on the latest research so that care can be evidence based.

MALIGNANT NEOPLASMS

Malignant neoplasms of the reproductive system include cancers of the endometrium, the cervix, the ovary, the vulva, the vagina, and the uterine tubes. In 2010 an estimated 83,750 women in the United States were diagnosed with a gynecologic cancer; an estimated 27,710 died (ACS, 2010a). Overweight and obesity are associated with increased risk for developing many cancers, including cancers of the endometrium, ovary, and cervix. Evidence also suggests that being overweight increases the risk for cancer recurrence and decreases the likelihood of survival for these cancers (ACS).

Cancer of the Endometrium

Incidence and Etiology

Endometrial cancer is the most common malignancy of the reproductive system (ACS, 2010a). It is most commonly seen in perimenopausal and postmenopausal women between ages 50 and 65. Certain risk factors have been associated with the development of endometrial cancer, including obesity, nulliparity, infertility, late onset of menopause, diabetes mellitus, hypertension, PCOS, and family history of ovarian or breast disease (ACS; Creasman, 2007a). There appears to be an increase in risk for endometrial cancer in families with hereditary nonpolyposis colorectal cancer (HNPCC). Hormone imbalance, however, seems to be the most significant risk factor (American College of Obstetricians and Gynecologists [ACOG], 2008). Numerous studies have correlated the use of exogenous estrogens (unopposed stimulation, i.e., absence of progesterone) in postmenopausal women with an increased incidence of uterine cancer. Tamoxifen taken by women for breast cancer also has been related to a slight increase in endometrial cancer (Creasman). Pregnancy and use of low-dose oral contraceptive pills appear to offer some protection (ACS). The incidence of endometrial cancer among Caucasian women is higher than that among African-American and Hispanic women; however, the mortality rates are more than one and one half times higher in African-American women (Ries, Melbert, Krapcho, Stinchcomb, Howlader, Horner, et al., 2008).

Endometrial cancer is slow growing and for that reason has a good prognosis if diagnosed at a localized stage. Most endometrial cancers are adenocarcinomas that develop from endometrial hyperplasia. The tumor usually develops in the fundus of the uterus and can spread directly to the myometrium and cervix, as well as to other reproductive organs. **Metastasis** (spread of cancer from its original site) is through the lymphatic system in the pelvis and through the blood to the liver, the lungs, and the brain.

CARE MANAGEMENT

ASSESSMENT AND NURSING DIAGNOSES

Assessment includes a history of physical symptoms. The cardinal sign of endometrial cancer is abnormal uterine bleeding (e.g., postmenopausal bleeding and premenopausal recurrent metrorrhagia). Thirty percent of postmenopausal bleeding is caused by carcinoma. Late signs include a mucosanguineous vaginal discharge, low back pain, or low pelvic pain. A pelvic examination may reveal the presence of a uterine enlargement or mass.

! NURSING ALERT

Women can be informed that they can identify their own risk for developing endometrial as well as ovarian, cervical, and breast cancers by filling out a confidential cancer risk assessment survey that is available at the American Cancer Society (ACS) website—www.cancer.org.

Histologic examination is used for diagnosis. A Pap smear of cellular material obtained by aspiration of the endocervix will identify only one third to one half of cases. Fractional curettage or endometrial biopsy yields the most accurate results. Fractional curettage involves scraping the endocervix and endometrium for histologic evaluation to determine the grade of neoplasm and its stage (extent). Perforation of the uterus is a possible complication of this procedure. Endometrial biopsy will identify about 90% of cases (Creasman, 2007a; Hacker, 2010a). It is usually done on an outpatient basis under local anesthesia. A suction-type curette is used to remove tissue for sampling. It is recommended that women at risk for HNPCC have an annual biopsy beginning at age 35 years (ACS, 2010a). Other diagnostic tests that may be useful include hysteroscopy (examination of the uterus through an endoscope) and vaginal ultrasonography. Tests to determine the spread of cancer include liver function tests, renal function tests, chest x-ray, intravenous pyelography (IVP), barium enema, computed tomography (CT), magnetic resonance imaging (MRI), bone scans, and biopsy of suggestive tissues. The International Federation of Gynecology and Obstetrics (FIGO) classification system is used to describe the stages of endometrial carcinoma (Table 11-1).

TABLE 11-1 FIGO CLASSIFICATION OF ENDOMETRIAL CARCINOMA*

STAGE	DESCRIPTION
Ia G1,2,3	Tumor limited to endometrium
Ib G1,2,3	Invasion of less than half of the myometrium
Ic G1,2,3	Invasion of more than half of the myometrium
IIa G1,2,3	Endocervical glandular involvement only
IIb G1,2,3	Cervical stromal invasion
IIIa G1,2,3	Tumor invades serosa and/or adnexae and/or positive peritoneal cytology
IIIb G1,2,3	Vaginal metastases
IIIc G1,2,3	Metastases to pelvic and/or paraaortic lymph nodes
IVa G1,2,3	Tumor invasion of bladder and/or bowel mucosa
IVb	Distant metastases, including intraabdominal and/or inguinal lymph nodes
Histopathology: degree of differentiation	
Cases of carcinoma of the corpus should be grouped according to the degree of differentiation of the adenocarcinoma as follows:	
GI = ≤5% of a nonsquamous or nonmorular solid growth pattern	
G2 = 6% to 50% of a nonsquamous or nonmorular solid growth pattern	
G3 = >50% of a nonsquamous or nonmorular solid growth pattern	

*Approved by FIGO, October 1988, Rio de Janeiro.
Source: Creasman, W. (2007a). Adenocarcinoma of the uterus. In P. DiSaia & W. Creasman (Eds.), *Clinical gynecologic oncology* (7th ed.). St. Louis: Mosby.

Possible nursing diagnoses that would apply to a woman with endometrial cancer include the following:

- *Deficient knowledge* related to:
  - diagnosis, treatment, and prognosis
- *Decisional conflict* related to:
  - treatment options
- *Fear/anxiety* related to:
  - diagnosis of cancer, loss of uterus
- *Impaired skin integrity* related to:
  - surgery or radiation therapy
- *Acute or chronic pain* related to:
  - cancer
  - surgical procedure
- *Disturbed body image* related to:
  - loss of uterus
- *Sexual dysfunction* related to:
  - anatomic and functional changes caused by cancer or its treatment

TABLE 11-2 COMMON SIDE EFFECTS OF CHEMOTHERAPY AGENTS USED FOR GYNECOLOGIC CANCERS*

AGENT	ALOPECIA	MYELOSUPPRESSION, LEUKOPENIA, THROMBOCYTOPENIA	NAUSEA AND VOMITING	STOMATITIS, MUCOSITIS	NEUROTOXICITY
Cisplatin	—	+	+	—	+
Doxorubicin	+	+	+	+	+
Paclitaxel	+	+	+	+	+
Bleomycin	+	+	+	+	+
5-fluorouracil (5-FU)	+	+	+	+	+
Carboplatin	—	+	+	+	+
Mitomycin	+	+	+	+	—
Ifosfamide	+	+	+	—	+
Cyclophosphamide	+	+	+	+	—
Methotrexate	+	+	+	+	+
Vincristine	+	+	+	+	+

*Incidence and seriousness of side effects may be dose related.

Sources: Chu, C., & Rubin, S. (2007). Basic principles of chemotherapy. In P. DiSaia & W. Creasman (Eds.), *Clinical gynecologic oncology* (7th ed.). St. Louis: Mosby; Facts and Comparisons. (2009). *Drug facts and comparisons.* St Louis: Wolters Kluwer; Kunos, C., & Waggoner, S. (2007). Principles of radiation therapy and chemotherapy in gynecologic cancer. In V. Katz, G., Lentz, R. Lobo, & D. Gershenson (Eds.), *Comprehensive gynecology* (5th ed.). Philadelphia: Mosby.

EXPECTED OUTCOMES OF CARE

Planning for care of the woman with endometrial cancer depends on the stage of cancer and the treatment selected. Examples of expected outcomes are that the woman will do the following:

- Demonstrate understanding of her diagnosis of endometrial cancer, the treatments available, and her prognosis.
- Make informed decisions about treatment options.
- Describe a decrease in anxiety and fear.
- Report that pain is reduced or manageable.
- Experience no skin breakdown or infection related to treatment.
- State that she understands the effects of cancer and treatment on her body image and that her concerns are reduced.
- Report that she and her partner expect to be able to resume mutually satisfying sexual relations after treatment.

PLAN OF CARE AND INTERVENTIONS

Therapeutic Management. Collaborative efforts from various health disciplines are needed to work with the woman with endometrial cancer. All must have an understanding of the treatments that may be used.

For stage I adenocarcinoma of the endometrium limited to the uterus, total abdominal hysterectomy (TAH) and bilateral salpingo-oophorectomy (BSO) is the usual treatment (Creasman, 2007a). Radiation use in stage I continues to be studied; it can reduce the risk of recurrence, but evidence does not demonstrate improved survival rates or reduce metastasis to distant sites. It can be used when the woman is a poor surgical risk (Lu & Slomovitz, 2007). A radical hysterectomy (abdominal hysterectomy with wide excision of parametrial tissue laterally and uterosacral ligaments posteriorly), BSO, and pelvic node dissection usually are performed for stage II endometrial cancer. If nodes are positive or if there is extensive uterine disease or metastasis outside the uterus, external pelvic radiation (see p. 257) is usually done postoperatively. Internal radiation therapy or brachytherapy (placement of an applicator loaded with a radiation source into the uterine cavity) (see p. 258) also may be used before surgery or combined with external radiation (Lu & Slomovitz). Treatment of advanced stages is individualized but usually includes a TAH-BSO plus chemotherapy or radiation, or both (Hacker, 2010a).

Chemotherapy is used to treat advanced and recurrent disease, although no effective treatment regimen has been established (Lu & Slomovitz, 2007). Agents that have been somewhat effective include cisplatin, doxorubicin, carboplatin, cyclophosphamide, 5-fluorouracil, and paclitaxel (Lu & Slomovitz). Chemotherapy may cause hair loss, anemia, and bone marrow depression, as well as other side effects (Table 11-2).

Progestational therapy—use of medroxyprogesterone (Depo-Provera) and megestrol (Megace)—may be effective for recurrent cancers, especially those that are estrogen receptor positive. These drugs usually do not cause acute side effects. Tamoxifen and raloxifene (see Medication Guide on pp. 226-227) are antiestrogens that have shown some effectiveness against recurrent endometrial cancer (Creasman, 2007a; Lu & Slomovitz, 2007).

Nursing Management. Nursing care is individualized to the woman and her specific situation and diagnosis. Interventions for the woman having surgery are directed by assessment of her perception of the anticipated surgery, her knowledge of what to expect after surgery, and any preoperative special procedures, such as cleansing enemas or douches. In today's practice of short hospital stays even for radical surgery, many of these preoperative procedures are performed at home before admission, so assessment of understanding becomes a critical nursing

CULTURAL CONSIDERATIONS

Meaning of Cancer

A woman's culture influences the meaning she attaches to cancer. Her response to the diagnosis must be appropriate to her cultural context for it to be acceptable to her. For example, body image issues (e.g., loss of uterus), the meaning of death, and pain responses (e.g., stoic or expressive) are influenced by cultural beliefs and values. In making assessments about these issues, the nurse takes into account the influence of culture before developing a plan of care.

action (see Cultural Considerations box). Nursing care for the woman having a TAH-BSO will be similar to that care for a woman having a hysterectomy for leiomyoma described earlier. The following section focuses on care of the woman having a radical hysterectomy.

Preoperative Care. The nurse working with the woman preparing for a radical hysterectomy and pelvic node dissection should explain any preoperative procedures to be done (see Box 11-2). Additional teaching is needed for the woman having a radical hysterectomy regarding possible postsurgical events (e.g., a suprapubic drain often remains in place for several days to a week).

Postoperative Care. Assessment of vital signs usually follows a postanesthesia protocol, gradually decreasing in frequency to two to four times a day. Intravenous fluids are maintained at a rate rapid enough to maintain hydration and electrolyte balance and are usually discontinued when the woman is taking oral fluids well and has no elevated temperature. A regular diet is resumed as tolerated. Intake and output are monitored. The Foley catheter is usually removed the morning after surgery and the first few voidings are measured.

The woman should turn and take deep breaths with assistance as needed. Breath sounds are assessed, and any deviations from normal are reported immediately. The most significant single cause of morbidity and prolonged hospitalization after major procedures is respiratory complications. Anesthesia and surgery alter breathing patterns and ability to cough. Atelectasis, pneumonia, and pulmonary embolus may occur.

To promote venous return and prevent deep vein thrombosis, the woman may wear antiembolic stockings or wear pneumonic pressure devices (i.e., boots) while she is in bed (Chard, 2010). Leg exercises and early ambulation are beneficial. Most women are encouraged to get out of bed the evening of or the day after surgery. Assistance in getting up and walking may be needed.

Hemorrhage is always a possible complication after surgery. The wound drainage tube is emptied as needed or every 4 hours, and the amount and character of drainage are recorded. Drainage from any tube is assessed for bleeding. Vaginal drainage, if any, should be serosanguineous. Hematuria is noted and recorded. The primary health care provider is kept apprised of any deviations from normal expectations.

Paralytic ileus may occur after surgery in which the intestines have been manipulated. Use of a nasogastric tube, limiting oral fluids, and early ambulation all support the return of gastrointestinal function. An enema or suppository may bring relief of flatus and stimulate the return of bowel function. Oral laxatives should not be given until lower bowel function has returned.

Narcotic analgesics and NSAIDs are used for postoperative pain. Patient-controlled analgesia pumps are commonly used to deliver the narcotic medications (Lowdermilk, 2008). Nursing measures such as massages, repositioning, and emotional support are all helpful adjuncts to pharmacologic control of discomfort.

Because the in-hospital convalescent period is generally short, close observation by the nurse and attention to detail are critical. Nursing actions appropriate to this period include monitoring for urinary retention after the catheter is removed, monitoring the woman's appetite and diet, monitoring bowel function, and encouraging progressive ambulation and self-care.

Discharge Planning and Teaching. Discharge planning and teaching are done throughout the preoperative and postoperative phases and culminate during the convalescent phase. Discharge teaching topics for the woman with a radical hysterectomy are similar to those that can be found in the Teaching for Self-Management box: Care After Myomectomy or Hysterectomy (see also Nursing Care Plan: Hysterectomy for Endometrial Cancer).

Care for the woman who has had external or internal radiation therapy is the same as that described for the woman with cervical cancer (see later discussion).

Nursing care for the woman undergoing chemotherapy will depend on the type of drug given. If alopecia is likely, the nurse can suggest wigs, scarves, or other kinds of head coverings. If the therapy affects the appetite or causes gastrointestinal side effects, suggestions such as those in Box 11-4 may be useful.

After discharge the woman may require continued nursing care or monitoring of her physical status or advice for management of effects of treatment or the cancer. The family is likely to have to provide much of the woman's care. Nurses must identify what families see as their greatest need so that interventions are planned that best use the family's resources.

Psychologic care for the woman with endometrial cancer is essential. A women needs to be able to discuss her concerns about having cancer and the potential for recurrence. She may have fears of death; permanent disfigurement and change in functioning; altered feelings of self as a woman; and concerns regarding her femininity, sexuality, and loss of reproductive capacity. She may have questions arising from things she has heard about posthysterectomy changes, radiation therapy, or chemotherapy. Significant others should be encouraged to express their questions and concerns as well. The woman and her significant others may benefit from a referral to a community cancer support group (see the ACS website, www.cancer.org).

EVALUATION

The nursing care of a woman with endometrial cancer is evaluated by using the expected outcomes and measurable criteria to ascertain the degree to which the outcomes were met.

Cancer of the Ovary

Incidence and Etiology

Cancer of the ovary is the second most frequently occurring reproductive cancer and causes more deaths than any other female genital tract cancer (ACS, 2010a). Because the symptoms of this type of cancer are vague and definitive screening tests do not exist, ovarian cancer is often diagnosed in an advanced stage. The 5-year survival rate for cancer diagnosed at a localized stage is about 94%; however, only about 15% of all ovarian cancers are found at this stage. For advanced stages, the rate is about 28% (ACS). Malignant neoplasia of the ovaries occurs at all ages, including in infants and children. However, cancer of the ovary is seen primarily in women older than age 50 with the greatest number of cases found in women ages 60 to 64 years (Copeland, 2007).

Major histologic cell types occur in different age-groups, with malignant germ cell tumors most common in women between 20 and 40 years of age and epithelial cancers occurring in the perimenopausal age-groups. The spread of ovarian cancer is by

NURSING CARE PLAN

Hysterectomy for Endometrial Cancer

NURSING DIAGNOSIS

Anxiety related to lack of understanding of diagnosis, treatment, and prognosis of endometrial cancer as evidenced by woman's questions and concerns

Expected Outcomes

Woman will identify source of anxiety and verbalize understanding of diagnosis, effects of hysterectomy, and prognosis.

Nursing Interventions/*Rationales*

- Assess woman's level of understanding of procedure and its effects *to correct any misunderstanding, provide clarification, and identify starting point for further information.*
- Provide information about cancer of the endometrium, individualizing information to woman's situation *to provide clarification concerning treatment regimen.*
- Provide preoperative and postoperative teaching *to give anticipatory guidance and rationales for upcoming events.*

NURSING DIAGNOSIS

Fear related to diagnosis of endometrial cancer as evidenced by woman's questions and concerns

Expected Outcome

Woman will be able to verbalize that fears have diminished after the procedure.

Nursing Interventions/*Rationales*

- Through therapeutic communication, encourage verbalization of fears *to provide clarification and validation of feelings.*
- Encourage woman to identify support system *to have resources readily available as needed.*

NURSING DIAGNOSIS

Acute pain related to surgical procedure as evidenced by woman's verbal and nonverbal behaviors

Expected Outcome

Woman will verbalize decrease in intensity and number of painful episodes after interventions.

Nursing Interventions/*Rationales*

- Assess the location and intensity of pain by using a pain scale *to use appropriate treatment.*
- Administer prescribed analgesics *to decrease perception of pain.*
- Use nonpharmacologic techniques such as distraction, relaxation, position changes, and heat *to decrease perception of pain.*
- Monitor effectiveness of interventions *to modify interventions if needed.*

NURSING DIAGNOSIS

Risk for infection related to surgical incision and impaired skin integrity

Expected Outcome

Woman will experience no infection after the procedure.

Nursing Interventions/*Rationales*

- Assess for clinical manifestations of infection: fever, drainage, redness, swelling at the incision site *to provide prompt treatment.*
- Encourage a diet high in protein, vitamin C, and calories *to promote wound healing.*
- Teach woman to maintain aseptic technique when performing dressing changes, such as good handwashing *to decrease chance of introducing microorganisms at the incision site.*

NURSING DIAGNOSIS

Disturbed body image related to loss of uterus as evidenced by woman's statements of fears or concerns

Expected Outcome

Woman will maintain a positive body image.

Nursing Interventions/*Rationales*

- Encourage expression of feelings through therapeutic communication *to provide clarification of and validity of feelings.*
- Encourage woman to share feelings with significant other *to obtain emotional support.*
- Assist woman to identify support systems *to be available in case she needs to ventilate feelings.*

NURSING DIAGNOSIS

Sexual dysfunction related to perceived loss of femininity

Expected Outcome

Woman will resume usual sexual relationship with partner.

Nursing Interventions/*Rationales*

- Encourage verbalization of feelings related to sexuality *to provide clarification.*
- Provide opportunity for role-playing *to alleviate fears about interactions with partner.*
- Encourage communication with partner *to address concerns about resumption of sexual relations.*
- Refer to sexual counselor *to provide in-depth intervention as needed.*

direct extension to adjacent organs, but distal spread can occur through lymphatic spread to the liver and the lungs.

The cause of ovarian cancer is unknown; however, a number of risk factors have been identified. These factors include nulliparity, infertility, previous breast cancer, family history of ovarian or breast cancer, and history of HNPCC. Inherited BRCA1 and BRCA2 mutations increase the risk, but 90% of women do not have inherited ovarian cancer (Coleman & Gershenson, 2007; Copeland, 2007). Women of North American or northern European descent have the highest incidence of ovarian cancers. Pregnancy and use of oral contraceptives seem to have some protective benefits against ovarian cancer, whereas use of postmenopausal estrogen may increase the risk (ACS, 2010a). Genital exposure to talc, a diet high in fat, lactose intolerance, and use of fertility drugs have been suggested as risk factors, but research findings are inconclusive (Berek, 2010; Coleman & Gershenson; Copeland).

Clinical Manifestations and Diagnosis

Ovarian cancer has been called a silent disease because early warning symptoms that would send a woman to her health care provider are absent (e.g., no bleeding or other discharge and no pain). Abdominal bloating, noticeable increase in abdominal girth, pelvic or abdominal pain, difficulty eating or feeling full quickly, and urinary urgency or frequency have been identified as the four most common symptoms of early ovarian cancer (Goff, Mandel, Drescher, Urban, Gough, Schurman, et al., 2007). The increase in abdominal girth (caused by ovarian

BOX 11-4 NUTRITIONAL MANAGEMENT FOR COMMON PROBLEMS RELATED TO GYNECOLOGIC CANCER OR TREATMENT

ALTERED TASTE
- Rinse mouth with baking soda solution
  - 1 teaspoon salt, 1 teaspoon baking soda to 1 quart (liter) water
- Use extra seasoning, spices
- Use sauces and marinades for meats
- Eat fish or chicken instead of red meat
- Eat tart foods to stimulate taste buds
- Try sugar-free mints, gum, hard sour candy

ANOREXIA
- Eat with family, friends
- Eat favorite foods anytime
- Try new foods, recipes
- Use smaller servings
- Eat high-calorie, high-protein snacks
- Drink nutritional supplements
- Exercise before meals to stimulate appetite

NAUSEA AND VOMITING
- Drink clear liquids
- Avoid carbonated fluids
- Avoid sweet, rich, fatty foods
- Eat cool foods rather than hot or warm foods
- Eat six to eight small meals a day
- Consume a high-calorie, high-protein diet
- Eat toast, bland foods
- Avoid lying down at least 1 hour after eating
- Take antiemetics before meals

STOMATITIS
- Eat small meals
- Eat soft, bland foods
- Avoid rough textured foods (e.g., chips, crackers)
- Drink 8 to 10 cups of fluids a day
- Avoid citrus fruits, spicy foods
- Avoid alcohol
- Avoid very hot or very cold foods
- Drink nutritional supplements, milkshakes
- Drink through a straw if mouth is sore
- Rinse mouth frequently with baking soda solution
- Eat liquid or pureed foods as needed

CONSTIPATION
- Increase fiber (bran, fresh fruits and vegetables)
- Drink 8 to 10 cups of fluids a day (2 to 2.4 L/day)
- Eat natural laxative foods (prunes, apples)
- Avoid cheese products
- Drink warm drinks with breakfast

DIARRHEA
- Limit milk to 2 cups a day (500 ml)
- Avoid high-fiber, spicy, fatty foods
- Eat foods high in potassium
- Increase fluid intake (3 L/day) (12.5 cups); avoid caffeine and carbonated fluids
- Add nutmeg to food to decrease gastric motility
- Eat a high-protein, high-carbohydrate diet
- Eat small meals and snacks

POSTOPERATIVE RECOVERY
- Eat food high in iron
- Eat high-protein foods
- Eat foods high in vitamins C, B complex, and K
- Drink 6 to 8 glasses of fluids a day (1.5 to 2 L a day)

Source: American Cancer Society. (2010). *Nutrition for the person with cancer during treatment: A guide for patients and families.* Available at www.cancer.org. Accessed June 17, 2010.

enlargement or ascites) is usually attributed to an increase in weight or a shift in weight that is seen commonly in women entering their middle years. An ovary enlarged 5 cm or more than normal that is found during routine examination requires careful diagnostic workup. Pelvic pain, anemia, and general weakness and malnutrition are signs of late-stage disease.

Early diagnosis of ovarian cancer is uncommon. Attempts at early detection have not proven to be reliable. Taking a family history is important because it may reveal cancer of the uterus or breast. Transvaginal ultrasound, CA-125 antigen (a tumor-associated antigen) testing, and frequent pelvic examinations have all been used without a great deal of success because these tests do not have high levels of sensitivity and specificity (Fields & Chevlen, 2006). Research continues on the use of proteomics (study of proteins in blood) to identify ovarian cancer in its earlier stages (ACS, 2010a; Cesario, 2010). Emerging technology includes tumor cell profiling and nanotechnology (use of microchips to sense biomarkers that are unique to a specific cancer).

Transvaginal ultrasound and CA-125 screening currently are not recommended for routine screening in the general population but are recommended for women who are at high risk (e.g., BRCA1 mutation carriers) (ACS, 2010a). Routine pelvic examination continues to be the only practical screening method for detecting early disease, even though few cancers are detected in women without symptoms. Any ovarian enlargement should be considered highly suggestive and needs further evaluation by laparoscopy or laparotomy. Responsibility for diagnosis rests with the pathologist. The size of the tumor is not indicative of the severity of disease. Clinical staging is done surgically and gives direction to treatment and prognosis (Copeland, 2007).

Therapeutic Management

Treatment is dictated by the stage of the disease at the time of initial diagnosis. Surgical removal of as much of the tumor as possible is the first step in therapy. This may involve just the removal of one ovary and tube or the radical excision of the uterus, ovaries, tubes, and omentum. Cytoreductive surgery (the debulking of the poorly vascularized larger tumors) also is done. The smaller the volume of tumor remaining, the better the response to adjuvant therapy. Because about three fourths of women are in stage II, III, or IV disease at the time of diagnosis, surgical cure is not possible; therefore, after tumor reduction surgery is performed, women with epithelial cell carcinoma will receive chemotherapy.

A combination of antineoplastic drugs such as paclitaxel and cisplatin or carboplatin and paclitaxel is recommended for most women with advanced disease. Women being treated with chemotherapy are followed up closely with laboratory and radiologic tests and CA-125 levels to monitor their response to the therapy (Copeland, 2007).

Second-look surgery is a technique used to determine the response of the disease to chemotherapy and to determine whether treatment should be continued; however, this procedure usually is not done unless it is part of a research protocol (Copeland, 2007).

Radiation has been used to treat early-stage disease, and some women have had long-term survival after debulking surgery followed by radiation therapy. It has also been used as a palliative measure in advanced disease (Coleman & Gershenson, 2007).

Nursing Implications

Lockwood-Rayermann, Donovan, Rambo, and Kuo (2009) reported on data analyzed from a survey conducted by the National Ovarian Cancer Coalition. These researchers concluded that awareness of the symptoms of and risk factors for ovarian cancer are low in the general population. Therefore, nurses need to be involved in raising the awareness of these risks and symptoms with the public and with women who are seeking care in health care settings such as clinics and physician offices (Cesario, 2010).

Goff and associates (2007) developed a symptom index to be used in identifying women at risk for ovarian cancer who might benefit from early screening. The index includes asking about symptoms (pelvic/abdominal pain, urinary urgency/frequency, increased abdominal size/bloating, and difficulty eating/feeling full) and the frequency and duration of the symptoms. The index is considered positive if any of the symptoms occurred more than 12 times per month and had been present for less than 1 year. Nursing can incorporate asking about these symptoms when women are seen for annual examinations or other gynecologic health visits and encouraging women to keep a symptom diary (Cesario, 2010).

The woman diagnosed with ovarian cancer has concerns similar to those described for the woman with endometrial and cervical cancer. Nursing interventions for the woman having surgery, chemotherapy, or external radiation therapy are described in other sections of this chapter.

Women with advanced ovarian cancer have a significant rate of recurrence. Follow-up for 5 years must be intensive. When a cure or remission cannot be achieved, palliative measures are initiated that alleviate symptoms of the progressing disease and provide comfort and maximal function. As the disease progresses, nutritional support, including enteral feedings and parenteral hyperalimentation, may be needed because of the effects on the gastrointestinal tract of both the disease and the treatments. The goal of nursing care is assisting the woman to maintain quality of life and to remain at home with her family as much as possible.

Because the period between a focus on cure and a focus on palliation is often prolonged, the woman with ovarian cancer is apt to experience most of the grief stages described by Kübler-Ross and to need support and encouragement through each stage. After diagnosis the woman often experiences denial and then anger. As treatment begins, she may "bargain" for a cure. If treatment is successful and death is forestalled by remission or cure, the process of adjustment to dying ceases, and the woman again focuses on life and its challenges. When treatment fails to secure a cure or remission ends, the woman must turn again to the task of adjustment (see Legal Tip).

> **LEGAL TIP: Advance Directives**
> Nurses who work with clients in hospitals with federal funding must know that because of the Patient Self-Determination Act, all clients must be asked if they have knowledge of advance directives and be provided with the information if desired. This is important to nurses working in gynecology-oncology settings, where decisions about living wills and "no codes" may be issues.

Family and friends also have diverse feelings. When grieving is prolonged, as it often is when the woman has cancer, the stress can be enormous and can interfere with other interpersonal relationships. If the woman is hospitalized, the environment may further intrude on relationships, limiting privacy and access to the woman and hindering opportunities for caring gestures. The nurse can assist the woman and her family to share their feelings with each other and help them to develop a support network. Referral to a cancer support group may be useful (see National Ovarian Cancer Coalition, www.ovarian.org).

Cancer of the Cervix

Incidence and Etiology

Cancer of the cervix is the third most common reproductive cancer. The accessible location of the cervix to both cell and tissue study and direct examination have led to a refinement of diagnostic techniques, contributing to improved diagnosis and management of these disorders. The incidence of invasive cancer has decreased over the last 30 years, reducing mortality rates. However, the incidence of preinvasive cancer has increased, and more women in their 20s and 30s are being diagnosed with preinvasive cervical lesions (ACS, 2010a).

Cancer of the cervix begins as neoplastic changes in the cervical epithelium. Terms that have been used to describe these epithelial changes or preinvasive lesions include **dysplasia** and **cervical intraepithelial neoplasia (CIN);** CIN is the term currently used. CIN 1 refers to abnormal cellular proliferation in the lower one third of the epithelium; this change tends to be self-limiting and generally regresses to normal. CIN 2 involves the lower two thirds of the epithelium and may progress to carcinoma in situ. CIN 3 involves the full thickness of the epithelium and often progresses to carcinoma in situ. **Carcinoma in situ (CIS)** is diagnosed when the full thickness of epithelium is replaced with abnormal cells (Creasman, 2007b) (Fig. 11-11). Terms used to describe neoplastic changes in abnormal cervical cytology reports are low-grade and high-grade **squamous intraepithelial lesions (SILs);** however, CIN continues to be a common term used in clinical practice.

Preinvasive lesions are limited to the cervix and usually originate in the squamocolumnar junction or **transformation zone** (Fig. 11-12). Intensive study of the cervix and the cellular changes that take place has shown that most cervical tumors have a gradual onset rather than an explosive one. Preinvasive conditions may exist for years before the development of invasive disease. These preinvasive conditions are highly treatable in many cases.

Invasive carcinoma is the diagnosis when abnormal cells penetrate the basement membrane and invade the stroma. There are two types of invasive carcinoma of the cervix: microinvasive

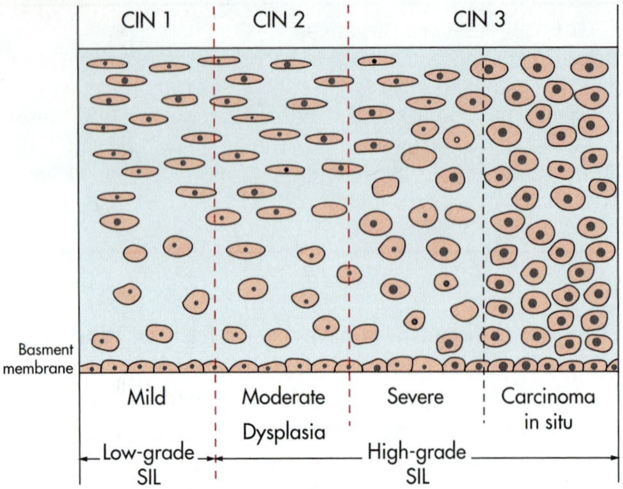

FIG. 11-11 Diagram of cervical epithelium showing progressive changes and various terminology.

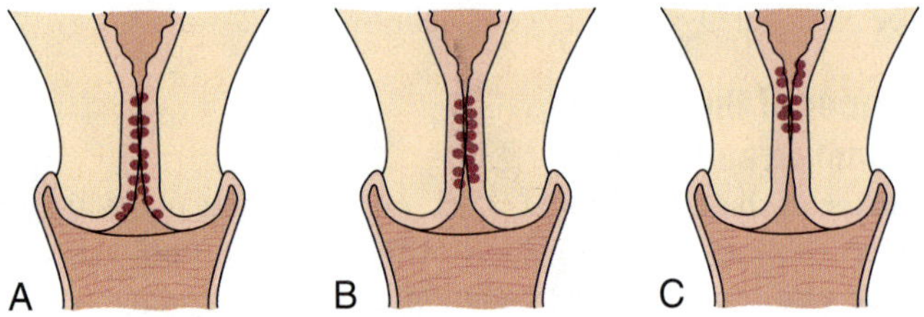

FIG. 11-12 Location of squamocolumnar junction according to age. The location where the endocervical glands meet the squamous epithelium becomes progressively higher with age. **A,** Puberty. **B,** Reproductive years. **C,** Postmenopausal.

and invasive. Microinvasive carcinoma is defined as one or more lesions that penetrate no more than 3 mm into the stroma below the basement membrane with no areas of lymphatic or vascular invasion (Creasman, 2007b). Invasive carcinoma describes invasion that goes beyond these parameters. The staging of invasive carcinoma extends from stage 0 (CIS) to stage IVb (distant metastasis or disease outside the true pelvis). A number of substages within each stage also exist. Clinical stages for cancer of the cervix are shown in Table 11-3.

Approximately 90% of cervical malignancies are squamous cell carcinomas; 10% are adenocarcinomas. Squamous cell carcinomas can spread by direct extension to the vaginal mucosa, the pelvic wall, the bowels, and the bladder. Metastasis usually occurs in the pelvis, but it can occur to the lungs and the brain through the lymphatic system.

The average age range for the occurrence of cervical cancer is 40 to 50 years; however, preinvasive conditions may exist for 10 to 15 years before the development of an invasive carcinoma. About 70% to 80% of cervical cancers are caused by human papillomavirus (HPV) (Creasman, 2007b). A strong link has been established between HPV types 16 and 18 and cervical neoplasia. Eighteen other types have been associated with genital tract infections and also may be associated with CIN (ACOG, 2008; Creasman). Other sexually transmitted infections that are identified as risk factors are herpes simplex virus 2 and possibly cytomegalovirus (Creasman). Risk factors include early age at first coitus (younger than 20 years); multiple sexual partners (more than two); a sexual partner with a history of multiple sexual partners; high parity, and belonging to a lower socioeconomic group. Potential factors include long-term use of oral contraceptives, cigarette smoking, and intrauterine exposure to diethylstilbestrol (DES) (ACS, 2010a; Creasman; Monk & Tewari, 2007). Low levels of beta-carotene, vitamin C, and folate are being investigated as potential risk factors (Monk & Tewari).

The incidence of cervical cancer in the United States is highest in Hispanic women and lowest in Native-American women, whereas the highest mortality occurs in African-American women (ACS, 2010a). Factors that may influence cervical screening behaviors for these groups include lack of a health promotion or disease prevention perspective, lack of knowledge about Pap tests and availability of services, financial barriers, and failure of health care providers to recommend screening (Giarratano, Bustamante-Forest, & Carter, 2005). There also is a high rate of CIN in human immunodeficiency virus–positive women, suggesting that altered immune status is a risk factor (Creasman, 2007b).

TABLE 11-3 FIGO CLASSIFICATION OF CERVICAL CARCINOMA

STAGE	DESCRIPTION
0	Carcinoma in situ, intraepithelial carcinoma
I	The carcinoma is strictly confined to the cervix (extension to the corpus should be disregarded)
Ia	Invasive cancer identified only microscopically; all gross lesions, even with superficial invasion, are stage Ib cancers. Invasion is limited to measured stromal invasion with maximum depth of 5 mm and no wider than 7 mm
Ia1	Measured invasion of stroma 3 mm in depth and no wider than 7 mm
Ia2	Measured invasion of stroma >3 mm and 5 mm in depth and no wider than 7 mm.
	The depth of invasion should not be >5 mm taken from the base of the epithelium, surface or glandular, from which it originates. Vascular space involvement, venous or lymphatic, should not alter the staging
Ib	Clinical lesions confined to the cervix or preclinical lesions greater than stage Ia
Ib1	Clinical lesions 4 cm or less
Ib2	Clinical lesions >4 cm
II	Involvement of the vagina but not the lower third, or infiltration of the parametria but not out to the side wall
IIa	Involvement of the vagina, but no evidence of parametrial involvement
IIb	Infiltration of the parametria, but not out to the side wall
III	Involvement of the lower third of the vagina or extension to the pelvic side wall. All cases with a hydronephrosis or nonfunctioning kidney should be included, unless they are known to be attributable to other cause
IIIa	Involvement of the lower third of the vagina but not out to the pelvic side wall if the parametria are involved
IIIb	Extension onto the pelvic side wall and/or hydronephrosis or nonfunctional kidney
IV	Extension outside the reproductive tract
IVa	Involvement of the mucosa of the bladder or the rectum
IVb	Distant metastasis or disease outside the true pelvis

Source: Monk, B., & Tewari, K. (2007). Invasive cervical cancer. In P. DiSaia & W. Creasman (Eds.), *Clinical gynecologic oncology* (7th ed.). St. Louis: Mosby.

Clinical Manifestations and Diagnosis

Preinvasive cancer of the cervix is often asymptomatic. Abnormal bleeding, especially postcoital bleeding, is the classic symptom of invasive cancer. Other late symptoms include rectal bleeding, hematuria, back pain, leg pain, and anemia. Diagnosis

BOX 11-5 2001 BETHESDA SYSTEM FOR REPORTING CERVICAL CYTOLOGY RESULTS

RESULTS/INTERPRETATIONS

Negative for Intraepithelial Malignancy
- Organisms (e.g., evidence of infections)
- Other nonneoplastic findings (e.g., inflammation, radiation changes, atrophy)
- Glandular cells status post hysterectomy
- Atrophy

Epithelial Cell Abnormalities
- Squamous cells
  - Atypical squamous cells (ASC)
  - Of undetermined significance (ASC-US)
  - Cannot exclude high-grade squamous intraepithelial lesion (HSIL) (ASC-H)
- Low-grade squamous intraepithelial lesion (LSIL)
  - Human papillomavirus (HPV), cervical intraepithelial neoplasia (CIN) 1
- HSIL
  - CIN 2, CIN 3
- Squamous cell carcinoma

Glandular Cell
- Atypical cells including endocervical, endometrial, and glandular or not otherwise specified
- Atypical cells including endocervical or glandular, suggestive of neoplasia (endocervical or not otherwise specified)
- Endocervical adenocarcinoma in situ
- Adenocarcinoma (endocervical, endometrial, extrauterine, or not otherwise specified)

Source: Creasman, W. (2007). Preinvasive disease of the cervix. In P. DiSaia,, & W. Creasman (Eds.), *Clinical gynecologic oncology* (7th ed.). St. Louis: Mosby.

includes taking a history that includes menstrual and sexual activity information, particularly sexually transmitted infections and abnormal bleeding episodes (Creasman, 2007b). A pelvic examination usually is normal except in late-stage cancer.

The single most reliable method to detect preinvasive cancer is the Pap test, which can detect 90% of early cervical changes. The U.S. Preventive Services Task Force (USPSTF) and the ACS recommend Pap tests to begin about 3 years after a woman becomes sexually active but not later than age 21. Annual screening is recommended to age 30 (with conventional Pap test; every 2 years if liquid-based Pap tests). After age 30 and three negative Pap tests, screening may be done every 2 to 3 years in consultation with the health care provider. Women ages 65 to 70 with no abnormal tests in the previous 10 years may choose to stop screenings. Women who have had total hysterectomies for benign disease can choose to stop having Pap tests (ACS, 2010a; USPSTF, 2009). Women in high risk categories should have more frequent Pap tests.

Pap test results in the past have been recorded by using several different classification systems. The reporting system most often used today is the Bethesda system, one that reports on gynecologic cytology as well as histology of cervical lesions (Box 11-5). Changes secondary to inflammation, treatment (e.g., radiation), and contraceptive devices can be reported, as well as changes caused by infections. Epithelial cell abnormalities are described in three categories: atypias, or atypical squamous cells

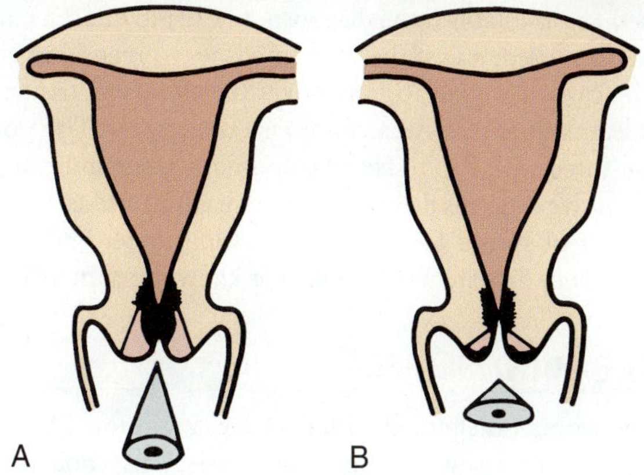

FIG. 11-13 A, Cone biopsy for endocervical disease. Limits of lesion were not seen colposcopically. **B,** Cone biopsy for cervical intraepithelial neoplasia of the exocervix. Limits of lesion were identified colposcopically. (Source: Creasman, W. (2007). Preinvasive disease of the cervix. In P. DiSaia & W. Creasman (Eds.), *Clinical gynecologic oncology* (7th ed.). St. Louis: Mosby.

(ASC); low-grade squamous intraepithelial lesions (LSILs); and high-grade squamous intraepithelial lesions (HSILs).

Several options for follow-up of a finding of ASC of undetermined significance (ASC-US) are suggested. These include immediate colposcopy, repeating cytology at 6 months and 12 months, or HPV testing and referral for colposcopy if test is positive. If the initial cytology test was obtained by a liquid-based method, HPV testing is preferred instead of follow-up with repeated cytology (ACOG, 2008). A finding of LSIL may include HPV and CIN 1. Colposcopy is recommended for evaluation of LSIL except in adolescents; teens can be followed with cytology tests at 6 and 12 months. HPV deoxyribonucleic acid (DNA) testing should not be used (ACOG). HSILs include lesions described as CIN 2, CIN 3, and carcinoma in situ (CIS). Follow-up for a report of HSIL includes colposcopy or loop electrosurgical excision (ACOG).

Colposcopy is the examination of the cervix with a stereoscopic binocular microscope that magnifies the view of the cervix. Usually a solution of 3% acetic acid is applied to the cervix for better visualization of the epithelium and to identify areas for biopsy. Colposcopy is not an invasive procedure and is usually well tolerated by the woman. However, the woman who is scheduled for colposcopy because of an abnormal Pap test may be anxious about the procedure and may need explanations or written information about what to expect during the procedure.

Biopsy is the removal of cervical tissue for study, and several techniques can be used. An endocervical curettage is an effective diagnostic tool in about 90% of cases. It can be performed as an outpatient procedure with little or no anesthesia. It may be uncomfortable, and interventions to help the woman relax and cope with the pain may be needed.

Conization and loop electrosurgical excision procedure (LEEP) (see later discussion) can be done as outpatient procedures, although neither is usually performed unless the biopsy is positive or the results of the colposcopy are unsatisfactory. Conization involves removal of a cone of tissue from the exocervix and endocervix (Fig. 11-13). It can be a cold knife procedure, a laser excision, or an electrosurgical excision (see later discussion). There are two advantages to a cone biopsy. It can be used (1) to establish the diagnosis and (2) to effect a cure. If CIS is diagnosed, and if the woman wishes to retain her childbearing capacity, conization removes the abnormal tissue; further treatment (e.g., hysterectomy) is unnecessary. The woman is monitored with Pap tests and colposcopy when indicated.

If invasive cancer is diagnosed, other diagnostic tests can assess the extent of spread (see earlier discussion under endometrial cancer). Once the extent of the cancer is known, treatment begins.

CARE MANAGEMENT

For the woman diagnosed with invasive carcinoma of the cervix, pretherapy assessment includes physical, psychologic, and educational components, regardless of whether surgery or radiation is the method of treatment. Physical assessment includes a review of current medications because medications for other medical problems may have to be continued. Skin is assessed to identify potential pressure points; respiratory and gastrointestinal status and state of nutrition are important factors to assess. Urinalysis and complete blood count also are commonly performed. An electrocardiogram and a chest x-ray examination may be done if use of a general anesthetic is anticipated for surgery or placement of internal applicators.

Psychologic assessment is important because frequently these women are emotionally distressed about the diagnosis and anticipated treatment (i.e., fear of being radioactive and fear of surgery and pain) and fear that family or significant others will become distant.

Educational assessment involves identifying the woman's current knowledge base regarding the diagnosis and proposed therapeutic regimen.

Nursing diagnoses for the woman having surgery for cervical cancer are similar to those identified for the woman having a hysterectomy for endometrial cancer (see Nursing Care Plan, p. 249). Nursing diagnoses for a woman having external or internal radiation therapy are listed in the Nursing Process box: Woman Having Radiation Therapy).

Medical and Surgical Management

Once a diagnosis has been identified, a course of treatment is planned. For preinvasive lesions, several techniques are used. As stated, because many preinvasive conditions are detected in

NURSING PROCESS

The Woman Having Radiation Therapy

ASSESSMENT

Women having radiation therapy for cervical cancer need the following assessments:

- Interview
  - Medical history to determine if other problems are present
  - Assessment of knowledge of treatment plan
  - Nutritional assessment
  - Psychologic assessment about concerns related to radiation or her cancer; sexual concerns related to treatment
  - Physical examination: skin assessment, respiratory and gastrointestinal status
- Laboratory test: hematocrit or hemoglobin for anemia

NURSING DIAGNOSES

Nursing diagnoses that might arise from an assessment for the woman who is to have external or internal radiation therapy for treatment of cervical cancer include:

Deficient Knowledge **related to:**
- treatment procedures

Fear/Anxiety **related to:**
- diagnosis
- anticipated pain
- concerns about radioactivity
- the response of the significant other or family

Disturbed Sensory Perception **related to:**
- internal radiation therapy
- restricted contact with visitors and nursing staff

Risk for Impaired Skin Integrity **related to:**
- external radiation exposure
- immobility and bed rest (internal radiation therapy)

Risk for Injury **related to:**
- dislodgment of radiation source

Acute Pain **related to:**
- internal applicators

Sexual Dysfunction **related to:**
- treatment or concerns of significant other

EXPECTED OUTCOMES OF CARE

Mutually determined outcomes for the woman undergoing radiation therapy for cervical cancer related to the identified nursing diagnoses might include that the woman will do the following:

- Verbalize an understanding of the proposed treatment and accompanying procedures.
- Verbalize her fears regarding diagnosis, treatment, and response of significant others and family.
- Identify methods to maintain skin hygiene.
- Remain free from skin breakdown.
- Verbalize control of pain.
- Maintain good nutrition by implementing interventions to cope with side effects of treatment.
- Resume a satisfactory sexual relationship with her partner.

PLAN OF CARE AND INTERVENTIONS

Interventions for caring for a woman undergoing external radiation are discussed on p. 257 and Teaching for Self-Management: Care After External Radiation Therapy box on p. 258.

- Provide information on skin care, nutrition, prevention of infection, and signs of complications.
- Interventions for caring for a woman undergoing internal radiation are discussed on p. 258 and in the Teaching for Self-Management: Care After Internal Radiation Therapy box.
- Provide information on preinsertion preparation, care during insertion phase, and postinsertion care.
- Provide information about the effects of radiation therapy on sexual functioning with the woman and her partner and offer suggestions for specific problems.
- Provide information on community resources and support groups as needed.

EVALUATION

The nurse can be reasonably assured that care was effective to the extent that the expected outcomes of care for the woman who has had radiation therapy have been achieved.

younger women who may wish to continue childbearing, treatment is geared toward eradicating abnormal cells while attempting to preserve the structure of the cervix. The techniques currently available for preinvasive lesions are cryotherapy, laser therapy, and LEEP, all of which have comparable success rates in treating CIN (ACOG, 2008).

Treatment for invasive cancer includes surgery, radiation therapy, and chemotherapy. Once the cancer is staged, treatment is begun. Microinvasive cancer is usually treated with conization, but a hysterectomy is often done if childbearing is not desired. The choice of treatment for early-stage invasive cancer is by either hysterectomy or chemoradiation therapy (Monk & Tewari, 2007). A radical hysterectomy is performed if the cancer has extended beyond the cervix but not to the pelvic wall. Locally advanced stages of cervical cancer usually are treated with radiation therapy, both external and internal, and chemotherapy. Late stages are usually treated with radiation and chemotherapy. Five-year survival rates are more than 97% when the cancer is localized (ACS, 2010a). Cisplatin is the most commonly used chemotherapy agent.

Cryosurgery. Cryosurgery uses a freezing technique that freezes abnormal cells, and when sloughing occurs, normal tissue is regenerated. Side effects occurring after treatment are usually few and not serious. A profuse watery discharge can

EVIDENCE-BASED PRACTICE — *Pat Gingrich*

Cervical Cancer Treatment Options: Conventional and Complementary

ASK THE QUESTION

What can I tell my clients with cervical cancer to expect with treatment? Are there any complementary or alternative treatments?

SEARCH FOR EVIDENCE

Search Strategies

Professional organization guidelines, meta-analyses, systematic reviews, randomized controlled trials, nonrandomized prospective studies and retrospective reviews since 2008.

Databases Searched

CINAHL, Cochrane, Medline, PUBMED, and the professional sites for the American College of Obstetricians and Gynecologists (ACOG) and the Association of Women's Health, Obstetric and Neonatal Nurses (AWHONN).

CRITICALLY ANALYZE THE DATA

Regular Papanicolaou smears and human papilloma virus (HPV) typing, combined with prophylactic HPV vaccines in girls and women (and perhaps men), have been shown to fight cervical cancer. In spite of these measures, cervical cancer still affects about 11,000 women and causes 4,000 deaths in the United States annually. Conventional therapy includes surgery, chemotherapy and radiation therapy, as well as some medical and complementary therapies. Three Cochrane Systematic Analyses present treatment options for cervical cancer:

- In one systematic review of 6 trials involving 1072 women, analysts revealed that in women with early (local) disease, chemotherapy given prior to surgery leads to longer than 5-year survival rates. It was unclear if it made surgery any easier, nor if it stopped recurrence or ultimately resulted in longer lifespan (Rydzewska, Tierney, Vale, & Symonds, 2010).
- While most cervical cancer is squamous cell carcinoma, which responds equally well to surgery or radiotherapy, the less common adenocarcinoma (glandular cell, which lines the cervical canal) responds more favorably to surgery, according to another meta-analysis of 12 studies. For women with lesions too large for surgery or suspected of spread to the lymph nodes, chemoradiation would be the first choice of treatment (Baalbergen, Veenstra, Stalpers, & Ansink, 2010).
- In a meta-analysis of 15 randomized controlled trials, women whose cervical cancer was inoperable or metastatic had a 6% greater 5-year survival rate with chemotherapy combined with radiation therapy (66%) than with radiation therapy alone (60%). The combined group also had fewer recurrences and less cancer spread. However, side effects, especially hematological and gastrointestinal toxicity, were increased with the combined therapy. Additional chemotherapy after the combined therapy may result in even longer survival (Chemoradiotherapy for Cervical Cancer Meta-analysis Collaboration, 2010).

IMPLICATIONS FOR PRACTICE

Women undergoing conventional treatment for cervical cancer can experience debilitating side effects from toxicity. Most common, besides systemic effects, are the vaginal (bladder dysfunction, abdominal pressure) and rectal complications (diarrhea, incontinence, pain, enteritis, ulceration, loss of elasticity). Many will seek out complementary or alternative therapies to increase the efficacy and safety of conventional treatments, and/or to ameliorate their toxic symptoms. A systematic review and meta-analysis of 18 randomized or clinical controlled trials involving 1657 women revealed that phytotherapy, or the use of natural herbs, significantly increased the survival rate at 1, 2, 3 and 10 years when added to conventional therapy such as surgery, radiation and chemotherapy. The most common herbs studied were Chinese combinations including *radix astragali*, ginseng, dong quai, licorice, cinnamon, and tangerine peel, among others. Tumor recession was also significantly better with phytotherapy plus conventional therapy, when compared to conventional therapy alone. In addition, phytotherapy significantly increased the efficacy of Western medicines (anti-infectives, vitamins and other symptomatic relief medications) for relieving vaginal and rectal symptoms (Xu, Deng, Qi, Deng, Zhao, Wong, et al., 2009).

Nurses who work with women with cervical cancer can help their patients by staying abreast of current cancer therapy and recommendations for symptomatic relief of sometimes debilitating side effects of therapy. Referrals to appropriate practitioners and anticipatory guidance about the course of treatments, tempered with empathy, listening and a positive outlook, can provide patients with emotional support at a very vulnerable time.

References

Baalbergen, A., Veenstra, Y., Stalpers, L, & Ansink, A. (2010). Primary surgery versus primary radiation therapy with or without chemotherapy for early adenocarcinoma of the uterine cervix. *The Cochrane Database of Systematic Reviews 2010,* 1, CD006248.

Chemoradiotherapy for Cervical Cancer Meta-analysis Collaboration. (2010). Reducing uncertainties about the effects of chemoradiotherapy for cervical cancer: Individual patient data meta-analysis. *The Cochrane Database of Systematic Reviews 2010,* 1, CD008285.

Rydzewska, L., Tierney, J., Vale, C., & Symonds, P. (2010). Neoadjuvant chemotherapy plus surgery versus surgery for cervical cancer. *The Cochrane Database of Systematic Reviews 2010,* 1, CD007406.

Xu, M., Deng, P., Qi, C., Deng, B., Zhao, Z., Wong, V., et al. (2009). Adjuvant phytotherapy in the treatment of cervical cancer: A systematic review and meta-analysis. *The Journal of Complementary and Alternative Medicine, 15*(12), 1347–1353.

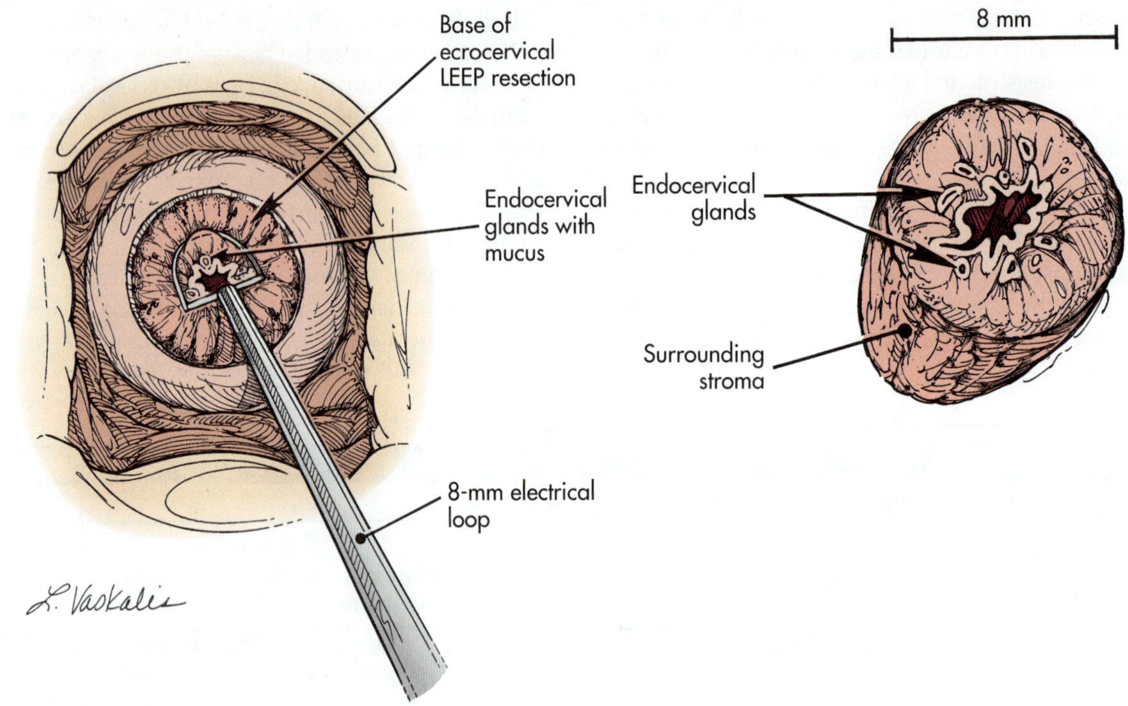

FIG. 11-14 Electrosurgical excision. The electric loop vaporizes quickly and removes cone of tissue. (From Nichols, D., & Clark-Pearson, D. [2000]. *Gynecologic, obstetric, and related surgery* [2nd ed.]. St. Louis: Mosby.)

persist for 2 to 4 weeks. Follow-up examination and a Pap test are scheduled in 4 to 6 months. Endocervical cells are thought to regenerate, leaving a normal cervical canal in most instances. Spotting and cervical stenosis are rare complications. Surveillance with frequent Pap tests and colposcopic examination must continue indefinitely after this type of conservative therapy. Persistent abnormal cells require reevaluation, and plans are made for repeated cryosurgery or other therapy.

Laser Ablation. Laser ablation uses a laser mounted on a colposcope that allows precise direction of a beam of light (heat) to remove diseased tissue. An endometrial sampling is recommended before ablation to avoid removal of unrecognized invasive cancer. For treatment of the cervix (relatively insensitive tissue), the woman may need no anesthesia. Some women complain of a burning or cramping sensation that is tolerable for most women. The cervix treated with CO_2 laser will show epithelial regrowth beginning by 2 days afterward. The site is usually healed in 4 to 6 weeks. The original architecture of the cervix is preserved, and the squamocolumnar junction remains visible; however, there can be more damage to normal tissues than with other treatments. Women usually have less vaginal discharge than with cryosurgery, but can have more discomfort after the procedure (Noller, 2007).

Electrosurgical Excision. The LEEP is a standard treatment for cervical intraepithelial neoplasia in the United States. This procedure uses a wire loop electrode that can excise and cauterize with minimal tissue damage (Fig. 11-14). Healing is rapid, and there is only a mild discharge afterward. Possible complications include bleeding, cervical stenosis, infertility, and loss of cervical mucus (ACOG, 2008).

Radical Hysterectomy. Radical hysterectomy involves removal of the uterus, the tubes, the ovaries, the upper third of the vagina, the entire uterosacral and uterovesical ligaments, and all of the parametrium on each side, along with pelvic node dissection encompassing the four major pelvic lymph node chains: ureteral, obturator, hypogastric, and iliac. Dissection serves to preserve the bladder, the rectum, and the ureters while removing as much of the remaining tissue of the pelvis as is feasible. Women with positive pelvic nodes usually receive postoperative whole pelvis irradiation (Monk & Tewari, 2007).

Nursing Management. Nursing care for the woman having a radical hysterectomy was discussed in the previous section on endometrial cancer (p. 248).

Radiation Therapy. Radiation may be delivered by internal radium applications to the cervix or external radiation therapy that includes lymphatics of the pelvic side wall. In preparation for radiation therapy the woman must maintain good nutritional status and a high-protein, high-vitamin, and high-calorie diet. Anemia, if present, should be corrected before initiating radiotherapy.

External radiation therapy and internal radiation therapy are given in various combinations for the best results and are tailored to each woman and her particular lesion. For example, external radiation may be given first to treat regional pelvic nodes and to shrink the tumor. External irradiation is usually an outpatient procedure given 5 days a week for 4 to 6 weeks. Internal radiation therapy consists of one or two intracavitary treatments at least 2 weeks apart (Monk & Tewari, 2007).

External irradiation is provided by megavoltage machines such as cobalt, and supervoltage machines such as linear accelerators and betatron, all of which have the distinct advantage of providing a more homogeneous dose to the pelvis. Before treatment begins, a localization procedure is done to determine the best way to deliver the treatments. Markings or small tattoos are placed on the body to make sure the woman is positioned correctly to get the treatment (Workman, 2010).

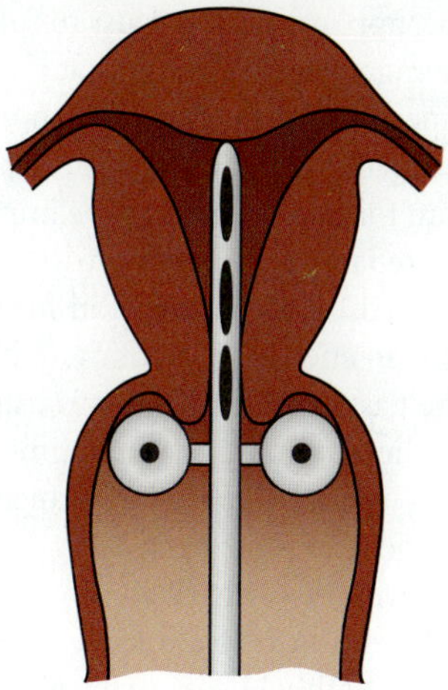

FIG. 11-15 Intracavitary implant. Applicator in place in uterus is loaded with radium source.

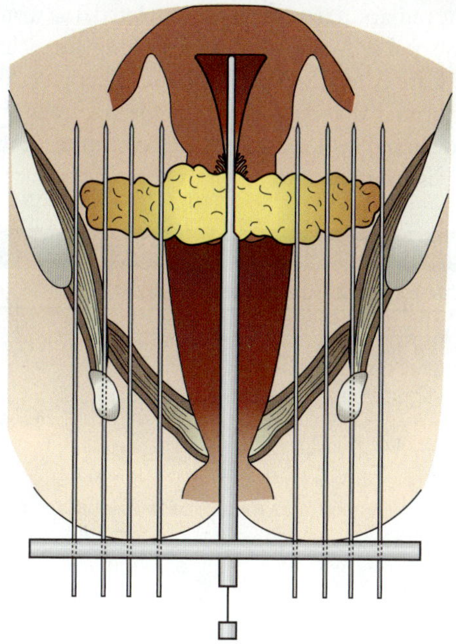

FIG. 11-16 Interstitial-intracavitary implant.

For internal radiation therapy, the woman may be treated in the hospital or in a special outpatient unit. If treatment is done in the hospital, the woman is taken to the operating room, and while she is under general or spinal anesthesia, a specially designed applicator is placed into her vagina and cervix. X-rays are taken to make sure the applicator is correctly placed. The woman is returned to her room, where the radioactive source is placed into the applicator (Fig. 11-15). The source remains in place from 12 hours to 3 days. If treatment is in the outpatient setting, the applicator is inserted into the uterus in a treatment room; use of high-dose implants shortens the treatment time and is being used more frequently than low-dose implants because no hospital stay is required (Monk & Tewari, 2007; Workman, 2010).

In advanced carcinoma of the cervix, conventional intracavitary applicators are not applicable. Interstitial therapy uses a template to guide the transperineal insertion of a group of 18 gauge hollow steel needles into the lesion (Fig. 11-16). After the needles are placed, the iridium wires are inserted when the woman is returned to her room.

Nursing Management. Nursing actions for external and internal radiation differ, so they are discussed separately.

External Therapy. Before external radiation therapy the woman's anxiety may be so high that information given by the radiologist may not be processed. The nurse should reinforce or fill in gaps, especially related to the following: the equipment, which is similar to that used for x-ray examination except larger; the hyperbaric oxygen chamber, which may be used to increase cellular oxygen and thus make tumor cells more radiosensitive; the radiotherapist, who will be behind a shield, but still close by and in communication with her; the position she will be put in and asked to maintain for some minutes; and the therapy, which is painless.

During the course of the therapy, the woman is counseled regarding maintaining general good health. To maintain good skin care the woman is taught to assess her skin often; avoid soaps, ointments, cosmetics, and deodorants if the axilla is being irradiated because these may contain metals that would alter the dose she receives and could lead to skin breakdown; wear loose clothing over the area and cotton underwear (or no underwear); use an air mattress or cover the mattress with foam pads or sheepskin; avoid exposing the irradiated areas to temperature extremes (e.g., hot tubs); and especially avoid removing the markings made by the radiologist. If her skin becomes red or itchy she can treat it with remedies recommended by the radiologist (e.g., aloe vera lotion, Aquaphor, or warm sitz baths). To treat skin that is broken or desquamating, the woman is shown how to use remedies prescribed by the radiologist (e.g., irrigation with warm water, application of antibiotic or lanolin ointment, exposure to air, and application of a loose dressing). The use of adhesive (or any) tape directly on the target area of skin should be avoided (Workman, 2010).

To maintain good nutrition the woman is reminded to keep a daily record of weight; use high-protein supplements; eat small, attractive, appetizing meals that are more bland than spicy; and keep the environment light, airy, clean, and quiet (especially before and after meals). A dietitian consult may be needed to help the woman and her family plan to meet the woman's nutritional needs. If the woman is ill enough to be hospitalized, she may need total parenteral nutrition or tube feedings. Nausea interferes with adequate intake; therefore, the woman may take antiemetics, as necessary. High daily fluid intake (2 to 3 L) should be suggested if not contraindicated. To increase her comfort, minimize infection, and promote adequate food intake, the woman is encouraged to perform frequent oral hygiene. Box 11-4 provides other suggestions for nutritional problems associated with radiation treatment.

The nurse explains, as necessary, the need for routine blood studies to monitor white blood cell count (to determine degree of immunosuppression). The woman and her family will need information about neutropenia, thrombocytopenia, and anemia and precautions to be taken. Because the woman is more vulnerable to infection, she is reminded of general measures to avoid infection (e.g., practice good hygiene, avoid people with infection, avoid large crowds, keep environment clean).

After the radiation treatment is completed, the woman needs information for self-care (see the Teaching for Self-Management box: Care After External Radiation Therapy). She should also be informed that side effects of the treatment, especially fatigue and altered taste sensations, can continue for weeks after the therapy is completed.

TEACHING FOR SELF-MANAGEMENT

Care After External Radiation Therapy

- Avoid infection and report symptoms of infection to health care provider immediately.
- Maintain good nutrition and fluid intake.
- Anticipate possible effects of radiation for 10 to 14 days after last treatment.
- Expect signs of healing to occur in about 3 weeks.
- Maintain good skin and mouth care to support a sense of well-being and prevent infection.
- Report the following symptoms to your health care provider:
  - Continued gastrointestinal symptoms (nausea, vomiting, anorexia, diarrhea)
  - Increasing skin irritation at the site of therapy (redness, swelling, pain, pruritus)
- Take medications as prescribed, and avoid any medications not prescribed or approved by health care provider.

Internal Therapy. Internal radiation therapy may require hospitalization or may be done in a special outpatient unit. Radiation safety officers determine the precautions to be observed in each situation. This discussion focuses on treatment in the hospital setting, but similar precautions would be used in the outpatient setting. Printed instruction sheets are usually available, stating precautions to be followed for each type of radiation substance used. A precaution sign is placed on the door of the woman's room.

SAFETY ALERT

Personnel who come into direct contact with anyone receiving radiation therapy should wear a film badge or other device to monitor the amount of exposure received.

Nurses must protect themselves from overexposure to radiation. Precautions include the following (Workman, 2010):

- Careful isolation techniques: wearing gloves while handling bodily fluids and observing good handwashing technique. These behaviors reflect knowledge that alpha and beta rays cannot pass through skin but may be in body fluids and excrement.
- Careful planning of nursing activity to limit time (to 30 minutes or less per 8 hours) spent in proximity to the woman to avoid exposure to gamma rays, which can penetrate several inches of lead.

Exposure to radiation is controlled in three ways: distance, time, and shielding (with lead). For the woman with sealed radiotherapy, a movable lead screen can be placed between the area in which the therapeutic applicator is located and the personnel. The lead screen also is used to protect visitors from radiation. Increasing the distance from the source also decreases exposure (Workman, 2010).

Familiarity with applicators is a must for all nurses working with people receiving radiotherapy so that if a "strange object" is found in the linen or on the floor, it is not touched. Today most hospital protocols include having a lead container and forceps in the room for use if a radioactive implant is dislodged.

The woman is prepared for insertion with the following care, which is accompanied by an explanation for each activity. To reduce the need for an enema or attention to bowel elimination for a few days, the gastrointestinal tract is usually prepared by using low-residue diet, enemas, and sometimes bowel sedation. The vaginal vault is usually prepared with an antiseptic douche, such as povidone-iodine.

An indwelling urinary catheter is inserted, as ordered, to prevent bladder distention that could dislodge the applicator. Food and fluids are withheld for a specified time before the procedure in anticipation of the use of general anesthesia. Preoperative medications may be ordered for the morning of the procedure. Deep-breathing exercises, range of motion (ROM) exercises, and positioning are all demonstrated before the procedure to minimize the effects of immobilization afterward. An intravenous (IV) solution will probably be started before the procedure, and IV therapy may be continued if nausea prevents good intake of oral fluids. The woman is assured that pain will be managed.

Explanations about restricted visitation of personnel and visitors also are given in the preinsertion phase. Women are often encouraged to bring reading materials to the hospital to combat the boredom that isolation imposes on them. In addition many units are equipped with television, CD, and video/DVD players.

The applicator is inserted into the woman's vaginal vault during surgery and after the usual postanesthesia recovery care, the woman is returned to her room, where the applicators are loaded with the radioactive substance.

A lead shield is placed next to the bed in line with the woman's pelvic area to protect the caregivers and visitors. Vital signs are monitored every 4 hours. Active ROM and deep-breathing exercises are encouraged every 2 hours; the woman is positioned on her back and may not be permitted to turn from side to side, although log-rolling may be done occasionally to relieve back pressure. The head of the bed may or may not be elevated slightly.

The woman's diet is changed from clear liquid to low residue, as ordered. Many individuals have difficulty eating while lying flat or even if the bed is elevated slightly. The nurse arranges the food so that it is easy to reach. Finger foods or liquids are generally more manageable. Parenteral or oral fluids are given, up to 3 L daily.

The urinary catheter remains in the bladder while the implant is in place. However, no perineal or catheter care is given. Intake and output are measured. The woman is given a partial bath, washing only above her waist. Massage is restricted to her shoulders and neck. Linen is changed only as absolutely necessary. Any linen or equipment used is retained in the room until therapy is complete to prevent loss of an applicator or seed. If vaginal or rectal bleeding or hematuria occurs, the physician is notified immediately.

Emotional support is provided by planning to be with the woman for short periods; encouraging her to verbalize concerns and needs; and encouraging family members, clergy, or others to visit for short periods daily or to communicate by telephone. Pregnant women and children are not permitted to visit.

Many women undergoing internal radiation treatment are given medication to prevent complications and to promote comfort during the procedure. Such medications might include antibiotics to prevent bladder infections, heparin injections to prevent thrombophlebitis, sedatives for relaxation, antiemetics for nausea, and narcotics for pain. The woman is considered radioactive during the time the internal sources are in place (Workman, 2010).

After the radium is removed the Foley catheter is removed, and the woman is assisted in getting out of bed the first time. She is usually discharged the same day. Discharge teaching can be found in the Teaching for Self-Management box: Care After Internal Radiation Therapy. The woman and her family are reassured that she is not radioactive after the treatment.

TEACHING FOR SELF-MANAGEMENT

Care After Internal Radiation Therapy

- Eat three balanced meals a day, and increase fluid to 3 L daily.
- Rest when tired, and resume normal activities as comfort permits.
- Maintain good hygiene (e.g., daily showers and daily douches until discharge stops).
- Use vaginal dilator if needed for vaginal stenosis. Sexual intercourse may be resumed in 7 to 10 days or as recommended by physician.
- Understand that sterility and cessation of menstruation usually occur with this procedure if you are premenopausal.
- Report any of the following to your health care provider: bleeding (vaginal, rectal, or in the urine), foul-smelling vaginal discharge, fever, abdominal distention, or pain.
- Take any prescribed medications as directed.
- Call your health care provider or clinic if there are concerns or problems.
- Plan follow-up visits to determine emotional as well as physical recovery.

Posttreatment complications range from those arising from immobilization, such as thrombophlebitis, pulmonary embolism, and pneumonia, to those arising from the treatment itself, such as hemorrhage, skin reactions (rashes or inflammation), diarrhea, cramping, dysuria, and vaginal stenosis. The woman is assessed for any of these complications before discharge.

The woman may experience altered patterns of sexuality related to treatment side effects. A decrease in vaginal secretions and sensation may occur, as well as vaginal stenosis. These can contribute to decreased sexual desire, because pain and discomfort during intercourse can affect the desire to resume sexual activities. The nurse can initiate a discussion with the woman and her partner, offer information about the effects of radiation on the ability to have sexual intercourse, and offer suggestions for specific problems, such as using a water-based lubricant for vaginal dryness and using a vaginal dilator as directed by her health care provider. If necessary, the couple can be referred to other resources.

Complications of Radiation Therapy. Morbidity as a direct result from properly conducted therapy is usually minimal. Some of the morbidity seen may be caused by the uncontrolled tumor and not by the therapy. Acute treatment complications occurring during or shortly after therapy include irritation of the rectum, the small bowel, and the bladder; reactions in the skinfolds; and mild bone marrow suppression. Dysuria and frequency may occur. Late complications, although not common, include genital fistulas and necrosis (Yashar, 2007).

Recurrent and Advanced Cancer of the Cervix

Approximately one third of women with invasive cervical cancer will have recurrent or persistent disease after therapy. The 5-year survival rate is approximately 17% (Monk & Tewari, 2007). Irradiation of metastatic areas is commonly successful in providing local control and symptomatic relief. Irradiation for recurrent disease may be considered for women who were initially treated with surgery. Further radiation may not be effective for those women who were initially treated with radiation.

Pelvic Exenteration. The woman who has recurrence only within the pelvis may be considered for **pelvic exenteration** if a cure is thought to be possible. A total exenteration involves removal of the perineum, the pelvic floor, the levator muscles, and all reproductive organs. Additionally, pelvic lymph nodes, rectum, sigmoid colon, urinary bladder, and distal ureters are removed, and a colostomy and ileal conduit are constructed (Monk & Tewari, 2007) (Fig. 11-17, *A*). In select cases the procedure can be modified to either an anterior or a posterior exenteration. In anterior pelvic exenteration all of the previously mentioned pelvic viscera are removed except the rectosigmoid, which is preserved. Urine is rerouted through an ileal conduit (see Fig. 11-17, *B*). In the posterior pelvic exenteration procedure, all pelvic viscera with the exception of the bladder are removed. The feces are rerouted through a colostomy (see Fig. 11-17, *C*). A neovagina (new vagina) may be constructed.

Women are carefully selected for this procedure; 5-year survival rates range from 20% to 62% (Monk & Tewari, 2007). Many of the complications that follow this surgery are those that follow any form of major surgery, for example, pulmonary embolism, pulmonary edema, myocardial infarction, and cerebrovascular accident. These complications are seen immediately after surgery. Infection originating in the pelvic cavity usually occurs later, if it occurs.

Nursing Management. Nursing care of the woman having a pelvic exenteration depends on what is removed. General preoperative considerations include assessments similar to those for a woman having a radical hysterectomy. Additionally, a thorough sexual assessment is needed because of the drastic changes involved. The woman needs information about the construction of a neovagina if that is an option. She will need to be assessed for stoma site selection and information about management of colostomy or ileal conduit if appropriate. Extensive preoperative bowel preparation is needed before surgery. Pain management is discussed, as is what to expect postoperatively (e.g., nasogastric tubes, arterial catheters). Significant others should be included in preoperative discussions when possible, because their postoperative support is essential.

Postoperative care usually begins in an intensive care unit until the woman's condition is stable. She is monitored for signs

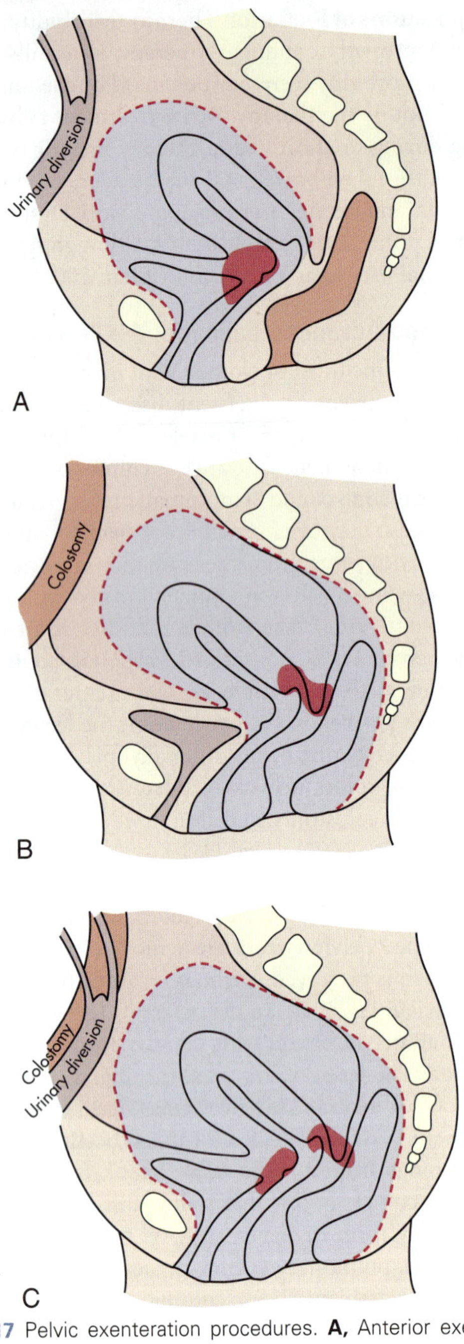

FIG. 11-17 Pelvic exenteration procedures. **A,** Anterior exenteration. **B,** Posterior exenteration. **C,** Total exenteration.

of complications, including shock, hemorrhage, pulmonary embolus and other pulmonary complications, fluid and electrolyte imbalance, and urinary complications (Monk & Tewari, 2007). Nursing care continues after the woman is stabilized and moved back to her room. Wound care consists of irrigation with half-strength normal saline, followed by drying of the area with either a hair dryer on cool setting or a heat lamp placed at least 12 inches from the perineal area. The woman is taught how to care for her colostomy or ileal conduit when she is able to begin self-care. Assessment for psychologic reactions is important. The woman will probably experience a grief reaction over her mutilated body. She may become depressed during the long convalescence.

The woman may be discharged to a long-term care facility or to her home. She will need assistance in her physical care for at least 6 months. Teaching needed for home care includes colostomy or ureterostomy care; dietary needs for healing; perineal care, including use of perineal pads to protect clothing from discharge; ROM exercises and physical activities permitted by her health care provider; and signs of complication, especially infection and bowel obstruction.

Because the woman will have sexual disruption and possibly be unable to have vaginal intercourse (if the vagina is not reconstructed), counseling about sexual activity is needed. Usually even with a vaginal reconstruction, vaginal intercourse is not advised until healing has taken place, usually in 12 to 18 months. Women with neovaginas may complain of decreased vaginal sensations or chronic discharge, or that the vagina is too short or too long. Women with colostomies or ureterostomies may worry about leakage or odors during sexual activities or may be concerned about their change in appearance. They may need counseling about alternative activities for sexual expression for themselves and their partners. The woman and her partner may need referral for further sexual counseling.

Chemotherapy. Chemotherapy may be used in advanced cancer of the cervix to reduce tumor size before surgery or as adjuvant therapy for poor-prognosis tumors. In general, no long-term benefits are derived with chemotherapy, although chemotherapy concurrent with radiation therapy can improve survival (Monk & Tewari, 2007). Cisplatin is the most effective; other chemotherapeutic agents used singly or in combination include 5-fluorouracil, carboplatin, cyclophosphamide, ifosfamide, methotrexate, mitomycin C, bleomycin, paclitaxel, and hydroxyurea (Chu & Rubin, 2007).

Cancer of the Vulva

Incidence and Etiology

Vulvar carcinoma accounts for about 4% of all female genital malignancies and is the fourth most commonly occurring gynecologic cancer. It appears most frequently in older women in their middle 60s to 70s; DNA testing of these women often shows mutation of the p53 tumor suppressor gene (ACS, 2010b). Vulvar cancers in older women do not appear to be etiologically related to HPV infection. The incidence of vulvar cancer, specifically vulvar intraepithelial neoplasia (VIN), is increasing in younger women. Almost 20% of vulvar cancers occur in women younger than 50 years of age, and most women are in their twenties. HPV infection is thought to be responsible for most of these cancers (ACS). Women who have a history of genital warts (condylomata acuminata) and who smoke have an increased risk of developing VIN (ACS).

By far the majority (90%) of vulvar carcinoma is squamous cell; other vulvar neoplasms are attributed to Paget's disease, adenocarcinoma of Bartholin glands, fibrosarcoma and melanoma, and basal cell carcinoma. VIN is the first neoplastic change, progressing over time to cancer in situ (CIS) and then to invasive cancer. Metastasis is by direct extension and lymphatic spread (Hacker, 2010b).

Prognosis depends on the size of the lesion and the tumor grade at the time of diagnosis. Fifty percent of women have symptoms for 2 to 16 months before seeking treatment. Fortunately, vulvar cancer grows slowly, extends slowly, and metastasizes fairly late. Even with a pattern of delayed diagnosis, survival rates are approximately 96% for all stages if nodes are negative. Survival rates drop to 66%, however, if lymph node metastasis has occurred (Stehman, 2007).

Clinical Manifestations and Diagnosis

Itching is the most common symptom of VIN; a lump or lesion is more common with invasive cancer (Hacker, 2010b). The most common site for vulvar lesions is on the labia majora. The vulvar lesion is usually asymptomatic until it is 1 to 2 cm in diameter. When it is symptomatic, women may complain of vulvar pruritus, burning, or pain. Necrosis and infection of the lesion result in ulceration with bleeding or watery discharge.

VINs are usually multifocal in young women. Unifocal lesions are associated with invasive cancer and are more common in older women. Initially, growth is superficial but later extends into the urethra, the vagina, and the anus. In approximately 50% of late cases, superficial inguinal and femoral lymph nodes become involved (Stehman, 2007).

Simple biopsy with histologic evaluation reveals the diagnosis. The areas of pathologic involvement are identified by staining the vulva with toluidine blue (1%), allowing an absorption time of 3 to 5 minutes, and then washing with acetic acid (2% to 3%); abnormal tissue retains the dye. Biopsy is necessary to rule out such conditions as sexually transmitted infections (e.g., chancroid, granuloma inguinale, syphilis), basal cell carcinoma, and CIS. In situ malignancies are initially small, red, white, or pigmented friable papules. In Paget's disease the lesions are red, moist, and elevated. Melanomas appear as bluish-black, pigmented, or papillary lesions. Melanomas metastasize through the bloodstream and lymphatics (Hacker, 2010b).

Collaborative Care

Therapeutic Management. Treatment varies, depending on the extent of the disease. Laser surgery, cryosurgery, or electrosurgical excision may be used to treat VIN. A disadvantage to these treatments is that healing is slow, and the treated area is painful. A local wide excision may be performed for localized lesions. Recurrence can occur after these treatments, so follow-up is important (Frumovitz & Bodurka, 2007).

Several types of vulvectomy procedures are used for CIS and invasive cancer. A *skinning vulvectomy* involves removal of the superficial vulvar skin; it is rarely performed.

A *simple vulvectomy* involves removal of all of the vulva (external genital organs including the mons pubis, labia majora and minora, and possibly the clitoris). The clitoris usually can be saved if cancer is not present.

For invasive disease, a *partial* or *complete radical vulvectomy* is performed. A partial vulvectomy is the removal of part of the vulva and deep tissues; a complete vulvectomy includes the removal of the whole vulva, deep tissues, and the clitoris (Fig. 11-18).

Skin grafts may be done if a large area of skin is removed during the vulvectomy; however, most surgeries can be closed without grafts. If grafts are needed, a surgeon who performs reconstruction surgery may be consulted (ACS, 2010b).

The inguinal nodes may be removed through an inguinal (groin) node dissection. Usually only lymph nodes on the same side as the cancer are removed; however, nodes on both sides may be removed if the cancer is in the middle (see Fig. 11-18). Swelling of the leg often is a problem after this surgery.

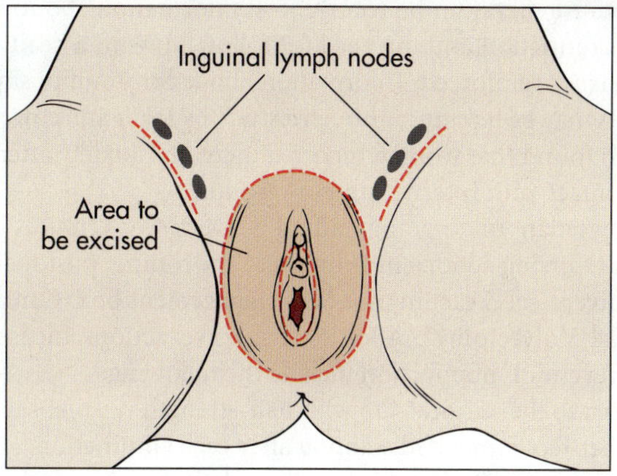

FIG. 11-18 Radical vulvectomy. Note dotted lines denoting vulvectomy incision and inguinal groin incisions.

A *sentinel node biopsy* may be done instead of the inguinal node dissection. This procedure involves injecting blue dye or radioactive material into the tumor site. A scan is performed to identify the sentinel (first) node to pick up the dye or radioactive material. The node is removed for microscopic study. If cancer cells are found, the rest of the lymph nodes will be removed, but if cancer is not found, further lymph node removal is not done. This procedure continues to be studied for use with vulvar cancers (ACS, 2010b).

External radiation therapy can be used to shrink tumors before surgery, but it is not the primary treatment. Postoperative external radiation therapy can be used for women who are at risk for recurrence. Radiation treatment causes dermatitis and ulceration that are uncomfortable for the woman.

Chemotherapy has not been very effective as a treatment except for the topical application of 5-fluorouracil for VIN or CIS. This treatment is painful and not used often. Chemotherapy continues to be investigated in combination with radiation as an adjunct to surgery in advanced cancer of the vulva (ACS, 2010b).

Nursing Management. Nursing care for the woman with vulvar cancer is similar to that for other gynecologic malignancies. A history of symptoms and a physical examination as well as an assessment of the woman's understanding of the surgical procedure and her emotional state should be done. Nursing diagnoses for women with vulvar cancer are similar to those for other gynecologic cancers; possible nursing diagnoses specific to problems with vulvar cancer treatment include the following:

- *Risk for infection* related to:
  - surgical incision
- *Sexual dysfunction* related to:
  - vulvectomy
- *Disturbed body image* related to:
  - loss of sexual organ
  - perceived or actual disfigurement
  - altered patterns of elimination as a result of surgery

Interventions for the woman treated with laser therapy include applying topical steroids to the area, administering sitz baths and drying the area with a hair dryer, applying local anesthetics, or giving oral pain medication as needed. Women need to be informed that pain may get worse 3 to 4 days after the treatment.

Because there can be recurrences, information about vulvar self-examination and the need for follow-up with a health care provider is reinforced. Information about community support groups may be helpful, although a study by Likes and coworkers (2008) found that women reported increased anxiety after having contact with Internet support groups.

A woman undergoing radical vulvectomy requires some special nursing actions in addition to the routine postoperative care given (see Teaching for Self-Management box: Care After Radical Vulvectomy). Additional nursing actions focused on the prevention of infection include the following:

- Irrigate the surgical site with half-strength normal saline or other recommended solution after each elimination.
- Dry the area thoroughly by using a hair dryer on cool setting or a heat lamp.
- Use a bed cradle or other means to lift the bed covers and allow air to circulate around the wound.
- Give stool softeners to decrease straining and disruption of the suture line.
- Note any change in color of the surgical site.
- Note any drainage or foul odor and, if present, notify primary health care provider.
- Perform catheter care as needed.
- Provide and instruct woman in the use of sitz baths.

TEACHING FOR SELF-MANAGEMENT

Care After Radical Vulvectomy

- Avoid sexual activity for 4 to 6 weeks or as health care provider directs.
- Rest frequently.
- Avoid crossing legs, sitting, or standing for long periods.
- Avoid tight, constricting clothing, and wear cotton underwear.
- Keep wound area clean and dry. Rinse area with warm water and pat dry after voiding.
- Continue wound care as prescribed (e.g., irrigate with solution of warm water; pack with gauze; dry using hair dryer on coolest setting. Report to your health care provider any swelling, redness, unusual tenderness, drainage, or foul odor of incision site.
- Report any temperature greater than 39° C.
- Eat a well-balanced diet to promote healing.
- Take all medications as prescribed.
- Elevate legs periodically to prevent pelvic congestion.
- Call your health care provider or clinic if there are concerns or problems.

The woman is at high risk for sexual dysfunction related to the effects of the surgery. For example, she may have concerns that her partner will be repulsed by the scarring and loss of the vulva. She also may have concerns about reaching orgasm and vaginal numbness or painful vaginal penetration. Nursing actions that focus on minimizing these risks include the following:

- Encouraging verbalization of feelings
- Providing privacy for discussion
- Encouraging open communication between the woman and her partner
- Discussing when sexual activity can be safely resumed
- Discussing alternative methods to achieve sexual satisfaction
- Providing information about use of vaginal dilators and water-soluble lubricants for painful vaginal intercourse
- Providing resources for counseling if necessary

Cancer of the Vagina

Vaginal carcinomas account for less than 2% of gynecologic malignancies, with a peak incidence between 50 and 70 years of age. Most lesions are squamous cell carcinomas, and are secondary rather than primary carcinomas of the vagina. Vaginal intraepithelial neoplasia (VAIN) is uncommon, and clear-cell adenocarcinoma is even rarer. It is found primarily in young women (ages 15 to 30 years) and is related to intrauterine exposure to DES. Sarcoma botryoides (embryonal rhabdomyosarcoma) occurs in infants and children (Dotters & Katz, 2007).

The etiology is unknown, but vaginal cancer may be caused by chronic vaginal irritation, vaginal trauma, and genital viruses (e.g., HPV). Women with VAIN often have had cancer or currently have cancer of another part of the genital tract (Slomovitz & Coleman, 2007). Vaginal lesions, usually seen in the upper one third of the vagina, often extend into the bladder and the rectum in late stages. Metastasis can occur early because of the rich lymphatic drainage in the vaginal area.

Some women with vaginal cancer are asymptomatic. Diagnosis often comes after an abnormal Pap test. Symptoms that have been associated with vaginal cancer include bleeding after coitus or examination, dyspareunia, and watery discharge. Bladder involvement results in urinary frequency or urgency; rectal extension causes painful defecation. A pelvic examination may reveal a single lesion, although multiple lesions are common (Hacker, 2010b).

Colposcopy examination and biopsy of Schiller-stained areas disclose the diagnosis. Therapy for vaginal cancer is directed by the extent of the lesion and the age and condition of the woman. Local excision is the preferred therapy for localized lesions. Topical application of 5-fluorouracil cream has been used with varying results. Laser surgery may be used to treat VAIN. Radical hysterectomy and removal of the upper vagina with dissection of the pelvic nodes or internal and external radiation are options for invasive cancer. Radiation therapy is the usual treatment of choice (Dotters & Katz, 2007). If a vaginectomy is performed, sexual function will be lost without reconstructive surgery. Chemotherapy has not been effective in treatment of vaginal cancer, although studies are ongoing on the effectiveness of chemotherapy in combination with radiation. In early-stage cancer, 5-year survival rates are greater than 80%, with stage II survival rates in the 50% range (Hacker, 2010b).

Nursing care for the woman with vaginal cancer is similar to that for other gynecologic cancers. Sexual counseling or referral may be needed.

Cancer of the Uterine Tubes

Primary carcinoma of the uterine (fallopian) tube (usually the distal one third) is one of the rarest cancers of the female genital tract (less than 1%), with a peak incidence between ages 50 and 60 years. The cause is unknown. Most women are asymptomatic in the early stages of tubal cancer. Vaginal bleeding is the most common symptom of tubal cancer, but clear vaginal discharge and lower abdominal pain also occur frequently. An enlarging unilateral pelvic mass or ascites may occur and is often misdiagnosed as ovarian carcinoma or endometrial carcinoma. Differential diagnosis of tubal cancer is usually made postoperatively. Because uterine tube cancer is so rare, there is no established management. Current therapy guidelines parallel those established for ovarian carcinoma; therefore, tumor-reducing surgery such as a total abdominal hysterectomy with BSO, omentectomy (removal of connective tissue covering the organs), and lymph node sampling are performed (Sunde, Kaplan, & Rose, 2007). Postoperative therapy consists of chemotherapy with cisplatin or other platinum-based drugs combined with paclitaxel, sometimes followed by second-look surgery to determine whether further treatment is needed. Radiation therapy is sometimes used if the disease is limited to the tube, ovary, and uterus, although reports of its effectiveness vary. Overall 5-year survival rates for all stages is 69%; 5-year survival rates for stages I and II are approximately 80% (Sunde et al.).

Nursing care for the woman with uterine tube cancer is similar to that of the woman with ovarian cancer.

Cancer and Pregnancy

Cancer occurs with relative infrequency during the reproductive years. Approximately 1 of every 1000 pregnant women will have cancer (Cohn, Ramaswamy, & Blum, 2009). These malignancies may be responsible for up to one third of maternal deaths. Although all forms of neoplasms have been documented in conjunction with pregnancy, the most frequently occurring types are breast cancer, cervical cancer, melanomas, ovarian cancer, leukemia and lymphomas, tubal cancers, and thyroid cancers. Bone, colorectal, vulvar, uterine, and vaginal cancers are rarely diagnosed during pregnancy. When pregnancy and cancer coincide, therapeutic issues are complex, and intense reactions occur in the woman, her family, and the health care team. Women are confronted with issues such as continuing or terminating the pregnancy. The selection and timing of therapies such as chemotherapy, radiation, and surgery are all affected by the pregnancy. Add to this the conflicting feelings the woman has (i.e., the joy of pregnancy versus the fear and anxiety associated with cancer), and the task of providing comprehensive care for the woman and her family presents a formidable challenge to the health care team. A brief discussion of the most frequent types of cancers that occur during pregnancy and the current therapies associated with them follows.

Cancer of the Breast

Approximately 1% to 2% of women are pregnant or lactating at the time of diagnosis of cancer of the breast (Tewari, 2007). Breast cancer complicates about 1 in 3000 pregnancies. The survival rate for women who are diagnosed with breast cancer while pregnant may be as low as 15% to 20% because the disease is generally in the advanced stages when first diagnosed (Tewari). Diagnosis is often delayed because breast engorgement may obscure the mass from palpation, and increased density of the tissue makes mammographic visualization more difficult. In addition, increased vascularity and lymphatic drainage in the breast of a pregnant woman may increase the speed of metastasis. Treatment is the same as for the nonpregnant woman, although surgery is usually the treatment of choice for breast cancer in pregnancy (Tewari). If an invasive tumor is found, it must be determined whether the tissue is positive or negative for estrogen receptors (ERs). ER-negative tumors spread more rapidly than ER-positive tumors and are more common in pregnancy.

Maternal-fetal management involves consideration of the gestational age of the fetus, the extent of disease, the tumor growth potential, and the proposed treatment. Termination of the pregnancy in early stages of the disease appears to have no effect on survival. There is little evidence to suggest that pregnancy affects the malignant process. Therapeutic abortion may become an issue in the presence of advanced disease and may be deemed necessary to achieve effective palliation. Lumpectomy or partial mastectomy is the most commonly used surgical procedure, but radical mastectomy is tolerated well in these women. For advanced disease in the second or third trimester, alkylating agents, 5-fluorouracil, doxorubicin, and vincristine are relatively safe for the fetus. Radiation therapy is avoided if at all possible until after the birth, because even with careful shielding the fetus may still receive sufficient radiation to produce detrimental effects (Tewari, 2007).

There is no agreement about whether a postpartum woman with breast cancer should breastfeed, although many surgeons recommend formula feeding. There are theoretic concerns that if one of the oncogenes for breast cancer is a virus, as many have postulated, the remaining breast may be contaminated, and the virus may be passed to the newborn, possibly acting as a latent inducer of breast carcinoma. Another reason is that lactation increases vascularity in the remaining breast, which may contain a neoplasm as well (Tewari, 2007).

Breastfeeding after lumpectomy is possible, but the site of the incision may interrupt the milk ducts or prevent the nipple from extending during feeding. Breastfeeding is contraindicated if the woman is receiving chemotherapy. Women receiving radiation will have diminished ability to lactate in the irradiated breast (Copeland & Landon, 2007; Tewari, 2007).

Pregnancy incidence after mastectomy is influenced by many factors, including prior treatment and duration of survival. About 7% of women will have one or more pregnancies within the first 5 years after mastectomy. In general, women with good prognoses (e.g., no positive nodes) are likely to be counseled to wait at least 2 years before attempting pregnancy (Cohn et al., 2009).

Cancer of the Cervix

The incidence of cervical cancer concurrent with pregnancy is reported to be 3% or about 1 in 2200 pregnancies, making it the most common reproductive tract cancer associated with pregnancy (Copeland & Landon, 2007). Birth can be accomplished by either the vaginal or the cesarean route; however, there is some concern regarding vaginal birth in the presence of invasive disease because the risk of hemorrhage and metastatic seeding from local trauma may be increased. The outcome for the woman with cervical cancer is roughly the same as that for the nonpregnant woman (Tewari, 2007).

Cervical abnormalities are diagnosed during pregnancy with an abnormal Pap test. If the report suggests that the pregnant woman has a squamous intraepithelial lesion, a colposcopy, possibly with directed biopsy, is done. If invasive disease is not found, treatment is delayed until after the woman gives birth. Colposcopy is often repeated every 6 to 8 weeks until the birth and again postpartum. Conization is not advised during pregnancy unless necessary to rule out invasive cancer because it is associated with bleeding, miscarriage, and preterm birth (Tewari, 2007).

The therapy of invasive carcinoma of the cervix during pregnancy is affected by many factors. The stage of the disease and the trimester in which the cancer is diagnosed are important. Equally important are the beliefs and desires of the woman and her family in terms of initiating therapy that can interrupt the pregnancy, as opposed to postponing the therapy until fetal viability is achieved. If the woman chooses not to continue the pregnancy, external radiation to the pelvis is done. Miscarriage usually occurs, and then internal radiation is done. If miscarriage does not occur, a modified radical hysterectomy may be performed. If the woman desires to continue the pregnancy, treatment of early-stage invasive cervical cancer can be delayed until fetal viability is reached, without harmful effects on the woman. Cesarean birth is usually performed, followed by radiation therapy (Copeland & Landon, 2007; Tewari, 2007).

Leukemia

The average age for pregnant women with acute leukemia is 28 years; incidence during pregnancy is about 1 in 75,000 (Cohn et al., 2009). Pregnancy seems to have no specific effect on the course of the disease, except that vigorous therapy is detrimental to early gestation. Preterm labor and postpartum hemorrhage are associated with acute leukemia (Tewari, 2007). Acute myelocytic leukemia (60% of cases) has a more fulminant course and requires immediate therapy; in the presence of chronic myelocytic leukemia, therapy can be delayed somewhat. Some pregnant women with the chronic form of the disease who had chemotherapy and radiation therapy directed at the spleen have given birth to apparently healthy infants. The decision to terminate the pregnancy rests with the woman and her family; however, prompt, aggressive therapy is always advisable if remission is to be achieved. Decisions may be influenced by the aggressiveness of the disease.

Hodgkin's Disease

Hodgkin's disease is a malignant lymphoma that affects many younger people and complicates about one in 6000 pregnancies. Younger women (younger than 40 years) have a better prognosis (Tewari, 2007).

Pregnancy appears to have no effect on the disease and vice versa, other than those effects resulting from therapy. Radiation therapy of the nodes and multiagent chemotherapy result in about a 90% cure rate. Unless gestation is well into the third trimester, delay in initiating therapy should be minimal, which brings up the dilemma of therapeutic abortion. Radiation therapy to diseased areas above the diaphragm can be initiated during the third trimester with proper shielding of the fetus (Cohn et al., 2009). Chemotherapy is strongly contraindicated during the first trimester but certain agents (antitumor antibiotics and antimicrotubule agents) appear safe to use in the second and third trimesters. Termination of the pregnancy during the course of the disease is not definitely indicated, although treatment decisions are easier (Tewari, 2007).

Melanoma

Malignant melanoma may be one of the rare cancers that can be affected by pregnancy. This is suggested by reports in which pregnancy has been shown to induce or exacerbate a melanoma. These suggestions are based on changes that occur naturally during pregnancy and include hyperpigmentation, an increase in melanocyte-stimulating hormone (MSH), and increased production of estrogen. ERs have been identified in about half of all melanomas (Tewari, 2007).

Although pregnancy has been implicated in the more rapid metastases to regional lymph nodes, stage for stage there does not seem to be a significant difference in the survival of pregnant and nonpregnant women. As a result, most authorities recommend that women who have histories of malignant melanoma delay pregnancy for 2 to 3 years after surgical excision, because this is the period of highest risk for recurrence (Copeland & Landon, 2007).

Diagnosis is established by biopsy. Therapy consists of radical local excision. For most other malignancies, the placenta is unexplainably resistant to invasion by maternal cancer. Although melanoma accounts for few cases of malignant disease during pregnancy, it is the most common cancer to metastasize to the placenta (Tewari, 2007).

Thyroid Cancer

The incidence of thyroid cancer in pregnancy is not established. Normally the thyroid gland enlarges during pregnancy, and an asymptomatic nodular mass is a common finding. Diagnosis is usually by cytologic testing of fine-needle aspirate. Thyroid suppression is the preferred treatment during pregnancy for a benign lesion. For a papillary or follicular malignancy found in the first or second trimester, the woman is advised to have a thyroidectomy in the second trimester followed by thyroid suppression (Tewari, 2007). If a tumor is found in the third trimester, surgery can be delayed until after the birth. With other thyroid malignancies, treatment is individualized based on the wishes of the woman and her family (Tewari).

! NURSING ALERT

Radioactive iodine is contraindicated in pregnancy and lactation.

Colon Cancer

The incidence of colon cancer in pregnancy is approximately 1 in 13,000 (Copeland & Landon, 2007). The signs and symptoms such as constipation, hemorrhoids, and backache are often attributed to pregnancy, resulting in diagnosis at a more advanced stage. Colonoscopy and biopsy are usually not done in pregnancy because these procedures can cause placental abruption and fetal injury from maternal hypoxia or hypotension.

Management of the cancer is based on the weeks of gestation and tumor stage. In a woman who is less than 20 weeks of gestation, surgery may be performed to remove the tumor. If she is more than 20 weeks of gestation, surgery may be delayed until after the birth. Chemotherapy and radiation are usually not used in pregnancy for colon cancer but may be used after the birth (Cohn et al.; Copeland & Landon).

Other Gynecologic Cancers

Cancer of the Vulva. The diagnosis of preinvasive (VIN) disease during pregnancy is becoming more common with the increase in the diagnosis of CIS of the vulva (Tewari, 2007).

Therapy is postponed until the postpartum period. If invasive disease (a rare occurrence) is diagnosed during the first trimester, vulvectomy with bilateral groin dissection may be done after the fourteenth week. When it is diagnosed in the third trimester, local wide excision is done, deferring definitive surgery until after birth. Pregnancy does not alter the course of the disease. Vaginal birth can be attempted if the surgical wounds are healed (Tewari).

After radical vulvectomy and bilateral inguinal node dissection, a woman who becomes pregnant again can carry the pregnancy to term and give birth vaginally. If vaginal stenosis is present and could impede birth, cesarean birth may be more appropriate (Tewari, 2007).

Cancer of the Vagina. Except for clear-cell adenocarcinoma of DES-exposed women, cancer of the vagina is rare. If clear-cell adenocarcinoma of the cervix and vagina or sarcoma is found in the upper vagina, the preferred surgery is radical hysterectomy, upper vaginectomy, and bilateral pelvic lymphadenectomy, followed by chemotherapy. Radiation is usually not advocated during pregnancy. Pregnancy does not seem to affect the course of the disease or the prognosis.

Cancer of the Uterus. Endometrial carcinoma during pregnancy is very rare. Diagnosis was usually an incidental finding after therapeutic abortion or surgery, and the lesions were minimally invasive or noninvasive. Recommended therapy is TAH-BSO and adjuvant radiotherapy (Tewari, 2007).

Cancer of the Uterine Tube. With a peak incidence between 50 and 55 years of age, concurrent pregnancy is only a remote possibility. Should it occur, the recommended therapy (TAH-BSO with postoperative radiotherapy or chemotherapy) is the same as that for the nonpregnant woman. Removal of the uterine tube is an alternative treatment (Tewari, 2007).

Cancer of the Ovary. Cancer of the ovary is the second most frequent reproductive cancer that occurs with pregnancy. Still, ovarian malignancy is relatively rare, being reported to occur in approximately 1 in 18,000 (Cohn et al., 2009).

Ovarian masses occur frequently during pregnancy. Because corpus luteum cysts account for a high percentage of these masses and because 99% of these resolve by the fourteenth week, any mass smaller than 5 cm may simply be observed until the end of the first trimester. Any mass larger than 5 cm, one that is growing, or one that does not resolve after the fourteenth week warrants further investigation. Abdominal palpation and ultrasound are the diagnostic tools of choice during pregnancy. However, in many cases, laparotomy is necessary to confirm the diagnosis. Laparotomy after 18 weeks of gestation has negligible fetal wastage associated with the procedure and is therefore considered safe (Tewari, 2007).

An ovarian tumor may be first diagnosed at birth or after birth because the enlarged uterus obscured its presence. Definitive diagnosis is needed before treatment is selected. For stage I tumors, treatment includes conservative surgery (unilateral oophorectomy and salpingectomy) and use of chemotherapy. If diagnosis occurs in the second or third trimester, treatment choices are difficult to make. They include interrupting the pregnancy and starting chemotherapy immediately, preserving pregnancy and starting chemotherapy with the fetus in utero (controversial), or delaying chemotherapy until the fetus is more mature and early scheduled birth is a low risk to the fetus (Tewari, 2007).

Cancer Therapy and Pregnancy

Decisions about the type and timing of therapy for cancer in the pregnant woman evoke moral and philosophic dilemmas, as well as complex medical judgments and intense emotional responses.

Ethical Considerations. When a pregnant woman has cancer and her survival is contingent on treatment that will harm the fetus, the health care team must work with the woman and her significant others to make decisions about how to proceed with her care. If a one-client model of ethical decision making is used, the risk-benefit analysis is applied to the maternal-fetal unit. The pregnant woman decides what is best for her and the fetus. The woman may accept or refuse treatment. If a two-client model is used for decision making, more weight is given to fetal well-being, but the pregnant woman cannot be forced to accept harm to herself for the sake of the fetus. Thus she could elect to accept treatment.

The fetus is at risk with either chemotherapy or radiation therapy. The effect of cancer therapy on the fetus can include death, miscarriage, teratogenesis, alteration in growth and development, alterations in function, and genetic mutation. The long-term effects on the fetus are unknown. These theoretic dangers must be weighed against the potential detrimental effects to the mother if treatment is withheld (Gilbert, 2011).

Timing of Therapy. Timing of therapy also is an important issue to discuss. Because most cancer therapy (except surgery) is geared toward having a differential and noxious effect on rapidly growing tissue, the fetus is most at risk during the first trimester, when organogenesis and rapid tissue growth occur. Surgery offers the least potential risk to the fetus; however, the risk of miscarriage and preterm labor may be increased.

Chemotherapy is avoided in the first trimester if at all possible. Although use of most chemotherapeutic agents has had isolated reports of fetal abnormalities, data on the agents used after the first trimester have recorded surprisingly few fetal abnormalities. The placenta may act as a barrier against the chemotherapeutic agents; therefore, although risk still exists, the judicious use of chemotherapy after the first trimester can result in live births with few congenital abnormalities. Acute drug toxicities may occur if treatment has occurred just before birth. Breastfeeding by women who are taking chemotherapeutic drugs is not recommended because most of these drugs may be excreted in breast milk (Copeland & Landon, 2007; Tewari, 2007).

Radiation therapy presents its own set of issues. During embryonic development, tissues are extremely radiosensitive. If cells are genetically altered or killed during this time, the child either will fail to survive or will be deformed. From a radiologic stance, there are three significant periods in embryonic development (Tewari, 2007):

1. Preimplantation: If irradiation does not destroy the fertilized egg, it probably does not affect it significantly.
2. Critical period of organogenesis: During this period, especially between days 18 and 38, the organism is most vulnerable; microcephaly, anencephaly, eye damage, growth restriction, spina bifida, and foot damage may occur.
3. After day 40: Large doses may still cause observable malformation and damage to the central nervous system.

Pregnancy After Cancer Treatment. If cancer therapy has not included the removal of the uterus, ovaries, or uterine (fallopian) tubes, there is a possibility that the woman may still be able to become pregnant. Although a woman's menstrual cycle may have resumed, pregnancy may be difficult to achieve. Therapy that has affected the pituitary or thyroid gland may make conception difficult. Radiation appears to have the most deleterious effects on the endocrine system. The use of chemotherapy may result in temporary or permanent sterility, depending on the drug, the dose, and the length of time since the therapy was completed. Rates of ovarian failure are increased with pelvic irradiation (Tewari, 2007).

Of growing concern is the increase in the number of childhood and adolescent cancer survivors. Long-term effects of therapy on fertility, including incidence of congenital anomalies, are not well known. Counseling issues to be discussed with the pregnant woman after cancer treatment include the risk of recurrence and the likely sites of recurrence, how the prior cancer treatment can affect fertility or reproductive outcome, and if a future pregnancy will adversely affect a tumor that is estrogen-receptor positive (Copeland & Landon, 2007).

For recovery from the disease and treatment to be complete, a delay of at least 2 years from the end of therapy to conception often is advised (Tewari, 2007). Before conception, a woman who has had cancer should have a complete physical examination to rule out complications that may place her or a fetus in jeopardy. Cardiac, pulmonary, hematologic, neurologic, renal, or gonadal function can be impaired. The woman and the potential father (if partnered) may be referred for reproductive and genetic counseling as well.

Gestational Trophoblastic Disease

Gestational trophoblastic disease (GTD) is a term that encompasses a spectrum of disorders arising from the placental trophoblast. It includes hydatidiform mole (see Chapter 28), invasive mole, and choriocarcinoma. **Gestational trophoblastic neoplasia (GTN)** refers to persistent trophoblastic tissue that is presumed to be malignant (Soper & Creasman, 2007).

Box 11-6 describes the clinical classifications of GTN. For several reasons, GTN is recognized as the most curable gynecologic malignancy. There is a sensitive marker produced by the tumor (hCG); the tumor is extremely sensitive to various chemotherapeutic agents; high risk factors in the disease process can be identified, allowing individualized therapy; and the aggressive use of multiple treatment methods is possible.

BOX 11-6 CLASSIFICATION OF GESTATIONAL TROPHOBLASTIC NEOPLASIA

I. Nonmetastatic disease: No evidence of disease outside uterus

II. Metastatic disease: Any disease outside uterus
- A. Good-prognosis metastatic disease
  1. Short duration (last pregnancy <4 months)
  2. Low pretreatment hCG titer (<100,000 International Units/24 hr or 40,000 milli-International Units/ml)
  3. No metastasis to brain or liver
  4. No significant prior chemotherapy
- B. Poor-prognosis metastatic disease
  1. Long duration (last pregnancy >4 months)
  2. High pretreatment hCG titer (>100,000 International Units/24 hr or >40,000 milli-International Units/ml)
  3. Brain or liver metastasis
  4. Significant prior chemotherapy
  5. Term pregnancy

Source: Soper, J., & Creasman, W. (2007). Gestational trophoblastic disease. In P. DiSaia & W. Creasman (Eds.), *Clinical gynecologic oncology* (7th ed.). St. Louis: Mosby.

Malignant disease follows normal pregnancy in about 30% to 50% of cases and hydatidiform mole in about 25% of cases. Miscarriage or ectopic pregnancy or another gestational event precedes about 25% of cases (Soper & Creasman, 2007). Metastasis occurs most often in the lungs, the vagina, the liver, and the brain.

Continued bleeding after evacuation of a hydatidiform mole is usually the most suggestive symptom of GTN. Other clinical signs include abdominal pain and uterine and ovarian enlargement. Signs of metastasis include pulmonary symptoms (e.g., dyspnea, cough). The diagnosis is usually confirmed by increasing or plateauing hCG levels after evacuation of a molar pregnancy. Once diagnosis is confirmed, other clinical studies (e.g., CT scan of lungs and brain, chest x-ray, pelvic ultrasound, and liver scan) are done to determine the extent of the disease (Soper & Creasman, 2007).

For women who wish to preserve their fertility and who have low risk nonmetastatic or low risk metastatic GTN, single-agent chemotherapy is chosen. Methotrexate has been the treatment of choice for years. High-dose methotrexate followed by folinic acid "rescue" within 24 hours also has shown excellent results and causes fewer toxic effects (Soper & Creasman, 2007). Dactinomycin also has been used with equally good results and is used for women with liver or renal disease, both of which are contraindications for methotrexate. Hysterectomy with adjuvant chemotherapy is often the choice of treatment for nonmetastatic tumors in women who have completed their childbearing (Soper & Creasman).

Women who have metastasis are classified as having either a good or poor prognosis, depending on the absence or presence of brain or liver metastasis, unsuccessful prior chemotherapy, symptoms lasting longer than 4 months, and serum β-hCG levels greater than 40,000 milli-International Units/ml. Treatment progresses from single-agent chemotherapy in the good-prognosis metastatic GTN to multiple-agent chemotherapy and multiple methods of treatment for the poor-prognosis group. Cure rates for the good-prognosis group are almost as positive as for those with nonmetastatic disease, both approaching 100% (Soper & Creasman, 2007).

Therapy is continued until negative hCG levels are obtained. After successful chemotherapy follow-up by serum hCG levels varies. One schedule is to obtain levels every 2 weeks for 3 months, every month for up to a year after completing therapy and every 6 to 12 months up to 3 to 5 years (Kavanagh & Gershenson 2007; Soper & Creasman, 2007). Physical examinations are done at least yearly as are chest radiographs if indicated. Contraception is needed until the woman has been in remission for 6 months to 1 year (Kavanagh & Gershenson; Soper & Creasman). Oral contraceptives are preferred, but barrier methods are acceptable if oral contraceptives are contraindicated; intrauterine devices (IUDs) are contraindicated (Gilbert, 2011). During a subsequent pregnancy, pelvic ultrasonography is recommended because the woman is at higher risk (1% to 2%) to develop another molar pregnancy. Serum hCG levels should be obtained 6 weeks after the birth (Kavanagh & Gershenson).

COMMUNITY ACTIVITY

- Visit the Women's Cancer Network website at www.wcn.org and select a gynecologic cancer. Review the client information about the cancer, statistics, treatment information (chemotherapy, radiation, hormone therapy, surgery), and quality of life issues. Is the information written to be easily understood by a lay person? What treatment facilities are located in your community?
- Research the availability of programs for women with cancer in your community, such as the Ovarian Cancer Survivor's Course and Endometrial Cancer Survivor's Course.

KEY POINTS

- Gynecologic disorders diminish the quality of life for affected women and their families.
- Structural disorders of the uterus and vagina related to pelvic relaxation and urinary incontinence can be a delayed result of childbearing, but they can be seen in young or childless women.
- Bladder training and pelvic muscle exercises can significantly decrease or relieve mild to moderate urinary incontinence.
- The development of neoplasms, whether benign or malignant, can have a significant physical and emotional effect on a woman and her family.
- Abnormal uterine bleeding is the most common symptom of leiomyomas or fibroid tumors.
- Various alternatives to hysterectomy exist for structural and benign disorders of the uterus; women need to be informed about the risks and benefits to make an informed decision about treatment.
- Endometrial cancer is the most common reproductive system malignancy.
- Hysterectomy is the usual treatment for early-stage endometrial cancer.
- Human papillomavirus infection is the primary cause of cervical cancer and is linked to vulvar cancer in women younger than 40 years of age.
- The squamocolumnar junction is an important landmark identified with neoplastic changes of the cervix.
- Preinvasive cancer of the cervix may be treated with techniques such as electrosurgical excision, cryotherapy, and laser therapy to save the structure of the cervix, particularly in women who desire to retain childbearing ability.
- External and internal radiation therapy in combination is as successful as surgery in treating early stages of cancer of the cervix.
- A Pap test will detect approximately 90% of early cervical dysplasias.
- Cancer of the ovary causes more deaths than any other female genital tract cancer.
- Nurses can control their exposure to radiation by increasing the distance from the radiation source, by limiting the time of exposure, and by using lead shielding.
- Cancer is relatively infrequent during pregnancy, occurring about once in every 1000 pregnancies.
- Radiation or chemotherapy treatment of the pregnant woman who has cancer places the fetus at risk for death, miscarriage, teratogenesis, and alterations in growth and development.
- Gestational trophoblastic neoplasms are highly curable but require close monitoring of hCG levels after treatment.

Audio Chapter Summaries Access an audio summary of these Key Points on evolve

REFERENCES

Agdi, M., & Tulandi, T. (2008). Endoscopic management of uterine fibroids. *Best Practices Research in Clinical Obstetrics and Gynaecology, 22*(4), 707–716.

American Cancer Society (ACS). (2010a). *Cancer facts and figures 2010*. New York: Author.

American Cancer Society (ACS). (2010b). Vulvar cancer. *Cancer reference information*. Available at www.cancer.org. Accessed June 15, 2010.

American College of Obstetricians and Gynecologists. (2008). ACOG Practice Bulletin No. 99: Management of abnormal cervical cytology and histology. *Obstetrics and Gynecology, 112*(6), 1419–1444.

Arnold, L., Bachmann, G., Rosen, R., & Rhoads, G. (2007). Assessment of vulvodynia symptoms in a sample of U.S. women: A prevalence survey with a nested case control sample. *American Journal of Obstetrics and Gynecology, 196*(2), 128e1-128e6.

Askew, J. (2009). A qualitative comparison of women's attitudes toward hysterectomy and myomectomy. *Health Care for Women International, 30*(8), 728–742.

Benson, S., Hahn, S., Tan, S., Janssen, O., Schedlowski, M., & Elsenbruch, S. (2010). *Journal of Obstetric, Gynecologic and Neonatal Nursing, 39*(1), 37–45.

Berek, J. (2010). Ovarian cancer. In N. Hacker, J. Gambone, & C. Hobel (Eds.), *Hacker and Moore's essentials of obstetrics and gynecology* (5th ed.). Philadelphia: Saunders.

Bergeron, S., Khalife, S., Glazer, H., & Binik, Y. (2008). Surgical and behavioral treatments for vestibulodynia: Two-and-one-half year follow-up and predictors of outcome. *Obstetrics and Gynecology, 111*(1), 159–166.

Bersuk, K. (2007). A strong pelvic floor: How nurses can spread the word. *Nursing for Women's Health, 11*(1), 54–62.

Cesario, S. (2010). Advances in the early detection of ovarian cancer: How to hear the whispers early. *Nursing for Women's Health, 14*(3), 222–234.

Chard, R. (2010). Care of preoperative patients. In D. Ignatavicius, & M. Workman (Eds.), *Medical-surgical nursing: Patient-centered collaborative care* (6th ed.). St. Louis: Saunders.

Chu, C., & Rubin, S. (2007). Basic principles of chemotherapy. In P. DiSaia, & W. Creasman (Eds.), *Clinical gynecologic oncology* (7th ed.). St. Louis: Mosby.

Cohn, D., Ramaswamy, B., & Blum, K. (2009). Malignancy and pregnancy. In R. Creasy, R. Resnik, J. Iams, C. Lockwood, & T. Moore (Eds.), *Creasy & Resnik's maternal-fetal medicine: Principles and practice* (6th ed.). Philadelphia: Saunders.

Coleman, R., & Gershenson, D. (2007). Neoplastic diseases of the ovary. Screening, benign and malignant epithelial cell neoplasms, sex-cord stromal tumors. In V. Katz, G. Lentz, R. Lobo, & D. Gershenson (Eds.), *Comprehensive gynecology* (5th ed.). Philadelphia: Mosby.

Copeland, L. (2007). Epithelial ovarian cancer. In P. DiSaia, & W. Creasman (Eds.), *Clinical gynecologic oncology* (7th ed.). St. Louis: Mosby.

Copeland, L., & Landon, M. (2007). Malignant disease and pregnancy. In S. Gabbe, J. Niebyl, & J. Simpson (Eds.), *Obstetrics: Normal and problem pregnancies* (5th ed.). Philadelphia: Churchill Livingstone.

Creasman, W. (2007a). Adenocarcinoma of the uterus. In P. DiSaia, & W. Creasman (Eds.), *Clinical gynecologic oncology* (7th ed.). St. Louis: Mosby.

Creasman, W. (2007b). Preinvasive disease of the cervix. In P. DiSaia & W. Creasman (Eds.), *Clinical gynecologic oncology* (7th ed.). St. Louis: Mosby.

Dotters, D., & Katz, V. (2007). Malignant diseases of the vagina. Intraepithelial neoplasia, carcinoma, sarcoma. In V. Katz, G. Lentz, R. Lobo, & D. Gershenson (Eds.), *Comprehensive gynecology* (5th ed.). Philadelphia: Mosby.

Dumoulin, C., & Hay-Smith, E. (2010). Pelvic floor muscle training versus no treatment, or inactive control treatments, for urinary incontinence in women. *The Cochrane Database of Systematic Reviews, 2010*, 1, CD005654.

Eckert, L., & Lentz, R. (2007). Infections of the lower genital tract: Vulva, vagina, cervix, toxic shock syndrome, HIV infections. In V. Katz, G. Lentz, R. Lobo, & D. Gershenson (Eds.), *Comprehensive gynecology* (5th ed.). Philadelphia: Mosby.

Fields, M., & Chevlen, E. (2006). Ovarian cancer screening: A look at the evidence. *Clinical Journal of Oncology Nursing, 10*(1), 77–81.

Frumovitz, M., & Bodurka, D. (2007). Neoplastic diseases of the vulva. Lichen sclerosus, intraepithelial neoplasia, Paget's disease, carcinoma. In V. Katz, G. Lentz, R. Lobo, & D. Gershenson (Eds.), *Comprehensive gynecology* (5th ed.). Philadelphia: Mosby.

Giarratano, G., Bustamante-Forest, R., & Carter, C. (2005). A multicultural and multilingual outreach program for cervical and breast cancer screening. *Journal of Obstetric, Gynecologic and Neonatal Nursing, 34*(3), 395–402.

Gilbert, E. (2011). *Manual of high risk pregnancy & delivery* (5th ed.). St. Louis: Mosby.

Goff, B., Mandel, L., Drescher, C., Urban, N., Gough, S., Schurman, K., et al. (2007). Development of an ovarian cancer symptom index: Possibilities for earlier detection. *Cancer, 109*(2), 221–227.

Goldstein, A., & Burrows, L. (2008). Vulvodynia. *Journal of Sexual Medicine, 5*(1), 5–15.

Hacker, N. (2010a). Uterine corpus cancer. In N. Hacker, J. Gambone, & C. Hobel (Eds.), *Hacker and Moore's essentials of obstetrics and gynecology* (5th ed.). Philadelphia: Saunders.

Hacker, N. (2010b). Vulvar and vaginal cancer. In N. Hacker, J. Gambone, & C. Hobel (Eds.), *Hacker and Moore's essentials of obstetrics and gynecology* (5th ed.). Philadelphia: Saunders.

Harlow, B., Vitonis, A., & Stewart, E. (2008). Influence of oral contraceptive use on the risk of adult-onset vulvodynia. *Journal of Reproductive Medicine, 53*(2), 103–105.

Harris, G., Horowitz, B., & Bordiga, A. (2007). Evaluation of gabapentin in the treatment of generalized vulvodynia, unprovoked. *Journal of Reproductive Medicine, 52*(2), 103–105.

Hartmann, D., Strauhal, M., & Nelson, C. (2007). Treatment of women in the United States with localized, provoked vulvodynia: Practice survey of women's health physical therapists. *Journal of Reproductive Medicine, 52*(1), 48–52.

Hiller, J., Miller, M., & Stavas, J. (2005). Uterine artery embolization: A minimally invasive option to end fibroid symptoms. *Advance for Nurse Practitioners, 13*(10), 20–26.

Istre, O. (2008). Management of symptomatic fibroids: Conservative surgical treatment modalities other than abdominal or laparoscopic myomectomy. *Best Practices Research in Clinical Obstetrics and Gynaecology, 22*(4), 735–737.

Katz, V. (2007). Benign gynecologic lesions: Vulva, vagina, cervix, uterus, oviduct, ovary. In V. Katz, G. Lentz, R. Lobo, & D. Gershenson (Eds.), *Comprehensive gynecology* (5th ed.). Philadelphia: Mosby.

Kavanagh, J., & Gershenson, D. (2007). Gestational trophoblastic disease: Hydatidiform mole, nonmetastatic and metastatic gestational trophoblastic tumor: Diagnosis and management. In V. Katz, G. Lentz, R. Lobo, & D. Gershenson (Eds.), *Comprehensive gynecology* (5th ed.). Philadelphia: Mosby.

Kingdon, J. (2009). Vulvodynia: A comprehensive review. *Nursing for Women's Health, 13*(1), 48–57.

Lentz, G. (2007). Anatomic defects of the abdominal wall and pelvic floor. In V. Katz, G. Lentz, R. Lobo, & D. Gershenson (Eds.), *Comprehensive gynecology* (5th ed.). Philadelphia: Mosby.

Leppert, P., Legro, R., & Kjerulff, K. (2007). Hysterectomy and loss of fertility: Implications for women's mental health. *Journal of Psychosometric Research, 63*(3), 269–274.

Likes, W., Russell, C., & Tillmanns, T. (2008). Women's experiences with vulvar intraepithelial neoplasia. *Journal of Obstetric, Gynecologic and Neonatal Nursing, 37*(6), 640–646.

Lobo, R. (2007). Hyerandrogenism: Physiology, etiology, differential diagnosis, management. In V. Katz, G. Lentz, R. Lobo, & D. Gershenson (Eds.), *Comprehensive gynecology* (5th ed.). Philadelphia: Mosby.

Lockwood-Rayermann, S., Donovan, H., Rambo, D., & Kuo, C. (2009). Women's awareness of ovarian cancer risks and symptoms. *American Journal of Nursing, 109*(9), 36–45.

Lowdermilk, D. (2008). Reproductive surgery. In C. Fogel, & N. Woods (Eds.), *Women's health care in advanced practice nursing*. New York: Springer.

Lu, K., & Slomovitz, B. (2007). Neoplastic diseases of the uterus. Endometrial hyperplasia, endometrial carcinoma, sarcoma: Diagnosis and management. In V. Katz, G. Lentz, R. Lobo, & D. Gershenson (Eds.), *Comprehensive gynecology* (5th ed.). Philadelphia: Mosby.

Monk, B., & Tewari, K. (2007). Invasive cervical cancer. In P. DiSaia & W. Creasman (Eds.), *Clinical gynecologic oncology* (7th ed.). St. Louis: Mosby.

Mueller, A., Renner, S., Haeberle, L., Lermann, J., Oppelt, P., Beckemann, M., & Thiel, F. (2009). Comparison of total laparoscopic hysterectomy (TLH) and laparoscopy-assisted supracervical hysterectomy (LASLH) in women with uterine leiomyoma. *European Journal of Obstetric and Gynecologic Reproductive Biology, 144*(1), 76–79.

Munday, P., Buchan, A., Ravenhill, G., Wiggs, A., & Brooks, E. (2007). A qualitative study of women with vulvodynia II. Response to a multidisciplinary approach to management. *Journal of Reproductive Medicine, 52*(1), 19–22.

Nieboer, T., Johnson, N., Lethaby, A., Tavender, E., Curr, E., Garry, R., et al. (2009). Surgical approach to hysterectomy for benign gynaecological disease. *The Cochrane Database of Systematic Reviews, 2009*, 3, CD003677.

Nelson, A., & Gambone, J. (2010). Congenital anomalies and benign conditions of the uterine corpus and cervix. In N. Hacker, J. Gambone, & C. Hobel (Eds.), *Hacker and Moore's essentials of obstetrics and gynecology* (5th ed.). Philadelphia: Saunders.

Noller, K. (2007). Intraepithelial neoplasia of the lower genital tract (cervix, culva): Etiology, screening, diagnostic techniques, management. In V. Katz, G. Lentz, R. Lobo, & D. Gershenson (Eds.), *Comprehensive gynecology* (5th ed.). Philadelphia: Mosby.

Peterson, J. (2008). Minimizing urinary incontinence: Maximize physical activity in women. *Urologic Nursing, 28*(5), 351–356.

Pisco, J., Bilhim, T., Duarte, M., & Santos, D. (2009). Management of uterine artery embolization for fibroids as an outpatient procedure. *Journal of Vascular and Interventional Radiology, 20*(6), 730–735.

Pukall, C., Kandyba, K., Amsel, R., Khalifé, S., & Binik, Y. (2007). Effectiveness of hypnosis for the treatment of vulvar vestibulitis syndrome: A preliminary investigation. *Journal of Sexual Medicine, 4*(2), 417–425.

Reed, B. (2006). Vulvodynia: Diagnosis and management. *American Family Physician, 73*(7), 1231–1238.

Reed, B., Caron, A., Gorenflo, D., & Haefner, H. (2006). Treatment of vulvodynia with tricyclic antidepressants: Efficacy and associated factors. *Journal of Lower Genital Tract Disease, 10*(4), 245–251.

Ries, L., Melbert, D., Krapcho, M., Stinchcomb, D., Howlader, N., Horner, M., et al. (Eds.), (2008). *SEER Cancer Statistics Review, 1975-2005*, Bethesda, MD: National Cancer Institute. Available at http://seer.cancer.gov/csr/1975_2005. Accessed January 28, 2010.

Sankaran, S., & Manyonda, I. (2008). Medical management of fibroids. *Best Practice and Research: Clinical Obstetrics and Gynaecology, 22*(4), 655–676.

Slomovitz, B., & Coleman, R. (2007). Invasive cancer of the vagina and urethra. In P. DiSaia & W. Creasman (Eds.), *Clinical gynecologic oncology* (7th ed.). St. Louis: Mosby.

Soper, J., & Creasman, W. (2007). Gestational trophoblastic disease. In P. DiSaia, & W. Creasman (Eds.), *Clinical gynecologic oncology* (7th ed.). St. Louis: Mosby.

Stehman, F. (2007). Invasive cancer of the vulva. In P. DiSaia, & W. Creasman (Eds.), *Clinical gynecologic oncology* (7th ed.). St. Louis: Mosby.

Sunde, J., Kaplan, K., & Rose, G. (2007). Fallopian tube cancer. In P. DiSaia, & W. Creasman (Eds.), *Clinical gynecologic oncology* (7th ed.). St. Louis: Mosby.

Sung, V., & Hampton, B. (2009). Epidemiology of pelvic floor dysfunction. *Obstetrics and Gynecology Clinics of North America, 36*(3), 421–443.

Sung, V., West, D., Hernandez, A., Wheeler, T., Myers, D., Subak, L., et al. (2009). Association between urinary incontinence and depressive symptoms in overweight and obese women. *American Journal of Obstetrics and Gynecology, 200*(5), 557. e1-557.e5.

Tarnay, C., & Bhatia, N. (2010). Genitourinary dysfunction: Pelvic organ prolapse, urinary incontinence, and infection. In N. Hacker, J. Gambone, & C. Hobel (Eds.), *Hacker and Moore's essentials of obstetrics and gynecology* (5th ed.). Philadelphia: Saunders.

Tewari, K. (2007). Cancer in pregnancy. In P. DiSaia, & W. Creasman (Eds.), *Clinical gynecologic oncology* (7th ed.). St. Louis: Mosby.

U.S. Preventive Services Task Force (USPTF). (2009). *The guide to clinical preventive services 2009. Screening for cervical cancer*. AHRQ Publication No. 09-IP 006, September 2009. Rockville, MD: Agency for Healthcare Research and Quality.

Waetjen, L., Laio, S., Johnson, W., Sampselle, C., Sternfield, B., Harlow, S., & Gold, E. (2007). Factors associated with prevalent and incident urinary incontinence in a cohort of midlife women; A longitudinal analysis of data: Study of women's health across the nation. *American Journal of Epidemiology, 165*(3), 309–318.

Wallner, L., Porten, S., Meenan, R., O'Keefe Rosetti, M., Calhoun, E., Sarma, A., & Clemens, J. (2009). Prevalence and severity of undiagnosed urinary incontinence in women. *American Journal of Medicine, 122*(11), 1037–1042.

Workman, M. (2010). Care of patients with cancer. In D. Ignatavicius & M. Workman (Eds.), *Medical-surgical nursing: Patient-centered collaborative care* (6th ed.). St Louis: Saunders.

Wu, J., Hundley, A., Fulton, R., & Myers, E. (2009). Forecasting the prevalence of pelvic floor disorders in U. S. women: 2020 to 2050. *Obstetrics and Gynecology, 114*(6), 1278–1283.

Wu, T., Chen, X., & Xie, L. (2007). Selective estrogen receptor modulators (SERMs) for uterine leiomyomas. *The Cochrane Database of Systematic Reviews, 2007*, 4, CD005287.

Yashar, C. (2007). Basic principles of gynecologic radiotherapy. In P. DiSaia & W. Creasman (Eds.), *Clinical gynecologic oncology* (7th ed.). St. Louis: Mosby.

Yen, J., Chen, Y., Long, C., Chang, Y., Yen, C., & Ko, C. (2008). Risk factors for major depressive disorder and the psychological impact of hysterectomy: A prospective investigation. *Psychosomatics, 49*(2), 137–142.

Zolnoun, D., Hartmann, K., Lamvu, G., As-Saine, S., Maixner, W., & Steege, J. (2006). A conceptual model for the pathophysiology of vulvar vestibulitis syndrome. *Obstetrical and Gynecological Survey, 61*(6), 395–401.

CHAPTER

12

Conception and Fetal Development

Shannon E. Perry

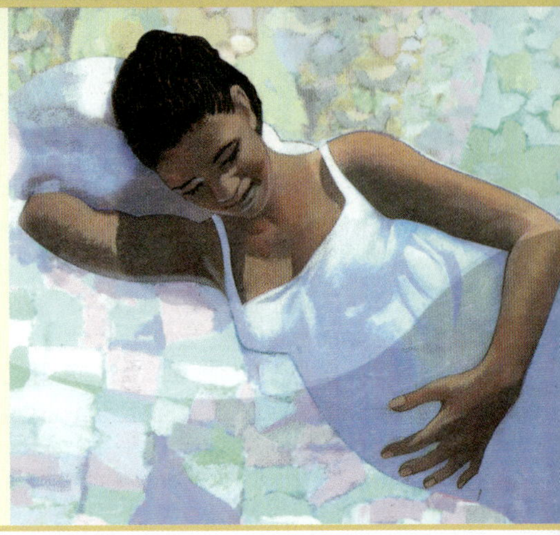

evolve WEBSITE

http://evolve.elsevier.com/Lowdermilk/MWHC/

Animations
- Female Accessory Sex Organs
- Female Reproductive Ducts
- Fertilization and Implantation
- First Trimester, Fetal Development
- Male Reproductive Ducts
- Male Accessory Sex Glands
- Male External Genitalia
- Maternal and Fetal Circulation
- Oogenesis and Meiosis
- Pathway of Ovum
- Pathway of Sperm
- Second Trimester, Fetal Development
- Spermatogenesis
- Spermatozoa
- Testes
- Third Trimester, Fetal Development

Audio Glossary
Audio Key Points
NCLEX Review Questions

LEARNING OBJECTIVES

- Summarize the process of fertilization.
- Describe the development, structure, and functions of the placenta.
- Describe the composition and functions of amniotic fluid.
- Identify three organs or tissues arising from each of the three primary germ layers.
- Summarize the growth and development of the embryo and fetus.
- Identify the potential effects of teratogens during vulnerable periods of embryonic and fetal development.
- Relate selected congenital defects to stage of fetal development.

This chapter presents an overview of the process of fertilization and the development of the normal embryo and fetus.

CONCEPTION

Conception, defined as the union of a single egg and sperm, marks the beginning of a pregnancy. Conception occurs not as an isolated event but as part of a sequential process. This sequential process includes **gamete** (egg and sperm) formation, ovulation (release of the egg), fertilization (union of the gametes), and implantation in the uterus.

Cell Division

Cells are reproduced by two different methods: mitosis and meiosis. In **mitosis,** body cells replicate to yield two cells with the same genetic makeup as the parent cell. First the cell makes a copy of its deoxyribonucleic acid (DNA), and then it divides; each daughter cell receives one copy of the genetic material. Mitotic division facilitates growth and development or cell replacement.

Meiosis, the process by which germ cells divide and decrease their chromosomal number by half, produces gametes (eggs and sperm). Each homologous pair of chromosomes contains one chromosome received from the mother and one from the father; thus meiosis results in cells that contain one of each of the 23 pairs of chromosomes. Because these germ cells contain 23 single chromosomes, half of the genetic material of a normal somatic cell, they are called haploid. This halving of the genetic material is accomplished by replicating the DNA once and then dividing twice. When the female gamete (egg or ovum) and the male gamete (spermatozoon) unite to form the zygote, the diploid number of human chromosomes (46, or 23 pairs) is restored.

The process of DNA replication and cell division in meiosis allows different alleles (genes on corresponding loci that code for variations of the same trait) for genes to be distributed at random by each parent and then rearranged on the paired chromosomes. The chromosomes then separate and proceed to different gametes. Many combinations of genes are possible on each chromosome because parents have genotypes derived from four different grandparents. This random mixing of alleles accounts for the variation of traits seen in the offspring of the same two parents.

Gametogenesis

Oogenesis, the process of egg (ovum) formation, begins during fetal life in the female. All the cells that may undergo meiosis in a woman's lifetime are contained in her ovaries at birth. The majority of the estimated 2 million primary oocytes (the cells that undergo the first meiotic division) degenerate spontaneously. Only 400 to 500 ova will mature during the approximately 35 years of a woman's reproductive life. The primary oocytes begin the first meiotic division (i.e., they replicate their DNA) during fetal life but remain suspended at this stage until puberty (Fig. 12-1, *A*). Then usually monthly, one primary oocyte matures and completes the first meiotic division, yielding two unequal cells: the secondary oocyte and a small polar body. Both contain 22 autosomes and one X sex chromosome.

At ovulation the second meiotic division begins; however, the ovum does not complete the second meiotic division unless fertilization occurs. At fertilization, when the sperm is united with the mature ovum, a second polar body and the **zygote** (the united egg and sperm) are produced (see Fig. 12-1, *C*). The three polar bodies degenerate.

When a male reaches puberty, his testes begin the process of **spermatogenesis.** The cells that undergo meiosis in the male are called spermatocytes. The primary spermatocyte, which undergoes the first meiotic division, contains the diploid number of chromosomes. The cell has already copied its DNA before division, so four alleles for each gene are present. The cell is still considered diploid because the copies are bound together (i.e., one allele plus its copy on each chromosome).

During the first meiotic division, two haploid secondary spermatocytes are formed. Each secondary spermatocyte contains 22 autosomes and one sex chromosome; one contains the X chromosome (plus its copy), and the other, the Y chromosome (plus its copy). During the second meiotic division, the male produces two gametes with an X chromosome and two gametes with a Y chromosome, all of which will develop into viable sperm (Fig. 12-1, *B*).

When homologous chromosomes fail to separate during gametogenesis (nondisjunction), some gametes have 24 chromosomes and others have 22 (Fig. 12-2). If a gamete with 24 chromosomes unites with a normal gamete with 23

Animations—Oogenesis and Meiosis, Spermatogenesis, Male External Genitalia

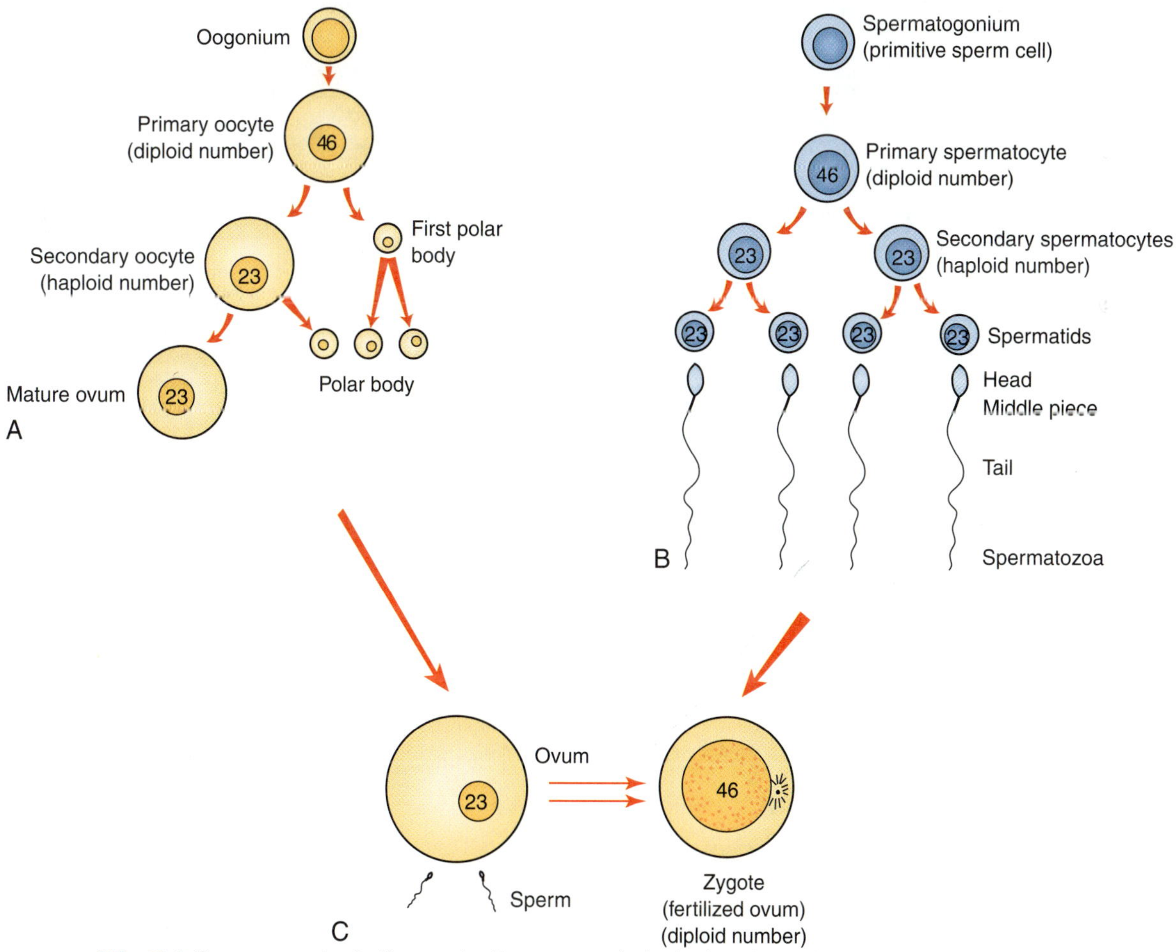

FIG. 12-1 Gametogenesis. **A,** Oogenesis. Gametogenesis in the female produces one mature ovum and three polar bodies. Note the relative difference in overall size between the ovum and sperm. **B,** Spermatogenesis. Gametogenesis of the male produces four mature gametes, the sperm. **C,** Fertilization results in the single-cell zygote and the restoration of the diploid number of chromosomes.

chromosomes, the resulting zygote has 47 chromosomes. This produces a trisomy as occurs in Down syndrome. When a gamete with 22 chromosomes unites with a normal gamete with 23 chromosomes, a zygote with 45 chromosomes results, producing a monosomy. Abnormal gametogenesis can occur in both sex chromosomes and in autosomes (Moore & Persaud, 2008).

Ovum

Meiosis occurs in the female in the ovarian follicles and produces an egg, or ovum. Each month, one ovum matures with a host of surrounding supportive cells. At ovulation the ovum is released from the ruptured ovarian follicle. High estrogen levels increase the motility of the uterine tubes so their cilia are able

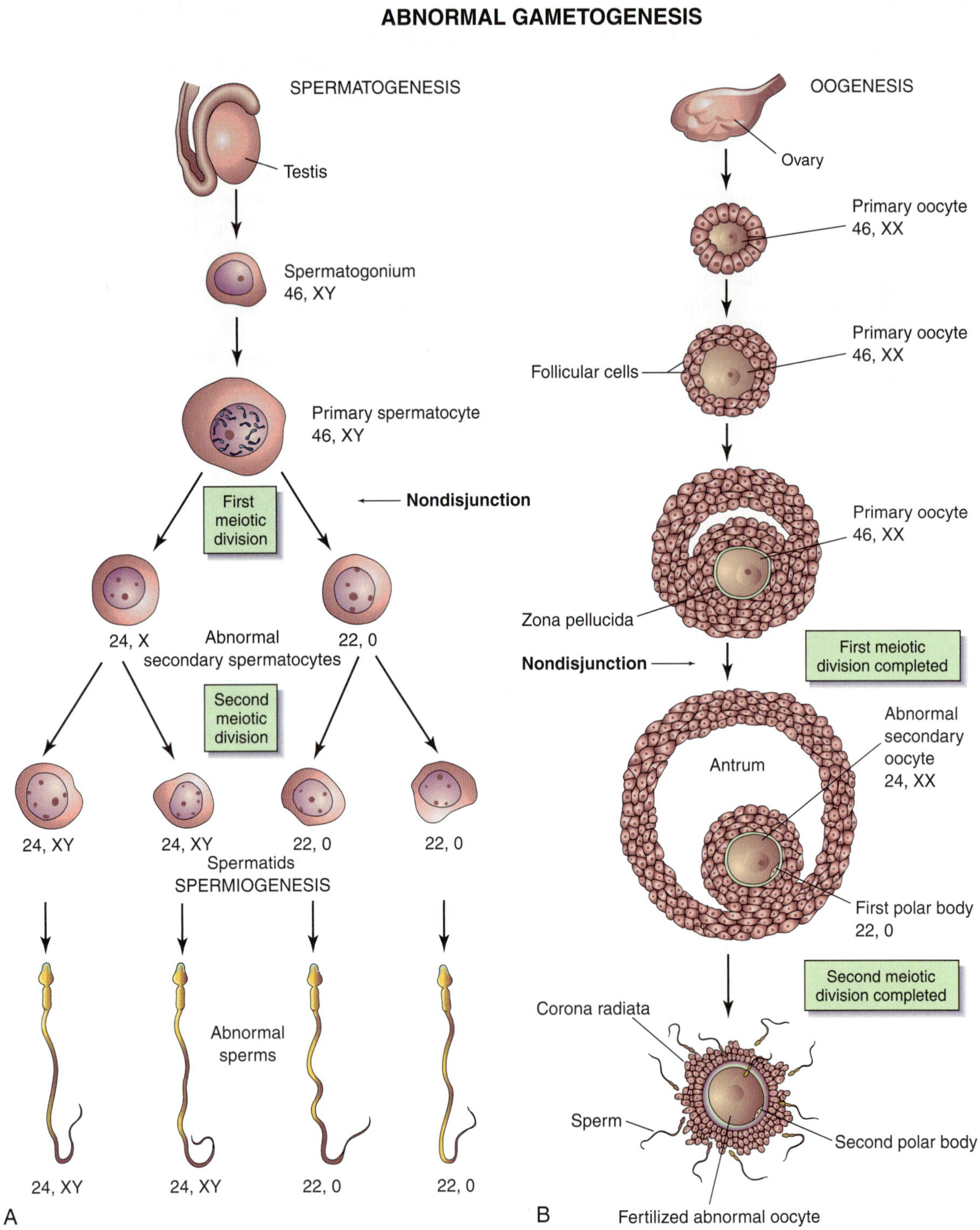

FIG. 12-2 Abnormal gametogenesis: nondisjunction. **A,** When nondisjunction occurs during the first meiotic division of spermatogenesis, one secondary spermatocyte contains 22 autosomes plus an X and a Y chromosome, whereas the other one contains 22 autosomes and no sex chromosomes. **B,** Nondisjunction during oogenesis may give rise to an oocyte with 22 autosomes and two X chromosomes (as shown) or one with 22 autosomes and no sex chromosome. (From Moore, K., & Persaud, T. [2008]. *Before we are born: Essentials of embryology and birth defects* [7th ed.]. Philadelphia: Saunders.)

Animations—Pathway of Ovum, Male Reproductive Ducts, Male Accessory Sex Glands

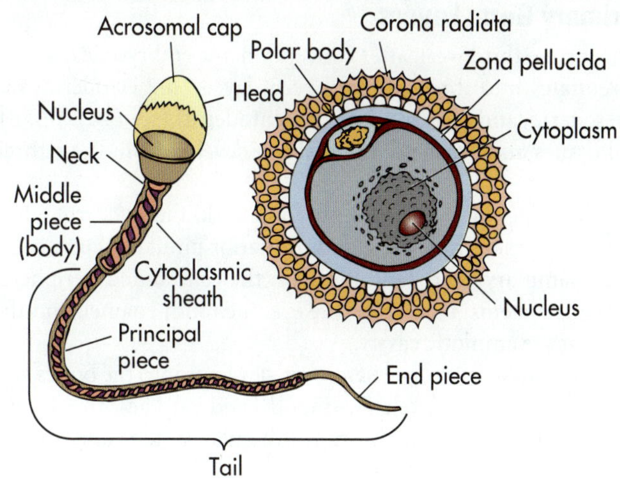

FIG. 12-3 Sperm and ovum.

to capture the ovum and propel it through the tube toward the uterine cavity. An ovum cannot move by itself.

Two protective layers surround the ovum (Fig. 12-3). The inner layer is a thick, acellular layer, the *zona pellucida.* The outer layer, the corona radiata, is composed of elongated cells.

Ova are considered fertile for about 24 hours after ovulation. If not fertilized by a sperm, the ovum degenerates and is resorbed.

Sperm

Ejaculation during sexual intercourse normally propels about a teaspoon of semen, containing as many as 200 to 500 million sperm, into the vagina. The sperm swim propelled by the flagellar movement of their tails. Some sperm can reach the site of fertilization within 5 minutes, but average transit time is 4 to 6 hours. Sperm remain viable within the woman's reproductive system for an average of 2 to 3 days. Most sperm are lost in the vagina, within the cervical mucus, or in the endometrium, or they enter the uterine tube that contains no ovum.

As the sperm travel through the female reproductive tract, enzymes are produced to aid in their capacitation. *Capacitation* is a physiologic change that removes the protective coating from the heads of the sperm. Small perforations then form in the acrosome (a cap on the sperm) and allow enzymes (e.g., hyaluronidase) to escape (see Fig. 12-3). These enzymes are necessary for the sperm to penetrate the protective layers of the ovum before fertilization.

Fertilization

Fertilization takes place in the ampulla (outer third) of the uterine tube. When a sperm successfully penetrates the membrane surrounding the ovum, both sperm and ovum are enclosed within the membrane, and the membrane becomes impenetrable to other sperm; this process is termed the zona reaction. The second meiotic division of the secondary oocyte is then completed, and the nucleus of the ovum becomes the female pronucleus. The head of the sperm enlarges to become the male pronucleus, and the tail degenerates. The nuclei fuse, and the chromosomes combine, restoring the diploid number (46) (Fig. 12-4). Conception, the formation of the zygote (the first cell of the new individual), has been achieved.

Mitotic cellular replication, called *cleavage,* begins as the zygote travels the length of the uterine tube into the uterus. This

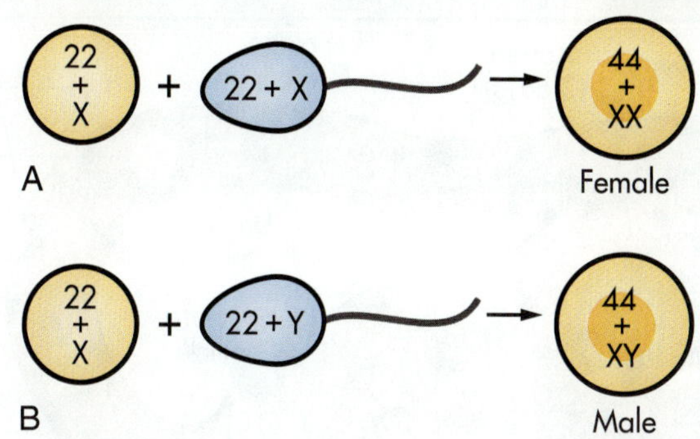

FIG. 12-4 Fertilization. **A,** Ovum fertilized by X-bearing sperm to form female zygote. **B,** Ovum fertilized by Y-bearing sperm to form male zygote.

transit takes 3 to 4 days. Because the fertilized egg divides rapidly with no increase in size, successively smaller cells, blastomeres, are formed with each division. A 16-cell **morula,** a solid ball of cells, is produced within 3 days and is still surrounded by the protective zona pellucida (Fig. 12-5, *A*). Further development occurs as the morula floats freely within the uterus. Fluid passes through the zona pellucida into the intercellular spaces between the blastomeres, separating them into two parts, the trophoblast (which gives rise to the placenta) and the embryoblast (which gives rise to the embryo). A cavity forms within the cell mass as the spaces come together, forming a structure called the blastocyst cavity. When the cavity becomes recognizable, the whole structure of the developing embryo is known as the **blastocyst.** Stem cells are derived from the inner cell mass of the blastocyst. The outer layer of cells surrounding the blastocyst cavity is the **trophoblast.** The trophoblast differentiates into villous and extravillous trophoblast (Fig. 12-6).

Implantation

The zona pellucida degenerates, the trophoblast cells displace endometrial cells at the implantation site, and the blastocyst embeds in the endometrium, usually in the anterior or posterior fundal region. Between 6 and 10 days after conception, the trophoblast secretes enzymes that enable it to burrow into the endometrium until the entire blastocyst is covered. This is termed **implantation.** Endometrial blood vessels erode, and some women have slight implantation bleeding (slight spotting or bleeding at the time of the first missed menstrual period). **Chorionic villi,** finger-like projections, develop out of the trophoblast and extend into the blood-filled spaces of the endometrium. These villi are vascular processes that obtain oxygen and nutrients from the maternal bloodstream and dispose of carbon dioxide and waste products into the maternal blood.

After implantation the endometrium is termed the *decidua.* The portion directly under the blastocyst, where the chorionic villi tap into the maternal blood vessels, is the **decidua basalis.** The portion covering the blastocyst is the *decidua capsularis,* and the portion lining the rest of the uterus is the *decidua vera* (Fig. 12-7).

EMBRYO AND FETUS

Pregnancy lasts approximately 10 lunar months, 9 calendar months, 40 weeks, or 280 days. Length of pregnancy is computed from the first day of the last menstrual period (LMP)

Animations— Fertilization and Implantation Pathway of Sperm, Spermatozoa, Testes

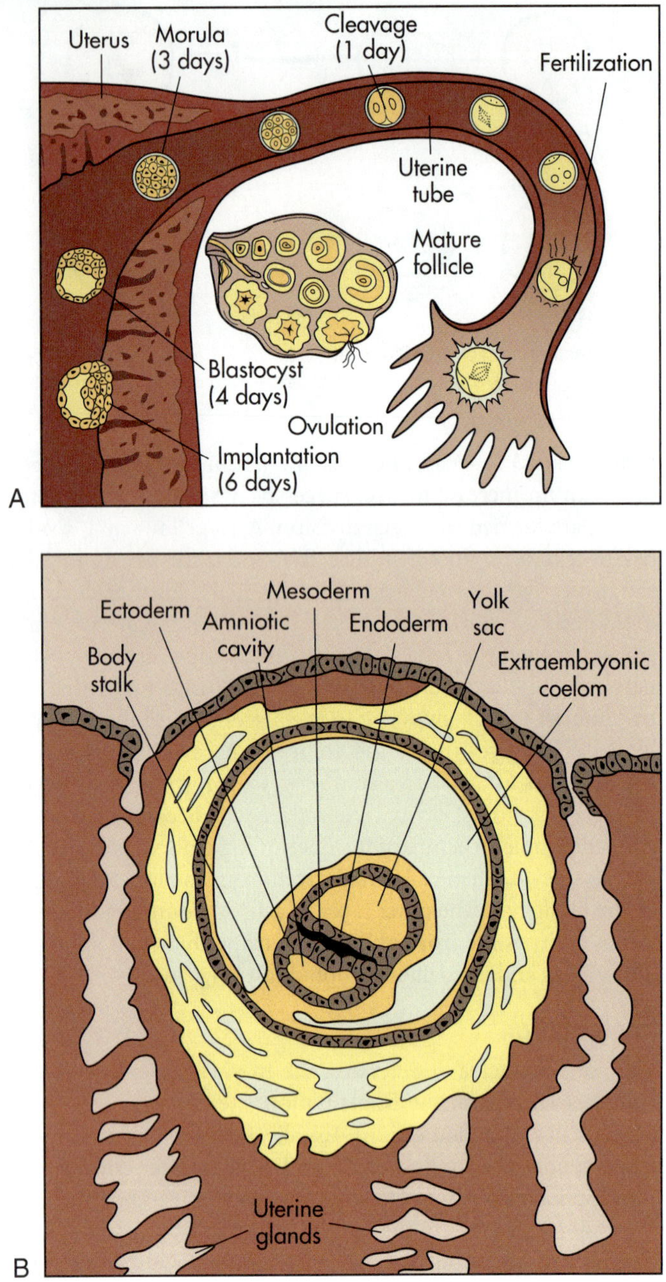

FIG. 12-5 First weeks of human development. **A,** Follicular development in the ovary, ovulation, fertilization, and transport of the early embryo down the uterine tube and into the uterus, where implantation occurs. **B,** Blastocyst embedded in endometrium. Germ layers forming. (**A** from Carlson, B. [2004]. *Human embryology and developmental biology* (3rd ed.). Philadelphia: Mosby; **B** adapted from Langley, L. [1980]. *Dynamic anatomy and physiology* [5th ed.]. New York: McGraw-Hill.)

until the day of birth. However, conception occurs approximately 2 weeks after the first day of the LMP; thus the postconception age of the fetus is 2 weeks less, for a total of 266 days or 38 weeks. Postconception age is used in the discussion of fetal development.

Intrauterine development is divided into three stages: ovum or preembryonic, embryo, and fetus (Fig. 12-8). The stage of the ovum lasts from conception until day 14. This period covers cellular replication, blastocyst formation, initial development of the embryonic membranes, and establishment of the primary germ layers.

Primary Germ Layers

During the third week after conception, the embryonic disk differentiates into three primary germ layers: the ectoderm, the mesoderm, and the endoderm (or entoderm) (see Fig. 12-5, *B*). All tissues and organs of the embryo develop from these three layers.

The upper layer of the embryonic disk, the *ectoderm,* gives rise to the epidermis, the glands (anterior pituitary, cutaneous, and mammary), the nails and hair, the central and peripheral nervous systems, the lens of the eye, the tooth enamel, and the floor of the amniotic cavity.

The middle layer, the *mesoderm,* develops into the bones and teeth, the muscles (skeletal, smooth, and cardiac), the dermis and connective tissue, the cardiovascular system and spleen, and the urogenital system.

The lower layer, the *endoderm,* gives rise to the epithelium lining the respiratory and digestive tracts, and the glandular cells of associated organs, including the oropharynx, the liver and pancreas, the urethra, the bladder, and the vagina. The endoderm forms the roof of the yolk sac.

Development of the Embryo

The stage of the **embryo** lasts from day 15 until approximately 8 weeks after conception, when the embryo measures 3 cm from crown to rump. This embryonic stage is the most critical time in the development of the organ systems and the main external features. Developing areas with rapid cell division are the most vulnerable to malformation caused by environmental **teratogens** (substances or exposure that causes abnormal development). At the end of the eighth week, all organ systems and external structures are present, and the embryo is unmistakably human (see Fig. 12-8 and Visible Embryo, www.visembryo.com/baby, for a pictorial view of normal and abnormal development).

Membranes

At the time of implantation, two fetal membranes that will surround the developing embryo begin to form. The **chorion** develops from the trophoblast and contains the chorionic villi on its surface. The villi burrow into the decidua basalis and increase in size and complexity as the vascular processes develop into the placenta. The chorion becomes the covering of the fetal side of the placenta. It contains the major umbilical blood vessels as they branch out over the surface of the placenta. As the embryo grows the decidua capsularis stretches. The chorionic villi on this side atrophy and degenerate, leaving a smooth chorionic membrane.

The inner cell membrane, the **amnion,** develops from the interior cells of the blastocyst. The cavity that develops between this inner cell mass and the outer layer of cells (trophoblast) is the amniotic cavity (see Fig. 12-5, *B*). As it grows larger, the amnion forms on the side opposite the developing blastocyst (see Figs. 12-5 and 12-7). The developing embryo draws the amnion around itself, forming a fluid-filled sac. The amnion becomes the covering of the umbilical cord and covers the chorion on the fetal surface of the placenta. As the embryo grows larger, the amnion enlarges to accommodate the embryo/fetus and the surrounding amniotic fluid. The amnion eventually comes into contact with the chorion surrounding the fetus.

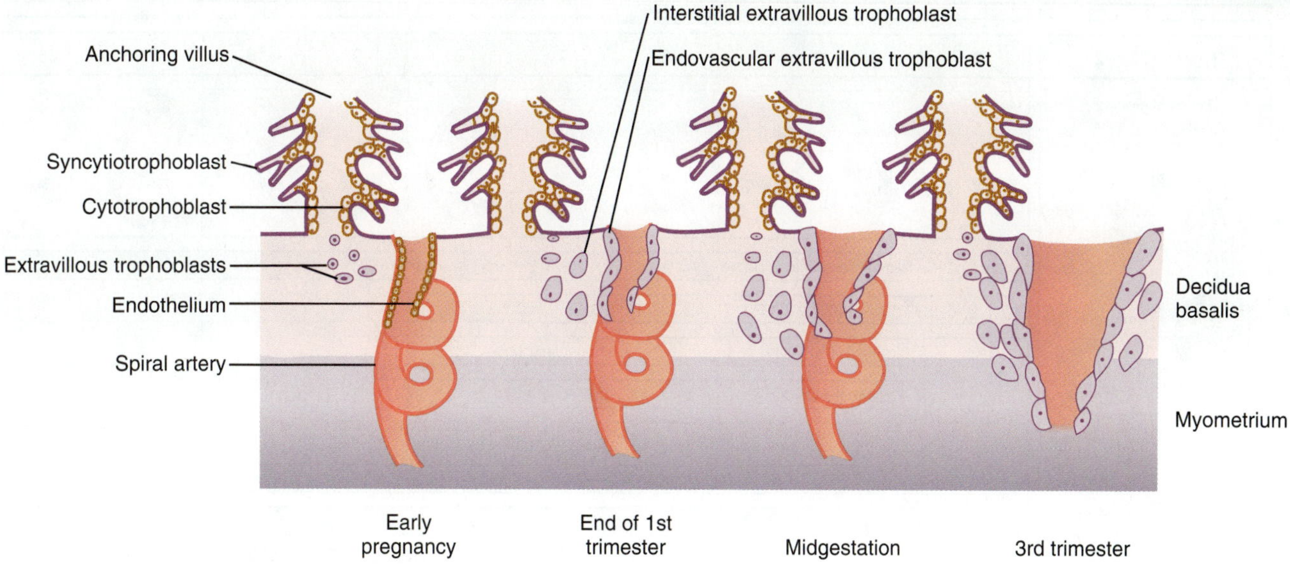

FIG. 12-6 Extravillous trophoblasts are found outside the villus and can be subdivided into endovascular and interstitial categories. Endovascular trophoblasts invade and transform spiral arteries during pregnancy to create low-resistance blood flow that is characteristic of the placenta. Interstitial trophoblasts invade the decidua and surround spiral arteries. (From Cunningham, F., Leveno, K., Bloom, S., Hauth, J., Rouse, D., & Spong, C. (2010). *Williams obstetrics* [23rd ed.]. New York: McGraw-Hill.)

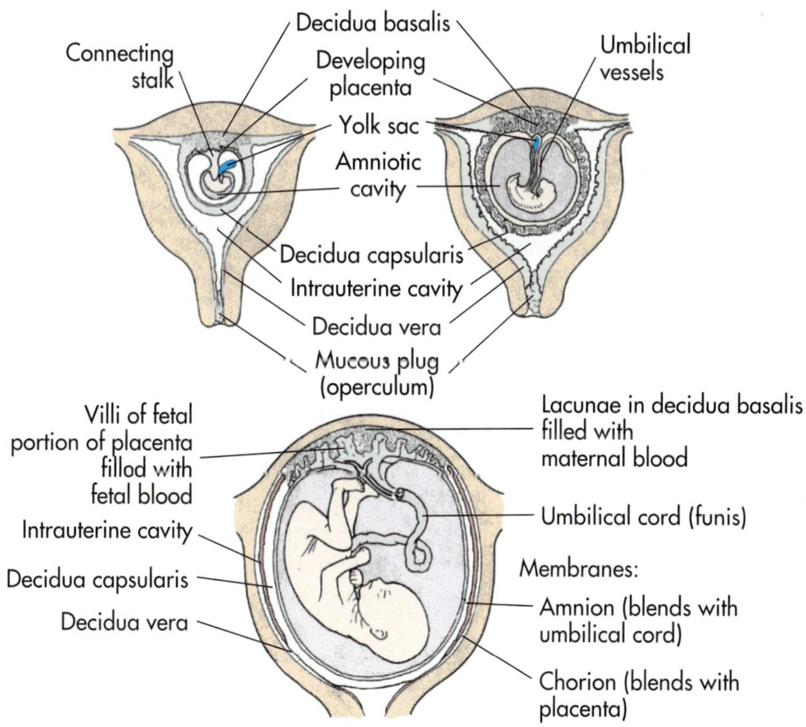

FIG. 12-7 Development of the fetal membranes. Note gradual obliteration of intrauterine cavity as decidua capsularis and decidua vera meet. Also note thinning of uterine wall. Chorionic and amniotic membranes are in apposition to each other but may be peeled apart.

Amniotic Fluid

The amniotic cavity initially derives its fluid by diffusion from the maternal blood. Fluid secreted by the respiratory and gastrointestinal tracts of the fetus also enters the amniotic cavity (Moore & Persaud, 2008). The amount of fluid increases weekly, and 700 to 1000 ml of transparent liquid is normally present at term. The amniotic fluid volume changes constantly. The fetus swallows fluid, and fluid flows into and out of the fetal lungs. Beginning in week 11, the fetus urinates into the fluid, increasing its volume.

Amniotic fluid serves many functions. It helps maintain a constant body temperature. It serves as a source of oral fluid and a repository for waste and assists in maintenance of fluid and electrolyte homeostasis. It allows freedom of movement for musculoskeletal development. It cushions the fetus from trauma by blunting and dispersing outside forces. It acts as a

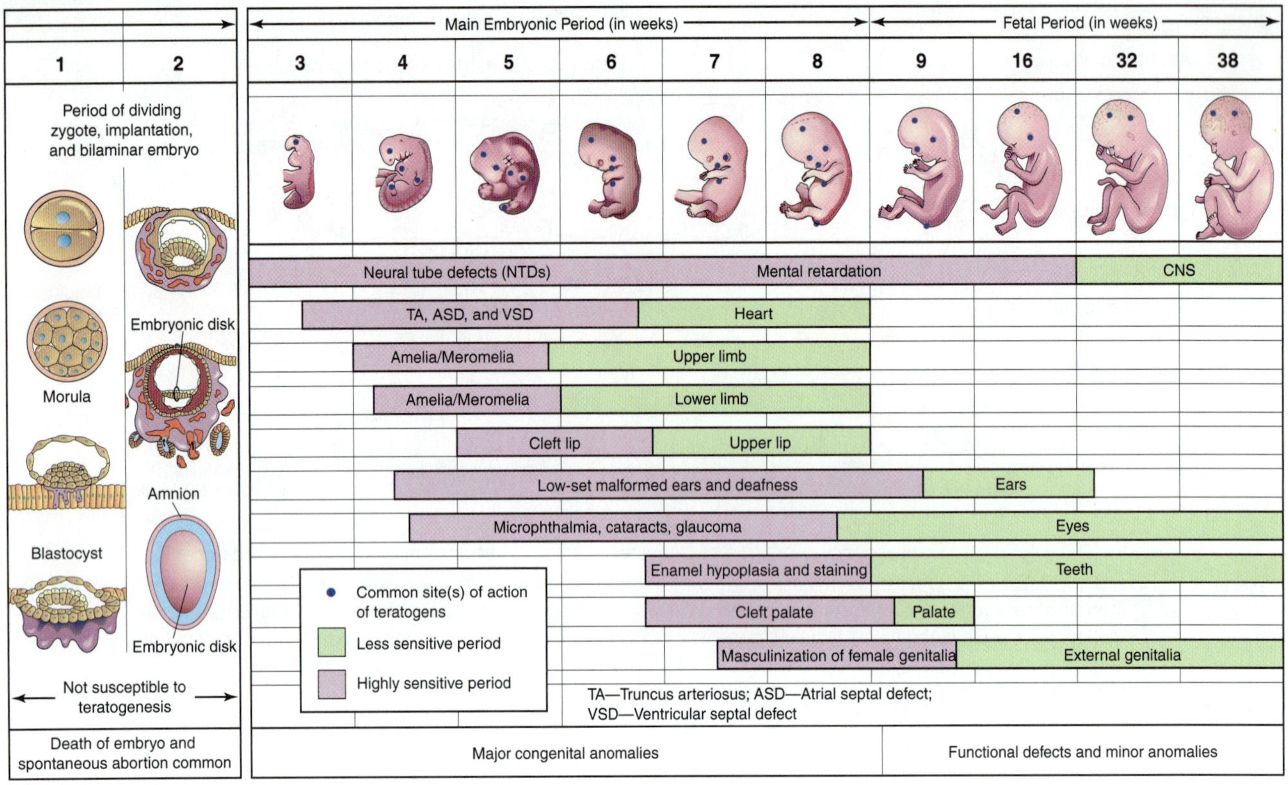

FIG. 12-8 Sensitive or critical periods in human development. During the first 2 weeks of development the embryo usually is not susceptible to teratogens. At that time a teratogen damages all or most of the cells, resulting in death of the embryo, or damages only a few cells, allowing the conceptus to recover and the embryo to develop without birth defects. The dark color denotes highly sensitive periods; the light color indicates stages that are less sensitive to teratogens. (From Moore, K., & Persaud, T. [2008]. *Before we are born: Essentials of embryology and birth defects* [7th ed.]. Philadelphia: Saunders.)

barrier to infection and allows fetal lung development (Moore & Persaud, 2008). The fluid keeps the embryo from tangling with the membranes, facilitating symmetric growth. If the embryo does become tangled with the membranes, amputations of extremities or other deformities can occur from constricting amniotic bands.

The volume of amniotic fluid is an important factor in assessing fetal well-being. Having less than 300 ml of amniotic fluid **(oligohydramnios)** is associated with fetal renal abnormalities. Having more than 2 L of amniotic fluid **(hydramnios)** is associated with gastrointestinal and other malformations.

Amniotic fluid contains albumin, urea, uric acid, creatinine, lecithin, sphingomyelin, bilirubin, fructose, fat, leukocytes, proteins, epithelial cells, enzymes, and lanugo hair. Study of fetal cells in amniotic fluid through amniocentesis yields much information about the fetus. Genetic studies (karyotyping) provide knowledge about the sex and the number and structure of chromosomes (see Chapter 3). Other studies, such as lecithin/sphingomyelin ratio, determine the health or maturity of the fetus (see Chapter 26).

Yolk Sac

When the amniotic cavity and amnion are forming, another blastocyst cavity forms on the other side of the developing embryonic disk (see Fig. 12-5, *B*). This cavity becomes surrounded by a membrane, forming the yolk sac. The yolk sac aids in transferring maternal nutrients and oxygen, which have diffused through the chorion, to the embryo. Blood vessels form to aid transport. Blood cells and plasma are manufactured in the yolk sac during the second and third weeks while uteroplacental circulation is being established and is forming primitive blood cells until hematopoietic activity begins. At the end of the third week the primitive heart begins to beat and circulate the blood through the embryo, the connecting stalk, the chorion, and the yolk sac.

The folding in of the embryo during the fourth week results in incorporation of part of the yolk sac into the embryo's body as the primitive digestive system. Primordial germ cells arise in the yolk sac and move into the embryo. The shrinking remains of the yolk sac degenerate (see Fig. 12-7). By the fifth or sixth week the remnant has separated from the embryo.

Umbilical Cord

By day 14 after conception, the embryonic disk, the amniotic sac, and the yolk sac are attached to the chorionic villi by the connecting stalk. During the third week the blood vessels develop to supply the embryo with maternal nutrients and oxygen. During the fifth week the embryo has curved inward on itself from both ends, bringing the connecting stalk to the ventral side of the embryo. The connecting stalk becomes compressed from both sides by the amnion and forms the narrower umbilical cord (see Fig. 12-7). Two arteries carry blood from the embryo to the chorionic villi, and one vein returns blood to the embryo. Approximately 1% of umbilical cords contain only two vessels: one artery and one vein. This occurrence is sometimes associated with congenital malformations.

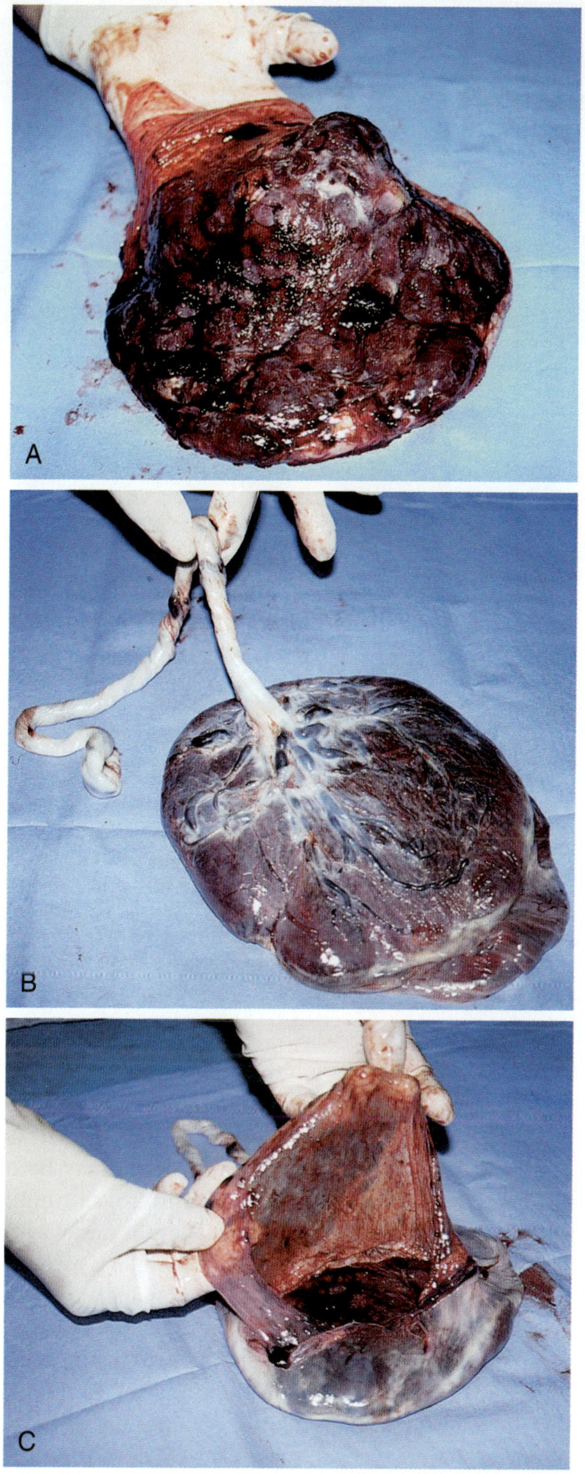

FIG. 12-9 Term placenta. **A,** Maternal (or uterine) surface, showing cotyledons and grooves. **B,** Fetal (or amniotic) surface, showing blood vessels running under amnion and converging to form umbilical vessels at attachment of umbilical cord. **C,** Amnion and smooth chorion are arranged to show that they are (1) fused and (2) continuous with margins of placenta. (Courtesy Marjorie Pyle, RNC, Lifecircle, Costa Mesa, CA.)

The cord rapidly increases in length. At term, the cord is 2 cm in diameter and ranges from 30 to 90 cm long (with an average of 55 cm). It twists spirally on itself and loops around the embryo/fetus. A true knot is rare, but false knots occur as folds or kinks in the cord and may jeopardize circulation to the fetus. Connective tissue called *Wharton's jelly* prevents compression

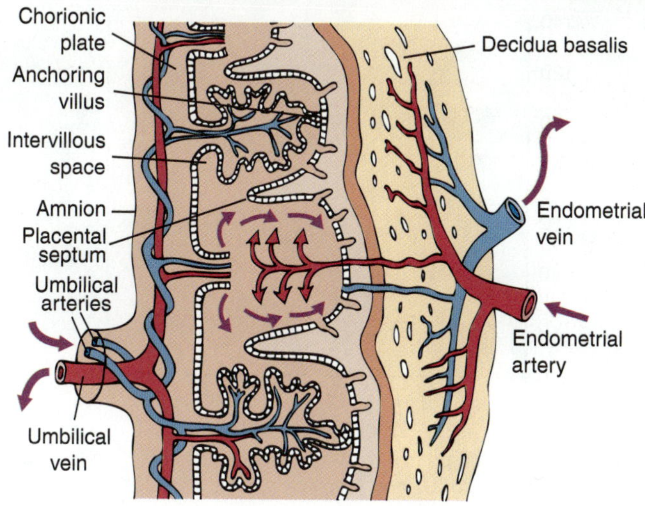

FIG. 12-10 Schematic drawing of the placenta illustrating how it supplies oxygen and nutrition to the embryo and removes its waste products. Deoxygenated blood leaves the fetus through the umbilical arteries and enters the placenta, where it is oxygenated. Oxygenated blood leaves the placenta through the umbilical vein, which enters the fetus via the umbilical cord.

of the blood vessels and ensures continued nourishment of the embryo/fetus. Compression can occur if the cord lies between the fetal head and the maternal pelvis or is twisted around the fetal body. When the cord is wrapped around the fetal neck, it is called a **nuchal cord.**

Because the placenta develops from the chorionic villi, the umbilical cord is usually located centrally. A peripheral location is less common and is termed *battledore placenta.* The blood vessels are arrayed out from the center to all parts of the placenta.

Placenta

Structure

The placenta begins to form at implantation. During the third week after conception, the trophoblast cells of the chorionic villi continue to invade the decidua basalis. As the uterine capillaries are tapped, the endometrial spiral arteries fill with maternal blood. The chorionic villi grow into the spaces with two layers of cells: the outer syncytium and the inner cytotrophoblast. A third layer develops into anchoring septa, dividing the projecting decidua into separate areas called cotyledons. In each of the 15 to 20 cotyledons, the chorionic villi branch out, and a complex system of fetal blood vessels forms. Each cotyledon is a functional unit. The whole structure is the **placenta** (Fig. 12-9).

The maternal-placental-embryonic circulation is in place by day 17, when the embryonic heart starts beating. By the end of the third week, embryonic blood is circulating between the embryo and the chorionic villi. In the intervillous spaces, maternal blood supplies oxygen and nutrients to the embryonic capillaries in the villi (Fig. 12-10). Waste products and carbon dioxide diffuse into the maternal blood.

The placenta functions as a means of metabolic exchange. Exchange is minimal at this time because the two cell layers of the villous membrane are too thick. Permeability increases as the cytotrophoblast thins and disappears; by the fifth month, only the single layer of syncytium is left between the maternal blood and the fetal capillaries. The syncytium is the functional

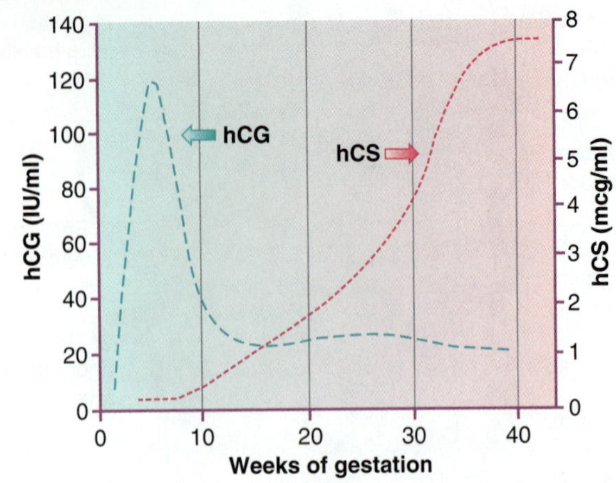

FIG. 12-11 Distinct profile for the concentrations of human chorionic gonadotropin (hCG) and human chorionic somatomammotropin (hCS) in serum of women through normal pregnancy. *IU,* International units. (Adapted from Cunningham, F., Leveno, K., Bloom, S., Hauth, J., Rouse, D., & Spong, C. [2010]. *Williams obstetrics* [23rd ed.]. New York: McGraw-Hill.)

layer of the placenta. By the eighth week, genetic testing may be done on a sample of chorionic villi by aspiration biopsy; however, limb defects have been associated with chorionic villus sampling done before 10 weeks. The structure of the placenta is complete by the twelfth week. The placenta continues to grow wider until 20 weeks, when it covers approximately half of the uterine surface. It then continues to grow thicker. The branching villi continue to develop within the body of the placenta, increasing the functional surface area.

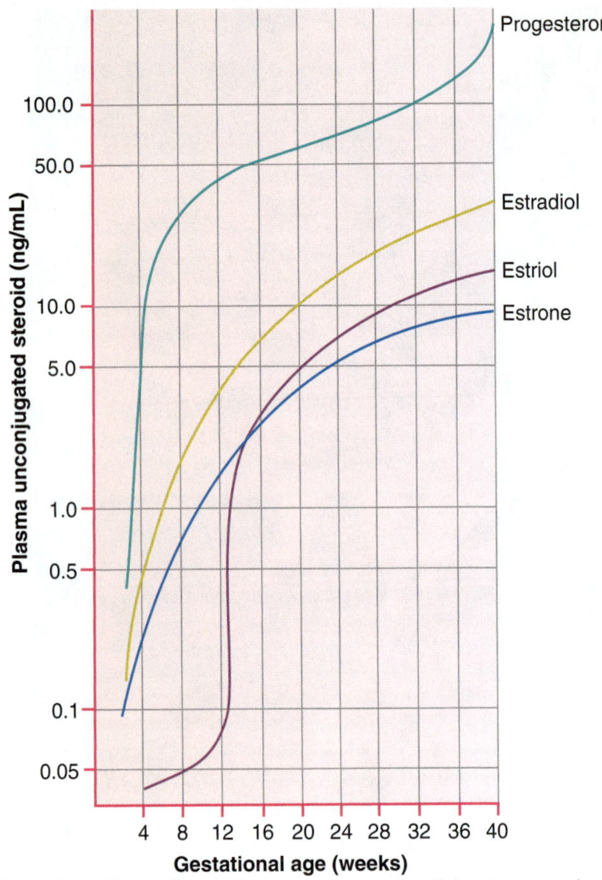

FIG. 12.12 Plasma level of progesterone, estradiol, estrone, and estriol in women during the course of gestation. (From Cunningham, F., Leveno, K., Bloom, S., Hauth, J., Rouse, D., & Spong, C. [2010]. *Williams obstetrics* [23rd ed.]. New York: McGraw-Hill.)

Functions

One of the early functions of the placenta is as an endocrine gland that produces hormones necessary to maintain the pregnancy and support the embryo and fetus. The hormones are produced in the syncytium.

The protein hormone **human chorionic gonadotropin (hCG)** can be detected in the maternal serum by 8 to 10 days after conception, shortly after implantation. This hormone is the basis for pregnancy tests. The hCG preserves the function of the ovarian corpus luteum, ensuring the continued supply of estrogen and progesterone needed to maintain the pregnancy. Miscarriage occurs if the corpus luteum stops functioning before the placenta is producing sufficient estrogen and progesterone. The amount of hCG reaches its maximal level at 50 to 70 days and then begins to decrease.

The other protein hormone produced by the placenta is human chorionic somatomammotropin (hCS) formerly known as human placental lactogen (hPL). This substance is similar to a growth hormone and stimulates the maternal metabolism to supply nutrients needed for fetal growth. This hormone increases the resistance to insulin, facilitates glucose transport across the placental membrane, and stimulates breast development to prepare for lactation (Fig. 12-11).

The placenta eventually produces more of the steroid hormone progesterone than the corpus luteum does during the first few months of pregnancy. Progesterone maintains the endometrium, decreases the contractility of the uterus, and stimulates maternal metabolism and development of breast alveoli.

By 7 weeks after fertilization the placenta is producing most of the maternal estrogens, which are steroid hormones. The major estrogen secreted by the placenta is estriol, whereas the ovaries produce mostly estradiol. Estriol levels may be measured to determine placental functioning. Estrogen stimulates uterine growth and uteroplacental blood flow. It causes a proliferation of the breast glandular tissue and stimulates myometrial contractility. Placental estrogen production increases greatly toward the end of pregnancy. One theory for the cause of the onset of labor is the decline in the ratio of circulating levels of progesterone to the increased levels of estrogen (Fig. 12-12).

The metabolic functions of the placenta are respiration, nutrition, excretion, and storage. Oxygen diffuses from the maternal blood across the placental membrane into the fetal blood, and carbon dioxide diffuses in the opposite direction. In this way the placenta functions as lungs for the fetus.

Carbohydrates, proteins, calcium, and iron are stored in the placenta for ready access to meet fetal needs. Water, inorganic salts, carbohydrates, proteins, fats, and vitamins pass from the maternal blood supply across the placental membrane into the fetal blood, supplying nutrition. Water and most electrolytes with a molecular weight below 500 readily diffuse through the membrane. Hydrostatic and osmotic pressures aid the flow of water and some solutions. Facilitated and active transport assist in the transfer of glucose, amino acids, calcium, iron, and substances with higher molecular weights. Amino acids and calcium are transported against the concentration gradient between the maternal blood and fetal blood.

The fetal concentration of glucose is lower than the glucose level in the maternal blood because of its rapid metabolism by the fetus. This fetal requirement demands larger concentrations of glucose than simple diffusion can provide. Therefore maternal glucose moves into the fetal circulation by active transport.

Pinocytosis is a mechanism used for transferring large molecules, such as albumin and gamma globulins, across the placental membrane. This mechanism conveys the maternal immunoglobulins that provide early passive immunity to the fetus.

Metabolic waste products of the fetus cross the placental membrane from the fetal blood into the maternal blood. The maternal kidneys then excrete them. Many viruses can cross the placental membrane and infect the fetus. Some bacteria and protozoa first infect the placenta and then infect the fetus. Drugs also can cross the placental membrane and may harm the fetus. Caffeine, alcohol, nicotine, carbon monoxide, and other toxic substances in cigarette smoke, as well as prescription and recreational drugs (such as cocaine and marijuana) readily cross the placenta (Box 12-1).

Although no direct link exists between the fetal blood in the vessels of the chorionic villi and the maternal blood in the intervillous spaces, only one cell layer separates them. Breaks occasionally occur in the placental membrane. Fetal erythrocytes then leak into the maternal circulation, and the mother may develop antibodies to the fetal red blood cells. This is often the way an Rh-negative mother becomes sensitized to the erythrocytes of her Rh-positive fetus. (See discussions of isoimmunization in Chapters 23 and 36.)

Although the placenta and the fetus are analogous to living tissue transplants, they are not destroyed by the host mother (Mor & Abrahams, 2009). Either the placental hormones suppress the immunologic response, or the tissue evokes no response.

Placental function depends on the maternal blood pressure supplying circulation. Maternal arterial blood, under pressure in the small uterine spiral arteries, spurts into the intervillous spaces (see Fig. 12-10). As long as rich arterial blood continues to be supplied, pressure is exerted on the blood already in the intervillous spaces, pushing it toward drainage by the low-pressure uterine veins. At term gestation 10% of the maternal cardiac output goes to the uterus.

If there is interference with the circulation to the placenta, the placenta cannot supply the embryo or fetus. Vasoconstriction, such as that caused by hypertension and cocaine use, diminishes uterine blood flow. Decreased maternal blood pressure or cardiac output also diminishes uterine blood flow.

When a woman lies on her back with the pressure of the uterus compressing the vena cava, blood return to the right atrium is diminished (see discussion of supine hypotension in Chapter 19 and Fig. 19-5). Excessive maternal exercise that diverts blood to the muscles away from the uterus compromises placental circulation. Optimal circulation is achieved when the woman is lying at rest on her side. Decreased uterine circulation may lead to intrauterine growth restriction of the fetus and to infants who are small for gestational age.

Braxton Hicks contractions appear to enhance the movement of blood through the intervillous spaces, aiding placental circulation. Prolonged contractions or too-short intervals between contractions during labor, however, reduce blood flow to the placenta.

BOX 12-1 DEVELOPMENTALLY TOXIC EXPOSURES IN HUMANS

- Aminopterin
- Androgens
- Angiotensin-converting enzyme inhibitors
- Carbamazepine
- Cigarette smoking
- Cocaine
- Coumarin anticoagulants
- Cytomegalovirus
- Diethylstilbestrol
- Ethanol (>1 drink/day)
- Etretinate
- Hyperthermia
- Iodides
- Ionizing radiation (>10 rad)
- Isotretinoin
- Lead
- Lithium
- Methimazole
- Methyl mercury
- Parvovirus B19
- Penicillamine
- Phenytoin
- Radioiodine
- Rubella
- Syphilis
- Tetracycline
- Thalidomide
- Toxoplasmosis
- Trimethadione
- Valproic acid
- Varicella

Fetal Maturation

The stage of the fetus lasts from 9 weeks (when the fetus becomes recognizable as a human being) until the pregnancy ends. Changes during the fetal period are not so dramatic, because refinement of structure and function are taking place. The fetus is less vulnerable to teratogens, except for those affecting central nervous system functioning.

Viability refers to the capability of the fetus to survive outside the uterus. With modern technology and advancements in maternal and neonatal care, infants who are 22 to 25 weeks of gestation are now considered to be on the threshold of viability (Cunningham, Leveno, Bloom, Hauth, Rouse, & Spong, 2010). The limitations on survival outside the uterus when an infant is born at this early stage are based on central nervous system function and the oxygenation capability of the lungs.

Fetal Circulatory System

Animation—Maternal and Fetal Circulation

The cardiovascular system is the first organ system to function in the developing human. Blood vessel and blood cell formation begins in the third week and supplies the embryo with oxygen and nutrients from the mother. By the end of the third week the tubular heart begins to beat, and the primitive cardiovascular system links the embryo, connecting stalk, chorion, and yolk sac. During the fourth and fifth weeks the heart develops into a four-chambered organ. By the end of the embryonic stage the heart is developmentally complete.

The fetal lungs do not function for respiratory gas exchange, so a special circulatory pathway, the **ductus arteriosus,** bypasses the lungs. Oxygen-rich blood from the placenta flows rapidly through the umbilical vein into the fetal abdomen (Fig. 12-13). When the umbilical vein reaches the liver, it divides into two branches; one branch circulates some oxygenated blood through the liver. Most of the blood passes through the **ductus venosus** into the inferior vena cava. There it mixes with the deoxygenated blood from the fetal legs and abdomen on its way to the right atrium. Most of this blood passes straight through

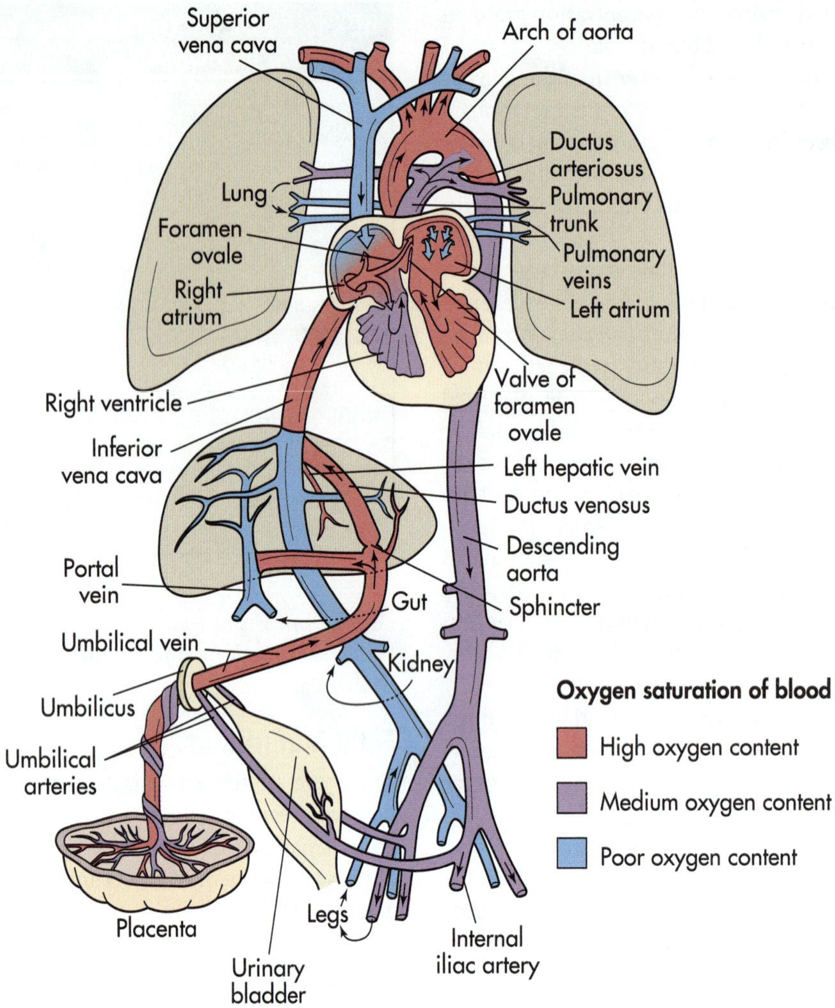

FIG. 12-13 Schematic illustration of the fetal circulation. The colors indicate the oxygen saturation of the blood, and the arrows show the course of the blood from the placenta to the heart. The organs are not drawn to scale. Observe that three shunts permit most of the blood to bypass the liver and lungs: (1) ductus venosus, (2) foramen ovale, and (3) ductus arteriosus. A small amount of highly oxygenated blood from the inferior vena cava remains in the right atrium and mixes with poorly oxygenated blood from the superior vena cava. This medium oxygenated blood then passes into the right ventricle. The poorly oxygenated blood returns to the placenta for oxygen and nutrients through the umbilical arteries. (Modified with permission from Moore, K., & Persaud, T. [2008]. *Before we are born: Essentials of embryology and birth defects* [7th ed.]. Philadelphia: Saunders).

the right atrium and through the **foramen ovale,** an opening into the left atrium. There it mixes with the small amount of deoxygenated blood returning from the fetal lungs through the pulmonary veins.

The blood flows into the left ventricle and is squeezed out into the aorta, where the arteries supplying the heart, head, neck, and arms receive most of the oxygen-rich blood. This pattern of supplying the highest levels of oxygen and nutrients to the head, neck, and arms enhances the cephalocaudal (head-to-rump) development of the embryo/fetus. Deoxygenated blood returning from the head and arms enters the right atrium through the superior vena cava. This blood is directed downward into the right ventricle, where it is squeezed into the pulmonary artery. A small amount of blood circulates through the resistant lung tissue, but the majority follows the path with less resistance through the ductus arteriosus into the aorta, distal to the point of exit of the arteries supplying the head and arms with oxygenated blood. The oxygen-poor blood flows through the abdominal aorta into the internal iliac arteries, where the umbilical arteries direct most of it back through the umbilical cord to the placenta. There the blood gives up its wastes and carbon dioxide in exchange for nutrients and oxygen. The blood remaining in the iliac arteries flows through the fetal abdomen and legs, ultimately returning through the inferior vena cava to the heart.

The following three special characteristics enable the fetus to obtain sufficient oxygen from the maternal blood:

- Fetal hemoglobin carries 20% to 30% more oxygen than maternal hemoglobin.
- The hemoglobin concentration of the fetus is about 50% greater than that of the mother.
- The fetal heart rate is 110 to 160 beats/min, making the cardiac output per unit of body weight higher than that of an adult.

Hematopoietic System

Hematopoiesis, the formation of blood, occurs in the yolk sac (see Fig. 12-5, *B*) beginning in the third week. Hematopoietic stem cells seed the fetal liver during the fifth week, and hematopoiesis begins there during the sixth week. This accounts for the relatively large size of the liver between the seventh and ninth weeks. Stem cells seed the fetal bone marrow, spleen, thymus, and lymph nodes between weeks 8 and 11 (for more information about stem cells see http://stemcells.nih.gov).

The antigenic factors that determine blood type are present in the erythrocytes soon after the sixth week. For this reason the Rh-negative woman is at risk for isoimmunization in any pregnancy that lasts longer than 6 weeks after fertilization.

Gastrointestinal System

During the fourth week the shape of the embryo changes from being almost straight to a C shape, as both ends fold in toward the ventral surface. A portion of the yolk sac is incorporated into the body from head to tail as the primitive gut (digestive system).

The foregut produces the pharynx, part of the lower respiratory tract, the esophagus, the stomach, the first half of the duodenum, the liver, the pancreas, and the gallbladder. These structures evolve during the fifth and sixth weeks. The malformations that can occur in these areas are esophageal atresia, hypertrophic pyloric stenosis, duodenal stenosis or atresia, and biliary atresia (see Chapter 36).

The midgut becomes the distal half of the duodenum, the jejunum and the ileum, the cecum and the appendix, and the proximal half of the colon. The midgut loop projects into the umbilical cord between weeks 5 and 10. A malformation (omphalocele) results if the midgut fails to return to the abdominal cavity, causing the intestines to protrude from the umbilicus (see Fig. 36-9, *A*). Meckel's diverticulum, the most common malformation of the midgut, occurs when a remnant of the yolk stalk that has failed to degenerate attaches to the ileum, leaving a blind sac.

The hindgut develops into the distal half of the colon, the rectum and parts of the anal canal, the urinary bladder, and the urethra. Anorectal malformations are the most common abnormalities of the digestive system.

The fetus swallows amniotic fluid beginning in the fifth month. Gastric emptying and intestinal peristalsis occur. Fetal nutrition and elimination needs are taken care of by the placenta. As the fetus nears term, fetal waste products accumulate in the intestines as dark green to black, tarry meconium. Normally this substance is passed through the rectum within 24 hours of birth. Sometimes with a breech presentation or fetal hypoxia, meconium is passed in utero into the amniotic fluid. The failure to pass meconium after birth may indicate atresia somewhere in the digestive tract, an imperforate anus (see Fig. 36-10), or meconium ileus, in which a firm meconium plug blocks passage (seen in infants with cystic fibrosis).

The metabolic rate of the fetus is relatively low, but the fetus has great growth and development needs. Beginning in week 9 the fetus synthesizes glycogen for storage in the liver. Between 26 and 30 weeks the fetus begins to lay down stores of brown fat in preparation for extrauterine cold stress. Thermoregulation in the neonate requires increased metabolism and adequate oxygenation.

The gastrointestinal system is mature by 36 weeks. Digestive enzymes (except pancreatic amylase and lipase) are present in sufficient quantity to facilitate digestion. The neonate cannot digest starches or fats efficiently. Little saliva is produced.

Hepatic System

The liver and biliary tract develop from the foregut during the fourth week of gestation. Hematopoiesis begins during the sixth week and requires that the liver be large. The embryonic liver is prominent, occupying most of the abdominal cavity. Bile, a constituent of meconium, begins to form in the twelfth week.

Glycogen is stored in the fetal liver beginning at week 9 or 10. At term, glycogen stores are twice those of the adult. Glycogen is the major source of energy for the fetus and neonate stressed by in utero hypoxia, extrauterine loss of the maternal glucose supply, the work of breathing, or cold.

Iron also is stored in the fetal liver. If the maternal intake is sufficient, the fetus can store enough iron to last for 5 months after birth.

During fetal life the liver does not have to conjugate bilirubin for excretion because the unconjugated bilirubin is cleared by the placenta. Therefore the glucuronyl transferase enzyme needed for conjugation is present in the fetal liver in amounts less than those required after birth. This predisposes the neonate, especially the preterm infant, to hyperbilirubinemia.

Coagulation factors II, VII, IX, and X cannot be synthesized in the fetal liver because of the lack of vitamin K synthesis in the sterile fetal gut. This coagulation deficiency persists after birth for several days and is the rationale for the prophylactic administration of vitamin K to the newborn.

Respiratory System

The respiratory system begins development during embryonic life and continues through fetal life and into childhood. The development of the respiratory tract begins in week 4 and continues through week 17 with formation of the larynx, the trachea, the bronchi, and the lung buds. Between 16 and 24 weeks the bronchi and terminal bronchioles enlarge, and vascular structures and primitive alveoli are formed. Between 24 weeks and term more alveoli form. Specialized alveolar cells, type I and type II cells, secrete pulmonary surfactants to line the interior of the alveoli. After 32 weeks sufficient surfactant is present in developed alveoli to provide infants with a good chance of survival.

Pulmonary Surfactants. The detection of the presence of pulmonary **surfactants,** surface-active phospholipids, in amniotic fluid has been used to determine the degree of fetal lung maturity, or the ability of the lungs to function after birth. Lecithin (L) is the most critical alveolar surfactant required for postnatal lung expansion. It is detectable at approximately 21 weeks and increases in amount after week 24. Another pulmonary phospholipid, sphingomyelin (S), remains constant in amount. Thus the measure of lecithin in relation to sphingomyelin, or the **L/S ratio,** is used to determine fetal lung maturity. When the L/S ratio reaches 2:1, the infant's lungs are considered to be mature. This occurs at approximately 35 weeks of gestation (Mercer, 2009).

Certain maternal conditions that cause decreased maternal blood flow, such as maternal hypertension, placental dysfunction, infection, or corticosteroid use, can accelerate fetal lung maturity. This apparently is caused by the resulting fetal hypoxia, which stresses the fetus and increases the blood levels of corticosteroids that accelerate alveolar and surfactant development.

Conditions such as gestational diabetes and chronic glomerulonephritis can retard fetal lung maturity. The use of intrabronchial synthetic surfactant in the treatment of respiratory distress syndrome in the newborn has greatly improved the chances of survival for preterm infants.

Fetal respiratory movements have been seen on ultrasound examination as early as week 11. These fetal respiratory movements may aid in development of the chest wall muscles and regulate lung fluid volume. The fetal lungs produce fluid that expands the air spaces in the lungs. The fluid drains into the amniotic fluid or is swallowed by the fetus.

Before birth, secretion of lung fluid decreases. The normal birth process squeezes out approximately one third of the fluid. Infants born by cesarean do not benefit from this squeezing process, thus they may have more respiratory difficulty at birth. The fluid remaining in the lungs at birth is usually reabsorbed into the infant's bloodstream within 2 hours of birth.

Renal System

The kidneys form during the fifth week and begin to function approximately 4 weeks later. Urine is excreted into the amniotic fluid and forms a major part of the amniotic fluid volume. Oligohydramnios is indicative of renal dysfunction. Because the placenta acts as the organ of excretion and maintains fetal water and electrolyte balance, the fetus does not need functioning kidneys while in utero. At birth, however, the kidneys are required immediately for excretory and acid-base regulatory functions.

A fetal renal malformation can be diagnosed in utero. Corrective or palliative fetal surgery may treat the malformation successfully, or plans can be made for treatment immediately after birth.

At term the fetus has fully developed kidneys. However, the glomerular filtration rate (GFR) is low, and the kidneys lack the ability to concentrate urine. This makes the newborn more susceptible to both overhydration and dehydration.

Most newborns void within 24 hours of birth. With the loss of the swallowed amniotic fluid and the metabolism of nutrients provided by the placenta, the amount voided for the first days of life is scanty until fluid intake increases.

Neurologic System

The nervous system originates from the ectoderm during the third week after fertilization. The open neural tube forms during the fourth week. It initially closes at what will be the junction of the brain and spinal cord, leaving both ends open. The embryo folds in on itself lengthwise at this time, forming a head fold in the neural tube at this junction. The cranial end of the neural tube closes, and then the caudal end closes. During week 5, different growth rates cause more flexures in the neural tube, delineating three brain areas: the forebrain, the midbrain, and the hindbrain.

The forebrain develops into the eyes (cranial nerve II) and the cerebral hemispheres. The development of all areas of the cerebral cortex continues throughout fetal life and into childhood. The olfactory system (cranial nerve I) and the thalamus also develop from the forebrain. Cranial nerves III and IV (oculomotor and trochlear) form from the midbrain. The hindbrain forms the medulla, the pons, the cerebellum, and the remainder of the cranial nerves. Brain waves can be recorded on an electroencephalogram by week 8.

The spinal cord develops from the long end of the neural tube. Another ectodermal structure, the neural crest, develops into the peripheral nervous system. By the eighth week, nerve fibers traverse throughout the body. By week 11 or 12 the fetus makes respiratory movements, moves all extremities, and changes position in utero. The fetus can suck his or her thumb and swim in the amniotic fluid pool, turn somersaults, and occasionally tie a knot in the umbilical cord. Sometime between 16 and 20 weeks, when the movements are strong enough to be perceived by the mother as "the baby moving," quickening has occurred. The perception of movement occurs earlier in the multipara than in the primipara. The mother also becomes aware of the sleep and wake cycles of the fetus.

Sensory Awareness. Purposeful movements of the fetus have been demonstrated in response to a firm touch transmitted through the mother's abdomen. Because it can feel, the fetus requires anesthesia when invasive procedures are done.

Fetuses respond to sound by 24 weeks. Different types of music evoke different movements. The fetus can be soothed by the sound of the mother's voice. Acoustic stimulation can be used to evoke a fetal heart rate response. The fetus becomes accustomed (i.e., habituates) to noises heard repeatedly. Hearing is fully developed at birth.

The fetus is able to distinguish taste. By the fifth month, when the fetus is swallowing amniotic fluid, a sweetener added to the fluid causes the fetus to swallow faster. The fetus also reacts to temperature changes. A cold solution placed into the amniotic fluid can cause fetal hiccups.

The fetus can see. Eyes have both rods and cones in the retina by the seventh month. A bright light shone on the mother's abdomen in late pregnancy causes abrupt fetal movements. During sleep time, rapid eye movements have been observed similar to those occurring in children and adults while dreaming.

At term the fetal brain is approximately one fourth the size of an adult brain. Neurologic development continues. Stressors on the fetus and neonate (e.g., chronic poor nutrition or hypoxia, drugs, environmental toxins, trauma, disease) cause damage to the central nervous system long after the vulnerable embryonic time for malformations in other organ systems. Neurologic insult can result in cerebral palsy, neuromuscular impairment, mental retardation, and learning disabilities.

Endocrine System

The thyroid gland develops along with structures in the head and neck during the third and fourth weeks. The secretion of thyroxine begins during the eighth week. Maternal thyroxine does not readily cross the placenta; therefore, the fetus who does not produce thyroid hormones will be born with congenital hypothyroidism. If untreated, hypothyroidism can result in severe mental retardation. Screening for hypothyroidism is typically included in the testing when screening for phenylketonuria (PKU) after birth.

The adrenal cortex is formed during the sixth week and produces hormones by the eighth or ninth week. As term approaches, the fetus produces more cortisol. This is believed to aid in initiation of labor by decreasing the maternal progesterone and stimulating production of prostaglandins.

The pancreas forms from the foregut during the fifth through eighth weeks. The islets of Langerhans develop during the twelfth week. Insulin is produced by week 20. In infants of mothers with uncontrolled diabetes, maternal hyperglycemia produces fetal hyperglycemia, stimulating hyperinsulinemia and islet cell hyperplasia. This results in a macrosomic (large) fetus. The hyperinsulinemia also blocks lung maturation, placing the neonate at risk for respiratory distress and hypoglycemia when the maternal glucose source is lost at birth. Control of the maternal glucose level before and during pregnancy minimizes problems for the fetus and infant.

Reproductive System

Sex differentiation begins in the embryo during the seventh week. Female and male external genitalia are indistinguishable until after the ninth week. Distinguishing characteristics appear around the ninth week and are fully differentiated by the twelfth week. When a Y chromosome is present, testes are formed. By the end of the embryonic period, testosterone is being secreted and causes formation of the male genitalia. By week 28 the testes begin descending into the scrotum. After birth low levels of testosterone continue to be secreted until the pubertal surge.

The female, with two X chromosomes, forms ovaries and female external genitalia. By the sixteenth week oogenesis has been established. At birth the ovaries contain the female's lifetime supply of ova. Most female hormone production is delayed until puberty. However, the fetal endometrium responds to maternal hormones, and withdrawal bleeding or vaginal discharge (pseudomenstruation) may occur at birth when these hormones are lost. The high level of maternal estrogen also stimulates mammary engorgement and secretion of fluid ("witch's milk") in newborn infants of both sexes.

Musculoskeletal System

Bones and muscles develop from the mesoderm by the fourth week of embryonic development. At that time the cardiac muscle is already beating. The mesoderm next to the neural tube forms the vertebral column and ribs. The parts of the vertebral column grow toward each other to enclose the developing spinal cord. Ossification, or bone formation, begins. If there is a defect in the bony fusion, various forms of spina bifida may occur. A large defect affecting several vertebrae may allow the membranes and spinal cord to pouch out from the back, producing neurologic deficits and skeletal deformity.

The flat bones of the skull develop during the embryonic period, and ossification continues throughout childhood. At birth connective tissue sutures exist where the bones of the skull meet. The areas where more than two bones meet (called *fontanels*) are especially prominent. The sutures and fontanels allow the bones of the skull to mold, or move during birth, enabling the head to pass through the birth canal.

The bones of the shoulders, arms, hips, and legs appear in the sixth week as a continuous skeleton with no joints. Differentiation occurs, producing separate bones and joints. Ossification will continue through childhood to allow growth. Beginning during the seventh week, muscles contract spontaneously. Arm and leg movements are visible on ultrasound examination, although the mother does not perceive them until sometime between 16 and 20 weeks.

CLINICAL REASONING

Ultrasound Examination During Pregnancy

Veronica is 16 weeks pregnant. She has taken a folic acid supplement since 3 months before she became pregnant. On ultrasound, a neural tube defect, myelomeningocele, was detected. Veronica is extremely upset and states that she took folic acid from before the time she was pregnant until now. She asks how this defect could have happened and what she should do about it. What information should the nurse provide Veronica?

1. Evidence—Is there sufficient evidence to draw conclusions about what information the nurse should provide Veronica?
2. Assumptions—What assumptions can be made about ultrasound about the following factors:
   a. Veronica's knowledge of folic acid and the cause of myelomeningocele
   b. Veronica's concern for her fetus
   c. Veronica's knowledge of myelomeningocele and its treatment
   d. Veronica's need for genetic counseling
3. What implications and priorities for nursing care can be made at this time?
4. Does the evidence objectively support your conclusion?
5. Are there alternative perspectives to your conclusion?

Integumentary System

The epidermis begins as a single layer of cells derived from the ectoderm at 4 weeks. By the seventh week there are two layers of cells. The cells of the superficial layer are sloughed and become mixed with the sebaceous gland secretions to form the white, cheesy **vernix caseosa,** the material that protects the skin of the fetus. The vernix is thick at 24 weeks but becomes scant by term.

The basal layer of the epidermis is the germinal layer, which replaces lost cells. Until 17 weeks the skin is thin and wrinkled, with blood vessels visible underneath. The skin thickens and all layers are present at term. After 32 weeks as subcutaneous fat is deposited under the dermis, the skin becomes less wrinkled and red in appearance.

By 16 weeks the epidermal ridges are present on the palms of the hands, the fingers, the bottom of the feet, and the toes. These handprints and footprints are unique to that infant.

Hairs form from hair bulbs in the epidermis that project into the dermis. Cells in the hair bulb keratinize to form the hair shaft. As the cells at the base of the hair shaft proliferate, the hair grows to the surface of the epithelium. Very fine hairs, called **lanugo,** appear first at 12 weeks on the eyebrows and upper lip. By 20 weeks they cover the entire body. At this time the eyelashes, eyebrows, and scalp hair are beginning to grow. By 28 weeks the scalp hair is longer than the lanugo, which thins and may disappear by term gestation.

Fingernails and toenails develop from thickened epidermis at the tips of the digits beginning during the tenth week. They grow slowly. Fingernails usually reach the fingertips by 32 weeks, and toenails reach toe tips by 36 weeks.

Immunologic System

During the third trimester albumin and globulin are present in the fetus. The only immunoglobulin that crosses the placenta, immunoglobulin G (IgG), provides passive acquired immunity to specific bacterial toxins. The fetus produces IgM by the end of the first trimester. These are produced in response to blood group antigens, gram-negative enteric organisms, and some viruses. IgA is not produced by the fetus; however, colostrum, the precursor to breast milk, contains large amounts of IgA and can provide passive immunity to the neonate who is breastfed.

The normal term neonate can fight infection but not so effectively as an older child. The preterm infant is at much greater risk for infection.

Table 12-1 summarizes embryonic and fetal development.

TABLE 12-1 MILESTONES IN HUMAN DEVELOPMENT BEFORE BIRTH SINCE LAST MENSTRUAL PERIOD

	4 WEEKS	8 WEEKS	12 WEEKS
EXTERNAL APPEARANCE	Body flexed, C-shaped; arm and leg buds present; head at right angles to body	Body fairly well formed; nose flat, eyes far apart; digits well formed; head elevating; tail almost disappeared; eyes, ears, nose, and mouth recognizable	Nails appearing; resembles a human; head erect but disproportionately large; skin pink, delicate
	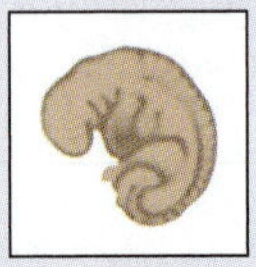	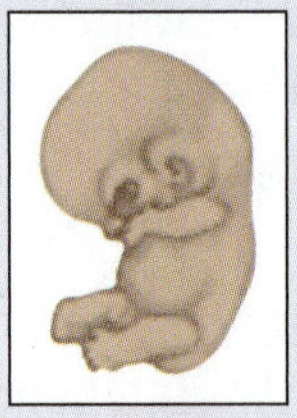	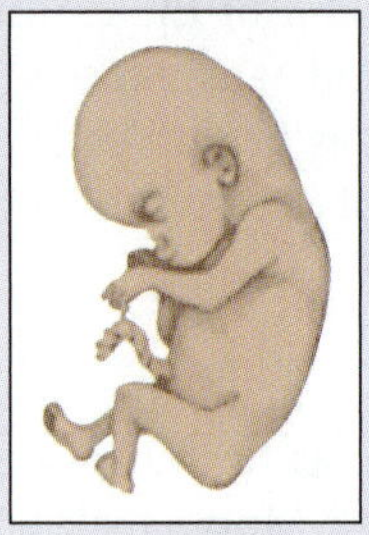
CROWN-TO-RUMP MEASUREMENT; WEIGHT	0.4-0.5 cm; 0.4 g	2.5-3 cm; 2 g	6-9 cm; 19 g
GASTROINTESTINAL SYSTEM	Stomach at midline and fusiform; conspicuous liver; esophagus short; intestine a short tube	Intestinal villi developing; small intestines coil within umbilical cord; palatal folds present; liver very large	Bile secreted; palatal fusion complete; intestines have withdrawn from cord and assume characteristic positions
MUSCULOSKELETAL SYSTEM	All somites present	First indication of ossification—occiput, mandible, and humerus; fetus capable of some movement; definitive muscles of trunk, limbs, and head well represented	Some bones well outlined, ossification spreading; upper cervical to lower sacral arches and bodies ossify; smooth muscle layers indicated in hollow viscera
CIRCULATORY SYSTEM	Heart develops, double chambers visible, begins to beat; aortic arch and major veins completed	Main blood vessels assume final plan; enucleated red cells predominate in blood	Blood forming in marrow
RESPIRATORY SYSTEM	Primary lung buds appear	Pleural and pericardial cavities forming; branching bronchioles; nostrils closed by epithelial plugs	Lungs acquire definite shape; vocal cords appear
RENAL SYSTEM	Rudimentary ureteral buds appear	Earliest secretory tubules differentiating; bladder-urethra separates from rectum	Kidney able to secrete urine; bladder expands as a sac
NERVOUS SYSTEM	Well-marked midbrain flexure; no hindbrain or cervical flexures; neural groove closed	Cerebral cortex begins to acquire typical cells; differentiation of cerebral cortex, meninges, ventricular foramina, cerebrospinal fluid circulation; spinal cord extends entire length of spine	Brain structural configuration almost complete; cord shows cervical and lumbar enlargements; fourth ventricle foramina are developed; sucking present
SENSORY ORGANS	Eye and ear appearing as optic vessel and otocyst	Primordial choroid plexuses develop; ventricles large relative to cortex; development progressing; eyes converging rapidly; internal ear developing; eyelids fuse	Earliest taste buds indicated; characteristic organization of eye attained
GENITAL SYSTEM	Genital ridge appears (fifth week)	Testes and ovaries distinguishable; external genitalia sexless but begin to differentiate	Sex recognizable; internal and external sex organs specific

	16 WEEKS	20 WEEKS	24 WEEKS
EXTERNAL APPEARANCE	Head still dominant; face looks human; eyes, ears, and nose approach typical appearance on gross examination; arm/leg ratio proportionate; scalp hair appears	Vernix caseosa appears; lanugo appears; legs lengthen considerably; sebaceous glands appear	Body lean but fairly well proportioned; skin red and wrinkled; vernix caseosa present; sweat glands forming
	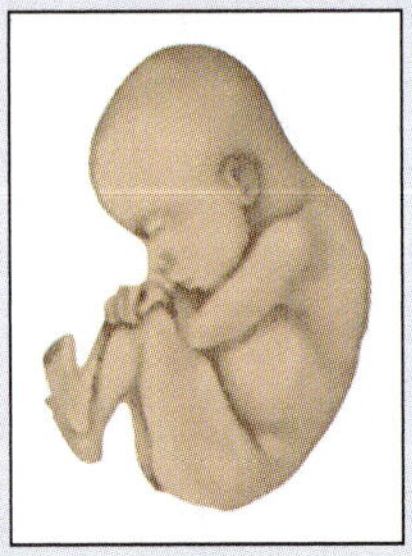	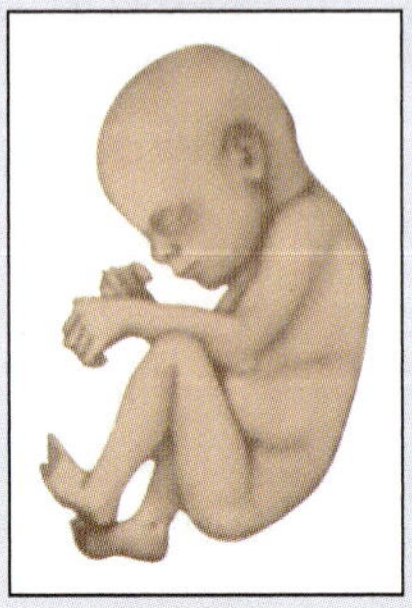	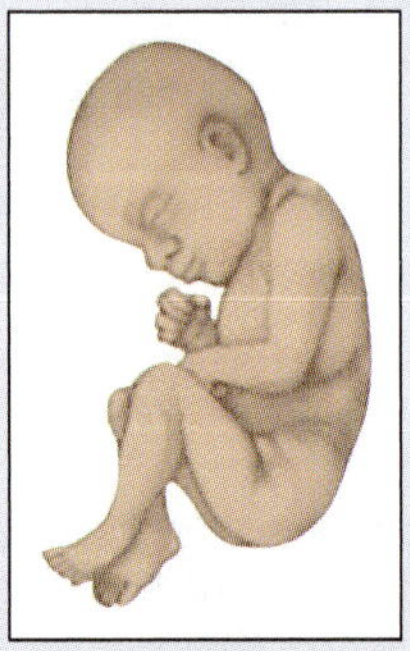

Animations—First Trimester, Fetal Development

TABLE 12-1 **MILESTONES IN HUMAN DEVELOPMENT BEFORE BIRTH SINCE LAST MENSTRUAL PERIOD—cont'd**

CROWN-TO-RUMP MEASUREMENT; WEIGHT		
11.5-13.5 cm; 100 g	16-18.5 cm; 300 g	23 cm; 600 g
GASTROINTESTINAL SYSTEM		
Meconium in bowel; some enzyme secretion; anus open	Enamel and dentine depositing; ascending colon recognizable	
MUSCULOSKELETAL SYSTEM		
Most bones distinctly indicated throughout body; joint cavities appear; muscular movements can be detected	Sternum ossifies; fetal movements strong enough for mother to feel	
CIRCULATORY SYSTEM		
Heart muscle well developed; blood formation active in spleen		Blood formation increases in bone marrow and decreases in liver
RESPIRATORY SYSTEM		
Elastic fibers appear in lungs; terminal and respiratory bronchioles appear	Nostrils reopen; primitive respiratory-like movements begin	Alveolar ducts and sacs present; lecithin begins to appear in amniotic fluid (weeks 26 to 27)
RENAL SYSTEM		
Kidney in position; attains typical shape and plan		
NERVOUS SYSTEM		
Cerebral lobes delineated; cerebellum assumes some prominence	Brain grossly formed; cord myelination begins; spinal cord ends at level of first sacral vertebra (S1)	Cerebral cortex layered typically; neuronal proliferation in cerebral cortex ends
SENSORY ORGANS		
General sense organs differentiated	Nose and ears ossify	Can hear
GENITAL SYSTEM		
Testes in position for descent into scrotum: vagina open		Testes at inguinal ring in descent to scrotum

28 WEEKS	**30–31 WEEKS**	**36–40 WEEKS**
EXTERNAL APPEARANCE		
Lean body, less wrinkled and red; nails appear	Subcutaneous fat beginning to collect; more rounded appearance; skin pink and smooth; has assumed birth position	36 weeks: Skin pink, body rounded; general lanugo disappearing; body usually plump 40 weeks: Skin smooth and pink; scant vernix caseosa; moderate to profuse hair; lanugo on shoulders and upper body only; nasal and alar cartilage apparent
	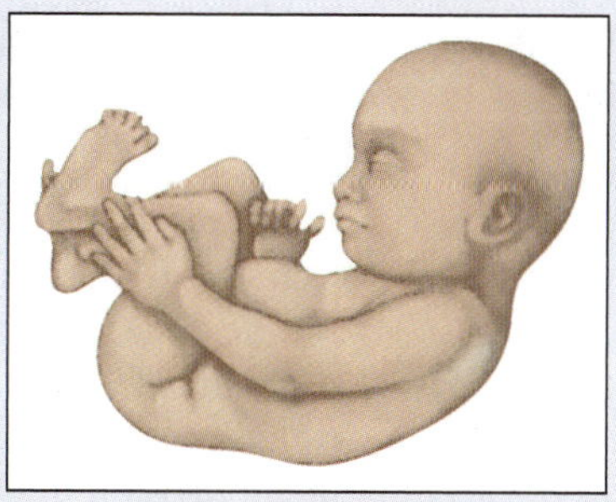	
CROWN-TO-RUMP MEASUREMENT; WEIGHT		
27 cm; 1100 g	31 cm; 1800-2100 g	36 weeks: 35 cm; 2200-2900 g 40 weeks: 40 cm; 3200+ g
MUSCULOSKELETAL SYSTEM		
Astragalus (talus, ankle bone) ossifies; weak, fleeting movements, minimum tone	Middle fourth phalanxes ossify; permanent teeth primordia seen; can turn head to side	36 weeks: Distal femoral ossification centers present; sustained, definite movements; fair tone; can turn and elevate head 40 weeks: Active, sustained movement; good tone; may lift head
RESPIRATORY SYSTEM		
Lecithin forming on alveolar surfaces	L/S ratio = 1.2:1	36 weeks: L/S ratio >2:1 40 weeks: Pulmonary branching only two thirds complete
RENAL SYSTEM		
		36 weeks: Formation of new nephrons ceases

Continued

Animations—Third Trimester, Fetal Development

TABLE 12-1 MILESTONES IN HUMAN DEVELOPMENT BEFORE BIRTH SINCE LAST MENSTRUAL PERIOD—cont'd

NERVOUS SYSTEM	Appearance of cerebral fissures, convolutions rapidly appearing; indefinite sleep-wake cycle; cry weak or absent; weak suck reflex		36 weeks: End of spinal cord at level of third lumbar vertebra (L3); definite sleep-wake cycle 40 weeks: Myelination of brain begins; patterned sleep-wake cycle with alert periods; strong suck reflex
SENSORY ORGANS	Eyelids reopen; retinal layers completed, light-receptive; pupils capable of reacting to light	Sense of taste present; aware of sounds outside mother's body	
GENITAL SYSTEM		Testes descending to scrotum	40 weeks: Testes in scrotum; labia majora well developed

L/S, Lecithin/spongomyelin.

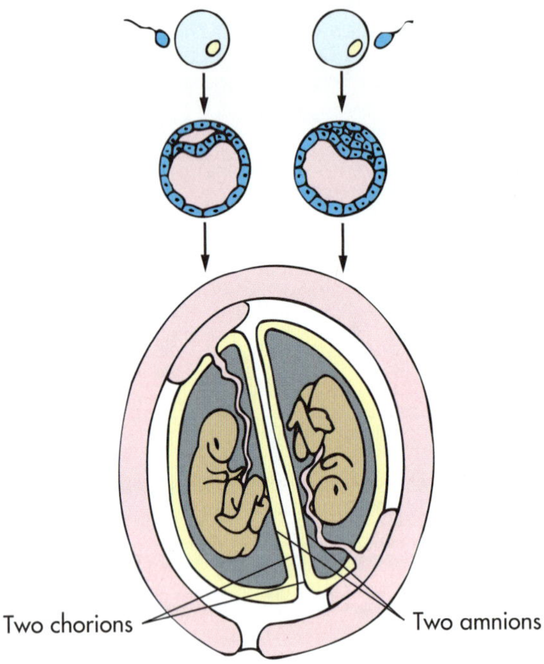

FIG. 12-14 Formation of dizygotic twins, with fertilization of two ova, two implantations, two placentas, two chorions, and two amnions.

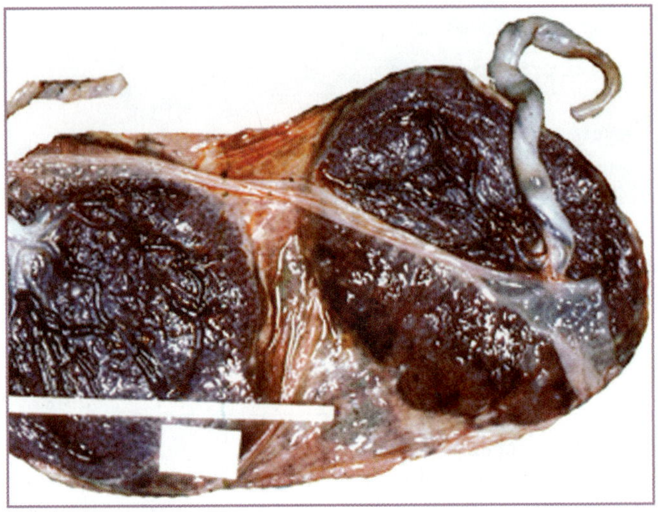

FIG. 12-15 Diamniotic dichorionic (separate) twin placenta. (From Benirschke, K. [2009]. Multiple gestation. The biology of twinning. In R. Creasy, R. Resnik, J. Iams, C. Lockwood, & T. Moore (Eds.), *Creasy and Resnik's maternal-fetal medicine: Principles and practice* (6th ed.). Philadelphia: Saunders.

Multifetal Pregnancy

Twins

The incidence of twinning is 1 in 30 pregnancies. There has been a steady rise in multiple births since 1973 (Benirschke, 2009). This is partly attributed to the availability of assisted reproductive technologies and the increasing age at which women give birth (Malone & D'Alton, 2009).

Dizygotic Twins. When two mature ova are produced in one ovarian cycle, both have the potential to be fertilized by separate sperm. This results in two zygotes, or dizygotic twins (Fig. 12-14). There are always two amnions, two chorions, and two placentas, which may be fused (Fig. 12-15). These dizygotic, or fraternal, twins can be the same sex or different sexes and are genetically no more alike than siblings born at different times. Dizygotic twinning occurs in families, more often among African-American women than among Caucasian women, and least often among Asian women. Dizygotic twinning increases in frequency with maternal age up to 35 years, with parity, and with the use of fertility drugs.

Monozygotic Twins. Identical or monozygotic twins develop from one fertilized ovum, which then divides (Fig. 12-16). They are the same sex and have the same genotype. If division occurs soon after fertilization, two embryos, two amnions, two chorions, and two placentas that can be fused will develop. Most often, division occurs between 4 and 8 days after fertilization, and there are two embryos, two amnions, one chorion, and one placenta. Rarely, division occurs after the eighth day after fertilization. In this case, there are two embryos within a common amnion and a common chorion with one placenta. This often causes circulatory problems because the umbilical cords may tangle together, and one or both fetuses may die. If division occurs very late, cleavage may not be complete, and conjoined twins could result. Monozygotic twinning occurs approximately 3.5 to 4 per 1000 births (Benirschke, 2009). There is no association with race, heredity, maternal age, or parity. Fertility drugs increase the incidence of monozygotic twinning.

Conjoined Twins. Conjoined twins are a type of monozygotic twins in which there is incomplete embryonic division at 13 to 15 days postconception (see Fig. 12-16). The estimated

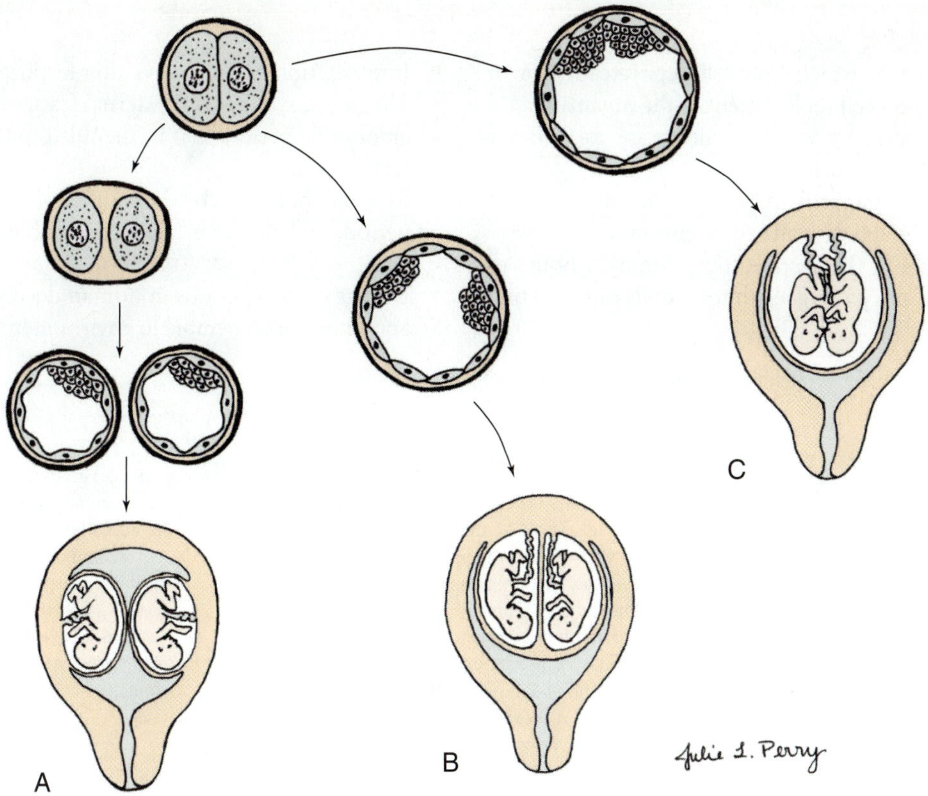

FIG. 12-16 Formation of monozygotic twins. **A,** One fertilization: blastomeres separate, resulting in two implantations, two placentas, and two sets of membranes. **B,** One blastomere with two inner cell masses, one fused placenta, one chorion, and separate amnions. **C,** One blastomere with incomplete separation of cell mass, resulting in conjoined twins.

frequency is 1 in 50,000 births (Malone & D'Alton, 2009). Prenatal diagnosis is possible with three-dimensional ultrasonography. Cesarean birth minimizes trauma to mother and fetuses.

Other Multifetal Pregnancies

The occurrence of multifetal pregnancies with three or more fetuses has increased with the use of fertility drugs and in vitro fertilization. Triplets occur in approximately 1 of 1341 pregnancies (Benirschke, 2009). They can occur from the division of one zygote into two, with one of the two dividing again, producing identical triplets. Triplets also can be produced from two zygotes, one dividing into a set of identical twins, and the second zygote developing as a single fraternal sibling, or from three zygotes. Quadruplets, quintuplets, sextuplets, and so on, likewise have similar possible derivations.

NONGENETIC FACTORS INFLUENCING DEVELOPMENT

Congenital disorders may be inherited, may be caused by environmental factors, or by inadequate maternal nutrition. Congenital means that the condition was present at birth. Some congenital malformations may be the result of teratogens, that is, environmental substances or exposures that result in functional or structural disability. In contrast to other forms of developmental disabilities, disabilities caused by teratogens are theoretically totally preventable. Known human teratogens are certain drugs and chemicals, infections, exposure to radiation, and certain maternal conditions such as diabetes and PKU (see Box 12-1). A teratogen has the greatest effect on the organs and parts of an embryo during its periods of rapid growth and differentiation. This occurs during the embryonic period, specifically from days 15 to 60. During the first 2 weeks of development, teratogens either have no effect or have effects so severe that they cause miscarriage. Brain growth and development continue during the fetal period, and teratogens can severely affect mental development throughout gestation (see Fig. 12-8).

In addition to the genetic makeup and the influence of teratogens, the adequacy of maternal nutrition influences development. The embryo and fetus must obtain the nutrients they need from the mother's diet; they cannot tap the maternal reserves. Malnutrition during pregnancy produces low-birth-weight newborns who are susceptible to infection. Malnutrition also affects brain development during the latter half of gestation and can result in learning disabilities in the child. Inadequate folic acid is associated with neural tube defects.

KEY POINTS

- Mitosis is the process by which body cells replicate for growth and development and cell replacement of the organism.
- Meiosis is the process by which gametes are formed for reproduction of the organism.
- Human gestation lasts approximately 280 days after the last menstrual period or 266 days after conception.
- Fertilization occurs in the uterine tube within 24 hours of ovulation. The zygote undergoes mitotic divisions, creating a 16-cell morula.
- Implantation begins 6 days after fertilization.
- The organ systems and external features develop during the embryonic period, that is, the third to the eighth week after fertilization.
- Refinement of structure and function occurs during the fetal period, and the fetus becomes capable of extrauterine survival.
- During critical periods in human development, the embryo and fetus are vulnerable to environmental teratogens.

Audio Chapter Summaries Access an audio summary of these Key Points on evolve

REFERENCES

Benirschke, K. (2009). Multiple gestation: The biology of twinning. In R. Creasy, R. Resnik, J. Iams, C. Lockwood, & T. Moore (Eds.), *Creasy and Resnik's maternal-fetal medicine: Principles and practice* (6th ed.). Philadelphia: Saunders.

Cunningham, F., Leveno, K., Bloom, S., Hauth, J., Rouse, D., & Spong, C. (2010). *Williams obstetrics* (23rd ed.). New York: McGraw-Hill.

Malone, F., & D'Alton, M. (2009). Multiple gestation: Clinical characteristics and management. In R. Creasy, R. Resnik, J. Iams, C. Lockwood, & T. Moore (Eds.), *Creasy and Resnik's maternal-fetal medicine: Principles and practice* (6th ed.). Philadelphia: Saunders.

Mercer, B. (2009). Assessment and induction of fetal pulmonary maturity. In R. Creasy, R. Resnik, J. Iams, C. Lockwood, & T. Moore (Eds.), *Creasy and Resnik's maternal-fetal medicine: Principles and practice* (6th ed.). Philadelphia: Saunders.

Moore, K., & Persaud, T. (2008). *Before we are born. Essentials of embryology and birth defects* (3rd ed.). Philadelphia: Saunders.

Mor, G., & Abrahams, V. (2009). The immunology of pregnancy. In R. Creasy, R. Resnik, J. Iams, C. Lockwood, & T. Moore (Eds.), *Creasy and Resnik's maternal-fetal medicine: Principles and practice* (6th ed.). Philadelphia: Saunders.

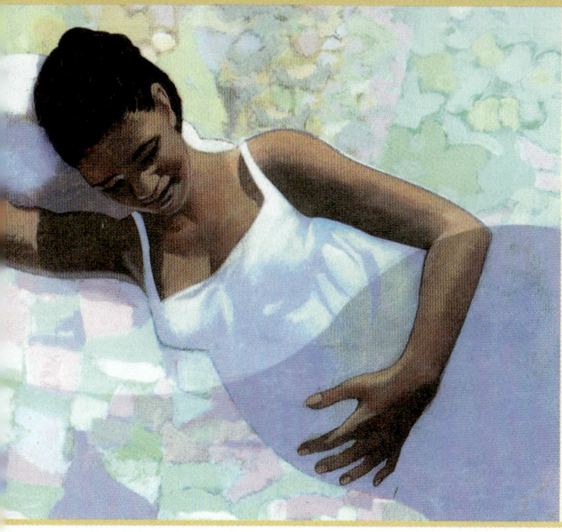

CHAPTER

13

Anatomy and Physiology of Pregnancy

Deitra Leonard Lowdermilk

evolve WEBSITE

http://evolve.elsevier.com/Lowdermilk/MWHC/
Audio Glossary
Audio Key Points
NCLEX Review Questions

LEARNING OBJECTIVES

- Determine obstetric history by using the five- and two-digit systems.
- Describe the various types of pregnancy tests including the timing of tests and interpretation of results.
- Explain the expected maternal anatomic and physiologic adaptations to pregnancy for each body system.
- Differentiate among presumptive, probable, and positive signs of pregnancy.
- Compare normal adult laboratory values with values for pregnant women.
- Compare the characteristics of the abdomen, the vulva, and the cervix of the nullipara and the multipara.
- Identify the maternal hormones produced during pregnancy, their target organs, and their major effects on pregnancy.

The goal of maternity care is a healthy pregnancy with a physically safe and emotionally satisfying outcome for mother, infant, and family. Consistent health supervision and surveillance are of utmost importance in achieving this outcome. However, many maternal adaptations are unfamiliar to pregnant women and their families. Helping the pregnant woman recognize the relation between her physical status and the plan for her care assists her in making decisions and encourages her to participate in her own care.

GRAVIDITY AND PARITY

An understanding of the following terms used to describe pregnancy and the pregnant woman is essential to the study of maternity care (Cunningham, Leveno, Bloom, Hauth, Rouse, & Spong, 2010):

- **gravida:** a woman who is pregnant
- **gravidity:** pregnancy
- **multigravida:** a woman who has had two or more pregnancies
- **multipara:** a woman who has completed two or more pregnancies to 20 or more weeks of gestation
- **nulligravida:** a woman who has never been pregnant
- **nullipara:** a woman who has not completed a pregnancy with a fetus or fetuses who have reached 20 weeks of gestation
- **parity:** the number of pregnancies in which the fetus or fetuses have reached 20 weeks of gestation when they are born, not the number of fetuses (e.g., twins) born. Whether the fetus is born alive or is stillborn (fetus who shows no signs of life at birth) does not affect parity
- **postdate or postterm:** a pregnancy that goes beyond 42 weeks of gestation
- **preterm:** a pregnancy that has reached 20 weeks of gestation but ends before completion of 37 weeks of gestation
- **primigravida:** a woman who is pregnant for the first time
- **primipara:** a woman who has completed one pregnancy with a fetus or fetuses who have reached 20 weeks of gestation
- **term:** a pregnancy from the completion of 37 weeks of gestation to the end of week 42 of gestation
- **viability:** capacity to live outside the uterus; there are no clear limits of gestational age or weight. Infants born at 22 to 25 weeks of gestation are considered to be on the threshold of viability and are especially vulnerable to brain injury if they survive. Survival rates for infants with birth weights of less than 500 g is approximately 45%.

TABLE 13-1 OBSTETRIC HISTORY USING FIVE-DIGIT SYSTEM AND TWO-DIGIT SYSTEM

CONDITION	G *Gravidity*	T *Term Births*	P *Preterm Births*	A *Abortions and Miscarriages*	L *Living Children*	G/P *Gravidity/ Parity*
Shauna is pregnant for the first time.	1	0	0	0	0	1/0
She carries the pregnancy to 34 weeks, and the neonate survives.	1	0	1	0	1	1/1
She becomes pregnant again.	2	0	1	0	1	2/1
Her second pregnancy ends in miscarriage at 10 weeks.	2	0	1	1	1	2/1
During her third pregnancy she gives birth at 38 weeks.	3	1	1	1	2	3/2
During her fourth pregnancy Shauna gives birth to twins at 36 weeks.	4	1	2	1	4	4/3

Gravidity and parity information is obtained during history-taking interviews. Obtaining and documenting this information accurately is important in making a plan of care for the pregnant woman.

! NURSING ALERT

Information may be recorded in client records in a variety of ways because no one standardized system exists. Until such a system is in place, the nurse should understand the documentation system used by the health care facility.

Two commonly used systems of summarizing the obstetric history are discussed here. Gravidity and parity is described with only two digits: the first digit represents the number of pregnancies the woman has had, including the present one; and parity is the number of pregnancies that have reached 20 or more weeks of gestation before the birth. For example, if the woman had twins at 36 weeks with her first pregnancy, parity would still be counted as one birth (gravida [G]1, para [P]1) (Cunningham et al., 2010). If the woman becomes pregnant a second time, she would still be G2P1 until she gives birth at 38 weeks when she would then become G2P2.

Another system that is commonly used consists of five digits separated with hyphens. This system provides more specific information about the woman's obstetric history, although it may not provide accurate information about parity because it provides information about births and not pregnancies reaching 20 weeks of gestation (Beebe, 2005). The first digit represents gravidity; the second digit represents the total number of term births; the third indicates the number of preterm births; the fourth identifies the number of abortions (miscarriage or elective termination of pregnancy); and the fifth is the number of children currently living. The acronym *GTPAL* (gravidity, term, preterm, abortions, living children) may be helpful in remembering this system of notation. For example, if a woman pregnant only once gives birth at week 34 and the infant survives, the abbreviation that represents this information is 1-0-1-0-1. During her next pregnancy, the abbreviation is 2-0-1-0-1. Additional examples are given in Table 13-1.

PREGNANCY TESTS

Early detection of pregnancy allows early initiation of care. **Human chorionic gonadotropin (hCG)** is the earliest biochemical marker for pregnancy, and pregnancy tests are based on the recognition of hCG or a beta (β) subunit of hCG. Production of β-hCG begins as early as the day of implantation and can be detected as early as 7 to 10 days after conception (Blackburn, 2007). The level of hCG increases until it peaks at about 60 to 70 days of gestation and then declines until about 80 days of pregnancy. It remains stable until about 30 weeks and then gradually increases until term. Higher than normal levels of hCG may indicate abnormal gestation (e.g., a fetus with Down syndrome) or multiple gestation; an abnormally slow increase or a decrease in hCG levels may indicate ectopic pregnancy or impending miscarriage (Burton, Sibley, & Jauniaux, 2007; Stewart, 2007).

Serum and urine pregnancy tests are performed in clinics, offices, women's health centers, and laboratory settings, and urine pregnancy tests may be performed at home. Both serum and urine tests can provide accurate results. A 7- to 10-ml sample of venous blood is collected for serum testing. Most urine tests require a first-voided morning urine specimen because it contains levels of hCG approximately the same as those in serum. Random urine samples usually have lower levels. Urine tests are less expensive and provide more immediate results than do serum tests (Stewart, 2007).

Many different pregnancy tests are available (Fig. 13-1). The wide variety of tests precludes discussion of each; however, several categories of tests are described here. The nurse should read the manufacturer's directions for the test to be used and determine if the woman understands the directions. A study by Wallace and associates (2009) reported that instructions for most home pregnancy tests do not meet the criteria recommended for compliance with the guidelines for use of plain language and that most instructions were written at a seventh grade level or above.

Radioimmunoassay (RIA) pregnancy tests for the beta subunit of hCG in serum or urine samples use radioactively labeled markers and are usually performed in a laboratory. These tests are accurate with low hCG levels (5 milli-International Units/ml) and can confirm pregnancy before the first menstrual period. Results are available within a few hours (Stewart, 2007).

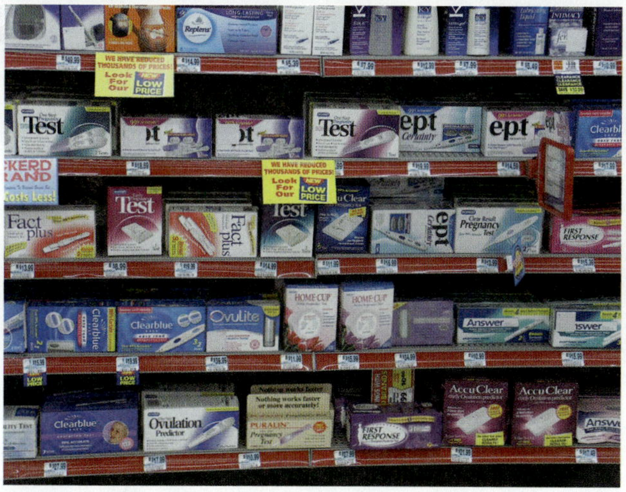

FIG. 13-1 Many pregnancy test products are available over the counter. (Courtesy Dee Lowdermilk, Chapel Hill, NC.)

CLINICAL REASONING

Pregnancy Testing

Joy, 34 years old, has been trying to get pregnant. Her menstrual periods are somewhat irregular but she is 7 days late. She bought a home pregnancy test, and the results were negative. At the clinic today she tells the nurse she is so depressed because the test was negative and she thinks she should see a fertility specialist.

1. Evidence—Is there sufficient evidence to draw conclusions about what advice would be appropriate for Joy?
2. Assumptions—What assumptions can be made about:
    a. hCG levels during pregnancy
    b. Accuracy of home pregnancy tests
    c. Irregular menstrual cycles and pregnancy testing
3. What are the implications and priorities for providing information to Joy?
4. Does the evidence objectively support your conclusion?
5. Are there alternative perspectives to your conclusion?

Radioreceptor assay (RRA) is a serum test that measures the ability of a blood sample to inhibit the binding of radiolabeled hCG to receptors. The test is 90% to 95% accurate from 6 to 8 days after conception (Pagana & Pagana, 2009).

Enzyme-linked immunosorbent assay (ELISA) testing is the most popular method of testing for pregnancy. It uses a specific monoclonal antibody (anti-hCG) with enzymes to bond with hCG in urine. As an office or home procedure, it requires minimal time and offers results in less than 5 minutes. A positive test result is indicated by a simple color-change reaction. Depending on the specific test, levels of hCG as low as 25 milli-International Units/ml can be detected as early as 7 days after conception (Stewart, 2007).

ELISA technology is the basis for most over-the-counter home pregnancy tests. With these one-step tests, the woman usually applies urine to a strip and reads the results. The test kits come with directions for collection of the specimen, the testing procedure, and reading of the results. A positive test result is indicated by a simple color change reaction or a digital reading. Most manufacturers of the kits provide a toll-free telephone number to call if users have concerns and questions about test procedures or results (see Teaching for Self-Management box). The most common error in home pregnancy tests is performing the test too early in pregnancy (Stewart, 2007).

TEACHING FOR SELF-MANAGEMENT

Home Pregnancy Testing

- Follow the manufacturer's instructions carefully. Do not omit steps.
- Review the manufacturer's list of foods, medications, and other substances that can affect the test results.
- Use a first-voided morning urine specimen.
- If the test done at the time of your missed period is negative, repeat the test in 1 week if you still have not had a period.
- If you have questions about the test, contact the manufacturer.
- Contact your health care provider for follow-up if the test result is positive, or if the test result is negative and you still have not had a period.

Interpreting the results of pregnancy tests requires some judgment. The type of pregnancy test and its degree of sensitivity (ability to detect low levels of a substance) and specificity (ability to discern the absence of a substance) must be considered in conjunction with the woman's history. This includes the date of her last menstrual period (LMP), her usual cycle length, and results of previous pregnancy tests. It is important to know if the woman is a substance abuser and what medications she is taking, because medications such as anticonvulsants and tranquilizers can cause false-positive results, whereas diuretics and promethazine can cause false-negative results (Pagana & Pagana, 2009). Improper collection of the specimen, hormone-producing tumors, and laboratory errors also can cause false results.

Depending on the specific test, levels of hCG as low as 6.3 milli-International Units/ml can be detected as early as the first day of a missed menstrual period as reported by Cole and coworkers (2005). These researchers found that most of the over-the-counter pregnancy tests in the study were less sensitive (25 to 100 milli-International Units/ml) and detected only a small percentage of pregnancies on the first day of a missed period even though most products claimed to be 99% accurate. Tomlinson and colleagues (2008) found that digital readings of low hCG levels (i.e., 25 milli-International Units/ml) were more accurately interpreted by consumers than nondigital tests.

Women who use a home pregnancy test should be advised about the variations in accuracy reporting and to use caution when interpreting results. Whenever there is any question, further evaluation or retesting is appropriate.

ADAPTATIONS TO PREGNANCY

Maternal physiologic adaptations are attributed to the hormones of pregnancy and to mechanical pressures arising from the enlarging uterus and other tissues. These adaptations protect the woman's normal physiologic functioning, meet the metabolic demands pregnancy imposes on her body, and provide a nurturing environment for fetal development and growth. Although pregnancy is a normal phenomenon, problems can occur.

TABLE 13-2 **SIGNS OF PREGNANCY**

TIME OF OCCURRENCE (GESTATIONAL AGE)	SIGN	OTHER POSSIBLE CAUSE
Presumptive Signs		
3-4 wk	Breast changes	Premenstrual changes, oral contraceptives
4 wk	Amenorrhea	Stress, vigorous exercise, early menopause, endocrine problems, malnutrition
4-14 wk	Nausea, vomiting	Gastrointestinal virus, food poisoning
6-12 wk	Urinary frequency	Infection, pelvic tumors
12 wk	Fatigue	Stress, illness
16-20 wk	Quickening	Gas, peristalsis
Probable Signs		
5 wk	Goodell sign	Pelvic congestion
6-8 wk	Chadwick sign	Pelvic congestion
6-12 wk	Hegar sign	Pelvic congestion
4-12 wk	Positive result of pregnancy test (serum)	Hydatidiform mole, choriocarcinoma
6-12 wk	Positive result of pregnancy test (urine)	False-positive results may be caused by pelvic infection, tumors
16 wk	Braxton Hicks contractions	Myomas, other tumors
16-28 wk	Ballottement	Tumors, cervical polyps
Positive Signs		
5-6 wk	Visualization of fetus by real-time ultrasound examination	No other causes
6 wk	Fetal heart tones detected by ultrasound examination	No other causes
16 wk	Visualization of fetus by radiographic study	No other causes
8-17 wk	Fetal heart tones detected by Doppler ultrasound stethoscope	No other causes
17-19 wk	Fetal heart tones detected by fetal stethoscope	No other causes
19-22 wk	Fetal movements palpated	No other causes
Late pregnancy	Fetal movements visible	No other causes

Signs of Pregnancy

Some of the physiologic adaptations are recognized as signs and symptoms of pregnancy. Three commonly used categories of signs and symptoms of pregnancy are presumptive (those changes noticed by the woman—e.g., amenorrhea, fatigue, nausea and vomiting, breast changes); probable (those changes observed by an examiner—e.g., Hegar sign, ballottement, pregnancy tests); and positive (those signs that are attributable only to the presence of the fetus—e.g., hearing fetal heart tones, visualization of the fetus, and palpating fetal movements). Table 13-2 summarizes these signs of pregnancy in relation to when they might occur and other causes for their occurrence.

Reproductive System and Breasts

Uterus

Changes in Size, Shape, and Position. The phenomenal uterine growth in the first trimester is stimulated by high levels of estrogen and progesterone. Early uterine enlargement results from increased vascularity and dilation of blood vessels, hyperplasia (production of new muscle fibers and fibroelastic tissue) and hypertrophy (enlargement of preexisting muscle fibers and fibroelastic tissue), and development of the decidua. By 7 weeks of gestation, the uterus is the size of a large hen's egg; by 10 weeks of gestation, it is the size of an orange (twice its nonpregnant size); and by 12 weeks of gestation, it is the size of a grapefruit. After the third month, uterine enlargement is primarily the result of mechanical pressure of the growing fetus.

As the uterus enlarges it also changes in shape and position. At conception the uterus is shaped like an upside-down pear. During the second trimester, as the muscular walls strengthen and become more elastic, the uterus becomes spherical or globular. Later, as the fetus lengthens, the uterus becomes larger and more ovoid and rises out of the pelvis into the abdominal cavity.

The pregnancy may "show" after the fourteenth week, although this depends to some degree on the woman's height and weight. Abdominal enlargement may be less apparent in the nullipara with good abdominal muscle tone (Fig. 13-2). Posture also influences the type and degree of abdominal enlargement that occurs. In normal pregnancies, the uterus enlarges at a predictable rate. As the uterus grows it may be palpated above the symphysis pubis some time between the twelfth and fourteenth weeks of pregnancy (Fig. 13-3). The uterus rises gradually to the level of the umbilicus at 22 to 24 weeks of gestation and nearly reaches the xiphoid process at term. Between weeks 38 and 40, fundal height drops as the fetus begins to descend and engage in the pelvis (lightening) (see Fig. 13-3, *dashed line*). Generally, lightening occurs in the nullipara about 2 weeks before the onset of labor and at the start of labor in the multipara.

Uterine enlargement is determined by measuring fundal height, a measurement commonly used to estimate the duration of pregnancy. However, variation in the position of the fundus or the fetus, variations in the amount of amniotic fluid present, the presence of more than one fetus, maternal obesity, and variation in examiner techniques can reduce the accuracy of this estimation of the duration of pregnancy (see Chapter 15).

The uterus normally rotates to the right as it elevates, probably because of the presence of the rectosigmoid colon on the left side, but the extensive hypertrophy (enlargement) of the round ligaments keeps the uterus in the midline. Eventually the growing uterus touches the anterior abdominal wall and displaces the intestines to either side of the abdomen (Fig. 13-4). Whenever

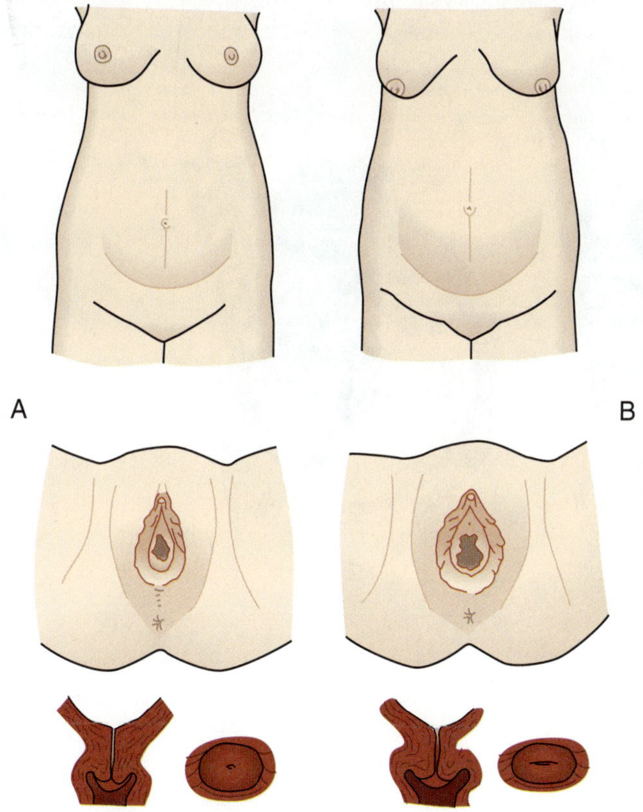

FIG. 13-2 Comparison of abdomen, vulva, and cervix in nullipara **(A),** and multipara **(B),** at the same stage of pregnancy.

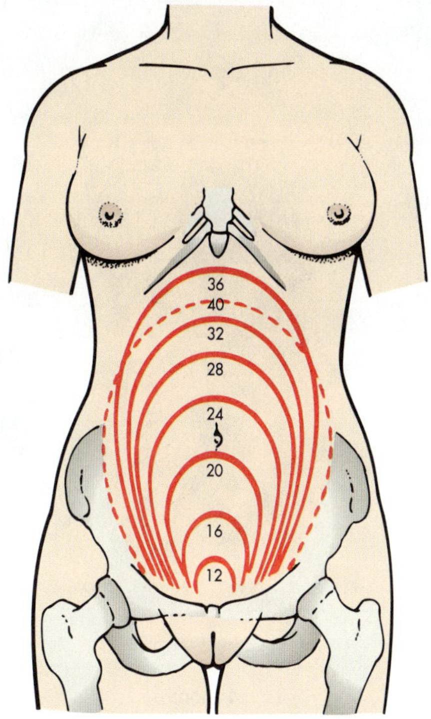

FIG. 13-3 Height of fundus by weeks of normal gestation with a single fetus. *Dashed line,* height after lightening. (From Seidel, H., Ball, J., Dains, J., Flynn, J., Solomon, B., & Stewart, R. [2011]. *Mosby's guide to physical examination* [7th ed.]. St. Louis: Mosby.)

a pregnant woman is standing, most of her uterus rests against the anterior abdominal wall, and this contributes to altering her center of gravity.

At approximately 6 weeks of gestation, softening and compressibility of the lower uterine segment (the uterine isthmus) occur **(Hegar sign)** (Fig. 13-5). This results in exaggerated uterine anteflexion during the first 3 months of pregnancy. In this position the uterine fundus presses on the urinary bladder, causing the woman to have urinary frequency.

Changes in Contractility. Soon after the fourth month of pregnancy, uterine contractions can be felt through the abdominal wall. These contractions are referred to as the **Braxton Hicks sign.** Braxton Hicks contractions are irregular and painless and occur intermittently throughout pregnancy. These contractions facilitate uterine blood flow through the intervillous spaces of the placenta and thereby promote oxygen delivery to the fetus. Although Braxton Hicks contractions are not painful, some women complain that they are annoying. After the twenty-eighth week these contractions become much more definite, but they usually cease with walking or exercise. Braxton Hicks contractions can be mistaken for true labor; however, they do not increase in intensity or frequency or cause cervical dilation.

Uteroplacental Blood Flow. Placental perfusion depends on the maternal blood flow to the uterus. Blood flow increases rapidly as the uterine size increases. Although uterine blood flow increases 20-fold, the fetoplacental unit grows more rapidly. Consequently, more oxygen is extracted from the uterine blood during the latter part of pregnancy (Cunningham et al., 2010). In a normal term pregnancy, one sixth of the total maternal blood volume is within the uterine vascular system. The rate of blood flow through the uterus ranges from 450 to 650 ml/min at term, and oxygen consumption of the gravid uterus increases to meet fetal needs. A low maternal arterial pressure, contractions of the uterus, and maternal supine position are three factors known to decrease blood flow. Estrogen stimulation may increase uterine blood flow. Doppler ultrasound examination can be used to measure uterine blood flow velocity, especially in pregnancies at risk because of conditions associated with decreased placental perfusion such as hypertension, intrauterine growth restriction, diabetes mellitus, and multiple gestation (Blackburn, 2007). By using an ultrasound device or a fetal stethoscope, the health care provider may hear the **uterine souffle** (sound made by blood in the uterine arteries that is synchronous with the maternal pulse) or the **funic souffle** (sound made by blood rushing through the umbilical vessels and synchronous with the fetal heart rate).

Cervical Changes. A softening of the cervical tip called **Goodell sign** can be observed at approximately the beginning of the sixth week in a normal, unscarred cervix. This sign is brought about by increased vascularity, slight hypertrophy, and hyperplasia (increase in number of cells) of the muscle and its collagen-rich connective tissue, which becomes loose, edematous, highly elastic, and increased in volume. The glands near the external os proliferate beneath the stratified squamous epithelium, giving the cervix the velvety appearance characteristic of pregnancy. *Friability* (tissue is easily damaged) is increased can cause slight bleeding after coitus with deep penetration or after vaginal examination. Pregnancy also can cause the squamocolumnar junction, the site for obtaining cells for cervical cancer screening, to be located away from the cervix. Because of all these changes, evaluation of abnormal Papanicolaou (Pap) tests during pregnancy can be complicated. However, careful

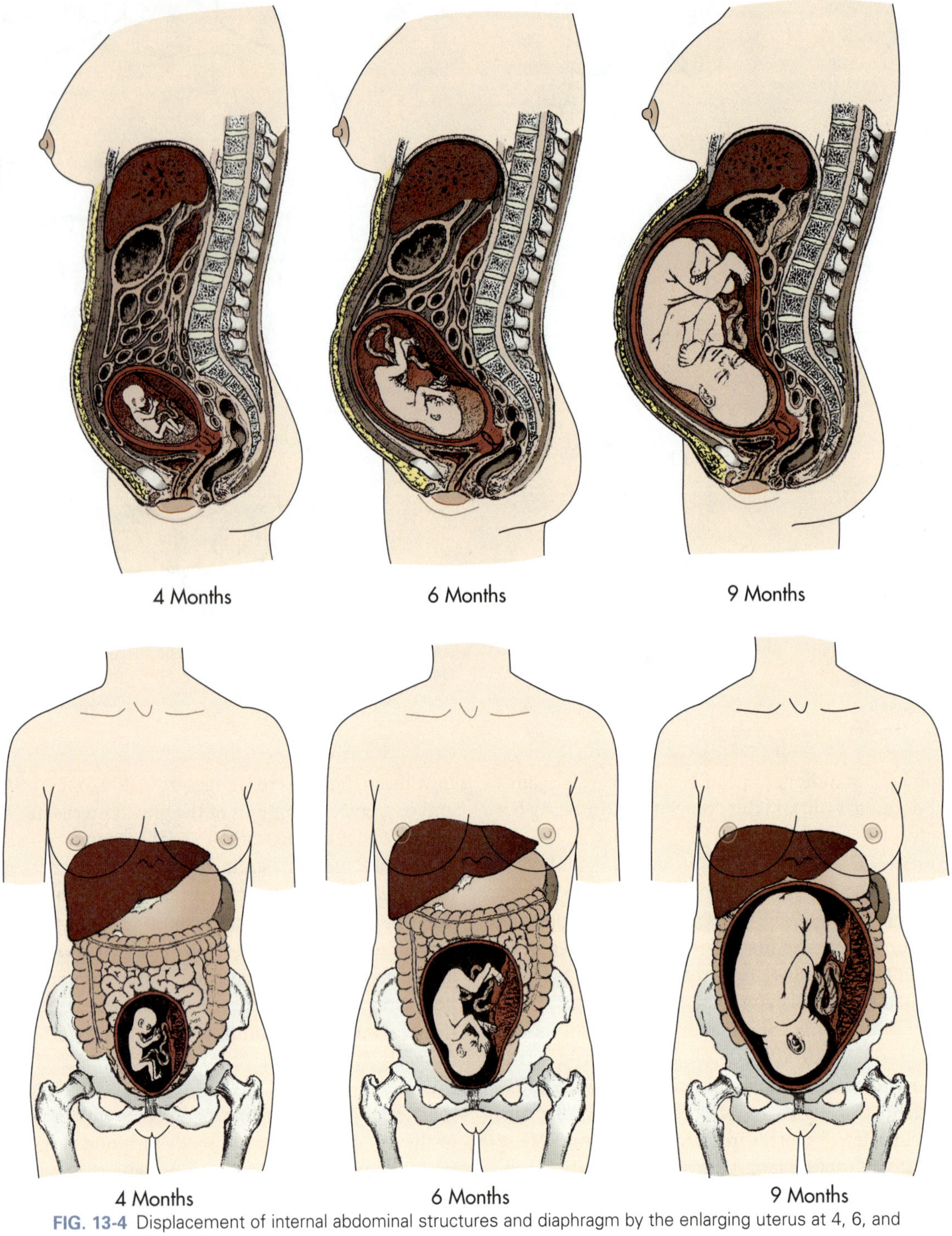

FIG. 13-4 Displacement of internal abdominal structures and diaphragm by the enlarging uterus at 4, 6, and 9 months of gestation.

assessment of all pregnant women is important, because about 3% of all cervical cancers are diagnosed during pregnancy (Copeland & Landon, 2007).

The cervix of the nullipara is rounded. Lacerations of the cervix almost always occur during the birth process. With or without lacerations, however, after childbirth the cervix becomes more oval in the horizontal plane, and the external os appears as a transverse slit (see Fig. 13-2).

Changes Related to the Presence of the Fetus. Passive movement of the unengaged fetus is called **ballottement** and can be identified generally between the sixteenth and eighteenth weeks. Ballottement is a technique of palpating a floating structure by bouncing it gently and feeling it rebound. In the technique used to palpate the fetus, the examiner places a finger in the vagina and taps gently upward, causing the fetus to rise. The fetus then sinks, and a gentle tap is felt on the finger (Fig. 13-6).

The first recognition of fetal movements, or "feeling life," by the multiparous woman may occur as early as the fourteenth to sixteenth weeks. The nulliparous woman may not notice these sensations until the eighteenth week or later. **Quickening** is commonly described as a flutter and is difficult to distinguish from peristalsis. Fetal movements gradually increase in intensity and frequency. The week when quickening occurs provides a tentative clue in dating the duration of gestation.

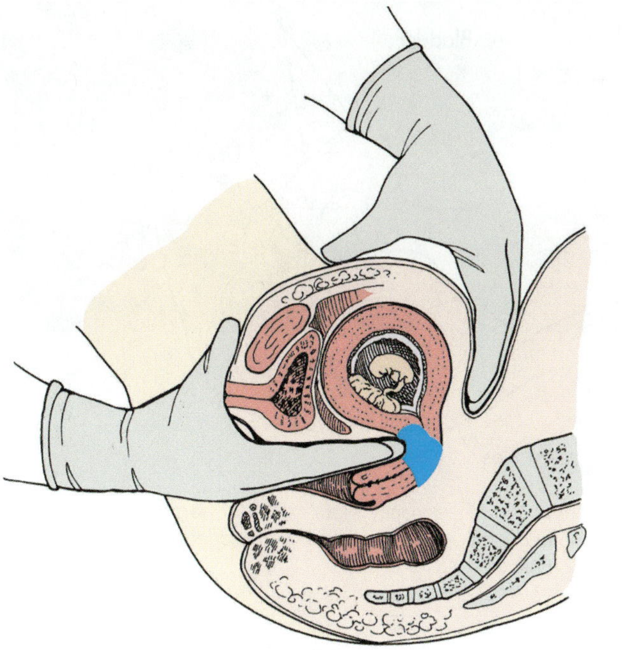

FIG. 13-5 Hegar sign. Bimanual examination for assessing compressibility and softening of the isthmus (lower uterine segment) while the cervix is still firm.

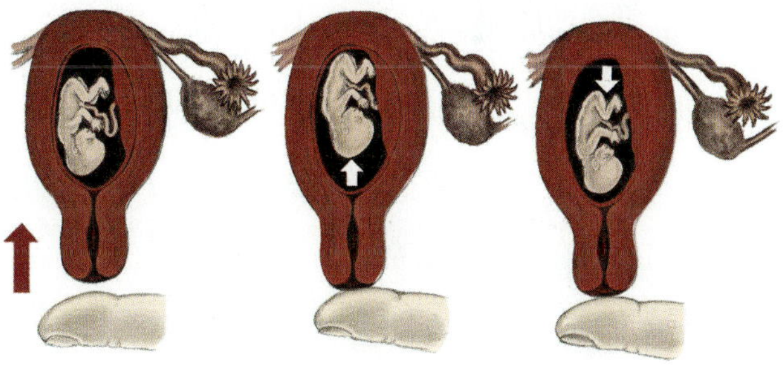

FIG. 13-6 Internal ballottement (18 weeks).

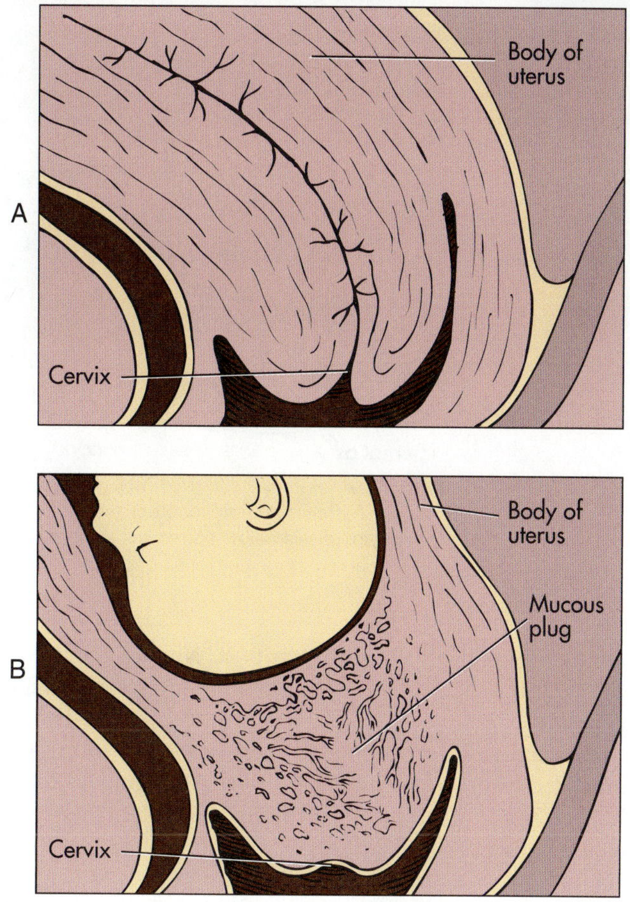

FIG. 13-7 **A,** Cervix in nonpregnant woman. **B,** Cervix during pregnancy.

Vagina and Vulva

Pregnancy hormones prepare the vagina for stretching during labor and birth by causing the vaginal mucosa to thicken, the connective tissue to loosen, the smooth muscle to hypertrophy, and the vaginal vault to lengthen. Increased vascularity results in a violet-bluish vaginal mucosa and cervix. The deepened color, termed the **Chadwick sign,** may be evident as early as the sixth week but is easily noted at the eighth week of pregnancy (Blackburn, 2007).

Leukorrhea is a white or slightly gray mucoid discharge with a faint musty odor. This copious mucoid fluid occurs in response to cervical stimulation by estrogen and progesterone. The fluid is whitish because of the presence of many exfoliated vaginal epithelial cells caused by the hyperplasia of normal pregnancy. This vaginal discharge is never pruritic or blood stained. Because of the progesterone effect, ferning usually does not occur in the dried cervical mucus smear as it would in a smear of amniotic fluid. Instead a beaded or cellular crystallizing pattern is seen in the dried mucus (Cunningham et al., 2010). The mucus fills the endocervical canal, resulting in the formation of the mucous plug **(operculum)** (Fig. 13-7). The operculum acts as a barrier against bacterial invasion during pregnancy.

During pregnancy the pH of vaginal secretions is more acidic than normal (ranging from approximately 3.5 to 6 [normal 4 to 5]) because of increased production of lactic acid (Cunningham et al., 2010). Although this acidic environment provides more protection from some organisms, the pregnant woman is more vulnerable to other infections, especially yeast infections because the glycogen-rich environment is more susceptible to *Candida albicans* (Duff, Sweet, & Edwards, 2009).

The increased vascularity of the vagina and other pelvic viscera results in a marked increase in sensitivity. The increased sensitivity may lead to a high degree of sexual interest and arousal, especially during the second trimester of pregnancy. The increased congestion plus the relaxed walls of the blood vessels and the heavy uterus may result in edema and varicosities of the vulva. The edema and varicosities usually resolve during the postpartum period.

External structures of the perineum are enlarged during pregnancy because of an increase in vasculature, hypertrophy of the perineal body, and deposition of fat (Fig. 13-8). The labia majora of the nullipara approximate and obscure the vaginal introitus; those of the parous woman separate and gape after childbirth and perineal or vaginal injury. Figure 13-2 compares the perineum of the nullipara and the multipara.

Breasts

Fullness, heightened sensitivity, tingling, and heaviness of the breasts occur in the early weeks of gestation in response to increased levels of estrogen and progesterone. Breast sensitivity

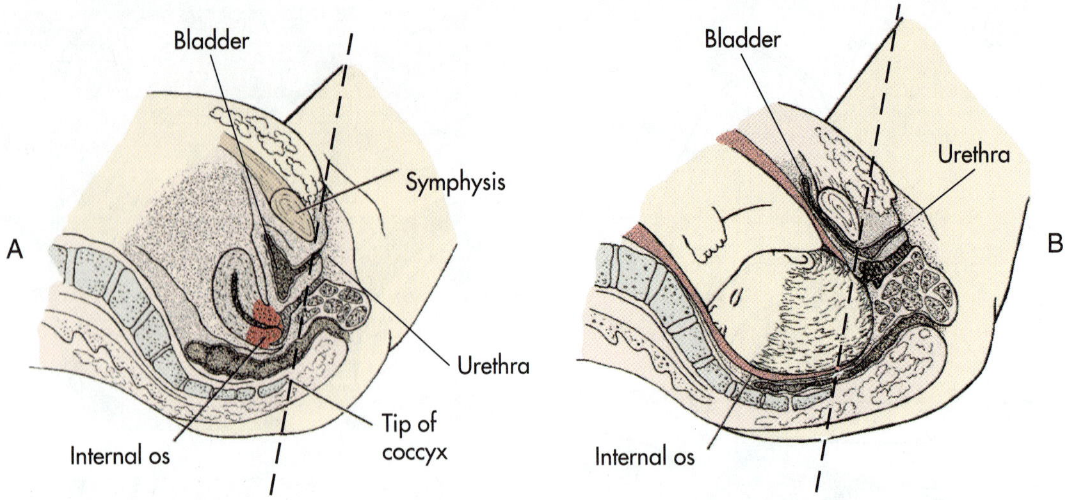

FIG. 13-8 **A,** Pelvic floor in nonpregnant woman. **B,** Pelvic floor at end of pregnancy. Note marked hypertrophy and hyperplasia below dotted line joining tip of coccyx and inferior margin of symphysis. Note elongation of bladder and urethra as a result of compression. Fat deposits are increased.

varies from mild tingling to sharp pain. Nipples and areolae become more pigmented, secondary pinkish areolae develop, extending beyond the primary areolae, and nipples become more erectile. Hypertrophy of the sebaceous (oil) glands embedded in the primary areolae, called **Montgomery tubercles** (see Fig. 4-6), may be seen around the nipples. These sebaceous glands may have a protective role in that they keep the nipples lubricated for breastfeeding.

The richer blood supply causes the vessels beneath the skin to dilate. Once barely noticeable, the blood vessels become visible, often appearing in an intertwining blue network beneath the surface of the skin. Venous congestion in the breasts is more obvious in primigravidas. Striae gravidarum may appear at the outer aspects of the breasts.

During the second and third trimesters, growth of the mammary glands accounts for the progressive breast enlargement. The high levels of luteal and placental hormones in pregnancy promote proliferation of the lactiferous ducts and lobule-alveolar tissue, so that palpation of the breasts reveals a generalized, coarse nodularity. Glandular tissue displaces connective tissue, and as a result, the tissue becomes softer and looser.

Although development of the mammary glands is functionally complete by midpregnancy, lactation is inhibited until a decrease in estrogen level occurs after the birth. A thin, clear, viscous secretory material (precolostrum) can be found in the acini cells by the third month of gestation. **Colostrum,** the creamy white-to-yellowish-to-orange premilk fluid, may be expressed from the nipples as early as 16 weeks of gestation (Blackburn, 2007). See Chapter 25 for discussion of lactation.

General Body Systems

Cardiovascular System

Maternal adjustments to pregnancy involve extensive changes in the cardiovascular system, both anatomic and physiologic. Cardiovascular adaptations protect the woman's normal physiologic functioning, meet the metabolic demands pregnancy imposes on her body, and provide for fetal developmental and growth needs.

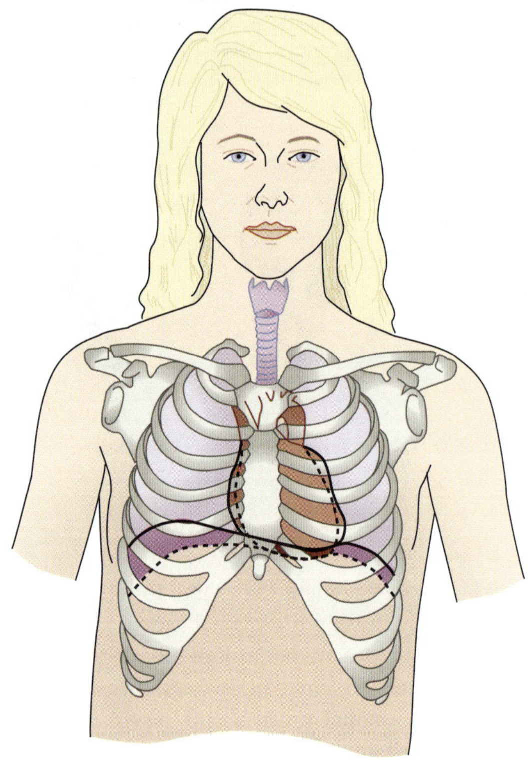

FIG. 13-9 Changes in position of heart, lungs, and thoracic cage in pregnancy. *Broken line,* nonpregnant; *solid line,* change that occurs in pregnancy.

Slight cardiac hypertrophy (enlargement) is probably secondary to the increased blood volume and cardiac output that occurs. The heart returns to its normal size after childbirth. As the diaphragm is displaced upward by the enlarging uterus, the heart is elevated upward and rotated forward to the left (Fig. 13-9). The apical impulse, a point of maximal intensity (PMI), is shifted upward and laterally about 1 to 1.5 cm. The degree of shift depends on the duration of pregnancy and the size and position of the uterus.

The changes in heart size and position and increases in blood volume and cardiac output contribute to auscultatory changes

BOX 13-1 BLOOD PRESSURE MEASUREMENT

- Use correct cuff size; cuff should cover approximately 80% of the upper arm or be 1.5 times the length of the upper arm.
- Measure BP after the woman sits for 5 minutes.
- Instruct the woman to refrain from tobacco or caffeine use 30 minutes before BP measurement.
- Measure blood pressure with the woman sitting or semi-reclining with her feet flat, not dangling.
- The arm should be supported on a desk at the level of the heart.
- Measurements with an automated device should be checked with a manual device.
- Diastolic pressure should be recorded at Korotkoff phase V (disappearance of sound).
- If the BP is elevated, have the woman rest for 5-10 minutes and then retake it.
- BP may vary by >10 mm Hg from one arm to the other; record the higher reading.
- Take the average of two readings at least 1 minute apart.

Source: Peters, R. (2008). High blood pressure in pregnancy. *Nursing for Women's Health, 12* (5), 412-421.

BOX 13-2 CALCULATION OF MEAN ARTERIAL PRESSURE

Blood pressure: 106/70 mm Hg

$$\text{Formula}: \frac{(\text{systolic}) + 2(\text{diastolic})}{3}$$

$$\frac{(106) + 2(70)}{3}$$

$$\frac{106 + 140}{3}$$

$$246/3 = 82 \text{ mm Hg}$$

common in pregnancy. There is more audible splitting of S_1 and S_2, and S_3 may be readily heard after 20 weeks of gestation. In addition, systolic and diastolic murmurs may be heard over the pulmonic area in some women. These are transient and disappear shortly after the woman gives birth (Cunningham et al., 2010).

Between 14 and 20 weeks of gestation, the pulse increases about 10 to 15 beats/min, which then persists to term. Palpitations may occur. In twin gestations the maternal heart rate increases significantly in the third trimester (Blackburn, 2007).

The cardiac rhythm may be disturbed. The pregnant woman may experience sinus arrhythmia, premature atrial contractions, and premature ventricular systole. In the healthy woman with no underlying heart disease, no therapy is needed; however, women with preexisting heart disease will need close medical and obstetric supervision during pregnancy (see Chapter 30).

Blood Pressure. Arterial blood pressure (brachial artery) is affected by age, activity level, presence of health problems, and circadian rhythm. Other factors include use of alcohol, smoking, and pain. Additional factors must be considered during pregnancy. These factors include maternal anxiety, maternal position, and size and type of blood pressure apparatus (Pickering, Hall, Appel, Falkner, Graves, Hill, et al., 2005).

Maternal anxiety can elevate readings. If an elevated reading is found, the woman is given time to rest, and the reading is repeated.

Maternal position affects readings. Brachial blood pressure is higher when the woman is sitting than when she is lying in the lateral recumbent position. The position of the arm can also make a difference in the measurement. If the arm is above the heart, the reading will be lower than the accurate reading; if held below the heart, the reading will be higher. Therefore at each prenatal visit the reading should be obtained in the same arm and with the woman in the same position with her back and arm supported and with her upper arm at the level of the right atrium (Monga, 2009; Pickering et al., 2005; Sibai, 2007). The position and arm used should be recorded along with the reading (Box 13-1).

The proper-size cuff is absolutely necessary for accurate readings. Too small a cuff yields a false high reading; too large a cuff yields a false low reading (Pickering et al., 2005).

Caution also should be used when comparing auscultatory and oscillatory blood pressure readings, because discrepancies can occur. Automated monitors may give inaccurate readings in women with hypertensive conditions (Gordon, 2007).

Systolic blood pressure usually remains the same as the prepregnancy level but may decrease slightly as pregnancy advances. Diastolic blood pressure begins to decrease in the first trimester, continues to drop until 24 to 32 weeks, then gradually increases and returns to prepregnancy levels by term (Blackburn, 2007).

Calculating the *mean arterial pressure (MAP)* (mean of the blood pressure in the arterial circulation) can increase the diagnostic value of the findings. Normal MAP readings in the nonpregnant woman are 86.4 mm Hg ± 7.5 mm Hg. MAP readings for a pregnant woman are slightly higher (Gordon, 2007). One way to calculate MAP is illustrated in Box 13-2.

Some degree of compression of the vena cava occurs in all women who lie flat on their backs during the second half of pregnancy (see Fig. 19-5). Some women experience a decrease in their systolic blood pressure of more than 30 mm Hg. After 4 to 5 minutes a reflex bradycardia is noted, cardiac output is reduced by half, and the woman feels faint. This condition is referred to as *supine hypotensive syndrome* (Cunningham et al., 2010).

Compression of the iliac veins and inferior vena cava by the uterus causes increased venous pressure and reduced blood flow in the legs (except when the woman is in the lateral position). These alterations contribute to the dependent edema, varicose veins in the legs and vulva, and hemorrhoids that develop in the latter part of term pregnancy (Fig. 13-10).

Blood Volume and Composition. The degree of blood volume expansion varies considerably. Blood volume increases by approximately 1500 ml, or 40% to 45% above nonpregnancy levels (Cunningham et al., 2010). This increase consists of 1000 ml plasma plus 450 ml red blood cells (RBCs). The blood volume starts to increase at about the tenth to twelfth week, peaks at about the thirty-second to thirty-fourth week, and then decreases slightly at the fortieth week. The increase in volume of a multiple gestation is greater than that for a pregnancy with a single fetus (Blackburn, 2007). Increased volume is a protective mechanism. It is essential for meeting the blood volume needs of the hypertrophied vascular system of

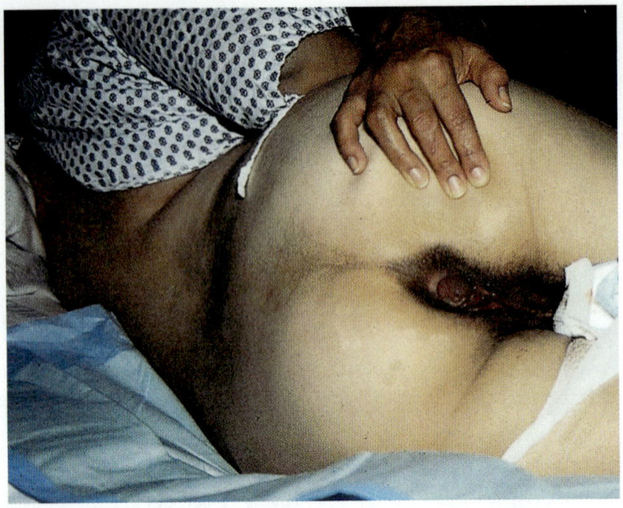

FIG. 13-10 Hemorrhoids. (Courtesy Marjorie Pyle, RNC, Lifecircle, Costa Mesa, CA.)

the enlarged uterus, for adequately hydrating fetal and maternal tissues when the woman assumes an erect or supine position, and for providing a fluid reserve to compensate for blood loss during birth and the puerperium. Peripheral vasodilation maintains a normal blood pressure despite the increased blood volume in pregnancy.

During pregnancy there is an accelerated production of RBCs (normal, 4.2 to 5.4 million/mm^3). The percentage of increase depends on the amount of iron available. The RBC mass increases by about 20% to 30% (Blackburn, 2007).

Because the plasma increase exceeds the increase in RBC production, a decrease occurs in normal hemoglobin values (12 to 16 g/dl blood [non-pregnant]) and hematocrit values (37% to 47% [non-pregnant]). This state of hemodilution is termed *physiologic anemia*. The decrease is more noticeable during the second trimester than at other times, when rapid expansion of blood volume takes place faster than RBC production. A hemoglobin value that drops below 11 g/dl should be considered abnormal and often is due to iron deficiency anemia (Samuels, 2007).

The total white cell count increases during the second trimester and peaks during the third trimester. This increase is primarily in the granulocytes; the lymphocyte count stays approximately the same throughout pregnancy. Table 13-3 lists the normal laboratory values during pregnancy.

Cardiac Output. Cardiac output increases from 30% to 50% over the nonpregnant rate by the thirty-second week of pregnancy; it declines to about a 20% increase at 40 weeks of gestation. This elevated cardiac output is caused by an increase in stroke volume and heart rate and occurs in response to increased tissue demands for oxygen (Monga, 2009). Cardiac output in late pregnancy is appreciably higher when the woman is in the lateral recumbent position than when she is supine. In the supine position the large, heavy uterus often impedes venous return to the heart and affects blood pressure. Cardiac output increases with any exertion, such as labor and birth. Table 13-4 summarizes cardiovascular changes in pregnancy.

Circulation and Coagulation Times. The circulation time decreases slightly by week 32. It returns to near normal close to term. There is a greater tendency for blood to coagulate (clot) during pregnancy because of increases in various clotting factors (factors VII, VIII, IX, X, and fibrinogen). This, combined with the fact that fibrinolytic activity (the splitting up or the dissolving of a clot) is depressed during pregnancy and the postpartum period, provides a protective function to decrease the chance of bleeding but also makes the woman more vulnerable to thrombosis, especially after cesarean birth.

Respiratory System

Structural and ventilatory adaptations occur during pregnancy to provide for maternal and fetal needs. Maternal oxygen requirements increase in response to the acceleration in the metabolic rate and the need to add to the tissue mass in the uterus and breasts. In addition, the fetus requires oxygen and a way to eliminate carbon dioxide.

Elevated levels of estrogen cause the ligaments of the rib cage to relax, permitting increased chest expansion (see Fig. 13-9). The transverse diameter of the thoracic cage increases by about 2 cm, and the circumference increases by 6 cm (Cunningham et al., 2010). The costal angle increases, and the lower rib cage appears to flare out. The chest may not return to its prepregnant state after birth (Seidel, Ball, Dains, Flynn, Solomon, & Stewart, 2011).

The diaphragm is displaced by as much as 4 cm during pregnancy. As pregnancy advances, thoracic (costal) breathing replaces abdominal breathing, and it becomes less possible for the diaphragm to descend with inspiration. Thoracic breathing is accomplished primarily by the diaphragm rather than by the costal muscles (Blackburn, 2007).

The upper respiratory tract becomes more vascular in response to elevated levels of estrogen. As the capillaries become engorged, edema and hyperemia develop within the nose, pharynx, larynx, trachea, and bronchi. This congestion within the tissues of the respiratory tract gives rise to several conditions commonly seen during pregnancy, including nasal and sinus stuffiness, epistaxis (nosebleed), changes in the voice, and a marked inflammatory response that can develop into a mild upper respiratory infection (Gordon, 2007).

Increased vascularity of the upper respiratory tract also can cause the tympanic membranes and eustachian tubes to swell, giving rise to symptoms of impaired hearing, earaches, or a sense of fullness in the ears.

Pulmonary Function. Respiratory changes in pregnancy are related to the elevation of the diaphragm and to chest wall changes. Changes in the respiratory center result in a lowered threshold for carbon dioxide. The actions of progesterone and estrogen are presumed responsible for the increased sensitivity of the respiratory center to carbon dioxide. (Table 13-5 summarizes respiratory changes in pregnancy.) Although pulmonary function is not impaired by pregnancy, diseases of the respiratory tract may be more serious during this time (Cunningham et al., 2010). One important factor responsible for this circumstance may be the increased oxygen requirement

Basal Metabolic Rate. The basal metabolic rate (BMR) increases during pregnancy. This increase varies considerably depending on the prepregnancy nutritional status of the woman and fetal growth (Blackburn, 2007). The BMR returns to nonpregnant levels by 5 to 6 days after birth. The elevation in BMR during pregnancy reflects increased oxygen demands

TABLE 13-3 LABORATORY VALUES FOR PREGNANT AND NONPREGNANT WOMEN

VALUES	NONPREGNANT	PREGNANT
Hematologic		
Complete Blood Count (CBC)		
Hemoglobin (g/dl)	12-16*	>11*
Hematocrit, PCV (%)	37-47	>33*
Red blood cell (RBC) volume (per ml)	1400	1650
Plasma volume (per ml)	2400	40%-60% increase
RBC count (million per mm^3)	4.2-5.4	5-6.25
White blood cells (total per mm^3)	5000-10,000	5000-15,000
Neutrophils (%)	55-70	60-85
Lymphocytes (%)	20-40	15-40
Erythrocyte sedimentation rate (mm/hr)	20	Elevated in second and third trimesters
Mean corpuscular hemoglobin concentration (MCHC) (g/dl packed RBCs)	32-36	No change
Mean corpuscular hemoglobin (MCH) (pg)	27-31	No change
Mean corpuscular volume (MCV), per mm^3	80-95	No change
Blood coagulation and fibrinolytic activity†		
Factor VII	65-140	Increase in pregnancy, return to normal in early puerperium
Factor VIII	55-145	Increases during pregnancy and immediately after birth
Factor IX	60-140	Same as factor VII
Factor X	45-155	Same as factor VII
Factor XI	65-135	Decrease in pregnancy
Factor XII	50-150	Same as factor VII
Prothrombin time (PT) (sec)	11-12.5	Slight decrease in pregnancy
Partial thromboplastin time (PTT) (sec)	60-70	Slight decrease in pregnancy and decrease during second and third stage of labor (indicates clotting at placental site)
Bleeding time (min)	1-9 (Ivy)	No appreciable change
Coagulation time (min)	6-10 (Lee/White)	No appreciable change
Platelets per (mm^3)	150,000-400,000	No significant change until 3-5 days after birth and then a rapid increase (may predispose woman to thrombosis) and gradual return to normal
Fibrinolytic activity	Normal	Decreases in pregnancy and then abruptly returns to normal (protection against thromboembolism)
Fibrinogen (mg/dl)	200-400	Increased levels late in pregnancy
Mineral and vitamin concentrations		
Vitamin B_{12}, folic acid, ascorbic acid	Normal	Moderate decrease
Serum proteins		
Total (g/dl)	6.4-8.3	5.5-7.5
Albumin (g/dl)	3.5-5	Slight increase
Globulin, total (g/dl)	2.3-3.4	3-4
Blood glucose		
Fasting (mg/dl)	70-105	Decreases
2-hr postprandial (mg/dl)	<140	<140 after a 100-g carbohydrate meal is considered normal
Acid-base values in arterial blood		
Po_2 (mm Hg)	80-100	104-108 (increased)
Pco_2 (mm Hg)	35-45	27-32 (decreased)
Sodium bicarbonate (HCO_3) (mEq/L)	21-28	18-31 (decreased)
Blood pH	7.35-7.45	7.40-7.45 (slightly increased, more alkaline)
Hepatic		
Bilirubin, total (mg/dl)	≤1	Unchanged
Serum cholesterol (mg/dl)	120-200	Increases from 16-32 weeks of pregnancy; remains at this level until after birth
Serum alkaline phosphatase, units/L	30-120	Increases from week 12 of pregnancy to 6 weeks after birth
Serum albumin (g/dl)	3.5-5	Slight decrease
Renal		
Bladder capacity (ml)	1300	1500
Renal plasma flow (RPF) (ml/min)	490-700	Increase by 25%-30%
Glomerular filtration rate (GFR) (ml/min)	88-128	Increase by 30%-50%
Nonprotein nitrogen (NPN) (mg/dl)	25-40	Decreases
Blood urea nitrogen (BUN) (mg/dl)	10-20	Decreases
Serum creatinine (mg/dl)	0.5-1.1	Decreases
Serum uric acid (mg/dl)	2.7-7.3	Decreases but returns to prepregnancy level by end of pregnancy
Urine glucose	Negative	Present in 20% of pregnant women
Intravenous pyelogram (IVP)	Normal	Slight to moderate hydroureter and hydronephrosis; right kidney larger than left kidney

*At sea level. Permanent residents of higher altitudes (e.g., Denver) require higher levels of hemoglobin.
†Pregnancy represents a hypercoagulable state.
ng, Nanogram; *pg*, picogram; *PCV*, packed cell volume.
Source: Blackburn, S. (2007). *Maternal, fetal, & neonatal physiology: A clinical perspective* (3rd ed.). St. Louis: Saunders; Gordon, M. (2007). Maternal physiology. In S. Gabbe, J. Niebyl, & J. Simpson (Eds.), *Obstetrics: Normal and problem pregnancies* (5th ed.). Philadelphia: Churchill Livingstone; Pagana, K., & Pagana, T. (2009). *Mosby's diagnostic and laboratory test reference* (9th ed.). St. Louis: Mosby.

TABLE 13-4 CARDIOVASCULAR CHANGES IN PREGNANCY

Heart rate	Increases 10-15 beats/min
Blood pressure	Systolic: slight or no decrease from prepregnancy levels Diastolic: slight decrease to midpregnancy (24-32 weeks) and gradually returns to prepregnancy levels by the end of pregnancy
Blood volume	Increases by 1500 ml or 40%-50% above prepregnancy level
Red blood cell mass	Increases 18%
Hemoglobin	Decreases
Hematocrit	Decreases
White blood cell count	Increases in second and third trimesters
Cardiac output	Increases 30%-50%

Source: Gordon, M. (2007). Maternal physiology. In S. Gabbe, J. Niebyl, & J. Simpson (Eds.), *Obstetrics: Normal and problem pregnancies* (5th ed.). Philadelphia: Churchill Livingstone.

TABLE 13-5 RESPIRATORY CHANGES IN PREGNANCY

Respiratory rate	Unchanged or slightly increased
Tidal volume	Increased 30%-40%
Vital capacity	Unchanged
Inspiratory capacity	Increased
Expiratory volume	Decreased
Total lung capacity	Unchanged to slightly decreased
Oxygen consumption	Increased 20%-40%

Source: Gordon, M. (2007). Maternal physiology. In S. Gabbe, J. Niebyl, & J. Simpson (Eds.), *Obstetrics: Normal and problem pregnancies* (5th ed.). Philadelphia: Churchill Livingstone.

of the uterine-placental-fetal unit and greater oxygen consumption because of increased maternal cardiac work. Peripheral vasodilation and acceleration of sweat gland activity help dissipate the excess heat resulting from the increased BMR during pregnancy. Pregnant women experience heat intolerance, which is annoying to some women. Lassitude and fatigability after only slight exertion are experienced by many women in early pregnancy. These feelings, along with a greater need for sleep, may persist and may be caused in part by the increased metabolic activity.

Acid-Base Balance. By about the tenth week of pregnancy, there is a decrease of about 5 mm Hg in the partial pressure of carbon dioxide (Pco_2). Progesterone may be responsible for increasing the sensitivity of the respiratory center receptors, so that tidal volume is increased, Pco_2 decreases, the base excess (HCO_3 or bicarbonate) decreases, and pH increases slightly. These alterations in acid-base balance indicate that pregnancy is a state of compensatory respiratory alkalosis (Gordon, 2007). These changes also facilitate the transport of CO_2 from the fetus and O_2 release from the mother to the fetus (see Table 13-3).

Renal System

The kidneys are responsible for maintaining electrolyte and acid-base balance, regulating extracellular fluid volume, excreting waste products, and conserving essential nutrients.

Anatomic Changes. Changes in renal structure during pregnancy result from hormonal activity (estrogen and progesterone), pressure from an enlarging uterus, and an increase in blood volume. As early as the tenth week of pregnancy, the renal pelves and the ureters dilate. Dilation of the ureters is more pronounced above the pelvic brim, in part because they are compressed between the uterus and the pelvic brim. In most women, the ureters below the pelvic brim are of normal size. The smooth-muscle walls of the ureters undergo hyperplasia, hypertrophy, and muscle tone relaxation. The ureters elongate, become tortuous, and form single or double curves. In the latter part of pregnancy, the renal pelvis and ureter are dilated more on the right side than on the left because the heavy uterus is displaced to the right by the sigmoid colon.

Because of these changes, a larger volume of urine is held in the pelves and ureters, and urine flow rate is slowed. The resulting urinary stasis or stagnation has the following consequences:

- A lag occurs between the time urine is formed and when it reaches the bladder. Therefore clearance test results may reflect substances contained in glomerular filtrate several hours before.
- Stagnated urine is an excellent medium for the growth of microorganisms. In addition, the urine of pregnant women contains more nutrients, including glucose, thereby increasing the pH (making the urine more alkaline). This makes pregnant women more susceptible to urinary tract infection.

Bladder irritability, nocturia, and urinary frequency and urgency (without dysuria) are commonly reported in early pregnancy. Near term, bladder symptoms may return, especially after lightening occurs.

Urinary frequency results initially from increased bladder sensitivity and later from compression of the bladder (see Fig. 13-8). In the second trimester, the bladder is pulled up out of the true pelvis into the abdomen. The urethra lengthens to 7.5 cm as the bladder is displaced upward. The pelvic congestion that occurs in pregnancy is reflected in hyperemia of the bladder and urethra. This increased vascularity causes the bladder mucosa to be traumatized and bleed easily. Bladder tone may decrease, which increases the bladder capacity to 1500 ml. At the same time, the bladder is compressed by the enlarging uterus, resulting in the urge to void even if the bladder contains only a small amount of urine.

Functional Changes. In normal pregnancy, renal function is altered considerably. Glomerular filtration rate (GFR) and renal plasma flow (RPF) increase early in pregnancy (Monga, 2009). These changes are caused by pregnancy hormones, an increase in blood volume, the woman's posture, physical activity, and nutritional intake. The woman's kidneys must manage the increased metabolic and circulatory demands of the maternal body and the excretion of fetal waste products. Renal function is most efficient when the woman lies in the lateral recumbent position and least efficient when the woman assumes a supine position. A side-lying position increases renal perfusion, which increases urinary output and decreases edema. When the pregnant woman is lying supine, the heavy uterus compresses the vena cava and the aorta, and cardiac output decreases. As a result, blood flow to the brain and heart is continued at the expense of other organs, including the kidneys and uterus.

Fluid and Electrolyte Balance. Selective renal tubular reabsorption maintains sodium and water balance regardless of changes in dietary intake and losses through sweat, vomitus, or diarrhea. From 500 to 900 mEq of sodium is normally retained during pregnancy to meet fetal needs. To prevent excessive sodium depletion, the maternal kidneys undergo a significant adaptation by increasing tubular reabsorption. Because of the need for increased maternal intravascular and extracellular fluid volume, additional sodium is needed to expand fluid volume and to maintain an isotonic state. As efficient as the renal system is, it can be overstressed by excessive dietary sodium intake or restriction or by use of diuretics. Severe hypovolemia and reduced placental perfusion are two consequences of using diuretics during pregnancy.

The capacity of the kidneys to excrete water during the early weeks of pregnancy is more efficient than it is later in pregnancy. As a result, some women feel thirsty in early pregnancy because of the greater amount of water loss. The pooling of fluid in the legs in the latter part of pregnancy decreases renal blood flow and GFR. This pooling of blood in the lower legs is sometimes referred to as *physiologic edema* or dependent edema and requires no treatment. The normal diuretic response to the water load is triggered when the woman lies down, preferably on her side, and the pooled fluid reenters general circulation.

Normally the kidney reabsorbs almost all of the glucose and other nutrients from the plasma filtrate. In pregnant women, however, tubular reabsorption of glucose is impaired, so that glucosuria occurs at varying times and to varying degrees. Normal values range from 0 to 20 mg/dl, meaning that during any day, the urine is sometimes positive and sometimes negative for glucose. In nonpregnant women, blood glucose levels must be at 160 to 180 mg/dl before glucose is "spilled" into the urine (not reabsorbed). During pregnancy, glucosuria (glycosuria) occurs when maternal glucose levels are lower than 160 mg/dl. Why glucose, as well as other nutrients such as amino acids, is wasted during pregnancy is not understood, nor has the exact mechanism been discovered. Although glucosuria may be found in normal pregnancies (2+ levels may be seen with increased anxiety states), the possibility of pregestational or gestational diabetes mellitus must be kept in mind.

Proteinuria usually does not occur in normal pregnancy except during labor or after birth (Cunningham et al., 2010). However, the increased amount of amino acids that must be filtered may exceed the capacity of the renal tubules to absorb it; thus small amounts of protein are then lost in the urine. The amount of protein excreted is not an indication of the severity of renal disease, nor does an increase in protein excretion in a pregnant woman with known renal disease necessarily indicate a progression in her disease. However, a pregnant woman with hypertension and proteinuria must be carefully evaluated because she may be at greater risk for an adverse pregnancy outcome (Gordon, 2007) (see Table 13-3).

Integumentary System

Alterations in hormonal balance and mechanical stretching are responsible for several changes in the integumentary system during pregnancy. Hyperpigmentation is stimulated by the anterior pituitary hormone melanotropin, which is increased during pregnancy. Darkening of the nipples, the areolae, the axillae, and the vulva occurs about the sixteenth week of gestation. Facial melasma, also called **chloasma** or mask of pregnancy, is a blotchy, brownish hyperpigmentation of the skin over the cheeks, nose, and forehead, especially in dark-complexioned pregnant women. Chloasma appears in 50% to 70% of pregnant women, beginning after the sixteenth week and increasing gradually until term. The sun intensifies this pigmentation in susceptible women. Chloasma caused by normal pregnancy usually fades after birth.

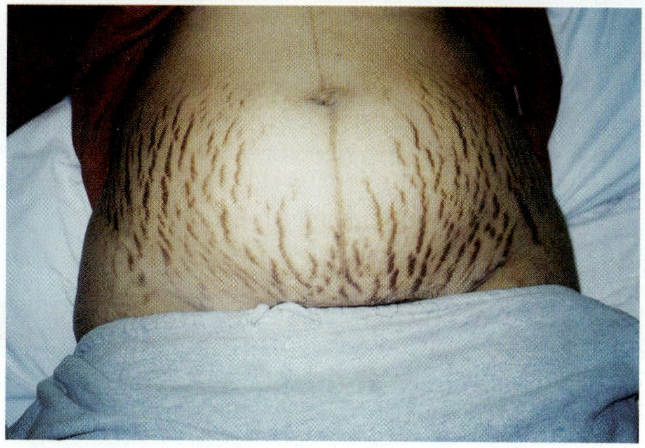

FIG. 13-11 Striae gravidarum and linea nigra in a dark-skinned woman. (Courtesy Shannon Perry, Phoenix, AZ.)

The **linea nigra** (Fig. 13-11) is a pigmented line extending from the symphysis pubis to the top of the fundus in the midline; this line is known as the *linea alba* before hormone-induced pigmentation. In primigravidas the extension of the linea nigra, beginning in the third month, keeps pace with the rising height of the fundus; in multigravidas, the entire line often appears earlier than the third month. Not all pregnant women develop linea nigra, and some women notice hair growth along the line with or without the change in pigmentation.

Striae gravidarum, or stretch marks (seen over lower abdomen in Fig. 13-11), which appear in 50% to 90% of pregnant women during the second half of pregnancy, may be caused by action of adrenocorticosteroids. Striae reflect separation within the underlying connective (collagen) tissue of the skin. These slightly depressed streaks tend to occur over areas of maximal stretch (i.e., abdomen, thighs, and breasts). The stretching sometimes causes a sensation that resembles itching. The tendency to develop striae may be familial. After birth they usually fade, although they never disappear completely. Color of striae varies depending on the pregnant woman's skin color. The striae appear pinkish on a woman with light skin and are lighter than surrounding skin in dark-skinned women. In the multipara, in addition to the striae of the present pregnancy, glistening silvery lines (in light-skinned women) or purplish lines (in dark-skinned women) are commonly seen. These represent the scars of striae from previous pregnancies.

Angiomas are commonly referred to as *vascular spiders.* They are tiny, star-shaped or branched, slightly raised and pulsating end-arterioles usually found on the neck, thorax, face, and arms. They occur as a result of elevated levels of circulating estrogen. The spiders are bluish in color and do not blanch with pressure. Vascular spiders appear during the second to the fifth month of pregnancy in almost 65% of Caucasian women and 10% of

African-American women. The spiders usually disappear after birth (Blackburn, 2007).

Pinkish-red, diffuse mottling or well-defined blotches are seen over the palmar surfaces of the hands in about 60% of Caucasian women and 35% of African-American women during pregnancy (Blackburn, 2007). These color changes, called **palmar erythema,** are related primarily to increased estrogen levels.

> **! NURSING ALERT**
>
> Because integumentary system changes vary greatly among women of different racial backgrounds, the color of a woman's skin should be noted along with any changes that may be attributed to pregnancy when performing physical assessments.

Some dermatologic conditions have been identified as unique to pregnancy or as having an increased incidence during pregnancy. Mild pruritus (pruritus gravidarum) is a relatively common dermatologic symptom in pregnancy. The problem usually resolves in the postpartum period (Papoutsis & Kroumpouzos, 2007). Systemic diseases can also cause pruritus, but these causes are uncommon or rare (Cappell, 2007). Preexisting skin diseases may complicate pregnancy or be improved. (See Chapter 30 for further discussion.)

Gum hypertrophy may occur. An **epulis** (gingival granuloma gravidarum) is a red, raised nodule on the gums that bleeds easily. This lesion may develop around the third month and usually continues to enlarge as pregnancy progresses. It is usually managed by avoiding trauma to the gums (e.g., using a soft toothbrush). An epulis usually regresses spontaneously after birth.

Nail growth may be accelerated. Some women may notice thinning and softening of the nails. Oily skin and acne vulgaris may occur during pregnancy. For some women, the skin clears and looks radiant. Hirsutism, the excessive growth of hair or growth of hair in unusual places, is commonly reported. An increase in fine hair growth may occur but tends to disappear after pregnancy; however, growth of coarse or bristly hair does not usually disappear. The rate of scalp hair loss slows during pregnancy, while increased hair loss may be noted in the postpartum period.

Increased blood supply to the skin leads to increased perspiration. Women feel hotter during pregnancy, a condition possibly related to a progesterone-induced increase in body temperature and the increased BMR.

Musculoskeletal System

The gradually changing body and increasing weight of the pregnant woman cause noticeable alterations in her posture (Fig. 13-12) and the way she walks. The great abdominal distention that gives the pelvis a forward tilt, decreased abdominal muscle tone, and increased weight bearing require a realignment of the spinal curvature late in pregnancy. The woman's center of gravity shifts forward. An increase in the normal lumbosacral curve (lordosis) develops, and a compensatory curvature in the cervicodorsal region (exaggerated anterior flexion of the head) develops to help her maintain her balance. Aching, numbness, and weakness of the upper extremities may result. Large breasts and a stoop-shouldered stance will further accentuate the lumbar and dorsal curves. Walking is more difficult, and the waddling gait of the pregnant woman, called "the proud walk of pregnancy" by Shakespeare, is commonly seen. The ligamentous and muscular structures of the middle and lower spine may be severely stressed. These and related changes often cause musculoskeletal discomfort, especially in older women or those with a back disorder or a faulty sense of balance.

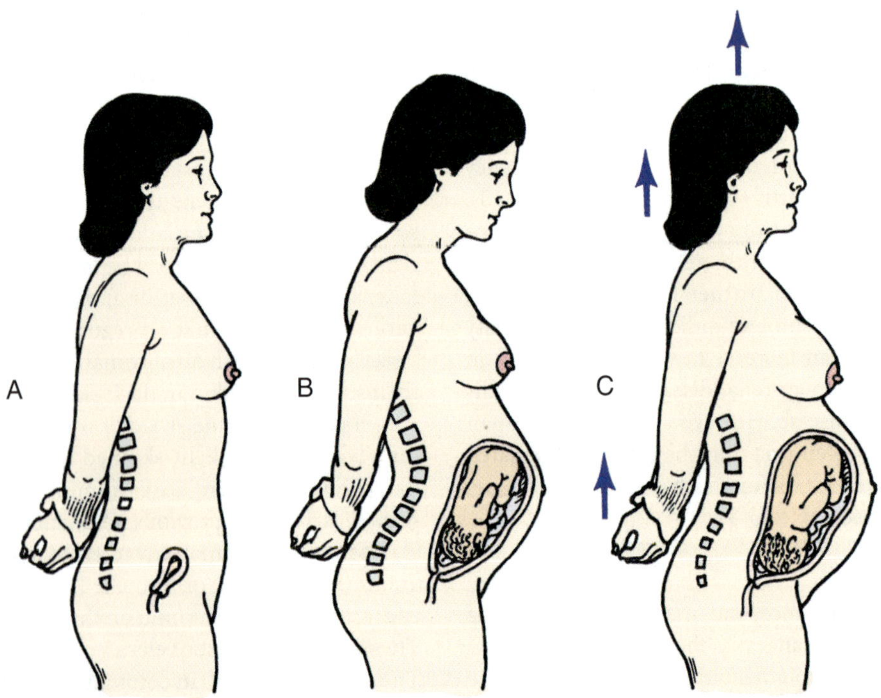

FIG. 13-12 Postural changes during pregnancy. **A,** Nonpregnant posture. **B,** Incorrect posture during pregnancy. **C,** Correct posture during pregnancy.

Slight relaxation and increased mobility of the pelvic joints are normal during pregnancy. These adaptations permit enlargement of pelvic dimensions to facilitate labor and birth. The degree of relaxation varies, but considerable separation of the symphysis pubis and the instability of the sacroiliac joints may cause pain and difficulty in walking. Obesity and multifetal pregnancy tend to increase the pelvic instability. Peripheral joint laxity also increases as pregnancy progresses, but the cause is not known (Murray & Hassall, 2009).

The muscles of the abdominal wall stretch and ultimately lose some tone. During the third trimester, the rectus abdominis muscles may separate (Fig. 13-13), allowing abdominal contents to protrude at the midline. The umbilicus flattens or protrudes. After birth, the muscles gradually regain tone; however, separation of the muscles **(diastasis recti abdominis)** may persist.

Neurologic System

Little is known regarding specific alterations in function of the neurologic system during pregnancy, aside from hypothalamic-pituitary neurohormonal changes. Specific physiologic alterations resulting from pregnancy may cause the following neurologic or neuromuscular symptoms:

- Compression of pelvic nerves or vascular stasis caused by enlargement of the uterus may result in sensory changes in the legs.
- Dorsolumbar lordosis may cause pain because of traction on nerves or compression of nerve roots.
- Edema involving the peripheral nerves may result in **carpal tunnel syndrome** during the last trimester (Samuels & Niebyl, 2007). The syndrome is characterized by paresthesia (abnormal sensation such as burning or tingling) and pain in the hand, radiating to the elbow. The sensations are caused by edema that compresses the median nerve beneath the carpal ligament of the wrist. Smoking and alcohol consumption can impair the microcirculation and may worsen the symptoms. The dominant hand is usually affected most, although as many as 80% of women experience symptoms in both hands. Symptoms usually regress after pregnancy. In some cases, surgical treatment may be necessary (Samuels & Niebyl).

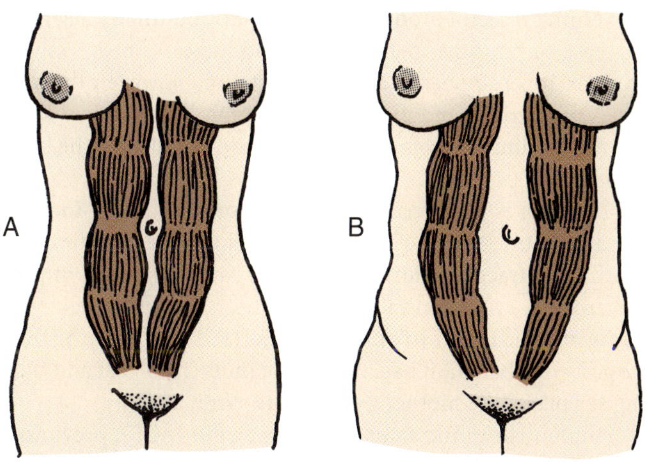

FIG. 13-13 Possible change in rectus abdominis muscles during pregnancy. **A,** Normal position in nonpregnant woman. **B,** Diastasis recti abdominis in pregnant woman.

- Acroesthesia (numbness and tingling of the hands) is caused by the stoop-shouldered stance (see Fig. 13-12, *B*) assumed by some women during pregnancy. The condition is associated with traction on segments of the brachial plexus.
- Tension headache is common when anxiety or uncertainty complicates pregnancy. However, vision problems, sinusitis, or migraine also may be responsible for headaches.
- "Light-headedness," faintness, and even syncope (fainting) are common during early pregnancy. Vasomotor instability, postural hypotension, or hypoglycemia may be responsible.
- Hypocalcemia can cause neuromuscular problems such as muscle cramps or tetany.

Gastrointestinal System

Appetite. During pregnancy, the woman's appetite and food intake fluctuate. Early in pregnancy, some women have nausea with or without vomiting (morning sickness), possibly in response to increasing levels of hCG and altered carbohydrate metabolism (Gordon, 2007). Morning sickness or nausea and vomiting of pregnancy (NVP) appears at about 4 to 6 weeks of gestation and usually subsides by the end of the third month (first trimester) of pregnancy (see Chapter 15). Severity varies from mild distaste for certain foods to more severe vomiting. The condition may be triggered by the sight or odor of various foods. By the end of the second trimester, the appetite increases in response to increasing metabolic needs. Rarely does NVP have harmful effects on the embryo, fetus, or the woman. Whenever the vomiting is severe or persists beyond the first trimester, or when it is accompanied by fever, pain, or weight loss, further evaluation is necessary, and medical intervention is likely (see Chapter 29).

Women also may have changes in their sense of taste, leading to cravings and changes in dietary intake. Some women have nonfood cravings (called *pica*), such as for ice, clay, and laundry starch. Usually the subjects of these cravings, if consumed in moderation, are not harmful to the pregnancy if the woman has adequate nutrition with appropriate weight gain (Gordon, 2007). See Chapter 14 for a discussion of nutrition in pregnancy.

Mouth. The gums become hyperemic, spongy, and swollen during pregnancy. They tend to bleed easily because the increasing levels of estrogen cause selective increased vascularity and connective tissue proliferation (a nonspecific gingivitis). Epulis (discussed in the section on the integumentary system) may develop at the gumline. Some pregnant women complain of **ptyalism** (excessive salivation), which may be caused by the decrease in unconscious swallowing by the woman when nauseated or from stimulation of salivary glands by eating starch (Cunningham et al., 2010).

Esophagus, Stomach, and Intestines. Herniation of the upper portion of the stomach (hiatal hernia) occurs after the seventh or eighth month of pregnancy in about 15% to 20% of pregnant women. This condition results from upward displacement of the stomach, which causes the hiatus of the diaphragm to widen. It occurs more often in multiparas and older or obese women.

Increased estrogen production causes decreased secretion of hydrochloric acid; therefore peptic ulcer formation or flare-up of existing peptic ulcers is uncommon during pregnancy and symptoms may improve (Gordon, 2007).

Increased progesterone production causes decreased tone and motility of smooth muscles, resulting in esophageal regurgitation, slower emptying time of the stomach, and reverse peristalsis. As a result, the woman may experience "acid indigestion" or heartburn (pyrosis) beginning as early as the first trimester and intensifying through the third trimester.

Iron is absorbed more readily in the small intestine in response to increased needs during pregnancy. Even when the woman is deficient in iron, it will continue to be absorbed in sufficient amounts for the fetus to have a normal hemoglobin level.

Increased progesterone (causing loss of muscle tone and decreased peristalsis) results in an increase in water absorption from the colon and may cause constipation. Constipation also may result from hypoperistalsis (sluggishness of the bowel), food choices, lack of fluids, iron supplementation, decreased activity level, abdominal distention by the pregnant uterus, and displacement and compression of the intestines. If the pregnant woman has hemorrhoids (see Fig. 13-10) and is constipated, the hemorrhoids may become everted or may bleed during straining at stool.

Gallbladder and Liver. The gallbladder is quite often distended because of its decreased muscle tone during pregnancy. Increased emptying time and thickening of bile caused by prolonged retention are typical changes. These features, together with slight hypercholesterolemia from increased progesterone levels, may account for the development of gallstones during pregnancy.

Hepatic function is difficult to appraise during pregnancy; however, only minor changes in liver function develop. Occasionally, *intrahepatic cholestasis* (retention and accumulation of bile in the liver, caused by factors within the liver) occurs late in pregnancy in response to placental steroids and may result in pruritus gravidarum (severe itching) with or without jaundice (Cappell, 2007) (see Chapter 30).

Abdominal Discomfort. Intraabdominal alterations that can cause discomfort include pelvic heaviness or pressure, round ligament tension, flatulence, distention and bowel cramping, and uterine contractions. In addition to displacement of intestines, pressure from the expanding uterus causes an increase in venous pressure in the pelvic organs. Although most abdominal discomfort is a consequence of normal maternal alterations, the health care provider must be constantly alert to the possibility of disorders such as bowel obstruction or an inflammatory process.

Appendicitis may be difficult to diagnose in pregnancy because the appendix is displaced upward and laterally, high and to the right, away from McBurney's point (Fig. 13-14).

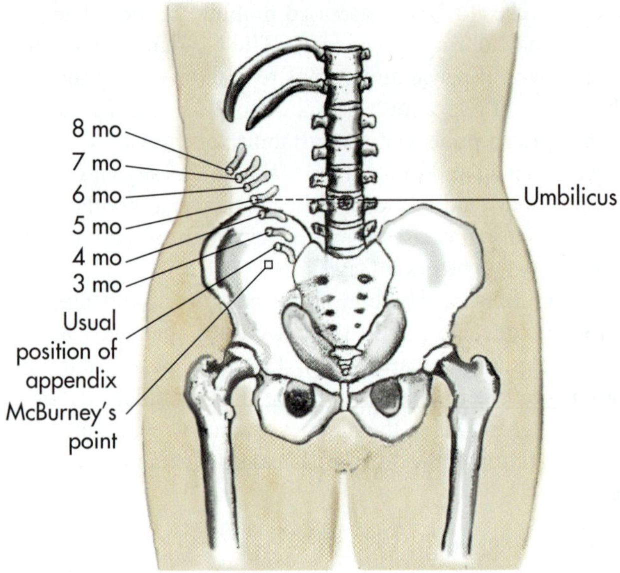

FIG. 13-14 Change in position of appendix in pregnancy. Note McBurney's point.

Endocrine System

Profound endocrine changes are essential for pregnancy maintenance, normal fetal growth, and postpartum recovery.

Pituitary and Placental Hormones. During pregnancy, the elevated levels of estrogen and progesterone (produced first by the corpus luteum in the ovary until about 14 weeks of gestation and then by the placenta) suppress secretion of follicle-stimulating hormone (FSH) and luteinizing hormone (LH) by the anterior pituitary. The maturation of a follicle and ovulation do not occur. Although the majority of women have amenorrhea (absence of menses), at least 20% have some slight, painless spotting during early gestation. Implantation bleeding and bleeding after intercourse related to cervical friability can occur. Most of the women experiencing slight gestational bleeding continue to term and have normal infants; however, all instances of bleeding should be reported and evaluated.

After implantation, the fertilized ovum and the chorionic villi produce hCG, which maintains the production by the corpus luteum of estrogen and progesterone until the placenta takes over production (Burton et al., 2007).

Progesterone is essential for maintaining pregnancy by relaxing smooth muscles, resulting in decreased uterine contractility and prevention of miscarriage. Progesterone and estrogen cause fat to deposit in subcutaneous tissues over the maternal abdomen, back, and upper thighs. This fat serves as an energy reserve for both pregnancy and lactation. Estrogen also promotes the enlargement of the genitals, the uterus, and the breasts and increases vascularity, causing vasodilation. Estrogen causes relaxation of pelvic ligaments and joints. It also alters metabolism of nutrients by interfering with folic acid metabolism, increasing the level of total body proteins, and promoting retention of sodium and water by kidney tubules. Estrogen may decrease secretion of hydrochloric acid and pepsin, which may be responsible for digestive upsets such as nausea.

Serum prolactin produced by the anterior pituitary begins to increase early in the first trimester and increases progressively to term. It is responsible for initial lactation; however, the high levels of estrogen and progesterone inhibit lactation by blocking the binding of prolactin to breast tissue until after the birth (Gordon, 2007).

Oxytocin is produced by the posterior pituitary in increasing amounts as the fetus matures. This hormone can stimulate uterine contractions during pregnancy, but high levels of progesterone prevent contractions until near term. Oxytocin also stimulates the let-down or milk-ejection reflex after the birth in response to the infant's sucking at the mother's breast and during sex play if the mother's nipples are stimulated .

Human chorionic somatomammotropin (hCS), previously called human placental lactogen, is produced by the placenta and has been suggested to act as a growth hormone and contribute to breast development. It also may decrease the maternal metabolism of glucose and increase the amount of fatty acids for metabolic needs; however, its function is poorly understood (Burton et al., 2007).

Thyroid Gland. During pregnancy, gland activity and hormone production increase. The increased activity is reflected in a moderate enlargement of the thyroid gland caused by hyperplasia of the glandular tissue and increased vascularity (Cunningham et al., 2010). Thyroxine-binding globulin (TBG) increases as a result of increased estrogen levels. This increase begins at about 20 weeks of gestation. The level of total (free and bound) thyroxine (T_4) increases between 6 and 9 weeks of gestation and plateaus at 18 weeks of gestation. Free thyroxine (T_4) and free triiodothyronine (T_3) return to nonpregnant levels after the first trimester. Despite these changes in hormone production, hyperthyroidism usually does not develop in the pregnant woman (Cunningham et al.).

Parathyroid Gland. Parathyroid hormone controls calcium and magnesium metabolism. Pregnancy induces a slight hyperparathyroidism, a reflection of increased fetal requirements for calcium and vitamin D. The peak level of parathyroid hormone occurs between 15 and 35 weeks of gestation, when the needs for growth of the fetal skeleton are greatest. Levels return to normal after birth.

Pancreas. The fetus requires significant amounts of glucose for its growth and development. To meet its need for fuel, the fetus not only depletes the store of maternal glucose but also decreases the mother's ability to synthesize glucose by siphoning off her amino acids. Maternal blood glucose levels decrease. Maternal insulin does not cross the placenta to the fetus. As a result, in early pregnancy the pancreas decreases its production of insulin.

As pregnancy continues, the placenta grows and produces progressively greater amounts of hormones (i.e., hCS, estrogen, and progesterone). Cortisol production by the adrenals also increases. Estrogen, progesterone, hCS, and cortisol collectively decrease the mother's ability to use insulin. Cortisol stimulates increased production of insulin but also increases the mother's peripheral resistance to insulin (i.e., the tissues cannot use the insulin). Decreasing the mother's ability to use her own insulin is a protective mechanism that ensures an ample supply of glucose for the needs of the fetoplacental unit. The result is an added demand for insulin by the mother that continues to increase at a steady rate until term. The normal beta cells of the islets of Langerhans in the pancreas can meet this demand for insulin.

Adrenal Glands. The adrenal glands change little during pregnancy. Secretion of aldosterone is increased, resulting in reabsorption of excess sodium from the renal tubules. Cortisol levels also are increased (Blackburn, 2007).

KEY POINTS

- The biochemical, physiologic, and anatomic adaptations that occur during pregnancy are profound and revert to the nonpregnant state after birth and lactation.
- Maternal adaptations are attributed to the hormones of pregnancy and to mechanical pressures exerted by the enlarging uterus and other tissues.
- ELISA testing, with monoclonal antibody technology, is the most popular method of pregnancy testing and is the basis for most over-the-counter home pregnancy tests.
- Presumptive, probable, and positive signs of pregnancy aid in the diagnosis of pregnancy; only positive signs (identification of a fetal heartbeat, verification of fetal movements, and visualization of the fetus) can establish the diagnosis of pregnancy.
- Adaptations to pregnancy protect the woman's normal physiologic functioning, meet the metabolic demands pregnancy imposes, and provide for fetal development and growth needs.
- Although the pH of the pregnant woman's vaginal secretions is more acidic, she is more vulnerable to some vaginal infections, especially yeast infections.
- Increased vascularity and sensitivity of the vagina and other pelvic viscera may lead to a high degree of sexual interest and arousal.
- Some adaptations to pregnancy result in discomforts such as fatigue, urinary frequency, nausea, and breast sensitivity.
- As pregnancy progresses, balance and coordination are affected by changes in the woman's joints and her center of gravity.

Audio Chapter Summaries Access an audio summary of these Key Points on evolve

REFERENCES

Beebe, K. (2005). The perplexing parity puzzle. *AWHONN Lifelines, 9*(5), 394–399.

Blackburn, S. (2007). *Maternal, fetal, & neonatal physiology: A clinical perspective* (3rd ed.). St. Louis: Saunders.

Burton, G., Sibley, C., & Jauniaux, E. (2007). Placental anatomy and physiology. In S. Gabbe, J. Niebyl, & J. Simpson (Eds.), *Obstetrics: Normal and problem pregnancies* (5th ed.). Philadelphia: Churchill Livingstone.

Cappell, M. (2007). Hepatic and gastrointestinal diseases. In S. Gabbe, J. Niebyl, & J. Simpson (Eds.), *Obstetrics: Normal and problem pregnancies* (5th ed.). Philadelphia: Churchill Livingstone.

Cole, L., Sutton-Riley, J., Khanlian, S., Borkovskaya, M., Rayburn, B., & Rayburn, W. (2005). Sensitivity of over-the-counter pregnancy tests: Comparison of utility and marketing messages. *Journal of the American Pharmacists Association, 45*(5), 608–615.

Copeland, L., & Landon, M. (2007). Malignant diseases and pregnancy. In S. Gabbe, J. Niebyl, & J. Simpson (Eds.), *Obstetrics: Normal and problem pregnancies* (5th ed.). Philadelphia: Churchill Livingstone.

Cunningham, F., Leveno, K., Bloom, S., Hauth, J., Rouse, D., & Spong, C. (2010). *Williams obstetrics* (23rd ed.). New York: McGraw-Hill.

Duff, P., Sweet, R., & Edwards, R. (2009). Maternal and fetal infections. In R. Creasy, R. Resnik, J. Iams, C. Lockwood, & T. Moore (Eds.), *Creasy & Resnik's maternal-fetal medicine: Principles and practice* (6th ed.). Philadelphia: Saunders.

Gordon, M. (2007). Maternal physiology. In S. Gabbe, J. Niebyl, & J. Simpson (Eds.), *Obstetrics: Normal and problem pregnancies* (5th ed.). Philadelphia: Churchill Livingstone.

Monga, M. (2009). Maternal cardiovascular, respiratory, and renal adaptations to pregnancy. In R. Creasy, R. Resnik, J. Iams, C. Lockwood, & T. Moore (Eds.), *Creasy & Resnik's maternal-fetal medicine: Principles and practice* (6th ed.). Philadelphia: Saunders.

Murray, I., & Hassall, J. (2009). Change and adaptation in pregnancy. In D. Fraser & M. Cooper (Eds.), *Myles textbook for midwives* (15th ed.). Edinburgh: Churchill Livingstone.

Pagana, K., & Pagana, T. (2009). *Mosby's diagnostic and laboratory test reference* (9th ed.). St. Louis: Mosby.

Papoutsis, J., & Kroumpouzos, G. (2007). Dermatologic disorders. In S. Gabbe, J. Niebyl, & J. Simpson (Eds.), *Obstetrics: Normal and problem pregnancies* (5th ed.). Philadelphia: Churchill Livingstone.

Pickering, T., Hall, J., Appel, L., Falkner, B., Graves, J., Hill, M., et al. (2005). Recommendations for blood pressure measurement in humans and experimental animals: Part 1: Blood pressure measurement in humans: A statement for professionals from the Subcommittee of Professional and Public Education of the American Heart Association Council on High Blood Pressure Research. *Hypertension, 45*(1), 142–161.

Samuels, P. (2007). Hematologic complications of pregnancy. In S. Gabbe, J. Niebyl, & J. Simpson (Eds.), *Obstetrics: Normal and problem pregnancies* (5th ed.). Philadelphia: Churchill Livingstone.

Samuels, P., & Niebyl, J. (2007). Neurologic disorders. In S. Gabbe, J. Niebyl, & J. Simpson (Eds.), *Obstetrics: Normal and problem pregnancies* (5th ed.). Philadelphia: Churchill Livingstone.

Seidel, H., Ball, J., Dains, J., Flynn, J., Solomon, B., & Stewart, R. (2011). *Mosby's guide to physical examination* (7th ed.). St. Louis: Mosby.

Sibai, B. (2007). Hypertension. In S. Gabbe, J. Niebyl, & J. Simpson (Eds.), *Obstetrics: Normal and problem pregnancies* (5th ed.). Philadelphia: Churchill Livingstone.

Stewart, F. (2007). Pregnancy testing and management of early pregnancy. In R. Hatcher, J. Trussell, F. Stewart, A. Nelson, W. Cates, F. Guest, et al. (Eds.), *Contraceptive technology* (19th rev. ed.). New York: Ardent Media.

Tomlinson, C., Marshall, J., & Ellis, J. (2008). Comparison of accuracy and certainty of results of six home pregnancy tests available over-the-counter. *Current Medical Research and Opinion, 24*(6), 1645–1649.

Wallace, L., Zite, N., & Homewood, V. (2009). Making sense of home pregnancy instructions. *Journal of Women's Health, 18*(3), 363–368.

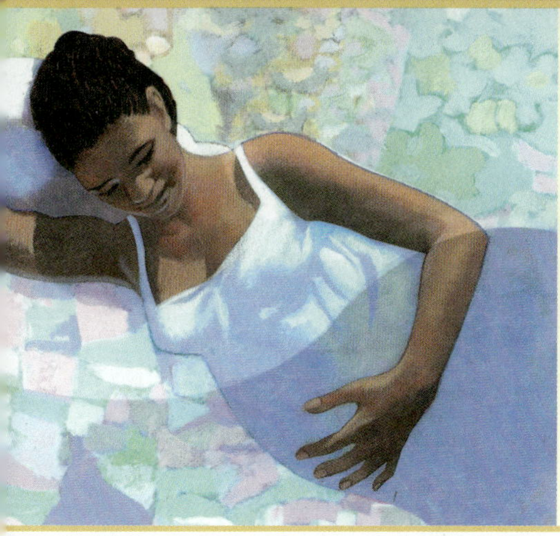

CHAPTER

14

Maternal and Fetal Nutrition

Mary Courtney Moore

evolve WEBSITE

http://evolve.elsevier.com/Lowdermilk/MWHC/

Audio Glossary
Audio Key Points
Critical Thinking Exercise
  Nutrition Education
NCLEX Review Questions
Nursing Care Plan
  Nutrition During Pregnancy
Spanish Guidelines
  Diet and Nutrition

LEARNING OBJECTIVES

- Explain recommended maternal weight gain during pregnancy.
- Compare the recommended level of intake of energy sources, protein, and key vitamins and minerals during pregnancy and lactation.
- Give examples of the food sources that provide the nutrients required for optimal maternal nutrition during pregnancy and lactation.
- Examine the role of nutritional supplements during pregnancy.
- List five nutritional risk factors during pregnancy.
- Compare the dietary needs of adolescent and mature pregnant women.
- Analyze examples of eating patterns of women from two different ethnic or cultural backgrounds, and identify potential dietary problems.
- Assess nutritional status during pregnancy.

Nutrition is one of many factors that influence the outcome of pregnancy (Fig. 14-1). However, maternal nutritional status is an especially significant factor, both because it is potentially alterable and because good nutrition before and during pregnancy is an important preventive measure for a variety of problems. These problems include birth of low-birth-weight (LBW; birth weight of 2500 g or less) and preterm infants. Evidence is growing that a mother's nutrition and lifestyle affect the long-term health of her children (Gardiner, Nelson, Shellhaas, Dunlop, Long, Andrist, & Jack, 2008). Thus the importance of good nutrition must be emphasized to all women of childbearing potential. Key components of nutrition care during the preconception period and pregnancy include:

- Nutrition assessment that includes appropriate weight for height and adequacy and quality of dietary intake and habits
- Diagnosis of nutrition-related problems or risk factors such as diabetes, phenylketonuria (PKU), and obesity
- Intervention based on an individual's dietary goals and plan to promote appropriate weight gain, ingestion of a variety of foods, appropriate use of dietary supplements, and physical activity
- Evaluation as an integral part of the nursing care provided to women during the preconception period and pregnancy, with referral to a nutritionist or dietitian as necessary (Gardiner et al.)

NUTRIENT NEEDS BEFORE CONCEPTION

The first trimester of pregnancy is crucial in terms of embryonic and fetal organ development. A healthful diet before conception is the best way to ensure that adequate nutrients are available for the developing fetus. Folate or folic acid intake is of particular concern in the periconception period. Folate is the form in which this vitamin is found naturally in foods, and folic acid is the form used in fortification of grain products and other

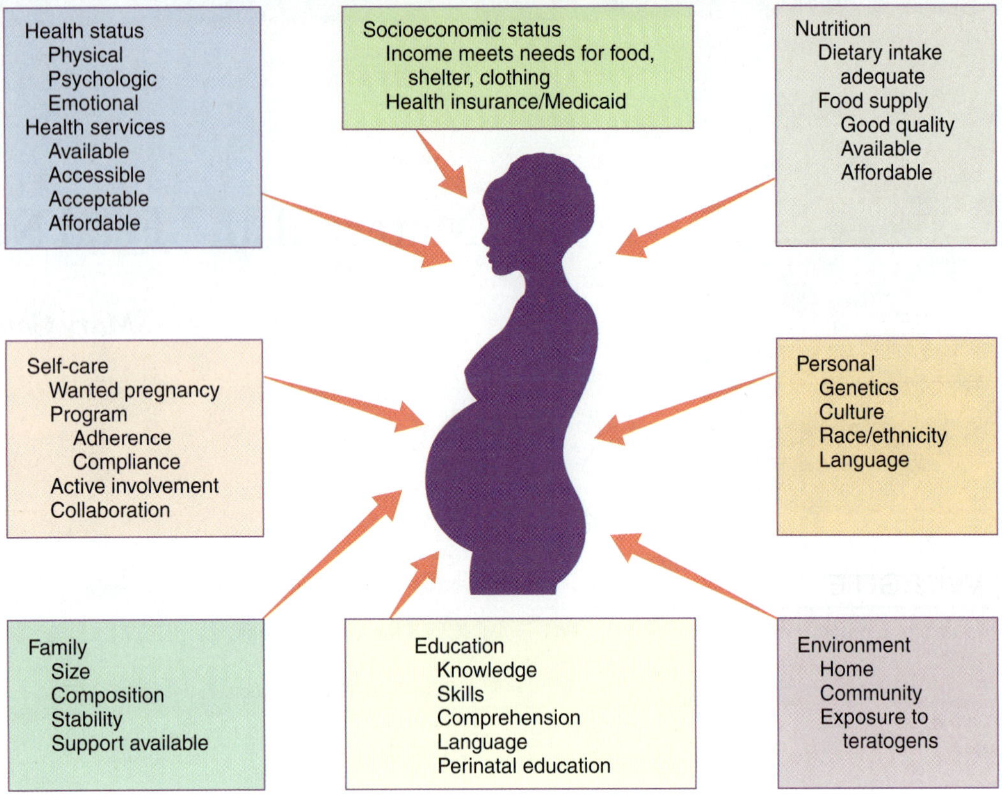

FIG. 14-1 Factors that affect the outcome of pregnancy.

foods and in vitamin supplements. **Neural tube defects,** or failures in closure of the neural tube, are more common in infants of women with poor folic acid intake. Proper closure of the neural tube is required for normal formation of the spinal cord, and the neural tube begins to close within the first month of gestation, often before the woman realizes that she is pregnant. It is estimated that the incidence of neural tube defects could be decreased 50% to 70% if all women had an adequate folate intake during the periconception period (National Center on Birth Defects and Developmental Disabilities, 2010; Wolff, Witkop, Miller, & Syed, 2009). All women capable of becoming pregnant are advised to consume 0.4 mg (400 mcg) of folic acid daily in fortified foods (ready-to-eat cereals and enriched grain products) or supplements, in addition to a diet rich in folate-containing foods: green leafy vegetables, whole grains, and fruits (Box 14-1) (Otten, Hellwig, & Meyers, 2006).

Maternal as well as fetal risks in pregnancy are increased when the mother is significantly underweight or overweight when pregnancy begins. Ideally all women would achieve their desirable body weights before conception.

NUTRIENT NEEDS DURING PREGNANCY

Nutrient needs are determined, at least in part, by the stage of gestation, in that the amount of fetal growth varies during the different stages of pregnancy. During the first trimester the synthesis of fetal tissues places relatively few demands on maternal nutrition; therefore, during the first trimester, when the embryo or fetus is very small, the needs are only slightly greater than those before pregnancy. In contrast, the last trimester is a period of noticeable fetal growth, when most of the fetal stores of energy and minerals are deposited. Therefore, as fetal growth progresses during the second and third trimesters, the pregnant woman's need for some nutrients increases greatly. Factors that contribute to the increase in nutrient needs include the following:

- The uterine-placental-fetal unit
- Maternal blood volume and constituents: During pregnancy the total blood volume increases by about 40% to 50% over the nonpregnant state.
- Maternal mammary development
- Metabolic needs: Basal metabolic rates, when expressed as kilocalories (kcal) per minute, are approximately 20% higher in pregnant women than in nonpregnant women. This increase includes the energy cost for tissue synthesis.

Dietary reference intakes (DRI)s (www.nap.edu) have been established for the people of the United States and Canada, and are updated regularly. The DRIs include recommendations for daily nutritional intakes that meet the needs of almost all (97% to 98%) of the healthy members of the population. They are divided into age, sex, and life-stage categories (e.g., infancy, pregnancy, and lactation), and they can be used as goals in planning individuals' diets (Table 14-1).

Energy Needs

Energy (kilocalories [kcal]) needs are met by carbohydrate, fat, and protein in the diet. No specific recommendations exist for the amount of carbohydrate and fat in the diet of the pregnant woman, but the intake of these nutrients should be adequate to support the recommended weight gain. Although protein can be used to supply energy, its primary role is to provide amino acids for the synthesis of new tissues (see discussion later in

BOX 14-1 FOOD SOURCES OF FOLATE

FOODS PROVIDING 500 MICROGRAMS OR MORE PER SERVING
Liver: chicken, turkey, goose (3.5 oz [100 g])

FOODS PROVIDING 200 MICROGRAMS OR MORE PER SERVING
Liver: lamb, beef, veal (3.5 oz [100 g])

FOODS PROVIDING 100 MICROGRAMS OR MORE PER SERVING
Legumes, cooked (½ cup)
- Peas: black-eyed, chickpea (garbanzo)
- Beans: black, kidney, pinto, red, navy
- Lentils

Vegetables (½ cup)
- Asparagus
- Spinach, cooked

Papaya (1 medium)
Breakfast cereal, ready-to-eat (½ to 1 cup)
Wheat germ (¼ cup)

FOODS PROVIDING 50 MICROGRAMS OR MORE PER SERVING
Vegetables (½ cup)
- Broccoli
- Beans: lima, baked, or pork and beans
- Greens: collard or mustard, cooked
- Spinach, raw

Fruits (½ cup)
- Avocado
- Orange or orange juice

Pasta, cooked (1 cup)
Rice, cooked (1 cup)

FOODS PROVIDING 20 MICROGRAMS OR MORE PER SERVING
Bread (1 slice)
Egg (1 large)
Corn (½ cup)

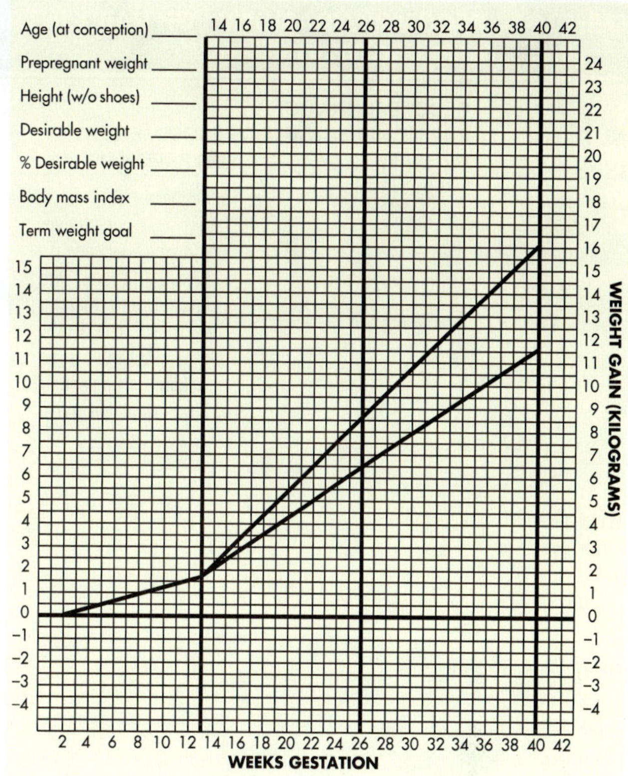

FIG. 14-2 Prenatal weight-gain chart for plotting weight gain of normal-weight women.

chapter). Longitudinal assessment of weight gain during pregnancy is the best way to determine whether the kcal intake is adequate; very underweight or active women may require more than the recommended increase in kcal to sustain the desired rate of weight gain.

Weight Gain

The desirable weight gain during pregnancy varies among women. The primary factor to consider in making a weight gain recommendation is the appropriateness of the prepregnancy weight for the woman's height, that is, whether the woman's weight was normal before pregnancy or whether she was underweight or overweight. Whenever possible the woman should achieve a weight in the normal range for her height before pregnancy. Maternal and fetal risks in pregnancy are increased when the mother is significantly underweight or overweight before pregnancy and when weight gain during pregnancy is either too low or too high. Severely underweight women are more likely to have preterm labor and to give birth to LBW infants. Both normal-weight and underweight women with inadequate weight gain have an increased risk of giving birth to an infant with intrauterine growth restriction (IUGR).

Greater-than-expected weight gain during pregnancy may occur for many reasons, including multiple gestation, edema, gestational hypertension, and overeating. When obesity is present (either preexisting obesity or obesity that develops during pregnancy), there is an increased likelihood of macrosomia and fetopelvic disproportion; operative vaginal birth; emergency cesarean birth; postpartum hemorrhage; wound, genital tract, or urinary tract infection; birth trauma; and late fetal death (Bhattacharya, Campbell, Liston, & Bhattacharya, 2007; Khashan & Kenny, 2009; Viswanathan, Siega-Riz, Moos, Deierlein, Mumford, Knaack, et al., 2008). Obese women are more likely than normal-weight women to have preeclampsia and gestational diabetes.

A commonly used method of evaluating the appropriateness of weight for height is the **body mass index (BMI)**, which is calculated by the following formula:

$$\text{BMI} = \text{Weight} \div \text{Height}^2$$

in which the weight is in kilograms and height is in meters. Thus for a woman who weighed 81 kg before pregnancy and is 1.68 m tall:

$$\text{BMI} = 81 \text{ kg} \div (1.68 \text{ m})^2 = 28.7$$

Prepregnant BMI can be classified into the following categories: less than 18.5, underweight; 18.5 to 24.9, normal; 25 to 29.9, overweight; and 30 or greater, obese (Institute of Medicine [IOM], 2009). A tool for estimating the BMI without the need for calculation can be found at www.nhlbi.nih.gov/guidelines/obesity/bmi_tbl.pdf.

At the first health care visit the pregnant woman should be helped to establish a weight gain goal for pregnancy that is

TABLE 14-1 **RECOMMENDATIONS FOR DAILY INTAKES OF SELECTED NUTRIENTS DURING PREGNANCY AND LACTATION**

NUTRIENT (UNITS)	RECOMMENDATION FOR NONPREGNANT WOMAN	RECOMMENDATION FOR PREGNANCY*	RECOMMENDATION FOR LACTATION*	ROLE IN RELATION TO PREGNANCY AND LACTATION	FOOD SOURCES
Energy (kilocalories [kcal] or kilojoules [kJ][†])	Variable	First trimester, same as nonpregnant; second trimester, nonpregnant needs + 340 kcal (1424 kJ); third trimester, nonpregnant needs + 452 kcal (1892 kJ)	First 6 months, nonpregnant needs + 330 kcal (1382 kJ); second 6 months, nonpregnant needs + 400 kcal (1675 kJ)	Growth of fetal and maternal tissues; milk production	Carbohydrate, fat, and protein
Protein (g)	46	First trimester, same as nonpregnant; second and third trimesters, nonpregnant needs + 25 g	Nonpregnant needs + 25 g	Synthesis of the products of conception; growth of maternal tissue and expansion of blood volume; secretion of milk protein during lactation	Meats, eggs, cheese, yogurt, legumes (dry beans and peas, peanuts), nuts, grains
Water (L) in food and beverages	2.7	3	3.8	Expansion of blood volume, excretion of wastes; milk secretion	Water and beverages made with water, milk, juices; all foods, especially frozen desserts, fruits, lettuce and other fresh vegetables
Fiber (g)	25	28	29	Promotes regular bowel elimination; reduces long-term risk of heart disease, diverticulosis, and diabetes	Whole grains, bran, vegetables, fruits, nuts and seeds
Minerals					
Calcium (mg)	1300/1000	1300/1000	1300/1000	Fetal skeleton and tooth formation; maintenance of maternal bone and tooth mineralization	Milk, cheese, yogurt, sardines or other fish eaten with bones left in, deep green leafy vegetables except spinach or Swiss chard, calcium-set tofu, baked beans, tortillas
Iron (mg)	15/18	30	10/9	Maternal hemoglobin formation, fetal liver iron storage	Liver, meats, whole grain or enriched breads and cereals, deep green leafy vegetables, legumes, dried fruits
Zinc (mg)	9/8	12/11	13/12	Component of numerous enzyme systems, possibly important in preventing congenital malformations	Liver, shellfish, meats, whole grains, milk
Iodine (mcg)	150	220	290	Increased maternal metabolic rate	Iodized salt, seafood, milk and milk products, commercial yeast breads, rolls, and doughnuts
Magnesium (mg)	360/310-320	400/350-360	360/310-320	Involved in energy and protein metabolism, tissue growth, muscle action	Nuts, legumes, cocoa, meats, whole grains
Fat-Soluble Vitamins					
A (mcg)	700	750/770	1200/1300	Essential for cell development, tooth bud formation, bone growth	Dark green leafy vegetables; dark yellow vegetables and fruits; liver, fortified margarine and butter
D (mcg)	5	5	5	Involved in absorption of calcium and phosphorus, improves mineralization	Fortified milk and breakfast cereals; salmon, tuna, and other oily fish; butter, liver
E (mg)	15	15	19	Antioxidant (protects cell membranes from damage), especially important for preventing breakdown of red blood cells (RBCs)	Vegetable oils, green leafy vegetables, whole grains, liver, nuts and seeds, cheese, fish

TABLE 14-1 **RECOMMENDATIONS FOR DAILY INTAKES OF SELECTED NUTRIENTS DURING PREGNANCY AND LACTATION—cont'd**

NUTRIENT (UNITS)	RECOMMENDATION FOR NONPREGNANT WOMAN	RECOMMENDATION FOR PREGNANCY*	RECOMMENDATION FOR LACTATION*	ROLE IN RELATION TO PREGNANCY AND LACTATION	FOOD SOURCES
Water-Soluble Vitamins					
C (mg)	65/75	80/85	115/120	Tissue formation and integrity, formation of connective tissue, enhancement of iron absorption	Citrus fruits, strawberries, melons, broccoli, tomatoes, peppers, raw dark green leafy vegetables
Folate (mcg)	400	600	500	Prevention of neural tube defects, increased maternal RBC formation	Fortified ready-to-eat cereals and other grain products, green leafy vegetables, oranges, broccoli, asparagus, artichokes, liver
B_6 or pyridoxine (mg)	1.2/1.3	1.9	2	Involved in protein metabolism	Meats, liver, dark green vegetables, whole grains
B_{12} (mcg)	2.4	2.6	2.8	Production of nucleic acids and proteins, especially important in formation of RBC and neural functioning	Milk and milk products, eggs, meats, liver, fortified soy milk

*When two values appear, separated by a diagonal slash, the first is for females younger than 19 years, and the second is for those 19 to 50 years of age.
†The international metric unit of energy measurement is the joule (J). 1 kcal = 4.184 kJ.
Source: Institute of Medicine. (2005). *Dietary reference intakes for energy, carbohydrate, fiber, fat, fatty acids, cholesterol, protein, and amino acids.* Washington, DC: National Academies Press; Institute of Medicine. (2006). *Dietary reference intakes: The essential guide.* Washington, DC: National Academies Press; Institute of Medicine. (2004). *Dietary reference intakes for water, potassium, sodium, chloride, and sulfate.* Washington, DC: National Academies Press.

suited to her prepregnancy weight. Progress toward this goal should be monitored at each visit.

For women with single fetuses, current recommendations are that women with normal BMI should gain 11.5 to 16 kg (25 to 35 lb) during pregnancy (Fig. 14-2). Box 14-2 lists recommended weight gain for pregnancies with single fetuses, twin gestations and multifetal (more than 2) gestations for women who are normal weight, underweight and overweight.

Pattern of Weight Gain

The optimal rate of weight gain depends on the stage of pregnancy. During the first and second trimesters, growth takes place primarily in maternal tissues, and during the third trimester, growth occurs primarily in fetal tissues. During the first trimester of singleton pregnancy, the average total weight gain is only 1 to 2 kg. Thereafter the recommended weight gain increases to approximately 0.5 kg per week for an underweight woman and 0.4 kg per week for a woman of normal weight (see Fig. 14-2). The recommended weekly weight gain for overweight women during the second and third trimesters is 0.3 kg, and for obese women, 0.2 kg.

The recommended energy (kcal) intake corresponds to the recommended pattern of gain (see Table 14-1). There is no increment for the first trimester; an additional 340 and 452 kcal per day over the prepregnant intake is recommended during the second and third trimesters, respectively. These recommendations are most appropriate for singleton pregnancy and may need to be adjusted in multiple gestation. The amount of food providing the needed increase in energy intake is not large. The

BOX 14-2 **WEIGHT GAIN DURING PREGNANCY**

- Progressive weight gain during pregnancy is essential to ensure normal fetal growth and development and the deposition of maternal stores that promote successful lactation.
- Recommended weight gain during pregnancy is determined largely by prepregnancy weight for height. The recommended total weight gain is as follows: underweight women, 12.5 to 18 kg (28 to 40 lb); normal-weight women, 11.5 to 16 kg (25 to 35 lb); overweight women, 7 to 11.5 kg (15 to 25 lb); and obese women 5 to 9 kg (11 to 20 lb). For twin gestations the recommended total weight gain is 21 to 28 kg (46 to 62 lb) for women who are underweight before conception, 17 to 25 kg (37 to 54 lb) for normal-weight women, 14 to 23 kg (31 to 50 lb) for overweight women, and 11 to 19 kg (25 to 42 lb) for obese women.
- There is not enough information available to make firm recommendations about optimal weight gain for women with more than 2 fetuses, but provisional recommendations have been made for all prepregnancy BMI categories except the underweight category (IOM, 2009). The provisional recommendations for a gestation with more than 2 fetuses suggest that normal-weight women gain 17 to 25 kg, overweight women gain 14 to 23 kg, and obese women gain 11 to 19 kg.
- Weight gain should be achieved through a balanced diet of regular foods chosen from all the different food groups (see Table 14-3).
- The pattern of weight gain is important: approximately 0.5 kg per week during the second and third trimesters for underweight women, 0.4 kg per week for normal-weight women, 0.3 kg per week for overweight women, and 0.2 kg per week for obese women.

340 additional kcal needed during the second trimester can be provided by one additional serving from each of the following groups: milk, yogurt, or cheese (all skim milk products); fruits; vegetables; and bread, cereal, rice, or pasta.

The reasons for an inadequate weight gain (less than 1 kg per month for normal-weight women or less than 0.5 kg per month for obese women during the last two trimesters) or excessive weight gain (more than 3 kg per month) should be thoroughly evaluated. Possible reasons for deviations from the expected rate of weight gain, besides inadequate or excessive dietary intake, include measurement or recording errors and differences in the weight of clothing or the time of day. An exceptionally high gain is likely to result from the accumulation of fluids, and a gain of more than 3 kg in a month, especially after the twentieth week of gestation, often indicates the development of preeclampsia.

Hazards of Restricting Adequate Weight Gain

An obsession with thinness and dieting pervades the North American culture. Figure-conscious women may find it difficult to make the transition from guarding against weight gain before pregnancy to valuing weight gain during pregnancy. In counseling these women the nurse can emphasize the positive effects of good nutrition as well as the adverse effects of maternal malnutrition (manifested by poor weight gain) on infant growth and development. This counseling includes information on the components of weight gain during pregnancy (Table 14-2) and the amount of this weight that will be lost after the birth. Because lactation can help to reduce maternal energy stores gradually, this also provides an opportunity to promote breastfeeding.

In the United States 20% of women who give birth are obese (Paul, 2008). Pregnancy is not a time for a weight reduction diet. Even overweight or obese pregnant women need to gain at least enough weight to equal the weight of the products of conception (fetus, placenta, and amniotic fluid). If they limit their energy intake to prevent weight gain, they also may excessively limit their intake of important nutrients. Moreover, dietary restriction results in the catabolism of fat stores, which in turn augments the production of ketones. The long-term effects of mild ketonemia during pregnancy are not known, but ketonuria is associated with the occurrence of preterm labor. It should be stressed to obese women, and all pregnant women for that matter, that the quality of the weight gain is important, with emphasis placed on the consumption of nutrient-dense foods and the avoidance of empty-calorie foods.

Excessive Weight Gain

Weight gain is important, but pregnancy is not an excuse for uncontrolled dietary indulgence. The old saying that the pregnant woman is "eating for two" should not be interpreted to mean that the food intake should be doubled. Instead the woman should place an emphasis on the quality of her food intake as she considers her needs and those of her fetus. Excessive weight gained during pregnancy may be difficult to lose after pregnancy, thus contributing to chronic overweight or obesity, an etiologic factor in a host of chronic diseases, including hypertension, diabetes mellitus, and arteriosclerotic heart disease. The woman who gains 18 kg or more is especially at

CLINICAL REASONING

Imbalanced Nutrition

Rosalia is a 16-year-old (G1,P0) who presents for her first appointment at 13 weeks of gestation. Her BMI places her in the underweight category. She reports that she has been nauseated during the first trimester and has lost 2-3 pounds (approximately 1-1.5 kg). Rosalia lives with her parents and three siblings. Her mother does most of the cooking at home, but Rosalia reports that she is often out with friends at meal time. She indicates that she is "excited but scared" about her pregnancy but feels that she wants to keep her baby.

1. Evidence—Is there sufficient evidence to draw conclusions about an appropriate nutrition plan?
2. Assumptions—What assumptions can be made about the following items?
   a. Possible nursing diagnoses for Rosalia
   b. Client history, physical assessment, laboratory tests, and diagnostic procedures that will be needed to make a diagnosis
   c. Rosalia's concern for her fetus
   d. Therapy for her problem
3. What implications and priorities for nursing care can be made at this time? What implications and priorities are likely to be relevant postpartum?
4. Does the evidence objectively support your conclusion?
5. Are there alternative perspectives to your conclusion?

TABLE 14-2 TISSUES CONTRIBUTING TO MATERNAL WEIGHT GAIN AT 40 WEEKS OF GESTATION

TISSUE	KILOGRAMS	POUNDS
Fetus	3.2-3.9	7-8.5
Placenta	0.9-1.1	2-2.5
Amniotic fluid	0.9	2
Increase in uterine tissue	0.9	2
Breast tissue	0.5-1.8	1-4
Increased blood volume	1.8-2.3	4-5
Increased tissue fluid	1.4-2.3	3-5
Increased stores (fat)	1.8-2.7	4-6

BOX 14-3 BARIATRIC OBSTETRIC CARE

Obstetricians today are seeing more morbidly obese pregnant women, those who weigh 400, 500, and even 600 pounds. Obesity creates many risks for pregnant women, including hypertension, diabetes, and prematurity. To manage their conditions and to meet their logistical needs, a new medical subspecialty—bariatric obstetrics—has arisen. Extra-wide blood pressure cuffs, scales that can accommodate up to 880 pounds, and extra-wide surgical tables designed to hold the weight of these women are used. Special techniques for ultrasound examination and longer surgical instruments for cesarean birth are required. In the bariatric obstetric clinic at St. Louis University in St. Louis, Missouri, women are counseled to avoid gaining weight and even to lose weight during pregnancy. New evidence indicates that when obese women maintain or lose weight during pregnancy, they have fewer complications and give birth to healthier babies (Paul, 2008).

risk (Box 14-3). Food energy intake and particularly intake of fat is likely to be high among pregnant women, especially low-income women.

Protein

Protein, with its essential constituent nitrogen, is the nutritional element basic to growth. An adequate protein intake is essential to meet increasing demands in pregnancy. These demands arise from the rapid growth of the fetus; enlargement of the uterus and its supporting structures, the mammary glands, and the placenta; increase in the maternal circulating blood volume and the subsequent demand for increased amounts of plasma protein to maintain colloidal osmotic pressure; and formation of amniotic fluid.

Milk, meat, eggs, and cheese are complete protein foods with a high biologic value. Legumes (dried beans and peas), whole grains, and nuts also are valuable sources of protein. In addition, these protein-rich foods are a source of other nutrients such as calcium, iron, and B vitamins; plant sources of protein often provide needed dietary fiber. The recommended daily food plan (Table 14-3) is a guide to the amounts of these foods that would supply the quantities of protein needed. The recommendations provide for only a modest increase in protein intake (25 g daily) over the prepregnant levels in adult women. Protein intake in many people in the United States is relatively high, and thus many women may not need to increase their protein intake at all during pregnancy. Three servings of milk, yogurt, or cheese (four for adolescents) and two servings (5 to 6 oz [140 to 168 g]) of meat, poultry, or fish would supply most of the recommended protein for a pregnant woman. Additional protein would be provided by vegetables and breads, cereals, rice, or pasta. Pregnant adolescents, women from impoverished backgrounds, and women adhering to unusual diets, such as a macrobiotic (highly restricted vegetarian) diet, are those whose protein intake is most likely to be inadequate. High-protein supplements are not recommended because they have been associated with an increased incidence of preterm births.

Pregnant and nursing women should be especially careful when choosing fish to select those that are low in mercury.

TABLE 14-3 DAILY FOOD GUIDE FOR PREGNANCY AND LACTATION

FOOD GROUP	DAILY AMOUNT OF FOOD RECOMMENDED FOR WOMEN*	SERVING SIZE
Grains	6- to 8-ounce equivalents At least half of grain servings should be whole grains. *Whole grains* are those that contain the entire grain kernel (bran, germ, endosperm) (e.g., whole wheat or cornmeal, oatmeal, and brown rice.) Refined grains have been milled to remove the bran and germ (e.g., white flour, white bread, degermed cornmeal, white rice, and corn or flour tortillas.)	1-ounce equivalent = 1 slice bread, 1 cup ready-to-eat cereal, or ½ cup cooked rice or pasta or cooked cereal
Vegetables Vary the vegetables consumed to take advantage of the different nutrients they offer	2½ to 3 cups Weekly intake should include at least the following: 3 cups dark green vegetables (e.g., spinach or greens, broccoli, bok choy, romaine lettuce); 2 cups orange vegetables (e.g., carrots; acorn, butternut, or Hubbard squash; sweet potatoes); 3 cups dry beans or peas (e.g., black, navy, or kidney beans; chickpeas; black-eyed peas; split peas; lentils; soybeans; tofu); 3 cups of starchy vegetables (corn, green peas, potatoes); and 6½ cups of other vegetables (e.g., artichokes, asparagus, bean sprouts, green beans, cauliflower, cucumber, tomatoes, iceberg or head lettuce).	1 cup = 2 cups raw leafy greens; 1 cup of other vegetables, raw or cooked; or 1 cup of vegetable juice
Fruits	2 cups	1 cup = 1 cup raw, frozen, or canned fruit; 1 cup 100% juice; or ½ cup dried fruit
Milk, yogurt, and cheese (milk group)	3 cups Most milk group choices should be fat free or low fat.	1 cup = 1 cup milk or yogurt; 1½ ounces natural cheese; 2 ounces processed cheese (such as American); 2 cups cottage cheese; 1½ cups ice cream (choose fat-free or low-fat most often)
Meat, poultry, fish, dry beans, eggs, and nuts (meat and beans† groups)	5½- to 6½-ounce equivalents Most meat and poultry choices should be lean or low fat. Fish, nuts, and seeds contain healthy oils, so choose these foods frequently instead of meat or poultry.	1 ounce-equivalent = 1 ounce (30 g) meat, poultry, or fish; ¼ cup cooked dried beans†; 1 egg; 1 tablespoon (15 ml) peanut butter; ½ ounce nuts or seeds
Oils	6 teaspoons (30 ml) Choose oils rather than solid fats. Solid fats are fats that are solid at room temperature, such as butter, shortening, stick margarine, and pork, chicken, or beef fat. Read the label: choose products with no *trans* fats, limit intake of saturated fats, and choose oils high in monounsaturated and polyunsaturated fats.	1 teaspoon = 1 teaspoon liquid oil (olive, canola, sunflower, safflower, peanut, soybean, cottonseed, etc.) or soft margarine (tub or squeeze bottle); 1 tablespoon mayonnaise or Italian salad dressing; ¾ tablespoon Thousand Island salad dressing; 8 large olives; ⅙ medium avocado; ⅓ ounce dry roasted peanuts, mixed nuts, cashews, sunflower seeds†

*These are approximate amounts, based on a relatively sedentary lifestyle, and should be individualized. Intake may have to be increased for women with a more active lifestyle or multiple gestation, those who are underweight before pregnancy, or those exhibiting poor gestational weight gain. Needs during lactation may also be greater than these recommendations.

†Beans are also part of the vegetable group; avocados are also part of the fruit group, and nuts and seeds are part of the meat and beans group.

SAFETY ALERT

High levels of mercury can harm the developing nervous system of the fetus or young child, and certain fish are especially high in mercury. Women who may become pregnant, women who are pregnant or nursing, and young children need to follow some precautions: (1) avoid eating shark, swordfish, king mackerel, and tilefish; (2) check local advisories about the safety of fish caught by family and friends in local bodies of water, but if no advisory is available, limit intake of these fish to 6 ounces and eat no other fish that week; and (3) eat as much as 12 ounces a week of a variety of commercially caught fish and shellfish low in mercury, such as shrimp, salmon, pollock, catfish, and canned light tuna (but limit intake of albacore or "white" tuna and tuna steaks, which contain more mercury, to 6 ounces per week). Additional information about mercury levels in a variety of commercial fish is available at www.cfsan.fda.gov/~frf/sea-mehg.html.

Fluids

Essential during the exchange of nutrients and waste products across cell membranes, water is the main substance of cells, blood, lymph, amniotic fluid, and other vital body fluids. It also aids in maintaining body temperature. A good fluid intake promotes regular bowel function, which is sometimes a problem during pregnancy. The recommended daily intake is about 8 to 10 glasses (2.3 L) of fluid. Water, milk, and decaffeinated tea are good sources. Foods in the diet should supply an additional 700 mL or more of fluid. Dehydration may increase the risk of cramping, contractions, and preterm labor.

The safety of caffeine use in pregnancy is an important issue. Some investigators (e.g., Weng, Odouli, & Li, 2008) but not others (e.g., Pollack, Louis, Sundaram, & Lum, 2010) have found that women who consume more than 200 mg of caffeine daily (equivalent to about 12 oz of coffee) may be at increased risk of miscarriage. There are also data suggesting that excess caffeine intake may contribute to IUGR. A recent review found that there is insufficient evidence to determine whether caffeine has any effect on pregnancy outcome (Jahanfar & Sharifah, 2009). Although the evidence about caffeine is far from conclusive, the March of Dimes recommends a daily intake of no more than 200 mg of caffeine (March of Dimes, 2008). Caffeine is found not only in coffee but also in tea, some soft drinks, and chocolate (Table 14-4).

TABLE 14-4 **CAFFEINE CONTENT OF COMMON BEVERAGES AND FOODS**

BEVERAGE OR FOOD	CAFFEINE (MG)
Coffee (8 oz [240 ml])	95
Espresso (1 oz [30 ml])	64
Tea, black, brewed (8 oz [240 ml])	47
Tea, ready-to-drink, with lemon (12 oz [360 ml])	7
Tea, green, brewed (8 oz [240 ml])	40
Tea, white, brewed (8 oz [240 ml])	35
Energy drink, Jolt, (23.5 oz [700 ml])	280
Energy drink, Red Bull (8.3 oz [250 ml])	80
Energy drink, Vault (12 oz [360 ml])	68
Vitamin water, Energy citrus (20 oz [600 ml])	50
Cola beverage, regular (12 oz [360 ml])	29
Hot chocolate, homemade or from mix (8 oz [240 ml])	5
Dark chocolate bar (1 oz [30 g])	27
Candy bar, milk chocolate with filling (1.5 oz [45 g])	6

Source: U.S. Department of Agriculture, Agricultural Research Service. (2009). *USDA National Nutrient Database for Standard Reference, Release 22.* Nutrient Data Laboratory Home Page. Available at www.ars.usda.gov/ba/bhnrc/ndl. Accessed August 18, 2010; Chin, J., Merves, M., Goldberger, B., Sampson-Cone, A., & Cone, E. (2008). Caffeine content of brewed teas. *Journal of Analytical Toxicology, 32*(8), 702-704; Reissig, C., Strain, E., & Griffiths, R. (2009). Caffeinated energy drinks—A growing problem. *Drug and Alcohol Dependence, 99*(1-3), 1-10.

Aspartame (NutraSweet, Equal), acesulfame potassium (Sunett), and sucralose (Splenda), artificial sweeteners commonly used in low- or no-calorie beverages and low-calorie food products, have not been found to have adverse effects on the normal mother and fetus and are therefore approved by the U.S. Food and Drug Administration (FDA) for use during pregnancy. Aspartame, which contains phenylalanine, should be avoided by the pregnant woman with PKU, however (Box 14-4). Stevia (stevioside) is a sweetener sold as a dietary supplement; no acceptable daily intake has been established for stevia.

Minerals and Vitamins

In general, the nutrient needs of pregnant women, with perhaps the exception of folate and iron, can be met through dietary sources. Counseling about the need for a varied diet rich in vitamins and minerals should be a part of the early prenatal care of every pregnant woman and should be reinforced throughout pregnancy. However, it has been suggested that taking a *micronutrient* supplement (including vitamins and trace minerals) before and during pregnancy reduces the risk of congenital defects, LBW, and preterm birth, as well as preeclampsia (Scholl, 2008). There is no conclusive evidence to support this suggestion, but further research is needed on maternal and fetal benefits of micronutrient supplementation (Peña-Rosas & Viteri, 2009). Supplements are especially advisable for women with known nutritional risk factors (Box 14-5). It is important that the pregnant woman understand that the use of a vitamin-mineral supplement does not lessen the need to consume a nutritious, well-balanced diet.

Iron

Iron is needed to allow transfer of adequate iron to the fetus and to permit expansion of the maternal RBC mass. During pregnancy, plasma volume increases more than RBC mass, with the difference between plasma and RBCs being greatest during the second trimester. The relative excess of plasma causes a modest decrease in the hemoglobin concentration and hematocrit, known as **physiologic anemia** of pregnancy. This is a normal adaptation during pregnancy.

However, poor iron status, which can result in iron deficiency anemia, is relatively common among women in the childbearing years. Iron deficiency (not necessarily anemia) is estimated to affect approximately 10% of nonpregnant women in the childbearing years in the United States. Anemic women are poorly prepared to tolerate hemorrhage at the time of birth. In addition, women who have iron deficiency anemia during early pregnancy are at increased risk of preterm birth. Iron deficiency during the third trimester apparently does not carry the same risk. In the United States, anemia is most common among adolescents, African-American women, and women of lower socioeconomic status.

BOX 14-4 USE OF ARTIFICIAL SWEETENERS DURING PREGNANCY

All of the following sweeteners are approved for use in all age groups, including pregnant women, in the United States:

Acesulfame K
- Brand names: Sunett, Sweet One
- Primary uses: baked goods, frozen desserts, candies, beverages
- Sweetness: 200 times sweeter than sugar
- Shelf life: long
- Suitability for cooking: good; does not break down when heated
- Health concerns: none known

Aspartame
- Brand names: Equal, NutraSweet, NatraTaste
- Primary uses: beverages, frozen desserts, dairy products, chewing gum, breakfast cereals, table-top sweetener
- Sweetness: 180 times sweeter than sugar
- Shelf life: relatively short (approximately 5 months in a soft drink)
- Suitability for cooking: breaks down and loses sweetness if cooked at high temperatures or for long periods
- Health concerns: contains phenylalanine, a consideration in the diets of people with phenylketonuria

Saccharin
- Brand name: Sweet'n Low
- Primary uses: fountain drinks, chewable vitamins and medications, tabletop sweetener
- Sweetness: 300 times sweeter than sugar
- Shelf life: long
- Suitability for cooking: good; does not lose sweetness during cooking
- Health concerns: linked to bladder cancer in rats

Sucralose
- Brand name: Splenda
- Primary uses: baked goods, beverages, frozen desserts, gelatins, tabletop sweetener
- Sweetness: 600 times sweeter than sugar
- Shelf life: long
- Suitability for cooking: very good; does not break down during cooking (maltodextrin is added to give products better bulk and texture)
- Health concerns: none known

Sugar alcohols (not technically artificial sweeteners; contain almost as many calories as sugar)
Types: sorbitol, xylitol, lactitol, mannitol, and maltitol
Primary uses: sugar-free candy, cookies, and chewing gum
Sweetness: most are approximately 70% as sweet as sugar; xylitol equals sugar in sweetness
Shelf life: long
Suitability for cooking: good
Advantages over sugar: Sugar alcohols do not promote tooth decay and are more slowly metabolized, thus they do not create a rapid peak in blood glucose.
Health concerns: Diarrhea can occur with large intakes.

Sugar is important for the volume and moisture of baked goods. Artificial sweeteners may produce a good-tasting product, but some sugar is necessary in many recipes to yield normal volume and texture.

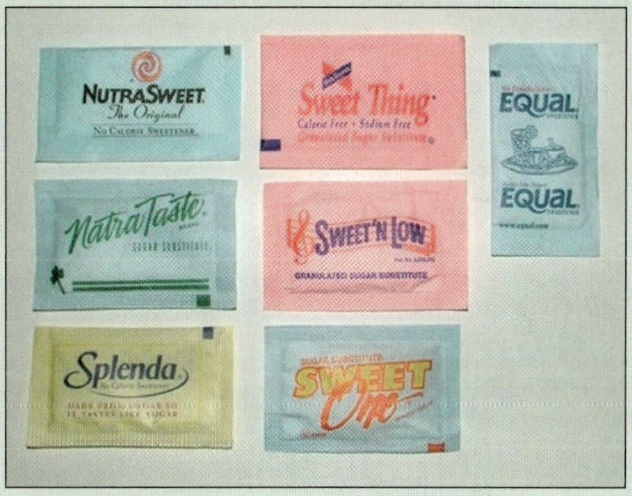

A supplement of 30 mg of ferrous iron daily, starting by 12 weeks of gestation, helps ensure an adequate iron intake. Iron supplements may be poorly tolerated during the nausea prevalent in the first trimester, and starting the supplement after this point may improve tolerance. If maternal iron deficiency anemia is present (preferably diagnosed by measurement of serum ferritin, a storage form of iron), increased iron dosages (60 to 120 mg daily) may be required. See the Teaching for Self-Management box regarding iron supplementation. Even when a woman is taking an iron supplement, however, she also should include good food sources of iron in her daily diet (see Table 14-1).

Calcium

There is no increase in the DRI of calcium during pregnancy and lactation, in comparison to the recommendation for the nonpregnant woman (see Table 14-1). The DRI (1000 mg daily for women 19 years and older and 1300 mg for those younger than 19 years) appears to provide sufficient calcium for fetal bone and tooth development to proceed while maintaining maternal bone mass. Milk and yogurt are especially rich

BOX 14-5 INDICATORS OF NUTRITIONAL RISK IN PREGNANCY

- Adolescence or less than 2 years postmenarche
- Frequent pregnancies: three within 2 years
- Poor fetal outcome in a previous pregnancy
- Poverty/food insecurity
- Poor diet habits with resistance to change
- Use of tobacco, alcohol, or drugs
- Weight at conception under or over normal weight
- Problems with weight gain
  - Any weight loss
  - Weight gain of less than 1 kg/month after the first trimester
  - Weight gain of more than 3 kg/month after the first trimester
- Multifetal pregnancy
- Low hemoglobin and/or hematocrit values
- Diabetes
- Chronic illness, including an eating disorder, that affects intake, absorption, or metabolism of nutrients

EVIDENCE-BASED PRACTICE

Pat Gingrich

What Else Should We Tell Our Pregnant Clients to Take, Besides Folic Acid?

ASK THE QUESTION

What other nutritional supplements, besides folic acid, provide optimal health during pregnancy?

SEARCH FOR EVIDENCE

Search Strategies

Professional organization guidelines, meta-analyses, systematic reviews, randomized controlled trials, nonrandomized prospective studies, and retrospective studies since 2006.

Databases Searched

CINAHL, Cochrane, Medline, the National Guideline Clearinghouse, and the websites for the Association of Women's Health, Obstetric and Neonatal Nurses, the Centers for Disease Control and Prevention, and the National Institute for Health and Clinical Excellence (NICE).

CRITICALLY ANALYZE THE EVIDENCE

The National Institute of Health and Clinical Evidence issued clinical guidelines for prenatal care that included the recommendation that all women be informed about the importance of vitamin D supplementation, especially for women with darker skin, low vitamin D diets, obesity, or low sun exposure (NICE, 2008). By facilitating the absorption of calcium, vitamin D prevents rickets, and may protect against preeclampsia.

Calcium is known to decrease the risk of preeclampsia by half, especially for women with low dietary calcium (Hofmeyr, Duley, & Atallah, 2007).

Since preeclampsia is a result of oxidative stress, it has been suggested that antioxidants may be protective. However, a Cochrane systematic review of 10 trials involving 6533 women found that neither vitamins C, E, selenium nor lycopene supplements caused any improvement in preeclampsia, preterm birth, small-for-gestational age status, or perinatal death (Rumbold, Duley, Crowther, & Haslam, 2008).

Another Cochrane review of 17 trials involving more than 9,000 women revealed that zinc supplementation in pregnancy may reduce preterm births in areas of high perinatal mortality, but showed no evidence of benefit in other settings (Mahomed, Bhutta, & Middleton, 2007). The reviewers recommend a more comprehensive approach to dietary nutrition in pregnancy, rather than focusing on specific micronutrients.

A systematic review by Shah and Ohlsson (2009) concluded that women who received multimicronutrient supplementation during pregnancy had a significant reduction in the risk of low birth-weight infants in comparison to women who took iron-folic acid supplementation.

IMPLICATIONS FOR PRACTICE

Good nutrition is essential to good health, especially in pregnancy. While certain micronutrients may go in and out of scientific favor, women from low-resource areas will most benefit themselves and their fetuses with comprehensive vitamin and mineral supplementation, and dietary adequacy and variety. Women at risk for certain conditions may then benefit from additional protective micronutrients, such as vitamin D and calcium for preeclampsia risk.

References

Hofmyer, G. J., Duley, L., & Atallah, A. (2007). Dietary calcium supplementation for prevention of pre-eclampsia and related problems: A systematic review and commentary. *BJOG: An International Journal of Obstetrics & Gynaecology, 114*(8), 933–943.

Mahomed, K., Bhutta, Z., & Middleton, P. (2007). Zinc supplementation for improving pregnancy and infant outcome. *The Cochrane Database of Systematic Reviews, 2007*, 2, CD000230.

National Institute for Health and Clinical Excellence. (2008). *Antenatal are: Routine care for the healthy pregnant woman.* Available at www.nice.org.uk/nicemedia/pdf/CG062NICEguideline.pdf. Accessed June 21, 2010.

Rumbold, A., Duley, L., Crowther, C., & Haslam, R. (2008). Antioxidants for preventing pre-eclampsia. *The Cochrane Database of Systematic Reviews, 2008*, 1, CD004227.

Shah, P., Ohlsson, A. Knowledge Synthesis Group on Determinants of Low Birth Weight and Preterm Births. (2009). Effects of prenatal multimicronutrient supplementation on pregnancy outcomes: A meta–analysis. *Canadian Medical Association Journal, 180*(12), E99–E108.

sources of calcium, providing approximately 300 mg per cup (240 ml). Nevertheless, many women do not consume these foods or do not consume adequate amounts to provide the recommended intakes of calcium. One problem that can interfere with milk consumption is **lactose intolerance,** the inability to digest milk sugar (lactose) because of the lack of the enzyme lactase in the small intestine. It is relatively common in adults, particularly African-Americans, Asians, Native Americans, and Inuits (Alaska Natives). Milk consumption may cause abdominal cramping, bloating, and diarrhea in such people, although many lactose-intolerant individuals can tolerate small amounts of milk without symptoms. Yogurt, sweet acidophilus milk, buttermilk, cheese, chocolate milk, and cocoa may be tolerated even when fresh fluid milk is not. Commercial lactase supplements (e.g., Lactaid) are widely available to consume with milk, and many supermarkets stock lactase-treated milk. The lactase in these products hydrolyzes, or digests, the lactose in the milk, making it possible for lactose-intolerant people to drink milk.

In some cultures it is uncommon for adults to drink milk. For example, Puerto Rican and other Hispanic people may use it only as an additive in coffee. Pregnant women from these cultures may need to consume nondairy sources of calcium (Box 14-6). If calcium intake appears low and the woman does not change her diet habits despite counseling, a supplement containing 600 mg of elemental calcium may be needed daily. Calcium supplements also may be recommended when a pregnant woman has leg cramps that are caused by an imbalance in the calcium-phosphorus ratio. Bone meal is not recommended as a calcium supplement because it may contain lead.

Other Minerals and Electrolytes

Magnesium. Diets of women in the childbearing years are likely to be low in magnesium, and as many as half of pregnant and lactating women may have inadequate intakes (IOM, 2006). Adolescents and low-income women are especially at risk. Dairy products, nuts, whole grains, and green leafy vegetables are good sources of magnesium.

Sodium. During pregnancy the need for sodium increases slightly, primarily because the body water is expanding (e.g., the expanding blood volume). Sodium is essential for maintaining body water balance. In the past, dietary sodium was routinely

BOX 14-6 CALCIUM SOURCES FOR WOMEN WHO DO NOT DRINK MILK

Each of the following provides approximately the same amount of calcium as 1 cup of milk:

FISH
3-oz can of sardines
4½-oz can of salmon (if bones are eaten)

BEANS AND LEGUMES
3 cups of cooked dried beans
2½ cups of refried beans
2 cups of baked beans with molasses
1 cup of tofu (calcium added in processing)

GREENS
1 cup of collards
1½ cups of kale or turnip greens

BAKED PRODUCTS
3 pieces of cornbread
3 English muffins
4 slices of French toast
2 (7-inch diameter) waffles

FRUITS
11 dried figs
1⅛ cups of orange juice with calcium added

SAUCES
3 oz of creamy pesto sauce
5 oz of cheese sauce

restricted in an effort to control the peripheral edema that commonly occurs during pregnancy. It is now recognized, however, that moderate peripheral edema is normal in pregnancy, occurring as a response to the fluid-retaining effects of elevated levels of estrogen. Sodium is not routinely restricted in pregnancy, and restriction has not proved effective in reducing the rates of preeclampsia. Severe sodium restriction also may make it difficult for pregnant women to achieve an adequate diet. Grain, milk, and meat products, which are good sources of the nutrients needed during pregnancy, are significant sources of sodium. Additionally, sodium restriction may stress the adrenal glands and kidneys as they attempt to retain adequate sodium. In general, sodium restriction is necessary only if the woman has a medical condition such as renal or liver failure or hypertension that warrants such a restriction.

On the other hand, excessive sodium intake is unwarranted because it may contribute to development of hypertension in salt-sensitive individuals. An adequate sodium intake for pregnant and lactating women, as well as nonpregnant women in the childbearing years, is estimated to be 1.5 g/day, with a recommended upper limit of intake of 2.3 g/day (Otten et al., 2006). Table salt (sodium chloride) is the richest source of sodium, with approximately 2.3 g sodium contained in 1 teaspoon (6 g) of salt. Most canned foods contain added salt, unless the label states otherwise. Large amounts of sodium also are found in many processed foods, including meats (e.g., smoked or cured meats, cold cuts, and corned beef), frozen entrees and meals, baked goods, mixes for casseroles or grain products, soups, and condiments. Products low in nutritive value and excessively high in sodium include pretzels, potato and other chips (except salt-free), pickles, catsup, prepared mustard, steak and Worcestershire sauces, some soft drinks, and bouillon. A moderate sodium intake can usually be achieved by salting food lightly during cooking, adding no additional salt at the table, and avoiding low-nutrient, high-sodium foods.

Potassium. Diets including adequate intakes of potassium are associated with reduced risk of hypertension. Potassium has been identified as one of the nutrients most likely to be lacking in the diets of women of childbearing age (IOM, 2006). A diet including 8 to 10 servings of unprocessed fruits and vegetables daily, along with moderate amounts of low-fat meats and dairy products, has been effective in reducing sodium intake while providing adequate amounts of potassium.

Zinc. Zinc is a constituent of numerous enzymes involved in major metabolic pathways. Zinc deficiency is associated with malformations of the central nervous system in infants. When large amounts of iron and folic acid are consumed, the absorption of zinc is inhibited, and the serum zinc levels are reduced as a result. Because iron and folic acid supplements are commonly prescribed during pregnancy, pregnant women should be encouraged to consume good sources of zinc daily (see Table 14-1). Women with anemia who receive high-dose iron supplements also need supplements of zinc and copper.

Fluoride. There is no evidence that prenatal fluoride supplementation reduces the child's likelihood of tooth decay during the preschool years. No increase in fluoride intake over the nonpregnant DRI is currently recommended during pregnancy (Otten et al., 2006).

Fat-Soluble Vitamins

The fat-soluble vitamins include vitamins A, D, E, and K. These are of special concern during pregnancy because vitamin E intake is among the nutrients most likely to be lacking in the diets of women of childbearing age, and intake of vitamins A and D is also low in the diets of some women (IOM, 2006). Fat-soluble vitamins are stored in the body tissues; in the event of prolonged overdoses, these vitamins can reach toxic levels. Because of the high potential for toxicity, pregnant women are advised to take fat-soluble vitamin supplements only as prescribed. Toxicity from dietary sources is very unlikely, however.

Vitamin E is needed for protection against oxidative stress, and pregnancy is associated with increased oxidative stress. Indeed, oxidative stress has been proposed as an explanation for the etiology of preeclampsia, although supplementation with vitamin E has not been effective in reducing rates of preeclampsia (Villar, Purwar, Merialdi, Zavaleta, Thi Nhu Ngoc, Anthony, et al., 2009). Vegetable oils and nuts are especially good sources of vitamin E, and whole grains and leafy green vegetables are moderate sources.

Adequate intake of vitamin A is needed so that sufficient amounts of the vitamin can be stored in the fetus; however, a well-chosen diet including adequate amounts of deep yellow and deep green vegetables and fruits such as leafy greens, broccoli, carrots, cantaloupe, and apricots provides sufficient amounts of carotenes that can be converted in the body to vitamin A. Congenital malformations have occurred in infants of mothers who took excessive amounts of preformed vitamin A (from supplements) during pregnancy, and thus supplements are not recommended routinely for pregnant women.

Vitamin A analogs (e.g., isotretinoin [Accutane]), which are prescribed for the treatment of cystic acne, when used during early pregnancy have been associated with an increased incidence of congenital defects, as well as an increased risk of miscarriage. Topical agents such as tretinoin (Retin-A) do not appear to enter the circulation in substantial amounts, but their safety in pregnancy has not been confirmed.

Vitamin D plays an important role in the absorption and metabolism of calcium. The main food sources of this vitamin are enriched or fortified foods such as milk and ready-to-eat cereals. Vitamin D also is produced in the skin by the action of ultraviolet light (in sunlight). A severe deficiency may lead to neonatal hypocalcemia and tetany, as well as to hypoplasia of the tooth enamel. Women with lactose intolerance and those who do not include milk in their diet for any reason are at risk for vitamin D deficiency. Other risk factors for deficiency are dark skin, with African-American women being at high risk of deficiency; habitual use of clothing that covers most of the skin (e.g., Muslim women with extensive body covering); and living in northern latitudes where sunlight exposure is limited, especially during the winter. Use of recommended amounts of sunscreen with a sun protection factor (SPF) rating of 15 or greater reduces skin vitamin D production by as much as 99%, thus bringing about a need for regular intake of fortified foods or a supplement.

Water-Soluble Vitamins

Body stores of water-soluble vitamins are much smaller than those of fat-soluble vitamins, and the water-soluble vitamins, in contrast to the fat-soluble ones, are readily excreted in the urine. Therefore, good sources of these vitamins must be consumed frequently, and toxicity with overdose is less likely than it is in people taking fat-soluble vitamins.

Folate/Folic Acid. Because of the increase in RBC production during pregnancy, as well as the nutritional requirements of the rapidly growing cells in the fetus and placenta, pregnant women should consume about 50% more folate than nonpregnant women, or about 0.6 mg (600 mcg) daily. In the United States, all enriched grain products (which include most white breads, flour, and pasta) must contain folic acid at a level of 1.4 mg/kg flour. This level of fortification is designed to supply approximately 0.1 mg folic acid daily in the average American diet and has significantly increased folic acid consumption in the population as a whole. All women of childbearing potential need careful counseling about including good sources of folate in their diets (see Box 14-1). Supplemental folic acid is usually prescribed to ensure that intake is adequate. Women who have borne a child with a neural tube defect are advised to consume 4 mg of folic acid daily, and a supplement is required for them to achieve this level of intake.

Pyridoxine. Pyridoxine, or vitamin B_6, is involved in protein metabolism. Although levels of a pyridoxine-containing enzyme have been reported to be low in women with preeclampsia, there is no evidence that supplementation prevents or eradicates the condition. Pyridoxine has been effective in reducing the nausea and vomiting of early pregnancy in some trials (Festin, 2007).

Vitamin C. Vitamin C, or ascorbic acid, plays an important role in tissue formation and enhances the absorption of iron.

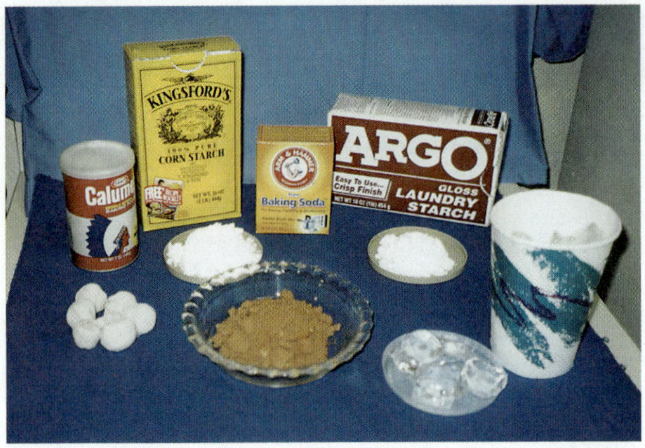

FIG. 14-3 Nonfood substances consumed in pica: red clay from Georgia, Nzu from East Nigeria, baking powder, cornstarch, baking soda, laundry starch, and ice. Some individuals practice *poly-pica*, consuming more than one of these or other nonfood substances. (Courtesy Shannon Perry, Phoenix, AZ.)

The vitamin C needs of most women are readily met by a diet that includes at least one or two daily servings of citrus fruit or juice or another good source of the vitamin (see Table 14-1), but women who smoke need more.

OTHER NUTRITIONAL ISSUES DURING PREGNANCY

Pica and Food Cravings

Pica, which is the practice of consuming nonfood substances (e.g., clay, soil, and laundry starch) or excessive amounts of foodstuffs low in nutritional value (e.g., ice or freezer frost, baking powder or soda, and cornstarch), often is influenced by the woman's cultural background (Fig. 14-3). In the United States it appears to be most common among African-American and Hispanic women, women from rural areas, and women with a family history of pica. In some U.S. studies pica has been reported in almost 40% of pregnant women, although it appears less common in homogeneous societies such as Denmark (Mikkelsen, Andersen, & Olsen, 2006). One problem with pica is that regular and heavy consumption of low-nutrient products may cause more nutritious foods to be displaced from the diet. As an example, cornstarch ingestion is popular among African-American women. It is a source of "empty" calories; half a cup (64 g) provides 240 kcal (57 kJ) but almost no vitamins, minerals, or protein. Overuse of cornstarch can contribute to development of gestational diabetes. In addition, the pica items consumed may interfere with the absorption of nutrients, especially minerals (Stokes, 2006). Women who practice pica have been found to have lower hemoglobin levels than do those who do not practice pica.

Moreover, there is a risk that nonfood items will be contaminated with heavy metals or other toxic substances. Among Mexican-American women, consumption of *tierra* includes both soil and pulverized Mexican pottery. Lead contamination of soils and soil-based products has caused high levels of lead in pregnant women and their newborns (Mills, 2007). Regular household use of Mexican pottery in cooking or serving food or ingestion of ground pottery must be included in interviews or questionnaires regarding nutritional intake of pregnant women. The possibility of pica must be considered when pregnant women are found to be anemic, and the nurse should provide counseling about the health risks associated with pica.

The existence of pica, as well as details of the types and amounts of products ingested, is likely to be discovered only by the sensitive interviewer who has developed a relationship of trust with the woman. It has been proposed that pica and food cravings (i.e., the urge to have ice cream, pickles, or pizza, for example) during pregnancy are caused by an innate drive to consume nutrients missing from the diet. However, research has not supported this hypothesis.

Adolescent Pregnancy Needs

Many adolescent females have diets that provide less than the recommended intakes of key nutrients, including calcium and iron. Pregnant adolescents and their infants are at increased risk of complications during pregnancy and parturition. Growth of the pelvis is delayed in comparison to growth in stature, and this helps to explain why cephalopelvic disproportion and other mechanical problems associated with labor are common among young adolescents. Competition between the growing adolescent and the fetus for nutrients also may contribute to some of the poor outcomes apparent in teen pregnancies. Recommended weight gain goals are not different from those of adult women. BMI is calculated as for adult women (IOM, 2009), rather than by using the adolescent BMI growth charts available from the Centers for Disease Control and Prevention (www.cdc.gov). Adolescent females that have given birth have greater percentages of total fat and visceral fat (associated with the metabolic syndrome and cardiovascular disease) than those that have never given birth (Gunderson, Striegel-Moore, Schreiber, Hudes, Biro, Daniels, et al., 2009); thus the adolescent mother needs careful teaching regarding nutritional intake and physical activity to control body weight in the postpartum period.

Efforts to improve the nutritional health of pregnant adolescents focus on improving the nutrition knowledge, meal planning, and food preparation and selection skills of young women; promoting access to prenatal care; developing nutrition interventions and educational programs that are effective with adolescents; and striving to understand the factors that create barriers to change in the adolescent population.

Preeclampsia

There has been speculation that the poor intake of various nutrients might contribute to development of preeclampsia, but there is no definitive evidence. At present, a diet adequate in the recommended nutrients (see Table 14-1), along with use of a supplement that provides micronutrients both before and during pregnancy, appears to be the best means of reducing the risk of preeclampsia (Scholl, 2008).

Physical Activity During Pregnancy

Moderate exercise during pregnancy yields numerous benefits, including improving muscle tone, potentially shortening the course of labor, and promoting a sense of well-being. Two nutritional concepts are especially important for women who choose to exercise during pregnancy. First, a liberal amount of fluid should be consumed before, during, and after exercise, because dehydration can trigger premature labor. Second, the calorie intake should be sufficient to meet the increased needs of pregnancy and the demands of exercise.

NUTRIENT NEEDS DURING LACTATION

Nutritional needs during lactation are similar in many ways to those during pregnancy. Needs for energy (calories), protein, calcium, iodine, zinc, the B vitamins (thiamine, riboflavin, niacin, pyridoxine, and vitamin B_{12}), and vitamin C remain greater than nonpregnant needs. The recommendations for some of these (e.g., vitamin C, zinc, and protein) are slightly to moderately higher than those during pregnancy (see Table 14-1). This allowance covers the amount of the nutrient released in the milk, as well as needs of the mother for tissue maintenance. In the case of iron and folic acid, the recommendation during lactation is lower than that during pregnancy. Both of these nutrients are essential for RBC formation and thus for maintaining the increase in the blood volume that occurs during pregnancy. With the decrease in maternal blood volume to nonpregnant levels after birth, maternal iron and folic acid needs also decrease. Many lactating women have a delay in the return of menses, which also conserves blood cells and reduces iron and folic acid needs. It is especially important that the calcium intake be adequate; if it is not, a supplement of 600 mg of calcium per day may be needed.

The recommended energy intake is an increase of 330 kcal per day for the first 6 months above the woman's nonpregnant daily requirement. It becomes difficult to obtain adequate nutrients for the maintenance of lactation if total intake is less than 1800 kcal. Because of the deposition of energy stores, the woman who has gained the optimal amount of weight during pregnancy is heavier after birth than at the beginning of pregnancy. As a result of the caloric demands of lactation, however, the lactating mother usually has a gradual but steady weight loss. Most women rapidly lose several kilograms during the first month after birth, whether they breastfeed or not. After the first month the average loss during lactation is 0.5 to 1 kg per month, and a woman who is overweight may be able to lose up to 2 kg without decreasing her milk supply.

Fluid intake also must be adequate to maintain milk production, but the mother's level of thirst is the best guide to the right amount. There is no need to consume more fluids than those needed to satisfy thirst.

Smoking, alcohol consumption, and excessive caffeine intake should be avoided during lactation. Smoking not only may impair milk production but also exposes the infant to the risk of passive smoking. It is speculated that the infant's psychomotor development may be affected by maternal alcohol use, and alcohol use may impair the milk-ejection reflex (Mennella & Pepino, 2008). Caffeine intake can lead to a reduced iron concentration in milk and consequently contribute to the development of anemia in the infant. The caffeine concentration in milk is only approximately 1% of the mother's plasma level, but caffeine levels build up in the infant. Breastfed infants of mothers who drink large amounts of coffee or caffeine-containing soft drinks may be unusually active and wakeful.

CARE MANAGEMENT

During pregnancy nutrition plays a key role in achieving an optimal outcome for the mother and her unborn baby. The motivation to learn about nutrition is usually greater during pregnancy because parents strive to "do what's right for the baby." Optimal nutrition cannot eliminate all the problems that may arise during pregnancy, but it does establish a good foundation for supporting the needs of the mother and her unborn baby (see the Nursing Process box).

Diet History

Assessment is based on a diet history (a description of the woman's usual food and beverage intake and factors affecting her nutritional status, such as medications being taken and the adequacy of income to allow her to purchase the necessary foods) obtained from an interview and review of the woman's health records, physical examination, and laboratory results. Ideally a nutritional assessment is performed before conception so that any recommended changes in diet, lifestyle, and weight can be accomplished before the woman becomes pregnant.

Obstetric and Gynecologic Effects on Nutrition

Nutritional reserves may be depleted in the multiparous woman or in the one who has had frequent pregnancies (especially three pregnancies within 2 years). A history of preterm birth or birth of an LBW or small-for-gestational-age (SGA) infant may indicate inadequate dietary intake. Birth of a large-for-gestational-age (LGA) infant often indicates the existence of maternal diabetes mellitus. Previous contraceptive methods also may affect reproductive health. Increased menstrual blood loss often occurs during the first 3 to 6 months after placement of an intrauterine contraceptive device; consequently the user may have low iron stores or even iron deficiency anemia. Oral contraceptive agents conversely are associated with decreased menstrual losses and increased iron stores; however, oral contraceptives may interfere with folic acid metabolism. The woman with polycystic ovary syndrome (PCOS) is likely to be

NURSING PROCESS

Excessive Gestational Weight Gain

ASSESSMENT

Assessment data include:

- History
  - Medical history of diabetes mellitus or hypertension; gestational diabetes during a previous pregnancy
  - Family history of type 2 diabetes mellitus, gestational diabetes, and overweight/obesity
  - Social history for marital status, family unit, cultural beliefs, activity level and lifestyle behaviors
  - Weight history (prepregnancy weight and body mass index [BMI], weight change over 6 to 12 months before conception, maximum prepregnant weight, rate and amount of weight gain during pregnancy)
- Physical examination
  - Current height, weight, and BMI
  - Blood pressure
  - Edema
  - Number of fetuses
- Laboratory tests
  - Chemistry panel (blood urea nitrogen [BUN], creatinine, glucose)

NURSING DIAGNOSES

Possible nursing diagnoses include:

***Imbalanced Nutrition: More than Body Requirements* related to:**

- excessive food intake for activity level and nutritional needs

***Deficient Knowledge* related to:**

- nutrition and physical activity needs during pregnancy
- effects of excessive weight gain on maternal and fetal health

***Risk for Injury (to the Fetus)* related to:**

- potential for fetal macrosomia with increased likelihood of shoulder dystocia, birth trauma, and operative birth

***Ineffective Health Maintenance* related to:**

- increased risk of developing diabetes during pregnancy
- risk for retention of excessive body fat after pregnancy with increased likelihood of development of diabetes, cardiovascular disease, and cancer

***Disturbed Body Image* related to:**

- excessive body weight

EXPECTED OUTCOMES OF CARE

Expected outcomes are that the woman will:

- Recognize the problems associated with excessive weight gain during pregnancy and set appropriate goals for weight gain for the remainder of the pregnancy.
- Plan a nutritionally adequate diet that is not excessive in calories and be able to adapt this skill in a variety of settings (e.g., restaurant eating, social events).
- Identify safe and effective measures of increasing physical activity during pregnancy and incorporate some of these measures into her daily routine.
- Develop no signs of complications related to overweight/obesity, including gestational diabetes mellitus and hypertension.
- Give birth to a healthy infant whose weight is appropriate for gestational age.
- Achieve a healthy weight after giving birth (e.g., one that will cause BMI to be in the range of 18.5 to 24.9).

PLAN OF CARE AND INTERVENTIONS

Home Care

- Evaluate current food intake and activity patterns.
- Review healthful dietary intake and activity levels with the woman and assess her ability to use this information.
- Establish with the woman an appropriate weekly weight gain goal for the remainder of pregnancy that will slow the rate of gain.
- Recommend that the woman weigh herself at least weekly and assess her progress toward her weight gain goal.
- Record weight gain at each visit with the health care provider and discuss progress toward the goal with the woman.
- Involve the family in the plan of care, evaluate their knowledge of healthy eating and activity patterns, and encourage them to participate with the woman in choosing a healthful diet and obtaining moderate physical activity most days of the week.

EVALUATION

The woman will improve her dietary and physical activity patterns so that the rate of weight gain will be slowed and she achieves the expected outcomes.

obese and insulin resistant and is prone to development of gestational diabetes (Rachoń & Teede, 2010).

Health History

Chronic maternal illnesses such as diabetes mellitus, renal disease, liver disease, cystic fibrosis or other malabsorptive disorders, seizure disorders and the use of anticonvulsant agents, hypertension, and PKU may affect a woman's nutritional status and dietary needs. In women with illnesses that have resulted in nutritional deficits or that require dietary treatment (e.g., diabetes mellitus or PKU), it is extremely important for nutritional care to be started and for the condition to be optimally controlled before conception. The registered dietitian can provide in-depth counseling for the woman who requires medical nutrition therapy during pregnancy and lactation.

Usual Maternal Diet

The woman's usual food and beverage intake, the adequacy of her income and other resources to meet her nutritional needs, any dietary modifications, food allergies and intolerances, and all medications and nutrition supplements being taken, as well as pica practice and cultural dietary requirements, should be ascertained. In addition, the presence and severity of nutrition-related discomforts of pregnancy such as morning sickness, constipation, and pyrosis (heartburn) should be determined. The nurse should be alert to any evidence of eating disorders such as anorexia nervosa, bulimia, and frequent and rigorous dieting before or during pregnancy.

The effect of food allergies and intolerances on nutritional status ranges from very important to almost nil. Lactose intolerance is of special concern in pregnant and lactating women because no other food group equals milk and milk products in terms of calcium content. If a woman has lactose intolerance, the interviewer should explore her intake of other calcium sources (see Box 14-6).

The assessment must include an evaluation of the woman's financial resources and her knowledge of sound dietary practices. The quality of the diet improves with increasing socioeconomic status and educational level. Poor women may not have access to adequate refrigeration and cooking facilities and may find it difficult to obtain adequate nutritious food. Food-borne illnesses may cause adverse effects in pregnancy, and the woman's understanding of safe food handling practices (cleansing hands, food preparation surfaces, and utensils frequently; avoiding contact between raw meat, fish, or poultry and other foods that will not be cooked before consumption; storing foods properly; and cooking foods to a safe temperature) should be assessed.

SAFETY ALERT

Pregnant women who contract listeriosis, a disease resulting from infection with the bacteria *Listeria,* are at increased risk of miscarriage, premature birth, and stillbirth. During pregnancy, women should not consume unpasteurized milk or products made with unpasteurized milk, including soft cheeses such as Brie, Camembert, and the soft Mexican cheeses queso blanco, queso fresco, panela, and asadero. Hot dogs, luncheon meats, bologna, and deli meats should be eaten only if they have been reheated to be steaming hot. Deli-made and other store bought salads such as egg, chicken, ham, and seafood should not be eaten.

Box 14-7 provides a simple tool for obtaining diet history information. When potential problems are identified, they should be followed up with a careful interview.

Physical Examination

Anthropometric measurements provide short- and long-term information on a woman's nutritional status and are thus essential to the assessment. At a minimum, the woman's height and weight must be determined at the time of her first prenatal visit, and her weight should be measured at every subsequent visit (see earlier discussion of BMI).

A careful physical examination can reveal objective signs of malnutrition (Table 14-5). It is important to note, however, that some of these signs are nonspecific, and the physiologic changes of pregnancy may complicate the interpretation of physical findings. For example, lower-extremity edema often occurs when caloric and protein deficiencies are present, but it also may be a normal finding in the third trimester. The interpretation of physical findings is made easier by a thorough health history and by laboratory testing, if indicated.

Laboratory Testing

The only nutrition-related laboratory test necessary for most pregnant women is a hematocrit or hemoglobin measurement to screen for the presence of anemia. Because of the physiologic anemia of pregnancy, the reference values for hemoglobin and hematocrit must be adjusted during pregnancy. The lower limit of the normal range for hemoglobin during pregnancy is 11 g/dl in the first and third trimesters and 10.5 g/dl in the second trimester (compared with 12 g/dl in the nonpregnant state). The lower limit of the normal range for hematocrit is 33% during the first and third trimesters and 32% in the second trimester (compared with 36% in the nonpregnant state) (Cunningham, Leveno, Bloom, Hauth, Rouse, & Spong, 2010; Pagana, & Pagana, 2009). Cutoff values for anemia are higher in women who smoke or live at high altitudes, because the decreased oxygen-carrying capacity of their RBCs causes them to produce more RBCs than other women.

A woman's history or physical findings may indicate the need for additional testing, such as a complete blood cell count with a differential to identify megaloblastic or macrocytic anemia and the measurement of levels of specific vitamins or minerals believed to be lacking in the diet.

Client Education

For many women with uncomplicated pregnancies, the nurse can serve as the primary source of nutrition education. The registered dietitian, who has specialized training in diet evaluation and planning, nutritional needs during illness, and ethnic and cultural food patterns, as well as in translating nutrient needs into food patterns, frequently serves as a consultant. Pregnant women with serious nutritional problems, those with intervening illnesses such as diabetes (either preexisting or gestational), and any others requiring in-depth nutrition counseling should be referred to the dietitian. The nurse, dietitian, physician, and nurse-midwife collaborate in helping the woman achieve nutrition-related expected outcomes. Nutritional care and teaching generally involve (1) acquainting the woman with the nutritional needs during pregnancy and the characteristics of an adequate diet, if necessary; (2) helping her to individualize her diet so that she achieves an adequate intake while

Critical Thinking Exercise—Nutrition Education

BOX 14-7 FOOD INTAKE QUESTIONNAIRE

Which of the following did you eat or drink yesterday? If the way you ate yesterday wasn't the way you usually eat, choose a recent day that was typical for you.

FOOD OR DRINK	NUMBER OF SERVINGS	FOOD OR DRINK	NUMBER OF SERVINGS
Beer, wine, other alcoholic drinks	_____	Orange or grapefruit juice	_____
Tea	_____	Fruit juice other than orange or grapefruit	_____
Coffee	_____	Soft drinks	_____
Caffeinated	_____	Milk	_____
Decaffeinated	_____	Cereal with milk	_____
Fruit drink	_____	Yogurt	_____
Water	_____	Pizza	_____
Cheese	_____	Melon (such as watermelon, cantaloupe,	_____
Macaroni and cheese	_____	honeydew)	_____
Other foods with cheese (such as lasagna,	_____	Berries (kind)	_____
enchiladas, cheeseburgers)	_____	Apples	_____
Orange or grapefruit	_____	Other fruit	_____
Bananas	_____	Broccoli	_____
Peaches or apricots	_____	Green beans	_____
Green salad	_____	Potatoes (other than fried)	_____
Spinach or greens	_____	Corn	_____
Green peas	_____	Other vegetables	_____
Sweet potatoes	_____	Chicken or turkey	_____
Carrots	_____	Egg	_____
Meat	_____	Nuts	_____
Fish	_____	Hot dog	_____
Peanut butter	_____	Cold cuts (e.g., bologna)	_____
Dried beans or peas	_____	Roll/bagel	_____
Bacon or sausage	_____	Noodles	_____
Bread	_____	Chips	_____
Rice	_____	Cake	_____
Spaghetti or other pasta	_____	Doughnut or pastry	_____
Tortillas	_____	Cookie	_____
French fries	_____	Pie	_____

Are you often bothered by any of the following? (Circle all that apply)
Nausea Vomiting Heartburn Constipation
Are you on a special diet? No _______ Yes _______
If yes, what kind? _______
Do you try to limit the amount or kind of food you eat to control your weight? No _______ Yes _______
Do you avoid any foods for health or religious reasons? No _______ Yes _______
If yes, what foods? _______
Do you take any prescribed drugs or medications? No _______ Yes _______
If yes, what are they? _______
Do you take any over-the-counter medications (such as aspirin, cold medicines, acetaminophen [Tylenol])? No _______ Yes _______
If yes, what are they? _______
Do you take any herbal supplements? No _______ Yes _______
If yes, what are they? _______
Do you ever have trouble affording the food you need? No _______ Yes _______
Do you have any help getting the food you need? No _______ Yes _______
If yes, what kind? Food stamps ____ WIC ____ School lunch or breakfast ____
Food from a food pantry, soup kitchen, or food bank _____ Other _______

conforming to her personal, cultural, financial, and health circumstances; (3) acquainting her with strategies for coping with the nutrition-related discomforts of pregnancy; (4) helping her use nutrition supplements appropriately; and (5) consulting with and making referrals to other professionals or services as indicated. Two programs that provide nutrition services are the food stamp program and the Special Supplemental Program for Women, Infants, and Children (WIC), which provides vouchers for selected foods to pregnant and lactating women, as well as infants and children at nutritional risk (see the Nursing Care Plan).

Adequate Dietary Intake

Nutrition teaching can take place in a one-on-one interview or in a group setting. In either case, teaching should emphasize the importance of choosing a varied diet composed of readily available foods (rather than specialized diet supplements). Good nutrition practices (and the avoidance of poor practices such as smoking and alcohol or drug use) are essential content for prenatal classes designed for women in early pregnancy.

MyPyramid (www.mypyramid.gov) can be used as a guide to making daily food choices during pregnancy and lactation, just

TABLE 14-5 **PHYSICAL ASSESSMENT OF NUTRITIONAL STATUS**

SIGNS OF GOOD NUTRITION	SIGNS OF POOR NUTRITION
General Appearance	
Alert, responsive, energetic, good endurance	Listless, apathetic, cachectic, easily fatigued, looks tired
Muscles	
Well developed, firm, good tone, some fat under skin	Flaccid, poor tone, tender, "wasted" appearance
Gastrointestinal Function	
Good appetite and digestion, normal regular elimination, no palpable organs or masses	Anorexia, indigestion, constipation or diarrhea, liver or spleen enlargement
Cardiovascular Function	
Normal heart rate and rhythm, no murmurs, normal blood pressure for age	Rapid heart rate, enlarged heart, abnormal rhythm, elevated blood pressure
Hair	
Shiny, lustrous, firm, not easily plucked, healthy scalp	Stringy, dull, brittle, dry, thin and sparse, depigmented, can be easily plucked
Skin (General)	
Smooth, slightly moist, good color	Rough, dry, scaly, pale, pigmented, irritated, easily bruised, petechiae
Face and Neck	
Skin color uniform, smooth, pink, healthy appearance; no enlargement of thyroid gland; lips not chapped or swollen	Scaly, swollen, skin dark over cheeks and under eyes, lumpiness or flakiness of skin around nose and mouth; thyroid enlarged; lips swollen, angular lesions or fissures at corners of mouth
Oral Cavity	
Reddish pink mucous membranes and gums; no swelling or bleeding of gums; tongue healthy pink or deep reddish in appearance, not swollen or smooth, surface papillae present; teeth bright and clean, no cavities, no pain, no discoloration	Gums spongy, bleed easily, inflamed or receding; tongue swollen, scarlet and raw, magenta color, beefy, hyperemic and hypertrophic papillae, atrophic papillae; teeth with unfilled caries, absent teeth, worn surfaces, mottled
Eyes	
Bright, clear, shiny, no sores at corners of eyelids, membranes moist and healthy pink color, no prominent blood vessels or mound of tissue (Bitot spots) on sclera, no fatigue circles beneath	Eye membranes pale, redness of membrane, dryness, signs of infection, redness and fissuring of eyelid corners, dryness of eye membrane, dull appearance of cornea, blue sclerae
Extremities	
No tenderness, weakness, or swelling; nails firm and pink	Edema, tender calves, tingling, weakness; nails spoon-shaped, brittle
Skeleton	
No malformations	Bowlegs, knock-knees, chest deformity at diaphragm, beaded ribs, prominent scapulas

COMMUNITY ACTIVITY

- Visit the Special Supplemental Nutrition Program for Women and Children (WIC) website at www.usda.gov/fns/wic.html. Review the client information regarding the application process for WIC, food packages, breastfeeding promotion and program data.
- Visit the website of the WIC program for your state. Review the eligibility for WIC, benefits, county directory, and health care provider resources. Research the location of a WIC office in your community or contact your local health department.

as it is during other stages of the life cycle. Additional individualized information and resources for professionals are available from the website. The importance of consuming adequate amounts from the milk, yogurt, and cheese group must be emphasized, especially for adolescents and women younger than 25 years who are still actively adding calcium to their skeletons; adolescents need at least three to four servings from the milk group daily.

Pregnancy. The pregnant woman must understand what an adequate weight gain during pregnancy means, recognize the reasons for its importance, and be able to evaluate her own gain in terms of the desirable pattern. Many women, particularly those who have worked hard to control their weight before pregnancy, may find it difficult to understand the reason the weight gain goal is so high when a newborn is so small. The nurse can explain that the maternal weight gain consists of increments in the weight of many tissues, not just the growing fetus (see Table 14-2).

Dietary overindulgence, conversely, which may result in excessive fat stores that persist after giving birth, should be discouraged. Nevertheless, it is best not to focus unduly on weight gain, which can result in feelings of stress and guilt in the woman who does not achieve the preferred pattern of gain. Teaching regarding weight gain during pregnancy is summarized in Box 14-2.

Postpartum. An important goal of postpartum nutrition is for the woman to lose the weight gained during pregnancy. Retention of this weight can contribute to overweight/obesity and the development of later health problems including metabolic syndrome, cardiovascular disease, and diabetes.

The need for a varied diet consisting of a representation of foods from all the food groups continues throughout lactation. The lactating woman should be advised to consume at least 1800 kcal daily, and she should receive counseling if her diet appears to be inadequate in any nutrients. Special attention should be given to her zinc, vitamin B_6, and folic acid

NURSING CARE PLAN

Nutrition During Pregnancy

NURSING DIAGNOSIS

Deficient knowledge related to nutritional requirements during pregnancy

Expected Outcomes

The woman will describe nutritional requirements and exhibit evidence of incorporating requirements into diet.

Nursing Interventions/*Rationales*

- Review basic nutritional requirements for a healthy diet by using recommended dietary guidelines and MyPyramid *to provide knowledge baseline for discussion.*
- Discuss increased nutrient needs (calories, protein, minerals, vitamins) that occur as a result of being pregnant *to increase knowledge needed about altered dietary requirements.*
- Discuss the relation between weight gain and fetal growth *to reinforce interdependence of fetus and mother.*
- Calculate the appropriate total weight gain range during pregnancy using the woman's body mass index as a guide, and discuss recommended rates of weight gain during the various trimesters of pregnancy *to provide concrete measures of dietary success.*
- Review food preferences, cultural eating patterns or beliefs, and prepregnancy eating patterns *to enhance integration of new dietary needs.*
- Discuss how to fit nutritional needs into usual dietary patterns and how to alter any identified nutritional deficits or excesses *to increase chances of success with dietary alterations.*
- Discuss food aversions or cravings that may occur during pregnancy and strategies to deal with these if they are detrimental to fetus (e.g., pica) *to ensure well-being of fetus.*
- Have woman keep a food diary delineating eating habits, dietary alterations, aversions, and cravings *to track eating habits and potential problem areas.*

NURSING DIAGNOSIS

Imbalanced nutrition: less than body requirements related to inadequate intake of needed nutrients

Expected Outcome

The woman's weekly weight gain will be increased to the appropriate rate using her BMI and recommended weight gain ranges as guidelines.

Nursing Interventions/*Rationales*

- Review recent diet history (including food aversions) using a food diary, 24-hour recall, or food frequency approach *to ascertain dietary inadequacies contributing to lack of sufficient weight gain.*
- Review normal activity and exercise routines *to determine level of energy expenditure;* discuss eating patterns and reasons that lead to decreased food intake (e.g., morning sickness, pica, fear of becoming fat, stress, boredom) *to identify habits that contribute to inadequate weight gain.*
- Review optimal weight gain guidelines and their rationale *to ensure that woman is knowledgeable about healthful weight gain rates.*
- Set target weight gains for the remaining weeks of the pregnancy *to establish set goals.*
- Review increased nutrient needs (calories, protein, minerals, vitamins) that occur as a result of being pregnant *to ensure woman is knowledgeable about altered dietary requirements.*
- Review relation between weight gain and fetal growth *to reinforce that adequate weight gain is needed to promote fetal well-being.*
- Discuss with woman what changes can be made in diet, activity, and lifestyle *to enhance chances of meeting set weight gain goals and nutrient needs of mother and fetus.*
- When a woman has fear of being fat, when symptoms of an eating disorder are evident, or when problems in adjusting to a changing body image surface, refer woman to the appropriate mental health professional for evaluation, *because intensive treatment and follow-up may be required to ensure fetal health.*

NURSING DIAGNOSIS

Nausea related to physiologic alterations of the first trimester of pregnancy

Expected Outcome

Nausea will not be so severe that it interferes with adequate nutrient intake or substantially reduces quality of life.

Nursing Interventions/*Rationales*

- Assess state of hydration to ensure that the woman does not have deficient fluid volume and assess pattern of weight gain during pregnancy *to ensure that nausea is not causing inadequate energy intake.*
- Review the nausea history (i.e., frequency of episodes of nausea, the likelihood of nausea progressing to vomiting, factors precipitating or associated with nausea, and any relief measures that the woman has tried) *to determine the severity of the problem and to begin to identify effective and ineffective measures for coping with nausea.*
- Review measures for prevention or relief of morning sickness *to ensure that the woman is knowledgeable about measures that are often effective in alleviating morning sickness.*
- Discuss with the woman what relief measures she will try *to determine whether she understands how to implement the measures.*

intake because the recommendations for these remain higher than those for nonpregnant women (see Table 14-1). Sufficient calcium is needed to allow for both milk formation and maintenance of maternal bone mass. It may be difficult for lactating women to consume enough of these nutrients without careful diet planning.

Obese women and normal-weight women who gain more than the recommended amount of weight during pregnancy are less likely to breastfeed than normal-weight women with appropriate weight gain (Viswanathan et al., 2008). Obese women who do choose to breastfeed have a statistically shorter period of lactation than normal-weight women (Viswanathan et al.). The woman who does not breastfeed can lose weight gradually if she consumes a balanced diet that provides slightly less than her daily energy expenditure, although overweight and obese women with excessive weight gain during pregnancy have an increased likelihood of failing to return to their prepregnancy weights (Siega-Riz, Viswanathan, Moos, Deierlein, Mumford, Knach, et al., 2009). A reasonable weight loss goal for nonlactating women is 0.5 to 0.9 kg per week; a loss of 1 kg per month is recommended for most lactating women. Those at risk for obesity and overweight need follow-up to ensure that they know how to make wise food choices, primarily from fruits, vegetables, whole grains, lean meats, and low-fat dairy products. An hour of moderately vigorous physical activity (walking, jogging, swimming, cycling, aerobic dance, etc.) most days of the week will improve the ability of the woman to lose weight gradually and maintain the weight loss.

Daily Food Guide and Menu Planning

The daily food plan (see Table 14-3) can be used as a guide for educating the woman about nutritional needs during pregnancy and lactation. This food plan is general enough to be used by women from a wide variety of cultures, including those who follow a vegetarian diet. One of the more helpful teaching strategies is to help the woman plan daily menus that follow the food plan and are affordable, are realistic in terms of preparation time, and are compatible with personal preferences and cultural practices. Information regarding cultural food patterns is provided later in this chapter.

Medical Nutrition Therapy

During pregnancy and lactation, the food plan for women receiving special medical nutrition therapy may have to be modified. The registered dietitian can instruct these women about their diets and assist them in meal planning. However, the nurse should understand the basic principles of the diet and be able to reinforce the teaching.

The nurse should be especially aware of the dietary modifications necessary for women with diabetes mellitus (gestational or preexisting) because this disease is relatively common and because fetal morbidity and mortality occur more often in pregnancies complicated by hyperglycemia or hypoglycemia. Every effort should be made to maintain blood glucose levels in the normal range throughout pregnancy. The food plan of the woman with diabetes usually includes four to six meals and snacks daily, with the daily carbohydrate intake distributed fairly evenly among the meals and snacks. The complex carbohydrates—fibers and starches—should be well represented in the diet. To maintain strict control of the blood glucose level, the pregnant woman with diabetes usually must monitor her own blood glucose daily (American Diabetes Association, 2006). The nurse must therefore teach the woman how to monitor her own blood glucose level, unless she has already been doing this before pregnancy (see Chapter 29).

Counseling About Iron Supplementation

The nutritional supplement most commonly needed during pregnancy is iron; however, a variety of dietary factors can affect the completeness of absorption of an iron supplement. The Teaching for Self-Management box summarizes important points regarding iron supplementation.

TEACHING FOR SELF-MANAGEMENT

Iron Supplementation

- A diet rich in vitamin C (in citrus fruits, tomatoes, melons, and strawberries) and heme iron (in meats) increase the absorption of iron supplement; therefore include these in the diet often.
- Bran, tea, coffee, milk, oxalates (in spinach and Swiss chard), and egg yolk decrease iron absorption. Avoid consuming them at the same time as the supplement.
- Iron is absorbed best if it is taken when the stomach is empty; that is, take it between meals with a beverage other than tea, coffee, or milk.
- Iron can be taken at bedtime if abdominal discomfort occurs when it is taken between meals.
- If an iron dose is missed, take it as soon as it is remembered if that is within 13 hours of the scheduled dose. Do not double up on the dose.
- Keep the supplement in a childproof container and out of the reach of any children in the household.
- The iron may cause stools to be black or dark green.
- Constipation is common with iron supplementation. A diet high in fiber with adequate fluid intake can help reduce constipation.

Spanish Guidelines—Diet and Nutrition

Coping with Nutrition-Related Discomforts of Pregnancy

The most common nutrition-related discomforts of pregnancy are nausea and vomiting or "morning sickness," constipation, and pyrosis.

Nausea and Vomiting. Nausea and vomiting of pregnancy (NVP) are most common during the first trimester. Most of the time NVP causes only mild to moderate problems nutritionally, although it may be a source of substantial discomfort. Antiemetic medications, vitamin B_6, ginger, or P6 acupressure may be effective in reducing the severity of symptoms, although the evidence supporting them is not strong (ACOG, 2004; Holst, Wright, Haavik, & Nordeng, 2009; Ozgoli, Goli, & Simbar, 2009). The dose of ginger tested is a total of 1 g daily, and there is no evidence that larger doses are safe or more effective than the 1-g dose (Holst et al.). The pregnant woman may find the suggestions in Box 14-8 helpful in alleviating NVP.

Hyperemesis gravidarum, or severe and persistent vomiting causing weight loss, dehydration, and electrolyte abnormalities, occurs in up to approximately 1% of pregnant women. (See Chapter 29 for further discussion.)

Constipation. Improved bowel function generally results from increasing the intake of fiber (e.g., bran and whole-grain products, popcorn, and raw or lightly cooked vegetables) in the diet, because fiber helps to create a bulky stool that stimulates intestinal peristalsis. The recommendation for fiber intake in pregnancy is 28 g daily. An adequate fluid intake (at least 50 ml/kg/day) helps to hydrate the fiber and increase the bulk of the stool. Making a habit of participating in physical activity that uses large muscle groups (walking, swimming, water aerobics) also helps to stimulate bowel motility.

Pyrosis. Pyrosis, or heartburn, is usually caused by the reflux of gastric contents into the esophagus. This condition can be minimized by the consumption of small, frequent meals, rather than two or three larger meals daily. Because fluids further distend the stomach they should not be consumed with foods. The woman needs to be sure to drink adequate amounts between meals, however. Avoiding spicy foods may help alleviate the problem. Lying down immediately after eating and wearing clothing that is tight across the abdomen can contribute to the problem of reflux.

Cultural Influences

Consideration of a woman's cultural food preferences enhances communication, providing a greater opportunity for compliance with the agreed-on pattern of intake. Women in most cultures are encouraged to eat a diet typical for them. The nurse needs to be aware of what constitutes a typical diet for different cultural or ethnic groups; however, within one cultural group, several variations may occur. Thus careful exploration of individual preferences is needed. Although ethnic and cultural food beliefs may seem at first glance to conflict with the dietary instruction provided by physicians, nurses, and dietitians, it is often possible for the empathic health care provider to identify cultural beliefs that are congruent with the modern understanding of pregnancy and fetal development. Many cultural food practices have some merit, or the culture would not have survived. Food cravings during pregnancy are considered normal by many cultures, but the kinds of cravings often are culturally specific. In most cultures women crave acceptable foods, such as chicken, fish, and greens among African-Americans. Cultural influences on food intake usually lessen as the woman and her family become more integrated into the dominant culture. Nutritional beliefs and the practices of selected cultural groups are summarized in Table 14-6.

BOX 14-8 SUGGESTIONS FOR MANAGING NAUSEA AND VOMITING DURING PREGNANCY

- Eat dry, starchy foods such as dry toast, melba toast, or crackers on awakening in the morning and at other times when nausea occurs.
- Avoid consuming excessive amounts of fluids early in the day or when nauseated (but compensate by drinking fluids at other times).
- Eat small amounts frequently (every 2 to 3 hours) and avoid large meals that distend the stomach.
- Avoid skipping meals and thus becoming extremely hungry, which may worsen nausea. Have a snack such as cereal with milk, a small sandwich, or yogurt before bedtime.
- Avoid sudden movements. Get out of bed slowly.
- Decrease intake of fried and other fatty foods. Try high-carbohydrate foods such as toast, rice, or potatoes. Some women find high-protein meals or snacks helpful.
- Breathe fresh air to help relieve nausea. Keep the environment well ventilated (e.g., open a window), go for a walk outside, or decrease cooking odors by using an exhaust fan.
- Eat foods served at cool temperatures and foods that give off little aroma. Avoid spicy foods.
- Avoid brushing teeth immediately after eating.
- Try salty and tart foods (e.g., potato chips and lemonade) during periods of nausea. Sucking a lemon slice may help.
- Try herbal teas such as those made with raspberry leaf or peppermint to decrease nausea.

Vegetarian Diets

Vegetarian diets represent another cultural effect on nutritional status. Foods basic to almost all vegetarian diets are vegetables, fruits, legumes, nuts, seeds, and grains, but with many variations. Lacto-vegetarians include milk products. Another type of vegetarian, lacto-ovovegetarians, consumes eggs and dairy products in addition to plant products. Vegans, or total vegetarians consume only plant products. All of these types of vegetarian diets, if they are well planned, can be nutritionally adequate for pregnant and lactating women (Craig & Mangels, 2009). Because vitamin B_{12} is found only in foods of animal origin, the vegan diet may be low in vitamin B_{12}. As a result, vegans should consume vitamin B_{12}-fortified foods such as fortified soy milk two or three times a day or take a supplement. Vitamin B_{12} deficiency can result in megaloblastic anemia, glossitis (inflamed red tongue), and neurologic deficits in the mother. Infants born to affected mothers are likely to have megaloblastic anemia and to exhibit neurodevelopmental delays. The diet should be carefully planned to include adequate minerals. Iron and zinc may not be as well absorbed from plant foods as they are from meats, and calcium intake can be low if milk products are avoided. Plant proteins tend to be "incomplete" in that they lack one or more amino acids required for growth and the maintenance of body tissues. However, the daily consumption of a variety of different plant proteins—grains, dried beans and peas, nuts, and seeds—can provide all of the essential amino acids.

TABLE 14-6 POPULAR FOODS OF VARIOUS CULTURAL AND ETHNIC GROUPS AND THEIR PLACE IN MYPYRAMID

CULTURAL OR ETHNIC GROUP OR EATING PATTERN	FOOD GROUPS				
	GRAINS	VEGETABLE	FRUIT	MILK	MEAT AND BEANS
Mexican	Tortilla Taco shell Posole (corn soup) Rice Postres (pastries)*	*Other vegetables:* Chayote (Mexican squash) Jicama (root vegetable) Nopales (cactus leaves) Tomato Corn	Avocado Mango Papaya Plantano (cooking banana) Zapote (sweet, yellowish fruit)	Queso blanco (white Mexican cheese) Custard (1 cup = 1 cup milk serving) Leche (milk)	Chorizo (sausage)* Chicken, beef, goat, or pork Beans, dried, cooked
African-American soul food (Southern-style cooking)	Biscuit Cornbread Grits, rice, macaroni, or noodles Hominy Crackers Hush puppies	*Dark green:* Collard, kale, mustard, or turnip greens *Orange:* Sweet potatoes *Other:* Okra Snap, pole (green), lima, and butter beans Turnips Summer squash (yellow or zucchini) Coleslaw	Blackberries Melons Muscadines (grapes) Peaches	Buttermilk	Pork (cured ham and uncured cuts), chicken, beef, fish Peas or beans (black-eyed, crowder, purple-hull, or cream)

TABLE 14-6 **POPULAR FOODS OF VARIOUS CULTURAL AND ETHNIC GROUPS AND THEIR PLACE IN MYPYRAMID—cont'd**

CULTURAL OR ETHNIC GROUP OR EATING PATTERN	FOOD GROUPS				
	GRAINS	VEGETABLE	FRUIT	MILK	MEAT AND BEANS
Vegetarian	Whole-grain bread Cereal, cooked or ready-to-eat Brown rice Whole-grain pasta Bagel	All	All	Milk and cheese (lacto-vegetarians) Soy milk, calcium-fortified Soy cheese	Cooked dried beans or peas Tofu (soybean curd) or tempeh (fermented soy) Nuts or seeds Peanut butter Egg (ovovegetarians)
Italian	Breadsticks, breads Gnocchi (dumplings) Polenta (cornmeal mush) Risotto (creamy rice dish) Pastas	*Dark green:* Spinach *Other:* Artichoke Eggplant Mushrooms Marinara sauce	Berries Figs Pomegranate	Cheeses (mozzarella, Parmesan, Romano, ricotta, etc.) Gelato (Italian ice cream)	Veal or beef Fish Sausage* Luncheon meats* Lentils Squid Almonds, pistachios
Chinese	Rice or millet Rice vermicelli (thin rice pasta) Cellophane noodles (bean thread) Steamed rolls Rice congee (soup) Rice sticks	*Other:* Pea pods Yard-long beans Baby corn Bamboo shoots Straw mushrooms Eggplant Bitter melon	Guava Lychee Persimmon Pummelo Kumquat Star fruit	Soy milk	Pork, fish, chicken Shrimp, crab, lobster Tofu or tempeh
Indian (south Asia)	Breads: roti (chapati), naan, paratha, batura, puris, dosa, idli Rice or rice pilau Pooha, upma, sabudana	*Dark green:* Saag (mixed greens and potatoes) Spinach *Other:* Green peppers Cabbage Eggplant Green beans Methi (fenugreek leaves) Cucumbers Chutney or vegetable pickles	Mango Dates Raisins Melons Figs Fruit juices and nectars	Yogurt	Dal (lentils, mung beans, other dried beans) Beef, chicken (some are vegetarian)
Native American†	Bread Fry bread Wild rice or oats Popcorn Tortilla Mush (cooked cereal)	*Orange:* Winter squash (hard outer shell) *Starchy:* Potato Corn *Other:* Rhubarb	Berries Cherries Plums Apples Peaches		Wild game (deer, rabbit, elk, beaver) Lamb Salmon and other fish Clams, mussels Crab Duck or quail
Middle Eastern	Rice or bulgur (cracked wheat) Couscous Bread Pita	*Yellow:* Pumpkin or winter squash (butternut) *Other:* Peppers Tomatoes Grape leaves Cucumbers Fava beans Eggplant	Apricots Grapes Melons Dried fruits: dates, raisins, apricots	Yogurt	Lamb, goat, fish Almonds Pistachio nuts Dried beans and peas, lentils Eggs

*High fat; use sparingly.
†Varies widely depending on tribal grouping and locale.

KEY POINTS

- A woman's nutritional status before, during, and after pregnancy contributes, to a significant degree, to her well-being and that of her developing fetus and newborn.
- Many physiologic changes occurring during pregnancy influence the need for additional nutrients and the efficiency with which the body uses them.
- Both the total maternal weight gain and the pattern of weight gain are important determinants of the outcome of pregnancy.
- The appropriateness of the mother's prepregnancy weight for height (BMI) is a major determinant of her recommended weight gain during pregnancy.
- Nutritional risk factors include adolescent pregnancy; bizarre or faddish food habits; abuse of nicotine, alcohol, or drugs; a low or high weight for height; and frequent pregnancies.
- Iron supplementation is usually recommended routinely during pregnancy, even though there is some controversy regarding its beneficial effects on successful outcome of pregnancy. Other supplements may be recommended when nutritional risk factors are present.
- The nurse and the woman are influenced by cultural and personal values and beliefs during nutrition counseling.
- Pregnancy complications that may be nutrition related include anemia, gestational hypertension, gestational diabetes, and IUGR.
- Dietary adaptation can be effective for some of the common discomforts of pregnancy, including nausea and vomiting, constipation, and heartburn.

Audio Chapter Summaries Access an audio summary of these Key Points on evolve

REFERENCES

American College of Obstetrics and Gynecology (ACOG). (2004). Practice bulletin: Nausea and vomiting of pregnancy. *Obstetrics and Gynecology, 103*(4), 803–814.

American Diabetes Association. (2006). Standards of medical care in diabetes—2006. *Diabetes Care, 29*(Suppl. 1), S4–S42.

Bhattacharya, S., Campbell, D., Liston, W., & Bhattacharya, S. (2007). Effect of body mass index on pregnancy outcomes in nulliparous women delivering singleton babies. *BMC Public Health, 7*, 168.

Cunningham, F., Leveno, K., Bloom, S., Hauth, J., Rouse, D., & Spong, C. (2010). *Williams obstetrics* (23rd ed.). New York: McGraw-Hill.

Craig, W., & Mangels, A. (2009). Position of the American Dietetic Association: Vegetarian diets. *Journal of the American Dietetic Association, 109*(7), 1266–1282.

Festin, M. (2007). Nausea and vomiting in early pregnancy. *Clinical Evidence (Online), 2007*(pii), 1405.

Gardiner, P., Nelson, L., Shellhaas, C., Dunlop, A., Long, R., Andrist, S., & Jack, B. (2008). The clinical content of preconception care: Nutrition and dietary supplements. *American Journal of Obstetrics and Gynecology, 199*(Suppl. 6), S345–S356.

Gunderson, E., Striegel-Moore, R., Schreiber, G., Hudes, M., Biro, F., Daniels, S., et al. (2009). Longitudinal study of growth and adiposity in parous compared with nulligravid adolescents. *Archives of Pediatrics and Adolescent Medicine, 163*(4), 349–356.

Holst, L., Wright, D., Haavik, S., & Nordeng, H. (2009). Safety and efficacy of herbal remedies in obstetrics—Review and clinical implications. *Midwifery*, Sept 24 EPub.

Institute of Medicine. (2006). *WIC food packages: Time for a change*. Washington, DC: National Academies Press.

Institute of Medicine. (2009). *Weight gain during pregnancy: Reexamining the guidelines*. Washington, DC: National Academies Press.

Jahanfar, S., & Sharifah, H. (2009). Effects of restricted caffeine intake by mother on fetal, neonatal and pregnancy outcome (Cochrane Review). *The Cochrane Database of Systematic Reviews, 2009*, 2, CD006965.

Khashan, A., & Kenny, L. (2009). The effects of maternal body mass index on pregnancy outcome. *European Journal of Epidemiology, 24*(11), 697–705.

March of Dimes. (2008). *Caffeine in pregnancy*. Available at www.marchofdimes.com/professionals/14332_1148.asp#miscarriage. Accessed June 21, 2010.

Mennella, J., & Pepino, M. (2008). Biphasic effects of moderate drinking on prolactin during lactation. *Alcoholism: Clinical and Experimental Research, 32*(11), 1899–1908.

Mikkelsen, T., Andersen, A., & Olsen, S. (2006). Pica in pregnancy in a privileged population: Myth or reality. *Acta Obstetrica et Gynecologica Scandinavica, 85*(10), 1265–1266.

Mills, M. (2007). Craving more than food: The implications of pica in pregnancy. *Nursing for Women's Health, 11*(3), 266–273.

National Center on Birth Defects and Developmental Disabilities. (2010). *Folic acid*. Available at www.cdc.gov/ncbddd/folicacid/index.html. Accessed June 21, 2010.

Otten, J., Hellwig, J., & Meyers, L. (Eds.), (2006). *Dietary reference intakes: The essential guide to nutrient requirements*. Washington, DC: National Academies Press.

Ozgoli, G., Goli, M., & Simbar, M. (2009). Effects of ginger capsules on pregnancy, nausea, and vomiting. *Journal of Alternative and Complementary Medicine, 15*(3), 243–246.

Pagana, K., & Pagana, T. (2009). *Mosby's diagnostic and laboratory test reference* (9th ed.). St. Louis: Mosby.

Paul, A. (2008). Too fat and pregnant. *New York Times*, July 13, 2008.

Peña-Rosas, J., & Viteri, F. (2009). Effects and safety of preventive oral iron or iron+folic acid supplementation for women during pregnancy. *The Cochrane Database of Systematic Reviews, 2009*, 4, CD004736.

Pollack, A., Louis, G., Sundaram, R., & Lum, K. (2010). Caffeine consumption and miscarriage: A prospective cohort study. *Fertility and Sterility, 93*(1), 304–306.

Rachoń, D., & Teede, H. (2010). Ovarian function and obesity—Interrelationship, impact on women's reproductive lifespan and treatment options. *Molecular and Cellular Endocrinology, 316*(2), 172–179.

Scholl, T. (2008). Maternal nutrition before and during pregnancy. *Nestle Nutrition Workshop Series: Pediatric Program, 61*, 79–89.

Siega-Riz, A., Viswanathan, M., Moos, M., Deierlein, A., Mumford, S., Knaack, J., et al. (2009). A systematic review of outcomes of maternal weight gain according to the Institute of Medicine recommendations: Birthweight, fetal growth, and postpartum weight retention. *American Journal of Obstetrics and Gynecology, 201*(4), 339, e1-e14.

Stokes, T. (2006). The earth-eaters. *Nature, 444*(7119), 543–544.

Villar, J., Purwar, M., Merialdi, M., Zavaleta, N., Thi Nhu Ngoc, N., Anthony, J., DeGreeff, A., Poston, L., Shennen, A., & WHO Vitamin C and Vitamin A Trial Group (2009). World Health Organisation multicentre randomised trial of supplementation with vitamins C and E among pregnant women at high risk for pre-eclampsia in populations of low nutritional status from developing countries. *BJOG: An International Journal of Obstetrics & Gynaecology, 116*(6), 780–788.

Viswanathan, M., Siega-Riz, A., Moos, M., Deierlein, A., Mumford, S., Knaack, J., Thieda, P., Lux, L., & Lohr, K. (2008). Outcomes of maternal weight gain. *Evidence Report Technology Assessment (Full Rep), 168*, 1–223.

Weng, X., Odouli, R., & Li, D. (2008). Maternal caffeine consumption during pregnancy and the risk of miscarriage: A prospective cohort study. *American Journal of Obstetrics and Gynecology, 198*(3), 279, e1-e8.

Wolff, T., Witkop, C., Miller, T., & Syed, S. (2009). Folic acid supplementation for the prevention of neural tube defects: An update of the evidence for the U.S. Preventive Services Task Force. *Annals of Internal Medicine, 150*(9), 632–639.

CHAPTER

15

Nursing Care of the Family During Pregnancy

Denise G. Link

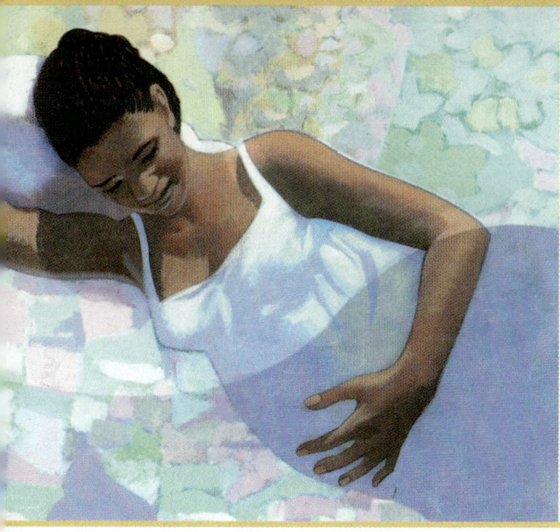

evolve WEBSITE

http://evolve.elsevier.com/Lowdermilk/MWHC/

- Audio Glossary
- Audio Key Points
- Case Studies
  - First Trimester
  - Second Trimester
  - Third Trimester
- Critical Thinking Exercises
  - Discomforts of Pregnancy
  - Teenage Pregnancy
- NCLEX Review Questions
- Nursing Care Plans
  - Adolescent Pregnancy
  - Discomforts of Pregnancy and Warning Signs
- Spanish Guidelines
  - Assessment of Respiratory Symptoms
  - Prenatal Interview
  - Prenatal Physical Examination
- Video—Assessment
  - Abdomen/Fundal Height
  - Breast
  - Chest Wall
  - Fetal Heart Rate
- Video—Nursing Skills
  - Assessing Fundal Height
  - Auscultating the Fetal Heart Rate

LEARNING OBJECTIVES

- Describe the process of confirming pregnancy and estimating the date of birth.
- Summarize the physical, psychosocial, and behavioral changes that usually occur as the mother and other family members adapt to pregnancy.
- Evaluate the benefits of prenatal care and problems of accessibility for some women.
- Outline the patterns of health care used to assess maternal and fetal health status at the initial and follow-up visits during pregnancy.
- Select the typical nursing assessments, diagnoses, interventions, and methods of evaluation in providing care for the pregnant woman.
- Plan education needed by pregnant women to understand physical discomforts related to pregnancy and to recognize signs and symptoms of potential complications.
- Examine the effect of culture, age, parity, and number of fetuses on the response of the family to the pregnancy and on the prenatal care provided.
- Describe the options for health care providers and birth setting choices that are available.

The prenatal period is a time of physical and psychologic preparation for birth and parenthood. Becoming a parent is considered one of the maturational milestones of adult life. It is a time of intense learning for parents and those close to them. The prenatal period provides a unique opportunity for nurses and other members of the health care team to influence family health. During this period essentially healthy women seek regular care and guidance. The nurse's health promotion interventions can affect the well-being of the woman, her unborn child, and the rest of her family for many years.

Regular prenatal visits, ideally beginning soon after the first missed menstrual period, offer opportunities to ensure the health of the expectant mother and her infant. Prenatal health care enables discovery, diagnosis, and treatment of preexisting maternal disorders and any disorders that develop during the pregnancy. Prenatal care is designed to monitor the growth and development of the fetus and to identify abnormalities that will interfere with the course of normal labor. Prenatal care also provides education and support for self-management and parenting.

Pregnancy spans 9 months, but health care providers do not use the familiar monthly calendar to determine fetal age or to discuss the pregnancy. Instead, they use lunar months, which last 28 days, or 4 weeks. Normal pregnancy, then, lasts about 10 lunar months, which is the same as 40 weeks or 280 days. Health care providers also refer to early, middle, and late pregnancy as **trimesters.** The first trimester lasts from weeks 1 through 13; the second, from weeks 14 through 26; and the third, from weeks 27 through 40. A pregnancy is considered to be at **term** if it advances to the completion of 37 weeks. The focus of this chapter is on meeting the health needs of the expectant family over the course of pregnancy, which is known as the prenatal period.

DIAGNOSIS OF PREGNANCY

Women suspect pregnancy when they miss a menstrual period. Many women come to the first prenatal visit after a positive home pregnancy test; however, the clinical diagnosis of pregnancy before the second missed period is difficult in some women. Physical variations, obesity, or tumors, for example, confound even the experienced examiner. Accuracy is important, however, because emotional, social, health, or legal consequences of an inaccurate diagnosis, either positive or negative, can be extremely serious.

Signs and Symptoms

The physical cues of pregnancy vary greatly; therefore, the diagnosis of pregnancy is uncertain for a time. Many of the indicators of pregnancy are clinically useful in the diagnosis of pregnancy, and they are classified as presumptive, probable, or positive (see Table 13-2).

Presumptive indicators of pregnancy include subjective symptoms and objective signs. Subjective symptoms are reported by the woman and include amenorrhea, nausea and vomiting **(morning sickness),** breast tenderness, urinary frequency, and fatigue. **Quickening,** the mother's first perception of fetal movement, is noted between weeks 16 and 20. Objective signs that are validated by the examiner include elevation of basal body temperature (BBT), breast and abdominal enlargement, and changes in the uterus and vagina. Other visible changes occur in the skin, such as striae gravidarum, deeper pigmentation of the areolae, chloasma (mask of pregnancy), and linea nigra (pigmented line on the abdomen).

The presumptive indicators of pregnancy can be caused by conditions other than gestation; therefore, these signs alone are not reliable for diagnosis of pregnancy.

Probable indicators of pregnancy are detected by an examiner and are related mainly to physical changes in the uterus. Objective signs include uterine enlargement, Braxton Hicks contractions, placental souffle (sound of blood passing through the placenta), ballottement (examiner is able to feel the fetus float during a vaginal examination), and a positive pregnancy test. When combined with presumptive signs and symptoms, they strongly suggest pregnancy, but they are not conclusive.

The positive indicators of pregnancy are directly attributed to the fetus and include the presence of a fetal heartbeat distinct from that of the mother, fetal movement felt by someone other than the mother, and visualization of the fetus with a technique such as ultrasound examination.

Case Study—First Trimester

BOX 15-1 USE OF NÄGELE'S RULE

December 10, 2011, is the first day of the last menstrual period (LMP).

	MONTH	DAY	YEAR
LMP	12	10	2011
	−3	+7	
Estimated day of birth:	9	17	2012

The estimated date of birth (EDB) is September 17, 2012.

Estimating Date of Birth

After the diagnosis of pregnancy the woman's first question usually concerns when she will give birth. This date has traditionally been termed the *estimated date of confinement (EDC),* although *estimated date of delivery (EDD)* also has been used. To promote a more positive perception of both pregnancy and birth, however, the term *estimated date of birth (EDB)* is suggested. Accurate dating of pregnancy and calculation of the EDB have implications for timing of specific prenatal screening tests, assessing fetal growth and critical decisions for managing pregnancy complications. Ultrasound dating of gestational age is accurate; however, researchers in the Routine Antenatal Diagnostic Imaging with Ultrasound Study (RADIUS) concluded that the cost associated with the routine use of ultrasound screening in the absence of clear clinical indications is prohibitive (Hunter, 2009).

Several formulas have been suggested for calculating the EDB based on the LMP. These rules assume regular 28-day ovulatory cycles and rely on a woman's accurate recall of her LMP. The most common of these methods is Nägele's rule, which is as follows: after determining the first day of the LMP, subtract 3 calendar months and add 7 days; or alternatively, add 7 days to the LMP and count forward 9 calendar months (Box 15-1). Only about 5% of women give birth spontaneously on the EDB as determined by Nägele's rule. Most women give birth during the period extending from 7 days before to 7 days after the EDB.

ADAPTATION TO PREGNANCY

Pregnancy affects all family members, and each family member must adapt to the pregnancy and interpret its meaning in light of his or her own needs. This process of family adaptation to pregnancy takes place within a cultural environment influenced by societal trends. Dramatic changes have occurred in Western society in recent years, and the nurse must be prepared to support not only traditional families in the childbirth experience but also single-parent families, reconstituted families, dual-career families, and alternative families.

Much of the research on family dynamics in pregnancy in the United States and Canada has been done with Caucasian, middle-class nuclear families. Therefore, the findings may not apply to families who do not fit the traditional North American model. Adaptation of terms is appropriate to avoid embarrassment to the nurse and offense to the family. Additional research is needed on a variety of families to determine if study findings generated in traditional families are applicable to others.

Maternal Adaptation

Women of all ages use the months of pregnancy to adapt to the maternal role, a complex process of social and cognitive learning. Early in pregnancy nothing seems to be happening, and a woman may spend much time sleeping secondary to the increased fatigue of this stage. With the perception of fetal movement in the second trimester, the woman turns her attention inward to her pregnancy and to relationships with her mother and other women who have been or who are pregnant.

Pregnancy is a maturational milestone that can be stressful but also rewarding as the woman prepares for a new level of caring and responsibility. Her self-concept changes in readiness for parenthood as she prepares for her new role. She moves gradually from being self-contained and independent to being committed to a lifelong concern for another human being. This growth requires mastery of certain developmental tasks: accepting the pregnancy, identifying with the role of mother, reordering the relationships between herself and her mother and between herself and her partner, establishing a relationship with the unborn child, and preparing for the birth experience. The partner's emotional support is an important factor in the successful accomplishment of these developmental tasks. Single women with limited support may have difficulty making this adaptation.

Accepting the Pregnancy

The first step in adapting to the maternal role is accepting the idea of pregnancy and assimilating the pregnant state into the woman's way of life. Mercer (1995) described this process as *cognitive restructuring* and credited Reva Rubin (1984) as the nurse theorist who pioneered our understanding of maternal role attainment. The degree of acceptance is reflected in the woman's emotional responses. Many women are upset initially at finding themselves pregnant, especially if the pregnancy is unintended. Eventual acceptance of pregnancy parallels the growing acceptance of the reality of a child. However, do not equate nonacceptance of the pregnancy with rejection of the child, for a woman may dislike being pregnant but feel love for the child to be born.

Women who are happy and pleased about their pregnancy often view it as biologic fulfillment and part of their life plan. They have high self-esteem and tend to be confident about outcomes for themselves, their babies, and other family members. Despite a general feeling of well-being, many women are surprised to experience *emotional lability*, that is, rapid and unpredictable changes in mood. These swings in emotions and increased sensitivity to others are disconcerting to the expectant mother and those around her. Increased irritability, explosions of tears, and anger can alternate with feelings of great joy and cheerfulness apparently with little or no provocation.

Profound hormonal changes that are part of the maternal response to pregnancy may be responsible for mood changes. Other reasons such as concerns about finances and changed lifestyle contribute to this seemingly erratic behavior.

Most women have ambivalent feelings during pregnancy whether the pregnancy was intended or not. Ambivalence—having conflicting feelings simultaneously—is considered a normal response for people preparing for a new role. During pregnancy women may, for example, feel great pleasure that they are fulfilling a lifelong dream, but they also may feel great regret that life as they now know it is ending.

Even women who are pleased to be pregnant may experience feelings of hostility toward the pregnancy or unborn child from time to time. Such incidents as a partner's chance remark about the attractiveness of a slim, nonpregnant woman or news of a colleague's promotion can give rise to ambivalent feelings. Body sensations, feelings of dependence, or the realization of the responsibilities of child care also can generate such feelings.

Intense feelings of ambivalence that persist through the third trimester may indicate an unresolved conflict with the motherhood role (Mercer, 1995). After the birth of a healthy child, memories of these ambivalent feelings usually are dismissed. If the child is born with a defect, however, a woman may look back at the times when she did not want the pregnancy and feel intensely guilty. She may believe that her ambivalence caused the birth defect. She then will need assurance that her feelings were not responsible for the problem.

Identifying with the Mother Role

The process of identifying with the mother role begins early in each woman's life when she is being mothered as a child. Her social group's perception of what constitutes the feminine role can subsequently influence her toward choosing between motherhood or a career, being married or single, being independent rather than interdependent, or being able to manage multiple roles. Practice roles, such as playing with dolls, babysitting, and taking care of siblings may increase her understanding of what being a mother involves.

Many women have always wanted a baby, liked children, and looked forward to motherhood. Their high motivation to become a parent promotes acceptance of pregnancy and eventual prenatal and parental adaptation. Other women apparently have not considered in any detail what motherhood means to them. During pregnancy these women must resolve conflicts such as not wanting the pregnancy and child-related or career-related decisions.

Reordering Personal Relationships

Close relationships of the pregnant woman undergo change during pregnancy as she prepares emotionally for the new role of mother. As family members learn their new roles, periods of tension and conflict may occur. An understanding of the typical patterns of adjustment can help the nurse reassure the pregnant woman and explore issues related to social support. Promoting effective communication patterns between the expectant mother and her own mother and between the expectant mother and her partner are common nursing interventions provided during the prenatal visits.

The woman's own relationship with her mother is significant in adaptation to pregnancy and motherhood. Important components in the pregnant woman's relationship with her mother are the mother's availability (past and present), her reactions to the daughter's pregnancy, respect for her daughter's autonomy, and the willingness to reminisce (Mercer, 1995).

The mother's reaction to the daughter's pregnancy signifies her acceptance of the grandchild and of her daughter. If the mother is supportive, the daughter has an opportunity to discuss pregnancy and labor with a knowledgeable and accepting

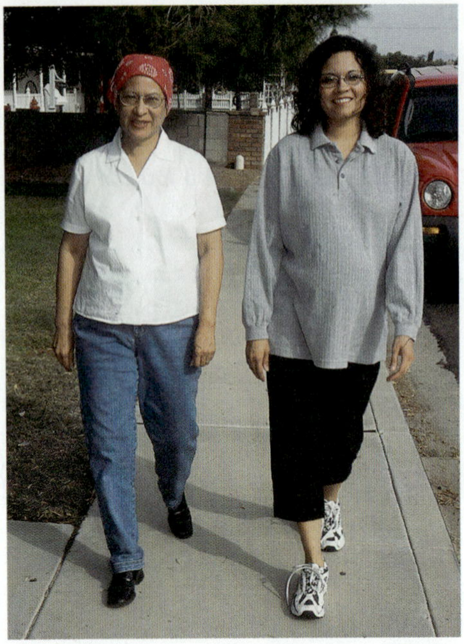

FIG. 15-1 A pregnant woman and her mother enjoying their walk together. (Courtesy Michael S. Clement, MD, Mesa, AZ.)

woman (Fig. 15-1). Reminiscing about the pregnant woman's early childhood and sharing the prospective grandmother's account of her childbirth experience help the daughter anticipate and prepare for labor and birth.

Although the woman's relationship with her mother is significant in considering her adaptation to pregnancy, the most important person to the pregnant woman is usually the father of her child. Women express two major needs within this relationship during pregnancy: feeling loved and valued and having the child accepted by the partner.

The marital or committed relationship is not static but evolves over time. The addition of a child changes forever the nature of the bond between partners. This may be a time when couples grow closer, and the pregnancy has a maturing effect on the partners' relationship as they assume new roles and discover new aspects of one another. Partners who trust and support each other are able to share mutual-dependency needs (Mercer, 1995).

Sexual expression during pregnancy is highly individual. The sexual relationship is affected by physical, emotional, and interactional factors, including misinformation about sex during pregnancy, sexual dysfunction, and physical changes in the woman. An individual may also inaccurately attribute anomalies, mental retardation, and other injuries to the fetus and mother to sexual relations during pregnancy. Some couples fear that the birth process will drastically change the woman's genitals. Some couples do not express their concerns to the health care provider because of embarrassment or because they do not want to appear foolish.

As pregnancy progresses, changes in body shape, body image, and levels of discomfort influence both partners' desire for sexual expression. During the first trimester the woman's sexual desire may decrease, especially if she has breast tenderness, nausea, fatigue, or sleepiness. As she progresses into the second trimester, however, her sense of well-being combined with the increased pelvic congestion that occurs at this time may increase her desire for sexual release. In the third trimester, somatic complaints and physical bulkiness may increase her physical discomfort and again diminish her interest in sex.

Partners need to feel free to discuss their sexual responses during pregnancy with each other and with their health care provider (see later discussion).

Establishing a Relationship with the Fetus

Emotional attachment—feelings of being tied by affection or love—begins during the prenatal period as women use fantasizing and daydreaming to prepare themselves for motherhood (Rubin, 1975). They think of themselves as mothers and imagine maternal qualities they would like to possess. Expectant parents desire to be warm, loving, and close to their child. They try to anticipate changes that the child will bring into their lives and wonder how they will react to noise, disorder, reduced freedom, and caregiving activities. The mother-child relationship progresses through pregnancy as a developmental process that unfolds in three phases.

In phase 1 the woman accepts the biologic fact of pregnancy. She needs to be able to state, "I am pregnant" and incorporate the idea of a child into her body and self-image. The woman's thoughts center around herself and the reality of her pregnancy. The child is viewed as part of herself, not a separate and unique person.

In phase 2 the woman accepts the growing fetus as distinct from herself, usually accomplished by the fifth month. She can now say, "I am going to have a baby." This differentiation of the child from the woman's self permits the beginning of the mother-child relationship that involves not only caring but also responsibility. Attachment of a mother to her child is enhanced by experiencing a planned pregnancy and it increases when ultrasound examination and quickening confirm the reality of the fetus.

With acceptance of the reality of the child (hearing the heartbeat and feeling the child move) and an overall feeling of well-being, the woman enters a quiet period and becomes more introspective. A fantasy child becomes precious to the woman. As the woman seems to withdraw and to concentrate her interest on the unborn child, her partner sometimes feels left out. If there are children in the family, they may become more demanding in their efforts to redirect the mother's attention to themselves.

During phase 3 of the attachment process, the woman prepares realistically for the birth and parenting of the child. She expresses the thought, "I am going to be a mother" and defines the nature and characteristics of the child. She may, for example, speculate about the child's sex (if unknown) and personality traits based on patterns of fetal activity.

Although the mother alone experiences the child within, both parents and siblings believe the unborn child responds in a very individualized, personal manner. Family members may interact a great deal with the unborn child by talking to the fetus and stroking the mother's abdomen, especially when the fetus shifts position (Fig. 15-2). The fetus may have a nickname used by family members.

Preparing for Childbirth

Many women actively prepare for birth by reading books, viewing films, attending parenting classes, and talking to other women. They seek the best caregiver possible for advice,

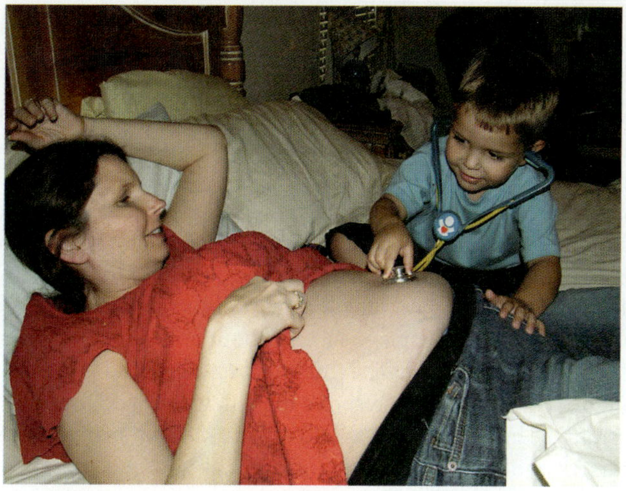

FIG. 15-2 Four-year-old likes to examine the pregnant abdomen of his mother. (Courtesy Kara George, Peoria, AZ.)

monitoring, and caring. The multiparous woman has her own history of labor and birth that influences her approach to preparation for this childbirth experience.

Anxiety can arise from concern about a safe passage for herself and her child during the birth process (Mercer, 1995; Rubin, 1975). Some women do not express this concern overtly, but they give cues to the nurse by making plans for care of the new baby and other children in case "anything should happen." These feelings persist despite statistical evidence about the safe outcome of pregnancy for mothers and their infants. Many women fear the pain of childbirth or mutilation because they do not understand anatomy and the birth process. Education can alleviate many of these fears. Women also express concern over what behaviors are appropriate during the birth process and whether caregivers will accept them and their actions.

Toward the end of the third trimester, breathing is difficult, and fetal movements become vigorous enough to disturb the woman's sleep. Backaches, frequency and urgency of urination, constipation, and varicose veins can become troublesome. The bulkiness and awkwardness of her body interfere with the woman's ability to care for other children, perform routine work-related duties, and assume a comfortable position for sleep and rest. By this time, most women become impatient for labor to begin, whether the birth is anticipated with joy, dread, or a mixture of both. A strong desire to see the end of pregnancy, to be over and done with it, makes women at this stage ready to move on to childbirth.

Paternal Adaptation

The father's beliefs and feelings about the ideal mother and father and his cultural expectation of appropriate behavior during pregnancy affect his response to his partner's need for him. One man may engage in nurturing behavior. Another may feel lonely and alienated as the woman becomes physically and emotionally engrossed in the unborn child. He may seek friends and relationships outside the home or become interested in a new hobby or involved with his work. Some men view pregnancy as proof of their masculinity and their dominant role. To others, pregnancy has no meaning in terms of responsibility to either mother or child. However, for most men, pregnancy can be a time of preparation for the parental role with intense learning.

Accepting the Pregnancy

The ways fathers adjust to the parental role has been the subject of considerable research. In older societies the man enacted the ritual couvade; that is, he behaved in specific ways and respected taboos associated with pregnancy and giving birth so his new status was recognized and endorsed. Now some men experience pregnancy-like symptoms, such as nausea, weight gain, and other physical symptoms. This phenomenon is known as the **couvade syndrome.** Changing cultural and professional attitudes have encouraged fathers' participation in the birth experience.

The man's emotional response to becoming a father, his concerns, and his informational needs change during the course of pregnancy. Phases of the developmental pattern become apparent. May (1982) described three phases characterizing the developmental tasks experienced by the expectant father:

- The *announcement phase* may last from a few hours to a few weeks. The developmental task is to accept the biologic fact of pregnancy. Men react to the confirmation of pregnancy with joy or dismay, depending on whether the pregnancy is desired, unplanned, or unwanted. Ambivalence in the early stages of pregnancy is common. If pregnancy is unplanned or unwanted, some men find the alterations in life plans and lifestyles difficult to accept. Some men engage in extramarital affairs for the first time during their partner's pregnancy. Others batter their wives for the first time or escalate the frequency of battering episodes (Krieger, 2008). Chapter 5 provides information about violence against women and offers guidance on assessment and intervention.
- The second phase, the *moratorium phase,* is the period when he adjusts to the reality of pregnancy. The developmental task is to accept the pregnancy. Men appear to put conscious thought of the pregnancy aside for a time. They become more introspective and engage in many discussions about their philosophy of life, religion, childbearing, and childrearing practices and their relationships with family members, particularly with their father. Depending on the man's readiness for the pregnancy, this phase may be relatively short or persist until the last trimester.
- The third phase, the *focusing phase,* begins in the last trimester and is characterized by the father's active involvement in both the pregnancy and his relationship with his child. The developmental task is to negotiate with his partner the role he is to play in labor and to prepare for parenthood. In this phase the man concentrates on his experience of the pregnancy and begins to think of himself as a father.

Identifying with the Father Role

Each man brings to pregnancy attitudes that affect the way in which he adjusts to the pregnancy and parental role. His memories of the fathering he received from his own father, the experiences he has had with child care, and the perceptions of the male and father roles within his social group will guide his selection of the tasks and responsibilities he will assume. Some men are highly motivated to nurture and love a child. They are excited and pleased about the anticipated role of father (Fig. 15-3). Others are more detached or even hostile to the idea of fatherhood.

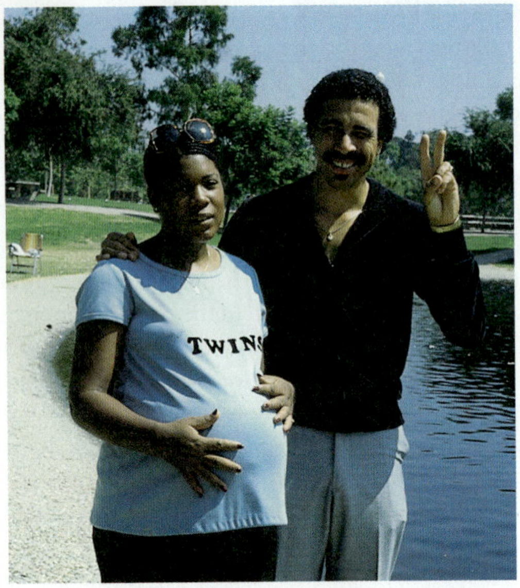

FIG. 15-3 A prospective mother and father walk together. Women respond positively to their partner's interest and concern. (Courtesy Marjorie Pyle, RNC, Lifecircle, Costa Mesa, CA.)

Reordering Personal Relationships

The partner's main role in pregnancy is to nurture and respond to the pregnant woman's feelings of vulnerability. The partner also must deal with the reality of the pregnancy. The partner's support indicates involvement in the pregnancy and preparation for attachment to the child.

Some aspects of a partner's behavior may indicate rivalry, and it may be especially evident during sexual activity. For example, some men protest that fetal movements prevent sexual gratification or feel that they are being watched by the fetus during sexual activity. However, feelings of rivalry are often unconscious and not verbalized, but expressed in subtle behaviors.

The woman's increased introspection may cause her partner to feel uneasy as she becomes preoccupied with thoughts of the child and of her motherhood, with her growing dependence on her health care provider, and with her reevaluation of the couple's relationship.

Establishing a Relationship with the Fetus

The father-child attachment can be as strong as the mother-child relationship, and fathers can be as competent as mothers in nurturing their infants. The father-child attachment also begins during pregnancy. A father may rub or kiss the maternal abdomen; try to listen, talk, or sing to the fetus; or play with the fetus as he notes movement. Calling the unborn child by name or nickname helps to confirm the reality of pregnancy and promote attachment.

Men prepare for fatherhood in many of the same ways as women do for motherhood—by reading and by fantasizing about the baby. Daydreaming about their role as father is common in the last weeks before the birth; however, men rarely describe their thoughts unless they are reassured that such daydreams are normal.

Nurses can help fathers identify concerns and prepare for the reality of a baby by asking questions such as the following:

- What do you expect the baby to look and act like?
- What do you think being a father will be like?
- Have you thought about the baby's crying? Changing diapers? Burping the baby? Being awakened at night? Sharing your partner with the baby?

Some fathers will not wish to answer such questions when they are asked but may need time to think them through or discuss them with their partners.

As the birth date approaches, men have more questions about fetal and newborn behaviors. Some men are shocked or amazed at the smallness of clothes and furniture for the baby. If an expectant father can imagine only an older child and has difficulty visualizing or talking about an infant, this situation must be explored. The nurse can tell the father about the unborn child's ability to respond to light, sound, and touch and encourage him to feel and talk to the fetus. A tour of a newborn nursery or discussions with new fathers, as in childbirth classes, may be welcomed.

Some men become involved by choosing the child's name and anticipating the child's sex, if it is not already known. Some couples select the name of the child as early as the first month of pregnancy. Family tradition, religious customs, and the continuation of the parent's name or names of relatives or friends are important in the selection process.

Preparing for Childbirth

The days and weeks immediately before the expected day of birth are characterized by anticipation and anxiety. Boredom and restlessness are common as the couple focuses on the birth process; however, during the last 2 months of pregnancy, many expectant fathers experience a surge of creative energy at home and on the job. They become dissatisfied with their present living space. If possible, they tend to act on the need to alter the environment (remodeling, painting, etc.). This activity is their way of sharing in the childbearing experience. They are able to channel the anxiety and other feelings experienced during the final weeks before birth into productive activities. This behavior earns recognition and compliments from friends, relatives, and their partners.

Major concerns for the man are getting the woman to a health care facility in time for the birth and not appearing ignorant. Many men want to be able to recognize labor and determine when it is appropriate to leave for the hospital or call the birth attendant. They fantasize different situations and plan what they will do in response to them, or rehearse taking various routes to the hospital, timing each route at different times of the day.

Some prospective fathers have questions about the labor suite's furniture and equipment, nursing staff, and location, as well as the availability of the birth attendant and anesthesia provider. Others want to know what is expected of them when their partners are in labor. The man also may have fears concerning safe passage of his child and partner and the possible death or complications of his partner and child. It is important he verbalize these fears, otherwise he cannot help his mate deal with her own spoken or unspoken apprehension.

With the exception of childbirth preparation classes, a man has few opportunities to learn ways to be an involved and active partner in this rite of passage into parenthood. Mothers often sense the tensions and apprehensions of the unprepared, unsupportive father and it often increases their fears.

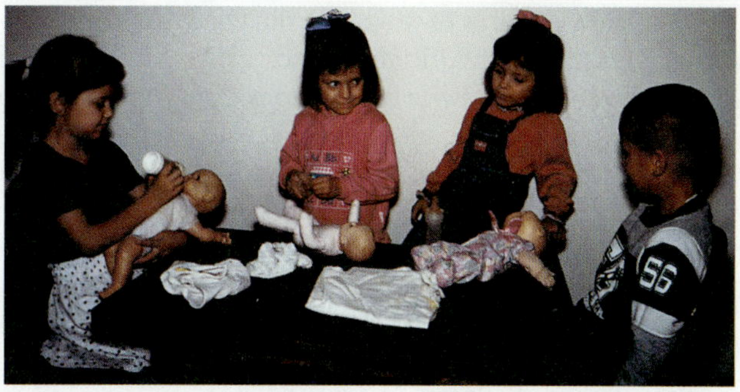

FIG. 15-4 A sibling class of preschoolers learns infant care using dolls. (Courtesy Marjorie Pyle, RNC, Lifecircle, Costa Mesa, CA.)

The same fears, questions, and concerns may affect birth partners who are not the biologic fathers. Birth partners need to be kept informed, supported, and included in all activities in which the mother desires their participation. Nurses can do much to promote pregnancy and birth as a family experience.

Sibling Adaptation

Sharing the spotlight with a new brother or sister may be the first major crisis for a child. The older child often experiences a sense of loss or feels jealous at being "replaced" by the new sibling. Some of the factors that influence the child's response are age, the parents' attitudes, the role of the father, the length of separation from the mother, the facility visitation policy, and the way the child has been prepared for the change.

A mother with other children must devote time and effort to reorganizing her relationships with them. She needs to prepare siblings for the birth of the baby (Fig. 15-4 and Box 15-2) and begin the process of role transition in the family by including the children in the pregnancy and being sympathetic to older children's concerns about losing their places in the family hierarchy. No child willingly gives up a familiar position.

Siblings' responses to pregnancy vary with their age and dependency needs. The 1-year-old infant seems largely unaware of the process, but the 2-year-old child notices the change in his or her mother's appearance and may comment that "Mommy's fat." Toddlers' need for sameness in the environment makes children aware of any change. They may exhibit more clinging behavior and sometimes regress in toilet training or eating.

By age 3 or 4 years, children like to be told the story of their own beginning and accept a comparison of their own development with that of the present pregnancy. They like to listen to the fetal heartbeat and feel the baby moving in utero (see Fig. 15-2). Sometimes they worry about how the baby is being fed and what it wears.

School-age children take a more clinical interest in their mother's pregnancy. They may want to know in more detail, "How did the baby get in there?" and "How will it get out?" Children in this age-group notice pregnant women in stores, churches, and schools and sometimes seem shy if they need to approach a pregnant woman directly. On the whole, they look forward to the new baby, see themselves as "mothers" or "fathers," and enjoy buying baby supplies and readying a place for the baby. Because they still think in concrete terms and base judgments on the here and now, they respond positively to their mother's current good health.

BOX 15-2 SIBLING ADAPTATION

TIPS FOR SIBLING PREPARATION

Prenatal

Take your child on a prenatal visit. Let the child listen to the fetal heart beat and feel the baby move.
Involve the child in preparations for the baby, such as helping decorate the baby's room.
Move the child to a bed (if still sleeping in a crib) at least 2 months before the baby is due.
Read books, show videos or DVDs, and/or take your child to sibling preparation classes, including a hospital tour.
Answer your child's questions about the coming birth, what babies are like, and any other questions.
Take your child to the homes of friends who have babies so that the child has realistic expectations of what babies are like.

During the Hospital Stay

Have someone bring the child to the hospital to visit you and the baby (unless you plan to have the child attend the birth).
Do not force interactions between the child and the baby. Often the child will be more interested in seeing you and being reassured of your love.
Help the child explore the infant by showing how and where to touch the baby.
Give the child a gift (from you or from you, the father, and baby).

Going Home

Leave the child at home with a relative or baby-sitter.
Have someone else carry the baby from the car so that you can hug the child first.

Adjustment After the Baby Is Home

Arrange for a special time for the child to be alone with each parent.
Do not exclude the child during infant feeding times. The child can sit with you and the baby and feed a doll or drink juice or milk or sit quietly with a game.
Prepare small gifts for the child so that when the baby gets gifts, the sibling won't feel left out. The child can also help open the baby gifts.
Praise the child for acting age appropriately (so that being a baby does not seem better than being older).

Early and middle adolescents preoccupied with the establishment of their own sexual identity may have difficulty accepting the overwhelming evidence of the sexual activity of their parents. They reason that if they are too young for such activity, certainly their parents are too old. They seem to take on a critical parental role and may ask, "What will people think?" or "How can you let yourself get so fat?" or "How can you let yourself get pregnant?" Many pregnant women with teenage children will confess that the attitudes of their teenagers are the most difficult aspect of their current pregnancy.

Late adolescents do not appear to be unduly disturbed. They are busy making plans for their own lives and realize that they soon will be gone from home. Parents usually report they are comforting and act more as other adults than as children.

Grandparent Adaptation

Every pregnancy affects all family relationships. For expectant grandparents a first pregnancy in a child is undeniable evidence that they are growing older. Many think of a grandparent as old, white-haired, and becoming feeble of mind and body; however, some people face grandparenthood while still in their 30s or 40s. Some individuals react negatively to the news that they will be grandparents, indicating that they are not ready for the new role.

In some family units, expectant grandparents are nonsupportive and may inadvertently decrease the self-esteem of the parents-to-be. Mothers may talk about their terrible pregnancies; fathers may discuss the endless cost of rearing children; and mothers-in-law may complain that their sons are neglecting them because their concern is now directed toward the pregnant daughters-in-law.

However, most grandparents are delighted at the prospect of a new baby in the family. It reawakens the feelings of their own youth, the excitement of giving birth, and their delight in the behavior of the parents-to-be when they were infants. They set up a memory store of the child's first smiles, first words, and first steps that they can use later for "claiming" the newborn as a member of the family. These behaviors provide a link between the past and present for the parents and grandparents-to-be.

In addition, the grandparent is the historian who transmits the family history, a resource person who shares knowledge based on experience; a role model; and a support person. The grandparent's presence and support can strengthen family systems by widening the circle of support and nurturance (Fig. 15-5).

CARE MANAGEMENT

The purpose of prenatal care is to identify existing risk factors and other deviations from normal so that pregnancy outcomes may be enhanced (Johnson, Gregory, & Niebyl, 2007). Major emphasis is placed on preventive aspects of care, primarily to motivate the pregnant woman to practice optimal self-management and to report unusual changes early so that problems can be prevented or minimized. If health behaviors must be modified in early pregnancy, nurses need to understand psychosocial factors that may influence the woman. In holistic care, nurses provide information and guidance about not only the physical changes but also the psychosocial impact of pregnancy on the woman and members of her family. The goals of prenatal nursing care, therefore, are to foster a safe birth for the infant and to promote satisfaction of the mother and family with the pregnancy and birth experience.

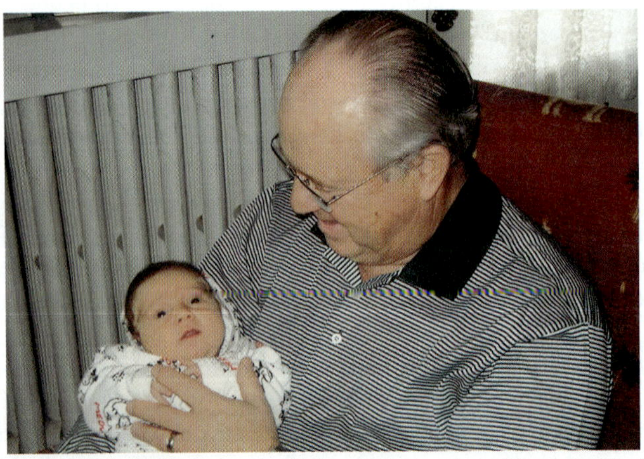

FIG. 15-5 A grandfather getting to know his grandson. (Courtesy Nicole Larson, Eden Prairie, MN.)

More than two thirds of women in the United States received care in the first trimester. African-American, Hispanic, and Native-American women were twice as likely to get late prenatal care or no care at all than were Caucasian women (Heron, Sutton, Xu, Ventura, Strobino, & Guyer, 2010). Although women of middle or high socioeconomic status routinely seek prenatal care, women living in poverty or who lack health insurance are not always able to use public health care services or gain access to private care. Lack of culturally sensitive care providers and barriers in communication resulting from differences in language also interfere with access to care (Darby, 2007). Likewise, immigrant women who come from cultures in which prenatal care is not emphasized may not know to seek routine prenatal care. Birth outcomes in these populations are less positive, with higher rates of maternal and fetal or newborn complications. Problems with low birth weight (LBW; less than 2500 g) and infant mortality have in particular been associated with lack of adequate prenatal care.

Barriers to obtaining health care during pregnancy include lack of transportation, unpleasant clinic facilities or procedures, inconvenient clinic hours, childcare problems, and personal attitudes (American College of Obstetricians and Gynecologists [ACOG] Committee on Health Care for Underserved Women, 2006; Daniels, Noe, & Mayberry, 2006; Johnson, Gregory, & Niebyl, 2007). The availability of advanced practice nurses (nurse practitioners and certified nurse-midwives) as independent providers of care or in collaborative practice with physicians improves the availability and accessibility of prenatal care. A regular schedule of home visiting by trained unlicensed health workers during pregnancy is effective in reducing barriers to prenatal care (Agency for Healthcare Research and Quality [AHRQ] Healthcare Innovations Exchange, 2009).

The current model for provision of prenatal care has been used for more than a century. The initial visit usually occurs in the first trimester, with monthly visits through week 28 of pregnancy. Thereafter, visits are scheduled every 2 weeks until week 36, and then every week until birth (American Academy of Pediatrics and ACOG, 2007) (Box 15-3). Research supports a model of fewer prenatal visits, and in some practices there is a growing tendency to have fewer visits with women who are at low risk for complications.

CenteringPregnancy is a care model that is gaining in popularity. This model is one of group prenatal care in which authority is shifted from the provider to the woman and other women who have similar due dates. The model creates an atmosphere

BOX 15-3 PRENATAL VISIT SCHEDULE

Traditional*	CenteringPregnancy†
• First visit within the first trimester (12 weeks)	• First visit within the first trimester (12 weeks)
• Monthly visits weeks 16 through 28	• Every 4 weeks—weeks 16 to 28
• Every two weeks from weeks 29 to 36	• Every 2 weeks—weeks 29 to 40
• Weekly visits week 36 to birth	

*Frequency of visits may be decreased in low risk women and increased in women with high risk pregnancies.

†Additional individual visits may be added as needed.

that facilitates learning, encourages discussion, and develops mutual support. Most care takes place in the group setting after the first visit and continues for ten 2-hour sessions (Moos, 2006). At each meeting, the first 30 minutes is spent in completing assessments (by the woman herself and by the healthcare provider), and the rest of the time is spent in group discussion of specific issues such as discomforts of pregnancy and preparation for labor and birth. Families and partners are encouraged to participate (Massey, Rising, & Ickovics, 2006; Reid, 2007) (see Box 15-3).

Prenatal care is ideally a multidisciplinary activity in which nurses work with nurse-midwives, nutritionists, physicians, social workers, and others. Collaboration among these individuals is necessary to provide holistic care. The case management model, which makes use of care maps and critical pathways, is one system that promotes comprehensive care with limited overlap in services. To emphasize the nursing role, care management for the initial visit and follow-up visits is organized around the central elements of the nursing process: assessment, nursing diagnoses, expected outcomes, plan of care and interventions, and evaluation (see the Nursing Process box).

In recent years the concept of preconception care has been recognized as an important contributor to good pregnancy outcomes (see Chapter 4). If women can be taught healthy lifestyle behaviors and then practice them before conception—specifically good nutrition, entering pregnancy with as healthy a weight as possible, adequate intake of folic acid, avoidance of alcohol and tobacco use, prevention of sexually transmitted infections (STIs) and other health hazards—a healthier pregnancy may result. Likewise, women who have health problems related to chronic diseases such as diabetes mellitus can be counseled regarding their special needs with the intent to minimize maternal and fetal complications.

Spanish Guidelines—Prenatal Interview

Initial Visit

Once the presence of pregnancy has been confirmed and the woman's desire to continue the pregnancy has been validated, prenatal care is begun. The assessment process begins at the initial prenatal visit and is continued throughout the pregnancy. Assessment techniques include the interview, physical examination, and laboratory tests. Because the initial visit and follow-up visits are distinctly different in content and process, they are described separately.

Prenatal Interview

The pregnant woman and family members who may be present should be told that the first prenatal visit is longer and more detailed than future visits. The initial evaluation includes a

NURSING PROCESS

Nursing Care During Pregnancy

ASSESSMENT

The assessment process begins at the initial prenatal visit and is continued throughout the pregnancy. Because the initial visit and follow-up visits are distinctly different in content and process, they are described separately (see text). Assessment techniques include:

- History (comprehensive health history, childbearing and reproductive system history, family history; physical abuse)
- Interview (psychosocial profile; mental status; risk assessment; symptoms she is experiencing)
- Physical examination (review of body systems; vital signs, weight; pelvic examination; fetal heart rate)
- Review of laboratory tests

NURSING DIAGNOSES

Nursing diagnoses that may be appropriate in the prenatal period include:

***Anxiety* related to:**
- physical discomforts of pregnancy
- ambivalent and labile emotions
- changes in family dynamics
- fetal well-being
- ability to manage anticipated labor

***Interrupted Family Processes* related to:**
- changing roles and responsibilities
- inadequate understanding of physical and emotional changes in pregnancy
- increased concern about labor

***Deficient Knowledge* related to:**
- posture and body mechanics
- rest and relaxation
- personal hygiene
- activity and exercise
- safety

***Disturbed Sleep Pattern* related to:**
- discomforts of late pregnancy
- anxiety about approaching labor

EXPECTED OUTCOMES OF CARE

Examples of outcomes of prenatal care include that the pregnant woman will:
- Indicate decreased anxiety about the health of her fetus and herself
- Describe improved family dynamics
- Show appropriate weight gain patterns
- Report signs and symptoms of complications
- Describe appropriate measures taken to relieve physical discomforts
- Develop a realistic birth plan

PLAN OF CARE AND INTERVENTIONS

A variety of educational materials are available to enhance the learning of the pregnant woman and her family. The following four topics are discussed in detail in the text (see detailed discussion starting on p. 344).
- Education about maternal and fetal changes
- Education for self-management
- Sexual counseling
- Psychosocial support

EVALUATION

Evaluation of the effectiveness of care of the woman during pregnancy is based on the previously stated outcomes.

comprehensive health history emphasizing the current pregnancy, previous pregnancies, the family, a psychosocial profile, a physical assessment, diagnostic testing, and an overall risk assessment. A prenatal history form (paper or electronic) is used to document information obtained.

The therapeutic relationship between the nurse and the woman is established during the initial assessment interview. Two types of data are collected: the woman's subjective appraisal of her health status and the nurse's objective observations.

One or more family members often will accompany the pregnant woman. With her permission, include those accompanying the woman in the initial prenatal interview. Observations and information about the woman's family are then included in the database. For example, if the woman has small children with her, the nurse can ask about her plans for child care during the time of labor and birth. Note any special needs at this time (e.g., wheelchair access, assistance in getting on and off the examining table, and cognitive deficits).

Reason for Seeking Care. Although pregnant women are scheduled for "routine" prenatal visits, they often come to the health care provider seeking information or reassurance about a particular concern. When the woman is asked a broad, open-ended question such as, "How have you been feeling?" she may reveal problems that could otherwise be overlooked. The woman's chief concerns should be recorded in her own words to alert other personnel to the priority of needs as identified by her. At the initial visit the desire for information about what is normal in the course of pregnancy is typical.

Current Pregnancy. The presumptive signs of pregnancy may be of great concern to the woman. A review of symptoms she is experiencing and how she is coping with them helps establish a database to develop a plan of care. Some early teaching may be provided at this time.

Childbearing and Female Reproductive System History. Data are gathered on the woman's age at menarche, menstrual history, and contraceptive history; the nature of any infertility or reproductive system conditions; a history of any STIs; a sexual history; and a detailed history of all her pregnancies, including the present pregnancy, and their outcomes. The date of the last Papanicolaou (Pap) test and the result are noted. The date of her LMP is obtained to calculate the EDB.

Health History. The health history includes those physical conditions or surgical procedures that may affect the pregnancy or that may be affected by the pregnancy. For example, a pregnant woman who has diabetes, hypertension, or epilepsy requires special care. Because most women are anxious during the initial interview, the nurse's reference to cues, such as a MedicAlert bracelet, prompts the woman to explain allergies, chronic diseases, or medications being taken (i.e., cortisone, insulin, or anticonvulsants).

The woman should also describe the nature of previous surgical procedures. If a woman has undergone uterine surgery or extensive repair of the pelvic floor, a cesarean birth may be necessary; appendectomy rules out appendicitis as a cause of right lower quadrant pain in pregnancy; and spinal surgery may contraindicate the use of spinal or epidural anesthesia. Note any injury involving the pelvis.

Women who have chronic or handicapping conditions often forget to mention them during the initial assessment because they have become so adapted to them. Special shoes or a limp may indicate the existence of a pelvic structural defect, which is an important consideration in pregnant women. The nurse who observes these special characteristics and inquires about them sensitively can obtain individualized data that will provide the basis for a comprehensive nursing care plan (Smeltzer, 2007). Observations are vital components of the interview process because they prompt the nurse and woman to focus on the specific needs of the woman and her family.

Nutritional History. The woman's nutritional history is an important component of the prenatal history because her nutritional status has a direct effect on the growth and development of the fetus. A dietary assessment can reveal special dietary practices, food allergies, eating behaviors, the practice of pica, and other factors related to her nutritional status (see Box 14-7). Obese women should receive counseling about weight gain, nutrition and food choices. They should also be advised about their risk for complications for themselves and increased risk for congenital abnormalities (Davies, Maxwell, McLeod, Gagnon, Basso, Bos, et al., 2010). Pregnant women are usually motivated to learn about good nutrition and respond well to nutritional advice generated by this assessment. Women who receive specific written and verbal information regarding nutrition, weight gain expectations, and exercise as well as weight gain reminders at each prenatal visit, are less likely to gain weight in excess of the IOM recommendations during pregnancy (Polley, Wing, & Sims, 2002).

History of Drug and Herbal Preparations Use. A woman's past and present use of drugs (legal over-the-counter [OTC] and prescription medications; herbal preparations; caffeine; alcohol; nicotine) and illegal (e.g., marijuana, cocaine, heroin) is assessed. This is because many substances cross the placenta and may therefore harm the developing fetus. See Chapter 32 for discussion of substance abuse during pregnancy. Increasing numbers of individuals are using herbal preparations, and this includes pregnant women. Therefore, it is important for health care providers to question prenatal women regarding the use of herbal preparations and document their responses.

Family History. The family history provides information about the woman's immediate family, including parents, siblings, and children. These data help identify familial or genetic disorders or conditions that could affect the present health status of the woman or her fetus.

Social, Experiential, and Occupational History. Situational factors such as the family's ethnic and cultural background and socioeconomic status are assessed while the history is obtained. The following information may be obtained in several encounters. The woman's perception of this pregnancy is explored by asking questions such as the following:

- Is this pregnancy planned or not, wanted or not?
- Is the woman pleased, displeased, accepting, or nonaccepting?
- What problems related to finances, career, or living accommodations will occur as a result of the pregnancy?

The family support system is determined by asking the following questions:

- What primary support is available to her?
- Are changes needed to promote adequate support?
- What are the existing relationships among the mother, father or partner, siblings, and in-laws?

- What preparations are being made for her care and that of dependent family members during labor and for the care of the infant after birth?
- Is financial, educational, or other support needed from the community?
- What are the woman's ideas about childbearing, her expectations of the infant's behavior, and her outlook on life and the female role?

Other questions that should be asked include the following:

- What does the woman think it will be like to have a baby in the home?
- How is her life going to change by having a baby?
- What plans are interrupted by having a baby?

During interviews throughout the pregnancy nurses should remain alert to the appearance of potential parenting problems, such as depression, lack of family support, and inadequate living conditions. Nurses must assess the woman's attitude toward health care, particularly during childbearing, her expectations of health care providers, and her view of the relationship between herself and the nurse.

Coping mechanisms and patterns of interacting are identified. Early in the pregnancy the nurse should determine the woman's knowledge in various areas: pregnancy, maternal changes, fetal growth, self-care, and care of the newborn, including feeding. Asking about attitudes toward unmedicated or medicated childbirth and about her knowledge of the availability of parenting skills classes is important. Before planning for nursing care, the nurse needs information about the woman's decision-making abilities and living habits (i.e., exercise, sleep, diet, diversional interests, personal hygiene, clothing). Common stressors during childbearing include the baby's welfare, labor and birth process, behaviors of the newborn, the woman's relationship with the baby's father and her family, changes in body image, and physical symptoms.

Explore attitudes concerning the range of acceptable sexual behavior during pregnancy by asking questions such as the following: What has your family (partner, friends) told you about sex during pregnancy? Give emphasis to the woman's sexual self-concept by asking questions such as the following: How do you feel about the changes in your appearance? How does your partner feel about your body now? How do you feel about wearing maternity clothes?

Women should be questioned regarding their occupation—past and present—because this may adversely affect maternal and fetal health. For some women, heavy lifting and exposure to chemicals and radiation may be part of their daily work, and these activities may negatively affect the pregnancy. Standing for long periods of time at a retail checkout line or in front of a classroom are associated with orthostatic hypotension. For others long hours of sitting at a desk working on a computer can contribute to carpal tunnel syndrome or circulatory stasis in the legs.

History of Physical Abuse. All women should be assessed for a history or risk of physical abuse, particularly because the likelihood of abuse increases during pregnancy. Although visual cues from the woman's appearance or behavior may suggest the possibility, no one profile of the battered woman exists. During pregnancy the target body parts change during abusive episodes. Women report physical blows directed to the head, breasts, abdomen, and genitalia. Sexual assault is common.

Battering and pregnancy in teenagers constitutes a particularly difficult situation. Adolescents may be trapped in the abusive relationship because of their inexperience. Routine screening for abuse and sexual assault is recommended for pregnant adolescents (Family Violence Prevention Fund, 2010). Because pregnancy in young adolescent girls is commonly the result of sexual abuse, the nurse should assess the desire to maintain the pregnancy (see Chapter 5 for further discussion).

Review of Systems. During this portion of the interview, ask the woman to identify and describe preexisting or concurrent problems in any of the body systems, and assess her mental status. Question the woman about physical symptoms she has experienced, such as shortness of breath or pain. Pregnancy affects and is affected by all body systems; therefore, information on the present status of the body systems is important in planning care. For each sign or symptom described, the following additional data should be obtained: body location, quality, quantity, chronology, aggravating or alleviating factors, and associated manifestations (onset, character, course) (Seidel, Ball, Dains, Flynn, Soloman, & Stewart, 2011).

Physical Examination

The initial physical examination provides the baseline for assessing subsequent changes. The nurse should determine the woman's needs for basic information regarding reproductive anatomy and provide this information, along with a demonstration of the equipment that may be used and an explanation of the procedure itself. The interaction requires an unhurried, sensitive, and gentle approach with a matter-of-fact attitude.

The physical examination begins with assessment of vital signs and height and weight (for calculation of body mass index [BMI]) (see Chapter 14). The bladder should be empty before pelvic examination. A urine specimen may be obtained to test for protein, glucose, or leukocytes or other tests.

Each examiner develops a routine for proceeding with the physical examination; most choose the head-to-toe progression. Heart and lung sounds are evaluated, and extremities are examined. Distribution, amount, and quality of body hair are of particular importance because the findings reflect nutritional status, endocrine function, and attention to hygiene. The thyroid gland is assessed carefully. The height of the fundus is noted if the first examination is done after the first trimester of pregnancy. During the examination the nurse must remain alert to the woman's cues that give direction to the remainder of the assessment and that indicate a potential threatening condition such as **supine hypotension**—low blood pressure (BP) that occurs while the woman is lying on her back, causing feelings of faintness. See Chapter 4 for a detailed description of the physical examination.

Whenever a pelvic examination is performed, the tone of the pelvic musculature and the woman's knowledge of Kegel exercises is assessed. Particular attention is paid to the size of the uterus because this is an indication of the duration of gestation. During the examination the nurse can coach the woman in breathing and relaxation techniques, as needed. One vaginal examination during pregnancy is recommended, but another is usually not performed unless medically indicated.

Spanish Guidelines—Assessment of Respiratory Symptoms, Prenatal Physical Examination

TABLE 15-1 **LABORATORY TESTS IN PRENATAL PERIOD**

LABORATORY TEST	PURPOSE
Hemoglobin, hematocrit, WBC, differential	Detects anemia; detects infection
Hemoglobin electrophoresis	Identifies women with hemoglobinopathies (e.g., sickle cell anemia, thalassemia)
Blood type, Rh, and irregular antibody	Identifies those fetuses at risk for developing erythroblastosis fetalis or hyperbilirubinemia in neonatal period
Rubella titer	Determines immunity to rubella
Tuberculin skin testing; chest film after 20 weeks of gestation in women with reactive tuberculin tests	Screens for exposure to tuberculosis
Urinalysis, including microscopic examination of urinary sediment; pH, specific gravity, color, glucose, albumin, protein, RBCs, WBCs, casts, acetone; hCG	Identifies women with glycosuria, renal disease, hypertensive disease of pregnancy; infection; occult hematuria
Urine culture	Identifies women with asymptomatic bacteriuria
Renal function tests: BUN, creatinine, electrolytes, creatinine clearance, total protein excretion	Evaluates level of possible renal compromise in women with a history of diabetes, hypertension, or renal disease
Pap test	Screens for cervical intraepithelial neoplasia; if a liquid-based test is used, may also screen for HPV
Cervical cultures for *Neisseria gonorrhoeae, Chlamydia*	Screens for asymptomatic infection at first visit
Vaginal/anal culture	GBS test done at 35-37 weeks for infection
RPR, VDRL, or FTA-ABS	Identifies women with untreated syphilis, done at first visit
HIV antibody, hepatitis B surface antigen, toxoplasmosis	Screens for the specific infections
1-hour glucose tolerance	Screens for gestational diabetes; done at initial visit for women with risk factors; done at 24-28 weeks for pregnant women at risk whose initial screen was negative; women with low risk usually not tested
3-hour glucose tolerance	Tests for gestational diabetes in women with elevated glucose level after 1-hour test; must have two elevated readings for diagnosis
Cardiac evaluation: ECG, chest x-ray, and echocardiogram	Evaluates cardiac function in women with a history of hypertension or cardiac disease

BUN, Blood urea nitrogen; *ECG,* electrocardiogram; *FTA-ABS,* fluorescent treponemal antibody absorption test; *GBS,* group B streptococci; *hCG,* human chorionic gonadotropin; *HIV,* human immunodeficiency virus; *HPV,* human papillomavirus; *RBC,* red blood cell; *RPR,* rapid plasma reagin; *VDRL,* Venereal Disease Research Laboratory; *WBC,* white blood cell.

Laboratory Tests

The laboratory data yielded by the analysis of the specimens obtained during the examination provide important information concerning the symptoms of pregnancy and the woman's health status.

Specimens are collected at the initial visit so that the cause of any abnormal findings can be treated (Table 15-1). Blood is drawn for a variety of tests. A sickle cell screen is recommended for women of African, Asian, or Middle Eastern descent, and testing for antibody to the human immunodeficiency virus (HIV) is strongly recommended for all pregnant women (Centers for Disease Control and Prevention [CDC], Workowski, & Berman, 2006) (Box 15-4). In addition, pregnant women and fathers with a family history of cystic fibrosis and of Caucasian ethnicity may elect to have blood drawn for testing to ascertain if they are a cystic fibrosis carrier (Norton, 2008). A urine specimen is collected for cultures and metabolic function tests. A purified protein derivative (PPD) tuberculin test may be administered to assess exposure to tuberculosis. During the pelvic examination, cervical and vaginal smears can be obtained for cytologic studies and for diagnosis of infection (e.g., gonorrhea, chlamydia).

The finding of risk factors during pregnancy may indicate the need to repeat some tests at other times. For example, exposure to tuberculosis or an STI would necessitate repeat testing after treatment. STIs are common in pregnancy and may have negative effects on mother and fetus. Careful assessment and screening are essential.

BOX 15-4 **HIV SCREENING**

- Pregnant women are ethically obligated to seek reasonable care during pregnancy and to avoid causing harm to the fetus. Women's health nurses should be advocates for the fetus while accepting of the pregnant woman's decision regarding testing and/or treatment for HIV.
- The incidence of perinatal transmission from an HIV-positive mother to her fetus is about 25%. Triple drug antiviral or highly active antiretroviral therapy (HAART) during pregnancy decreases perinatal transmission and the risk of infant death. Elective cesarean birth and avoidance of breastfeeding combined with HAART reduce transmission to the neonate to less than 2%.

Testing has the potential to identify HIV-positive women who can then be treated. Health care providers have an obligation to ensure that pregnant women are well informed about HIV symptoms, testing, and methods of decreasing maternal-fetal transmission. The Centers for Disease Control and Prevention and the American College of Obstetricians and Gynecologists recommend universal opt-out screening, which means that all pregnant women are offered HIV screening but have the opportunity to opt out if desired (ACOG Committee on Obstetric Practice, 2004; Branson, Handsfield, Lampe, Janssen, Taylor, Lyss, et al., 2006). The Association of Women's Health, Obstetric and Neonatal Nurses (AWHONN) supports this system of HIV screening that allows all pregnant women to be offered screening (2008).

Sources: American College of Obstetricians and Gynecologists Committee on Obstetric Practice. (2004). Prenatal and perinatal human immunodeficiency virus testing: Expanded recommendations. ACOG Committee Opinion No. 304. *Obstetrics and Gynecology, 104*(5 Part 1), 1119-1124; AWHONN (2008). *HIV screening procedures for pregnant women and newborns.* Policy position statement. Washington, DC: AWHONN. Available at www.awhonn.org. Accessed June 22, 2010. Branson, B., Handsfield, H., Lampe, M., Janssen, R., Taylor, A., Lyss, S., et al. (2006). Revised recommendations for HIV testing of adults, adolescents, and pregnant women in health-care settings. *MMWR Morbidity and Morbidity Weekly Report, 55*(RR-14), 1-17.

Follow-up Visits

In traditional prenatal care, monthly visits are scheduled routinely during the first and second trimesters, although clients can make additional appointments as the need arises. During the third trimester, however, the possibility for complications increases, and closer monitoring is necessary. Starting with week 28, maternity visits are scheduled every 2 weeks until week 36 and then every week until birth, unless the health care provider individualizes the schedule. Visits can occur more or

Video—Assessment: Chest Wall

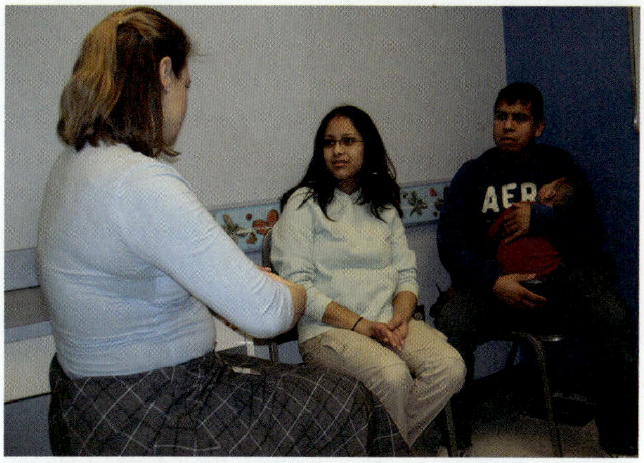

FIG. 15-6 A prenatal interview. (Courtesy Dee Lowdermilk, Chapel Hill, NC.)

less frequently, often depending on individual needs, complications, and risks of the pregnant woman. The pattern of interviewing the woman first and then assessing physical changes and performing laboratory tests continues.

In prenatal care models that use a reduced frequency screening schedule or in CenteringPregnancy, the timing of follow-up visits will be different, but assessments and care will be similar.

Interview

Follow-up visits are less intensive than the initial prenatal visit. At each of these follow-up visits, the woman is asked to summarize relevant events that have occurred since the previous visit. She is asked about her general emotional and physiologic well-being, complaints, problems, and questions she may have. Personal and family needs also are identified and explored (Fig. 15-6).

Emotional changes are common during pregnancy, and therefore asking whether the woman has experienced any mood swings, reactions to changes in her body image, bad dreams, or worries is reasonable. Note any positive feelings (her own and those of her family). Record the reactions of family members to the pregnancy and the woman's emotional changes.

During the third trimester, assess current family situations and their effect on the woman. For example, assess siblings' and grandparents' responses to the pregnancy and the coming child. In addition, assess the woman and her family's knowledge of warning signs of emergencies; signs of preterm and term labor; the labor process and concerns about labor; and fetal development and methods to assess fetal well-being. The nurse should ask if the woman is planning to attend childbirth preparation classes and what she knows about pain management during labor.

A review of the woman's physical systems is appropriate at each prenatal visit, and any suspicious signs or symptoms are assessed in depth. Identify any discomforts reflecting adaptations to pregnancy. Inquire about success with self-care measures as well as outcomes of prescribed therapy.

Physical Examination

Reevaluation is a constant aspect of a pregnant woman's care. Physiologic changes are documented as the pregnancy progresses and reviewed for possible deviations from normal progress.

EMERGENCY

Supine Hypotension

SIGNS AND SYMPTOMS

- Pallor
- Dizziness, faintness, breathlessness
- Tachycardia
- Nausea
- Clammy (damp, cool) skin; sweating

INTERVENTIONS

- Position woman on her side until her signs and symptoms subside and vital signs stabilize within normal limits (WNL).

At each visit physical parameters are measured. BP is measured using the same arm at every visit (see Box 13-1). The woman's weight is assessed, and the appropriateness of the gestational weight gain is evaluated in relationship to her BMI. Urine may be checked by dipstick, and the presence and degree of edema are noted. For examination of the abdomen, the woman lies on her back with her arms by her side and head supported by a pillow. The bladder should be empty. Abdominal inspection is followed by measurement of the height of the fundus (see Fig. 15-7). While the woman lies on her back, the nurse should be alert for the occurrence of supine hypotension. When a pregnant woman is lying in this position, the weight of the abdominal contents may compress the vena cava and aorta, causing a decrease in BP and a feeling of faintness (see the Emergency box).

The information provided through the interview and the physical examination reflects the status of maternal adaptations. When any of the findings are suspicious, an in-depth examination is performed. For example, careful interpretation of BP is important in the risk factor analysis of all pregnant women. Signs and symptoms other than hypertension also may be present that indicate potential complications (see the Signs of Potential Complications box).

Fetal Assessment

Listening for Fetal Heart Tones. Toward the end of the first trimester, before the uterus is an abdominal organ, the fetal heart tones (FHTs) can be heard with an ultrasound fetoscope or an ultrasound stethoscope (see Fig. 15-8). To hear the FHTs, place the instrument in the midline, just above the symphysis pubis, and apply firm pressure. Offer the woman and her family the opportunity to listen to the FHTs.

Measuring Fundal Height. During the second trimester the uterus becomes an abdominal organ. The fundal height (measurement of the height of the uterus above the symphysis pubis) is used as one indicator of fetal growth. The measurement also provides a gross estimate of the duration of pregnancy. From gestational weeks (GW) 18 to 32, the height of the fundus in centimeters is approximately the same as the number of weeks of gestation (± 2 GW), if the woman's bladder is empty at the time of measurement. As much as a 3-cm variation is possible if the bladder is full (Cunningham, Leveno, Bloom, Hauth, Rouse, & Spong, 2010). For example, a woman of 28 weeks of gestation, with an empty bladder, would measure from 26 to 30 cm. In addition, the fundal height measurement may aid in the identification of high risk factors. A stable or decreased fundal height

Video—Assessment: Abdomen Fundal Height, Fetal Heart Rate

SIGNS OF POTENTIAL COMPLICATIONS

First, Second, and Third Trimesters

SIGNS AND SYMPTOMS	POSSIBLE CAUSES
FIRST TRIMESTER	
Severe vomiting	Hyperemesis gravidarum
Chills, fever	Infection
Burning on urination	Infection
Diarrhea	Infection
Abdominal cramping; vaginal bleeding	Miscarriage, ectopic pregnancy
SECOND AND THIRD TRIMESTERS	
Persistent, severe vomiting	Hyperemesis gravidarum, hypertension, preeclampsia
Sudden discharge of fluid from vagina before 37 weeks	Premature rupture of membranes (PROM)
Vaginal bleeding, severe abdominal pain	Miscarriage, placenta previa, abruptio placentae
Chills, fever, burning on urination, diarrhea	Infection
Severe backache or flank pain	Kidney infection or stones; preterm labor
Change in fetal movements: absence of fetal movements after quickening, any unusual change in pattern or amount	Fetal jeopardy or intrauterine fetal death
Uterine contractions; pressure; cramping before 37 weeks	Preterm labor
Visual disturbances: blurring, double vision, or spots	Hypertensive conditions, preeclampsia
Swelling of face or fingers and over sacrum	Hypertensive conditions, preeclampsia
Headaches: severe, frequent, or continuous	Hypertensive conditions, preeclampsia
Muscular irritability or convulsions	Hypertensive conditions, preeclampsia
Epigastric or abdominal pain (perceived as heartburn or severe stomachache)	Hypertensive conditions, preeclampsia, abruptio placentae
Glycosuria, positive glucose tolerance test reaction	Gestational diabetes mellitus

may indicate the presence of intrauterine growth restriction (IUGR); an excessive increase could indicate the presence of multifetal gestation (more than one fetus) or polyhydramnios.

A disposable paper metric tape measure is preferred for measuring fundal height; plastic retractable tape measures should be cleaned after use and prior to retraction. To increase the reliability of the measurement, the same person examines the pregnant woman at each of her prenatal visits, but often this is not possible. All clinicians who examine a particular pregnant woman should be consistent in their measurement technique. Ideally, a protocol should be established for the health care setting in which the measurement technique is explicitly set forth, and the woman's position on the examining table, the measuring device, and method of measurement used are specified. Conditions under which the measurements are taken also can be described in the woman's records, including whether the bladder was empty and whether the uterus was relaxed or contracted at the time of measurement.

Video—Nursing Skill: Assessing Fundal Height

Various positions for measuring fundal height have been described. The woman can be supine, have her head elevated, have her knees flexed, or have both her head elevated and knees flexed. Measurements obtained with the woman in the various positions differ, making it even more important to standardize the fundal height measurement technique.

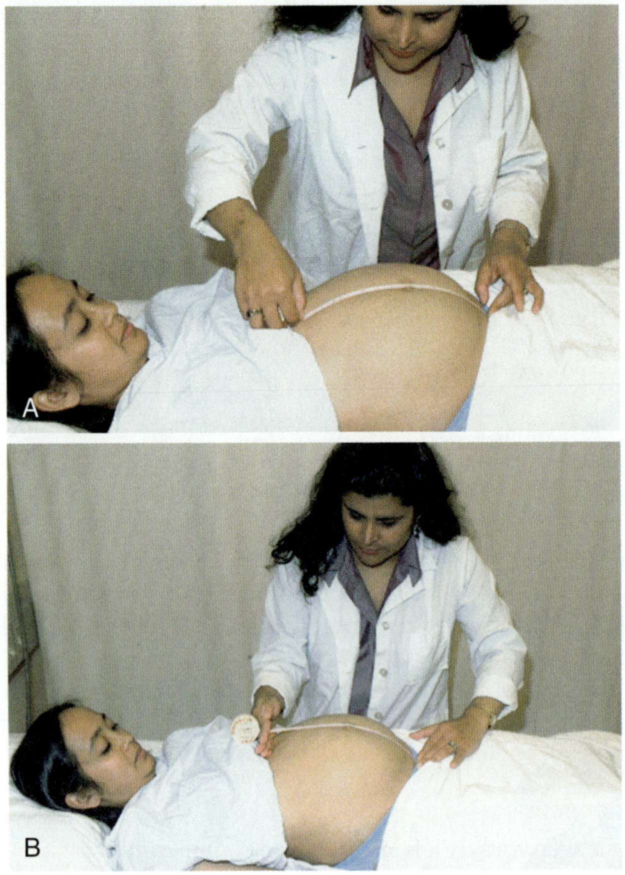

FIG. 15-7 Measurement of fundal height from symphysis that **(A)**, includes the upper curve of the fundus and **(B)**, does not include the upper curve of the fundus. Note position of hands and measuring tape. (Courtesy Chris Rozales, San Francisco, CA.)

Placement of the tape measure also can vary. The tape can be placed in the middle of the woman's abdomen and the measurement made from the upper border of the symphysis pubis to the upper border of the fundus, with the tape measure held in contact with the skin for the entire length of the uterus (Fig. 15-7, *A*). In another measurement technique, the upper curve of the fundus is not included in the measurement. Instead, one end of the tape measure is held at the upper border of the symphysis pubis with one hand, and the other hand is placed at the upper border of the fundus. The tape is placed between the middle and index fingers of the other hand, and the point where these fingers intercept the tape measure is taken as the measurement (see Fig. 15-7, *B*).

Gestational Age. In an uncomplicated pregnancy fetal gestational age is estimated after the duration of pregnancy and the EDB are determined. Fetal gestational age is determined from the menstrual history, contraceptive history, pregnancy test result, and the following findings obtained during the clinical evaluation:

- First uterine evaluation: date, size
- Fetal heart first heard: date, method (Doppler stethoscope, fetoscope)
- Date of quickening

Video—Nursing Skill: Auscultating the Fetal Heart Rate

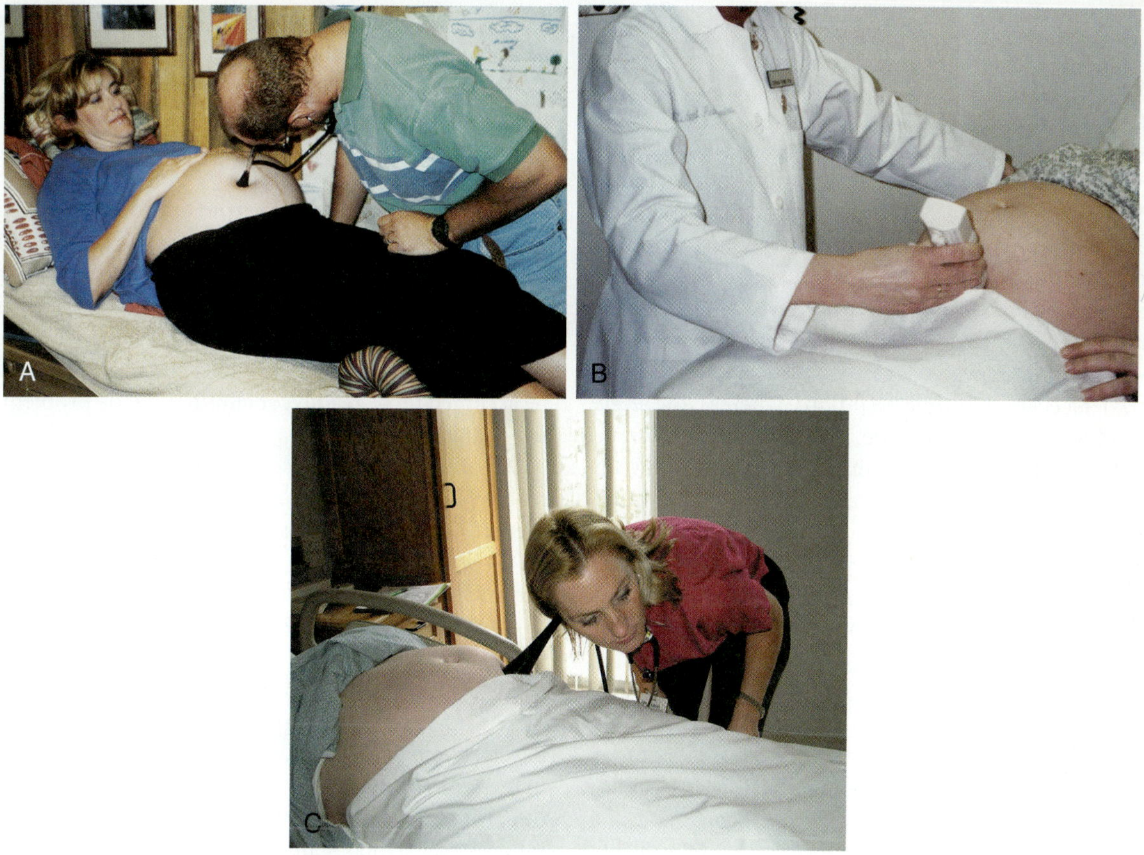

FIG. 15-8 Detecting fetal heart rate. **A,** Father listens to the fetal heart (first detectable around 18 to 20 weeks) with a fetoscope. **B,** Doppler ultrasound stethoscope (fetal heartbeat detectable at 12 weeks). **C,** Pinard fetoscope. Note: Hands should not touch fetoscope while listening. **(A,** Courtesy Shannon Perry, Phoenix, AZ; **B,** courtesy Dee Lowdermilk, Chapel Hill, NC; **C,** courtesy Julie Perry Nelson, Loveland, CO.)

- Current fundal height, estimated fetal weight (EFW)
- Current week of gestation by history of LMP and/or ultrasound examination
- Ultrasound examination: date, week of gestation, biparietal diameter (BPD)
- Reliability of dates

Quickening usually occurs between 16 and 20 weeks of gestation and is initially experienced as a fluttering sensation. The mother's report should be recorded. Multiparas often perceive fetal movement earlier than primigravidas.

The use of ultrasound examination (also called a *sonogram*) in early pregnancy has become routine, and many health care providers have this equipment available in the office. This procedure may be used to establish the duration of pregnancy if the woman cannot give a precise date for her LMP or if the size of the uterus does not conform to the EDB as calculated by Nägele's rule. Ultrasound also provides information about the well-being of the fetus (see Chapter 26 for further discussion). However, the routine use of ultrasound has not been found to substantively improve fetal outcome (Hunter, 2009).

Health Status. The assessment of fetal health status includes consideration of fetal movement. The mother is instructed to note the extent and timing of fetal movements and to report immediately if the pattern changes or if movement ceases. Regular movement has been found to be a reliable indicator of fetal health (Frøen, Heazell, Tveit, Saastad, Fretts, & Flenday, 2008) (see Chapter 26).

The fetal heart rate (FHR) is checked on routine visits once it has been heard (Fig. 15-8). Early in the second trimester, the heartbeat may be heard with a Doppler stethoscope (see Fig. 15-8, *B*). To detect the heartbeat before the fetal position can be palpated by Leopold maneuvers (see Chapter 19), the scope is moved around the abdomen until the heartbeat is heard. Each nurse develops a set pattern for searching the abdomen for the heartbeat—for example, starting first in the midline about 2 to 3 cm above the symphysis, then moving to the left lower quadrant, and so on. The heartbeat is counted for 1 minute, and the quality and rhythm noted. Later in the second trimester, the FHR can be determined with a fetoscope or a Pinard fetoscope (see Fig. 15-8, *A* and *C*). A normal rate and rhythm are other good indicators of fetal health. Once the heartbeat is noted, its absence is cause for immediate investigation.

Fetal health status is investigated intensively if any maternal or fetal complications arise (e.g., gestational hypertension, IUGR, premature rupture of membranes [PROM], irregular or absent FHR, or decreased/absent fetal movements after quickening). Careful, precise, and concise recording of client responses and laboratory results contributes to the continuous supervision vital to ensuring the well-being of the mother and fetus.

Laboratory Tests

The number of routine laboratory tests done during follow-up visits in pregnancy is limited. A clean-catch urine specimen is obtained to test for glucose, protein, nitrites, and leukocytes at each visit. Urine specimens for culture and sensitivity are obtained, and cervical and vaginal smears and blood tests are repeated as necessary.

First-trimester screening for chromosomal abnormalities is offered as an option between 11 and 14 weeks. This multiple marker screen includes sonographic evaluation of nuchal translucency (NT) and biochemical markers—pregnancy-associated placental protein (PAPP-A) and free beta-human chorionic gonadotropin (β-hCG).

Maternal serum alpha-fetoprotein (MSAFP) screening is recommended between 15 and 22 GW, ideally between 16 and 18 weeks of gestation. Elevated levels are associated with open neural tube defects and multiple gestations, whereas low levels are associated with Down syndrome. The multiple-marker, or triple-screen, blood test is also recommended. Done between 16 and 18 weeks of gestation, it measures the MSAFP, hCG, and unconjugated estriol, the levels of which are combined to yield one value. Maternal serum marker levels that are higher or lower than normal are associated with chromosomal abnormalities (see Chapter 26). If not done earlier in pregnancy, a glucose screen is obtained for women at high risk for gestational diabetes between 24 and 28 weeks of gestation. GBS testing is done between 35 and 37 weeks of gestation; cultures collected earlier will not accurately predict GBS status at time of birth (Van Dyke, Phares, Lynfield, Thomas, Arnold, Craig, et al., 2009).

Other diagnostic tests, such as amniocentesis, are available to assess the health status of both the pregnant woman and the fetus (See Chapter 26 for further discussion).

Collaborative Care

After obtaining information through the assessment process, the data are analyzed to identify deviations from the norm and unique needs of the pregnant woman and her family.

The nurse-client relationship is critical in setting the tone for further interaction. The techniques of listening with an attentive expression, touching, and using eye contact have their place, as does recognizing the woman's feelings and her right to express these feelings. The interaction may occur in various formal or informal settings. A clinical setting, home visits, or telephone conversations all provide opportunities for contact and can be used effectively.

In supporting a woman, the nurse must remember that both the nurse and the woman are contributing to the relationship. The nurse has to accept the woman's responses as a factor in trying to be of help. An example of one nurse-client relationship is as follows:

> Keisha has been very forthright in saying that this pregnancy was unplanned but had countered this observation with comments such as, "All things happen for the best," and "Children bring their own love." Over time, as our relationship developed to one of mutual trust, she complained increasingly of her fear of pain, of hating to wear maternity clothes, and of having to give up helping the family. Finally I ventured to say, "Sometimes when a pregnancy is unplanned, women resent it and are angry about it." Her relief was evident. She said, "You don't know how angry I've been." As a result, the whole tenor of support being offered changed, and the plan was adjusted to meet her real needs.

The nurse also must accept that the woman must be a willing partner in a purely voluntary relationship. As such, the relationship can be refused or terminated at any time by the pregnant woman or her family.

Supportive care involves developing, augmenting, or changing the mechanisms used by women and their families in coping with stress. The nurse tries to promote active participation by the family in the solution of their own problems. The nurse can help a woman gather pertinent information, explore options, decide on a course of action, and assume responsibility for the outcomes. These outcomes may include living with a problem as it is, easing the effects of a problem so that it can be accepted more readily, or eliminating the problem by effecting change.

At other times a successful outcome can be documented readily. For example, a woman who early in her pregnancy had predicted a severe depressive state in the post-birth period was elated when such a state did not materialize. She remarked to the nurse who had provided support during the labor and birth, "You're the best nerve medicine I've ever had!"

Education About Maternal and Fetal Changes

Expectant parents are typically curious about the growth and development of the fetus and the subsequent changes that occur in the mother's body. Mothers in particular are sometimes more tolerant of the discomforts related to the continuing pregnancy if they understand the underlying causes. Educational literature that describes fetal and maternal changes is available and can be used in explaining changes as they occur. The nurse's familiarity with any material shared with pregnant families is essential to effective client education. Educational material may include electronic and written materials appropriate to the pregnant woman's or couple's literacy level and experience and the agency's resources. It is important that available educational materials reflect the pregnant woman's or couple's ethnicity, culture, and literacy level to be most effective.

Education for Self-Management

The expectant mother needs information about many subjects. The nurse who is observant, listens, and knows typical concerns of expectant parents can anticipate questions that will be asked and prompt mothers and partners to discuss what is on their minds. Many times, printed literature can be given to supplement the individualized teaching the nurse provides, and women often avidly read books and pamphlets related to their own experience. When nurses read the literature before they distribute it, they can point out areas that may not correspond with local health care practices. Because family members are common sources for health information, it is also important to include them in the health education endeavors (Yamashita, 2009). In addition, as more individuals use the computer for information, the pregnant woman or couple may have questions from their Internet reviews. Nurses may also share recommended electronic sites from reliable sources.

Pregnant women who receive conflicting advice or instruction are likely to grow increasingly frustrated with members of the health care team and the care provided. Several topics that may cause concerns in pregnant women are discussed in the following sections.

Nutrition. Good nutrition is important for the maintenance of maternal health during pregnancy and the provision of adequate nutrients for embryonic and fetal development (American Dietetic Association [ADA], 2008). Assessing a woman's nutritional status and providing information on nutrition are part of the nurse's responsibilities in providing prenatal care. This includes assessment of weight gain during pregnancy as well as prenatal nutrition. Teaching may include discussion about foods high in iron, encouragement to take prenatal vitamins, and recommendations to moderate or limit caffeine intake. In some settings a registered dietitian conducts classes for pregnant women on the topics of nutritional status and nutrition during pregnancy, or interviews them to assess their knowledge of these topics. Nurses can refer women to a registered dietitian if a need is revealed during the nursing assessment. (For detailed information concerning maternal and fetal nutritional needs and related nursing care, see Chapter 14.)

Personal Hygiene. During pregnancy the sebaceous (sweat) glands are highly active because of hormonal influences, and women often perspire freely. They may be reassured that the increase is normal and that their previous patterns of perspiration will return after the postpartum period. Baths and warm showers can be therapeutic because they relax tense, tired muscles, help counter insomnia, and make the pregnant woman feel fresh. Tub bathing is permitted even in late pregnancy because little water enters the vagina unless under pressure. However, late in pregnancy, when the woman's center of gravity lowers, she is at risk for falling. Tub bathing is contraindicated after rupture of the membranes.

Prevention of Urinary Tract Infections. Because of physiologic changes that occur in the renal system during pregnancy (see Chapter 13), urinary tract infections (UTIs) are common but they may be asymptomatic. Women should be instructed to inform their health care provider if blood or pain occurs with urination. UTIs pose a risk to the mother and fetus; therefore, the prevention or early treatment of these infections is essential.

The nurse can assess the woman's understanding and use of good handwashing techniques before and after urinating and the importance of wiping the perineum from front to back. Soft, absorbent toilet tissue, preferably white and unscented, should be used; harsh, scented, or printed toilet paper may cause irritation. Bubble bath or other bath oils should be avoided because these may irritate the urethra. Women should wear cotton-crotch underpants and pantyhose and avoid tight-fitting slacks or jeans for long periods; anything that allows a buildup of heat and moisture in the genital area may foster the growth of bacteria.

Some women do not consume enough fluid and food. After discovering the woman's food preferences, the nurse should advise her to drink at least 2 L (eight glasses) of liquid a day, preferably water, to maintain an adequate fluid intake that ensures frequent urination. Pregnant women should not limit fluids in an effort to reduce the frequency of urination. Women need to know that if urine looks dark (concentrated), they must increase their fluid intake. The consumption of yogurt and acidophilus milk may help prevent urinary tract and vaginal infections. The nurse should review healthy urination practices with the woman. Women are told not to ignore the urge to urinate because holding urine lengthens the time bacteria are in the bladder and allows them to multiply. Women should plan ahead when they are faced with situations that may normally require them to delay urination (e.g., a long car ride). They always should urinate before going to bed at night. Bacteria can be introduced during intercourse; therefore, women are advised to urinate before and after intercourse, and then drink a large glass of water to promote additional urination. Although frequently recommended, there is conflicting evidence regarding the effectiveness of cranberry juice and, in particular, the effective dosage in the prevention of urinary tract infections (Jepson & Craig, 2008).

Kegel Exercises. Kegel exercises (deliberate contraction and relaxation of the pubococcygeus muscle) strengthen the muscles around the reproductive organs and improve muscle tone. Many women are not aware of the muscles of the pelvic floor until it is pointed out that these are the muscles used during urination and sexual intercourse that can be consciously controlled. The muscles of the pelvic floor encircle the vaginal outlet, and they need to be exercised because an exercised muscle can then stretch and contract readily at the time of birth. Practice of pelvic muscle exercises during pregnancy also results in fewer complaints of urinary incontinence in late pregnancy and postpartum (Lentz, 2007).

Several ways of performing Kegel exercises have been described. The method described in the Teaching for Self-Management box on p. 91. demonstrates evidence-based nursing care. This method was developed by nurses involved in a research utilization project for continence in women. Teaching has been effective if the woman reports an increased ability to control urine flow and greater muscular control during sexual intercourse.

Preparation for Breastfeeding. Pregnant women are usually eager to discuss their plans for feeding the newborn. Breast milk is the food of choice, in part because breastfeeding is associated with a decreased incidence of perinatal morbidity and mortality. The American Academy of Pediatrics recommends breastfeeding for at least a year. However, a deep-seated aversion to breastfeeding on the part of the woman or partner, the woman's need for certain medications or use of street drugs, and certain life-threatening illnesses and medical complications, such as HIV infection, are contraindications to breastfeeding (Lawrence & Lawrence, 2005). Although hepatitis B surface antigen (HBsAg) has not been shown to be transmitted through breast milk, as an added precaution, it is recommended that infants born to HBsAg-positive women receive the hepatitis B vaccine and hepatitis B immune globulin (HBIg) immediately after birth. In developed countries, women who are HIV positive are discouraged from nursing because the risk of HIV transmission outweighs the risk of the infant dying from another cause (Lawrence & Lawrence).

A woman's decision about the method of infant feeding often is made before pregnancy; therefore, educating women of childbearing age about the benefits of breastfeeding is essential. If undecided, the pregnant woman and her partner are given information about the advantages and disadvantages of bottle feeding and breastfeeding so they can make an informed choice. Health care providers support their decisions and provide any needed teaching,

Women with inverted nipples need special consideration if they are planning to breastfeed. The **pinch test** is done to

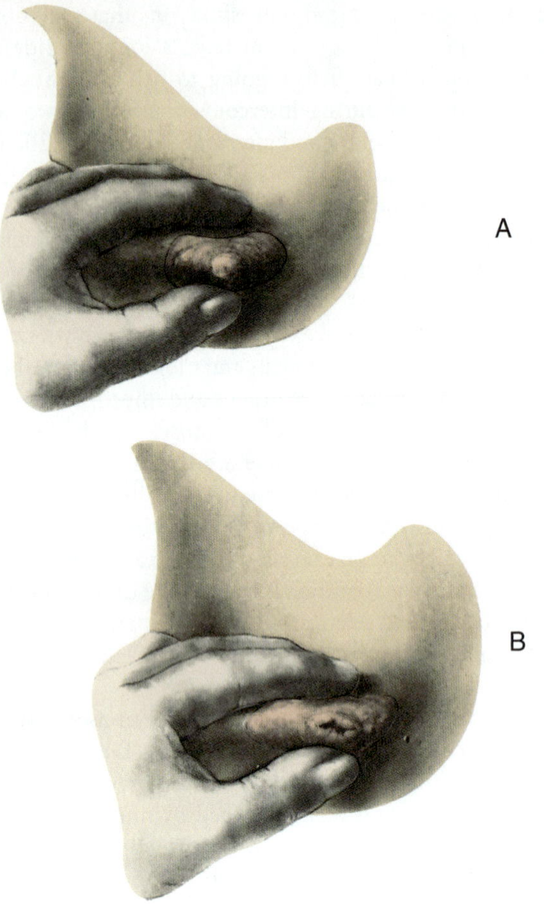

FIG. 15-9 **A,** Normal nipple everts with gentle pressure. **B,** Inverted nipple inverts with gentle pressure. (Modified from Lawrence, R., & Lawrence, R. [2005]. *Breastfeeding: A guide for the medical profession* [6th ed.]. Philadelphia: Mosby.)

determine whether the nipple is everted or inverted (Fig. 15-9). The nurse shows the woman the way to perform the pinch test. It involves having the woman place her thumb and forefinger on her areola and gently press inward. This action will cause her nipple either to stand erect or to invert. Most nipples will stand erect.

Exercises to break the adhesions that cause the nipple to invert do not work and may precipitate uterine contractions (Lawrence & Lawrence, 2005). Breast shells, small plastic devices that fit over the nipples, may be recommended for women who have flat or inverted nipples (Fig. 15-10). Breast shells work by exerting a continuous, gentle pressure around the areola that pushes the nipple through a central opening in the inner shield. The shells should be worn for 1 to 2 hours daily during the last trimester of pregnancy and for gradually increasing lengths of time (Lawrence & Lawrence). Breast stimulation is contraindicated in women at risk for preterm labor; therefore, the decision to suggest the use of breast shells to women with flat or inverted nipples must be made judiciously.

Video—Assessment: Breast

The woman is taught to cleanse the nipples with warm water to keep the ducts from being blocked with dried colostrum. Soap, ointments, alcohol, and tinctures should not be applied because they remove protective oils that keep the nipples supple. The use of these substances may cause the nipples to crack during early lactation (Lawrence & Lawrence, 2005).

The woman who plans to breastfeed should purchase a nursing bra that will accommodate her increased breast size during

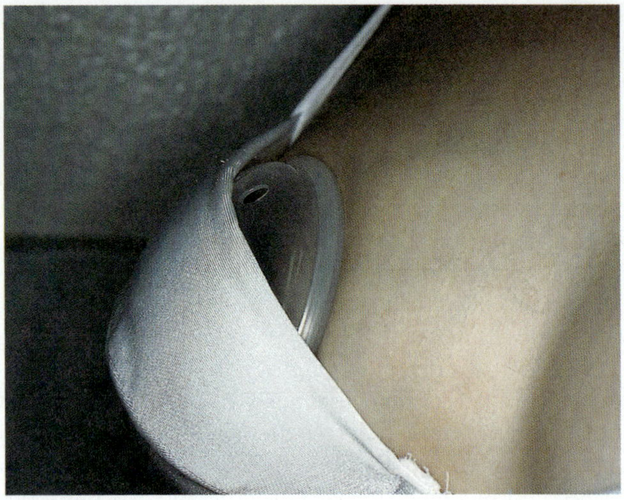

FIG. 15-10 Breast shell in place inside bra to evert nipple. (Courtesy Michael S. Clement, MD, Mesa, AZ.)

the last few months of pregnancy and during lactation. If her breasts are very heavy, or if the woman feels uncomfortable with the weight unsupported, the bra can be worn day and night.

Dental Care. Dental care during pregnancy is especially important because nausea during pregnancy may lead to poor oral hygiene, allowing dental caries to develop. A fluoride toothpaste should be used daily. Inflammation and infection of the gingival and periodontal tissues may occur (Russell & Mayberry, 2008). Research links periodontal disease with preterm births and LBW (Lopez, 2005) and an increased risk for preeclampsia (Boggess & Edelstein, 2006; Dasanayake, Gennaro, Hendricks-Munoz, & Chhun, 2008).

Because calcium and phosphorus in the teeth are fixed in enamel, the old adage "for every child a tooth" is not true. There is no scientific evidence to support the belief that filling teeth or even dental extraction involving the administration of local or nitrous oxide–oxygen anesthesia precipitates miscarriage or premature labor. However, antibacterial therapy should be considered for sepsis, especially in pregnant women who have had rheumatic heart disease or nephritis. Emergency dental surgery is not contraindicated during pregnancy. However, explain the risks and benefits of dental surgery to the woman. The American Dental Association (2006) recommends that elective dental treatment not be scheduled in the first trimester or last half of the third trimester. The woman will be most comfortable during the second trimester because the uterus is now outside the pelvis but not so large as to cause discomfort while she sits in a dental chair (Russell & Mayberry, 2008).

Physical Activity. Physical activity promotes a feeling of well-being in the pregnant woman. It improves circulation, promotes relaxation and rest, and counteracts boredom, as it does in the nonpregnant woman (ACOG, 2002). Detailed exercise tips for pregnancy are presented in the Teaching for Self-Management box: Exercise Tips for Pregnant Women. Exercises that help relieve the low back pain that often arises during the second trimester because of the increased weight of the fetus are demonstrated in Figure 15-11.

Posture and Body Mechanics. Skeletal and musculature changes and hormonal changes (relaxin) in pregnancy may

TEACHING FOR SELF-MANAGEMENT

Exercise Tips for Pregnant Women

- *Consult your health care provider* when you know or suspect you are pregnant. Discuss your health and pregnancy history, your current exercise regimen, and the exercises you would like to continue throughout pregnancy.
- *Seek help* in determining an exercise routine that is well within your limit of tolerance, especially if you have not been exercising regularly.
- *Consider decreasing weight-bearing exercises* (jogging, running) and concentrating on non–weight-bearing activities such as swimming, cycling, or stretching. If you are a runner, starting in your seventh month, you may wish to walk instead.
- *Avoid risky activities* such as surfing, mountain climbing, skydiving, and racquetball because such activities, which require precise balance and coordination, may be dangerous. Avoid activities that require holding your breath and bearing down (Valsalva maneuver). Jerky, bouncy motions also should be avoided.
- *Exercise regularly* every day if possible, as long as you are healthy, to improve muscle tone and increase or maintain your stamina. Exercising sporadically may put undue strain on your muscles. Thirty minutes of moderate physical exercise is recommended. This activity can be broken up into shorter segments with rest in between. For example, exercise for 10 to 15 minutes, rest for 2 to 3 minutes, then exercise for another 10 to 15 minutes.
- *Decrease your exercise level* as your pregnancy progresses. The normal alterations of advancing pregnancy, such as decreased cardiac reserve and increased respiratory effort, may produce physiologic stress if you exercise strenuously for a long time.
- *Take your pulse* every 10 to 15 minutes while you are exercising. If it is more than 140 beats/min, slow down until it returns to a maximum of 90 beats/min. You should be able to converse easily while exercising. If you cannot, you need to slow down.
- *Avoid becoming overheated* for extended periods. It is best not to exercise for more than 35 minutes, especially in hot, humid weather. As your body temperature rises, the heat is transmitted to your fetus. Prolonged or repeated elevation of fetal temperature may result in birth defects, especially during the first 3 months of pregnancy. Your temperature should not exceed 38° C.
- *Avoid the use of hot tubs and saunas.*
- *Warm-up and stretching exercises* prepare your joints for more strenuous exercise and lessen the likelihood of strain or injury to your joints. After the fourth month of gestation you should not perform exercises flat on your back.
- *A cool-down period* of mild activity involving your legs after an exercise period will help bring your respiration, heart, and metabolic rates back to normal and prevent the pooling of blood in the exercised muscles.
- *Rest for 10 minutes after exercising,* lying on your side. As the uterus grows it puts pressure on a major vein in your abdomen that carries blood to your heart. Lying on your side removes the pressure and promotes return circulation from your extremities and muscles to your heart, thereby increasing blood flow to your placenta and fetus. You should rise gradually from the floor to prevent dizziness or fainting (orthostatic hypotension).
- *Drink two or three 8-ounce glasses of water* after you exercise to replace the body fluids lost through perspiration. While exercising, drink water whenever you feel the need.
- *Increase your caloric intake* to replace the calories burned during exercise and provide the extra energy needs of pregnancy. (Pregnancy alone requires an additional 340-452 kcal/day.) Choose such high-protein foods as fish, milk, cheese, eggs, and meat.
- *Take your time.* This is not the time to be competitive or train for activities requiring speed or long endurance.
- *Wear a supportive bra.* Your increased breast weight may cause changes in posture and put pressure on the ulnar nerve.
- *Wear supportive shoes.* As your uterus grows your center of gravity shifts and you compensate for this by arching your back. These natural changes may make you feel off balance and more likely to fall.
- *Stop exercising immediately* if you experience shortness of breath, dizziness, numbness, tingling, pain of any kind, more than four uterine contractions per hour, decreased fetal activity, or vaginal bleeding, and consult your health care provider.

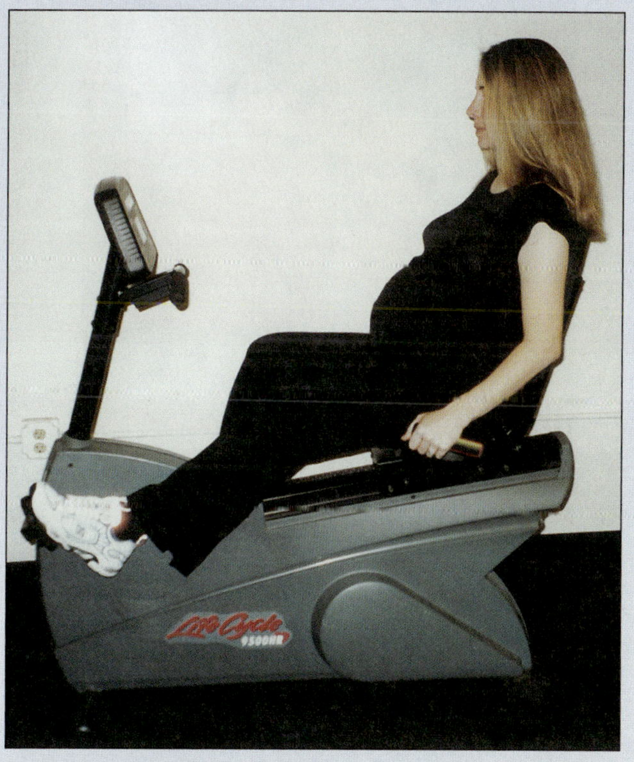

Riding a recumbent bicycle provides exercise while supplying back support. (Courtesy Shannon Perry, Phoenix, AZ.)

Sources: American College of Obstetricians and Gynecologists (ACOG). (2002). Exercise during pregnancy and the postpartum period. ACOG Committee Opinion No. 267. *Obstetrics & Gynecology, 77*(1), 79-81; Kramer, M., & McDonald, S. (2006). Aerobic exercise for women during pregnancy. *Cochrane Database of Systematic Reviews, 2006,* 2, CD000180; Morris, S., & Johnson, N. (2005). Exercise in pregnancy: A critical appraisal of the literature. *Journal of Reproductive, 50*(3), 181-188.

predispose the woman to backache and possible injury. As pregnancy progresses, the pregnant woman's center of gravity changes, pelvic joints soften and relax, and stress is placed on abdominal musculature. Poor posture and body mechanics contribute to the discomfort and potential for injury. To minimize these problems, women can learn good body posture and body mechanics (Fig. 15-12). Strategies to prevent or relieve backache are presented in the Teaching for Self-Management box: Posture and Body Mechanics.

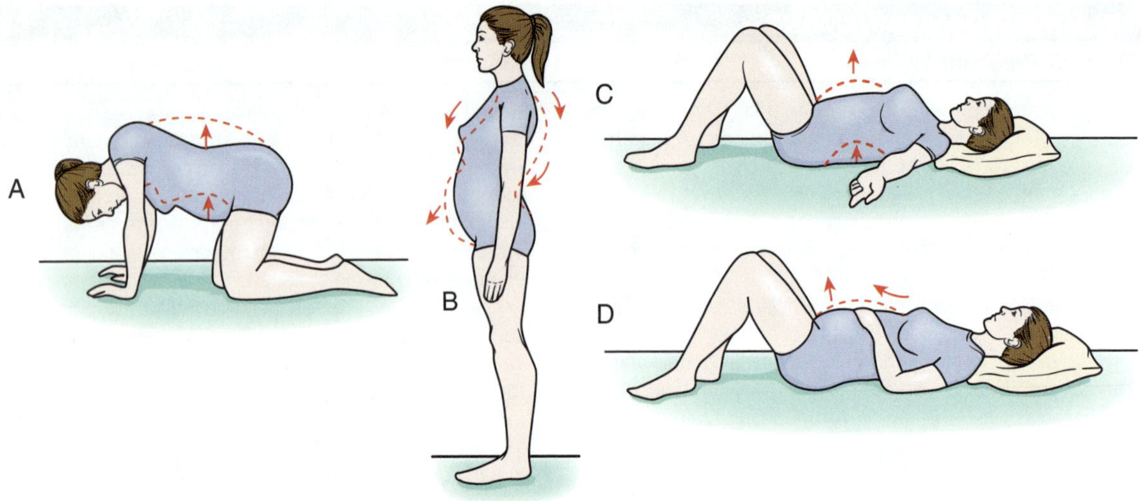

FIG. 15-11 Exercises. **A-C,** Pelvic rocking relieves low backache (excellent for relief of menstrual cramps as well). **D,** Abdominal breathing aids relaxation and lifts abdominal wall off uterus.

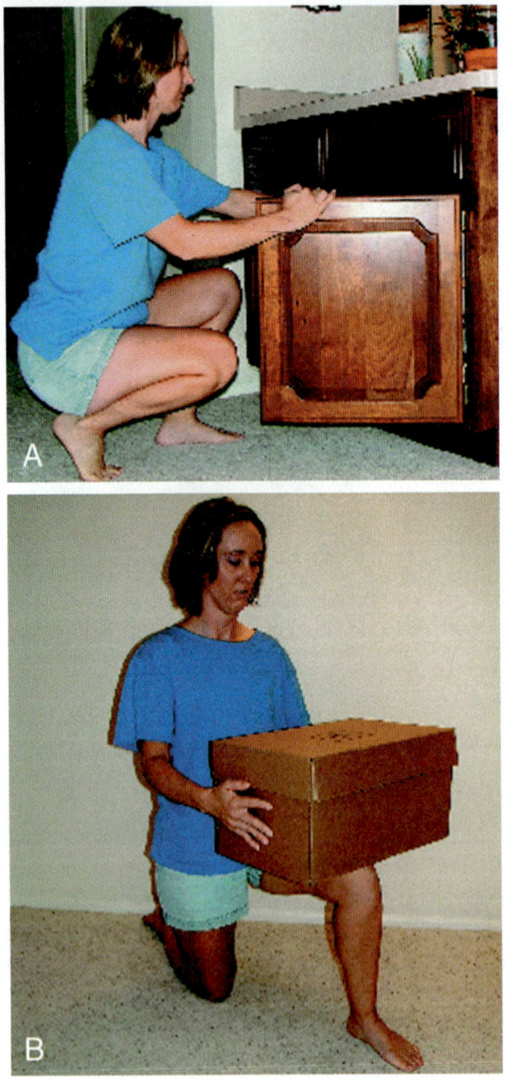

FIG. 15-12 Correct body mechanics. **A,** Squatting. **B,** Lifting. (Courtesy Julie Perry Nelson, Loveland, CO).

TEACHING FOR SELF-MANAGEMENT

Posture and Body Mechanics

TO PREVENT OR RELIEVE BACKACHE

Do pelvic tilt:

- Pelvic tilt (rock) on hands and knees (see Fig. 15-11, *A*) and while sitting in straight-back chair.
- Pelvic tilt (rock) in standing position against a wall, or lying on floor (see Fig. 15-11, *B* and *C*).
- Perform abdominal muscle contractions during pelvic tilt while standing, lying, or sitting to help strengthen rectus abdominis muscle (see Fig. 15-11, *D*).
- Use good body mechanics.
- Use leg muscles to reach objects on or near floor. Bend at the knees, not from the back. Knees are bent to lower body to squatting position. Feet are kept 12 to 18 inches apart to provide a solid base to maintain balance (see Fig. 15-12, *A*).
- Lift with the legs. To lift a heavy object (e.g., young child) one foot is placed slightly in front of the other and kept flat as woman lowers herself onto one knee. She lifts the weight, holding it close to her body and never higher than her chest. To stand up or sit down she places one leg slightly behind the other as she raises or lowers herself (see Fig. 15-12, *B*).

TO RESTRICT THE LUMBAR CURVE

- For prolonged standing (e.g., ironing, employment), place one foot on low footstool or box; change positions often.
- Move car seat forward so that knees are bent and higher than hips. If needed, use a small pillow to support low back area.
- Sit in chairs low enough to allow both feet to be placed on floor, preferably with knees higher than hips.

TO PREVENT ROUND LIGAMENT PAIN AND STRAIN ON ABDOMINAL MUSCLES

- Implement suggestions given in Table 15-2.

Case Study—Second Trimester

Rest and Relaxation. Nurses encourage women to plan regular rest periods, particularly as pregnancy advances. The side-lying position is recommended because it promotes uterine perfusion and fetoplacental oxygenation by eliminating pressure on the ascending vena cava and descending aorta, which can lead to supine hypotension (Fig. 15-13). Show the woman how to rise slowly from a side-lying position to prevent placing strain on the back and to minimize the orthostatic hypotension caused by changes in position common in the latter part of pregnancy. To stretch and rest back muscles at home or work, the nurse can show the woman the way to do the following exercises:

- Stand behind a chair. Support and balance self by using the back of the chair (Fig. 15-14). Squat for 30 seconds; stand for 15 seconds. Repeat 6 times, several times per day, as needed.
- While sitting in a chair, lower head to knees for 30 seconds. Raise head. Repeat 6 times, several times per day, as needed.

Conscious relaxation is the process of releasing tension from the mind and body through deliberate effort and practice. The ability to relax consciously and intentionally is beneficial for the following reasons:

- To relieve the normal discomforts related to pregnancy
- To reduce stress and therefore diminish pain perception during the childbearing cycle
- To heighten self-awareness and trust in one's own ability to control responses and functions
- To help cope with stress in everyday life situations, whether the woman is pregnant or not

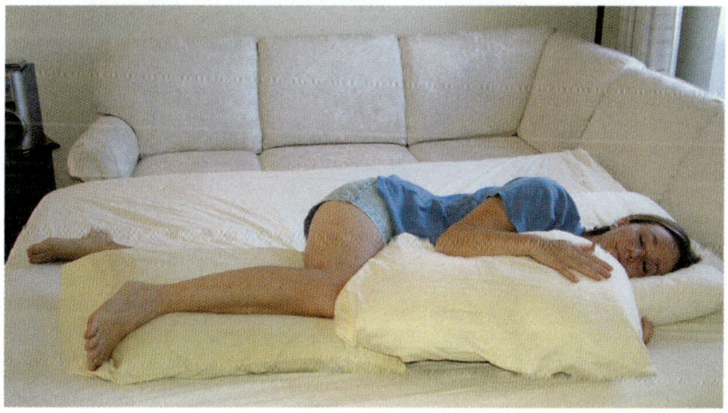

FIG. 15-13 Side-lying position for rest and relaxation. Some women prefer to support upper part of leg with pillows. (Courtesy Julie Perry Nelson, Loveland, CO.)

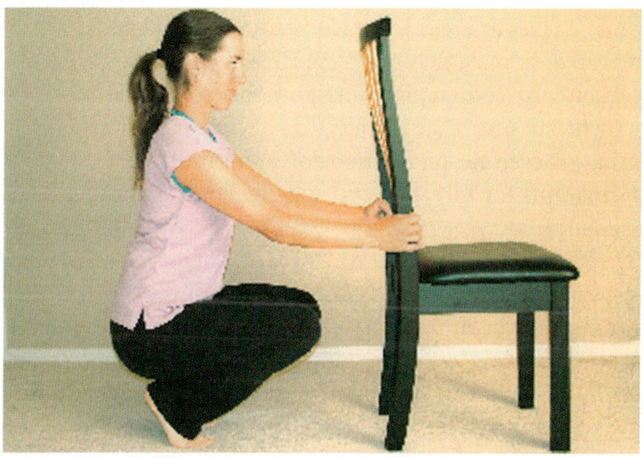

FIG. 15-14 Squatting for muscle relaxation and strengthening and for keeping leg and hip joints flexible. (Courtesy Julie Perry Nelson, Loveland, CO).

The techniques for conscious relaxation are numerous and varied. Box 15-5 gives some guidelines.

Employment. Employment of pregnant women usually has no adverse effects on pregnancy outcomes. Job discrimination that is based strictly on pregnancy is illegal. However, some job environments pose potential risk to the fetus (e.g., dry-cleaning plants, chemistry laboratories, parking garages). Excessive fatigue is usually the deciding factor in the termination of employment. Strategies to improve safety during pregnancy are described in the Teaching for Self-Management box: Safety During Pregnancy.

BOX 15-5 CONSCIOUS RELAXATION TIPS

- *Preparation:* Loosen clothing, assume a comfortable sitting or side-lying position with all parts of body well supported with pillows.
- *Beginning:* Allow yourself to feel warm and comfortable. Inhale and exhale slowly, and imagine peaceful relaxation coming over each part of the body, starting with the neck and working down to the toes. Often people who learn conscious relaxation speak of feeling relaxed even if some discomfort is present.
- *Maintenance:* Use imagery (fantasy or daydream) to maintain the state of relaxation. Using active imagery, imagine yourself moving or doing some activity and experiencing its sensations. Using passive imagery, imagine yourself watching a scene, such as a lovely sunset.
- *Awakening:* Return to the wakeful state gradually. Slowly begin to take in stimuli from the surrounding environment.
- *Further retention and development of the skill:* Practice regularly for some periods each day, for example, at the same hour for 10 to 15 minutes each day, to feel refreshed, revitalized, and invigorated.

TEACHING FOR SELF-MANAGEMENT

Safety During Pregnancy

Changes in the body resulting from pregnancy include relaxation of the joints, alteration to the center of gravity, faintness, and discomforts. Problems with coordination and balance are common. Therefore, the woman should follow these guidelines:

- Use good body mechanics.
- Use safety features on tools and vehicles (e.g., safety seat belts, shoulder harnesses, headrests, goggles, helmets) as specified.
- Avoid activities requiring coordination, balance, and concentration.
- Take rest periods; reschedule daily activities to meet rest and relaxation needs.

Embryonic and fetal development is vulnerable to environmental teratogens. Many potentially dangerous chemicals—cleaning agents, paints, sprays, herbicides, and pesticides—are present in the home, yard, and workplace. The soil and water supply may be unsafe. Therefore, the woman should follow these guidelines:

- Read all labels for ingredients and proper use of product.
- Ensure adequate ventilation with clean air.
- Dispose of wastes appropriately.
- Wear gloves when handling chemicals.
- Change job assignments or workplace as necessary.
- Avoid travel to high-altitude regions, which could jeopardize oxygen intake.

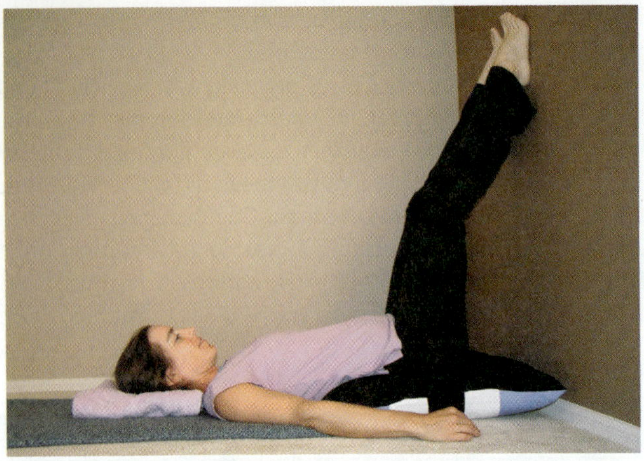

FIG. 15-15 Position for resting legs and for reducing edema and varicosities. Encourage woman with vulvar varicosities to include pillow under her hips. (Courtesy Julie Perry Nelson, Loveland, CO.)

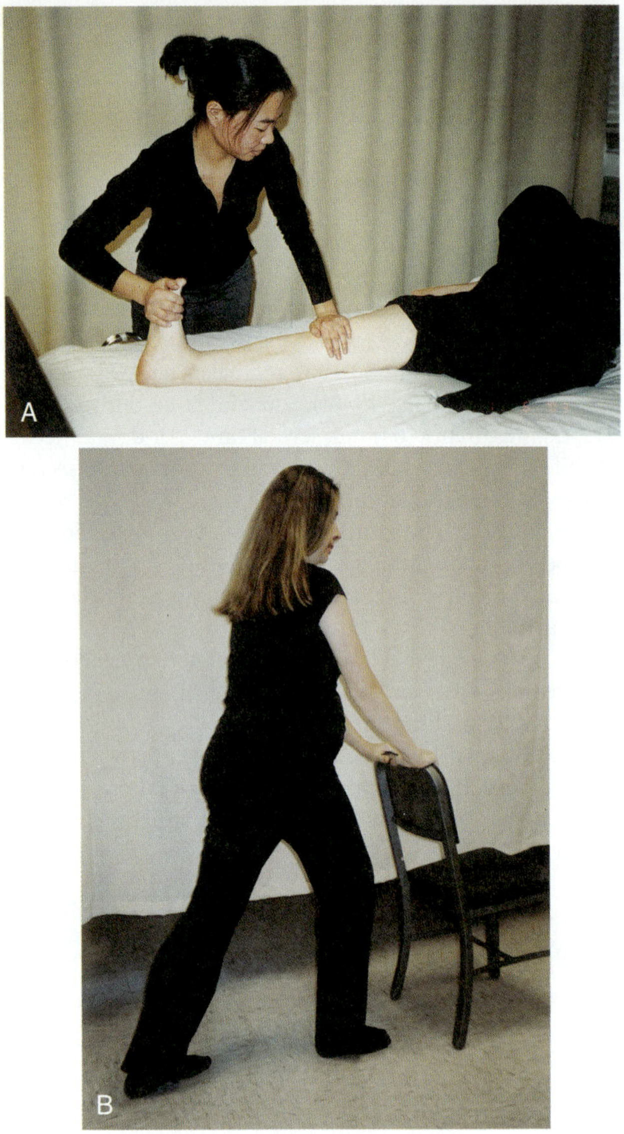

FIG. 15-16 Relief of muscle spasm (leg cramps). **A,** Another person dorsiflexes foot with knee extended. **B,** Woman stands and leans forward, thereby dorsiflexing foot of affected leg. (Courtesy Shannon Perry, Phoenix, AZ.)

Women with sedentary jobs need to walk around at intervals to counter the usual sluggish circulation in the legs. They also should neither sit nor stand in one position for long periods, and they should avoid crossing their legs at the knees, because all of these activities can foster the development of varices and thrombophlebitis. Standing for long periods also increases the risk of preterm labor. The pregnant woman's chair should provide adequate back support. Use of a footstool can prevent pressure on veins, relieve strain on varicosities, minimize edema of feet, and prevent backache.

Clothing. Some women continue to wear their usual clothes during pregnancy as long as they fit and feel comfortable. If maternity clothing is needed, outfits may be purchased new or found at thrift shops or garage sales in good condition. Comfortable, loose clothing is recommended. Tight bras and belts, stretch pants, garters, tight-top knee socks, panty girdles, and other constrictive clothing should be avoided because tight clothing over the perineum encourages vaginitis and miliaria (heat rash), and impaired circulation in the legs can cause varicosities.

Maternity bras are constructed to accommodate the increased breast weight, chest circumference, and the size of breast tail tissue (under the arm). These bras also have drop-flaps over the nipples to facilitate breastfeeding. A good bra can help prevent neckache and backache.

Maternal support hose give considerable comfort and promote greater venous emptying in women with large varicose veins. Ideally, support stockings should be put on before the woman gets out of bed in the morning. Figure 15-15 demonstrates a position for resting the legs and reducing swelling and varicosities.

Comfortable shoes that provide firm support and promote good posture and balance also are advisable. Very high heels and platform shoes are not recommended because of the changes in the pregnant woman's center of gravity, and the hormone relaxin, which softens pelvic joints in later pregnancy, all of which can cause her to lose her balance. In addition, in the third trimester, the woman's pelvis tilts forward, and her lumbar curve increases. The resulting leg aches and cramps are aggravated by nonsupportive shoes. Exercises to relieve leg cramps are depicted in Figure 15-16.

Travel. Travel is not contraindicated in low risk pregnant women. However, women with high risk pregnancies are advised to avoid long-distance travel after fetal viability has been reached to avert possible economic and psychologic consequences of giving birth to a preterm infant far from home. Travel to areas in which medical care is poor, water is untreated, or malaria is prevalent should be avoided if possible. Women who contemplate foreign travel should be aware that many health insurance carriers do not cover a birth in a foreign setting or even hospitalization for preterm labor. In addition, vaccinations for foreign travel may be contraindicated during pregnancy.

Pregnant women who travel for long distances should schedule periods of activity and rest. While sitting, the woman can practice deep breathing, foot circling, and alternately contracting and relaxing different muscle groups. She should avoid becoming fatigued. Although travel in itself is not a cause of adverse outcomes such as miscarriage or preterm labor, certain precautions are recommended while traveling in a car. For example, women riding in a car should wear automobile restraints and stop to walk every hour.

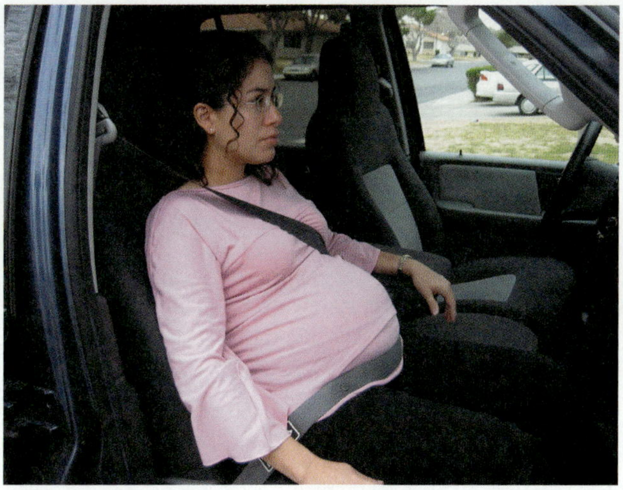

FIG. 15-17 Proper use of seat belt and headrest. (Courtesy Brian and Mayannyn Sallee, Anchorage, AK.)

Maternal death as a result of injury is the most common cause of fetal death. The next most common cause is placental separation that occurs because body contours change in reaction to the force of a collision. The uterus as a muscular organ can adapt its shape to that of the body, but the placenta is not resilient. At the impact of collision, placental separation can occur. A combination lap belt and shoulder harness is the most effective automobile restraint, and both should be used (Fig. 15-17). The lap belt should be worn low across the pelvic bones and as snug as is comfortable. The shoulder harness should be worn above the gravid uterus and below the neck to prevent chafing. The pregnant woman should sit upright. The headrest should be used to prevent whiplash injury. Airbags if present should remain engaged, but the steering wheel should be tilted upward, away from the abdomen and the seat moved back away from the steering wheel as much as possible (Cesario, 2007).

A pregnant woman traveling in high-altitude regions has lowered oxygen levels that may cause fetal hypoxia, especially if she is anemic. However, the current information on this condition is limited, and recommendations are not standardized.

Airline travel in large commercial jets usually poses little risk to the pregnant woman, but policies vary from airline to airline. The pregnant woman is advised to inquire about restrictions or recommendations from her carrier. Most health care providers allow air travel up to 36 weeks of gestation in women without health or pregnancy complications. Metal detectors used at airport security checkpoints are not harmful to the fetus. The 8% humidity at which the cabins of commercial airlines are maintained may result in some water loss; hydration (with water) should therefore be maintained under these conditions. Sitting in the cramped seat of an airliner for prolonged periods may increase the risk of superficial and deep thrombophlebitis; therefore, the woman is encouraged to take a walk around the aircraft during each hour of travel to minimize this risk. A review of the literature reveals that cosmic radiation exposure for flight crews is well below the annual limit recommended by the International Commission on Radiological Protection (Health Physics Society, 2009).

Medications and Herbal Preparations. Although much has been learned in recent years about fetal drug toxicity, the possible teratogenicity of many medications, both prescription and OTC, is still unknown. This is especially true for new medications and combinations of drugs. Moreover, certain subclinical errors or deficiencies in intermediate metabolism in the fetus may cause an otherwise harmless drug to be converted into a hazardous one. The greatest danger of drug-caused developmental defects in the fetus extends from the time of fertilization through the first trimester, a time when the woman may not realize she is pregnant. Self-treatment must be discouraged.

! NURSING ALERT

Although complementary and alternative medicine (CAM) may benefit the woman during pregnancy, some practices should be avoided because they may increase risk for complications. It is important to ask the woman what OTC products (including herbals and vitamins) she may be using.

Immunizations. Some individuals have raised concern over the safety of various immunization practices during pregnancy. Immunization with live or attenuated live viruses is contraindicated during pregnancy because of its potential teratogenicity but should be part of postpartum care. Live-virus vaccines include those for measles (rubeola and rubella), chickenpox, and mumps, as well as the Sabin (oral) poliomyelitis vaccine (no longer used in the United States). Vaccines that can be administered during pregnancy include tetanus, diphtheria, recombinant hepatitis B, and influenza (inactivated) vaccines (CDC, 2008; www.cdc.gov/vaccines).

SAFETY ALERT

Pregnant women who become ill with seasonal respiratory influenza (flu) are more likely than other persons to develop serious complications, such as pneumonia. All women whose pregnancy will take place from November through March should be offered a flu vaccination.

Alcohol, Cigarette Smoke, Caffeine, and Drugs. A safe level of alcohol consumption during pregnancy has not been established. Complete abstinence is strongly advised in order to avoid any risk of pregnancy complications. Maternal alcoholism is associated with high rates of miscarriage and fetal alcohol spectrum disorders (FASD); the risk for miscarriage in the first trimester is dose related (three or more drinks per day) (CDC, 2009). Cigarette smoking or continued exposure to secondhand smoke (even if the mother does not smoke) is associated with IUGR and an increase in perinatal and infant morbidity and mortality. Smoking is associated with an increased frequency of preterm labor, PROM, abruptio placentae, placenta previa, and fetal death, possibly resulting from decreased placental perfusion. Smoking cessation activities should be incorporated into routine prenatal care (ACOG Committee on Obstetric Practice, 2005). All women who smoke should be strongly encouraged to quit or at least reduce the number of cigarettes they smoke. Most studies of human pregnancy have revealed no association between caffeine consumption and birth defects or LBW. Some studies have documented an increased risk for miscarriage with caffeine intake greater than 200 mg/day (Weng, Odouli, & Li, 2008).

EVIDENCE-BASED PRACTICE

Pat Gingrich

Perinatal Smoking Cessation

ASK THE QUESTION

What interventions can I use to encourage and support my pregnant patients who smoke to quit?

SEARCH FOR EVIDENCE

Search Strategies

Professional organization guidelines, meta-analyses, systematic reviews, randomized controlled trials, nonrandomized prospective studies and retrospective reviews since 2009.

Databases Searched

CINAHL, Cochrane, Medline, PUBMED, and the American College Obstetricians and Gynecologists and the Association of Women's Health, Obstetric and Neonatal Nurses websites.

CRITICALLY ANALYZE THE DATA

Smoking causes harm in pregnancy and is associated with low birth weight (less than 2500 grams), prematurity, perinatal death, and sudden infant death syndrome. In addition, smoking is associated with low breastfeeding initiation and shorter duration, as well as high rates of childhood lung disease, ear infections, asthma and possible behavioral disorders. Approximately one out of eight pregnant women smoke. Smoking is more prevalent for women of lower income and education, young age, single, poor social support, depression, and increased parity.

A Cochrane Database of Systematic Review of 72 trials, involving over 20,000 pregnant women, found that interventions to promote smoking cessation resulted in a significant reduction in smoking in late pregnancy over control groups who received only usual care. The interventions used included individual counseling, cognitive behavioral and motivational counseling; offering incentives; evaluation for readiness for change; education on fetal health status; serum nicotine measurement; and pharmacological therapy such as bupropion and nicotine replacement. The interventions reduced low birth weight and preterm birth. No significant differences were noted for stillbirths, perinatal mortality, or admission to intensive care. The authors recommend implementing interventions in all maternity settings, with special attention to at-risk populations (Lumley, Chamberlain, Dowswell, Oliver, Oakley, & Watson, 2009).

The authors of a review of 64 nurse-led qualitative and quantitative research studies on smoking cessation in pregnancy found four themes regarding barriers to quitting and risks for relapse postpartum: addiction, social stressors, physiologic aversion to smoking during pregnancy which reverses postpartum, and reluctance to request partner support or partner cessation. Women considered interventions such as home visits and resource material to be helpful, but found support groups and phone quit lines to be less helpful. Since the relapse rate postpartum was 60-70%, the authors recommended that interventions continue past 6 weeks postpartum, to include the stressful times of transition to parenthood, infant irritability, and postpartum depression. Even though office time is very limited, the authors suggested the use of medical records that encourage smoking cessation by prompting the health care provider to identify barriers and quit strategies at every visit. Finally, the authors recommended the resolution of underlying social stressors, including family, financial, transition to parenthood and intimate partner violence, for which the smoking may be a coping mechanism (Gaffney, Baghi, & Sheehan, 2009).

IMPLICATIONS FOR PRACTICE

The U.S. Preventive Services Task Force issued a guideline (2009) that recommends that clinicians ask all pregnant women at every visit about tobacco use. Individual counseling and self-help information tailored for pregnant women's perceived barriers increases abstinence rates during pregnancy. Women should hear that cessation of smoking at any point during pregnancy results in substantial health benefits for mother and baby. A dose-related effect of counseling (more counseling equals greater abstinence) is noted up to about 90 total minutes, but even brief targeted counseling is beneficial. The most helpful counseling targets developing a quit plan, overcoming barriers, and providing social support. Complementary strategies include motivational interviewing, assessing readiness, more intensive counseling and telephone quit lines.

Finally, although smokers may feel helpless against addiction, they can have their cognitions changed in a short period of time by media campaigns (Vallone, Duke, Mowery, McCausland, Xiao, & Constantino, 2010). A longitudinal study of 212 smokers tracked their perceptions of a branded media campaign that used empathy and humor to disassociate smoking from common triggers and "relearn" living smoke-free. The American Legacy Foundation's "EX" campaign has self-help material tailored to pregnant women available at www.becomeanex.org/pregnant-smokers.php.

References

Gaffney, K., Baghi, H., & Sheehan, S. (2009). Two decades of nurse-led research on smoking during pregnancy and postpartum: Concept development to intervention trials. Annual Review of Nursing Research (27), 195–219.

Lumley, J., Chamberlain, C., Dowswell, T., Oliver, S., Oakley, L., & Watson, L. (2009). Interventions for promoting smoking cessation during pregnancy. *The Cochrane Database of Systematic Reviews 2009, 3,* Chichester, UK: John Wiley & Sons.

United States Preventive Services Task Force. (2009). Counseling and interventions to prevent tobacco use and tobacco-caused disease in adults and pregnant women: U.S. Preventive Services Task Force reaffirmation recommendation statement. *Annals of Internal Medicine, 150*(8), 1–46.

Vallone, D., Duke, J., Mowery, P., McCausland, K., Xiao, H., Constantino, J., et al. (2010). The impact of EX: Results from a pilot smoking-cessation media campaign. *American Journal of Preventive Medicine, 38*(3 Suppl), S312–S318.

Because other effects are unknown, however, pregnant women are advised to limit their caffeine intake, particularly coffee intake because it has high caffeine content per unit of measure.

Any drug or environmental agent that enters the pregnant woman's bloodstream has the potential to cross the placenta and harm the fetus. Marijuana, heroin, and cocaine are common examples. Although the problem of substance abuse in pregnancy is considered a major public health concern and comprehensive care of drug-addicted women improves maternal and neonatal outcomes, few facilities are available for treatment of these women (see Chapters 32 and 35).

Normal Discomforts. Pregnant women have physical symptoms that would be considered abnormal in the nonpregnant state. Women pregnant for the first time have an increased need for explanations of the causes of the discomforts and for advice on ways to relieve them. The discomforts of the first trimester are fairly specific. Information about the physiology and prevention of and self-management for discomforts experienced during the three trimesters is given in Table 15-2. Box 15-6 lists alternative and complementary therapies and why they might be used in pregnancy (see also Fig. 15-18). Nurses can do much to allay a first-time mother's anxiety about such symptoms by

CLINICAL REASONING

Nausea in Pregnancy

Meka is 10 weeks pregnant with her first baby. She is complaining of nausea every morning. She has heard that ginger is good for nausea and wants to know if she should take it. What is your response?

1. Evidence—Is evidence sufficient to draw conclusions about the effectiveness of ginger on nausea and vomiting of pregnancy?
2. Assumptions—Describe the underlying assumptions for each of the following issues:
   a. Causes of nausea and vomiting of pregnancy
   b. Self-medicating during pregnancy
   c. Evidence for herbal use in pregnancy
3. What implications and priorities for nursing care can be drawn at this time?
4. Does the evidence objectively support your conclusion?
5. Are there alternative perspectives to your conclusion?

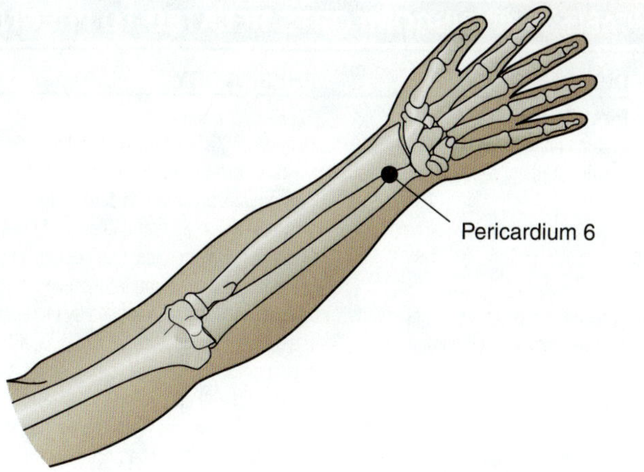

FIG. 15-18 Pericardium 6 (p6) acupressure point for nausea.

BOX 15-6 COMPLEMENTARY AND ALTERNATIVE THERAPIES USED IN PREGNANCY

MORNING SICKNESS AND HYPEREMESIS

- Acupuncture
- Acupressure (Fig. 15-18)
- Shiatzu
- Herbal remedies*
  - Peppermint
  - Spearmint
  - Ginger root

RELAXATION AND MUSCLE-ACHE RELIEF

- Yoga
- Biofeedback
- Reflexology
- Therapeutic touch
- Massage

*Some herbs can cause miscarriage, preterm labor, or fetal or maternal injury. Pregnant women should discuss use with pregnancy health care provider, as well as an expert qualified in the use of the herb.

Source: Born, D., & Barron, M. (2005). Herb use in pregnancy: What nurses should know. *MCN American Journal of Maternal/Child Nursing, 30*(3), 201-208; Smith, C., Crowther, C., Willson, K., Hotham, N., & McMillian, V. (2004). A randomized controlled trial of ginger to treat nausea and vomiting in pregnancy. *Obstetrics and Gynecology, 103*(4), 639-645; Tiran, D., & Mack, S. (2000). *Complementary therapies for pregnancy and childbirth* (2nd ed.). Edinburgh: Baillière Tindall.

TEACHING FOR SELF-MANAGEMENT

Sexuality in Pregnancy

- Be aware that maternal physiologic changes, such as breast enlargement, nausea, fatigue, abdominal changes, perineal enlargement, leukorrhea, pelvic vasocongestion, and orgasmic responses may affect sexuality and sexual expression.
- Discuss responses to pregnancy with your partner.
- Keep in mind that cultural prescriptions ("do's") and proscriptions ("dont's") may affect your responses.
- Although your libido may be depressed during the first trimester, it often increases during the second and third trimesters.
- Discuss and explore with your partner:
  - Alternative behaviors (e.g., mutual masturbation, foot massage, cuddling)
  - Alternative positions (e.g., female superior, side-lying) for sexual intercourse
- Intercourse is safe as long as it is not uncomfortable. There is no correlation between intercourse and miscarriage, but observe the following precautions:
  - Abstain from intercourse if you experience uterine cramping or vaginal bleeding; report event to your caregiver as soon as possible.
  - Abstain from intercourse (or any activity that results in orgasm) if you have a history of cervical insufficiency, until the problem is corrected.
- Continue to use risk-reducing sexual behaviors. Women at risk for acquiring or conveying sexually transmitted infections are encouraged to use condoms during sexual intercourse throughout pregnancy.

telling her about them in advance and using terminology that the woman (or couple) can understand. Understanding the rationale for treatment promotes their participation in their care. Interventions should be individualized, with attention given to the woman's lifestyle and culture (see Nursing Care Plan: Discomforts of Pregnancy and Warning Signs).

Recognizing Potential Complications. One of the most important responsibilities of care providers is to alert the pregnant woman to signs and symptoms that indicate a potential complication of pregnancy. The woman needs to know how and to whom to report such warning signs. Therefore, the pregnant woman and her family can be reassured if they receive and use a printed form written at the appropriate literacy level, in their language and reflective of their culture, listing the signs and symptoms that warrant an investigation and the telephone numbers to call if they have questions or an emergency.

The nurse must answer questions honestly as they arise during pregnancy. Pregnant women often have difficulty deciding when to report signs and symptoms. The mother is encouraged to refer to the printed list of potential complications and to listen to her body. If the woman senses that something is wrong, she should call her care provider. Several signs and symptoms must be discussed more extensively. These include vaginal bleeding, alteration in fetal movements, symptoms of gestational hypertension, rupture of membranes, and preterm labor.

TABLE 15-2 **DISCOMFORTS RELATED TO PREGNANCY**

DISCOMFORT	PHYSIOLOGY	EDUCATION FOR SELF-MANAGEMENT
First Trimester		
Breast changes, new sensations: pain, tingling, tenderness	Hypertrophy of mammary glandular tissue and increased vascularization, pigmentation, and size and prominence of nipples and areolae caused by hormonal stimulation	Wear supportive maternity bras with pads to absorb discharge, may be worn at night; wash with warm water and keep dry; breast tenderness may interfere with sexual expression or foreplay but is temporary
Urgency and frequency of urination	Vascular engorgement and altered bladder function caused by hormones; bladder capacity reduced by enlarging uterus and fetal presenting part	Empty bladder regularly; perform Kegel exercises; limit fluid intake before bedtime; wear perineal pad; report pain or burning sensation to primary health care provider
Languor and malaise; fatigue (early pregnancy, most common)	Unexplained; may be caused by increasing levels of estrogen, progesterone, and hCG or by elevated BBT; psychologic response to pregnancy and its required physical and psychologic adaptations	Rest as needed; eat well-balanced diet to prevent anemia
Nausea and vomiting, morning sickness—occurs in 50%-75% of pregnant women; starts between first and second missed periods and lasts until about fourth missed period; may occur any time during day; fathers also may have symptoms	Cause unknown; may result from hormonal changes, possibly hCG; may be partly emotional, reflecting pride in, ambivalence about, or rejection of pregnant state	Avoid empty or overloaded stomach; maintain good posture—give stomach ample room; stop smoking; eat dry carbohydrate on awakening; remain in bed until feeling subsides, or alternate dry carbohydrate every other hour with fluids such as hot herbal decaffeinated tea, milk, or clear coffee until feeling subsides; eat five or six small meals per day; avoid fried, odorous, spicy, greasy, or gas-forming foods; consult primary health care provider if intractable vomiting occurs
Ptyalism (excessive salivation) may occur starting 2 to 3 weeks after first missed period	Possibly caused by elevated estrogen levels; may be related to reluctance to swallow because of nausea	Use astringent mouthwash, chew gum, eat hard candy as comfort measures
Gingivitis and epulis (hyperemia, hypertrophy, bleeding, tenderness of the gums); condition will disappear spontaneously 1 to 2 months after birth	Increased vascularity and proliferation of connective tissue from estrogen stimulation	Eat well-balanced diet with adequate protein and fresh fruits and vegetables; brush teeth gently and observe good dental hygiene; avoid infection; see dentist
Nasal stuffiness; epistaxis (nosebleed)	Hyperemia of mucous membranes related to high estrogen levels	Use humidifier; avoid trauma; normal saline nose drops or spray may be used
Leukorrhea: often noted throughout pregnancy	Hormonally stimulated cervix becomes hypertrophic and hyperactive, producing abundant amount of mucus	Not preventable; do not douche; wear perineal pads; perform hygienic practices such as wiping front to back; report to primary health care provider if accompanied by pruritus, foul odor, or change in character or color
Psychosocial dynamics, mood swings, mixed feelings	Hormonal and metabolic adaptations; feelings about female role, sexuality, timing of pregnancy, and resultant changes in life and lifestyle	Participate in pregnancy support group; communicate concerns to partner, family, and health care provider; request referral for supportive services if needed (financial assistance)
Second Trimester		
Pigmentation deepens; acne, oily skin	Melanocyte-stimulating hormone (from anterior pituitary)	Not preventable; usually resolves during puerperium
Spider nevi (angiomas) appear over neck, thorax, face, and arms during second or third trimester	Focal networks of dilated arterioles (end arteries) from increased concentration of estrogens	Not preventable; they fade slowly during late puerperium; rarely disappear completely
Pruritus (noninflammatory)	Unknown cause; various types: nonpapular; closely aggregated pruritic papules	Keep fingernails short and clean; contact primary health care provider for diagnosis of cause
	Increased excretory function of skin and stretching of skin possible factors	Not preventable; use comfort measures for symptoms such as Keri baths; distraction; tepid baths with sodium bicarbonate or oatmeal added to water; lotions and oils; change of soaps or reduction in use of soap; loose clothing; see health care provider if mild sedation is needed
Palpitations	Unknown; should not be accompanied by persistent cardiac irregularity	Not preventable; contact primary health care provider if accompanied by symptoms of cardiac decompensation
Supine hypotension (vena cava syndrome) and bradycardia	Induced by pressure of gravid uterus on ascending vena cava when woman is supine; reduces uteroplacental and renal perfusion	Side-lying position or semi-sitting posture, with knees slightly flexed (see Emergency box; Supine Hypotension, p. 341)
Faintness and, rarely, syncope (orthostatic hypotension) may persist throughout pregnancy	Vasomotor lability or postural hypotension from hormones; in late pregnancy may be caused by venous stasis in lower extremities	Moderate exercise, deep breathing, vigorous leg movement; avoid sudden changes in position and warm crowded areas; move slowly and deliberately; keep environment cool; avoid hypoglycemia by eating five or six small meals per day; wear elastic hose; sit as necessary; if symptoms are serious, contact primary health care provider
Food cravings	Cause unknown; craving influenced by culture or geographic area	Not preventable; satisfy craving unless it interferes with well-balanced diet; report unusual cravings to primary health care provider
Heartburn (pyrosis or acid indigestion): burning sensation, occasionally with burping and regurgitation of a little sour-tasting fluid	Progesterone slows GI tract motility and digestion, reverses peristalsis, relaxes cardiac sphincter, and delays emptying time of stomach; stomach displaced upward and compressed by enlarging uterus	Limit or avoid gas-producing or fatty foods and large meals; maintain good posture; sip milk for temporary relief; drink hot herbal tea; primary health care provider may prescribe antacid between meals; contact primary health care provider for persistent symptoms

e Nursing Care Plan—Discomforts of Pregnancy and Warning Signs

TABLE 15-2 DISCOMFORTS RELATED TO PREGNANCY—cont'd

DISCOMFORT	PHYSIOLOGY	EDUCATION FOR SELF-MANAGEMENT
Constipation	GI tract motility slowed because of progesterone, resulting in increased resorption of water and drying of stool; intestines compressed by enlarging uterus; predisposition to constipation because of oral iron supplementation	Drink 8 to 10 glasses of water per day; include roughage in diet; engage in moderate exercise; maintain regular schedule for bowel movements; use relaxation techniques and deep breathing; do not take stool softener, laxatives, mineral oil, other drugs, or enemas without first consulting primary health care provider
Flatulence with bloating and belching	Reduced GI motility because of hormones, allowing time for bacterial action that produces gas; swallowing air	Chew foods slowly and thoroughly; avoid gas-producing foods, fatty foods, large meals; exercise; maintain regular bowel habits
Varicose veins (varicosities): may be associated with aching legs and tenderness; may be present in legs and vulva; hemorrhoids are varicosities in perianal area	Hereditary predisposition; relaxation of smooth muscle walls of veins because of hormones causing tortuous dilated veins in legs and pelvic vasocongestion; condition aggravated by enlarging uterus, gravity, and bearing down for bowel movements; thrombi from leg varices rare but may occur in hemorrhoids	Avoid lengthy standing or sitting, constrictive clothing, and constipation and bearing down with bowel movements; moderate exercise; rest with legs and hips elevated (see Fig. 15-15); wear support stockings; thrombosed hemorrhoid may be evacuated; relieve swelling and pain with warm sitz baths, local application of astringent compresses
Leukorrhea: often noted throughout pregnancy	Hormonally stimulated cervix becomes hypertrophic and hyperactive, producing abundant amount of mucus	Not preventable; do not douche; maintain good hygiene; wear perineal pads; report to primary health care provider if accompanied by pruritus, foul odor, or change in character or color
Headaches (through week 26)	Emotional tension (more common than vascular migraine headache); eye strain (refractory errors); vascular engorgement and congestion of sinuses resulting from hormone stimulation	Conscious relaxation; contact primary health care provider for constant "splitting" headache to assess for preeclampsia
Carpal tunnel syndrome (involves thumb, second, and third fingers, lateral side of little finger)	Compression of median nerve resulting from changes in surrounding tissues; pain, numbness, tingling, burning; loss of skilled movements (typing); dropping of objects	Not preventable; elevate affected arms; splinting of affected hand may help; regressive after pregnancy; surgery is curative
Periodic numbness, tingling of fingers (acrodysesthesia) occurs in 5% of pregnant women	Brachial plexus traction syndrome resulting from drooping of shoulders during pregnancy (occurs especially at night and early morning)	Maintain good posture; wear supportive maternity bra; condition will disappear after childbirth if lifting and carrying baby does not aggravate it
Round ligament pain (tenderness)	Stretching of ligament caused by enlarging uterus	Not preventable; rest, maintain good body mechanics to avoid overstretching ligament; relieve cramping by squatting or bringing knees to chest; sometimes heat helps
Joint pain, backache, and pelvic pressure; hypermobility of joints	Relaxation of symphyseal and sacroiliac joints because of hormones, resulting in unstable pelvis; exaggerated lumbar and cervicothoracic curves caused by change in center of gravity resulting from enlarging abdomen	Maintain good posture and body mechanics; avoid fatigue; wear low-heeled shoes; abdominal supports may be useful; conscious relaxation; sleep on firm mattress; apply local heat or ice; get back rubs; do pelvic tilt exercises; rest; condition will disappear 6 to 8 weeks after the birth
Third Trimester		
Shortness of breath and dyspnea occur in 60% of pregnant women	Expansion of diaphragm limited by enlarging uterus; diaphragm is elevated about 4 cm; some relief after lightening	Good posture; sleep with extra pillows; avoid overloading stomach; stop smoking; contact health care provider if symptoms worsen to rule out anemia, emphysema, and asthma
Insomnia (later weeks of pregnancy)	Fetal movements, muscle cramping, urinary frequency, shortness of breath, or other discomforts	Reassurance; conscious relaxation; back massage or effleurage; support of body parts with pillows; warm milk or warm shower before retiring
Psychosocial responses: mood swings, mixed feelings, increased anxiety	Hormonal and metabolic adaptations; feelings about impending labor, birth, and parenthood	Reassurance and support from significant other and health care providers; improved communication with partner, family, and others
Urinary frequency and urgency return	Vascular engorgement and altered bladder function caused by hormones; bladder capacity reduced by enlarging uterus and fetal presenting part	Empty bladder regularly; Kegel exercises; limit fluid intake before bedtime; reassurance; wear perineal pad; contact health care provider for pain or burning sensation
Perineal discomfort and pressure	Pressure from enlarging uterus, especially when standing or walking; multifetal gestation	Rest, conscious relaxation, and good posture; contact health care provider for assessment and treatment if pain is present
Braxton Hicks contractions	Intensification of uterine contractions in preparation for work of labor	Reassurance; rest; change of position; practice breathing techniques when contractions are bothersome; effleurage; differentiate from preterm labor
Leg cramps (gastrocnemius spasm), especially when reclining	Compression of nerves supplying lower extremities because of enlarging uterus; reduced level of diffusible serum calcium or elevation of serum phosphorus; aggravating factors: fatigue, poor peripheral circulation, pointing toes when stretching legs or when walking, drinking more than 1 L (1 qt) of milk per day	Check for Homans sign; if negative, use massage and heat over affected muscle; dorsiflex foot until spasm relaxes (see Fig. 15-16); stand on cold surface; oral supplementation with calcium carbonate or calcium lactate tablets; aluminum hydroxide gel, 30 ml, with each meal removes phosphorus by absorbing it (consult primary health care provider before taking these remedies)
Ankle edema (nonpitting) to lower extremities	Edema aggravated by prolonged standing, sitting, poor posture, lack of exercise, constrictive clothing, or hot weather	Ample fluid intake for natural diuretic effect; put on support stockings before arising; rest periodically with legs and hips elevated (see Fig. 15-15); exercise moderately; contact health care provider if generalized edema develops; diuretics are contraindicated

BBT, Basal body temperature; *GI,* gastrointestinal; *hCG,* human chorionic gonadotropin.

NURSING CARE PLAN

Discomforts of Pregnancy and Warning Signs

FIRST TRIMESTER

NURSING DIAGNOSIS

Anxiety related to deficient knowledge about schedule of prenatal visits throughout pregnancy as evidenced by woman's questions and concerns

Expected Outcome

Woman will verbalize correct appointment schedule for the duration of the pregnancy and feelings of being "in control."

Nursing Interventions/*Rationales*

- Provide information regarding schedule of visits, tests, and other assessments and interventions that will be provided throughout the pregnancy *to empower woman to function in collaboration with the caregiver and diminish anxiety.*
- Allow woman time to describe level of anxiety *to establish basis for care.*
- Provide information to woman regarding prenatal classes and labor area tours *to decrease feelings of anxiety about the unknown.*

NURSING DIAGNOSIS

Imbalanced nutrition: less than body requirements related to nausea and vomiting as evidenced by woman's report and weight loss

Expected Outcome

Woman will gain 1 to 2.5 kg during the first trimester.

Nursing Interventions/*Rationales*

- Verify prepregnant weight *to plan a realistic diet according to individual woman's nutritional needs.*
- Obtain diet history *to identify current meal patterns and foods that may be implicated in nausea.*
- Advise woman to consume small frequent meals and avoid having empty stomach *to avoid further nausea episodes.*
- Suggest that woman eat a simple carbohydrate such as dry crackers before arising in the morning *to avoid empty stomach and decrease incidence of nausea and vomiting.*
- Advise woman to call health care provider if vomiting is persistent and severe *to identify possible incidence of hyperemesis gravidarum.*

NURSING DIAGNOSIS

Fatigue related to hormonal changes in the first trimester as evidenced by woman's complaints

Expected Outcome

Woman will report a decreased number of episodes of fatigue.

Nursing Interventions/*Rationales*

- Rest as needed *to avoid increasing feeling of fatigue.*
- Eat a well-balanced diet *to meet increased metabolic demands and avoid anemia.*
- Discuss the use of support systems to help with household responsibilities *to decrease workload at home and decrease fatigue.*
- Reinforce to woman the transitory nature of first trimester *fatigue to provide emotional support.*
- Explore with the woman a variety of techniques to prioritize roles *to decrease family expectations.*

SECOND TRIMESTER

NURSING DIAGNOSIS

Constipation related to progesterone influence on GI tract as evidenced by woman's report of altered patterns of elimination

Expected Outcome

Woman will report a return to normal bowel elimination pattern after implementation of interventions.

Nursing Interventions/*Rationales*

- Provide information to woman regarding pregnancy-related causes: progesterone slowing gastrointestinal motility, growing uterus compressing intestines, and influence of iron supplementation *to provide basic information for self-management during pregnancy.*
- Assist woman to plan a diet that will promote regular bowel movements, such as increasing amount of oral fluid intake to at least 8 glasses of water a day, increasing the amount of fiber in daily diet, and maintaining moderate exercise program *to promote self-management care.*
- Reinforce for woman that she should not take any laxatives, stool softeners, or enemas without first consulting the health care provider *to prevent any injuries to woman or fetus.*

NURSING DIAGNOSIS

Anxiety related to deficient knowledge about course of first pregnancy as evidenced by woman's questions regarding possible complications of second and third trimesters

Expected Outcomes

Woman will correctly list signs of potential complications that can occur during the second and third trimesters and exhibit no overt signs of stress.

Nursing Interventions/*Rationales*

- Provide information concerning the potential complications or warning signs that can occur during the second and third trimesters, including possible causes of signs and the importance of calling the health care provider immediately, *to ensure identification and treatment of problems in a timely manner.*
- Provide a written list of complications *to have a reference list for emergencies.*

THIRD TRIMESTER

NURSING DIAGNOSIS

Fear related to deficient knowledge regarding onset of labor and the processes of labor related to inexperience as evidenced by woman's questions and statement of concerns

Expected Outcomes

Woman will verbalize basic understanding of signs of labor onset and when to call the health care provider, identify resources for childbirth education, and express increasing confidence in readiness to cope with labor.

Nursing Interventions/*Rationales*

- Provide information regarding signs of labor onset, when to call the health care provider, and give written information regarding local childbirth education classes *to empower and promote self-management.*

NURSING CARE PLAN—cont'd

Discomforts of Pregnancy and Warning Signs

- Promote ongoing effective communication with health care provider *to promote trust and decrease fear of unknown.*
- Provide the woman with decision-making opportunities *to promote effective coping.*
- Provide opportunity for woman to verbalize fears regarding childbirth *to assist in decreasing fear through discussion.*

NURSING DIAGNOSIS

Disturbed sleep patterns related to discomforts or insomnia of third trimester as evidenced by woman's report of inadequate rest

Expected Outcome

Woman will report an improvement of quality and quantity of rest and sleep.

Nursing Interventions/*Rationales*

- Assess current sleep pattern and review need for increased requirement during pregnancy *to identify need for change in sleep patterns.*
- Suggest change of position to side-lying with pillows between legs or to semi-Fowler's position *to increase support and decrease any problems with dyspnea or heartburn.*
- Reinforce the possibility of the use of various sleep aids such as relaxation techniques, reading, and decreased activity before bedtime *to decrease the possibility of anxiety or physical discomforts before bedtime.*

NURSING DIAGNOSIS

Ineffective sexuality patterns related to changes in comfort level and fatigue

Expected Outcomes

Woman will verbalize feelings regarding changes in sexual desire, and woman and her partner will express satisfaction with sexual activities.

Nursing Interventions/*Rationales*

- Assess couple's usual sexuality patterns *to determine how patterns have been altered by pregnancy.*
- Provide information regarding expected changes in sexuality patterns during pregnancy *to correct any misconceptions.*
- Allow the couple to express feelings in a nonjudgmental atmosphere *to promote trust.*
- Refer couple for counseling as appropriate *to assist the couple to cope with sexuality pattern changes.*
- Suggest alternative sexual positions *to decrease pressure on enlarging abdomen of woman and increase sexual comfort and satisfaction of couple.*

Recognizing Preterm Labor. Teaching each expectant mother to recognize preterm labor is necessary for early diagnosis and treatment. Preterm labor occurs after the twentieth week but before the thirty-seventh week of pregnancy and consists of uterine contractions that if untreated cause the cervix to open earlier than normal and result in preterm birth. Warning signs and symptoms of preterm labor are discussed in Chapter 33.

Sexual Counseling

Sexual counseling of expectant couples includes countering misinformation, providing reassurance of normality, and suggesting alternative behaviors. The uniqueness of each couple is considered within a biopsychosocial framework (see the Teaching for Self-Management box: Sexuality in Pregnancy). Nurses can initiate discussion about sexual adaptations that must be made during pregnancy, but they themselves need a sound knowledge base about the physical, social, and emotional responses to sex during pregnancy. Not all maternity nurses are comfortable dealing with the sexual concerns of their clients. Be aware of your personal strengths and limitations in dealing with sexual content and be prepared to make referrals if necessary.

Many women merely need permission to be sexually active during pregnancy. Many other women, however, need to be given information about the physiologic changes that occur during pregnancy, have the myths that are associated with sex during pregnancy dispelled, and participate in open discussions of positions for intercourse that decrease pressure on the gravid abdomen. Such tasks are within the purview of the nurse and should be an integral component of the health care rendered.

Some couples need to be referred for sex therapy or family therapy. Couples with long-standing problems with sexual dysfunction that are intensified by pregnancy are candidates for sex therapy. Whenever a sexual problem is a symptom of a more serious relationship problem, the couple would benefit from family therapy.

Using the History. The couple's sexual history provides a basis for counseling, but history taking also is an ongoing process. The couple's receptivity to changes in attitudes, body image, partner relationships, and physical status are relevant topics throughout pregnancy. The history reveals the woman's knowledge of female anatomy and physiology and her attitudes about sex during pregnancy, as well as her perceptions of the pregnancy, the health status of the couple, and the quality of their relationship.

Countering Misinformation. Many myths and much of the misinformation related to sex and pregnancy are masked by seemingly unrelated issues. For example, a discussion about the baby's ability to hear and see in utero may be prompted by questions about the baby being an "unseen observer" of the couple's lovemaking. The counselor must be extremely sensitive to the questions behind such questions when counseling in this highly charged emotional area.

Suggesting Alternative Behaviors. Research has not demonstrated that coitus and orgasm are contraindicated at any time during pregnancy for the obstetrically and medically healthy woman (Cunningham et al., 2010). However, a history of more than one miscarriage; a threatened miscarriage in the first trimester; impending miscarriage in the second trimester; and PROM, bleeding, or abdominal pain during the third trimester warrant caution when it comes to coitus and orgasm.

Solitary and mutual masturbation and oral-genital intercourse may be used by couples as alternatives to penile-vaginal intercourse. Partners who enjoy cunnilingus (oral stimulation of the clitoris or vagina) may feel "turned off" by the normal increase in the amount and odor of vaginal discharge during pregnancy. Couples who practice cunnilingus should be cautioned against the blowing of air into the vagina, particularly during the last few weeks of pregnancy when the cervix may be slightly open. An air embolism can occur if air is forced between the uterine wall and the fetal membranes and enters the maternal vascular system through the placenta.

Showing the woman or couple pictures of possible variations of coital position often is helpful (Fig. 15-19). The female-superior, side-by-side, rear-entry, and side-lying are possible alternative positions to the traditional male-superior position. The woman astride (superior position) allows her to control the angle and depth of penile penetration, as well as to protect her breasts and abdomen. The side-by-side position or any position that places less pressure on the pregnant abdomen and requires less energy may be preferred during the third trimester.

Multiparous women sometimes have significant breast tenderness in the first trimester. A coital position that avoids direct pressure on the woman's breasts and decreased breast fondling during love play can be recommended to such couples. The woman also should be reassured that this condition is normal and temporary.

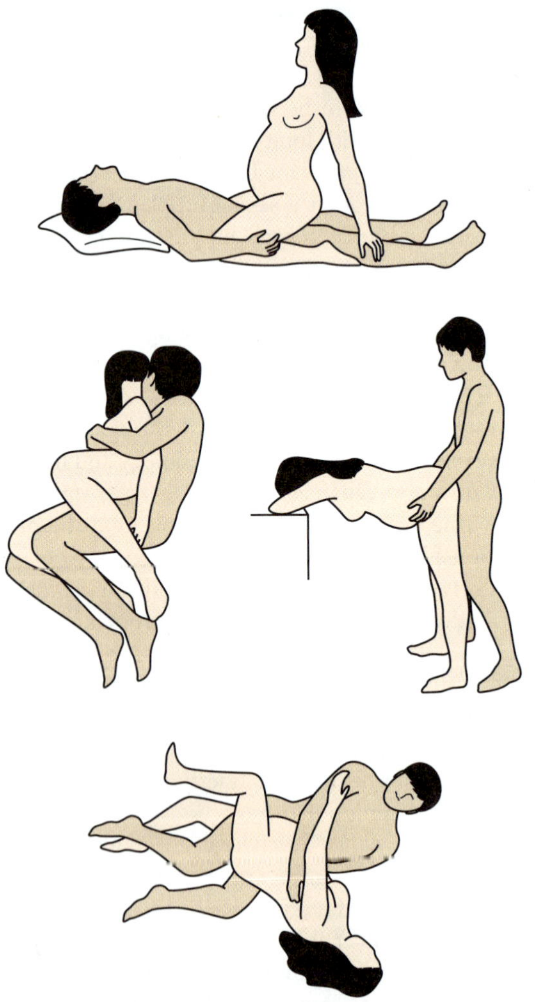

FIG. 15-19 Positions for sexual intercourse during pregnancy. **A,** Female superior. **B,** Side by side. **C,** Rear entry. **D,** Side-lying, facing each other.

Some women complain of lower abdominal cramping and backache after orgasm during the first and third trimesters. A back rub can often relieve some of the discomfort and provide a pleasant experience. A tonic uterine contraction, often lasting up to a minute, replaces the rhythmic contractions of orgasm during the third trimester. Changes in the FHR without fetal distress also have been reported.

The objective of risk-reduction measures is to provide prophylaxis against the acquisition and transmission of STIs (e.g., herpes simplex virus [HSV], HIV). Because these diseases may be transmitted to the woman and her fetus, the use of condoms is recommended throughout pregnancy if the woman is at risk for acquiring an STI.

Psychosocial Support

Esteem, affection, trust, concern, consideration of cultural and religious responses, and listening are all components of the emotional support given to the pregnant woman and her family. The woman's satisfaction with her relationships—partner and familial—and their support, her feeling of competence, and her sense of being in control are important issues to be addressed in the third trimester. A discussion of fetal responses to stimuli, such as sound and light, as well as patterns of sleeping and waking, can be helpful. Other issues of concern that may arise for the pregnant woman and couple include fear of pain, loss of control, and possible birth of the infant before reaching the hospital; anxieties about parenthood; parental concerns about the safety of the mother and unborn child; siblings and their acceptance of the new baby; social and economic responsibilities; and parental concerns arising from conflicts in cultural, religious, or personal value systems. In addition, the father's or partner's commitment to the pregnancy and to the couple's relationship and concerns about sexuality and its expression are topics for discussion for many couples. Providing the prospective parents with an opportunity to discuss their concerns and validating the normality of their responses can meet their needs to varying degrees. Anticipatory guidance and health promotion strategies can help partners cope with their concerns. Health care providers can stimulate and encourage open dialogue between the expectant mother and her partner.

VARIATIONS IN PRENATAL CARE

The course of prenatal care described thus far may seem to suggest that the experiences of childbearing women are similar and that nursing interventions are uniformly consistent across all populations. Although typical patterns of response to pregnancy are easily recognized and many aspects of prenatal care indeed are consistent, pregnant women enter the health care system with individual concerns and needs. The nurse's ability to assess unique needs and to tailor interventions to the individual is the hallmark of expertise in providing care. Variations that influence prenatal care include culture, age, and number of fetuses.

Cultural Influences

Prenatal care as we know it is a phenomenon of Western medicine. In the U.S. biomedical model of care, women are encouraged to seek prenatal care as early as possible in their pregnancy by visiting a physician and/or a nurse-midwife. This model not only is unfamiliar but also seems strange to women of other cultures.

Many cultural variations are found in prenatal care. Even if the prenatal care described is familiar to a woman, some practices may conflict with the beliefs and practices of a subculture group to which she belongs. Because of these and other factors, such as lack of money, lack of transportation, and language barriers, women from diverse cultures may not participate in the prenatal care system, for instance by keeping prenatal appointments. Such behavior may be misinterpreted by nurses as uncaring, lazy, or ignorant.

A concern for modesty also is a deterrent to many women seeking prenatal care. For some women, exposing body parts, especially to a man, is considered a major violation of their modesty. For many women, invasive procedures, such as a vaginal examination, may be so threatening that they cannot be discussed even with their own husbands; therefore, many women prefer a female health care provider. Too often, health care providers assume women lose this modesty during pregnancy and labor, but actually most women value and appreciate efforts to maintain their modesty.

For many cultural groups a physician is deemed appropriate only in times of illness. Because pregnancy is considered a normal process and the woman is in a state of health, the services of a physician are considered inappropriate. Even if what are considered problems with pregnancy by standards of Western medicine develop, they may not be perceived as problems by members of other cultural groups.

Although pregnancy is considered normal by many, certain practices are expected of women of all cultures to ensure a good outcome. **Cultural prescriptions** tell women what to do, and **cultural proscriptions** establish taboos. The purposes of these practices are to prevent maternal illness resulting from a pregnancy-induced imbalanced state and to protect the vulnerable fetus. Prescriptions and proscriptions regulate the woman's emotional response, clothing, activity and rest, sexual activity, and dietary practices. Exploration of the woman's beliefs, perceptions of the meaning of childbearing, and health care practices may help health care providers foster her self-actualization, promote attainment of the maternal role, and positively influence her relationship with her partner.

To provide culturally responsive care, nurses must be knowledgeable about practices and customs, although it is not possible to know all there is to know about every culture and subculture or the many lifestyles that exist. It is important to learn about the varied cultures in the community where you practice (Cooper, Grywalski, Lamp, Newhouse, & Studlien, 2007). When exploring cultural beliefs and practices related to childbearing, the nurse can support and nurture those beliefs that promote physical or emotional adaptation. However, if you identify potentially harmful beliefs or activities, provide education and propose modifications.

Emotional Response

Virtually all cultures emphasize the importance of maintaining a socially harmonious and agreeable environment for a pregnant woman. A lifestyle with minimal stress is important in ensuring a successful outcome for the mother and baby. Harmony with other people must be fostered, and visits from extended family members may be required to demonstrate pleasant and noncontroversial relationships. If discord exists in a relationship, it is usually dealt with in culturally prescribed ways.

Besides proscriptions regarding food, other proscriptions involve forms of magic. For example, some Mexicans believe that pregnant women should not witness an eclipse of the moon because it may cause a cleft palate in the infant. They also believe that exposure to an earthquake may precipitate preterm birth, miscarriage, or even a breech presentation. In some cultures a pregnant woman must not ridicule someone with an affliction for fear her child might be born with the same handicap. A mother should not hate a person lest her child resemble that person, and dental work should not be done because it may cause a baby to have a "harelip." A widely held folk belief in some cultures is that the pregnant woman should refrain from raising her arms above her head, because such movement ties knots in the umbilical cord and may cause it to wrap around the baby's neck. Another belief is that placing a knife under the bed of a laboring woman will "cut" her pain.

Clothing

Although most cultural groups do not prescribe specific clothing to be worn during pregnancy, modesty is an expectation of many. Some Mexican women of the Southwest and women of Central America wear a cord beneath the breasts and knotted over the umbilicus. This cord, called a muñeco, is thought to prevent morning sickness and ensure a safe birth (Fig. 15-20). Amulets, medals, and beads also may be worn to ward off evil spirits.

Physical Activity and Rest

Norms that regulate the physical activity of mothers during pregnancy vary tremendously. Many groups, including Native Americans and some Asian groups, encourage women to be

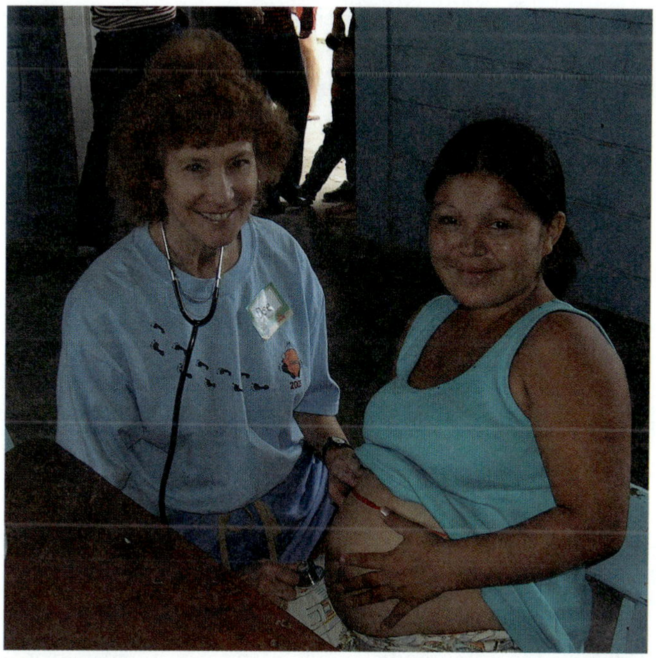

FIG. 15-20 A young woman from Honduras wearing a muñeco given to her by her mother to ensure a safe birth. (Courtesy Dee Lowdermilk, Chapel Hill, NC)

active, to walk, and to engage in normal, although not strenuous, activities to ensure that the baby is healthy and not too large. Conversely, other groups such as Filipinos believe that any activity is dangerous, and others willingly take over the work of the pregnant woman. Some Filipinos believe that this inactivity protects the mother and child. The mother is encouraged simply to produce the succeeding generation. If health care providers do not know of this belief, they could misinterpret this behavior as laziness or nonadherence with the desired prenatal health care regimen. It is important for the nurse to find out the way each pregnant woman views activity and rest.

Sexual Activity

In most cultures sexual activity is not prohibited until the end of pregnancy. Some Hispanics view sexual activity as necessary to keep the birth canal lubricated. Conversely, some Vietnamese may have definite proscriptions against sexual intercourse, requiring abstinence throughout the pregnancy because it is thought that sexual intercourse may harm the mother and fetus.

Diet

Nutritional information given by Western health care providers also may be a source of conflict for many cultural groups. Such a conflict commonly is not known by health care providers unless they understand the dietary beliefs and practices of the people for whom they are caring. For example, Muslims have strict regulations regarding preparation of food, and if meat cannot be prepared as prescribed, they may omit meats from their diets. Many cultures permit pregnant women to eat only warm foods.

Age Differences

The age of the childbearing couple may have a significant influence on their physical and psychosocial adaptation to pregnancy. Normal developmental processes that occur in both very young and older mothers are interrupted by pregnancy and require a different type of adaptation to pregnancy than that of the woman of typical childbearing age. Although the individuality of each pregnant woman is recognized, special needs of expectant mothers 15 years of age or younger or those 35 years of age or older are summarized.

Adolescents

Critical Thinking Exercise—Teenage Pregnancy

Teenage pregnancy is a worldwide problem. About 1 million adolescent females in the United States, or 4 out of every 10 girls, become pregnant each year. Most of the pregnancies are unintended. Adolescents are responsible for almost 450,000 births in the United States annually. Hispanic adolescents currently have the highest birth rate, although the rate for African-American adolescents also is high (Heron et al., 2010). Most of these young women are unmarried, and many are not ready for the emotional, psychosocial, and financial responsibilities of parenthood.

Numerous adolescent pregnancy-prevention programs have had varying degrees of success. Characteristics of programs that make a difference are those that have sustained commitment to adolescents over a long time, involve the parents and other adults in the community, promote abstinence and personal responsibility, and assist adolescents to develop a clear strategy for reaching future goals such as a college education or a career.

When adolescents do become pregnant and decide to give birth, they are much less likely than older women to receive adequate prenatal care, with many receiving no care at all. These young women also are more likely to smoke and less likely to gain adequate weight during pregnancy. As a result of these and other factors, babies born to adolescents are at greatly increased risk of LBW, of serious and long-term disability, and of dying during the first year of life (Chedraui, 2008).

Delayed entry into prenatal care may be the result of late recognition of pregnancy, denial of pregnancy, or confusion about the available services. Such a delay in care may leave an inadequate time before birth to attend to correctable problems. The very young pregnant adolescent is at higher risk for each of the variables associated with poor pregnancy outcomes (e.g., socioeconomic factors) and for those conditions associated with a first pregnancy regardless of age (e.g., gestational hypertension). The role of the nurse in reducing the risks and consequences of adolescent pregnancy is very important as adolescents often see the nurse as trustworthy and someone who will keep their confidence as well as provide them with accurate information. Therefore, effective communication is essential in providing care to the pregnant adolescent (King-Jones, 2008) (Fig. 15-21) (see Nursing Care Plan: Adolescent Pregnancy).

Women Older Than 35 Years

Two groups of older parents have emerged in the population of women having a child late in their childbearing years. One group consists of women who have many children or who have an additional child during the menopausal period. The other group consists of women who have deliberately delayed childbearing until their late 30s or early 40s.

Multiparous Women. Multiparous women may have never used contraceptives because of personal choice or lack of knowledge concerning contraceptives. They also may be women who have used contraceptives successfully during the childbearing years, but as menopause approaches they may cease menstruating regularly or stop using contraceptives and consequently become pregnant. The older multiparous woman may feel that pregnancy separates her from her peer group and that her age

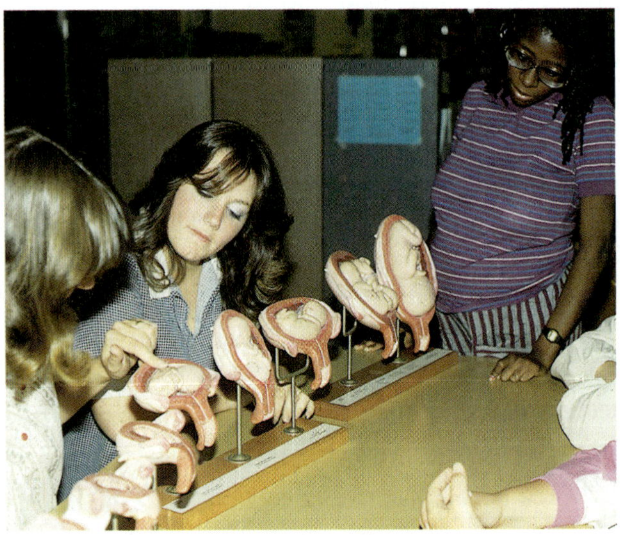

FIG. 15-21 Pregnant adolescents reviewing fetal development. (Courtesy Marjorie Pyle, RNC, Lifecircle, Costa Mesa, CA.)

NURSING CARE PLAN

Adolescent Pregnancy

NURSING DIAGNOSIS

Imbalanced nutrition: less than body requirements related to intake insufficient to meet metabolic needs of fetus and adolescent client

Expected Outcome

Adolescent will gain weight as prescribed, take prenatal vitamins and iron as prescribed, and maintain normal hematocrit and hemoglobin values.

Nursing Interventions/*Rationales*

- Assess current diet history and intake *to determine prescriptions for additions or changes in present dietary pattern.*
- Compare prepregnancy weight with current weight *to determine if pattern is consistent with appropriate fetal growth and development.*
- Provide information concerning food prescriptions for appropriate weight gain, considering preferences for fast food and peer influences *to correct any misconceptions and increase chances for compliance with diet.*
- Include adolescent's immediate family or support system during instruction *to ensure that person preparing family meals receives information.*

NURSING DIAGNOSIS

Risk for injury, maternal or fetal, related to inadequate prenatal care and screening

Expected Outcomes

Adolescent will experience uncomplicated pregnancy and give birth to a healthy fetus at term.

Nursing Interventions/*Rationales*

- Provide information using therapeutic communication and confidentiality *to establish relationship and build trust.*
- Discuss importance of ongoing prenatal care and possible risks to adolescent client and fetus *to reinforce that ongoing assessment is crucial to health and well-being of client and fetus, even if client feels well.* The adolescent client is at greater risk for certain complications that may be avoided or managed early if prenatal visits are maintained.
- Discuss risks of alcohol, tobacco, and recreational drug use during pregnancy *to minimize risks to the adolescent and fetus,* because the adolescent client has a higher substance abuse rate than the rest of the pregnant population.
- Assess for evidence of sexually transmitted infection (STI) and provide information regarding sexual practices *to minimize risk to client and fetus,* because adolescent is at greater risk for STIs.
- Screen for preeclampsia on an ongoing basis *to minimize risk,* because adolescent population is at greater risk for preeclampsia.

NURSING DIAGNOSIS

Social isolation related to body image changes of pregnant adolescent as evidenced by client statements and concerns

Expected Outcomes

Adolescent will identify support systems and report decreased feelings of social isolation.

Nursing Interventions/*Rationales*

- Establish a therapeutic relationship *to listen objectively and establish trust.*
- Discuss with adolescent any changes in relationships that have occurred as a result of the pregnancy *to determine extent of isolation from family, peers, and father of the baby.*
- Provide referrals and resources appropriate for developmental stage of adolescent *to give information and support.*
- Provide information regarding parenting classes, breastfeeding classes, and childbirth-preparation classes *to give further information and group support, which lessens social isolation.*

NURSING DIAGNOSIS

Interrupted family processes related to adolescent pregnancy

Expected Outcome

Adolescent will reestablish relationship with her mother and father of the baby.

Nursing Interventions/*Rationales*

- Encourage communication with mother *to clarify roles and relationships related to birth of infant.*
- Encourage communication with father of baby (if she desires continued contact) *to ascertain level of support to be expected from the father of the baby.*
- Refer to support group *to learn more effective ways of problem solving and reduce conflict within the family.*

NURSING DIAGNOSIS

Disturbed body image related to situational crisis of pregnancy

Expected Outcome

Pregnant adolescent will verbalize positive comments regarding her body image during the pregnancy.

Nursing Interventions/*Rationales*

- Assess pregnant adolescent's perception of self related to pregnancy *to provide basis for further interventions.*
- Give information regarding expected body changes occurring during pregnancy *to provide a realistic view of these temporary changes.*
- Provide opportunity to discuss personal feelings and concerns *to promote trust and support.*

NURSING DIAGNOSIS

Risk for impaired parenting related to immaturity and lack of experience in new role of adolescent mother

Expected Outcome

Parents will demonstrate parenting roles with confidence.

Nursing Interventions/*Rationales*

- Provide information on growth and development *to enhance knowledge so that adolescent mother can have basis for caring for her infant.*
- Refer to parenting classes *to enhance knowledge and obtain support for providing appropriate care to newborn and infant.*
- Initiate discussion of child care *to assist adolescent in problem solving for future needs.*
- Assess parenting abilities of adolescent mother and father *to provide baseline for education.*
- Provide information on parenting classes that are appropriate for parents' developmental stage *to give opportunity to share common feelings and concerns.*
- Assist parents to identify pertinent support systems *to give assistance with parenting as needed.*

is a hindrance to close associations with young mothers. Other parents welcome the unexpected infant as evidence of continuing maternal and paternal roles.

Primiparous Women. The number of first-time pregnancies in women between the ages of 35 and 40 years has increased significantly over the past three decades (Heron et al., 2010). Seeing women in their late 30s or 40s during their first pregnancy is no longer unusual for health care providers. Reasons for delaying pregnancy include a desire to obtain advanced education, career priorities, and use of better contraceptive measures. Women who are infertile do not delay pregnancy deliberately but may become pregnant at a later age as a result of fertility studies and therapies.

These women choose parenthood. They often are successfully established in a career and a lifestyle with a partner that includes time for self-attention, the establishment of a home with accumulated possessions, and freedom to travel. When asked the reason they chose pregnancy later in life, many reply, "Because time is running out."

The dilemma of choice includes the recognition that being a parent will have positive and negative consequences. Couples should discuss the consequences of childbearing and childrearing before committing themselves to this lifelong venture. Partners in this group seem to share the preparation for parenthood, planning for a family-centered birth, and desire to be loving and competent parents; however, the reality of child care may prove difficult for such parents.

First-time mothers older than 35 years select the "right time" for pregnancy; this time is influenced by their awareness of the increasing possibility of infertility or of genetic defects in the infants of older women. Such women seek information about pregnancy from books, friends, and electronic resources. They actively try to prevent fetal disorders and are careful in searching for the best possible maternity care. They identify sources of stress in their lives. They have concerns about having enough energy and stamina to meet the demands of parenting and their new roles and relationships.

If older women become pregnant after treatment for infertility, they may suddenly have negative or ambivalent feelings about the pregnancy. They may experience a multifetal pregnancy that may create emotional and physical problems. Adjusting to parenting two or more infants requires adaptability and additional resources.

During pregnancy parents explore the possibilities and responsibilities of changing identities and new roles. They must prepare a safe and nurturing environment during pregnancy and after birth. They must integrate the child into an established family system and negotiate new roles (parent roles, sibling roles, grandparent roles) for family members.

Adverse perinatal outcomes are more common in older primiparas than in younger women, even when they receive good prenatal care. Suplee and associates (2007) reported that women ages 35 years and older are more likely than are younger primiparas to have LBW infants, premature birth, and multiple births. The occurrence of these complications is quite stressful for the new parents, and nursing interventions that provide information and psychosocial support are needed, as well as care for physical needs. In addition, in women ages 35 years or older there is an increased risk of maternal mortality. Pregnancy-related deaths are from hemorrhage, infection, embolisms, hypertensive disorders of pregnancy, cardiomyopathy, and strokes (Johnson et al., 2007).

Multifetal Pregnancy

When the pregnancy involves more than one fetus, both the mother and fetuses are at increased risk for adverse outcomes. The maternal blood volume is increased, resulting in an increased strain on the maternal cardiovascular system. Anemia often develops because of a greater demand for iron by the fetuses. Marked uterine distention and increased pressure on the adjacent viscera and pelvic vasculature and diastasis of the two rectus abdominis muscles (see Fig. 13-13) may occur. Placenta previa develops more commonly in multifetal pregnancies because of the large size or placement of the placentas (Gilbert, 2011). Premature separation of the placenta may occur before the second and any subsequent fetuses are born.

Twin pregnancies often end in prematurity. Spontaneous rupture of membranes before term is common. Congenital malformations are twice as common in monozygotic twins as in singletons, although there is no increase in the incidence of congenital anomalies in dizygotic twins. In addition, two-vessel cords—that is, cords with a vein and a single umbilical artery instead of two—occur more often in twins than in singletons, but this abnormality is most common in monozygotic twins. The clinical diagnosis of multifetal pregnancy is accurate in about 90% of cases. The likelihood of a multifetal pregnancy is increased if any one or a combination of the following factors is noted during a careful assessment:

- History of dizygotic twins in the female lineage
- Use of fertility drugs
- More rapid uterine growth for the number of weeks of gestation
- Polyhydramnios
- Palpation of more than the expected number of small or large parts
- Asynchronous fetal heartbeats or more than one fetal electrocardiographic tracing
- Ultrasonographic evidence of more than one fetus

The diagnosis of multifetal pregnancy can come as a shock to many expectant parents, and they may need additional support and education to help them cope with the changes they face. The mother needs nutrition counseling so that she gains more weight than that needed for a singleton birth, counseling that maternal adaptations will probably be more uncomfortable, and information about the possibility of a preterm birth.

If the presence of more than three fetuses is diagnosed, the parents may receive counseling regarding selective reduction to reduce the incidence of premature birth and improve the opportunities for the remaining fetuses to grow to term gestation (Cleary-Goldman, Chitkara, & Berkowitz, 2007). This situation may pose an ethical dilemma for many couples, especially those who have worked hard to overcome problems with infertility and have strong values regarding right to life. Initiating a discussion to identify what resources could help the couple (e.g., a minister, priest, or mental health counselor) to make the decision is important because the decision-making process and the procedure itself may be stressful. Most women will have feelings of guilt, anger, and sadness but most will come to terms with the loss and will bond with the remaining fetus or fetuses (Cleary-Goldman, et al.).

The prenatal care given women with multifetal pregnancies includes changes in the pattern of care and modifications in other aspects such as the amount of weight gained and the nutritional intake necessary. The prenatal visits of these women are scheduled at least every 2 weeks in the second trimester and weekly thereafter. Ultrasound evaluations are scheduled at 18 to 20 weeks and then every 3 to 4 weeks to monitor the fetal growth and amniotic fluid volume (Cleary-Goldman, et al., 2007). In twin gestations the recommended weight gain is 16 to 20 kg. Iron and vitamin supplementation is desirable. As the risk for preeclampsia and eclampsia increases in multifetal pregnancies, nurses aggressively work to identify and treat these complications of pregnancy.

The considerable uterine distention involved can cause the backache commonly experienced by pregnant women to be even worse. Maternal support hose may be worn to control leg varicosities. If risk factors such as premature dilation of the cervix or bleeding are present, abstinence from orgasm and nipple stimulation during the last trimester is recommended to help avert preterm labor. Frequent ultrasound examinations, nonstress tests, and FHR monitoring will be performed. Some practitioners recommend bed rest beginning at 20 weeks in women carrying multiple fetuses to prevent preterm labor. Other practitioners question the value of prolonged bed rest. If bed rest is recommended, the mother assumes a lateral position to promote increased placental perfusion. If birth is delayed until after the thirty-sixth week, the risk of morbidity and mortality decreases for the neonates.

Multiple newborns will likely place a strain on finances, space, workload, and the woman's and family's coping capability. Lifestyle changes may be necessary. Parents will need assistance in making realistic plans for the care of the babies (e.g., whether to breastfeed and whether to raise them as "alike" or as separate persons). Parents should be referred to national organizations such as Parents of Twins and Triplets (www.potatonet.org), Mothers of Twins (www.nomotc.org), and the La Leche League (www.lalecheleague.org) for further support.

CHILDBIRTH AND PERINATAL EDUCATION

The goal of childbirth and perinatal education is to assist individuals and their family members to make informed, safe decisions about pregnancy, birth, and early parenthood. It also is to assist them to comprehend the long-lasting potential that empowering birth experiences have in the lives of women and that early experiences have on the development of children and the family. The perinatal education program is an expansion of the earlier childbirth education movement that originally offered a set of classes in the third trimester of pregnancy to prepare parents for birth. Today perinatal education programs consist of a menu of class series and activities from preconception through the early months of parenting.

Health-promoting education should be provided in a context that emphasizes how a healthy body is best able to adapt to the changes that accompany pregnancy. Without this context of health, routine care and testing for risks may contribute to a mindset of families that pregnancy is a pathologic as opposed to a healthy mind-body-spirit event.

Some of the decisions the childbearing family must consider are the decision to have a baby, followed by choices of a care provider and type of care (a midwifery model [natural oriented] versus a medical [intervention oriented] model); the place for birth (hospital, birthing center, home); and the type of infant feeding (breast or bottle) and infant care. If a woman has had a cesarean birth, she may consider having a vaginal birth. Perinatal education can provide information to help childbearing families make informed decisions about these issues.

Previous pregnancy and childbirth experiences are important elements that influence current learning needs. The woman's (and support person's) age, cultural background, personal philosophy with regard to childbirth, socioeconomic status, spiritual beliefs, and learning styles are assessed to develop the best plan to help the woman meet her needs.

For the most part, the pregnant woman and her partner attend childbirth education classes, although sometimes a friend, teenage daughter, or parent is the designated support person (Fig. 15-22). There are also classes for grandparents and siblings to prepare them for their attendance at birth and/or the arrival of the baby. Siblings often see a film about birth and learn ways they can help welcome the baby. They also learn to cope with changes that include a reduction in parental time and attention. Grandparents learn about current child care practices and how to help their adult children adapt to parenting in a supportive way.

Childbirth Education Programs

Childbirth, when one is prepared and well supported, presents to women a unique and powerful opportunity to find their core strength in a manner that forever changes their self-perception. Expectant parents and their families have different interests and information needs as the pregnancy progresses.

Early pregnancy ("early bird") classes provide fundamental information. Classes are developed around the following areas: (1) early fetal development, (2) physiologic and emotional changes of pregnancy, (3) human sexuality, and (4) the nutritional needs of the mother and fetus. The classes often address environmental and workplace hazards. Exercises, nutrition, warning signs, drugs, and self-medication also are topics of interest and concern.

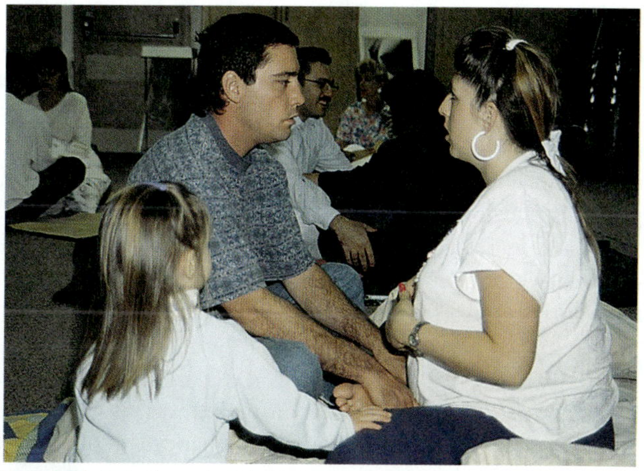

FIG. 15-22 Learning relaxation exercises with the whole family. (Courtesy Marjorie Pyle, RNC, Lifecircle, Costa Mesa, CA.)

Mid-pregnancy classes emphasize the woman's participation in self-management. Classes provide information on preparation for breastfeeding and formula feeding, infant care, basic hygiene, common complaints and simple safe remedies, infant health, parenting, and updating and refining the birth plans.

Late pregnancy classes emphasize labor and birth. There are different methods of coping with labor and birth and these are often the basis for various prenatal classes. These include Lamaze, Bradley, and Dick-Read. These classes usually include a hospital tour.

Current Practices in Childbirth Education

A variety of approaches to childbirth education have evolved as childbirth educators attempt to meet learning needs. In addition to classes designed specifically for pregnant adolescents, their partners, and/or parents, classes exist for other groups with special learning needs. These include classes for first-time mothers older than age 35, single women, adoptive parents, and parents of multiples or women with handicaps such as those who are visually impaired or deaf. Refresher classes for parents with children not only review coping techniques for labor and birth but also help couples prepare for sibling reactions and adjustments to a new baby. Cesarean birth classes are available for couples who have this kind of birth scheduled because of breech presentation or other risk factors. Other classes focus on vaginal birth after cesarean (VBAC) because many women can successfully give birth vaginally after previous cesarean birth.

Throughout the series of classes there is discussion of support systems that people can use during pregnancy and after birth. Such support systems help parents function independently and effectively. During all the classes the open expression of feelings and concerns about any aspect of pregnancy, birth, and parenting is welcomed.

Pain Management

Fear of pain in labor is a key issue and the reason many women give for attending childbirth education classes. Numerous studies show that women who have received childbirth preparation later report no less pain but do report greater ability to cope with the pain during labor and birth and more birth satisfaction than unprepared women. Therefore, although pain management strategies are an essential component of childbirth education, total pain eradication is not the primary source of birth satisfaction or a goal. Eliminating suffering is a realistic goal. Control in childbirth, meaning participation in decision making, has repeatedly been the primary source of birth satisfaction.

Couples need information about the advantages and disadvantages of pain medication and about other techniques for coping with labor. An emphasis on nonpharmacologic pain management strategies helps couples manage the labor and birth with dignity and increased comfort. Most instructors teach a flexible approach, which helps couples learn and master many techniques to use during labor (see Chapter 17 for further discussion).

Perinatal Care Choices

Often the first decision the woman makes is who will be her primary health care provider for the pregnancy and birth. This decision is doubly important because it usually affects where the birth will take place. The nurse can provide information about the different types of health care providers and what kind of care to expect from each type.

The Coalition to Improve Maternity Services (CIMS, 2000), a group of more than 50 nursing and maternity care–oriented organizations, produced a document to assist women in selecting their perinatal care. After some explanation of choices, encourage women to ask potential care providers the following questions:

- Who can be with me during labor and birth?
- What happens during a normal labor and birth in your setting?
- How do you allow for differences in culture and beliefs?
- May I walk and move around during labor? What position do you suggest for birth?
- How do you make sure everything goes smoothly when my nurse, doctor, nurse-midwife, or agency works with one another?
- What things do you normally do to a woman in labor?
- How do you help mothers stay as comfortable as they can be? Besides drugs, how do you help mothers relieve the pain of labor?
- What if my baby is born early or has special problems?
- Do you circumcise babies?
- How do you help mothers who want to breastfeed?

Physicians

Physicians (obstetricians, family medicine physicians) attend 91.6% of births in the United States and Canada (Heron et al., 2010). They see low and high risk clients. Care often includes pharmacologic and medical management of problems as well as use of technologic procedures. Family medicine physicians may need backup by obstetricians if a specialist is needed for a problem (e.g., a cesarean birth). Most physicians manage births in a hospital setting.

Nurse-Midwives

Most midwives are certified nurse midwives (CNMs). They provide care for more than 8% of the births in the United States and Canada (Martin, Hamilton, Sutton, Ventura, Menacker, Kirmeyer, et al., 2009). They usually see low risk obstetric clients. Care is often noninterventionist, and they often encourage the woman and her family to be active participants in the care. Nurse-midwives refer patients to physicians for complications. Most births (about 94%) are managed in hospital settings or alternative birth centers; a small number are managed in a home setting.

Direct-Entry Midwives

Direct-entry midwives and independent (lay) midwives manage slightly less than 1% of births in the United States; most are in the home setting.

Doulas

A doula is professionally trained to provide labor support, including physical, emotional, and informational support to women and their partners during labor and birth. The doula does not become involved with clinical tasks (Doulas of North America [DONA], 2008). Today many couples, no matter which type of childbirth classes they take, also employ a doula for labor support.

COMMUNITY ACTIVITY

- Visit the website childbirth.org, which provides educational and informational links for families. Review the information in the labor and childbirth section, about childbirth classes and the role of the doula.
- Locate a childbirth class in your community. Contact the Instructor and try to attend a class. Compare and contrast the educational content of a class for expectant families versus a lecture in nursing school on the same subject.
- Research midwifery care options in your community, including hospital-based midwives and home birth midwives. Visit the website of a hospital-based midwifery service. What types of services do the midwives provide? How is the care by a nurse midwife different than that of an obstetrician?

A Cochrane synopsis of 16 trials involving 13,391 women found that "continuous labor support like that provided by doulas reduces a woman's likelihood of having pain medication, increases her satisfaction and chances for spontaneous birth, and has no known risks" (Hodnett, Gates, Hofmeyr, & Sakala, 2007).

A doula typically meets with the woman and her husband or partner before labor. At this meeting she ascertains the woman's expectations and desires for the birth experience. With this information as her guide during labor and birth, the doula focuses her efforts on assisting the woman to achieve her goals. Doulas work collaboratively with other health care providers and the husband or other supportive individuals, but their primary goal is to assist the woman.

Doulas may be found through community contacts, other health care providers, or childbirth educators; a number of organizations offer information or referral services. It is important that the expectant mother be comfortable with the doula who will be attending her. See Box 15-7 for a list of questions to ask when arranging for a doula. Doulas of North America (DONA) is an organization that certifies doulas (www.dona.org). Although the doula role originally developed as an assistant during labor, some women benefit from assistance during the postpartum period. There are small but growing numbers of postnatal doulas who provide assistance to the new mother as she develops competence with infant care, feeding, and other maternal tasks.

Birth Plans

Once the maternity care provider is chosen, there are numerous other decisions to be made over the course of the perinatal year. Many prenatal care providers and childbirth educators encourage expectant parents to develop a birth plan to identify their options and set priorities. The **birth plan** is a tool with which parents can explore their childbirth options and choose those that are most important to them. The plan must be viewed as tentative because the realities of what is feasible may change as the actual labor and birth unfold. It is understood to be a preference list based on a best case scenario (see Chapter 19).

Birth Setting Choices

With careful thought, the concept of natural or family- or woman-centered maternity care can be implemented in any setting. The three primary options for birth settings are the hospital, birth center, and home. Women consider several factors in choosing a setting for childbirth, including the preference of their health care provider, characteristics of the birthing unit, and preference of their third-party payer. Approximately 99% of all births in the United States take place in a hospital setting (Martin et al., 2009). However, the types of labor and birth services vary greatly, from the traditional labor and delivery rooms with separate postpartum and newborn units, to in-hospital birthing centers, where all or almost all care takes place in a single unit.

BOX 15-7 QUESTIONS TO ASK WHEN CHOOSING A DOULA

To discover the specific training, experience, and services offered by anyone who provides labor support, potential patients, nursing supervisors, physicians, midwives, and others should ask the following questions of that person:

- What training have you had?
- Tell me about your experience with birth, personally and as a doula.
- What is your philosophy about childbirth and supporting women and their partners through labor?
- May we meet to discuss our birth plans and the role you will play in supporting me through childbirth?
- May we call you with questions or concerns before and after the birth?
- When do you try to join women in labor? Do you come to our home or meet us at the hospital?
- Do you meet with us after the birth to review the labor and answer questions?
- Do you work with one or more backup doulas for times when you are not available? May we meet them?
- What is your fee?

Source: Doulas of North America (DONA). (2008). *Doulas of North America position paper: The doula's contribution to modern maternity care.* Available at www.dona.org/PDF/QuestionsToAskADoula.pdf. Accessed June 23, 2010.

Labor, Delivery, Recovery, Postpartum (Birthing) Rooms

Labor, delivery, and recovery (LDR), and labor, delivery, recovery, and postpartum (LDRP) rooms offer families a comfortable, private space for childbirth (Fig. 15-23). Women are admitted to LDR units, labor and give birth, and spend the first 1 to 2 hours postpartum there for immediate recovery and to have time with their families to bond with their newborns. After this period of recovery, the mothers and newborns move to a postpartum unit and nursery or mother-baby unit for the duration of their stay.

In LDRP units, the same nursing staff usually provides total care from admission through postpartum discharge. The woman and her family may stay in this unit for 6 to 48 hours after giving birth. The units are furnished to provide a homelike atmosphere, as LDR units are, but have accommodations for family members to stay overnight.

Both units have fetal monitors, emergency resuscitation equipment for mother and newborn, and heated cribs or warming units for the newborn. Often this equipment is out of sight in cabinets or closets when it is not being used.

Birth Centers

Free-standing birth centers are usually built in locations separate from the hospital but are often located nearby in case transfer of the woman or newborn is needed. These birth centers

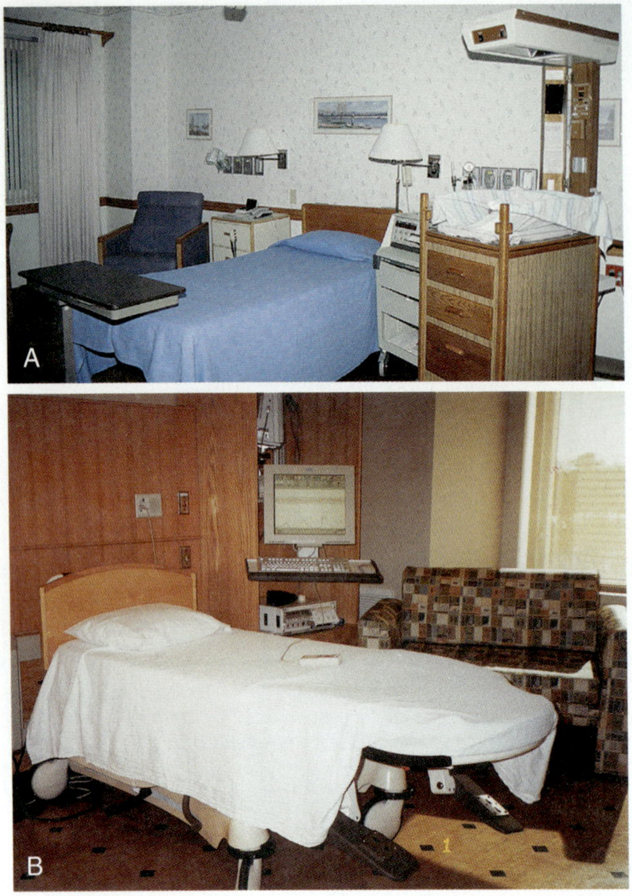

FIG. 15-23 **A,** Labor, delivery, and recovery (LDR) unit. **B,** Labor, delivery, recovery, and postpartum (LDRP) unit. Note sofa in background that converts to a bed. **(A,** Courtesy Julie Perry Nelson, Loveland, CO; **B,** Courtesy Dee Lowdermilk, Chapel Hill, NC.)

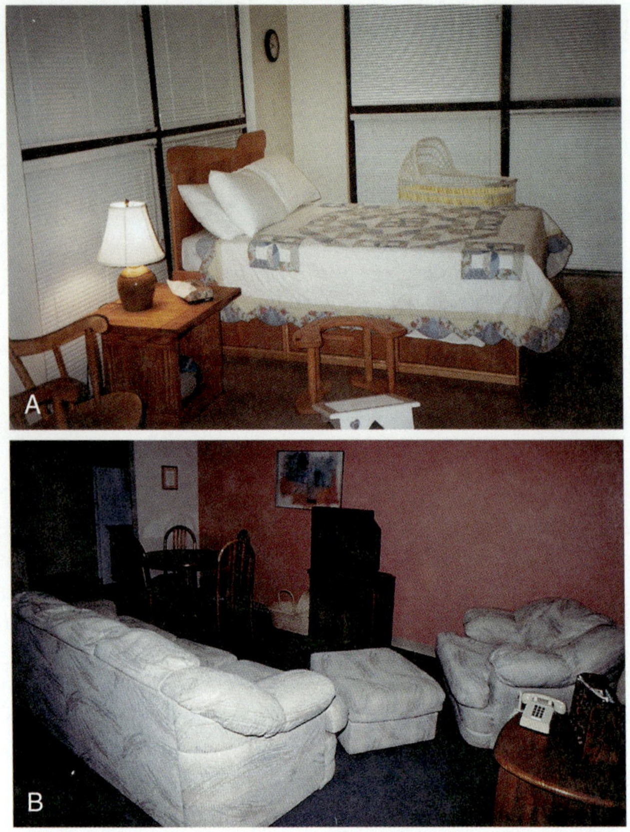

FIG. 15-24 Birth center. **A,** Note double bed, baby crib, and birthing stool. **B,** Lounge and kitchen. **(A,** Courtesy Dee Lowdermilk, Chapel Hill, NC. Photo location: The Women's Birth and Wellness Center, Chapel Hill, NC; **B,** Courtesy Michael S. Clement, MD, Mesa, AZ. Photo location: Bethany Birth Center, Phoenix, AZ.)

offer families a safe and cost-effective alternative to hospital or home birth. About one fourth of the 1% of out-of-hospital births are in birthing centers (Martin et al., 2009). The centers are usually staffed by nurse-midwives or physicians who also have privileges at the local hospital. Only women at low risk for complications are included for care. Attendance at childbirth and parenting classes is required of all clients. The family is admitted to the birth center for labor and birth and will remain there until discharge, which often takes place within 6 hours of the birth.

Birth centers typically have homelike accommodations, including a double bed for the couple and a crib for the newborn (Fig. 15-24). Emergency equipment and drugs are usually in cabinets, out of view but easily accessible. Private bathroom facilities are incorporated into each birth unit. There may be an early labor lounge or a living room and small kitchen.

Services provided by the free-standing birth centers include those necessary for safe management during the childbearing cycle. Clients must understand that some situations require transfer to a hospital, and they must agree to abide by those guidelines.

Birth centers as well as a hospital with a comprehensive birthing program may have resources for parents such as a lending library that includes books and videotapes; reference files on related topics; recycled maternity clothes, baby clothes, and equipment; and supplies and reference materials for childbirth educators. The centers may also have referral files for community resources that offer services relating to childbirth and early parenting, including support groups (e.g., for single parents, for postbirth support, and for parents of twins), genetic counseling, women's issues, and consumer action.

A birth center should be located close to a major hospital so that quick transfer to that institution is possible if necessary for the birth. Ambulance service and emergency procedures must be readily available. Fees vary with the services provided by birthing centers but typically are less than or equal to those charged by local hospitals. Some base fees on the ability of the family to pay (a reduced-fee sliding scale). Several third-party payers, as well as Medicaid and the Civilian Health and Medical Programs of the Uniformed Services (TRICARE/CHAMPUS), recognize and reimburse these centers.

Home Birth

Home birth has always been popular in certain countries, such as Sweden and The Netherlands. In developing countries, hospitals or adequate lying-in facilities often are unavailable to most pregnant women, and home birth is a necessity. In North America home births account for about two thirds of the less than 1% of births outside the hospital setting (Martin et al., 2009).

Although home births are considered countercultural by many in the United States, there is no evidence base to discourage low risk couples who desire a carefully planned out-of-the-hospital birth (Johnson & Daviss, 2005). National groups

Case Study—Third Trimester

supporting home birth are the Home Oriented Maternity Experience (HOME) and the National Association of Parents for Safe Alternatives in Childbirth (NAPSAC). These groups work to foster more humane childbearing practices at all levels, integrating the alternatives for childbirth to meet the needs of the total population.

One advantage of home birth is that the family is in control of the experience. Another is that the birth may be more physiologically normal in familiar surroundings. The mother may be more relaxed than she would be in the hospital environment. Care providers who participate in home births tend to be more support oriented and less intervention oriented. The family can assist in and be a part of the happy event, and contact with the newborn is immediate and sustained. In addition, home birth may be less expensive than a hospital confinement. Serious infection may be less likely, assuming strict aseptic principles are followed, because people generally are relatively immune to their own home bacteria.

KEY POINTS

- The prenatal period is a preparatory one both physically, in terms of fetal growth and parental adaptations, and psychologically, in terms of anticipation of parenthood.
- Pregnancy affects parent-child, sibling-child, and grandparent-child relationships.
- Discomforts and changes of pregnancy can cause anxiety to the woman and her family and require sensitive attention and a plan for teaching self-management measures.
- Education about healthy ways of using the body (e.g., exercise, body mechanics) is essential given maternal anatomic and physiologic responses to pregnancy.
- Important components of the initial prenatal visit include detailed and carefully recorded findings from the interview, a comprehensive physical examination, and selected laboratory tests.
- Follow-up visits are shorter than the initial visit and are important for monitoring the health of the mother and fetus and providing anticipatory guidance as needed.
- Even in normal pregnancy the nurse must remain alert to hazards such as supine hypotension, signs and symptoms of potential complications, and signs of family maladaptations.
- Blood pressure is evaluated based on absolute values and length of gestation and interpreted in light of modifying factors.
- Each pregnant woman needs to know how to recognize and report signs of potential complications such as preterm labor.
- The likelihood of physical abuse increases during pregnancy.
- Culture, age, parity, and multiple pregnancy can have a significant effect on the course and outcome of the pregnancy.
- Nurses must be knowledgeable about practices and customs related to childbearing to provide culturally sensitive care.
- Childbirth education teaches tuning in to the body's inner wisdom and coping strategies that enhance women's ability to know how to give birth.
- Childbirth education strives to promote healthier pregnancies and family lifestyles.

Audio Chapter Summaries Access an audio summary of these Key Points on evolve

REFERENCES

Agency for Healthcare Research and Quality (AHRQ) Healthcare Innovations Exchange. (2009). *Inter-agency collaborative provides home visits, specialized support to at-risk families, leading to better prenatal care, less child abuse, and fewer early childhood deaths.* Available at www.innovations.ahrq.gov/content.aspx?id=2295. Accessed June 22, 2010.

American Academy of Pediatrics and American College of Obstetricians and Gynecologists (ACOG.). (2007). *Guidelines for perinatal care* (6th ed.). Washington, DC: Author.

American College of Obstetricians and Gynecologists (ACOG). (2002). Exercise during pregnancy and the postpartum period, ACOG Committee Opinion No. 267. *Obstetrics and Gynecology, 99*(1), 171–173.

American College of Obstetricians and Gynecologists (ACOG). (2003). Immunization during pregnancy, ACOG Committee Opinion No. 282. *Obstetrics and Gynecology, 101*(1), 207–212.

American College of Obstetricians and Gynecologists Committee on Health Care for Underserved Women. (2006). Psychosocial risk factors: Perinatal screening and intervention. ACOG Committee Opinion No. 343. *Obstetrics and Gynecology, 108*(2), 469–477.

American College of Obstetricians and Gynecologists Committee on Obstetric Practice. (2004). ACOG Committee Opinion No. 304. Prenatal and perinatal human immunodeficiency virus testing: Expanded recommendations. *Obstetrics and Gynecology, 104*(5 Part 1), 1119–1124.

American College of Obstetricians and Gynecologists Committee on Obstetric Practice. (2005). Smoking cessation during pregnancy. ACOG Committee Opinion No. 316, October, 2005. *Obstetrics and Gynecology, 106*(4), 883–888.

American Dental Association. (2006). *Women's oral health issues: Pregnancy.* Available at www.ada.org/prof/resources/topics/healthcare_pregnancy.pdf. Accessed June 22, 2010.

American Dietetic Association (ADA). (2008). Position of the American Dietetic Association: Nutrition and lifestyle for a healthy pregnancy. *Journal of the American Dietetic Association, 108*(3), 553–561.

Association of Women's Health, Obstetric and Neonatal Nurses. (2008). *HIV screening procedures for pregnant women and newborns.* Policy position statement. Washington, DC: AWHONN. Available at www.awhonn.org. Accessed June 22, 2010.

Boggess, K., & Edelstein, B. (2006). Oral health in women during preconception and pregnancy: Implications for birth outcomes and infant oral health. *Maternal and Child Health Journal, 10*(Suppl. 5), S169–S174.

Branson, B., Handsfield, H., Lampe, M., Janssen, R., Taylor, A., Lyss, S., et al. (2006). Revised recommendations for HIV testing of adults, adolescents, and pregnant women in health-care settings. *MMWR Morbidity and Mortality Weekly Report, 55*(RR-14), 1–17.

Centers for Disease Control and Prevention, Workowski, K., & Berman, S. (2006). Sexually transmitted diseases treatment guidelines, 2006. *MMWR Morbidity and Mortality Weekly Report, 55*(RR-11), 1–94.

Centers for Disease Control and Prevention. (2008). *AICP: Guidance for vaccine recommendations in pregnant and breastfeeding women.* Available at www.cdc.gov/vaccines. Accessed June 22, 2010.

Centers for Disease Control and Prevention. (2009). *Fetal alcohol spectrum disorders.* Available at www.cdc.gov/ncbddd/fasd/alcohol-use.html. Accessed June 22, 2010.

Cesario, S. (2007). Seat belt use in pregnancy: History, misconceptions, and the need for education. *Nursing for Women's Health, 11*(5), 474–481.

Chedraui, P. (2008). Pregnancy among young adolescents: Trends, risk factors, and maternal-perinatal outcome. *Journal of Perinatal Medicine, 36*(3), 256–259.

Cleary-Goldman, J., Chitkara, U., & Berkowitz, R. (2007). Multiple gestation. In S. Gabbe, J. Niebyl, & J. Simpson (Eds.), *Obstetrics: Normal and problem pregnancies* (5th ed.). Philadelphia: Churchill Livingstone.

Coalition to Improve Maternity Services. (2000). *Having a baby? Ten questions to ask.* Available at www.motherfriendly.org. Accessed June 22, 2010.

Cooper, M., Grywalski, M., Lamp, J., Newhouse, L., & Studlien, R. (2007). Enhancing cultural competence: A model for nurses. *Nursing for Women's Health, 11*(2), 148–159.

Cunningham, F., Leveno, K., Bloom, S., Hauth, J., Rouse, D., & Spong, C. (2010). *Williams obstetrics* (23rd ed.). New York: McGraw Hill.

Daniels, P., Noe, G., & Mayberry, R. (2006). Barriers to prenatal care among black women of low socioeconomic status. *American Journal of Health Behavior, 30*(2), 188–198.

Darby, S. (2007). Pre- and perinatal care of Hispanic families. *Nursing for Women's Health, 11*(2), 160–169.

Dasanayake, A., Gennaro, S., Hendricks-Munoz, K., & Chhun, N. (2008). Maternal periodontal disease, pregnancy, and neonatal outcomes. *MCN The American Journal of Maternal/Child Nursing, 33*(1), 45–49.

Davies, G., Maxwell, C., McLeod, L., Gagnon R., Basso, M., Bos, H., et al. (2010). Obesity in pregnancy. *Journal of Obstetrics and Gynecology,* Canada, 32(2), 165–173.

Doulas of North America (DONA). (2008). *Doulas of North America position paper: The doula's contribution to modern maternity care.* Available at www.dona.org. Accessed June 22, 2010.

Driggers, R., & Siebert, D. (2008). Prenatal screening: New guidelines, new challenges. *The Journal for Nurse Practitioners, 4*(5), 351–356.

Family Violence Prevention Fund. (2010). *The facts on adolescent pregnancy, reproductive risk, and exposure to dating and family violence.* Available at http://endabuse.org/userfiles/file/HelathCare/Adolescent%20Pregnancy%20HealthReproductive%20Risk%FINAL%202-10.pdf. Accessed June 22, 2010.

Frøen, J., Heazell, A., Tveit, J., Saastad, E., Fretts, R., & Flenady, V. (2008). Fetal movement assessment. *Seminars in Perinatology, 32*(4), 243–246.

Gilbert, E. (2011). *Manual of high risk pregnancy & delivery* (5th ed.). St. Louis: Mosby.

Health Physics Society. (2009). *Radiation exposure during commercial airline flights.* Available at www.hps.org/publicinformation/ate/faqs/commercialflights.html. Accessed June 22, 2010.

Heron, M., Sutton, P., Xu, J., Ventura, S., Strobino, D., & Guyer, B. (2010). Annual summary of vital statistics—2007. *Pediatrics, 125*(1), 4–15.

Hodnett, E., Gates, S., Hofmeyr, G., & Sakala, C. (2007). Continuous support for women during childbirth. *The Cochrane Database of Systematic Reviews, 2007,* 3, CD003766.

Hunter, L. (2009). Issues in pregnancy dating: Revisiting the evidence. *Journal of Midwifery & Women's Health, 54*(3), 184–190.

Jepson, R., & Craig, J. (2008). Cranberries for preventing urinary tract infections (Cochrane Review). *The Cochrane Database of Systematic Reviews, 2008,* 1, CD001231.

Johnson, K., & Daviss., B. (2005). Outcomes of planned home births and certified professional midwives: Large prospective study in North America. *British Medical Journal, 330*(7505), 1416.

Johnson, T., Gregory, K., & Niebyl, J. (2007). Preconception and prenatal care: Part of the continuum. In S. Gabbe, J. Niebyl, & J. Simpson (Eds.). *Obstetrics: Normal and problem pregnancies* (5th ed.). Philadelphia: Churchill Livingstone.

King-Jones, T. (2008). Caring for the pregnant adolescent: Perils and pearls of communication. *Nursing for Women's Health, 12*(2), 114–119.

Krieger, C. (2008). Intimate partner violence: A review for nurses. *Nursing for Women's Health, 12*(3), 224–234.

Lawrence, R., & Lawrence, R. (2005). *Breastfeeding: A guide for the medical profession* (6th ed.). Philadelphia: Mosby.

Lentz, G. (2007). Physiology of micturition, diagnosis of voiding dysfunction, and incontinence: Surgical and nonsurgical treatment. In V. Katz, G. Lentz, R. Lobo, & D. Gershenson (Eds.), *Comprehensive gynecology* (5th ed.). Philadelphia: Mosby.

Lopez, R. (2005). Periodontal disease, preterm birth, and low birth weight. *Evidence-Based Dentistry, 6*(4), 90–91.

Martin, J., Hamilton, B., Sutton, P., Ventura, S., Menacker, F., Kirmeyer, S., et al. (2009). Births: Final data for 2006. *National Vital Statistics Reports, 57*(7), 1–102.

Massey, Z., Rising, S., & Ickovics, J. (2006). CenteringPregnancy group prenatal care: Promoting relationship-centered care. *Journal of Obstetric, Gynecologic and Neonatal Nursing, 35*(2), 286–294.

May, K. (1982). Three phases of father involvement in pregnancy. *Nursing Research, 31*(6), 337–342.

Mercer, R. (1995). *Becoming a mother.* New York: Springer.

Moos, M. (2006). Prenatal care: Limitations and opportunities. *Journal of Obstetric, Gynecologic and Neonatal Nursing, 35*(2), 278–285.

Norton, M. (2008). Genetic screening and counseling. *Current Opinion in Obstetrics and Gynecology, 20*(2), 157–163.

Polley, B., Wing, R., & Sims, C. (2002). Randomized controlled trial to prevent excess weight gain in pregnant women. *International Journal of Obesity, 26*(11), 1494–1502.

Reid, J. (2007). CenteringPregnacy: A model for group prenatal care. *Nursing for Women's Health, 11*(4), 382–388.

Rubin, R. (1975). Maternal tasks in pregnancy. *Maternal and Child Nursing Journal, 4*(3), 143–153.

Rubin, R. (1984). *Maternal identity and the maternal experience.* New York: Springer.

Russell, S., & Mayberry, L. (2008). Pregnancy and oral health: A review and recommendation to reduce gaps in practice and research. *MCN The American Journal of Maternal/Child Nursing, 33*(1), 32–37.

Seidel, H., Ball, J., Dains, J., Flynn, J., Solomon, B., & Stewart, R. (2011). *Mosby's guide to physical examination* (7th ed.). St. Louis: Mosby.

Smeltzer, S. (2007). Pregnancy in women with physical disabilities. *Journal of Obstetric, Gynecologic and Neonatal Nursing, 36*(1), 88–96.

Suplee, P., Dawley, K., & Bloch, J. (2007). Tailoring peripartum nursing care for women of advanced maternal age. *Journal of Obstetric, Gynecologic and Neonatal Nursing, 36*(6), 616–623.

Van Dyke, M., Phares, C., Lynfield, R., Thomas, A., Arnold, K., Craig, A., et al. (2009). Evaluation of universal antenatal screening for group B Streptococcus. *New England Journal of Medicine, 360*(25), 2626–2636.

Weng, X., Odouli, R., & Li, D. (2008). Maternal caffeine consumption during pregnancy and the risk of miscarriage: A prospective cohort study. *American Journal of Obstetrics and Gynecology, 198*(3), 279, e-1–e-8.

Yamashita, E. (2009). *Information seeking during pregnancy: Investigating health information-seeking behaviors among low-income pregnant women in rural California.* Saarbrücken, Germany: VDM Publishing.

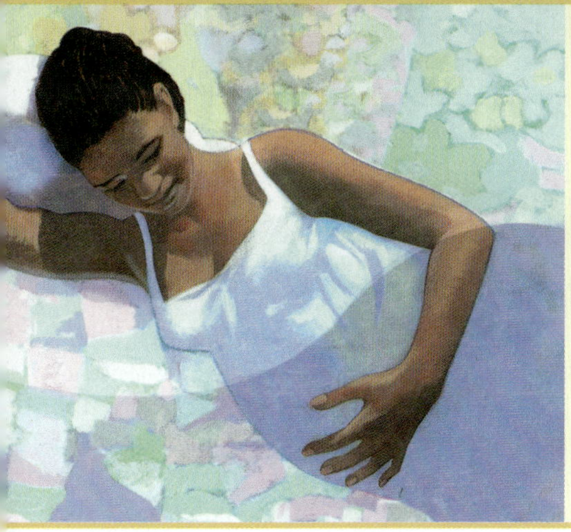

CHAPTER

16

Labor and Birth Processes

Deitra Leonard Lowdermilk

evolve WEBSITE

http://evolve.elsevier.com/Lowdermilk/MWHC/

Audio Glossary
Audio Key Points
Critical Thinking Exercise
  Fetal Presentation
NCLEX Review Questions
Video—Assessment
  Fetal Lie
  Position
  Presentation

LEARNING OBJECTIVES

- Explain the five major factors that affect the labor process.
- Describe the anatomic structure of the bony pelvis.
- Recognize the normal measurements of the diameters of the pelvic inlet, cavity, and outlet.
- Explain the significance of the size and position of the fetal head during labor and birth.
- Summarize the cardinal movements of the mechanism of labor for a vertex presentation.
- Examine the maternal anatomic and physiologic adaptations to labor.
- Describe factors thought to contribute to the onset of labor.
- Describe fetal adaptations to labor.

During late pregnancy a woman and fetus prepare for the labor process. The fetus has grown and developed in preparation for extrauterine life. The woman has undergone various physiologic adaptations during pregnancy that prepare her for birth and motherhood. Labor and birth represent the end of pregnancy, the beginning of extrauterine life for the newborn, and a change in the lives of the family. This chapter discusses the factors affecting labor, the process involved, the normal progression of events, and the adaptations made by both the woman and fetus.

FACTORS AFFECTING LABOR

At least five factors affect the process of labor and birth. These are easily remembered as the five P's: *p*assenger (fetus and placenta), *p*assageway (birth canal), *p*owers (contractions), *p*osition of the mother, and *p*sychologic response. The first four factors are presented here as the basis of understanding the physiologic process of labor. The fifth factor is discussed in Chapter 17. Other factors that may be a part of the woman's labor experience may be important as well. VandeVusse (1999) identified external forces including place of birth, preparation, type of provider (especially nurses), and procedures. Physiology (sensations) was identified as an internal force. These factors are discussed generally in Chapter 19 as they relate to nursing care during labor. Further research investigating essential forces of labor is recommended.

Passenger

The way the passenger, or fetus, moves through the birth canal is determined by several interacting factors: the size of the fetal head, fetal presentation, fetal lie, fetal attitude, and fetal position. Because the placenta also must pass through the birth canal, it can be considered a passenger along with the fetus; however, the placenta rarely impedes the process of labor in normal vaginal birth, except in cases of placenta previa.

Size of the Fetal Head

Because of its size and relative rigidity, the fetal head has a major effect on the birth process. The fetal skull is composed of two parietal bones, two temporal bones, the frontal bone, and the occipital bone (Fig. 16-1, *A*). These bones are united by membranous sutures: sagittal, lambdoidal, coronal, and frontal (see Fig. 16-1, *B*). Membrane-filled spaces called **fontanels** are located where the sutures intersect. During labor, after rupture of membranes, palpation of fontanels and sutures during

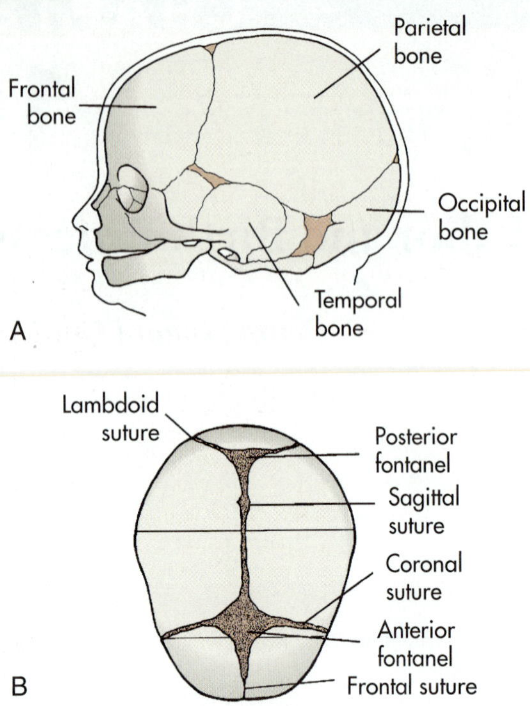

FIG. 16-1 Fetal head at term. **A,** Bones. **B,** Sutures and fontanels.

vaginal examination reveals fetal presentation, position, and attitude.

The anterior and posterior fontanels are the two most important (see Fig. 16-1, *B*). The larger of these, the anterior fontanel, is diamond shaped, is about 3 cm by 2 cm, and lies at the junction of the sagittal, coronal, and frontal sutures. It closes by 18 months after birth. The posterior fontanel lies at the junction of the sutures of the two parietal bones and the occipital bone, is triangular, and is about 1 cm by 2 cm. It closes 6 to 8 weeks after birth.

Sutures and fontanels make the skull flexible to accommodate the infant brain, which continues to grow for some time after birth. However, because the bones are not firmly united, slight overlapping of the bones, or **molding** of the shape of the head, occurs during labor. This capacity of the bones to slide over one another also permits adaptation to the various diameters of the maternal pelvis. Molding can be extensive, but the heads of most newborns assume their normal shape within 3 days after birth.

Although the size of the fetal shoulders may affect passage, their position can be altered relatively easily during labor, so one shoulder may occupy a lower level than the other. This creates a shoulder diameter that is smaller than the skull, facilitating passage through the birth canal. The circumference of the fetal hips is usually small enough not to create problems.

Video—Assessment: Fetal Lie, Position, Presentation

Fetal Presentation

Presentation refers to the part of the fetus that enters the pelvic inlet first and leads through the birth canal during labor. The three main presentations are **cephalic presentation** (head first), occurring in 96% of births (Fig. 16-2); **breech presentation** (buttocks, feet, or both first), occurring in 3% of births (Fig. 16-3, *A-C*); and **shoulder presentation,** seen in 1% of births (see Fig. 16-3, *D*). The **presenting part** is that part of the fetus that lies closest to the internal os of the cervix. It is the part of the fetal body first felt by the examining finger during a vaginal examination. In a cephalic presentation the presenting part is usually the occiput; in a breech presentation it is the sacrum; in the shoulder presentation it is the scapula. When the presenting part is the occiput, the presentation is noted as **vertex** (see Fig. 16-2). Factors that determine the presenting part include fetal lie, fetal attitude, and extension or flexion of the fetal head.

Fetal Lie

Lie is the relation of the long axis (spine) of the fetus to the long axis (spine) of the mother. The two primary lies are longitudinal, or vertical, in which the long axis of the fetus is parallel with the long axis of the mother (see Fig. 16-2); and transverse, horizontal, or oblique, in which the long axis of the fetus is at a right angle diagonal to the long axis of the mother (see Fig. 16-3, *D*). Longitudinal lies are either cephalic or breech presentations, depending on the fetal structure that first enters the mother's pelvis. Vaginal birth cannot occur when the fetus stays in a transverse lie. An oblique lie, one in which the long axis of the fetus is lying at an angle to the long axis of the mother, is less common and usually converts to a longitudinal or transverse lie during labor (Cunningham, Leveno, Bloom, Hauth, Rouse, & Spong, 2010).

Fetal Attitude

Attitude is the relation of the fetal body parts to each other. The fetus assumes a characteristic posture (attitude) in utero partly because of the mode of fetal growth and partly because of the way the fetus conforms to the shape of the uterine cavity. Normally the back of the fetus is rounded so that the chin is flexed on the chest, the thighs are flexed on the abdomen, and the legs are flexed at the knees. The arms are crossed over the thorax, and the umbilical cord lies between the arms and the legs. This attitude is termed **general flexion** (see Fig. 16-2).

Deviations from the normal attitude may cause difficulties in childbirth. For example, in a cephalic presentation, the fetal head may be extended or flexed in a manner that presents a head diameter that exceeds the limits of the maternal pelvis, leading to prolonged labor, forceps or vacuum-assisted birth, or cesarean birth.

Certain critical diameters of the fetal head are usually measured. The **biparietal diameter,** which is about 9.25 cm at term, is the largest transverse diameter and an important indicator of fetal head size (Fig. 16-4, *B*). In a well-flexed cephalic presentation, the biparietal diameter is the widest part of the head entering the pelvic inlet. Of the several anteroposterior diameters, the smallest and the most critical one is the **suboccipitobregmatic diameter** (about 9.5 cm at term). When the head is in complete flexion, this diameter allows the fetal head to pass through the true pelvis easily (see Fig. 16-4, *A*; Fig. 16-5, *A*). As the head is more extended, the anteroposterior diameter widens, and the head may not be able to enter the true pelvis (see Fig. 16-5, *B* and *C*).

Fetal Position

The presentation or presenting part indicates that portion of the fetus that overlies the pelvic inlet. **Position** is the relationship of a reference point on the presenting part (occiput, sacrum,

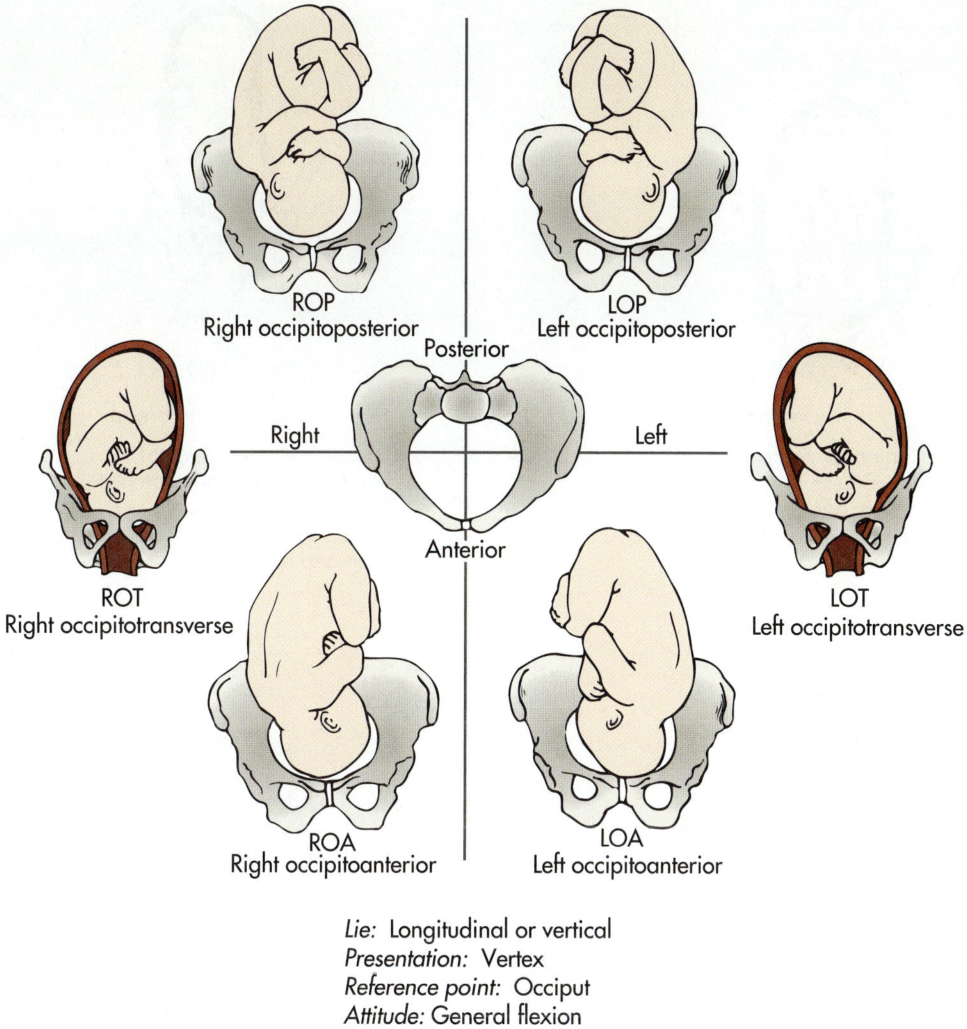

FIG. 16-2 Examples of fetal vertex (occiput) presentations in relation to front, back, or side of maternal pelvis.

mentum [chin], or sinciput [deflexed vertex]) to the four quadrants of the mother's pelvis (see Fig. 16-2). Position is denoted by a three-part abbreviation. The first letter of the abbreviation denotes the location of the presenting part in the right (R) or left (L) side of the mother's pelvis. The middle letter(s) stands for the specific presenting part of the fetus (O for occiput, S for sacrum, M for mentum [chin], and Sc for scapula [shoulder]). The final letter stands for the location of the presenting part in relation to the anterior (A), posterior (P), or transverse (T) portion of the maternal pelvis. For example, ROA means that the occiput is the presenting part and is located in the right anterior quadrant of the maternal pelvis (see Fig. 16-2). LSP means that the sacrum is the presenting part and is located in the left posterior quadrant of the maternal pelvis (see Fig. 16-3).

Station is the relationship of the presenting fetal part to an imaginary line drawn between the maternal ischial spines and is a measure of the degree of descent of the presenting part of the fetus through the birth canal. The placement of the presenting part is measured in centimeters above or below the ischial spines (Fig. 16-6). For example, when the lowermost portion of the presenting part is 1 cm above the spines, it is noted as being minus (−) 1. At the level of the spines, the station is said to be 0 (zero). When the presenting part is 1 cm below the spines, the station is said to be plus (+) 1. Birth is imminent when the presenting part is at +4 to +5 cm. The station of the presenting part should be determined when labor begins so that the rate of descent of the fetus during labor can be accurately determined.

Engagement is the term used to indicate that the largest transverse diameter of the presenting part (usually the biparietal diameter) has passed through the maternal pelvic brim or inlet into the true pelvis and usually corresponds to station 0. Engagement often occurs in the weeks just before labor begins in nulliparas and may occur before labor or during labor in multiparas. Engagement can be determined by abdominal or vaginal examination.

Passageway

The passageway, or birth canal, is composed of the mother's rigid bony pelvis and the soft tissues of the cervix, the pelvic floor, the vagina, and the introitus (the external opening to the vagina). Although the soft tissues, particularly the muscular layers of the pelvic floor, contribute to vaginal birth of the fetus, the maternal pelvis plays a far greater role in the labor process because the fetus must successfully accommodate itself to this relatively rigid passageway. The determination of the size and shape of the pelvis can be done at the initial prenatal visit or on admission in labor. This information can then be used in the assessment of labor progress (Thorp 2009).

A

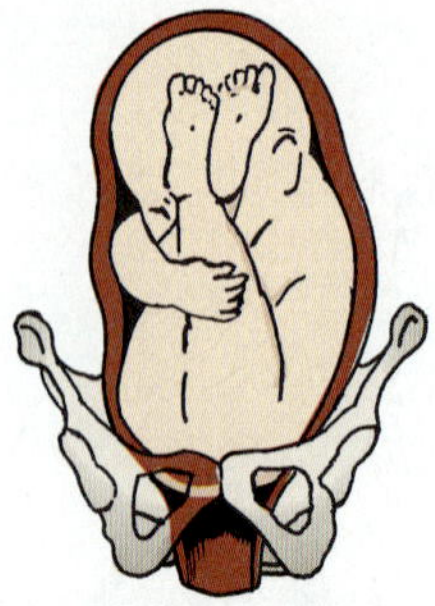

Frank breech

Lie: Longitudinal or vertical
Presentation: Breech (incomplete)
Presenting part: Sacrum
Attitude: Flexion, except for legs at knees

B

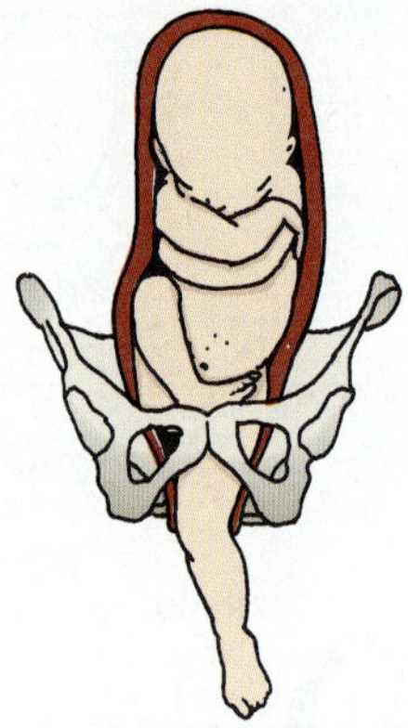

Single footling breech

Lie: Longitudinal or vertical
Presentation: Breech (incomplete)
Presenting part: Sacrum
Attitude: Flexion, except for one leg extended at hip and knee

C

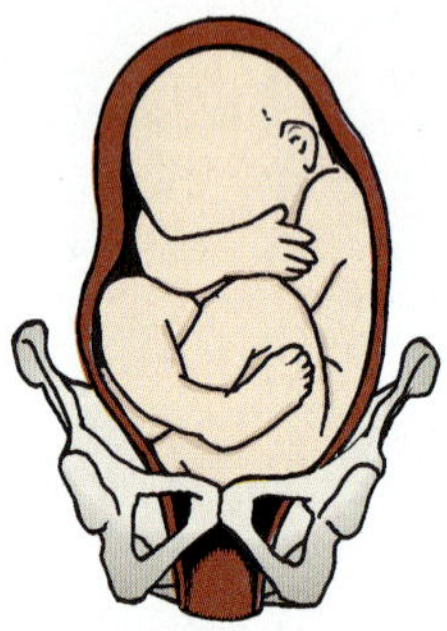

Complete breech

Lie: Longitudinal or vertical
Presentation: Breech (sacrum and feet presenting)
Presenting part: Sacrum (with feet)
Attitude: General flexion

D

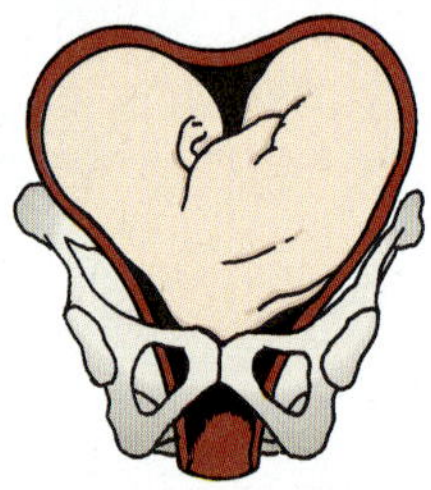

Shoulder presentation

Lie: Transverse or horizontal
Presentation: Shoulder
Presenting part: Scapula
Attitude: Flexion

FIG. 16-3 Fetal presentations. **A** through **C,** Breech (sacral) presentations. **D,** Shoulder presentation.

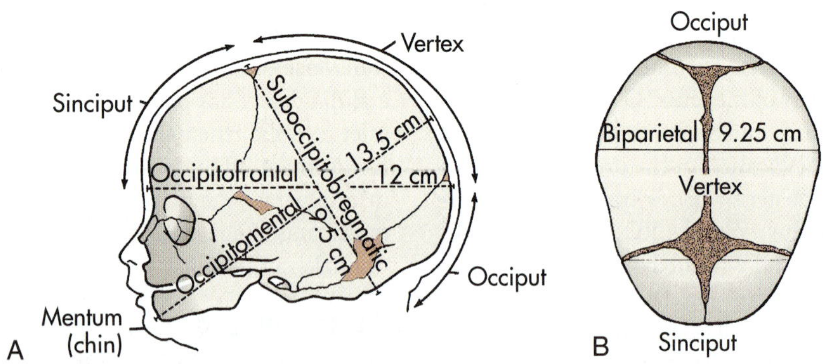

FIG. 16-4 Diameters of the fetal head at term. **A,** Cephalic presentations: occiput, vertex, and sinciput; and cephalic diameters: suboccipitobregmatic, occipitofrontal, and occipitomental. **B,** Biparietal diameter.

Bony Pelvis

The anatomy of the bony pelvis is described in Chapter 4. The following discussion focuses on the importance of pelvic configurations as they relate to the labor process. (It may be helpful to refer to Fig. 4-4.)

The bony pelvis is formed by the fusion of the ilium, the ischium, the pubis, and the sacral bones. The four pelvic joints are the symphysis pubis, the right and left sacroiliac joints, and the sacrococcygeal joint (Fig. 16-7, *A*). The bony pelvis is separated by the brim, or inlet, into two parts: the false pelvis and the true pelvis. The false pelvis is the part above the brim and plays no part in childbearing. The true pelvis, the part involved in birth, is divided into three planes: the inlet, or brim; the midpelvis, or cavity; and the outlet.

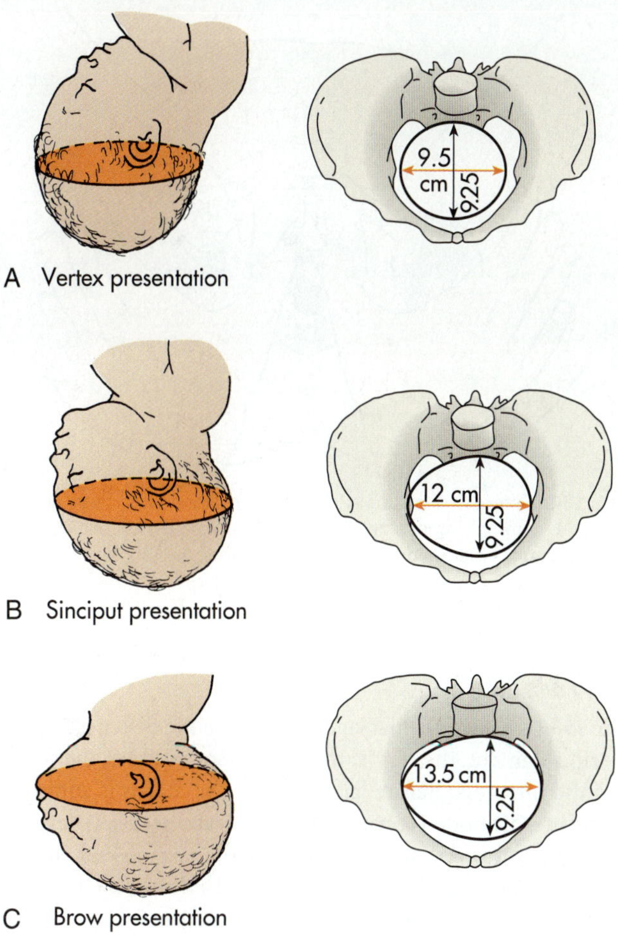

FIG. 16-5 Head entering pelvis. Biparietal diameter is indicated with shading (9.25 cm). **A,** Suboccipitobregmatic diameter: complete flexion of head on chest so that smallest diameter enters. **B,** Occipitofrontal diameter: moderate extension (military attitude) so that large diameter enters. **C,** Occipitomental diameter: marked extension (deflection), so that the largest diameter, which is too large to permit head to enter pelvis, is presenting.

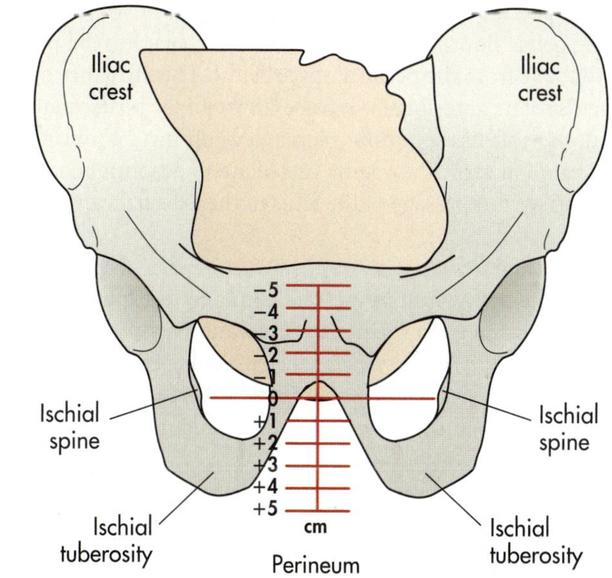

FIG. 16-6 Stations of presenting part, or degree of descent. The lowermost portion of the presenting part is at the level of the ischial spines, station 0.

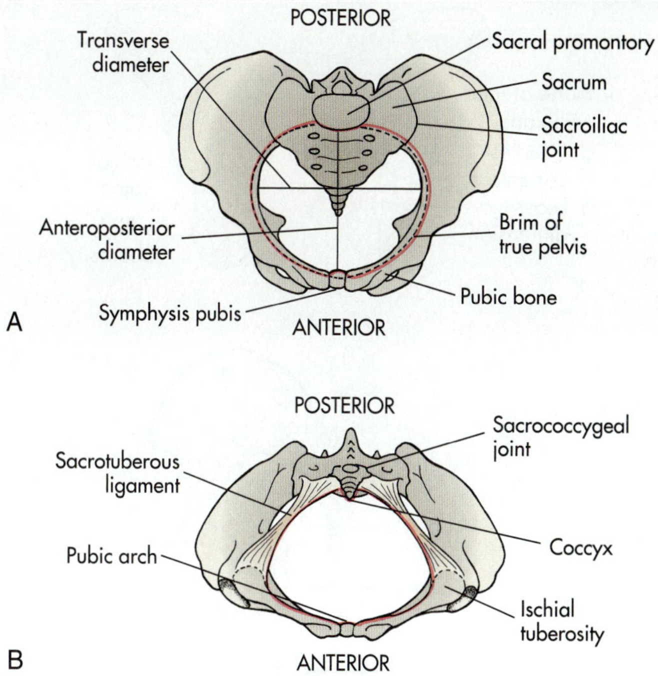

FIG. 16-7 Female pelvis. **A,** Pelvic brim from above. **B,** Pelvic outlet from below.

The pelvic inlet, which is the upper border of the true pelvis, is formed anteriorly by the upper margins of the pubic bone, laterally by the iliopectineal lines along the innominate bones, and posteriorly by the anterior, upper margin of the sacrum and the sacral promontory.

The pelvic cavity, or midpelvis, is a curved passage with a short anterior wall and a much longer concave posterior wall. It is bounded by the posterior aspect of the symphysis pubis, the ischium, a portion of the ilium, the sacrum, and the coccyx.

The pelvic outlet is the lower border of the true pelvis. Viewed from below it is ovoid, somewhat diamond shaped, and bounded by the pubic arch anteriorly, the ischial tuberosities laterally, and the tip of the coccyx posteriorly (see Fig. 16-7, *B*). In the latter part of pregnancy the coccyx is movable (unless it has been broken in a fall during skiing or skating, for example, and has fused to the sacrum during healing).

The pelvic canal varies in size and shape at various levels. The diameters at the plane of the pelvic inlet, midpelvis, and outlet, plus the axis of the birth canal (Fig. 16-8), determine whether vaginal birth is possible and the manner by which the fetus may pass down the birth canal.

The subpubic angle, which determines the type of pubic arch, together with the length of the pubic rami and the intertuberous diameter, is of great importance. Because the fetus must first pass beneath the pubic arch, a narrow subpubic angle will be less accommodating than a rounded, wide arch. The method of measurement of the subpubic arch is shown in Fig. 16-9. A summary of obstetric measurements is given in Table 16-1.

The four basic types of pelvis are classified as follows:

1. Gynecoid (the classic female type)
2. Android (resembling the male pelvis)
3. Anthropoid (resembling the pelvis of anthropoid apes)
4. Platypelloid (the flat pelvis)

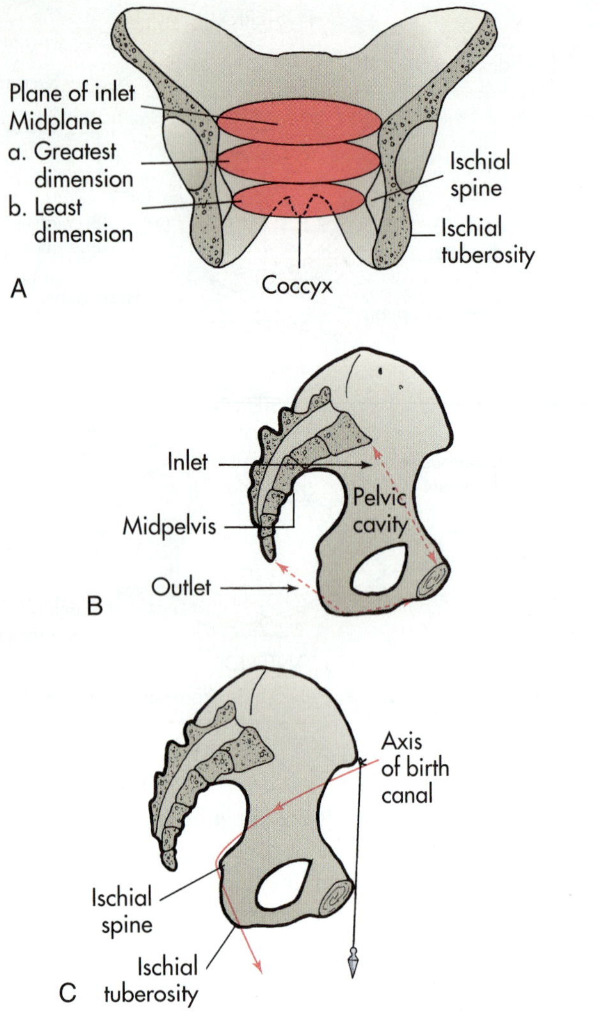

FIG. 16-8 Pelvic cavity. **A,** Inlet and midplane. Outlet not shown. **B,** Cavity of true pelvis. **C,** Note curve of sacrum and axis of birth canal.

The gynecoid pelvis is the most common, with major gynecoid pelvic features present in 50% of all women. Anthropoid and android features are less common, and platypelloid pelvic features are the least common. Mixed types of pelves are more common than are pure types (Cunningham et al., 2010). Examples of pelvic variations and their effects on mode of birth are given in Table 16-2.

Assessment of the bony pelvis can be performed during the first prenatal evaluation and need not be repeated if the pelvis is of adequate size and suitable shape. In the third trimester of pregnancy, the examination of the bony pelvis may be more thorough and the results more accurate because there is relaxation and increased mobility of the pelvic joints and ligaments owing to hormonal influences. Widening of the joint of the symphysis pubis and the resulting instability may cause pain in any or all of the pelvic joints.

Because the examiner does not have direct access to the bony structures and because the bones are covered with varying amounts of soft tissue, size and shape are estimated. Precise bony pelvis measurements can be determined by use of computed tomography, ultrasound, or x-ray films. However, radiographic examination is rarely done during pregnancy because the x-rays may damage the developing fetus.

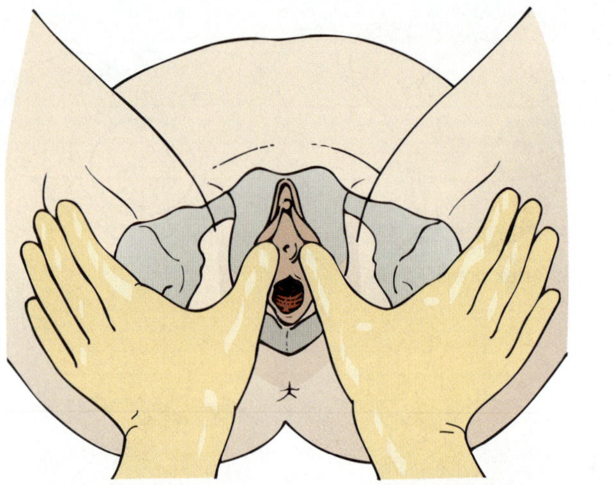

FIG. 16-9 Estimation of angle of subpubic arch. With both thumbs, examiner externally traces descending rami down to tuberosities. (From Barkauskas, V., Baumann, L., & Darling-Fisher, C. [2002]. *Health and physical assessment* [3rd ed.]. St. Louis: Mosby.)

Soft Tissues

The soft tissues of the passageway include the distensible lower uterine segment, the cervix, the pelvic floor muscles, the vagina, and the introitus. Before labor begins, the uterus is composed of the uterine body (corpus) and the cervix (neck). After labor has begun, uterine contractions cause the uterine body to have a thick and muscular upper segment and a thin-walled, passive, muscular lower segment. A *physiologic retraction ring* separates the two segments (Fig. 16-10). The lower uterine segment gradually distends to accommodate the intrauterine contents as the wall of the upper segment thickens and its accommodating capacity is reduced. The contractions of the uterine body thus exert downward pressure on the fetus, pushing it against the cervix.

The cervix effaces (thins) and dilates (opens) sufficiently to allow the first fetal portion to descend into the vagina. As the fetus descends, the cervix is actually drawn upward and over this first portion.

The pelvic floor is a muscular layer that separates the pelvic cavity above from the perineal space below. This structure helps the fetus rotate anteriorly as it passes through the birth canal. As noted, the soft tissues of the vagina develop throughout pregnancy until at term the vagina can dilate to accommodate the fetus and permit passage of the fetus to the external world.

Powers

Involuntary and voluntary powers combine to expel the fetus and the placenta from the uterus. Involuntary uterine contractions, called the *primary powers,* signal the beginning of labor. Once the cervix has dilated, voluntary bearing-down efforts by the woman, called the *secondary powers,* augment the force of the involuntary contractions.

Primary Powers

The involuntary contractions originate at certain pacemaker points in the thickened muscle layers of the upper uterine segment. From the pacemaker points, contractions move downward over the uterus in waves, separated by short rest periods.

TABLE 16-1 OBSTETRIC MEASUREMENTS

PLANE	DIAMETER	MEASUREMENTS
Inlet (superior strait)		
Conjugates		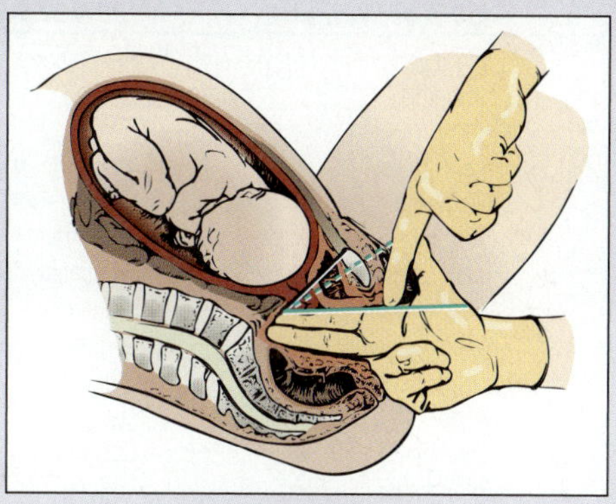 Length of diagonal conjugate (solid colored line), obstetric conjugate (broken colored line), and true conjugate (blue line)*
Diagonal	12.5-13 cm	
Obstetric: measurement that determines whether presenting part can engage or enter superior strait	1.5-2 cm less than diagonal (radiographic)	
True (vera) (anteroposterior)	≥11 cm (12.5) (radiographic)	
Midplane		
Transverse diameter (interspinous diameter)	10.5 cm	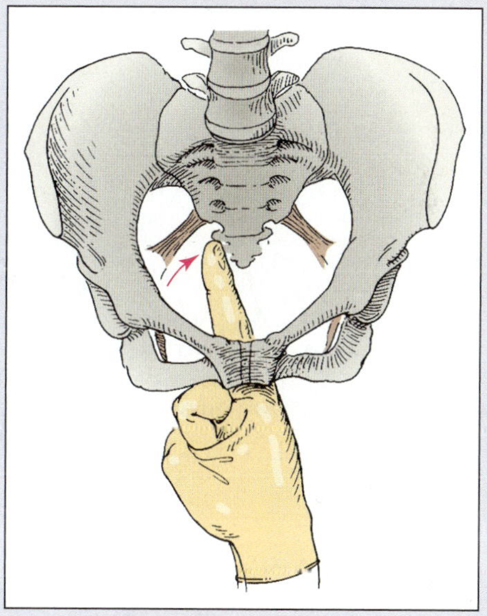 Measurement of interspinous diameter*
The midplane of the pelvis normally is its largest plane and the one of greatest diameter		
Outlet		
Transverse diameter (intertuberous diameter) (biischial)	≥8 cm	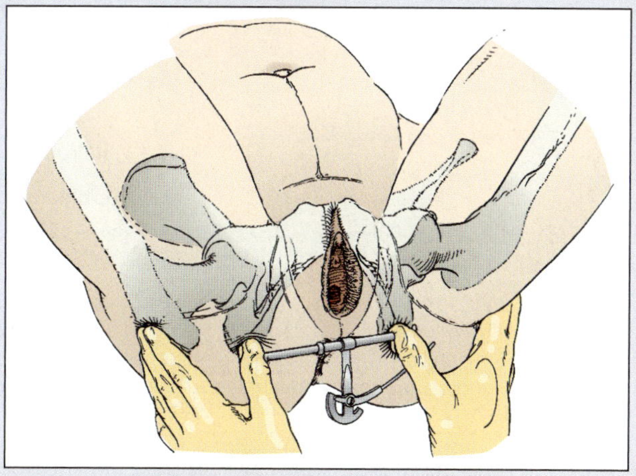 Use of Thom's pelvimeter to measure intertuberous diameter*
The outlet presents the smallest plane of the pelvic canal		

*From Seidel, H., Ball, J., Dains, J., Flynn, J., Solomon, B., and Stewart, R. (2011). *Mosby's guide to physical examination* (7th ed.). St. Louis: Mosby.

TABLE 16-2 COMPARISON OF PELVIC TYPES

	GYNECOID *(50% of Women)*	ANDROID *(23% of Women)*	ANTHROPOID *(24% of Women)*	PLATYPELLOID *(3% of Women)*
Brim	Slightly ovoid or transversely rounded	Heart shaped, angulated	Oval, wider anteroposteriorly	Flattened anteroposteriorly, wide transversely
Shape	Round	Heart	Oval	Flat
Depth	Moderate	Deep	Deep	Shallow
Side walls	Straight	Convergent	Straight	Straight
Ischial spines	Blunt, somewhat widely separated	Prominent, narrow interspinous diameter	Prominent, often with narrow interspinous diameter	Blunted, widely separated
Sacrum	Deep, curved	Slightly curved, terminal portion often beaked	Slightly curved	Slightly curved
Subpubic arch	Wide	Narrow	Narrow	Wide
Usual mode of birth	Vaginal Spontaneous Occipitoanterior position	Cesarean Vaginal Difficult, with forceps	Vaginal Forceps Spontaneous Occipitoposterior or occipitoanterior position	Vaginal Spontaneous

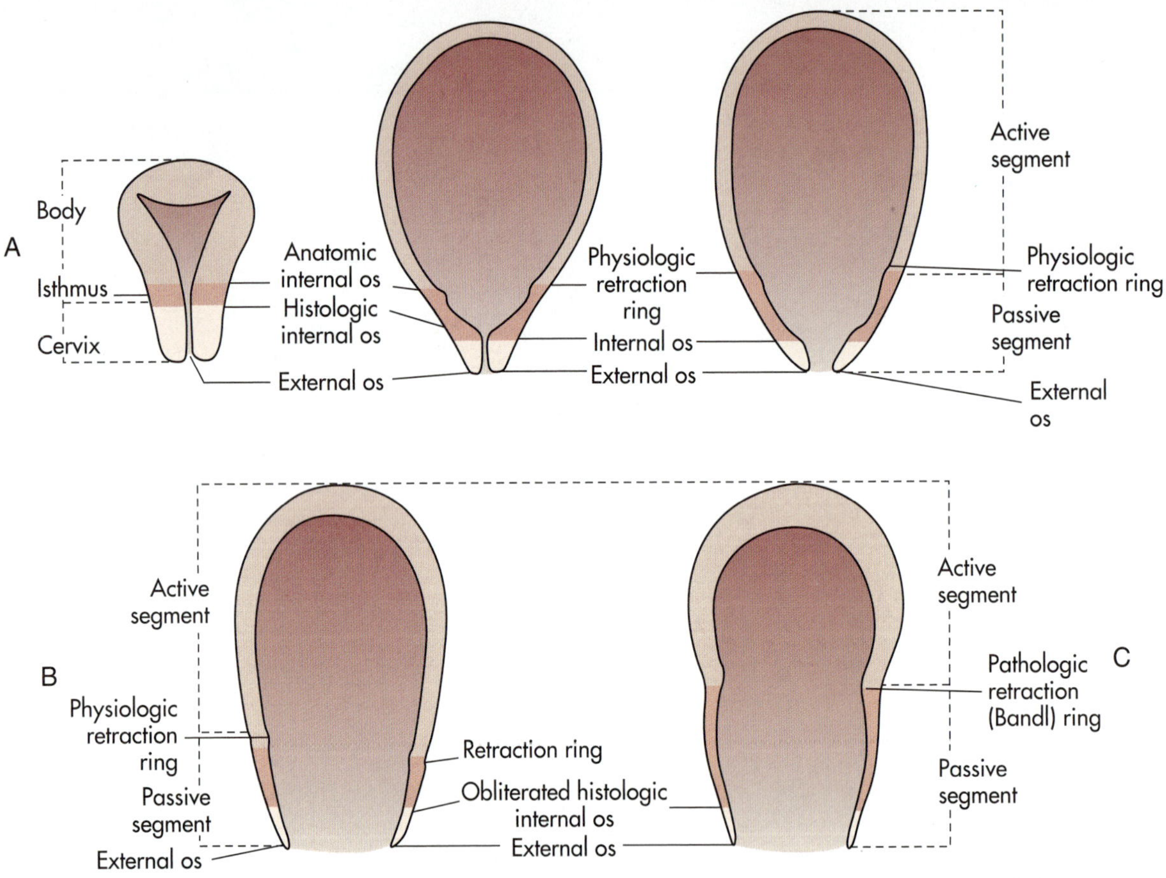

FIG. 16-10 **A,** Uterus in normal labor in early first stage, and **B,** in second stage. Passive segment is derived from lower uterine segment (isthmus) and cervix, and physiologic retraction ring is derived from anatomic internal os. **C,** Uterus in abnormal labor in second-stage dystocia. Pathologic retraction (Bandl) ring that forms under abnormal conditions develops from the physiologic ring.

Terms used to describe these involuntary contractions include *frequency* (the time from the beginning of one contraction to the beginning of the next), *duration* (length of contraction), and *intensity* (strength of contraction at its peak).

The primary powers are responsible for the effacement and dilation of the cervix and descent of the fetus. **Effacement** of the cervix means the shortening and thinning of the cervix during the first stage of labor. The cervix, normally 2 to 3 cm long and about 1 cm thick, is obliterated or "taken up" by a shortening of the uterine muscle bundles during the thinning of the lower uterine segment that occurs in advancing labor. Only a thin edge of the cervix can be palpated when effacement is complete. Effacement generally is advanced in first-time term pregnancy before more than slight dilation occurs. In subsequent pregnancies,

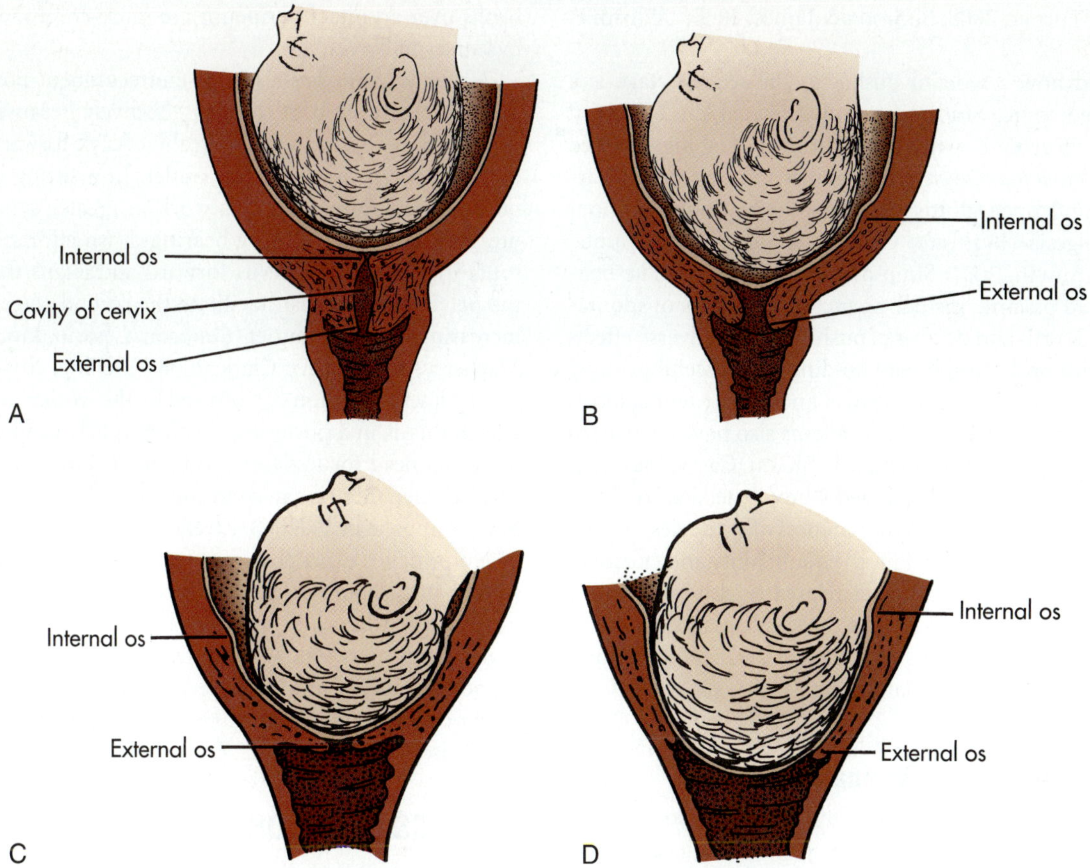

FIG. 16-11 Cervical effacement and dilation. Note how cervix is drawn up around presenting part (internal os). Membranes are intact, and head is not well applied to cervix. **A,** Before labor. **B,** Early effacement. **C,** Complete effacement (100%). Head is well applied to cervix. **D,** Complete dilation (10 cm). Cranial bones overlap somewhat, and membranes are still intact.

effacement and dilation of the cervix tend to progress together. Degree of effacement is expressed in percentages from 0% to 100% (e.g., a cervix is 50% effaced) (Fig. 16-11, *A-C*).

Dilation of the cervix is the enlargement or widening of the cervical opening and the cervical canal that occurs once labor has begun. The diameter of the cervix increases from less than 1 cm to full dilation (approximately 10 cm) to allow birth of a term fetus. When the cervix is fully dilated (and completely retracted), it can no longer be palpated (see Fig. 16-11, *D*). Full cervical dilation marks the end of the first stage of labor.

Dilation of the cervix occurs by the drawing upward of the musculofibrous components of the cervix, caused by strong uterine contractions. Pressure exerted by the amniotic fluid while the membranes are intact or by the force applied by the presenting part also can promote cervical dilation. Scarring of the cervix as a result of prior infection or surgery may slow cervical dilation.

In the first and second stages of labor, increased intrauterine pressure caused by contractions exerts pressure on the descending fetus and the cervix. When the presenting part of the fetus reaches the perineal floor, mechanical stretching of the cervix occurs. Stretch receptors in the posterior vagina cause release of endogenous oxytocin that triggers the maternal urge to bear down, or the *Ferguson reflex.*

Uterine contractions are usually independent of external forces. For example, laboring women who are paralyzed because of spinal cord lesions above the twelfth thoracic vertebra will have normal but painless uterine contractions (Cunningham et al., 2010). However, uterine contractions may decrease temporarily in frequency and intensity if narcotic analgesic medication is given early in labor. Studies of effects of epidural analgesia have demonstrated prolonged length of labor for nulliparas both in the active phase of first-stage labor and in the second stage (Salim, Nachum, Moscovici, Lavee, & Shalev, 2005; Schiessl, Janni, Jundt, Rammel, Peschers, & Kainer, 2005).

Secondary Powers

As soon as the presenting part reaches the pelvic floor, the contractions change in character and become expulsive. The laboring woman experiences an involuntary urge to push. She uses secondary powers (bearing-down efforts) to aid in expulsion of the fetus as she contracts her diaphragm and abdominal muscles and pushes. These bearing-down efforts result in increased intraabdominal pressure that compresses the uterus on all sides and adds to the power of the expulsive forces.

The secondary powers have no effect on cervical dilation, but they are of considerable importance in the expulsion of the infant from the uterus and vagina after the cervix is fully dilated. Studies have shown that pushing in the second stage is more effective and the woman is less fatigued when she begins to push only after she has the urge to do so rather than beginning to push when she is fully dilated without an urge to do so

(Jacobson & Turner, 2008; Simpson & James, 2005; Yildirim & Beji, 2008).

When and how a woman pushes in the second stage is a much-debated topic. Studies have investigated the effects of spontaneous bearing-down efforts, directed pushing, delayed pushing, *Valsalva maneuver* (closed glottis and prolonged bearing down), and open-glottis pushing both with and without epidural analgesia (Brancato, Church, & Stone, 2008; Gupta, Hofmeyr, & Smyth, 2004; Simpson & James, 2005). The benefits of delayed pushing include an increased chance of spontaneous vaginal birth and decreased pushing time. Adverse effects associated with prolonged breath holding and forceful pushing efforts include increased fetal hypoxia and subsequent acidosis (Simpson & James). Pelvic floor problems also have been associated with directed pushing (Schaffer, Bloom, Casey, McIntire, Nihira, & Leveno, 2005). Continued study is needed to determine the effectiveness and appropriateness of strategies used by nurses to teach pushing techniques, the suitability and effectiveness of various pushing techniques related to abnormal (nonreassuring) fetal heart patterns, and the standards for length of duration of pushing in terms of maternal and fetal outcomes (Gennaro, Mayberry, & Kafulafula, 2007). (See Chapter 19 for further discussion.)

Position of the Laboring Woman

Position affects the woman's anatomic and physiologic adaptations to labor. Frequent changes in position relieve fatigue, increase comfort, and improve circulation. Therefore, a laboring woman should be encouraged to find positions that are most comfortable for her (Fig. 16-12, *A*).

An upright position (walking, sitting, kneeling, or squatting) offers a number of advantages. Gravity can promote the descent of the fetus. Uterine contractions are generally stronger and more efficient in effacing and dilating the cervix, resulting in a shorter labor (Gupta et al., 2004; Lawrence, Lewis, Hofmeyr, Dowswell, & Styles, 2009; Zwelling, 2010).

An upright position also is beneficial to the mother's cardiac output, which normally increases during labor as uterine contractions return blood to the vascular bed. The increased cardiac output improves blood flow to the uteroplacental unit and the maternal kidneys. Cardiac output is compromised if the descending aorta and ascending vena cava are compressed during labor (see Fig. 19-5). Compression of these major vessels may result in supine hypotension that decreases placental perfusion. With the woman in an upright position, pressure on the maternal vessels is reduced, and compression is prevented. If the woman wishes to lie down, a lateral position is suggested (Blackburn, 2007; Zwelling, 2010).

The "all fours" position (hands and knees) may be used to relieve backache if the fetus is in an occipitoposterior position and may assist in anterior rotation of the fetus and in cases of shoulder dystocia (Hunter, Hofmeyr & Kulier, 2007; Zwelling, 2010).

Positioning for second-stage labor (see Fig. 16-12, *B*) may be determined by the woman's preference, but it is constrained by the condition of the woman and fetus, the environment, and the health care provider's confidence in assisting with a birth in a specific position. The predominant position in the United States in physician-attended births is the lithotomy position. Alternative positions and position changes that result in more births over an intact perineum are more commonly practiced by nurse-midwives.

A woman who pushes in a semirecumbent position needs adequate body support to push effectively because her weight will be on her sacrum, moving the coccyx forward and causing a reduction in the pelvic outlet. In a sitting or squatting position, abdominal muscles work in greater synchrony with uterine contractions during bearing-down efforts. Kneeling or squatting moves the uterus forward and aligns the fetus with the pelvic inlet and can facilitate the second stage of labor by increasing the pelvic outlet (Simpson, Cesario, Morin, Trapani, Mayberry, & Snelgrove-Clark, 2008; Zwelling, 2010).

The lateral position can be used by the woman to help rotate a fetus that is in a posterior position. It also can be used when there is a need for less force to be used during bearing down, such as when there is a need to control the speed of a precipitate birth (Simpson et al., 2008; Zwelling, 2010).

No evidence exists that any of these positions suggested for second-stage labor increases the need for use of operative techniques (e.g., forceps or vacuum-assisted birth, cesarean birth, episiotomy) or causes perineal trauma. No evidence has been found that use of any of these positions adversely affects the newborn (Lawrence et al., 2009; Roberts, Algert, Cameron, & Torvaldsen, 2005).

PROCESS OF LABOR

The term *labor* refers to the process of moving the fetus, placenta, and membranes out of the uterus and through the birth canal. Various changes take place in the woman's reproductive system in the days and weeks before labor begins. Labor itself can be discussed in terms of the mechanisms involved in the process and the stages the woman moves through.

Signs Preceding Labor

In first-time pregnancies the uterus sinks downward and forward about 2 weeks before term, when the fetus's presenting part (usually the fetal head) descends into the true pelvis. This settling is called **lightening,** or "dropping," and usually happens gradually. After lightening, women feel less congested and breathe more easily, but usually more bladder pressure results from this shift, and consequently a return of urinary frequency occurs. In a pregnancy in a multiparous woman, lightening may not take place until after uterine contractions are established and true labor is in progress.

The woman may complain of persistent low backache and sacroiliac distress as a result of relaxation of the pelvic joints. She may identify strong and frequent but irregular uterine (Braxton Hicks) contractions.

The vaginal mucus becomes more profuse in response to the extreme congestion of the vaginal mucous membranes. The thick mucus that has obstructed the cervical canal since conception is passed (commonly referred to as the mucous plug). Brownish or blood-tinged cervical mucus may be passed *(bloody show)*. The cervix becomes soft (ripens) and partially effaced and may begin to dilate. The membranes may rupture spontaneously.

Other phenomena are common in the days preceding labor: (1) loss of 0.5 to 1.5 kg in weight, caused by water loss resulting

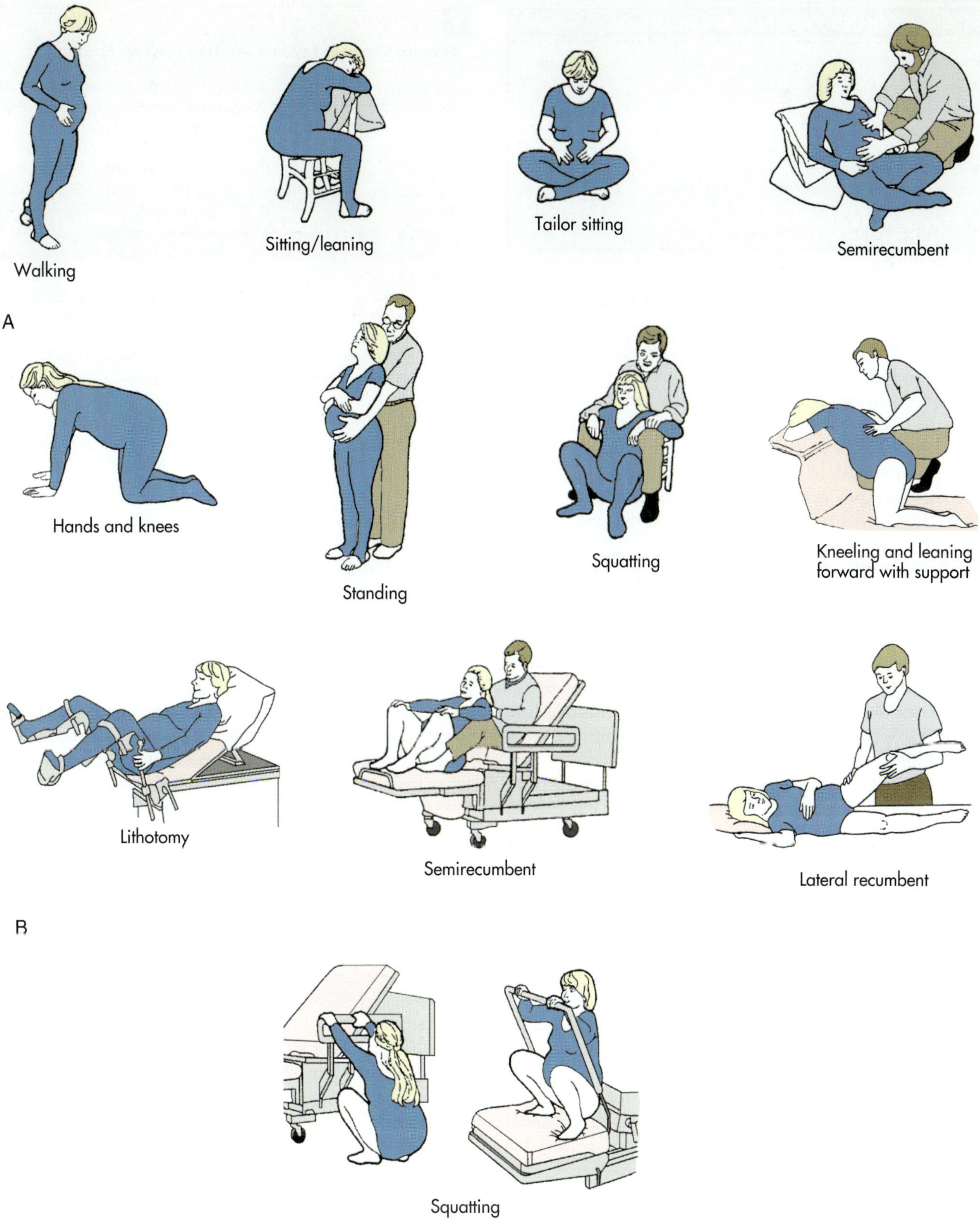

FIG. 16-12 Positions for labor and birth. **A,** Positions for labor. **B,** Positions for birth.

from electrolyte shifts that in turn are produced by changes in estrogen and progesterone levels; and (2) a surge of energy. Women speak of having a burst of energy that they often use to clean the house and put everything in order. Less commonly, some women have diarrhea, nausea, vomiting, and indigestion. Box 16-1 lists signs that may precede labor.

Onset of Labor

The onset of true labor cannot be ascribed to a single cause. Many factors, including changes in the maternal uterus, cervix, and pituitary gland, are involved. Hormones produced by the normal fetal hypothalamus, pituitary, and adrenal cortex probably contribute to the onset of labor. Progressive uterine distention,

BOX 16-1 SIGNS PRECEDING LABOR

- Lightening
- Return of urinary frequency
- Backache
- Stronger Braxton Hicks contractions
- Weight loss of 0.5 to 1.5 kg
- Surge of energy
- Increased vaginal discharge; bloody show
- Cervical ripening
- Possible rupture of membranes

increasing intrauterine pressure, and aging of the placenta seem to be associated with increasing myometrial irritability. This is a result of increased concentrations of estrogen and prostaglandins, as well as decreasing progesterone levels. The mutually coordinated effects of these factors result in the occurrence of strong, regular, rhythmic uterine contractions (Kilpatrick & Garrison, 2007). The outcome of these factors working together is normally the birth of the fetus and the expulsion of the placenta; however, how certain alterations trigger others and how proper checks and balances are maintained is not known.

Stages of Labor

The course of labor at or near term gestation in a woman without complications and a fetus in vertex presentation consists of: (1) regular progression of uterine contractions, (2) effacement and progressive dilation of the cervix, and (3) progress in descent of the presenting part. Four stages of labor are recognized. An overview of these stages is discussed here. These stages are discussed in greater detail, along with nursing care for the laboring woman and family, in Chapter 19.

The *first stage* of labor is considered to last from the onset of regular uterine contractions to full effacement and dilation of the cervix. Commonly the onset of labor is difficult to establish because the woman may be admitted to the labor unit just before birth, and the beginning of labor may be only an estimate. The first stage is much longer than the second and third stages combined. Great variability is the rule, however, depending on the factors discussed previously in this chapter. Parity has a strong effect on the duration of first-stage labor (Gross, Drobnic, & Keirse, 2005). Full dilation may occur in less than 1 hour in some multiparous pregnancies. In first-time pregnancy, complete dilation of the cervix can take 20 hours or more. Variations may reflect differences in the client population (e.g., risk status, age) or in clinical management of the labor and birth.

The first stage of labor is divided into three phases: a latent phase, an active phase, and a transition phase. During the latent phase there is more progress in effacement of the cervix and little increase in descent. During the active phase and the transition phase, there is more rapid dilation of the cervix and increased rate of descent of the presenting part. Maternal prepregnancy overweight and obesity can cause the active phase of labor to be longer than for women of normal weight; specifically arrest of dilation can occur (Liao, Buhimschi, & Norwitz, 2005; Verdiales, Pacheco, & Cohen, 2009).

The *second stage of labor* lasts from the time the cervix is fully effaced and dilated to the birth of the fetus. The second stage takes an average of 20 minutes for a multiparous woman and 50

CLINICAL REASONING

Second Stage Labor in a Woman with an Epidural

During your clinical experience in the labor and birth unit, you are assigned to Heather, a 28-year-old having her first baby. She has epidural analgesia. Her cervix is 10 cm dilated and 100% effaced, the fetus is in a vertex presentation, and the presenting part is at station 0. Although she really does not feel her contractions, she has been pushing for about 45 minutes with no noticeable fetal descent. She has been in a semirecumbent position. What nursing interventions would be appropriate?

1. Evidence—Is there sufficient evidence to draw conclusions about what interventions are needed?
2. Assumptions—Describe underlying assumptions about the following issues:
   a. Positions for second-stage labor
   b. Immediate versus delayed pushing (laboring down)
   c. Effects of epidural analgesia during second stage labor
3. What implications and priorities for nursing care can be made at this time?
4. Does the evidence objectively support your conclusion?
5. Are there alternative perspectives to your conclusion?

minutes for a nulliparous woman. Labor of up to 2 hours (up to 3 hours with use of regional anesthesia) has been considered within the normal range for the second stage, but Cesario (2004) found a wider range of normal was associated with no adverse effects on the mother or infant. Ethnicity may play a role in length of second-stage labor. Greenberg and associates (2006) found that nulliparous Asian women had a longer second stage than nulliparous Caucasian women, whereas African-American and Hispanic women had shorter second stages of labor than Caucasian women.

The second stage of labor is composed of two phases: the latent phase and the active pushing (descent) phase. During the latent phase the fetus continues to descend passively through the birth canal and rotate to an anterior position as a result of ongoing uterine contractions. The urge to bear down during this phase is not strong and some women do not experience it at all. During the active pushing phase the woman has strong urges to bear down as the presenting part of the fetus descends and presses on the stretch receptors of the pelvic floor.

The *third stage of labor* lasts from the birth of the fetus until the placenta is delivered. The placenta normally separates with the third or fourth strong uterine contraction after the infant has been born. After it has separated the placenta can be delivered with the next uterine contraction. The placenta is usually expelled within 10 to 15 minutes after birth of the baby. The third stage of labor is normally completed within 30 minutes. The risk of hemorrhage increases as the length of the third stage increases (Battista & Wing, 2007).

The *fourth stage of labor* arbitrarily lasts 1 to 2 hours after delivery of the placenta. It is the period of immediate recovery, when homeostasis is reestablished. It is an important period of observation for complications, such as abnormal bleeding (see Chapter 19).

Mechanism of Labor

As discussed, the female pelvis has varied contours and diameters at different levels, and the presenting part of the passenger is large in proportion to the passage. Therefore, for vaginal birth to

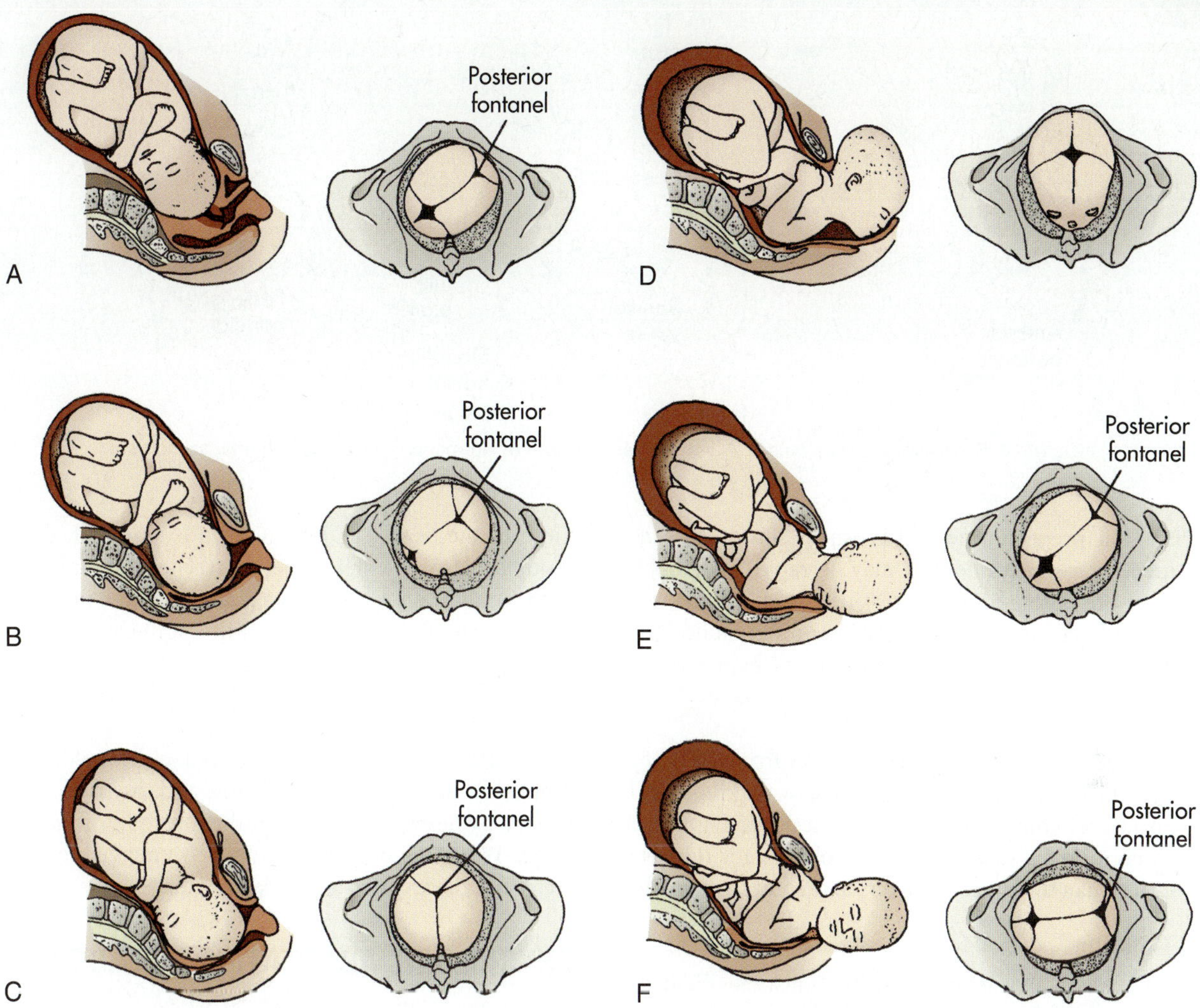

FIG. 16-13 Cardinal movements of the mechanism of labor. Left occipitoanterior (LOA) position. Pelvic figures show the position of the fetal head as seen by the birth attendant. **A,** Engagement and descent. **B,** Flexion. **C,** Internal rotation to occipitoanterior position (OA). **D,** Extension. **E,** External rotation beginning (restitution). **F,** External rotation.

occur, the fetus must adapt to the birth canal during the descent. The turns and other adjustments necessary in the human birth process are termed the **mechanism of labor** (Fig. 16-13). The seven cardinal movements of the mechanism of labor that occur in a vertex presentation are engagement, descent, flexion, internal rotation, extension, external rotation (restitution), and finally birth by expulsion. Although these movements are discussed separately, in actuality a combination of movements occurs simultaneously. For example, engagement involves both descent and flexion.

Engagement

When the biparietal diameter of the head passes the pelvic inlet, the head is said to be engaged in the pelvic inlet (see Fig. 16-13, *A*). In most nulliparous pregnancies, this occurs before the onset of active labor because the firmer abdominal muscles direct the presenting part into the pelvis. In multiparous pregnancies, in which the abdominal musculature is more relaxed, the head often remains freely movable above the pelvic brim until labor is established.

Asynclitism. The head usually engages in the pelvis in a synclitic position—one that is parallel to the anteroposterior plane of the pelvis. Frequently **asynclitism** occurs (the head is deflected anteriorly or posteriorly in the pelvis), which can facilitate descent because the head is being positioned to accommodate to the pelvic cavity (Fig. 16-14). Extreme asynclitism can cause cephalopelvic disproportion, even in a normal-size pelvis, because the head is positioned so that it cannot descend.

Descent

Descent refers to the progress of the presenting part through the pelvis. Descent depends on at least four forces: (1) pressure exerted by the amniotic fluid, (2) direct pressure exerted by the contracting fundus on the fetus, (3) force of the contraction of the maternal diaphragm and abdominal muscles in the second stage of labor, and (4) extension and straightening of the fetal body. The effects of these forces are modified by the size and shape of the maternal pelvic planes and the size of the fetal head and its capacity to mold.

The degree of descent is measured by the station of the presenting part (see Fig. 16-6). As mentioned, little descent occurs during the latent phase of the first stage of labor. Descent accelerates in the active phase when the cervix has dilated to 4 to 7 cm. It is especially apparent when the membranes have ruptured.

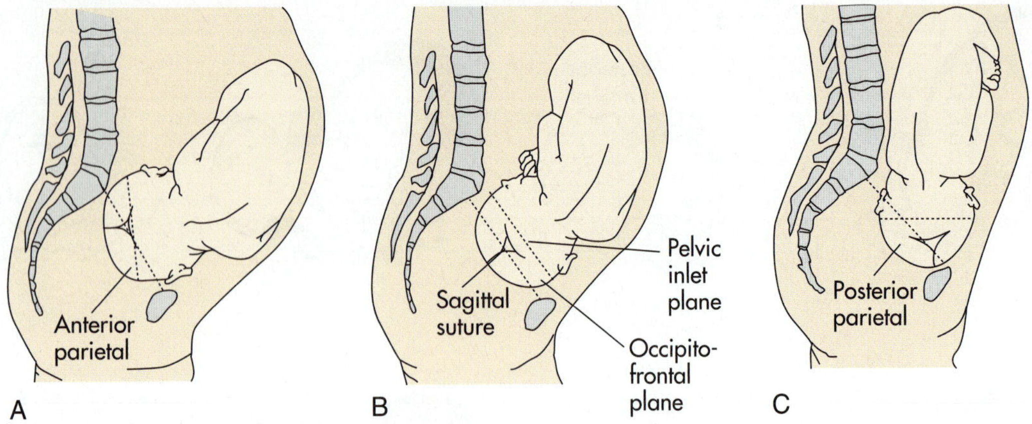

FIG. 16-14 Synclitism and asynclitism. **A,** Anterior asynclitism. **B,** Normal synclitism. **C,** Posterior asynclitism.

In a first-time pregnancy descent is usually slow but steady; in subsequent pregnancies descent may be rapid. Progress in descent of the presenting part is determined by abdominal palpation (Leopold maneuvers) and vaginal examination until the presenting part can be seen at the introitus (see Chapter 19).

Flexion

As soon as the descending head meets resistance from the cervix, pelvic wall, or pelvic floor, it normally flexes, so that the chin is brought into closer contact with the fetal chest (see Fig. 16-13, *B*). Flexion permits the smaller suboccipitobregmatic diameter (9.5 cm) rather than the larger diameters to present to the outlet.

Internal Rotation

The maternal pelvic inlet is widest in the transverse diameter; therefore the fetal head passes the inlet into the true pelvis in the occipitotransverse position. The outlet is widest in the anteroposterior diameter; for the fetus to exit, the head must rotate. Internal rotation begins at the level of the ischial spines but is not completed until the presenting part reaches the lower pelvis. As the occiput rotates anteriorly, the face rotates posteriorly. With each contraction the fetal head is guided by the bony pelvis and the muscles of the pelvic floor. Eventually the occiput will be in the midline beneath the pubic arch. The head is almost always rotated by the time it reaches the pelvic floor (see Fig. 16-13, *C*). Both the levator ani muscles and the bony pelvis are important for achieving anterior rotation. A previous childbirth injury or regional anesthesia may compromise the function of the levator sling.

Extension

When the fetal head reaches the perineum for birth, it is deflected anteriorly by the perineum. The occiput passes under the lower border of the symphysis pubis first, and then the head emerges by extension: first the occiput, then the face, and finally the chin (see Fig. 16-13, *D*).

Restitution and External Rotation

After the head is born it rotates briefly to the position it occupied when it was engaged in the inlet. This movement is referred to as *restitution* (see Fig. 16-13, *E*). The 45-degree turn realigns the infant's head with her or his back and shoulders. The head can then be seen to rotate further. This external rotation occurs as the shoulders engage and descend in maneuvers similar to those of the head (see Fig. 16-13, *F*). As noted, the anterior shoulder descends first. When it reaches the outlet, it rotates to the midline and is delivered from under the pubic arch. The posterior shoulder is guided over the perineum until it is free of the vaginal introitus.

Expulsion

After birth of the shoulders, the head and shoulders are lifted up toward the mother's pubic bone and the trunk of the baby is born by flexing it laterally in the direction of the symphysis pubis. When the baby has completely emerged, birth is complete, and the second stage of labor ends.

PHYSIOLOGIC ADAPTATION TO LABOR

In addition to the maternal and fetal anatomic adaptations that occur during birth, physiologic adaptations must occur. Accurate assessment of the laboring woman and fetus requires knowledge of these expected adaptations.

Fetal Adaptation

Several important physiologic adaptations occur in the fetus. These changes occur in fetal heart rate, fetal circulation, respiratory movements, and other behaviors.

Fetal Heart Rate

Fetal heart rate (FHR) monitoring provides reliable and predictive information about the condition of the fetus related to oxygenation. The average FHR at term is 140 beats/min. The normal range is 110 to 160 beats/min. Earlier in gestation the FHR is higher, with an average of approximately 160 beats/min at 20 weeks of gestation. The rate decreases progressively as the maturing fetus reaches term. However, temporary accelerations and slight early decelerations of the FHR can be expected in response to spontaneous fetal movement, vaginal examination, fundal pressure, uterine contractions, abdominal palpation, and fetal head compression. Stresses to the uterofetoplacental unit result in characteristic FHR patterns (see Chapter 18 for further discussion).

Fetal Circulation

Fetal circulation can be affected by many factors, including maternal position, uterine contractions, blood pressure, and umbilical cord blood flow. Uterine contractions during labor tend to decrease circulation through the spiral arterioles and subsequent perfusion through the intervillous space. Most healthy fetuses are well able to compensate for this stress and exposure to increased pressure while moving passively through the birth canal during labor. Usually umbilical cord blood flow is undisturbed by uterine contractions or fetal position (Tucker, Miller, & Miller, 2009).

Fetal Respiration

Certain changes stimulate chemoreceptors in the aorta and carotid bodies to prepare the fetus for initiating respirations immediately after birth (Blackburn, 2007; Rosenberg, 2007). These changes occur during labor and include the following:

- Fetal lung fluid is cleared from the air passages during labor and (vaginal) birth.
- Fetal oxygen pressure (Po_2) decreases.
- Fetal arterial carbon dioxide pressure (Pco_2) increases.
- Fetal arterial pH decreases.
- Fetal bicarbonate level decreases.
- Fetal respiratory movements decrease during labor.

Maternal Adaptation

As the woman progresses through the stages of labor, various body system adaptations cause her to exhibit both objective signs and subjective symptoms (Box 16-2).

BOX 16-2 MATERNAL PHYSIOLOGIC CHANGES DURING LABOR

- Cardiac output increases 10% to 15% in first stage; 30% to 50% in second stage.
- Heart rate increases slightly in first and second stages.
- Systolic blood pressure increases during uterine contractions in first stage; systolic and diastolic pressures increase during uterine contractions in second stage.
- White blood cell (WBC) count increases.
- Respiratory rate increases.
- Temperature may be slightly elevated.
- Proteinuria may occur.
- Gastric motility and absorption of solid food is decreased; nausea and vomiting may occur during transition to second-stage labor.
- Blood glucose level decreases.

Cardiovascular Changes

During each contraction an average of 400 mL of blood is emptied from the uterus into the maternal vascular system. This increases cardiac output by about 12% to 31% in the first stage and by about 50% in the second stage of labor. The heart rate increases slightly (Gordon, 2007).

Changes in blood pressure also occur. Blood flow, which is reduced in the uterine artery by contractions, is redirected to peripheral vessels. As a result, peripheral resistance increases, and blood pressure increases (Gordon, 2007). During the first stage of labor, uterine contractions cause systolic readings to increase by about 10 mm Hg; assessing blood pressure between contractions therefore provides more accurate readings. During the second stage contractions may cause systolic pressures to increase by 30 mm Hg and diastolic readings to increase by 25 mm Hg, with both systolic and diastolic pressures remaining somewhat elevated even between contractions (Gordon). Therefore, the woman already at risk for hypertension is at increased risk for complications such as cerebral hemorrhage.

Supine hypotension (see Fig. 19-5, p. 444) occurs when the ascending vena cava and descending aorta are compressed. The laboring woman is at greater risk for supine hypotension if the uterus is particularly large because of multifetal pregnancy, hydramnios, or obesity or if the woman is dehydrated or hypovolemic. In addition, anxiety and pain, as well as some medications, can cause hypotension.

The woman should be discouraged from using the Valsalva maneuver (holding one's breath and tightening abdominal muscles) for pushing during the second stage. This activity increases intrathoracic pressure, reduces venous return, and increases venous pressure. The cardiac output and blood pressure increase and the pulse slows temporarily. During the Valsalva maneuver fetal hypoxia may occur. The process is reversed when the woman takes a breath.

The white blood cell (WBC) count can increase (Blackburn, 2007). Although the mechanism leading to this increase in WBCs is unknown, it may be secondary to physical or emotional stress or to tissue trauma. Labor is strenuous, and physical exercise alone can increase the WBC count.

Some peripheral vascular changes occur, perhaps in response to cervical dilation or to compression of maternal vessels by the fetus passing through the birth canal. Flushed cheeks, hot or cold feet, and eversion of hemorrhoids may result.

Respiratory Changes

Increased physical activity with greater oxygen consumption is reflected in an increase in the respiratory rate. Hyperventilation may cause respiratory alkalosis (an increase in pH), hypoxia, and hypocapnia (decrease in carbon dioxide). In the unmedicated woman in the second stage of labor, oxygen consumption almost doubles. Anxiety also increases oxygen consumption.

Renal Changes

During labor, spontaneous voiding may be difficult for various reasons: tissue edema caused by pressure from the presenting part, discomfort, analgesia, and embarrassment. Proteinuria of 1+ is a normal finding because it can occur in response to the breakdown of muscle tissue from the physical work of labor.

Integumentary Changes

The integumentary system changes are evident, especially in the great distensibility (stretching) in the area of the vaginal introitus. The degree of distensibility varies with the individual. Despite this ability to stretch, even in the absence of episiotomy or lacerations, minute tears in the skin around the vaginal introitus do occur.

Musculoskeletal Changes

The musculoskeletal system is stressed during labor. Diaphoresis, fatigue, proteinuria (1+), and possibly an increased temperature accompany the marked increase in muscle activity. Backache and joint aches (unrelated to fetal position) occur as a result of increased joint laxity at term. The labor process itself and the woman's pointing her toes can cause leg cramps.

Neurologic Changes

Sensorial changes occur as the woman moves through the phases of the first stage of labor and as she moves from one stage to the next. Initially she may be euphoric. Euphoria gives way to increased seriousness, then to amnesia between contractions during the second stage, and finally to elation or fatigue after giving birth. Endogenous endorphins (morphine-like chemicals produced naturally by the body) raise the pain threshold and produce sedation. In addition, physiologic anesthesia of perineal tissues, caused by pressure of the presenting part, decreases perception of pain.

Gastrointestinal Changes

During labor, gastrointestinal motility and absorption of solid foods are decreased, and stomach-emptying time is slowed. Nausea and vomiting of undigested food eaten after onset of labor are common. Nausea and belching also occur as a reflex response to full cervical dilation. The woman may state that diarrhea accompanied the onset of labor, or the nurse may palpate the presence of hard or impacted stool in the rectum.

Endocrine Changes

The onset of labor may be triggered by decreasing levels of progesterone and increasing levels of estrogen, prostaglandins, and oxytocin (Norwitz & Lye, 2009). Metabolism increases, and blood glucose levels may decrease with the work of labor.

Accurate assessment of the mother and fetus during labor and birth depends on knowledge of these expected adaptations so that appropriate interventions can be implemented.

KEY POINTS

- Labor and birth are affected by the five P's: *p*assenger, *p*assageway, *p*owers, *p*osition of the woman, and *p*sychologic responses.
- Because of its size and relative rigidity, the fetal head is a major factor in determining the course of birth.
- The diameters at the plane of the pelvic inlet, the midpelvis, and the outlet, plus the axis of the birth canal, determine whether vaginal birth is possible and the manner in which the fetus passes down the birth canal.
- Involuntary uterine contractions act to expel the fetus and placenta during the first stage of labor; these are augmented by voluntary bearing-down efforts of the woman during the second stage.
- The first stage of labor lasts from the time dilation begins to the time when the cervix is fully effaced and dilated.
- The second stage of labor lasts from the time of full cervical effacement and dilation to the birth of the infant.
- The third stage of labor lasts from the infant's birth to the expulsion of the placenta.
- The fourth stage is the first 1 to 2 hours after birth.
- The cardinal movements of the mechanism of labor are engagement, descent, flexion, internal rotation, extension, restitution and external rotation, and expulsion of the infant.
- Although the events precipitating the onset of labor are unknown, many factors, including changes in the maternal uterus, cervix, and pituitary gland, are thought to be involved.
- A healthy fetus with an adequate uterofetoplacental circulation will be able to compensate for the stress of uterine contractions.
- As the woman progresses through labor, various body systems adapt to the birth process.

Audio Chapter Summaries Access an audio summary of these Key Points on evolve

REFERENCES

Battista, L., & Wing, D. (2007). Abnormal labor and induction of labor. In S. Gabbe, J. Niebyl, & J. Simpson (Eds.), *Obstetrics: Normal and problem pregnancies* (5th ed.). New York: Churchill Livingstone.

Blackburn, S. (2007). *Maternal, fetal, and neonatal physiology: A clinical perspective* (3rd ed.). St. Louis: Saunders.

Brancato, R., Church, S., & Stone, P. (2008). A meta-analysis of passive descent versus immediate pushing in nulliparous women with epidural analgesia in the second stage of labor. *Journal of Obstetric, Gynecologic and Neonatal Nursing, 37*(1), 4–12.

Cesario, S. (2004). Reevaluation of Friedman's labor curve: A pilot study. *Journal of Obstetric, Gynecologic and Neonatal Nursing, 33*(6), 713–722.

Cunningham, F., Leveno, K., Bloom, S., Hauth, J., Rouse, D., & Spong, C. (2010). *Williams obstetrics* (23rd ed.). New York: McGraw-Hill.

Gennaro, S., Mayberry, L., & Kafulafula, U. (2007). The evidence supporting nursing management of labor. *Journal of Obstetric, Gynecologic and Neonatal Nursing, 36*(6), 598–604.

Gordon, M. (2007). Maternal physiology. In S. Gabbe, J. Niebyl, & J. Simpson (Eds.), *Obstetrics: Normal and problem pregnancies* (5th ed.). New York: Churchill Livingstone.

Greenberg, M., Cheng, Y., Hopkins, L., Stotland, N., Bryant, A., & Caughey, A. (2006). Are there ethnic differences in the length of labor? *American Journal of Obstetrics and Gynecology, 195*(3), 743–748.

Gross, M., Drobnic, S., & Keirse, M. (2005). Influence of fixed and time-dependent factors on duration of normal first stage labor. *Birth, 32*(1), 27–33.

Gupta, J., Hofmeyr, G., & Smyth, R. (2004). Position in the second stage of labor of women with epidural analgesia. *The Cochrane Database of Systematic Reviews, 2004*, 1, CD002006.

Hunter, S., Hofmeyr, G., & Kulier, R. (2007). Hands and knees posture in late pregnancy or labour for fetal malposition (lateral or posterior). *The Cochrane Database of Systematic Reviews, 2007*, 4, CD001063.

Jacobson., P., & Turner, L. (2008). Management of the second stage of labor in women with epidural analgesia. *Journal of Midwifery & Women's Health, 53*(10), 82–85.

Kilpatrick, S., & Garrison, E. (2007). Normal labor and delivery. In S. Gabbe, J. Niebyl, & J. Simpson (Eds.), *Obstetrics: Normal and problem pregnancies* (5th ed.). Philadelphia: Churchill Livingstone.

Lawrence, A., Lewis, L., Hofmeyr, G., Dowswell., T., & Styles, C. (2009). Maternal positions and mobility during first stage labour. *The Cochrane Database of Systematic Reviews, 2009*, 2, CD003934.

Liao, J., Buhimschi, D., & Norwitz, E. (2005). Normal labor: Mechanism and duration. *Obstetric and Gynecologic Clinics of North America, 32*(2), 145–164.

Norwitz, E., & Lye, S. (2009). Biology of parturition. In R. Creasy, R. Resnik, J. Iams, C. Lockwood, & T. Moore (Eds.), *Creasy & Resnik's maternal-fetal medicine: Principles and practice* (6th ed.). Philadelphia: Saunders.

Roberts, C., Algert, C., Cameron, C., & Torvaldsen, S. (2005). A meta-analysis of upright positions in the second stage to reduce instrumental deliveries in women with epidural analgesia. *Acta Obstetricia et Gynecologica Scandinavica, 84*(8), 794–798.

Rosenberg, A. (2007). The neonate. In S. Gabbe, J. Niebyl, & J. Simpson (Eds.). *Obstetrics: Normal and problem pregnancies* (5th ed.). Philadelphia: Churchill Livingstone.

Salim, R., Nachum, Z., Moscovici, R., Lavee, M., & Shalev, E. (2005). Continuous compared with intermittent epidural infusion on progress of labor and patient satisfaction. *Obstetrics and Gynecology, 106*(2), 301–306.

Schaffer, J., Bloom, S., Casey, B., McIntire, D., Nihira, M., & Leveno, K. (2005). A randomized trial of the effects of coached vs. uncoached maternal pushing during the second stage of labor on postpartum pelvic floor structure and function. *American Journal of Obstetrics and Gynecology, 192*(5), 1692–1696.

Schiessl, B., Janni, W., Jundt, K., Rammel, G., Peschers, U., & Kainer, F. (2005). Obstetrical parameters influencing the duration of second stage labor. *European Journal of Obstetric and Gynecologic Reproductive Biology, 118*(1), 17–20.

Simpson, K., Cesario, S., Morin, K., Trapani, K., Mayberry, L., & Snelgrove-Clark, E. (2008). *Nursing management of the second stage of labor: Evidence-based clinical practice guidelines*. Washington, DC: Association of Women's Health, Obstetric and Neonatal Nurses.

Simpson, K., & James, D. (2005). Effects of immediate versus delayed pushing during second-stage labor on fetal well-being: A randomized clinical trial. *Nursing Research, 54*(3), 149–157.

Thorp, J. (2009). Clinical aspects of normal and abnormal labor. In R. Creasy, R. Resnik, J. Iams, C. Lockwood, & T. Moore (Eds.), *Creasy & Resnik's maternal-fetal medicine: Principles and practice* (6th ed.). Philadelphia: Saunders.

Tucker, S., Miller, L., & Miller, D. (2009). *Mosby's pocket guide to fetal monitoring: A multidisciplinary approach* (6th ed.). St. Louis: Mosby.

VandeVusse, L. (1999). The essential forces of labor revisited: 13 Ps reported in women's birth stories. *MCN The American Journal of Maternal/Child Nursing, 24*(4), 176–184.

Verdiales, M., Pacheco, C., & Cohen, W. (2009). The effect of maternal obesity on the course of labor. *Journal of Perinatal Medicine, 37*(6), 651–655.

Yildirim, G., & Beji, N. (2008). Effects of pushing techniques in birth on mother and fetus: A randomized study. *Birth, 35*(10), 25–30.

Zwelling, E. (2010). Overcoming the challenges: Maternal movement and positioning to facilitate labor progress. *MCN The American Journal of Maternal/Child Nursing, 35*(2), 72–78.

CHAPTER

17

Pain Management

Karen A. Piotrowski

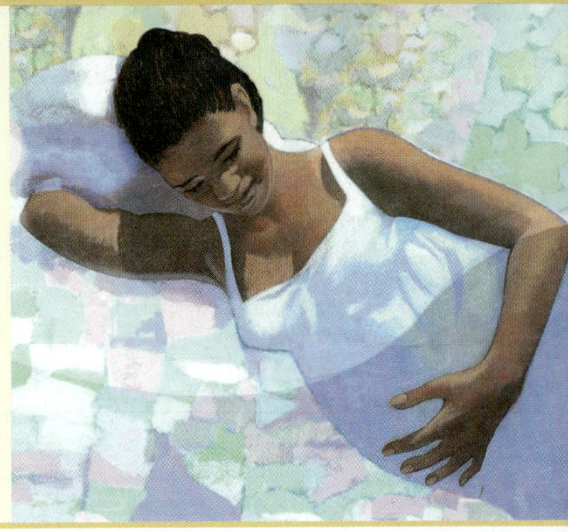

evolve WEBSITE

http://evolve.elsevier.com/Lowdermilk/MWHC

Audio Glossary
Audio Key Points
Critical Thinking Exercise
  Client Receiving Epidural Block
NCLEX Review Questions
Nursing Care Plan
  Epidural Block During Labor
  Nonpharmacologic Pain Management
Spanish Guidelines
  Pain Management
Video—Nursing Skills
  Assisting with an Epidural

LEARNING OBJECTIVES

- Describe breathing and relaxation techniques used for each stage of labor.
- Analyze nonpharmacologic strategies used to enhance relaxation and decrease discomfort during labor.
- Compare pharmacologic methods used to relieve discomfort in different stages of labor and for vaginal or cesarean birth.
- Discuss the use of naloxone (Narcan).
- Create an evidence-based plan to manage the discomfort a woman experiences during childbirth.
- Apply the nursing process to pain management for a woman in labor.
- Summarize the nursing responsibilities appropriate in providing care for a woman receiving analgesia or anesthesia during labor.

Pain is an unpleasant, complex, highly individualized phenomenon with sensory and emotional components. Pregnant women commonly worry about the pain they will experience during labor and birth and about how they will react to and deal with that pain. A variety of nonpharmacologic and pharmacologic methods can help the woman or the couple cope with the discomfort of labor. The methods selected depend on the situation, availability, and the preferences of the woman and her health care provider.

PAIN DURING LABOR AND BIRTH

Neurologic Origins

The pain and discomfort of labor have two origins, visceral and somatic. During the first stage of labor, uterine contractions cause cervical dilation and effacement. Uterine ischemia (decreased blood flow and therefore local oxygen deficit) results from compression of the arteries supplying the myometrium during uterine contractions. Pain impulses during the first stage of labor are transmitted via the T1 to T12 spinal nerve segment and accessory lower thoracic and upper lumbar sympathetic nerves. These nerves originate in the uterine body and cervix (Blackburn, 2007).

The pain from distention of the lower uterine segment, stretching of cervical tissue as it effaces and dilates, pressure and traction on adjacent structures (e.g., uterine tubes, ovaries, ligaments) and nerves, and uterine ischemia during the first stage of labor is visceral pain. It is located over the lower portion of the abdomen. Referred pain occurs when pain that originates in the uterus radiates to the abdominal wall, lumbosacral area of the back, iliac crests, gluteal area, thighs, and lower back (Blackburn, 2007; Zwelling, Johnson, & Allen, 2006).

During most of the first stage of labor the woman usually has discomfort only during contractions and is free of pain between contractions. Some women, especially those whose fetus is in a posterior position, experience continuous contraction-related low back pain, even in the interval between contractions. As labor progresses and pain becomes more intense and persistent, women become fatigued and discouraged, often experiencing difficulty coping with contractions (Blackburn, 2007; Creehan, 2008; Zwelling et al., 2006).

During the second stage of labor the woman has somatic pain, which is often described as intense, sharp, burning, and well localized. This pain results from stretching and distention of perineal tissues and the pelvic floor to allow passage of the fetus, from distention and traction on the peritoneum and uterocervical supports during contractions, from pressure against the bladder and rectum, and from lacerations of soft tissue (e.g., cervix, vagina, and perineum). As women concentrate on the work of bearing down to give birth to their baby, they may report a decrease in pain intensity (Creehan, 2008). Pain impulses during the second stage of labor are transmitted via the pudendal nerve through S2 to S4 spinal nerve segments and the parasympathetic system (Blackburn, 2007).

Pain experienced during the third stage of labor and the afterpains of the early postpartum period are uterine, similar to the pain experienced early in the first stage of labor. Areas of discomfort during labor are shown in Figure 17-1.

Perception of Pain

Although the pain threshold is remarkably similar in everyone regardless of gender, social, ethnic, or cultural differences, these differences play a definite role in the person's perception of and behavioral responses to pain. The effects of factors such as culture, counterstimuli, and distraction in coping with pain are not fully understood. The meaning of pain and the verbal and nonverbal expressions given to pain are apparently learned from interactions within the primary social group. Cultural influences may impose certain behavioral expectations regarding acceptable and unacceptable behavior when experiencing pain.

Pain tolerance refers to the level of pain a laboring woman is willing to endure. When this level is exceeded, she will seek measures to relieve the pain. Factors that influence her pain tolerance level and her request for pharmacologic pain relief measures include a woman's desire for a natural, vaginal birth; her preparation for childbirth; the nature of her support during labor; and her willingness and ability to participate in nonpharmacologic measures for comfort (Creehan, 2008).

Expression of Pain

Pain results in physiologic effects and sensory and emotional (affective) responses. During childbirth pain gives rise to identifiable physiologic effects. Sympathetic nervous system activity is stimulated in response to intensifying pain, resulting in increased catecholamine levels. Blood pressure and heart rate increase. Maternal respiratory patterns change in response to an increase in oxygen consumption. Hyperventilation, sometimes accompanied by respiratory alkalosis, can occur as pain intensifies and more rapid, shallow breathing techniques are used during contractions. Pallor and diaphoresis may be seen. Gastric acidity increases, and nausea and vomiting are common in the active and transition phases of the first stage of labor. Placental perfusion may decrease, and uterine activity may diminish, potentially prolonging labor and affecting fetal well-being.

Certain emotional (affective) expressions of pain often are seen. Such changes include increasing anxiety with lessened perceptual field, writhing, crying, groaning, gesturing (hand clenching and wringing), and excessive muscular excitability throughout the body.

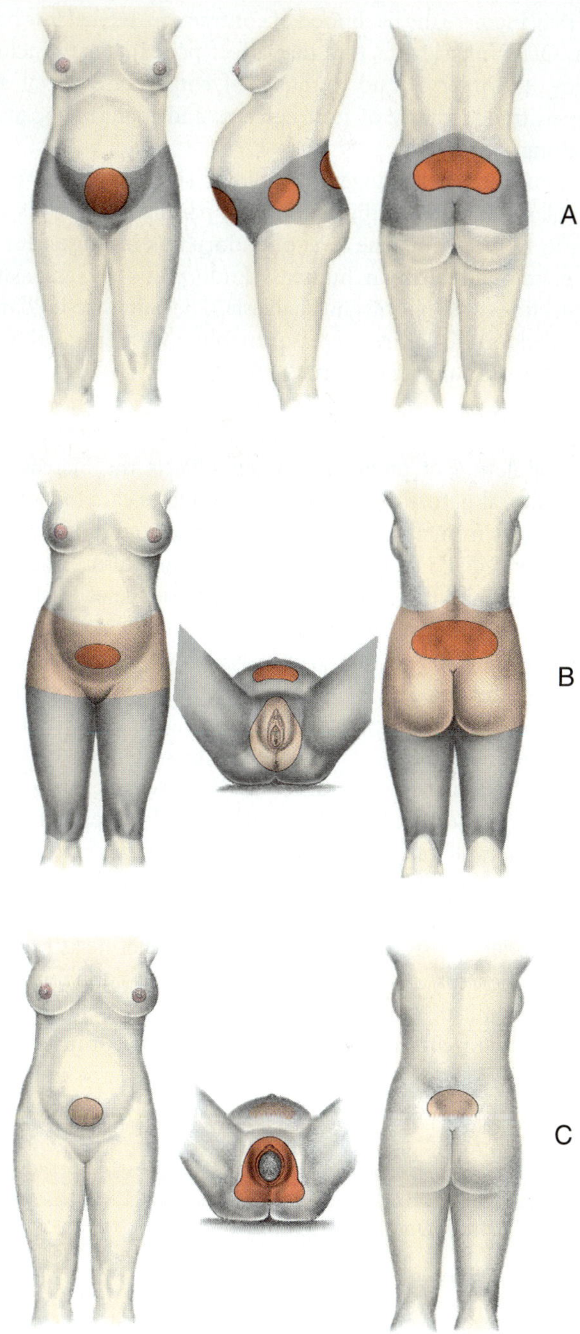

FIG. 17-1 Discomfort during labor. **A,** Distribution of labor pain during first stage. **B,** Distribution of labor pain during transition and early phase of second stage. **C,** Distribution of pain during late second stage and actual birth. (*Gray areas* indicate mild discomfort; *light pink areas* indicate moderate discomfort; *dark red areas* indicate intense discomfort.)

Factors Influencing Pain Response

Pain during childbirth is unique to each woman. How she perceives or interprets that pain is influenced by a variety of physiologic, psychologic, emotional, social, cultural, and environmental factors (Zwelling et al., 2006).

Physiologic Factors

A variety of physiologic factors can affect the intensity of childbirth pain. Women with a history of dysmenorrhea may experience increased pain during childbirth as a result of higher prostaglandin levels. Back pain associated with menstruation also may increase the likelihood of contraction-related low back pain. Other physical factors that affect pain intensity include fatigue, the interval and duration of contractions, fetal size and position, rapidity of fetal descent, and maternal position (Zwelling et al., 2006).

Endorphins are endogenous opioids secreted by the pituitary gland that act on the central and peripheral nervous systems to reduce pain. The level of endorphins increases during pregnancy and birth in humans. Endorphins are associated with feelings of euphoria and analgesia. The pain threshold may rise as endorphin levels increase, enabling women in labor to tolerate acute pain (Blackburn, 2007).

Culture

The population of pregnant women reflects the increasingly multicultural nature of U.S. society. As nurses care for women and families from a variety of cultural backgrounds, they must have knowledge and understanding of how culture mediates pain. Although all women expect to experience at least some pain and discomfort during childbirth, it is their culture and religious belief system that determines how they will perceive, interpret, and respond to and manage the pain. For example, women with strong religious beliefs often accept pain as a necessary and inevitable part of bringing a new life into the world (Callister, Khalaf, Semenic, Kartchner, & Vehvilainen-Julkunen, 2003). An understanding of the beliefs, values, expectations, and practices of various cultures will narrow the cultural gap and help the nurse to assess the laboring woman's pain experience more accurately. The nurse can then provide appropriate, culturally sensitive care by using pain relief measures that preserve the woman's sense of control and self-confidence (see Cultural Considerations box: Some Cultural Beliefs About Pain). Recognize that although a woman's behavior in response to pain may vary according to her cultural background, it may not accurately reflect the intensity of the pain she is experiencing. Assess the woman for the physiologic effects of pain and listen to the words she uses to describe the sensory and affective qualities of her pain.

CULTURAL CONSIDERATIONS

Some Cultural Beliefs About Pain

The following examples demonstrate how women of different cultural backgrounds may react to pain. Because they are generalizations, the nurse must assess each woman experiencing pain related to childbirth.

- Chinese women may not exhibit reactions to pain, although exhibiting pain during childbirth is acceptable. They consider accepting something when it is first offered as impolite; therefore, pain interventions must be offered more than once. Acupuncture may be used for pain relief.
- Arab or Middle Eastern women may be vocal in response to labor pain. They may prefer medication for pain relief.
- Japanese women may be stoic in response to labor pain, but they may request medication when pain becomes severe.
- Southeast Asian women may endure severe pain before requesting relief.
- Hispanic women may be stoic until late in labor, when they may become vocal and request pain relief.
- Native-American women may use medications or remedies made from indigenous plants. They are often stoic in response to labor pain.
- African-American women may express pain openly. Use of medication for pain relief varies.

Anxiety

Anxiety is commonly associated with increased pain during labor. Mild anxiety is considered normal for a woman during labor and birth. However, excessive anxiety and fear cause more catecholamine secretion, which increases the stimuli to the brain from the pelvis because of decreased blood flow and increased muscle tension. This action, in turn, magnifies pain perception (Zwelling et al., 2006). Thus as anxiety and fear heighten, muscle tension increases, the effectiveness of uterine contractions decreases, the experience of discomfort increases, and a cycle of increased fear and anxiety begins. Ultimately this cycle will slow the progress of labor. The woman's confidence in her ability to cope with pain will be diminished, potentially resulting in reduced effectiveness of the pain relief measures being used.

Previous Experience

Previous experience with pain and childbirth may affect a woman's description of her pain and her ability to cope with the pain. Childbirth, for a healthy young woman, may be her first experience with significant pain, and as a result she may not have developed effective pain coping strategies. She may describe the intensity of even early labor pain as pain "as bad as it can be." The nature of previous childbirth experiences also may affect a woman's responses to pain. For women who have had a difficult and painful previous birth experience, anxiety and fear from this past experience may lead to increased pain perception.

Sensory pain for nulliparous women is often greater than that for multiparous women during early labor (dilation less than 5 cm) because their reproductive tract structures are less supple. During the transition phase of the first stage of labor and during the second stage of labor, multiparous women may experience greater sensory pain than nulliparous women because their more supple tissue increases the speed of fetal descent and thereby intensifies pain. The firmer tissue of nulliparous women results in a slower, more gradual descent. Affective pain is usually greater for nulliparous women throughout the first stage of labor but decreases for both nulliparous and multiparous women during the second stage of labor (Lowe, 2002).

Parity may affect perception of labor pain because nulliparous women often have longer labors and therefore greater fatigue. Because fatigue magnifies pain, the combination of increased pain, fatigue, and reduced ability to cope may lead to a greater reliance on pharmacologic support.

Gate-Control Theory of Pain

Even particularly intense pain stimuli can at times be ignored. This is possible because certain nerve cell groupings within the spinal cord, brainstem, and cerebral cortex have the ability to modulate the pain impulse through a blocking mechanism. This **gate-control theory of pain** helps explain the way hypnosis and the pain relief techniques taught in childbirth preparation classes work to relieve the pain of labor. According to this theory, pain sensations travel along sensory nerve pathways to the brain, but only a limited number of sensations, or messages, can travel through these nerve pathways at one time. Using distraction techniques such as massage or stroking, music, focal points, and imagery reduces or completely blocks the capacity of nerve pathways to transmit pain. These distractions are thought to work by closing down a hypothetic gate in the spinal cord, thus preventing pain signals from reaching the brain. The perception of pain is thereby diminished.

In addition, when the laboring woman engages in neuromuscular and motor activity, activity within the spinal cord itself further modifies the transmission of pain. Cognitive work involving concentration on breathing and relaxation requires selective and directed cortical activity that activates and closes the gating mechanism as well. As labor intensifies, more complex cognitive techniques are required to maintain effectiveness. The gate-control theory underscores the need for a supportive birth setting that allows the laboring woman to relax and use various higher mental activities.

Comfort

Although the predominant medical approach to labor is that it is painful, and the pain must be removed, an alternative view is that labor is a natural process, and women can experience comfort and transcend the discomfort or pain to reach the joyful outcome of birth. Having needs and desires met promotes a feeling of comfort. The most helpful interventions in enhancing comfort are a caring nursing approach and a supportive presence.

Support. Current evidence indicates that a woman's satisfaction with her labor and birth experience is determined by how well her personal expectations of childbirth were met and the quality of support and interaction she received from her caregivers (Box 17-1). In addition, satisfaction is influenced by the degree to which she was able to stay in control of her labor and to participate in decision making regarding her labor, including the pain relief measures to be used (Albers, 2007; Zwelling et al., 2006).

BOX 17-1 SUGGESTED MEASURES FOR SUPPORTING A WOMAN IN LABOR

- Provide companionship and reassurance.
- Offer positive reinforcement and praise for her efforts.
- Encourage participation in distracting activities and nonpharmacologic measures for comfort.
- Give nourishment.
- Assist with personal hygiene.
- Offer information and advice.
- Involve the woman in decision making regarding her care.
- Interpret the woman's wishes to other health care providers and to her support group.
- Create a relaxing environment.
- Use a calm and confident approach.
- Support and encourage the woman's family members by role modeling labor support measures and providing time for breaks.

Source: Creehan, P. (2008). Pain relief and comfort measures in labor. In K. Rice Simpson & P. Creehan. (Eds.), *AWHONN's perinatal nursing* (3rd ed.). Philadelphia: Lippincott Williams & Wilkins.

The value of the continuous supportive presence of a person (e.g., doula, childbirth educator, family member, friend, nurse, or partner) during labor who provides physical comforting, facilitates communication, and offers information and guidance to the woman in labor has long been known. Emotional support is demonstrated by giving praise and reassurance and conveying a positive, calm, and confident demeanor when caring for the woman in labor (Creehan, 2008). Women who have continuous support beginning early in labor are less likely to use pain medications or epidurals and are more likely to experience a spontaneous vaginal birth and express satisfaction with their childbirth experience. Interestingly, research findings concluded that a more positive effect was achieved when the continuous support was provided by people who were not hospital staff members (Albers, 2007; Berghella, Baxter, & Chauhan, 2008; Hodnett, Gates, Hofmeyr, & Sakala, 2007).

Environment. The quality of the environment can influence pain perception and the laboring woman's ability to cope with her pain. Environment includes the individuals present (e.g., how they communicate, their philosophy of care including a belief in the value of nonpharmacologic pain relief measures, practice policies, and quality of support) and the physical space in which the labor occurs (Creehan, 2008; Zwelling et al., 2006). Women usually prefer to be cared for by familiar caregivers in a comfortable, homelike setting. The environment should be safe and private, allowing a woman to feel free to be herself as she tries out different comfort measures. Stimuli such as light, noise, and temperature should be adjusted according to her preferences. The environment should have space for movement and equipment such as birth balls. Comfortable chairs, tubs, and showers should be readily available to facilitate participation in a variety of nonpharmacologic pain relief measures. The familiarity of the environment can be enhanced by bringing items from home such as pillows, objects for a focal point, music, and DVDs.

NONPHARMACOLOGIC PAIN MANAGEMENT

The alleviation of pain is important. Commonly it is not the amount of pain the woman experiences, but whether she meets the goals she set for herself to cope with the pain, that influences her perception of the birth experience as good or bad. The observant nurse looks for clues to the woman's desired level of control in the management of pain and its relief.

Nonpharmacologic measures are often simple and safe, with few if any major adverse reactions, relatively inexpensive, and can be used throughout labor. Additionally, they provide the woman with a sense of control over her childbirth as she makes choices about the measures that are best for her. During the prenatal period she should explore a variety of nonpharmacologic measures. Techniques she usually finds helpful in relieving stress and enhancing relaxation (e.g., music, meditation, massage, warm baths) may be very effective as components of a plan for managing labor pain. The woman should be encouraged to communicate to her health care providers her preferences for relaxation and pain relief measures and to actively participate in their implementation.

Many of the nonpharmacologic methods for relief of discomfort are taught in different types of prenatal preparation classes, or the woman or couple may have read various books

Spanish Guidelines—Pain Management

and magazine articles on the subject in advance. Many of these methods require practice for best results (e.g., hypnosis, patterned breathing and controlled relaxation techniques, biofeedback), although the nurse may use some of them successfully without the woman or couple having prior knowledge (e.g., slow-paced breathing, massage and touch, effleurage, counterpressure). Women should be encouraged to try a variety of methods and to seek alternatives, including pharmacologic methods, if the measure being used is no longer effective.

With increasing use of epidural analgesia, nurses may be less likely to encourage women to use nonpharmacologic measures, in part because these methods may be viewed as more complex and time consuming than monitoring a woman receiving an epidural. Additionally, new nurses may not have had the opportunity to develop skill in the implementation of these methods. It is imperative that perinatal nurses develop a commitment to and expertise in using a variety of nonpharmacologic pain relief strategies in order for women in labor to be comfortable using them. Although there are limited research data to support the effectiveness of many of these nonpharmacologic measures, there are sufficient reports of their benefits from women and health care providers to recommend that nurses encourage their use (Creehan, 2008). (See Evidence-Based Practice box and Clinical Reasoning box.) The analgesic effect of many nonpharmacologic measures is comparable to or even superior to opioids that are administered parenterally (Box 17-2).

EVIDENCE-BASED PRACTICE

Pat Gingrich

Complementary and Alternative Pain Management in Labor

ASK THE QUESTION

Is it beneficial to use nonpharmacologic measures to decrease or eliminate the use of medications in labor? What therapies are safe for mother and baby?

SEARCH FOR EVIDENCE

Search Strategies

Professional organization guidelines, meta-analyses, systematic reviews, randomized controlled trials, nonrandomized prospective studies and retrospective reviews since 2008.

Databases Searched

CINAHL, Cochrane, Medline, PUBMED, and the professional website for the Association of Women's Health, Obstetric and Neonatal Nurses (AWHONN).

CRITICALLY ANALYZE THE DATA

Critics of Western childbirth claim that use of opioid and/or neuraxial (epidural or spinal) medication leads to immobility, prolonged labor, increased cesarean rates, and birth trauma. A meta-analysis of 21 RCTs involving 3706 women revealed that walking or assuming an upright position can decrease the duration of first stage labor by an hour, and decrease the use of epidural analgesia (Lawrence, Lewis, Hofmyer, Dowswell, & Styles, 2009). The ideal pain relief intervention would allow for position changes and mobility, decrease time in labor, cause no side effects for mother or baby, be safe and easy to administer, and have a low cost. Anecdotally, nonpharmacologic complementary and alternative therapies may offer pain relief, but is there evidence that they are beneficial and safe?

Immersion in water: A Cochrane Database Systematic Review of 11 trials involving 3146 women found that water immersion significantly reduced the use of neuraxial analgesia. There were no adverse effects on length of labor, operative delivery rates, perineal tears, maternal infection, or APGAR scores (Cluett & Burns, 2009).

Sterile Water Injections: It is estimated that about one third of laboring women experience painful "back labor." A meta-analysis of 8 RCTs involving 828 women found that sterile water injected superficially lateral to the lumbar spine was beneficial. Originally developed as a pain relief measure for kidney stones, the sterile water injections were found to reduce pain and decrease the rate of cesarean birth from 9.9% in the control group to 4.6% in the experimental group (Hutton, Kasperink, Rutten, Reitsma, & Wainman, 2009).

Transcutaneous nerve stimulation (TENS): A patient-controlled low voltage current may alleviate pain by blocking spinal pain pathways. It may be applied to the back, the head, or acupuncture points. A Cochrane Database Systematic Review of 19 studies involving a total of 1671 women found evidence that use of TENS at acupuncture points led to less severe pain. There were no adverse outcomes noted for labor duration, interventions, nor maternal or neonatal well-being (Dowsdell, Bedwell, Lavender, & Neilson, 2009). The researchers concluded that this pain-relief measure should be offered to women in labor.

Acupuncture: A randomized controlled trial of 607 women found that acupuncture use in labor leads to significantly less use of pharmacologic pain relief and/or invasive (neuraxial) analgesia, when compared to TENS or usual care (control). Acupuncture points included lower back, forearm, ankle, and/or ear pina. While pain scores, labor duration and oxytocin use were comparable between all groups, the acupuncture group had significantly higher umbilical pH (less acidosis) and better APGAR scores at 5 minutes (Borup, Wurlitzer, Hedegaard, Kesmodel, & Hvidman, 2009).

IMPLICATIONS FOR PRACTICE

When researchers verify the safety and efficacy of complementary and alternative therapies, health care providers have more pain relief management options available for laboring women. Complementary and alternative methods may provide sufficient pain relief during labor, or may allow lower doses of pain medications, which would allow for the benefits of greater mobility and fewer side effects. Most complementary and alternative therapies are inexpensive and can be administered in low-resource facilities. The relaxation that comes from pain relief may stimulate the parasympathetic nervous system, decreasing the "cascade of intervention" and increasing the chance of spontaneous vaginal birth.

References

Borup, L., Wurlitzer, W., Hedegaard, M., Kesmodel, U., & Hvidman, L. (2009). Acupuncture as pain relief during delivery: a randomized controlled trial. *Birth, 36*(1), 5–12.

Cluett, E., & Burns, E. (2009). Immersion in water in labour and birth. *The Cochrane Database of Systematic Reviews, 2009*, 2, CD00011.

Dowsdell, T., Bedwell, C., Lavender, T., & Neilson, J. (2009). Transcutaneous electrical nerve stimulation (TENS) for pain relief in labour. *The Cochrane Database of Systematic Reviews, 2009*, 2, CD007214.

Hutton, E., Kasperink, M., Rutten, M., Reitsma, A., & Wainman, B. (2009). Sterile water injection for labour pain: A systematic review and meta-analysis of randomized controlled trials. *British Journal of Obstetrics and Gynaecology, 116*(9), 1158–1166.

Lawrence, A., Lewis, L., Hofmyer, G., Dowsdell, T., & Styles, C. (2009). Maternal positions and mobility during first stage labor. *The Cochrane Database of Systematic Reviews, 2009*, 2, CD003934.

CLINICAL REASONING

Making Decisions Regarding Pain Management for Labor

Andrea, a primigravid woman at 28 weeks of gestation, discusses her fear of the pain she will experience during labor at a routine prenatal visit where you are participating in a clinical experience as a nursing student. She tells you that she knows the pain will be "awful" based on what her friends have told her about their labors. Andrea says that her friends all had epidurals, which were very helpful, but they had to wait until they were in labor for several hours. In addition, her friends told her not to bother with any of the "breathing and relaxation stuff" that everyone learns in classes because it does not work. She asks you if epidurals are safe and tells you how afraid she is to have anything inserted into her spine because she has had some lower back pain since her third trimester began. She is also very concerned about using medications that can harm her baby.

1. Evidence—Is there sufficient evidence regarding nonpharmacologic and pharmacologic pain relief measures for you to make recommendations to Andrea?
2. Assumptions—Describe the underlying assumptions about each of the following issues:
   a. Timing for epidural administration
   b. Effectiveness of relaxation and stress reduction on the labor process
   c. Approaches that are proven to reduce the use of pharmacologic measures
   d. Modifiable factors that can reduce the severity of the pain experienced during labor
3. What approach should you use to address Andrea's concerns and provide recommendations for pain relief during labor?
4. Does the evidence objectively support your conclusion?
5. Are there alternative perspectives to your conclusion?

Childbirth Preparation Methods

The childbirth education movement began in the 1950s. Today most health care providers recommend or offer childbirth preparation classes for expectant parents. Historically, popular childbirth methods taught in the United States were the Dick-Read method, the Lamaze (psychoprophylaxis) method, and the Bradley (husband-coached childbirth) method (see Community Activity box). Although these three organizations continue to exist, they are now less focused on a "method" approach. Rather, women are assisted to develop their birth philosophy and inner knowledge and then choose from a variety of skills to use to cope with the labor process. Many childbirth educators teach a variety of techniques that originated in several different organizations or publications. Women are encouraged to choose the techniques that work best for them.

Gaining popularity are methods developed and promoted by Birthing From Within, Birthworks, Association of Labor Assistants and Childbirth Educators (ALACE), Childbirth and Postpartum Professional Association (CAPPA), and HypnoBirthing, to name a few. These methods offer classes and other services that focus on fostering a woman's confidence in her innate ability to give birth. The woman or couple is helped to recognize the uniqueness of their pregnancy and childbirth experience (see Resources on the Evolve website).

BOX 17-2 NONPHARMACOLOGIC STRATEGIES TO ENCOURAGE RELAXATION AND RELIEVE PAIN

CUTANEOUS STIMULATION STRATEGIES
- Counterpressure
- Effleurage (light massage)
- Therapeutic touch and massage
- Walking
- Rocking
- Changing positions
- Application of heat or cold
- Transcutaneous electrical nerve stimulation (TENS)
- Acupressure
- Water therapy (showers, whirlpool baths)
- Intradermal water block

SENSORY STIMULATION STRATEGIES
- Aromatherapy
- Breathing techniques
- Music
- Imagery
- Use of focal points

COGNITIVE STRATEGIES
- Childbirth education
- Hypnosis
- Biofeedback

COMMUNITY ACTIVITY

- Visit the Lamaze International website at www.lamaze-childbirth.com and click on the New & Expectant Parents link. Review the information about the Lamaze method of preparation for childbirth and healthy birth practices. Locate a Lamaze class in your community. Contact the instructor and try to attend a class.
- Visit the website of a hospital that provides maternity services in your community. Review the client information about the Birth Center. Do any of the labor and birth rooms have whirlpool bathtubs for pain management and comfort during labor? Are cordless fetal and maternal monitors available, so that the women can walk during labor or sit in a chair?

Relaxation and Breathing Techniques

Focusing and Relaxation Techniques

By reducing tension and stress, focusing and relaxation techniques allow a woman in labor to rest and to conserve energy for the task of giving birth. *Attention-focusing* and *distraction* techniques are forms of care that are effective to some degree in relieving labor pain (Albers, 2007). Some women bring a favorite object such as a photograph or stuffed animal to the labor room and focus their attention on this object during contractions. Others choose to fix their attention on some object in the labor room. As the contraction begins, they focus on their chosen object and perform a breathing technique to reduce their perception of pain.

With *imagery* the woman focuses her attention on a pleasant scene, a place where she feels relaxed, or an activity she enjoys. She can imagine walking through a restful garden or breathing

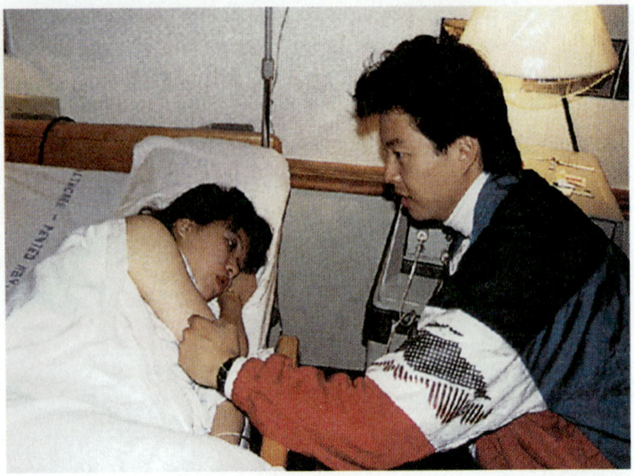

FIG. 17-2 A laboring woman using focusing and breathing techniques during a uterine contraction with coaching from her partner. (Courtesy Marjorie Pyle, RNC, Lifecircle, Costa Mesa, CA.)

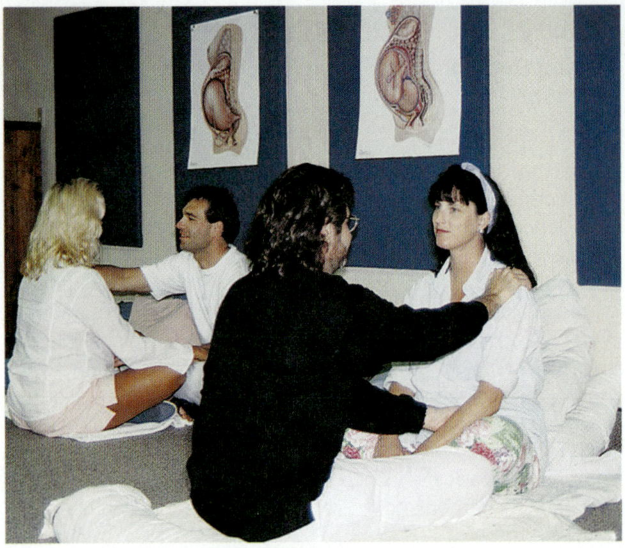

FIG. 17-3 Expectant parents learning relaxation techniques. (Courtesy Marjorie Pyle, RNC, Lifecircle, Costa Mesa, CA.)

in light, energy, and healing color and breathing out worries and tension. Choosing the subject for the imagery and practicing the technique during pregnancy enhances effectiveness during labor.

During childbirth preparation classes the coach can learn how to palpate a woman's body to detect tense and contracted muscles. The woman then learns how to relax the tense muscle in response to the gentle stroking of the muscle by the coach (Fig. 17-2). In a common feedback mechanism, the woman and her coach say the word "relax" at the onset of each contraction and throughout it as needed. With practice, the coach can effectively use support, feedback, and touch to facilitate the woman's relaxation and thereby reduce tension and stress and enhance the progress of labor (Humenick, Schrock, & Libresco, 2000).

Women may find that drinking herb tea during labor can help them to relax (e.g., chamomile), to reduce nausea (e.g., lemon balm, peppermint), and to enhance energy and reduce fatigue (e.g., ginger, ginseng). Drinking tea can have the additional benefit of maintaining fluid balance (Walls, 2009).

The nurse can assist the woman by providing a quiet and relaxed environment, offering cues as needed, and recognizing signs of tension (e.g., frowning, change in tone of voice, clenching of fists). A relaxed environment for labor is created by controlling sensory stimuli (e.g., light, noise, temperature), and reducing interruptions. Nurses should remain calm and unhurried in their approach and sit rather than stand at the bedside whenever possible (Creehan, 2008).

Breathing Techniques

Different approaches to childbirth preparation stress varying breathing techniques to provide distraction, thereby reducing the perception of pain and helping the woman maintain control throughout contractions. In the first stage of labor such breathing techniques can promote relaxation of the abdominal muscles and thereby increase the size of the abdominal cavity. This lessens discomfort generated by friction between the uterus and abdominal wall during contractions. Because the muscles of the genital area also become more relaxed, they do not interfere with fetal descent. In the second stage, breathing is used to increase abdominal pressure and thereby assist in expelling the fetus. Breathing also can be used to relax the pudendal muscles to prevent precipitate expulsion of the fetal head (Fig. 17-3).

For couples who have prepared for labor by practicing relaxing and breathing techniques, a simple review with occasional reminders may be all that is necessary to help them along. For those who have had no preparation, instruction and practice in simple breathing and relaxation techniques can be given early in labor and often is surprisingly successful. Nurses can also model breathing techniques and breathe in synchrony with the woman and her partner. Motivation is high, and readiness to learn is enhanced by the reality of labor.

Various breathing techniques can be used for controlling pain during contractions (Box 17-3). The nurse needs to determine what, if any, techniques the laboring couple knows before giving them instruction. Simple patterns are more easily learned. Paced breathing is most associated with prepared childbirth and includes slow-paced, modified-paced, and patterned-paced breathing (pant-blow) techniques. Each labor is different, and nursing support includes assisting couples to adapt breathing techniques to their individual labor experience.

All patterns begin with a deep, relaxing, cleansing breath to "greet the contraction" and end with another deep breath exhaled to "gently blow the contraction away." These deep breaths ensure adequate oxygen for mother and baby and signal that a contraction is beginning or has ended. As the breath is exhaled, respiratory and voluntary muscles relax (Creehan, 2008). In general, *slow-paced breathing* is performed at approximately half the woman's normal breathing rate and is initiated when she can no longer walk or talk through contractions. The woman should take no fewer than three or four breaths per minute. Slow-paced breathing aids in relaxation and provides optimum oxygenation. The woman should continue to use this technique for as long as it is effective in reducing the perception of pain and maintaining control. As contractions increase in frequency and intensity, the woman often needs to change to a more complex breathing technique, which is shallower and faster than her normal rate of breathing, but should not exceed twice her resting respiratory rate. This *modified-paced breathing*

BOX 17-3 PACED BREATHING TECHNIQUES

CLEANSING BREATH

- Relaxed breath in through nose and out through mouth. Used at the beginning and end of each contraction.

SLOW-PACED BREATHING (APPROXIMATELY 6 TO 8 BREATHS PER MINUTE)

- Performed at approximately half the normal breathing rate (number of breaths per minute divided by 2)
- IN-2-3-4/OUT-2-3-4/IN-2-3-4/OUT-2-3-4 ...

MODIFIED-PACED BREATHING (APPROXIMATELY 32 TO 40 BREATHS PER MINUTE)

- Performed at about twice the normal breathing rate (number of breaths per minute multiplied by 2)
- IN-OUT/IN-OUT/IN-OUT/IN-OUT ...
- For more flexibility and variety, the woman may combine the slow and modified breathing by using the slow breathing for beginnings and ends of contractions and modified breathing for more intense peaks. This technique conserves energy, lessens fatigue, and reduces risk for hyperventilation.

PATTERNED-PACED OR PANT-BLOW BREATHING (SAME RATE AS MODIFIED)

- Enhances concentration
  3:1 Patterned breathing IN-OUT/IN-OUT/IN-OUT/IN-BLOW (repeat through contraction)
  4:1 Patterned breathing IN-OUT/IN-OUT/IN-OUT/IN-OUT/IN-BLOW (repeat through contraction)

Source: Nichols, F. (2000). Paced breathing techniques. In F. Nichols & S. Humenick (Eds.), *Childbirth education: Practice, research, and theory* (2nd ed.). Philadelphia: Saunders; Perinatal Education Associates. (2008). *Breathing.* Available at www.birthsource.com/scripts/article.asp?articleid=211. Accessed July 2, 2010.

pattern requires that she remain alert and concentrate more fully on breathing, thus blocking more painful stimuli than the simpler slow-paced breathing pattern (Perinatal Education Associates, 2008 [www.birthsource.com]).

The most difficult time to maintain control during contractions comes during the transition phase of the first stage of labor, when the cervix dilates from 8 cm to 10 cm. Even for the woman who has prepared for labor, concentration on breathing techniques is difficult to maintain. *Patterned-paced (pant-blow) breathing* is suggested during this phase. It is performed at the same rate as modified-paced breathing and consists of panting breaths combined with soft blowing breaths at regular intervals. The patterns may vary (i.e., *pant, pant, pant, pant, blow* [4:1 pattern] or *pant, pant, pant, blow* [3:1 pattern]) (Perinatal Education Associates, 2008). An undesirable reaction to this type of breathing is hyperventilation. The woman and her support person must be aware of and watch for symptoms of the resultant respiratory alkalosis: lightheadedness, dizziness, tingling of the fingers, or circumoral numbness. Respiratory alkalosis may be eliminated by having the woman breathe into a paper bag held tightly around her mouth and nose. This enables her to rebreathe carbon dioxide and replace the bicarbonate ions. The woman also can breathe into her cupped hands if no bag is available. Maintaining a breathing rate that is no more than twice the normal rate will lessen chances of hyperventilation. The partner can help the woman maintain her breathing rate with visual, tactile, or auditory cues.

As the fetal head reaches the pelvic floor, the woman may feel the urge to push and may automatically begin to exert downward pressure by contracting her abdominal muscles. During second-stage pushing, the woman should find a breathing pattern that is relaxing and feels good to her and is safe for her baby. Any regular or rhythmic breathing that avoids prolonged breath holding during pushing should maintain a good oxygen flow to the fetus (Perinatal Education Associates, 2008).

The woman can control the urge to push by taking panting breaths or by slowly exhaling through pursed lips (as though blowing out a candle). This type of breathing can be used to overcome the urge to push when the cervix is not fully prepared (e.g., less than 8 cm dilated, not retracting) and to facilitate a slow birth of the fetal head.

Effleurage and Counterpressure

Effleurage (light massage) and counterpressure have brought relief to many women during the first stage of labor. The gate-control theory may supply the reason for the effectiveness of these measures. **Effleurage** is light stroking, usually of the abdomen, in rhythm with breathing during contractions. It is used to distract the woman from contraction pain. Often the presence of monitor belts makes it difficult to perform effleurage on the abdomen; therefore, a thigh or the chest may be used. As labor progresses, hyperesthesia may make effleurage uncomfortable and thus less effective.

Counterpressure is steady pressure applied by a support person to the sacral area with a firm object (e.g., tennis ball) or the fist or heel of the hand. Pressure can also be applied to both hips (double hip squeeze) or to the knees (Creehan, 2008). Application of counterpressure helps the woman cope with the sensations of internal pressure and pain in the lower back. It is especially helpful when back pain is caused by pressure of the occiput against spinal nerves when the fetal head is in a posterior position. Counterpressure lifts the occiput off these nerves, thereby providing pain relief. The support person will need to be relieved occasionally because application of counterpressure is hard work.

Music

Music, recorded or live, can provide a distraction, enhance relaxation, and lift spirits during labor, thereby reducing the woman's level of stress, anxiety, and perception of pain. It can be used to promote relaxation in early labor and to stimulate movement as labor progresses. Music can help to create a more relaxed atmosphere in the birth room, leading to a more relaxed approach by health care providers (Creehan, 2008; Zwelling, et al., 2006). Women should be encouraged to prepare their musical preferences in advance and to bring a CD player or mP3 player (e.g., iPod) to the hospital or birthing center. They should choose familiar music that is associated with pleasant memories, which can also facilitate the process of guided imagery. Use of a headset or earphones may increase the effectiveness of the music because other sounds will be shut out. Live music provided at the bedside by a support person may be very helpful in transmitting energy that decreases tension and elevates mood. Changing the tempo of the music to coincide with the rate and rhythm of each breathing technique may facilitate proper pacing. Although promising, there is insufficient evidence at the present time to support the effectiveness of music as a method

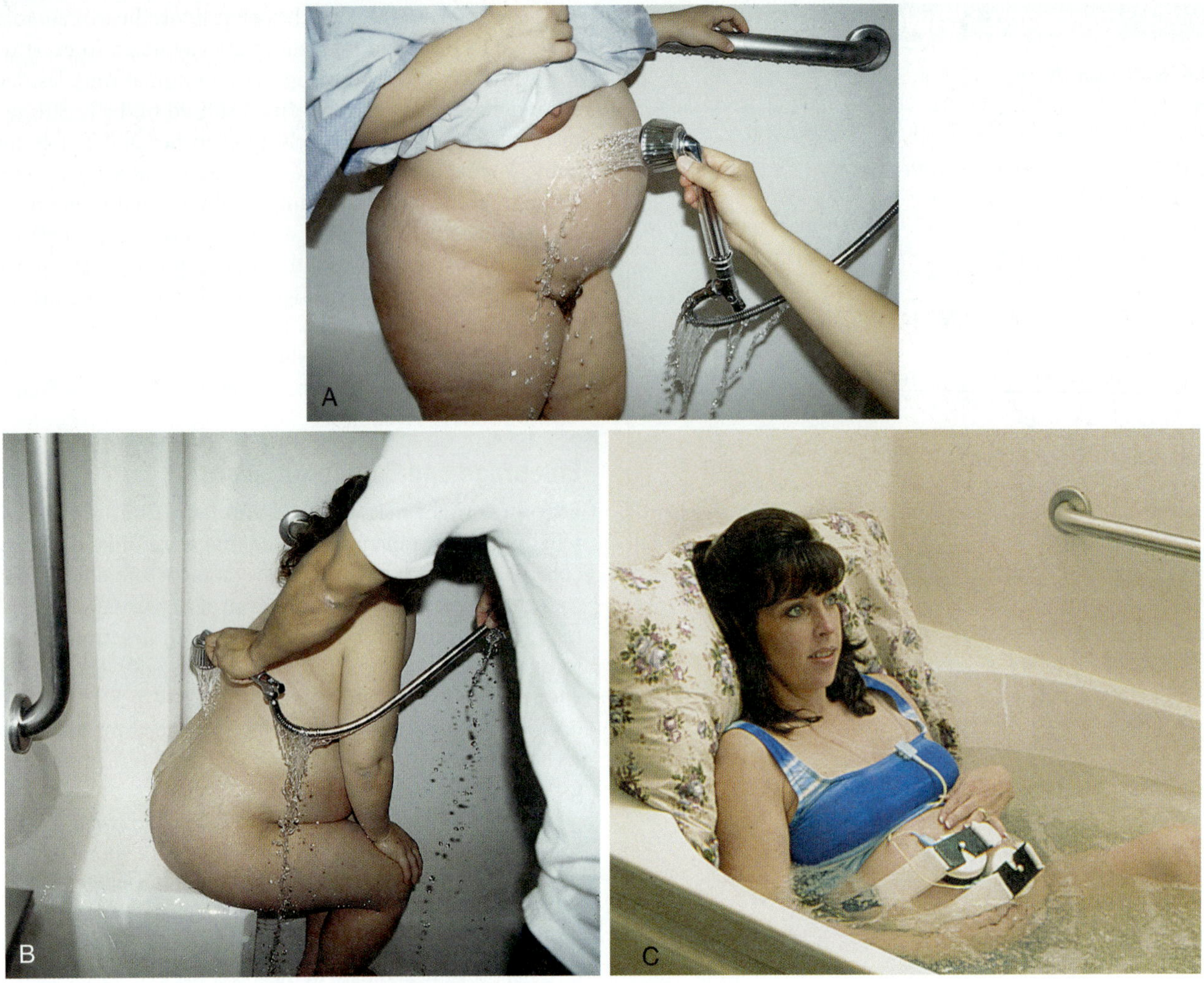

FIG. 17-4 Water therapy during labor. **A,** Use of shower during labor. **B,** Woman experiencing back labor relaxes as partner sprays warm water on her back. **C,** Laboring woman relaxes in Jacuzzi. Note that fetal monitoring can continue during time in the Jacuzzi. (**A** and **B,** Courtesy Marjorie Pyle, RNC, Lifecircle, Costa Mesa, CA; **C,** courtesy Spacelabs Medical, Redmond, WA.)

of pain relief during labor. Further research is recommended (Smith, Collins, Cyna, & Crowther, 2006).

Water Therapy (Hydrotherapy)

Bathing, showering, and jet hydrotherapy (whirlpool baths) with warm water (e.g., at or below body temperature) are nonpharmacologic measures that can promote comfort and relaxation during labor (Fig. 17-4). The warm water stimulates the release of endorphins, relaxes fibers to close the gate on pain, promotes better circulation and oxygenation and helps to soften the perineal tissues. Most women find immersion in water to be soothing, relaxing, and comforting. While immersed, they may find it easier to let go and allow labor to take its course (Gilbert, 2011). Women in labor often report that pain and discomfort subside while in the water (Albers, 2007).

Prior to initiating hydrotherapy measures, agency policy should be consulted to determine if the approval of the laboring woman's primary health care provider is required and if criteria need to be met in terms of the status of the maternal and fetal unit (e.g., stable vital signs and fetal heart rate [FHR] and pattern, stage of labor, etc.). In order to reduce the risk of a prolonged labor, hydrotherapy is usually initiated when the woman is in active labor, at approximately 5 cm. It is at this time that she may be getting discouraged and will welcome the change that hydrotherapy offers. Remember to preserve her modesty because she may be shy about the exposure of her body when getting into a tub or shower (Creehan, 2008).

In addition to pain relief and relaxation, hydrotherapy offers other benefits. If a woman is having "back labor" as the result of an occiput posterior or transverse position, assuming a hands-and-knees or a side-lying position in the tub enhances spontaneous fetal rotation to the occiput anterior position as a result of increased buoyancy. Because less effort is needed to change positions while in the water, women are encouraged to assume upright positions and to alter positions more frequently, facilitating the progress of their labors and helping them cope with labor-associated stressors (Stark, Rudell, & Haus, 2008). Additionally, hydrotherapy results in less use of pharmacologic pain relief measures, fewer forceps- or vacuum-assisted births, fewer episiotomies, less perineal trauma, and increased maternal satisfaction with the birth experience (Zwelling et al., 2006) (see Community Activity box.)

When hydrotherapy is in use, FHR monitoring is done by Doppler, fetoscope, or wireless external monitor (see Fig. 17-4, *C*). Placement of internal electrodes is contraindicated for jet hydrotherapy. Several studies have investigated the risks of using hydrotherapy with ruptured membranes. Findings have shown no increases in chorioamnionitis, postpartum endometritis, neonatal infections, or antibiotic use. However, care must be taken to use tubs that can be cleansed easily and thoroughly. A unit protocol should be developed for cleaning the tubs (Tournaire & Theau-Yonneau, 2007; Zwelling et al., 2006).

There is no limit to the time women can stay in the bath, and often they are encouraged to stay in it as long as desired. However, most women use jet hydrotherapy for 30 to 60 minutes at a time. During the bath, if the woman's temperature and the FHR increase, if the labor process becomes less effective (e.g., slows or becomes too intense), or if relief of pain is reduced, the woman can come out of the bath and return at a later time. Repeated baths with occasional breaks may be more effective in relieving pain in long labors than extended amounts of time in the water. The temperature of the water should be maintained at 36° to 37° C with the water covering the woman's abdomen to gain maximum effect from the hydrostatic pressure and buoyancy of the water. Her shoulders should remain out of the water to facilitate the dissipation of heat (Creehan, 2008).

Using a shower provides comfort through the application of heat as the handheld shower head is directed to areas of discomfort (see Fig. 17-4, *A* and *B*). The coach or partner can participate in this comfort measure by holding and directing the shower head.

SAFETY ALERT

Because warm water can cause dizziness, a shower stool should be used, and the woman should be assisted when getting in and out of the tub.

Transcutaneous Electrical Nerve Stimulation

Transcutaneous electrical nerve stimulation (TENS) involves the placing of two pairs of flat electrodes on either side of the woman's thoracic and sacral spine (Fig. 17-5). These electrodes provide continuous low-intensity electrical impulses or stimuli from a battery-operated device. During a contraction the woman increases the stimulation from low to high intensity by turning control knobs on the device. High intensity should be maintained for at least 1 minute to facilitate release of endorphins. Women describe the resulting sensation as a tingling or buzzing. TENS is most useful for lower back pain during the early first stage of labor. Women tend to rate the device as helpful although its use does not decrease pain. It appears that the electrical impulses or stimuli somehow make the pain less disturbing. There are no serious safety concerns associated with the use of TENS (Hawkins, Goetzl, & Chestnut, 2007).

Acupressure and Acupuncture

Acupressure and acupuncture can be used in pregnancy, in labor, and postpartum to relieve pain and other discomforts. Pressure, heat, or cold is applied to acupuncture points called *tsubos*. These points have an increased density of neuroreceptors and increased electrical conductivity. Acupressure is said to promote circulation of blood, the harmony of yin and yang,

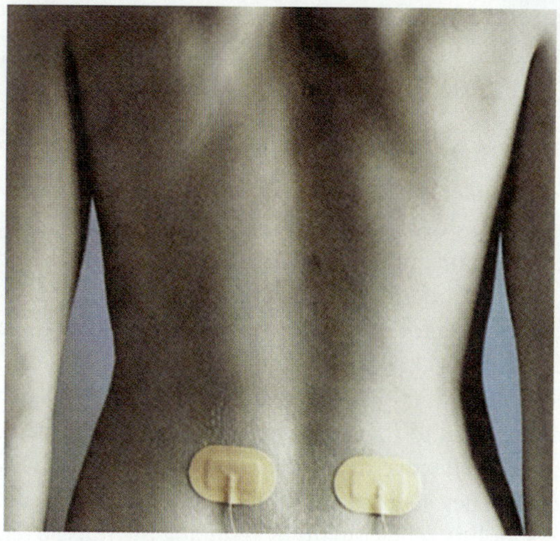

FIG. 17-5 Placement of transcutaneous electrical nerve stimulation (TENS) electrodes on back for relief of labor pain.

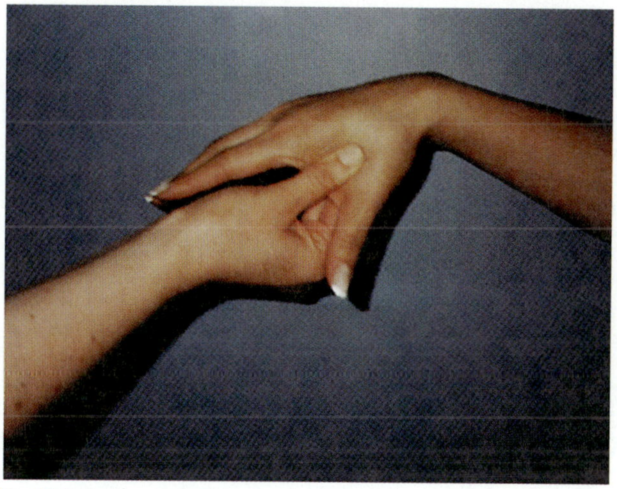

FIG. 17-6 Ho-Ku acupressure point (back of hand where thumb and index finger come together) used to enhance uterine contractions without increasing pain. (Courtesy Julie Perry Nelson, Loveland, CO.)

and the secretion of neurotransmitters, thus maintaining normal body functions and enhancing well-being (Tournaire & Theau-Yonneau, 2007). Acupressure is best applied over the skin without using lubricants. Pressure is usually applied with the heel of the hand, fist, or pads of the thumbs and fingers (Fig. 17-6). Tennis balls or other devices also may be used. Pressure is applied with contractions initially and then continuously as labor progresses to the transition phase at the end of the first stage of labor (Tournaire & Theau-Yonneau). Synchronized breathing by the caregiver and the woman is suggested for greater effectiveness. Acupressure points are found on the neck, the shoulders, the wrists, the lower back including sacral points, the hips, the area below the kneecaps, the ankles, the nails on the small toes, and the soles of the feet.

Acupuncture is the insertion of fine needles into specific areas of the body to restore the flow of *qi* (energy) and to decrease pain, which is thought to be obstructing the flow of energy. Effectiveness may be attributed to the alteration of chemical neurotransmitter levels in the body or to the release of endorphins as a result of hypothalamic activation. Acupuncture should be done by a trained certified therapist. Current evidence indicates that acupuncture may be beneficial for relief of labor pain; however, further study is indicated (Hawkins et al., 2007; Smith et al., 2006; Tournaire & Theau-Yonneau, 2007).

Application of Heat and Cold

Warmed blankets, warm compresses, heated rice bags, a warm bath or shower, or a moist heating pad can enhance relaxation and reduce pain during labor. Heat relieves muscle ischemia and increases blood flow to the area of discomfort. Heat application is effective for back pain caused by a posterior presentation or general backache from fatigue.

Cold application such as cold cloths, frozen gel packs, or ice packs applied to the back, the chest, and/or the face during labor may be effective in increasing comfort when the woman feels warm. They also may be applied to areas of musculoskeletal pain. Cooling relieves pain by reducing the muscle temperature and relieving muscle spasms (Creehan, 2008). A woman's culture may make the use of cold during labor unacceptable, however.

Heat and cold may be used alternately for a greater effect. Neither heat nor cold should be applied over ischemic or anesthetized areas because tissues can be damaged. One or two layers of cloth should be placed between the skin and a hot or cold pack to prevent damage to the underlying integument.

Touch and Massage

Touch and massage have been an integral part of the traditional care process for women in labor. A variety of massage techniques have been shown to be safe and effective during labor (Gilbert, 2011; Zwelling et al., 2006).

Touch can be as simple as holding the woman's hand, stroking her body, and embracing her. When using touch to communicate caring, reassurance, and concern, it is important that the woman's preferences for touch (e.g., who can touch her, where they can touch her, and how they can touch her) and responses to touch be determined. A woman with a history of sexual abuse or certain cultural beliefs may be uncomfortable with touch. Women who perceive touch during labor as positive have less pain, anxiety, and need for pain medication (Tournaire & Theau-Yonneau, 2007). Touch also can involve very specialized techniques that require manipulation of the human energy field.

Therapeutic touch (TT) uses the concept of energy fields within the body called *prana*. Prana are thought to be deficient in some people who are in pain. TT uses laying-on of hands by a specially trained person to redirect energy fields associated with pain. Research has demonstrated the effectiveness of TT to enhance relaxation, reduce anxiety, and relieve pain (Aghabati, Mohammadi, & Pour Esmaiel, 2010); however, little is known about the use or effectiveness of TT for relieving labor pain.

Head, hand, back, and foot massage may be very effective in reducing tension and enhancing comfort. Hand and foot massage may be especially relaxing in advanced labor when hyperesthesia limits a woman's tolerance for touch on other parts of her body. Combining massage with aromatherapy oil or lotion enhances relaxation both during and between contractions. The woman and her partner should be encouraged to experiment with different types of massage during pregnancy to determine what might feel best and be most relaxing during labor.

Hypnosis

Hypnosis is a form of deep relaxation, similar to daydreaming or meditation (see www.hypnobirthing.com). While under hypnosis women are in a state of focused concentration and the subconscious mind can be more easily accessed. Hypnosis techniques used for labor and birth place an emphasis on enhancing relaxation and diminishing fear, anxiety, and perception of pain. Current evidence suggests that hypnosis seems to reduce fear, tension, and pain during labor and to raise the pain threshold. Women using this technique report a greater sense of control over painful contractions and a higher level of satisfaction with their childbirth experience. Because it reduces the need for pain medication, hypnosis can be helpful when used with other interventions during labor. A few negative effects of hypnosis have been reported, including mild dizziness, nausea, and headache. These negative effects seem to be associated with failure to dehypnotize the woman properly (Tournaire & Theau-Yonneau, 2007).

Biofeedback

Biofeedback may provide another relaxation technique that can be used for labor. Biofeedback is based on the theory that if a person can recognize physical signals, certain internal physiologic events can be changed (i.e., whatever signs the woman has that are associated with her pain). For biofeedback to be effective, the woman must be educated during the prenatal period to become aware of her body and its responses and how to relax. The woman must learn how to use thinking and mental processes (e.g., focusing) to control body responses and functions. Informational biofeedback helps couples develop awareness of their bodies and use strategies to change their responses to stress. If the woman responds to pain during a contraction with tightening of muscles, frowning, moaning, and breath holding, her partner uses verbal and touch feedback to help her relax. Formal biofeedback, which uses machines to detect skin temperature, blood flow, or muscle tension, also can prepare women to intensify their relaxation responses. Biofeedback-assisted relaxation techniques are not always successful in reducing labor pain. Using these techniques effectively requires the strong support of caregivers (Tournaire & Theau-Yonneau, 2007).

Aromatherapy

Aromatherapy uses oils distilled from plants, flowers, herbs, and trees to promote health and to treat and balance the mind, body, and spirit. These essential oils are highly concentrated, complex essences, and are mixed with lotions or creams before they are applied to the skin (e.g., for a back massage). Certain essential oils can tone the uterus, encourage contractions, reduce pain, relieve tension, diminish fear and anxiety, and enhance the feeling of well-being. Lavender, rose, and jasmine oils can promote relaxation and reduce pain. Rose oil also acts as an antidepressant and uterine tonic, while jasmine oil strengthens contractions and decreases feelings of panic in addition to reducing pain. Essential oils of bergamot or rosemary can be diffused or used in a massage oil to relieve exhaustion (Gilbert, 2011; Tournaire & Theau-Yonneau, 2007; Walls, 2009). Oils may also be used by adding a few drops to a warm bath, to warm water used for soaking compresses that can be applied to the body, or to

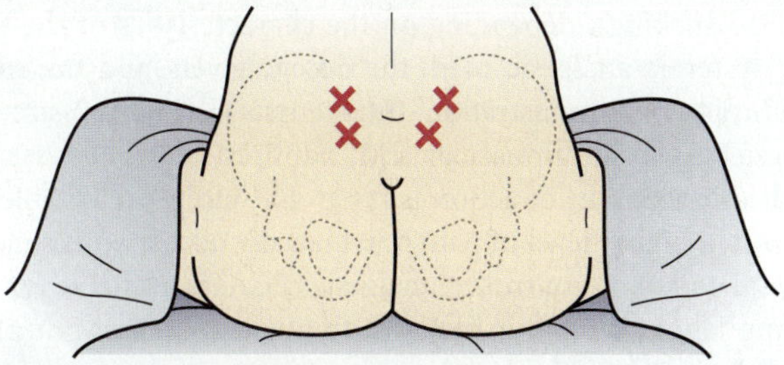

FIG. 17-7 Intradermal injections of 0.1 ml of sterile water in the treatment of women with back pain during labor. Sterile water is injected into four locations on the lower back, two over each posterior superior iliac spine (PSIS) and two 3 cm below and 1 cm medial to the PSIS. The injections should raise a bleb on the skin. Simultaneous injections administered by two clinicians will decrease the pain of the injections. (Source: Leeman, L., Fontaine, P., King, V., Klein, M., & Ratcliffe, S. [2003]. The nature and management of labor pain: Part I. Nonpharmacologic pain relief. *American Family Physician 68*[6], 1109-1112.)

an aromatherapy lamp to vaporize a room. Drops of essential oils can be put on a pillow or on a woman's brow or palms, or used as an ingredient in creating massage oil (Simkin & Bolding, 2004; Walls; Zwelling et al., 2006). Certain odors or scents can evoke pleasant memories and feelings of love and security. As a result, it would be helpful for a woman to choose the scents that she will use (Trout, 2004). Currently there is insufficient evidence to support the effectiveness of aromatherapy for pain relief in labor although its use has elicited promising results (Berghella et al., 2008; Smith et al., 2006; Zwelling et al.).

Intradermal Water Block

An intradermal water block involves the injection of small amounts of sterile water (e.g., 0.05 to 0.1 ml) by using a fine needle (e.g., 25 gauge) into four locations on the lower back to relieve low back pain (Fig. 17-7). It is a simple procedure that can be performed by the nurse and is effective in early labor and in an effort to delay the initiation of pharmacologic pain relief measures (Hawkins et al., 2007). Intense stinging will occur for about 20 to 30 seconds after injection, but relief of back pain for up to 2 hours has been reported. The procedure can be repeated although the woman may find that the stinging that occurs with administration creates too much discomfort (Creehan, 2008). Effectiveness of this method is probably related to the mechanisms of counterirritation (i.e., reducing localized pain in one area by irritating the skin in an area nearby), gate control, or an increase in the level of endogenous opioids (endorphins). When the effect wears off, the treatment can be repeated, or another method of pain relief can be used (Fogarty, 2008; Tournaire & Theau-Yonneau, 2007).

PHARMACOLOGIC PAIN MANAGEMENT

Pharmacologic measures for pain management should be implemented before pain becomes so severe that catecholamines increase and labor is prolonged. It is unacceptable for women in labor to endure severe pain when safe and effective relief measures are available (American College of Obstetricians and Gynecologists [ACOG], 2004). Pharmacologic and nonpharmacologic measures, when used together, increase the level of pain relief and create a more positive labor experience for the woman and her family. Nonpharmacologic measures can be used for relaxation and pain relief, especially in early labor. Pharmacologic measures can be implemented as labor becomes more active and discomfort and pain intensify. Less pharmacologic intervention often is required because nonpharmacologic measures enhance relaxation and potentiate the analgesic effect. However, women are increasingly using pharmacologic measures, especially epidural analgesia, to relieve their pain during labor and birth.

Sedatives

Sedatives relieve anxiety and induce sleep. They may be given to a woman experiencing a prolonged latent phase of labor when there is a need to decrease anxiety or promote sleep. They may also be given to augment analgesics and reduce nausea when an opioid is used.

Barbiturates such as secobarbital sodium (Seconal) can cause undesirable side effects including respiratory and vasomotor depression affecting the woman and newborn. Because of the potential for neonatal central nervous system (CNS) depression, barbiturates should be avoided if birth is anticipated within 12 to 24 hours. The depressant effects are increased if a barbiturate is administered with another CNS depressant such as an opioid analgesic. However, pain will be magnified if a barbiturate is given without an analgesic to women experiencing pain because normal coping mechanisms may be blunted. As a result of these disadvantages, barbiturates are seldom used during labor (Creehan, 2008; Hawkins et al., 2007).

Phenothiazines (e.g., promethazine [Phenergan], hydroxyzine [Vistaril]) do not relieve pain but are often given with opioids to decrease anxiety and apprehension, increase sedation, and reduce nausea and vomiting. Promethazine is probably the most widely used drug in this class. It causes significant sedation and has been shown to impair the analgesic efficacy of opioids. Using opioids with less potential to cause nausea and vomiting should make the routine use of promethazine unnecessary Metoclopramide (Reglan) is an antiemetic that causes little sedation and may potentiate the effects of analgesics, Ondansetron (Zofran) is another very effective antiemetic that has few side effects. Whenever possible, it should be used instead of promethazine (Hawkins et al., 2007).

Benzodiazepines (e.g., diazepam [Valium], lorazepam [Ativan]), when given with an opioid analgesic, seem to enhance pain relief and reduce nausea and vomiting. Because benzodiazepines cause significant maternal amnesia, however, their use should be avoided during labor. A major disadvantage of diazepam is that it disrupts thermoregulation in newborns, making them less able to maintain body temperature (Hawkins et al., 2007).

Analgesia and Anesthesia

The use of analgesia and anesthesia was not generally accepted as part of obstetric management until Queen Victoria used chloroform during the birth of her son in 1853. Since then much study has gone into the development of pharmacologic measures for controlling discomfort during the birth period. The goal of researchers is to develop methods that will provide adequate pain relief to women without increasing maternal or fetal risk or affecting the progress of labor.

Nursing management of obstetric analgesia and anesthesia combines the nurse's expertise in maternity care with a

BOX 17-4 PHARMACOLOGIC CONTROL OF DISCOMFORT BY STAGE OF LABOR AND METHOD OF BIRTH

FIRST STAGE
- Systemic analgesia
- Opioid agonist analgesics
- Opioid agonist-antagonist analgesics
- Epidural (block) analgesia
- Combined spinal-epidural (CSE) analgesia
- Nitrous oxide

SECOND STAGE
- Nerve block analgesia and anesthesia
- Local infiltration anesthesia
- Pudendal block
- Spinal (block) anesthesia
- Epidural (block) analgesia
- CSE analgesia
- Nitrous oxide

VAGINAL BIRTH
- Local infiltration anesthesia
- Pudendal block
- Epidural (block) analgesia and anesthesia
- Spinal (block) anesthesia
- CSE analgesia and anesthesia
- Nitrous oxide

CESAREAN BIRTH
- Spinal (block) anesthesia
- Epidural (block) anesthesia
- General anesthesia

knowledge and understanding of anatomy and physiology and of medications and their therapeutic effects, adverse reactions, and methods of administration.

Anesthesia encompasses analgesia, amnesia, relaxation, and reflex activity. Anesthesia abolishes pain perception by interrupting the nerve impulses to the brain. The loss of sensation may be partial or complete, sometimes with the loss of consciousness.

The term **analgesia** refers to the alleviation of the sensation of pain or the raising of the threshold for pain perception without loss of consciousness.

The type of analgesic or anesthetic chosen is determined in part by the stage of labor of the woman and by the method of birth planned (Box 17-4).

Systemic Analgesia

Use of **systemic analgesia** for relieving the pain of labor has been declining, although it still remains the major pharmacologic method for relieving the pain of labor when personnel trained in regional analgesia (e.g., epidural analgesia) are not available (Bucklin, Hawkins, Anderson, & Ullrich, 2005). Systemic analgesics cross the maternal blood-brain barrier to provide central analgesic effects. They also cross the placenta. Once transferred to the fetus, analgesics cross the fetal blood-brain barrier more readily than the maternal blood-brain barrier. The duration of action also will be longer because the systemic analgesics used during labor have a significantly longer half-life in the fetus and newborn. Effects on the fetus and newborn can be profound (e.g., respiratory depression, decreased alertness, delayed sucking), depending on the characteristics of the specific systemic analgesic used, the dosage given, and the route and timing of administration. Intravenous (IV) administration is preferred to intramuscular (IM) administration because the medication's onset of action is faster and more predictable; as a result, a higher level of pain relief usually occurs with smaller doses. IV patient-controlled analgesia (PCA) is available for use during labor. With this method, the woman self-administers small doses of an opioid analgesic by using a pump programmed for dose and frequency. Overall, a lower total amount of analgesic is used, and women appreciate the sense of autonomy provided by this method of pain relief (Hawkins et al., 2007).

Classifications of analgesic drugs used to relieve the pain of childbirth include opioid (narcotic) agonists and opioid (narcotic) agonist-antagonists. Choice of which medication to use often depends on the primary health care provider's preferences and the characteristics of the laboring woman. The type of systemic analgesics used therefore often varies among obstetric units.

Opioid Agonist Analgesics. **Opioid (narcotic) agonist analgesics** such as hydromorphone hydrochloride (Dilaudid), meperidine (Demerol), fentanyl (Sublimaze), and sufentanil citrate (Sufenta) are effective for relieving severe, persistent, or recurrent pain by blunting the perception of pain, though not eliminating it completely. As pure opioid agonists they stimulate major opioid receptors, mu and kappa. They have no amnesic effect but create a feeling of well-being or euphoria and enhance a woman's ability to rest between contractions. Because opioids can inhibit uterine contractions, they should not be administered until labor is well established unless they are being used to enhance therapeutic rest during a prolonged latent phase of labor (Creehan, 2008). These analgesics decrease gastric emptying and increase nausea and vomiting. Bladder and bowel elimination can be inhibited. Because heart rate (e.g., bradycardia, tachycardia), blood pressure (e.g., hypotension), and respiratory effort (e.g., depression) can be adversely affected, opioid analgesics should be used cautiously in women with respiratory and cardiovascular disorders. Safety precautions should be taken because sedation and dizziness can occur after administration, increasing the risk for injury.

SAFETY ALERT

Opioids decrease maternal heart and respiratory rate and blood pressure, which affects fetal oxygenation. Therefore maternal vital signs and FHR and pattern must be assessed and documented prior to and after administration of opioids for pain relief.

Hydromorphone hydrochloride (Dilaudid) is a potent opioid agonist analgesic that can be administered by IV or IM route during labor. After IV administration the onset of action occurs within 10 to 15 minutes, the peak effect is reached in 15 to 30 minutes, and the duration of action is approximately 2 to 3 hours. IM administration has an onset of action in 15 minutes, with a peak in 30 to 60 minutes and a duration of action of approximately 4 to 5 hours.

Meperidine hydrochloride (Demerol) used to be the most commonly used opioid agonist analgesic for women in labor, but is no longer the preferred choice because other medications have fewer side effects. In particular, the accumulation of normeperidine, a toxic metabolite of meperidine, causes prolonged neonatal sedation and neurobehavioral changes that are evident for the first 2 to 3 days of life (Hawkins et al., 2007). When it is used, the onset of action after IV administration is almost immediate and the duration of action is approximately 1.5 to 2 hours. The onset of action begins in 10 to 20 minutes after an IM injection of meperidine and the duration is 2 to 3 hours (Hawkins et al.).

Fentanyl citrate (Sublimaze) and sufentanil citrate (Sufenta) are potent short-acting opioid agonist analgesics. Sufentanil use is increasing because it has a more potent analgesic action than fentanyl when given through an epidural catheter. Also less sufentanil will cross the placenta, resulting in reduced fetal exposure. Onset of action after IV injection occurs within 2 to 5 minutes, the action peaks in 3 to 5 minutes, and the duration of action is approximately 30 to 60 minutes. Onset of the medication action occurs in 7 to 8 minutes after IM injection, reaches its peak effect in 20 to 30 minutes, and lasts for 1 to 2 hours. More frequent dosing is required with fentanyl and sufentanil because of their relatively short duration of action (Hawkins et al., 2007). As a result, these opioids are most commonly administered intrathecally or epidurally, alone or in combination with a local anesthetic agent (e.g., bupivacaine [Marcaine]) (see the Medication Guide: Opioid Agonist Analgesics).

Ideally, birth should occur less than 1 hour or more than 4 hours after administration of an opioid agonist analgesic so that neonatal CNS depression resulting from the opioid is minimized.

Opioid (Narcotic) Agonist-Antagonist Analgesics. An agonist is an agent that activates or stimulates a receptor to act; an antagonist is an agent that blocks a receptor or a medication designed to activate a receptor. **Opioid (narcotic) agonist-antagonist analgesics** such as butorphanol (Stadol) and nalbuphine (Nubain) are agonists at kappa opioid receptors and are either antagonists or weak agonists at mu opioid receptors. In the doses used during labor, these mixed opioids provide adequate analgesia without causing significant respiratory depression in the mother or neonate. They are less likely to cause nausea and vomiting, but sedation may be as great or greater when compared with pure opioid agonists. As a result of these effects, parenteral opioid agonist-antagonist analgesics are used more commonly during labor than the opioid agonist analgesics. Intramuscular, subcutaneous, and intravenous routes of administration can be used, but the IV route is preferred. This classification of opioid analgesics, especially nalbuphine, is not suitable for women with an opioid dependence because the antagonist activity could precipitate withdrawal symptoms (abstinence syndrome) in both the mother and her newborn (Hawkins et al., 2007) (see the Medication Guide: Opioid Agonist-Antagonist Analgesics and Signs of Potential Complications box: Maternal Opioid Abstinence Syndrome).

MEDICATION GUIDE

Opioid Agonist Analgesics

Fentanyl Citrate (Sublimaze)
Sufentanil Citrate (Sufenta)

ACTION

Opioid agonist analgesics that stimulate both mu and kappa opioid receptors to decrease the transmission of pain impulses, rapid action with short duration (0.5 to 1 hour IV; 1 to 2 hours epidural); sufentanil citrate has a more potent analgesic action than fentanyl citrate with less passage across the placenta to the fetus.

INDICATION

Because of their short duration of action when given intravenously, they are most commonly administered epidurally or intrathecally, alone or in combination with a local anesthetic agent, to relieve moderate to severe labor pain and postoperative pain after cesarean birth.

DOSAGE AND ROUTE

Fentanyl citrate: 25 to 50 mcg IV; 1 to 2 mcg with 0.125% bupivacaine at rate of 8 to 10 ml/hr epidurally
Sufentanil citrate: 10 to 15 mcg with 0.125% bupivacaine at rate of 10 ml/hr epidurally

ADVERSE EFFECTS

Dizziness, drowsiness, allergic reactions, rash, pruritus, maternal and fetal or neonatal respiratory depression, nausea and vomiting, urinary retention

NURSING CONSIDERATIONS

Assess for respiratory depression; naloxone should be available as an antidote.

MEDICATION GUIDE

Opioid Agonist-Antagonist Analgesics

Butorphanol Tartrate (Stadol)
Nalbuphine Hydrochloride (Nubain)

ACTION

Mixed agonist-antagonist analgesics that stimulate kappa opioid receptors and block or weakly stimulate mu opioid receptors, resulting in good analgesia but with less respiratory depression and nausea and vomiting when compared with opioid agonist analgesics

INDICATION

Moderate to severe labor pain and postoperative pain after cesarean birth

DOSAGE AND ROUTE

Butorphanol tartrate: 1 mg (range 0.5 to 2 mg) IV every 3 to 4 hours as needed; 2 mg (range 1 to 4 mg) IM every 3-4 hours as needed
Nalbuphine hydrochloride: 5 to 10 mg IV every 3 hours as needed; 10 to 20 mg IM every 3 to 4 hours as needed

ADVERSE EFFECTS

Confusion, sedation, hallucinations, "floating" feeling, drowsiness, headache, dizziness, nervousness, sweating; maternal palpitations and tachycardia or bradycardia; transient nonpathologic sinusoidal-like fetal heart rate rhythm; respiratory depression; nausea and vomiting; difficulty with urination (retention, urgency)

NURSING CONSIDERATIONS

May precipitate withdrawal symptoms in opioid-dependent women and their newborns. Assess maternal vital signs, degree of pain, FHR, and uterine activity before and after administration; observe for maternal respiratory depression, notifying primary health care provider if maternal respirations are ≤12 breaths/min; encourage voiding every 2 hours and palpate for bladder distention; if birth occurs within 1 to 4 hours of dose administration, observe newborn for respiratory depression; implement safety measures as appropriate, including use of side rails and assistance with ambulation; continue use of nonpharmacologic pain-relief measures.

SIGNS OF POTENTIAL COMPLICATIONS

Maternal Opioid Abstinence Syndrome (Opioid/Narcotic Withdrawal)

- Yawning, rhinorrhea (runny nose), sweating, lacrimation (tearing), mydriasis (dilation of pupils)
- Anorexia
- Irritability, restlessness, generalized anxiety
- Tremors
- Chills and hot flashes
- Piloerection ("gooseflesh" or "chill bumps")
- Violent sneezing
- Weakness, fatigue, and drowsiness
- Nausea and vomiting
- Diarrhea, abdominal cramps
- Bone and muscle pain, muscle spasms, kicking movements

Opioid (Narcotic) Antagonists. Opioids such as hydromorphone, meperidine, and fentanyl can cause excessive CNS depression in the mother, the newborn, or both, although the current practice of giving lower doses of opioids intravenously has reduced the incidence and severity of opioid-induced CNS depression. **Opioid (narcotic) antagonists** such as naloxone (Narcan) can promptly reverse the CNS depressant effects, especially respiratory depression. In addition, the antagonist counters the effect of the stress-induced levels of endorphins. An opioid antagonist is especially valuable if labor is more rapid than expected and birth is anticipated when the opioid is at its peak effect. The antagonist may be given through an IV line, or it can be administered intramuscularly (see the Medication Guide: Opioid Antagonist). The woman should be told that the pain that was relieved with the use of the opioid analgesic will return with the administration of the opioid antagonist.

! NURSING ALERT

An opioid antagonist (e.g., naloxone [Narcan]) is contraindicated for opioid-dependent women because it may precipitate abstinence syndrome (withdrawal symptoms). For the same reason, opioid agonist-antagonist analgesics such as butorphanol (Stadol) and nalbuphine (Nubain) should not be given to opioid-dependent women (see the Signs of Potential Complications box: Maternal Opioid Abstinence Syndrome).

An opioid antagonist can be given to the newborn as one part of the treatment for **neonatal narcosis,** which is a state of CNS depression in the newborn produced by an opioid. Prophylactic administration of naloxone is controversial. Affected infants may exhibit respiratory depression, hypotonia, lethargy, and a delay in temperature regulation. Risk for hypoxia, hypercarbia, and acidosis increases if neonatal narcosis is not treated promptly. Treatment involves ventilation, administration of oxygen, and gentle stimulation. Naloxone is administered, if still required, to reverse CNS depression. More than one dose of naloxone may be required because its half-life is shorter than the half-life of opioids. Alterations in neurologic and behavioral responses may be evident in the newborn for as long as 2 to 4 days after birth. The significance of these neurobehavioral changes is unknown (Hawkins et al., 2007).

MEDICATION GUIDE

Opioid Antagonist

Naloxone Hydrochloride (Narcan)

ACTION

Opioid antagonist that blocks both mu and kappa opioid receptors from the effects of opioid agonists

INDICATION

Reverses opioid-induced respiratory depression in woman or newborn; may be used to reverse pruritus from epidural opioids

DOSAGE AND ROUTE

Adult

Opioid overdose: 0.4 to 2 mg IV, may repeat IV at 2- to 3-min intervals up to 10 mg; if IV route unavailable, IM or subcutaneous administration may be used

Postoperative opioid depression: Initial dose 0.1 to 0.2 mg IV at 2- to 3-min intervals up to 3 doses until desired degree of reversal obtained; may repeat dose in 1 to 2 hours if needed

Newborn

Opioid-induced depression: Initial dose is 0.1 mg/kg IV, IM, or subcutaneously; may be repeated at 2- to 3-min intervals up to 3 doses until desired degree of reversal obtained

ADVERSE EFFECTS

Maternal hypotension or hypertension, tachycardia, hyperventilation, nausea and vomiting, sweating, and tremulousness

NURSING CONSIDERATIONS

Woman should delay breastfeeding until medication is out of her system; do not give to woman or the newborn if the woman is opioid dependent—may cause abrupt withdrawal in the woman and newborn; if given to woman for reversal of respiratory depression caused by opioid analgesic, pain will return suddenly.

Nerve Block Analgesia and Anesthesia

A variety of local anesthetic agents are used in obstetrics to produce regional analgesia (some pain relief and motor block) and anesthesia (complete pain relief and motor block). Most of these agents are related chemically to cocaine and end with the suffix *-caine.* This helps to identify a local anesthetic.

The principal pharmacologic effect of local anesthetics is the temporary interruption of the conduction of nerve impulses, notably pain. Examples of common agents given are bupivacaine (Marcaine), chloroprocaine (Nesacaine), lidocaine (Xylocaine), ropivacaine (Naropin), and mepivacaine (Carbocaine). Rarely, people are sensitive (allergic) to one or more local anesthetics. Such a reaction may include respiratory depression, hypotension, and other serious adverse effects. Epinephrine, antihistamines, oxygen, and supportive measures should reverse these effects. Sensitivity may be identified by administering minute amounts of the drug to test for an allergic reaction.

Local Perineal Infiltration Anesthesia. **Local perineal infiltration anesthesia** may be used when an episiotomy is to be performed or when lacerations must be sutured after birth in a woman who does not have regional anesthesia. Rapid anesthesia is produced by injecting approximately 10 to 20 ml of 1% lidocaine or 2% chloroprocaine into the skin and then subcutaneously into the region to be anesthetized. Epinephrine often is added to the solution to localize and intensify the effect of the anesthesia in a region and to prevent excessive bleeding and

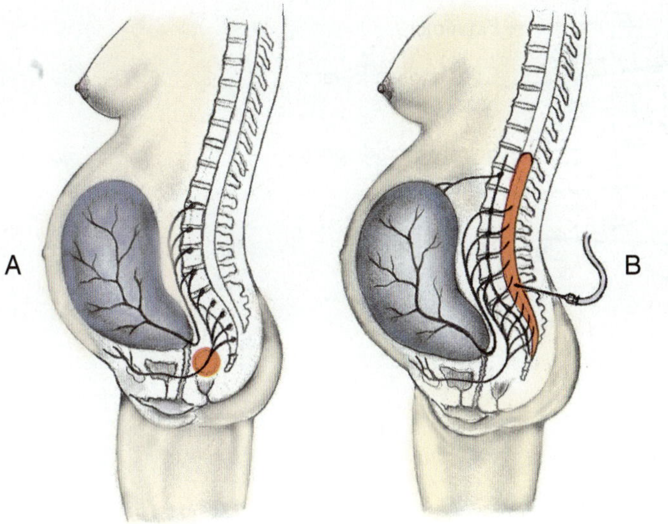

FIG. 17-8 Pain pathways and sites of pharmacologic nerve blocks. **A,** Pudendal nerve block: suitable during second and third stages of labor and for repair of episiotomy or lacerations. **B,** Epidural block: suitable for all stages of labor and types of birth, and for repair of episiotomy and lacerations.

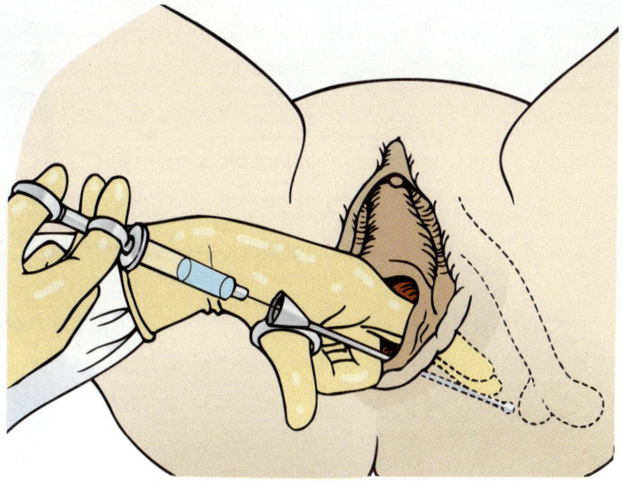

FIG. 17-9 Pudendal nerve block. Use of needle guide (Iowa trumpet) and Luer-Lok syringe to inject medication.

systemic absorption by constricting local blood vessels. Injections can be repeated to keep the woman comfortable while postbirth repairs are completed.

Pudendal Nerve Block. Pudendal nerve block, administered late in the second stage of labor, is useful if an episiotomy is to be performed or if forceps or a vacuum extractor are to be used to facilitate birth. It can also be administered during the third stage of labor if an episiotomy or lacerations must be repaired (American Academy of Pediatrics [AAP] & ACOG, 2007). A pudendal nerve block is considered to be reasonably effective for pain relief, simple to perform, and very safe (Cunningham, Leveno, Bloom, Hauth, Rouse, & Spong, 2010; Hawkins et al., 2007). Although a pudendal nerve block does not relieve the pain from uterine contractions, it does relieve pain in the lower vagina, the vulva, and the perineum (Fig. 17-8, *A*). A pudendal nerve block should be administered 10 to 20 minutes before perineal anesthesia is needed.

The pudendal nerve traverses the sacrosciatic notch just medial to the tip of the ischial spine on each side. Injection of an anesthetic solution at or near these points anesthetizes the pudendal nerves peripherally (Fig. 17-9). The transvaginal approach is generally used because it is less painful for the woman, has a higher rate of success in blocking pain, and tends to cause fewer fetal complications (Hawkins et al., 2007). Pudendal block does not change maternal hemodynamic or respiratory functions, vital signs, or the FHR. However, the bearing-down reflex is lessened or lost completely.

Spinal Anesthesia. In spinal anesthesia (block), an anesthetic solution containing a local anesthetic alone or in combination with an opioid agonist analgesic is injected through the third, fourth, or fifth lumbar interspace into the subarachnoid space (Fig. 17-10, *A* and *B*), where the anesthetic solution mixes with cerebrospinal fluid (CSF). The use of this technique has increased for both elective and emergent cesarean births and is more common than epidural anesthesia for these types of births (Bucklin et al., 2005). Low spinal anesthesia (block) may be used for vaginal birth, but it is not suitable for labor. Spinal anesthesia (block) used for cesarean birth provides anesthesia from the nipple (T6) to the feet. If it is used for vaginal birth, the anesthesia level is from the hips (T10) to the feet (see Fig. 17-10, *C*).

For spinal anesthesia (block), the woman sits or lies on her side (e.g., modified Sims position) with back curved to widen the intervertebral space to facilitate insertion of a small-gauge spinal needle and injection of the anesthetic solution into the spinal canal. The nurse supports the woman and encourages her to use breathing and relaxation techniques because she must remain still during the placement of the spinal needle. The needle is inserted and the anesthetic injected between contractions. After the anesthetic solution has been injected, the woman may be positioned upright to allow the heavier (hyperbaric) anesthetic solution to flow downward to obtain the lower level of anesthesia suitable for a vaginal birth. To obtain the higher level of anesthesia desired for cesarean birth she will be positioned supine with head and shoulders slightly elevated. In order to prevent supine hypotensive syndrome, the uterus is displaced laterally by tilting the operating table or placing a wedge under one of her hips. Usually the level of the block will be complete and fixed within 5 to 10 minutes after the anesthetic solution is injected but it can continue to creep upward for 20 minutes or longer. The anesthetic effect will last 1 to 3 hours, depending on the type of agent used (Hawkins et al., 2007) (Fig. 17-11).

SAFETY ALERT

To reduce the risk for transmission of pathogens, it is recommended that masks be worn during the induction of intrathecal and epidural anesthesia/analgesia.

Marked hypotension, impaired placental perfusion, and an ineffective breathing pattern may occur during spinal anesthesia. Before induction of the spinal anesthetic, maternal vital signs are assessed and a 20- to 30-minute EFM strip is obtained and evaluated. In addition, the woman's fluid balance is assessed. A bolus of IV fluid (usually 500 to 1000 ml of lactated Ringer's or

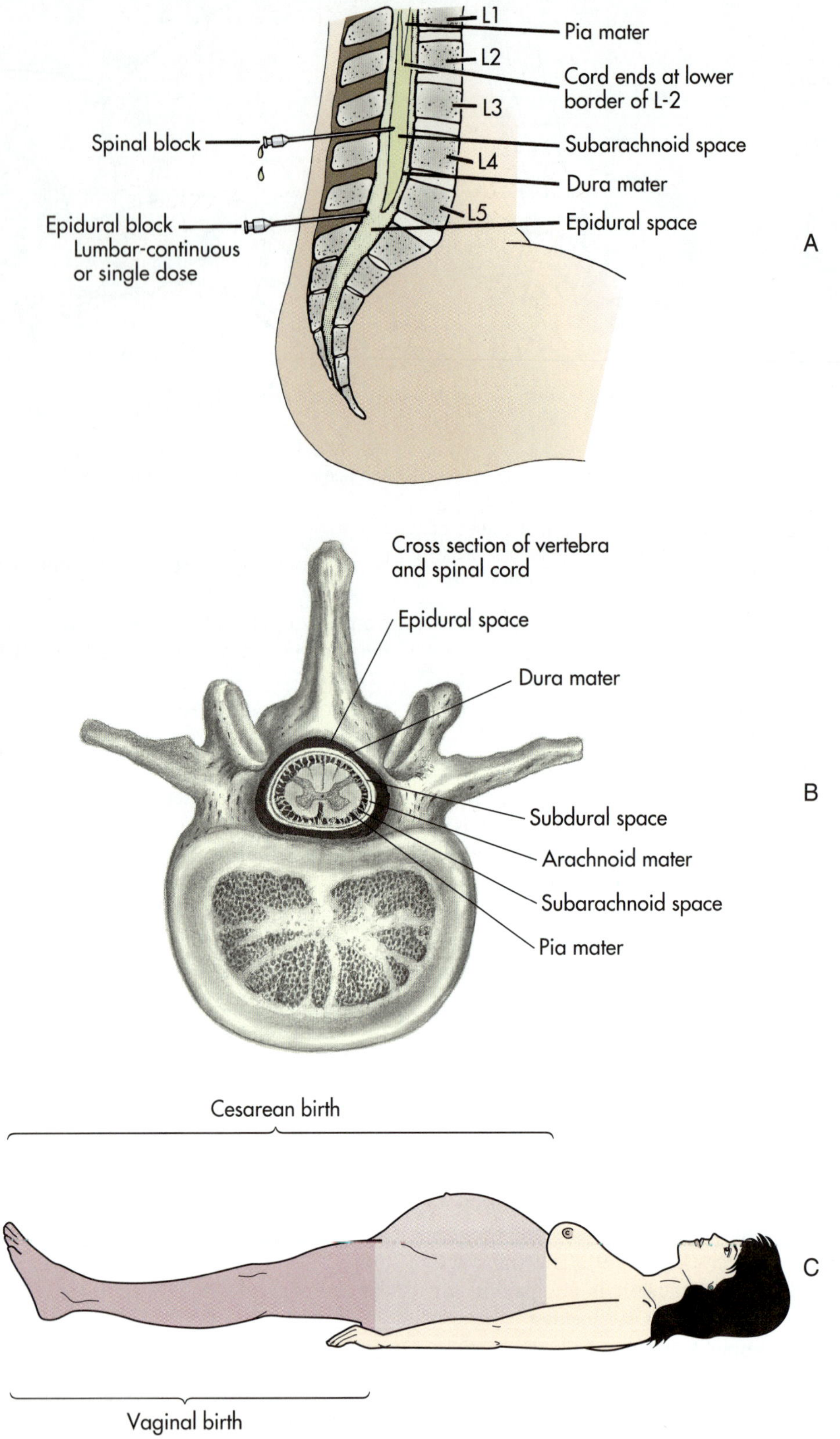

FIG. 17-10 A, Membranes and spaces of spinal cord and levels of sacral, lumbar, and thoracic nerves. **B,** Cross section of vertebra and spinal cord. **C,** Level of anesthesia necessary for cesarean birth and for vaginal births.

normal saline solution) may be administered 15 to 30 minutes prior to induction of the anesthetic to decrease the potential for hypotension caused by sympathetic blockade (vasodilation with pooling of blood in the lower extremities decreases cardiac output). Although the practice guidelines for obstetric anesthesia published by the American Society of Anesthesiologists (2007) state that this preanesthetic fluid bolus is not required, it is still usually administered in most clinical settings.

After induction of the anesthetic, maternal blood pressure, pulse, and respirations and fetal heart rate and pattern

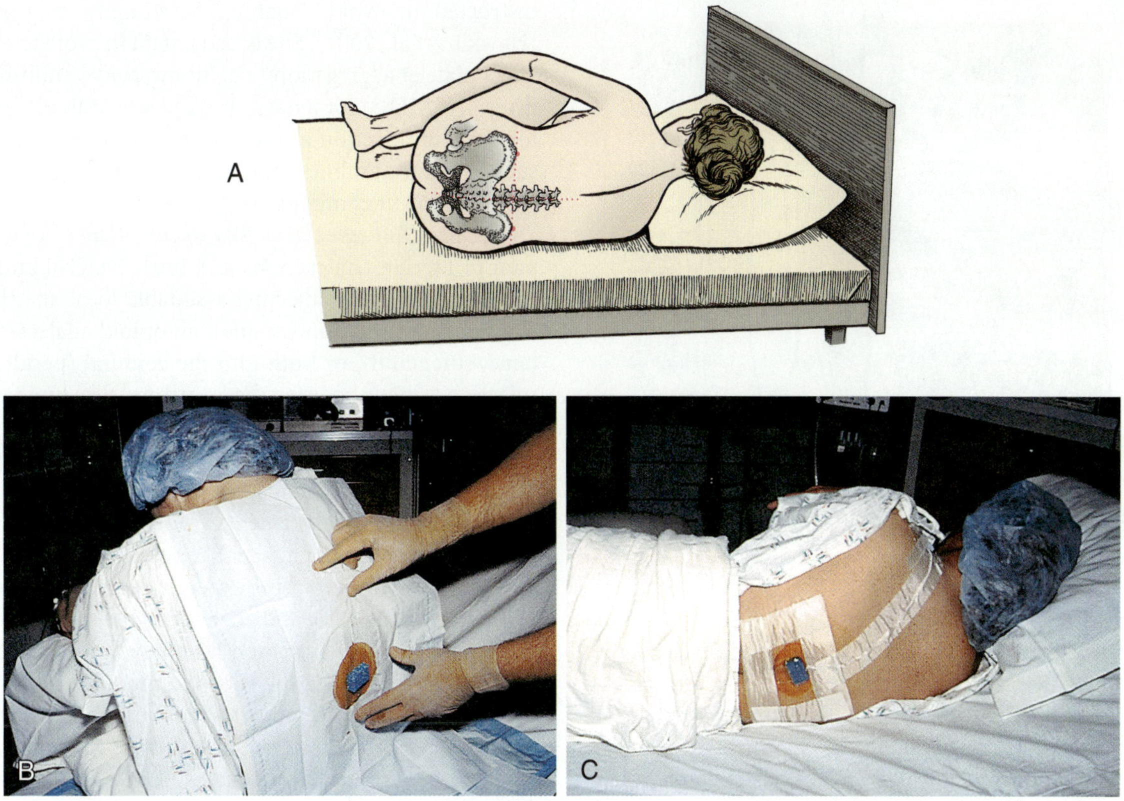

FIG. 17-11 Positioning for spinal and epidural blocks. **A,** Lateral position. **B,** Upright position. **C,** Catheter for epidural is taped to woman's back with port segment located near her shoulder. **(B** and **C,** Courtesy Michael S. Clement, MD, Mesa, AZ.)

must be checked and documented every 5 to 10 minutes. If signs of serious maternal hypotension (e.g., a drop in systolic blood pressure to 100 mm Hg or less or below 20% of the baseline blood pressure) or fetal distress (e.g., bradycardia, minimal or absent variability, late decelerations) develop, emergency care must be given (Creehan, 2008) (see the Emergency box: Maternal Hypotension with Decreased Placental Perfusion).

Because the woman is unable to sense her contractions, she must be instructed when to bear down during a vaginal birth. Use of a combination of local anesthetic agent and an opioid reduces the degree of motor function loss, enhancing a woman's ability to push effectively. If the birth occurs in a delivery room (rather than a labor-delivery-recovery room), the woman will need assistance in the transfer to a recovery bed after expulsion of the placenta and perineal repair if required.

Advantages of spinal anesthesia include ease of administration and absence of fetal hypoxia with maintenance of maternal blood pressure within a normal range. Maternal consciousness is maintained, excellent muscular relaxation is achieved, and blood loss is not excessive.

Disadvantages of spinal anesthesia include possible medication reactions (e.g., allergy), hypotension, and an ineffective breathing pattern; cardiopulmonary resuscitation may be needed. When a spinal anesthetic is given, the need for operative birth (e.g., episiotomy, forceps-assisted birth, or vacuum-assisted birth) tends to increase because voluntary expulsive efforts are reduced or eliminated. After birth, the incidence of bladder and uterine atony, as well as postdural puncture headache, is higher.

EMERGENCY

Maternal Hypotension with Decreased Placental Perfusion

SIGNS AND SYMPTOMS

- Maternal hypotension (20% decrease from preblock baseline level or ≤100 mm Hg systolic)
- Fetal bradycardia
- Absent or minimal FHR variability

INTERVENTIONS

- Turn woman to lateral position or place pillow or wedge under hip to displace uterus.
- Maintain IV infusion at rate specified, or increase administration per hospital protocol.
- Administer oxygen by nonrebreather face mask at 10 to 12 L/min or per protocol.
- Elevate the woman's legs.
- Notify the primary health care provider, anesthesiologist, or nurse anesthetist.
- Administer IV vasopressor (e.g., ephedrine 5 to 10 mg or phenylephrine 50 to 100 mcg) per protocol if previous measures are ineffective.
- Remain with woman; continue to monitor maternal blood pressure and FHR every 5 minutes until her condition is stable or per primary health care provider's order.

Leakage of CSF from the site of puncture of the dura mater (membranous covering of the spinal cord) is thought to be the major causative factor in *postdural puncture headache* (PDPH), commonly referred to as a spinal headache. Spinal headache is much more likely to occur when the dura is accidentally

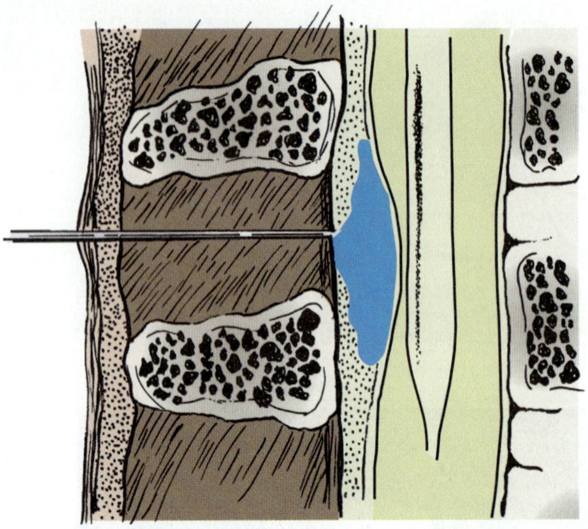

FIG. 17-12 Blood-patch therapy for spinal headache.

punctured during the process of administering an epidural block. The needle used for an epidural block has a much larger gauge than the one used for spinal anesthesia and thus creates a bigger opening in the dura, resulting in a greater loss of CSF. Presumably postural changes cause the diminished volume of CSF to exert traction on pain-sensitive CNS structures. Characteristically, assuming an upright position triggers or intensifies the headache, whereas assuming a supine position achieves relief (Hawkins et al., 2007). The resulting headache, auditory problems (e.g., tinnitus) and visual problems (e.g., blurred vision, photophobia) begin within 2 days of the puncture and may persist for days or weeks.

The likelihood of headache after dural puncture can be reduced, however, if the anesthesia care provider uses a small-gauge spinal needle and avoids making multiple punctures of the meninges. Passing an epidural catheter through the dural opening at the time of puncture to provide continuous spinal anesthesia, with removal of the catheter 24 hours later, may help prevent spinal headache. Injecting preservative-free saline through the spinal catheter before removing it also may decrease the incidence of headache. Hydration and bed rest in the prone position have been recommended as preventive measures, but have not been proven to be of much value (Hawkins et al., 2007).

Conservative management for a PDPH includes administration of oral analgesics and methylxanthines (e.g., caffeine or theophylline). Methylxanthines cause constriction of cerebral blood vessels and may provide symptomatic relief. An autologous **epidural blood patch** is the most rapid, reliable, and beneficial relief measure for PDPH. The woman's blood (i.e., 20 ml) is injected slowly into the lumbar epidural space, creating a clot that patches the tear or hole in the dura mater. Treatment with a blood patch is considered if the headache is severe or debilitating or does not resolve after conservative management. The blood patch is remarkably effective and is nearly complication free (Hawkins et al., 2007) (Fig. 17-12).

The woman should be observed for alteration in vital signs, pallor, clammy skin, and leakage of CSF for 1 to 2 hours after the blood patch is performed. If no complications occur, she may then resume normal activity. She should, however, be instructed to avoid coughing or straining for several days (Hawkins et al., 2007). She is also taught to avoid analgesics that affect platelet aggregation (e.g., nonsteroidal antiinflammatory drugs [NSAIDs]) for 2 days, drink plenty of fluids, and observe for signs of infection at the site and for neurologic symptoms such as pain, numbness and tingling in the legs, and difficulty with walking or elimination.

Epidural Anesthesia or Analgesia (Block). Relief from the pain of uterine contractions and birth (vaginal and cesarean) can be achieved by injecting a suitable local anesthetic agent (e.g., bupivacaine, ropivacaine), an opioid analgesic (e.g., fentanyl, sufentanil), or both into the epidural (peridural) space. Injection is made between the fourth and fifth lumbar vertebrae for a lumbar **epidural block** (see Figs. 17-8, *B*, and 17-10, *A*). Depending on the type, amount, and number of medications used, an anesthetic or analgesic effect will occur with varying degrees of motor impairment. The combination of an opioid with the local anesthetic agent reduces the dose of anesthetic required, thereby preserving a greater degree of motor function.

Epidural anesthesia and analgesia is the most effective pharmacologic pain relief method for labor that is currently available. As a result, it is the most commonly used method for relieving pain during labor in the United States, and its use has been increasing. Nearly two thirds of American women in labor choose epidural analgesia (AAP & ACOG, 2007; Bucklin et al., 2005; Hawkins et al., 2007). For relieving the discomfort of labor and vaginal birth, a block from T10 to S5 is required. For cesarean birth, a block from at least T8 to S1 is essential. The diffusion of epidural anesthesia depends on the location of the catheter tip, the dose and volume of the anesthetic agent used, and the woman's position (e.g., horizontal or head-up). The woman must cooperate and maintain her position without moving during the insertion of the epidural catheter in order to prevent misplacement, neurologic injury, or hematoma formation.

! NURSING ALERT

Epidural anesthesia effectively relieves the pain caused by uterine contractions. For most women, however, it does not completely remove the pressure sensations that occur as the fetus descends in the pelvis.

For the induction of an epidural block, the woman is positioned as for a spinal block. She may sit with her back curved or assume a modified Sims position with her shoulders parallel, legs slightly flexed, and back arched. It is important to avoid severe spinal flexion because it could compress the epidural space, increasing the risk for dural puncture (Creehan, 2008) (see Fig. 17-11). A large-bore needle is inserted into the epidural space. A catheter is then threaded through the needle until its tip rests in the epidural space. The needle is then removed and the catheter is taped in place. After the epidural catheter is inserted and secured, a small amount of medication, called a test dose, is injected to be sure that the catheter has not been accidentally placed in the subarachnoid (spinal) space or in a blood vessel (Hawkins et al., 2007).

It is often more difficult to insert an epidural catheter when the woman is obese. Morbidly obese patients are more likely to have failed epidural placement, and accidental dural puncture (Valleyo, 2007). While epidural catheter placement can present technical challenges, use of regional anesthesia can provide adequate pain management for the obese woman during labor and birth. Problems may be encountered when assisting her into a proper position and identifying the required landmarks to ensure location of the appropriate insertion site. Placing the catheter in early labor when the woman is more comfortable and is able to fully cooperate is a recommended solution (Creehan, 2008; Saravanakumar, Rao, & Cooper, 2006). Early placement of a functioning epidural may reduce the potential complications associated with intubation during an emergent delivery. Note that epidural anesthesia presents less risk for the obese woman than does general anesthesia (AAP & ACOG, 2007).

After the epidural has been initiated, the woman is positioned preferably on her side so that the uterus does not compress the ascending vena cava and descending aorta, which can impair venous return, reduce cardiac output and blood pressure, and decrease placental perfusion. Her position should be alternated from side to side every hour. Upright positions and ambulation may be possible, depending on the degree of motor impairment. Oxygen should be available if hypotension occurs despite maintenance of hydration with IV fluid and displacement of the uterus to the side. Ephedrine or phenylephrine (vasopressors used to increase maternal blood pressure) and increased IV fluid infusion may be needed (see the Emergency box on p. 403). The fetal heart rate and pattern, contraction pattern, and progress in labor must be monitored carefully because the woman may not be aware of changes in the strength of the uterine contractions or the descent of the presenting part.

Several methods can be used for an epidural block. An intermittent block is achieved by using repeated injections of anesthetic solution; it is the least common method. The most common method is the continuous block, achieved by using a pump to infuse the anesthetic solution through an indwelling plastic catheter. Patient-controlled epidural analgesia (PCEA) is the newest method; it uses an indwelling catheter and a programmed pump that allows the woman to control the dosing. This method has been found to provide optimal analgesia with higher maternal satisfaction and enhanced sense of control during labor while decreasing the total amount of medication, including local anesthetic, used (Saito, Okutomi, Kanai, Mochizuki, Tani, Amano, et al., 2005). Women using PCEA experience less sedation and nausea when compared with women using patient-controlled intravenous opioid analgesia (Halpern, Muir, Breen, Campbell, Barrett, Liston, et al., 2004).

The advantages of an epidural block are numerous: the woman remains alert and is more comfortable and able to participate, good relaxation is achieved, airway reflexes remain intact, only partial motor paralysis develops, gastric emptying is not delayed, and blood loss is not excessive. Fetal complications are rare but may occur in the event of rapid absorption of the medication or marked maternal hypotension. The dose, volume, type, and number of medications used can be modified to allow the woman to push, to assume upright positions and even to walk, to produce perineal anesthesia, and to permit forceps-assisted, vacuum-assisted, or cesarean birth if required.

BOX 17-5 SIDE EFFECTS OF EPIDURAL AND SPINAL ANESTHESIA

- Hypotension
- Local anesthetic toxicity
  - Lightheadedness
  - Dizziness
  - Tinnitus (ringing in the ears)
  - Metallic taste
  - Numbness of the tongue and mouth
  - Bizarre behavior
  - Slurred speech
  - Convulsions
  - Loss of consciousness
- High or total spinal anesthesia
- Fever
- Urinary retention
- Pruritus (itching)
- Limited movement
- Longer second stage labor
- Increased use of oxytocin
- Increased likelihood of forceps- or vacuum-assisted birth

Video—Nursing Skills: Assisting with an Epidural

The disadvantages of epidural block also are numerous. The woman's ability to move freely and to maintain control of her labor is limited, related to the use of numerous medical interventions (e.g., an intravenous infusion and electronic monitoring) and the occurrence of orthostatic hypotension and dizziness, sedation, and weakness of the legs. CNS effects (Box 17-5) can occur if a solution containing a local anesthetic agent is accidentally injected into a blood vessel or if excessive amounts of local anesthetic are given. High spinal or "total spinal" anesthesia, resulting in respiratory arrest, can occur if the relatively high dosage used with an epidural block is accidentally injected into the subarachnoid space. Women who receive an epidural have a higher rate of fever (i.e., intrapartum temperature of 38° C or higher), especially when labor lasts longer than 12 hours; the temperature elevation most likely is related to thermoregulatory changes, although infection cannot be ruled out. The elevation in temperature can result in fetal tachycardia and neonatal workup for sepsis, whether or not signs of infection are present (see Box 17-5).

Severe hypotension (systolic blood pressure 100 mm Hg or less or more than a 20% decrease from the baseline blood pressure) as a result of sympathetic blockade can be an outcome of an epidural block (Anim-Somuah, Smyth, & Howell, 2008) (see the Emergency box on p. 403). It can result in a significant decrease in uteroplacental perfusion and oxygen delivery to the fetus. Urinary retention and stress incontinence can occur in the immediate postpartum period. This temporary difficulty in urinary elimination could be related not only to the effects of the epidural block but also to the increased duration of labor and need for forceps- or vacuum-assisted birth associated with the block. Pruritus (itching) is a side effect that often occurs with the use of an opioid, especially fentanyl. A relationship between epidural analgesia and longer second-stage labor, use of oxytocin, and forceps- or vacuum-assisted birth has been documented. Research findings have been unable to demonstrate a significant increase in cesarean birth associated with epidural analgesia (Cunningham et al., 2010). For some women, the epidural block is not effective, and a second form of analgesia is required to establish effective pain relief. When women progress rapidly in labor, pain relief may not be obtained before birth occurs.

Combined Spinal-Epidural (CSE) Analgesia. In the CSE analgesia technique, sometimes referred to as a "walking epidural," an epidural needle is inserted into the epidural space. Before the epidural catheter is placed, a smaller-gauge spinal needle is inserted through the bore of the epidural needle into the subarachnoid space. A small amount of opioid or combination of opioid and local anesthetic is then injected intrathecally to rapidly provide analgesia. Afterward the epidural catheter is inserted as usual. The CSE technique is an increasingly popular approach that can be used to block pain transmission without compromising motor ability. The concentration of opioid receptors is high along the pain pathway in the spinal cord, in the brainstem, and in the thalamus. Because these receptors are highly sensitive to opioids, a small quantity of an opioid-agonist analgesic produces marked pain relief lasting for several hours. If additional pain relief is needed, medication can be injected through the epidural catheter (see Fig. 17-10, *A*). The most common side effects of CSE are pruritus, urinary retention, immediate or delayed respiratory depression, and nausea. Naloxone can be given intravenously to manage these side effects without decreasing the degree of analgesia achieved (Cunningham et al., 2010; Hawkins et al., 2007). CSE analgesia is also associated with a greater incidence of FHR abnormalities than is epidural analgesia alone, necessitating close assessment of fetal heart rate and pattern (Cunningham et al.).

Although women can walk (hence the term "walking epidural"), they often choose not to do so because of sedation and fatigue, abnormal sensations in and weakness of the legs, and a feeling of insecurity. Often health care providers are reluctant to encourage or assist women to ambulate for fear of injury. However, women can be assisted to change positions and use upright positions during labor and birth. Upright positioning is associated with less pain and more efficient labor progress. Enhanced motor function facilitates more effective bearing-down efforts, thereby reducing the risk for forceps- or vacuum-assisted birth (Albers, 2007; Berghella et al., 2008; Zwelling, 2010). Laboring upright also conveys a sense of normalcy, autonomy, and personal control (Albers).

Epidural and Intrathecal (Spinal) Opioids. Opioids also can be used alone, eliminating the effect of a local anesthetic altogether. The use of epidural or intrathecal opioids without the addition of a local anesthetic agent during labor has several advantages. Opioids administered in this manner do not cause maternal hypotension or affect vital signs. The woman feels contractions but not pain. Her ability to bear down during the second stage of labor is preserved because the pushing reflex is not lost, and her motor power remains intact.

Fentanyl, sufentanil, or preservative-free morphine can be used. Fentanyl and sufentanil produce short-acting analgesia (i.e., 1.5 to 3.5 hours), and morphine can provide pain relief for 4 to 7 hours. Morphine can be combined with fentanyl or sufentanil. Using short-acting opioids with multiparous women and morphine with nulliparous women or women with a history of long labors is appropriate. Because opioids alone usually do not provide adequate analgesia, however, they are most often given in combination with a local anesthetic (Cunningham et al., 2010).

A more common indication for the administration of epidural or intrathecal analgesics is the relief of postoperative pain. For example, a woman who gives birth by cesarean can receive fentanyl or morphine through a catheter. The catheter can then be removed, and the woman is usually free of pain for 24 hours. Occasionally the catheter is left in place in the epidural space in case another dose is needed.

Women receiving epidurally administered morphine after a cesarean birth can ambulate sooner than women who do not. The early ambulation and freedom from pain also facilitate bladder emptying, enhance peristalsis, and prevent clot formation in the lower extremities (e.g., thrombophlebitis). Women may require additional medication for breakthrough pain during the first 24 hours after surgery. If so, they will usually be given an NSAID such as ketorolac (Toradol), indomethacin (Indocin), or ibuprofen (Motrin) rather than a narcotic.

Side effects of opioids administered by the epidural and intrathecal routes include nausea, vomiting, diminished peristalsis, pruritus, urinary retention, and delayed respiratory depression. These effects are more common when morphine is administered. Antiemetics, antipruritics, and opioid antagonists are used to relieve these symptoms. For example, naloxone, promethazine, or metoclopramide may be administered. Hospital protocols or detailed physician orders should provide specific instructions for the treatment of these side effects. Use of epidural opioids is not without risk. Respiratory depression is a serious concern; for this reason the woman's respiratory status should be assessed and documented every hour for 24 hours, or as designated by hospital protocol. Naloxone should be readily available for use if the respiratory rate decreases to less than 10 breaths per minute or if the oxygen saturation rate decreases to less than 89%. Administration of oxygen by nonrebreather face mask also can be initiated, and the anesthesia care provider should be notified.

Contraindications to Subarachnoid and Epidural Blocks. Contraindications to epidural analgesia (Creehan, 2008; Cunningham et al., 2010; Hawkins et al., 2007) include the following:

- Active or anticipated serious maternal hemorrhage. Acute hypovolemia leads to increased sympathetic tone to maintain the blood pressure. Any anesthetic technique that blocks the sympathetic fibers can produce significant hypotension that can endanger the mother and fetus.
- Maternal hypotension
- Coagulopathy: If a woman is receiving anticoagulant therapy (e.g., last dose of low-molecular-weight heparin within 12 hours) or has a bleeding disorder, injury to a blood vessel may cause the formation of a hematoma that may compress the cauda equina or the spinal cord and lead to serious CNS complications.
- Infection at the injection site. Infection can be spread through the peridural or subarachnoid spaces if the needle traverses an infected area.
- Increased intracranial pressure caused by a mass lesion
- Allergy to the anesthetic drug.
- Maternal refusal or inability to cooperate.
- Some types of maternal cardiac conditions
- Abnormal (nonreassuring) FHR and pattern requiring immediate birth.

Epidural Block Effects on Newborn. Analgesia or anesthesia during labor and birth has little or no lasting effect on the physiologic status of the newborn. Currently, there is no evidence that the administration of maternal analgesia or anesthesia during labor and birth has a significant effect on the child's later mental and neurologic development (AAP & ACOG, 2007).

Nitrous Oxide for Analgesia

Nitrous oxide mixed with oxygen can be inhaled in a low concentration (50% or less) to reduce, but not eliminate, pain during the first and second stages of labor. At the lower doses used for analgesia, the woman remains awake, and the danger of aspiration is avoided because the laryngeal reflexes are unaffected. Nitrous oxide can be used in combination with other nonpharmacologic and pharmacologic measures for pain relief. Many women report significant analgesia with nitrous oxide use and would use it again for a subsequent labor (Tournaire & Theau-Yonneau, 2007).

A face mask or mouthpiece is used to self-administer the gas. The woman places the mask over her mouth and nose or inserts the mouthpiece 30 seconds before the onset of a contraction (if regular) or as soon as a contraction begins (if irregular). When she inhales, a valve opens and the gas is released. She should continue to inhale the gas slowly and deeply until the contraction starts to subside. When inhalation stops, the valve closes. Between contractions the woman should remove the device and breathe normally (Cunningham et al., 2010).

Because it can be difficult to coordinate adequate inhalation and placement of the mask or mouthpiece, the woman may initially require the assistance of the nurse to obtain maximum effectiveness from the method. In addition, the nurse should observe the woman for nausea and vomiting, drowsiness, dizziness, hazy memory, and loss of consciousness. Loss of consciousness is more likely to occur if opioids are used with the nitrous oxide (Cunningham et al., 2010). The use of nitrous oxide does not appear to depress uterine contractions or cause adverse reactions in the fetus and newborn.

General Anesthesia

General anesthesia rarely is used for uncomplicated vaginal birth and is infrequently used for elective cesarean birth. It may be necessary if there is a contraindication to a spinal or epidural block or if indications necessitate rapid birth (vaginal or emergent cesarean) without sufficient time or available personnel to perform a block (Bucklin et al., 2005). In addition, being awake and aware during major surgery may be unacceptable for some women having a cesarean birth. The major risks associated with general anesthesia are difficulty with or inability to intubate and aspiration of gastric contents (Cunningham, et al., 2010; Hawkins et al., 2007). Anesthesia care providers are more likely to encounter difficulty with intubating morbidly obese clients, especially in an emergency situation, than women of normal weight (Valleyo, 2007).

If general anesthesia is being considered, give the woman nothing by mouth and ensure that an IV infusion is in place. If time allows, premedicate the woman with a nonparticulate (clear) oral antacid (e.g., sodium citrate [Bicitra], Alka-Seltzer) to neutralize the acidic contents of the stomach. Aspiration of highly acidic gastric contents will damage lung tissue. Some anesthesia care providers also order the administration of a histamine (H_2)-receptor blocker such as cimetidine (Tagamet) or ranitidine (Zantac) to decrease the production of gastric acid and metoclopramide (Reglan) to accelerate gastric emptying (Hawkins et al., 2007). Before the anesthesia is given, a wedge should be placed under one of the woman's hips to displace the uterus. Uterine displacement prevents compression of the aorta and vena cava, which maintains cardiac output and placental perfusion.

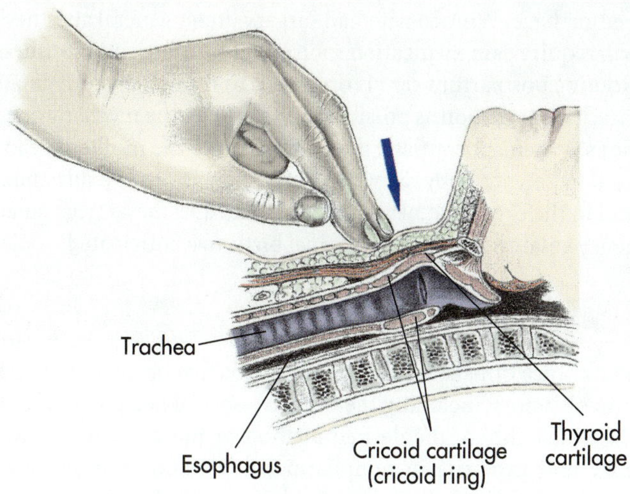

FIG. 17-13 Technique of applying pressure on cricoid cartilage to occlude esophagus to prevent pulmonary aspiration of gastric contents during induction of general anesthesia.

Prior to the induction of anesthesia, the woman will be preoxygenated with 100% oxygen by nonrebreather face mask for 2 to 3 minutes. This is especially important in pregnant women, who are more likely than other adults to rapidly become hypoxemic if there is a delay in successful intubation. Thiopental, a short-acting barbiturate, or ketamine is administered intravenously to render the woman unconscious. Next, succinylcholine, a muscle relaxer, is administered to facilitate passage of an endotracheal tube (Cunningham et al., 2010; Hawkins et al., 2007). Sometimes the nurse is asked to assist with applying cricoid pressure before intubation as the woman begins to lose consciousness. This maneuver blocks the esophagus and prevents aspiration should the woman vomit or regurgitate (Fig. 17-13). Pressure is released once the endotracheal tube is securely in place.

After the woman is intubated, nitrous oxide and oxygen in a 50:50 mixture are administered. A low concentration of a volatile halogenated agent (e.g., isoflurane) also may be administered to increase pain relief and to reduce maternal awareness and recall (Cunningham et al., 2010; Hawkins et al., 2007). In higher concentrations, isoflurane or methoxyflurane relaxes the uterus quickly and facilitates intrauterine manipulation, version, and extraction. However, at higher concentrations, these agents cross the placenta readily and can produce narcosis in the fetus and could reduce uterine tone after birth, increasing the risk for hemorrhage. Because of this risk of neonatal narcosis, it is critical that the baby be delivered as soon as possible after the induction of the anesthetic to reduce the degree of fetal exposure to the anesthetic agents and the CNS depressants administered.

Priorities for recovery room care are to maintain an open airway and cardiopulmonary function and to prevent postpartum hemorrhage. Women who had surgery under general anesthesia will require pain medication soon after regaining consciousness. Routine postpartum care is organized to facilitate parent-infant attachment as soon as possible and to answer the mother's questions. When appropriate, the nurse assesses the mother's readiness to see her baby, as well as her response to the anesthesia and to the event that necessitated general anesthesia (e.g., emergency cesarean birth when vaginal birth was anticipated).

CARE MANAGEMENT

The choice of pain relief interventions depends on a combination of factors, including the woman's special needs and wishes, the availability of the desired method or methods, the knowledge and expertise in nonpharmacologic and pharmacologic methods of the health care providers involved in the woman's care, and the phase and stage of labor. The nurse is responsible for assessing maternal and fetal status, establishing mutual goals with the woman (and her family as appropriate), formulating nursing diagnoses, planning and implementing nursing care, and evaluating the effects of care (see the Nursing Process box).

Nonpharmacologic Interventions

The nurse supports and assists the woman as she uses nonpharmacologic interventions for pain relief and relaxation. During labor the nurse should ask the woman how she feels to evaluate the effectiveness of the specific pain management techniques used. Appropriate interventions can then be planned or continued for effective care, such as trying other nonpharmacologic methods or combining nonpharmacologic methods with medications (see the Nursing Care Plan).

The woman's perception of her behavior during labor is of utmost importance. If she planned an unmedicated birth but then needs and accepts medication, her self-esteem may falter. Verbal and nonverbal acceptance of her behavior is given as necessary by the nurse and reinforced by discussion and reassurance after birth. Providing explanations about the fetal response to maternal discomfort, the effects of maternal stress and fatigue on the progress of labor, and the medication itself is a supportive measure. The woman may also experience anxiety and stress related to anticipated or actual pain. Stress can cause increased maternal catecholamine production. Increased levels of catecholamines have been linked to dysfunctional labor and fetal and neonatal distress and illness. Nurses must be able to implement strategies aimed at reducing this stress.

Pharmacologic Interventions

Informed Consent

Pregnant women have the right to be active participants in determining the best pain care approach to use during labor and birth. The primary health care provider and anesthesia care provider are responsible for fully informing women of the alternative methods of pharmacologic pain relief available in the hospital. A description of the various anesthetic techniques and what they entail is essential to informed consent, even if the woman received information about analgesia and anesthesia earlier in her pregnancy. The initial discussion of pain management options ideally should take place in the third trimester so the woman has time to consider alternatives. Nurses play a part in the informed consent by clarifying and describing procedures or by acting as the woman's advocate and asking the primary health care provider for further explanations. There are three essential components of an informed consent. First, the procedure and its advantages and disadvantages must be thoroughly explained. Second, the woman must agree with the plan of labor pain care as explained to her. Third, her consent must be given freely without coercion or manipulation from her health care provider.

LEGAL TIP: Informed Consent for Anesthesia

The woman receives (in an understandable manner) the following:

- Explanation of alternative methods of anesthesia and analgesia available
- Description of the anesthetic, including its effects and the procedure for its administration
- Description of the benefits, discomforts, risks, and consequences for the mother, the fetus, and the newborn
- Explanation of how complications can be treated
- Information that the anesthetic is not always effective
- Indication that the woman may withdraw consent at any time
- Opportunity to have any question answered
- Opportunity to have components of the consent explained in the woman's own words

The consent form will:

- Be written or explained in the woman's primary language
- Have the woman's signature
- Have the date of consent
- Carry the signature of the anesthetic care provider, certifying that the woman has received and expresses understanding of the explanation

Timing of Administration

It is often the nurse who notifies the primary health care provider that the woman is in need of pharmacologic measures to relieve her discomfort. Orders are often written for the administration of pain medication as needed by the woman and based on the nurse's clinical judgment. In the past, pharmacologic measures for pain relief were usually not implemented until labor had advanced to the active phase of the first stage of labor and the cervix had dilated approximately 4 to 5 cm, to avoid suppressing the progress of labor. However, it is now known that epidural anesthesia in early labor does not increase the rate of cesarean birth and may shorten the duration of labor. Consequently, women in labor must no longer reach a certain level of cervical dilation or fetal station before receiving epidural anesthesia (AAP & ACOG, 2007; Cunningham et al., 2010). It is still recommended that the administration of systemic opioid analgesics be delayed until labor is well established (Creehan, 2008). Nonpharmacologic measures can be used to relieve pain and stress and enhance progress at any time in labor.

Preparation for Procedures

The methods of pain relief available to the woman are reviewed and information is clarified as necessary. The procedure and what will be asked of the woman (e.g., to maintain flexed position during insertion of epidural needle) must be explained.

NURSING PROCESS

Pain Management

ASSESSMENT

- History
  - Review prenatal record for relevant data (e.g., parity, EDB, health problems, medications)
  - Changes noted since last prenatal visit (e.g., infections, diarrhea, bleeding, change in fetal activity pattern)
  - History of smoking; neurologic or spinal disorders
  - Time of woman's last meal; type of food and fluid consumed
  - Nature of existing respiratory condition (e.g., cold, flu, asthma, rhinitis)
  - Allergies to medications, cleansing agents (e.g., povidone-iodine [Betadine]), latex, or tape
  - Childbirth preparation, knowledge and preferences for management of discomfort; birth plan
  - Persons who will be present to provide support during labor (e.g., doula, partner, family member)
  - Type of analgesia or anesthesia chosen (see Box 17-4)
  - If evidence of substance abuse, identify type of drug, last time drug taken, and method of administration. Urine drug screen may be ordered.
  - Determine if woman wears contact lenses or dentures
- Pain assessment
  - Characteristics of pain experienced including location, intensity, sensory quality (e.g., prickling, stabbing, burning, cramping, etc.), frequency, duration
  - Physiologic effects of pain (e.g., alteration in vital signs, pallor, diaphoresis, nausea and vomiting, fatigue)
  - Emotional (affective) responses to pain (e.g., increasing anxiety, restlessness, fist clenching, groaning, writhing)
  - Effectiveness of pain relief measures used
- Physical examination
  - Character and status of labor
  - Fetal response (e.g., alteration in fetal heart rate and pattern)
  - Hydration status; intake and output, moisture of mucous membranes, skin turgor
  - Integrity of integument including over potential epidural catheter insertion site
- Amount and characteristics of urine; presence of bladder distention
- Obtain current weight for calculating medication doses
- Review results of laboratory tests ordered
- Anesthesia assessment (should be completed by a member of the anesthesia care team immediately following the woman's admission to the labor and birth unit)
  - Time of woman's last meal; type of food and fluid consumed
  - Nature of existing respiratory condition (e.g., cold, allergy)
  - Allergies to medications, cleansing agents, latex, or tape
  - Personal or family history of problems with anesthesia (e.g., history of malignant hypertension)
  - Past or current neurologic or spinal disorders
  - Current medical problems that could affect her choice of anesthesia for labor and birth (e.g., thrombocytopenia, low hematocrit [e.g., <25%], vaginal bleeding, rash or infection on lower back, fever of unknown origin)
  - Type of analgesia or anesthesia chosen (see Box 17-4)
  - Brief physical exam, focusing especially on the woman's airway and respiratory status

NURSING DIAGNOSES

Possible nursing diagnoses include:

Acute Pain **related to:**
- processes of labor and birth

Risk for Ineffective Tissue Perfusion **related to:**
- effects of analgesia or anesthesia
- maternal position

Situational Low Self-esteem **related to:**
- negative perception of the woman's (or her family's) behavior

Anxiety or Fear **related to:**
- procedure for epidural analgesia
- expected sensations during nerve block analgesia

Risk for Fetal Injury **related to:**
- maternal hypotension
- maternal position (aortocaval compression)

Risk for Maternal Injury **related to:**
- effects of analgesia and anesthesia on sensation and motor control

EXPECTED OUTCOMES OF CARE

The woman will:
- Promptly report the characteristics of her pain and discomfort.
- Verbalize understanding of her needs and rights with regard to pain relief management that uses a variety of nonpharmacologic and pharmacologic methods reflecting her preferences.
- Experience adequate pain relief without adding to maternal risk or fetal risk (e.g., through the use of appropriate nonpharmacologic methods and appropriate medication, including the appropriate dose, timing, and route of administration).
- Give birth to a neonate who adjusts to extrauterine life without problems related to the management of maternal pain.

PLAN OF CARE AND INTERVENTIONS

- Assist woman in use of nonpharmacologic interventions.
- Provide explanations of fetal response to maternal discomfort and effects of maternal stress and fatigue on the progress of labor.
- Ensure informed consent to procedures and anesthesia.
- Administer pharmacologic measures as ordered and, if possible, as determined by woman or expressed in her birth plan.
- Prepare woman for procedures, such as epidural catheter insertion and IV administration of analgesics.
- Monitor for signs of potential problems.
- Protect from injury.
- Monitor and record response to interventions.

EVALUATION

Evaluation of the effectiveness of care related to pain management is based on the previously stated expected outcomes.

The woman also can benefit from knowing the way that the medication is to be given, the interval before the medication takes effect, and the expected pain relief from the medication. Skin-preparation measures are described, and an explanation is given for the need to empty the bladder before the analgesic or anesthetic is administered and the reason for keeping the bladder empty. When an indwelling catheter is to be threaded into the epidural space, the woman should be told that she may have a momentary twinge down her leg, hip, or back, and that this feeling is not a sign of injury (Box 17-6).

NURSING CARE PLAN

Nonpharmacologic Pain Management

NURSING DIAGNOSIS

Anxiety related to lack of confidence in ability to cope effectively with pain during labor

Expected Outcomes

Woman will express decrease in anxiety and experience satisfaction with her labor and birth performance.

Nursing Interventions/*Rationales*

- Assess whether woman and significant other have attended childbirth classes, their knowledge of the labor process, and their current level of anxiety *to plan supportive strategies that address the couple's specific needs.*
- Encourage support person to remain with woman in labor *to provide support and increase probability of positive response to comfort measures.*
- Teach or review nonpharmacologic techniques available to decrease anxiety and pain during labor (e.g., focusing, relaxation and breathing techniques, effleurage, and sacral pressure) *to enhance chances of success in using techniques.*
- Explore other techniques that the woman or significant other may have learned in childbirth classes (e.g., hypnosis, hydrotherapy, acupressure, biofeedback, therapeutic touch, aromatherapy, imaging, music) *to provide more options for coping strategies.*
- Explore the use of transcutaneous nerve stimulation if ordered by the primary health care provider *to provide an increased perception of control over pain and an increase in release of endogenous opiates (endorphins).*
- Assist the woman to change positions and to use pillows *to reduce stiffness, aid circulation, and promote comfort.*
- Assess the bladder for distention and encourage voiding often *to avoid bladder distention, subsequent discomfort, and potential for suppression of uterine contractions.*
- Encourage rest between contractions *to minimize fatigue.*
- Keep woman and significant other informed about progress *to allay anxiety.*
- Guide couple through the labor stages and phases, helping them use and modify comfort techniques that are appropriate to each phase, *to ensure the greatest effectiveness of the techniques used.*
- Support the couple if pharmacologic measures are required to increase pain relief, explaining safety and effectiveness, *to reduce anxiety and maintain self-esteem and sense of control over labor process.*

NURSING DIAGNOSIS

Health-seeking behavior (labor) related to desire for a healthy outcome of labor and birth

Expected Outcome

Woman will participate in planning care for labor.

Nursing Interventions/*Rationales*

- Discuss the woman's birth plan and knowledge about the birth process *to collect data for the nursing plan of care.*
- Provide information about the labor process *to correct any misconceptions.*
- Inform the woman about her labor status and the fetus's well-being *to promote comfort and confidence.*
- Discuss rationales for all interventions *to incorporate the woman into the plan of care.*
- Incorporate nonpharmacologic interventions into the plan of care *to increase the woman's sense of control during labor.*
- Provide emotional support and ongoing positive feedback *to enhance positive coping mechanisms.*

Administration of Medication

Accurate monitoring of the progress of labor forms the basis for the nurse's judgment that a woman needs pharmacologic control of discomfort. Knowledge of the medications used during childbirth is essential. The most effective route of administration is selected for each woman; then the medication is prepared and administered correctly.

Any medication can cause a minor or severe allergic reaction. As part of the assessment for such allergic reactions, the nurse should monitor the woman's vital signs, respiratory rate and effort, cardiovascular status, integument, and platelet and white blood cell count. The woman is observed for side effects of drug therapy, especially drowsiness and dyspnea. Minor reactions can consist of rash, rhinitis, fever, shortness of breath, or pruritus. Management of the less acute allergic response is not an emergency.

Severe allergic reactions (anaphylaxis) may occur suddenly and lead to shock or death. The most dramatic form of anaphylaxis is sudden, severe bronchospasm, upper airway obstruction, and/or hypotension (Brown, Mullins, & Gold, 2006). Signs of anaphylaxis are largely caused by contraction of smooth muscles and may begin with irritability, extreme weakness, nausea, and vomiting. This may lead to dyspnea, cyanosis, convulsions, and cardiac arrest. Anaphylaxis must be diagnosed and treated immediately. Initial treatment usually consists of placing the woman in a supine position, injecting epinephrine intramuscularly, administering fluid intravenously, supporting the airway with ventilation if necessary, and giving oxygen. If response to these measures is inadequate, intravenous epinephrine should be given (Brown et al.). Cardiopulmonary resuscitation may be necessary.

Intravenous Route. The preferred route of administration of medications such as hydromorphone, butorphanol, fentanyl, or nalbuphine is through IV tubing, administered into the port nearest the point of insertion of the infusion (proximal port). The medication is given slowly, in small doses, during a contraction. It may be given over a period of three to five consecutive contractions if needed to complete the dose. It is given during contractions to decrease fetal exposure to the medication because uterine blood vessels are constricted during contractions and the medication stays within the maternal vascular system for several seconds before the uterine blood vessels reopen.

Intramuscular Route. The maternal plasma level of the medication necessary to bring pain relief usually is reached 45 minutes after IM injection, followed by a decline in plasma levels. The maternal medication levels (after IM injections) also are unequal because of uneven distribution (maternal uptake) and metabolism. The advantage of using the IM route is quick administration by the health care provider. IM injections given in the upper arm (deltoid muscle) seem to result in more rapid absorption and higher blood levels of the medication (Bricker &

BOX 17-6 NURSING INTERVENTIONS FOR THE WOMAN RECEIVING EPIDURAL OR SPINAL ANESTHESIA

PRIOR TO THE BLOCK
- Assist primary health care provider and/or anesthesia care provider with explaining the procedure and obtaining the woman's informed consent.
- Assess maternal vital signs, level of hydration, labor progress, and FHR and pattern.
- Start an intravenous line and infuse a bolus of fluid (Ringer's lactate or normal saline) if ordered (e.g., 500 to 1000 ml 15 to 20 minutes prior to induction of the anesthesia).
- Obtain laboratory results (hematocrit or hemoglobin level, other tests as ordered).
- Assess the woman's level of pain using a pain scale (from 0 [no pain] to 10 [pain as bad as it could possibly be]).
- Assist the woman to void.

DURING INITIATION OF THE BLOCK
- Assist the woman with assuming and maintaining proper position.
- Verbally guide the woman through the procedure, explaining sounds and sensations as she experiences them.
- Assist the anesthesia care provider with documentation of vital signs, time and amount of medications given, etc.
- Monitor maternal vital signs (especially blood pressure) and FHR as ordered.
- Have oxygen and suction readily available.
- Monitor for signs of local anesthetic toxicity (see Box 17-5) as the test dose of medication is administered.

WHILE THE BLOCK IS IN EFFECT
- Continue to monitor maternal vital signs and FHR as ordered (continuous monitoring of maternal heart rate [electrocardiogram (ECG)] and blood pressure may be ordered to monitor for accidental intravenous injection of medication).
- Continue to assess the woman's level of pain with every check of vital signs using a pain scale (from 0 [no pain] to 10 [pain as bad as it could possibly be]).
- Monitor for bladder distention.
  - Assist with spontaneous voiding on bedpan or toilet.
  - Insert urinary catheter if necessary.
- Encourage or assist the woman to change positions from side to side every hour.
- Promote safety.
  - Keep side rails up on the bed.
  - Place telephone and call light within easy reach.
  - Instruct woman not to get out of bed without help.
  - Make sure there is no prolonged pressure on anesthetized body parts.
- Keep the catheter insertion site clean and dry.
- Continue to monitor for anesthetic side effects (see Box 17-5).

WHILE THE BLOCK IS WEARING OFF AFTER BIRTH
- Assess regularly for the return of sensory and motor function.
- Continue to monitor maternal vital signs as ordered.
- Monitor for bladder distention.
  - Assist with spontaneous voiding on bedpan or toilet.
  - Insert urinary catheter if necessary.
- Promote safety.
  - Keep side rails up on the bed.
  - Place telephone and call light within easy reach.
  - Instruct woman not to get out of bed without help.
  - Make sure there is no prolonged pressure on anesthetized body parts.
- Keep the catheter insertion site clean and dry.
- Continue to monitor for anesthetic side effects (see Box 17-5).

Lavender, 2002). If regional anesthesia is planned later in labor, the autonomic blockade from the regional (e.g., epidural) anesthesia increases blood flow to the gluteal region and accelerates absorption of medication that may be sequestered there. Administration of opioids, including nalbuphine, subcutaneously in the upper arm avoids this risk and as a result is often used as an alternative to IM injection.

Regional (Epidural or Spinal) Anesthesia. An IV infusion is established before the induction of regional anesthesia (epidural, subarachnoid). Anesthesia protocols will likely include the prophylactic administration of IV fluid before epidural and spinal anesthesia for blood volume expansion to prevent maternal hypotension. Hypotension is one of the most common complications of regional anesthesia (see Box 17-5) (AAP & ACOG, 2007; Cunningham et al., 2010).

Lactated Ringer's or normal saline solutions are commonly used infusion solutions. Infusion solutions without dextrose are preferred, especially when the solution must be infused rapidly (e.g., to treat dehydration or to maintain blood pressure) because solutions containing dextrose rapidly increase maternal blood glucose levels. The fetus responds to high blood glucose levels by increasing insulin production; neonatal hypoglycemia may result. In addition, dextrose changes the osmotic pressure so that fluid is excreted from the kidneys more rapidly.

According to professional standards (Association of Women's Health, Obstetric and Neonatal Nurses [AWHONN], 2007), the nonanesthetist registered nurse is permitted to monitor the status of the woman, the fetus and the progress of labor, replace empty infusion syringes or bags with the same medication and concentration, stop the infusion and initiate emergency measures if the need arises, and remove the catheter if properly educated to do so. Only qualified, licensed anesthesia care providers are permitted to insert a catheter and initiate epidural anesthesia, verify catheter placement, inject medication through the catheter, or alter the medication or medications, including the type, the amount, or the rate of infusion.

! NURSING ALERT

Complications may occur with epidural analgesia, including injection-related emergencies and compression problems. These complications can require immediate interventions. Nurses must be prepared to provide safe and effective care during the emergency situation. Clear procedures or protocols should be in place in labor and birth units delineating responsibilities and actions needed (Mahlmeister, 2003).

Because spinal nerve blocks can reduce bladder sensation, resulting in difficulty voiding, the woman should empty her bladder before the induction of the block and should be encouraged to void at least every 2 hours thereafter. The nurse should palpate for bladder distention and measure urinary

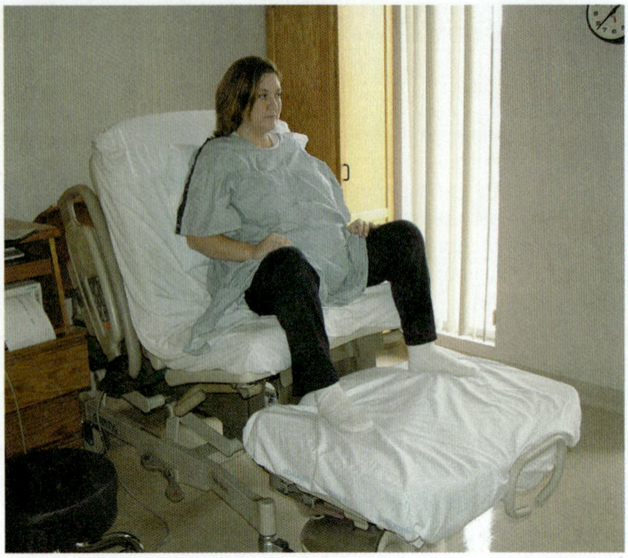

FIG. 17-14 Modified throne position for labor. (Courtesy Julie Perry Nelson, Loveland, CO.)

output to ensure that the bladder is being completely emptied. A distended bladder can inhibit uterine contractions and fetal descent, resulting in a slowing of the progress of labor. For this reason, an indwelling urinary catheter (Foley) is often routinely inserted immediately after epidural or spinal anesthesia is initiated and left in place for the remainder of the first stage of labor.

The status of the maternal-fetal unit and the progress of labor must be established before the block is performed. The nurse must assist the woman to assume and maintain the correct position for induction of epidural and spinal anesthesia (see Fig. 17-11, *A* and *B*).

Depending on the level of motor blockade, the woman should be assisted to remain as mobile as possible. When in bed, her position should be alternated from side to side every hour to ensure adequate distribution of the anesthetic solution and to maintain circulation to the uterus and placenta. Assisting the woman to assume upright positions such as sitting (e.g., modified throne position in which the woman sits on the bed with the bottom part lowered to place her feet below her body) (Fig. 17-14), tug-of-war position (woman tugs on towel or sheet that is tied to the bar on the bed or held by the nurse), and squatting (see Figs. 19-12 and 19-16, *E*) will facilitate fetal descent and

SAFETY ALERT

After receiving an epidural block or opioid intravenously for pain, the woman should not be allowed to ambulate alone. She must either remain in bed or request assistance before attempting to get out of bed. The nurse assesses the woman for signs of orthostatic hypotension and return of sensation and motor function of the lower extremities prior to ambulation.

enhance bearing-down efforts (Gilder, Mayberry, Gennaro, & Clemmons, 2002; Zwelling, 2010). Upright positions are very important in the prevention of operative births (e.g., forceps or vacuum-assisted birth) and should be encouraged when the woman has a low-dose epidural or CSE (Mayberry, Strange, Suplee, & Gennaro, 2003).

Health care providers should recognize that the second stage of labor may be prolonged in women who use epidural analgesia for pain management. Research evidence indicates that as long as the well-being of the maternal-fetal unit is established, a period of passive descent or "laboring down" can be implemented to allow the fetus to descend and rotate with uterine contractions until the woman perceives the urge to bear down (Brancato, Church, & Stone, 2008; Simpson & James, 2005). Fetal well-being, along with less maternal fatigue, fever, and perineal trauma and fewer operative vaginal births, are beneficial outcomes of this approach for the management of the second stage of labor for women with epidural analgesia. Evidence is insufficient to support the practice of discontinuing epidural analgesia during the second stage in an effort to enhance the effectiveness of bearing-down efforts and decrease the risk for forceps or vacuum-assisted birth. This practice results in an increase in the woman's level of pain (Torvaldsen, Roberts, Bell, & Raynes-Greenow, 2010). (See Chapter 19 for a full discussion of second stage labor management.) Box 17-6 summarizes the nursing interventions for women receiving epidural or spinal anesthesia.

Safety and General Care

The nurse monitors and records the woman's response to nonpharmacologic pain relief methods and to medication(s). This includes the degree of pain relief, the level of apprehension, the return of sensations and perception of pain, and allergic or adverse reactions (e.g., hypotension, respiratory depression, fever, pruritus, and nausea and vomiting). The nurse continues to monitor maternal vital signs and fetal heart rate and pattern at frequent intervals, the strength and frequency of uterine contractions, changes in the cervix and station of the presenting part, the presence and quality of the bearing-down reflex, bladder filling, and state of hydration. Determining the fetal response after administration of analgesia or anesthesia is vital. The woman is asked if she (or the family) has any questions. The nurse also assesses the woman's and her family's understanding of the need for ensuring her safety (e.g., keeping side rails up, calling for assistance as needed).

The time that elapses between the administration of an opioid and the baby's birth is documented. Medications given to the newborn to reverse opioid effects are recorded. After birth, the woman who has had spinal, epidural, or general anesthesia is assessed for return of sensory and motor function in addition to the usual postpartum assessments. Both the nurse and the anesthesia provider are responsible for documenting assessments and care in relation to the epidural (Mahlmeister, 2003).

KEY POINTS

- Nonpharmacologic pain and stress management strategies are valuable for managing labor discomfort alone or in combination with pharmacologic methods.
- The gate-control theory of pain and the stress response are the bases for many of the nonpharmacologic methods of pain relief.
- The type of analgesic or anesthetic to be used is determined in part by the stage of labor and the method of birth.
- Sedatives may be appropriate for women in prolonged early labor when there is a need to decrease anxiety or to promote sleep or therapeutic rest.
- Naloxone is an opioid antagonist that can reverse opioid effects, especially respiratory depression.
- Pharmacologic control of discomfort during labor requires collaboration among the health care providers and the laboring woman.
- The nurse must understand medications, their expected effects, their potential adverse reactions, and their methods of administration.
- Maintenance of maternal fluid balance is essential during spinal and epidural nerve blocks.
- Maternal analgesia or anesthesia potentially affects initial neonatal neurobehavioral response.
- The use of opioid agonist-antagonist analgesics in women with preexisting opioid dependence may cause symptoms of abstinence syndrome (opioid withdrawal).
- Epidural anesthesia and analgesia is the most effective pharmacologic pain relief method for labor that is currently available. As a result, it is the most commonly used method for relieving pain during labor in the United States.
- General anesthesia is rarely used for vaginal birth but may be used for cesarean birth or whenever rapid anesthesia is needed in an emergency.

Audio Chapter Summaries Access an audio summary of these Key Points on evolve

REFERENCES

Aghabati, N., Mohammadi, E., & Pour Esmaiel, Z. (2010). The effect of therapeutic touch on pain and fatigue of cancer patients undergoing chemotherapy. *Evidence-based Complementary and Alternative Medicine, 7*(3), 375–381.

Albers, L. (2007). The evidence for physiologic management of the active phase of the first stage of labor. *Journal of Midwifery and Women's Health, 52*(3), 207–215.

American Academy of Pediatrics (AAP) & American College of Obstetricians and Gynecologists (ACOG). (2007). *Guidelines for perinatal care* (6th ed.). Washington, DC: ACOG.

American College of Obstetricians and Gynecologists (ACOG). (2004). *Pain relief during labor.* Committee Opinion No. 295. Washington, DC: ACOG.

American Society of Anesthesiologists. (2007). *Guidelines for regional anesthesia in obstetrics.* Available at www.asahq.org/publicationsandservices/standards/45.pdf. Accessed August 22, 2010.

Anim-Somuah, M., Smyth, R., & Howell, C. (2008). Epidural versus non-epidural or no analgesia in labor. *The Cochrane Database of Systematic Reviews, 2005*, 4, CD000331.

Association of Women's Health, Obstetric and Neonatal Nurses (AWHONN). (2007). *The role of the registered nurse (RN) in the care of pregnant women receiving analgesia/anesthesia by catheter techniques (epidural, intrathecal, spinal, PCEA catheters).* Clinical position statement. Available at www.awhonn.org. Accessed July 2, 2010.

Berghella, V., Baxter, J., & Chauhan, S. (2008). Evidence-based labor and delivery management. *American Journal of Obstetrics and Gynecology, 199*(5), 445–454.

Blackburn, S. (2007). *Maternal, fetal, and neonatal physiology: A clinical perspective* (3rd ed.). St. Louis: Mosby.

Brancato, R., Church, S., & Stone, P. (2008). A meta-analysis of passive descent versus immediate pushing in nulliparous women with epidural analgesia in the second stage of labor. *Journal of Obstetric, Gynecologic and Neonatal Nursing, 37*(1), 4–12.

Bricker, L., & Lavender, T. (2002). Parenteral opioids for labor pain relief: A systematic review. *American Journal of Obstetrics and Gynecology, 186*(5), S94–S109.

Brown, S., Mullins, R., & Gold, M. (2006). Anaphylaxis: Diagnosis and management. *Medical Journal of Australia, 185*(5), 283–289.

Bucklin, B., Hawkins, J., Anderson, J., & Ullrich, F. (2005). Obstetric anesthesia workforce survey. *Anesthesiology, 103*(3), 645–653.

Callister, L., Khalaf, I., Semenic, S., Kartchner, R., & Vehvilainen-Julkunen, K. (2003). The pain of childbirth: Perceptions of culturally diverse women. *Pain Management Nursing, 4*(4), 145–154.

Creehan, P. (2008). Pain relief and comfort measures in labor. In K. Rice Simpson & P. Creehan (Eds.), *AWHONN's perinatal nursing* (3rd ed.). Philadelphia: Lippincott Williams & Wilkins.

Cunningham, F., Leveno, K., Bloom, S., Hauth, J., Rouse, D., & Spong, C. (2010). *Williams obstetrics* (23rd ed.). New York: McGraw-Hill.

Fogarty, V. (2008). Intradermal sterile water injections for the relief of low back pain in labour—A systematic review of the literature. *Women and Birth, 21*(4), 157–163.

Gilbert, E. (2011). *Manual of high risk pregnancy & delivery* (5th ed.). St. Louis: Mosby.

Gilder, K., Mayberry, L., Gennaro, S., & Clemmons, D. (2002). Maternal positions in labor with epidural analgesia: Results from a multi-site survey. *AWHONN Lifelines, 6*(1), 40–45.

Halpern, S., Muir, H., Breen, T., Campbell, D., Barrett, J., Liston, R., et al. (2004). A multicenter randomized controlled trial comparing patient-controlled epidural with intravenous analgesia for pain relief in labor. *Anesthesia & Analgesia, 99*(5), 1532–1538.

Hawkins, J., Goetzl, L., & Chestnut, D. (2007). Obstetric anesthesia. In S. Gabbe, J. Niebyl, & J. Simpson (Eds.), *Obstetrics: Normal and problem pregnancies* (5th ed.). Philadelphia: Churchill Livingstone.

Hodnett, E., Gates, S., Hofmeyr, G., & Sakala, C. (2007). Continuous support for women during childbirth. *The Cochrane Database of Systematic Reviews, 2007*, 3, CD003766.

Humenick, S., Schrock, P., & Libresco, M. (2000). Relaxation. In F. Nichols & S. Humenick (Eds.), *Childbirth education: Practice, research, and theory* (2nd ed.). Philadelphia: Saunders.

Lowe, N. (2002). The nature of labor pain. *American Journal of Obstetrics and Gynecology, 186*(5), S16–S24.

Mahlmeister, L. (2003). Nursing responsibilities in preventing, preparing for, and managing epidural emergencies. *Journal of Perinatal and Neonatal Nursing, 17*(1), 19–32.

Mayberry, L., Strange, L., Suplee, P., & Gennaro, S. (2003). Use of upright positioning with epidural analgesia: Findings from an observational study. *MCN The American Journal of Maternal/Child Nursing, 28*(3), 152–159.

Perinatal Education Associates. (2008). *Breathing.* Available at www.birthsource.com. Accessed July 2, 2010.

Saito, M., Okutomi, T., Kanai, Y., Mochizuki, J., Tani, A., Amano, K., et al. (2005). Patient-controlled epidural analgesia during labor using ropivacaine and fentanyl provides better maternal satisfaction with less local anesthetic requirement. *Journal of Anesthesia, 19*(3), 208–212.

Saravanakumar, K., Rao, S., & Cooper, G. (2006). The challenges of obesity and obstetric anesthesia. *Current Opinion in Obstetrics and Gynecology, 18*(6), 631–635.

Simkin, P., & Bolding, A. (2004). Update on nonpharmacologic approaches to relieve labor pain and prevent suffering. *Journal of Midwifery & Women's Health, 49*(6), 489–504.

Simpson, K., & James, D. (2005). Effects of immediate versus delayed pushing during second-stage labor on fetal well-being: A randomized clinical trial. *Nursing Research, 54*(3), 149–157.

Smith, C., Collins, C., Cyna, A., & Crowther, C. (2006). Complementary and alternative therapies for pain management in labour. *The Cochrane Database of Systematic Reviews, 2006*, 4, CD003521.

Stark, M., Rudell, B., & Haus, G. (2008). Observing position and movements in hydrotherapy: A pilot study. *Journal of Obstetric, Gynecologic and Neonatal Nursing, 37*(1), 116–122.

Torvaldsen, S., Roberts, C., Bell, J., & Raynes-Greenow, C. (2004). Discontinuation of epidural analgesia late in labour for reducing the adverse delivery outcomes associated with epidural analgesia. *The Cochrane Database of Systematic Reviews, 2004*, 4, CD004457.

Tournaire, M., & Theau-Yonneau, A. (2007). Complementary and alternative approaches to pain relief during labor. *Evidence-based Complementary and Alternative Medicine, 4*(4), 409–417.

Trout, K. (2004). The neuromatrix theory of pain: Implications for selected nonpharmacologic methods of pain relief for labor. *Journal of Midwifery & Women's Health, 49*(6), 482–488.

Valleyo, M. (2007). Anesthetic management of the morbidly obese parturient. *Current Opinions in Anaesthesiology, 20*(3), 175–180.

Walls, D. (2009). Herbs and natural therapies for pregnancy, birth, and breastfeeding. *International Journal of Childbirth Education, 24*(2), 29–37.

Zwelling, E. (2010). Overcoming the challenges: Maternal movement and positioning to facilitate labor progress. *MCN The American Journal of Maternal/Child Nursing, 35*(2), 72–78.

Zwelling, E., Johnson, K., & Allen, J. (2006). How to implement complementary therapies for laboring women. *MCN The American Journal of Maternal/Child Nursing, 30*(6), 364–372.

CHAPTER

18

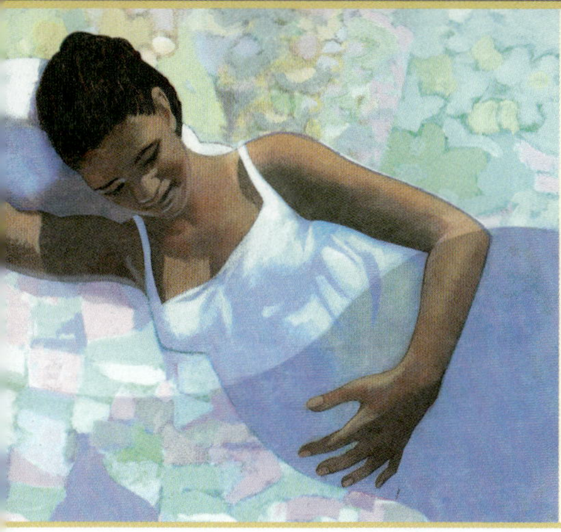

Fetal Assessment During Labor

Linda Fowler Shahzad

evolve WEBSITE

http://evolve.elsevier.com/Lowdermilk/MWHC/

Audio Glossary
Audio Key Points
Critical Thinking Exercise
  Fetal Monitoring
NCLEX Review Questions
Nursing Care Plan
  Electronic Fetal Monitoring During Labor
Spanish Guidelines
  Fetal Monitoring

LEARNING OBJECTIVES

- Identify typical signs of normal (reassuring) and abnormal (nonreassuring) fetal heart rate (FHR) patterns.
- Compare FHR monitoring performed by intermittent auscultation with external and internal electronic methods.
- Explain the baseline FHR and evaluate periodic changes.
- Describe nursing measures that can be used to maintain FHR patterns within normal limits.
- Differentiate among the nursing interventions used for managing specific FHR patterns, including tachycardia and bradycardia, absent or minimal variability, and late and variable decelerations.
- Review the documentation of the monitoring process necessary during labor.

The ability to assess the fetus by auscultation of the fetal heart was initially described more than 300 years ago. With the advent of the fetoscope and stethoscope after the turn of the twentieth century the listener could hear clearly enough to count the FHR. When electronic FHR monitoring made its debut for clinical use in the early 1970s, the anticipation was that its use would result in fewer cases of cerebral palsy and be more sensitive than stethoscopic auscultation in predicting and preventing fetal compromise (Garite, 2007). Consequently, the use of electronic fetal monitoring rapidly expanded. However, the rate of cerebral palsy has not declined since that time and is not likely to improve, because more preterm infants are surviving and because these infants have an increased risk for congenitally acquired neurologic damage (Gilbert, 2011). Moreover, in 2008 the cesarean birth rate in the United States reached an all-time high of 32.3% (Hamilton, Martin, & Ventura, 2010).

Still, **electronic fetal monitoring (EFM)** is a useful tool for visualizing FHR patterns on a monitor screen or printed tracing. It continues to be the primary mode of intrapartum fetal assessment in the United States and is the most commonly performed obstetric procedure in that country (American College of Obstetricians and Gynecologists [ACOG], 2009; Tucker, Miller, & Miller, 2009). Pregnant women should be informed about the equipment and procedures used and the risks, benefits, and limitations of intermittent auscultation and EFM. This chapter discusses the basis for intrapartum fetal monitoring, the types of monitoring, and nursing assessment and management of abnormal fetal status.

BASIS FOR MONITORING

Fetal Response

Because labor is a period of physiologic stress for the fetus, frequent monitoring of fetal status is part of the nursing care during labor. The fetal oxygen supply must be maintained during labor to prevent fetal compromise and to promote newborn health after birth. The fetal oxygen supply can decrease in a number of ways:

- Reduction of blood flow through the maternal vessels as a result of maternal hypertension (chronic hypertension, preeclampsia, or gestational hypertension), hypotension (caused by supine maternal position, hemorrhage, or epidural analgesia or anesthesia), or hypovolemia (caused by hemorrhage)
- Reduction of the oxygen content in the maternal blood as a result of hemorrhage or severe anemia

- Alterations in fetal circulation, occurring with compression of the umbilical cord (transient, during uterine contractions [UCs], or prolonged, resulting from cord prolapse), placental separation or complete abruption, or head compression (head compression causes increased intracranial pressure and vagal nerve stimulation with an accompanying decrease in the FHR)
- Reduction in blood flow to the intervillous space in the placenta secondary to uterine hypertonus (generally caused by excessive exogenous oxytocin) or secondary to deterioration of the placental vasculature associated with maternal disorders such as hypertension or diabetes mellitus

Fetal well-being during labor can be measured by the response of the FHR to UCs. A group of fetal monitoring experts recommended that FHR tracings demonstrating certain reassuring characteristics be described as *normal* (category I) (Box 18-1).

BOX 18-1 THREE-TIER FETAL HEART RATE CLASSIFICATION SYSTEM

CATEGORY I

Category I fetal heart rate (FHR) tracings include all of the following:

- Baseline rate 110 to 160 beats/min (bpm)
- Baseline FHR variability: moderate
- Late or variable decelerations: absent
- Early decelerations: either present or absent
- Accelerations: either present or absent

CATEGORY II

Category II FHR tracings include all FHR tracings not categorized as category I or category III. Examples of category II tracings include any of the following:

- Baseline rate
  - Bradycardia not accompanied by absent baseline variability
  - Tachycardia
- Baseline FHR variability
  - Minimal baseline variability
  - Absent baseline variability not accompanied by recurrent decelerations
  - Marked baseline variability
- Accelerations
  - No acceleration produced in response to fetal stimulation
- Periodic or episodic decelerations
  - Recurrent variable decelerations accompanied by minimal or moderate baseline variability
  - Prolonged decelerations (≥2 minutes but <10 minutes)
  - Recurrent late decelerations with moderate baseline variability
  - Variable decelerations with other characteristics, such as slow return to baseline, "overshoots" or "shoulders"

CATEGORY III

Category III FHR tracings include either:

- Absent baseline variability and any of the following:
  - Recurrent late decelerations
  - Recurrent variable decelerations
  - Bradycardia
- Sinusoidal pattern

Source: Macones, G., Hankins, G., Spong, C., Hauth, J., & Moore, T. (2008). The 2008 National Institute of Child Health and Human Development workshop report on electronic fetal monitoring: Update on definitions, interpretation, and research guidelines. *Journal of Obstetric, Gynecologic and Neonatal Nursing, 37*(5), 510-515.

Uterine Activity

Table 18-1 describes normal uterine activity (UA) during labor.

Fetal Compromise

The goals of intrapartum FHR monitoring are to identify and differentiate the normal (reassuring) patterns from the abnormal (nonreassuring) patterns, which can be indicative of fetal compromise. Although the 2008 National Institute of Child Health and Human Development workshop (Macones, Hankins, Spong, Hauth, & Moore, 2008) and ACOG (2009) both recommend use of the terms *normal* and *abnormal* to describe FHR tracings, the terms *reassuring* and *nonreassuring* are still frequently used clinically.

Abnormal FHR patterns are those associated with fetal **hypoxemia,** which is a deficiency of oxygen in the arterial blood. If uncorrected, hypoxemia can deteriorate to severe fetal **hypoxia,** which is an inadequate supply of oxygen at the cellular level. See Box 18-1 for examples of abnormal (category III) FHR tracings.

MONITORING TECHNIQUES

The ideal method of fetal assessment during labor continues to be debated. Research findings support the use of both intermittent auscultation (IA) of the FHR and electronic FHR monitoring (Gilbert, 2011). Although IA is a high-touch, low-technology method of assessing fetal status during labor that places fewer restrictions on maternal activity, more than 85% of laboring

TABLE 18-1 NORMAL UTERINE ACTIVITY DURING LABOR

CHARACTERISTIC	DESCRIPTION
Frequency	Contraction frequency overall generally ranges from two to five per 10 minutes during labor, with lower frequencies seen in the first stage of labor and higher frequencies (up to five contractions in 10 minutes) seen during the second stage of labor.
Duration	Contraction duration remains fairly stable throughout the first and second stages, ranging from 45-80 seconds, not generally exceeding 90 seconds.
Intensity (peak less resting tone)	Intensity of uterine contractions generally range from 25-50 mm Hg in the first stage of labor and may rise to over 80 mm Hg in second stage. Contractions palpated as "mild" would likely peak at less than 50 mm Hg if measured internally, whereas contractions palpated as "moderate" or greater would likely peak at 50 mm Hg or greater if measured internally.
Resting tone	Average resting tone during labor is 10 mm Hg; if using palpation, should palpate as "soft" (i.e., easily indented, no palpable resistance).
Montevideo units (MVUs)	Ranges from 100-250 MVUs in the first stage, may rise to 300-400 in the second stage. Contraction intensities of 40 mm Hg or more and MVUs of 80-120 are generally sufficient to initiate spontaneous labor. MVUs are used only with internal monitoring of contractions.

Sources: Tucker, S., Miller, L., & Miller, D. (2009). *Mosby's pocket guide to fetal monitoring: A multidisciplinary approach* (6th ed.). St. Louis: Mosby; Macones, G., Hankins, G, Spong, C., Hauth, J., & Moore, T. (2008). The 2008 National Institute of Child Health and Human Development Workshop Report on Electronic Fetal Monitoring: Update on definitions, interpretation, and research guidelines. *Journal of Obstetric, Gynecologic and Neonatal Nursing, 37*(5), 510-515.

women in the United States are monitored electronically for at least part of their labor (ACOG, 2009; Tucker et al., 2009). The continued use of EFM in place of IA is thought to be due to concerns about liability and the increased nurse-client ratio required with IA. Because all surveillance methods including EFM have limitations, some feel the evidence supports a return to the use of IA for low risk laboring women (ACOG; Tucker et al.).

Intermittent Auscultation

Intermittent auscultation involves listening to fetal heart sounds at periodic intervals to assess the FHR. IA of the fetal heart can be performed with a Pinard stethoscope, Doppler ultrasound (Fig.18-1, *A*), an ultrasound stethoscope (see Fig. 18-1, *B*), or a DeLee-Hillis fetoscope (see Fig. 18-1, *C*). The fetoscope is applied to the listener's forehead because bone conduction amplifies the fetal heart sounds for counting. Doppler ultrasound and ultrasound stethoscopes transmit ultra high-frequency sound waves, reflecting movement of the fetal heart, and convert these sounds into an electronic signal that can be counted. Box 18-2 describes how to perform IA.

IA is easy to use, inexpensive, and less invasive than EFM. It is often more comfortable for the woman and gives her more freedom of movement. Other care measures, such as ambulation and the use of baths or showers, are easier to carry out when IA is used. However, IA may be difficult to perform in women who are obese. Because IA is intermittent, significant events may occur during a time when the FHR is not being auscultated. Also IA does not provide a permanent documented visual record of the FHR and cannot be used to assess visual patterns of the FHR variability or periodic changes (Albers, 2007; Tucker et al., 2009). By using IA the nurse can assess the baseline FHR, rhythm, and increases and decreases from baseline.

EVIDENCE-BASED PRACTICE

Pat Gingrich

Fetal Monitoring and the Machine That Goes "Beep"

ASK THE QUESTION

Does electronic fetal monitoring (EFM) make a difference in perinatal outcomes?

SEARCH FOR EVIDENCE

Search Strategies

Professional organization guidelines, meta-analyses, systematic reviews, randomized controlled trials, nonrandomized prospective studies, and retrospective studies since 2008.

Databases Searched

CINAHL, Cochrane, Medline, National Guideline Clearinghouse, TRIP Database Plus, and the websites for American College of Obstetricians and Gynecologists, Association of Women's Health, Obstetric and Neonatal Nurses, and National Institute of Health and Clinical Excellence.

CRITICALLY ANALYZE THE EVIDENCE

The electronic fetal heart monitor has been standard equipment in the labor and birth setting for many decades, especially in the United States. It has been suggested that EFM is not necessary for the low-risk woman in labor, and that it may even present a risk of false abnormal readings leading to high rates of cesarean births.

A meta-analysis of trials measuring fetal outcomes and use of EFM revealed there was no significant difference in APGAR scores for women who had EFM on admission for labor, when compared to women who were not monitored at admission. However, there was a statistically increased risk for cesarean birth in the monitored women (Gourounti & Sandall, 2007). A Cochrane Systematic Database Review of 6 studies involving 2105 pregnant women at increased risk for complications found that use of EFM made no difference in outcomes of perinatal mortality or cesarean rate, when compared to no EFM use (Grivell, Alfirevic, Gyte & Devane, 2010). The reviewers call for more research, particularly of computerized EFM (where the computer analyzes and alerts the practitioner about abnormal patterns).

The National Institute of Health and Clinical Excellence (NICE) issued professional guidelines for intrapartum care that do not recommend EFM for the low-risk laboring woman (NICE, 2007). Instead, the guidelines recommend intermittent auscultation at admission and during labor, using a stethoscope or Doppler. Use of continuous EFM should begin in the presence of meconium, bleeding, abnormal fetal heart rate (<110 bpm, or >160 bpm), oxytocin use, or client request.

IMPLICATIONS FOR PRACTICE

Health care providers, including nurses, can use the mnemonic DR C BRAVADO to remember the systematic and holistic interpretation of EFM:

- DR = Determine Risk factors of mother and fetus
- C = Contraction number in a 10 minute window, averaged over 30 minutes
- BRA = Baseline Rate of fetal heart in a 10 minute window
- V = Variability
- A = Accelerations
- D = Deceleration
- O = Overall assessment (Bailey, 2009)

EFM is here to stay, but it is only a tool. Women and providers have come to expect the constant feedback, and busy nurses have come to rely on the remote screens as they move from room to room. However, the risks of false alarms, and the legal vulnerability of ambiguous patterns, may be contributing to the soaring cesarean rate, which carries its own risks. Continuous monitoring of low-risk women restricts client mobility, which may prolong labor and increase discomfort. In high-risk situations, EFM can be valuable for identifying some fetal stress early, but also may be inaccurate, ambiguous, and cause needless anxiety. Women who expect routine monitoring need explanations about the risks and benefits of continuous monitoring versus intermittent auscultation, and to be given informed choices. The health care team may also need to become more proficient and familiar with auscultation as an assessment tool.

References

Bailey, R. (2009). Intrapartum fetal monitoring. *American Family Physician, 80*(12), 1388–1396.

Gourounti, K., & Sandall, J. (2007). Admission cardiotocography versus intermittent auscultation of fetal heart rate: Effects on neonatal Apgar score, on the rate of caesarean sections and on the rate of instrumental delivery—A systematic review. *International Journal of Nursing Studies, 44*(6), 1029–1035.

Grivell, R., Alfirevic, Z., Gyte, G., & Devane, D. (2010). Antenatal cardiotocography for fetal assessment. *The Cochrane Database of Systematic Reviews 2010*, 1, CD007863.

National Institute of Health and Clinical Excellence. (2007). Intrapartal care: Care for healthy women and their babies during childbirth. *NICE Clinical Guideline 55*. London, NICE. Available at www.nice.org.uk/nicemedia/pdf/IPCNICEGuidance.pdf. Accessed July 5, 2010.

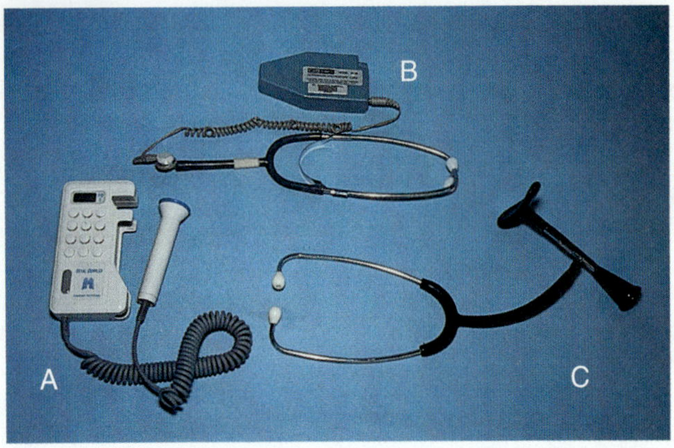

FIG. 18-1 **A,** Ultrasound fetoscope. **B,** Ultrasound stethoscope. **C,** DeLee-Hillis fetoscope. (Courtesy Michael S. Clement, MD, Mesa, AZ.)

BOX 18-2 PROCEDURE FOR INTERMITTENT AUSCULTATION OF THE FETAL HEART RATE

1. Palpate the maternal abdomen to identify fetal presentation and position.
2. Apply ultrasonic gel to the device if using a Doppler ultrasound. Place the listening device (see Fig. 18-1) over the area of maximal intensity and clarity of the fetal heart sounds to obtain the clearest and loudest sound, which is easiest to count. This location will usually be over the fetal back. If using the fetoscope, firm pressure may be needed.
3. Count the maternal radial pulse while listening to the FHR to differentiate it from the fetal rate.
4. Palpate the abdomen for the presence or absence of UA so as to count the FHR between contractions.
5. Count the FHR for 30 to 60 seconds between contractions to identify the auscultated rate, best assessed in the absence of UA.
6. Auscultate the FHR before, during, and after a contraction to identify the FHR during the contraction, as a response to the contraction, and to assess for the absence or presence of increases or decreases in FHR.
7. When distinct discrepancies in the FHR are noted during listening periods, auscultate for a longer period during, after, and between contractions to identify significant changes that may indicate the need for another mode of FHR monitoring.

FHR, Fetal heart rate; *UA,* uterine activity.
Source: Tucker, S., Miller, L., & Miller, D. (2009). *Mosby's pocket guide to fetal monitoring: A multidisciplinary approach* (6th ed.). St. Louis: Mosby.

The American College of Nurse-Midwives reviewed references from the United States, Great Britain, and Canada regarding the recommended frequency of IA in low risk women and found consistent recommendations for every 15 minutes in the active phase of the first stage of labor and every 5 minutes in the second stage of labor (Tucker et al., 2009). ACOG (2009) concurs that these time frames are acceptable for IA in low risk women. The Association of Women's Health, Obstetric and Neonatal Nurses (AWHONN) recommends different IA frequencies: every hour in the latent phase of first stage labor, every 30 minutes in the active phase of first stage labor, and every 15 minutes in the second stage of labor (AWHONN, 2009). However, the optimal frequency for IA in low risk women during labor has not been determined (Nageotte & Gilstrap, 2009).

! NURSING ALERT

When the FHR is auscultated and documented, it is inappropriate to use the descriptive terms associated with EFM (e.g., moderate variability, variable deceleration) because most of the terms are visual descriptions of the patterns produced on the monitor tracing. Terms that are numerically defined, however, such as bradycardia and tachycardia, can be used. FHR when auscultated should be described as a baseline number or range, and as having a regular or irregular rhythm. The presence or absence of accelerations or decelerations both during and after contractions should also be noted (AWHONN, 2009).

Every effort should be made to use the method of fetal assessment the woman desires, if possible. However, auscultation of the FHR in accordance with the frequency guidelines suggested earlier may be difficult in today's busy labor and birth units. When used as the primary method of fetal assessment, auscultation requires a one-to-one nurse-to-client staffing ratio. If acuity and census change so that auscultation standards are no longer met, the nurse must inform the physician or nurse-midwife that continuous EFM will be used until staffing can be arranged to meet the standards.

The woman can become anxious if the examiner cannot readily count the fetal heartbeats. It often takes time for the inexperienced listener to locate the heartbeat and find the area of maximal intensity. To allay the mother's concerns, she can be told that the nurse is "finding the spot where the sounds are loudest." If it takes considerable time to locate the fetal heartbeats, the examiner can reassure the mother by offering her an opportunity to listen to them, too. If the examiner cannot locate the fetal heartbeat, assistance should be requested. In some cases ultrasound can be used to help locate the fetal heartbeat. Seeing the FHR on the ultrasound screen will be reassuring to the mother if there was initial difficulty in locating the best area for auscultation.

When using IA, uterine activity is assessed by palpation. The examiner should keep his or her fingertips placed over the fundus before, during, and after contractions. The contraction intensity is usually described as mild, moderate, or strong. The contraction duration is measured in seconds, from the beginning to the end of the contraction. The frequency of contractions is measured in minutes, from the beginning of one contraction to the beginning of the next contraction. The examiner should keep his or her hand on the fundus after the contraction is over to evaluate uterine resting tone or relaxation between contractions. Resting tone between contractions is usually described as soft or relaxed (AWHONN, 2009).

Accurate and complete documentation of fetal status and uterine activity is especially important when IA and palpation are being used because no paper tracing record or computer storage of these assessments is provided as is the case with continuous EFM. Labor flow records or computer charting systems that prompt notations of all assessments are useful for ensuring such comprehensive documentation.

Electronic Fetal Monitoring

The purpose of electronic FHR monitoring is the ongoing assessment of fetal oxygenation. FHR tracings are analyzed for characteristic patterns that suggest fetal hypoxic events and metabolic acidosis during labor. When hypoxia or metabolic acidosis is suspected in labor, interventions to resolve the problem can be implemented in a timely manner before permanent damage or death occurs (Garite, 2007). The two modes of electronic fetal monitoring include the external mode, which uses external transducers placed on the maternal abdomen to assess FHR and uterine activity, and the internal mode, which uses a **spiral electrode** applied to the fetal presenting part to assess the FHR and an **intrauterine pressure catheter (IUPC)** to assess UA and uterine resting tone. The differences between the external and internal modes of EFM are summarized in Table 18-2.

External Monitoring

Separate transducers are used to monitor the FHR and UCs (Fig. 18-2). The **ultrasound transducer** works by reflecting high-frequency sound waves off a moving interface: in this case, the fetal heart and valves. It is sometimes difficult to reproduce a continuous and precise record of the FHR because of artifact introduced by fetal and maternal movement. Maternal obesity, occiput posterior position of the fetus, and anterior attachment of the placenta can cause weak or absent signals (AWHONN, 2009). The FHR is printed on specially formatted monitor paper. The standard paper speed used in the United States is 3 cm/min. Once the area of maximal intensity of the FHR has been located, conductive gel is applied to the surface of the ultrasound transducer, and the transducer is then positioned over this area and held securely in place using an elastic belt.

The **tocotransducer** (tocodynamometer) measures UA transabdominally. The device is placed over the fundus above the umbilicus and held securely in place using an elastic belt (see Fig. 18-2, *B*). UCs or fetal movements depress a pressure-sensitive surface on the side next to the abdomen. The tocotransducer can measure and record the frequency and approximate duration of UCs but not their intensity. This method is especially valuable for measuring UA during the first stage of labor in women with intact membranes or for antepartum testing. If the woman is obese, the tocotransducer may be unable to detect the exact frequency and duration of UA.

Because the tocotransducer of most electronic fetal monitors is designed for assessing UA in the term pregnancy, it may not be sensitive enough to detect preterm UA. When monitoring the woman in preterm labor, remember that the fundus may be located below the level of the umbilicus. The nurse may need to rely on the woman to indicate when UA is occurring and to use palpation as an additional way of assessing contraction frequency and validating the monitor tracing.

The external transducers are easily applied by the nurse, but often must be repositioned as the woman or fetus changes position. The woman is asked to assume a semi-Fowler's or lateral position. Use of external transducers confines the woman to bed or chair. Portable telemetry monitors allow observation of the FHR and UC patterns by means of centrally located electronic display stations. These portable units permit the woman to walk around during electronic monitoring.

Internal Monitoring

The technique of continuous internal FHR or UA monitoring provides a more accurate appraisal of fetal well-being during labor than external monitoring because it is not interrupted by fetal or maternal movement or affected by maternal size (Fig. 18-3). For this type of monitoring, the membranes must be ruptured, the cervix sufficiently dilated (at least 2 to 3 cm), and the presenting part low enough to allow placement of the spiral electrode or intrauterine pressure catheter or both. Internal and external modes of monitoring may be combined (i.e., internal FHR with external UA or external FHR with internal UA) without difficulty.

TABLE 18-2 EXTERNAL AND INTERNAL MODES OF MONITORING

EXTERNAL MODE	INTERNAL MODE
Fetal Heart Rate	
Ultrasound transducer: High-frequency sound waves reflect mechanical action of the fetal heart. Noninvasive. Does not require rupture of membranes or cervical dilation. Used during both the antepartum and intrapartum periods.	*Spiral electrode:* Converts the fetal ECG as obtained from the presenting part to the FHR via a cardiotachometer. Can be used only when membranes are ruptured and the cervix is sufficiently dilated during the intrapartum period. Electrode penetrates into fetal presenting part by 1.5 mm and must be attached securely to ensure a good signal.
Uterine Activity	
Tocotransducer: Monitors frequency and duration of contractions by means of a pressure-sensing device applied to the maternal abdomen. Used during both the antepartum and intrapartum periods.	*Intrauterine pressure catheter (IUPC):* Monitors the frequency, duration, and intensity of contractions. The two types of IUPCs are a fluid-filled system and a solid catheter. Both measure intrauterine pressure at the catheter tip and convert the pressure into millimeters of mercury on the uterine activity panel of the strip chart. Both can be used only when membranes are ruptured and the cervix is sufficiently dilated during the intrapartum period.

ECG, Electrocardiogram; *FHR,* fetal heart rate.

Internal monitoring of the FHR is accomplished by attaching a small spiral electrode to the presenting part. For UA to be monitored internally an IUPC is introduced into the uterine cavity. The catheter has a pressure-sensitive tip that measures changes in intrauterine pressure. As the catheter is compressed during a contraction, pressure is placed on the pressure transducer. This pressure is then converted into a pressure reading in millimeters of mercury (mm Hg). The IUPC can objectively measure the frequency, duration, and intensity of UC, as well as uterine resting tone.

Because it can precisely measure the intensity of individual UCs, the IUPC can be used to evaluate the adequacy of UA for achieving progress in labor. **Montevideo units (MVUs)** are calculated by subtracting the baseline uterine pressure from the peak contraction pressure for each contraction that occurs in a 10 minute window, and then adding together the pressures generated by each contraction that occurs during that period of time. Spontaneous labor usually begins when MVUs are between 80 and 120. Uterine activity during normal labor rarely exceeds 250 MVUs (see Table 18-1) (Cunningham, Leveno, Bloom, Hauth, Rouse, & Spong, 2010; Tucker et al., 2009).

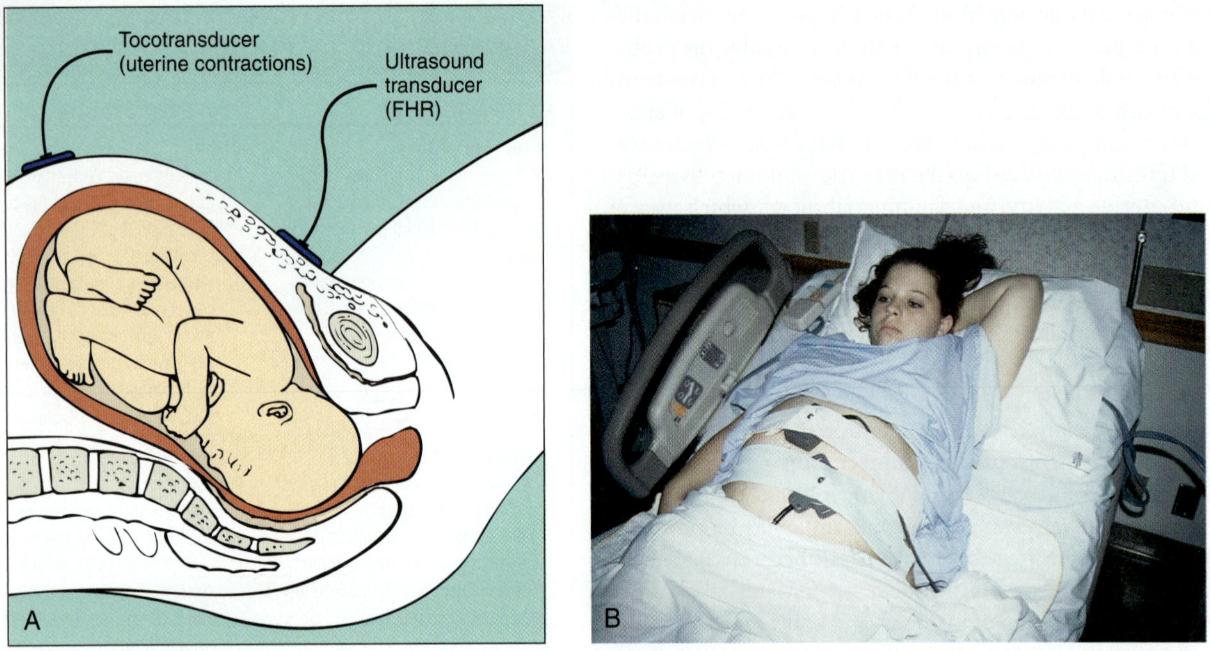

FIG. 18-2 **A,** External noninvasive fetal monitoring with tocotransducer and ultrasound transducer. **B,** Ultrasound transducer is placed below umbilicus, over the area where fetal heart rate is best heard, and tocotransducer is placed on uterine fundus. (**B,** Courtesy Marjorie Pyle, RNC, Lifecircle, Costa Mesa, CA.)

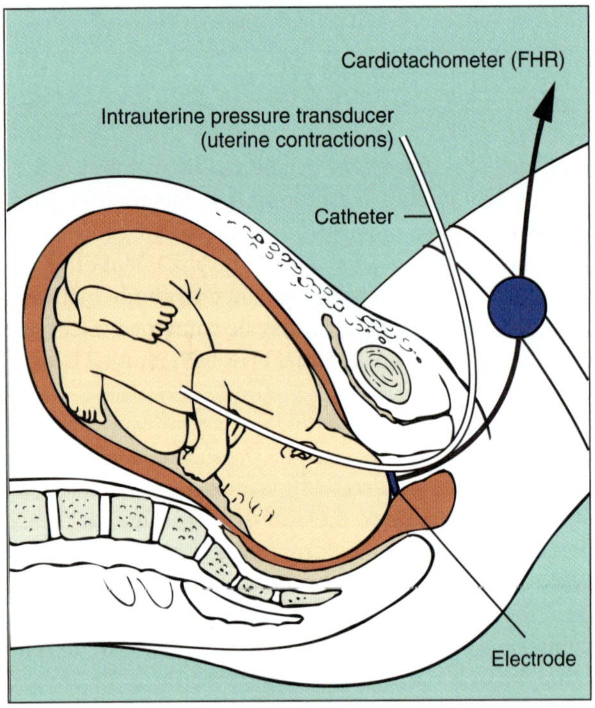

FIG. 18-3 Diagrammatic representation of internal invasive fetal monitoring with intrauterine pressure catheter and spiral electrode in place (membranes ruptured and cervix dilated).

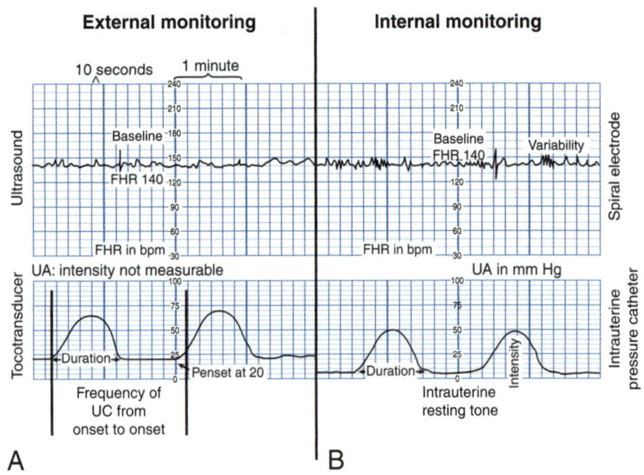

FIG. 18-4 Display of fetal heart rate and uterine activity on monitor paper. **A,** External mode with ultrasound and tocotransducer as signal source. **B,** Internal mode with spiral electrode and intrauterine catheter as signal source. Frequency of contractions is measured from the beginning of one contraction to the beginning of the next. (From Tucker, S., Miller, L., & Miller, D. [2009]. *Mosby's pocket guide to fetal monitoring: A multidisciplinary approach* [6th ed.]. St. Louis: Mosby.)

Display

The FHR and UA are displayed on the monitor paper or computer screen, with the FHR in the upper section and UA in the lower section. Figure 18-4 contrasts the internal and external modes of electronic monitoring. Note that each small square on the monitor paper or screen represents 10 seconds; each larger box of six squares equals 1 minute (when paper is moving through the monitor at the rate of 3 cm/min).

FETAL HEART RATE PATTERNS

Characteristic FHR patterns are associated with fetal and maternal physiologic processes and have been identified for many years. Because EFM was introduced into clinical practice before consensus was reached in regard to standardized terminology, however, variations in the description and interpretation of common fetal heart rate patterns were often great. In 1997 the National Institute of Child Health and Human Development (NICHD) published a proposed nomenclature system for EFM interpretation with standardized definitions for FHR monitoring. The NICHD recommendations were not widely incorporated into clinical practice, however, until they were endorsed by

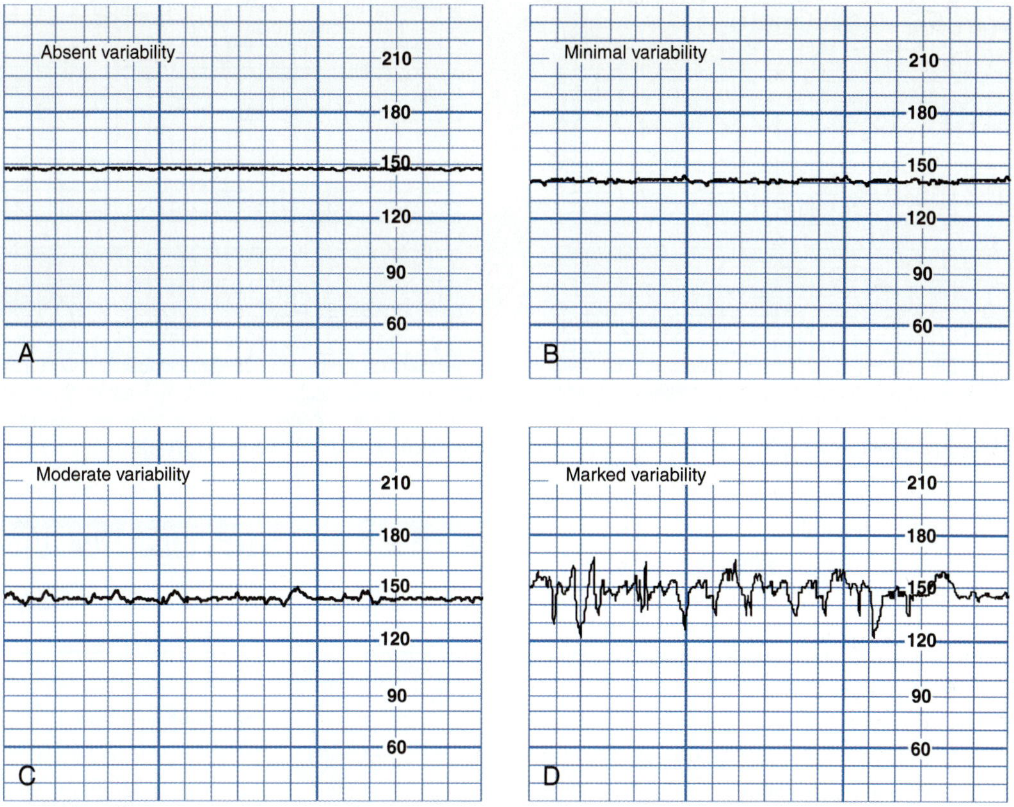

FIG. 18-5 Fetal heart rate variability. **A,** Absent variability; amplitude range undetectable. **B,** Minimal variability; amplitude range detectable up to and including 5 beats/min. **C,** Moderate variability; amplitude range 6 to 25 beats/min. **D,** Marked variability; amplitude range >25 beats/min. (From Tucker, S., Miller, L., & Miller, D. [2009]. *Mosby's pocket guide to fetal monitoring: A multidisciplinary approach* [6th ed.]. St. Louis: Mosby.)

ACOG in 2005. Shortly thereafter, use of the NICHD standard terminology was also endorsed by AWHONN and the American College of Nurse-Midwives (ACNM) (Tucker et al., 2009). All three organizations cited concerns regarding client safety and the need for improved communication among caregivers as reasons for using standard EFM definitions in clinical practice.

In April 2008 the NICHD, ACOG, and the Society for Maternal-Fetal Medicine partnered to sponsor another workshop to revisit the FHR definitions recommended by the NICHD in 1997. The 1997 FHR definitions were reaffirmed at this workshop. In addition, new definitions related to UA were recommended, as well as a three-tier system of FHR pattern interpretation and categorization (Macones et al., 2008).

Baseline Fetal Heart Rate

The intrinsic rhythmicity of the fetal heart, the central nervous system (CNS), and the fetal autonomic nervous system control the FHR. An increase in sympathetic response results in acceleration of the FHR, whereas an increase in parasympathetic response produces a slowing of the FHR. Usually a balanced increase of sympathetic and parasympathetic response occurs during contractions, with no observable change in the baseline FHR.

The **baseline fetal heart rate** is the average rate during a 10-minute segment that excludes periodic or episodic changes, periods of marked variability, and segments of the baseline that differ by more than 25 beats/min. There must be at least 2 minutes of interpretable baseline data in a 10-minute segment of tracing in order to determine the baseline FHR (Macones et al, 2008). After 10 minutes of tracing is observed the approximate mean rate is rounded to the closest 5-beats/min interval (AWHONN, 2009). For example, if the FHR rate varies between 130 and 140 beats/min over a 10-minute period, the baseline is recorded as 135 beats/min. The normal range at term is 110 to 160 beats/min. In the preterm fetus the baseline rate is slightly higher.

Variability

Variability of the FHR can be described as irregular waves or fluctuations in the baseline FHR of two cycles per minute or greater (Macones et al., 2008). It is a characteristic of the baseline FHR and does not include accelerations or decelerations of the FHR. Variability is quantified in beats per minute and is measured from the peak to the trough of a single cycle. Four possible categories of variability have been identified: absent, minimal, moderate, and marked (Fig. 18-5). In the past, variability was described as either long term or short term (beat to beat). The NICHD definitions do not distinguish between long- and short-term variability, however, because in actual practice they are visually determined as a unit (NICHD, 1997).

Depending on other characteristics of the FHR tracing, absent or minimal variability is classified as either abnormal or indeterminate (Macones et al., 2008) (see Fig. 18-5, *A* and *B*). It can result from fetal hypoxemia and metabolic acidemia. Other possible causes of absent or minimal variability include congenital anomalies and preexisting neurologic injury. CNS depressant medications, including analgesics, narcotics (meperidine [Demerol]), barbiturates (secobarbital [Seconal] and pentobarbital [Nembutal]), tranquilizers (diazepam [Valium]), ataractics (promethazine [Phenergan]), and general anesthetics are other

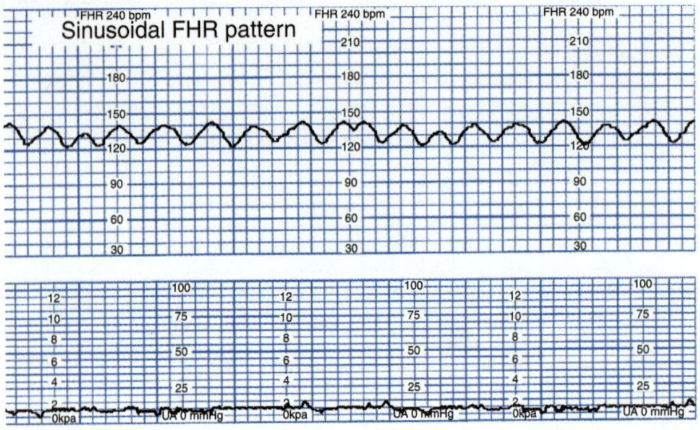

FIG. 18-6 Sinusoidal FHR pattern. (From Tucker, S., Miller, L., & Miller, D. [2009]. *Mosby's pocket guide to fetal monitoring: A multidisciplinary approach* [6th ed.]. St. Louis: Mosby.)

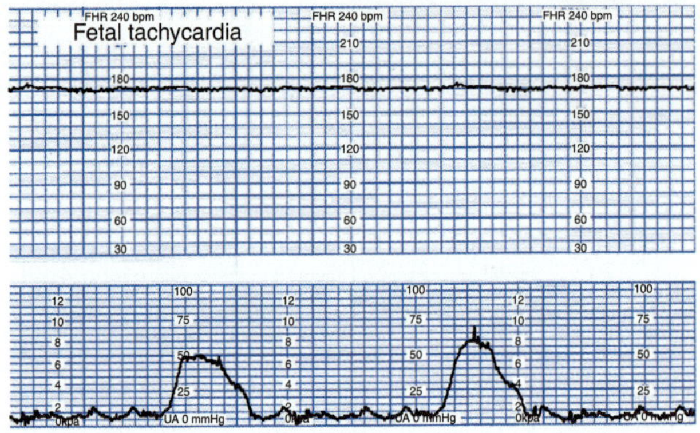

FIG. 18-7 Fetal tachycardia. (From Tucker, S., Miller, L., & Miller, D. [2009]. *Mosby's pocket guide to fetal monitoring: A multidisciplinary approach* [6th ed.]. St. Louis: Mosby.)

possible causes of minimal variability. In addition, minimal variability can occur with tachycardia, extreme prematurity, or when the fetus is temporarily in a sleep state (Tucker et al., 2009). These sleep states do not usually last longer than 30 minutes.

Moderate variability, however, is considered normal (see Fig. 18-5, *C*). Its presence is highly predictive of a normal fetal acid-base balance (absence of fetal metabolic acidemia). Moderate variability indicates that FHR regulation is not significantly affected by fetal sleep cycles, tachycardia, prematurity, congenital anomalies, preexisting neurologic injury, or CNS depressant medications (Macones et al., 2008; Tucker et al., 2009).

The significance of marked variability (see Fig. 18-5, *D*) is unclear (Macones et al., 2008). A sinusoidal pattern—a regular smooth, undulating wavelike pattern—is not included in the definition of FHR variability. This uncommon pattern classically occurs with severe fetal anemia (Fig. 18-6) (Tucker et al., 2009).

Tachycardia

Tachycardia is a baseline FHR greater than 160 beats/min for 10 minutes or longer (Fig. 18-7). It can be considered an early sign of fetal hypoxemia, especially when associated with late decelerations and minimal or absent variability. Fetal tachycardia can result from maternal or fetal infection, such as prolonged rupture of membranes with amnionitis; from maternal hyperthyroidism or fetal anemia; or in response to medications such as atropine, hydroxyzine (Vistaril), terbutaline (Brethine), or illicit drugs such as cocaine or methamphetamines. Table 18-3 lists causes, clinical significance, and nursing interventions for tachycardia.

Bradycardia

Bradycardia is a baseline FHR less than 110 beats/min for 10 minutes or longer (Fig. 18-8). True bradycardia occurs rarely and is not specifically related to fetal oxygenation. True bradycardia must be distinguished from a prolonged deceleration because the causes and management of these two conditions are very different. Bradycardia is often caused by some type of fetal cardiac problem such as structural defects involving the pacemakers or conduction system or fetal heart failure. Other causes of bradycardia include viral infections (e.g., cytomegalovirus), maternal hypoglycemia, and maternal hypothermia. The clinical significance of the bradycardia depends on the underlying cause and accompanying FHR patterns, including variability and the presence of accelerations or decelerations (Tucker et al., 2009). (See Table 18-3 for a list of causes, clinical significance, and nursing interventions for bradycardia.)

TABLE 18-3 TACHYCARDIA AND BRADYCARDIA

TACHYCARDIA	BRADYCARDIA
DEFINITION	
FHR 160 beats/min lasting >10 min	FHR <110 beats/min lasting >10 min
POSSIBLE CAUSES	
Early fetal hypoxemia Fetal cardiac arrhythmias Maternal fever Infection (including chorioamnionitis) Parasympatholytic drugs (atropine, hydroxyzine) β-Sympathomimetic drugs (terbutaline) Maternal hyperthyroidism Fetal anemia Drugs (caffeine, cocaine, methamphetamines)	Atrioventricular dissociation (heart block) Structural defects Viral infections (e.g., cytomegalovirus) Medications Fetal heart failure Maternal hypoglycemia Maternal hypothermia
CLINICAL SIGNIFICANCE	
Persistent tachycardia in absence of periodic changes does not appear serious in terms of neonatal outcome (especially true if tachycardia is associated with maternal fever); tachycardia is abnormal when associated with late decelerations, severe variable decelerations, or absent variability.	Baseline bradycardia alone is not specifically related to fetal oxygenation. The clinical significance of bradycardia depends on the underlying cause and the accompanying FHR patterns, including variability, accelerations, or decelerations.
NURSING INTERVENTIONS	
Dependent on cause; reduce maternal fever with antipyretics as ordered and cooling measures; oxygen at 8 to 10 L/min by nonrebreather face mask may be of some value; carry out health care provider's orders based on alleviating cause.	Dependent on cause

FHR, Fetal heart rate.

Periodic and Episodic Changes in Fetal Heart Rate

Changes in FHR from the baseline are categorized as periodic or episodic. **Periodic changes** are those that occur with UCs. **Episodic changes** are those that are not associated with UCs.

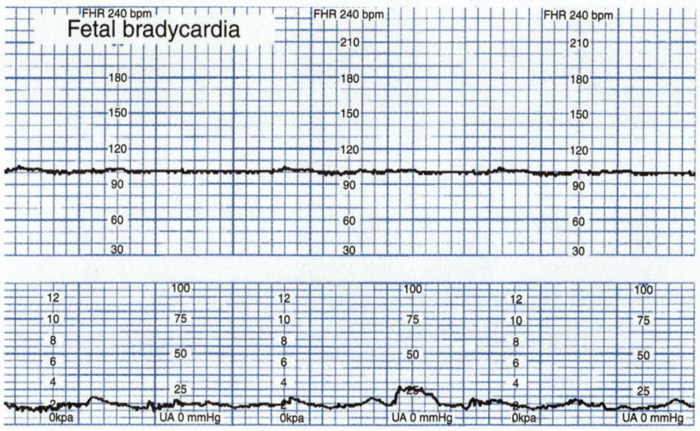

FIG. 18-8 Fetal bradycardia. (From Tucker, S., Miller, L., & Miller, D. [2009]. *Mosby's pocket guide to fetal monitoring: A multidisciplinary approach* [6th ed.]. St. Louis: Mosby.)

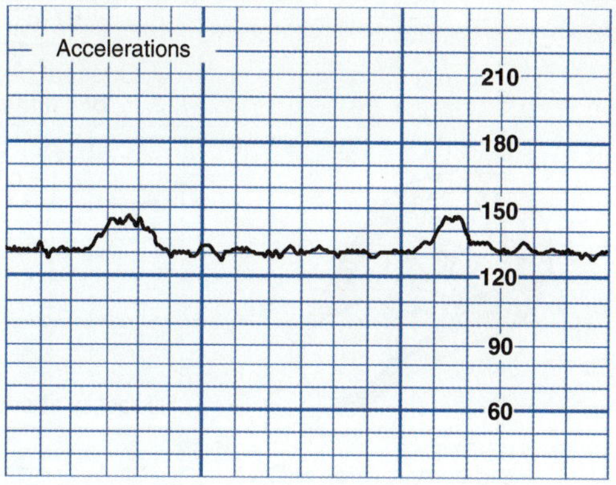

FIG. 18-9 Fetal accelerations. (From Tucker, S., Miller, L., & Miller, D. [2009]. *Mosby's pocket guide to fetal monitoring: A multidisciplinary approach* [6th ed.]. St. Louis: Mosby.)

These patterns include both accelerations and decelerations (Macones et al., 2008).

Accelerations

Acceleration of the FHR is defined as a visually apparent abrupt (onset to peak less than 30 seconds) increase in FHR above the baseline rate (Fig. 18-9). The peak is at least 15 beats/min above the baseline, and the acceleration lasts 15 seconds or more, with the return to baseline less than 2 minutes from the beginning of the acceleration. Before 32 weeks of gestation the definition of an acceleration is a peak of 10 beats/min or more above the baseline and a duration of at least 10 seconds. Acceleration of the FHR for more than 10 minutes is considered a change in baseline rate (Tucker et al., 2009).

Accelerations can be periodic or episodic. They may occur in association with fetal movement or spontaneously. If accelerations do not occur spontaneously, they can be elicited by fetal scalp stimulation or vibroacoustic stimulation. Similar to moderate variability, accelerations are considered an indication of fetal well-being. Their presence is highly predictive of a normal fetal acid-base balance (absence of fetal metabolic acidemia) (Tucker et al., 2009). Box 18-3 lists causes, clinical significance, and nursing interventions for accelerations.

BOX 18-3 ACCELERATIONS

CAUSES
- Spontaneous fetal movement
- Vaginal examination
- Electrode application
- Fetal scalp stimulation
- Fetal reaction to external sounds
- Breech presentation
- Occiput posterior position
- Uterine contractions
- Fundal pressure
- Abdominal palpation

CLINICAL SIGNIFICANCE

Normal pattern. Acceleration with fetal movement signifies fetal well-being representing fetal alertness or arousal states

NURSING INTERVENTIONS

None required

Decelerations

A deceleration (caused by dominance of a parasympathetic response) may be benign or abnormal (nonreassuring). FHR decelerations are categorized as early, late, variable, or prolonged. They are described by their visual relation to the onset and end of a contraction and by their shape.

Early Decelerations. **Early deceleration** of the FHR is a visually apparent gradual (onset to lowest point ≥30 seconds) decrease in and return to baseline FHR associated with UCs. They are thought to be caused by transient fetal head compression and are considered a normal and benign finding (Macones et al., 2008; Tucker et al., 2009). Generally the onset, nadir, and recovery of the deceleration correspond to the beginning, peak, and end of the contraction (Fig. 18-10). For this reason, early decelerations are sometimes called the "mirror image" of a contraction.

Early decelerations may occur during uterine contractions, during vaginal examinations, as a result of fundal pressure, and during placement of the internal mode of fetal monitoring. When present, they usually occur during the first stage of labor when the cervix is dilated 4 to 7 cm. Early decelerations are also sometimes seen during the second stage when the woman is pushing.

Because early decelerations are considered to be benign, interventions are not necessary. The value of identifying early decelerations is so that they can be distinguished from late or variable decelerations, which can be abnormal (nonreassuring) and for which interventions are appropriate. Box 18-4 lists causes, clinical significance, and nursing interventions for early decelerations.

Late Decelerations. **Late deceleration** of the FHR is a visually apparent gradual decrease in and return to baseline FHR associated with UCs (Macones et al., 2008). The deceleration begins after the contraction has started, and the lowest point of the deceleration occurs after the peak of the contraction. The deceleration usually does not return to baseline until after the contraction is over (Fig. 18-11).

Uteroplacental insufficiency causes late decelerations. Persistent and repetitive late decelerations usually indicate the presence of fetal hypoxemia stemming from insufficient placental perfusion during UCs. If recurrent or sustained, late decelerations can lead to metabolic acidemia (Tucker et al., 2009). They should be considered an ominous sign when

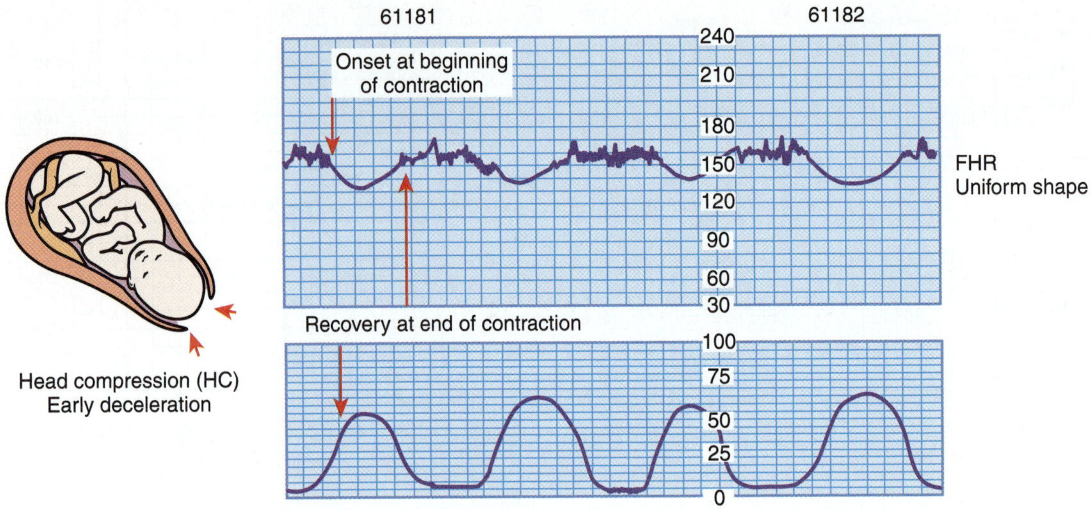

FIG. 18-10 Early decelerations. (From Tucker, S. [2004]. *Pocket guide to fetal monitoring and assessment* [5th ed.]. St. Louis: Mosby.)

BOX 18-4 EARLY DECELERATIONS

CAUSE

Head compression resulting from the following:

- Uterine contractions
- Vaginal examination
- Fundal pressure
- Placement of internal mode of monitoring

CLINICAL SIGNIFICANCE

Normal pattern; not associated with fetal hypoxemia, acidemia, or low Apgar scores

NURSING INTERVENTIONS

None required

they are uncorrectable, especially if they are associated with absent or minimal variability and tachycardia. Several factors can disrupt oxygen transfer to the fetus, including maternal hypotension, uterine tachysystole (e.g., more than five contractions in 10 minutes, averaged over a 30-minute window), preeclampsia, postdate or postterm pregnancy, amnionitis, small-for-gestational-age fetuses, maternal diabetes, placenta previa, placental abruption, conduction anesthetics, maternal cardiac disease, and maternal anemia. The clinical significance and nursing interventions for late decelerations are described in Box 18-5.

Variable Decelerations. Variable deceleration of the FHR is defined as a visually abrupt (onset to lowest point less than 30 seconds) decrease in FHR below the baseline. The decrease is at least 15 beats/min or more below the baseline, lasts at least 15 seconds, and returns to baseline in less than 2 minutes from the time of onset (Macones et al., 2008). Variable decelerations occur any time during the uterine contraction phase and are caused by compression of the umbilical cord (Fig. 18-12).

The appearance of variable decelerations differs from those of early and late decelerations, which closely approximate the shape of the corresponding UC. Instead, variable decelerations have a U, V, or W shape, characterized by a rapid descent and ascent to and from the nadir (lowest point) of the deceleration (see Fig. 18-12). Some variable decelerations are preceded and followed by brief accelerations of the FHR, known as "shoulders," which is an appropriate compensatory response to compression of the umbilical cord.

Occasional variables have little clinical significance. Recurrent variable decelerations, however, indicate repetitive disruption in the fetus's oxygen supply. This can result in hypoxemia and metabolic acidemia (Tucker et al., 2009). Variable decelerations are most commonly found during the transition phase of first stage labor or the second stage of labor as a result of umbilical cord compression and stretching during fetal descent (Garite, 2007). Box 18-6 lists causes, clinical significance, and nursing interventions for variable decelerations.

CLINICAL REASONING

Admission of an Emergency Client to Labor and Delivery

Your client, Rina, 35 years old, G1 P0, arrives via wheelchair to the Labor and Birth Unit in active labor from the emergency department. Rina is at 41 weeks and 3 days of gestation. She states she is scheduled for induction of labor in 2 days. There is moderate vaginal bleeding on the towel in the chair. Rina states her membranes ruptured about 30 minutes ago and "there was not much water, mostly blood." Now the baby is "not moving much." This is your second day in the Labor and Birth Unit with an RN mentor. She applies ultrasound and a tocodynamometer for fetal monitoring. You are asked to assist your mentor by taking vital signs. Rina's vital signs are temperature 37° C, pulse 98, respirations 22, blood pressure 100/54, and oxygen saturation 91%. The fetal heart baseline rate is between 170 and 180 beats per minite, the tracing looks "smooth," and the fetal heart is decreasing after every contraction with return to baseline after the contraction is over. Contractions are occuring every 2 minutes. Rina's pain score is 8/10.

1. Evidence—Is there evidence that Rina and her fetus are at risk?
2. Assumptions—Describe the findings from Rina's admission assessment data presented that support decisions for care based on NICHD terminology.
3. What priorities for Rina's care can be drawn at this time?
4. Does the evidence objectively support your conclusion?
5. Are there alternative perspectives to your conclusion?

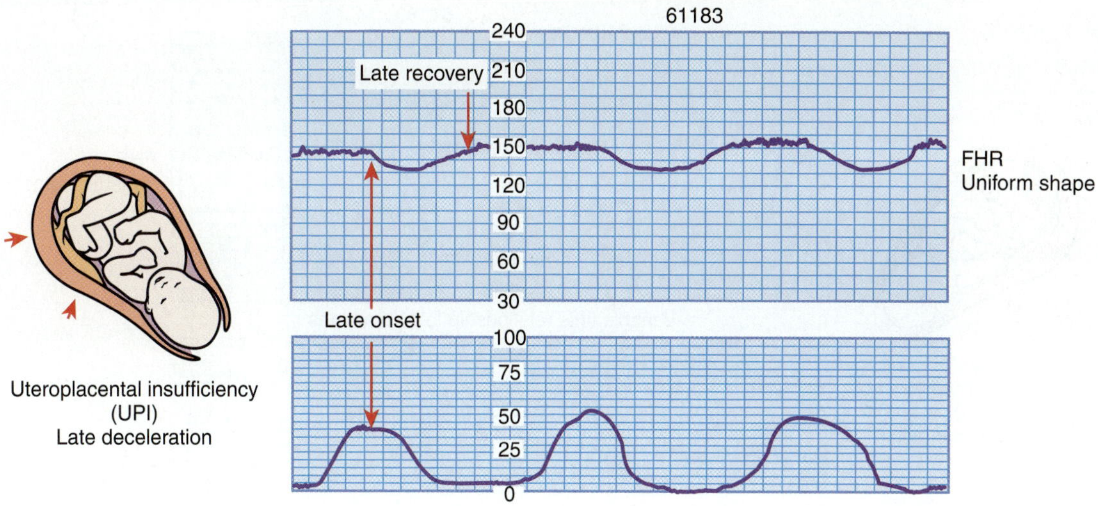

FIG. 18-11 Late decelerations. (From Tucker, S. [2004]. *Pocket guide to fetal monitoring and assessment* [5th ed.]. St. Louis: Mosby.)

BOX 18-5 LATE DECELERATIONS

CAUSE

Uteroplacental insufficiency caused by the following:

- Uterine tachysystole
- Maternal supine hypotension
- Epidural or spinal anesthesia
- Placenta previa
- Placental abruption
- Hypertensive disorders
- Postmaturity
- Intrauterine growth restriction
- Diabetes mellitus
- Intraamniotic infection

CLINICAL SIGNIFICANCE

Abnormal pattern associated with fetal hypoxemia, acidemia, and low Apgar scores; considered ominous if persistent and uncorrected, especially when associated with fetal tachycardia and loss of variability

NURSING INTERVENTIONS

The usual priority is as follows:

1. Change maternal position (lateral).
2. Correct maternal hypotension by elevating legs.
3. Increase rate of maintenance IV solution.
4. Palpate uterus to assess for tachysystole.
5. Discontinue oxytocin if infusing.
6. Administer oxygen at 8 to 10 L/min by nonrebreather face mask.
7. Notify physician or nurse-midwife.
8. Consider internal monitoring for a more accurate fetal and uterine assessment.
9. Assist with birth (cesarean or vaginal assisted) if pattern cannot be corrected.

IV, Intravenous.

Prolonged Decelerations. A **prolonged deceleration** is a visually apparent decrease (may be either gradual or abrupt) in FHR of at least 15 beats/min below the baseline and lasting more than 2 minutes but less than 10 minutes. A deceleration lasting more than 10 minutes is considered a baseline change (Macones et al., 2008) (Fig. 18-13).

Prolonged decelerations are caused by a disruption in the fetal oxygen supply. They usually begin as a reflex response to hypoxia. If the disruption continues, however, the fetal cardiac tissue itself will become hypoxic, resulting in direct myocardial depression of the FHR (Tucker et al., 2009). Prolonged decelerations may be caused by prolonged cord compression, profound uteroplacental insufficiency, or perhaps sustained head compression. The presence and degree of hypoxia present are thought to correlate with the depth and duration of the deceleration, how abruptly it returns to the baseline, how much variability is lost during the deceleration, and whether rebound tachycardia and loss of variability occur after the deceleration (Garite, 2007).

Significant stimuli that may result in prolonged decelerations are a prolapsed umbilical cord or other forms of prolonged cord compression, prolonged uterine tachysystole, hypotension after spinal or epidural anesthesia or analgesia, placental abruption, eclamptic seizure, and rapid fetal descent through the birth canal. Other more benign causes of prolonged decelerations include pelvic examination, application of a spiral electrode, and sustained maternal Valsalva maneuver (Garite, 2007).

! NURSING ALERT

Nurses should notify the physician or nurse-midwife immediately and initiate appropriate treatment of abnormal patterns when they see a prolonged deceleration.

CARE MANAGEMENT

Care of the woman receiving EFM in labor begins with evaluation of the EFM equipment. The nurse must ensure that the monitor is recording FHR and UA accurately and that the tracing is interpretable. If external monitoring is not adequate, changing to a fetal spiral electrode or IUPC may be necessary. A checklist for fetal monitoring equipment can be used to evaluate the equipment functions (Box 18-7).

After ensuring that the monitor is recording properly, the FHR and UA tracings are evaluated regularly throughout labor.

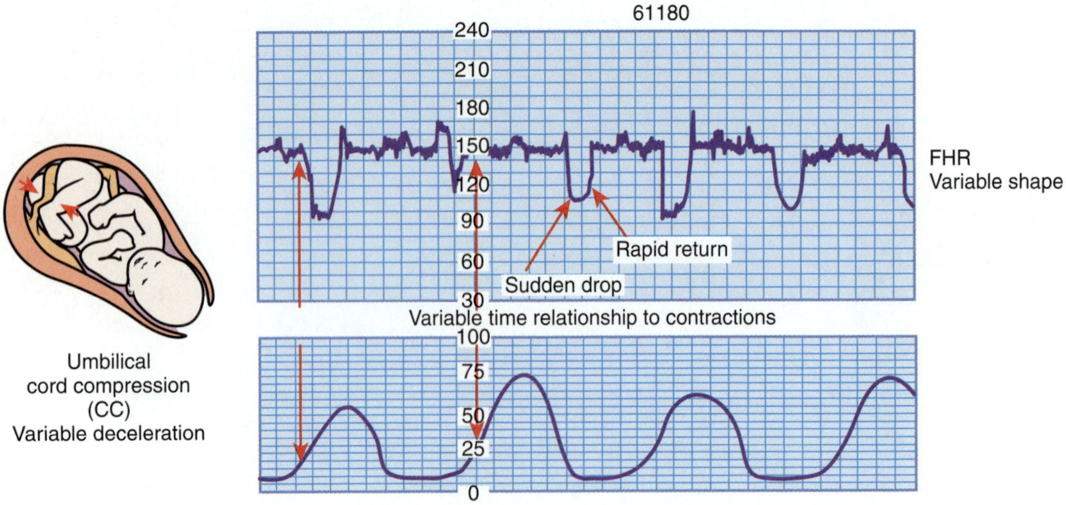

FIG. 18-12 Variable decelerations. (From Tucker, S. [2004]. *Pocket guide to fetal monitoring and assessment* [5th ed.]. St. Louis: Mosby.)

BOX 18-6 VARIABLE DECELERATIONS

CAUSE

Umbilical cord compression caused by the following:

- Maternal position with cord between fetus and maternal pelvis
- Cord around fetal neck, arm, leg, or other body part
- Short cord
- Knot in cord
- Prolapsed cord

CLINICAL SIGNIFICANCE

Variable decelerations occur in approximately 50% of all labors and usually are transient and correctable

NURSING INTERVENTIONS

The usual priority is as follows:

1. Change maternal position (side to side, knee chest).
2. Discontinue oxytocin if infusing.
3. Administer oxygen at 8 to 10 L/min by nonrebreather face mask.
4. Notify physician or nurse-midwife.
5. Assist with vaginal or speculum examination to assess for cord prolapse.
6. Assist with amnioinfusion if ordered.
7. Assist with birth (vaginal assisted or cesarean) if pattern cannot be corrected.

Guidelines for Perinatal Care, published jointly by the American Academy of Pediatrics (AAP) and ACOG (2007), recommends that the FHR tracing be evaluated at least every 30 minutes during the first stage of labor and every 15 minutes during the second stage of labor in low risk women. If risk factors are present, then the FHR tracing should be evaluated more frequently: every 15 minutes in the first stage of labor and every 5 minutes in the second stage of labor.

Based on assessment findings the nurse identifies relevant nursing diagnoses and expected outcomes of care, implements appropriate interventions, and evaluates the care provided (see the Nursing Process box). Assessing FHR and UA patterns, implementing independent nursing interventions, documenting observations and actions according to the established standard of care, and reporting abnormal patterns

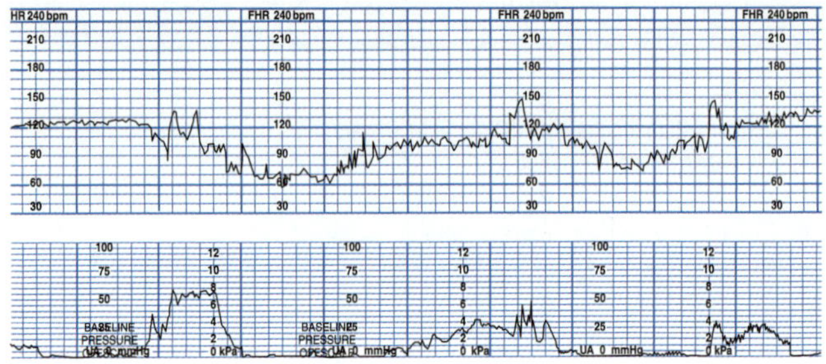

FIG. 18-13 Prolonged decelerations. (From Tucker, S., Miller, L., & Miller, D. [2009]. *Mosby's pocket guide to fetal monitoring: A multidisciplinary approach* [6th ed.]. St. Louis: Mosby.)

to the primary care provider (e.g., physician, certified nurse-midwife) are the responsibilities of the nurse providing care to women in labor.

Electronic Fetal Monitoring Pattern Recognition and Interpretation

Nurses must evaluate many factors to determine whether an FHR pattern is normal (reassuring) or abnormal (nonreassuring) (see the Nursing Process box). Nurses evaluate these factors based on the presence of other obstetric complications, progress in labor, and use of analgesia or anesthesia. They also must consider the estimated time interval until birth. Interventions are therefore based on clinical judgment of a complex, integrated process (Simpson & James, 2005).

Categorizing FHR Tracings

As previously mentioned, a three tier system of categorizing FHR tracings is recommended (see Box 18-1). Category I FHR tracings are normal and strongly predictive of normal fetal acid-base status at the time of observation. These tracings may be followed in a routine manner and do not require any specific action. Category II FHR tracings are indeterminate. This category includes all tracings that do not meet category I or category III criteria. Category II tracings require continued observation and evaluation. Category III FHR tracings are abnormal. Immediate evaluation and prompt intervention is required when these patterns are identified (Macones et al., 2008).

BOX 18-7 CHECKLIST FOR FETAL MONITORING EQUIPMENT

PREPARATION OF MONITOR

1. Is the paper inserted correctly?
2. Are transducer cables plugged securely into the appropriate port on the monitor?
3. Is the paper speed set to 3 cm/min?
4. Was the monitor date and time verified (when using electronic documentation)?

ULTRASOUND TRANSDUCER

1. Has ultrasound transmission gel been applied to the transducer?
2. Was the fetal heart rate (FHR) tested and noted on the monitor strip?
3. Was the FHR compared with the maternal pulse and noted?
4. Does a signal light flash or an audible beep occur with each heartbeat?
5. Is the belt secure and snug but comfortable for the laboring woman?

TOCOTRANSDUCER

1. Is the tocotransducer firmly positioned at the site of the least maternal tissue?
2. Has it been applied without gel or paste?
3. Was the uterine activity (UA) baseline adjusted between contractions to print at the 20 mm Hg line?
4. Is the belt secure and snug but comfortable for the laboring woman?

SPIRAL ELECTRODE

1. Is the connector attached firmly to the electrode pad (on the leg plate or abdomen)?
2. Is the spiral electrode attached to the presenting part of the fetus?
3. Is the inner surface of the electrode pad pre-gelled or covered with electrode gel?
4. Is the electrode pad properly secured to the woman's thigh or abdomen?

INTERNAL CATHETER OR STRAIN GAUGE

1. Is the length line on the catheter visible at the introitus?
2. Is it noted on the monitor paper that a UA test or calibration was performed?
3. Has the monitor been set to zero according to manufacturer's directions?
4. Is the intrauterine pressure catheter properly secured to the woman?
5. Is the baseline resting tone of the uterus documented?

Source: Tucker, S., Miller, L., & Miller, D. (2009). *Mosby's pocket guide to fetal monitoring: A multidisciplinary approach* (6th ed.). St. Louis: Mosby.

NURSING PROCESS

Electronic Fetal Heart Rate Monitoring

ASSESSMENT

Assessment should be performed at least every 30 minutes during the first stage of labor and every 15 minutes during the second stage of labor in low risk women. If risk factors are present, assessment should be performed every 15 minutes in the first stage of labor and every 5 minutes in the second stage of labor.

- Fetal heart rate (FHR) tracing
  - Baseline rate
  - Baseline variability (absent, minimal, moderate, or marked)
  - Presence of accelerations
  - Presence of early, late, variable, or prolonged decelerations
  - Changes in the FHR and pattern over time
- Uterine activity (UA)
  - Contraction frequency
  - Contraction duration
  - Contraction intensity
  - Uterine resting tone
- Maternal vital signs (usually assessed at the same time as the FHR and UA)
  - Blood pressure
  - Pulse
  - Respirations

NURSING DIAGNOSES

Possible nursing diagnoses include:

Decreased Maternal Cardiac Output **related to:**

- supine hypotension secondary to maternal position or regional (epidural) anesthesia

Anxiety **related to:**

- lack of knowledge concerning fetal monitoring during labor
- restriction of mobility or movement during EFM

Impaired Fetal Gas Exchange **related to:**

- umbilical cord compression
- placental insufficiency

Risk for Fetal Injury **related to:**

- unrecognized hypoxemia or metabolic acidemia
- maternal hypotension
- maternal position (aortocaval compression)

EXPECTED OUTCOMES OF CARE

Expected outcomes for the pregnant woman, her family, and the fetus include:

- The pregnant woman and family will verbalize their understanding of the need for monitoring.
- The pregnant woman and family will recognize and avoid situations that compromise maternal and fetal circulation.
- The fetus will not develop hypoxemia or metabolic acidemia.
- Should fetal compromise occur, it will be identified promptly, and appropriate interventions such as intrauterine resuscitation will be initiated.

PLAN OF CARE AND INTERVENTIONS

Implement basic corrective actions immediately whenever one of the essential components of the FHR tracing (see Assessment, above) is determined to be abnormal (see Boxes 18-5, 18-6, 18-8, and Table 18-3 for specific interventions).

EVALUATION

Evaluation of the effectiveness of care of the woman and fetus during electronic FHR and UA monitoring is based on the previously stated expected outcomes.

Source: American Academy of Pediatrics (AAP) and American College of Obstetricians and Gynecologists (ACOG). (2007). *Guidelines for perinatal care* (6th ed.). Washington, DC: ACOG.

LEGAL TIP: Fetal Monitoring Standards

Nurses who care for women during childbirth are legally responsible for correctly interpreting FHR patterns, initiating appropriate nursing interventions based on those patterns, and documenting the outcomes of those interventions. Perinatal nurses are responsible for the timely notification of the physician or nurse-midwife in the event of abnormal FHR patterns. Perinatal nurses also are responsible for initiating the institutional chain of command should differences in opinion arise among health care providers concerning the interpretation of the FHR pattern and the intervention required.

Nursing Management of Abnormal Patterns

The five essential components of the fetal heart rate tracing that must be evaluated regularly are baseline rate, baseline variability, accelerations, decelerations, and changes or trends over time. Whenever one of these five essential components is assessed as abnormal, corrective measures must immediately be taken (see the Nursing Process box). The purpose of these actions is to improve fetal oxygenation (Tucker et al., 2009). The term *intrauterine resuscitation* is sometimes used to refer to specific interventions initiated when an abnormal FHR pattern is noted. Basic corrective measures include providing supplemental oxygen, instituting maternal position changes, and increasing intravenous fluid administration. These interventions are implemented to improve uterine and intervillous space blood flow and increase maternal oxygenation and cardiac output (Simpson & James, 2005). Box 18-8 lists basic interventions to improve maternal and fetal oxygenation status.

Depending on the underlying cause of the abnormal FHR pattern, other interventions, such as correcting maternal hypotension, reducing uterine activity, and altering second stage pushing techniques, also may be instituted (Tucker et al., 2009). Box 18-8 lists interventions for these specific problems. Some of the items listed are not independent nursing interventions. Any medications administered, for example, must be authorized either through inclusion in a specific unit protocol or by a specific order. Some interventions are specific to the FHR pattern. (See Table 18-3 and Boxes 18-5 and 18-6 for nursing interventions for tachycardia, late decelerations, and variable decelerations.) Based on the FHR response to these interventions the primary health care provider decides whether additional interventions should be instituted or whether immediate vaginal or cesarean birth should be performed.

OTHER METHODS OF ASSESSMENT AND INTERVENTION

A major shortcoming of EFM is its high rate of false-positive results. Even the most abnormal patterns are poorly predictive of neonatal morbidity. Therefore, other methods of assessment have been developed to evaluate fetal status. Fetal scalp stimulation and vibroacoustic stimulation and umbilical cord acid-base determination are frequently performed assessments. However, fetal scalp blood sampling and fetal pulse oximetry are rarely performed in the United States. Amnioinfusion and tocolytic therapy are interventions often used in an attempt to improve abnormal FHR patterns.

BOX 18-8 MANAGEMENT OF ABNORMAL FETAL HEART RATE PATTERNS

BASIC INTERVENTIONS

- Administer oxygen by nonrebreather face mask at a rate of 8 to 10 L/min.
- Assist the woman to a side-lying (lateral) position.
- Increase maternal blood volume by increasing the rate of the primary IV infusion.

INTERVENTIONS FOR SPECIFIC PROBLEMS

- Maternal hypotension
    - Increase the rate of the primary IV infusion.
    - Change to lateral or Trendelenburg positioning.
    - Administer ephedrine or phenylephrine if other measures are unsuccessful in increasing blood pressure.
- Uterine tachysystole
    - Reduce or discontinue the dose of any uterine stimulants in use (e.g., oxytocin [Pitocin]).
    - Administer a uterine relaxant (tocolytic) (e.g., terbutaline [Brethine]).
- Abnormal fetal heart rate pattern during the second stage of labor
    - Use open-glottis pushing.
    - Use fewer pushing efforts during each contraction.
    - Make individual pushing efforts shorter.
    - Push only with every other or every third contraction.
    - Push only with a perceived urge to push (in women with regional anesthesia).

IV, Intravenous.

ASSESSMENT TECHNIQUES

Fetal Scalp Stimulation and Vibroacoustic Stimulation

Several research studies undertaken in the 1980s found that an FHR acceleration in response to digital or vibroacoustic stimulation was highly predictive of a normal scalp blood pH. The two methods of fetal stimulation used most often in clinical practice are scalp stimulation (using digital pressure during a vaginal examination) and vibroacoustic stimulation (using an artificial larynx or fetal acoustic stimulation device on the maternal abdomen over the fetal head for 1 to 5 seconds). The desired result of both methods of stimulation is an acceleration in the FHR of at least 15 beats/min for at least 15 seconds (Tucker et al., 2009). An FHR acceleration indicates the absence of metabolic acidemia. If the fetus does not respond to stimulation with an acceleration, fetal compromise is not necessarily indicated; however, further evaluation of fetal well-being is needed. Fetal stimulation should be performed at times when the FHR is at baseline. Neither fetal scalp stimulation nor vibroacoustic stimulation should be instituted if FHR decelerations or bradycardia is present (Tucker et al.).

Umbilical Cord Acid-Base Determination

In assessing the immediate condition of the newborn after birth, a sample of cord blood is a useful adjunct to the Apgar score. The procedure is generally performed by withdrawing blood from both the umbilical artery and the umbilical vein. Both samples are then tested for pH, carbon dioxide pressure (Pco_2), oxygen pressure (Po_2), and base deficit or base excess (Garite, 2007; Tucker et al., 2009). Umbilical arterial values reflect fetal condition, whereas umbilical vein values indicate placental function (Tucker et al.).

TABLE 18-4 APPROXIMATE NORMAL VALUES FOR CORD BLOOD

CORD BLOOD	PH	CARBON DIOXIDE PRESSURE (Pco_2) (mm Hg)	OXYGEN PRESSURE (Po_2) (mm Hg)	BASE DEFICIT (mmol/L)
Artery	7.2-7.3	45-55	15-25	<12
Vein	7.3-7.4	35-45	25-35	<12

From: Tucker, S., Miller, L., & Miller, D. (2009). *Mosby's pocket guide to fetal monitoring: A multidisciplinary approach* (6th ed.). St. Louis: Mosby.

TABLE 18-5 TYPES OF ACIDEMIA

BLOOD GASES	RESPIRATORY	METABOLIC	MIXED
pH	<7.20	<7.20	<7.20
Carbon dioxide pressure (Pco_2)	Elevated	Normal	Elevated
Base deficit	<12 mmol/L	≥12 mmol/L	≥12 mmol/L

From: Tucker, S., Miller, L. & Miller, D. (2009). *Mosby's pocket guide to fetal monitoring: A multidisciplinary approach* (6th ed.). St. Louis: Mosby.

ACOG (2006a) suggests obtaining cord blood values in the following clinical situations: cesarean birth for fetal compromise, low 5-minute Apgar score, severe intrauterine growth restriction, abnormal FHR tracing, maternal thyroid disease, intrapartum fever, and multifetal gestation. Normal umbilical artery and vein cord blood values are listed in Table 18-4. Normal findings preclude the presence of acidemia at, or immediately before, birth. If acidemia is present (e.g., pH less than 7.20), then the type of acidemia is determined (respiratory, metabolic, or mixed) by analyzing the blood gas values (Table 18-5) (Tucker et al., 2009).

Fetal Scalp Blood Sampling

Sampling of the fetal scalp blood for pH determination was first described in the 1960s and performed extensively in the 1970s. The procedure is performed by obtaining a sample of fetal scalp blood through the dilated cervix after the membranes have ruptured. Its use is limited by many factors, including the requirement for cervical dilation and membrane rupture, technical difficulty of the procedure, need for repetitive pH determinations, and uncertainty regarding interpretation and application of results. This procedure is now seldom used in the United States but remains a common practice in other countries (Tucker et al., 2009).

Fetal Pulse Oximetry

Fetal pulse oximetry or continuous monitoring of fetal oxygen saturation levels is a fetal assessment that indirectly measures the oxygen saturation of hemoglobin in fetal blood. An intrauterine sensor placed in contact with the fetal cheek or temple area provides a continuous estimation of fetal oxygen saturation. Fetal pulse oximetry was approved for clinical use by the U.S. Food and Drug Administration in May 2000. The hope was that this technology would help to interpret abnormal (nonreassuring) FHR patterns more accurately and perhaps decrease the number of cesarean births performed for nonreassuring FHR tracings (Garite, 2007). Several studies, however, found that although fetal pulse oximetry did decrease the incidence of cesarean births for fetal indications, it had no consistent effect on overall cesarean birth rates or newborn outcomes. Therefore, fetal pulse oximetry has not proven to be a clinically useful test for determining fetal status (ACOG, 2009). Because the manufacturer no longer distributes the sensors, the product has in effect been taken off the market (Tucker et al., 2009).

INTERVENTIONS

Amnioinfusion

Amnioinfusion is infusion of room-temperature isotonic fluid (usually normal saline or lactated Ringer's solution) into the uterine cavity if the volume of amniotic fluid is low. Without the buffer of amniotic fluid the umbilical cord can easily become compressed during contractions or fetal movement, diminishing the flow of blood between the fetus and placenta. The purpose of amnioinfusion is to relieve intermittent umbilical cord compression that results in variable decelerations and transient fetal hypoxemia by restoring the amniotic fluid volume to a normal or near-normal level (Tucker et al., 2009). Women with an abnormally small amount of amniotic fluid (oligohydramnios) or no amniotic fluid (anhydramnios) are candidates for this procedure. Conditions that can result in oligohydramnios or anhydramnios are uteroplacental insufficiency and premature rupture of membranes.

In the past, amnioinfusion was also used to dilute moderate to thick meconium in an attempt to prevent meconium aspiration syndrome. However, a large research study found that amnioinfusion did not significantly reduce the incidence of meconium aspiration syndrome or perinatal death (Fraser, Hofmeyr, Lede, Faron, Alexander, Goffinet, et al., 2005). Therefore routine amnioinfusion for meconium-stained amniotic fluid without the presence of variable decelerations is not recommended by ACOG (2006b).

Risks of amnioinfusion are overdistention of the uterine cavity and increased uterine tone. Fluid is administered through an IUPC either by gravity flow or by an infusion pump. Usually a bolus of fluid is administered over 20 to 30 minutes, then the infusion is slowed to a maintenance rate. Likely no more than 1000 ml of fluid will need to be administered. The fluid may be warmed for the preterm fetus by infusing it through a blood warmer (Tucker et al., 2009).

Intensity and frequency of UCs should be continually assessed during the procedure. The recorded uterine resting tone during amnioinfusion will appear higher than normal because of resistance to outflow and turbulence at the end of the catheter. Uterine resting tone should not exceed 40 mm Hg during the procedure. The amount of fluid return must be estimated and documented during amnioinfusion to prevent overdistention of the uterus. The volume of fluid returned should be approximately the same as the amount infused (Tucker et al., 2009).

Tocolytic Therapy

Tocolysis (relaxation of the uterus) can be achieved through the administration of drugs that inhibit UCs. This therapy can be used as an adjunct to other interventions in the management of fetal stress when the fetus is exhibiting abnormal patterns

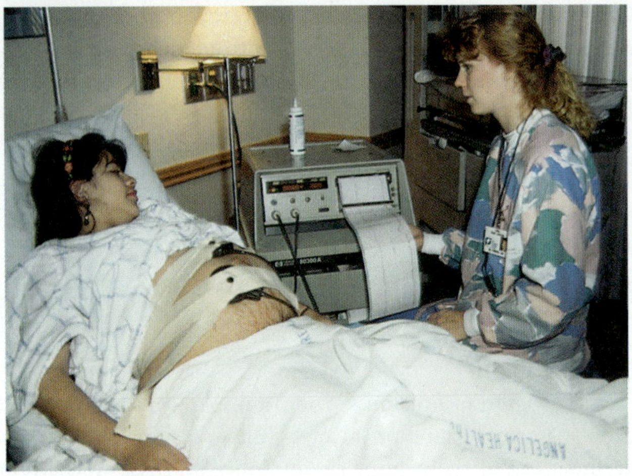

FIG. 18-14 A nurse explains electronic fetal monitoring as ultrasound transducer monitors the fetal heart rate. (Courtesy Marjorie Pyle, RNC, Lifecircle, Costa Mesa, CA.)

associated with increased UA. Tocolysis improves blood flow through the placenta by inhibiting UCs. Tocolysis may be implemented by the primary health care provider when other interventions to reduce UA, such as maternal position change and discontinuance of an oxytocin infusion, have no effect on diminishing the UCs. Tocolytics are often administered when women are having excessive UCs spontaneously. Tocolytics are also frequently administered after a decision for cesarean birth has been made while preparations for surgery are under way. The most commonly used tocolytic in these situations is terbutaline (Brethine), given subcutaneously. Terbutaline works quickly and has been demonstrated to improve Apgar scores and cord pH values without apparent complications (Garite, 2007). If the FHR and UC patterns improve, the woman may be allowed to continue labor; if no improvement is seen, immediate cesarean birth may be needed.

CLIENT AND FAMILY TEACHING

Although the use of EFM can be reassuring to many parents, it can be a source of anxiety to some. Therefore, the nurse must be particularly sensitive and respond appropriately to the emotional, informational, and comfort needs of the woman in labor and those of her family (Fig. 18-14 and Box 18-9).

Part of the nurse's role includes acting as a partner with the woman to achieve a high-quality birthing experience. In addition to teaching and supporting the woman and her family with understanding of the laboring and birth process, breathing techniques, use of equipment, and pain management techniques, the nurse can assist with two factors that have an effect on fetal status: positioning and pushing. The nurse should solicit the woman's cooperation in avoiding the supine position. Instead, the woman should be encouraged to maintain a side-lying position or semi-Fowler's position with a lateral tilt to the uterus. In addition, the nurse should instruct the woman to keep her mouth and glottis open and to let air escape from her lungs during the pushing process. Both of these interventions will help to improve fetal oxygenation. See Chapter 19 for further discussion of maternal positioning and pushing techniques.

Spanish Guidelines—Fetal Monitoring

BOX 18-9 CLIENT AND FAMILY TEACHING WHEN ELECTRONIC FETAL MONITOR IS USED

The following guidelines relate to client teaching and the functioning of the monitor.

- Explain the purpose of monitoring.
- Explain each procedure.
- Provide rationale for maternal position other than supine.
- Explain that fetal status can be continuously assessed by electronic fetal monitoring (EFM), even during contractions.
- Explain that the lower tracing on the monitor strip paper shows uterine activity; the upper tracing shows the fetal heart rate (FHR).
- Reassure woman and partner that prepared childbirth techniques can be implemented without difficulty.
- Explain that during external monitoring effleurage can be performed on sides of abdomen or upper portion of thighs.
- Explain that breathing patterns based on the time and intensity of contractions can be enhanced by the observation of uterine activity on the monitor strip, which shows the onset of contractions.
- Note peak of contraction; knowing that contraction will not get stronger and is halfway over is usually helpful.
- Note diminishing intensity.
- Coordinate with appropriate breathing and relaxation techniques.
- Reassure woman and partner that the use of internal monitoring does not restrict movement, although she is confined to bed.*
- Explain that use of external monitoring usually requires the woman's cooperation during positioning and movement.
- Reassure woman and partner that use of monitoring does not imply fetal jeopardy.

*Portable telemetry monitors allow the FHR and uterine contraction patterns to be observed on centrally located display stations. These portable units permit ambulation during electronic monitoring.

DOCUMENTATION

Clear and complete documentation in the woman's medical record is essential. Each FHR and UA assessment must be completely documented in the woman's medical record. More and more hospitals are moving to use of the electronic medical record and computerized charting. With computerized charting, each required component usually appears on the screen so that it will routinely be addressed. Computerized charting often includes forced choices that greatly increase the use of standardized FHR terminology by all members of the health care team. In the past, nurses were often encouraged to chart both on the monitor strip and in the medical record. However, charting directly on the monitor strip is unnecessary when an electronic medical record is used. Any information that is handwritten on the monitor strip will not be recorded in the computer record. Furthermore, given that the EFM tracing is stored on computer, the paper strips are destroyed after the woman is discharged. No permanent record of the handwritten charting exists.

In institutions that still use a paper chart, documentation on the woman's monitor strip is started before the initiation of monitoring and consists of identifying information plus other relevant data. This documentation is continued and updated according to institutional protocol as monitoring progresses. See Box 18-10 for a checklist that can be used for documentation in a paper medical record. In some institutions, observations

BOX 18-10 CHECKLIST FOR FETAL HEART RATE AND UTERINE ACTIVITY ASSESSMENT WITH ELECTRONIC FETAL MONITORING

Client's name ____________________

Date/time ____________________

1. What is the baseline fetal heart rate (FHR)?
   _____ Beats/min
   Check one of the following as observed on the monitor strip:
   _____ Average baseline FHR (110-160 beats/min)
   _____ Tachycardia (>160 beats/min)
   _____ Bradycardia (<110 beats/min)
2. What is the baseline variability?
   _____ Absent variability
   _____ Minimal variability (detectable up to 5 beats/min)
   _____ Moderate variability (6-25 beats/min)
   _____ Marked variability (>25 beats/min)
3. Any periodic or episodic changes in FHR?
   _____ Accelerations with fetal movement
   _____ Accelerations with contractions
   _____ Early decelerations (head compression)
   _____ Late decelerations (uteroplacental insufficiency)
   _____ Variable decelerations (cord compression)
   _____ Prolonged deceleration (>2 minutes up to 10 minutes)
4. What is the uterine activity or contraction pattern?
   _____ Frequency (beginning to end of uterine contraction [UC])
   _____ Duration (beginning of one UC to beginning of the next UC)
   Abdominal palpation method
   _____ Strength (mild, moderate, strong)
   _____ Resting tone (from end of one contraction to beginning of next one)
   Internal monitoring (intrauterine pressure catheter)
   _____ Intensity (mm Hg pressure)
   _____ Resting tone (mm Hg pressure)

Comments: ____________________

____

Panel Number: ____________________

____

What can be or should have been done?

____

____

____

Modified from Tucker, S. (2004). *Pocket guide to fetal monitoring and assessment* (5th ed.). St. Louis: Mosby.

noted and interventions implemented are recorded on the monitor strip to produce a comprehensive document that chronicles the course of labor and the care rendered. In other institutions, this documentation is confined to the labor flow record. Advocates of documenting on both the medical record and the EFM strip cite as advantages of this approach the ease of writing directly on the strip while at the bedside and the improved accuracy in documenting critical events and the interventions implemented. Others believe that charting on the EFM strip constitutes duplicate documentation of the same information noted in the medical record, and thus it is unnecessary additional paperwork for the nurse.

A disadvantage of documenting on both the EFM strip and the medical record is that the times noted for events and interventions on the EFM strip frequently do not correlate with what is later documented in the medical record. These inaccuracies can lead persons involved in the retrospective review process carried out during litigation to infer that documentation errors have occurred. Therefore, if institutional policy mandates documentation both on the monitor strip and in the medical record, the nurse must make sure the times and notations of events and interventions recorded in each place agree. Many of the aspects of care and events that can be documented on the client's medical record or the monitor strip are listed in Box 18-10.

KEY POINTS

- Fetal well-being during labor is gauged by the response of the FHR to UCs.
- Standardized definitions for many common FHR patterns have been adopted for use in clinical practice by ACNM, ACOG, and AWHONN.
- The five essential components of the fetal heart rate tracing are baseline rate, baseline variability, accelerations, decelerations, and changes or trends over time.
- The monitoring of fetal well-being includes FHR and UA assessment, as well as assessment of maternal vital signs.
- Assessing FHR and UA patterns, implementing independent nursing interventions, and reporting abnormal patterns to the physician or nurse-midwife are the nurse's responsibilities.
- AWHONN and ACOG have established and published health care provider standards and guidelines for FHR monitoring.
- The emotional, informational, and comfort needs of the woman and her family must be addressed when the mother and her fetus are being monitored.
- Documentation of fetal assessment is initiated and updated according to institutional protocol.

Audio Chapter Summaries Access an audio summary of these Key Points on Evolve

REFERENCES

Albers, L. (2007). The evidence for physiologic management of the active phase of the first stage of labor. *Journal of Midwifery & Women's Health, 52*(3), 207–215.

American Academy of Pediatrics (AAP) and American College of Obstetricians and Gynecologists (ACOG). (2007). *Guidelines for perinatal care* (6th ed.). Washington, DC: ACOG.

American College of Obstetricians and Gynecologists (ACOG). (2006a). *Umbilical cord blood gas and acid-base analysis. ACOG Committee Opinion*. Washington, DC: ACOG.

American College of Obstetricians and Gynecologists (ACOG). (2006b). *Amnioinfusion does not prevent meconium aspiration syndrome. ACOG Committee Opinion No. 346*. Washington, DC: ACOG.

American College of Obstetricians and Gynecologists (ACOG). (2009). *Intrapartum fetal heart rate monitoring: Nomenclature, interpretation, and general management principles. ACOG Practice Bulletin No. 106*. Washington, DC: ACOG.

Association of Women's Health, Obstetric and Neonatal Nurses. (2009). *Fetal heart monitoring principles and practice* (4th ed.). Dubuque, IA: Kendall/Hunt.

Cunningham, F., Leveno, K., Bloom, S., Hauth, J., Rouse, D., & Spong, C. (2010). *Williams obstetrics* (23rd ed.). New York: McGraw-Hill.

Fraser, W., Hofmeyr, J., Lede, R., Faron, G., Alexander, S., Goffinet, F., et al. (2005). Amnioinfusion trial group: Amnioinfusion for the prevention of the meconium aspiration syndrome. *New England Journal of Medicine, 353*(9), 909–917.

Garite, T. (2007). Intrapartum fetal evaluation. In S. Gabbe, J. Niebyl, & J. Simpson (Eds.), *Obstetrics: Normal and problem pregnancies* (5th ed.). Philadelphia: Churchill Livingstone.

Gilbert, E. (2011). *Manual of high risk pregnancy & delivery* (5th ed.). St. Louis: Mosby.

Hamilton, B., Martin, J., & Ventura, S. (2010). Births: Preliminary data for 2008. *National Vital Statistics Reports, 58*(16), 1–18.

Macones, G., Hankins, G., Spong, C., Hauth, J., & Moore, T. (2008). The 2008 National Institute of Child Health and Human Development Workshop Report on Electronic Fetal Monitoring: Update on definitions, interpretation, and research guidelines. *Journal of Obstetric, Gynecologic and Neonatal Nursing, 37*(5), 510–515.

Nageotte, M., & Gilstrap, L. (2009). Intrapartum fetal surveillance. In R. Creasy, R. Resnik, J. Iams, C. Lockwood, & T. Moore (Eds.), *Creasy & Resnik's maternal-fetal medicine: Principles and practice* (6th ed.). Philadelphia: Saunders.

National Institute of Child Health and Human Development Research Planning Workshop. (1997). Electronic fetal heart rate monitoring: Research guidelines for interpretation. *American Journal of Obstetrics and Gynecology, 177*(6), 1385–1390.

Simpson, K., & James, D. (2005). Efficacy of intrauterine resuscitation techniques in improving fetal oxygen status during labor. *Obstetrics and Gynecology, 105*(6), 1362–1368.

Tucker, S., Miller, L., & Miller, D. (2009). *Mosby's pocket guide to fetal monitoring: A multidisciplinary approach* (6th ed.). St. Louis: Mosby.

CHAPTER

19

Nursing Care of the Family During Labor and Birth

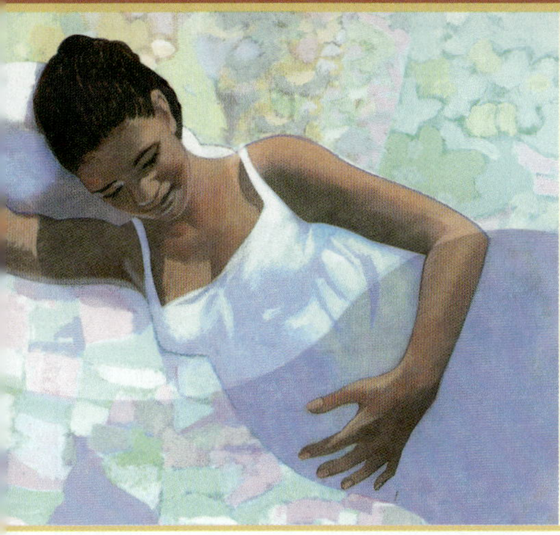

Karen A. Piotrowski

evolve WEBSITE

http://evolve.elsevier.com/Lowdermilk/MWHC/

- Animation
  - Vaginal Birth
- Audio Glossary
- Audio Key Points
- Case Studies
  - First Stage of Labor
  - Second/Third Stages of Labor
- Critical Thinking Exercise
  - Positioning During Labor
  - Postpartum Home Care
- NCLEX Review Questions
- Nursing Care Plan
  - Labor and Birth
- Spanish Guidelines
  - Care During Labor
  - Labor Assessment
- Video—Assessment
  - Leopold Maneuvers
- Video—Childbirth
  - Vaginal
- Video—Nursing Skills
  - Performing Leopold Maneuvers
  - Positioning and Assisting with Comfort Measures in Labor

LEARNING OBJECTIVES

- Review the factors included in the initial assessment of the woman in labor.
- Describe the ongoing assessment of maternal progress during the first, second, third, and fourth stages of labor.
- Recognize the physical and psychosocial findings indicative of maternal progress during labor.
- Describe fetal assessment during labor.
- Identify signs of developing complications during labor and birth.
- Incorporate evidence-based nursing interventions into a comprehensive plan of care relevant to each stage of labor.
- Recognize the importance of support (family, partner, doula, nurse) in fostering maternal confidence and facilitating the progress of labor and birth.
- Analyze the influence of cultural and religious beliefs and practices on the process of labor and birth.
- Describe the role and responsibilities of the nurse during emergency childbirth.
- Evaluate the effect of perineal trauma on the woman's reproductive and sexual health.

The labor process is an exciting and anxious time for the woman and her significant others (support persons, family). In a relatively short period they experience one of the most profound changes in their lives.

For most women labor begins with the first uterine contraction, continues with hours of hard work during cervical dilation and birth, and ends as the woman begins to recover physically from birth and she and her significant others begin the attachment process with the newborn. Nursing care management focuses on assessment and support of the woman and her significant others throughout labor and birth, with the goal of ensuring the best possible outcome for all involved.

A woman often has lingering impressions of her childbirth experience. Satisfaction with childbirth hinges on her ability to maintain a sense of control. Caregivers who encourage a woman to be actively involved in decision making and who are respectful, supportive, protective, patient, and calm help the woman to remember her childbirth experience in positive terms. Other factors cited by women as influencing their satisfaction with their childbirth experience include degree of awareness of what is occurring, support from their partner, being together with their baby immediately after birth, type of birth (e.g., vaginal or emergency cesarean birth), and degree to which expectations were met and pain was managed (Bryanton, Gagnon, Johnston, & Hatem, 2008). A satisfactory view of childbirth contributes to a woman's self-esteem and sense of accomplishment with her performance. Adaptation to her role as a mother may also be enhanced.

Frustrations a woman feels regarding her childbirth experience generally stem from factors such as unmet expectations, poorly managed pain, loss of control, lack of knowledge, or the negative behaviors of some caregivers. A woman who perceives her childbirth to be unsatisfactory or traumatic could be at risk for postpartum depression, posttraumatic stress disorder (PTSD), low self-esteem, impaired attachment with the newborn, and fear leading to no further pregnancies or cesarean birth for a subsequent pregnancy (Bryanton et al., 2008). It is critical that nurses recognize the factors that influence maternal satisfaction as they plan care for women and their families during childbirth.

FIRST STAGE OF LABOR

CARE MANAGEMENT

The **first stage of labor** begins with the onset of regular uterine contractions and ends with full cervical effacement and dilation. The first stage of labor consists of three phases: the **latent phase** (through 3 cm of dilation), the **active phase** (4 to 7 cm of dilation), and the **transition phase** (8 to 10 cm of dilation). Most nulliparous women seek admission to the hospital in the latent phase because they have not experienced labor before and are unsure of the "right" time to come in. Multiparous women usually do not come to the hospital until they are in the active phase of the first stage of labor. Even though no two labors are identical, women who have given birth before often are less anxious about the process, unless their previous experience has been negative.

Case Study—First Stage of Labor

TEACHING FOR SELF-MANAGEMENT

How to Distinguish True Labor from False Labor

TRUE LABOR

- Contractions
  - Occur regularly, becoming stronger, lasting longer, and occurring closer together
  - Become more intense with walking
  - Are usually felt in the lower back, radiating to lower portion of the abdomen
  - Continue despite use of comfort measures
- Cervix (by vaginal examination)
  - Shows progressive change (softening, effacement, and dilation signaled by the appearance of bloody show)
  - Moves to an increasingly anterior position
- Fetus
  - Presenting part usually becomes engaged in the pelvis, which results in increased ease of breathing; at the same time, the presenting part presses downward and compresses the bladder, resulting in urinary frequency

FALSE LABOR

- Contractions
  - Occur irregularly or become regular only temporarily
  - Often stop with walking or position change
  - Can be felt in the back or abdomen above the navel
  - Can often be stopped through the use of comfort measures
- Cervix (by vaginal examination)
  - May be soft but with no significant change in effacement or dilation or evidence of bloody show
  - Is often in a posterior position
- Fetus
  - Presenting part is usually not engaged in the pelvis

ASSESSMENT

Assessment begins at the first contact with the woman, whether by telephone or in person. Many women call the hospital or birthing center first for validation that it is all right for them to come in for evaluation or admission or if it is all right for them to remain home. Many hospitals, however, discourage the nurse from giving advice regarding what to do because of legal liability. Nurses are often instructed to tell women who call with questions to call their primary health care provider or to come to the hospital if they feel the need to be checked. The nature of the telephone conversation including any advice or instructions given should be documented in the client's record (Gilbert, 2011).

A pregnant woman may first call her primary care provider or come to the hospital while in false labor or early in the latent phase of the first stage of labor. She may feel discouraged, angry, or confused on learning that the contractions that feel so strong and regular to her are not true contractions because they are not causing cervical dilation, or that they are still not strong or frequent enough for admission. During the third trimester of pregnancy, women should be instructed regarding the stages of labor and the signs indicating its onset. They should be informed of the possibility that they will not be admitted if they are 3 cm or less dilated (see the Teaching for Self-Management box).

If the woman lives near the hospital and has adequate support and transportation, she may be encouraged to stay home or return home to allow labor to progress (i.e., until the uterine contractions are more frequent and intense). The ideal setting for the low risk woman at this time usually is the familiar environment of her home. The woman who lives at a considerable distance from the hospital, who lacks adequate support and transportation, or who has a history of rapid labors in the past, however, may be admitted in latent labor. The same measures used by the woman at home should be offered to the hospitalized woman in early labor.

A warm shower is often relaxing during early labor. However, warm baths before labor is well established could inhibit uterine contractions and prolong the labor process (Waterbirth International, 2009). Soothing back, foot, and hand massage or a warm drink of preferred liquids such as tea or milk can help the woman to rest and even to sleep, especially if false or early labor is occurring at night. Diversional activities such as walking outdoors or in the house, reading, watching television, knitting, or talking with friends can reduce the perception of early discomfort, help the time pass, and reduce anxiety.

When the woman arrives at the perinatal unit, assessment is the top priority (Fig. 19-1). The nurse first performs a screening assessment by using the techniques of interview and physical assessment and reviews the laboratory and diagnostic test findings to determine the health status of the woman and her fetus and the progress of her labor. The nurse also notifies the primary health care provider and if the woman is admitted, a detailed systems assessment is done.

When the woman is admitted, she is usually moved from an observation area to the labor room; the labor, delivery, and recovery (LDR) room; or the labor, delivery, recovery, and postpartum (LDRP) room. If the woman wishes, include her partner in the assessment and admission process. The nurse can direct

LEGAL TIP: Obstetric Triage and EMTALA

The Emergency Medical Treatment and Active Labor Act (EMTALA) is a federal regulation enacted to ensure that a woman gets emergency treatment or active labor care whenever such treatment is sought. According to the EMTALA, true labor is considered to be an emergency medical condition. Nurses working in labor and birth units must be familiar with their responsibilities according to the EMTALA regulations, which include providing services to pregnant women when they experience an urgent pregnancy problem (e.g., labor, decreased fetal movement, rupture of membranes, recent trauma) and fully documenting all relevant information (e.g., assessment findings, interventions implemented, client responses to care measures provided). A pregnant woman presenting in an obstetric triage is considered to be in "true" labor until a qualified health care provider certifies that she is not. Agencies need to have specific policies and procedures in place so that compliance with the EMTALA regulations is achieved while safe and efficient care is provided (Angelini & Mahlmeister, 2005; Tucker, Miller, & Miller, 2009).

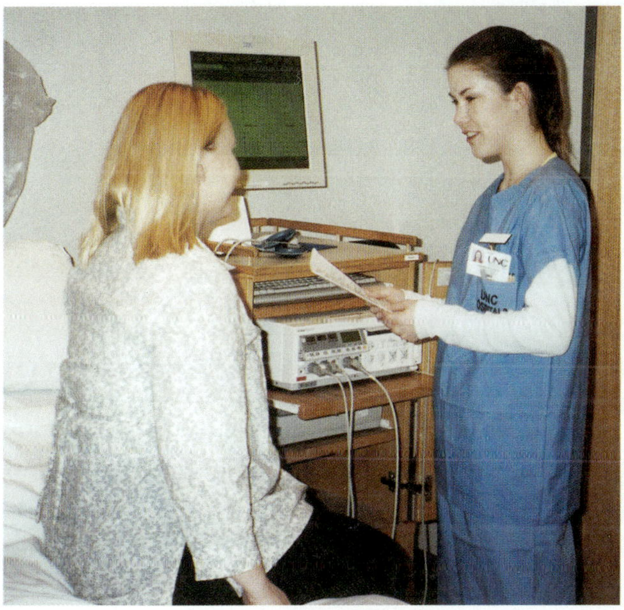

FIG. 19-1 Woman being assessed for admission to the labor and birth unit. (Courtesy Dee Lowdermilk, Chapel Hill, NC.)

significant others not participating in this process to the appropriate waiting area. The woman undresses and puts on her own gown or a hospital gown. The nurse places an identification band on the woman's wrist. Her personal belongings are put away safely or given to family members, according to agency policy. Women who participate in expectant parents classes often bring a birth bag or Lamaze bag with them. The nurse then shows the woman and her partner the layout and operation of the unit and room, how to use the call light and telephone system, and how to adjust lighting in the room and the different bed positions.

The nurse reassures the woman that she is in competent, caring hands and that she and persons to whom she gives permission can ask questions related to her care and status and that of her fetus at any time during labor. The nurse can minimize the woman's anxiety by explaining terms commonly used during labor. The woman's interest, response, and prior experience guide the depth and breadth of these explanations.

COMMUNITY ACTIVITY

- Visit the website of a hospital that provides maternity services in your community. Review the client information about the Labor and Birth Unit. Is the model of care LDR or LDRP? Are the rooms designed in a more home-like setting versus a hospital setting? Is emergency equipment available but hidden from view?
- Visit the website of a free-standing birth center in your state. What is the mission of the center? Is the center staffed by nurse-midwives or obstetricians? What types of services do they provide? How soon after birth are the mothers usually discharged? Are postpartum home visits routinely done? To what hospital would the women be transferred if that became necessary? Compare and contrast the care at a free standing birth center versus a hospital birth center.

Most hospitals have specific forms, whether paper or electronic, which are used to obtain important assessment information when a woman in labor is being evaluated or admitted (Fig. 19-2). More and more hospitals now use an electronic medical record—almost all charting is done on computer. Sources of data include the prenatal record, the initial interview, physical examination to determine baseline physiologic parameters (e.g., vital signs), laboratory and diagnostic test results, expressed psychosocial and cultural factors, and the clinical evaluation of labor status.

Prenatal Data

The nurse reviews the prenatal record to identify the woman's individual needs and risks. Copies of prenatal records are generally filed in the perinatal unit at some time during the woman's pregnancy (usually in the third trimester) or accessed by computer so that they are readily available on admission. If the woman has had no prenatal care or her prenatal records are unavailable, the nurse must obtain certain baseline information. If the woman is having discomfort, the nurse should ask questions between contractions when the woman can concentrate more fully on her answers. At times the partner or support person(s) may need to be secondary sources of essential information. According to the Health Insurance Portability and Accountability Act (HIPAA), the woman must give permission for other persons to be involved in the exchange of information regarding her care. This permission should be obtained during pregnancy and a signed form included in her health records.

Knowing the woman's age is important so that the nurse can individualize the nursing care plan to the needs of her age-group. For example, a 14-year-old girl and a 40-year-old woman have different but specific needs, and their ages place them at risk for different problems. Accurate height and weight measurements are important. A pregnancy weight gain greater than recommended may place the woman at a higher risk for cephalopelvic disproportion and cesarean birth. This is especially true for women who are petite and have gained 16 kg or more. A prepregnancy body mass index (BMI) greater than 30 is also a cause for concern. Other factors to consider are the woman's general health status, current medical conditions or allergies, respiratory status, and previous surgical procedures.

The nurse should carefully review the woman's prenatal records, taking note of her obstetric and pregnancy history

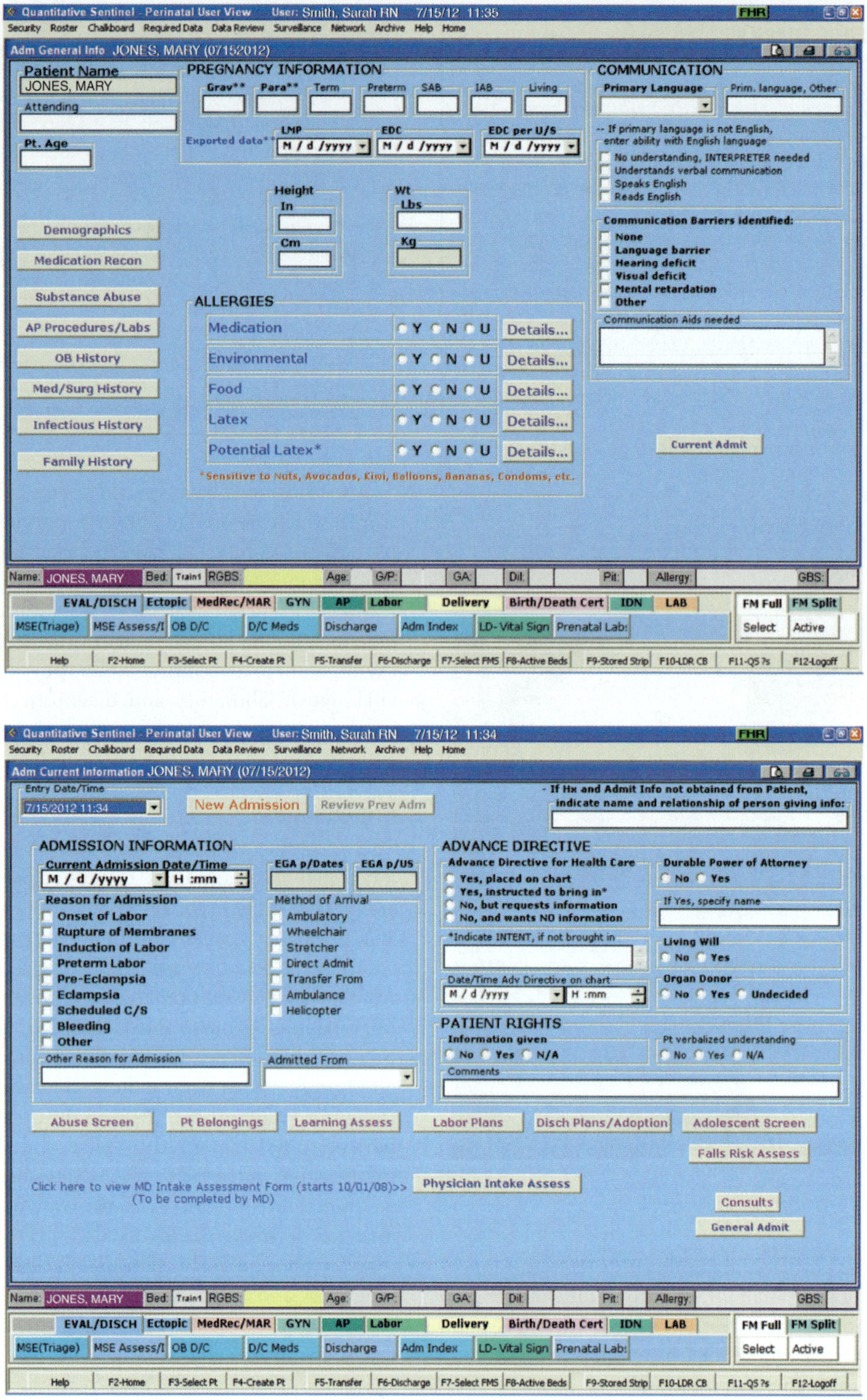

FIG. 19-2 Admission screens in an electronic medical record. **A**, General admission screen. **B**, Current admission screen. (Courtesy Kitty Cashion, Memphis, TN).

including gravidity, parity, and problems such as history of vaginal bleeding, gestational hypertension, anemia, pregestational or gestational diabetes, infections (e.g., bacterial, viral, sexually transmitted), and immunodeficiency status. In addition, the expected date of birth (EDB) should be confirmed. Other important data found in the prenatal record include patterns of maternal weight gain; physiologic measurements such as maternal vital signs (blood pressure, temperature, pulse, respirations); fundal height; baseline fetal heart rate (FHR); and laboratory and diagnostic test results. See Table-15-1 for a list of common prenatal laboratory tests. Common diagnostic and fetal assessment tests performed prenatally include amniocentesis, nonstress test (NST), biophysical profile (BPP), and ultrasound examination. See Chapter 26 for more information.

If this labor and birth experience is not the woman's first, the nurse needs to note the characteristics of her previous experiences. This information includes the duration of previous labors, the type of anesthesia used, the kind of birth (e.g., spontaneous vaginal, forceps-assisted, vacuum-assisted, or cesarean birth), and the condition of the newborn. Explore the woman's perception of her previous labor and birth experiences because this perception may influence her attitude toward her current experience.

Interview

The woman's primary reason for coming to the hospital is determined in the interview. Her primary reason may be, for example, that her bag of waters (BOW, amniotic membranes) ruptured, with or without contractions. The woman may have come in for an obstetric check, which is a period of observation reserved for women who are unsure about the onset of their labor. This check allows time on the unit for the diagnosis of labor without official admission and minimizes or avoids cost to the woman when used by the hospital and approved by her health insurance plan.

Even the experienced woman may have difficulty determining the onset of labor. The woman is asked to recall the events of the previous days and to describe the following:

- Time and onset of contractions and progress in terms of frequency, duration, and intensity
- Location and character of discomfort from contractions (e.g., back pain, abdominal or suprapubic discomfort)
- Persistence of contractions despite changes in maternal position and activity (e.g., walking or lying down)
- Presence and character of vaginal discharge or "show"
- The status of amniotic membranes, such as a gush or seepage of fluid **(spontaneous rupture of membranes [SROM])**. If there has been a discharge that may be amniotic fluid, she is asked the date and time the fluid was first noted and the fluid's characteristics (e.g., amount, color, unusual odor). In many instances, a sterile speculum examination and a **Nitrazine** (pH) and **fern test** can confirm that the membranes are ruptured (see the Procedure box: Tests for Rupture of Membranes).

These descriptions help the nurse assess the degree of progress in the process of labor. **Bloody show** is distinguished from bleeding by the fact that it is pink and feels sticky because of its mucoid nature. There is very little bloody show in the beginning, but the amount increases with effacement and dilation of the cervix. A woman may report a small amount of brownish to bloody discharge that may be attributed to cervical trauma resulting from vaginal examination or coitus (intercourse) within the last 48 hours.

Assessing the woman's respiratory status is important in case general anesthesia is needed in an emergency. The nurse determines this status by asking the woman if she has a "cold" or related symptoms (e.g., "stuffy nose," sore throat, or cough). The status of allergies, including allergies to latex and tape, and medications routinely used in obstetrics, such as opioids (e.g., hydromorphone [Dilaudid], butorphanol [Stadol], fentanyl [Sublimaze], nalbuphine [Nubain]), anesthetic agents (e.g., bupivacaine, lidocaine, ropivacaine), and antiseptics (Betadine) is reviewed. Some allergic responses cause swelling of the mucous membranes of the respiratory tract, which could interfere with breathing and the administration of inhalation anesthesia. Because vomiting and subsequent aspiration into the respiratory tract can complicate an otherwise normal labor, the nurse records the time and type of the woman's most recent solid and liquid intake.

The nurse obtains any information not found in the prenatal record during the admission assessment. Pertinent data include the birth plan (Box 19-1), the choice of infant feeding method, the type of pain management preferred, and the name of the pediatric health care provider. Obtain a client profile that identifies the woman's preparation for childbirth, the support person or family members desired during childbirth and

PROCEDURE

Tests for Rupture of Membranes

NITRAZINE TEST FOR pH

- Explain procedure to the woman or couple.

Procedure

- Wash hands.
- Use a cotton-tipped applicator impregnated with Nitrazine dye for determining pH (differentiates amniotic fluid, which is slightly alkaline, from urine and purulent material [pus], which are acidic).
- Dip the cotton-tipped applicator deep into the vagina to pick up fluid. (Procedure may be performed during speculum examination.)

Read Results

- Membranes probably intact: identifies vaginal and most body fluids that are acidic:

Yellow	pH 5.0
Olive-yellow	pH 5.5
Olive-green	pH 6.0

- Membranes probably ruptured: identifies amniotic fluid that is alkaline:

Blue-green	pH 6.5
Blue-gray	pH 7.0
Deep blue	pH 7.5

- Realize that false test results are possible because of presence of bloody show, insufficient amniotic fluid, or semen.
- Provide pericare as needed.
- Remove gloves and wash hands.

Document Results

- Results are positive or negative.

TEST FOR FERNING OR FERN PATTERN

- Explain procedure to woman or couple.
- Wash hands, apply sterile gloves, obtain specimen of fluid (usually during sterile speculum examination).
- Spread a drop of fluid from the vagina on a clean glass slide with a sterile cotton-tipped applicator.
- Allow fluid to dry.
- Examine the slide under microscope; observe for appearance of ferning (a frondlike crystalline pattern) (do not confuse with cervical mucus test, when high levels of estrogen cause the ferning).
- Observe for absence of ferning (alerts staff to possibility that amount of specimen was inadequate or that specimen was urine, vaginal discharge, or blood).
- Provide pericare as needed.
- Remove gloves and wash hands.

Document Results

- Results are positive or negative.

BOX 19-1 THE BIRTH PLAN

The birth plan should include the woman's or couple's preferences related to:

- Presence of birth companions such as the partner, older children, parents, friends, and doula, and the role each will play
- Presence of other persons such as students, male attendants, and interpreters
- Clothing to be worn
- Environmental modifications such as lighting, music, privacy, focal point, items from home such as pillows
- Labor activities such as preferred positions for labor and for birth, ambulation, birth balls, showers and whirlpool baths, oral food and fluid intake
- List of comfort and relaxation measures
- Labor and birth medical interventions such as pharmacologic pain relief measures, intravenous therapy, electronic monitoring, induction or augmentation measures, and episiotomy
- Care and handling of the newborn immediately after birth such as cutting of the cord, eye care, breastfeeding
- Cultural and religious requirements related to the care of the mother, newborn, and placenta

The childbirth website—www.childbirth.org—provides couples with an interactive birth plan along with examples of birth plans and descriptions of the options that can be included.

their availability, and ethnic or cultural expectations and needs. Determine the woman's use of alcohol, drugs, and tobacco before or during pregnancy.

The nurse reviews the birth plan. If no written plan has been prepared, then the nurse helps the woman formulate a birth plan by describing options available and determining the woman's wishes and preferences. As caregiver and advocate the nurse integrates the woman's desires into the nursing care plan as much as possible. The nurse also prepares the woman for the possibility of change in her plan as labor progresses and assures her that the staff will provide information so that she can make informed decisions. The woman must also realize, however, that the longer her list of "wishes" is, the greater the likelihood that her expectations will not be met.

The nurse should discuss with the woman and her partner their plans for preserving childbirth memories through the use of photography and videotaping. Information should be provided about the agency's policies regarding these practices and under what circumstances they are allowed. Protection of privacy and safety and infection control are major concerns for the expecting parents and the agency. To avoid future embarrassment and distress, the nurse should clarify with the woman exactly what parts of her childbirth she wishes to have photographed and the degree of detail. The woman's record should reflect that the childbirth was recorded. Some hospitals and health care providers do not allow videotaping of the birth because of concerns related to legal liability.

Psychosocial Factors

The woman's general appearance and behavior (and that of her partner) provide valuable clues to the type of supportive care she will need. However, keep in mind that general appearance and behavior may vary, depending on the stage and phase of labor (Table 19-1 and Box 19-2).

Women with a History of Sexual Abuse. Labor can trigger memories of sexual abuse, especially during intrusive procedures such as vaginal examinations. Monitors, intravenous (IV) lines, and epidurals can make the woman feel a loss of control or feel as if she is being confined to bed and "restrained." Being observed by students and having intense sensations in the uterus and genital area, especially at the time when she must push the baby out, can also trigger memories.

The nurse can help the abuse survivor to associate the sensations she is experiencing with the process of childbirth and not with her past abuse. Help maintain her sense of control by explaining all procedures and why they are needed, validating her needs, and paying close attention to her requests. Wait for the woman to give permission before touching her, and accept her often extreme reactions to labor (Simpson, 2008). Avoid words and phrases that can cause the woman to recall the words of her abuser (e.g., "open your legs," "relax and it won't hurt so much"). Limit the number of procedures that invade her body (e.g., vaginal examinations, urinary catheter, internal monitor, forceps or vacuum extractor) as much as possible. Encourage her to choose a person (e.g., doula, friend, family member) to be with her during labor to provide continuous support and comfort and to act as her advocate. Nurses are advised to care for all laboring women in this manner because it is not unusual for a woman to choose not to reveal a history of sexual abuse. These care measures can help a woman perceive her childbirth experience in positive terms.

Stress in Labor

The way in which women and their support person or family members approach labor is related to the manner in which they have been socialized to the childbearing process. Their reactions reflect their life experiences regarding childbirth–physical, social, cultural, and religious. Society communicates its expectations regarding acceptable and unacceptable maternal behaviors during labor and birth. These expectations may be used by some women as the basis for evaluating their own actions during childbirth. An idealized perception of labor and birth may be a source of guilt and cause a sense of failure if the woman finds the process less than joyous, especially when the pregnancy is unplanned or is the product of a dysfunctional or terminated relationship. Often women have heard horror stories or have seen friends or relatives going through labors that appear anything but easy. Multiparous women will often base their expectations of the present labor on their previous childbirth experiences.

Discuss the feelings a woman has about her pregnancy and fears regarding childbirth. This discussion is especially important if the woman is a primigravida who has not attended childbirth classes or is a multiparous woman who has had a previous negative childbirth experience. Women in labor usually have a variety of concerns that they will voice if asked but rarely volunteer. Major fears and concerns relate to the process and effects of childbirth, maternal and fetal well-being, and the attitude and actions of the health care staff. Unresolved fears increase a woman's stress and can slow the process of labor as a result of the inhibiting effects of catecholamines associated with the stress response on uterine contractions (Zwelling, Johnson, & Allen, 2006).

TABLE 19-1 **EXPECTED MATERNAL PROGRESS IN FIRST STAGE OF LABOR**

	PHASES MARKED BY CERVICAL DILATION*		
CRITERION	**LATENT (0-3 CM)**	**ACTIVE (4-7 CM)**	**TRANSITION (8-10 CM)**
Duration†	***About 6-8 Hours***	***About 3-6 Hours***	***About 20-40 Minutes***
Contractions			
• Strength	Mild to moderate	Moderate to strong	Strong to very strong
• Rhythm	Irregular	More regular	Regular
• Frequency	5-30 minutes apart	3-5 minutes apart	2-3 minutes apart
• Duration	30-45 seconds	40-70 seconds	45-90 seconds
Descent			
• Station of presenting part	Nulliparous: 0		Varies: +1 to +3 cm
			Varies: +2 to +3 cm
	Multiparous: −2 cm to 0		Varies: +1 to +2 cm
			Varies: +2 to +3 cm
Show			
• Color	Brownish discharge mucous plug, or pale pink mucus	Pink to bloody mucus	Bloody mucus
• Amount	Scant	Scant to moderate	Copious
Behavior and appearance‡	Excited; thoughts center on self, labor, and baby; fairly confident; may be talkative or silent, calm or tense; some apprehension; pain controlled fairly well—able to talk and ambulate through contractions; alert, follows directions readily; open to instructions	Becomes more serious, more quiet, doubtful of control of pain, more apprehensive; desires companionship and encouragement; attention more inwardly directed; fatigue evidenced; malar (cheeks) flush; has some difficulty following directions but accepts coaching; describes increasing discomfort	Pain described as severe; backache common; frustration, fear of loss of control, and irritability may be voiced; expresses doubt about ability to continue; vague in communications; amnesia between contractions; writhing with contractions; nausea and vomiting, especially if hyperventilating; hyperesthesia; circumoral pallor, perspiration of forehead and upper lips; shaking tremor of thighs; feeling of need to defecate, pressure on anus

*In the nullipara, effacement is often complete before dilation begins; in the multipara, it occurs simultaneously with dilation.
†Duration of each phase is influenced by such factors as parity, maternal emotions, position, level of activity, and fetal size, presentation, and position. For example, the labor of a nullipara tends to last longer, on average, than the labor of a multipara. Women who ambulate and assume upright positions or change positions frequently during labor tend to experience a shorter first stage. Descent is often prolonged in breech presentations and occiput posterior positions.
‡Women who have epidural analgesia for pain relief may not demonstrate some of these behaviors.

BOX 19-2 **PSYCHOSOCIAL ASSESSMENT OF THE LABORING WOMAN**

VERBAL INTERACTIONS
- Does the woman ask questions?
- Can she ask for what she needs?
- Does she talk to her support person(s)?
- Does she talk freely with the nurse or respond only to questions?

BODY LANGUAGE
- Does she change positions or lie rigidly still?
- What is her anxiety level?
- How does she react to being touched by the nurse or support person?
- Does she avoid eye contact?
- Does she look tired? If she appears tired, ask her how much rest she has had in the past 24 hours.

PERCEPTUAL ABILITY
- Is there a language barrier?
- Are repeated explanations necessary because her anxiety level interferes with her ability to comprehend?
- Can she repeat what she has been told or otherwise demonstrate her understanding?

DISCOMFORT LEVEL
- To what degree does the woman describe what she is experiencing including her pain experience?
- How does she react to a contraction?
- How does she react to assessment and care measures?
- Are any nonverbal pain messages noted?
- Can she ask for comfort measures?

The father, coach, or significant other also experiences stress during labor. The nurse can assist and support these individuals by identifying their needs and expectations and by helping make sure these are met. The nurse can determine what role the support person intends to fulfill and whether he or she is prepared for that role by making observations and asking herself or himself such questions as, "Has the couple attended childbirth classes?" "What role does this person expect to play?" "Does he or she do all the talking?" "Is he or she nervous, anxious, aggressive, or hostile?" "Does he or she look hungry, tired, worried, or confused?" "Does he or she watch television, sleep, or stay out of the room instead of paying attention to the woman?" "Where does he or she sit?" "Does he or she touch the woman; what is the character of the touch?" Be sensitive to the needs of support persons and provide teaching and support as appropriate. In many instances the support these persons provide to the laboring woman is in direct proportion to the support they receive from the nurses and other health care providers.

Cultural Factors

Currently more than 30% of the population in the United States comes from cultural groups other than non-Hispanic whites compared with only 9% of registered nurses (Callister, 2008). As the population in the United States and Canada becomes more diverse, it is increasingly important to note the woman's ethnic or cultural and religious values, beliefs, and practices in order to anticipate nursing interventions to add or eliminate from an individualized, mutually acceptable plan of care

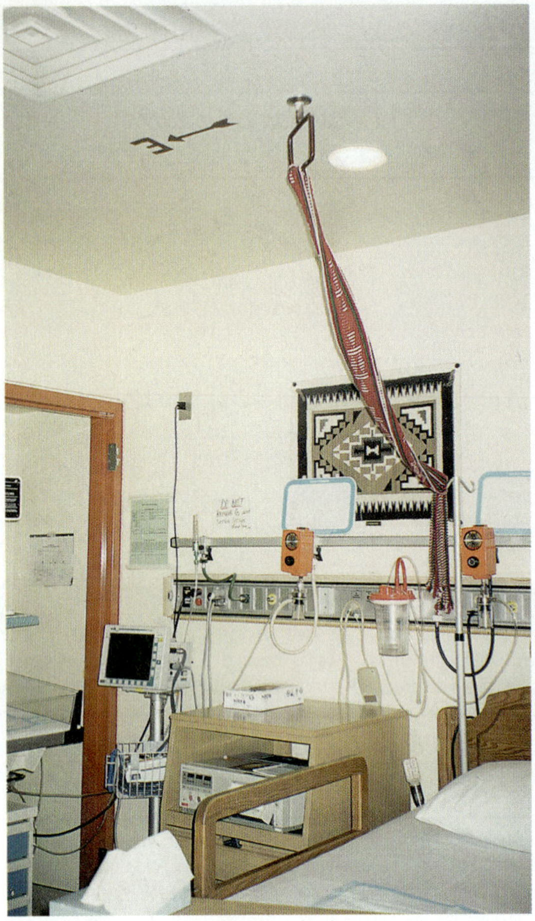

FIG. 19-3 Birthing room specific to a Native-American population. Note the arrow pointing east, the rug on the wall, and the rope or sash belt hanging from the ceiling. (Courtesy Patricia Hess, San Francisco, CA; Chinle Comprehensive Health Care Center, Chinle, AZ.)

that provides a feeling of safety and control (Fig. 19-3). Nurses should be committed to providing culturally sensitive care and to developing an appreciation and respect for cultural diversity (Callister, 2005; 2008). Encourage the woman to request specific caregiving behaviors and practices that are important to her. If a special request contradicts usual practices in that setting, the woman or the nurse can ask the woman's primary health care provider to write an order to accommodate the special request. For example, in many cultures, it is unacceptable to have a male caregiver examine a pregnant woman. In some cultures, it is traditional to take the placenta home; in others, the woman has only certain nourishments during labor. Some women believe that cutting her body, as with an episiotomy, allows her spirit to leave her body and that rupturing the membranes prolongs, not shortens, labor. It is important to explain the rationale for required care measures carefully (see the Cultural Considerations box).

Within cultures, women may have an idea of the "right" way to behave in labor and may react to the pain experienced in that way. These behaviors can range from total silence to moaning or screaming, but they do not necessarily indicate the degree of pain. A woman who moans with contractions may not be in as much physical pain as a woman who is silent but winces during contractions. Some women believe that screaming or crying out in pain is shameful if a man is present. If the woman's support person is her mother, she may perceive the need to "behave" more strongly than if her support person is the father of the baby. She will perceive herself as failing or succeeding based on her ability to follow these "standards" of behavior. Conversely, a woman's behavior in response to pain may influence the support received from significant others. In some cultures, women who lose control and cry out in pain may be scolded, whereas in other cultures, support persons will become more helpful (D'Avanzo, 2008).

CULTURAL CONSIDERATIONS

Birth Practices in Different Cultures

SOUTH KOREA
Stoic response to labor pain; fathers usually not present

JAPAN
Natural childbirth methods practiced; may labor silently; may eat during labor; father may be present

CHINA
Stoic response to pain; fathers usually not present; side-lying position preferred for labor and birth because this position is thought to reduce infant trauma

INDIA
Natural childbirth methods preferred; father is usually not present; female relatives usually present

IRAN
Father not present; female support and female caregivers preferred

MEXICO
May be stoic about discomfort until second stage, then may request pain relief; fathers and female relatives may be present

LAOS
May use squatting position for birth; fathers may or may not be present; female attendants preferred

Source: D'Avanzo, C. (2008). *Mosby's pocket guide to cultural health assessment* (4th ed.). St. Louis: Mosby.

Culture and Father Participation. A companion is an important source of support, encouragement, and comfort for women during childbirth. The woman's cultural and religious background influences her choice of birth companion as do trends in the society in which she lives. For example, in Western societies the father is viewed as the ideal birth companion. For European-American couples, attending childbirth classes together has become a traditional, expected activity. Laotian (Hmong) husbands also traditionally participate actively in the labor process. In some other cultures the father may be available, but his presence in the labor room with the mother may not be considered appropriate, or he may be present but resist active involvement in her care. Such behavior could be perceived by the nursing staff to indicate a lack of concern, caring, or interest. Women from many cultures prefer female caregivers and want to have at least one female companion present during labor and birth. They also are usually very concerned about modesty. If couples from these cultures immigrate to the United States or Canada, their roles may change. The nurse needs to talk to the woman and her support persons to determine the roles they will assume.

The Non–English-Speaking Woman in Labor. A woman's level of anxiety in labor increases when she does not understand what is happening to her or what is being said. Non–English-speaking women often feel a complete loss of control over their situation if no health care provider is present who speaks their language. They can panic and withdraw or become physically abusive when someone tries to do something they perceive might harm them or their babies. A support person is sometimes able to serve as an interpreter. However, caution is warranted because the interpreter may not be able to convey exactly what the nurse or others are saying or what the woman is saying, which can increase the woman's stress level even more.

Ideally, a bilingual nurse will care for the woman. Alternatively a hospital employee or volunteer interpreter may be contacted for assistance (see Box 2-2). Ideally, the interpreter is from the woman's culture. For some women a female is more acceptable than a male interpreter. If no one in the hospital is able to interpret, call a service so that interpretation can take place over the telephone. Even when the nurse has limited ability to communicate verbally with the woman, in most instances the woman appreciates the nurse's efforts to do so. Speaking slowly and avoiding complex words and medical terms can help a woman and her partner understand. Often the woman understands English much better than she speaks it.

Physical Examination

Spanish Guidelines—Labor Assessment

The initial physical examination includes a general systems assessment and an assessment of fetal status. During the examination uterine contractions are assessed and a vaginal examination is performed. The findings of the admission physical examination serve as a baseline for assessing the woman's progress from that point. See Chapter 4 for information regarding physical examination of women with disabilities.

The information obtained from a complete and accurate assessment during the initial examination serves as the basis for determining whether the woman should be admitted and what her ongoing care should be. Expected maternal progress and minimal assessment guidelines during the first stage of labor are presented in Table 19-1 and the Nursing Process Box: First Stage of Labor.

Birth is a time when nurses and other health care providers are exposed to a great deal of maternal and newborn blood and body fluids. Therefore, Standard Precautions should guide all assessment and care measures (Box 19-3). Hand hygiene

NURSING PROCESS

First Stage of Labor

ASSESSMENT

Assessment begins at the first contact with the woman, whether by telephone or in person.

- History (use secondary sources if permission is given by woman):
  - Review prenatal data from the chart and from the woman.
  - Discuss her current health status including any health problems.
  - Discuss status of her labor: when did it start, characteristics of contractions, status of amniotic membranes, signs of prodromal labor (e.g., lightening, passage of mucous plug, etc.).
  - Assess psychosocial and cultural factors; determine her support persons.
  - Review birth plan if woman has one or discuss preferences for her labor, if she does not.
- Physical examination: frequency of assessment is determined by phase of labor and condition of maternal-fetal unit including whether the pregnancy is classified as low risk or high risk. More frequent assessments are required for the high risk mother or if problems arise during labor:
  - Admission: general systems assessment along with maternal vital signs, FHR and pattern, and status of labor (e.g., uterine contractions, cervical changes, status of membranes, show)
  - Latent phase:
    - Perform every 30 to 60 minutes: maternal blood pressure, pulse, and respirations
    - Perform every 30 to 60 minutes: FHR and pattern, uterine activity, vaginal show
    - Assess temperature every 4 hours until membranes rupture, then every 2 hours
    - Perform vaginal examination as needed to identify progress
    - Observe every 30 minutes: changes in maternal appearance, mood, affect, energy level and condition of partner/coach
  - Active phase:
    - Perform every 30 minutes: maternal blood pressure, pulse, and respirations
    - Perform every 15 to 30 minutes: FHR and pattern, uterine activity, vaginal show
    - Assess temperature every 4 hours until membranes rupture, then every 2 hours
    - Perform vaginal examination as needed to identify progress
    - Observe every 15 minutes: changes in maternal appearance, mood, affect, energy level and condition of partner/coach
  - Transition phase:
    - Perform every 15 to 30 minutes: maternal blood pressure, pulse, and respirations
    - Perform every 15 to 30 minutes: FHR and pattern
    - Assess every 10 to 15 minutes: uterine activity, vaginal show
    - Assess temperature every 4 hours until membranes rupture, then every 2 hours
    - Perform vaginal examination as needed to identify progress
    - Observe every 5 minutes: changes in maternal appearance, mood, affect, energy level and condition of partner/coach

NURSING DIAGNOSES

Possible nursing diagnoses include:

***Acute Pain* related to:**
- effects of uterine contractions and fetal descent

***Anxiety* related to:**
- negative experience with a previous childbirth
- cultural differences
- triggering of memories associated with history of sexual abuse

***Impaired Urinary Elimination* related to:**
- reduced intake of oral fluids
- decreased sensation of bladder fullness associated with epidural anesthesia or analgesia

Continued

NURSING PROCESS

First Stage of Labor—cont'd

***Impaired Gas Exchange (Fetal)* related to:**
- decreased placental perfusion associated with maternal hypertension or hypotension
- maternal position
- intense and frequent uterine contractions
- compression of the umbilical cord

***Situational Low Self-esteem (Maternal)* related to:**
- inability to meet self-expectations regarding performance during childbirth
- loss of control during labor

***Situational Low Self-esteem (Father or Partner)* related to:**
- unrealistic expectations regarding role as labor coach
- perceived ineffectiveness in meeting the needs of the laboring woman

EXPECTED OUTCOMES OF CARE

Expected outcomes are that the woman will:
- Accept comfort and support measures from significant others and health care providers as needed.
- Actively participate in the labor process, with no evidence of injury to her or her fetus.
- Maintain adequate hydration status through oral or intravenous fluid intake.
- Empty bladder (by spontaneous voiding or catheterization) at least every 2 hours to prevent bladder distention.
- Verbalize discomfort and indicate the need for measures that help reduce discomfort and promote relaxation.
- Express satisfaction with her performance during labor.

PLAN OF CARE AND INTERVENTIONS

Latent phase
- Teach woman to:
  - Stay at home as long as possible
  - Use relaxation measures; rest and sleep (at night)
  - Remain active: change positions frequently, ambulate, engage in diversional activities (during the day)
  - Eat light foods and drink liquids in moderation
  - Void every 2 hours
  - Perform basic hygiene measures
- Discuss process of labor and what to expect
- Monitor the progress of labor and fetal status at recommended intervals
- Keep woman/partner informed regarding progress
- Demonstrate breathing and relaxation techniques and comfort measures as needed
- Create a calm, relaxing, safe environment

Active and transition phase
- Monitor the progress of labor and fetal status at recommended intervals
- Keep woman/partner informed regarding progress
- Encourage and assist with nonpharmacologic measures to enhance progress and relieve discomfort
- Provide pharmacologic measures for pain relief as ordered by the primary health care provider and as requested by the woman
- Offer fluids as desired and ordered to maintain hydration; initiate intravenous fluids if ordered
- Assist with activity and position changes emphasizing upright positions and movement
- Help to rest and relax between contractions
- Encourage voiding every 2 hours
- Assist with hygienic measures: oral care, perineal cleansing
- Provide emotional support and encouragement; provide positive reinforcement of her efforts

EVALUATION

Evaluation of the effectiveness of care of the woman in the first stage of labor is based on the previously stated expected outcomes.

BOX 19-3 STANDARD PRECAUTIONS DURING CHILDBIRTH

- Wash hands before and after putting on gloves and performing procedures; cleansing alcohol rubs can be used if hands are not visibly soiled.
- Wear gloves (clean or sterile, as appropriate) when performing procedures that require contact with the woman's genitalia and body fluids, including bloody show (e.g., during vaginal examination, amniotomy, hygienic care of the perineum, insertion of an internal scalp electrode and intrauterine pressure monitor, and urinary catheterization).
- Wear a mask that has a shield or protective eyewear, and cover gown when assisting with the birth. Cap and shoe covers are worn for cesarean birth but are optional for vaginal birth in a birthing room. Gowns worn by the primary health care provider who is attending the birth should have a waterproof front and sleeves and should be sterile. Mask also should be worn during spinal puncture or insertion of an epidural catheter.
- Drape the woman with sterile towels and sheets as appropriate. Explain to the woman what can and cannot be touched.
- Help the woman's partner put on appropriate coverings for the type of birth, such as cap, mask, gown, and shoe covers. Show the partner where to stand and what can and cannot be touched.
- Wear gloves and gown when handling the newborn immediately after birth.
- Use an appropriate method to suction the newborn's airway, such as a bulb syringe, or mechanical wall suction.

(e.g., washing hands with soap or application of an alcohol-based antiseptic rub) before and after assessing the woman and providing care is a critical step in the prevention of infection transmission. The nurse should explain assessment findings to the woman and her partner whenever possible. Throughout labor, accurate documentation, following agency policy, is done as soon as possible after a procedure has been performed (Fig. 19-4).

General Systems Assessment. On admission, the nurse should perform a brief systems assessment. This includes an assessment of the heart, lungs, and skin and an examination to determine the presence and extent of edema of the face, hands, sacrum, and legs. It also includes testing of deep tendon reflexes and for clonus if indicated. Also note the woman's weight. Increasing numbers of women are overweight or obese.

Excessive size can make nursing care during labor and birth more difficult and places the woman at risk for complications such as operative birth, infection, and blood clots. See Chapter 33 for further information.

Vital Signs. Assess vital signs (temperature, pulse, respirations, and blood pressure, using a correct-size cuff) on admission. The initial values are used as the baseline for comparison for all future measurements. If the blood pressure is elevated, reassess it 30 minutes later, between contractions, to obtain a reading after the woman has relaxed. Encourage the woman to lie on her side to prevent supine hypotension and fetal distress (Fig. 19-5). Monitor her temperature so that you can identify signs of infection or a fluid deficit (e.g., dehydration associated with inadequate intake of fluids).

Leopold Maneuvers (Abdominal Palpation). Leopold maneuvers are performed with the woman briefly lying on her back (see the Procedure box: Leopold Maneuvers). These maneuvers help identify the (1) number of fetuses; (2) presenting part, fetal lie, and fetal attitude; (3) degree of the presenting part's descent into the pelvis; and (4) expected location of the point of maximal intensity (PMI) of the FHR on the woman's abdomen.

Assessment of Fetal Heart Rate and Pattern. The PMI of the FHR is the location on the maternal abdomen at which the FHR is heard the loudest. It is usually directly over the fetal back (Fig. 19-6). In a vertex presentation, you can usually hear the FHR below the mother's umbilicus in either the right or the left lower quadrant of the abdomen. In a breech presentation you usually hear the FHR above the mother's umbilicus. The Nursing Process Box: First Stage of Labor summarizes assessments recommended for determining fetal status. In addition, you must assess the FHR after ROM because this is the most common time for the umbilical cord to prolapse, after any change in the contraction pattern or maternal status, and before and after the woman receives medication or a procedure is performed (Tucker et al., 2009).

Assessment of Uterine Contractions. A general characteristic of effective labor is regular uterine activity (i.e., contractions becoming more frequent with increased duration), but uterine activity is not directly related to labor progress. Uterine contractions are the primary powers that act involuntarily to expel the fetus and the placenta from the uterus. Several methods are used to evaluate uterine contractions, including the woman's subjective description, palpation and timing of contractions by a health care provider, and electronic monitoring.

Video—Assessment: Leopold Maneuvers

PROCEDURE

Leopold Maneuvers

- Wash hands.
- Ask woman to empty bladder.
- Position woman supine with one pillow under her head and with her knees slightly flexed.
- Place small rolled towel under woman's right or left hip to displace uterus off major blood vessels (prevents supine hypotensive syndrome; see Fig. 19-5, *D*).
- *If right-handed, stand on woman's right, facing her:*
  1. Identify fetal part that occupies the fundus. The head feels round, firm, freely movable, and palpable by ballottement; the breech feels less regular and softer. This maneuver identifies fetal lie (longitudinal or transverse) and presentation (cephalic or breech) (Fig. A).
  2. Using palmar surface of one hand, locate and palpate the smooth convex contour of the fetal back and the irregularities that identify the small parts (feet, hands, elbows). This maneuver helps identify fetal presentation (Fig. B).
  3. With right hand, determine which fetal part is presenting over the inlet to the true pelvis. Gently grasp the lower pole of the uterus between the thumb and fingers, pressing in slightly (Fig. C). If the head is presenting and not engaged, determine the attitude of the head (flexed or extended).
  4. Turn to face the woman's feet. Using both hands, outline the fetal head (Fig. D) with the palmar surface of the fingertips. When the presenting part has descended deeply, only a small portion of it may be outlined. Palpation of the cephalic prominence helps identify the attitude of the head. If the cephalic prominence is found on the same side as the small parts, this means that the head must be flexed and the vertex is presenting (see Fig. D). If the cephalic prominence is on the same side as the back, this indicates that the presenting head is extended and the face is presenting.
- Document fetal presentation, position, and lie and whether presenting part is flexed or extended, engaged, or free floating. Use agency's protocol for documentation (e.g., "Vtx, LOA, floating").

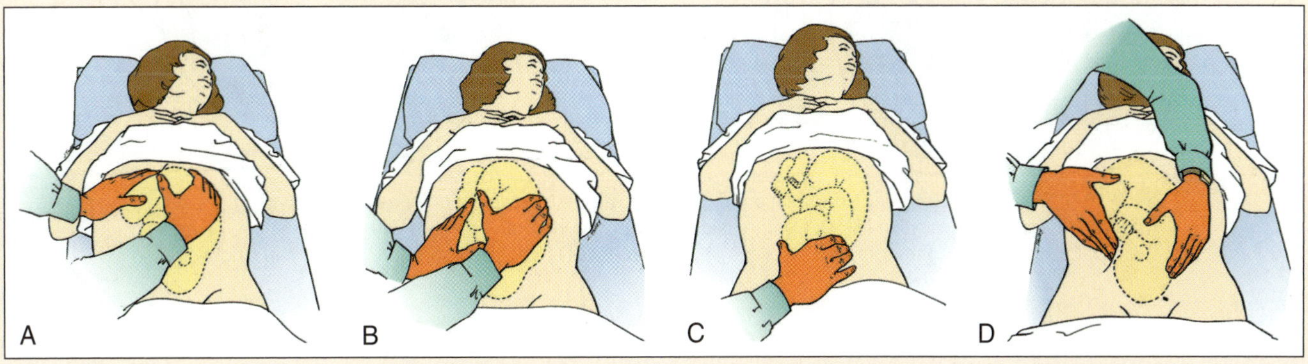

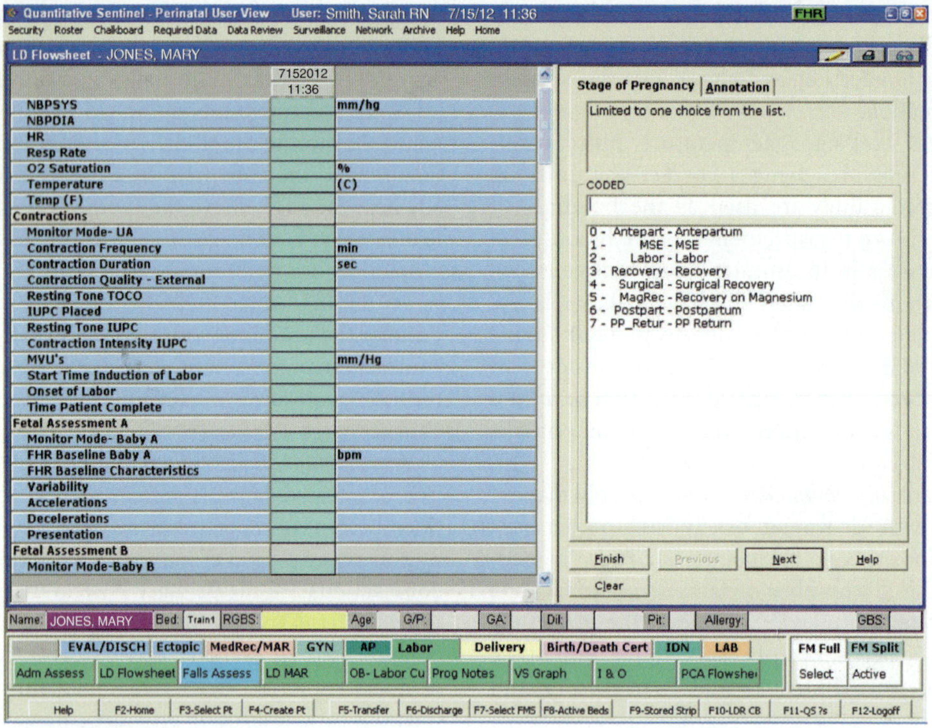

FIG. 19-4 Portion of the labor flowsheet screen in an electronic medical record. (Courtesy Kitty Cashion, Memphis, TN).

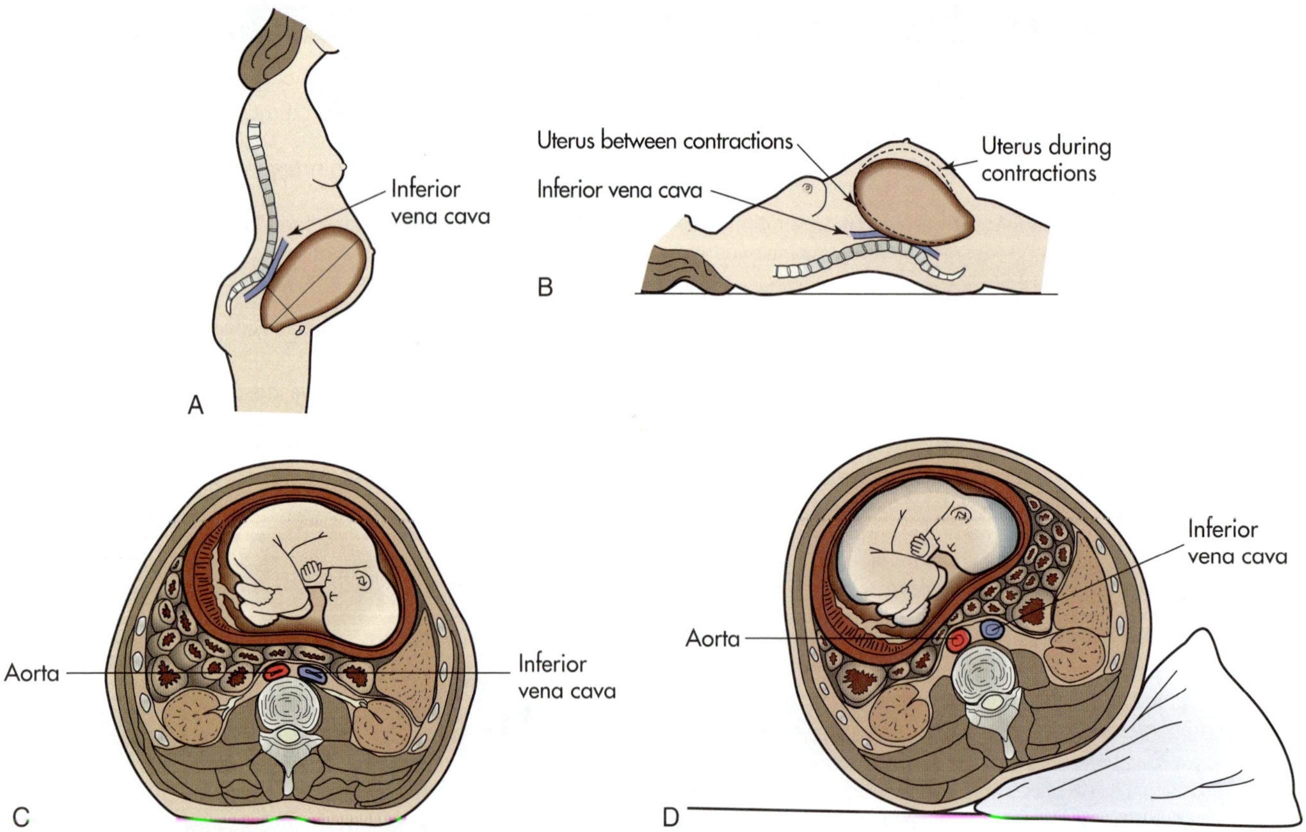

FIG. 19-5 Supine hypotension. Note relation of pregnant uterus to ascending vena cava in standing position **(A)**, and in the supine position **(B)**. **C,** Compression of aorta and inferior vena cava with woman in supine position. **D,** Compression of these vessels is relieved by placement of a wedge pillow under the woman's right side.

Video—Nursing Skills: Performing Leopold Maneuvers

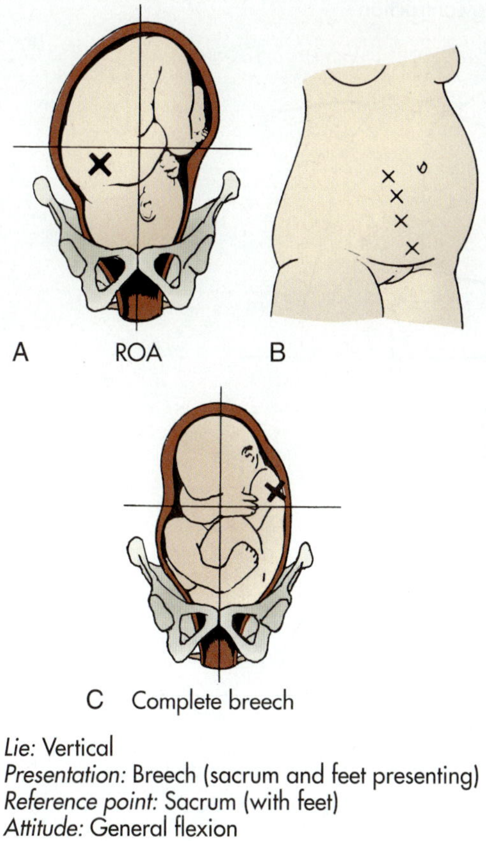

FIG. 19-6 Location of the fetal heart tones (FHTs). **A,** FHTs with fetus in right occipitoanterior (ROA) position. **B,** Changes in location of point of maximal intensity of FHTs as fetus undergoes internal rotation from ROA to OA and descent for birth. **C,** FHTs with fetus in left sacrum posterior position. (**A** and **C,** Courtesy Ross Laboratories, Columbus, OH.)

Each contraction exhibits a wavelike pattern. It begins with a slow increment (the "building up" of a contraction from its onset), gradually reaches a peak, and then diminishes rapidly (decrement, the "letting down" of the contraction). An interval of rest ends when the next contraction begins. The outward appearance of the woman's abdomen during and between contractions and the pattern of a typical uterine contraction are shown in Figure 19-7.

A uterine contraction is described in terms of the following characteristics:

- *Frequency:* How often uterine contractions occur; the time that elapses from the beginning of one contraction to the beginning of the next contraction
- *Intensity:* The strength of a contraction at its peak
- *Duration:* The time that elapses between the onset and the end of a contraction
- *Resting tone:* The tension in the uterine muscle between contractions; relaxation of the uterus

Uterine contractions are assessed by palpation or by using an external or internal electronic monitor (see Chapter 18 for further discussion). Frequency and duration can be measured by all three methods of uterine activity monitoring. The accuracy of determining intensity and resting tone varies by the method used. The woman's description and palpation are more subjective and less precise ways of determining the intensity of uterine contractions and resting tone than is the electronic fetal monitor. The following terms describe what is felt on palpation:

- *Mild:* Slightly tense fundus that is easy to indent with fingertips (feels like touching finger to tip of nose)
- *Moderate:* Firm fundus that is difficult to indent with fingertips (feels like touching finger to chin)
- *Strong:* Rigid boardlike fundus that is almost impossible to indent with fingertips (feels like touching finger to forehead)

Women in labor tend to describe the pain of contractions in terms of the sensations they are experiencing in the lower abdomen or back, which are sometimes unrelated to the firmness of the uterine fundus. Therefore, their assessment of the strength of their contractions can be less accurate than that of the health care provider, although the amount of discomfort reported is valid.

External electronic monitoring provides some information about the strength of uterine contractions when the appearance of contractions on admission is compared to those that occur later in labor. Internal electronic monitoring with an intrauterine pressure catheter, however, is the most accurate way of assessing the intensity of uterine contractions and resting tone.

On admission, at least a 20- to 30-minute baseline monitoring period of uterine contractions and the fetal heart rate and pattern commonly is done using electronic monitors. The minimal times for assessing uterine activity during the various phases of labor are given in the Nursing Process boxes for the First Stage of Labor; the Second Stage of Labor and the findings expected as labor progresses are summarized in Tables 19-1 and 19-3.

! NURSING ALERT

If you find the characteristics of contractions to be abnormal, either exceeding or falling below what is considered acceptable in terms of the standard characteristics, report this finding to the primary health care provider.

You must consider uterine activity in the context of its effect on cervical effacement and dilation and on the degree of descent of the presenting part (see Chapter 16). You must also consider the effect on the fetus. You can verify the progress of labor effectively through the use of graphic charts (partograms) on which you plot cervical dilation and station (descent). This type of graphic charting assists in early identification of deviations from expected labor patterns. Figure 19-8 provides examples of partograms. Hospitals and birthing centers may develop their own assessment graphs that may include data not only on dilation and descent but also maternal vital signs, FHR, and uterine activity.

! NURSING ALERT

The nurse should recognize that active labor can actually last longer than the expected labor patterns because all women are different. This finding is not a cause for concern unless the maternal-fetal unit exhibits signs of stress (e.g., abnormal fetal heart rate patterns, maternal fever).

Vaginal Examination. The vaginal examination reveals whether the woman is in true labor and enables the examiner to determine whether the membranes have ruptured (Fig. 19-9). Because this examination is often stressful and uncomfortable

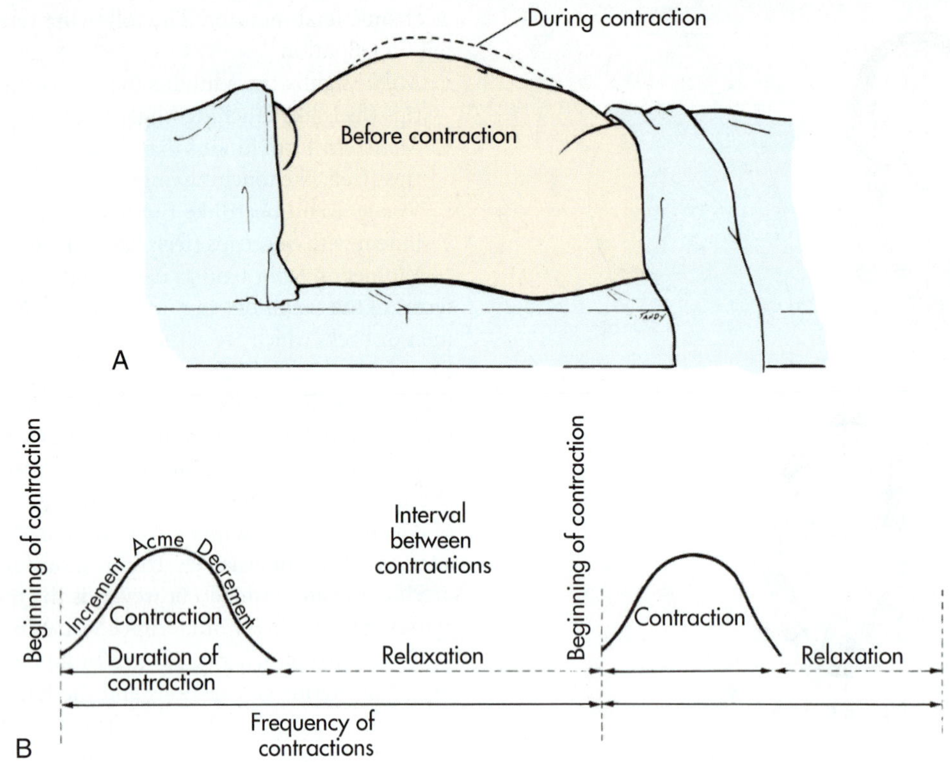

FIG. 19-7 Assessment of uterine contractions. **A,** Abdominal contour before and during uterine contraction. **B,** Wavelike pattern of contractile activity.

for the woman, perform it only when indicated by the status of the woman and her fetus. For example, you should perform a vaginal examination on admission, prior to administering medications (e.g., analgesics, increasing oxytocin infusion), when significant change has occurred in uterine activity, on maternal perception of perineal pressure or the urge to bear down, when membranes rupture, or when you note variable decelerations of the FHR. A full explanation of the examination and support of the woman are important in reducing the stress and discomfort associated with the examination (Simpson, 2008) (see the Procedure box: Vaginal Examination of the Laboring Woman.)

PROCEDURE

Vaginal Examination of the Laboring Woman

- Use a sterile glove and antiseptic solution or soluble gel for lubrication.
- Position the woman to prevent supine hypotension. Drape to ensure privacy.
- Cleanse the perineum and vulva if needed.
- After obtaining the woman's permission to touch her, gently insert the index and middle fingers into the woman's vagina.
- Determine:
  - Cervical dilation, effacement, and position (e.g., posterior, mid, anterior)
  - Presenting part, position, and station; molding of the head with development of caput succedaneum (may effect accuracy of determination of station)
  - Status of membranes (intact, bulging, or ruptured)
  - Characteristics of amniotic fluid (e.g., color, clarity, and odor) if membranes are ruptured
- Explain findings of the examination to the woman.
- Document findings and report to primary health care provider.

Laboratory and Diagnostic Tests

Analysis of Urine Specimen. A clean-catch urine specimen may be obtained to gather further data about the pregnant woman's health. Analysis of the specimen is a convenient and simple procedure that can provide information about her hydration status (e.g., specific gravity, color, amount), nutritional status (e.g., ketones), infection status (e.g., leukocytes), or the status of possible complications such as preeclampsia, shown by finding protein in the urine. In most hospitals this test must be done in the laboratory rather than at the bedside, even if a urine "dipstick" is used.

Blood Tests. The blood tests performed vary with the hospital protocol and the woman's health status. Currently, all blood tests must be performed in the hospital laboratory rather than on the perinatal unit. Often blood samples are obtained from the hub of the catheter when an IV is started. A hematocrit will likely be ordered. More comprehensive blood assessments such as white blood cell count, red blood cell count, hemoglobin level, hematocrit, and platelet values are included in a complete blood count (CBC). A CBC may be ordered for women with a history of infection, anemia, gestational hypertension, or other disorders. Any woman whose human immunodeficiency virus (HIV) status is undocumented at the time of labor should be screened with a rapid HIV test unless she declines (opts out) of testing (Centers for Disease Control and Prevention [CDC], Branson, Handsfield, Lampe, Janssen, & Taylor, et al., 2006).

Most hospitals require that a "type and screen," to determine the woman's blood type and Rh status, be performed on admission. Even if these tests have already been performed during pregnancy, the hospital's laboratory or blood bank must verify

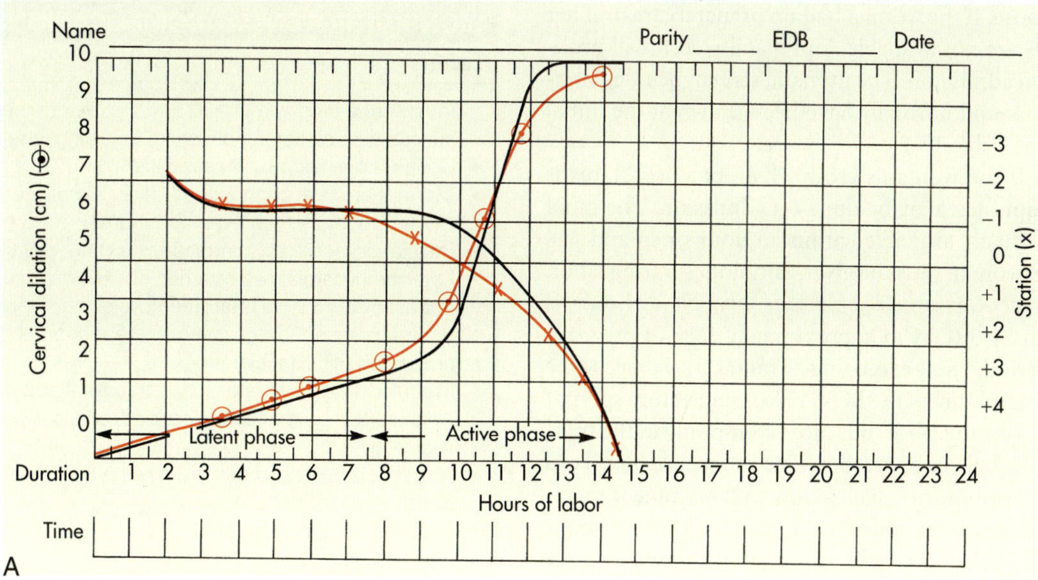

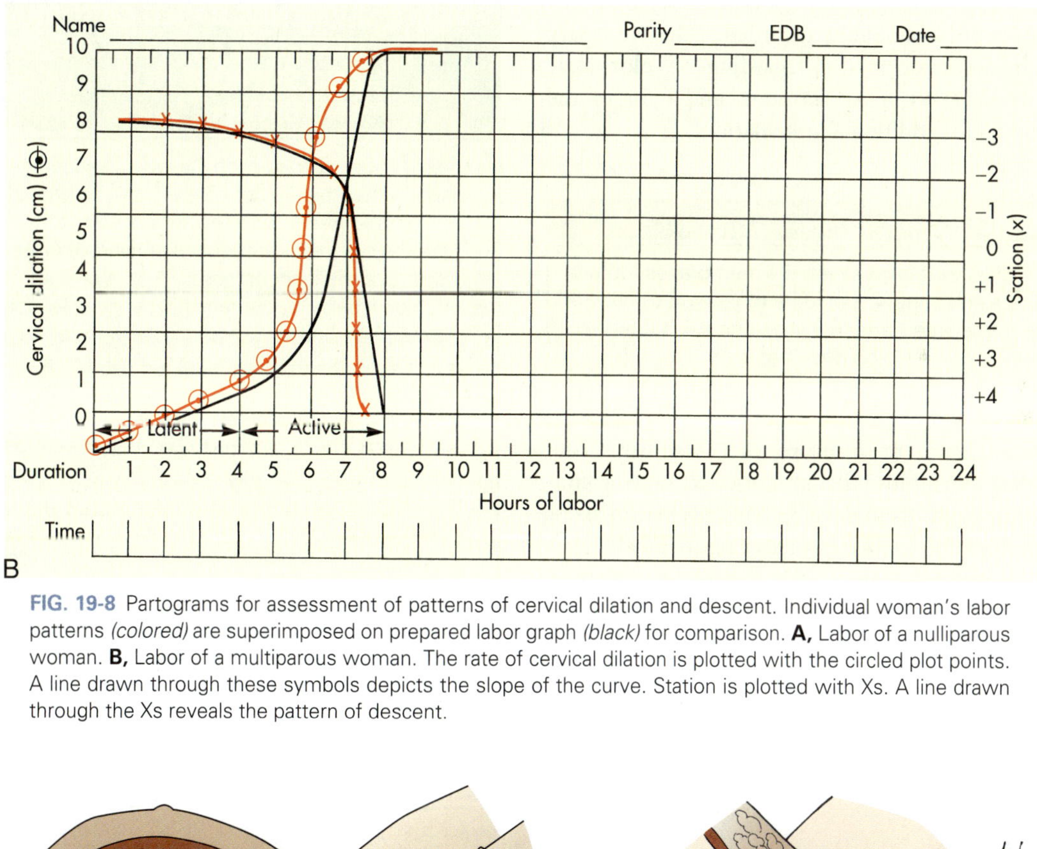

FIG. 19-8 Partograms for assessment of patterns of cervical dilation and descent. Individual woman's labor patterns *(colored)* are superimposed on prepared labor graph *(black)* for comparison. **A,** Labor of a nulliparous woman. **B,** Labor of a multiparous woman. The rate of cervical dilation is plotted with the circled plot points. A line drawn through these symbols depicts the slope of the curve. Station is plotted with Xs. A line drawn through the Xs reveals the pattern of descent.

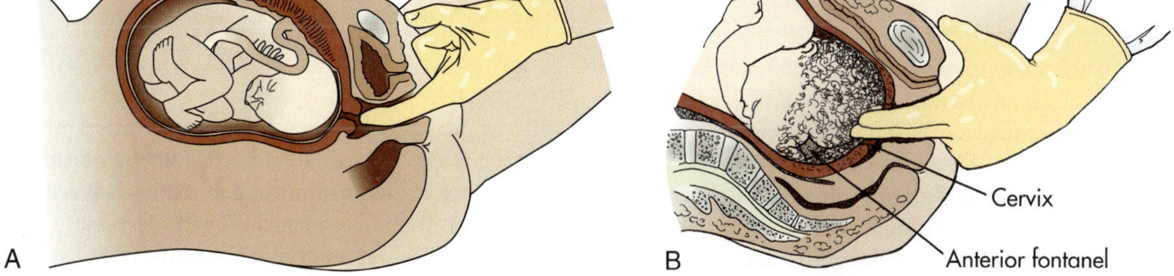

FIG. 19-9 Vaginal examination. **A,** Undilated, uneffaced cervix; membranes intact. **B,** Palpation of sagittal suture line. Cervix effaced and partially dilated.

the results in-house. If the woman had no prenatal care or if her prenatal records are not available, a prenatal screen will probably be drawn on admission. The prenatal screen includes laboratory tests that would normally have been drawn at the initial prenatal visit (see Table 15-2).

Other Tests. If the woman's group B streptococci status is not known, a rapid test may be done on admission. The rapid test results are usually available within an hour or so and will determine if the woman must be given antibiotics during labor.

Assessment of Amniotic Membranes and Fluid. Labor is initiated at term by SROM in approximately 25% of pregnant women. A lag period, rarely exceeding 24 hours, may precede the onset of labor. Membranes (the BOW) also can rupture spontaneously any time during labor, but most commonly in the transition phase of the first stage of labor. The Procedure box: Tests for Rupture of Membranes explains how to determine if membranes are ruptured. If the membranes do not rupture spontaneously, the BOW will likely be ruptured artificially at some time during labor. Artificial rupture of membranes (AROM), called an **amniotomy,** is performed by the physician or certified nurse-midwife using a plastic AmniHook or a surgical clamp.

Whether the membranes rupture spontaneously or artificially, the time of rupture should be recorded. Other necessary documentation includes information regarding the color (clear or meconium-stained), estimated amount, and odor of the fluid. See Chapter 33 for additional information.

! NURSING ALERT

The umbilical cord may prolapse when the membranes rupture. The fetal heart rate and pattern should be monitored closely for several minutes immediately after ROM to determine fetal well-being, and the findings should be documented.

Infection. When membranes rupture, microorganisms from the vagina can then ascend into the amniotic sac, causing chorioamnionitis and placentitis to develop. For this reason assess maternal temperature and vaginal discharge frequently (at least every 2 hours) so that you can quickly identify an infection developing after ROM. Even when membranes are intact, however, microorganisms may ascend and cause infection.

Assessment findings serve as a baseline for evaluating the woman's subsequent progress during labor. Although some problems can be anticipated, others may appear unexpectedly during the clinical course of labor (see the Signs of Potential Complications box).

Nursing Care

The nursing process provides the framework for the nursing care management of women in labor. The physical nursing care given to a woman in labor is an essential component of her care. The current emphasis on evidence-based practice supports the management of care by using this approach to enhance the safety, effectiveness, and acceptability of the physical care measures chosen to support the woman during labor and birth (Box 19-4). The various physical needs, the necessary nursing actions, and the rationale for care are presented in Table 19-2, the Nursing Care Plan and the Nursing Process box: First Stage of Labor.

SIGNS OF POTENTIAL COMPLICATIONS

Labor

- Intrauterine pressure of ≥80 mm Hg (determined by intrauterine pressure catheter monitoring) or resting tone of ≥20 mm Hg
- Contractions lasting ≥90 seconds
- More than five contractions in a 10-minute period (occur more frequently than every 2 minutes)
- Relaxation between contractions lasting <30 seconds
- Fetal bradycardia; tachycardia; absent or minimal variability not associated with fetal sleep cycle or temporary effects of CNS depressant drugs given to the woman; late, variable, or prolonged FHR decelerations
- Irregular fetal heart rate; suspected fetal arrhythmias
- Appearance of meconium-stained or bloody fluid from the vagina
- Arrest in progress of cervical dilation or effacement, descent of the fetus, or both
- Maternal temperature of ≥38° C
- Foul-smelling vaginal discharge
- Persistent bright or dark red vaginal bleeding

BOX 19-4 EVIDENCE-BASED CARE PRACTICES DESIGNED TO PROMOTE, PROTECT, AND SUPPORT NORMAL LABOR AND BIRTH

- Allow labor to begin on its own: encourage spontaneous labor rather than fostering elective labor inductions.
- Encourage freedom of movement throughout labor to facilitate the progress of labor and enhance maternal comfort and control of the labor process.
- Provide labor support beginning early in labor and continuing throughout the process of childbirth to relieve maternal anxiety and stress and decrease the risk for epidural anesthesia and cesarean birth; support should be provided by someone not employed by the hospital (e.g., doula).
- Avoid routine implementation of interventions (e.g., intravenous fluids, oral intake restrictions, continuous electronic fetal monitoring, labor augmentation measures [e.g., amniotomy, oxytocin administration], and epidural anesthesia).
- Support the practice of spontaneous, nondirected pushing in nonsupine positions (e.g., lateral, squatting, standing, kneeling, and semisitting) to facilitate the progress of fetal descent and shorten the second stage of labor.
- Avoid separation of the mother from her healthy baby after birth by encouraging skin-to-skin contact of mother and baby to keep newborn warm, prevent neonatal infection, enhance the newborn's physiologic adjustment to extrauterine life, and foster early breastfeeding.

Source: Romano, A. & Lothian, J. (2008). Promoting, protecting, and supporting normal birth: A look at the evidence. *Journal of Obstetric, Gynecologic and Neonatal Nursing, 37*(1), 94-105.

General Hygiene

Offer women in labor the use of showers or warm-water baths, if they are available, to enhance the feeling of well-being and to minimize the discomfort of contractions. Water immersion during active labor is associated with decreases in the use of analgesia and in reported maternal pain (Berghella, Baxter, & Chauhan, 2008). Also encourage women to wash their hands or use cleansing foam after voiding and to perform self-hygiene

NURSING CARE PLAN

Labor and Birth

NURSING DIAGNOSIS

Anxiety related to labor and the birthing process

Expected Outcome

Woman exhibits decreased signs of anxiety.

Nursing Interventions/*Rationales*

- Orient woman and significant others to labor and birth unit and explain admission protocol *to allay initial feelings of anxiety.*
- Assess woman's knowledge, experience, and expectations of labor; note any signs or expressions of anxiety, nervousness, or fear *to establish a baseline for intervention.*
- Discuss the expected progression of labor and describe what to expect during the process *to decrease anxiety associated with the unknown.*
- Actively involve the woman in care decisions during labor, interpret sights and sounds of environment (monitor sights and sounds, unit activities), and share information on progression of labor (vital signs, fetal heart rate [FHR], dilation, effacement) *to increase her sense of control and lessen fears.*

NURSING DIAGNOSIS

Acute pain related to increasing frequency and intensity of contractions

Expected Outcome

Woman exhibits signs of ability to cope with discomfort.

Nursing Interventions/*Rationales*

- Assess woman's level of pain and strategies that she has used to cope with pain *to establish a baseline for intervention.*
- Encourage significant other to remain as support person during labor process *to assist with support and comfort measures, because measures are often more effective when delivered by a familiar person.*
- Instruct woman and support person in use of specific techniques such as conscious relaxation, focused breathing, effleurage, massage, and application of sacral pressure *to increase relaxation, decrease intensity of contractions, and promote use of controlled thought and direction of energy.*
- Provide comfort measures such as frequent mouth care *to prevent dry mouth,* application of damp cloth to forehead, and changing of damp gown or bed covers *to relieve discomfort associated with diaphoresis.*
- Help woman to change position *to reduce stiffness, promote comfort, and facilitate progress of birth.*
- Explain what analgesics and anesthesia are available for use during labor and birth *to provide knowledge to help woman make decisions about pain control.*
- Administer analgesics and/or assist with regional anesthesia (e.g., epidural) as ordered or desired *to provide effective pain relief during labor and birth.*

NURSING DIAGNOSIS

Risk for impaired urinary elimination related to sensory impairment secondary to labor

Expected Outcome

Woman does not show signs of bladder distention.

Nursing Interventions/*Rationales*

- Palpate the bladder superior to the symphysis on a frequent basis (at least every 2 hours) *to detect a full bladder that occurs from increased fluid intake and inability to feel urge to void.*
- Encourage frequent voiding (at least every 2 hours) and catheterize if necessary *to avoid bladder distention, because it impedes progress of fetus down birth canal and may result in trauma to the bladder.*
- Assist woman to bathroom or commode to void, if appropriate; provide privacy, and use techniques to stimulate voiding such as running water *to facilitate bladder emptying with an upright position (natural) and relaxation.*

NURSING DIAGNOSIS

Risk for ineffective individual coping related to birthing process

Expected Outcome

Woman actively participates in the birth process with no evidence of injury to her or her fetus.

Nursing Interventions/*Rationales*

- Constantly monitor events of labor and birth, including physiologic responses of woman and fetus and emotional responses of woman and partner *to ensure maternal, partner, and fetal well-being.*
- Provide ongoing feedback to woman and partner *to decrease anxiety and enhance participation.*
- Continue to provide comfort measures and minimize distractions *to decrease discomfort and aid in focus on the birth process.*
- Encourage woman to experiment with various positions *to assist downward movement of the fetus.*
- Ensure that woman takes deep cleansing breaths before and after each contraction *to enhance gas exchange and oxygen transport to the fetus.*
- Encourage woman to push spontaneously when urge to bear down is perceived during a contraction *to aid the descent and rotation of the fetus.*
- Encourage woman to exhale, holding breath for short periods while bearing down *to avoid holding breath and triggering the Valsalva maneuver, thereby increasing intrathoracic and cardiovascular pressure and decreasing perfusion of placental oxygen, placing the fetus at risk.*
- Have woman take deep breaths and relax between contractions *to reduce fatigue and increase effectiveness of pushing efforts.*
- Have mother pant as fetal head crowns *to control birth of head and reduce risk for perineal trauma or fetal head injury.*
- Explain to woman and labor partner what is expected in the third stage of labor *to enlist cooperation.*
- Have woman maintain her position *to facilitate delivery of the placenta.*

NURSING DIAGNOSIS

Fatigue related to energy expenditure required during labor and birth

Expected Outcome

Woman's energy levels are restored.

Nursing Interventions/*Rationales*

- Educate woman and partner about need for rest and help them plan strategies (e.g., restricting visitors, increasing role of support systems performing functions associated with daily routines) that allow specific times for rest and sleep *to ensure that woman can restore depleted energy levels in preparation for caring for a new infant.*
- Monitor woman's fatigue level and the amount of rest received *to ensure restoration of energy.*
- Group care activities as much as possible *to allow for periods of uninterrupted rest.*

TABLE 19-2 PHYSICAL NURSING CARE DURING LABOR

NEED	NURSING ACTIONS	RATIONALE
	GENERAL HYGIENE	
Showers or bed baths, Jacuzzi bath	Assess for progress in labor	Determines appropriateness of the activity
	Supervise showers closely if woman is in true labor	Prevents injury from fall; labor may be accelerated
	Suggest allowing warm water to flow over back	Aids relaxation; increases comfort
Perineum	Cleanse frequently, especially after rupture of membranes and when show increases	Enhances comfort and reduces risk of infection
Oral hygiene	Offer toothbrush or mouthwash, or wash the teeth with an ice-cold wet washcloth as needed	Refreshes mouth; helps counteract dry, thirsty feeling
Hair	Brush, braid per woman's wishes	Improves morale; increases comfort
Handwashing	Offer washcloths or cleansing foam before and after voiding and as needed	Maintains cleanliness; prevents infection
Face	Offer cool washcloth	Provides relief from diaphoresis; cools and refreshes
Gowns and linens	Change as needed	Improves comfort; enhances relaxation
	NUTRIENT AND FLUID INTAKE	
Oral	Offer fluids and solid foods as ordered by primary health care provider and desired by laboring woman	Provides hydration and calories; enhances positive emotional experience and maternal control
Intravenous (IV)	Establish and maintain IV line as ordered	Maintains hydration; provides venous access for medications
	ELIMINATION	
Voiding	Encourage voiding at least every 2 hours	A full bladder may impede descent of presenting part; overdistention may cause bladder atony and injury, as well as postpartum voiding difficulty
Ambulatory woman	Allow ambulation to bathroom according to orders of primary health care provider, if:	
	The presenting part is engaged	Reinforces normal process of urination
	The membranes are not ruptured	Precautionary measure to protect against prolapse of umbilical cord
	The woman is not medicated	Precautionary measure to protect against injury
Woman on bed rest	Offer bedpan	Prevents complications of bladder distention and ambulation
	Encourage upright position on bedpan, allow tap water to run; place woman's hands in warm water; pour warm water over the vulva; give positive suggestion	Encourages voiding
	Provide privacy	Shows respect for woman
	Put up side rails on bed	Prevents injury from fall
	Place call bell and telephone within reach	Reinforces safe care
	Offer washcloth or cleansing foam for hands	Maintains cleanliness; prevents infection
	Wash vulvar area	Maintains cleanliness; enhances comfort; prevents infection
Catheterization	Catheterize according to orders of primary health care provider or hospital protocol if measures to facilitate voiding are ineffective	Prevents complications of bladder distention
	Insert catheter between contractions	Minimizes discomfort
	Avoid force if obstacle to insertion is noted	"Obstacle" may be caused by compression of urethra by presenting part
Bowel elimination—sensation of rectal pressure	Perform vaginal examination	Prevents misinterpretation of rectal pressure from the presenting part as the need to defecate Determines degree of descent of presenting part
	Help the woman ambulate to bathroom, or offer bedpan if rectal pressure is not from presenting part	Reinforces normal process of bowel elimination and safe care
	Cleanse perineum immediately after passage of stool	Reduces risk of infection and sense of embarrassment

measures. Change the linen if it becomes wet or stained with blood, and use linen savers (Chux), changing them as needed.

Nutrient and Fluid Intake

Oral Intake. Prior to the 1940s women were allowed to eat and drink during labor to maintain the energy required to sustain labor and the stamina required to give birth. This practice changed, allowing the laboring woman only clear liquids or ice chips or nothing by mouth during the active phase of labor when concern arose regarding the risk of anesthesia complications and their secondary effects if general anesthesia were required in an emergency. These secondary effects include the aspiration of gastric contents and resultant compromise in oxygen perfusion, which could endanger the lives of the mother and fetus (Simpson, 2008). There have been no randomized trials evaluating the ingestion of solid foods in labor, so current management is based mostly on expert opinions. Ice chips and sips of clear liquids are still the only oral intake recommended during labor in the United States by the American Society of Anesthesiologists Task Force on Obstetrical Anesthesia (Berghella et al., 2008). This practice is being challenged by some health care providers, however, because regional anesthesia is used more often than general anesthesia, even for emergency cesarean births. Women are awake during regional anesthesia and are able to participate in their own care and protect their airway.

An adequate intake of fluids and calories is required to meet the energy demands and fluid losses associated with childbirth. The progress of labor slows, with a more rapid development of hypoglycemia and ketosis if these demands are not met and fat is metabolized. Reduced energy for bearing-down efforts (pushing) increases the risk for a forceps- or vacuum-assisted birth. This is most likely to occur in women who begin to labor early in the morning after a night without caloric intake. When women are permitted to consume fluids and food freely, they typically regulate their own oral intake, eating light foods (e.g., eggs, yogurt, ice cream, dry toast and jelly, fruit) and drinking fluids during early labor and tapering off to the intake of clear fluids and sips of water or ice chips as labor intensifies and the second stage approaches (Parsons, Bidwell, & Nagy, 2006).

Common practice is to allow clear liquids (e.g., water, tea, fruit juices without pulp, clear sodas, coffee, sports drinks, fruit ice, Popsicles, gelatin, broth) during early labor, tapering off to ice chips and sips of water as labor progresses and becomes more active. Herbal teas can provide not only hydration but also other beneficial effects. Chamomile tea can enhance relaxation, lemon balm or peppermint tea can reduce nausea, and teas of ginger or ginseng root are energizing (Walls, 2009). A woman's culture may influence what she will eat and drink during labor. In addition, women who use nonpharmacologic pain relief measures and labor at home or in birthing centers are more likely to eat and drink during labor. The amount of solid and liquid carbohydrates to offer a woman in labor is still unclear. Though it is known that energy needs increase as labor becomes prolonged, there is limited evidence regarding the effect of oral carbohydrate intake in enhancing the progress of labor and reducing the risk for dystocia (Tranmer, Hodnett, Hannah, & Stevens, 2005).

Withholding food and fluids in labor is unlikely to be beneficial, and offering oral fluids is demonstrably useful and should be encouraged (Hofmeyr, 2005). Nurses should follow the orders of the woman's primary health care provider when offering the woman food or fluids during labor. As advocates, however, nurses can facilitate change by informing others of the current research findings that support the safety and effectiveness of the oral intake of food and fluid during labor and by initiating such research themselves.

Intravenous Intake. Fluids are administered intravenously to the laboring woman to maintain hydration, especially when a labor is long and the woman is unable to ingest a sufficient amount of fluid orally or if she is receiving epidural or intrathecal anesthesia. In most cases an electrolyte solution without glucose (e.g., Ringer's lactate or normal saline) is adequate and does not introduce excess glucose into the bloodstream. The latter is important because an excessive maternal glucose level results in fetal hyperglycemia and fetal hyperinsulinism. After birth the neonate's high level of insulin will reduce his or her glucose stores, and hypoglycemia will result. Infusions containing glucose can also reduce sodium levels in the woman and the fetus, leading to transient neonatal tachypnea. If maternal ketosis occurs, the primary health care provider may order an IV solution containing a small amount of dextrose to provide the glucose needed to assist in fatty acid metabolism.

! NURSING ALERT

Nurses should carefully monitor the intake and output of laboring women receiving IV fluids because they face an increased danger of hypervolemia as a result of the fluid retention that occurs during pregnancy.

Elimination

Voiding. Encourage voiding every 2 hours. A distended bladder may impede descent of the presenting part, slow or stop uterine contractions, and lead to decreased bladder tone or uterine atony after birth. Women who receive epidural analgesia or anesthesia are especially at risk for the retention of urine. Therefore, the need to void should be assessed more frequently with them.

Assist the woman to the bathroom to void or use a bedside commode, unless any of the following apply: the primary health care provider has ordered bed rest; the woman is receiving epidural analgesia or anesthesia; internal monitoring is being used; or ambulation will compromise the status of the laboring woman or her fetus. External monitoring can usually be interrupted long enough for the woman to go to the bathroom.

If using a bedpan is necessary, encourage spontaneous voiding by providing privacy and having the woman sit upright (as she would on a toilet). Other interventions to encourage urination, either in the bathroom or on the bedpan, are having the woman listen to the sound of water slowly running from a faucet, placing her hands in warm water, having her blow bubbles into a glass of water using a straw, or pouring warm water over the vulva and perineum using a peri bottle.

Catheterization. If the woman is unable to void and her bladder is distended, she may need to be catheterized. Many hospitals have protocols that rely on the nurse's judgment concerning the need for catheterization. Before performing the catheterization, clean the vulva and perineum because vaginal show and amniotic fluid may be present. If an obstacle that prevents advancement of the catheter is present, this obstacle is most likely the presenting part. If you cannot advance the catheter, stop the procedure and notify the primary health care provider of the difficulty.

Bowel Elimination. Most women do not have bowel movements during labor because of decreased intestinal motility. Stool that has formed in the large intestine often moves downward toward the anorectal area as a result of pressure exerted by the fetal presenting part as it descends. This stool is often expelled during second-stage pushing and birth. However, the passage of stool with bearing-down efforts increases the risk of infection and may embarrass the woman, thereby reducing the effectiveness of her pushing efforts. To prevent these problems, the nurse should immediately cleanse the perineal area to remove any stool, while reassuring the woman that the passage of stool at this time is a normal and expected event, because the same muscles used to expel the baby also expel stool.

Routine use of enemas on admission for women at term has shown only modest benefits. There is a trend toward lower infection rates and the newborns have fewer lower respiratory tract infections and less need for antibiotics. However, because enemas cause discomfort for women and increase the costs of giving birth, the small benefits do not outweigh the disadvantages of this practice (Berghella et al., 2008). In addition, a recent Cochrane review of this topic found that the evidence does not support the routine use of enemas during labor (Reveiz, Gaitan, & Cuervo, 2007).

When the presenting part is deep in the pelvis, even in the absence of stool in the anorectal area, the woman may feel rectal pressure and think she needs to defecate. If the woman expresses the urge to defecate, the nurse should perform a vaginal examination to assess cervical dilation and station. When a multiparous woman experiences the urge to defecate, this often means birth will follow quickly.

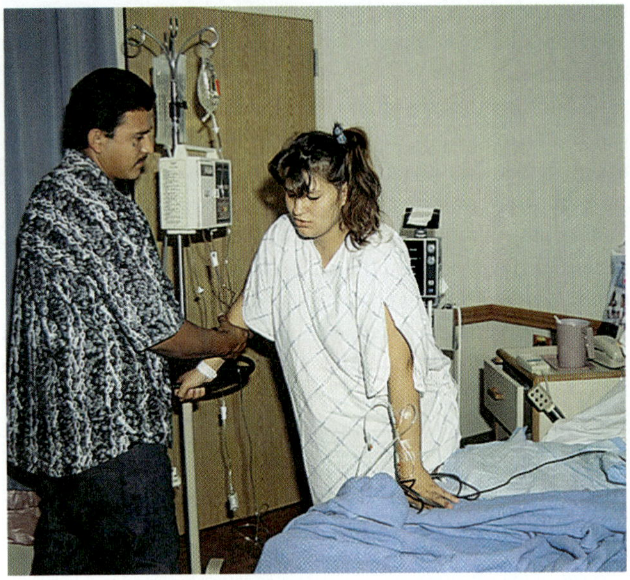

FIG. 19-10 Woman preparing to walk with partner. (Courtesy Marjorie Pyle, RNC, Lifecircle, Costa Mesa, CA.)

Ambulation and Positioning

Confinement to bed is the norm for labor management in the United States. The increased use of epidurals during childbirth accompanied by multiple medical interventions (e.g., monitors, intravenous infusions) and reduced motor control contribute to this practice, thereby interfering with a woman's freedom of movement. Upright positions and mobility during labor, however, may be more pleasant for laboring women. These practices have also been associated with improved uterine contraction intensity and shorter labors, less need for pain medications, reduced rate of operative birth (e.g., cesarean birth, forceps- and vacuum-assisted birth), increased maternal autonomy and control, distraction from labor's discomforts, and an opportunity for close interaction with the woman's partner and care provider as they assist her to assume upright positions and remain mobile. No harmful effects have been observed from maternal activity and position changes (Albers, 2007; Simpson, 2008; Zwelling, 2010).

Encourage ambulation if membranes are intact, if the fetal presenting part is engaged after ROM, and if the woman has not received medication for pain (Fig. 19-10). The woman also may find it comfortable to stand and lean forward on her partner, doula, or nurse for support at times during labor (Fig. 19-11, *A*). Ambulation may be contraindicated, however, because of maternal or fetal status.

When the woman lies in bed, she will usually change her position spontaneously as labor progresses. If she does not change position every 30 to 60 minutes, assist her to do so. The side-lying (lateral) position is preferred because it promotes optimal uteroplacental and renal blood flow and increases fetal oxygen saturation (Fig. 19-12, *B*). If the woman wants to lie supine, the nurse should place a pillow under one hip as a wedge to prevent the uterus from compressing the

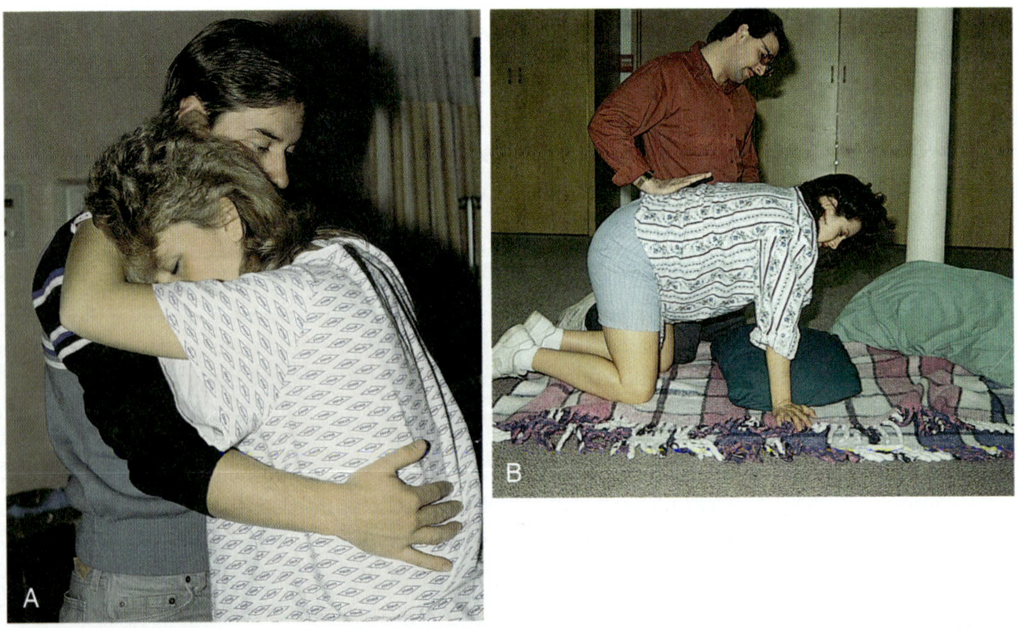

FIG. 19-11 **A,** Woman standing and leaning forward with support. **B,** Woman in hands-and-knees position. (Courtesy Marjorie Pyle, RNC, Lifecircle, Costa Mesa, CA.)

Critical Thinking Exercises—Positioning During Labor

aorta and vena cava (see Fig. 19-5). Sitting is not contraindicated unless it adversely affects fetal status, which you can determine by checking the FHR and pattern. If the fetus is in the occiput posterior position, it may be helpful to encourage the woman to squat during contractions because this position increases the pelvic diameter, allowing the head to rotate to a more anterior position (see Fig. 19-12, *A*). A hands-and-knees position during contractions or a lateral position on the same side as the fetal spine also are recommended to facilitate the rotation of the fetal occiput from a posterior to an anterior position, as gravity pulls the fetal back forward. These positions also provide access to the back for application of counterpressure by the partner, doula, or nurse (Hanson, 2009; Simpson, Cesario, Morin, Trapani, Mayberry, & Snelgrove-Clark, 2008; Zwelling, 2010) (see Fig. 19-11, *B*). Women with epidural anesthesia may not be able to squat or assume a hands-and-knees position depending on the degree of motor involvement resulting from the epidural.

Much research continues to focus on acquiring a better understanding of the physiologic and psychologic effects of maternal position in labor. Box 19-5 describes a variety of positions that are commonly used and recommended.

The woman can use a birth ball (gymnastic ball, physical therapy ball) to support her body as she assumes a variety of labor and birth positions (Fig. 19-13). She can sit on the ball while leaning over the bed, or lean over the ball to support her upper body and reduce stress on her arms and hands when she assumes a hands-and-knees position. The birth ball can encourage pelvic mobility and pelvic and perineal relaxation when the woman sits on the firm yet pliable ball and rocks in rhythmic movements. Warm compresses applied to the perineum and lower back can maximize this relaxation and comfort effect. The birth ball should be large enough so that when the woman sits, her knees are bent at a 90-degree angle and her feet are flat on the floor and approximately 2 feet apart.

SAFETY ALERT

A woman may experience dizziness as she changes upright positions during labor. It is essential that the nurse or support person be present to provide assistance should dizziness occur.

Supportive Care During Labor and Birth

Support during labor and birth involves emotional support, physical care and comfort measures, and advice and information. The value of the continuous supportive presence of a person (e.g., doula, childbirth educator, family member, friend, nurse, partner) during labor has long been known. Women who have continuous support beginning in early labor are less likely to use pain medication or epidurals, more likely to have a spontaneous vaginal birth, and less likely to report dissatisfaction with their birth experience. No harmful effects from continuous labor support have been identified. To the contrary, there is good evidence that labor support improves important health outcomes (Albers, 2007; Berghella et al., 2008; Hodnett, Gates, Hofmeyer, & Sakala, 2007).

Labor rooms should be airy, clean, and homelike. The laboring woman should feel safe in this environment and free to be herself and to use the comfort and relaxation measures she prefers. To enhance relaxation, turn off bright overhead lights when not needed, and keep noise and intrusions to a

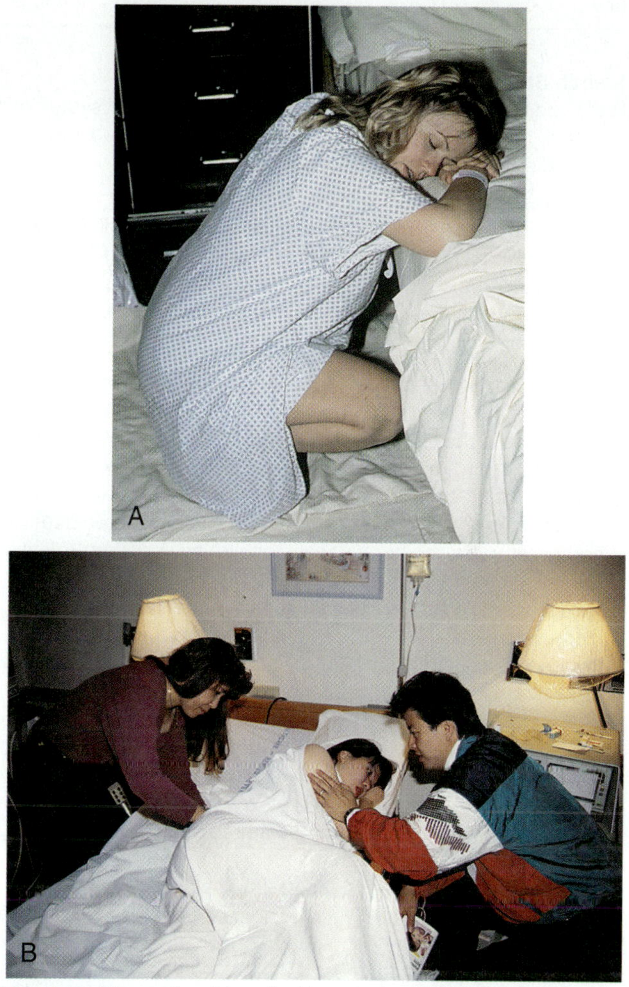

FIG. 19-12 Maternal positions for labor. **A,** Squatting. **B,** Lateral position. Support person is applying sacral pressure while partner provides encouragement. (Courtesy Marjorie Pyle, RNC, Lifecircle, Costa Mesa, CA.)

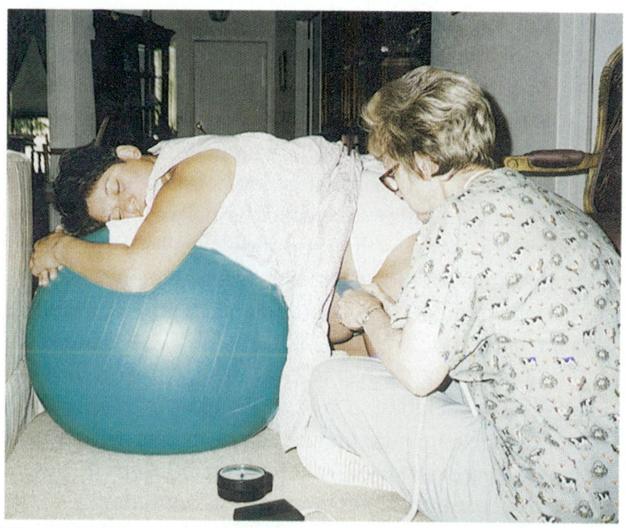

FIG. 19-13 Woman laboring using birth ball. (Courtesy Polly Perez, Cutting Edge Press, Johnson, VT.)

Video—Nursing Skills: Positioning and Assisting with Comfort Measures in Labor

EVIDENCE-BASED PRACTICE

Pat Gingrich

Benefits of Continuous Labor Support

ASK THE QUESTION

How does continuous labor support benefit laboring women? Who should provide this support? Is this type of support a nursing role?

SEARCH FOR EVIDENCE

Search Strategies

Professional organization guidelines, meta-analyses, systematic reviews, randomized controlled trials, nonrandomized prospective studies and retrospective reviews since 2008.

Databases Searched

CINAHL, Cochrane, Medline, PUBMED, National Guideline Clearinghouse, and the websites for the Association of Women's Health, Obstetric and Neonatal Nurses (AWHONN) and the Society of Obstetricians and Gynaecologists of Canada (SOGC).

CRITICALLY ANALYZE THE EVIDENCE

For millennia, women have labored in the company of other women, usually family or friends who have experienced birth themselves. In the last century, Western women in labor became more isolated in institutional, high-technology settings. Loss of dedicated labor support coincided with increasing technology, pain management, and operative birth. Observers now question whether returning the human touch of birthing assistants, such as doulas, could improve outcomes.

In a randomized controlled trial of 420 women, continuous labor support was associated with decreased cesarean and instrumental birth, decreased need for pain medication or regional analgesia, and 100% positive feelings about birth (McGrath & Kennell, 2008).

A Cochrane Database Systematic Review examined an active labor management protocol that included continuous labor support, as well as artificial rupture of membranes and strict management of slow labor progress by use of oxytocin. In 7 trials involving 5390 women, the protocol group had fewer cesarean births and shorter labors than the group with usual care. The two groups showed no difference in assisted births or complications (Brown, Paranjothy, Dowswell, & Thomas, 2008). While the protocol appeared safe, the contribution of continuous labor support to the results was not addressed.

In a joint policy statement, five Canadian medical professional groups with an interest in birth recommended continuous labor support be used in all birth settings, as a way of decreasing the risks resulting from interventions such as cesarean birth and operative (assisted) birth (SOGC, AWHONN Canada, Canadian Association of Midwives, the College of Family Physicians of Canada, & the Society of Rural Physicians of Canada, 2008).

In addition to shorter second stage labors and fewer assisted births, a prospective study of 141 low-income women found that doula care also significantly increased the initiation of breastfeeding and the number of women still breastfeeding at 6 weeks postpartum (Nommsen-Rivers, Mastergeorge, Hansen, Cullum, & Dewey, 2009). The potential for benefit is great, as low-income mothers are usually less likely to breastfeed, and the benefits of breastfeeding may decrease the prevalence of obesity in low-income populations.

IMPLICATIONS FOR PRACTICE

Nurses and nurse midwives provide attentive care for laboring women, but their workload usually precludes their continuous presence at the bedside. Partners might be well intentioned but may find the powerful reality of birth to be overwhelming. An experienced doula or birth attendant can keep the laboring woman calm and comfortable, which not only improves the experience emotionally, but also reduces pain, stress hormones, and muscular tension, thereby facilitating vaginal birth. Doulas are not there to replace the nurse or the partner but rather to provide support as needs arise. In addition, the rapport the doulas build may provide a "teachable moment" to encourage breastfeeding with all its documented benefits, especially in low-income populations where breastfeeding is less common. Insurance companies and institutions that see the measurable benefits of doulas are wise to value and encourage their contribution.

References

Brown, H., Paranjothy, S., Dowswell, T., & Thomas, J. (2008). Package of care for active management in labour for reducing caesarean section rates in low-income women. *The Cochrane Database of Systematic Reviews, 2008*, 4, CD004907.

McGrath, S., & Kennell, J. (2008). A randomized controlled trial of continuous labor support: Effect on cesarean delivery rates. *Birth, 35*(2), 92–97.

Nommsen-Rivers, L., Mastergeorge, A., Hansen, R., Cullum, A., & Dewey, K. (2009). Doula care, early breastfeeding, and breastfeeding status at 6 weeks postpartum among low-income primiparae. *Journal of Obstetric, Gynecologic and Neonatal Nursing, 38*(2), 157–173.

Society of Obstetricians and Gynaecologists of Canada, the Association of Women's Health, Obstetric and Neonatal Nurses of Canada, the Canadian Association of Midwives, the College of Family Physicians of Canada, & the Society of Rural Physicians of Canada. (2008). Joint policy statement on normal childbirth. *Journal of Obstetrics and Gynaecology of Canada, 30*(12), 1163–1165.

Spanish Guidelines—Care During Labor

minimum. Control the temperature to ensure the laboring woman's comfort. The room should be large enough to accommodate a comfortable chair for the woman's partner, the monitoring equipment, and hospital personnel. Encourage women to bring their own pillows to make the hospital surroundings more homelike and to facilitate position changes. Environmental modifications should reflect the preferences of the woman, including the number of visitors and availability of a telephone, television, and music.

Labor Support by the Nurse. Supportive nursing care for a woman in labor includes:

- Helping the woman maintain control and participate to the extent she wishes in the birth of her infant
- Providing continuity of care that is nonjudgmental and respectful of her cultural and religious values and beliefs
- Meeting the woman's expected outcomes for her labor
- Listening to the woman's concerns and encouraging her to express her feelings
- Acting as the woman's advocate, supporting her decisions and respecting her choices as appropriate, and relating her wishes as needed to other health care providers
- Helping the woman conserve her energy and cope effectively with her pain and discomfort by using a variety of comfort measures that are acceptable to her
- Helping control the woman's discomfort
- Acknowledging the woman's efforts during labor including her strength and courage, as well as those of her partner, and providing positive reinforcement
- Protecting the woman's privacy, modesty, and dignity

Women who have attended childbirth education programs that teach the psychoprophylactic (Lamaze) approach will know something about the labor process, coaching techniques, and comfort measures. The nurse plays a supportive role and keeps the woman and her partner informed of the labor progress. If necessary, review the methods learned in class and practiced at home because it may be difficult for the woman to effectively use these methods and techniques now that she is in labor and in an unfamiliar setting.

Even when a laboring woman has not attended childbirth classes, the nurse can teach her simple breathing and relaxation techniques during the early phase of labor. In this case the nurse provides more of the coaching and supportive care until the support person feels ready to take on a more active coaching role (see Chapter 17). The nurse can demonstrate comfort

CLINICAL REASONING

Encouraging Evidence-Based Birth Practices

After attending a professional seminar for perinatal nurses, a nurse becomes concerned that the care approaches used on her labor and birth unit do not support the concept of normal birth but instead reflect a more traditional "we have always done it this way and it works" approach. Many of the women receive oxytocin [Pitocin] some time during labor. It is rare for a woman to have doula support because most feel that an epidural, as early as possible, is just fine. The cesarean birth rate on this unit reflects the national norm of approximately 30%. Although the unit has spacious birthing rooms with Jacuzzis, laboring women spend most of their labor in bed as a result of the use of blood pressure and electronic fetal monitoring, and intravenous infusions to support the implementation of epidural anesthesia. The nurse approaches her unit manager to discuss what she learned at the seminar regarding evidence-based practices that promote, protect, and support normal birth. The manager expresses great interest, and asks the nurse to present an in-service program for the medical and nursing staff regarding this issue as a first step in trying to implement a more evidence-based care approach. What should this nurse include in her in-service program to convince the medical and nursing staff that there is evidence to support more natural approaches to birth that are safer and more effective for women and their newborns?

1. Evidence—Is there sufficient evidence to support the safety and effectiveness of normal birth?
2. Assumptions—What assumptions can be made about the following issues related to normal birth?
   a. Benefits of an approach that promotes, protects, and supports normal birth
   b. Management approaches that should be emphasized during the labor
   c. Why it is essential to include and gain the support of both the medical and nursing staff to effect the change in care focus on this unit
3. What are the nursing priorities for teaching pregnant women about labor preparation if a more evidence-based approach to care is adapted by the unit?
4. Does the evidence objectively support your conclusion?
5. Are there alternative perspectives to your conclusion?

BOX 19-5 COMMON MATERNAL POSITIONS* DURING LABOR AND BIRTH

SEMIRECUMBENT POSITION (See Figs. 19-15, *B*; Fig. 19-16, *B*)

With woman sitting with her upper body elevated to at least a 30-degree angle, place wedge or small pillow under hip to prevent vena cava compression and reduce likelihood of supine hypotension (see Fig. 19-5).

- The greater the angle of elevation, the more gravity or pressure is exerted that promotes fetal descent, the progress of contractions, and the widening of pelvic dimensions.
- Position is convenient for rendering care measures and for external fetal monitoring.

LATERAL POSITION (See Figs. 19-12, *B*, and 19-15, *A*)

Have woman alternate between left and right side-lying position, and provide abdominal and back support as needed for comfort.

- Removes pressure from the vena cava and back, enhances uteroplacental perfusion, and relieves backache.
- Facilitates internal rotation of fetus in a posterior position to an anterior position (woman should lie on same side as fetal spine).
- Makes it easier to perform back massage or counterpressure.
- Associated with less frequent, but more intense, contractions.
- Obtaining good external fetal monitor tracings may be more difficult.
- May be used as a birthing position.
- Takes pressure off perineum, allowing it to stretch gradually.
- Reduces risk for perineal trauma.

UPRIGHT POSITION

The gravity effect enhances the contraction cycle and fetal descent: the weight of the fetus places increasing pressure on the cervix; the cervix is pulled upward, facilitating effacement and dilation; impulses from the cervix to the pituitary gland increase, causing more oxytocin to be secreted; and contractions are intensified, thereby applying more forceful downward pressure on the fetus, but they are less painful.

- Fetus is aligned with pelvis, and pelvic diameters are widened slightly.
- Effective upright positions include:
  - Ambulation (see Fig. 19-10)
  - Standing and leaning forward with support provided by coach (see Fig. 19-11, *A*), end of bed, back of chair, or birth ball; relieves backache and facilitates application of counterpressure or back massage
  - Sitting up in bed, chair, birthing chair, on toilet, or bedside commode (see Fig. 19-15, *B*)
  - Squatting (see Fig. 19-12, *A*, and Fig. 19-16, *E*)

HANDS-AND-KNEES POSITION—POSITION FOR POSTERIOR POSITIONS OF THE PRESENTING PART (See Figs. 19-11, *B*; Fig. 19-13)

Assume an "all fours" position or lean over an object (e.g., birth ball) while on knees in bed or on a covered floor; allows for pelvic rocking.

- Relieves backache characteristic of "back labor."
- Facilitates internal rotation of the fetus by increasing mobility of the coccyx, increasing the pelvic diameters, and using gravity to turn the fetal back and rotate the head (NOTE: A side-lying position, double hip squeeze, or knee squeeze can also facilitate internal rotation.)

*Assess the effect of each position on the laboring woman's comfort and anxiety level, progress of labor, and fetal heart rate and pattern. Alternate positions every 30 to 60 minutes, allowing the woman to take control of her position changes.

measures while encouraging the support person to assist and the laboring woman to express her needs and feelings. Observing the comforting approaches of the nurse can help the partner to learn effective comfort measures.

Comfort measures vary with the situation (Fig. 19-14). The nurse can draw on the woman's list of comfort measures and relaxation techniques learned during the pregnancy and through life experiences. Such measures include maintaining a comfortable, calm, supportive atmosphere in the labor and birth area; using touch therapeutically (e.g., heat or cold applied to the lower back in the event of back labor, a cool cloth applied to the forehead, massage); providing nonpharmacologic measures to relieve discomfort (e.g., hydrotherapy); and most important, just being there (MacKinnon, McIntyre, & Quance, 2005) (see Tables 19-1 and 19-2). See Chapter 17 for a full discussion of pharmacologic and nonpharmacologic comfort measures.

Most women in labor respond positively to touch, but you should obtain permission before using any touching measures. Women appreciate gentle handling by staff members. Back rubs and counterpressure may be offered, especially if the woman is experiencing back labor. Teach the support person to exert counterpressure against the woman's sacrum over the occiput of the head of a fetus in a posterior position (see Fig. 19-12, *B*). Double hip or knee squeezes can also be helpful in reducing back pain. The back pain is caused by the occiput pressing on spinal nerves, and counterpressure lifts the occiput off these nerves, providing some relief from pain. The partner will need to be relieved after a while, however, because exerting counterpressure is hard work. Hand and foot massage also can be soothing and relaxing.

The woman's perception of the soothing qualities of touch may change as labor progresses. Many women become more sensitive to touch (hyperesthesia) as labor progresses. This is a typical response during the transition phase (see Table 19-1). They may tell their coach to leave them alone or not to touch them. The partner who is unprepared for this normal response may feel rejected and may react by withdrawing active support. The nurse can reassure him or her that this response is a positive indication that the first stage is ending and the second stage is approaching. Women with increased sensitivity to touch may tolerate it better on surfaces of the body where hair does not grow, such as the forehead, the palms of the hands, and the soles of the feet.

Labor Support by the Father or Partner. Although another woman or a man other than the father may be the woman's partner, the father of the baby is usually the support person during labor. He is often able to provide the comfort measures and touch that the laboring woman needs. When the woman becomes focused on her pain, sometimes the partner can persuade her to try nonpharmacologic variations of comfort measures. In addition, he usually is able to interpret the woman's needs and desires for staff members.

The feelings of a first-time father change as labor progresses. Although he is often calm at the onset of labor, feelings of fear and helplessness begin to dominate as labor becomes more active and the father realizes that labor is more work than he anticipated. Capogna, Camorcia, and Stirparo (2007) found that fathers whose partners received epidural analgesia during labor reported less anxiety and stress and more satisfaction with their childbirth experience than fathers whose partners did not.

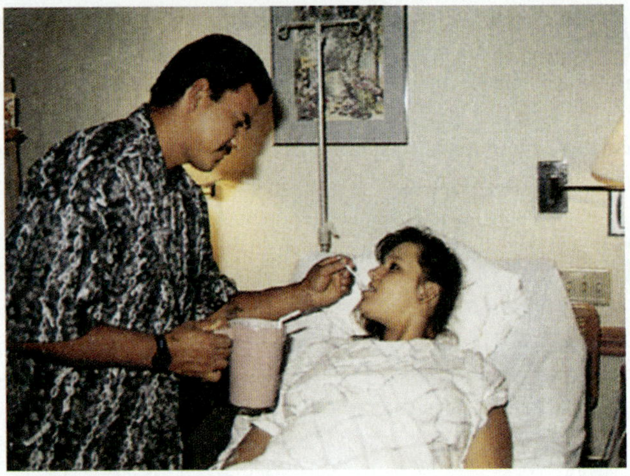

FIG. 19-14 Partner providing comfort measures. (Courtesy Marjorie Pyle, RNC, Lifecircle, Costa Mesa, CA.)

Staff members should tell the father that his presence is helpful and encourage him to be involved in the care of the woman to the extent to which he and his partner are comfortable. He should be reassured that he is not assuming the responsibility for observation and management of his partner's labor, but that his responsibility is to support her as the labor progresses. The nurse can suggest alternative comfort measures when those he is using are no longer helpful or are rejected by his partner.

The first-time father may feel excluded as birth preparations begin during the transition phase. Once the second stage begins and birth nears, the father's focus changes from the woman to the baby who is about to be born. The father will be exposed to many sights and smells he may never have experienced. Therefore, the nurse needs to tell him what to expect and to make him comfortable about leaving the room to regain his composure should something occur that surprises him, but make sure that someone else is available to support the woman during his absence.

Nursing actions that support the father convey several important concepts: first, that he is a person of value; second, that he can be a partner in the woman's care; and third, that childbearing is a team effort. Box 19-6 details ways in which the nurse can support the father-partner. A well-informed father can make an important contribution to the health and well-being of the mother and child, their family interrelationship, and his self-esteem.

Labor Support by Doulas. Continuity of care has been cited by women as a critical component of a satisfying childbirth experience. A specially trained, experienced female labor attendant called a **doula** can meet this need. The doula provides a continual one-on-one caring presence throughout the labor and birth of the woman she is attending (Pascali-Bonaro & Kroeger, 2004). The primary role of the doula is to focus on the laboring woman and to provide physical and emotional support by using soft, reassuring words of praise and encouragement; touching; stroking; and hugging. The doula also administers comfort measures to reduce pain and enhance relaxation and coping, walks with the woman, helps her to change positions, and coaches her bearing-down efforts. Doulas provide information about labor progress and explain procedures and events. They advocate for the woman's right to participate actively in the management of her labor.

BOX 19-6 GUIDELINES FOR SUPPORTING THE FATHER*

- Orient him to the labor room and the unit; explain location of the cafeteria, toilet, waiting room, and nursery; give information about visiting hours; introduce personnel present by name and describe their functions.
- Inform him of sights and smells he can expect to encounter; encourage him to leave the room if necessary.
- Respect his or the couple's decision about the degree of his involvement. Offer them freedom to make decisions.
- Tell him when his presence has been helpful, and continue to reinforce this throughout labor.
- Offer to teach him comfort measures; demonstrate or role model performance of these measures.
- Inform him frequently of the progress of the labor and the woman's needs. Keep him informed about procedures to be performed.
- Prepare him for changes in the woman's behavior and physical appearance.
- Remind him to eat; offer him snacks and fluids if possible.
- Relieve him of the job of support person as necessary. Offer him blankets if he is to sleep in a chair by the bedside.
- Acknowledge the stress experienced by each partner during labor and birth, and identify normal responses.
- Attempt to modify or eliminate unsettling stimuli, such as extra noise and extra light; create a relaxing and calm environment.

*These guidelines are appropriate for any support person or partner.

The doula also supports the woman's partner, who often feels unqualified to be the sole labor support and may find it difficult to watch the woman when she is experiencing pain. The doula can encourage and praise the partner's efforts, create a partnership as caregivers, and provide respite care. Doulas also facilitate communication between the laboring woman and her partner, as well as between the couple and the health care team (Simkin & Way, 2008).

Doula support during labor is associated with decreased use of analgesia, decreased incidence of operative birth, increased incidence of spontaneous vaginal birth, and increased maternal satisfaction with the childbirth experience (Berghella et al., 2008).

The roles of the nurse and the doula are complementary. They should work together as a team, recognizing and respecting the role each plays in supporting and caring for the woman and her partner during the childbirth process. The doula provides supportive nonmedical care measures while the nurse focuses on monitoring the status of the maternal-fetal unit, implementing clinical care protocols (including pharmacologic interventions), and documenting assessment findings, actions, and responses (Adams & Bianchi, 2004; Simkin & Way, 2008).

Labor Support by Grandparents. When grandparents act as labor coaches, it is especially important to support and treat them with respect. They may have a way to deal with pain relief based on their experience. Grandparents should be encouraged to help as long as their actions do not compromise the status of the mother or the fetus. The nurse treats grandparents with dignity and respect by acknowledging the value of their contributions to parental support, and by recognizing the difficulty parents have in witnessing the woman's discomfort or crisis. If they have never witnessed a birth, the nurse may need to provide explanations of what is happening. Many of the activities used to support fathers also are appropriate for grandparents.

Siblings During Labor and Birth

Preparing siblings for acceptance of the new child helps promote the attachment process and may help the older children accept this change. The older child or children who know themselves to be important to the family become active participants. Rehearsal for the event before labor is essential.

The age and developmental level of children influence their responses; therefore, preparation for the children to be present during labor is adjusted to meet each child's needs. The child younger than 2 years shows little interest in pregnancy and labor. However, for the older child, such preparation may reduce fears and misconceptions. Parents need to be prepared for labor and birth themselves and feel comfortable about the process and the presence of their children. Most parents have a "feel" for their children's maturational level and their physical and emotional ability to observe and cope with the events of the labor and birth process. Preparation can include a description of the anticipated sights, events (e.g., ROM, monitors, IV infusions), smells, and sounds; a labor and birth demonstration; a tour of the birthing unit; and an opportunity to be around a real newborn. Storybooks about the birth process can be read to or by children to prepare them for the event. Films are available for preparing preschool and school-age children to participate in the labor and birth experience. Children must learn that their mother will be working hard during labor and birth. She will not be able to talk to them during contractions. She may groan, scream, grunt, and pant at times as well as say things she would not say otherwise (e.g., "I can't take this anymore," "Take this baby out of me," or "This pain is killing me"). You can tell them that labor is uncomfortable, but that their mother's body is made for the job.

Most agencies require that a specific person be designated to watch over the children who are participating in their mother's childbirth experience, to provide them with support, explanations, diversions, and comfort as needed. Health care providers involved in attending women during birth must be comfortable with the presence of children and the unpredictability of their questions, comments, and behaviors.

Emergency Interventions

Emergency conditions that require immediate nursing intervention can arise with startling speed. The Emergency box outlines the care management required for an abnormal FHR, inadequate uterine relaxation, vaginal bleeding, infection, and prolapse of the cord.

SECOND STAGE OF LABOR

The **second stage of labor** is the stage in which the infant is born. This stage begins with full cervical dilation (10 cm) and complete effacement (100%) and ends with the baby's birth. The force exerted by uterine contractions, gravity, and maternal bearing-down efforts facilitates achievement of the expected outcome of a spontaneous, uncomplicated vaginal birth. The median duration of second stage labor is

50 minutes in nulliparous women and 20 minutes in multiparous women. In addition to parity, maternal size and fetal weight, position, and descent influence the length of this stage. The use of epidural anesthesia during labor often increases the length of the second stage of labor because the epidural blocks or reduces the woman's urge to bear down and limits her ability to attain an upright position to push. The upper limits for the duration of normal second stage labor are (Battista & Wing, 2007):

- Nulliparous women: 2 hours with no regional anesthesia use; 3 hours with use of regional anesthesia
- Multiparous women: 1 hour with no regional anesthesia use; 2 hours with regional anesthesia

A prolonged second stage is diagnosed after these time limits are reached. A thorough assessment of the status of the maternal-fetal unit should be made as well as a determination regarding the likely effectiveness and safety of further bearing-down efforts (Simpson et al., 2008).

The second stage of labor is composed of two phases: the latent phase and the active pushing (descent) phase. Maternal verbal and nonverbal behaviors, uterine activity, the urge to bear down, and fetal descent characterize these phases (Hanson, 2009; Simpson et al., 2008).

The *latent phase* is a period of rest and relative calm (i.e., "laboring down"). During this early phase the fetus continues to descend passively through the birth canal and rotate to an anterior position as a result of ongoing uterine contractions. The woman is quiet and often relaxes with her eyes closed between contractions. The urge to bear down is not strong and some women do not experience it at all or only during the acme (peak) of a contraction. Allowing a woman to rest during this phase, and waiting until the urge to push intensifies, reduces maternal fatigue, conserves energy for bearing-down efforts, and provides optimal maternal and fetal outcomes (Simpson, 2005). Although *delayed pushing* is associated with a longer second stage of labor, it results in a significantly higher incidence of spontaneous vaginal birth. Other benefits of delayed pushing include less FHR decelerations, fewer forceps- and vacuum-assisted births, and less perineal damage (lacerations and episiotomies). Careful monitoring with assurance of normal fetal status should be used during delayed pushing. If descent is slow and the woman becomes anxious, she should be encouraged to change positions frequently or to stand by the bedside to use the advantage of gravity and movement to facilitate descent and progress to the active pushing phase signaled by a perception of the need to bear down (Hanson, 2009). The longer length of second stage labor is not associated with poor neonatal outcome, as long as the fetal status during this time is normal (Berghella et al., 2008; Brancato, Church, & Stone, 2008; Roberts & Hanson, 2007; Simpson & James, 2005).

During the phase of active pushing (descent) the woman has strong urges to bear down as the **Ferguson reflex** is activated when the presenting part presses on the stretch receptors of the pelvic floor. At this point, the fetal station is usually +1 and the position is anterior. This stimulation causes the release of oxytocin from the posterior pituitary gland, which provokes stronger expulsive uterine contractions. The woman becomes more focused on bearing-down efforts, which become rhythmic. She changes positions frequently to find a more comfortable pushing position. The woman often announces the onset of contractions and becomes more vocal as she bears down. The urge to bear down intensifies as descent progresses and the presenting part reaches the perineum. The woman may be more verbal about the pain she is experiencing; she may scream or swear and may act out of control.

The nurse encourages the woman to "listen" to her body as she progresses through the phases of the second stage of labor. When a woman listens to her body to tell her when to bear down, she is using an internal locus of control and often feels more satisfied with her efforts to give birth to her baby. This enhances her sense of self-esteem and accomplishment and her efforts become more effective. Always encourage the woman's trust in her own body and her ability to give birth to her baby. Validate the woman's experience of pressure, stretching, and straining as normal and a signal that the descent of the fetus is progressing and that her body is capable of withstanding birth. Honestly explain what is happening and describe the progress being made.

CARE MANAGEMENT

The only certain objective sign that the second stage of labor has begun is the inability to feel the cervix during vaginal examination, indicating that the cervix is fully dilated and effaced. The precise moment that this occurs is not easily determined because it depends on when a vaginal examination is performed to validate full dilation and effacement. This makes timing of the actual duration of the second stage difficult. Other signs that suggest the onset of the second stage include the urge to push or feeling the need to have a bowel movement. These signs commonly appear at the time the cervix reaches full dilation. However, they can appear earlier in labor. Women with an epidural block may not exhibit such signs.

Women can begin to experience an irresistible urge to bear down before full dilation. For some, this occurs as early as 5 cm dilation. This is most often related to the station of the presenting part below the level of the ischial spines of the maternal pelvis. This occurrence creates a conflict between the woman, whose body is telling her to push, and her health care providers, who believe that pushing the fetal presenting part against an incompletely dilated cervix will result in cervical edema and lacerations, as well as slow the labor progress. Evaluate the premature urge to bear down as a sign of labor progress, possibly indicating the onset of the second stage of labor. Base the timing of when a woman pushes in relation to whether her cervix is fully dilated on research evidence rather than on tradition or routine practice. Pushing with the urge to bear down at the acme of a contraction may be safe and effective for a woman if her cervix is soft, retracting, and 8 cm or more dilated and if the fetus is at +1 station and rotating to an anterior position (Roberts, 2002).

Assessment is continuous during the second stage of labor. Professional standards and agency policy determine the specific type and timing of assessments, as well as the way in which findings are documented. Signs and symptoms of impending birth (Table 19-3) may appear unexpectedly, requiring immediate action by the nurse (Box 19-7). As with the first stage of

Case Study—Second/Third Stages of Labor

EMERGENCY

Interventions for Emergencies During Labor

SIGNS	INTERVENTIONS (PRIORITIES ARE BASED ON WHAT SIGN IS PRESENT)*
NONREASSURING OR ABNORMAL FETAL HEART RATE AND PATTERN	
• Fetal bradycardia (FHR <110 beats/min for >10 minutes) • Fetal tachycardia (FHR >160 beats/min for >10 minutes in term pregnancy) • Irregular FHR, abnormal sinus rhythm shown by internal monitor • Absent or minimal baseline FHR variability without an identified cause • Late, variable, and prolonged deceleration patterns • Absence of FHTs	• Notify primary health care provider.[†] • Change maternal position. Discontinue oxytocin (Pitocin) infusion, if tachysystole is occurring. • Start an IV line if one is not in place. • Increase IV fluid rate, if fluid is being infused, per protocol or order. • Administer oxygen at 8 to 10 L/min by nonrebreather face mask. • Check maternal temperature for elevation. • Assist with amnioinfusion if ordered. • Perform fetal scalp stimulation or vibroacoustic stimulation as ordered or per protocol.
INADEQUATE UTERINE RELAXATION	
• Intrauterine pressure ≥80 mm Hg (shown by intrauterine pressure catheter monitoring) • Contractions consistently lasting >90 seconds • Contractions occurring more frequently than every 2 minutes (>5 contractions in 10 minutes)	• Notify primary health care provider.[†] • Discontinue oxytocin infusion, if being infused. • Change woman to side-lying position. • Start an IV line if one is not in place. • Increase IV fluid rate, if fluid is being infused. • Administer oxygen at 8 to 10 L/min by nonrebreather face mask. • Palpate and evaluate contractions. • Give tocolytic (terbutaline [Brethine]), as ordered or per protocol.
VAGINAL BLEEDING	
• Vaginal bleeding (bright red, dark red, or in an amount in excess of that expected during normal cervical dilation) • Continuous vaginal bleeding with FHR changes • Pain may or may not be present	• Notify primary health care provider.[†] • Assist with ultrasound examination if performed. • Start an IV line if one is not in place. • Begin continuous FHR and contraction monitoring, if not already in progress. • Anticipate emergency (stat) cesarean birth. • *Do NOT perform a vaginal examination.*
INFECTION	
• Foul-smelling amniotic fluid • Maternal temperature >38° C in presence of adequate hydration (straw-colored urine) • Fetal tachycardia >160 beats/min for >10 minutes	• Notify primary health care provider.[†] • Institute cooling measures for laboring woman. • Start an IV line if one is not in place. • Assist with or perform collection of catheterized urine specimen and amniotic fluid sample and send to the laboratory for urinalysis and cultures. • Administer antibiotics as ordered.
PROLAPSE OF CORD	
• Fetal bradycardia with variable deceleration during uterine contraction • Woman reports feeling the cord after membranes rupture • Cord lies alongside or below the presenting part of the fetus; can be seen or felt in or protruding from the vagina • Major predisposing factors: — Rupture of membranes with a gush — Loose fit of presenting part in lower uterine segment — Presenting part not yet engaged — Breech presentation	• Call for assistance. Do not leave woman alone. • Have someone notify the primary health care provider immediately.[†] • Glove the examining hand quickly and insert two fingers into the vagina to the cervix; with one finger on either side of the cord or both fingers to one side, exert upward pressure against the presenting part to relieve compression of the cord. • Place a rolled towel under the woman's hip. • Place woman in extreme Trendelenburg or modified Sims position or knee-chest position. • If the cord is protruding from the vagina, wrap the cord loosely in a sterile towel saturated with warm sterile normal saline. • Administer oxygen at 8 to 10 L/min by nonrebreather face mask until birth is accomplished. • Start IV fluids or increase existing drip rate. • Continue to monitor FHR by internal fetal scalp electrode, if possible. • Do not attempt to replace cord into cervix. • Prepare for immediate birth (vaginal or cesarean).

FHR, Fetal heart rate; *FHT,* fetal heart tones; *IV,* intravenous.

*In an emergency situation, assistance from other nurses on the unit will be available to help provide care. Because emergency situations are often frightening events, it is important for the nurse to explain to the woman and her support person what is happening and how it is being managed.

†In most emergency situations, nurses take immediate action, following a protocol and standards of nursing practice. Another person can notify the primary health care provider, or this can be done by the nurse as soon as possible.

TABLE 19-3 EXPECTED MATERNAL PROGRESS IN THE SECOND STAGE OF LABOR

Criterion	LATENT PHASE *(Average Duration, 10-30 minutes)*	ACTIVE PUSHING (DESCENT) PHASE *(Average Duration Varies)**
Contractions		
Intensity	Period of physiologic lull for all criteria; period of peace and rest; "laboring down"	Significant increase becoming overwhelmingly strong and expulsive
Frequency		Every 2 to 2.5 minutes progressing to every 1 to 2 minutes
Duration		90 sec
Descent, station	0 to +2	+2 to +4; Rate of descent increases and Ferguson reflex† is activated; fetal head becomes visible at introitus and birth occurs
Show: color and amount		Significant increase in dark red bloody show; bloody show accompanies emergence of head
Spontaneous bearing-down efforts	Slight to absent, except during acme of strongest contractions	Increased urge to bear down; becomes stronger as fetus descends to vaginal introitus and reaches perineum
Vocalization	Quiet; concern over progress	Grunting sounds or expiratory vocalizations; announces contractions; may scream or swear
Maternal behavior	Experiences sense of relief that transition to second stage is finished Feels fatigued and sleepy Feels a sense of accomplishment and optimism, because the "worst is over" Feels in control	Senses increased urge to push and describes increasing pain; describes *ring of fire* (burning sensation of acute pain as vagina stretches and fetal head crowns) Expresses feeling of powerlessness Shows decreased ability to listen or concentrate on anything but giving birth Alters respiratory pattern: has short 4- to 5-second breath holds with regular breaths in between, 5 to 7 times per contraction Frequent repositioning Often shows excitement immediately after birth of head

*Duration of descent phase can vary depending on maternal parity, effectiveness of bearing-down effort, and presence of spinal anesthesia or epidural analgesia.
†Pressure of presenting part on stretch receptors of pelvic floor stimulates release of oxytocin from posterior pituitary, resulting in more intense uterine contractions.
Sources: Hanson, L. (2009). Second-stage labor care. *Journal of Perinatal and Neonatal Nursing, 23*(1), 31-39; Simpson, K., Cesario, S., Morin, K., Trapani, K., Mayberry, L., & Snelgrove-Clark, E. (2008). *Nursing care and management of the second stage of labor: Evidence-based clinical practice guideline.* (2nd ed.). Washington, DC: Association of Women's Health, Obstetric & Neonatal Nurses; Roberts, J. (2002). The "push" for evidence: Management of the second stage. *Journal of Midwifery & Women's Health, 47*(1), 2-15; Simkin, P., & Ancheta, R. (2000). *The labor progress handbook.* Malden, MA: Blackwell Science.

labor, care management is guided by the nursing process (see the Nursing Process box: Second Stage of Labor).

The nurse continues to monitor maternal-fetal status and events of the second stage and provide comfort measures for the mother. This includes helping her change position; providing mouth care; maintaining clean, dry bedding; and keeping extraneous noise, conversation, and other distractions (e.g., laughing, talking of attending personnel in or outside the labor area) to a minimum. The woman is encouraged to indicate other support measures she would like (Table 19-2; Nursing Care Plan).

In the hospital, birth may occur in an LDR, LDRP, or delivery room. If the mother is to be transferred to the delivery room for birth, perform the transfer early enough to avoid rushing her. The birth area also is readied.

Preparing for Birth

Maternal Position

No single position for childbirth exists. Labor is a dynamic, interactive process involving the woman's uterus, pelvis, and voluntary muscles. In addition, angles between the baby and the woman's pelvis constantly change as the infant turns and flexes down the birth canal. The woman may want to assume various positions for childbirth. She should be encouraged to change positions frequently and assisted in attaining and maintaining her position(s) of choice (Figs. 19-15 and 19-16). Supine, semirecumbent, or lithotomy positions are still widely used in Western societies despite evidence that women prefer upright positions for their bearing-down efforts and birth (Roberts & Hanson, 2007).

Birth attendants play a major role in influencing a woman's choice of positions for birth, with nurse-midwives tending to advocate nonlithotomy positions (e.g., upright, lateral) for the second stage of labor. The use of upright and lateral positions is associated with a shorter interval to birth, less pain and perineal damage, fewer episiotomies and abnormal FHR patterns, and fewer operative vaginal births (Berghella et al., 2008; Roberts & Hanson, 2007; Simpson et al., 2008; Zwelling, 2010). The benefits of upright positions may be related to:

- Straightening of the longitudinal axis of the birth canal and improvement in the alignment of the fetus for passage through the pelvis
- Application of gravity to direct the fetal head toward the pelvic inlet, thereby facilitating descent
- Enlargement of pelvic dimensions and restriction of the encroachment of the sacrum and coccyx into the pelvic outlet
- Increased uteroplacental circulation, resulting in more intense, efficient uterine contractions
- Enhancement of the woman's ability to bear down effectively, thereby minimizing maternal exhaustion

Squatting is highly effective in facilitating the descent and birth of the fetus. It is one of the best and most natural positions for second stage labor and has been associated with the same benefits of other upright and lateral positions (Roberts, 2002; Simpson et al., 2008). Women should assume a modified, supported squat until the fetal head is engaged, at which time a deep squat can be used. A firm surface is required for this position, and the woman will need side support (see Fig. 19-12, *A*). In a birthing bed, a squat bar is available that she can use to help support herself (Fig. 19-16, *E*). A birth ball can also be used to

NURSING PROCESS

Second Stage of Labor

ASSESSMENT

- Signs that suggest the onset of the second stage:
  - Feeling an urge to push or need to have a bowel movement
  - Sudden appearance of sweat on upper lip
  - An episode of vomiting
  - Increased bloody show
  - Shaking of extremities
  - Increased restlessness; verbalization (e.g., "I can't go on")
  - Involuntary bearing-down efforts
- Physical assessment:
  - Perform every 5 to 30 minutes: maternal blood pressure, pulse, and respirations
  - Assess every 5 to 15 minutes: FHR and pattern
  - Assess every 10 to 15 minutes: vaginal show, signs of fetal descent, and changes in maternal appearance, mood, affect, energy level and condition of partner/coach
  - Assess every contraction and bearing-down effort

NURSING DIAGNOSES

Possible nursing diagnoses include:

***Risk for Injury (to Mother and Fetus)* related to:**
- persistent use of Valsalva maneuver during bearing-down efforts

***Acute Pain* related to:**
- bearing-down efforts and distention of the perineum

***Anxiety* related to:**
- inability to control defecation during bearing-down efforts
- deficient knowledge regarding perineal sensations associated with the urge to bear down
- coaching that contradicts woman's physiologic urge to push

***Risk for Infection* related to:**
- prolonged rupture of membranes
- use of invasive measures (e.g., forceps, vacuum) to facilitate birth
- perineal trauma (e.g., lacerations, episiotomy) associated with vaginal birth

***Situational Low Self-esteem (Maternal)* related to:**
- deficient knowledge of normal, beneficial effects of vocalization during bearing-down efforts
- inability to carry out plan for birth

EXPECTED OUTCOMES OF CARE

Expected outcomes for the woman in the second stage of labor are that the woman will:
- Actively participate in the process of giving birth.
- Sustain no injury to herself or her fetus during the birth process.
- Accept support measures from significant others and health care providers as needed during bearing-down efforts.
- Express satisfaction with her performance during labor and birth.
- Initiate, along with her partner and family, the process of bonding and attachment with the newborn.

PLAN OF CARE AND INTERVENTIONS

- Latent phase
  - Assist to rest in a position of comfort; encourage relaxation to conserve energy
  - Promote progress of fetal descent and onset of the urge to bear down by encouraging position changes, pelvic rock, ambulation, showering
- Stage of active pushing (descent)
  - Assist to change position and encourage spontaneous bearing-down efforts
  - Help to relax and conserve energy between contractions
  - Provide comfort and pain relief measures as needed
  - Cleanse perineum promptly if fecal material is expelled
  - Coach to pant during contractions and to gently push between contractions when head is being delivered
  - Provide emotional support, encouragement, and positive reinforcement of efforts
  - Keep informed regarding progress
  - Create a calm and quiet environment
  - Offer mirror to watch birth

EVALUATION

Evaluation of the effectiveness of care of the woman and her family during the second stage of labor is based on the previously stated expected outcomes.

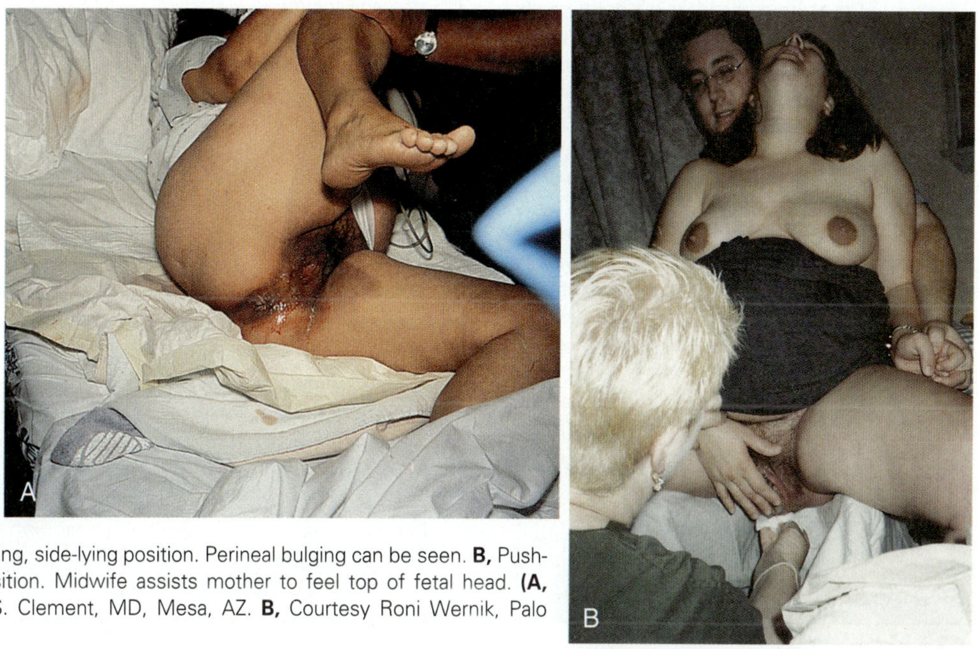

FIG. 19-15 **A,** Pushing, side-lying position. Perineal bulging can be seen. **B,** Pushing, semisitting position. Midwife assists mother to feel top of fetal head. **(A,** Courtesy Michael S. Clement, MD, Mesa, AZ. **B,** Courtesy Roni Wernik, Palo Alto, CA.)

help a woman maintain the squatting position. The fetus will be aligned with the birth canal, and pelvic and perineal relaxation is facilitated as she sits on the ball or holds it in front of her for support as she squats (see Box 19-5).

When a woman uses the supported standing position for bearing down, her weight is borne on both femoral heads, allowing the pressure in the acetabulum to cause the transverse diameter of the pelvic outlet to increase by up to 1 cm. This can be helpful if descent of the head is delayed because the occiput has not rotated from the lateral (transverse diameter of pelvis) to the anterior position. Birthing chairs or rocking chairs may be used to provide women with a good physiologic position to

BOX 19-7 GUIDELINES FOR ASSISTANCE AT THE EMERGENCY BIRTH OF A FETUS IN THE VERTEX PRESENTATION

1. The woman usually assumes the position most comfortable for her. A lateral position is often recommended to facilitate a controlled birth of the head, thereby minimizing the risk for perineal trauma and neonatal head injury.
2. Reassure the woman that birth is usually uncomplicated in these situations. Use eye-to-eye contact and a calm, relaxed manner. If there is someone else available, such as the partner, that person could help support the woman in the position, assist with coaching, and provide positive reinforcement and praise of her efforts.
3. Wash your hands and put on gloves, if available.
4. Place under woman's buttocks whatever clean material is available.
5. Avoid touching the vaginal area to decrease the possibility of infection.
6. As the head begins to crown, you should perform the following tasks:
   a. Tear the amniotic membranes if they are still intact.
   b. Instruct the woman to pant or pant-blow, thus minimizing the urge to push.
   c. Place the flat side of your hand on the exposed fetal head and apply *gentle* pressure toward the vagina to prevent the head from "popping out." The mother may participate by placing her hand under yours on the emerging head. NOTE: Rapid birth of the fetal head must be prevented because a rapid change of pressure within the molded fetal skull follows, which may result in dural or subdural tears. Rapid birth also may cause vaginal or perineal lacerations.
7. After the birth of the head, check for the umbilical cord. If the cord is around the baby's neck, try to slip it over the baby's head or pull it *gently* to get some slack so that you can slip it over the shoulders.
8. Support the fetal head as external rotation occurs. Then with one hand on each side of the baby's head, exert *gentle* pressure downward so that the anterior shoulder emerges under the symphysis pubis and acts as a fulcrum; then, as *gentle* pressure is exerted in the opposite direction, the posterior shoulder, which has passed over the sacrum and coccyx, emerges.
9. Be alert! Hold the baby securely because the rest of the body may emerge quickly. The baby will be slippery!
10. Cradle the baby's head and back in one hand and the buttocks in the other. Keep the baby's head down to drain away the mucus. Use a bulb syringe, if one is available, to remove mucus from the baby's mouth and then from the nose.
11. Dry the baby quickly to prevent rapid heat loss. Keep the baby at the same level as the mother's uterus until the end of the cord stops pulsating. NOTE: The baby should be kept at the same level as the mother's uterus to prevent the baby's blood from flowing to or from the placenta and the resultant hypovolemia or hypervolemia. Also, do not "milk" the cord.
12. Place the baby on the mother's abdomen, cover the baby (remember to keep the head warm, too) with the mother's clothing, and have her cuddle the baby. Compliment her (them) on a job well done, and on the baby, if appropriate.
13. Wait for the placenta to separate. *Do not* tug on the cord. NOTE: Inappropriate traction may tear the cord, separate the placenta, or invert the uterus. Signs of placental separation include a slight gush of dark blood from the introitus, lengthening of the cord, and change in the uterine contour from a discoid to globular shape.
14. Instruct the mother to push to deliver the separated placenta. Gently ease out the placental membranes using an up-and-down motion until the membranes are removed. If birth occurs outside a hospital setting, to minimize complications, do not cut the cord without proper clamps and a sterile cutting tool. Inspect the placenta for intactness. Place the baby on the placenta and wrap the two together for additional warmth.
15. Check the firmness of the uterus. Gently massage the fundus and demonstrate to the mother how she can massage her own fundus properly.
16. If supplies are available, clean the mother's perineal area and apply a peripad.
17. In addition to gentle massage of the fundus, the following measures can be taken to prevent or minimize hemorrhage:
   a. Put the baby to the mother's breast as soon as possible. Sucking or nuzzling and licking the nipple stimulates the release of oxytocin from the posterior pituitary. NOTE: If the baby does not or cannot nurse, manually stimulate the mother's nipples.
   b. Do not allow the mother's bladder to become distended. Assess the bladder for fullness and encourage her to void if fullness is found.
   c. Expel any clots from the mother's uterus after ensuring that the fundus is firm.
18. Comfort or reassure the mother and her family or friends. Keep the mother and the baby warm. Give her fluids if available and tolerated.
19. If this birth is multifetal, identify the infants in order of birth (using letters *A*, *B*, etc.).
20. Make notations regarding the following aspects of the birth:
   a. Fetal presentation and position
   b. Presence of cord around neck (nuchal cord) or other parts and number of times cord encircled part
   c. Color, character, and estimated amount of amniotic fluid, if rupture of membranes occurs immediately before birth
   d. Time of birth
   e. Estimated time of determination of Apgar score (e.g., 1 and 5 minutes after birth), resuscitation efforts implemented, and ultimate condition of baby
   f. Gender of baby
   g. Time of placental expulsion, as well as the appearance and completeness of the placenta
   h. Maternal condition: affect, behavior, and demeanor, amount of bleeding, and status of uterine tonicity
   i. Any unusual occurrences during the birth (e.g., maternal or paternal response, verbalizations, or gestures in response to birth of baby)

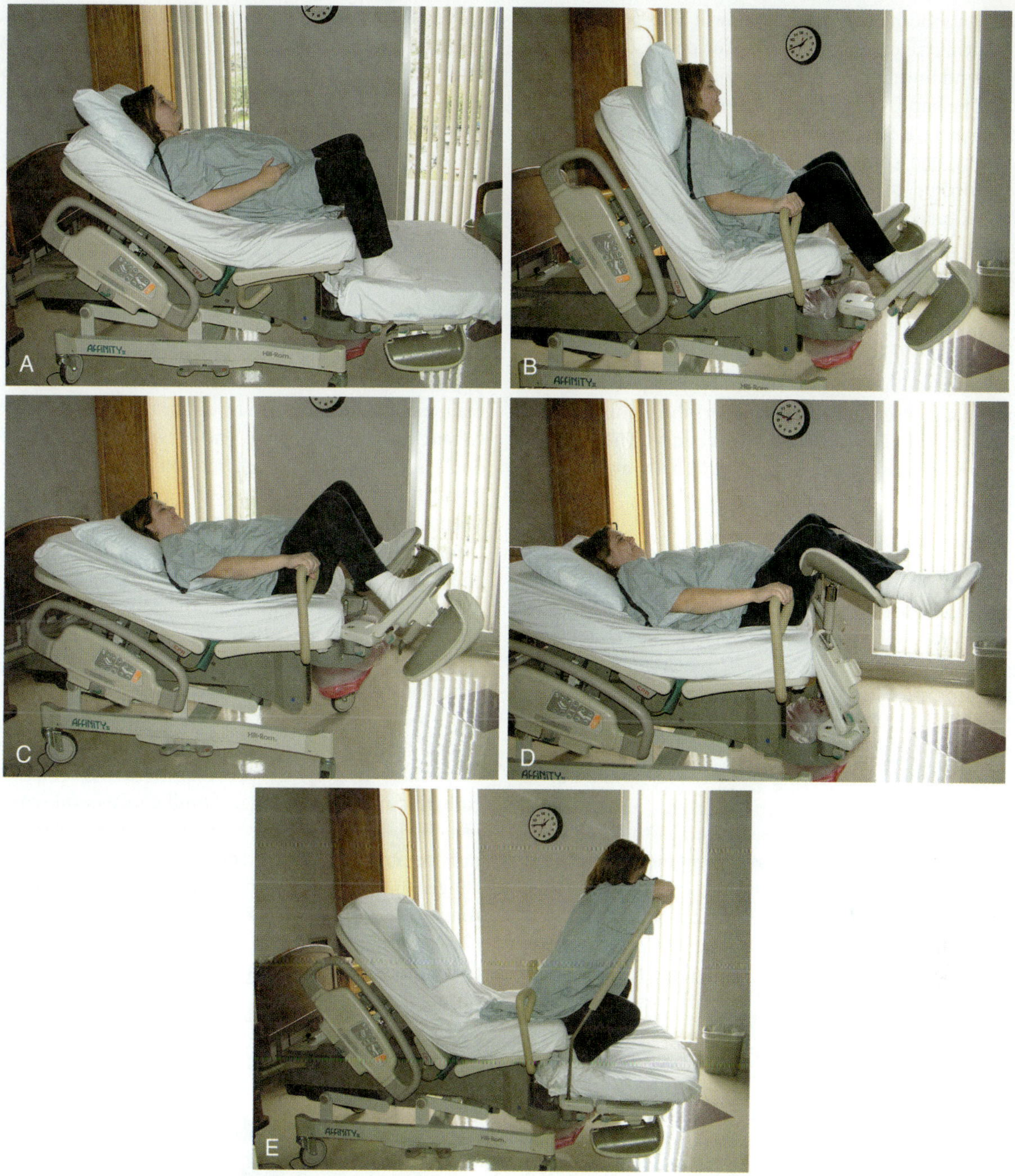

FIG. 19-16 The versatility of today's birthing bed makes it practical in a variety of settings. Note: OB table used for lithotomy position. **A,** Labor bed. **B,** Birth chair. **C,** Birth bed. **D,** OB table. **E,** Squatting or birth bar. (Courtesy Julie Perry Nelson, Loveland, CO.)

enhance bearing-down efforts during childbirth (see Box 19-5), although some women feel restricted by a chair. The upright position also provides a potential psychologic advantage in that it allows the mother to see the birth as it occurs and to maintain eye contact with the attendant.

Oversized beanbag chairs and large floor pillows may be used for both labor and birth. They can mold around and support the mother in whatever position she selects. These chairs are of particular value for mothers who wish to be actively involved in the birth process. Birthing stools can be used to support the woman in an upright position similar to squatting. Some women may feel more comfortable sitting on the toilet or commode during pushing because they are concerned about stool incontinence during this stage. Encourage them to empty their bladder to avoid the effects of a distended bladder. You must closely monitor these women, however, and remove them from the toilet before birth becomes imminent. Because sitting on chairs, stools, toilets, or commodes can increase perineal edema and blood loss, assist the woman to change her position frequently (e.g., every 10 to 15 minutes).

The side-lying, or lateral, position, with the upper part of the woman's leg held by the nurse or coach or placed on a pillow, is an effective position for the second stage of labor (see Fig. 19-15, *A* and Box 19-5). Some women prefer a semisitting (semirecumbent) position instead (see Fig. 19-16, *B* and Box 19-5). If the semirecumbent position is used, do not force the woman's legs against her abdomen as she bears down. This position will increase perineal stretching and the risk for perineal trauma as well as spinal and lower extremity neurologic injuries (Simpson et al., 2008). The hands-and-knees position is yet another effective position for birth (see Fig. 19-11, *B* and Box 19-5).

The birthing bed commonly used can be set for different positions according to the woman's needs (Figs. 19-16 and 19-17). The woman can squat, kneel, sit, recline, or lie on her side, choosing the position most comfortable for her without having to climb into bed for the birth. At the same time, the birthing bed provides excellent exposure for examinations, electrode placement, and birth. You can position the bed for the administration of anesthesia and it is ideal to help women receiving an epidural to assume different positions to facilitate birth. You can also use the bed to transport the woman to the operating room if a cesarean birth is necessary. The woman can use squat bars, over-the-bed tables, birth balls, and pillows for support.

Bearing-Down Efforts

As the fetal head reaches the pelvic floor, most women experience the urge to bear down. Reflexively the woman will begin to exert downward pressure by contracting her abdominal muscles while relaxing her pelvic floor. This bearing down is an involuntary response to the Ferguson reflex. A strong expiratory grunt or groan (vocalization) often accompanies pushing when the woman exhales as she pushes. This natural vocalization by women during open-glottis bearing-down efforts should not be discouraged.

When coaching women to push, encourage them to push as they feel like pushing (instinctive, spontaneous pushing) rather than to give a prolonged push on command (directed, closed-glottis pushing). Prolonged breath-holding, or sustained, directed bearing down is still a common practice often beginning at 10 cm dilation and before the urge to bear down is perceived. The woman is coached to hold her breath, closing her glottis, and to push while the nurse or partner counts to 10. This method of bearing down may trigger the **Valsalva maneuver,** which occurs when the woman closes her glottis (closed-glottis pushing), which increases intrathoracic and cardiovascular pressure. This reduces cardiac output and decreases perfusion of the uterus and the placenta. Adverse effects associated with prolonged breath-holding and forceful pushing efforts include fetal hypoxia and subsequent acidosis, increased risk for pelvic floor damage (structural and neurogenic), and perineal trauma (Schaffer, Bloom, Casey, McIntire, Nihira, & Leveno, 2005; Simpson & James, 2005; Simpson et al., 2008). The benefits of spontaneous pushing efforts rather than sustained Valsalva pushes include less hypoxic stress for the fetus and less pelvic or perineal damage for the woman, reducing her risk for future incontinence and pelvic organ prolapse (Roberts & Hanson, 2007). In addition, these more effective bearing-down efforts conserve maternal energy and reduce the risk for operative vaginal births (Roberts, 2002; Sampselle, Miller, Luecha, Fischer, & Rosten, 2005; Simpson & James, 2005). Based on this evidence, it is essential that perinatal nurses advocate for the practice of delayed and spontaneous bearing-down efforts with the woman in an upright or lateral position (Hanson, 2009).

A woman can become confused and anxious when she is being told to do something in conflict with what her body is telling her. Using phrases such as "You are doing so well, do it again," "You are moving the baby down," and "Follow what your body is telling you," rather than "Push, push, push," encourages a woman to feel confident in her body and what she is feeling (Hanson, 2009; Sampselle et al., 2005).

Monitor the woman's breathing so that she does not hold her breath for more than 6 to 8 seconds at a time followed by a slight exhale (a combination of open-glottis and voluntary closed-glottis pushing). Remind her to ventilate her lungs fully by taking deep cleansing breaths before and after each contraction. Bearing down while exhaling (open-glottis pushing) and taking breaths between bearing-down efforts help to maintain adequate oxygen levels for the mother and fetus, thus enhancing fetal well-being. The active pushing phase of the second stage of labor is considered to be the most physiologically stressful part of labor. Therefore, every effort should be made to ensure that women use nondirected spontaneous pushing to conserve energy and maximize the effect of each bearing-down effort. A woman's bearing-down efforts naturally will become more forceful and frequent as the second stage progresses to birth (Simpson et al., 2008).

A woman may reach the second stage of labor and then experience a lack of readiness to complete the process and give birth to her child. She may have doubts about her readiness to be a mother or may desire to wait for her support person or primary health care provider to arrive. Fear, anxiety, or embarrassment regarding unfamiliar or painful sensations and behaviors during pushing (e.g., sounds made, passage of stool) may be other inhibiting factors. Fear that the baby will be in danger once it emerges from the protective intrauterine environment also may be present. By recognizing that a woman may experience a need to hold back the birth of her baby, you can address the woman's concerns and effectively coach her during this stage of labor.

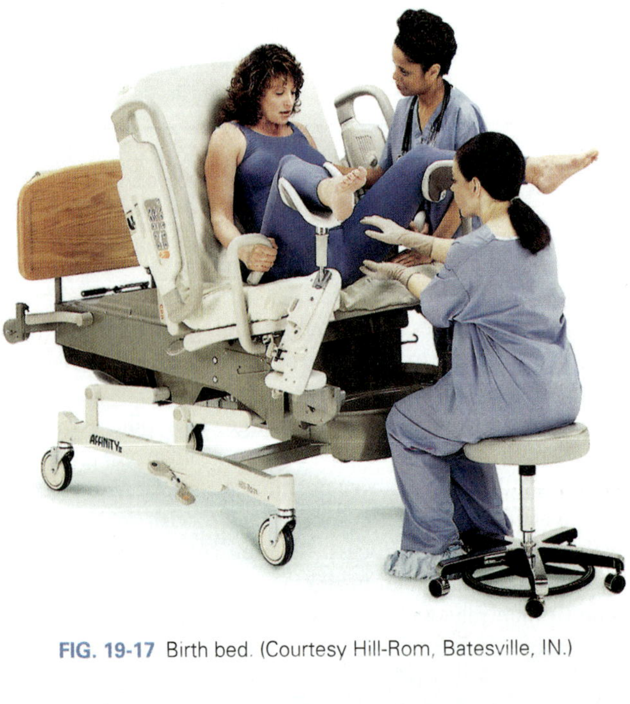

FIG. 19-17 Birth bed. (Courtesy Hill-Rom, Batesville, IN.)

To ensure the slow birth of the fetal head, encourage the woman to control the urge to bear down by coaching her to take panting breaths or exhale slowly through pursed lips as the baby's head crowns. At this point the woman needs simple, clear directions from one person. Amnesia between contractions often occurs in the second stage; therefore, you may have to rouse the woman to get her to cooperate in the bearing-down process. Parents who have attended childbirth education classes may have devised a set of verbal cues for the laboring woman to follow.

Fetal Heart Rate and Pattern

As noted, you must check the fetal heart rate regularly (see Chapter 18 for further discussion). If the baseline rate begins to slow, if a loss of variability occurs, or if deceleration patterns develop (e.g., late, variable, or prolonged), initiate interventions promptly. Turn the woman onto her side to reduce the pressure of the uterus against the ascending vena cava and descending aorta (see Fig. 19-5). Oxygen can be administered by nonrebreather mask at 8 to 10 L/min (Tucker et al., 2009). These interventions are often all that is necessary to restore a normal pattern. If the FHR and pattern do not become normal immediately, notify the primary health care provider because the woman may need medical intervention to give birth. See the Emergency box for more interventions related to abnormal FHR.

Support of the Father or Partner

During the second stage the woman needs continuous support and coaching (see Table 19-3). Because the coaching process is often physically and emotionally tiring for support persons, the nurse offers them nourishment and fluids and encourages them to take short breaks as needed (see Box 19-6). If birth occurs in an LDR or LDRP room, the support person usually wears street clothes. Instruct the support person who attends the birth in a delivery room to put on a cover gown or scrub clothes, mask, hat, and shoe covers, if required by agency policy. The nurse also specifies support measures that can be used for the laboring woman and points out areas of the room in which the partner can move freely.

Encourage partners to be present at the birth of their infants if doing so is in keeping with their cultural and personal expectations and beliefs. The presence of partners maintains the psychologic closeness of the family unit, and the partner can continue to provide the supportive care given during labor. The woman and her partner need to have an equal opportunity to initiate the attachment process with the baby.

Supplies, Instruments, and Equipment

To prepare for birth in any setting, the birthing table is usually set up during the transition phase for nulliparous women and during the active phase for multiparous women.

Prepare the birthing bed or table, and arrange instruments on the instrument table or delivery cart (Fig. 19-18). Follow standard procedures for gloving, identifying and opening sterile packages, adding sterile supplies to the instrument table, unwrapping sterile instruments, and handing them to the primary health care provider. Ready the crib or radiant warmer and equipment for the support and stabilization of the infant (Fig. 19-19).

The items used for birth may vary among different facilities; therefore, consult each facility's procedure manual to determine the protocols specific to that facility.

The nurse estimates the time until the birth will occur and notifies the primary health care provider if he or she is not in the woman's room. Even the most experienced nurse can miscalculate the time left before birth occurs; therefore, every nurse who attends a woman in labor must be prepared to assist with an emergency birth if the primary health care provider is not present (see Box 19-7).

Birth in a Delivery Room or Birthing Room

The woman will need assistance if she must move from the labor bed to the delivery table (Fig. 19-20). The various positions assumed for birth in a delivery room are the Sims or lateral position in which the attendant supports the upper part of the woman's leg, the dorsal position (supine position with one hip elevated), and the lithotomy position.

The **lithotomy position** makes dealing with complications that arise more convenient for the primary health care provider (see Fig. 19-16, *D*). To place the woman in this position, bring her buttocks to the edge of the bed or table and place her legs in stirrups. Take care to pad the stirrups, to raise and place both legs simultaneously, and to adjust the shanks of the stirrups so that the calves of the legs are supported. No pressure should be placed on the popliteal space. Stirrups that are not the same height will strain ligaments in the woman's back as she bears down, leading to considerable discomfort in the postpartum period. The lower portion of the table may be dropped down and rolled back under the table.

The maternal position for birth in a birthing room varies from a lithotomy position with the woman's feet in stirrups or resting on footrests or with her legs held and supported by the nurse or support person, to one in which her feet rest on footrests while she holds on to a squat bar, to a side-lying position with the woman's upper leg supported by the coach, nurse, or squat bar. Once the woman is positioned, the foot of the bed is removed so that the primary health care provider attending the birth can gain better perineal access for performing an episiotomy, delivering a large baby, using forceps or vacuum extractor, or getting access to the emerging head to facilitate suctioning. Alternately, the foot of the bed can be left in place and lowered slightly to form a ledge that allows access

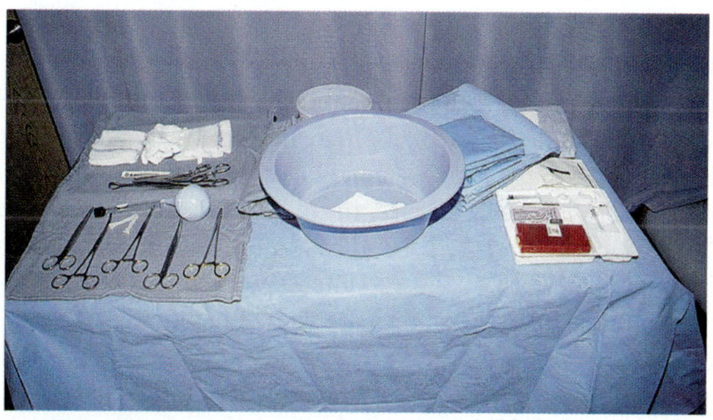

FIG. 19-18 Instrument table. (Courtesy Marjorie Pyle, RNC, Lifecircle, Costa Mesa, CA.)

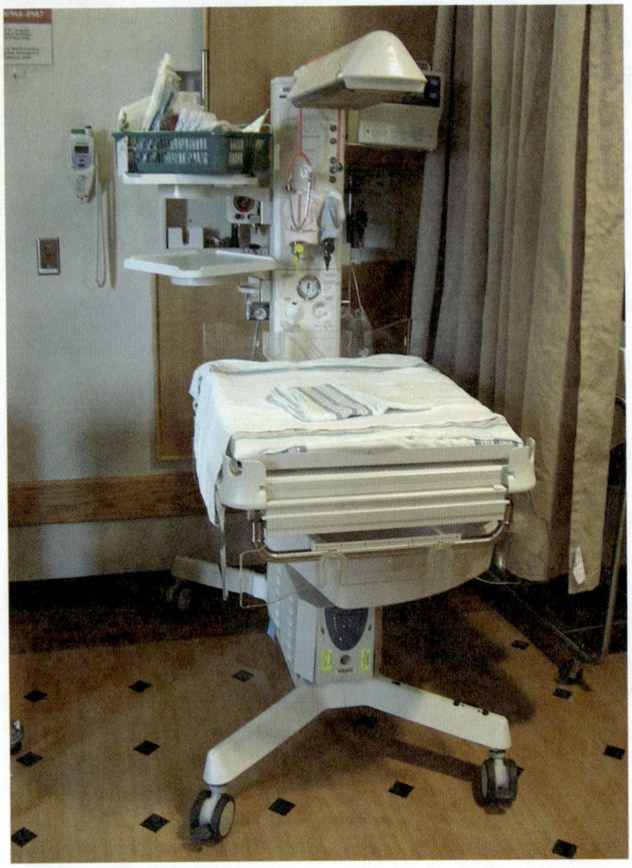

FIG. 19-19 Radiant warmer for newborn. (Courtesy Dee Lowdermilk, Chapel Hill, NC.)

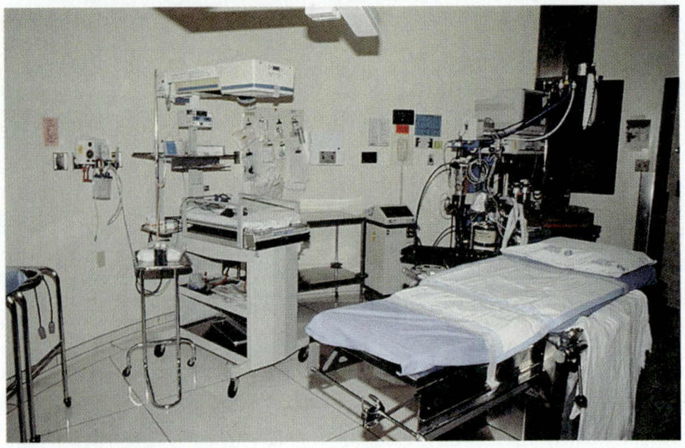

FIG. 19-20 Delivery room. (Courtesy Michael S. Clement, MD, Mesa, AZ.)

for birth and that also serves as a place to lay the newborn (see Fig. 19-16, *A*).

Once the woman is positioned for birth either in a delivery room or birthing room, the vulva and perineum are cleansed. Hospital protocols and the preferences of primary health care providers for cleansing may vary.

The nurse continues to coach and encourage the woman and monitor the fetal status (see the Nursing Process Box: Second Stage of Labor). Keep the primary health care provider informed of the fetal heart rate and pattern (Tucker et al., 2009). Prepare or obtain an oxytocic medication such as oxytocin (Pitocin) so that it is ready to be administered immediately after expulsion of the placenta. Always follow Standard Precautions as care is administered during the process of labor and birth (see Box 19-3).

In the delivery room, the primary health care provider puts on a cap, a mask that has a shield or protective eyewear, and shoe covers. After washing hands, the provider puts on a sterile gown (with waterproof front and sleeves) and sterile gloves. Nurses attending the birth also may need to wear caps, protective eyewear, masks, gowns, and gloves. The woman may then be draped with sterile drapes. In the birthing room, Standard Precautions are observed, but the amount and types of protective coverings worn by those in attendance may vary.

Maintain contact with the parents by touching, verbal comforting, describing progress, explaining the reasons for care, and sharing in the parents' joy at the birth of their child.

Mechanism of Birth: Vertex Presentation. The three phases of the spontaneous birth of a fetus in a vertex presentation are (1) birth of the head, (2) birth of the shoulders, and (3) birth of the body and extremities (see Chapter 16).

With voluntary bearing-down efforts, the head appears at the introitus (Fig. 19-21). **Crowning** occurs when the widest part of the head (the biparietal diameter) distends the vulva just before birth. Immediately before birth, the perineal musculature becomes greatly distended. If an episiotomy (incision into the perineum to enlarge vaginal outlet) is necessary, it is done at this time to minimize soft-tissue damage. A local anesthetic may be administered if necessary before performing an episiotomy. Box 19-8 shows the process of normal vaginal childbirth using a series of photographs.

The physician or nurse-midwife may use a hands-on approach to control the birth of the head, believing that guarding the perineum results in a gradual birth that will prevent fetal intracranial injury, protect maternal tissues, and reduce postpartum perineal pain. This approach involves: (1) applying pressure against the rectum, drawing it downward to aid in flexing the head as the back of the neck catches under the symphysis pubis; (2) then applying upward pressure from the coccygeal region (modified **Ritgen maneuver**) (Fig. 19-22) to extend the head during the actual birth, thereby protecting the musculature of the perineum; and (3) assisting the mother with voluntary control of the bearing-down efforts by coaching her to pant while letting uterine forces expel the fetus.

Some health care providers use a hands-poised (hands-off) approach when attending a birth. In this approach, hands are prepared to place light pressure on the fetal head to prevent rapid expulsion. The provider does not place hands on the perineum or use them to assist with birth of the shoulders and body.

The hands-on and hands-poised approaches have similar results in terms of perineal and vaginal tears, but the hands-on technique is associated with a higher incidence of third-degree tears and episiotomies. In one study, the hands-poised approach resulted in fewer third-degree tears (Berghella, Baxter, & Chauhan, 2008). However, the hands-on approach may result in less perineal pain.

The umbilical cord often encircles the neck **(nuchal cord)** but rarely so tightly as to cause hypoxia. After the head is born, gentle palpation is used to feel for the cord. If present, the health care provider slips the cord gently over the head if possible. If the loop is tight or if there is a second loop, he or she will probably clamp the cord twice, cut between the clamps, and unwind

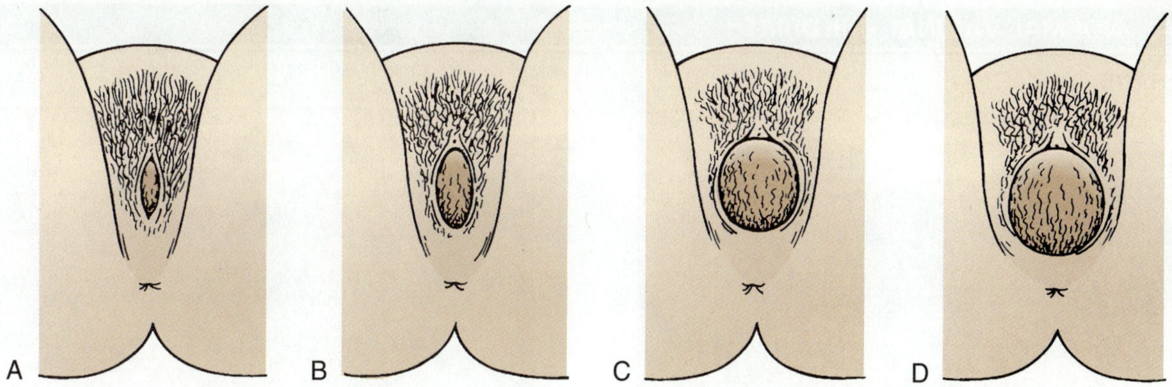

FIG. 19-21 Beginning birth with vertex presenting. **A,** Anteroposterior slit. **B,** Oval opening. **C,** Circular shape. **D,** Crowning.

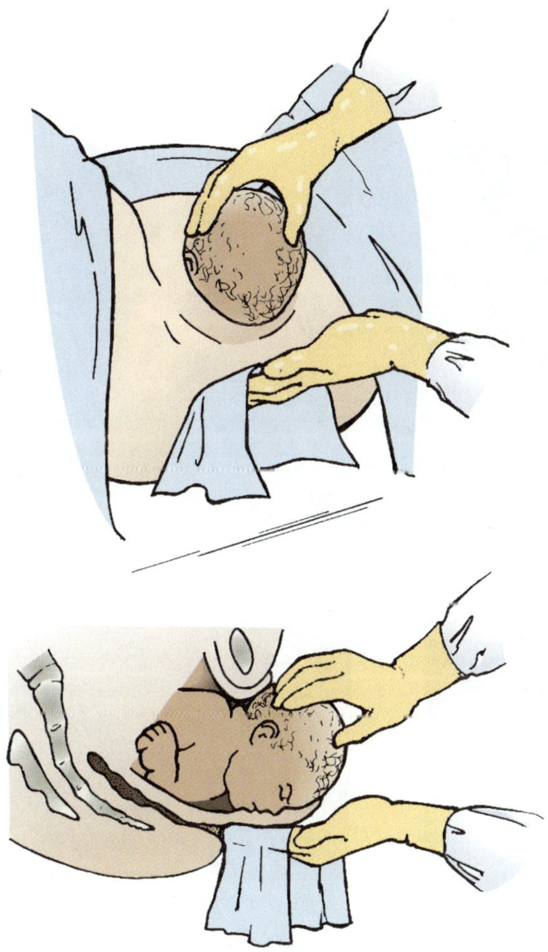

FIG. 19-22 Birth of head with modified Ritgen maneuver. Note control to prevent too-rapid birth of head.

the cord from around the neck before the birth is allowed to continue. Mucus, blood, or meconium in the nasal or oral passages may prevent the newborn from breathing. To eliminate this problem, moist gauze sponges are used to wipe the nose and mouth. A bulb syringe will be inserted first into the mouth and oropharynx and then into both nares to aspirate contents.

Fundal Pressure. Fundal pressure is the application of gentle, steady pressure against the fundus of the uterus to facilitate the vaginal birth. Historically it has been used when the administration of analgesia and anesthesia decreased the woman's ability to push during the birth, in cases of shoulder dystocia, and when second-stage fetal bradycardia or other abnormal FHR patterns were present. Use of fundal pressure by nurses is not advised because there is no standard technique available for this maneuver. Also no current legal, professional, or regulatory standards exist for its use and no evidence related to its effectiveness in facilitating a safe vaginal birth is available (Simpson et al., 2008).

Immediate Assessments and Care of the Newborn

The time of birth is the precise time when the entire body is out of the mother; you must record the time of birth. In the case of multiple births, each birth would be noted in the same way. If the newborn's condition is not compromised, he or she may be placed on the mother's abdomen immediately after birth and covered with a warm, dry blanket. The cord may be clamped at this time, and the primary health care provider may ask if the woman's partner would like to cut the cord. If so, the partner is given a sterile pair of scissors and instructed to cut the cord 1 inch (2.5 cm) above the clamp.

The care given immediately after the birth focuses on assessing and stabilizing the newborn. The nurse's main responsibility at this time is the infant, because the primary health care provider is involved with the delivery of the placenta and the care of the mother. The nurse must watch the infant for any signs of distress and initiate appropriate interventions should any appear.

Perform a brief assessment of the newborn immediately, even while the mother is holding the infant. This assessment includes assigning Apgar scores at 1 and 5 minutes after birth (see Table 24-1). Maintaining a patent airway, supporting respiratory effort, and preventing cold stress by drying and covering the newborn with a warmed blanket or placing him or her under a radiant warmer are the major priorities in terms of the newborn's immediate care. You can postpone further examination, identification procedures, and care until later in the third stage of labor or early in the fourth stage.

LEGAL TIP: Documentation

Documentation of all observations (e.g., maternal vital signs, FHR and pattern, progress of labor) and nursing interventions, including the woman's response, should be done concurrent with care. The course of labor and the maternal-fetal response may change without warning. All documentation must be accurate, complete, timely, and according to agency policy.

BOX 19-8 NORMAL VAGINAL CHILDBIRTH

FIRST STAGE

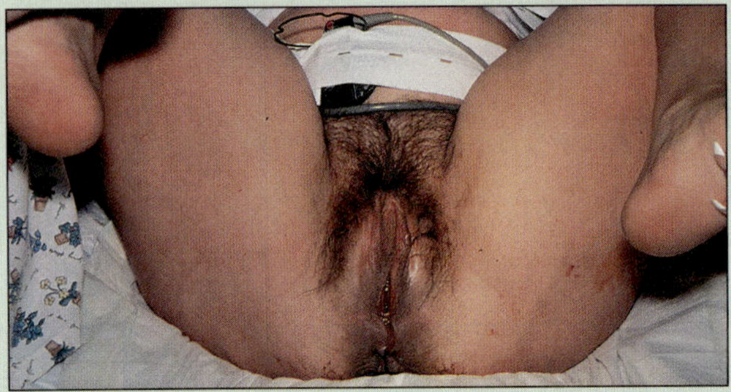

Anteroposterior slit. Vertex visible during contraction.

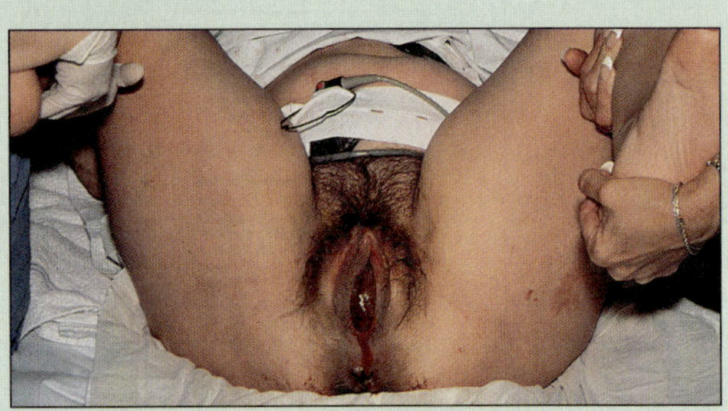

Oval opening. Vertex presenting. NOTE: Nurse *(on left)* is wearing gloves, but support person *(on right)* is not.

SECOND STAGE

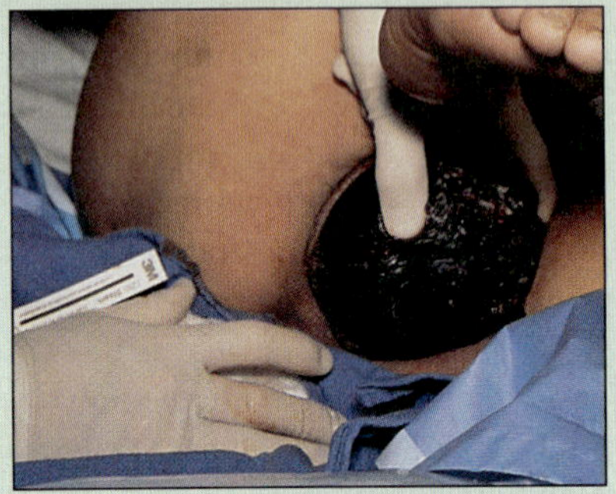

Crowning.

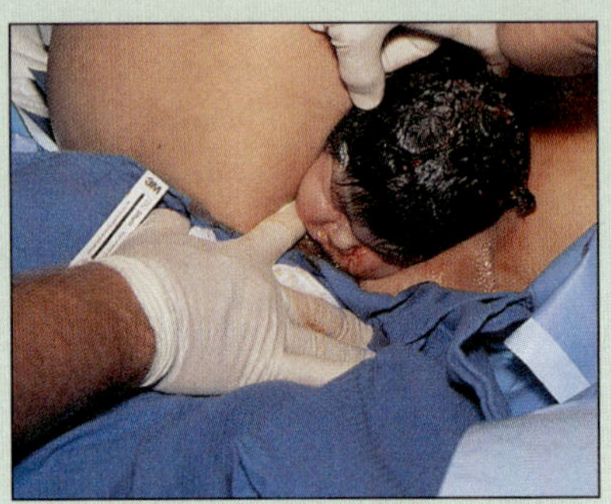

Nurse-midwife using Ritgen maneuver as head is born by extension.

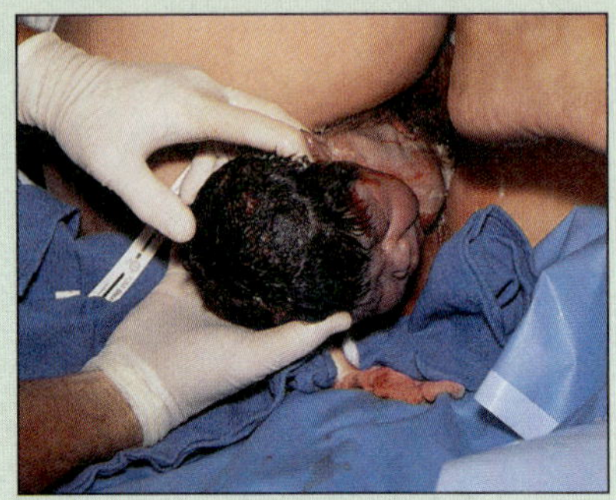

After nurse-midwife checks for nuchal cord, she supports head during external rotation and restitution.

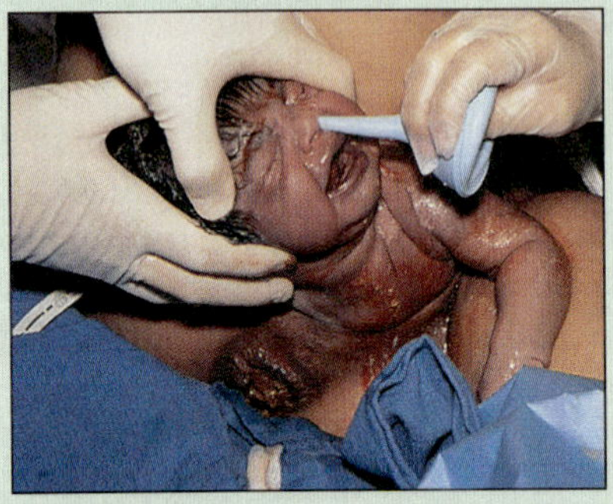

Use of bulb syringe to suction mucus.

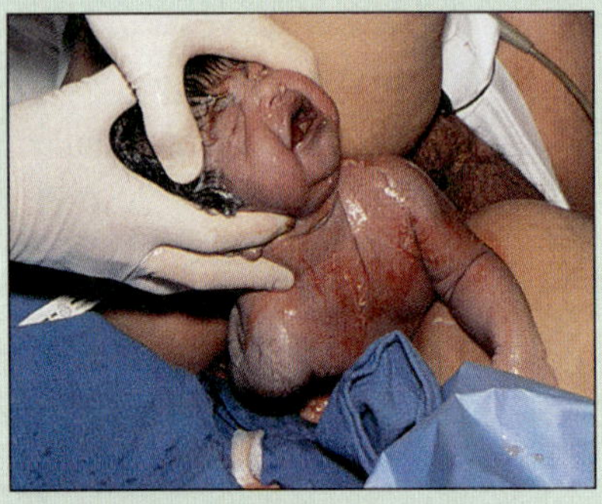

Birth of posterior shoulder.

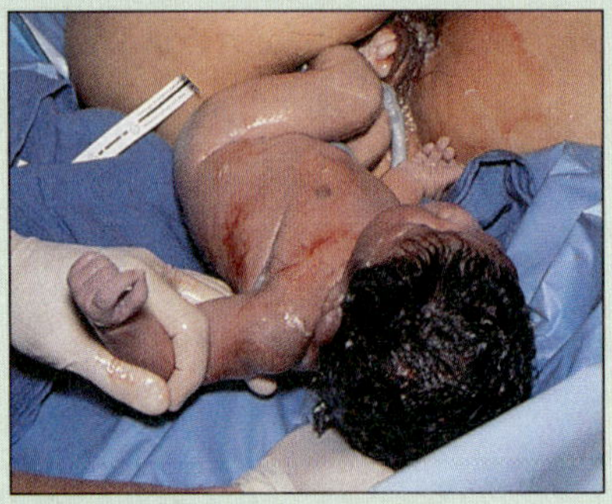

Birth of newborn by slow expulsion.

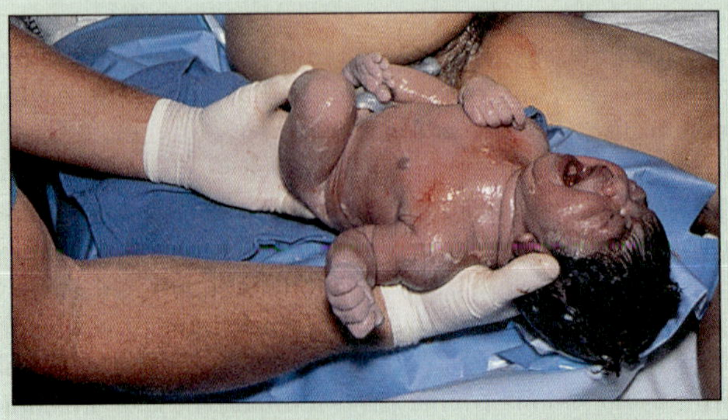

Second stage complete. Note that newborn is not completely pink yet.

Video—Childbirth: Vaginal

Animation—Vaginal Birth

BOX 19-8 **NORMAL VAGINAL CHILDBIRTH—cont'd**

THIRD STAGE

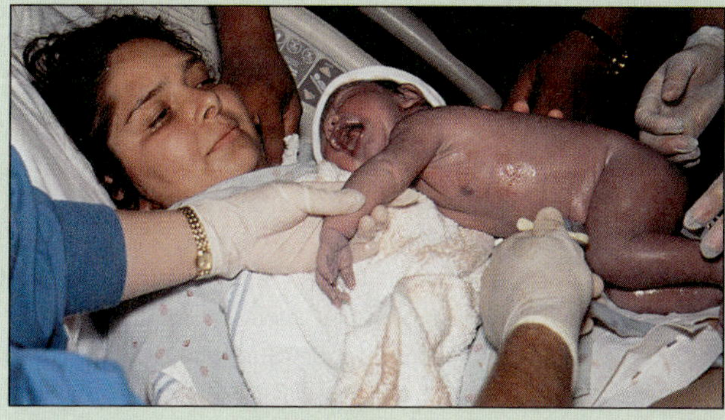

Newborn placed on mother's abdomen while cord is clamped and cut.

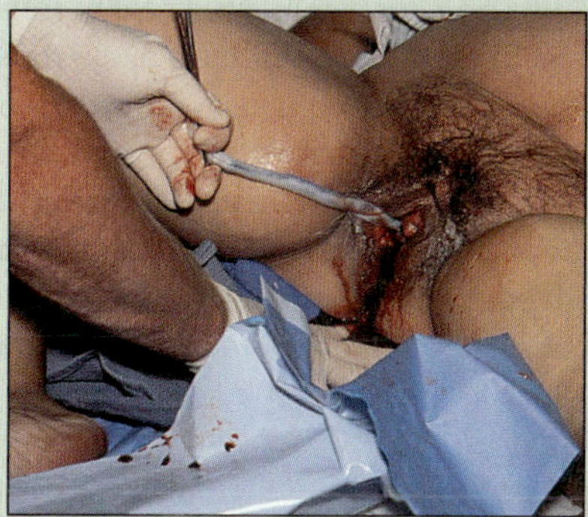

Note increased bleeding as placenta separates.

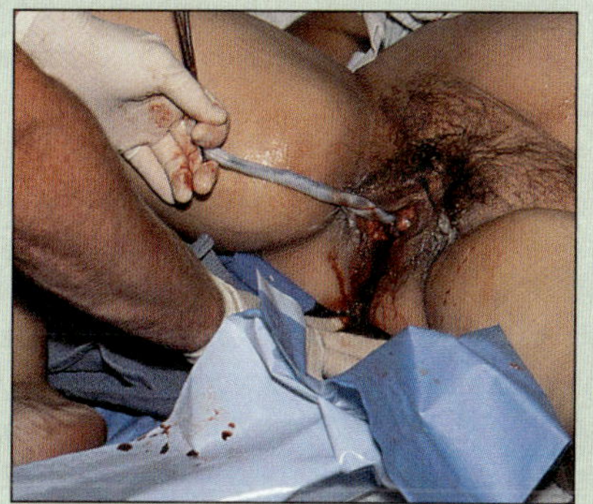

Expulsion of placenta.

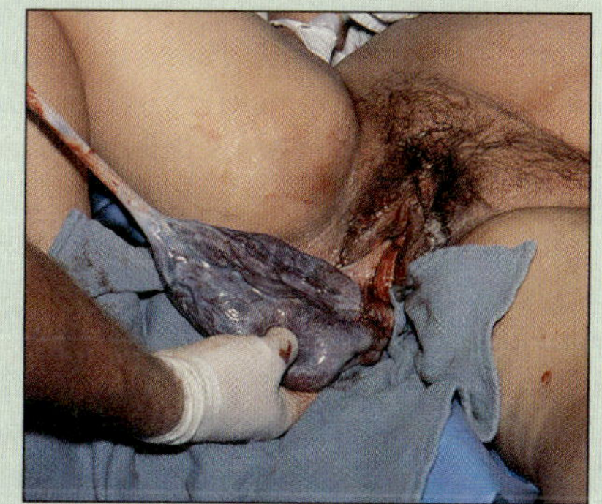

Expulsion is complete, marking the end of the third stage.

THE NEWBORN

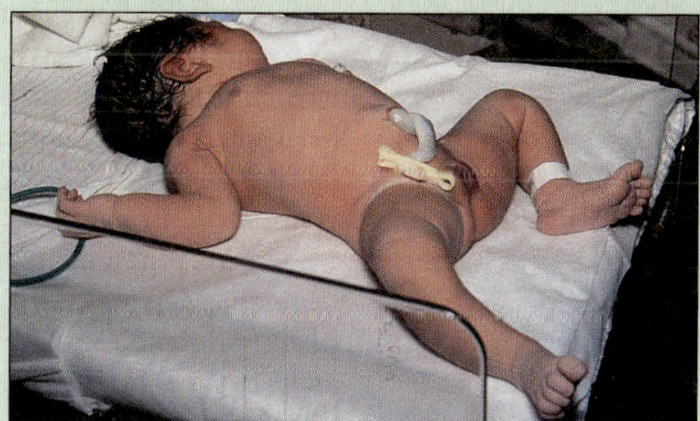

Newborn awaiting assessment. Note that color is almost completely pink.

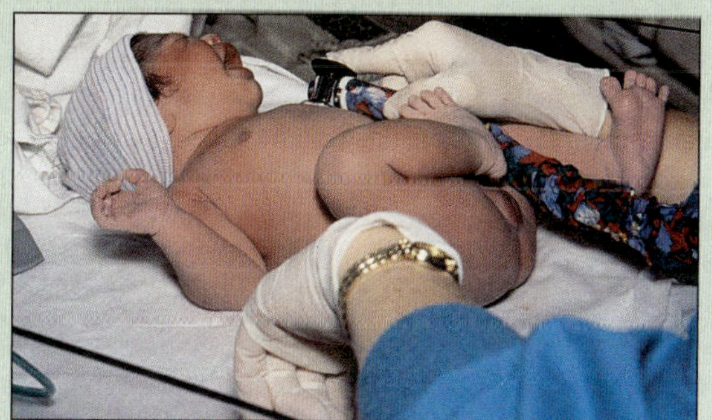

Newborn assessment under radiant warmer.

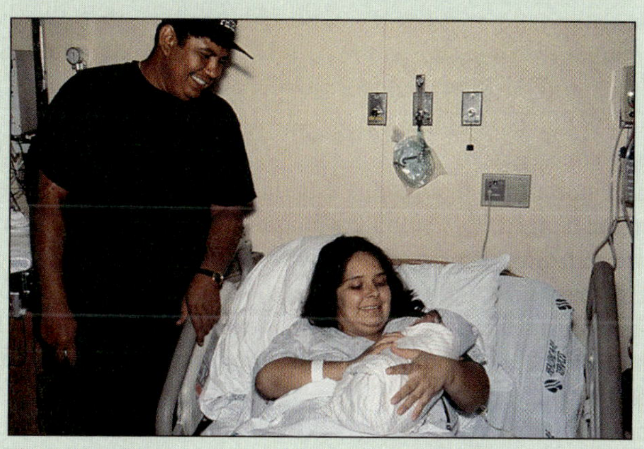

Parents admiring their newborn.

Courtesy Michael S. Clement, MD, Mesa, AZ.

Perineal Trauma Related to Childbirth

Most acute injuries and lacerations of the perineum, vagina, uterus, and their support tissues occur during childbirth. Alternative measures for perineal management, such as application of warm compresses and gentle perineal massage and stretching have been suggested to lessen the degree of perineal lacerations and trauma. Perineal massage during pregnancy has been shown to be somewhat effective for the primigravida (Beckmann & Garret, 2006). There has been limited evidence, however, for the benefit of perineal measures used during the second stage of labor. In fact, research findings are mixed with some studies indicating an increased risk for perineal trauma when using these measures, whereas other studies indicate that these measures may lessen the degree of perineal lacerations (Simpson et al., 2008). Therefore, these measures should be avoided during labor until further research can provide evidence of their benefit (Albers, Sedler, Bedrick, Teaf, & Peralta, 2005; Berghella et al., 2008).

Some degree of damage occurs during every birth to the soft tissues of the birth canal and adjacent structures. The tendency to sustain lacerations varies with each woman; that is, the soft tissue in some women may be less distensible. Damage usually is more pronounced in nulliparous women because the tissues are firmer and more resistant than are those in multiparous women. Heredity is also a factor. For example, the tissue of light-skinned women, especially those with reddish hair, is not as readily distensible as that of darker-skinned women, and healing may be less efficient. Other risk factors associated with perineal trauma include maternal position, pelvic inadequacy (e.g., narrow subpubic arch with a constricted outlet), fetal malpresentation and position (e.g., breech, occiput posterior position), large (macrosomic) infants, use of forceps or vacuum to facilitate birth, prolonged second stage of labor, and rapid labor in which there is insufficient time for the perineum to stretch.

Some injuries to the supporting tissues, whether they are acute or nonacute and whether they were repaired or not, may lead to genitourinary and sexual problems later in life (e.g., pelvic relaxation, uterine prolapse, cystocele, rectocele, dyspareunia, urinary and bowel dysfunction) (See Chapter 11). Use of Kegel exercises in the prenatal and postpartum periods improves and restores the tone and strength of the perineal muscles (see p. 91). Health practices, including good nutrition and appropriate hygienic measures, help maintain the integrity and suppleness of the perineal tissues, enhance healing, and prevent infection.

Perineal Lacerations. Perineal lacerations usually occur as the fetal head is being born. The extent of the laceration is defined in terms of its depth:

First degree: Laceration that extends through the skin and structures superficial to muscles

Second degree: Laceration that extends through muscles of the perineal body

Third degree: Laceration that continues through the anal sphincter muscle

Fourth degree: Laceration that also involves the anterior rectal wall

Perineal injury often is accompanied by small lacerations on the medial surfaces of the labia minora below the pubic rami and to the sides of the urethra (periurethral) and clitoris. Lacerations in this highly vascular area often result in profuse bleeding. Third- and fourth-degree lacerations must be carefully repaired so that the woman retains fecal continence. Simple perineal injuries usually heal without permanent disability, regardless of whether they were repaired. However, repairing a new perineal injury to prevent future complications is easier than correcting long-term damage.

Vaginal and Urethral Lacerations. Vaginal lacerations often occur in conjunction with perineal lacerations. Vaginal lacerations tend to extend up the lateral walls (sulci) and, if deep enough, involve the levator ani muscle. Additional injury may occur high in the vaginal vault near the level of the ischial spines. Vaginal vault lacerations are often circular and may result from use of forceps to rotate the fetal head, rapid fetal descent, or precipitous birth.

Cervical Injuries. Cervical injuries occur when the cervix retracts over the advancing fetal head. These cervical lacerations occur at the lateral angles of the external os. Most lacerations are shallow and bleeding is minimal. Larger lacerations may extend to the vaginal vault or beyond it into the lower uterine segment; serious bleeding may occur. Extensive lacerations may follow hasty attempts to enlarge the cervical opening artificially or to deliver the fetus before full cervical dilation is achieved. Injuries to the cervix can have adverse effects on future pregnancies and childbirths.

Episiotomy. An **episiotomy** is an incision made in the perineum to enlarge the vaginal outlet (Fig. 19-23). It is performed more commonly in the United States and Canada than in Europe. The side-lying position for birth, used routinely in Europe, causes less tension on the perineum, making possible a gradual stretching of the perineum with fewer indications for episiotomies.

Different types of episiotomies are performed, depending on the site and direction of the incision (see Fig. 19-23); the type that provides the best outcome is unknown (Berghella et al., 2008). Midline (median) episiotomy is most commonly used in the United States. It is effective, easily repaired, and generally the least painful. However, midline episiotomies also are associated with a higher incidence of third- and fourth-degree lacerations. Sphincter tone is usually restored after primary healing and a good repair. Mediolateral episiotomy is used in operative births when the need for posterior extension is likely. Although a fourth-degree laceration may be prevented, a third-degree laceration may occur. The blood loss is also greater and the repair more difficult and painful than with midline episiotomies. It is also more painful in the postpartum period, and the pain lasts longer.

Routine use of episiotomies has declined in the United States from 55.6% in 1990 to 19.3% in 2005 (DeFrances, Cullen, & Kozak, 2007). The practice in many settings now is to support the perineum manually during birth and allow the perineum to tear rather than perform an episiotomy. Tears are often smaller than an episiotomy, are repaired easily or not at all, and heal quickly. Episiotomies are associated with more posterior perineal trauma, suturing and healing complications, and later pain with intercourse. Therefore,

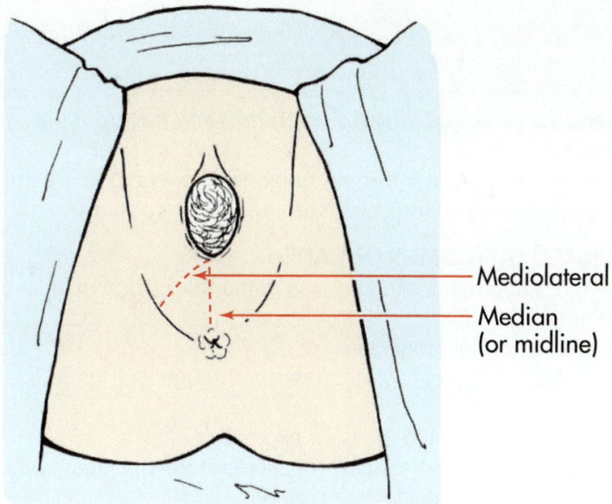

FIG. 19-23 Types of episiotomies.

episiotomy should be avoided if at all possible (Berghella et al., 2008).

THIRD STAGE OF LABOR

The **third stage of labor** lasts from the birth of the baby until the placenta is expelled. The goal in the management of the third stage of labor is the prompt separation and expulsion of the placenta, achieved in the easiest, safest manner. The third stage is generally by far the shortest stage of labor (see the Nursing Process box: Third Stage of Labor). The placenta is usually expelled within 10 to 15 minutes after the birth of the baby. If the third stage has not been completed within 30 minutes, the placenta is considered to be retained and interventions to hasten its separation and expulsion are usually instituted (Battista & Wing, 2007).

Under normal circumstances the placenta is attached to the decidual layer of the basal plate's thin endometrium by numerous fibrous anchor villi—much in the same way a postage stamp is attached to a sheet of postage stamps. After the birth of the fetus, strong uterine contractions and the sudden decrease in uterine size cause the placental site to shrink. This causes the anchor villi to break and the placenta to separate from its attachments. Normally the first few strong contractions that occur after the baby's birth cause the placenta to shear away from the basal plate. A placenta cannot detach itself from a flaccid (relaxed) uterus because the placental site is not reduced in size.

Placental Separation and Expulsion

Depending on preference, the primary health care provider may use either a passive or an active approach to manage the third stage of labor. Passive management involves patiently watching for signs that the placenta has spontaneously separated from the uterine wall (see Nursing Process box: Third Stage of Labor). Active management of third stage labor involves administering oxytocic medication (e.g., oxytocin [Pitocin]) to hasten placental separation in order to decrease the incidence of postpartum hemorrhage and reduce total blood loss. However, the active approach has not been found to be superior in all studies of third stage labor management (Kilpatrick & Garrison, 2007).

To assist in the delivery of the placenta, the woman is instructed to push when signs of separation have occurred (Fig. 19-24). If possible, the woman should expel the placenta during a uterine contraction. Alternate compression and elevation of the fundus, plus minimal, controlled traction on the umbilical cord, may also be used to facilitate delivery of the placenta and amniotic membranes. Oxytocics are usually administered after the placenta is removed because they stimulate the uterus to contract, thereby helping to prevent hemorrhage (see the Nursing Process box: Third Stage of Labor.)

Whether the placenta first appears by its shiny fetal surface (Schultze mechanism) or turns to show its dark roughened maternal surface first (Duncan mechanism) is of no clinical importance.

After the placenta and the amniotic membranes emerge, the primary health care provider examines them for intactness to ensure that no portion remains in the uterine cavity (i.e., no fragments of the placenta or membranes are retained) (Fig. 19-25).

When the third stage of labor has been completed the primary health care provider examines the woman for any perineal, vaginal, or cervical lacerations requiring repair. If an episiotomy was performed, it will be sutured. Immediate repair promotes healing, limits residual damage, and decreases the possibility of infection. The woman usually feels some discomfort while the primary health care provider carries out the postbirth vaginal examination. Help the woman to use breathing and relaxation or distraction techniques to assist her in dealing with the discomfort. During this time the nurse performs a quick assessment of the newborn's physical condition, weighs the baby, and places matching identification bands on baby and mother. The baby may also receive eye prophylaxis and a vitamin K injection at this time.

After any necessary repairs have been completed, cleanse the vulvar area gently with warm water or normal saline, and apply a perineal pad or an ice pack to the perineum. Reposition the birthing bed or table, and lower the woman's legs simultaneously from the stirrups if she gave birth in a lithotomy position. Remove any drapes, and place dry linen under the woman's buttocks. Provide the woman with a clean gown and a blanket, which is warmed, if needed.

The nursing process continues to be used as a framework to manage nursing care during the third stage of labor (see the Nursing Process box: Third Stage of Labor).

Some women and their families may have culturally based beliefs regarding the care of the placenta and the manner of its disposal after birth, viewing the care and disposal of the placenta as a way of protecting the newborn from bad luck and illness. In Spanish the placenta is referred to as *el compañero* or "the companion of the child" (Callister, 2008). Requests by the woman to take the placenta home and dispose of it according to her customs sometimes conflict with health care agency policies, especially those related to infection control and the disposal of biologic wastes. Many cultures follow specific rules regarding the disposal of the placenta in terms of method (burning, drying, burying, eating), site for disposal (in or near the home), and timing of disposal (immediately after birth, time of day, astrologic signs). Disposal rituals may vary according to the gender of the child and the length of time before another child is desired. Some cultures believe that eating the placenta is a means of restoring a woman's well-being after birth or ensuring high-quality breast milk. Health care providers can provide

NURSING PROCESS

Third Stage of Labor

ASSESSMENT

- Signs that suggest the onset of the third stage
  - A firmly contracting fundus
  - A change in the uterus from a discoid to a globular ovoid shape as the placenta moves into the lower uterine segment
  - A sudden gush of dark blood from the introitus
  - Apparent lengthening of the umbilical cord as the placenta descends to the introitus
  - The finding of vaginal fullness (the placenta) on vaginal or rectal examination or of fetal membranes at the introitus
- Physical assessment
  - Perform every 15 minutes: maternal blood pressure, pulse, and respirations
  - Assess for signs of placental separation and amount of bleeding
  - Assist with determination of Apgar score at 1 and 5 minutes after birth
  - Assess maternal and paternal response to completion of childbirth process and their reaction to the newborn

NURSING DIAGNOSES

Possible nursing diagnoses include:

***Risk for Deficient Fluid Volume* related to:**

- blood loss occurring after placental separation and expulsion
- ineffective contraction of the uterus
- unrepaired perineal trauma (e.g., lacerations, episiotomy) associated with vaginal birth

***Risk for Infection* related to:**

- perineal trauma (e.g., lacerations, episiotomy) associated with vaginal birth

***Anxiety* related to:**

- lack of knowledge regarding the separation and expulsion of the placenta
- occurrence of perineal trauma and the need for repair

***Fatigue* related to:**

- energy expenditure associated with childbirth and the bearing-down efforts of the second stage of labor

***Compromised Family Coping* related to:**

- birth of infant whose gender was not preferred by the parents
- unexpected birth of an infant with serious congenital anomalies

***Situational Low Self-esteem (maternal and paternal)* related to:**

- perceived inability to meet personal expectations regarding performance during childbirth

EXPECTED OUTCOMES OF CARE

Expected outcomes for the woman in the third stage of labor are that the woman will:

- Continue normal progression of labor.
- Maintain adequate hydration status through oral or IV intake (or both).
- Actively participate in the labor and birth process.
- Accept comfort and support measures from significant others and health care providers as needed.
- Expel the placenta with a blood loss of less than 500 ml.
- Continue, along with the partner and family, the processes of bonding and attachment with the newborn.
- Express satisfaction with her performance during labor and birth.

PLAN OF CARE AND INTERVENTIONS

- Assist the woman to bear down to facilitate delivery of the separated placenta.
- Administer an oxytocic medication as ordered to insure adequate contraction of the uterus thereby preventing hemorrhage.
- Provide nonpharmacologic and pharmacologic comfort and pain relief measures.
- Perform hygienic cleansing measures.
- Keep woman informed of progress of placental separation and expulsion and of perineal repair if appropriate.
- Explain purpose of medications administered.
- Introduce parents to their baby and facilitate the attachment process by delaying eye prophylaxis; wrap mother and baby together for skin-to-skin contact.
- Provide private time for parents to bond with new baby; help them to create memories.
- Encourage breastfeeding if desired.

EVALUATION

Evaluation of the effectiveness of care of the woman and her family during the third stage of labor is based on the previously stated expected outcomes.

culturally sensitive health care by encouraging women and their families to express their wishes regarding the care and disposal of the placenta and by establishing a policy to fulfill these requests (D'Avanzo, 2008).

FOURTH STAGE OF LABOR

CARE MANAGEMENT

The first 1 to 2 hours after birth, sometimes called the fourth stage of labor, is a crucial time for mother and newborn. Both are not only recovering from the physical process of birth but are also becoming acquainted with each other and additional family members. During this time maternal organs undergo their initial readjustment to the nonpregnant state, and the functions of body systems begin to stabilize.

In most hospitals the mother remains in the labor and birth area during this recovery time. In an institution where LDR rooms are used, the woman stays in the same room where she gave birth. In traditional settings, women are taken from the delivery room to a separate recovery area for observation. Arrangements for care of the newborn vary during the fourth stage of labor. In many settings the baby remains at the mother's bedside, and the labor or birth nurse cares for both of them. In other institutions the baby is taken to the nursery for several hours of observation after an initial bonding period with the parents, siblings, and perhaps other family members (Fig. 19-26).

ASSESSMENT

If the recovery nurse has not previously cared for the new mother, she begins with an oral report from the nurse who attended the woman during labor and birth and a review of the prenatal, labor, and birth records. Of primary importance are conditions that could predispose the mother to hemorrhage,

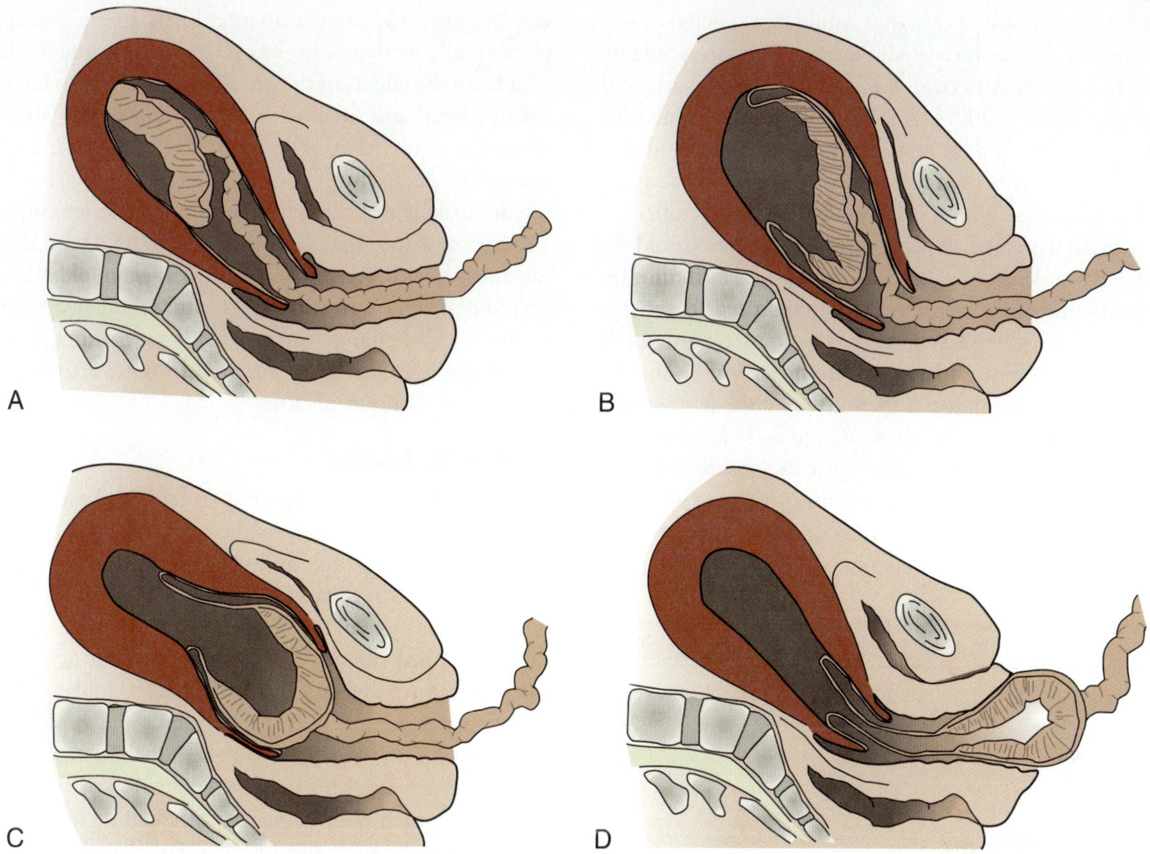

FIG. 19-24 Third stage of labor. **A,** Placenta begins to separate in central portion, accompanied by retroplacental bleeding. Uterus changes from discoid to globular shape. **B,** Placenta completes separation and enters lower uterine segment. Uterus has globular shape. **C,** Placenta enters vagina, cord is seen to lengthen, and there may be an increase in bleeding. **D,** Expulsion (delivery) of placenta and completion of third stage.

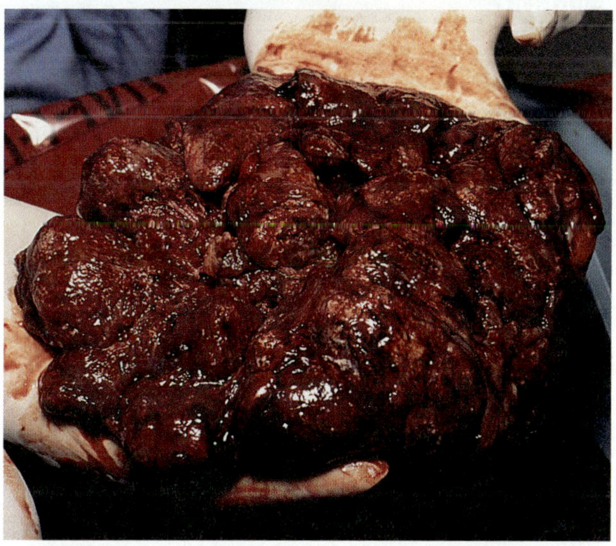

FIG. 19-25 Examination of the placenta. (Courtesy Michael S. Clement, MD, Mesa, AZ.)

such as precipitous labor, a large baby, grand multiparity (i.e., having given birth to six or more viable infants), induced labor, or a magnesium infusion during labor. For healthy women, hemorrhage is the most dangerous potential complication during the fourth stage of labor.

During the first hour following birth, the mother is assessed frequently. Box 19-9 describes the physical assessment of the mother during the fourth stage of labor. All factors except

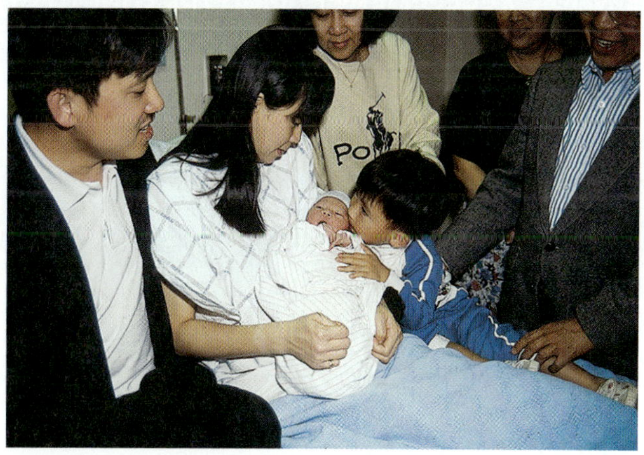

FIG. 19-26 Big brother becomes acquainted with new baby sister. (Courtesy Marjorie Pyle, RNC, Lifecircle, Costa Mesa, CA.)

temperature are assessed every 15 minutes for 1 hour. Temperature is assessed at the beginning and after the first hour of the recovery period. After the fifth 15-minute assessment (which completes the first hour of recovery) if all parameters have stabilized within the normal range, the process is usually repeated once in the second hour.

Postanesthesia Recovery

The woman who has given birth by cesarean or has received regional anesthesia for a vaginal birth requires special attention during the recovery period. Obstetric recovery areas are held to the same standard of care that would be expected of any other postanesthesia recovery (PAR) unit (American Academy of Pediatrics [AAP] & American College of Obstetricians and Gynecologists [ACOG], 2007). A PAR score is determined for each woman on arrival and is updated as part of every 15-minute assessment. Components of the PAR score include activity, respirations, blood pressure, level of consciousness, and color.

If the woman received general anesthesia, she should be awake and alert and oriented to time, place, and person. Her respiratory rate should be within normal limits, and her oxygen saturation level at least 95%, as measured by a pulse oximeter. If the woman received epidural or spinal anesthesia, she should be able to raise her legs, extended at the knees, off the bed, or flex her knees, place her feet flat on the bed, and raise her buttocks well off the bed. The numb or tingling, prickly sensation should be entirely gone from her legs. The length of time required to recover from regional anesthesia varies greatly. Often it takes several hours for these anesthetic effects to disappear completely.

> **! NURSING ALERT**
>
> Regardless of her obstetric status, no woman should be discharged from the recovery area until she has completely recovered from the effects of anesthesia.

Care of the New Mother

Restriction of food and fluid intake and the loss of fluids (blood, perspiration, or emesis) during labor cause many women to be very hungry and thirsty soon after birth. In the absence of complications, a woman who has given birth vaginally; has recovered from the effects of the anesthetic; and has stable vital signs, a firm uterus, and small to moderate lochial flow may have fluids and a regular diet as desired (AAP & ACOG, 2007). In the immediate postpartum period, women who give birth by cesarean are usually restricted to clear liquids and ice chips.

As soon as they have had a chance to bond with the baby and eat, most new mothers are ready for a nap, or at least a quiet period of rest. Following this rest period, the woman may want to shower and change clothes. Most new mothers are capable of self-management or are assisted in these activities by family members or support persons.

Care of the Family

Most parents enjoy being able to handle, hold, explore, and examine the baby immediately after birth. Both parents can assist with the thorough drying of the infant. Usually the infant is wrapped in a receiving blanket and given to the mother or father/partner to hold. If skin-to-skin contact is desired, place the unwrapped infant on the woman's chest or abdomen and then cover the baby with a warm blanket. Holding the newborn next to her skin helps the mother maintain the baby's body heat and provides skin-to-skin contact. Stockinette caps are often used to keep the newborn's head warm and prevent heat loss.

Many women wish to begin breastfeeding their newborns at this time to take advantage of the infant's alert state *(first period of reactivity)* and to stimulate the production of oxytocin that promotes contraction of the uterus and prevents hemorrhage.

BOX 19-9 ASSESSMENT DURING THE FOURTH STAGE OF LABOR

BLOOD PRESSURE
- Measure blood pressure every 15 minutes for the first hour.

PULSE
- Assess rate and regularity. Measure every 15 minutes for the first hour.

TEMPERATURE
- Determine temperature at the beginning of the recovery period and after the first hour of recovery.

FUNDUS
- Position woman with knees flexed and head flat.
- Just below umbilicus, cup hand and press firmly into abdomen. At the same time, stabilize the uterus at the symphysis with the opposite hand (see Fig. 21-3).
- If fundus is firm (and bladder is empty), with uterus in midline, measure its position relative to woman's umbilicus. Lay fingers flat on abdomen under umbilicus; measure how many fingerbreadths (fb) or centimeters (cm) fit between umbilicus and top of fundus. Fundal height is documented according to agency guidelines. For example, if the fundus is 1 fb or 1 cm above the umbilicus, fundal height may be recorded as either +1, u+1, or 1/u. If the fundus is 1 fb or 1 cm below the umbilicus, fundal height may be recorded as either -1, u-1, or u/1.
- If fundus is not firm, massage it gently to contract and expel any clots before measuring distance from umbilicus.
- Place hands appropriately; massage gently only until firm.
- Expel clots while keeping hands placed as in Fig. 21-3. With upper hand, firmly apply pressure downward toward vagina; observe perineum for amount and size of expelled clots.

BLADDER
- Assess distention by noting location and firmness of uterine fundus and by observing and palpating bladder. A distended bladder is seen as a suprapubic rounded bulge that is dull to percussion and fluctuates like a water-filled balloon. When the bladder is distended, the uterus is usually boggy in consistency, well above the umbilicus, and to the woman's right side.
- Assist woman to void spontaneously. Measure amount of urine voided.
- Catheterize as necessary.
- Reassess after voiding or catheterization to make sure the bladder is not palpable and the fundus is firm and in the midline.

LOCHIA
- Observe lochia on perineal pads and on linen under the mother's buttocks. Determine amount and color; note size and number of clots; note odor.
- Observe perineum for source of bleeding (e.g., episiotomy, lacerations).

PERINEUM
- Ask or assist woman to turn on her side and flex upper leg on hip.
- Lift upper buttock.
- Observe perineum in good lighting.
- Assess episiotomy or laceration repair for redness (erythema), edema, ecchymosis (bruising), drainage, and approximation (REEDA).
- Assess for presence of hemorrhoids.

In Baby Friendly Hospitals, breastfeeding is initiated within the first hour after birth. Some women prefer to wait to breastfeed until they have time to rest. In some cultures, however (e.g., Vietnamese and Hispanic), breastfeeding is not acceptable to some women until the milk comes in.

Family-Newborn Relationships

The woman's reaction to the sight of her newborn may range from excited outbursts of laughing, talking, and even crying to apparent apathy. A polite smile and nod may be her only acknowledgment of the comments of nurses and the primary health care provider. Occasionally the reaction is one of anger or indifference; the woman turns away from the baby, concentrates on her own pain, and sometimes makes hostile comments. These varied reactions can arise from pleasure, exhaustion, or deep disappointment. When evaluating parent-newborn interactions after birth, the nurse should consider the cultural characteristics of the woman and her family and the expected behaviors of that culture. In some cultures the birth of a male child is preferred, and women may grieve when a female child is born (D'Avanzo, 2008).

Whatever the reaction and its cause, the woman needs continuing acceptance and support from all staff. Make a notation regarding the parents' reaction to the newborn in the recovery record. Assess this reaction by asking yourself such questions as, "How do the parents look?" "What do they say?" "What do they do?" Conduct further assessment of the parent-newborn relationship as you give care during the period of recovery. This assessment is especially important if you notice warning signs (e.g., passive or hostile reactions to the newborn, disappointment with gender or appearance of the newborn, absence of eye contact, or limited interaction of parents with each other) immediately after birth. Nurses often find it helpful to discuss warning signs with the woman's primary health care provider.

Siblings, who may have appeared only remotely interested in the final phases of the second stage, tend to experience renewed interest and excitement when the newborn appears. They can be encouraged to hold the baby (see Fig. 19-26).

Parents usually respond to praise of their newborn. Many need to be reassured that the dusky appearance of their baby's extremities immediately after birth is normal until circulation is well established. If appropriate, explain the reason for the molding of the newborn's head. Communicate information about hospital routine. Recognize, however, that the cultural background of the parents may influence their expectations regarding the care and handling of their newborn immediately after birth. For example, some traditional Southeast Asians believe that the head should not be touched because it is the most sacred part of a person's body. They also believe that praise of the baby is dangerous because jealous spirits may then cause the baby harm or take it away (D'Avanzo, 2008). Hospital staff members, by their interest and concern, can provide the environment for making this a satisfying experience for parents, family, and significant others.

KEY POINTS

- The onset of labor may be difficult to determine for both nulliparous and multiparous women.
- The familiar environment of her home is most often the ideal place for a woman during the latent phase of the first stage of labor.
- The nurse assumes much of the responsibility for assessing the progress of labor and for keeping the primary health care provider informed about progress in labor and deviations from expected findings.
- The fetal heart rate and pattern reveal the fetal response to the stress of the labor process.
- Assessment of the laboring woman's urinary output and bladder is critical to ensure her progress and to prevent injury to the bladder.
- Regardless of the actual labor and birth experience, the woman's or couple's perception of the birth experience is most likely to be positive when events and performances are consistent with expectations, especially in terms of maintaining control and adequacy of pain relief.
- The woman's level of anxiety may increase when she does not understand what is being said to her about her labor because of the medical terminology used or because of a language barrier.
- Coaching, emotional support, and comfort measures assist the woman to use her energy constructively in relaxing and working with the contractions.
- The progress of labor is enhanced when a woman changes her position frequently during the first stage of labor.
- Doulas provide a continuous, supportive presence during labor that can have a positive effect on the process of childbirth and its outcome.
- The cultural beliefs and practices of a woman and her significant others, including her partner, can have a profound influence on their approach to labor and birth.
- Siblings present for labor and birth need preparation and support for the event.
- Women with a history of sexual abuse often experience profound stress and anxiety during childbirth.
- Inability to palpate the cervix during vaginal examination indicates that complete effacement and full dilation have occurred and is the only certain, objective sign that the second stage has begun.
- Women may have an urge to bear down at various times during labor; for some it may be before the cervix is fully dilated and for others it may not occur until the active phase of the second stage of labor.
- When encouraged to respond to the rhythmic nature of the second stage of labor, the woman normally changes body positions, bears down spontaneously, and vocalizes (open-glottis pushing) when she perceives the urge to push (Ferguson reflex).
- Women should bear down several times during a contraction using the open-glottis pushing method. They should avoid sustained closed-glottis pushing because this will inhibit oxygen transport to the fetus.

KEY POINTS—cont'd

- Nurses can use the role of advocate to prevent routine use of episiotomy and to reduce the incidence of lacerations by empowering women to take an active role in their birth and by educating health care providers about approaches to managing childbirth that reduce the incidence of perineal trauma.
- Objective signs indicate that the placenta has separated and is ready to be expelled; excessive traction (pulling) on the umbilical cord before the placenta has separated can result in maternal injury.
- During the fourth stage of labor, the woman's fundal tone, lochial flow, and vital signs should be assessed frequently to ensure that she is physically recovering well after giving birth.
- Most parents/families enjoy being able to handle, hold, explore, and examine the baby immediately after the birth.

Audio Chapter Summaries Access an audio summary of these Key Points on evolve

REFERENCES

Adams, E., & Bianchi, A. (2004). Can a nurse and a doula exist in the same room? *International Journal of Childbirth Education, 19*(4), 12–15.

Albers, L. (2007). The evidence for physiologic management of the active phase of the first stage of labor. *Journal of Midwifery & Women's Health, 52*(3), 207–215.

Albers, L., Sedler, K., Bedrick, E., Teaf, D., & Peralta, P. (2005). Midwifery care measures in the second stage of labor and reduction of genital tract trauma at birth: A randomized trial. *Journal of Midwifery & Women's Health, 50*(5), 365–372.

American Academy of Pediatrics (AAP) & American College of Obstetricians and Gynecologists (ACOG). (2007). *Guidelines for perinatal care* (6th ed.). Washington, DC: ACOG.

Angelini, D., & Mahlmeister, L. (2005). Liability in triage: Management of EMTALA regulations and common obstetric risks. *Journal of Midwifery & Women's Health, 50*(6), 472–478.

Battista, L., & Wing, D. (2007). Abnormal labor and induction of labor. In S. Gabbe, J. Niebyl, & J. Simpson (Eds.), *Obstetrics: Normal and problem pregnancies* (5th ed.). Philadelphia: Churchill Livingstone.

Beckmann, M., & Garrett, A. (2006). Antenatal perineal massage for reducing perineal trauma. *The Cochrane Database of Systematic Reviews, 2006*, 1, CD005123.

Berghella, V., Baxter, J., & Chauhan, S. (2008). Evidence-based labor and delivery management. *American Journal of Obstetrics & Gynecology, 199*(5), 445–454.

Brancato, R., Church, S., & Stone, P. (2008). A meta-analysis of passive descent versus immediate pushing in nulliparous women with epidural analgesia in the second stage of labor. *Journal of Obstetric, Gynecologic and Neonatal Nursing, 37*(1), 4–12.

Bryanton, J., Gagnon, A., Johnston, C., & Hatem, M. (2008). Predictors of women's perceptions of the childbirth experience. *Journal of Obstetric, Gynecologic and Neonatal Nursing, 37*(1), 24–34.

Callister, L. (2005). What has the literature taught us about culturally competent care of women and children? *MCN American Journal of Maternal/Child Nursing, 30*(6), 380–388.

Callister, L. (2008). Integrating cultural beliefs and practices when caring for childbearing women and familes. In K. Rice Simpson, & P. Creehan (Eds.), *AWHONN's perinatal nursing* (3rd ed.). Philadelphia: Lippincott Williams & Wilkins.

Capogna, G., Camorcia, M., & Stirparo, S. (2007). Expectant fathers' experience during labor with or without epidural analgesia. *International Journal of Obstetric Anesthesia, 16*(2), 110–115.

Centers for Disease Control and Prevention, Branson, B., Handsfield, H., Lampe, M., Janssen, R., Taylor, A., Lyss, S., & Clark, J. (2006). Revised recommendations for HIV testing of adults, adolescents, and pregnant women in health-care settings. *MMWR Morbidity and Mortality Weekly Report, 55*(RR-14), 1–17.

D'Avanzo, C. (2008). *Mosby's pocket guide to cultural health assessment* (4th ed.). St. Louis: Mosby.

DeFrances, C., Cullen, K., & Kozak, L. (2007). National hospital discharge survey: 2005 annual summary with detailed diagnosis and procedure data. National Center for Health Statistics. *Vital and Health Statistics, 13*(165), 1–218.

Gilbert, E. (2011). *Manual of high risk pregnancy & delivery* (5th ed.). St. Louis: Mosby.

Hanson, L. (2009). Second-stage labor care: Challenges in spontaneous bearing down. *Journal of Perinatal and Neonatal Nursing, 23*(1), 31–39.

Hodnett, E., Gates, S., Hofmeyr, G., & Sakala, C. (2007). Continuous support for women during childbirth. *The Cochrane Database of Systematic Reviews, 2007*, 3, CD003766.

Hofmeyr, G. (2005). Evidence-based intrapartum care. *Best Practices Research in Clinical Obstetrics and Gynaecology, 19*(1), 103–115.

Kilpatrick, S., & Garrison, E. (2007). Normal labor and delivery. In S. Gabbe, J. Niebyl, & J. Simpson (Eds.), *Obstetrics: Normal and problem pregnancies* (5th ed.). Philadelphia: Churchill Livingstone.

MacKinnon, K., McIntyre, M., & Quance, M. (2005). The meaning of the nurse's presence during childbirth. *Journal of Obstetric, Gynecologic and Neonatal Nursing, 34*(1), 28–36.

Parsons, M., Bidwell, J., & Nagy, S. (2006). Natural eating behavior in latent labor and its effect on outcomes in active labor. *Journal of Midwifery & Women's Health, 51*(1), e1–e6.

Pascali-Bonaro, D., & Kroeger, M. (2004). Continuous female companionship during childbirth: A crucial resource in times of stress or calm. *Journal of Midwifery & Women's Health, 49*(4 Suppl. 1), 19–27.

Reveiz, L., Gaitan, H., & Cuervo, L. (2007). Enemas during labour. *The Cochrane Database of Systematic Reviews, 2007*, 4, CD000330.

Roberts, J. (2002). The "push" for evidence: Management of the second stage. *Journal of Midwifery & Women's Health, 47*(1), 2–15.

Roberts, J., & Hanson, L. (2007). Best practices in second stage labor care: Maternal bearing down and positioning. *Journal of Midwifery & Women's Health, 52*(3), 238–245.

Sampselle, C., Miller, J., Luecha, Y., Fischer, K., & Rosten, L. (2005). Provider support of spontaneous pushing during the second stage of labor. *Journal of Obstetric, Gynecologic and Neonatal Nursing, 34*(6), 695–702.

Schaffer, J., Bloom, S., Casey, B., McIntire, D., Nihira, M., & Leveno, K. (2005). A randomized trial of the effects of coached vs uncoached maternal pushing during the second-stage of labor on postpartum pelvic floor structure and function. *American Journal of Obstetrics & Gynecology, 192*(5), 1692–1696.

Simkin, P., & Way, K. (2008). *Doulas of North America (DONA) international position paper: The birth doula's contribution to modern maternity care.* Available at www.DONA.org. Accessed July 5, 2010.

Simpson, K. (2005). The context and clinical evidence for common nursing practices during labor. *MCN American Journal of Maternal/Child Nursing, 30*(6), 356–363.

Simpson, K. (2008). Labor and birth. In K. Rice Simpson, & P. Creehan (Eds.), *AWHONN's perinatal nursing* (3rd ed.). Philadelphia: Lippincott Williams & Wilkins.

Simpson, K., Cesario, S., Morin, K., Trapani, K., Mayberry, L., & Snelgrove-Clark, E. (2008). *Nursing care and management of the second stage of labor: Evidence-based clinical practice guideline* (2nd ed.). Washington, DC: Association of Women's Health, Obstetric and Neonatal Nurses.

Simpson, K., & James, D. (2005). Effects of immediate versus delayed pushing during second stage labor on fetal well-being: A randomized clinical trial. *Nursing Research, 54*(3), 149–157.

Tranmer, J., Hodnett, E., Hannah, M., & Stevens, B. (2005). The effect of unrestricted oral carbohydrate intake on labor progress. *Journal of Obstetric, Gynecologic and Neonatal Nursing, 34*(3), 319–328.

Tucker, S., Miller, L., & Miller, D. (2009). *Mosby's pocket guide to fetal monitoring: A multidisciplinary approach* (6th ed.). St. Louis: Mosby.

Walls, D. (2009). Herbs and natural therapies for pregnancy, birth, and breastfeeding. *International Journal of Childbirth Education, 24*(2), 29–37.

Waterbirth International. (2009). *Frequently asked questions.* Available at http://waterbirth.org. Accessed July 5, 2010.

Zwelling, E. (2010). Overcoming the challenges: Maternal movement and positioning to facilitate labor progress. *MCN American Journal of Maternal/Child Nursing, 35*(2), 72–78.

Zwelling, E., Johnson, K., & Allen, J. (2006). How to implement complementary therapies for laboring women. *MCN American Journal of Maternal/Child Nursing, 31*(6), 364–372.

CHAPTER

20

Postpartum Physiology

Shannon E. Perry

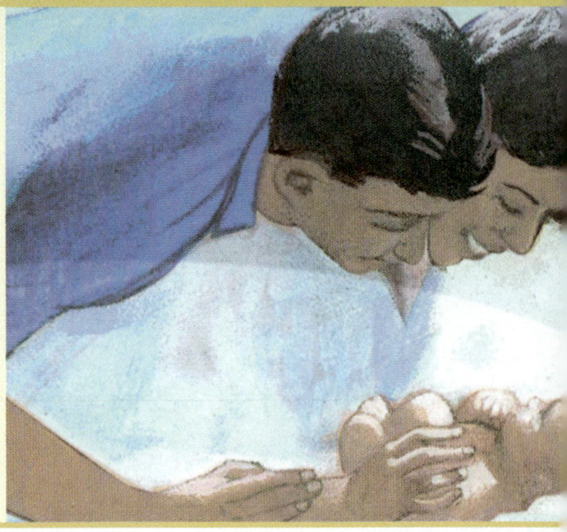

evolve WEBSITE

http://evolve.elsevier.com/Lowdermilk/MWHC/

Audio Glossary

Audio Key Points

NCLEX Review Questions

Spanish Guidelines

Postpartum Physical Assessment

Video—Nursing Skills

Assessing the Fundus Postpartum

LEARNING OBJECTIVES

- Describe the anatomic and physiologic changes that occur during the postpartum period.
- Identify characteristics of uterine involution and lochial flow and describe ways to measure them.
- List expected values for vital signs, deviations from normal findings, and probable causes of the deviations.

The postpartum period is the interval between the birth of the newborn and the return of the reproductive organs to their normal nonpregnant state. This period is sometimes known as the **puerperium,** or fourth trimester of pregnancy. Although the puerperium has traditionally been considered to last 6 weeks, this time frame varies among women. The distinct physiologic changes that occur as the processes of pregnancy are reversed are normal. To provide care during the recovery period that is beneficial to the mother, her infant, and her family, the nurse must synthesize knowledge of maternal anatomy and physiology, the newborn's physical and behavioral characteristics, infant care activities, and the family response to the birth of the child. This chapter focuses on anatomic and physiologic changes that occur in the woman during the postpartum period.

REPRODUCTIVE SYSTEM AND ASSOCIATED STRUCTURES

Uterus

Involution Process

The return of the uterus to a nonpregnant state after birth is known as **involution.** This process begins immediately after expulsion of the placenta with contraction of the uterine smooth muscle.

At the end of the third stage of labor, the uterus is in the midline, approximately 2 cm below the level of the umbilicus, with the fundus resting on the sacral promontory. At this time the uterus weighs approximately 1000 g (Cunningham, Leveno, Bloom, Hauth, Rouse, & Spong, 2010).

Within 12 hours the fundus rises to approximately the level of the umbilicus (Fig. 20-1). The fundus descends 1 to 2 cm every 24 hours. By 1 week after birth the fundus is normally located halfway between the umbilicus and the symphysis pubis. The uterus should not be palpable abdominally after 2 weeks and should have returned to its nonpregnant location by 6 weeks after birth (Blackburn, 2007).

The uterus, which at full term weighs approximately 11 times its prepregnancy weight, involutes to approximately 500 g by 1 week after birth and to 350 g by 2 weeks after birth. At 6 weeks postpartum, it weighs 60 to 80 g.

Increased estrogen and progesterone levels are responsible for stimulating the massive growth of the uterus during pregnancy. Prenatal uterine growth results from both hyperplasia, an increase in the number of muscle cells, and hypertrophy, enlargement of the existing cells. Postpartally the decrease in the secretion of these hormones causes **autolysis,** the self-destruction of excess hypertrophied tissue. The additional cells laid down during pregnancy remain, however, and account for the slight increase in uterine size after each pregnancy.

Subinvolution is the failure of the uterus to return to a nonpregnant state. The most common causes of subinvolution are retained placental fragments and infection (see Chapter 34).

Contractions

Postpartum hemostasis is achieved primarily by compression of intramyometrial blood vessels as the uterine muscle contracts, rather than by platelet aggregation and clot formation. The hormone oxytocin, released from the posterior pituitary

Video—Nursing Skills: Assessing the Fundus Postpartum

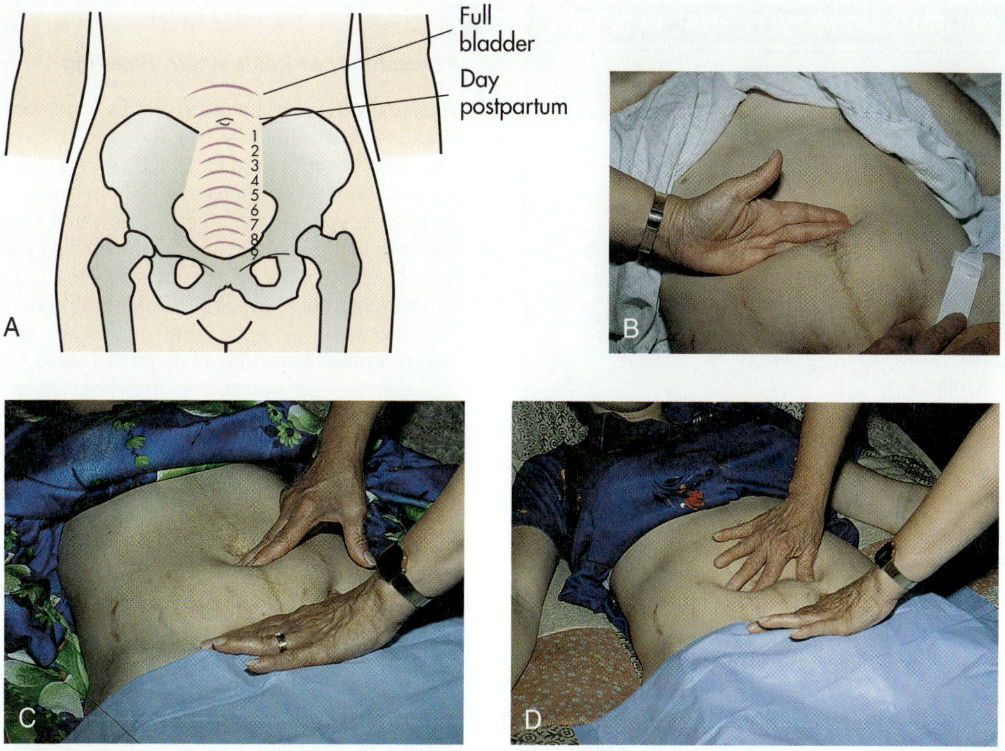

FIG. 20-1 Assessment of involution of uterus after childbirth. **A,** Normal progress, days 1 through 9. **B,** Size and position of uterus 2 hours after childbirth. **C,** Two days after childbirth. **D,** Four days after childbirth. (**B, C,** and **D,** Courtesy Marjorie Pyle, RNC, Lifecircle, Costa Mesa, CA.)

gland, strengthens and coordinates these uterine contractions, which compress blood vessels and promote hemostasis. During the first 1 to 2 postpartum hours, uterine contractions may decrease in intensity and become uncoordinated. Because the uterus must remain firm and well contracted, exogenous oxytocin (Pitocin) is usually administered intravenously or intramuscularly immediately after expulsion of the placenta. Women who plan to breastfeed can be encouraged to put the baby to her breast immediately after birth because suckling stimulates oxytocin release.

Afterpains

In first-time mothers, uterine tone is good, the fundus generally remains firm, and the woman usually perceives only mild uterine cramping. Periodic relaxation and vigorous contraction are more common in subsequent pregnancies and may cause uncomfortable cramping called **afterpains (afterbirth pains)** that persist throughout the early puerperium. Afterpains are more noticeable after births in which the uterus was overdistended (e.g., large baby, multifetal gestation, polyhydramnios). Breastfeeding and exogenous oxytocic medication usually intensify these afterpains, because both stimulate uterine contractions.

Placental Site

Immediately after the placenta and membranes are expelled, vascular constriction and thromboses reduce the placental site to an irregular nodular and elevated area. Upward growth of the endometrium causes sloughing of necrotic tissue and prevents the scar formation that is characteristic of normal wound healing. This unique healing process enables the endometrium to resume its usual cycle of changes and to permit implantation and placentation in future pregnancies. Endometrial regeneration is completed by postpartum day 16, except at the placental site. Regeneration at the placental site occurs gradually and is not usually complete until 6 weeks after birth (Blackburn, 2007).

Lochia

Uterine discharge after childbirth, commonly called **lochia,** is initially bright red (lochia rubra) and may contain small clots. For the first 2 hours after birth the amount of uterine discharge should be approximately that of a heavy menstrual period. After that time the lochial flow should steadily decrease.

Lochia rubra consists mainly of blood and decidual and trophoblastic debris. The flow pales, becoming pink or brown (lochia serosa) after 3 to 4 days. **Lochia serosa** consists of old blood, serum, leukocytes, and tissue debris. The median duration of lochia serosa discharge is 22 to 27 days (Katz, 2007). In most women, approximately 10 days after childbirth the drainage becomes yellow to white (lochia alba). **Lochia alba** consists primarily of leukocytes and decidual cells but also contains epithelial cells, mucus, serum, and bacteria. Lochia alba usually continues for 10 to 14 days but may last longer and still be normal. Thus lochia persists up to 4 to 8 weeks after birth (Cunningham et al., 2010).

If the woman receives an oxytocic medication, regardless of the route of administration, the flow of lochia is often scant until the effects of the medication wear off. The amount of lochia typically is less after cesarean births because the surgeon suctions the blood and fluids from the uterus or wipes the uterine lining before closing the incision. Flow of lochia usually

TABLE 20-1 LOCHIAL AND NONLOCHIAL BLEEDING

LOCHIAL BLEEDING	NONLOCHIAL BLEEDING
Lochia usually trickles from the vaginal opening. The steady flow increases as the uterus contracts. A gush of lochia may result as the uterus is massaged. If the lochia is dark in color, it has pooled in the relaxed vagina, and the amount soon lessens to a trickle of bright red lochia (in the early puerperium). Excess lochia can be due to uterine atony and can lead to postpartum hemorrhage.	If the bloody discharge spurts from the vagina, damage to a blood vessel may have occurred during birth. This bleeding is not just normal lochial flow. If the amount of bleeding continues to be excessive and bright red, a vaginal or cervical tear may be the source.

increases with ambulation and breastfeeding. Lochia tends to pool in the vagina when the woman is lying in bed; on standing, the woman may experience a gush of blood. This gush should not be confused with hemorrhage.

Persistence of lochia rubra early in the postpartum period suggests continued bleeding as a result of retained fragments of the placenta or membranes. Recurrence of bleeding approximately 7 to 14 days after birth is from the healing placental site. Approximately 10% to 15% of women will still be experiencing normal lochia serosa discharge at their 6-week postpartum examination (Katz, 2007). In the majority of women, however, a continued flow of lochia serosa or lochia alba by 3 to 4 weeks after birth may indicate endometritis, particularly if fever, pain, or abdominal tenderness is associated with the discharge. Lochia should smell like normal menstrual flow; an offensive odor usually indicates infection.

Not all postpartal bleeding is lochia; bleeding after birth may be a result of unrepaired vaginal or cervical lacerations or uterine atony (see Chapter 34). Table 20-1 distinguishes between lochial and nonlochial bleeding.

Cervix

The cervix is soft immediately after birth. The ectocervix (portion of the cervix that protrudes into the vagina) appears bruised and has some small lacerations—optimal conditions for the development of infection. Over the next 12 to 18 hours it shortens and becomes firmer. The cervical os, which dilated to 10 cm during labor, closes gradually. Within 2 to 3 days postpartum it has shortened, become firm, and regained its form. The cervix up to the lower uterine segment remains edematous, thin, and fragile for several days after birth. By the second or third postpartum day the cervix is dilated 2 to 3 cm, and by 1 week after birth it is approximately 1 cm dilated (Blackburn, 2007). The external cervical os never regains its prepregnancy appearance; it no longer has a circular shape but appears as a jagged slit often described as a "fish mouth" (see Fig. 13-2). Lactation delays the production of cervical and other estrogen-influenced mucus and mucosal characteristics.

Vagina and Perineum

Postpartum estrogen deprivation is responsible for the thinness of the vaginal mucosa and the absence of rugae. The greatly distended smooth-walled vagina gradually decreases in size and regains tone, although it never completely returns to its prepregnancy state (Cunningham et al., 2010). Rugae reappear within 3 to 4 weeks, but they are never as prominent as they are in the nulliparous woman. Most rugae are permanently flattened. The hymen remains as small tags of tissue that scar and form the myrtiform caruncles (Cunningham et al.). The mucosa remains atrophic in the lactating woman, at least until menstruation resumes. Thickening of the vaginal mucosa occurs with the return of ovarian function. Estrogen deficiency is also responsible for a decreased amount of vaginal lubrication. Localized dryness and coital discomfort (dyspareunia) may persist until ovarian function returns and menstruation resumes. The use of a water-soluble lubricant during sexual intercourse is usually recommended.

Immediately after birth the introitus is erythematous and edematous, especially in the area of the episiotomy or laceration repair. It is usually barely distinguishable from that of a nulliparous woman if lacerations and an episiotomy have been carefully repaired, hematomas are prevented or treated early, and the woman observes good hygiene during the first 2 weeks after birth.

Most episiotomies and laceration repairs are visible only if the woman is lying on her side with her upper buttock raised or if she is placed in the lithotomy position. A good light source is essential for visualization of some repairs. Healing of an episiotomy or laceration is the same as that of any surgical incision. Signs of infection (pain, redness, warmth, swelling, or discharge) or the loss of approximation (separation of the incision edges) may occur. Initial healing occurs within 2 to 3 weeks, but 4 to 6 months can be required for the repair to heal completely (Blackburn, 2007).

Hemorrhoids (anal varicosities) are commonly seen (see Fig. 13-10). Internal hemorrhoids can evert while the woman is pushing during birth. Women often experience associated

CLINICAL REASONING

Assessment of Postpartum Bleeding

You are the nurse assigned to care for Maria Rosa, a G7, now P7, who gave birth vaginally 1 hour ago to twins. Twin A weighed 6 pounds, 4 ounces (2835 g), and Twin B weighed 6 pounds, 8 ounces (2948 g). The babies were born over an intact perineum, that is, Maria Rosa had no episiotomy and sustained no lacerations requiring repair. You are at the nurse's station when Maria Rosa calls and asks for her nurse to "come quick!" When you arrive in her room, you find Maria Rosa lying in a pool of blood. The disposable pad underneath her, as well as her perineal pad, are completely soaked with bright red blood.

1. Evidence—Is the evidence sufficient to draw conclusions about what immediate assesments are necessary to determine the cause and management of Maria Rosa's excessive bleeding?
2. Assumptions—can be made about the following issues:
   a. Normal amount of lochia expected at this time (1 hour after birth)
   b. Maria Rosa's risk factors for uterine atony
   c. Immediate nursing interventions for Maria Rosa
   d. Other possible causes for Maria Rosa's excessive bleeding
3. What implications and priorities for nursing care can be made a this time? Use the situation background assessment recommendation (SBAR) technique to report Maria Rosa's primary health care provider about her current status.
4. Does the evidence objectively support your conclusion?
5. Are there alternative perspectives to your conclusion?

symptoms such as itching, discomfort, and bright red bleeding with defecation. Hemorrhoids usually decrease in size within 6 weeks of childbirth.

Pelvic Muscular Support

The supporting structure of the uterus and vagina may be injured during childbirth and contributes to later gynecologic problems. Supportive tissues of the pelvic floor that are torn or stretched during childbirth may require up to 6 months to regain tone. Kegel exercises, which help to strengthen perineal muscles and encourage healing, are recommended after childbirth (see the Teaching for Self-Management box, p. 91). Later in life, women can experience **pelvic relaxation,** the lengthening and weakening of the fascial supports of pelvic structures. These structures include the uterus, the upper posterior vaginal wall, the urethra, the bladder, and the rectum. Although pelvic relaxation can occur in any woman, it is usually a direct but delayed complication of childbirth (see Chapter 11).

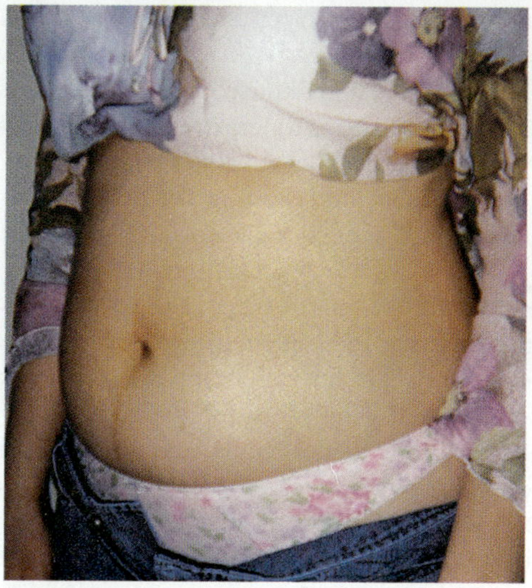

FIG. 20-2 Abdominal wall 6 weeks after vaginal birth is almost back to prepregnancy appearance. Note that the linea nigra is still visible. (Courtesy Jodi Brackett, Phoenix, AZ.)

ENDOCRINE SYSTEM

Placental Hormones

Significant hormonal changes occur during the postpartal period. Expulsion of the placenta results in dramatic decreases of the hormones produced by that organ. Decreases in human chorionic somatomammotropin, estrogens, cortisol, and the placental enzyme insulinase reverse the diabetogenic effects of pregnancy, resulting in significantly lower blood sugar levels in the immediate puerperium. For several days after birth, mothers with type 1 diabetes will likely require much less insulin than they did at the end of pregnancy. Because these normal hormonal changes make the puerperium a transitional period for carbohydrate metabolism, interpreting glucose tolerance tests is difficult at this time.

Estrogen and progesterone levels decrease markedly after expulsion of the placenta and reach their lowest levels 1 week after childbirth. Decreased estrogen levels are associated with breast engorgement and with the diuresis of excess extracellular fluid accumulated during pregnancy. In nonlactating women, estrogen levels begin to rise by 2 weeks after birth and by postpartum day 17 are higher than in women who breastfeed (Katz, 2007).

Human chorionic gonadotropin (hCG) disappears fairly quickly from maternal circulation. However, because removing hCG from the extravascular and intracellular spaces takes additional time, the hormone can be detected in the maternal system for 3 to 4 weeks after birth (Blackburn, 2007).

Pituitary Hormones and Ovarian Function

Lactating and nonlactating women differ considerably in the time when the first ovulation occurs and when menstruation resumes. The persistence of elevated serum prolactin levels in breastfeeding women appears to be responsible for suppressing ovulation (Katz, 2007). Prolactin levels in blood rise progressively throughout pregnancy and remain elevated in women who breastfeed (Lawrence & Lawrence, 2009). The duration of anovulation is influenced by the frequency of breastfeeding, the duration of each feeding, and the degree to which supplementary feedings are used (Katz). Individual differences in the strength of an infant's sucking stimulus probably also affect prolactin levels. In women who breastfeed, the mean length of time to initial ovulation is approximately 6 months (Blackburn, 2007; Katz).

In nonlactating women, prolactin levels decline after birth and reach the prepregnant range by the third postpartum week (Katz, 2007). Ovulation occurs as early as 27 days after birth in nonlactating women, with a mean time of approximately 70 to 75 days. Menstruation usually resumes by 4 to 6 weeks postpartum after childbirth. Some women ovulate before their first postpartum menstrual period occurs; therefore, contraceptive options should be discussed early in the puerperium (Blackburn, 2007; Cunningham et al., 2010).

The first menstrual flow after childbirth is usually heavier than usual. Within three or four cycles, the amount of menstrual flow returns to the woman's prepregnancy volume.

ABDOMEN

When the woman stands up during the first days after birth, her abdomen protrudes and gives her a still-pregnant appearance. During the first 2 weeks after birth the abdominal wall is relaxed. Approximately 6 weeks are required for the abdominal wall to approximate its prepregnancy state (Fig. 20-2). The skin regains most of its previous elasticity, but some striae may persist. The return of muscle tone depends on previous tone, proper exercise, and the amount of adipose tissue present. Occasionally, with or without overdistention because of a large fetus or multiple fetuses, the abdominal wall muscles separate, a condition termed **diastasis recti abdominis** (see Fig. 13-13b). Persistence of this defect may be disturbing to the woman, but surgical correction is rarely necessary. With time, the defect becomes less apparent.

URINARY SYSTEM

The hormonal changes of pregnancy (i.e., high steroid levels) contribute to an increase in renal function; diminishing steroid levels after birth may partly explain the reduced renal function that occurs during the puerperium. Kidney function returns to normal within 1 month after birth. From 2 to 8 weeks are required for the pregnancy-induced hypotonia and dilation of the ureters and renal pelves to return to the nonpregnant state (Cunningham et al., 2010). In a small percentage of women, dilation of the urinary tract can persist for 3 months, which increases the chance of developing a urinary tract infection.

Urine Components

The renal glycosuria induced by pregnancy disappears by 1 week postpartum (Blackburn, 2007), but lactosuria can occur in lactating women. The blood urea nitrogen (BUN) level increases during the puerperium as autolysis of the involuting uterus occurs. This breakdown of excess protein in the uterine muscle cells also contributes to pregnancy-associated proteinuria, which resolves by 6 weeks after birth. The BUN returns to a nonpregnant level by 2 to 3 months after childbirth (Blackburn). Ketonuria can occur in women with an uncomplicated birth or after a prolonged labor with dehydration.

Postpartal Diuresis

Within 12 hours of birth, women begin to lose the excess tissue fluid accumulated during pregnancy. Profuse diaphoresis often occurs, especially at night, for the first 2 or 3 days after childbirth. Postpartal diuresis, caused by decreased estrogen levels, removal of increased venous pressure in the lower extremities, and loss of the remaining pregnancy-induced increase in blood volume, also aids the body in ridding itself of excess fluid. Fluid loss through perspiration and increased urinary output accounts for a weight loss of approximately 2.25 kg during the early puerperium.

Urethra and Bladder

Birth-induced trauma, increased bladder capacity after childbirth, and the effects of conduction anesthesia combine to cause a decreased urge to void. In addition, pelvic soreness caused by the forces of labor, vaginal lacerations, or an episiotomy reduces or alters the voiding reflex. Decreased voiding, combined with postpartal diuresis, can result in bladder distention.

Immediately after birth excessive bleeding can occur if the bladder becomes distended because it pushes the uterus up and to the side and prevents it from contracting firmly. Later in the puerperium overdistention can make the bladder increasingly susceptible to infection and impede the resumption of normal voiding (Cunningham et al., 2010). With adequate emptying of the bladder, bladder tone is usually restored 5 to 7 days after childbirth.

GASTROINTESTINAL SYSTEM

Appetite

The mother is usually hungry shortly after giving birth and can tolerate a light diet. Most new mothers are very hungry after full recovery from analgesia, anesthesia, and fatigue. Requests for extra portions of food and frequent snacks are common.

Bowel Evacuation

A spontaneous bowel evacuation may not occur for 2 to 3 days after childbirth. This delay can be explained by decreased muscle tone in the intestines during labor and the immediate puerperium, prelabor diarrhea, lack of food, or dehydration. The mother often anticipates discomfort during the bowel movement because of perineal tenderness as a result of an episiotomy, lacerations, or hemorrhoids and resists the urge to defecate. Regular bowel habits should be reestablished when bowel tone returns.

Operative vaginal birth (forceps use) and anal sphincter lacerations are associated with an increased risk of postpartum anal incontinence. Women with this problem are more often incontinent of flatus than of stool. If anal incontinence lasts more than 6 months, studies should be conducted to determine the specific cause and appropriate treatment (Katz, 2007).

BREASTS

Promptly after birth a decrease occurs in the concentrations of hormones (i.e., estrogen, progesterone, hCG, prolactin, cortisol, and insulin) that stimulated breast development during pregnancy. The time required for these hormones to return to prepregnancy levels is determined in part by whether the mother breastfeeds her infant.

Breastfeeding Mothers

During the first 24 hours after birth, little if any change occurs in the breast tissue. Colostrum or early milk, a clear yellow fluid, may be expressed from the breasts. The breasts gradually become fuller and heavier as the colostrum transitions to mature milk by approximately 72 to 96 hours after birth; this breast change is often referred to as the "milk coming in." The breasts may feel warm, firm, and somewhat tender. Bluish-white milk with a skim-milk appearance (mature milk) can be expressed from the nipples. As milk glands and milk ducts fill with milk, breast tissue may feel somewhat nodular or lumpy. Unlike the lumps associated with fibrocystic breast disease or cancer (which may be palpated consistently in the same location), the nodularity associated with milk production tends to shift in position. Some women experience engorgement, but with frequent breastfeeding and proper care, this condition is temporary and typically lasts only 24 to 48 hours (see Chapter 25).

Nonbreastfeeding Mothers

The breasts generally feel nodular in contrast to the granular feel of breasts in nonpregnant women. The nodularity is bilateral and diffuse. Prolactin levels drop rapidly. Colostrum is present for the first few days after childbirth. Palpation of the breasts on the second or third day, as milk production begins, may reveal tissue tenderness in some women. On the third or fourth postpartum day, engorgement may occur. The breasts are distended (swollen), firm, tender, and warm to the touch (because of vasocongestion). Breast distention is caused primarily by the temporary congestion of veins and lymphatics rather than by an accumulation of milk. Milk is present but should not be expressed. Axillary breast tissue (the tail of Spence) and any accessory breast or nipple tissue along the milk line may be involved. Engorgement resolves spontaneously, and discomfort usually decreases within 24 to 36 hours. A breast binder or well-fitted, supportive bra, ice packs, fresh cabbage leaves (see Fig. 25-15), and mild analgesics may be used to relieve discomfort. Nipple stimulation is avoided. If suckling or expression of milk (pumping) is never begun (or is discontinued), lactation ceases within a few days to a week.

TABLE 20-2 **VITAL SIGNS AFTER CHILDBIRTH**

NORMAL FINDINGS	DEVIATIONS FROM NORMAL FINDINGS AND PROBABLE CAUSES
Temperature	
Temperature during first 24 hours may rise to 38° C as a result of dehydrating effects of labor or a consequence of epidural anesthesia. After 24 hours the woman should be afebrile.	A diagnosis of puerperal sepsis is suggested if a rise in maternal temperature to 38° C is noted after the first 24 hours after childbirth and recurs or persists for 2 days. Other possible diagnoses are mastitis, endometritis, urinary tract infection, and other systemic infections.
Pulse	
Pulse returns to nonpregnant levels within a few days postpartum, although the rate of return varies among individual women.	A rapid pulse rate or one that is increasing may indicate hypovolemia as a result of hemorrhage.
Respirations	
Respirations should decrease to within the woman's normal prepregnancy range by 6 to 8 weeks after birth.	Hypoventilation may follow an unusually high subarachnoid (spinal) block or epidural narcotic after a cesarean birth.
Blood Pressure	
Blood pressure is altered slightly if at all. Orthostatic hypotension, as indicated by feelings of faintness or dizziness immediately after standing up, can develop in the first 48 hours as a result of the splanchnic engorgement that can occur after birth.	A low or decreasing blood pressure may reflect hypovolemia secondary to hemorrhage. It is a late sign, however, and other symptoms of hemorrhage usually alert the staff. An increased reading may result from excessive use of vasopressor or oxytocic medications. Because preeclampsia can persist into or occur first in the postpartum period, routine evaluation of blood pressure is needed. If a woman complains of headache, hypertension must be ruled out as a cause before analgesics are administered.

CARDIOVASCULAR SYSTEM

Blood Volume

Changes in blood volume after birth depend on several factors, such as blood loss during childbirth and the amount of extravascular water (physiologic edema) mobilized and excreted. Pregnancy-induced hypervolemia (an increase in blood volume of at least 35% more than prepregnancy values near term) allows most women to tolerate considerable blood loss during childbirth. The average blood loss for a vaginal birth of a single fetus ranges from 300 ml to 500 ml (10% of blood volume). The typical blood loss for women who give birth by cesarean is 500 ml to 1000 ml (15% to 30% of blood volume). During the first few days after birth the plasma volume decreases further as a result of diuresis (Blackburn, 2007).

The woman's response to blood loss during the early puerperium differs from that in a nonpregnant woman. Three postpartum physiologic changes protect the woman by increasing the circulating blood volume: (1) elimination of uteroplacental circulation reduces the size of the maternal vascular bed by 10% to 15%, (2) loss of placental endocrine function removes the stimulus for vasodilation, and (3) mobilization of extravascular water stored during pregnancy occurs. By the third postpartum day the plasma volume has been replenished as extravascular fluid returns to the intravascular space (Katz, 2007).

Cardiac Output

Pulse rate, stroke volume, and cardiac output increase throughout pregnancy. Cardiac output remains increased for at least the first 48 hours postpartum because of an increase in stroke volume. This increased stroke volume is caused by the return of blood to the maternal systemic venous circulation, a result of a rapid decrease in uterine blood flow and mobilization of extravascular fluid (Blackburn, 2007). Cardiac output decreases by 30% by 2 weeks after childbirth and then gradually decreases to nonpregnant values by 6 to 12 weeks in most women. Stroke volume, end diastolic volume, cardiac output, and systemic vascular resistance remain elevated in some women over nonpregnant values for up to 12 weeks or longer (Blackburn).

Vital Signs

Few alterations in vital signs are seen under normal circumstances. Heart rate and blood pressure return to nonpregnant levels within a few days (Katz, 2007) (Table 20-2). Respiratory function rapidly returns to nonpregnant levels after birth (Blackburn, 2007). After the uterus is emptied, the diaphragm descends, the normal cardiac axis is restored, and the point of maximal impulse and the electrocardiogram are normalized.

Blood Components

Hematocrit and Hemoglobin

After childbirth the total blood volume decreases by approximately 16% from its prebirth value, resulting in a transient anemia. After 8 weeks, however, the number of red blood cells has increased and the majority of women have a normal hematocrit (Katz, 2007).

White Blood Cell Count

Normal leukocytosis of pregnancy averages approximately 12,000/mm^3. During the first 10 to 12 days after childbirth, values between 20,000 and 25,000/mm^3 are common. Neutrophils are the most numerous white blood cells. Leukocytosis, coupled with the normal increase in erythrocyte sedimentation rate, can obscure the diagnosis of acute infection at this time.

Coagulation Factors

Clotting factors and fibrinogen are normally increased during pregnancy and remain elevated in the immediate puerperium. When combined with vessel damage and immobility, this hypercoagulable state causes an increased risk of thromboembolism, especially after a cesarean birth. Fibrinolytic activity also increases during the first few days after childbirth (Katz, 2007). Factors I, II, VII, VIII, IX, and X decrease to nonpregnant levels within a few days. Fibrin split products, probably released from the placental site, also can be found in maternal blood.

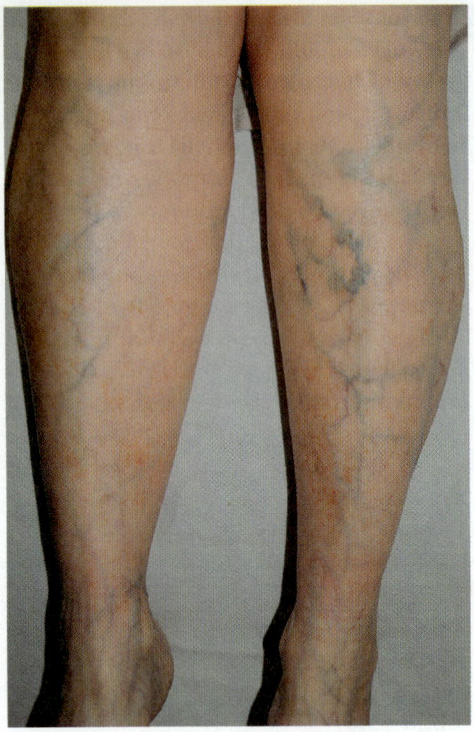

Fig. 20-3 Varicosities in legs. (Courtesy Cheryl Briggs, RNC, Annapolis, MD.)

Varicosities

Varicosities (varices) of the legs (Fig. 20-3) and around the anus (hemorrhoids) are common during pregnancy. Varices, even the less common vulvar varices, regress (empty) rapidly immediately after childbirth. Surgical repair of varicosities is not considered during pregnancy. Total or nearly total regression of varicosities is expected after childbirth.

NEUROLOGIC SYSTEM

Neurologic changes during the puerperium are those that result from a reversal of maternal adaptations to pregnancy and those resulting from trauma during labor and childbirth.

Pregnancy-induced neurologic discomforts disappear after birth. Elimination of physiologic edema through the diuresis that follows childbirth relieves carpal tunnel syndrome by easing the compression of the median nerve. The periodic numbness and tingling of fingers that afflict 5% of pregnant women usually disappear after childbirth unless lifting and carrying the baby aggravate the condition. Headache requires careful assessment. Postpartum headaches can be caused by various conditions, including postpartum-onset preeclampsia, stress, and leakage of cerebrospinal fluid into the extradural space during placement of the needle for epidural or spinal anesthesia. Depending on the cause and effectiveness of the treatment, the duration of the headaches can vary from 1 to 3 days to several weeks.

MUSCULOSKELETAL SYSTEM

Adaptations of the mother's musculoskeletal system that occur during pregnancy are reversed in the puerperium. These adaptations include the relaxation and subsequent hypermobility of the joints and the change in the mother's center of gravity in response to the enlarging uterus. The joints are completely stabilized by 6 to 8 weeks after birth. Although all other joints return to their normal prepregnancy state, those in the parous woman's feet do not. The new mother may notice a permanent increase in her shoe size.

INTEGUMENTARY SYSTEM

Chloasma (mask) of pregnancy usually disappears at the end of pregnancy. Hyperpigmentation of the areolae and linea nigra may not regress completely after childbirth. Some women will have permanent darker pigmentation of those areas (see Fig. 13-11). Striae gravidarum (stretch marks) on the breasts, the abdomen, the hips, and the thighs may fade but usually do not disappear.

Vascular abnormalities such as spider angiomas (nevi), palmar erythema, and an epulis generally regress in response to the rapid decline in estrogen levels after pregnancy. Spider nevi persist indefinitely in some women.

Hair growth slows during the postpartum period. Some women may actually experience hair loss because the amount of hair lost is temporarily more than the amount regrown. The abundance of fine hair seen during pregnancy usually disappears after birth; however, any coarse or bristly hair that appears during pregnancy usually remains. Fingernails return to their nonpregnant consistency and strength.

IMMUNE SYSTEM

No significant changes in the maternal immune system occur during the postpartum period. The mother's need for a rubella, varicella, or tetanus-diphtheria-acellular pertussis vaccination or for prevention of Rh isoimmunization is determined (see Chapter 21).

KEY POINTS

- Uterine involution begins immediately after birth and is complete in approximately 6 weeks.
- The rapid drop in estrogen and progesterone levels after expulsion of the placenta is responsible for triggering many of the anatomic and physiologic changes in the puerperium.
- The return of ovulation and menses is determined in part by whether the woman breastfeeds her infant.
- Assessment of lochia and fundal height is essential to monitor the progress of normal involution and to identify potential problems.
- Under normal circumstances, few alterations in vital signs are seen after childbirth.
- Hypercoagulability, vessel damage, and immobility predispose the woman to thromboembolism.
- Marked diuresis, decreased bladder sensitivity, and overdistention of the bladder can lead to problems with urinary elimination.
- Pregnancy-induced hypervolemia and several postpartum physiologic changes allow the woman to tolerate considerable blood loss at birth.

Audio Chapter Summaries Access an audio summary of these Key Points on evolve

REFERENCES

Blackburn, S. (2007). *Maternal, fetal, and neonatal physiology: A clinical perspective* (3rd ed.). St. Louis: Saunders.

Cunningham, F., Leveno, K., Bloom, S., Hauth, J., Rouse, D., & Spong, C. (2010). *Williams obstetrics* (23rd ed.). New York: McGraw-Hill.

Katz, V. (2007). Postpartum care. In S. Gabbe, J. Niebyl, & J. Simpson (Eds.), *Obstetrics: Normal and problem pregnancies* (5th ed). Philadelphia: Churchill Livingstone.

Lawrence, R., & Lawrence, R. (2009). The breast and the physiology of lactation. In R. Creasy, R. Resnik, J. Iams, C. Lockwood, & T. Moore (Eds.), *Creasy and Resnik's maternal-fetal medicine: Principles and practice* (6th ed.). Philadelphia: Saunders.

CHAPTER

21

Nursing Care of the Family During the Postpartum Period

Shannon E. Perry

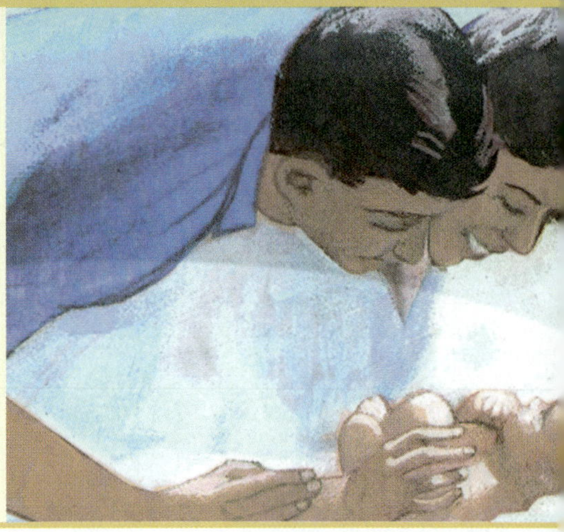

evolve WEBSITE

http://evolve.elsevier.com/Lowdermilk/MWHC/

Audio Glossary
Audio Key Points
Case Study
- Fourth Trimester

Critical Thinking Exercise
- Priority Nursing Care: Postpartum Unit

NCLEX Review Questions
Nursing Care Plan
- Postpartum Care: Vaginal Birth

Spanish Guidelines
- Assessing for Hemorrhage
- Assessing for Infection
- Discharge Teaching
- Postpartum Adjustment

Video—Nursing Skills
- Assisting with a Sitz Bath

LEARNING OBJECTIVES

- Describe components of a systematic postpartum assessment.
- Recognize signs of potential complications in the postpartum woman.
- Identify common selection criteria for safe early postpartum discharge.
- Explain the influence of cultural beliefs and practices on postpartum care.
- Identify psychosocial needs of the woman in the early postpartum period.
- Prepare a plan for postpartum teaching for self-management.
- Describe the nurse's role in these postpartum follow-up strategies: home visits, telephone follow-up, warm lines and help lines, support groups, and referrals to community resources.
- Formulate a nursing care plan for a woman in the postpartum period.

At no other time is family-centered maternity care more important than in the postpartum period. Nursing care is provided in the context of the family unit and focuses on assessment and support of the woman's physiologic and emotional adaptation after birth. During the early postpartum period, components of nursing care include assisting the mother with rest and recovery from the process of labor and birth, assessment of physiologic and psychologic adaptation after birth, prevention of complications, education regarding self-management and infant care, and support of the mother and her partner during the initial transition to parenthood. In addition, the nurse considers the needs of other family members and includes strategies in the nursing care plan to assist the family in adjusting to the new baby.

The approach to the care of women after birth is wellness oriented. In the United States most women remain hospitalized no more than 1 or 2 days after vaginal birth, and some for as few as 6 hours. Because so much important information needs to be shared with these women in a very short time, their care must be thoughtfully planned and provided. This chapter discusses nursing care of the woman and her family in the postpartum period extending into the fourth trimester—the first 3 months after birth.

Transfer from the Recovery Area

After the initial recovery period has been completed, and provided that her condition is stable, the woman may be transferred to a postpartum room in the same or another nursing unit. In facilities with labor, delivery, recovery, postpartum (LDRP) rooms, the woman is not moved and the nurse who provides care during the recovery period usually continues caring for the woman. In many settings, women who have received general or regional anesthesia must be cleared for transfer from the recovery area by a member of the anesthesia care team. In other settings, a nurse makes the determination.

In preparing the transfer report, the recovery nurse uses information from the records of admission, birth, and recovery

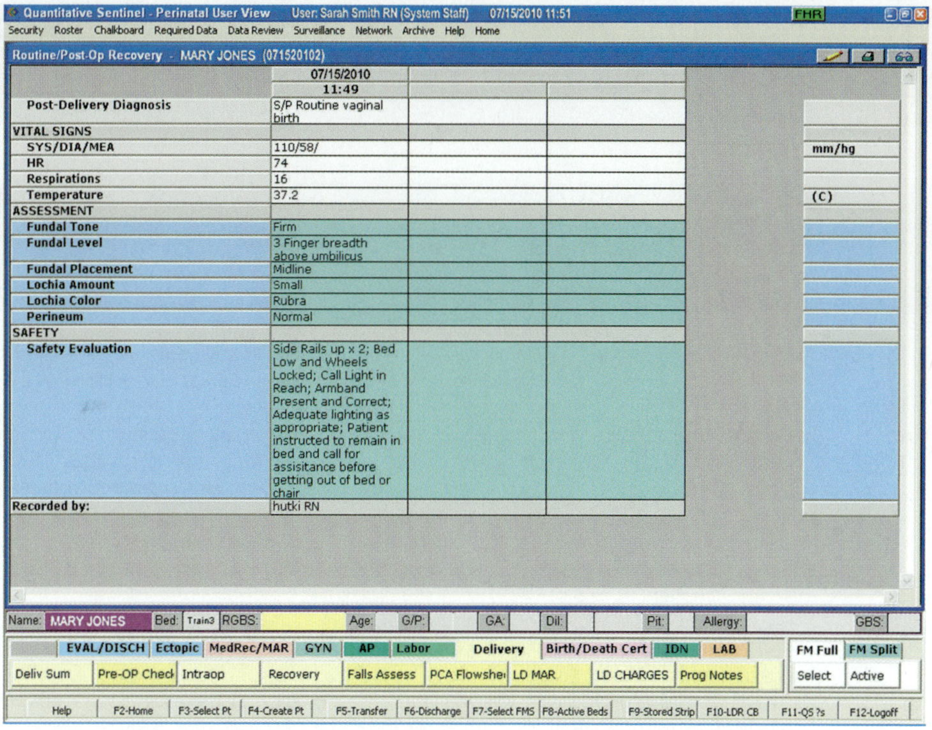

FIG. 21-1 Portion of a vaginal birth recovery screen in an electronic record. (Courtesy Kitty Cashion, Memphis, TN.)

(Fig. 21-1). Information that must be communicated to the postpartum nurse includes identity of the health care provider; gravidity and parity; age; anesthetic used; any medications given; duration of labor and time of rupture of membranes; whether labor was induced or augmented; type of birth and repair; blood type and Rh status; group B streptococci (GBS) status; status of rubella immunity; human immunodeficiency virus (HIV) and hepatitis B serology test results; other infections identified during pregnancy (e.g., syphilis, gonorrhea, chlamydia), and whether these were treated; intravenous infusion of any fluids; physiologic status since birth; description of fundus, lochia, bladder, and perineum; sex and weight of infant; time of birth; chosen method of feeding; any abnormalities noted; and assessment of initial parent-infant interaction.

Most of this information is also documented for the nursing staff in the newborn nursery if the infant is transferred to that unit (in some settings, the newborn never leaves the mother's room). In addition, specific information should be provided regarding the newborn's Apgar scores (see Chapter 24), weight, voiding, stooling, whether fed since birth, and the name of the pediatric care provider. Nursing interventions that have been completed (e.g., eye prophylaxis, vitamin K injection) as well as identification procedures done (e.g., footprints, armbands) must be recorded.

Table 21-1 gives examples for documenting this information before the transfer of the woman from the recovery area.

PLANNING FOR DISCHARGE

From their initial contact with the postpartum woman, nurses prepare the new mother for the time when she will return home. The length of hospital stay after giving birth depends on many factors, including the physical condition of the mother and the newborn, mental and emotional status of the mother, social support at home, client education needs for self-management and infant care, and financial constraints.

Women who give birth in birthing centers may be discharged within a few hours, after the woman's and infant's conditions are stable. Mothers and newborns who are at low risk for complications may be discharged from the hospital within 24 to 36 hours after vaginal birth. This short time frame is often called early postpartum discharge, shortened hospital stay, and 1-day maternity stay. The trend of shortened hospital stays is based largely on efforts to reduce health care costs coupled with consumer demands to have less medical intervention and more family-focused experiences. Although there are advantages to early postpartum discharge, disadvantages also exist (Box 21-1).

Laws Relating to Discharge

Health care providers have expressed concern with shortened stays because some medical problems do not show up in the first 24 hours after birth. The greatest risk associated with early discharge is for the infant who may develop jaundice, feeding difficulties, infection, or unrecognized respiratory or cardiac problems (Cargill, Martel, & Society of Obstetricians and Gynaecologists of Canada, 2007). In addition, new mothers may not have had sufficient time to learn how to care for their newborns, and breastfeeding may not be well established. The concern for the potential increase in adverse maternal-infant outcomes from hospital early-discharge practices led the American College of Obstetricians and Gynecologists (ACOG), the American Academy of Pediatrics (AAP), and other professional health care organizations in the U.S. to promote the enactment of federal and state maternity length-of-stay bills to ensure adequate

TABLE 21-1 **RECOVERY NURSE'S REPORT**

ITEM	EXAMPLE OF DOCUMENTATION OF MOTHER	EXAMPLE OF DOCUMENTATION OF NEWBORN
Type of labor and birth: unusual observations, if any, of the placenta	Spontaneous or assisted (forceps) vaginal birth; vertex presentation	Spontaneous or assisted (forceps, vacuum) vaginal birth in vertex presentation; time of ROM
Gravidity and parity, age	G1, P1, age 22 years; 39 weeks of gestation	G1, P1, age 22 years; 39 weeks of gestation
Anesthesia and analgesia used	None; epidural, low spinal, local	None; epidural, low spinal, or local
Condition of perineum	Episiotomy; repair of lacerations; intact	
Events since birth	Vital signs, BP, fundus, lochia, intake and output, medications (including dosage, time of administration, and results), response to newborn, observation of family interactions, including siblings, if present	Breastfed eagerly for 10 minutes Voided × 1; meconium stool × 1 Eye prophylaxis given Vitamin K injection given Held by siblings who are happy (or have other response to newborn)
Condition and sex of newborn; other information	Time of birth; Apgar at 1 and 5 minutes; weight; whether breastfeeding or bottle-feeding; sex of baby	Time of birth: Apgar scores at 1 and 5 minutes Sex; weight; name of pediatrician; breastfeeding or bottle-feeding whether or not mother received magnesium sulfate; time of last systemic analgesia
Relevant information from prenatal record	Need for rubella vaccination; presence of infections; hepatitis B status; HIV status; blood type; Rh status; GBS status and treatment if positive	Unremarkable pregnancy Mother's hepatitis B status and GBS status
Miscellaneous information: IV drip	If IV drip is infusing, type of fluid, rate of infusion, medication added (e.g., oxytocin [Pitocin]), whether to keep open or discontinue after completion of bag that is hung	
Social factors	If woman is releasing baby for adoption, whether or not she wants to see the baby, breastfeed, allow visitors, or other preferences she may have	Baby up for adoption; to stay in NBN until discharge

BP, Blood pressure; *GBS,* group B streptococci; *HIV,* human immunodeficiency virus; *IV,* intravenous; *NBN,* newborn nursery; *ROM,* rupture of membranes.

BOX 21-1 **CRITERIA FOR EARLY DISCHARGE**

MOTHER
- Uncomplicated pregnancy, labor, vaginal birth, and postpartum course
- No evidence of premature rupture of membranes
- Blood pressure and temperature stable and within normal limits
- Ambulating unassisted
- Voiding adequate amounts without difficulty
- Hemoglobin >10 g
- No significant vaginal bleeding: perineum intact or no more than second-degree episiotomy or laceration repair; uterus is firm
- Received instructions on postpartum self-management

INFANT
- Term infant (38 to 42 weeks) with weight appropriate for gestational age
- Normal findings on physical assessment
- Temperature, respirations, and heart rate within normal limits and stable for the 12 hours preceding discharge
- At least two successful feedings completed (normal sucking and swallowing)
- Urination and stooling have occurred at least once
- No evidence of significant jaundice in the first 24 hours after birth
- No excessive bleeding at the circumcision site for at least 2 hours
- Screening tests performed according to state regulations; tests to be repeated at follow-up visit if done before the infant is 24 hours old
- Initial hepatitis B vaccine given or scheduled for first follow-up visit
- Laboratory data reviewed: maternal syphilis and hepatitis B status; infant or cord blood type and Coombs' test results if indicated

GENERAL
- No social, family, or environmental risk factors identified
- Family or support person available to assist mother and infant at home
- Follow-up scheduled within 1 week if discharged before 48 hours after birth
- Documentation of skill of mother in feeding (breastfeeding or bottle-feeding), cord care, skin care, perineal care, infant safety (use of car seat, sleeping positions), and recognizing signs of illness and common infant problems

Source: American Academy of Pediatrics (AAP) Committee on Fetus and Newborn. (2004). Hospital stay for healthy term infants. *Pediatrics, 113*(5), 1434-1436.

care for mother and newborn. The passage of the Newborns' and Mothers' Health Protection Act of 1996 provided minimum federal standards for health plan coverage for mothers and their newborns. Under this act, all health plans are required to allow the new mother and newborn to remain in the hospital for a minimum of 48 hours after a normal vaginal birth and for 96 hours after a cesarean birth unless the attending provider, in consultation with the mother, decides on early discharge (AAP Committee on Fetus and Newborn, 2004).

Criteria for Discharge

Early discharge with postpartum home care can be a safe and satisfying option for women and their families when the plan is comprehensive and based on individual needs (AAP Committee on Fetus and Newborn, 2004) and when follow-up takes place (see Box 21-1). Effective follow-up within 72 hours after discharge can significantly decrease infant readmissions and maternal postpartum depression (Goulet, D'Amour, & Pineault, 2007).

TABLE 21-2 **POSTPARTUM ASSESSMENT AND SIGNS OF POTENTIAL COMPLICATIONS**

ASSESSMENT	NORMAL FINDINGS	SIGNS OF POTENTIAL COMPLICATIONS
Blood pressure (BP)	Consistent with BP baseline during pregnancy; can have orthostatic hypotension for 48 hours	Hypertension: anxiety, preeclampsia, essential hypertension Hypotension: hemorrhage
Temperature	36.2°-38° C	>38° C after 24 hours: infection
Pulse	50-90 beats/min	Tachycardia: pain, fever, dehydration, hemorrhage
Respirations	16-24 breaths/min	Bradypnea: effects of narcotic medications Tachypnea: anxiety; may be sign of respiratory disease
Breath sounds	Clear to auscultation	Crackles: possible fluid overload
Breasts	Days 1-2: soft Days 2-3: filling Days 3-5: full, soften with breastfeeding (milk is "in")	Firmness, heat, pain: engorgement Redness of breast tissue, heat, pain, fever, body aches: mastitis
Nipples	Skin intact; no soreness reported	Redness, bruising, cracks, fissures, abrasions, blisters: usually associated with latching problems
Uterus (fundus)	Firm, midline; first 24 hours at level of umbilicus; involutes ~1 cm/day	Soft, boggy, higher than expected level: uterine atony Lateral deviation: distended bladder
Lochia	Days 1-3: rubra (dark red) Days 4-10: serosa (brownish red or pink) After 10 days: alba (yellowish white) Amount: scant to moderate Few clots Fleshy odor	Large amount of lochia: uterine atony, vaginal or cervical laceration Foul odor: infection
Perineum	Minimal edema Laceration or episiotomy: edges approximated Pain minimal to moderate: controlled by analgesics, nonpharmacologic techniques, or both	Pronounced edema, bruising, hematoma Redness, warmth, drainage: infection Excessive discomfort first 1-2 days: hematoma; after day 3: infection
Rectal area	No hemorrhoids; if hemorrhoids are present, soft and pink	Discolored hemorrhoidal tissue, severe pain: thrombosed hemorrhoid
Bladder	Able to void spontaneously; no distention; able to empty completely; no dysuria Diuresis begins ~12 hours after birth; may void 3000 ml/day	Overdistended bladder possibly causing uterine atony, excessive lochia Dysuria, frequency, urgency: infection
Abdomen and bowels	Abdomen soft, active bowel sounds in all quadrants Bowel movement by day 2 or 3 after birth Cesarean: incision dressing clean and dry; suture line intact	 No bowel movement by day 3 or 4: constipation; diarrhea Abdominal incision—redness, edema, warmth, drainage: infection
Legs	Deep tendon reflexes (DTRs) 1+ to 2+ Peripheral edema possibly present Homans sign negative	DTRs ≥3+: preeclampsia Redness, tenderness, pain, positive Homans sign: thrombophlebitis
Energy level	Able to care for self and infant; able to sleep	Lethargy, extreme fatigue, difficulty sleeping: postpartum depression
Emotional status	Excited, happy, interested or involved in infant care	Sad, tearful, disinterested in infant care: postpartum blues or depression

Ideally, hospital stays are long enough to identify problems and ensure that the woman is sufficiently recovered and is prepared to care for herself and the baby at home. Nurses must consider the medical needs of the woman and her baby and provide care that is coordinated to meet those needs so as to provide timely physiologic interventions and treatment to prevent morbidity and hospital readmission.

Hospital-based maternity nurses continue to play invaluable roles as caregivers, teachers, and advocates for mothers, newborn, and families in developing and implementing effective home-care strategies. Postpartum order sets and maternal-newborn teaching checklists can be used to accomplish client care tasks and educational outcomes. With coordination, clinical care and education can be planned and provided throughout pregnancy, during the hospital stay, and in the home after discharge to ensure the family's continued well-being.

LEGAL TIP: Early Discharge
Whether or not the woman and her family have chosen early discharge, the nurse and the primary health care provider are held responsible if the woman is discharged before her condition has stabilized within normal limits. If complications occur, the medical and nursing staff could be sued for abandonment.

CARE MANAGEMENT: PHYSICAL NEEDS

The nursing care plan includes both the postpartum woman and her newborn, even if the nursery nurse retains primary responsibility for the infant. In many hospitals, **couplet care** (also called mother-baby care or single-room maternity care) is practiced. Nurses in these settings have been educated in both mother and infant care and function as primary nurses for both mother and infant, even if the infant is kept in the nursery. This approach is a variation of rooming-in, in which the mother and infant room together and mother and nurse share the care of the infant. The organization of the mother's care must take the newborn into consideration. The day actually revolves around the baby's feeding and care times (see Nursing Process: Postpartum Physical Concern).

ONGOING PHYSICAL ASSESSMENT

Ongoing assessments are performed throughout hospitalization. In addition to vital signs, physical assessment of the postpartum woman focuses on evaluation of the breasts, uterine fundus, lochia, perineum, bladder and bowel function, vital signs, and legs (Table 21-2).

NURSING PROCESS

Postpartum Physical Concerns

ASSESSMENT

Initial assessment

- Obtain information from the nursing staff report and medical record regarding gravidity, parity, length and difficulty of labor, type of birth (i.e., vaginal or cesarean), presence of perineal lacerations or episiotomy, and whether the mother plans to breastfeed or bottle-feed.
- Assess vital signs.
- Conduct a general systems assessment, including a systematic postpartum assessment.
- For cesarean birth assess the abdominal dressing over the incision.
- Assess discomfort, emotional status, fatigue, energy level, hunger, and thirst.
- Monitor intake and output.
- Assess knowledge regarding self-management, breastfeeding, and infant care.

Ongoing assessment

- Assess vital signs every 4 to 8 hours or once each shift per hospital protocol.
- Perform focused postpartum assessment every 4 to 8 hours or once each shift per hospital protocol.
- Assess discomfort, fatigue, and emotional status.
- Assess breastfeeding technique.
- Monitor intake and output.
- Monitor laboratory values, especially hemoglobin and hematocrit; collect urine for routine urinalysis and culture or sensitivity; note rubella and Rh status.

NURSING DIAGNOSES

Examples of nursing diagnoses for meeting physical needs in the postpartum period include:

***Risk for Constipation* related to:**

- post-childbirth discomfort
- childbirth trauma to tissues
- decreased intake of solid food or fluids
- side effects of narcotic analgesics

***Acute Pain* related to:**

- uterine involution
- trauma to perineum (laceration or episiotomy)
- hemorrhoids
- sore nipples
- engorged breasts

***Ineffective Breastfeeding* related to:**

- maternal discomfort
- insufficient knowledge regarding breastfeeding techniques
- lack of support from spouse, partner, family, or friends
- lack of maternal self-confidence, anxiety, and fear of failure
- difficult latching or infant sucking problems
- difficulty waking the sleepy baby

EXPECTED OUTCOMES OF CARE

Expected outcomes for the postpartum period are based on the nursing diagnoses identified for the woman and her family. Examples of expected outcomes are:

- Vital signs are within normal limits.
- Fundus is firm, midline, and demonstrates normal involution.
- Lochia has changed color and decreased in amount; no foul odor is noted.
- Bowel function will return to normal (bowel movement in 2 or 3 days after vaginal birth, by 3 to 5 days after cesarean).
- Bladder function will return to normal; no dysuria is noted; bladder feels empty after voiding.
- Pain is relieved or controlled by oral analgesic medications; pain gradually resolves completely.
- Woman verbalizes or demonstrates knowledge of self-management, breastfeeding, signs of potential complications, and when to notify health care provider.
- The newborn is integrated into the family.

PLAN OF CARE AND INTERVENTIONS

Many of the interventions in the postpartum period are focused on preventing potential complications through thorough assessment and client education. Major areas of focus include:

- preventing infection
- preventing excessive bleeding
- maintaining uterine tone
- preventing bladder distention
- promoting rest, comfort, and ambulation, and exercise
- promoting nutrition
- promoting normal bladder and bowel patterns
- promoting and supporting breastfeeding
- promoting healthy future pregnancies and children (see text)

EVALUATION

The nurse can be reasonably assured that care was effective when the expected outcomes of care for physical needs have been achieved.

Routine Laboratory Tests

Several laboratory tests may be performed in the immediate postpartum period. Hemoglobin and hematocrit values are often evaluated on the first postpartum day to assess blood loss during childbirth, especially after cesarean birth. In some hospitals a clean-catch or catheterized urine specimen may be obtained and sent for routine urinalysis or culture and sensitivity, especially if an indwelling urinary catheter was inserted during the intrapartum period. In addition, if the woman's rubella and Rh status are unknown, tests to determine her status and need for possible treatment should be performed at this time.

Nursing Interventions

Once the nursing diagnoses are formulated, the nurse plans with the woman what nursing measures are appropriate and which are to be given priority. The nursing care plan includes periodic assessments to detect deviations from normal physical changes, measures to relieve discomfort or pain, safety measures to prevent injury and infection, and teaching and counseling measures designed to promote the woman's feelings of competence in self-management and infant care. The spouse or partner and other family members who are present can be included in the teaching. The nurse evaluates continually and is ready to change the plan if indicated. Almost all hospitals use standardized care plans or care paths as a basis for planning. Nurses individualize care of the postpartum woman and neonate according to their specific needs (see the Nursing Care Plan). Signs of potential problems that may be identified during the assessment process are listed in Table 21-2.

Nurses assume many roles while implementing the nursing care plan. They provide direct physical care, teach mother-baby care, and provide anticipatory guidance and counseling.

NURSING CARE PLAN

Postpartum Care—Vaginal Birth

NURSING DIAGNOSIS

Risk for deficient fluid volume related to uterine atony and hemorrhage

Expected Outcome

Fundus is firm, lochia is moderate, and there is no evidence of hemorrhage.

Nursing Interventions/*Rationales*

- Monitor lochia (color, amount, consistency), and count and weigh sanitary pads if lochia is heavy *to evaluate amount of bleeding.*
- Monitor and palpate fundus for location and tone *to determine status of uterus and dictate further interventions because uterine atony is the most common cause of postpartum hemorrhage.*
- Monitor intake and output, assess for bladder fullness, and encourage voiding *because a full bladder interferes with involution of the uterus.*
- Monitor vital signs (increased pulse and respirations, decreased blood pressure) and skin temperature and color *to detect signs of hemorrhage or shock.*
- Monitor postpartum hematology studies *to assess effects of blood loss.*
- If fundus is boggy, apply gentle massage and assess tone response *to promote uterine contractions and increase uterine tone.* (Do not overstimulate because doing so can cause fundal relaxation.)
- Express uterine clots *to promote uterine contraction.*
- Explain to the woman the process of involution and teach her to assess and massage the fundus and to report any persistent bogginess *to involve her in self-management and increase her sense of control.*
- Administer oxytocic agents per physician or nurse-midwife order and evaluate effectiveness *to promote continued uterine contraction.*
- Administer fluids, blood, blood products, or plasma expanders as ordered *to replace lost fluid and restore blood volume.*

NURSING DIAGNOSIS

Acute pain related to postpartum physiologic changes (hemorrhoids, episiotomy, breast engorgement, sore nipples)

Expected Outcome

Woman exhibits signs of decreased discomfort.

Nursing Interventions/*Rationales*

- Assess location, type, and quality of pain *to direct intervention.*
- Explain to the woman the source and reasons for the pain, its expected duration, and treatments *to decrease anxiety and increase sense of control.*
- Administer prescribed pain medications *to provide pain relief.*
- If pain is perineal (episiotomy or lacerations, hemorrhoids), apply ice packs in the first 24 hours *to reduce edema and vulvar irritation and reduce discomfort;* encourage sitz baths using cool water for first 24 hours *to reduce edema* and warm water thereafter *to promote circulation;* apply witch hazel compresses *to reduce edema;* teach woman to use prescribed perineal creams, sprays, or ointments *to depress response of peripheral nerves;* teach woman to tighten buttocks before sitting and to sit on flat, hard surfaces *to compress buttocks and reduce pressure on the perineum.* (Avoid donuts and soft pillows as they separate the buttocks and decrease venous blood flow, increasing pain.)
- If nipples are sore and woman is breastfeeding, have the woman rub breast milk into nipples after feeding and air-dry nipples, apply purified lanolin or other nipple creams as prescribed or hydrogel pads, and wear breast shells in her bra *to minimize nipple irritation.* Assist the woman to correct latch problem *to prevent further nipple soreness.*
- If breasts are engorged, have the woman apply ice packs to breasts (15 minutes on, 45 minutes off) and apply cabbage leaves in the same manner *to relieve discomfort* (use only two or three times). Use warm compresses or take a warm shower before breastfeeding *to stimulate milk flow and relieve stasis.* Hand-express or pump milk *to relieve discomfort if infant is unable to latch on and feed.*
- If pain is from breast and the woman is not breastfeeding, encourage use of a well-fitted, supportive bra and application of ice packs *to suppress milk production and decrease discomfort.*

NURSING DIAGNOSIS

Disturbed sleep patterns related to excitement, discomfort, and environmental interruptions

Expected Outcome

Woman sleeps for uninterrupted periods of time and feels rested after waking.

Nursing Interventions/*Rationales*

- Establish the woman's routine sleep patterns and compare with current sleep patterns, exploring factors that interfere with sleep, *to determine scope of problem and direct interventions.*
- Individualize nursing routines to fit the woman's natural body rhythms (i.e., sleep-wake cycles), provide a sleep-promoting environment (i.e., darkness, quiet, adequate ventilation, appropriate room temperature), prepare for sleep using the woman's usual routines (i.e., back rub, soothing music, warm milk), and teach the use of guided imagery and relaxation techniques *to promote optimum conditions for sleep.*
- Avoid circumstances or routines that may interfere with sleep (i.e., caffeine, foods that induce heartburn, fluids, strenuous mental or physical activity) *to promote healthy sleep patterns.*
- Administer sedation or pain medication as prescribed *to enhance quality of sleep.*
- Advise the woman or partner to limit visitors and activities *to prevent further fatigue.*
- Teach woman to use infant nap time as a time for her also *to nap and replenish energy and decrease fatigue.*

NURSING DIAGNOSIS

Impaired urinary elimination related to perineal trauma and effects of anesthesia

Expected Outcome

Woman will void within 6 to 8 hours after birth and will empty bladder completely.

Nursing Interventions/*Rationale*

- Assess position and character of uterine fundus and bladder *to determine if any further interventions are indicated because of displacement of the fundus or distention of the bladder.*
- Measure intake and output *to assess for evidence of dehydration and subsequent anticipated decrease in urine output.*
- Encourage voiding by assisting the woman to walk to the bathroom, pouring running water over the perineum, running water in the sink, and providing privacy *to encourage voiding.*
- Encourage oral intake *to replace fluids lost during birth and prevent dehydration.*
- Catheterize as necessary by indwelling or straight method *to ensure bladder emptying and allow uterine involution.*

Perhaps most important, they nurture the woman by providing encouragement and support as she begins to assume the many tasks of motherhood. Nurses who take the time to "mother the mother" do much to increase feelings of self-confidence in new mothers.

The first step in providing individualized care is to confirm the woman's identity by checking her wristband. At the same time, the infant's identification number is matched with the corresponding band on the mother's wrist, and in some instances the father's or partner's wrist. The nurse determines how the mother wishes to be addressed, then notes her preference in her record and in her nursing care plan.

The woman and her family are oriented to their surroundings. Familiarity with the unit, routines, resources, and personnel reduces one potential source of anxiety—the unknown. The mother is reassured through knowing whom and how she can call for assistance and what she can expect in the way of supplies and services. If the woman's usual daily routine before admission differs from the facility's routine, the nurse works with the woman to develop a mutually acceptable routine.

Infant abduction from hospitals in the United States has increased over the past several years. As a result, many units have special limited-entry systems. Nurses teach mothers to check the identity of any person who comes to remove the baby from their room. Hospital personnel usually wear picture identification badges. On some units all staff members wear matching scrubs or special badges. Other units use closed-circuit television, computer monitoring systems, or fingerprint identification pads. As a rule, the infant is never carried in a staff member's arms between the mother's room and the nursery but is always wheeled in a bassinet, which also contains baby care supplies. New mothers and nurses must work together to ensure the safety of newborns in the hospital environment.

Prevention of Infection

Nurses in the postpartum setting are acutely aware of the importance of preventing infection in their clients. One important means of preventing infection is by maintaining a clean environment. Bed linens should be changed as needed. Disposable pads and draw sheets are changed frequently. Women should wear shoes when walking about to prevent contamination of the linens when they return to bed. Personnel must be conscientious about their hand hygiene to prevent cross-infection. Standard Precautions must be practiced. Staff members with colds, coughs, or skin infections (e.g., a cold sore on the lip [herpes simplex virus, type 1]) must follow hospital protocol when in contact with postpartum women. In many hospitals, staff members with open herpetic lesions, strep throat, conjunctivitis, upper respiratory infections, or diarrhea are

BOX 21-2 INTERVENTIONS FOR EPISIOTOMY, LACERATIONS, AND HEMORRHOIDS

Explain procedure and rationale before implementation.

CLEANSING

- Wash hands before and after cleansing perineum and changing pads.
- Wash perineum with mild soap and warm water at least once daily.
- Cleanse from symphysis pubis to anal area.
- Apply peripad from front to back, protecting inner surface of pad from contamination.
- Wrap soiled pad and place in covered waste container.
- Change pad with each void or defecation or at least four times per day.
- Assess amount and character of lochia with each pad change.

ICE PACK

Apply a covered ice pack to perineum from front to back:

- During first 24 hours to decrease edema formation and increase comfort
- After the first 24 hours following the birth as needed to provide anesthetic effect

SQUEEZE BOTTLE

- Demonstrate use and assist woman as needed; explain rationale.
- Fill bottle with tap water warmed to approximately 38° C (comfortably warm on the wrist).
- Instruct woman to position nozzle between her legs so that squirts of water reach perineum as she sits on toilet seat. Explain that it will take the whole bottle of water to cleanse perineum.
- Remind her to blot dry with toilet paper or clean wipes.
- Remind her to avoid contamination from anal area.
- Apply clean pad.

SITZ BATH

Built-in Type

- Prepare bath by thoroughly scrubbing with cleaning agent and rinsing.
- Pad with towel before filling.
- Fill one half to one third with water of correct temperature, 38° to 40.6° C. Some women prefer cool sitz baths. Ice is added to water to lower the temperature to a comfortable level.
- Encourage woman to use at least twice a day for 20 minutes.
- Place call light within easy reach.
- Teach woman to enter bath by tightening gluteal muscles, keeping them tightened, then relaxing them after she is in the bath.
- Place dry towels within reach.
- Ensure privacy.
- Check woman in 15 minutes; assess pulse as needed.

Disposable Type

- Clamp tubing and fill bag with warm water.
- Raise toilet seat, place bath in bowl with overflow opening directed toward back of toilet.
- Place container above toilet bowl.
- Attach tube into groove at front of bath.
- Loosen tube clamp to regulate rate of flow: fill bath to about one half full; continue as above for built-in sitz bath.

TOPICAL APPLICATIONS

- Apply anesthetic cream or spray after cleansing perineal area: use sparingly three or four times per day.
- Apply witch hazel pads after voiding or defecating; woman pats perineum dry from front to back, then applies witch hazel pads.
- Apply hemorrhoidal cream as ordered to anal area after cleansing.

Spanish Guidelines—Assessing for Infection

encouraged to avoid contact with mothers and infants by staying home until the condition is no longer contagious. Visitors with signs of illness are not permitted to enter the postpartum unit.

Perineal lacerations and episiotomies can increase the risk of infection as a result of interruption in skin integrity. Proper perineal care helps prevent infection in the genitourinary area and aids the healing process. Educating the woman to wipe from front to back (urethra to anus) after voiding or defecating is a simple first step. In many hospitals a squeeze bottle filled with warm water or an antiseptic solution is used after each voiding to cleanse the perineal area. The woman should change her perineal pad from front to back each time she voids or defecates and wash her hands thoroughly before and after doing so (Box 21-2).

Prevention of Excessive Bleeding

A moderate amount of vaginal bleeding (lochia) is expected in the immediate postpartum period. Nurses need to assess and prevent excessive bleeding, the most frequent cause of which is **uterine atony,** failure of the uterine muscle to contract firmly. The two most important interventions for preventing excessive bleeding are maintaining good uterine tone and preventing bladder distention. If uterine atony occurs, the relaxed uterus distends with blood and clots, blood vessels in the placental site are not clamped off, and excessive bleeding results. Although the cause of uterine atony is not always clear, it often results from retained placental fragments.

Excessive blood loss after childbirth can also be caused by vaginal or vulvar hematomas or unrepaired lacerations of the vagina or cervix. These potential sources might be suspected if excessive vaginal bleeding occurs in the presence of a firmly contracted uterus.

> **! NURSING ALERT**
>
> A perineal pad saturated in 15 minutes or less and pooling of blood under the buttocks are indications of excessive blood loss, requiring immediate assessment, intervention, and notification of the primary health care provider.

Accurate visual estimation of blood loss is an important nursing responsibility. Blood loss is usually described subjectively as scant, light, moderate, or heavy (profuse). Figure 21-2 shows examples of perineal pad saturation corresponding to each of these descriptions.

Although postpartal blood loss may be estimated by observing the amount of staining on a perineal pad, judging the amount of lochial flow is difficult if based only on observation of perineal pads. More objective estimates of blood loss include measuring serial hemoglobin or hematocrit values; weighing blood clots and items saturated with blood (1 ml equals 1 g); and establishing how many milliliters are required to saturate perineal pads being used. In general nurses tend to overestimate, rather than underestimate, blood loss.

Any estimation of lochial flow is inaccurate and incomplete without consideration of the time factor. The woman who saturates a perineal pad in 1 hour or less is bleeding much more heavily than the woman who saturates one perineal pad in 8 hours.

Different brands of perineal pads vary in their saturation volume and soaking appearance. For example, blood placed on some brands tends to soak down into the pad, whereas on other brands it tends to spread outward. Nurses should determine saturation volume and soaking appearance for the brands used in their institution so that they may improve accuracy of blood loss estimation.

> **! NURSING ALERT**
>
> The nurse always checks for blood under the mother's buttocks as well as on the perineal pad. Although the amount on the perineal pad may be slight, blood may flow between the buttocks onto the linens under the mother. When this happens, excessive bleeding can go undetected.

When excessive bleeding occurs, vital signs are monitored closely. Blood pressure is not a reliable indicator of impending shock from early postpartum hemorrhage because compensatory mechanisms prevent a significant drop in blood pressure until the woman has lost 30% to 40% of her blood volume (see Chapter 34). Respirations, pulse, skin condition, urinary output, and level of consciousness are more sensitive means of identifying shock (see the Emergency box). The frequent physical assessments performed during the fourth stage of labor are designed to provide prompt identification of excessive bleeding. Nurses maintain vigilance for excessive bleeding throughout the hospital stay as they perform periodic assessment of the uterine fundus and lochia.

Maintenance of Uterine Tone. A major intervention to alleviate uterine atony and restore uterine muscle tone is stimulation by gently massaging the fundus until firm (Fig. 21-3). Fundal massage can cause a temporary increase in the amount of vaginal bleeding seen as pooled blood leaves the uterus. Clots can also be expelled. The uterus can remain boggy even after massage and expulsion of clots.

Fundal massage can be a very uncomfortable procedure. If the nurse explains the purpose of fundal massage as well as the causes and dangers of uterine atony, the woman will likely be more cooperative. Teaching the woman to massage her own fundus enables her to maintain some control and decreases her anxiety.

When uterine atony and excessive bleeding occur, additional interventions likely to be used are administration of intravenous fluids and oxytocic medications (drugs that stimulate contraction of the uterine smooth muscle). (See Medication Guide in Chapter 34 for information about common oxytocic medications.)

Prevention of Bladder Distention. Uterine atony and excessive bleeding after birth can be the result of bladder distention. A full bladder causes the uterus to be displaced above the

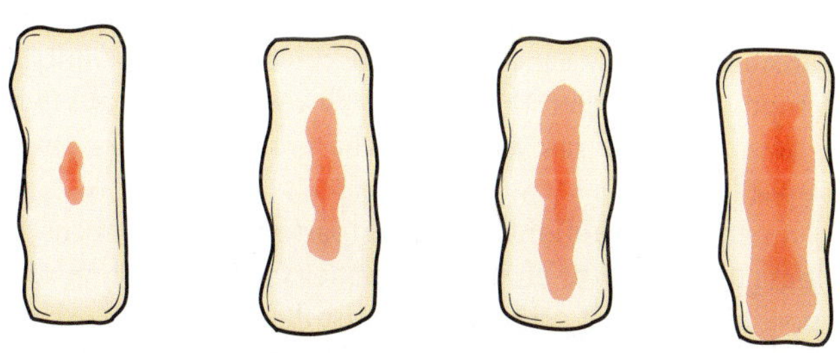

FIG. 21-2 Blood loss after birth is assessed by the extent of perineal pad saturation as *(from left to right)* scant (<2.5 cm), light (<10 cm), moderate (>10 cm), or heavy (one pad saturated within 2 hours).

EMERGENCY

Hypovolemic Shock

SIGNS AND SYMPTOMS

- Persistent significant bleeding occurs—perineal pad is soaked within 15 minutes; may not be accompanied by a change in vital signs or maternal color or behavior.
- Woman states she feels weak, lightheaded, "funny," or nauseated or that she "sees stars."
- Woman begins to act anxious or exhibits air hunger.
- Woman's skin color turns ashen or grayish.
- Skin feels cool and clammy.
- Pulse rate increases.
- Blood pressure decreases.

INTERVENTIONS

- Notify primary health care provider.
- If uterus is atonic, massage gently and expel clots to cause uterus to contract; compress uterus manually, as needed, using two hands. Add oxytocic agent to intravenous drip, as ordered.
- Give oxygen by non-rebreather face mask or nasal prongs at 8 to 10 L/min.
- Tilt the woman onto her side or elevate the right hip; elevate her legs to at least a 30-degree angle.
- Provide additional or maintain existing intravenous infusion of lactated Ringer's solution or normal saline solution to restore circulatory volume (woman should have two patent IV lines; insert second IV using 16-18 gauge IV catheter).
- Administer blood or blood products, as ordered.
- Monitor vital signs.
- Insert an indwelling urinary catheter to monitor perfusion of kidneys.
- Administer emergency drugs, as ordered.
- Prepare for possible surgery or other emergency treatments or procedures.
- Chart incident, medical and nursing interventions instituted, and the woman's response to interventions.

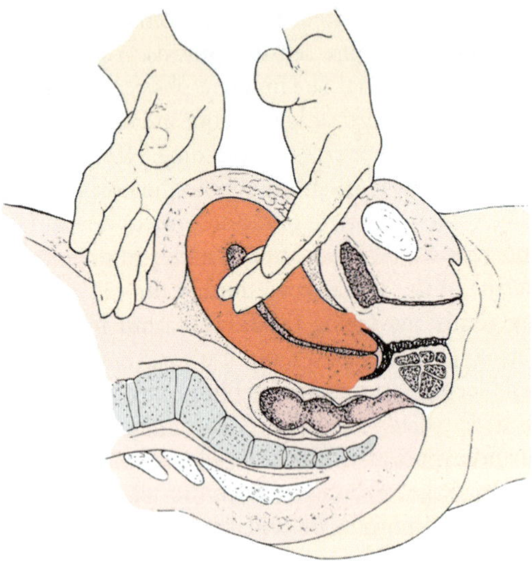

FIG. 21-3 Palpating fundus of uterus during the postpartum period. Note that upper hand is cupped over fundus; lower hand dips in above symphysis pubis and supports uterus while it is massaged gently.

umbilicus and well to one side of midline in the abdomen. It also prevents the uterus from contracting normally.

Women may be at risk of bladder distention resulting from urinary retention based on intrapartum factors. These risk factors include epidural anesthesia, episiotomy, extensive vaginal or perineal lacerations, instrument-assisted birth, or prolonged labor. Women who have had indwelling catheters, such as with cesarean birth, may experience some difficulty as they initially attempt to void after the catheter is removed. Nurses who are aware of these risk factors can be proactive in preventing complications.

Nursing interventions for a postpartum woman focus on helping the woman to empty her bladder spontaneously as soon as possible. The first priority is to assist the woman to the bathroom or onto a bedpan if she is unable to ambulate. Having the woman listen to running water, placing her hands in warm water, or pouring water from a squeeze bottle over her perineum may stimulate voiding. Other techniques include assisting the woman into the shower or sitz bath and encouraging her to void; relaxation techniques can also be helpful. Administering analgesics, if ordered, may be indicated because some women fear voiding because of anticipated pain. If these measures are unsuccessful, a sterile catheter may be inserted to drain the urine.

Video—Nursing Skills: Assisting with a Sitz Bath

Promotion of Comfort, Rest, Ambulation, and Exercise

Comfort. Most women experience some degree of discomfort during the postpartum period. Common causes of discomfort include pain from uterine contractions (afterpains), perineal lacerations or episiotomy, hemorrhoids, sore nipples, and breast engorgement. Women likely to experience the greatest perineal discomfort are those who had forceps- or vacuum-assisted operative birth, and those who have an episiotomy (Declercq, Cunningham, Johnson, & Sakala, 2008). Multiparous and breastfeeding women have the most discomfort from afterpains.

The woman's description of the location, type, and severity of her pain is the best guide in choosing an appropriate intervention. To confirm the location and extent of discomfort, the nurse inspects and palpates areas of pain as appropriate for redness, swelling, discharge, and heat and observes for body tension, guarded movements, and facial tension. Blood pressure, pulse, and respirations may be elevated in response to acute pain. Diaphoresis may accompany severe pain. A lack of objective signs does not necessarily mean there is no pain because there can be a cultural component to the expression of pain. Nursing interventions are intended to eliminate the pain sensation entirely or reduce it to a tolerable level that allows the woman to care for herself and her baby. Nurses may use nonpharmacologic and pharmacologic interventions to promote comfort. Pain relief is enhanced by using more than one method or route.

Nonpharmacologic Interventions. A variety of nonpharmacologic measures is used to reduce postpartum discomfort. These include distraction, imagery, therapeutic touch, relaxation, acupressure, aromatherapy, hydrotherapy, massage therapy, music therapy, and transcutaneous electrical nerve stimulation (TENS).

For women who are experiencing discomfort associated with uterine contractions, application of warmth (e.g., heating pad) or lying prone may be helpful. Interaction with the infant may also provide distraction and decrease this discomfort. Because afterpains are more severe during and after breastfeeding, the timing of interventions are planned to provide the most timely and effective relief.

Simple interventions that can decrease the discomfort associated with an episiotomy or perineal lacerations include encouraging the woman to lie on her side whenever possible. Other interventions include application of an ice pack; topical application (if ordered) of anesthetic spray or cream; dry heat; cleansing with water from a squeeze bottle; and a cleansing shower, tub bath, or sitz bath. Many of these interventions are also effective for hemorrhoids, especially ice packs, sitz baths, and topical applications (such as witch hazel pads). Box 21-2 gives additional specific information about these interventions.

Sore nipples in breastfeeding mothers are most likely related to ineffective latch technique. Assessment and assistance with feeding can help alleviate the cause. To ease discomfort associated with sore nipples the mother may apply topical preparations such as purified lanolin or hydrogel pads (see Chapter 25).

Breast engorgement can occur whether the woman is breastfeeding or formula feeding. The discomfort associated with engorged breasts may be reduced by applying ice packs or cabbage leaves (or both) to the breasts, and wearing a well-fitted support bra. Antiinflammatory medications can also be helpful in relieving some of the discomfort. Decisions about specific interventions for engorgement are based on whether the woman chooses breastfeeding or bottle-feeding (see Chapter 25).

Pharmacologic Interventions. Pharmacologic interventions are commonly used to relieve or reduce postpartum discomfort. Most health care providers routinely order a variety of analgesics to be administered as needed, including both narcotic and nonnarcotic (e.g., nonsteroidal antiinflammatory drugs [NSAIDs]). In some hospitals NSAIDs are administered on a scheduled basis, especially if the woman had perineal repair. Topical application of antiseptic or anesthetic ointment or spray can be used for perineal pain. Patient-controlled analgesia (PCA) pumps and epidural analgesia are commonly used to provide pain relief after cesarean birth.

> **! NURSING ALERT**
>
> The nurse should carefully monitor all women receiving opioids because respiratory depression and decreased intestinal motility are side effects.

Many women want to participate in decisions about analgesia. Severe pain, however, may interfere with active participation in choosing pain relief measures. If an analgesic is to be given, the nurse must make a clinical judgment of the type, appropriate dosage, and frequency from the medications ordered. The woman is informed of the prescribed analgesic and its common side effects; this teaching is documented.

Breastfeeding mothers often have concerns about the effects of an analgesic on the infant. Although nearly all drugs present in maternal circulation are also found in breast milk, many analgesics commonly used during the postpartum period are considered relatively safe for breastfeeding mothers and infants. Often the timing of medications can be adjusted to minimize infant exposure. A mother may be given pain medication immediately after breastfeeding so that the interval between medication administration and the next nursing period is as long as possible. The decision to administer medications of any kind to a breastfeeding mother must always be made by carefully weighing the woman's need against actual or potential risks to the infant.

If acceptable pain relief has not been obtained in 1 hour and there is no change in the initial assessment, the nurse may need to contact the primary care provider for additional pain relief orders or further directions. Unrelieved pain results in fatigue, anxiety, and a worsening perception of the pain. It might also indicate the presence of a previously unidentified or untreated problem.

Rest. Postpartum fatigue (PPF) is more than just feeling tired; it is a complex phenomenon affected by a combination of physiologic, psychologic, and situational variables. Fatigue is common in the early postpartum period and involves physiologic as well as psychologic components. Physical fatigue or exhaustion may be associated with long labors or cesarean birth; hospital routines and infant care demands such as breastfeeding also contribute to maternal fatigue. Fatigue can also be associated with anemia, infection, or thyroid dysfunction (Corwin & Arbour, 2007). The excitement and exhilaration experienced after the birth of the infant makes resting difficult. Physical discomfort can interfere with sleep. Well-intentioned visitors can interrupt periods of rest in the hospital and at home. Mothers can also experience psychologic fatigue related to anxiety or depression. PPF is a recognized risk factor for postpartum depression (Corwin, Brownstead, Barton, Heckard, & Morin, 2005).

Fatigue is likely to worsen over the first 6 weeks after birth, often because of situational factors. After discharge from the hospital, fatigue increases as the woman provides care and feeding for the newborn in combination with other family and household responsibilities such as caring for other children, preparing meals, and doing laundry. Many women have partners, family members, or friends to provide much-needed assistance, whereas others can be without any help at all. The nurse needs to inquire about resources available to the woman after discharge and help her plan accordingly (Runquist, 2007).

Interventions are planned to meet the woman's individual needs for sleep and rest while she is in the hospital. Back rubs, other comfort measures, and medication for sleep may be necessary. The side-lying position for breastfeeding minimizes fatigue in nursing mothers. Support and encouragement of mothering behaviors help reduce anxiety. Hospital and nursing routines can be adjusted to meet needs of individual mothers. In addition, the nurse can help the family limit visitors and provide a comfortable chair or bed for the partner or other family member who is staying with the new mother.

Because PPF can be very debilitating, follow-up after hospital discharge is important. Screening for PPF can be accomplished with a nurse-initiated telephone call at 2 weeks, as well as at the routine 6-week postpartum visit with the primary health care provider (Corwin & Arbour, 2007).

Physiologic factors contributing to postpartum fatigue are amenable to intervention and may be identified even before birth. Women with anemia, infection or inflammation, or thyroid dysfunction can be identified as having increased risk for postpartum fatigue. Other physical conditions and psychologic or situational factors that might contribute to PPF can be identified during the prenatal period. The medical records of women with known risk factors can be flagged to alert hospital staff to their special needs (Corwin & Arbour, 2007).

Ambulation. Early ambulation is associated with a reduced incidence of venous thromboembolism (VTE); it also promotes the return of strength. Free movement is encouraged once anesthesia wears off unless a narcotic analgesic has been administered. After the initial recovery period the mother is encouraged to ambulate frequently.

In the early postpartum period, women can feel lightheaded or dizzy when standing. The rapid decrease in intraabdominal pressure after birth results in a dilation of blood vessels supplying the intestines (splanchnic engorgement) and causes blood to pool in the viscera. This condition contributes to the development of orthostatic hypotension when the woman who has recently given birth sits or stands up, first ambulates or takes a warm shower or sitz bath. When assisting a woman to ambulate, the nurse needs to consider the baseline blood pressure, amount of blood loss, and type, amount, and timing of analgesic or anesthetic medications administered.

Women who have had epidural anesthesia may have slow return of sensory and motor function in their lower extremities, increasing the risk of falls with early ambulation. Careful assessment by the postpartum nurse can prevent falls. Factors that the nurse should consider are the time lapse since epidural medication was given; the woman's ability to bend both knees, place both feet flat on the bed, and lift buttocks off the bed without assistance; medications since birth; vital signs; and estimated blood loss with birth. Before allowing the woman to ambulate the nurse assesses the ability of the woman to stand unassisted beside her bed, simultaneously bending both knees slightly, and then standing with knees locked. If the woman is unable to balance herself, she can be safely eased back into bed without injury (Frank, Lane, & Hokanson, 2009).

SAFETY ALERT

To promote patient safety and prevent injury, it is important to have hospital personnel present the first time the woman gets out of bed after birth because she can feel weak, dizzy, faint, or lightheaded.

Prevention of venous thromboembolism is important. Women who must remain in bed after giving birth are at increased risk for the development of a thromboembolism. Antiembolic stockings (TED hose) or a sequential compression device (SCD boots) can be ordered prophylactically. If a woman remains in bed longer than 8 hours (e.g., for postpartum magnesium sulfate therapy for preeclampsia), exercise to promote circulation in the legs is indicated, using the following routine:

- Alternating flexion and extension of feet
- Rotating the ankles in a circular motion
- Alternating flexion and extension of legs
- Pressing the back of the knees to the bed surface; relax

If the woman is susceptible to thromboembolism, she is encouraged to walk about actively for true ambulation and is discouraged from sitting immobile in a chair. Women with varicosities are encouraged to wear support hose. If a thrombus is suspected, as evidenced by complaint of pain in calf muscles or warmth, redness, or tenderness in the suspected leg, or a positive **Homans sign** (dorsiflexing the foot sharply with the knee flexed; may cause pain in the calf in the presence of deep vein thrombosis), the primary health care provider should be notified; meanwhile the woman should be confined to bed, with the affected limb elevated on pillows.

Exercise. Postpartum exercise can begin soon after birth, although the woman should be encouraged to start with simple exercises and gradually progress to more strenuous ones. Figure 21-4 illustrates a number of exercises appropriate for the new mother. Abdominal exercises are postponed until approximately 4 weeks after cesarean birth.

Kegel exercises to strengthen muscle tone are extremely important, particularly after vaginal birth. Kegel exercises help women regain the muscle tone that is often lost as pelvic tissues are stretched and torn during pregnancy and birth. Women who maintain muscle strength benefit years later by retaining urinary continence.

Women must learn to perform Kegel exercises correctly (see Teaching for Self-Management box on p. 91). Some women perform them incorrectly and may increase their risk of incontinence, which can occur when inadvertently bearing down on the pelvic floor muscles, thrusting the perineum outward. The woman's technique can be assessed during the pelvic examination at her checkup by inserting two fingers intravaginally and noting whether the pelvic floor muscles correctly contract and relax.

Promotion of Nutrition

During the hospital stay most women display a good appetite and eat well. They can request that family members bring favorite or culturally appropriate foods. Cultural dietary preferences must be respected. This interest in food presents an ideal opportunity for nutritional counseling on dietary needs after pregnancy, with specific information related to breastfeeding, preventing constipation and anemia, promoting weight loss, and promoting healing and well-being (see Chapter 14). Prenatal vitamins and iron supplements are often continued until 6 weeks after childbirth or until the ordered supply has been used.

The recommended caloric intake for the moderately active, nonlactating postpartum woman is 1800 to 2200 kcal/day. According to the Institute of Medicine (2005) the estimated energy requirement (EER) for a lactating woman during the first 6 months is 2700 kcal/day; during the next 6 months it is 2768 kcal/day. Higher-than-normal caloric intake is recommended for lactating women who are underweight or who exercise vigorously and those who are breastfeeding more than one infant. See Chapter 14 for recommendations for weight loss for the obese woman. Although most women desire to return to their prepregnancy weight as soon as possible, gradual weight loss is recommended (Becker & Scott, 2008).

Promotion of Normal Bladder and Bowel Patterns

Bladder Function. The mother should void spontaneously within 6 to 8 hours after giving birth. The first several voidings should be measured to document adequate emptying of the bladder. A volume of at least 150 ml is expected for each

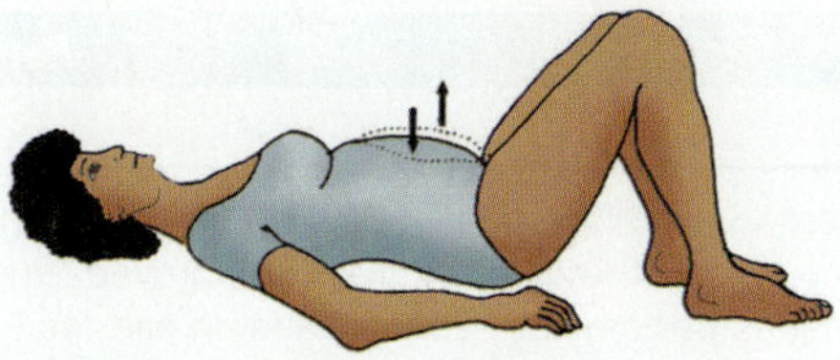

Abdominal Breathing. Lie on back with knees bent. Inhale deeply through nose. Keep ribs stationary and allow abdomen to expand upward. Exhale slowly but forcefully while contracting the abdominal muscles; hold for 3 to 5 seconds while exhaling. Relax.

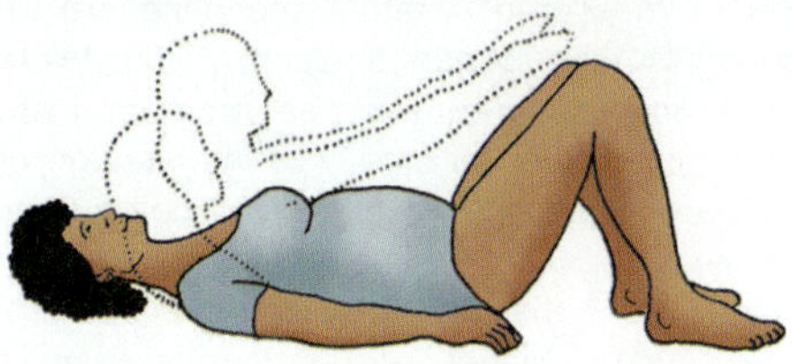

Reach for the Knees. Lie on back with knees bent. While inhaling, deeply lower chin onto chest. While exhaling, raise head and shoulders slowly and smoothly and reach for knees with arms outstretched. The body should rise only as far as the back will naturally bend while waist remains on floor or bed (about 6 to 8 inches). Slowly and smoothly lower head and shoulders back to starting position. Relax.

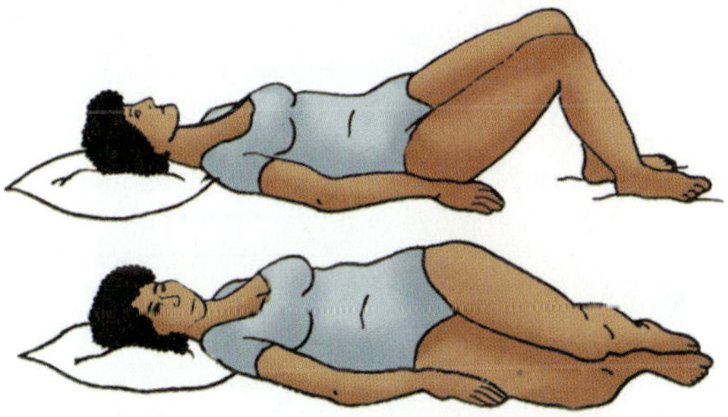

Double Knee Roll. Lie on back with knees bent. Keeping shoulders flat and feet stationary, slowly and smoothly roll knees over to the left to touch floor or bed. Maintaining a smooth motion, roll knees back over to the right until they touch floor or bed. Return to starting position and relax.

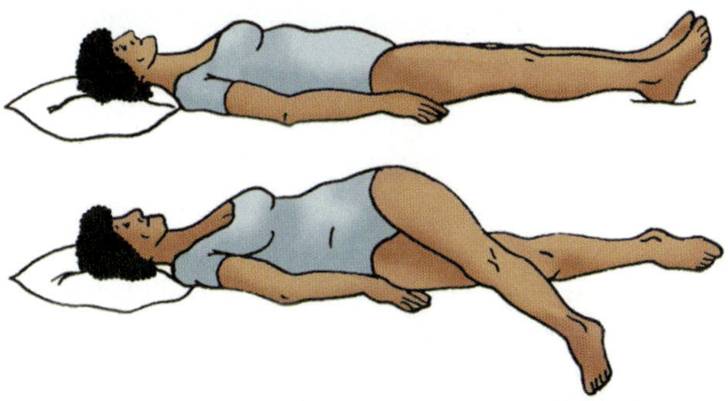

Leg Roll. Lie on back with legs straight. Keeping shoulders flat and legs straight, slowly and smoothly lift left leg and roll it over to touch the right side of floor or bed and return to starting position. Repeat, rolling right leg over to touch left side of floor or bed. Relax.

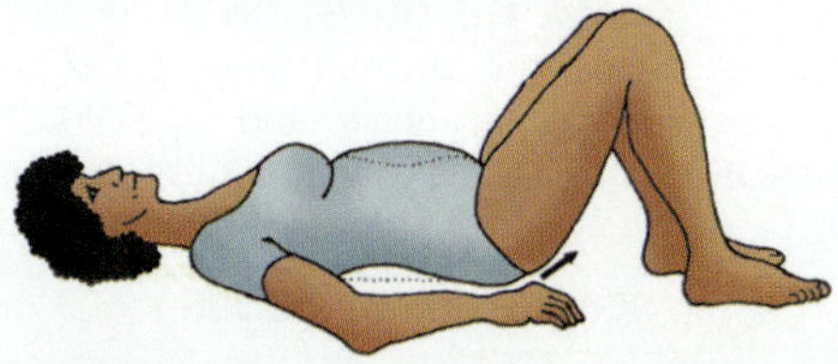

Combined Abdominal Breathing and Supine Pelvic Tilt (Pelvic Rock). Lie on back with knees bent. While inhaling deeply, roll pelvis back by flattening lower back on floor or bed. Exhale slowly but forcefully while contracting abdominal muscles and tightening buttocks. Hold for 3 to 5 seconds while exhaling. Relax.

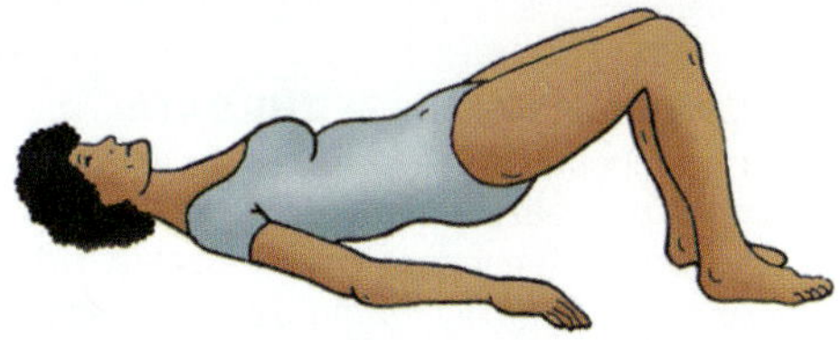

Buttocks Lift. Lie on back with arms at sides, knees bent, and feet flat. Slowly raise buttocks and arch back. Return slowly to starting position.

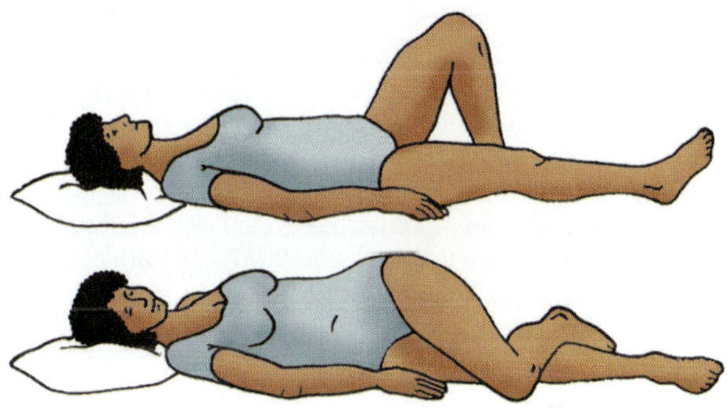

Single Knee Roll. Lie on back with right leg straight and left leg bent at the knee. Keeping shoulders flat, slowly and smoothly roll left knee over to the right to touch floor or bed and then back to starting position. Reverse position of legs. Roll right knee over to the left to touch floor or bed and return to starting position. Relax.

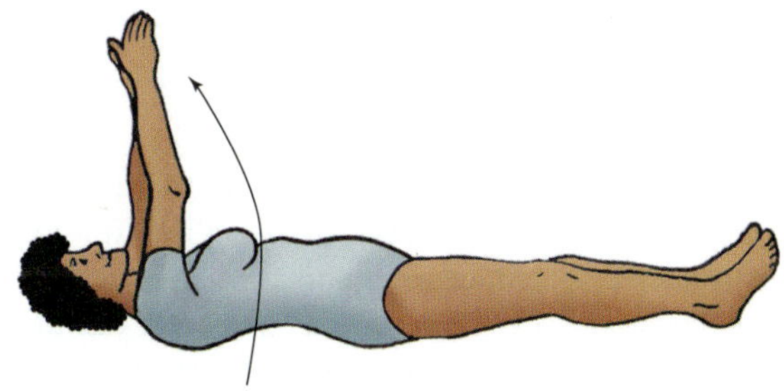

Arm Raises. Lie on back with arms extended at 90-degree angle from body. Raise arms so they are perpendicular and hands touch. Lower slowly.

FIG. 21-4 Postpartum exercise should begin as soon as possible. The woman should start with simple exercises and gradually progress to more strenuous ones.

EVIDENCE-BASED PRACTICE

Pat Gingrich

Kegel, Kegel, Kegel!

ASK THE QUESTION

Does teaching postpartum women how to do pelvic floor muscle exercises prevent urinary and fecal incontinence? How long should we recommend that our clients continue the exercises?

SEARCH FOR EVIDENCE

Search Strategies

Professional organization guidelines, meta-analyses, systematic reviews, randomized controlled trials since 2008.

Databases Searched

CINAHL, Cochrane, Medline, PUBMED, National Guideline Clearinghouse, and National Institute for Health and Clinical Evidence (NICE).

CRITICALLY ANALYZE THE DATA

Stress urinary incontinence is the loss of urine as a result of the pressure of a cough or sneeze. It may result from trauma or weakened pelvic floor and/or urinary sphincter muscles. Urinary leakage is the involuntary contraction of the bladder, resulting in loss of urine before the person can get to a toilet. Incontinence is a common complaint for postpartum women, and may persist for years. In midlife, bladder tone may further weaken due to loss of estrogen, causing incontinence symptoms in up to one third of women. Fecal incontinence affects 10% of women, and has a profoundly negative effect on quality of life.

Two Cochrane Database Systematic Reviews confirm that teaching women pelvic floor muscle training exercises (PFMT, commonly called "Kegel" exercises) can be beneficial. Hay-Smith, Morkved, Fairbrother, and Herbison (2008) analyzed 15 studies involving 6181 women. Women were randomized into groups that received some instructions on PFMT or sham/placebo or usual care. Measures of urinary and/or fecal incontinence up to 12 months postbirth showed 20% less urinary incontinence and up to half the amount of fecal incontinence in the educational intervention group, compared to the usual care or the sham groups. Reviewers noted a dose-related effect: the more intense the treatment, the greater the effect. The reviewers suggest that the effect is greater in high-risk populations, such as women with a history of incontinence, large baby, early pregnancy or forceps-assisted birth.

This recommendation was confirmed when reviewers analyzed 12 trials involving 672 women (Dumoulin & Hay-Smith, 2010). Women who practiced PFMT were significantly more likely to report that they were cured or improved (fewer incontinent episodes per day and less leakage on pad test) than nonpracticers. The PFMT practice group reported increased quality of life. One study confirmed a dose-related effect. The authors note greater benefit in women who exercise for at least three months.

Another systematic review of 4 trials involving 3295 postpartum women measured whether the beneficial effects are maintained across time (Wagg & Bunn, 2007). Women were randomized to individualized exercise program instruction in a variety of settings or usual care. The intervention group was intensively taught to clench or tighten their pelvic floor muscles using specific exercises ("unassisted," meaning without any special equipment). Some trials also provided the intervention group with reminders such as diaries, posters, or educational materials. Some interventions were taught over 5 to 6 days, and followed up with 3 visits in 9 months. All trials showed less incontinence of the intensive intervention group at 3 months, but the effect had faded by 12 months. In addition, the regular use of the exercise declined across time, although the intervention group was more likely to exercise than the control group.

IMPLICATIONS FOR PRACTICE

Urinary and fecal incontinence are distressing symptoms, sometimes suffered in silence and shame. Teaching PFMT to pregnant and postpartum women improves continence. It is relatively easy to teach, requires no equipment, and can be done in absolute privacy by any woman. The goal is to get the woman to believe that the exercise will improve or prevent incontinence, and then to remember to exercise. Individualizing the program and providing reminders can improve compliance and benefits, as does reinforcing and encouraging regular pelvic floor muscle exercises at each visit.

References

Dumoulin, C., & Hay-Smith, J. (2010). Pelvic floor muscle training versus no treatment, or inactive control treatments, for urinary incontinence in women. *The Cochrane Database of Systematic Reviews 2001*, 1, CD005654.

Hay-Smith, J., Morkved, S., Fairbrother, K., & Herbison, G. (2008). Pelvic floor muscle training for prevention and treatment of urinary and faecal incontinence in antenatal and postnatal women. *The Cochrane Database of Systematic Reviews 2008*, 4, CD007471.

Wagg, A., & Bunn, F. (2007). Unassisted pelvic floor exercises for postnatal women: A systematic review. *Journal of Advanced Nursing, 58*(5), 407–417.

voiding. Some women experience difficulty in emptying the bladder, possibly as a result of diminished bladder tone, edema from trauma, or fear of discomfort. Nursing interventions for inability to void and bladder distention are discussed on p. 494.

Bowel Function. After birth, women may be at risk for constipation related to side effects of medications (narcotic analgesics, iron supplements, magnesium sulfate), dehydration, immobility, or the presence of episiotomy, perineal lacerations, or hemorrhoids. The woman may fear pain with the first bowel movement.

Nursing interventions to promote normal bowel elimination include educating the woman about measures to prevent constipation, such as ensuring adequate intake of roughage and fluids and promoting exercise. Alerting the woman to side effects of medications such as narcotic analgesics (e.g., decreased gastrointestinal tract motility) may encourage her to implement measures to reduce the risk of constipation. Stool softeners or laxatives may be necessary during the early postpartum period. With early discharge, a new mother may be home before having a bowel movement.

! NURSING ALERT

Rectal suppositories and enemas should not be administered to women with third- or fourth-degree perineal lacerations. These measures to treat constipation can be very uncomfortable and can cause hemorrhage or damage to the suture line. They can also predispose the woman to infection (Association of Women's Health, Obstetric, and Neonatal Nurses [AWHONN], 2006).

Some mothers experience gas pains; this is more common following cesarean birth. Antigas medications may be ordered.

Ambulation or rocking in a rocking chair may stimulate passage of flatus and relief of discomfort.

Breastfeeding Promotion and Lactation Suppression

Breastfeeding Promotion. The ideal time to initiate breastfeeding is within the first 1 to 2 hours after birth. Baby-friendly hospitals mandate that the infant be put to breast within the first hour after birth (Baby-Friendly Hospital Initiative USA, 2010). At this time, most infants are alert and ready to nurse. Breastfeeding aids in the contraction of the uterus and prevention of maternal hemorrhage. The first hour after birth is also an opportune time to assist the mother with breastfeeding, assess her basic knowledge of breastfeeding, and assess the physical appearance of the breasts and nipples. Throughout the hospital stay, nurses provide teaching and assistance for the breastfeeding mother, making appropriate referrals to lactation consultants as needed and available. (See Chapter 25 for further information on assisting the breastfeeding woman.)

Lactation Suppression. Suppression of lactation is necessary when the woman has decided not to breastfeed or in the case of neonatal death. Wearing a well-fitted support bra continuously for at least the first 72 hours after giving birth is important. Women should avoid breast stimulation, including running warm water over the breasts, newborn suckling, or pumping of the breasts. Some nonbreastfeeding mothers experience severe breast **engorgement** (swelling of breast tissue caused by increased blood and lymph supply to the breasts as the body produces milk, occurring at about 72 to 96 hours after birth). Breast engorgement can usually be managed satisfactorily with nonpharmacologic interventions.

Ice packs to the breasts help decrease the discomfort associated with engorgement. The woman should use a 15 minutes on, 45 minutes off schedule (to prevent the rebound swelling that can occur if ice is used continuously). While there is lack of scientific evidence to support effectiveness, cabbage leaves are often recommended to help relieve the engorgement; formula-feeding mothers may be told to place fresh green cabbage leaves over their breasts and to replace the leaves when they are wilted. A mild analgesic or antiinflammatory medication can aid in decreasing the discomfort associated with engorgement. Medications that were once prescribed for lactation suppression (e.g., estrogen, estrogen and testosterone, and bromocriptine) are no longer used.

Health Promotion for Future Pregnancies and Children

Rubella Vaccination. For women who have not had rubella (10% to 20% of all women) or women who are serologically not immune (titer of 1:8 or enzyme immunoassay level less than 0.8), a subcutaneous injection of rubella vaccine is recommended in the postpartum period to prevent the possibility of contracting rubella in future pregnancies. Seroconversion occurs in approximately 90% of women vaccinated after birth. The live attenuated rubella virus is not communicable in breast milk; therefore, breastfeeding mothers can be vaccinated. However, because the virus is shed in urine and other body fluids, the vaccine should not be given if the mother or other household members are immunocompromised. The most common side effects are fever, lymphadenopathy, and arthralgia.

Varicella Vaccination. The Centers for Disease Control and Prevention (CDC) recommend that varicella vaccine be administered before discharge in women who have no immunity. A second dose is given at the postpartum follow-up visit (4 to 8 weeks) (CDC, 2007).

> **LEGAL TIP: Rubella and Varicella Vaccination**
> Informed consent for rubella and varicella vaccination in the postpartum period includes information about possible side effects and the risk of teratogenic effects. Women must understand that they must practice contraception to prevent pregnancy for 1 month after being vaccinated (ACOG, 2002; CDC, 2007).

Tetanus-Diphtheria-Acellular Pertussis Vaccine. Tetanus-diphtheria-acellular pertussis (Tdap) vaccine is recommended for postpartum women who have not previously received the vaccine; it is given before discharge from the hospital or as early as possible in the postpartum period to protect women from pertussis and to decrease the risk of infant exposure to pertussis. For women whose most recent tetanus-diphtheria (Td) vaccine was given more than 2 years before the pregnancy, the Tdap vaccine can also be given in the early postpartum period (CDC, 2008).

Prevention of Rh Isoimmunization. Injection of Rh immune globulin (a solution of gamma globulin that contains Rh antibodies) within 72 hours after birth prevents sensitization in the Rh-negative woman who has had a fetomaternal transfusion of Rh-positive fetal red blood cells (RBCs) (see the Medication Guide). Rh immune globulin promotes lysis of fetal Rh-positive blood cells before the mother forms her own antibodies against them.

> **! NURSING ALERT**
> After birth, Rh immune globulin is administered to all Rh-negative, antibody (Coombs')–negative women who give birth to Rh-positive infants. Rh immune globulin is administered to the mother intramuscularly (RhoGAM, Gamulin RH, HypRho-D, Rhophylac) or intravenously (Rhophylac). It should never be given to an infant.

The administration of 300 mcg (1 vial) of Rh immune globulin is usually sufficient to prevent maternal sensitization. If a large fetomaternal transfusion is suspected, however, the dosage needed should be determined by performing a Kleihauer-Betke test, which detects the amount of fetal blood in the maternal circulation. If more than 15 ml of fetal blood is present in maternal circulation, the dosage of Rh immune globulin must be increased.

A 1:1000 dilution of Rh immune globulin is crossmatched to the mother's RBCs to ensure compatibility. Because Rh immune globulin is usually considered a blood product, precautions similar to those used for transfusing blood are necessary. The identification number on the woman's hospital wristband should correspond to the identification number found on the laboratory slip. The nurse must also check to see that the lot number on the laboratory slip corresponds to the lot number on the vial. Finally, the expiration date on the vial should be checked to be certain of a usable product.

MEDICATION GUIDE

Rh Immune Globulin, RhoGAM, Gamulin Rh, HypRho-D, Rhophylac

ACTION

Suppression of immune response in nonsensitized women with Rh-negative blood who receive Rh-positive blood cells because of fetomaternal hemorrhage, transfusion, or accident

INDICATIONS

Routine antepartum prevention at 28 weeks of gestation in women with Rh-negative blood; suppress antibody formation after birth, miscarriage, or pregnancy termination, abdominal trauma, ectopic pregnancy, amniocentesis, version, or chorionic villus sampling

DOSAGE AND ROUTE

Standard dose 1 vial (300 mcg) IM in deltoid or gluteal muscle; microdose 1 vial (50 mcg) IM in deltoid muscle; Rhophylac can be given IM or IV (available in prefilled syringes)

ADVERSE EFFECTS

Myalgia, lethargy, localized tenderness and stiffness at injection site, mild and transient fever, malaise, headache; rarely nausea, vomiting, hypotension, tachycardia, possible allergic response

NURSING CONSIDERATIONS

Give standard dose to mother at 28 weeks of gestation as prophylaxis, or after an incident or exposure risk that occurs after 28 weeks of gestation (e.g., amniocentesis, second-trimester miscarriage or abortion, after version) and within 72 hours after birth if baby is Rh positive. Give microdose for first trimester miscarriage or abortion, ectopic pregnancy, chorionic villus sampling.

Verify that the woman is Rh negative and has not been sensitized, that Coombs' test is negative, and that baby is Rh positive. Provide explanation to the woman about procedure, including the purpose, possible side effects, and effect on future pregnancies. Have the woman sign a consent form if required by agency. Verify correct dosage and confirm lot number and woman's identity before giving injection (verify with another registered nurse or other procedure per agency policy); document administration per agency policy. Observe woman for allergic response for at least 20 minutes after administration.

The medication is made from human plasma (a consideration if woman is a Jehovah's Witness). The risk of transmitting infectious agents, including viruses, cannot be completely eliminated.

Rh immune globulin suppresses the immune response. Therefore, the woman who receives both Rh immune globulin and rubella vaccine must be tested at 3 months to see if she has developed rubella immunity. If not, she will need another dose of rubella vaccine.

There is some disagreement about whether Rh immune globulin should be considered a blood product. Health care providers need to discuss the most current information about this issue with women whose religious beliefs conflict with having blood products administered to them (e.g., Jehovah's Witnesses).

CARE MANAGEMENT: PSYCHOSOCIAL NEEDS

Meeting the psychosocial needs of new mothers involves assessing the parents' reactions to the birth experience, feelings about themselves, and interactions with the new baby and other family members. Specific interventions are planned to increase the parents' knowledge and self-confidence as they assume the care and responsibility of the new baby and integrate this new member into their existing family structure in a way that meets their cultural expectations (see Chapters 22 and 24 and the Nursing Process box: Postpartum Pyschosocial Concerns).

There is evidence that nurses and other health care providers do not adequately address maternal psychosocial needs, instead focusing their attention on postpartum physical changes and medically based care (Cheung, Fowles, & Walker, 2006). Taking time to assess maternal emotional needs and to address concerns before discharge may promote better psychologic health and adjustment to parenting. Ongoing support for postpartum women is also needed. Even though issues such as fatigue are often evident during the hospital stay, clearly this type of support will likely be an ongoing concern after discharge when the woman is providing care for the newborn, herself, and other family members. Postpartum support is especially beneficial to at-risk populations such as low-income primiparas, those at risk for family dysfunction and child abuse, and those at risk for postpartum depression (Shaw, Levitt, Wong, & Kaczorowski, 2006).

Sometimes the psychosocial assessment indicates serious actual or potential problems that must be addressed. The Signs of Potential Complications box identifies psychosocial characteristics and behaviors that may warrant ongoing evaluation after hospital discharge. Women exhibiting these needs should be referred to appropriate community resources for assessment and management.

SIGNS OF POTENTIAL COMPLICATIONS

Postpartum Psychosocial Concerns

The following signs may suggest potentially serious complications and should be reported to the health care provider or clinic (these may be noticed by the partner or other family members):

- Unable or unwilling to discuss labor and birth experience
- Refers to self as ugly and useless
- Excessively preoccupied with self (body image)
- Markedly depressed
- Lacks a support system
- Partner or other family members react negatively to the baby
- Refuses to interact with or care for baby; for example, does not name baby, does not want to hold or feed baby, is upset by vomiting and wet or soild diapers (cultural appropriateness of actions must be considered)
- Expresses disappointment over baby's sex
- Sees baby as messy or unattractive
- Baby reminds mother of family member or friend she does not like
- Has difficulty sleeping
- Experiences loss of appetite

Effect of the Birth Experience

Many women indicate a need to examine the birth process itself and look retrospectively at their own intrapartal behavior. Their partners may express similar desires. If their birth experience was different from their birth plan (e.g., induction, epidural anesthesia, cesarean birth), both partners may need to mourn the loss of their expectations before they can adjust to the reality

NURSING PROCESS

Postpartum Psychosocial Concerns

ASSESSMENT

- Obtain information from the medical record and nursing staff regarding any risk factors for psychologic problems after birth (e.g., history of depression, anxiety, panic disorders); review the history and current list of medications to identify any that are used for psychologic conditions.
- Assess emotional status.
- Assess reaction to the labor and birth.
- Observe interactions with the neonate.
- Observe interactions with the partner and family members.
- Identify cultural beliefs and practices.
- Assess maternal self-concept and body image.
- Assess the support system.

NURSING DIAGNOSES

Examples of nursing diagnoses for meeting psychosocial needs during the postpartum period include:

***Readiness for Enhanced Family Processes* related to:**
- excitement about newborn

***Risk for Impaired Parenting* related to:**
- long, difficult labor
- unmet expectations of labor and birth

***Risk for Situational Low Self-esteem* related to:**
- body image changes

***Risk for Caregiver Role Strain* related to:**
- postpartum fatigue

***Risk for Ineffective Coping* related to:**
- lack of support
- postpartum fatigue

EXPECTED OUTCOMES OF CARE

Examples of common expected outcomes include that the mother (family) will:

- Identify measures that promote a healthy personal adjustment in the postpartum period.
- Maintain healthy family functioning based on cultural norms and personal expectations.
- Discuss the events of the birth experience.
- Demonstrate an attachment to the newborn.
- Express positive feelings about the birth, her role, or the newborn.
- Indicates that she feels safe at home.
- Rests or sleeps between infant feedings.
- Identifies sources of support and assistance at home.
- Demonstrates knowledge of resources to call after discharge (physician, clinic, lactation consultant, social worker, etc.).

PLAN OF CARE AND INTERVENTIONS

The nurse provides education, encouragement, and support while implementing the psychosocial plan of care for a postpartum woman. Implementation of the psychosocial care plan involves carrying out specific activities to achieve the expected outcome of care planned for each individual woman. Topics that should be included in the psychosocial nursing care plan include promotion of parenting skills and family member adjustment to the newborn infant (see text).

EVALUATION

The nurse can be reasonably assured that care was effective if expected outcomes of care for psychosocial concerns have been met.

of their actual birth experience. Inviting them to review the events and describe how they feel helps the nurse assess how well they understand what happened and how well they have been able to put their childbirth experience into perspective.

Maternal Self-Image

An important assessment concerns the woman's self-concept, body image, and sexuality. How the new mother feels about herself and her body during the postpartum period may affect her behavior and adaptation to parenting. The woman's self-concept and body image can also affect her sexuality.

Feelings related to sexual adjustment after childbirth are often a cause of concern for new parents. Women who have recently given birth may be reluctant to resume sexual intercourse for fear of pain or may worry that coitus could damage healing perineal tissue. Because many new parents are anxious for information but reluctant to bring up the subject, postpartum nurses should matter-of-factly include the topic of postpartum sexuality during their routine physical assessment and teaching. Partners often have questions and concerns as well; it is helpful to include them in teaching sessions or discussions regarding sexuality in the postpartum period.

Adaptation to Parenthood and Parent-Infant Interactions

The psychosocial assessment also includes evaluating adaptation to parenthood. This task is accomplished by observing maternal and paternal reactions to the newborn and their interactions with the infant. Clues indicating successful adaptation begin to appear soon after birth as parents react positively to the newborn infant and continue the process of establishing a relationship with their infant. In nontraditional families, such as lesbian couples, it is important to observe the partner's reactions and interactions with the neonate.

Parents are adapting well to their new roles when they exhibit a realistic perception and acceptance of their newborn's needs and limited abilities, immature social responses, and helplessness. Examples of positive parent-infant interactions include taking pleasure in the infant and in providing care, responding appropriately to infant cues, and providing comfort (see Chapter 24). Should these indicators be missing, the nurse needs to investigate further what is hindering the normal adaptation process.

Family Structure and Functioning

A woman's adjustment to her role as mother is affected greatly by her relationships with her partner, her mother and other relatives, and any other children (Fig. 21-5). Nurses can help ease the new mother's return home by identifying possible conflicts among family members and helping the woman plan strategies for dealing with these problems before discharge. Such a conflict could arise when couples have very different ideas about parenting. Dealing with the stresses of sibling rivalry and unsolicited grandparent advice also can affect the woman's psychologic well-being. Only by asking about other nuclear and extended family members can the nurse discover potential problems in such relationships and help plan workable solutions for them.

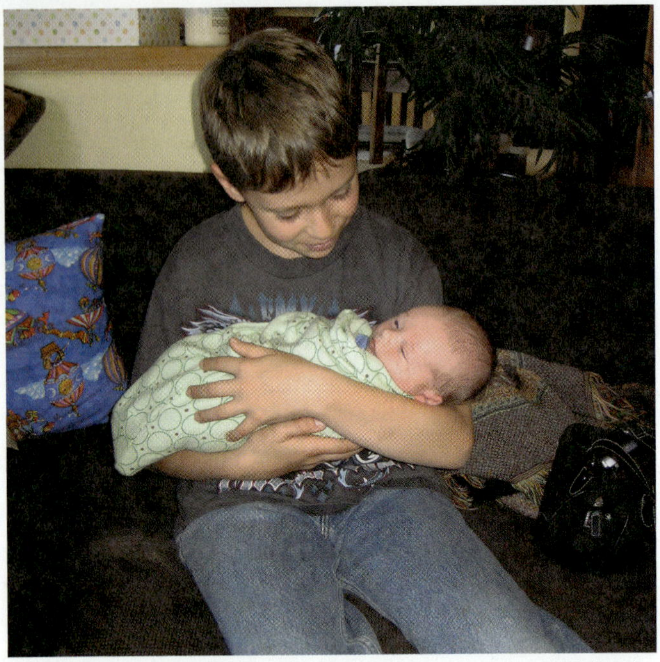

FIG. 21-5 A mother's adjustment is eased with acceptance of infant by other children. Smile indicates acceptance of the baby. (Courtesy Kody Skaggs, Morrison, CO.)

Effect of Cultural Diversity

The final component of a complete psychosocial assessment is the woman's cultural beliefs, values, and practices. Much of a woman's behavior during the postpartum period is strongly influenced by her cultural background. Nurses are likely to come into contact with women from many different countries and cultures. Within the North American population, varied traditional health beliefs and practices can be found. All cultures have developed safe and satisfying methods of caring for new mothers and babies. Only by understanding and respecting the values and beliefs of each woman can the nurse design a plan of care to meet the individual's needs.

To identify cultural beliefs and practices when planning and implementing care, the nurse conducts a cultural assessment. This assessment is ongoing; it is ideally begun during pregnancy and continued into the postpartum period. It can be accomplished most easily through conversation with the mother and her partner. Some hospitals have assessment tools designed to identify cultural beliefs and practices that may influence care (Cooper, Grywalski, Lamp, Newhouse, & Studlien, 2007). Components of the cultural assessment include the ability to read and write English, primary language spoken, family involvement and support, dietary preferences, infant care, attachment, circumcision, religious or cultural beliefs, folk medicine practices, nonverbal communication, and personal space preferences.

Women from various cultures view health as a balance between opposing forces (e.g., cold versus hot; yin versus yang), being in harmony with nature, or just "feeling good." Traditional practices may include the observance of certain dietary restrictions, clothing, or taboos for balancing the body; participation in certain activities such as sports and art for maintaining mental health; and use of silence, prayer, or meditation for developing spiritually. Practices (e.g., using religious objects or eating garlic) are used to protect oneself from illness and can involve avoiding people who are believed to create hexes or spells or who have an "evil eye." Restoration of health can involve taking folk medicines (e.g., herbs, animal substances) or using a traditional healer.

Childbirth occurs within this sociocultural context. Rest, seclusion, dietary restraints, and ceremonies honoring the mother are all common traditional practices that are followed for the promotion of the health and well-being of the mother and baby.

During the postpartum period there are several common traditional health practices used and beliefs held by women and their families. In Asia, for example, pregnancy is considered to be a "hot" state, and childbirth results in a sudden loss of this state. Therefore, balance must be restored by facilitating the return of the hot state, which is present physically or symbolically in hot food, hot water, and warm air.

Another common belief is that the mother and baby remain in a weak and vulnerable state for several weeks after birth. During this time the mother may remain in a passive role, taking no baths or showers, and may stay in bed to prevent cold air from entering her body.

Women who have immigrated to the United States or other Western nations without their extended families may have little help at home, making it difficult for them to observe these activity restrictions. The Cultural Considerations box lists some common cultural beliefs about the postpartum period and family planning.

It is important that nurses consider all cultural aspects when planning care and avoid using their own cultural beliefs as the framework for that care. Although the beliefs and behaviors of other cultures seem different or strange, they should be encouraged as long as the mother wants to conform to them and she and the baby suffer no ill effects. The nurse needs to determine whether a woman is using any folk medicine during the postpartum period because active ingredients in folk medicine can have adverse physiologic effects when used in combination with prescribed medicines. The nurse should not assume that a mother desires to use traditional health practices that represent a particular cultural group merely because she is a member of that culture. Many young women who are first- or second-generation Americans follow their cultural traditions only when older family members are present, or not at all.

DISCHARGE TEACHING

Self-Management and Signs of Complications

Discharge planning begins at the time of admission to the unit and should be reflected in the nursing care plan developed for each individual woman. For example, a great deal of time during the hospital stay is usually spent in teaching about maternal self-management and care of the newborn because the goal is for all women to be capable of providing basic care for themselves and their infants at the time of discharge. In addition, every woman must be taught to recognize physical and psychologic signs and symptoms that might indicate problems and how to obtain advice and assistance quickly if these signs appear. Table 21-2 and the Signs of Potential Complications box on pp. 489 and 500, respectively, list several common indications of maternal physical and psychosocial problems in the

Spanish Guidelines—Discharge Teaching

CULTURAL CONSIDERATIONS

Postpartum Period and Family Planning

POSTPARTUM CARE

- *Chinese, Mexican, Korean, and Southeast Asian women* may wish to consume only warm foods and hot drinks to replace blood loss and restore the balance of hot and cold in their bodies. These women may also wish to stay warm and avoid bathing, exercises, and hair washing for 7 to 30 days after childbirth. Self-management may not be a priority; care by family members is preferred. The woman has respect for elders and authority. These women may wear abdominal binders. They may prefer not to give their babies colostrum.
- *Arabic women* eat special meals designed to restore their energy. They are expected to stay at home for 40 days after birth to avoid illness resulting from exposure to the outside air.
- *Haitian women* may request to take the placenta home to bury or burn.
- *Muslim women* follow strict religious laws on modesty and diet. A Muslim woman must keep her hair, body, arms to the wrist, and legs to the ankles covered at all times. She cannot be alone in the presence of a man other than her husband or a male relative. Observant Muslims will not eat pork or pork products and are obligated to eat meat slaughtered according to Islamic laws (halal meat). If halal meat is not available, kosher meat, seafood, or a vegetarian diet is usually accepted.

FAMILY PLANNING

- Birth control is government mandated in mainland *China*. Most *Chinese women* will have an intrauterine device (IUD) inserted after the birth of their first child. Women do not want hormonal methods of contraception because they fear putting these medications into their bodies.
- *Hispanic women* may choose the rhythm method or natural family planning because most are Catholic.
- *(East) Indian men* are encouraged to have voluntary sterilization by vasectomy.
- *Muslim couples* may practice contraception by mutual consent as long as its use is not harmful to the woman. Acceptable contraceptive methods include foam and condoms, the diaphragm, and natural family planning.
- *Hmong women* highly value and desire large families, which limits birth control practices.
- *Arabic women* value large families, and sons are especially prized.

postpartum period. (See Chapter 34 for more information on postpartum complications.) Before discharge, women need basic instruction regarding a variety of self-management topics such as nutrition, exercise, family planning, the resumption of sexual intercourse, prescribed medications, and routine mother-baby follow-up care.

Because of the limited time available for teaching, nurses must target their teaching on expressed needs of the woman. Giving the woman a list of topics and asking her to indicate her learning needs helps the nurse maximize teaching efforts and can increase retention of information. Providing written materials on postpartum self-management, breastfeeding, and infant care that the woman can consult after discharge is helpful.

Just before the time of discharge the nurse reviews the woman's chart to see that laboratory reports, medications, signatures, and other items are in order. Some hospitals have a checklist to use before the woman's discharge. The nurse verifies that medications, if ordered, have arrived on the unit; that any valuables kept secured during the woman's stay have been returned to her and that she has signed a receipt for them; and that the infant is ready to be discharged. The woman's and the baby's identification bands are carefully checked.

No medication that can cause drowsiness should be administered to the mother before discharge if she is the one who will be holding the baby on the way out of the hospital. In most instances, the woman is seated in a wheelchair and is given the baby to hold. Some families leave unescorted and ambulatory, depending on hospital protocol. The newborn must be secured in a car seat for the drive home.

In many hospitals, new mothers (breastfeeding and formula feeding) are routinely presented with gift bags that contain samples of infant formula.

NURSING ALERT

Prepackaged formula should not be given to mothers who are breastfeeding. Such "gifts" are associated with earlier cessation of breastfeeding.

Sexual Activity and Contraception

Discussing sexual activity with the woman and her partner and family planning with heterosexual couples is important before they leave the hospital because many couples resume sexual activity before the traditional postpartum checkup 6 weeks after childbirth. For most women the risk of hemorrhage or infection is minimal by approximately 2 weeks postpartum. Couples may be anxious about the topic but uncomfortable and unwilling to bring it up. The nurse needs to discuss the physical and psychologic effects that giving birth can have on sexual activity (see the Teaching for Self-Management box). Contraceptive options should also be discussed with heterosexual women (and their partners, if present) before discharge so that they can make informed decisions about fertility management before resuming sexual activity. Waiting to discuss contraception at the 6-week checkup may be too late. Ovulation can occur as soon as 1 month after birth, particularly in women who bottle-feed. Breastfeeding mothers should be informed that breastfeeding is not a reliable means of contraception and that other methods should be used; nonhormonal methods are best because oral contraceptives can interfere with milk production. Women who are undecided about contraception at the time of discharge need information about using condoms with foam or creams until the first postpartum checkup. Contraceptive options are discussed in detail in Chapter 8.

Prescribed Medications

Women routinely continue to take their prenatal vitamins during the postpartum period. Breastfeeding mothers usually continue prenatal vitamins for the duration of breastfeeding. Supplemental iron can be prescribed for mothers with lower than normal hemoglobin levels. Women with extensive episiotomies or perineal lacerations (third or fourth degree) are usually prescribed stool softeners to take at home. Pain medications (analgesics or NSAIDs) may be prescribed, especially for

TEACHING FOR SELF-MANAGEMENT

Resumption of Sexual Activity

- You can safely resume sexual activity by the second to fourth week after birth, when bleeding has stopped and the episiotomy or laceration has healed. For the first 6 weeks to 6 months, vaginal lubrication is decreased.
- Your physical reactions to sexual stimulation for the first 3 months after birth will likely be slower and less intense than before birth. The strength of the orgasm may be reduced.
- A water-soluble gel, cocoa butter, or a contraceptive cream or jelly is recommended for lubrication. If some vaginal tenderness is present, your partner can be instructed to insert one or more clean, lubricated fingers into the vagina and rotate them within the vagina to help relax it and to identify possible areas of discomfort. A position in which you have control of the depth of the insertion of the penis also is useful. The side-by-side or female-on-top position may be more comfortable than other positions.
- The presence of the baby influences postbirth lovemaking. Parents hear every sound the baby makes; conversely you may be concerned that the baby hears every sound you make. In either case, any phase of the sexual response cycle may be interrupted by hearing the baby cry or move, leaving both of you frustrated and unsatisfied. In addition, the amount of psychologic energy expended by you in child care activities may lead to fatigue. Newborns require a great deal of attention and time.
- Some women have reported feeling sexual stimulation and orgasms when breastfeeding their babies. Breastfeeding mothers often are interested in returning to sexual activity before nonbreastfeeding mothers.
- You should be instructed to perform Kegel exercises correctly to strengthen your pubococcygeal muscle. This muscle is associated with bowel and bladder function and with vaginal feeling during intercourse.

CLINICAL REASONING

Family Planning and Contraceptive Use

Victoria, a 36-year-old Hispanic Roman Catholic, has just given birth to her sixth child. During a discharge teaching session, Victoria hesitantly tells the nurse that she and her husband, Martin, just cannot afford any more children but her church does not allow her to use birth control. She is afraid to discuss this with Martin because he feels that having many sons is important. She asks the nurse what she can do. She is concerned about her family, her husband, and the teachings of her church.

1. Evidence—Is evidence sufficient to draw conclusions about counseling women with regard to family planning that fits with their culture and religious faith?
2. Assumptions—What assumptions can be made about the following issues?
   a. Victoria's statement that her church does not allow her to use birth control
   b. Effective methods of family planning that are acceptable to the Roman Catholic Church
   c. The necessity of communication between Victoria and Martin regarding family planning
   d. Resources to learn alternative methods of family planning
3. What implications and priorities for nursing care can be drawn at this time?
4. Does the evidence objectively support your conclusion?
5. Are there alternative perspectives to your conclusion?

women who had cesarean births. The nurse should make certain that the woman knows the route, dosage, frequency, and common side effects of all medications that she will be taking at home. Written information about the medications is usually included in the discharge instructions.

FOLLOW-UP AFTER DISCHARGE

Routine Mother and Baby Follow-up Care

Women who have experienced uncomplicated vaginal births are commonly scheduled for the traditional 6-week postpartum examination. Women who have had a cesarean birth are often seen in the health care provider's office or clinic within 2 weeks after hospital discharge. The date and time for the follow-up appointment should be included in the discharge instructions. If an appointment has not been made before the woman leaves the hospital, she should be encouraged to call the health care provider's office or clinic to schedule an appointment.

Parents who have not already done so need to make plans for newborn follow-up at the time of discharge. Breastfeeding infants are routinely seen by the pediatric health care provider or clinic within 3 to 5 days after discharge and again at approximately 2 weeks of age. Formula-feeding infants may be seen for the first time at 2 weeks of age. If an appointment for a specific date and time was not made for the infant before leaving the hospital, the parents should be encouraged to call the office or clinic soon after their arrival home.

Home Visits

Home visits to mothers and babies within a few days of discharge can help bridge the gap between hospital care and routine visits to health care providers. Nurses can assess the mother, the infant, and the home environment; answer questions and provide education and emotional support; and make referrals to community resources if necessary. Home visits have been shown to reduce the need for more expensive health care, such as emergency department visits and rehospitalization; they can also reduce the incidence of postpartum depression in women who are at risk (Goulet et al., 2007).

The support provided by nurses and other trained community health workers can enhance parent-infant interaction and parenting skills; home visits also help to promote mutual support between the mother and her partner (De La Rosa, Perry, & Johnson, 2009). Breastfeeding outcomes can be enhanced through home visitation programs (Mannan, Rahman, Sania, Seraji, Arifeen, Winch, et al., 2008).

Home nursing care may not be available, even if needed, because no agencies are available to provide the service or no coverage is in place for payment by third-party payers. If care is available, a referral form containing information about the mother and baby should be completed at hospital discharge and sent immediately to the home care agency.

The home visit is most commonly scheduled on the woman's second day home from the hospital, but it can be scheduled on any of the first 4 days at home, depending on the individual family's situation and needs. Additional visits are planned throughout the first week, as needed. The home visits may be extended beyond that time if the family's needs warrant it and i a home visit is the most appropriate option for carrying out the follow-up care required to meet the specific needs identified.

During the home visit the nurse conducts a systematic assessment of mother and newborn to determine physiologic adjustment and to identify any existing complications, The assessment also focuses on the mother's emotional adjustment and her knowledge of self-management and infant care. Conducting the assessment in a private area of the home provides an opportunity for the mother to ask questions on potentially sensitive topics such as breast care, constipation, sexual activity, or family planning. Family adjustment to the newborn is assessed and concerns are addressed during the home visit.

During the newborn assessment the nurse can demonstrate and explain normal newborn behavior and capabilities and encourage the mother and family to ask questions or express concerns they have. The home care nurse verifies if the newborn screen for phenylketonuria and other inborn errors of metabolism has been drawn. If the baby was discharged from the hospital before 24 hours of age, a blood sample for the newborn screen can be drawn by the home care nurse or the family will need to take the infant to the health care provider's office or clinic.

Telephone Follow-up

In addition to or instead of a home visit, many providers are implementing one or more postpartum telephone follow-up calls to their clients for assessment, health teaching, and identification of complications to effect timely intervention and referrals. Telephone follow-up may be among the services offered by hospitals, private physicians, clinics, or private agencies. It may be either a separate service or combined with other strategies for extending postpartum care. Telephone nursing assessments are frequently used as follow-up to postpartum home visits.

Warm Lines

The **warm line** is another type of telephone link between the new family and concerned caregivers or experienced parent volunteers. A warm line is a help line or consultation service, not a crisis intervention line. The warm line is appropriately used for dealing with less extreme concerns that seem urgent at the time the call is placed but are not actual emergencies. Calls to warm lines commonly relate to infant feeding, prolonged crying, or sibling rivalry. Families are encouraged to call when concerns arise. Telephone numbers for warm lines should be given to parents before hospital discharge.

Support Groups

The woman adjusting to motherhood may desire interaction and conversation with other women who are having similar experiences. Postpartum women who have met earlier in prenatal clinics or on the hospital unit may begin to associate for mutual support. Members of childbirth classes who attend a postpartum reunion may decide to extend their relationship during the fourth trimester. Fathers or partners also benefit from participation in support groups.

A postpartum support group enables mothers and partners/fathers to share with and support each other as they adjust to parenting. Many new parents find it reassuring to discover that they are not alone in their feelings of confusion and uncertainty. An experienced parent can often impart concrete information that is valuable to other group members. Inexperienced parents can imitate the behavior of others in the group whom they perceive as particularly capable.

Referral to Community Resources

To develop an effective referral system the nurse should have an understanding of the needs of the woman and family and of the organization and community resources available for meeting those needs. Locating and compiling information about available community services contributes to the development of a referral system. The nurse also needs to develop his or her own resource file of local and national services that are commonly used by health care providers (see Resources on this book's Evolve website).

COMMUNITY ACTIVITY

- Visit the website of a hospital that provides maternity services in your community. Review the information about the Mother/Baby or Postpartum unit. How does the hospital support family-centered care? Are infants allowed to room in with the mother 24 hours a day? What is the visitation policy for the father of the baby (or significant other) and other family members? What types of infant security measures are in place to prevent abductions?
- Contact a hospital-based lactation consultant (LC). Try to schedule a shadow experience. Due to health and safety requirements, select the same hospital where you currently have Maternal/Newborn clinical. How soon after birth does the LC visit the mother? What hours of the day is the LC available?

KEY POINTS

- Postpartum care is family centered and modeled on the concept of health.
- Cultural beliefs and practices affect the maternal and family response to the postpartum period.
- The nursing care plan includes assessments to detect deviations from normal, comfort measures to relieve discomfort or pain, and safety measures to prevent injury or infection.
- Common nursing interventions in the postpartum period focus on prevention of excessive bleeding, bladder distention, infection; nonpharmacologic and pharmacologic relief of discomfort associated with the episiotomy, lacerations, or breastfeeding; and instituting measures to promote or suppress lactation.
- Teaching and counseling measures are designed to promote the woman's feelings of competence in self-management and infant care.
- Meeting the psychosocial needs of new mothers involves taking into consideration the composition and functioning of the entire family.
- Early postpartum discharge will continue as a result of consumer demand, medical necessity, discharge criteria for low risk childbirth, and cost-containment measures.
- Early discharge classes, telephone follow-up, home visits, warm lines, and support groups are effective means of facilitating physiologic and psychologic adjustments in the postpartum period.

Audio Chapter Summaries Access an audio summary of these Key Points on evolve

REFERENCES

American Academy of Pediatrics (AAP) Committee on Fetus and Newborn. (2004). Hospital stay for healthy term infants. *Pediatrics, 113*(5), 1434–1436.

American Academy of Pediatrics (AAP) & American College of Obstetricians and Gynecologists (ACOG). (2007). *Guidelines for perinatal care* (6th ed.). Elk Grove Village, IL: AAP.

American College of Obstetricians and Gynecologists (ACOG). (2002). ACOG Committee Opinion #281. Rubella vaccine. *Obstetrics and Gynecology, 100*(6), 1417.

Association of Women's Health, Obstetric and Neonatal Nurses (AWHONN). (2006). *The compendium of postpartum care.* Washington, DC: AWHONN.

Baby-Friendly Hospital Initiative USA. (2010). *The ten steps to successful breastfeeding.* Available at www.babyfriendlyusa.org/eng/10steps.html. Accessed January 20, 2010.

Becker, G., & Scott, M. (2008). Nutrition for lactating women. In R. Mannel, P. Martens, & M. Walker (Eds.), *Core curriculum for lactation consultant practice* (2nd ed.). Sudbury, MA: Jones and Bartlett.

Cargill, Y., Martel, M. (2007). Society of Obstetricians and Gynaecologists of Canada: Postpartum maternal and newborn discharge. SGOC Policy Statement No. 190. *Journal of Obstetrics and Gynaecology Canada, 29*(4), 357–363.

Centers for Disease Control and Prevention (CDC). (2007). Prevention of varicella: Recommendations of the Advisory Committee on Immunization Practices (ACIP). *MMWR Morbidity and Mortality Weekly Recommendations and Report, 56*(RR04), 1–40.

Centers for Disease Control and Prevention (CDC). (2008). Prevention of pertussis, tetanus, and diphtheria among pregnant and postpartum women and their infants: Recommendations of the Advisory Committee on Immunization Practices (ACIP). *MMWR Morbidity and Mortality Weekly Report, 57*(RR-4), 1–51.

Cheung, C., Fowles, E., & Walker, L. (2006). Postpartum maternal health care in the United States: A critical review. *Journal of Perinatal Education, 15*(3), 34–42.

Cooper, M., Grywalski, M., Lamp, J., Newhouse, L., & Studlien, R. (2007). Enhancing cultural competence: A model for nurses. *Nursing for Women's Health, 11*(2), 148–160.

Corwin, E., & Arbour, M. (2007). Postpartum fatigue and evidence-based interventions. *MCN American Journal of Maternal/Child Nursing, 32*(4), 215–220.

Corwin, E., Brownstead, J., Barton, N., Heckard, S., & Morin, K. (2005). The impact of fatigue on the development of postpartum depression. *Journal of Obstetric, Gynecologic and Neonatal Nursing, 34*(5), 577–586.

Declercq, E., Cunningham, D., Johnson, C., & Sakala, C. (2008). Mothers' reports of postpartum pain associated with vaginal and cesarean deliveries: Results of a national survey. *Birth, 35*(1), 16–24.

De La Rosa, I., Perry, J., & Johnson, V. (2009). Benefits of increased home-visitation services: Exploring a case management model. *Family and Community Health, 32*(10), 58–75.

Frank, B., Lane, C., & Hokanson, H. (2009). Designing a postepidural fall risk assessment score for the obstetric patient. *Journal of Nursing Care Quality, 24*(1), 50–54.

Goulet, L., D'Amour, D., & Pineault, R. (2007). Type and timing of services following postnatal discharge: Do they make a difference? *Women & Health, 45*(4), 19–39.

Institute of Medicine. (2005). *Dietary reference intakes for energy, carbohydrate, fiber, fatty acids, cholesterol, protein, and amino acids.* Washington, DC: Food and Nutrition Board, Institute of Medicine, National Academies Press.

Mannan, I., Rahman, S., Sania, A., Seraji, H., Arifeen, S., Winch, P., et al. (2008). Can early postpartum visits by trained community health workers improve breastfeeding of newborns? *Journal of Perinatology, 28*(9), 632–640.

Runquist, J. (2007). Persevering through postpartum fatigue. *Journal of Obstetric, Gynecologic and Neonatal Nursing, 36*(1), 28–37.

Shaw, E., Levitt, C., Wong, S., & Kaczorowski, J. (2006). Systematic review of the literature on postpartum care: Effectiveness of postpartum support to improve maternal parenting, mental health, quality of life, and physical health. *Birth, 33*(3), 210–220.

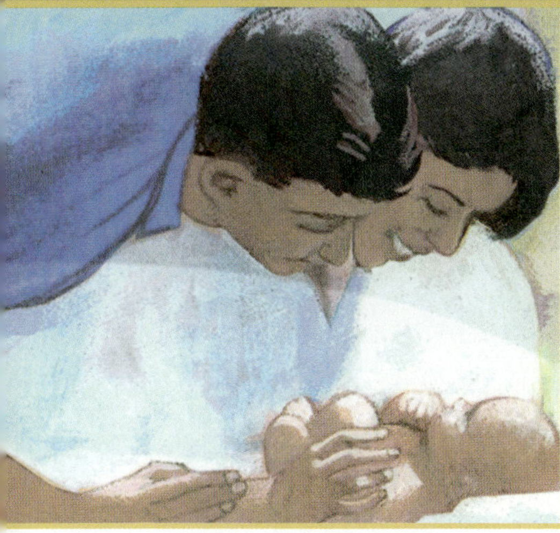

CHAPTER 22

Transition to Parenthood

Kathryn Rhodes Alden

Evolve WEBSITE

http://evolve.elsevier.com/Lowdermilk/MWHC/

Audio Glossary
Audio Key Points
NCLEX Review Questions
Nursing Care Plans
- Home Care Follow-Up: Transition to Parenthood
- The Multiparous Woman and Family

LEARNING OBJECTIVES

- Identify parental and infant behaviors that facilitate and those that inhibit parental attachment.
- Describe sensual responses that strengthen attachment.
- Examine the process of becoming a mother and becoming a father.
- Compare maternal adjustment and paternal adjustment to parenthood.
- Describe how the nurse can facilitate parent-infant adjustment.
- Examine the effects of the following on parenting responses and behavior: parental age (i.e., adolescence and older than 35 years), social support, culture, socioeconomic conditions, personal aspirations, and sensory impairment.
- Describe sibling adjustment.
- Discuss grandparent adaptation.

Becoming a parent creates a period of change and instability for men and women who decide to have children. This period occurs whether parenthood is biologic or adoptive and whether the parents are married husband-wife couples, cohabiting couples, single mothers, single fathers, lesbian couples with one woman as biologic mother, or gay male couples who adopt a child. Parenting is a process of role attainment and role transition. The transition is an ongoing process as the parents and infant develop and change.

PARENTAL ATTACHMENT, BONDING, AND ACQUAINTANCE

The process by which a parent comes to love and accept a child and a child comes to love and accept a parent is known as **attachment.** Attachment occurs through the process of bonding. In their **bonding** theory, Klaus and Kennell (1976) proposed that there is a sensitive period during the first few minutes or hours after birth when mothers and fathers must have close contact with their infants to optimize the child's later development. Klaus and Kennell (1982) later revised their theory of parent-infant bonding, modifying their claim of the critical nature of immediate contact with the infant after birth. They acknowledged the adaptability of human parents, stating that more than minutes or hours were needed for parents to form an emotional relationship with their infants. The terms *attachment* and *bonding* continue to be used interchangeably.

Attachment is developed and maintained by proximity and interaction with the infant, through which the parent becomes acquainted with the infant, identifies the infant as an individual, and claims the infant as a member of the family. Positive feedback between the parent and the infant through social, verbal, and nonverbal responses (whether real or perceived) facilitates the attachment process. Attachment occurs through a mutually satisfying experience. A mother commented on her son's grasp reflex, "I put my finger in his hand, and he grabbed right on. It is just a reflex, I know, but it felt good anyway" (Fig. 22-1).

The concept of attachment includes **mutuality;** that is, the infant's behaviors and characteristics elicit a corresponding set of parental behaviors and characteristics. The infant displays signaling behaviors such as crying, smiling, and cooing that initiate the contact and bring the caregiver to the child. These behaviors are followed by executive behaviors such as rooting, grasping, and postural adjustments that maintain the contact. Most caregivers are attracted to an alert, responsive, cuddly infant and repelled by an irritable, apparently disinterested

TABLE 22-1 INFANT BEHAVIORS AFFECTING PARENTAL ATTACHMENT

FACILITATING BEHAVIORS	INHIBITING BEHAVIORS
Visually alert; eye-to-eye contact; tracking or following of parent's face	Sleepy; eyes closed most of the time; gaze aversion
Appealing facial appearance; randomness of body movements reflecting helplessness	Resemblance to person parent dislikes; hyperirritability or jerky body movements when touched
Smiles	Bland facial expression; infrequent smiles
Vocalization; crying only when hungry or wet	Crying for hours on end; colicky
Grasp reflex	Exaggerated motor reflex
Anticipatory approach behaviors for feedings; sucks well; feeds easily	Feeds poorly; regurgitates; vomits often
Enjoys being cuddled and held	Resists holding and cuddling by crying, stiffening body
Easily consolable	Inconsolable; unresponsive to parenting, caretaking tasks
Activity and regularity somewhat predictable	Unpredictable feeding and sleeping schedule
Attention span sufficient to focus on parents	Inability to attend to parent's face or offered stimulation
Differential crying, smiling, and vocalizing; recognizes and prefers parents	Shows no preference for parents over others
Approaches through locomotion	Unresponsive to parent's approaches
Clings to parent; puts arms around parent's neck	Seeks attention from any adult in room
Lifts arms to parents in greeting	Ignores parents

Source: Gerson, E. (1973). *Infant behavior in the first year of life.* New York: Raven Press.

TABLE 22-2 PARENTAL BEHAVIORS AFFECTING INFANT ATTACHMENT

FACILITATING BEHAVIORS	INHIBITING BEHAVIORS
Looks; gazes; takes in physical characteristics of infant; assumes en face position; eye contact	Turns away from infant; ignores infant's presence
Hovers; maintains proximity; directs attention to, points to infant	Avoids infant; does not seek proximity; refuses to hold infant when given opportunity
Identifies infant as unique individual	Identifies infant with someone parent dislikes; fails to recognize any of infant's unique features
Claims infant as family member; names infant	Fails to place infant in family context or identify infant with family member; has difficulty naming
Touches; progresses from fingertip to fingers to palms to encompassing contact	Fails to move from fingertip touch to palmar contact and holding
Smiles at infant	Maintains bland countenance or frowns at infant
Talks to, coos, or sings to infant	Wakes infant when infant is sleeping; handles roughly; hurries feeding by moving nipple continuously
Expresses pride in infant	Expresses disappointment, displeasure in infant
Relates infant's behavior to familiar events	Does not incorporate infant into life
Assigns meaning to infant's actions and sensitively interprets infant's needs	Makes no effort to interpret infant's actions or needs
Views infant's behaviors and appearance in positive light	Views infant's behavior as exploiting, deliberately uncooperative; views appearance as distasteful, ugly

Source: Mercer, R. (1983). Parent-infant attachment. In L. Sonstegard, K. Kowalski, & B. Jennings (Eds.), *Women's Health* (Vol. 2). New York: Grune & Stratton.

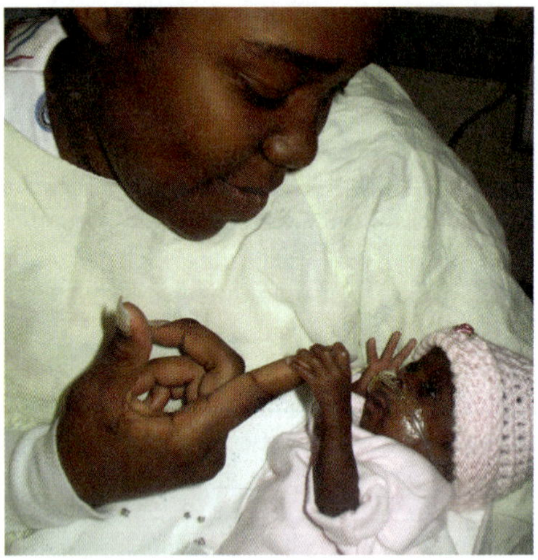

FIG. 22-1 Hands. (Courtesy Cheryl Briggs, RNC, Annapolis, MD.)

infant. Attachment occurs more readily with the infant whose temperament, social capabilities, appearance, and sex fit the parent's expectations. If the infant does not meet these expectations, the parent's disappointment can delay the attachment process. Table 22-1 presents a comprehensive list of classic infant behaviors affecting parental attachment. Table 22-2 presents a corresponding list of parental behaviors that affect infant attachment.

An important part of attachment is **acquaintance.** Parents use eye contact (Fig. 22-2), touching, talking, and exploring to become acquainted with their infant during the immediate postpartum period. Adoptive parents undergo the same process when they first meet their new child. During this period families engage in the **claiming process,** which is the identification of the new baby (Fig. 22-3). The child is first identified in terms of "likeness" to other family members, then in terms of "differences," and finally in terms of "uniqueness." The unique newcomer is thus incorporated into the family. Mothers and fathers examine their infant carefully and point out characteristics that the child shares with other family members and that are indicative of a relationship between them. Maternal comments such as the following reveal the claiming process: "Everyone says, 'He's the image of his father,' but I found one part like me—his toes are shaped like mine."

On the other hand, some mothers react negatively. They "claim" the infant in terms of the discomfort or pain the baby causes. The mother interprets the infant's normal responses as being negative toward her and reacts to her child with dislike or indifference. She does not hold the child close or touch the child to be comforting. For example, "The nurse put the baby into Lydia's arms. She promptly laid him across her knees and glanced up at the television. 'Stay still until I finish watching; you've been enough trouble already.'"

Nursing interventions related to the promotion of parent-infant attachment are numerous and varied (Table 22-3). They can enhance positive parent-infant contacts by heightening

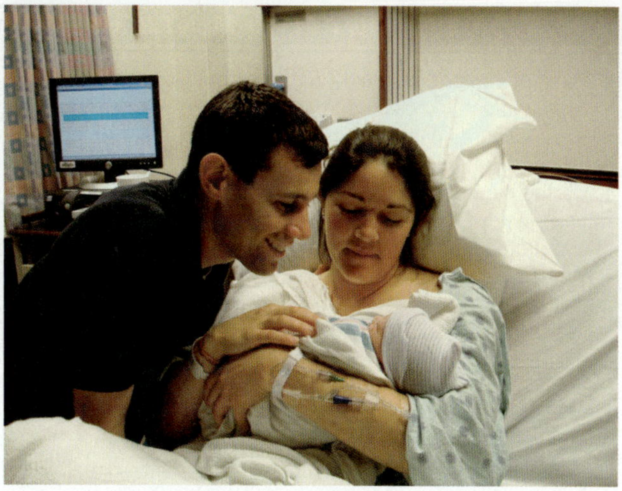

FIG. 22-2 Early acquaintance between parents and newborn as mother holds infant in en face position. (Courtesy Kathryn Alden, Chapel Hill, NC.)

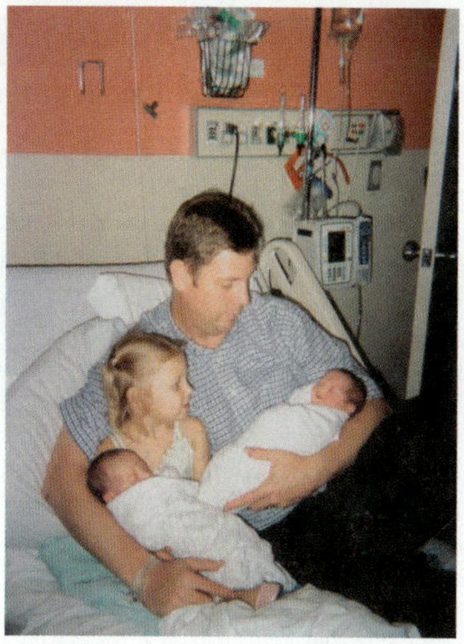

FIG. 22-3 Father looks for resemblance between newborns and older daughter. (Courtesy Cheryl Briggs, RNC, Annapolis, MD.)

TABLE 22-3 **EXAMPLES OF PARENT-INFANT ATTACHMENT INTERVENTIONS**

INTERVENTION LABEL AND DEFINITION	ACTIVITIES
Attachment Promotion Facilitation of development of parent-infant relationship	Provide opportunity for parent or parents to see, hold, and examine newborn immediately after birth. Encourage parent or parents to hold infant close to body. Assist parent or parents to participate in infant care. Provide rooming-in while in hospital.
Environmental Management: Attachment Process Manipulation of individuals' surroundings to facilitate development of parent-infant relationship	Create environment that fosters privacy. Individualize daily routine to meet parents' needs. Permit father or significant other to sleep in room with mother. Develop policies that permit presence of significant others as much as desired.
Family Integrity Promotion: Childbearing Family Facilitation of growth of individuals or families who are adding infant to family unit	Prepare parent or parents for expected role changes involved in becoming a parent. Prepare parent or parents for responsibilities of parenthood. Monitor effects of newborn on family structure. Reinforce positive parenting behaviors.
Lactation Counseling Use of interactive helping process to assist in achieving and maintaining successful breastfeeding	Correct misconceptions, misinformation, and inaccuracies about breastfeeding. Assess feeding techniques and assist as needed. Evaluate parents' understanding of infant's feeding cues (e.g., rooting, sucking, alertness). Determine frequency of feedings in relation to infant's needs. Demonstrate breast massage and discuss its advantages to increasing milk supply. Provide education, encouragement, and support.
Parent Education: Infant Instruction on nurturing and physical care needed during first year of life	Determine parents' knowledge, readiness, and ability to learn about infant care. Provide anticipatory guidance about developmental changes during first year of life. Teach parent or parents skills to care for newborn. Demonstrate ways in which parent or parents can stimulate infant's development. Discuss infant's capabilities for interaction. Demonstrate quieting techniques.
Risk Identification: Childbearing Family Identification of individual or family likely to experience difficulties in parenting and assigning priorities to strategies to prevent parenting problems	Determine developmental stage of parent or parents. Review prenatal history for factors that predispose individuals or family to complications. Ascertain understanding of English or other language used in community. Monitor behavior that may indicate problem with attachment. Plan for risk-reduction activities in collaboration with individual or family.

Modified from Bulechek, G., Butcher, H., & Dochterman, J. (2008). *Nursing interventions classification (NIC)* (5th ed.). St. Louis: Mosby.

CULTURAL CONSIDERATIONS

Fostering Bonding in Women of Varying Ethnic and Cultural Groups

Childbearing practices and rituals of other cultures are not always congruent with standard practices associated with bonding in the Anglo-American culture. For example, Chinese families traditionally use extended family members to care for the newborn so that the mother can rest and recover, especially after a cesarean birth. Some Native-American, Asian, and Hispanic women do not initiate breastfeeding until their breast milk comes in. Haitian families do not name their babies until after the confinement month. The amount of eye contact varies among cultures as well. Yup'ik Eskimo mothers almost always position their babies so that they can make eye contact.

Nurses should become knowledgeable about the childbearing beliefs and practices of diverse cultural and ethnic groups. Because individual cultural variations exist within groups, nurses need to clarify with the client and family members or friends what cultural norms they follow. Incorrect judgments can be made about parent-infant bonding if nurses do not practice culturally sensitive care.

Modified from D'Avanzo, C. (2008). *Mosby's pocket guide to cultural health assessment* (4th ed.). St. Louis: Mosby.

parental awareness of an infant's responses and ability to communicate. As the parent attempts to become competent and loving in that role, nurses can bolster the parent's self-confidence and ego. Nurses can identify actual and potential problems and collaborate with other health care professionals who will provide care for the parents after discharge. Nursing considerations for fostering maternal-infant bonding among special populations may vary (see the Cultural Considerations box).

Assessment of Attachment Behaviors

One of the most important areas of assessment is careful observation of specific behaviors thought to indicate the formation of emotional bonds between the newborn and the family, especially the mother. Unlike physical assessment of the neonate, which has concrete guidelines to follow, assessment of parent-infant attachment relies more on skillful observation and interviewing. Rooming-in of mother and infant and liberal visiting privileges for father or partner, siblings, and grandparents provide nurses with excellent opportunities to observe interactions and identify behaviors that demonstrate positive or negative attachment. Attachment behaviors can be easily observed during infant feeding sessions. Box 22-1 presents guidelines for assessment of attachment behaviors.

During pregnancy, and often even before conception occurs, parents develop an image of the "ideal" or "fantasy" infant. At birth the fantasy infant becomes the real infant. How closely the dream child resembles the real child influences the bonding process. Assessing such expectations during pregnancy and at the time of the infant's birth allows identification of discrepancies in the parents' view of the fantasy child versus the real child.

The labor process significantly affects the immediate attachment of mothers to their newborn infants. Factors such as a long labor, feeling tired or "drugged" after birth, and problems with breastfeeding can delay the development of initial positive feelings toward the newborn.

BOX 22-1 ASSESSING ATTACHMENT BEHAVIOR

- When the infant is brought to the parents, do they reach out for the infant and call the infant by name? (Recognize that in some cultures parents may not name the infant in the early newborn period.)
- Do the parents speak about the infant in terms of identification—whom the infant resembles, and what appears special about their infant over other infants?
- When parents are holding the infant, what kind of body contact is seen—do parents feel at ease in changing the infant's position, are fingertips or whole hands used, and does the infant have parts of the body they avoid touching or parts of the body they investigate and scrutinize?
- When the infant is awake, what kinds of stimulation do the parents provide—do they talk to the infant, to each other, or to no one, and how do they look at the infant—direct visual contact, avoidance of eye contact, or looking at other people or objects?
- How comfortable do the parents appear in terms of caring for the infant? Do they express any concern regarding their ability or disgust for certain activities, such as changing diapers?
- What type of affection do they demonstrate to the newborn, such as smiling, stroking, kissing, or rocking?
- If the infant is fussy, what kinds of comforting techniques do the parents use, such as rocking, swaddling, talking, or stroking?

PARENT-INFANT CONTACT

Early Contact

Early close contact can facilitate the attachment process between parent and child. Although a delay in contact does not necessarily mean that attachment will be inhibited, additional psychologic energy may be necessary to achieve the same effect. To date, no scientific evidence has demonstrated that immediate contact after birth is essential for the human parent-child relationship.

Early skin-to-skin contact between the mother and newborn immediately after birth and during the first hour facilitates maternal affectionate and attachment behaviors (Moore, Anderson, & Bergman, 2009). The newborn is placed in the prone position on the mother's bare chest; the baby and mother's chest are covered with a warm, dry blanket and the infant's head is covered with a cap to prevent heat loss. This practice promotes early and effective breastfeeding and increases breastfeeding duration. It is also associated with less infant crying, improved thermoregulation (especially in low-birth-weight infants), and improved cardiorespiratory stability in late preterm infants (Moore et al.).

Parents who are unable to have early contact with their newborn (e.g., the infant was transferred to the intensive care nursery) can be reassured that such contact is not essential for optimal parent-infant interactions. Otherwise, adopted infants would not form affectionate ties with their parents. Nurses need to stress that the parent-infant relationship is a process that occurs over time.

Extended Contact

Rooming-in is common in family-centered care. With this practice the infant stays in the room with the mother. In some facilities the newborn never leaves the mother's presence; nursery nurses perform the initial assessment and care in the room with the parents. In other hospitals the infant is transferred to the postpartum or mother-baby unit from the transitional nursery (if the facility uses one) after showing satisfactory extrauterine adjustment. Nurses encourage the father or partner to participate in caring for the infant in as active a role as they desire. They can also encourage siblings and grandparents to visit and become acquainted with the infant. Whether the method of family-centered care is rooming-in, mother-baby or couplet care, or a family birth unit, mothers, their partners, and family members are equal and integral parts of the developing family.

Extended contact with the infant should be available for all parents but especially for those at risk for parenting inadequacies, such as adolescents and low-income women. Postpartum nurses need to consider and encourage activities that optimize family-centered care.

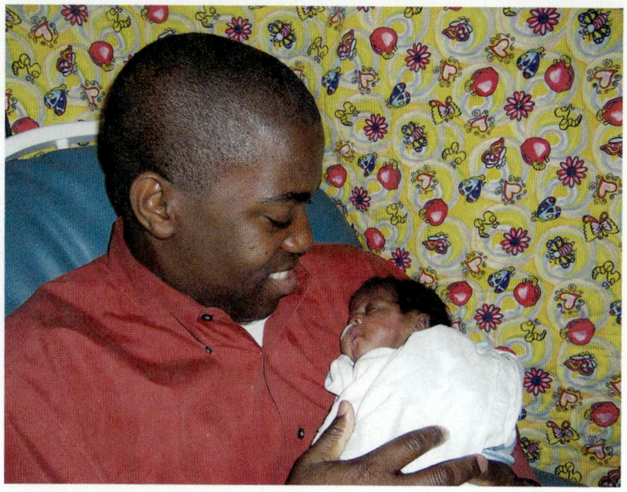

FIG. 22-4 Father interacts with his newborn son. (Courtesy Cheryl Briggs, RNC, Annapolis, MD.)

COMMUNICATION BETWEEN PARENT AND INFANT

The parent-infant relationship is strengthened through the use of sensual responses and abilities by both partners in the interaction. The nurse should keep in mind that cultural variations are often seen in these interactive behaviors.

The Senses

Touch

Touch, or the tactile sense, is used extensively by parents as a means of becoming acquainted with the newborn. Many mothers reach out for their infants as soon as they are born and the cord is cut. Mothers lift their infants to their breasts, enfold them in their arms, and cradle them. Once the infant is close, the mother begins the exploration process with her fingertips, one of the most touch-sensitive areas of the body. Within a short time she uses her palm to caress the baby's trunk and eventually enfolds the infant. Similar progression of touching is demonstrated by fathers, partners, and other caregivers. Gentle stroking motions are used to soothe and quiet the infant; patting or gently rubbing the infant's back is a comfort after feedings. Infants also pat the mother's breast as they nurse. Both seem to enjoy sharing each other's body warmth. Parents seem to have an innate desire to touch, pick up, and hold the infant (Fig. 22-4). They comment on the softness of the baby's skin and note details of the baby's appearance. As parents become increasingly sensitive to the infant's like or dislike for different types of touch, they draw closer to the baby.

Touching behaviors by mothers vary in different cultural groups. For example, minimal touching and cuddling is a traditional Southeast Asian practice thought to protect the infant from evil spirits. Because of tradition and spiritual beliefs, women in India and Bali have practiced infant massage since ancient times.

Eye Contact

Parents repeatedly demonstrate interest in having eye contact with the baby. Some mothers remark that once their babies have looked at them, they feel much closer to them. Parents spend much time getting their babies to open their eyes and look at them. In the United States, eye contact appears to reinforce the development of a trusting relationship and is an important factor in human relationships at all ages. In other cultures, eye contact is perceived differently. For example, in Mexican culture, sustained direct eye contact is considered rude, immodest, and dangerous for some. This danger may arise from the *mal de ojo* (evil eye), resulting from excessive admiration. Women and children are thought to be more susceptible to *mal de ojo* (D'Avanzo, 2008).

As newborns become functionally able to sustain eye contact with their parents, they spend time in mutual gazing, often in the **en face** position, a position in which the parent's and infant's faces are approximately 20 cm apart and on the same plane (see Fig. 22-2). Nurses and physicians or midwives can facilitate eye contact immediately after birth by positioning the infant on the mother's abdomen or breasts with the mother's and the infant's faces on the same plane. Dimming the lights encourages the infant's eyes to open. To promote eye contact, instillation of prophylactic antibiotic ointment in the infant's eyes can be delayed until the infant and parents have had some time together in the first hour after birth.

Voice

The shared response of parents and infants to each other's voices is remarkable. Parents wait tensely for the first cry. Once that cry has reassured them of the baby's health, they begin comforting behaviors. As the parents speak, the infant is alerted and turns toward them. Infants respond to higher-pitched voices and can distinguish their mother's voice from others soon after birth.

Odor

Another behavior shared by parents and infants is a response to each other's odor. Mothers comment on the smell of their babies when first born and have noted that each infant has a unique odor. Infants learn rapidly to distinguish the odor of their mother's breast milk.

Entrainment

Newborns move in time with the structure of adult speech, which is termed **entrainment.** They wave their arms, lift their heads, and kick their legs, seemingly "dancing in tune"

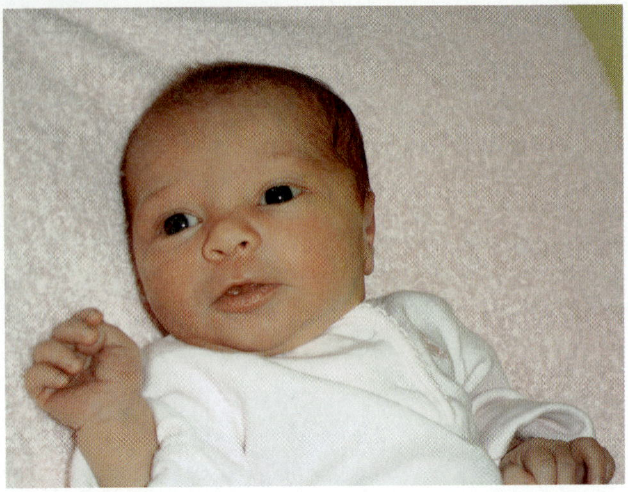

FIG. 22-5 Infant in alert state. (Courtesy Kathryn Alden, Chapel Hill, NC.)

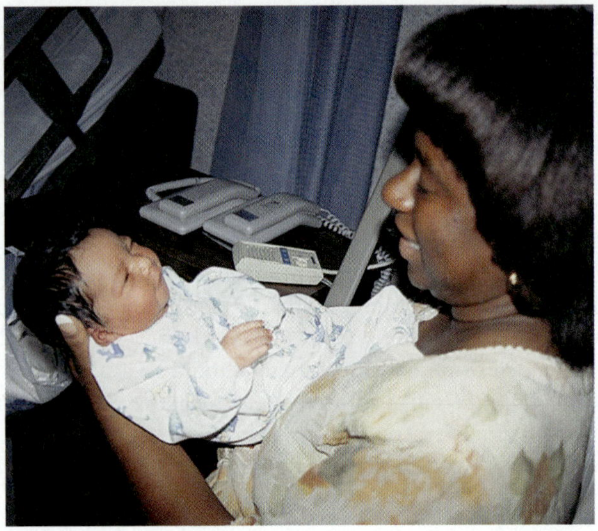

FIG. 22-6 Sharing a smile: an example of synchrony. (Courtesy Marjorie Pyle, RNC, Lifecircle, Costa Mesa, CA.)

to a parent's voice. Culturally determined rhythms of speech are ingrained in the infant long before he or she uses spoken language to communicate. This shared rhythm also gives the parent positive feedback and establishes a positive setting for effective communication.

Biorhythmicity

Biorhythmicity refers to the infant being in tune with the mother's natural rhythms. The mother's heartbeat or a recording of a heartbeat can soothe a crying infant. One of the newborn's tasks is to establish a personal biorhythm. Parents can help in this process by giving consistent loving care and using their infant's alert state to develop responsive behavior and increase social interactions and opportunities for learning (Fig. 22-5). The more quickly parents become competent in child care activities, the more quickly they can direct their psychologic energy toward observing and responding to the communication cues the infant gives them.

Reciprocity and Synchrony

Reciprocity is a type of body movement or behavior that provides the observer with cues. The observer or receiver interprets those cues and responds to them. Reciprocity often takes several weeks to develop with a new baby. For example, when the newborn fusses and cries, the mother responds by picking up and cradling the infant; the baby becomes quiet and alert and establishes eye contact; the mother verbalizes, sings, and coos while the baby maintains eye contact. The baby then averts the eyes and yawns; the mother decreases her active response. If the parent continues to stimulate the infant, the baby may become fussy.

The term **synchrony** refers to the "fit" between the infant's cues and the parent's response. When parent and infant experience a synchronous interaction, it is mutually rewarding (Fig. 22-6). Parents need time to interpret the infant's cues correctly. For example, the infant develops a specific cry in response to different situations such as boredom, loneliness, hunger, and discomfort. The parent may need assistance in interpreting these cries, along with trial and error interventions, before synchrony develops.

PARENTAL ROLE AFTER BIRTH

Adaptation involves a stabilizing of tasks, a coming to terms with commitments. Parents demonstrate growing competence in child care activities and become increasingly more attuned to their infant's behavior. Typically, the period from the decision to conceive through the first months of having a child is termed the **transition to parenthood.**

Transition to Parenthood

Historically, the transition to parenthood was viewed as a crisis. The current perspective is that parenthood is a developmental transition rather than a major life crisis. The transition to parenthood is a time of disorder and disequilibrium, as well as satisfaction, for mothers and their partners. Usual methods of coping often seem ineffective during this time. Some parents are so distressed that they are unable to be supportive of each other. Because men typically identify their spouses as their primary or only source of support, the transition can be comparatively harder for the fathers. They often feel deprived when the mothers, who are also experiencing stress, cannot provide their usual level of support. Many parents are unprepared for the strong emotions such as helplessness, inadequacy, and anger that arise when dealing with a crying infant. However, parenthood allows adults to develop and display a selfless, warm, and caring side of themselves that may not be expressed in other adult roles.

For the majority of mothers and their partners the transition to parenthood is an opportunity rather than a time of danger. Parents try new coping strategies as they work to master their new roles and reach new developmental levels. As they work through the transition, they often find personal strength and resourcefulness.

Parental Tasks and Responsibilities

Parents need to reconcile the actual child with the fantasy and dream child. This process means coming to terms with the infant's physical appearance, sex, innate temperament, and physical status. If the real child differs greatly from the fantasy child, some parents delay acceptance of the child. In some instances, they never accept the child.

NURSING CARE PLAN

Home Care Follow-up: Transition to Parenthood

NURSING DIAGNOSIS

Deficient knowledge of infant care related to lack of experience or lack of support

Expected Outcomes

The parents provide safe and adequate care and the infant appears healthy.

Nursing Interventions/*Rationales*

- Observe infant care routines (bathing, diapering, feeding, play) *to evaluate parental ease with care and adequacy of techniques.*
- Observe the infant's appearance (height-weight ratio, head circumference, fontanels, skin tone and turgor), and assess the vital signs, overall tone, reflexes, and age-appropriate developmental skills *to evaluate for signs indicative of inadequate care.*
- Explore available support systems for infant care *to determine the adequacy of existing system.*
- Demonstrate care routines that pose difficulties, and have involved family members return the demonstration *to facilitate improvements in care.*
- Provide ongoing follow-up and referrals as needed *to ensure that identified potential and actual care deficits are addressed and resolved.*

NURSING DIAGNOSIS

Disturbed sleep pattern related to infant demands and environmental interruptions

Expected Outcomes

Woman sleeps for uninterrupted periods and states that she feels rested on waking.

Nursing Interventions/*Rationales*

- Discuss the woman's routine, and specify factors that interfere with sleep *to determine the scope of the problem and direct interventions.*
- Explore ways the woman and significant others can make the environment more conducive to sleep (e.g., privacy, darkness, quiet, back rubs, soothing music, warm milk), and teach the use of guided imagery and relaxation techniques *to promote optimal conditions for sleep.*
- Eliminate factors or routines (e.g., caffeine, foods that induce heartburn, strenuous mental or physical activity) *that may interfere with sleep.*
- Advise the family to limit visitors and activities *to prevent further stress and fatigue.*
- Have the family plan specific times to care for the newborn *to allow mother time to sleep;* have the mother learn to use infant nap time as a time for her to nap as well *to replenish energy and decrease fatigue.*
- Assist the family to identify persons such as family members or friends who can provide help with household tasks, infant care, and care of other children *to allow the mother more time to rest.*

NURSING DIAGNOSIS

Risk for impaired home maintenance related to addition of new family member, inadequate resources, or inadequate support systems

Expected Outcome

Home exhibits signs of safe and functional environment.

Nursing Interventions/*Rationales*

- Observe the home environment (e.g., available living space and sleeping arrangements; adequacy of facilities for food preparation and storage, hygiene, and toileting; overall state of repair; cleanliness; presence of safety hazards) *to determine the adequacy and effective use of resources.*
- Observe arrangements for the newborn, such as sleeping space, care equipment, and supplies (bathing, changing, feeding, transportation) *to determine the adequacy of resources.*
- Explore who is responsible for cooking, cleaning, child care, and newborn care, and determine whether the mother seems adequately rested *to determine the adequacy of support systems.*
- Identify and arrange referrals to needed social agencies (e.g., Temporary Assistance for Needy Families [TANF]; Special Supplemental Nutrition Program for Women, Infants, and Children [WIC] program; food pantries) *to address resource deficits (finances, supplies, equipment).*

NURSING DIAGNOSIS

Risk for interrupted family processes related to inclusion of the new family member

Expected Outcome

Infant is successfully incorporated into the family structure.

Nursing Interventions/*Rationales*

- Explore with the family the ways that the birth and neonate have changed the family structure and function *to evaluate functional and role adjustment.*
- Observe the family's interaction with the newborn, and note degree of bonding, evidence of sibling rivalry, and involvement in newborn care *to evaluate the acceptance of the newest family member.*
- Clarify identified misinformation and misperceptions *to promote clear communication.*
- Assist the family in exploring options for solutions to identified problems *to promote effective problem resolution.*
- Support the family's efforts as they move toward adjusting and incorporating the new member *to reinforce new functions and roles.*
- If needed, make referrals to appropriate social services or community agencies *to ensure ongoing support and care.*

Many parents know the sex of the infant before birth because of the use of ultrasound assessments. For those who do not have this information, disappointment over the baby's sex can take time to resolve. The parents may provide adequate physical care but have difficulty in being sincerely involved with the infant until this internal conflict has been resolved. As one mother remarked, "I really wanted a boy. I know it is silly and irrational, but when they said, 'She's a lovely little girl,' I was so disappointed and angry—yes, angry—I could hardly look at her. Oh, I looked after her okay, her feedings and baths and things, but I couldn't feel excited. To tell the truth, I felt like a monster not liking my child. Then one day, she was lying there and she turned her head and looked right at me. I felt a flooding of love for her come over me, and we looked at each other a long time. It's okay now. I wouldn't change her for all the boys in the world."

The normal appearance of the neonate—size, color, molding of the head, or bowed appearance of the legs—is startling for some parents. Nurses can encourage parents to examine their babies and to ask questions about newborn characteristics.

Parents need to become adept in the care of the infant, including caregiving activities, noting the communication cues given by the infant to indicate needs, and responding appropriately to the infant's needs. Self-esteem grows with competence. Breastfeeding helps mothers believe that they are contributing in a unique way to the welfare of the infant. The parent may interpret the infant's response to the parental care and attention as a comment on the quality of that care. Infant behaviors that parents interpret as positive responses to their care include being consoled easily, enjoying being cuddled, and making eye contact. Spitting up frequently after feedings, crying, and being unpredictable are often perceived as negative responses to parental care. Continuation of these infant responses that parents view as negative can result in alienation of parent and infant.

Some people view assistance, including advice by husbands, partners, wives, mothers, mothers-in-law, and health care professionals, as supportive. Others view advice as criticism or an indication of how inept these people judge the new parents to be. Criticism, real or imagined, of the new parents' ability to provide adequate physical care, nutrition, or social stimulation for the infant can be devastating. By providing encouragement and praise for parenting efforts, nurses can bolster the new parents' confidence.

Parents must establish a place for the newborn within the family group. Whether the infant is the firstborn or the last born, all family members must adjust their roles to accommodate the newcomer.

Becoming a Mother

Rubin (1961) identified three phases of maternal role attainment in which the mother adjusts to her parental role. These phases extend over the first several weeks and are characterized by dependent behavior, dependent-independent behavior, and interdependent behavior (Table 22-4). Rubin's research was conducted when the length of stay in the hospital was for a longer period (3 to 5 or more days). With today's early discharge, women seem to move through the phases faster.

Mercer (2004) suggested that the concept of *maternal role attainment,* be replaced with *becoming a mother* to signify the transformation and growth of the mother's identity. Becoming a mother implies more than attaining a role. It includes learning new skills and increasing her confidence in herself as she meets new challenges in caring for her child or children.

Mercer (2004) identified four stages in the process of becoming a mother: "[a] commitment, attachment to the unborn baby, and preparation for delivery and motherhood during pregnancy; [b] acquaintance/attachment to the infant, learning to care for the infant, and physical restoration during the first 2 to 6 weeks following birth; [c] moving toward a new normal; and [d] achievement of a maternal identity through redefining self to incorporate motherhood (around 4 months)" (Mercer & Walker, 2006, pp. 568-569). The time of achievement of the stages is variable and the stages may overlap. Achievement is influenced by mother and infant variables and the social environment.

Maternal sensitivity or maternal responsiveness is an important determinant of the maternal-infant relationship. It can be defined as the quality of a mother's sensitive behaviors that are based on her awareness, perception, and responsiveness to infant cues and behaviors. Maternal sensitivity significantly influences the infant's physical, psychologic, and cognitive development. Maternal qualities inherent to this sensitivity include awareness and responsiveness to infant cues, affect, timing, flexibility, acceptance, and conflict negotiation. Maternal sensitivity is dynamic and develops over time in a reciprocal give-and-take with the infant (Shin, Park, Ryu, & Seomun, 2008).

TABLE 22-4 PHASES OF MATERNAL POSTPARTUM ADJUSTMENT

PHASE	CHARACTERISTICS

Dependent: taking-in phase	• First 24 hours (range, 1 to 2 days)
	• Focus: self and meeting of basic needs:
	  • Reliance on others to meet needs for comfort, rest, closeness, and nourishment
	  • Excited and talkative
	  • Desire to review birth experience

Dependent-independent: taking-hold phase	• Starts second or third day; lasts 10 days to several weeks
	• Focus: care of baby and competent mothering:
	  • Desire to take charge
	  • Still has need for nurturing and acceptance by others
	  • Eagerness to learn and practice—optimal period for teaching by nurses
	  • Handling of physical discomforts and emotional changes
	  • Possible experience with "blues"

Interdependent: letting-go phase	• Focus: forward movement of family as unit with interacting members:
	  • Reassertion of relationship with partner
	  • Resumption of sexual intimacy
	  • Resolution of individual roles

Source: Rubin, R. (1961). Basic maternal behavior. *Nursing Outlook, 9(11),* 683-686.

The transition to motherhood requires adjustment for the mother and her family. Disruption is inherent in that adjustment. Circumstances such as problems in postpartum recovery or giving birth to a high risk infant add to the disruption (Lutz & May, 2007).

Nelson (2003) identified two social processes in maternal transition. The primary process is engagement, which is making a commitment to being a mother, actively caring for her child, and experiencing his or her presence. The secondary process is experiencing herself as a mother, which leads to growth and transformation. During this process she must learn how to mother and adapt to a changed relationship with her partner, family, and friends. The woman must examine herself in relation to the past and her present and come to view herself as a mother. She must make important decisions such as whether to return to work and, if so, when.

Not all mothers experience the transition to motherhood in the same way. For some women becoming a mother entails multiple losses. For example, for a single woman a loss of the family of origin may occur when the family does not accept her decision to have the child. There may be loss of a relationship with the father of the baby, with friends, and with her own sense of self. Some women describe a loss of dreams that includes loss of job, financial security, and a future profession. Accompanying these losses is a loss of support.

Reality-based perinatal education programs are necessary to prepare mothers better and decrease their anxiety. Live classes allow time for questions to be answered and for mothers to lend support to one another. Mothers need to know that during the first months of parenthood it is common to feel overwhelmed and insecure and to experience physical and mental fatigue. They need to be assured that this situation is temporary and that 3 to 6 months may be needed to become comfortable in caregiving and in being a mother. Maternal support by professionals should not end with hospital discharge but extend over the next 4 to 6 months; long-term interventions tend to be more successful than one-time encounters. Nurses can advocate for the extension of such support services well into the postpartum period (Mercer & Walker, 2006).

During pregnancy and after birth nurses can discuss the usual postpartum concerns that mothers experience. They can provide anticipatory guidance on coping strategies, such as resting when the infant sleeps and planning with an extended family member or friend to do the housework for the first week or two after the baby is born. Once a mother is home, periodic telephone calls from a nurse who cared for her in the birth setting can provide the mother with an opportunity to vent her concerns and get support and advice from "her" nurse. Nurses should plan additional supportive counseling for first-time mothers inexperienced in child care, women whose careers had provided outside stimulation, women who lack friends or family members with whom to share delights and concerns, and adolescent mothers. When possible, postpartum home visits are included in the plan of care.

Postpartum "Blues"

The "pink" period surrounding the first day or two after birth, characterized by heightened joy and feelings of well-being, is often followed by a "blue" period. Approximately 50% to 80% of women of all ethnic and racial groups experience the **postpartum blues** or "baby blues." During the blues, women are emotionally labile and often cry easily for no apparent reason. This lability seems to peak around the fifth day and subside by the tenth day. Other symptoms of postpartum blues include depression, a let down feeling, restlessness, fatigue, insomnia, headache, anxiety, sadness, and anger. Biochemical, psychologic, social, and cultural factors have been explored as possible causes of postpartum blues; however, the cause remains unknown.

Whatever the cause, the early postpartum period appears to be one of emotional and physical vulnerability for new mothers, who are often psychologically overwhelmed by the reality of parental responsibilities. Mothers feel deprived of the supportive care they received from family members and friends during pregnancy. Some mothers regret the loss of the mother–unborn child relationship and mourn its passing. Still others experience a let-down feeling when labor and birth are complete. The majority of women experience fatigue after childbirth, which is compounded by the around-the-clock demands of the new baby. Postpartum fatigue increases the risk of postpartum depressive symptoms and can have a negative effect on maternal role attainment (Corwin & Arbour, 2007). To help mothers cope with postpartum blues, nurses can suggest various strategies (see the Teaching for Self-Management box).

A few questions on a discharge checklist can help mothers assess their level of "blues" and decide when to seek advice from their nurse, nurse-midwife, or physician. Home visits and telephone follow-up calls by a nurse are important to assess the mother's pattern of "blue" feelings and behavior over time.

Although the postpartum blues are usually mild and short lived, approximately 10% to 15% of women experience a more severe syndrome termed *postpartum depression* (PPD). Symptoms of PPD can range from mild to severe, with women having good days and bad days. Fathers can also experience PPD. Screening for PPD should be performed with both mothers and fathers. PPD can go undetected because new parents generally do not voluntarily admit to this kind of emotional distress out of embarrassment, guilt, or fear. Nurses need to include teaching about how to differentiate symptoms of the "blues" and PPD and urge parents to report depressive symptoms promptly if they occur (see Chapter 32).

TEACHING FOR SELF-MANAGEMENT

Coping with Postpartum Blues

- Remember that the "blues" are normal and that both the mother and the father or partner may experience them.
- Get plenty of rest; nap when the baby does if possible. Go to bed early and let friends and family know when to visit and how they can help. (Remember, you are not "Supermom.")
- Use relaxation techniques learned in childbirth classes (or ask the nurse to teach you and your partner some techniques).
- Do something for yourself. Take advantage of the time your partner or family members care for the baby—soak in the tub (a 20-minute soak can be the equivalent of a 2-hour nap), or go for a walk.
- Plan a day out of the house—go to the mall with the baby, being sure to take a stroller or carriage, or go out to eat with friends without the baby. Many communities have churches or other agencies that provide child care programs such as Mothers' Morning Out.
- Talk to your partner about the way you feel—for example, about feeling tied down, how the birth met your expectations, and things that will help you (do not be afraid to ask for specifics).
- If you are breastfeeding, give yourself and your baby time to learn.
- Seek out and use community resources such as La Leche League or community mental health centers. One nationally recognized resource is:
  Postpartum Support International
  927 North Kellogg Ave.
  Santa Barbara, CA 93111
  (805) 967-7636
  www.postpartum.net

Becoming a Father

Research on paternal adjustment to parenthood indicates that men go through predictable phases during their transition to parenthood as they seek to become involved fathers (Goodman, 2005). In the first phase, men enter parenthood with intentions of being an emotionally involved father with deep connections to the infant. Many desire to parent differently than their own fathers. The second phase is a time of confronting reality, when men realize that their expectations were inconsistent with the realities of life with a newborn during the first few weeks. During this period fathers experience intense emotions. Many

TABLE 22-5 EARLY DEVELOPMENT OF THE INVOLVED FATHER ROLE

PHASES	CHARACTERISTICS
Expectations and intentions	Desire for emotional involvement and deep connection with infant
Confronting reality	Dealing with unrealistic expectations, frustration, disappointment, feelings of guilt, helplessness, and inadequacy
Creating the role of involved father	Altering expectations, establishing new priorities, redefining role, negotiating changes with partner, learning to care for infant, increasing interaction with infant, struggling for recognition
Reaping rewards	Infant smile, sense of meaning, completeness and immortality

Source: Goodman, J. (2005). Becoming an involved father of an infant. *Journal of Obstetric, Gynecologic and Neonatal Nursing, 34*(2), 190-200.

acknowledge that their expectations were of limited value once they were immersed in the reality of parenthood. Feelings that often accompany this reality are sadness, ambivalence, jealousy, frustration at not being able to participate in breastfeeding, and an overwhelming desire to be more involved. Some men are surprised that establishing a relationship with the infant is more gradual than expected. Fathers often feel alone, having no one with whom to discuss their feelings during this time. Mothers are preoccupied with infant care and their own transition to parenting. However, some fathers are pleasantly surprised at the ease and fun of parenting and take an active role. Many fathers of breastfeeding infants find ways to be involved in infant care other than feeding. The third phase is working to create the role of involved father. The realities of the first few weeks at home with a newborn cause fathers to change their expectations, set new priorities, and redefine their role. They develop strategies for balancing work, their own needs, and the needs of their partner and infant. Men become increasingly more comfortable with infant care. During this time they may struggle for recognition and positive feedback from their partner, the infant, and others. They may feel excluded from support and attention by health care providers. The final phase of becoming an involved father is one of reaping rewards, the most significant being reciprocity from the infant, such as a smile. This phase typically occurs around 6 weeks to 2 months. Increased sociability of the infant enhances the father infant relationship (Goodman) (Table 22-5).

First-time fathers perceive the first 4 to 10 weeks of parenthood in much the same way that mothers do. It is a period characterized by uncertainty, increased responsibility, disruption of sleep, and inability to control time needed to care for the infant and reestablish the couple's relationship. Fathers express concerns about decreased attention from their partners relative to their personal relationship, the mother's lack of recognition of the father's desire to participate in decision making for the infant, and limited time available to establish a relationship with the infant. These concerns can precipitate feelings of jealousy of the infant. The father should discuss his individual concerns and needs with the mother and become more involved with the infant. This effort can help alleviate feelings of jealousy.

In North American culture neonates have a powerful effect on their fathers who become intensely involved with their babies.

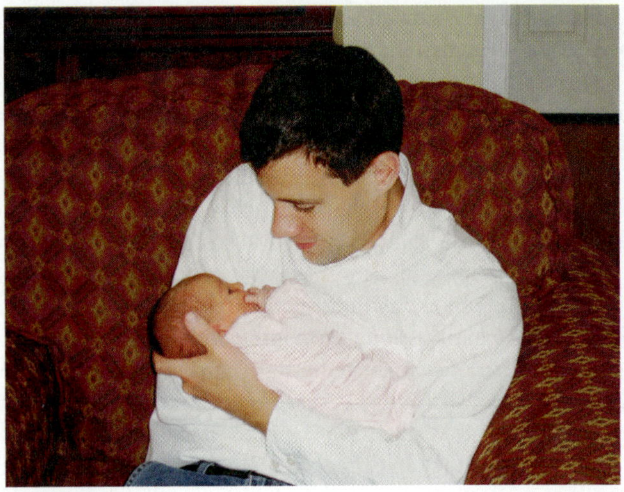

FIG. 22-7 Engrossment. Father is absorbed in looking at his newborn. (Courtesy Kathryn Alden, Chapel Hill, NC.)

The term used for the father's absorption, preoccupation, and interest in the infant is **engrossment.** Characteristics of engrossment include some of the sensual responses relating to touch and eye-to-eye contact that were discussed earlier and the father's keen awareness of features both unique and similar to himself that validate his claim to the infant. An outstanding response is one of strong attraction to the newborn. Fathers spend considerable time "communicating" with the infant and taking delight in the infant's response to them (Fig. 22-7). Fathers experience increased self-esteem and a sense of being proud, bigger, more mature, and older after seeing their baby for the first time.

Fathers spend less time than mothers with infants, and their interactions with infants tend to be characterized by stimulating social play rather than caretaking. The variations in infant stimulation from both parents provide a wider social experience for the infant.

Fathers lack interpersonal and professional support compared with mothers and can feel excluded from antenatal appointments and antenatal classes. They need information and encouragement during pregnancy and in the postnatal period related to infant care, parenting, and relationship changes. During the postpartum hospital stay, nurses can arrange to teach infant care when the father is present and provide anticipatory guidance for fathers about the transition to parenthood. Separate prenatal and parenting classes and parenting support groups for fathers can provide them with an opportunity to discuss their concerns and have some of their needs met. Postpartum telephone calls and home visits by the nurse should include time for assessment of the father's adjustment and needs (Deave, Johnson, & Ingram, 2008; Fletcher, Vimpani, Russell, & Sibbritt, 2008; Halle, Dowd, Fowler, Rissel, Hennessy, MacNevin, et al., 2008; St. John, Cameron, & McVeigh, 2005).

Adjustment for the Couple

The transition to parenthood brings about changes in the relationship between the mother and her partner. A strong, healthy marriage or couple relationship is the best foundation for parenthood, although even the best relationships are often shaken with the addition of a new baby. During the first few weeks after birth, parents experience a plethora of emotions. Even though they may feel an overwhelming love and a sense of amazement toward their newborn, they also feel a great responsibility. Even if the mother and her partner have been to prenatal classes, read books, or sought advice from family or friends, they are usually surprised by the realities of life with a new baby and the changes in their relationship (Deave et al., 2008). Because men and women experience pregnancy and birth differently, the expectation is that they will also vary in their adjustment to parenthood.

Common issues that couples face as they become parents include changes in their relationship with one another, division of household and infant care responsibilities, financial concerns, balancing work and parental responsibilities, and social activities. To assist new parents in their transition, nurses can encourage them during pregnancy and in the postpartum period to share personal expectations with each other and to assess their relationship periodically. Couples need to schedule time into their busy lives for one-on-one conversation and try to have regular "dates" or time apart from the infant. The mother and her partner need to express appreciation for one another and for their baby. Support from family, friends, and community health professionals should be identified early and used as needed during pregnancy and in the postpartum period and beyond. The couple who is willing to experiment with new approaches to their lifestyle and habits can find the transition to parenthood less difficult (Brotherson, 2007).

Resuming Sexual Intimacy

Nurses can provide opportunities for parents to discuss concerns and ask questions about resuming sexual intimacy. The couple may begin to engage in sexual intercourse during the second to fourth week after the baby is born. Some couples begin earlier, as soon as it can be accomplished without discomfort, depending on factors such as timing, amount of vaginal dryness, and breastfeeding status. Sexual intimacy enhances the adult aspect of the family, and the adult pair shares a closeness denied to other family members. Changes in a woman's sexuality after childbirth are related to hormonal shifts, increased breast size, uneasiness with a body that has yet to return to a prepregnant size, chronic fatigue related to sleep deprivation, and physical exhaustion. Many new fathers speak of feeling alienated when they observe the intimate mother-infant relationship, and some are frank in expressing feelings of jealousy toward the infant. The resumption of sexual intimacy seems to bring the parents' relationship back into focus. Before and after birth, nurses should review with new parents their plans for other pregnancies and their preferences for contraception.

Infant-Parent Adjustment

It has long been recognized that newborns participate actively in shaping their parents' reaction to them. Behavioral characteristics of the infant influence parenting behaviors. The infant and the parent each have unique rhythms, behaviors, and response styles that are brought to every interaction. Infant-parent interactions can be facilitated in any of three ways: (1) modulation of rhythm, (2) modification of behavioral repertoires, and (3) mutual responsivity. Nurses can teach parents about these three aspects of infant-parent interaction through discussions, written materials, and videotapes describing infant capabilities. A creative approach is to videotape the parent-infant pair during an interaction and then use the individualized tape to discuss the pair's rhythm, behavioral repertoire, and responsivity.

Rhythm. To modulate **rhythm,** both parent and infant must be able to interact. Therefore the infant must be in the alert state, one of the most difficult of the sleep-wake states to maintain. The alert state (Fig. 22-8) occurs most often during a feeding or in face-to-face play. The parent must work hard to help the infant maintain the alert state long enough and often enough for interactions to take place. The *en face* position is usually assumed (Fig. 22-8, *D*). Multiparous mothers in particular are very sensitive and responsive to the infant's feeding rhythms.

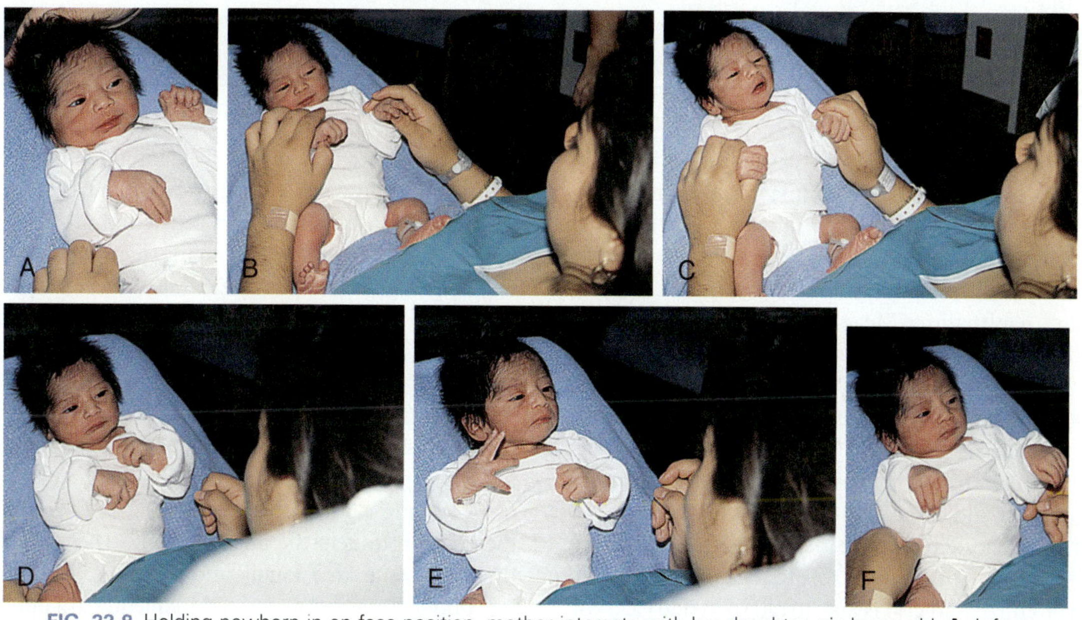

FIG. 22-8 Holding newborn in en face position, mother interacts with her daughter, six hours old. **A,** Infant is quiet and alert. **B,** Mother begins talking to daughter. **C,** Infant responds, opens mouth like her mother. **D,** Infant gazes at her mother. **E,** Infant waves hand. **F,** Infant glances away, resting; hands relax. (Courtesy Marjorie Pyle, RNC, Lifecircle, Costa Mesa, CA.)

EVIDENCE-BASED PRACTICE

Pat Gingrich

Education for Family Planning

ASK THE QUESTION

What are the most effective interventions for educating new families about contraception?

SEARCH FOR EVIDENCE

Search Strategies

Professional organization guidelines, meta-analyses, systematic reviews, randomized controlled trials since 2008.

Databases Searched

CINAHL, Cochrane, Medline, PUBMED.

CRITICALLY ANALYZE THE DATA

It is assumed that new families are highly motivated to delay a subsequent pregnancy. Unfortunately, much contraception teaching is scattered, depending very much on the nurse's knowledge base and willingness to overcome the sensitive nature of the topic. However, even a brief discussion on the subject can improve client commitment to use contraception. In a Cochrane Database Systematic Review, Lopez, Hiller, and Grimes (2010) examined eight postpartum contraception education interventions from Australia, Nepal, Pakistan and the U.S. In-hospital counseling interventions resulted in greater contraception use in the short term. More comprehensive programs with multiple visits resulted in fewer pregnancies and births among adolescents, and home-visit programs resulted in greater contraceptive use. Interestingly, the longer-term intervention may not be more costly than the single visit program.

A systematic analysis of educational strategies for presenting contraceptive counseling concluded that women found audiovisual materials more helpful than just talking (Lopez, Steiner, Grimes, & Schulz, 2008). Written materials were easier to understand if they used categories, graphs and charts, rather than just numbers. Comprehensive counseling resulted in choosing highly reliable methods or sterilization.

Theory-based interventions have been used successfully in HIV and STI prevention, as well as quit-smoking programs, but have not typically been the basis for contraceptive teaching. To examine the efficacy of theory-based family planning counseling, a Cochrane Review team examined 26 trials addressing contraceptive counseling (Lopez, Tolley, Grimes, & Chen-Mok, 2009). Many of the theories used were based on Albert Bandura's social cognitive model. An example of a social cognitive model is the transtheoretical model, in which the person must go through several stages of increasing commitment towards a goal of behavior change (many quit-smoking interventions use this). The Health Belief Model identifies motivators within individuals that prompt health behavior: a feeling of susceptibility, the belief that consequences of illness are severe, and that the benefits of a health behavior outweigh the costs. Another example commonly used in nursing is the concept of self-efficacy. The authors of the review found that contraceptive counseling was more successful when using these models for intervention development. Using theoretical models fosters improved outcomes by encouraging researchers to be able to use the same language and build upon previous work.

IMPLICATIONS FOR PRACTICE

Postpartum women have proven fertility. Among the long list of other teaching goals that must be addressed during the short hospital stay, it can be a challenge for nurses to offer comprehensive contraceptive counseling. In addition, discomfort with intimate topics or lack of privacy may be a barrier to good communication. However, to adequately limit or space childbearing, and give new parents all the time they need to adjust as a family, it is important that they have a contraceptive plan in place when they go home from the hospital. This is especially true for adolescents, many of whom are likely to give birth again within a year. The nurse should determine the couple's interest and previous knowledge, and then use developmentally appropriate and evidence-based educational materials. To reinforce and reassess, the nurse should address the topic of contraception at every follow-up visit. Finally, the nurse who understands the theoretical basis of interventions can better apply and build upon the teaching principles involved.

References

Lopez, L., Hiller, J., & Grimes, D. (2010). Education for contraceptive use by women after childbirth. *The Cochrane Database of Systematic Reviews 2010, 1,* CD001863.

Lopez, L., Steiner, M., Grimes, D., & Schulz, K. (2008). Strategies for communicating contraceptive effectiveness. *The Cochrane Database of Systematic Reviews 2008, 2,* CD006964.

Lopez, L., Tolley, E., Grimes, D., & Chen-Mok, M. (2009). Theory-based interventions for contraception. *The Cochrane Database of Systematic Reviews 2009, 1,* CD007249.

Mothers learn to reserve stimulation for pauses in sucking activity and not to talk or smile excessively while the infant is sucking because the infant will stop feeding to interact with her. With maturity the infant can sustain longer interactions by modulating activity rhythms, that is, limb movement, sucking, gaze alternation, and habituation. Meanwhile, the parent becomes more attuned to the infant's rhythms and learns to modulate the rhythms, facilitating a rhythmic turn-taking interaction.

Behavioral Repertoires. Both the infant and the parent have a repertoire of behaviors they can use to facilitate interactions. Fathers and mothers engage in these behaviors depending on the extent of contact and caregiving of the infant.

The infant's behavioral repertoire includes gazing, vocalizing, and facial expressions. The infant is able to focus and follow the human face from birth and also is able to alternate the gaze voluntarily, looking away from the parent's face when understimulated or overstimulated (Fig. 22-8, *F*). One of the key responses for the parents to learn is to be sensitive to the infant's capacity for attention and inattention. Developing this sensitivity is especially important when interacting with preterm infants.

Body gestures form a part of the infant's "early language." Babies greet parents with waving hands (Fig. 22-8, *E*) or a reaching out of hands. They can raise an eyebrow or soften their expression to elicit loving attention. Game playing can stimulate them to smile or laugh. Pouting or crying, arching of the back, and general squirming usually signal the end of an interaction.

The parents' repertoire includes various types of interactive behaviors such as constantly looking at the infant and noting the infant's response. New parents often remark that they are exhausted from looking at the baby and smiling. Adults also "infantilize" their speech to help the infant "listen." They do this by slowing the tempo, speaking loudly and rhythmically, and emphasizing key words. Phrases are repeated frequently. Infantilizing does not mean using "baby talk," which involves distortion of sounds.

To communicate emotions to the infant, parents often use facial expressions such as slow and exaggerated looks of surprise, happiness, and confusion. Games such as "peek-a-boo" and imitation of the infant's behaviors are other means of interaction. For example, if the baby smiles, so does the parent; if the baby frowns, the parent responds in kind.

Responsivity. Contingent responses (responsivity) are those that occur within a specific time and are similar in form to a stimulus behavior. The adult has the feeling of having an influence on the interaction. Infant behaviors such as smiling, cooing, and sustained eye contact, usually in the en face position, are viewed as contingent responses. The infant's responses act as rewards to the initiator and encourage the adult to continue with the game when the infant responds positively. When the adult imitates the infant, the infant appears to enjoy it. A progression occurs in the types of behaviors that parents present for the baby to imitate; for example, in early interactions, the parent will grimace rather than laugh, which is in keeping with the infant's developmental level. Such "turnabout" behaviors sustain interactions and promote harmony in the relationship.

DIVERSITY IN TRANSITIONS TO PARENTHOOD

Various factors, including age, social networks, socioeconomic conditions, and personal aspirations for the future, influence how parents respond to the birth of a child. Cultural beliefs and practices also affect parenting behaviors. Factors that are recognized to increase the risk of parenting problems include age (adolescent or older than 35 years), lesbian parenting, social support, culture, socioeconomic conditions, and personal aspirations.

Age

Maternal age has a definite effect on the transition to parenting. The mother, fetus, and newborn are at highest risk when the mother is an adolescent or older than 35 years.

The Adolescent Mother

Although becoming a parent is biologically possible for the adolescent female, her egocentricity and concrete thinking often interfere with the ability to parent effectively. Adolescent mothers are more likely to give birth to preterm and/or low-birth-weight infants. Mortality rates are higher among infants of adolescent mothers. This can be related to inherent problems associated with preterm birth or other conditions, but it is also influenced by the mother's inexperience, lack of knowledge, and immaturity. Nevertheless, in most instances, with adequate support and developmentally appropriate teaching, adolescents can learn effective parenting skills. Strong social and functional support promotes positive outcomes for adolescent mothers.

Contrary to popular beliefs related to the detrimental effects of adolescent pregnancy, research evidence suggests that the life course for adolescent mothers is similar to that of their socioeconomic peers (Beers & Hollo, 2009). In some families or communities, adolescent parenthood is considered a normal or positive life event. Even so, adolescent pregnancy and parenting are important public health concerns.

The transition to parenthood can be difficult for adolescent parents. Because many adolescents have their own unmet developmental needs, coping with the developmental tasks of parenthood is often difficult. Some young parents experience difficulty accepting a changing self-image and adjusting to new roles related to the responsibilities of infant care. Adolescent mothers are at increased risk for postpartum depression; this is often associated with a lack of social support and poor relations with their partner (Beers & Hollo, 2009).

As adolescent parents move through the transition to parenthood, they can feel "different" from their peers, excluded from "fun" activities, and prematurely forced to enter an adult social role. The conflict between their own desires and the infant's demands, in addition to the low tolerance for frustration that is typical of adolescence, further contribute to the normal psychosocial stress of childbirth and parenting. Maintaining a relationship with the baby's father is beneficial for the teen mother and her infant, although adolescent pregnancy often heralds the departure of the young father from the relationship (Herrman, 2008).

Adolescent mothers provide warm and attentive physical care; however, they use less verbal interaction than older parents, and adolescents tend to be less responsive and to interact less positively with their infants than older mothers. Interventions emphasizing verbal and nonverbal communication skills between mother and infant are important. Such intervention strategies must be concrete and specific because of the cognitive level of adolescents. Although some observers suggest that some adolescents may use more aggressive behaviors, a higher than normal incidence of child abuse has not been documented. In comparison to older mothers, teenage mothers have a limited knowledge of child development. They tend to expect too much of their infants too soon and often characterize their infants as being fussy. This limited knowledge may cause teenagers to respond to their infants inappropriately.

CLINICAL REASONING

Transition to Parenthood for the Adolescent Couple

As a mother-baby nurse you are assigned the care of Tamika, a 16-year-old, who is being discharged from the hospital 72 hours after giving birth by cesarean to a 5-pound baby girl. Tamika has been trying to breastfeed, but the baby has lost 8% of her birth weight, and the pediatrician ordered formula supplementation after breastfeeding. Her breasts are engorged and painful. Tamika says she slept very little last night because she was trying to feed the baby. She is tearful and says it hurts too much to breastfeed. She asks you to take the baby back to the nursery and give her a bottle. Her mother is staying with her. The baby's father, Thomas, 16 years of age, is in the room with Tamika. He has come to take Tamika and the baby home. Thomas has been to visit a few times but is trying to go to school and work his evening job at the local grocery store.

1. Evidence—Is evidence sufficient to draw conclusions about the education and care these new parents need?
2. Assumptions—What assumptions can be made about the following factors?
    a. The relationship of maternal age and postpartum adjustment
    b. The need for social support in the postnatal period
    c. The need for perinatal education
    d. Long-term prognosis for positive outcomes
3. What implications and priorities for nursing care can be drawn at this time?
4. Does the evidence objectively support your conclusion?
5. Are there alternative perspectives to your conclusion?

Many young mothers pattern their maternal role on what they themselves experienced. Therefore, nurses need to determine the type of support that people close to the young mother are able and prepared to give, as well as the kinds of community assistance available to supplement this support. Many teen mothers can identify a source of social support, with the predominant source being their own mothers.

The need for continued assessment of the new mother's parenting abilities during this postbirth period is essential. Continued support is facilitated by involving the grandparents and other family members, as well as through home visits and group sessions for discussion of infant care and parenting problems. Community-based programs for pregnant adolescents and adolescent parents improve access to health care, education, and other support services. Serious problems can be prevented through outreach programs concerned with self-management, parent-child interactions, infant development, child injuries, and failure to thrive. As the adolescent performs her mothering role within the framework of her family, she may need to address dependency versus independency issues. The adolescent's family members also need help adapting to their new roles. Some mothers and fathers of adolescents feel they are too young and unprepared to be grandparents.

The Adolescent Father

The adolescent father and mother face immediate developmental crises, which include completing the developmental tasks of adolescence, making a transition to parenthood, and sometimes adapting to marriage. These transitions are often stressful. The nurse can initiate interaction with the adolescent father if he is present during prenatal visits or if he is with his partner during labor and birth. During the hospital stay the nurse can include the adolescent father in teaching sessions about infant care and parenting. The nurse can ask him to be present during postpartum home visits and to accompany the mother and the baby to well-baby checkups at the clinic or pediatrician's office. With the adolescent mother's agreement the nurse may contact the father directly. Adolescent fathers need support to discuss their emotional responses to the pregnancy, birth, and fatherhood. The nurse needs to be aware of the father's feelings of guilt, powerlessness, or bravado because these feelings may have negative consequences for both the parents and the child. Counseling of adolescent fathers needs to be reality oriented and should include topics such as finances, child care, parenting skills, and the father's role in the parenting experience. Teenage fathers also need to know about reproductive physiology and birth control options, as well as sex practices that lower the risk of pregnancy and sexually transmitted infections.

The adolescent father may continue to be involved in an ongoing relationship with the young mother and his baby. In those instances he plays an important role in the decisions about child care and raising the child. He may need help to develop realistic perceptions of his role as "father to a child" and is encouraged to use coping mechanisms that are not harmful to his own, his partner's, or his child's well-being. The nurse enlists support systems, parents, and professional agencies on his behalf.

Maternal Age Older Than 35 Years

Women older than 35 years have always continued their childbearing either by choice or because of a lack of or a failure of contraception during the perimenopausal years. Added to this group are women who have postponed pregnancy because of careers or other reasons, as well as women of infertile couples who finally become pregnant with the aid of technologic advances.

Support from partners aids in the adjustment of older mothers to changes involved in becoming a parent and seeing themselves as competent. Support from other family members and friends is also important for positive self-evaluation of parenting, a sense of well-being and satisfaction, and help in dealing with stress. Women of advanced maternal age can experience social isolation. Older mothers may have less family and social support than younger mothers. They are less likely to live near family, and their own parents, if still living, can be unable to provide assistance or support because of age or health issues. Mothers of advanced maternal age are often caught in the "sandwich generation," taking on responsibility for care of aging parents while parenting young children. Social support may be lacking because their peers are probably busy with their careers and have limited time to help. Their friends are likely to have older children and have less in common with the new mother (Suplee, Dawley, & Bloch, 2007).

Changes in the sexual aspect of a relationship can create stress for new midlife parents. Mothers report that it is difficult to find time and energy for a romantic rendezvous. They attribute much of this difficulty to the reality of caring for an infant, but the decreasing libido that normally accompanies getting older also contributes.

Work and career issues are sources of conflict for older mothers. Conflicts emerge over being disinterested in work, worrying about giving enough attention to work with the distractions of a new baby, and anticipating what returning to work will entail. Child care is a major factor in causing stress about work.

Another major issue for older mothers with careers is the perception of loss of control. Mothers older than 35 years, when compared with younger mothers, are at a different stage in their careers, having attained high levels of education, career, and income. The loss of control experienced when going from the consistency of a work role to the inconsistency of the parent role comes as a surprise to many older women. Helping the older mother have realistic expectations of herself and of parenthood is essential.

New mothers who are also perimenopausal may have difficulty distinguishing fatigue, loss of sleep, decreased libido, or other physiologic symptoms as the causes of the change in their sex lives. Although many women view menopause as a natural stage of life, for midlife mothers, this cessation of menstruation coincides with the state of parenthood. The changes of midlife and menopause can add more emotional and physical stress to older mothers' lives because of the time- and energy-consuming aspects of raising a young child.

Paternal Age Older Than 35 Years

Although many older fathers describe their experience of midlife parenting as wonderful, they also recognize drawbacks. Positive aspects of fatherhood in older years include increased love and commitment between the two parents, a reinforcement of why one married in the first place, a feeling of being complete, experiencing of "the child" again in oneself, more financial stability than in younger years, and more freedom to focus on parenting rather than on career. A common drawback of midlife parenting is the change that it brings about in the relationships with their partners.

Parenting in the Lesbian Couple

The transition to parenting for lesbian couples is unique in that there are two women with maternal status, one who gave birth and the other who may be referred to as "the other mother," "nonbiologic mother," "co-parent," or other term preferred by the couple. It is important for health care providers to determine the couple's preference about how they wish to be identified (McManus, Hunter, & Renn, 2006).

Among lesbian couples the decision to conceive is intentional. There are several methods to achieve a pregnancy. One woman can be artificially inseminated and conceive a child who is genetically related to her. The fertilized egg of one partner can be implanted into the uterus of the other who carries the pregnancy. Alternatively, one woman can be implanted with the fertilized egg from a donor so that the child is not biologically related to either partner. Research evidence suggests that the birth mother has chosen to be the one to carry the baby because of a greater desire to experience the pregnancy and birth and to be genetically related to the child. Other factors that influence the decision are age, health, infertility, and career considerations (Goldberg, 2006).

Health care providers demonstrate a variety of reactions to lesbian couples ranging from rejection and exclusion to complete acceptance and inclusion. Judgmental attitudes, confusion, or lack of understanding can affect the quality of care provided to these families. Although the traditional roles of the mother and father in heterosexual relationships are well recognized, the role of the lesbian co-parent can be questioned, misunderstood, and ignored by society and by health care providers. Intentionally or accidentally, health care providers can exclude partners or fail to acknowledge their roles in pregnancy, birth, and parenting (McManus et al., 2006; Renaud, 2007).

Integration of the nonchildbearing partner into care includes offering opportunities afforded male partners of heterosexual women such as "cutting the cord" and rooming in with the mother and baby during hospitalization. An option not available to male partners is to actually breastfeed the infant. The nonchildbearing female partner can stimulate milk production through induced lactation using medications and regular pumping. A supplemental feeding device containing expressed breast milk or formula can be used to provide additional milk to the breastfeeding infant. Women who choose not to induce lactation yet desire to have the breastfeeding experience can put the baby to breast using a supplemental feeding device (McManus et al., 2006; Riordan & Wambach, 2010).

Similar to heterosexual parents, lesbian couples face challenges in adjusting to life with a new baby. After birth the birth mother tends to be the one most responsible for child care as she is likely to be working fewer hours than her partner. Couples who are intentional about creating opportunities for bonding between the baby and the mother who did not give birth report success in minimizing the effects of biologic motherhood (Goldberg & Perry-Jenkins, 2007). Tensions can arise between the partners in relation to their roles. For example, the birth mother can feel that she has a greater role in parenting because she considers herself more primary. This can be compounded by the lack of a formal, recognized relationship of the co-parent to the infant and the issues surrounding her legal rights in relation to her partner and the infant (McManus et al., 2006).

Lesbian couples face strong social sanctions regarding pregnancy and parenting. Their families may not have resolved the initial dismay and guilt over learning of their daughters' homosexuality, or they may disagree with the lesbian couple's decision to conceive and be parents. Lesbian parents deal with public ignorance, social and legal invisibility, and the lack of biologic connection to the child by using various techniques. These techniques include carefully planning and accomplishing their transition to parenthood, displaying public acts of equal mothering, sharing parenting at home, establishing a distinct parenting role within the family, and supporting each partner's sense of identity as a mother. In situations in which family support is limited or absent the nurse can help lesbian couples locate supportive social groups, lesbian or heterosexual.

Social Support

Social support is strongly related to positive adaptation by new parents, including adolescent parents, during the transition to parenthood. Social support is multidimensional and includes the number of members in a person's social network, types of support, perceived general support, actual support received, and satisfaction with support available and received. The type and satisfaction of support seems to be more important than the total number of support network members.

Across cultural groups, families and friends of new parents form an important dimension of the parent's social network. Through seeking help within the social network, new mothers learn culturally valued practices and develop role competency.

Social networks provide a support system on which parents can rely for assistance, but they also can be a source of conflict. Sometimes a large network can cause problems because it results in conflicting advice that comes from numerous people. Grandparents or in-laws are most appreciated when they assist with household responsibilities and do not intrude into the parents' privacy or judge them critically.

Because of the extent of restructuring and reorganization that occurs in a family with the birth of another child, the mothers' moods and fatigue in the postpartum period can be helped more by situation-specific support from family and friends than by general support. General support addresses feeling loved, respected, and valued. Situation-specific support relates to practical concerns such as physical needs and child care. For example, the practical support of a grandparent bathing the infant can help lessen a second-time mother's feelings of loss by providing her time to be with her firstborn child.

Culture

Cultural beliefs and practices are important determinants of parenting behaviors. Culture influences the interactions with the baby, as well as the parents' or the family's caregiving style.

For example, the provision for a period of rest and recuperation for the mother after birth is prominent in several cultures. Asian mothers must remain at home with the baby up to 30 days after birth and are not supposed to engage in household chores, including care of the baby. Many times the grandmother takes over the baby's care immediately, even before discharge from the hospital. Jordanian mothers have a 40-day lying-in after birth during which their mothers or sisters care for the baby. Japanese mothers rest for the first 2 months after childbirth. Hispanics practice an intergenerational family ritual, *la cuarentena*. For 40 days after birth the mother is expected to recuperate and get acquainted with her infant. Traditionally this process involves many restrictions concerning food (spicy or cold foods, fish, pork, and citrus are avoided; tortillas and chicken soup are encouraged), exercise, and activities, including sexual intercourse. Many women avoid bathing and washing their hair. Traditional Hispanic husbands do not expect to see their wives or infants until both have been cleaned and dressed after birth. *La cuarentena* incorporates individuals into the family, instills parental responsibility, and integrates the family during a critical life event (D'Avanzo, 2008).

All cultures place importance on desiring and valuing children. In Asian families, children are a source of family strength and stability, are perceived as wealth, and are objects of parental love and affection. Infants are almost always given an affectionate "cradle" name that is used during the first years of life; for example, a Filipino girl might be called "Ling-Ling" and a boy "Bong-Bong."

Differing cultural values can influence parents' interactions with health care professionals. For example, Asians are taught to be humble and obedient; to be outspoken is frowned upon. They are brought up to refrain from questioning authority figures (e.g., a nurse), to avoid confrontation, and to respect the yin/yang balance in nature. Because of these learned values, an Asian mother might not confront the nurse about the length of time taken to receive the medication requested for her episiotomy pain. A mother may nod and say, "Yes," in response to the nurse's directions for using an iced sitz bath but then will not use the sitz bath. The "yes," in this case, is a gesture of courtesy, meaning, "I'm listening"; it is not an indication of agreement to comply. The mother does not use the iced sitz bath because of her traditional avoidance of bathing and cold after birth. Because not all members of a cultural group adhere to traditional practices, it is necessary to validate which cultural practices are important to individual parents.

Knowledge of cultural beliefs can help the nurse make more accurate assessments and diagnoses of observed parenting behaviors. For example, nurses may become concerned when they observe cultural practices that appear to reflect poor maternal-infant bonding. Algerian mothers may not unwrap and explore their infants as part of the acquaintance process because in Algeria, babies are wrapped tightly in swaddling clothes to protect them physically and psychologically (D'Avanzo, 2008). The nurse may observe a Vietnamese woman who gives minimal care to her infant but refuses to cuddle or further interact with her baby. This apparent lack of interest in the newborn is this cultural group's attempt to ward off "evil spirits" and actually reflects an intense love and concern for the infant. An Asian mother might be criticized for almost immediately relinquishing the care of the infant to the grandmother and not even attempting to hold her baby when it is brought to her room. However, in Asian extended families, members show their support for a new mother's rest and recuperation by assisting with the care of the baby. Contrary to the guidance that is sometimes given to mothers in the United States about "nipple confusion," a mix of breastfeeding and bottle-feeding is standard practice for Japanese mothers. This tradition is related to concern for the mother's rest during the first 2 to 3 months and does not usually lead to problems with lactation; breastfeeding is widespread and successful among Japanese women.

Cultural beliefs and values give perspective to the meaning of childbirth for a new mother. Nurses can provide an opportunity for a new mother to talk about her perception of the meaning of childbearing. In helping new families adjust to parenthood, nurses must provide culturally sensitive care by following principles that facilitate nursing practice within transcultural situations.

Socioeconomic Conditions

Socioeconomic conditions often determine access to available resources. Parents whose economic condition is made worse with the birth of each child and who are unable to use an effective method of fertility management can find childbirth complicated by concern for their own health and a sense of helplessness. Mothers who are single, separated, or divorced from their husbands or without a partner, family, and friends can view the birth of a child with dread. Serious financial problems may negatively affect mothering behaviors. Similarly, fathers who are overwhelmed with financial stresses may lack effective parenting skills and behaviors.

Personal Aspirations

For some women, parenthood interferes with or blocks plans for personal freedom or career advancement. Unresolved resentment will affect caregiving activities and adjustment to parenting. This situation may result in indifference and neglect of the infant or in excessive concerns; the mother may set impossibly high standards for her own behavior or the child's performance.

Nursing interventions include providing opportunities for mothers to express their feelings freely to an objective listener, to discuss measures to permit personal growth, and to learn about the care of their infant. Referring the woman to a support group of other mothers "in the same situation" may also be helpful.

Nurses can be proactive in influencing changes in work policies related to maternity and paternity leaves, varying models of work sharing and family-friendly work environments. Some corporations already structure their worksites to support new mothers (e.g., by providing on-site daycare facilities and lactation rooms).

PARENTAL SENSORY IMPAIRMENT

In early interactions between the parent and child, each one uses all senses—sight, hearing, touch, taste, and smell—to initiate and sustain the attachment process. A parent who has an impairment of one or more of the senses needs to maximize use of the remaining senses. Mothers with disabilities tend to value the importance of performing parenting tasks in the perceived culturally usual way.

Visually Impaired Parent

Visual impairment alone does not seem to have a negative effect on parents' early parenting experiences. These parents, just as sighted parents, express the wonders of parenthood and encourage other visually impaired persons to become parents.

Although visually impaired parents initially feel a pressure to conform to traditional, sighted ways of parenting, they soon adapt these ways and develop methods better suited to themselves. Examples of activities that visually impaired parents perform differently include preparation of the infant's nursery, clothes, and supplies. Some parents put an entire clothing outfit together and hang it in the closet rather than keeping items separate in drawers. Some develop a labeling system for the infant's clothing and put diapering, bathing, and other care supplies where they will be easy to locate. A strength that visually impaired parents have is a heightened sensitivity to other sensory outputs. Visually impaired parents can tell when their infant is facing them because they notice the baby's breath on their faces.

One of the major difficulties that visually impaired parents experience is the skepticism, open or hidden, of health care professionals. Visually impaired people sense reluctance on the part of others to acknowledge that they have a right to be parents. All too often, nurses and physicians lack the experience to deal with the childbearing and childrearing needs of visually impaired parents, as well as parents with other disabilities, such as the hearing impaired, physically impaired, and mentally challenged. The nurse's best approach is to assess the parents' capabilities and to use that information as a basis for making plans to assist the parent, often in much the same way as for a parent without impairments. Visually impaired mothers have made suggestions for providing care for women such as themselves during childbearing (Box 22-2). Such approaches can help avoid a sense of increased vulnerability on the parent's part.

Eye contact is important in U.S. culture. With a parent who is visually impaired, this critical factor in the parent-child attachment process is obviously missing. However, the blind parent, who may never have experienced this method of strengthening relationships, does not miss it. The infant will need other sensory input from that parent. An infant looking into the eyes of a parent who is blind may be unaware that the eyes are unseeing. Other people in the newborn's environment can also participate in active eye-to-eye contact to supply this need. A problem may arise, however, if the visually impaired parent has little facial expression. The infant, after making repeated unsuccessful attempts to engage in face play with the mother, will abandon the behavior with her and intensify it with the father or other people in the household. Nurses can provide anticipatory guidance regarding this situation and help the mother learn to nod and smile while talking and cooing to the infant.

BOX 22-2 NURSING APPROACHES FOR WORKING WITH VISUALLY IMPAIRED PARENTS

- Parents who are blind need verbal teaching by health care providers because pregnancy and childbirth information is usually not accessible to blind people.
- A visually impaired parent needs an orientation to the hospital room that allows the parent to move about the room independently. For example, "Go to the left of the bed and trail the wall until you feel the first door. That is the bathroom."
- Parents who are blind need explanations of routines.
- Parents who are blind need to feel devices (e.g., portable sitz bath equipment, breast pump) and to hear descriptions of the devices.
- Visually impaired parents need a chance to ask questions.
- Visually impaired parents need the opportunity to hold and touch the baby after birth.
- Nurses need to demonstrate baby care by touch and to follow with, "Now show me how you would do it."
- Nurses need to give instructions such as, "I'm going to give you the baby. The head is to your left side."

Hearing-Impaired Parent

A parent who has a hearing impairment faces challenges in caregiving and parenting, particularly if the deafness dates from birth or early childhood. Whether one or both parents are hearing impaired, they are likely to have established an independent household. Devices that transform sound into light flashes can be fitted into the infant's room to permit immediate detection of crying. Even if the parent is not speech trained, vocalizing can serve as both a stimulus and a response to the infant's early vocalizing. Deaf parents can provide additional vocal training by use of recordings and television so that from birth the child is aware of the full range of the human voice. Young children acquire sign language readily, and the first sign used is as varied as the first word.

Section 504 of the Rehabilitation Act of 1973 requires that hospitals and other institutions receiving funds from the U.S. Department of Health and Human Services use various communication techniques and resources with the deaf, including having staff members or certified interpreters who are proficient in sign language. For example, provision of written materials with demonstrations and having nurses stand where the parent can read their lips (if the parent practices lip reading) are two techniques that can be used. A creative approach is for the nursing unit to develop videos in which information on postpartum care, infant care, and parenting issues is signed by an interpreter and spoken by a nurse. A videotape in which a nurse signs while speaking would be ideal. With the advent of the Internet, many resources are available to deaf parents. Box 22-3 lists suggestions for working with hearing-impaired parents.

SIBLING ADAPTATION

Because the family is an interactive, open unit, the addition of a new family member affects everyone in the family. Siblings have to assume new positions within the family hierarchy. Parents often face the task of caring for a new child while not neglecting the others and need to distribute their attention equitably. When the newborn was born prematurely or has special needs, this task can be difficult.

BOX 22-3 NURSING APPROACHES FOR WORKING WITH HEARING-IMPAIRED PARENTS

- Before initiating communication, the nurse needs to be aware of the parents' preferences and capabilities: Do they wear a hearing aid? Do they read lips? Do they wish to have an interpreter?
- The nurse should make certain that the parent(s) sees the nurse approaching to avoid startling the parent.
- Before speaking, the nurse needs to be directly in front of the parent and should have that person's full attention.
- When speaking, the nurse should face the parent directly and should be at the same level.
- It is best to avoid standing in front of a light or a window while speaking to the parent.
- Keep hands away from the face while speaking to minimize distractions.
- If the parent relies on lip reading, the nurse should sit close enough so that the parent can easily visualize lip movements.
- The nurse should speak clearly with a regular voice volume and lip movements, while maintaining eye contact.
- Speak in short, simple sentences to facilitate understanding.
- If the parent does not understand something, it is better to find a different way to say what needs to be communicated rather than repeating the same words over and over.
- Written messages aid in communication. A small white or black erasable board can be useful.
- Educational materials should be given to hearing-impaired parents and they should be asked to read the materials prior to doing client teaching. They can refer to the materials after discharge.
- Visual aids such as pictures, diagrams, or other devices should be used when doing client teaching.
- When doing parent teaching, it is helpful for a hearing person (partner or family member) to be present.
- The nurse should allow ample time to communicate with the hearing-impaired parent; being in a rush can evoke stress and create barriers to effective communication.

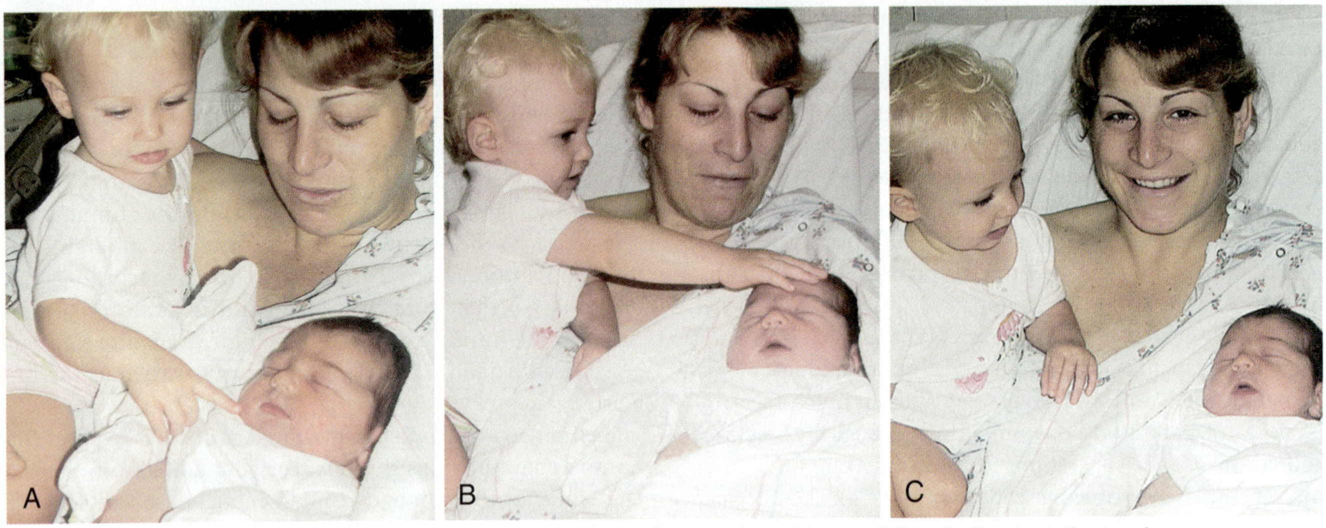

FIG. 22-9 First meeting. Sister with mother during first meeting with new sibling. **A,** First tentative touch with fingertip. **B,** Relationship is more secure; touching with whole hand is now okay. **C,** Smiles indicate acceptance. (Courtesy Sara Kossuth, Los Angeles, CA.)

Reactions of siblings result from temporary separation from the mother, changes in the mother's or father's behavior, or the infant coming home. Positive behavioral changes of siblings include interest in and concern for the baby (Fig. 22-9) and increased independence. Regression in toileting and sleep habits, aggression toward the baby, and increased seeking of attention and whining are examples of negative behaviors.

The parents' attitudes toward the arrival of the baby can set the stage for the other children's reactions. Because the baby absorbs the time and attention of the important people in the other children's lives, jealousy (**sibling rivalry**) is common once the initial excitement of having a new baby in the home is over.

Parents, especially mothers, spend much time and energy promoting sibling acceptance of a new baby. Participating in sibling preparation classes makes a difference in the ability of mothers to cope with sibling behavior. Older children are actively involved in preparing for the infant, and this involvement intensifies after the birth of the child. Parents have to manage the feeling of guilt that the older children are being deprived of parental time and attention and monitor the behavior of older children toward the more vulnerable infant and divert aggressive behavior. Box 22-4 presents strategies that parents have used to facilitate acceptance of a new baby by siblings.

Siblings demonstrate acquaintance behaviors with the newborn. The acquaintance process depends on the information given to the child before the baby is born and on the child's cognitive development level. The initial behaviors of siblings with the newborn include looking at the infant and touching the head (see Fig. 22-9). The initial adjustment of older children to a newborn takes time, and parents should allow children to interact at their own pace rather than forcing them to interact. To expect a young child to accept and love a rival for the parents' affection assumes an unrealistic level of maturity. Sibling love grows as does other love, that is, by being with another person and sharing experiences. The bond between siblings

BOX 22-4 STRATEGIES FOR FACILITATING SIBLING ACCEPTANCE OF A NEW BABY

- Take your older child (or children) on a tour of your hospital room and point out similarities between this birth and his or her birth. "This is like the room I was in with you, and the baby is in the same kind of bassinet that you were in."
- Have a small gift from the baby to give to your older child each day he or she visits in the hospital.
- Give the older child a T-shirt that says "I'm a big brother" [or "sister"].
- Arrange for your children to be among the first to see the newborn. Let them hold the baby in the hospital. One mother and father arranged for their firstborn son to be present at the births of his three brothers and to be the first one to hold them.
- When the older child visits for the first time, make sure you are not holding the new baby. Your arms need to be open and available for the older child. Instruct the person accompanying the older child to call ahead or give a warning knock to give you time to lay the baby down or have someone else hold the baby.
- Plan individual time with each child. The father or partner can spend time with the older siblings while the mother is taking care of the baby and vice versa. Siblings like to have time and attention from both parents.
- Give preschool and early school-age siblings a newborn doll as "their baby." Give the sibling a photograph of the new baby to take to school to show off "his" or "her" baby. Older siblings may enjoy the responsibility of helping care for the newborn, such as learning how to give the baby a bottle or change a diaper. Remember to supervise interactions between the siblings and new baby.

involves a secure base in which one child provides support for the other, is missed when absent, and is looked to for comfort and security.

GRANDPARENT ADAPTATION

Becoming a grandparent is most often associated with great joy and happiness. Yet it is a time of transition as roles and relationships are changing and new opportunities arise. Emotions are varied and can change from day to day; feelings of joy, anticipation, and excitement are often intermingled with some degree of anxiety and uncertainty. Circumstances surrounding the pregnancy and birth influence the feelings, reactions, and responses of grandparents.

Pregnancy and birth necessitate redefining of intergenerational roles and relationships within the family. A primary role of the grandparents is to support, nurture, and empower their children in the parenting role. Grandparents must acknowledge that things have changed since they first became parents as they deal with changes in practices and attitudes toward childbirth, childrearing, and men's and women's roles at home and in the workplace. The degree to which grandparents understand and accept current practices can influence how supportive they are to their adult children.

At the same time that they are adjusting to grandparenthood, the majority of grandparents are experiencing typical life-transitions and events, such as retirement and a move to smaller housing, and need support from their adult children. Some may feel regret about their limited involvement because of poor health or geographic distance.

The extent of grandparent involvement in the care of the newborn depends on many factors such as the willingness of the grandparents to become involved, the proximity of the grandparents, and cultural expectations of the grandparents' role. For example, if the new parents live in the United States, Asian grandparents typically come to the United States to care for the baby and the mother after birth and to care for the children once the parents return to work. In the United States, paternal grandparents, in contrast to those in other cultures, frequently consider themselves secondary to the maternal grandparents. Less seems expected of them, and they are initially less involved. Nevertheless, these grandparents are eager to help and express great pleasure in their son's fatherhood and his involvement with the baby (Fig. 22-10).

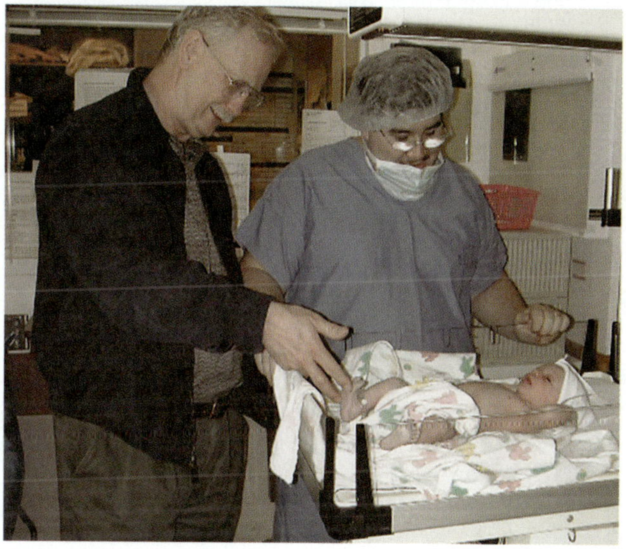

FIG. 22-10 Father, grandfather, and new grandson get acquainted. (Courtesy Sharon Johnson, Petaluma, CA.)

Relationships between grandparents and parents may change with the birth of a new baby. For first-time parents, pregnancy and parenthood can reawaken old issues related to dependence versus independence. Couples often do not plan on their parents' help immediately after the baby arrives. They want time "to be a family," implying a couple-baby unit, not the intergenerational family network. Contrary to their expectations, however, new parents do call on their parents for help, especially the maternal grandmother. Many grandparents are aware of their adult children's wishes for autonomy, respect these wishes, and remain available to help when asked.

Grandparents' classes can be used to bridge the generation gap and to help the grandparents understand their adult children's parenting concepts. The classes include information on up-to-date childbearing practices; family-centered care; infant care, feeding, and safety (car seats); and exploration of roles that grandparents play in the family unit.

Increasing numbers of grandparents are providing permanent care for their grandchildren as a result of divorce,

NURSING PROCESS

Transition to Parenthood

ASSESSMENT

Assessment should include a psychosocial assessment focusing on:

- Parent-infant attachment
- Adjustment to the parental role
- Sibling adjustment
- Social support
- Education needs
- Mother's and baby's physical adaptation
- Beginnings of positive or negative parenting behaviors

NURSING DIAGNOSES

Examples of nursing diagnoses related to transition to parenthood include:

Readiness for Enhanced Family Coping **related to:**

- positive attitude and realistic expectations for newborn and adapting to parenthood
- nurturing behaviors with newborn
- verbalizing positive factors in lifestyle change

Risk for Impaired Parenting **related to:**

- lack of knowledge of infant care
- feelings of incompetence or lack of confidence
- unrealistic expectations of newborn or infant
- fatigue from interrupted sleep

Parental Role Conflict **related to:**

- role transition and role attainment
- unwanted pregnancy
- lack of resources to support parenting (e.g., no paid leave)

Risk for Impaired Parent/Child Attachment **related to:**

- difficult labor and birth
- postpartum complications
- neonatal complications or anomalies

Readlines for Enhanced Family Processes **related to:**

- Birth of infant following planned pregnancy
- Ability of parents to express their needs
- Adequate support from family and friends

EXPECTED OUTCOMES OF CARE

Expected outcomes for effective transition to parenthood include that the parents will:

- Demonstrate behaviors that reflect appreciation of sensory and behavioral capacities of the infant.
- Verbalize increasing confidence and competence in feeding, diapering, dressing, and sensory stimulation of the infant.
- Identify deviations from normal in the infant that should be brought to the immediate attention of the primary health care provider.
- Relate effectively to the newborn's siblings and grandparents.

PLAN OF CARE AND INTERVENTIONS

A plan of care is formulated in collaboration with the family, incorporating their priorities and preferences, to meet their specific needs.

- Provide opportunities for parent-infant interaction.
- Implement strategies to facilitate sibling acceptance of infant (see Box 22-4).
- Provide practical suggestions for infant care (see Chapter 24).
- Provide anticipatory guidance on what to expect as newborn grows and develops.
  - Sleep-wake cycles
  - Interpretation of crying and quieting techniques
  - Infant developmental milestones
  - Sensory enrichment/infant stimulation
  - Recognizing signs of illness
  - Well-baby follow-up and immunizations
- Provide positive reinforcement for loving and nurturing behaviors with the infant.
- Closely monitor parents who interact in inappropriate or abusive ways with their infants, and notify an appropriate mental health practitioner or professional social worker.

EVALUATION

Evaluation is based on the expected outcomes of care. The plan is revised as needed based on the evaluation findings.

substance abuse, child abuse or neglect, abandonment, teenage pregnancy, death, human immunodeficiency virus and acquired immunodeficiency syndrome, unemployment, incarceration, and mental health problems. This emerging trend requires the nurse to evaluate the role of the grandparent in parenting the infant. Educational and financial considerations must be addressed and available support systems identified for these families.

CARE MANAGEMENT

Numerous changes occur during the first weeks of parenthood. Nursing care management should be directed toward helping parents cope with infant care, role changes, altered lifestyle, and change in family structure resulting from the addition of a new baby. Developing skill and confidence in caring for an infant can be anxiety provoking. Anticipatory guidance can help prevent a shock of reality in the transition from hospital or birthing center to home that might negate the parents' joy or cause them undue stress (see Nursing Process box).

COMMUNITY ACTIVITY

- Visit the website of a hospital that provides maternity services in your community. Does the hospital offer prepared child birth, parenting, sibling or infant/child CPR classes? Are group tours of the birthing center provided for expectant parents?
- Visit the website babycenter.com, which provides information for parents about pregnancy, parenting and children's health. Review the information about postpartum emotional health, causes and treatments of baby blues, and baby blues versus postpartum depression.
- Visit the FamilyandHomeNetwork.com website, and research the availability of support groups for parents in your community.

Through education, support, and encouragement, nurses are instrumental in assisting mothers and their partners in the transition to parenthood, whether they are first-time parents or parents of several other children. Early and ongoing assessment and intervention promotes positive outcomes for parents, infants, and family members.

KEY POINTS

- The birth of a child necessitates changes in the existing interactional structure of a family.
- Attachment is the process by which the parent and infant come to love and accept each other.
- Attachment is strengthened through the use of sensual responses or interactions by both partners in the parent-infant interaction.
- Women go through predictable stages in becoming a mother.
- Many mothers exhibit signs of postpartum blues (baby blues).
- Fathers experience emotions and adjustments during the transition to parenthood that are similar to, and also distinctly different from, those of mothers.
- Modulation of rhythm, modification of behavioral repertoires, and mutual responsivity facilitate infant-parent adjustment.
- Many factors influence adaptation to parenthood (e.g., age, culture, socioeconomic level, expectations of what the child will be like).
- A parent who has a sensory impairment needs to maximize use of the remaining senses.
- Sibling adjustment to a new baby requires creative parental interventions.
- Grandparents can have a positive influence on the postpartum family.

Audio Chapter Summaries Access an audio summary of these Key Points on evolve

REFERENCES

Beers, L., & Hollo, R. (2009). Approaching the adolescent-headed family: A review of teen parenting. *Current Problems in Pediatric and Adolescent Health Care, 39*(9), 216–233.

Brotherson, S. (2007). From partners to parents: Couples and the transition to parenthood. *International Journal of Childbirth Education, 22*(2), 7–12.

Corwin, E., & Arbour, M. (2007). Postpartum fatigue and evidence-based interventions. *MCN The American Journal of Maternal/Child Nursing, 32*(4), 215–220.

Deave, T., Johnson, D., & Ingram, J. (2008). Transition to parenthood: The needs of parents in pregnancy and early parenthood. *BMC Pregnancy and Childbirth, 8*(30), 1–11. Available at www.biomedcentral.com/1471-2393/8/30. Accessed July 6, 2010.

D'Avanzo, C. (2008). *Mosby's pocket guide to cultural health assessment* (4th ed.). St. Louis: Mosby.

Fletcher, R., Vimpani, G., Russell, G., & Sibbritt, D. (2008). Psychosocial assessment of expectant fathers. *Archives of Women's Mental Health, 11*(1), 27–32.

Goldberg, A. (2006). The transition to parenthood for lesbian couples. *Journal of Gay, Lesbian, Bisexual, and Transgender Family Studies, 2*(1), 13–42.

Goldberg, A., & Perry-Jenkins, M. (2007). The division of labor and perceptions of parental roles: Lesbian couples across the transition to parenthood. *Journal of Social and Personal Relationships, 24*(2), 297–318.

Goodman, J. (2005). Becoming an involved father of an infant. *Journal of Obstetric, Gynecologic and Neonatal Nursing, 34*(2), 190–200.

Halle, C., Dowd, T., Fowler, C., Rissel, K., Hennessy, K., MacNevin, R., et al. (2008). Supporting fathers in the transition to parenthood. *Contemporary Nurse, 31*(1), 57–70.

Herrman, J. (2008). Adolescent perceptions of teen births. *Journal of Obstetric, Gynecologic and Neonatal Nursing, 37*(1), 42–50.

Klaus, M., & Kennell, J. (1976). *Maternal-infant bonding*. St. Louis: Mosby.

Klaus, M., & Kennell, J. (1982). *Parent-infant bonding* (2nd ed.). St. Louis: Mosby.

Lutz, K., & May, K. (2007). The impact of high-risk pregnancy on the transition to parenthood. *International Journal of Childbirth Education, 22*(3), 20–22.

McManus, A., Hunter, L., & Renn, H. (2006). Lesbian experiences and needs during childbirth: Guidance for health care providers. *Journal of Obstetric, Gynecologic and Neonatal Nursing, 35*(1), 13–26.

Mercer, R. (2004). Becoming a mother versus maternal role attainment. *Journal of Nursing Scholarship, 36*(3), 226–232.

Mercer, R., & Walker, L. (2006). A review of nursing interventions to foster becoming a mother. *Journal of Obstetric, Gynecologic and Neonatal Nursing, 35*(5), 568–582.

Moore, E., Anderson, G., & Bergman, N. (2009). Early skin-to-skin contact for mothers and their healthy newborn infants. *The Cochrane Database of Systematic Reviews, 2007*, 3, CD003519.

Nelson, A. (2003). Transition to motherhood. *Journal of Obstetric, Gynecologic and Neonatal Nursing, 32*(4), 465–477.

Renaud, M. (2007). We are mothers too: Childbearing experiences of lesbian families. *Journal of Obstetric, Gynecologic and Neonatal Nursing, 36*(2), 190–199.

Riordan, J., & Wambach, K. (2010). *Breastfeeding and human lactation* (4th ed.). Boston: Jones and Bartlett.

Rubin, R. (1961). Basic maternal behavior. *Nursing Outlook, 9*(11), 683–686.

Shin, H., Park, Y., Ryu, H., & Seomun, G. (2008). Maternal sensitivity: A concept analysis. *Journal of Advanced Nursing, 64*(3), 304–314.

St. John, W., Cameron, C., & McVeigh, C. (2005). Meeting the challenge of new fatherhood during the early weeks. *Journal of Obstetric, Gynecologic and Neonatal Nursing, 34*(2), 180–189.

Suplee, P., Dawley, K., & Bloch, J. (2007). Tailoring peripartum nursing care for women of advanced maternal age. *Journal of Obstetric, Gynecologic and Neonatal Nursing, 36*(6), 616–623.

CHAPTER

23

Physiologic and Behavioral Adaptations of the Newborn

Kathryn Rhodes Alden

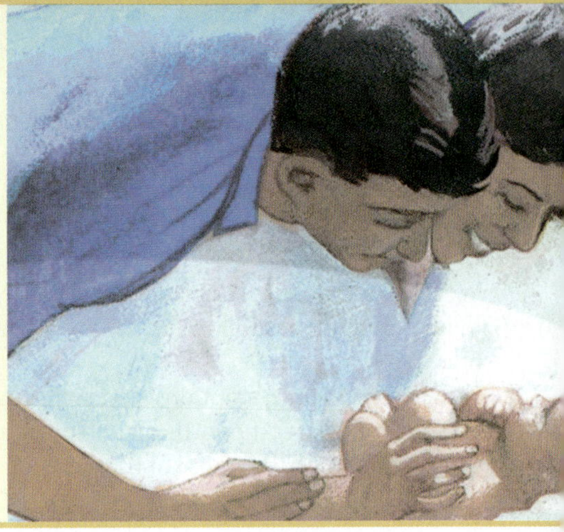

evolve WEBSITE

http://evolve.elsevier.com/Lowdermilk/MWHC/

Anatomy Review
- Sutures and Fontanels

Audio Glossary

Audio Key Points

Case Study
- Newborn Health Problems

NCLEX Review Questions

Nursing Skill
- Thermoregulation

Video—Assessment
- Male Breasts (Supine Position)
- Cremasteric Reflex
- Buttocks
- Neck (Posterior)
- Upper Extremities
- Legs (Symmetry, Length)
- Moro Reflex
- Plantar Grasp
- Rooting and Sucking

Video—Nursing Skills
- Assessing a Newborn's Reflex
- Ausculating Newborn Heart Sounds

LEARNING OBJECTIVES

- Discuss the physiologic adaptations that the neonate must make during the period of transition from the intrauterine to the extrauterine environment.
- Describe the behavioral adaptations that are characteristic of the newborn during the transition period.
- Explain the mechanisms of thermoregulation in the neonate and the potential consequences of hypothermia and hyperthermia.
- Recognize newborn reflexes and differentiate characteristic responses from abnormal responses.
- Discuss the sensory and perceptual functioning of the neonate.
- Identify signs that the neonate is at risk related to problems with each body system.

The neonatal period includes the time from birth through day 28 of life. During this time the neonate must make many physiologic and behavioral adaptations to extrauterine life. Physiologic adjustment tasks are those that involve: (1) establishing and maintaining respirations; (2) adjusting to circulatory changes; (3) regulating temperature; (4) ingesting, retaining, and digesting nutrients; (5) eliminating waste; and (6) regulating weight. Behavioral tasks include: (1) establishing a regulated behavioral tempo independent of the mother, which involves self-regulation of arousal, self-monitoring of changes in state, and patterning of sleep; (2) processing, storing, and organizing multiple stimuli; and (3) establishing a relationship with caregivers and the environment. The term infant usually makes these adjustments with little or no difficulty.

TRANSITION TO EXTRAUTERINE LIFE

The major adaptations associated with transition from intrauterine to extrauterine life occur during the first 6 to 8 hours after birth. The predictable series of events during transition are mediated by the sympathetic nervous system and result in changes that involve heart rate, respirations, temperature, and gastrointestinal function. This transition period represents a time of vulnerability for the neonate and warrants careful observation by nurses. To detect disorders in adaptation soon after birth, nurses must be aware of normal features of the transition period.

In their classic work on newborn adaptation to extrauterine life, Desmond and associates (1966) proposed three stages of newborn transition. The stages are still considered valid today. (Desmond, Rudolph, & Phitaksphraiwan, 1966).

The first stage of the transition period lasts up to 30 minutes after birth and is called the *first period of reactivity*. The newborn's heart rate increases rapidly to 160 to 180 beats/min but gradually falls after 30 minutes or so to a baseline rate of 100 to 120 beats/min. Respirations are irregular, with a rate between 60 and 80 breaths/min. Fine crackles can be present on auscultation. Audible grunting, nasal flaring, and retractions of the chest also can be present, but these should cease within the first hour of birth. The infant is alert and may have spontaneous startles, tremors, crying, and head movement from side to side. Bowel sounds are audible, and meconium may be passed.

After the first period of reactivity the newborn either sleeps or has a marked decrease in motor activity. This *period of decreased responsiveness* lasts from 60 to 100 minutes. During this time the infant is pink and respirations are rapid and shallow (up to 60 breaths/min), but unlabored. Bowel sounds are audible and peristaltic waves may be noted over the rounded abdomen.

The *second period of reactivity* occurs roughly between 2 and 8 hours after birth and lasts from 10 minutes to several hours. Brief periods of tachycardia and tachypnea occur, associated with increased muscle tone, changes in skin color, and mucus production. Meconium is commonly passed at this time. Most healthy newborns experience this transition regardless of gestational age or type of birth; extremely and very preterm infants do not because of physiologic immaturity.

PHYSIOLOGIC ADAPTATIONS

Respiratory System

As the infant emerges from the intrauterine environment and the umbilical cord is severed, profound adaptations are necessary for survival. The most critical of these adaptations is the establishment of effective respirations. Most newborns breathe spontaneously after birth and are able to maintain adequate oxygenation. Preterm infants often encounter respiratory difficulties related to immaturity of the lungs.

Initiation of Breathing

During intrauterine life, oxygenation of the fetus occurs through transplacental gas exchange. However, at birth the lungs must be established as the site of gas exchange. In utero, fetal blood was shunted away from the lungs, but when birth occurs, the pulmonary vasculature must be fully perfused for this purpose. Clamping the umbilical cord causes a rise in blood pressure, which increases circulation and lung perfusion.

It has been recognized that there is no one single trigger for newborn respiratory function. The initiation of respirations in the neonate is the result of a combination of chemical, mechanical, thermal, and sensory factors.

Chemical Factors. The activation of chemoreceptors in the carotid arteries and the aorta results from the relative state of hypoxia associated with labor. With each labor contraction, there is a temporary decrease in uterine blood flow and transplacental gas exchange resulting in transient fetal hypoxia and hypercarbia. Although the fetus is able to recover between contractions, there appears to be a cumulative effect that results in progressive decline in Po_2, increased Pco_2, and lowered blood pH. Decreased levels of oxygen and increased levels of carbon dioxide seem to have a cumulative effect that is involved in initiating neonatal breathing by stimulating the respiratory center in the medulla. Another chemical factor may also play a role; it is thought that as a result of clamping the cord, there is a drop in levels of a prostaglandin that can inhibit respirations.

Mechanical Factors. Respirations in the newborn can be stimulated by changes in intrathoracic pressure resulting from compression of the chest during vaginal birth. As the infant passes through the birth canal, the chest is compressed. With birth this pressure on the chest is released and the negative intrathoracic pressure helps draw air into the lungs. Crying increases the distribution of air in the lungs and promotes expansion of the alveoli. The positive pressure created by crying helps to keep the alveoli open.

Thermal Factors. With birth the newborn enters the extrauterine environment, in which the temperature is significantly lower. The profound change in environmental temperature stimulates receptors in the skin, resulting in stimulation of the respiratory center in the medulla.

Sensory Factors. Sensory stimulation occurs in a variety of ways with birth. Some of these include handling the infant by the physician or midwife, suctioning the mouth and nose, and drying by the nurses. Pain associated with birth can also be a factor. The lights, sounds, and smells of the new environment can also be involved in stimulation of the respiratory center.

At term the lungs hold approximately 20 ml of fluid per kilogram. Air must be substituted for the fluid that filled the fetal respiratory tract. It has been traditionally thought that the thoracic squeeze occurring during normal vaginal birth resulted in significant clearance of lung fluid. However, it appears that this event plays a minor role. In the days preceding labor, there is reduced production of fetal lung fluid and concomitant decreased alveolar fluid volume. Shortly before the onset of labor, there is a catecholamine surge that seems to promote fluid clearance from the lungs. The movement of lung fluid from the air spaces occurs through active transport into the interstitium, with drainage occurring through the pulmonary circulation and lymphatic system. Retention of lung fluid can interfere with the infant's ability to maintain adequate oxygenation, especially if other factors (e.g., meconium aspiration, congenital diaphragmatic hernia, esophageal atresia with fistula, choanal atresia, congenital cardiac defect, immature alveoli) that compromise respirations are present. Infants born by cesarean in which labor did not occur prior to birth can experience some lung fluid retention, although it typically clears without deleterious effects on the infant. These infants are also more likely to develop transient tachypnea of the newborn (TTNB) due to the lower levels of catecholamines (Jain & Eaton, 2006).

The alveoli of the term infant's lungs are lined with **surfactant,** a protein manufactured in type II cells of the lungs. Lung expansion is largely dependent on chest wall contraction and adequate secretion of surfactant. Surfactant lowers surface tension, therefore reducing the pressure required to keep the alveoli open with inspiration, and prevents total alveolar collapse on exhalation, thereby maintaining alveolar stability. The decreased surface tension results in increased lung compliance, helping to establish the functional residual capacity of the lungs. With absent or decreased surfactant, more pressure must be generated for inspiration, which can soon tire or exhaust preterm or sick term infants.

Breathing movements that began in utero as intermittent become continuous after birth, although the mechanism for this is not well understood. Once respirations are established, breaths are shallow and irregular, ranging from 30 to 60 breaths/min, with periods of breathing that include pauses in respirations lasting less than 20 seconds. These episodes of periodic breathing occur most often during the active (rapid eye movement [REM]) sleep cycle and decrease in frequency and duration with age. Apneic periods longer than 20 seconds are indicative of a pathologic process and should be thoroughly evaluated.

! NURSING ALERT

Newborn infants are by preference nose breathers. The reflex response to nasal obstruction is to open the mouth to maintain an airway. This response is not present in most infants until 3 weeks after birth; therefore, cyanosis or asphyxia can occur with nasal blockage.

In the majority of newborn infants, auscultation of the chest reveals loud, clear breath sounds that seem very near, because little chest tissue intervenes. Breath sounds should be clear and equal bilaterally. The ribs of the infant articulate with the spine at a horizontal rather than a downward slope; consequently, the rib cage cannot expand with inspiration as readily as that of an adult. Because neonatal respiratory function is largely a matter of diaphragmatic contraction, abdominal breathing is characteristic of newborns. The newborn infant's chest and abdomen rise simultaneously with inspiration. Characteristics of the respiratory system of the neonate and the effects of these characteristics on respiratory function are listed in Table 23-1.

TABLE 23-1 CHARACTERISTICS OF THE RESPIRATORY SYSTEM OF THE NEONATE

CHARACTERISTIC	EFFECT ON FUNCTION
Decreased lung elastic tissue and recoil	Decreased lung compliance requiring higher pressures and more work to expand; increased risk of atelectasis
Reduced diaphragm movement and maximal force potential	Less effective respiratory movement; difficulty generating negative intrathoracic pressures; risk of atelectasis
Tendency to nose breathe; altered position of larynx and epiglottis	Enhanced ability to synchronize swallowing and breathing; risk of airway obstruction; possibly more difficult to intubate
Small compliant airway passages with higher airway resistance; immature reflexes	Risk of airway obstruction and apnea
Increased pulmonary vascular resistance with sensitive pulmonary arterioles	Risk of ductal shunting and hypoxemia with events such as hypoxia, acidosis, hypothermia, hypoglycemia, and hypercarbia
Increased oxygen consumption	Increased respiratory rate and work of breathing; risk of hypoxia
Increased intrapulmonary right-left shunting	Increased risk of atelectasis with wasted ventilation; lower Pco_2
Immaturity of pulmonary surfactant system in immature infants	Increased risk of atelectasis and respiratory distress syndrome; increased work of breathing
Immature respiratory control	Irregular respirations with periodic breathing; risk of apnea; inability to rapidly alter depth of respirations

Pco_2, Partial pressure of carbon dioxide.
Source: Blackburn, S. (2007). *Maternal, fetal, & neonatal physiology: A clinical perspective* (3rd ed.). St. Louis: Saunders.

Signs of Respiratory Distress

Signs of respiratory distress can include nasal flaring, intercostal or subcostal retractions (in-drawing of tissue between the ribs or below the rib cage), or grunting with respirations. Suprasternal or subclavicular retractions with stridor or gasping most often represent an upper airway obstruction. Seesaw or paradoxical respirations (exaggerated rise in abdomen, with respiration, as the chest falls) instead of abdominal respirations are abnormal and should be reported. A respiratory rate of less than 30 or greater than 60 breaths/min with the infant at rest must be thoroughly evaluated. The respiratory rate of the infant can be slowed, depressed, or absent due to the effects of analgesics or anesthetics administered to the mother during labor and birth. Apneic episodes can be related to several events (rapid increase in body temperature, hypothermia, hypoglycemia, or sepsis) that require thorough evaluation. Tachypnea can result from inadequate clearance of lung fluid, or it can be an indication of newborn respiratory distress syndrome.

Changes in the infant's color can indicate respiratory distress. Acrocyanosis, the bluish discoloration of hands and feet is a normal finding in the first 24 hours after birth. Transient periods of duskiness while crying are not uncommon immediately after birth; however, central cyanosis is abnormal and signifies hypoxemia. With central cyanosis, the lips and mucous membranes are bluish. Central cyanosis can be the result of inadequate delivery of oxygen to the alveoli, poor perfusion of the lungs that inhibits gas exchange, or cardiac dysfunction. Because central cyanosis is a late sign of distress, newborns usually have significant hypoxemia when cyanosis appears (Askin, 2009).

Infants who experience mild TTNB often have signs of respiratory distress during the first 1 to 2 hours after birth as they transition to extrauterine life. Tachypnea with rates up to 100 breaths/min can be present along with intermittent grunting, nasal flaring, and mild retractions. Supplemental oxygen may be needed.

In neonates with more serious respiratory problems, symptoms of distress are more pronounced and tend to last beyond the first 2 hours after birth. Respiratory rates can exceed 120 breaths/min. Moderate to severe retractions, grunting, pallor, and central cyanosis can occur. The respiratory symptoms can be accompanied by hypotension, temperature instability, hypoglycemia, acidosis, and signs of cardiac problems. Common respiratory complications affecting neonates include respiratory distress syndrome (RDS), meconium aspiration, pneumonia, and persistent pulmonary hypertension of the newborn (PPHN) (Askin, 2009) (see Chapter 35).

Cardiovascular System

The cardiovascular system changes significantly after birth. The infant's first breaths, combined with increased alveolar capillary distention, inflate the lungs and reduce pulmonary vascular resistance to the pulmonary blood flow from the pulmonary

e Case Study—Newborn Health Problems

Video—Nursing Skills: Auscullating newborn Heart Sounds

TABLE 23-2 **CARDIOVASCULAR CHANGES AT BIRTH**

PRENATAL STATUS	POSTBIRTH STATUS	ASSOCIATED FACTORS
Primary Changes		
Pulmonary circulation: high pulmonary vascular resistance, increased pressure in right ventricle and pulmonary arteries	Low pulmonary vascular resistance; decreased pressure in right atrium, ventricle, and pulmonary arteries	Expansion of collapsed fetal lung with air
Systemic circulation: low pressures in left atrium, ventricle, and aorta	High systemic vascular resistance; increased pressure in left atrium, ventricle, and aorta	Loss of placental blood flow
Secondary Changes		
Umbilical arteries: patent, carrying of blood from hypogastric arteries to placenta	Functionally closed at birth; obliteration by fibrous proliferation possibly taking 2 to 3 months, distal portions becoming lateral vesicoumbilical ligaments, proximal portions remaining open as superior vesicle arteries	Closure preceding that of umbilical vein, probably accomplished by smooth muscle contraction in response to thermal and mechanical stimuli and alteration in oxygen tension, mechanically severed with cord at birth
Umbilical vein: patent, carrying of blood from placenta to ductus venosus and liver	Closed, becoming ligamentum teres hepatis after obliteration	Closure shortly after umbilical arteries, hence blood from placenta possibly entering neonate for short period after birth, mechanically severed with cord at birth
Ductus venosus: patent, connection of umbilical vein to inferior vena cava	Closed, becoming ligamentum venosum after obliteration	Loss of blood flow from umbilical vein
Ductus arteriosus: patent, shunting of blood from pulmonary artery to descending aorta	Functionally closed almost immediately after birth, anatomic obliteration of lumen by fibrous proliferation requiring 1 to 3 months, becoming ligamentum arteriosum	Increased oxygen content of blood in ductus arteriosus creating vasospasm of its muscular wall High systemic resistance increasing aortic pressure; low pulmonary resistance reducing pulmonary arterial pressure
Foramen ovale: formation of a valve opening that allows blood to flow directly to left atrium (shunting of blood from right to left atrium)	Functionally closed at birth, constant apposition gradually leading to fusion and permanent closure within a few months or years in majority of persons	Increased pressure in left atrium and decreased pressure in right atrium causing closure of valve over foramen

arteries. Pulmonary artery pressure drops, and pressure in the right atrium declines. Increased pulmonary blood flow from the left side of the heart increases pressure in the left atrium, which causes a functional closure of the foramen ovale. During the first few days of life, crying can reverse the flow through the foramen ovale temporarily and lead to mild cyanosis.

In utero, fetal Po_2 is 27 mm Hg. After birth, when the Po_2 level in the arterial blood approximates 50 mm Hg, the ductus arteriosus constricts in response to increased oxygenation. Circulating levels of the hormone prostaglandin E_2 (PGE_2) also have an important role in closure of the ductus arteriosus. In term infants it functionally closes within the first hours after birth; permanent closure usually occurs within 3 to 4 weeks and the ductus arteriosus becomes a ligament. The ductus arteriosus can open in response to low oxygen levels in association with hypoxia, asphyxia, or prematurity. With auscultation of the chest a patent ductus arteriosus can be detected as a heart murmur.

There is rapid constriction of the umbilical vein and arteries within the first 2 minutes after birth. It is thought that this is related to exposure of the cord to the cooler extrauterine environment and to increased oxygenation as the infant begins to breathe. With the clamping and severing of the cord, the umbilical arteries, the umbilical vein, and the ductus venosus are functionally closed; they are converted into ligaments within 2 to 3 months. The hypogastric arteries also occlude and become ligaments. Table 23-2 summarizes the cardiovascular changes at birth.

Heart Rate and Sounds

The term newborn has a resting heart rate between 100 and 160 beats/min, with brief fluctuations above and below these values, usually noted during sleeping and waking states. Shortly after the first cry the infant's heart rate can accelerate as high as 180 beats/min. The range of the heart rate in the term infant is about 85 to 100 beats/min during deep sleep and 120 to 160 beats/min while the infant is awake. A heart rate of 180 beats/min is not unusual when the infant cries. A heart rate that is either high (more than 160 beats/min) or low (fewer than 100 beats/min) should be reevaluated within 30 minutes to 1 hour or when the activity of the infant changes. Immediately after birth the heart rate can be palpated by grasping the base of the umbilical cord.

By term the infant's heart lies midway between the crown of the head and the buttocks, and the axis is more transverse than that in an adult. The apical impulse (point of maximal impulse [PMI]) in the newborn is at the fourth intercostal space and to the left of the midclavicular line. The PMI is often visible because of the thin chest wall.

Apical pulse rates should be determined for all infants. Auscultation should be for a full minute, preferably when the infant is asleep. An irregular heart rate is not uncommon in the first few hours of life. After this time an irregular heart rate not attributed to changes in activity or respiratory pattern should be further evaluated.

Heart sounds during the neonatal period are of higher pitch, shorter duration, and greater intensity than those during adult life. The first sound (S_1) is typically louder and duller than the second sound (S_2), which is sharp. The third and fourth heart sounds are not auscultated in newborns. Most heart murmurs heard during the first few days of life have no pathologic significance, and more than one half of the murmurs disappear by 6 months. However, the presence of a murmur and accompanying signs such as poor feeding, apnea, cyanosis, or pallor are considered abnormal and should be further investigated. There can be significant cardiac defects without symptoms in the early newborn period. This reinforces the importance of ongoing assessment (Askin, 2009).

Blood Pressure

Blood pressure varies according to weight and gestational age. The newborn infant's average systolic blood pressure (BP) is 60 to 80 mm Hg, and the average diastolic pressure is 40 to 50 mm Hg. The BP increases by the second day of life, with minor variations noted during the first month of life. A drop in systolic BP (approximately 15 mm Hg) in the first hour of life is common. Crying and movement usually cause increased systolic pressure. The measurement of BP is best accomplished with an oscillometric device while the infant is at rest. A correctly sized cuff must be used for accurate measurement of an infant's BP.

Unless a specific indication exists, BP is not usually measured in the newborn on a routine basis except as a baseline. In some institutions nurses obtain four extremity blood pressures in the presence of any cardiovascular symptoms such as tachycardia, persistent murmur, abnormal pulses, poor perfusion, or abnormal precordial activity. The value of four extremity BPs in the early newborn period to detect coarctation of the aorta (COA) has been questioned (Razmus & Lewis, 2006). This is based on evidence that COA defects do not occur in the immediate postbirth period but more typically at approximately 12 to 14 days of age, a time when the ductus arteriosus closes.

Blood Volume

The blood volume of the newborn is approximately 80 to 85 ml/kg of body weight. Immediately after birth the total blood volume averages 300 ml, but this can increase by as much as 100 ml, depending on the length of time before the cord is clamped and cut. The preterm infant has a relatively greater blood volume than the term newborn because the preterm infant has a proportionately greater plasma volume, not a greater red blood cell (RBC) mass.

Early or late clamping of the umbilical cord changes the circulatory dynamics of the newborn. Late clamping expands the blood volume from the so-called placental transfusion of blood to the newborn. Delayed cord clamping (≥2 minutes after birth) has been reported to be beneficial in improving hematocrit and iron status and in decreasing anemia; such benefits can last up to 6 months. Polycythemia that occurs with delayed clamping is usually not harmful, although there can be an increased risk of jaundice that requires phototherapy (Arca, Botet, Palacio, & Carbonell-Estrany, 2010; Hutton & Hassan, 2007; McDonald & Middleton, 2008).

Signs of Risk for Cardiovascular Problems

Close monitoring of the infant's vital signs is important for early detection of impending problems. Persistent tachycardia (more than 160 beats/min) can be associated with anemia, hypovolemia, hyperthermia, or sepsis. Persistent bradycardia (less than 100 beats/min) can be a sign of a congenital heart block or hypoxemia.

The newborn's skin color can be reflective of cardiovascular problems. Pallor in the immediate postpartum period is often symptomatic of underlying problems such as anemia or marked peripheral vasoconstriction as a result of intrapartum asphyxia or sepsis. Any prolonged cyanosis other than in the hands or feet can indicate respiratory and/or cardiac problems. The presence of jaundice can indicate ABO or Rh factor incompatibility problems (see Chapter 36).

Congenital heart defects are the most common type of congenital malformations (see Chapter 36). Although the more serious defects such as tetralogy of Fallot are likely to have clinical manifestations such as cyanosis, dyspnea, and hypoxia, others such as small ventricular septal defects can be asymptomatic. The prenatal history can provide information regarding risk factors for congenital heart defects so that the nurse knows to be more alert for symptoms. Maternal illness such as rubella, metabolic disease such as diabetes, and drug ingestion are associated with an increased risk of cardiac defects.

Hematopoietic System

The hematopoietic system of the newborn exhibits certain variations from that of the adult. Levels of RBCs and leukocytes differ, but platelet levels are relatively the same.

Red Blood Cells

Because fetal circulation is less efficient at oxygen exchange than the lungs, the fetus needs additional RBCs for transport of oxygen in utero. Therefore, at birth the average levels of RBCs, hemoglobin, and hematocrit are higher than those in the adult; these levels fall slowly over the first month. At birth the RBC count ranges from 4.8 to 7.1 × 10^6/mcl. The term newborn may have a hemoglobin concentration of 14 to 24 g/dl, decreasing gradually to 12 to 20 g/dl during the first 2 weeks. On the first day, the hematocrit ranges from 44% to 64% and by 8 weeks, it is between 39% and 59% (Pagana & Pagana, 2009). Polycythemia (central venous hematocrit greater than 65%) can occur in term and preterm infants as a result of delayed cord clamping, maternal hypertension or diabetes, or intrauterine growth restriction.

The source of the sample is a significant factor in levels of RBCs, hemoglobin, and hematocrit because capillary blood yields higher values than venous blood. The timing of blood sampling is also significant; the slight rise in RBCs after birth is followed by a substantial drop. At birth the infant's blood contains an average of 70% fetal hemoglobin, but because of the shorter life span of the cells containing fetal hemoglobin, the percentage falls to 55% by 5 weeks and to 5% by 20 weeks. Iron stores generally are sufficient to sustain normal RBC production for 4 to 5 months in the term infant, at which time a transient physiologic anemia can occur.

Leukocytes

Leukocytosis, with a white blood cell (WBC) count of approximately 18,000 cells/mm^3 (range, 9000 to 30,000 cells/mm^3), is normal at birth (Pagana & Pagana, 2009). The number of WBCs increases to 23,000 to 24,000 cells/mm^3 during the first day after birth. This initial high WBC count of the newborn decreases rapidly, and a resting level of 12,000 cells/mm^3 is normally maintained during the neonatal period. Serious infection is not well tolerated by the newborn; leukocytes are slow to recognize foreign protein and to localize and fight infection early in life. Sepsis can be accompanied by a concomitant rise in WBCs (neutrophilia); however, some infants exhibit clinical signs of sepsis without a significant elevation in WBCs. In addition, events other than infection can cause neutrophilia in the newborn. These events include prolonged crying, maternal hypertension, asymptomatic hypoglycemia, hemolytic disease, meconium aspiration syndrome, labor induction with oxytocin, surgery, difficult labor, high altitude, and maternal fever.

Platelets

The platelet count ranges between 150,000 and 300,000 cells/mm^3 and is essentially the same in newborns as in adults (Pagana & Pagana, 2009). The levels of factors II, VII, IX, and X, found in the liver, are decreased during the first few days of life because the newborn cannot synthesize vitamin K. However, bleeding tendencies in the newborn are uncommon, and unless the vitamin K deficiency is great, clotting is sufficient to prevent hemorrhage.

Blood groups

The infant's blood group is genetically determined and established early in fetal life. However, during the neonatal period the strength of the agglutinogens present in the RBC membrane gradually increases. Cord blood samples can be used to identify the infant's blood type and Rh status.

Thermogenic System

Next to establishing respirations and adequate circulation, heat regulation is most critical to the newborn's survival. During the first 12 hours after birth the neonate attempts to achieve thermal balance in adjusting to the extrauterine environmental temperature. **Thermoregulation** is the maintenance of balance between heat loss and heat production. Newborns attempt to stabilize their core body temperatures within a narrow range. Hypothermia from excessive heat loss is a common and dangerous problem.

Anatomic and physiologic characteristics of neonates place them at risk for heat loss. Newborns have a thin layer of subcutaneous fat. The blood vessels are closer to the surface of the skin. Changes in environmental temperature alter the temperature of the blood, thereby influencing temperature regulation centers in the hypothalamus. Newborns have larger body surface-to-body weight (mass) ratios than do children and adults (Sedin, 2006).

Heat Loss

The body temperature of newborn infants is dependent on the heat transfer between the infant and the external environment. Factors that influence heat loss to the environment include the temperature and humidity of the air, the flow and velocity of the air, and the temperature of surfaces in contact with and around the infant. The goal of care is to maintain a **neutral thermal environment** for the neonate in which heat balance is maintained. The neutral thermal environment is the ideal environmental temperature that allows the neonate to maintain a normal body temperature to minimize oxygen and glucose consumption.

Heat loss in the newborn occurs by four modes:

- *Convection* is the flow of heat from the body surface to cooler ambient air. Because of heat loss by convection the ambient temperature in the nursery or mother's room is kept at approximately 24° C, and newborns in open bassinets are wrapped to protect them from the cold.
- *Radiation* is the loss of heat from the body surface to a cooler solid surface not in direct contact but in relative proximity. To prevent this type of loss, newborn cribs and examining tables are placed away from outside windows, and care is taken to avoid direct air drafts.

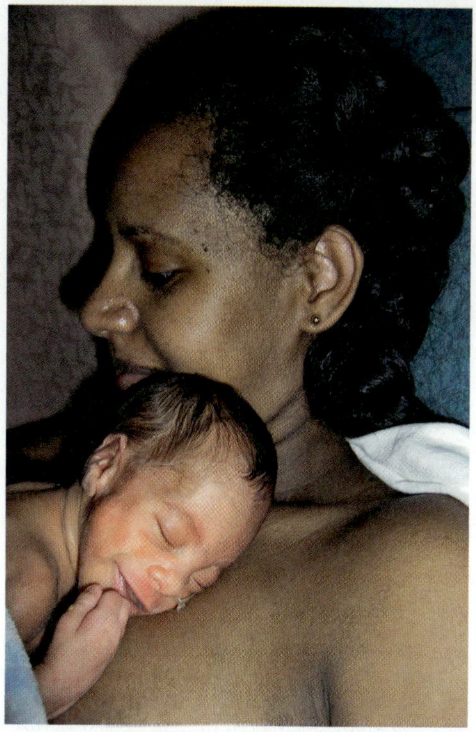

FIG. 23-1 Infant in skin-to-skin contact with mother. (Courtesy Cheryl Briggs, RNC, Annapolis, MD.)

- *Evaporation* is the loss of heat that occurs when a liquid is converted to a vapor. In the newborn, heat loss by evaporation occurs as a result of vaporization of moisture from the skin. This heat loss can be intensified by failure to dry the newborn directly after birth or by drying the infant too slowly after a bath. The less mature the newborn is, the more severe the evaporative heat loss will be. Evaporative heat loss, as a component of insensible water loss, is the most significant cause of heat loss in the first few days of life.
- *Conduction* is the loss of heat from the body surface to cooler surfaces in direct contact. Soon after birth, if or when the infant is placed in a warmer or crib, it should be pre-warmed to prevent heat loss. The scales used for weighing the newborn should have a protective cover to minimize conductive heat loss as well.

Loss of heat must be controlled to protect the infant. Control of such modes of heat loss is the basis of caregiving policies and techniques. One method for promoting maternal-newborn interaction is to place the naked healthy newborn on the mother's bare chest or abdomen and cover both with a blanket. This skin-to-skin contact promotes stabilization of newborn temperature while enhancing mother-infant attachment (Fig. 23-1).

Thermogenesis

In response to cold the neonate attempts to generate heat **(thermogenesis)** by increasing muscle activity. Cold infants may cry and appear restless. Because of vasoconstriction the skin can feel cool to touch, and acrocyanosis can be present. There is an increase in cellular metabolic activity, primarily in the brain, heart, and liver; this also increases oxygen and glucose consumption.

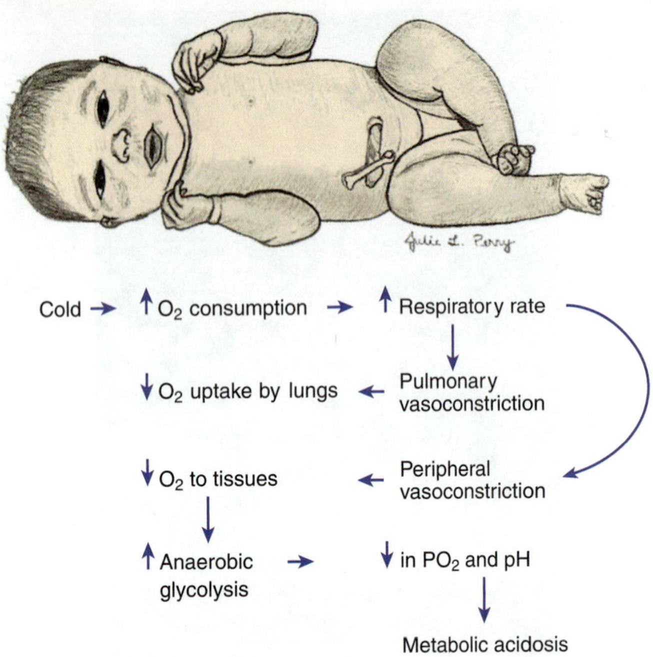

FIG. 23-2 Effects of cold stress. When an infant is stressed by cold, oxygen consumption increases, and pulmonary and peripheral vasoconstriction occurs, thereby decreasing oxygen uptake by the lungs and oxygen to the tissues; anaerobic glycolysis increases; and the Po_2 and pH decrease, leading to metabolic acidosis.

In an effort to conserve heat, term newborns assume a position of flexion that helps guard against heat loss because it diminishes the amount of body surface exposed to the environment. Infants also can reduce the loss of internal heat through the body surface by constricting peripheral blood vessels.

Whereas adults are able to produce heat through shivering, the shivering mechanism of heat production is rarely operable in the newborn. Nonshivering thermogenesis is accomplished primarily by metabolism of **brown fat,** which is unique to the newborn, and secondarily by increased metabolic activity in the brain, heart, and liver. Brown fat is located in superficial deposits in the interscapular region and axillae, as well as in deep deposits at the thoracic inlet, along the vertebral column, and around the kidneys. Brown fat has a richer vascular and nerve supply than ordinary fat. Heat produced by intense lipid metabolic activity in brown fat can warm the newborn by increasing heat production as much as 100%. Reserves of brown fat, usually present for several weeks after birth, are rapidly depleted with cold stress. The amount of brown fat reserve increases with the weeks of gestation. A full-term newborn has greater stores than a preterm infant.

Cold Stress

Cold stress imposes metabolic and physiologic demands on all infants, regardless of gestational age and condition. The respiratory rate increases in response to the increased need for oxygen. In the cold-stressed infant, oxygen consumption and energy are diverted from maintaining normal brain and cardiac function and growth to thermogenesis for survival. If the infant cannot maintain an adequate oxygen tension, vasoconstriction follows and jeopardizes pulmonary perfusion. As a consequence, the Po_2 is decreased, and the blood pH drops. These changes can prompt a transient respiratory distress or aggravate existing respiratory distress syndrome. Moreover, decreased pulmonary perfusion and oxygen tension can maintain or reopen the right-to-left shunt across the ductus arteriosus.

The basal metabolic rate increases with cold stress. If cold stress is protracted, anaerobic glycolysis occurs, resulting in increased production of acids. Metabolic acidosis develops, and if a defect in respiratory function is present, respiratory acidosis also develops (Fig. 23-2). Excessive fatty acids can displace the bilirubin from the albumin-binding sites and exacerbate hyperbilirubinemia.

Hypoglycemia is another metabolic consequence of cold stress. The process of anaerobic glycolysis uses approximately three to four times the amount of blood glucose, thereby depleting existing stores. If the infant is sufficiently stressed and low glucose stores are not replaced, hypoglycemia, which can be asymptomatic in the newborn, can develop.

Hyperthermia

Although occurring less frequently than hypothermia, **hyperthermia** can occur and must be corrected. A body temperature greater than 37.5° C is considered to be abnormally high and is typically caused by excess heat production related to sepsis or to a decrease in heat loss. The clinical appearance of the infant who is hyperthermic often indicates the causative mechanism. Infants who are overheated due to environmental factors such as being swaddled in too many blankets, exhibit signs of heat-losing mechanisms: skin vessels dilate, skin appears flushed, hands and feet are warm to touch, and the infant assumes a posture of extension. The newborn who is hyperthermic because of sepsis will appear stressed: vessels in the skin are constricted, color is pale, and hands and feet are cool. Hyperthermia develops more rapidly in a newborn than in an adult because of the relatively larger surface area of an infant. Sweat glands do not function well. Serious overheating of the newborn can cause cerebral damage from dehydration or even heat stroke and death (Sedin, 2006).

Renal System

At term gestation the kidneys occupy a large portion of the posterior abdominal wall. The bladder lies close to the anterior abdominal wall and is an abdominal organ and a pelvic organ. In the newborn almost all palpable abdominal masses are renal.

A small quantity (approximately 40 ml) of urine is usually present in the bladder of a full-term infant at birth. Voiding at the time of birth often occurs. During the first 30 hours after birth, 98% of newborns will void. If a newborn has not voided within 48 hours, it can be a sign of renal impairment (Vogt, Dell, & Davis, 2006).

! NURSING ALERT

Noting and recording the first voiding is important. An infant who has not voided by 24 hours should be assessed for adequacy of fluid intake, bladder distention, restlessness, and symptoms of pain. The pediatrician or neonatal nurse practitioner should be notified.

The frequency of voiding varies from 2 to 6 times per day during the first and second days of life and from 5 to 25 times per day thereafter. Approximately 6 to 8 voidings per day of pale straw-colored urine are indicative of adequate fluid intake after the first 3 to 4 days. Generally, term infants void 15 to 60 ml of urine/kg/day.

Full-term infants have limited capacity to concentrate urine; therefore the specific gravity of the urine can range from 1.001 to 1.020. The ability to concentrate urine fully is attained by approximately 3 months of age. After the first voiding the infant's urine can appear cloudy (because of mucus content) and have a much higher specific gravity. This level decreases as fluid intake increases. Normal urine during early infancy is usually straw colored and almost odorless. During the first days after birth, urine contains an abundance of uric acid crystals that can appear as pink or orange stains ("brick dust") on the diaper. If this occurs after the first week, it can be an indication of insufficient intake and dehydration.

Fluid and Electrolyte Balance

In the term neonate 75% of body weight consists of water. At birth approximately 40% of the body weight is held within the extracellular fluid compartment. A reduction in extracellular fluid occurs with diuresis during the first few days after birth.

The daily fluid requirement for full-term neonates during the first 2 days of life is 60 to 80 ml/kg. From 3 to 7 days the requirement is 100 to 150 ml/kg/day; and from 8 to 30 days it is 120 to 180 ml/kg/day (Dell & Davis, 2006).

At birth, the glomerular filtration rate (GFR) of a newborn is approximately 30% to 50% that of the adult. This results in a decreased ability to remove nitrogenous and other waste products from the blood. The GFR rapidly increases during the first month of life as a result of postnatal physiologic changes including decreased renal vascular resistance, increased renal blood flow, and increased filtration pressure.

Sodium reabsorption is decreased as a result of a lowered sodium- or potassium-activated adenosine triphosphatase activity. The decreased ability to excrete excessive sodium results in hypotonic urine compared with plasma, leading to a higher concentration of sodium, phosphates, chloride, and organic acids and a lower concentration of bicarbonate ions. The infant has a higher renal threshold for glucose than adults.

Bicarbonate concentration and buffering capacity are decreased. This can lead to acidosis and electrolyte imbalance.

Signs of Risk for Renal System Problems

The renal system has a wide range of functions. Dysfunction resulting from physiologic abnormalities can range from the lack of a steady stream of urine to gross anomalies such as hypospadias and exstrophy of the bladder, which can be identified easily at birth. Enlarged or cystic kidneys can be identified as masses during abdominal palpation. Some kidney anomalies also can be detected by ultrasound examination during pregnancy (see Chapter 36).

Gastrointestinal System

The term newborn is capable of swallowing, digesting, metabolizing, and absorbing proteins and simple carbohydrates and emulsifying fats. With the exception of pancreatic amylase the characteristic enzymes and digestive juices are present even in low-birth-weight neonates.

In the adequately hydrated infant the mucous membrane of the mouth is moist and pink. The hard and soft palates are intact. The presence of moderate to large amounts of mucus is common in the first few hours after birth. Small whitish areas (Epstein pearls) may be found on the gum margins and at the juncture of the hard and soft palate. The cheeks are full because of well-developed sucking pads. These pads, like the labial tubercles (sucking calluses) on the upper lip, disappear around the age of 12 months, when the sucking period is over.

Even though fetal sucking motions have been recorded by ultrasound, these motions are not coordinated with swallowing in any infant born before 32 to 33 weeks of gestation. Sucking behavior is influenced by factors such as neuromuscular maturity, physiologic status, sleep-wake state, and the type of feeding (e.g., breast, bottle, or orogastric).

A special mechanism in healthy term newborns coordinates the breathing, sucking, and swallowing reflexes necessary for oral feeding. Sucking takes place in small bursts of 3 or 4 and up to 8 to 10 sucks at a time, with a brief pause in between bursts. The infant is unable to move food from the lips to the pharynx; therefore, placing the nipple (breast or bottle) well inside the baby's mouth is necessary. Peristaltic activity in the esophagus is uncoordinated in the first few days of life but quickly becomes coordinated in healthy full-term infants, and they swallow easily.

Teeth begin developing in utero, with enamel formation continuing until approximately age 10 years. Tooth development is influenced by neonatal or infant illnesses, medications, and maternal illnesses or medications taken by the mother during pregnancy. The fluoride level in the water supply also influences tooth development. Occasionally an infant is born with one or more teeth. These natal teeth have poorly formed roots and as they loosen place the infant at risk of aspiration. Therefore, they are usually extracted.

Bacteria are not present in the infant's gastrointestinal tract at birth. Soon after birth, oral and anal orifices permit entry of bacteria and air. Generally the highest bacterial concentration is found in the lower portion of the intestine, particularly in the large intestine. Normal colonic bacteria are established within the first week after birth, and normal intestinal flora help synthesize vitamin K, folate, and biotin. Bowel sounds can usually be heard shortly after birth.

The capacity of the newborn stomach varies widely depending on the size of the infant from less than 30 ml on day one to more than 90 ml on day 3. After birth the newborn stomach becomes increasingly more compliant and relaxed to accommodate larger volumes (Spangler, Randenberg, Brenner, & Howett, 2008). Emptying time for the stomach is highly variable and can be affected by several factors such as time and volume of feedings or type and temperature of food. The cardiac sphincter and nervous control of the stomach are immature, thus some regurgitation can occur. Regurgitation during the first day or two of life can be decreased by avoiding overfeeding, by burping the infant, and by positioning the infant with the head slightly elevated.

Digestion

The infant's ability to digest carbohydrates, fats, and proteins is regulated by the presence of certain enzymes. Most of these enzymes are functional at birth except for amylase and lipase.

Amylase is produced by the salivary glands after approximately 3 months and by the pancreas at approximately 6 months of age. This enzyme is necessary to convert starch into maltose and occurs in high amounts in colostrum. The other exception is lipase, also secreted by the pancreas; it is necessary for the digestion of fat. Therefore, the normal newborn is capable of digesting simple carbohydrates and proteins but has a limited ability to digest fats.

Further digestion and absorption of nutrients occur in the small intestine in the presence of pancreatic secretions, secretions from the liver through the common bile duct, and secretions from the duodenal portion of the small intestine.

Stools

Meconium fills the lower intestine at birth. It is formed during fetal life from the amniotic fluid and its constituents, intestinal secretions (including bilirubin), and cells (shed from the mucosa). Meconium is greenish black and viscous and contains occult blood. The first meconium passed is usually sterile, but within hours all meconium passed contains bacteria. The majority of healthy term infants pass meconium within the first 12 to 24 hours of life, and almost all do so by 48 hours (Blackburn, 2007). The number of stools passed varies during the first week, being most numerous between the third and sixth days. Newborns fed early pass stools sooner. Progressive changes in the stooling pattern indicate a properly functioning gastrointestinal tract (Box 23-1).

Feeding Behaviors

Variations occur among infants regarding interest in food, signs of hunger, and amount ingested at one time. The amount of food that the infant takes in at any feeding depends on the size, hunger level, and alertness of the infant. When put to breast some infants feed immediately, whereas others require a longer learning period. Random hand-to-mouth movement and sucking of fingers are well developed at birth and intensify when the infant is hungry. Caregivers should be alert and responsive to these hunger cues (Lawrence & Lawrence, 2005).

Signs of Risk for Gastrointestinal Problems

The time, color, and character of the infant's first stool should be noted. Failure to pass meconium can indicate bowel obstruction related to conditions such as an inborn error of metabolism (e.g., cystic fibrosis) or a congenital disorder (e.g., Hirschsprung disease or an imperforate anus). An active rectal "wink" reflex (contraction of the anal sphincter muscle in response to touch) is a sign of good sphincter tone.

Fullness of the abdomen above the umbilicus can be due to problems such as hepatomegaly, duodenal atresia, or distention. Abdominal distention at birth usually indicates a serious disorder such as a ruptured viscus (from abdominal wall defects) or tumors. Distention that occurs later can be the result of overfeeding or can signal gastrointestinal disorders. A scaphoid (sunken) abdomen, with bowel sounds heard in the chest and signs of respiratory distress indicate a diaphragmatic hernia. Fullness below the umbilicus can indicate a distended bladder.

Some infants are intolerant of certain commercial infant formulas. If an infant is allergic to or unable to digest a formula, the stools can become very soft with a high water content that is signaled by a distinct water ring around the stool on the diaper. Forceful ejection of stool and a water ring around the stool are signs of diarrhea. Care must be taken to avoid misinterpreting transitional stools for diarrhea. The loss of fluid in diarrhea can rapidly lead to fluid and electrolyte imbalance. Passage of meconium from the vagina or urinary meatus is a sign of a possible fistulous tract from the rectum.

The amount and frequency of regurgitation ("spitting up") after feedings should be documented. Color change, gagging, and projectile (very forceful) vomiting occur in association with esophageal and tracheoesophageal anomalies (see Chapter 36).

BOX 23-1 CHANGE IN STOOLING PATTERNS OF NEWBORNS

MECONIUM

- Infant's first stool is composed of amniotic fluid and its constituents, intestinal secretions, shed mucosal cells, and possibly blood (ingested maternal blood or minor bleeding of alimentary tract vessels).
- Passage of meconium should occur within the first 24 to 48 hours, although it may be delayed up to 7 days in very low-birth-weight infants.

TRANSITIONAL STOOLS

- Usually appear by the third day after initiation of feeding; greenish brown to yellowish brown, thin, and less sticky than meconium; may contain some milk curds

MILK STOOL

- Usually appears by the fourth day
- Breastfed infants: stools yellow to golden, pasty in consistency, resemble mixture of mustard and cottage cheese, with an odor similar to that of sour milk
- Formula-fed infants: stools pale yellow to light brown, firmer in consistency, with a more offensive odor

Hepatic System

The liver and gallbladder are formed by the fourth week of gestation. In the newborn the liver can be palpated approximately 1 cm below the right costal margin because it is enlarged and occupies approximately 40% of the abdominal cavity. The infant's liver plays an important role in iron storage, carbohydrate metabolism, conjugation of bilirubin, and coagulation.

Iron Storage

The fetal liver, which serves as the site for production of hemoglobin after birth, begins storing iron in utero. The infant's iron store is proportional to total body hemoglobin content and length of gestation. At birth the term infant has an iron store sufficient to last 4 to 6 months. Iron stores of preterm and small-for-gestational age infants are often lower and are depleted sooner than in healthy term infants. Although both breast milk and cow's milk contain iron, the bioavailability of iron in breast milk is far superior. Full-term infants who are breastfed do not need supplemental iron for 6 months, whereas formula-fed infants should receive a formula that contains supplemental iron (Luchtman-Jones, Schwartz, & Wilson, 2006).

Carbohydrate Metabolism

At birth the newborn is cut off from the maternal glucose supply and, as a result, has an initial decrease in serum glucose levels. The newborn's increased energy needs, decreased hepatic release of glucose from glycogen stores, increased RBC volume, and increased brain size can initially contribute to the rapid depletion of stored glycogen within the first 24 hours after birth. In most healthy term newborns blood glucose levels stabilize at 50 to 60 mg/dl during the first several hours after birth; by the third day of life the blood glucose levels should be approximately 60 to 70 mg/dl. The initiation of feedings assists in the stabilization of the newborn's blood glucose levels. In general, blood glucose levels less than 40 mg/dl are considered abnormal and warrant intervention. The hypoglycemic infant can display the classic symptoms of jitteriness, lethargy, apnea, feeding problems, or seizures, or the infant can be asymptomatic. Hypoglycemia in the initial newborn period is most often transient and easily corrected through feeding. Persistent or recurrent hypoglycemia necessitates intravenous glucose therapy and possible pharmacologic intervention.

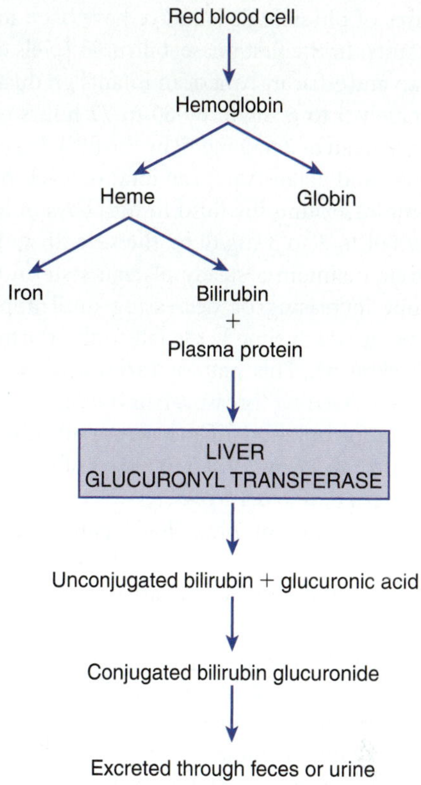

FIG. 23-3 Formation and excretion of bilirubin.

Conjugation of Bilirubin and Newborn Jaundice

Jaundice, the visible yellowish color of the skin and sclera, is due to elevated serum levels of bilirubin (hyperbilirubinemia). The liver is responsible for the conjugation of bilirubin, which results from the breakdown of red blood cells. When RBCs reach the end of their life span, their membranes rupture and hemoglobin is released. The hemoglobin is phagocytosed by macrophages; it then splits into heme and globin. The heme is broken down by the reticuloendothelial cells, converted to bilirubin, and released in an unconjugated form. The unconjugated (indirect) bilirubin is relatively insoluble and almost entirely bound to circulating albumin, a plasma protein. Bilirubin that is not bound to albumin, or free bilirubin, can easily cross the blood-brain barrier and cause neurotoxicity (Bagwell, 2007; Wong, DeSandre, Sibley, & Stevenson, 2006).

The unconjugated bilirubin must be conjugated so that it becomes soluble and excretable. In the liver the unbound bilirubin is conjugated with glucuronic acid in the presence of the enzyme glucuronyl transferase. The conjugated form of bilirubin (direct bilirubin) is soluble and is excreted from liver cells as a constituent of bile. Along with other components of bile, direct bilirubin is excreted into the biliary tract system that carries the bile into the duodenum. Bilirubin is converted to urobilinogen and stercobilinogen within the duodenum through the action of the bacterial flora. Urobilinogen is excreted in urine and feces; stercobilinogen is excreted in the feces (Fig. 23-3). The effectiveness of bilirubin excretion through the feces depends on the stooling pattern of the newborn and on the substances in the intestine that break down conjugated bilirubin. In the newborn intestine the enzyme β-glucuronidase is able to convert conjugated bilirubin into the unconjugated form, which is subsequently reabsorbed by the intestinal mucosa and transported to the liver; this is called enterohepatic circulation. Feeding is important in reducing serum bilirubin levels because it stimulates peristalsis and produces more rapid passage of meconium, thus diminishing the amount of reabsorption of unconjugated bilirubin. Feeding also introduces bacteria to aid in the reduction of bilirubin to urobilinogen. Colostrum, a natural laxative, facilitates meconium evacuation.

When levels of unconjugated bilirubin exceed the liver's ability for conjugation, plasma levels of bilirubin increase and jaundice appears. Jaundice is generally noticeable first in the head, especially in the sclera and mucous membranes, then progresses gradually to the thorax, abdomen, and extremities. The degree of jaundice is determined by serum total bilirubin measurements. Jaundice is likely to appear when bilirubin levels exceed 2.5 mg/dl (Bagwell, 2007).

The newborn is at risk for hyperbilirubinemia because of distinctive aspects of normal neonatal physiology. The higher red blood cell mass at birth and shorter life span of neonatal red blood cells mean that there is the need for greater bilirubin synthesis. The liver's ability to conjugate bilirubin is reduced during the first few days after birth; it can metabolize and excrete only about two thirds of the circulating bilirubin. In addition, there are fewer bilirubin binding sites because newborns have lower serum albumin levels. In the intestines, conjugated bilirubin becomes unconjugated and recirculated through the enterohepatic circulation, which increases serum bilirubin levels.

Traditionally newborn jaundice has been categorized as either physiologic or pathologic (nonphysiologic) depending primarily on the time it appears and on the serum bilirubin levels. Controversy surrounds the definitions of normal or physiologic ranges of total serum bilirubin. Total serum bilirubin levels in newborns are affected by variables such as length of gestation, age, weight, race, nutritional status, and mode of feeding (Wong et al., 2006).

Physiologic Jaundice. Physiologic jaundice or nonpathologic unconjugated hyperbilirubinemia occurs in as many as 60% of newborn infants and in 80% of preterm newborns. Physiologic jaundice usually resolves without treatment.

Two phases of physiologic jaundice have been identified in full-term infants. In the first phase, bilirubin levels of formula-fed Caucasian and African-American infants gradually increase to approximately 5 to 6 mg/dl by 60 to 72 hours of life, then decrease to a plateau of 2 to 3 mg/dl by the fifth day (Blackburn, 2007). In Asian and Asian-American infants, levels reach a peak of 10 to 14 mg/dl around the third to fifth days of life; the levels gradually fall to 2 to 3 mg/dl by the seventh to tenth days. Bilirubin levels maintain a steady plateau state in the second phase without increasing or decreasing until approximately 12 to 14 days, at which time levels fall to the normal value of 1 mg/dl (Blackburn). This pattern varies according to racial group, method of feeding (breast versus bottle), and gestational age. In preterm formula-fed infants, serum bilirubin levels can peak as high as 10 to 12 mg/dl at 5 to 6 days of life and decrease slowly over a period of 2 to 4 weeks.

Some characteristics of physiologic jaundice include the following:

- The infant is otherwise well relative to cardiorespiratory status, neurologic status, carbohydrate metabolism, feeding pattern, and elimination.
- In term infants, jaundice first appears after 24 hours and disappears by the end of the seventh day.
- In preterm infants, jaundice is first evident after 48 hours and disappears by the ninth or tenth day.
- The infant's predischarge total serum bilirubin falls below the high risk category (less than the 95th percentile) on the hour-specific nomogram (see Fig. 24-8).
- The serum concentration of unconjugated bilirubin usually does not exceed 12 mg/dl in term infants and 15 mg/dl in preterm infants.
- Direct bilirubin does not exceed 1 to 1.5 mg/dl.
- Indirect or unconjugated bilirubin concentration does not increase by more than 5 mg/dl per day.

! NURSING ALERT

The appearance of jaundice during the first 24 hours of life or persistence beyond the ages previously delineated usually indicates a potential pathologic process that requires further investigation.

Table 23-3 lists the varying causes of neonatal indirect hyperbilirubinemia.

Pathologic Jaundice. Although physiologic jaundice is usually considered benign, unconjugated bilirubin (indirect) can accumulate to hazardous levels and lead to a pathologic condition. **Pathologic** or **nonphysiologic jaundice** is unconjugated hyperbilirubinemia that is either pathologic in origin or severe enough to warrant further evaluation and treatment (see Chapter 36). Jaundice is usually considered pathologic or nonphysiologic if it appears within 24 hours of birth, if total serum bilirubin levels increase by more than 5 mg/dl in 24 hours, and if the serum bilirubin level exceeds 15 mg/dl at any time. High levels of unconjugated bilirubin are usually due to excessive production of bilirubin through hemolysis, Hemolytic disease of the newborn, caused by maternal/newborn blood group incompatibility is the most common cause of hyperbilirubinemia. Other causes are listed in Table 23-3.

TABLE 23-3 CAUSES OF NEONATAL UNCONJUGATED (INDIRECT) HYPERBILIRUBINEMIA

BASIS	CAUSES
INCREASED PRODUCTION OF BILIRUBIN	
Increased hemoglobin destruction	Fetomaternal blood group incompatibility (Rh, ABO) Congenital red blood cell abnormalities Congenital enzyme deficiencies (G6PD, galactosemia) Sepsis Enclosed hemorrhage (cephalhematoma, bruising)
Increased amount of hemoglobin	Polycythemia (maternal-fetal or twin-twin transfusion, SGA) Delayed cord clamping
Increased enterohepatic circulation	Delayed passage of meconium, meconium ileus, or plug Fasting or delayed initiation of feeding Intestinal atresia or stenosis
ALTERED HEPATIC CLEARANCE OF BILIRUBIN	
Alteration in uridine diphosphoglucuronyl transferase production or activity	Immaturity Metabolic/endocrine disorders (e.g., Crigler-Najjar disease, hypothyroidism, disorders of amino acid metabolism)
Alteration in hepatic function and perfusion (and thus conjugating ability)	Sepsis (also causes inflammation) Asphyxia, hypoxia, hypothermia, hypoglycemia Drugs and hormones (e.g., novobiocin, pregnanediol)
Hepatic obstruction (associated with direct hyperbilirubinemia)	Congenital anomalies (biliary atresia, cystic fibrosis) Biliary stasis (hepatitis, sepsis) Excessive bilirubin load (often seen with severe hemolysis)

G6PD, Glucose-6-phosphate dehydrogenase; *SGA,* small for gestational age.
Source: Blackburn, S. (2007). *Maternal, fetal, and neonatal physiology: A clinical perspective* (3rd ed.). St. Louis: Saunders.

If increased levels of unconjugated bilirubin are left untreated, neurotoxicity can result as bilirubin is transferred into the brain cells. **Acute bilirubin encephalopathy** refers to the acute manifestations of bilirubin toxicity that occur during the first weeks after birth. This can include a range of symptoms such as lethargy, hypotonia, irritability, seizures, coma, and death. **Kernicterus** refers to the irreversible, long-term consequences of bilirubin toxicity such as hypotonia, delayed motor skills, hearing loss, cerebral palsy, and gaze abnormalities (American Academy of Pediatrics [AAP], 2004; Bradshaw, 2010).

Jaundice Related to Breastfeeding. Two forms of breastfeeding-related jaundice are recognized: breastfeeding-associated jaundice and breast milk jaundice. These typically occur in otherwise healthy infants. Both types can occur in the same infant and are not easily differentiated (Blackburn, 2007).

Breastfeeding-associated jaundice (early-onset jaundice) begins at 2 to 4 days of age and occurs in approximately 10% to 25% of breastfed newborns. Breastfeeding does not cause the jaundice; instead, it is a lack of effective breastfeeding that contributes to the hyperbilirubinemia. If the infant is not feeding effectively, there is less caloric and fluid intake and possible dehydration. Hepatic clearance of bilirubin is reduced. With less intake, there are fewer stools. As a result, bilirubin is reabsorbed from the intestine back into the bloodstream and must be conjugated again so that it can be excreted (Blackburn, 2007; Page-Goertz, 2008).

Breast-milk jaundice (late-onset jaundice) can initially begin as the early-onset variety or can begin at age 4 to 6 days and occurs in 2% to 3% of breastfed infants. Infants are usually feeding well and gaining weight appropriately. Rising levels of bilirubin peak during the second week and gradually diminish. Despite high levels of bilirubin that may persist for 3 to 12 weeks, these infants have no signs of hemolysis or liver dysfunction. The etiology of breast milk jaundice is uncertain. However, it seems to be related to factors in the breast milk (e.g., pregnanediol, fatty acids, and β-glucuronidase) that either inhibit the conjugation or decrease the excretion of bilirubin (Blackburn, 2007). (See Chapter 25 for a discussion of these conditions in relation to newborn nutrition.)

Coagulation

The liver plays an important role in blood coagulation. Coagulation factors, which are synthesized in the liver, are activated by vitamin K. The lack of intestinal bacteria needed to synthesize vitamin K results in transient blood coagulation deficiency between the second and fifth days of life. The levels of coagulation factors slowly increase to reach adult levels by age 9 months. The administration of intramuscular vitamin K shortly after birth helps prevent clotting problems. Any bleeding problems noted in the newborn should be reported immediately, and tests for clotting ordered (Luchtman-Jones et al., 2006).

Signs of Risk for Hepatic System Problems

Preterm infants are at greater risk for hepatic system problems such as hyperbilirubinemia and hypoglycemia because of their immaturity. The hematologic status of all newborns should be assessed for anemia. Because infants can develop a coagulation deficiency, a male neonate who has been circumcised must be observed closely for signs of hemorrhage. Hemorrhage also can be caused by a clotting defect, indicating a serious problem such as hemophilia (see Chapter 36).

Immune System

Beginning early in gestation, the immune system of the fetus is developing the capacity to respond to foreign antigens. The development of the immune system is necessary to equip the neonate to meet the numerous environmental challenges (microorganisms) associated with life in the extrauterine world.

At birth most of the circulating antibodies in the newborn are immunoglobulin G (IgG) antibodies that were transported across the placenta from the maternal circulation. This transfer of antibodies from the mother begins as early as 14 weeks of gestation and is greatest during the third trimester. By term, the IgG levels in the cord blood of the infant are higher than those in maternal blood. The passive immunity afforded the infant through the placental transfer of IgG usually provides sufficient antimicrobial protection during the first 3 months of life. Production of adult concentrations of IgG is reached by 4 to 6 years of age (Kapur, Yoder, & Polin, 2006).

The fetus is capable of producing IgM by the eighth week of gestation, and low levels are present at term (less than 10% of adult levels). By the age of 2 years, IgM reaches adult levels. The production of IgA, IgD and IgE is much more gradual, and maximal levels are not attained until early childhood (Kapur et al., 2006).

Natural barrier mechanisms such as the acidity of the stomach and the production of pepsin and trypsin, which maintain sterility of the small intestine, are not fully developed until age 3 to 4 weeks.

The membrane-protective IgA is missing from the respiratory and urinary tracts, and unless the newborn is breastfed, it also is absent from the gastrointestinal tract. Breast milk provides the newborn with important immunity. The secretory IgA in human milk acts locally in the intestines to neutralize bacterial and viral pathogens. It may also lessen the risk of allergy and food intolerance through modulation of exposure to foreign milk protein antigens.

The newborn is capable of producing a protective immune response to vaccines, given as early as a few hours after birth. For example, when hepatitis B vaccine is administered at birth to the infant born to a mother with hepatitis B, there is an excellent immune response. This holds true even if the infant does not receive additional hepatitis B immunoglobulins.

The white blood cells of the newborn display a delayed response to invading bacteria. The influx of phagocytic cells to areas of inflammation is somewhat slowed, although the ability of these cells to attack and destroy bacteria is equivalent to that of adults (Kapur et al., 2006).

Risk for Infection

All newborns, and preterm newborns especially, are at high risk for infection during the first several months of life. During this period infection is one of the leading causes of morbidity and mortality. The newborn cannot limit the invading pathogen to the portal of entry because of the generalized hypofunctioning of the inflammatory and immune mechanisms.

Early signs of infection must be recognized so that prompt diagnosis and treatment can occur. Temperature instability or hypothermia can be symptomatic of serious infection; newborns do not typically exhibit fever, although hyperthermia can occur (temperature greater than 38° C). Lethargy, irritability, poor feeding, vomiting or diarrhea, decreased reflexes, and pale or mottled skin color are some of the clinical signs that are suggestive of infection. Respiratory symptoms such as apnea, tachypnea, grunting, or retracting can be associated with infection such as pneumonia (Lott, 2010).

Any unusual discharge from the infant's eyes, nose, mouth, or other orifice must be investigated. If a rash appears it must be evaluated closely; many normal rashes in the newborn are not associated with any infection. Infants must be protected from infections by the use of good hand hygiene techniques.

The greatest risk factor for neonatal infection is prematurity because of immaturity of the immune system. Other risk factors include premature rupture of membranes, chorioamnionitis, maternal fever, antenatal or intrapartal asphyxia, invasive procedures, stress, and congenital anomalies (Lott, 2010).

Integumentary System

All skin structures are present at birth. The epidermis and dermis are loosely bound and extremely thin. After 35 weeks of gestation, the skin is covered by **vernix caseosa** (a cheeselike, whitish substance) that is fused with the epidermis and serves as a protective covering. Vernix caseosa is a product of the sebaceous glands. The amount of vernix decreases with age and is shed into the amniotic fluid. In the term newborn, vernix is present in the creases of the neck, the axilla, and the groin. Post-term infants have little vernix.

The term infant has erythematous (red) skin for a few hours after birth, after which it fades to its normal color. The skin often appears blotchy or mottled, especially over the extremities. The hands and feet appear slightly cyanotic **(acrocyanosis)**; this is caused by vasomotor instability, capillary stasis, and a high hemoglobin level. Acrocyanosis is normal and can appear intermittently over the first 7 to 10 days, especially with exposure to cold.

The healthy term newborn usually appears plump. Subcutaneous fat accumulated during the last trimester acts as insulation. Fine lanugo hair may be noted over the face, shoulders, and back. Edema of the face and ecchymosis (bruising) or petechiae can be present as a result of face presentation, forceps-assisted birth, or vacuum extraction (see Fig. 24-6). Petechiae appearing on areas of the skin other than the face or neck can be associated with serious infection or hematologic problems (Lissauer, 2006).

Creases are located on the palms of the hands and on the soles of the feet. The simian line, a single palmar crease, is often seen in Asian infants or in infants with Down syndrome. The soles of the feet should be inspected for the number of creases during the first few hours after birth; as the skin dries, more creases appear. Increasing numbers of creases correlate with a greater maturity rating. Premature newborns have few if any creases.

Sweat Glands

Sweat glands are present at birth but do not respond to increases in ambient or body temperature. Some fetal sebaceous gland hyperplasia and secretion of sebum result from the hormonal influences of pregnancy. Distended, small, white sebaceous glands **(milia)** may be noticeable on the newborn's face.

Desquamation

Desquamation (peeling) of the skin of the term infant does not usually occur until a few days after birth. Large generalized areas of skin desquamation present at birth may be an indication of postmaturity.

Mongolian Spots

Mongolian spots, bluish black areas of pigmentation, can appear over any part of the exterior surface of the body, including the extremities. They are more commonly noted on the back and buttocks (Fig. 23-4). These pigmented areas are most frequently noted in newborns whose ethnic origins are in the Mediterranean area, Latin America, Asia, or Africa. They are more common in dark-skinned individuals but occur in 5% to 13% of Caucasians as well (Blackburn, 2007). They fade gradually over months or years.

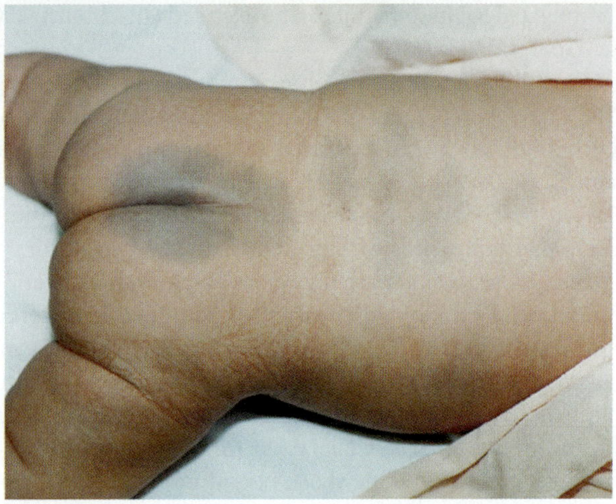

FIG. 23-4 Mongolian spot.

Nevi

Telangiectatic nevi, known as "stork bites," are pink and easily blanched (Fig. 23-5, *A*). They appear on the upper eyelids, nose, upper lip, lower occipital area, and nape of the neck. They have no clinical significance and fade by the second year of life.

The nevus vasculosus is a common type of capillary hemangioma. It consists of dilated newly formed capillaries occupying the entire dermal and subdermal layers, with associated connective tissue hypertrophy. The typical lesion is a raised, sharply demarcated, bright red or dark red, rough-surfaced swelling. As the infant grows the hemangioma may proliferate and become more vascular, thus often called a *strawberry hemangioma*. Lesions are usually single but may be multiple, with 75% occurring on the head. These lesions can remain until the child is of school age or sometimes even longer but can be removed successfully with pulsed dye laser therapy and prednisone administration. In some cases, subcutaneous injections of interferon alfa-2a or interferon alfa-2b may be required if prednisone therapy and the pulsed dye laser fail to control a problematic hemangioma.

A port-wine stain, or nevus flammeus, when present, is usually observed at birth and is composed of a plexus of newly formed capillaries in the papillary layer of the corium. It is red to purple; varies in size, shape, and location; and is not elevated. True port-wine stains do not blanch with pressure or disappear. They are most commonly found on the face and neck.

Erythema Toxicum

A transient rash, **erythema toxicum,** is also called *erythema neonatorum, newborn rash,* or *flea bite dermatitis*. It is found in term neonates during the first 3 weeks of life. Erythema toxicum produces lesions in different stages: erythematous macules, papules, and small vesicles (see Fig. 23-5, *B*). The lesions may appear suddenly anywhere on the body. The rash is thought to be an inflammatory response. Eosinophils, which help decrease inflammation, are found in the vesicles. Although the appearance is alarming, the rash has no clinical significance and requires no treatment.

Signs of Risk for Integumentary Problems

Close observation of the newborn's skin color can lead to early detection of potential problems. Any pallor, plethora (deep purplish color from increased circulating RBCs), petechiae, central cyanosis, or jaundice should be noted and described. The skin should be examined for signs of birth injuries, such as forceps marks and lesions related to fetal monitoring. Bruises

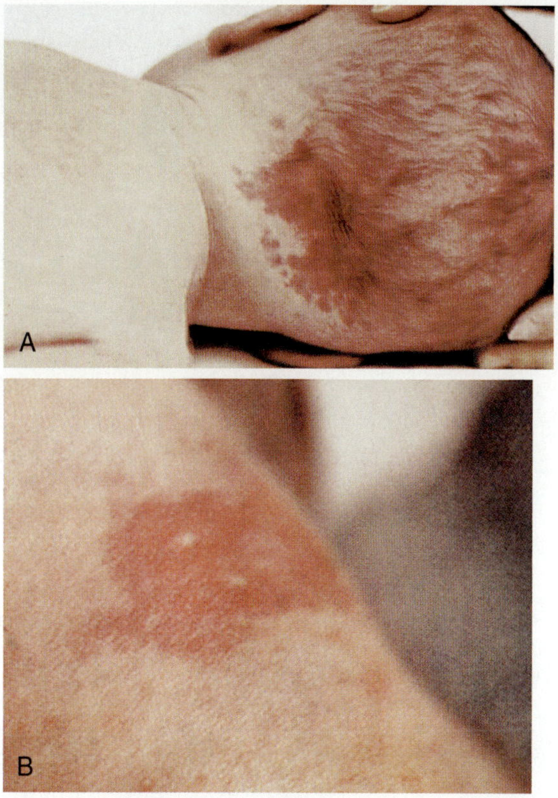

FIG. 23-5 **A,** Telangiectatic nevi (stork bite). **B,** Erythema toxicum (flea bite dermatitis). (Courtesy Mead Johnson & Co., Evansville, IN.)

or petechiae may be present on the head, neck, and face of an infant born with a nuchal cord (cord around the neck) or in an infant who had a face presentation at birth. Bruising can increase the risk of hyperbilirubinemia. Petechiae can be present if increased pressure was applied to an area. Petechiae scattered over the infant's body should be reported to the pediatrician because their presence can indicate underlying problems such as low platelet count or infection. Unilateral or bilateral periauricular papillomas (skin tags) occur fairly frequently. Their occurrence is usually a family trait and of no consequence.

Reproductive System

Female

At birth the ovaries contain thousands of primitive germ cells. These cells represent the full complement of potential ova; no oogonia form after birth in term infants. The ovarian cortex, which is made up primarily of primordial follicles, occupies a larger portion of the ovary in the newborn female than in the adult female. From birth to sexual maturity the number of ova decreases by approximately 90%.

An increase of estrogen during pregnancy followed by a decrease after birth results in a mucoid vaginal discharge and even some slight bloody spotting (pseudomenstruation). External genitals (i.e., labia majora and minora) are usually edematous with increased pigmentation. In term infants the labia majora and minora cover the vestibule (Fig. 23-6, *A*). In preterm infants, the clitoris is prominent, and the labia majora are small and widely separated. Vaginal or hymenal tags are common findings and have no clinical significance. Vernix caseosa can be present between the labia and should not be forcibly removed during bathing.

If the infant was born in the breech position, the labia can be edematous and bruised. The edema and bruising resolve in a few days.

Male

The foreskin completely covers the glans. The urethral opening may be completely covered by the prepuce, which is not retractable for 3 to 4 years. The position of the urethra should be at the tip of the penis. With hypospadias, the urethral opening is located in an abnormal position, on or adjacent to the glans, although it can be placed on the penile shaft or perineum. Small, white, firm lesions called *epithelial pearls* may be seen at the tip of the prepuce. By 28 to 36 weeks of gestation, the testes can be palpated in the inguinal canal, and a few rugae appear on the scrotum. At 36 to 40 weeks of gestation, the testes are palpable in the upper scrotum, and rugae appear on the anterior portion. After 40 weeks the testes can be palpated in the scrotum, and rugae cover the scrotal sac. The postterm neonate has deep rugae and a pendulous scrotum. Hydroceles, caused by an accumulation of fluid around the testes, may be present. They can be easily transilluminated with a light and usually resolve without treatment.

The scrotum is usually more deeply pigmented than the rest of the skin (see Fig. 23-6, *B*), particularly in darker-skinned infants. A bluish discoloration of the scrotum suggests testicular torsion, which needs immediate attention. If the male infant is born in a breech presentation, the scrotum can be very edematous and bruised (Fig. 23-7). The swelling and discoloration subside within a few days.

Swelling of Breast Tissue

Swelling of the breast tissue in term infants of both sexes is caused by the hyperestrogenism of pregnancy. In a few infants a thin discharge (witch's milk) can be seen. This finding has no clinical significance, requires no treatment, and subsides within a few days as the maternal hormones are eliminated from the infant's body.

The nipples should be symmetric on the chest. Breast tissue and areola size increase with gestation. The areola appears slightly elevated at 34 weeks of gestation. By 36 weeks a breast bud of 1 to 2 mm is palpable and increases to 12 mm by 42 weeks.

Signs of Risk for Reproductive System Problems

The infant must be closely inspected for ambiguous genitalia and other abnormalities. Normally in a female infant the urethral opening is located behind the clitoris. Any deviation from this can incorrectly suggest that the clitoris is a small penis, which can occur in conditions such as adrenal hyperplasia. Nearly all female infants are born with hymenal tags; absence of such tags can indicate vaginal agenesis. Fecal discharge from the vagina indicates a rectovaginal fistula. Any of these findings must be reported to the physician or neonatal nurse practitioner for further evaluation.

Hypospadias, undescended or maldescended testes, and other abnormalities of the male genitalia must be reported. Circumcision is contraindicated in the presence of hypospadias since the foreskin is used in repair of this anomaly.

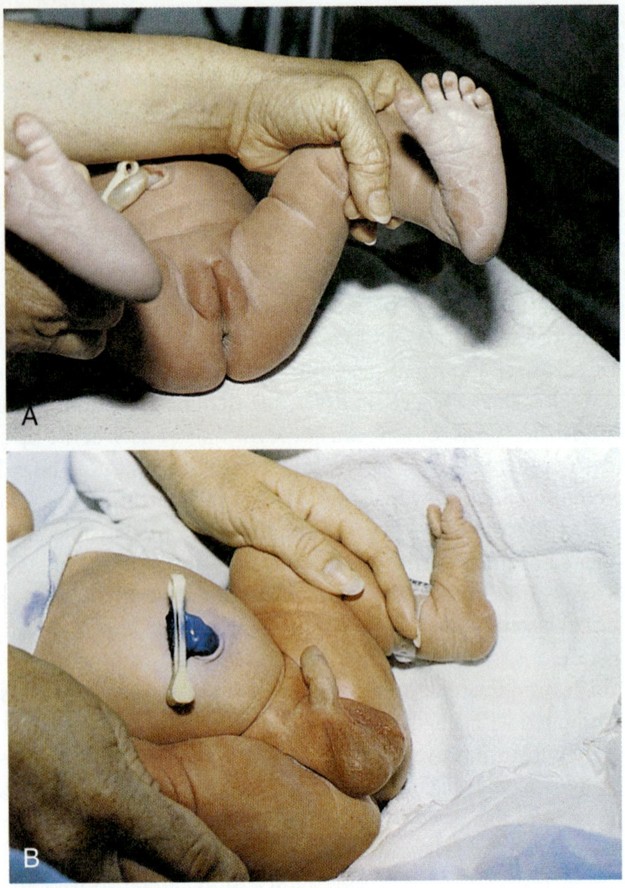

FIG. 23-6 External genitalia. **A**, Genitals in female term infant. Note mucoid vaginal discharge. **B**, Genitals in male infant. Uncircumcised penis. Rugae cover scrotum, indicating term gestation. Cord has been swabbed with ethylene blue to prevent infection. (Courtesy Marjorie Pyle, RNC, Lifecircle, Costa Mesa, CA.)

Inguinal hernias can be present and become more obvious when the infant cries. They are common, especially in African-American neonates, and usually require no treatment because they resolve with time (Lissauer, 2006).

Skeletal System

The infant's skeletal system undergoes rapid development during the first year of life. At birth more cartilage is present than ossified bone. Because of cephalocaudal (head-to-rump) development the newborn appears somewhat out of proportion.

At term the head is one fourth of the total body length. The arms are slightly longer than the legs. In the newborn the legs are one third of the total body length but only 15% of the total body weight. As growth proceeds the midpoint in head-to-toe measurements gradually descends from the level of the umbilicus at birth to the level of the symphysis pubis at maturity.

The face appears small in relation to the skull, which appears large and heavy. Cranial size and shape can be distorted by **molding** (the shaping of the fetal head by the overlapping of cranial bones to facilitate movement through the birth canal during labor) (Fig. 23-8). It is not uncommon to see edematous areas on the newborn's head after birth, especially following a prolonged second stage of labor. Caput succedaneum and cephalhematoma are seen most often; these are usually self-limiting and resolve without treatment. A more serious injury is subgaleal hemorrhage (Fig. 23-9, *C*), which is discussed in Chapter 35.

Anatomy Review—Sutures and Fontanels

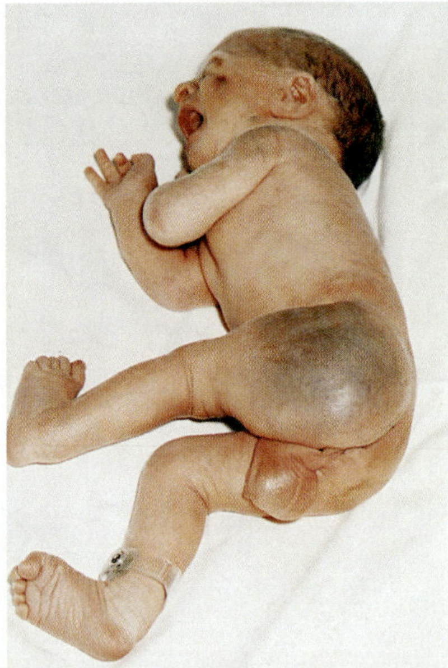

FIG. 23-7 Swelling of the genitals and bruising of the buttocks after a breech birth. (From O'Doherty, N. [1986]. *Neonatology: Micro atlas of the newborn.* Nutley, NJ: Hoffman-LaRoche.)

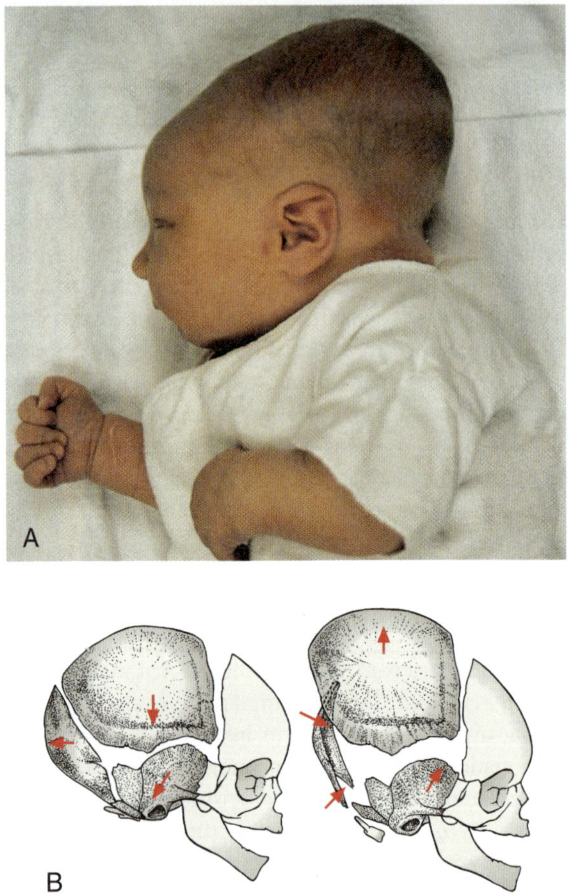

FIG. 23-8 Molding. **A**, Significant molding, soon after birth. **B**, Schematic of bones of skull when molding is present. (**A**, Courtesy Kim Molloy, Knoxville, IA.)

Caput succedaneum is a generalized, easily identifiable edematous area of the scalp, most commonly found on the occiput (Fig. 23-9, *A*). With vertex presentation the sustained pressure of the presenting vertex against the cervix results in compression of local vessels, slowing venous return. The slower

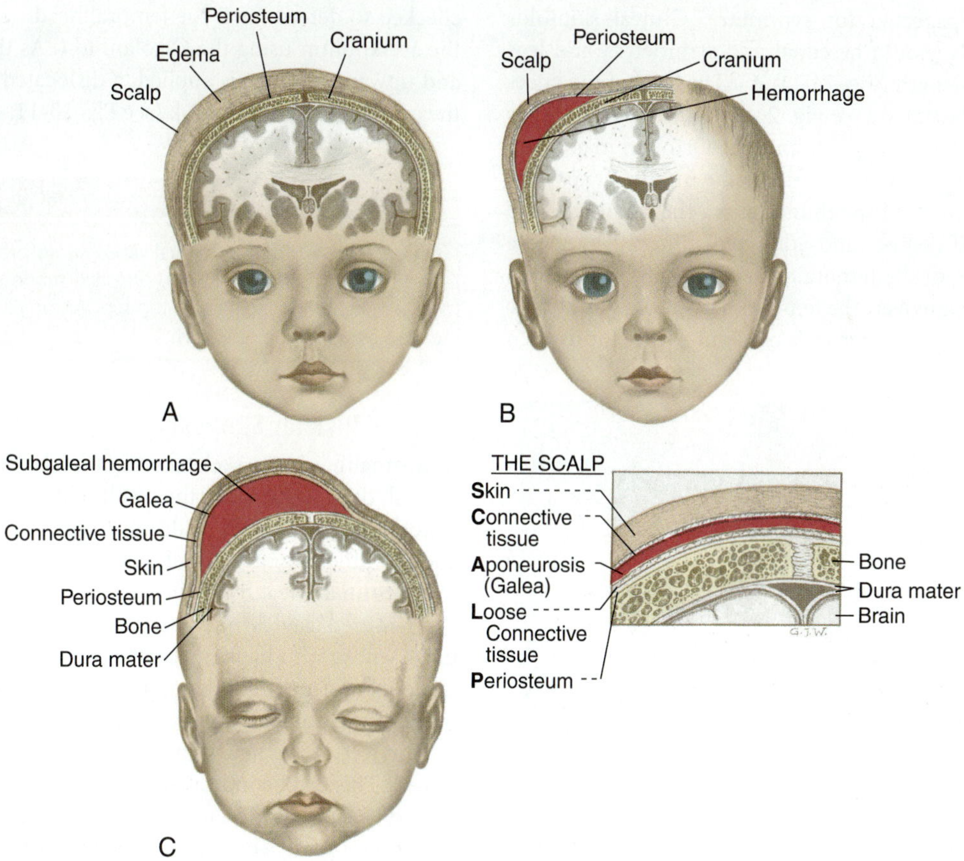

FIG. 23-9 Differences between caput succedaneum, cephalhematoma, and subgaleal hemorrhage. **A**, Caput succedaneum: edema of scalp noted at birth; crosses suture lines. **B**, Cephalhematoma: bleeding between periosteum and skull bone appearing within first 2 days; does not cross suture lines. **C**, Subgaleal hemorrhage: bleeding into the subgaleal compartment; bleeding extends beyond bone, often posteriorly into the neck and continues after birth. (From Seidel, H., Ball, J., Dains, J., & Benedict, G. [2006]. *Mosby's guide to physical examination* [6th ed.]. St. Louis: Mosby.)

venous return causes an increase in tissue fluids within the skin of the scalp, and an edematous swelling develops. This edematous swelling, present at birth, extends across suture lines of the skull and disappears spontaneously within 3 to 4 days. Infants who are born with the assistance of vacuum extraction usually have a caput in the area where the cup was applied. Bruising of the scalp is often seen in the presence of caput succedaneum.

Cephalhematoma is a collection of blood between a skull bone and its periosteum; therefore, a cephalhematoma does not cross a cranial suture line (see Fig. 23-9, *B*). Caput succedaneum and cephalhematoma often occur simultaneously.

Bleeding can occur with spontaneous birth from pressure against the maternal bony pelvis. Low forceps birth and difficult forceps rotation and extraction can also cause bleeding. This soft, fluctuating, irreducible fullness does not pulsate or bulge when the infant cries. It appears several hours or the day after birth and may not become apparent until a caput succedaneum is absorbed. A cephalhematoma is usually largest on the second or third day, by which time the bleeding stops. The fullness of a cephalhematoma spontaneously resolves in 3 to 6 weeks. It is not aspirated because infection can develop if the skin is punctured. As the hematoma resolves, hemolysis of RBCs occurs, and jaundice can result. Hyperbilirubinemia and jaundice can occur after the newborn is discharged home.

The bones in the vertebral column of the newborn form two primary curvatures—one in the thoracic region and one in the sacral region. Both are forward, concave curvatures. As the infant gains head control at approximately age 3 months, a secondary curvature appears in the cervical region. The newborn's spine appears straight and can be easily flexed. The newborn can lift the head and turn it from side to side when prone. The vertebrae should appear straight and flat. If a pilonidal dimple is noted, further inspection is required to determine whether a sinus is present. A pilonidal dimple, especially with a sinus and nevus pilosis (hairy nevus), is significant because it can be associated with spina bifida.

The infant's extremities should be symmetric and of equal length. Fingers and toes should be equal in number (five fingers on each hand and five toes on each foot) and should have nails present. Digits may be missing (oligodactyly). Extra digits (polydactyly) are sometimes found on hands or feet. Fingers or toes may be fused (syndactyly).

The infant is examined for developmental dysplasia of the hips (DDH). At birth the hip is rarely dislocated, but instead is dislocatable. Postnatal factors determine whether the hip dislocates, subluxates, or remains stable. DDH occurs more often in female infants, in breech presentations (Fig. 23-10), and in infants with family history of DDH (Lissauer, 2006). If the hip is dislocated, the femoral head is above and lateral to the acetabulum. With subluxation or laxity of ligaments, the femoral head is within the acetabulum, but it can be manipulated to the edge of the acetabulum. The majority of unstable hips will become clinically normal by one month of age.

The hips are inspected for symmetry. Gluteal skinfolds and thigh skinfolds should be equal and symmetric, and legs should be of equal length (Fig. 23-11, *A*). The level of the knees in flexion should be equal (see Fig. 23-11, *C*). Hip integrity is assessed by using the Barlow test and the Ortolani maneuver. For the Barlow test the examiner places the middle finger over the greater trochanter and the thumb along the midthigh. The hip is flexed to 90 degrees and adducted followed by gentle downward pushing of the femoral head. If the hip can be dislocated with this maneuver, the femoral head moves out of the acetabulum and the examiner feels a "clunk." The hip is then checked to determine if the femoral head can be returned into the acetabulum using the Ortolani test. As the hip is abducted and upward leverage is applied, a dislocated hip will return to the acetabulum with a clunk (see Fig. 23-11, *B* and *D*).

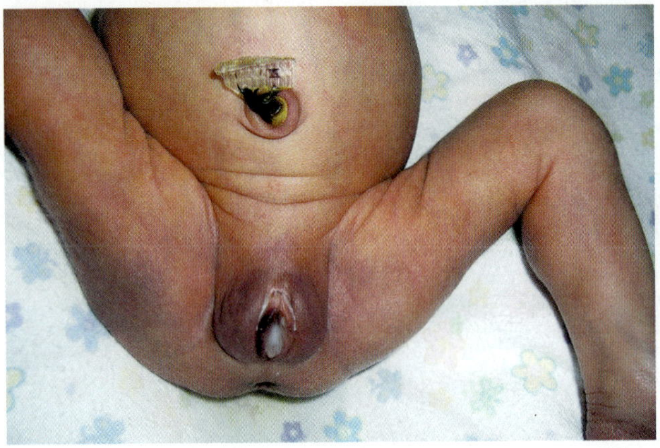

FIG. 23-10 Position of infant's legs after breech birth. (Courtesy Cheryl Briggs, RNC, Annapolis, MD.)

SAFETY ALERT

Only expert examiners (physicians, nurse practitioners) should perform the Barlow test and Ortolani maneuver to assess for developmental dysplasia of the hip. An unskilled examiner can cause injury to the newborn.

Signs of Risk for Skeletal Problems

Abnormalities of the skeletal system can be congenital, developmental, drug induced, or the result of intrapartum or postnatal factors. Signs of DDH, additional digits or webbing of digits, and any other abnormality should be documented and reported to the primary health care provider.

Fractured clavicle often occurs in macrosomic infants and in those whose who had a difficult birth (e.g., shoulder dystocia). Unequal movement of the upper extremities or a crepitant feeling over the clavicular area can indicate fracture.

The feet of the newborn can appear to be abnormally positioned. This can be indicative of congenital deformity or can be related to fetal positioning in utero. For example, clubfoot (talipes equinovarus), a deformity in which the foot turns inward and

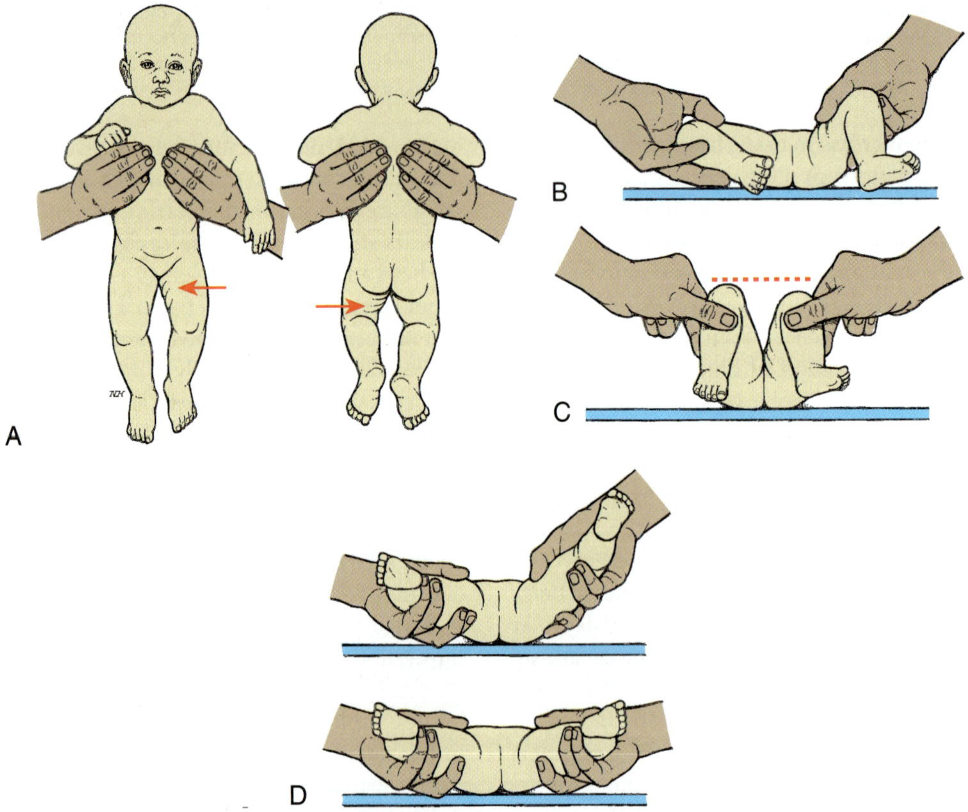

FIG. 23-11 Signs of developmental dysplasia of the hip. **A**, Asymmetry of gluteal and thigh folds with shortening of the thigh (Galeazzi sign). **B**, Limited hip abduction, as seen in flexion (Ortolani maneuver). **C**, Apparent shortening of the femur, as indicated by the level of the knees in flexion (Allis sign). **D**, Ortolani maneuver with femoral head moving in and out of acetabulum (in infants 1 to 2 months of age). (From Hockenberry, M., & Wilson, D. [2009]. *Wong's essentials of pediatric nursing* [8th ed.]. St. Louis: Mosby.)

is fixed in a plantar-flexion position, is a congenital condition that warrants attention. If the foot is turned inward in the plantar-flexion position but can be moved into the normal position, it is likely due to fetal positioning and should gradually resolve.

Neuromuscular System

The neuromuscular system is almost completely developed at birth. The term newborn is a responsive and reactive being with remarkable capacity for social interaction and self-organization.

Growth of the brain after birth follows a predictable pattern of rapid growth during infancy and early childhood, and growth becomes more gradual during the remainder of the first decade and minimal during adolescence. By the end of the first year the cerebellum ends its growth spurt, which began at approximately 30 gestational weeks.

The brain requires glucose as a source of energy and a relatively large supply of oxygen for adequate metabolism. Such requirements signal a need for careful assessment of the infant's respiratory status. The necessity for glucose requires attentiveness to those neonates who are at risk for hypoglycemia (e.g., infants of mothers who have diabetes, infants who are macrosomic or small for gestational age, and newborns experiencing prolonged birth, hypoxia, or preterm birth).

Spontaneous motor activity can be seen as transient tremors of the mouth and chin, especially during crying episodes, and of the extremities, notably the arms and hands. Transient tremors are normal and can be observed in nearly every newborn. These tremors should not be present when the infant is quiet and should not persist beyond 1 month of age. Persistent tremors or tremors involving the total body can indicate pathologic conditions. Normal tremors, tremors of hypoglycemia, and central nervous system (CNS) disorders must be differentiated so corrective care can be instituted as necessary.

The posture of the term newborn demonstrates flexion of the arms at the elbows and the legs at the knees. Hips are abducted and partially flexed. Intermittent fisting of the hands is common.

Muscle tone and strength are directly related. The infant with normal tone and strength exhibits some resistance to passive movement, such as when being pulled to sit, or when the arm or leg is extended by the examiner. The hypotonic neonate shows little resistance and can feel like a "rag doll." Hypertonia is evidenced by increased resistance to passive movement.

Neuromuscular control, although very limited, can be noted. If newborns are placed face down on a firm surface, they will turn their heads to the side. They attempt to hold their heads in line with their bodies if they are raised by their arms. Various reflexes serve to promote safety and adequate food intake.

Newborn Reflexes

The newborn has many primitive reflexes. The times at which these reflexes appear and disappear reflect the maturity and intactness of the developing nervous system. The most common reflexes found in the normal newborn are described in Table 23-4.

Signs of Risk for Neuromuscular Problems

Any absence of a newborn reflex can indicate major neurologic problems. Birth trauma can cause nerve damage that results in facial asymmetry and paralysis. CNS depression resulting from maternal medications received during labor and birth also will influence neuromuscular functioning.

The cry of the healthy term newborn is strong and "lusty." A weak cry is often associated with prematurity, neuromuscular disease, or sepsis. A high-pitched or shrill cry can suggest CNS abnormality. A low-pitched, husky cry can be related to hypothyroidism. Stridor with crying can indicate airway obstruction.

Observation of the neonate for any abnormalities must be documented. A thorough physical examination of the newborn assists in detecting any potential complications (see Table 24-2).

BEHAVIORAL CHARACTERISTICS

The healthy infant must accomplish behavioral and biologic tasks to develop normally. Behavioral characteristics form the basis of the social capabilities of the infant. Healthy newborns differ in their activity levels, feeding patterns, sleeping patterns, and responsiveness. Parents' reactions to their newborns are often determined by these differences. Showing parents the unique characteristics of their infant assists parents to develop a more positive perception of the infant with increased interaction between infant and parent.

Behavioral responses, as well as physical characteristics, change during the period of transition. The Brazelton Neonatal Behavioral Assessment Scale (BNBAS) can be used to assess the infant's behavior systematically (Brazelton, 1999; Brazelton & Nugent, 1996). The BNBAS is an interactive examination that assesses the infant's response to 28 areas organized according to the clusters in Box 23-2. It is generally used as a research or diagnostic tool and requires special training.

In addition to use as initial and ongoing tools to assess neurologic and behavioral responses, the scales can assess initial parent-infant relationships and help parents focus on their infant's individuality and develop a deeper attachment to their child. See Chapter 22 for further discussion of attachment.

BOX 23-2 CLUSTERS OF NEONATAL BEHAVIORS IN THE BRAZELTON NEONATAL BEHAVIORAL ASSESSMENT SCALE (BNBAS)

- *Habituation:* Ability to respond to and then inhibit responding to discrete stimuli (light, rattle, bell, pinprick) while asleep
- *Orientation:* Quality of alert states and ability to attend to visual and auditory stimuli while alert
- *Motor performance:* Quality of movement and tone
- *Range of state:* Measure of general arousal level or arousability of infant
- *Regulation of state:* How infant responds when aroused
- *Autonomic stability:* Signs of stress (tremors, startles, skin color) related to homeostatic (self-regulator) adjustment of the nervous system
- *Reflexes:* Assessment of several neonatal reflexes

From: Brazelton, T., & Nugent, K. (1996). *Neonatal behavioural assessment scale* (3rd ed.). London: MacKeith.

TABLE 23-4 ASSESSMENT OF NEWBORN'S REFLEXES*

REFLEX	ELICITING THE REFLEX	CHARACTERISTIC RESPONSE	COMMENTS
Sucking and rooting	Touch infant's lip, cheek, or corner of mouth with nipple	Infant turns head toward stimulus, opens mouth, takes hold, and sucks	Response is difficult if not impossible to elicit after infant has been fed; if response is weak or absent, consider prematurity or neurologic defect Parental guidance: Avoid trying to turn head toward breast or nipple, allow infant to root; response disappears after 3 to 4 months but may persist up to 1 year If response is weak or absent, may indicate prematurity or neurologic defect
Swallowing	Feed infant; swallowing usually follows sucking and obtaining fluids	Swallowing is usually coordinated with sucking and usually occurs without gagging, coughing, or vomiting	Sucking and swallowing are often uncoordinated in preterm infant
Grasp			
Palmar	Place finger in palm of hand	Infant's fingers curl around examiner's fingers	Palmar response lessens by 3 to 4 months; parents enjoy this contact with infant.
Plantar	Place finger at base of toes	Toes curl downward (see Fig. 16-12)	Plantar response lessens by 8 months
Extrusion	Touch or depress tip of tongue	Newborn forces tongue outward	Response disappears about fourth month of life
Glabellar (Myerson sign)	Tap over forehead, bridge of nose, or maxilla of newborn whose eyes are open	Newborn blinks for first four or five taps	Continued blinking with repeated taps is consistent with extrapyramidal disorder
Tonic neck or "fencing"	With infant falling asleep or sleeping, turn head quickly to one side	With infant facing left side, arm and leg on that side extend; opposite arm and leg flex (turn head to right, and extremities assume opposite postures)	Responses in leg are more consistent Complete response disappears by 3 to 4 months, incomplete response may be seen until third or fourth year After 6 weeks, persistent response is sign of possible cerebral palsy
Moro	Hold infant in semisitting position, allow head and trunk to fall backward to an angle of at least 30 degrees Place infant on flat surface, strike surface to startle infant Perform sharp hand clap	Symmetric abduction and extension of arms are seen; fingers fan out and form a C with thumb and forefinger; slight tremor may be noted; arms are adducted in embracing motion and return to relaxed flexion and movement Legs may follow similar pattern of response Preterm infant does not complete "embrace"; instead, arms fall backward because of weakness	Response is present at birth; complete response may be seen until 8 weeks; body jerk is seen only between 8 and 18 weeks; response is absent by 6 months if neurologic maturation is not delayed; response may be incomplete if infant is deeply asleep; give parental guidance about normal response Asymmetric response may connote injury to brachial plexus, clavicle, or humerus Persistent response after 6 months indicates possible brain damage

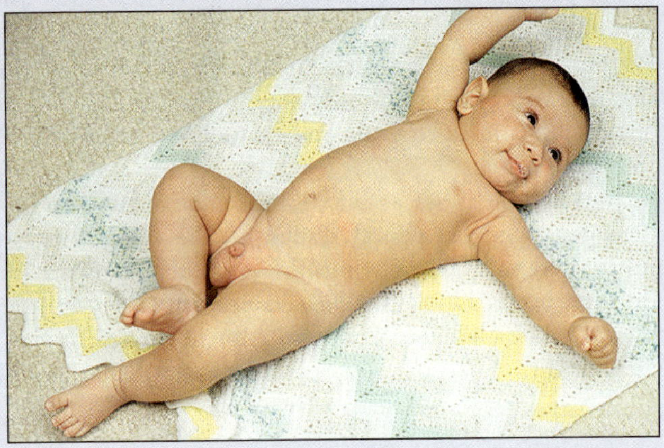

Classic pose in spontaneous tonic neck reflex. (Courtesy Marjorie Pyle, RNC, Lifecircle, Costa Mesa, CA.)

*All durations for persistence of reflexes are based on time elapsed after 40 weeks of gestation; that is, if this newborn was born at 36 weeks of gestation, add 1 month to all time limits given.

Video—Nursing Skills: Assessing a Newborn's Reflexes

TABLE 23-4 **ASSESSMENT OF NEWBORN'S REFLEXES—cont'd**

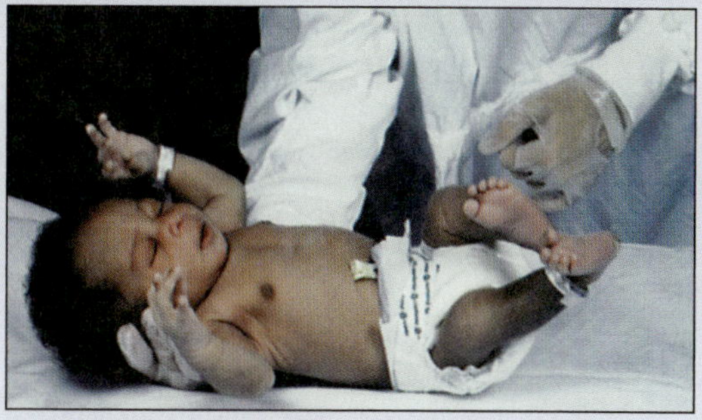

Moro reflex. (From Dickason, E., Silverman, B., & Kaplan, J. [1998]. *Maternal-infant nursing care* [3rd ed.]. St. Louis: Mosby.)

REFLEX	ELICITING THE REFLEX	CHARACTERISTIC RESPONSE	COMMENTS
Stepping or "walking"	Hold infant vertically, allowing one foot to touch table surface	Infant will simulate walking, alternating flexion and extension of feet; term infants walk on soles of their feet, and preterm infants walk on their toes	Response is normally present for 3 to 4 weeks

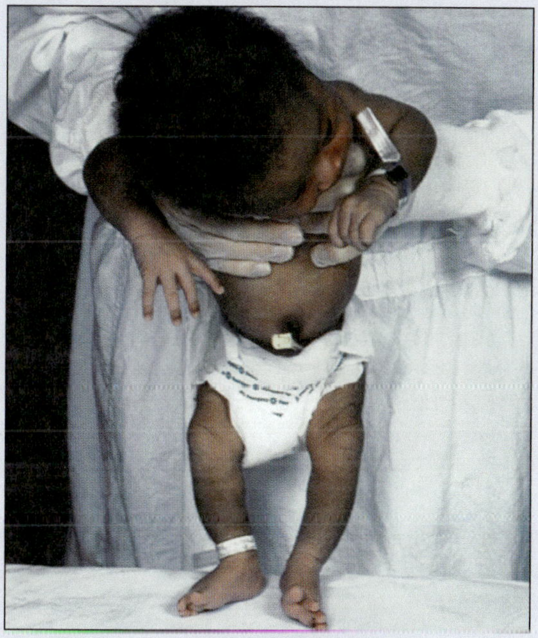

Stepping reflex. (From Dickason, E., Silverman, B., & Kaplan, J. [1998]. *Maternal-infant nursing care* [3rd ed.]. St. Louis: Mosby.)

REFLEX	ELICITING THE REFLEX	CHARACTERISTIC RESPONSE	COMMENTS
Crawling	Place newborn on abdomen	Newborn makes crawling movements with arms and legs	Response should disappear about 6 weeks of age
Deep tendon	Use finger instead of percussion hammer to elicit patellar, or knee jerk, reflex; newborn must be relaxed	Reflex jerk is present; even with newborn relaxed, nonselective overall reaction may occur	
Crossed extension	Infant should be supine; extend one leg, press knee downward, stimulate bottom of foot; observe opposite leg	Opposite leg flexes, adducts, and then extends	This reflex should be present during newborn period

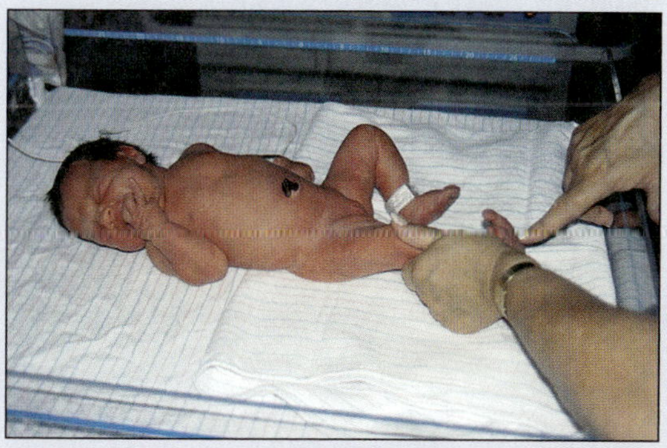

Crossed extension reflex. (Courtesy Marjorie Pyle, RNC, Lifecircle, Costa Mesa, CA.)

Continued

Video—Newborn Assessment

TABLE 23-4 **ASSESSMENT OF NEWBORN'S REFLEXES*—cont'd**

REFLEX	ELICITING THE REFLEX	CHARACTERISTIC RESPONSE	COMMENTS
Babinski sign (plantar)	On sole of foot, beginning at heel, stroke upward along lateral aspect of sole, then move finger across ball of foot	All toes hyperextend, with dorsiflexion of big toe; recorded as a positive sign	Absence requires neurologic evaluation, should disappear after 1 year of age

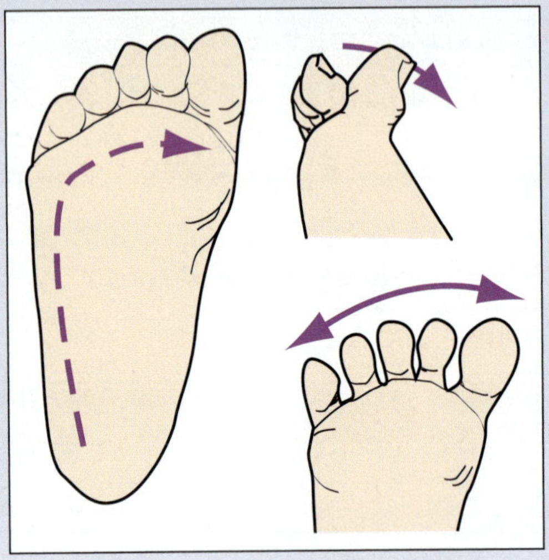

Babinski reflex. (From Hockenberry, M. & Wilson, D. [2011]. *Wong's nursing care of infants and children* [9th ed.]. St. Louis: Mosby.)

REFLEX	ELICITING THE REFLEX	CHARACTERISTIC RESPONSE	COMMENTS
Pull-to-sit (traction)	Pull infant up by wrists from supine position with head in midline	Head will lag until infant is in upright position, then head will be held in same plane with chest and shoulder momentarily before falling forward; infant will attempt to right head	Response depends on general muscle tone and maturity and condition of infant
Trunk incurvation (Galant)	Place infant prone on flat surface, run finger down back about 4 to 5 cm lateral to spine, first on one side and then down other	Trunk is flexed, and pelvis is swung toward stimulated side	Response disappears by fourth week Response may vary but should be obtainable in all infants, including preterm ones. Absence suggests general depression of nervous system With transverse lesions of cord, no response below the level of the lesion is present.

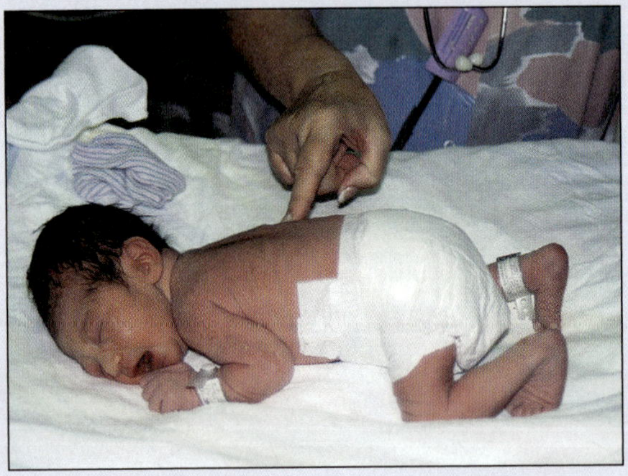

Trunk incurvation reflex. (Courtesy Marjorie Pyle, RNC, Lifecircle, Costa Mesa, CA.)

TABLE 23-4 ASSESSMENT OF NEWBORN'S REFLEXES—cont'd

REFLEX	ELICITING THE REFLEX	CHARACTERISTIC RESPONSE	COMMENTS
Magnet	Place infant in supine position, partially flex both lower extremities, and apply pressure to soles of feet *(A)*	Both lower limbs should extend against examiner's pressure *(B)*	Absence suggests damage to spinal cord or malformation Reflex may be weak or exaggerated after breech birth
Additional newborn responses: yawn, stretch, burp, hiccup, sneeze	These responses are spontaneous behaviors	May be slightly depressed temporarily because of maternal analgesia or anesthesia, fetal hypoxia, or infection	Parental guidance: most of these behaviors are pleasurable to parents Parents need to be assured that behaviors are normal Sneeze is usually response to lint, etc., in nose and not an indicator of a cold No treatment is needed for hiccups; sucking may help

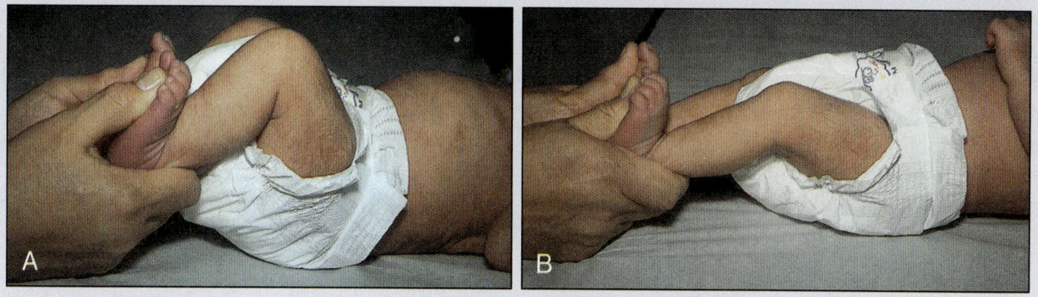

Magnet reflex. (Courtesy Michael S. Clement, MD, Mesa, AZ.)

Sleep-Wake States

Variations in the state of consciousness of infants are called **sleep-wake states.** The six states form a continuum from deep sleep to extreme irritability (Fig. 23-12): two sleep states (deep sleep and light sleep) and four wake states (drowsy, quiet alert, active alert, and crying) (Blackburn, 2007). Each state has specific characteristics and state-related behaviors. The optimal state of arousal is the quiet alert state. During this state infants smile, vocalize, move in synchrony with speech, watch their parents' faces, and respond to people talking to them. Infants respond to internal and external environmental factors by controlling sensory input and regulating the sleep-wake states; the ability to make smooth transitions between states is called *state modulation.* The ability to regulate sleep-wake states is essential in the infant's neurobehavioral development. As infants approach term gestation, they are better able to cope with external or internal factors that affect the sleep-wake patterns.

Infants use purposeful behavior to maintain the optimal arousal state as follows: (1) actively withdrawing by increasing physical distance, (2) rejecting by pushing away with hands and feet, (3) decreasing sensitivity by falling asleep or breaking eye contact by turning the head, or (4) using signaling behaviors, such as fussing and crying. These behaviors permit infants to quiet themselves and reinstate readiness to interact.

The first 6 weeks of life involve a steady decrease in the proportion of active REM sleep to total sleep. A steady increase in the proportion of quiet sleep to total sleep also occurs. Periods of wakefulness increase. For the first few weeks the wakeful periods seem dictated by hunger but soon a need for socializing appears as well. The newborn sleeps on average approximately 17 hours a day, with periods of wakefulness gradually increasing. By the fourth week of life, some infants stay awake from one feeding to the next.

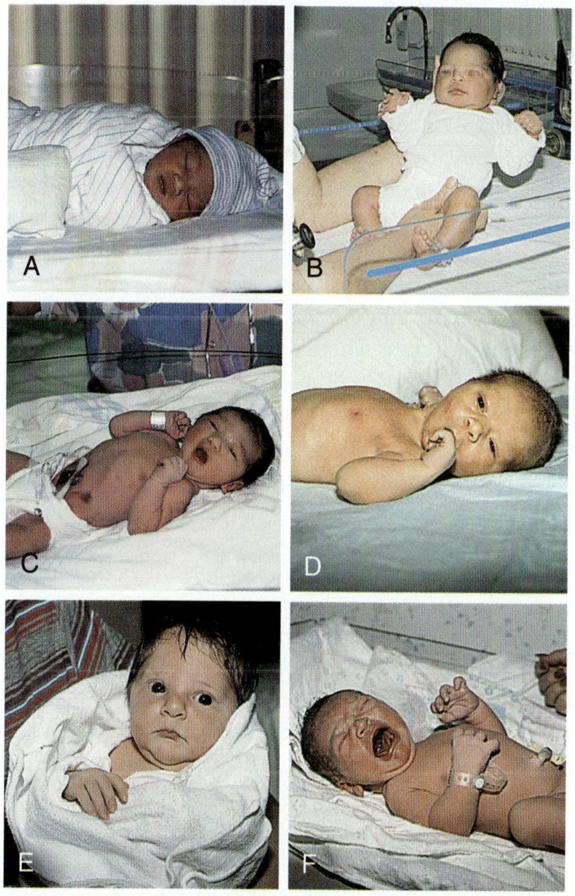

FIG. 23-12 Summary of newborn sleep-wake states. States of consciousness: **A**, Deep sleep. **B**, Light sleep. **C**, Drowsy. **D**, Quiet alert. **E**, Active alert. **F**, Crying. (Courtesy Marjorie Pyle, RNC, Lifecircle, Costa Mesa, CA.)

Other Factors Influencing Newborn Behavior

Gestational Age

The gestational age of the infant and level of CNS maturity affect the observed behavior. In an infant with an immature CNS (preterm) the entire body responds to a pinprick of the foot although the response may not be observed by an untrained observer. The more mature infant withdraws only the foot. CNS immaturity is reflected in reflex development, sleep-wake states, and ability (or lack thereof) to regulate or modulate a smooth transition between different states. Preterm infants have brief periods of alertness but have difficulty maintaining alertness without becoming overstimulated, which leads to autonomic instability unless intervention is implemented. Premature or sick infants show signs of fatigue or physiologic stress sooner than full-term healthy infants.

Time

The time elapsed since birth affects the behavior of infants as they attempt to become organized initially. Time elapsed since the previous feeding and time of day also can influence infants' responses.

Stimuli

Environmental events and stimuli affect the behavioral responses of infants. The newborn responds to animate and inanimate stimuli. Nurses in intensive care nurseries observe that infants respond to loud noises, bright lights, monitor alarms, and tension in the unit. If a mother is tense, nervous, or uncomfortable while feeding her infant, the infant may sense her tension and demonstrate difficulty feeding.

Medication

There is no conclusive evidence regarding the effects of maternal analgesia or anesthesia during labor on neonatal behavior. Some researchers note that infants of mothers given certain analgesic medications can have disturbances in newborn behavior such as more crying, an increase in temperature, and some difficulty in breastfeeding (Ransjö-Arvidson, Matthiesen, Lilja, Nissen, Widström, & Uvnäs-Moberg, 2001). Other researchers maintain that the effect on infant behavior is negligible. Researchers who have studied the effects of epidural medications on breastfeeding behaviors have been unable to show a cause-and-effect relationship (Chang & Heaman, 2006; Devroe, De Coster, & Van de Velde, 2009; Torvaldsen, Roberts, Simpson, Thompson, & Ellwood, 2006).

Sensory Behaviors

From birth, infants possess sensory capabilities that indicate a state of readiness for social interaction. Infants effectively use behavioral responses in establishing their first dialogues. These responses, coupled with the newborns' "baby appearance" (e.g., facial proportions of forehead, eyes larger than the lower portion of the face) and their small size and helplessness, rouse feelings of wanting to hold, protect, and interact with them.

Vision

At birth the eye is structurally incomplete and the muscles are immature. The process of accommodation is not present but improves over the first 3 months of life. The pupils react to light, the blink reflex is easily stimulated, and the corneal reflex is activated by light touch. Term newborns can see objects as far away as 50 cm (2.5 feet). The clearest visual distance is 17 to 20 cm (8 to 12 inches), which is approximately the distance between the mother's face and the infant's face during breastfeeding or cuddling. Infants are sensitive to light; they will frown if a bright light is flashed in their eyes, and will turn toward a soft, red light. If the room is darkened, they will open their eyes wide and look about. By 2 months of age they can detect color; but at 5 days of age and younger, they seem more attracted by black-and-white patterns.

Response to movement is noticeable. If a bright light is shown to newborns (even at 15 minutes of age), they will follow it visually; some will even turn their heads to do so. Because human eyes are bright shiny objects, newborns will track their parents' eyes. Parents often comment on their excitement in observing this behavior. The development of eye-to-eye contact is very important for parent-infant attachment. Children of blind parents, and parents who have blind children, must circumvent this obstacle for the formation of a relationship.

Visual acuity is surprising. Even at 2 weeks of age infants can distinguish patterns with stripes 3 mm apart. By 6 months their vision is as acute as that of an adult. They prefer to look at patterns rather than plain surfaces, even if the latter are brightly colored. Infants prefer more complex patterns to simple ones. They prefer novelty (changes in pattern) by 2 months of age. The infant of a few weeks of age is therefore capable of responding actively to an enriched environment.

Hearing

As soon as the amniotic fluid drains from the ears the infant's hearing is similar to that of an adult. Loud sounds of approximately 90 decibels cause the infant to respond with a Mono reflex. The newborn responds to low-frequency sounds such as a heartbeat or lullaby by decreasing motor activity or stopping crying. High-frequency sound elicits an alerting reaction.

The infant responds readily to the mother's voice. Studies indicate a selective listening to maternal voice sounds and rhythms during intrauterine life that prepares newborns for recognition and interaction with their primary caregivers—their mothers. Newborns are accustomed in the uterus to hearing the regular rhythm of the mother's heartbeat. As a result, they respond by relaxing and ceasing to fuss and cry if a regular heartbeat simulator is placed in their cribs.

The internal and middle portions of the ear are larger at birth, but the external canal is small. The mastoid process and bony parts of the external canal have not developed; therefore, the tympanic membrane and facial nerve are very close to the surface and can be easily damaged. Hearing loss is common at birth; 1 in 1000 newborn infants is afflicted with a sensorineural hearing loss significant enough to affect speech and language development. Approximately half of those are due to hereditary loss and the other half are due to an acquired loss. The most common cause of acquired hearing loss is infection that is transmitted from the mother to the fetus transplacentally (Arnold & Sprecher, 2006). To identify affected infants the hearing of all infants is screened before discharge from the birth institution (Fig. 24-9).

Smell

Newborns have a highly developed sense of smell and can detect and discriminate distinct odors. It has been shown that preterm infants as early as 28 weeks are capable of reacting to odors.

Newborns react to strong odors such as alcohol or vinegar by turning their heads away, but are attracted to sweet smells. By the fifth day of life, newborn infants can recognize their mother's smell (Brazelton, 1999). Breastfed infants are able to smell breast milk and can differentiate their mothers from other lactating women (Lawrence & Lawrence, 2005).

Taste

The newborn can distinguish among tastes, and various types of solutions elicit differing facial expressions. A tasteless solution produces no response; a sweet solution elicits eager sucking. A sour solution causes a puckering of the lips, and a bitter liquid produces a grimace.

Young infants are particularly oriented toward the use of their mouths, both for meeting their nutritional needs for rapid growth and for releasing tension through sucking. The early development of circumoral sensation, muscle activity, and taste would seem to be preparation for survival in the extrauterine environment.

Touch

The infant is responsive to touch on all parts of the body. The face (especially the mouth), the hands, and the soles of the feet seem to be the most sensitive. Reflexes can be elicited by stroking the infant. The newborn's responses to touch suggest that this sensory system is well prepared to receive and process tactile messages. Touch and motion are essential to normal growth and development. However, each infant is unique, and variations can be seen in newborns' responses to touch. Birth trauma or stress and depressant drugs taken by the mother decrease the infant's sensitivity to touch or painful stimuli.

Response to Environmental Stimuli

Temperament

Classic studies (Thomas, Birch, Chess, & Robbins, 1961; Thomas, Chess, & Birch, 1970) identified individual variations in the primary reaction pattern of newborns and described them as temperament. Their style of behavioral response to stimuli is guided by the temperament affecting the newborn's sensory threshold, ability to habituate, and response to maternal behaviors. The newborn possesses individual characteristics that affect selective responses to various stimuli present in the internal and external environment.

Habituation

Habituation is a protective mechanism that allows the infant to become accustomed to environmental stimuli. Habituation is a psychologic and physiologic phenomenon in which the response to a constant or repetitive stimulus is decreased. In the term newborn, habituation can be demonstrated in several ways. Shining a bright light into a newborn's eyes will cause a startle or squinting the first two or three times. The third or fourth flash will elicit a diminished response, and by the fifth or sixth flash the infant ceases to respond (Brazelton, 1999; Brazelton & Nugent, 1996). The same response pattern holds true for the sounds of a rattle or a pinprick to the heel.

The ability to habituate also allows the newborn to select stimuli that promote continued learning about the social world, thus preventing overload. The intrauterine experience seems to have programmed the newborn to be especially responsive to human voices, soft lights, soft sounds, and sweet tastes.

The newborn quickly learns the sounds in the home environment and is able to sleep in their midst. The selective responses of the newborn indicate cerebral organization capable of memory and making choices. The ability to habituate depends on state of consciousness, hunger, fatigue, and temperament. These factors also affect consolability, cuddliness, irritability, and crying.

Consolability

Newborns vary in their ability to console themselves or to be consoled. In the crying state, most newborns initiate one of several methods for reducing their distress. Hand-to-mouth movements are common, with or without sucking, as well as alerting to voices, noises, or visual stimuli.

Cuddliness

Cuddliness is especially important to parents because they often gauge their ability to care for the child by the child's responses to their actions. Variability is noted in the degree to which newborns will mold into the contours of the persons holding them. Babies are soothed and become alert with the vestibular stimulation of being picked up and moved.

Irritability

Some newborns cry longer and harder than others. For some infants the sensory threshold seems low. They are readily upset by unusual noises, hunger, wetness, or new experiences and respond intensely to these stimuli. Others with a high sensory threshold require a great deal more stimulation and variation to reach the active, alert state.

Crying

Crying in an infant may signal hunger, pain, desire for attention, or fussiness. Most mothers learn to distinguish among the cries. The duration of crying is highly variable in each infant; newborns may cry for as little as 5 minutes or as much as 2 hours or more per day. The amount of crying peaks in the second month and then decreases. A diurnal rhythm of crying can be noted, with more crying in the evening hours. Crying does not seem to differ with different caregivers.

KEY POINTS

- By full term the infant's various anatomic and physiologic systems have reached a level of development and functioning that permits a physical existence apart from the mother.
- The healthy term infant has sensory capabilities that indicate a state of readiness for social interaction.
- Several significant differences exist among the respiratory, renal, and thermogenic systems of the newborn and those of an adult.
- Physiologic jaundice occurs in approximately 60% of term newborns and 80% of preterm newborns.

- Jaundice is considered pathologic or nonphysiologic if it appears within the first 24 hours of life, if serum bilirubin levels increase by more than 5 mg/dl in 24 hours, or if the serum bilirubin level exceeds 15 mg/dl at any time.
- Heat loss in the healthy term newborn can exceed the capacity to produce heat, causing cold stress which can lead to metabolic and respiratory complications that threaten the newborn's well-being.
- Some reflex behaviors are important for the newborn's survival.
- Individual personalities and behavioral characteristics of infants play major roles in their ultimate relationships with their parents.
- Sleep-wake states and other factors influence the newborn's behavior.
- Each full-term newborn has a predisposed capacity to handle the multitude of stimuli in the external world.

Audio Chapter Summaries Access an audio summary of these Key Points on evolve

REFERENCES

American Academy of Pediatrics (AAP) Subcommittee on Hyperbilirubinemia. (2004). Clinical practice guideline: Management of hyperbilirubinemia in the newborn infant 35 or more weeks of gestation. *Pediatrics, 114*(1), 297–316.

Arca, G., Botet, F., Palacio, M., & Carbonell-Estrany, X. (2010). Timing of umbilical cord clamping: New thoughts on an old discussion. *The Journal of Maternal-Fetal and Neonatal Medicine.* Available at http://informahealthcare.com/doi/abs/10.3109/14767050903551475. Accessed July 8, 2010.

Arnold, J., & Sprecher, R. (2006). Hearing loss in the newborn infant. In R. Martin, A. Fanaroff, & M. Walsh (Eds.), *Fanaroff and Martin's neonatal-perinatal medicine: Diseases of the fetus and infant* (8th ed.). Philadelphia: Mosby.

Askin, D. (2009). Fetal-to-neonatal transition—What is normal and what is not? Part II: Red flags. *Neonatal Network, 28*(3), e37–e40. Available at www.metapress.com/content/V471277271677852. Accessed July 8, 2010.

Bagwell, G. (2007). Hematologic system. In C. Kenner & J. Lott (Eds.), *Comprehensive neonatal care: An interdisciplinary approach* (4th ed.). St. Louis: Saunders.

Blackburn, S. (2007). *Maternal, fetal, & neonatal physiology: A clinical perspective* (3rd ed.). St. Louis: Saunders.

Bradshaw, W. (2010). Gastrointestinal disorders. In M. Verklan & M. Walden (Eds.), *Core curriculum for neonatal intensive care nursing* (4th ed.). St. Louis: Saunders.

Brazelton, T. (1999). Behavioral competence. In G. Avery, M. Fletcher, & M. MacDonald (Eds.), *Neonatology: Pathophysiology and management of the newborn* (5th ed.). Philadelphia: Lippincott Williams & Wilkins.

Brazelton, T., & Nugent, K. (1996). *Neonatal behavioural assessment scale* (3rd ed.). London: MacKeith.

Chang, Z., & Heaman, M. (2006). Epidural analgesia during labor and delivery: Effects on the initiation and continuation of effective breastfeeding. *Journal of Human Lactation, 21*(3), 305–314.

Dell, K., & Davis, I. (2006). Fluid, electrolyte, and acid-base homeostasis. In R. Martin, A. Fanaroff, & M. Walsh (Eds.), *Fanaroff and Martin's neonatal-perinatal medicine: Diseases of the fetus and infant* (8th ed.). Philadelphia: Mosby.

Desmond, M., Rudolph, A., & Phitaksphraiwan, P. (1966). The transitional care nursery: A mechanism for preventive medicine in the newborn. *Pediatric Clinics of North America, 13*(3), 651–668.

Devroe, S., De Coster, J., & Van de Velde, M. (2009). Breastfeeding and epidural analgesia during labour. *Current Opinion in Anaesthesiology, 22*(3), 327–329.

Hutton, E., & Hassan, E. (2007). Late vs early clamping of the umbilical cord in full-term neonates: Systematic review and meta-analysis of controlled trials. *Journal of the American Medical Association, 297*(11), 1241–1252.

Jain, L., & Eaton, D. (2006). Physiology of fetal lung fluid clearance and the effect of labor. *Seminars in Perinatology, 30*(1), 34–43.

Kapur, R., Yoder, M., & Polin, R. (2006). Developmental immunology. In R. Martin, A. Fanaroff, & M. Walsh (Eds.), *Fanaroff and Martin's neonatal-perinatal medicine: Diseases of the fetus and infant* (8th ed.). Philadelphia: Mosby.

Lawrence, R., & Lawrence, R. (2005). *Breastfeeding: A guide for the medical profession* (6th ed.). Philadelphia: Mosby.

Lissauer, T. (2006). Physical examination of the newborn. In R. Martin, A. Fanaroff, & M. Walsh (Eds.), *Fanaroff and Martin's neonatal-perinatal medicine: Diseases of the fetus and infant* (8th ed.). Philadelphia: Mosby.

Lott, J. (2010). Immunology and infectious disease. In M. Verklan & M. Walden (Eds.), *Core curriculum for neonatal intensive care nursing* (4th ed.). St. Louis: Saunders.

Luchtman-Jones, L., Schwartz, A., & Wilson, D. (2006). Hematologic problems in the fetus and neonate. In R. Martin, A. Fanaroff, & M. Walsh (Eds.), *Fanaroff and Martin's neonatal-perinatal medicine: Diseases of the fetus and infant* (8th ed.). Philadelphia: Mosby.

McDonald, S., & Middleton, P. (2008). Effect of timing of umbilical cord clamping of term infants on maternal and neonatal outcomes. *The Cochrane Database of Systematic Reviews, 2008*, 2, CD004074.

Pagana, K., & Pagana, T. (2009). *Mosby's diagnostic and laboratory test reference* (9th ed.). St. Louis: Mosby.

Page-Goertz, S. (2008). Hyperbilirubinemia and hypoglycemia. In R. Mannel, P. Martens, & M. Walker (Eds.), *Core curriculum for lactation consultant practice* (2nd ed.). Sudbury, MA: Jones and Bartlett.

Ransjö-Arvidson, A., Matthiesen, A., Lilja, G., Nissen, E., Widström, A., & Uvnäs-Moberg, K. (2001). Maternal analgesia during labor disturbs newborn behavior: Effects on breastfeeding temperature, and crying. *Birth, 28*(1), 5–12.

Razmus, I., & Lewis, L. (2006). Using four limb blood pressures as a screening tool in normal newborns. *Society of Pediatric Nursing News, 15*(6), 5–7.

Sedin, G. (2006). Physical environment: Part 1: The thermal environment of the newborn infant. In R. Martin, A. Fanaroff, & M. Walsh (Eds.), *Fanaroff and Martin's neonatal-perinatal medicine: Diseases of the fetus and infant* (8th ed.). Philadelphia: Mosby.

Spangler, A., Randenberg, A., Brenner, M., & Howett, M. (2008). Belly models as teaching tools: What is their utility? *Journal of Human Lactation, 24*(2), 199–205.

Thomas, A., Birch, H., Chess, S., & Robbins, L. (1961). Individuality in responses of children to similar environmental situations. *American Journal of Psychiatry, 117*(9), 798–803.

Thomas, A., Chess, S., & Birch, H. (1970). The origin of personality. *Scientific American, 223*(2), 102–109.

Torvaldsen, S., Roberts, C., Simpson, J., Thompson, J., & Ellwood, D. (2006). Intrapartum epidural analgesia and breastfeeding: A prospective cohort study. *International Breastfeeding Journal, 1*(24), 1–7. Available at www.internationalbreastfeedingjournal.com/content/1/1/24. Accessed July 8, 2010.

Vogt, B., Dell, K., & Davis, I. (2006). The kidney and urinary tract. In R. Martin, A. Fanaroff, & M. Walsh (Eds.), *Fanaroff and Martin's neonatal-perinatal medicine: Diseases of the fetus and infant* (8th ed.). Philadelphia: Mosby.

Wong, R., DeSandre, G., Sibley, E., & Stevenson, D. (2006). Neonatal jaundice and liver disease. In R. Martin, A. Fanaroff & M. Walsh (Eds.), *Fanaroff and Martin's neonatal-perinatal medicine: Diseases of the fetus and infant* (8th ed.). Philadelphia: Mosby.

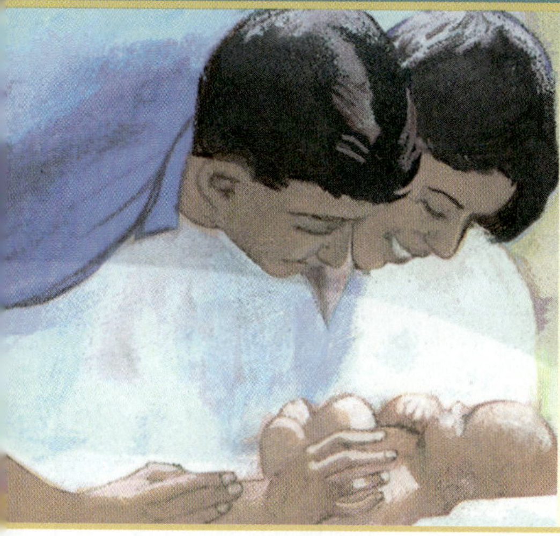

CHAPTER

24

Nursing Care of the Newborn and Family

Kathryn Rhodes Alden

evolve WEBSITE

http://evolve.elsevier.com/Lowdermilk/MWHC/

- Audio Glossary
- Audio Key Points
- Case Study
    - The Normal Newborn
- Critical Thinking Exercises
    - Circumcision
    - Jaundice
- NCLEX Review Questions
- Nursing Care Plans
    - Immediate Care of the Newborn
    - The Normal Newborn and Family
- Nursing Skills
    - Changing a Diaper
    - Infant Bathing
    - Pain Assessment
    - Swaddling
- Spanish Guidelines
    - Daily Care
    - General Advice
    - Infant Quieting Techniques
- Video—Assessment
    - Circumcision
    - Crying Female Neonate
- Video—Nursing Skills
    - Administering Intramuscular Injections to a Newborn
    - Assisting with a Circumcision
    - Obtaining an Apgar Score
    - Performing Newborn Cord Care
    - Suctioning with a Bulb Syringe or Mechanical Apparatus
    - Weighing and Measuring a Newborn

LEARNING OBJECTIVES

- Explain the purpose and components of the Apgar score.
- Describe how to perform a physical assessment of a newborn.
- Describe how to perform a gestational age assessment of a newborn.
- Compare the characteristics of the preterm, late preterm, term, and postterm neonate.
- Explain the elements of a safe environment.
- Discuss phototherapy and the guidelines for teaching parents about this treatment.
- Explain the purposes and methods for circumcision, the postoperative care of the circumcised infant, and parent teaching regarding circumcision.
- Review the procedures for performing a heelstick, collecting urine specimens, and assisting with venipuncture.
- Evaluate pain in the newborn based on physiologic changes and behavioral observations.
- Review anticipatory guidance nurses provide to parents before discharge.

Although most infants make the necessary biopsychosocial adjustments to extrauterine existence without undue difficulty, their well-being depends on the care they receive from others. This chapter describes the assessment and care of the infant immediately after birth until discharge, as well as important anticipatory guidance related to ongoing infant care. A discussion of pain in the neonate and its management is included.

CARE MANAGEMENT: BIRTH THROUGH THE FIRST 2 HOURS

Care begins immediately after birth and focuses on assessing and stabilizing the newborn's condition. The nurse has the primary responsibility for the infant during this period because the physician or midwife is involved with care of the mother. The nurse must be alert for any signs of distress and initiate appropriate interventions.

With the possibility of transmission of viruses such as hepatitis B virus (HBV) and human immunodeficiency virus (HIV) through maternal blood and blood-stained amniotic fluid, the newborn must be considered a potential contamination source until proved otherwise. As part of Standard Precautions, nurses wear gloves when handling the newborn until blood and amniotic fluid are removed by bathing.

The foundation for providing comprehensive, family-centered newborn care is awareness of the mother's preconception and prenatal history as well as intrapartal events. Recognition of risk factors (Box 24-1) enables the nurse to be more astute in observations and assessments and more likely to identify early signs of complications. This allows for earlier intervention and promotes positive outcomes.

It is important for the nurse to have as much information as possible related to the prenatal and intrapartum history before starting to assess and provide nursing care for the newborn. Essential information is most often communicated from nurse to nurse through oral reports (see Table 21-1). The newborn's medical record is a primary source of information. Data from the mother's medical record provide insights into potential risk factors that can affect the newborn's health. Through interaction with the mother and family, the nurse gains a greater understanding of neonatal and family needs. Assessment is ongoing throughout the hospital stay and extends into follow-up care.

ASSESSMENT

Initial Assessment and Apgar Scoring

The initial assessment of the neonate is performed immediately after birth using the Apgar score (Table 24-1) and a brief physical examination (Box 24-2). A gestational age assessment is completed within the first hours of birth in a stable newborn (Fig. 24-1). A more comprehensive physical assessment is completed within 24 hours of birth (see Table 24-2).

BOX 24-1 ASSESSMENT OF PRECONCEPTION, PRENATAL, AND INTRAPARTUM RISK FACTORS

PRECONCEPTION
- Age
- Preexisting medical conditions: Diabetes, hypertension, cardiac disease, anemia, thyroid disorder, renal disease, obesity
- Genetic factors: Family history
- Obstetric history: Gravidity, parity, number of living children and their ages, history of stillbirth, previous infant with congenital anomalies, habitual abortion, use of assisted-reproductive technology, interpregnancy spacing
- Blood type and Rh status

PRENATAL
- Prenatal care: When started
- Nutrition: Weight gain, diet, obesity, eating disorders
- Health-compromising behaviors: Smoking, alcohol use, substance abuse
- Blood group or Rh sensitization
- Medications: Prescription, over-the-counter, and complementary/alternative medications
- History of infection: Sexually-transmitted infections, TORCH, group B streptococci status

INTRAPARTUM
- Length of gestation: Preterm, late preterm, term, or postterm
- First stage of labor: length, electronic fetal monitoring—internal or external, rupture of membranes (time, presence of meconium), abnormal (nonreassuring) fetal signs (decelerations)
- Group B streptococci status: Treatment during labor
- Second stage of labor: Length, vaginal or cesarean, instrument assisted—forceps or vacuum extractor, complications (shoulder dystocia, bleeding [abruptio placentae or placenta previa), cord prolapse, maternal analgesia and/or anesthesia

Adapted from Broussard, A., & Hurst, H. (2010). Antepartum-intrapartum complications. In T. Verklan & M. Walden (Eds.), *AWHONN core curriculum for neonatal intensive care nursing* (4th ed.). St Louis: Saunders.

Video—Nursing Skills: Obtaining an Apgar Score

Apgar Score

The Apgar score permits a rapid assessment of the newborn's transition to extrauterine existence based on five signs that indicate the physiologic state of the neonate: (1) heart rate, based on auscultation with a stethoscope or palpation of the umbilical cord; (2) respiratory effort, based on observed movement of the chest wall; (3) muscle tone, based on degree of flexion and movement of the extremities; (4) reflex irritability, based on response to suctioning of the nares or nasopharynx; and (5) generalized skin color, described as pallid, cyanotic, or pink (see Table 24-1). Evaluations are made at

TABLE 24-1 APGAR SCORE

SIGN	SCORE 0	1	2
Heart rate	Absent	Slow (<100)	>100
Respiratory effort	Absent	Slow, weak cry	Good cry
Muscle tone	Flaccid	Some flexion of extremities	Well flexed
Reflex irritability	No response	Grimace	Cry
Color	Blue, pale	Body pink, extremities blue	Completely pink

BOX 24-2 INITIAL PHYSICAL ASSESSMENT OF THE NEWBORN

General appearance
[ ] Color pink
[ ] Acrocyanosis present
[ ] Flexed posture
[ ] Alert
[ ] Active

Respiratory system
[ ] Airway patent
[ ] No upper airway congestion
[ ] No retractions or nasal flaring
[ ] Respiratory rate, 30-60 breaths/min
[ ] Lungs clear to auscultation bilaterally
[ ] Chest expansion symmetric

Cardiovascular system
[ ] Heart rate strong and regular
[ ] No murmurs heard
[ ] Pulses strong and equal bilaterally

Neurologic system
[ ] Moves extremities
[ ] Normotonic
[ ] Symmetric features, movement
[ ] Reflexes present:
  [ ] Sucking
  [ ] Rooting
  [ ] Moro
  [ ] grasp
[ ] Anterior fontanel soft and flat

Gastrointestinal system
[ ] Abdomen soft, no distention
[ ] Cord attached and clamped
[ ] Anus appears patent

Eyes, nose, mouth
[ ] Eyes clear
[ ] Palates intact
[ ] Nares patent

Skin
[ ] No signs of birth trauma
[ ] No lesions or abrasions

Genitourinary system
[ ] Normal genitalia

Other
[ ] No obvious anomalies

Comments:
___
___
___

1 and 5 minutes after birth and can be completed by the nurse or birth attendant. Scores of 0 to 3 indicate severe distress, scores of 4 to 6 indicate moderate difficulty, and scores of 7 to 10 indicate that the infant is having minimal or no difficulty adjusting to extrauterine life. Apgar scores do not predict future neurologic outcome but are useful for describing the newborn's transition to the extrauterine environment (Box 24-3). If resuscitation is required it should be initiated before the 1-minute Apgar score (American Academy of Pediatrics [AAP] and American College of Obstetricians and Gynecologists [ACOG], 2007).

Initial Physical Assessment

The initial examination of the newborn (see Box 24-2) can occur while the nurse is drying and wrapping the infant, or observations can be made while the infant is lying on the mother's abdomen or in her arms immediately after birth. Efforts should be directed toward minimizing interference in the initial parent-infant acquaintance process. If the infant is breathing effectively, is pink, and has no apparent life-threatening anomalies or risk factors requiring immediate attention (e.g., infant of a mother with diabetes), further examination can be delayed until after the parents have had an opportunity to interact with the infant. Routine procedures and the admission process can be carried out in the mother's room or in a separate nursery.

Physical Assessment

Although the initial assessment following birth can reveal significant anomalies, birth injuries, and cardiopulmonary problems that have immediate implications, a more detailed, thorough physical examination should follow within 12 to 18 hours after birth (Box 24-4; see Table 24-2). The parents' presence during this and other examinations encourages discussion of their concerns and actively involves them in the health care of their infant from birth. It also affords the nurse an opportunity to observe parental interactions with the infant. The findings provide a database for implementing the nursing process with newborns and providing anticipatory guidance for the parents. Ongoing assessments are made throughout the hospital stay; another detailed physical examination is performed before discharge.

General Appearance

The neonate's maturity level can be gauged by assessment of general appearance. Features to assess in the general survey include posture, activity, any overt signs of anomalies that can cause initial distress, presence of bruising or other consequences of birth, and state of alertness. The normal resting position of the neonate is one of general flexion.

Vital Signs

The temperature, heart rate, and respiratory rate are always obtained. BP is not assessed unless cardiac problems are suspected. An irregular, very slow, or very fast heart rate can indicate a need for further evaluation of circulatory status including BP measurement.

The axillary temperature is a safe, accurate measurement of temperature. Electronic thermometers have expedited this task and provide a reading within 1 minute. Temporal artery, tympanic, and oral routes for measuring temperature in the newborn are not considered accurate (Asher & Northington, 2008). Taking an infant's temperature can cause the infant to cry and struggle against the placement of the thermometer in the axilla. Before taking the temperature the examiner can determine the apical heart rate and respiratory rate while the infant is quiet and at rest. The normal axillary temperature averages 37° C with a range from 36.5° to 37.2° C.

Text continued on p. 565.

BOX 24-3 SIGNIFICANCE OF THE APGAR SCORE

The Apgar score was developed to provide a systematic method of assessing an infant's condition at birth. Researchers have tried to correlate Apgar scores with various outcomes such as intelligence and neurologic development. In some instances researchers have attempted to attribute causality to the Apgar score, that is, to suggest that the low Apgar score caused or predicted later problems. This use of the Apgar score is inappropriate. Instead the score should be used to ensure that infants are systematically observed at birth to ascertain the need for immediate care. Either a physician or a nurse may assign the score; however, to avoid the real or perceived appearance of bias, the person assisting with the birth should not assign the score. Lack of consistency in the assigned scores limits studies of the Apgar's long-term predictive value. Prospective parents and the public need education on the significance of the Apgar score, as well as its limits. Because infants often do not receive the maximal score of 10, parents need to know that scores of 7 to 10 are within normal limits. Attorneys involved in litigation related to injury of an infant at birth or negative outcomes, either short term or long term, also need education about the Apgar score, its significance, and its limits. This useful tool needs to be used appropriately; health care providers, parents, and the public may need education to ensure appropriate use of the score.

Source: Montgomery, K. (2000). Apgar scores: Examining the long-term significance. *Journal of Perinatal Education, 9*(3), 5-9.

BOX 24-4 PERFORMING A PHYSICAL EXAMINATION OF THE NEWBORN

- Provide a normothermic and nonstimulating examination area.
- Check that equipment and supplies are working properly and are accessible.
- Undress only the body area to be examined to prevent heat loss.
- Proceed in an orderly sequence (usually head to toe) with the following exceptions:
  - Perform all procedures that require quiet first, such as observing respirations, position, skin color, tone, and condition.
  - Next, auscultate the lungs, heart, and abdomen.
  - Perform more disturbing procedures, such as testing reflexes, last.
  - Measure head and length at same time to compare results.
- Proceed quickly to prevent stressing the infant.
- Comfort the infant during and after the examination; involve the parent in the following:
  - Talk softly.
  - Hold the infant's hands against his or her chest.
  - Swaddle and hold.
  - Give a pacifier or gloved finger to suck.

TABLE 24-2 PHYSICAL ASSESSMENT OF NEWBORN

AREA ASSESSED AND APPRAISAL PROCEDURE	NORMAL FINDINGS: AVERAGE FINDINGS	NORMAL FINDINGS: NORMAL VARIATIONS	DEVIATIONS FROM NORMAL RANGE: POSSIBLE PROBLEMS (ETIOLOGY)
Posture			
Inspect newborn before disturbing for assessment Refer to maternal chart for fetal presentation, position, and type of birth (vaginal, surgical), given that newborn readily assumes in utero position	Vertex: arms, legs in moderate flexion; fists clenched Resistance to having extremities extended for examination or measurement, crying possible when attempted Cessation of crying when allowed to resume curled-up fetal position (lateral) Normal spontaneous movement bilaterally asynchronous (legs moving in bicycle fashion) but equal extension in all extremities	Frank breech: legs straighter and stiff, newborn assuming intrauterine position in repose for a few days Prenatal pressure on limb or shoulder possibly causing temporary facial asymmetry or resistance to extension of extremities	Hypotonia, relaxed posture while awake (preterm or hypoxia in utero, maternal medications, neuromuscular disorder such as spinal muscular atrophy) Hypertonia (chemical dependence, central nervous system [CNS] disorder) Limitation of motion in any of extremities
Vital Signs			
Check heart rate and pulses: Thorax (chest) Inspection Palpation	Visible pulsations in left midclavicular line, fifth intercostal space Apical pulse, fourth intercostal space 120-160 beats/min when awake	80-100 beats/min (sleeping) to 180 beats/min (crying); possibly irregular for brief periods, especially after crying	Tachycardia: persistent, ≥180 beats/min (respiratory distress syndrome [RDS]; pneumonia) Bradycardia: persistent, ≤80 beats/min (congenital heart block, maternal lupus)
Auscultation Apex: mitral valve Second interspace, left of sternum: pulmonic valve Second interspace, right of sternum: aortic valve Junction of xiphoid process and sternum: tricuspid valve	Quality: *first sound* (closure of mitral and tricuspid valves) and *second sound* (closure of aortic and pulmonic valves) sharp and clear	Murmur, especially over base or at left sternal border in interspace 3 or 4 (foramen ovale anatomically closing at approximately 1 yr)	Murmur (possibly functional) Arrhythmias: irregular rate Sounds: Distant (pneumopericardium) Poor quality Extra Heart on right side of chest (dextrocardia, often accompanied by reversal of intestines)
Peripheral pulses: femoral, brachial, popliteal, posterior tibial	Peripheral pulses equal and strong		Weak or absent peripheral pulses (decreased cardiac output, thrombus, possible coarctation of aorta if weak on left and strong on right) Bounding
Obtain temperature: Axillary: method of choice Temporal and intraauricular thermometers are not effective in measuring newborn temperature.	Axillary: 37° C Temperature stabilized by 8-10 hr of age	36.5°-37.2° C Heat loss: from evaporation, conduction, convection, radiation	Subnormal (preterm birth, infection, low environmental temperature, inadequate clothing, dehydration) Increased (infection, high environmental temperature, excessive clothing, proximity to heating unit or in direct sunshine, chemical dependence, diarrhea and dehydration) Temperature not stabilized by 6-8 hr after birth (if mother received magnesium sulfate, newborn less able to conserve heat by vasoconstriction; maternal analgesics possibly reducing thermal stability in newborn)
Observe and monitor respiratory rate and effort:			
Observe respirations when infant is at rest Observe respiratory effort Count respirations for full minute Auscultate breath sounds Listen for sounds audible without stethoscope	40/min Tendency to be shallow and irregular in rate, rhythm, and depth when infant is awake Crackles may be heard after birth No adventitious sounds audible on inspiration and expiration Breath sounds: bronchial; loud, clear	30-60/min Short periodic breathing episodes and no evidence of respiratory distress or apnea (>20 sec); periodic breathing First period (reactivity): 50-60/min Second period: 50-70/min Stabilization (1-2 days): 30-40/min Crackles (fine)	Apneic episodes: >20 sec (preterm infant: rapid warming or cooling of infant; CNS or blood glucose instability) Bradypnea: <25/min (maternal narcosis from analgesics or anesthetics, birth trauma) Tachypnea: >60/min (RDS, transient tachypnea of the newborn, congenital diaphragmatic hernia) Breath sounds: Crackles (coarse), rhonchi, wheezing Expiratory grunt (narrowing of bronchi) Distress evidenced by nasal flaring, grunting, retractions, labored breathing Stridor (upper airway occlusion)

TABLE 24-2 **PHYSICAL ASSESSMENT OF NEWBORN—cont'd**

AREA ASSESSED AND APPRAISAL PROCEDURE	NORMAL FINDINGS: AVERAGE FINDINGS	NORMAL FINDINGS: NORMAL VARIATIONS	DEVIATIONS FROM NORMAL RANGE: POSSIBLE PROBLEMS (ETIOLOGY)
Vital Signs, cont'd			
Obtain blood pressure (BP) (usually not done in normal term infant) Check oscillometric monitor BP cuff: BP cuff width affects readings, use appropriately sized cuff and palpate brachial, popliteal, or posterior tibial pulse (depending on measurement site)	80-90/40-50 (approximate ranges) At birth Systolic: 60-80 mm Hg Diastolic: 40-50 mm Hg At 10 days Systolic: 95-100 mm Hg Diastolic: 45-75 mm Hg	Variation with change in activity level: awake, crying, sleeping	Difference between upper and lower extremity pressures (coarctation of aorta) Hypotension (sepsis, hypovolemia) Hypertension (coarctation of aorta, renal involvement, thrombus)
Weight*			
Put protective liner cloth or paper in place and adjust scale to 0 g or pounds and ounces Weigh at same time each day Protect newborn from heat loss	Female: 3400 g Male: 3500 g Regaining of birth weight within first 2 weeks	2500-4000 g Acceptable weight loss: 10% or less in first 3-5 days Second baby weighing more than first (on average)	Weight ≤2500 g (preterm, small for gestational age, rubella syndrome) Weight ≥4000 g (large for gestational age, maternal diabetes, heredity—normal for these parents) Weight loss more than 10% to 15% (growth failure, dehydration); assess breastfeeding success

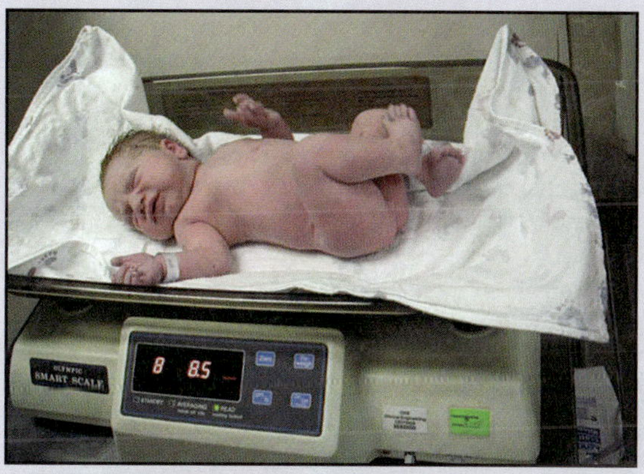

Weighing the infant. The nurse never leaves the infant alone on a scale. The scale is covered to protect against cross-infection. (Courtesy Wendy and Marwood Larson-Harris, Roanoke, VA.)

AREA ASSESSED AND APPRAISAL PROCEDURE	NORMAL FINDINGS: AVERAGE FINDINGS	NORMAL FINDINGS: NORMAL VARIATIONS	DEVIATIONS FROM NORMAL RANGE: POSSIBLE PROBLEMS (ETIOLOGY)
Length			
Measure length from top of head to heel; measuring is difficult in term infant because of presence of molding, incomplete extension of knees	50 cm	45-55 cm	<45 cm or >55 cm (chromosomal abnormality, heredity—normal for these parents); some syndromes present shorter than average limb length (skeletal dysplasias, achondroplasia)

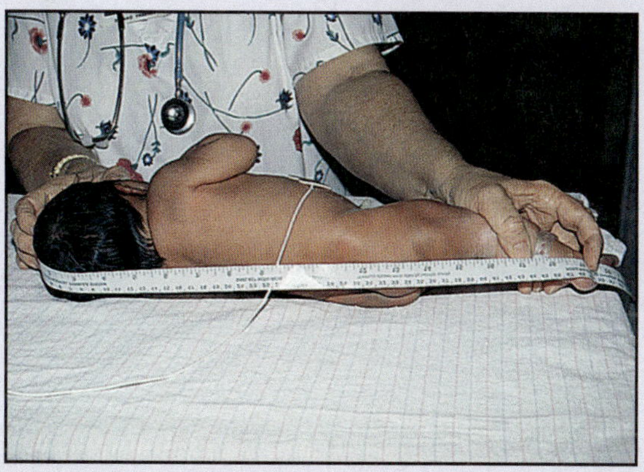

Measuring length crown to heel. To determine total length, include length of legs. If measurements are taken before the infant's initial bath, wear gloves. (Courtesy Marjorie Pyle, RNC, Lifecircle, Costa Mesa, CA.)

NOTE: Weight, length, and head circumference should all be close to the same percentile for any child.

Continued

TABLE 24-2 PHYSICAL ASSESSMENT OF NEWBORN—cont'd

AREA ASSESSED AND APPRAISAL PROCEDURE	NORMAL FINDINGS: AVERAGE FINDINGS	NORMAL FINDINGS: NORMAL VARIATIONS	DEVIATIONS FROM NORMAL RANGE: POSSIBLE PROBLEMS (ETIOLOGY)
Head Circumference			
Measure head at greatest diameter: occipitofrontal circumference May need to remeasure on second or third day after resolution of molding and caput succedaneum	33-35 cm Circumference of head and chest approximately the same for first 1 or 2 days after birth; chest rarely measured on routine basis	32-36.8 cm	Microcephaly, head ≤32 cm: (maternal rubella, toxoplasmosis, cytomegalovirus, fused cranial sutures [craniosynostosis]) Hydrocephaly: sutures widely separated, circumference ≥4 cm more than chest circumference (infection) Increased intracranial pressure (hemorrhage, space-occupying lesion)

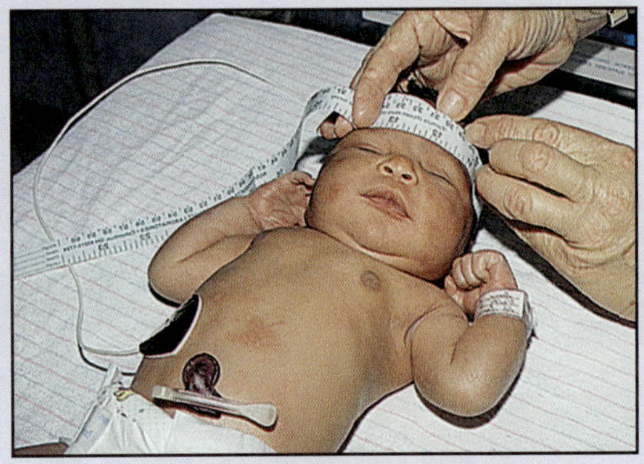

Measuring circumference of head. (Courtesy Marjorie Pyle, RNC, Lifecircle, Costa Mesa, CA.)

AREA ASSESSED AND APPRAISAL PROCEDURE	NORMAL FINDINGS: AVERAGE FINDINGS	NORMAL FINDINGS: NORMAL VARIATIONS	DEVIATIONS FROM NORMAL RANGE: POSSIBLE PROBLEMS (ETIOLOGY)
Chest Circumference			
Measure at nipple line	2-3 cm less than head circumference; averages between 30 and 33 cm	≤30 cm	Prematurity

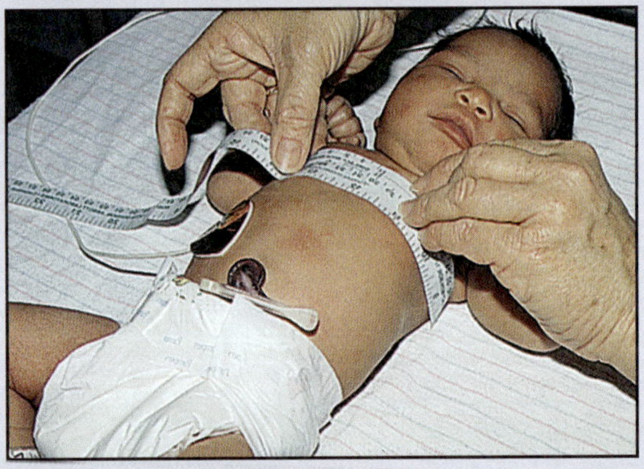

Measuring circumference of chest. (Courtesy Marjorie Pyle, RNC, Lifecircle, Costa Mesa, CA.)

AREA ASSESSED AND APPRAISAL PROCEDURE	NORMAL FINDINGS: AVERAGE FINDINGS	NORMAL FINDINGS: NORMAL VARIATIONS	DEVIATIONS FROM NORMAL RANGE: POSSIBLE PROBLEMS (ETIOLOGY)
Skin			
Check color Inspect and palpate Inspect semi-naked newborn in well-lighted, warm area without drafts; natural daylight best Inspect newborn when quiet and alert	Generally pink Varies with ethnic origin, skin pigmentation beginning to deepen right after birth in basal layer of epidermis Acrocyanosis common after birth	Mottling Harlequin sign Plethora Telangiectases ("stork bites" or capillary hemangiomas) (see Fig. 23-5, *A*) Erythema toxicum/neonatorum ("newborn rash") (see Fig. 23-5, *B*) Milia Petechiae over presenting part Ecchymoses from forceps in vertex births or over buttocks, genitalia, and legs in breech births	Dark red (preterm, polycythemia) Gray (hypotension, poor perfusion) Pallor (cardiovascular problem, CNS damage, blood dyscrasia, blood loss, twin-to-twin transfusion, infection) Cyanosis (hypothermia, infection, hypoglycemia, cardiopulmonary diseases, neurologic, or respiratory malformations) Generalized petechiae (clotting factor deficiency, infection) Generalized ecchymoses (hemorrhagic disease)

TABLE 24-2 **PHYSICAL ASSESSMENT OF NEWBORN—cont'd**

AREA ASSESSED AND APPRAISAL PROCEDURE	NORMAL FINDINGS: AVERAGE FINDINGS	NORMAL FINDINGS: NORMAL VARIATIONS	DEVIATIONS FROM NORMAL RANGE: POSSIBLE PROBLEMS (ETIOLOGY)
Skin, cont'd			
Observe for jaundice	None at birth	Physiologic jaundice in up to 60% of term infants in first week of life	Jaundice within first 24 hr (increased hemolysis, Rh isoimmunization, ABO incompatibility)
Observe for birthmarks or bruises: Inspect and palpate for location, size, distribution, characteristics, color, if obstructing airway or oral cavity		Mongolian spot (see Fig. 23-4) in infants of African-American, Asian, and Native-American origin	Hemangiomas Nevus flammeus: port-wine stain Nevus vasculosus: strawberry mark Cavernous hemangioma
Check skin condition: Inspect and palpate for intactness, smoothness, texture, edema, pressure points if ill or immobilized	Edema confined to eyelid (result of eye prophylaxis) Opacity: few large blood vessels visible indistinctly over abdomen	Slightly thick; superficial cracking, peeling, especially of hands, feet No visible blood vessels, a few large vessels clearly visible over abdomen Some fingernail scratches	Edema on hands, feet; pitting over tibia; periorbital (overhydration; hydrops) Texture thin, smooth, or of medium thickness; rash or superficial peeling visible (preterm, postterm) Numerous vessels very visible over abdomen (preterm) Texture thick, parchment-like; cracking, peeling (postterm) Skin tags, webbing Papules, pustules, vesicles, ulcers, maceration (impetigo, candidiasis, herpes, diaper rash)
Weigh infant routinely Inspect and palpate Gently pinch skin between thumb and forefinger over abdomen and inner thigh to check for turgor Note presence of subcutaneous fat deposits (adipose pads) over cheeks, buttocks	Dehydration: loss of weight best indicator After pinch released, skin returns to original state immediately	Normal weight loss after birth: up to 10% of birth weight Possibly puffy Variation in amount of subcutaneous fat	Loose, wrinkled skin (prematurity, postmaturity, dehydration: fold of skin persisting after release of pinch) Tense, tight, shiny skin (edema, extreme cold, shock, infection) Lack of subcutaneous fat, prominence of clavicle or ribs (preterm, malnutrition)
Check for vernix caseosa: Observe color, amount, and odor before bath or removing clothing	Whitish, cheesy, odorless	Usually more found in creases, folds	Absent or minimal (postmature infant) Abundant (preterm) Green color (possible in utero release of meconium or presence of bilirubin) Odor (possible intrauterine infection)
Assess lanugo: Inspect for thin, fine, downy hair, amount and distribution	Over shoulders, pinnas of ears, forehead	Variation in amount	Absent (postmature) Abundant (preterm, especially if lanugo abundant, long and thick over back)
Head			
Palpate skin	(See Skin)	Caput succedaneum, possibly showing some ecchymosis (see Fig. 23-9, *A*)	Cephalhematoma (see Fig. 23-9, *B*)
Inspect shape, size	Making up one fourth of body length Molding (see Fig. 23-8)	Slight asymmetry from intrauterine position Lack of molding (preterm, breech presentation, cesarean birth)	Severe molding (birth trauma) Indentation (fracture from trauma)
Palpate, inspect, and note size and status of fontanels (open vs. closed)	Anterior fontanel 5-cm diamond, increasing as molding resolves Posterior fontanel triangle, smaller than anterior	Variation in fontanel size with degree of molding Difficulty in feeling fontanels possible because of molding	Fontanels: Full, bulging (tumor, hemorrhage, infection) Large, flat, soft (malnutrition, hydrocephaly, delayed bone age, hypothyroidism) Depressed (dehydration)
Palpate sutures	Palpable and separated sutures	Possible overlap of sutures with molding	Sutures: Widely spaced (hydrocephaly) Premature closure (fused) (craniosynostosis)
Inspect pattern, distribution, amount of hair; feel texture	Silky, single strands lying flat; growth pattern toward face and neck	Variation in amount	Fine, wooly (preterm) Unusual swirls, patterns, or hairline; or coarse, brittle (endocrine or genetic disorders)

Continued

TABLE 24-2 **PHYSICAL ASSESSMENT OF NEWBORN—cont'd**

AREA ASSESSED AND APPRAISAL PROCEDURE	NORMAL FINDINGS: AVERAGE FINDINGS	NORMAL FINDINGS: NORMAL VARIATIONS	DEVIATIONS FROM NORMAL RANGE: POSSIBLE PROBLEMS (ETIOLOGY)
Eyes			
Check placement on face	Eyes and space between eyes each one third the distance from outer-to-outer canthus	Epicanthal folds: characteristic in some ethnicities	Epicanthal folds when present with other signs (chromosomal disorders such as Down, cri-du-chat syndromes)

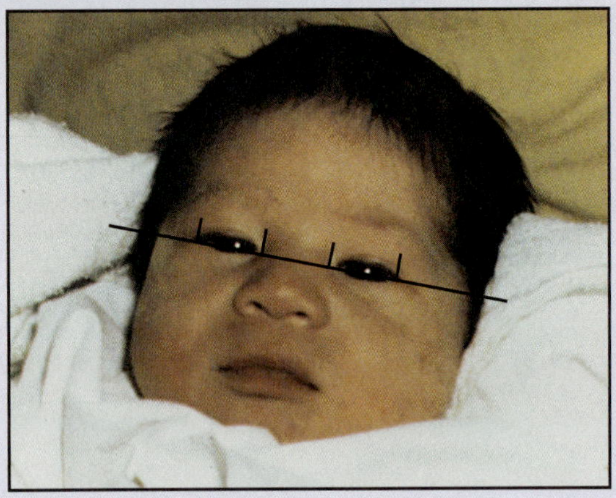

Eyes. In pseudostrabismus, inner epicanthal folds cause the eyes to appear misaligned; however, corneal light reflexes are perfectly symmetric. Eyes are symmetric in size and shape and are well placed.

AREA ASSESSED AND APPRAISAL PROCEDURE	NORMAL FINDINGS: AVERAGE FINDINGS	NORMAL FINDINGS: NORMAL VARIATIONS	DEVIATIONS FROM NORMAL RANGE: POSSIBLE PROBLEMS (ETIOLOGY)
Check for symmetry in size, shape	Symmetric in size, shape		
Check eyelids for size, movement, blink	Blink reflex	Edema if eye prophylaxis drops or ointment instilled	
Assess for discharge	None No tears	Some discharge if silver nitrate used Occasional presence of some tears	Discharge: purulent (infection) Chemical conjunctivitis from eye medication is common—requires no treatment
Evaluate eyeballs for presence, size, shape	Both present and of equal size, both round, firm	Subconjunctival hemorrhage	Agenesis or absence of one or both eyeballs Lens opacity or absence of red reflex (congenital cataracts, possibly from rubella, retinoblastoma [cat's eye reflex]) Lesions: coloboma, absence of part of iris (congenital) Pink color of iris (albinism) Jaundiced sclera (hyperbilirubinemia)
Check pupils	Present, equal in size, reactive to light		Pupils: unequal, constricted, dilated, fixed (intracranial pressure, medications, tumor)
Evaluate eyeball movement	Random, jerky, uneven, focus possible briefly, following to midline	Transient strabismus or nystagmus until third or fourth month	Persistent strabismus Doll's eyes (increased intracranial pressure) Sunset (increased intracranial pressure)
Assess eyebrows: amount of hair, pattern	Distinct (not connected in midline)		Connection in midline (Cornelia de Lange syndrome)
Nose			
Observe shape, placement, patency, configuration	Midline Some mucus but no drainage Preferential nose breather Sneezing to clear nose	Slight deformity (flat or deviated to one side) from passage through birth canal	Copious drainage (rarely congenital syphilis); blockage membranous or bone with cyanosis at rest and return of pink color with crying (choanal atresia) Malformed (congenital syphilis, chromosomal disorder) Flaring of nares (respiratory distress)

TABLE 24-2 **PHYSICAL ASSESSMENT OF NEWBORN—cont'd**

AREA ASSESSED AND APPRAISAL PROCEDURE	NORMAL FINDINGS: AVERAGE FINDINGS	NORMAL FINDINGS: NORMAL VARIATIONS	DEVIATIONS FROM NORMAL RANGE: POSSIBLE PROBLEMS (ETIOLOGY)
Ears			
Observe size, placement on head, amount of cartilage, open auditory canal	Correct placement line drawn through inner and outer canthi of eyes reaching to top notch of ears (at junction with scalp) Well-formed, firm cartilage	Size: small, large, floppy Darwin's tubercle (nodule on posterior helix)	Agenesis Lack of cartilage (preterm) Low placement (chromosomal disorder, mental retardation, kidney disorder) Preauricular tag or sinus Size: possibly overly prominent or protruding ears

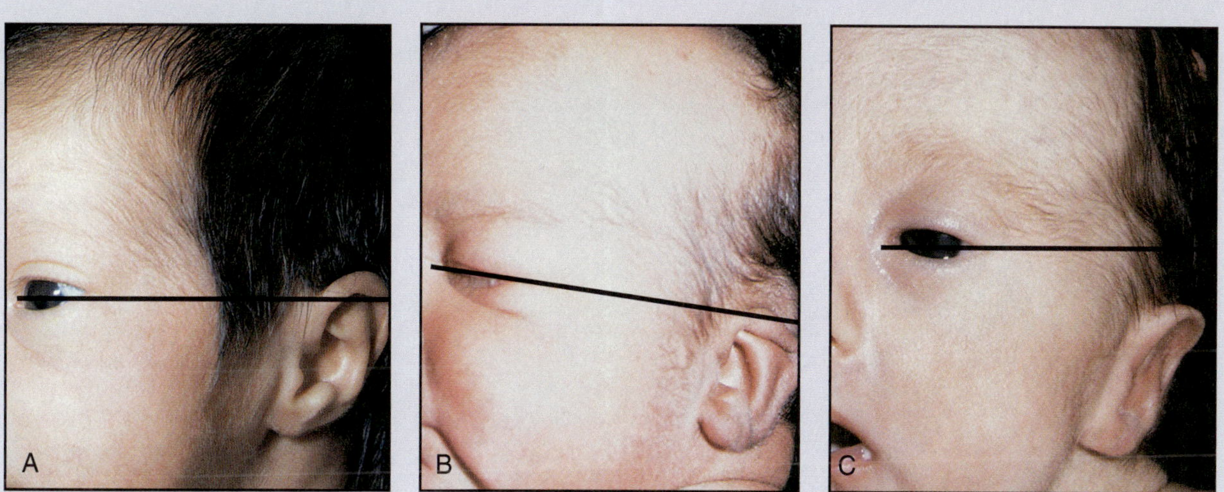

Placement of ears on the head in relation to a line drawn from the inner to the outer canthus of the eye. **A**, Normal position. **B**, Abnormally angled ear. **C**, True low-set ear. (Courtesy Mead Johnson Nutritionals, Evansville, IN.)

AREA ASSESSED AND APPRAISAL PROCEDURE	NORMAL FINDINGS: AVERAGE FINDINGS	NORMAL FINDINGS: NORMAL VARIATIONS	DEVIATIONS FROM NORMAL RANGE: POSSIBLE PROBLEMS (ETIOLOGY)
Assess hearing	Responds to voice and other sounds	State (e.g., alert, asleep) influencing response	Lack of response to loud noise *should not* imply deafness
Perform universal newborn hearing screening to identify deficits (see Fig. 24-9).	Both ears pass		One or both ears fail
Facies			
Observe overall appearance and symmetry of face	Rounded and symmetric; influenced by birth type, molding, or both	Positional deformities	Usually accompanied by other features such as low-set ears, other structural disorders (hereditary, chromosomal aberration)
Mouth			
Inspect and palpate Assess buccal mucosa Dry or moist Pink Status intact Assess lips for color, configuration, movement	Symmetry of lip movement	Transient circumoral cyanosis	Gross anomalies in placement, size, shape (cleft lip or palate [or both], gums) Cyanosis, circumoral pallor (respiratory distress, hypothermia) Asymmetry in movement of lips (seventh cranial nerve paralysis)
Check gums	Pink gums	Inclusion cysts (Epstein pearls—Bohn nodules, whitish, hard nodules on gums or roof of mouth)	Teeth: predeciduous or deciduous (hereditary)
Assess tongue for color, mobility, movement, size	Tongue not protruding, freely movable, symmetric in shape, movement Sucking pads inside cheeks	Short lingual frenulum (ankyloglossia)	Macroglossia (preterm, chromosomal disorder) Thrush: white plaques on cheeks or tongue that bleed if touched *(Candida albicans)*
Assess palate (soft, hard): Arch Uvula	Soft and hard palates intact Uvula in midline	Anatomic groove in palate to accommodate nipple, disappearance by 3 to 4 yr of age Epstein pearls	Cleft hard or soft palate
Assess chin	Distinct chin		Micrognathia—recessed chin with prominent overbite (Pierre Robin or other syndrome)
Evaluate saliva for amount, character	Mouth moist, pink		Excessive salivation and choking or turning blue (esophageal atresia, tracheoesophageal fistula)

Continued

TABLE 24-2 **PHYSICAL ASSESSMENT OF NEWBORN—cont'd**

AREA ASSESSED AND APPRAISAL PROCEDURE	NORMAL FINDINGS: AVERAGE FINDINGS	NORMAL FINDINGS: NORMAL VARIATIONS	DEVIATIONS FROM NORMAL RANGE: POSSIBLE PROBLEMS (ETIOLOGY)
Mouth, cont'd			
Check reflexes: Rooting Sucking Extrusion	Reflexes present	Reflex response dependent on state of wakefulness and hunger	Absent (preterm)
Neck			
Inspect and palpate for movement, flexibility, masses, bruising	Short, thick, surrounded by skin folds; no webbing		Webbing (Turner syndrome)
Check sternocleidomastoid muscles, movement and position of head	Head held in midline (sternocleidomastoid muscles equal), no masses Freedom of movement from side to side and flexion and extension, no movement of chin past shoulder	Transient positional deformity apparent when newborn is at rest: passive movement of head possible	Restricted movement, holding of head at angle (torticollis [wryneck], opisthotonos) Absence of head control (preterm birth, Down syndrome, hypotonia [spinal muscular atrophy])
Assess trachea for position and thyroid gland	Thyroid not palpable		Masses (enlarged thyroid) Distended veins (cardiopulmonary disorder) Skin tags
Chest			
Inspect and palpate			
Shape	Almost circular, barrel shaped	Tip of sternum possibly prominent	Bulging of chest, unequal movement (pneumothorax, pneumomediastinum) Malformation (funnel chest—pectus excavatum)
Observe respiratory movements	Symmetric chest movements, chest and abdominal movements synchronized during respirations	Occasional retractions, especially when crying	Retractions with or without respiratory distress (preterm, RDS) Paradoxical breathing
Evaluate clavicles	Clavicles intact		Fracture of clavicle (trauma); crepitus
Assess ribs	Rib cage symmetric, intact; moves with respirations		Poor development of rib cage and musculature (preterm)
Assess nipples for size, placement, number	Nipples prominent, well formed; symmetrically placed		Nipples Supernumerary, along nipple line Malpositioned or widely spaced
Check breast tissue	Breast nodule: approximately 6 mm in term infant	Breast nodule: 3-10 mm Secretion of witch's milk	Lack of breast tissue (preterm) Sounds: bowel sounds may be heard in diaphragmatic hernia (see Abdomen)
Auscultate: Heart sounds and rate and breath sounds (see Vital Signs)			
Abdomen			
Inspect and palpate umbilical cord	Two arteries, one vein Whitish gray Definite demarcation between cord and skin, no intestinal structures within cord Dry around base, drying Odorless Cord clamp in place for 24 hr		One artery (renal anomaly) Meconium stained (intrauterine distress) Bleeding or oozing around cord (hemorrhagic disease) Redness or drainage around cord (infection, possible persistence of urachus)
		Reducible umbilical hernia	Hernia: herniation of abdominal contents through cord opening (e.g., omphalocele); defect covered with thin, friable membrane, possibly extensive
Inspect size of abdomen and palpate contour	Rounded, prominent, dome shaped because abdominal musculature not fully developed Liver possibly palpable 1-2 cm below right costal margin No other masses palpable No distention Few visible veins on abdominal surface	Some diastasis recti (separation) of abdominal musculature	Gastroschisis: herniation of abdominal contents to the side or above the cord, contents not covered by membranous tissue and may include liver Distention at birth: Ruptured viscus, genitourinary masses or malformations: hydronephrosis, teratomas, abdominal tumors Mild (overfeeding, high gastrointestinal tract obstruction) Marked (lower gastrointestinal tract obstruction, anorectal malformation, anal stenosis), often with bilious emesis Intermittent or transient (overfeeding) Partial intestinal obstruction (stenosis of bowel) Visible peristalsis (obstruction) Malrotation of bowel or adhesions Sepsis (infection)

TABLE 24-2 **PHYSICAL ASSESSMENT OF NEWBORN—cont'd**

AREA ASSESSED AND APPRAISAL PROCEDURE	NORMAL FINDINGS: AVERAGE FINDINGS	NORMAL FINDINGS: NORMAL VARIATIONS	DEVIATIONS FROM NORMAL RANGE: POSSIBLE PROBLEMS (ETIOLOGY)
Abdomen, cont'd			
Auscultate bowel sounds and note number, amount, and character of stools	Sounds present within minutes after birth in healthy term infant Meconium stool passing within 24-48 hr after birth		Scaphoid, with bowel sounds in chest and severe respiratory distress (congenital diaphragmatic hernia)
Assess color		Linea nigra possibly apparent and caused by hormone influence during pregnancy	
Observe movement with respiration	Respirations primarily diaphragmatic, abdominal and chest movement synchronous		Decreased or absent abdominal movement with breathing (phrenic nerve palsy, congenital diaphragmatic hernia)
Genitalia			
Female (see Fig. 23-6, A)			
Inspect and palpate General appearance Clitoris Labia majora	Female genitals: Usually edematous Usually edematous, covering labia minora in term newborns	Increased pigmentation caused by pregnancy hormones Edema and ecchymosis after breech birth Some vernix caseosa between labia possible	Ambiguous genitalia—wide variation (small phallus not well distinguished from enlarged clitoris) Virilized female—extremely large clitoris (congenital adrenal hyperplasia)
Labia minora	Possible protrusion over labia majora		Enlarged clitoris with urinary meatus on tip, absent scrotum, micropenis, fused labia
Discharge Vagina	Smegma Open orifice Mucoid discharge Hymenal/vaginal tag	Blood-tinged discharge from pseudomenstruation caused by pregnancy hormones	Stenosed meatus Labia majora widely separated and labia minora prominent (preterm) Absence of vaginal orifice Fecal discharge (fistula)
Urinary meatus	Beneath clitoris, difficult to see		Bladder exstrophy (bladder outside abdominal cavity and turned inside out)
Check urination	Voiding 2-6 times per 24 hrs for first 1-2 days; voiding 6-10 times per 24 hrs by day 4 or 5	Rust-stained urine (uric acid crystals)	No void within first 24 hours (renal agenesis; Potter syndrome)
Male (see Fig. 23-6, B)			
Inspect and palpate General appearance Penis Urinary meatus appearance Prepuce (foreskin)—do not forcibly retract foreskin if uncircumcised	Male genitals: Foreskin covers glans (if uncircumcised), meatus at tip of penis Prepuce covering glans penis and not retractable	Increased size and pigmentation caused by pregnancy hormones, (wide variation in size of genitals) Prepuce removed if circumcised	Ambiguous genitalia Micropenis Urinary meatus not on tip of glans penis (hypospadias, epispadias, foreskin may be retracted or absent) Round meatal opening
Scrotum: Rugae (wrinkles)	Large, edematous, pendulous in term infant; covered with rugae	Scrotal edema and ecchymosis if breech birth Hydrocele, small, noncommunicating	Scrotum smooth and testes undescended (preterm, cryptorchidism) Bifid scrotum Hydrocele Inguinal hernia
Testes	Palpable on each side	Bulge palpable in inguinal canal	Undescended (preterm)
Check urination	Voiding within 24 hr, stream adequate	Rust-stained urine (uric acid crystals)	No void in first 24 hr (renal agenesis; Potter syndrome)
Check reflexes: Cremasteric	Testes retracted, especially when newborn is chilled		
Extremities			
Make a general check: Inspect and palpate Degree of flexion Range of motion Symmetry of motion Muscle tone	Assuming of position maintained in utero Attitude of general flexion Full range of motion, spontaneous movements	Transient positional deformities	Limited motion (malformations) Poor muscle tone (preterm, maternal medications, CNS anomalies)
Check arms and hands: Inspect and palpate Color Intactness Appropriate placement	Longer than legs in newborn period Contours and movements symmetric	Slight tremors sometimes apparent Some acrocyanosis	Asymmetry of movement (fracture/crepitus, brachial nerve trauma, malformations) Asymmetry of contour (malformations, fracture) Amelia or phocomelia (teratogens) Palmar creases Simian line with short, incurved little fingers (Down syndrome)

Continued

TABLE 24-2 **PHYSICAL ASSESSMENT OF NEWBORN—cont'd**

AREA ASSESSED AND APPRAISAL PROCEDURE	NORMAL FINDINGS: AVERAGE FINDINGS	NORMAL FINDINGS: NORMAL VARIATIONS	DEVIATIONS FROM NORMAL RANGE: POSSIBLE PROBLEMS (ETIOLOGY)
Extremities, cont'd			
Count number of fingers	Five on each hand Fist often clenched with thumb under fingers		Webbing of fingers: syndactyly Absence or excess of fingers Strong, rigid flexion; persistent fists; positioning of fists in front of mouth constantly (CNS disorder) Yellowed nailbeds (meconium staining)
Evaluate joints Shoulder Elbow Wrist Fingers	Full range of motion, symmetric contour		Increased tonicity, clonus, prolonged tremors (CNS disorder)
Check Reflex: Grasp (Palmar and Plantar)			
Check legs and feet: Inspect and palpate Color Intactness Length in relation to arms and body and to each other	Appearance of bowing because lateral muscles more developed than medial muscles	Feet appearing to turn in but can be easily rotated externally, positional defects tending to correct while infant is crying Acrocyanosis	Amelia, phocomelia (chromosomal defect, teratogenic effect) Temperature of one leg differing from that of the other (circulatory deficiency, CNS disorder)
Number of toes	Five on each foot		Webbing, syndactyly (chromosomal defect) Absence or excess of digits (chromosomal defect, familial trait)
Femur	Intact femur		Femoral fracture (difficult breech birth)
Head of femur as legs are flexed and abducted, placement in acetabulum (see Fig. 23-11)			Developmental dysplasia of the hip
Major gluteal folds	Major gluteal folds even		Gluteal folds uneven: DDT
Soles of feet	Soles well lined (or wrinkled) over two thirds of foot in term infants Plantar fat pad giving flat-footed effect		Soles of feet: Few creases (preterm) Covered with creases (postmature) Congenital clubfoot
Evaluate joints Hip Knee Ankle Toes	Full range of motion, symmetric contour		Hypermobility of joints (Down syndrome)
Check reflexes (see Table 23-4)			Asymmetric movement (trauma, CNS disorder)
Back			
Assess anatomy: Inspect and palpate Spine Shoulders Scapulae Iliac crests	Spine straight and easily flexed Infant able to raise and support head momentarily when prone Shoulders, scapulae, and iliac crests lining up in same plane	Temporary minor positional deformities, correction with passive manipulation	Limitation of movement (fusion or deformity of vertebra)
Base of spine—pilonidal dimple or sinus			Spina bifida cystica (meningocele, myelomeningocele) Pigmented nevus with tuft of hair, location anywhere along the spine, often associated with spina bifida occulta Sinus (opening to spinal cord)
Check Reflexes (Spinal Related)			
Test trunk incurvation reflex	Trunk flexed and pelvis swings to stimulated side	May not be apparent in first few days but is usually present in 5-6 days	If transverse lesion is present, no response below lesion; absence of response: central nervous system abnormality or CNS depression

Continued

TABLE 24-2 **PHYSICAL ASSESSMENT OF NEWBORN—cont'd**

AREA ASSESSED AND APPRAISAL PROCEDURE	NORMAL FINDINGS: AVERAGE FINDINGS	NORMAL FINDINGS: NORMAL VARIATIONS	DEVIATIONS FROM NORMAL RANGE: POSSIBLE PROBLEMS (ETIOLOGY)
Back, cont'd			
Test magnet reflex	Lower limbs extend as pressure applied to feet with legs in semiflexed position	Weak or exaggerated response with breech presentation	Absence: suggestive of CNS damage or malformation
Anus			
Inspect and palpate	One anus with good sphincter tone	Passage of meconium within 48 hr of birth	Imperforate anus without fistula
Placement	Passage of meconium within 24 hr after birth		Rectal atresia and stenosis
Patency			Absence of anal opening; drainage of fecal material from vagina in female or urinary meatus in male (rectal fistula) or along perineal raphe (midline area between base of penis and anus)—anorectal malformation
Test for sphincter response (active "wink" reflex)	Anal "wink" present, anal opening patent		
Observe for the following:			
Abdominal distention			
Passage of meconium from anal opening			
Fecal drainage from perineum, penis, vagina			
Stools			
Observe frequency, color, consistency	Meconium followed by transitional and soft yellow stool		No stool (obstruction) Frequent watery stools (infection, phototherapy)

The respiratory rate varies with the state of alertness and activity after birth. Respirations are abdominal in nature and can be counted by observing or lightly feeling the rise and fall of the abdomen. Neonatal respirations are shallow and irregular. The respirations should be counted for a full minute to obtain an accurate count because there are periods when respirations can cease for seconds (≤20) and resume again. The examiner should also observe for symmetry of chest movement. The average respiratory rate is 40 breaths/min but will vary between 30 and 60 breaths/min; respiratory rate can exceed 60 breaths/min if the newborn is very active or crying.

An apical pulse rate should be obtained on all newborns. Auscultation should be for a full minute, preferably when the infant is asleep or in a quiet alert state. The infant may need to be held and comforted during assessment. Heart rate can increase with birth and remain higher during the first hour. When the infant's condition has stabilized, the normal heart rate ranges from 120 to 160 beats/min (Blackburn, 2007). Brachial and femoral pulses are assessed for equality and strength.

If BP is measured, an oscillometric monitor calibrated for neonatal pressures is preferred. An appropriate sized cuff (width-to-arm or calf ratio of 0.45 to 0.70 or approximately one half to three quarters) is essential for accuracy. Neonatal BP is usually highest immediately after birth and falls to a minimum by 3 hours after birth. It then begins to rise steadily and reaches a plateau between 4 and 6 days after birth. This measurement is usually equal to that of the immediate postbirth BP. The BP varies with the neonate's activity; accurate measurement is best obtained while the newborn is at rest.

Prior to the infant's discharge from the birth institution a baseline pulse oximetry measurement may be obtained along with palpation of peripheral pulses (brachial, femoral, pedal), especially if a congenital cardiac defect is suspected.

Baseline Measurements of Physical Growth

Baseline measurements are taken and recorded to help assess the progress and determine the growth patterns of the neonate. These measurements may be recorded on growth charts. The following measurements are made when the neonate is assessed.

Weight. The newborn is usually weighed shortly after birth. This assessment can be performed in the labor and birthing area, the mother's room, or on admission to the nursery. Care must be taken to ensure that the scales are balanced. The totally unclothed neonate is placed in the center of the scale, which is usually covered with a disposable pad or cloth to prevent heat loss via conduction and to prevent cross-infection. The nurse should place one hand over (but not touching) the neonate to prevent the infant from falling off the scales. Weighing the infant at the same time every day is common during the hospital stay. Birth weight of a term infant typically ranges from 2500 to 4000 g.

Head Circumference and Body Length. The head is measured at the widest part, which is the occipitofrontal diameter. The tape measure is placed around the head just above the infant's eyebrows. The term neonate's head circumference ranges from 32 to 36.8 cm.

The length may be difficult to obtain because of the flexed posture of the newborn. The examiner places the newborn on a flat surface and extends the leg until the knee is flat against the surface. Placing the head against a perpendicular surface and extending the leg may assist with obtaining this measurement. In the term neonate, head-to-heel length ranges from 45 to 55 cm.

Neurologic Assessment

The physical examination includes a neurologic assessment of newborn reflexes (see Table 23-3). This assessment provides useful information about the infant's nervous system and state

NURSING CARE PLAN

The Normal Newborn

NURSING DIAGNOSIS

Risk for ineffective airway clearance related to excess mucus production or improper positioning

Expected Outcomes

Neonate's airway remains patent; breath sounds are clear, and no respiratory distress is evident.

Nursing Interventions/*Rationales*

- Teach the parents that gagging, coughing, and sneezing are normal neonatal responses *that assist the neonate in clearing the airways.*
- Teach the parents feeding techniques that prevent overfeeding and distention of the abdomen and to burp the neonate frequently *to prevent regurgitation and aspiration.*
- Position the neonate on the back when sleeping *to prevent suffocation.*
- Suction the mouth and nasopharynx with a bulb syringe as needed; clean the nares of crusted secretions *to clear the airway and prevent aspiration and airway obstruction.*

NURSING DIAGNOSIS

Risk for imbalanced body temperature related to larger body surfaces relative to mass

Expected Outcome

Neonate temperature remains in range of 36.5° to 37.2° C.

Nursing Interventions/*Rationales*

- Maintain a neutral thermal environment *to identify any changes in the neonate's temperature that may be related to other causes.*
- Monitor the neonate's axillary temperature frequently *to identify any changes promptly and ensure early interventions.*
- Bathe the neonate efficiently when temperature is stable, using warm water, drying carefully, and avoiding exposing neonate to drafts *to avoid heat losses from evaporation and convection.*
- Report any alterations in temperature findings promptly *to assess and treat for possible infection.*

NURSING DIAGNOSIS

Risk for infection related to immature immunologic defenses and environmental exposure

Expected Outcome

The neonate will be free from signs of infection.

Nursing Interventions/*Rationales*

- Review the maternal record for evidence of any risk factors *to ascertain whether the neonate may be predisposed to infection.*
- Monitor vital signs *to identify early possible evidence of infection, especially temperature instability.*
- Have all care providers, including parents, perform proper hand hygiene before handling the newborn *to prevent the spread of infection.*
- Provide the prescribed eye prophylaxis *to prevent infection.*
- Keep the genital area clean and dry using proper cleansing techniques *to prevent skin irritation, cross-contamination, and infection.*
- Keep the umbilical stump clean and dry, and keep it exposed to the air *to promote drying and to minimize the chance of infection.*
- If the infant is circumcised, keep the site clean *to prevent infection,* and apply the diaper loosely *to prevent trauma.*
- Teach the parents to keep the neonate away from crowds and environmental irritants *to reduce potential sources of infection.*

NURSING DIAGNOSIS

Risk for injury related to sole dependence on caregiver

Expected Outcome

Neonate remains free of injury.

Nursing Interventions/*Rationales*

- Monitor the environment for hazards such as sharp objects (e.g., long fingernails, and jewelry of the caretaker) *to prevent injury.*
- Handle the neonate gently and support the head, ensure the use of a car seat by parents, teach parents to avoid placing the neonate on a high surface unsupervised and to supervise pet and sibling interactions *to prevent injury.*
- Assess the neonate frequently for any evidence of jaundice *to identify rising bilirubin levels, treat promptly, and prevent complications such as acute bilirubin encephalopathy and kernicterus.*

NURSING DIAGNOSIS

Readiness for enhanced family coping related to anticipatory guidance regarding responses to the neonate's crying

Expected Outcomes

Parents will verbalize their understanding of the methods of coping with the neonate's crying, and describe increased success in interpreting the neonate's cries.

Nursing Interventions/*Rationales*

- Alert the parents to crying as the neonate's form of communication and that cries can be differentiated to indicate hunger, wetness, pain, and loneliness *to provide reassurance that crying is not indicative of the neonate's rejection of parents and that parents will learn to interpret the different cries of their child.*
- Differentiate self-consoling behaviors from fussing or crying *to give parents concrete examples of interventions.*
- Discuss methods of consoling a neonate who has been crying, such as checking and changing diapers, talking softly to the neonate, holding the neonate's arms close to the body, swaddling, picking the neonate up, rocking, using a pacifier, feeding, or burping *to provide anticipatory guidance.*

of neurologic maturation. Many reflex behaviors (e.g., sucking, rooting) are important for proper development. Other reflexes such as gagging and sneezing act as primitive safety mechanisms. The assessment needs to be carried out as early as possible because abnormal signs present in the early neonatal period may require further investigation before the newborn is discharged home.

Gestational Age Assessment

Assessment of gestational age is important because perinatal morbidity and mortality rates are related to gestational age and birth weight. A frequently used method of determining gestational age is the simplified Assessment of Gestational Age scale (Ballard, Novak, & Driver, 1979) (see Fig. 24-1, *A*). This scale, an abbreviated version of the Dubowitz scale, can be used to measure gestational ages of infants between 35 and 42 weeks. It assesses six external physical and six neuromuscular signs. Each sign has a numerical score, and the cumulative score correlates with a maturity rating of 26 to 44 weeks of gestation.

The New Ballard Score, a revision of the original scale, can be used with newborns as young as 20 weeks of gestation. The tool has the same physical and neuromuscular sections but includes −1 to −2 scores that reflect signs of extremely premature infants, such as fused eyelids; imperceptible breast tissue; sticky, friable, transparent skin; no lanugo; and square-window (flexion of wrist) angle greater than 90 degrees (see Fig. 24-1, *A*). The examination of infants with a gestational age of 26 weeks or less should be performed at a postnatal age of less than 12 hours. For infants with a gestational age of at least 26 weeks the examination can be performed up to 96 hours after birth. To ensure accuracy, experts recommend that the initial examination be performed within the first 48 hours of life. Neuromuscular adjustments after birth in extremely immature neonates require that a follow-up examination be performed to further validate neuromuscular criteria (Ballard, Khoury, Wedig, Wang, Eilers-Walsman, & Lipp, 1991). Box 24-5 highlights specific maneuvers used in gestational age assessment.

Classification of Newborns by Gestational Age and Birth Weight. Classification of infants at birth by both birth weight and gestational age provides a more satisfactory method for predicting mortality risks and providing guidelines for management of the neonate than estimating gestational age or birth weight alone. The infant's birth weight, length, and head circumference are plotted on standardized graphs that identify normal values for gestational age. A normal range of birth weights exists for each gestational week (see Fig. 24-1, *B*).

Intrauterine growth curves developed by Battaglia and Lubchenco (1967) have been used to classify infants according to birth weight and gestational age. Other intrauterine growth charts have been developed to reflect a more heterogeneous sample population than previously described. The primary

NEUROMUSCULAR MATURITY

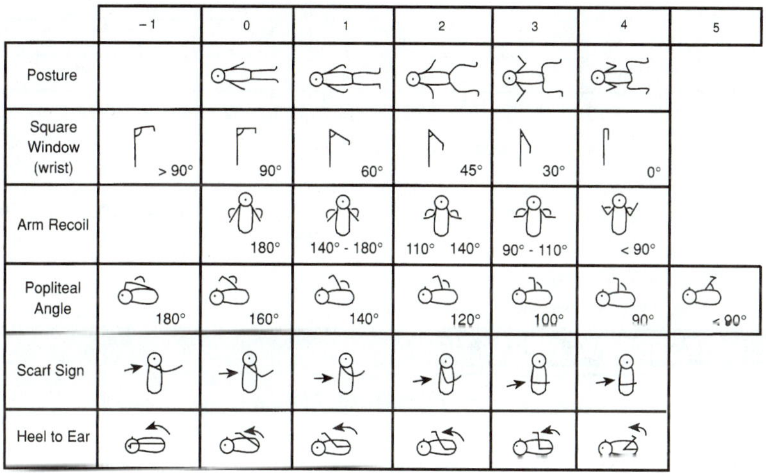

PHYSICAL MATURITY

Skin	sticky friable transparent	gelatinous red, translucent	smooth pink, visible veins	superficial peeling or rash, few veins	cracking pale areas rare veins	parchment deep cracking no vessels	leathery cracked wrinkled
Lanugo	none	sparse	abundant	thinning	bald areas	mostly bald	
Plantar Surface	heel-toe 40-50 mm: -1 <40 mm: -2	>50 mm no crease	faint red marks	anterior transverse crease only	creases ant. 2/3	creases over entire sole	
Breast	imperceptible	barely perceptible	flat areola no bud	stippled areola 1-2 mm bud	raised areola 3-4 mm bud	full areola 5-10 mm bud	
Eye/Ear	lids fused loosely: -1 tightly: -2	lids open pinna flat stays folded	sl. curved pinna; soft; slow recoil	well-curved pinna; soft but ready recoil	formed & firm instant recoil	thick cartilage ear stiff	
Genitals (male)	scrotum flat, smooth	scrotum empty faint rugae	testes in upper canal rare rugae	testes descending few rugae	testes down good rugae	testes pendulous deep rugae	
Genitals (female)	clitoris prominent labia flat	prominent clitoris small labia minora	prominent clitoris enlarging minora	majora & minora equally prominent	majora large minora small	majora cover clitoris & minora	

MATURITY RATING

score	weeks
-10	20
-5	22
0	24
5	26
10	28
15	30
20	32
25	34
30	36
35	38
40	40
45	42
50	44

A

FIG. 24-1 Estimation of gestational age. **A**, New Ballard Score for newborn maturity rating. Expanded scale includes extremely premature infants and has been refined to improve accuracy in more mature infants. (From Ballard, J., Khoury, J., Wang, L., Eilers-Walsman, B., & Lipp, R. [1991]. New Ballard score, expanded to include extremely premature infants, *Journal of Pediatrics, 119*[3], 424.)

Continued

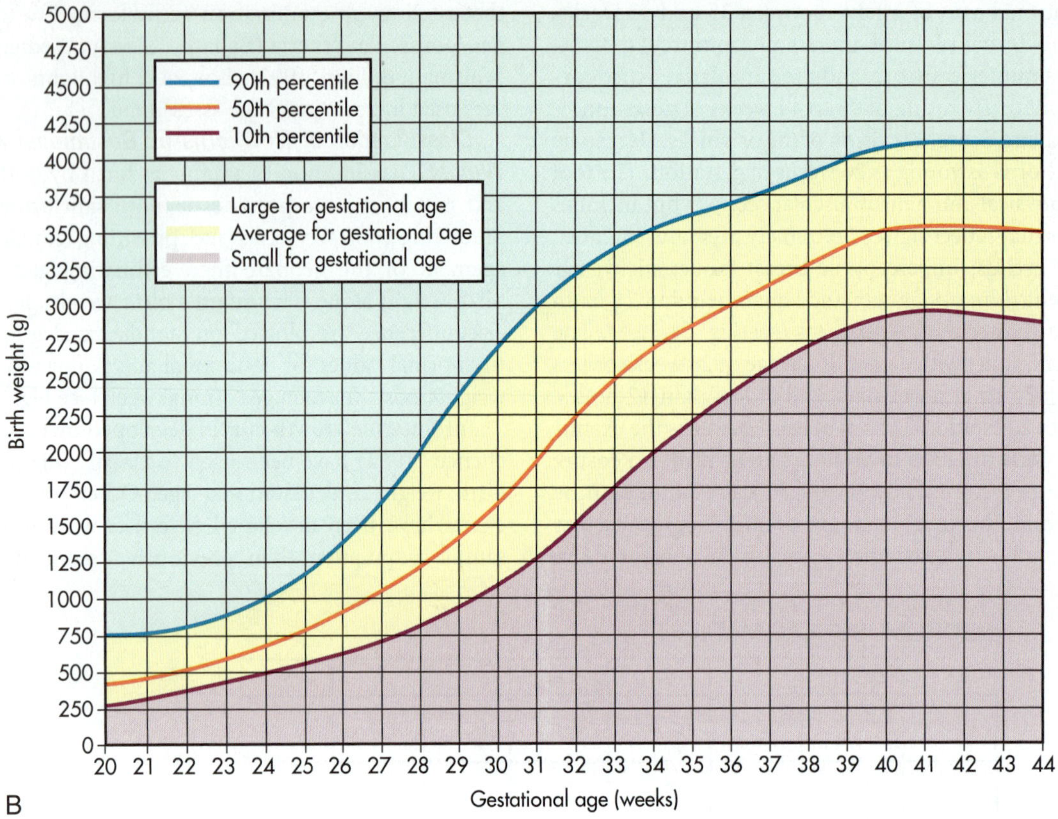

FIG. 24-1, cont'd B, Intrauterine growth: birth weight percentiles based on live single births at gestational ages 20 to 44 weeks. (Data from Alexander, G., Himes, J., Kaufman, R., Mor, J., & Kogan, M. [1996]. A United States national reference for fetal growth. *Obstetrics and Gynecology, 87*[2], 163-168.)

BOX 24-5 MANEUVERS USED IN ASSESSING GESTATIONAL AGE

POSTURE
With infant quiet and in a supine position, observe degree of flexion in arms and legs. Muscle tone and degree of flexion increase with maturity. Full flexion of the arms and legs = score 4.*

SQUARE WINDOW
With thumb supporting back of arm below wrist, apply gentle pressure with index and third fingers on dorsum of hand without rotating infant's wrist. Measure angle between base of thumb and forearm. Full flexion (hand lies flat on ventral surface of forearm) = score 4.*

ARM RECOIL
With infant supine, fully flex both forearms on upper arms and hold for 5 seconds; pull down on hands to extend fully, and rapidly release arms. Observe rapidity and intensity of recoil to a state of flexion. A brisk return to full flexion = score 4.*

POPLITEAL ANGLE
With infant supine and pelvis flat on a firm surface, flex lower leg on thigh and then flex thigh on abdomen. While holding knee with thumb and index finger, extend lower leg with index finger of other hand. Measure degree of angle behind knee (popliteal angle). An angle of less than 90 degrees = score 5.*

SCARF SIGN
With infant supine, support head in midline with one hand; use other hand to pull infant's arm across the shoulder so that infant's hand touches shoulder. Determine location of elbow in relation to midline. Elbow does not reach midline = score 4.*

HEEL TO EAR
With infant supine and pelvis flat on a firm surface, pull foot as far as possible (without using force) up toward ear on same side. Measure distance of foot from ear and degree of knee flexion (same as popliteal angle). Knees flexed with a popliteal angle of less than 10 degrees = score 4.*

*See Figure 24-1 for scale and interpretation of scores.
Source: Hockenberry, M., & Wilson, D. (2007). *Wong's nursing care of infants and children* (8th ed.). St Louis: Mosby.

intrauterine growth charts that provide national reference data include the work of Alexander and associates (1996), which is representative of more than 3.1 million live births in the United States; the work of Thomas and colleagues (2000); Arbuckle and coworkers (1993); and Kramer and colleagues (2001), which are representative of intrauterine growth among the Canadian population. Thomas and colleagues concluded that intrauterine growth measured by head circumference, birth weight, and length varies according to race and sex. These researchers also found that altitude did not seem to affect birth weight significantly, as has been suggested by other authors. In one study, Asian and Hispanic newborns had lower mean birth weights, shorter mean lengths, and smaller mean head circumferences than Caucasian newborns (Madan, Holland, Humbert, & Benitz, 2002). The reader should access and use the most current intrauterine growth chart specific to the referent population being evaluated, especially when considering multiples such as twins.

The infant whose weight is appropriate for gestational age (AGA) (between the 10th and 90th percentiles) can be presumed to have grown at a normal rate regardless of the length of gestation—preterm, term, or postterm. The infant who is large for gestational age (LGA) (more than the 90th percentile) can be presumed to have grown at an accelerated rate during fetal life; the small-for-gestational-age (SGA) infant (less than the 10th percentile) can be presumed to have grown at a restricted rate during intrauterine life. When gestational age is determined according to the New Ballard Score, the newborn will fall into one of the following nine possible categories for birth weight and gestational age: AGA—term, preterm, postterm; SGA—term, preterm, postterm; or LGA—term, preterm, postterm. Birth weight influences mortality: the lower the birth weight, the higher the mortality. The same is true for gestational age: the lower the gestational age, the higher the mortality (Stoll, 2007).

Infants may also be classified in the following ways according to gestation:

- *Preterm or premature*—born before completion of 37 weeks of gestation, regardless of birth weight
- *Late preterm*—born between 34 0/7 and 36 6/7 weeks
- *Term*—born between the end of week 37 and the end of week 42 of gestation
- *Postterm (postdate)*—born after completion of week 42 of gestation
- *Postmature*—born after completion of week 42 of gestation and showing the effects of progressive placental insufficiency

NURSING PROCESS

Care of the Newborn and Family

ASSESSMENT

A brief initial assessment is performed to detect problems that can interfere with effective newborn transition. After the infant is stabilized and mother-infant contact has occurred, a gestational assessment (see Fig. 24-1 and Box 24-5) and a complete examination can be performed (see Table 24-2 and Box 24-4).

Assessment should include a review of the prenatal and intrapartal history for risk factors, psychosocial assessment focusing on parent-infant attachment, adjustment to the parental role, sibling adjustment, social support, and education needs, as well as the mother's and the baby's physical adaptation.

NURSING DIAGNOSES

Nursing diagnoses for the newborn are established after analyzing the findings of the physical assessment and can include:

***Ineffective Airway Clearance* related to:**
- airway obstruction with mucus, blood, and amniotic fluid
- inability to clear mucus by cough or expectoration

***Impaired Gas Exchange* related to:**
- airway obstruction
- ineffective breathing pattern

***Risk for Imbalanced Body Temperature* related to:**
- imbalance between body heat loss and heat production

***Acute Pain* related to:**
- heelstick, circumcision, venipuncture

Possible nursing diagnoses for the parents are:

***Readiness for Enhanced Parenting* related to:**
- knowledge of newborn's social capabilities and dependency needs
- knowledge of newborn's biologic and behavioral characteristics

***Readiness for Enhanced Family Coping* related to:**
- positive attitude and realistic expectations for newborn and adapting to parenthood
- nurturing behaviors with newborn
- verbalizing positive factors in lifestyle change

***Risk for Impaired Parent-Infant Attachment* related to:**
- difficult labor and birth
- postpartum complications
- neonatal complications or anomalies

***Situational Low Self-Esteem* related to:**
- misinterpretation of newborn's behavioral cues

EXPECTED OUTCOMES OF CARE

Expected outcomes can apply to both the infant and the caregiver. Expected outcomes for the newborn during the immediate recovery period include that the infant will:
- Maintain an effective breathing pattern
- Maintain effective thermoregulation
- Remain free from infection
- Receive necessary nutrition for growth
- Establish adequate elimination patterns
- Experience minimal pain
- Remain injury free

Expected outcomes for the parents include that they will:
- Attain knowledge, skill, and confidence relevant to infant care activities
- State understanding of biologic and behavioral characteristics of the newborn
- Identify deviations from normal that should be brought to the attention of the primary health care provider
- Have opportunities to intensify their relationship with the infant
- Begin to integrate the infant into the family

PLAN OF CARE AND INTERVENTIONS

- The nurse provides therapeutic interventions to prevent injury and to assist the newborn with:
  - maintaining a patent airway and adequate gas exchange (p. 570)
  - achieving and maintaining a stable body temperature (pp. 571-572)
  - establishing effective feeding at the breast or by bottle
- The nurse employs Standard Precautions and careful hand hygiene practices to prevent neonatal infection (p. 582)
- The nurse provides anticipatory guidance for parents on relevant topics including infant care, feeding, safety, immunizations, follow-up care, and signs of illness (pp. 591-604).

EVALUATION

Evaluation is based on the expected outcomes of care. The plan is revised as needed based on the evaluation findings.

Late Preterm Infant. Attention has been focused on infants who are considered "late preterm." These infants are often the size and weight of term infants and may be admitted to the healthy newborn nursery and treated as healthy newborns. Late preterm infants, born at 34 0/7 to 36 6/7 weeks of gestation, have risk factors resulting from their physiologic immaturity that require close attention by nurses working with such infants (Bakewell-Sachs, 2007). These risk factors include the tendency to develop respiratory distress, temperature instability, hypoglycemia, apnea, feeding difficulties, jaundice, and hyperbilirubinemia. Nurses working with healthy term infants must be cognizant of the risk factors for late preterm infants and be continually vigilant for the development of problems related to the infant's immaturity. The late preterm infant's care is further addressed in Chapter 37.

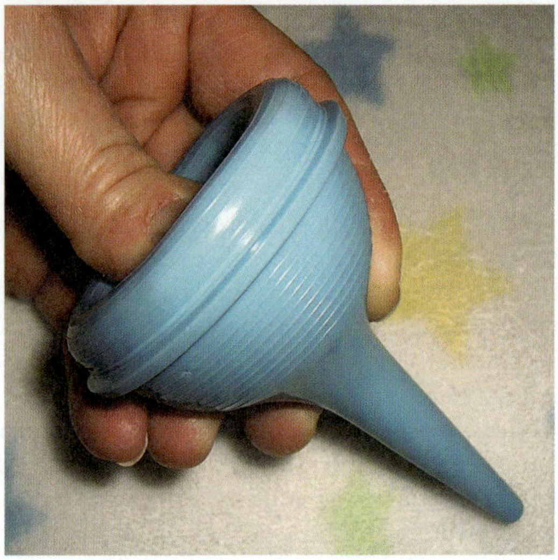

FIG. 24-2 Bulb syringe. Bulb must be compressed before insertion. (Courtesy Cheryl Briggs, RNC, Annapolis, MD.)

INTERVENTIONS

Changes can occur quickly in newborns immediately after birth. Assessment must be followed by the implementation of appropriate care. The nursing process in the immediate care of the newborn and family is outlined in the Nursing Process box.

Airway Maintenance

Generally the healthy term infant born vaginally has little difficulty clearing the airway. Most secretions are moved by gravity and brought by the cough reflex to the oropharynx to be drained or swallowed. The infant is often maintained in a side-lying position (head stabilized, not in the Trendelenburg position) with a rolled blanket at the back to facilitate drainage.

If the infant has excess mucus in the respiratory tract, the mouth and nasal passages can be gently suctioned with a bulb syringe (see the Procedure box: Suctioning with a Bulb Syringe; Fig. 24-2). Routine chest percussion and suctioning of healthy term or late preterm infants is avoided; evidence is insufficient to support anything other than gentle nasopharyngeal and oropharyngeal suctioning to clear secretions (Hagedorn, 2006). The nurse should listen to the infant's respirations and lung sounds with a stethoscope to determine if crackles or inspiratory stridor is present. Fine crackles may be auscultated for several hours after birth. If the bulb syringe does not clear mucus interfering with respiratory effort, mechanical suction can be used.

If the newborn has an obstruction that is not cleared with suctioning, the health care provider should be notified. Further investigation must occur to determine if a mechanical defect (e.g., tracheoesophageal fistula, choanal atresia [see Chapter 36]) is causing the obstruction.

Deeper suctioning may be needed to remove mucus from the newborn's nasopharynx or posterior oropharynx. However, this type of suctioning should be performed only after an assessment of the risks involved. This procedure can be repeated until the infant has a clear airway (see the Procedure box: Suctioning with a Nasopharyngeal Catheter with Mechanical Suction Apparatus).

Video—Nursing Skills: Suctioning with a Bulb Syringe or Mechanical Apparatus

PROCEDURE

Suctioning with a Bulb Syringe

- The bulb syringe should always be kept in the infant's crib.
- The mouth is suctioned first to prevent the infant from inhaling pharyngeal secretions by gasping as the nares are touched.
- The bulb is compressed (see Fig. 24-2) and inserted into one side of the mouth. The center of the infant's mouth is avoided because the gag reflex can be stimulated.
- The nasal passages are suctioned one nostril at a time.
- When the infant's cry does not sound as though it is through mucus or a bubble, suctioning can be stopped.
- The parents should be given demonstrations on how to use the bulb syringe and asked to perform a return demonstration.

PROCEDURE

Suctioning with a Nasopharyngeal Catheter with Mechanical Suction Apparatus

To remove excessive or tenacious mucus from the infant's nasopharynx:

- If wall suction is used, adjust the pressure to less than 80 mm Hg. Proper tube insertion and suctioning for 5 seconds per tube insertion help prevent laryngospasms and oxygen depletion.
- Lubricate the catheter in sterile water and then insert either orally along the base of the tongue or up and back into the nares.
- After the catheter is properly placed, create suction by intermittently placing your thumb over the control as the catheter is carefully rotated and gently withdrawn.
- Repeat the procedure until the infant's cry sounds clear and air entry into the lungs is heard by stethoscope.

SIGNS OF POTENTIAL COMPLICATIONS

Abnormal Newborn Breathing

- Bradypnea (≤30 respirations/min)
- Tachypnea (≥60 respirations/min)
- Abnormal breath sounds: coarse or fine crackles, wheezes, expiratory grunt
- Respiratory distress: nasal flaring, retractions, stridor, gasping, chin tug
- Seesaw or paradoxical respirations
- Skin color: cyanosis, mottling
- Pulse oximetry value: <95%

Maintaining an Adequate Oxygen Supply

Four conditions are essential for maintaining an adequate oxygen supply:

- A clear airway
- Effective establishment of respirations
- Adequate circulation, adequate perfusion, and effective cardiac function
- Adequate thermoregulation (exposure to cold stress increases oxygen and glucose needs.)

Newborns who encounter respiratory problems are likely to exhibit signs and symptoms that indicate some degree of distress. Preterm infants are at greatest risk for respiratory distress (see the Signs of Potential Complications box; see also Chapter 37).

Maintaining Body Temperature

Effective neonatal care includes maintenance of a neutral thermal environment (see Chapter 23). Cold stress increases the need for oxygen and can deplete glucose stores. The infant may react to exposure to cold by increasing the respiratory rate and may become cyanotic. Ways to stabilize the newborn's body temperature include placing the infant directly on the mother's chest and covering with a warm blanket (skin-to-skin contact), drying and wrapping the newborn in warmed blankets immediately after birth, keeping the head well covered, and keeping the ambient temperature of the nursery or mother's room at 22° to 26° C (AAP & ACOG, 2007).

If the infant does not remain with the mother during the first 1 to 2 hours after birth, the nurse places the thoroughly dried

EVIDENCE-BASED PRACTICE — *Pat Gingrich*

Hypothermia Prevention and Skin-to-Skin Contact

ASK THE QUESTION

What interventions to prevent hypothermia in the newborn immediately after birth are safe and effective?

SEARCH FOR EVIDENCE

Search Strategies

Professional organization guidelines, meta-analyses, systematic reviews, randomized controlled trials, nonrandomized prospective studies and retrospective reviews since 2008.

Databases Searched

CINAHL, Cochrane, Medline, PUBMED, and the National Guideline Clearinghouse.

CRITICALLY ANALYZE THE DATA

One of the biggest initial challenges in providing nursing care for newborns is the risk of hypothermia. Term infants may take 6-12 hours to thermoregulate, while preterm and low birthweight babies are at greater risk, due to immaturity, less body fat and greater surface-to-body mass ratio. Hypothermia causes newborns to burn more brown fat, leading to metabolic acidosis, poor feeding, and even death.

A Cochrane Database Systematic Review of seven trials involving 391 preterm or low birthweight babies examined delivery room care by measuring temperature upon admission to the neonatal intensive care unit. The reviewers found that plastic (polyethylene) caps and plastic wraps or bags were equally effective in reducing heat losses in very preterm (less than 29 weeks) newborns, while stockinette caps were not effective. As for external heat sources, the authors found that skin-to-skin contact (SSC) and transwarmer mattresses were more effective at reducing hypothermia than conventional incubator care (McCall, Alderdice, Halliday, Jenkins, & Vohra, 2010). Another single randomized control trial of 96 very preterm infants confirmed the superiority of plastic caps or plastic wraps/bags over conventional care for preventing hypothermia (Trevisanuto, Doglioni, Cavallin, Parotti, Micaglio, and Zanardo, 2010).

"Kangaroo care" is an intervention that includes SSC (usually in an upright position, with the baby's head up), exclusive breastfeeding, and frequent neonatal assessment. In a systematic analysis of 15 studies of low birthweight infants receiving kangaroo care, meta-analysis showed substantially reduced mortality and morbidity. In particular, the rate of infection was reduced (Lawn, Mwansa-Kambafwile, Horta, Barros, & Cousens, 2010). SSC is also beneficial for term babies. The Academy of Breastfeeding Medicine Protocol Committee (2008) recommends that newborns be given SSC with their mother immediately after birth until after the first feeding. To promote physiologic stability and opportunities for breastfeeding, the recommendations include all newborn assessment and care being carried out without separating the baby and mother. Some culturally diverse populations may be at risk for stopping breastfeeding early, but this also improves with early SSC, according to a prospective exploratory study of 48 mother-infant pairs. The researchers recommend that the SSC should be provided early postpartum with warmth and sensitivity (Chiu, Anderson, & Burkhammer, 2008).

IMPLICATIONS FOR PRACTICE

In some of the trials analyzed, "preterm" was defined as less than 37 weeks and "low birth weight" was less than 2500 grams. Most newborn nurseries routinely care for late preterm babies that meet these criteria. Term babies may not need the additional insulation from plastic caps or wraps, but they are still vulnerable to hypothermia and so will benefit from SSC. The advantages for thermoregulation, early breastfeeding and bonding are important enough that keeping mother and baby together in SSC should be the normal routine for nursing care. Measuring, weighing and medications can be delayed up to an hour, or until the first feeding is complete. The nurse sets a family-centered tone by being sensitive and positive. Encouraging SSC is low-cost, pleasing for families, and can be used in low-technology settings. Families will appreciate staying together, and the infants will benefit from comfort, warmth, and a good start to breastfeeding. In turn, these early practices may strengthen and prolong breastfeeding, which can especially benefit at-risk mothers and babies.

References

Academy of Breastfeeding Medicine Protocol Committee. (2008). ABM clinical protocol #5: Peripartum breastfeeding management for the healthy mother and infant at term. *Breastfeeding Medicine, 3*(2), 129–132.

Chiu, S., Anderson, G., & Burkhammer, M. (2008). Skin-to-skin contact for culturally diverse women having breastfeeding difficulties during early postpartum. *Breastfeeding Medicine, 3*(4), 231–237.

Lawn, J., Mwansa-Kambafwile, J., Horta, B., Barros, F., & Cousens, S. (2010). 'Kangaroo mother care' to prevent neonatal deaths due to preterm birth complications. *International Journal of Epidemiology, 39*(Supp. 1), i144–i154.

McCall, E., Alderdice, F., Halliday, H., Jenkins, J., & Vohra, S. (2010). Interventions to prevent hypothermia at birth in preterm and/or low birthweight infants. *The Cochrane Database of Systematic Reviews, 2010*, 3, CD004210.

Trevisanuto, D., Doglioni, N., Cavallin, F., Parotti, M., Micaglio, M., & Zanardo, V. (2010). Heat loss prevention in very preterm infants in delivery rooms: A prospective, randomized, controlled trial of polyethylene caps. *Journal of Pediatrics, 156*(6), 914–917.

infant under a radiant warmer or in a warm incubator until the body temperature stabilizes. The infant's skin temperature is used as the point of control in a warmer with a servo-controlled mechanism. The control panel is usually maintained between 36° and 37° C. This setting should maintain the healthy term newborn's skin temperature at approximately 36.5° to 37° C. A thermistor probe (automatic sensor) is usually placed on the upper quadrant of the abdomen immediately below the right or left costal margin (never over a bone). A reflector adhesive patch can be used over the probe to provide adequate warming. This probe will ensure detection of minor temperature changes resulting from external environmental factors or neonatal factors (peripheral vasoconstriction, vasodilation, or increased metabolism) before a dramatic change in core body temperature develops. The servo-controller adjusts the temperature of the warmer to maintain the infant's skin temperature within the preset range. The sensor needs to be checked periodically to make sure it is securely attached to the infant's skin. The axillary temperature of the newborn is checked every hour (or more often as needed) until the newborn's temperature stabilizes. The length of time to stabilize and maintain body temperature varies; each newborn should therefore be allowed to achieve thermal regulation as necessary, and care should be individualized.

During all procedures, heat loss must be avoided or minimized for the newborn; therefore, examinations and activities are performed with the newborn under a heat panel. The initial bath is postponed until the newborn's skin temperature is stable and can adjust to heat loss from a bath. The exact and optimal timing of the bath for each newborn remains unknown.

Even a healthy term infant can become hypothermic. Inadequate drying and wrapping immediately after birth, a cold birthing room, or birth in a car on the way to the hospital can cause the newborn's temperature to fall below the normal range (hypothermia). The hypothermic infant should be warmed gradually because rapid warming can cause apneic spells and acidosis. Therefore, the warming process is monitored to progress slowly over 2 to 4 hours.

Immediate Interventions

One of the nurse's responsibilities is to perform certain interventions soon after birth to provide for the safety and well-being of the newborn.

Eye Prophylaxis

The instillation of a prophylactic agent in the eyes of all neonates (Fig. 24-3) is mandatory in the United States. This is a precautionary measure against ophthalmia neonatorum, which is an inflammation of the eyes resulting from gonorrheal or chlamydial infection contracted by the newborn during passage through the mother's birth canal. In the United States, if parents object to this treatment, they can be asked to sign an informed refusal form, and their refusal is documented in the neonate's record. The agent used for prophylaxis varies according to hospital protocols, but usually includes forms of erythromycin, tetracycline, or silver nitrate (see the Medication Guide: Eye Prophylaxis). Canadian hospitals have not recommended the use of silver nitrate since 1986. Its use in the United States is minimal because silver nitrate does not protect against chlamydial infection and can cause chemical conjunctivitis.

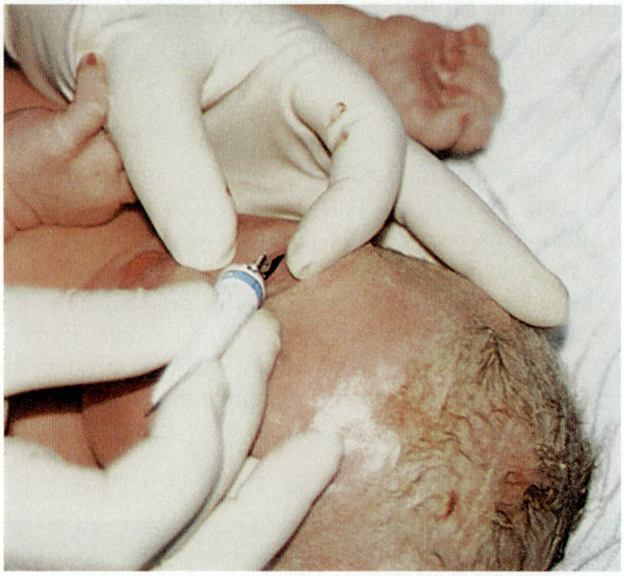

FIG. 24-3 Instillation of medication into eye of newborn. Thumb and forefinger are used to open the eye; medication is placed in the lower conjunctiva from the inner to the outer canthus. (Courtesy Marjorie Pyle, RNC, Lifecircle, Costa Mesa, CA.)

MEDICATION GUIDE

Eye Prophylaxis: Erythromycin Ophthalmic Ointment, 0.5%, and Tetracycline Ophthalmic Ointment, 1%

ACTION

These antibiotic ointments are both bacteriostatic and bactericidal. They provide prophylaxis against ophthalmia neonatorum.

INDICATION

These medications are applied to prevent ophthalmia neonatorum in newborns of mothers who are infected with gonorrhea and chlamydia.

NEONATAL DOSAGE

Apply a 1- to 2-cm ribbon of ointment to the lower conjunctival sac of each eye; can also be used in drop form.

ADVERSE REACTIONS

Can cause chemical conjunctivitis that lasts 24 to 48 hours; vision can be blurred temporarily.

NURSING CONSIDERATIONS

- Administer within 1 to 2 hours of birth. Wear gloves. Cleanse the eyes if necessary before administration. Open the eyes by putting a thumb and finger at the corner of each lid and gently pressing on the periorbital ridges. Squeeze the tube and spread the ointment from the inner canthus of the eye to the outer canthus. Do not touch the tube to the eye. After 1 minute, excess ointment may be wiped off. Observe eyes for irritation. Explain the treatment to the parents.
- Eye prophylaxis for ophthalmia neonatorum is required by law in all states of the United States.

Instillation of eye prophylaxis can be delayed until an hour or so (up to 2 hours in Canada) after birth so that eye contact and parent-infant attachment and bonding are facilitated.

Topical antibiotics such as tetracycline and erythromycin, silver nitrate, and a 2.5% povidone-iodine solution are not

MEDICATION GUIDE

Vitamin K: Phytonadione (AquaMEPHYTON, Konakion)

ACTION
This intervention provides vitamin K because the newborn does not have the intestinal flora to produce this vitamin in the first week after birth. It also promotes formation of clotting factors (II, VII, IX, X) in the liver.

INDICATION
Vitamin K is used for the prevention and treatment of hemorrhagic disease in the newborn.

NEONATAL DOSAGE
Administer a 0.5- to 1-mg (0.25- to 0.5-ml) dose intramuscularly within 2 hours of birth; can be repeated if the newborn shows bleeding tendencies.

ADVERSE REACTIONS
Edema, erythema, and pain at the injection site occur rarely; hemolysis, jaundice, and hyperbilirubinemia have been reported, particularly in preterm infants.

NURSING CONSIDERATIONS
Wear gloves. Administer in the middle third of the vastus lateralis muscle by using a 25-gauge, 5/8-inch needle. Inject into skin that has been cleaned, or allow alcohol to dry on puncture site for 1 minute to remove organisms and prevent infection. Stabilize the leg firmly, and grasp the muscle between the thumb and fingers. Insert the needle at a 90-degree angle; release the muscle; and inject the medication slowly if no blood return occurs. Massage the site with a dry gauze square after removing needle to increase absorption. Observe for signs of bleeding from the site.

effective in the treatment of chlamydial conjunctivitis. A 14-day course of oral erythromycin or an oral sulfonamide can be given for chlamydial conjunctivitis (AAP Committee on Infectious Diseases, 2009).

Vitamin K Prophylaxis

Administering vitamin K intramuscularly is routine in the newborn period in the United States. A single intramuscular injection of 0.5 to 1 mg of vitamin K is given soon after birth to prevent hemorrhagic disease of the newborn. Administration can be delayed until after the first breastfeeding in the birthing room (AAP & ACOG, 2007). Vitamin K is synthesized by intestinal flora, which are not present at birth. The introduction of bacteria begins with the first feedings and by the age of seven days, healthy newborns are able to produce their own vitamin K (see the Medication Guide: Vitamin K).

SAFETY ALERT

Vitamin K is never administered by the intravenous route for the prevention of hemorrhagic disease of the newborn except in some cases of a preterm infant who has no muscle mass. In such cases the medication should be diluted and given over 10 to 15 minutes while closely monitoring the infant with a cardiorespiratory monitor. Rapid bolus administration of vitamin K can cause cardiac arrest.

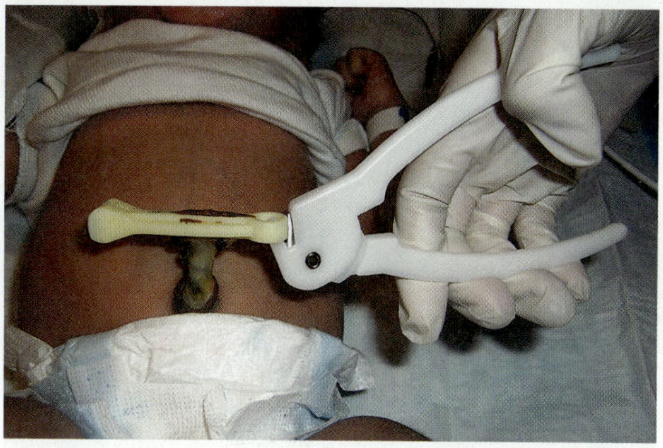

FIG. 24-4 With special tool, remove clamp after cord dries (approximately 24 hours). (Courtesy Cheryl Briggs, RNC, Annapolis, MD.)

Video—Nursing Skills: Performing Newborn Cord Care

Umbilical Cord Care

The cord is clamped immediately after birth. The cord clamp is removed once the stump has started drying and is no longer bleeding (Fig. 24-4), typically in 24 hours.

The goal of cord care is to prevent or decrease the risk of hemorrhage and infection. The umbilical cord stump is an excellent medium for bacterial growth and can easily become infected. Hospital protocol determines the technique for routine cord care. Common methods include the use of an antimicrobial agent such as bacitracin or triple dye, although some experts advocate the use of alcohol alone, soap and water, sterile water, povidone-iodine, or no treatment (natural healing). A one-time application of triple dye has been shown to be superior to alcohol, povidone-iodine, or topical antibiotics in reducing colonization or infection; the use of alcohol is associated with prolonged cord drying and separation (McConnell, Lee, Couillard, & Sherrill, 2004; Zupan, Garner, & Omari, 2004). Current recommendations for cord care by the Association of Women's Health, Obstetric and Neonatal Nurses (AWHONN, 2007) include cleaning the cord with sterile water initially and subsequently with plain water.

The stump and base of the cord should be assessed for edema, redness, and purulent drainage with each diaper change. The nurse or parent cleanses the cord and skin area around the base of the cord with the prescribed preparation (e.g., sterile water, erythromycin solution, or triple dye). The stump deteriorates through the process of dry gangrene; therefore odor alone is not a positive indicator of omphalitis (infection of the umbilical stump). Cord separation time is influenced by several factors, including type of cord care, type of birth, and other perinatal events. The average cord separation time is 10 to 14 days. Some dried blood may be seen in the umbilicus at separation (Fig. 24-5).

Promoting Parent-Infant Interaction

Today's childbirth practices promote the family as the focus of care. Parents generally desire to share in the birth process and to have early contact with their infants. The infant can be put to breast soon after birth. Early contact between mother and newborn can be important in developing future relationships; it also has a positive effect on the initiation and duration of breastfeeding. Early mother-infant contact produces physiologic benefits for the mother and neonate. Maternal levels of oxytocin and prolactin rise with early breastfeeding.

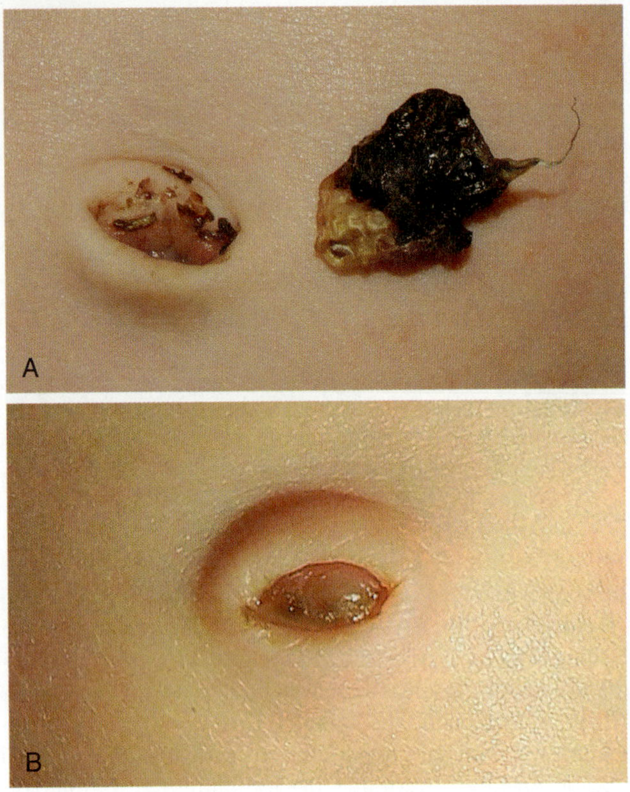

FIG. 24-5 Cord separation. **A**, Cord separated with some dried blood still in the umbilicus. **B**, Umbilicus cleansed and beginning to heal. (Courtesy Cheryl Briggs, RNC, Annapolis, MD.)

The process of developing active immunity begins as the infant ingests antibodies from the mother's colostrum.

CARE MANAGEMENT: FROM 2 HOURS AFTER BIRTH UNTIL DISCHARGE

In an effort to provide more family-centered care, many hospitals have adopted variations of single-room maternity care (SRMC) or mother-baby (couplet) care in which the same nurse provides care for the mother and newborn. SRMC allows the infant to remain with the parents after the birth. Many of the procedures, such as assessment of weight and measurement of head circumference and length, instillation of eye medication, administration of vitamin K, and physical assessment, are carried out in the labor and birth unit. Nurses who work in an SRMC unit; a labor, delivery, and recovery (LDR) unit; or a labor, delivery, recovery, and postpartum (LDRP) unit must be educated and competent in providing intrapartal, neonatal, and postpartum nursing care. If an infant is transferred to the nursery, the nurse receiving the newborn verifies the infant's identification, places the baby in a warm environment, and begins the admission process.

Critical Thinking Exercise—Jaundice

Common Newborn Problems

Birth Injuries

Birth trauma includes any physical injury sustained by a newborn during labor and birth. Although most injuries are minor and resolve during the neonatal period without treatment, some types of trauma require intervention; a few are serious enough to be fatal. (See Chapter 35 for more information on birth injuries.)

Soft Tissue Injuries

Subconjunctival and retinal hemorrhages result from rupture of capillaries caused by increased pressure during birth. These hemorrhages usually clear within 5 days after birth and present no further problems. Parents need explanation and reassurance that these injuries are harmless.

Erythema, ecchymoses, petechiae, abrasions, lacerations, or edema of the buttocks and extremities can be present. Localized discoloration can appear over the presenting part as a result of forceps- or vacuum-assisted birth. Ecchymoses and edema can appear anywhere on the body. Petechiae (pinpoint hemorrhagic areas) acquired during birth can extend over the upper trunk and face. These lesions are benign if they disappear within 2 or 3 days of birth and no new lesions appear. Ecchymoses and petechiae can be signs of a more serious disorder, such as thrombocytopenic purpura. To differentiate hemorrhagic areas from a skin rash or discolorations, try to blanch the skin with two fingers. Petechiae and ecchymoses will not blanch because extravasated blood remains within the tissues, whereas skin rashes and discolorations do blanch.

Trauma can occur during labor and birth to the presenting fetal part. Caput succedaneum and cephalhematoma are discussed in Chapter 23 (see Fig. 23-9). Forceps injury and bruising from the vacuum cup occur at the site of application of the instruments. A forceps injury commonly produces a linear mark across both sides of the face in the shape of the blades of the forceps. The affected areas are kept clean to minimize the risk of infection. These injuries usually resolve spontaneously within several days with no specific therapy. With the increased use of the vacuum extractor and the use of padded forceps blades, the incidence of these lesions can be significantly reduced.

Bruises over the face can be the result of face presentation (Fig. 24-6). In a breech presentation, bruising and swelling may be seen over the buttocks or genitalia (see Fig. 23-7). The skin over the entire head can be ecchymotic and covered with petechiae caused by a tight nuchal cord. If the hemorrhagic areas do

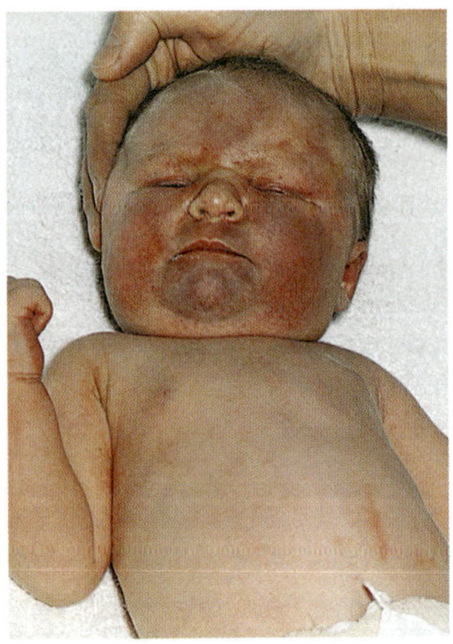

FIG. 24-6 Marked bruising on the entire face of an infant born vaginally after face presentation. Less severe ecchymoses were present on the extremities. Phototherapy was required for treatment of jaundice resulting from the breakdown of accumulated blood. (From O'Doherty, N. [1986]. *Neonatology: Micro atlas of the newborn.* Nutley, NJ: Hoffman-LaRoche.)

not disappear spontaneously in 2 days, or if the infant's condition changes, the primary health care provider is notified.

Accidental lacerations can be inflicted with a scalpel during a cesarean birth. These cuts may occur on any part of the body but are most often found on the scalp, buttocks, and thighs. They are usually superficial and need only to be kept clean. Butterfly adhesive strips will hold together the edges of more serious lacerations. Rarely are sutures needed.

Physiologic Problems

Jaundice

Physiologic Jaundice. Every newborn is assessed for jaundice. To differentiate cutaneous jaundice from normal skin color, the nurse applies pressure with a finger over a bony area (e.g., the nose, forehead, sternum) for several seconds to empty all the capillaries in that spot. If jaundice is present, the blanched area will appear yellow before the capillaries refill. The conjunctival sacs and buccal mucosa also are assessed, especially in darker-skinned infants. Assessing for jaundice in natural light is recommended because artificial lighting and reflection from nursery walls can distort the actual skin color. Visual assessment of jaundice does not, however, provide an accurate assessment of the level of serum bilirubin.

Noninvasive monitoring of bilirubin using cutaneous reflectance measurements (transcutaneous bilirubinometry [TcB]) allows for repetitive estimations of bilirubin (Fig. 24-7). These devices work well on both dark- and light-skinned infants and demonstrate linear correlation with serum determinations of bilirubin levels in full-term infants. TcB monitors can be used to screen clinically significant jaundice and decrease the need for serum bilirubin measurements. The new TcB monitors provide accurate measurements within 2 to 3 mg/dl in most neonatal populations at serum levels below 15 mg/dl (AAP Subcommittee on Hyperbilirubinemia, 2004). After phototherapy has been initiated, TcB is no longer useful as a screening tool.

The use of hour-specific serum bilirubin levels to predict term newborns at risk for rapidly rising levels is an official recommendation by the American Academy of Pediatrics (AAP) Subcommittee on Hyperbilirubinemia (2004) for the monitoring of healthy neonates at 35 weeks of gestation or greater before discharge from the hospital. Using a nomogram (Fig. 24-8) with three levels (high, intermediate, or low risk) of rising total serum bilirubin values assists in the determination of which newborns might need further evaluation after discharge. Universal bilirubin screening based on hour-specific total serum bilirubin can be performed at the same time as the routine newborn profile (phenylketonuria [PKU], galactosemia, and others) (AAP Subcommittee on Hyperbilirubinemia). The hour-specific bilirubin risk nomogram is used to determine the infant's risk for development of hyperbilirubinemia requiring medical treatment or closer screening. Studies have demonstrated the accuracy of the nomogram in predicting rapidly rising bilirubin levels requiring evaluation or treatment (Keren, Luan, Friedman, Saddlemire, Cnaan, & Bhutani, 2008).

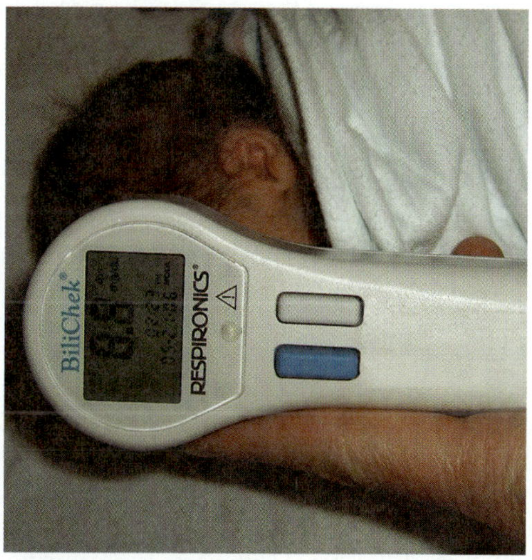

FIG. 24-7 Transcutaneous monitoring of bilirubin with a transcutaneous bilirubinometry (TcB) monitor. (Courtesy Cheryl Briggs, RNC, Annapolis, MD.)

The degree of jaundice is determined by serum bilirubin measurements. Normal values of unconjugated (indirect) bilirubin are 0.2 to 1.4 mg/dl. Normal values for total serum bilirubin range from 1 to 12 mg/dl (Pagana & Pagana, 2009).

An important point to remember is that the evaluation of jaundice is based not only on serum bilirubin and transcutaneous bilirubin levels but also on the timing of the appearance of clinical jaundice, gestational age at birth, age in hours since birth, family history that includes maternal blood type and Rh status and history of hyperbilirubinemia in a sibling, evidence of hemolysis, feeding method, the infant's physiologic status, and the progression of serial serum bilirubin levels.

Factors recognized to place infants in the high risk category include gestational age less than 38 weeks, breastfeeding, previous sibling with significant jaundice, and jaundice appearing before discharge (AAP Subcommittee on Hyperbilirubinemia, 2004). Experts recommend that healthy infants (35 weeks or greater) receive follow-up care and assessment of bilirubin within 3 days of discharge if discharged at less than 24 hours and a risk assessment with tools such as the hour-specific nomogram. Newborns discharged at 24 to 47.9 hours should receive follow-up evaluation within 4 days (96 hours), and those discharged between 48 and 72 hours should receive follow-up within 5 days (AAP Subcommittee on Hyperbilirubinemia).

Hypoglycemia

Hypoglycemia in a term infant during the early newborn period is defined as a blood glucose concentration less than adequate to support neurologic, organ, and tissue function; however, the precise level at which this concentration occurs in every neonate is not known. Hypoglycemia that warrants treatment is usually defined as blood glucose levels less than 40 mg/dl, although some experts recommend treatment for levels less than 50 mg/dl (Sperling, 2007).

At birth the maternal source of glucose is cut off with the clamping of the umbilical cord. Most healthy term newborns experience a transient decrease in glucose levels, with a subsequent mobilization of free fatty acids and ketones to help maintain adequate glucose levels (Blackburn, 2007). Infants who are asphyxiated or have other physiologic stress can experience hypoglycemia as a result of a decreased glycogen supply, inadequate gluconeogenesis, or overutilization of glycogen stored during fetal life. There is concern about neurologic injury as a

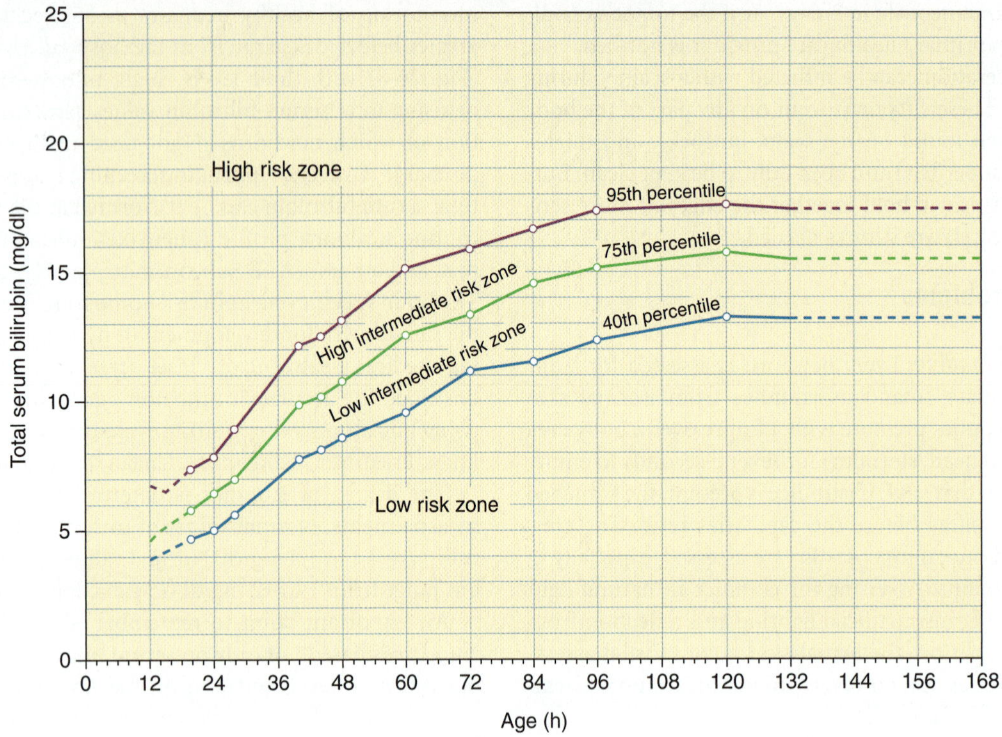

FIG. 24-8 Nomogram for designation of risk in 2840 well newborns at 36 or more weeks of gestational age with birth weight of 2000 g or more or 35 or more weeks of gestational age and birth weight of 2500 g or more based on the hour-specific serum bilirubin values. (This nomogram should not be used to represent the natural history of neonatal hyperbilirubinemia.) (From Bhutani, V., Johnson, L., & Sivieri, E. [1999]. Predictive ability of a predischarge hour-specific serum bilirubin for subsequent significant hyperbilirubinemia in healthy term and near-term newborns. *Pediatrics, 103*[1], 6-14.)

result of severe or prolonged hypoglycemia, especially in combination with ischemia (Volpe, 2008).

For the healthy full-term infant born after an uneventful pregnancy and birth, recommendations are to assess glucose levels only when risk factors are present or when there are clinical manifestations of hypoglycemia. The clinical signs of hypoglycemia can be transient or recurrent and include jitteriness, lethargy, poor feeding, hypotonia, temperature instability (hypothermia), respiratory distress, apnea, and seizures. It is important to remember that hypoglycemia can be present in the absence of clinical manifestations.

For infants who are at risk for hypoglycemia, close monitoring of blood glucose levels is recommended. Glucose levels should be measured within the first hour after birth and frequently thereafter until levels stabilize. Hospital protocols vary in the time intervals recommended for glucose monitoring. Risk factors for hypoglycemia include maternal diabetes, gestational hypertension, and tocolytic therapy. Neonatal risk factors include prematurity, LGA, SGA, perinatal hypoxia, infection, hypothermia, and congenital malformations.

! NURSING ALERT

Late preterm infants are at increased risk for hypoglycemia. They have decreased glycogen stores and lack hepatic enzymes for gluconeogenesis and glycogenolysis. Their hormonal regulation and insulin secretion are immature. The increased risk of cold stress and feeding difficulties adds to the risk for hypoglycemia (Ramachandrappa & Jain, 2009).

Hypoglycemia in the low risk term infant is usually treated by feeding the infant a source of carbohydrate (i.e., human milk or formula). If the newborn has a blood glucose level less than 40 mg/dl and is asymptomatic, breastfeeding or bottle-feeding should be instituted. If levels remain low despite feeding, intravenous dextrose is warranted. In such infants the treatment should be aimed at maintaining the blood glucose levels above 45 mg/dl (2.5 mmol/L). For the neonate with clinical signs of hypoglycemia, regardless of cause or age, some experts recommend parenteral glucose infusion (Kalhan & Parimi, 2006). Experts further recommend that emphasis be placed less on an absolute glucose value but rather on promoting normoglycemia with interventions for less optimal values (Blackburn, 2007).

Hypocalcemia

Hypocalcemia is defined as serum calcium levels of less than 7.8 to 8 mg/dl in term infants and slightly lower (7 mg/dl) in preterm infants; ideally, ionized fraction levels reflect the biologically active form and levels range from 3 to 4.4 mg/dl depending on the measurement method (Blackburn, 2007). Hypocalcemia can occur in infants of mothers with diabetes or in those who had perinatal asphyxia or trauma, and in low-birth-weight and preterm infants. Early-onset hypocalcemia usually occurs within the first 24 to 48 hours after birth. Signs of hypocalcemia include jitteriness, high-pitched cry, irritability, apnea, intermittent cyanosis, abdominal distention, and laryngospasm, although some hypocalcemic infants are asymptomatic (Blackburn). Jitteriness is a symptom of both hypoglycemia and hypocalcemia; therefore, hypocalcemia must be considered if the therapy for hypoglycemia proves ineffective.

In most instances, early-onset hypocalcemia is self-limiting and resolves within 1 to 3 days. Treatment usually includes early feeding of an appropriate source of calcium such as fortified human milk or a preterm infant formula.

Laboratory and Diagnostic Tests

Because newborns experience many transitional events in the first 28 days of life, laboratory samples are often collected to determine adequate physiologic adaptation and to identify disorders that can adversely affect the child's life beyond the neonatal period. Blood samples for most laboratory tests can be obtained from the neonate with a heel puncture. Tests commonly performed other than blood glucose and bilirubin levels include newborn screening tests and serum drug levels. Standard laboratory values for a term newborn are given in Box 24-6.

Mandated by U.S. law, newborn genetic screening is an important public health program aimed at early detection of genetic diseases that result in severe health problems if

BOX 24-6 STANDARD LABORATORY VALUES IN THE NEONATAL PERIOD

			NEONATAL	
1. HEMATOLOGIC VALUES				
Clotting factors				
Bleeding time (Ivy)			2 to 7 minutes	
Fibrinogen			125 to 300 mg/dl*	
		TERM		**PRETERM**
Hemoglobin (g/dl)		14.5 to 22.5		15 to 24
Hematocrit (%)		48 to 69		45 to 55
Reticulocytes (%)		0.4 to 6		Up to 10
Fetal hemoglobin (% of total)		40 to 70		80 to 90
Red blood cells (RBCs)/mcl		4.8×10^6 to 7.1×10^6		
Platelet count/mm³		150,000 to 300,000		120,000 to 180,000
White blood cells (WBCs)/mcl		9000 to 30,000		10,000 to 20,000
Neutrophils ("segs") (%)		54-62		47
Eosinophils (%)		1 to 3		
Basophils (%)		0 to .75		
Lymphocytes (%)		25 to 33		33
Monocytes (%)		3 to 7		4
Immature WBCs (%)		10		16
			NEONATAL	
2. BIOCHEMICAL VALUES				
Bilirubin, direct			0 to 1 mg/dl	
Bilirubin, total	Cord:		<2 mg/dl	
	Peripheral blood:	0 to 1 day	6 mg/dl	
		1 to 2 days	8 mg/dl	
		2 to 5 days	12 mg/dl	
Serum glucose			40 to 60 mg/dl	
Blood gases		Arterial:	pH 7.31 to 7.49	
			Pco_2 26 to 41 mm Hg	
			Po_2 60 to 70 mm Hg	
		Venous:	pH 7.31 to 7.41	
			Pco_2 40 to 50 mm Hg	
			Po_2 40 to 50 mm Hg	
3. URINALYSIS				
Color			Clear, straw	
Specific gravity			1.001 to 1.020	
pH			5 to 7	
Protein			Negative	
Glucose			Negative	
Ketones			Negative	
RBCs			0 to 2	
WBCs			0 to 4	
Casts			None	

*1 dl = 100 ml; this conforms to the standardized international (SI) system measurements.
Volume: 24 to 72 ml/kg excreted daily in the first few days; by week 1, 24-hour urine volume close to 200 ml.
Protein: may be present in first 2 to 4 days.
Osmolarity (mOsm/l): 100 to 600.
Pco_2, Partial pressure of carbon dioxide; *Po_2,* partial pressure of oxygen; *RBCs,* red blood cells; *WBCs,* white blood cells.
Source: Hockenberry, M., & Wilson, D. (2007). *Wong's nursing care of infants and children* (8th ed.). St. Louis: Mosby; Pagana, K. & Pagana, T. (2009). *Mosby's manual of diagnostic and laboratory tests* (4th ed.). St. Louis: Mosby.

not treated early. Using tandem mass spectrometry, all states screen for PKU and hypothyroidism, but each state determines whether other tests are performed. Other genetic defects that are included in some screening programs include galactosemia, cystic fibrosis, maple syrup urine disease, and sickle cell disease. Experts recommend that the screening test be repeated at age 1 to 2 weeks if the initial specimen was obtained when the infant was younger than 24 hours (Zinn, 2006).

Families should be educated regarding the availability of metabolic tests routinely screened in their state of residence. Tandem mass spectrometry has the potential for identifying more than 30 disorders in addition to the standard inborn errors of metabolism (IEMs). With tandem mass spectrometry, earlier identification of IEMs can prevent further developmental delays and morbidities in affected children.

Information about which tests are required in a state can be obtained from state health departments (see Resources on this book's website). Some of the major disorders for which infants are screened are described in Table 24-3.

Newborn Hearing Screening

Significant hearing loss occurs in approximately 1 in 1000 births, often when there is no other identifiable problem. Hearing loss is difficult to detect during the first 2 to 3 years of life until the child demonstrates problems with speech and language development. When hearing loss is identified early, interventions can

TABLE 24-3 NEWBORN SCREENING SUMMARY

DISORDER/EVIDENCE	SYMPTOMS	SCREENING INCIDENCE	TREATMENT
PKU (classic) Elevated phenylalanine (plasma concentrations >20 mg/dl)	Severe mental retardation if early detection and treatment not started; eczema, seizures, behavior disorders, decreased pigmentation, distinctive musty or mouselike odor	1:13,500 to 1:20,000 More common in Caucasians and Native Americans	Lifelong dietary management with low-phenylalanine diet; possible tyrosine supplementation
Congenital hypothyroidism (primary) Low T_4, elevated TSH	Asymptomatic at birth; mental and motor delays (although neonatal detection and treatment have decreased incidence of mental retardation), short stature, coarse, dry skin and hair, hoarse cry, constipation	1:3600 to 1 in 5000 live births with some ethnic variation 1:32,000 African-American births 1:2000 Hispanic and Native American births	Maintain L-thyroxine levels in upper half of normal range; periodic bone age to monitor growth
Galactosemia (transferase deficiency) Elevated galactose; low or absent fluorescence	Hypotonia, lethargy, vomiting, diarrhea, metabolic acidosis, *Escherichia coli* sepsis, or liver dysfunction; mental retardation, jaundice, blindness, cataracts, long-term behavioral problems, and neurologic impairment	1:60,000 to 1:250,000	Eliminate galactose and lactose from the diet; soy formulas in infancy; lactose-free solid foods
Maple syrup urine disease (MSUD) Elevated leucine	Poor feeding, lethargy, hypotonia, vomiting, ketoacidosis, and seizures; sweet maple syrup odor may occur in urine, cerumen, or sweat	1:90,000 to 1:100,000; higher in certain Mennonite (Older Order) populations, 1 in 246 to 1 in 358	Branched-chain amino acid–free formula with added protein-based formula; thiamine supplement in some individuals; lifelong treatment and monitoring necessary
Homocystinuria Elevated methionine and homocysteine	Infancy: nonspecific growth failure; developmental delay; more commonly diagnosed around 3 yr—mental retardation, seizures, behavioral disorders, early-onset thromboses, dislocated lenses, tall lanky body habitus	1:150,000 to 1:200,000; more prevalent in Ireland and New South Wales, Australia (1 in 60,000)	Methionine-restricted diet; vitamin B_6 supplement if responsive
Congenital adrenal hyperplasia (CAH) Elevated 24-hydroxyprogesterone; abnormal electrolytes	Hyponatremia, hyperkalemia, hypoglycemia, dehydration; weight loss; hypotension; shock in "salt wasting" type; female virilization; progressive virilization in both sexes	1:10,000 to 1:20,000; higher in Native Alaskans, 1 in 300	Reduce excessive corticotropins; replace glucocorticoids and mineral corticoids; corrective surgery for ambiguous genitalia (intersex assignment is controversial)
Sickle cell/hemoglobin SC (thalassemias)	Repeated infections, growth failure , pallor, hemolytic anemia; sickle cell crisis	Sickle cell anemia (SCA), 1 in 647 in non–African-Americans; 1 in 375 African-Americans; 1 in 36,000 Hispanics	Preventive care: treatment of meningococcal and pneumococcal infections; hydroxyurea (antisickling agent); prevent human parvovirus B19 infection (limits production of reticulocytes)
Biotinidase deficiency Deficient or absent activity of biotinidase on colorimetric assay	Myoclonic seizures, hypotonia, feeding difficulties, organic aciduria, fungal infections, ataxia, skin rash, hearing loss, alopecia, optic nerve atrophy, developmental delay, coma, and death	1:60,000 to 1:137,000	5-20 mg biotin daily; less with partial deficiency

PKU, Phenylketonuria; T_4, thyroxine, *TSH,* thyroid-stimulating hormone.

Source: DeBaun, M., & Vichinsky, E. (2007). Hemoglobinopathies. In R. Kliegman, R. Behrman, H. Jenson, & B. Stanton (Eds.), *Nelson textbook of pediatrics* (18th ed.). Philadelphia: Saunders; LaFranchini, S. (2007). Disorders of the thyroid gland. In R. Kliegman, R. Behrman, H. Jenson, & B. Stanton (Eds.), *Nelson textbook of pediatrics* (18th ed.). Philadelphia: Saunders; Lashley, F. (2002). Newborn screening: New opportunities and new challenges. *Newborn & Infant Nursing Reviews, 2*(4), 228-242; Rezvani, I. (2007). Metabolic diseases. In R. Kliegman, R. Behrman, H. Jenson, & B. Stanton (Eds.), *Nelson textbook of pediatrics* (18th ed.). Philadelphia: Saunders.

help prevent early developmental delays. To address this problem, the majority of states have enacted legislation mandating universal hearing screening. It is performed routinely in other states. The majority (95%) of newborns are screened for hearing loss in the United States before leaving the hospital (Joint Committee on Infant Hearing, 2007).

Two tests commonly are used to assess hearing function in the newborn. Initial screening is done with the evoked otoacoustic emissions (EOAE) test. The auditory brainstem response (ABR) test is used as follow-up if the initial screening is abnormal. Neither test is definitive in diagnosing hearing loss; they are used to determine whether further, more accurate hearing testing is needed through audiologic evaluation.

For the EOAE test, a soft rubber earpiece that makes a soft clicking noise is placed in the baby's outer ear (Fig. 24-9, *A*). A healthy ear will "echo" the click sound back to a microphone inside the earpiece that is in the baby's ear. The ABR test is performed by attaching sensors to the baby's forehead and behind each ear. An earphone is placed in the baby's outer ear and sends a series of quiet sounds into the sleeping baby's ear (Fig. 24-9, *B*). The sensors measure the responses of the baby's acoustic nerve. The responses are recorded and stored in a computer.

The Joint Committee on Infant Hearing (2007) recommends routine hearing screening for all newborns before hospital discharge or no later than 1 month of age. Through early hearing detection and intervention (EHDI) programs, the outcome for infants who are deaf or hard of hearing can be maximized. Using noninvasive technology, newborn hearing screening provides information about the pathways from the external ear to the cerebral cortex. Newborns who do not pass the initial screening test should have a comprehensive audiologic evaluation by 3 months of age. Regardless of the outcome of hearing testing, all infants should have regular and ongoing surveillance of developmental, hearing, and speech-language skills through regular well-child visits beginning at the age of 2 months so that any hearing loss may be promptly identified and treated (Joint Committee on Infant Hearing).

Collection of Specimens

Ongoing evaluation and screening of a newborn often requires obtaining blood by heelstick or venipuncture or the collection of a urine specimen. The nurse is responsible for collecting the necessary specimens in a manner that minimizes pain and trauma to the infant and maximizes the accuracy of test results.

Heelstick. Most blood specimens are drawn by laboratory technicians. Nurses, however, may be required to perform heelsticks to obtain blood for glucose monitoring or newborn screening. The same technique is used to obtain a blood sample or to test for PKU, galactosemia, hypothyroidism, or other IEMs (see Table 24-3).

Warming the heel before the sample is taken is often helpful; application of heat for 5 to 10 minutes helps dilate the vessels in the area. A cloth soaked with warm water and wrapped loosely around the foot provides effective warming. Disposable heel warmers also are available from a variety of companies but should be used with care to prevent burns. Nurses should wear gloves when collecting any specimen. The nurse cleanses the area with an appropriate skin antiseptic, restrains the infant's foot with a free hand, and then punctures the site. A spring-loaded automatic puncture device causes less pain and requires fewer punctures than a manual lance blade.

The most serious complication of an infant heelstick is necrotizing osteochondritis resulting from lancet penetration of the bone. To prevent this problem the stick should be made at the outer aspect of the heel and should penetrate no deeper than 2.4 mm. To identify the appropriate puncture site the nurse should draw an imaginary line from between the fourth and fifth toes and parallel to the lateral aspect of the foot to the heel where the stick should be made; a second line can be drawn from the great toe to the medial aspect of the heel (Fig. 24-10). Repeated trauma to the walking surface of the heel can cause fibrosis and scarring that can lead to problems with walking later in life.

After the specimen has been collected, pressure should be applied with a dry gauze square. No further skin cleanser should be applied because it will cause the site to continue to bleed. The site is then covered with an adhesive bandage. The nurse ensures proper disposal of equipment used, reviews the laboratory requisition for correct identification, and checks the specimen for accurate labeling and routing.

A heelstick is traumatic for the infant and causes pain. After several heelsticks, infants have been observed to withdraw their feet when they are touched. To reassure the infant and promote feelings of safety the neonate should be cuddled and

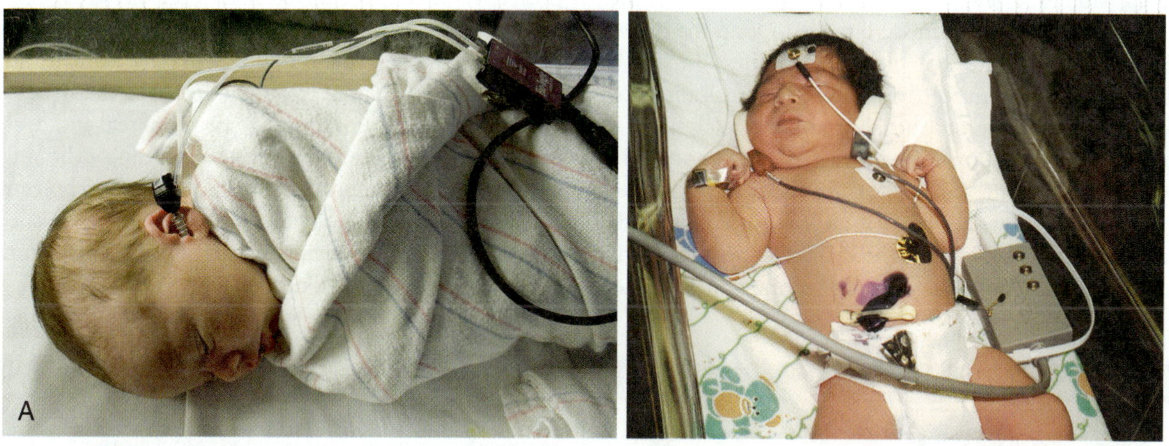

FIG. 24-9 Newborn hearing screening. **A,** Evoked otoacoustic emissions (EOAE) test. **B,** Auditory brain response (ABR)) test. (**A,** Courtesy Julie and Darren Nelson, Loveland, CO; **B,** courtesy Dee Lowdermilk, Chapel Hill, NC.)

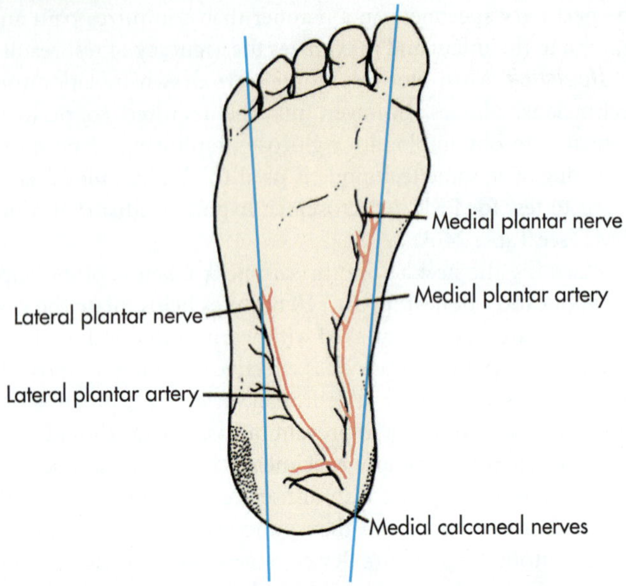

FIG. 24-10 Heelstick sites *(shaded areas)* on infant's foot for obtaining samples of capillary blood.

comforted when the procedure is complete and appropriate pain management measures taken to minimize the pain.

Venipuncture. Venous blood samples can be drawn from antecubital, saphenous, superficial wrist, and rarely, scalp veins. If an existing intravenous site is used to obtain a blood specimen, the type of infusion fluid is an important consideration; contamination of the blood sample with the fluid can alter the results.

When venipuncture is required, positioning of the needle is extremely important. Although regular venipuncture needles can be used, butterfly needles are sometimes preferred (Fig. 24-11). A 25-gauge needle is adequate for blood sampling in neonates, with minimal hemolysis occurring when the proper procedure is followed. Patience is required during the procedure because the blood return in small veins is slow, and consequently the small needle must remain in place longer than a larger needle. A tourniquet is optional but can help increase blood flow with venipuncture. The mummy restraint is commonly used to help secure the infant (Fig. 24-12). Other methods of restraint are illustrated in Figure 24-13.

If venipuncture or arterial puncture is being performed for blood gas studies, crying, fear, and agitation will affect the values; therefore, every effort must be made to keep the infant quiet during the procedure. For blood gas studies, the blood sample tubes are packed in ice (to reduce blood cell metabolism) and taken immediately to the laboratory for analysis.

Pressure must be maintained over an arterial or femoral vein puncture with a dry gauze square for at least 3 to 5 minutes to prevent bleeding from the site. For an hour after any venipuncture the nurse should observe the infant frequently for evidence of bleeding or hematoma formation at the puncture site.

> **! NURSING ALERT**
>
> Only venous or capillary blood samples can be used for newborn screening and genetic studies; cord blood is not used for such samples.

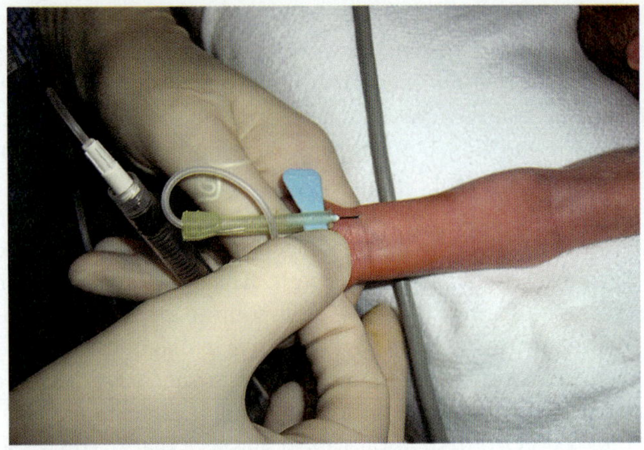

FIG. 24-11 Venipuncture using a butterfly needle. (Courtesy Cheryl Briggs, RNC, Annapolis, MD.)

The nurse assesses and documents the infant's tolerance of the procedure. The infant should be cuddled and comforted (e.g., rocked, given a pacifier) when the procedure is completed and appropriate pain management measures taken.

Obtaining a Urine Specimen. Analysis of urine is a valuable laboratory tool for infant assessment; the way in which the specimen is collected can influence the results. The urine sample should be fresh and analyzed within 1 hour of collection.

A variety of urine collection bags are available (Fig. 24-14). These containers are clear plastic, single-use bags with an adhesive material around the opening at the point of attachment.

To prepare the infant the nurse removes the diaper and places the infant in a supine position. The genitalia, perineum, and surrounding skin are washed and thoroughly dried because the adhesive on the bag will not stick to moist, powdered, or oily skin surfaces. The protective paper is removed to expose the adhesive (see Fig. 24-14, *A*). In female infants the perineum is stretched to flatten skinfolds; then the adhesive area on the bag is pressed firmly to the skin all around the urinary meatus and vagina. (NOTE: Start with the narrow portion of the butterfly-shaped adhesive patch.) Starting the application at the bridge of skin separating the rectum from the vagina and working upward is most effective (see Fig. 24-14, *B*). In male infants the penis (and scrotum, depending on the size of the collection device) is tucked through the opening into the collector before the protective paper is removed from the adhesive; the protective paper is then removed, and the flaps are pressed firmly onto the perineum, making sure the entire adhesive is firmly attached to skin and the edges of the opening do not pucker (see Fig. 24-14, *C*). This method helps ensure a leakproof seal and decreases the chance of contamination from stool. Cutting a slit in the diaper and pulling the bag through the slit can also help prevent leaking.

The diaper is carefully replaced, and the bag is checked frequently. When a sufficient amount of urine (this amount varies according to the test done) appears, the bag is removed. The infant's skin is observed for signs of irritation while the bag is in place. The specimen can be aspirated with a syringe or drained directly from the bag. For draining the bag is held in one hand and tilted to keep urine away from the tab. The tab is then removed and the urine is drained into a clean receptacle.

Collection of a 24-hour specimen from an infant can be a challenge; the infant may need light restraint with elbow

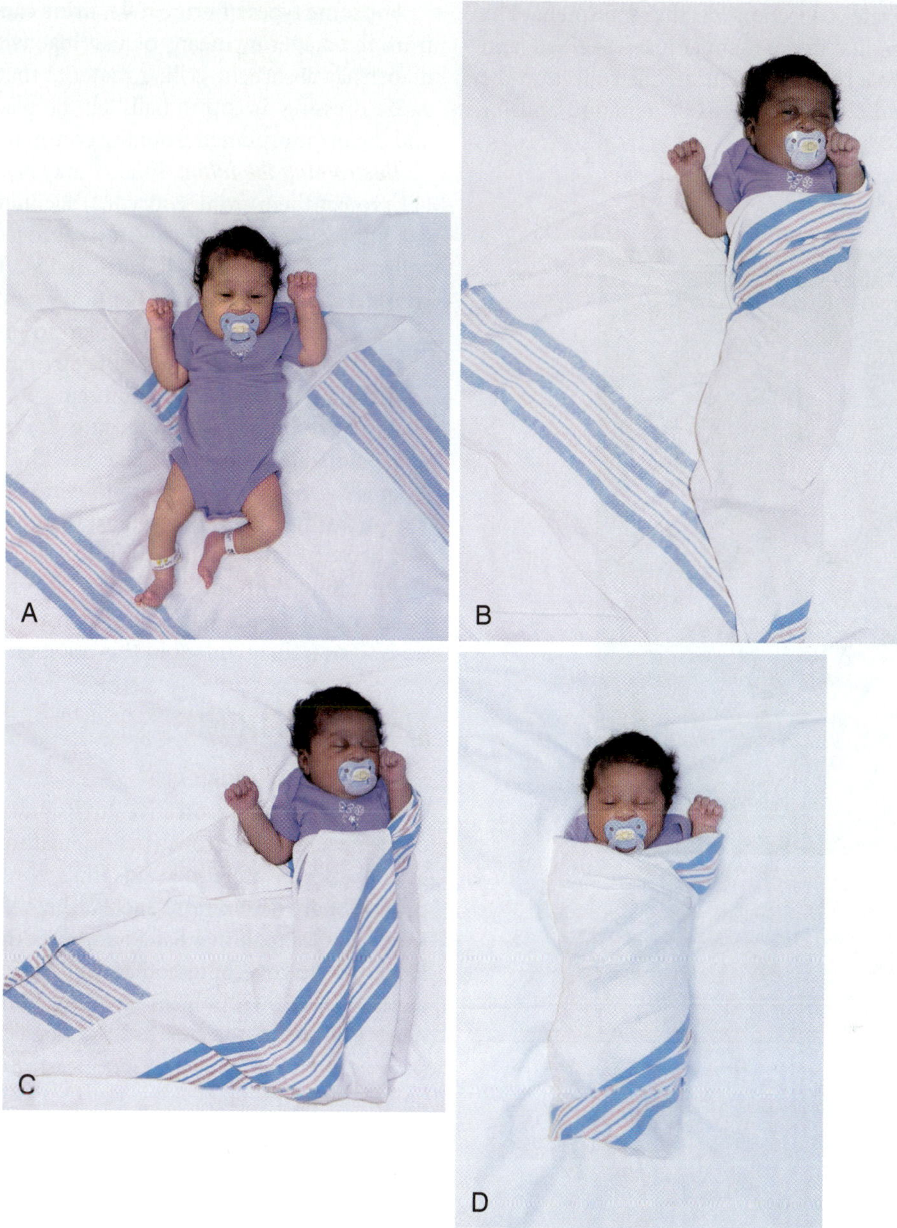

FIG. 24-12 Application of mummy restraint (swaddling). **A**, Infant is placed on folded corner of blanket. **B**, One corner of blanket is brought across body and secured beneath the body. **C**, Lower corner is folded and tucked and second corner is brought across body and secured. **D**, Modified mummy restraint with one hand uncovered. (Courtesy Cheryl Briggs, RNC, Annapolis, MD.)

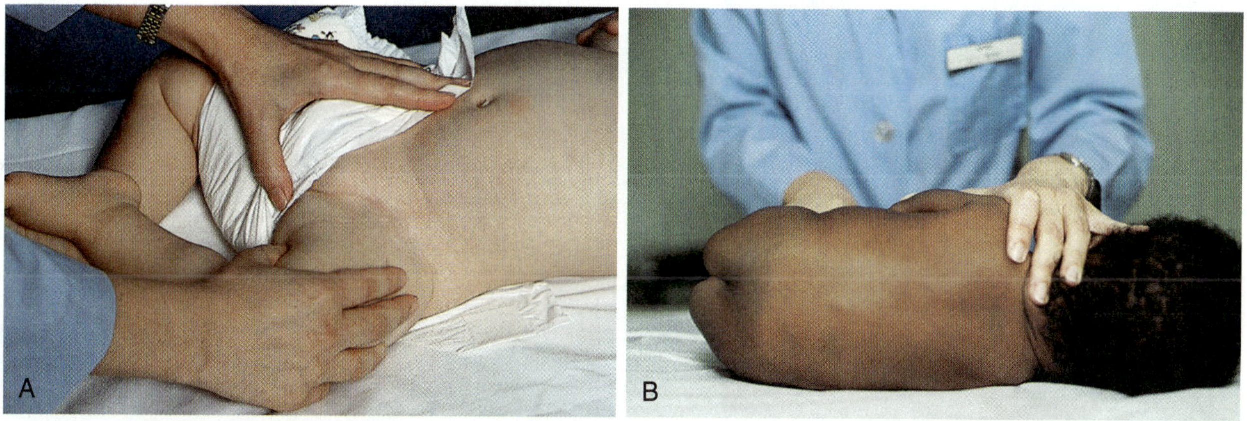

FIG. 24-13 Alternate methods of infant restraint. **A**, Restraining infant for femoral vein puncture. **B**, Modified side-lying position for lumbar puncture. (From Hockenberry, M. & Wilson, D. [2007]. *Wong's nursing care of infants and children* [8th ed.]. St. Louis: Mosby.)

restraints for appropriate collection of the specimen. The 24-hour urine bag is applied in the manner just described, and the urine is drained into a receptacle. During the collection the infant's skin is observed closely for signs of irritation and for lack of a proper seal.

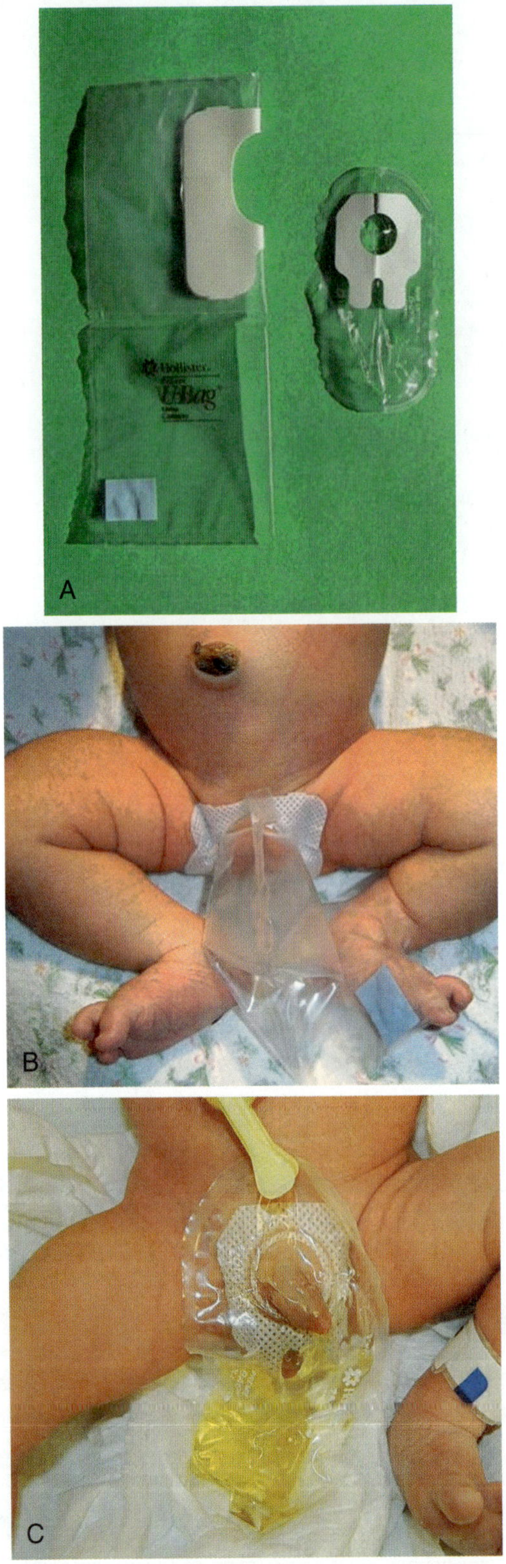

FIG. 24-14 Collection of urine specimen. **A**, Protective paper is removed from the adhesive surface. **B**, Applied to female infant. **C**, Applied to male infant. (Courtesy Cheryl Briggs, RNC, Annapolis, MD.)

For some types of urine tests, urine can be aspirated directly from the diaper by means of a syringe without a needle. If the diaper has absorbent gelling material that traps urine, a small gauze dressing or cotton balls can be placed inside the diaper and the urine aspirated from the cotton or gauze.

Restraining the Infant. Infants may need to be restrained to: (1) protect them from injury, (2) facilitate examinations, and (3) limit discomfort during tests, procedures, and specimen collections (see Figs. 24-12 and 24-13). The following special considerations must be kept in mind when restraining an infant:

- Apply restraints and check them to make sure they are not irritating the skin or impairing circulation.
- Maintain proper body alignment.
- Apply restraints without using knots or pins if possible. If knots are necessary, make the kind that can be released quickly. Use pins with care to eliminate the danger of their puncturing or pressing against the infant's skin.
- Check the infant hourly, or more frequently if indicated.

Restraint Without Appliance. The nurse can restrain the infant by using the hands and body. Figure 24-13 illustrates ways to restrain an infant in this manner.

INTERVENTIONS

Protective Environment

The provision of a protective environment is basic to the care of the newborn. The construction, maintenance, and operation of nurseries in accredited hospitals is monitored by national professional organizations such as the AAP, The Joint Commission, the Occupational Safety and Health Administration, and local or state governing bodies. In addition, hospital personnel develop their own policies and procedures for protecting the newborns under their care. Prescribed standards cover areas such as environmental factors, measures to control infection, and safety factors.

Environmental Factors. Environmental factors include provision of adequate lighting, elimination of potential fire hazards, safety of electrical appliances, adequate ventilation, and controlled temperature (i.e., warm and free of drafts) and humidity (i.e., 40% to 60%) (AAP & ACOG, 2007).

Infection Control Factors. Measures to control infection include adequate floor space to permit the positioning of bassinets at least 3 feet apart in all directions, handwashing facilities, and areas for cleaning and storing equipment and supplies. Only specified personnel directly involved in the care of mothers and infants are allowed in these areas, thereby reducing the opportunities for the transmission of pathogenic organisms.

> **! NURSING ALERT**
>
> Proper hand hygiene is essential to preventing the spread of health care associated infection. Personnel should wash hands with soap and water or use an alcohol-based handrub in accordance with hospital infection control policies. Hand hygiene should be performed before and after touching the infant, before an invasive procedure or medication administration, after contact with potentially contaminated objects (e.g., computer keyboards, telephone, countertop surfaces), and after removing sterile or nonsterile gloves (World Health Organization [WHO], 2009).

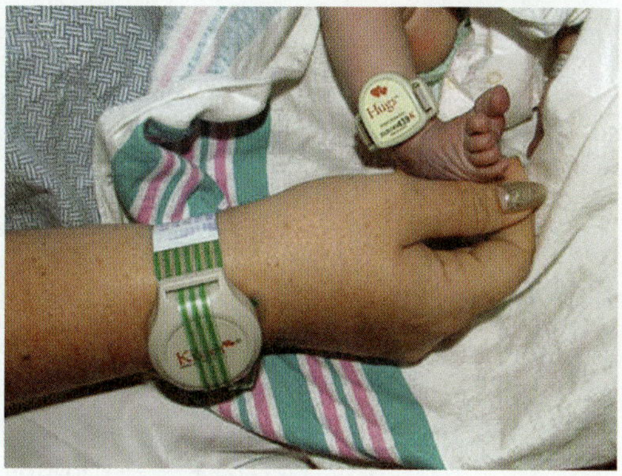

FIG. 24-15 Neonatal safety device. (Courtesy Shannon Perry, Phoenix, AZ.)

Health care workers must wear gloves when handling infants until blood and amniotic fluid have been removed from the skin, when drawing blood (e.g., heelstick), when caring for a fresh wound (e.g., circumcision), and during diaper changes.

Visitors such as siblings and grandparents are expected to perform hand hygiene before having contact with infants or equipment. Individuals with infectious conditions are excluded from contact with newborns or must take special precautions when working with infants. This group includes persons with upper respiratory tract infections, gastrointestinal tract infections, and infectious skin conditions.

Safety Factors. Health care institutions must be proactive in protecting newborns from abductions. Examples of measures taken include placing matching identification bracelets on infants and their parents, using identification bands with radiofrequency transmitters (Fig. 24-15) that set off an alarm if the bracelet is removed or if a certain threshold is crossed (doorway to exit the unit or building), and footprinting or taking identification pictures immediately after birth, before the infant leaves the mother's side. In addition, agencies must conduct periodic unit- and hospital-wide drills aimed at preventing newborn abductions. Personnel caring for newborns must be clearly identified by photo identification, and parents must be educated regarding measures to prevent abduction from the mother's room (i.e., be certain they know the identity of anyone who cares for the infant and never to release the infant to anyone who is not wearing the appropriate identification). Parents are educated before discharge regarding measures to minimize the risk for abduction from the home setting.

Therapeutic and Surgical Procedures

Intramuscular Injection. Administering a single dose of 0.5 to 1 mg of vitamin K intramuscularly to an infant is routine soon after birth (see the Medication Guide box on p. 573).

Hepatitis B (HB) vaccination is recommended for all infants. Infants at highest risk for contracting HB are those born to women who have hepatitis or whose HB status is unknown. If the infant is born to an infected mother or to a mother who is a chronic carrier, HB vaccine and HB immune globulin (HBIG) should be administered within 12 hours of birth (see the Medication Guides: Hepatitis B Vaccine, and Hepatitis B Immune Globulin). The HB vaccine is given in one site and the HBIG in another. For infants born to HB-negative women the first dose of the vaccine can be given at birth or at 1 month of age. Parental consent should be obtained before administering these vaccines.

MEDICATION GUIDE

Hepatitis B Vaccine (Recombivax HB, Engerix-B)

ACTION

Hepatitis B vaccine induces protective antihepatitis B antibodies in 95% to 99% of healthy infants who receive the recommended three doses. The duration of protection of the vaccine is unknown.

INDICATION

Hepatitis B vaccine is for immunization against infection caused by all known subtypes of hepatitis B virus (HBV).

NEONATAL DOSAGE

The usual dosage is Recombivax HB, 5 mg/0.5 ml, or Engerix-B, 10 mg/0.5 ml, at 0, 1, and 6 months. An alternate dosing schedule is 0, 1, 2, and 12 months and is usually for newborns whose mothers were hepatitis B surface antigen (HBsAg) positive.

ADVERSE REACTIONS

Common adverse reactions are rash, fever, erythema, swelling, and pain at injection site.

NURSING CONSIDERATIONS

Parental consent must be obtained before administration. Wear gloves. Administer in the middle third of the vastus lateralis muscle by using a 25-gauge, 5/8-inch needle. Inject into skin that has been cleaned, or allow alcohol to dry on puncture site for 1 minute to remove organisms and prevent infection. Stabilize the leg firmly and grasp the muscle between the thumb and fingers. Insert the needle at a 90-degree angle; release the muscle; aspirate, and inject the medication slowly if no blood return occurs. Massage the site with a dry gauze square after removing the needle to increase absorption. If the infant was born to HBsAg positive mother, hepatitis B immune globulin (HBIG) should be given within 12 hours of birth in addition to the hepatitis B vaccine. Separate sites must be used.

Selection of the appropriate equipment and site for injection is important. In most cases a 25-gauge, 5/8-inch needle should be used for the vitamin K and HB vaccine injections. Injections must be given in muscles large enough to accommodate the medication, and major nerves and blood vessels must be avoided. The muscles of newborns may not tolerate more than a 0.5 ml per intramuscular injection. The preferred injection site for newborns is the vastus lateralis (Fig. 24-16). The dorsogluteal muscle is very small, poorly developed, and dangerously close to the sciatic nerve, which occupies a proportionately larger area in infants than in older children. Therefore, it is not recommended as an injection site in small children. The newborn's deltoid muscle has an inadequate amount of muscle for intramuscular administration. A key factor in preventing and minimizing local reaction to intramuscular injections is adequate deposition of the medication deep within the muscle; therefore, muscle size, needle length, and amount of medication injected should be carefully considered.

The nurse wears nonsterile gloves when administering an injection. The neonate's leg should be stabilized. The nurse cleanses the injection site with an appropriate skin antiseptic, then stabilizes the infant's muscle between the thumb and forefinger. The needle is inserted into the vastus lateralis at a 90-degree angle. The plunger of the syringe is gently withdrawn, and if no blood is aspirated, the medication is injected. If blood

Video— Nursing Skill: Administering Intramuscular Injections to a Newborn

MEDICATION GUIDE

Hepatitis B Immune Globulin

ACTION

Hepatitis B immune globulin (HBIG) provides a high titer of antibody to hepatitis B surface antigen (HBsAg).

INDICATION

The HBIG vaccine provides prophylaxis against infection in infants born of HBsAg-positive mothers.

NEONATAL DOSAGE

Administer one 0.5-mL dose intramuscularly within 12 hours of birth.

ADVERSE REACTIONS

Hypersensitivity may occur.

NURSING CONSIDERATIONS

The HBIG vaccine must be given within 12 hours of birth. Wear gloves. Administer in the middle third of the vastus lateralis muscle by using a 25-gauge, 5/8-inch needle. Inject the vaccine into skin that has been cleaned, or allow alcohol to dry on puncture site for 1 minute to remove organisms and prevent infection. Stabilize the leg firmly, and grasp the muscle between the thumb and fingers. Insert the needle at a 90-degree angle; release the muscle; and inject the medication slowly if no blood return occurs. Massage the site with a dry gauze square after removing needle to increase absorption. The HBIG vaccine can be given at the same time as the hepatitis B vaccine but at a different site.

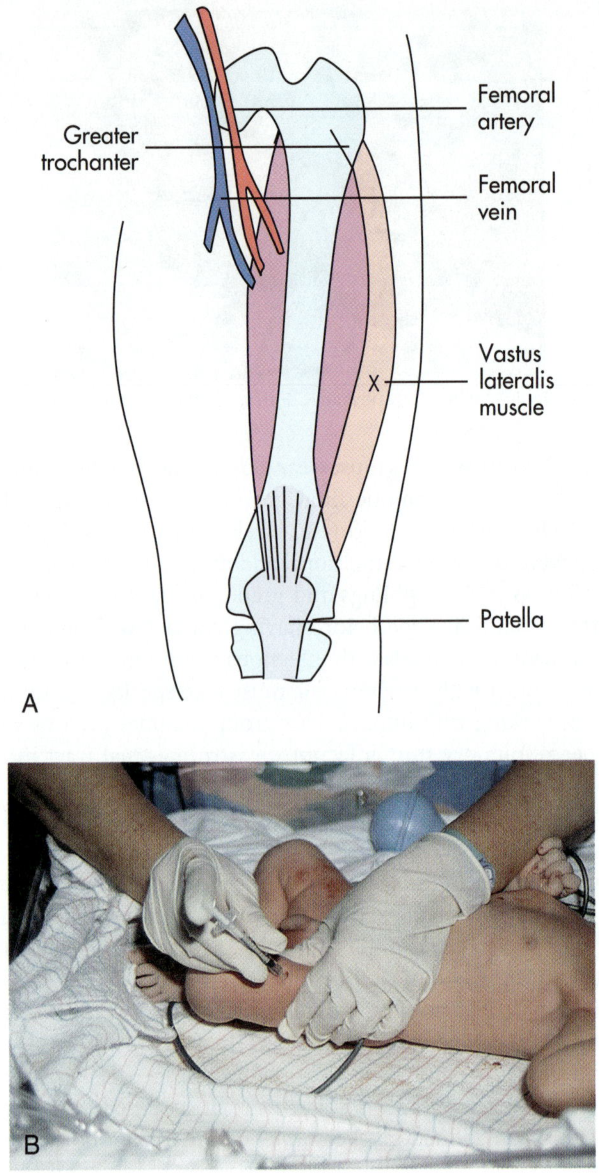

FIG. 24-16 Intramuscular injection. **A**, Acceptable intramuscular injection site for newborn infant. *X*, Injection site. **B**, Infant's leg stabilized for intramuscular injection. Nurse is wearing gloves to give injection. (**B**, Courtesy Marjorie Pyle, RNC, Lifecircle, Costa Mesa, CA.)

is aspirated, the needle is withdrawn. A new needle is used and the injection is given in another site after proper cleansing and checking for aspiration of blood. After the medication is injected, the nurse withdraws the needle quickly and applies gentle pressure at the site to minimize pain and bleeding.

The nurse should always remember to comfort the infant after an injection and to discard equipment properly. Needles should never be recapped but should be properly discarded in an appropriate safety container. The name of the medication, date and time, amount, route, and site of injection must be recorded in the newborn's record.

Therapy for Hyperbilirubinemia. The best therapy for hyperbilirubinemia is prevention. Because bilirubin is excreted in meconium, prevention can be facilitated by early feeding, which stimulates the passage of meconium. However, despite early passage of meconium, the term infant can have trouble conjugating the increased amount of bilirubin derived from disintegrating fetal RBCs. As a result, the serum levels of unconjugated bilirubin can rise beyond normal limits, causing hyperbilirubinemia. The goal of treatment of hyperbilirubinemia is to help reduce the newborn's serum levels of unconjugated bilirubin. The two principal ways of reaching this goal are phototherapy and, rarely, exchange blood transfusion. Exchange transfusion is used to treat infants whose levels of serum bilirubin are rising rapidly despite the use of intensive phototherapy (see Chapter 36).

Phototherapy. The purpose of phototherapy is to reduce the level of circulating unconjugated bilirubin or to keep it from increasing. Phototherapy uses light energy to change the shape and structure of unconjugated bilirubin and convert it to molecules that can be excreted. The dose and effectiveness of phototherapy are affected by the source of light. Phototherapy units vary in the spectrum of light they deliver and in the filters that are used. Most units use daylight, cool white, blue, or special blue fluorescent bulbs. The most effective therapy is achieved with the special blue light or a specially designed light-emitting diode (LED) light. Phototherapy lights do not emit significant ultraviolet radiation; the small amount that is emitted does not cause erythema. Most of the ultraviolet light is absorbed by the glass wall of the fluorescent tube and by the plastic cover of the light (AAP Subcommittee on Hyperbilirubinemia, 2004; Maisels & McDonagh, 2008).

Phototherapy is usually effective for treatment of hyperbilirubinemia that has not reached levels associated with acute bilirubin encephalopathy or kernicterus. Guidelines for the use of phototherapy were developed by the AAP Subcommittee on Hyperbilirubinemia (2004).

The effectiveness of phototherapy is related to the distance between the light and the neonate and on the area of skin that

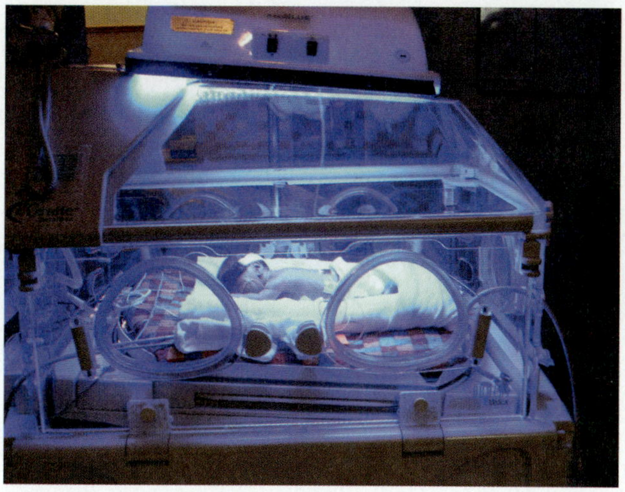

FIG. 24-17 Infant under phototherapy lights while in incubator. (Courtesy Randi and Jacob Wills, Clayton, NC.)

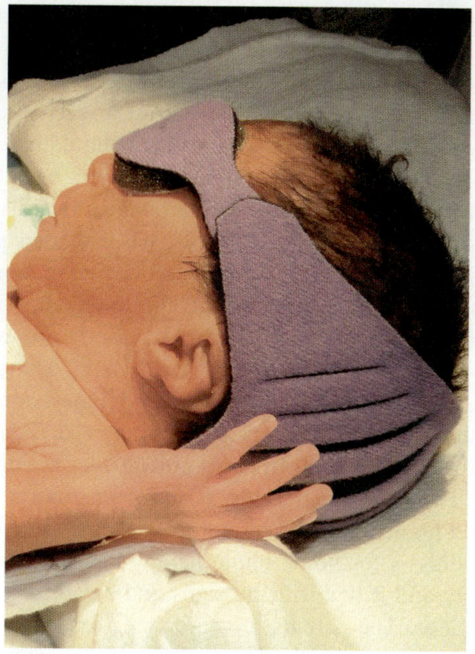

FIG. 24-18 Infant with eyes covered while receiving phototherapy. (Courtesy Cheryl Briggs, RNC, Annapolis, MD.)

is exposed. During phototherapy the unclothed infant is placed under a bank of lights approximately 45 to 50 cm from the light source. Phototherapy can be used for the infant in an incubator (Fig. 24-17) or in an open crib. The distance varies according to unit protocol and type of light used. The lamp's energy output should be monitored routinely with a photometer during treatment to ensure efficacy of therapy. Phototherapy is used until the infant's serum bilirubin level decreases to within an acceptable range. The decision to discontinue therapy is based on the observation of a definite downward trend in the bilirubin values.

The infant's eyes must be protected by an opaque mask to prevent overexposure to the light. The eye shield should cover the eyes completely but not occlude the nares. Before the mask is applied the infant's eyes should be closed gently to prevent excoriation of the corneas. The mask should be removed periodically and during infant feedings so that the eyes can be checked and cleansed with water and the parents can have visual contact with the infant (Fig. 24-18).

It is usually unnecessary to remove the newborn's diaper during phototherapy, although with rising bilirubin levels the diaper may need to be removed until levels show a significant decline (Maisels & McDonagh, 2008). To promote optimal skin exposure during phototherapy a "string bikini" made from a disposable face mask is often used instead of a diaper, which allows optimal skin exposure and provides protection for the genitals and the bedding. Before use the metal strip must be removed from the mask to prevent burning the infant. Lotions and ointments should not be used during phototherapy because they absorb heat and can cause burns.

Phototherapy can cause changes in the infant's temperature, depending partially on the bed used: bassinet, incubator, or radiant warmer. The infant's temperature should be closely monitored. Phototherapy lights can increase the rate of insensible water loss, which contributes to fluid loss and dehydration. Therefore, the infant must be adequately hydrated. Hydration maintenance in the healthy newborn is accomplished with human milk or infant formula; administering glucose water or plain water has no advantage or benefit because these liquids do not promote excretion of bilirubin in the stools and may actually perpetuate enterohepatic circulation, thus delaying bilirubin excretion.

It is important to closely monitor urinary output while the infant is receiving phototherapy. Urine output can be decreased or unaltered; the urine can have a dark gold or brown appearance.

The number and consistency of stools are monitored. Bilirubin breakdown increases gastric motility, which results in loose stools that can cause skin excoriation and breakdown. The infant's buttocks must be cleaned after each stool to help maintain skin integrity. A fine maculopapular rash can appear during phototherapy, but this condition is transient.

In addition to phototherapy lights other systems are used for phototherapy. A bassinet system provides special blue light above and beneath the infant. A bilirubin blanket is a woven fiberoptic blanket pad connected to a light source. The blanket is flexible and can be placed around the infant's torso or underneath the infant in the bassinet. There are also bilirubin beds with LED lights in a pad that covers the surface of the bassinet. The LEDs do not produce heat and can be used with radiant warmers. These devices are usually less effective when used alone as compared with conventional phototherapy lights. They can be very useful in combination with overhead phototherapy lights. In certain instances the infant's bilirubin levels are increasing rapidly and intensive phototherapy is required; this situation involves the use of a combination of conventional lights and fiberoptic blankets to maximize bilirubin reduction. Although fiberoptic lights do not produce heat as do conventional lights, staff should ensure that a covering pad is placed between the infant's skin and the fiberoptic device to prevent skin burns, especially in preterm infants. The newborn can remain in the mother's room in an open crib or in her arms during treatment. The use of eye patches depends on whether the devices are used alone or in combination with phototherapy lights.

Parent Education. Serum levels of bilirubin in the newborn continue to rise until the fifth day of life. Many parents leave the hospital within 24 hours of birth, and some as early as 6 hours after birth. Therefore, parents must receive education regarding jaundice and its treatment. They should have written instructions for assessing the infant's condition and the name of a contact person for reporting their findings and raising their concerns. Some institutions or third-party providers pay for a home visit to evaluate the infant's condition and to monitor the mother's health. If measuring serum bilirubin levels proves necessary after discharge from the hospital, a health care technician or nurse may draw the blood for the specimen, or the parents may take the baby to a laboratory to have blood drawn for a serum bilirubin. In some cases, parents may take the newborn to an outpatient clinic or physician's office to be evaluated.

Home Phototherapy. Healthy term infants may at times be discharged home and need phototherapy for hyperbilirubinemia. Candidates for home phototherapy include infants who are healthy and active with no signs and symptoms of other complications. The parents or other caregivers must be willing and able to assume the responsibility for therapy maintenance and monitoring, and the home environment should be adequate with a telephone, heat, and electricity. Fiberoptic bilirubin blankets are often used for home phototherapy.

The company that provides the home therapy equipment is responsible for setting up the phototherapy unit and teaching the parents or caregivers how to use the equipment. The home care nurse schedules home visits to assess the infant's response to therapy, including weight, feeding, output, and temperature stability. Additional education of parents may be necessary; their understanding of the therapy and their responsibilities is assessed. Blood may be drawn for laboratory work and results reported to the primary health care provider. When therapy is discontinued, follow-up visits for monitoring may be ordered. The equipment company is called to arrange for pick-up of the phototherapy unit.

Video—Nursing Skills: Assisting with a Circumcision

Video—Assessment: Circumcision

Circumcision. Circumcision is the removal of all or part of the foreskin (prepuce) of the penis. Most often it is performed during the first few days of life, but is sometimes done at a later time for religious or cultural reasons.

Circumcision was the third most common inpatient surgical procedure in the United States in 2005. Approximately 56% of male newborns were circumcised prior to hospital discharge; this is a decline from a high of 65% in 1980 (Merrill, Nagamine, & Steiner, 2008).

The AAP Task Force on Circumcision issued a policy statement on newborn circumcision in 1999 and reaffirmed the policy in 2005 (AAP, 2005; AAP Task Force on Circumcision, 1999). The policy states that "existing scientific evidence demonstrates potential medical benefits of newborn male circumcision; however, these data are not sufficient to recommend routine neonatal circumcision" (AAP Task Force on Circumcision, p. 686). The task force further recommended that if circumcision is performed, procedural analgesia should be used. ACOG (2001) issued similar recommendations regarding newborn circumcision.

There is ongoing discussion and controversy among health care experts related to newborn circumcision as scientific evidence emerges. Proponents of circumcision cite health advantages such as decreased incidence of urinary tract infection in infants less than 1 year of age; reduced risk of penile cancer, phimosis, paraphimosis, and balanitis; and decreased risk for sexually transmitted infections including HIV and human papillomavirus. They note a low rate of complications and no substantial negative effect on sexual function. Opponents of circumcision feel that the procedure is unnatural and unnecessary. They cite risks related to acute complications such as hemorrhage, infection, and penile injury (removal of excessive skin, damage to the meatus or glans) and long-term implications such as adverse effects on sexual function and pleasure. Other negative aspects of newborn circumcision are acute pain and long-term psychologic effects (Brady, 2010).

Recent evidence from well-designed, well-controlled studies in Africa indicates that male circumcision can prevent acquisition of HIV, herpes simplex 2, and human papillomavirus (Auvert, Taljaard, Lagarde, Sobngwi-Tambekou, Sitta, & Puren, 2005; Bailey, Moses, Parker, Agot, Maclean, Krieger, et al., 2007; Gray, Kigozi, Serwadda, Makumbi, Watya, Nalugoda, et al., 2007; Siegfried, Muller, Deeks, & Volmink, 2009). Whereas it is clear that prevalence rates for HIV are lower in the United States, the studies provide evidence that newborn circumcision can reduce the risk of HIV by about 16% (Sansom, Prabhu, Hutchinson, An, Hall, Shrestha, et al., 2010). The World Health Organization (WHO) recognizes male circumcision as an important intervention in reducing the risk of heterosexually acquired HIV in men (Joint United Nations Programme on HIV/AIDS, 2007).

Circumcision is a matter of personal parental choice. Parents usually decide to have their newborn circumcised for one or more of the following reasons: hygiene, religious conviction, tradition, culture, or social norms. Cost and insurance coverage are considerations in the parents' decision-making process. Some private insurance companies no longer cover circumcision. Medicaid does not cover the cost of circumcision in 16 states. Interestingly, in those states circumcision rates are 24% lower than in states with Medicaid coverage (Leibowitz, Desmond, & Belin, 2009). This is another point of controversy because the lack of Medicaid coverage unfairly affects disadvantaged minorities; as adults, they have the highest risk of sexually transmitted infections (STIs) and HIV. Parents need to make an informed choice regarding newborn circumcision based on the most current evidence and recommendations. Health care providers and nurses who care for childbearing families should provide factual, unbiased information regarding circumcision and give parents opportunities to discuss the benefits and risks of the procedure.

Circumcision is not performed immediately after birth because of the danger of cold stress and decreased clotting factors, but is usually done in the hospital before discharge. The circumcision of a Jewish male infant is commonly performed on the eighth day after birth at home in a ceremony called a bris. This timing is logical from a physiologic standpoint because clotting factors decrease somewhat immediately after birth and do not return to prebirth levels until the end of the first week.

Feedings are usually withheld up to 2 to 3 hours before the circumcision to prevent vomiting and aspiration. To prepare the infant for the circumcision, he is positioned on a plastic restraint form (Fig. 24-19), and the penis is cleansed with soap and water or a preparatory solution such as povidone-iodine.

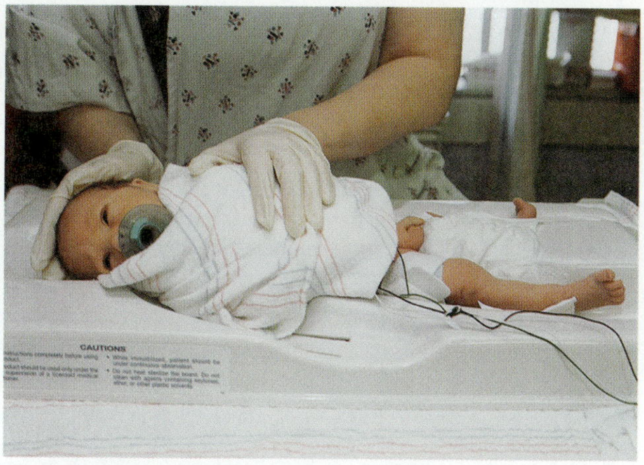

FIG. 24-19 Proper positioning of infant for circumcision. (Photo by Paul Vincent Kuntz, Texas Children's Hospital, Houston, TX.)

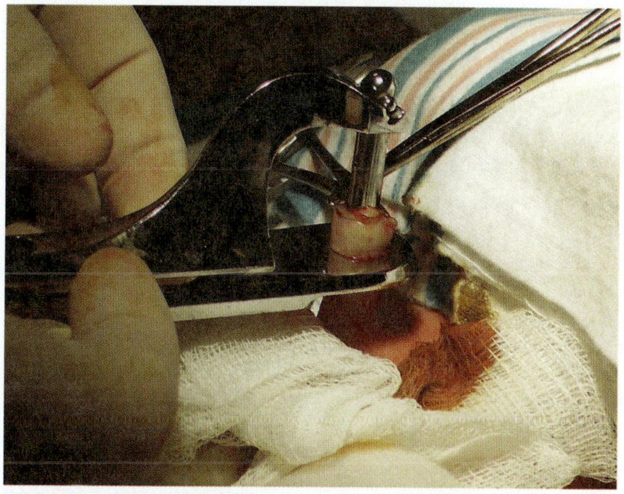

FIG. 24-20 Circumcision with Yellen clamp. After hemostasis occurs, the prepuce (over cone) will be cut away. (Courtesy Cheryl Briggs, RNC, Annapolis, MD.)

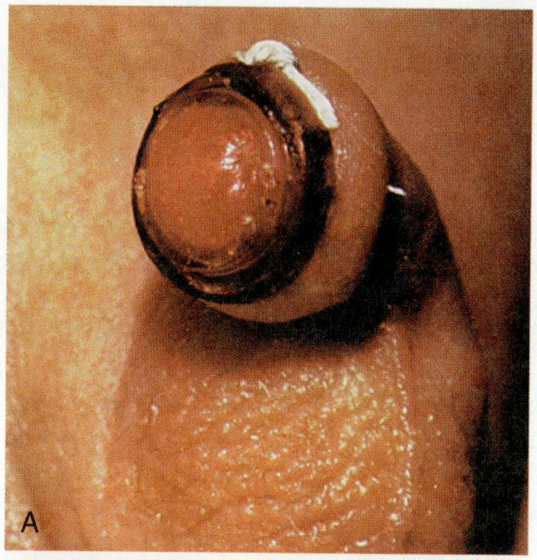

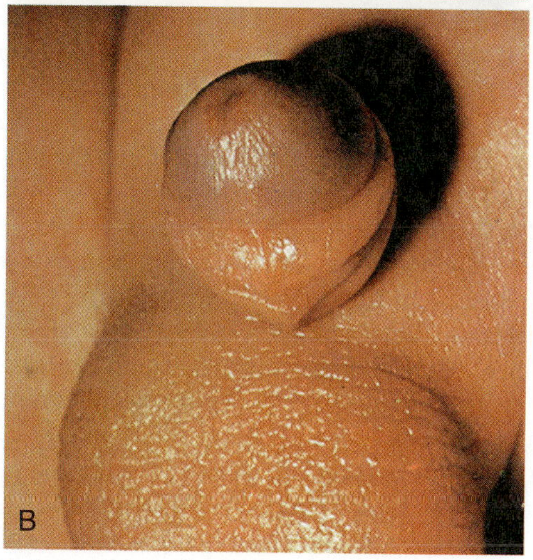

FIG. 24-21 Circumcision using Hollister PlastiBell. **A**, Suture around rim of PlastiBell controls bleeding. **B**, Plastic rim and suture drop off in 7 to 10 days. (Permission to use or reproduce this copyrighted material has been granted by the owner, Hollister, Inc., Libertyville, IL.)

The infant is draped to provide warmth and a sterile field, and the sterile equipment is readied for use.

The circumcision procedure itself takes only a few minutes. Although some circumcision procedures require no special equipment or appliances, the most common procedures for newborn circumcision involve the use of specific devices: the Yellen (Gomco) clamp or the PlastiBell device. The Mogen clamp is often used by Jewish mohels for ceremonial circumcision.

With the Yellen (Gomco) clamp technique, a metal bell is placed over the glans and the foreskin is pulled over the bell, which is then fit into a metal baseplate. The device crushes the foreskin between the bell and the baseplate. The foreskin is then excised with a scalpel (Fig. 24-20). Following the procedure, a small petrolatum gauze dressing is applied to the glans. Thereafter, petroleum gauze or a generous amount of petrolatum ointment is applied to the penis for the first few days to prevent the diaper from adhering to the glans. It may be necessary to gently retract the skin of the penile shaft if it starts to encroach on the glans. Some health care providers recommend doing this with each diaper change to prevent adhesions from forming.

When the PlastiBell device is used for circumcision, a plastic bell is placed between the glans and the foreskin; the foreskin is pulled forward over the bell and suture is tied around the rim of the bell, leaving a plastic rim in place. Excess foreskin is usually excised. The suture cuts off blood supply to the foreskin, causing it to wither. Within 5 to 7 days, the plastic rim falls off, along with the foreskin (Fig. 24-21). Petrolatum is not usually needed when the PlastiBell is used.

Procedural Pain Management. Circumcision is painful. The pain is characterized by both physiologic and behavioral changes in the infant (see discussion that follows). Four types of anesthesia and analgesia are used in newborns who undergo circumcisions: ring block, dorsal penile nerve block (DPNB), topical anesthetic such as eutectic mixture of local anesthetic (EMLA) (prilocaine-lidocaine) or LMX4 (4% lidocaine), and concentrated oral sucrose. Nonpharmacologic methods such as nonnutritive sucking, containment, and swaddling can be used to enhance pain management. The Cochrane group exploring pain relief for neonatal circumcision (Brady-Fryer, Wiebe, & Lander, 2004) found that DPNB was the most effective intervention for decreasing the pain of circumcision. A DPNB includes subcutaneous injections of buffered lidocaine at the 2 o'clock and 10 o'clock positions at the base of the penis. A ring block is the injection of buffered lidocaine administered subcutaneously on each side of the penile shaft. The circumcision should not be performed for at least 5 minutes after these injections.

A topical cream containing prilocaine-lidocaine such as EMLA can be applied to the base of the penis at least 1 hour before the circumcision. The area where the prepuce attaches to the glans is well coated with 1 g of the cream and then covered with a transparent occlusive dressing or finger cot. Just before the procedure, the cream is removed. Blanching or redness of the skin may occur.

After the circumcision the infant is comforted until he is quieted. If the parents were not present during the procedure, the infant is returned to them. The infant can be fussy for several hours and can have disturbed sleep-wake states and disorganized feeding behaviors. Oral liquid acetaminophen may be administered after the procedure every 4 hours (as ordered by the practitioner) for a maximum of five doses in 24 hours or a maximum of 75 mg/kg/day.

Care of the Newly Circumcised Infant. Postcircumcision protocols vary. In many settings, the circumcision site is assessed for bleeding every 15 to 30 minutes for the first hour and then hourly for the next 4 to 6 hours. The nurse monitors the infant's urinary output, noting the time and amount of the first voiding after the circumcision.

If bleeding occurs from the circumcision site, the nurse applies gentle pressure with a folded sterile gauze square. A hemostatic agent such as Gelfoam® powder or sponge can be applied to help control bleeding. If bleeding is not easily controlled, a blood vessel may need to be ligated. In this event, one nurse notifies the physician and prepares the necessary equipment (i.e., circumcision tray and suture material), while another nurse maintains intermittent pressure until the physician arrives.

Nurses provide education for parents related to care of the circumcised infant, which includes observing for complications such as bleeding or infection (see Box 24-7). Parents need support and encouragement as they perform postcircumcision care. Newborns typically cry when the diaper is changed and when petrolatum gauze is removed and reapplied. This can make new parents feel anxious because they do not want to inflict pain on the infant. Nurses can inform parents that the discomfort is usually temporary and will soon subside.

Nursing actions are planned and implemented to prevent infection. Prepackaged commercial wipes should not be used because they contain alcohol, which delays healing and causes discomfort. Instead, the nurse washes the penis gently with water to remove urine and feces and, if necessary, applies fresh petrolatum around the glans after each diaper change. The glans penis, normally dark red during healing, becomes covered with a yellow exudate in about 24 hours, which is part of normal healing, not an infective process. No attempt should be made to remove the exudate, which persists for 2 to 3 days. Parents should be taught to apply the diaper so that it does not press on the circumcised area. They should be encouraged to change the diaper at least every 4 hours to prevent it from sticking to the penis.

BOX 24-7 CARE OF THE CIRCUMCISED NEWBORN AT HOME

- Wash hands before touching the newly circumcised penis.

CHECK FOR BLEEDING

- Check circumcision for bleeding with each diaper change.
- If bleeding occurs, apply gentle pressure with a folded sterile gauze square. If bleeding does not stop with pressure, notify primary health care provider.

OBSERVE FOR URINATION

- Check to see that the infant urinates after being circumcised.
- Infant should have a wet diaper 2 to 6 times per 24 hours the first 1 to 2 days after birth, then at least 6 to 8 times per 24 hours after 3 to 4 days.

KEEP AREA CLEAN

- Change the diaper and inspect the circumcision at least every 4 hours.
- Wash the penis gently with warm water to remove urine and feces. Apply petrolatum to the glans with each diaper change (omit petrolatum if a PlastiBell was used).
- Do not wash the penis with soap until the circumcision is healed (5 to 6 days).
- Apply the diaper loosely over the penis to prevent pressure on the circumcised area.

CHECK FOR INFECTION

- Glans penis is dark red after circumcision, then becomes covered with yellow exudate in 24 hours, which is normal and will persist for 2 to 3 days. Do not attempt to remove it.
- Redness, swelling, discharge, or odor indicates infection. Notify the primary health care provider if you think the circumcision area is infected.

PROVIDE COMFORT

- Circumcision is painful. Handle the area gently.
- Provide extra holding, feeding, and opportunities for nonnutritive sucking for a day or two.

Neonatal Pain

Pain has physiologic and psychologic components. Its psychologic component and the diffuse total body response to pain exhibited by the neonate led many health care providers in the past to believe that infants, especially preterm infants, do not experience pain. The central nervous system is well developed, however, as early as 24 weeks of gestation. The peripheral and spinal structures that transmit pain information are present and functional between the first and second trimesters. The pituitary-adrenal axis is also well developed at this time, and a fight-or-flight reaction is observed in response to the catecholamines released in response to stress.

The physiologic response to pain in neonates can be life threatening. Pain response can decrease tidal volume, increase demands on the cardiovascular system, increase metabolism, and cause neuroendocrine imbalance. The hormonal-metabolic response to pain in a term infant has greater magnitude and shorter duration than that in adults. The newborn's sympathetic response to pain is less mature and therefore less predictable than an adult's.

Neonatal Responses to Pain. Pain response is influenced by a variety of factors such as characteristics of the painful stimulus, gestational age, biologic factors, and behavioral state. The source, location, and timing of the pain affect the response; newborns respond differently to acute pain than to prolonged or recurrent pain. In general, infants of younger gestational ages seem to display less vigorous pain responses. There can be

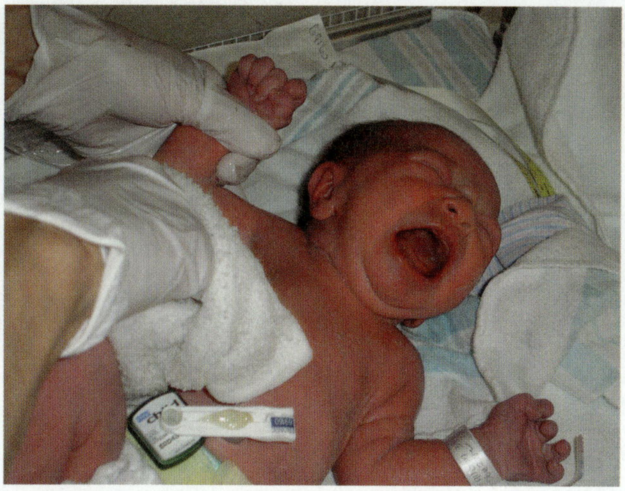

FIG. 24-22 Signs of discomfort: note eye squeeze, brow bulge, nasolabial furrow, and wide-spread mouth (Courtesy Kathryn Alden, Chapel Hill, NC.)

genetic differences in pain responses related to the amount and type of neurotransmitters and receptors available to mediate pain. The behavioral state of the neonate also affects the pain response. Those who are more awake tend to have more robust pain responses than those in sleep states (Walden, 2007).

The most common behavioral sign of pain is a vocalization or crying, ranging from a whimper to a distinctive high-pitched, shrill cry. Facial expressions include grimacing, eye squeeze, brow contraction, deepened nasolabial furrows, a taut and quivering tongue, and an open mouth (Fig. 24-22). The infant will flex and adduct the upper body and lower limbs in an attempt to withdraw from the painful stimulus. The preterm infant has a lower than normal threshold for initiation of this flex response. An infant who receives a muscle-paralyzing agent such as vecuronium will be unable to mount a behavioral or visible pain response.

Pain can result in significant changes in heart rate, blood pressure (increased or decreased), intracranial pressure, vagal tone, respiratory rate, and oxygen saturation. Neonates respond to painful stimuli with release of epinephrine, norepinephrine, glucagon, corticosterone, cortisol, 11-deoxycorticosterone, lactate, pyruvate, and glucose (Walden & Gibbins, 2008).

Assessment of Neonatal Pain. In assessing pain the nurse needs to consider the health of the neonate, the type and duration of the painful stimulus, environmental factors, and the infant's state of alertness. For example, severely compromised neonates may be unable to generate a pain response, although they are in fact experiencing pain.

Every client should have an initial pain assessment, as well as a pain management plan; this mandate includes newborns. The National Association of Neonatal Nurses (NANN) developed practice guidelines stating that all nurses who care for newborns should have education and competency validation in pain assessment. Pain should be assessed and documented on a regular basis (Walden & Gibbins, 2008).

Several pain assessment tools have been developed for use with neonates. A combination of behavioral and physiologic indicators of pain is used to diagnose and differentiate infant pain levels. Tools that have been shown to have validity and reliability include the Neonatal Infant Pain Scale (NIPS) (Lawrence, Alcock, McGrath, Kay, MacMurray, & Dulberg, 1993) and the Premature Infant Pain Profile (PIPP) (Stevens, Johnston, Petryshen, & Taddio, 1996). A pain assessment tool used by nurses in the NICU is CRIES (Krechel & Bildner, 1995) (Table 24-4). This tool was developed for use by nurses who work with preterm and term infants. CRIES is an acronym for the physiologic and behavioral indicators of pain used in the tool: *c*rying, *r*equiring increased oxygen, *i*ncreased vital signs, *e*xpression, and *s*leeplessness. Each indicator is scored from 0 to 2. The total possible pain score, which represents the worst pain, is 10. A pain score greater than 4 should be considered significant. This tool can be used on infants between 32 weeks of gestation and 20 weeks after birth.

Management of Neonatal Pain. The goals of the management of neonatal pain are to: (1) minimize the intensity, duration, and physiologic cost of the pain, and (2) maximize the neonate's ability to cope with and recover from the pain. Nonpharmacologic and pharmacologic strategies are used.

Nonpharmacologic Management. Containment, also known as *swaddling,* is effective in reducing excessive immature motor responses (Fig. 24-23). Containment can provide comfort through other senses, such as thermal, tactile, and proprioceptive senses. Nonnutritive sucking on a pacifier is a common comfort measure used with newborns. Oral sucrose, with or without nonnutritive sucking is safe and effective in reducing pain during single events (Stevens, Yamada, & Ohlsson, 2010). Skin-to-skin contact with the mother during a painful procedure can help to reduce pain (Chermont, Falcão, de Sousa Silva, de Cássia Xavier Balda, & Guinsburg, 2009). Breastfeeding helps reduce pain during heel lancing and blood collection (Leite, Lander, Linhares, Castral, dos Santos, & Silvan Scochi, 2009; Weissman, Aranovitch, Blazer, & Zimmer, 2009). Combining these nonpharmacologic methods results in more effective pain reduction. Distraction with visual, oral, auditory, or tactile stimulation can be helpful in term or older infants.

Pharmacologic Management. Pharmacologic agents are used to alleviate pain in neonates associated with procedures. Local anesthesia is routinely used during procedures such as chest tube insertion and circumcision. Topical anesthesia is used for circumcision, lumbar puncture, venipuncture, and heelsticks. Nonopioid analgesia (oral liquid acetaminophen) is effective for mild to moderate pain from inflammatory conditions. Morphine and fentanyl are the most widely used opioid analgesics for pharmacologic management of neonatal pain. Continuous or bolus intravenous infusion of opioids provides effective and safe pain control. Ketorolac (Toradol) has been shown to be effective in the management of postoperative neonatal pain. Other methods for managing neonatal pain are epidural infusion, local and regional nerve blocks, and intradermal or topical anesthetics.

Promoting Parent-Infant Interaction

Nurses play an important role in promoting early social interaction between parents and their newborn infant. From birth throughout the hospital stay, nurses assess attachment behaviors (see Chapter 22) and provide support and education to parents as they become acquainted with the neonate. Nurses working in outpatient settings or home care provide

Nursing Skill—Pain Assessment

TABLE 24-4 **CRIES NEONATAL POSTOPERATIVE PAIN SCALE***

	0	1	2
Crying	No	High pitched	Inconsolable
Requires oxygen for saturation >95%	No	<30%	>30%
Increased vital signs	Heart rate and blood pressure equal to or less than preoperative state	Heart rate and blood pressure <20% of preoperative state	Heart rate and blood pressure >20% of preoperative state
Expression	None	Grimace	Grimace and grunt
Sleepless	No	Wakes at frequent intervals	Constantly awake

Coding Tips for Using Cries

Crying	The characteristic cry of pain is high pitched. If no cry or cry that is not high pitched, score 0. If cry is high pitched but infant is easily consoled, score 1. If cry is high pitched and infant is inconsolable, score 2.
Requires oxygen for saturation >95%	Look for changes in oxygenation. Infants experiencing pain manifest decreases in oxygenation as measured by total carbon dioxide or oxygen saturation. (Consider other causes of changes in oxygenation, such as atelectasis, pneumothorax, oversedation.) If no oxygen is required, score 0. If <30% oxygen is required, score 1. If >30% oxygen is required, score 2.
Increased vital signs	NOTE: Measure blood pressure last because this may wake the infant, causing difficulty with other assessments. Use baseline preoperative parameters from a nonstressed period. Multiply baseline heart rate (HR) × 0.2, then add this to baseline HR to determine the HR that is 20% over baseline. Do likewise for blood pressure (BP). Use mean BP. If HR and BP are both unchanged or less than baseline, score 0. If HR or BP is increased but increase is <20% of baseline, score 1. If either one is increased >20% over baseline, score 2.
Expression	The facial expression most often associated with pain is a grimace. This may be characterized by brow lowering, eyes squeezed shut, deepening of the nasolabial furrow, open lips and mouth. If no grimace is present, score 0. If grimace alone is present, score 1. If grimace and noncry vocalization grunt is present, score 2.
Sleepless	This is scored based on the infant's state during the hour preceding this recorded score. If the child has been continuously asleep, score 0. If he or she has awakened at frequent intervals, score 1. If he or she has been awake constantly, score 2.

*Neonatal pain assessment tool developed at the University of Missouri–Columbia.
Source: Krechel, S., & Bildner, J. (1995). CRIES: A new neonatal postoperative pain measurement score: Initial testing of validity and reliability. *Paediatric Anaesthesia, 5*(1), 53-61.

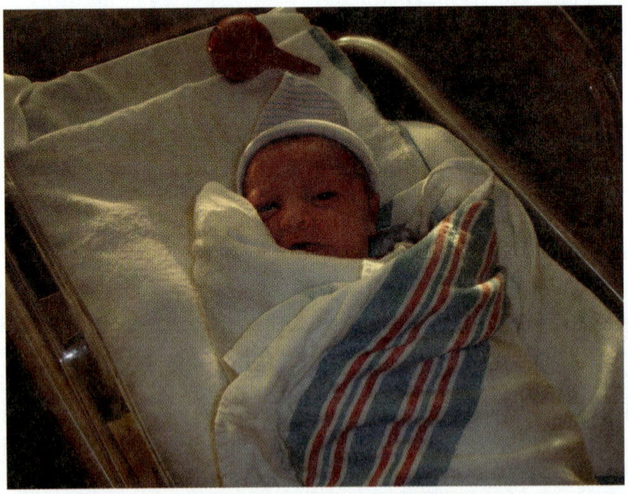

FIG. 24-23 Baby swaddled snugly with one hand near face and other held close to body. (Courtesy Kathryn Alden, Chapel Hill, NC.)

follow-up assessments and care related to parent-child interactions. By teaching parents to recognize infant cues and respond appropriately, the nurse facilitates development of the parents' confidence in meeting the needs of their newborn.

The sensitivity of the parent to the social responses of the infant is basic to the development of a mutually satisfying parent-child relationship. Sensitivity increases over time as parents become more aware of their infant's social capabilities. In supporting parents, nurses need to consider cultural beliefs and traditions that influence parenting behaviors and infant care practices (see the Cultural Considerations box).

CULTURAL CONSIDERATIONS

Cultural Beliefs and Practices Related to Infant Care

Nurses working with childbearing families from other cultures and ethnic groups must be aware of cultural beliefs and practices that are important to individual families. People with a strong sense of heritage may hold on to traditional health beliefs long after adopting other U.S. lifestyle practices. These health beliefs may involve practices regarding the newborn. For example, some Asians, Hispanics, eastern Europeans, and Native Americans delay breastfeeding because they believe that colostrum is "bad." Some Hispanics and African-Americans place a belly band over the infant's umbilicus. The birth of a male child is generally preferred by Asians and Eastern Indians, and some Asians and Haitians delay naming their infants (D'Avanzo, 2008).

The activities of daily care during the neonatal period are the best times for infant and family interactions. While caring for their newborn the mother and father can talk to the infant, play

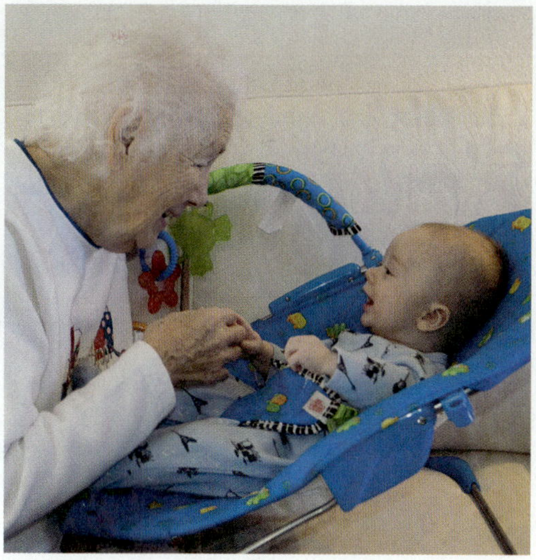

FIG. 24-24 Great-grandmother and infant enjoying social interaction. (Courtesy Freida Belding, Bird City, KS.)

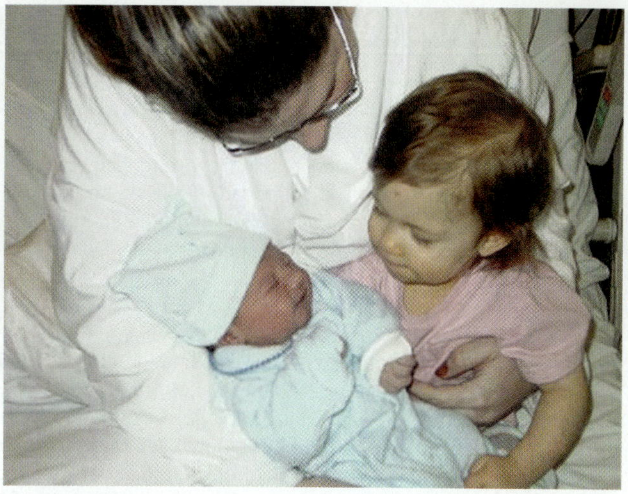

FIG. 24-25 Mother supervising contact of older sibling with newborn. (Courtesy Rebekah Vogel, Fort Collins, CO.)

baby games, caress and cuddle the baby, and perhaps use infant massage. Feeding is an optimal time for interaction because the infant is usually awake and alert, at least at the beginning of the feeding. In Figure 24-24 a great-grandmother and infant are shown engaging in arousal, imitation of facial expression, and smiling. Too much stimulation should be avoided after feeding and before a sleep period. Older children's contact with a newborn is encouraged and supervised based on the developmental level of the child (Fig. 24-25). Parents often keep memento books that record the birth, the hospital stay, and their infant's progress. Other parents create blogs (e.g., www.wordpress.com) to share their development as a family.

Discharge Planning and Teaching

Infant care activities can cause anxiety for new parents. Support from nursing staff members can be an important factor in determining whether new parents seek and accept help in the future. Whether this child is the woman's or the couple's first newborn or an adolescent whose mother will be the primary caregiver, and whether or not the parents attended parenthood preparation classes, parents appreciate anticipatory guidance in the care of their infant. The nurse should avoid trying to cover all the content at one time because the parents can be overwhelmed by too much information and become more anxious. However, because early discharge of new mothers is common practice, teaching all the content that is necessary can be a challenge for the nurse because of time constraints. As a result, many institutions have developed home visitation programs that take the necessary teaching to the new parents, although the hospital nurse still provides most of the essential information for newborn care.

To set priorities for teaching, the nurse follows parental cues. Knowledge deficits or gaps should be identified before beginning to teach. Normal growth and development and the changing needs of the infant (e.g., for personal interaction and stimulation, growth milestones, exercise, injury prevention, and social contacts), as well as the topics that follow, should be included during discharge planning with parents. Safety issues should be addressed (Box 24-8).

Temperature

Parents need to understand practical information related to thermoregulation. The nurse discusses the following topics in parent teaching:

- The causes of elevation in body temperature (e.g., overwrapping, cold stress with resultant vasoconstriction, or minimal response to infection) and the body's response to extremes in environmental temperature
- Ways to promote normal body temperature, such as dressing the infant appropriately for the environmental air temperature and protecting the infant from exposure to direct sunlight
- Use of warm wraps or extra blankets in cold weather
- Technique for taking the newborn's axillary temperature, and normal values for axillary temperature
- Signs to be reported to the primary health care provider such as high or low temperatures with accompanying fussiness, lethargy, irritability, poor feeding, and crying

Respirations

The nurse provides information to parents regarding the normal characteristics of newborn respirations, emergency procedures, and measures to protect the infant. It is helpful to discuss signs of the common cold and to offer suggestions related to care of the infant who experiences this type of illness. Review the following points:

- Normal variations in the rate and rhythm of respirations
- Reflexes such as sneezing to clear the airway
- Use of the bulb syringe
- Steps to take if the infant appears to be choking (see the Emergency box, p. 599)
- The need to protect the infant from the following:
  - Exposure to people with upper respiratory tract infections and respiratory syncytial virus
  - Exposure to secondhand tobacco smoke
  - Suffocation from loose bedding, water beds, and beanbag chairs; drowning (in bath water); entrapment under excessive bedding or in soft bedding; anything tied around the infant's neck; poorly constructed playpens, bassinets, or cribs

BOX 24-8 INFANT SAFETY

- Never leave your baby alone on a bed, couch, or table. Even newborns can move enough to eventually reach the edge and fall off.
- Never put your baby on a cushion, pillow, beanbag, or waterbed to sleep. Your baby may suffocate. Also, do not keep pillows, large floppy toys, or loose plastic sheeting in the crib.
- The back-lying position is recommended for sleep. Do not place your infant on his or her stomach to sleep during the first few months of life.
- When using an infant carrier, stay within arm's reach when the carrier is on a high place, such as a table, sofa, or store counter. If at all possible, place the carrier on the floor near you.
- Infant carriers do not keep your baby safe in a car. Always place your baby in an approved car safety seat when traveling in a motor vehicle (car, truck, bus, or van). Car safety seats are recommended for travel on trains and airplanes as well. Use the car safety seat for *every* ride. Your baby should be in a rear-facing infant car safety seat from birth for as long as possible up to the weight or height limit of the seat. At a minimum, the infant should ride in a rear-facing car seat until he or she reaches one year of age *and* a weight of 20 pounds; the car safety seat should be in the back seat of the car (see Fig. 24-28). This precaution is especially important in vehicles with front passenger air bags because when air bags inflate they can be fatal for infants and toddlers. If an infant must ride in the front seat, disable the airbag.
- When bathing your baby, never leave him or her alone. Newborns and infants can drown in 1 to 2 inches of water.
- Be sure that your hot water heater is set at 120° F or less. Always check bathwater temperature with your elbow before putting your baby in the bath.
- Do not tie anything around your baby's neck. Pacifiers, for example, tied around the neck with a ribbon or string may strangle your baby.
- Check your baby's crib for safety. Slats should be no more than 2¼ inches apart. The space between the mattress and sides should be less than 2 fingerwidths. The bedposts should have no decorative knobs.
- Keep the crib or playpen away from window blind and drapery cords; your baby could strangle on them.
- Keep the crib and playpen well away from radiators, heat vents, and portable heaters. Linens in the crib or playpen can catch fire if they come into contact with these heat sources.
- Install smoke detectors on every floor of your home. Check them once a month to be sure they are working properly. Change batteries twice a year.
- Avoid exposing your baby to cigarette or cigar smoke in your home or other places. Passive exposure to tobacco smoke greatly increases the likelihood that your infant will have respiratory symptoms and illnesses.
- Be gentle with your baby. Do not pick your baby up or swing your baby by the arms or throw him or her up in the air. Never shake the baby.

- Sleep position—on back when put to sleep
- Avoid the use of baby powder, which is a commonly aspirated substance. If parents desire to use a powder, a cornstarch preparation can be substituted. Whenever a powder is used, it should be placed in the caregiver's hand and then applied to the skin, never sprinkled directly onto the skin.
- Notify the health care provider if the infant develops symptoms such as difficulty breathing or swallowing, nasal congestion, excess drainage of mucus, coughing, sneezing, decreased interest in feeding, or fever.
- If the infant has a respiratory illness such as the "common cold," the following suggestions can be helpful:
  - Feed smaller amounts more often to prevent overtiring the infant.
  - Hold the baby in an upright position to feed.
  - For sleeping, raise the infant's head and chest by raising the mattress 30 degrees. (Do *not* use a pillow.)
  - Avoid drafts; do not overdress the baby.
  - Use only medications prescribed by a physician. (Over-the-counter "cold" remedy medications are not appropriate for infants and should be avoided [Sharfstein, North, & Serwint, 2007]).
  - Use nasal saline drops in each nostril and suction well with bulb syringe to decrease and relieve secretions.

Feeding Patterns

Nurses instruct parents about infant feeding and provide assistance based on whether they have chosen breastfeeding or formula feeding. Feeding patterns and practices for newborns are discussed in Chapter 25.

Elimination

Awareness of the normal elimination patterns of newborns helps parents to recognize problems related to voiding or stooling. The following points are included in teaching about elimination:

- Color of normal urine and number of voidings to expect each day: at least two to six for the first one to three days, then a minimum of six to eight voidings per day thereafter
- Changes to be expected in the color and consistency of the stool (i.e., meconium to transitional to soft yellow or golden yellow) and the number of bowel evacuations, plus the odor of stools for breastfed or bottle-fed infants (see Chapter 25)
- Formula-fed infants may have as few as one stool every other day after the first few weeks of life; stools are pasty to semiformed
- Breastfed infants should have at least three stools every 24 hours for the first few weeks; the stools are looser and resemble mustard mixed with cottage cheese; the odor is less offensive than that of formula stools

Positioning and Holding

The AAP Task Force on Infant Sleep Position and Sudden Infant Death Syndrome (SIDS) (2005) continues to recommend placing the infant in the supine position during the first few months of life to prevent SIDS. The prone position has been associated with an increased incidence of SIDS. Since the original sleep position statement was made in 1992 recommending supine sleep position for all newborns, death rates from SIDS have decreased by more than 40% in the United States.

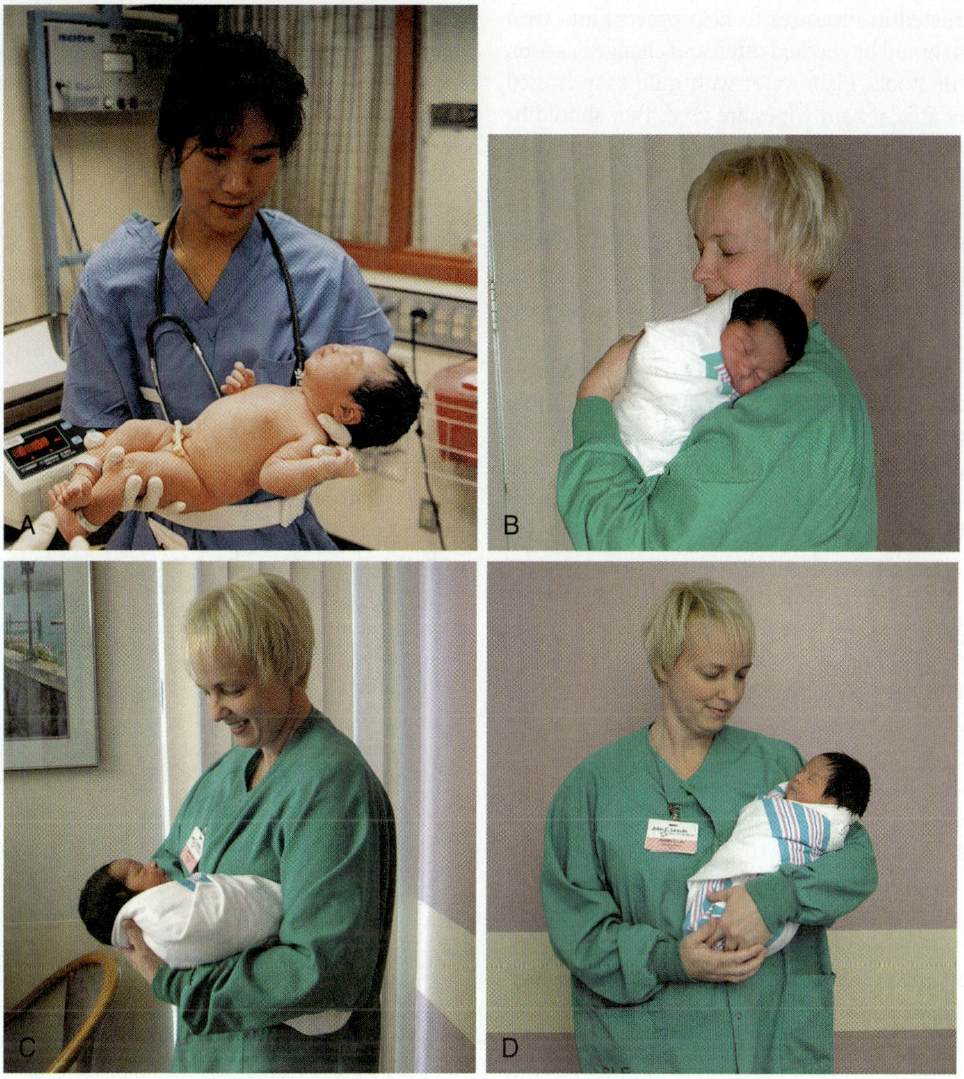

FIG. 24-26 Holding baby securely with support for head. **A**, Holding infant while moving infant from one place to another. Baby is undressed to show posture. **B**, Holding baby upright in "burping" position. **C**, "Football" (under the arm) hold. **D**, Cradling hold. (**A**, Courtesy Kim Molloy, Knoxville, IA. **B**, **C**, and **D**, Courtesy Julie Perry Nelson, Loveland, CO.)

Infants should sleep on a firm surface, specifically on a firm crib mattress covered by a sheet. Soft materials such as comforters, quilts, pillows, or sheepskins should not be placed under the sleeping infant. These same objects should be kept out of the infant's sleeping environment. Loose bedding such as sheets and blankets can be dangerous and if used, should be tucked securely around the crib mattress to prevent the infant's face from being covered by the bedding. Sleep clothing such as infant sleep sacks are useful to keep the infant covered without the danger of covering the head. It is important to avoid overheating the infant during sleep. Bed sharing is not recommended during infant sleep. Infants may be brought into the parent's bed for comforting or for breastfeeding, but should be returned to the crib or bassinet before the parent goes to sleep. Room sharing (infant sleeping in the parent's room) is associated with a decreased risk of SIDS (AAP Task Force on Infant Sleep Position and Sudden Infant Death Syndrome, 2005).

Anatomically, the infant's shape—a barrel chest and flat, curveless spine—facilitates the infant to roll from the side to the prone position; therefore, the side-lying position for sleep is not recommended. When the infant is awake, "tummy time" can be provided under parental supervision so the infant can begin to develop appropriate muscle tone for eventual crawling; this tummy time is also effective in the prevention of a misshaped head (positional plagiocephaly). Care must be taken to prevent the infant from rolling off flat, unguarded surfaces. When an infant is on such a surface the parent or nurse who must turn away from the infant even for a moment should always keep one hand placed securely on the infant. The infant is always held securely with the head supported because newborns are unable to maintain an erect head posture for more than a few moments. Figure 24-26 illustrates various positions for holding an infant with adequate support.

Rashes

Diaper Rash. The majority of infants develop a diaper rash at some time. This dermatitis or skin inflammation appears as redness, scaling, blisters, or papules. Various factors contribute to diaper rash including infrequent diaper changes, diarrhea, use of plastic pants to cover the diaper, a change in the infant's diet such as when solid foods are added, or when breastfeeding mothers eat certain foods.

Parents are instructed in measures to help prevent and treat diaper rash. Diapers should be checked often and changed as soon as the infant voids or stools. Plain water with mild soap is used to cleanse the diaper area; if baby wipes are used, they should be unscented and contain no alcohol. The infant's skin should be allowed to dry completely before applying another diaper. Exposing the buttocks to air can help dry up diaper rash. Because bacteria thrive in moist dark areas, exposing the skin to dry air decreases bacterial proliferation. Zinc oxide ointments can be used to protect the infant's skin from moisture and further excoriation.

Although diaper rash can be alarming to parents and annoying to babies, most cases resolve within a few days with simple home treatments. There are instances when diaper rash is more serious and can require medical treatment.

The warm, moist atmosphere in the diaper area provides an optimal environment for *Candida albicans* growth; dermatitis appears in the perianal area, inguinal folds, and lower abdomen. The affected area is intensely erythematous with a sharply demarcated, scalloped edge, often with numerous satellite lesions that extend beyond the larger lesion. The usual source of infection is from handling by persons who do not practice good hand hygiene. It may also appear 2 to 3 days after an oral infection (thrush).

Therapy consists of applications of an anticandidal ointment, such as clotrimazole or miconazole, with each diaper change. Sometimes the infant is given an oral antifungal preparation such as nystatin or fluconazole to eliminate any gastrointestinal source of infection.

Other Rashes. A rash on the cheeks can result from the infant's scratching with long unclipped fingernails or from rubbing the face against the crib sheets, particularly if regurgitated stomach contents are not washed off promptly. The newborn's skin begins a natural process of peeling and sloughing after birth. Dry skin may be treated with a neutral pH lotion, but this should be used sparingly. Newborn rash, erythema toxicum, is a common finding (see Fig. 23-5, *B*) and needs no treatment.

Clothing

Parents commonly ask how warmly they should dress their infant. A simple suggestion is to dress the child as they dress themselves, adding or subtracting clothes and wraps for the child as necessary. A cotton shirt and diaper may be sufficient clothing for the young infant in warm weather. A cap or bonnet is needed to protect the scalp and minimize heat loss if the weather is cool or to protect against sunburn. Wrapping the infant snugly in a blanket maintains body temperature and promotes a feeling of security. Overdressing in warm temperatures can cause discomfort, as can underdressing in cold weather. Parents are encouraged to dress the infant at all times in flame-retardant clothing. The eyes should be shaded if it is sunny and hot. Infant sunglasses are available to protect the infant's eyes when outdoors (Fig. 24-27).

Car Seat Safety

Infants should travel only in federally approved rear-facing safety seats secured in the rear seat (Fig. 24-28).

To secure the infant in the rear-facing car safety seat, shoulder harnesses are placed in the slots at or below the level of the infant's shoulders. The harness is snug, and the retainer clip is placed at the level of the infant's armpits as opposed to on the abdomen or neck area. The car seat is secured by using the vehicle seat belts.

SAFETY ALERT

Infants should use a rear-facing car seat for as long as possible up to the weight and height limit for their particular car seat. At a minimum, infants should ride in a rear-facing car seat until they are one year of age and weigh at least 20 pounds. The safest area of the car is the back seat. A car safety seat that faces the rear gives the best protection for the disproportionately weak neck and heavy head of an infant. In this position the force of a frontal crash is spread over the head, neck, and back; the back of the car safety seat supports the spine (AAP, 2010; National Highway and Traffic Safety Administration [NHTSA], 2010).

In cars equipped with air bags, rear-facing infant seats should not be placed in the front seat. Serious injury can occur if the air bag inflates because these types of infant seats fit close to the dashboard. If the infant must ride in the front seat, the air bag must be turned off (AAP, 2010; NHTSA, 2010).

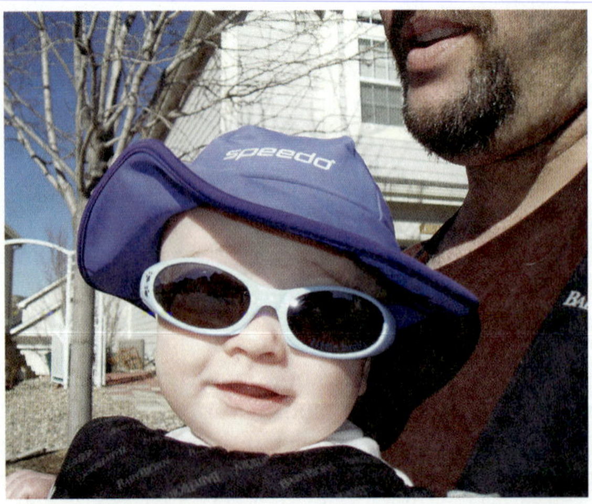

FIG. 24-27 Sunglasses protect the infant's eyes. (Courtesy Julie Perry Nelson, Loveland, CO.)

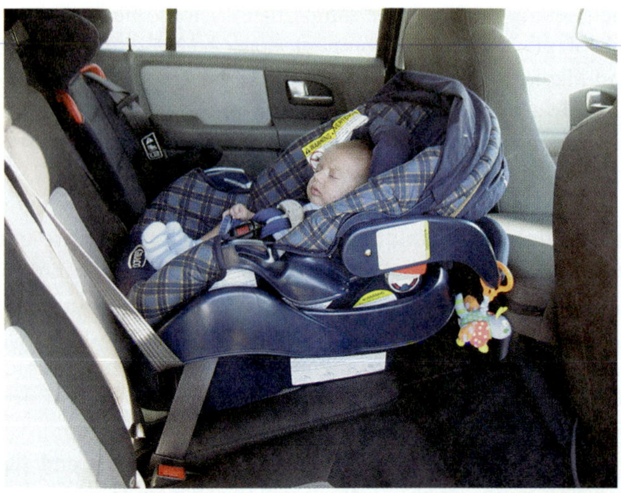

FIG. 24-28 Rear-facing car seat in rear seat of car. Infant is placed in seat when going home from the hospital. (Courtesy Brian and Mayannyn Sallee, Anchorage, AK.)

Infants are positioned at a 45-degree angle in a car seat to prevent slumping and subsequent airway obstruction. Many seats allow for adjustment of the seat angle. For seats that are not adjustable, a tightly rolled newspaper, a solid-core Styrofoam roll, or a firm roll of fabric can be placed under the car safety seat to place the infant at a 45 degree angle (Bull; Engle; Committee on Injury, Violence, and Poison Prevention; & Committee on Fetus and Newborn; 2009).

Prior to discharge from the birth institution, infants born at less than 37 weeks of gestation should be observed in a car seat (preferably their own) for at least 90 to 120 minutes or a period of time equal to the length of the car ride home. The infant is monitored for apnea, bradycardia, and a decrease in oxygen saturation. If the infant exhibits any of these clinical signs, travel home should be in an FMVSS 213-approved car bed (Bull et al., 2009).

If the parents do not have a car safety seat, arrangements should be made to make an appropriate seat available for purchase, loan, or donation. Parents need to be cautioned about purchasing a secondhand car safety seat without knowing the seat's history. They should never use a car seat that was involved in a moderate to severe crash, is too old, has visible cracks, does not have a label with the model number and manufacture date, does not come with instructions, is missing parts, or was recalled (AAP, 2010).

Nonnutritive Sucking

Sucking is the infant's chief pleasure. However, sucking needs may not be satisfied by breastfeeding or bottle-feeding alone. In fact, sucking is such a strong need that infants who are deprived of sucking, such as those with a cleft lip, will suck on their tongues. Some newborns are born with sucking pads on their fingers that developed during in utero sucking. Several benefits of nonnutritive sucking have been demonstrated, such as an increased weight gain in preterm infants, increased ability to maintain an organized state, and decreased crying.

There is compelling evidence that pacifiers help to prevent SIDS. The AAP Task Force on Infant Sleep Position and Sudden Infant Death Syndrome (2005) suggested that parents consider offering a pacifier for naps and bedtime. The pacifier should be used when the infant is placed down for sleep and it should not be reinserted once the infant falls asleep. No infant should be forced to take a pacifier. Pacifiers are to be cleaned often and replaced regularly and should not be coated with any type of sweet solution. Pacifier use should be delayed until the age of 1 month for breastfeeding infants to ensure that breastfeeding is well established (AAP Task Force on Infant Sleep Position and Sudden Infant Death Syndrome).

Problems arise when parents are concerned about the sucking of fingers, thumb, or pacifier and try to restrain this natural tendency. Before giving advice, nurses should investigate the parents' feelings and base the guidance they give on the information solicited. For example, some parents see no problem with the use of a finger but find the use of a pacifier objectionable. In general, either practice need not be restrained unless thumb sucking or pacifier use persists past 4 years of age or past the time when the permanent teeth erupt. Parents are advised to consult with their pediatrician, pediatric dentist, or pediatric nurse practitioner about this topic.

A parent's excessive use of the pacifier to calm the infant should also be explored, however. Placing a pacifier in the infant's mouth as soon as the infant begins to cry can reinforce a pattern of distress and relief.

If parents choose to let their infant use a pacifier, they need to be aware of certain safety considerations before purchasing one. A homemade or poorly designed pacifier can be dangerous because the entire object can be aspirated if it is small, or a portion can become lodged in the pharynx. Improvised pacifiers, such as those made from a padded nipple, also pose dangers because the nipple can separate from the plastic collar and be aspirated. Safe pacifiers are made of one piece that includes a shield or flange large enough to prevent entry into the mouth and a handle that can be grasped (Fig. 24-29).

Bathing, Cord Care, and Skin Care

Bathing. Bathing serves several purposes. It provides opportunities for (1) completely cleansing the infant, (2) observing the infant's condition, (3) promoting comfort, and (4) parent-child-family socializing.

An important consideration in skin cleansing is the preservation of the skin's acid mantle, which is formed from the uppermost horny layer of the epidermis, sweat, superficial fat, metabolic products, and external substances such as amniotic fluid and microorganisms. To protect the pH of the newborn's skin, alkaline soaps (such as Ivory®) and oils, powder, and lotions should not be used during this time because they alter the acid mantle, thus providing a medium for bacterial growth.

Sponge baths are usually used until the infant's umbilical cord falls off and the umbilicus is healed. However, bathing the newborn by immersion has been found to allow less heat loss and provoke less crying. Immersion bathing is a safe alternative to sponge bathing, provided that the infant's condition is stable (no temperature instability, respiratory or cardiac illness) and that the infant is dried off immediately thereafter and kept warm (AWHONN, 2007). A daily bath is not necessary for achieving cleanliness and can do harm by disrupting the integrity of the newborn's skin; cleansing the perineum after a soiled diaper and daily cleansing of the face is usually sufficient. Until the initial bath is completed, personnel must wear gloves to handle the newborn.

The infant bath time provides a wonderful opportunity for parent-infant social interaction (Fig. 24-30). While bathing the baby, parents can talk to the infant, caress and cuddle the infant,

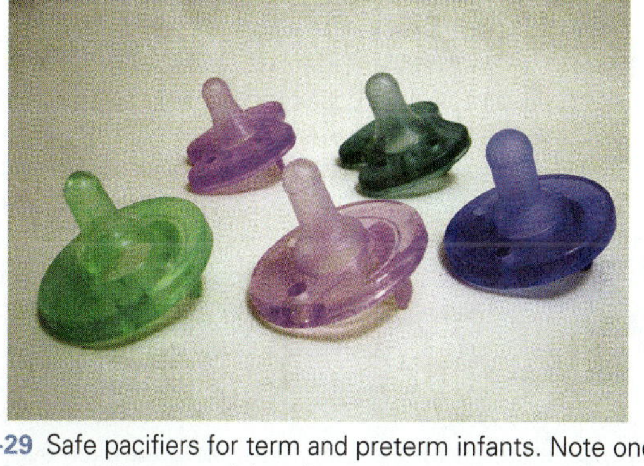

FIG. 24-29 Safe pacifiers for term and preterm infants. Note one-piece construction, easily grasped handle, and large shield with ventilation holes. (Courtesy Julie Perry Nelson, Loveland, CO.)

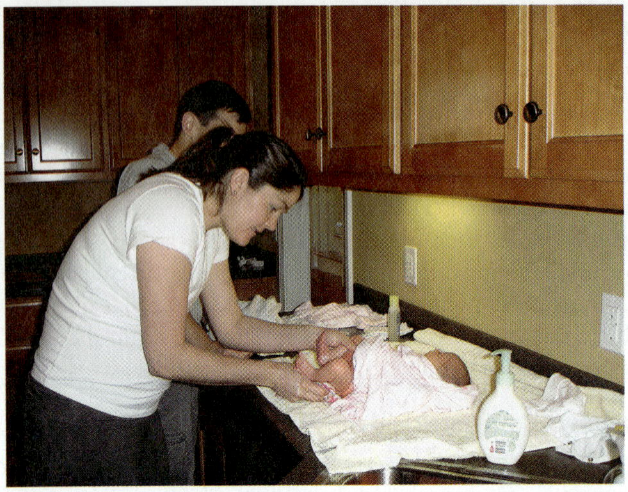

FIG. 24-30 Mother giving newborn a sponge bath at home. (Courtesy Kathryn Alden, Chapel Hill, NC.)

and engage in arousal and imitation of facial expressions and smiling. Parents can pick a time for the bath that is easy for them and when the baby is awake, usually before a feeding.

Cord Care. The umbilical cord begins to dry, shrivel, and blacken by the second or third day of life, depending in part on the cleansing method used. The umbilicus should be inspected often for signs of infection (e.g., foul odor, redness, purulent discharge), granuloma (i.e., small, red, raw-appearing polyp where the umbilical cord separates), bleeding, and discharge. The cord clamp is removed when the cord is dry in approximately 24 hours (see Fig. 24-4). The cord normally falls off in 10 to 14 days after birth but can remain attached for as long as 3 weeks in some cases. Parents are instructed in appropriate home cord care (per practitioner or institution protocol) and the expected time of cord separation.

Box 24-9 contains information regarding sponge bathing, skin care, cord care, cutting nails, and dressing the infant.

BOX 24-9 BATHING, CORD CARE, SKIN CARE, AND NAIL CARE

FIT BATHS INTO THE FAMILY'S SCHEDULE

- Give a bath at any time convenient to you but not immediately after a feeding period because the increased handling may cause regurgitation.

PREVENT HEAT LOSS

- The temperature of the room should be 24° C (75° F), and the bathing area should be free of drafts.
- Control heat loss during the bath to conserve the infant's energy. Bathing the infant quickly, exposing only a portion of the body at a time, and drying thoroughly are all parts of the bathing technique.

GATHER SUPPLIES AND CLOTHING BEFORE STARTING

- Clothing suitable for wearing indoors: diaper, shirt; stretch suit or nightgown optional
- Unscented, mild soap
- Pins, if needed for diaper, closed and placed well out of the baby's reach
- Cotton balls
- Towels for drying the infant and a clean washcloth
- Receiving blanket
- Tub for water; fill only to 3 to 4 inches of water

BATHE THE BABY

- Bring the infant to the bathing area when all supplies are ready.
- Never leave the infant alone on bath table or in the bath water, not even for a second! If you have to leave, take the infant with you, or place the infant back into the crib.
- Test the temperature of the water. It should feel pleasantly warm to the inner wrist—36.6° to 37.2° C (98°-99° F).
- Do not hold the infant under running water—the water temperature can change, and the infant can be scalded or chilled rapidly. The baby can be tub bathed after the cord drops off and the umbilicus and circumcised penis are completely healed.
- If sponge bathing is to be performed, undress the baby and wrap in a towel with the head exposed. Uncover the parts of the body you are washing, taking care to keep the rest of the baby covered as much as possible to prevent heat loss.
- Begin by washing the baby's face with water; do not use soap on the face. Cleanse the eyes from the inner canthus outward using separate parts of a clean washcloth for each eye. For the first 2 to 3 days a discharge may result from the reaction of the conjunctiva to the substance (erythromycin) used as a prophylactic measure against infection. Any discharge should be considered abnormal and reported to the health care provider.
- Cleanse the ears and nose with twists of moistened cotton or a corner of the washcloth. Do not use cotton-tipped swabs because they can cause injury. The areas behind the ears need daily cleansing.
- Wash the body with mild soap; rinse and dry to decrease heat loss. Place your hand under the baby's shoulders and lift gently to expose the neck, lift the chin, and wash the neck, taking care to cleanse between the skinfolds. Wash between the fingers and toes, then rinse and dry thoroughly. Wash the genital area last.
- If the hair is to be washed, begin by wrapping the infant in a towel with the head exposed. Hold the infant in a football position (under the arm) with one hand, using the other hand to wash the hair. Wash the scalp with water, mild soap, and a soft brush; rinse well and dry thoroughly. Scalp desquamation, called *cradle cap,* can often be prevented by removing any scales with a fine-toothed comb or brush after washing. If the condition persists, the health care provider may prescribe a medicated shampoo to massage into the scalp. A blow dryer is never used on an infant because the temperature is too hot for a baby's skin.

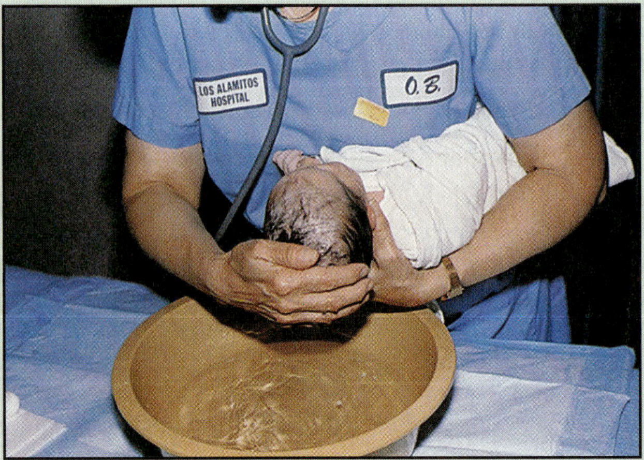

Wash hair with baby wrapped to limit heat loss. (Courtesy Marjorie Pyle, RNC, Lifecircle, Costa Mesa, CA.)

Nursing Skill—Infant Bathing

BOX 24-9 BATHING, CORD CARE, SKIN CARE, AND NAIL CARE—cont'd

SKIN CARE

- The skin of a newborn is sensitive and should be cleaned only with water between baths. Soap has drying properties, and its use is limited to bathing. Creams, lotions, ointments, or powders are not recommended. If the skin seems excessively dry during the first 2 to 3 weeks after birth, an unscented, non–alcohol-based lotion may be used; checking with the health care provider for suggestions on skin care products is best. Experts advise that baby clothes be laundered separately using a mild laundry detergent (Dreft or Ivory Snow); clothes should be rinsed twice with plain water.
- The fragile skin can be injured by too vigorous cleansing. If stool or other debris has dried and caked on the skin, soak the area to remove it. Do not attempt to rub it off because abrasion may result. Gentleness, patting dry rather than rubbing, and using a mild soap without perfumes or coloring are recommended. Chemicals in the coloring and perfume can cause rashes on sensitive skin.
- Babies are very prone to sunburn and should be kept out of direct sunlight. Use of sunscreens should be discussed with the health care provider.
- Babies often develop rashes that are normal. Neonatal acne resembles pimples and may appear at 2 to 4 weeks of age, resolving without treatment by 6 to 8 months. Heat rash is common in warm weather, which appears as a fine red rash around creases or folds where the baby sweats.

CORD CARE

- Cleanse with soap and water around base of the cord where it joins the skin. Notify the health care provider of any odor, discharge, or skin inflammation around the cord. The clamp is removed when the cord is dry (approximately 24 hours). The diaper should not cover the cord because a wet or soiled diaper will slow or prevent drying of the cord and foster infection. When the cord drops off after 10 to 14 days, small drops of blood may be seen when the baby cries. This bleeding will heal by itself. It is not dangerous.

NAIL CARE

- Do not cut fingernails and toenails immediately after birth. The nails have to grow out far enough from the skin so that the skin is not cut by mistake. If the baby scratches him or herself, apply loosely fitted mitts over each of the baby's hands. Do so as a last resort, however, because it interferes with the baby's ability for self-consolation sucking on thumb or finger. When the nails have grown, the fingernails and toenails can be trimmed with manicure scissors or clippers; nails should be cut straight across. The ideal time to trim the nails is when the infant is sleeping. Soft emery boards may be used to file the nails. Nails should be kept short.

CLEAN GENITALS

- Cleanse the genitals of infants daily and after voiding or defecating. For girls the genitals are cleansed by separating the labia and gently washing from the pubic area to the anus. For uncircumcised boys, gently pull back (retract) the foreskin. Stop when resistance is felt. In most newborns the inner layer of the foreskin adheres to the glans, and the foreskin cannot be retracted. Wash and rinse the tip (glans) with soap and warm water, and replace the foreskin. The foreskin must be returned to its original position to prevent constriction and swelling. By age 3 years in 90% of boys the foreskin can be retracted easily without causing pain or trauma. For others the foreskin is not retractable until adolescence. As soon as the foreskin is partly retractable and the child is old enough, he can be taught self-care. Once healed the circumcised penis does not require any special care other than cleansing with diaper changes.
- The infant's skin should be allowed to dry completely before applying another diaper. Exposing the buttocks to air can help dry up diaper rash. Because bacteria thrive in moist dark areas, exposing the skin to dry air decreases bacterial proliferation. Zinc oxide ointments can be used to protect the infant's skin from moisture and further excoriation.

Infant Follow-up Care

Follow-up care after hospital discharge usually occurs within 72 hours at the clinic or health care provider's office. This is especially important for breastfed newborns for monitoring their weight and hydration status. When infants are discharged at less than 48 hours of age, home care follow-up is an essential component of care. Home care may be provided either by a nurse as part of the routine follow-up care of clients or through a visiting nurse or community health nurse referral service. The home care nurse provides information to parents to help them recognize signs that the newborn is progressing satisfactorily after early discharge (see Box 24-10).

Parents should plan for their infant's follow-up health care at the following ages: within 3 days if discharged early or breastfeeding to check for status of jaundice, feeding, and elimination; 2 to 3 weeks of age for breastfeeding babies; 2 to 4 weeks of age for formula feeding babies; then every 2 months until 6 to 7 months of age; then every 3 months until 18 months; at 2 years; at 3 years; at preschool; and every 2 years thereafter.

Immunizations

The schedule for immunizations should be reviewed with parents (Table 24-5); HB vaccine is currently administered to newborns before hospital discharge (depending on maternal HB status) or within 1 month of birth.

Nurses should become familiar with this schedule and provide written instructions to the parents about when and where to obtain immunizations. (Immunization schedules change periodically and the nurse can update any information needed by checking with the website www.cdc.gov.) An infant's ability to protect him- or herself against antigens by the formation of antibodies develops sequentially; therefore, the infant must be developmentally capable of responding to these antibodies, which is the reason for planning sequential immunizations for infants.

Cardiopulmonary Resuscitation

All personnel working with infants must have current infant cardiopulmonary resuscitation (CPR) certification. Parents should receive instruction in relieving airway obstruction (see the Emergency box: Relieving Airway Obstruction) and CPR (see the Emergency box: Cardiopulmonary Resuscitation (CPR) for Infants). Classes are often offered in hospitals and clinics during the prenatal period or to parents of newborns. Such instruction is especially important for parents whose infants were preterm or had cardiac or respiratory problems. Some grandparents take CPR classes. Babysitters should also learn CPR.

Practical Suggestions for the First Weeks at Home

Numerous changes occur during the first weeks of parenthood. Care management should be directed toward helping parents

BOX 24-10 NEWBORN PROGRESS AFTER EARLY DISCHARGE

- Wet diapers: minimum of six to eight per day after 3 or 4 days
- Breastfeeding: successful latch and feeding every 1.5 to 3 hours daily (8-12 times in 24 hours)
- Formula-feeding: successfully, voiding as noted above, taking approximately 3 to 4 ounces every 3 to 4 hours
- Circumcision: wash with warm water only; yellow exudate forming, nonbleeding, PlastiBell intact for 48 hours
- Stools: at least one every 48 hours for formula-fed infants and at least three per day for breastfeeding infants
- Color: pink to ruddy when crying; pink centrally when at rest or asleep
- Activity: has four or five wakeful periods per day and alerts to environmental sounds and voices
- Jaundice: physiologic jaundice (not appearing in first 24 hours), feeding, voiding, and stooling as noted above, or practitioner notification for suspicion of pathologic jaundice (appears within 24 hours of birth, ABO/Rh problem suspected; hemolysis); decreased activity; poor feeding; dark orange skin persisting beyond fifth day in light-skinned newborn
- Cord: kept above diaper line; drying; periumbilical area skin pink (drainage, odor, or erythematous circle at umbilical site can be sign of omphalitis)
- Vital signs: heart rate 120 to 160 beats/min when awake; respiratory rate 30 to 55 breaths/min without evidence of retractions, grunting, or nasal flaring; temperature 36.5° to 37.2° C axillary
- Position of sleep: back

Any deviation from the above or suspicion of poor newborn adaptation should be reported to the primary health care provider at once.

cope with infant care, role changes, altered lifestyle, and change in family structure resulting from the addition of a new baby. Developing skill and confidence in caring for an infant can be especially anxiety provoking. Anticipatory guidance can help prevent a reality shock in the transition from hospital or birthing center to home that might negate the parents' joy or cause them undue stress. For example, the nurse can teach parents several strategies that help quiet a fussy baby, prevent crying, and induce quiet attention or sleep.

Parents must be helped to anticipate events during the transition from hospital to home. This is especially important for first-time parents. Even the simplest strategies can provide enormous support. Written information reinforcing education topics is helpful, as is a list of available community resources, both local and national, and websites that provide reliable information about child care. Classes in the prenatal period or during the postpartum stay are helpful. Instructions for the first days at home should minimally include activities of daily living, dealing with visitors, and activity and rest.

Activities of Daily Living. Given the demands of a newborn, the mother's discomfort or fatigue associated with giving birth, and a busy homecoming day, even small details of daily life can become stressful. Measures such as using disposable diapers, preparing frozen or microwave dinners during pregnancy, or getting takeout meals can decrease stress by eliminating at least one or two parental responsibilities during the first few days at home.

TABLE 24-5 IMMUNIZATION SCHEDULE—2010*

IMMUNIZATION	AGE GIVEN
HBV (hepatitis B)	3 injections: before hospital discharge, 1 or 2 months, final dose no earlier than age 24 weeks
HBIG (hepatitis B immune globulin—if mother is HBsAg positive)	Within 12 hours after birth
Rotavirus	2, 4 months
DTaP (diphtheria, tetanus, acellular pertussis)	2, 4, 6 months
Hib (*Haemophilus influenzae* b conjugate vaccine)	2, 4 months
Pneumococcus	2, 4, 6 months
IPV (inactivated polio vaccine—injectable)	2, 4, 6-18 months
Influenza ("flu shot")	Yearly after 6 months
MMR (measles, mumps, rubella)	12 to 18 months
Varicella (chickenpox)	12 to 15 months
Hepatitis A	12-23 months (2 doses at least 6 months apart)

*This is the schedule for the first 18 months. For the full schedule, go to *www.cdc.gov*.
Source: U.S. Department of Health and Human Services, Centers for Disease Control and Prevention. (2010). *Recommended immunization schedule for persons aged 0 through 6 years—United States 2010.* Available at http://www.cdc.gov/vaccines/recs/schedules/downloads/child/2010/10_0-6yrs-schedule-pr.pdf. Accessed July 18, 2010.

It is best to plan for hospital discharge to occur soon after an infant feeding. This increases the likelihood that the couple will have adequate time to get home and relatively settled before the next feeding. Offering a sample carton of premixed bottles for the formula-fed infant prevents the need for rushed preparation of formula.

Visitors. New parents are often inadequately prepared for the reality of bringing a new infant home because they romanticize the homecoming. One mother stated, "By the time we drove an hour through traffic, my stitches were hurting, and all I wanted was a warm sitz bath and some private time with Bill and the baby, in that order. Instead, a carload of visitors pulled into the driveway as we were unbuckling the baby from his car seat. I thought I would surely cry."

The nurse can help parents explore ways, in advance, to assert their need to limit visitors. Parents can work out a signal for alerting the partner that the mother is getting tired or uncomfortable and needs the partner to invite the visitors to another room or to leave. Some mothers find that wearing a robe and not appearing ready for company leads visitors to stay a shorter time. A sign on the front door saying "Mother and baby resting—please do not disturb" may be useful.

Activity and Rest. Because mothers often report that fatigue is a major problem during the first few weeks after giving birth, they need to be encouraged to limit their activities and be realistic about their level of fatigue. Activities should not be sustained for long periods. Family, friends, and neighbors can be solicited for support and help with meals, housecleaning, picking up other children, and so on. Rest periods throughout the day are important. Mothers can nap when the baby sleeps. Adequate nutrition is also important for postpartum recovery and in dealing with fatigue.

Anticipatory guidance helps prepare new parents for what to expect as their newborn grows and develops. Parents with

EMERGENCY

Relieving Airway Obstruction

- Back blow and chest thrusts are used to clear an airway obstructed by a foreign body.

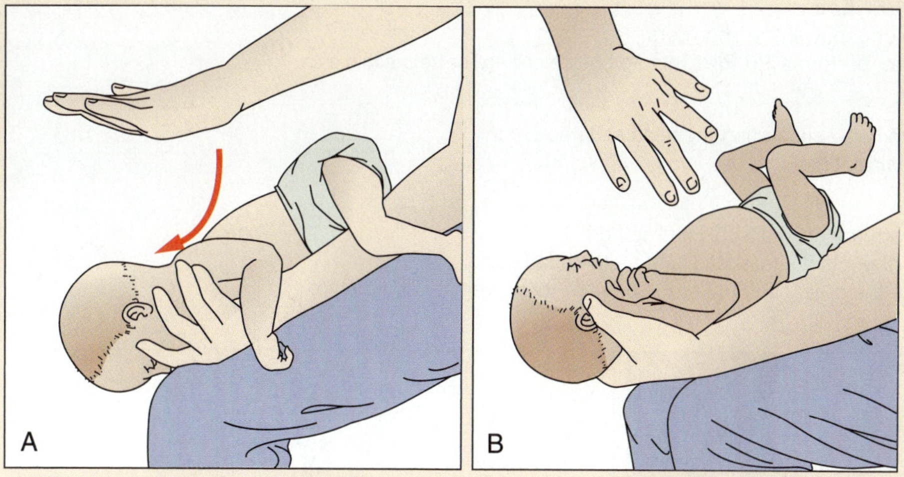

Back blows and chest thrust in infant to clear airway obstruction. **A**, Back blow. **B**, Chest thrust.

BACK BLOWS
- Position the infant prone over the forearm with the infant's head down and the jaw firmly supported.
- Rest the supporting arm on the thigh.
- Deliver four back blows forcefully between the infant's shoulder blades with the heel of the free hand.

TURN THE INFANT
- Place the free hand on the infant's back to sandwich the baby between both hands; one hand supports the neck, jaw, and chest, while the other supports the back.
- Turn the infant over, and place the infant's head lower than the chest, supporting the head and neck.
- Alternative position: Place the infant face down on your lap with the head lower than the trunk; firmly support the head. Apply back blows, and then turn the infant as a unit.

CHEST THRUSTS
- Provide four downward chest thrusts on the lower third of the sternum.
- Remove the foreign body, if it is visible.

OPEN THE AIRWAY
- Open the airway with the head tilt–chin lift maneuver, and attempt to ventilate.
- Repeat the sequence of back blows, turning, and chest thrusts.
- Continue these emergency procedures until signs of recovery occur:
  - Palpable peripheral pulses return.
  - The pupils become normal in size and are responsive to light.
  - Mottling and cyanosis disappear.
- Record the time and duration of the procedure and the effects of this intervention.

realistic expectations of infant needs and behavior are better prepared to adjust to the demands of a new baby and to parenthood itself.

New parents can be overwhelmed by a large volume of information and become anxious. Anticipatory guidance should include the following: newborn sleep-wake cycles, interpretation of crying and quieting techniques, infant developmental milestones, sensory enrichment and infant stimulation, recognizing signs of illness, and well-baby follow-up and immunizations. Printed materials and audiotapes, videotapes, or DVDs for parents to take home are helpful. Parents can also be given a list of reliable websites to access for information.

Development of Day-Night Routines. Nurses can help prepare new parents for the fact that most newborns cannot tell the difference between night and day and must learn the rhythm of day-night routines. Nurses should provide basic suggestions for settling a newborn and for helping him or her develop a predictable routine. Examples of such suggestions include the following:

- In the late afternoon, bring the baby out to the center of family activity. Keep the baby there for the rest of the evening. If the baby falls asleep, let the baby do so in the infant seat or in someone's arms. Save the crib or bassinet for nighttime sleep.
- Give the baby a bath right before bedtime. This activity soothes the baby and helps him or her expend energy.
- Feed the baby for the last evening time around 11 o'clock, and put him or her to bed in the crib or bassinet.
- For nighttime feedings and diaper changes, keep a small night-light on to avoid turning on bright lights. Talk in soft whispers (if at all), and handle the baby gently and only as absolutely necessary to feed and diaper. Nighttime feedings should be all business and no play! Babies usually go back to sleep if the room is quiet and dark.

EMERGENCY

Cardiopulmonary Resuscitation (CPR) for Infants

- Wash hands before and after touching infant and equipment. Wear gloves, if possible.

ASSESS RESPONSIVENESS

- Observe color; tap or gently shake shoulders.
- Yell for help; if alone, perform CPR for 1 minute before calling for help again.

POSITION INFANT

- Turn the infant onto back, supporting the head and neck.
- Place the infant on firm, flat surface.

AIRWAY

- Open the airway with the head tilt–chin lift method.
- Place one hand on the infant's forehead, and tilt the head back.
- Place the fingers of the other hand under the bone of the lower jaw at the chin.

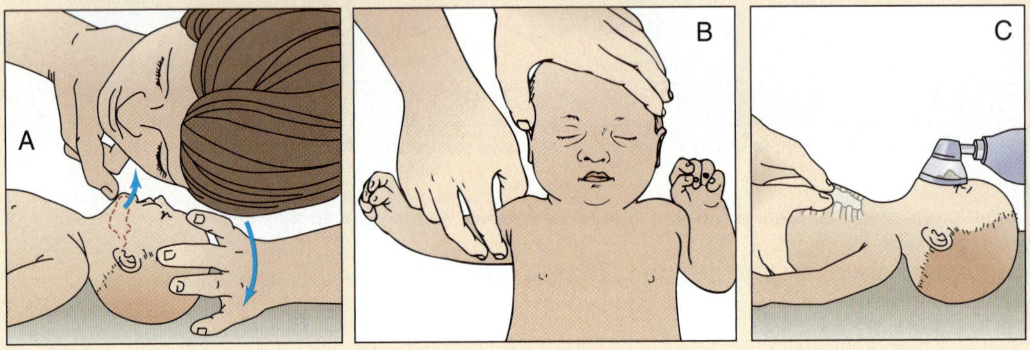

A, Opening airway with head tilt–chin lift method. **B**, Checking pulse of brachial artery. **C**, Side-by-side thumb placement for chest compression in newborn.

BREATHING

- Assess for evidence of breathing:
  - Observe for chest movement.
  - Listen for exhaled air.
  - Feel for exhaled air flow.
- To breathe for infant:
  - Take a breath.
  - Place your mouth over the infant's nose and mouth to create a seal. NOTE: When available, a mask with a one-way valve should be used.
  - Give two slow breaths (1 to 1.5 seconds for each breath), pausing to inhale between breaths. NOTE: Gently puff the volume of air in your cheeks into infant. Do not force air.
- The infant's chest should rise slightly with each puff; keep fingers on the chest wall to sense air entry.

CIRCULATION

- Assess circulation:
  - Check pulse of the brachial artery while maintaining the head tilt.
  - If the pulse is present, initiate rescue breathing. Continue procedure at 40 to 60 breaths/min until spontaneous breathing resumes.
  - If the pulse is absent, initiate chest compressions and coordinate them with breathing.
- Chest compression: Two systems of chest compression can be used. Nurses should know both methods.
- Maintain the head tilt and:
  1. Place thumbs side-by-side in the middle third of the sternum with fingers around the chest and supporting the back. Compress the sternum one third the depth of the chest.
  2. Place index finger of hand just under an imaginary line drawn between the nipples. Place the middle and ring fingers on the sternum adjacent to the index finger. Using the middle and ring fingers, compress the sternum approximately one third the depth of the chest.
- Avoid compressing the xiphoid process.
- Release pressure without moving the thumbs and fingers from the chest.
- Use a 30:2 compression-ventilation ratio for one-rescuer CPR and 15:2 compression-ventilation ratio for two-rescuer CPR.
- Provide 100 compressions per minute.
- Provide five cycles of three compressions and two ventilations of CPR (about 2 minutes) before leaving to call 911.
- After the cycles, check the brachial artery to determine whether a pulse can be felt.
- Discontinue compressions when the infant's spontaneous heart rate reaches or exceeds 80 beats/min.
- Record the time and duration of the procedure and the effects of intervention.

Source: American Heart Association. (2005). 2005 American Heart Association guidelines for cardiopulmonary resuscitation and emergency cardiovascular care. *Circulation, 112*(24) (Suppl) IV12-IV18.

A predictable, stable routine gradually develops for *most* babies; however, some babies *never* develop one. New parents will cope better if they are willing to be flexible and to give up some control during the early weeks.

Interpretation of Crying and Use of Quieting Techniques. Crying is an infant's first social communication. Some babies cry more than others, but all babies cry. They cry to communicate that they are hungry, uncomfortable, wet, ill, or bored and sometimes for no apparent reason at all. The longer parents are around their infants, the easier the task becomes of interpreting what a cry means. Many infants have a fussy period during the day, often in the late afternoon or early evening when everyone is naturally tired. Environmental tension adds to the length and intensity of crying spells. Babies also have periods of vigorous crying when no comforting can help. These periods of crying can last for long stretches until the infants seem to cry themselves to sleep. Possibly the infants are trying to discharge enough energy so they can settle themselves down. The nurse needs to reinforce for new parents that time and infant maturation will take care of these types of cries. Many hospitals distribute a DVD on infant crying to new parents. The "Period of Purple Crying" is an example. It is intended to help parents understand that crying is normal and help them cope with infant crying. If parents have greater understanding of infant crying, they may be less likely to inflict harm such as occurs with "shaken-baby" syndrome.

Crying because of colic is a common concern of new parents. Babies with colic cry inconsolably for several hours, pull their legs up to their stomach, and pass large amounts of gas. No one really knows what colic is or why babies get it. Parents can be encouraged to contact the infant's health care provider if they are concerned that their baby has colic.

Certain types of sensory stimulation can calm and quiet infants and help them get to sleep. Important characteristics of this sensory stimulation—whether tactile, vestibular, auditory, or visual—appear to be that the stimulation is mild, slow, and rhythmic, and consistently and regularly presented. Tactile stimulation can include warmth, patting, back rubbing, and covering the skin with textured cloth. Swaddling (see Fig. 24-23) to keep arms and legs close to the body (as in utero) provides widespread and constant tactile stimulation and a sense of security. Vestibular stimulation is especially effective and can be accomplished by mild rhythmic movement such as rocking or by holding the infant upright, as on the parent's shoulder. The nurse can teach parents several strategies that help quiet a fussy baby, prevent crying, and induce quiet attention or sleep (Box 24-11).

BOX 24-11 INFANT QUIETING TECHNIQUES

- Many newborns feel insecure in the center of a large crib. They prefer a small, warm, soft space that reminds them of intrauterine life. Try a smaller bed, such as a bassinet, portable crib, buggy, or cradle.
- Carry your baby in a front pack or backpack.
- Swaddle your newborn snugly in a receiving blanket. Swaddling keeps your newborn's arms and legs close to his or her body, similar to the intrauterine position; it also makes the newborn feel more secure.
- Prewarm the crib sheets with a hot water bottle or heating pad set on low that you remove before putting your baby to bed. Some babies startle when placed on a cold sheet.
- Some newborns need extra sucking to soothe themselves to sleep. Babies may enjoy sucking on a pacifier. However, pacifier use is not recommended for breastfeeding infants until one month of age when breastfeeding is well-established. Breastfeeding mothers may prefer to let their infant suckle at the breast as a soothing technique. Around 3 months of age, infants become able to consistently find and suck their thumbs as a way of self-consoling.
- A rhythmic, monotonous noise simulating the intrauterine sounds of your heartbeat and blood flow may help your infant settle down. Some parents have found that putting the baby in a portable crib beside the dishwasher or washing machine helps settle a fussy baby.
- Movement often helps quiet a baby. Take your baby for a ride in the car, or take your baby for an outing in a stroller or carriage. Rock your baby in a rocking chair or cradle.
- Place your baby on his or her stomach across your lap; pat and rub his or her back while gently bouncing your legs or swaying them from left to right.
- Babies enjoy close skin-to-skin contact. A combination of this and warm water often helps soothe a fussy baby. Fill your tub with warm water. Get in and let the baby lie on your chest so that the baby is immersed in the water up to his or her neck. Cuddle the baby close.
- Let your baby see your face. Talk to your baby in a soothing voice.
- Your baby may simply be bored. Bring him or her into the room where you and the rest of the family are. Change your baby's position; many babies like to be upright, for example, by being held up on your shoulder.

Spanish Guidlines—Infant Quieting Techniques

Developmental Milestones

Knowledge of infant growth and development helps parents have realistic expectations of what an infant can do. When parents understand and appreciate the limitations and developing abilities of their infant, adjustment to parenthood can go more smoothly. Emphasizing the individuality of the infant enhances the capacity of the family to offer their infant an optimally nurturing environment.

Brazelton (1995) suggests the concept of "touch-points" for intervention, that is, points at which a change in the system (baby, parent, and family) is brought about by the baby's spurts in development (cognitive, motor, or emotional). Immediately before each spurt in development is a predictable short period of disorganization in the baby. Parents are likely to feel disorganized and stressed as well. Because these periods of disorganization are predictable, nurses can offer parents anticipatory guidance to help them understand what happens with infant development and to prepare them for the subsequent spurts in development.

The nurse should provide parents with information on month-by-month infant growth and development. Written information that parents can consult later is especially helpful. Table 24-6 provides a summary of infant growth and development during the first 3 months.

Video—Assessment: Crying Female Neonate

Infant Stimulation

Interacting with their parents is an important way in which infants learn about themselves and their environment. Nurses can teach parents a variety of ways to stimulate their infant's development and to enrich the infant's learning environment. Home health nurses can evaluate the home environment and make suggestions to parents for promotion of their baby's physical, cognitive, and emotional development. Suggestions

TABLE 24-6 **GROWTH AND DEVELOPMENT DURING INFANCY**

1 MONTH	2 MONTHS	3 MONTHS
Physical		
Weight gain of 5 to 7.5 oz (150-210 g) weekly for first 6 mo Height gain of 1 in (2.5 cm) monthly for first 6 mo Head circumference increases by 0.6 in (1.5 cm) monthly for first 6 mo Primitive reflexes present and strong Doll's-eye reflex and dance reflex fading Preferential nose breathing (most infants)	Posterior fontanel closed Crawling reflex disappears	Primitive reflexes fading
Gross Motor		
Assumes flexed position with pelvis high but knees not under abdomen when prone (at birth, knees flexed under abdomen)* Can turn head from side to side when prone, lifts head momentarily from bed† Has marked head lag, especially when pulled from lying to sitting position Holds head momentarily parallel and in midline when suspended in prone position Assumes asymmetric tonic neck reflex position when supine In sitting position, back is uniformly rounded; absence of head control	Assumes less flexed position when prone—hips flat, legs extended, arms flexed, head to side† Less head lag when pulled to sitting position Can maintain head in same plane as rest of body when held in ventral suspension When prone, can lift head almost 45 degrees off table When held in sitting position, head is held up but bobs forward Assumes asymmetric tonic neck reflex position intermittently	Has only slight head lag when pulled to sitting position Assumes symmetric body positioning Able to raise head and shoulders from prone position to a 45- to 90-degree angle from table; bears weight on forearms When held in standing position, able to bear slight fraction of weight on legs Able to hold head more erect when sitting, but still bobs forward When held in standing position, body limp at knees and hips Regards own hand
Fine Motor		
Hands predominantly closed Grasp reflex strong Hand clenches on contact with rattle	Hands often open Grasp reflex fading	Actively holds rattle but will not reach for it† Grasp reflex absent Hands kept loosely open Clutches own hand; pulls at blanket and clothes
Sensory		
Able to fixate on moving object in range of 45 degrees when held at a distance of 8-10 in. Visual acuity approaches 20/100*† Follows light to midline Quiets when hears a voice	Binocular fixation and convergence to near objects beginning When supine, follows dangling toy from side to point beyond midline Visually searches to locate sounds Turns head to side when sound is made at level of ear	Follows object to periphery (180 degrees)† Locates sound by turning head to side and looking in same direction† Begins to have ability to coordinate stimuli from various sense organs
Vocalization		
Cries to express displeasure Makes small throaty sounds Makes comfort sounds during feeding	Vocalizes, distinct from crying† Crying becomes differentiated Coos Vocalizes to familiar voice	Squeals aloud to show pleasure† Coos, babbles, chuckles Vocalizes when smiling "Talks" a great deal when spoken to Less crying during periods of wakefulness
Socialization and Cognition		
Is in sensorimotor phase—stage I, use of reflexes (birth-1 mo), and stage II, primary circular reactions (1-4 mo) Watches parent's face intently as she or he talks to infant	Demonstrates social smile in response to various stimuli†	Displays considerable interest in surroundings Ceases crying when parent enters room Can recognize familiar faces and objects, such as feeding bottle Shows awareness of strange situations

*Degree of visual acuity varies according to vision measurement procedure used.
†Milestones represent essential integrative aspects of development that lay the foundation for the achievement of more advanced skills.
Source: Hockenberry, M. (2011). *Wong's nursing care of infants and children* (9th ed.). St. Louis: Mosby.

for teaching infants during the first few months are presented in Boxes 24-12 and 24-13. Table 24-7 presents suggestions for visual, auditory, tactile, and kinetic stimulation.

Recognizing Signs of Illness

In addition to explaining the need for well-baby follow-up visits, the nurse should discuss with parents the signs of illness in newborns (Box 24-14). Of particular importance is the parents' assessment of jaundice in newborns discharged early. Parents should be advised to call their nurse-practitioner or pediatrician immediately if they notice increasing jaundice or signs of illness and to ask about over-the-counter medications, such as acetaminophen for infants, to keep at home.

BOX 24-12 TEACHING YOUR NEWBORN

- Newborns learn things every day. You can teach your newborn by playing with him or her and giving your newborn toys that help him or her to learn.
- Talk to your baby a lot. Tell your baby what is going on in the room ("Listen to the dog barking"). Label objects that you see or use ("Here's the washcloth"), and describe things you are doing ("Let's put the shirt over Kerry's head").
- Look at your baby's face and make eye contact. Play face-making games: smile, stick out your tongue, open your eyes wide. As your baby gets older, he or she will try to imitate these facial expressions.
- Babies like music and rhythmic movement. Rock or swing your baby as you sing to him or her in a gentle voice.
- Acknowledge your baby's attempts to "answer" your talking and singing. He or she will respond to you by looking in your direction, making eye contact, moving his or her arms and legs, and making sounds.
- Babies like bright colors and vivid contrasts. Show your baby pictures and objects that are black and white, or bright primary colors (red, blue, yellow), and have large patterns. Keep colorful mobiles and toys where your baby can see them.
- Babies like to be held upright. Holding your newborn on your shoulder lets your baby look around his or her world and provides vestibular stimulation. Let your baby lift his or her head for a few seconds. Keep your hand ready to support your baby's head.

BOX 24-13 TEACHING YOUR 1-MONTH-OLD

At 1 to 2 months of age your infant is gaining more control of his or her movements; the infant has more head control and may even hold an object briefly in his or her hand. Your baby is also becoming more social. He or she demonstrates behaviors to engage you in interaction: smiling, cooing, making longer eye contact, and following you with his or her eyes.

During these months, you can help your baby learn if you:

- Put your baby on his or her stomach on a blanket on the floor. Lie on your stomach facing your baby. Talk to your baby to get him or her to raise his or her head to see you.
- Roll your baby onto his or her back and play with your baby's legs. Move the baby's legs in a bicycle-riding motion. Try to get your baby to kick his or her legs.
- Play hand games, such as pat-a-cake, with your baby; kiss your baby's fingers; place your baby's hands on your face. Bring your baby's hands in front of his or her eyes as you play; get your baby to look at his or her hands.
- Encourage your baby to watch and follow objects with his or her eyes. Use a noise-making toy, such as a rattle or a chime, or a brightly colored object approximately 12 inches from his or her eyes; move it slowly to one side and then the other. Objects hanging from a play frame are good for your baby to watch while he or she is on his or her back or sitting in an infant seat.
- Continue to talk and sing a lot to your baby. Continue to tell your baby what you are doing with him or her and what is going on in the immediate environment.
- Keep your baby near you during times when the family usually is together, such as at mealtimes. Infant seats, especially ones that bounce or rock, and infant swings are good to use at these times.

TABLE 24-7 PLAY DURING INFANCY: SUGGESTED ACTIVITIES FOR BIRTH THROUGH 3 MONTHS

AGE	VISUAL STIMULATION	AUDITORY STIMULATION	TACTILE STIMULATION	KINETIC STIMULATION
Birth-1	Look at infant at close range Hang bright, shiny object within 9 to 10 inches of infant's face and in midline Hang mobiles with black-and-white contrast designs	Talk to infant, sing in soft voice Play music box, radio, television Have ticking clock or metronome nearby	Hold, caress, cuddle Keep infant warm Infant may like to be swaddled	Rock infant, place in cradle Use carriage for walks
2-3	Provide bright objects Make room bright with pictures or mirrors on walls Take infant to various rooms while doing chores Place infant in infant seat for vertical view of environment	Talk to infant Include in family gatherings Expose to various environmental noises other than those of home Use rattles, wind chimes	Caress infant while bathing, at diaper change Comb hair with a soft brush	Use infant swing Take in car for rides Exercise body by moving extremities in swimming motion Use cradle gym

Source: Hockenberry, M. (2011). *Wong's nursing care of infants and children* (9th ed.). St. Louis: Mosby.

BOX 24-14 SIGNS OF ILLNESS

- Fever: temperature above 38° C (100.4° F) axillary (under arm for 3 to 4 minutes); also a continual rise in temperature
- Hypothermia: temperature below 36.5° C (97.7° F) axillary
- Poor feeding or little interest in food: refusal to eat for two feedings in a row
- Vomiting: more than one episode of forceful vomiting or frequent vomiting (over a 6-hour period)
- Diarrhea: two consecutive green, watery stools (NOTE: Stools of breastfed infants are normally looser than stools of formula-fed infants. Diarrhea will leave a water ring around the stool, whereas breastfed stools will not.)
- Decreased bowel movement: in a breastfed infant, less than three stools per day; in a formula-fed infant, less than one stool every other day
- Decreased urination: less than six to eight wet diapers per day after 3 to 4 days of age
- Breathing difficulties: labored breathing with flared nostrils or absence of breathing for more than 15 seconds (NOTE: A newborn's breathing is normally irregular and between 30 to 40 breaths/min. Count the breaths for a full minute.)
- Cyanosis (bluish skin color) whether accompanying a feeding or not
- Lethargy: sleepiness, difficulty waking, or periods of sleep longer than 6 hours (most newborns sleep for short periods, usually from 1 to 4 hours, and wake to be fed)
- Inconsolable crying (attempts to quiet not effective) or continuous high-pitched cry
- Bleeding or purulent (yellowish) drainage from umbilical cord or circumcision
- Drainage from the eyes

COMMUNITY ACTIVITY

- Visit the National Newborn Screening and Genetics Resource Center (NNSGRC) website (http://genes-r-us.uthscsa.edu). Review the information for parents and family about resources, disorders tested, and screening programs. What types of disorders are screened in your state? Is the screening for the condition required by law and fully implemented?
- At the NNSGRC website, visit the newborn screening program website for your state. Does your state require newborn hearing screening? Review the information for parents about diagnostic testing and community support services.

KEY POINTS

- Assessment of the newborn requires data from the prenatal, intrapartal, and postnatal periods.
- The immediate assessment of the newborn includes Apgar scoring and a general evaluation of physical status.
- Knowledge of biologic and behavioral characteristics is essential for guiding assessment and interpreting data.
- Gestational age assessment is important for predicting mentality risks and providing guidelines for care management.
- Nursing care immediately after birth includes maintaining an open airway, preventing heat loss, and promoting parent-infant interaction.
- Providing a protective environment is a key responsibility of the nurse and includes such measures as careful identification procedures, support of physiologic functions, ways to prevent infection, and restraining techniques.
- The newborn has social and physical needs.
- Circumcision is an elective surgical procedure.
- Pain in neonates must be assessed and managed.
- Anticipatory guidance an topics such as feeding and elimination patterns; positioning and holding; car seat safety, bathing, cord care, and skin care; and signs of illness helps to prepare new parents for what to expect after hospital discharge.
- All parents should have instruction in infant CPR.

Audio Chapter Summaries Access an audio summary of these Key Points on evolve

REFERENCES

Alexander, G., Himes, J., Kaufman, R., Mor, J., & Kogan, M. (1996). A United States national reference for fetal growth. *Obstetrics and Gynecology*, *87*(2), 163–168.

American Academy of Pediatrics. (2005). AAP publications retired and reaffirmed. *Pediatrics*, *116*(3), 796.

American Academy of Pediatrics. (2010). *Car safety seats: A guide for families 2010*. Elk Grove Village, IL: AAP. Available at http://www.healthychildren.org/English/safety-prevention/on-the-go/pages/Car-Safety-Seats-Information-for-Families-2010.aspx. Accessed July 12, 2010.

American Academy of Pediatrics (AAP) & American College of Obstetricians and Gynecologists (ACOG). (2007). *Guidelines for perinatal care* (6th ed.). Elk Grove Village, IL: AAP.

American Academy of Pediatrics (AAP) Committee on Infectious Diseases. (2009). *Red book: 2009 report of the committee on infectious diseases* (28th ed.). Elk Grove Village, IL: AAP.

American Academy of Pediatrics (AAP) Subcommittee on Hyperbilirubinemia. (2004). Clinical practice guideline: Management of hyperbilirubinemia in the newborn infant 35 or more weeks of gestation. *Pediatrics*, *114*(1), 297–316.

American Academy of Pediatrics (AAP) Task Force on Circumcision. (1999). Circumcision policy statement. *Pediatrics*, *103*(3), 686–693.

American Academy of Pediatrics (AAP) Task Force on Infant Sleep Position and Sudden Infant Death Syndrome. (2005). The changing concept of sudden infant death syndrome: Diagnostic coding shifts, controversies regarding the sleeping environment, and new variables to consider in reducing risk. *Pediatrics*, *116*(5), 1245–1255.

American College of Obstetricians and Gynecologists (ACOG). (2001). Circumcision. ACOG Committee opinion no. 260. *Obstetrics and Gynecology, 98*(4), 707–708.

Arbuckle, T., Wilkins, R., & Sherman, G. (1993). Birth weight percentiles by gestational age in Canada. *Obstetrics and Gynecology, 81*(1), 39–48.

Asher, C., & Northington, L. (2008). Position statement for measurement of temperature/fever in children. *Journal of Pediatric Nursing, 23*(3), 234–236.

Association of Women's Health, Obstetric, and Neonatal Nurses (AWHONN). (2007). *Neonatal skin care: Evidence-based clinical practice guideline* (2nd ed.). Washington, DC: AWHONN.

Auvert, B., Taljaard, D., Lagarde, E., Sobngwi-Tambekou, J., Sitta, R., & Puren, A. (2005). Randomized, controlled intervention trial of male circumcision for reduction of HIV infection risk: The ANRS 1265 trial. *PLoS Medicine, 2*(11), e298.

Bailey, R., Moses, S., Parker, C., Agot, K., Maclean, I., Krieger, J., et al. (2007). Male circumcision for HIV prevention in young men in Kisumu, Kenya: A randomised controlled trial. *Lancet, 369*(9562), 643–656.

Bakewell-Sachs, S. (2007). Near-term/late preterm infants. *Newborn & Infant Nursing Reviews, 7*(2), 67–71.

Ballard, J., Khoury, J., Wedig, K., Wang, L., Eilers-Walsman, B., & Lipp, R. (1991). New Ballard score, expanded to include extremely premature infants. *Journal of Pediatrics, 119*(3), 417–423.

Ballard, J., Novak, K., & Driver, M. (1979). A simplified score for assessment of fetal maturity of newly born infants. *Journal of Pediatrics, 95*(5 Pt 1), 769–774.

Battaglia, F., & Lubchenco, L. (1967). A practical classification of newborn infants by weight and gestational age. *Journal of Pediatrics, 71*(2), 159–163.

Blackburn, S. (2007). *Maternal, fetal, and neonatal physiology: A clinical perspective* (3rd ed.). St. Louis: Saunders.

Brady, M. (2010). Newborn circumcision: Routine or not routine, that is the question. *Archives of Pediatric and Adolescent Medicine, 164*(1), 94–96.

Brady-Fryer, B., Wiebe, N., & Lander, J. (2004). Pain relief for neonatal circumcision. *The Cochrane Database of Systematic Reviews, 2004*, 3, CD004217.

Brazelton, T. (1995). Working with families: Opportunities for early intervention. *Pediatric Clinics of North America, 42*(1), 1.

Bull, M., Engle, W., & Committee on Injury, Violence, and Poison Prevention, & Committee on Fetus and Newborn. (2009). Safe transportation of preterm and low birth weight infants at hospital discharge. *Pediatrics, 123*(5), 1424–1429.

Chermont, A., Falcão, L., de Souza Silva, E., de Cássia Xavier Balda, R., & Guinsburg, R. (2009). Skin-to-skin contact and/or oral 25% sucrose for procedural pain relief for term newborn infants. *Pediatrics, 124*(6), e1101–e1107.

D'Avanzo, C. (2008). *Mosby's pocket guide to cultural health assessment* (4th ed.). St. Louis: Mosby.

Furdon, S., Eastman, M., Benjamin, K., & Horgan, M. (1998). Outcome measures after standardized pain management strategies in postoperative patients in the NICU. *Journal of Perinatal and Neonatal Nursing, 12*(1), 58–69.

Gray, R., Kigozi, G., Serwadda, D., Makumbi, F., Watya, S., Nalugoda, F., et al. (2007). Male circumcision for HIV prevention in men in Rakai, Uganda: A randomised trial. *Lancet, 369*(9562), 657–666.

Hagedorn, M. (2006). Respiratory distress. In G. Merenstein, & S. Gardner (Eds.), *Handbook of neonatal intensive care* (6th ed.). St. Louis: Mosby.

Joint Committee on Infant Hearing. (2007). Year 2007 position statement: Principles and guidelines for early hearing detection and intervention programs. *Pediatrics, 120*(4), 898–921.

Joint United Nations Programme on HIV/AIDS. (2007). *New data on male circumcision and HIV prevention: Policy and programme implications*. Montreux, Switzerland: Joint United Nations Programme on HIV/AIDS.

Kalhan, S., & Parimi, P. (2006). Metabolic and endocrine disorders. In R. Martin, A. Fanaroff, & M. Walsh (Eds.), *Fanaroff and Martin's neonatal-perinatal medicine: Diseases of the fetus and infant* (8th ed.). Philadelphia: Mosby.

Keren, R., Luan, X., Friedman, S., Saddlemire, S., Cnaan, A., & Bhutani, V. (2008). A comparison of alternative risk-assessment strategies for predicting significant neonatal hyperbilirubinemia in term and near-term infants. *Pediatrics, 121*(1), e170–e179.

Kramer, M., Platt, R., Wen, S., Joseph, K., Allen, A., Abrahamowicz, M., et al. (2001). A new and improved population-based Canadian reference for birth weight for gestational age. *Pediatrics, 108*(2), e35.

Krechel, S., & Bildner, J. (1995). CRIES: A new neonatal postoperative pain measurement score—Initial testing of validity and reliability. *Paediatric Anaesthesia, 5*(1), 53–61.

Lawrence, J., Alcock, D., McGrath, P., Kay, J., MacMurray, S., & Dulberg, C. (1993). The development of a tool to assess neonatal pain. *Neonatal Network, 12*(6), 59–66.

Leibowitz, A., Desmond, K., & Belin, T. (2009). Determinants and policy implications of male circumcision in the United States. *American Journal of Public Health, 99*(1), 138–145.

Leite, A., Linhares, M., Lander, J., Castral, T., dos Santos, C., & Silvan Scochi, C. (2009). Effects of breastfeeding on pain relief in full-term newborns. *Clinical Journal of Pain, 25*(9), 827–832.

Madan, A., Holland, S., Humbert, J., & Benitz, W. (2002). Racial differences in birth weight of term infants in a northern California population. *Journal of Perinatology, 22*(3), 230–235.

Maisels, M., & McDonagh, A. (2008). Phototherapy for neonatal jaundice. *New England Journal of Medicine, 358*(9), 920–928.

McConnell, T., Lee, C., Couillard, M., & Sherrill, W. (2004). Trends in umbilical cord care: Scientific evidence for practice. *Newborn & Infant Nursing Reviews, 4*(4), 211–222.

Merrill, C., Nagamine, M., & Steiner, C. (2008). Circumcisions performed in U.S. community hospitals, 2005. Statistical brief #45. *Healthcare cost and utilization project (HCUP)*. Rockville, MD: Agency for Healthcare Research and Quality. Available at www.hcup-us.ahrq.gov/reports/statbriefs/sb45.jsp. Accessed July 12, 2010.

National Highway Traffic Administration. (2010). *Child passenger safety: A parent's primer*. Washington, DC: NHTSA. Available at www.nhtsa.gov/DOT/NHTSA/TrafficInjuryControl/Articles/AssociatedFiles/4StepsFlyer.pdf. Accessed July 20, 2010.

Pagana, K., & Pagana, T. (2009). *Mosby's diagnostic and laboratory test reference* (9th ed.). St. Louis: Mosby.

Ramachandrappa, A., & Jain, L. (2009). Health issues of the late preterm infant. *Pediatric Clinics of North America, 56*(3), 565–577.

Sansom, S., Prabhu, V., Hutchinson, A., An, Q., Hall, I., Shrestha, R., et al. (2010). Cost-effectiveness of newborn circumcision in reducing lifetime HIV risk among U.S. males. *PLoS ONE, 5*(1), e8723.

Sharfstein, J., North, M., & Serwint, J. (2007). Over the counter but no longer under the radar—Pediatric cough and cold medications. *New England Journal of Medicine, 357*(23), 2321–2324.

Siegfried, N., Muller, M., Deeks, J., & Volmink, J. (2009). Male circumcision for prevention of heterosexual acquisition of HIV in men. *The Cochrane Database of Systematic Reviews, 2009*, 2, CD003362.

Sperling, M. (2007). Hypoglycemia. In R. Kliegman, R. Behrman, H. Jenson, & B. Stanton (Eds.), *Nelson textbook of pediatrics* (18th ed.). Philadelphia: Saunders.

Stevens, B., Johnston, C., Petryshen, P., & Taddio, A. (1996). Premature infant pain profile: Development and initial validation. *Clinical Journal of Pain, 12*(1), 13–22.

Stevens, B., Yamada, J., & Ohlsson, A. (2010). Sucrose for analgesia in newborn infants undergoing painful procedures. *The Cochrane Database of Systematic Reviews, 2010*, 1, CD001069.

Stoll, B. (2007). The fetus and the neonatal infant. In R. Kliegman, R. Behrman, H. Jenson, & B. Stanton (Eds.), *Nelson textbook of pediatrics* (18th ed.). Philadelphia: Saunders.

Thomas, P., Peabody, J., Turnier, V., & Clark, R. (2000). A new look at intrauterine growth and the impact of race, altitude, and gender. *Pediatrics, 106*(2), e21.

Volpe, J. (2008). *Neurology of the newborn* (5th ed.). Philadelphia: Saunders.

Walden, M. (2007). Pain management in the newborn and infant. In C. Kenner, & J. Lott (Eds.), *Comprehensive neonatal care: An interdisciplinary approach* (4th ed.). St. Louis: Saunders.

Walden, M., & Gibbins, S. (2008). *Pain assessment & management guideline for practice* (2nd ed.). Glenview, IL: National Association of Neonatal Nurses.

Weissman, A., Aranovitch, M., Blazer, S., & Zimmer, E. (2009). Heel-lancing in newborns: Behavioral and spectral analysis assessment of pain control methods. *Pediatrics, 124*(5), e921–e926.

World Health Organization. (2009). *WHO guidelines on hand hygiene in health care: A summary*. Geneva, Switzerland: WHO Press.

Zinn, A. (2006). Inborn errors of metabolism. In R. Martin, A. Fanaroff, & M. Walsh (Eds.), *Fanaroff and Martin's neonatal-perinatal medicine: Diseases of the fetus and infant* (8th ed.). Philadelphia: Mosby.

Zupan, J., Garner, P., & Omari, A. (2004). Topical umbilical cord care at birth. *The Cochrane Database of Systematic Reviews, 2004*, 3, CD001057.

CHAPTER

25

Newborn Nutrition and Feeding

Kathryn Rhodes Alden

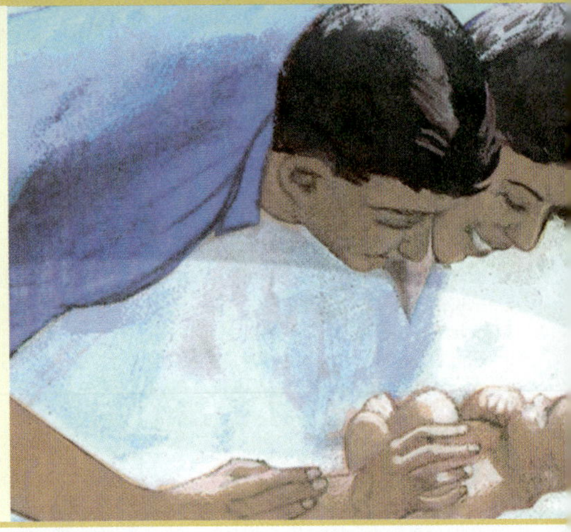

evolve WEBSITE

http://evolve.elsevier.com/Lowdermilk/MWHC/

Audio Glossary
Audio Key Points
Case Study
- Breastfeeding

Critical Thinking Exercises
- Breastfeeding
- Formula Preparation

NCLEX Review Questions
Nursing Care Plans
- Breastfeeding and Infant Nutrition
- The Newborn with Insufficient Intake of Nutrients

Nursing Skill
- Infant Feeding

Spanish Guidelines
- Breastfeeding: Latch
- Burping

Video—Nursing Skills
- Teaching Breastfeeding

LEARNING OBJECTIVES

- Describe current recommendations for infant feeding.
- Explain the nurse's role in helping families choose an infant feeding method.
- Discuss benefits of breastfeeding for infants, mothers, families, and society.
- Describe nutritional needs of infants.
- Describe anatomic and physiologic aspects of breastfeeding.
- Recognize newborn feeding-readiness cues.
- Explain maternal and infant indicators of effective breastfeeding.
- Examine nursing interventions to facilitate and promote successful breastfeeding.
- Analyze common problems associated with breastfeeding and interventions to help resolve them.
- Compare powdered, concentrated, and ready-to-use forms of commercial infant formula.
- Develop a teaching plan for the formula-feeding family.

Good nutrition in infancy fosters optimal growth and development. Infant feeding is more than the provision of nutrition; it is an opportunity for social, psychologic, and even educational interaction between parent and infant. It can also establish a basis for developing good eating habits that last a lifetime.

Through preconception and prenatal education and counseling, nurses play an instrumental role in assisting parents with the selection of an infant feeding method. Scientific evidence is clear that human milk provides the best nutrition for infants, and parents should be strongly encouraged to choose breastfeeding (American Academy of Pediatrics [AAP] Section on Breastfeeding, 2005; Ip, Chung, Raman, Chew, Magula, DeVine, et al., 2007). Although many health care providers and the general public consider commercial infant formula to be equivalent to breast milk, this belief is erroneous. Human milk is species-specific, uniquely designed to meet the needs of human infants. The composition of human milk changes to meet the nutritional needs of growing infants. It is highly complex, with antiinfective and nutritional components combined with growth factors, enzymes that aid in digestion and absorption of nutrients, and fatty acids that promote brain growth and development. Infant formulas are usually adequate in providing nutrition to maintain infant growth and development within normal limits, but they are not equivalent to human milk.

Breastfeeding is defined as the transfer of human milk from mother to child; the infant receives milk directly from the mother's breast. *Breast milk feeding* is the provision of mother's milk to the infant; the mother expresses her milk and feeds it to the infant. *Human milk feeding* refers to feeding of breast milk from another individual or from a milk bank. *Exclusive breastfeeding* means that the infant is fed no other liquid or solid food (Academy of Breastfeeding Medicine [ABM] Board of Directors, 2008).

Whether the parents choose breastfeeding, breast milk feeding, human milk feeding, or feeding with commercial infant formula, nurses provide support and ongoing education. Parent education is necessarily based on current research findings and standards of practice.

This chapter focuses on meeting nutritional needs for normal growth and development from birth to 6 months, with emphasis on the neonatal period, when feeding practices and patterns are established. Breastfeeding and formula feeding are addressed. Information on breastfeeding is focused on the direct transfer of milk from mother to infant.

RECOMMENDED INFANT NUTRITION

The American Academy of Pediatrics (AAP) recommends exclusive breastfeeding or human milk feeding for the first 6 months of life and that breastfeeding or human milk feeding continue as the sole source of milk for the first year. During the second 6 months of life, appropriate complementary foods (solids) are added to the infant diet. If infants are weaned from breast milk before 12 months of age, they should receive iron-fortified infant formula, not cow's milk (AAP Section on Breastfeeding, 2005). According to the Global Strategy for Infant and Young Child Feeding, endorsed by the World Health Organization (WHO) and United Nations Children's Fund (UNICEF), infants should be exclusively breastfed for 6 months, and breastfeeding should continue for up to 2 years and beyond (WHO/UNICEF, 2003).

Exclusive breastfeeding for the first 6 months of life is also recommended by other professional health care organizations such as the American Academy of Family Physicians (AAFP) (2007), Academy of Breastfeeding Medicine (ABM Board of Directors, 2008), the American College of Obstetricians and Gynecologists (ACOG) (ACOG Committee on Health Care for Underserved Women & Committee on Obstetric Practice, 2007), and the American Dietetic Association (ADA) (2009). The Association of Women's Health, Obstetric and Neonatal Nurses (AWHONN) (2007) actively supports breastfeeding as the ideal form of infant nutrition and provides guidelines for nurses in promoting breastfeeding and supporting breastfeeding families.

BREASTFEEDING RATES

Data from the Centers for Disease Control and Prevention (CDC) National Immunization Survey (2009) indicate that breastfeeding rates in the United States have risen steadily over the past decade. In 2006, the percent of infants ever breastfed was 73.9%, falling short of the *Healthy People 2010* goal of 75%. However, 28 states had breastfeeding initiation rates that met or exceeded the *Healthy People* goal. The 6-month breastfeeding rate was 43.4% and the 12-month rate was 22.7%. The *Healthy People 2010* goals of 50% at 6 months and 25% at 12 months were not achieved. Exclusive breastfeeding rates were 33.1% at 3 months and 13.6% at 6 months; the *Healthy People* goals were 40% and 17%, respectively (CDC, 2009; U.S. Department of Health and Human Services [USDHHS], 2000).

Among a birth cohort group of 434 infants in the National Health and Nutrition Examination Survey (McDowell, Wang, & Kennedy-Stephenson, 2008), the percentage who were ever breastfed rose to a record level of 77% for 2005-2006. This was an increase from 60% among infants born from 1993 to 1994. There were no significant changes in breastfeeding rates at 6 months of age—the highest breastfeeding rates were reported among Mexican-Americans (40%) and non-Hispanic white infants (35%). Breastfeeding initiation rates increased significantly to 65% among non-Hispanic black women. Results of the survey showed that certain breastfeeding trends continue: those most likely to breastfeed are Caucasian, older than age 30, with higher incomes.

The proposed objective for *Healthy People 2020* is retained from the 2010 objectives: to "increase the proportion of mothers who breastfeed their babies." The proposed goals related to breastfeeding rates remain the same as for *Healthy People 2010* (USDHHS, 2009).

BENEFITS OF BREASTFEEDING

Numerous research studies have identified the beneficial effects of human milk for infants during the first year of life. Long-term epidemiologic studies have shown that these benefits do not cease when the infant is weaned; instead, they extend into childhood and beyond. Breastfeeding has many advantages for mothers, for families, and for society in general (AAP Section on Breastfeeding, 2005; Horta, Bahl, Martines, & Victora, 2007; Ip et al., 2007; Stuebe, 2009). To discuss breastfeeding with parents, nurses and other health care professionals must have a thorough understanding of its benefits from both a physiologic and a psychosocial perspective (Table 25-1).

CHOOSING AN INFANT FEEDING METHOD

Breastfeeding is a natural extension of pregnancy and childbirth; it is much more than simply a means of supplying nutrition for infants. Women most often breastfeed their babies because they are aware of the benefits to the infant. Many women seek the unique bonding experience between mother and infant that is characteristic of breastfeeding. Women tend to select the same method of infant feeding for each of their children. If the first child was breastfed, subsequent children will likely also be breastfed (Taylor, Geller, Risica, Kirtania, & Cabral, 2008).

The support of the partner and family is a major factor in the mother's decision to breastfeed. Women who perceive their partners to prefer breastfeeding are more likely to choose this method (Scott, Binns, Graham, & Oddy, 2006). Women are more likely to breastfeed successfully when partners and family members are positive about breastfeeding and have the skills to support breastfeeding (Clifford & McIntyre, 2008).

Parents who choose to formula feed often make this decision without complete information and understanding of the benefits of breastfeeding. Even women who are educated about the advantages of breastfeeding may still decide to formula feed. Cultural beliefs, as well as myths and misconceptions about breastfeeding, influence women's decision making. Many women see bottle feeding as more convenient or less embarrassing than breastfeeding. Some view formula feeding as a way to ensure that the father, other family members, and daycare providers can feed the baby. Some women lack confidence in their ability to produce breast milk of adequate quantity or quality. Women who have had

TABLE 25-1 **BENEFITS OF BREASTFEEDING**

BENEFITS FOR THE INFANT	BENEFITS FOR THE MOTHER	BENEFITS TO FAMILIES AND SOCIETY
Decreased incidence and severity of infectious diseases: bacterial meningitis, bacteremia, diarrhea, respiratory infection, necrotizing enterocolitis, otitis media, urinary tract infection, late-onset sepsis in preterm infants Reduced postneonatal infant mortality Decreased rates of SIDS Decreased incidence of type 1 and type 2 diabetes Decreased incidence of lymphoma, leukemia, Hodgkin disease Reduced risk of obesity and hypercholesterolemia Decreased incidence and severity of asthma and other allergies Possible enhanced cognitive development Enhanced jaw development and decreased problems with malocclusions and malalignment of teeth Analgesic effect for infants undergoing painful procedures such as venipuncture	Decreased postpartum bleeding and more rapid uterine involution Reduced risk of ovarian cancer and premenopausal breast cancer Lower risk of hypertension, hypercholesterolemia, and cardiovascular disease Earlier return to prepregnancy weight Decreased risk of postmenopausal osteoporosis Unique bonding experience Increased maternal role attainment	Convenient; ready to feed No bottles or other necessary equipment Less expensive than infant formula Reduced annual health care costs Less parental absence from work because of ill infant Reduced environmental burden related to disposal of formula cans

SIDS, Sudden infant death syndrome.

Sources: American Academy of Pediatrics Section on Breastfeeding. (2005). Breastfeeding and the use of human milk. Policy statement. *Pediatrics, 115*(23), 496-506; Horta, B., Bahl, R., Martines, J., & Victora, C. (2007). *Evidence of the long-term effects of breastfeeding.* Geneva: World Health Organization; Ip, S., Chung, M., Raman, G., Chew, P., Magula, N., DeVine, D., et al. (2007). *Breastfeeding and maternal and infant health outcomes in developed countries.* Evidence report/technology assessment No. 153. (Prepared by Tufts-New England Medical Center Evidence-Based Practice Center under contract No. 290-02-0022). AHRQ publication No. 07-E007. Rockville, MD: Agency for Healthcare Research and Quality; Stuebe, A. (2009). The risks of not breastfeeding for mothers and infants. *Reviews in Obstetrics and Gynecology, 2*(4), 222-231.

previous unsuccessful breastfeeding experiences may choose to formula feed subsequent infants. Some women see breastfeeding as incompatible with an active social life, or they think that it will prevent them from going back to work. Modesty issues and societal barriers exist against breastfeeding in public. A major barrier for many women is the influence of family and friends.

Breastfeeding is contraindicated in a few situations. Newborns who have galactosemia should not be breastfed. Mothers with active tuberculosis and those who are positive for human T-cell lymphotropic virus type I or type II should not breastfeed.

In the United States, maternal HIV infection is considered a contraindication for breastfeeding (AAP Section on Breastfeeding, 2005). However, that is not true in other countries. In developing countries where HIV is prevalent, the benefits of breastfeeding for infants outweigh the risk of contracting HIV from infected mothers. In 2010, The World Health Organization (2010) published revised guidelines on HIV and infant feeding. The guidelines indicate that national or sub-national health authorities should decide which feeding practice for HIV-infected mothers will be promoted and supported by Maternal and Child Health services: avoiding all breastfeeding or breastfeeding and receiving antiretroviral (ARV) medications. HIV-infected mothers who are taking ARV therapy should breastfeed until infants are 12 months of age. If ARVs are not available, breastfeeding can improve the chances of HIV-free survival for infants born to HIV-infected mothers. Therefore, for HIV-infected mothers who do not have access to ARVs, exclusive breastfeeding for the first six months is recommended; complementary foods can be introduced thereafter, and breastfeeding should continue until the infant is one year old. Furthermore, breastfeeding should continue until a safe and nutritionally adequate diet without breastmilk can be provided for the infant (WHO, United Nations Children's Fund [UNICEF], United Nations Population Fund [UNFPA], & Joint United Nations Programme on HIV/AIDS [UNAIDS], 2010).

Video—Nursing Skills: Teaching Breastfeeding

Breastfeeding is not recommended when mothers are receiving chemotherapy or radioactive isotopes (e.g., with diagnostic procedures). Maternal use of mood-altering drugs ("street drugs") is incompatible with breastfeeding (AAP Section on Breastfeeding, 2005). In addition, women who are taking certain medications such as bromocriptine, reserpine, high-dose corticosteroids, or cyclosporine should not breastfeed (WHO, 2009).

SUPPORTING BREASTFEEDING MOTHERS

The key to encouraging mothers to breastfeed is education and anticipatory guidance, beginning as early as possible during and even before pregnancy. Each encounter with an expectant mother is an opportunity to educate, dispel myths, clarify misinformation, and address concerns. Prenatal education and preparation for breastfeeding influence feeding decisions, breastfeeding success, and the amount of time that women breastfeed (Rosen, Krueger, Carney, & Graham, 2008). Prenatal preparation ideally includes the father of the baby, partner, or another significant support person, providing information about benefits of breastfeeding and how he or she can participate in infant care and nurturing.

Connecting expectant mothers with women from similar backgrounds who are breastfeeding or have successfully breastfed is often helpful. Nursing mothers' support groups provide information about breastfeeding along with opportunities for breastfeeding mothers to interact with one another and share concerns (Fig. 25-1). Peer counseling programs, such as those instituted by Special Supplemental Nutrition Program for Women, Infants, and Children (WIC) programs, are beneficial.

For women with limited access to health care, the postpartum period may provide the first opportunity for education about breastfeeding. Even women who have indicated the desire to formula-feed can benefit from information about the

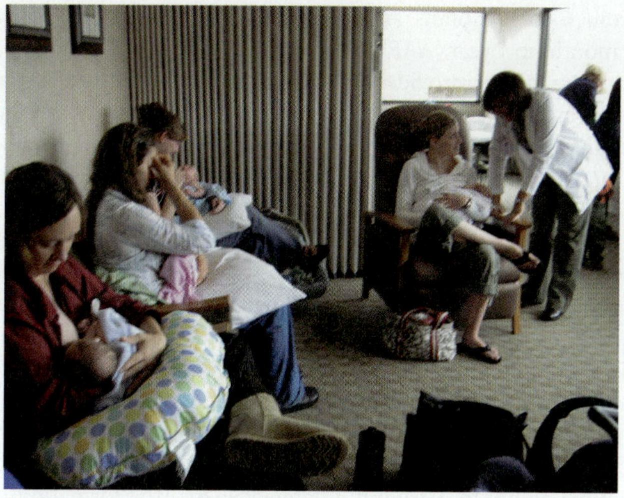

FIG. 25-1 Breastfeeding mothers support group with lactation consultant. (Courtesy Shannon Perry, Phoenix, AZ.)

benefits of breastfeeding. Offering these women the chance to try breastfeeding with the assistance of a nurse or lactation consultant may influence a change in infant feeding practices.

Promoting feelings of competence and confidence in the breastfeeding mother and reinforcing the unequaled contribution she is making toward the health and well-being of her infant are the responsibility of the nurse and other health care professionals. Women who are optimistic, with a sense of breastfeeding self-efficacy, and faith in breast milk as the best nutrition for the infant are likely to breastfeed longer (O'Brien, Buikstra, & Hegney, 2008). The most common reasons for breastfeeding cessation are insufficient milk supply, painful nipples, and problems getting the infant to feed (Lewallen, Dick, Flowers, Powell, Zickefoose, Wall, et al., 2006). Early and ongoing assistance and support from health care professionals to prevent and address problems with breastfeeding can help promote a successful and satisfying breastfeeding experience for mothers and infants (Renfrew & Hall, 2008). Many health care agencies have certified lactation consultants on staff. These health care professionals, who are usually nurses, have specialized training and experience in assisting breastfeeding mothers and infants. Evidence-based guidelines for supporting breastfeeding are available for use by health care professionals (AWHONN, 2007; International Lactation Consultant Association [ILCA], 1999; Overfield, Ryan, Spangler, & Tully, 2005).

All parents are entitled to a birthing environment in which breastfeeding is promoted and supported. The Baby Friendly Hospital Initiative (BFHI), sponsored by the WHO and United Nations Children's Fund (UNICEF), was founded in 1991 to encourage institutions to offer optimal levels of care for lactating mothers. When a hospital achieves the "Ten Steps to Successful Breastfeeding for Hospitals," it is recognized as a Baby Friendly Hospital (Box 25-1) (BFHI USA, 2010).

CULTURAL INFLUENCES ON INFANT FEEDING

Cultural beliefs and practices are significant influences on infant feeding methods. Although recognized cultural norms exist, one cannot assume that generalized observations about any cultural group hold true for all members of that group.

BOX 25-1 TEN STEPS TO SUCCESSFUL BREASTFEEDING FOR HOSPITALS

1. Have a written breastfeeding policy that is routinely communicated to all health care staff.
2. Train all health care staff in skills necessary to implement this policy.
3. Inform all pregnant women about the benefits and management of breastfeeding.
4. Help mothers initiate breastfeeding within ½ hour of birth.
5. Show mothers how to breastfeed and maintain lactation, even if they should be separated from their infants.
6. Give newborn infants no food or drink other than breast milk, unless medically indicated.
7. Practice rooming-in—that is, allow mothers and infants to remain together 24 hours a day.
8. Encourage breastfeeding on demand.
9. Give no artificial teats or pacifiers (also called dummies or soothers) to breastfeeding infants.
10. Foster the establishment of breastfeeding support groups and refer mothers to them on discharge from the hospital or clinic.

Source: Baby-Friendly USA. (2010). *BFHI USA: Implementing the UNICEF/WHO baby friendly hospital initiative in the U.S.* Sandwich, MA: BFUSA. Available at www.babyfriendlyusa.org. Accessed July 12, 2010.

Many regional and ethnic cultures are found within the United States. Dealing effectively with these groups requires that nurses are knowledgeable and sensitive to the cultural factors influencing infant feeding practices.

In general, people who have immigrated to the United States from poorer countries often choose to formula feed their infants because they believe it is a better, more "modern" method or because they want to adapt to U.S. culture and perceive that formula feeding is the custom. However, this notion is not always true. For example, Hispanic women born in the United States are less likely to breastfeed, whereas those women who have recently immigrated tend to choose the social norm of breastfeeding that is characteristic of their homeland (Gill, 2009). Women from Mexico are accustomed to breastfeeding as the expected method of infant feeding. Mexico has federal guidelines that support breastfeeding and include standards to promote and protect exclusive breastfeeding. Federal regulations in Mexico restrict commercial infant formula distribution in hospitals (Castrucci, Piña Carrizales, D'Angelo, McDonald, Foulkes, Ahluwalia, et al., 2008).

Breastfeeding beliefs and practices vary across cultures. For example, among the Muslim culture, breastfeeding for 24 months is customary. Before the first feeding, rubbing a small piece of softened date on the newborn's palate is a ritual practice. Because of the cultural emphasis on privacy and modesty, Muslim women may choose to bottle-feed formula or expressed breast milk while in the hospital (Shaikh & Ahmed, 2006).

Because of beliefs about the harmful nature or inadequacy of colostrum, some cultures apply restrictions on breastfeeding for a period of days after birth. Such is the case for many cultures in Southern Asia, the Pacific Islands, and parts of sub-Saharan Africa. Before the mother's milk is deemed to be "in," babies are fed prelacteal food such as honey or clarified butter, in the belief that these substances will help clear out meconium (Laroia & Sharma, 2006; Shaikh & Ahmed, 2006). Other cultures begin breastfeeding immediately and offer the breast each time the infant cries.

A common practice among Mexican women is *los dos*. This refers to combining breastfeeding and commercial infant formula. It is based on the belief that by combining the two methods, the mother and infant receive the benefits of breastfeeding, and the infant also receives the additional vitamins from infant formula (Rios, 2009). This practice can result in problems with milk supply and babies refusing to latch on to the breast, which can lead to early termination of breastfeeding (Bunik, Clark, Zimmer, Jimenez, O'Connor, Crane et al., 2006).

Some cultures have specific beliefs and practices related to the mother's intake of foods that foster milk production. Korean mothers often eat seaweed soup and rice to enhance milk production. Hmong women believe that boiled chicken, rice, and hot water are the only appropriate nourishments during the first postpartum month. The balance between energy forces, hot and cold, or yin and yang is integral to the diet of the lactating mother. Hispanics, Vietnamese, Chinese, East Indians, and Arabs often use this belief in choosing foods. "Hot" foods are considered best for new mothers. This belief does not necessarily relate to the temperature or spiciness of foods. For example, chicken and broccoli are considered "hot," whereas many fresh fruits and vegetables are considered "cold." Families often bring desired foods into the health care setting.

NUTRIENT NEEDS

Fluids

During the first 2 days of life the fluid requirement for healthy infants (more than 1500 g) is 60 to 80 ml of water per kilogram of body weight per day. From day 3 to 7 the requirement is 100 to 150 ml/kg/day and from day 8 to day 30, 120 to 180 ml/kg/day (Dell & Davis, 2006). In general, neither breastfed nor formula-fed infants need to be given water, not even those living in very hot climates. Breast milk contains 87% water, which easily meets fluid requirements. Feeding water to infants may only decrease caloric consumption at a time when they are growing rapidly.

Infants have room for little fluctuation in fluid balance and should be monitored closely for fluid intake and water loss. They lose water through excretion of urine and insensibly through respiration. Under normal circumstances, they are born with some fluid reserve, and some of the weight loss during the first few days is related to fluid loss. In some cases, however, they do not have this fluid reserve, possibly because of inadequate maternal hydration during labor or birth.

Energy

Infants require adequate caloric intake to provide energy for growth, digestion, physical activity, and maintenance of organ metabolic function. Energy needs vary according to age, maturity level, thermal environment, growth rate, health status, and activity level. For the first 3 months the infant needs 110 kcal/kg/day. From 3 months to 6 months the requirement is 100 kcal/kg/day. This level decreases slightly to 95 kcal/kg/day from 6 to 9 months and increases to 100 kcal/kg/day from 9 months to 1 year (AAP, 2008).

Human milk provides 67 kcal/100 ml or 20 kcal/oz. The fat portion of the milk provides the greatest amount of energy. Infant formulas simulate the caloric content of human milk. Usually a standard formula contains 20 kcal/oz, though the composition differs among brands.

Carbohydrate

According to the Institute of Medicine (IOM) (2005), the adequate dietary reference intake (DRI) for carbohydrate in the first 6 months of life is 60 g/day and 95 g/day for the second 6 months. Because newborns have only small hepatic glycogen stores, carbohydrates should provide at least 40% to 50% of the total calories in the diet. Moreover, newborns may have a limited ability to carry out gluconeogenesis (the formation of glucose from amino acids and other substrates) and ketogenesis (the formation of ketone bodies from fat), the mechanisms that provide alternative sources of energy.

As the primary carbohydrate in human milk and commercially prepared infant formula, lactose is the most abundant carbohydrate in the diet of infants up to age 6 months. Lactose provides calories in an easily available form. Its slow breakdown and absorption also increase calcium absorption. Corn syrup solids or glucose polymers are added to infant formulas to supplement the lactose in the cow's milk and thereby provide sufficient carbohydrates.

Oligosaccharides, another form of carbohydrate found in breast milk, are critical in the development of microflora in the intestinal tract of the newborn. These prebiotics promote an acidic environment in the intestines, preventing the growth of gram-negative and other pathogenic bacteria, thus increasing the infant's resistance to gastrointestinal (GI) illness.

Fat

The average recommended DRI of fat for infants younger than 6 months is 31 g/day (IOM, 2005). For infants to acquire adequate calories from human milk or formula, at least 15% of the calories provided must come from fat (triglycerides).

The fat content of human milk is composed of lipids, triglycerides, and cholesterol; cholesterol is an essential element for brain growth. Human milk contains the essential fatty acids (EFAs), linoleic acid, and linolenic acid, as well as the long-chain polyunsaturated fatty acids, arachidonic acid (ARA), and docosahexaenoic acid (DHA). Fatty acids are important for growth, neurologic development, and visual function. Cow's milk contains fewer of the EFAs and no polyunsaturated fatty acids. Most formula companies add DHA and ARA to their products. Studies of infants receiving supplements of DHA and ARA have shown inconclusive results in terms of visual acuity and cognitive function (Heird, 2007; Simmer, Patole, & Rao, 2008).

Modified cow's milk is used in most infant formulas, but the milk fat is removed, and another fat source such as corn oil, which the infant can digest and absorb, is added in its place. If whole milk or evaporated milk without added carbohydrate is fed to infants, the resulting fecal loss of fat (and therefore loss of energy) can be excessive because the milk moves through the infant's intestines too quickly for adequate absorption to take place. This can lead to poor weight gain.

Protein

High-quality protein from breast milk, infant formula, or other complementary foods is necessary for infant growth. The protein requirement per unit of body weight is greater in the newborn than at any other time of life. For infants younger than 6 months the average DRI for protein is 9.1 g/day (IOM, 2005).

Human milk contains the two proteins, whey (lactalbumin) and casein (curd), in a ratio of approximately 60:40, as compared with the ratio of 80:20 in most cow's milk–based formula. This whey/casein ratio in human milk makes it more easily digested and produces the soft stools seen in breastfed infants. The whey protein lactoferrin in human milk has iron-binding capabilities and bacteriostatic properties, particularly against gram-positive and gram-negative aerobes, anaerobes, and yeasts. The casein in human milk enhances the absorption of iron, thus preventing iron-dependent bacteria from proliferating in the GI tract (Lawrence & Lawrence, 2005).

The amino acid components of human milk are uniquely suited to the newborn's metabolic capabilities. For example, cystine and taurine levels are high, whereas phenylalanine and methionine levels are low.

Vitamins

Human milk contains all of the vitamins required for infant nutrition, with individual variations based on maternal diet and genetic differences. Vitamins are added to cow's-milk formulas to resemble levels found in breast milk. Although cow's milk contains adequate amounts of vitamin A and vitamin B complex, vitamin C (ascorbic acid), vitamin E, and vitamin D must be added.

Vitamin D facilitates intestinal absorption of calcium and phosphorus, bone mineralization, and calcium resorption from bone. According to the AAP, all infants who are breastfed or partially breastfed should receive 400 International Units of vitamin D daily, beginning the first few days of life. Nonbreastfeeding infants and older children who consume less than 1 quart per day of vitamin D–fortified milk should also receive 400 International Units of vitamin D each day (Wagner, Grier, & AAP Section on Breastfeeding, & Committee on Nutrition, 2008).

Vitamin K, required for blood coagulation, is produced by intestinal bacteria. However, the gut is sterile at birth, and a few days are required for intestinal flora to become established and produce vitamin K. To prevent hemorrhagic problems in the newborn an injection of vitamin K is given at birth to all newborns, regardless of feeding method (AAP Section on Breastfeeding, 2005).

The breastfed infant's vitamin B_{12} intake is dependent on the mother's dietary intake and stores. Mothers who are on strict vegetarian (vegan) diets and those who consume few dairy products, eggs, or meat are at risk of vitamin B_{12} deficiency. Breastfed infants of vegan mothers should be supplemented with vitamin B_{12} from birth.

Minerals

The mineral content of commercial infant formula is designed to reflect that of breast milk. Unmodified cow's milk is much higher in mineral content than human milk, which also makes it unsuitable for infants during the first year of life. Minerals are typically highest in human milk during the first few days after birth and decrease slightly throughout lactation.

The ratio of calcium to phosphorus in human milk is 2:1, an optimal proportion for bone mineralization. Although cow's milk is high in calcium, the calcium/phosphorus ratio is low, resulting in decreased calcium absorption. Consequently, young infants fed unmodified cow's milk are at risk for hypocalcemia, seizures, and tetany. The calcium/phosphorus ratio in commercial infant formula is between that of human milk and cow's milk. The average DRI for calcium is 210 mg/day for infants younger than 6 months and 270 mg/day for infants between 7 months and 1 year (IOM, 2005).

Iron levels are low in all types of milk; however, iron from human milk is better absorbed than iron from cow's milk, iron-fortified formula, or infant cereals. Breastfed infants draw on iron reserves deposited in utero and benefit from the high lactose and vitamin C levels in human milk that facilitate iron absorption. The infant who is entirely breastfed usually maintains adequate hemoglobin levels for the first 6 months. After that time, iron-fortified cereals and other iron-rich foods are added to the diet. Infants who are weaned from the breast before 6 months of age and all formula-fed infants should receive an iron-fortified commercial infant formula until 12 months of age. Infants should not be fed low-iron formula (AAP Section on Breastfeeding, 2005).

Fluoride levels in human milk and commercial formulas are low. This mineral, which is important in preventing dental caries, can cause spotting of the permanent teeth (fluorosis) in excess amounts. Experts recommend that no fluoride supplements be given to infants younger than 6 months. From 6 months to 3 years, fluoride supplements are based on the concentration of fluoride in the water supply (AAP Section on Breastfeeding, 2005).

ANATOMY AND PHYSIOLOGY OF LACTATION

Anatomy of the Lactating Breast

Each female breast is composed of approximately 15 to 20 segments (lobes) embedded in fat and connective tissues and well supplied with blood vessels, lymphatic vessels, and nerves (Fig. 25-2). Within each lobe is glandular tissue consisting of alveoli, the milk-producing cells, surrounded by myoepithelial cells that contract to send the milk forward to the nipple during milk ejection. Each nipple has multiple pores that transfer milk to the suckling infant. The ratio of glandular tissue to adipose tissue in the lactating breast is approximately 2:1 compared with a 1:1 ratio in the nonlactating breast. Within each breast is a complex, intertwining network of milk ducts that transport milk from the alveoli to the nipple. The milk ducts dilate and expand at milk ejection. Previous thinking held that the milk ducts converged behind the nipple in lactiferous sinuses, which acted as reservoirs for milk. However, research based on ultrasonography of lactating breasts has shown that these sinuses do not exist, and in fact glandular tissue can be found directly beneath the nipple (Geddes, 2007; Ramsay, Kent, Hartmann, & Hartmann, 2005) (Fig. 25-3).

The size and shape of the breast are not accurate indicators of its ability to produce milk. Although nearly every woman can lactate, a small number have insufficient mammary gland

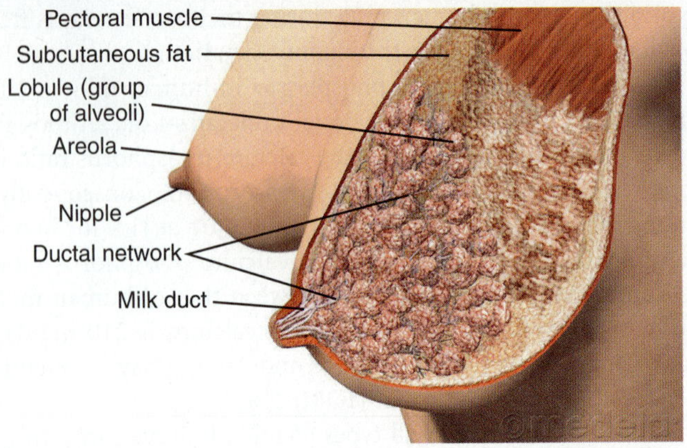

FIG. 25-2 Anatomy of the lactating breast. (Courtesy Medela, Inc., McHenry, IL.)

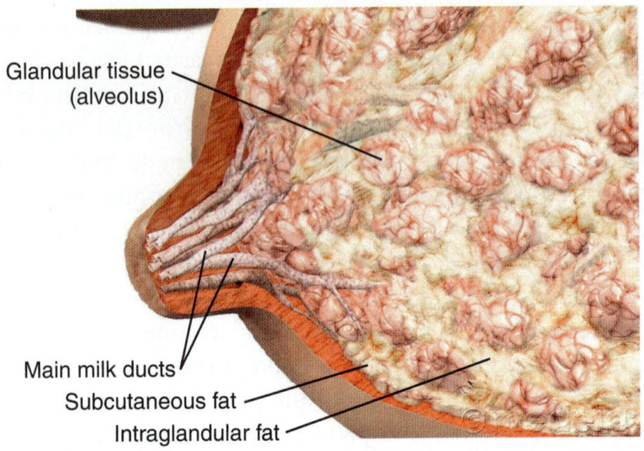

FIG. 25-3 Enhanced view of milk glands and milk ducts. (Courtesy Medela, Inc., McHenry, IL.)

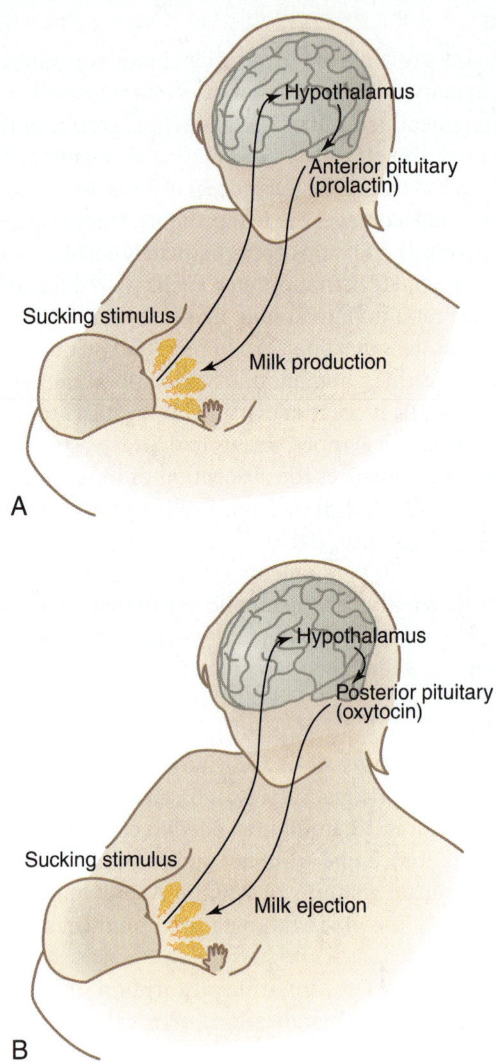

FIG. 25-4 Maternal breastfeeding reflexes. **A,** Milk production. **B,** Milk ejection (let-down).

development to breastfeed their infants exclusively. Typically these women experience few breast changes during puberty or early pregnancy. In some cases they are still able to produce some breast milk, although the quantity is not likely to be sufficient to meet the nutritional needs of the infant. These mothers can offer supplemental nutrition to support optimal infant growth. Devices are available to allow mothers to offer supplements while the baby is nursing at the breast.

Because of the effects of estrogen, progesterone, human placental lactogen, and other hormones of pregnancy, changes occur in the breasts in preparation for lactation. Breasts increase in size corresponding to growth of glandular and adipose tissue. Blood flow to the breasts nearly doubles during pregnancy. Sensitivity of the breasts increases, and veins become more prominent. The nipples become more erect, and the areola darken. Nipples and areola may enlarge. Around week 16 of gestation the alveoli begin producing colostrum (early milk). Montgomery glands on the areola enlarge. The oily substance secreted by these sebaceous glands helps provide protection against the mechanical stress of sucking and invasion by pathogens. The odor of the secretions can be a means of communication with the infant (Geddes, 2007).

Lactogenesis

After the mother gives birth a precipitous fall in estrogen and progesterone levels triggers the release of prolactin from the anterior pituitary gland. During pregnancy, prolactin prepares the breasts to secrete milk and, during lactation, to synthesize and secrete milk. Prolactin levels are highest during the first 10 days after birth, gradually declining over time but remaining above baseline levels for the duration of lactation. Prolactin is produced in response to infant suckling and emptying of the breasts (Fig. 25-4, *A*). Milk production is a **supply-meets-demand system;** that is, as milk is removed from the breast, more is produced. Incomplete removal of milk from the breasts can lead to decreased milk supply.

Oxytocin is the other hormone essential to lactation. As the nipple is stimulated by the suckling infant, the posterior pituitary is prompted by the hypothalamus to produce oxytocin. This hormone is responsible for the **milk ejection reflex (MER),** or let-down reflex (see Fig. 25-4, *B*). The myoepithelial cells surrounding the alveoli respond to oxytocin by contracting and sending the milk forward through the ducts to the nipple. Many let-downs can occur with each feeding session. Thoughts, sights, sounds, or odors that the mother associates with her baby (or other babies), such as hearing the baby cry, can trigger the MER. Many women report a tingling "pins and needles" sensation in the breasts as milk ejection occurs, although some mothers can detect milk ejection only by observing the sucking and swallowing of the infant. The milk ejection reflex also can occur during sexual activity because oxytocin is released during orgasm. The reflex can be inhibited by fear, stress, and alcohol consumption.

> **! NURSING ALERT**
>
> Be cautious in referring to the milk ejection reflex as "let-down." Some women may interpret let-down as being associated with feelings of depression.

Oxytocin is the same hormone that stimulates uterine contractions during labor. Consequently, the MER can be triggered during labor, as evidenced by leakage of colostrum. This reflex readies the breast for immediate feeding by the infant after birth. Oxytocin has the important function of contracting the mother's uterus after birth to control postpartum bleeding and promote uterine involution. Thus mothers who breastfeed are at decreased risk for postpartum hemorrhage. These uterine contractions, or "afterpains," that occur with breastfeeding are often painful during and after feeding for the first 3 to 5 days, particularly in multiparas, although they resolve within 1 week after birth.

Prolactin and oxytocin have been called the "mothering hormones" because they affect the postpartum woman's emotions, as well as her physical state. Many women report feeling thirsty or very relaxed during breastfeeding, probably as a result of these hormones.

The nipple-erection reflex is an important part of lactation. When the infant cries, suckles, or rubs against the breast, the nipple becomes erect, which assists in the propulsion of milk through the ducts to the nipple pores. Nipple sizes, shapes, and ability to become erect vary with individuals. Some women have flat or inverted nipples that do not become erect with stimulation; these women will likely need assistance with effective latch. These infants should not be offered bottles or pacifiers until breastfeeding is well established.

Uniqueness of Human Milk

Human milk is the ideal food for human infants. It is a dynamic substance with a composition that changes to meet the changing nutritional and immunologic needs of the infant's growth and development. Breast milk is specific to the needs of each newborn; for example, the milk produced by mothers of preterm infants differs in composition from that of mothers who give birth at term.

Human milk contains immunologically active components that provide some protection against a broad spectrum of bacterial, viral, and protozoal infections. Secretory IgA is the major immunoglobulin in human milk; IgG, IgM, IgD, and IgE are also present. Human milk also contains T and B lymphocytes, epidermal growth factor, cytokines, interleukins, bifidus factor, complement (C3 and C4), and lactoferrin, all of which have a specific role in preventing localized and systemic bacterial and viral infections (Lawrence & Lawrence, 2005).

Human milk composition and volumes vary according to the stage of lactation. In **lactogenesis** stage I, beginning at approximately 16 to 18 weeks of pregnancy, the breasts are preparing for milk production by producing colostrum. **Colostrum,** a clear yellowish fluid, is more concentrated than mature milk and is extremely rich in immunoglobulins. It has higher concentrations of protein and minerals but less fat than mature milk. The high protein level of colostrum facilitates binding of bilirubin, and the laxative action of colostrum promotes early passage of meconium. Colostrum gradually changes to mature milk which quickly increases in volume; this transition is called "the milk coming in" or lactogenesis stage II. By day 3 to 5 after birth, most women have had this onset of copious milk secretion. Breast milk continues to change in composition for approximately 10 days, when the mature milk is established in stage III of lactogenesis (Lawrence & Lawrence, 2005).

Composition of mature milk changes during each feeding. As the infant nurses the fat content of breast milk increases. Initially, a bluish white foremilk is released that is part skim milk (approximately 60% of the volume) and part whole milk (approximately 35% of the volume). It provides primarily lactose, protein, and water-soluble vitamins. The hindmilk, or cream (approximately 5%), is usually released 10 to 20 minutes into the feeding, although it can occur sooner. It contains the denser calories from fat necessary for ensuring optimal growth and contentment between feedings. Because of this changing composition of human milk during each feeding, breastfeeding the infant long enough to supply a balanced feeding is important.

Milk production gradually increases as the baby grows. Infants have fairly predictable **growth spurts** (at approximately 10 days, 3 weeks, 6 weeks, 3 months, and 6 months), when more frequent feedings stimulate increased milk production. These growth spurts usually last 24 to 48 hours, and then the infants resume their usual feeding pattern.

CARE MANAGEMENT: THE BREASTFEEDING MOTHER AND INFANT

Effective management of the breastfeeding mother and infant requires that caregivers are knowledgeable about the benefits, as well as the basic anatomic and physiologic aspects, of breastfeeding. Caregivers also need to know how to assist the mother with feedings and interventions for common problems. Ongoing support of the mother enhances her self-confidence and promotes a satisfying and successful breastfeeding experience. During the time in the hospital the mother is encouraged to view each breastfeeding session as a "feeding lesson" or "practice session" that will foster her self-confidence and promote a satisfying experience for herself and her infant.

The mother needs to understand infant behaviors in relation to breastfeeding. When newborns feel hunger, they usually cry vigorously until their needs are met. Some infants, however, will withdraw into sleep because of discomfort associated with hunger. Babies exhibit **feeding-readiness cues** that a knowledgeable caregiver can recognize. Instead of waiting to feed until the infant is crying in a distraught manner or withdrawing into sleep, beginning a feeding when the baby exhibits some of these cues (even during light sleep) is preferable:

- Hand-to-mouth or hand-to-hand movements
- Sucking motions
- **Rooting reflex**—infant moves toward whatever touches the area around the mouth and attempts to suck
- Mouthing

Babies normally consume small amounts of milk during the first 3 days of life. As the baby adjusts to extrauterine life and the digestive tract is cleared of meconium, milk intake increases from 15 to 30 ml per feeding in the first 24 hours to 60 to 90 ml by the end of the first week.

At birth and for several months thereafter, all of the secretions of the infant's digestive tract contain enzymes especially suited to the digestion of human milk. The ability to digest foods other than milk depends on the physiologic development of the infant. The capacities for salivary, gastric, pancreatic, and intestinal digestion increase with age, indicating that the natural time for introduction of solid foods is around 6 months of age.

Babies are born with a tongue extrusion reflex that causes them to push out of the mouth anything placed on the tongue. This reflex disappears by 6 months—another indication of physiologic readiness for solids.

Early introduction of solids can make the infant more prone to food allergies. It can also lead to decreased intake of breast milk or formula and is associated with earlier cessation of breastfeeding.

In the early postpartum period, interventions focus on helping the mother and the newborn initiate breastfeeding and achieve some degree of success and satisfaction before discharge from the hospital or birthing center. Interventions to promote successful breastfeeding include basics such as latch and positioning, signs of adequate feeding, and self-care measures such as prevention of engorgement. It is important to provide the parents with a list of resources that they may contact after discharge from the hospital.

The ideal time to begin breastfeeding is immediately after birth. Newborns without complications should be allowed to remain in direct skin-to-skin contact with the mother until the baby is able to breastfeed for the first time (AAP Section on Breastfeeding, 2005). Each mother should receive instruction, assistance, and support in positioning and latching-on until she is able to do so independently (see the Nursing Process box).

Positioning

The four basic positions for breastfeeding are the football or clutch hold (under the arm), cradle, modified cradle or across-the-lap, and side-lying (Fig. 25-5). Initially it is advisable to

NURSING PROCESS

Breastfeeding Mother-Infant Pair

ASSESSMENT

In preparation for breastfeeding, the nurse assesses infant feeding cues and the mother's physical and psychologic readiness to breastfeed.

Infant

- Feeding readiness: stable vital signs, unlabored respirations, active bowel sounds, no abdominal distention
- Feeding cues: hand-to-mouth or hand-to-hand movements, sucking motions, rooting, mouthing

Mother

- Previous experience, knowledge, and feelings about breastfeeding
- Physical features: breast fullness, protractility of nipples, previous breast surgery
- Comfort level: pain, fatigue
- Support from partner, family, and friends

During breastfeeding, the nurse assesses:

- Positioning and latch
- Infant sucking and milk transfer (swallowing)
- Mother's confidence and comfort with breastfeeding

The nurse also assesses the mother's learning needs related to breastfeeding.

If the father of the baby, partner, or other family member is present, the nurse observes his or her involvement in supporting the breastfeeding mother.

NURSING DIAGNOSES

Nursing diagnoses for the breastfeeding woman and infant can include the following:

***Effective Breastfeeding* related to:**

- mother's knowledge of breastfeeding techniques
- mother's appropriate response to infant's feeding readiness cues
- mother's ability to facilitate efficient breastfeeding

***Risk for Ineffective Breastfeeding* related to:**

- insufficient knowledge regarding newborn's reflexes and breastfeeding techniques
- lack of support by infant's father, partner, family, friends
- lack of maternal self-confidence; presence of anxiety, fear of failure
- poor infant suckling reflex
- difficulty waking sleepy newborn

***Risk for Imbalanced Nutrition: Less than Body Requirements* related to:**

- increased caloric and nutrient needs for breastfeeding (mother)
- incorrect latch and inability to transfer milk (infant)

***Risk for Deficient Fluid Volume* related to:**

- ineffective suckling (infant)

EXPECTED OUTCOMES OF CARE

Infant

- Latch and feed effectively at least eight times per 24 hr
- Gain weight appropriately
- Remain well hydrated (have two to six wet diapers per 24 hr until the fourth day of life and then six to eight wet diapers and at least three bowel movements every 24 hours)
- Sleep or seem contented between feedings

Mother

- Verbalize and demonstrate understanding of breastfeeding techniques, including positioning and latch, signs of adequate feeding, and self-care
- Report no nipple discomfort with breastfeeding
- Express satisfaction with the breastfeeding experience
- Consume a nutritionally balanced diet with appropriate caloric and fluid intake to support breastfeeding

PLAN OF CARE AND INTERVENTIONS

The nurse provides assistance, support, and education for the breastfeeding mother as she is learning how to breastfeed her newborn. Anticipatory guidance includes the following: signs of effective feeding, maternal diet, breast care, engorgement, and sore nipples. Discussion of interventions begins on p. 613.

EVALUATION

Evaluation is based on the expected outcomes, and the care plan is revised as needed based on the evaluation.

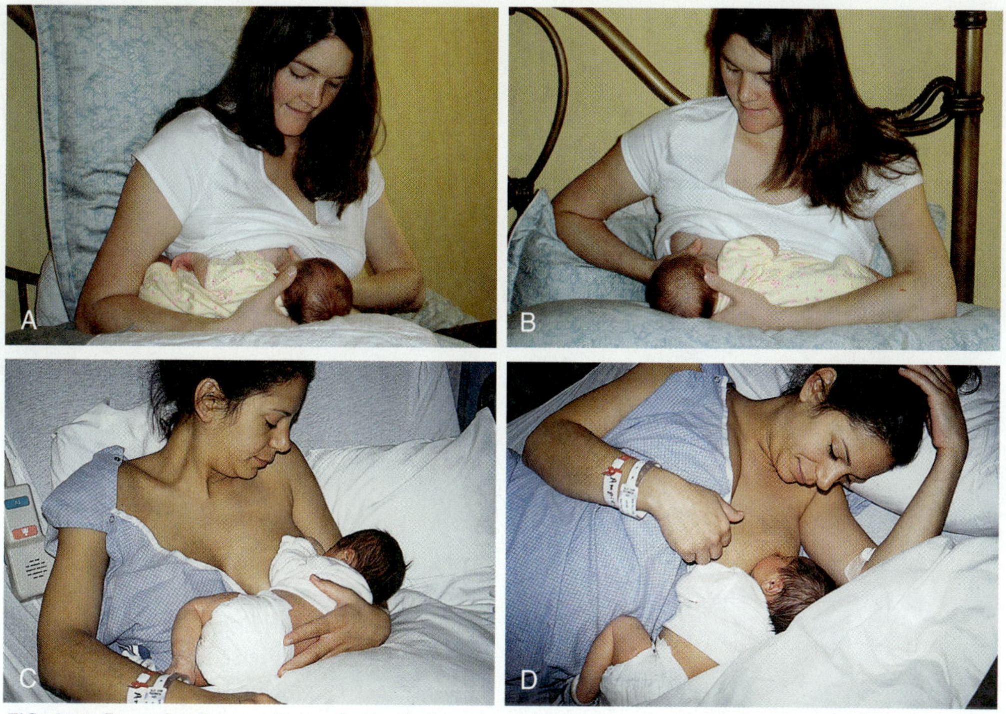

FIG. 25-5 Breastfeeding positions. **A,** Football or clutch (under the arm) hold. **B,** Across the lap (modified cradle). **C,** Cradling. **D,** Lying down. (**A** and **B,** Courtesy Kathryn Alden, Chapel Hill, NC; **C** and **D,** courtesy Marjorie Pyle, RNC, Lifecircle, Costa Mesa, CA.)

use the position that most easily facilitates latch while allowing maximal comfort for the mother. The football or clutch hold is often recommended for early feedings because the mother can easily see the baby's mouth as she guides the infant onto the nipple.

! NURSING ALERT

To avoid confusion and misunderstanding, when working with Hispanic women, avoid the term "football hold" to describe the under-the-arm or clutch position for breastfeeding—"football" refers to soccer in their culture.

Mothers who gave birth by cesarean often prefer the football or clutch hold. The modified cradle or across-the-lap hold also works well for early feedings, especially with smaller babies. The side-lying position allows the mother to rest while breastfeeding. Women with perineal pain and swelling often prefer this position. Cradling is the most common breastfeeding position for infants who have learned to latch easily and feed effectively. Before discharge from the birth institution the nurse can assist the mother to try all of the positions so that she will feel confident in trying these positions at home.

During breastfeeding the mother should be as comfortable as possible. The nurse might suggest that the mother take time to empty her bladder and attend to other needs before starting a feeding session. The mother should place the infant at the level of the breast, supported by firm pillows or folded blankets, turn the infant completely onto his or her side, facing the mother so that the infant is "belly to belly," with the arms "hugging" the breast. The baby's mouth is directly in front of the nipple. The mother should support the baby's neck and shoulders with her hand and not push on the occiput. The baby's body is held in correct alignment (ears, shoulders, and hips are in a straight line) during latch and feeding.

Latch

Latch is defined as placement of the infant's mouth over the nipple, areola, and breast, making a seal between the mouth and breast to create adequate suction for milk removal. In preparation for latch during early feedings the mother should manually express a few drops of colostrum or milk and spread it over the nipple. This action lubricates the nipple and entices the baby to open the mouth as the milk is tasted.

To facilitate latch the mother supports her breast in one hand with the thumb on top and four fingers underneath at the back edge of the areola. The breast is compressed slightly, as one might compress a large sandwich in preparing to take a bite, so that an adequate amount of breast tissue is taken into the mouth with latch. Most mothers need to support the breast during feeding for at least the first days until the infant is adept at feeding.

With the baby held close to the breast and the mouth directly in front of the nipple the mother tickles the baby's lower lip with her nipple, stimulating the mouth to open. When the mouth is open wide and the tongue is down the mother quickly "hugs" the baby to the breast, bringing the baby onto the nipple. She brings the infant to the breast, not the breast to the infant (Fig. 25-6).

The amount of areola in the baby's mouth with correct latch depends on the size of the baby's mouth and the size of the areola and the nipple. In general, the baby's mouth should cover the nipple and an areolar radius of approximately 2 to 3 cm all around the nipple. If breastfeeding is painful, the baby likely has

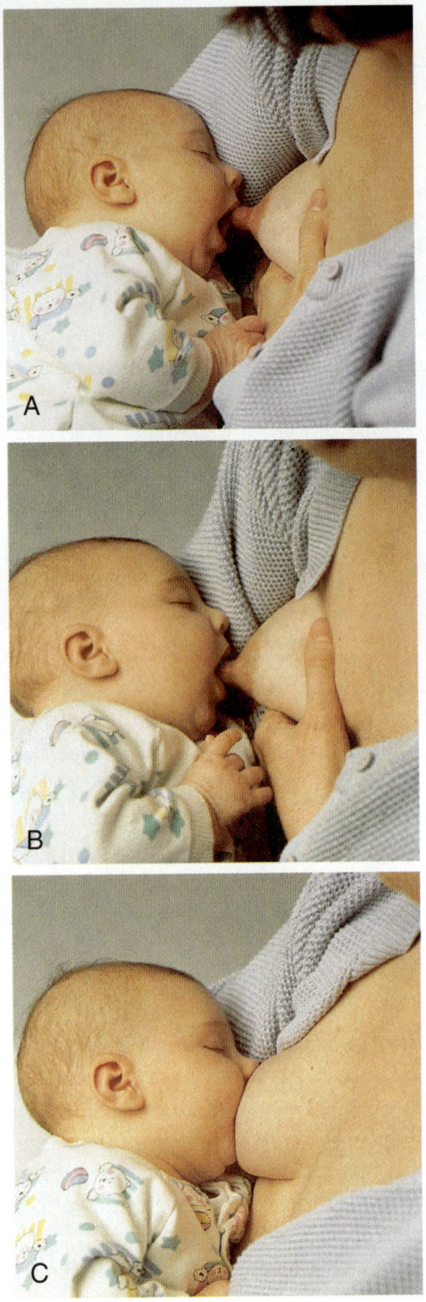

FIG. 25-6 Latch. **A,** The mother tickles baby's lower lip with the nipple until he or she opens wide. **B,** Once baby's mouth is opened wide, she quickly "hugs" the baby to the breast. **C,** Baby should have as much areola (dark area around nipple) in his or her mouth as possible, not just the nipple. (Courtesy Medela, Inc., McHenry, IL.)

not taken enough of the breast into the mouth, and the tongue is pinching the nipple.

When latched correctly, the baby's cheeks and chin are touching the breast. Depressing the breast tissue around the baby's nose to create breathing space is not necessary. If the mother is worried about the baby's breathing, she can raise the baby's hips slightly to change the angle of the baby's head at the breast. If the baby's nostrils happen to become occluded by the breast, reflexes will prompt the newborn to move the head and pull back to breathe.

If the baby is nursing appropriately, (1) the mother reports a firm tugging sensation on her nipples but feels no pinching or pain, (2) the baby sucks with cheeks rounded, not dimpled, (3) the baby's jaw glides smoothly with sucking, and (4) swallowing is usually audible. Sucking creates a vacuum in the intraoral cavity as the breast is compressed between the tongue and the palate. If the mother feels pinching or pain after the initial sucks or does not feel a strong tugging sensation on the nipple, the latch and positioning are evaluated. Any time the signs of adequate latch and sucking are not present the baby should be taken off the breast and latch attempted again. To prevent nipple trauma as the baby is taken off the breast the mother is instructed to break the suction by inserting a finger in the side of the baby's mouth between the gums and leaving it there until the nipple is completely out of the baby's mouth (Fig. 25-7). (See Nursing Care Plan.)

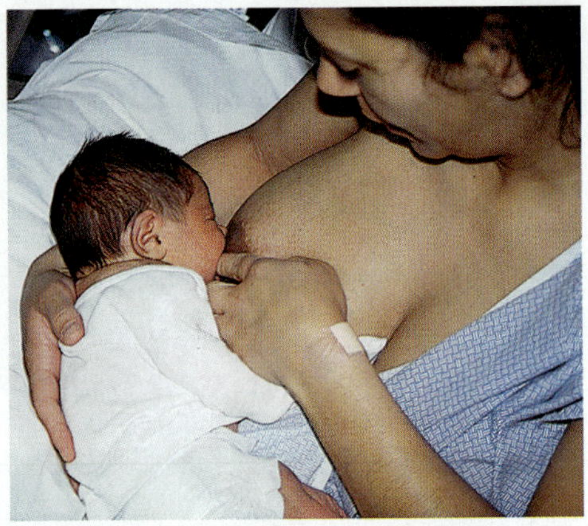

FIG. 25-7 Removing infant from the breast. (Courtesy Marjorie Pyle, RNC, Lifecircle, Costa Mesa, CA.)

Milk Ejection or Let-Down

As the baby begins sucking on the nipple the milk ejection, or let-down, reflex is stimulated (see Fig. 25-4, *B*). The following signs indicate that milk ejection has occurred:

- The mother may feel a tingling sensation in the nipples and in the breasts, although many women never feel when milk ejection (let down) occurs.
- The baby's suck changes from quick, shallow sucks to a slower, more drawing, sucking pattern.
- Audible swallowing is present as the baby sucks.
- In the early days the mother feels uterine cramping and can have increased lochia during and after feedings.
- The mother feels relaxed or drowsy during feedings.
- The opposite breast may leak.

Frequency of Feedings

Newborns need to breastfeed at least 8 to 12 times in a 24-hour period. Feeding patterns are variable because every baby is unique. Some infants will breastfeed every 2 to 3 hours throughout a 24-hour period. Others may cluster-feed, breastfeeding every hour or so for three to five feedings and then sleeping for 3 to 4 hours between clusters. During the first 24 to 48 hours after birth, most babies do not awaken this often to feed. Parents need to understand that they should awaken the baby to feed at least every 3 hours during the day and at least every 4 hours at night. (Feeding frequency is determined by counting from the beginning of one feeding to the beginning of the next.) Once the infant is feeding well and gaining weight adequately, going to **demand feeding** is appropriate, in which case the infant determines the frequency of feedings. (With demand feeding the infant should still receive at least eight feedings in 24 hours.) Caregivers should caution parents against attempting to place newborn infants on strict feeding schedules.

Infants should be fed whenever they exhibit feeding cues. Keeping the baby close is the best way to observe and respond to infant feeding cues. Newborns should remain with mothers during the recovery period after birth and room-in during the hospital stay. At home, babies should be kept nearby so that parents can observe signs that the baby is ready to feed. One recommendation is that mother and breastfeeding infant sleep in proximity to promote breastfeeding (AAP Section on Breastfeeding, 2005). The issue of bed-sharing (co-bedding) has raised concerns because of the association between a higher incidence of sudden infant death syndrome (SIDS) and bed-sharing with an adult. Experts recommend that the breastfeeding infant be placed in a bassinet near the mother, which would then allow for more convenient breastfeeding and at the same time prevent continuous bed-sharing (AAP Task Force on SIDS, 2005).

Duration of Feedings

The duration of breastfeeding sessions is highly variable because the timing of milk transfer differs for each mother-baby pair. The average time for early feedings is 30 to 40 minutes or approximately 15 to 20 minutes per breast. As infants grow, they become more efficient at breastfeeding, and consequently the length of feedings decreases.

Some mothers prefer one-sided nursing, in which case the baby nurses only one breast at each feeding. The first breast offered should be alternated at each feeding to ensure that each breast receives equal stimulation and emptying. In reality, instructing mothers to feed for a set number of minutes is inappropriate. Mothers can determine when a baby has finished a feeding. The baby's sucking and swallowing pattern has slowed, the breast is softened, and the baby appears content and may fall asleep or release the nipple.

If a baby seems to be feeding effectively and the urine output is adequate but the weight gain is not satisfactory, the mother may be switching to the second breast too soon. The high-lactose, low-fat foremilk can cause the baby to have explosive stools, gas pains, and inconsolable crying. Feeding on the first breast until it softens ensures that the baby receives the higher fat hindmilk, which usually results in increased weight gain.

Indicators of Effective Breastfeeding

In the newborn period, when breastfeeding is becoming established, parents should be taught about the signs that breastfeeding is going well. Awareness of these signs will help them recognize when problems arise so that they can seek appropriate assistance (Box 25-2).

During the early days of breastfeeding, keeping a feeding diary can be helpful, recording the time and length of feedings, as well as infant urine output and bowel movements. The data from the diary provide evidence of the effectiveness of breastfeeding and are useful to health care providers in assessing adequacy of feeding. Parents are instructed to take this feeding diary to the follow-up visit with the pediatric care provider.

BOX 25-2 SIGNS OF EFFECTIVE BREASTFEEDING

MOTHER

- Onset of copious milk production (milk is "in") by day 3 or 4
- Firm tugging sensation on nipple as infant sucks, but no pain
- Uterine contractions and increased vaginal bleeding while feeding (first week or less)
- Feels relaxed and drowsy while feeding
- Increased thirst
- Breasts soften or lighten while feeding
- With milk ejection (let-down), can feel warm rush or tingling in breasts, leaking of milk from opposite breast

INFANT

- Latches without difficulty
- Has bursts of 15 to 20 sucks/swallows at a time
- Audible swallowing is present
- Easily releases breast at end of feeding
- Infant appears contented after feeding
- Has at least three substantive bowel movements and six to eight wet diapers every 24 hours after day 4

Although the number of wet diapers and bowel movements is highly indicative of feeding adequacy, it is also important that parents are aware of the expected changes in the characteristics of urine output and bowel movements during the early newborn period. As the volume of breast milk increases, urine becomes more dilute and should be light yellow; dark, concentrated urine can be associated with inadequate intake and possible dehydration. (NOTE: Infants with jaundice often have darker urine as bilirubin is excreted.) The first 1 to 2 days after birth, newborns pass meconium stools, which are greenish black, thick, and sticky. By day 2 or 3, the stools become greener, thinner, and less sticky. If the mother's milk has come in by day 3 or 4, the stools will start to appear greenish yellow and are looser. By the end of the first week, breast milk stools are yellow, soft, and seedy (they resemble a mixture of mustard and cottage cheese). If an infant is still passing meconium stool by day 3 or 4, breastfeeding effectiveness and milk transfer should be assessed.

For approximately the first month, breastfed infants typically have 5 to 10 bowel movements per day, often associated with feedings. The stooling pattern gradually changes; breastfed infants can continue to stool more than once per day or they may stool only every 2 to 3 days. As long as the baby continues to gain weight and appears healthy, this decrease in the number of bowel movements is normal.

Supplements, Bottles, and Pacifiers

Unless a medical indication exists, no supplements should be given to breastfeeding infants (AAP Section on Breastfeeding, 2005; ABM Protocol Committee, 2009). With sound breastfeeding knowledge and practice, supplements are rarely needed. If a supplement is deemed necessary, giving the baby expressed breast milk is best. Prior to supplementation, it is important to perform a careful evaluation of the mother-infant dyad.

Possible indications for supplementary feeding include infant factors such as hypoglycemia, dehydration, weight loss of 8% to 10% associated with delayed lactogenesis, delayed passage of bowel movements or meconium stool continued to day 5, poor milk transfer, or hyperbilirubinemia. Maternal

Critical Thinking Exercise: Breastfeeding

NURSING CARE PLAN

Breastfeeding and Infant Nutrition

NURSING DIAGNOSIS

Ineffective breastfeeding related to knowledge deficit of the mother as evidenced by ongoing incorrect latch technique

Expected Outcomes

Mother will demonstrate the correct latch technique. Infant will latch correctly and suck with gliding jaw movements and audible swallowing. Mother will report "tugging" but no nipple pain with infant suckling. Mother will express increased satisfaction with breastfeeding, and neonate will exhibit satisfaction of hunger and sucking needs.

Nursing Interventions/*Rationales*

- Assess the mother's knowledge and motivation for breastfeeding *to provide a starting point for teaching.*
- Observe a breastfeeding session *to provide a baseline assessment for positive reinforcement and problem identification.*
- Describe and demonstrate ways to stimulate the sucking reflex, various positions for breastfeeding, and the use of pillows during a session *to promote maternal and neonatal comfort and effective latch.*
- Monitor the position of the infant's mouth on the areola and position of the head and body *to give positive reinforcement for correct latch position* or *to correct poor latch position.*
- Teach the mother ways to stimulate neonate to maintain an awake state by diapering, unwrapping, massaging, or burping *to complete a breastfeeding session thoroughly and satisfactorily.*
- Give the mother information regarding lactation diet, expression of milk by hand or pump, and storage of expressed breast milk *to provide basic information.*
- Make sure the mother has written information on all aspects of breastfeeding *to reinforce oral instructions and demonstrations.*
- Refer to support groups, lactation consultant, or both, if needed, *to provide further information and group support.*

NURSING DIAGNOSIS

Ineffective infant feeding pattern related to inability to coordinate sucking and swallowing

Expected Outcome

Neonate will coordinate sucking and swallowing to accomplish an effective feeding pattern.

Nursing Interventions/*Rationales*

- Assess for factors that can contribute to ineffective sucking and swallowing *to provide a basis for a plan of care.*
- Teach the mother to observe feeding readiness cues *to enhance effective feeding.*
- Modify feeding methods as needed *to maintain hydration status and nutritional requirements.*
- Promote a calm, relaxed atmosphere *to provide a pleasant breastfeeding experience for the mother and neonate.*
- Refer to lactation consultant *to provide specialized support.*

NURSING DIAGNOSIS

Anxiety related to ineffective infant feeding pattern

Expected Outcomes

Mother will report a decrease in the anxiety level and express satisfaction with breastfeeding.

Nursing Interventions/*Rationales*

- Monitor the maternal anxiety level during feeding sessions *to provide a basis for care planning.*
- Provide positive reinforcement for feeding pattern improvement *to decrease anxiety.*
- Monitor weight, intake, and output of the neonate *to provide information regarding effective feeding.*
- Enlist assistance of support persons *to provide positive feedback for increasing skill.*
- Provide information for lactation support *to decrease anxiety after discharge.*
- Initiate follow-up (telephone calls, follow-up with health care provider, outpatient lactation consultant) as needed *to assess progress, detect problems, and provide support.*

Nursing Care Plan—Breastfeeding and Infant Nutrition

indications for possible supplementation include delayed lactogenesis, and intolerable pain during feedings. Women who have had previous breast surgery such as augmentation or reduction may need to provide supplementary feedings for their infants (ABM Protocol Committee, 2009).

Offering formula to a baby after breastfeeding just to "make sure the baby is getting enough" is normally unnecessary and should be avoided. This action can contribute to low milk supply because the baby becomes overly full and does not breastfeed often enough. Supplementation interferes with the supply-meets-demand system of milk production. The parents can interpret the baby's willingness to take a bottle to mean that the mother's milk supply is inadequate. They need to know that a baby will automatically suck from a bottle, as the easy flow of milk from the nipple triggers the suck-swallow reflex.

Newborns can become confused going from breast to bottle or bottle to breast when breastfeeding is first being established. Breastfeeding and bottle feeding require different oral motor skills. The way newborns use their tongues, cheeks, and lips, as well as the swallowing patterns, are very different. Even though some newborns can transition easily between breast and bottle, others experience considerable difficulty. Because predicting which infants will adapt well and which ones will not is impossible, it is best to avoid bottles until breastfeeding is well established, usually after 3 to 4 weeks.

If the baby needs additional breast milk or formula, parents can use supplemental nursing devices, in which case the baby can be supplemented while breastfeeding (see Fig. 25-8). Infants can also be fed using a spoon, dropper, cup, or syringe. If parents choose to use bottles, a slow-flow nipple is recommended. Although some parents combine breastfeeding and bottle feeding, many babies never take a bottle and go directly from the breast to a cup.

Pacifier use with breastfeeding infants is usually discouraged until breastfeeding is well established. However, evidence does not support an adverse relationship between pacifier use and the exclusivity or duration of breastfeeding (Jenik, Vain, Gorestein, Jacobi, & Pacifier and Breastfeeding Trial Group, 2009; O'Connor, Tanabe, Siadaty, & Hauck, 2009). Because a correlation has been identified between pacifier use at bedtime and a decreased risk of SIDS, experts recommend that the caregiver consider offering the infant a pacifier at naptime or

EVIDENCE-BASED PRACTICE

Pat Gingrich

Supplemental Feeding

ASK THE QUESTION

My newly postpartum patient has indicated she wants to feed her baby using both breast and bottle. What can I tell her to encourage exclusive breastfeeding?

SEARCH FOR EVIDENCE

Search Strategies

Professional organization guidelines, meta-analyses, systematic reviews, randomized controlled trials, nonrandomized prospective studies and retrospective reviews since 2008.

Databases Searched

CINAHL, Cochrane, Medline, PUBMED, National Guideline Clearinghouse, Zynx Health, and the website for the Academy of Breastfeeding Medicine (ABM), American Academy of Pediatrics (AAP), and American Congress of Obstetricians and Gynecologists (ACOG).

CRITICALLY ANALYZE THE DATA

There is no question that breastfeeding provides numerous advantages for babies (reduced incidence of otitis media, gastroenteritis, respiratory illness, sudden infant death, obesity, hypertension, and necrotizing enterocolitis) and mothers (reduced incidence of breast and ovarian cancer, type 2 diabetes, postpartum depression), as well as being less costly (James, Lessen, & American Dietetic Association, 2009). Currently, about 75% of postpartum women try breastfeeding, but only about 13% are still exclusively breastfeeding by 6 months, the recommended interval before introducing complementary (solid) foods. Sometimes family or cultural beliefs can cause women to lack confidence that their milk supply is adequate. They may start with the intention of exclusive breastfeeding, but when their baby cries and seems hungry while going through that first growth spurt, these new mothers are overwhelmed and may reach for supplemental feeding. In a randomized controlled trial of 341 low-income, Latina primiparas whose babies received supplemental feedings in the hospital, researchers tried, and failed, to overcome the perception that formula was a good alternative to feeding difficulties. Breastfeeding education and daily telephone support did not improve the rate of exclusive breastfeeding. Inadequate milk supply was the main reason given for stopping breastfeeding in both groups (Bunik, Shobe, O'Connor, Beaty, Langendoerfer, Crane, et al., 2010).

The Academy of Breastfeeding Medicine Protocol Committee defines *supplemental feeding* as feedings that replace breastfeeding (2009). For the majority of newborns who are breastfeeding, supplementation is not necessary. During the first 24 hours, the amount of colostrum is sufficient in quantity for the newborn's nutritional and fluid needs, even in hot climates. As long as the newborn's weight loss does not exceed 7% of birth weight and there are not extenuating medical issues (asymptomatic hypoglycemia, significant dehydration, delayed bowel movement, breastmilk jaundice, or poor/absent milk production or transfer), the baby should be placed skin-to-skin, room in, feedings observed, and the mother should be taught early hunger cues and to awaken the baby for feeding about every 3 hours. If breastmilk transfer is documented to be low by infant weight, the mother can express or pump her breasts after breastfeeding sessions, to stimulate milk production. In the protocol regarding jaundice in late preterm or term infants, the ABM Protocol Committee (2010) recommends frequent breastfeeding. If supplementation is required, the first choice is the mother's own expressed milk; after that, the best choice is banked human milk.

IMPLICATIONS FOR PRACTICE

Exclusive breastfeeding for six months is unquestionably the gold standard for healthy newborns. Early supplementation by hospital staff undermines a new mother's confidence and models behavior that is counterproductive to prolonging breastfeeding. Therefore, supplemental feedings, even with water, are not recommended for healthy term newborns. Nurses caring for mother-baby dyads should observe entire breastfeeding sessions in order to assess, teach, and make suggestions about feeding cues, positioning, and latch. Even with a good start, the breastfeeding relationship is not static, but rather evolves from the first sleepy 24 hours, through the period of possible engorgement (experienced by 2 out 3 women), transitioning as milk supply and feeding patterns are established, and adjusting as the baby grows. The nurse can give education and anticipatory guidance to the family about these changes, and suggest ongoing community support resources.

References

Academy of Breastfeeding Medicine Protocol Committee. (2009). ABM Clinical protocol #3: Hospital guidelines for the use of supplementary feedings in the healthy term breastfed neonate, revised 2009. *Breastfeeding Medicine, 4*(3), 175–179.

Academy of Breastfeeding Medicine Protocol Committee. (2010). ABM Clinical protocol #22: Guideline for management of jaundice in the breastfed equal to or greater than 35 weeks gestation. *Breastfeeding Medicine, 5*(2), 87–93.

Bunik, M., Shobe, P., O'Connor, M., Beaty, B., Langendoerfer, S., Crane, L., et al. (2010). Are 2 weeks of daily breastfeeding support insufficient to overcome the influences of formula? *Academic Pediatrics, 10*(1), 21–28.

James, D., Lessen, R., & American Dietetic Association (2010). Position of the American Dietetic Association: Promoting and supporting breastfeeding. *Journal of the American Dietetic Association, 109*(11), 1926–1942.

regular bedtime. In the breastfeeding infant the pacifier is not offered until after 1 month, at which time breastfeeding should be well established (AAP Task Force on Sudden Infant Death Syndrome, 2005; AWHONN, 2007).

Special Considerations

Sleepy Baby

During the first few days of life, some babies need to be awakened for feedings. Parents are instructed to be alert for behavioral signs or feeding cues. If the infant is awakened from a sound sleep, attempts at feeding are more likely to be unsuccessful. Unwrapping the baby, changing the diaper, sitting the baby upright, talking to the baby with variable pitch, gently massaging the baby's chest or back, and stroking the palms or soles may bring the baby to an alert state. It is helpful to place the sleepy baby skin-to-skin with the mother; she can move the infant to the breast when feeding readiness cues are apparent (Box 25-3).

Fussy Baby

Babies sometimes awaken from sleep crying frantically. Although they are hungry, they cannot focus on feeding until they are calmed. Parents can swaddle the baby, hold the baby close, talk soothingly, and allow the baby to suck on a clean

BOX 25-3 WAKING THE SLEEPY NEWBORN

- Lay the baby down and unwrap.
- Change the diaper.
- Hold the baby upright, turn from side to side.
- Talk to the baby.
- Gently, but firmly, massage the chest and back.
- Rub the baby's hands and feet.
- Gently rock the baby from a lying to sitting position and back again until the eyes open.
- Place the baby skin-to-skin on mother's chest.
- Adjust lighting up for stimulation or down to encourage the baby to open the eyes.

finger until calm enough to latch on to the breast. Placing the baby skin-to-skin with the mother can be very effective in calming a fussy infant (Box 25-4).

Infant fussiness during feeding can be the result of birth injury such as bruising of the head or fractured clavicle. Changing the feeding position can help alleviate this problem.

Infants who were suctioned extensively or intubated at birth can demonstrate an aversion to oral stimulation. The baby may scream and stiffen if anything approaches the mouth. Parents need to spend time holding and cuddling the baby before attempting to breastfeed.

An infant can become fussy and appear discontented when sucking if the nipple does not extend far enough into the mouth. The feeding can begin with well-organized sucks and swallows, but the infant soon begins to pull off the breast and cry. The mother should support her breast throughout the feeding so that the nipple stays in the same position as the feeding proceeds and the breast softens.

Fussiness can be related to GI distress (e.g., cramping, gas pains). It can occur in response to an occasional feeding of infant formula, or it can be related to something the mother has ingested, although most women are able to eat a normal diet without causing GI distress to the breastfeeding infant. No standard foods should be avoided by all mothers when breastfeeding because each mother-baby couple responds individually. However, an important point to note is that the flavor of breast milk changes according to the foods and spices ingested by the mother. If a food is suspected to cause GI problems in the infant, the mother should eliminate it from her diet for 2 weeks, reintroduce the food, and see if symptoms reappear. When a strong family history of milk protein intolerance exists, the baby may develop colic-like symptoms. Similarly, if the risk of allergy is high, breastfeeding mothers may be advised to avoid peanuts and other potent allergens (Becker & Scott, 2008).

Persistent crying or refusing to breastfeed can indicate illness, and parents are instructed to notify the health care provider if either circumstance occurs. Ear infections, sore throat, or oral thrush can cause the infant to be fussy and not breastfeed well.

Slow Weight Gain

Newborn infants typically lose 5% to 6% of body weight before they gain weight. Weight loss of 7% or more in a breastfeeding infant during the first 3 days of life needs to be investigated. After the early milk has transitioned to mature milk, infants should gain approximately 110 to 200 g/week or 20 to 28 g/day

e Nursing Care Plan—The Newborn with Insufficient Intake of Nutrients

BOX 25-4 CALMING THE FUSSY BABY

- Swaddle the baby.
- Hold closely.
- Move or rock gently.
- Talk soothingly.
- Reduce environmental stimuli.
- Place the baby skin-to-skin on mother's chest.
- Allow baby to suck on adult finger.

BOX 25-5 WARNING SIGNS OF INEFFECTIVE BREASTFEEDING

- Baby has fewer than six wet diapers per day after the fourth day of life.
- Baby is having fewer than three stools per day after the fourth day of life.
- Stools are still meconium (black, tarry) by the fourth day of life.
- Mother's nipples are painful throughout feeding.
- Mother's nipples are damaged (bruised, cracked, bleeding).
- Milk supply has not increased (no breast fullness) by day 4.
- Baby seems to be feeding constantly.
- Baby is losing weight after the fourth day of life.
- Baby is gaining less than 0.5 ounce (14 grams) per day after the fourth day of life.
- Baby has not regained birth weight by the tenth day of life.

for the first 3 months. (Breastfed infants usually do not gain weight as quickly as formula-fed infants.) Health care providers should evaluate and monitor infants who continue to lose weight after 5 days, who do not regain birth weight by 14 days, or whose weight is below the 10th percentile by 1 month.

Parents are taught the warning signs of ineffective breastfeeding, including inadequate weight gain, minimal output, and feeding constantly (Box 25-5). If any of these warning signs are present, the parent should notify the health care provider.

At times, slow weight gain is related to inadequate breastfeeding. Feedings can be short or infrequent, or the infant can be latching incorrectly or sucking ineffectively or inefficiently. Other possibilities are illness or infection, malabsorption, or circumstances that increase the baby's energy needs, such as congenital heart disease, cystic fibrosis, or simply being small for gestational age. Slow weight gain must be differentiated from failure to thrive; this can be a serious problem that warrants medical intervention.

Maternal factors can be the cause of slow weight gain. The mother can have a problem with inadequate emptying of the breasts, pain with feeding, or inappropriate timing of feedings. Inadequate glandular breast tissue or previous breast surgery can affect milk supply. Severe intrapartum or postpartum hemorrhage, illness, or medications can decrease milk supply. Stress and fatigue also negatively affect milk production.

In most instances, the solution to slow weight gain is to improve the feeding technique. Positioning and latch are evaluated and adjustments are made. Adding a feeding or two in a 24-hour period can help. If the problem is a sleepy baby, parents are instructed in waking techniques.

Using alternate breast massage during feedings can help increase the amount of milk going to the infant. With this technique the mother massages her breast from the chest wall to

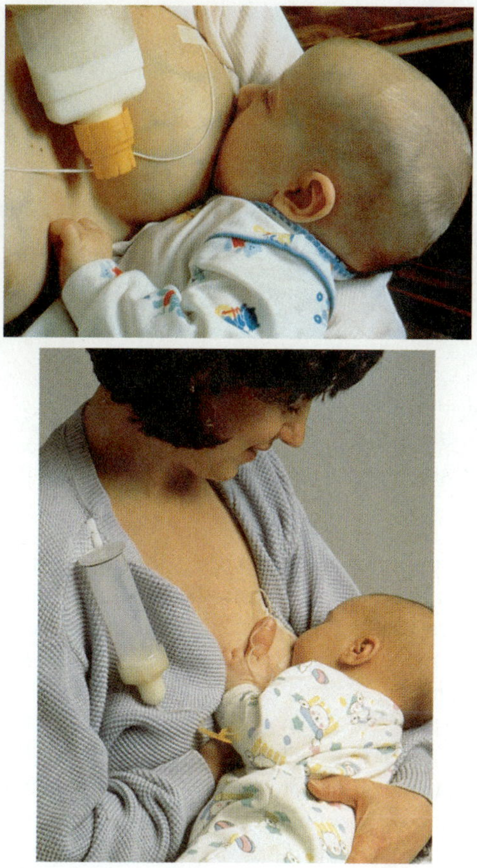

FIG. 25-8 Supplemental nursing system. (Courtesy Medela, Inc., McHenry, IL.)

the nipple whenever the baby has sucking pauses. This technique also can increase the fat content of the milk, which aids in weight gain.

When babies are calorie deprived and need supplementation, they can receive expressed breast milk or formula with a nursing supplementer (Fig. 25-8), spoon, cup, syringe, or bottle. In most cases, supplementation is necessary only for a short time until the baby gains weight and is feeding adequately.

Jaundice

Chapter 23 discusses jaundice (hyperbilirubinemia) in the newborn in detail. The type of jaundice most often seen in term newborns is physiologic jaundice. Hyperbilirubinemia is caused by bilirubin levels that rise steadily over the first 3 to 4 days, peak around day 5, and decrease thereafter. This condition has been called **early-onset jaundice** or **breastfeeding-associated jaundice,** which in the breastfed infant can be associated with insufficient feeding and infrequent stooling. Colostrum has a natural laxative effect and promotes early passage of meconium. Bilirubin is excreted from the body primarily through the intestines. Infrequent stooling allows bilirubin in the stool to be reabsorbed into the infant's system, thus promoting hyperbilirubinemia. Infants who receive water or glucose water supplements are more likely to have hyperbilirubinemia because only small amounts of bilirubin are excreted through the kidneys. Decreased caloric intake (less milk) is associated with decreased stooling and increased jaundice.

To prevent early-onset, breastfeeding-associated jaundice, newborns should be breastfed frequently during the first several days of life. Increased frequency of feedings is associated with decreased bilirubin levels.

To treat early-onset jaundice, breastfeeding is evaluated in terms of frequency and length of feedings, positioning, latch, and milk transfer. Factors such as a sleepy or lethargic infant or maternal breast engorgement can interfere with effective breastfeeding and should be corrected. If the infant's intake of milk needs to be increased, a supplemental feeding device can deliver additional breast milk or formula while the infant is nursing. Hyperbilirubinemia may reach levels that require treatment with phototherapy (see Chapter 24).

Late-onset jaundice or **breast milk jaundice** affects a few breastfed infants and develops in the second week of life, peaking between 6 and 14 days. Affected infants are typically thriving, gaining weight, and stooling normally; all pathologic causes of jaundice have been ruled out. In the presence of other risk factors, hyperbilirubinemia may be severe enough to require phototherapy. In most cases of breast milk jaundice, no intervention is necessary. Some health care providers recommend temporary interruption of breastfeeding for 12 to 24 hours to allow bilirubin levels to decrease, although this approach is not preferred (Blackburn, 2007; Page-Goertz, 2008).

Any breastfeeding infant who develops jaundice should be carefully evaluated for weight loss greater than 7%, decreased milk intake, infrequent stooling (fewer than three stools per day by day 4), and decreased urine output (fewer than four to six wet diapers per day). Bilirubin levels should be assessed by serum testing or transcutaneous monitoring (AAP Section on Breastfeeding, 2005).

Preterm Infants

Human milk is the ideal food for preterm infants, with benefits that are unique and in addition to those received by term, healthy infants. Breast milk enhances retinal maturation in the preterm infant and improves neurocognitive outcomes; it also decreases the risk of necrotizing enterocolitis. Greater physiologic stability occurs with breastfeeding as compared with bottle feeding.

Initially, preterm milk contains higher concentrations of energy, fat, protein, sodium, chloride, potassium, iron, and magnesium than term milk. The milk is more similar to term milk by approximately 4 to 6 weeks. Human milk fortifier may be added to expressed breast milk if growth of the preterm infant is inadequate (Lanese & Cross, 2008).

Depending on gestational age and physical condition, many preterm infants are capable of breastfeeding for at least some feedings each day. Mothers of preterm infants who are not able to breastfeed their infants should begin pumping their breasts as soon as possible after birth with a hospital-grade electric pump (Fig. 25-9). To establish optimal milk supply the mother should use a dual collection kit, pumping both breasts simultaneously 8 to 12 times daily for the first 10 to 14 days. These women are taught proper handling and storage of breast milk to minimize bacterial contamination and growth. Kangaroo care (skin-to-skin contact) is advised until the baby is able to breastfeed, and while breastfeeding is established, because it enhances milk production (Lanese & Cross, 2008).

The mothers of preterm infants often receive specific emotional benefits in breastfeeding or providing breast milk for

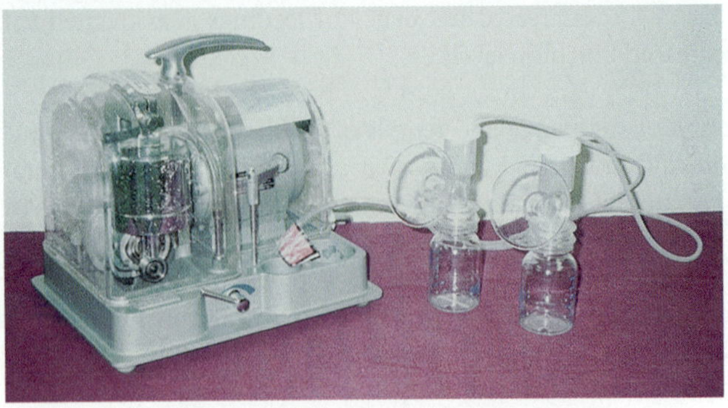

FIG. 25-9 Hospital-grade electric breast pump.

their babies. They find rewards in knowing they can provide the healthiest nutrition for the infant and believe that breastfeeding enhances feelings of closeness to the infant.

Late Preterm Infants

Neonates born at 34 0/7 to 36 6/7 weeks of gestation are categorized as *late preterm infants.* These newborns are at risk of feeding difficulties because of their low energy stores and high energy demands. They tend to be sleepy, with minimal and short wakeful periods. Late preterm infants often tire easily while feeding, have a weak suck, and low tone; these factors can contribute to inadequate milk intake. Early and extended skin-to-skin contact promotes breastfeeding and helps prevent hypothermia. Because these infants are more prone to positional apnea than term infants, mothers are advised to use the clutch (under the arm or football) hold for feeding, and to avoid flexing the head, which can impede breathing. Supplementation is often needed; expressed breast milk is the optimal supplement, preferably at the breast using a supplementer system (see Fig. 25-8) (Cleveland, 2010; Walker 2008a).

Breastfeeding Multiple Infants

Breastfeeding is especially beneficial to twins, triplets, and other higher-order multiples because of the immunologic and nutritional advantages, as well as the opportunity for the mother to interact with each baby frequently. Most mothers are capable of producing an adequate milk supply for multiple infants. Parenting multiples can be overwhelming, and mothers, as well as fathers, need extra support and assistance learning how to manage feedings (Fig. 25-10).

Expressing and Storing Breast Milk

Breast milk expression is a common practice, typically performed to obtain breast milk for someone else to feed to the baby. It is most often associated with maternal employment (Labiner-Wolfe, Fein, Shealy, & Wang, 2008). In some situations, expression of breast milk is necessary or desirable, such as when engorgement occurs, when the mother's nipples are sore or damaged, when the mother and baby are separated as in the case of a preterm infant who remains in the hospital after the mother is discharged, or when the mother leaves the infant with a caregiver and will not be present for feeding. Some women express milk to have an emergency supply (Labiner-Wolfe et al.). Some women choose to pump exclusively, providing breast milk for their infants, but never allowing the baby to suckle at the breast (Shealy, Scanlon, Labiner-Wolfe, Fein, & Grummer-Strawn, 2008).

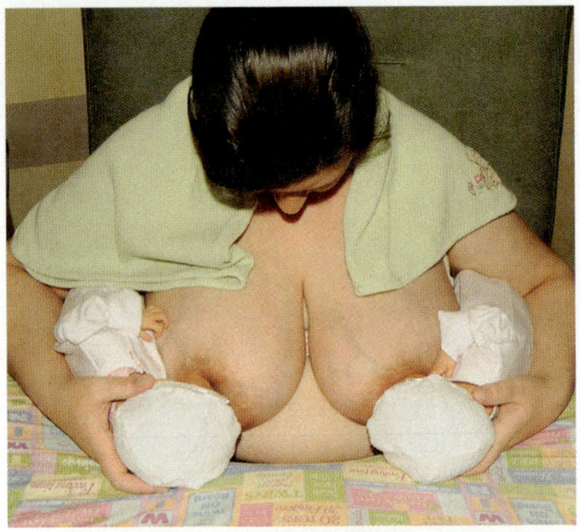

FIG. 25-10 Breastfeeding twins. (Courtesy Cheryl Briggs, RNC, Annapolis, MD.)

Because pumping and hand expression are rarely as efficient as a baby in removing milk from the breast, the milk supply is never judged based solely on the volume expressed. Milk volume can be more accurately assessed using pre- and postfeeding infant weights.

Hand Expression. All mothers should be instructed in hand expression. After thoroughly washing her hands, the mother places one hand on her breast at the edge of the areola. With her thumb above and fingers below, she presses in toward her chest wall and gently compresses the breast while rolling her thumb and fingers forward toward the nipple. She repeats these motions rhythmically until the milk begins to flow. The mother simply maintains steady, light pressure while the milk is flowing easily. The thumb and fingers should not pinch the breast or slip down to the nipple, and the mother should rotate her hand to reach all sections of the breast.

Mechanical Expression (Pumping). For most women, recommendations are to initiate pumping only after the milk supply is well established and the infant is latching and breastfeeding well. However, when breastfeeding is delayed after birth, such as when babies are ill or preterm, mothers should begin pumping with an electric breast pump as soon as possible and continue to pump regularly until the infant is able to breastfeed effectively.

Numerous approaches to pumping can be used. Some women pump on awakening in the morning or after feedings. Others choose to pump one breast while the baby is feeding from the other; this is usually done if the baby typically feeds from only one breast at each feeding. Double pumping (pumping both breasts at the same time) saves time and can stimulate the milk supply more effectively than single pumping (Fig. 25-11).

The amount of milk obtained when pumping depends on the type of pump being used, the time of day, the time since the baby breastfed, the mother's milk supply, how practiced she is at pumping, and her comfort level (pumping is uncomfortable for some women). Breast milk can vary in color and consistency, depending on the time of day, the age of the baby, and foods the mother has eaten.

Types of Pumps. Many types of breast pumps are available, varying in price and effectiveness. Before purchasing or renting a breast pump the mother will benefit from counseling by a nurse or lactation consultant to determine which pump best

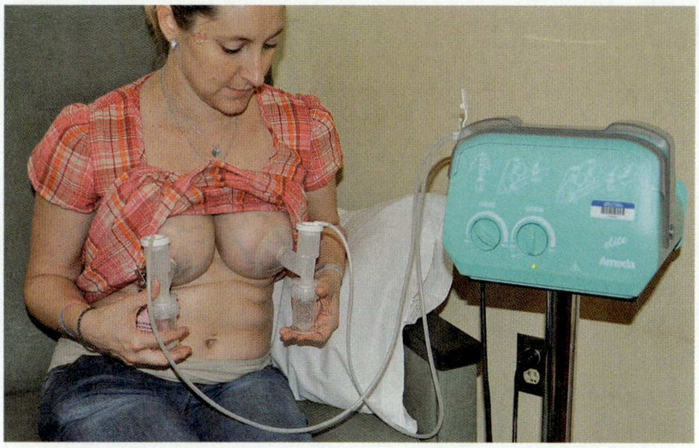

FIG. 25-11 Bilateral breast pumping. (Courtesy Cheryl Briggs, RNC, Annapolis, MD.)

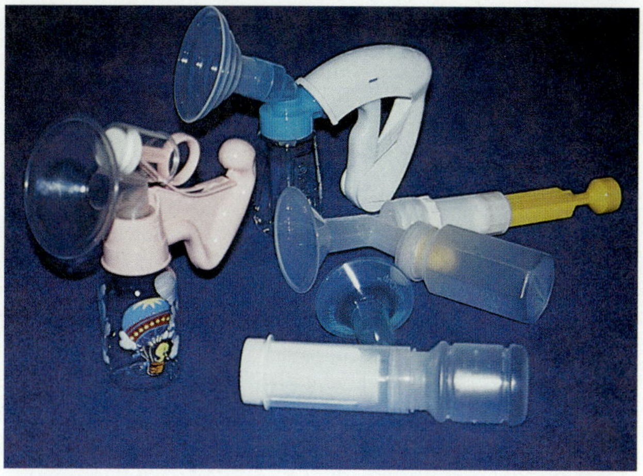

FIG. 25-12 Manual breast pumps. (Courtesy Marjorie Pyle, RNC, Lifecircle, Costa Mesa, CA.)

suits her needs. The flange (funnel-shaped device that fits over the nipple or areola) should fit the nipple to prevent nipple pain, trauma, and possible reduction in milk supply. Mothers are advised to use the lowest suction setting on electric pumps, increasing gradually if needed. Breast massage before and during pumping can increase the amount of milk obtained (Mannel, 2008).

Manual or hand pumps are the least expensive and can be the most appropriate where portability and quietness of operation are important. These pumps are most often used by mothers who are pumping for an occasional bottle (Fig. 25-12).

Full-service electric pumps, or hospital-grade pumps (see Figs. 25-9 and 25-11), most closely duplicate the sucking action and pressure of the breastfeeding infant. When breastfeeding is delayed after birth (e.g., preterm or ill newborn), or when the mother and baby are separated for lengthy periods, these pumps are most appropriate. Because hospital-grade breast pumps are very heavy and expensive, portable versions of these pumps are available to rent for home use.

Electric self-cycling double pumps are efficient and easy to use. These pumps are designed for working mothers. Some of these pumps come with carry bags containing coolers to store pumped milk.

Smaller electric or battery-operated pumps are typically used when pumping is performed occasionally, but some models are satisfactory for working mothers or others who pump on a regular basis.

Storage of Breast Milk. The preferred containers for long-term storage of breast milk are hard sided, such as hard plastic or glass, with an airtight seal. For short-term storage (less than 72 hours), plastic bags designed for human milk can be safely used.

For full-term healthy infants, under very clean conditions, freshly expressed breast milk can be safely stored at room temperature (16-29° C [60-85° F]) for up to 8 hours and can be refrigerated (≤4° C, 39° F) safely for up to 8 days. Milk can be frozen for up to 6 months in the freezer compartment of a two door refrigerator (<-5° C [23° F]) and up to 12 months in a freezer (<-4° C [24° F]). When breast milk is stored, the container should be dated, and the oldest milk should be used first (ABM Protocol Committee, 2010; Jones & Tully, 2006).

Frozen milk is thawed by placing the container in the refrigerator for gradual thawing or in warm water for faster thawing. It cannot be refrozen and should be used within 24 hours. After thawing, the container needs to be shaken so as to mix the layers that have separated (ABM Protocol Committee, 2010; Jones & Tully, 2006) (see Teaching Guidelines box: Breast Milk Storage Guidelines for Home Use for Full-Term Infants).

SAFETY ALERT

Breast milk is never thawed or heated in a microwave oven. Microwaving does not heat evenly and can cause encapsulated boiling bubbles to form in the center of the liquid, which may not be detected when drops of milk are checked for temperature. Babies have sustained severe burns to the mouth, throat, and upper GI tract as a result of microwaved milk. In addition, microwaving significantly decreases the antiinfective properties and vitamin C content. The safety of low-temperature microwaving is questionable (ABM Protocol Committee, 2010; Lawrence & Lawrence, 2005).

Being Away from the Baby

Although returning to work is a common reason for early weaning, many women are able to combine breastfeeding successfully with employment, attending school, or other commitments. If feedings are missed, the milk supply can be affected. Some women's bodies adjust the milk supply to the times they are with their infants for feedings, whereas other women find they must pump, otherwise the milk supply diminishes rapidly.

Maternal Employment. Returning to work after birth is associated with a decrease in the duration of breastfeeding. Women who return to work often face workplace challenges in breastfeeding such as lack of flexibility in work schedules, inadequate breaks to allow time for pumping, lack of privacy, lack of space for pumping, and lack of support from supervisors or coworkers. Increasing numbers of women are working from home and are likely to resume their jobs earlier than the traditional 6-week to 3-month maternity leave. Issues that can challenge continued breastfeeding while working include fatigue, child care concerns, competing demands, and household responsibilities (Walker, 2006).

Employed mothers can continue breastfeeding with appropriate guidance and support. They are encouraged to set realistic goals for employment and breastfeeding, with accurate information regarding the costs, risks, and benefits of available feeding options.

TEACHING FOR SELF-MANAGEMENT

Breast Milk Storage Guidelines for Home Use for Full-Term Infants

- Before expressing or pumping breast milk, wash your hands.
- Containers for storing milk should be washed in hot, soapy water and rinsed thoroughly; they can also be washed in a dishwasher. If the water supply may not be clean, boil the containers after washing. Plastic bags designed specifically for breast milk storage can be used for short-term storage (<72 hours).
- Write the date of expression on the container before storing the milk. A waterproof label is best.
- Store milk in serving sizes of 2 to 4 ounces to prevent waste.
- Storing breast milk in the refrigerator or freezer with other food items is acceptable.
- When storing milk in a refrigerator or freezer, place the containers in the middle or back of the freezer, not on the door.
- When filling a storage container that will be frozen, fill only three quarters full, allowing space at the top of the container for expansion.
- To thaw frozen breast milk, place the container in the refrigerator for gradual thawing, or place the container under warm, running water for quicker thawing. Never boil or microwave.
- Milk thawed in the refrigerator can be stored for 24 hours.
- Thawed breast milk should never be refrozen.
- Shake the milk container before feeding baby, and test the temperature of the milk on the inner aspect of your wrist.
- Any unused milk left in the bottle after feeding is discarded.

HUMAN MILK STORAGE GUIDELINES FOR FULL-TERM INFANTS

Location of Storage	Temperature	Recommended Safe Duration for Storage
Room temperature	16-29° C (60-85° F)	3-4 hours optimal 6-8 hours acceptable*
Refrigerator	4° C (39° F) or lower	72 hours optimal 5-8 days acceptable*
Freezer	Less than -4° C (24° F)	6 months optimal 12 months acceptable

*Under very clean conditions.

Source: Academy of Breastfeeding Medicine Protocol Committee. (2010). ABM clinical protocol No. 8: Human milk storage information for home use for full-term infants. *Breastfeeding Medicine, 5*(3), 127-130.

Women who are able to breastfeed their infants during the workday tend to breastfeed longer. With increasing numbers of women having the option of working from home, this situation is becoming more common. Many working mothers pump their milk while they are at work and save the milk for later feedings. Working mothers who are unable to pump or breastfeed their infants during the workday have the shortest duration of breastfeeding (Fein, Mandal, & Roe, 2008).

Because women are a significant proportion of the workforce, many companies make provisions for breastfeeding women returning to work. Breastfeeding programs typically include on-site lactation rooms and/or education and consulting services. Lactation rooms that provide space and privacy for pumping are available at many worksites and on college campuses (Fig. 25-13). In some instances, breastfeeding women bring their babies to work. Since 1999, by law, women may breastfeed in federal buildings and on federal property. Some states have enacted legislation to ensure that mothers may breastfeed their babies in public places. These efforts can help mothers breastfeed longer.

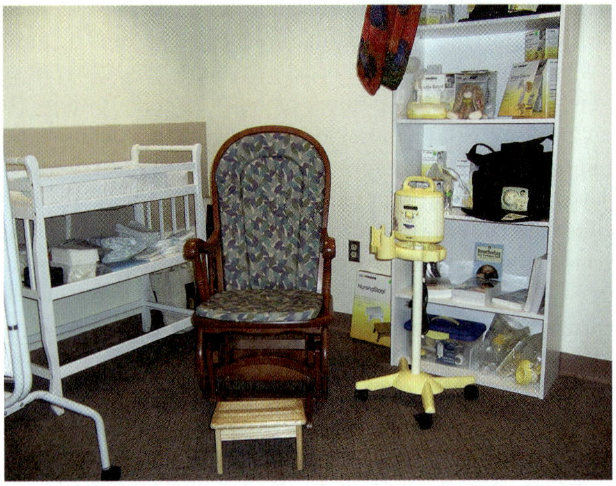

FIG. 25-13 Lactation room. Note the breast pump, rocking chair, nursing foot stool, changing table, books, and supplies. (Courtesy Cheryl Briggs, RNC, Annapolis, MD.)

Workplace support for breastfeeding mothers has improved significantly. However, further efforts are needed to educate employers about the importance of supporting their breastfeeding employees. Employers need to realize that breastfeeding programs can provide short- and long-term cost savings with significant health benefits for mothers, infants, and families (Tuttle & Slavit, 2009). The Health Resources and Services Administration offers a free toolkit for employers: the "Business Case for Breastfeeding" outlines steps that employers can take to support breastfeeding employees (www.womenshealth.gov/breastfeeding/programs/business-case/tool-kit.cfm://aks/hrsa/gov).

Weaning

Weaning is initiated when babies are introduced to foods other than breast milk and concludes with the last breastfeeding. Gradual weaning, over weeks or months, is easier for mothers and infants than abrupt weaning. Abrupt weaning is likely to be distressing for mother and baby, as well as physically uncomfortable for the mother.

Weaning is initiated by either the infant or the mother. With infant-led weaning the infant moves at his or her own pace in omitting feedings, which usually facilitates a gradual decrease in the mother's milk supply. Mother-led weaning means that the mother decides which feedings to drop. This approach is most easily undertaken by omitting the feeding of least interest to the baby or the one through which the infant is most likely to sleep. Every few days thereafter the mother drops another feeding, and so on, until the infant is gradually weaned from the breast.

Infants can be weaned directly from the breast to a cup. Bottles are usually offered to infants younger than 6 months. If the infant is weaned before age 1 year, the infant should receive iron-fortified formula instead of cow's milk (AAP Section on Breastfeeding, 2005).

If abrupt weaning is necessary, breast engorgement often occurs. To relieve the discomfort the mother can take mild analgesics, wear a supportive bra, apply ice packs or cabbage leaves to the breasts, and pump small amounts if needed. When possible, it is best to avoid pumping because the breasts should remain full enough to promote a decrease in the milk supply.

Weaning is often a very emotional time for mothers; many feel that it is the end to a special, satisfying relationship with the infant and benefit from time to adapt to the changes. Sudden weaning can evoke feelings of guilt and disappointment. Some women go through a grieving period after weaning. Nurses and others can assist the mother by discussing other ways to continue this nurturing relationship with the infant, such as skin-to-skin contact while bottle feeding or holding and cuddling the baby. Support from the father of the baby and other family members is essential at this time.

Milk Banking

For infants who cannot be breastfed but who also cannot survive except on human milk, banked donor milk is critically important. Because of the antiinfective and growth-promoting properties of human milk, as well as its superior nutrition, donor milk is used in many neonatal intensive care units for preterm or sick infants when the mother's own milk is not available. Donor milk also is used therapeutically in other situations such as for infants with short gut syndrome, for infants with IgA deficiency who are not breastfed, and for older children or adults with IgA deficiency (Tully & Jones, 2010).

The Human Milk Banking Association of North America (HMBANA) (www.hmbana.org) has established annually reviewed guidelines for the operation of donor human milk banks. The milk banks collect, screen, process, and distribute the milk donated by breastfeeding mothers who are feeding their own infants and pumping a few ounces extra each day for the milk bank. All donors are screened both by interview and serologically for communicable diseases. Donor milk is stored frozen until it is heat processed to kill potential pathogens; it is then refrozen for storage until it is dispensed for use. The heat processing adds a level of protection for the recipient that is not possible with any other donor tissue or organ. Banked milk is dispensed only by prescription. A per-ounce fee is charged by the bank to pay for the processing costs, but the HMBANA guidelines prohibit payment to donors (Tully & Jones, 2010).

Care of the Mother

Diet. In general, the breastfeeding mother should eat a healthy, well-balanced diet. Caloric intake during lactation should be sufficient to achieve the goal of balancing energy intake and expenditure. Most women are able to achieve that balance by adding 300 to 500 calories per day. Even with the increased caloric intake, women who are breastfeeding tend to lose weight more quickly than those who are formula feeding (Becker & Scott, 2008).

No specific foods have been identified that the breastfeeding mother must consume or avoid. In most cases the woman can consume a normal diet, according to her personal preferences and cultural practices. The ideal diet for the lactating mother is well balanced, consisting of nutrient-dense foods. The intake of calcium, minerals, and fat-soluble vitamins should be adequate. Women may be told to continue taking their prenatal vitamins as long as they are breastfeeding.

Mothers are encouraged to drink to quench thirst. Consumption of water by the mother does not increase milk supply, and overhydration can actually decrease milk production.

Weight Loss. Medications or diets that promote weight loss are not recommended for breastfeeding mothers. Many women will experience a gradual weight loss while lactating as fat stores deposited during pregnancy are used. This factor can be an added incentive for breastfeeding. Rapid loss of large amounts of weight can be detrimental, given that fat-soluble contaminants to which the mother has been exposed are stored in body fat reserves, and these can be released into the breast milk. Another potential consequence of weight loss is reduced milk production. For most women, weight loss of 1 to 2 kg per month is safe; however, if weight loss exceeds this amount, careful evaluation of infant weight and feeding pattern is recommended. The mother's diet is also evaluated.

Rest. The breastfeeding mother should rest as much as possible, especially in the first 1 or 2 weeks after birth. Fatigue, stress, and worry can negatively affect milk production and milk ejection (let-down). The nurse can encourage the mother to sleep when the baby sleeps. Breastfeeding in a side-lying position promotes rest for the mother. Assistance with household chores and caring for other children can be done by the father, partner, grandparents or other relatives, and friends.

Breast Care. The breastfeeding mother's normal routine bathing is all that is necessary to keep her breasts clean. Soap can have a drying effect on nipples; therefore, the mother should avoid washing the nipples with soap.

Breast creams should not be used routinely because they can block the natural oil secreted by the Montgomery glands on the areola. Modified lanolin with reduced allergens is safe to use on dry or sore nipples. Because lanolin is made from wool, women with wool allergies should be cautioned against its use. Lanolin is not recommended if nipple soreness is possibly related to monilial infection.

The mother with flat or inverted nipples will likely benefit from wearing breast shells in her bra. These hard plastic devices exert mild pressure around the base of the nipple to encourage nipple eversion. Breast shells are also useful for sore nipples to keep the mother's bra or clothing from touching the nipples (Fig. 25-14).

If a mother needs breast support, she will likely be uncomfortable unless she wears a bra because the ligament that supports the breast (Cooper's ligament) will otherwise stretch and be painful. Bras should fit well and provide nonbinding support. Underwire bras or improperly fitting bras can cause clogged milk ducts.

If leakage of milk between feedings is a problem, mothers can wear breast pads (disposable or washable) inside the bra. Plastic-lined breast pads are not recommended because they trap moisture and can contribute to sore nipples.

Sexual Sensations. Some women experience rhythmic uterine contractions during breastfeeding. Such sensations are not unusual because uterine contractions and milk ejection are both triggered by oxytocin; however, they are disturbing to some mothers who perceive them to resemble orgasm.

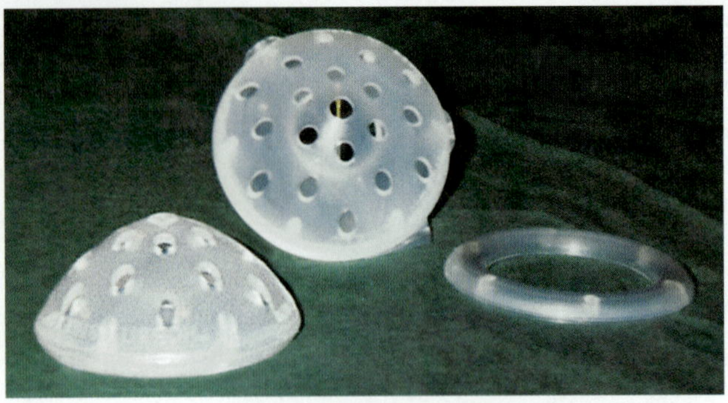

FIG. 25-14 Breast shells.

Breastfeeding and Contraception. Although breastfeeding confers a period of infertility, it is not considered an effective method of contraception. Breastfeeding delays the return of ovulation and menstruation; however, ovulation can occur before the first menstrual period after birth.

The contraceptive methods least likely to affect lactation are the lactational amenorrhea method, natural family planning, barrier methods (diaphragm/cap, spermicides, condoms), and intrauterine devices. Hormonal methods including combined oral contraceptives (pill, patch, or ring) and progestin-only contraceptives (pill, injection, or implant), are usually not recommended for use during the first four weeks after birth (CDC, 2010). The Academy of Breastfeeding Medicine cautions that hormonal contraceptives should be avoided in women with low milk supply, history of lactation failure, history of breast surgery, multiple birth, preterm birth, and in instances when the health of the mother or infant is compromised (ABM Protocol Committee, 2006). (See Chapter 8)

Breastfeeding During Pregnancy. Breastfeeding women can conceive and continue breastfeeding throughout the pregnancy if there are no medical contraindications (e.g., risk of preterm labor). For pregnant women who are breastfeeding, adequate nutrition is especially important to promote normal fetal growth.

Nipple tenderness associated with early pregnancy may cause discomfort when nursing the older child. The taste and composition of breast milk are altered during pregnancy, which may prompt some children to self-wean. Milk production can decrease about the fourth or fifth month of pregnancy (Mohrbacher, 2008).

When the baby is born, colostrum is produced. The practice of breastfeeding a newborn and an older child is called **tandem nursing.** The nurse should remind the mother always to feed the infant first to ensure that the newborn is receiving adequate nutrition. The supply-meets-demand principle works in this situation, just as with breastfeeding multiples.

Breastfeeding After Breast Surgery. Previous breast surgery can affect the ability to produce breast milk and transfer breast milk to the infant. Before undergoing breast surgery, all women should discuss their lactation potential with their surgeon. Surgical procedures can damage nerves and interrupt milk ducts. Women who have had augmentation mammoplasty (breast implants) should be able to breastfeed successfully, particularly if the implants are placed underneath the chest wall muscle. Reduction mammoplasty is more likely to cause problems with the ability to successfully lactate due to interference with milk ducts, removal of glandular tissue, and nerve damage. Even so, many women are still able to breastfeed completely or partially. Mothers with a history of breast surgery are instructed to carefully monitor their infants for signs of adequate feeding.

Women with a history of breast cancer who give birth can usually breastfeed. However, treatment for breast cancer (surgery, radiation, chemotherapy) can result in reduced milk supply or absence of lactation in the affected breast. Breastfeeding is contraindicated for women who are taking Tamoxifen (Riordan & Wambach, 2010).

Medications and Breastfeeding. Although much concern exists about the compatibility of drugs and breastfeeding, few drugs are absolutely contraindicated during lactation. Considerations in evaluating the safety of a specific medication during breastfeeding include the pharmacokinetics of the drug in the maternal system, as well as the absorption, metabolism, distribution, storage, and excretion in the infant. The gestational and chronologic age of the infant, body weight, and breastfeeding pattern are also considered. Breastfeeding mothers should be cautioned about taking any medications except those that are deemed essential. They are advised to check with their physician before taking any medication. References are available with specific information about medications and breastfeeding (Hale, 2010).

Drugs that are absolutely contraindicated for breastfeeding mothers include antimetabolite and cytotoxic medications and drugs of abuse such as cocaine, heroin, amphetamines, and phencyclidine. Other medications that are generally contraindicated are amiodarone, chloramphenicol, doxepin, lithium, and radiopharmaceuticals (Hale, 2010).

Certain medications can reduce maternal milk production and should be avoided. These include ergot alkaloids (bromocriptine, cabergoline, ergotamine), and pseudoephedrine (Hale, 2010).

As the use of antidepressant medications rises among childbearing women, there are increasing concerns about the effects of these medications on breastfeeding infants. A review of psychotropic medications indicates that the safest antidepressant drugs for breastfeeding mothers are sertraline, paroxetine, and fluvoxamine because there is minimal transfer into human milk. Antidepressants that are contraindicated while breastfeeding include citalopram, escitalopram, and fluoxetine because of the high levels excreted in breast milk, their long half-life, and adverse effects on the infant (Fortinguerra, Clavenna, & Bonati, 2009).

Alcoholic beverages are not recommended for breastfeeding mothers. Alcohol passes freely into breast milk with peak levels occurring in 30 to 60 minutes on an empty stomach and 60 to 90 minutes when consumed with food (Becker & Scott, 2008). The milk ejection reflex and milk production can be adversely affected by maternal alcohol intake.

Smoking can impair milk production; it also exposes the infant to the risks of secondhand smoke. Nicotine is transferred to the infant in breast milk, whether the mother smokes or uses a nicotine patch, although the effect on the infant is uncertain. Lactating mothers who continue to smoke should be advised not to smoke within 2 hours before breastfeeding and never to smoke in the same room with the infant.

Caffeine intake can be associated with reduced iron concentration in milk and subsequent anemia in the infant. Maternal intake of caffeine can cause infant irritability and poor sleeping patterns. For most women, two servings of caffeine a day does not cause untoward effects; however, some infants are sensitive to even small amounts. Mothers of such infants should limit caffeine intake. Caffeine is found in coffee, tea, chocolate, and many soft drinks.

Herbs and herbal teas are becoming more widely used during lactation. Although some herbs are considered safe, others contain pharmacologically active compounds that may have unfavorable effects. A thorough maternal history should include the use of any herbal remedies. Each remedy should then be evaluated for its compatibility with breastfeeding. The regional poison control center can provide information on the active properties of herbs.

Environmental Contaminants. Human milk is often used to measure community exposure to environmental contaminants because there is a close correlation between milk levels and the levels in fat stores. Except under unusual circumstances, breastfeeding is not contraindicated because of exposure to environmental contaminants such as dichlorodiphenyltrichloroethane (DDT; an insecticide) and tetrachloroethylene (used in dry-cleaning plants) (Lawrence & Lawrence, 2005).

Common Concerns of the Breastfeeding Mother

The breastfeeding mother can experience some common problems. In the majority of cases, these complications are preventable if the mother receives appropriate education about breastfeeding. Early recognition and prompt resolution of these problems is important to prevent interruption of breastfeeding and to promote the mother's comfort and sense of well-being. Emotional support provided by the nurse or lactation consultant is essential to help allay the mother's frustration and anxiety and to prevent early cessation of breastfeeding.

Engorgement. Engorgement is a common response of the breasts to the sudden change in hormones and the onset of significantly increased milk volume. It usually occurs 3 to 5 days after birth when the milk "comes in" and lasts approximately 24 hours. Blood supply to the breasts increases and causes swelling of tissues surrounding the milk ducts. The milk ducts may be pinched shut so that milk cannot flow from the breasts. The breasts are firm, tender, and hot and may appear shiny and taut. The areolae are firm, and the nipples may flatten, creating difficulty for the infant in latching on to the breast. Because back pressure on full milk glands inhibits milk production, if milk is not removed from the breasts, the milk supply can diminish.

When engorgement occurs, it is a temporary condition that is usually resolved within 24 hours. The mother is instructed to feed every 2 hours, softening at least one breast, and pumping the other breast as needed to soften it. Pumping during engorgement will not cause a problematic increase in milk supply.

A variety of interventions are used to treat engorgement. There is a lack of research evidence confirming the effectiveness of any specific intervention. Frequently used treatments for engorgement include the use of cold (ice packs, gel packs, cold compresses) after breastfeeding, chilled cabbage leaves, warmth (warm compresses, warm showers) before breastfeeding, antiinflammatory medications, breast massage, and pumping.

Because of the swelling of breast tissue surrounding the milk ducts, ice packs are often recommended in a 15- to 20-minutes on, 45 minutes off rotation between feedings. The ice packs should cover both breasts. Large bags of frozen peas or niblet corn make easy packs and can be refrozen between uses.

Fresh, raw cabbage leaves placed over the breasts between feedings can help reduce the swelling. (It is unclear how the leaves act to reduce engorgement; it is thought that the effect may be related to the cool temperature of the leaves or possibly related to a substance contained in the leaves.) The cabbage leaves are washed, chilled in the refrigerator or freezer, and then placed over the breasts for 15 to 20 minutes (Fig. 25-15). Some experts recommend crushing the leaves before placing them on the breasts. This treatment can be repeated for two or three sessions. Frequent application of cabbage leaves can decrease milk supply. Cabbage leaves are often very effective for formula-feeding mothers who want their milk to "dry up"; they are advised to wear the cabbage leaves constantly while engorged, replacing the leaves with fresh ones as they become wilted. Cabbage leaves should not be used if the mother is allergic to cabbage or develops a skin rash.

Antiinflammatory medications, such as ibuprofen, can help reduce the pain and swelling associated with engorgement. Ibuprofen also helps reduce fever and aching in the breasts that are often associated with engorgement.

Because heat increases blood flow, application of heat to an already congested breast is usually counterproductive.

CLINICAL REASONING

Breastfeeding: Engorgement and Nipple Soreness

The home care nurse visits Mary, a 35 year old primipara who was discharged from the hospital 24 hours after giving birth to Matthew, a 3400 g (7.5 lb) baby boy who is now three days old. When Mary answers the door, she is tearful and appears very tired. The baby is asleep in the arms of Mary's mother. Mary tells the nurse that when she awakened this morning her breasts were very firm and "achy." She tried to latch the baby on to the breast, but the nipple was too flat and he could not get it in his mouth; he was crying so hard that her mother gave him some formula. Mary's nipples appear irritated and cracked; she says "it hurts too much to feed him anyway." The baby has had only two wet diapers and no bowel movements in the last 24 hours. Mary says he cries much of the time and never seems to settle down to sleep for very long. Mary states, "I think it would be easier if I switch to formula."

1. Evidence—Does the nurse have sufficient evidence at this time to draw conclusions about the feeding difficulties experienced by this mother and infant?
2. Assumptions—What assumptions can be made about the following issues?
   a. Mary's milk supply
   b. Mary's sore nipples
   c. Matthew's urinary output and bowel elimination pattern
   d. Mary's commitment to breastfeeding
3. What implications and priorities for nursing care can be identified at this time?
4. Does the evidence objectively support your conclusion?
5. Are there alternative perspectives to your conclusion?

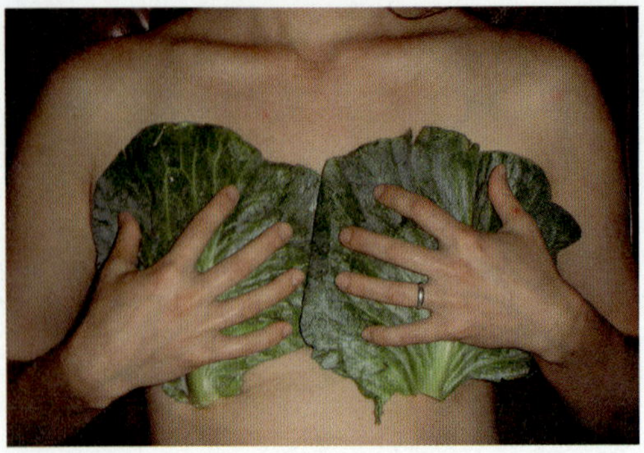

FIG. 25-15 Cabbage leaves to treat engorgement. (Courtesy Kathryn Alden, Chapel Hill, NC.)

Occasionally, however, standing in a warm shower will start the milk leaking, or the mother may be able to manually express enough milk to soften the areola sufficiently to allow the baby to latch and breastfeed.

When engorgement occurs or as a result of excessive intravenous fluids during labor, the nipple and areola can become distended, making it difficult for the newborn to latch successfully. This can also occur in mothers who have received oxytocin for labor induction or augmentation. A technique called *reverse pressure softening* manually displaces the areolar interstitial fluid inward, softening the areola, and making it easier for the infant's mouth to grasp the nipple and areola with latch (Cotterman, 2004). (Information on reverse pressure softening is available at http://www.perinatalprofessionals.org/images/Reverse_Pressure_Softening_for_Hidden_Barriers_Presentation.pdf.)

Sore Nipples. Mild nipple tenderness during the first few days of breastfeeding is common. Severe soreness or painful, abraded, cracked, or bleeding nipples are not normal and most often result from poor positioning, incorrect latch, improper suck, or monilial infection. Severe nipple pain can be related to vasospasm or Raynaud's phenomenon (Walker, 2008b). The key to preventing sore nipples is correct breastfeeding technique. Limiting the time at the breast will not prevent sore nipples. Sore nipples are often the result of the mother allowing the baby to latch onto the breast before the mouth is open wide.

For the first few days after birth the mother can experience some mild discomfort with the infant's initial sucks. This should quickly dissipate as the milk begins to flow and acts as a lubricant. To make the initial sucks less painful the mother can express a few drops of colostrum or milk to moisten the nipple and areola before latch. If the mother continues to experience nipple pain or discomfort after the first few sucks, the nurse or lactation consultant helps the mother evaluate the latch and baby's position at the breast. If the nipple pain continues, the mother needs to remove the baby from the breast, breaking suction with her finger in the baby's mouth. Repositioning the mother or infant may be helpful in resolving the nipple discomfort. The mother then proceeds to attempt latch again, making sure the baby's mouth is open wide before the baby is pulled quickly to the breast (see Fig. 25-6).

The nurse or lactation consultant can assess the infant's suck by inserting a clean, gloved finger into the mouth and stimulating the infant to suck. If the tongue is not extruding over the lower gum and the mother reports pain or pinching with sucking, the baby may have ankyloglossia, which is a short or tight frenulum (commonly known as tongue-tie). In some instances, this condition is corrected surgically to free the tongue for less painful, more effective breastfeeding (Dollberg, Botzer, Grunis, & Mimouni, 2006).

The treatment for sore nipples is first to identify the cause and then attempt to correct the problem. Early assessment and intervention are essential to increase the likelihood that the mother will continue to breastfeed. Once the problem is identified and corrected, sore nipples should heal within a few days, even though the baby continues to breastfeed regularly. When sore nipples occur, the woman is advised to start the feeding on the least sore nipple. After feeding, the mother can wipe the nipples with water to remove the baby's saliva. A few drops of milk can be expressed, rubbed into the nipple, and allowed to air dry. Sore nipples should be open to air as much as possible. Breast shells worn inside the bra allow air to circulate while keeping clothing off sore nipples (see Fig. 25-14).

Rapid healing of sore nipples is critical to relieve the mother's discomfort, maintain breastfeeding, and prevent mastitis. Although numerous creams, ointments, and gels have been used to treat sore nipples, warm water, purified lanolin, and hydrogel are the only treatments that have been shown to have some effect. Women may find that these treatments increase their comfort, but there is a lack of research evidence to support their value in promoting healing of sore nipples. Purified lanolin helps sore nipples by retaining the skin's natural moisture and protecting the nipple from further abrasion. It is applied to nipples after feeding. Hydrogel dressings, applied to nipples between feedings, create a soothing, moist environment by using a glycerin-based gel or saline-based hydrophilic polymer. An antibiotic ointment may be recommended if nipples are cracked, abraded, or bleeding, but it must be washed off before feeding (Smith & Riordan, 2010; Walker, 2008b).

If nipples are extremely sore or damaged, and if the mother cannot tolerate breastfeeding, she may need to use an electric breast pump for 24 to 48 hours to allow the nipples to begin healing before resuming breastfeeding. The mother should use a pump that will effectively empty the breasts (see Figs. 25-9 and 25-11).

Candidiasis. Sore nipples that occur after the newborn period are often the result of a candidal infection. The mother usually reports sudden onset of severe nipple pain and tenderness, burning, or stinging; some women have sharp, shooting, burning pains into the breasts during and after feedings. The nipples appear somewhat pink and shiny; they can also be scaly or flaky. A visible rash, small blisters, or thrush can be present. Most often the pain is out of proportion to the appearance of the nipple. Candidal infections of the nipples and breast are excruciatingly painful and can lead to early cessation of breastfeeding if not recognized and treated promptly.

Infants may or may not exhibit symptoms of candidiasis. Oral thrush and a red, raised diaper rash are common signs of a yeast infection. An affected infant is usually very fussy and gassy. When feeding, the infant is likely to pull off the breast soon after starting to feed, crying with apparent pain.

The most common predisposing factors for candidal infections of the breast include vaginal yeast infections, previous antibiotic use, and nipple damage. Oral thrush in the infant is a common cause of candidiasis in maternal nipples and breasts.

Mothers and infants must be treated simultaneously, even if the infant has no visible signs of infection. Treatment for the mother is typically an antifungal cream such as miconazole applied to the nipples after feedings and, in some cases, a systemic antifungal medication such as fluconazole, taken for approximately 2 weeks. Most pediatricians prescribe an oral antifungal medication, such as nystatin, miconazole, or fluconazole, for infants. Treatment should continue for at least 7 days after symptoms begin to improve. Careful hand hygiene is essential to prevent the spread of a candidal infection (Walker, 2008b).

Plugged Milk Ducts. A milk duct can become plugged or clogged, causing an area of the breast to become swollen and tender. This area typically does not empty or soften with feeding or pumping. A small white pearl may also be visible on the tip of the nipple; this pearl is the curd of milk blocking the flow. The mother is afebrile and has no generalized symptoms.

Plugged milk ducts are most often the result of inadequate removal of milk from the breast, which can be caused by clothing that is too tight, a poorly fitting or underwire bra, or always using the same position for feeding. Application of warm compresses to the affected area and to the nipple before feeding helps promote emptying of the breast and release of the plug. (A disposable diaper filled with warm water makes an easy compress.)

Frequent feeding is recommended, with the baby beginning the feeding on the affected side to foster more complete emptying. The mother is advised to massage the affected area while the infant nurses or while she is pumping. Varying feeding positions and feeding without wearing a bra may be useful in resolving a plugged duct.

Plugged milk ducts may increase susceptibility to breast infection. For recurrent plugged ducts, taking lecithin, a fat emulsifier, may be useful for the mother (Walker, 2008b).

Mastitis. Although the term **mastitis** means inflammation of the breast, it is most often used to refer to infection of the breast. Mastitis is characterized by the sudden onset of influenza-like symptoms, including fever, chills, body aches, and headache. Localized breast pain and tenderness and a hot, reddened area on the breast, often resembling the shape of a pie wedge, are noted (see Fig. 34-4). Mastitis most commonly occurs in the upper outer quadrant of the breast; one or both breasts can be affected. The majority of cases occur during the first 6 weeks of breastfeeding, but mastitis can occur at any time (ABM Protocol Committee, 2008).

Certain factors can predispose a woman to mastitis. Inadequate emptying of the breasts is common, which can be related to engorgement, plugged ducts, a sudden decrease in the number of feedings, abrupt weaning, or wearing underwire bras. Sore, cracked nipples can lead to mastitis by providing a portal of entry for causative organisms (*Staphylococcus, Streptococcus,* and *Escherichia coli* being most common). Stress and fatigue, maternal illness, ill family members, breast trauma, and poor maternal nutrition also are predisposing factors for mastitis. Women with insulin-dependent diabetes may be at increased risk of mastitis (ABM Protocol Committee, 2008).

Breastfeeding mothers should be taught the signs of mastitis before they are discharged from the hospital after birth, and they need to know to call the health care provider promptly if the symptoms occur. Treatment includes antibiotics such as cephalexin or dicloxacillin for 10 to 14 days and analgesic and antipyretic medications such as ibuprofen. The mother is advised to rest as much as possible and to breastfeed the baby or pump frequently, striving to empty the affected side adequately. Warm compresses to the breast before feeding or pumping can be useful. Adequate fluid intake and a balanced diet are important for the mother with mastitis (ABM Protocol Committee, 2008).

Complications of mastitis include breast abscess, chronic mastitis, and fungal infections of the breast. Most complications can be prevented by early recognition and treatment.

Follow-up After Hospital Discharge

Problems with sore nipples, engorgement, and jaundice are likely to occur after discharge from the birth institution. One of the nurse's roles is to educate and prepare the mother for problems she may encounter once she is home. The mother should be given a list of resources for help with breastfeeding concerns. Community resources for breastfeeding mothers include lactation consultants in hospitals, physician offices, or in private practice; nurses in pediatric or obstetric offices; support groups such as La Leche League; and peer counseling programs (e.g., those offered through WIC). The Internet has many websites containing current and correct information about breastfeeding (e.g., www.breastfeeding.com).

Telephone follow-up by hospital, birth center, or office nurses within the first day or two after discharge can help identify problems and offer needed advice and support. Breastfeeding infants should be seen by a health care provider at 3 to 5 days of age and again at 2 to 3 weeks to assess weight gain and offer encouragement and support to the mother (AAP Section on Breastfeeding, 2005).

FORMULA FEEDING

Parent Education

The majority of infants receive at least some amount of commercial infant formula during their first year of life. Some parents choose formula feeding instead of breastfeeding; others combine the two methods. If the infant is weaned from breastfeeding before the first birthday, iron-fortified infant formula should be given (AAP Section on Breastfeeding, 2005).

For some mothers, formula feeding is associated with a variety of negative emotions, especially if they had intentions of breastfeeding. Mothers who are unable to breastfeed or decide to switch to formula feeding after attempting to breastfeed can experience a sense of failure along with feelings of guilt, shame, and worry. Others have a sense of relief once they start formula feeding. Mothers who decide prenatally to formula feed can feel guilty about not doing what they know is best for the baby—breastfeeding (Lakshman, Ogilvie, & Ong, 2009).

Mothers have reported that they do not get sufficient information from health care professionals about formula feeding (Labiner-Wolfe, Fein, & Shealy, 2008; Lakshman et al., 2009). In a large sample of formula-feeding mothers from the Infant Feeding Practices Study II, 77% of women with the youngest infants said they did not receive instruction from a health care professional about formula preparation, and 73% said they received no information about formula storage. More than half of the mothers reported that they did not always wash their hands with soap before preparing formula, 32% did not adequately clean bottle nipples between uses, and 35% used a microwave oven to heat formula (Labiner-Wolfe et al.).

Because of the lack of clear information about the practical aspects of formula feeding, parents often rely on advice from friends and family. If that advice is incorrect and the parents use unsafe practices for formula preparation and feeding, the infant is at risk for foodborne illness and burns.

It is important for nurses and other health care professionals to be intentional about providing education for parents related to formula preparation, feeding, and common problems they can encounter (Hancock & Brown, 2010). For women who are experiencing feelings of failure, guilt, shame, or worry, nurses can use the teaching sessions as opportunities for mothers to express their feelings. Some parents who are formula feeding express concern that the baby will suffer as a result of their decision to formula feed. Emphasis on the beneficial use of feeding times for close contact and socializing with the infant can help relieve some of this concern.

Readiness for Feeding

The first feeding of formula is ideally given after the neonate's initial transition to extrauterine life. Feeding-readiness cues include stability of vital signs, effective breathing pattern, presence of bowel sounds, an active sucking reflex, and those signs described earlier for breastfed infants.

Feeding Patterns

In the first 24 to 48 hours of life a newborn will typically consume 15 to 30 ml of formula at a feeding. Intake gradually increases during the first week of life. Most newborns are drinking 90 to 150 ml at a feeding by the end of the second week, or sooner. The newborn infant should be fed at least every 3 to 4 hours, even if waking the newborn is required for the feedings; rigid feeding schedules, however, are not recommended. The infant showing an adequate weight gain can be allowed to sleep at night and be fed only on awakening. Most newborns need six to eight feedings in 24 hours, and the number of feedings decreases as the infant matures and consumes more at each feeding. By 3 to 4 weeks after birth a fairly predictable feeding pattern has usually developed. Scheduling feedings arbitrarily at predetermined intervals may not meet a newborn's needs, but initiating feedings at convenient times often moves the newborn's feedings to times that work for the family.

Mothers will usually notice increases in the infant's appetite at the age of approximately 10 days, 3 weeks, 6 weeks, 3 months, and 6 months. These appetite spurts correspond to growth spurts. Mothers should increase the amount of formula per feeding by approximately 30 ml to meet the baby's needs at these times.

Feeding Technique

Infants should be held for all feedings. During feedings, parents are encouraged to sit comfortably, holding the infant closely in a semi-upright position with good head support. Feedings provide opportunities to bond with the baby through touching, talking, singing, or reading to the infant. Parents should consider feedings a time of peaceful relaxation with the infant.

Nursing Skill—Infant Feeding

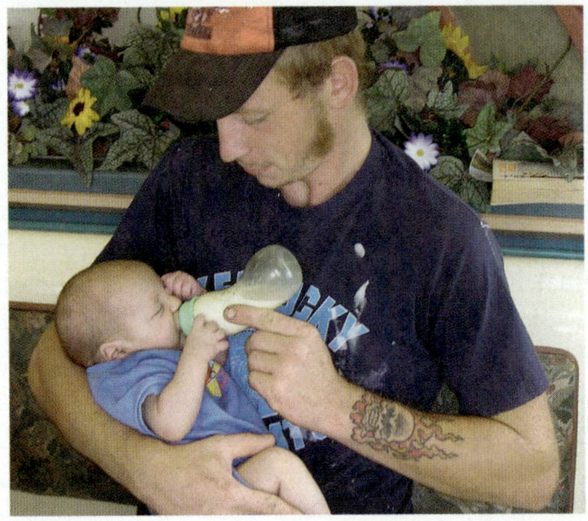

FIG. 25-16 Father bottle feeding infant son. Note angled bottle that ensures that milk covers nipple area. (Courtesy Eugene Doerr, Leitchfield, KY.)

SAFETY ALERT

A bottle should never be propped with a pillow or other inanimate object and left with the infant. This practice can result in choking, and it deprives the infant of important interaction during feeding. Moreover, propping the bottle has been implicated in causing nursing-bottle caries or decay of the first teeth resulting from continuous bathing of the teeth with carbohydrate-containing fluid as the infant sporadically sucks the nipple.

The bottle should be held so that fluid fills the nipple and none of the air in the bottle is allowed to enter the nipple (Fig. 25-16). If the infant falls asleep, turns the head, or ceases to suck, it usually indicates that the baby has consumed enough formula to feel satiated. Teach parents to look for these cues and avoid overfeeding, which can contribute to obesity.

Most infants swallow air when fed from a bottle and need a chance to burp several times during a feeding. Parents are taught various positions that can be used for burping (Fig. 25-17).

Common Concerns

Parents need to know what to do if the infant spits up. They may need to decrease the amount of feeding or feed smaller amounts more frequently. Burping the infant several times during a feeding, such as when the infant's sucking slows down or stops, can decrease spitting. Holding the baby upright for 30 minutes after feeding and avoiding bouncing or placing the infant on the abdomen soon after the feeding is finished can also help. Spitting can be a result of overfeeding or it can be symptomatic of gastroesophageal reflux. Parents should report vomiting one third or more of the feeding at most feeding sessions or projectile vomiting to the health care provider and should be cautioned to refrain from changing the infant's formula without consulting the health care provider.

Bottles and Nipples

Various brands and styles of bottles and nipples are available. Most babies will feed well with any bottle and nipple. The bottles, nipples, rings, and caps should be washed in warm soapy water, using a bottle and nipple brush to facilitate thorough cleansing. They should be placed in boiling water for 5 minutes

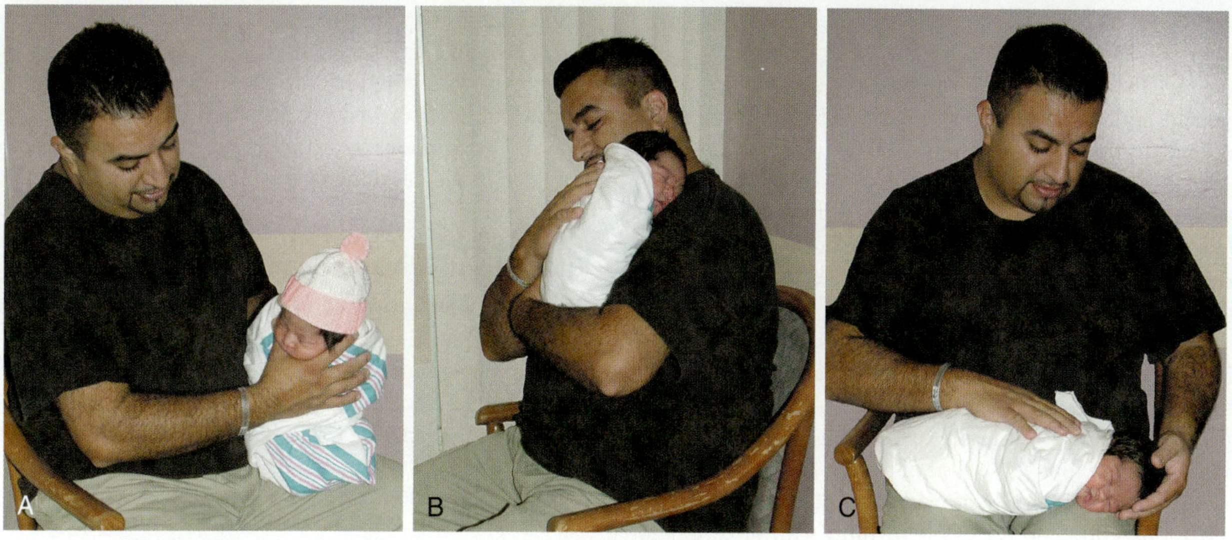

FIG. 25-17 Positions for burping an infant. **A,** Sitting. **B,** On the shoulder. **C,** Across the lap. (Courtesy Julie Perry Nelson, Loveland, CO.)

and allowed to air dry; this should be done at least prior to the first use and thereafter unless they are cleaned in a dishwasher (see Teaching for Self-Management box: Formula Preparation and Feeding). Boiling of feeding equipment is recommended if the infant has oral thrush. An angled bottle can be preferable to a straight bottle because it encourages more physiologic positioning of the infant, improves the infant's comfort level, and decreases the need for burping (see Fig. 25-16).

Infant Formulas

Commercial Formulas

Commercial infant formulas are designed to resemble human milk as closely as possible, although none has ever duplicated it. The exact composition of infant formula varies with the manufacturer, but all must meet specific standards.

Infants who are not breastfed should be given commercial iron-fortified formulas. Families with limited income may be eligible for services through the WIC program, which provides iron-fortified infant formula.

Commercially prepared formulas are cow's milk–based formulas that have been modified to closely resemble the nutritional content of human milk. These formulas are altered from cow's milk by removing butterfat, decreasing the protein content, and adding vegetable oil and carbohydrate. Some have demineralized whey added to yield a whey/casein ratio of 60:40. The standard cow's milk–based formulas, regardless of the commercial brand, have essentially the same compositions of vitamins, minerals, protein, carbohydrates, and essential amino acids, with minor variations such as the source of carbohydrate; nucleotides to enhance immune function; and long-chain polyunsaturated fatty acids, DHA, and arachidonic acid, which are thought to improve visual and cognitive function. Furthermore, the U.S. Food and Drug Administration regulates the manufacture of infant formula in the United States to ensure product safety. Standard cow's milk–based formulas are sold as low-iron and iron-fortified formulas; however, only the iron-fortified formulas meet infants' requirements.

Four main categories of commercially prepared infant formulas are available: (1) cow's milk–based formulas, (2) soy-based formulas, commonly used for children who are lactose or cow's milk protein intolerant; (3) casein- or whey-hydrolysate formulas, used primarily for children who cannot tolerate or digest cow's milk or soy-based formulas; and (4) amino acid formulas, used for infants with multiple food protein intolerances.

The AAP Committee on Nutrition indicates that few solid indications exist for the use of soy protein–based formulas instead of cow's milk–based formulas (Bhatia, Greer, & AAP Committee on Nutrition, 2008). Soy-based formulas are recommended for infants with galactosemia and congenital lactase deficiency; infants with secondary lactase deficiency may benefit as well. Infants with documented IgE allergies caused by cow's milk should be fed an extensively hydrolyzed protein formula because approximately 10% to 14% of infants with cow's milk–based intolerance also have a soy protein allergy. Soy protein–based formulas have not been proved to be effective against colic or in the prevention of allergy in healthy or high risk infants.

Alternate milk sources such as goat's milk, skim or low-fat milk, condensed milk, or raw, unpasteurized milk from any animal source should not be fed to infants because they are inadequate to support growth and may contain excess protein or an inadequate calcium/phosphorus ratio, which may cause seizures.

SAFETY ALERT

Because of concerns about potential harmful effects of bisphenol A (BPA), parents should be cautioned about using hard plastic polycarbonate baby bottles or containers. BPA is a chemical that is used to harden plastics, to prevent bacterial contamination of foods, and to prevent can rusting. It is in many food and liquid containers, including baby bottles. The AAP (2009) recommends avoiding clear plastic bottles or containers imprinted with the recycling number 7 and the letters PC, and purchasing bottles that are certified or identified as BPA-free. Glass bottles are an alternative, but parents must be aware of the risk for injury if the bottle is dropped or broken. Because heat can cause the release of BPA from plastic, polycarbonate bottles should never be boiled, heated in the microwave, or washed in a dishwasher (AAP).

Spanish Guidelines—Burping

Formula Preparation

Commercial formulas are available in three forms: powder, concentrate, and ready-to-feed. All forms are equivalent in terms of nutritional content, but they vary considerably in cost.

- Ready-to-feed formula is the most expensive but the easiest to use. The desired amount is poured into the bottle. The opened can is safely refrigerated for 48 hours. This type of formula can be purchased in individual disposable bottles for the most convenient feeding.
- Concentrated formula is less expensive than ready-to-feed. It is diluted with equal parts of water and can be stored in the refrigerator for 48 hours after opening.
- Powdered formula is the least expensive. It is easily mixed by using one scoop for every 60 ml of water.

The commercial infant formula must include label directions for preparation and use of the formula with pictures and symbols for the benefit of individuals who cannot read. Some manufacturers translate the directions into languages such as Spanish, French, Vietnamese, Chinese, and Arabic to prevent misunderstanding and errors in formula preparation.

SAFETY ALERT

An important aspect to impress on families is that the proportions must not be altered—that is, neither diluted to extend the amount of formula nor concentrated to provide more calories. The newborn's kidneys are immature; giving the infant overly concentrated formula can provide protein and minerals in amounts that exceed the kidneys' excretory ability. In contrast, if the formula is diluted too much (sometimes done to save money), the infant does not consume sufficient calories and does not grow appropriately.

The water used to mix either powdered or concentrated liquid formula need not contain any fluoride, especially in the first 6 months of life. Excess fluoride can permanently stain the teeth once they do appear.

Sterilization of formula rarely is recommended when families have access to a safe public water supply. Instead, formula is prepared with attention to cleanliness. When water from a private well is used, parents should be advised to contact the health department to have a chemical and bacteriologic analysis of the water performed before using the water in formula preparation. The presence of nitrates, excess fluoride, or bacteria may be harmful to the infant.

It is usually safe to mix infant formula with cold tap water that has been boiled for 1-2 minutes and allowed to cool. Bottled water that is labeled as "sterile" is safe for mixing formula. However, non-sterile bottled water should be boiled for 1-2 minutes and cooled.

If the conditions in the home appear unsanitary, the nurse should recommend the use of ready-to-feed formula or teach the mother to sterilize the formula. The two traditional methods for sterilization are terminal heating and the aseptic method. In the terminal heating method the prepared formula is placed in the bottles, which are topped with the nipples placed upside down and covered with the caps, and then sealed loosely with the rings. The bottles are then boiled together in a water bath for 25 minutes. In the aseptic method the bottles, rings, caps, nipples, and any other necessary equipment, such as a funnel, are boiled separately, after which the formula is poured into the bottles. Any formula left in the bottle after the feeding should be discarded because the infant's saliva has mixed with it. (Instructions for formula preparation and feeding are provided in the Teaching Guidelines box: Formula Preparation and Feeding).

Critical Thinking Exercise—Formula Preparation

Vitamin and Mineral Supplementation

Commercial iron-fortified formula has all of the nutrients that infants need for the first 6 months of life. After 6 months, fluoride supplementation of 0.25 mg/day is required if the local water supply is not fluoridated. Nonbreastfeeding infants who consume less than 1 quart per day of vitamin D–fortified milk should receive 400 International Units of vitamin D each day (Wagner et al., 2008).

Weaning

The bottle-fed infant will gradually learn to use a cup, and the parents will find that they are preparing fewer bottles. The bottle feeding before bedtime is often the last one to remain. Babies have a strong need to suck, and the baby who has the bottle taken away too early or abruptly will compensate with nonnutritive sucking on his or her fingers, thumb, a pacifier, or even his or her own tongue. Weaning from a bottle should therefore be attempted gradually because the baby has learned to rely on the comfort that sucking provides.

Complementary Feeding: Introducing Solid Foods

Complementary feedings are defined as foods or liquids given to the infant in addition to breast milk or formula. The AAP Committee on Nutrition (2008) recommends introducing solid foods after 4 months of age, and preferably after 6 months of age. First foods should include a source of iron such as iron-fortified cereal or meat. New foods should be introduced slowly to assess for any allergic reaction or intolerance. It is best to offer no more than three new foods per week. Fruits and vegetables should be offered to infants daily starting at 6 to 8 months. Fruit juices are not recommended before 6 months of age due to the possibility that the infant who drinks juice will consume less breast milk or formula. Infants should be limited in the consumption of low-nutrient foods such as fatty or sugary foods or restaurant foods.

In spite of the recommendations from the AAP, many parents begin complementary feedings earlier than 4 months. In a recent large scale study of feeding practices, more than half of the infants had received solid foods before the age of 4 months (Grummer-Strawn, Scanlon, & Fein, 2008). The infant receives the right balance of nutrients from breast milk or formula during the first 4 to 6 months. The notion that the feeding of solids will help the infant sleep through the night is not true. Parents should not put cereal into the infant's bottle. Introduction of solid foods before the infant is 4 to 6 months of age can result in overfeeding and decreased intake of breast milk or formula.

Cultural beliefs and traditions affect complementary feeding practices. First foods given to infants vary widely. For example, first foods for Egyptian infants include bread soaked in milk and tea or yogurt sweetened with honey. Chinese and Vietnamese infants are sometimes fed prechewed rice paste, rice, or sweetened porridge (Pak-Gorstein, Haq, & Graham, 2009).

TEACHING FOR SELF-MANAGEMENT

Formula Preparation and Feeding

FORMULA PREPARATION

- Using warm, soapy water, wash your hands, arms, and under your nails; rinse well. Clean and sanitize the surface where you will be preparing the bottles.
- Thoroughly wash bottles, nipples, rings, caps, can opener, and other preparation utensils in hot soapy water and rinse thoroughly. Squeeze water through nipples to make sure the holes are open.
- Place bottles, nipples, rings, and caps in a pot and cover with water; boil for 5 minutes; remove items from pot with sanitized tongs and allow them to air dry. (Do this at least before using items the first time; thereafter, you can continue to do this, or place items in the dishwasher.)
- Note the expiration date on the formula container. It should be used before the expiration date. Any unopened expired formula should be returned to the place of purchase.
- Read the label on the container of formula and mix it exactly according to the directions.
- Mix formula with tap water deemed safe by the local health department. Allow cold water to run for 2 minutes before collecting it. Then, bring it to a rolling boil and continue boiling for 1-2 minutes. If using bottled water, make sure it is labeled as "sterile"; unsterile bottled water must be boiled. After boiling, allow water to cool before mixing the formula, but not longer than 30 minutes.
- If using a can of ready-to-feed or concentrated formula, wash the top of the can with hot, soapy water and rinse well. Shake the can before opening.
- Mixing formula
  - *Ready-to-feed:* no mixing is needed; do not add water. Pour desired amount of formula into clean bottle, add nipple and ring.
  - *Concentrate:* pour desired amount of formula into a clean bottle and add equal amount of cooled boiled water. Add nipple and ring and shake well.
  - *Powder:* when first opening the container of powder, write the date on the lid. Using the scoop from the container, add 1 scoop of powdered formula for each 2 ounces of boiled, cooled water in a clean bottle. For example, if 6 ounces of water is in the bottle, add three scoops of powder. Add nipple and ring and shake well.
- If preparing multiple bottles at the same time, place nipple right side up on each bottle and cover with a clean nipple cap. Use bottles within 48 hours.
- Opened cans of ready-to-feed or concentrated formula should be covered and refrigerated. Any unused portions must be discarded after 48 hours.
- Bottles or cans of unopened formula can be stored at room temperature.
- If the formula is refrigerated, warm it by placing the bottle in a pan of hot water. Never use a microwave to warm any food to be given to a baby. Test the temperature of the formula by letting a few drops fall on the inside of your wrist. If the formula feels comfortably warm to you, the temperature is correct.

FEEDING TECHNIQUES AND TIPS

- Newborns should be fed at least every 3 to 4 hours and should never go longer than 4 hours without feeding until a satisfactory pattern of weight gain is established. This period may be as long as 2 weeks. If a baby cries or fusses between feedings, check to see if the diaper should be changed and if the baby needs to be picked up and cuddled. If the baby continues to cry and acts hungry, then feed the baby. Babies do not get hungry on a regular schedule.
- Infants gradually increase the amount of milk they drink with each feeding. The first day or so, most newborns consume 15 to 30 ml (0.5 to 1 ounce) with each feeding. This amount increases as the infant grows. If any formula remains in the bottle as the feeding ends, that milk must be thrown away because saliva from the baby's mouth can cause the formula to spoil.
- Keep a feeding diary, writing down the amount of formula the infant drinks with each feeding for the first week or so. Also record the wet diapers and bowel movements the baby is having. Take this diary with you when you take the baby for the first follow-up visit with the primary health care provider.
- For feeding, hold the infant close in a semi-reclining position. Talk to the baby during the feeding. This time is ideal for social interaction and cuddling.
- Place the nipple in the infant's mouth on the tongue. It should touch the roof of the mouth to stimulate the baby's sucking reflex. Hold the bottle like a pencil. Keep the bottle tipped so that the nipple stays filled with milk and the baby does not suck in air.
- Taking a few sucks and then pausing briefly before continuing to suck again is normal for infants. Some infants take longer to feed than others. Be patient. Keeping the baby awake and encouraging sucking may be necessary. Moving the nipple gently in the infant's mouth may stimulate sucking.
- Newborns are apt to swallow air when sucking. Give the infant opportunities to burp several times during a feeding. As the infant gets older, you will know better when to stop for burping.
- After the first 2 or 3 days the stools of a formula-fed infant are yellow and soft but formed. The infant may have a stool with each feeding in the first 2 weeks, although this amount may decrease to one or two stools each day. It is not abnormal for formula fed infants to have a stool every other day.

SAFETY TIPS

- Infants should be held and never left alone while feeding. Never prop the bottle. The infant might inhale formula or choke on any that was spit up. Infants who fall asleep with a propped bottle of milk or juice may be prone to cavities when the first teeth come in.
- Know how to use the bulb syringe and how to help an infant who is choking.

Sources: World Health Organization & Food and Agriculture Organization of the United Nations. (2007). Safe preparation, storage, and handling of powdered infant formula: Guidelines. Geneva: World Health Organization. Available at www.who.int/foodsafety/publications/micro/pif_guidelines.pdf. Accessed July 18, 2010; United States Department of Agriculture. (2008). Infant nutrition and feeding. Washington, DC: USDA. Available at www.nal.usda.gov/wicworks/Topics/FG/CompleteIFG.pdf. Accessed July 18, 2010.

In some cultures it is common to feed the infant premasticated foods. This is not considered to be a safe practice because of the risk of transferring illness to the infant.

Nurses and other health care professionals provide education to parents regarding complementary feedings. This most often occurs during well-baby supervision visits with the pediatric health care provider. Early feeding practices have implications for long-term dietary patterns; therefore, it is essential to teach parents about proper nutrition.

COMMUNITY ACTIVITY

- Visit the International Lactation Consultant Association (ILCA) website (www.ilca.org). What is the mission and vision of the association? Locate a board certified lactation consultant in your community. What other resources are available for breastfeeding mothers after discharge from the hospital in your community?
- Visit the La Leche League International website (www.llli.org). What is the mission of the La Leche League? Locate a La Leche League group in your community.

KEY POINTS

- Human breast milk is species specific and is the recommended form of infant nutrition. It provides immunologic protection against many infections and diseases.
- Breast milk changes in composition with each stage of lactation, during each feeding, and as the infant grows.
- During the prenatal period, expectant parents should be informed of the benefits of breastfeeding for infants, mothers, families, and society.
- Infants should be breastfed as soon as possible after birth and at least 8 to 12 times per day thereafter.
- Specific, measurable indicators have been identified to show that the infant is breastfeeding effectively.
- Breast milk production is based on a supply-meets-demand principle: The more the infant nurses, the greater the milk supply.
- Infants go through predictable growth spurts.
- Sore nipples are most often caused by incorrect latch.
- Commercial infant formulas provide satisfactory nutrition for most infants.
- Infants should be held for feedings.
- Parents should be instructed about the types of commercial infant formulas, proper preparation for feeding, and correct feeding technique.
- Solid foods should be started after age 4 to 6 months.
- Unmodified cow's milk is inappropriate during the first year of life.
- Nurses must be knowledgeable about feeding methods and provide education and support for families.

Audio Chapter Summaries Access an audio summary of these Key Points on evolve

REFERENCES

Academy of Breastfeeding Medicine (ABM) Board of Directors. (2008). Position on breastfeeding. *Breastfeeding Medicine, 3*(4), 267–270.

Academy of Breastfeeding Medicine Protocol Committee. (2010). ABM clinical protocol #8: Human milk storage information for home use for full-term infants. *Breastfeeding Medicine, 5*(3), 127–130.

Academy of Breastfeeding Medicine Protocol Committee. (2006). ABM clinical protocol No. 13: Contraception during breastfeeding. *Breastfeeding Medicine, 1*(1), 43–51.

Academy of Breastfeeding Medicine Protocol Committee. (2008). ABM clinical protocol #4: Mastitis. *Breastfeeding Medicine, 3*(3), 177–180.

Academy of Breastfeeding Medicine Protocol Committee. (2009). ABM clinical protocol #3: Hospital guidelines for the use of supplementary feedings in the healthy term breastfed infant, revised 2009. *Breastfeeding Medicine, 4*(3), 175–182.

American Academy of Family Physicians. (2007). *Family physicians supporting breastfeeding.* Available at www.aafp.org/online/en/home/policies/b/breastfeedingpositionpaper.html. Accessed February 26, 2010.

American Academy of Pediatrics (AAP) (2009). *Caring for your baby and young child: Ages birth to age 5.* Available at www.healthychildren.org/English/ages-stages/baby/feeding-nutrition/pages/Baby-Bottles-And-Bisphenol-A-BPA.aspx. Accessed July 20, 2010.

American Academy of Pediatrics (AAP) Committee on Nutrition. (2008). *Pediatric nutrition handbook* (6th ed.). Elk Grove Village, IL: AAP.

American Academy of Pediatrics (AAP) Section on Breastfeeding. (2005). Breastfeeding and the use of human milk. Policy statement. *Pediatrics, 115*(23), 496–506.

American Academy of Pediatrics (AAP) Task Force on Sudden Infant Death Syndrome. (2005). The changing concept of sudden infant death syndrome: Diagnostic coding shifts, controversies regarding the sleeping environment, and new variables to consider in reducing risk. *Pediatrics, 116*(5), 1245–1255.

American College of Obstetricians and Gynecologists (ACOG) Committee on Health Care for Underserved Women & Committee on Obstetric Practice. (2007). Breastfeeding: Maternal and infant aspects. *ACOG Clinical Review, 12*(1), 1S–16S.

American Dietetic Association (ADA) (2009). Position of the American Dietetic Association: Promoting and supporting breastfeeding. *Journal of the American Dietetic Association (ADA). 109*(11), 1926–1942.

Association of Women's Health, Obstetric and Neonatal Nurses (AWHONN). (2007). *Breastfeeding and the role of the nurse in the promotion of breastfeeding.* Washington, DC: AWHONN.

Baby-Friendly USA. (2010). *BFHI USA: Implementing the UNICEF/WHO baby friendly hospital initiative in the U.S.* Sandwich, MA: BFUSA. Available at www.babyfriendlyusa.org. Accessed July 12, 2010.

Becker, G., & Scott, M. (2008). Nutrition for lactating women. In R. Mannel, P. Martens, & M. Walker (Eds.), *Core curriculum for lactation consultant practice* (2nd ed.). Sudbury, MA: Jones and Bartlett.

Bhatia, J., Greer, F., & American Academy of Pediatrics (AAP) Committee on Nutrition. (2008). Use of soy protein-based formulas in infant feeding. *Pediatrics, 121*(5), 1062–1068.

Blackburn, S. (2007). *Maternal, fetal, and neonatal physiology: A clinical perspective* (3rd ed.). St. Louis: Saunders.

Bunik, M., Clark, L., Zimmer, L., Jimenez, L., O'Connor, M., Crane, L., et al. (2006). Early infant feeding decisions in low-income Latinas. *Breastfeeding Medicine, 1*(4), 225–235.

Castrucci, B., Piña Carrizales, L., D'Angelo, D., McDonald, J., Foulkes, H., Ahluwalia, I., et al. (2008). Attempted breastfeeding before hospital discharge on both sides of the US-Mexico border, 2005: The Brownsville-Matamoros sister city project for women's health. *Preventing Chronic Disease, 5*(4). Available at www.cdc.gov/pcd/issues/2008/oct/08_0058.htm. Accessed July 21, 2010.

Centers for Disease Control and Prevention (CDC). (2009). *Breastfeeding report card—United States, 2009*. Available at www.cdc.gov/breastfeeding/data/report_card.htm. Accessed July 21, 2010.

Centers for Disease Control and Prevention. (2010). U.S. medical eligibility criteria for contraceptive use, 2010: Adapted from the World Health Organization medical eligibility criteria for contraceptive use (4th ed.). *MMRW Morbidity and Mortality Weekly Report, Recommendations and Reports, 59*(RR4), 1–86.

Cleveland, K. (2010). Feeding challenges in the late preterm infant. *Neonatal Network, 29*(1), 37–41.

Clifford, J., & McIntyre, E. (2008). Who supports breastfeeding? *Breastfeeding Review, 16*(2), 9–19.

Cotterman, J. (2004). Reverse pressure softening: A simple tool to prepare areola for easier latching during engorgement. *Journal of Human Lactation, 20*(2), 227–237.

Dell, K., & Davis, I. (2006). Fluid, electrolyte, and acid-base homeostasis. In R. Martin, A. Fanaroff, & M. Walsh (Eds.), *Fanaroff and Martin's neonatal-perinatal medicine: Diseases of the fetus and infant* (8th ed.). St. Louis: Mosby.

Dollberg, S., Botzer, E., Grunis, E., & Mimouni, F. (2006). Immediate nipple pain relief after frenotomy in breast-fed infants with ankyloglossia: A randomized, prospective study. *Journal of Pediatric Surgery, 41*(9), 1598–1600.

Fein, S., Mandal, B., & Roe, B. (2008). Success of strategies for combining employment and breastfeeding. *Pediatrics, 122*(Suppl. 2), S56–S62.

Fortinguerra, F., Clavenna, A., & Bonati, M. (2009). Psychotropic drug use during breastfeeding: A review of the evidence. *Pediatrics, 124*(4), e547–e556.

Geddes, D. (2007). Inside the lactating breast: The latest anatomy research. *Journal of Midwifery and Women's Health, 52*(6), 556–563.

Gill, S. (2009). Breastfeeding by Hispanic women. *Journal of Obstetric, Gynecologic and Neonatal Nursing, 38*(2), 244–252.

Grummer-Strawn, L., Scanlon, K., & Fein, S. (2008). Infant feeding and feeding transitions during the first year of life. *Pediatrics, 122*(Suppl. 2), S36–S42.

Hale, T. (2010). Drug therapy and breastfeeding. In J. Riordan & K. Wambach (Eds.), *Breastfeeding and human lactation* (4th ed.). Boston: Jones and Bartlett.

Hancock, M., & Brown, J. (2010). Formula-feeding safety: What nurses need to teach parents who choose to formula-feed. *Nursing for Women's Health, 14*(4), 303-309.

Heird, W. (2007). The feeding of infants and children. In R. Kliegman, R. Behrman, H. Jenson, & B. Stanton (Eds.), *Nelson textbook of pediatrics* (18th ed.). Philadelphia: Saunders.

Horta, B., Bahl, R., Martines, J., & Victora, C. (2007). *Evidence on the long-term effects of breastfeeding: Systematic reviews and meta-analyses*. Geneva: World Health Organization. Available at http://whqlibdoc.who.int/publications/2007/9789241595230_eng.pdf. Accessed July 21, 2010.

Institute of Medicine. (2005). *Dietary reference intakes for energy, carbohydrate, fiber, fatty acids, cholesterol, protein, and amino acids*. Washington, DC: Food and Nutrition Board, Institute of Medicine, National Academies Press.

International Lactation Consultant Association (ILCA). (1999). *Evidence-based guidelines for breastfeeding management during the first fourteen days*. Raleigh, NC: ILCA.

Ip, S., Chung, M., Raman, G., Chew, P., Magula, N., DeVine, D., et al. (2007). *Breastfeeding and maternal and infant health outcomes in developed countries*. Evidence report/technology assessment No. 153. (Prepared by Tufts-New England Medical Center Evidence-Based Practice Center under contract no. 290-02-0022). AHRQ Publication No. 07-E007. Rockville, MD: Agency for Healthcare Research and Quality. Available at http://www.ahrq.gov/downloads/pub/evidence/pdf/brfout/brfout.pdf. Accessed July 21, 2010.

Jenik, A., Vain, N., Gorestein, A., Jacobi, N., & Pacifier and Breastfeeding Trial Group. (2009). Does the recommendation to use a pacifier influence the prevalence of breastfeeding? *Journal of Pediatrics, 155*(3), 350–354.

Jones, F., & Tully, M. (2006). *Best practices for expressing, storing, and handling human milk in hospitals, homes, and child care settings* (2nd ed.). Raleigh, NC: Human Milk Banking Association of America.

Labiner-Wolfe, J., Fein, S., & Shealy, K. (2008). Infant formula handling education and safety. *Pediatrics, 122*(Suppl. 2), S85–S90.

Labiner-Wolfe, J., Fein, S., Shealy, K., & Wang, C. (2008). Prevalence of breast milk expression and associated factors. *Pediatrics, 122*(Suppl. 2), S63–S68.

Lakshman, R., Ogilvie, D., & Ong, K. (2009). Mothers' experiences of bottle-feeding: A systematic review of qualitative and quantitative studies. *Archives of Disease in Childhood, 94*(8), 596–601.

Lanese, M., & Cross, M. (2008). Breastfeeding a preterm infant. In R. Mannel, P. Martens, & M. Walker (Eds.), *Core curriculum for lactation consultant practice* (2nd ed.). Sudbury, MA: Jones and Bartlett.

Laroia, N., & Sharma, D. (2006). The religious and cultural bases for breastfeeding practices among the Hindus. *Breastfeeding Medicine, 1*(2), 94–98.

Lawrence, R., & Lawrence, R. (2005). *Breastfeeding: A guide for the medical profession* (6th ed.). St. Louis: Mosby.

Lewallen, L., Dick, M., Flowers, J., Powell, W., Zickefoose, K., Wall, Y., et al. (2006). Breastfeeding support and early cessation. *Journal of Obstetric, Gynecologic and Neonatal Nursing, 35*(2), 166–172.

Mannel, R. (2008). Milk expression, storage, and handling. In R. Mannel, P. Martens, & M. Walker (Eds.), *Core curriculum for lactation consultant practice* (2nd ed.). Sudbury, MA: Jones and Bartlett.

McDowell, M., Wang, C., & Kennedy-Stephenson, J. (2008). Breastfeeding in the United States: Findings from the national health and nutrition examination surveys, 1999-2006. *National Center for Health Statistics (NCHS) Data Brief, 5*, 1–7.

Mohrbacher, N. (2008). Breastfeeding and growth: Birth through weaning. In R. Mannel, P. Martens, & M. Walker (Eds.), *Core curriculum for lactation consultant practice* (2nd ed.). Sudbury, MA: Jones and Bartlett.

O'Brien, M., Buikstra, E., & Hegney, D. (2008). The influence of psychological factors on breastfeeding duration. *Journal of Advanced Nursing, 63*(4), 397–408.

O'Connor, N., Tanabe, K., Siadaty, M., & Hauck, F. (2009). Pacifiers and breastfeeding: A systematic review. *Archives of Pediatric and Adolescent Medicine, 163*(4), 378–382.

Overfield, M., Ryan, C., Spangler, A., & Tully, M. (2005). *Clinical guidelines for the establishment of exclusive breastfeeding* (2nd ed.). Raleigh, NC: ILCA.

Page-Goertz, S. (2008). Hyperbilirubinemia and hypoglycemia. In R. Mannel, P. Martens, & M. Walker (Eds.), *Core curriculum for lactation consultant practice* (2nd ed.). Sudbury, MA: Jones and Bartlett.

Pak-Gorstein, S., Haq, A., & Graham, E. (2009). Cultural influences on infant feeding practices. *Pediatrics in Review, 30*(3), e11–e21.

Ramsay, D., Kent, J., Hartmann, R., & Hartmann, P. (2005). Anatomy of the lactating human breast redefined with ultrasound imaging. *Journal of Anatomy, 206*(6), 525–534.

Renfrew, M., & Hall, D. (2008). Enabling women to breastfeed. *British Medical Journal, 337*, a1570.

Riordan, J., & Wambach, K. (2010). Breast-related problems. In J. Riordan & K. Wambach (Eds.), *Breastfeeding and human lactation* (4th ed.). Boston: Jones and Bartlett.

Rios, E. (2009). Promoting breastfeeding in the Hispanic community. *Breastfeeding Medicine, 4*(Suppl. 1), S69–S70.

Rosen, I., Krueger, M., Carney, L., & Graham, J. (2008). Prenatal breastfeeding education and breastfeeding outcomes. *MCN: The American Journal of Maternal/Child Nursing, 33*(5), 315–319.

Scott, J., Binns, C., Graham, K., & Oddy, W. (2006). Temporal changes in the determinants of breastfeeding initiation. *Birth, 33*(1), 37–45.

Shaikh, U., & Ahmed, O. (2006). Islam and infant feeding. *Breastfeeding Medicine, 1*(3), 164–167.

Shealy, K., Scanlon, K., Labiner-Wolfe, J., Fein, S., & Grummer-Strawn, L. (2008). Characteristics of breastfeeding practice among U.S. mothers. *Pediatrics, 122*(2), S50–S55.

Simmer, K., Patole, S., & Rao, S. (2008). Long chain polyunsaturated fatty acid supplementation in infants born at term. *The Cochrane Database of Systematic Reviews, 2008*, 1, CD000376.

Smith, L., & Riordan, J. (2010). Postpartum care. In J. Riordan & K. Wambach (Eds.), *Breastfeeding and human lactation* (4th ed.). Boston: Jones and Bartlett.

Stuebe, A. (2009). The risks of not breastfeeding for mothers and infants. *Reviews in Obstetrics and Gynecology, 2*(4), 222–231.

Taylor, J., Geller, L., Risica, P., Kirtania, U., & Cabral, H. (2008). Birth order and breastfeeding initiation: Results of a national survey. *Breastfeeding Medicine, 3*(1), 20–27.

Tully, M., & Jones, F. (2010). Donor milk banking. In J. Riordan & K. Wambach (Eds.), *Breastfeeding and human lactation* (4th ed.). Boston: Jones and Bartlett.

Tuttle, C., & Slavit, W. (2009). Establishing the business case for breastfeeding. *Breastfeeding Medicine, 4*(Suppl. 1), S59–S62.

U.S. Department of Health and Human Services. (2000). Maternal, infant, and child health. In *Healthy People 2010* (2nd ed.). (Vol. 2). Washington, DC: Department of Health and Human Services. Available at www.healthypeople.gov/Document/pdf/Volume2/16MICH.pdf. Accessed July 21, 2010.

U.S. Department of Health and Human Services. (2009). *Healthy People 2020: The road ahead.* Washington, DC: Department of Health and Human Services. Available at. www.healthypeople.gov/hp2020/default.asp. Accessed July 21, 2010.

Wagner, C., Grier, F., & AAP Section on Breastfeeding, & Committee on Nutrition (2008). Prevention of rickets and vitamin D deficiency in infants, children and adolescents. *Pediatrics, 122*(5), 1142–1152.

Walker, M. (2006). *Breastfeeding management for the clinician: Using the evidence.* Sudbury, MA: Jones and Bartlett.

Walker, M. (2008a). Breastfeeding the late preterm infant. *Journal of Obstetric, Gynecologic and Neonatal Nursing, 37*(6), 692–701.

Walker, M. (2008b). Conquering common breastfeeding problems. *Journal of Perinatal Nursing, 22*(4), 267–274.

World Health Organization (WHO) & UNICEF. (2003). *Global strategy for infant and young child feeding.* Geneva: WHO. Available at www.who.int/child_adolescent_health/documents/9241562218/en. Accessed July 21, 2010.

World Health Organization (WHO) (2009). *Medical eligibility criteria for contraceptive use* (4th ed.). Geneva: WHO.

WHO, UNICEF, UNFPA, & UNAIDS. (2010). *Guidelines on HIV and infant feeding.* Geneva: WHO. Available at http://whqlibdoc.who.int/publications/2010/9789241599535_eng.pdf. Accessed July 15, 2010.

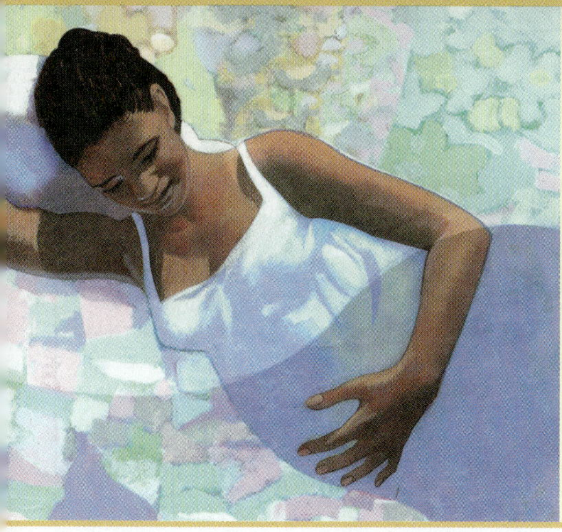

CHAPTER 26

Assessment for Risk Factors in Pregnancy

Kitty Cashion

evolve WEBSITE

http://evolve.elsevier.com/Lowdermilk/MWHC/

Audio Glossary
Audio Key Points
NCLEX Review Questions
Spanish Guidelines
  High Risk Factors
Video—Nursing Skills
  Assisting During Amniocentesis

LEARNING OBJECTIVES

- Explore the biophysical, psychosocial, sociodemographic, and environmental influences on high risk pregnancy.
- Examine risk factors identified through history, physical examination, and diagnostic techniques.
- Discuss psychologic considerations for the woman and her family experiencing a high risk pregnancy.
- Differentiate among screening and diagnostic techniques, including when they are used in pregnancy and for what purposes.
- Develop a teaching plan to explain screening and diagnostic techniques and implications of findings to women and their families.

Approximately 500,000 of the 4 million births that occur in the United States each year are categorized as high risk because of maternal or fetal complications. A *high risk* pregnancy is one in which the life or health of the mother or fetus is jeopardized by a disorder coincidental with or unique to pregnancy. Care of these high risk women requires the combined efforts of medical and nursing personnel. Factors associated with a high risk pregnancy are identified in this chapter. Screening and diagnostic techniques often used to monitor the maternal-fetal unit at risk are also described.

ASSESSMENT OF RISK FACTORS

Pregnancies can be designated as high risk for any of several undesirable outcomes. Those considered to be at risk for **uteroplacental insufficiency (UPI),** the gradual decline in delivery of needed substances by the placenta to the fetus, carry a serious threat for fetal growth restriction, intrauterine fetal death, intrapartum fetal distress, and various types of neonatal morbidity.

In the past, risk factors were evaluated only from a medical standpoint. Therefore, only adverse medical, obstetric, or physiologic conditions were considered to place the woman at risk. Today a more comprehensive approach to high risk pregnancy is used, and the factors associated with high risk childbearing are grouped into broad categories based on threats to health and pregnancy outcome. Categories of risk are biophysical, psychosocial, sociodemographic, and environmental (Box 26-1). Risk factors are interrelated and cumulative in their effects.

Biophysical risks include factors that originate within the mother or fetus and affect the development or functioning of either one or both. Examples include genetic disorders, nutritional and general health status, and medical or obstetric-related illnesses. Box 26-2 lists common risk factors for several pregnancy-related problems.

Psychosocial risks consist of maternal behaviors and adverse lifestyles that have a negative effect on the health of the mother or fetus. These risks may include emotional distress and disturbed interpersonal relationships, as well as inadequate social support and unsafe cultural practices.

Sociodemographic risks arise from the mother and her family. These risks may place the mother and fetus at risk. Examples include lack of prenatal care, low income, marital status, and ethnicity (see Box 26-1). Environmental factors include hazards in the workplace and the woman's general environment and may include environmental chemicals (e.g., lead, mercury), anesthetic gases, and radiation (Chambers & Weiner, 2009; Cunningham, Leveno, Bloom, Hauth, Rouse, & Spong, 2010).

BOX 26-1 CATEGORIES OF HIGH RISK FACTORS

BIOPHYSICAL FACTORS

- *Genetic considerations.* Genetic factors may interfere with normal fetal or neonatal development, result in congenital anomalies, or create difficulties for the mother. These factors include defective genes, transmissible inherited disorders and chromosomal anomalies, multiple pregnancy, large fetal size, and ABO incompatibility.
- *Nutritional status.* Adequate nutrition, without which fetal growth and development cannot proceed normally, is one of the most important determinants of pregnancy outcome. Conditions that influence nutritional status include the following: young age; three pregnancies in the previous 2 years; tobacco, alcohol, or drug use; inadequate dietary intake because of chronic illness or food fads; inadequate or excessive weight gain; and hematocrit value less than 33%.
- *Medical and obstetric disorders.* Complications of current and past pregnancies, obstetric-related illnesses, and pregnancy losses put the woman at risk (see Box 26-2).

PSYCHOSOCIAL FACTORS

- *Smoking.* A strong, consistent, causal relation has been established between maternal smoking and reduced birth weight. Risks include low-birth-weight infants, higher neonatal mortality rates, increased rates of miscarriage, and increased incidence of premature rupture of membranes. These risks are aggravated by low socioeconomic status, poor nutritional status, and concurrent use of alcohol.
- *Caffeine.* Birth defects in humans have not been related to caffeine consumption. However, pregnant women who consume more than 200 mg of caffeine daily (equivalent to about 12 ounces of coffee per day) may be at increased risk for miscarriage or for giving birth to infants with intrauterine growth restriction (IUGR).
- *Alcohol.* Although the exact effects of alcohol in pregnancy have not been quantified and its mode of action is largely unexplained, it exerts adverse effects on the fetus, resulting in fetal alcohol syndrome, fetal alcohol effects, learning disabilities, and hyperactivity.
- *Drugs.* The developing fetus may be adversely affected by drugs through several mechanisms. They can be teratogenic, cause metabolic disturbances, produce chemical effects, or cause depression or alteration of central nervous system (CNS) function. This category includes medications prescribed by a health care provider or bought over the counter, as well as commonly abused drugs such as heroin, cocaine, and marijuana. (See Chapter 32 for more information about drug and alcohol abuse.)
- *Psychologic status.* Childbearing triggers profound and complex physiologic, psychologic, and social changes, with evidence to suggest a relationship between emotional distress and birth complications. This risk factor includes conditions such as specific intrapsychic disturbances and addictive lifestyles; a history of child or spouse abuse; inadequate support systems; family disruption or dissolution; maternal role changes or conflicts; noncompliance with cultural norms; unsafe cultural, ethnic, or religious practices; and situational crises.

SOCIODEMOGRAPHIC FACTORS

- *Low income.* Poverty underlies many other risk factors and leads to inadequate financial resources for food and prenatal care, poor general health, increased risk of medical complications of pregnancy, and greater prevalence of adverse environmental influences.
- *Lack of prenatal care.* Failure to diagnose and treat complications early is a major risk factor arising from financial barriers or lack of access to care; depersonalization of the system resulting in long waits, routine visits, variability in health care personnel, and unpleasant physical surroundings; lack of understanding of the need for early and continued care or cultural beliefs that do not support the need; and fear of the health care system and its providers.
- *Age.* Women at both ends of the childbearing age spectrum have an increased incidence of poor outcomes; however, age may not be a risk factor in all cases. Physiologic and psychologic risks should be evaluated.
  - *Adolescents.* More complications are seen in young mothers (younger than 15 years), who have a 60% higher mortality rate than those older than 20 years and in pregnancies occurring less than 6 years after menarche. Complications include anemia, preeclampsia, prolonged labor, and contracted pelvis and cephalopelvic disproportion. Long-term social implications of early motherhood are lower educational status, lower income, increased dependence on government support programs, higher divorce rates, and higher parity.
  - *Mature mothers.* The risks to older mothers are not from age alone but from other considerations such as number and spacing of previous pregnancies, genetic disposition of the parents, and medical history, lifestyle, nutrition, and prenatal care. The increased likelihood of chronic diseases and complications that arise from more invasive medical management of a pregnancy and labor combined with demographic characteristics put an older woman at risk. Conditions more likely to be experienced by mature women include chronic hypertension and preeclampsia, diabetes, extended labor, cesarean birth, placenta previa, abruptio placentae, and death. Her fetus is at greater risk for low birth weight and macrosomia, chromosomal abnormalities, congenital malformations, and neonatal death.
- *Parity.* The number of previous pregnancies is a risk factor associated with age and includes all first pregnancies, especially a first pregnancy at either end of the childbearing age continuum. The incidence of preeclampsia and dystocia is increased with a first birth.
- *Marital status.* The increased mortality and morbidity rates for unmarried women, including an increased risk for preeclampsia, are often related to inadequate prenatal care and a young childbearing age.
- *Residence.* The availability and quality of prenatal care vary widely with geographic residence. Women in metropolitan areas have more prenatal visits than those in rural areas who have fewer opportunities for specialized care and consequently a higher incidence of maternal mortality. Health care in the inner city, where residents are usually poorer and begin childbearing earlier and continue longer, may be of lower quality than in a more affluent neighborhood.
- *Ethnicity.* Although ethnicity by itself is not a major risk, race is an indicator of other sociodemographic risk factors. Non-Caucasian women are more than three times as likely as Caucasian women to die of pregnancy-related causes. African-American babies have the highest rates of prematurity and low birth weight, with the infant mortality rate among African-Americans being more than double that among Caucasians.

ENVIRONMENTAL FACTORS

- Various environmental substances can affect fertility and fetal development, the chance of a live birth, and the child's subsequent mental and physical development. Environmental influences include infections, radiation, chemicals such as mercury and lead, therapeutic drugs, illicit drugs, industrial pollutants, cigarette smoke, stress, and diet. Paternal exposure to mutagenic agents in the workplace has been associated with an increased risk of miscarriage.

BOX 26-2 SPECIFIC PREGNANCY PROBLEMS AND RELATED RISK FACTORS

POLYHYDRAMNIOS
- Diabetes mellitus
- Fetal congenital anomalies (e.g., gastrointestinal obstruction, twin-twin transfusion syndrome)

INTRAUTERINE GROWTH RESTRICTION

Maternal causes
- Hypertensive disorders
- Diabetes
- Chronic renal disease
- Collagen vascular disease
- Thrombophilia
- Cyanotic heart disease
- Poor weight gain
- Smoking, alcohol use, illicit drug use
- Living at a high altitude
- Multiple gestation

Fetoplacental causes
- Chromosomal abnormalities
- Congenital malformations
- Intrauterine infection
- Genetic syndromes (e.g., trisomy 13 and trisomy 18)
- Abnormal placental development

OLIGOHYDRAMNIOS
- Renal agenesis (Potter syndrome)
- Premature rupture of membranes
- Prolonged pregnancy
- Uteroplacental insufficiency
- Maternal hypertensive disorders

CHROMOSOMAL ABNORMALITIES
- Maternal age 35 years or older
- Balanced translocation (maternal and paternal)

Sources: Baschat, A., Galan, H., Ross, M., & Gabbe, S. (2007). Intrauterine growth restriction. In S. Gabbe, J. Niebyl, & J. Simpson (Eds.), *Obstetrics: Normal and problem pregnancies* (5th ed.). Philadelphia: Churchill Livingstone; Gilbert, W. (2007). Amniotic fluid disorders. In S. Gabbe, J. Niebyl, & J. Simpson (Eds.), *Obstetrics: Normal and problem pregnancies* (5th ed.). Philadelphia: Churchill Livingstone; Resnik, R., & Creasy, R. (2009). Intrauterine growth restriction. In R. Creasy, R. Resnik, J. Iams, C. Lockwood, & T. Moore (Eds.), *Creasy and Resnik's maternal-fetal medicine: Principles and practice* (6th ed.). Philadelphia: Saunders; Simpson, J., & Otano, L. (2007). Prenatal genetic diagnosis. In S. Gabbe, J. Niebyl, & J. Simpson (Eds.), *Obstetrics: Normal and problem pregnancies* (5th ed.). Philadelphia: Churchill Livingstone.

PSYCHOLOGIC CONSIDERATIONS RELATED TO HIGH RISK PREGNANCY

Once a pregnancy has been identified as high risk, the pregnant woman and her fetus will be monitored carefully throughout the remainder of the pregnancy. All women who undergo antepartal assessments are at risk for real and potential problems and may feel anxious. In most instances the tests are ordered because of suspected fetal compromise, deterioration of a maternal condition, or both. In the third trimester, pregnant women are most concerned about protecting themselves and their fetuses and consider themselves most vulnerable to outside influences. The label of high risk often increases this sense of vulnerability.

When a woman is diagnosed with a high risk pregnancy, she and her family will likely experience stress related to the diagnosis. The woman may exhibit various psychologic responses including anxiety, low self-esteem, guilt, frustration, and inability to function. A high risk pregnancy can also affect parental attachment, accomplishment of the tasks of pregnancy, and family adaptation to the pregnancy. If the woman is fearful for her own well-being, she may continue to feel ambivalence about the pregnancy or may not accept the reality of the pregnancy. She may not be able to complete preparations for the baby or go to childbirth classes if she is placed on restricted activity at home or is hospitalized. The family may become frustrated because they cannot engage in activities that prepare them for parenthood. The nurse can help the woman and her family regain control and balance in their lives by providing support and encouragement, information about the pregnancy problem and its management, and opportunities to make as many choices as possible about the woman's care.

BOX 26-3 COMMON INDICATIONS FOR ANTEPARTUM TESTING

OBSTETRIC INDICATIONS
- Postterm pregnancy
- Previous unexplained stillbirth
- Suspected fetal growth restriction
- Decreased fetal movement
- Preeclampsia
- Oligohydramnios

MEDICAL INDICATIONS
- Diabetes
- Chronic hypertension
- Cyanotic cardiac disease
- Renal disease
- Thyroid disease
- Pulmonary disease (severe asthma)
- Collagen vascular disease
- Hemoglobinopathy
- Substance abuse

Source: Tucker, S., Miller, L., & Miller, D. (2009). *Mosby's pocket guide to fetal monitoring: A multidisciplinary approach* (6th ed.). St. Louis: Mosby.

ANTEPARTUM TESTING

The major expected outcome of all antepartum testing is the detection of potential fetal compromise. Ideally the technique used identifies fetal compromise before intrauterine asphyxia occurs so that the health care provider can take measures to prevent or minimize adverse perinatal outcomes. Antepartum testing is used primarily in pregnant women at risk for disrupted fetal oxygenation. In most cases, monitoring begins by 32 to 34 weeks of gestation and continues regularly until birth. Assessment tests should be selected based on their effectiveness, and the results must be interpreted in light of the complete clinical picture. Box 26-3 lists common obstetric and medical indications for antepartum testing (Tucker, Miller, & Miller, 2009).

The remainder of this chapter describes maternal and fetal assessment tests that are often used to monitor high risk pregnancies.

BIOPHYSICAL ASSESSMENT

Daily Fetal Movement Count

Assessment of fetal activity by the mother is a simple yet valuable method for monitoring the condition of the fetus. The **daily fetal movement count (DMFC)** (also called *kick count*) can be assessed at home and is noninvasive, inexpensive, simple to understand, and usually does not interfere with a daily routine. The DFMC is frequently used to monitor the fetus in pregnancies complicated by conditions that may affect fetal oxygenation (see Box 26-2). The presence of movements is generally a reassuring sign of fetal health.

Several different protocols are used for counting. One recommendation is to count once a day for 60 minutes. Another common recommendation is that mothers count fetal activity two or three times daily for 60 minutes each time. Except for establishing a very low number of daily fetal movements or a trend toward decreased motion, the clinical value of the absolute number of fetal movements has not been established, other than in the situation in which fetal movements cease entirely for 12 hours (the so-called *fetal alarm signal*). A count of fewer than three fetal movements within 1 hour warrants further evaluation by a nonstress test (NST) or a contraction stress test (CST) (oxytocin challenge test [OCT]), biophysical profile, or a combination of these (see later discussion). Women should be taught the significance of the presence or absence of fetal movements (or both), the procedure for counting that is to be used, how to record findings on a daily fetal movement record, and when to notify the health care provider.

> **! NURSING ALERT**
>
> In assessing fetal movements it is important to remember that they are usually not present during the fetal sleep cycle and that they may be temporarily reduced if the woman is taking depressant medications, drinking alcohol, or smoking a cigarette. They do not decrease as the woman nears term. Obesity decreases the ability of the mother to perceive fetal movement.

Ultrasonography

Sound is a form of wave energy that causes small particles in a medium to oscillate. The frequency of sound, which refers to the number of peaks or waves that move over a given point per unit of time, is expressed in hertz (Hz). Sound with a frequency of 1 cycle, or one peak per second, has a frequency of 1 Hz. When directional beams of sound strike an object, an echo is returned. The time delay between the emission of the sound and the return of the echo and the direction of the echo are noted. From these data the distance and location of an object can be calculated. Ultrasound is sound frequency higher than that detectable by humans (greater than 20,000 Hz). Ultrasound images are a reflection of the strength of the sending beam, the strength of the returning echo, and the density of the medium (e.g., muscle [uterus], bone, tissue [placenta], fluid, or blood) through which the beam is sent and returned.

Diagnostic ultrasonography is an important, safe technique in antepartum fetal surveillance. It provides critical information to health care providers regarding fetal activity and gestational age, normal versus abnormal fetal growth curves, visual assistance with which invasive tests may be performed more safely, fetal and placental anatomy, and fetal well-being (Richards, 2007). Ultrasound examination can be performed abdominally or transvaginally during pregnancy. Both methods produce a three-dimensional view from which a pictorial image is obtained. Newer machines produce a four-dimensional view (Fig. 26-1, *A* and *B*). Abdominal ultrasonography is more useful after the first trimester, when the pregnant uterus becomes an abdominal organ. During the procedure the woman should have a full bladder to displace the uterus upward to provide a better image of the fetus. Transmission gel or paste is applied to the woman's abdomen before a transducer is moved over the skin to enhance transmission and reception of the sound waves. She is positioned with small pillows under her head and knees. The display panel is positioned so that she or her partner (or both) can observe the images on the screen if they desire.

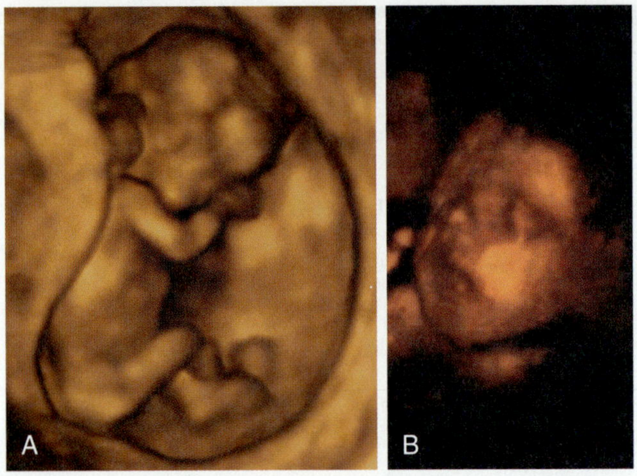

FIG. 26-1 Fetus seen on three-dimensional ultrasound. **A,** Full body view of fetus at 11 weeks and 6 days of gestation. **B,** Close-up view of fetal face later in pregnancy. (**A,** Courtesy Shannon Perry, Phoenix, AZ; **B,** courtesy Margaret Spann, New Johnsonville, TN.)

Transvaginal ultrasonography, in which the probe is inserted into the vagina, allows pelvic anatomic features to be evaluated in greater detail and intrauterine pregnancy to be diagnosed earlier. A transvaginal ultrasound examination is well tolerated by most pregnant women because it removes the need for a full bladder. It is especially useful in obese women whose thick abdominal layers cannot be penetrated adequately with an abdominal approach. A transvaginal ultrasound may be performed with the woman in a lithotomy position or with her pelvis elevated by towels, cushions, or a folded pillow. This pelvic tilt is optimal to image the pelvic structures. A protective cover such as a condom, the finger of a clean surgical glove, or a special probe cover provided by the manufacturer is used to cover the transducer probe. The probe is lubricated with a water-soluble gel and placed in the vagina either by the examiner or by the woman herself. During the examination the position of the probe or the tilt of the examining table may be changed so that the complete pelvis is in view. The procedure is not physically painful, although the woman will feel pressure as the probe is moved. Transvaginal ultrasonography is optimally used in the first trimester to detect ectopic pregnancies, monitor the developing embryo, help identify abnormalities, and help establish gestational age. In some instances it may be used as an adjunct

TABLE 26-1 MAJOR USES OF ULTRASONOGRAPHY DURING PREGNANCY

FIRST TRIMESTER	SECOND TRIMESTER	THIRD TRIMESTER
Confirm pregnancy Confirm viability Determine gestational age Rule out ectopic pregnancy Detect multiple gestation Determine the cause of vaginal bleeding Use for visualization during chorionic villus sampling Detect maternal abnormalities such as bicornuate uterus, ovarian cysts, fibroids	Establish or confirm dates Confirm viability Detect polyhydramnios, oligohydramnios Detect congenital anomalies Detect intrauterine growth restriction (IUGR) Assess placental placement Use for visualization during amniocentesis	Confirm gestational age Confirm viability Detect macrosomia Detect congenital anomalies Detect IUGR Determine fetal position Detect placenta previa or abruptio placentae Use for visualization during amniocentesis, external version Biophysical profile Amniotic fluid volume assessment Doppler flow studies Detect placental maturity

to abdominal scanning to evaluate preterm labor in second- and third-trimester pregnancies.

Levels of Ultrasonography

The American College of Obstetricians and Gynecologists (ACOG) (2004) described three levels of ultrasonography. The *standard* examination is used most frequently and can be performed by ultrasonographers or other heath care professionals, including nurses, who have had special training. Indications for standard ultrasonography are described in detail in the next section. Its primary use is to detect fetal viability, determine the presentation of the fetus, assess gestational age, locate the placenta, examine the fetal anatomic structures for malformations, and determine amniotic fluid volume (AFV). *Limited* examinations are performed for specific indications such as identifying fetal presentation during labor or evaluating fetal heart rate (FHR) activity when it is not detected by other methods (ACOG). *Specialized* or targeted examinations are performed if a woman is suspected of carrying an anatomically or a physiologically abnormal fetus. Indications for this comprehensive examination include abnormal findings on clinical examination, especially with polyhydramnios or oligohydramnios, elevated alpha-fetoprotein (AFP) levels, and a history of offspring with anomalies that can be detected by ultrasound examination. Specialized ultrasonography is performed by highly trained and experienced personnel (ACOG).

Indications For Use

Major indications for obstetric sonography are listed by trimester in Table 26-1. During the first trimester ultrasound examination is performed to obtain information regarding the number, size, and location of gestational sacs; the presence or absence of fetal cardiac and body movements; the presence or absence of uterine abnormalities (e.g., bicornuate uterus or fibroids) or adnexal masses (e.g., ovarian cysts or an ectopic pregnancy); and pregnancy dating (by measuring the crown-rump length).

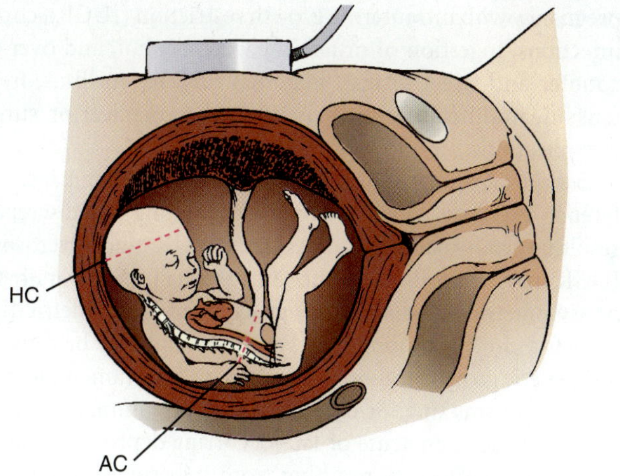

FIG. 26-2 Appropriate planes of sections *(dotted lines)* for head circumference *(HC)* and abdominal circumference *(AC)*.

During the second and third trimesters information regarding the following conditions is sought: fetal viability, number, position, gestational age, growth pattern, and anomalies; AFV; placental location and maturity; presence of uterine fibroids or anomalies; presence of adnexal masses; and cervical length.

Ultrasonography provides earlier diagnoses, allowing therapy to be instituted sooner in the pregnancy, thereby decreasing the severity and duration of morbidity, both physical and emotional, for the family. For instance, early diagnosis of a fetal anomaly gives the family choices such as intrauterine surgery or other therapy for the fetus, termination of the pregnancy, or preparation for the care of an infant with a disorder.

Fetal Heart Activity. Fetal heart activity can be demonstrated as early as 6 to 7 weeks of gestation by real-time echo scanners and at 10 to 12 weeks by Doppler mode. By 9 to 10 weeks, gestational trophoblastic disease can be diagnosed. Fetal death can be confirmed by lack of heart motion, the presence of fetal scalp edema, and maceration and overlap of the cranial bones.

Gestational Age. Gestational dating by ultrasonography is indicated for conditions such as uncertain dates for the last normal menstrual period, recent discontinuation of oral contraceptives, a bleeding episode during the first trimester, uterine size that does not agree with dates, and other high risk conditions. In fact, growing evidence suggests that pregnancies should be dated by an ultrasound performed before 22 weeks of gestation rather than by menstrual dates because the ultrasound dating is more accurate than even "sure" menstrual dates (Richards, 2007). The methods of fetal age estimation used include determination of gestational sac dimensions (at approximately 8 weeks), measurement of crown-rump length (between 7 and 12 weeks), measurement of the biparietal diameter (BPD) (after 12 weeks), and measurement of femur length (after 12 weeks) (Fig. 26-2). An ultrasound examination performed for pregnancy dating between 14 and 22 weeks of gestation is comparable to one performed during the first trimester in terms of accuracy. After that time, however, ultrasound dating is less reliable because of variability in fetal size (Richards).

Fetal Growth. Fetal growth is determined by both intrinsic growth potential and environmental factors. Conditions that require ultrasound assessment of fetal growth include poor maternal weight gain or pattern of weight gain, previous pregnancy with intrauterine growth restriction (IUGR), chronic infections, ingestion of drugs (tobacco, alcohol, and over-the-counter and street drugs), maternal diabetes mellitus, hypertension, multifetal pregnancy, and other medical or surgical complications.

Serial evaluations of BPD, limb length, and abdominal circumference (AC) can allow differentiation among size discrepancy resulting from inaccurate dates, true IUGR, and macrosomia. IUGR may be symmetric (the fetus is small in all parameters) or asymmetric (head and body growth vary). Symmetric IUGR reflects a chronic or long-standing insult and may be caused by low genetic growth potential, intrauterine infection, undernutrition, heavy smoking, or chromosomal aberration. Asymmetric growth suggests an acute or late-occurring deprivation, such as placental insufficiency resulting from hypertension, renal disease, or cardiovascular disease. Reduced fetal growth is still one of the most frequent conditions associated with stillbirth. Macrosomic infants (those weighing 4000 g or more) are at increased risk for traumatic injury and asphyxia during birth. Macrosomia may also be characterized as symmetric or asymmetric.

Fetal Anatomy. Anatomic structures that can be identified by ultrasonography (depending on the gestational age) include the following: head (including ventricles and blood vessels), neck, spine, heart, stomach, small bowel, liver, kidneys, bladder, and limbs. Ultrasonography permits the confirmation of normal anatomy, as well as the detection of major fetal malformations. The presence of an anomaly may influence the location of birth (e.g., a subspecialty center versus a basic care center) and the method of birth (vaginal versus cesarean) to optimize neonatal outcomes. For example, plans are often made for a fetus with a condition that will require immediate surgery to be born in or near a hospital able to provide that care, rather than in a small community hospital that is totally unequipped to meet the newborn's needs.

The number of fetuses and their presentations also may be assessed by ultrasonography, allowing plans for therapy and mode of birth to be made in advance.

Fetal Genetic Disorders and Physical Anomalies. A prenatal screening technique called *nuchal translucency* (NT) screening uses ultrasound measurement of fluid in the nape of the fetal neck between 10 and 14 weeks of gestation to identify possible fetal abnormalities (Fig. 26-3). A fluid collection that is greater than 3 mm is considered abnormal. When combined with low maternal serum marker levels, elevated NT indicates a possible increased risk of certain chromosomal abnormalities in the fetus, including trisomies 13, 18, and 21. An elevated NT alone indicates an increased risk of fetal cardiac disease. If the NT is abnormal, diagnostic genetic testing is recommended (ACOG, 2007; Gilbert, 2011).

Placental Position and Function. The pattern of uterine and placental growth and the fullness of the maternal bladder influence the apparent location of the placenta by ultrasonography. During the first trimester, differentiation between the endometrium and small placenta is difficult. By 14 to 16 weeks the placenta is clearly defined; but if it is seen to be low lying, its relationship to the internal cervical os can sometimes be dramatically altered by varying the fullness of the maternal bladder. In approximately 4% to 6% of all pregnancies in which ultrasound scanning is performed during the second trimester, the placenta seems to be overlying the os. However, more than 90% of cases of placenta previa diagnosed during the second trimester will have resolved by term, primarily because of the elongation of the lower uterine segment as pregnancy advances. Therefore, if placenta previa is diagnosed before 24 weeks of gestation, an ultrasound examination should be repeated between 28 and 32 weeks of gestation to confirm the diagnosis (Francois & Foley, 2007).

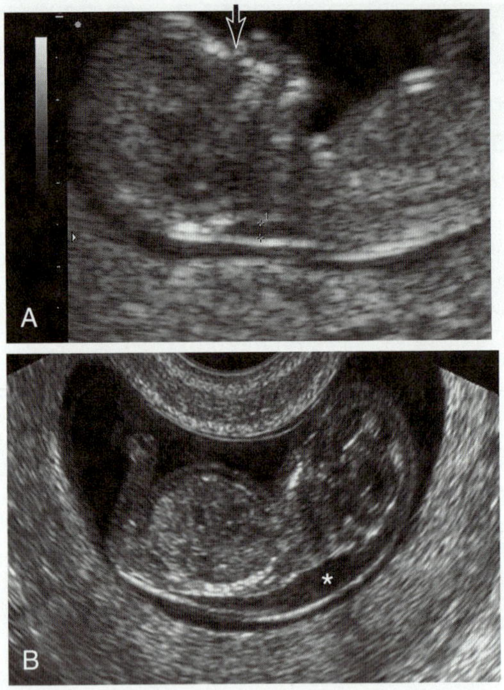

FIG. 26-3 Fetal nuchal translucency. **A,** Nuchal lucency (calipers) and nasal bone *(arrow)* in 12-week fetus. **B,** Increased nuchal translucency. Transvaginal ultrasound performed at 12 weeks demonstrates a sonolucent area *(asterisk)* over the posterior neck and upper thorax. (From Martin, R., Fanaroff, A., & Walsh, M. [2006]. *Fanaroff and Martin's neonatal-perinatal medicine: Diseases of the fetus and infant* [8th ed.]. Philadelphia: Mosby.)

Another use for ultrasonography is grading of placental aging. Calcium and fibrin deposits in an aging placenta result in intervillous hemorrhagic infarcts. Also as blood vessels in the placenta age and thicken, oxygen transport is affected. Whether these placental changes adversely affect fetal outcomes in post-term pregnancies is unknown, however, given that most fetuses continue to grow (Gilbert, 2011).

Adjunct to Other Invasive Tests. The safety of amniocentesis is increased when the positions of the fetus, placenta, and pockets of amniotic fluid can be identified accurately. Ultrasound scanning has reduced risks previously associated with amniocentesis, such as fetomaternal hemorrhage from a pierced placenta. Percutaneous umbilical blood sampling and chorionic villus sampling also are guided by ultrasonography to identify the cord and chorion frondosum accurately.

Fetal Well-being. Physiologic parameters of the fetus that can be assessed with ultrasound scanning include AFV, vascular waveforms from the fetal circulation, heart motion, fetal breathing movements (FBMs), fetal urine production, and fetal limb and head movements. Assessment of these parameters, alone or in combination, yields a fairly reliable picture of fetal well-being. The significance of these findings is discussed in the following sections.

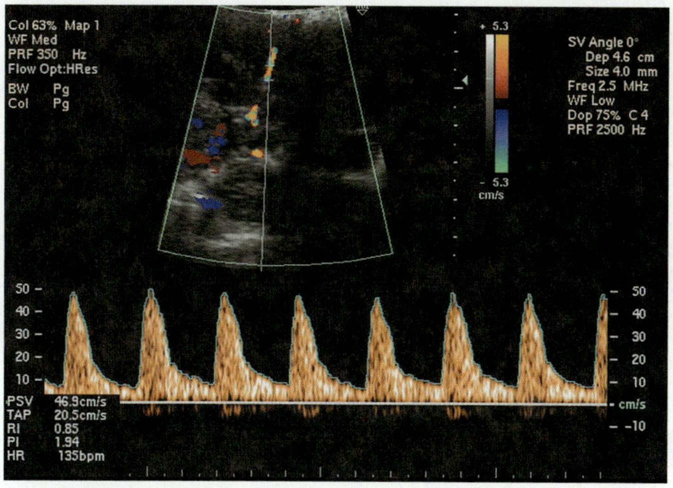

FIG. 26-4 Umbilical artery velocity waveform. (From Callen, P. [2000]: *Ultrasonography in obstetrics and gynecology* [4th ed.]. Philadelphia: Saunders.)

Doppler Blood Flow Analysis. One of the major advances in perinatal medicine is the ability to study blood flow noninvasively in the fetus and placenta with ultrasound. **Doppler blood flow analysis** is a helpful adjunct in the management of pregnancies at risk because of hypertension, IUGR, diabetes mellitus, multiple fetuses, and preterm labor.

When a sound wave is reflected from a moving target, a change occurs in the frequency of the reflected wave relative to the transmitted wave, called the *Doppler effect*. An ultrasound beam scattered by a group of red blood cells (RBCs) is an example of this effect. The velocity of the RBCs can be determined by measuring the change in the frequency of the sound wave reflected off the cells (Fig. 26-4).

The shifted frequencies can be displayed as a plot of velocity versus time, and the shape of these waveforms can be analyzed to give information about blood flow and resistance in a given circulation. Velocity waveforms from umbilical and uterine arteries, reported as systolic/diastolic (S/D) ratios, can be first detected at 15 weeks of pregnancy. Because of the progressive decline in resistance in both the umbilical and uterine arteries, this ratio normally decreases as pregnancy advances. IUGR is seen more often in fetuses whose ratios remain elevated for their gestational age (Druzin, Smith, Gabbe, & Reed, 2007). Severely restricted uterine artery blood flow is indicated by absent or reversed flow during diastole (Tucker et al., 2009). In postterm pregnancies evaluated by Doppler umbilical flow studies an elevated S/D ratio indicates a poorly perfused placenta. Abnormal results also are seen with certain chromosome abnormalities (trisomy 13 and 18) in the fetus and with lupus erythematosus in the mother. Exposure to nicotine from maternal smoking also has been reported to increase the S/D ratio (see Fig. 26-4).

Amniotic Fluid Volume. Abnormalities in AFV are frequently associated with fetal disorders. Subjective determinants of oligohydramnios (decreased fluid) include the absence of fluid pockets in the uterine cavity and the impression of crowding of small fetal parts. An objective criterion of decreased AFV is met if the largest pocket of fluid measured in two perpendicular planes is less than 2 cm (Harman, 2009). Increased amniotic fluid is called *polyhydramnios* or sometimes just *hydramnios*. Subjective criteria for polyhydramnios include multiple large pockets of fluid, the impression of a floating fetus, and free movement of fetal limbs. Hydramnios is usually defined as pockets of amniotic fluid measuring more than 8 cm (Gilbert, 2007).

The total AFV can be evaluated by a method in which the vertical depths (in centimeters) of the largest pocket of amniotic fluid in all four quadrants surrounding the maternal umbilicus are totaled, providing an **amniotic fluid index (AFI)**. A normal AFI is 10 cm or greater, with the upper range of normal around 25 cm. AFI values between 5 and 10 cm are considered to be low normal, whereas an AFI of less than 5 cm indicates oligohydramnios. With polyhydramnios the AFI would be above 25 cm (Tucker et al., 2009). Oligohydramnios is associated with congenital anomalies (e.g., renal agenesis), growth restriction, and fetal distress during labor. Polyhydramnios is associated with neural tube defects (NTDs), obstruction of the fetal gastrointestinal tract, multiple fetuses, and fetal hydrops.

Biophysical Profile. Real-time ultrasound permits detailed assessment of the physical and physiologic characteristics of the developing fetus and cataloging of normal and abnormal biophysical responses to stimuli. The **biophysical profile (BPP)** is a noninvasive dynamic assessment of a fetus that is based on acute and chronic markers of fetal disease. The BPP includes AFV, FBMs, fetal movements, and fetal tone determined by ultrasound and FHR reactivity determined by means of NST. The BPP may therefore be considered a physical examination of the fetus, including determination of vital signs. FHR reactivity, FBMs, fetal movement, and fetal tone reflect current central nervous system (CNS) status, whereas the AFV demonstrates

TABLE 26-2 BIOPHYSICAL PROFILE SCORING

BIOPHYSICAL VARIABLE	NORMAL (SCORE = 2)	ABNORMAL (SCORE = 0)
Fetal breathing movements	At least one episode of >30 seconds' duration in 30 minutes' observation	Absent or no episode of ≥30 seconds' duration in 30 minutes
Gross body movement	At least three discrete body/limb movements in 30 minutes (episodes of active continuous movement considered a single movement)	Up to two episodes of body/limb movements in 30 minutes
Fetal tone	At least one episode of active extension with return to flexion of fetal limb(s) or trunk, opening and closing of hand considered normal tone	Either slow extension with return to partial flexion or movement of limb in full extension or absent fetal movement
Reactive fetal heart rate	At least two episodes of acceleration of ≥15 beats/min and 15 seconds' duration associated with fetal movement in 30 minutes	Fewer than two accelerations or acceleration <15 beats/min in 30 minutes
Qualitative amniotic fluid volume	At least one pocket of amniotic fluid measuring 2 cm in two perpendicular planes	Either no amniotic fluid pockets or a pocket <2 cm in two perpendicular planes

Source: Druzin, M., Smith, J., Gabbe, S., & Reed, K. (2007). Antepartum fetal evaluation. In S. Gabbe, J. Niebyl, & J. Simpson (Eds.), *Obstetrics: Normal and problem pregnancies* (5th ed.). Philadelphia: Churchill Livingstone.

TABLE 26-3 **BIOPHYSICAL PROFILE MANAGEMENT**

SCORE	INTERPRETATION	MANAGEMENT
10	Normal infant; low risk of chronic asphyxia	Repeat testing at weekly intervals; repeat twice weekly in women with diabetes and women at 41 weeks of gestation
8	Normal infant; low risk of chronic asphyxia	Repeat testing at weekly intervals; repeat testing twice weekly in women with diabetes and women at 41 weeks of gestation; oligohydramnios is an indication for delivery
6	Suspect chronic asphyxia	If 36 weeks of gestation and conditions are favorable, deliver; if at >36 weeks and L/S <2, repeat test in 4-6 hours; deliver if oligohydramnios is present
4	Suspect chronic asphyxia	If 36 weeks of gestation, deliver; if <32 weeks of gestation, repeat test
0-2	Strongly suspect chronic asphyxia	Extend testing time to 120 minutes; if persistent score ≤4, deliver, regardless of gestational age

L/S, Lecithin/sphingomyelin.
Source: Druzin, M., Smith, J., Gabbe, S., & Reed, K. (2007). Antepartum fetal evaluation. In S. Gabbe, J. Niebyl, & J. Simpson (Eds.), *Obstetrics: Normal and problem pregnancies* (5th ed.). Philadelphia: Churchill Livingstone.

EVIDENCE-BASED PRACTICE

Pat Gingrich

"How's My Baby Doing?"

ASK THE QUESTION

What method of antepartal assessment fetal well-being is the gold standard?

SEARCH FOR EVIDENCE

Search Strategies

Professional organization guidelines, meta-analyses, systematic reviews, randomized controlled trials, nonrandomized prospective studies and retrospective reviews since 2008.

Databases Searched

CINAHL, Cochrane, Medline, PUBMED, and the Association of Women's Health, Obstetric and Neonatal Nurses (AWHONN).

CRITICALLY ANALYZE THE DATA

Fetal assessment tests should give useful data that allow the practitioner to make clinical decisions leading to positive outcomes. Tests that fail to detect a problem (low sensitivity) or that falsely indicate a problem exists when there is none (low specificity) may result in incorrect treatment that could harm mother and baby.

Ultrasound has proven its worth throughout pregnancy and labor. In early pregnancy, ultrasound offers more accurate gestational dating than in later pregnancy, according to a Cochrane Database Systematic Review (Whitworth, Bricker, Neilson, & Dowswell, 2010). More accurate gestational dating may help to avoid postmaturity. In addition, early ultrasound detects multiple gestation, which helps to place the mother into high-risk prenatal care earlier.

Ultrasound testing for amniotic fluid level is a screening test for oligohydramnios (low amniotic fluid), which is associated with fetal anomalies, post-term pregnancy, preeclampsia and intrauterine growth restriction. Two methods are used: the amniotic fluid index (AFI), which adds up the deepest pockets in the 4 quadrants of the pregnant abdomen, or the single deepest vertical pocket (SDVP), which measures the largest area with no fetal parts nor cord in it. A Cochrane Database Systematic Review of five trials involving 3226 women revealed that the two methods were similar for the prevention of poor fetal outcomes such as admission to neonatal intensive care, cord blood pH less than 7.1 (acidosis), APGAR score less than 7 at 5 minutes, meconium in the amniotic fluid, and abnormal (nonreassuring) fetal heart rate. However, the use of AFI increased the diagnosis of oligohydramnios, which led to more inductions and cesarean births for fetal distress. The authors therefore recommended the SDVP method, to avoid the risk of overtreatment (Nabhan & Abdelmoula, 2008).

In an effort to detect poor oxygenation and fetal distress, a test called a biophysical profile (BPP) uses ultrasound to assess for fetal movement, tone, breathing and amniotic fluid level, plus a 20-minute electronic fetal monitor (EFM) strip. A variation, called the modified BPP, screens with EFM and amniotic fluid level, and follows up with the movement assessments only if there is a problem. In five trials involving 2974 women with high-risk pregnancies authors of a systematic review compared BPP to EFM alone. Combined data showed no differences between the groups in fetal deaths or low APGAR scores. However, BPP was associated with an increase in inductions and cesarean births. Once again, the screening test might be leading to overdiagnosis and subsequent risks of overly aggressive treatment. The authors did not find sufficient evidence yet to support the use of BPP (Lalor, Fawole, Alfirevic, & Devane, 2008.)

IMPLICATIONS FOR PRACTICE

The nurse should be familiar with the evidence for these fetal assessment tests, in order to offer accurate information and reassurance to the worried woman and family. The nurse may be called upon to accompany the woman or assist in the procedure. Knowing the limitations of testing can guide the nurse to advocate for the client. In addition, the nurse should remain aware that tests may have upsetting results, and can provide anticipatory guidance, and realistic but positive support for the family.

References

Lalor, J., Fawole, B., Alfirevic, Z., & Devane, D. (2008). Biophysical profile for fetal assessment in high risk pregnancies. *The Cochrane Database of Systematic Reviews, 2008*, 1, CD000038.

Nabhan, A., & Abdelmoula, Y. (2008). Amniotic fluid index versus single deepest vertical pocket as a screening test for preventing adverse pregnancy outcome. *The Cochrane Database of Systematic Reviews, 2008*, 3, CD006593.

Whitworth, M., Bricker, L., Neilson, J., & Dowswell, T. (2010). Ultrasound for fetal assessment in early pregnancy. *The Cochrane Database of Systematic Reviews, 2010*, 4, CD007058.

the adequacy of placental function over a longer period (Tucker et al., 2009). BPP scoring and management are detailed in Tables 26-2 and 26-3.

The BPP is used very frequently for antepartum fetal testing because it is a reliable predictor of fetal well-being. A BPP of 8 to 10 with a normal AFV is considered normal. Advantages of the test include excellent sensitivity and a low false-negative rate (Tucker et al., 2009). One limitation of the test is that if the fetus is in a quiet sleep state, the BPP can require a long period of observation. Also unless the ultrasound examination is videotaped, it cannot be reviewed (Druzin et al., 2007).

Nursing Role

Although a growing number of nurses perform ultrasound scans and BPPs in certain centers, the main role of nurses is in counseling and educating women about the procedure. Ultrasound is

CLINICAL REASONING

Fetal Assessment Using the Biophysical Profile

LaTonya is a 30-year-old G5 T2 P1 A1 L3 who is now 35 weeks of gestation. Because she has chronic hypertension, her physician has scheduled her to have a biophysical profile (BPP) twice each week. LaTonya's BPP score today is 6. No fetal breathing movements and no pockets of amniotic fluid were seen on ultrasound. In addition, she had a nonreactive nonstress test. After learning the results of today's BPP, LaTonya's physician wants to admit her immediately to the labor and birth unit for prolonged monitoring followed by a repeat BPP in 6 hours. LaTonya begins to cry and says, "I can't stay. I don't have anyone to take care of my children. Why can't I just come back in a couple of days and have the test redone?"

1. Is there sufficient evidence to support performing fetal assessment tests, such as the BPP late in pregnancy?
2. What assumptions can be made about the following?
   a. Physiologic principles on which the BPP is based
   b. Advantages of the BPP
   c. Disadvantages of the BPP
   d. The desired result of the BPP
3. What implications and priorities for nursing care can be drawn at this time?
4. Does the evidence objectively support your conclusion?
5. Are there alternative perspectives to your conclusion?

widely used and in fact is considered a standard part of current prenatal care. Unlike many diagnostic tests, most women look forward to and enjoy their prenatal ultrasound. In the 30 years that diagnostic ultrasonography has been used, no evidence of any harmful effects on humans has emerged (Richards, 2007).

Magnetic Resonance Imaging

Magnetic resonance imaging (MRI) is a noninvasive radiologic technique used for obstetric and gynecologic diagnosis. Similar to computed tomography (CT), MRI provides excellent pictures of soft tissue. Unlike CT, ionizing radiation is not used. Therefore, vascular structures within the body can be visualized and evaluated without injecting an iodinated contrast medium, thus eliminating any known biologic risk. Similar to sonography, MRI is noninvasive and can provide images in multiple planes, but no interference occurs from skeletal, fatty, or gas-filled structures, and imaging of deep pelvic structures does not require a full bladder.

With MRI the examiner can evaluate fetal structure (CNS, thorax, abdomen, genitourinary tract, musculoskeletal system) and overall growth, the placenta (position, density, and presence of gestational trophoblastic disease), and the quantity of amniotic fluid. Maternal structures (uterus, cervix, adnexa, and pelvis), the biochemical status (pH, adenosine triphosphate content) of tissues and organs, and soft-tissue, metabolic, or functional anomalies can also be evaluated.

The woman is placed on a table in the supine position and moved into the bore of the main magnet, which is similar in appearance to a CT scanner. Depending on the reason for the study the procedure may take from 20 to 60 minutes, during which time the woman must be perfectly still except for short respites. Because of the long time needed to produce MRIs, the fetus will probably move, which will obscure anatomic details. The only way to ensure that this problem does not occur is to administer a sedative to the mother, but this approach should be reserved for selected cases in which visualization of fetal detail is critical.

MRI has little effect on the fetus. Concerns that the FHR or fetal movement would decrease have not been supported.

Video—Nursing Skills: Assisting During Amniocentesis

BIOCHEMICAL ASSESSMENT

Biochemical assessment involves biologic examination (e.g., as chromosomes in exfoliated cells) and chemical determinations (e.g., lecithin/sphingomyelin [L/S] ratio, surfactant/albumin [S/A] ratio [TDX FLM assay], and bilirubin level) (Table 26-4). Procedures used to obtain the needed specimens include amniocentesis, percutaneous umbilical blood sampling, chorionic villus sampling, and maternal sampling (Box 26-4).

Amniocentesis

Amniocentesis is performed to obtain amniotic fluid, which contains fetal cells. Under direct ultrasonographic visualization, a needle is inserted transabdominally into the uterus, amniotic fluid is withdrawn into a syringe, and the various assessments are performed (Fig. 26-5). Amniocentesis is possible after week 14 of pregnancy, when the uterus becomes an abdominal organ, and sufficient amniotic fluid is available for testing. Indications for the procedure include prenatal diagnosis of genetic disorders or congenital anomalies (NTDs in particular), assessment of pulmonary maturity, and diagnosis of fetal hemolytic disease.

Complications in the mother and fetus occur in less than 1% of the cases and include the following:

- *Maternal:* hemorrhage, fetomaternal hemorrhage with possible maternal Rh isoimmunization, infection, labor, placental abruption, inadvertent damage to the intestines or bladder, and anaphylactoid syndrome of pregnancy (amniotic fluid embolism)
- *Fetal:* death, hemorrhage, infection (amnionitis), direct injury from the needle, miscarriage or preterm labor, and leakage of amniotic fluid

Many of the complications have been minimized or eliminated by using ultrasonography to direct the procedure.

NURSING ALERT

Because of the possibility of fetomaternal hemorrhage, administering Rh_oD immune globulin to the woman who is Rh negative is standard practice after an amniocentesis.

Indications for Use

Genetic Concerns. Historically, prenatal assessment of genetic disorders focused on women older than 35 years (Box 26-5), with a previous child with a chromosomal abnormality, or with a family history of chromosomal anomalies. Inherited errors of metabolism (such as Tay-Sachs disease), hemophilia, and thalassemia and other disorders for which marker genes are known also can be detected by prenatal screening. Fetal cells can be cultured for karyotyping of chromosomes (see Chapter 3). Karyotyping also permits determination of fetal sex, which is important if an X-linked disorder (occurring almost always in a male fetus) is suspected.

TABLE 26-4 SUMMARY OF BIOCHEMICAL MONITORING TECHNIQUES

TEST	POSSIBLE FINDINGS	CLINICAL SIGNIFICANCE
Maternal Blood		
Coombs test	Titer of 1:8 and increasing	Significant Rh incompatibility
AFP	See below	
Amniotic Fluid Analysis		
Lung profile:		Fetal lung maturity
L/S ratio	2:1	
Phosphatidylglycerol	Present	
S/A ratio (TDx FLM assay)	≥55 mg/g	
Creatinine	>2 mg/dl	Gestational age >36 weeks
Bilirubin (ΔOD, 450/nm)	<0.015	Gestational age >36 weeks, normal pregnancy
	High levels	Fetal hemolytic disease in Rh isoimmunized pregnancies
Lipid cells	>10%	Gestational age >35 weeks
AFP	High levels after 15 weeks gestation	Open neural tube or other defect
Osmolality	Declines after 20 weeks gestation	Advancing gestational age
Genetic disorders: Sex-linked, Chromosomal, Metabolic	Dependent on cultured cells for karyotype and enzymatic activity	Counseling possibly required

AFP, Alpha-fetoprotein; *L/S,* lecithin/sphingomyelin; S/A, surfactant/albumin; *TDx FLM assay,* name of specific test used to determine S/A ratio.

BOX 26-4 FETAL RIGHTS

Amniocentesis, percutaneous umbilical blood sampling (PUBS), and chorionic villus sampling (CVS) are prenatal tests used for diagnosing fetal defects in pregnancy. They are invasive and carry risks to the mother and fetus. A consideration of induced abortion is linked to the performance of these tests because no treatment for genetically affected fetuses has been developed; therefore, the issue of fetal rights is a key ethical concern in prenatal testing for fetal defects.

BOX 26-5 ELIMINATION OF MATERNAL AGE AS AN INDICATION FOR INVASIVE PRENATAL DIAGNOSIS

Maternal age of 35 years and older has been a standard indication for invasive prenatal testing since 1979. However, because most genetically abnormal children are born to parents of varying ages who have no history of abnormality, genetic screening is now recommended for all women, regardless of age (Gilbert, 2011). In January 2007, the American College of Obstetricians and Gynecologists (ACOG) published new guidelines stating that no specific age should be used as a threshold for invasive or noninvasive screening. Furthermore, all women, regardless of age, should have the option of invasive testing without first having screening (ACOG, 2007).

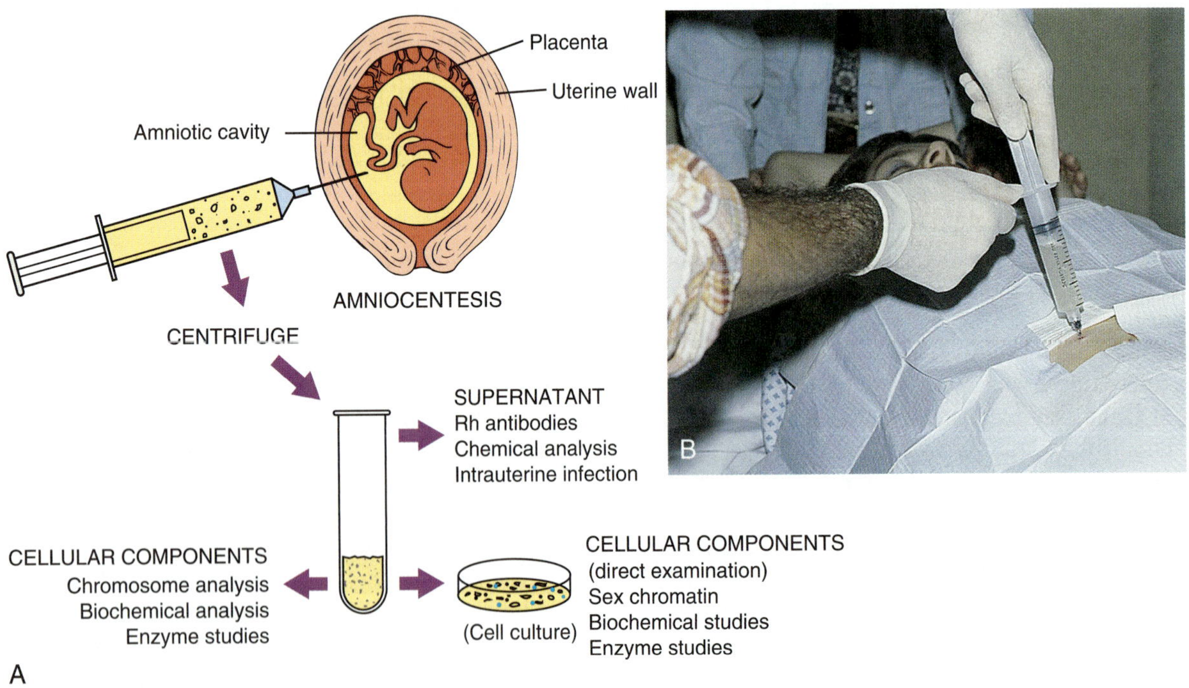

FIG. 26-5 **A,** Amniocentesis and laboratory use of amniotic fluid aspirant. **B,** Transabdominal amniocentesis. (**B,** Courtesy Marjorie Pyle, RNC, Lifecircle, Costa Mesa, CA.)

Biochemical analysis of enzymes in amniotic fluid can detect inborn errors of metabolism. For example, AFP levels in amniotic fluid are assessed as a follow-up for elevated levels in maternal serum. High AFP levels in amniotic fluid help confirm the diagnosis of an NTD such as spina bifida or anencephaly or an abdominal wall defect such as omphalocele. The elevation results from the increased leakage of cerebrospinal fluid into the amniotic fluid through the closure defect. AFP levels may also be elevated in a normal multifetal pregnancy and with intestinal atresia, presumably caused by lack of fetal swallowing.

A concurrent test that finds the presence of acetylcholinesterase almost always indicates a fetal defect (Wapner, Jenkins, & Khalek, 2009). In such instances, follow-up ultrasound examination is recommended.

Fetal Maturity. Late in pregnancy, accurate assessment of fetal lung maturity is possible by examining amniotic fluid for the presence of phosphatidylglycerol (PG). Determination of the lecithin/sphingomyelin (L/S) ratio and the surfactant/albumin (S/A) ratio [TDx FLM assay] are other methods to determine fetal lung maturity. The FLM assay is often used as the primary test for determining fetal lung maturity in clinical practice because it is simple to perform and accurate. FLM test results are similar to those of the PG test and the L/S ratio in terms of predicting pulmonary maturity (Mercer, 2009) (see Table 26-4).

Fetal Hemolytic Disease. Another indication for amniocentesis is the identification and follow-up of fetal hemolytic disease in cases of isoimmunization. The procedure is usually not performed until the mother's antibody titer reaches 1:8 and is increasing. Although percutaneous umbilical blood sampling is still the procedure of choice to treat fetal hemolytic disease, it is used less frequently for evaluating this condition. Instead, doppler velocimetry of the fetal middle cerebral artery is used to predict anemia associated with fetal hemolytic disease accurately and noninvasively (Tucker et al., 2009).

Chorionic Villus Sampling

The combined advantages of earlier diagnosis and rapid results have made **chorionic villus sampling (CVS)** a popular technique for genetic studies in the first trimester, although some risks to the fetus exist. Indications for CVS are similar to those for amniocentesis, although CVS cannot be used for maternal serum marker screening because no fluid is obtained. CVS performed in the second trimester carries no greater risk of pregnancy loss than amniocentesis and is considered equal to amniocentesis in diagnostic accuracy (Simpson & Otano, 2007).

The procedure can be performed in the first or second trimester, ideally between 10 and 13 weeks of gestation and involves the removal of a small tissue specimen from the fetal portion of the placenta (Figs. 26-6 and 26-7). Because chorionic villi originate in the zygote, this tissue reflects the genetic makeup of the fetus (Gilbert, 2011).

CVS procedures can be accomplished transcervically or transabdominally. In transcervical sampling a sterile catheter is introduced into the cervix under continuous ultrasonographic guidance, and a small portion of the chorionic villi is aspirated with a syringe. The aspiration cannula and obturator must be placed at a suitable site, and rupture of the amniotic sac must be avoided (see Fig 26-6). The transcervical procedure is contraindicated if a cervical infection, such as chlamydia or herpes, is present (Gilbert, 2011).

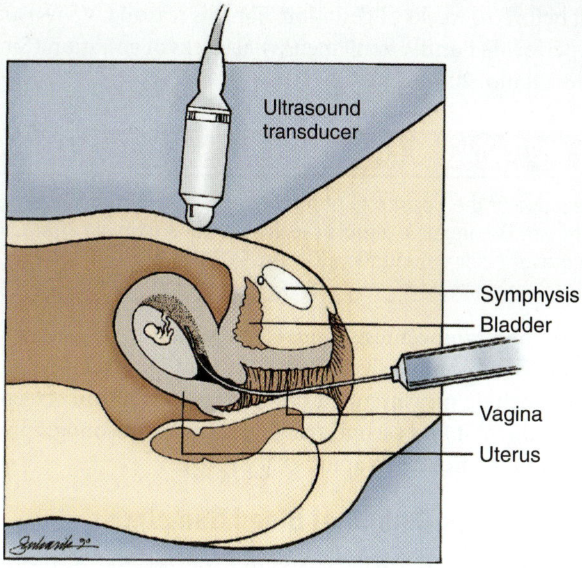

FIG. 26-6 Transcervical chorionic villus sampling. (From Gabbe, S., Niebyl, J., & Simpson, J. [2007]. *Obstetrics: Normal and problem pregnancies* [5th ed.]. Philadelphia: Churchill Livingstone.)

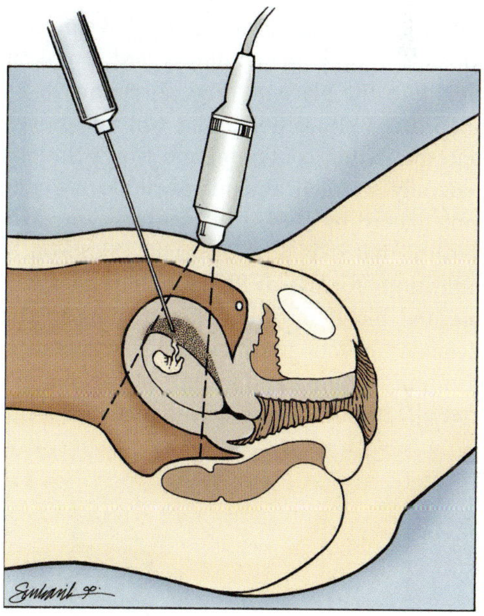

FIG. 26-7 Transabdominal chorionic villus sampling. (From Gabbe, S., Niebyl, J., & Simpson, J. [2007]. *Obstetrics: Normal and problem pregnancies* [5th ed.]. Philadelphia: Churchill Livingstone.)

If the abdominal approach is used, an 18-gauge spinal needle with stylet is inserted under sterile conditions through the abdominal wall into the chorion frondosum under ultrasound guidance. The stylet is then withdrawn, and the chorionic tissue is aspirated into a syringe (see Fig. 26-7).

Complications of the procedure include vaginal spotting or bleeding immediately afterward, miscarriage (0.3% of cases), rupture of membranes (0.1% of cases), and chorioamnionitis (0.5% of cases). Controversy exists concerning fetal limb reduction defects associated with CVS. Any increased risk appears to exist before 10 weeks of gestation. For this reason CVS is usually not performed until after 9 menstrual weeks of gestation (Simpson & Otano, 2007).

! NURSING ALERT

Because of the possibility of fetomaternal hemorrhage, women who are Rh negative should receive immune globulin after CVS to prevent isoimmunization (Gilbert, 2011).

Use of amniocentesis and CVS is declining because of advances in noninvasive screening techniques. These techniques include measurement of NT, maternal serum screening tests in the first and second trimesters, and ultrasonography in the second trimester (Wapner et al., 2009).

Percutaneous Umbilical Blood Sampling

Direct access to the fetal circulation during the second and third trimesters is possible through **percutaneous umbilical blood sampling (PUBS) (also called *cordocentesis*),** which is the most widely used method for fetal blood sampling and transfusion. PUBS involves the insertion of a needle directly into a fetal umbilical vessel, preferably the vein, under ultrasound guidance. Ideally, the umbilical cord is punctured near its insertion into the placenta (Figs. 26-8 and 26-9). At this point the cord is well anchored and will not move, and the risk of maternal blood contamination (from the placenta) is slight. Generally, a small amount of blood is removed and tested immediately by the Kleihauer-Betke procedure (Apt test) to ensure that it is fetal in origin (Simpson & Otano, 2007). Indications for use of PUBS include prenatal diagnosis of inherited blood disorders, karyotyping of malformed fetuses, detection of fetal infection, and assessment and treatment of isoimmunization and thrombocytopenia in the fetus (Wapner et al., 2009). Complications that can occur include loss of the pregnancy, hematomas, bleeding from the puncture site in the umbilical cord, transient fetal bradycardia, and fetomaternal hemorrhage. Maternal complications are rare, but include hemorrhage and transplacental hemorrhage (Simpson & Otano).

In fetuses at risk for isoimmune hemolytic anemia, PUBS permits precise identification of fetal blood type and RBC count and may prevent the need for further intervention. If the fetus is positive for the presence of maternal antibodies, a direct blood test can confirm the degree of anemia resulting from hemolysis. Intrauterine transfusion of severely anemic fetuses can be performed 4 to 5 weeks earlier than through the intraperitoneal route.

Follow-up includes continuous FHR monitoring for 1 to 2 hours after the procedure. Women should also be taught to do fetal movement counting at home (Gilbert, 2011).

Maternal Assays

Alpha-Fetoprotein

Maternal serum alpha-fetoprotein (MSAFP) levels are used as a screening tool for NTDs in pregnancy. Through this technique, approximately 80% to 85% of all open NTDs and open abdominal wall defects can be detected early in pregnancy. Screening is recommended for all pregnant women.

The cause of NTDs is not well understood, but 95% of all affected infants are born to women with no family history of similar anomalies (Wapner et al., 2009). The defect occurs in approximately 2 of 1000 births in the United States. The rate of NTDs is decreasing as a result of the use of folate preconceptionally and during early pregnancy for prevention of this condition (Manning, 2009).

Alpha-Fetoprotein (AFP) is produced by the fetal liver, and increasing levels are detectable in the serum of pregnant women from 14 to 34 weeks of gestation. Although amniotic fluid AFP measurement is diagnostic for NTD, MSAFP is a screening tool only and identifies candidates for the more definitive procedures of amniocentesis and ultrasound examination. MSAFP screening can be performed with reasonable reliability any time between 15 and 20 weeks of gestation (16 to 18 weeks being ideal) (Wapner et al., 2009).

Once the maternal level of AFP is determined, it is compared with normal values for each week of gestation. Values also

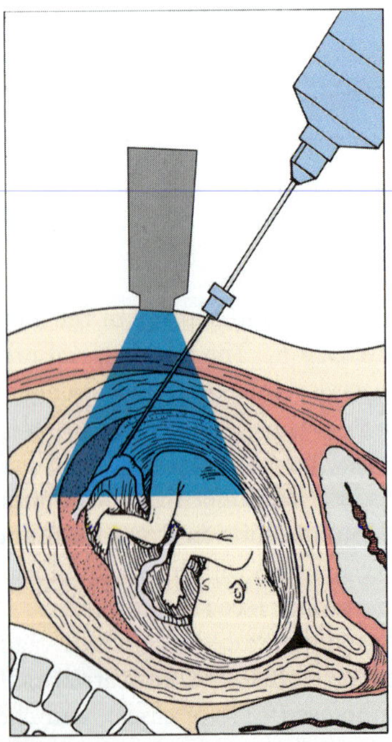

FIG. 26-8 Technique for percutaneous umbilical blood sampling guided by ultrasound.

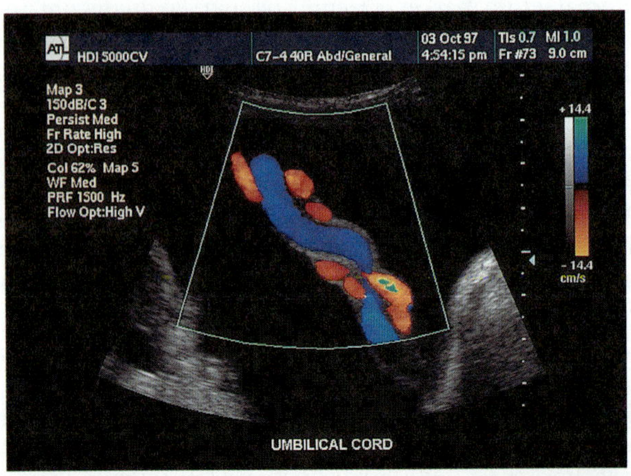

FIG. 26-9 Umbilical cord as seen on ultrasound at 26 weeks of gestation. (Courtesy Advanced Technology Laboratories, Bothell, WA.)

should be correlated with maternal age, weight, race, presence of a multifetal pregnancy, and whether the woman has insulin-dependent diabetes. If findings are abnormal, follow-up procedures include genetic counseling for families with a history of NTD, repeated AFP, specialized ultrasound examination, and possibly, amniocentesis (Cunningham et al., 2010).

Multiple Marker Screens

Screening to detect fetal chromosomal abnormalities, particularly Trisomy 21 (Down syndrome) is now available, beginning in the first trimester of pregnancy. This first trimester screen is done at 11 to 14 weeks of gestation. It includes measurement of two maternal biochemical markers, pregnancy-associated placental protein (PAPP-A) and human chorionic gonadotropin (hCG) or the free beta-human chorionic gonadotropin (β-hCG) subunit, and evaluation of fetal NT, or a combination of both. In the first trimester, hCG levels are higher than normal while PAPP-A levels are lower than normal in the presence of a fetus with Trisomy 21. First trimester screening using PAPP-A and hCG or β-hCG levels has been shown to be as accurate for detecting fetuses with Trisomy 21 as triple screening in the second trimester (Cunningham et al., 2010; Wapner, et al., 2009).

About one third of all fetuses with an increased NT will have a chromosome abnormality; half of these are Trisomy 21. Combining the serum marker and NT values results in the detection of Down syndrome in 79% to 87% of cases. These results are comparable to those obtained with quad screening in the second trimester (Cunningham et al., 2010).

In the second trimester, triple and quad screening is available to screen for fetuses with Trisomy 21 and Trisomy 18. The *triple-marker screen*, performed at 16 to 18 weeks of gestation, measures the levels of three maternal serum markers: MSAFP, unconjugated estriol, and hCG. In the presence of a fetus with Trisomy 21 the MSAFP and unconjugated estriol levels are low, whereas the hCG level is elevated. Low values in all three markers are associated with Trisomy 18 (Cunningham et al., 2010; Gilbert, 2011).

The *quad-screen* adds an additional marker, a placental hormone called *inhibin A*, to increase the accuracy of screening for Down syndrome in women less than 35 years of age. Low inhibin A levels indicate the possibility of Down syndrome (Gilbert, 2011). The addition of inhibin A to the other three markers increases the detection rate for Down syndrome in the entire population from 70% to 80% (Simpson & Otano, 2007). Similar to triple marker screening, the optimal time to perform the quad-screen is between 16 and 18 weeks of gestation (Gilbert).

The ability of multiple marker tests to detect chromosomal abnormalities depends on the accuracy of gestational age assessment. These tests are screening procedures only and are not diagnostic. A positive screening test result indicates an increased risk but is not diagnostic of Trisomy 21 or another chromosomal abnormality. Women with positive results should be offered diagnostic testing by amniocentesis or fetal blood sampling for fetal karyotyping (Cunningham et al., 2010).

Coombs Test

The indirect Coombs test is a screening tool for Rh incompatibility. If the maternal titer for Rh antibodies is greater than 1:8, amniocentesis for determination of bilirubin in amniotic fluid is indicated to establish the severity of fetal hemolytic anemia. The Coombs test can also detect other antibodies that may place the fetus at risk for incompatibility with maternal antigens.

ANTEPARTAL ASSESSMENT USING ELECTRONIC FETAL MONITORING

Indications

First- and second-trimester antepartal assessment is directed primarily at the diagnosis of fetal anomalies. The goal of third-trimester testing is to determine whether the intrauterine environment continues to be supportive to the fetus. The testing is often used to determine the timing of childbirth for women at risk for UPI. Gradual loss of placental function results first in inadequate nutrient delivery to the fetus, leading to IUGR. Subsequently, respiratory function also is compromised, resulting in fetal hypoxia. Common indications for both the **nonstresss test (NST)** and the **contraction stress test CST,** sometimes called the **oxytocin challenge test (OCT),** are listed in Box 26-6.

No clinical contraindications exist for the NST, but results may not be conclusive if gestation is 26 weeks or less. In general the CST cannot be performed on women who should not give birth vaginally at the time the test is performed. Absolute contraindications for the CST are the following: preterm labor, placenta previa, vasa previa, cervical incompetence, multiple gestation, and previous classic incision for cesarean birth (Tucker et al., 2009).

Nonstress Test

The NST is the most widely applied technique for antepartum evaluation of the fetus. It is an ideal screening test and is the primary method of antepartum fetal assessment at most sites. The basis for the NST is that the normal fetus will produce characteristic heart rate patterns in response to fetal movement. In the term fetus, accelerations are associated with movement more than 85% of the time (Druzin et al., 2007). The most common reason for the absence of FHR accelerations is the quiet fetal sleep state. However, medications such as narcotics, barbiturates, and beta-blockers, maternal smoking, and the

BOX 26-6 INDICATIONS FOR ELECTRONIC FETAL MONITORING ASSESSMENT USING THE NONSTRESS TEST AND THE CONTRACTION STRESS TEST

- Maternal diabetes mellitus
- Chronic hypertension
- Hypertensive disorders in pregnancy
- Intrauterine growth restriction
- Sickle cell disease
- Maternal cyanotic heart disease
- Postmaturity
- History of previous stillbirth
- Decreased fetal movement
- Isoimmunization
- Hyperthyroidism
- Collagen disease
- Chronic renal disease

presence of fetal malformations can also adversely affect the test (Druzin et al.; Gilbert, 2011). The NST can be performed easily and quickly in an outpatient setting because it is noninvasive, is relatively inexpensive, and has no known contraindications. Disadvantages include the requirement for twice-weekly testing and a high false-positive rate. The test also is slightly less sensitive in detecting fetal compromise than the CST or BPP (Tucker et al., 2009).

Procedure

The woman is seated in a reclining chair (or in semi-Fowler position) with a slight lateral tilt to optimize uterine perfusion and prevent supine hypotension. The FHR is recorded with a Doppler transducer, and a tocodynamometer is applied to detect uterine contractions or fetal movements. The tracing is observed for signs of fetal activity and a concurrent acceleration of FHR. If evidence of fetal movement is not apparent on the tracing, the woman may be asked to depress a button on a handheld event marker connected to the monitor when she feels fetal movement. The movement is then noted on the tracing. Because almost all accelerations are accompanied by fetal movement, the movements need not be recorded for the test to be considered reactive. The test is usually completed within 20 to 30 minutes, but more time may be required if the fetus must be awakened from a sleep state.

Caregivers sometimes suggest that the woman drink orange juice or be given glucose to increase her blood sugar level and thereby stimulate fetal movements. Although this practice is common, research has not proven it to be effective (Druzin et al., 2007).

Vibroacoustic stimulation is often used to stimulate fetal activity if the initial NST result is nonreactive and thus hopefully shortens the time required to complete the test (Druzin et al., 2007).

Interpretation

NST results are either reactive (Fig. 26-10) or nonreactive (Fig. 26-11). Box 26-7 lists criteria for both results.

A nonreactive test requires further evaluation. The testing period is often extended, usually for an additional 20 minutes, with the expectation that the fetal sleep state will change and the test will become reactive. During this time, vibroacoustic stimulation (see later discussion) may be used to stimulate fetal activity. If the test does not meet the criteria after 40 minutes, a CST or BPP will usually be performed. Once NST testing is initiated, it is usually repeated once or twice weekly for the

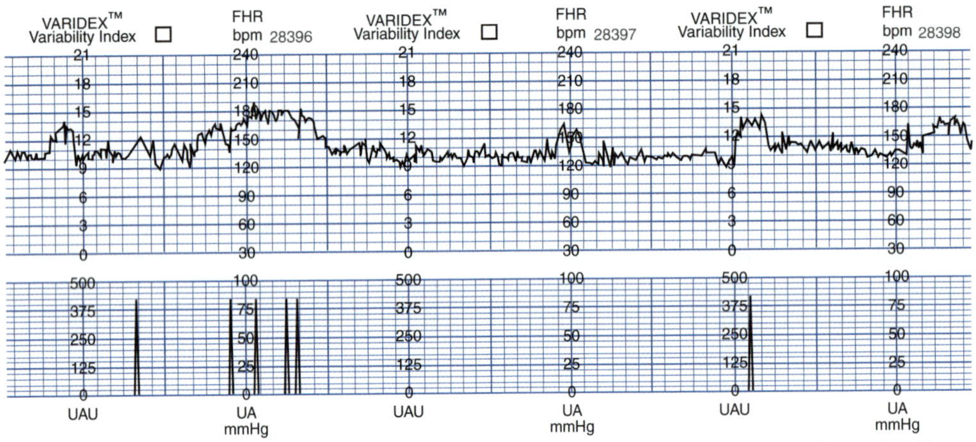

FIG. 26-10 Reactive nonstress test. (From Gabbe, S., Niebyl, J., & Simpson, J. [2007]. *Obstetrics: Normal and problem pregnancies* [5th ed.]. Philadelphia: Churchill Livingstone.)

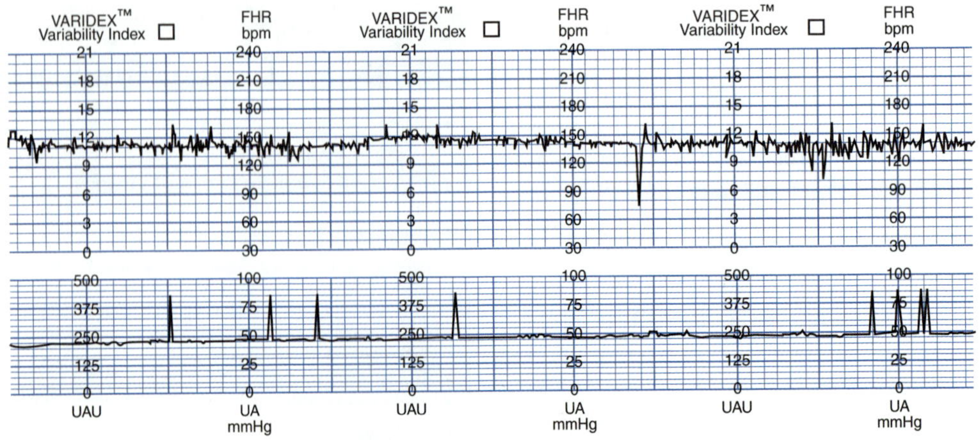

FIG. 26-11 Nonreactive nonstress test. (From Gabbe, S., Niebyl, J., & Simpson, J. [2007]. *Obstetrics: Normal and problem pregnancies* [5th ed.]. Philadelphia: Churchill Livingstone.)

remainder of the pregnancy (Druzin et al., 2007; Tucker et al., 2009).

Vibroacoustic Stimulation

Vibroacoustic stimulation (also called the *fetal acoustic stimulation test*) is another method of testing antepartum FHR response. This test is generally performed in conjunction with the NST and uses a combination of sound and vibration to stimulate the fetus. Whether the acoustic or the vibratory component alters the fetal state is unclear. The test takes approximately 15 minutes to complete, with the fetus monitored for 5 to 10 minutes before stimulation to obtain a baseline FHR. If the fetal baseline pattern is nonreactive, the sound source (usually a laryngeal stimulator) is then activated for 3 seconds on the maternal abdomen over the fetal head. Monitoring continues for another 5 minutes, after which the monitor tracing is assessed. The desired result is a reactive NST. The accelerations produced may have a significant increase in duration (Fig 26-12). The test may be repeated at 1-minute intervals up to three times when no response is noted. Further evaluation is needed with BPP or CST if the pattern is still nonreactive (Druzin et al., 2007).

Contraction Stress Test

The CST (or OCT) was the first widely used electronic fetal assessment test. It was devised as a graded stress test of the fetus, and its purpose was to identify the jeopardized fetus that was stable at rest but showed evidence of compromise after stress. Uterine contractions decrease uterine blood flow and placental perfusion. If this decrease is sufficient to produce hypoxia in the fetus, a deceleration in FHR will result.

BOX 26-7 INTERPRETATION OF THE NONSTRESS TEST

Reactive test: Two accelerations in a 20-minute period, each lasting at least 15 seconds and peaking at least 15 beats/min above the baseline. (Before 32 weeks of gestation, an acceleration is defined as an increase of at least 10 beats/min and lasting at least 10 seconds.)

Nonreactive test: A test that does not produce two or more qualifying accelerations in a 20-minute period.

Source: Tucker, S., Miller, L., & Miller, D. (2009). *Mosby's pocket guide to fetal monitoring: A multidisciplinary approach* (6th ed.). St. Louis: Mosby.

! NURSING ALERT

In a healthy fetoplacental unit, uterine contractions do not usually produce late decelerations, whereas, if underlying UPI exists, contractions will produce late decelerations.

The CST provides an earlier warning of fetal compromise than the NST and with fewer false-positive results. However, in addition to the contraindications described earlier the CST is more time consuming and expensive than the NST. It is also an invasive procedure if oxytocin stimulation is required. Because of these disadvantages, the CST is used infrequently.

Procedure

The woman is placed in semi-Fowler position or sits in a reclining chair with a slight lateral tilt to optimize uterine perfusion and avoid supine hypotension. She is monitored electronically with the fetal ultrasound transducer and uterine tocodynamometer. The tracing is observed for 10 to 20 minutes for baseline rate and variability and the possible occurrence of spontaneous contractions. The two methods of CST are the nipple-stimulated contraction test and the more commonly used oxytocin-stimulated contraction test.

Nipple-Stimulated Contraction Test. Several methods of nipple stimulation have been described. In one approach the woman applies warm, moist washcloths to both breasts for several minutes. The woman is then asked to massage one nipple for 10 minutes. Massaging the nipple causes a release of oxytocin from the posterior pituitary. An alternative approach is for her to massage one nipple through her clothes for 2 minutes, rest for 5 minutes, and repeat the cycles of massage and rest as necessary to achieve adequate uterine activity. When adequate contractions or hyperstimulation (defined as uterine contractions lasting more than 90 seconds or five or more contractions

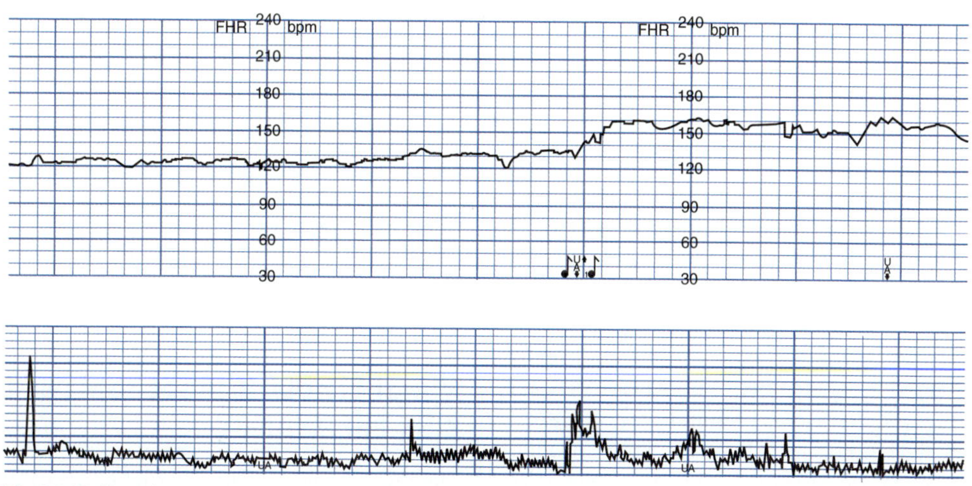

FIG. 26-12 Reactive nonstress test after vibroacoustic stimulation. The stimulus was applied at the point marked by the musical notes. A sustained fetal heart rate acceleration was produced. (From Gabbe, S., Niebyl, J., & Simpson, J. [2007]. *Obstetrics: Normal and problem pregnancies* [5th ed.]. Philadelphia: Churchill Livingstone.)

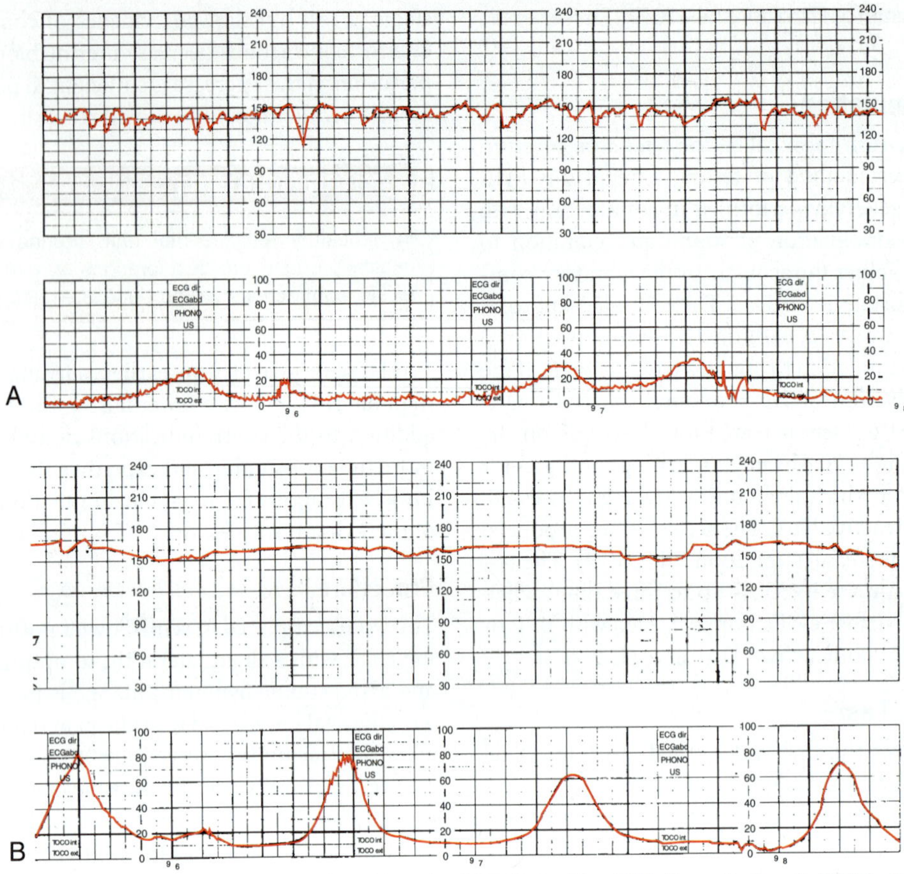

FIG. 26-13 Contraction stress test (CST). **A,** Negative CST. **B,** Positive CST. (From Tucker, S. [2004]. *Pocket guide to fetal monitoring and assessment* [5th ed.]. St. Louis: Mosby.)

in 10 minutes) occurs, stimulation should be stopped (Druzin et al., 2007).

Oxytocin-Stimulated Contraction Test. Exogenous oxytocin also can be used to stimulate uterine contractions. An intravenous (IV) infusion is begun, and a dilute solution of oxytocin (e.g., 30 units in 500 ml of fluid) is infused into the tubing of the main IV device through a piggyback port and delivered by an infusion pump to ensure an accurate dose. One method of oxytocin infusion is to begin at 0.5 milliunits/min and double the dose every 20 minutes until three uterine contractions of good quality, each lasting 40 to 60 seconds, are observed within a 10-minute period. A rate of 10 milliunits/min is usually adequate to elicit uterine contractions (Druzin et al., 2007).

Interpretation

CST results are either negative, positive, equivocal, suspicious, or unsatisfactory. If no late decelerations are observed with the contractions, the findings are considered negative (Fig. 26-13, *A*). Repetitive late decelerations render the test results positive (see Fig. 26-13, *B*). Box 26-8 lists criteria for each possible test result.

The desired CST result is negative because it has consistently been associated with good fetal outcomes. With a negative result the test is repeated in 1 week. Positive CST results have been associated with intrauterine fetal death, late FHR decelerations in labor, IUGR, and meconium-stained amniotic fluid. A positive CST result usually leads to hospitalization for further close observation or birth. Unsatisfactory, suspicious, and equivocal tests must be repeated within 24 hours (Druzin et al., 2007; Tucker et al., 2009).

BOX 26-8 INTERPRETATION OF THE CONTRACTION STRESS TEST

Negative test: At least three uterine contractions occur in a 10-minute period, with no late or significant variable decelerations.

Positive test: Late decelerations occur with 50% or more of contractions (even if fewer than three contractions occur in 10 minutes).

Equivocal-suspicious test: Prolonged decelerations, variable decelerations, or late decelerations occur with less than 50% of contractions.

Equivocal-hyperstimulatory test: Decelerations occur in the presence of contractions more frequent than every 2 minutes or lasting longer than 90 seconds.

Unsatisfactory test: Fewer than three uterine contractions in a 10-minute period or inability to obtain a continuous tracing of the fetal heart rate.

Source: Tucker, S., Miller, L., & Miller, D. (2009). *Mosby's pocket guide to fetal monitoring: A multidisciplinary approach* (6th ed.). St. Louis: Mosby.

NURSES' ROLE IN ASSESSMENT OF THE HIGH RISK PREGNANCY

The nurse's role is primarily that of educator and support person when the woman is undergoing such examinations as ultrasonography, MRI, CVS, PUBS, and amniocentesis. In some instances the nurse may assist the physician with the procedure.

In many settings, nurses perform NSTs, CSTs, and BPPs; conduct an initial assessment; and begin necessary interventions for nonreassuring results. These nursing procedures are accomplished after additional education and training, under guidance of established protocols, and in collaboration with obstetric providers. Client teaching, which is an integral component of this role, involves preparing the woman for the procedure, interpreting the findings, and providing psychosocial support when needed.

KEY POINTS

- A high risk pregnancy is one in which the life or well-being of the mother or infant is jeopardized by a biophysical or psychosocial disorder coincidental with or unique to pregnancy.
- Biophysical, sociodemographic, psychosocial, and environmental factors place the pregnancy and fetus or neonate at risk.
- Biophysical assessment techniques include DFMCs, ultrasonography, and MRI.
- Biochemical monitoring techniques include amniocentesis, PUBS, CVS, MSAFP, and multiple marker screens.
- Reactive NSTs and negative CSTs suggest fetal well-being.
- Most assessment tests have some degree of risk for the mother and fetus and usually cause some anxiety for the woman and her family.
- The nurse's role in assessment of the high risk pregnancy is primarily that of educator and support person.

Audio Chapter Summaries Access an audio summary of these Key Points on evolve

REFERENCES

American College of Obstetricians and Gynecologists (ACOG). (2007). *Screening for fetal chromosomal abnormalities.* Practice Bulletin No. 77. Washington, DC: ACOG.

American College of Obstetricians and Gynecologists (ACOG). (2004). *Ultrasonography in pregnancy.* Practice Bulletin No. 58. Washington, DC: ACOG.

Chambers, C., & Weiner, C. (2009). Teratogenesis and environmental exposure. In R. Creasy, R. Resnik, J. Iams, C. Lockwood, & T. Moore (Eds.), *Creasy and Resnik's maternal-fetal medicine: Principles and practice* (6th ed). Philadelphia: Saunders.

Cunningham, F., Leveno, K., Bloom, S., Hauth, J., Rouse, D., & Spong, C. (Eds.). (2010). *Williams obstetrics* (23rd ed.). New York: McGraw-Hill.

Druzin, M., Smith, J., Gabbe, S., & Reed, K. (2007). Antepartum fetal evaluation. In S. Gabbe, J. Niebyl, & J. Simpson (Eds.), *Obstetrics: Normal and problem pregnancies* (5th ed.). Philadelphia: Churchill Livingstone.

Francois, K., & Foley, M. (2007). Antepartum and postpartum hemorrhage. In S. Gabbe, J. Niebyl, & J. Simpson (Eds.), *Obstetrics: Normal and problem pregnancies* (5th ed.). Philadelphia: Churchill Livingstone.

Gilbert, E. (2011). *Manual of high risk pregnancy & delivery* (5th ed.). St. Louis: Mosby.

Gilbert, W. (2007). Amniotic fluid disorders. In S. Gabbe, J. Niebyl, & J. Simpson (Eds.), *Obstetrics: Normal and problem pregnancies* (5th ed.). Philadelphia: Churchill Livingstone.

Harman, C. (2009). Assessment of fetal health. In R. Creasy, R. Resnik, J. Iams, C. Lockwood, & T. Moore (Eds.), *Creasy and Resnik's maternal-fetal medicine: Principles and practice* (6th ed.). Philadelphia: Saunders.

Manning, F. (2009). Imaging in the diagnosis of fetal anomalies. In R. Creasy, R. Resnik, J. Iams, C. Lockwood, & T. Moore (Eds.), *Creasy and Resnik's maternal-fetal medicine: Principles and practice* (6th ed.). Philadelphia: Saunders.

Mercer, B. (2009). Assessment and induction of fetal pulmonary maturity. In R. Creasy, R. Resnik, J. Iams, C. Lockwood, & T. Moore (Eds.), *Creasy and Resnik's maternal-fetal medicine: Principles and practice* (6th ed.). Philadelphia: Saunders.

Richards, D. (2007). Ultrasound for pregnancy dating, growth, and the diagnosis of fetal malformations. In S. Gabbe, J. Niebyl, & J. Simpson (Eds.), *Obstetrics: Normal and problem pregnancies* (5th ed.). Philadelphia: Churchill Livingstone.

Simpson, J., & Otano, L. (2007). Prenatal genetic diagnosis. In S. Gabbe, J. Niebyl, & J. Simpson (Eds.), *Obstetrics: Normal and problem pregnancies* (5th ed.). Philadelphia: Churchill Livingstone.

Tucker, S., Miller, L., & Miller, D. (2009). *Mosby's pocket guide to fetal monitoring: A multidisciplinary approach* (6th ed.). St. Louis: Mosby.

Wapner, R., Jenkins, T., & Khalek, N. (2009). Prenatal diagnosis of congenital disorders. In R. Creasy, R. Resnik, J. Iams, C. Lockwood, & T. Moore (Eds.), *Creasy and Resnik's maternal-fetal medicine: Principles and practice* (6th ed.). Philadelphia: Saunders.

CHAPTER

27

Hypertensive Disorders in Pregnancy

Dusty Dix

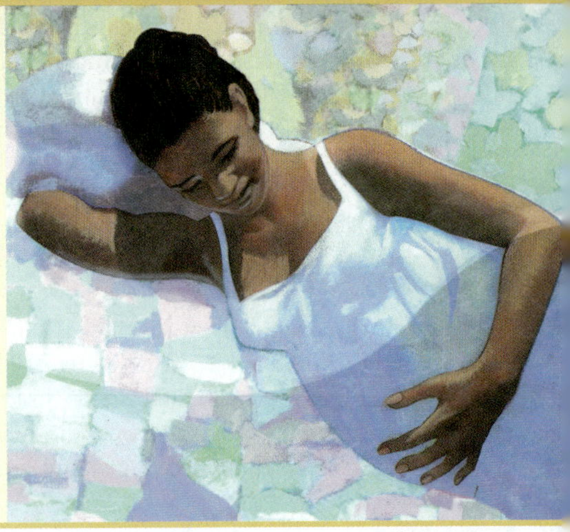

evolve WEBSITE

http://evolve.elsevier.com/Lowdermilk/MWHC/

Audio Glossary
Audio Key Points
Case Studies
- Nursing Care of the Obese Pregnant Woman with Chronic Hypertension
  - First Trimester
  - Second and Third Trimesters
- Preeclampsia

Critical Thinking Exercise
- Preeclampsia

NCLEX Review Questions
Nursing Care Plans
- Mild Preeclampsia
- Severe Preeclampsia

Video—Nursing Skills
- Assessing Deep Tendon Reflexes

LEARNING OBJECTIVES

- Describe the characteristics of gestational hypertension, preeclampsia, eclampsia, and chronic hypertension.
- Identify the maternal-fetal complications associated with hypertensive disorders in pregnancy.
- List risk factors for preeclampsia.
- Describe the pathophysiologic mechanisms of preeclampsia and eclampsia.
- Explain how the abnormal laboratory values present in HELLP syndrome are produced by the pathophysiology that occurs with severe preeclampsia.
- Differentiate the antepartum, intrapartum, and postpartum management of the woman with mild or severe preeclampsia and mild or severe gestational hypertension.
- Describe appropriate nursing actions during and after an eclamptic seizure.
- Discuss the preconception, antepartum, intrapartum, and postpartum management of the woman with chronic hypertension.

Gestational hypertensive disorders develop during pregnancy, labor, or after birth. These disorders include gestational hypertension, preeclampsia, and eclampsia. Chronic hypertensive disorders precede pregnancy or develop before 20 weeks of gestation. Women with chronic hypertension can also develop superimposed preeclampsia or eclampsia. The classification, pathophysiologic changes, assessment and management of hypertensive disorders of pregnancy are discussed in this chapter with a primary focus on preeclampsia. The care of women with hypertensive disorders during the perinatal period requires a collaborative effort, including early detection, thorough assessment, and timely intervention.

SIGNIFICANCE AND INCIDENCE

Hypertensive disorders complicate 5% to 10% of all pregnancies and are a common medical complication during pregnancy. The incidence varies among hospitals, regions, and countries (Gilbert, 2011; Sibai, 2007). In the United States, the rate of pregnancy-associated hypertension for all ages and ethnic groups has increased by approximately 1% each year since 2000, reaching the rate of 39.1 per 1000 live births in 2006. The annual rate of increase for chronic hypertension has risen at an even faster pace, from 2% per year in the 1990s to 6% annually since 2000, reaching the rate of 10.8 in 2006. The rate of chronic hypertension in mothers ages 40 and older is nearly ten times higher than for those younger than age 20 (30.4 compared with 3.9 per 1000 live births) (Martin, Hamilton, Sutton, Ventura, Menacker, Kirmeyer, & Mathews, 2009).

MORBIDITY AND MORTALITY

Hypertensive disorders contribute significantly to maternal and infant morbidity and mortality worldwide (Sibai, 2007). Maternal complications associated with hypertensive disorders include placental abruption (abruptio placentae), acute

TABLE 27-1 **CLASSIFICATION OF HYPERTENSIVE STATES OF PREGNANCY**

TYPE	DESCRIPTION
Gestational Hypertensive Disorders	
Gestational hypertension	Development of mild hypertension after 20 weeks of pregnancy in previously normotensive woman without proteinuria
Preeclampsia	Development of hypertension and proteinuria in previously normotensive woman after 20 weeks of gestation or in early postpartum period; in presence of trophoblastic disease, preeclampsia can develop before 20 weeks of gestation
Eclampsia	Development of convulsions or coma not attributable to other causes in preeclamptic woman
Chronic Hypertensive Disorders	
Chronic hypertension	Hypertension in pregnant woman present before pregnancy or diagnosed before 20 weeks of gestation and persistent after 6 weeks postpartum
Superimposed preeclampsia or eclampsia	In women with hypertension before 20 weeks of gestation: new-onset proteinuria (≥0.5 g protein in a 24-hr collection) In women with both hypertension and proteinuria before 20 weeks of gestation: significant increase in hypertension, plus one of the following: new onset of symptoms, thrombocytopenia, or elevated liver enzymes

Sources: American College of Obstetricians and Gynecologists (ACOG). (2002). *Diagnosis and management of preeclampsia and eclampsia.* ACOG Practice Bulletin No. 33. Washington DC: ACOG; Sibai, B. (2007). Hypertension. In S. Gabbe, J. Niebyl, & J. Simpson (Eds.), *Obstetrics: Normal and problem pregnancies* (5th ed.). Philadelphia: Churchill Livingstone.

TABLE 27-2 **DIFFERENTIATION BETWEEN MILD AND SEVERE PREECLAMPSIA**

	MILD PREECLAMPSIA	SEVERE PREECLAMPSIA
Maternal Effects		
Blood pressure (BP)	BP reading ≥140/90 mm Hg × two, at least 4-6 hr apart but within a maximum of a 1-wk period	Rise to ≥160/110 mm Hg on two separate occasions 6 hr apart with pregnant woman on bed rest
Proteinuria		
Qualitative dipstick	≥1+ on dipstick	≥3+ on dipstick
Quantitative 24-hr analysis	Proteinuria of ≥300 mg in a 24-hr specimen	Proteinuria of ≥5 g in 24-hr specimen
Urine output	Output matching intake, ≥25-30 ml/hr	<400-500 ml/24 hr
Headache	Absent or transient	Persistent or severe
Visual problems	Absent	Blurred, photophobia
Irritability or changes in affect	Transient	May be severe
Epigastric or right upper quadrant pain, nausea, and vomiting	Absent	May be present
Thrombocytopenia	Absent	May be present
Impaired liver function	Normal	May be present
Pulmonary edema	Absent	May be present
Fetal Effects		
Placental perfusion	Reduced	Decreased perfusion expressing as IUGR in fetus; abnormal (nonreassuring) fetal status on antepartum testing

FHR, Fetal heart rate; *IUGR*, Intrauterine growth restriction.
Sources: American College of Obstetricians and Gynecologists (ACOG). (2002). *Diagnosis and management of preeclampsia and eclampsia.* ACOG Practice Bulletin No. 33. Washington, DC: ACOG; Sibai, B. (2007). Hypertension. In S. Gabbe, J. Niebyl, & J. Simpson (Eds.), *Obstetrics: Normal and problem pregnancies* (5th ed.). Philadelphia: Churchill Livingstone.

respiratory distress syndrome (ARDS), stroke, cerebral hemorrhage, hepatic or renal failure, disseminated intravascular coagulation (DIC), and pulmonary edema. Most perinatal complications are related to placental insufficiency which causes intrauterine growth restriction (IUGR), prematurity associated with indicated preterm birth, hypoxia/acidosis, or placental abruption (Gilbert, 2011).

Pregnancy associated hypertension accounts for 10% to 15% of maternal deaths worldwide (Askie, Duley, Henderson-Smart, & Stewart, 2007). Preeclampsia is the second leading cause of maternal mortality in the United States (Hawfield & Freedman, 2009). The majority of maternal deaths result from complications of hepatic rupture, placental abruption, or eclampsia (Roberts & Funai, 2009).

CLASSIFICATION

The classification of hypertensive disorders in pregnancy is confusing because standard definitions are not used consistently by all health care providers. The classification system most commonly used in the United States is based on reports from the American College of Obstetricians and Gynecologists (ACOG) (2002) and the National High Blood Pressure Education Program Working Group on High Blood Pressure in Pregnancy (Working Group) (2000). This classification system is summarized in Table 27-1.

Gestational Hypertension

Gestational hypertension is the onset of hypertension without proteinuria after week 20 of pregnancy (ACOG, 2002; Working Group, 2000). Hypertension is defined as a systolic blood pressure (BP) greater than 140 mm Hg or a diastolic BP greater than 90 mm Hg. The hypertension should be recorded on at least two separate occasions at least 4 to 6 hours apart and within a 1-week period (ACOG, 2002; Sibai, 2007; Working Group, 2000).

Gestational hypertension is the most frequent cause of hypertension during pregnancy, with an incidence of 6% to 17% in primigravidas and 2% to 4% in multiparous women. It occurs much more frequently in women with multifetal pregnancies (Sibai, 2007). While gestational hypertension can occur at any time after 20 weeks of pregnancy, it usually develops at or after 37 weeks of gestation. Women with gestational hypertension have no evidence of preexisting hypertension, and their BPs return to normal levels within 6 weeks after giving birth. Gestational hypertension is further classified as either mild or severe. The definitions of mild and severe gestational hypertension are the same as the definitions for blood pressure readings for mild and severe preeclampsia (Table 27-2). Women with mild gestational hypertension usually have good pregnancy outcomes. Some women who are initially thought to have gestational hypertension will eventually be diagnosed with chronic hypertension instead. Others will go on to develop proteinuria, thereby changing their diagnosis to preeclampsia. Women who are diagnosed with gestational hypertension before 35 weeks of gestation are more likely to progress to preeclampsia than women whose onset of hypertension occurs closer to term (Sibai).

TABLE 27-3 **COMMON LABORATORY CHANGES IN PREECLAMPSIA**

	NORMAL NONPREGNANT	PREECLAMPSIA	HELLP
Hemoglobin, hematocrit	12-16 g/dl, 37%-47%	May ↑	↓
Platelets (cells/mm³)	150,000-400,000/mm³	Unchanged or <100,000/mm³	<100,000/mm³
Prothrombin time (PT), partial thromboplastin time (PTT)	12-14 sec, 60-70 sec	Unchanged	Unchanged
Fibrinogen	200-400 mg/dl	300-600 mg/dl	↓
Fibrin split products (FSPs)	Absent	Absent or present	Present
Blood urea nitrogen (BUN)	10-20 mg/dl	↑	↑
Creatinine	0.5-1.1 mg/dl	>1.2 mg/dl	↑
Lactate dehydrogenase (LDH)*	45-90 units/L	↑	↑ (>600 units/L)
Aspartate aminotransferase (AST)	4-20 units/L	Elevated	↑ (>70 units/L)
Alanine aminotransferase (ALT)	3-21 units/L	Elevated	↑
Creatinine clearance	80-125 ml/min	130-180 ml/min	↓
Burr cells or schistocytes	Absent	Absent	Present
Uric acid	2-6.6 mg/dl	>5.9 mg/dl	>10 mg/dl
Bilirubin (total)	0.1-1 mg/dl	Unchanged or ↑	↑ (>.1.2 mg/dl)

*LDH values differ according to the test or assays being performed.

Sources: American College of Obstetricians and Gynecologists (ACOG). (2002). *Diagnosis and management of preeclampsia and eclampsia.* ACOG Practice Bulletin No. 33. Washington, DC: AGOG; Cunningham, F., Leveno, K., Bloom, S., Hauth, J., Rouse, D., & Spong, C. (Eds.). (2010). *Williams obstetrics* (23rd ed.). New York: McGraw-Hill; Dildy, G. (2004). Complications of preeclampsia. In G. Dildy, M. Belfort, G. Saade, J. Phelan, G. Hankins, & S. Clark (Eds.), *Critical care obstetrics* (4th ed.). Malden, MA: Blackwell Science; Sibai, B. (2007). Hypertension. In S. Gabbe, J. Niebyl, & J. Simpson (Eds.), *Obstetrics: Normal and problem pregnancies* (5th ed.). Philadelphia: Churchill Livingstone.

Preeclampsia

Preeclampsia is a pregnancy-specific condition in which hypertension and proteinuria develop after 20 weeks of gestation in a previously normotensive woman. A significant contributor to maternal and perinatal morbidity and mortality, preeclampsia complicates approximately 3% to 7% of all pregnancies (American Academy of Pediatrics [AAP] & ACOG, 2007). Preeclampsia is a vasospastic, systemic disorder and is usually categorized as mild or severe for purposes of management (ACOG, 2002; Working Group, 2000). Table 27-2 lists criteria for mild and severe preeclampsia, and Table 27-3 gives common laboratory changes that occur in mild and severe preeclampsia.

Eclampsia

Eclampsia is the onset of seizure activity or coma in a woman with preeclampsia, with no history of preexisting pathology, which can result in seizure activity (Roberts & Funai, 2009; Sibai, 2007). Eclamptic seizures can occur before, during, or after birth. Approximately one third of eclamptic seizures occur after birth, almost always within the first 48 hours postpartum (Roberts & Funai).

Case Study—Nursing Care of the Obese Pregnant Woman with Chronic Hypertension

COMMUNITY ACTIVITY

- Visit the Preeclampsia Foundation website, which provides education and support for women with preeclampsia and other hypertensive disorders of pregnancy. What is the mission of the foundation? Review the information about preeclampsia and related links.
- Research the availability of a perinatologist or maternal-fetal medicine specialist in your community. What types of maternal-fetal complications are referred to a maternal-fetal medicine specialist? If a maternal-fetal medicine specialist is not available in your community, how and where are women referred for care? What other types of services are available, such as prenatal diagnostic techniques, genetic counseling, or complicated maternal/fetal surgery?

Chronic Hypertension

Chronic hypertension is defined as hypertension that is present before the pregnancy or develops before 20 weeks of gestation (Roberts & Funai, 2009). Hypertension initially diagnosed during pregnancy that persists longer than 6 weeks postpartum is also classified as chronic hypertension (Sibai, 2007). Other authorities believe that a diagnosis of chronic hypertension can be made only if the BP has not returned to normal levels by 12 weeks after birth (Roberts & Funai). Most women with mild chronic hypertension experience uncomplicated pregnancies. However, those with severe chronic hypertension have an increased risk of perinatal mortality (Gilbert, 2011).

Chronic Hypertension with Superimposed Preeclampsia

Women with chronic hypertension may develop superimposed preeclampsia, which increases the morbidity for mother and fetus. A diagnosis of **chronic hypertension with superimposed preeclampsia** is made with the following findings (Sibai, 2007):

- In women with hypertension before 20 weeks of gestation
  - New-onset proteinuria (≥0.5 g protein in a 24-hour collection)
- In women with both hypertension and proteinuria before 20 weeks of gestation
  - Significant increase in hypertension, plus one of the following:
    - New onset of symptoms
    - Thrombocytopenia
    - Elevated liver enzymes

PREECLAMPSIA

Etiology

Preeclampsia is a condition unique to human pregnancy. Signs and symptoms develop only during pregnancy and disappear soon after birth of the fetus and placenta. Common risk factors associated with the development of preeclampsia are listed in Box 27-1. Preeclampsia occurs most often with primigravid women or multiparous women with a new partner. Age distribution remains U-shaped; women younger than 19 years and older than 40 years have the highest rates of occurrence (Gilbert, 2011).

The cause of preeclampsia is unknown. Many theories have been suggested to explain the etiology of preeclampsia. Current

BOX 27-1 RISK FACTORS FOR PREECLAMPSIA

- First pregnancy or new partner with this pregnancy
- Extremes of maternal age: younger than 19 or older than 40 years
- Obesity
- Personal or family history of preeclampsia
- Exposure to abundance of trophoblast tissue
  - Multifetal gestation
  - Hydatidiform mole
- Poor outcome in previous pregnancy:
  - Intrauterine growth restriction
  - Placental abruption (abruptio placentae)
  - Fetal death
- Preexisting medical or genetic conditions
  - Chronic hypertension
  - Renal disease
  - Type 1 diabetes mellitus
  - Collagen disease
- Thrombophilias
  - Antiphospholipid antibody syndrome
  - Protein C, protein S, antithrombin deficiency
  - Factor V Leiden mutation
- Periodontal disease

Sources: Gilbert, E. (2011). *Manual of high risk pregnancy & delivery* (5th ed.). St. Louis: Mosby; Sibai, B. (2007). Hypertension. In S. Gabbe, J. Niebyl, & J. Simpson (Eds.), *Obstetrics: Normal and problem pregnancies* (5th ed.). Philadelphia: Churchill Livingstone.

theories that are still being considered include abnormal trophoblast invasion, coagulation abnormalities, vascular endothelial damage, cardiovascular maladaptation, and dietary deficiencies or excesses. Immunologic factors and genetic predisposition may also play important roles (Sibai, 2007).

Pathophysiology

Preeclampsia can progress along a continuum from mild to severe preeclampsia to eclampsia. Current thought is that the pathologic changes that occur in the woman with preeclampsia are caused by disruptions in placental perfusion and endothelial cell dysfunction (Gilbert, 2011; Peters, 2008). These changes are present long before the clinical diagnosis of preeclampsia is made (Roberts & Funai, 2009). Normally in pregnancy the spiral arteries in the uterus widen from thick-walled muscular vessels to thinner, saclike vessels with much larger diameters. This change increases the capacity of the vessels, allowing them to handle the increased blood volume of pregnancy. Because this vascular remodeling does not occur or only partially develops in women with preeclampsia, decreased placental perfusion and hypoxia result (Peters). Placental ischemia is thought to cause endothelial cell dysfunction by stimulating the release of a substance that is toxic to endothelial cells. This anomaly causes generalized vasospasm, which results in poor tissue perfusion in all organ systems, increased peripheral resistance and BP, and increased endothelial cell permeability, leading to intravascular protein and fluid loss and ultimately to less plasma volume. The main pathogenic factor is not an increase in BP but poor perfusion as a result of vasospasm and reduced plasma volume (Fig. 27-1) (Gilbert; Peters; Roberts & Funai). Figure 27-2 demonstrates how endothelial cell dysfunction causes many of the common signs and symptoms of preeclampsia.

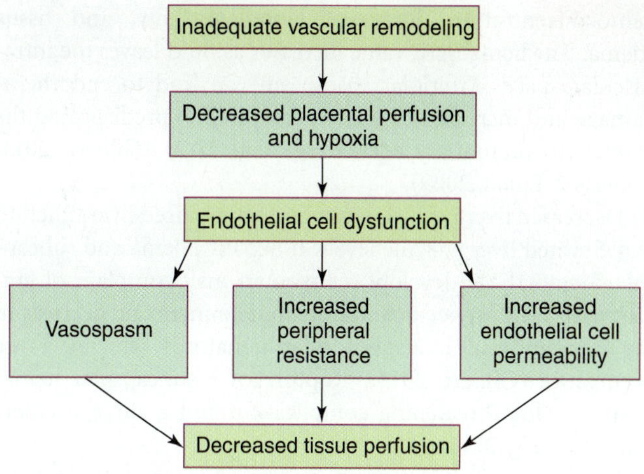

FIG. 27-1 Etiology of preeclampsia: disruptions in placental perfusion and endothelial cell dysfunction

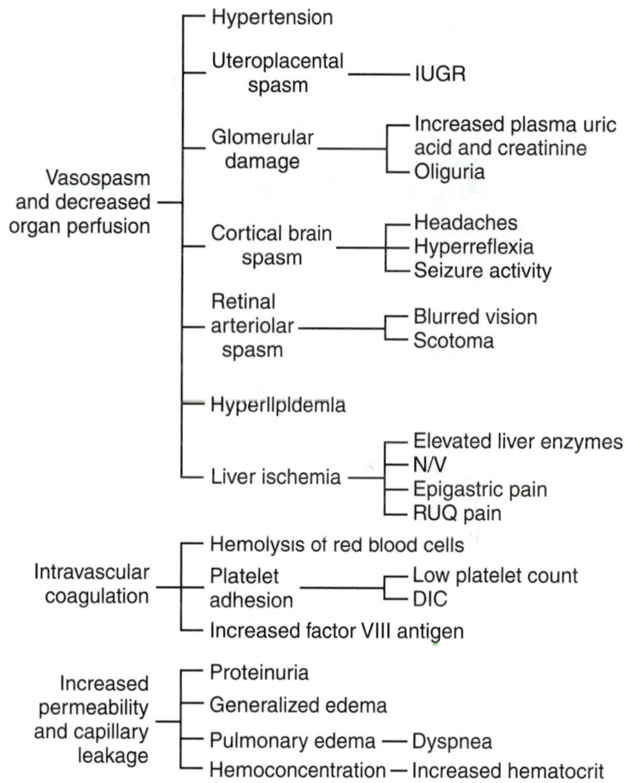

FIG. 27-2 Consequences of endothelial cell dysfunction. *DIC*, Disseminated vascular coagulation; *IUGR*, intrauterine growth restriction, *N/V*, nausea/vomiting; *RUQ*, right upper quadrant. (From Gilbert, E. [2011]. *Manual of high risk pregnancy & delivery* [5th ed.]. St. Louis: Mosby.)

Reduced kidney perfusion decreases the glomerular filtration rate and can lead to degenerative glomerular changes and oliguria. Pathologic changes in the endothelial cells of the glomeruli (glomerular endotheliosis) are uniquely characteristic of preeclampsia. Protein, primarily albumin, is lost in the urine. Uric acid clearance is decreased. Serum uric acid levels, however, increase. Sodium and water are retained. Acute tubular necrosis and renal failure may occur (Gilbert, 2011; Peters, 2008; Roberts & Funai, 2009).

Plasma colloid osmotic pressure decreases as serum albumin levels decrease. Intravascular volume is reduced as fluid moves out of the intravascular compartment, resulting in hemoconcentration, increased blood viscosity, and tissue edema. The hematocrit value increases as fluid leaves the intravascular space. Arteriolar vasospasm can lead to endothelial damage and increased capillary permeability, predisposing the woman to pulmonary edema (see Fig. 27-2) (Gilbert, 2011; Roberts & Funai, 2009).

Decreased liver perfusion can lead to impaired liver function and elevated liver enzyme levels. If hepatic edema and subcapsular hemorrhage develop, the woman may complain of epigastric or right upper quadrant pain. Hemorrhagic necrosis in the liver can result in a subcapsular hematoma, which is a rare occurrence (Gilbert, 2011). Rupture of a subcapsular hematoma is a life-threatening complication and a surgical emergency (see Fig. 27-2).

Neurologic complications associated with preeclampsia include cerebral edema and hemorrhage and increased central nervous system (CNS) irritability. CNS irritability manifests as headaches, hyperreflexia, positive ankle clonus, and seizures. Arteriolar vasospasms and decreased blood flow to the retina can lead to visual disturbances such as scotoma (dim vision or blind or dark spots in the visual field) and blurred or double vision (Gilbert, 2011; Roberts & Funai, 2009).

Decreased placental perfusion contributes significantly to restriction of fetal growth and the increased incidence of placental abruption, premature birth, and early degenerative aging of the placenta. The rate of fetal complications is directly related to the severity of the disease (Peters, 2008; Sibai, 2007).

HELLP Syndrome

HELLP syndrome is a laboratory diagnosis for a variant of severe preeclampsia that involves hepatic dysfunction, characterized by hemolysis (H), elevated liver enzymes (EL), and low platelet count (LP). It is not a separate illness. No consensus has been reached, however, regarding which laboratory tests should be used to diagnose HELLP syndrome or what values should be considered abnormal (Sibai, 2007). Table 27-3 lists laboratory changes that occur in HELLP syndrome.

The pathophysiologic changes of HELLP syndrome occur as a result of arteriolar vasospasm, endothelial cell dysfunction with fibrin deposits, and adherence of platelets in blood vessels. Red blood cells are damaged as they pass through narrowed blood vessels and become hemolyzed, resulting in a decreased red blood cell and platelet count, as well as hyperbilirubinemia. Endothelial damage and fibrin deposits in the liver lead to impaired liver function and can cause hemorrhagic necrosis. Liver enzymes are elevated when hepatic tissue is damaged (Gilbert, 2011)

HELLP syndrome usually develops in the third trimester of pregnancy, or within 48 hours after birth. The clinical presentation of HELLP syndrome is often nonspecific. Most women with the disorder report a history of malaise, influenza-like symptoms, epigastric or right upper quadrant abdominal pain, nausea, vomiting, and headaches. A small number of women may exhibit symptoms related to thrombocytopenia, such as bruising or hematuria (Peters, 2008; Sibai, 2007).

Because no agreement has been reached regarding the diagnostic criteria for HELLP syndrome, its reported incidence varies. It has been reported to occur in anywhere from 5% to 20% of women with preeclampsia (Emery, 2005; Gilbert, 2011). HELLP syndrome appears to occur more frequently in Caucasian women than women of other races. A diagnosis of HELLP syndrome is associated with an increased risk for adverse perinatal outcomes, including pulmonary edema, acute renal failure, DIC, placental abruption, liver hemorrhage or failure, ARDS, sepsis, and stroke (Sibai, 2007). Perinatal mortality rates range from 7.4% to 20.4% with a maternal mortality of approximately 1% (Sibai). The rate of preterm birth in women with HELLP syndrome is approximately 70%, with 15% of these occurring before 28 weeks of gestation. Most of the perinatal deaths occur before 28 weeks of gestation, in association with placental abruption or severe IUGR (Sibai).

CLINICAL REASONING

Severe Complications of Preeclampsia

Donna is a 35-year-old primigravida at 33 weeks of gestation, who arrives at her doctor's office for a prenatal visit. Donna is seen in the office twice a week for evaluation of her BP, fetal status, and laboratory studies. At 30 weeks of gestation, Donna developed signs of mild preeclampsia: BP of 140/90 mm Hg, with 2+ proteinuria and generalized edema. She was hospitalized for 2 days for a thorough assessment of maternal/fetal status and diagnostic/laboratory tests. Donna has been home on modified bed rest. A home health nurse visits her twice a week and calls her daily.

When you ask Donna how she is feeling, she replies that she does not feel well and is very tired. She also states, "I have been nauseated for several days, my stomach hurts all the time, and I have a headache." Donna thinks she might have the flu. The physician examines Donna and decides to admit her to the labor and birth unit immediately. Laboratory tests demonstrate an abnormal peripheral smear, liver enzymes—AST >70 International Units/L and LDH >600 International Units/L, and a platelet count of 80,000/mm^3.

1. Evidence—Is there sufficient evidence to draw conclusions about Donna's diagnosis?
2. Assumptions—Describe the rationale for each of the following:
   a. Probable diagnosis
   b. Signs and symptoms associated with this diagnosis
   c. Laboratory values associated with this diagnosis
   d. Risk factors associated with the diagnosis
3. What implications and priorities for nursing care can be drawn at this time?
4. Does the evidence objectively support your conclusion?
5. Are there alternative perspectives to your conclusion?

! NURSING ALERT

An extremely important point to understand is that many women with HELLP syndrome may not have signs or symptoms of severe preeclampsia. For example, although most women have hypertension, BP may be only mildly elevated in 50% of cases. Proteinuria may be absent. As a result, women with HELLP syndrome are often misdiagnosed with a variety of other medical or surgical disorders (Sibai, 2007).

CARE MANAGEMENT

Identifying and Preventing Preeclampsia

Numerous clinical trials have examined various interventions to prevent preeclampsia such as low-dose aspirin, antioxidants, calcium, magnesium, zinc, restricted protein or sodium intake,

EVIDENCE-BASED PRACTICE

Pat Gingrich

Preeclampsia Risk Factors and Prevention

ASK THE QUESTION

What risk factors predict preeclampsia? Once risk is identified, can anything prevent its onset?

SEARCH FOR EVIDENCE

Search Strategies

Professional organization guidelines, meta-analyses, systematic reviews, randomized controlled trials since 2008.

Databases Searched

CINAHL, Cochrane, Medline, National Guideline Clearinghouse, and the websites for the Association of Women's Health, Obstetric and Neonatal Nurses; the National Institute for Health and Clinical Excellence; and the Society of Obstetricians and Gynaecologists of Canada.

CRITICALLY ANALYZE THE DATA

Preeclampsia can endanger the fetus by impeding uteroplacental perfusion while risking maternal harm from hypertension and seizures. In high-risk women, uterine Doppler ultrasound detection of placental abnormalities can predict preeclampsia as early as the first trimester, well before symptoms start. In addition to established risk factors based on medical history, a systematic review of the association between maternal infections and the occurrence of preeclampsia revealed that periodontal disease and urinary tract infection were risk factors (Conde-Agudelo, Villar, & Lindheimer, 2008). Another systematic analysis of 16 studies found that maternal bacterial or viral infections were associated with twice the risk of preeclampsia when compared with similar women who had no infection (Rustveld, Kelsey, & Sharma, 2008). The authors suggest that this association is related to the inflammation of preeclampsia.

Prevention of preeclampsia in women at increased risk for the disease has had variable success. Professional guidelines of the SOGC (2008) recommend low-dose aspirin started before 16 weeks of gestation, plus calcium supplementation for women with low calcium intake. The evidence for aspirin therapy was strengthened by a meta-analysis of nine trials, involving 1317 pregnant women with abnormal Doppler findings: earlier treatment (less than 16 weeks of gestation) with low-dose aspirin was associated with less preeclampsia and hypertension, and less intrauterine growth restriction (Bujold, Morency, Roberge, Lacasse, Forest, & Giguere, 2009). A Cochrane meta-analysis of 10 randomized controlled trials involving 65,000 women found that antioxidant vitamins A and E are not effective at decreasing the risk of preeclampsia (Rumbold, Duley, Crowther, & Haslam, 2008). The SOGC guidelines specifically do not recommend calorie or sodium restrictions during pregnancy, or treatment with prostaglandins or thiazide diuretics. Evidence reinforces the importance for pregnant women at risk for preeclampsia to avoid alcohol and smoking, engage in regular exercise, and take multivitamins with folate. Women may reduce the risk for preeclampsia by avoiding interpregnancy weight gain, increasing rest and decreasing stress during the third trimester (SOGC, 2008).

IMPLICATIONS FOR PRACTICE

The woman at risk for preeclampsia, especially severe or early preeclampsia, may suffer harm to her own health and compromise of the growing fetus, resulting in preterm birth or a small-for-gestational-age infant. Screening for risk factors enables more diligent observation for the onset of preeclampsia, screening and perhaps even prevention. Women at risk need education about any prescription or over-the-counter supplements and the signs and symptoms of the disease. Women who have experienced infections, especially periodontal disease and urinary tract infection, should be thoroughly assessed at prenatal visits for any sign of preeclampsia. It may be protective to decrease free-radical production by avoiding alcohol, smoking, and stress. Some treatments, such as low-dose aspirin, work best if started before 16 weeks of gestation or even before conception. Women should be aware of the increased risk of bleeding with aspirin therapy.

Health care workers will need to keep informed about the evidence, which can sometimes be contradictory. Finally, women at risk for preeclampsia and especially those who have been diagnosed should have the opportunity to ask questions and voice their fears about this poorly understood disease.

References

Bujold, E., Morency, A., Roberge, S., Lacasse, Y., Forest, J., & Giguere, Y. (2009). Acetylsalicylic acid for the prevention of preeclampsia and intra-uterine growth restriction in women with abnormal uterine artery Doppler: A systematic review and analysis. *Journal of Obstetrics and Gynaecology Canada, 31*(9), 818–826.

Conde-Agudelo, A., Villar, J., & Lindheimer, M. (2008). Maternal infections and risk of preeclampsia: Systematic review and metaanalysis. *American Journal of Obstetrics and Gynecology, 198*(1), 7–22.

Rumbold, A., Duley, L., Crowther, C., & Haslam, R. (2008). Antioxidants for preventing pre-eclampsia. *The Cochrane Database of Systematic Reviews, 2008*, 1, CD004227.

Rustveld, L., Kelsey, S., & Sharma, R. (2008). Association between maternal infections and preeclampsia: A systematic review of epidemiological studies. *Maternal Child Health Journal, 12*(2), 223–242.

Society of Obstetricians and Gynaecologists of Canada (SOCG). (2008). Diagnosis, evaluation, and management of the hypertensive disorders of pregnancy. *Journal of Obstetrics and Gynaecology Canada, 30*(3), s1–s6.

and fish oil supplements. None of these interventions demonstrated a significant benefit in preventing or reducing the severity of preeclampsia (Sibai, 2007).

No reliable test has been developed that can be used as a routine screening tool for predicting preeclampsia (Peters, 2008). Several studies found that women with high levels of two proteins in their blood (soluble endoglin and fms-like tyrosine kinase 1) were more likely to develop preeclampsia. These proteins reduce levels of placental growth factor (PIGF) (Hellwig, 2007). Another study found a correlation between preeclampsia and very low levels of 25-hydroxyvitamin D (Ravin, 2008).

Although research offers future promise, much work remains before a screening test for preeclampsia is available for widespread clinical use. Nurses should be aware of what strategies are being studied and use the most valid results, so that they can counsel pregnant women about interventions that are evidence based. Meanwhile, the best preeclampsia prevention methods include early prenatal care for the identification of women at risk and early detection of the disease.

Health Assessment and Screening

Health assessment and screening begins with a systemic evaluation, which includes history taking, physical examination, and laboratory testing. (See the Nursing Process box for more details.)

Interview. The woman's personal health profile is reviewed during the first prenatal visit. (See Chapter 15 for additional information.) The risk factors associated with the development of preeclampsia are also evaluated during the interview (see Box 27-1).

NURSING PROCESS

Mild Preeclampsia

ASSESSMENT

History

- Medical history for diabetes mellitus, renal disease, and hypertension
- History of preeclampsia in a previous pregnancy
- Family history for hypertensive disorders, diabetes mellitus, and other chronic conditions
- Social history for marital status, cultural beliefs, activity level, and lifestyle behaviors (smoking; alcohol and drug use)
- Current symptoms: presence of headache, epigastric pain, or visual disturbances

Physical examination

- Blood pressure
- Edema
- Deep tendon reflexes
- Uterine tone and tenderness; presence of vaginal bleeding

Laboratory tests

- Weekly blood tests: hematocrit, platelet count, and liver function tests (lactate dehydrogenase [LDH], aspartate aminotransferase [AST], alanine aminotransferase [ALT])
- Weekly 24-hour urine collection for protein
- Twice weekly urine dipstick determination of urine protein by health care professional (or daily testing at home by the woman)

Fetal testing

- Daily fetal movement counts
- Nonstress test or biophysical profile once or twice weekly

NURSING DIAGNOSES

Possible nursing diagnoses include:

***Anxiety* related to:**

- preeclampsia and its effect on woman and fetus

***Ineffective Individual and Family Coping* related to:**

- the woman's restricted activity and concern over a complicated pregnancy
- the woman's inability to work outside the home

***Powerlessness* related to:**

- inability to prevent or control condition and outcomes

***Ineffective Tissue Perfusion* related to:**

- hypertension
- cyclic vasospasms
- cerebral edema
- hemorrhage

***Risk for Injury (to fetus)* related to:**

- uteroplacental insufficiency
- preterm birth
- placental abruption (abruptio placentae)

EXPECTED OUTCOMES OF CARE

Expected outcomes are that the woman will:

- Recognize and immediately report abnormal signs and symptoms indicative of worsening condition.
- Adhere to the medical regimen to minimize risk to herself and her fetus.
- Identify and use available support systems.
- Verbalize her fears and concerns to cope with the condition and situation.
- Develop no signs of eclampsia and its complications.
- Give birth to a healthy infant.
- Develop no adverse sequelae from her condition or its management.

PLAN OF CARE AND INTERVENTIONS

Care for women managed at home includes:

- Reinforce the need to keep appointments at home or at the clinic or office for health care personnel to collect blood and urine specimens for testing.
- Teach how to do self assessments including blood pressure, urine dipstick testing, and daily fetal movement counts.
- Emphasize the need to keep appointments for antepartum testing (ultrasound, nonstress test, biophysical profile) to evaluate fetal growth and well-being and amniotic fluid volume.

Other care measures include the following:

- Teach how to cope with restricted activity (see the Teaching for Self-Management box: Coping with Activity Restriction).
- Recommend a nutritious, balanced diet (see the Teaching for Self-Management box: Diet for Preeclampsia).
- Review clinical signs to report (see the Teaching for Self-Management box: Assessing and Reporting Clinical Signs of Preeclampsia).
- Involve woman and family in plan of care.
- Provide emotional and psychologic support.
- Evaluate support systems.

EVALUATION

Evaluation of the effectiveness of care of the woman with mild preeclampsia is based on the expected outcomes.

Physical Examination. Accurate measurement of BP is essential in the early detection of hypertensive disorders. Personnel caring for pregnant women need to be consistent in taking and recording BP measurements in a standardized manner (see Box 13-1).

Assessment for edema is another component of the physical examination, although the presence of edema is no longer included in the definition of preeclampsia. Edema is assessed for distribution, degree, and pitting. Dependent edema is edema of the lowest or most dependent parts of the body, where hydrostatic pressure is greatest. If a pregnant woman is ambulatory, the edema may first be evident in the feet and ankles. If she is confined to bed, the edema is more likely to occur in the sacral region. Pitting edema leaves a small depression or pit after finger pressure is applied to the swollen area. The pit, which is caused by movement of fluid to adjacent tissue away

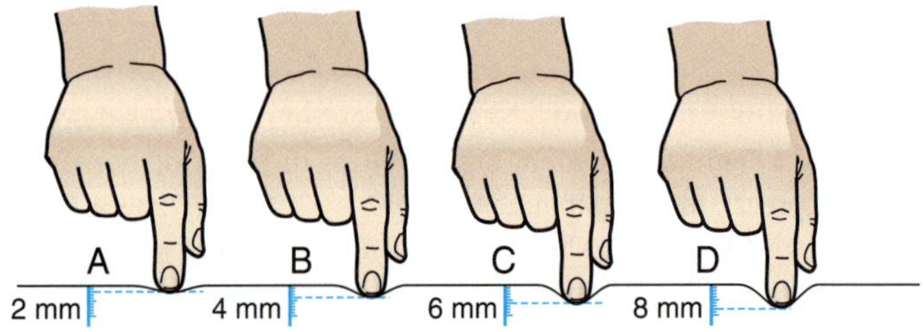

FIG. 27-3 Assessment of pitting edema of lower extremities. **A**, +1; **B**, +2; **C**, +3; **D**, +4.

from the point of pressure, normally disappears within 10 to 30 seconds. Although the amount of edema is difficult to quantify, the method shown in Figure 27-3 may be used to record relative degrees of edema formation.

Deep tendon reflexes (DTRs) reflect the balance between the cerebral cortex and spinal cord. They are evaluated as a baseline

Video—Nursing Skills: Assessing Deep Tendon Reflexes

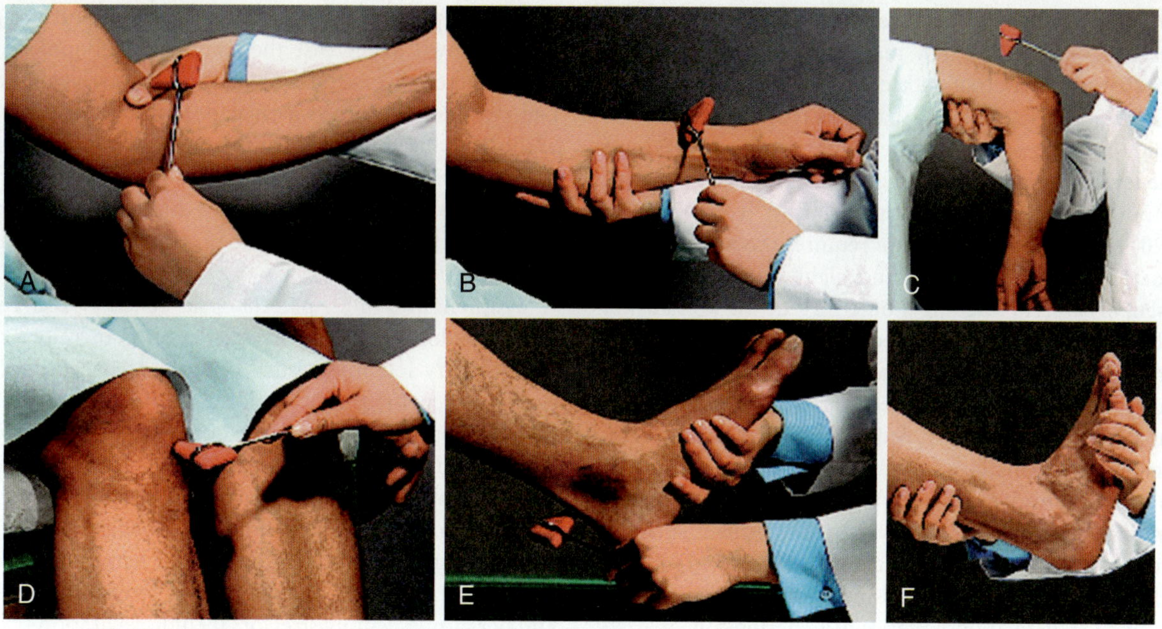

FIG. 27-4 Location of tendons for evaluation of deep tendon reflexes. **A**, Biceps. **B**, Brachioradial. **C**, Triceps. **D**, Patellar. **E**, Achilles, **F**, Evaluation of ankle clonus. (From Seidel, H., Ball, J., Dains, J., Flynn, J., Solomon, B., & Stewart, R. [2011]. *Mosby's guide to physical examination* [7th ed.]. St. Louis: Mosby.)

TABLE 27-4 ASSESSING DEEP TENDON REFLEXES

GRADE	DEEP TENDON REFLEX RESPONSE
0	No response
1+	Sluggish or diminished
2+	Active or expected response
3+	More brisk than expected, slightly hyperactive
4+	Brisk, hyperactive, with intermittent or transient clonus

Source: Seidel, H., Ball, J., Dains, J., Flynn, J., Solomon, B., & Stewart, R. (2011). *Mosby's guide to physical examination* (7th ed.). St. Louis: Mosby.

and to detect any changes. The biceps and patellar reflexes are assessed and the findings recorded (Fig. 27-4 and Table 27-4). To elicit the biceps reflex, the examiner strikes a downward blow over the thumb, which is situated over the biceps tendon (see Fig. 27-4, *A*). Normal response is flexion of the arm at the elbow, described as a 2+ response. The patellar reflex is elicited with the woman's legs hanging freely over the end of the examining table or with the woman lying on her side with the knee slightly flexed (see Fig. 27-4, *D*). The patellar tendon (inferior to the patella) is tapped with a percussion hammer. Normal response is the extension or kicking out of the leg.

To assess for hyperactive reflexes **(clonus)** at the ankle joint, the examiner supports the leg with the knee flexed (see Fig. 27-4, *F*). With one hand the examiner sharply dorsiflexes the foot, maintains the position for a moment, and then releases the foot. Normal (negative clonus) response is elicited when no rhythmic oscillations (jerks) are felt while the foot is held in dorsiflexion. When the foot is released, no oscillations are seen as the foot drops to the plantar-flexed position. Abnormal (positive clonus) response is recognized by rhythmic oscillations of one or more "beats" felt when the foot is in dorsiflexion and seen as the foot drops to the plantar-flexed position.

The presence of proteinuria is determined from dipstick testing on a clean-catch or a catheterized urine specimen or evaluation of a 24-hour urine collection. Proteinuria is defined as a concentration at or greater than 30 mg/dl (≥1+ on dipstick measurement) in at least two random urine specimens collected at least 6 hours apart. In a 24-hour specimen, proteinuria is defined as a concentration at or greater than 300 mg/24 hours. A diagnosis of severe preeclampsia requires a concentration of ≥5 g protein in a 24-hour urine collection or a value of ≥3+ on dipstick (ACOG, 2002; Sibai, 2007). Because a 24-hour collection to measure the quantity of protein and creatinine clearance is more reflective of true renal status, it is preferred over dipstick testing. Alkaline, concentrated, or dilute urine can yield a false reading. Urine contaminated with bacteria, blood, and amniotic fluid also can yield a false positive for proteinuria (Gilbert, 2011; Peters 2008).

During the examination the woman is evaluated for signs and symptoms of severe preeclampsia such as severe headaches (usually frontal), epigastric pain (heartburn), right upper quadrant abdominal pain, or visual disturbances such as scotoma, photophobia, or double vision. The signs and symptoms of mild versus severe preeclampsia are summarized in Table 27-2.

Mild Gestational Hypertension and Mild Preeclampsia

The goals of therapy for women with mild gestational hypertension and mild preeclampsia are to ensure maternal safety and to have the woman give birth to a healthy newborn as close to term as possible. At or near term the plan of care for a woman with mild gestational hypertension or mild preeclampsia is most likely to be the induction of labor, preceded, if necessary, by cervical ripening. When mild gestational hypertension or mild preeclampsia is suspected earlier in gestation the woman should be hospitalized for several days for a thorough evaluation of maternal-fetal status. After the evaluation is completed, a multidisciplinary plan of care is developed with the woman and her family. Immediate birth may not be in the best interest of the fetus. Women with mild gestational hypertension or mild preeclampsia that are less than 36 weeks of gestation may be discharged with close maternal and fetal surveillance (expectant management) (Barton & Sibai, 2008; Gilbert, 2011).

Home Care. Women with mild gestational hypertension and mild preeclampsia can be safely managed at home, provided they have frequent maternal and fetal evaluation. Criteria for home health care include BP less than 150/100; proteinuria less than 500 mg per day; normal platelet count, liver enzymes, and creatinine levels; normal (reassuring) fetal status; and no signs or symptoms of severe preeclampsia (Barton & Sibai, 2008; Gilbert, 2011). Successful home care requires the woman to be well educated about preeclampsia and highly motivated to follow the plan of care. All teaching should include the woman and her family, and time must be allowed for them to absorb information, ask questions, and voice concerns. Methods for enhancing learning include visual aids, videotapes or DVDs, handouts, and demonstrations with return demonstrations. Furthermore, the effects of illness, language, age, cultural beliefs, and support systems must be considered (see the Nursing Process box).

Maternal and Fetal Assessment. Maternal assessment includes measurement of hematocrit, platelet count, liver function tests, and a 24-hour urine protein assessment once each week. In addition, women with mild gestational hypertension or mild preeclampsia are usually seen twice weekly for the evaluation of BP and urine protein by dipstick. Women may also be asked to take their BP and perform urine dipstick testing each day (see the Teaching for Self-Management box: Assessing and Reporting Clinical Signs of Preeclampsia). Fetal evaluation usually includes daily fetal movement counts and nonstress testing or a biophysical profile once or twice weekly until birth. (See Chapter 26 for more information on fetal assessment tests.) Ultrasound evaluation of amniotic fluid volume and determination of estimated fetal weight are performed at the time mild preeclampsia is diagnosed and serially thereafter, depending on findings (Sibai, 2007).

Activity Restriction. Complete or partial bed rest for the duration of the pregnancy is still frequently recommended. However, no evidence has been found that this practice improves pregnancy outcome. Moreover, prolonged bed rest is known to increase the risk of thrombophlebitis (Sibai, 2007). Other adverse physiologic outcomes related to complete bed rest include cardiovascular deconditioning; diuresis with accompanying fluid, electrolyte, and weight loss; muscle atrophy; and psychologic stress. These changes begin on the first day of bed rest and continue for the duration of therapy. Therefore, restricted activity, rather than complete bed rest, is recommended (Sibai).

Women with mild preeclampsia generally feel reasonably well; boredom from activity restriction is therefore common. Diversionary activities, visits from friends, telephone conversations, and creation of a comfortable and convenient environment are ways to cope with the boredom. Gentle exercise (e.g., range of motion exercises, stretching, Kegel exercises, pelvic tilts) is important in maintaining muscle tone, blood flow, regularity of bowel function, and a sense of well-being (see the Teaching for Self-Management box: Coping with Activity Restriction).

A high risk pregnancy can be very stressful for the woman and her family. Family stressors include separation from family members when hospitalized, need for activity restriction, financial concerns, ability to manage the household, family activities, and child care. The family will need to use coping mechanisms and support systems to help them through this crisis. An excellent web-based support group for pregnant women on bed rest is Sidelines (www. sidelines.org) (Gilbert, 2011). Relaxation techniques can also help to reduce stress and prepare the woman for labor and birth.

Diet. Women with mild preeclampsia may have a regular diet with adequate protein (60 to 70 g), calcium (1200 mg), 400 mcg of folic acid, and adequate zinc and sodium (2 to 6 g). Adequate fluid intake (six to eight 8-ounce glasses of water per day) is encouraged to enhance renal perfusion and bowel function (Gilbert, 2011). (See the Teaching for Self-Management box: Diet for Preeclampsia.)

TEACHING FOR SELF-MANAGEMENT

Assessing and Reporting Clinical Signs of Preeclampsia

- Take your blood pressure as directed. Use the same arm in a sitting position each time for consistent and accurate readings. Support the arm on a table in a horizontal position at heart level.
- Report to your health care provider immediately any increase in your blood pressure.
- Dipstick test your clean-catch urine sample as directed to assess proteinuria.
- Report to your health care provider if proteinuria is 2+ or more or if you have a decrease in urine output.
- Assess your baby's activity daily. Decreased activity (four or fewer movements per hour) may indicate fetal compromise and should be reported.
- Be sure to keep your scheduled prenatal appointments so that any changes in your or your baby's condition can be detected.
- Keep a daily log or diary of your assessments for your home health care nurse, or bring it with you to your next prenatal visit.
- Report to your health care provider immediately any headache, dizziness, blurring of vision, or muscular irritability (seizures).

Severe Gestational Hypertension and Severe Preeclampsia

Women with severe gestational hypertension are at greater risk for pregnancy complications than are women with mild preeclampsia. Therefore, women with severe gestational hypertension should be managed as if they have severe preeclampsia. Women diagnosed with severe gestational hypertension or severe preeclampsia should be hospitalized immediately for a thorough evaluation of maternal-fetal status (Sibai, 2007; Sibai & Barton, 2008). Maternal assessments include monitoring of BP, urine output, cerebral status, and the presence of epigastric pain, abdominal tenderness, signs of labor, or placental abruption. Laboratory evaluation includes a platelet count, liver enzymes, and serum creatinine (see Table 27-3). Fetal assessment consists of continuous fetal heart rate (FHR) monitoring, a biophysical profile, and ultrasound assessment of fetal growth and amniotic fluid volume (Sibai).

A multidisciplinary plan of care is developed with the woman and her family. The goals of care management are to ensure maternal safety, assess the degree of maternal and fetal risk, formulate a plan for giving birth, and prevent eclampsia and other serious complications. If the pregnancy is 34 weeks of gestation or greater, birth might be accomplished promptly, either by

TEACHING FOR SELF-MANAGEMENT

Coping with Activity Restriction

AT HOME

- Clarify with your health care provider: What is bed rest? Question your activity level, positioning, bathroom privileges, children's visits, activities, personal hygiene, mobility, diet, and visitors.
- Have your computer or smart phone available at your bedside. Both devices can be used for communication with friends, to conduct business, and to shop as necessary. Also use your computer or smart phone to communicate with Internet support groups and obtain information.
- Have a television and DVD player to watch movies and a radio, CD player, or MP3 player to listen to music.
- Delegate responsibilities to family members or friends as much as possible—attend to the laundry, pick up groceries, drop off and pick up dry cleaning, meet repair people, attend to child care, organize meals.
- Have a telephone at your bedside—schedule appointments, parent teacher conferences, call friends and family.
- Egg crate mattress
- Pillows and more pillows (body pillow)
- Big trash basket
- Place a box or crate near the bed/sofa to store items such as:
  - Post-it notes
  - Cups with lids and flexible straws
  - Paper plates
  - Plastic forks, spoons, and knives
  - Baby monitor or walkie-talkies
  - Wet wipes
  - Notebook to record questions for providers, telephone numbers, to-do lists
  - Envelopes and stationery
  - Take-out menus
  - Reading materials
  - Books
  - Audio books
  - Magazines
- Stock mini-refrigerator or cooler with water or other beverages or healthy snacks.
- Plan for family time—visits and interaction, particularly with small children (see the Teaching for Self-Management box: Activities for Children of Women on Activity Restriction in Chapter 33).
- Explore your interest in a new hobby.
  - Work crossword puzzles or jigsaw puzzles.
  - Learn to embroider, smock, crochet, or knit.
  - Do mending or sewing.
- Do craft projects; make something for the baby.
- Identify relaxation exercises and activities (music) and implement.
- Arrange to have a facial, manicure/pedicure, neck massage, or other special treat when you need a lift.

IN THE HOSPITAL

- Clarify with your health care provider: What is bed rest? Question your activity level, positioning, bathroom privileges, children's visits, activities, personal hygiene, mobility, diet, and visitors.
- In addition to survival tips for the home, the following may be useful in the hospital setting:
  - Bring your own pillow, shampoo, and conditioner.
  - Have wheelchair for outside visits or visiting other antepartal women if allowed.
  - If possible, bring a laptop computer with DVD capabilities to allow you to watch movies.
  - Ask friends to bring healthy food and snacks when visiting rather than flowers.
  - Explore your interest in handheld games.
  - Work with staff regarding scheduling—obstetrics provider examinations, vital signs, nursing assessments, etc.
  - Bring earplugs to block the hospital noise.
  - Ask for a room with a view.
  - Have a large calendar and clock for easy viewing. Record significant events on the calendar.

TEACHING FOR SELF-MANAGEMENT

Diet for Preeclampsia

- Eat a nutritious, balanced diet (60-70 g protein, 1200 mg calcium, 400 mcg of folic acid, and 2 to 6 g of zinc and sodium). Consult with registered dietitian on the diet best suited for you as an individual.
- Salt foods to taste. Limiting excessively salty foods (luncheon meats, pretzels, chips, pickles, and sauerkraut) will likely be necessary to avoid a sodium intake of more than 6 g per day.
- Eat foods with roughage (whole grains, raw fruits, and vegetables).
- Drink six to eight 8-ounce glasses of water per day.
- Avoid alcohol and tobacco, and limit caffeine intake.

cesarean or after labor induction. By 34 weeks of gestation, the risks of continuing the pregnancy are considered greater than the risks of preterm birth (Sibai, 2007; Sibai & Barton, 2008).

If the pregnancy is less than 34 weeks of gestation, the plan includes pharmacologic therapy to prevent seizures and control BP, and continuous maternal-fetal surveillance for indicators of worsening condition (Sibai, 2007; Sibai & Barton, 2008). Corticosteroids (betamethasone) will be ordered to enhance fetal lung maturation. The dose is 12.5 mg intramuscularly (IM), repeated in 24 hours. Optimal benefit begins 24 hours after the first dose is administered and lasts for 7 days (Gilbert, 2011).

Women who are less than 34 weeks of gestation can be monitored closely and allowed to continue the pregnancy, if their BP is adequately controlled and fetal testing is normal (reassuring). The woman should be hospitalized in a tertiary-care center that is able to provide both maternal and neonatal intensive care. Most women managed with close observation will develop a maternal or fetal indication for giving birth within 2 weeks. Immediate birth is indicated (regardless of the gestational age) if signs of fetal stress, placental abruption, HELLP syndrome, oliguria, pulmonary edema, eclampsia, or uncontrolled high blood pressure develop (Sibai, 2007; Sibai & Barton, 2008).

Intrapartum Care. Intrapartum nursing care is directed toward the early identification of FHR abnormalities and the prevention of maternal complications. Continuous FHR and uterine contraction monitoring are initiated and the woman should be assessed for signs of placental abruption such as hypertonic contractions or vaginal bleeding. Other maternal assessments include review of the central nervous, cardiovascular, pulmonary, and renal systems. Vital signs and assessments are performed as ordered and per hospital policy (see the Nursing Care Plan). Client and family education and

NURSING CARE PLAN

Severe Preeclampsia

NURSING DIAGNOSIS

Risk for injury to woman and fetus related to CNS irritability (seizures)

Expected Outcome

Woman will show diminished signs of CNS irritability (e.g., deep tendon reflexes [DTRs] ≤2+, absence of clonus) and have no seizure activity.

Nursing Interventions/*Rationales*

- Establish baseline data (e.g., DTRs, clonus) *to use as a basis for evaluating effectiveness of treatment.*
- Administer IV magnesium sulfate per physician's orders *to decrease hyperreflexia and minimize risk of seizure activity.*
- Monitor maternal vital signs, level of consciousness, FHR, urine output, DTRs, IV flow rate, and serum levels of magnesium sulfate *to assess for and prevent magnesium sulfate toxicity (e.g., drowsiness, lethargy, slurred speech, depressed respirations, oliguria, sudden drop in blood pressure, hyporeflexia, fetal distress).*
- Have calcium gluconate or calcium chloride on the unit *to be available if needed as an antidote for magnesium sulfate toxicity.*
- Maintain a quiet, darkened environment *to avoid stimuli that may precipitate seizure activity.*

NURSING DIAGNOSIS

Ineffective tissue perfusion related to preeclampsia secondary to arteriolar vasospasm

Expected Outcome

Woman will exhibit signs of adequate tissue perfusion (i.e., adequate urine output and normal FHR tracing).

Nursing Interventions/*Rationales*

- Administer intravenous magnesium sulfate per physician order *to relax vasospasms and increase renal perfusion.*
- Place the woman on bed rest in a side-lying position *to maximize uteroplacental blood flow, reduce blood pressure, and promote diuresis.*
- Monitor the fetal heart for rate, baseline variability, and absence of late decelerations *to assess for evidence of adequate uteroplacental oxygenation.*

OTHER POSSIBLE NURSING DIAGNOSES

- *Risk for excess fluid volume* related to increased sodium retention secondary to administration of magnesium sulfate
- *Risk for impaired gas exchange* related to pulmonary edema secondary to increased vascular resistance
- *Risk for decreased cardiac output* related to use of antihypertensive drugs
- *Risk for injury* to fetus related to uteroplacental insufficiency secondary to use of antihypertensive medications

EXPECTED OUTCOMES

Woman will exhibit signs of normal fluid volume (i.e., balanced intake and output, normal serum creatinine levels, normal breath sounds), adequate oxygenation (i.e., normal respirations, full orientation to person, time, and place), normal range of cardiac output (i.e., normal pulse rate and rhythm), and fetal well-being (i.e., adequate fetal movement, normal FHR).

Nursing Interventions/*Rationales*

- Monitor the woman for signs of fluid volume excess (increased edema, decreased urine output, elevated serum creatinine level, weight gain, dyspnea, crackles) *to detect potential complications.*
- Monitor the woman for signs of impaired gas exchange (increased respirations, dyspnea, altered blood gases, hypoxemia) *to detect potential complications.*
- Monitor the woman for signs of decreased cardiac output (altered pulse rate and rhythm) *to detect potential complications.*
- Monitor the fetus for abnormal (nonreassuring) signs (decreased fetal activity, decreased FHR) *to prevent complications.*
- Record findings and report signs of increasing problems to the physician *to enable timely interventions.*

Nursing Care Plan—Severe Preeclampsia

supportive measures are also initiated (Gilbert, 2011; Simpson & Creehan, 2008).

The woman with severe preeclampsia is maintained on bed rest with the side rails up in a quiet, darkened environment. Emergency drugs, oxygen, and suction equipment should be checked and readily available (Box 27-2). In order to reduce the risk of pulmonary edema, total intravenous (IV) and oral fluids should not exceed 125 ml/hr. Intensive hemodynamic monitoring is not a routine standard of care and is indicated only in the presence of pulmonary edema or oliguria unresponsive to fluid challenge or severe hypertension unresponsive to medications. A pulmonary artery (Swan-Ganz) catheter can be inserted to evaluate central venous and pulmonary artery pressures (Gilbert, 2011; Simpson & Creehan, 2008) (see Chapter 31).

Pharmacologic Therapy

Magnesium Sulfate. Magnesium sulfate is the drug of choice in the prevention and treatment of seizure activity caused by severe preeclampsia or eclampsia. Magnesium sulfate is almost always administered intravenously as a secondary infusion (piggyback) by a volumetric infusion pump. Per protocol or physician's order, an initial loading dose of 4 to 6 g of magnesium sulfate is infused over 15 to 30 minutes. This dose is followed by a maintenance dose of magnesium sulfate that is diluted in an IV solution (e.g., 40 g of magnesium sulfate in 1000 ml of lactated Ringer's solution [1 g = 25 ml]) and administered by an infusion pump at 2 g/hr. This dose should maintain a therapeutic serum magnesium level of 4 to 7 mEq/l. After the loading

BOX 27-2 HOSPITAL PRECAUTIONARY MEASURES

- Environment:
  - Quiet
  - Nonstimulating
  - Lighting subdued
- Seizure precautions:
  - Suction equipment tested and ready to use
  - Oxygen administration equipment tested and ready to use
- Call button within easy reach
- Emergency medications available on the unit:
  - Hydralazine
  - Labetalol
  - Nifedipine
  - Magnesium sulfate
  - Calcium gluconate or calcium chloride
- Emergency birth pack accessible

dose, transient lowering of the arterial BP may occur secondary to relaxation of smooth muscle (Cunningham, Leveno, Bloom, Hauth, Rouse, & Spong, 2010; Gilbert, 2011; Sibai, 2007).

Magnesium sulfate is rarely given intramuscularly because the absorption rate cannot be controlled, injections are painful, and tissue necrosis may occur. However, the IM route may be used with some women who are being transported to a tertiary-care center. The IM dose is 4 to 5 g given in each buttock, a total of 10 g (local anesthetic can be added to the solution to reduce injection pain), and can be repeated at 4-hour intervals. The Z-track technique should be used for the deep IM injection, followed by gentle massage at the site.

! NURSING ALERT

High serum levels of magnesium can cause relaxation of smooth muscle, such as the uterus. When administered as a 4 to 6 g loading dose followed by a 1 to 2 g/hr maintenance dose, however, magnesium sulfate has not been shown to significantly affect the need for oxytocin (Pitocin) stimulation of labor. Other than a brief period of uterine muscle relaxation during and immediately after administration of the loading dose, no evidence of decreased uterine contractility has been observed (Cunningham et al., 2010).

Magnesium sulfate interferes with the release of acetylcholine at the synapses, decreasing neuromuscular irritability, depressing cardiac conduction, and decreasing CNS irritability. Because magnesium is excreted in the urine, accurate recordings of maternal urine output must be obtained. If renal function declines, all of the magnesium sulfate will not be adequately excreted resulting in magnesium toxicity. Expected side effects of magnesium sulfate are a feeling of warmth, flushing, diaphoresis, and burning at the IV site. Symptoms of mild toxicity include lethargy, muscle weakness, decreased or absent DTRs, double vision, and slurred speech. Increasing toxicity may be indicated by maternal hypotension, bradycardia, bradypnea, and cardiac arrest (Gilbert, 2011). Blood can be drawn to precisely determine the serum magnesium level if mild or severe toxicity is suspected (Box 27-3).

! NURSING ALERT

If magnesium toxicity is suspected, prompt actions are needed to prevent respiratory or cardiac arrest. The magnesium infusion should be discontinued immediately. Calcium gluconate or calcium chloride (antidotes for magnesium sulfate) can be given intravenously (Cunningham et al., 2010).

Critical Thinking Exercise—Preeclampsia

BOX 27-3 CARE OF THE WOMAN WITH PREECLAMPSIA RECEIVING MAGNESIUM SULFATE

CLIENT AND FAMILY TEACHING

- Explain technique, rationale, and reactions to expect
  - Route and rate
  - Purpose of "piggyback" infusion
- Reasons for use:
  - Tailor information to woman's readiness to learn.
  - Explain that magnesium sulfate is used to prevent disease progression.
  - Explain that magnesium sulfate is used to prevent seizures, *not* to decrease blood pressure.
- Reactions to expect from medication
  - Initially the woman will appear flushed and will feel hot, sedated, and nauseated. She may experience burning at the IV site, especially during the bolus.
  - Sedation will continue.
- Monitoring to anticipate:
  - *Maternal:* blood pressure, pulse, respiratory rate, DTRs, level of consciousness, urine output (indwelling catheter), presence of headache, visual disturbances, epigastric pain
  - *Fetal:* FHR and activity

ADMINISTRATION

- Verify physician's order.
- Position woman in side-lying position.
- Prepare solution and administer with an infusion control device (pump).
- Piggyback a solution of 40 g of magnesium sulfate in 1000 ml lactated Ringer's solution with an infusion control device at the ordered rate: loading dose—initial bolus of 4 to 6 g over 15 to 30 min; maintenance dose—2 g/hr, according to unit protocol or specific physician's order.

MATERNAL AND FETAL ASSESSMENTS

Vital signs and assessments are performed as ordered by the health care provider and per hospital protocol.

- Monitor blood pressure, pulse, respiratory rate every 15 to 30 minutes, depending on woman's condition.
- Monitor FHR and contractions continuously.
- Monitor intake and output, proteinuria, DTRs, presence of headache, visual disturbances, level of consciousness, and epigastric pain at least hourly.
- Restrict hourly fluid intake to a total of no more than 125 ml/hr; urinary output should be at least 25 to 30 ml/hr.

REPORTABLE CONDITIONS

- Blood pressure: systolic ≥160 mm Hg or diastolic ≥110 mm Hg
- Respiratory rate: ≤12 breaths/min
- Urinary output <25 to 30 ml/hr
- Presence of headache, visual disturbances, decrease in level of consciousness, or epigastric pain
- Increasing severity or loss of DTRs, increasing edema, proteinuria
- Any abnormal laboratory values (magnesium levels, platelet count, creatinine clearance, levels of uric acid, AST, ALT, prothrombin time, partial thromboplastin time, fibrinogen, fibrin split products)
- Any other significant change in maternal or fetal status

EMERGENCY MEASURES

- Keep emergency drugs and intubation equipment immediately available.
- Keep side rails up.
- Keep lights dimmed, and maintain a quiet environment.

DOCUMENTATION

- All of the above

ALT, Alanine aminotransferase; *AST,* aspartate aminotransferase; *DTRs,* deep tendon reflexes; *FHR,* fetal heart rate; *IV,* intravenous.

Magnesium sulfate does not seem to affect the FHR in a healthy term fetus. Doses of magnesium sulfate that prevent maternal seizures have been determined to be safe for the fetus. Neonatal serum magnesium levels approximate the levels of the mother (Roberts & Funai, 2009). Findings from several research studies suggest that magnesium sulfate administration during labor may provide a protective effect against the development of cerebral palsy in preterm very low birthweight infants (Cunningham et al., 2010).

SAFETY ALERT

Magnesium sulfate is considered a high-alert medication because it can cause client harm when administered incorrectly. Measures to improve the safe use of this medication include developing detailed policies, procedures, protocols, and standing orders, as well as thorough assessment and documentation. *Never* abbreviate magnesium sulfate as $MgSO_4$ anywhere in the medical record (Institute for Safe Medication Practices [ISMP], 2008).

Antihypertensive Medications. Antihypertensive medications are indicated when the systolic BP exceeds 160 mm Hg, or the diastolic BP exceeds 110 mm Hg. Maternal risks associated with severe hypertension include left ventricular failure and cerebral hemorrhage. In order to maintain uteroplacental perfusion, antihypertensive therapy must not decrease the arterial pressure too much or too rapidly. Hydralazine, labetalol, and nifedipine are effective drugs for treating hypertension intrapartum. They may also be used during pregnancy or in the postpartum period for BP control (Cunningham et al., 2010; Gilbert, 2011; Sibai, 2007). Table 27-5 compares antihypertensive agents used to treat hypertension in pregnancy.

Postpartum Care. Throughout the postpartum period the woman will need careful assessment of her vital signs, intake and output, DTRs, and level of consciousness. The magnesium sulfate infusion is continued after birth for seizure prophylaxis as ordered, usually for 12 to 24 hours. Assessments for effects and side effects continue until the medication is discontinued. Given that magnesium sulfate potentiates the action of narcotics, CNS depressants, and calcium channel blockers, these drugs must be administered with caution.

The symptoms of preeclampsia or eclampsia usually resolve within 48 hours after birth. However, approximately 30% of cases of eclampsia and HELLP syndrome occur postpartum. The nurse should regularly assess the woman for any symptoms of preeclampsia such as headaches, visual disturbances, or epigastric pain. Clinical signs that demonstrate resolution of

TABLE 27-5 PHARMACOLOGIC CONTROL OF HYPERTENSION IN PREGNANCY

ACTION	TARGET TISSUE	MATERNAL EFFECTS	FETAL EFFECTS	NURSING ACTIONS
Hydralazine (Apresoline, Neopresol)				
Arteriolar vasodilator	Peripheral arterioles: to decrease muscle tone, decrease peripheral resistance; hypothalamus and medullary vasomotor center for minor decrease in sympathetic tone	Headache, flushing, palpitation, tachycardia, some decrease in uteroplacental blood flow, increase in heart rate and cardiac output, increase in oxygen consumption, nausea and vomiting	Tachycardia; late decelerations and bradycardia if maternal diastolic pressure <90 mm Hg	Assess for effects of medication; alert mother (family) to expected effects of medication; assess blood pressure frequently because precipitous drop can lead to shock and perhaps placental abruption (abruptio placentae); if giving multiple doses, wait at least 20 minutes after the first dose is given to administer an additional dose to allow time to assess the effects of the initial dose; assess urinary output; maintain bed rest in a lateral position with side rails up; use with caution in presence of maternal tachycardia.
Labetalol Hydrochloride (Normodyne, Trandate)				
Combined alpha- and beta-blocking agent causing vasodilation without significant change in cardiac output	Peripheral arterioles (see hydralazine)	Minimal: flushing, tremulousness, orthostatic hypotension; minimal change in pulse rate	Minimal, if any	See hydralazine; less likely to cause excessive hypotension and tachycardia; less rebound hypertension than hydralazine.
Methyldopa (Aldomet)				
Maintenance therapy if needed: 250-500 mg orally every 8 hr (α_2-receptor agonist)	Postganglionic nerve endings: interferes with chemical neurotransmission to reduce peripheral vascular resistance; causes CNS sedation	Sleepiness, postural hypotension, constipation; rare: drug-induced fever in 1% of women and positive Coombs test result in 20% of women	After 4 months of maternal therapy, positive Coombs test result in infant	See hydralazine.
Nifedipine (Adalat, Procardia)				
Calcium channel blocker	Arterioles: to reduce systemic vascular resistance by relaxation of arterial smooth muscle	Headache, flushing; possible potentiation of effects on CNS if administered concurrently with magnesium sulfate; may interfere with labor	Minimal	See hydralazine; use caution if woman is also receiving magnesium sulfate

CNS, Central nervous system.

preeclampsia include diuresis and decreased edema (Barton & Sibai, 2008; Gilbert, 2011).

The preeclamptic woman is unable to tolerate excessive postpartum blood loss because of hemoconcentration. Oxytocin or prostaglandin products are used to control bleeding. Ergot products (e.g., Ergotrate, Methergine) are contraindicated because they increase BP.

Severe preeclampsia and HELLP syndrome contribute to small-for-gestational age infants and premature birth (Peters, 2008; Sibai, 2007). Nursing care that facilitates bonding and attachment includes providing the family with photographs of the infant, keeping the family informed of the infant's status, encouraging the father to visit the neonatal intensive care unit (NICU) and taking the woman to the NICU by wheelchair after her condition has stabilized (Gilbert, 2011). Postpartum recovery may be prolonged as a result of the physiologic consequences of prolonged activity restriction. The nurse should accompany the woman when she ambulates and assess for weakness, dizziness, shortness of breath, and muscle soreness.

Hypertension may persist for days or weeks after birth. Women with severe gestational hypertension or severe preeclampsia are frequently discharged from the hospital on an antihypertensive medication such as labetalol or nifedipine. If this is the case, the BP needs to be checked frequently either at home or at the health care provider's office. Often BP returns to normal within a few weeks after birth and antihypertensive medications can be discontinued.

Future Health Care. The woman with preeclampsia has a sevenfold increased risk of developing preeclampsia or eclampsia in a future pregnancy. She also has an increased risk of adverse perinatal outcomes such as preterm labor and birth, fetal growth restriction, placental abruption, and fetal death. Care management during a future pregnancy is directed toward increased maternal surveillance and frequency of prenatal visits, close monitoring for signs of severe hypertension and preeclampsia, serial ultrasound evaluation for fetal growth and amniotic fluid volume, and home blood pressure monitoring (Barton & Sibai, 2008).

Women with preeclampsia (especially early onset and severe preeclampsia) have an increased risk of chronic hypertension and cardiovascular disease later in life. The postpartum period provides an excellent opportunity to educate women about lifestyle changes that may decrease their risk for developing future health problems (Gilbert, 2011; Sibai, 2007).

ECLAMPSIA

Eclampsia is usually preceded by premonitory signs and symptoms, including persistent headache, blurred vision, severe epigastric or right upper quadrant abdominal pain, and altered mental status. However, convulsions can appear suddenly and without warning in a seemingly stable woman with only minimal BP elevations (Sibai, 2007). The convulsions that occur in eclampsia are frightening to observe. Tonic contraction of all body muscles (seen as arms flexed, hands clenched, legs inverted) precedes the tonic-clonic convulsion. During this stage muscles alternately relax and contract. Respirations are halted and then begin again with long, deep, stertorous inhalations. Hypotension follows, and muscular twitching, disorientation, and amnesia persist for a while after the convulsion.

EMERGENCY

Eclampsia

TONIC-CLONIC CONVULSION SIGNS

- Stage of invasion: 2-3 seconds, eyes are fixed, twitching of facial muscles occurs
- Stage of contraction: 15-20 seconds, eyes protrude and are bloodshot, all body muscles are in tonic contraction
- Stage of convulsion: muscles relax and contract alternately (clonic), respirations are halted and then begin again with long, deep, stertorous inhalation; coma ensues

INTERVENTION

- Keep airway patent: turn head to one side, place pillow under one shoulder or back if possible.
- Call for assistance. Do not leave the bedside.
- Protect with padded side rails up.
- Observe and record convulsion activity.

AFTER CONVULSION

- Do not leave unattended until fully alert.
- Observe for postconvulsion confusion, coma, incontinence.
- Use suction as needed.
- Administer oxygen via nonrebreather face mask at 10 L/min.
- Start intravenous fluids, and monitor for potential fluid overload.
- Give magnesium sulfate or other anticonvulsant drug as ordered.
- Insert indwelling urinary catheter.
- Monitor blood pressure.
- Monitor fetal and uterine status.
- Expedite laboratory work as ordered to monitor kidney function, liver function, coagulation system, and drug levels.
- Provide hygiene and a quiet environment.
- Support and keep woman and family informed.
- Be prepared for assisting with birth when woman is in stable condition.

Immediate Care

Nursing actions during a convulsion are directed toward ensuring a patent airway and client safety (see the Emergency box.) It is important to note the time of onset and duration of the seizure. Call for help but do not leave the bedside. Make certain that the side rails on the bed are raised; pad them with a folded blanket or pillow if possible. Women with eclampsia have been known to sustain fractures from falling out of bed during the seizure. Immediately after the convulsion, lower the head of the bed and turn the woman onto her side. This helps prevent aspiration of vomitus (Gilbert, 2011).

Nursing actions after a convulsion are directed toward maternal stabilization. First assess the status of the woman's airway, breathing, and pulse. Suction secretions from her glottis to clear the airway, insert an oral airway, and administer oxygen at 10 L/min by nonrebreather face mask. If an IV infusion is not in place, insert one with an 18-gauge needle. If an IV line was in place before the seizure, it may have infiltrated and will need to be restarted immediately. As soon as IV access is obtained, administer magnesium sulfate as ordered (Gilbert, 2011).

If eclampsia develops after initiating magnesium sulfate therapy, additional magnesium sulfate or another anticonvulsant (e.g., diazepam [Valium]) may be administered. Fetal and neonatal effects of diazepam include decreased (absent or minimal) FHR variability, neonatal hypotonia, decreased respirations, and depressed sucking reflex. However, with adequate blood magnesium levels, the eclamptic woman will rarely continue to have seizures (Chan & Winkle, 2006, Sibai, 2007).

A rapid assessment of uterine activity, cervical status, and fetal status is performed after the convulsion. During a convulsion the uterus becomes hypercontractile and hypertonic. As a result, the membranes may have ruptured or the cervix may have dilated rapidly, and birth may be imminent. The fetal heart rate tracing may demonstrate bradycardia, late decelerations, minimal baseline variability, or any combination. These findings usually resolve within a few minutes after the convulsion ends and the woman's hypoxia is corrected (Sibai, 2007). Assist the woman with hygiene and a change of linens and gown because she may have been incontinent of urine or stool during the convulsion.

! NURSING ALERT

Immediately after a seizure a woman may be very confused and can be combative. Restraints may be necessary temporarily. Several hours may be needed for the woman to regain her usual level of mental functioning so she should not be left alone. Provide emotional support to the family and discuss with them the rationale of management and the woman's progress.

Laboratory tests to evaluate liver enzymes and platelet count are ordered to assess for HELLP syndrome. Other tests include determination of electrolyte levels and clotting profile for DIC (see Table 27-3). Blood is typed and crossmatched for administration of packed red blood cells as needed.

After stabilization of the woman and fetus, a decision will be made regarding timing and method of birth. Eclampsia alone is not an indication for immediate cesarean birth. The route of birth (induction of labor versus cesarean birth) depends on maternal and fetal condition, fetal gestational age, and the cervical Bishop score. Regional anesthesia is not recommended for eclamptic women with coagulopathy or a platelet count less than 50,000/mm^3 (Sibai, 2007).

CHRONIC HYPERTENSION

Chronic hypertension affects approximately 4% to 5% of all pregnancies (Gilbert, 2011). Approximately 90% of women with chronic hypertension have primary or essential hypertension. In the remaining 10%, the hypertension is secondary to a medical condition such as renal or collagen disease (Sibai, 2007). Chronic hypertension in pregnancy is associated with an increased incidence of placental abruption, superimposed preeclampsia, and increased perinatal mortality (three- or fourfold). Fetal effects include fetal growth restriction and preterm birth (Cunningham et al., 2010).

Ideally the management of chronic hypertension in pregnancy begins before conception. An evaluation is performed to assess the cause and severity of the hypertension, and the presence of any target organ damage (e.g., heart, eye, and kidney). Moreover, the woman should be encouraged to make lifestyle changes prior to conception such as smoking and alcohol cessation, participating in aerobic exercise, and losing weight if indicated. A diet that includes a maximum of 2.4 g sodium per day is recommended (Gilbert, 2011). These lifestyle modifications should continue throughout the pregnancy.

Based on the history and physical findings, women with chronic hypertension are classified as either high or low risk for pregnancy complications. Women who are high risk are managed with antihypertensive medication and frequent assessments of maternal and fetal well-being. Methyldopa (Aldomet) is most often recommended for treating chronic hypertension in pregnancy. However, because it is rarely used for treating chronic hypertension in nonpregnant women, it may not be practical to switch medications because of pregnancy. Labetalol and nifedipine are other antihypertensive medications used during pregnancy (see Table 27-5). Women with low risk chronic hypertension may not require any antihypertensive medication at all during pregnancy (Cunningham et al., 2010; Sibai, 2007).

Women who are high risk are monitored closely, and the method and timing of the birth are dependent on the maternal and fetal status. After giving birth the woman should be monitored closely for complications such as pulmonary edema, renal failure, heart failure, and encephalopathy. Women with chronic hypertension can breastfeed if they desire. All antihypertensive medications are present to some degree in breast milk. Levels of methyldopa in breast milk appear to be low and are considered safe. Labetalol also has a low concentration in breast milk. Little is known about the transfer of calcium channel blockers, such as nifedipine, in breast milk, but no apparent side effects have been noted in infants (Sibai, 2007).

There is a need for improved prenatal screening, prevention, and treatment strategies to reduce the incidence and severity of hypertensive disorders in pregnancy and improve the health of women long term (Wagner, Barac, & Garovic, 2007).

KEY POINTS

- Hypertensive disorders during pregnancy are a leading cause of maternal and infant morbidity and mortality worldwide.
- The cause of preeclampsia is unknown. No reliable test has yet been developed that can be used as a routine screening tool for predicting preeclampsia.
- Preeclampsia is a multisystem disease. The pathophysiologic changes associated with preeclampsia are present long before clinical manifestations such as hypertension become evident.
- HELLP syndrome is a variant of severe preeclampsia, not a separate illness.
- Once preeclampsia becomes clinically evident, therapeutic interventions may slow the progression of the disease, allowing the pregnancy to continue, but the underlying pathology continues.
- Magnesium sulfate, the anticonvulsant of choice for preventing or controlling eclamptic seizures, requires careful monitoring of reflexes, respirations, and urinary output. The antidote, calcium gluconate or calcium chloride, should be on the unit.
- Nursing actions during a convulsion are directed toward ensuring a patent airway and client safety.
- Complications associated with chronic hypertension in pregnancy include placental abruption, superimposed preeclampsia, fetal growth restriction, and increased perinatal mortality.
- Women with preeclampsia have an increased risk of adverse perinatal outcomes in a future pregnancy and are at risk of developing chronic hypertension and cardiovascular disease later in life.

Audio Chapter Summaries Access an audio summary of these Key Points on evolve

REFERENCES

American Academy of Pediatrics (AAP) & American College of Obstetricians and Gynecologists (ACOG). (2007). *Guidelines for perinatal care* (6th ed.). Washington, DC: ACOG.

American College of Obstetricians and Gynecologists (ACOG). (2002). *Diagnosis and management of preeclampsia and eclampsia.* ACOG Practice Bulletin No. 33. Washington, DC: ACOG.

Askie, L., Duley, L., Henderson-Smart, D., & Stewart, L. (2007). Anti-platelet agents for prevention of preeclampsia: A meta-analysis of individual patient data. *Lancet, 369*(9575), 1791–1798.

Barton, J., & Sibai, B. (2008). Prediction and prevention of recurrent preeclampsia. *Obstetrics and Gynecology, 112*(2 Pt 1), 359–372.

Chan, P., & Winkle, C. (2006). *Gynecology and obstetrics: Current clinical strategies.* Laguna Hills, CA: CCS Publishing.

Cunningham, F., Leveno, K., Bloom, S., Hauth, J., Rouse, D., & Spong, C. (Eds.). (2010). *Williams obstetrics* (23rd ed.). New York: McGraw-Hill.

Emery, S. (2005). Hypertensive disorders of pregnancy: Overdiagnosis is appropriate. *Cleveland Clinic Journal of Medicine, 72*(4), 345–352.

Gilbert, E. (2011). *Manual of high risk pregnancy & delivery* (5th ed.). St. Louis: Mosby.

Hawfield, A., & Freedman, B. (2009). Preeclampsia: The pivotal role of the placenta in its pathophysiology and markers for early detection. *Therapeutic Advances in Cardiovascular Disease, 3*(1), 65–73.

Hellwig, J. (2007). Predicting preeclampsia. *AWHONN Lifelines, 10*(6), 456.

Institute for Safe Medication Practices (ISMP). (2008). *ISMP's list of high-alert medications.* Available at www.ismp.org. Accessed July 16, 2010.

Martin, J., Hamilton, B., Sutton, P., Ventura, S., Menacker, F., Kirmeyer, S., & Mathews, T. (2009). Births: Final data for 2006. *National Vital Statistics Reports, 57*(7), 1–102.

National High Blood Pressure Education Program Working Group on High Blood Pressure in Pregnancy. (2000). Report of the national high blood pressure education program working group on high blood pressure in pregnancy. *American Journal of Obstetrics and Gynecology, 183*(1), S1–S22.

Peters, R. (2008). High blood pressure in pregnancy. *Nursing for Women's Health, 12*(5), 412–421.

Ravin, C. (2008). Vitamin D and health. What does the latest research show? *Nursing for Women's Health, 12*(1), 70–74.

Roberts, J., & Funai, E. (2009). Pregnancy-related hypertension. In R. Creasy, R. Resnik, J. Iams, C. Lockwood, & T. Moore (Eds.), *Creasy and Resnik's maternal-fetal medicine: Principles and practice* (6th ed.). Philadelphia: Saunders.

Sibai, B. (2007). Hypertension. In S. Gabbe, J. Niebyl, & J. Simpson (Eds.), *Obstetrics: Normal and problem pregnancies* (5th ed.). Philadelphia: Churchill Livingstone.

Sibai, B., & Barton, J. (2008). Expectant management of severe preeclampsia remote from term: Patient selection, treatment, and delivery indications. *American Journal of Obstetrics and Gynecology, 196*(6), 514, e1-e9.

Simpson, K., & Creehan, P. (2008). *AWHONN's perinatal nursing* (3rd ed.). Philadelphia: Lippincott Williams & Wilkins.

Wagner, S., Barac, S., & Garovic, V. (2007). Hypertensive pregnancy disorders: Current concepts. *Journal of Clinical Hypertension, 9*(7), 560–566.

CHAPTER

28 Antepartum Hemorrhagic Disorders

Kitty Cashion

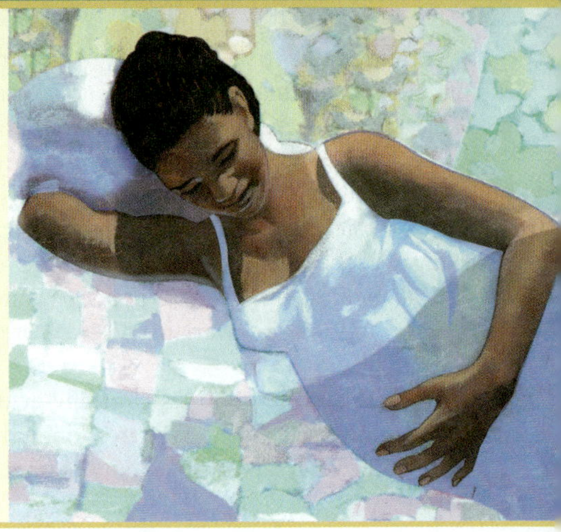

evolve WEBSITE

http://evolve.elsevier.com/Lowdermilk/MWHC/

Audio Glossary
Audio Key Points
NCLEX Review Questions
Nursing Care Plan
  Placenta Previa
Spanish Guidelines
  Assessment of Bleeding in Early Pregnancy

LEARNING OBJECTIVES

- Differentiate among causes of early pregnancy bleeding, including miscarriage, ectopic pregnancy, premature dilation of the cervix, and hydatidiform mole.
- Discuss signs and symptoms, possible complications, and management of miscarriage, ectopic pregnancy, premature dilation of the cervix, and hydatidiform mole.
- Compare and contrast placenta previa and abruptio placentae (placental abruption) in relation to signs and symptoms, complications, and management.
- Discuss the diagnosis and management of disseminated intravascular coagulation.
- Examine the role of the nurse in the health care team approach to the treatment of bleeding disorders.

Bleeding in pregnancy may jeopardize maternal and fetal well-being. Maternal blood loss decreases oxygen-carrying capacity, which places the woman at increased risk for hypovolemia, anemia, infection, and preterm labor, and adversely affects oxygen delivery to the fetus. Fetal risks from maternal hemorrhage include blood loss or anemia, hypoxemia, hypoxia, anoxia, and preterm birth. Hemorrhagic disorders in pregnancy are medical emergencies. The incidence and type of bleeding vary by trimester. Ruptured ectopic pregnancy and abruptio placentae (placental abruption) have the highest incidence of maternal mortality. Prompt assessment and intervention by the health care team is essential to save the lives of both the woman and her fetus.

EARLY PREGNANCY BLEEDING

Bleeding during early pregnancy is alarming to the woman and of concern to health care providers. The common bleeding disorders of early pregnancy include miscarriage (spontaneous abortion), premature dilation of the cervix (incompetent cervix), ectopic pregnancy, and hydatidiform mole (molar pregnancy).

Miscarriage (Spontaneous Abortion)

A pregnancy that ends as a result of natural causes before 20 weeks of gestation is defined as a **miscarriage (spontaneous abortion).** This 20-week marker is considered to be the point of viability, when a fetus may survive in an extrauterine environment. A fetal weight less than 500 g also may be used to define an abortion (Cunningham, Leveno, Bloom, Hauth, Rouse, & Spong, 2010). The term *miscarriage* is used throughout this discussion because this term is more appropriate than abortion to use with clients. Abortion may be perceived as an insensitive term to use with families who are grieving a pregnancy loss. Therapeutic or elective induced abortion is discussed in Chapter 8.

Incidence and Etiology

Approximately 10% to 15% of all clinically recognized pregnancies end in miscarriage (Simpson & Jauniaux, 2007). The majority—greater than 80% of miscarriages—are early pregnancy losses, occurring before 12 weeks of gestation (Cunningham et al., 2010). Of all clinically recognized pregnancy losses, at least 50% result from chromosomal

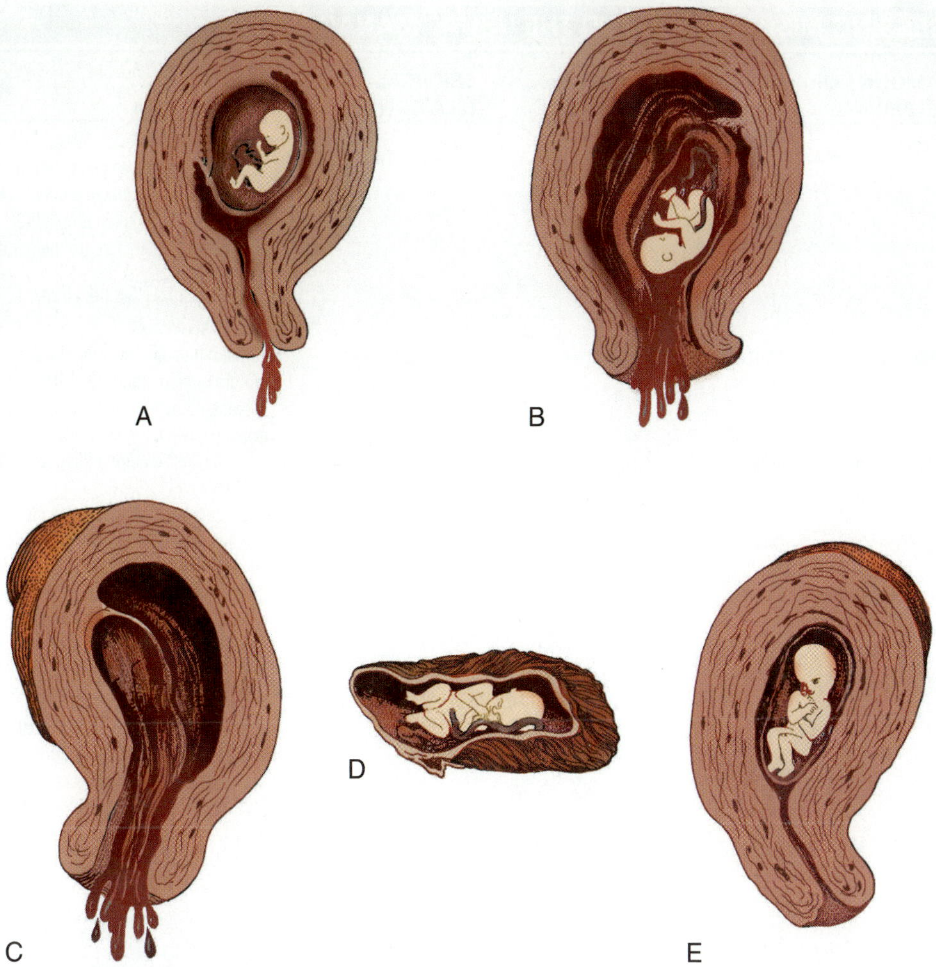

FIG. 28-1 Miscarriage. **A,** Threatened. **B,** Inevitable. **C,** Incomplete. **D,** Complete. **E,** Missed.

abnormalities (Cunningham et al.; Simpson & Jauniaux). Other possible causes of early miscarriage include endocrine imbalance (as in women who have luteal phase defects, hypothyroidism, or insulin-dependent diabetes mellitus with high blood glucose levels in the first trimester), immunologic factors (e.g., antiphospholipid antibodies), systemic disorders (e.g., lupus erythematosus), and genetic factors. Infections are not a common cause of early miscarriage (Cunningham et al.), but there is an increased risk for a spontaneous abortion with varicella infection in the first trimester (Gilbert, 2011).

A late miscarriage, sometimes called a second-trimester loss, occurs between 12 and 20 weeks of gestation. It usually results from maternal causes, such as advancing maternal age and parity, premature dilation of the cervix and other anomalies of the reproductive tract, inadequate nutrition, tobacco, alcohol, and caffeine use (Cunningham et al., 2010), obesity, and stressful life events (Gilbert, 2011). Little can be done to prevent genetically caused pregnancy loss, but correction of maternal disorders, a healthy lifestyle, adequate early prenatal care, and treatment of pregnancy complications can do much to prevent other causes of miscarriage.

Types

The types of miscarriage include threatened, inevitable, incomplete, complete, and missed. All types of miscarriage can recur in subsequent pregnancies. All types except the threatened miscarriage can lead to infection (Fig. 28-1).

Clinical Manifestations

Signs and symptoms of miscarriage depend on the duration of pregnancy. The presence of uterine bleeding, uterine contractions, or abdominal pain is an ominous sign during early pregnancy and must be considered a threatened miscarriage until proven otherwise.

If miscarriage occurs before the sixth week of pregnancy, the woman may report what she believes is a heavy menstrual flow. Miscarriage that occurs between weeks 6 and 12 of pregnancy causes moderate discomfort and blood loss. After week 12, miscarriage is typified by severe pain, similar to that of labor, because the fetus must be expelled. Diagnosis of the type of miscarriage is based on the signs and symptoms present (Table 28-1).

Symptoms of a *threatened* miscarriage (see Fig. 28-1, *A*) include spotting of blood but with the cervical os closed. Mild uterine cramping may be present.

Inevitable (see Fig. 28-1, *B*) and *incomplete* (see Fig. 28-1, *C*) miscarriages involve a moderate to heavy amount of bleeding with an open cervical os. Tissue may be present with the bleeding. Mild to severe uterine cramping may be present. An inevitable miscarriage is often accompanied by rupture of membranes (ROM) and cervical dilation. Passage of the products of conception will occur. An incomplete miscarriage involves the expulsion of the fetus with retention of the placenta.

TABLE 28-1 **ASSESSING MISCARRIAGE AND THE USUAL MANAGEMENT**

TYPE OF MISCARRIAGE	AMOUNT OF BLEEDING	UTERINE CRAMPING	PASSAGE OF TISSUE	CERVICAL DILATION	MANAGEMENT
Threatened	Slight, spotting	Mild	No	No	Bed rest is often ordered, but has not proven to be effective in preventing progression to actual miscarriage. Repetitive transvaginal ultrasounds and assessment of human chorionic gonadotropin (hCG) and progesterone levels may be done to determine if the fetus is still alive and in the uterus. Further treatment depends on whether progression to actual miscarriage occurs.
Inevitable	Moderate	Mild to severe	No	Yes	Bed rest if no pain, fever, or bleeding. If rupture of membranes (ROM), bleeding, pain or fever is present, then prompt termination of pregnancy is accomplished usually by dilation and curettage.
Incomplete	Heavy, profuse	Severe	Yes	Yes, with tissue in cervix	May or may not require additional cervical dilation before curettage. Suction curettage may be performed.
Complete	Slight	Mild	Yes	No (cervix has already closed after tissue passed)	No further intervention may be needed if uterine contractions are adequate to prevent hemorrhage and no infection is present. Suction curettage may be performed to ensure no retained fetal or maternal tissue.
Missed	None, spotting	None	No	No	If spontaneous evacuation of the uterus does not occur within 1 month, pregnancy is terminated by method appropriate to duration of pregnancy. Blood clotting factors are monitored until uterus is empty. Disseminated intravascular coagulation (DIC) and incoagulability of blood with uncontrolled hemorrhage may develop in cases of fetal death after the twelfth week, if products of conception are retained for longer than 5 weeks. May be treated with dilation and curettage or misoprostol (Cytotec) given orally or vaginally.
Septic	Varies, usually malodorous	Varies	Varies	Yes, usually	Immediate termination of pregnancy by method appropriate to duration of pregnancy. Cervical culture and sensitivity studies are performed, and broad-spectrum antibiotic therapy (e.g., ampicillin) is started. Treatment for septic shock is initiated if necessary.
Recurrent (generally defined as three or more consecutive miscarriages)	Varies	Varies	Yes	Yes, usually	Varies; depends on type. Prophylactic cerclage may be performed if premature cervical dilation is the cause. Tests of value include: parental cytogenetic analysis and lupus anticoagulant and anticardiolipin antibodies assays on the woman.

Source: Cunningham, F., Leveno, K., Bloom, S., Hauth, J., Rouse, D., & Spong, C. (2010), *Williams obstetrics* (23rd ed.). New York: McGraw-Hill; Gilbert, E. (2011). *Manual of high risk pregnancy & delivery* (5th ed.). St. Louis: Mosby.

In a *complete* miscarriage (see Fig. 28-1, *D*), the cervix has already closed after all fetal tissue was expelled. Slight bleeding may occur and mild uterine cramping may be present, as well.

The term *missed* miscarriage (see Fig. 28-1, *E*) refers to a pregnancy in which the fetus has died, but the products of conception are retained in utero for up to several weeks. It may be diagnosed by ultrasonic examination after the uterus stops increasing in size or even decreases in size. There may be no bleeding or cramping, and the cervical os remains closed.

Recurrent early (habitual) miscarriage is three or more spontaneous pregnancy losses before 20 weeks of gestation. The causes of recurrent miscarriage are the same as those discussed earlier in this section. Another possible cause of recurrent pregnancy loss is parental chromosomal abnormalities. The evaluation of couples experiencing recurrent pregnancy loss usually includes karyotyping of both partners and evaluating the woman's uterine cavity and testing for antiphospholipid antibody syndrome. No cause can be identified in approximately half of all couples who experience recurrent pregnancy loss. However, 60% to 70% of these couples will go on to have a successful pregnancy with no treatment (Cunningham et al., 2010).

Miscarriages can become septic, although this is uncommon. Symptoms of a septic miscarriage include fever and abdominal tenderness. Vaginal bleeding, which may be slight to heavy, is usually malodorous.

Management

Initial Care. Management depends on the classification of the miscarriage and on signs and symptoms (see Table 28-1). Traditionally, threatened miscarriages have been managed expectantly with supportive care. However, there

NURSING PROCESS

Miscarriage

ASSESSMENT

- History
  - Pregnancy history: last menstrual period, previous pregnancies, pregnancy losses
- Interview
  - Pain (type, location)
  - Bleeding (quantity, appearance)
  - Allergies
  - Emotional status
- Physical examination
  - Vital signs
  - Speculum vaginal examination
  - Ultrasonography
- Laboratory tests
  - β-hCG and progesterone levels (pregnancy)
  - Hemoglobin level (anemia)
  - White blood cell count (infection)

NURSING DIAGNOSES

Possible nursing diagnoses include:

***Anxiety or Fear* related to:**

- unknown outcome and unfamiliarity with medical procedures

***Deficient Fluid Volume* related to:**

- excessive bleeding secondary to miscarriage

***Acute Pain* related to:**

- uterine contractions

***Anticipatory Grieving* related to:**

- unexpected pregnancy outcome

***Situational Low Self-esteem* related to:**

- inability to successfully carry a pregnancy to term gestation

***Risk for Infection* related to:**

- surgical treatment
- dilated cervix

EXPECTED OUTCOMES OF CARE

Expected outcomes are that the woman will:

- Discuss the effect of the loss on her and her family.
- Identify and use available support systems.
- Develop no physiologic or psychologic complications (e.g., hemorrhage, infection, depression).
- Verbalize relief from pain.

PLAN OF CARE AND INTERVENTIONS

- Physiologic stabilization:
  - Initiate an intravenous line.
  - Initial laboratory tests: blood type and Rh, hemoglobin, hematocrit.
- Administer medications as ordered (antiemetics, uterotonics, antibiotics, analgesics).
- Prepare woman for manual or surgical evacuation of uterus if products of conception have not passed.
- Explain procedures.
- Offer the option of seeing the products of conception.
- Provide education on recognition of grief responses and how to manage these responses.
- Provide discharge teaching (medications, need for rest, normal physical findings, resumption of sexual activity, family planning). (See the Teaching for Self-Management box: Discharge Teaching for the Woman After Early Miscarriage.)
- Refer to support group or counseling as necessary.
- Follow up with telephone calls.

EVALUATION

Evaluation is based on the predetermined woman-centered outcomes.

are no proven effective therapies for this condition. Bed rest, although often prescribed, does not prevent progression to actual miscarriage. Repetitive transvaginal ultrasounds and measurement of human chorionic gonadotropin (hCG) and progesterone levels may be performed to determine if the fetus is alive and within the uterus (Cunningham et al., 2010).

Follow-up treatment depends on whether the threatened miscarriage progresses to actual miscarriage or symptoms subside and the pregnancy remains intact (see the Nursing Process box: Miscarriage). If bleeding and infection do not occur, expectant management is a reasonable option. In approximately half of all threatened miscarriages managed in this way, the pregnancy continues (Cunningham et al., 2010).

Once the cervix begins to dilate the pregnancy cannot continue and miscarriage becomes inevitable. If all the products of conception are passed, no surgical intervention is necessary. If heavy bleeding, excessive cramping, or infection is present, however, the remaining embryonic, fetal or placental tissue must be removed from the uterus, usually by suction curettage. In women who are clinically stable, expectant management to allow spontaneous resolution of an incomplete miscarriage is another treatment option (Cunningham et al., 2010; Gilbert, 2011).

Most missed miscarriages eventually end spontaneously. Women may be offered expectant management at the time the pregnancy loss is diagnosed. Expectant management results in eventual spontaneous miscarriage in 16% to 76% of cases (Gilbert, 2011).

Medical management is another treatment option if bleeding and infection are not present. Prostaglandin medications (e.g., misoprostol [Cytotec]) may be given orally or vaginally and is usually effective in completing the miscarriage within 7 days (Cunningham et al., 2010). If medical management is chosen, nursing care is similar to the care for any woman whose labor is being induced (see Chapter 33). Special care may be needed for management of side effects of prostaglandin, such as nausea, vomiting, and diarrhea. If the products of conception are not passed completely, the woman may be prepared for manual or surgical evacuation of the uterus.

A third management option, and one that is often chosen, is dilation and curettage (D&C), a surgical procedure in which the cervix is dilated and a suction curette is inserted to scrape the uterine walls and remove uterine contents (Cunningham et al., 2010). Before a surgical procedure is performed, a full history should be obtained and general and pelvic examinations conducted. General preoperative and postoperative care is appropriate for the woman requiring surgical intervention for miscarriage. Analgesics and anesthesia that are appropriate to the

EVIDENCE-BASED PRACTICE

Pat Gingrich

The Precarious First Trimester

ASK THE QUESTION

Are any treatments effective for preventing first trimester miscarriages? What are the recommendations for management after a miscarriage?

SEARCH FOR EVIDENCE

Search Strategies

Professional organization guidelines, meta-analyses, systematic reviews, randomized controlled trials, nonrandomized prospective studies and retrospective reviews since 2008.

Databases Searched

CINAHL, Cochrane, Medline, PUBMED.

CRITICALLY ANALYZE THE DATA

Miscarriage in the first trimester occurs in about 10% to 15% of all pregnancies. It is commonly thought to result from probable chromosomal abnormalities. Evidence suggests that placental problems are also associated with first-trimester miscarriage. A systematic review of 14 studies where pregnancy remained viable after early bleeding found that threatened miscarriages during the first trimester were associated with significantly increased antepartal hemorrhage due to placenta previa. In addition, the gestations were more at risk for preterm premature rupture of membranes, preterm birth, intrauterine growth restriction, perinatal mortality, and low birth weight (Saraswat, Bhattacharya, Maheshwari, & Bhattacharya, 2010).

Since progesterone is necessary to maintain the uterine lining, it has been suggested that inadequate progesterone could be one cause of early miscarriage. To determine whether administering progestogen (synthetic progesterone) to pregnant women could prevent miscarriage, Cochrane Database reviewers analyzed 15 trials involving 2118 women given routine progestogen in early pregnancy. Progestogen use did not prevent miscarriages except in women with a history of recurrent (3 or more) miscarriages. The reviewers found no evidence of adverse effects from the progestogen on mother or baby (Haas & Ramsey, 2008).

If miscarriage is inevitable, incomplete or missed, management has conventionally been surgical interventions to empty the uterus (curettage or vacuum aspiration), which is quick. However, medical management using misoprostol (a prostaglandin that causes uterine contractions) may be as effective and carry less risk of infection. A third option is expectant care, which involves watching and waiting for nature to take its course. A Cochrane Database Review of 15 studies involving 2750 women found that medical treatment with misoprostol and expectant care were equally successful (80% to 99%). In addition, the women were equally satisfied, and future fertility was not affected (Neilson, Gyte, Hickey, Vazquez, & Dou, 2010). Another systematic review of 21 studies found that in women who had experienced induced abortion or miscarriage, subsequent pregnancies were at greater risk for preterm birth (Swingle, Colaizy, Zimmerman, & Morriss, 2009).

IMPLICATIONS FOR PRACTICE

First-trimester bleeding can be very upsetting and frightening for newly pregnant women. Just when they were starting to develop a sense of being pregnant and imagining the future, bleeding and the possibility of miscarriage throws that future into doubt. It may be unsettling to women to have few treatment options, and to have to surrender to "nature taking its course." The all-or-nothing of first trimester miscarriages may be due to profound chromosomal changes incompatible with development. This may not be a comfort, as women may wonder if this will repeat in a later pregnancy.

If the bleeding persists and assessment reveals that the pregnancy cannot continue, women will need to be fully informed about their options: watchful waiting, medical management causing uterine contractions, or surgical emptying of remaining uterine contents. As with elective abortions, some women prefer the slower pace, lower technology and lesser risk of infection of watchful waiting or medical management. Others want to get it over with as soon as possible with dilation and suction or curettage. The surgical option is preferable in an emergent situation of rapid blood loss.

Each pregnancy is unique. Nursing care for women who are experiencing miscarriage should include assessment for the meaning that this pregnancy carries for the woman and her partner. For many women, a miscarriage is the emotional equivalent of the loss of a living child. They may feel that their body has failed them, or feel responsible and guilty. They will probably have questions about the risks for future pregnancies. Nurses are in the best position to offer support, information, and anticipatory guidance. In addition, the nurse can offer the family resources for grief, such as www.resolve.org.

References

Haas, D., & Ramsey, P. (2008). Progestogen for preventing miscarriage. *The Cochrane Database of Systematic Reviews, 2008*, 2, CD003511.

Neilson, J., Gyte, G., Hickey, M., Vazquez, J., & Dou, L. (2010). Medical treatments for incomplete miscarriage (less than 24 weeks). *The Cochrane Database of Systematic Reviews, 2010*, 1, CD007223.

Saraswat, L., Bhattacharya, S., Maheshwari, A., & Bhattacharya, S. (2010). Maternal and perinatal outcome in women with threatened miscarriage in the first trimester: A systematic review. *British Journal of Obstetrics and Gynaecology, 117*(3), 245–557.

Swingle, H., Colaizy, T., Zimmerman, M., & Morriss, F. (2009). Abortion and the risk of subsequent preterm birth: A systematic review with meta-analyses. *Journal of Reproductive Medicine, 54*(2), 95–108.

procedure are used. The nurse reinforces explanations, answers any questions or concerns, and prepares the woman for surgery.

After evacuation of the uterus, oxytocin is often given to prevent hemorrhage. For excessive bleeding after the miscarriage, ergot products such as methylergonovine (Methergine) or a prostaglandin derivative such as carboprost tromethamine (Hemabate) may be given to contract the uterus. (See the Medication Guide: Drugs Used to Manage Postpartum Hemorrhage, on p. 827 in Chapter 34). Antibiotics are given as necessary. Analgesics, such as antiprostaglandin agents (e.g., nonsteroidal anti-inflammatory drugs [NSAIDS]), may decrease discomfort from cramping. Transfusion therapy may be required for shock or anemia. The woman who is Rh negative and is not isoimmunized is given $Rh_o(D)$ immune globulin (Cunningham et al., 2010).

Psychosocial aspects of care focus on what the pregnancy loss means to the woman and her family. Grief from perinatal loss is complex and unique to each individual. Explanations are provided regarding the nature of the miscarriage, expected procedures, and possible future implications for childbearing.

As with other fetal or neonatal losses, the woman should be offered the option of seeing the products of conception. She may also want to know what the hospital does with the products of conception or whether she needs to make a decision about final disposition of fetal remains.

! NURSING ALERT

Procedures for disposition of the fetal remains vary from hospital to hospital and state to state. The nurse should know what the usual procedures are in his or her setting.

Follow-up Care at Home. The woman will likely be discharged home within a few hours after a D&C or as soon as her vital signs are stable, vaginal bleeding remains minimal, and she has recovered from anesthesia. Discharge teaching emphasizes the need for rest. If significant blood loss has occurred, iron supplementation may be ordered. Teaching includes information about normal physical findings, such as cramping, type and amount of bleeding, resumption of sexual activity, and family planning (see the Teaching for Self-Management box). Frequently the woman and her partner want to know when she may become pregnant again. Discuss with them the importance of completely resolving the loss before attempting another pregnancy (Gilbert, 2011). Follow-up care should assess the woman's physical and emotional recovery. Referrals to local support groups should be provided as needed. Share Pregnancy and Infant Loss Support, Inc. (www.nationalshare.org) is an excellent online resource for families that have experienced an early pregnancy loss.

TEACHING FOR SELF-MANAGEMENT

Discharge Teaching for the Woman After Early Miscarriage

- Clean the perineum after each voiding or bowel movement and change perineal pads often.
- Shower (avoid tub baths) for 2 weeks.
- Avoid tampon use, douching, and vaginal intercourse for 2 weeks.
- Notify physician if an elevated temperature or a foul-smelling vaginal discharge develops.
- Eat foods high in iron and protein to promote tissue repair and red blood cell replacement.
- Seek assistance from support groups, clergy, or professional counseling as needed.
- Allow yourself (and your partner) to grieve the loss before becoming pregnant again.

Follow-up telephone calls after a loss are important. The woman may appreciate a telephone call on what would have been her due date. These calls provide opportunities for the woman to ask questions, seek advice, and receive information to help process her grief.

COMMUNITY ACTIVITY

- Visit the Miscarriage Support website, which provides assistance for families who have experienced the loss of a child by miscarriage. Review the information about the stages of grief and resources. What resources are available for women that experience a perinatal loss in your community?
- Visit the American Pregnancy Association website, and go to the pregnancy complications link. Select an antepartum hemorrhagic disorder such as miscarriage, ectopic pregnancy, molar pregnancy, placental abruption, or placenta previa and evaluate the accuracy and comprehensiveness of the information in regard to causes, risk factors, symptoms, diagnosis, and treatment.

Recurrent Premature Dilation of the Cervix (Incompetent Cervix)

One cause of late miscarriage is recurrent **premature dilation of the cervix (incompetent cervix),** which has traditionally been defined as passive and painless dilation of the cervix during the second trimester. This definition assumes an all-or-nothing role for the cervix: it is either competent or incompetent. Current thinking is that cervical competence is variable and exists as a continuum that is determined in part by cervical length. Other related causative factors include composition of the cervical tissue and the individual circumstances associated with the pregnancy in terms of maternal stress and lifestyle. Iams (2009) refers to this condition as *cervical insufficiency.*

Etiology

Etiologic factors include a history of previous cervical trauma such as lacerations during childbirth, excessive cervical dilation for curettage or biopsy, or ingestion of diethylstilbestrol (DES) by the woman's mother while pregnant with the woman. Because DES has not been used since the early 1970s, however, this risk factor should soon be of only historic interest. Multiple gestation alone does not produce reduced cervical competency or justify prophylactic cervical cerclage (Ludmir & Owen, 2007). Other causes are a congenitally short cervix and cervical or uterine anomalies.

Diagnosis

Reduced cervical competence is a clinical diagnosis, based on history. Short labors, recurring loss of the pregnancy at progressively earlier gestational ages, advanced cervical dilation at the time of first presentation for care, and a history of prior cervical surgery or trauma suggest reduced cervical competence (Iams, 2009). Ultrasound examination during pregnancy is used to diagnose this condition objectively. A short cervix (less than 25 mm) is indicative of reduced cervical competence. Often the short cervix is accompanied by **cervical funneling** (beaking) or effacement of the internal cervical os (Cunningham et al., 2010; Iams; Ludmir & Owen, 2007).

Management

Medical management consists of bed rest, pessaries, antibiotics, antiinflammatory drugs, and progesterone supplementation (Iams, 2009). Surgical management, with placement of a cervical **cerclage,** may be chosen instead. During pregnancy the McDonald technique is often the procedure of choice. In this procedure suture is placed around the cervix beneath the mucosa to constrict the internal os of the cervix (Fig. 28-2) (Cunningham et al., 2010). A cerclage may be placed prophylactically or as a rescue procedure once the cervix has been found to be effaced or dilated (Cunningham et al.; Gilbert, 2011).

A prophylactic cerclage is usually placed at 11 to 15 weeks of gestation. The cerclage is electively removed (usually an office or a clinic procedure) when the woman reaches 37 weeks of gestation, or it may be left in place until spontaneous labor begins. Occasionally the cerclage is left in place and a cesarean birth performed. The best treatment for reduced cervical competence is uncertain at this time. Research results indicate that selective cerclage placement during pregnancy based on

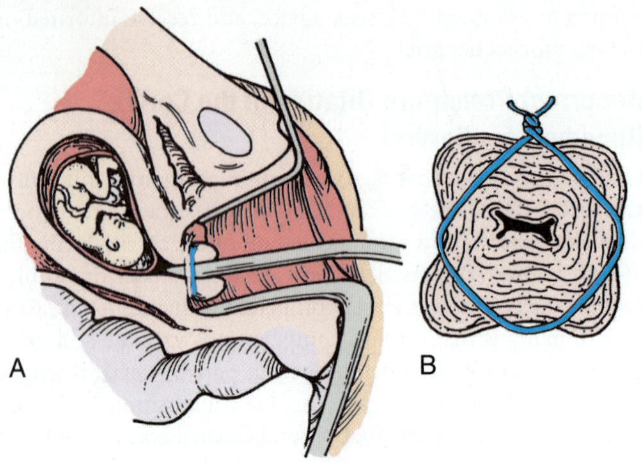

FIG. 28-2 **A,** Cerclage correction of premature dilation of the cervical os. **B,** Cross-sectional view of closed internal os.

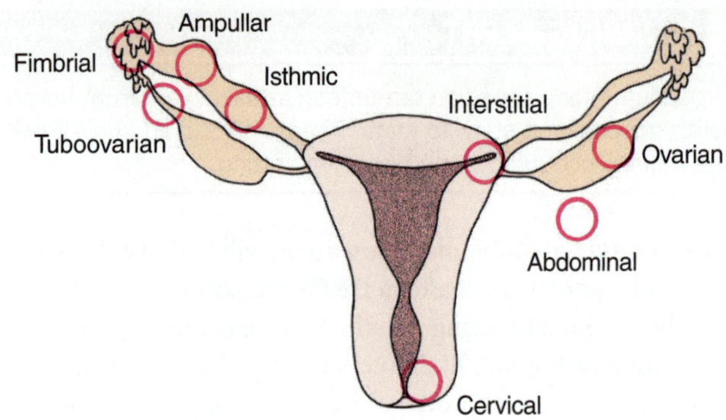

FIG. 28-3 Sites of implantation of ectopic pregnancies. Order of frequency of occurrence is ampulla, isthmus, interstitium, fimbria, tubo-ovarian ligament, ovary, abdominal cavity, and cervix (external os).

repeated ultrasound examination of the cervix may produce pregnancy outcomes that are just as good as those obtained after prophylactic cerclage placement. Ultrasound surveillance begins at 15 to 16 weeks of gestation. Cerclage placement is offered if the cervical length falls to less than 20 to 25 mm before 23 to 24 weeks (Iams, 2009). Risks of the procedure include premature rupture of membranes (PROM), preterm labor, and chorioamnionitis. Although no consensus has been reached, 24 weeks is often used as the upper gestational age limit for cerclage placement (Iams).

The nurse assesses the woman's feelings about her pregnancy and her understanding of reduced cervical competence. Evaluating the woman's support systems is also important. Because the diagnosis of reduced cervical competence is usually not made until the woman has lost one or more pregnancies, she may feel guilty or to blame for this impending loss. Assessing for previous reactions to stresses and appropriateness of coping responses is therefore important. The woman needs the support of her health care providers, as well as that of her family.

Follow-up Care at Home

The woman will likely be on bed rest for a least a few days immediately following cerclage placement. She will also probably be advised to avoid sexual intercourse until after a postoperative check. Thereafter, decisions about physical activity and intercourse are individualized, based on the status of the woman's cervix, as determined by digital and ultrasound examination (Ludmir & Owen, 2007). The woman must understand the importance of initial activity restriction at home and the need for close observation and supervision. Tocolytic medications may be prescribed to prevent uterine contractions and further dilation of the cervix. If so, the woman must be instructed on the expected response and possible side effects. Additional instruction includes the need to watch for and report signs of preterm labor, ROM, and infection. Finally, the woman should know the signs that would warrant an immediate return to the hospital, including strong contractions less than 5 minutes apart, ROM, severe perineal pressure, and an urge to push. If management is unsuccessful and the fetus is born before viability, appropriate grief support should be provided. If the fetus is born prematurely, appropriate anticipatory guidance and support will be necessary.

Ectopic Pregnancy

Incidence and Etiology

An **ectopic pregnancy** is one in which the fertilized ovum is implanted outside the uterine cavity (Fig. 28-3). Two percent of all first-trimester pregnancies in the United States are ectopic, and these account for 9% of all pregnancy-related maternal deaths. Women are less likely to have a successful subsequent pregnancy after an ectopic pregnancy (Cunningham et al., 2010; Gilbert, 2011). Ectopic pregnancy is also a leading cause of infertility.

Ectopic pregnancies are often called *tubal pregnancies* because approximately 95% are located in the uterine tube (Cunningham et al., 2010). Although they are much less common, ectopic pregnancies can also occur in the abdominal cavity, on an ovary, or on the cervix. Of all tubal ectopic pregnancies, more than half (approximately 55%) are located in the ampulla, or largest portion of the tube (Gilbert, 2011).

The reported incidence of ectopic pregnancy rose through 1990 in the United States. Since then, because more cases are managed medically, reliable data on the actual number of ectopic pregnancies have not been available (Cunningham et al., 2010). Some of the increased incidence is likely because of improved diagnostic techniques, such as more sensitive β-hCG measurement and transvaginal ultrasound, resulting in the identification of more cases. Other causes for the rise include an increased incidence of sexually transmitted infections, tubal infection and damage, popularity of contraceptive methods that predispose failures to be ectopic (e.g., the intrauterine device [IUD]), use of tubal sterilization methods that increase the chance of ectopic pregnancy, increased use of assisted reproductive techniques, and increased use of tubal surgery (Cunningham et al.; Gilbert, 2011).

Ectopic pregnancy is classified according to site of implantation (e.g., tubal, ovarian, or abdominal). The uterus is the only organ capable of containing and sustaining a term pregnancy. Only approximately 5% of abdominal pregnancies reach viability. Surgery to remove the embryo or fetus is usually performed as soon as an abdominal pregnancy is identified, however, because of the high risk for hemorrhage at any time during the pregnancy (Cunningham et al., 2010; Gilbert, 2011). The chance of fetal survival in an abdominal pregnancy depends on gestational age at birth. The risk for fetal deformity in an abdominal pregnancy is high as a result of pressure deformities

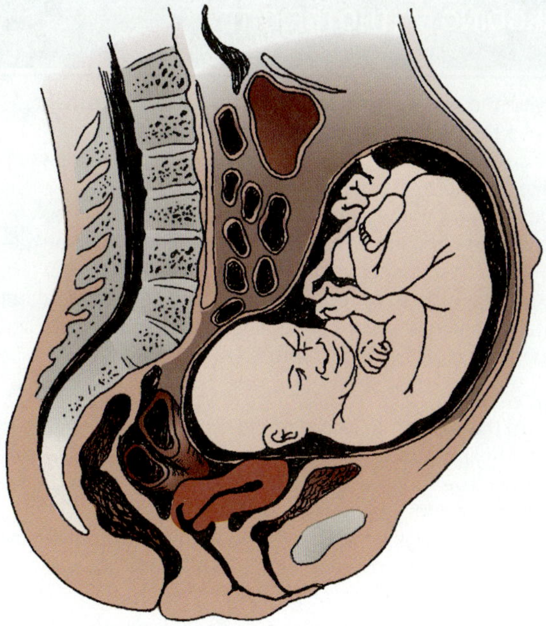

FIG. 28-4 Ectopic pregnancy, abdominal.

caused by oligohydramnios. The most common problems include facial or cranial asymmetry, various joint deformities, limb deficiency, and central nervous system anomalies (Fig. 28-4) (Cunningham et al.; Gilbert).

Clinical Manifestations

Most cases of ectopic (tubal) pregnancy are diagnosed before rupture based on the three most classic symptoms: (1) abdominal pain, (2) delayed menses, and (3) abnormal vaginal bleeding (spotting) that occurs approximately 6 to 8 weeks after the last normal menstrual period (Gilbert, 2011). Abdominal pain occurs in almost every case. It usually begins as a dull, lower quadrant pain on one side. The discomfort can progress from a dull pain to a colicky pain when the tube stretches, to sharp, stabbing pain (Cunningham et al., 2010; Gilbert). It progresses to a diffuse, constant, severe pain that is generalized throughout the lower abdomen (Gilbert). Up to 90% of women with an ectopic pregnancy report a period that is delayed 1 to 2 weeks or is lighter than usual, or an irregular period. Mild to moderate dark red or brown intermittent vaginal bleeding occurs in up to 80% of women (Gilbert).

If the ectopic pregnancy is not diagnosed until after rupture has occurred, referred shoulder pain may be present in addition to generalized, one-sided, or deep lower quadrant acute abdominal pain. Referred shoulder pain results from diaphragmatic irritation caused by blood in the peritoneal cavity. The woman may exhibit signs of shock, such as faintness and dizziness, related to the amount of bleeding in the abdominal cavity and not necessarily related to obvious vaginal bleeding. An ecchymotic blueness around the umbilicus (Cullen sign), indicating hematoperitoneum, may also develop in an undiagnosed, ruptured intraabdominal ectopic pregnancy.

Tubal Pregnancy Management

The differential diagnosis of ectopic pregnancy involves consideration of numerous disorders that share many signs and symptoms. Many of these women come to the emergency department experiencing first-trimester bleeding or pain. Miscarriage, ruptured corpus luteum cyst, appendicitis, salpingitis, ovarian cysts, torsion of the ovary, and urinary tract infection are possible diagnoses. The key to early detection of ectopic pregnancy is having a high index of suspicion for this condition. Every woman with abdominal pain, vaginal spotting or bleeding, and a positive pregnancy test should undergo screening for ectopic pregnancy.

The most important screening tools for ectopic pregnancy are quantitative β-hCG levels and transvaginal ultrasound examination. When β-hCG levels are greater than 1500 to 2000 milli-International Units/ml, a normal intrauterine pregnancy should be visible on transvaginal ultrasound. Therefore, if β-hCG levels are greater than 1500 milli-International Units/ml but no intrauterine pregnancy is seen on transvaginal ultrasound, an ectopic pregnancy is very likely. β-hCG levels will probably be redrawn every 48 hours to determine if the pregnancy is viable. A transvaginal ultrasound may also be repeated to determine if the pregnancy is inside the uterus. Sometimes the location of an ectopic pregnancy will be visible on transvaginal ultrasound (Cunningham et al., 2010; Gilbert, 2011).

Another laboratory test that can be ordered to decide if the pregnancy is developing normally is a progesterone level. A progesterone level greater than 25 ng/ml almost always rules out the presence of an ectopic pregnancy. However, a progesterone level less than 5 ng/ml suggests either an ectopic pregnancy or an abnormal intrauterine pregnancy (Cunningham et al., 2010).

The woman should also be assessed for the presence of active bleeding, which is associated with tubal rupture. If internal bleeding is present, assessment may reveal vertigo, shoulder pain, hypotension, and tachycardia. A vaginal examination should be performed only once, and then with great caution. Approximately 20% of women with a tubal pregnancy have a palpable mass on examination. Rupturing the mass is possible during a bimanual examination, thus a gentle touch is critical.

Initial Care

Medical Management. Medical management involves giving methotrexate to dissolve the tubal pregnancy. Methotrexate is an antimetabolite and folic acid antagonist that destroys rapidly dividing cells. The woman must be hemodynamically stable to be eligible for medical management. The best results following methotrexate therapy are usually obtained if the mass is unruptured and measures less than 3.5 cm in diameter by ultrasound, if no fetal cardiac activity is noted on ultrasound, and if the serum β-hCG level is less than 5000 milli-International Units/ml (Cunningham et al., 2010). To be a candidate for medical management, the woman must also be willing to comply with posttreatment lifestyle restrictions and monitoring. Methotrexate therapy avoids surgery and is a safe, effective, and cost-effective way of managing many cases of tubal pregnancy. The woman is informed of how the medication works, possible side effects, whom to call if she has concerns or if problems develop, and the importance of follow-up care (Box 28-1).

> **! NURSING ALERT**
>
> The woman on methotrexate therapy who drinks alcohol and takes vitamins containing folic acid (such as prenatal vitamins) increases her risk of having side effects of the drug or exacerbating the ectopic rupture.

BOX 28-1 NURSING CONSIDERATIONS FOR WOMEN UNDERGOING METHOTREXATE TREATMENT FOR ECTOPIC PREGNANCY

ADMINISTRATION

- Obtain woman's height and weight.
- Check to make sure laboratory and diagnostic tests have been completed, including:
  - Complete blood cell count and blood type and Rh-antibody status
  - Liver and renal function tests
  - Serum β-hCG levels (Should be < 5000 milli-international Units/ml)
  - Transvaginal ultrasound confirming size of mass and absence of fetal cardiac activity
- Administer methotrexate 50 mg/m² intramuscular (IM)
- Administer Rh_o(D) immune globulin (150 mcg to 300 mcg IM as ordered if woman has Rh-negative blood).

CLIENT AND FAMILY TEACHING

- Review how methotrexate works.
- Inform the woman of possible side effects—gas pain, stomatitis and conjunctivitis are common; rare effects include pleuritis, gastritis, diarrhea, oral ulcers, dermatitis, alopecia, enteritis, increased liver enzymes, and bone marrow suppression.
- Advise the woman to discontinue folic acid supplements.
- Advise the woman to avoid "gas-forming" foods.
- Advise the woman to avoid sun exposure because the drug will make her more photosensitive.
- Advise the woman to refrain from strenuous activities.
- Advise the woman to avoid putting anything in her vagina—no tampons, douches, or vaginal intercourse.
- Advise the woman to report to her health care provider immediately if she has severe abdominal pain that may be a sign of impending or actual tubal rupture.

FOLLOW-UP

- Inform the woman to return to the clinic or office as instructed by her health care provider for measurement of β-hCG level.
- If β-hCG level does not drop appropriately, a second dose of methotrexate may be necessary.
- Advise the woman that she will need to return to the clinic or office for weekly measurements of β-hCG until the level is less than 15 milli-International Units/ml. Weekly follow-up visits may be required for several months until the desired β-hCG level is reached.

Sources: Gilbert, E. (2011). *Manual of high risk pregnancy & delivery* (5th ed.). St. Louis: Mosby; Murray, H., Baakdah, H., Bardell, T., & Tulandi, T. (2005). Diagnosis and treatment of ectopic pregnancy. *Canadian Medical Association Journal, 173*(8), 905-912.

Surgical Management. Surgical management depends on the location and cause of the ectopic pregnancy, the extent of tissue involvement, and the woman's desires regarding future fertility. One option is removal of the entire tube (salpingectomy). If the tube has not ruptured and the woman desires future fertility, salpingostomy may be performed instead. In this procedure an incision is made over the pregnancy site in the tube and the products of conception are gently and very carefully removed. The incision is not sutured but left to close by secondary intention instead, given that this method results in less scarring.

If surgery is planned, general preoperative and postoperative care is appropriate for the woman with an ectopic pregnancy. Before surgery, vital signs (pulse, respirations, and blood pressure [BP]) are assessed every 15 minutes or as needed, according to the severity of the bleeding and the woman's condition. Preoperative laboratory tests include determination of blood type and Rh factor, complete blood cell count, and serum quantitative β-hCG level. Ultrasonography is used to confirm an extrauterine pregnancy. Blood replacement may be necessary. The nurse verifies the woman's Rh and antibody status and administers Rh_o(D) immune globulin postoperatively if appropriate.

Follow-up Care. The woman and her family should be encouraged to share their feelings and concerns related to the loss. Future fertility should be discussed. A contraceptive method should be used for at least three menstrual cycles to allow time for the woman's body to heal (Gilbert, 2011). Every woman who has been diagnosed with an ectopic pregnancy should be instructed to contact her health care provider as soon as she suspects that she might be pregnant because of the increased risk for recurrent ectopic pregnancy. These women may need referral to grief or infertility support groups. In addition to the loss of the current pregnancy, they are faced with the possibility of future pregnancy losses or infertility.

Hydatidiform Mole (Molar Pregnancy)

Hydatidiform mole (molar pregnancy) is a benign proliferative growth of the placental trophoblast in which the chorionic villi develop into edematous, cystic, avascular transparent vesicles that hang in a grapelike cluster. Hydatidiform mole is a gestational trophoblastic disease. Gestational trophoblastic disease (GTD) is a group of pregnancy-related trophoblastic proliferative disorders without a viable fetus. In addition to hydatidiform mole, GTD includes invasive mole, gestational choriocarcinoma, placental site trophoblastic tumor, and gestational trophoblastic neoplasia (GTN) (American College of Obstetricians and Gynecologists [ACOG], 2004). (See Chapter 11 for a discussion of GTN.)

Incidence and Etiology

Hydatidiform mole occurs in 1 in 1000 pregnancies in the United States (Cohn, Ramaswamy, & Blum, 2009). The cause is unknown, although it may be related to an ovular defect or a nutritional deficiency. Women at increased risk for hydatidiform mole formation are those who have had ovulation stimulation with clomiphene (Clomid) and those who are in their early teens or older than 40 years of age. Other risk factors include history of miscarriage and nutritional factors (e.g., deficient intake of carotene and animal fats) (Bess & Wood, 2006; Cohn et al.).

Types

A hydatidiform mole may be further categorized as a complete or partial mole. The complete mole results from fertilization of an egg in which the nucleus has been lost or inactivated (Fig. 28-5, *A*). The nucleus of a sperm (23,X) duplicates itself (resulting in the diploid number 46,XX) because the ovum has no genetic material or the material is inactive. It is also possible for an "empty" egg to be fertilized by two normal sperm, thereby

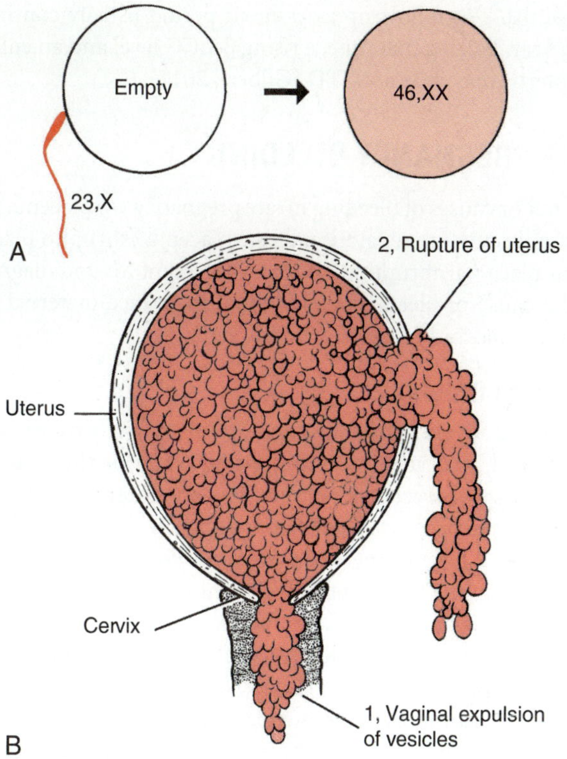

FIG. 28-5 **A,** Chromosomal origin of complete mole. Single sperm *(color)* fertilizes an "empty" ovum. Reduplication of sperm's 23,X set gives completely homozygous diploid 46,XX. **B,** Uterine rupture with hydatidiform mole. *1,* Vaginal expulsion of mole through cervix. *2,* Rupture of uterus and spillage of mole into peritoneal cavity (rare).

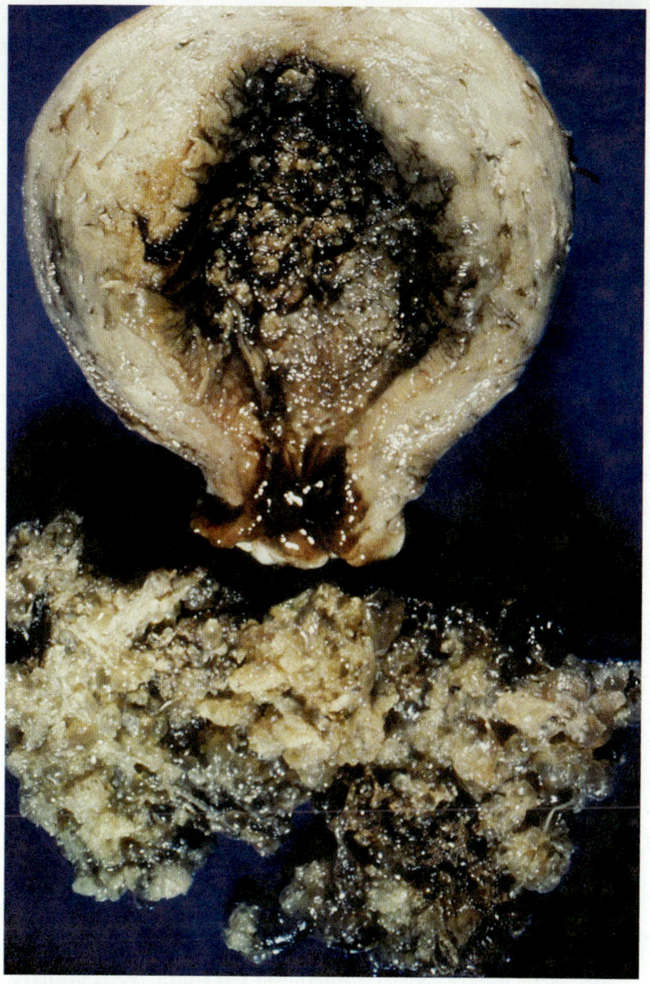

FIG. 28-6 Gross specimen in a woman treated for complete hydatidiform mole with primary hysterectomy. (Courtesy John Soper, M.D.) (From DiSaia P., & Creasman W. [2007]: *Clinical gynecologic oncology* [7th ed.]. Philadelphia: Mosby.)

producing either a 46,XX or 46,XY karyotype. The mole resembles a bunch of white grapes (see Fig. 28-5, *B*). The hydropic (fluid-filled) vesicles grow rapidly, causing the uterus to be larger than expected for the duration of the pregnancy. Usually the complete mole contains no fetus, placenta, amniotic membranes, or fluid (Fig. 28-6). Maternal blood has no placenta to receive it; therefore, hemorrhage into the uterine cavity and vaginal bleeding occur. Approximately 15% to 20% of women with a complete mole have evidence of persistent GTD (Cunningham et al., 2010).

For a partial mole, chromosomal studies often show a karyotype of 69,XXY; 69,XXX; or rarely 69,XYY. This arrangement occurs as a result of two sperm fertilizing an apparently normal ovum (Fig. 28-7). Partial moles often have embryonic or fetal parts and an amniotic sac. Congenital anomalies are usually present. The risk of persistent GTD is much less than with a complete mole. If persistent GTD does occur, it is usually not a choriocarcinoma (Cunningham et al., 2010).

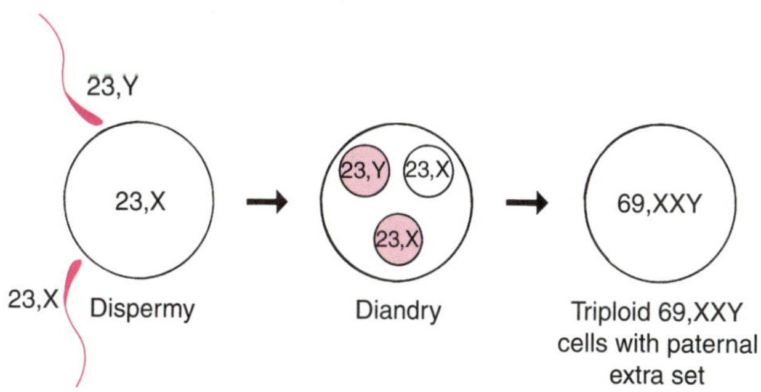

FIG. 28-7 Chromosomal origin of triploid partial mole. Normal ovum with 23,X haploid set is fertilized by two sperms to give total of 69 chromosomes. Sex configuration of XXY, XXX, or XYY is possible.

Clinical Manifestations

In the early stages the clinical manifestations of a complete hydatidiform mole cannot be distinguished from those of normal pregnancy. Later, vaginal bleeding occurs in almost 95% of cases. The vaginal discharge may be dark brown (resembling prune juice) or bright red and either scant or profuse. It may continue for only a few days or intermittently for weeks. Early in pregnancy the uterus in approximately one half of affected women is significantly larger than expected from menstrual dates. The percentage of women with an excessively enlarged uterus increases as length of time since the last menstrual period increases. Approximately 25% of affected women have a uterus smaller than would be expected from menstrual dates.

Anemia from blood loss, excessive nausea and vomiting (hyperemesis gravidarum), and abdominal cramps caused by uterine distention are relatively common findings. Women may also pass vesicles, which are frequently avascular edematous villi, from the uterus. Preeclampsia occurs in approximately

70% of women with large, rapidly growing hydatidiform moles and occurs earlier than usual in the pregnancy. If preeclampsia is diagnosed before 24 weeks of gestation, hydatidiform mole should be suspected and ruled out. Hyperthyroidism is another serious complication of hydatidiform mole. Usually treatment of the hydatidiform mole restores thyroid function to normal. Partial moles cause few of these symptoms and may be mistaken for an incomplete or missed miscarriage (Cohn et al., 2009; Nader, 2009; Roberts & Funai, 2009).

Diagnosis

Transvaginal ultrasound and serum hCG levels are used for diagnosis. Transvaginal ultrasound is the most accurate tool for diagnosing a hydatidiform mole. A characteristic pattern of multiple diffuse intrauterine masses, often called a *snowstorm pattern,* is seen in place of, or along with, an embryo or a fetus. The trophoblastic tissue secretes the hCG hormone. In a molar pregnancy, hCG levels are persistently high or rising beyond 10 to 12 weeks of gestation, the time they would begin to decline in a normal pregnancy (Gilbert, 2011).

Management

Although most moles abort spontaneously, suction curettage offers a safe, rapid, and effective method of evacuating a hydatidiform mole if necessary (Cunningham et al., 2010; Gilbert, 2011). Induction of labor with oxytocic agents or prostaglandin is not recommended because of the increased risk of embolization of trophoblastic tissue. Post-evacuation administration of Rh_o(D) immune globulin to women who are Rh negative is necessary to prevent isoimmunization (Gilbert).

The nurse provides the woman and her family with information about the disease process, the necessity for a long course of follow-up, and the possible consequences of the disease. The nurse also helps the woman and her family cope with the pregnancy loss and recognize that the pregnancy was not normal. In addition, the woman and her family are encouraged to express their feelings, and information is provided about local support groups or counseling resources as needed. Internet resources such as Share: Pregnancy and Infant Loss Support, Inc., at www.nationalshare.org and the International Society for the Study of Trophoblastic Disease at www.isstd.org may also be useful. Explanations about the importance of postponing a subsequent pregnancy and contraceptive counseling are provided to emphasize the need for consistent and reliable use of the method chosen.

> **! NURSING ALERT**
>
> To avoid confusion in regard to rising levels of hCG that are normal in pregnancy but could indicate GTD, pregnancy should be avoided during the follow-up assessment period. Any contraceptive method except an IUD is acceptable. Oral contraceptives are preferred because they are highly effective.

Follow-up Care

Follow-up care includes frequent physical and pelvic examinations along with weekly measurements of the β-hCG level until the level decreases to normal and remains normal for 3 consecutive weeks. Monthly measurements are then taken for 6 months. The follow-up assessment period usually continues for a year. During that time, a rising β-hCG level and an enlarging uterus may indicate GTD (Gilbert, 2011).

LATE PREGNANCY BLEEDING

The major causes of bleeding in late pregnancy are placenta previa and premature separation of the placenta (abruptio placentae or placental abruption). Rapid assessment for and diagnosis of the cause of bleeding are essential to reduce maternal and perinatal morbidity and mortality (Table 28-2).

Placenta Previa

Because of advances in ultrasonography, especially transvaginal ultrasound, and an increased understanding of the changing relationship between the placenta and the internal cervical os as pregnancy progresses, definitions and classifications of placenta previa have changed. In **placenta previa** the placenta is implanted in the lower uterine segment such that it completely or partially covers the cervix or is close enough to the cervix to cause bleeding when the cervix dilates or the lower uterine segment effaces (Fig. 28-8) (Hull & Resnik, 2009). When transvaginal ultrasound is used, the placenta is classified as a *complete placenta previa* if it totally covers the internal cervical os. In a *marginal placenta previa* the edge of the placenta is seen on transvaginal ultrasound to be 2.5 cm or closer to the internal cervical os. When the exact relationship of the placenta to the internal cervical os has not been determined or in the case of apparent placenta previa in the second trimester, the term *low-lying placenta* is used (Hull & Resnik).

Incidence and Etiology

Placenta previa affects approximately 1 in 200 pregnancies at term. Some evidence suggests that the incidence of placenta previa is increasing, perhaps as a result of the increasing cesarean birth rate. In addition to a history of previous cesarean birth, other risk factors for placenta previa include advanced maternal age (more than 35 to 40 years of age), multiparity, history of prior suction curettage, and smoking (Hull & Resnik, 2009). Cigarette smoking leads to a decrease in uteroplacental oxygenation and thus a need for increased placental surface area. Placenta previa is more likely to occur in women with multiple gestations because of the larger placental area associated with these pregnancies. Women who had placenta previa in a previous pregnancy are more likely than others to develop the problem in a subsequent pregnancy, perhaps as a result of a genetic predisposition. Previous cesarean birth and curettage in the past for miscarriage or induced abortion are risk factors for placenta previa because both result in endometrial damage and uterine scarring (Francois & Foley, 2007; Hull & Resnik).

Clinical Manifestations

Placenta previa is typically characterized by painless bright red vaginal bleeding during the second or third trimester. In the past, placenta previa was usually diagnosed after an episode of bleeding. Currently, however, most cases are diagnosed by ultrasound before significant vaginal bleeding occurs. This bleeding is associated with the disruption of placental blood vessels that occurs with stretching and thinning of the lower

TABLE 28-2 **SUMMARY OF FINDINGS: ABRUPTIO PLACENTAE AND PLACENTA PREVIA**

	ABRUPTIO PLACENTAE			
	GRADE 1 MILD SEPARATION (10%-20%)	GRADE 2 MODERATE SEPARATION (20%-50%)	GRADE 3 SEVERE SEPARATION (>50%)	PLACENTA PREVIA
Bleeding, external, vaginal	Minimal	Absent to moderate	Absent to moderate	Minimal to severe and life threatening
Total amount of blood loss	<500 ml	1000-1500 ml	>1500 ml	Varies
Color of blood	Dark red	Dark red	Dark red	Bright red
Shock	Rare; none	Mild shock	Common, often sudden, profound	Uncommon
Coagulopathy	Rare, none	Occasional DIC	Frequent DIC	None
Uterine tonicity	Normal	Increased, may be localized to one region or diffuse over uterus, uterus fails to relax between contractions	Tetanic, persistent uterine contractions, boardlike uterus	Normal
Tenderness (pain)	Usually absent	Present	Agonizing, unremitting uterine pain	Absent
Ultrasonographic Findings				
Location of placenta	Normal, upper uterine segment	Normal, upper uterine segment	Normal, upper uterine segment	Abnormal, lower uterine segment
Station of presenting part	Variable to engaged	Variable to engaged	Variable to engaged	High, not engaged
Fetal position	Usual distribution*	Usual distribution*	Usual distribution*	Commonly transverse, breech, or oblique
Gestational or chronic hypertension	Usual distribution*	Commonly present	Commonly present	Usual distribution*
Fetal effects	Normal fetal heart rate and pattern	Abnormal (nonreassuring) fetal heart rate and pattern	Abnormal (nonreassuring) fetal heart rate and pattern; fetal death can occur	Normal fetal heart rate and pattern

*Usual distribution refers to the expected variations of incidence seen when there is no concurrent problem.
DIC, Disseminated intravascular coagulation.

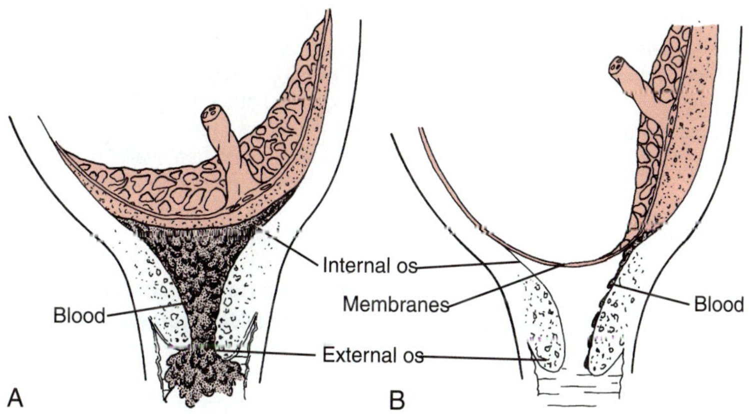

FIG. 28-8 Types of placenta previa. **A,** Complete. **B,** Marginal.

uterine segment (Francois & Foley, 2007). The initial bleeding is usually a small amount and stops as clots form. It can recur, however, at any time (Gilbert, 2011).

Vital signs may be normal, even with heavy blood loss, because a pregnant woman can lose up to 40% of her blood volume without showing signs of shock. Clinical presentation and decreasing urinary output may be better indicators of acute blood loss than vital signs alone. The fetal heart rate (FHR) is normal (reassuring) unless a major detachment of the placenta occurs.

Abdominal examination usually reveals a soft, relaxed, nontender uterus with normal tone. The presenting part of the fetus usually remains high because the placenta occupies the lower uterine segment. Thus the fundal height is often greater than expected for gestational age. Because of the abnormally located placenta, fetal malpresentation (breech and transverse or oblique lie) is common.

Maternal and Fetal Outcomes

The major maternal complication associated with placenta previa is hemorrhage. Another serious complication is development of an abnormal placental attachment (e.g., *placenta accreta*, *increta*, or *percreta*) (see Chapter 34). If excessive bleeding cannot be controlled, hysterectomy may be necessary (Cunningham et al., 2010; Hull & Resnik, 2009). Because most women with placenta previa give birth by cesarean, surgery-related trauma to structures adjacent to the uterus and anesthesia complications are also possible. In addition, blood transfusion reactions, anemia, thrombophlebitis, and infection may occur.

The greatest risk of fetal death is caused by preterm birth. Other fetal risks include stillbirth, malpresentation and fetal anemia. Intrauterine growth restriction (IUGR) has also been associated with placenta previa. This association can be related to poor placental exchange (Gilbert, 2011). One study found an increased incidence of fetal anomalies in pregnancies complicated by placenta previa (Cunningham et al., 2010).

Diagnosis

All women with painless vaginal bleeding after 20 weeks of gestation should be assumed to have a placenta previa until proven otherwise. A transabdominal ultrasound examination should be performed initially followed by a transvaginal scan, unless the transabdominal ultrasound clearly shows that the placenta is not located in the lower uterine segment. A transvaginal ultrasound is better than a transabdominal scan for accurately determining placental location (Hull & Resnik, 2009). If ultrasonographic scanning reveals a normally implanted placenta, a speculum examination may be performed to rule out local causes of bleeding (e.g., cervicitis, polyps, carcinoma of the cervix), and a coagulation profile is obtained to rule out other causes of bleeding.

Management

Once placenta previa has been diagnosed, a management plan is developed. The woman will be managed either expectantly or actively, depending on the gestational age, amount of bleeding, and fetal condition (see the Nursing Process box: Placenta Previa).

Expectant Management. Expectant management (observation and bed rest) is implemented if the fetus is at less than 36 weeks of gestation and has a normal (reassuring) FHR tracing, the bleeding is mild (<250 ml) and stops, and the woman is not in labor. The purpose of expectant management is to allow the fetus time to mature (Gilbert, 2011). The woman will initially be hospitalized in a labor and birth unit for continuous FHR and contraction monitoring. Large-bore intravenous (IV) access should be initiated immediately. Initial laboratory tests include hemoglobin, hematocrit, platelet count, and coagulation studies. A "type and screen" blood sample should be maintained at all times in the hospital's transfusion services department to allow for immediate crossmatch of blood component therapy if necessary. If the woman is at less than 34 weeks of gestation, antenatal corticosteroids should be administered (Francois & Foley, 2007; Gilbert).

If the bleeding stops, the woman will most likely be placed on bed rest with bathroom privileges and limited activity (able to use the bathroom, shower, and move around her hospital room for 15 to 30 minutes at a time, four times a day). No vaginal or rectal examinations are performed, and the woman is placed on "pelvic rest" (nothing in the vagina). Ultrasonographic examinations may be performed every 2 to 3 weeks. Fetal surveillance may include a nonstress test (NST) or biophysical profile

NURSING PROCESS

Placenta Previa

ASSESSMENT

- History
  - Pregnancy (gravidity, parity, estimated date of birth)
- Interview
  - General status
  - Bleeding (quantity, precipitating event, associated pain)
- Physical examination
  - Vital signs
  - Fetal status
  - Abdominal exam (soft, relaxed, nontender, with normal tone)
- Laboratory tests
  - Complete blood cell count
  - Blood type and Rh factor
  - Coagulation profile
  - Possible type and cross match
- Abdominal or transvaginal ultrasound or both

NURSING DIAGNOSES

Possible nursing diagnoses include:

***Decreased Cardiac Output* related to:**
- excessive blood loss secondary to placenta previa

***Deficient Fluid Volume* related to:**
- excessive blood loss secondary to placenta previa

***Ineffective Peripheral Tissue Perfusion* related to:**
- hypovolemia and shunting of blood to central circulation

***Anxiety or Fear* related to:**
- maternal condition and pregnancy outcome

***Grieving* related to:**
- actual or perceived threat to self, pregnancy, or infant

EXPECTED OUTCOMES OF CARE

Expected outcomes are that the woman will:
- Verbalize understanding of her condition and its management.
- Identify and use available support systems.
- Demonstrate compliance with prescribed activity limitations.
- Develop no complications related to bleeding.
- Give birth to a healthy term infant.

PLAN OF CARE AND INTERVENTIONS

Expected Management
- Place on bed rest with bathroom privileges and limited activity.
- Monitor maternal vital signs.
- Monitor blood loss:
  - Estimate and record amount of blood on disposable pads, perineal pads, and bed linens.
  - Obtain serial hematocrit or hemoglobin levels.
- Maintain a "type and screen" sample in the hospital's transfusion services department at all times.
- Monitor fetal condition: Perform a nonstress test or biophysical profile once or twice per week as ordered.
- Place on "pelvic rest."
  - No vaginal examinations!
  - No douching.
  - No vaginal intercourse.
- Provide emotional support to the woman and her family.
- Administer medications as ordered.
- Provide diversionary activities.
- Notify hospital chaplain or other support services as desired by the woman.
- Be prepared for an emergency cesarean birth at any time.

EVALUATION

The expected outcomes of care are used to evaluate the care for the woman with placenta previa.

Nursing Care Plan—Placenta Previa

(BPP) once or twice weekly. Bleeding is assessed by checking the amount of bleeding on perineal pads, bed pads, and linens. Serial laboratory values are evaluated for decreasing hemoglobin and hematocrit levels and changes in coagulation values. The woman should also be monitored for signs of preterm labor. Magnesium sulfate can be given for tocolysis if uterine contractions are identified (Francois & Foley, 2007; Gilbert, 2011).

The woman with placenta previa should always be considered a potential emergency because massive blood loss with resulting hypovolemic shock can occur quickly if bleeding resumes. The possibility always exists that she will require an emergency cesarean for birth. Placenta previa in a preterm gestation may be an indication for transfer to a tertiary-care perinatal center, given that a neonatal intensive care unit may be necessary for care of the preterm infant. Also, because many community hospitals are not prepared to perform emergency surgery 24 hours per day, 7 days per week, transfer to a tertiary-care center may be necessary to ensure constant access to cesarean birth.

Home Care. Sometimes women with placenta previa are discharged from the hospital before giving birth to be managed at home. The woman's condition should be stable, and she should have experienced no vaginal bleeding for at least 48 hours before discharge (Hull & Resnik, 2009). A candidate for home care must meet other strict criteria as well. She should be willing and able to comply with activity restrictions (bed rest with bathroom privileges and pelvic rest), have access to a telephone, close supervision by family or friends in the home, and constant access to transportation. If bleeding resumes, she will need to return to the hospital immediately. She must also be able to keep all appointments for fetal testing, laboratory assessments, and prenatal care. Visits by a perinatal home care nurse may be arranged.

If hospitalization or home care with activity restriction is prolonged, the woman may have concerns about her work- or family-related responsibilities or may become bored with inactivity. She should be encouraged to participate in her own care and decisions about care as much as possible. Provision of diversionary activities or encouragement to participate in activities she enjoys and can perform during bed rest is needed. Participation in a support group made up of other women on bed rest while hospitalized or online if at home may be a helpful coping mechanism. (See the Teaching for Self-Management box: Coping with Activity Restriction on page 663 in Chapter 27.)

Active Management. If the woman is at or beyond 36 weeks of gestation or bleeding is excessive or persistent, immediate cesarean birth is indicated (Hull & Resnik, 2009). Expectant management will be terminated as soon as the fetus is mature, if excessive bleeding develops, active labor begins, or any other obstetric reason to terminate the pregnancy (e.g., chorioamnionitis) develops (Gilbert, 2011). Cesarean birth is indicated in all women with ultrasound evidence of placenta previa. An asymptomatic woman whose placenta lies more than 2 cm from the cervical os, however, can labor safely (Francois & Foley, 2007; Hull & Resnik).

If cesarean birth is planned, the nurse continuously assesses maternal and fetal status while preparing the woman for surgery. Maternal vital signs are assessed frequently for decreasing BP, increasing pulse rate, changes in level of consciousness, and oliguria. Fetal assessment is maintained by continuous electronic fetal monitoring (EFM) to assess for signs of hypoxia.

Blood loss may not cease with the birth of the infant. The large vascular channels in the lower uterine segment may continue to bleed because of that segment's diminished muscle content. The natural mechanism to control bleeding so characteristic of the upper part of the uterus—the interlacing muscle bundles, the "living ligature" contracting around open vessels—is absent in the lower part of the uterus. Postpartum hemorrhage may therefore occur even if the fundus is contracted firmly (see Chapter 34).

Emotional support for the woman and her family is extremely important. The actively bleeding woman is concerned not only for her own well-being but also for the well-being of her fetus. All procedures should be explained, and a support person should be present. The woman should be encouraged to express her concerns and feelings. If the woman and her support person or family desire pastoral support, the nurse can notify the hospital chaplain service or provide information about other supportive resources.

Premature Separation of Placenta (Abruptio Placentae [Placental Abruption])

Premature separation of the placenta, or **abruptio placentae,** is the detachment of part or all of a normally implanted placenta from the uterus (Fig. 28-9). Separation occurs in the area of the decidua basalis after 20 weeks of gestation and before the birth of the infant.

Incidence and Etiology

Premature separation of the placenta is a serious complication that accounts for significant maternal and fetal morbidity and mortality. Approximately 1 in 75 to 1 in 226 pregnancies is complicated by placental abruption. The range in incidence likely reflects both variable criteria for diagnosis and an increased recognition of milder forms of abruption. Approximately one third of all antepartum bleeding is caused by placental abruption (Francois & Foley, 2007).

Maternal hypertension, whether chronic or pregnancy related, is the most consistently identified risk factor for abruption. Cocaine use is also a risk factor because it causes vascular disruption in the placental bed. Blunt external abdominal trauma, most often the result of motor vehicle accidents (MVAs)

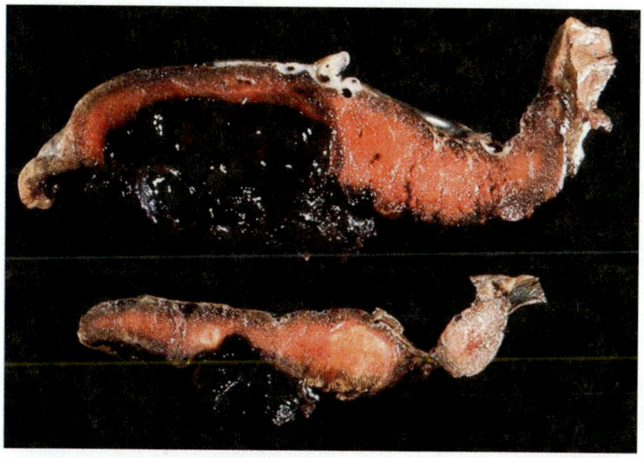

FIG. 28-9 Abruptio placentae. Premature separation of normally implanted placenta. A large retroplacental clot is present. (From Creasy, R., Resnik, R., Iams, J., Lockwood, C., & Moore, T. [2009]. *Creasy & Resnik's maternal-fetal medicine: Principles and practice* [6th ed.]. Philadelphia: Saunders.)

CLINICAL REASONING

Third-Trimester Vaginal Bleeding

Ashley is a 29-year-old G6 P5 who presents to the emergency department with heavy vaginal bleeding and contractions. She has had no prenatal care, but is approximately 33 weeks of gestation by her LMP. During her medical screening examination Ashley admitted to past cocaine use and reported that her boyfriend punched her in the abdomen earlier in the day.

1. Evidence—Is there sufficient evidence at this time to diagnose the cause of Ashley's bleeding?
2. What assumptions can be made about the following:
   a. Possible diagnoses for Ashley
   b. Laboratory and diagnostic tests necessary to diagnose the cause of Ashley's bleeding
   c. Management options for Ashley
3. What implications and priorities for nursing care can be drawn at this time?
4. Does the evidence objectively support your conclusion?
5. Are there alternative perspectives to your conclusions?

or maternal battering, is another frequent cause of placental abruption (Cunningham et al., 2010; Francois & Foley, 2007). Other risk factors include cigarette smoking, a history of abruption in a previous pregnancy, preterm PROM, and the presence of inherited or acquired thrombophilias (e.g., factor V Leiden mutation or protein S deficiency) (Cunningham et al.; Hull & Resnik, 2009; Paidas & Hossain, 2009). Abruption is more likely to occur in twin gestations than in singletons (Francois & Foley). Women who have had two previous abruptions have a recurrence risk of 25% in the next pregnancy (Hull & Resnik).

Classification

The most common classification of placental abruption is according to type and severity. This classification system is summarized in Table 28-2.

Clinical Manifestations

The separation may be partial or complete, or only the margin of the placenta may be involved. Bleeding from the placental site may dissect (separate) the membranes from the decidua basalis and flow out through the vagina (70% to 80%), it may remain concealed (retroplacental hemorrhage) (10% to 20%), or both (Fig. 28-10) (Francois & Foley, 2007; Gilbert, 2011). Clinical symptoms vary with degree of separation (see Table 28-2). If cesarean birth is performed, blood clots may be noted on entry into the uterus. A blood clot often will be attached to the posterior surface of the placenta (referred to as a retroplacental clot) (see Fig 28-9).

Classic symptoms of placental abruption include vaginal bleeding, abdominal pain, and uterine tenderness and contractions (Cunningham et al., 2010; Hull & Resnik, 2009). Bleeding may result in maternal hypovolemia (i.e., shock, oliguria, anuria) and coagulopathy. Mild to severe uterine hypertonicity is present. Pain is mild to severe and localized over one region of the uterus or diffuse over the uterus with a boardlike abdomen.

Extensive myometrial bleeding damages the uterine muscle. If blood accumulates between the separated placenta and the uterine wall, it may produce a **couvelaire uterus.** The uterus appears purple or blue, rather than its usual "bubble-gum pink" color, and contractility is lost. Shock may occur and is out of proportion

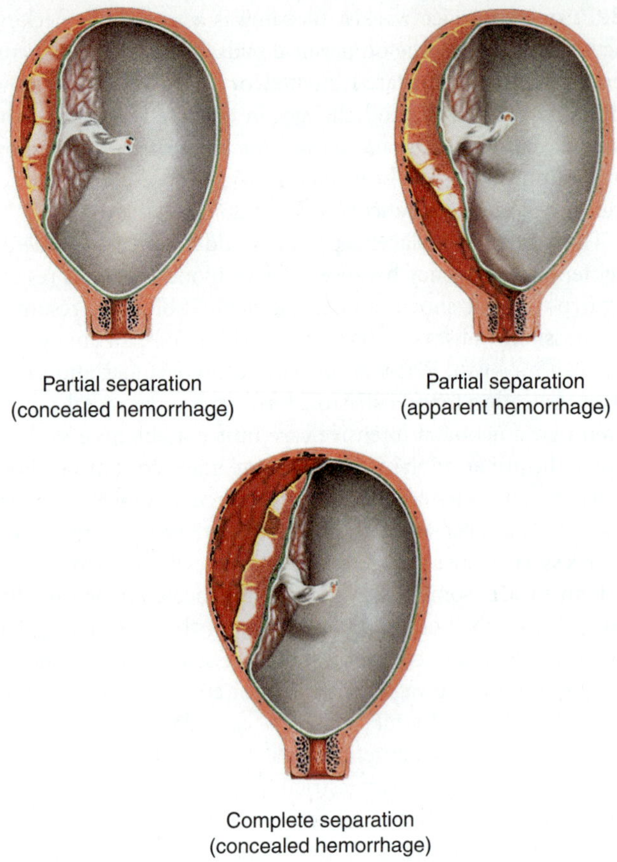

FIG. 28-10 Abruptio placentae, showing partial and complete placental separation.

to blood loss. Laboratory findings include a positive Apt test result (blood in the amniotic fluid); a decrease in hemoglobin and hematocrit levels, which may appear later; and a decrease in coagulation factor levels. Clotting defects (e.g., disseminated intravascular coagulation) are present in approximately 40% of women who develop a large abruption (Francois & Foley, 2007). A Kleihauer-Betke (KB) test may be ordered to determine the presence of fetal-to-maternal bleeding (transplacental hemorrhage), although this test appears to have no value in the general workup of women with abruption. The KB test may be useful to guide Rh_o(D) immune globulin therapy in Rh-negative women who have had an abruption (Hull & Resnik, 2009).

Maternal and Fetal Outcomes

The mother's prognosis depends on the extent of placental detachment, overall blood loss, degree of coagulopathy present and time between placental detachment and birth. Maternal complications are associated with the abruption or its treatment. Hemorrhage, hypovolemic shock, hypofibrinogenemia, and thrombocytopenia are associated with severe abruption. Renal failure and pituitary necrosis may result from ischemia. In rare cases, women who are Rh negative can become sensitized if fetal-to-maternal hemorrhage occurs and the fetal blood type is Rh positive.

Placental abruption is associated with a perinatal mortality rate of 20% to 30%. If more than 50% of the placenta is involved, fetal death is likely to occur. Other fetal and neonatal risks include IUGR and preterm birth (Francois & Foley, 2007; Hull & Resnik, 2009). Risks for neurologic defects, cerebral palsy, and death from sudden infant death syndrome are also increased in newborns following placental abruption (Cunningham et al., 2010; Francois & Foley).

Diagnosis

Placental abruption is primarily a clinical diagnosis. Although ultrasound can be used to rule out placenta previa, it cannot detect all cases of abruption. A retroplacental mass may be detected with ultrasonographic examination, but negative findings do not rule out a life-threatening abruption. In fact, at least 50% of abruptions cannot be identified on ultrasound (Hull & Resnik, 2009). Hypofibrinogenemia and evidence of DIC support the diagnosis, but many women with placental abruption do not develop coagulopathy. The diagnosis of abruption is confirmed after birth by visual inspection of the placenta. Adherent clot on the maternal surface of the placenta and depression of the underlying placental surface are usually present (see Fig. 28-9) (Francois & Foley, 2007; Gilbert, 2011).

Placental abruption should be highly suspected in the woman who experiences a sudden onset of intense, usually localized, uterine pain, with or without vaginal bleeding. Initial assessment is much the same as for placenta previa. Physical examination usually reveals abdominal pain, uterine tenderness, and contractions. The fundal height may be measured over time because an increasing fundal height indicates concealed bleeding. Approximately 60% of live fetuses exhibit abnormal (nonreassuring) FHR patterns, and elevated uterine resting tone may also be noted on the monitor tracing (Francois & Foley, 2007). Coagulopathy, as evidenced by abnormal clotting studies (fibrinogen, platelet count, partial thromboplastin time [PTT], fibrin split products), may be present if a large or complete abruption has occurred.

Management

Expectant Management. Management depends on the severity of blood loss and fetal maturity and status. If the fetus is less than 34 weeks of gestation and both the woman and fetus are stable, expectant management can be implemented. The woman is monitored closely because the abruption may extend at any time. The fetus will be regularly assessed for evidence of appropriate growth, because there is risk for IUGR. In addition, assessments of fetal well-being (e.g., NST and BPP) are performed regularly. See Chapter 26 for further discussion of these tests. Corticosteroids will be given to accelerate fetal lung maturity (Hull & Resnik, 2009).

Active management. Immediate birth is the management of choice if the fetus is at term gestation or if the bleeding is moderate to severe and the mother or fetus is in jeopardy. At least one large-bore (16- to 18-gauge) IV line should be started. Maternal vital signs are monitored frequently to observe for signs of declining hemodynamic status, such as increasing pulse rate and decreasing BP. Serial laboratory studies include hematocrit or hemoglobin determinations and clotting studies. Continuous EFM is mandatory. An indwelling catheter is inserted for continuous assessment of urine output, an excellent indirect measure of maternal organ perfusion. Blood and fluid volume replacement may be necessary, along with administering blood products to correct any coagulation defects.

Vaginal birth is usually feasible and is desirable, especially in cases of fetal death. Labor induction or augmentation may be initiated so long as the mother and fetus are closely monitored for any evidence of compromise. Cesarean birth should be reserved for cases of fetal distress or other obstetric complications. Cesarean birth should not be attempted when the women has severe and uncorrected coagulopathy because it can result in uncontrollable bleeding (Francois & Foley, 2007).

Nursing care of women experiencing moderate to severe abruption is demanding because it requires constant close monitoring of the maternal and fetal condition. Information about placental abruption, including the cause, treatment, and expected outcome, is given to the woman and her family. Emotional support is also extremely important because the woman and her family may be experiencing fetal loss in addition to the woman's critical illness.

Cord Insertion and Placental Variations

Velamentous insertion of the cord *(vasa previa)* is a rare placental anomaly associated with placenta previa and multiple gestation. The cord vessels begin to branch at the membranes and then course onto the placenta (Fig. 28-11). ROM or traction on the cord may tear one or more of the fetal vessels. As a result the fetus may rapidly bleed to death. *Battledore* (marginal) insertion of the cord (Fig. 28-12, *A*) increases the risk of fetal hemorrhage, especially after marginal separation of the placenta.

In rare instances the placenta may be divided into two or more separate lobes, resulting in *succenturiate* placenta (see Fig. 28-12, *B*). Each lobe has a distinct circulation. The vessels collect at the periphery, and the main trunks eventually unite to form the vessels of the cord. Blood vessels joining the lobes may be supported only by the fetal membranes and are therefore in danger of tearing during labor, birth, or expulsion of the placenta. During placental expulsion, one or more of the separate lobes may remain attached to the decidua basalis, preventing uterine contraction and increasing the risk of postpartum hemorrhage.

Clotting Disorders in Pregnancy

Normal Clotting

Normally a delicate balance (homeostasis) exists between the opposing hemostatic and fibrinolytic systems. The hemostatic system stops the flow of blood from injured vessels, first by a platelet plug, which is followed by the formation of a fibrin clot. The coagulation process involves an interaction of the coagulation factors that constantly circulate in the bloodstream in which each factor sequentially activates the factor next in line, the "cascade effect" sequence. The fibrinolytic system is the process through which the fibrin clot is split into fibrinolytic degradation products and circulation is restored.

Clotting Problems

Disseminated Intravascular Coagulation. **Disseminated vascular coagulation (DIC),** or consumptive coagulopathy, is a pathologic form of clotting that is diffuse and consumes large amounts of clotting factors, causing widespread external bleeding, internal bleeding, or both, and clotting (Cunningham et al., 2010). DIC is never a primary diagnosis. Instead it results from some problem that triggered the clotting cascade, either extrinsically, by the release of large amounts of tissue thromboplastin, or intrinsically, by widespread damage to vascular integrity.

In the obstetric population, DIC is most often triggered by the release of large amounts of tissue thromboplastin, which

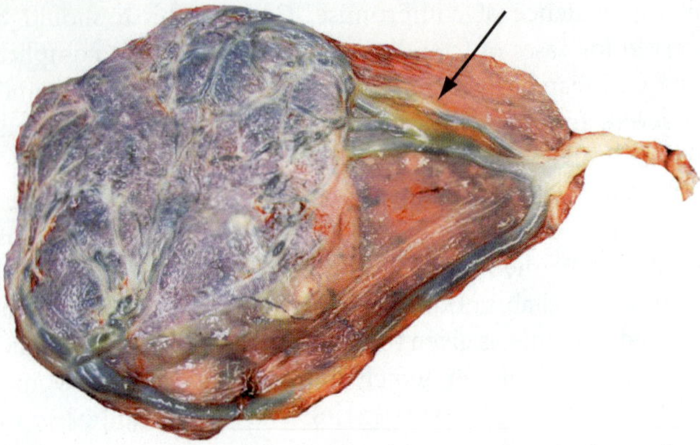

FIG. 28-11 Vasa previa (velamentous insertion of cord). *Arrow* shows velamentous cord insertion in the placenta. (From Creasy, R., Resnik, R., Iams, J., Lockwood, C., & Moore, T. [2009]. *Creasy & Resnik's maternal-fetal medicine: Principles and practice* [6th ed.]. Philadelphia: Saunders.)

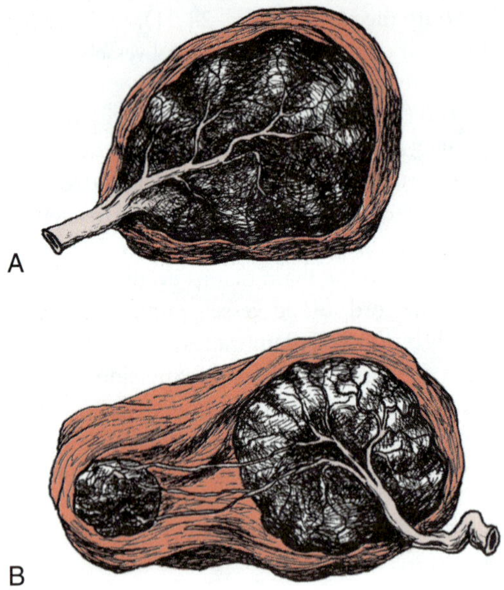

FIG. 28-12 Cord insertion and placental variations **A,** Battledore placenta. **B,** Placenta succenturiate.

occurs in placental abruption (the most common cause of severe consumptive coagulopathy in obstetrics) and in the retained dead fetus syndrome and the anaphylactoid syndrome of pregnancy (amniotic fluid embolus). Severe preeclampsia, HELLP syndrome, and gram-negative sepsis are examples of conditions that can trigger DIC because of widespread damage to vascular integrity (Cunningham et al., 2010; Gilbert, 2011). DIC is an overactivation of the clotting cascade and the fibrinolytic system, resulting in depletion of platelets and clotting factors, which results in the formation of multiple fibrin clots throughout the body's vasculature, even in the microcirculation. Blood cells are destroyed as they pass through these fibrin choked vessels. Thus DIC results in a clinical picture of clotting, bleeding, and ischemia (Cunningham et al.). Clinical manifestations and laboratory test results are summarized in Box 28-2.

Management. Medical management in all cases of DIC involves correction of the underlying cause (e.g., removal of the dead fetus, treatment of existing infection or of preeclampsia or eclampsia, or removal of an abrupted placenta).

BOX 28-2 CLINICAL MANIFESTATIONS AND LABORATORY SCREENING RESULTS FOR WOMEN WITH DISSEMINATED INTRAVASCULAR COAGULATION

POSSIBLE PHYSICAL EXAMINATION FINDINGS

- Spontaneous bleeding from gums, nose
- Oozing, excessive bleeding from venipuncture site, intravenous access site, or site of insertion of urinary catheter
- Petechiae, for example, on the arm where blood pressure cuff was placed
- Other signs of bruising
- Hematuria
- Gastrointestinal bleeding
- Tachycardia
- Diaphoresis

LABORATORY COAGULATION SCREENING TEST RESULTS

- Platelets—decreased
- Fibrinogen—decreased
- Factor V (proaccelerin)—decreased
- Factor VIII (antihemolytic factor)—decreased
- Prothrombin time—prolonged
- Partial prothrombin time—prolonged
- Fibrin degradation products—increased
- D-dimer test (specific fibrin degradation fragment)—increased
- Red blood smear—fragmented red blood cells

Sources: Cunningham, F., Leveno, K., Bloom, S., Hauth, J., Rouse, D., & Spong, C. (2010). *Williams obstetrics* (23rd ed.). New York: McGraw-Hill; Labelle, C., & Kitchens, C. (2005). Disseminated intravascular coagulation: Treat the cause, not the lab values. *Cleveland Clinic Journal of Medicine, 72*(5), 377-397; Roberts, J., & Funai, E. (2009). Pregnancy-related hypertension. In R. Creasy, R. Resnik, J. Iams, C. Lockwood, & T. Moore (Eds.), *Creasy and Resnik's maternal-fetal medicine: Principles and practice* (6th ed.). Philadelphia: Saunders.

Volume replacement, blood component therapy, optimization of oxygenation and perfusion status, and continued reassessment of laboratory parameters are the usual forms of treatment. Vitamin K administration and recombinant activated factor VIIa may be considered as additional therapies (Francois & Foley, 2007).

Nursing interventions include assessment for signs of bleeding (see Box 28-2) and signs of complications from the administration of blood and blood products, administering fluid or blood replacement as ordered, cardiac and hemodynamic monitoring, and protecting the woman from injury. Because renal failure is one consequence of DIC, urinary output is closely monitored by using an indwelling catheter. Urinary output must be maintained at more than 30 ml/hr (Gilbert, 2011). Vital signs are assessed frequently. If DIC develops before birth, continuous electronic fetal monitoring is necessary. The woman should be maintained in a side-lying tilt to maximize blood flow to the uterus. Oxygen may be administered through a nonrebreather face mask at 8 to 10 L/min or per hospital protocol or physician order. DIC usually is "cured" with the birth and as coagulation abnormalities resolve.

The woman and her family will be anxious and concerned about her condition and prognosis. The nurse offers explanations about care and provides emotional support to the woman and her family through this critical time.

KEY POINTS

- Blood loss during pregnancy should always be regarded as a warning sign until the cause is determined.
- Some miscarriages occur for unknown reasons, but fetal or placental maldevelopment and maternal factors account for many others.
- The type of miscarriage and signs and symptoms direct care management.
- Recurrent premature dilation of the cervix (incompetent cervix) may be treated with a cervical cerclage; the woman is instructed on recognizing the warning signs of preterm labor, ROM, and infection.
- Ectopic pregnancy is a significant cause of maternal morbidity and mortality, even in developed countries.
- Both complete and partial hydatidiform moles can progress to become gestational trophoblastic neoplasias, one of several types of gestational trophoblastic disease.
- Premature separation of the placenta (placental abruption) and placenta previa are differentiated by type of bleeding, uterine tonicity, and presence or absence of pain.
- Management of late-pregnancy bleeding requires immediate evaluation; care is based on gestational age, amount of bleeding, and fetal condition.
- Disseminated intravascular coagulation is a pathologic form of clotting that causes widespread bleeding and clotting. It is never a primary diagnosis, but always results from some problem that triggered the clotting cascade.

Audio Chapter Summaries Access an audio summary of these Key Points on evolve

REFERENCES

American College of Obstetricians and Gynecologists (ACOG). (2004). Diagnosis and treatment of gestational trophoblastic disease. ACOG Practice Bulletin No. 53. *Obstetrics and Gynecology, 103*(6), 1365–1377.

Bess, K., & Wood, T. (2006). Understanding gestational trophoblastic disease: How nurses can help those dealing with a diagnosis. *AWHONN Lifelines, 10*(4), 320–326.

Cohn, D., Ramaswamy, B., & Blum, K. (2009). Malignancy and pregnancy. In R. Creasy, R. Resnik, J. Iams, C. Lockwood, & T. Moore (Eds.), *Creasy and Resnik's maternal-fetal medicine: Principles and practice* (6th ed.). Philadelphia: Saunders.

Cunningham, F., Leveno, K., Bloom, S., Hauth, J., Rouse, D., & Spong, C. (2010). *Williams obstetrics* (23rd ed.). New York: McGraw-Hill.

Francois, K., & Foley, M. (2007). Antepartum and postpartum hemorrhage. In S. Gabbe, J. Niebyl, & J. Simpson (Eds.), *Obstetrics: Normal and problem pregnancies* (5th ed.). Philadelphia: Churchill Livingstone.

Gilbert, E. (2011). *Manual of high risk pregnancy & delivery* (5th ed.). St. Louis: Mosby.

Hull, A., & Resnik, R. (2009). Placenta previa, placenta accrete, abruptio placentae, and vasa previa. In R. Creasy, R. Resnik, J. Iams, C. Lockwood, & T. Moore (Eds.), *Creasy and Resnik's maternal-fetal medicine: Principles and practice* (6th ed.). Philadelphia: Saunders.

Iams, J. (2009). Cervical insufficiency. In R. Creasy, R. Resnik, J. Iams, C. Lockwood, & T. Moore (Eds.), *Creasy and Resnik's maternal-fetal medicine: Principles and practice* (6th ed.). Philadelphia: Saunders.

Ludmir, J., & Owen, J. (2007). Cervical incompetence. In S. Gabbe, J. Niebyl, & J. Simpson (Eds.), *Obstetrics: Normal and problem pregnancies* (5th ed.). Philadelphia: Churchill Livingstone.

Nader, S. (2009). Thyroid disease and pregnancy. In R. Creasy, R. Resnik, J. Iams, C. Lockwood, & T. Moore (Eds.), *Creasy and Resnik's maternal-fetal medicine: Principles and practice* (6th ed.). Philadelphia: Saunders.

Paidas, M., & Hossain, N. (2009). Embryonic and fetal demise. In R. Creasy, R. Resnik, J. Iams, C. Lockwood, & T. Moore (Eds.), *Creasy and Resnik's maternal-fetal medicine: Principles and practice* (6th ed.). Philadelphia: Saunders.

Roberts, J., & Funai, E. (2009). Pregnancy-related hypertension. In R. Creasy, R. Resnik, J. Iams, C. Lockwood, & T. Moore (Eds.), *Creasy and Resnik's maternal-fetal medicine: Principles and practice* (6th ed.). Philadelphia: Saunders.

Simpson, J., & Jauniaux, E. (2007). Pregnancy loss. In S. Gabbe, J. Niebyl, & J. Simpson (Eds.), *Obstetrics: Normal and problem pregnancies* (5th ed.). Philadelphia: Churchill Livingstone.

CHAPTER

29

Endocrine and Metabolic Disorders in Pregnancy

Kitty Cashion

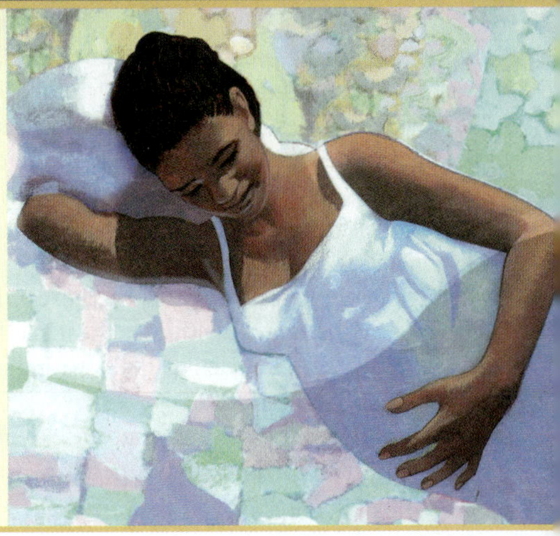

evolve WEBSITE

http://evolve.elsevier.com/Lowdermilk/MWHC/

Audio Glossary
Audio Key Points
Case Study
- Pregestational Diabetes

Critical Thinking Exercise
- Gestational Diabetes

NCLEX Review Questions
Nursing Care Plans
- Hyperemesis Gravidarum
- The Pregnant Woman with Gestational Diabetes

LEARNING OBJECTIVES

- Differentiate the types of diabetes mellitus and their respective risk factors in pregnancy.
- Compare insulin requirements during pregnancy, postpartum, and with lactation.
- Identify maternal and fetal risks or complications associated with diabetes in pregnancy.
- Develop a plan of care for the pregnant woman with pregestational or gestational diabetes.
- Explain the effects of hyperemesis gravidarum on maternal and fetal well-being.
- Discuss the management of the woman with hyperemesis gravidarum in the hospital and at home.
- Explain the effects of thyroid disorders on pregnancy.
- Compare the management of a pregnant woman with hyperthyroidism with one who has hypothyroidism.
- Discuss care management for the woman with phenylketonuria during the perinatal period.
- Examine the effects of maternal phenylketonuria on pregnancy outcome.

This chapter discusses the care of women for whom pregnancy represents a significant risk because it is superimposed on an endocrine or metabolic disorder. Specific disorders covered in this chapter include diabetes mellitus, hyperemesis gravidarum, hyper- and hypothyroidism, and phenylketonuria. Providing safe and effective care for women with these disorders and their fetuses is a challenge. Although unique needs related to the specific endocrine or metabolic condition are present, these women also experience the feelings, needs, and concerns associated with a normal pregnancy. The primary objective of nursing care is to achieve optimal outcomes for both the pregnant woman and the fetus. With the active participation of well-motivated women in the treatment plan and careful management from a multidisciplinary health care team, positive outcomes are often possible.

DIABETES MELLITUS

Around the world the incidence of diabetes mellitus is increasing at a rapid rate. In 2009 an estimated 23.6 million people in the United States (7.8% of the total population) have diabetes. Of these, 5.7 million are undiagnosed (National Center for Chronic Disease Prevention and Health Promotion, 2009). In the United States, experts predict a marked increase in the number of women with preexisting diabetes who will become pregnant (Moore & Catalano, 2009). Diabetes mellitus is currently the most common endocrine disorder associated with pregnancy, occurring in approximately 4% to 14% of pregnant women (Gilbert, 2011). The perinatal mortality rate for well-managed diabetic pregnancies, excluding major congenital malformations, is approximately the same as for any other pregnancy (Landon, Catalano, & Gabbe, 2007). The key to an optimal pregnancy outcome is strict maternal glucose control before conception, as well as throughout the gestational period. Consequently, for women with diabetes, much emphasis is placed on preconception counseling.

Pregnancy complicated by diabetes is still considered high risk. It is most successfully managed by a multidisciplinary approach involving the obstetrician, perinatologist, internist or endocrinologist, ophthalmologist, nephrologist, neonatologist, nurse, nutritionist or dietitian, and social worker, as needed. A favorable outcome requires commitment and active participation by the pregnant woman and her family.

Pathogenesis

Diabetes mellitus refers to a group of metabolic diseases characterized by hyperglycemia resulting from defects in insulin secretion, insulin action, or both (American Diabetes Association [ADA], 2008). Insulin, produced by the beta cells in the islets of Langerhans in the pancreas, regulates blood glucose levels by enabling glucose to enter adipose and muscle cells, where it is used for energy. When insulin is insufficient or ineffective in promoting glucose uptake by the muscle and adipose cells, glucose accumulates in the bloodstream, and hyperglycemia results. Hyperglycemia causes hyperosmolarity of the blood, which attracts intracellular fluid into the vascular system, resulting in cellular dehydration and expanded blood volume. Consequently the kidneys function to excrete large volumes of urine (polyuria) in an attempt to regulate excess vascular volume and to excrete the unusable glucose (glycosuria). Polyuria, along with cellular dehydration, causes excessive thirst (polydipsia).

The body compensates for its inability to convert carbohydrate (glucose) into energy by burning proteins (muscle) and fats. However, the end products of this metabolism are ketones and fatty acids, which, in excess quantities, produce ketoacidosis and acetonuria. Weight loss occurs as a result of the breakdown of fat and muscle tissue. This tissue breakdown causes a state of starvation that compels the individual to eat excessive amounts of food (polyphagia).

Over time, diabetes causes significant changes in the microvascular and macrovascular circulations. These structural changes affect a variety of organ systems, particularly the heart, the eyes, the kidneys, and the nerves. Complications resulting from diabetes include premature atherosclerosis, retinopathy, nephropathy, and neuropathy.

Diabetes may be caused either by impaired insulin secretion, when the beta cells of the pancreas are destroyed by an autoimmune process, or by inadequate insulin action in target tissues at one or more points along the metabolic pathway. Both of these conditions are commonly present in the same person, and determining which, if either, abnormality is the primary cause of the disease is difficult (ADA, 2008). For additional information on diabetes, visit the American Diabetes Association's website at www.diabetes.org.

Classification

The current classification system includes four groups: type 1 diabetes, type 2 diabetes, other specific types (e.g., diabetes caused by genetic defects in beta cell function or insulin action, disease or injury of the pancreas, or drug-induced diabetes), and gestational diabetes mellitus (GDM) (ADA, 2008; Moore & Catalano, 2009). Almost 90% of all pregnant women with diabetes have GDM (Gilbert, 2011). Of the women with pregestational diabetes, the majority (65%) have type 2 diabetes (Chan & Johnson, 2006).

Type 1 diabetes includes cases that are caused primarily by pancreatic islet beta cell destruction and that are prone to ketoacidosis. People with type 1 diabetes usually have an abrupt onset of illness at a young age and an absolute insulin deficiency. Type 1 diabetes includes cases thought to be caused by an autoimmune process, as well as those for which the cause is unknown (ADA, 2008; Landon et al., 2007).

Type 2 diabetes is the most prevalent form of the disease and includes individuals who have insulin resistance and usually relative (rather than absolute) insulin deficiency. Specific causes of type 2 diabetes are unknown at this time. Type 2 diabetes often goes undiagnosed for years because hyperglycemia develops gradually and is often not severe enough for the client to recognize the classic signs of polyuria, polydipsia, and polyphagia. Most people who develop type 2 diabetes are obese or have an increased amount of body fat distributed primarily in the abdominal area. Other risk factors for the development of type 2 diabetes include aging, a sedentary lifestyle, family history and genetics, puberty, hypertension, and prior gestational diabetes. Type 2 diabetes often has a strong genetic predisposition (ADA, 2008; Moore & Catalano, 2009).

Pregestational diabetes mellitus is the label sometimes given to type 1 or type 2 diabetes that existed before pregnancy.

Gestational diabetes mellitus (GDM) is any degree of glucose intolerance with the onset or first recognition occurring during pregnancy. This definition is appropriate whether or not insulin is used for treatment or the diabetes persists after pregnancy. It does not exclude the possibility that the glucose intolerance preceded the pregnancy or that medication might be required for optimal glucose control. Women experiencing gestational diabetes should be reclassified 6 weeks or more after the pregnancy ends (ADA, 2008; Moore & Catalano, 2009).

White's Classification of Diabetes in Pregnancy

Dr. Priscilla White, a physician who worked with pregnant women with diabetes during the 1940s, developed a classification system specifically for use with this group of women (Table 29-1). White's system was based on age at diagnosis, duration of illness, and presence of vascular disease (Landon et al., 2007; Moore & Catalano, 2009). Her classification system has been modified through the years but is still frequently used to assess both maternal and fetal risk. Women in classes A through C generally have good pregnancy outcomes as long as their blood glucose levels are well controlled. Women in classes D through T, however, usually have poorer pregnancy outcomes because they have already developed the vascular damage that often accompanies long-standing diabetes.

Metabolic Changes Associated with Pregnancy

Normal pregnancy is characterized by complex alterations in maternal glucose metabolism, insulin production, and metabolic homeostasis. During normal pregnancy, adjustments in maternal metabolism allow for adequate nutrition for the mother and the developing fetus. Glucose, the primary fuel used by the fetus, is transported across the placenta through the process of carrier-mediated facilitated diffusion, meaning that the glucose levels in the fetus are directly proportional to maternal levels. Although glucose crosses the placenta, insulin does not. Around the tenth week of gestation the fetus begins to secrete its own insulin at levels adequate to use the glucose obtained from the mother. Therefore, as maternal glucose levels rise, fetal glucose levels are increased, resulting in increased fetal insulin secretion.

TABLE 29-1 WHITE'S CLASSIFICATION OF DIABETES IN PREGNANCY (MODIFIED)

Gestational Diabetes	
Class A_1	Client has two or more abnormal values on the OGTT with a normal fasting blood sugar. Blood glucose levels are diet controlled.
Class A_2	Client was not known to have diabetes before pregnancy but requires medication for blood glucose control.
Pregestational Diabetes	
Class B	Onset of disease occurs after age 20 and duration of illness <10 years.
Class C	Onset of disease occurs between 10 and 19 years of age or duration of illness for 10 to 19 years or both.
Class D	Onset of disease occurs <10 years of age or duration of illness >20 years or both.
Class F	Client has developed diabetic nephropathy.
Class R	Client has developed retinitis proliferans.
Class T	Client has had a renal transplant.

OGTT, Oral glucose tolerance test.
Sources: Landon, M., Catalano, P., & Gabbe, S. (2007). Diabetes mellitus complicating pregnancy. In S. Gabbe, J. Niebyl, & J. Simpson (Eds.), *Obstetrics: Normal and problem pregnancies* (5th ed.). Philadelphia: Churchill Livingstone; Moore, T., & Catalano, P. (2009). Diabetes in pregnancy. In R. Creasy, R. Resnik, J. Iams, C. Lockwood, & T. Moore (Eds.), *Creasy and Resnik's maternal-fetal medicine: Principles and practice* (6th ed.). Philadelphia: Saunders.

During the first trimester of pregnancy the pregnant woman's metabolic status is significantly influenced by the rising levels of estrogen and progesterone. These hormones stimulate the beta cells in the pancreas to increase insulin production, which promotes increased peripheral use of glucose and decreased blood glucose, with fasting levels being reduced by approximately 10% (Fig. 29-1, *A*). At the same time, an increase in tissue glycogen stores and a decrease in hepatic glucose production occur, which further encourage lower fasting glucose levels. As a result of these normal metabolic changes of pregnancy, women with insulin-dependent diabetes are prone to hypoglycemia during the first trimester.

During the second and third trimesters, pregnancy exerts a "diabetogenic" effect on the maternal metabolic status. Because of the major hormonal changes, decreased tolerance to glucose, increased insulin resistance, decreased hepatic glycogen stores, and increased hepatic production of glucose occur. Rising levels of human chorionic somatomammotropin, estrogen, progesterone, prolactin, cortisol, and insulinase increase insulin resistance through their actions as insulin antagonists. Insulin resistance is a glucose-sparing mechanism that ensures an abundant supply of glucose for the fetus. Maternal insulin requirements gradually increase from approximately 18 to 24 weeks of gestation to approximately 36 weeks of gestation. Maternal insulin requirements may double or quadruple by the end of the pregnancy (see Fig. 29-1, *B* and *C*).

At birth, expulsion of the placenta prompts an abrupt drop in levels of circulating placental hormones, cortisol, and insulinase (see Fig. 29-1, *D*). Maternal tissues quickly regain their prepregnancy sensitivity to insulin. For the nonbreastfeeding mother the prepregnancy insulin-carbohydrate balance usually returns in approximately 7 to 10 days (see Fig. 29-1, *E*). Lactation uses maternal glucose; therefore, the breastfeeding mother's insulin requirements remain low during lactation. On completion of weaning the mother's prepregnancy insulin requirement is reestablished (see Fig. 29-1, *F*).

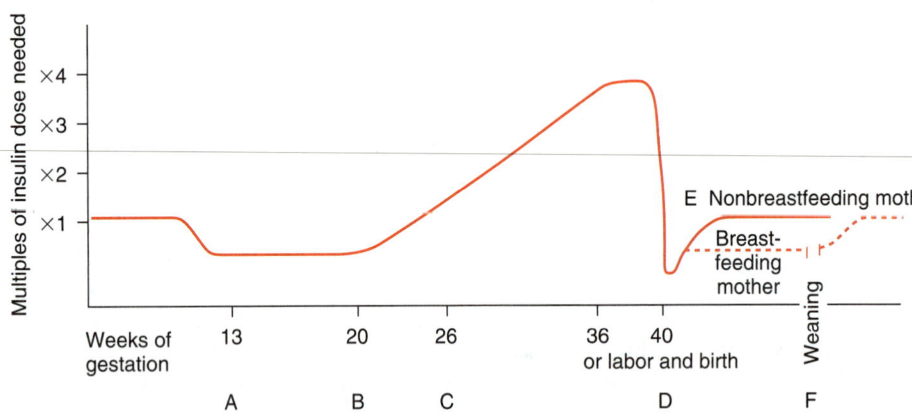

FIG. 29-1 Changing insulin needs during pregnancy. *A,* First trimester: Insulin need is reduced because of increased insulin production by pancreas and increased peripheral sensitivity to insulin; nausea, vomiting, and decreased food intake by mother and glucose transfer to embryo or fetus contribute to hypoglycemia. *B,* Second trimester: Insulin needs begin to increase as placental hormones, cortisol, and insulinase act as insulin antagonists, decreasing insulin's effectiveness. *C,* Third trimester: Insulin needs may double or even quadruple but usually level off after 36 weeks of gestation. *D,* Day of birth: Maternal insulin requirements decrease drastically to approach prepregnancy levels. *E,* Breastfeeding mother maintains lower insulin requirements, as much as 25% less than those of prepregnancy; insulin needs of nonbreastfeeding mother return to prepregnancy levels in 7 to 10 days. *F,* Weaning of breastfeeding infant causes mother's insulin needs to return to prepregnancy levels.

PREGESTATIONAL DIABETES MELLITUS

Approximately 2 per 1000 pregnancies are complicated by preexisting diabetes. Women who have **pregestational diabetes mellitus** may have either type 1 or type 2 diabetes, which may be complicated by vascular disease, retinopathy, nephropathy, or other diabetic sequelae. Type 2 is a more common diagnosis than type 1. Almost all women with pregestational diabetes are insulin dependent during pregnancy. According to White's classification system, these women fall into classes B through T (see Table 29-1).

The diabetogenic state of pregnancy imposed on the compromised metabolic system of the woman with pregestational diabetes has significant implications. The normal hormonal adaptations of pregnancy affect glycemic control, and pregnancy may accelerate the progress of vascular complications.

During the first trimester, when maternal blood glucose levels are normally reduced and the insulin response to glucose is enhanced, glycemic control is improved. The insulin dose for the woman with well-controlled diabetes may have to be reduced to prevent hypoglycemia. Nausea, vomiting, and cravings typical of early pregnancy result in dietary fluctuations that influence maternal glucose levels and may also necessitate a reduction in the insulin dose.

Because insulin requirements steadily increase after the first trimester, the insulin dose must be adjusted accordingly to prevent hyperglycemia. Insulin resistance begins as early as 14 to 16 weeks of gestation and continues to rise until it stabilizes during the last few weeks of pregnancy.

Preconception Counseling

Preconception counseling is recommended for all women of reproductive age who have diabetes because it is associated with less perinatal mortality and fewer congenital anomalies (Moore & Catalano, 2009). Under ideal circumstances, women with pregestational diabetes are counseled before the time of conception to plan the optimal time for pregnancy, establish glycemic control before conception, and diagnose any vascular complications of diabetes. However, estimates indicate that less than 20% of women with diabetes in the United States participate in preconception counseling (Landon et al., 2007).

The woman's partner should be included in the counseling to assess the couple's level of understanding related to the effects of pregnancy on the diabetic condition and of the potential complications of pregnancy as a result of diabetes. The couple should also be informed of the anticipated alterations in management of diabetes during pregnancy and the need for a multidisciplinary team approach to health care. Financial implications of diabetic pregnancy and other demands related to frequent maternal and fetal surveillance should be discussed. Contraception is another important aspect of preconception counseling to assist the couple in planning effectively for pregnancy.

COMMUNITY ACTIVITY

- Visit the American Diabetes Association website at www.diabetes.org. Review the client information about gestational diabetes and treatment. Research the importance of preconception counseling for women with type 1 diabetes. Are any community based programs sponsored by the ADA available in your community?
- Visit the Hyperemesis Gravidarum (HG) Education and Research (HER) Foundation website. Review the client information about hyperemesis gravidarum, nutritional strategies, and treatment. Locate a health care professional experienced in treating HG, and hospitals with treatment programs for HG in your state.

Maternal Risks and Complications

Although maternal morbidity and mortality rates have improved significantly, the pregnant woman with diabetes remains at risk for the development of complications during pregnancy. Poor glycemic control around the time of conception and in the early weeks of pregnancy is associated with an increased incidence of miscarriage. Women with good glycemic control before conception and in the first trimester are no more likely to miscarry than women who do not have diabetes (Moore & Catalano, 2009).

Poor glycemic control later in pregnancy, particularly in women without vascular disease, increases the rate of fetal macrosomia. **Macrosomia** has been defined in several different ways, including a birth weight more than 4000 to 4500 g, a birth weight greater than the 90th percentile, and estimates of neonatal adipose tissue. Macrosomia occurs in approximately 40% of pregestational diabetic pregnancies and in up to 50% of pregnancies complicated by GDM (Landon et al., 2007; Moore & Catalano, 2009). Infants born to women with diabetes tend to have a disproportionate increase in shoulder, trunk, and chest size. Because of this tendency the risk of shoulder dystocia is greater in these babies than in other macrosomic infants. Women with diabetes therefore face an increased likelihood of cesarean birth because of failure of fetal descent or labor progress or of operative vaginal birth (birth involving the use of episiotomy, forceps, or vacuum extractor) (Landon et al.; Moore & Catalano).

Women with preexisting diabetes are at risk for several obstetric and medical complications. In general, the risk of developing these complications increases with the duration and severity of the woman's diabetes. In one study the rates of preeclampsia, preterm birth, cesarean birth, and maternal mortality were much higher in women with preexisting diabetes than in women who did not have this disease. Approximately a third of women who have had diabetes for more than 20 years, for example, develop preeclampsia. Women with nephropathy and hypertension in addition to diabetes are also increasingly likely to develop preeclampsia. The rate of hypertensive disorders in all types of pregnancies complicated by diabetes is 15% to 30%. Chronic hypertension occurs in 10% to 20% of all pregnant women with diabetes, and in up to 40% of those women who have preexisting renal or retinal vascular disease (Moore & Catalano, 2009).

Hydramnios (polyhydramnios) frequently develops during the third trimester of pregnancy in women with diabetes. Its cause is unknown. One theory is that hydramnios in women with diabetes is caused by an increased glucose concentration in amniotic fluid resulting from maternal and fetal hyperglycemia. The complications most frequently associated with hydramnios (usually defined as an amniotic fluid index [AFI] greater than 24 to 25 cm) are placental abruption (abruptio placentae), uterine dysfunction, and postpartum hemorrhage (Cunningham, Leveno, Bloom, Hauth, Rouse, & Spong, 2010).

Infections are more common and more serious in pregnant women with diabetes than in pregnant women without the disease. Disorders of carbohydrate metabolism alter the body's normal resistance to infection. The inflammatory response, leukocyte function, and vaginal pH are all affected. Vaginal infections, particularly monilial vaginitis, are more common. Urinary tract infections (UTIs) are also more prevalent. Infection is serious because it causes increased insulin resistance and may result in ketoacidosis.

Ketoacidosis (accumulation of ketones in the blood resulting from hyperglycemia and leading to metabolic acidosis) occurs most often during the second and third trimesters, when the diabetogenic effect of pregnancy is the greatest. When the maternal metabolism is stressed by illness or infection, the woman is at increased risk for diabetic ketoacidosis (DKA). DKA can also be caused by poor client compliance with treatment or the onset of previously undiagnosed diabetes (Moore & Catalano, 2009). The use of beta-mimetic drugs such as terbutaline for tocolysis to arrest preterm labor or corticosteroids given to enhance fetal lung maturation may also contribute to the risk for hyperglycemia and subsequent DKA (Cunningham et al., 2010; Iams, Romero, & Creasy, 2009).

DKA may occur with blood glucose levels barely exceeding 200 mg/dl, as compared with 300 to 350 mg/dl in the nonpregnant state. In response to stress factors such as infection or illness, **hyperglycemia** occurs as a result of increased hepatic glucose production and decreased peripheral glucose use. Stress hormones, which act to impair insulin action and further contribute to insulin deficiency, are released. Fatty acids are mobilized from fat stores to enter the circulation. As they are oxidized, ketone bodies are released into the peripheral circulation. The woman's buffering system is unable to compensate, and metabolic acidosis develops. The excessive blood glucose and ketone bodies result in osmotic diuresis with subsequent loss of fluid and electrolytes, volume depletion, and cellular dehydration. DKA is a medical emergency. Prompt treatment is necessary to prevent maternal coma or death. Ketoacidosis occurring at any time during pregnancy can lead to intrauterine fetal death. The incidence of DKA has decreased in recent years. Currently it affects only about 1% of pregnant women with diabetes (Cunningham et al., 2010). The rate of intrauterine fetal demise (IUFD) with DKA, formerly approximately 35%, is 10% or less (Moore & Catalano, 2009) (Table 29-2).

TABLE 29-2 DIFFERENTIATION OF HYPOGLYCEMIA (INSULIN SHOCK) AND HYPERGLYCEMIA (DIABETIC KETOACIDOSIS)

CAUSES	ONSET	SYMPTOMS	INTERVENTIONS
HYPOGLYCEMIA (INSULIN SHOCK)			
Excess insulin Insufficient food (delayed or missed meals) Excessive exercise or work Indigestion, diarrhea, vomiting	Rapid (regular insulin) Gradual (modified insulin or oral hypoglycemic agents)	Irritability Hunger Sweating Nervousness Personality change Weakness Fatigue Blurred or double vision Dizziness Headache Pallor; clammy skin Shallow respirations Rapid pulse Laboratory values Urine: Negative for sugar and acetone Blood glucose: ≤60 mg/dl	Check blood glucose level when symptoms first appear. Eat or drink 15 g fast sugar (simple carbohydrate) immediately. Recheck blood glucose level in 15 minutes, and eat or drink another 15 g fast sugar (simple carbohydrate) if glucose remains low. Recheck blood glucose level in 15 minutes. Notify primary health care provider if no change in glucose level. If woman is unconscious, administer 50% dextrose IV push, 5% to 10% dextrose in water IV drip, or 1 mg glucagon subcutaneously. Obtain blood and urine specimens for laboratory testing.
HYPERGLYCEMIA (DKA)			
Insufficient insulin Excess or wrong kind of food Infection, injuries, illness Emotional stress Insufficient exercise	Slow (hours to days)	Thirst Nausea or vomiting Abdominal pain Constipation Drowsiness Dim vision Increased urination Headache Flushed, dry skin Rapid breathing Weak, rapid pulse Acetone (fruity) breath odor Laboratory values Urine: Positive for sugar and acetone Blood glucose: ≥200 mg/dl	Notify primary health care provider. Administer insulin in accordance with blood glucose levels. Give IV fluids such as normal saline solution or one-half normal saline solution; potassium when urinary output is adequate; bicarbonate for pH <7. Monitor laboratory testing of blood and urine.

DKA, Diabetic ketoacidosis; *IV*, intravenous.

The risk of **hypoglycemia** (a less than normal amount of glucose in the blood) is also increased. Early in pregnancy, when hepatic production of glucose is diminished and peripheral use of glucose is enhanced, hypoglycemia occurs frequently, often during sleep. Later in pregnancy, hypoglycemia may also result as insulin doses are adjusted to maintain euglycemia (a normal blood glucose level). Women with a prepregnancy history of severe hypoglycemia are at increased risk for severe hypoglycemia during gestation. Mild to moderate hypoglycemic episodes do not appear to have significant damaging effects on fetal well-being (see Table 29-2).

Fetal and Neonatal Risks and Complications

From the moment of conception the infant of a woman with diabetes faces an increased risk of complications that may occur during the antepartum, intrapartum, or neonatal periods. Infant morbidity and mortality rates associated with diabetic pregnancy are significantly reduced with strict control of maternal glucose levels before and during pregnancy.

Despite the improvements in care of pregnant women with diabetes, IUFD (sometimes called *stillbirth*) remains a major concern. Approximately 2% to 5% of all fetal deaths occur in women whose pregnancies are complicated by preexisting diabetes. Hyperglycemia, ketoacidosis, congenital anomalies, infections, and maternal obesity are thought to be reasons for fetal death. In the third trimester, fetal acidosis is the most likely cause of fetal death (Paidas & Hossain, 2009).

The most important cause of perinatal loss in diabetic pregnancy is congenital malformations, which account for 30% to 50% of all perinatal loss (Lindsay, 2006). The incidence of congenital malformations is related to the severity and duration of the diabetes. Hyperglycemia during the first trimester of pregnancy, when organs and organ systems are forming, is the main cause of diabetes-associated birth defects. Anomalies commonly seen in infants affect primarily the cardiovascular system, the central nervous system (CNS), and the skeletal system (Cunningham et al., 2010; Moore & Catalano, 2009) (see Chapter 35).

The fetal pancreas begins to secrete insulin at 10 to 14 weeks of gestation. The fetus responds to maternal hyperglycemia by secreting large amounts of insulin (hyperinsulinism). Insulin acts as a growth hormone, causing the fetus to produce excess stores of glycogen, protein, and adipose tissue and leading to increased fetal size, or macrosomia. Birth injuries are more common in infants born to mothers with diabetes compared with mothers who do not have diabetes, and macrosomic fetuses have the highest risk for this complication. Common birth injuries associated with diabetic pregnancies include brachial plexus palsy, facial nerve injury, humerus or clavicle fracture, and cephalhematoma. Most of these injuries are associated with difficult vaginal birth and shoulder dystocia (Moore & Catalano, 2009). Hypoglycemia at birth is also a risk for infants born to mothers with diabetes (for further discussion of neonatal complications related to maternal diabetes, see Chapter 35).

CARE MANAGEMENT

Antepartum

When a pregnant woman with diabetes initiates prenatal care, a thorough evaluation of her health status is completed. At the initial visit a complete physical examination is performed to assess the woman's health status. In addition to the routine prenatal examination, specific efforts are made to assess the effects of the diabetes, specifically retinopathy, nephropathy, peripheral and autonomic neuropathy, peripheral vascular, and cardiac involvement (Gilbert, 2011) (see the Nursing Process box).

In addition to routine prenatal laboratory tests, baseline renal function may be assessed with a 24-hour urine collection for total protein excretion and creatinine clearance. Urinalysis and culture are performed to assess for the presence of a urinary tract infection (UTI), which is common in diabetic pregnancy. Because of the risk of coexisting thyroid disease, thyroid function tests may also be performed (see later discussion of thyroid disorders). The **glycosylated hemoglobin A_{1c}** level may be measured to assess recent glycemic control. With prolonged hyperglycemia, some of the hemoglobin remains saturated with glucose for the life of the red blood cell (RBC). Therefore, a test for glycosylated hemoglobin provides a measure of glycemic control over time, specifically over the previous 4 to 6 weeks. Hemoglobin A_{1c} levels greater than 6 indicate elevated glucose during the previous 4 to 6 weeks (Gilbert, 2011). Fasting blood glucose or random (1 to 2 hours after eating) glucose levels may be assessed during antepartum visits (Fig. 29-2). Self-monitoring blood glucose records may also be reviewed.

Because of her high risk status, a woman with diabetes is monitored much more frequently and thoroughly than other pregnant women. During the first and second trimesters of pregnancy, her routine prenatal care visits will be scheduled every 1 to 2 weeks. In the last trimester she will likely be seen one or two times each week. In the past, routine hospitalization for management of the diabetes, such as insulin dose changes, was common. With the availability of improved home glucose monitoring and the growing reluctance of third-party payers to reimburse for hospitalization, pregnant women with diabetes are now generally managed as outpatients. Some client and family education and maternal and fetal assessment may be performed in the home, depending on the woman's insurance coverage and care provider preference.

Achieving and maintaining constant euglycemia, with plasma glucose levels in the range of 65 to 95 mg/dl preprandially and no higher than 130 to 140 mg/dl when measured 1 hour postprandially (Table 29-3), is the primary goal of medical therapy (Moore & Catalano, 2009). Euglycemia is achieved through a combination of diet, insulin, and exercise. Providing the woman with the knowledge, skill, and motivation she needs to achieve and maintain excellent blood glucose control is the primary nursing goal.

Achieving euglycemia requires commitment on the part of the woman and her family to make the necessary lifestyle changes, which can sometimes seem overwhelming. Maintaining tight blood glucose control necessitates that the woman follow a consistent daily schedule. She must get up and go to bed, eat, exercise, and take insulin at the same time each day. Blood glucose measurements are taken frequently to determine how well the major components of therapy (diet, insulin, and exercise) are working together to control blood glucose levels. The pregnant woman with diabetes should wear a medical identification bracelet at all times and carry insulin, syringes, and sources of fast sugar (simple carbohydrate) with her whenever she is away from home.

NURSING PROCESS

Pregestational Diabetes

ASSESSMENT

When a pregnant woman with diabetes initiates prenatal care, a thorough evaluation of her health status is completed. The assessment includes the following areas.

History

- Routine prenatal history
- Onset and course of diabetes
- Degree of glycemic control before pregnancy

Interview

- Learning needs
  - Diabetes in pregnancy
  - Potential fetal complications
  - Plan of care
- Emotional status
  - Coping with pregnancy superimposed on preexisting diabetes
  - Dealing with high risk status
  - Fear of maternal and fetal complications
  - Major changes in patterns of daily living so as to comply with plan of care
  - Support system
- Identifying significant persons and their roles
  - Assess their reactions to the pregnancy and the management plan.
  - Assess their involvement in the treatment regimen.

Physical Examination

- Assess current health status.
- Perform routine prenatal examination.
- Determine effects of diabetes on pregnancy.
  - Perform a baseline electrocardiogram to assess cardiovascular status.
  - Evaluate for retinopathy with follow-up as needed by an ophthalmologist each trimester and more often if retinopathy is diagnosed.
- Monitor blood pressure.
- Monitor weight gain.
- Assess fundal height.

Laboratory Tests

- Glycosylated hemoglobin (hemoglobin A_{1c})
- 24-hour urine collection for total protein excretion and creatinine clearance
- Urinalysis and culture: Initial prenatal visit and throughout the pregnancy as needed
- Urine dipstick for ketones
- Thyroid function tests

NURSING DIAGNOSES

Nursing diagnoses for the woman with pregestational diabetes include:

Deficient Knowledge **related to:**
- diabetic pregnancy, management, and potential effects on the pregnant woman and fetus

Anxiety, Fear, Dysfunctional Grieving, Powerlessness, Disturbed Body Image, Situational Low Self-esteem, Spiritual Distress, Ineffective Role Performance, and Interrupted Family Processes **related to:**
- diagnosis of *diabetes* and consequently being considered *high risk*
- effects of diabetes and its potential sequelae on the pregnant woman and the fetus
- lack of understanding by partner of effects of diabetes on pregnancy

Risk for Injury (to Fetus) **related to:**
- uteroplacental insufficiency
- birth trauma

Risk for Injury (to Mother) **related to:**
- failure to follow a diabetic diet
- improper insulin administration
- hypoglycemia and hyperglycemia
- cesarean or operative vaginal birth
- postpartum infection

EXPECTED OUTCOMES OF CARE

Expected outcomes of care for the pregnant woman with pregestational diabetes include that she will:

- Demonstrate or verbalize understanding of pregnancy complicated by diabetes, the plan of care, and the importance of glycemic control.
- Achieve and maintain glycemic control.
- Demonstrate effective coping.
- Experience no complications (maternal morbidity or mortality).
- Give birth to a healthy infant at term.

PLAN OF CARE AND INTERVENTIONS

Antepartum

- Routine prenatal visits every 1 to 2 weeks in first and second trimester and one to two times per week in the third trimester
- Provide education for the following:
  - Home glucose monitoring
  - Importance of a consistent daily schedule to maintain tight glucose control
  - Importance of good foot care and general skin care
- Diet
  - Nutrition counseling by a registered dietitian
- Insulin therapy
- Exercise as prescribed by the primary health care provider
- Fetal surveillance:
  - Ultrasound examinations throughout pregnancy to determine gestational age, monitor fetal growth, and assess for hydramnios and anomalies
  - Maternal serum alpha-fetoprotein determination to screen for neural tube defects
  - Daily fetal movement counts (beginning at 28 weeks of gestation)
  - Nonstress tests, contraction stress tests, or biophysical profiles once or twice weekly (beginning at 34 weeks of gestation or sooner)

Intrapartum

- Determine blood glucose hourly.
- Administer rapid- or short-acting insulin by intravenous drip as needed to maintain blood glucose levels in desired range.
- Monitor fetal heart rate (FHR) continuously.
- Observe for fetal dystocia.
- Ensure that a neonatal care provider is present at birth.

Postpartum

- Monitor blood glucose levels and adjust insulin dose as appropriate.
- Observe for complications (preeclampsia, hemorrhage, infection).
- Encourage breastfeeding.
- Provide family planning education.

EVALUATION

Evaluation of the effectiveness of care is based on the expected outcomes, which are closely associated with the degree of maternal metabolic control during pregnancy.

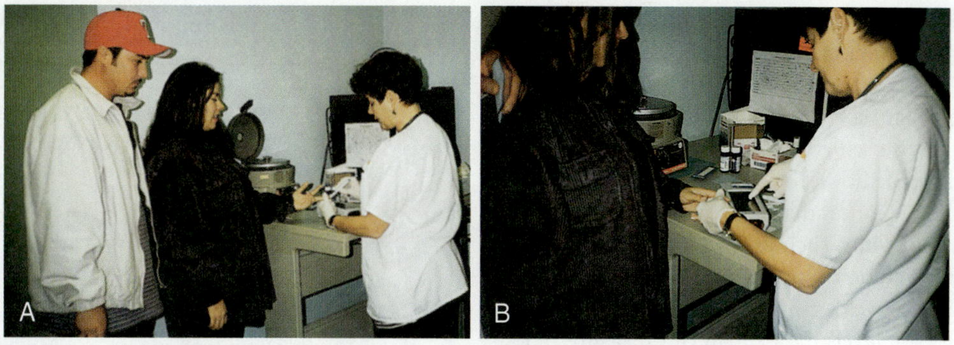

FIG. 29-2 **A,** Clinic nurse collects blood to determine glucose level. **B,** Nurse interprets glucose value displayed by monitor. (Courtesy Dee Lowdermilk, UNC Ambulatory Care Clinics, Chapel Hill, NC.)

TABLE 29-3 TARGET BLOOD GLUCOSE LEVELS DURING PREGNANCY

TIME OF DAY	TARGET PLASMA GLUCOSE LEVEL (mg/dl)
Premeal or fasting	>65 but <95
Postmeal (1 hr)	<130-140
Postmeal (2 hr)	<120

Sources: Landon, M., Catalano, P., & Gabbe, S. (2007). Diabetes mellitus complicating pregnancy. In S. Gabbe, J. Niebyl, & J. Simpson (Eds.), *Obstetrics: Normal and problem pregnancies* (5th ed.). Philadelphia: Churchill Livingstone; Moore, T., & Catalano, P. (2009). Diabetes in pregnancy. In R. Creasy, R. Resnik, J. Iams, C. Lockwood, & T. Moore (Eds.), *Creasy and Resnik's maternal-fetal medicine: Principles and practice* (6th ed.). Philadelphia: Saunders.

Because the woman with diabetes is at increased risk for infections, eye problems, and neurologic changes, foot care and general skin care are important. A daily bath that includes good perineal care and foot care is important. For dry skin, lotions, creams, or oils can be applied. Tight clothing should be avoided. Shoes or slippers that fit properly should be worn at all times and are best worn with socks or stockings. Feet should be inspected regularly; toenails should be cut straight across, and professional help should be sought for any foot problems. Extremes of temperature should be avoided.

Diet. The woman with pregestational diabetes has usually had nutritional counseling regarding management of her diabetes. However, because pregnancy produces special nutritional concerns and needs, the woman must be educated to incorporate these changes into dietary planning. For the woman who has "controlled" her diabetes for several years the changes in her insulin and dietary needs mandated by pregnancy may be difficult. Nutritional counseling is usually provided by a registered dietitian.

Dietary management during diabetic pregnancy must be based on blood (not urine) glucose levels. The diet is individualized to allow for increased fetal and metabolic requirements, with consideration of such factors as prepregnancy weight and dietary habits, overall health, ethnic background, lifestyle, stage of pregnancy, knowledge of nutrition, and insulin therapy. The dietary goals are to provide weight gain consistent with a normal pregnancy, to prevent ketoacidosis, and to minimize wide fluctuation of blood glucose levels.

For nonobese women, dietary counseling based on preconception body mass index (BMI) is 30 to 35 kcal/kg/day (Cunningham et al., 2010). In contrast, for obese women with a BMI greater than 30, experts recommend that the caloric intake total 25 kcal/kg/day (Moore & Catalano, 2009). The average diet includes 2200 calories (first trimester) to 2500 calories (second and third trimesters). Total calories may be distributed among three meals and one evening snack or, more commonly, three meals and two or three snacks. Meals should be eaten on time and never skipped. Going more than 4 hours without food intake increases the risk for episodes of hypoglycemia. Snacks must be carefully planned in accordance with insulin therapy to prevent fluctuations in blood glucose levels. A large bedtime snack of at least 25 g of carbohydrate with some protein or fat is recommended to help prevent hypoglycemia and starvation ketosis during the night (Moore & Catalano).

The ideal diet is composed of 55% carbohydrate, 20% protein, and 25% fat, with less than 10% as saturated fat (Cunningham et al., 2010) (see the Teaching for Self-Management box: Dietary Management of Diabetic Pregnancy). Simple carbohydrates are limited. Complex carbohydrates that are high in fiber content are recommended because the starch and protein in such foods help regulate the blood glucose level by more sustained glucose release (Gilbert, 2011; Moore & Catalano, 2009).

TEACHING FOR SELF-MANAGEMENT

Dietary Management of Diabetic Pregnancy

- Follow the prescribed diet plan.
- Eat a well-balanced diet, including daily food requirements for a normal pregnancy.
- Divide daily food intake among three meals and two or three snacks, depending on individual needs.
- Eat a substantial bedtime snack to prevent a severe drop in blood glucose level during the night.
- Take daily vitamins and iron as prescribed by the health care provider.
- Avoid foods high in refined sugar.
- Eat consistently each day; never skip meals or snacks.
- Eat foods high in dietary fiber.
- Avoid alcohol, nicotine, and caffeine.

Exercise. Although studies have shown that exercise enhances the use of glucose and decreases insulin need in women without diabetes, data regarding exercise in women with pregestational diabetes are limited. Any prescription of exercise during pregnancy for women with diabetes should be given by the primary health care provider and should be monitored closely to prevent complications. Regular exercise may be contraindicated in women with diabetes who also have uncontrolled hypertension, advanced retinopathy, or severe autonomic or peripheral neuropathy (Gilbert, 2011).

When exercise is prescribed by the health care provider as part of the treatment plan, specific instructions are given to the woman. Aerobic exercise with resistance training for at least 30 minutes most days of the week is the best type of exercise (Gilbert, 2011). Other exercises that may be recommended are non–weight-bearing activities such as arm exercises or use of a recumbent bicycle. The best time for exercise is after meals, when the blood glucose level is rising. To monitor the effect of insulin on blood glucose levels the woman can measure blood glucose before, during, and after exercise.

! NURSING ALERT

Uterine contractions may occur during exercise. The woman should be advised to stop exercising immediately if they are detected, drink two to three glasses of water, and lie down on her side for an hour. If the contractions continue, she should contact her health care provider.

Insulin Therapy. Adequate insulin is the primary factor in the maintenance of euglycemia during pregnancy, thus ensuring proper glucose metabolism of the woman and fetus. Insulin requirements during pregnancy change dramatically as the pregnancy progresses, necessitating frequent adjustments in the dose. In the first trimester, from weeks 3 to 7 of gestation, insulin requirements are increased followed by a decrease between weeks 7 and 15 of gestation. The commonly prescribed dose is 0.7 units/kg in the first trimester for women with type 1 diabetes. During the second and third trimesters, because of insulin resistance, the dose must be increased significantly to maintain target glucose levels. Insulin requirements normally plateau after 35 weeks of gestation and often drop significantly after 38 weeks (Moore & Catalano, 2009).

For the woman with type 1 pregestational diabetes who has typically been accustomed to one injection per day of intermediate-acting insulin, multiple daily injections of mixed insulin are a new experience. The woman with type 2 diabetes previously treated with oral hypoglycemics is faced with the task of learning to self-administer injections of insulin. The nurse is instrumental in the education and support of women with pregestational diabetes in regard to insulin administration and adjustment of the insulin dose to maintain euglycemia (see the Teaching for Self-Management box: Self-Administration of Insulin and Box 29-1).

Since 1982, most insulin preparations have been produced by inserting portions of deoxyribonucleic acid (DNA) ("recombinant DNA") into special laboratory-cultivated bacteria or yeast cells. The cells then produce synthetic human insulin (Humulin), which is less likely to cause antibody formation than animal-derived (beef or pork) insulin. More recently, insulin products called *insulin analogs*, in which the structure differs slightly from human insulin, have been produced. This small alteration in insulin structure results in changes in the onset and peak of action of the medication. The most commonly used insulin preparations include rapid-acting, short-acting, intermediate-acting, and long-acting (Landon et al., 2007) (Table 29-4). Mixtures of short- and intermediate-acting insulins in several proportions are also available.

TEACHING FOR SELF-MANAGEMENT

Self-Administration of Insulin

PROCEDURE FOR MIXING NPH (INTERMEDIATE-ACTING) AND REGULAR (SHORT-ACTING) INSULIN

- Wash hands thoroughly and gather supplies. Be sure the insulin syringe corresponds to the concentration of insulin you are using.
- Check the insulin bottle to be certain it is the appropriate type, and check the expiration date.
- Gently rotate (do not shake) the insulin vial to mix the insulin.
- Wipe off rubber stopper of each vial with alcohol.
- Draw into syringe the amount of air equal to total dose.
- Inject air equal to NPH dose into NPH vial. Remove syringe from vial.
- Inject air equal to regular insulin dose into regular insulin vial.
- Invert regular insulin bottle and withdraw regular insulin dose.
- Without adding more air to NPH vial, carefully withdraw NPH dose.

PROCEDURE FOR SELF-INJECTION OF INSULIN

- Select proper injection site.
- Injection site should be clean. No need to use alcohol. If alcohol is used, let it dry before injecting.
- Pinch the skin up to form a subcutaneous pocket and, holding the syringe as you would hold a pencil, puncture the skin at a 45- to 90-degree angle. If a great deal of fatty tissue is at the site, spread the skin taut and inject the syringe at a 90-degree angle.
- Slowly inject the insulin.
- As you withdraw the needle, cover the injection site with sterile gauze and apply gentle pressure to prevent bleeding.
- Record insulin dose and time of injection.

BOX 29-1 HELPFUL HINTS FOR USING INSULIN

- The most common type of insulin used during pregnancy is a biosynthetic human insulin (Humulin) made by programming *Escherichia coli* bacteria to produce insulin.
- Insulin is classified either as rapid acting, short acting, intermediate acting, or long acting (see Table 29-4).
- Unused vials of insulin should be stored in the refrigerator until reaching their expiration date. Insulin should not be frozen. Vials currently in use can be stored at room temperature for up to a month. They should not be stored in direct sunlight.
- Regular insulin can be mixed with NPH insulin in the same syringe. Lispro insulin can also be mixed in a syringe with NPH or Ultralente insulin. Once mixed, the syringe can be used immediately or stored for future use. If it is used later, the syringe should be rotated 20 times before injection.
- Glargine insulin is administered at bedtime. It cannot be mixed with any other insulin in the same syringe. Prepared syringes are stable for 2 weeks in the refrigerator.
- Insulin may be administered by pen injector, jet injector, or insulin pump, in addition to syringe.
- The abdomen is the preferred injection site because insulin is best absorbed there. Other possible injection sites are the upper outer arm (not the deltoid area), the thighs, and the buttocks.
- Each injection should be given 1 inch from the previous injection. Each individual injection site should not be used more often than once in 30 days.

Source: Gilbert, E. (2007). *Manual of high risk pregnancy & delivery* (4th ed.). St. Louis: Mosby.

TABLE 29-4 COMMON INSULIN PREPARATIONS

TYPE OF INSULIN	GENERIC (TRADE) NAME	ONSET OF ACTION	PEAK OF ACTION	DURATION OF ACTION
Rapid-acting	Lispro (Humalog)	15 min	30-90 min	4-5 hr
	Aspart (NovoLog)	15 min	1-3 hr	3-5 hr
Short-acting	Humulin R	30 min	2-4 hr	5-7 hr
	Novolin R	30 min	2.5-5 hr	6-8 hr
Intermediate-acting	Humulin NPH	1-2 hr	6-12 hr	18-24 hr
	Novolin N	1.5 hr	4-20 hr	24 hr
	Humulin Lente	1-3 hr	6-12 hr	18-24 hr
	Novolin L	2.5 hr	7-15 hr	22 hr
Long-acting	Humulin Ultralente	4-6 hr	8-20 hr	>36 hr
	Glargine (Lantus)	1 hr	None	24 hr

R, Regular.
Source: Landon, M., Catalano, P., & Gabbe, S. (2007). Diabetes mellitus complicating pregnancy. In S. Gabbe, J. Niebyl, & J. Simpson (Eds.), *Obstetrics: Normal and problem pregnancies* (5th ed.). Philadelphia: Churchill Livingstone.

Lispro (Humalog) and aspart (NovoLog) are commonly prescribed rapid-acting insulins with a shorter duration of action than regular insulin. Advantages of rapid-acting insulins include convenience because they are injected immediately before mealtime, less hyperglycemia after meals, and fewer hypoglycemic episodes in some people. Because their effects last only 3 to 5 hours, most clients require a longer-acting insulin in addition to the rapid-acting insulin to maintain optimal blood glucose levels (Landon et al., 2007; Moore & Catalano, 2009) (see Table 29-4).

Glargine (Lantus) is a long-acting insulin lasting approximately 24 hours. Small amounts of glargine insulin are slowly released, with no pronounced peak. This preparation is most often used with women who have insulin-resistant diabetes (type 2) requiring high doses of long-acting insulin. Glargine insulin is combined with a rapid-acting insulin to prevent hypoglycemia. Concerns associated with this medication include the need for monitoring for nocturnal hypoglycemia (Moore & Catalano, 2009) and a possible increase in the progression of retinopathy in some women (Landon et al., 2007) (see Table 29-4).

Most women with insulin-dependent diabetes are managed with two or three injections per day (Landon et al., 2007). Usually two thirds of the daily insulin dose, with intermediate-acting and short-acting insulin combined in a 2:1 ratio, is given before breakfast. The remaining one third, again a combination of longer- and short-acting insulin, is administered in the evening before dinner. To reduce the risk of hypoglycemia during the night, separate injections often are administered, with short-acting insulin given before dinner followed by longer-acting insulin at bedtime. An alternative insulin regimen that works well for some women is to administer short-acting insulin before each meal and longer-acting insulin at bedtime (Moore & Catalano, 2009).

Continuous subcutaneous insulin infusion (CSII) systems are increasingly used during pregnancy. The insulin pump is designed to mimic more closely the function of the pancreas in secreting insulin (Fig. 29-3). This portable battery-powered device is worn, similar to a pager, during most daily activities. The pump infuses regular insulin at a set basal rate and has the capacity to deliver up to four different basal rates in 24 hours. It also delivers bolus doses of insulin before meals to control postprandial blood glucose levels. A fine-gauge plastic catheter is inserted into subcutaneous tissue, usually in the abdomen, and attached to the pump syringe by connecting tubing. The subcutaneous catheter and connecting tubing are changed every 2 to 3 days, although the infusion tubing can be left in place for several weeks without local complications. Although the insulin pump is convenient and generally provides good glycemic control, complications such as pump failure, precipitation of insulin inside the pump mechanism, abscess formation, and poor uptake from the infusion site can still occur. Therefore, use of the insulin pump requires a knowledgeable, motivated woman; skilled health care providers; and prompt 24-hour availability of emergency assistance (Moore & Catalano, 2009).

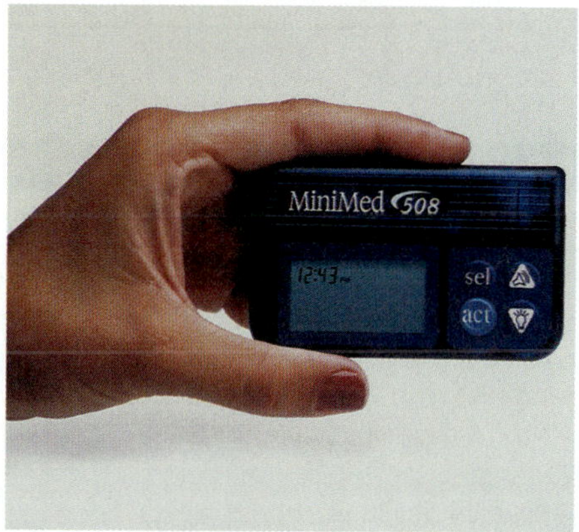

FIG. 29-3 Insulin pump shows basal rate for pregnant women with diabetes. (Courtesy MiniMed, Inc., Sylmar, CA.)

Monitoring Blood Glucose Levels. Blood glucose testing at home with a glucose reflectance meter is considered the standard of care for monitoring blood glucose levels during pregnancy. It provides the most important tool available to the woman to assess her degree of glycemic control. Most of the newer reflectance meters are calibrated to provide plasma (rather than whole blood) glucose values. Plasma glucose values are 10% to 15% lower than those measured in whole blood from the same sample (Moore & Catalano, 2009).

SAFETY ALERT

The nurse must be knowledgeable about the specific glucose reflectance meter that the client uses because target glucose values depend on the type of meter used (Moore & Catalano, 2009).

To perform blood glucose monitoring a drop of blood is obtained by means of a fingerstick and placed on a test strip. After a specified amount of time the glucose level is displayed by the meter (see the Teaching for Self-Management box: Self-Testing of Blood Glucose Level). Blood glucose levels are routinely measured at various times throughout the day, such as before breakfast, lunch, and dinner; 2 hours after each meal; at bedtime; and in the middle of the night. When any readjustment in the insulin dose or diet is made, more frequent measurement of blood glucose is warranted. If nausea, vomiting, or diarrhea occurs, or if any infection is present, the woman will be asked to monitor her blood glucose levels more closely than usual.

! NURSING ALERT

Hyperglycemia is most likely to be identified in 2-hour postprandial values because blood glucose levels peak approximately 2 hours after a meal.

TEACHING FOR SELF-MANAGEMENT

Self-Testing of Blood Glucose Level

- Gather supplies, check expiration date, and read instructions on testing materials. Prepare glucose reflectance meter for use according to manufacturer's directions.
- Wash hands in warm water (warmth increases circulation).
- Select site on side of any finger (all fingers should be used in rotation).
- Pierce site with lancet (may use automatic spring-loaded, puncturing device). Cleaning the site with alcohol is not necessary.
- Drop hand down to side; with other hand gently squeeze finger from hand to fingertip.
- Allow blood to drop onto testing strip. Be sure to cover entire testing area.
- Determine blood glucose value using the glucose reflectance meter following manufacturer's instructions.
- Record results.
- Repeat as instructed by the health care provider and as needed for signs of hypoglycemia or hyperglycemia.

Target levels of blood glucose during pregnancy are lower than nonpregnant values (see Table 29-3). Acceptable fasting levels are generally between 65 and 95 mg/dl, and 1-hour postprandial levels should be less than 130 to 140 mg/dl (Moore & Catalano, 2009). Two-hour postprandial levels should be less than 120 mg/dl (Landon et al., 2007). The woman should be told to report episodes of hypoglycemia (less than 60 mg/dl) and hyperglycemia (more than 200 mg/dl) immediately to her health care provider so that adjustments in diet or insulin therapy can be made.

Pregnant women with diabetes are much more likely to develop hypoglycemia than hyperglycemia. Most episodes of mild or moderate hypoglycemia can be treated with oral intake of 15 g of simple carbohydrate (fast sugar) (see the Teaching for Self-Management box: Treatment for Hypoglycemia). If severe hypoglycemia occurs, in which case the woman experiences a decrease in or loss of consciousness or an inability to swallow, she will require a parenteral injection of glucagon or intravenous (IV) glucose. Because hypoglycemia can develop rapidly, and because impaired judgment can be associated with even moderate episodes, family members, friends, and work colleagues must be able to recognize signs and symptoms quickly and initiate proper treatment if necessary.

TEACHING FOR SELF-MANAGEMENT

Treatment for Hypoglycemia

- Be familiar with signs and symptoms of hypoglycemia (nervousness, headache, fatigue, shaking, irritability, tachycardia, hunger, blurred vision, sweaty skin, tingling of mouth or extremities).
- Check blood glucose level immediately when hypoglycemic symptoms occur.
- If blood glucose is less than 60 mg/dl, immediately eat or drink something that contains 15 g of fast sugar (simple carbohydrate). Examples are:
    - ½ cup (4 ounces) unsweetened orange juice
    - ½ cup (4 ounces) regular (not diet) soda
    - 5 or 6 hard candies
    - 1 cup (8 ounces) skim milk
    - 2 or 3 glucose tablets
- Rest for 15 minutes, then recheck blood glucose.
- If glucose level is greater than 60 mg/dl, eat a meal to stabilize the sugar level.
- If glucose level is still less than 60 mg/dl, eat or drink another serving of one of the fast sugars listed above.
- Wait 15 minutes, then recheck blood glucose. If the level is still less than 60 mg/dl, notify your health care provider immediately.

Hyperglycemia is less likely than hypoglycemia to occur, but it can rapidly progress to DKA, which is associated with an increased risk of fetal death (Cunningham et al., 2010; Moore & Catalano, 2009). Women and family members should be particularly alert for signs and symptoms of hyperglycemia, especially when infections or other illnesses occur (see the Teaching for Self-Management box: What to Do When Illness Occurs).

TEACHING FOR SELF-MANAGEMENT

What to Do When Illness Occurs

- Be sure to take insulin even if unable to eat or appetite is less than normal. (Insulin needs are increased with illness or infection.)
- Call the health care provider and relay the following information:
    - Symptoms of illness (e.g., nausea, vomiting, diarrhea)
    - Elevated temperature
    - Most recent blood glucose level
    - Urine ketones
    - Time and amount of last insulin dose
- Increase oral intake of fluids to prevent dehydration.
- Rest as much as possible.
- If you are unable to reach your health care provider and blood glucose exceeds 200 mg/dl with urine ketones present, seek emergency treatment at the nearest health care facility. Do not attempt to self-treat for this condition.

Urine Testing. Urine testing for glucose is not beneficial during pregnancy. Because of the lowered renal threshold for glucose, the degree of glycosuria does not accurately reflect the blood glucose level. Urine testing for ketones, however, continues to have a place in diabetic management. Monitoring for urine ketones may detect inadequate caloric or carbohydrate intake or skipped meals or snacks. Testing may also be performed when illness occurs, or when the blood glucose level is greater than 200 mg/dl (Gilbert, 2011).

Complications Requiring Hospitalization. Occasionally, hospitalization is necessary to regulate insulin therapy and stabilize glucose levels. Infection, which can lead to hyperglycemia and DKA, is an indication for hospitalization, regardless of gestational age. Hospitalization during the third trimester for close maternal and fetal observation may be indicated for women whose diabetes is poorly controlled. In addition, women with diabetes are 10% to 20% more likely than women who do not have diabetes to also have preexisting hypertension or develop preeclampsia, which may necessitate hospitalization (Moore & Catalano, 2009).

Fetal Surveillance. Diagnostic techniques for fetal surveillance are often performed to assess fetal growth and well-being. The goals of fetal surveillance are to detect fetal compromise as early as possible and to prevent intrauterine fetal death or unnecessary preterm birth.

Early in pregnancy the estimated date of birth is determined. A baseline sonogram is obtained during the first trimester to assess gestational age. Follow-up ultrasound examinations are usually performed during the pregnancy (as often as every 4 to 6 weeks) to monitor fetal growth, estimate fetal weight, and detect hydramnios, macrosomia, and congenital anomalies.

Because the fetus of a woman with diabetes is at increased risk for neural tube defects (e.g., spina bifida, anencephaly, microcephaly), measurement of maternal serum alpha-fetoprotein is performed between 15 and 20 weeks of gestation (ideally between 16 and 18 weeks of gestation) (Wapner, Jenkins, & Khalek, 2009). This assessment is often performed in conjunction with a detailed ultrasound study to examine the fetus for neural tube defects.

Fetal echocardiography may be performed between 20 and 22 weeks of gestation to detect cardiac anomalies, especially in women who had less-than-desirable glucose control early in pregnancy, as demonstrated by a hemoglobin A_{1c} level above 6% at the first prenatal visit (Gilbert, 2011; Moore & Catalano, 2009). Some practitioners repeat this fetal surveillance test at 34 weeks of gestation. Doppler studies of the umbilical artery may be performed in women with vascular disease to detect placental compromise.

The majority of fetal surveillance measures are concentrated in the third trimester, when the risk of fetal compromise is greatest. The goals of antepartum testing during the third trimester are to prevent IUFD and maximize the opportunity for the woman to safely give birth vaginally. Pregnant women should be taught how to make daily fetal movement counts, beginning at 28 weeks of gestation (see Chapter 26) (Moore & Catalano, 2009).

Biophysical testing (nonstress testing, contraction stress testing, or biophysical profile) once or twice weekly to evaluate fetal well-being, is typically begun around 34 weeks of gestation. This testing should begin around 28 weeks in women who have poor glucose control or significant hypertension (Moore & Catalano, 2009) (see Chapter 26).

Determination of Birth Date and Mode of Birth. The optimal time for birth is between 38.5 and 40 weeks of gestation, as long as good metabolic control is maintained and parameters of antepartum fetal surveillance remain within normal limits. Reasons to proceed with birth before term include poor metabolic control, worsening hypertensive disorders, fetal macrosomia, or fetal growth restriction (Moore & Catalano, 2009).

Many practitioners plan for elective labor induction between 38 and 40 weeks of gestation. To confirm fetal lung maturity an amniocentesis should be performed when birth will occur before 38.5 weeks of gestation. For the pregnancy complicated by diabetes, fetal lung maturation is best predicted by the amniotic fluid phosphatidylglycerol (greater than 3%). If the fetal lungs are still immature, birth should be postponed until 40 weeks of gestation as long as fetal assessment test results remain reassuring. After that time, however, the benefits of conservative management are outweighed by the increasing risk of fetal compromise if the pregnancy is allowed to continue. Birth, despite poor fetal lung maturity, may be necessary when testing suggests fetal compromise or worsening maternal condition, such as deteriorating renal function or severe preeclampsia (Moore & Catalano, 2009).

Although vaginal birth is expected for most women with pregestational diabetes, the cesarean rate for these women ranges from 50% to 80% (Cunningham et al., 2010). The American College of Obstetricians and Gynecologists (ACOG) recommends that cesarean birth be considered when the estimated fetal weight is expected to be greater than 4500 g in an attempt to reduce the risk of shoulder dystocia. This recommendation appears to result in a small improvement in neonatal outcome (Moore & Catalano, 2009). Fetal distress and induction failures before term also contribute to the high rate of cesarean birth in these women (Gilbert, 2011).

Intrapartum

During the intrapartum period the woman with pregestational diabetes must be monitored closely to prevent complications related to dehydration, hypoglycemia, and hyperglycemia. An IV line is inserted for infusion of a maintenance fluid. Initially this infusion may be normal saline or lactated Ringer's solution. The IV fluid will be changed to one containing 5% dextrose during active labor to provide the energy (calories) necessary for the woman to accomplish the work and manage the stress of labor and birth. Most commonly, insulin is administered by continuous infusion, piggybacked into the main IV line. Only rapid- or short-acting insulin may be administered intravenously. Determinations of blood glucose levels are made every hour, and fluids and insulin are adjusted to maintain the blood glucose level at less than 140 mg/dl (Landon et al., 2007). Maintaining this target glucose level is essential because hyperglycemia during labor can cause metabolic problems in the neonate, particularly hypoglycemia.

During labor continuous fetal heart monitoring is necessary. The woman should assume an upright or side-lying position during bed rest in labor to prevent supine hypotension because of a large fetus or polyhydramnios. Labor (spontaneous or induced) is allowed to progress as long as expected rates of cervical dilation and fetal descent are maintained, and fetal well-being is evident. Failure to progress may indicate a macrosomic infant and cephalopelvic disproportion, necessitating a cesarean birth. The woman is observed and treated during labor for complications of diabetes such as hyperglycemia, ketosis, and ketoacidosis. During second-stage labor, shoulder dystocia may occur with birth of a macrosomic infant (see Chapter 33). A neonatologist, pediatrician, or neonatal nurse practitioner will likely be present at the birth to initiate assessment and neonatal care.

If a cesarean birth is planned, it should be scheduled in the early morning to facilitate glycemic control. Women should take their full dose of insulin the night before surgery. No morning insulin is given on the day of surgery, and the woman is given nothing by mouth. Epidural anesthesia is recommended because hypoglycemia can be detected earlier if the woman is awake. After surgery, glucose levels should be monitored carefully. Generally sliding scale insulin is used to control blood glucose levels until the woman resumes a regular diet (Moore & Catalano, 2009).

Postpartum

During the first 24 hours postpartum, insulin requirements decrease substantially because the major source of insulin resistance, the placenta, has been removed. Women with type 1 diabetes may require only one third to one half of their last pregnancy insulin dose on the first postpartum day, provided that they are eating a full diet (Landon et al., 2007). These women who give birth by cesarean may require an IV infusion of glucose and insulin until they resume a regular diet (Moore & Catalano, 2009). Several days after birth may be required to reestablish carbohydrate homeostasis (see Fig. 29-1, *D* and *E*). Blood glucose levels are carefully monitored in the postpartum period and the insulin dose is adjusted, often using a sliding scale. The woman who has insulin-dependent diabetes must realize the importance of eating on time even if the baby needs feeding or other pressing demands exist. Women with type 2 diabetes often require only 30% to 50% of their pregnancy insulin dose in the postpartum period (Moore & Catalano).

Possible postpartum complications include preeclampsia or eclampsia, hemorrhage, and infection. Hemorrhage is a possibility if the mother's uterus was overdistended (hydramnios, macrosomic fetus) or overstimulated (oxytocin induction). Postpartum infections such as endometritis are more likely to occur in women with diabetes than in women who do not have diabetes.

Mothers are encouraged to breastfeed. In addition to the advantages of maternal satisfaction and pleasure, breastfeeding has an antidiabetogenic effect for the children of women with diabetes and for women with gestational diabetes (Lindsay, 2006; Moore & Catalano, 2009). This effect is important because a child born to a mother with type 2 diabetes has a 70% chance of also developing type 2 diabetes later in life. In addition, children who were exposed to hyperglycemia prenatally have an increased risk for obesity in childhood (Gilbert, 2011).

Insulin requirements in breastfeeding women may be one half of prepregnancy levels because of the carbohydrate used in human milk production. Because glucose levels are lower than normal, breastfeeding women are at increased risk for hypoglycemia, especially in the early postpartum period and after breastfeeding sessions, particularly after late-night nursing (Gilbert, 2011; Moore & Catalano, 2009). Breastfeeding mothers with diabetes may be at increased risk for mastitis and yeast infections of the breast. The insulin dose, which is decreased during lactation, must be recalculated at weaning (see Fig. 29-1, *F*).

The mother may have early breastfeeding difficulties. Poor metabolic control may delay lactogenesis and contribute to decreased milk production (Moore & Catalano, 2009). Initial contact with and opportunity to breastfeed the infant may be delayed for mothers who gave birth by cesarean or if infants are placed in neonatal intensive care units or special care nurseries for observation during the first few hours after birth. Support and assistance from nursing staff and lactation specialists can facilitate the mother's early experience with breastfeeding and encourage her to continue.

The new mother needs information about family planning and contraception. Although family planning is important for all women, it is essential for the woman with diabetes so as to safeguard her own health and to promote optimal outcomes in future pregnancies. The risks and benefits of contraceptive methods should be discussed with the mother and her partner before discharge from the hospital. Barrier methods are often recommended as safe, inexpensive options that have no inherent risks for women with diabetes. The intrauterine device (IUD) may also be used without concerns about an increased risk of infection (Landon et al., 2007).

Use of oral contraceptives by women with diabetes is controversial because of the risk of thromboembolic and vascular complications and the effect on carbohydrate metabolism. In non-smoking women who are less than 35 years old and do not have vascular disease, combination low-dose oral contraceptives can be prescribed. Progestin-only oral contraceptives can also be used because they affect minimally, if at all, carbohydrate metabolism (Cunningham et al., 2010). Close monitoring of blood pressure and lipid levels is necessary to detect complications (Landon et al., 2007).

Opinion is divided about the use of long-acting parenteral progestins, such as Depo-Provera. Some health care providers recommend their use, particularly in women who are noncompliant with daily dosing oral contraceptives. In contrast, other health care providers believe this method may adversely affect glycemic control.

Transdermal (patch) and transvaginal (vaginal ring) administration are newer contraceptive methods, particularly effective in women who prefer weekly or every-third-week dosing, respectively. For women weighing more than 90 kg the contraceptive failure rate with transdermal administration is higher than in normal-weight women. Therefore, this method would be contraindicated in obese women. In addition, women who choose the patch as their contraceptive method should have no risk factors for cardiovascular or thromboembolic disease (Cunningham et al., 2010).

The risks associated with pregnancy increase with the duration and severity of diabetes. In addition, pregnancy may contribute to the vascular changes associated with diabetes. This information needs to be thoroughly discussed with the woman and her partner. Sterilization is often recommended for the woman who has completed her family, who has poor metabolic control, or who has significant vascular problems.

GESTATIONAL DIABETES MELLITUS

GDM complicates approximately 3% to 9% of all pregnancies (Moore & Catalano, 2009) and accounts for more than 90% of all cases of diabetic pregnancy (Landon et al., 2007). According to White's classification system, these women fall into classes A_1 and A_2 (see Table 29-1). GDM is more likely to occur among Hispanic, Native American, Asian, and African-American women than in Caucasians and is likely to recur in future pregnancies; the risk for development of overt diabetes in later life is also increased (Moore & Catalano). This tendency is especially true of women whose GDM is diagnosed early in pregnancy or who are obese (Landon et al.). Classic risk factors for GDM include maternal age older than 25 years, previous macrosomic infant, previous unexplained IUFD, previous pregnancy with GDM, strong immediate family history of type 2 diabetes or GDM, obesity (weight more than 90 kg), and fasting blood glucose greater than 140 mg/dl or random blood glucose greater than 200 mg/dl. Women at high risk for developing GDM should have glucola screening at the first prenatal visit and again at 24 to 28 weeks of gestation if the initial screen is negative (Landon et al.).

GDM is usually diagnosed during the second half of pregnancy. As fetal nutrient demands rise during the late second and the third trimesters, maternal nutrient ingestion induces greater and more sustained levels of blood glucose. At the same time, maternal insulin resistance is also increasing because of the insulin-antagonistic effects of the placental hormones, cortisol, and insulinase. Consequently, maternal insulin demands rise as much as threefold. Most pregnant women are capable of increasing insulin production to compensate for insulin resistance and to maintain euglycemia. When the pancreas is unable to produce sufficient insulin or the insulin is not used effectively, however, gestational diabetes can result.

Fetal Risks

No increase in the incidence of birth defects has been found among infants of women who develop gestational diabetes after the first trimester because the critical period of organ formation has already passed by that time (Moore & Catalano, 2009). However, Anderson and associates (2005) found that women who were obese before conception (BMI more than 30 kg/m^2) and developed gestational diabetes were at greater risk to give birth to infants with CNS defects.

Screening for Gestational Diabetes Mellitus

All pregnant women not known to have pregestational diabetes should be screened for GDM by history, clinical risk factors, or laboratory screening of blood glucose levels. Based on history and clinical risk factors, some women are at low risk for the development of GDM. Therefore, glucose testing for this low risk population is not cost effective (ADA, 2008). This group includes normal-weight women younger than 25 years of age who have no family history of diabetes, are not members of an ethnic or a racial group known to have a high prevalence of the disease, and have no history of abnormal glucose tolerance or adverse obstetric outcomes usually associated with GDM (ADA).

The screening test (glucola screening) most often used consists of a 50-g oral glucose load followed by a plasma glucose measurement 1 hour later. The woman need not be fasting. A glucose value of 130 to 140 mg/dl is considered a positive screen and should be followed by a 3-hour (100-g) oral glucose tolerance test (OGTT). The OGTT is administered after an overnight fast and at least 3 days of unrestricted diet (at least 150 g of carbohydrate) and physical activity. The woman is instructed to avoid caffeine because it will increase glucose levels and to abstain from smoking for 12 hours before the test. The 3-hour OGTT requires a fasting blood glucose level, which is drawn before giving a 100-g glucose load. Blood glucose levels are then drawn 1, 2, and 3 hours later. The woman is diagnosed with gestational diabetes if two or more values are met or exceeded (Moore & Catalano, 2009) (Fig. 29-4).

Nursing diagnoses and expected outcomes of care for women with GDM are basically the same as those for women with pregestational diabetes except that the time frame for planning may be shortened with GDM because the diagnosis is usually made later in pregnancy (see the Nursing Care Plan).

Critical Thinking Exercise—Gestational Diabetes

CARE MANAGEMENT

Antepartum

When the diagnosis of gestational diabetes is made, treatment begins immediately, allowing little or no time for the woman and her family to adjust to the diagnosis before they are expected to participate in the treatment plan. With each step of the treatment plan the nurse and other health care providers should educate the woman and her family, providing detailed and comprehensive explanations to ensure understanding, participation, and adherence to the necessary interventions. Potential complications should be discussed, and the need for maintenance of euglycemia throughout the remainder of the pregnancy reinforced. Knowing that gestational diabetes typically disappears when the pregnancy is over may be reassuring for the woman and her family.

As with pregestational diabetes, the aim of therapy in women with GDM is strict blood glucose control. Fasting blood glucose levels should range from 65 to 95 mg/dl, and 1-hour postprandial blood glucose levels should be less than 130 to 140 mg/dl (Moore & Catalano, 2009).

Diet. Dietary modification is the mainstay of treatment for GDM. The woman with GDM is placed on a standard diabetic diet. The usual prescription is 30 kcal/kg/day based on a normal preconception weight. For obese women the usual prescription is up to 25 kcal/kg/day, which translates into 1500 to 2000 kcal/day. Carbohydrate intake is restricted to approximately 50% of caloric intake (Moore & Catalano, 2009). Dietary counseling by a registered dietician is recommended.

Exercise. Several studies have examined the benefits of exercise in women with GDM. Three randomized trials found that exercise improved cardiovascular fitness without improving pregnancy outcome. Another study found that exercise decreased the need for insulin in overweight women with GDM (Cunningham et al., 2010).

EVIDENCE-BASED PRACTICE

Pat Gingrich

Stricter Glucose Tolerance Test in Pregnancy Will Mean Increased Diagnoses of Gestational Diabetes

ASK THE QUESTION

Does screening for gestational diabetes contribute to better outcomes for mother and baby?

SEARCH FOR EVIDENCE

Search Strategies

Professional organization guidelines, meta-analyses, systematic reviews, randomized controlled trials, nonrandomized prospective studies and retrospective studies since 2008.

Databases Searched

CINAHL, Cochrane, Medline, and the websites for the National Guideline Clearinghouse, TRIP Database, and American College of Obstetricians and Gynecologists.

CRITICALLY ANALYZE THE DATA

During pregnancy, hormonal changes, insulin resistance, and a growing fetus cause frequent shifts in glycemic control. Approximately 7% of all pregnancies will be affected by gestational diabetes mellitus (GDM), which is defined as any glucose intolerance that initially manifests during pregnancy. Fetal risks associated with GDM include macrosomia leading to birth trauma and hypoglycemia. Maternal risks include injury from operative or cesarean birth, and the development of overt diabetes later in life.

In pregnancy, some practitioners have screened women for GDM based on risk factors, while others have screened universally. The American Diabetes Association has issued practice standards (2010) calling for screening of all women who have moderate to high risk factors for GDM. Low-risk women who do not need screening include those who are less than 25 years old, normal pre-pregnancy weight, member of low-risk ethnic group, no diabetes history in close relatives, no personal history of glucose intolerance or previous poor obstetrical outcome. The Hyperglycemic and Adverse Pregnancy Outcome study was an international, large scale epidemiological study of around 25,000 women to evaluate diagnostic criteria. The researchers recommended universal glucose tolerance tests at 24-28 weeks, and raising the threshold glucose results. This increases the sensitivity of the test, and thus will include more women under the diagnosis of GDM (Coustan, Lowe, Metzger, Dyer, & the International Association of Diabetes and Pregnancy Study Groups, 2010).

Whether or not the stricter guidelines for glucose tolerance testing are accepted as standard practice, some interventions for women diagnosed with GDM have been found to contribute to better outcomes for the woman and newborn. A Cochrane Systematic Review of five trials involving 1255 women found that intensive treatment that included nutrition and medical therapy (oral hypoglycemics or insulin) for even mild GDM reduced perinatal mortality, shoulder dystocia, bone fracture, nerve palsy and macrosomia. However, intensive treatment was also associated with a higher incidence of labor induction (Alwan, Tuffnell, & West, 2009). This was confirmed in a systematic review and meta-analysis of five randomized, controlled trials that found screening and treating women for GDM resulted in significantly less shoulder dystocia, preeclampsia, and macrosomia. The review found a dose-related effect (the more intensive the treatments, the greater the benefit) (Horvath, Koch, Jeitler, Matyas, Bender, Bastian, et al., 2010).

All persons with GDM should be counseled about the benefits of a low-glycemic diet. Low-glycemic foods slow down the digestion of food and moderate the postprandial glucose spike. The prevention of glucose extremes is especially important in pregnancy. A Cochrane Database meta-analysis found that women with GDM can benefit themselves and their babies by eating low-glycemic foods such as fruits, vegetables, whole grains, and legumes (Tieu, Crowther, & Middleton, 2008).

IMPLICATIONS FOR PRACTICE

Nurses are in an ideal position to counsel their patients at risk for GDM about the importance of glucose control and healthy habits before pregnancy. Screenings following the evidence-based guidelines are likely to identify more women as having GDM. Women and their babies benefit from the skills that women learn about diet and exercise, as well as medical management of GDM. Of particular benefit is the instruction in the low-glycemic diet. Women should be given the information they need to make informed decisions about their health and empowered by the knowledge to self-manage their care in partnership with the health team. Nurses should offer a positive message about their pregnancy and constant support, as well as frequent monitoring and follow-up. Women need emergency telephone numbers and other resources they can access anytime they have questions. Nurses can offer frequent encouragement and praise that pregnant women with GDM are giving their babies the best possible start in life.

References

Alwan, N., Tuffnell, D., & West, J. (2009). Treatment for gestational diabetes. *The Cochrane Database of Systematic Reviews, 2009*, 3, CD003395.

American Diabetes Association. (2010). Standards of medical care in diabetes-2010. *Diabetes Care, 33*(supplement), S11–S61.

Coustan, D., Lowe, L., Metzger, B., Dyer, A., and the International Association of Diabetes and Pregnancy Study Groups. (2010). The Hyperglycemic and Adverse Pregnancy Outcome (HAPO) study: Paving the way for new diagnostic criteria for gestational diabetes mellitus. *American Journal of Obstetrics and Gynecology, 202*(6), e1–e6.

Horvath, K., Koch, K., Jeitler, K., Matyas, E., Bender, R., Bastian, H., et al. (2010). Effects of treatment in women with gestational diabetes mellitus: Systematic review and meta-analysis. *British Medical Journal, 340*, 1395.

Tieu, J., Crowther, C., & Middleton, P. (2008). Dietary advice in pregnancy for preventing gestational diabetes mellitus. *The Cochrane Database of Systematic Reviews, 2008*, 2, CD006674.

Monitoring Blood Glucose Levels. Blood glucose monitoring is necessary to determine whether euglycemia can be maintained by diet and exercise. Women are instructed to monitor their blood sugar daily. The frequency and timing of blood glucose monitoring should be individualized for each woman. A typical schedule for monitoring blood glucose is on rising in the morning, after breakfast, before and after lunch, after dinner, and at bedtime (Moore & Catalano, 2009). Women with GDM usually perform self-monitoring with additional monitoring at the clinic or office visit.

Medications for Controlling Blood Glucose Levels. Up to 20% of women with GDM will require insulin during the pregnancy to maintain adequate blood glucose levels, despite compliance with the prescribed diet. In contrast to women with insulin-dependent diabetes, women with gestational diabetes are initially managed with diet and exercise alone. If fasting plasma glucose levels are greater than 95 mg/dl or 2-hour postprandial levels are greater than 120 mg/dl, then insulin therapy is begun (Cunningham et al., 2010) (see Table 29-3). Glyburide, an oral hypoglycemic agent, is being used more frequently with women with GDM instead of insulin. The fact that only minimal amounts of glyburide cross the placenta to the fetus makes it a good drug for use during pregnancy. It has also been used in women with type 2 diabetes who required large amounts of insulin to achieve glucose control with smaller insulin doses. Studies have shown that glyburide should be taken at least

NURSING CARE PLAN

The Pregnant Woman with Gestational Diabetes

NURSING DIAGNOSIS

Deficient knowledge related to gestational diabetes as evidenced by the woman's questions and concerns

Expected Outcome

The woman will be able to verbalize important information regarding gestational diabetes, its management, and potential effects on the pregnancy and fetus.

Nursing Interventions/*Rationales*

- Assess the woman's current knowledge base regarding the disease process, management, effects on pregnancy and fetus, and potential complications *to provide a database for further teaching.*
- Explain the pathophysiologic aspects of diabetes, effects on pregnancy and the fetus, and potential complications *to promote compliance with the treatment plan.*
- Explain the principles of the diabetic diet and have the woman plan her meals for 1 day, following these principles, *to promote self-management and compliance with the treatment plan.*
- Demonstrate the procedure for blood glucose monitoring and obtain a return demonstration *to establish the woman's comfort and competence with the procedure.*
- Demonstrate the procedure for insulin administration, should this become necessary, and obtain a return demonstration *to establish the woman's comfort and competence with the procedure.*
- Explain the importance of correctly taking oral hypoglycemic medication (right dose, right time), should this become necessary, *to promote self-management and compliance with the treatment plan.*
- Review signs and symptoms of hypoglycemia and hyperglycemia and appropriate interventions for both *to promote prompt recognition of complications and self-management.*
- Provide contact numbers for the health care team for prompt interventions and answers to questions on an ongoing basis *to promote comfort.*
- Review the expected plan of care *to allay anxiety and enlist cooperation of the woman in her care.*

NURSING DIAGNOSIS

Risk for fetal injury related to elevated maternal glucose levels

Expected Outcomes

The fetus will remain free of injury and be born at term in a healthy state.

Nursing Interventions/*Rationales*

- Assess the woman's current diabetic control *to identify the risk for fetal macrosomia.*
- Monitor fundal height during each prenatal visit *to identify appropriate fetal growth.*
- Assess fetal movement and heart rate during each prenatal visit and perform fetal assessment tests as ordered during the third trimester *to assess fetal well-being.*

NURSING DIAGNOSIS

Anxiety related to threat to maternal and fetal well-being as evidenced by the woman's verbal expressions of concern

Expected Outcomes

The woman will identify sources of anxiety and report feeling less anxious.

Nursing Interventions/*Rationales*

- Through therapeutic communication, promote an open relationship with woman *to promote trust.*
- Listen to the woman's feelings and concerns *to assess for any misconception or misinformation that may be contributing to anxiety.*
- Review potential dangers by providing factual information *to correct any misconceptions or misinformation.*
- Encourage the woman to share concerns with her health care team *to promote collaboration in her care.*

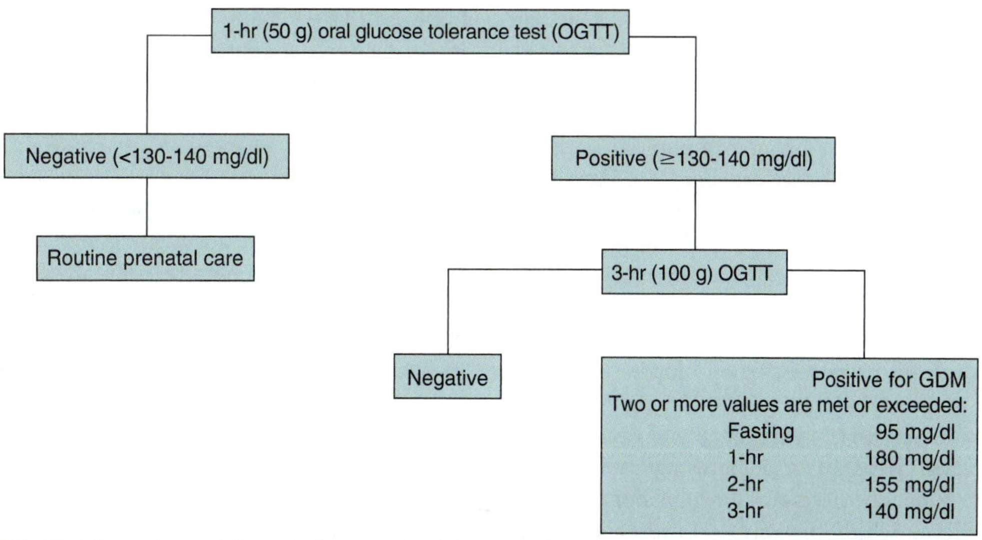

FIG. 29-4 Screening and diagnosis for gestational diabetes. (Sources: American Diabetes Association. [2008]. Position statement: Diagnosis and classification of diabetes mellitus. *Diabetes Care, 31*[Suppl.], S55-S60; Moore, T., & Catalano, P. [2009]. Diabetes in pregnancy. In R. Creasy, R. Resnik, J. Iams, C. Lockwood, & T. Moore [Eds.], *Creasy and Resnik's maternal-fetal medicine: Principles and practice* [6th ed.]. Philadelphia: Saunders.)

CLINICAL REASONING

Causes of Hyperglycemia in a Woman with Gestational Diabetes Mellitus (GDM)

Heather, a 26-year-old G1 P0, was diagnosed with gestational diabetes at 28 weeks of gestation and placed on a 2000-calorie ADA diet. She returns for a routine prenatal visit today at 32 weeks of gestation. You have just performed a blood glucose assessment, which was 180 mg/dl. On learning the result, Heather bursts into tears and sobs, "I don't know *why* my blood sugar would be that high! I have not eaten even one piece of candy since I was told I have diabetes!"

1. Evidence—Is there sufficient evidence to determine the cause of Heather's hyperglycemia at this time?
2. Assumptions—What assumptions can be made about the following issues related to hyperglycemia in a woman with GDM?
   a. Possible causes of hyperglycemia
   b. Possible management of hyperglycemia
   c. Significance of GDM in terms of future (after the pregnancy ends) health
3. What implications and priorities for nursing care can be drawn at this time?
4. Does the evidence objectively support your conclusion?
5. Are there alternative perspectives to your conclusion?

30 minutes (preferably 1 hour) before a meal so that its peak effect covers the 2-hour postprandial blood glucose level. Because episodes of hypoglycemia can occur between meals, women taking glyburide should always carry with them sources of fast sugar (Moore & Catalano, 2009). Women with diabetes who are unable or unwilling to take insulin by injection or are cognitively impaired also may be candidates for glyburide use.

Fetal Surveillance. No standard recommendation has been formulated for fetal surveillance in pregnancies complicated by GDM. Women whose blood glucose levels are well controlled by diet are at low risk for fetal complications. Limited antepartum fetal testing is performed in women with gestational diabetes as long as their fasting and 2-hour postprandial blood glucose levels remain within normal limits and they have no other risk factors. Women with hypertension, a prior IUFD, or suspected macrosomia or those who require insulin for blood glucose control may have twice-weekly nonstress testing beginning at 32 weeks of gestation (Landon et al., 2007). In general, women with GDM can continue pregnancy until 40 weeks of gestation and the spontaneous onset of labor. However, fetal growth should be monitored carefully because the risk for macrosomia as the pregnancy approaches 40 weeks of gestation is apparently increased (Landon et al.).

Intrapartum

During the labor and birth process, blood glucose levels are monitored hourly to maintain levels at 80 to 120 mg/dl (Moore & Catalano, 2009). Levels within this range will decrease the incidence of neonatal hypoglycemia. Infusing rapid-acting insulin intravenously may be necessary during labor to maintain blood glucose levels within this range. However, it is usually possible to maintain excellent glucose control in women with Class A_1 GDM during labor by simply avoiding dextrose intravenous fluids (Gilbert, 2011; Moore & Catalano, 2009). Although gestational diabetes is not an indication for cesarean birth, this procedure may be necessary in the presence of preeclampsia or macrosomia.

Postpartum

Most women with GDM will return to normal glucose levels after childbirth. However, the recurrence risk for GDM in the next pregnancy is 35% to 75%. In addition, women who have had GDM have a 35% to 60% risk for developing type 2 diabetes mellitus within the next twenty years (Gilbert, 2011). Assessment for carbohydrate intolerance with a 75-g OGTT should be performed at 6 to 12 weeks postpartum and a random or fasting blood glucose level should be checked each year (Cunningham et al., 2010; Gilbert). Obesity is a major risk factor for the later development of diabetes. Women with a history of GDM, particularly those who are overweight, should be encouraged to make lifestyle changes that include weight loss and exercise to reduce this risk (Gilbert). Children born to women with GDM are also at risk for becoming obese in childhood or adolescence (Lindsay, 2006).

HYPEREMESIS GRAVIDARUM

Nausea and vomiting complicate as many as 80% of all pregnancies beginning typically at 4 weeks of gestation. These symptoms are usually confined to the first 20 weeks of gestation (Kelly & Savides, 2009). Although nausea and vomiting are distressing, they are typically benign, with no significant metabolic alterations or risks to the mother or fetus. The cause of nausea and vomiting in pregnancy is not well understood, although it may involve relaxation of the smooth muscle of the stomach and increasing levels of estrogen, progesterone, and human chorionic gonadotropin (hCG). Pregnancies complicated by nausea and vomiting generally have a more favorable outcome than those without these symptoms (Gordon, 2007).

When vomiting during pregnancy becomes excessive enough to cause weight loss, electrolyte imbalance, nutritional deficiencies, and ketonuria, the disorder is termed **hyperemesis gravidarum.** This disorder occurs in approximately 0.5% of all live births. Hyperemesis gravidarum usually begins during the first trimester, but approximately 10% of women with the disorder continue to have symptoms throughout the pregnancy (Kelly & Savides, 2009). It has been associated with women who are nulliparous, have increased body weight, have a history of migraines (Davis, 2004), have a multiple gestation, have gestational trophoblastic disease, or are carrying a fetus with a chromosomal abnormality such as triploidy or trisomy 21 (Kelly & Savides). For unknown reasons, women carrying a female fetus are more likely than those carrying a male fetus to develop hyperemesis (Cunningham et al., 2010; Kelly & Savides). A family history of hyperemesis may also be present (Gilbert, 2011). In some cases, there is also an interrelated psychologic component (Cunningham et al.).

Complications accompanying severe hyperemesis gravidarum include esophageal rupture and deficiencies of vitamin K and thiamine with resulting Wernicke encephalopathy (CNS involvement) (Cunningham et al., 2010; Kelly & Savides, 2009). Fetal and neonatal complications include small-for-gestational-age fetuses, low birth weight, prematurity, and 5-minute Apgar scores less than 7 (Kelly & Savides).

Nursing Care Plan—Hyperemesis Gravidarum

Etiology

The cause of hyperemesis gravidarum remains obscure. Several theories have been proposed as to the cause, although none of them adequately explains the disorder. Hyperemesis gravidarum may be related to high levels of estrogen or hCG and may be associated with transient hyperthyroidism during pregnancy. Gastric dysrhythmias, esophageal reflux, and reduced gastric motility may also contribute to the development of hyperemesis gravidarum (Kelly & Savides, 2009).

Psychosocial factors may play a part in the development of hyperemesis gravidarum for some women. Ambivalence toward the pregnancy and increased stress may be associated with this condition (Davis, 2004). Conflicting feelings regarding prospective motherhood, body changes, and lifestyle alterations may contribute to episodes of vomiting, particularly if these feelings are excessive or unresolved. Women with associated psychosocial factors usually improve dramatically while in the hospital but may resume vomiting after discharge (Cunningham et al., 2010).

Clinical Manifestations

The woman with hyperemesis gravidarum usually has significant weight loss and dehydration. She may have dry mucous membranes, decreased blood pressure (BP), increased pulse rate, and poor skin turgor. She is frequently unable to keep down even clear liquids taken by mouth. Laboratory tests may reveal electrolyte imbalances.

CARE MANAGEMENT

ASSESSMENT

Whenever a pregnant woman has nausea and vomiting, the first priority is a thorough assessment to determine the severity of the problem. In most cases the woman should be told to come immediately to the health care provider's office or to the emergency department because the severity of the illness is often difficult to determine by telephone conversation.

The assessment should include frequency, severity, and duration of episodes of nausea and vomiting. If the woman reports vomiting, then the assessment should also include the approximate amount and color of the vomitus. Other symptoms such as diarrhea, indigestion, and abdominal pain or distention also are identified. The woman is asked to report any precipitating factors relating to the onset of her symptoms. Any pharmacologic or nonpharmacologic treatment measures used should be recorded. Prepregnancy weight and documented weight gain or loss during pregnancy is important to note.

The woman's weight and vital signs are measured, and a complete physical examination is performed, with attention to signs of fluid and electrolyte imbalance and nutritional status. The most important initial laboratory test to be obtained is a determination of ketonuria. Other laboratory tests that may be ordered are a urinalysis, a complete blood cell count, electrolytes, liver enzymes, and bilirubin levels. These tests help rule out the presence of underlying diseases such as gastroenteritis, pyelonephritis, pancreatitis, cholecystitis, peptic ulcer, and hepatitis (Cunningham et al., 2010). Because of the recognized association between hyperemesis gravidarum and hyperthyroidism, thyroid levels may also be measured (Nader, 2009).

Psychosocial assessment includes asking the woman about anxiety, fears, and concerns related to her own health and the effects on pregnancy outcome. Family members should be assessed both for anxiety and in regard to their role in providing support for the woman.

Initial Care

Initially the woman who is unable to keep down clear liquids by mouth will require IV therapy for correction of fluid and electrolyte imbalances. In the past, women requiring IV therapy were admitted to the hospital. Today, however, they may be, and often are, successfully managed at home, even if on enteral therapy. Medications may be used if nausea and vomiting are uncontrolled. Frequently prescribed drugs include pyridoxine (vitamin B_6), doxylamine (Unisom), promethazine (Phenergan), and metoclopramide (Reglan) (Kelly & Savides, 2009). Other antiemetic medication options include prochlorperazine (Compazine) and ondansetron (Zofran) (Gordon, 2007). Chlorpromazine (Thorazine) given rectally may be effective in difficult to treat cases (Kelly & Savides). Corticosteroids (methylprednisolone [Medrol] or hydrocortisone) may be prescribed, although there is little evidence that their use is effective (Cunningham et al., 2010). Lastly, enteral or parenteral nutrition may be used for women who are nonresponsive to other medical therapies (Kelly & Savides).

Nursing care of the woman with hyperemesis gravidarum involves implementing the medical plan of care, whether this care is given in the hospital or home setting. Interventions may include initiating and monitoring IV therapy, administering drugs and nutritional supplements, and monitoring the woman's response to interventions. The nurse observes the woman for any signs of complications such as metabolic acidosis (secondary to starvation), jaundice, or hemorrhage and alerts the physician should these occur. Monitoring includes assessment of the woman's nausea, retching without vomiting, and vomiting, given that these symptoms, although related, are separate. Intake and output, including the amount of emesis, should be accurately measured and recorded. Oral hygiene while the woman is receiving nothing by mouth, and after episodes of vomiting, helps allay associated discomforts. Assistance with positioning and providing a quiet, restful environment that is free from odors may increase the woman's comfort.

Once the vomiting has stopped, feedings are started in small amounts at frequent intervals. In the beginning, limited amounts of oral fluids and bland foods such as crackers, toast, or baked chicken are offered. The diet is progressed slowly as tolerated by the woman until she is able to consume a nutritionally sound diet. Because sleep disturbances may accompany hyperemesis gravidarum, promoting adequate rest is important. The nurse can assist in coordinating treatment measures and periods of visitation to provide opportunity for rest periods.

Follow-up Care

Most women are able to take nourishment by mouth after several days of treatment. They should be encouraged to eat small, frequent meals and to eat foods that sound appealing, often nongreasy, dry, sweet, and salty foods. In many instances, women discover that foods they normally like have no appeal at

TEACHING FOR SELF-MANAGEMENT

Diet for Hyperemesis

- Eat frequently, at least every 2 to 3 hours. Separate liquids from solids and alternate every 2 to 3 hours.
- Eat a snack at bedtime.
- Eat dry, bland, low-fat, and high-protein foods. Cold foods may be better tolerated than those served at a warm temperature.
- In general, eat what sounds good to you, rather than trying to balance your meals.
- Follow the salty and sweet approach; even so-called junk foods are okay.
- Eat protein after sweets.
- Dairy products may stay down more easily than other foods.
- If you vomit even when your stomach is empty, try sucking on a Popsicle.
- Try ginger tea. Peel and finely dice a knuckle-sized piece of ginger and place it in a mug of boiling water. Steep for 5 to 8 minutes and add brown sugar to taste.
- Try warm ginger ale (with sugar, not artificial sweetener) or water with a slice of lemon.
- Drink liquids from a cup with a lid.

all during this time (see the Teaching for Self-Management box: Diet for Hyperemesis for more suggestions). Many pregnant women find exposure to cooking odors nauseating. Having other family members cook may lessen the woman's nausea and vomiting, even if only temporarily. The woman is counseled to contact her health care provider immediately if the nausea and vomiting recur.

The woman with hyperemesis gravidarum needs calm, compassionate, and sympathetic care, with recognition that the manifestations of hyperemesis can be physically and emotionally debilitating to her and stressful for her family. Irritability, tearfulness, and mood changes are often consistent with this disorder. Fetal well-being is a primary concern of the woman. The nurse can provide an environment conducive to discussion of concerns and assist the woman in identifying and mobilizing sources of support. The family should be included in the plan of care whenever possible. Their participation may help alleviate some of the emotional stress associated with this disorder.

THYROID DISORDERS

Hyperthyroidism

Hyperthyroidism in pregnancy is rare, occurring in approximately 1 of every 1000 to 2000 pregnancies (Cunningham et al., 2010). In 90% to 95% of pregnant women, hyperthyroidism is caused by Graves' disease (Nader, 2009). Clinical manifestations of hyperthyroidism include heat intolerance, diaphoresis, fatigue, anxiety, emotional lability, and tachycardia. Many of these symptoms also occur with pregnancy; thus the disorder can be difficult to diagnose. Signs that may help differentiate hyperthyroidism from normal pregnancy changes include weight loss, goiter, and a pulse rate greater than 100 beats/min (Nader). Laboratory findings include elevated free thyroxine (T_4) and triiodothyronine (T_3) levels and greatly suppressed thyroid-stimulating hormone (TSH) levels (Cunningham et al.; Nader). Moderate and severe hyperthyroidism must be treated during pregnancy. Untreated or inadequately treated women have an increased risk of miscarriage, preterm birth, and giving birth to stillborn infants or infants with goiter, hyperthyroidism, or hypothyroidism. Most neonates born to women with hyperthyroidism, however, will have normal thyroid function. Women with hyperthyroidism are at increased risk for developing severe preeclampsia and heart failure (Cunningham et al.; Nader).

The primary treatment of hyperthyroidism during pregnancy is drug therapy. The medication most often prescribed in the United States is propylthiouracil (PTU). The usual starting dose is 100 to 150 mg every 8 hours, with higher doses required for some women. Women generally show clinical improvement within 2 weeks of beginning therapy, but the medication requires 6 to 8 weeks to reach full effectiveness. During therapy the woman's free T_4 levels are measured monthly, and the results are used to taper the drug to the smallest effective dose to prevent development of unnecessary fetal or neonatal hypothyroidism. In many women the medication can be discontinued by 32 to 36 weeks of gestation. PTU readily crosses the placenta and may cause fetal hypothyroidism, which is characterized by goiter, bradycardia, and intrauterine growth restriction (IUGR) (Mestman, 2007; Nader, 2009).

PTU is well tolerated by most women. Maternal side effects include pruritus, skin rash, drug-related fever, hepatitis, bronchospasm, and a lupus-like syndrome. The most severe side effect is agranulocytosis, which occurs rarely and usually develops only in older women and in those taking high doses of PTU. Symptoms of agranulocytosis are fever and unexpected sore throat, which should be reported immediately to the health care provider, and the woman should stop taking the PTU. Leukopenia of a transient and benign nature may occur as a result of PTU therapy (Cunningham et al., 2010; Nader, 2009); liver toxicity is another rare but serious complication (Cunningham et al.). Beta-adrenergic blockers such as propranolol (Inderal) or atenolol (Tenormin) may be used in severe hyperthyroidism to control maternal symptoms, especially heart rate. Long-term use of these medications is not recommended because of the potential for IUGR, bradycardia, and hypoglycemia (Nader).

After birth, women taking PTU who choose to breastfeed should be informed that the medication is not significantly concentrated in breast milk and does not appear to adversely affect the neonate's thyroid function. The woman should take her antithyroid medication just after breastfeeding, thus allowing a 3- to 4-hour period before nursing again (Nader, 2009).

Radioactive iodine must not be used in diagnosis or treatment of hyperthyroidism in pregnancy because therapeutic doses given to treat maternal thyroid disease may also destroy the fetal thyroid (Cunningham et al., 2010). In severe cases, surgical treatment of hyperthyroidism, subtotal thyroidectomy, can be performed during pregnancy. Surgery is best performed during the second trimester of pregnancy, although it can be performed during the first or third trimester if necessary. Surgery is usually reserved for women with severe disease, those for whom drug therapy proves toxic, and those who are unable to follow the prescribed medical regimen. Risks associated with the surgery are hypoparathyroidism, recurrent laryngeal nerve paralysis, and anesthesia-related complications (Nader, 2009).

! NURSING ALERT

A serious but uncommon complication of undiagnosed or partially treated hyperthyroidism is thyroid storm, which can occur in response to stress such as labor and vaginal birth, infection, preeclampsia, or surgery. A woman with this emergency disorder may have fever, restlessness, tachycardia, vomiting, hypotension, or stupor. Prompt treatment is essential. IV fluids and oxygen are administered, along with high doses of PTU. After administration of PTU, iodide is given. Other medications include antipyretics, dexamethasone, and beta-blockers (Cunningham et al., 2010; Nader, 2009).

Hypothyroidism

Hypothyroidism occurs in 2 to 3 pregnancies per 1000. Because severe hypothyroidism is often associated with infertility and an increased risk of miscarriage, it is not often seen during pregnancy (Cunningham et al., 2010). Although iodine deficiency is rare in the United States, it is a common cause of maternal, fetal, and neonatal hypothyroidism in the world (Nader, 2009). Adult hypothyroidism is usually caused by glandular destruction by autoantibodies, most commonly because of Hashimoto's thyroiditis. Characteristic symptoms of hypothyroidism include weight gain, lethargy, decrease in exercise capacity, and cold intolerance. Women who are moderately symptomatic can also develop constipation, hoarseness, hair loss, brittle nails, and dry skin. Laboratory values in pregnancy include elevated levels of TSH, with or without low T_4 levels (Nader).

Pregnant women with untreated hypothyroidism are at increased risk for miscarriage, preeclampsia, gestational hypertension, placental abruption, preterm birth, and stillbirth. Infants born to mothers with hypothyroidism may also be of low birth weight (Cunningham et al., 2010; Nader, 2009). These outcomes can be improved with early treatment (Nader).

Thyroid hormone supplements are used to treat hypothyroidism. Levothyroxine (e.g., thyroxine [Synthroid]) is most often prescribed during pregnancy. The usual beginning dosage is 0.1 to 0.15 mg per day, with adjustment by 25 to 50 mcg every 4 to 6 weeks as necessary based on the maternal TSH level (Cunningham et al., 2010; Nader, 2009). The aim of drug therapy is to maintain the TSH level at the lower end of the normal range for pregnant women. Women with little or no functioning thyroid tissue will require higher doses of levothyroxine. Also, as pregnancy progresses, increased doses of thyroid hormone are usually required. This increased demand during pregnancy is probably related to increased estrogen levels (Cunningham et al.; Nader).

! NURSING ALERT

If taking iron supplementation, pregnant women should be told to take levothyroxine at a different time of day than their iron tablets because ferrous sulfate decreases absorption of T_4 (Nader, 2009).

The fetus depends on maternal thyroid hormones until approximately 18 weeks of gestation, when fetal production begins. Normal maternal thyroxine levels early in pregnancy are important for proper fetal brain development. Studies have shown that even mild maternal hypothyroidism during the first trimester has been associated with long-term neuropsychologic damage in their children. More research needs to be conducted on this topic (Mestman, 2007).

Nursing Care

Education of the pregnant woman with thyroid dysfunction is essential to promote compliance with the plan of treatment. Important points to discuss with the woman and her family include the disorder and its potential effect on her, her family, and her fetus; the medication regimen and possible side effects; the need for continuing medical supervision; and the importance of compliance.

The woman often needs assistance from the nurse in coping with the discomforts and frustrations associated with symptoms of the disorder. For example, the woman with hyperthyroidism who has nervousness and hyperactivity along with weakness and fatigue may benefit from suggestions to channel excess energies into quiet diversional activities such as reading or crafts. Discomfort associated with hypersensitivity to heat (hyperthyroidism) or cold intolerance (hypothyroidism) can be minimized by appropriate clothing and regulation of environmental temperatures, and by avoiding temperature extremes.

Nutritional counseling with a registered dietitian may provide guidance in selecting a well-balanced diet. The woman with hyperthyroidism who has increased appetite and poor weight gain and the hypothyroid woman who has anorexia and lethargy need counseling to ensure adequate intake of nutritionally sound foods to meet both maternal and fetal needs.

MATERNAL PHENYLKETONURIA

Phenylketonuria (PKU), a recognized cause of mental retardation, is an inborn error of metabolism caused by an autosomal recessive trait that creates a deficiency in the enzyme phenylalanine hydrolase. Absence of this enzyme impairs the body's ability to metabolize the amino acid phenylalanine, found in all protein foods. Consequently, toxic accumulation of phenylalanine in the blood occurs, which interferes with brain development and function. Individuals with this disorder also have hypopigmentation of hair, eyes, and skin because phenylalanine inhibits melanin production. PKU affects 1 in every 10,000 to 15,000 Caucasian newborns (Cunningham et al., 2010).

PKU was the first inborn error of metabolism to be universally screened for in the United States. Since 1961, all newborns have been tested soon after birth for this disorder. Prompt diagnosis and therapy with a phenylalanine-restricted diet significantly decreases the incidence of mental retardation (Aminoff, 2009). The special diet should be followed indefinitely because individuals who do not continue phenylalanine restriction have been reported to have significantly lower IQs (Cunningham et al., 2010).

The keys to the prevention of fetal anomalies caused by PKU are the identification of women in their reproductive years with the disorder and dietary compliance for women who are diagnosed. Screening for undiagnosed homozygous maternal PKU at the first prenatal visit may be warranted, especially in individuals with a family history of the disorder, with low intelligence of uncertain origin, or who have given birth to microcephalic infants. Ideally women with PKU begin dietary phenylalanine restriction before conception and continue it throughout pregnancy. The dietary modification normally excludes all high-protein foods such as meat, milk, eggs, and nuts, as well as wheat products. Phenylalanine levels are monitored at least once and preferably twice a week throughout pregnancy (Gilbert, 2011). Experts recommend that maternal phenylalanine levels be less than 6 mg/dl for a least 3 months before conception and range between 2 and 6 mg/dl throughout pregnancy. These levels are associated with a decrease in fetal sequelae (Cunningham et al., 2010; Gilbert). High maternal phenylalanine levels are associated with microcephaly, mental retardation, and congenital heart defects in their children (Aminoff, 2009; Cunningham et al.). Ultrasound examinations are used for fetal surveillance beginning in the first trimester. A spontaneous vaginal birth is anticipated.

Women with PKU should be advised against breastfeeding because their milk will contain a high concentration of phenylalanine (Aminoff, 2009). If these women choose to breastfeed despite the risk, their phenylalanine blood levels must be monitored closely (Lawrence & Lawrence, 2005).

KEY POINTS

- In pregnant women with pregestational diabetes, lack of glycemic control before conception and in the first trimester of pregnancy may be responsible for fetal congenital malformations.
- For pregnant women who have diabetes and are insulin dependent, insulin requirements increase as the pregnancy progresses and may quadruple by term as a result of insulin resistance created by placental hormones, insulinase, and cortisol. After birth, levels decrease dramatically; breastfeeding affects insulin needs.
- Poor glycemic control before and during pregnancy in women who have diabetes can lead to maternal complications such as miscarriage, infection, and dystocia (difficult labor) caused by fetal macrosomia.
- Careful glucose monitoring, insulin administration when necessary, and dietary counseling are used to create a normal intrauterine environment for fetal growth and development in the pregnancy complicated by diabetes mellitus.
- Because GDM is asymptomatic in most cases, all women who do not have pregestational diabetes undergo routine screening by history, clinical risk factors, or glucola administration during pregnancy.
- The woman with hyperemesis gravidarum may have significant weight loss and dehydration. Management focuses on restoring fluid and electrolyte balance and preventing recurrence of nausea and vomiting.
- Thyroid dysfunction, hyperthyroidism or hypothyrodism, during pregnancy requires close monitoring of thyroid hormone levels to regulate therapy and prevent fetal insult.
- High levels of phenylalanine in the maternal bloodstream cross the placenta and are teratogenic to the developing fetus. Damage can be prevented or minimized by dietary restriction of phenylalanine before and during pregnancy.

Audio Chapter Summaries Access an audio summary of these Key Points on evolve

REFERENCES

American Diabetes Association (ADA). (2008). Position statement: Diagnosis and classification of diabetes mellitus. *Diabetes Care, 31*(Suppl.), S55–S60.

Aminoff, M. (2009). Neurologic disorders. In R. Creasy, R. Resnik, J. Iams, C. Lockwood, & T. Moore (Eds.), *Creasy and Resnik's maternal-fetal medicine: Principles and practice* (6th ed.). Philadelphia: Saunders.

Anderson, J., Waller, D., Canfield, M., Shaw, G., Watkins, M., & Werler, M. (2005). Maternal obesity, gestational diabetes, and central nervous system birth defects. *Epidemiology, 16*(1), 87–92.

Chan, P., & Johnson, S. (2006). *Gynecology and obstetrics: Current clinical strategies*. Laguna Hills, CA: CCS Publishing.

Cunningham, F., Leveno, K., Bloom, S., Hauth, J., Rouse, D., & Spong, C. (Eds.). (2010). *Williams obstetrics* (23rd ed.). New York: McGraw-Hill.

Davis, M. (2004). Nausea and vomiting of pregnancy: An evidence-based review. *Journal of Perinatal and Neonatal Nursing, 18*(4), 312–328.

Gilbert, E. (2011). *Manual of high risk pregnancy & delivery* (5th ed.). St. Louis: Mosby.

Gordon, M. (2007). Maternal physiology. In S. Gabbe, J. Niebyl, & J. Simpson (Eds.), *Obstetrics: Normal and problem pregnancies* (5th ed.). Philadelphia: Churchill Livingstone.

Iams, J., Romero, R., & Creasy, R. (2009). Preterm labor and birth. In R. Creasy, R. Resnik, J. Iams, C. Lockwood, & T. Moore (Eds.), *Creasy and Resnik's maternal-fetal medicine: Principles and practice* (6th ed.). Philadelphia: Saunders.

Kelly, T., & Savides, T. (2009). Gastrointestinal disease in pregnancy. In R. Creasy, R. Resnik, J. Iams, C. Lockwood, & T. Moore (Eds.), *Creasy and Resnik's maternal-fetal medicine: Principles and practice* (6th ed.). Philadelphia: Saunders.

Landon, M., Catalano, P., & Gabbe, S. (2007). Diabetes mellitus complicating pregnancy. In S. Gabbe, J. Niebyl, & J. Simpson (Eds.), *Obstetrics: Normal and problem pregnancies* (5th ed.). Philadelphia: Churchill Livingstone.

Lawrence, R., & Lawrence, R. (2005). *Breastfeeding: A guide for the medical profession* (6th ed.). St. Louis: Mosby.

Lindsay, C. (2006). Pregnancy complicated by diabetes mellitus. In R. Martin, A. Fanaroff, & M. Walsh (Eds.), *Fanaroff and Martin's neonatal-perinatal medicine: Diseases of the fetus and infant* (8th ed.). Philadelphia: Mosby.

Mestman, J. (2007). Thyroid and parathyroid diseases in pregnancy. In S. Gabbe, J. Niebyl, & J. Simpson (Eds.), *Obstetrics: Normal and problem pregnancies* (5th ed.). Philadelphia: Churchill Livingstone.

Moore, T., & Catalano, P. (2009). Diabetes in pregnancy. In R. Creasy, R. Resnik, J. Iams, C. Lockwood, & T. Moore (Eds.), *Creasy and Resnik's maternal-fetal medicine: Principles and practice* (6th ed.). Philadelphia: Saunders.

Nader, S. (2009). Thyroid disease and pregnancy. In R. Creasy, R. Resnik, J. Iams, C. Lockwood, & T. Moore (Eds.), *Creasy and Resnik's maternal-fetal medicine: Principles and practice* (6th ed.). Philadelphia: Saunders.

National Center for Chronic Disease Prevention and Health Promotion. (2009). *Diabetes successes and opportunities for population-based prevention and control*. Available at www.cdc.gov/nccdphp/publications/aag/pdf/diabetes.pdf. Accessed July 15, 2010.

Paidas, M., & Hossain, N. (2009). Embryonic and fetal demise. In R. Creasy, R. Resnik, J. Iams, C. Lockwood, & T. Moore (Eds.), *Creasy and Resnik's maternal-fetal medicine: Principles and practice* (6th ed.). Philadelphia: Saunders.

Wapner, R., Jenkins, T., & Khalek, N. (2009). Prenatal diagnosis of congenital disorders. In R. Creasy, R. Resnik, J. Iams, C. Lockwood, & T. Moore (Eds.), *Creasy and Resnik's maternal-fetal medicine: Principles and practice* (6th ed.). Philadelphia: Saunders.

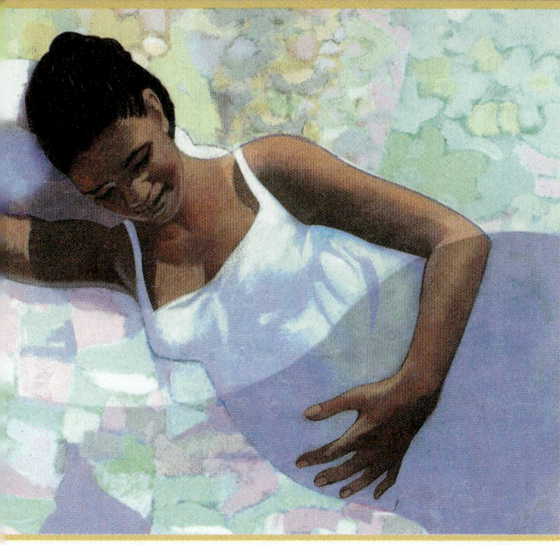

CHAPTER

30

Medical-Surgical Problems in Pregnancy

Jane McAteer

evolve WEBSITE

http://evolve.elsevier.com/Lowdermilk/MWHC/

Audio Glossary
Audio Key Points
Case Study
    Class III Cardiac Disorder
NCLEX Review Questions
Nursing Care Plan
    The Pregnant Woman with Heart Disease

LEARNING OBJECTIVES

- Describe the management of cardiovascular disorders in pregnant women.
- Identify nursing interventions for a pregnant woman with a cardiovascular disorder.
- Discuss anemia during pregnancy.
- Explain the care of pregnant women with pulmonary disorders.
- Examine the effect of a gastrointestinal disorder on gastrointestinal function during pregnancy.
- Identify the effects of neurologic disorders on pregnancy.
- Describe the care of women whose pregnancies are complicated by autoimmune disorders.
- Differentiate signs and symptoms and management during pregnancy of urinary tract infections.
- Explain the basic principles of care for a pregnant woman having surgery.

For most women, pregnancy represents a normal part of life. This chapter discusses the care of women for whom pregnancy represents a significant risk because it is superimposed on a preexisting medical condition. Care of women with normal pregnancies who develop medical or surgical problems that could happen to anyone at any time of life but occur during pregnancy is also discussed. With the active participation of well-motivated women in the treatment plan and careful management from a multidisciplinary health care team, positive pregnancy outcomes are often possible in both of these situations.

This chapter focuses on cardiovascular disorders, along with selected respiratory, integumentary, neurologic, autoimmune, gastrointestinal, and urinary tract diseases. Care of the pregnant woman undergoing surgery is also discussed.

CARDIOVASCULAR DISORDERS

During a normal pregnancy the maternal cardiovascular system undergoes many changes that place a physiologic strain on the heart. The major cardiovascular changes that occur during a normal pregnancy and that affect the woman with cardiac disease are increased intravascular volume, decreased systemic vascular resistance, cardiac output changes occurring during labor and birth, and the intravascular volume changes that occur just after childbirth. These physiologic changes are present during pregnancy and continue for a few weeks after birth. The normal heart can compensate for the increased workload so that pregnancy, labor, and birth are generally well tolerated, but the diseased heart is hemodynamically challenged.

If the cardiovascular changes are not well tolerated, cardiac failure can develop during pregnancy, labor, or the postpartum period. In addition, if myocardial disease develops, valvular disease exists, or a congenital heart defect is present, *cardiac decompensation* (inability of the heart to maintain a sufficient cardiac output) may occur.

About 1% of pregnancies are complicated by serious heart disease. The risk of maternal morbidity and mortality ranges from low to high, depending on the cardiac defect (Tomlinson, 2006). Congenital diseases and mitral valve disease are increasing in women of childbearing age, whereas the incidence of rheumatic fever has diminished. The presence of a maternal congenital cardiac defect increases the risk to the fetus for a

BOX 30-1 MATERNAL CARDIAC DISEASE RISK GROUPS

GROUP I (LOW RISK)
- Corrected tetralogy of Fallot
- Pulmonic/tricuspid disease
- Mitral stenosis (New York Heart Association [NYHA] classes I, II)
- Patent ductus arteriosus
- Ventricular septal defect
- Atrial septal defect
- Corrected congenital heart disease without residual cardiac dysfunction

GROUP II (MODERATE RISK)
- Mitral stenosis with atrial fibrillation
- Artificial heart valves
- Mitral stenosis (NYHA classes III, IV)
- Uncorrected tetralogy of Fallot
- Aortic coarctation (uncomplicated)
- Aortic stenosis
- Marfan syndrome with normal aorta
- Previous myocardial infarction
- Moderate to severe systemic ventricular dysfunction
- History of peripartum cardiomyopathy with no residual ventricular dysfunction

GROUP III (HIGH RISK)
- Aortic coarctation (complicated)
- History of peripartum cardiomyopathy with residual ventricular dysfunction
- Marfan syndrome with aortic involvement
- Pulmonary hypertension
- Any condition with NYHA class III or IV

Source: Tomlinson, M. (2006).Cardiac disease. In D. James, P. Steer, C. Weiner, & B. Gonik (Eds.), *High risk pregnancy: Management options* (3rd ed.). Philadelphia: Saunders.

congenital heart defect from 1% to about 4% to 6% (Easterling & Stout, 2007). A perinatal mortality of up to 50% is anticipated with persistent cardiac decompensation. Box 30-1 lists maternal cardiac disease risk groups.

The degree of disability experienced by the woman with cardiac disease is often more important in the treatment and prognosis of cardiac disease complicating pregnancy than is the diagnosis of cardiovascular disease. The New York Heart Association's (NYHA) functional classification of organic heart disease is a widely accepted standard:

- Class I: asymptomatic without limitation of physical activity
- Class II: symptomatic with slight limitation of activity
- Class III: symptomatic with marked limitation of activity
- Class IV: symptomatic with inability to carry on any physical activity without discomfort

No classification of heart disease can be considered rigid or absolute, but the NYHA classification offers a basic practical guide for treatment, assuming that frequent prenatal visits, good client cooperation, and appropriate obstetric care occur. The functional classification may change for the pregnant woman because of the hemodynamic changes that occur in the cardiovascular system during pregnancy. A 30% to 45% increase in cardiac output occurs compared with nonpregnancy resting values, with most of the increase in the first trimester and the peak at 20 to 26 weeks of gestation (Blanchard & Shabetai, 2009). The functional classification of the disease is determined at 3 months and again at 7 or 8 months of gestation. Pregnant women may progress from class I or II to III or IV during the pregnancy. Women with cyanotic congenital heart disease do not fit into the NYHA classification because their exercise-induced symptoms have causes unrelated to heart failure.

A diagnosis of cardiac disease depends on the history, physical examination, radiographic and electrocardiographic findings, Holter monitoring, and, if indicated, ultrasonographic results. Most diagnostic studies are noninvasive and can be safely performed during pregnancy. The differential diagnosis of heart disease also involves ruling out respiratory problems and other potential causes of chest pain.

The maternal mortality rate in women with cardiac events is higher than that for abortion, genital tract sepsis, and hemorrhage (Setaro & Caulin-Glaser, 2004). The highest risk of complications or death occurs in women with pulmonary hypertension, complicated coarctation of the aorta, and Marfan syndrome with aortic involvement (Tomlinson, 2006).

Cardiac diseases vary in their effect on pregnancy depending on whether they are acute or chronic conditions. The following discussion focuses on selected congenital and acquired cardiac conditions and other cardiac disorders. A review of the care of the pregnant woman who has had a heart transplant concludes this section.

Congenital Cardiac Disease

Septal Defects

Atrial Septal Defect. Atrial septal defect (ASD) (an abnormal opening between the atria), one of the causes of a left-to-right shunt, is one of the most common congenital defects seen during pregnancy. This defect may go undetected because the woman usually is asymptomatic. The pregnant woman with an ASD will most likely have an uncomplicated pregnancy. Some women may have right-sided heart failure or arrhythmias as the pregnancy progresses as a result of increased plasma volume. The risk to the fetus of a woman with ASD for congenital heart disease is 3% to 10% (Tomlinson, 2006).

Ventricular Septal Defect. Ventricular septal defect (VSD) (an abnormal opening between the right and left ventricles), another cause of a left-to-right shunt, is usually diagnosed and corrected early in life. As a result, a VSD is not very common in pregnancy. Women with small, uncomplicated VSDs usually do not have pregnancy complications. For women with a large VSD, there is a higher risk for arrhythmias, heart failure, and pulmonary hypertension. Medical management includes rest and decreased physical activity, as well as administration of anticoagulants, if indicated. The fetus has a 6% to 10% risk of a congenital heart defect (Tomlinson, 2006).

Patent Ductus Arteriosus. Patent ductus arteriosus (PDA) is another cause of a left-to-right shunt that is usually diagnosed and corrected during infancy. Possible complications of a PDA include those of VSD as well as endocarditis and pulmonary emboli. Medical management is the same as for VSD.

Acyanotic Lesions

Coarctation of the Aorta. Coarctation of the aorta (localized narrowing of the aorta near the insertion of the ductus) is an example of an acyanotic congenital heart lesion. If at all possible, the lesion should be corrected surgically before pregnancy.

Case Study—Class III Disorder

However, pregnancy is usually relatively safe for the woman with uncomplicated, uncorrected, coarctation. Maternal mortality is about 3% for uncorrected defects (Blanchard & Shabetai, 2009). Complications that can occur include hypertension, congestive heart failure, aortic dissection, aneurysm, and rupture. The mainstays of treatment for uncorrected coarctation of the aorta during pregnancy are rest and antihypertensive medications, preferably beta-adrenergic blocking agents. Vaginal birth is preferable, with epidural anesthesia and shortening of the second stage with vacuum extraction or use of forceps, if necessary. Beta-blockers should be continued throughout labor. Because of the risk of endocarditis, antibiotic prophylaxis is recommended at birth (see later discussion).

Cyanotic Lesions

Tetralogy of Fallot. Tetralogy of Fallot is by far the most common cyanotic heart disease observed during pregnancy (Blanchard & Shabetai, 2009). Components of tetralogy of Fallot include a VSD, pulmonary stenosis, overriding aorta, and right ventricular hypertrophy, leading to a right-to-left shunt. Women with tetralogy of Fallot are encouraged to have surgical repair before conception because pregnancy does not cause a significant risk once the VSD and pulmonary stenosis have been repaired. Women with uncorrected tetralogy of Fallot, however, experience more right-to-left shunting during pregnancy, resulting in reduced blood flow through the pulmonary circulation and increasing hypoxemia, which can cause syncope or death. Maintenance of venous return in women with uncorrected tetralogy of Fallot is critical. Therefore, the most dangerous time for these women is the late third trimester of pregnancy and the early postpartum period, when venous return is reduced by the large pregnant uterus and by peripheral venous pooling after birth. Use of pressure-graded support hose is recommended. Blood loss during birth may also adversely affect venous return, thus blood volume must be adequately maintained. Prophylactic antibiotics should be given during the intrapartum period (Blanchard & Shabetai).

Acquired Cardiac Disease

Mitral Valve Stenosis

Mitral valve stenosis (narrowing of the opening of the mitral valve caused by stiffening of valve leaflets, which obstructs blood flow from the left atrium to the left ventricle) is the characteristic lesion resulting from rheumatic heart disease (RHD) (Tomlinson, 2006). As the mitral valve narrows, dyspnea worsens, occurring first on exertion and eventually at rest. A tight stenosis plus the increase in blood volume and cardiac output of normal pregnancy may cause pulmonary edema, atrial fibrillation, right-sided heart failure, infective endocarditis, pulmonary embolism, and massive hemoptysis (Blanchard & Shabetai, 2009; Cunningham, Leveno, Bloom, Hauth, Rouse, & Spong, 2010). Maternal mortality is related to functional capacity. Almost all maternal deaths related to mitral stenosis occur in women who are classified as NYHA class III or class IV (Cunningham et al.).

Pharmacologic treatment for women with a history of rheumatic heart disease includes beta-blockers or calcium channel blockers to prevent tachycardia (Easterling & Stout, 2007). A combination of drugs will most likely be needed. Cardioversion may be needed for new-onset atrial fibrillation. Women who have chronic atrial fibrillation may require digoxin or beta-blockers to control the heart rate. In addition, anticoagulant therapy may be needed to prevent embolism (Blanchard & Shabetai, 2009). About 25% of women with mitral valve stenosis experience cardiac failure for the first time during pregnancy (Cunningham et al., 2010). The care of the woman with mitral stenosis typically is managed by reducing her activity, restricting dietary sodium, and monitoring weight. The pregnant woman with mitral stenosis should be assessed clinically for symptoms and with echocardiograms to monitor the atrial and ventricular size, as well as heart valve function. Prophylaxis for intrapartum endocarditis and pulmonary infections may be provided for women at high risk (Blanchard & Shabetai; Easterling & Stout) (Box 30-2).

BOX 30-2 PROPHYLAXIS FOR BACTERIAL ENDOCARDITIS DURING LABOR AND BIRTH

HIGH RISK CLIENTS

In active labor: Ampicillin 2 g IV or IM plus gentamicin 1.5 mg/kg (not to exceed 120 mg)

6 hours later: Ampicillin 1 g IV or IM or amoxicillin 1 g PO

Penicillin-Allergic Clients

In active labor: Vancomycin 1 g IV over 1-2 hr plus gentamicin as above

MODERATE RISK CLIENTS

In active labor: Amoxicillin 2 g PO or ampicillin 2 g IV or IM

Penicillin-Allergic Clients

In active labor: Vancomycin 1 g IV over 1-2 hr

IM, Intramuscular; *IV,* intravenous; *PO,* by mouth.
Source: Easterling, T., & Stout, K. (2007). Heart disease. In S. Gabbe, J. Niebyl, & J. Simpson (Eds.), *Obstetrics: Normal and problem pregnancies* (5th ed.). Philadelphia: Churchill Livingstone.

During labor adequate pain control is required to prevent tachycardia. Epidural analgesia for labor is preferred (Tomlinson, 2006). Shortening the second stage of labor is also important to decrease the cardiac workload. Even with close monitoring, the woman with moderate to severe mitral stenosis is at risk for pulmonary edema, right-sided heart failure, and hypotension. Central hemodynamic monitoring may be necessary for some women during labor, birth, and the postpartum period because fluid shifts can place the woman at risk for pulmonary edema.

For women with NYHA class III or IV cardiac disease, percutaneous balloon mitral valvuloplasty can be performed, but this procedure should be considered only when symptoms cannot be controlled by standard means. Mitral balloon valvuloplasty is optimally performed after the first trimester to decrease radiation risks to the fetus. This relatively safe nonsurgical procedure is now performed more frequently during pregnancy than surgical valvotomy. The balloon procedure is just as successful as surgical repair but is associated with a lower perinatal mortality rate (Cunningham et al., 2010).

Mitral Valve Prolapse

Mitral valve prolapse (MVP) is a fairly common, usually benign, condition. More specific echocardiographic diagnostic criteria have resulted in significantly reduced prevalence estimates for

MVP (perhaps 1% of the female population) than previously thought (Blanchard & Shabetai, 2009). The mitral valve leaflets prolapse into the left atrium during ventricular systole, allowing some backflow of blood. Midsystolic click and late systolic murmur are hallmarks of this syndrome. Most cases are asymptomatic. A few women have atypical chest pain (sharp and located in the left side of the chest) that occurs at rest and does not respond to nitrates. They may also have anxiety, palpitations, dyspnea on exertion, and syncope. Specific treatment usually is not necessary except for symptomatic tachyarrhythmias and rarely, heart failure. Women usually are treated with beta-adrenergic blockers such as atenolol or metoprolol (Lopressor) (Blanchard & Shebetai). Pregnancy and its associated hemodynamic changes may change or alleviate the murmur and click of MVP, as well as symptoms. Antibiotic prophylaxis is usually given before birth to prevent bacterial endocarditis (see Box 30-2). Pregnancy usually is well tolerated unless bacterial endocarditis occurs (Cunningham et al. 2010; Easterling & Stout, 2007).

Aortic Stenosis

Aortic stenosis (narrowing of the opening of the aortic valve leading to an obstruction to left ventricular ejection) is rarely encountered as a complication of pregnancy because most women who develop this condition do so after their childbearing years are over. In the past, the maternal mortality rate was reported to be as high as 17%, but it has decreased over the last several decades (Easterling & Stout, 2007). Medical management is similar to that for mitral stenosis.

Ischemic Heart Disease

Myocardial Infarction

Myocardial infarction (MI) (an acute ischemic event) is a rare event in women of childbearing age, usually occurring in the third trimester with a maternal mortality rate of 20% (Tomlinson, 2006). It is estimated to occur in only 1 in 10,000 women during pregnancy and usually in women older than 33 years of age (Blanchard & Shabetai, 2009). It is anticipated that the incidence of MIs will rise, however, considering the increase in the age of childbearing women. No cardiac risk factors are present in approximately 40% of women (Tomlinson). One study, however, found that the three most likely predictors of MI were chronic hypertension, advancing age, and diabetes. Women with intrapartum diagnoses were most likely to have severe preeclampsia or eclampsia. Prenatal or postpartal MIs were most likely related to diabetes, coronary artery disease, and lipid disorders (Martin & Foley, 2007). Women who have MIs during pregnancy or the postpartum period should be assessed for thrombophilias (deficiency of proteins involved in coagulation inhibition), such as antiphospholipid antibody.

Medical management for pregnant women after MI is the same as for nonpregnant women and includes the administration of oxygen, aspirin, beta-blockers, nitrates, and heparin. Labor should be postponed for at least 2 weeks, if possible, in order to allow the myocardium to heal (Martin & Foley, 2007). Women who have had symptomatic cardiac disease during the pregnancy should continue cardiac medications and receive oxygen during labor. Because pain can lead to tachycardia and increased cardiac demands, pain control during labor is crucial. The side-lying position is preferred to avoid pressure on the vena cava. Vaginal birth is preferable, with avoidance of maternal pushing and a vacuum- or forceps-assisted birth (Easterling & Stout, 2007).

Other Cardiac Diseases and Conditions

Primary Pulmonary Hypertension

Women with primary pulmonary hypertension (PPH) have constriction of the arteriolar vessels in the lungs, leading to an increase in the pulmonary artery pressure. As a result of this pathology, there is right ventricular hypertension, right ventricular hypertrophy and dilation, and finally, right ventricular failure with tricuspid regurgitation and systemic congestion. The major physiologic difficulty in PPH is maintaining blood flow to the lungs. Any event that significantly decreases venous return to the heart, such as hypotension, impairs the ability of the right ventricle to pump blood through the pulmonary vessels with their high, fixed vascular resistance. Because hypotension can occur quickly and is often unresponsive to medical therapy, it must be avoided at all costs (Blanchard & Shabetai, 2009).

Symptoms may be nonspecific, such as fatigue and shortness of breath. Dyspnea on exertion is the most common symptom (Cunningham et al., 2010).

PPH is diagnosed by electrocardiography. The diagnosis is confirmed by right-sided cardiac catheterization, which may be deferred during pregnancy (Cunningham et al., 2010). Mortality rates reported during pregnancy are as high as 50%, so pregnancy is not advised in women with this condition (Blanchard & Shabetai, 2009). The most dangerous times for women with this condition are the intrapartal and early postpartal periods because of increases in cardiac output and fluid shifts.

Medical management of pregnant women with PPH during pregnancy includes limiting activity and avoiding supine positioning. Diuretics, supplemental oxygen, and vasodilator medications will also be ordered. During labor and birth hypotension must be avoided by carefully establishing epidural analgesia and preventing blood loss (Cunningham et al., 2010).

Marfan Syndrome

Marfan syndrome is an autosomal dominant genetic disorder characterized by generalized weakness of the connective tissue, resulting in joint deformities, ocular lens dislocation, and weakness of the aortic wall and root. Associated cardiovascular changes include mitral valve prolapse, mitral regurgitation, aortic regurgitation, aortic root dilation, and possible dissection or rupture of the aortic root (Easterling & Stout, 2007). Excruciating chest pain is the most common symptom of aortic dissection. Aortic dissection most often occurs in the third trimester or postpartum. Preconception genetic counseling is recommended to make women aware of the risks of pregnancy with this condition. Because the condition is inherited, each child born to a woman with Marfan syndrome has a 50% chance of having the disorder (Martin & Foley, 2007). Baseline data should be gathered about the aortic root before pregnancy or at the first prenatal visit by noninvasive imaging with transesophageal echocardiography, computed tomography (CT), or magnetic resonance imaging (MRI).

Management during pregnancy includes restricted activity and use of beta-blockers; surgery may be indicated in some women. Vaginal birth is considered safe for women with aortic root diameters less than 4 cm. Some authorities, however, recommend that women with larger aortic root diameters give birth by elective cesarean because of concerns about increased pressure in the aorta during labor (Blanchard & Shabetai, 2009; Easterling & Stout, 2007).

Infective Endocarditis

Infective endocarditis is inflammation of the innermost lining—the endocardium—of the heart, caused by invasion of microorganisms. Children and adults who have had corrective surgery for congenital heart disease are at greatest risk for developing infective endocarditis. The disease may also be seen in women who use street drugs intravenously (Cunningham et al., 2010). Bacterial endocarditis, leading to incompetence of heart valves and thus congestive heart failure and cerebral emboli, can result in death. Treatment is with antibiotics. Prophylactic treatment with antibiotics is used only for women at highest risk for this condition.

Eisenmenger Syndrome

Eisenmenger syndrome is a right-to-left or bidirectional shunting that can occur either at the atrial or the ventricular level of the heart and is combined with elevated pulmonary vascular resistance (Blanchard & Shabetai, 2009). The syndrome is associated with high mortality (50% in mothers and 50% in fetuses). Because of the risk for poor pregnancy outcomes, pregnancy should be avoided by women with Eisenmenger syndrome (Blanchard & Shabetai).

In women who continue pregnancy despite the risks, physical activity is strictly limited. Hospitalization may be necessary to provide optimal care, which includes oxygen administration, rest, and fetal monitoring. During labor and birth, intrathecal or epidural morphine sulfate is recommended in order to maintain hemodynamic stability. Hypotension must be avoided at all costs because it results in more right-to-left shunting (Easterling & Stout, 2007). Pulse oximetry is a useful assessment tool to guide the treatment plan during labor and birth. Cesarean birth should be performed only for obstetric indications and avoided whenever possible (Easterling & Stout).

Peripartum Cardiomyopathy

Peripartum cardiomyopathy (PCM) is congestive heart failure with cardiomyopathy. The classic criteria for the diagnosis of PCM include development of congestive heart failure in the last month of pregnancy or within the first 5 postpartum months, absence of heart disease before the last month of pregnancy, and, most important, lack of another cause for heart failure. The cause of the disease is unknown. The incidence is 1 in 3000 to 4000 live births in the United States (Blanchard & Shabetai, 2009).

Associated risk factors for PCM include maternal age older than 35 years, multifetal gestation, preeclampsia, gestational hypertension, multiparity, African descent, and prolonged tocolytic therapy (Klein & Galan, 2004). Maternal mortality has been estimated in the range of 30% to 40% (Martin & Foley, 2007). Clinical findings are those of congestive heart failure (left ventricular failure). Clinical manifestations include dyspnea, fatigue, and edema, as well as radiologic findings of cardiomegaly.

Medical management of PCM includes a regimen used for congestive heart failure: diuretics, sodium and fluid restriction, afterload-reducing agents, and digoxin. Anticoagulation may be necessary if the cardiac chambers are significantly dilated and contract poorly because of the increased risk for clot formation. During labor epidural anesthesia is often used for pain control to decrease the cardiac workload and reduce tachycardia. Cesarean birth should be performed only for obstetric indications (Easterling & Stout, 2007).

In half of all women with PCM, left ventricular dysfunction resolves within 6 months. These women generally do well. If left ventricular dysfunction does not resolve within 6 months, however, approximately 85% of women with PCM will die in the next 4 to 5 years. Death is usually the result of progressive congestive heart failure, arrhythmia, or thromboembolism (Easterling & Stout, 2007). The recurrence rate for cardiomyopathy in a subsequent pregnancy is high—anywhere from 20% to 50%. The risk of recurrence is increased in women who did not have complete recovery of left ventricular function after the initial episode of PCM (Blanchard & Shabetai, 2009).

Valve Replacement

Pregnant women with mechanical or bioprosthetic heart valves require specialized care for this high risk situation. The primary medical management, anticoagulation, is both controversial and complicated. A high risk for thromboembolism exists because of the hypercoagulability of pregnancy. At the same time, the use of anticoagulants during pregnancy presents the possibility of maternal and fetal hemorrhage. Some oral anticoagulants pose a significant risk to the fetus for abnormalities and intracranial hemorrhage. Prosthetic heart valve thrombosis is a life-threatening emergency during pregnancy and requires clot removal surgery, which carries a high mortality rate (Tomlinson, 2006).

Women with bioprosthetic heart valves usually do not require anticoagulation during pregnancy. This type of valve is an ideal replacement for women of childbearing age. A disadvantage of this valve, however, is premature failure, which may occur within 10 to 15 years of placement. Premature valve failure may be exacerbated by pregnancy (Tomlinson, 2006).

The recommendations for pregnant women with mechanical prosthetic valves who need anticoagulation therapy include several different treatment regimens. Because the most effective and safest management has not been determined through controlled trials, the decision regarding choice of therapy should be made between the physician and the woman, who should be fully informed about the potential risks of the various options to her and her unborn child. One option is to use subcutaneous heparin for the first 12 weeks of gestation. Warfarin (Coumadin) then is used until week 35 of gestation, followed by a return to heparin (intravenous) until after the birth. If prothrombin time (PT) results are reported in international normalized ratio (INR) values, then the desired range is between 2 and 4.9 (Tomlinson, 2006). A second option is to use warfarin for the entire pregnancy up to 35 weeks of gestation followed by intravenous heparin until labor begins. Data are inconclusive regarding the use of low-molecular-weight heparin (Lovenox). Anticoagulation therapy should be discontinued during active labor and resumed in the postpartum period. Warfarin does not adversely affect breastfeeding.

Heart Transplantation

Increasing numbers of heart recipients are successfully completing pregnancies. It is recommended that pregnancy be avoided for at least 1 year after the transplant (Blanchard & Shabetai, 2009). Before conception the woman should be assessed for quality of ventricular function and potential rejection of the transplant. She also should be considered to be stabilized on her immunosuppressant regimen. Women who have no evidence of rejection and have normal cardiac function at the beginning of the pregnancy appear to do well during pregnancy, labor, and birth. Risks to the woman include hypertension, preeclampsia, preterm birth, and mild rejection episodes (Martin & Foley, 2007).

CARE MANAGEMENT

The presence of cardiac disease is a significant influencing factor in the decision-making process for or against becoming pregnant. Couples planning a pregnancy must understand the risks involved in their situation. If the pregnancy is unplanned, the nurse should explore the couple's desire to continue the pregnancy in light of the risks involved. Pregnancy termination is one option, depending on the severity of the cardiac defect. The family may need further information in order to make an informed decision regarding the future of the pregnancy.

The pregnant woman with a cardiac disorder is in a high risk situation. Her care will be provided by a multidisciplinary team, including a cardiologist, obstetrician, perinatologist, and registered nurse experienced in the care of women with high risk pregnancies. If she chooses to continue the pregnancy, the woman's condition may be assessed as often as weekly (see the Nursing Process box: Cardiac Disease). For additional information on cardiac disease, visit the American Heart Association's website at www.americanheart.org.

Antepartum

Therapy for the pregnant woman with heart disease is focused on minimizing stress on the heart, which is greatest between 28 and 32 weeks of gestation as the hemodynamic changes reach their maximum. Factors that increase the risk of cardiac decompensation are avoided. The workload of the cardiovascular system is reduced by appropriate treatment of any coexisting emotional stress, hypertension, anemia, hyperthyroidism, or obesity.

Signs and symptoms of cardiac decompensation are taught at the first prenatal visit and reviewed at each subsequent visit (see the Signs of Potential Complications box; see also the Nursing Process box: Cardiac Disease for other information to include in client teaching).

Infections are treated promptly because respiratory, urinary, or gastrointestinal (GI) tract infections can complicate the condition by accelerating the heart rate and by direct spread of organisms (e.g., streptococci) to the heart structure. The woman should notify her physician at the first sign of infection or exposure to an infection. Vaccination against influenza and pneumococci can be given.

Nutrition counseling is necessary, optimally with the woman's family present. The pregnant woman needs a well-balanced diet with iron and folic acid supplementation, high protein levels, and adequate calories to gain weight. Iron supplements tend to cause constipation so the woman should increase her intake of fluids and fiber. A stool softener may also be prescribed. It is important that the woman with a cardiac disorder avoid straining during defecation, thus causing the Valsalva maneuver (forced expiration against a closed airway, which when released, causes blood to rush to the heart and overload the cardiac system). A referral to a registered dietitian may be necessary for a nutritional plan of care.

Cardiac medications are prescribed as needed, with attention to fetal well-being. The hemodynamic changes that occur during pregnancy, such as increased plasma volume and increased renal clearance of drugs, can alter the amount of medication needed to establish and maintain a therapeutic drug level. Therefore, monitoring drug levels during pregnancy is crucial in order to maintain effective therapy for the woman while minimizing risk to the fetus. Table 30-1 lists information on medications that are often used to treat cardiac disorders during pregnancy.

Anticoagulant therapy may be prescribed during pregnancy for several conditions, such as recurrent venous thrombosis, pulmonary embolus, rheumatic heart disease, prosthetic valves, or cyanotic congenital heart defects. If anticoagulant therapy is required during pregnancy a number of various regimens may be recommended. (See the section on valve disorders for more discussion of anticoagulant therapy.) The nurse should be aware of the goals of therapy and monitor the PT and INR accordingly. The woman may need to learn to self-administer injectable agents such as heparin or low-molecular-weight heparin. A woman taking warfarin (Coumadin) requires specific nutritional teaching to avoid foods high in vitamin K, such as raw, dark green leafy vegetables, which counteract the effects of warfarin. In addition, she will require a folic acid supplement.

Tests for fetal maturity and well-being and placental sufficiency may be necessary. Other therapy is directly related to the functional classification of heart disease. The nurse must reinforce the need for close medical supervision (see the Nursing Care Plan).

SIGNS OF POTENTIAL COMPLICATIONS

Cardiac Decompensation

PREGNANT WOMAN: SUBJECTIVE SYMPTOMS

- Increasing fatigue or difficulty breathing, or both, with her usual activities
- Feeling of smothering
- Frequent cough
- Palpitations; feeling that her heart is "racing"
- Generalized edema: swelling of face, feet, legs, fingers (e.g., rings do not fit anymore)

NURSE: OBJECTIVE SIGNS

- Irregular, weak, rapid pulse (≥100 beats/min)
- Progressive, generalized edema
- Crackles at base of lungs after two inspirations and exhalations that do not clear after coughing
- Orthopnea; increasing dyspnea
- Rapid respirations (≥25 breaths/min)
- Moist, frequent cough
- Cyanosis of lips and nailbeds

NURSING PROCESS

Cardiac Disease

ASSESSMENT

The assessment of a pregnant woman with cardiac disease may include the following:

Interview

- Personal and family medical history: diseases of cardiovascular significance, including congenital heart disease, streptococcal infections, rheumatic fever, valvular disease, endocarditis, congestive heart failure, angina, or myocardial infarction
- Factors that would increase stress on the heart:
  - Anemia
  - Infection
  - Edema
- Symptoms of cardiac decompensation (see the Signs of Potential Complications box)
- Current medications
- Current stressors

Physical Examination

- Monitor
  - Amount and pattern of edema
  - Vital signs
  - Amount and pattern of weight gain
- Observe for signs of cardiac decompensation (see the Signs of Potential Complications box)

Laboratory and Diagnostic Tests

- Review results of laboratory and diagnostic tests:
  - Routine urinalysis and blood work (complete blood count and blood chemistry)
  - Perform baseline 12-lead electrocardiogram at the beginning of the pregnancy, if not before pregnancy
  - Perform echocardiograms and pulse oximetry studies as indicated

NURSING DIAGNOSES

Possible nursing diagnoses include:

PRENATAL PERIOD

***Fear* related to:**

- increased peripartum risk

***Deficient Knowledge* related to:**

- cardiac condition
- pregnancy and how it affects cardiac condition
- requirements to alter self-management activities

***Activity Intolerance* related to:**

- cardiac condition

***Risk for Self-care Deficit (bathing, grooming, and dressing)* related to:**

- fatigue or activity intolerance
- need for bed rest

***Impaired Home Maintenance* related to:**

- woman's confinement to bed or limited activity level

INTRAPARTUM PERIOD

***Anxiety* related to:**

- fear for infant's safety during birth

Fear related to:

- possibility of dying
- perceived physiologic inability to cope with stress of labor

***Risk for Impaired Gas Exchange* related to:**

- cardiac condition

POSTPARTUM PERIOD

***Risk for Impaired Gas Exchange* related to:**

- cardiac condition

***Risk for Excess Fluid Volume* related to:**

- extravascular fluid shifts

***Ineffective Breastfeeding* related to:**

- fatigue from cardiac condition

EXPECTED OUTCOMES OF CARE

Expected outcomes are that the woman (and family, if appropriate) will:

- Verbalize understanding of the disorder, management, and probable outcome.
- Describe her role in management, including when and how to take medication, adjust diet, and prepare for and participate in treatment.
- Cope with emotional reactions to pregnancy and an infant at risk.
- Adapt to the physiologic stressors of pregnancy, labor, and birth.
- Identify and use support systems.
- Carry her fetus to viability or to term.

PLAN OF CARE AND INTERVENTIONS

- Assist the pregnant woman and her family to identify signs and symptoms of cardiac decompensation.
- Provide client teaching as follows, based on the woman's NYHA classification:

The woman with class I or II heart disease:

- Needs 10 hours of sleep every night and should take 30 minutes of rest after meals
- Should restrict activities (limit housework, shopping, and exercise) to the amount recommended for the functional classification of her heart disease

The woman with class II cardiac disease:

- Should avoid heavy exertion; stop any activity that causes even minor signs and symptoms of cardiac decompensation
- Will likely be admitted to the hospital near term (or earlier if signs of cardiac overload or arrhythmia develop) for evaluation and treatment

The woman with class III cardiac disease:

- Needs bed rest for much of the day

Other considerations

- Treat infections promptly; administer prophylactic antibiotics against bacterial endocarditis as ordered.
- Provide nutrition counseling. Refer to a registered dietitian as necessary.
- Teach the woman how to avoid constipation and resulting straining with bowel movements (Valsalva maneuver).
- Teach the importance of daily weighing. A sudden weight gain indicates fluid retention.
- Teach the woman to take cardiac medications as prescribed.
- Teach signs and symptoms of preterm labor because most of the cardiac medications used in pregnancy are reported to increase uterine contractility.
- Monitor drug levels.
- Monitor the woman's blood work.
- Review results of tests for fetal maturity and well-being and placental sufficiency.
- Reinforce the need for close medical supervision.

EVALUATION

The nurse uses the previously stated expected outcomes as criteria to evaluate the care of the woman with cardiac disease.

TABLE 30-1 **SELECTED DRUGS USED IN TREATMENT OF CARDIAC DISORDERS IN THE PREGNANT WOMAN**

GENERIC (TRADE) NAME	CROSSES PLACENTA	CONSIDERATIONS
Digoxin (Lanoxin)	Yes	Blood levels should be monitored to ensure adequate levels
Procainamide (Procanbid, Pronestyl)	Yes	No known teratogenic effects Caution needed with use
Verapamil (Calan, Isoptin)	Yes	Considered safe for use in pregnancy but can produce maternal hypotension with decreased uterine blood flow No controlled human studies on fetal effects
Propranolol (Inderal)	Yes	Considered safe for use in pregnancy No known teratogenic effects Associated with neonatal bradycardia, IUGR
Heparin	No	If anticoagulant therapy needed, heparin usually used (see discussion of use in pregnant women with valve replacement on p. 713)
Warfarin (Coumadin)	Yes	Warfarin embryopathy, fetal hemorrhage, CNS abnormalities Maternal hemorrhage Contraindicated in first trimester and at term
Furosemide (Lasix)	Yes	Fetal levels estimated to be equal to maternal levels No known teratogenic effects Limit use in first trimester Necessary to monitor for decreased plasma volume
Atenolol (Tenormin)	Yes	Reduced fetal growth; decreased placental growth and weight
Lidocaine (Xylocaine)	Yes	Safe as long as toxic levels avoided Toxic dose—fetal CNS depression
Quinidine (Quinidex)	Yes	Toxic dose may induce preterm labor and cause transient damage to the fetal eighth cranial nerve Transient neonatal thrombocytopenia reported
Nifedipine (Procardia, Adalat)	Yes	Fetal distress as a result of maternal hypotension May inhibit labor
ACE inhibitors (a class of drugs)	Yes	Oligohydramnios, fetal limb contractures, craniofacial deformities, hypoplastic lung development
Sodium nitroprusside	Yes	Low dose does not appear to cause toxic cyanide levels (fetal cyanide toxicity possibly occurring with higher doses)

ACE, Angiotensin-converting enzyme; *CNS*, central nervous system; *IUGR*, intrauterine growth restriction.

Sources: Blanchard, D., & Shabetai, R. (2009). Cardiac diseases. In R. Creasy, R. Resnik, J. Iams, C. Lockwood, & T. Moore (Eds.), *Maternal-fetal medicine: Principles and practice* (6th ed.). Philadelphia: Saunders; Klein, L., & Galan, H. (2004). Cardiac disease in pregnancy. *Obstetrics and Gynecology Clinics of North America, 31*(2), 429-459.; Niebyl, J., & Simpson, J. (2007). Drugs and environmental agents in pregnancy and lactation: Embryology, teratology, epidemiology. In S. Gabbe, J. Niebyl, & J. Simpson (Eds.), *Obstetrics: Normal and problem pregnancies* (5th ed.). Philadelphia: Churchill Livingstone.

Heart Surgery During Pregnancy. Ideally surgery to correct a cardiac lesion should be performed prior to pregnancy. In some women, however, cardiac disease is diagnosed for the first time during pregnancy. The maternal mortality risk does not increase, but there is a fetal mortality risk of 10% to 15% if heart surgery is performed, especially if cardiopulmonary bypass is used. If possible, surgery should be postponed until the third trimester of pregnancy, when the risk to the fetus is considerably decreased (Blanchard & Shabetai, 2009).

The woman, the fetus, and uterine activity must be monitored carefully during surgery. Electrocardiographic monitoring and intraarterial and Swan-Ganz catheters are usually recommended for intraoperative and postoperative assessment. In some cases, transesophageal echocardiography may be required (Blanchard & Shabetai, 2009). Closed cardiac surgery, such as release of a stenotic mitral valve, can be accomplished with little risk to mother or fetus. Open heart surgery, however, requires extracorporeal circulation, and fetal bradycardia may occur as a result of low blood-flow rates. Periods of hypoxemia for the fetus can lead to various kinds of neurologic insults. Increase in flow rates on cardiopulmonary bypass as well as intravenous nitroprusside may correct fetal bradycardia. Preterm labor occurs more frequently in women having cardiac surgery (Blanchard & Shabetai).

Intrapartum

For all pregnant women, the intrapartum period is the one that evokes the most apprehension in clients and caregivers. The woman with impaired cardiac function has additional reasons to be anxious because labor and giving birth place an additional burden on her already compromised cardiovascular system.

Assessments include the routine assessments for all laboring women, as well as assessments for cardiac decompensation. In addition, arterial blood gases (ABGs) may be needed to assess for adequate oxygenation. A pulmonary artery catheter may be inserted to monitor hemodynamic status accurately during labor and birth (see Chapter 31). ECG monitoring and

! NURSING ALERT

A pulse rate of 100 beats/min or greater or a respiratory rate of 25 breaths/min or greater is a concern. Check the respiratory status frequently for developing dyspnea, coughing, or crackles at the base of the lungs. Note the color and temperature of the skin as well. Pale, cool, clammy skin may indicate cardiac shock.

NURSING CARE PLAN

The Pregnant Woman with Heart Disease

NURSING DIAGNOSIS

Activity intolerance related to effects of pregnancy on the woman with rheumatic heart disease with mitral valve stenosis

Expected Outcome

Woman will verbalize a plan to change lifestyle throughout pregnancy so as to reduce the risk of cardiac decompensation.

Nursing Interventions/*Rationales*

- Assist the woman in identifying factors that decrease activity tolerance and explore extent of limitations *to establish a baseline for evaluation.*
- Help the woman develop an individualized program of activity and rest, taking into account the living and working environment, as well as support of family and friends, *to maintain sufficient cardiac output.*
- Teach the woman to monitor physiologic responses to activity (e.g., pulse rate, respiratory rate) and reduce activity that causes fatigue or pain *to maintain sufficient cardiac output and prevent potential injury to the fetus.*
- Enlist the woman's family and friends to assist her in pacing activities and to provide support in performing role functions and self-management activities that are too strenuous *to increase the chances of compliance with activity restrictions.*
- Suggest that the woman maintain an activity log that records activities, time, duration, intensity, and physiologic response *to evaluate effectiveness of and adherence to the activity program.*
- Discuss various quiet diversional activities that the woman can or may perform *to decrease the potential for boredom during rest periods.*

NURSING DIAGNOSIS

Risk for ineffective therapeutic regimen management related to the woman's first pregnancy and perceived sense of wellness

Expected Outcome

Woman will participate in an effective therapeutic regimen for pregnancy complicated by heart disease.

Nursing Interventions/*Rationales*

- Identify factors such as insufficient knowledge about the effect of cardiac disease on pregnancy that might inhibit the woman from participating in a therapeutic regimen *to promote early interventions, such as teaching about the importance of rest.*
- Teach the woman and her family about factors such as lack of rest or not taking prescribed medications that might adversely affect the pregnancy *to provide information and promote empowerment over the situation.*
- Encourage expression of feelings about the disease and its potential effect on the pregnancy *to promote a sense of trust.*
- Identify resources in the community *to provide a shared sense of common experiences.*
- Encourage the woman to verbalize her plan for carrying out the regimen of care *to evaluate the effects of teaching.*

NURSING DIAGNOSIS

Decreased cardiac output related to increased circulatory volume secondary to pregnancy and cardiac disease

Expected Outcome

Woman will exhibit signs of adequate cardiac output (i.e., normal pulse and blood pressure; normal heart and breath sounds; normal skin color, tone, and turgor; normal capillary refill; normal urine output; no evidence of edema).

Nursing Interventions/*Rationales*

- Reinforce the importance of activity and rest cycles *to prevent cardiac complications.*
- Reinforce the importance of the frequent visit schedule to the caregiver *to provide adequate surveillance of the high risk pregnancy.*
- Teach the woman and her family members the signs of cardiac decompensation *to provide information about when to contact the health care provider.*
- Teach the woman to lie on her side *to increase uteroplacental blood flow* and to elevate legs while sitting *to promote venous return.*
- Monitor intake and output and check for edema *to assess for renal complications or venous return problems.*
- Monitor fetal heart rate and fetal activity and perform a nonstress test as indicated *to assess fetal status and detect uteroplacental insufficiency.*

continuous monitoring of blood pressure and oxygen saturation (pulse oximetry) are usually instituted for the woman, and continuous fetal monitoring is used to monitor the fetus.

Nursing care during labor and birth focuses on the promotion of cardiac function. Minimize anxiety by maintaining a calm atmosphere in the labor and birth rooms. Provide anticipatory guidance by keeping the woman and her family informed of labor progress and events that will probably occur, as well as answering any questions they have. Support the woman's childbirth preparation method to the degree it is feasible for her cardiac condition. Nursing techniques that promote comfort, such as back massage, are also used.

Cardiac function is supported by keeping the woman's head and shoulders elevated and body parts resting on pillows. The side-lying position usually facilitates positive hemodynamics during labor. Discomfort is relieved with medication and supportive care. Epidural regional analgesia provides better pain relief than narcotics and causes fewer alterations in hemodynamics (Easterling & Stout, 2007).

LEGAL TIP: Cardiac and Metabolic Emergencies
The management of emergencies such as maternal cardiopulmonary distress or arrest or maternal metabolic crisis should be documented in policies, procedures, and protocols. Any independent nursing actions appropriate to the emergency should be clearly identified.

Beta-adrenergic agents such as terbutaline (Brethine) are associated with various side effects, including tachycardia, irregular pulse, myocardial ischemia, and pulmonary edema. Therefore, these medications should not be used in women with known or suspected heart disease (Gilbert, 2011; Iams & Romero, 2007; Iams, Romero, & Creasy, 2009). A synthetic oxytocin (Syntocinon) can be used to induce labor. This drug does not appear to cause significant coronary artery constriction in doses prescribed for labor induction or control of postpartum uterine atony. Cervical ripening agents containing prostaglandin are usually tolerated well, but should be used cautiously.

If no obstetric problems exist, vaginal birth is recommended and may be accomplished with the woman in the side-lying position to facilitate uterine perfusion. If the supine position is used, position a pad under one hip to displace the uterus laterally and minimize the danger of supine hypotension. Have the woman flex her knees and place her feet flat on the bed. To prevent compression of popliteal veins and an increase in blood volume in the chest and trunk as a result of the effects of gravity, do not use stirrups. Open-glottis pushing is recommended. The woman should avoid the Valsalva maneuver when pushing in the second stage of labor because it reduces diastolic ventricular filling and obstructs left ventricular outflow. Mask oxygen is important. Episiotomy and vacuum extraction or outlet forceps can be used to decrease the length of the second stage of labor and decrease the workload of the heart in second stage labor. Cesarean birth is not routinely recommended for women who have cardiovascular disease because of the risks of dramatic fluid shifts, sustained hemodynamic changes, and increased blood loss.

Penicillin prophylaxis may be ordered for nonallergic pregnant women with class II or higher cardiac disease to protect against bacterial endocarditis in labor and during the early puerperium (see Box 30-2). Oxytocin is usually given immediately after birth to prevent hemorrhage. Ergot products should not be used because they increase blood pressure. Fluid balance should be maintained and blood loss replaced. If tubal sterilization is desired, surgery is delayed at least several days to ensure homeostasis.

Postpartum

Monitoring for cardiac decompensation in the postpartum period is essential. The first 24 to 48 hours after birth are the most hemodynamically difficult for the woman. Hemorrhage or infection, or both, may worsen the cardiac condition. The woman with a cardiac disorder may continue to require a pulmonary artery catheter and ABG monitoring.

! NURSING ALERT

The immediate postbirth period is hazardous for a woman whose heart function is compromised. Cardiac output increases rapidly as extravascular fluid is remobilized into the vascular compartment. At the moment of birth, intraabdominal pressure is reduced drastically; pressure on veins is removed, the splanchnic vessels engorge, and blood flow to the heart is increased.

Care in the postpartum period is tailored to the woman's functional capacity. Postpartum assessment of the woman with cardiac disease includes vital signs, oxygen saturation levels, lung and heart auscultation, presence and degree of edema, amount and character of bleeding, uterine tone and fundal height, urinary output, pain (especially chest pain), the activity-rest pattern, dietary intake, mother-infant interactions, and emotional state. The head of the bed is elevated, and the woman is encouraged to lie on her side. Bed rest may be ordered, with or without bathroom privileges. Progressive ambulation may be permitted as tolerated. The nurse may help the woman meet her grooming and hygiene needs and other activities. Bowel movements without stress or strain for the woman are promoted with stool softeners, diet, and fluids.

The woman may need a family member to help in the care of the infant. Breastfeeding is not contraindicated, but some women with heart disease (particularly those with life-threatening disease) may be unable to breastfeed. The woman who chooses to breastfeed will need the support of her family and the nursing staff to be successful. For example, she may need assistance in positioning herself and/or the infant for feeding. To further conserve the woman's energy, the infant can be brought to the mother and taken from her after the feeding. Most medications used to manage cardiac disorders are compatible with breastfeeding. Thiazide diuretics, however, may suppress lactation (Blanchard & Shabetai, 2009). Because diuretics can cause neonatal diuresis that can lead to dehydration, lactating women must be monitored closely to determine if medication doses can be reduced and still be effective.

If the woman is unable to breastfeed and her energies do not allow her to bottle feed the infant, the baby can be kept at the bedside so she can look at and touch her baby to establish an emotional bond, with a low expenditure of energy. The infant should be held at the mother's eye level and near her lips and brought to her fingers. At the same time, involving the mother passively in her infant's care helps the mother feel vitally important—as she is—to the infant's well-being (e.g., "You can offer something no one else can: you can provide your baby with your sounds, touch, and rhythms that are so comforting"). Perhaps the woman can be encouraged to make a tape recording of her talking, singing, or whispering, which can be played for the baby in the nursery to help the infant feel her presence and be in contact with her voice. This also enhances maternal-infant bonding.

Preparation for discharge is carefully planned with the woman and family. Provision of help for the woman in the home by relatives, friends, and others must be addressed. If necessary, the nurse refers the family to community resources (e.g., for assistance with household activities). Rest and sleep periods, activity, and diet must be planned. The couple may need information about reestablishing sexual relations and contraception or sterilization.

Women with congenital heart disease should be offered contraceptive counseling. In general, for women with congenital heart disease, the complications associated with pregnancy are usually greater than the risks associated with any form of contraception (Easterling & Stout, 2007). Women at particular risk for thromboembolism should avoid combined estrogen-progestin oral contraceptives, but progestin-only pills may be used. Parenteral progestins (e.g., Depo-Provera) are safe and effective for women with cardiac disease. An intrauterine device (IUD) may be used by some women with congenital heart lesions. Although a theoretical risk exists for developing endocarditis, the actual risk for women using an IUD is probably very minimal (Easterling & Stout).

Monitoring for cardiac decompensation continues through the first few weeks after birth because of hormonal shifts that affect hemodynamics. Maternal cardiac output is usually stabilized by 2 weeks postpartum (Easterling & Stout, 2007).

Men and women with congenital heart disease are at increased risk for having children who also have congenital heart disease. The risk for affected mothers is greater, approximately two to more than three times that of affected fathers. Children born with congenital heart disease to parents with congenital heart defects appear to inherit the risk for cardiac maldevelopment in general because they often do not have the same defect as the parent (Easterling & Stout, 2007). Therefore preconception counseling and genetic counseling before a subsequent pregnancy are essential.

Cardiopulmonary Resuscitation of the Pregnant Woman

Trauma, cardiac abnormalities, embolism, magnesium overdose, sepsis, intracranial hemorrhage, anesthetic complications, eclampsia, and uterine rupture are the most common causes of cardiac arrest in a pregnant woman (Martin & Foley, 2009). Special modifications are necessary when cardiopulmonary resuscitation (CPR) is performed during the second half of pregnancy. In nonpregnant women, chest compressions produce a cardiac output of only about 30% of normal. Cardiac output in pregnant women may be even less due to aortocaval compression caused by the gravid uterus. Therefore, uterine displacement during resuscitation efforts is critical (Cunningham et al., 2010). The uterus may be displaced laterally either manually or by placing a wedge, rolled blanket, or towel under one of the woman's hips. If defibrillation is needed, the paddles must be placed one rib interspace higher than usual because the heart is displaced slightly by the enlarged uterus (see the Emergency box).

If CPR is not effective within 4 to 5 minutes, perimortem cesarean birth is often recommended if the fetus is viable and maternal cardiopulmonary arrest appears to be untreatable. According to one study, 98% of infants born within 5 minutes of maternal cardiac arrest were neurologically normal. The rate of intact neonatal survival decreases, however, as the time from maternal arrest to birth increases (Cunningham et al., 2010; Lu & Curet, 2007). Cesarean birth may also facilitate maternal resuscitative efforts. Therefore, the American College of Obstetricians and Gynecologists (ACOG) recommends that performing a cesarean birth be considered within 4 minutes of cardiac arrest in the third trimester of pregnancy (ACOG, 2009).

Complications may be associated with CPR on a pregnant woman. These complications may include laceration of the liver, rupture of the spleen or uterus, hemothorax, hemopericardium, or fracture of ribs or the sternum. Fetal complications, including cardiac arrhythmia or asystole related to maternal defibrillation and medications, and central nervous system (CNS) depression related to antiarrhythmic drugs and inadequate uteroplacental perfusion, with possible fetal hypoxemia and acidemia, also may occur.

If the resuscitation is successful, the woman must be carefully monitored afterward. She remains at increased risk for recurrent cardiac arrest and arrhythmias (e.g., ventricular tachycardia, supraventricular tachycardia, bradycardia). Therefore, her cardiovascular, pulmonary, and neurologic status should be assessed continuously. If the pregnancy remains intact, uterine activity and resting tone must be monitored. Fetal status and gestational age should also be determined and used in decision making regarding the continuation of the pregnancy or the timing and route of birth.

Another common reason for performing CPR on a pregnant woman is airway obstruction caused by choking. Clearing an airway obstruction is usually accomplished by performing abdominal thrusts (formerly known as the Heimlich maneuver). During the second and third trimesters of pregnancy, however, chest thrusts, rather than abdominal thrusts, should be used (see the Emergency box and Fig. 30-1).

EMERGENCY

Cardiopulmonary Resuscitation (CPR) for the Pregnant Woman

AIRWAY

- Determine unresponsiveness.
- Activate emergency medical system and get the automated external defibrillator (AED) if available.
- Position the woman on flat, firm surface with uterus displaced laterally with a wedge (e.g., a rolled towel placed under her hip) or manually, or place her in a lateral position.
- Open airway with head tilt–chin lift maneuver.

BREATHING

- Determine breathlessness (look, listen, feel).
- If the woman is not breathing, give two breaths, 1 second each.

CIRCULATION

- Determine pulselessness by feeling carotid pulse.
- If no pulse is detectable, begin chest compressions at a rate of 100 per minute. Chest compressions may be performed slightly higher on the sternum if the uterus is enlarged enough to displace the diaphragm into a higher position.
- After five cycles of 30 compressions and two breaths (or ~2 min), check her pulse. If no pulse, continue cardiopulmonary resuscitation.

DEFIBRILLATION

- Use an AED according to standard protocol to analyze heart rhythm and deliver shock if indicated.

RELIEF OF FOREIGN BODY AIRWAY OBSTRUCTION

- If the pregnant woman is unable to speak or cough, perform chest thrusts. Stand behind the woman and place your arms under her armpits to encircle her chest. Press backward with quick thrusts until the foreign body is expelled (see Fig. 30-1). If the woman becomes unresponsive, follow the steps for victims who become unresponsive, but use chest thrusts instead of abdominal thrusts.

Source: American Heart Association (AHA). (2005). American Heart Association guidelines for cardiopulmonary resuscitation and emergency cardiovascular care. Part 10.8: Cardiac arrest associated with pregnancy. *Circulation, 112*(24 Suppl), IV-150-153.

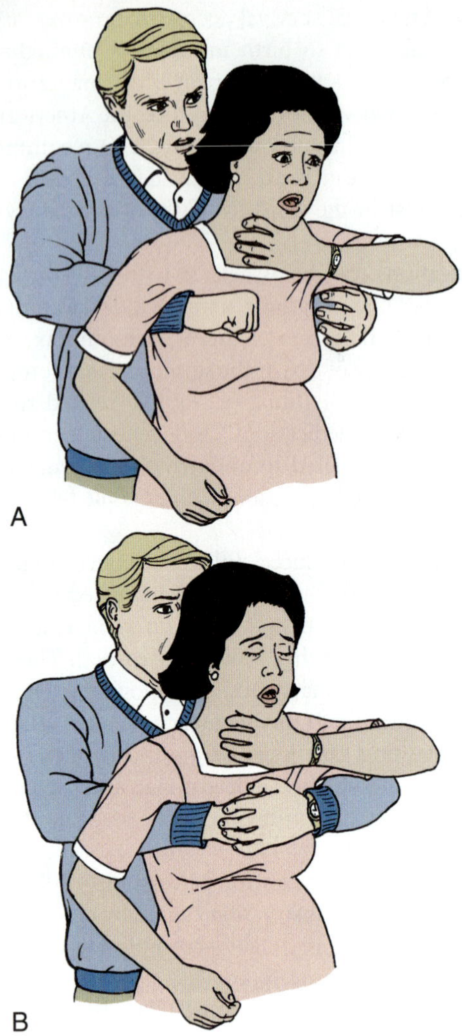

FIG. 30-1 Abdominal thrust maneuver (formerly known as the Heimlich maneuver). Clearing airway obstruction in woman in late stage of pregnancy (can also be used in markedly obese victim). **A,** Standing behind victim, place your arms under woman's armpits and across chest. Place thumb side of your clenched fist against middle of sternum, and place other hand over fist. **B,** Perform backward chest thrusts until foreign body is expelled or woman becomes unconscious. If pregnant woman becomes unconscious because of foreign body airway obstruction, place her on her back and kneel close to her side. (Be sure uterus is displaced laterally by using, for example, a rolled blanket under her hip.) Open mouth with tongue-jaw lift, perform finger sweep, and attempt rescue breathing. If unable to ventilate, position hands as for chest compression. Deliver five chest thrusts firmly to remove obstruction. Repeat this sequence of abdominal thrust maneuver, finger sweep, and attempt to ventilate. Continue sequence until pregnant woman's airway is clear of obstruction or help has arrived to relieve you. If the woman is unconscious, give chest compressions as for a woman without pulse (American Heart Association [AHA]. [2005]. American Heart Association guidelines for cardiopulmonary resuscitation and emergency cardiovascular care. Part 10.8: Cardiac arrest associated with pregnancy. *Circulation, 112*(24 Suppl), IV-150-153.)

OTHER MEDICAL DISORDERS IN PREGNANCY

Anemia

Anemia is a common medical disorder of pregnancy, affecting from 20% to 60% of pregnant women (Kilpatrick, 2009). Anemia results in a reduction of the oxygen-carrying capacity of the blood. Because the oxygen-carrying capacity of the blood is decreased, the heart tries to compensate by increasing the cardiac output. This effort increases the workload of the heart and stresses ventricular function. Therefore, anemia that occurs with any other complication (e.g., preeclampsia) may result in congestive heart failure.

An indirect index of the oxygen-carrying capacity is the packed red blood cell (RBC) volume, or hematocrit level. The normal hematocrit range in nonpregnant women is 37% to 47%. However, normal values for pregnant women with adequate iron stores may be as low as 33%. According to the Centers for Disease Control and Prevention (CDC), anemia in pregnancy is defined as hemoglobin less than 11 g/dl in the first and third trimesters and less than 10.5 g/dl in the second trimester (Kilpatrick, 2009). A hemoglobin level less than 6 to 8 mg/dl is considered severe anemia (Blackburn, 2007).

When a woman has anemia during pregnancy, the loss of blood at birth, even if minimal, is not well tolerated. She is at an increased risk for requiring blood transfusions. Women with anemia have a higher incidence of puerperal complications, such as infection, than pregnant women with normal hematologic values.

Care of the anemic pregnant woman requires that the health care provider distinguish between the normal physiologic anemia of pregnancy and disease states. The majority of cases of anemia in pregnancy are caused by iron deficiency. The other types include a considerable variety of acquired and hereditary anemias, such as folic acid deficiency, sickle cell anemia, and thalassemia.

Iron Deficiency Anemia

Iron deficiency anemia is the most common anemia of pregnancy. It is diagnosed by checking the woman's serum ferritin level in addition to her hemoglobin and hematocrit levels. The serum ferritin level reflects iron reserves. A serum ferritin value less than 12 mcg/dl in the presence of a low hemoglobin value indicates iron deficiency anemia. An association appears to exist between maternal iron deficiency anemia, especially severe anemia, and preterm birth and low-birth-weight infants, although whether these poor pregnancy outcomes are caused by iron deficiency anemia is uncertain (Samuels, 2007). Usually even the fetus of an anemic woman will receive adequate iron stores from the mother, at the cost of further depleting the mother's iron level (Blackburn, 2007).

Generally iron deficiency anemia is preventable or easily treated with iron supplements. Because of the increased amounts of iron needed for fetal development and maternal stores, pregnant women are often encouraged to take prophylactic iron supplementation (Blackburn, 2007; Gilbert, 2011). Most women with iron deficiency anemia can absorb as much iron as they need by taking one 325-mg tablet of ferrous sulfate twice each day (Samuels, 2007). An important aspect to teach the pregnant woman is the significance of the iron therapy. Some pregnant women cannot tolerate the prescribed oral iron because of nausea and vomiting associated with the pregnancy and as a side effect of iron therapy. In such cases the woman may be given parenteral iron therapy by intramuscular or intravascular injection. Women who are severely anemic may require blood transfusions (Samuels).

Teach the importance of iron supplements for preventing or treating iron deficiency anemia (see the Teaching for

Self-Management box: Iron Supplementation in Chapter 14, p. 325). In addition, teach dietary ways to decrease the GI side effects of iron therapy.

Folate Deficiency Anemia

Folate is a water-soluble vitamin found naturally in dark green leafy vegetables, citrus fruits, eggs, legumes, and whole grains. Even in well-nourished women, folate deficiency is common. Poor diet, cooking with large volumes of water, and increased alcohol use may contribute to folate deficiency. During pregnancy the need for folate increases, both because of fetal demands and because folate is less well absorbed from the GI tract during gestation. Folic acid is the form of the vitamin used in vitamin supplements. The recommended daily intake of folic acid for pregnant women is 600 mcg. Both prescription and nonprescription prenatal vitamins contain more than this amount of folic acid and should be sufficient to prevent and treat folate deficiency. Women at particular risk for folate deficiency include those who have significant hemoglobinopathies, take anticonvulsant medication, or are pregnant with a multifetal gestation. These women will require larger than usual doses of folic acid (Samuels, 2007).

Folate deficiency is the most common cause of megaloblastic anemia during pregnancy, but a vitamin B_{12} deficiency must also be considered. Megaloblastic anemia rarely occurs before the third trimester of pregnancy (Kilpatrick, 2009; Samuels, 2007). Women with megaloblastic anemia caused by folic acid deficiency have the usual presenting symptoms and signs of anemia: pallor, fatigue, and lethargy, as well as glossitis and skin roughness, which are associated specifically with megaloblastic anemia (Kilpatrick). Folate deficiency usually improves rapidly with folic acid therapy. It rarely occurs in the fetus and is not a significant cause of perinatal morbidity. Iron deficiency often occurs along with folate deficiency (Samuels).

Sickle Cell Hemoglobinopathy

Sickle cell hemoglobinopathy is a disease caused by the presence of abnormal hemoglobin in the blood. Sickle cell trait (SA hemoglobin pattern) is sickling of the RBCs but with a normal RBC life span. Most people with sickle cell trait are asymptomatic. Approximately 1 in 12 African-American adults in the United States have sickle cell trait (Samuels, 2007). Women with sickle cell trait require genetic counseling and partner testing to determine their risk of producing children with sickle cell trait or disease.

Women with sickle cell trait usually do well in pregnancy. However, they are at increased risk for preeclampsia, intrauterine fetal death, preterm birth and low-birth-weight infants, and postpartum endometritis. They are also at increased risk for urinary tract infections (UTIs) and may be deficient in iron (Kilpatrick, 2009; Samuels, 2007).

Sickle cell anemia (sickle cell disease) is a recessive, hereditary, familial hemolytic anemia that affects persons of African or Mediterranean ancestry. These individuals usually have abnormal hemoglobin types (SS or SC). The average life span of RBCs in a person with sickle cell anemia is only 5 to 10 days, in comparison to the 120-day life span of a normal RBC. Sickle cell anemia occurs in 1 in 708 African-Americans in the United States (Samuels, 2007). Persons with sickle cell anemia have recurrent attacks (crises) of fever and pain, most often in the abdomen, joints, or extremities, although virtually all organ systems can be affected. These attacks are attributed to vascular occlusion when RBCs assume a characteristic sickled shape. Crises are usually triggered by dehydration, hypoxia, or acidosis (Samuels).

Women with sickle cell anemia require genetic counseling before pregnancy. All children born to a woman with sickle cell anemia will be affected in some way by the disease. The woman's partner must be tested to determine the couple's risk of producing children with sickle cell disease rather than sickle cell trait. Women with sickle cell anemia are at risk for poor pregnancy outcomes, including miscarriage, IUGR, and stillbirth. Although maternal mortality is rare, maternal morbidity is significant and includes an increased risk for preeclampsia and infection, particularly in the urinary tract and in the lungs. The frequency of painful crises also appears to be increased during pregnancy (Samuels, 2007).

The woman will be monitored carefully during pregnancy for the development of urinary tract infection or preeclampsia. In addition, she will have serial ultrasound examinations to monitor fetal growth and will likely have antepartum fetal testing performed regularly during the third trimester. Infections are treated aggressively with antibiotics. If crises occur they are managed with analgesia, oxygen, and hydration. Some authorities recommend prophylactic transfusions as a way to improve oxygen-carrying capacity and suppress the synthesis of sickle hemoglobin. Others, however, believe that prophylactic transfusions do not improve fetal or neonatal outcome (Samuels, 2007).

SAFETY ALERT

Women with sickle cell anemia are not iron deficient. Therefore, routine iron supplementation, even that found in prenatal vitamins, should be avoided because these women can develop iron overload (Samuels, 2007).

If no complications occur, pregnancy can continue until term. Intrapartum, women with sickle cell disease should be encouraged to labor in a side-lying position. They may require supplemental oxygen. Adequate hydration should be

COMMUNITY ACTIVITY

- Select a medical disorder such as sickle cell anemia, epilepsy or multiple sclerosis. Visit the website of the national organization. Review the client information about the disorder and treatment options. Research the importance of preconception counseling for women with medical disorders. Are any community-based programs sponsored by the national organization available in your community?
- Research the availability of obstetrical home health care services for women with a high-risk pregnancy in your community. What types of pregnancy complications are cared for in the home setting? Does the company provide both around the clock telephone and home nursing services? Visit the Alere Women's and Children's Health website. Alere is a home health agency that manages and monitors pregnant women with medical or pregnancy-related problems.

maintained while preventing fluid overload. Conduction anesthesia (e.g., epidural or combined spinal-epidural anesthesia) is recommended because it provides excellent pain relief. Vaginal birth is preferred. Cesarean birth should be performed only for obstetric indications (Samuels, 2007).

Thalassemia

Thalassemia is a relatively common anemia in which an insufficient amount of hemoglobin is produced to fill the RBCs. Thalassemia is a hereditary disorder that involves the abnormal synthesis of the alpha or beta chains of hemoglobin. Beta thalassemia is the more common variety in the United States and usually occurs in persons of Mediterranean, North African, Middle Eastern, and Asian descent (Kilpatrick, 2009).

Beta thalassemia minor is the heterozygous form of this disorder. Persons with heterozygous beta thalassemia are carriers of the disorder and are usually asymptomatic (Samuels, 2007). They can expect to have a normal life span despite a moderately reduced hemoglobin level. Pregnancy will not worsen beta thalassemia minor. Neither does the disorder adversely affect pregnancy. Women with beta thalassemia minor do not require antepartum fetal testing (Samuels). Iron therapy should only be prescribed for women who are iron deficient, although folic acid supplementation is recommended for all women with beta thalassemia minor.

The homozygous form of beta thalassemia is known as thalassemia major, or Cooley anemia. Persons with this form of the disease usually have hepatosplenomegaly and bone deformities caused by massive marrow tissue expansion. These individuals usually die of infection or cardiovascular complications fairly early in life. If women live to reach childbearing age, infertility is common. If women with this disorder do become pregnant, they usually experience severe anemia and congestive heart failure, although successful full-term pregnancies have been reported. Women with beta thalassemia major are managed much like those with sickle cell anemia during pregnancy (Samuels, 2007).

Pulmonary Disorders

As pregnancy advances and the uterus presses on the thoracic cavity, any pregnant woman may have increased respiratory difficulty. This difficulty will be compounded by pulmonary disease. A pulmonary disorder in pregnancy requires assessment, planning, and interventions specific to the disease process, in addition to routine peripartum care.

Asthma

Asthma is a chronic inflammatory disorder involving the tracheobronchial airways, with increased airway responsiveness to a variety of stimuli. It is characterized by periods of exacerbations and remissions. Exacerbations are usually triggered by stimuli such as allergens, upper respiratory infection, medications (i.e., aspirin, beta-blockers), environmental pollutants, occupational exposures, exercise, cold air, or emotional stress (Powrie, 2006). In many cases the actual cause may be unknown, although a family history of allergy is common in people with asthma. In response to stimuli, there is widespread but reversible narrowing of the hyperreactive airways, making it difficult to breathe. The clinical manifestations are expiratory wheezing, productive cough, thick sputum, dyspnea, or any combination.

From 4% to 8% of pregnant women have asthma (Whitty & Dombroski, 2009), making it one of the most common preexisting conditions of pregnancy. The effect of pregnancy on asthma is unpredictable. The severity of the disease is unchanged in one third, improved in one third, and worsened in one third of pregnant women. If asthma worsens, the more severe symptoms usually occur between 17 and 24 weeks of gestation (Gilbert, 2011). Asthma appears to be associated with uteroplacental insufficiency, IUGR, and preterm birth (Gilbert; Whitty & Dombrowski).

The ultimate goal of asthma therapy in pregnancy is maintaining adequate oxygenation of the fetus by preventing hypoxic episodes in the mother. Achieving this goal requires monitoring lung function objectively (e.g., peak expiratory flow rate and forced expiratory volume in 1 second), avoiding or controlling asthma triggers (e.g., dust mites, animal dander, pollen, wood smoke), educating clients about the importance of controlling asthma during pregnancy, and drug therapy. Current drug therapy for asthma emphasizes treatment of airway inflammation to decrease airway hyperresponsiveness and prevent asthma symptoms. Decreasing airway inflammation with inhaled corticosteroids is the preferred treatment for managing persistent asthma during pregnancy (Whitty & Dombrowski, 2009) (see the Nursing Process box: Asthma).

Although asthma exacerbations during labor are very rare, medications for asthma are continued during labor and the postpartum period. Pulse oximetry should be instituted during labor. Epidurals are recommended for pain relief. Morphine and meperidine are histamine-releasing narcotics and should be avoided. Fentanyl may be used as an alternative for pain relief because it is less likely to cause histamine release (Powrie, 2006). Table 30-2 lists information on medications used in women with asthma during the intrapartum and postpartum periods.

During the postpartum period, women who have asthma are at increased risk for hemorrhage. If excessive bleeding occurs, oxytocin is the recommended drug (see Table 30-2). Asthma medications are usually safe for administration during the postpartum period and lactation. The woman usually returns to her prepregnancy asthma status within 3 months after giving birth.

Cystic Fibrosis

Cystic fibrosis is a common autosomal recessive genetic disorder in which the exocrine glands produce excessive viscous secretions, which causes problems with both respiratory and digestive functions. Most persons with cystic fibrosis have chronic obstructive pulmonary disease, pancreatic exocrine insufficiency, and elevated sweat electrolytes. Morbidity and mortality are usually caused by progressive chronic bronchial pulmonary disease (Whitty & Dombrowski, 2009).

Because the gene for cystic fibrosis was identified in 1989, data can be collected for the purposes of genetic counseling for couples regarding carrier status. In the United States, approximately 4% of the Caucasian population are carriers of the cystic fibrosis gene. Cystic fibrosis occurs in 1 in 3200 live

NURSING PROCESS

Asthma

ASSESSMENT

The assessment of a pregnant woman with asthma may include:

History

- Medical history of respiratory disorders
- Allergy history and testing
- Previous response to treatment
- Previous pregnancies and outcomes
- Exposure to potential environmental triggers (i.e., cigarette smoke, mold, dander)

Physical examination

- Respiratory rate and effort
- Breath sound auscultation
- Symmetric respiratory effort
- Signs of distress
- Skin color

Laboratory tests

- Peak expiratory flow rate as measured by peak flowmeter
- Pulse oximetry
- Chest x-ray
- Complete blood count
- Arterial blood gases

NURSING DIAGNOSES

Possible nursing diagnoses include:

***Risk for Injury (to the fetus)* related to:**

- episodes of maternal hypoxia, leading to inadequate fetal oxygenation

***Anxiety* related to:**

- asthma and its potential effect on the pregnancy and the fetus

***Ineffective Airway Clearance* related to:**

- bronchial inflammation
- bronchial spasm

***Deficient Knowledge* related to:**

- asthma triggers
- use of peak flowmeter
- use of inhaled agents
- when to call care provider

EXPECTED OUTCOMES OF CARE

Expected outcomes are that the woman will:

- Verbalize her concerns related to the effect of asthma on the pregnancy and fetus.
- Use available coping mechanisms and support systems.
- Experience no adverse pregnancy or fetal effects due to asthma.
- Maintain control of asthma throughout the pregnancy.
- Verbalize situations in which she should notify her health care provider.
- Demonstrate accurate use of the peak flowmeter and knowledge of her personal best numbers.
- Demonstrate correct use of prescribed inhaler medications (both maintenance and rescue inhalers).
- Maintain the treatment regimen as prescribed.
- Verbalize a plan to avoid personal asthma triggers.

PLAN OF CARE AND INTERVENTIONS

Home care

Teach the woman to:

- Avoid asthma triggers.
- Use inhalers and/or oral medications as prescribed.
- Use peak flowmeter daily or more often as prescribed. Record numbers for care provider to review.
- Maintain prenatal visit schedule.
- Call care provider when necessary.
- Use support systems as necessary.

EVALUATION

Evaluation of the effectiveness of care of the woman with asthma is based on the expected outcomes.

TABLE 30-2 MEDICATIONS USED IN PREGNANCY IN WOMEN WITH ASTHMA

STAGE/CONDITION OF PREGNANCY	PREFERRED MEDICATION	MEDICATION(S) TO AVOID (RATIONALE)
Labor	Continue asthma medications	
Induction	Prostaglandin E_1 (Misoprostol [Cytotec]) and E_2 (Dinoprostone [Cervidil; Prepidil] may be used for cervical ripening) Oxytocin (Pitocin)	15-methyl prostaglandin $F_{2\alpha}$ (Prostin/15m; Carboprost; Hemabate) (may cause bronchoconstriction or bronchospasm)
Pain relief	Fentanyl (Sublimaze) Epidural anesthesia	Morphine and meperidine (Demerol) (release histamine)
Preterm labor	Magnesium sulfate	Beta-agonist (e.g., terbutaline [Brethine]) if woman is already taking one for her asthma (may cause respiratory distress) Indomethacin (Indocin) may cause bronchospasm NSAIDs (may exacerbate asthma)
Postpartum hemorrhage	Oxytocin	Methylergonovine (Methergine) and 15-methyl prostaglandin $F_{2\alpha}$ (Prostin/15m; Carboprost; Hemabate) (may worsen asthma)

NSAIDs, Nonsteroidal antiinflammatory drugs.

Source: Whitty, J., & Dombrowski, M. (2009). Respiratory diseases in pregnancy. In R. Creasy, R. Resnik, J. Iams, C. Lockwood, & T. Moore (Eds.), *Maternal-fetal medicine: Principles and practice* (6th ed.). Philadelphia: Saunders.

EVIDENCE-BASED PRACTICE

Pat Gingrich

The 2009 Influenza A (H1N1) Pandemic and Pregnancy

ASK THE QUESTION

What are the risks for women who contract influenza during pregnancy?

SEARCH FOR EVIDENCE

Search Strategies

Professional organization guidelines, meta-analyses, systematic reviews, randomized controlled trials, nonrandomized prospective studies and retrospective reviews since 2008.

Databases Searched

CINAHL, Cochrane, Medline, PUBMED, and the websites for the Agency for Healthcare Research and Quality (AHRQ) and the Centers for Disease Control and Prevention (CDC).

CRITICALLY ANALYZE THE DATA

Immune suppression in pregnancy is an adaptive mechanism to keep the maternal antibodies from attacking the foreign protein of the fetus. However, this mildly immunocompromised state leaves pregnant women more vulnerable to infections. The 2009 pandemic of influenza A (H1N1), which was more serious in younger adults, caused severe respiratory disease. Pregnant women already have increased demands for oxygenation from pregnancy, so respiratory impairment becomes magnified. In addition, febrile illness can cause fetal distress. Antiviral treatment works best if started within 48 hours of the onset of symptoms. The CDC noted that between April and December of 2009, 953 women were reported to have influenza A (H1N1) (Siston, Rasmussen, Honein, Fry, Seib, Callaghan, et al., 2010). Of those identified, 280 were admitted to an intensive care unit (ICU). Pregnant women were found to have a disproportionately high risk of mortality: 56 died, or 6% of all reported H1N1 deaths. Of those deaths, 7% died in the first trimester, 27% in the second trimester, and 64% during the third trimester of pregnancy. Early (less than 48 hours) antiviral treatment was much more successful at preventing ICU admission than treatment started after 4 days (9.4% vs 56.9%). Only one death occurred in the early treatment group.

A population based cohort study conducted in New Zealand and Australia from 6/1/09 to 8/31/09 noted that 64 pregnant or postpartum women were admitted to the ICU. Compared with non-pregnant women of childbearing age, the pregnant women were 7.4 times more likely to be admitted to the ICU, and 13 times more likely if they were more than 20 weeks of gestation. Of the women in the ICU, 69% were on mechanical ventilation and 19% were on extracorporeal mechanical oxygenation. There were 22 preterm births (39%), and 32 admissions to neonatal ICU (57%). In addition, there were 7 maternal deaths, 4 stillbirths, and 3 neonatal deaths (ANZIC Influenza Investigators and Australasian Maternity Outcomes Surveillance System, 2010).

The evidence available from the H1N1 pandemic has not yet developed to the level of systematic nor meta-analyses. However, a review of published and unpublished literature found that pregnant women were at a much greater risk for pneumonitis (inflammation of the lung tissue) and respiratory failure during influenza infection, especially during pandemics (Lapinsky, 2010). Fetal distress results from hypoxemia and fever. During early pregnancy, fever can cause neural tube defects, while late in pregnancy and in labor, maternal fever can cause neonatal outcomes such as seizures, encephalopathy, cerebral palsy, and death. Oseltamivir (Tamiflu) or zanamivir (Relenza) were effective at decreasing the severity of the influenza symptoms, but amantadine and rimantadine were not recommended (CDC, 2009).

IMPLICATIONS FOR PRACTICE

All pregnant women need to be evaluated promptly if they develop flu-like symptoms (fever, chills, headache, upper respiratory symptoms, shortness of breath, myalgias, fatigue, vomiting or diarrhea). Practice guidance from 2010 recommends that pregnant women receive vaccination (non-live) for both seasonal and A (H1N1) influenza. Symptomatic pregnant women should be kept on voluntary home quarantine, using all recommended hand and cough/sneeze hygiene, face masks and respirators. Women with symptoms should wear a face mask in labor, birth and postpartum. Since newborns have little resistance to infections, neonates should be kept separately from their mother, either in an isolette or an open crib at least 6 feet away (out of the droplet zone), although they may room-in and be cared for by a healthy family member or nurse. Exposed neonates should not return to the nursery, to avoid exposing other babies. Because the maternal antibodies in the colostrum will greatly benefit the newborn's immunities, women should be encouraged to pump their breasts, to be given to the newborn by the healthy caretaker. Breast milk does not transmit the virus, and the mother's antiviral medication passed through the milk is not harmful to the newborn. These precautions in effect should remain until the mother has been on antiviral medication for at least 48 hours, afebrile without antipyretics for 24 hours, and can control coughing and secretions. After meeting these criteria, the mother may breastfeed and care for the baby, but must wear a face mask until 7 days after symptom onset or 24 hours after symptoms have resolved. The nurse should also teach the family careful handwashing, including the baby's hands, as well as environmental cleaning and cough hygiene. No sick people should be allowed contact with the newborn. In addition, the nurse can teach the family to monitor closely and bring the baby in at the first sign of infection. Updates may be found at cdcinfo@cdc.gov.

References

ANZIC Influenza Investigators and Australasian Maternity Outcomes Surveillance System. (2010). Critical illness due to 2009 A/H1N1 influenza in pregnant and postpartum women: Population based cohort study. *British Medical Journal, 340*, c1279, doi: 10.1136/bmj.c.1279.

Centers for Disease Control and Prevention (CDC). (2009). *Interim guidance: Considerations regarding 2009 H1N1 influenza in intrapartum and postpartum hospital settings.* Atlanta, GA: Centers for Disease Control and Prevention.

Lapinsky, S. (2010). H1N1 novel influenza A in pregnant and immunocompromised patients. *Critical Care Medicine, 38*(Suppl.4), e52–e57.

Siston, A., Rasmussen, S., Honein, M., Fry, A., Seib, K., Callaghan, W., et al. (2010). Pandemic 2009 influenza A (H1N1) virus illness among pregnant women in the United States. *Journal of the American Medical Association, 303*(15), 1517–1525.

Caucasian births (Whitty & Dombrowski, 2009). Persons with cystic fibrosis now live longer than they did in the past because of earlier diagnosis of the disease and advances in antibiotic therapy and nutritional support. Men tend to live a little longer (median age of survival is 29.6 years) as compared with women, whose median age of survival is 27.3 years. Although most men with cystic fibrosis are infertile, women with the disease are often fertile and thus able to become pregnant (Whitty & Dombrowski, 2007).

Preconception counseling is essential for women with cystic fibrosis. Women should be advised of the risks of pregnancy, depending on their status. If possible, a woman should lose or gain weight to be at 90% of her ideal body weight before conception (Cunningham et al., 2010; Whitty & Dombrowski, 2009).

Pulmonary function studies are the best predictor of both pregnancy and long term maternal outcome. Women with good nutrition, mild obstructive lung disease, and minimal lung impairment generally tolerate pregnancy well (Cunningham et al., 2010; Whitty & Dombrowski, 2009).

In women with severe disease, pregnancy is often complicated by chronic hypoxia and frequent pulmonary infections. Women with cystic fibrosis show a decrease in their residual volume during pregnancy, as do normal pregnant women, and are unable to maintain vital capacity. Presumably the pulmonary vasculature cannot accommodate the increased cardiac output of pregnancy. The result is decreased oxygen supply to the myocardium, decreased cardiac output, and increased hypoxemia. A pregnant woman with less than 50% of expected vital capacity usually has a difficult pregnancy. Increased maternal and perinatal mortality is related to severe pulmonary infection. There is an increased incidence of preterm birth, IUGR, and uteroplacental insufficiency (Cunningham et al., 2010; Whitty & Dombrowski, 2009).

In addition to respiratory problems, women with cystic fibrosis may also develop gestational diabetes and liver disease. Pancreatic insufficiency may put the woman at risk for malnutrition because she cannot meet the increased nutritional requirements of pregnancy. Fat-soluble vitamins may not be absorbed as well, resulting in deficiency in those nutrients. A weight gain of 11 to 12 kg is recommended during pregnancy. Women who are unable to achieve the recommended weight gain through oral supplements may require nasogastric tube feedings at night. If malnutrition is severe, parenteral hyperalimentation may be necessary (Whitty & Dombrowski, 2009).

Throughout pregnancy, frequent monitoring of the woman's weight, blood glucose, hemoglobin, total protein, serum albumin, PT, and fat-soluble vitamins A and E is suggested. Her pancreatic enzyme prescription may need to be adjusted. Baseline pulmonary function tests should be completed before pregnancy ideally and repeated as necessary during pregnancy. Inhaled recombinant human deoxyribonuclease I may be given to improve lung function by decreasing sputum viscosity. Inhaled 7% saline is also beneficial in this regard (Cunningham et al., 2010). Early detection and treatment of infection are critical. Management of infection includes intravenous, inhaled, or oral antibiotics along with chest physiotherapy and bronchial drainage (Cunningham et al.; Whitty and Dombrowski, 2009).

Fetal assessment is essential, given that the fetus is at risk for uteroplacental insufficiency, which can result in IUGR. Maternal nutritional status and weight gain during pregnancy significantly affect fetal growth. Fundal height should be measured routinely and ultrasound examinations performed to evaluate fetal growth and amniotic fluid volume. Fetal movement counts are often recommended, starting at 28 weeks of gestation. Nonstress tests should be initiated at 32 weeks of gestation or sooner if there is evidence of fetal compromise (see Chapter 26) (Whitty & Dombrowski, 2009).

During labor, monitoring for fluid and electrolyte balance is required. Increased cardiac output could lead to cardiopulmonary failure in the woman with pulmonary hypertension or cor pulmonale. The amount of sodium lost through sweat can be significant, and hypovolemia can occur. Conversely, if any degree of cor pulmonale is present, fluid overload is a concern. Oxygen is given by nonrebreather face mask during labor, and monitoring by pulse oximetry is recommended. Diuretics may be prescribed for fluid overload. Epidural or local analgesia is the preferred analgesic for birth, with vaginal birth recommended. Cesarean birth should be reserved for obstetric indications.

Breastfeeding appears to be safe as long as the sodium content of the milk is not abnormal (Lawrence & Lawrence, 2005). Pumping and discarding the milk are done until the sodium content has been determined. Milk samples should be tested periodically for sodium, chloride, and total fat, and the infant's growth pattern should be monitored.

Acute Respiratory Distress Syndrome

Acute respiratory distress syndrome (ARDS), or shock lung, occurs when the lungs are unable to maintain levels of oxygen and carbon dioxide within normal limits. Severe hypoxemia, in spite of high levels of inspired oxygen, is accompanied by an increase in pulmonary capillary permeability, a decrease in lung volume, and shunting of blood.

ARDS is not specific to pregnancy; it also can result from trauma, pneumonia, sepsis, aspiration of gastric contents, fat emboli, acute pancreatitis, and drug overdose. When ARDS is associated with pregnancy, the precipitating factors can also be amniotic fluid embolism, air embolism, tocolytic therapy, asthma, thromboembolism, disseminated intravascular coagulopathy, pyelonephritis, preeclampsia, eclampsia, severe hemorrhage, blood transfusion reactions, or peripartum cardiomyopathy (Curran, 2006). An initial intervention is to find and correct the underlying cause, if possible. To provide the best fetal environment, early intubation and mechanical ventilation are recommended. With severe lung injury, positive end-expiratory pressure (PEEP) may be necessary. Sedatives may be prescribed for intubation and ventilation. The administration of vasoactive agents, inotropic agents, and corticosteroids may be necessary. Maintaining fluid balance is a challenge and a key component of management. For the woman who is hypovolemic, administration of blood may help increase cardiac output. For the woman who is hypervolemic, diuretics may be necessary to maintain adequate cardiac output. Whether birth of the fetus improves maternal oxygenation remains controversial (Cunningham et al., 2010).

The postpartum incidence of ARDS is affected not by the method of birth but by the amount of trauma occurring during pregnancy and birth. ARDS can also occur after miscarriage or therapeutic abortion.

Laboratory results are important in identifying the origin of acute pulmonary problems. Chest radiographs can indicate the presence of infiltrates in the lungs, and ABGs identify the status of acid-base balance. The priority assessments are vital signs, oxygen saturation levels, and signs and symptoms of thrombophlebitis and hemorrhage. During the postpartum period, apprehension, distended neck veins, cyanosis, diaphoresis, or pallor may indicate hypoxemia. Mental confusion or disorientation also may be noted.

The pulse rate increases to compensate for respiratory insufficiency of any origin. The severity of the pulmonary problem increases as the pulse rate increases. An initial increase in blood pressure occurs as cardiac output increases in an attempt to supply the tissue with oxygen. When lung damage is severe, blood pressure decreases.

Respiratory changes are the most important indicators of ARDS. The rate and depth of respirations, respiratory pattern, symmetry of chest movement, and use of accessory muscles should be noted; therefore, observation of respiratory characteristics after activity is important.

! NURSING ALERT

If there is any indication of abnormality, respirations are counted for a full minute; an error in rate of plus or minus four respirations per minute may be highly significant.

On auscultation, crackles, rhonchi, wheezes, or a pleural friction rub should be reported, especially when they are present after an earlier assessment with normal findings. The pregnant woman should be positioned for breathing comfort. Oxygen and emergency equipment should be available. The woman should be reassured and coached in relaxation techniques to lessen her anxiety.

Although they are usually younger and healthier than most adults who develop ARDS, pregnant women with this condition still experience mortality rates of 25% to 40%. With pulmonary injury, the clinical condition is determined by the degree of damage, the ability to compensate for it, and the stage of the disease. Ideally, lung injury will be detected at an early stage and the underlying disease process promptly identified and treated. The long-term prognosis for pulmonary function in survivors is surprisingly good, even for women who experienced severe lung damage (Cunningham et al., 2010).

Integumentary Disorders

Dermatologic disorders induced by pregnancy include melasma (chloasma), vascular "spiders," palmar erythema, and striae gravidarum. A number of chronic skin disorders may complicate pregnancy. These disorders may be present prior to pregnancy or appear for the first time during pregnancy. The course of these disorders varies during pregnancy. Acne, for example, may improve. Psoriasis improves in 40% of women, remains unchanged in 40% of women, and worsens in 20% of women during pregnancy. Lesions from neurofibromatosis may increase in size and number during pregnancy (Cunningham et al., 2010). Explanation, reassurance, and commonsense measures should suffice for normal skin changes. In contrast, disease processes during and soon after pregnancy may be extremely difficult to diagnose and treat.

SAFETY ALERT

Isotretinoin (Accutane), commonly prescribed for cystic acne, is highly teratogenic. There is a risk for craniofacial, cardiac, and CNS malformations in exposed fetuses. This drug should not be taken during pregnancy.

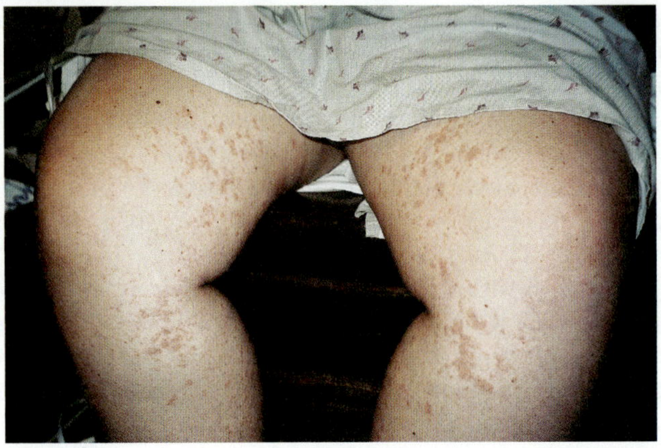

FIG. 30-2 Woman with pruritic urticarial papules and plaques of pregnancy. Lesions also are present on her arms, back, abdomen, and buttocks. (Courtesy Shannon Perry, Phoenix, AZ.)

Pruritus is a major symptom in several pregnancy-related skin diseases. *Pruritus gravidarum,* generalized itching without the presence of a rash, develops in up to 14% of pregnant women. It is often limited to the abdomen and is usually caused by skin distention and development of striae. Pruritus gravidarum is not associated with poor perinatal outcomes. It is treated symptomatically with skin lubrication, topical antipruritics, and oral antihistamines. Ultraviolet light and careful exposure to sunlight decrease itching. Pruritus gravidarum usually disappears shortly after birth but can recur in approximately half of all subsequent pregnancies (Rapini, 2009).

Another common pregnancy-specific cause of pruritus is *pruritic urticarial papules and plaques of pregnancy (PUPPP)* (Fig. 30-2), also known as polymorphic eruption of pregnancy. PUPPP classically appears in primigravidas during the third trimester. The abdomen is usually affected, but lesions can spread to the arms, the thighs, the back, and the buttocks. PUPPP almost always causes pruritus, and the itching is severe in 80% of cases. It is not, however, associated with poor maternal or fetal outcomes. Therefore, the goal of therapy is simply to relieve maternal discomfort. Antipruritic topical medications, topical steroids, and oral antihistamines usually provide relief. Women with severe symptoms may require oral prednisone. PUPPP usually resolves before birth or within several weeks after birth. Rarely, however, it may persist or even begin after birth. PUPPP does not usually recur in subsequent pregnancies (Papoutsis & Kroumpouzos, 2007; Rapini, 2009).

Intrahepatic cholestasis of pregnancy (ICP) is a liver disorder unique to pregnancy that is characterized by generalized pruritus. The itching commonly affects the palms and soles but can occur on any part of the body. No skin lesions are present. Women with ICP have elevated serum bile acids and elevated liver function tests. Jaundice may or may not be present. Up to one half of women with ICP develop dark urine and light-colored stools. The cause of ICP is unknown, but approximately half of women have a family history of the disorder. ICP occurs more frequently during the winter months. A geographic variance in the prevalence of the disease also occurs. ICP occurs most often in Southeast Asia, Chile, Bolivia, and Scandinavia, although it is seen less frequently now in Chile and in Scandinavia than in the past (Cappell, 2007; Williamson & Mackillop, 2009).

The major risks associated with ICP are meconium staining, stillbirth, and preterm birth. The cause of these complications is likely related to increased levels of fetal serum bile levels. Treatment consists of giving ursodeoxycholic acid, which effectively controls the pruritus and laboratory abnormalities associated with ICP, and continued monitoring of liver function tests and bile acids (Cappell, 2007; Williamson & Mackillop, 2009). Antepartum fetal testing is essential. If liver function tests do not improve, induction of labor is considered at 36 to 37 weeks of gestation if the fetal lungs are mature. Symptoms usually disappear and laboratory abnormalities resolve within 2 to 4 weeks postpartum. ICP can recur in subsequent pregnancies, however, or with oral contraceptive use (Cappell).

Neurologic Disorders

The pregnant woman with a neurologic disorder must deal with potential teratogenic effects of prescribed medications, changes of mobility during pregnancy, and impaired ability to care for the baby. The nurse should be aware of all drugs the woman is taking and the associated potential for producing congenital anomalies. As the pregnancy progresses, the woman's center of gravity shifts and causes balance and gait changes. The nurse should advise the woman of these expected changes and suggest safety measures as appropriate. Family and community resources may be needed to assist in providing infant care for the neurologically impaired woman.

Epilepsy

Epilepsy (often called seizure disorder) is a disorder of the brain that causes recurrent seizures and is the most common major neurologic disorder accompanying pregnancy. Less than 1% of all pregnant women have a seizure disorder (Aminoff, 2009). Seizure disorders are either acquired (less than 15% of all cases) or idiopathic (more than 85% of all cases), which means that a specific cause for the seizures cannot be identified. The majority of women with a seizure disorder who become pregnant have an uneventful pregnancy with an excellent outcome (Samuels & Niebyl, 2007).

Women with epilepsy should receive preconception counseling if at all possible. A detailed history of medication use and seizure frequency should be obtained. If the woman has frequent seizures before conception, she is likely to continue this pattern during pregnancy; therefore, achieving effective seizure control is extremely important before conception, even if changing medications is required. Many studies have reported an increased incidence of congenital anomalies, including cleft lip and palate, congenital heart disease, and neural tube defects (NTDs), in infants born to women taking anticonvulsant medications.

SAFETY ALERT

Carbamazepine (Tegretol) and valproate (Depakote) should be avoided if possible during pregnancy because their use is associated with NTDs in the fetus.

Several new anticonvulsant medications have been developed for use within the last decade. More information is needed regarding the fetal effects of these medications. Any anticonvulsant medication required to achieve good seizure control in a woman with epilepsy should be used, however, regardless of the increased risk of fetal anomalies because the most important goal during pregnancy is the prevention of seizures (Samuels & Niebyl, 2007).

Pregnant women with epilepsy are advised to take a folic acid supplement of 4 mg daily, which may decrease the incidence of NTDs. They are also encouraged to take a prenatal vitamin containing vitamin D daily because anticonvulsant medications can interfere with production of the active form of this vitamin (Cunningham et al., 2010; Samuels & Niebyl, 2007).

During pregnancy, only one anticonvulsant medication—at the lowest dose level that is effective at keeping the woman seizure free—should be prescribed. The increase in plasma volume that is a normal pregnancy change can affect drug metabolism and distribution. Therefore, blood levels of anticonvulsant medications should be checked and drug dosages adjusted as necessary. With client cooperation and close monitoring, most women with epilepsy should experience no change or even have fewer seizures during pregnancy. An increase in seizure frequency is usually related either to noncompliance with taking prescribed anticonvulsant medications or with sleep deprivation (Samuels & Niebyl, 2007). If an increase in seizure activity does occur during pregnancy, it is usually in women who had frequent seizures (more than one per month) before pregnancy (Aminoff, 2009).

In addition to congenital anomalies, the fetus of a woman with epilepsy is also at risk for IUGR. Determining an accurate gestational age as early as possible is important. This information will decrease any confusion later in pregnancy in regard to fetal growth issues. Maternal serum screening around 16 weeks of gestation and ultrasound examination at 18 to 22 weeks of gestation should be performed to assess for the presence of an NTD or other fetal anomalies. Nonstress testing later in pregnancy is not necessary, unless the woman has other medical or obstetric factors that increase the risk for stillbirth (Samuels & Niebyl, 2007).

Management of anticonvulsant therapy during prolonged labor is challenging. During labor, absorption of medications given orally is unpredictable, especially if vomiting occurs. Women who are maintained on phenytoin (Dilantin) or phenobarbital may be given these medications parenterally during labor. No parenteral form of carbamazepine has been developed; therefore, women maintained on this medication may be given phenytoin intravenously instead to carry them through labor. Vaginal birth is preferred (Samuels & Niebyl, 2007).

After birth the levels of anticonvulsant medications must be monitored frequently for the first few weeks because they can rise rapidly. If medication dose levels were increased during pregnancy, they will need to be decreased quickly to prepregnancy levels. All of the major anticonvulsant medications are found in breast milk, but the use of these medications is not a contraindication to breastfeeding. Neonatal sedation may be a side effect of carbamazepine, primidone (Mysoline), and phenobarbital (Samuels & Niebyl, 2007).

During the neonatal period infants can have a hemorrhagic disorder associated with exposure to anticonvulsant medications in utero, which causes vitamin K deficiency. Some authorities recommend giving vitamin K daily during the last few weeks of pregnancy to women taking anticonvulsant medications, but this practice is not considered the standard of care (Samuels & Niebyl, 2007).

All methods of contraception can be used by women with an idiopathic seizure disorder. Commonly prescribed anticonvulsant medications such as carbamazepine, primidone, phenobarbital, and phenytoin, however, reduce the effectiveness of oral contraceptives. Women taking low-dose oral contraceptives especially may have more breakthrough bleeding and be at risk for an unplanned pregnancy (Cunningham et al., 2010; Samuels & Niebyl, 2007). Valproic acid and the newer anticonvulsant medications have not been reported to cause oral contraceptive failure (Aminoff, 2009). In terms of planning for future childbearing, couples should be informed that children born to women with a seizure disorder of unknown cause have a four times greater chance of developing an idiopathic seizure disorder compared with the general population. Epilepsy in the father does not appear to increase a child's risk for developing a seizure disorder (Samuels & Niebyl).

Multiple Sclerosis

Multiple sclerosis (MS), a patchy demyelinization of the spinal cord and CNS, may be a viral disorder. MS occurs equally in men and women. Onset of symptoms, which include weakness of one or both lower extremities, visual complaints, and loss of coordination, is subtle and usually occurs between the ages of 20 and 40 years. The disease is characterized by exacerbations and remissions. Pregnancy does not seem to worsen the disease (Samuels & Niebyl, 2007).

Remissions during pregnancy are common. If an exacerbation occurs, it is more likely to do so during the third trimester of pregnancy or postpartum. Treatment may include corticosteroids and immunosuppressive agents. Several new drugs and biopharmaceuticals are available for treating MS. These agents should be used during pregnancy only if the benefits clearly appear to outweigh the potential risks as their effects on pregnancy and the fetus are unknown (Samuels & Niebyl, 2007).

Women who have become paraplegic or have lumbosacral lesions as a result of MS may have little pain during labor. Determining when labor begins may be difficult for them. Uterine contractions occur normally, but these women may have difficulty pushing effectively during the second stage of labor. Therefore, vacuum- or forceps-assisted birth may be necessary (Samuels & Niebyl, 2007). Breastfeeding is encouraged.

Bell Palsy

Bell palsy is an acute idiopathic facial paralysis. The cause is unknown, but it may be related to the reactivation of herpesvirus infection or acute human immunodeficiency virus type 1 (HIV-1) retroviral infections. Bell palsy occurs fairly often, especially in women of reproductive age. Women are affected two to four times more often than men (Cunningham et al., 2010). An association between Bell palsy and pregnancy was first cited by Bell in 1830. Pregnant women are affected three to four times more often than nonpregnant women. The incidence usually peaks during the third trimester and the puerperium. Women who develop Bell palsy during pregnancy have an increased risk for gestational hypertension as well (Cunningham et al.).

The clinical manifestations of Bell palsy include the sudden development of a unilateral facial weakness, with maximal weakness within 48 hours after onset, pain surrounding the ear, difficulty closing the eye on the affected side, hyperacusis (abnormal acuteness of the sense of hearing), and occasionally a loss of taste (Aminoff, 2009; Cunningham et al., 2010).

No effects of maternal Bell palsy have been observed in infants. Maternal outcome is generally good unless a complete block in nerve conduction occurs. Steroid therapy may improve outcome, although its benefits have not always been proven in past research studies. To be effective, steroids should be administered within the first 5 to 6 days after the paralysis develops (Aminoff, 2009). Supportive care includes prevention of injury to the constantly exposed cornea, facial muscle massage, careful chewing and manual removal of food from inside the affected cheek, and reassurance. Although 80% of affected men and nonpregnant women recover to a satisfactory level within a year, only approximately half of women who develop the disorder during pregnancy do so (Cunningham et al., 2010).

Autoimmune Disorders

Autoimmune disorders make up a large group of diseases that disrupt the function of the immune system of the body. In these types of disorders the body's immune system is unable to distinguish "self" from "nonself." As a result, antibodies develop that attack its normally present antigens, causing tissue damage. Autoimmune disorders can occur during pregnancy because a large percentage of women with an autoimmune disease are women of childbearing age (Gilbert, 2011). Common autoimmune diseases include systemic lupus erythematosus, myasthenia gravis, antiphospholipid syndrome, rheumatoid arthritis, and systemic sclerosis (Cunningham et al., 2010; Holmgren & Branch, 2007).

Systemic Lupus Erythematosus

Systemic lupus erythematosus (SLE) is a chronic, multisystem inflammatory disease that affects the skin, joints, kidneys, lungs, nervous system, liver, and other body organs. The exact cause is unknown but probably involves the interaction of several factors, including immunologic, environmental, hormonal, and genetic factors. SLE is the most common serious autoimmune disease affecting women of reproductive age. It occurs 2 to 4 times more often in African-American and Hispanic women than in Caucasian women and is 10 times more common in women than in men. Most cases of SLE occur in adolescence or young adulthood (Gilbert, 2011; Holmgren & Branch, 2007).

The most common presenting symptoms of SLE include fatigue, weight loss, arthralgias, arthritis, and myalgias. Although a diagnosis of SLE is suspected based on clinical signs and symptoms, it is confirmed by laboratory testing that demonstrates the presence of circulating autoantibodies. As is the case with other autoimmune diseases, SLE is characterized by a series of exacerbations (flares) and remissions (Holmgren & Branch, 2007).

If the diagnosis has been established and the woman desires a child, she is advised to wait until she has been in remission for at least 6 months before attempting to become pregnant (Gilbert,

2011). A lupus flare occurs during pregnancy or postpartum in 15% to 60% of women with SLE. In addition to an exacerbation, other maternal risks include an increased rate of miscarriage, nephritis, preeclampsia, possible need to give birth at a preterm gestation, and an increased risk of cesarean birth. Fetal risks include stillbirth, IUGR, and preterm birth (Holmgren & Branch, 2007).

Medical therapy during pregnancy is kept to a minimum in women who are in remission or who have a mild form of SLE. Immunosuppressive medications should be discontinued before conception. Nonsteroidal antiinflammatory drugs and aspirin are ordinarily the most commonly used antiinflammatory drugs, but they are not recommended for use during pregnancy. Aspirin should not be used after 24 weeks of gestation because of an increased risk of premature closure of the fetal ductus arteriosus (Cunningham et al., 2010). Maintenance therapy with hydroxychloroquine or low doses of glucocorticoids can continue. Hydroxychloroquine, an antimalarial drug, may be the best medication for maintenance SLE therapy during pregnancy because it significantly reduces SLE disease activity but appears to cause no adverse effects on the fetus (Holmgren & Branch, 2007).

Prenatal care otherwise focuses on close monitoring to detect common pregnancy complications, such as hypertension, proteinuria, and IUGR. Ultrasound examinations are performed frequently to monitor fetal growth. Fetal assessment tests, including daily fetal movement counts, nonstress tests, and amniotic fluid volume assessment, will likely begin at 30 to 32 weeks of gestation (see Chapter 26). More frequent ultrasound examinations and fetal testing are necessary if the woman develops a SLE flare, hypertension, proteinuria, or evidence of IUGR (Holmgren & Branch, 2007).

Women with SLE can develop an exacerbation during labor. Even if a flare does not occur, all women who have received chronic steroid therapy within the year will need larger (stress) doses of steroids during labor (Holmgren & Branch, 2007). Vaginal birth is preferred, but cesarean birth is common because of maternal and fetal complications.

Because determining which, if any, women are at risk for a SLE flare after birth is difficult, close follow-up with all of these women during the postpartum period is necessary. Any maintenance medications that were discontinued during the intrapartum period should be restarted immediately at doses similar to those used during pregnancy (Holmgren & Branch, 2007).

Women with SLE and chronic vascular or renal disease should limit the number of their pregnancies because of maternal complications associated with the illness, as well as increased adverse perinatal outcomes (Cunningham et al., 2010). If desired, the safest time for tubal sterilization is during the postpartum period or when the disease is in remission. Estrogen-containing oral contraceptives may increase the risk of thromboembolism (Gilbert, 2011). Progestin-only implants and injections provide effective contraception with no known effects on lupus flares (Cunningham et al.). Barrier methods, in addition to progestin-only contraceptive options, are the least risky forms of contraception for women with SLE (Gilbert). Evidence does not support concerns regarding an increased risk of infection when IUDs are prescribed for women receiving immunosuppressive therapy (Cunningham et al.).

Myasthenia Gravis

Myasthenia gravis (MG), an autoimmune motor (muscle) end-plate disorder that involves acetylcholine use, affects the motor function at the myoneural junction. Muscle weakness results, particularly of the eyes, the face, the tongue, the neck, the limbs, and the respiratory muscles. In addition, women may experience ptosis, diplopia, and dysphagia. Women are affected twice as often as men, and the incidence peaks between the ages of 20 and 30 years (Porter & Branch, 2006). Because the greatest period of risk is during the first year after diagnosis, pregnancy should probably be avoided until symptomatic improvement occurs (Cunningham et al., 2010). The response of women with MG to pregnancy is unpredictable; remission, exacerbation, or continued stability during pregnancy can occur.

Pregnancy does not appear to affect the overall course of MG, but as the uterus enlarges respirations may be compromised. Also the normal fatigue experienced by many pregnant women may be tolerated poorly by those with MG (Cunningham et al., 2010). Treatment during pregnancy is the same as for nonpregnant women. Usual medications include glucocorticoids and acetylcholinesterase inhibitors. Monitoring blood glucose values is important because hyperglycemia may result from corticosteroid therapy. Thymectomy may result in remission of the disease but is best performed before or after pregnancy, if at all possible. For severe weakness, plasmapheresis or intravenous (IV) immunoglobulin therapy may be needed.

Because MG does not affect smooth muscle, most women usually tolerate labor well. Vaginal birth is desired, but vacuum or forceps assistance may be required because of muscle weakness. Oxytocin may be given, but all medications that cause muscular relaxation should be avoided if at all possible. Magnesium sulfate should not be administered to these women because it inhibits the release of acetylcholine and can trigger myasthenic crisis. Narcotics must be used cautiously because they may cause respiratory depression, and women with MG are already at risk for respiratory muscle weakness. Regional analgesia is preferred (Aminoff, 2009; Cunningham et al., 2010). After birth, women must be carefully supervised because relapses often occur during the puerperium.

Approximately 10% to 15% of neonates born to women with MG develop neonatal myasthenia. This transient disorder results from the transfer of maternal antibody against acetylcholine receptors across the placenta. Symptoms, including a poor cry, respiratory difficulties, weakness in suckling, a weak Moro reflex, and feeble limb movements, usually appear within the first 72 hours after birth. Neonatal myasthenia can be treated with anticholinesterase medications and usually resolves by 6 weeks after birth (Aminoff, 2009).

Gastrointestinal Disorders

Compromise of gastrointestinal (GI) function during pregnancy is a concern. Obvious physiologic alterations, such as the greatly enlarged uterus, and less apparent changes, such as hormonal differences and hypochlorhydria (deficiency of hydrochloric acid in the stomach's gastric juice), require understanding for proper diagnosis and treatment. Gallbladder disease and inflammatory bowel disease are examples of GI disorders that may occur during pregnancy.

Cholelithiasis and Cholecystitis

Cholelithiasis (the presence of gallstones in the gallbladder) occurs more often in women than in men. Its incidence increases during pregnancy, probably because of increased hormone levels, along with pressure from the enlarged uterus that interferes with the normal circulation and drainage of the gallbladder. In fact, the second most common nonobstetric condition requiring surgery during pregnancy is symptomatic cholelithiasis, occurring in 1 of 1600 pregnancies (Blackburn, 2007; Lu & Curet, 2007).

Cholecystitis (inflammation of the gallbladder), although rare, also occurs more often during pregnancy and the postpartum period. The incidence of acute cholecystitis is about 4 cases per 10,000 pregnancies. It most often occurs in multiparous women who have a history of previous attacks. Acute cholecystitis is the third most common indication for nonobstetric surgical intervention in pregnancy (Blackburn, 2007; Cappell, 2007). Women with acute cholecystitis usually have fatty food intolerance along with colicky abdominal pain radiating to the back or shoulder, nausea, and vomiting. Fever may also be present. Ultrasound is often used to detect the presence of stones or dilation of the common bile duct (Lu & Curet, 2007).

Often gallbladder surgery is postponed until the puerperium. The woman can usually be managed conservatively for the remainder of the pregnancy. Initial therapy generally includes intravenous hydration, bowel rest with nasogastric suction and no oral intake, and narcotics. Morphine should not be used as an analgesic because it may cause ductal spasm. Antibiotics are given if evidence of cholecystitis or infection exists (Lu & Curet, 2007). See the Teaching for Self-Management box: Nutritional Counseling for the Pregnant Woman with Cholecystitis or Cholelithiasis for diet suggestions once the woman is able to resume oral intake. Currently, however, cholecystitis is increasingly being managed surgically during pregnancy. If cholecystitis is treated conservatively, there is a high risk for recurrent problems during the pregnancy. Also if cholecystitis recurs later in pregnancy, preterm labor is more likely, and if surgery is necessary it is technically more difficult to perform (Cunningham et al., 2010).

Women with obstructive jaundice, gallstone pancreatitis, suspected peritonitis or those for whom conservative (medical) management has not been successful should be treated surgically with cholecystectomy or cholecystotomy (Lu & Curet, 2007). Although the second trimester has traditionally been considered the safest time for this surgery, it is increasingly performed at any time during pregnancy because of improved surgical outcomes. Both laparoscopic and open cholecystectomy procedures are acceptable during pregnancy (Cappell, 2007; Cunningham et al., 2010). Preoperative care includes IV fluids, discontinuing oral intake, analgesia, and administration of antibiotics.

TEACHING FOR SELF-MANAGEMENT

Nutritional Counseling for the Pregnant Woman with Cholecystitis or Cholelithiasis

- Assess your diet for foods that cause discomfort and flatulence, and omit foods that trigger episodes.
- Reduce dietary fat intake to 40 to 50 g/day.
- Limit protein to 10% to 12% of total calories.
- Choose foods so that most of the calories come from carbohydrates.
- Prepare food without adding fats or oils as much as possible.
- Avoid fried foods.

Inflammatory Bowel Disease

Inflammatory bowel disease, particularly ulcerative colitis and Crohn disease, is relatively common in young women, so these disorders are seen during pregnancy. The incidence of an inflammatory bowel disease flare is not increased in pregnancy and no evidence suggests that pregnancy significantly affects either ulcerative colitis or Crohn disease (Cunningham et al., 2010). Women with ulcerative colitis and Crohn disease usually have healthy babies at the same rate as the general population, although some studies have suggested a higher risk for preterm birth and low-birth-weight infants (Kelly & Savides, 2009). Active disease early in pregnancy increases the risk for a poor pregnancy outcome (Cunningham et al.).

Treatment of inflammatory bowel disease is usually the same for the pregnant woman as it is for the nonpregnant woman. Sulfasalazine, 5-aminosalicylate drugs, and corticosteroids are often prescribed for treatment of inflammatory bowel disease. These drugs appear to be safe for use during pregnancy (Kelly & Savides, 2009). Fat-soluble vitamin and folic acid supplementation is especially important because of problems with intestinal malabsorption. Calcium supplementation is also necessary because osteoporosis is common. Some women may require parenteral nutrition. With complications, such as hemorrhage, or if there is no response to medical therapy, surgery may be indicated (Cunningham et al., 2010).

Urinary Tract Infections

Urinary tract infections (UTIs) are a common medical complication of pregnancy, occurring in approximately 20% of all pregnancies. They are also responsible for 10% of all hospitalizations during pregnancy (Duff, Sweet, & Edwards, 2009). UTIs include asymptomatic bacteriuria, cystitis, and pyelonephritis. UTIs are usually caused by coliform organisms that are a normal part of the perineal flora. By far the most common cause is *Escherichia coli,* a gram-negative bacteria responsible for 85% of cases. Another gram-negative bacterium that causes UTIs is *Klebsiella pneumoniae.* The gram-positive organisms group B streptococci, enterococci, and staphylococci account for approximately 3% to 7% of all infections (Gilbert, 2011).

Asymptomatic Bacteriuria

Asymptomatic bacteriuria refers to the persistent presence of bacteria within the urinary tract of women who have no symptoms. A clean-voided urine specimen containing more than 100,000 organisms per ml is diagnostic. If asymptomatic bacteriuria is not treated, up to 40% of infected women will subsequently develop symptomatic infection during the pregnancy (Colombo & Samuels, 2007). Therefore, the ACOG recommends that all women be screened for asymptomatic bacteriuria at their first prenatal visit (Colombo & Samuels). Asymptomatic bacteriuria has been associated with preterm birth and low-birth-weight infants (American Academy of Pediatrics [AAP] & ACOG, 2007; Cunningham et al., 2010).

Asymptomatic bacteriuria should be treated with an antibiotic. Antibiotics that are often prescribed include amoxicillin, ampicillin, cephalexin (Keflex), ciprofloxacin (Cipro), levofloxacin (Levaquin), nitrofurantoin (Macrodantin), and trimethoprim-sulfamethoxazole (Bactrim DS). Several different regimens, including single dose, 3-, 7-, and 10-day treatment may be used (Cunningham et al., 2010). A repeat urine culture is usually ordered 1 to 2 weeks after completing therapy because approximately 15% of women will not respond to therapy or will have a reinfection (Colombo & Samuels, 2007). Women who have persistent or frequent recurrences of bacteriuria may be placed on suppressive therapy, often nitrofurantoin each night at bedtime, for the remainder of the pregnancy (Cunningham et al.).

Cystitis

Cystitis (bladder infection) is characterized by dysuria, urgency, and frequency, along with lower abdominal or suprapubic pain. Usually white blood cells, as well as bacteria, will be found in the urine. Microscopic or gross hematuria may also be present. Typically, symptoms are confined to the bladder rather than becoming systemic. Cystitis is usually uncomplicated, but it may lead to ascending UTI if untreated. Approximately 40% of pregnant women with pyelonephritis experienced symptoms of bladder infection before developing pyelonephritis (Cunningham et al., 2010).

Cystitis is often treated with a 3-day course of antibiotic therapy, which is usually 90% effective in curing the infection. Antibiotics often prescribed include amoxicillin, ampicillin, cephalexin (Keflex), ciprofloxacin (Cipro), levofloxacin (Levaquin), nitrofurantoin (Macrodantin), and trimethoprim-sulfamethoxazole (Bactrim DS) (Cunningham et al., 2010). Phenazopyridine (Pyridium), a urinary analgesic, is often prescribed along with an antibiotic for relief of symptoms caused by irritation of the urinary tract. Although phenazopyridine is effective at relieving dysuria, urgency, and frequency, women should be taught that the medication colors urine and tears orange. Therefore, they should be instructed to avoid wearing contact lenses while taking this medication and warned that it will stain underwear.

CLINICAL REASONING

Asymptomatic Bacteriuria

Emily is a 23-year-old G1 P0 who has her initial prenatal visit at 8 weeks of gestation. During the visit a routine urine sample is collected and sent to the lab. Two days later Emily receives a call at work from her health care provider, telling her that she needs to pick up a prescription for an antibiotic because her lab results indicated that she has a urinary tract infection (UTI). Emily asks, "Why do I need an antibiotic? I feel fine! I thought that it would hurt to urinate if I had a urinary tract infection."

1. Evidence—Is there sufficient evidence to determine the type of UTI that Emily has?
2. What assumptions can be made about the following issues:
   a. Risks associated with asymptomatic bacteriuria
   b. Management plan for treating asymptomatic bacteriuria
3. What are the priorities for nursing care at this time?
4. Does the evidence objectively support your conclusion?
5. Are there alternative perspectives to your conclusions?

Pyelonephritis

Renal infection (pyelonephritis) is a common serious medical complication of pregnancy and the second most common nondelivery reason for hospitalization (Cunningham et al., 2010). The most common maternal complications associated with pyelonephritis include anemia, septicemia, transient renal dysfunction, and pulmonary insufficiency. Women with pyelonephritis can develop urosepsis, sepsis syndrome, and renal dysfunction. In addition, pulmonary injury resembling ARDS can occur in pregnant women with acute pyelonephritis, most likely the result of damage to alveolar tissue caused by the release of endotoxins from gram-negative bacteria (Colombo & Samuels, 2007; Cunningham et al.). Recurrent pyelonephritis is thought to cause fetal death and IUGR. Acute pyelonephritis is associated with preterm labor (Colombo & Samuels).

Pyelonephritis develops most often during the second trimester of pregnancy and is usually caused by the *E. coli* organism. Infection develops only in the right kidney in more than half of all cases. The onset of pyelonephritis is often abrupt, with fever, shaking chills, and aching in the lumbar area of the back. Anorexia and nausea and vomiting also can be present. Usually one or both costovertebral angles will be tender to palpation.

Women diagnosed with pyelonephritis are admitted to the hospital immediately. Treatment with IV antibiotics is started as soon as urine and blood samples for culture and sensitivity have been collected. Ampicillin, gentamicin, cefazolin (Ancef), or ceftriaxone (Rocephin) are often ordered initially because they are broad-spectrum antibiotics that are usually effective. The woman must be monitored closely for the possible development of sepsis (Cunningham et al., 2010).

Clinical symptoms generally resolve within a couple of days after antibiotic therapy is begun. The antibiotic may need to be changed based on the results of the initial culture and sensitivity testing, or if the woman has not responded to therapy within 48 hours (Gilbert, 2011). Most women become afebrile within 72 hours. If no clinical improvement is seen within 48 to 72 hours, an ultrasound should be performed to assess for a urinary tract obstruction. Once the woman is afebrile, she will be changed from IV to oral antibiotics (Cunningham et al., 2010).

Usually antibiotic therapy is continued for 7 to 14 days after the woman is discharged from the hospital. A urine culture will likely be repeated 1 to 2 weeks after antibiotic therapy has been completed. Recurrent infection develops in 30% to 40% of women after completion of treatment for pyelonephritis. Therefore, urine cultures should be obtained each trimester for the remainder of the pregnancy. Many women are maintained on a prophylactic antibiotic (often nitrofurantoin once or twice daily) for the remainder of the pregnancy (Colombo & Samuels, 2007; Cunningham et al., 2010).

Client Education

Nurses are often responsible for teaching pregnant women about taking medications safely and effectively. This education is especially important in regard to antibiotics because this type of medication is so often misused by the general public. The woman should be instructed to finish the entire course of prescribed antibiotic therapy rather than stopping the medication as soon as she feels better. Failure to do so can lead to the creation of additional drug-resistant organisms. Antibiotics should

TEACHING FOR SELF-MANAGEMENT

Prevention of Urinary Tract Infections

- Wipe from front to back after voiding or having a bowel movement.
- Choose underwear or hosiery with a cotton crotch.
- Avoid tight-fitting clothing, especially jeans.
- Limit time spent in damp exercise clothes (especially swimsuits and leotards or tights).
- Avoid bath salts or bubble bath.
- Avoid colored or scented toilet tissue.
- If sensitive, discontinue use of feminine hygiene deodorant sprays.
- Don't ignore the urge to void.
- Void before and after intercourse and before going to bed at night.
- Drink at least 8 glasses of fluid (especially water) every day.

be taken on time and around the clock so that medication levels in the body remain constant. Finally, many women will develop a yeast infection while taking antibiotics because the medication kills normal flora in the genitourinary tract, as well as pathologic organisms. Therefore, they should be encouraged to include yogurt, cheese, or milk containing active acidophilus cultures in their diet while on antibiotics.

Woman should also be taught simple ways to prevent urinary tract infections. See the Teaching for Self-Management box: Prevention of Urinary Tract Infections for several suggestions.

SURGERY DURING PREGNANCY

The need for abdominal surgery occurs as frequently among pregnant women as among nonpregnant women of comparable age. However, pregnancy may make the diagnosis more difficult. An enlarged uterus and displaced internal organs may make abdominal palpation more difficult, alter the position of an affected organ, and/or change the usual signs and symptoms associated with a particular disorder. The most common nongynecologic condition necessitating abdominal surgery during pregnancy is appendicitis.

Appendicitis

Appendicitis occurs approximately once in 1000 pregnancies. The incidence is 30%, 45%, and 25% in the first, second, and third trimesters, respectively (Mahomed, 2006). The diagnosis of appendicitis is often delayed because the usual signs and symptoms mimic some normal changes of pregnancy such as nausea and vomiting and increased white blood cell (WBC) count. As pregnancy progresses, the appendix is pushed upward and to the right from its usual anatomic location (see Fig. 13-14) (Cunningham et al., 2010). Because of these changes, rupture of the appendix and the subsequent development of peritonitis occur two to three times more often in pregnant women than in nonpregnant women.

The most common symptom of appendicitis in pregnant women is right lower quadrant abdominal pain, regardless of gestational age. Nausea and vomiting are often present, but loss of appetite is not a reliable indicator of appendicitis. Fever, tachycardia, a dry tongue, and localized abdominal tenderness are commonly found in nonpregnant persons with appendicitis, but they are less likely indicators for the disorder in pregnant women. Because of the physiologic increase in WBCs that occurs in pregnancy, this test is not helpful in making the diagnosis. A urinalysis and a chest x-ray should be performed to rule out UTI and right lower lobe pneumonia, given that both of these conditions can cause lower abdominal pain (Kelly & Savides, 2009). Appendicitis can also be confused with other disorders such as cholecystitis, preterm labor, pyelonephritis, or placental abruption (abruptio placentae) (Cunningham et al., 2010).

Ultrasound is useful during the first and second trimesters of pregnancy for diagnosing appendicitis. It is less accurate during the third trimester than earlier in pregnancy because it is technically more difficult to perform. In the third trimester of pregnancy, helical CT scanning may be more useful than other imaging modalities (Lu & Curet, 2007). MRI may be used if appendicitis has not been confirmed by other imaging techniques (Kelly & Savides, 2009).

Prompt surgical intervention to remove the appendix is still the standard treatment (Kelly & Savides, 2009). Appendectomy before rupture usually does not require either antibiotic or tocolytic therapy. If surgery is delayed until after rupture, multiple antibiotics are ordered. Rupture is likely to result in preterm labor and perhaps fetal loss.

CARE MANAGEMENT

Initial assessment of the pregnant woman requiring surgery focuses on her presenting signs and symptoms. A thorough history and physical examination are performed. Laboratory testing includes, at a minimum, a complete blood count with differential and a urinalysis. Additional laboratory and other diagnostic tests may be necessary to reach a diagnosis. In addition, fetal heart rate (FHR) and activity, along with uterine activity, should be monitored, and constant vigilance for symptoms of impending obstetric complications maintained. The extent of presurgery assessment is determined by the immediacy of surgical intervention and the specific disorder that requires surgery.

Hospital Care

When surgery becomes necessary during pregnancy, the woman and her family are concerned about the effects of the procedure and medication on fetal well-being and the course of pregnancy. An important aspect of preoperative nursing care is encouraging the woman to express her fears, concerns, and questions.

Preoperative care for a pregnant woman differs from that for a nonpregnant woman in one significant aspect: the presence of at least one other person, the fetus. Continuous FHR and uterine contraction monitoring should be performed if the fetus is considered viable. Procedures such as preparation of the operative site and time of insertion of IV lines and urinary retention catheters vary with the physician and the facility. However, in every instance, there is a total restriction of solid foods and liquids or a clear specification of the type, amount, and time at which clear liquids may be taken before surgery. Some bowel preparation such as clear liquids and laxatives may be required before surgery. Food by mouth is restricted for several hours before a scheduled procedure. Even if she has had nothing by mouth—but more important, if surgery is unexpected—the woman is in danger of vomiting and aspirating, and special precautions are taken before anesthetic is administered (e.g., administering an antacid).

Intraoperatively, perinatal nurses may collaborate with the surgical staff to increase their knowledge about the special needs of pregnant women undergoing surgery. One intervention to improve fetal oxygenation is positioning the woman on the operating table with a lateral tilt to avoid compression of the maternal vena cava. Continuous fetal and uterine monitoring during the procedure is recommended because of the risk for preterm labor. Monitoring may be accomplished by using sterile aquasonic gel and a sterile sleeve for the transducer. During abdominal surgery, uterine contractions may be manually palpated.

In the immediate recovery period, general observations and care pertinent to postoperative recovery are initiated. Frequent assessments are carried out for several hours after surgery. Whether the woman is cared for in the surgical postanesthesia recovery area or in a labor and birth unit, continuous fetal and uterine monitoring will likely be initiated or resumed because of the potential risk for preterm labor. Tocolysis may be necessary if preterm labor occurs (see Chapter 33).

Home Care

Plans for the woman's return home and for convalescent care should be completed as early as possible before discharge. Depending on her insurance coverage, nursing care may be provided through a home health agency. If not, the woman and other support persons must be taught necessary skills and procedures, such as wound care. Ideally the woman and other caregivers should have opportunities for supervised practice before discharge so that they can feel comfortable with their knowledge and ability before being totally responsible for providing care. Box 30-3 lists information that should be included in discharge teaching for the postoperative client. The woman also may need referrals to various community agencies for evaluation of the home situation, child care, home health care, and financial or other assistance.

BOX 30-3 DISCHARGE TEACHING FOR HOME CARE AFTER SURGERY

- Care of incision site
- Diet and elimination related to gastrointestinal (GI) function
- Signs and symptoms of developing complications: wound infection, thrombophlebitis, pneumonia
- Equipment needed and technique for assessing temperature
- Recommended schedule for resumption of activities of daily living
- Treatments and medications ordered
- List of resource persons and their telephone numbers
- Schedule of follow-up visits

If birth has not occurred:

- Assessment of fetal activity (kick counts)
- Signs of preterm labor

KEY POINTS

- The normal hemodynamic values are significantly altered as a result of pregnancy.
- The stress of the normal maternal adaptations to pregnancy on a heart whose function is already taxed may cause cardiac decompensation.
- Maternal morbidity and mortality are significant risks in a pregnancy complicated by mitral stenosis.
- In the case of a cardiac arrest in a pregnant woman, the standard advanced cardiac life support guidelines should be implemented with a few slight modifications: the uterus must be displaced laterally, and the defibrillation paddles should be placed one rib interspace higher.
- Anemia, a common medical disorder of pregnancy, affects at least 20% of pregnant women.
- Asthma is a common medical condition to complicate pregnancy, and the prevalence and morbidity from this disorder are increasing.
- Pruritus is a common symptom in pregnancy-specific inflammatory skin diseases.
- A pregnant woman with epilepsy should take only one anticonvulsant medication at the lowest dose level that is effective at keeping her seizure-free.
- Autoimmune disorders can occur during pregnancy because a large percentage of persons with an autoimmune disorder are women of childbearing age. Common autoimmune diseases include SLE and MG.
- Cholecystitis and cholelithiasis are common GI problems in pregnancy.
- UTIs are a common medical complication of pregnancy.
- Pyelonephritis is a very serious medical complication of pregnancy and the second most common nondelivery reason for hospitalization.
- In the pregnant woman, an enlarged uterus, displaced internal organs, and altered laboratory values may confuse the diagnosis when the need for immediate abdominal surgery occurs.
- Perioperative care for a pregnant woman differs from that for a nonpregnant woman in one significant aspect: the presence of at least one other person, the fetus.

Audio Chapter Summaries Access an audio summary of these Key Points on evolve

REFERENCES

American Academy of Pediatrics (AAP) & American College of Obstetricians and Gynecologists (ACOG). (2007). *Guidelines for perinatal care* (6th ed.). Washington, DC: ACOG.

American College of Obstetricians and Gynecologists (ACOG). (2009). *Critical care in pregnancy.* ACOG Practice Bulletin No. 100. Washington, DC: ACOG.

Aminoff, M. (2009). Neurologic disorders. In R. Creasy, R. Resnik, J. Iams, C. Lockwood, & T. Moore (Eds.), *Creasy and Resnik's maternal-fetal medicine: Principles and practice* (6th ed.). Philadelphia: Saunders.

Blackburn, S. (2007). *Maternal, fetal, and neonatal physiology: A clinical perspective* (3rd ed.). St. Louis: Saunders.

Blanchard, D., & Shabetai, R. (2009). Cardiac diseases. In R. Creasy, R. Resnik, J. Iams, C. Lockwood, & T. Moore (Eds.), *Creasy and Resnik's maternal-fetal medicine: Principles and practice* (6th ed.). Philadelphia: Saunders.

Cappell, M. (2007). Hepatic and gastrointestinal diseases. In S. Gabbe, J. Niebyl, & J. Simpson (Eds.), *Obstetrics: Normal and problem pregnancies* (5th ed.). Philadelphia: Churchill Livingstone.

Colombo, D., & Samuels, P. (2007). Renal disease. In S. Gabbe, J. Niebyl, & J. Simpson (Eds.), *Obstetrics: Normal and problem pregnancies* (5th ed.). Philadelphia: Churchill Livingstone.

Cunningham, F., Leveno, K., Bloom, S., Hauth, J., Rouse, D., & Spong, C. (2010). *Williams obstetrics* (23rd ed.). New York: McGraw-Hill.

Curran, C. (2006). The effects of rhinitis, asthma & acute respiratory distress syndrome as acute or chronic pulmonary conditions during pregnancy. *Journal of Perinatal and Neonatal Nursing, 20*(2), 147–154.

Duff, P., Sweet, R., & Edwards, R. (2009). Maternal and fetal infections. In R. Creasy, R. Resnik, J. Iams, C. Lockwood, & T. Moore (Eds.), *Creasy and Resnik's maternal-fetal medicine: Principles and practice* (6th ed.). Philadelphia: Saunders.

Easterling, T., & Stout, K. (2007). Heart disease. In S. Gabbe, J. Niebyl, & J. Simpson (Eds.), *Obstetrics: Normal and problem pregnancies* (5th ed.). New York: Churchill Livingstone.

Gilbert, E. (2011). *Manual of high risk pregnancy & delivery* (5th ed.). St. Louis: Mosby.

Holmgren, C., & Branch, D. (2007). Collagen vascular diseases. In S. Gabbe, J. Niebyl, & J. Simpson (Eds.), *Obstetrics: Normal and problem pregnancies* (5th ed.). Philadelphia: Churchill Livingstone.

Iams, J., & Romero, R. (2007). Preterm birth. In S. Gabbe, J. Niebyl, & J. Simpson (Eds.), *Obstetrics: Normal and problem pregnancies* (5th ed.). Philadelphia: Churchill Livingstone.

Iams, J., Romero, R., & Creasy, R. (2009). Preterm labor and birth. In R. Creasy, R. Resnik, J. Iams, C. Lockwood, & T. Moore (Eds.), *Creasy and Resnik's maternal-fetal medicine: Principles and practice* (6th ed.). Philadelphia: Saunders.

Kelly, T., & Savides, T. (2009). Gastrointestinal disease in pregnancy. In R. Creasy, R. Resnik, J. Iams, C. Lockwood, & T. Moore (Eds.), *Creasy and Resnik's maternal-fetal medicine: Principles and practice* (6th ed.). Philadelphia: Saunders.

Kilpatrick., S. (2009). Anemia in pregnancy. In R. Creasy, R. Resnik, J. Iams, C. Lockwood, & T. Moore (Eds.), *Creasy and Resnik's maternal-fetal medicine: Principles and practice* (6th ed.). Philadelphia: Saunders.

Klein, L., & Galan, H. (2004). Cardiac disease in pregnancy. *Obstetrics and Gynecology Clinics of North America, 31*(2), 429–459.

Lawrence, R., & Lawrence, R. (2005). *Breastfeeding: A guide for the medical profession* (6th ed.). Philadelphia: Mosby.

Lu, E., & Curet, M. (2007). Surgical procedures in pregnancy. In S. Gabbe, J. Niebyl, & J. Simpson (Eds.), *Obstetrics: Normal and problem pregnancies* (5th ed.). Philadelphia: Churchill Livingstone.

Mahomed, K. (2006). Abdominal pain. In D. James, P. Steer, C. Weiner, & B. Gonik (Eds.), *High risk pregnancy: Management options* (3rd ed.). Philadelphia: Saunders.

Martin, S., & Foley, M. (2007). Cardiac disease in pregnancy. In J. Queenan, C. Spong, & C. Lockwood (Eds.), *Management of high-risk pregnancy: An evidenced-based approach* (5th ed.). Malden, MA: Blackwell.

Martin, S., & Foley, M. (2009). Intensive care monitoring of the critically ill pregnant patient. In R. Creasy, R. Resnik, J. Iams, C. Lockwood, & T. Moore (Eds.), *Creasy and Resnik's maternal-fetal medicine: Principles and practice* (6th ed.). Philadelphia: Saunders.

Papoutsis, J., & Kroumpouzos, G. (2007). Dermatologic disorders of pregnancy. In S. Gabbe, J. Niebyl, & J. Simpson (Eds.), *Obstetrics: Normal and problem pregnancies* (5th ed.). Philadelphia: Churchill Livingstone.

Porter, T., & Branch, D. (2006). Autoimmune diseases. In D. James, P. Steer, C. Weiner, & B. Gonik (Eds.), *High risk pregnancy: Management options* (3rd ed.). Philadelphia: Saunders.

Powrie, R. (2006). Respiratory diseases. In D. James, P. Steer, C. Weiner, & B. Gonik (Eds.), *High risk pregnancy: Management options* (3rd ed.). Philadelphia: Saunders.

Rapini, R. (2009). The skin and pregnancy. In R. Creasy, R. Resnik, J. Iams, C. Lockwood, & T. Moore (Eds.), *Creasy and Resnik's maternal-fetal medicine: Principles and practice* (6th ed.). Philadelphia: Saunders.

Samuels, P. (2007). Hematologic complications of pregnancy. In S. Gabbe, J. Niebyl, & J. Simpson (Eds.), *Obstetrics: Normal and problem pregnancies* (5th ed.). Philadelphia: Churchill Livingstone.

Samuels, P., & Niebyl, J. (2007). Neurologic disorders. In S. Gabbe, J. Niebyl, & J. Simpson (Eds.), *Obstetrics: Normal and problem pregnancies* (5th ed.). Philadelphia: Churchill Livingstone.

Setaro, J., & Caulin-Glaser, T. (2004). Pregnancy and cardiovascular disease. In G. Burrow, T. Duffy, & J. Copel (Eds.), *Medical complications during pregnancy* (6th ed.). Philadelphia: Saunders.

Tomlinson, M. (2006). Cardiac disease. In D. James, P. Steer, C. Weiner, & B. Gonik (Eds.), *High risk pregnancy: Management options* (3rd ed.). Philadelphia: Saunders.

Whitty, J., & Dombrowski, M. (2007). Respiratory diseases in pregnancy. In S. Gabbe, J. Niebyl, & J. Simpson (Eds.), *Obstetrics: Normal and problem pregnancies* (5th ed.). Philadelphia: Churchill Livingstone.

Whitty, J., & Dombrowski, M. (2009). Respiratory diseases in pregnancy. In R. Creasy, R. Resnik, J. Iams, C. Lockwood, & T. Moore (Eds.), *Creasy and Resnik's maternal-fetal medicine: Principles and practice* (6th ed.). Philadelphia: Saunders.

Williamson, C., & Mackillop, L. (2009). Diseases of the liver, biliary system, and pancreas. In R. Creasy, R. Resnik, J. Iams, C. Lockwood, & T. Moore (Eds.), *Creasy and Resnik's maternal-fetal medicine: Principles and practice* (6th ed.). Philadelphia: Saunders.

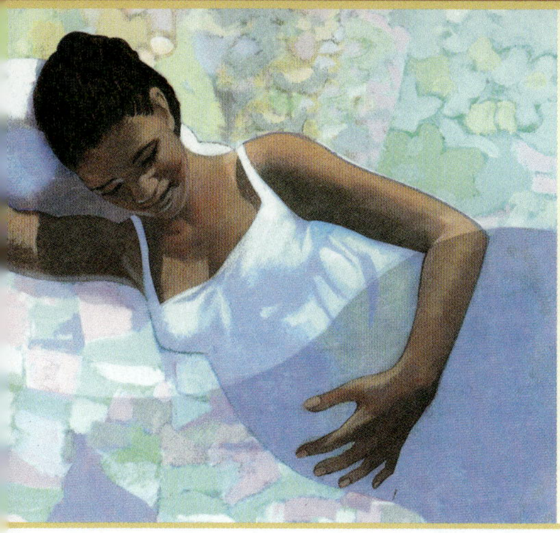

CHAPTER

31

Obstetric Critical Care

Karen F. Dorman

evolve WEBSITE

http://evolve.elsevier.com/Lowdermilk/MWHC/

Audio Glossary

Audio Key Points

NCLEX Review Questions

LEARNING OBJECTIVES

- Discuss factors that have contributed to the development of the specialty of critical care obstetrics.
- Describe conditions that may place a pregnant woman in a critically ill state.
- Examine factors that affect the provision of obstetric critical care when a pregnant woman becomes critically ill.
- Describe significant cardiovascular, pulmonary, and hematologic alterations during pregnancy that affect critical care for the pregnant woman.
- Describe the parameters measured and state normal values for pulmonary artery and arterial pressure monitoring.
- Identify treatment strategies based on interpretation of hemodynamic profiles.
- Identify physiologic alterations of pregnancy that affect stabilization and treatment of the pregnant woman who has undergone trauma.
- Describe immediate assessment and stabilization measures for the pregnant victim of trauma.
- Compare components of the primary and secondary surveys for the pregnant woman who has undergone trauma.
- Discuss inclusion of the components of family-centered maternity care for the critically ill pregnant woman.
- Examine the effect of maternal death on families and nursing staff members who cared for the woman.

Obstetric and critical care units are equally challenged whenever presented with the multiple, complex needs of a critically ill pregnant woman and her fetus. Optimal outcome for mother and fetus depends on: (1) swift recognition of severe complications, and (2) delivery of critical care therapies adjusted for the physiologic alterations of pregnancy. Fetal effects of therapies also must be considered. Management of the critically ill pregnant woman includes assessing maternal and fetal status continuously, selecting therapeutic interventions appropriate for mother and fetus, and carefully choosing the timing of birth.

Providing critical care and hemodynamic monitoring for the seriously ill pregnant woman has developed slowly in many institutions because of two factors: (1) obstetric nurses and physicians, expert in the care of pregnant women, can feel threatened by pressure transducers, alarms, hemodynamic monitoring, and ventilators; and (2) critical care nurses and physicians, expert in hemodynamic monitoring and mechanical ventilation, can feel threatened by the pregnant uterus, labor, birth, the fetus, and fetal monitoring. The result is that few institutions have been able to provide optimal care whenever a sudden, acute, life-threatening complication has occurred in a pregnant woman.

OBSTETRIC INTENSIVE CARE UNIT

Critical care obstetrics evolved as a subspecialty of perinatal medicine in response to the need for optimal care for the critically ill pregnant woman and her fetus. This subspecialty prepares the obstetric team, which has in-depth knowledge of pregnancy, to use critical care techniques in the management of the critically ill pregnant woman and her fetus. Some centers have developed obstetric intensive care units (OBICUs) so that specific equipment and individuals with special training and expertise in obstetric care and critical care are available to provide this care.

Complications may develop during pregnancy that are so severe and life threatening that optimal maternal and fetal outcome, and many times survival, depends on the woman receiving critical care that meets her specific needs. Maternal adaptations that are normal for the pregnancy state alter physiologic status and make the pregnant woman hemodynamically different from the nonpregnant woman.

Before the development of OBICUs, care for the critically ill pregnant woman was usually provided in an ICU for adults, where management modalities were based on hemodynamic values that are normal for the nonpregnant individual but resulted in less than desirable outcomes for pregnant women. Research in some of the first OBICUs reported on physical and hemodynamic differences during the pregnant state. Normal hemodynamic values for pregnancy were identified. Maternal and fetal outcomes improved when management of care was based on the enhanced hemodynamic state that accompanies normal pregnancy and care was provided in the specialized units.

Anyone providing care for pregnant women may encounter the pregnant woman with a life-threatening complication and be challenged to recognize the need for immediate, critical care and to provide such care. This care may be delivered in a variety of ways. Problems can be decreased by developing a viable plan to provide care for the critically ill pregnant woman, adequately educating nursing, medical, and ancillary staff, providing necessary equipment at the bedside, and encouraging frequent consultation between the obstetric and critical care units.

The most practical, efficient, and economic method to provide care for the critically ill obstetric client who requires invasive hemodynamic monitoring, mechanical ventilation, or both depends primarily on the numbers of pregnant women cared for annually and the referral patterns in a specific facility. The ideal method to provide care for the pregnant woman is a specially trained team of obstetricians and obstetric nurses in an OBICU, augmented by anesthesiologists, pulmonologists, cardiologists, and intensivists. A larger tertiary center is more likely to have this type of unit because the census of pregnant women cared for annually in the referral center would support development of the service. OBICUs are often small and may consist of one bed. Admissions may be limited only to the very sickest women and may not include all women eligible for a bed in the OBICU.

However, even in many large, tertiary centers, the number of truly critically ill pregnant women is not large enough to warrant such an investment in equipment and training of medical and nursing staff. In these centers, collaborative practice between obstetrics and intensive care has been successful in providing the best care for these women (Zeeman, 2006). If the woman remains pregnant, the optimal place for her is the labor and birth unit, with a critical care nurse in attendance. The American College of Obstetricians and Gynecologists (ACOG, 2009) reports that 75% of admissions to the ICU occur in the postpartum period, after consideration of the fetal condition and management decisions regarding birth are no longer a concern. However, there are still situations before birth in which the ICU is the best site for this collaborative care. In this instance, obstetric practitioners serve a vital role in monitoring the woman as well as assessing the fetus. The institution must develop policies and procedures so that care is provided where it is most advantageous. Some institutions provide dual training for selected nurses (i.e., an ICU nurse receives advanced education in obstetrics or an obstetric nurse receives advanced education in intensive care nursing).

> **LEGAL TIP: Nursing Assignments**
> Continual assignment of an obstetric and an intensive care nurse, or one nurse experienced in both specialties, is required in the care of the critically ill woman with a viable pregnancy.

In still other institutions, an obstetric service may be established to provide care during the low risk pregnancy. The plan for the smaller unit or the low risk unit may be for the nursing and medical team to recognize the critical illness immediately, stabilize the woman, and initiate measures for transport to the tertiary center and/or the OBICU. The *Standards and Guidelines for Professional Nursing Practice in the Care of Women and Newborns* (Association of Women's Health, Obstetric and Neonatal Nurses [AWHONN], 2009) includes guidelines for the care of the pregnant woman requiring critical care. Obstetric clients requiring critical care are at risk for undesirable pregnancy outcomes because of the severity of complications, including decreased oxygen transport and multiple system organ failure and the possibility of long-term residual physical effects of the illness.

> **LEGAL TIP: Client Care Standards**
> Client care standards established for obstetric and intensive care must be met within the plan developed by an institution to provide complex, critical care for the critically ill pregnant woman. Standards of care from both specialties must be followed.

Equipment and Expertise

The usual equipment for a labor, birth, and recovery suite is mandatory for an ICU or surgical suite where a woman may be admitted for care. Staff and equipment for neonatal resuscitation must also be available. The usual equipment for intensive care, including hemodynamic monitoring and mechanical ventilation, is equally necessary whenever the critically ill woman is in the labor and birth unit.

A severe complication of pregnancy may prompt the need for obstetric critical care with hemodynamic monitoring or mechanical ventilation. See Box 31-1 for a list of complications that indicate a need for critical care.

> **LEGAL TIP: Legal Review**
> Because an optimal outcome is uncertain when the pregnant woman is critically ill, the medical records, with documentation of the medical and nursing care that mother, fetus, and neonate received, are more likely to be subjected to legal review than are medical records of other clients.

The number of pregnant women who need obstetric critical care has increased in recent years as the result of many factors: women are surviving childhood illnesses because of advances in pediatric care which include the development of pediatric ICUs; improved surgical procedures for infants with congenital defects, such as cardiac lesions; and advanced knowledge in pediatric care for children with chronic health problems, including diabetes, cystic fibrosis, and pulmonary disorders. The desire to become a parent is not eliminated by a chronic health problem, and numerous women each year risk their lives to have a baby. Many women have had successful pregnancies

BOX 31-1 COMPLICATIONS OF PREGNANCY THAT INDICATE THE NEED FOR CRITICAL CARE

- Severe preeclampsia or eclampsia with complications
  - Refractory pulmonary edema
  - Refractory oliguria
  - Hypertensive crisis
  - Severe hemorrhage or disseminated intravascular coagulation (DIC)
  - Renal failure
- Hemorrhage or DIC that requires multiple transfusions
- Cardiac problems
- Chronic health problems
  - Systemic lupus erythematosus
  - Diabetic ketoacidosis
  - Sickle cell disease
  - Diabetes complicated by vascular changes
  - Others
- Trauma victim
  - Motor vehicle crash
  - Violence, battering

after kidney transplants (Davison & Bailey, 2003), after thoracic organ transplant such as heart, lung and heart and lung (Wu, Wilt, & Restaino, 2007), and after liver transplants (Christopher, Al-Chalabi, Richardson, Muiesan, Rela, Heaton, et al., 2006). Most transplant clients do very well with pregnancy, provided the new organ is functioning well. Another reason for the increase in critically ill pregnant women is that more are waiting to become pregnant at a later age, thus increasing the occurrence of heart disease and other age-related factors.

Other pregnant women need critical care because of trauma resulting from motor vehicle crashes or violence and battering. These account for most of the traumatic injuries during pregnancy. There has been an increase in the number of women with respiratory compromise as a result of the H1N1 flu outbreak because pregnant women are more susceptible to the virus and also become sicker than women in the same age-group who are not pregnant. Pregnant women were at increased risk for severe complications such as pneumonia, acute respiratory distress syndrome (ARDS), and even death from the 2009 H1N1 influenzavirus (ACOG, 2009).

Since 2004, there has been little new information written about the care of critically ill pregnant women and critical care obstetrics in the United States. Admission of an obstetric client to the intensive care unit occurs in approximately 1% to 3% of pregnant women requiring critical care services (40,000 to 120,000/year) (ACOG, 2009). Zeeman (2006) reported that the most common diagnosis for admission to an OBICU is severe preeclampsia with complications including refractory pulmonary edema, refractory oliguria, hypertensive crisis, severe hemorrhage or disseminated intravascular coagulation (DIC), and renal failure. Massive hemorrhage or DIC is reported as the second most common reason for admission. Reports from other developed countries report similar incidences of ICU admission with regard to frequency and diagnosis (Anwari, Butt, & Al-Dar, 2004; Baskett & O'Connell, 2009; Keizer, Zwart, Meerman, Harinck, Feuth, & Roosmalen, 2006; Saravanakumar, Davies, Lewis, & Cooper, 2008; Selo-Ojeme, Omosaiye, Battacharjee, & Kadir, 2005).

Conditions that classify the parturient as critically ill and indicate the need for a pulmonary artery catheter include the following (ACOG, 1992):

- Sepsis with refractory hypotension or oliguria
- Unexplained or refractory pulmonary edema, congestive heart failure, or oliguria
- Severe preeclampsia with pulmonary edema or refractory oliguria
- Intraoperative or intrapartum cardiovascular decompensation
- Massive blood loss or volume replacement needs
- ARDS
- Shock of undefined source
- Chronic disease, particularly when associated with labor or major surgery

The identification of women needing OBICU services merits careful consideration. It is important not to visualize just the "sickest client scenario"—that dramatic case, never to be forgotten. Instead the typical picture of a critically ill pregnant woman is one with severe preeclampsia, whose condition has worsened and now has headache, high blood pressure (BP), oliguria, and low platelets. Or the woman may have been referred from a level I center with a preexisting cardiac lesion exacerbated by pregnancy that has gradually deteriorated from class I to class III cardiac disease. Her presenting complaint may be "feeling extremely tired."

PHYSIOLOGIC CHANGES IN PREGNANCY

The normal physiologic adaptations that accompany pregnancy and produce profound hemodynamic changes are the primary factors that make the pregnant woman a different type of critical care client and merit a separate critical care facility. Knowledge of the effects of the physiologic alterations during pregnancy is essential for optimal critical care management. Normal maternal alterations during pregnancy affect the major systems: cardiovascular, pulmonary, renal, and hematologic (Norwitz, Robinson, & Malone, 2004).

Cardiovascular Changes

The cardiovascular system changes dramatically during pregnancy. Because it is a state of high flow and low resistance, pregnancy is hemodynamically similar to early sepsis. Hypervolemia is the result of the influence of estrogen and progesterone on aldosterone, which produces an increase in circulating blood volume. The expansion in maternal blood volume begins with a 22% increase by 8 weeks of gestation and progresses to a maximum increase of 45% by 32 to 34 weeks of gestation. This represents an increase of approximately 1570 ml for a singleton gestation and includes a 40% to 50% increase in plasma volume and a 20% to 30% increase in red blood cell mass. This disproportional increase results in a state of hemodilution. An increase in total body water of 6 to 8 L in the extravascular compartment, accompanied by an accumulation of 500 to 900 mEq of sodium, also occurs during pregnancy. Heart rate (HR) increases 20% (10 to 15 beats/min) with the major increase in the third trimester, and stroke volume increases to accommodate the increased circulating volume. See Table 31-1 for a summary of cardiovascular adaptations.

TABLE 31-1 **CARDIOVASCULAR CHANGES DURING PREGNANCY**

PARAMETER	CHANGE
Blood volume	40%-50% increase
Plasma volume	40%-50% increase (1200-1300 ml)
Red blood cell mass	20%-30% increase (250-450 ml)
Heart	Displaced to the left and upward
Point of maximal intensity (PMI)	Fourth intercostal space and lateral
Rate	20% increase (10-15 beats/min)
Sounds	Exaggerated splitting first sound
	Systolic murmur usually present
	Third sound present
Stroke volume	32% increase by 20-24 wks
Cardiac output	Increases by 30%-50%
	22% increase by 28 wks
	43% increase by term
	Increases during labor
	≤3 cm, 17% increase
	4-7 cm, 23% increase
	≥8 cm, 34% increase

Source: Norwitz, E., Robinson, J., & Malone, F. (2004). Pregnancy-induced physiologic alterations. In G. Dildy, M. Belfort, G. Saade, J. Phelan, G. Hankins, & S. Clark (Eds.), *Critical care obstetrics* (4th ed.). Malden, MA: Blackwell Science.

Colloid Osmotic Pressure

Colloid osmotic pressure (COP) is the gradient controlling whether fluid remains inside the capillary or moves into the interstitial space. The force to keep the fluid inside the vessel is the pulling pressure of the colloids, or proteins, present in the plasma. The most important plasma proteins are albumin, globulin, and fibrinogen. Pregnancy produces a decrease in COP values resulting from the hemodilutional state that reduces the concentration of plasma proteins. Severe preeclampsia usually produces renal damage, with a subsequent loss of proteins in the urine, further reducing the COP. The force exerted to push fluids through the membrane is the capillary hydrostatic pressure and is measured as the pulmonary capillary wedge pressure (PCWP). Colloid osmotic (oncotic) values in pregnancy are shown in Table 31-2. Though not routinely evaluated and not available in many institutions, knowledge of this key concept is helpful in understanding one of the basic differences between pregnant and nonpregnant women. Pulmonary edema tends to develop in pregnant women at a lower PCWP than in those who are not pregnant and have a normal COP.

The lower the COP and the higher the PCWP, the more likely it is for pulmonary edema to develop, as reflected by a lower COP to PCWP gradient. The gradient is the difference between the COP and the PCWP. COP to PCWP gradient values are as follows: nonpregnant, 14.5 ± 2.5; pregnant, 10.5 ± 2.7.

Pulmonary edema is more likely to develop in pregnancy. For example, the normal PCWP is 6 to 10 mm Hg during pregnancy and 4 to 9 mm Hg in the nonpregnant state (Clark, Cotton, Lee, Bishop, Hill, Southick, et al., 1989). With a PCWP of 8, calculations of the COP-PCWP gradient show:

- Nonpregnant woman: COP of 25 – PCWP of 8 = 17 mm Hg
- Pregnant woman with severe preeclampsia: COP of 13 – PCWP of 8 = 5 mm Hg

Lower COP to PCWP gradients during pregnancy are usually caused by lower COP values occurring during pregnancy.

TABLE 31-2 **COLLOID OSMOTIC (ONCOTIC) PRESSURE VALUES**

Nonpregnant	25.4 ± 2.3 mm Hg
Pregnant, antepartum	22.4 ± 0.54 mm Hg
Pregnant, postpartum	15.4 ± 2.1 mm Hg
Preeclampsia, antepartum	17.9 ± 0.68 mm Hg
Preeclampsia, postpartum	13.7 ± 0.46 mm Hg

Respiratory Changes

Anatomic and physiologic alterations during pregnancy are necessary to adequately oxygenate the mother and fetus. A relative hyperventilation of pregnancy begins in the first trimester and increases 42% by term. Respiratory rate increases only slightly. Tidal volume and minute ventilations increase approximately 50% by term to meet increased oxygen consumption needs. The enlarging uterus pushes the diaphragm upward approximately 4 to 7 cm, reducing lung volume. Compensation is necessary to meet increased ventilatory demands, and the transverse diameter of the thorax increases 2 to 4 cm as the rib cage flares out. The functional residual capacity decreases 25% because more of the inhaled air is used, resulting in decreased reserve. Pregnant women become short of breath easily, as seen in walking or light exercise. This can become critical if the oxygen demands of the pregnant woman increase. The hyperventilation of pregnancy is associated with a resting arterial carbon dioxide tension of less than 30 mm Hg. Maternal alkalosis is prevented by the compensatory decrease in serum bicarbonate of about 4 mEq/L, from 26 to 22 mEq. During gestation respiratory acidosis and metabolic acidosis develop more rapidly than in the nonpregnant state.

Normal arterial blood gas (ABG) values for pregnancy reflect a chronic state of compensated respiratory alkalosis, represented by a right shift in the oxyhemoglobin dissociation curve caused by the increased levels of 2,3-diphosphoglycerate from the high progesterone and estrogen levels present. Normal ABG values for pregnant women as compared to those for nonpregnant women are listed in Table 13-3, p. 299.

Hematologic Changes

Pregnancy is a hypercoagulable state, as preparation is made for the blood loss that accompanies childbirth. Table 13-3, p. 299, gives a summary of alterations that enhance coagulation.

Bleeding and clotting times remain unchanged even when hypervolemia and hemodilution are present. The critically ill pregnant woman is at increased risk for thrombus formation whenever hemoconcentration develops, as occurs with severe preeclampsia or dehydration.

Systemic Vascular Resistance

Systemic vascular resistance (SVR) is a measure of the tension required for the ejection of blood into the circulation (afterload). To describe the physiologic relations between pressure and flow, measurements are made by the following formula as a ratio of pressure to flow:

$$SVR = \frac{[(MAP - CVP) \times 80]}{CO}$$

where MAP is mean arterial pressure (in millimeters of mercury), CVP is central venous pressure (in millimeters of mercury), and CO is cardiac output (in liters per minute).

Vasodilation of arterial vessels, a result of hormonal influences, and development of the uteroplacental circulation result in a decrease in SVR of 20% to 25% and a decrease in pulmonary vascular resistance of 40% during pregnancy. Blood pressure, especially diastolic pressure, decreases during pregnancy, reaching the nadir at 24 to 32 weeks of gestation, with a gradual return to prepregnancy values by term (Blackburn, 2007).

HEMODYNAMIC MONITORING

Anatomic and Physiologic Characteristics of Circulation

An in-depth knowledge of normal functioning and hemodynamics of the cardiovascular system is the basis for understanding hemodynamic monitoring; therefore, a review of these functions is included. The purpose of the cardiopulmonary system is to deliver oxygenated blood to the tissues throughout the body and to remove waste products through the dynamics of normal circulation as follows).

Deoxygenated blood flows from the capillaries into the veins and the right side of the heart through the superior vena cava, draining the upper part of the body, and from the inferior vena cava, draining the lower part of the body. Venous blood flows into the right atrium, a holding chamber for the right side of the heart. When the atrium is filled, the tricuspid valve opens, and blood flows through this valve into the right ventricle.

When the right ventricle is filled, its muscles (myocardium) contract, and blood is ejected through the pulmonic valve into the pulmonary artery. Blood is pushed through the pulmonary artery and its branches to the capillary beds (pulmonary beds) in both lungs. Gas exchange occurs in the capillary beds as carbon dioxide is released and oxygen enters the circulation across the alveolar membrane.

Oxygenated blood drains from the pulmonary beds into the pulmonary veins, two from each lung, into the left atrium, the holding chamber for the left side of the heart. When the left atrium is filled, the mitral valve opens, and blood flows through this valve into the left ventricle. After the left ventricle is filled, the muscles of the left ventricle contract, and the oxygenated blood is ejected through the aortic valve into the aorta and then pumped throughout the systemic arterial circulation so that oxygen is supplied to the organs and tissues of the body.

Synchronization by the electrical conduction system of the myocardium causes the right and left atrial and ventricular contractions to occur simultaneously. The period of the cardiac cycle when both ventricles are relaxed and filling is termed *diastole,* and the period of the cardiac cycle when both ventricles contract is termed *systole.*

Left ventricle contractions must generate enough force to pump blood throughout the systemic circulation. Force required for right ventricular work is less because the right ventricle has to exert only enough force for blood to flow through the pulmonary circulation. Therefore, the left ventricle is referred to as the *hemodynamic ventricle,* and the left side of the heart is referred to as the *hemodynamic heart.* Hemodynamic monitoring with a pulmonary artery catheter provides

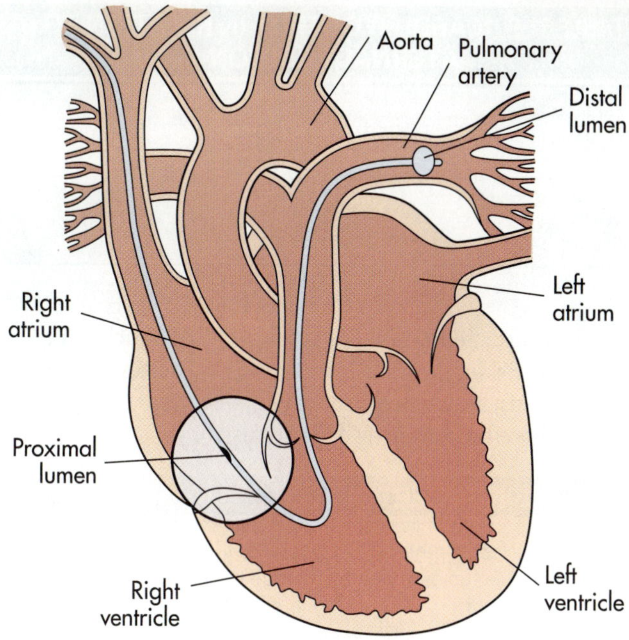

FIG. 31-1 Diagram of heart with position of pulmonary artery catheter.

left heart values, and during a critical illness, values of left heart function are more significant than are values of right heart function (Fig. 31-1).

Cardiac Output

Cardiac output (CO) is the volume of blood ejected from the left ventricle in 1 minute; it is measured in liters per minute. CO is the product of **stroke volume (SV),** the volume of blood ejected from the left ventricle during one cardiac cycle, and HR; thus CO = HR × SV. Because HR and SV increase during pregnancy, CO increases. The normal prepregnancy range of CO is 3 to 5 L/min. CO increases 40% to 50% during pregnancy, to produce a normal CO in the last trimester of 6 to 7 L/min at rest. Labor produces an additional 40% increase in CO because of catecholamine release in response to pain perception and the shunting of blood from the placental-fetal unit with uterine contractions, for a CO range during labor of 8 to 10 L/min. CO increases further after birth because of significant hemodynamic fluctuations that reflect the net effect of blood loss at birth and the autotransfusion with approximately 1000 ml of blood that occurs after the uterus is emptied. Soon after birth the accumulated 6 to 8 L of extravascular fluid is mobilized into the intravascular compartment. The large increase in CO remains for 7 to 10 days after birth in the healthy woman but will continue longer if the usual diuresis fails to occur because of a complication.

Positional Changes

Maternal CO in the last trimester is position dependent. Clark and colleagues (1991) showed the effect of maternal position on CO output (Table 31-3).

The right or left lateral recumbent position provides the optimal CO for the critically ill pregnant woman. Whenever maternal CO is decreased, compensatory mechanisms are initiated. The first compensatory response is to shunt blood away from the peripheral circulation to the central circulation, to

TABLE 31-3 CARDIAC OUTPUT IN RELATION TO MATERNAL POSITION

Position	Cardiac output
Knee-chest	6.9 L/min (±2.1)
Right lateral	6.8 L/min (±1.3)
Left lateral	6.6 L/min (±1.4)
Sitting	6.2 L/min (±2.0)
Supine	6.0 L/min (±1.4)
Standing	5.4 L/min (±2.0)

save the heart and brain. Peripheral circulation includes circulation to the skin, the renal system, the gastrointestinal system, the lung beds, and the reproductive system. Enhancing maternal CO, therefore, enhances fetal perfusion.

! NURSING ALERT

During the last trimester, CO decreases so significantly when the woman is supine that a hip wedge under one hip or manual displacement of the uterus to one side is necessary to prevent a sudden decrease in CO and a subsequent decrease in fetal perfusion.

Cardiac Output Determinants

The four determinants of CO are reflected in the calculation for cardiac output (CO = HR × SV) because SV is the result of preload, afterload, and contractility.

Preload is defined as the volume of blood in the ventricles at the end of diastole; it is determined by intraventricular pressure and volume. Right preload is assessed by right atrial or CVP, and left preload is assessed by PCWP. The volume of blood in the ventricles stretches the myocardial muscle fibers and produces the intraventricular pressure. Measurements are made at end diastole, the time immediately preceding systole when the ventricles reach maximal stretch because of the extra amount of blood delivered into the ventricles when the tricuspid and mitral valves snap closed.

Right preload reflects the blood circulating through the right side of the heart, and left preload reflects the amount of blood circulating in the left side of the heart. The two sides of the heart are not equal when cardiac or pulmonary complications are present; therefore, they are measured separately.

Preload must be adequate to maintain CO, and plotting of CO against preload gives a cardiac function curve (Fig. 31-2). As preload increases, CO increases up to the point of failure. The cardiac function curve shows that a heart in failure requires a higher preload than the healthy heart to produce the same CO. Bedside manipulations of preload are possible with continuous hemodynamic monitoring to determine effects on CO. A low preload can be increased by the administration of fluids, including crystalloids, colloids, or blood, and by positioning with legs elevated. A high preload can be decreased by the administration of a vasodilator or diuretic or by phlebotomy and upright positioning.

Afterload is defined as the ventricular wall tension during systole, or the resistance the blood meets as blood is ejected from the ventricles. Afterload is dependent on the end-diastolic radius of the ventricle, the aortic pressure, and the thickness of

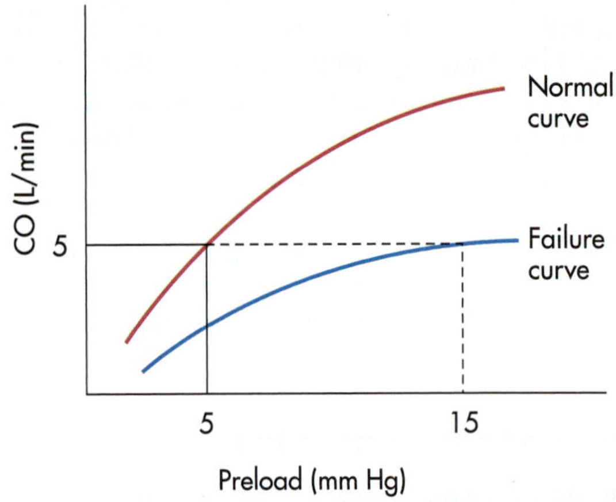

FIG. 31-2 Relation of preload to cardiac output. Ventricular function (Starling) curve for heart, showing both normal function and during failure.

the ventricle wall. As afterload increases, CO decreases. Bedside manipulation of afterload is possible to achieve optimal cardiac output (Fig. 31-3). Right afterload is assessed by the **pulmonary vascular resistance (PVR),** and left afterload is assessed by the SVR. Arterial BP measurement does not give as accurate an indication of left ventricular work as the SVR but is used clinically as reflecting left afterload. Therefore, control of the woman's blood pressure is used to control left afterload.

Afterload must be adequate for circulation and CO; extremes of afterload may decrease CO. Increased left afterload occurs with hypertensive disease caused by the systemic arterial vasoconstriction. Increased right afterload occurs with pulmonary hypertension resulting from vasoconstriction in the pulmonary circulation.

Increased afterload can be corrected by the administration of vasodilator drugs. Hydralazine is commonly used as the first-line drug for hypertension. It is an arterial vasodilator that is usually effective and safe for mother and fetus. As an added bonus, the majority of obstetric personnel are comfortable with its use. However, others believe that the calcium channel blockers (such as nifedipine, orally) and the beta-blockers (such as labetalol) cause less hypotension (Magee & von Dadelszen, 2009) (see Table 27-5, p. 666). Sodium nitroprusside is rarely used in pregnancy because it produces cyanide as a metabolite; fetal cyanide toxicity must be a concern if this drug is administered during pregnancy. Of paramount importance is the correction of hypovolemia before administration of any antihypertensive to prevent acute hypotension.

SAFETY ALERT

Sodium nitroprusside by continuous intravenous infusion is the vasodilator drug used most commonly in the adult intensive care setting, but it is saved for emergency use for pregnant women.

Severe vasodilation and loss of arterial resistance with a decreased afterload impedes venous return of blood to the right side of the heart and decreases CO. This situation is seen with septic shock. Decreased afterload can be corrected by fluid administration to fill the vascular space or by the administration of vasopressor medications such as dopamine or dobutamine (Martin &

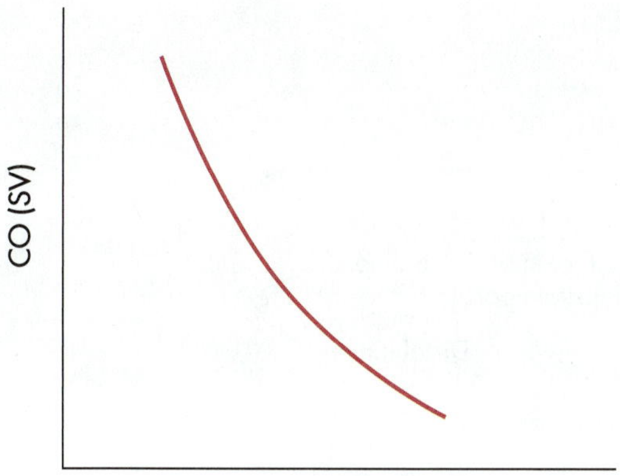

FIG. 31-3 Relation of afterload to cardiac output when preload is maintained constant. As afterload increases, cardiac output decreases.

Foley, 2009). **Contractility** (inotropic state of the heart) is defined as the force and velocity of ventricular contractions when preload and afterload are held constant. Contractility is governed by the Frank-Starling law, which states that the greater the length of the muscle fibers before contraction, the greater will be the contraction of the fibers, up to the point of failure. Fiber length is related to the maximal stretch of preload, because as more blood volume enters the ventricles, the more the fibers in the myocardium stretch to accommodate the increased volume.

Decreased contractility results in decreased CO. The first response to correct this problem is bedside manipulation to optimize both preload and afterload. If this fails to increase CO to the desired level, medications to increase myocardial contractility are indicated. Inotropic drugs such as dopamine hydrochloride or dobutamine are administered. Digitalis therapy also may be necessary.

Heart rate is the fourth determinant of cardiac output. The rate at which the ventricles fill and contract affects CO. Extremes of HR may decrease CO.

Sustained tachycardia can decrease CO as a result of myo cardial ischemia or the decreased time for adequate filling of the ventricles during diastole and shortened systolic ejection times. The cause, such as fever, hypoxia, pain, hypovolemia, or hyperthyroidism, should be determined and treated. Drugs to correct tachycardia are seldom necessary for obstetric clients. However, propranolol, digoxin, or calcium channel blockers such as verapamil are effective agents to decrease HR if needed.

Bradycardia can compromise CO when the number of ventricular contractions per minute that occur are inadequate to deliver the circulating volume needed to perfuse and oxygenate the body. If treatment is necessary for this problem, atropine or cardiac pacing is used.

Invasive Hemodynamic Monitoring

Invasive hemodynamic monitoring provides continuous measurements of preload, afterload, myocardial contractility, and HR in the critically ill pregnant woman so that therapeutic manipulations may be made quickly at the bedside in response to changes in client status. Monitoring may be done by use of a **pulmonary artery catheter (PAC)** (a balloon-tipped, multilumen catheter) or by CVP.

Although few adequate clinical studies demonstrate the benefit of pulmonary artery catheterization for the critically ill client, most critical care bedside clinicians use the PAC to direct their therapy modalities. They believe that use of the PAC does improve outcomes in selected critically ill clients (Fujitani & Baldisseri, 2005).

Use of a PAC allows the management of care to be based on immediate recognition of changes in hemodynamic values from the left ventricle. Immediate information is obtained, calculations are made, and management is adjusted quickly as needed. Results of therapeutic strategies can be calculated and evaluated (ACOG, 1992). The continuous hemodynamic measurements obtained will reinforce therapies in use or show that therapy should be changed. Use of a PAC in combination with an arterial pressure catheter and a pulse oximeter provides adequate data to assess the cardiac, fluid, and pulmonary status continuously. Indications for the use of invasive hemodynamic monitoring are the same in obstetrics as in any other area of medicine.

It is essential to evaluate risks and benefits of any procedure before its use, especially because there are risks associated with invasive techniques. The information obtained from hemodynamic monitoring is essential for management of critical, complex cases and is unavailable by other means; thus the benefits outweigh the risks in most cases. The overall complication rate in the obstetric population is low, approximately 1%. This low rate of complications is related to three factors: (1) the pregnant woman usually needs the device because of an acute event, (2) the duration of use is usually short, and (3) the majority of pregnant women requiring its use are young and healthy before the acute event.

It is essential that meticulous attention be paid to each step and detail of all procedures to decrease problems with the technique itself. The rate of complications associated with PAC insertion decreases as the experience level of the clinician increases. Therefore, only properly trained personnel should insert catheters for invasive hemodynamic monitoring (Martin & Foley, 2009).

Although the PAC remains the gold standard for measuring hemodynamic status in the critically ill client, transesophageal echocardiography (TEE) is sometimes used as a noninvasive bedside method for assessing the hemodynamic status of nonpregnant adults. A few studies in obstetric clients have found that CO measured with TEE correlates well with CO measured by PAC. More research is needed, but TEE may prove useful in the care of critically ill pregnant women (Martin & Foley, 2009).

Pulmonary Artery Catheter

A PAC, commonly called the Swan-Ganz catheter, provides continuous measurements of **pulmonary artery pressure (PAP)** and right atrial pressure (RAP) or CVP. Intermittent measurements of PCWP and CO also are possible. The standard flow-directed thermodilution PAC has three lumina and a thermistor connector (Fig. 31-4). The distal lumen or port is located in the pulmonary artery after insertion. It is connected to a transducer with a heparinized pressure line to measure a continuous PAP when the balloon is deflated and intermittent PCWP when the balloon is inflated. A continuous flush of 3 ml/hr of heparinized solution maintains patency of the lumen.

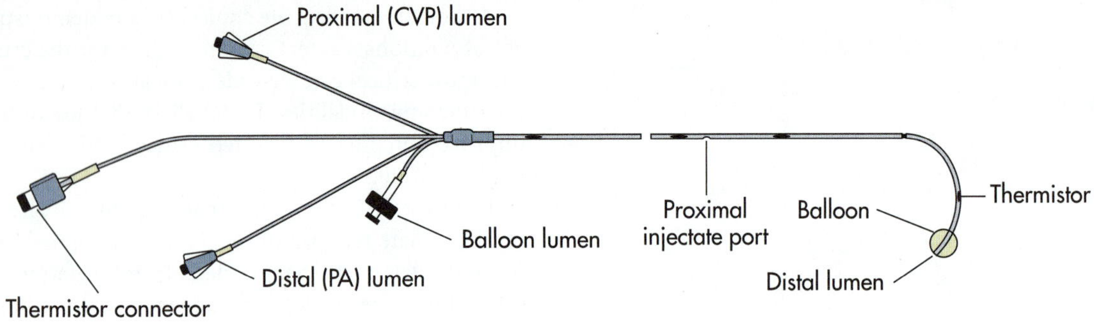

FIG. 31-4 Standard triple-lumen flow-directed pulmonary artery catheter.

The proximal lumen or port exits approximately 30 cm from the tip of the catheter and is located in the right atrium after insertion. This port also is connected to a transducer with a heparinized line and can be used to measure continuous RAP, which is comparable to the CVP, or to administer fluid or drugs. Both the proximal and distal lumina of the catheter can be used to withdraw blood samples for laboratory studies.

The balloon lumen ends in a small latex balloon, located 0.5 inch from the tip of the PAC. Inflation of the balloon is used to assist in the insertion of the catheter and to obtain PCWP readings.

The thermodilution port is connected to a thermistor, a temperature sensor, located 5 cm proximal to the tip of the PAC. The thermistor continuously measures the temperature of the blood in the pulmonary artery.

Other types of PACs are available in addition to the standard PAC. Some have an extra right atrial port for intracardiac infusions. The small size of the ports makes them more effective for the administration of vasopressors or drugs such as antibiotics, than for the rapid administration of large volumes of blood or fluids. A fiberoptic PAC includes a sensor that can continuously measure the hemoglobin saturation of mixed venous blood, the Svo_2, in the pulmonary artery and is useful in cases of decreased oxygen transport, such as with preeclampsia and eclampsia.

Venous Access

The internal or external jugular vein or the subclavian vein is most commonly used for venous access for invasive hemodynamic monitoring during pregnancy. The right internal jugular vein is usually the preferred site because it offers the shortest and most direct entry into the right heart (Martin & Foley, 2009). Access with femoral or antecubital veins is not used as frequently for pregnant women because of the greater difficulty in positioning the catheter when this route is accessed. Furthermore, with use of a vein in the inguinal area, birth of the infant at a critical time can limit access to and manipulation of the catheter.

The flow-directed PAC is usually inserted at the bedside after preparations are complete. Meticulous attention to detail is critical when the equipment is prepared. Flushing the pressure tubing to eliminate any air, establishing a zero reference point, and both zeroing and calibrating the pressure transducer are done carefully before insertion. See the Procedure box that explains how to set up a pressure line and how to zero-reference and calibrate a pressure transducer. Box 31-2 describes nursing care during insertion and continuing care for a woman with a PAC.

PROCEDURE

How to Set Up, Calibrate, and Zero-Reference Pressure Lines

1. Connect pressure tubing to sterile disposable pressure transducer.
2. Check all connections for a tight fit to prevent leakage.
3. Heparinize flush solution of normal saline solution. Heparin is necessary for the pregnant woman to prevent thrombus formation.
4. Connect the pressure tubing to the intravenous bag of heparinized solution.
5. Gently flush both pressure tubing and transducer to remove all air. Cap stopcocks with nonvented covers.
6. Connect transducer to hemodynamic monitor.
7. Place a pressure bag on the heparinized solution. Inflate to 300 mm Hg of pressure. (This allows a continuous rate of 3 ml/hr of heparinized solution to flow as a flush solution.) The heparinized solution and continuous flow of fluid prevent clot formation on the tip of the catheter.
8. Calibrate the pressure transducer by zeroing the line.
9. Zero-reference the transducer by positioning the woman supine with a hip wedge under one hip, locating the phlebostatic axis at the fourth intercostal space at the midaxillary line, and marking on the chest wall.
10. Open stopcock to air. Push zero button on the monitor to identify zero. The transducer negates atmospheric pressure and establishes a baseline for subsequent readings. Close the stopcock to air.

NOTE: The phlebostatic axis is the physiologic reference point used when measuring pulmonary and arterial line pressures (Fig. 31-5 illustrates this procedure).

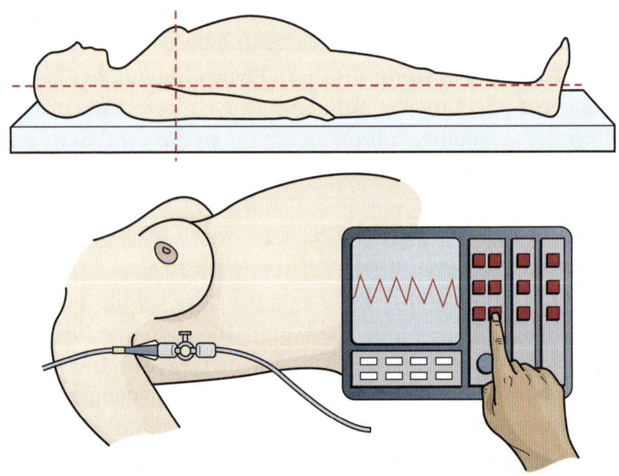

FIG. 31-5 Location of phlebostatic axis and zeroing.

BOX 31-2 PULMONARY ARTERY CATHETER (PAC) PROTOCOL

SETUP
- Prepare two pressure lines for the distal and proximal ports as described in the Procedure box on p. 742, How to Set Up, Calibrate, and Zero-Reference Pressure Lines.
- Connect an intravenous line of normal saline solution, per infusion pump, to the introducer.
- Check PAC balloon for symmetric inflation, absence of air leak, and ease of spontaneous deflation.

CLIENT PREPARATION FOR INSERTION
- Assess woman's knowledge level and explain procedure to ensure her understanding, cooperation, and acceptance of the procedure.
- Confirm that informed consent form is signed and placed in medical record.
- Provide support and encouragement throughout the procedure.
- Initiate electrocardiographic (ECG) monitoring. Obtain baseline ECG pattern.

NURSING MANAGEMENT DURING INSERTION
- Monitor ECG continuously as catheter passes through right ventricle to recognize any ventricular ectopy (premature beats) present.
- Use a slight Trendelenburg position with a hip wedge. This position engorges the neck veins and facilitates placement of the catheter. When the internal jugular approach is used, tilt head to the side away from the site of cannulation.
- Be available to provide assistance to the physician throughout the procedure.
- Adjust intravenous line connected to the introducer to maintain patency.
- Observe waveform patterns on the monitor screen and record pressures as the catheter advances through the chambers in the heart.
- Have lidocaine hydrochloride available for arrhythmias.
- Ensure that balloon is deflated. Deflate balloon passively.
- Anticipate orders for chest radiograph film to verify catheter placement.
- Apply dressing after physician secures introducer.
- Observe monitor screen for continuous tracing of pulmonary artery pressures.

NURSING ASSESSMENTS
- Verify that alarms are set at all times.
- Observe monitor screen closely for pressures and waveforms that denote placement of catheter. Be prepared to intervene when necessary (see Box 31-3).
- Record hemodynamic parameters according to client status and unit care protocols. Follow the procedure for obtaining a pulmonary capillary wedge pressure reading (see Procedure box, p. 744).
- Inspect all connection sites every 2 hours and entire monitor system for presence of air or blood clots.
- Examine insertion site frequently for bleeding or signs of infection. Perform site care every shift or daily, according to unit infection control policy.
- Change pressure and intravenous lines every 24 to 48 hours, according to unit infection control policy.
- Monitor heparinized pressure flush for continuous correct pressure (300 mm Hg).
- Rezero and calibrate transducer every shift and as necessary.

NURSING MANAGEMENT FOR CATHETER REMOVAL
- Document vital signs and ECG pattern.
- Monitor for ECG arrhythmias during removal.
- After catheter removal, pressure to site must be applied for 5 minutes. Anticipate that physician may request application of pressure. Ensure that bleeding has stopped completely before pressure is removed.
- Apply pressure dressing to site, per unit protocol. Keep pressure dressing in place for 8 hours.

DOCUMENTATION
- Presence of signed informed consent form in medical record
- Date, time, site of insertion, type of introducer, and name of physician who performed procedure
- Type of pulmonary catheter, number of attempts, confirmation of placement by x-ray studies, and any ventricular ectopy
- Woman's tolerance of procedure
- Zeroing and calibration of transducers and verification of alarm settings
- Hemodynamic parameters obtained according to client status
- Pertinent nursing assessments and medical and nursing care
- Site assessments and care
- Changes of pressure and intravenous lines
- Date and time of removal of intact catheter, date and time of removal of introducer
- Nursing care and assessments after catheter removal

Hemodynamic monitoring systems have three major components: (1) a pressure transducer that converts physiologic pressures into electrical energy, (2) an amplifier to magnify the volume of the signal being measured, and (3) a monitor screen to display in digital and graphic form the converted physiologic signal (Fig. 31-6).

Waveforms and Pressure Readings

The basis of interpretation of assessments obtained by hemodynamic monitoring is to understand the relation to cardiovascular status of the waveforms observed on the monitor screen and the pressure readings obtained.

Specific chambers in the heart have different pressures that are reflected by changing waveform patterns, and placement of the PAC is evaluated through the pressure and waveform changes that appear on the monitor screen to reflect the position of the catheter. Figure 31-7 displays pressure waveforms in different chambers of the heart.

Because the right atrium is a holding chamber with relatively small muscle mass, the waveform pattern for this chamber has a low amplitude. Right atrium pressures reflect intravascular volume and compliance of the right ventricle. Mean right atrium pressures in pregnancy are relatively low, 0 to 7 mm Hg.

When the catheter is inserted into the right ventricle, pressures change, and a distinct spiking waveform appears. The low-amplitude waveform of the right atrium converts to a high-amplitude waveform with distinct systolic and diastolic components in the right ventricle, with a baseline pressure of 0 mm Hg. Right ventricular pressures are measured as systolic and diastolic. Normal right ventricle systolic pressure is 18 to 30 mm Hg, and the normal diastolic pressure is 0 to 7 mm Hg.

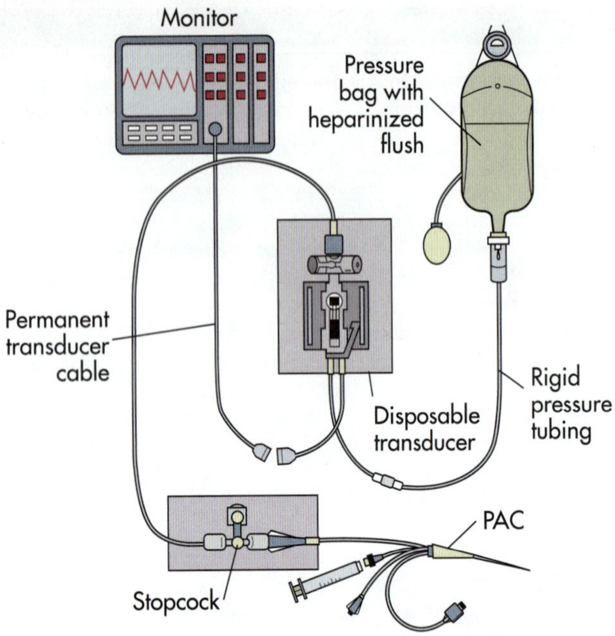

FIG. 31-6 Components of hemodynamic monitoring system: pressurized tubing, pressure transducer, and hemodynamic monitor.

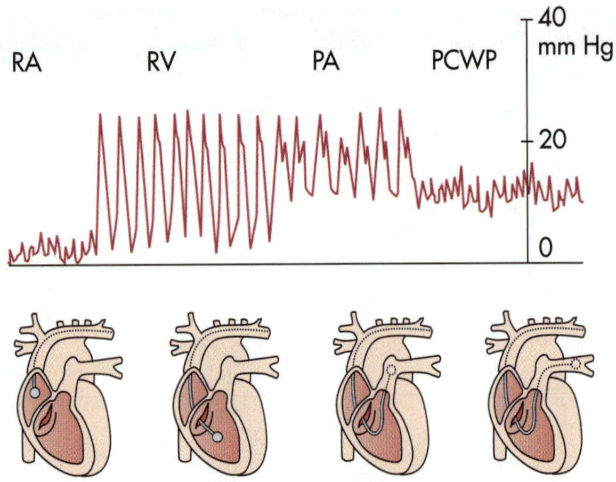

FIG. 31-7 Pressure waveform in relation to catheter position from right atrium *(RA)*, to right ventricle *(RV)*, to pulmonary artery *(PA)*, to pulmonary capillary wedge pressure *(PCWP)*.

The catheter is then advanced into the pulmonary artery. This is reflected by a different spiking waveform with baseline pressures greater than 0 mm Hg. Pulmonary artery systolic pressures are equal to the systolic pressures in the right ventricle, but pulmonary artery diastolic pressures abruptly increase to the range of 6 to 10 mm Hg.

The catheter advances through the pulmonary artery as far as possible and becomes "wedged" in the vessel. This wedging is reflected by a distinct waveform of a dampened tracing with respiratory variation. This relatively low amplitude reflects the low pressures in the capillary beds of the lungs.

The PCWP is obtained when the balloon is inflated, with all pressures from the right side of the heart obstructed, so that the distal port now reads pressures from the left side of the heart across the lungs, because there are no valves in the pulmonary circulation. The PCWP measures left atrial filling pressures or left-sided preload. During right ventricular diastole, the pulmonic valve is closed, with the mitral valve open; the diastolic PAP is measured. In the absence of a problem, such as mitral valve disease or pulmonary edema, PAP diastolic readings reflect PCWP or left ventricular preload. The diastolic PAP is therefore used clinically to reflect left preload (Darovic, 2002). See the Procedure box that explains how to obtain a PCWP reading.

The normal PCWP during pregnancy is 6 to 10 mm Hg. Pressures higher than 20 mm Hg are usually caused by abnormal left ventricular performance, such as left ventricular failure, mitral valve stenosis, or fluid volume overload. Lower than normal readings are seen usually with hypovolemia (see Fig. 31-7).

Box 31-3 describes nursing measures for managing selected problems that may arise with a PAC.

Arterial Pressure Catheter

Percutaneous arterial catheterization, in which a Teflon intravenous catheter, usually 20 gauge, is placed in an artery and connected to a hemodynamic monitor by a pressure line, provides continuous measurements of the systolic, diastolic, and mean arterial blood pressures. The **arterial pressure catheter** produces a waveform and provides access for ABG sampling and analysis.

Indications for use of this type of hemodynamic monitoring include situations in which frequent and accurate BP measurements are needed, such as the administration of potent drugs (e.g., dopamine to treat septic shock or nitroprusside to treat severe hypertensive disease), or when frequent ABG determinations are needed. Characteristics of desirable arteries for an arterial line are: (1) a vessel that has a diameter large enough for accurate measurement of pressure without occlusion of the artery by the catheter, (2) adequate collateral circulation, (3) ease of access to the site for care, and (4) a site not prone to infection. The most common vessels used in the pregnant woman are the radial, axillary, and pedal arteries, in that order.

In preparation for insertion of the arterial line into the radial artery, explain the procedure to the woman in simple terms. Obtain her informed consent and perform Allen's test to confirm collateral circulation into the hand by demonstrating a patent ulnar artery. Box 31-4 describes the steps to perform Allen's test.

PROCEDURE

Obtaining a Pulmonary Capillary Wedge Pressure Reading

1. Inflate balloon slowly while observing waveform on monitor screen. Stop inflation as soon as pulmonary artery waveform changes to pulmonary capillary wedge pressure waveform.
2. Note amount of air necessary to achieve capillary wedge waveform. Do *not* inflate balloon further than necessary to obtain capillary wedge waveform.
3. Keep balloon inflated only long enough to obtain pressure reading, about 5 seconds. Complications associated with sustained wedging (more than 10 seconds) are pulmonary infarction and pulmonary rupture.
4. Release syringe and allow balloon to deflate passively. Do *not* aspirate air from syringe. (Passive deflation of the balloon correlates with an intact balloon.)
5. Note return of pulmonary artery waveform after deflation of balloon.
6. Document assessments made.

BOX 31-3 TROUBLESHOOTING PULMONARY ARTERY CATHETER PROBLEMS

SPONTANEOUS WEDGING: PCWP WAVEFORM APPEARS ON MONITOR SCREEN

- Assess syringe. Determine if balloon is inflated or deflated.
- Have the woman turn her head, cough deeply two or three times, and then take a few deep breaths while observing monitor screen for return of pulmonary artery waveform.
- If wedge waveform continues, call physician immediately to the bedside to reposition catheter. (Catheter will need to be pulled back into larger-diameter vessel.)
- Monitor screen for return of pulmonary artery waveform.

MIGRATION OF CATHETER BACKWARD: RIGHT VENTRICULAR WAVEFORM ON SCREEN

- Call physician immediately to bedside to reposition catheter. (Balloon must be reinflated for catheter to flow back into the pulmonary artery.)
- Monitor electrocardiogram (ECG) pattern for ventricular ectopy, especially premature ventricular contractions if catheter tip irritates wall of right ventricle.
- Have lidocaine hydrochloride available.

SUSPECTED BALLOON RUPTURE: ABSENCE OF RESISTANCE FELT WHEN INFLATING BALLOON OR INABILITY TO OBTAIN PCWP READING

- Confirm tight attachment of syringe. Do *not* inject air. Slowly withdraw plunger.
- Rupture may be assumed if unable to aspirate blood or fluid because of absence of resistance in syringe. Do *not* inject any air. Tape closed and label balloon inflation port, "balloon rupture."
- Notify physician.
- Usually does not necessitate change of catheter, especially if diastolic PAP and PCWP readings have been similar. Diastolic PAP will be monitored to reflect left preload values.

PAP, Pulmonary artery pressure; *PCWP,* pulmonary capillary wedge pressure.

BOX 31-4 ALLEN'S TEST PROCEDURE

1. Determine the woman's dominant hand. Use opposite extremity.
2. Elevate woman's hand and occlude both radial and ulnar arteries.
3. Have woman clench and unclench fist to facilitate venous drainage.
4. Observe that palm is blanched.
5. Release pressure on the ulnar artery only. Radial artery remains occluded.
6. Observe and time the palm for capillary refill (normal time is ≤5 seconds).
7. If it takes more than 5 seconds, collateral circulation may be impaired.

The most common risk associated with an intraarterial line is infection. More serious but less common risks include hemorrhage, thrombus formation, and embolization. The heparinized continuous flush solution of the pressure line helps prevent thrombus formation. Once the line is in place, a transparent occlusive dressing is applied. The transducer is then rezeroed, and an armboard is used to prevent movement of the wrist.

The hemodynamic monitor displays an arterial waveform and the systolic, diastolic, and MAPs for the health care team to interpret. Normal versus abnormal waveforms must be recognized at the bedside, and immediate intervention must be available if indicated. The normal waveform should include the following (Fig. 31-8):

- Rapid upstroke to systole
- Clear dicrotic notch, which denotes closure of the aortic valve
- Definite end-diastolic wave

A blood pressure taken with a sphygmomanometer should be ascertained periodically to verify accuracy of the hemodynamic monitor.

Continuing assessments and documentation include the following:

- Systolic and diastolic arterial pressures
- Cuff pressure readings
- Intraarterial strip recording
- Site care
- Dressing and line changes
- Transducer zeroing and calibration
- Description of the circulation in the extremity

Pressure Lines

All pressure lines use a specialized high-pressure tubing to transmit the physiologic signal to the transducer and monitor. The pressure tubing is rigid to prevent the dampening or absorption of pressure itself, so that the physiologic pressures are transmitted directly from the catheter tip to the transducer through the fluid that fills the length of the tubing. The line includes a continuous flushing mechanism to ensure patency (see Fig. 31-6).

Data Collection

Continuous measurements of the CVP and PAPs and intermittent PCWPs are obtained from the PAC. CO is also calculated intermittently by the use of a PAC with the thermodilution technique (see the Procedure box that explains how to make and record hemodynamic assessments). Electrocardiographic (ECG) monitoring permits continuous evaluation of HR and rhythm. Newer ECG monitors with sensitive leads connected to the chest wall also monitor respiratory rate. Systemic arterial BP can be evaluated by a manual or an automatic sphygmomanometer or by an arterial pressure line. Placement of an arterial

PROCEDURE

Making and Recording Hemodynamic Assessments

1. Position the woman in supine position with a hip wedge.
2. Rezero all pressure transducers.
3. Print a strip recording of the PAC and arterial line blood pressures. Observe oscilloscope for mean values.
4. Record findings of the PAP, central venous pressure, and arterial BP.
5. Calibrate PCWP according to the Procedure box for obtaining a PCWP reading. Record the mean determination.
6. Calibrate CO according to the Procedure box outlining the thermodilution procedure for measuring CO.
7. Document all findings and woman's tolerance of procedures.

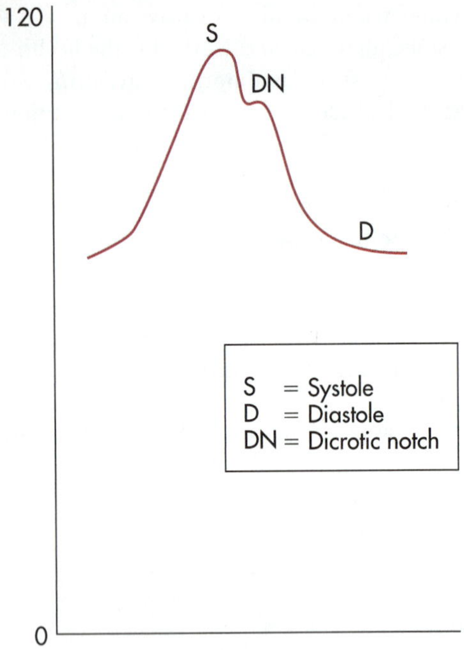

FIG. 31-8 Arterial waveform.

pressure line also permits ready access for frequent arterial blood sampling and analysis, especially for ABGs.

The PCWP is reported as a mean value, determined by the average of its maximal and minimal deflections on the monitor screen or oscilloscope. Reading values from the oscilloscope is usually adequate for clinical management at the bedside; however, for complex cases, strip chart recordings are recommended (see the Procedure box on p. 745 that explains how to make and record hemodynamic assessments).

When the thermodilution procedure to calculate CO in a pregnant woman is performed, the injectate should be chilled to obtain an accurate reading because of the high COs normal for pregnancy (Wallace & Winslow, 1993). The thermistor at the tip of the PAC measures the speed with which the blood temperature cools and returns to normal after the chilled fluid is injected. The time required for the temperature changes is computed, and a CO readout is given. See the Procedure box that describes the thermodilution procedure for measuring CO.

PROCEDURE

Thermodilution Procedure for Measuring Cardiac Output

1. Enter the CO coefficient into the computer.
2. Chill injectate in ice bath.
3. Use insulated syringe.
4. Flush coiled tubing with injectate solution to remove all air.
5. Connect syringe to three-way stopcock at the proximal port.
6. Draw injectate (5 or 10 ml per unit protocol) into insulated syringe.
7. Depress the CO control on the computer.
8. Inject the injectate as rapidly as possible with both hands. Observe oscilloscope for a smooth curve.
9. Repeat the procedure twice. Calculate results. If readings are within 15% of each other, average the three to determine CO. If not, omit the highest and lowest.

Oxygenation

Oxygen delivery to and use by the peripheral tissues must be adequate. Determination of oxygen transport is essential in the care of the critically ill pregnant woman. Oxygen delivery is directly proportional to CO; if CO decreases 50%, oxygen delivery decreases 50%. Conversely, increasing CO 50% doubles oxygen delivery. Oxygen delivery also can be improved by increasing the hemoglobin value, which can be accomplished by the administration of red blood cells.

Sao$_2$ Monitoring. Oxygen is transported to the tissues in two ways: dissolved in plasma and bound to hemoglobin. The oxygen dissolved in plasma (Pao$_2$) makes up only 1% to 2% of the total oxygen content, whereas the oxygen bound to hemoglobin (Sao$_2$) makes up 98% to 99% of the total oxygen content. Results of arterial blood gas determination reflect the dissolved oxygen according to the Pao$_2$ value. The Pao$_2$ reflects the partial pressure that oxygen exerts when it is dissolved in blood; it is measured in millimeters of mercury. The normal Pao$_2$ for the pregnant state is 100 to 106 mm Hg. The adequacy of maternal oxygenation for delivery to the fetus can be evaluated by the usual methods of fetal well-being assessment such as electronic fetal monitoring or biophysical profile. The partial pressure of the oxygen tension is important because circulation transports the higher Pao$_2$ blood to organs with a lower Pao$_2$, and gas exchange occurs as gases move from the higher concentration to the lower concentration. The higher tension (Pao$_2$) pushes the oxygen molecule off the hemoglobin molecule through the cell membrane so that tissues receive a supply of oxygen.

The oxygen that cells can use is the oxygen molecules bound to hemoglobin (Sao$_2$). Each molecule of hemoglobin has four binding sites for oxygen. When all four sites are bound, an oxyhemoglobin molecule results. The saturation of hemoglobin with oxygen (Sao$_2$) is evaluated with the pulse oximeter (Sao$_2$ monitoring). The normal range for Sao$_2$ is 95% to 100%, and normal Sao$_2$ values for pregnancy are 97% to 100%. Critically ill pregnant women benefit from continuous Sao$_2$ monitoring.

Svo$_2$ Monitoring. The percentage of saturation of hemoglobin with oxygen in mixed venous and arterial blood is reflected as an Svo$_2$ value. Svo$_2$ monitoring involves insertion of a fiberoptic PAC that is connected to a bedside microprocessor to give a continuous Svo$_2$ value. Mixed venous blood saturation reflects the balance between oxygen delivery and oxygen use. It reflects tissue perfusion, the variation in oxygen requirements for different organs, and the affinity of hemoglobin to accept and then release oxygen. The normal value of Svo$_2$ is 60% to 80%. Values less than 60% are interpreted as abnormally low.

Fiberoptic PACs and bedside microprocessors provide the technology to plot the mixed venous blood oxygen saturation continuously. Plotting of mixed venous oxygen content is used as an early warning system because values may decrease before any other evidence of hemodynamic instability is seen (Fujitani & Baldisseri, 2005).

Use of pulse oximetry permits evaluation of the Sao$_2$, arterial blood saturation. Arterial blood usually has a saturation of 90% or greater. Because of the shape of the oxyhemoglobin dissociation curve, fluctuations at the high levels of oxygen tension, 90% and higher, are reflected by a small change in arterial oxygen saturation (Sao$_2$). However, the lower levels of oxygen tension in mixed venous blood (40% or less) produce a linear relation between saturation and tension, resulting in the Svo$_2$ becoming a sensitive alarm to detect physiologic instability.

Arterial blood analysis evaluates pulmonary oxygen exchange and ventilation but does not evaluate overall adequacy of oxygen delivery to the peripheral tissues. However, mixed venous blood analysis (Svo_2) reflects the end product of supply and demand and is used to evaluate overall adequacy of oxygen delivery to the peripheral tissues. This technique provides additional data and can be especially useful to support or change management strategies when used in conjunction with thermodilution CO calculations.

Continuous monitoring of Svo_2 is recommended for titration of vasoactive or inotropic drugs, during adjustments of positive end-expiratory pressure, evaluation of fluid administration, and routine care of critically ill pregnant women.

! NURSING ALERT

Stable CO measurements in conjunction with an improvement in Svo_2 readings are associated with clinical improvement and are a good prognostic sign. The same improved Svo_2 readings in conjunction with a 100% increase in CO are a common first sign of the development of sepsis.

Central Venous Pressure Lines

Before the development of the flow-directed PAC in the early 1970s, CVP lines were used for the critically ill. Two primary problems with the use of CVP lines became apparent. First,

BOX 31-5 CASE STUDIES

CASE 1

Jessica is a 24-year-old, G4P2 client at 35 weeks of gestation, diagnosed with severe preeclampsia. She is scheduled for labor induction today because of the increasing severity of the disease.

Everything went well for the first 5 hours after admission. However, this hour's urine output is only 22 ml. The physician orders a fluid challenge of 1000 ml of lactated Ringer's (LR) solution. One hour after this fluid infusion is completed, urine output is 24 ml.

This is a failed fluid challenge. A Swan-Ganz catheter (PAC) is inserted to determine the volume status and to help determine the cause of the oliguria. The hemodynamic profile is the following:

CVP	2 mm Hg
PAP	15/5 mm Hg
PCWP	4 mm Hg
CO	6.1 L/min

Evaluation

Evaluation of this profile shows a low PCWP of 4 mm Hg, which denotes decreased left preload and reflects hypovolemia. The low PAP reflects the decreased pulmonary circulating volume. CO is low for a laboring woman, probably as a result of the decreased preload. Her CO at 6.1 L/min is probably being maintained by her elevated heart rate; however, she is not in danger of dying with a CO of 6 L/min. This hemodynamic profile correlates with hypovolemia as the reason for oliguria. Urine is not being produced because the renal system is not adequately perfused. Additional fluids are needed rapidly. The oliguria is due to compensatory mechanisms that shunt the blood from the peripheral circulation to the central circulation in response to the extremely low preload. The 1000 ml of fluid given in the fluid challenge was not adequate to correct the hypovolemia. Additional fluid should be administered until left preload is adequate.

CASE 2

Ashley is an 18-year-old G1P0 client at 34 weeks of gestation with a diagnosis of severe preeclampsia. She is scheduled for induction of labor today because of the increasing severity of the disease.

Everything went well for the first 5 hours after admission. However, this hour's urine output is only 23 ml. The physician orders a fluid challenge of 1000 ml of LR. One hour after this fluid is infused, urine output is 24 ml.

This is a failed fluid challenge. A Swan-Ganz catheter (PAC) is inserted to determine the volume status and to help determine the cause of the oliguria. The hemodynamic profile is the following:

CVP	2 mm Hg
PAP	22/9 mm Hg
PCWP	8 mm Hg
CO	7.8 L/min

Evaluation

Evaluation of this profile shows a normal PCWP of 8 mm Hg, a normal PAP, and a CO of 7.8 L/min. A normal hemodynamic profile in conjunction with refractory oliguria is associated with renal artery spasm that decreases perfusion and oxygenation to the kidneys and results in decreased urine output. Renal dose (low-dose) dopamine is used as the first-line management strategy to correct this type of oliguria. An arterial pressure line will be used during administration of the drug to monitor blood pressure closely. Relaxation of the renal artery will improve renal system perfusion and correct the oliguria.

CASE 3

Bonnie is a 32-year-old G5 P4 client, at 36 weeks of gestation with a diagnosis of severe preeclampsia. She is scheduled for labor induction today because of the increasing severity of the disease.

Everything went well for the first 5 hours after admission. However, this hour's urine output is only 20 ml. The physician orders a fluid challenge of 1000 ml of LR. One hour after this fluid infusion is completed, urine output is 22 ml.

This is a failed fluid challenge. A Swan-Ganz catheter (PAC) is inserted to determine the volume status and to help determine the cause of the oliguria. The hemodynamic profile is the following:

CVP	2 mm Hg
PAP	44/20 mm Hg
PCWP	18 mm Hg
CO	6.6 L/min

Evaluation

Evaluation of this profile shows a high PCWP of 18 mm Hg, which denotes an increased left preload. CO is adequate. This profile correlates with oliguria in the hypervolemic pregnant woman. Lack of urine excretion is probably due to renal damage from the ischemia accompanying the severe hypertensive disease. Intravenous fluids should be restricted to 50 ml/hr. The high wedge pressure correlates with pulmonary edema during pregnancy. With such severe preeclampsia, pulmonary edema is usually a combined cardiogenic and noncardiogenic type. Cardiogenic pulmonary edema is a result of the increased SVR, which increases the resistance that the left ventricle must overcome to eject blood. This can lead to congestive heart failure. The noncardiogenic pulmonary edema is a result of an extremely low COP, a result of renal disease and protein excretion. Reduction of left afterload with hydralazine is the initial management strategy to correct the pulmonary edema. CO is adequate, probably because of the increased heart rate and circulating volume. The high PAP reflects the increased pressures in the pulmonary circulation because of the excessive fluid that is present, produced by the increased left afterload. Immediate delivery by cesarean birth will permit further renal studies to evaluate renal function. Dialysis may be indicated.

CO, Cardiac output; *COP,* colloid osmotic pressure; *CVP,* central venous pressure; *PAC,* pulmonary artery catheter; *PAP,* pulmonary artery pressure; *PCWP,* pulmonary capillary wedge pressure; *SVR,* systemic vascular resistance.

CVP monitoring provides right-sided heart information only, the right preload. When a cardiac or pulmonary complication is present, right- and left-sided values are not equal. CVP monitoring gives no information about left ventricular function. Second, changes in CVP values occur much later with left ventricular dysfunction. This type of monitoring does not permit rapid assessment of the effects of treatment modalities. Additionally, several studies reported disparities in the relationship between CVP and PCWP in preeclampsia (Martin & Foley, 2009). Considering that the risks for insertions are similar, when invasive hemodynamic monitoring is required, use of the PAC is preferred.

Interpretation of Hemodynamic Data

Data obtained with hemodynamic monitoring techniques include values that reflect blood volume in the pulmonary and systemic circulations, which profoundly affect cardiac performance, in the following ways:

- Right atrial pressure or CVP indicates right end-diastolic pressure and reflects right preload.
- PAP: PVR is the calculation for right afterload. Clinically, mean PAP reflects right afterload.
- Diastolic PAP approximates PCWP and reflects left preload.
- PCWP indicates left end-diastolic pressure and reflects left preload.
- CO refers to the volume of blood ejected from the left ventricle in liters per minute.
- SVR is the calculation for left afterload; arterial BP reflects left afterload.

Hemodynamic profiles provide valuable data for evaluating the status of the woman and changing treatment strategies as needed. Normal hemodynamic values in pregnancy to be used for calculations in the cases described in the following material are shown in Table 31-4. Table 31-5 compares normal nonpregnant hemodynamic values with normal values during pregnancy.

TABLE 31-4 NORMAL HEMODYNAMIC VALUES IN PREGNANCY

Right atrial pressure (RAP) or central venous pressure (CVP)	0-7 mm Hg
Pulmonary artery pressure (PAP)	18-30 mm Hg (systolic) 6-10 mm Hg (diastolic)
Pulmonary capillary wedge pressure (PCWP)	6 10 mm Hg
Cardiac output (CO)	6-7 L/min
Systemic vascular resistance (SVR)	1210 ± 266
Pulmonary vascular resistance (PVR)	78 ±22

TABLE 31-5 CENTRAL HEMODYNAMIC NORMAL VALUES

PARAMETER	NONPREGNANT	PREGNANT
CO (L/min)	4.3 ± 0.9	6.2 ± 1
HR (beats/min)	71 ± 10	83 ± 10
SVR (dynes/cm/sec^{-5})	1530 ± 520	1210 ± 266
PVR (dynes/cm/sec^{-5})	119 ± 47	78 ± 22
PCWP (mm Hg)	6.3 ± 2.1	7.5 ± 1.8
CVP (mm Hg)	3.7 ± 2.6	3.6 ± 2.5
Left ventricular work index	41 ± 8	48 ± 6

Source: Clark, S., et al. (1989). Central hemodynamic assessment of normal term pregnancy. *American Journal of Obstetrics and Gynecology, 16*(6), 1439-1442.

Oliguria is diagnosed if urine output is less than 20 to 30 ml for 2 consecutive hours. It may indicate severe renal dysfunction (Roberts & Funai, 2009). If oliguria is not corrected with fluid challenge, the woman is diagnosed as having oliguria refractory to conservative therapy.

Refractory oliguria caused by preeclampsia may be associated with three different hemodynamic subsets: hypovolemia, hypervolemia, and renal artery spasm. Treatment strategies for correction of oliguria are different for each hemodynamic subset. Noninvasive assessments do not differentiate the type of treatment that would be appropriate for the pregnant woman. Recognition of which hemodynamic subset has produced the refractory oliguria is obtained only by the use of a PAC. Failure to use a PAC when refractory oliguria is present can result in inappropriate treatment.

Examples of three different pregnant women with preeclampsia complicated by refractory oliguria are included in Box 31-5 to demonstrate how useful hemodynamic monitoring is in determining the appropriate care for the individual woman with this complication. These three women, all with severe preeclampsia with similar noninvasive assessment findings, illustrate the need for use of a PAC when the pregnant woman with hypertensive disease and oliguria fails a fluid challenge test. Noninvasive parameters do not reflect volume status. Completely different treatment modalities to correct oliguria are indicated for each of these three women.

? CLINICAL REASONING

Nursing Care of the Critically Ill Pregnant Woman

Celesta, a 34-year-old G3 P1, is brought to the hospital by ambulance with complaints of severe epigastric pain that she had when she awoke that morning. She is at 31 weeks of gestation. Her blood pressure (BP) is 190/110 mm Hg. An intravenous (IV) line is started and blood drawn to rule out preeclampsia. Urine dipstick shows 4+ proteinuria, and magnesium sulfate is started for seizure prophylaxis. An indwelling catheter is inserted to assess urine output. The laboratory results are indicative of severe preeclampsia with elevated liver enzymes. Induction of labor is started with oxytocin. She has been on oxytocin for 4 hours. Her last hourly urine output was 20 ml. The physician orders a fluid challenge of 1000 ml lactated Ringer's solution (LR). In 1 hour, her urine output is 24 ml. A pulmonary artery catheter is inserted to determine volume status and the cause of oliguria.

Her hemodynamic profile is as follows:

CVP	3 mm Hg
PAP	15/4 mm Hg
PCWP	5 mm Hg
CO	6.5 L/min

1. Evidence—Is there sufficient information to determine what action is needed?
2. Assumptions—What assumptions can be made about the following?
   a. Fluid challenge as treatment for hypovolemia
   b. Hemodynamic values in pregnancy
3. What implications and priorities for nursing care can be made at this time?
4. Does the evidence objectively support your conclusion?
5. Are there alternative perspectives to your conclusion?

Pulmonary Edema. One of the most common uses of the PAC during pregnancy is the differentiation of cardiogenic (heart failure or hydrostatic) pulmonary edema from noncardiogenic (permeability or lung failure) pulmonary edema (Mabie, 2004). Optimal therapies for the two types of pulmonary edema are dramatically different; however, the correct diagnosis can be determined only by evaluation of the hemodynamic profile.

Cardiogenic or heart failure pulmonary edema develops as a result of left ventricular failure or acute fluid overload. The PCWP is elevated because of the increased volume of fluid in the pulmonary circulation. Therapy is focused on improvement of myocardial contractility with an inotropic drug, decreasing left afterload, if elevated, with an arterial vasodilator and reducing preload to a normal range with a diuretic drug. This type of pulmonary edema usually responds to therapy within a few hours, and a normal PCWP is restored.

Pulmonary edema also may result from damage to the pulmonary alveolar capillary membrane by numerous factors, the most common being sepsis. Disturbance of membrane permeability results in the leakage of both protein and fluid into the pulmonary interstitium and alveoli, in the presence of normal cardiac function and ventricular filling pressures (Mabie, 2004). The PCWP is normal. Alveolar membranes require days to heal, and ARDS may develop if the source of injury is not found and eradicated. The focus of therapy is to maintain the PCWP in the low-normal range to minimize transudation of protein and fluid into the lung and to eliminate the source of injury.

When radiography reveals pulmonary edema, evaluation of the hemodynamic profile is the only way to correctly diagnose the type of pulmonary edema present, as illustrated in the following two hemodynamic profiles (refer to Table 31-4 for the normal values):

Case I

CVP	4 mm Hg
PAP	44/21 mm Hg
PCWP	20 mm Hg
CO	6.1 L/min

The high wedge pressure reflects a high left preload and correlates with cardiogenic pulmonary edema. Treatment includes an inotropic drug such as dobutamine, a vasodilator such as hydralazine if hypertension is present, and a diuretic such as furosemide (Lasix) because CO is adequate.

Case II

CVP	2 mm Hg
PAP	23/8 mm Hg
PCWP	7 mm Hg
CO	7.1 L /min

All readings are in the normal range, although pulmonary edema is present. This correlates with noncardiogenic pulmonary edema. A diuretic should not be administered. Preload is in the low-normal range. Reducing the preload with a diuretic drug could decrease CO and jeopardize the woman's status. Instead, sepsis should be suspected, and treatment should focus on antibiotic therapy and elimination of foci of infection, continuing assessments, and support of vital systems while lung membranes heal.

TRAUMA DURING PREGNANCY

Trauma continues to be a common complication during pregnancy because of the continuation of usual activities by the majority of pregnant women in the United States.

Significance

Approximately 8% of pregnancies have been reported to be complicated by physical trauma (Brown, 2009). As pregnancy progresses, the risk of trauma seems to increase because more cases of trauma are reported in the third trimester than earlier in gestation. Most maternal injuries are a result of motor vehicle accidents and falls. Other sources of trauma include intimate partner violence, assaults, and suicide attempts (Martin & Foley, 2009).

Trauma is the leading nonobstetric cause of maternal mortality (Brown, 2009). Motor vehicle accidents account for more than 50% of maternal trauma incidents. About 50% of fetal deaths are associated with maternal trauma, and most of these are due to motor vehicle accidents. Maternal death caused by trauma is usually the result of head injury or hemorrhagic shock. Fetal death usually occurs as a result of maternal death or because of placental abruption (abruptio placentae). Fortunately the majority of trauma injuries during pregnancy are minor and have no effect on pregnancy outcome. However, each case of trauma during pregnancy must be evaluated carefully because pregnancy can mask signs of severe injury.

Multisystem trauma during pregnancy is usually the result of a serious motor vehicle crash, especially if the woman is not wearing a seat belt with a shoulder harness and is ejected from the vehicle. To improve chances of survival for mother and fetus, pregnant women should wear properly positioned restraints at all times when in a motor vehicle (see Fig. 15-17) (Cunningham, Leveno, Bloom, Hauth, Rouse, & Spong, 2010).

The effect of trauma on pregnancy is influenced by the length of gestation, type and severity of the trauma, and degree of disruption of uterine and fetal physiologic features. Trauma increases the incidence of preterm labor and birth, placental abruption, and fetal or neonatal death (Martin & Foley, 2009). Other common fetal effects of trauma include premature rupture of membranes (PROM), fetomaternal transfusion, skull injuries, and hypoxia because of maternal respiratory compromise. Trauma results in fetal death more often than in maternal death (Gilbert, 2011).

Special considerations for mother and fetus are necessary when trauma occurs during pregnancy because of the physiologic alterations that accompany pregnancy and because of the presence of the fetus. Fetal survival depends on maternal survival; therefore, the pregnant woman must receive immediate stabilization and appropriate care for optimal fetal outcome.

Maternal Physiologic Characteristics

Optimal care for the pregnant woman after trauma is dependent on understanding the physiologic state of pregnancy and its effects on trauma. The pregnant woman's body will exhibit responses different from those of a nonpregnant person to the same traumatic insults. Because of the different responses to injury during pregnancy, management strategies must be adapted for appropriate resuscitation, fluid therapy, positioning, assessments, and most other interventions. Significant maternal adaptations and the relation to trauma are summarized in Table 31-6.

The uterus and bladder are confined to the bony pelvis during the first trimester of pregnancy and are at reduced risk for injury in cases of abdominal trauma. After pregnancy progresses beyond the fourteenth week, the uterus becomes an abdominal organ, and the risk for injury in cases of abdominal trauma increases. During the second and third trimesters, the distended bladder becomes an abdominal organ and is at increased risk for injury and rupture. Bowel injuries occur less often during pregnancy because of the protection provided by the enlarged uterus.

The elevated levels of progesterone that accompany pregnancy relax smooth muscle and profoundly affect the gastrointestinal tract. Gastrointestinal motility decreases, with a resultant increased time required for gastric emptying, whereas the production of hydrochloric acid increases in the last trimester, and the gastroesophageal sphincter relaxes (Norwitz et al., 2004). Airway management of the unconscious pregnant woman is of critical importance.

! NURSING ALERT

The unconscious pregnant woman is at increased risk for regurgitation of gastric contents and aspiration whenever her head is positioned lower than her stomach or if abdominal pressure is applied.

A pregnant woman has decreased tolerance for hypoxia and apnea because of her decreased functional residual capacity and increased renal loss of bicarbonate. Acidosis develops more quickly in the pregnant than in the nonpregnant state.

CO increases 44% to 50% over prepregnancy values and is position dependent in the third trimester. Because of compression of the inferior vena cava and descending aorta by the pregnant uterus, CO will decrease dramatically if the woman is placed in the supine position. The supine position must be avoided, even in women with cervical spine injuries. It is a primary priority that lateral uterine displacement be accomplished without any head movement. As soon as the neck is immobilized, the stretcher should be tilted laterally.

Circulating blood volume increases 40% to 50% during gestation, and pregnant women can tolerate a 1000 ml blood loss readily without demonstrating clinical signs. Hemodynamic instability that indicates the need for transfusion may not be apparent until blood loss exceeds 1500 ml (Martin & Foley, 2009). Clinical signs of hemorrhage do not appear until after a 30% loss of circulating volume occurs. Although HR increases with pregnancy, a maternal HR greater than 100 beats/min should be considered abnormal.

TABLE 31-6 **MATERNAL ADAPTATIONS DURING PREGNANCY AND RELATION TO TRAUMA**

SYSTEM	ALTERATION	CLINICAL RESPONSES
Respiratory	↑ Oxygen consumption	↑ Risk of acidosis
	↑ Tidal volume	↑ Risk of respiratory mismanagement
	↓ Functional residual capacity	
	Chronic compensated alkalosis ↓ $Paco_2$ ↓ Serum bicarbonate	↓ Blood-buffering capacity
Cardiovascular	↑ Circulating volume, 1600 ml	Can lose 1000 ml blood
	↑ CO	No signs of shock until blood loss >30% total blood volume
	↑ Heart rate	
	↓ SVR	↓ Placental perfusion in supine position
	↓ Arterial blood pressure	
	Heart displaced upward to left	Point of maximal impulse, fourth intercostal space
Renal	↑ Renal plasma flow	
	Dilation of ureters and urethra	↑ Risk of stasis, infection
	Bladder displaced forward	↑ Risk of bladder trauma
Gastrointestinal	↓ Gastric motility	↑ Risk of aspiration
	↑ Hydrochloric acid production	
	↓ Competency of gastroesophageal sphincter	Passive regurgitation of stomach acids if head lower than stomach
Reproductive	↑ Blood flow to organs	↑ Source of increased blood loss
	Uterine enlargement	Vena caval compression in supine position
Musculoskeletal	Displacement of abdominal viscera	↑ Risk of injury, altered rebound response
	Pelvic venous congestion	Altered pain referral
	Cartilage softened	↑ Risk of pelvic fracture Center of gravity changed
	Fetal head in pelvis	↑ Risk of fetal injury
Hematologic	↑ Clotting factors	↑ Risk of thrombus formation
	↓ Fibrinolytic activity	

CO, Cardiac output; *$Paco_2$*, arterial partial pressure of carbondioxide; *SVR*, systemic vascular resistance.

Fetal Physiologic Characteristics

Perfusion of the uterine arteries, which provide the primary blood supply to the uteroplacental unit, depends on adequate maternal arterial pressure, because these vessels lack autoregulation. Therefore maternal hypotension decreases uterine and fetal perfusion. Maternal shock results in splanchnic and uterine artery vasoconstriction, which decreases blood flow and oxygen transport to the fetus. Electronic fetal monitoring (EFM) tracings can assist in the evaluation of maternal status after trauma. EFM tracings reflect fetal cardiac responses to hypoxia and hypoperfusion, including tachycardia or bradycardia, minimal or absent baseline variability, and late decelerations.

Careful monitoring of fetal status assists greatly in maternal assessment, because the fetal monitor tracing works as an "oximeter" of internal maternal well-being. Hypoperfusion may be present in the pregnant woman before the onset of clinical signs of shock. The EFM tracings show the first signs of maternal compromise, such as when maternal HR, BP, and color appear normal, yet the EFM printout shows signs of fetal hypoxia (Murray, 2007).

Mechanisms of Trauma

Blunt Abdominal Trauma

Blunt abdominal trauma is most commonly the result of motor vehicle crashes but also may be the result of battering or falls. Maternal and fetal mortality and morbidity rates are directly correlated with whether the mother remains inside the vehicle or is ejected. Maternal death is usually the result of a head injury or exsanguination from a major vessel rupture. Serious retroperitoneal hemorrhage after lower abdominal and pelvic trauma is reported more frequently during pregnancy. Serious maternal abdominal injuries are usually the result of splenic rupture or liver or renal injury.

When the mother survives, placental abruption is the most common cause of fetal death (Gilbert, 2011). Placental separation is thought to be a result of deformation of the elastic myometrium around the relatively inelastic placenta. Shearing of the placental edge from the underlying decidua basalis results and is worsened by the increased intrauterine pressure resulting from the impact. It is critical that all pregnant victims be carefully evaluated for signs and symptoms of placental abruption after even minor blunt abdominal trauma.

! NURSING ALERT

Signs and symptoms of placental abruption include uterine tenderness or pain, uterine irritability, uterine contractions, vaginal bleeding, leaking of amniotic fluid, or a change in FHR characteristics.

Pelvic fracture may result from severe injury and may produce bladder trauma or retroperitoneal bleeding with the two-point displacement of pelvic bones that usually occurs. One point of displacement is commonly at the symphysis pubis, and the second point is posterior, because of the structure of the pelvis. Careful evaluation for clinical signs of internal hemorrhage is indicated.

Direct fetal injury as a complication of trauma during pregnancy most often involves the fetal skull and brain. Most commonly this injury accompanies maternal pelvic fracture in late gestation, after the fetal head becomes engaged. When the force of the impact is great enough to fracture the maternal pelvis, the fetus will often sustain a skull fracture. Evaluation for fetal skull fracture or intracranial hemorrhage is indicated.

Uterine rupture as a result of trauma is rare, occurring in less than 1% of severe cases. Rupture is more likely in a previously scarred uterus. When uterine rupture occurs, it is usually associated with a direct blow delivered with substantial force (Cunningham et al., 2010). Fetal death is common with traumatic uterine rupture. However, maternal death occurs less than 10% of the time, and when it occurs, it is usually the result of massive injuries sustained from an impact severe enough to rupture the uterus.

Penetrating Abdominal Trauma

Bullet wounds are the most frequent cause of penetrating abdominal injury, followed by stab wounds. When the uterus sustains penetrating wounds, the fetus is more likely than the mother to be seriously injured. The enlarged uterus may protect other maternal organs, particularly the bowel, but the fetus is more vulnerable (Cunningham et al., 2010; Martin & Foley, 2009).

Numerous factors determine the extent and severity of maternal and fetal injury from a bullet wound, including size and velocity of the bullet, anatomic region penetrated, angle of entry, path of the bullet, organs damaged, gestational age, and exit wound. Once the bullet enters the body, it may ricochet several times as it encounters organs or bone, or it may sever a large blood vessel. During the second half of pregnancy, the fetus usually sustains a direct injury from the bullet. Gunshot wounds require surgical exploration to determine the extent of injury and repair damage as needed.

Stab wounds are limited by the length and width of the penetrating object and are usually confined to the pathway of the weapon. Maternal and fetal injury is less if the stab wound is located in the upper abdomen and from movement of the penetrating object from above the head downward toward the abdomen than from movement of the penetrating object from the ground upward toward the lower abdomen. Stab wounds usually require surgical exploration to clean out debris, determine extent of injury, and repair damage.

Thoracic Trauma

Thoracic trauma is reported to produce 25% of all trauma deaths. Pulmonary contusion results from nearly 75% of blunt thoracic trauma and is a potentially life-threatening condition. Pulmonary contusion can be difficult to recognize, especially if flail chest also is present or if there is no evidence of thoracic injury. Pulmonary contusion should be suspected in cases of thoracic injury, especially after blunt acceleration or deceleration trauma, such as that occurring when a rapidly moving vehicle crashes into an immovable object.

Penetrating wounds into the chest can result in pneumothorax or hemothorax. This type of injury is usually caused by a vehicular crash that results in impalement by the steering column or a loose article in the vehicle that became a projectile with the force of impact. Stab wounds into the chest also may occur as a result of violence.

Immediate Stabilization

Immediate priorities for stabilization of the pregnant woman after trauma should be identical to those of the nonpregnant trauma client. Pregnancy should not result in any restriction of the usual diagnostic, pharmacologic, or resuscitative procedures or maneuvers (American Academy of Pediatrics [AAP] & ACOG, 2007). The initial response of many trauma team members when caring for the pregnant woman is to assess fetal status first because of the concern for a healthy neonate. Instead, the trauma team should follow a methodical evaluation of maternal status to ensure complete assessment and stabilization of the mother. Fetal survival depends on maternal survival, and stabilization of the mother improves the chance of fetal survival.

! NURSING ALERT

Priorities of care for the pregnant woman after trauma must be to resuscitate the woman and stabilize her condition first, and then consider fetal needs.

Primary Survey

The systematic evaluation begins with a *primary survey* and the initial *ABCDs* of resuscitation: establishment of and maintaining an *airway*, ensuring adequate *breathing*, maintenance of an adequate *circulatory volume*, and *defibrillation*. If defibrillation is needed, the paddles need to be placed one rib interspace higher than usual because the heart is displaced slightly by the enlarged uterus.

Increased oxygen needs during gestation necessitate a rapid response. The presence of a cervical spine injury is always assumed.

> **! NURSING ALERT**
>
> Hyperextension of the neck is avoided; instead jaw thrust is used to establish an airway for the trauma victim.

Once an airway is established, assessment should focus on adequacy of oxygenation. The chest wall is observed for movement. If breathing is absent, ventilations and endotracheal intubation are initiated. Supplemental oxygen should be administered with a tight-fitting, nonrebreathing face mask at 10 to 12 L/min to maintain adequate oxygen availability to the fetus. The chest wall is assessed for penetrating chest wound or flail chest. Breathing with a flail chest will be rapid and labored; chest wall movements will be uncoordinated and asymmetric; crepitus from bony fragments may be palpated.

Rapid placement of two large-bore (14- to 16-gauge) intravenous lines is necessary in the majority of seriously injured clients. It is important to place the lines while veins are still distended. Cardiac arrest during the immediate stabilization period is usually the result of profound hypovolemia, necessitating massive fluid resuscitation. Infusion of crystalloids such as Ringer's solution or normal saline solution should be given as a 3:1 ratio; that is, 3 ml of crystalloid replacement to 1 ml of the estimated blood loss is given over the first 30 to 60 minutes of acute resuscitation (ACOG, 2006). Because of the 50% increase in blood volume during pregnancy, published formulas for nonpregnant adults used for estimating crystalloid and blood replacement to counter blood loss must be adjusted upward for pregnancy.

Replacement of red blood cells and other blood components is anticipated, and blood is drawn for type, crossmatch, complete blood cell count, and platelet count. Infusion of type-specific whole blood or packed red blood cells is usually necessary to improve fetal oxygenation status and to replace blood loss. During an extreme emergency, type O Rh-negative blood may be administered without matching.

Vasopressor drugs to restore maternal arterial BP should be avoided if possible until volume replacement is administered. Although vasopressor agents result in decreased perfusion to the uterus, they should be given if needed for successful resuscitation of the mother (Lu & Curet, 2007).

After 20 weeks of gestation venous return to the heart is best accomplished by positioning the uterus to one side to eliminate the weight of the uterus compressing the inferior vena cava or the descending aorta. This facilitates efforts to establish the forward flow of blood through resuscitation and stabilization. If a lateral position is not possible because of resuscitative efforts or cervical spine immobilization, the uterus can be manually deflected, or a wedge should be inserted underneath one side of the backboard or stretcher.

Signs of bleeding may be more difficult to recognize in the pregnant woman because a 30% to 35% loss of maternal blood volume may produce only a minimal change in maternal MAP. Hypovolemia can be detrimental for the fetus because the vascular bed of the uterus is a low-resistance system that depends on adequate maternal arterial pressure to maintain uterine and fetal perfusion. Maternal hypovolemia can be fatal for the fetus (Friese & Wojciehoski, 2005).

Establishing a baseline neurologic status (level of consciousness, pupil size and reactivity) is essential. The Glasgow Coma Scale is commonly used at the scene of the accident to help determine the extent of the head injury. The scale is simple and easy to use (Box 31-6).

Secondary Survey

After immediate resuscitation and successful stabilization measures, a more detailed *secondary survey* of the mother and fetus should be accomplished. A complete physical assessment including all body systems is performed (Box 31-7).

The maternal abdomen should be evaluated carefully because a large percentage of serious injuries involve the uterus, intraperitoneal structures, and the retroperitoneum. The pregnant woman's stomach is assumed to be full. A nasogastric tube can be used to empty the stomach to help prevent acid aspiration syndrome. An empty stomach facilitates respiratory efforts. The uterus should be evaluated for evidence of gross deformity, tenderness, or contractions (ACOG, 2006).

The greatest clinical concern after vehicular crashes is placental abruption because up to 40% of these women have an abruption (Brown, 2009). Assessments should focus on recognition of this complication, with careful evaluation of fetal monitor tracings, uterine tenderness, labor, or vaginal bleeding. Ultrasound examination may be performed to determine gestational age, viability of the fetus, and placental location. However, ultrasound studies cannot exclude placental abruption. Most cases of abruption that occur as a result of trauma are associated with relatively minor injuries (Cunningham et al., 2010; Martin & Foley, 2009).

If trauma is the result of a penetrating wound, the woman should be completely undressed and carefully examined for all entrance and exit wounds. Ultrasonography and computed tomography (CT) scan should be performed to assess for the likelihood of intraabdominal bleeding. Peritoneal lavage can be performed on hemodynamically stable women if ultrasound and CT findings do not provide a clear diagnosis. Under direct visualization, the peritoneum is incised, and a peritoneal dialysis catheter is positioned. If aspiration yields free-flowing blood, the test is considered positive, and a laparotomy is warranted (Cunningham et al., 2010; Martin & Foley, 2009).

Exploratory laparotomy is necessary after a gunshot wound to explore the abdominal cavity for organ damage and to repair any damage, with careful examination of all organs, the entire bowel, and posterior vessels. If uterine injury is found, a careful evaluation of the risks and benefits of cesarean birth is quickly accomplished. A cesarean birth is desirable if the fetus is alive

BOX 31-6 GLASGOW COMA SCALE

Eyes	Open	Spontaneously	4
		To verbal command	3
		To pain	2
		No response	1
Best motor response	To verbal command	Obeys	6
	To painful stimulus	Localizes pain	5
		Flexion-withdrawal	4
		Flexion-abnormal (decorticate rigidity)	3
		Extension (decerebrate rigidity)	2
		No response	1
Best verbal response		Oriented and converses	5
		Disoriented and converses	4
		Inappropriate words	3
		Incomprehensible sounds	2
		No response	1
Total			3-15

A score of 3 = deepest coma. A score of 15 = optimal level of consciousness.

and near term and may be necessary for the preterm fetus because of the high incidence of fetal injury in these cases. The fetus usually tolerates surgery and anesthesia if adequate uterine perfusion and oxygenation are maintained. Tetanus prophylaxis guidelines are not changed by pregnancy.

Trauma may affect numerous systems in the maternal body and may affect more than the pregnancy. External signs of maternal trauma should suggest the possibility of internal trauma. Back and neck pain suggest spine injury, abrasions on the chest suggest chest injury, and limb pain and malposition suggest limb fractures. If head injury results in nonresponsiveness, suspect spinal, thoracic, and abdominal injuries. Hypovolemic shock can occur with internal hemorrhage, fracture of long bones, ruptured liver or spleen, hemothorax, or arterial dissection.

Once immediate stabilization is achieved, obstetric clients with severe trauma and massive blood loss that merits vigorous fluid resuscitation will usually benefit from the use of hemodynamic monitoring with a fiberoptic pulmonary catheter to determine cardiac and pulmonary function more precisely and to calculate volume and oxygen needs. The hemodynamic profile permits precise fluid resuscitation volumes. Oxygenation status calculations, including oxygen content, delivery, and consumption, will demonstrate which fluids are needed to enhance oxygen transport. Precise determinations can help prevent the potential sequelae of too little or too much fluid administration. With massive trauma, this care may be best provided in a regional trauma center with the obstetric team working closely with the trauma team, the obstetric team providing the obstetric care while the trauma team provides the trauma care.

All female trauma victims of childbearing age should be considered pregnant until proven otherwise. Determination of the health history and a history of the events preceding the trauma are important components of care. If the pregnant woman was involved in a vehicular crash, it should be determined whether she was the driver or a passenger and if she was ejected from the vehicle or used a restraining device and remained within the vehicle.

The physical examination should be performed in a systematic manner (see Box 31-7).

BOX 31-7 PHYSICAL EXAMINATION OF THE PREGNANT TRAUMA VICTIM

HEAD
- Check scalp for signs of cuts, bruises, or edema. Examine skull for deformities, depressions, or lumps. Examine eyes and eyelids. Evaluate pupils for size, equality, and reaction to light. If contact lenses are present, remove them. Examine nose and ears, and observe for serous or bloody fluid. Open the mouth and look for blood, vomitus, loose teeth, and dentures.
- Neurologic function should be evaluated frequently because the most frequent cause of death in women not using seat belts is head trauma (ACOG, 2006). If neurologic checks show a possible head trauma, a complete neurologic consultation and examination should be obtained quickly, including skull films and computed tomographic examination.

NECK
- Palpate for tenderness over the cervical spine area. Immobilize with a cervical collar and backboard if complaints of tenderness are present or any injury is suspected. Tilt backboard to side as soon as the pregnant woman is placed on backboard.

CHEST
- Observe for lacerations, contusions, wounds, or impaled objects. Observe chest wall movement for symmetry and equal expansion. Assess breath sounds and quality and rate of respirations. Observe for deviated trachea, sounds of sucking wounds, and flail chest. Palpate ribs, sternum, and clavicles.

ABDOMEN
- Observe for lacerations, contusions, wounds, or impaled objects. Perform light and then deep palpation. Apply electronic fetal monitoring (EFM) devices—ultrasound Doppler and tocodynamometer. Palpate for intensity of uterine contractions and determine uterine resting tone. Observe fetal heart rate tracing for normal (reassuring) or abnormal (nonreassuring) characteristics.

LOWER BACK
- Palpate for tenderness. Observe for contusions, deformities, or other signs of injury.

EXTREMITIES
- Examine for deformities, edema, dislocation, bleeding, contusions, and fractures. Palpate for tenderness. Assess radial and pedal pulses. Ask pregnant woman to move extremities; observe response.

VAGINA
- Use digital examination for term gestation without vaginal bleeding; use sterile speculum examination for preterm gestation or if vaginal bleeding is present. Assess for signs of labor, injuries to tissues, or evidence of ruptured membranes.

URINARY TRACT
- Observe for the presence of blood in the urine. Trauma to the lower urinary tract is usually accompanied by a fractured pelvis, requiring use of a Foley catheter. Rupture of the bladder may occur in late pregnancy without a pelvic fracture because the full bladder becomes an abdominal organ. Maintain accurate documentation of intake and output and observe color of urine.

Electronic Fetal Monitoring

External FHR and contraction monitoring is recommended after blunt trauma in a viable gestation for a minimum of 4 hours, regardless of injury severity. Fetal monitoring should be initiated soon after the woman is stable (Cunningham et al., 2010; Martin & Foley, 2009). Continuous EFM may show early signs of placental abruption, including a change in baseline rate, loss of accelerations, or the presence of late decelerations, especially when accompanied by absent or minimal variability. The external device to monitor uterine activity, the tocodynamometer, is unable to measure pressures, and the pattern made with this device shows the frequency and duration of contractions only. Palpation is required to evaluate the intensity of contractions and the uterine resting tone. It is important to palpate between contractions to verify that the uterus is well relaxed. If the uterus does not relax between contractions, placental abruption could be present.

The exact duration of FHR and contraction monitoring required after blunt abdominal trauma is not known. Monitoring should be continued indefinitely if uterine contractions, abnormal (nonreassuring) FHR characteristics, vaginal bleeding, uterine tenderness or irritability, serious maternal injury, or ruptured membranes are present. Most physicians recommend continuous monitoring for at least 24 hours. Most abruptions develop soon after the traumatic event, although in rare cases abruption has developed days afterward (Cunningham et al., 2010; Martin & Foley, 2009).

> **LEGAL TIP: Care of the Pregnant Woman Involved in a Minor Trauma Situation**
>
> After minor trauma the pregnant woman may be discharged after an adequate period of EFM that demonstrates a normal (reassuring, category I) tracing (see Chapter 18) and absence of uterine contractions. However, clear instructions must be given for immediate return if vaginal bleeding, leaking of amniotic fluid, decreased fetal movement, or severe abdominal pain occurs (ACOG, 2006).

Fetal-Maternal Hemorrhage

The potential for fetal-maternal hemorrhage exists after trauma. Hemorrhage can lead to fetal anemia, distress, or even death. If the pregnant trauma victim is Rh negative, fetal-maternal hemorrhage can result in sensitization and hemolytic disease of the neonate. The Kleihauer-Betke assay is often performed in women following blunt abdominal trauma to estimate the amount of fetal blood within the maternal circulation. Because most cases have less than 30 ml of hemorrhage, however, Kleihauer-Betke test results seldom alter management (Cunningham et al., 2010; Martin & Foley, 2009). Usually the routine administration of 300 mcg (one ampule) of $Rh_o(D)$ immunoglobulin is sufficient to protect almost all pregnant trauma clients negative for $Rh_o(D)$ from isoimmunization.

Ultrasound

Ultrasonography after trauma is not as sensitive as EFM for diagnosing placental abruption. Ultrasound may be useful to help establish gestational age, locate the placenta, evaluate cardiac activity (to determine whether the fetus is alive), and determine amniotic fluid volume. Ultrasound may also be used to evaluate the presence of intraabdominal fluid that would suggest the presence of intraabdominal hemorrhage.

Radiation Exposure

If the pregnant woman has sustained serious injuries, any necessary radiographic examination should be performed, regardless of fetal exposure. If radiographic examination would be performed for the nonpregnant trauma victim, it also should be performed for the pregnant woman. Abdominal or pelvic CT scanning can be used to visualize extraperitoneal and retroperitoneal structures and the genitourinary tract. Radiation exposure of less than 5 rads has not been associated with fetal abnormalities or pregnancy loss, and the radiation level associated with abdominal or pelvic CT scans is far below this amount (Martin & Foley, 2009). Blunt head trauma and loss of consciousness necessitate skull films and CT assessment with neurosurgical consultation. Magnetic resonance imaging also can be safely used to assess injuries because it does not produce ionizing radiation (Martin & Foley, 2009).

Perimortem Cesarean Birth

In the presence of multisystem trauma, *perimortem cesarean birth* may be indicated. Removal of the stressor of pregnancy early in the process of resuscitation may increase the chance for maternal survival. Fetal survival is unlikely if cesarean birth is accomplished more than 20 minutes after maternal cardiac arrest. Therefore, to facilitate resuscitative efforts, a cesarean birth should be performed after 4 minutes of resuscitative efforts if there is no evidence of a maternal pulse (Martin & Foley, 2009). It should be emphasized that this procedure is rarely successful.

FAMILY-CENTERED OBSTETRIC CRITICAL CARE

Obstetric critical care should include the components of family-centered maternity care because the critically ill woman also is experiencing pregnancy and birth.

Family-centered critical care includes the following components:

- Open visitation so that spouse, significant other, or family members are present and provide support during labor, birth, and the postpartum period.
- Facilitation of parent-infant contact and attachment. The neonate should be brought to the bedside frequently if the condition permits. When the infant's condition does not permit leaving the neonatal intensive care unit (NICU), pictures of the infant should be placed within focus of the mother's eyes. Staff and family can talk about the infant and keep her updated on the infant's condition.
- Sibling visitation, reassuring the mother that the older child is included in the experience.
- Family visitation as the mother desires. This can be arranged around necessary care procedures. The critically ill mother needs this support, perhaps even more than the healthy mother does.

Obstetric nurses have become accustomed to family-centered maternity care. When the critically ill mother receives care in an OBICU, there seem to be fewer problems for inclusion of the components of family-centered care than when the mother has to be transported to the adult ICU, probably because the obstetric staff is accustomed to this care and the nursery is more readily available to the labor and birth unit than to the ICU. Obstetric and critical care nurses can work together to include the components of family-centered care. Many ICUs are adopting the family-centered care philosophy, which ranges from open visitation to more inclusion of the family in the woman's care—depending mainly on her condition (Henneman & Cardin, 2002).

Never assume that the mother is too ill to see and hold her infant. Encourage this and observe her body language to determine how much contact with the infant she desires. If perinatal loss occurs as a result of severe illness, provide grief support. Initiate all the components of grief support as usual for the institution. Burial plans can be delayed until the mother's condition improves so that her concerns are addressed (see Chapter 38).

MATERNAL DEATH

It is extremely rare for a woman to die in childbirth, but it does happen. The yearly occurrence of maternal deaths in the United States is 12.7 per 100,000 live births (Xu, Kochanek, Murphy, & Tejada-Vera, 2010). The leading causes of maternal death are embolism and preeclampsia. Older women (≥35) and those without prenatal care are at greatest risk. A higher mortality ratio exists in African-American women compared with Caucasian women. The father and extended family who are faced with mourning not only the death of a wife and mother but also the death of a baby have a particularly difficult time. Conversely, the father may be faced with parenting a baby without a surviving mother. Death of a mother disrupts the family structure and leaves the father with the care of a baby when he is greatly distressed. Thus the father and extended family, especially other children and grandparents, need supportive grief counseling at the time of death and after discharge for them to heal after such a devastating loss.

The nursing care of families at this time is similar to that described in Chapter 38. Options need to be offered, memories made, and mementos obtained and held for the family until they are ready for them. These families are at risk for complicated bereavement and altered parenting of the surviving baby and other children in the family. Referral to social services to help the family mobilize support systems and for counseling can help combat problems before they develop. Such a referral may be beneficial not only at the time of the loss but also in the future.

The emotional toll that a maternal death can take on the nursing and medical staff also must be addressed. Guilt, anger, fear, sadness, and depression are common responses to a maternal death. The staff may want to review the situation surrounding the events, the chart, and their responses in the forum of a morbidity-mortality review and a critical incident debriefing to help in coping with the feelings and emotions that result after a maternal death. Attending memorial or funeral services may benefit staff and family.

KEY POINTS

- The numbers of critically ill pregnant women are increasing, paralleling improvements in pediatric and neonatal care.
- Any nurse providing care for pregnant women may encounter the critically ill pregnant woman and must be able to initiate appropriate care.
- Nurses must recognize early signs of severe complications and expedite the institution's plan for the critically ill pregnant woman to receive necessary complex care.
- The institutional plan may consist of actual implementation of critical care procedures in a labor and birth unit or stabilization and preparation for transport to a tertiary center or adult ICU, with obstetric consultation after transport.
- Normal physiologic alterations during pregnancy produce profound hemodynamic changes. The critical care team should base care on knowledge of normal hemodynamic values for the pregnant state.
- Pregnancy is not a contraindication for hemodynamic monitoring.
- Invasive hemodynamic monitoring is associated with potential complications. However, the benefits usually outweigh the risks when the woman is critically ill.
- Pulmonary artery catheterization provides continuous information about left ventricular function; this information is not available from any other method.
- Use of a PAC in combination with an arterial pressure catheter and pulse oximeter provides adequate data to assess continuously both cardiac and pulmonary status.
- The fiberoptic PAC provides a continuous Svo_2, which is a sensitive marker of physiologic instability because it reflects overall adequacy of oxygen delivery to the tissues.
- The active roles assumed by most pregnant women today place them at risk for vehicular crashes, falls, violence, and other injuries.
- Pregnancy does not limit or restrict resuscitative, diagnostic, or pharmacologic treatment after trauma.
- Fetal survival depends on maternal survival. After trauma the first priority, before consideration of fetal concerns, is resuscitation and stabilization of the mother.
- Optimal care for the pregnant victim of trauma depends on knowledge of the physiologic state of pregnancy.
- Minor trauma can be associated with major complications for the pregnancy, including placental abruption, fetomaternal hemorrhage, preterm labor and birth, and fetal death.
- Trauma from accidents is the most common cause of death in women of childbearing age.
- Care of the critically ill pregnant woman should include the components of family-centered childbirth.
- Death of a woman in childbirth is rare; it disrupts family structure, and the family needs supportive grief counseling. Medical and nursing staff also can benefit from debriefing and counseling sessions.

Audio Chapter Summaries Access an audio summary of these Key Points on evolve

REFERENCES

American Academy of Pediatrics (AAP) & American College of Obstetricians and Gynecologists (ACOG). (2007). *Guidelines for perinatal care* (6th ed.). Elk Grove Village, IL: Authors.

American College of Obstetricians and Gynecologists (ACOG). (1992). *Invasive hemodynamic monitoring in obstetrics and gynecology.* ACOG Technical Bulletin No. 175. Washington, DC: Author.

American College of Obstetricians and Gynecologists (ACOG). (2006). *Obstetric aspects of trauma management.* ACOG Educational Bulletin No. 251. Washington, DC: Author.

American College of Obstetricians and Gynecologists (ACOG). (2009). *Critical care in pregnancy.* ACOG Clinical Management Guidelines for Obstetrician-Gynecologist. No. 100. Washington, DC: Author.

Anwari, J., Butt, A., & Al-Dar, M. (2004). Obstetric admissions to the intensive care unit. *Saudi Medical Journal, 25*(10), 1394–1399.

Association of Women's Health, Obstetric and Neonatal Nurses (AWHONN). (2009). *Standards and guidelines for professional nursing practice in the care of women and newborns* (6th ed.). Washington, DC: Author.

Baskett, T., & O'Connell, C. (2009). Maternal critical care in obstetrics. *Journal of Obstetrics and Gynaecology Canada, 31*(3), 218–221.

Berg, C., Chang, J., Callaghan, W., & Whitehead, S. (2003). Pregnancy-related mortality in the United States, 1991-1997. *Obstetrics and Gynecology, 101*(2), 289–296.

Blackburn, S. (2007). *Maternal, fetal, & neonatal physiology: A clinical perspective* (3rd ed.). St. Louis: Saunders.

Brown, H. (2009). Trauma in pregnancy. *Obstetrics and Gynecology, 114*(1), 147–160.

Christopher, V., Al-Chalabi, T., Richardson, P., Muiesan, P., Rela, M., Heaton, N., et al. (2006). Pregnancy outcome after liver transplantation: A single-center experience of 71 pregnancies in 45 recipients. *Liver Transplantation, 12*(7), 1138–1143.

Clark, S., Cotton, D., Lee, W., Bishop, C., Hill, T., Southick, J., et al. (1989). Central hemodynamic assessment of normal term pregnancy. *American Journal of Obstetrics and Gynecology, 161*(6), 1439–1442.

Cunningham, F., Leveno, K., Bloom, S., Hauth, J., Rouse, D., & Spong, C. (Eds.). (2010). *Williams obstetrics (23rd ed.).* New York: McGraw-Hill.

Darovic, G. (2002). *Hemodynamic monitoring: Invasive and noninvasive clinical application.* Philadelphia: Saunders.

Davison, J., & Bailey, D. (2003). Pregnancy following renal transplantation. *Journal of Obstetrics and Gynaecology Research, 29*(4), 227–233.

Friese, G., & Wojciehoski, R. (2005). Fetal trauma from motor vehicle collisions. *Journal of Emergency Medical Services, 30*(5), 110–127.

Fujitani, S., & Baldisseri, M. (2005). Hemodynamic assessment in a pregnant and peripartum patient. *Critical Care Medicine, 33*(Suppl.), S354–S361.

Gilbert, E. (2011). *Manual of high risk pregnancy & delivery* (5th ed.). St. Louis: Mosby.

Henneman, E., & Cardin, S. (2002). Family-centered critical care: A practical approach to making it happen. *Critical Care Nursing, 22*(6), 12–19.

Keizer, J., Zwart, J., Meerman, R., Harinck, B., Feuth, H., & Roosmalen, J. (2006). Obstetric intensive care admissions: A 12-year review in a tertiary care centre. *European Journal of Obstetrics, Gynecology, and Reproductive Biology, 128*(1-2), 152–156.

Lu, E., & Curet, M. (2007). Surgical procedures in pregnancy. In S. Gabbe, J. Niebyl, & J. Simpson (Eds.), *Obstetrics: Normal and problem pregnancies (5th ed.).* Philadelphia: Churchill Livingstone.

Mabie, W. (2004). Pulmonary edema. In G. Dildy, M. Belfort, G. Saade, J. Phelan, G. Hankins, & S. Clark (Eds.), *Critical care obstetrics* (4th ed.). Malden, MA: Blackwell Science.

Magee, L., & von Dadelszen, P. (2009). The management of severe hypertension. *Seminars in Perinatology, 33*(3), 138–142.

Martin, S., & Foley, M. (2009). Intensive care monitoring of the critically ill pregnant patient. In R. Creasy, R. Resnik, J. Iams, C. Lockwood, & T. Moore (Eds.), *Creasy & Resnik's Maternal-fetal medicine: Principles and practice* (6th ed.). Philadelphia: Saunders.

Murray, M. (2007). *Antepartal and intrapartal fetal monitoring* (3rd ed.). New York: Springer, Publishing Co.

Norwitz, E., Robinson, J., & Malone, F. (2004). Pregnancy-induced physiologic alterations. In G. Dildy, M. Belfort, G. Saade, J. Phelan, G. Hankins, & S. Clark (Eds.), *Critical care obstetrics* (4th ed.). Malden, MA: Blackwell Science.

Roberts, J., & Funai, E. (2009). Pregnancy-related hypertension. In R. Creasy, R. Resnik, J. Iams, C. Lockwood, & T. Moore (Eds.), *Creasy & Resnik's Maternal-fetal medicine: Principles and practice* (6th ed.). Philadelphia: Saunders.

Saravanakumar, K., Davies, L., Lewis, M., & Cooper, G. (2008). High dependency care in an obstetric setting in the UK. *Anaesthesia, 63*(10), 1081–1086.

Selo-Ojeme, D., Omosaiye, M., Battacharjee, P., & Kadir, R. (2005). Risk factors for obstetric admissions to the intensive care unit in a tertiary hospital: A case-control study. *Archives of Gynecology and Obstetrics, 272*(3), 207–210.

Wallace, D., & Winslow, E. (1993). Effects of iced and room temperature injectate on cardiac output measurements in critically ill patients with low and high cardiac outputs. *Heart and Lung, 32*(1), 2–12.

Wu, D., Wilt, J., & Restaino, S. (2007). Pregnancy after thoracic organ transplantation. *Seminars in Perinatology, 31*(6), 354–362.

Xu, J., Kochanek, K., Murphy, S., & Tejada-Vera, B. (2010). Deaths: Final data for 2007. *National Vital Statistics Report, 58*(19), 1–135.

Zeeman, G. (2006). Obstetric critical care: A blueprint for improved outcomes. *Critical Care Medicine, 34*(Suppl. 9), S208–S214.

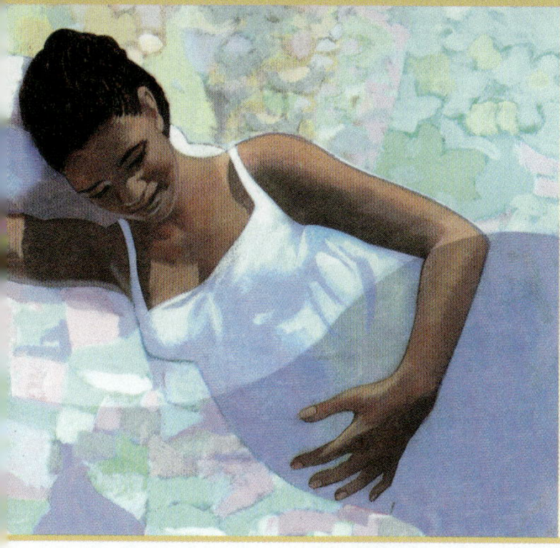

CHAPTER

32

Mental Health Disorders and Substance Abuse in Pregnancy

Anne Hopkins Fishel

evolve WEBSITE

http://evolve.elsevier.com/Lowdermilk/MWHC/

Audio Glossary
Audio Key Points
Critical Thinking Exercise
    Postpartum Depression
NCLEX Review Questions
Nursing Care Plan
    Postpartum Depression
    Substance Abuse During Pregnancy

LEARNING OBJECTIVES

- Delineate emotional complications during pregnancy, including management of anxiety disorders and mood disorders.
- Examine substance abuse during pregnancy, including dual diagnosis, prevalence, risk factors, legal considerations, treatment programs, barriers to treatment, and care management.
- Identify postpartum emotional complications, including incidence, risk factors, signs and symptoms, and management.
- Evaluate the role of the nurse in assessing and managing care of women with emotional complications during pregnancy and postpartum.
- Develop a nursing care plan for a woman with an anxiety disorder, such as panic disorder.

Management of mental health disorders takes place primarily in community settings. Compared with births in the general non-mentally ill population, women with mental illness who give birth have a higher risk of obstetric complications (Thornton, Guendelman, & Hosang, 2009). However, mentally ill women who were treated were at lower risk than women not treated. Twelve-month prevalence rates for women with psychiatric disorders range from 22.6% (anxiety disorders) to 14.1% (mood disorders) to 6.6% (substance abuse) (Hendrick, 2006). In a cross-national study of the association between gender and mental disorders, the World Health Organization reported that in all age cohorts and countries, women had more anxiety and mood disorders than men; however, men had more substance disorders (Seedat, Scott, Angermeyer, Berglund, Bromet, Brugha, et al., 2009). The symptoms and treatment can complicate pregnancy, childbirth, and the postpartum period.

MENTAL HEALTH DISORDERS DURING PREGNANCY

Women are at the greatest risk for developing a psychiatric disorder between the ages of 18 and 45 years—the childbearing years (Hendrick, 2006). Women who have serious mental disorders may be engaging in sexual activities that can result in pregnancy. The pregnant woman may have a history of disorder in mood, anxiety, substance use, schizophrenia, personality, or development. Assessment throughout pregnancy and the postpartum period is critical to the mother's and the baby's health. With a history or current symptoms of mental illness, referral to a mental health specialist for evaluation is recommended. Mental health disorders have implications for the pregnant woman, the fetus, the newborn, and the entire family.

Mood Disorders

Women who are being treated for depression may become pregnant, either intentionally or accidentally. In a review of 21 research articles, the prevalence of depression during pregnancy was cited as being 7.4% during the first trimester, 12.8% during the second trimester, and 12% during the third trimester (Bennett, Einarson, Toddio, Koren, & Einarson, 2004). Of all pregnant women treated for depression, approximately one third have a first occurrence during pregnancy (Pigarelli, Kraus, & Potter, 2005). These findings dispel the myth that pregnancy is a "pleasant and happy event" for all women.

Mood disorders are defined as disorders that have as their dominant feature a disturbance in the prevailing emotional state. To be diagnosed with major depression, at least five of the following signs or symptoms must be present nearly every day: depressed mood, often with spontaneous crying; markedly diminished interest in all activities; insomnia or hypersomnia; weight changes (increases or decreases); psychomotor retardation or agitation; fatigue or loss of energy; feelings of worthlessness or inappropriate guilt; diminished ability to concentrate; and suicidal ideation with or without a suicidal plan (American Psychiatric Association [APA], 2000). The 10-item Edinburgh Postnatal Depression Scale accurately identifies depression in pregnant and postpartum women (Sadock, Sadock, & Ruiz, 2009).

! NURSING ALERT

Diagnostic assessment for depression in pregnant women is difficult because many of the symptoms of pregnancy mimic depression. Critical cues are the presence of psychologic symptoms, a suicide plan, and major disruptions in sleep pattern. Risk factors for developing depression in pregnancy include a prior history in self or family, a lack of social support, stressful life events, partner discord, and history of premenstrual syndrome (PMS).

Collaborative Care

Medical management of depression is usually a combination of antidepressants and cognitive-behavioral or interpersonal psychotherapy. Self-help strategies such as exercise, respite from caregiving, self-help groups, and making time for one's self can be helpful. Nursing strategies include educating the woman about depression as an illness, about treatment success, and about antidepressant medications. For the woman who refuses medications during pregnancy, the nurse should discuss alternative treatments and respect her choice. The nurse also can be effective by maintaining a caring relationship, which includes being hopeful. The nurse can ask about a time when the woman was coping well and how she was able to combat the depression then.

Antidepressant Medications. No consensus exists regarding safety in the use of antidepressant medications with pregnant women. To date, the U.S. Food and Drug Administration (FDA) has not approved any psychotropic medication for use during pregnancy. None of these medications is rated as an FDA Category A drug (controlled studies show no risk to the fetus) (see Table 32-1 for FDA pregnancy risk categories of most common antidepressant medications). The commonly used antidepressant drugs are often divided into four groups: selective serotonin reuptake inhibitors (SSRIs), serotonin/norepinephrine reuptake inhibitors (SNRIs), tricyclic antidepressants (TCAs), and monoamine oxidase inhibitors (MAOIs).

Amitriptyline, imipramine, and nortriptyline (TCAs), along with paroxetine (an SSRI) and MAOIs are the most risky antidepressant medications (Schatzberg, Cole, & DeBattista, 2007). Because the majority of women are not aware of their pregnancy until at least 6 weeks of gestation, psychotropic medications may not be discontinued until after the period of greatest potential risk to the fetus has passed. Risk-benefit analyses of depression treatment options should consider the potential risks that may accrue if depressive episodes go untreated in the pregnant woman (Sadock et al., 2009). Risks include severe psychologic distress, suicide, financial hardships, and inability to plan for transition to parenthood. Most women who discontinue antidepressant medications relapse during pregnancy. The majority of relapses occur in the first trimester, and relapse is more prevalent in women with histories of more chronic depression (Schatzberg et al.). Because randomized clinical trial data regarding the relative safety of available psychotropic medications are unavailable, clinical decision making is particularly complicated (Sadock et al.).

Concerns regarding the safety of antidepressant medications are common. However, untreated depression may also cause adverse effects on the developing fetus and neonate, such as preterm birth, small head circumference, and low Apgar scores.

TABLE 32-1 ANTIDEPRESSANT MEDICATIONS

	PREGNANCY RISK CATEGORY*	LACTATION RISK CATEGORY*
Selective Serotonin Reuptake Inhibitors (SSRIs)		
Citalopram (Celexa)	C	L3
Escitalopram (Lexapro)	C	L3 in older infants
Fluoxetine (Prozac)	C	L2 in older infants; L3 in neonates
Fluvoxamine (Luvox)	C	L2
Paroxetine (Paxil)	D	L2
Sertraline (Zoloft)	C	L2
Serotonin/Norepinephrine Reuptake Inhibitors (SNRIs)		
Bupropion (Wellbutrin) IR & SR	B	L3
Maprotiline (Ludiomil)	B	L3
Mirtazapine (Remeron)	C	L3
Trazodone (Desyrel)	C	L2
Venlafaxine (Effexor)	C	L3
Tricyclics (TCAs)		
Amitriptyline (Elavil)	D	L2
Amoxapine (Asendin)	C	L2
Clomipramine (Anafranil)	C	L2
Desipramine (Norpramin)	C	L2
Doxepin (Sinequan)	C	L5
Imipramine (Tofranil)	D	L2
Nortriptyline (Pamelor)	D	L2
Monoamine Oxidase Inhibitors (MAOIs)		
Phenelzine (Nardil)	C	Unknown
Tranylcypromine (Parnate)	C	Unknown

B = Animal studies have not shown fetal risk, but no controlled studies in pregnant women *or* animal studies showed adverse effect that was not confirmed in controlled studies in women in first trimester—no risk in later trimesters.
C = Animal studies show adverse effects on fetus and no controlled studies in pregnant women *or* no studies available.
D = Positive evidence of human fetal risk.
L2 = Drug studied in limited number of breastfeeding women with no adverse effects in infant *or* evidence is remote.
L3 = No controlled studies *or* studies show minimal nonthreatening effects.
L5 = Contraindicated because studies have shown significant and documented risk to infant.
IR, Intermediate release; *SR,* sustained release.
*Sources: Hale, T. (2004). *Medications and mother's milk* (11th ed.). Amarillo, TX: Pharmasoft; Schatzberg, A., Cole, J., & DeBattista, C. (2007). *Manual of clinical psychopharmacology.* Washington, DC: American Psychiatric Publishing.

For women with a diagnosis of major depression, treatment with antidepressants is appropriate. Depression in the first trimester, if it is not moderate to severe, may be treated by supportive measures such as psychotherapy. Several studies have found interpersonal psychotherapy effective in significantly reducing depression during pregnancy (Sadock et al., 2009). Use of antidepressants, including SSRIs, is indicated for vegetative signs accompanying a major depressive episode that do not resolve with supportive intervention. The data show no evidence for a statistically significant association between fetal exposure and high rates of congenital malformations in fetuses exposed to tricyclic or other antidepressant drugs, although isolated cases of abnormalities have been reported. Paroxetine has been associated with ventricular septal defects for first-trimester exposure; venlafaxine has been associated with a poor neonatal adaptation syndrome, and mirtazapine with greater risk of preterm birth (Sadock et al.).

Although less information is known regarding the use of SSRIs during pregnancy compared with the use of TCAs, this class of drugs is emerging as first-line agents in treatment (Sadock et al., 2009). They are relatively safe and carry fewer side effects than the TCAs. However, if an SSRI is taken with dextromethorphan, an agent found in cough syrup, the combination could trigger the serotonin syndrome (e.g., mental status changes, agitation, hyperreflexia, shivering, and diarrhea). The most frequent side effects with the SSRIs are gastrointestinal (GI) disturbances (e.g., nausea and diarrhea), headache, and insomnia. In about one third of clients, the SSRIs reduce libido, arousal, or orgasmic function (Schatzberg et al., 2007). SSRIs also can inhibit specific P-450 isoenzymes, resulting in a marked elevation in drug concentration and a reduction in drug clearance. An epidemiologic study by the Centers for Disease Control and Prevention on the causes of birth defects found no association between SSRI use and birth defects. However, the study did find an association between SSRI use and a slightly increased risk for three specific birth defects: a defect of the brain, one type of abnormal skull development, and a GI abnormality. These increases in risk were minimal and have not been found before or since (Sadock et al.).

The TCAs cause many central nervous system (CNS) and peripheral nervous system side effects. Although some are simply annoying, others are significant or even dangerous (Schatzberg et al., 2007). In overdose, these medications can cause death. A common CNS effect is sedation. Other side effects include weight gain, tremors, grand mal seizures, nightmares, agitation or mania, and extrapyramidal side effects. Anticholinergic side effects include dry mouth, blurred vision (usually temporary), difficulty voiding, constipation, sweating, and difficulty with orgasm (Schatzberg et al.). The use of MAOIs during pregnancy is contraindicated because of risk for fetal growth restriction. In animals, hypertension with subsequent placental hypoperfusion and complications with anesthesia during labor have been reported (Sadock et al., 2009).

Anxiety Disorders

Anxiety disorders are the most common mental disorder. They include phobias (irrational fears that lead a person to avoid common objects, events, or situations), panic disorder (repeated, unprovoked episodes of intense fear that develop without warning and are not related to any specific event), generalized anxiety disorder (constant worry unrelated to any event), obsessive-compulsive disorder (OCD), and posttraumatic stress disorder (PTSD) (APA, 2000).

OCD symptoms include recurrent, persistent, and intrusive thoughts that cause anxiety, which a person tries to control by performing repetitive behaviors or "compulsions" (APA, 2000). The pregnant woman may have persistent thoughts that something is wrong with the fetus. Treatment usually includes antidepressant medication (SSRIs), cognitive-behavioral therapy, and education about how to manage the symptoms of the illness (Sadock et al., 2009).

PTSD can occur as a result of rape (see Chapter 5). Symptoms include reexperiencing the traumatic event, persistent avoidance of stimuli, and numbing, as well as difficulty sleeping, irritability or angry outbursts, difficulty concentrating, hypervigilance, and exaggerated startle response (APA, 2000). Nurses can support the healing process of individuals with PTSD by being alert to what the woman is experiencing during pregnancy and labor.

If the current pregnancy is a result of rape, the woman may be extremely ambivalent about the baby. If the rape occurred some time ago, the whole experience of pregnancy with prenatal examinations can trigger memories of the original trauma. She may avoid prenatal examinations because of the anxiety triggered by bodily touch and vaginal examinations. Some pregnant women with PTSD may feel more comfortable with a female nurse-midwife or a female physician. Giving birth can trigger memories of being out of control, and she may lose contact with reality. The nurse can verbalize understanding of the anxiety and orient to current reality by saying, "You're having an examination to make sure the baby is okay," or, "You're in labor preparing to give birth to your baby. I am your nurse. You're in the hospital. I will check on you frequently. You are safe here." Treatment usually includes psychotherapy and referral to support groups.

Collaborative Care

Benzodiazepines and antidepressants are the most commonly used drugs for the treatment of anxiety disorders (see Table 32-1 and Table 32-2 for FDA categories for these medications). Although benzodiazepines are the most widely prescribed, antidepressant medications are the treatments of choice. Some pregnant women who have been using benzodiazepines for "anxiety," "nervousness," or insomnia may not realize that these medications may be teratogenic (with consequences including cleft lip and palate), and that their use during pregnancy is not advised, particularly during the first trimester (Schatzberg et al., 2007). Note that most of the antianxiety medications are FDA Category D (evidence of human fetal risk) or Category X (demonstrated fetal abnormalities and use is contraindicated). However, benzodiazepines should not be abruptly discontinued during pregnancy, and they should be tapered sufficiently before the birth to limit neonatal withdrawal syndrome. Nurses should educate women about the dangers of benzodiazepines during pregnancy, assess for use during pregnancy, and help pregnant women find other ways to handle their anxiety and insomnia, or refer them to a psychiatrist who specializes in psychiatric disorders in pregnancy. Nursing strategies to reduce anxiety include

TABLE 32-2 **ANTIANXIETY MEDICATIONS**

ANTIANXIETY MEDICATIONS	PREGNANCY RISK CATEGORY*	LACTATION RISK CATEGORY*
Alprazolam (Xanax)	D	L3
Buspirone (BuSpar)	C	L3
Chlordiazepoxide (Librium)	D	L3
Clonazepam (Klonopin)	C	L3
Clorazepate (Tranxene)	D	L3
Diazepam (Valium)	D	L3; L4 if used chronically
Flurazepam (Dalmane)	X	L3
Lorazepam (Ativan)	D	L3
Midazolam (Versed)	D	L3
Temazepam (Restoril)	X	L3
Triazolam (Halcion)	X	L3

C = Animal studies show adverse effects on fetus but no controlled studies in pregnant women *or* no studies available.
D = Positive evidence of human fetal risk.
X = Contraindicated because studies have shown significant and documented risk to fetus.
L3 = No controlled studies *or* studies show minimal nonthreatening effects.
L4 = Possibly hazardous.
*Sources: Hale, T. (2004). *Medications and mother's milk* (11th ed.). Amarillo, TX: Pharmasoft; Schatzberg, A., Cole, J., & DeBattista, C. (2007). *Manual of clinical psychopharmacology*. Washington, DC: American Psychiatric Publishing.

TABLE 32-3 **MOOD STABILIZERS**

MOOD STABILIZERS	PREGNANCY RISK CATEGORY*	LACTATION RISK CATEGORY*
Carbamazepine (Tegretol XR)	C	L2
Clonazepam (Klonopin)	C	L3
Gabapentin (Neurontin)	C	L3
Lamotrigine (Lamictal)	C	L3
Lithium carbonate (Eskalith)	C	L4
Topiramate (Topamax)	C	L3
Valproic acid (Depakene, Depakote, Depakote ER)	D	L2

C = Animal studies show adverse effects on fetus but no controlled studies in pregnant women *or* no studies available.
D = Positive evidence of human fetal risk.
L2 = Drug studied in limited number of breastfeeding women with no adverse effects in infant *or* evidence is remote.
L3 = No controlled studies *or* studies show minimal nonthreatening effects.
L4 = Possibly hazardous.
ER, XR, Extended release.
*Sources: Hale, T. (2004). *Medications and mother's milk* (11th ed.). Amarillo, TX: Pharmasoft; Schatzberg, A., Cole, J., & DeBattista, C. (2007). *Manual of clinical psychopharmacology*. Washington, DC: American Psychiatric Publishing.

empowerment through education; sensory interventions such as music therapy and aromatherapy; behavioral interventions such as breathing exercises, progressive muscle relaxation, guided imagery, and medication (see Table 32-2); and cognitive strategies such as encouraging positive self-talk and questioning negative thinking.

Special Considerations for Medications During Pregnancy. Even though the basic rule is to avoid administering any medication to a woman who is pregnant, particularly during the first trimester, decisions about the use of medications during pregnancy should be made jointly by the woman, her partner, and her health care providers. If the woman is stable and appears likely to remain well while not taking medication, then discontinuation before pregnancy is a viable option. For those women with a history of relapse after medication discontinuation, remaining on the drug during pregnancy is advised. Although a pregnant woman should be receiving the lowest therapeutic dose, psychotropic medications may have to be increased over the course of pregnancy to maintain adequate therapeutic serum concentrations and response (Sadock et al., 2009). The administration of psychotherapeutic medications at or near birth may cause a baby to be overly sedated at birth and require ventilatory support, or to be physically dependent on the drug and to require detoxification and treatment of a withdrawal syndrome.

If a woman becomes psychotic during pregnancy, it is usually either because she has stopped taking mood stabilizers or antipsychotics, or because she has a history of schizophrenia. Psychosis is a medical emergency. To treat a psychotic state, antipsychotic medication or electroconvulsive therapy (ECT) can be used (Bozkurt, Karlidere, Isintas, Ozmenier, Ozsahin, & Yanarates, 2007; Sadock et al., 2009). Lithium is currently considered the first-line medication for the treatment of psychosis during pregnancy (Roy & Payne, 2009).

Most of the mood-stabilizing medications such as lithium carbonate, carbamazepine (Tegretol), gabapentin (Neurontin), lamotrigine (Lamictal), and divalproex sodium (Depakote) are Category D (see Table 32-3 for FDA categories of mood stabilizers). In women with preexisting illness, there is a high recurrence of mania during pregnancy that may present as psychosis, thus maintenance on lithium is important to deter the development of adverse effects in the mother and infant. In reviews of epidemiologic data, the risk of Epstein's anomaly (congenital cardiac defect involving the tricuspid valve) is lower than was previously thought (Sadock et al., 2009). Other side effects in the newborn include muscular hypotonia with impaired breathing and cyanosis ("floppy baby syndrome"), neonatal hypothyroidism, nephrogenic diabetes insipidus, atrial flutter, tricuspid regurgitation, and congestive heart failure (Schatzberg et al., 2007). A 2008 study reported that discontinuing mood stabilizer treatment presents high risks of illness recurrence among pregnant women diagnosed with bipolar disorder. The researchers also reported that lamotrigine may afford protective effects with comparable fetal safety to other agents used to manage bipolar disorder (Newport, Stowe, Viguera, Calamaras, Juric, Knight, et al., 2008). Mood stabilizers are often taken over the life span by women with bipolar disorder. Women with this disorder should receive prepregnancy counseling. Those who have experienced a single manic episode may elect to have the medication tapered gradually and make an attempt to have a lithium-free pregnancy, or, if indicated, reinstitution of lithium after the first trimester.

No conclusive evidence indicates that antipsychotic medications (either typical or atypical) are teratogenic (Sadock et al., 2009). Atypical antipsychotics (except clozapine) are currently classed as Category C agents simply because data do not exist to define a risk (Schatzberg et al., 2007). Some health care providers are more comfortable with the older typical antipsychotics because so many women have been treated with them with no clear evidence of a teratogenic effect. "At this time, it probably [is] preferable to employ high potency typical agents during pregnancy rather than either atypical agents, whose risks are unknown, or low-potency agents with significant anticholinergic properties" (Schatzberg et al., p. 555).

If the pregnant woman is receiving pharmacologic treatment, the nurse must make sure that she is being treated by a psychiatrist or an advanced practice psychiatric nurse. No woman should withdraw abruptly from any psychotropic medication because of the risk of withdrawal symptoms.

COMMUNITY ACTIVITY

- What resources are available to help women with mood and anxiety disorders in your community? Visit the Postpartum Support International website at www.postpartum.net. Review the client information about the different types of mood and anxiety disorders, screening tools and resources.
- Visit the Substance Abuse Treatment Facility Locater website. Locate a substance abuse treatment program for pregnant/postpartum women in your community. What is the mission of the organization? What types of services do they provide, such as education, drug treatment, and counseling? Is the program out-patient or residential?

SUBSTANCE ABUSE DURING PREGNANCY

Substance abuse refers to the continued use of substances despite related problems in physical, social, or interpersonal areas (APA, 2000). Recurrent abuse results in failure to fulfill major role obligations, and there may be substance-related legal problems. Any use of alcohol or illicit drugs during pregnancy is considered abuse (APA). **Dual diagnosis** is the coexistence of substance abuse and another disorder. Major depression and anxiety disorders are the psychiatric disorders that commonly occur with substance abuse.

The damaging effects of alcohol and illicit drugs on pregnant women and their fetuses are well documented (Gilbert, 2011; Wisner, Sit, Reynolds, Altemus, Bogen, Sunder, et al., 2007). Alcohol and other drugs easily pass from a mother to her fetus through the placenta. Smoking during pregnancy may have serious health risks, including bleeding complications, miscarriage, stillbirth, prematurity, low birth weight, and sudden infant death syndrome (SIDS). Prenatal exposure to nicotine may lead to dysregulation in the neurodevelopment of the child and higher risk for behavioral problems (Gilbert; Wisner et al.). Congenital abnormalities have occurred in infants of mothers who have taken drugs. The safest pregnancy is one in which the mother is totally drug and alcohol-free, with one exception. For pregnant women addicted to opiates, methadone maintenance is safer for the fetus than acute opiate detoxification (Wisner et al.).

Prevalence

Because many pregnant women are reluctant to reveal their use of substances or the extent of their use, data on prevalence are highly variable. Approximately 15% of all mothers have a substance abuse problem (Gilbert, 2011). Among pregnant women responding to a national survey, 10% reported alcohol use, 4% reported binge alcohol use, and almost 1% reported heavy alcohol use in the month before the survey. The Pregnancy Risk Assessment Monitoring System (PRAMS) estimated that the prevalence of alcohol use during pregnancy ranged from 3% to 10% (Brady & Ashley, 2005). Blinded urine drug screens conducted at hospitals across the United States revealed that similar rates of substance use during pregnancy occurred in women of different ages, races, and social classes, although the specific substances used differed by race and social class. African-American and poor women were more likely to use illicit substances, particularly cocaine, whereas Caucasian women were more likely to use alcohol (Wisner et al., 2007). The National Pregnancy and Health Survey found that 19% of females used alcohol during pregnancy, and 5% used an illicit drug at least once during pregnancy, including marijuana (3%) and cocaine (1%) (Brady & Ashley).

Risk Factors

Many factors contribute to substance abuse. Women have a clearer pattern of self-medication and are more likely than men to use a combination of alcohol and prescription drugs. Women begin to use drugs during periods of depression, to relax, to feel more adequate, to lose weight, to decrease stress, or to help them sleep at night. Many pregnant abusers encounter multiple socioenvironmental risk factors including unstable home environments (Miotto, Suti, Hernandez, & Pham, 2006). Major risk factors for substance abuse in women include a history of childhood sexual or physical abuse and a spouse or partner who abuses substances. In a national sample, substance use in pregnant women was significantly lower than in nonpregnant women. The pregnant women who were more vulnerable to substance use were unemployed, unmarried, and experiencing psychiatric disorders (Havens, Simmons, Shannon, & Hansen, 2009). Another important risk factor for substance abuse is intimate partner violence; victims are significantly more likely to abuse substances during pregnancy (Miotto et al.).

Barriers to Treatment

Less than 10% of pregnant women who are substance abusers receive treatment for their addictions. Social stigma, labeling, and guilt are significant barriers to treatment (Brady & Ashley, 2005). Women often do not seek help because they fear losing custody of their child or children or criminal prosecution. Pregnant women who abuse substances commonly have little understanding of the ways in which these substances affect them, their pregnancies, or their babies. Pregnant women who are substance abusers may not seek prenatal care until labor begins. Often pregnant women who use psychoactive substances receive negative feedback from society, as well as from health care providers, who not only may condemn them for endangering the life of their fetuses, but also may even withhold support as a result. Barriers within the drug treatment system can deter these women as well. Traditionally, substance-abuse treatment programs have not addressed issues that affect pregnant women, such as the concurrent need for obstetric care and child care for other children. Long waiting lists and lack of health insurance present further barriers to treatment. Pregnant women with coexisting substance abuse and psychiatric disorders face unique barriers because of the social stigma attached to both conditions along with providers' insufficient knowledge and training to manage coexisting disorders (Brady & Ashley).

Legal Considerations

Because of the risks to the unborn children and financial concerns, pregnant women who abuse substances may face criminal charges in several states under expanded interpretations of child abuse and drug trafficking statutes. South Carolina is the only state that has passed specific legislation criminalizing pregnant women who abuse substances. However, many states have modified their civil child protection laws by mandating reports to child welfare authorities or defining child neglect to include cases in which a newborn is physically dependent, tests positive for, or has been harmed by substances of abuse. In 25 states, cases of maternal drug or alcohol use are referred to a hospital social worker, who evaluates and determines whether it is safe for the child to be taken home (Miotto et al., 2006). Nurses who screen for substance abuse in pregnancy and encourage prenatal care, counseling, and treatment will be of greater benefit to the mother and child than will prosecution.

> **LEGAL TIP: Drug Testing During Pregnancy**
> There is no requirement in the United States for a health care provider to test either the pregnant woman or the newborn for the presence of drugs. However, nurses need to know the practices of the states in which they are working. In some states a woman whose urine drug screen is positive at the time of labor and birth must be referred to child protective services. If the mother is not in a drug treatment program or is judged unable to provide care, the infant may be placed in foster care. The U.S. Supreme Court has ruled that in all states it is unlawful to test for drug use without the pregnant woman's permission (Harris & Paltrow, 2003).

Commonly Abused Drugs

Nicotine and Caffeine

Nicotine and caffeine are two examples of legal substances that can be addicting or harmful to the pregnant woman, fetus, and newborn. Effects of nicotine and caffeine on the fetus and newborn are discussed in Chapter 35. Tobacco contains nicotine, which is an addictive substance that creates both a physical and a psychologic dependence. Cigarette smoking is a major preventable cause of death and illness. Smoking is linked to cardiovascular disease, various types of cancers (especially lung and cervical), and chronic lung disease.

Smoking during pregnancy is known to cause a decrease in placental perfusion and is a cause of low birth weight (Bandestra & Accornero, 2006; Pichler, Heinzinger, Klaritsch, Zotter, Wilheim, & Uriesberger, 2008). The oxygen-carrying capacity of hemoglobin is decreased when carbon monoxide passes through the placenta. Furthermore, nicotine causes vasoconstriction, and smokers generally have a nutrient-poor diet. A 2009 study reported that the maternal use of tobacco while pregnant is associated with an increased risk for psychotic symptoms such as hallucinations and delusions in their children (Zammit, Thomas, Thompson, Horwood, Menezes, Gunnell, et al. 2009).

Caffeine is found in society's most popular drinks: coffee, tea, chocolate, energy drinks, and soft drinks. It is a stimulant that can affect mood and interrupt bodily functions by producing anxiety and sleep disruptions. Although maternal caffeine consumption during pregnancy may have adverse effects on fetal, neonatal and maternal outcomes, a rigorous review of literature reported that there is insufficient evidence to confirm or refute the effectiveness of caffeine avoidance on birth weight or other pregnancy outcomes (Jahanfar & Sharifah, 2009). The March of Dimes, however, recommends a daily intake of no more than 200 mg (March of Dimes, 2008).

Alcohol

Despite warnings, prenatal exposure to alcohol far exceeds exposure to illicit drugs. Women give birth each year to more than 2.6 million infants who have been exposed to alcohol (Miotto et al., 2006). Disorders associated with prenatal alcohol exposure include fetal alcohol syndrome (FAS), alcohol-related birth defects (ARBDs), and alcohol-related neurodevelopmental disorder. FAS is the most severe condition that affects the fetus. In fact FAS is the most common cause of preventable mental retardation and birth defects. It affects between 1.3 and 2.2 children per 1000 live births annually in North America (Miotto et al.). See Chapter 35 for information on newborn consequences of prenatal alcohol exposure.

Accurate data about alcohol abuse are difficult to obtain. Because alcohol is rapidly absorbed in the small intestine and metabolized in the liver, testing for its presence in blood is difficult. Underdiagnosing and underreporting alcohol use in pregnancy are major concerns of health care providers. Alcohol-dependent women who suddenly cease drinking may experience withdrawal symptoms that could be threatening to the mother and cause fetal distress (Miotto et al., 2006). Alcohol withdrawal in pregnant women is usually treated with benzodiazepines. Brief fetal exposure to benzodiazepines does not seem to increase the risk of major malformations or oral cleft. However, they can cause neonatal hypotonia, hypothermia, and mild neonatal respiratory distress when taken in late pregnancy (Miotto et al.).

Disulfiram (Antabuse), a medication that acts as a deterrent to alcohol ingestion because it produces a dramatic, unpleasant reaction when small amounts of alcohol are consumed, is contraindicated during pregnancy because it is teratogenic (Doering, 2005). Two other medications, naltrexone and acamprosate, have proven effective for decreasing alcohol intake. However, because they have not been tested in pregnant women, their use should be avoided (Doering).

Marijuana

Marijuana, a substance derived from the cannabis plant, is the most frequently used illicit drug in the United States (Miotto et al., 2006). It is usually rolled into a cigarette and smoked, but it also may be mixed into food and eaten. Marijuana produces a "high," relaxation, increased appetite, and reduced inhibition. Prolonged use may lead to apathy, lack of energy, loss of desire to work or be productive, diminished concentration, poor personal hygiene, and preoccupation with marijuana—the amotivational syndrome (Gold, Roytberg, Frost-Pineda, Jacobs, & Teitelbaum, 2007). Marijuana causes increased carbon monoxide levels in the mother's blood, which readily cross the placenta and reduce the oxygen supply to the fetus. Marijuana use during pregnancy can significantly affect the size of the neonate at birth, but research findings regarding the effects of maternal marijuana use on later child development are inconsistent (Miotto et al.).

Cocaine and Methamphetamine

Cocaine and methamphetamine are powerful CNS stimulants that block the reuptake of norepinephrine and dopamine at the nerve endings. Because more neurotransmitter is present at the synapse, the receptors are continuously activated. It is believed that this causes the euphoric effect for which both drugs are well known. At the same time, presynaptic supplies of dopamine and norepinephrine are depleted. This causes the "crash" that happens when the effect of the drug wears off (Andreasen & Black, 2007). The euphoria is short-lived, starting with a 10- to 20-second rush and followed by 15 to 20 minutes of less intense euphoria. A person who is high on cocaine feels euphoric, energetic, self-confident, and sociable. Stimulant intoxication can induce aggression, agitation, and impaired judgment. Unlike other stimulants, cocaine intoxication can cause tactile hallucinations and other psychotic symptoms including delusions, bizarre behavior, and paranoia (Andreasen & Black). The relapse rate for clients who try to discontinue cocaine use is very high.

Cocaine may be smoked, inhaled, or injected. The smokable form of cocaine is produced by a process called freebasing. Crack is cocaine mixed with baking soda and heated until it reaches its purest form. It is sold in the form of "rocks," which are smoked in pipes (Miotto et al., 2006). Crack is used by people from all cultures. Its low cost and easy availability make it the drug of choice among the economically disadvantaged. In one study, cocaine was the primary substance of abuse for 17% of admissions to treatment among pregnant women (Miotto et al.). Because crack is highly psychologically addictive, it poses management problems for health care providers who care for pregnant addicts.

Medical complications of cocaine use in pregnancy range from mild to severe. Some of the less serious medical problems are lack of energy, insomnia, sinusitis, nosebleeds, sore throat, and decreased libido. More serious problems develop as the person's general health deteriorates. These include perforation of the nasal septum, increased cardiovascular stress, tachycardia, systemic hypertension, ventricular arrhythmias, sudden coronary artery spasm, and myocardial infarction (Miotto et al., 2006). Needle-borne diseases such as hepatitis B and human immunodeficiency virus (HIV) are common among cocaine users. The tachycardia and subsequent increase in blood pressure are caused by the increasing levels of catecholamines produced by the cocaine (Sadock et al., 2009). During pregnancy uterine blood vessels are normally maximally dilated, but they vasoconstrict in the presence of catecholamines. The placental separation (abruption) or the acute onset of preterm labor with long, hard contractions and precipitate birth sometimes seen in pregnant women after they have used cocaine is probably secondary to acute spasm of uterine blood vessels.

At birth some infants show signs of cocaine exposure, including tremulousness, irritability, hyperactivity to environmental stimuli, and poor feeding (Sadock et al., 2009). Although infants with histories of prenatal cocaine exposure have higher rates of SIDS, it is unknown whether this is related to cocaine exposure itself or to co-occurring risk factors. Developmental problems in a range of physical and behavioral areas have been attributed to prenatal cocaine exposure, although the evidence for most remains inconclusive (Sadock et al.).

One of the promising treatments for cocaine abuse in pregnancy is acupuncture. A component of traditional Chinese medicine, acupuncture is used to redirect energy flow (chi) within the body, reduce cravings, and enhance well-being. The pace and location of the flow of chi can be influenced by the insertion of needles at certain points along the meridians to facilitate harmony (Otto, 2003). Evidence from controlled studies of the effectiveness of acupuncture alone or in combination with other therapies, however, has been inconsistent.

Methamphetamine use is a major problem in the United States. Approximately 12 million Americans have tried "meth," and 1.5 million are regular users (Schatzberg et al., 2007). Relatively cheap, the highly addictive stimulant is hooking more and more people across the socioeconomic spectrum. Meth makes many users feel hypersexual and uninhibited, thus leading to more sexual activity with less protection from pregnancy.

The active metabolite of methamphetamine is amphetamine. Agents used as appetite suppressants or diet pills are closely related substances. The crystalline form of methamphetamine is known as "ice." When smoked it produces a potent, long-lasting high. Ice enables a person to go without rest or food for 24 hours, only to "crash" for the next 24 hours. Clinical manifestations of methamphetamine use are euphoria, abrupt awakening, increased energy, talkativeness, elation, agitation, hyperactivity, irritability, grandiosity, diaphoresis, weight loss, insomnia, hypertension, increased temperature, ectopic heartbeat, urinary retention, constipation, dry mouth, paranoid delusions, and violent behavior. Seizures, heart attacks, strokes, and death may occur as a result of overdose (Miotto et al., 2006).

Although fewer maternal and neonatal complications have been attributed to this class of substances than to cocaine (APA, 2000), the rates of preterm birth and of intrauterine growth restriction with smaller head circumference are higher in methamphetamine-exposed pregnant women than in pregnant women who abuse other substances (see Chapter 35). Another complication of methamphetamine use is an increased incidence of placental abruption. As with cocaine, methamphetamine dependence is best managed in an inpatient treatment setting, with follow-up substance abuse treatment (Miotto et al., 2006).

Opiates

Opiates include opium, heroin, morphine, codeine, and methadone. Methadone is used to treat addiction to other opiates. It can be used either to aid withdrawal or to provide maintenance at a stable dose. Women taking methadone may work and live normally, although they are still addicted to narcotics. Heroin is one of the most commonly abused drugs of this class. It is usually taken by intravenous injection but can be smoked or "snorted" (Miotto et al., 2006). The signs and symptoms of heroin use are euphoria, relaxation, relief from pain, "nodding out" (apathy, detachment from reality, impaired judgment, and drowsiness), constricted pupils, nausea, constipation, slurred speech, and respiratory depression (APA, 2000).

BOX 32-1 CAGE QUESTIONNAIRE

C Have you ever felt you ought to **C**UT DOWN on your drinking?
A Have people **A**NNOYED you by criticizing your drinking?
G Have you ever felt bad or **G**UILTY about your drinking?
E Have you ever had a drink first thing in the morning to steady your nerves or get rid of a hangover? (**E**YE OPENER)

Source: Ewing, J. (1984). Detecting alcoholism: The CAGE questionnaire. *Journal of the American Medical Association, 22*(14), 1905-1907.

BOX 32-2 SCREENING WITH THE 4P's PLUS

Parents: Did either of your parents ever have a problem with alcohol or drugs?
Partner: Does your partner have a problem with alcohol or drugs?
Past: Have you ever had any beer or wine or liquor?
Pregnancy: In the month before you knew you were pregnant, how many cigarettes did you smoke? In the month before you knew you were pregnant, how much beer, wine, or liquor did you drink?

Sources: Chasnoff, I., McGourty, R.., Bailey, G., Hutchins, E., Lightfoot, S., Pawson, L., et al. (2005). The 4 P's Plus screen for substance use in pregnancy: Clinical application and outcomes. *Journal of Perinatology, 25*(6), 368-374; Wisner, K., Sit, D., Reynolds, S., Altemus, M., Bogen, D., Sunder, K., et al. (2007). Psychiatric disorders. In S. Gabbe, J. Niebyl, & J. Simpson (Eds.), *Obstetrics: Normal and problem pregnancies* (5th ed.). Philadelphia: Churchill Livingstone.

The incidence of heroin use among pregnant women is unknown; however, those women with a dependency on heroin may use multiple drugs. Possible effects on pregnancy include preeclampsia, IUGR, miscarriage, premature rupture of membranes, infections, breech presentation, and preterm labor. Adverse outcomes for the neonate include low birth weight, prematurity, neonatal abstinence syndrome, stillbirth, and SIDS (Miotto et al., 2006).

The recommended treatment for opiate dependence during pregnancy is methadone maintenance combined with psychotherapy. This well-documented approach improves outcomes for both woman and fetus (Miotto et al., 2006). Another treatment method is slow medical withdrawal with methadone, but the safety of this second approach is questionable. During pregnancy methadone is metabolized more rapidly, leading to withdrawal symptoms in less than 24 hours in many women. These symptoms can include fetal hyperactivity and, if severe, preterm labor or fetal death. Women may resort to heroin use to alleviate the uncomfortable symptoms. If higher doses of methadone are required during the course of pregnancy, twice-daily medication administration (morning and evening) is the most effective way to prevent withdrawal and subsequent heroin use (Miotto et al.).

CARE MANAGEMENT

Screening

The care of the substance-dependent pregnant woman is based on historical data, symptoms, physical findings, and laboratory results. All pregnant women should be asked screening questions for alcohol and drug abuse in the overall assessment at the first prenatal visit. Any judgmental attitude on the part of the health care provider will be evident to the woman and will interfere with the development of trust and with an accurate report of consumption. Information about drug use should be obtained by first asking about the woman's intake of over-the-counter and prescribed medications. Next, her use of legal drugs such as caffeine, nicotine, and alcohol should be determined. Finally, she should be questioned about her use of illicit drugs, such as cocaine, heroin, and marijuana. The approximate frequency and amount should be documented for each drug used (Seidel, Ball, Dains, Flynn, Solomon, & Stewart, 2011).

A variety of screening tests are available to screen for alcohol abuse. The CAGE questionnaire (Ewing, 1984) (Box 32-1) and the Brief Michigan Alcoholism Screening Test (MAST) (Pokorny, Miller, & Kaplan, 1972) are two well-known screens for alcohol use that are often administered by the nurse or included in the written previsit questionnaire. The CAGE is the most popular test used in primary care. Both the CAGE and MAST questionnaires, however, focus on alcohol dependency and may not be sensitive enough to detect the levels of drinking that are considered harmful in pregnancy. The 4P's Plus (Box 32-2) is a screening tool designed specifically to identify pregnant women who need in-depth assessment. It consists of five questions and takes less than a minute to complete (Chasnoff, McGourty, Bailey, Hutchins, Lightfoot, Pawson, et al., 2005). Because pregnant women frequently deny or greatly underreport usage, asking about substance use prior to pregnancy is often a more effective screening method (Wisner et al., 2007).

Urine toxicology testing is often performed to screen for illicit drug use. Drugs may be found in urine days to weeks after ingestion, depending on how quickly they are metabolized and excreted from the body. Meconium (from the neonate) and hair can also be analyzed to determine past drug use over a longer period (Gilbert, 2011).

In addition to screening for alcohol and drug abuse, the nurse should also screen for physical and sexual abuse and history of psychiatric illness because these are risk factors in women who abuse substances. Substance-abusing women feel much stigma, shame, and guilt, which leads to denial of the abuse. If the nurse can help reduce those feelings, the woman will be more apt to confide in the nurse—the first step in receiving help. Asking about how a spouse or partner feels about using substances can reveal whether there are family supports or barriers (see Box 32-2).

ASSESSMENT

After screening results indicate that substance abuse is a problem for an individual woman, the nursing process is used to deal with that problem (see the Nursing Process box). Because of the lifestyle often associated with drug use, substance-abusing women are at risk for sexually transmitted infections (STIs), including HIV. Laboratory assessments will likely include screening for syphilis, hepatitis B and C, and HIV. A skin test to screen for tuberculosis may also be ordered. Initial and serial ultrasound studies are usually performed to determine gestational age because the woman may have had amenorrhea as a result of her drug use or may have no idea when her last menstrual period occurred.

NURSING PROCESS

Substance Abuse

ASSESSMENT

The assessment of a pregnant woman who is a substance abuser may include the following:

- Interview:
  - Screen for current alcohol and drug abuse during the first prenatal visit. Document approximate frequency and amount for each drug used. Ask in this order:
    - Over-the-counter and prescribed medications
    - Legal drugs (e.g., caffeine, nicotine, alcohol)
    - Illicit drugs (e.g., marijuana, cocaine, methamphetamines, heroin, etc.)
  - Assess for past or current physical abuse.
  - Assess for past or current sexual abuse.
  - Assess for history of psychiatric illness.
  - Assess for barriers to care, such as peer pressure, socioeconomic status, psychologic stress, or other environmental factors.
- Comprehensive physical examination
- Laboratory tests:
  - Complete blood cell count
  - Syphilis
  - Hepatitis B and C serology
  - Human immunodeficiency virus
  - Tuberculosis
  - Urine toxicologic testing for suspected drugs used or drugs commonly abused in the community
  - Liver function tests if alcohol abuse is suspected
- Pregnancy and fetal assessment:
  - Ultrasound to determine gestational age and fetal weight
  - Nonstress testing

NURSING DIAGNOSES

Nursing diagnoses for the woman who is a substance abuser may include the following:

***Risk for Imbalanced Nutrition: Less than Body Requirements* related to:**
- effects of excessive use of psychoactive drugs

***Risk for Injury (to self, fetus, or newborn)* related to:**
- sensory effects of drug

***Risk for Infection* related to:**
- lifestyle
- malnutrition
- method of drug administration

***Self-care Deficit (bathing or hygiene)* related to:**
- effects of substance used

***Ineffective Coping* related to:**
- lack of support system
- low self-esteem
- denial
- lack of anger management techniques

***Risk for Impaired Parent-infant Attachment* related to:**
- guilt
- continued substance abuse

***Hopelessness* related to:**
- inability to stop using substances

***Powerlessness* related to:**
- lack of resources
- relationship with one or more abusive partners

***Risk for Suicide* related to:**
- depression
- impulsivity while using substances

EXPECTED OUTCOMES OF CARE

The ideal long-term outcome is total abstinence, but this outcome may not be possible. The woman should participate in setting short-term outcomes such as the following:

- The woman will keep appointments for prenatal and postpartum care for herself and well-baby care for the infant.
- Fetal effects related to maternal substance abuse will be minimized.
- The infant will be cared for in a safe environment.
- The woman's physiologic symptoms will stabilize, and she will be able to care for herself and her infant.
- The woman will develop an attachment to her infant.
- The woman will become involved in a substance abuse treatment program.

PLAN OF CARE AND INTERVENTIONS

- Develop a trusting relationship.
- Maintain a nonjudgmental, nonpunitive attitude.
- Determine the woman's readiness for change.
- Motivate the woman to make lifestyle changes by providing her with information about health risks and the effects of substance abuse on her fetus.
- Enlist the support of family members or friends if possible.
- Refer to community and social services as needed.
- Refer to local clinics dealing with pregnant substance abusers when the woman is ready for treatment.
- Provide ongoing encouragement and support.
- Reinforce importance of keeping prenatal appointments.
- Promote maternal-infant bonding after the birth.

EVALUATION

Evaluation is difficult in pregnant women with substance abuse problems because the long-range effects cannot be projected. Short-term positive achievements are indicative of some success.

Collaborative Care

Intervention with women who have substance abuse problems begins with education about specific effects on pregnancy, the fetus, and the newborn for each drug used. Consequences of perinatal drug use should be clearly communicated and abstinence recommended as the safest course of action, unless the woman is abusing opioids. Women are frequently more receptive to making lifestyle changes during pregnancy than at any other time in their lives. The casual, experimental or recreational drug user is frequently able to achieve and maintain abstinence when she receives education, support, and continued monitoring throughout the remainder of the pregnancy.

Treatment for substance abuse will be individualized for each woman, depending on the type of drug used and the frequency and amount of use. Women are more likely to attempt to stop smoking during pregnancy than at any other time in their lives. Quitting before conception is ideal but even quitting before 16 weeks of gestation significantly decreases the risks. Smoking cessation programs during pregnancy are effective and should be offered to all pregnant smokers (see Box 4-11).

These programs should continue throughout the postpartum period as well, because many women resume smoking after the birth. Many smoking cessation resources are available, both in print and online (Gilbert, 2011; Wisner et al., 2007). For more information on smoking cessation, visit the American Lung Association's website at www.lungusa.org.

National concern regarding the problem of alcohol and drug use during pregnancy has brought attention to not only the lack of treatment programs specifically targeted to pregnant women, but also the need for high quality randomized controlled trials to determine the effectiveness of interventions (Lui, Terplan, & Smith, 2008). Any discussion of treatment programs must start with the understanding that substance abuse in women is a complex problem surrounded by multiple individual, familial, and social issues that require many levels of intervention and treatment (Worley, Conners, Crone, Williams, & Bokony, 2005). The powerlessness of the alcoholic condition and the powerlessness of the female condition act on each other, reinforcing the impotence and hopelessness of both and leaving the woman with few resources to regain control of her life. In comparing women-only with mixed-gender substance abuse treatment programs, pregnant women treated in a women-only program demonstrated greater severity in drug use, legal problems, and psychiatric problems than those treated in the mixed-gender group (Hser & Niv, 2006). The women in the women-only group were less likely to be employed and more likely to be homeless, more likely to need child care, children's psychologic services, and HIV testing. The greater problem severity of pregnant women treated in women-only programs suggests that these specialized services are filling an important gap in addiction services, although further expansion is warranted (Hser & Niv).

Methadone maintenance treatment (MMT) is currently considered the standard of care for pregnant women dependent on heroin or other narcotics. Birth weight and head circumference are increased in infants born to women receiving MMT. However, 30% to 80% of infants exposed to opioids, including methadone, in utero require treatment for neonatal abstinence syndrome (see Chapter 35) (Wisner et al., 2007). Higher doses of maternal methadone are associated with an increase in diagnosis and longer duration of neonatal abstinence syndrome (Lim, Prasad, Samuels, Gardner, & Cordero, 2009). Pregnant women who use stimulants should be advised to stop using immediately, but they will need a great deal of assistance to do so and the rate of relapse is very high (Miotto et al., 2006).

There is little empirical evidence as to what treatment program is best for substance-using mothers; however, two studies are notable. Greenfield and associates (2004) found a strong association between length of stay in residential treatment and posttreatment abstinence. Terplan and Lui (2007) reported that "contingency management" was effective in improving the retention of pregnant women in illicit drug treatment programs, but it had only a minimal effect on abstinence and did not affect birth or neonatal outcomes. There is general agreement that programs should include a cognitive-behavioral approach and mostly female staff. Programs also need to address issues of stigmatization, the high probability of sexual and physical abuse, lack of social support, need for social services and child care, need for transportation, family support services, medical (particularly women's health) and mental health services, child development services, family planning, respite care, life skills management, pharmacologic services, self-help groups and stress management, and need for support and education in the mothering role. Drug-free public housing or residential communities may offer an ideal route to stabilization in a safe environment. Treatment must demonstrate cultural sensitivity and responsiveness to recognize ethnicity and culture as an important part of a woman's identity. Many women also need relationship counseling and vocational and legal assistance.

Women for Sobriety may be a more helpful organization for women than Alcoholics Anonymous (AA) or Narcotics Anonymous (NA), which are based on the 12-step program. The emphasis on powerlessness over addiction and avoidance of codependency found in 12-step programs may further disempower and isolate women, particularly women of color (Saulnier, 1996). The confrontational techniques of the 12-step program, developed to break down denial in men, may be especially threatening to women, who often feel unworthy and full of shame and guilt. In addition, women may be vulnerable to "thirteenth-stepping"—a euphemistic term referring to men who target new, more vulnerable women for dates or sex. In one study, 50% of the women experienced thirteenth-stepping behaviors, and two had been raped by men in AA (Bogart & Pearce, 2003). Especially vulnerable women, such as those with histories of sexual abuse, should be referred to female-only groups.

Whereas the treatment approach of male substance abusers tends to be oriented toward the individual, substance-abusing women should be viewed within the context of their relationships to others. Women tend to find satisfaction, pleasure, and a sense of worth if they experience their life activities as arising from and leading back to a sense of connection with others. Women who use illicit drugs are likely to be introduced to and supplied with these drugs by men as part of an intimate or sexual relationship.

An interdisciplinary, comprehensive model is essential when planning the care for women who abuse substances. Pregnancy presents a window of opportunity for motivating women to stop their abuse of substances, but what specifically can a nurse do?

First, nurses must be knowledgeable about how to screen and identify women who abuse substances while pregnant. They also must maintain a nonjudgmental, nonpunitive attitude. Nurses can advocate for access to woman-centered drug treatment and harm reduction measures to minimize the damage caused by alcohol and drugs (Lester & Twomey, 2008). Collaboration with advanced practice psychiatric nurses will enable nurses to deal with their feelings and provide better care for this challenging group of women. Until the nurse can approach the woman with caring and concern, the therapeutic alliance, which is so important for any change to take place, will not occur. The nurse's role is aimed not only at promoting abstinence but also providing a caring, nurturing, and empowering environment in which women can rediscover their values and become authentic, independent decision makers. Use of the contingency management model, which includes an abstinence-based incentive program and substance monitoring contract, may be useful with adolescent abusers (Stanger, Budney, Kamon, & Thostensen, 2009).

Second, the nurse should determine the individual's readiness for change. One model for doing this was developed by Prochaska and DiClemente (1992). The five stages of the model illustrate the readiness of women to change. *Precontemplation* is the earliest stage, in which individuals are unaware, unwilling, or discouraged about changing substance use behavior. They will be least responsive to interventions focused on change activities. First they need to take ownership of the problem. *Contemplation* involves an active consideration of the prospects of change. Women engage in information seeking and begin to reevaluate themselves in light of their substance abuse behavior. *Preparation* indicates a readiness to change. They intend to change in the near future and have learned valuable lessons from past change attempts and failures. *Action* involves the overt modification of the problem behavior, and individuals must have the skills to carry out the changes. *Maintenance* is the final stage. Environmental supports are particularly important in this stage, as well as supportive relationships with health care providers.

When working with pregnant adolescents with addictions, the nurse also must consider their developmental stage. A part of normal adolescence often includes experimenting with drugs or alcohol, so how does the nurse know when alcohol or drug use is a problem? Certain patterns, such as drinking to escape reality or drinking to "get wasted," are more dangerous than others. Drinking alone and being secretive about drugs and alcohol also are unhealthy patterns.

Third, the nurse uses supportive nursing interventions such as mutuality and avoidance of confrontation. In mutuality, the nurse conveys to women drug users that their perspective on their life situation is as valid as that of the nurse. Women should be encouraged to describe their views on the role of drug use in their lives, the degree of impairment they are experiencing, and the feasibility of change at this time. Avoiding confrontation is important because it can be damaging to the nurse-client relationship. The likely consequences of continued drug use can be presented in a warmly concerned, factual manner rather than as threats.

Fourth, the nurse uses principles of motivational interviewing (Miller & Rollnick, 1991) to effect change. These principles include the following:

- Displaying empathy
- Developing the discrepancy between individuals' perceptions of where they are and where they want to be
- Avoiding argumentation
- Rolling with resistance
- Supporting the woman's sense of self-efficacy

When problematic drug use is suspected, the nurse might ask in a noncritical way, "Are drugs or alcohol any part of this situation you have been describing?" By asking about the role of drugs in self-medication for stressors, the nurse can help the woman reflect on the degree of the problem and avenues for change. The woman can be helped to express the positive aspects of drug use that lead her to continue using and the harmful consequences that she has observed. She can be asked about times she tried to reduce or quit using her drug of choice. What interfered with her success? What times was she successful? What enabled her to succeed at those times? Praise can be given for being able to be successful at some time and optimism expressed that she can be successful again.

Doggett and colleagues (2005) reviewed six studies that provided home visit services to postpartum women who had drug or alcohol problems. Home visitors in these studies included community health nurses, pediatric nurses, trained counselors, paraprofessional advocates, midwives, and lay African-American women. Although the home visits did increase the women's involvement in drug treatment services, there was insufficient evidence to show that they improved the health of mothers or babies. Additional research is recommended, particularly with the home visits beginning during pregnancy.

Intrapartum and Postpartum Care Considerations. Although women who abuse substances may be difficult to care for at any time, they are often particularly challenging during the intrapartum and postpartum periods because of manipulative and demanding behavior. Typically, these women display poor control over their behavior and a low threshold for pain. Increased dependency needs and poor parenting skills may also be apparent.

Nurses must understand that substance abuse is an illness and that these women deserve to be treated with patience, kindness, consistency, and firmness when necessary. Even women who are actively abusing drugs will experience pain during labor and after giving birth and may need pain medication, as well as nonpharmacologic interventions. Developing a standardized plan of care so that clients have limited opportunities to play staff members against one another is helpful. Mother-infant attachment should be promoted by identifying the woman's strengths and reinforcing positive maternal feelings and behaviors. Staffing should be sufficient to ensure strict surveillance of visitors and prevent unsupervised drug use.

Advice regarding breastfeeding must be individualized. Although all abused substances appear in breast milk, some in greater amounts than others (Lawrence & Lawrence, 2005), breastfeeding is definitely contraindicated in women who use amphetamines, alcohol, cocaine, heroin, or marijuana. Methadone use, however, is not a contraindication to breastfeeding. The baby's nutrition and safety needs are of primary importance in this consideration. For some women a desire to breastfeed may provide strong motivation to achieve and maintain abstinence.

Smoking can interfere with the let-down reflex. Women who smoke in the postpartum period and breastfeed should avoid smoking for 2 hours before a feeding to minimize the nicotine content in the milk and improve the let-down reflex. All smokers should be discouraged from smoking in the same room with the infant because exposure to secondhand smoke can increase the likelihood that the infant will experience behavioral and respiratory health problems (Lawrence & Lawrence, 2005).

Before a woman who is a known substance abuser is discharged with her baby, the home situation must be assessed to determine that the environment is safe and that someone will be available to meet the infant's needs if the mother proves unable to do so. The hospital's social services department will usually be involved in interviewing the mother before discharge to ensure that the infant's needs will be met. Family members or friends will sometimes be asked to become actively involved with the mother and infant after discharge. A home care or public health nurse may be asked to make home visits to assess the mother's ability to care for the baby and provide guidance and support. If serious questions about the infant's well-being exist, the case will probably be referred to the state's child protective services agency for further action.

POSTPARTUM PSYCHOLOGIC COMPLICATIONS

The weeks following the birth are a time of vulnerability to psychiatric disorders for many women, causing significant distress for the mother, disrupting family life, and, if prolonged, negatively affecting the child's emotional and social development (Hendrick, 2006). Mood and anxiety disorders are particularly likely to recur or worsen during these weeks. Such conditions can interfere with attachment to the newborn and family integration, and some may threaten the safety and well-being of the mother, the newborn, and other children. Because birth is usually thought to be a happy event, a new mother's emotional distress may puzzle and immobilize family and friends. When she most needs the caring attention of loved ones, they may either criticize or withdraw because of their anxiety. Nurses can offer anticipatory guidance, assess the mental health of new mothers, offer therapeutic interventions, and make referrals when necessary. Failure to do so may result in tragic consequences. In the rarest of cases, a disturbed mother may kill her infant, other family members, or herself.

Mood Disorders

Mood disorders are the predominant mental health disorder in the postpartum period (APA, 2000). Up to 60% of women experience a mild depression or "baby blues" after the birth of a child; however, functioning of the woman is usually not impaired. Serious depression, experienced by 10% to 15% of postpartum women, can eventually incapacitate them to the point of being unable to care for themselves or their babies (Sadock et al., 2009). Postpartum depression occurs in a variety of countries, though the manifestations may vary by culture (Goldbort, 2006). In a community sample of postpartum Spanish mothers, 18% were found to have postpartum psychiatric disorders (Navarro, Garcia-Esteve, Ascasco, Aguardo, Gelabert, & Martin-Santos, 2008).

The *Diagnostic and Statistical Manual of Mental Disorders (DSM-IV)* contains the official guidelines for the assessment and diagnosis of psychiatric illness (APA, 2000). However, specific criteria for postpartum depression (PPD) are not listed. Instead, postpartum onset can be specified for any mood disorder either without psychotic features (i.e., PPD) or with psychotic features (i.e., postpartum psychosis) if the onset occurs within 4 weeks of childbirth (APA).

Etiology and Risk Factors

The cause of PPD may be biologic, psychologic, situational, or multifactorial. Several studies suggest that estrogen fluctuations and postpartum hypogonadism (the change from the high levels of estrogen and progesterone at the end of pregnancy to the much lower levels of both hormones that are present after birth) are important etiologic factors. Of women who present with PPD, 20% to 30% have a previous episode of major depressive disorder (MDD) (Epperson & Ballew, 2006). Other risk factors include a personal history of severe premenstrual dysphoria, family history of mood disorder, marital discord, lack of a confiding relationship, and stressful life events in the previous year (Epperson & Ballew; Milgrom, Gemmill, Bilszta, Hayes, Barnett, Brooks, et al., 2008). Mood and anxiety symptoms during pregnancy and postpartum blues increase the risk for PPD (APA, 2000). Neurotransmitter deficiencies and psychosocial and marital adjustments in the postpartum period have been related to PPD (APA). Although personal and family history of psychiatric disorders are the major risk factors for PPD, the potential role of psychosocial variables as risk factors for depression onset during the postpartum period should not be underestimated (Sadock et al., 2009). In a comprehensive review of the literature, Bina (2008) found that cultural practices could positively or negatively affect the development of PPD. Women facing multiple or severe psychosocial problems or chronic interpersonal difficulties are at increased risk of experiencing a major depressive episode.

Critical Thinking Exercise—Postpartum Depression

BOX 32-3 RISK FACTORS FOR POSTPARTUM DEPRESSION

- Prenatal depression
- Low self-esteem
- Stress of child care
- Prenatal anxiety
- Life stress
- Lack of social support
- Marital relationship problems
- History of depression
- "Difficult" infant temperament
- Postpartum blues
- Single status
- Low socioeconomic status
- Unplanned/unwanted pregnancy

Sources: Beck, C. (2002). Revision of the Postpartum Depression Predictors Inventory. *Journal of Obstetric, Gynecologic and Neonatal Nursing, 31*(4), 394-402; Beck, C. (2001). Predictors of postpartum depression: An update. *Nursing Research, 50*(5), 275-282.

The occurrence of PPD is higher among younger women, those with lower educational attainment, and those receiving Medicaid (Centers for Disease Control and Prevention [CDC], 2008). African-American mothers were twice as likely as Caucasian mothers to experience PPD. Mothers who had no one to talk to about their problems after giving birth had a high rate of PPD and a low rate of seeking help (Sword, Busser, Ganann, McMillan, & Swinton, 2008).

Beck (2008a, 2008b) published an integrative review of 141 studies of what nurse researchers internationally have contributed to the state of the science on postpartum depression. One aspect was in identifying risk factors. Beck described at least five instruments that have been developed since 1990 to assess risk factors or symptoms of PPD. The most common risk factors are listed in Box 32-3.

Postpartum Depression Without Psychotic Features

PPD is an intense and pervasive sadness with severe and labile mood swings and is more serious and persistent than postpartum blues. Intense fears, anger, anxiety, and despondency that persist past the baby's first few weeks of life are not a normal part of postpartum blues. Occurring in approximately 10% to 15% of new mothers, these symptoms rarely disappear without outside help (CDC, 2008; Sadock et al., 2009). Approximately 50% of these mothers, however, do not seek help from any source (Dennis & Chung-Lee, 2006). The occurrence of PPD among teenage mothers is approximately 50% more than that for older mothers (Driscoll, 2006). Young mothers (younger than 20 years) and those with a high school education or less are less likely to seek help and have higher rates of PPD than other women (Mayberry, Horowitz, & Declercq, 2007).

The symptoms of postpartum major depression do not differ from the symptoms of nonpostpartum mood disorders, except that the mother's feelings of guilt and inadequacy feed her worries about being an incompetent and inadequate parent. In PPD, the woman may have odd food cravings (often, sweet desserts) and binges with abnormal appetite and weight gain. New mothers report an increased yearning for sleep, sleeping heavily but awakening instantly with any infant noise, and an inability to go back to sleep after infant feedings. Determining difficulty falling asleep is a relevant screening question to ascertain risk for PPD (Goyal, Gay, & Lee, 2007).

A distinguishing feature of PPD is irritability. These episodes of irritability may flare up with little provocation, and they may sometimes escalate to violent outbursts or dissolve into uncontrollable sobbing. Many of these outbursts are directed against significant others ("He never helps me") or the baby ("She cries all the time, and I feel like hitting her"). Women with postpartum major depressive episodes often have severe anxiety, panic attacks, and spontaneous crying long after the usual duration of baby blues.

Many women feel especially guilty about having depressive feelings at a time when they believe they should be happy. They may be reluctant to discuss their symptoms or their negative feelings toward the infant. A prominent feature of PPD is rejection of the infant, often caused by abnormal jealousy (APA, 2000). The mother may be obsessed by the notion that the offspring may take her place in her partner's affections. Attitudes toward the infant may include disinterest, annoyance with care demands, and blaming because of her lack of maternal feeling. When observed, she may appear awkward in her responses to the baby. Obsessive thoughts about harming the child are very frightening to her. Often she does not share these thoughts because of embarrassment, but when she does, other family members may be frightened.

Medical Management. The natural course of PPD is one of gradual improvement over the 6 months after birth. However, supportive treatment alone is not efficacious for major PPD. Pharmacologic intervention is needed in most instances. Treatment options include antidepressants, antianxiety agents (shorter acting), mood stabilizers, antipsychotics, and ECT (Epperson & Ballew, 2006). A number of nonpharmacologic options have shown some success in investigations. Alternative therapies such as herbs, dietary supplements, massage, aromatherapy, bright light therapy, and acupuncture may be helpful.Women should be encouraged to take time for themselves, to rest and relax, and to ask friends and family for help as needed. Exercise, proper nutrition, and adequate sleep also contribute to symptom alleviation. Psychotherapy focuses on the woman's fears and concerns regarding her new responsibilities and roles, as well as monitoring for suicidal or homicidal thoughts. Support groups and marital counseling may be helpful (Epperson & Ballew). For some women, hospitalization is necessary.

Postpartum Depression with Psychotic Features

The most severe of the perinatal mood disorders, **postpartum psychosis** is rare, affecting approximately 0.1% to 0.2% of postpartum women (Sadock et al., 2009). Once a woman has had one episode of postpartum psychosis, she has a 30% to 50% likelihood of recurrence with each subsequent birth (APA, 2000). This disorder tends to show onset within 2 weeks postpartum; however, it may present later in the course of the illness as depression (Sadock et al.).

Episodes of postpartum psychosis are typified by auditory or visual hallucinations, paranoid or grandiose delusions, elements of delirium or disorientation, and extreme deficits in judgment accompanied by high levels of impulsivity that may contribute to increased risks of suicide or infanticide (in 5% of psychotic women) (Sadock et al., 2009). Characteristically the woman begins to complain of fatigue, insomnia, and restlessness and may have episodes of tearfulness and emotional lability. Complaints regarding the inability to move, stand, or work also are common. Later, suspiciousness, confusion, incoherence, irrational statements, and obsessive concerns about the baby's health and welfare may be present. Delusions may be present in 50% of women with postpartum psychosis, and hallucinations in approximately 25% of women with this disorder. Auditory hallucinations that command the mother to kill the infant can occur in severe cases. When delusions are present, they are often related to the infant. The mother may think the infant is possessed by the devil, has special powers, or is destined for a terrible fate (APA, 2000). Grossly disorganized behavior may be manifested as a disinterest in the infant or an inability to provide care. Some women will insist that something is wrong with the baby or accuse nurses or family members of hurting or poisoning their child.

! NURSING ALERT

Nurses are advised to be alert for mothers who are agitated, overactive, confused, complaining, or suspicious.

Postpartum psychosis is most commonly associated with the diagnosis of **bipolar (or manic-depressive) disorder** (Sadock et al.; Sharma, Burt, & Ritchie, 2009). This mood disorder is defined by the presence of one or more episodes of abnormally elevated energy levels, cognition, and mood and one or more depressive episodes. The elevated moods are clinically referred to as mania. Clinical manifestations of a manic episode include at least three of the following: grandiosity, decreased need for sleep, pressured speech, flight of ideas, distractibility, psychomotor agitation, and excessive involvement in pleasurable activities without regard for negative consequences (APA, 2000). While in a manic state, mothers need constant supervision when caring for their infant. Usually, however, they are too preoccupied to provide child care. Individuals who experience manic episodes also commonly experience depressive episodes or symptoms, or mixed episodes, in which features of both mania and depression are present at the same time. These episodes are usually separated by periods of "normal" mood, but in some individuals, depression and mania may rapidly alternate. These rapid changes in mood are known as rapid cycling.

Medical Management. Postpartum psychosis carries a relatively good prognosis with early detection and aggressive treatment, but if left untreated it may progress to the second postpartum year and become more refractory to treatment (Sadock et al., 2009). Postpartum psychosis is a psychiatric emergency, and the mother will probably need psychiatric hospitalization. Antipsychotics and mood stabilizers such as lithium are the treatments

TABLE 32-4 ANTIPSYCHOTIC MEDICATIONS

ANTIPSYCHOTIC MEDICATIONS	*PREGNANCY RISK CATEGORY	*LACTATION RISK CATEGORY
Traditional Antipsychotics		
Chlorpromazine (Thorazine)	C	L3
Fluphenazine (Prolixin)	C	L3
Haloperidol (Haldol)	C	L2
Perphenazine (Trilafon)	C	L3
Thioridazine (Mellaril)	C	L4
Thiothixene (Navane)	C	L4
Trifluoperazine (Stelazine)	Unknown	Unknown
Atypical Antipsychotics		
Aripiprazole (Abilify)	C	L3
Clozapine (Clozaril)	C	L3
Loxapine (Loxitane)	C	L4
Olanzapine (Zyprexa)	C	L2
Quetiapine (Seroquel)	C	L4
Risperidone (Risperdal)	C	L3
Ziprasidone (Geodon)	C	L4

C = Animal studies show adverse effects on fetus but no controlled studies in pregnant women *or* no studies available.
L2 = Drug studied in limited number of breastfeeding women with no adverse effects in infant *or* evidence is remote.
L3 = No controlled studies *or* studies show minimal nonthreatening effects.
L4 = Possibly hazardous.
*Source: Hale, T. (2004). *Medications and mother's milk* (11th ed.). Amarillo, TX: Pharmasoft.

of choice (see Table 32-3 and Table 32-4 for FDA categories of risk). Antidepressants should be used very cautiously in treating postpartum psychosis, even when depressive symptoms are present, because of the risk of precipitating rapid cycling. Given that 43.4% of women breastfeed for at least the first 6 weeks after birth, informed consent regarding the risks and benefits of exposing the newborn to a psychotropic agent and maternal mental illness must be discussed and documented (see additional discussion of lactation and psychotropic medications later in this chapter). ECT, especially when bilaterally administered, has also been shown to be highly effective in the treatment of postpartum psychosis (Epperson & Ballew, 2006). It is usually advantageous for the mother to have contact with her baby if she so desires, but visits must be closely supervised. Psychotherapy is indicated after the period of acute psychosis has passed.

CARE MANAGEMENT

Even though the prevalence of PPD is fairly well established, it often remains undetected because women are hesitant to report symptoms of depression to their own health care providers or to seek help from a mental health provider (McQueen, Montgomery, Lappan-Gracon, Evans, & Hunter, 2008). Primary health care providers can usually recognize severe PPD or postpartum psychosis but may miss milder forms; even if it is recognized, the woman may be treated inappropriately or subtherapeutically. Identification and treatment of maternal depression must be continued beyond the immediate post-birth period to prevent negative effects of maternal depression on the children of these mothers (McCue Horwitz, Briggs-Gowan, Storfer-Isser, & Carter, 2007). The following discussion identifies ways to assess for symptoms of PPD and describes the treatment options (see the Nursing Care Plan: Postpartum Depression and the Nursing Process box: Postpartum Depression).

To recognize symptoms of PPD as early as possible, the nurse should be an active listener and demonstrate a caring attitude. Nurses cannot depend on women volunteering unsolicited information about their depression or asking for help. The nurse should observe for signs of depression and ask appropriate questions to determine moods, appetite, sleep, energy, and fatigue levels, and ability to concentrate. Examples of ways to initiate conversation include the following: "Now that you have had your baby, how are things going for you?" "Have you had to change many things in your life since having the baby?" and "How much time do you spend crying?" If the nurse assesses that the new mother is depressed, she or he must ask if the mother has thought about hurting herself or the baby. The woman may be more willing to answer honestly if the nurse says, "Lots of women feel depressed after having a baby, and some feel so bad that they think about hurting themselves or the baby. Have you had these thoughts?"

SAFETY ALERT

Because mothers with PPD with psychotic features may harm their infants, extra caution is needed in assessment and intervention. The nurse needs to ask specifically if the mother has had thoughts about harming her baby.

Postpartum Depression Screening Tools

Nurses can use screening tools in assessing whether the depressive symptoms have progressed from postpartum blues to PPD. Examples of screening tools are the Edinburgh Postnatal Depression Scale (EPDS), the Postpartum Depression Predictors Inventory (PDPI), and the Postpartum Depression Screening Scale (PDSS). The EPDS is a self-report assessment designed specifically to identify women experiencing PPD. It has been used and validated in studies in numerous cultures and is viewed as a valid screening tool for PPD (Lintner & Gray, 2006). The assessment tool asks the woman to respond to 10 statements about the common symptoms of depression. The woman is asked to choose the response that is closest to describing how she has felt for the past week (Cox, Holden, & Sagovsky, 1987).

Through focused research over at least a decade, Beck has developed and continues to refine the PDPI (PDPI-R [Revised]) (Beck, 2001, 2002) and the PDSS (Beck & Gable, 2002). The PDPI-R consists of 13 risk factors related to PPD. The PDSS is a 35-item Likert response scale that assesses for seven dimensions of depression: sleeping or eating disturbances, anxiety or insecurity, emotional lability, mental confusion, loss of self, guilt or shame, and suicidal thoughts (Beck, 2008a). Both published tools are designed to be used by nurses and other health care providers to elicit information from the woman during an interview to assess risk. Areas assessed include the predictors of depression as listed in Box 32-3.

In addition, a simple two-item tool has been shown to be effective in identifying women at risk for PPD. Ask, "Are you sad and depressed?" and "Have you had a loss of pleasurable activities?" An affirmative answer to both questions suggests that depression is likely (Jesse & Graham, 2005).

If the initial interaction with the woman or analysis of her self-report reveals some question that she might be depressed,

NURSING CARE PLAN

Postpartum Depression (PPD)

NURSING DIAGNOSIS

Risk for injury (to the woman and/or newborn) related to woman's emotional state and/or treatment

Expected Outcomes

The mother and newborn will remain free of injury. The woman's family will verbalize understanding of the need for maternal and infant supervision and have a plan to provide that supervision.

Nursing Interventions/*Rationales*

- Assess the postpartum woman for risk factors for depression (before discharge) *to determine if she is at risk and in need of prompt interventions or referral.*
- Provide information about signs of PPD to woman and family *to promote prompt recognition of problems.*
- Observe maternal-infant interactions before discharge *to determine appropriateness.*
- Maintain frequent contact with woman by telephone calls and home visits after discharge *to determine if further interventions are necessary.*
- Counsel woman and family to telephone health care provider if behaviors indicating depression, such as crying, increase *to provide prompt care and referral if necessary and avoid injury to newborn and mother.*
- Provide opportunities for woman and family to verbalize feelings and concerns in a nonjudgmental setting *to promote a trusting relationship.*
- Assess woman for any suicidal thoughts or plans *to provide for safety of woman and infant.*
- Assist family to develop a plan for maternal and infant supervision *to provide for safety of woman and infant.*
- Provide information about community resources for assistance *to ensure care if woman is unable to care for herself or infant.*
- Reinforce teaching or refer breastfeeding mother to lactation consultant *to obtain information regarding effects of antidepressant and antipsychotic medications.*

NURSING DIAGNOSIS

Disabled family coping related to postpartum maternal depression as evidenced by family members' denial of woman's illness

Expected Outcomes

Family will identify positive coping mechanisms and initiate a plan to cope with the woman's depression.

Nursing Interventions/*Rationales*

- Provide opportunity for family and significant others to verbalize feelings and concerns *to establish a trusting relationship.*
- Give information regarding postpartum depression to the family *to clarify any misconceptions or misinformation.*
- Assist family to identify positive coping mechanisms that have been effective during past crises *to promote active participation in care.*
- Assist family to identify community sources of support *to provide additional resources as needed.*
- Refer family to mental health counselor as needed *to provide further expertise from a mental health professional.*

NURSING DIAGNOSIS

Risk for impaired parenting related to inability of mother to attach to infant

Expected Outcomes

Woman demonstrates appropriate attachment behaviors in infant interactions. Woman expresses satisfaction with infant.

Nursing Interventions/*Rationales*

- Observe maternal-infant interactions *to assess quality of interactions and to determine need for interventions.*
- Encourage woman to express her anxiety, fears, or other feelings *to allow woman to ventilate her concerns and have them accepted.*
- Encourage woman to have as much contact with infant as possible *to minimize separation and to promote attachment.*
- Encourage family participation in care of infant *to promote attachment.*
- Demonstrate infant care and explain infant behaviors *to enhance mother's care abilities and understanding of infant's abilities.*
- Make referrals as needed to community resources *to assist the woman in developing parenting skills or promoting confidence in infant care.*

a formal screening is helpful in determining the urgency of the referral and the type of provider. Also important is the need to assess the woman's family because they may be able to offer valuable information, as well as need to express how they have been affected by the woman's emotional disorder.

Nursing Care on the Postpartum Unit

The postpartum nurse must observe the new mother carefully for any signs of tearfulness and conduct further assessments as necessary. Nurses must discuss PPD to prepare new parents for potential problems in the postpartum period (see the Teaching for Self-Management box and Chapter 21). The family must be able to recognize the symptoms and know where to go for help. Written materials that explain what the woman can do to prevent depression could be used as part of discharge planning.

Mothers are often discharged from the hospital before the blues or depression occurs. If the postpartum nurse is concerned about the mother, a mental health consult should be requested before the mother leaves the hospital. Routine instructions regarding PPD should be given to the person who comes to take the woman home; for example, "If you notice that your wife [or daughter] is upset or crying a lot, please call the postpartum care provider immediately—don't wait for the routine postpartum appointment."

TEACHING FOR SELF-MANAGEMENT

Activities to Prevent Postpartum Depression

- Educate close family and friends about postpartum emotional problems.
- Take care of yourself: eat a balanced diet, exercise on a regular basis, and get enough sleep. Ask someone to take care of the baby so that you can get a full night's sleep.
- Share your feelings with someone close to you; don't isolate yourself at home.
- Don't overcommit yourself or feel like you need to be a superwoman.
- Don't place unrealistic expectations on yourself.
- Don't be ashamed of having emotional problems after your baby is born—it happens to approximately 15% of women.

NURSING PROCESS

Postpartum Depression

ASSESSMENT

- Be an active listener and demonstrate a caring attitude because women may not volunteer unsolicited information about their depression.
- Observe for signs of depression.
- Ask appropriate questions to determine moods, appetite, sleep, energy and fatigue levels, and ability to concentrate. An example of how to initiate a conversation is, "Now that you have had your baby, how are things going for you?"
- Use a screening tool to assess whether the depressive symptoms have progressed from postpartum blues to postpartum depression (PPD) (see text).
- If depression is identified, ask if the mother has thought about hurting herself or the baby.

NURSING DIAGNOSES

Possible nursing diagnoses for the woman with postpartum depression include:

***Risk for Self-directed (mother) or Other-directed (children) violence* related to:**

- PPD

***Situational Low Self-esteem (in the mother)* related to:**

- stresses associated with role changes

***Disabled Family Coping* related to:**

- increased care needs of mother and infant

***Risk for Impaired Parenting* related to:**

- inability of depressed mother to attach to infant

***Risk for Injury (to the newborn)* related to:**

- mother's depression (inattention to infant's needs for hygiene, nutrition, safety) and psychotropic medications via breast milk

EXPECTED OUTCOMES OF CARE

Specific measurable criteria can be developed based on the following general outcomes:

- The mother will no longer be depressed.
- The mother's and infant's physical well-being will be maintained.
- The family will cope effectively.
- Family members will demonstrate continued healthy growth and development.
- The infant will be fully integrated into the family.

PLAN OF CARE AND INTERVENTIONS

- Teach signs and symptoms of PPD to woman and family.
- Provide information about community resources for PPD, including mental health therapists and support groups.
- Refer woman and family to mental health therapists or support groups as needed.
- Provide teaching about psychotropic medications if ordered, including risks of breastfeeding (see text discussion).
- Provide information on alternative therapies as needed or requested (see text discussion).
- Provide periodic follow-up telephone calls.

EVALUATION

The expected outcomes of care are used to evaluate the care for the woman with PPD.

! NURSING ALERT

Because the newborn may be scheduled for a checkup before the mother's 6-week checkup, nurses in well-baby clinics or pediatrician's offices should be alert for signs of PPD in new mothers and be knowledgeable about community referral resources.

Nursing Care in the Home and Community

Postpartum home visits can reduce the incidence of or complications from depression. A brief home visit or phone call at least once a week until the new mother returns for her postpartum visit may save the life of a mother and her infant; however, home visits may not be feasible or available. Supervision of the mother with emotional complications may become a prime concern. Because depression can greatly interfere with her mothering functions, family and friends may need to participate in the infant's care. This is a time for the extended family and friends to determine what they can do to help, and the nurse can work with them to ensure adequate supervision of and their understanding of the woman's mental illness (Lintner & Gray, 2006).

When the woman has PPD, a partner often reacts with confusion, shock, denial, and anger and feels neglected and blamed. The nurse can explain to the woman that her partner is probably very worried about her, and that sometimes people withdraw or criticize when they are deeply worried about their significant others. The nurse can provide nonjudgmental opportunities for the partner to verbalize feelings and concerns, help the partner identify positive coping strategies, and be a source of encouragement for the partner to continue supporting the woman. Suggestions for partners of women with PPD include helping around the house, setting limits with family and friends, going with her to doctors' appointments, educating themselves, writing down concerns and questions to take to doctor or therapist appointments, and just being with her—sitting quietly, hugging her, and expressing their love. Both the woman and her partner need an opportunity to express their needs, fears, thoughts, and feelings in a nonjudgmental environment.

Even if the mother is severely depressed, hospitalization can be avoided if adequate resources can be mobilized to ensure safety for both mother and infant. The nurse in home health care will need to make frequent phone calls or home visits to do assessment and counseling. Community resources that may be helpful are temporary child care or foster care, homemaker service, Meals on Wheels, parenting guidance centers, mother's-day-out programs, and telephone support groups such as Postpartum Support International (www.chss.iup.edu/postpartum) and Depression after Delivery (www.depressionafterdelivery.com).

Referral. Women with moderate to severe PPD should be referred to a mental health therapist, such as an advanced practice psychiatric nurse or psychiatrist, for evaluation and therapy to prevent the effects that PPD can have on the woman and on her relationships with her partner, baby, and other children. Inpatient psychiatric hospitalization may be necessary. This decision is made when the safety needs of the mother or children are threatened.

EVIDENCE-BASED PRACTICE

Pat Gingrich

Assessing for Postpartum Depression

ASK THE QUESTION

Who is at risk for postpartum depression? What is the best way to assess for it?

SEARCH FOR EVIDENCE

Search Strategies

Professional organization guidelines, meta-analyses, systematic reviews, randomized controlled trials, nonrandomized prospective studies, and retrospective studies since 2008.

Databases Searched

CINAHL, Cochrane, Medline, National Guideline Clearinghouse, TRIP Database Plus, and the websites for the Association of Women's Health, Obstetric and Neonatal Nurses, the Centers for Disease Control and Prevention, and the Society of Obstetricians and Gynaecologists of Canada.

CRITICALLY ANALYZE THE EVIDENCE

Postpartum depression (PPD) is an insidious disease that can rob a new family of valuable nurturing time. Using data on U.S. women from the Pregnancy Risk Assessment Monitoring System (PRAMS), the Centers for Disease Control and Prevention (CDC) reported a prevalence of PPD in the first year after birth ranging from 11.7% to 20.4% (CDC, 2008). Risk factors for PPD included young age, low socioeconomic status, and use of Medicaid benefits. The CDC recommends incorporating PPD information into existing programs for high risk women, such as intimate partner violence services.

A large prospective study of 40,000 Australian women found risk factors for PPD that included low partner support and previous history of depression, especially current or antenatal anxiety or depression (Milgrom, Gemmill, Bilszta, Hayes, Barnett, Brooks, et al., 2008). The authors recommend interventions targeted to women with current depression or anxiety and low social support.

Underscoring the bidirectional and compounding nature of depression in relationships, a meta-analysis of 43 studies involving 28,000 participants found an incidence of paternal depression in about 10% of the new fathers. Paternal depression was highest at 3-6 months postpartum, and was more likely in the presence of maternal depression (Paulson & Bazemore, 2010).

IMPLICATIONS FOR PRACTICE

In an update on the evidence-based guidelines of the Registered Nurses' Association of Ontario, nurses are encouraged to give individualized, flexible care. Women should be assessed early and often. There are several assessment tools available. The Edinburgh Postnatal Depression Score (EPDS) is the most well-tested screening tool for client self-testing. Intervene swiftly for a score greater than 12 on the EPDS, or if there is any evidence of self-harm ideation (on score item #10) or in clinical judgment; and encourage peer support group participation (McQueen, Montgomery, Lappan-Gracon, Evans, & Hunter, 2008).

A systematic review of telephone support revealed that proactive telephone support decreases the symptoms of PPD. Other postpartum benefits included preventing smoking relapse and promoting breastfeeding (Dennis & Kingston, 2008).

Depression affects the entire family unit, and may be magnified by partner symptoms. Nurses can help by teaching women and men psychological self-care, especially symptoms and risk factors for PPD, helping them to feel safe and empowered in discussing their mental and social health, and facilitating adequate social and partner support. Women and their families should be given written resources in their native language and emergency telephone numbers to call. Last but not least, follow-up is a powerful tool for detection and deterrence of PPD, and should include assessment of the partner and children for symptoms.

References

Centers for Disease Control and Prevention. (2008). Prevalence of self-reported postpartum depression symptoms—17 states, 2004-2005. *MMWR Morbidity and Mortality Weekly Report, 57*(14), 361–366.

Dennis, C., & Kingston, D. (2008). A systematic review of telephone support for women during pregnancy and the early postpartum period. *Journal of Obstetric, Gynecologic and Neonatal Nursing, 37*(3), 301–314.

Milgrom, J., Gemmill, A., Bilszta, J., Hayes, B., Barnett, B., Brooks, J., et al. (2008). Antenatal risk factors for postnatal depression: A large prospective study. *Journal of Affective Disorders, 108*(1-2), 147–157.

McQueen, K., Montgomery, P., Lappan-Gracon, S., Evans, M., & Hunter, J. (2008). Evidence-based recommendations for depressive symptoms in postpartum women. *Journal of Obstetric, Gynecologic and Neonatal Nursing, 37*(2), 127–136.

Paulson, P., & Bazemore, S. (2010). Prenatal and postpartum depression in fathers and its association with maternal depression: A meta-analysis. *Journal of the American Medical Association, 303*(19), 1961–1969.

Providing Safety. If delusional thinking about the baby is suspected, the nurse asks, "Have you thought about hurting your baby?" When depression is suspected, the nurse asks, "Have you thought about hurting yourself?" Four criteria can used to measure the seriousness of a suicidal plan: method, availability, specificity, and lethality. Has the woman specified a method? Is the method of choice available? How specific is the plan? If the method is concrete and detailed, with access to it right at hand, the suicide risk increases. How lethal is the method? The most lethal method is shooting, with hanging a close second. The least lethal is slashing one's wrists.

SAFETY ALERT

Medication overdose with TCAs does cause death. Therefore, avoid the use of TCA medications in suicidal women because of this danger.

! NURSING ALERT

Suicidal thoughts or attempts are among the most serious symptoms of PPD and require immediate assessment and intervention.

Psychiatric Hospitalization

Women with postpartum psychosis must be referred immediately to a psychiatrist who is experienced in working with women with PPD, who can prescribe medication and other forms of therapy, and who can assess the need for hospitalization.

LEGAL TIP: Commitment for Psychiatric Care

If a woman with PPD is experiencing active suicidal ideation or harmful delusions about the baby and is unwilling to seek treatment, legal intervention may be necessary to commit the woman to an inpatient psychiatric setting for treatment.

If allowed within the inpatient psychiatric setting, the reintroduction of the baby to the mother can occur at the mother's own pace. A schedule is set for increasing the number of hours the mother cares for the baby over several days, culminating in the infant's staying overnight in the mother's room. This method allows the mother to experience meeting the infant's needs and giving up sleep for the baby, a situation difficult for new mothers even under ideal conditions. The mother's readiness for discharge and caring for the baby is assessed. Her interactions with her baby also are carefully supervised and guided. A postpartum nurse is often asked to assist the psychiatric nursing staff in assessment of the mother-infant interactions.

Nurses also should observe the mother for signs of bonding with the baby. Attachment behaviors are defined as eye-to-eye contact; physical contact that involves holding, touching, cuddling, and talking to the baby and calling the baby by name; and the initiation of appropriate care. A staff member is assigned to keep the baby in sight at all times. Indirect teaching, praise, and encouragement are designed to bolster the mother's self-esteem and self-confidence.

Psychotropic Medications

PPD is usually treated with antidepressant medications. If the woman with PPD is not breastfeeding, antidepressants can be prescribed without special precautions. In addition to TCAs, SSRIs, and SNRIs, MAOIs, mood stabilizers, and antipsychotic medications may be prescribed for nonbreastfeeding women (American College of Obstetricians and Gynecologists [ACOG], 2008).

Hypertensive crisis is the main reason that MAOIs are not prescribed more frequently than other psychotropic medications. The woman should be taught to watch for signs of hypertensive crisis—a throbbing, occipital headache, stiff neck, chills, nausea, flushing, retroorbital pain, apprehension, pallor, sweating, chest pain, and palpitations (Schatzberg et al., 2007). This crisis is brought on by the woman taking any of a large variety of over-the-counter medications or eating foods that contain tyramine, which normally is broken down by the enzyme monoamine oxidase. The nurse must do extensive teaching about absolute avoidance of foods and medications that contain tyramine such as pseudoephedrine-containing medications, aged cheese, red wine, fava or Italian green beans, brewer's yeast, smoked fish, chicken or beef livers, preserved meats, and tap beers (Anaizi, 2006; Schatzberg et al.). Foods that may cause problems in large amounts include alcohol, ripe avocados, yogurt, ripe bananas, and soy sauce (Schatzberg et al.).

The woman taking mood stabilizers (see Table 32-3) must be taught about the many side effects, and especially, for those taking lithium, the need to have serum lithium levels determined every 6 months. Women with severe psychiatric syndromes such as schizophrenia, bipolar disorder, or psychotic depression will probably require antipsychotic medications (see Table 32-4). Most of these antipsychotic medications can cause sedation and orthostatic hypotension—both of which could interfere with the mother being able to care safely for her baby. They also can cause peripheral nervous system (PNS) effects such as constipation, dry mouth, blurred vision, tachycardia, urinary retention, weight gain, and agranulocytosis. CNS effects may include akathisia, dystonias, parkinsonian-like symptoms, tardive dyskinesia (irreversible), and neuroleptic malignant syndrome (potentially fatal) (Schatzberg et al., 2007). Medication education is especially important when caring for women who are taking antipsychotic medications. The nurse should use discretion in selecting the content to be shared because of the women's altered thought processes and the large number of side/toxic effects. The nurse may choose to do more extensive education with a close family member. The newer, atypical antipsychotic medications such as aripiprazole, olanzapine, quetiapine, risperidone, and ziprasidone are usually safer and have fewer side effects than the older, more traditional antipsychotics. Their safety in breastfeeding women, however, has not been established (Epperson & Ballew, 2006).

Psychotropic Medications and Lactation

In the past, women were told to choose between psychotropic medication and breastfeeding. Current beliefs are that although most drugs will diffuse into breast milk, there are very few instances in which breastfeeding must be discontinued (Epperson & Ballew, 2006). Several factors influence the amount of drug an infant will receive through breastfeeding: the amount of milk produced, the composition of the milk (mature milk versus colostrum), the concentration of the medication, and the extent to which the breast was emptied during a previous feeding (Menon, 2008). The practice of pumping and then discarding breast milk either in the morning after a bedtime dose or when the medication is expected to peak in breast milk can limit the degree of infant exposure to medications. The point at which the drug peaks in breast milk is known only for sertraline, paroxetine, and fluoxetine (Epperson & Ballew). Some women may find that pumping is either impractical because of other responsibilities or raises their anxiety level about the infant's medication exposure. Some mothers may enjoy partial breastfeeding, particularly once feeding has been well established. Infants also vary in their ability to absorb, metabolize, and excrete ingested medication. Premature infants may not have optimal liver function, and kidney function does not reach maturity until 2 to 4 months of age (Epperson & Ballew).

The FDA has not approved any psychotropic medication for use during lactation. However, most of the medications listed in the position statement from the American Academy

CLINICAL REASONING

Postpartum Depression

Jenna, 31, gave birth to a 7 lbs 6 oz boy 4 weeks ago. She has been diagnosed with postpartum depression, and an SSRI (sertraline [Zoloft]) medication has been prescribed. Jenna is breastfeeding and has concerns about taking the medication.

1. Evidence—Is there sufficient evidence regarding the safety of psychotropic medications and lactation?
2. Assumptions—What assumptions can be made about the following?
   a. Lactation risk categories of SSRI medications
   b. Timing of feeding and medication administration
   c. Risks of discontinuing medications while breastfeeding
3. What is the nursing priority in this situation?
4. Does the evidence objectively support your conclusion?
5. Are there alternative perspectives to your conclusion?

of Pediatrics (AAP) are compatible with breastfeeding (AAP, 2001) (see Tables 32-1 through 32-4 for risk of taking common psychotropic medications during lactation). Long-term effects on the newborn are unknown (AAP). Because all psychotropic medications pass through breast milk to the infant, the risks associated with the use of such medications must be weighed against the benefits associated with breastfeeding for mother and infant. Almost all of the psychotropic medications are drugs for which the effects on the breastfeeding newborn are unknown but still may be of concern (AAP).

The relatively extensive literature focusing on SSRIs in breastfeeding indicates that infants can continue to nurse when their mothers are prescribed these agents without risk of adverse events (Epperson & Ballew, 2006). According to a pooled analysis of available data, breastfeeding infants exposed to paroxetine or sertraline are least likely to demonstrate detectable or elevated plasma drug levels, whereas infants exposed to fluoxetine appear to be at higher risk of developing elevated levels (Sadock et al., 2009). Of the SSRIs, fluoxetine is the most extensively studied in breastfed infants. One study reported reduced growth curves in children, and there is one case report of transient seizure activity. Although the majority of studies focusing on the use of fluoxetine during breastfeeding suggest no apparent adverse effects, long-term developmental and behavioral effects have not been investigated (Epperson & Ballew). If treatment with an SSRI is started during the postpartum period, fluoxetine should not be the first choice (Sadock et al.). Less is known about venlafaxine or bupropion in breastfeeding infants. Most TCAs appear to be safe during breastfeeding, with the exception of doxepin, which is associated with respiratory depression. Although TCAs have been the treatment of choice in the past, SSRIs are gaining popularity because of their superior safety profiles (Epperson & Ballew). MAOIs are usually avoided. The lowest effective dose of antidepressant medication should be used in a breastfeeding mother. When the use of an SSRI is clearly indicated in a breastfeeding mother, the data generally indicate that the positive effects of breastfeeding outweigh the risks for adverse effects in the infant (Sadock et al.).

Benzodiazepines, mood stabilizers, and antipsychotic medications are all used frequently in the treatment of postpartum psychiatric disorders, despite the lack of research in this population (Epperson & Ballew, 2006). No long-term effects have been reported in exclusively breastfed infants whose mothers were taking benzodiazepines on a regular basis. The shorter acting agents (alprazolam, lorazepam) are favored over those with longer half-lives (clonazepam, diazepam) (Epperson & Ballew).

Mood-stabilizing medications are present in breast milk. Lithium has been the most extensively studied. Lithium has been linked to several serious adverse effects in breastfeeding infants, including hypotonia, hypothermia, cyanosis, and electrocardiogram abnormalities. Therefore, its use is not recommended in breastfeeding mothers. Valproic acid and carbamazepine are considered reasonably safe for use while breastfeeding, although careful monitoring for infant hepatotoxicity is recommended (Epperson & Ballew, 2006). The benefits of breastfeeding and the potential risks must be carefully considered before using lithium or other mood stabilizers (Fankhauser & Freeman, 2005).

In summary, all psychotropic medications studied to date are excreted in breast milk. When selecting psychotropic medications for breastfeeding women, choose those with the greatest documentation of prior use, lower FDA risk category, few or no metabolites, and fewer side effects (ACOG, 2008).

When breastfeeding women have emotional complications and need psychotropic medications, referral to a mental health care provider who specializes in postpartum disorders is preferred. The woman should be informed of the risks and benefits to her and her infant of the medications to be taken. Depressed women will need the nurse to reinforce the need to take antidepressants as ordered. Because antidepressants do not exert any effect for approximately 2 weeks and usually do not reach full effect for 4 to 6 weeks, many women discontinue taking the medication on their own. Client and family teaching should reinforce the schedule for taking medications in conjunction with the infant's feeding schedule and to continue taking the medication until therapeutic effects occur.

Other Treatments for PPD

Other treatments for PPD include complementary or alternative therapies (e.g., yoga, massage, relaxation techniques), ECT, and psychotherapy (group or individual). ECT may be used for women with PPD who have not improved with antidepressant therapy. Psychotherapy in the form of group therapy or individual (interpersonal) therapy also has been used with positive results alone and in conjunction with antidepressant therapy; however, more studies are needed to determine what types of professional support are most effective (Dennis & Hodnett, 2007). Alternative therapies may be used alone but often are used with other treatments for PPD. Safety and efficacy studies of these alternative therapies are needed to ensure that care and advice is based on evidence.

! NURSING ALERT

St. John's wort is often used to treat depression. It has not been proven safe for women who are breastfeeding.

Postpartum Onset of Anxiety Disorders

In a metaanalysis, anxiety disorders were noted to be common during the perinatal period, with reported rates of OCD and generalized anxiety disorder being higher in postpartum women than in the general population (Ross & McLean, 2006). In one study, 147 community women completed an interview and self-report inventories about 8 weeks after childbirth (Wenzel, Haugen, Jackson, & Brendle, 2005). In approximately 3% to 5% of women, panic disorder or OCD develops in the postpartum period. It is very important to distinguish between the symptoms of OCD in the postpartum client and those of postpartum psychosis because either may involve ideation regarding harming the newborn (Abramowitz, Larsen, & Moore, 2006). Delusions such as "the baby is born of the Devil" are typical in psychosis and dangerous for the baby, but not found in OCD. Postpartum obsessions such as the woman fearing that she will throw the baby out the window are not associated with an increased risk of harm to the baby (Abramowitz et al.).

Panic attacks are discrete periods of sudden onset of intense apprehension, fearfulness, or terror (APA, 2000). During these attacks, symptoms such as shortness of breath, palpitations, chest pain, choking, smothering sensations, and fear of losing control are present. Women have reported having intrusive thoughts about terrible injury done to the infant, such as stabbing or burns, sometimes by themselves. Rarely do the women harm the baby. Nurses need only to listen to the mother to hear symptoms of panic disorder. Usually these women are so distraught that they will share with whoever will listen. Often the family has tried to tell them that what they are experiencing is normal, but they know differently. Potential nursing diagnoses for women experiencing postpartum anxiety disorders include the following:

- *Anxiety* related to:
  - postpartum adaptations and expectations
- *Fear* related to:
  - obsessions
  - thoughts about harming others
- *Powerlessness* related to:
  - feelings of losing control
- *Deficient Knowledge* related to:
  - postpartum mental health problems

Medical Management

There are effective treatments for anxiety disorders, and this fact should be communicated to clients (Abramowitz et al., 2006). Cognitive-behavioral therapy (CBT) is an attractive option because of its substantial benefits, limited duration, no drug exposure to the infant, and durability of effect. Pharmacotherapy, primarily in the form of SSRIs, is useful. The widespread availability and ease of administration make SSRIs an appealing option (Abramowitz et al.). Antidepressants such as SSRIs are the treatment of choice, rather than benzodiazepines. Much remains unknown regarding the effects of SSRIs on the fetus and breastfeeding baby. Each woman should be approached on an individualized basis, assessing the severity of symptoms, obtaining the history and response to any previous treatments, understanding the woman's preferences, and educating the woman about the potential benefits and potential risk of each treatment (Abramowitz et al.). Treatment is usually a combination of medications, education, psychotherapy, and CBT, along with an attempt to identify any medical or physiologic contributors.

Nursing Considerations

The following nursing interventions are suggested:

Education is a crucial nursing intervention. New mothers should be provided with anticipatory guidance concerning the possibility of anxiety disorders during the postpartum period. Preparing for the attacks may help offset their unexpected, terrifying nature (Beck, 1998; Driscoll, 2006).

Empowerment conveys to the woman that she can sort through her fears and expectations and take charge of her life. Women can be reassured that it is common to feel a sense of impending doom and fear of insanity during panic attacks.

Nurses can help women identify panic triggers that are particular to their own lives. Keeping a diary can help identify the triggers.

Family and social supports are helpful. The new mother is encouraged to put usual chores on hold and to ask for and accept help.

Support groups allow these mothers to feel comfort in seeing others in similar circumstances.

Sensory interventions such as music therapy and aromatherapy are nonintrusive and inexpensive.

Behavioral interventions such as breathing exercises and progressive muscle relaxation can be helpful (Peeke, 2008).

Cognitive interventions such as positive self-talk training, reframing and redefining, and reassurance can help a woman learn to change the way she feels or acts even in situations that do not change (National Women's Health Resource Center, 2008)

Exercise may be helpful for some women, particularly if they have low levels of gamma aminobutyric acid (Peeke, 2008).

KEY POINTS

- Because pregnant women may have a history of mental disorder or substance abuse, careful assessment is extremely important at the first and each subsequent prenatal and postnatal visit.
- Identification of women at greatest risk for substance abuse during pregnancy and depression in the postpartum period can be facilitated by use of various screening tools.
- Values clarification for health care workers may be necessary to assist them in providing nonjudgmental care for woman who abuse substances.
- Alcohol abuse during pregnancy is the leading cause of mental retardation in the United States, and it is entirely preventable.
- Treatment programs must start with an understanding that substance abuse in women is a complex problem surrounded by multiple individual, familial, and social issues that require many levels of intervention and treatment.
- Mood disorders account for most mental health disorders in the postpartum period.
- Suicidal thoughts or attempts are among the most serious symptoms of PPD.
- Antidepressant medications are the usual treatment for PPD; however, specific precautions are needed for breastfeeding women.
- Treatment of postpartum onset of panic disorder requires a combination of medication, education, supportive measures, and psychotherapy.

Audio Chapter Summaries Access an audio summary of these Key Points on evolve

REFERENCES

Abramowitz, J., Larsen, K., & Moore, K. (2006). Treatment of anxiety disorders in pregnancy and the postpartum. In V. Hendrick (Ed.), *Psychiatric disorders in pregnancy and the postpartum*. Totowa, NJ: Humana Press.

American Academy of Pediatrics (AAP) Committee on Drugs. (2001). The transfer of drugs and other chemicals into human milk. *Pediatrics, 108*(3), 776–789.

American College of Obstetricians and Gynecologists (ACOG). (2008). *Use of psychiatric medications during pregnancy and lactation.* ACOG Practice Bulletin No. 92. Washington, DC: ACOG.

American Psychiatric Association. (2000). *Diagnostic and statistical manual of mental disorders* (4th ed., rev.). Washington, DC: American Psychiatric Association Press.

Anaizi, N. (2006). Food-drug interactions. *The drug monitor*. Available at www.thedrugmonitor.com. Accessed July 20, 2010.

Andreasen, N., & Black, D. (2007). *Introductory textbook of psychiatry*. Washington, DC: American Psychiatric Publishing, Inc.

Bandestra, E., & Accornero, V. (2006). Infants of substance-abusing mothers. In A. Fanaroff, R. Martin, & M. Walsh (Eds.), *Fanaroff and Martin's neonatal-perinatal medicine: Diseases of the fetus and infant* (8th ed.). Philadelphia: Mosby.

Beck, C. (2002). Revision of the Postpartum Depression Predictors Inventory. *Journal of Obstetric, Gynecologic and Neonatal Nursing, 31*(4), 394–402.

Beck, C. (2008a). State of the science on postpartum depression: What nurse researchers have contributed—part 1. *MCN The American Journal of Maternal/Child Nursing, 33*(2), 122–126.

Beck, C. (2008b). State of the science on postpartum depression: What nurse researchers have contributed—part 2. *MCN The American Journal of Maternal/Child Nursing, 33*(3), 151–156.

Beck, C., & Gable, R. (2002). *Postpartum depression screening scale manual.* Los Angeles: Western Psychological Services.

Bennett, H., Einarson, A., Toddio, A., Koren, G., & Einarson, T. (2004). Prevalence of depression during pregnancy: Systematic review. *Obstetrics and Gynecology, 103*(4), 698–709.

Bina, R. (2008). The impact of cultural factors upon postpartum depression: A literature review. *Health Care for Women International, 29*(6), 568–592.

Bogart, C., & Pearce, C. (2003). "13th stepping": Why Alcoholics Anonymous is not always a safe place for women. *Journal of Addictions Nursing, 14*(1), 43–47.

Bozkurt, A., Karlidere, T., Isintas, M., Ozmenier, N., Ozsahin, A., & Yanarates, O. (2007). Acute and maintenance electroconvulsive therapy for treatment of psychotic depression in a pregnant patient. *The Journal of ECT, 23*(3), 185–187.

Brady, T., & Ashley, O. (2005). *Women in substance abuse treatment: Results from alcohol and drug services study (ADSS)*. USDHHS publication no. SMA 04-3968 analytic series A 26. Rockville, MD: Substance and Mental Health Services Administration, Office of Applied Studies.

Centers for Disease Control and Prevention (CDC). (2008). Prevalence of self-reported postpartum depressive symptoms—17 states, 2004-2005. *MMWR Morbidity and Mortality Weekly Report, 57*(14), 361–366.

Chasnoff, I., McGourty, R., Bailey, G., Hutchins, E., Lightfoot, S., Pawson, L., et al. (2005). The 4Ps Plus screen for substance use in pregnancy: Clinical application and outcomes. *Journal of Perinatology, 25*(6), 368–374.

Cox, J., Holden, J., & Sagovsky, R. (1987). Detection of postnatal depression. Development of the 10 item Edinburgh Postnatal Depression Scale. *British Journal of Psychiatry, 150*(6), 782–786.

Dennis, C., & Chung-Lee, L. (2006). Postpartum depression helpseeking barriers and maternal treatment preferences: A qualitative systematic review. *Birth, 33*(4), 323–331.

Dennis, C., & Hodnett, E. (2007). Psychosocial and psychological interventions for treating postpartum depression. *The Cochrane Database of Systematic Reviews, 2007*, 4, CD006116.

Doering, P. (2005). Substance-related disorders: Alcohol, nicotine, and caffeine. In J. DiPiro, R. Talbert, G. Yee, G. Matzke, B. Wells, & M. Posey (Eds.), *Pharmacotherapy: A pathophysiologic approach* (6th ed.). New York: McGraw-Hill.

Doggett, C., Burrett, S., & Osborn, D. (2005). Home visits during pregnancy and after birth for a woman with a drug or alcohol problem. *The Cochrane Database of Systematic Reviews, 2005*, 4, CD004456.

Driscoll, J. (2006). Postpartum depression: How nurses can identify and care for women grappling with this disorder. *AWHONN Lifelines, 10*(5), 400–409.

Epperson, C., & Ballew, J. (2006). Postpartum depression: A common complication of childbirth. In V. Hendrick (Ed.), *Psychiatric disorders in pregnancy and the postpartum.* Totowa, NJ: Humana Press.

Ewing, J. (1984). Detecting alcoholism: The CAGE questionnaire. *Journal of the American Medical Association, 22*(14), 1905–1907.

Fankhauser, M., & Freeman, M. (2005). Bipolar disorder. In J. DiPiro, R. Talbert, G. Yee, G. Matzke, B. Wells, & M. Posey (Eds.), *Pharmacotherapy: A pathophysiologic approach* (6th ed.). New York: McGraw-Hill.

Gilbert, E. (2011). *Manual of high risk pregnancy & delivery* (5th ed.). St. Louis: Mosby.

Gold, M., Roytberg, A., Frost-Pineda, K., Jacobs, W., & Teitelbaum, S. (2007). Marijuana. In G. Gabbard (Ed.), *Gabbard's treatments of psychiatric disorders* (4th ed.). Washington, DC: American Psychiatric Publishing, Inc.

Goldbort, J. (2006). Transcultural analysis of postpartum depression. *MCN The American Journal of Maternal/Child Nursing, 31*(2), 121–126.

Goyal, D., Gay, C., & Lee, K. (2007). Patterns of sleep disruption and depressive symptoms in new mothers. *Journal of Perinatal and Neonatal Nursing, 21*(2), 323–329.

Greenfield, L., Burgdorf, K., Porowski, A., Roberts, T., & Herrell, J. (2004). Effectiveness of long-term residential substance abuse treatment for women: Findings from three national studies. *American Journal of Drug and Alcohol Abuse, 30*(3), 537–550.

Harris, L., & Paltrow, L. (2003). The status of pregnant women and fetuses in U.S. criminal law. *Journal of the American Medical Association, 289*(13), 1697–1699.

Hendrick, V. (2006). General considerations in treating psychiatric disorders during pregnancy and following delivery. In V. Hendrick (Ed.), *Psychiatric disorders in pregnancy and the postpartum*. Totowa, NJ: Humana Press.

Hser, Y., & Niv, N. (2006). Pregnant women in women-only and mixed-gender substance abuse treatment programs: A comparison of client characteristics and program services. *Journal of Behavioral Health Services Research, 33*(4), 431–432.

Jahanfar, S., & Sharifah, H. (2009). Effects of restricted caffeine intake by mother on fetal, neonatal and pregnancy outcome. *The Cochrane Database of Systematic Reviews, 2009*, 2, CD006965.

Jesse, D., & Graham, M. (2005). Are you sad and depressed? Brief measures to identify women at risk for depression in pregnancy. *MCN The American Journal of Maternal/Child Nursing, 30*(1), 40–45.

Lawrence, R., & Lawrence, R. (2005). *Breastfeeding: A guide for the medical profession* (6th ed.). St. Louis: Mosby.

Lester, B., & Twomey, J. (2008). Treatment of substance abuse during pregnancy. *Women's Health (London, England), 4*(1), 67–77.

Lim, S., Prasad, M., Samuels, P., Gardner, D., & Cordero, L. (2009). High-dose methadone in pregnant women and its effect on duration of neonatal abstinence syndrome. *American Journal of Obstetrics and Gynecology, 200*(1), 70.e1-e5.

Lintner, N., & Gray, B. (2006). Childbearing and depression: What nurses need to know. *AWHONN Lifelines, 10*(1), 50–57.

Lui, S., Terplan, M., & Smith, E. (2008). Psychosocial interventions for women enrolled in alcohol treatment during pregnancy. *The Cochrane Database of Systematic Reviews, 2008*, 3, CD006753.

March of Dimes. (2008). *Caffeine in pregnancy*. from www.marchofdimes.com/professionals/14332_1148.asp#miscarriage.

Mayberry, L., Horowitz, J., & Declercq, E. (2007). Depression symptom prevalence and demographic risk factors among U.S. women during the first 2 years postpartum. *Journal of Obstetric, Gynecologic and Neonatal Nursing, 36*(6), 542–549.

McCue Horwitz, S., Briggs-Gowan, M., Storfer-Isser, A., & Carter, A. (2007). Prevalence, correlates, and persistence of maternal depression. *Journal of Women's Health, 16*(5), 678–691.

McQueen, K., Montgomery, P., Lappan-Gracon, S., Evans, E., & Hunter, J. (2008). Evidence-based recommendations for depressive symptoms in postpartum women. *Journal of Obstetric, Gynecologic and Neonatal Nursing, 37*(2), 127–136.

Menon, S. (2008). Psychotropic medication during pregnancy and lactation. *Archives of Gynecology and Obstetrics, 277*(1), 1–13.

Milgrom, J., Gemmill, A., Bilszta, J., Hayes, B., Barnett, B., Brooks, J., et al. (2008). Antenatal risk factors for postnatal depression: A large prospective study. *Journal of Affective Disorders, 108*(1-2), 147–157.

Miller, W., & Rollnick, S. (1991). *Motivational interviewing: Preparing people to change addictive behaviour.* New York: Guilford Press.

Miotto, K., Suti, E., Hernandez, M., & Pham, P. (2006). Pregnancy and substance abuse. In V. Hendrick (Ed.), *Psychiatric disorders in pregnancy and the postpartum.* Totowa, NJ: Humana Press.

National Women's Health Resource Center. (2008). Women and anxiety disorders. *National Women's Health Report, 30*(1), 1–7.

Navarro, P., Garcia-Esteve, L., Ascasco, C., Aguardo, J., Gelabert, E., & Martin-Santos, R. (2008). Non-psychotic psychiatric disorders after childbirth: Prevalence and comorbidity in a community sample. *Journal of Affective Disorders, 109*(1-2), 171–176.

Newport, D., Stowe, Z., Viguera, A., Calamaras, M., Juric, S., Knight, B., et al. (2008). Lamotrigine in bipolar disorder: Efficacy during pregnancy. *Bipolar Disorders, 10*(3), 432–436.

Otto, K. (2003). Acupuncture and substance abuse: A synopsis with indications for further research. *American Journal of Addictions, 12*(1), 43–51.

Peeke, P. (2008). Anxiety: Things you can do to beat it. *National Women's Health Report, 30*(1), 8.

Pichler, G., Heinzinger, J., Klaritsch, P., Zotter, H., Wilheim, M., & Uriesberger, B. (2008). Impact of smoking during pregnancy on peripheral tissue oxygenation in term neonates. *Neonatology, 93*(2), 132–137.

Pigarelli, J., Kraus, C., & Potter, B. (2005). Pregnancy and lactation: Therapeutic considerations. In J. DiPiro, R. Talbert, G. Yee, G. Matzke, B. Wells, & M. Posey (Eds.), *Pharmacotherapy: A pathophysiologic approach* (6th ed.). New York: McGraw-Hill.

Pokorny, A., Miller, B., & Kaplan, H. (1972). The Brief MAST: A shortened version of the Michigan Alcoholism Screening Test. *American Journal of Psychiatry, 129*(3), 342–345.

Prochaska, J., & DiClemente, C. (1992). Stages of change in the modification of problem behaviors. In M. Hersen, R. Eisler, & P. Miller (Eds.), *Progress in behavior modification* Vol. 28. Sycamore, IL: Sycamore.

Ross, L., & McLean, L. (2006). Anxiety disorders during pregnancy and the postpartum period: A systematic review. *Journal of Clinical Psychiatry, 67*(8), 1285–1298.

Roy, P., & Payne, J. (2009). Treatment of bipolar disorder during and after pregnancy. In C. Zarate, & K. Husseini (Eds.), *Bipolar depression: Molecular neurobiology, clinical diagnosis and pharmacotherapy.* Cambridge, MA: Birkhauser.

Sadock, B., Sadock, V., & Ruiz, P. (2009). *Kaplan & Sadock's comprehensive textbook of psychiatry,* Vol. 2. (9th ed.). Philadelphia: Lippincott Williams & Wilkins.

Saulnier, C. (1996). African-American women in an alcohol intervention group: Addressing personal and political problems. *Substance Use and Misuse, 31*(10), 1259–1278.

Schatzberg, A., Cole, J., & DeBattista, C. (2007). *Manual of clinical psychopharmacology.* Washington, DC: American Publishing, Inc.

Seedat, S., Scott, K., Angermeyer, M., Berglund, P., Bromet, E., Brugha, T., et al. (2009). Cross-national associations between gender and mental disorders in the World Health Organization World Mental Health Surveys. *Archives of General Psychiatry, 66*(7), 785–795.

Seidel, H., Ball, J., Dains, J., Flynn, J., Solomon, B., & Stewart, R. (2011). *Mosby's guide to physical examination* (7th ed.). St. Louis: Mosby.

Sharma, V., Burt, V., & Ritchie, H. (2009). Bipolar II postpartum depression: Detection, diagnosis, and treatment. *American Journal of Psychiatry, 166*(11), 1201–1204.

Stanger, C., Budney, A., Kamon, J., & Thostensen, J. (2009). A randomized trial of contingency management of adolescent marijuana abuse and dependence. *Drug and Alcohol Dependence, 105*(3), 240–247.

Sword, W., Busser, D., Ganann, R., McMillan, T., & Swinton, M. (2008). Women's care seeking experiences after referral for postpartum depression. *Qualitative Research Health, 18*(9), 1161–1173.

Terplan, M., & Lui, S. (2007). Psychosocial interventions for pregnant women in outpatient illicit drug treatment programs compared to other interventions. *The Cochrane Database of Systematic Reviews, 2007*, 4, CD006037.

Thornton, D., Guendelman, S., & Hosang, N. (2009). Obstetric complications in women with diagnosed mental illness: The relative success of California's county mental health system. *Health Services Research, 45*(1), 246–264.

Wenzel, A., Haugen, E., Jackson, D., & Brendle, J. (2005). Anxiety symptoms and disorders at eight weeks postpartum. *Journal of Anxiety Disorders, 19*(3), 295–311.

Wisner, K., Sit, D., Reynolds, S., Altemus, M., Bogen, D., Sunder, K., et al. (2007). Psychiatric disorders. In S. Gabbe, J. Niebyl, & J. Simpson (Eds.), *Obstetrics: Normal and problem pregnancies* (5th ed.). Philadelphia: Churchill Livingstone.

Worley, L., Conners, N., Crone, C., Williams, V., & Bokony, P. (2005). Building a residential treatment program for dually diagnosed women with their children. *Archives of Women's Mental Health, 8*(2), 105–111.

Zammit, S., Thomas, K., Thompson, A., Horwood, J., Menezes, P., Gunnell, D., et al. (2009). Maternal tobacco, cannabis and alcohol use during pregnancy and risk of adolescent psychotic symptoms in offspring. *British Journal of Psychiatry, 195*(4), 294–300.

CHAPTER

33

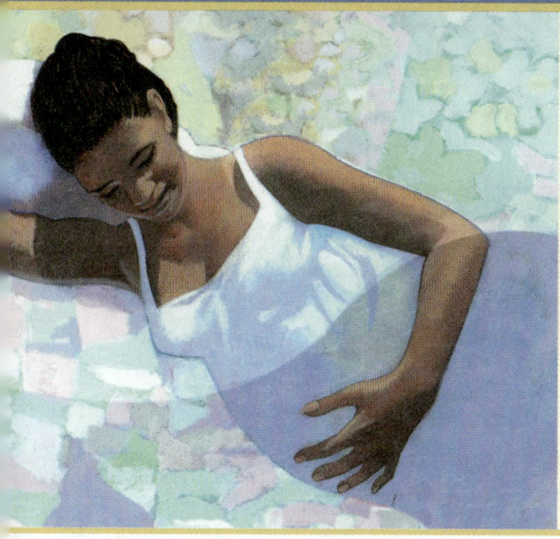

Labor and Birth Complications

Karen A. Piotrowski

evolve WEBSITE

http://evolve.elsevier.com/Lowdermilk/MWHC/

- Animations
  - Breech Birth
  - Breech Examination
  - Cord Prolapse
  - Shoulder Dystocia
- Audio Glossary
- Audio Key Points
- Case Studies
  - Preterm Labor
  - Postdate Pregnancy
- Critical Thinking Exercise
  - Preterm Labor
- NCLEX Review Questions
- Nursing Care Plans
  - Dysfunctional Labor: Hypotonic Uterus Dysfunction with Protracted Active Phase
  - Preterm Labor
- Spanish Guidelines
  - Cesarean Birth
  - Induction of Labor
- Video—Childbirth
  - Cesarean

LEARNING OBJECTIVES

- Differentiate between preterm birth and low birth weight.
- Identify major risk factors associated with preterm labor.
- Analyze current interventions to prevent spontaneous preterm birth.
- Discuss the use of tocolytics and antenatal glucocorticoids in preterm labor.
- Evaluate the effects of prescribed bed rest on pregnant women and their families.
- Design a nursing care plan for women with preterm premature rupture of the membranes (preterm PROM).
- Explain the challenge of caring for obese women during labor and birth.
- Summarize the nursing care for a trial of labor, the induction and augmentation of labor, forceps- and vacuum-assisted birth, cesarean birth, and vaginal birth after a cesarean birth (VBAC).
- Explain the care of a woman with postterm pregnancy.
- Discuss obstetric emergencies and their appropriate management.

When complications arise during labor and birth, risk for perinatal morbidity and mortality increases. Some complications are anticipated, especially if the woman is identified to be at high risk during the antepartum period; other complications are unexpected or unforeseen. It is crucial for nurses to understand the normal birth process to prevent and detect deviations from normal labor and birth and to promptly implement nursing measures when complications arise. Optimal care of the laboring woman, fetus, and family experiencing complications is possible only when the nurse and other members of the obstetric team use their knowledge and skills in a concerted effort to provide competent and compassionate care. This chapter focuses on the problems of preterm labor and birth, dystocia, obesity, postterm pregnancy, and obstetric emergencies.

PRETERM LABOR AND BIRTH

Preterm labor is defined as cervical changes and uterine contractions occurring between 20 and 37 weeks of pregnancy. **Preterm birth** is any birth that occurs before the completion of

37 weeks of pregnancy (Iams & Romero, 2007). More than 33% of infant mortality is associated with prematurity. In 2008 the preterm birth rate for all races in the United States was 12.3%, an increase of 20% since 1990 (Hamilton, Martin, & Ventura, 2010).

About 75% of all preterm births in the United States are termed **late preterm** because they occur between 34 and 36 weeks of gestation. The steady increase in the preterm birth rate has been attributed to the rise in the rate of late preterm births, which has increased 25% since 1990. Late preterm infants are at increased risk for early death and long-term health problems when compared with infants who are born full term. Although late preterm babies do experience significant problems, the great majority of infant deaths and the most serious morbidity and mortality occur among the 16% of all preterm infants who are born before 32 weeks of gestation **(very preterm birth).** The very preterm birth rate is approximately 2%, representing only a slight increase from the rate in 1981, which was 1.81% (Iams, Romero, & Creasy, 2009; Martin, Hamilton, Sutton, Ventura, Menacker, Kirmeyer, et al., 2009).

In the United States the incidence of preterm birth has been increasing for the three largest racial and ethnic groups. Non-Hispanic black women have the highest rate. Hispanic woman have the next highest, and non-Hispanic white women have the lowest rate of preterm birth. The extremely preterm birth (less than 28 weeks of gestation) rate has decreased for non-Hispanic black women, but the rate is still three times higher than the rates for non-Hispanic white and Hispanic women (Martin et al., 2009). The incidence of preterm birth in developed countries has also been increasing, mainly due to more late preterm births and multifetal gestations. An increased rate of assisted reproductive technologies and more births to women older than the age of 35, which increases the risk for twinning, has led to the rise in multifetal gestations. More willingness on the part of health care providers to proceed to birth when maternal or obstetric conditions threaten the health of the mother or fetus after 32 to 34 weeks of gestation also contributes to the rise in preterm births (Iams et al., 2009).

Preterm Birth Versus Low Birth Weight

Although they have distinctly different meanings, the terms *preterm birth* or *prematurity* and *low birth weight* are often interchanged. Preterm birth describes length of gestation (i.e., less than 37 weeks regardless of the weight of the infant), whereas **low birth weight** describes only weight at the time of birth (i.e., 2500 g or less). Because birth weight was far easier to determine than gestational age, in many settings and publications low birth weight was used as a substitute term for preterm birth. Preterm birth, however, is a more dangerous health condition for an infant because less time in the uterus correlates with immaturity of body systems. Low-birth-weight babies can be, but are not necessarily, preterm; low birth weight can be caused by conditions other than preterm birth, such as **intrauterine growth restriction (IUGR),** a condition of inadequate fetal growth not necessarily correlated with initiation of labor. Pregnant women who have various complications of pregnancy that interfere with uteroplacental perfusion, such as gestational hypertension or poor nutrition, may give birth to a baby at term who is low birth weight because of IUGR. However, infants born at a preterm gestation can weigh more that 2500 g at birth. Today, thanks to advances in pregnancy dating, outcomes related to gestational age can increasingly be distinguished from outcomes related to birth weight (Iams et al., 2009).

Critical Thinking Exercise—Preterm Labor

Preterm births are divided into two categories: spontaneous and indicated. Spontaneous preterm births occur following an early initiation of the labor process and comprise nearly 75% of all preterm births in the United States. Conditions such as preterm labor with intact membranes, preterm premature rupture of membranes (preterm PROM), cervical insufficiency, or amnionitis often result in preterm birth (Iams et al., 2009). Box 33-1 lists risk factors for the development of spontaneous preterm labor.

Indicated preterm births occur as a means to resolve maternal or fetal risk related to continuing the pregnancy. About 25% of all preterm births in the United States are indicated because of medical or obstetric conditions that affect the mother, the fetus, or both. An increase in the number of indicated preterm births accounts for much of the recent rise in late preterm births (Iams et al., 2009). Box 33-2 lists common causes of indicated preterm births.

The remainder of this section deals with spontaneous preterm labor and birth.

BOX 33-1 RISK FACTORS FOR SPONTANEOUS PRETERM LABOR

- Genital tract infection
- Non-Caucasian race
- Multifetal gestation
- Second trimester bleeding
- Low prepregnancy weight
- History of previous spontaneous preterm birth

Source: Iams, J., Romero, R., & Creasy, R. (2009). Preterm labor and birth. In R. Creasy, R. Resnik, J. Iams, C. Lockwood, & T. Moore (Eds.), *Creasy and Resnik's maternal-fetal medicine: Principles and practice* (6th ed.). Philadelphia: Saunders.

BOX 33-2 COMMON CAUSES OF INDICATED PRETERM BIRTH

- Preeclampsia
- Fetal distress
- Intrauterine growth restriction
- Placental abruption
- Intrauterine fetal demise
- Pregestational and gestational diabetes
- Renal disease
- Rh sensitization
- Congenital malformations

Source: Iams, J., Romero, R., & Creasy, R. (2009). Preterm labor and birth. In R. Creasy, R. Resnik, J. Iams, C. Lockwood, & T. Moore (Eds.), *Creasy and Resnik's maternal-fetal medicine: Principles and practice* (6th ed.). Philadelphia: Saunders.

Predicting Spontaneous Preterm Labor and Birth

Major risk factors associated with preterm labor and birth are a history of preterm birth, current multifetal pregnancy, cervical or uterine abnormalities, bleeding after the first trimester of pregnancy, and a low or a high maternal body mass index

(BMI). Non-white race (especially non-Hispanic black), low socioeconomic and educational status, living with chronic stress, intimate partner violence, lack of social support, smoking, substance abuse, and physically demanding working conditions also have been identified as risk factors (Bowers, Curran, Freda, Krening, Poole, Slocum, et al., 2008; Iams et al., 2009). A study by nurse researchers found that perceived levels of stress measured at 28 weeks of gestation in black women experiencing preterm labor were higher in those who gave birth prematurely than in those whose pregnancies reached term (Gennaro, Shults, & Garry, 2008). In addition, the risk of preterm birth appears to be genetically related. Relatives of women who were born prematurely or gave birth prematurely also have an increased risk for spontaneous preterm birth. Research has found links between preterm birth and singleton pregnancies conceived through assisted reproductive technologies (ART) (Bowers et al.; Iams et al.).

Researchers have developed many risk scoring systems in an attempt to determine which women might go into labor prematurely. No risk scoring system has been very successful in lowering the preterm birth rate, however, because at least 50% of all women who ultimately give birth prematurely have no identifiable risk factors (Iams & Romero, 2007; Iams et al., 2009). Therefore, it is important that all women be educated about prematurity, not only in early pregnancy but also in the preconception period. Unless all women are included in prevention efforts, a widespread reduction of preterm birth rates cannot be expected (Maloni & Damato, 2004).

Biochemical Marker

Fetal fibronectin has been studied extensively and is marketed in the United States as a diagnostic test for preterm labor. Fetal fibronectin is a glycoprotein "glue" found in plasma and produced during fetal life. The test is performed by collecting fluid from the woman's vagina using a swab during a speculum examination. Fetal fibronectin normally appears in cervical and vaginal secretions early in pregnancy, and then again in late pregnancy.

The presence of fetal fibronectin during the late second and early third trimesters of pregnancy may be related to placental inflammation, which is thought to be one cause of spontaneous preterm labor. The presence of fetal fibronectin is not very sensitive as a predictor of preterm birth, however. Before 35 weeks of gestation, a positive fetal fibronectin test predicts preterm birth only about 25% of the time. The test's sensitivity may be better earlier in pregnancy. In one study, the fetal fibronectin test predicted 65% of preterm births occurring before 28 weeks when it was performed between 22 and 24 weeks. Often the test is used to predict who will *not* go into preterm labor because preterm labor is very unlikely to occur in women with a negative result. Use of the fetal fibronectin test in women who are at low risk for preterm birth as a screening tool is not recommended (Iams et al., 2009).

Cervical Length

Another possible predictor of preterm labor is endocervical length. Changes in cervical length occur before uterine activity, so cervical measurement can identify women in whom the labor process has begun. However, because preterm cervical shortening occurs over a period of weeks, neither digital nor ultrasound cervical examination is very sensitive at predicting imminent preterm birth (Iams et al., 2009). Women whose cervical length is greater than 30 mm are unlikely to give birth prematurely even if they have symptoms of preterm labor (Iams & Romero, 2007; Iams et al.).

Case Study—Preterm Labor

Causes of Preterm Labor and Birth

Infection is the only factor definitely shown to cause preterm labor. When bacterial cervical or urinary tract infections are present, the risk of preterm birth increases. Thus early, continuous, and comprehensive prenatal care, which can detect and treat infections, is essential in dealing with this aspect of preterm birth prevention. Evidence has demonstrated a link between periodontal infection and preterm labor and birth as a result of the release of prostaglandins by the causative pathogens. Although research is ongoing, recommendations for all pregnant women should include regular dental care before and during pregnancy, oral assessment as part of prenatal care, and strict oral hygiene measures (e.g., brushing teeth, using dental floss, rinsing with baking soda and water after vomiting) (Bowers et al., 2008; Wener and Lavigne, 2004).

Another proposed cause of preterm labor and birth is bleeding at the site of placental implantation in the uterus in the first or second trimester of pregnancy. The resulting uteroplacental ischemia or hemorrhage at the decidual layer of the placenta may somehow activate the preterm labor process. Intrauterine inflammation is associated with infection, uterine vascular compromise, and decidual hemorrhage, and may contribute to preterm labor. Maternal and fetal stress, uterine overdistention, allergic reaction, and a decrease in progesterone are other factors that may play a part in initiating preterm labor. It is becoming increasingly clear that preterm labor is caused by multiple pathologic processes that eventually result in uterine contractions, cervical changes, and membrane rupture (Iams et al., 2009, Romero & Lockwood, 2009).

Two research studies suggest that recurrent preterm birth can be prevented in some women by administering prophylactic progesterone supplementation. In one study, women were given vaginal suppositories daily; in the other, women received weekly intramuscular injections of 17-alpha hydroxyprogesterone caproate. In both studies the risk of recurrent preterm birth was reduced by about one third. Exactly how progesterone works to prevent recurrent preterm birth is unclear, so more study is necessary. It is also important to note that prophylactic supplemental progesterone administration is recommended only for women who have previously given birth prematurely (Meis & Society for Maternal-Fetal Medicine, 2005; Romero & Lockwood, 2009).

Sociodemographic factors such as poverty, low educational level, lack of social support, smoking, little or no prenatal care, intimate partner violence, and stress are thought to contribute to the 50% of preterm births that may be preventable (Gennaro & Hennessy, 2003; Iams et al., 2009). If prenatal care programs are to be effective in reducing the rate of preterm labor and birth, they must address these sociodemographic factors and develop strategies to attract all women to participate, including those at high risk for preterm labor. Addressing the factors that contribute to preterm labor and birth can produce significant results (Maloni & Damato, 2004).

NURSING CARE PLAN

Preterm Labor

NURSING DIAGNOSIS

Deficient knowledge related to recognition of preterm labor

Expected Outcome

Woman and partner describe the signs and symptoms of preterm labor.

Nursing Interventions/*Rationales*

- Assess what the woman and partner know about preterm labor and birth and how to recognize its presence *to identify areas of deficit.*
- Discuss signs and symptoms that serve as warning signs of preterm labor so that the woman or her partner has adequate information *to identify problems early.*
- Provide written supplemental materials that include a list of warning signs and instructions regarding what to do if any of the listed signs occur *so that the couple can reinforce and review learning and act swiftly and appropriately should a sign occur.*
- Discuss and demonstrate how to assess and time the contractions *to provide needed skills to assess the signs of labor.*

NURSING DIAGNOSIS

Risk for injury (maternal/fetal) related to recurrence of preterm labor

Expected Outcomes

Woman demonstrates ability to assess self for signs of recurring labor; maternal-fetal well-being is maintained.

Nursing Interventions/*Rationales*

- Teach the woman and partner how to monitor uterine contraction activity daily *to provide immediate evidence of a worsening condition.*
- Have the woman and partner report rupture of membranes, vaginal bleeding, cramping, pelvic pressure, or low backache to appropriate health care resource immediately *because such symptoms are signs of labor.*
- Have the woman monitor her weight, diet, fluid intake, and vital signs on a daily basis *to evaluate for potential problems.*
- Have the woman limit activities to those recommended in a restricted activity plan *to decrease the likelihood of onset of labor.*
- Encourage the woman to use a side-lying position when reclining *to enhance placental perfusion.*
- Teach the woman signs and symptoms of thrombophlebitis and encourage gentle exercise of lower extremities *because pregnancy and limited activity increase risk for clot formation.*
- Counsel the woman to abstain from sexual intercourse and nipple stimulation if symptoms of preterm labor occur *because such activities may stimulate uterine contractions.*
- Encourage the woman to practice relaxation techniques *to decrease uterine tone and decrease anxiety and stress.*
- Teach the woman to take tocolytic or other medications per physician's orders *to inhibit uterine contractions.*
- Teach the woman and partner about and have them report any medication side effects immediately *to prevent medication-induced complications.*
- Have the family arrange for alternative strategies in carrying out the woman's usual roles and functions *to decrease stress and limit temptations to increase activity.*
- If small children are part of the household, encourage the family to make alternative arrangements for child care *to enhance woman's adherence to her restricted activity protocol.*

NURSING DIAGNOSIS

Anxiety related to preterm labor and potentially premature neonate

Expected Outcome

Feeling and symptoms of anxiety are reduced.

Nursing Interventions/*Rationales*

- Provide a calm, soothing atmosphere and encourage the family to provide emotional support *to facilitate coping.*
- Encourage verbalization of fears *to decrease intensity of emotional response.*
- Involve the woman and family in the home management of her condition *to promote a greater sense of control.*
- Help the woman identify and use appropriate coping strategies and support systems *to reduce fear/anxiety.*
- Explore the use of desensitization strategies such as progressive muscle relaxation, visual imagery, or thought stopping *to reduce fear-related emotions and related physical symptoms.*
- Provide information about online support groups *to reduce fear and anxiety.*

NURSING DIAGNOSIS

Deficient diversional activity related to modified bed rest

Expected Outcome

The woman will verbalize diminished feelings of boredom.

Nursing Interventions/*Rationales*

- Assist the woman to creatively explore personally meaningful activities that can be pursued from the bed *to ensure activities that have meaning, purpose, and value to the individual.*
- Maintain an emphasis on personal choices of the woman *because doing so promotes control and minimizes the imposition of routines by others.*
- Evaluate the support and system resources that are available in the environment *to assist in providing diversional activities.*
- Explore ways for the woman to remain an active participant in home management and decision making *to promote control.*
- Engage the support of family and friends in carrying out chosen activities and making necessary environmental alterations *to ensure success.*
- Encourage the woman to use the Internet to communicate with other women on bed rest *to obtain support and share feelings.*
- Teach the woman about stress management and relaxation techniques *to help manage tension of confinement.*

Nursing Care Plan—Preterm Labor

CARE MANAGEMENT

Because all pregnant women must be considered at risk for preterm labor, nursing assessment for factors that contribute to this risk begins early in pregnancy and continues throughout the prenatal period. The onset of preterm labor is often insidious and can be easily mistaken for normal discomforts of pregnancy. Nursing diagnoses, expected outcomes of care, and evidence-based interventions are established for each woman based on her assessment findings (see the Nursing Care Plan).

Prevention

Primary prevention strategies that address risk factors associated with preterm labor and birth are less costly in human and financial terms than the high-tech and often lifelong care required by preterm infants and their families. Programs aimed at health promotion and disease prevention that encourage healthy lifestyles for the population in general and women of childbearing age in particular should be developed. Preconception counseling and care for women, especially those with a history of preterm birth, may identify correctable risk factors and provide a means to encourage women to participate in health promoting activities. Smoking cessation, for example, has been shown to prevent preterm labor and birth (Freda, 2006; Iams et al., 2009). Many interventions intended to prevent spontaneous preterm birth have been recommended in the past and are still often prescribed. However, some of these interventions have not been shown to reduce the rate of preterm birth. Ongoing research is needed, especially since our understanding of the pathophysiology of preterm birth is increasing (Iams et al.).

Early Recognition and Diagnosis

Although preterm birth is often not preventable, early recognition of preterm labor is still essential to implement interventions that have been demonstrated to reduce neonatal morbidity and mortality. These interventions include transfer of the mother prior to birth to a hospital equipped to care for her preterm infant, giving antibiotics in labor to prevent neonatal group B streptococci infection, and administering glucocorticoids to the woman in labor in order to prevent or reduce neonatal morbidity and mortality from health problems including respiratory distress syndrome, intraventricular hemorrhage, and necrotizing enterocolitis (Iams & Romero, 2007).

Although maternal transport helps ensure a better health outcome for the mother and the baby, it also has a downside. Women may be transported to tertiary centers far from home, making visits by family and friends difficult and increasing the anxiety levels of the woman and her family. Attention to the needs of the woman and her family before, during, and after the transport is essential to comprehensive nursing care.

Because more than half of preterm births occur in women without obvious risk factors, it is essential that all pregnant women be taught the symptoms of preterm labor (Box 33-3). The nurse caring for women in a prenatal setting should use modalities that are known to be successful for teaching pregnant women about how to recognize these symptoms and then assess for these symptoms at each prenatal visit. Women also must be taught the significance of these symptoms of preterm labor and what to do should they occur (see the Teaching for Self-Management box: What to Do If Symptoms of Preterm Labor Occur).

In particular, client education regarding any symptoms of uterine contractions or cramping between 20 and 27 weeks of gestation must emphasize that these symptoms are not just normal discomforts of pregnancy, but indications of possible preterm labor (Fig. 33-1). Waiting too long to see a health care provider could result in inevitable preterm birth without sufficient time to administer antenatal corticosteroids (i.e., medication given to accelerate fetal lung maturity) and to transfer the woman to a hospital capable of providing care for her preterm infant.

BOX 33-3 SIGNS AND SYMPTOMS OF PRETERM LABOR

UTERINE ACTIVITY
- Uterine contractions occurring more frequently than every 10 minutes persisting for 1 hour or more
- Uterine contractions may be painful or painless

DISCOMFORT
- Lower abdominal cramping similar to gas pains; may be accompanied by diarrhea
- Dull, intermittent low back pain (below the waist)
- Painful, menstrual-like cramps
- Suprapubic pain or pressure
- Pelvic pressure or heaviness; feeling that "baby is pushing down"
- Urinary frequency

VAGINAL DISCHARGE
- Change in character or amount of usual discharge: thicker (mucoid) or thinner (watery), bloody, brown or colorless, increased amount, odor
- Rupture of amniotic membranes

TEACHING FOR SELF-MANAGEMENT

What to Do If Symptoms of Preterm Labor Occur

- Empty your bladder.
- Drink two to three glasses of water or juice.
- Lie down on your side for 1 hour.
- Palpate for contractions.
- If symptoms continue, call your health care provider or go to the hospital.
- If symptoms go away, resume light activity, but not what you were doing when the symptoms began.
- If symptoms return, call your health care provider or go to the hospital.
- If any of the following symptoms occur, call your health care provider immediately:
  - Uterine contractions every 10 minutes or less for 1 hour or more
  - Vaginal bleeding
  - Odorous vaginal discharge
  - Fluid leaking from the vagina

The diagnosis of preterm labor is based on three major diagnostic criteria:

- Gestational age between 20 and 37 weeks
- Uterine activity (e.g., contractions)
- Progressive cervical change (e.g., effacement of 80%, or cervical dilation of 2 cm or greater)

If the presence of fetal fibronectin is used as another diagnostic criterion, a sample of cervical and vaginal secretions for testing should be obtained before an examination for cervical changes because the lubricant used to examine the cervix can reduce the accuracy of the test for fetal fibronectin. The presence of vaginal bleeding or ruptured membranes, or a history of intercourse within the past 24 hours can also reduce the accuracy of the test results.

The pregnant woman at 30 weeks with an irritable uterus but no documented cervical change is not in preterm labor, though she should be carefully evaluated during follow-up care to determine whether she has progressed to active preterm labor (e.g., effacement, dilation, or both). Misdiagnosis of preterm

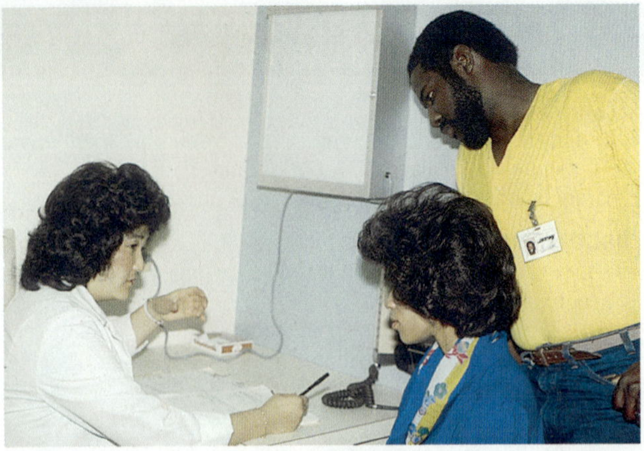

FIG. 33-1 A nurse teaching a couple signs and symptoms of preterm labor. (Courtesy Marjorie Pyle, RNC, Lifecircle, Costa Mesa, CA.)

labor can lead to inappropriate use of pharmacologic agents that can be dangerous to the health of the woman, the fetus, or both (Bowers et al., 2008).

COMMUNITY ACTIVITY

- Visit the website of KeepEmCookin.com, which provides education for pregnant women to prevent preterm birth and online community support. Review the information about the symptoms, causes, prevention and treatment of preterm birth, coping with bed rest and resources.
- What resources are available to help women with a high-risk pregnancy and their families in your community? Visit the Sidelines National Support Network website at sidelines.org, which provides support for women experiencing complicated pregnancies.

Lifestyle Modifications

Activity Restriction. Activity restriction, including bed rest and limited work, is a commonly prescribed intervention for the prevention of preterm birth. Bed rest, however, is not a benign intervention, and no evidence has been published in the literature to support the effectiveness of this intervention in reducing preterm birth rates (Iams et al., 2009). In fact, the American College of Obstetricians and Gynecologists (ACOG) (2003) states in its practice bulletin on management of preterm labor that bed rest should not be routinely recommended. Research indicates that bed rest causes adverse physical effects, including risk of thrombus formation, muscle atrophy, osteoporosis, and cardiovascular deconditioning (Iams & Romero, 2007). In many instances these symptoms are not resolved by 6 weeks postpartum (Maloni & Park, 2005). Additionally, bed rest affects women and their families psychologically, emotionally, socially, and financially. Box 33-4 lists adverse effects of bed rest.

Restriction of Sexual Activity. Restriction of sexual activity is frequently recommended for women at risk for preterm birth. This intervention has not been shown to be effective at preventing preterm birth. However, sexual abstinence has not been studied in women with specific risk factors for preterm birth, such as a short cervix. Therefore, more research is indicated (Iams et al., 2009). If, however, symptoms of preterm labor occur after sexual activity, then that activity may need to be curtailed until 37 weeks of gestation.

BOX 33-4 ADVERSE EFFECTS OF BED REST

MATERNAL EFFECTS (PHYSICAL)
- Weight loss; indigestion; loss of appetite
- Muscle wasting, weakness; aching muscles
- Bone demineralization and calcium loss
- Decreased plasma volume and cardiac output
- Increased clotting tendency; risk for thrombophlebitis
- Cardiac deconditioning
- Alteration in bowel function
- Sleep disturbance, fatigue
- Prolonged postpartum recovery

MATERNAL EFFECTS (PSYCHOSOCIAL)
- Loss of control associated with role reversals
- Dysphoria—anxiety, depression, hostility, and anger
- Guilt associated with difficulty complying with activity restriction and inability to meet role responsibilities
- Boredom, loneliness
- Emotional lability (mood swings); difficulty concentrating
- Increased stress

EFFECTS ON SUPPORT SYSTEM
- Stress associated with role reversals, increased responsibilities, and disruption of family routines
- Financial strain associated with loss of maternal income and cost of treatment
- Fear and anxiety regarding the well-being of the mother and fetus

Home Care. Women who are at high risk for preterm birth commonly are told that it would be best for them to "take it easy" at home for weeks or months. Many health care providers now recommend only modified bed rest because strict bed rest has not been shown to be effective at preterm birth prevention. Home care of the woman at risk for preterm birth is a challenge, however, for the nurse, who must assist the woman and her family in dealing with the many difficulties faced by families in which one member is unable to fulfill usual role responsibilities.

The woman's environment can be modified for convenience by using tables and storage units around her bed to keep essential items within reach (e.g., cell phone, television, radio, MP3 player, CD player, computer with Internet access, snacks, books, magazines, newspapers, and items for hobbies) (Fig. 33-2). Ensuring that the bed or couch is near a window and the bathroom is also helpful. Covering the bed with an eggcrate mattress can relieve discomfort. Women often find that a daily schedule of smaller, more frequent meals, activities (e.g., paying bills, planning and helping with meal preparation, hobbies), limited naps, and hygiene and grooming (e.g., shower, dressing in street clothes, applying makeup) reduces boredom and helps them maintain control and normalcy. See the Teaching for Self-Management box: Coping with Activity Restriction on p. 663 for more information.

Also see the Teaching for Self-Management box: Activities for Children of Women on Activity Restriction for additional ideas and suggestions. With modified bed rest, women are usually allowed bathroom privileges for toileting and showering and can be up to the table for meals.

EVIDENCE-BASED PRACTICE

Pat Gingrich

Preterm Labor: Is Bed Rest (Especially in the Hospital) Really Best?

ASK THE QUESTION

In women at risk for preterm birth, does bed rest, particularly in the hospital, result in any differences in maternal and neonatal outcomes?

SEARCH FOR EVIDENCE

Search Strategies

Professional organization guidelines, meta-analyses, systematic reviews, randomized controlled trials, nonrandomized prospective studies and retrospective reviews since 2008.

Databases Searched

CINAHL, Cochrane, Medline, and PUBMED.

CRITICALLY ANALYZE THE DATA

Bed rest for prevention of preterm birth is a widely known cautionary treatment, dating from a time when there was very little else that could be done. Intended to provide maternal rest and decrease stress, bed rest may instead cause more maternal distress as it disrupts family function. This may be intensified if accompanied by hospitalization.

One cost-effective and less disruptive solution might be for women to attend an antenatal day care unit. A Cochrane Database Review of three trials involving 504 women found that when hospitalized women who had either hypertension or preterm prelabor rupture of membranes (preterm PROM) were compared to similar women who attended a day care unit, there were no major differences in outcomes for mothers or babies, and modes of birth (vaginal versus cesarean) were similar. In one trial, women who attended day care were less likely to have their labor induced. Although cost comparisons were mixed, the women preferred going home each night to hospitalization (Dowswell, Middleton, & Weeks, 2009).

Likewise, a review of two trials involving 116 women with preterm PROM compared those assigned to either home or hospital care after a period of monitoring. Women with preterm PROM are at risk for infection as they have lost the natural barrier of the amniotic membrane. The fetus may continue developing in utero, as long as infection does not pose a risk. While the trials were too few and small to draw conclusions, the authors noted there were no differences between groups for neonatal outcomes of chorioamnionitis, gestational age at birth, birth weight, or admission to intensive care. Home-care mothers spent approximately 10 days less in the hospital, with reduced costs and increased satisfaction. There was some evidence that cesarean birth was more likely in the hospitalized women (Abou El Senoun, Dowswell & Mousa, 2010).

In the past, women pregnant with multiples might typically have expected to go onto bed rest in later pregnancy. A Cochrane Database Review of seven trials involving 713 women and 1452 babies found no benefit from routine bed rest in hospital for the outcomes of preterm birth or perinatal morbidity or mortality. There was a nonsignificant increase in birth weight in the hospitalized group. Only one trial inquired about the women's feelings; most found hospitalization distressing. The authors did not find enough evidence to recommend routine hospitalization for bed rest (Crowther & Han, 2010).

IMPLICATIONS FOR PRACTICE

Hospitalized bed rest is such a culturally accepted and expected practice for women at risk for preterm birth that women and their families may be alarmed if it is not prescribed. However, for many women, antepartal bed rest (even at home) puts considerable strain on family functioning in regard to childcare, housework, finances and job for both patient and spouse. Hospitalization far from family can be traumatic and isolating. In addition, confinement can be boring. Nurses should routinely identify and address family difficulties. Families can benefit from referral for increased instrumental support, financial and childcare management. Support groups and visitation can provide emotional support and stimulation. Antenatal day care units allow monitoring and rest, without the inconvenience and cost of hospitalization. Nurses can reassure women and their families that they are not putting their baby at risk by remaining at home and out of bed. Finally, while some women may have psychological or social issues that make hospitalization the best option, most women will find remaining at home to be more satisfactory.

References

Abou El Senoun, G., Dowswell, T., & Mousa, H. (2010). Planned home versus hospital care for preterm prelabour rupture of the membranes (PPROM) prior to 37 weeks' gestation. *The Cochrane Database of Systematic Reviews 2010,* 4, CD008053.

Crowther, C., & Han, S. (2010). Hospitalisation and bed rest for multiple pregnancy. *The Cochrane Database of Systematic Reviews 2010,* 7, CD000110.

Dowswell, T., Middleton, P., & Weeks, A. (2009). Antenatal day care units versus hospital admission for women with complicated pregnancy. *The Cochrane Database of Systematic Reviews 2009,* 4, CD001803.

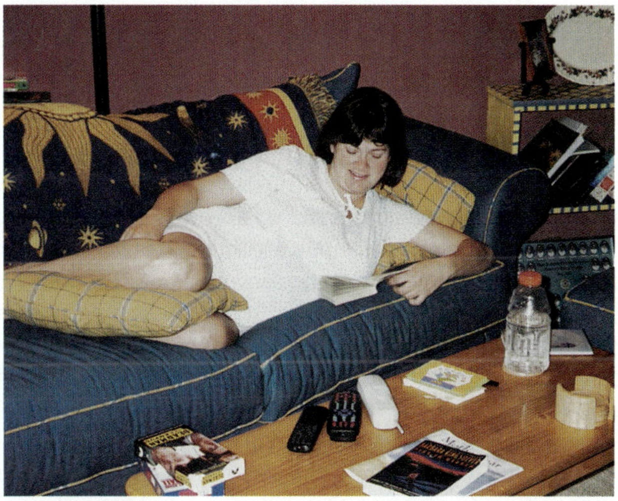

FIG. 33-2 Woman at home on restricted activity for preterm labor prevention. Note how she has arranged her daytime resting area so that needed items are close at hand. (Courtesy Amy Turner, Cary, NC.)

TEACHING FOR SELF-MANAGEMENT

Activities for Children of Women on Activity Restriction

- Schedule brief play periods throughout the day.
- Keep a few favorite toys in a box or basket close to the bed or couch.
- Read to the children.
- Put puzzles together.
- Watch videos, play video games (remote control for television is ideal).
- Play card or board games.
- Color in coloring books.
- Cut out pictures from magazines and paste on cardboard.
- Play bed basketball with a soft (sponge) ball or rolled up sock and a trash can or empty laundry basket.

Sources: McCann, M. (2006). *Days in waiting: A guide to surviving bedrest* (3rd ed.). St. Paul, MN: A Place to Remember; Tracy, A. (2001). *The pregnancy bedrest book: A survival guide for expectant mothers and their families.* New York: Berkley Publishing Group.

BOX 33-5 CONTRAINDICATIONS TO TOCOLYSIS

MATERNAL
- Hypertension
- Significant vaginal bleeding
- Cardiac disease

FETAL
- Gestational age of 36 weeks or more
- Fetal demise
- Lethal fetal anomaly
- Chorioamnionitis
- Evidence of acute or chronic fetal compromise

Source: Iams, J., Romero, R., & Creasy, R. (2009). Preterm labor and birth. In R. Creasy, R. Resnik, J. Iams, C. Lockwood, & T. Moore (Eds.), *Creasy and Resnik's maternal-fetal medicine: Principles and practice* (6th ed.). Philadelphia: Saunders.

Suppression of Uterine Activity

Tocolytics are medications given to arrest labor after uterine contractions and cervical change have occurred. Tocolytic therapy usually will not prolong the pregnancy long enough for further fetal growth or maturation to occur; rather, the goal is to delay birth long enough to institute interventions that reduce neonatal morbidity and mortality (Iams et al., 2009). Maternal and fetal contraindications to tocolytic therapy are listed in Box 33-5. Box 33-6 describes nursing care for women receiving tocolytic therapy.

Selecting the appropriate tocolytic medication requires consideration of each drug's effectiveness, risks, and side effects. Currently only one medication, (ritodrine [Yutopar]), in the United States has been approved by the U.S. Food and Drug Administration (FDA) for the purpose of arresting preterm labor. It is very rarely used, however, because of adverse reactions associated with its stimulation of beta-receptors. Drugs marketed for other purposes, such as treatment of asthma or hypertension, or as antiinflammatory or analgesic agents, are used on an "off-label" basis (i.e., drugs known to be effective for a specific purpose, although not specifically developed and tested for this purpose) to suppress preterm labor (Iams et al., 2009). Important contraindications exist to the use of all tocolytics (see Box 33-5).

Magnesium sulfate is the most commonly used tocolytic agent because maternal and fetal or neonatal adverse reactions are less common than with the beta-adrenergic agonists. Clinicians are familiar with its use as a treatment of preeclampsia and believe it is safer to use when compared with the beta-adrenergic agonists. Evidence for its effectiveness as a tocolytic is weak, however (Grimes & Nanda, 2006). Magnesium sulfate apparently promotes relaxation of smooth muscles by competing with calcium in cells (Iams & Romero, 2007; Rideout, 2005). Magnesium sulfate is administered intravenously. It may be a good choice for use in women in whom other tocolytic agents are contraindicated (see the Medication Guide: Tocolytic Therapy for Preterm Labor) (Iams & Romero; Iams et al., 2009).

SAFETY ALERT

Because magnesium sulfate depresses function of the central nervous system (CNS), it is essential that the nurse frequently assess the woman's respiratory status, deep tendon reflexes, and level of consciousness to identify signs that the serum level of magnesium sulfate is reaching toxic levels.

BOX 33-6 NURSING CARE FOR THE WOMAN RECEIVING TOCOLYTIC THERAPY

- Explain the purpose and side effects of the tocolytic medication(s) ordered to the woman and her family.
- Position the woman on her side to enhance placental perfusion and reduce pressure on the cervix.
- Monitor maternal vital signs including lung sounds and respiratory effort, fetal heart rate and pattern, and labor status according to hospital protocol and professional standards.
- Assess mother and fetus for signs of adverse reactions related to the tocolytic medication(s) being administered (see the Medication Guide: Tocolytic Therapy for Preterm Labor).
- Determine maternal fluid balance by measuring daily weight and intake and output.
- Limit fluid intake to 2500 to 3000 ml/day, especially if a beta-adrenergic agonist or magnesium sulfate is being administered.
- Provide psychosocial support and opportunities for the woman and family to express feelings and concerns.
- Offer comfort measures as needed.
- Encourage diversional activities and relaxation techniques.

Beta$_2$-adrenergic agonists (e.g., ritodrine and terbutaline [Brethine]) have been widely used in the past as tocolytics. They have many maternal and fetal adverse reactions, however, including beta$_1$-stimulated cardiopulmonary (e.g., tachycardia) effects and beta$_2$-stimulated metabolic (e.g., hyperglycemia) effects. Therefore, beta$_2$-adrenergic agonists are increasingly being replaced by medications that are safer and have fewer adverse reactions. They should not be used in women with known or suspected heart disease, severe preeclampsia or eclampsia, pregestational or gestational diabetes, or hyperthyroidism (Iams et al., 2009; Iams & Romero, 2007). Use of beta$_2$-adrenergic agonists is also contraindicated in women with migraine headaches (Gilbert, 2011).

Terbutaline, the most commonly administered beta-adrenergic agonist used for tocolysis, works by relaxing uterine smooth muscle as a result of stimulation of beta$_2$-receptors in the uterine smooth muscle. A single dose of terbutaline given subcutaneously may help diagnose preterm labor. In one study, women whose contractions persisted or recurred after a single injection of terbutaline were more likely to actually be in preterm labor than those whose contractions ceased. Terbutaline is often given subcutaneously to facilitate maternal transfer to a tertiary center or to initiate tocolytic therapy while another agent with a slower onset of action is administered concurrently. Additionally, a subcutaneous injection of 0.25 mg may be given to suppress uterine tachysystole during labor induction or augmentation or to suppress contractions prior to cesarean birth. Long-term oral or subcutaneous administration (e.g., terbutaline pump) as maintenance therapy to suppress preterm labor has not been proven to be effective at reducing prematurity or neonatal morbidity (Bowers et al., 2008; Gilbert, 2011; Iams & Romero, 2007; Iams et al., 2009) (see the Medication Guide: Tocolytic Therapy for Preterm Labor).

Nifedipine (Adalat, Procardia), a calcium channel blocker, is another tocolytic agent that can suppress contractions. It works by inhibiting calcium from entering smooth muscle cells, thus reducing uterine contractions. Because of its ease of

MEDICATION GUIDE

Tocolytic Therapy for Preterm Labor

MEDICATION AND ACTION	DOSAGE AND ROUTE	ADVERSE EFFECTS	NURSING CONSIDERATIONS
Magnesium Sulfate CNS depressant; relaxes smooth muscles including uterus	Intravenous fluid should contain 40 g in 1000 ml, piggyback to primary infusion, and administer using controller pump: Loading dose: 4-6 g over 20-30 min Maintenance dose: 1-4 g/hr Use for stabilization only Discontinue within 24-48 hr at the maintenance dose or if intolerable adverse effects occur	Maternal: • Hot flushes, sweating, burning at the IV insertion site, nausea and vomiting, dry mouth, drowsiness, blurred vision, diplopia, headache, ileus, generalized muscle weakness, lethargy, dizziness • Hypocalcemia • SOB • Transient hypotension • Some reactions may subside when loading dose is completed Intolerable: • Respiratory rate fewer than 12 breaths/min • Pulmonary edema • Absent DTRs • Chest pain • Severe hypotension • Altered level of consciousness • Extreme muscle weakness • Urine output less than 25-30 ml/hr or less than 100 ml/4 hr • Serum magnesium level of 10 mEq/L (9 mg/dl) or greater Fetal (uncommon): • Decreased breathing movement • Reduced FHR variability • Nonreactive NST	Assess woman and fetus to obtain baseline before beginning therapy and then before and after each increment; follow frequency of agency protocol Monitor serum magnesium levels with higher doses; therapeutic range is between 4 and 7.5 mEq/L or 5-8 mg/dl Discontinue infusion and notify physician if intolerable adverse effects occur Ensure that calcium gluconate 1 g (10 ml of 10% solution) or calcium chloride (normal dose is 500 mg IV infused over 30 min) is available for emergency administration to reverse magnesium sulfate toxicity Should not be given to women with myasthenia gravis Total IV intake should be limited to 125 ml/hr

Continued

administration and low incidence of significant maternal and fetal side effects, nifedipine's use is increasing. The drug is rapidly absorbed after oral administration. Maternal side effects, which include headache, flushing, dizziness, and nausea, are generally mild and relate primarily to hypotension and reflex tachycardia that occurs with administration. The decrease in blood pressure that occurs may be helpful for women who are also diagnosed with gestational hypertension or preeclampsia. However, at least one myocardial infarction has been reported in a healthy young woman who received a second dose of nifedipine. Concerns regarding adverse fetal effects have been reduced. Safety is achieved by following recommended dosages, avoiding concurrent use with magnesium sulfate, and maintaining maternal blood pressure, thereby preserving effective uteroplacental perfusion. Administering both nifedipine and magnesium sulfate can cause skeletal muscle blockade. Additionally, nifedipine should not be given along with or immediately following a $beta_2$-adrenergic agonist (Iams & Romero, 2007; Iams et al., 2009) (see the Medication Guide: Tocolytic Therapy for Preterm Labor).

SAFETY ALERT

Because using a calcium channel blocker can result in orthostatic hypotension and dizziness, it is essential to instruct women to slowly change position from supine to upright and then sit before standing until any dizziness disappears. Additionally, it is important to maintain adequate fluid balance to reduce the drop in blood pressure that can occur with the drug-related vasodilation.

Indomethacin (Indocin), a nonsteroidal antiinflammatory drug (NSAID), has been shown in some trials to suppress preterm labor by blocking the production of prostaglandins. Serious maternal side effects are uncommon and indomethacin is usually well tolerated. However, three serious fetal or neonatal side effects have caused major concerns about its use as a tocolytic. These side effects include constriction of the ductus arteriosus, oligohydramnios, and neonatal pulmonary hypertension. Therefore, limiting the use of indomethacin to a short duration of treatment in women with preterm labor at less than 32 weeks of gestation is

MEDICATION GUIDE

Tocolytic Therapy for Preterm Labor—cont'd

MEDICATION AND ACTION	DOSAGE AND ROUTE	ADVERSE EFFECTS	NURSING CONSIDERATIONS
BETA-ADRENERGIC AGONIST (BETA-MIMETIC)			
Terbutaline (Brethine)			
Relaxes smooth muscles, inhibiting uterine activity and causing bronchodilation	Subcutaneous injection of 0.25 mg every 4 hr Treatment should last no longer than 24 hr Discontinue use if intolerable adverse effects occur	Maternal (most are mild and of limited duration): • Tachycardia, chest discomfort, palpitations, arrhythmias • Tremors, dizziness, nervousness • Headache • Nasal congestion • Nausea and vomiting • Hypokalemia • Hyperglycemia • Hypotension Intolerable: • Tachycardia greater than 130 beats/min • BP less than 90/60 • Chest pain • Cardiac arrhythmias • Myocardial infarction • Pulmonary edema Fetal: • Tachycardia • Hyperinsulinemia • Hyperglycemia	Should not be used in women with a history of cardiac disease, pregestational or gestational diabetes, severe gestational hypertension, preeclampsia or eclampsia, migraine headaches, or hyperthyroidism, or with significant hemorrhage Myocardial infarction leading to death has been reported after use Validate that woman is in PTL and is >20 wk and <35 wk of gestation Assess woman and fetus according to agency protocol, being alert for adverse effects Assess maternal glucose and potassium levels before treatment is initiated and periodically during treatment. Significant hyperglycemia (greater than 180 mg/dl) and hypokalemia (less than 2.5 mEq/L) may occur. Notify physician if the woman exhibits the following: • Maternal heart rate greater than 130 beats/min; arrhythmias, chest pain • BP less than 90/60 mm Hg • Signs of pulmonary edema (e.g., dyspnea, crackles, decreased Sao_2) • Fetal heart rate greater than 180 beats/min Hyperglycemia occurs more frequently in women who are being treated simultaneously with corticosteroids Ensure that propranolol (Inderal) is available to reverse adverse effects related to cardiovascular function

MEDICATION GUIDE

Tocolytic Therapy for Preterm Labor—cont'd

MEDICATION AND ACTION	DOSAGE AND ROUTE	ADVERSE EFFECTS	NURSING CONSIDERATIONS
PROSTAGLANDIN SYNTHETASE INHIBITORS (NSAIDs)			
Indomethacin (Indocin)			
Relaxes uterine smooth muscle by inhibiting prostaglandins	Loading dose: 50 mg orally, then 25-50 mg orally every 6 hr for 48 hr	Maternal (common): • Nausea and vomiting • Heartburn Less common, but more serious: • Gastrointestinal bleeding • Prolonged bleeding time • Thrombocytopenia • Asthma in aspirin-sensitive clients Fetal: • Constriction of ductus arteriosus • Oligohydramnios, caused by reduced fetal urine production • Neonatal pulmonary hypertension	The long acting formulations decrease the incidence of adverse effects Used when other methods fail only if gestational age is less than 32 wk Administer for 48 hr or less Do not use in women with renal or hepatic disease, active peptic ulcer disease, poorly controlled hypertension, asthma, or coagulation disorders Can mask maternal fever Assess woman and fetus according to agency policy, being alert for adverse effects Determine amniotic fluid volume and function of fetal ductus arteriosus before initiating therapy and within 48 hr of discontinuing therapy; assessment is critical if therapy continues for more than 48 hr Administer with food to decrease GI distress Monitor for signs of postpartum hemorrhage
CALCIUM CHANNEL BLOCKERS			
Nifedipine (Adalat, Procardia)			
Relaxes smooth muscles including the uterus by blocking calcium entry	Initial dose: 10-20 mg, orally, every 3 to 6 hr until contractions are rare, followed by long-acting formulations of 30 or 60 mg every 8-12 hr for 48 hr while corticosteroids are being given (however, the ideal dose has not been established)	Maternal (most effects are mild): • Hypotension • Headache • Flushing • Dizziness • Nausea Fetal: • Hypotension (questionable)	Avoid concurrent use with magnesium sulfate because skeletal muscle blockade can result Should not be given simultaneously with or immediately after terbutaline because of effects on heart rate and blood pressure Assess woman and fetus according to agency protocol, being alert for adverse effects Do not use sublingual route of administration

NOTE: There are variations in recommended administration protocols; always consult agency protocol, which should be evidence based.

BP, Blood pressure; *CNS,* central nervous system; *DTRs,* deep tendon reflexes; *FHR,* fetal heart rate; *GI,* gastrointestinal; *NSAIDs,* nonsteroidal antiinflammatory drugs; *NST,* nonstress test; *PTL,* preterm labor; *Sao_2,* arterial oxygen saturation; *SOB,* shortness of breath.

Sources: Gilbert, E. (2011). *Manual of high risk pregnancy & delivery* (5th ed.). St. Louis: Mosby; Iams, J., & Romero, R. (2007). Preterm birth. In S. Gabbe, J. Niebyl, & J. Simpson (Eds.), *Obstetrics: Normal and problem pregnancies* (5th ed.). Philadelphia: Churchill Livingstone; Iams, J., Romero, R., & Creasy, R. (2009). Preterm labor and birth. In R. Creasy, R. Resnik, J. Iams, C. Lockwood, & T. Moore (Eds.), *Creasy and Resnik's maternal-fetal medicine: Principles and practice* (6th ed.). Philadelphia: Saunders.

MEDICATION GUIDE

Antenatal Glucocorticoid Therapy with Betamethasone or Dexamethasone

ACTION

Stimulates fetal lung maturation by promoting release of enzymes that induce production or release of lung surfactant. NOTE: The U.S. Food and Drug Administration has not approved these medications for this use (i.e., this is an unlabeled use for obstetrics).

INDICATION

To prevent or reduce the severity of neonatal respiratory distress syndrome by accelerating lung maturity in fetuses between 24 and 34 weeks of gestation

DOSAGE AND ROUTE

- Betamethasone: 12 mg intramuscularly (IM) for two doses 24 hours apart
- Dexamethasone: 6 mg IM for four doses 12 hours apart

ADVERSE EFFECTS

- Pulmonary edema (if given with beta-adrenergic medications)
- May worsen maternal condition (diabetes, hypertension)

NURSING CONSIDERATIONS

- Give deep IM in ventral gluteal or vastus lateralis muscle.
- Teach signs of pulmonary edema.
- Assess blood glucose levels and lung sounds.

recommended (Iams & Romero, 2007; Iams et al., 2009) (see the Medication Guide: Tocolytic Therapy for Preterm Labor).

Promotion of Fetal Lung Maturity

Antenatal glucocorticoids, given as intramuscular injections to the mother to accelerate fetal lung maturity by stimulating fetal surfactant production, are now considered one of the most effective and cost-efficient interventions for preventing morbidity and mortality associated with preterm labor. Antenatal glucocorticoids have been shown to significantly reduce the incidence of respiratory distress syndrome, intraventricular hemorrhage, necrotizing enterocolitis, and death in neonates, without increasing the risk of infection in either mothers or newborns (Mercer, 2009a). The National Institutes of Health (NIH) consensus panel recommended that all women between 24 and 34 weeks of gestation be given a single course of antenatal glucocorticoids when preterm birth is threatened, unless evidence indicates that glucocorticoids will have an adverse effect on the mother or birth is imminent. In general, women who are candidates for tocolytic therapy are also candidates for antenatal glucocorticoids (Mercer). The regimen for administration of antenatal glucocorticoids is given in the Medication Guide: Antenatal Glucocorticoid Therapy with Betamethasone or Dexamethasone.

! NURSING ALERT

All women between 24 and 34 weeks of gestation who are at risk for preterm birth within 7 days should receive treatment with a single course of antenatal glucocorticoids. Because optimal benefit begins 24 hours after the first injection, timely administration is essential (Mercer, 2009a).

Management of Inevitable Preterm Birth

Labor that has progressed to a cervical dilation of 4 cm or more is likely to lead to inevitable preterm birth. If birth appears imminent, preparations to care for a small, immature neonate should be made. Women in preterm labor may rapidly progress to birth and a very small fetus may be born through a partially dilated cervix. Also malpresentation (e.g., breech presentation) occurs much more frequently in preterm than in term fetuses. Therefore, nurses must be prepared to handle the emergency birth of a preterm infant, from either cephalic or breech presentation, without the woman's primary health care provider being present. Personnel skilled at neonatal resuscitation should be present at the time of birth. Equipment, supplies, and medications used for neonatal resuscitation should be gathered in advance and prepared for immediate use. If birth occurs in a hospital that is not prepared to provide continuing care for a preterm neonate, plans should be made for transfer of the baby to a higher level of care as soon as possible.

Fetal and Early Neonatal Loss

Preterm birth or the presence of congenital anomalies or genetic disorders incompatible with life are major reasons for intrauterine fetal demise (stillbirth) or early neonatal death. In many of these situations the parents will have already been told that the fetus has died or that the baby has a condition that is incompatible with life and will most likely die very soon after birth. Sometimes, however, the fetal death will be unexpected, diagnosed only after the woman has been admitted to the labor and birth unit. Whatever the case, labor and birth nurses must be prepared to provide sensitive care to these women and their families.

If fetal or early neonatal death is expected, the parents and members of the health care team need to discuss the situation before the birth and decide on a management plan that is acceptable to everyone. Despite counseling about the likelihood of a poor outcome, some parents want "everything possible," including cesarean birth for an abnormal fetal heart rate (FHR) tracing, to be done for the baby. If such intervention is not desired, usually the FHR will not be monitored during labor.

Another major decision is whether to attempt neonatal resuscitation, and to what lengths resuscitation should go. Sometimes the feasibility of neonatal resuscitation cannot be determined until the baby's size and physical appearance have been assessed. If the baby is too small, too immature, or too malformed for effective resuscitation, comfort care can be provided instead. The baby is kept warm and comfortable, either at the mother's bedside or in the nursery, depending on the parents' desires, until death occurs. Parents can choose to view and hold the baby as they wish.

After the birth, the woman should be given the opportunity to decide if she wants to stay on the maternity unit or be moved to another hospital unit. She may prefer to be away from the sound of crying babies and exposure to other families who have had healthy infants. However, postpartum care and grief support may not be as good on another hospital unit where the staff is not experienced in postpartum and bereavement care.

Whether death occurs in utero or after birth, parents are faced with the same needs. See Chapter 38 for additional information on dealing with families experiencing a perinatal loss.

PREMATURE RUPTURE OF MEMBRANES

Premature rupture of membranes (PROM) is the spontaneous rupture of the amniotic sac and leakage of amniotic fluid beginning before the onset of labor at any gestational age. **Preterm premature rupture of membranes (preterm PROM)** (i.e., membranes rupture before the completion of 37 weeks of gestation) is responsible for about one third of all preterm births (Mercer, 2007). Preterm PROM most likely results from pathologic weakening of the amniotic membranes caused by inflammation, stress from uterine contractions, or other factors that cause increased intrauterine pressure. Infection of the urogenital tract is a major risk factor associated with preterm PROM (Mercer, 2007; 2009b). PROM or preterm PROM are diagnosed after the woman reports either a sudden gush of fluid or a slow leak of fluid from the vagina.

Chorioamnionitis is the most common maternal complication of preterm PROM, making it a major complication of pregnancy (see later discussion). Other less common but serious maternal complications include placental abruption, sepsis, and death (Mercer, 2007; 2009b). Fetal complications from preterm PROM are primarily related to intrauterine infection, cord prolapse, umbilical cord compression associated with oligohydramnios, and placental abruption. Another possible fetal complication when preterm PROM occurs prior to 20 weeks of gestation is pulmonary hypoplasia (Mercer, 2009b).

CARE MANAGEMENT

Management of PROM is determined for each woman based on an assessment of the estimated risk of maternal, fetal, and neonatal complications if pregnancy is allowed to continue or immediate labor and birth are attempted. At term, because infection is the greatest maternal, fetal, and neonatal risk, birth is the best option. Labor will most likely be induced if it does not begin spontaneously soon after PROM occurs (Mercer, 2009b).

Preterm PROM is often managed expectantly or conservatively if the risks to the fetus and newborn associated with preterm birth are considered to be greater than the risks of infection. Women with preterm PROM may be hospitalized in an attempt to prolong pregnancy and allow additional time for fetal maturation unless intrauterine infection, significant vaginal bleeding, placental abruption, preterm labor, or fetal compromise occurs (Mercer, 2009b). Nursing support of the woman and her family is critical at this time. They are often anxious about the health of the baby and the woman may fear that she was responsible in some way for the membrane rupture. The nurse can reassure the woman that in most cases the cause of PROM is unknown (Gilbert, 2011). Other nursing interventions include encouraging expression of feelings and concerns, providing information, and making referrals as needed.

Conservative management of preterm PROM includes fetal assessment by nonstress test (NST) and biophysical profile (BPP). The woman should also be taught how to assess her fetus using daily fetal movement counts (DFMC) because a slowing of fetal movement has been shown to be a precursor to severe fetal compromise. (See Chapter 26 for further discussion of these tests.) In addition, the woman will be monitored for signs of labor, placental abruption, and the development of intrauterine infection. Antenatal glucocorticoids will be administered to women who are less than 32 weeks of gestation because they have been proven to decrease the risk of several neonatal complications. In addition, a 7-day course of broad-spectrum antibiotics (e.g., ampicillin, erythromycin) will be administered to treat or prevent intrauterine infection (Mercer, 2007; 2009b).

Vigilance for signs of infection is a major part of the nursing care and client education after preterm PROM. The woman must be taught how to keep her genital area clean and that nothing should be introduced into her vagina. Signs of infection (e.g., fever, foul-smelling vaginal discharge, maternal and fetal tachycardia) should be reported to the primary health care provider immediately (see the Teaching for Self-Management box: The Woman with Preterm Premature Rupture of Membranes). If chorioamnionitis develops, labor will be induced. Should preterm labor occur, tocolytic medications may be administered in an attempt to gain time for transporting the woman to a hospital capable of providing care to a preterm infant or for antenatal corticosteroids or antibiotics to reach effective levels (Gilbert, 2011; Mercer, 2007).

TEACHING FOR SELF-MANAGEMENT

Home Care Instructions for the Woman with Preterm Premature Rupture of Membranes

- Take your temperature and assess pulse every 4 hours when awake.
- Report temperature of more than 38° C (100.4° F).
- Remain on modified bed rest.
- Insert nothing into the vagina.
- Do not engage in sexual activity.
- Assess for uterine contractions.
- Do fetal movement counts daily.
- Do not take tub baths.
- Watch for foul-smelling vaginal discharge or if uterus becomes tender or sore when touched.
- Wipe from front to back after urinating or having a bowel movement.
- Take antibiotics, if prescribed, on an around-the-clock schedule; be sure to complete the entire course of treatment.
- See primary health care provider as scheduled.

CHORIOAMNIONITIS

Chorioamnionitis, bacterial infection of the amniotic cavity, is a major cause of complications for both mothers and newborns at any gestational age. It occurs in 0.5% to 10% of pregnancies. Other terms for this condition include *clinical chorioamnionitis, amnionitis, intrapartum infection, amniotic fluid infection,* and *intraamniotic infection.* Chorioamnionitis is usually diagnosed by the clinical findings of maternal fever, maternal and fetal tachycardia, uterine tenderness, and foul odor of amniotic fluid (Duff, Sweet, & Edwards, 2009).

Chorioamnionitis most often occurs after membranes rupture or labor begins, as organisms that are part of the normal vaginal flora ascend into the amniotic cavity. Many of the risk factors for chorioamnionitis are associated with a long labor, such as prolonged membrane rupture, multiple vaginal examinations, and use of internal FHR and contraction monitoring modes (Duff et al., 2009). Other risk factors include young maternal age, low socioeconomic status, nulliparity, and preexisting infections of the lower genital tract (Duff, 2007).

Women with chorioamnionitis can develop bacteremia. They are also more likely to have dysfunctional labor, which can result in the need for cesarean birth (see later discussion). If cesarean birth is necessary, wound infection or pelvic abscess are complications that can occur. Neonatal risks include pneumonia, bacteremia, and sepsis. Death is more likely to occur in preterm than in term infants (Duff, 2007; Duff et al., 2009). An association between chorioamnionitis and long-term neurologic development in the newborn, including cerebral palsy, has been reported (Duff et al.).

In order to prevent maternal and neonatal complications, prompt treatment with intravenous broad-spectrum antibiotics and birth of the fetus are necessary. Ampicillin or penicillin and gentamicin are the antibiotics most often used to treat chorioamnionitis during labor. After cesarean birth, an antibiotic that provides coverage for anaerobic organisms, such as clindamycin (Cleocin) or metronidazole (Flagyl) should be added. Antibiotics can usually be discontinued soon after birth (Duff, 2007).

The increased use of intrapartum antibiotic prophylaxis during labor in women who are group B streptococci positive has decreased the incidence of chorioamnionitis. Other measures that have proven to be effective in decreasing the frequency of chorioamnionitis are active management of labor (see later discussion) and induction of labor, rather than expectant management, following rupture of membranes at term (Duff et al., 2009).

DYSFUNCTIONAL LABOR (DYSTOCIA)

Dysfunctional labor (dystocia) is defined as a long, difficult, or abnormal labor caused by various conditions associated with the five factors affecting labor. It is estimated that dysfunctional labor occurs in approximately 8% to 11% of all births and it is the most common indication for cesarean birth (Gilbert, 2011). Dysfunctional labor is responsible for approximately 60% of all primary cesarean births in the United States (Cunningham, Leveno, Bloom, Hauth, Rouse, & Spong, 2010). It can be caused by any of the following:

- Ineffective uterine contractions or maternal bearing-down efforts (the powers)
- Alterations in the pelvic structure (the passage)
- Fetal causes, including abnormal presentation or position, anomalies, excessive size, and number of fetuses (the passenger)
- Maternal position during labor and birth
- Psychologic responses of the mother to labor related to past experiences, preparation, culture and heritage, and support system

These five factors are interdependent. In assessing the woman for an abnormal labor pattern, the nurse must consider the way in which these factors interact and influence labor progress. Dysfunctional labor is suspected when there is an alteration in the characteristics of uterine contractions, a lack of progress in the rate of cervical dilation, or a lack of progress in fetal descent and expulsion.

Nursing Care Plan—Dysfunctional Labor: Hypotonic Uterine Dysfunction

Gilbert (2011) cited several factors that seem to increase a woman's risk for dysfunctional labor including the following:

- Overweight
- Short stature
- Advanced maternal age
- Infertility difficulties
- Prior version
- Masculine characteristics
- Uterine abnormalities (e.g., congenital malformations; overdistention, as with multiple gestation; or polyhydramnios)
- Malpresentations and positions of the fetus
- Cephalopelvic disproportion (CPD) (or fetopelvic disproportion [FPD])
- Uterine overstimulation with oxytocin
- Maternal fatigue, dehydration and electrolyte imbalance, and fear
- Administration of an analgesic too early in labor or use of continuous epidural analgesia

Abnormal Uterine Activity

Abnormal uterine activity can be further described as being *hypertonic or hypotonic*. Contractions may be frequent and painfully strong with hypertonic uterine activity, but ineffective at promoting cervical effacement and dilation. With hypotonic uterine activity, the rise in uterine pressure generated during contractions is insufficient to promote cervical effacement and dilation (Gilbert, 2011).

Hypertonic Uterine Dysfunction

The woman experiencing **hypertonic uterine dysfunction,** or primary dysfunctional labor, often is an anxious first-time mother who is having painful and frequent contractions that are ineffective in causing cervical dilation or effacement to progress. These contractions usually occur in the latent phase of first stage labor (cervical dilation of less than 4 cm) and are usually uncoordinated. The force of the contractions may be in the midsection of the uterus rather than in the fundus; therefore, the uterus is unable to apply downward pressure to push the presenting part against the cervix. The uterus may not relax completely between contractions.

Women with hypertonic uterine dysfunction may be exhausted and express concern about loss of control because of the intense pain they are experiencing and the lack of progress. **Therapeutic rest,** which is achieved with a warm bath or shower and the administration of an analgesic such as morphine, to inhibit uterine contractions, reduce pain, and encourage sleep, is usually prescribed to manage hypertonic uterine dysfunction. In the absence of pain, zolpidem (Ambien) may be used to facilitate rest and sleep. After a 4- to 6-hour rest, these women are likely to awaken in active labor with a normal uterine contraction pattern (Battista & Wing, 2007; Gilbert, 2011).

Hypotonic Uterine Dysfunction

The second and more common type of uterine dysfunction is **hypotonic uterine dysfunction,** or secondary uterine inertia. The woman initially makes normal progress into the active phase of first stage labor but then the contractions become weak and inefficient or stop altogether. The uterus is easily indented, even at the peak of contractions. Intrauterine pressure (IUP)

TABLE 33-1 DYSFUNCTIONAL LABOR: PRIMARY AND SECONDARY POWERS

PRIMARY POWERS		SECONDARY POWERS
HYPERTONIC UTERINE DYSFUNCTION	**HYPOTONIC UTERINE DYSFUNCTION**	**INADEQUATE VOLUNTARY EXPULSIVE FORCES**
Description		
Usually occurs before 4 cm dilation; cause unknown, may be related to fear and tension	Cause is usually cephalopelvic disproportion or fetal malposition	Involves abdominal and levator ani muscles Occurs in second stage of labor; cause may be related to nerve block anesthetic, analgesia, exhaustion
Change in Pattern of Progress		
Pain out of proportion to intensity of contractions and to effectiveness of contractions in effacing and dilating the cervix Contractions increase in frequency and are uncoordinated Uterus is contracted between contractions, cannot be indented	Contractions decrease in frequency and intensity Uterus easily indentable even at peak of contractions Uterus relaxed between contractions (normal)	No voluntary urge to push or bear down or inadequate or ineffective pushing
Potential Maternal Effects		
Loss of control related to intensity of pain and lack of progress Exhaustion Fear regarding unexpected nature of labor	Infection Exhaustion Stress regarding change in progress	Spontaneous vaginal birth prevented; assisted birth likely
Potential Fetal Effects		
Fetal asphyxia with meconium aspiration	Fetal infection Fetal and neonatal death	Fetal asphyxia
Care Management		
Initiate therapeutic rest measures Administer analgesic (e.g., morphine) if membranes intact and pelvic adequacy is confirmed Relieve pain to permit mother to rest Assist with measures to enhance rest and relaxation (e.g., hydrotherapy, massage, music, distracting activities)	Rule out cephalopelvic disproportion Augment labor with oxytocin (Pitocin) Perform amniotomy Assist with measures to enhance the progress of labor (e.g., position changes, ambulation, hydrotherapy)	Coach mother in bearing down with contractions; assist with relaxation between contractions Position mother in favorable position for pushing Reduce epidural infusion rate Assist with forceps- or vacuum-assisted birth Prepare for cesarean birth if abnormal (nonreassuring) fetal status occurs

during the contraction (usually less than 25 mm Hg) is insufficient for progress of cervical effacement and dilation. CPD and malposition are common causes of this type of uterine dysfunction.

A woman with hypotonic uterine dysfunction may become exhausted and be at increased risk for infection. Management usually consists of ruling out CPD and assessing the FHR and pattern, characteristics of amniotic fluid if membranes are ruptured, and maternal well-being. An intrauterine pressure catheter (IUPC) may be inserted to accurately evaluate uterine activity. If findings are normal, labor augmentation measures may be implemented (e.g., ambulation, hydrotherapy, rupture of membranes, nipple stimulation, oxytocin infusion).

Secondary Powers

Secondary powers, or bearing-down efforts, are compromised when large amounts of analgesia are given. Anesthesia may also block the bearing-down reflex and, as a result, alter the effectiveness of voluntary bearing-down efforts. Exhaustion resulting from lack of sleep or long labor, and fatigue resulting from inadequate hydration and food intake reduce the effectiveness of the woman's voluntary bearing-down efforts. Maternal position can work against the forces of gravity and decrease the strength and efficiency of the contractions. Table 33-1 summarizes the characteristics of dysfunctional labor.

Abnormal Labor Patterns

Six abnormal labor patterns were identified and classified by Friedman (1989) according to the nature of the cervical dilation and fetal descent. These patterns include: (1) prolonged latent phase, (2) protracted active phase dilation, (3) secondary arrest: no change, (4) protracted descent, (5) arrest of descent, and (6) failure of descent. Table 33-2 further describes these abnormal labor patterns. These patterns may result from a variety of causes, including ineffective uterine contractions, pelvic contractures, CPD, abnormal fetal presentation or position, early use of analgesics, nerve block analgesia or anesthesia, and anxiety and stress. Progress in either the first or the second stage of labor can be protracted (prolonged) or arrested (stopped). Abnormal progress can be identified by plotting cervical dilation and fetal descent on a labor graph (partogram) at various intervals after the onset of labor and comparing the resulting curve with the expected labor curve for a nulliparous or multiparous labor. If a woman exhibits an abnormal labor pattern, the primary health care provider should be notified.

TABLE 33-2 ABNORMAL LABOR PATTERNS

PATTERN	NULLIPARAS	MULTIPARAS
Prolonged latent phase	>20 hr	>14 hr
Protracted active phase dilation	<1.2 cm/hr	<1.5 cm/hr
Secondary arrest: no change	≥2 hr	≥2 hr
Protracted descent	<1 cm/hr	<2 cm/hr
Arrest of descent	≥1 hr	≥½hr
Failure of descent	No change during deceleration phase and second stage	
Precipitous labor	>5 cm/hr	10 cm/hr

Health care providers must be careful when diagnosing a labor pattern as prolonged and when intervening based on this diagnosis. Cesario (2004) found that although the average length of labor today is similar to that found by Friedman, a wider range of normal occurs. Parameters to determine if labor is progressing normally may have to be expanded. Criteria defining the differences between false, latent, and active labor should be established. Using hospital admission areas to evaluate a woman's labor status is helpful in preventing the premature implementation of labor interventions such as administration of systemic opioid analgesics or induction of epidural analgesia or anesthesia. If a woman is found to be in false (prelabor) or latent (early) labor, she can be sent home if she lives near the hospital or remain in the admissions area until labor becomes active. Only when they are in active labor should women be admitted to the labor and birth unit.

Maternal morbidity and mortality from uterine rupture, infection, severe dehydration, and postpartum hemorrhage are higher for women experiencing dysfunctional labor. The fetus is at increased risk for hypoxia. A long and difficult labor also can have an adverse psychologic effect on the mother, father, and family.

Precipitous Labor

Precipitous labor is defined as labor that lasts less than 3 hours from the onset of contractions to the time of birth. This abnormal labor pattern occurs in approximately 2% of all births in the United States. Precipitous birth alone is not usually associated with significant maternal or infant morbidity or mortality (Battista & Wing, 2007).

Precipitous labor may result from hypertonic uterine contractions that are tetanic in intensity. Conditions often associated with this type of uterine contractions include placental abruption, an excessive number of uterine contractions, and recent cocaine use (Battista & Wing, 2007). Maternal complications can include uterine rupture, lacerations of the birth canal, anaphylactoid syndrome of pregnancy (amniotic fluid embolism), and postpartum hemorrhage. Fetal complications include hypoxia caused by decreased periods of uterine relaxation between contractions and, in rare instances, intracranial trauma related to rapid birth (Cunningham et al., 2010).

Women who have experienced precipitous labor often describe feelings of disbelief that their labor began so quickly, alarm that their labor progressed so rapidly, panic about the possibility they would not make it to the hospital in time to give birth, and finally, relief when they arrived at the hospital. In addition, women have expressed frustration when nurses did not believe them when they reported their readiness to push. Progress can be so rapid in some women that they may have difficulty remembering the details of their childbirth. They should be provided with an opportunity to discuss their labor and birth with caregivers.

Alterations in Pelvic Structure

Pelvic Dystocia

Pelvic dystocia can occur whenever there are contractures of the pelvic diameters that reduce the capacity of the bony pelvis, including the inlet, the midpelvis, outlet, or any combination of these planes. Pelvic contractures may be caused by congenital abnormalities, maternal malnutrition, neoplasms, or lower spinal disorders. An immature pelvic size predisposes some adolescent mothers to pelvic dystocia. Pelvic deformities also may be the result of automobile or other accidents or trauma.

Soft-Tissue Dystocia

Soft-tissue dystocia results from obstruction of the birth passage by an anatomic abnormality other than that involving the bony pelvis. The obstruction may result from placenta previa (low-lying placenta) that partially or completely obstructs the internal cervical os. Other causes, such as leiomyomas (uterine fibroids) in the lower uterine segment, ovarian tumors, and a full bladder or rectum, may prevent the fetus from entering the pelvis. Occasionally cervical edema occurs during labor when the cervix is caught between the presenting part and the symphysis pubis or when the woman begins bearing-down efforts prematurely, thereby inhibiting complete dilation. Sexually transmitted infections (e.g., human papillomavirus) can alter cervical tissue integrity and thus interfere with adequate effacement and dilation.

Fetal Causes

Dystocia of fetal origin may be caused by anomalies, excessive fetal size (macrosomia), malpresentation, malposition, or multifetal pregnancy. Complications associated with dystocia of fetal origin include neonatal asphyxia, fetal injuries or fractures, and maternal vaginal lacerations. Although spontaneous vaginal birth is possible in these instances, a forceps-assisted, vacuum-assisted, or cesarean birth often is necessary.

Anomalies

Gross ascites, large tumors, open neural tube defects (e.g., myelomeningocele), and hydrocephalus are examples of fetal anomalies that can cause dystocia. The anomalies affect the relationship of the fetal anatomy to the maternal pelvic capacity, with the result that the fetus is unable to descend through the birth canal.

Cephalopelvic Disproportion

Cephalopelvic disproportion (CPD), also called FPD, is disproportion between the size of the fetus and the size of the mother's pelvis. With CPD the fetus cannot fit through the maternal pelvis to be born vaginally. Although CPD is often related to excessive fetal size, or macrosomia (i.e., 4000 g or more), the problem in many cases is malposition of the fetal presenting part rather than true CPD (Battista & Wing, 2007). Fetal macrosomia is associated with maternal diabetes mellitus, obesity, multiparity, or the large size of one or both parents. If the maternal pelvis is too small, abnormally shaped, or deformed, CPD may be of maternal origin. In this case, the fetus may be of average size or even smaller. CPD cannot be accurately predicted (Battista & Wing).

Malposition

The most common fetal malposition is persistent occipitoposterior position (i.e., right occipitoposterior [ROP] or left occipitoposterior [LOP]; see Chapter 16), occurring in approximately 15% of all labors during the latent phase of the first stage of labor. About 5% of all fetuses are in this position at birth (Gilbert, 2011). Labor, especially the second stage, is prolonged. The woman typically complains of severe back pain from the

BOX 33-7 MEASURES TO REDUCE BACK PAIN AND FACILITATE ROTATION OF FETAL HEAD DURING BACK LABOR—OCCIPUT POSTERIOR POSITION

MEASURES TO REDUCE BACK PAIN DURING A CONTRACTION

- *Counterpressure:* Apply fist or heel of the hand to sacral area.
- *Heat or cold applications:* Apply to sacral area.
- *Double hip squeeze:*
  - Woman assumes a position with hip joints flexed, such as the knee-chest position.
  - Partner, nurse, or doula places hands over gluteal muscles and presses with palms of hands up and inward toward the center of the pelvis.
- *Knee press:*
  - Woman assumes a sitting position with knees a few inches apart and feet flat on the floor or on a stool.
  - Partner, nurse, or doula cups a knee in each hand with heels of hands on top of tibia then presses the knees straight back toward the woman's hips while leaning forward toward the woman.

MEASURES TO FACILITATE THE ROTATION OF THE FETAL HEAD (MAY ALSO REDUCE BACK PAIN)

- *Lateral abdominal stroking:* Stroke the abdomen in the direction that the fetal head should rotate.
- *Hands-and-knees position (all-fours):* Can also be accomplished by kneeling while leaning forward over a birth ball, padded chair seat, bed, or over-the-bed table.
- *Squatting*
- *Pelvic rocking*
- *Stair climbing*
- *Lateral position (Sims):* Lie on same side as fetal back (spine).
- *Lunges:* Widens pelvis on side toward which woman lunges:
  - Woman stands, facing forward, next to or alongside a chair, so that she can lunge toward the side the fetal back is on or in the direction of the fetal occiput.
  - Woman places foot on seat of chair with toes pointed toward the back of the chair, then lunges.
  - Alternative position for lunge: kneeling.

pressure of the fetal head (occiput) pressing against her sacrum. Box 33-7 identifies suggested measures to relieve back pain and encourage rotation of the fetal occiput to an anterior position, which will facilitate birth (Gilbert; Stremler, Hodnett, Petryshen, Stevens, Weston, & Willan, 2005). Evidence provides support for encouraging women whose fetus is in an occiput posterior position to assume and maintain a Sims position on the same side as the fetal spine as much as possible during labor. There is limited evidence to support the commonly used hands-and-knees position (Ridley, 2007).

Malpresentation

Malpresentation (the fetal presentation is something other than cephalic or head first) is another commonly reported complication of labor and birth. Breech presentation is the most common form of malpresentation, occurring in 3% to 4% of all labors (Lanni & Seeds, 2007). The three types of breech presentation are frank breech (hips flexed, knees extended), complete breech (hips and knees flexed), and footling breech (when one foot [single footling] or both feet [double footling] present before the buttocks) (Gilbert, 2011) (Fig. 33-3). Breech presentations are associated with multifetal gestation, preterm birth, fetal and maternal anomalies, hydramnios, and oligohydramnios. High rates of breech presentation are also noted in fetuses with certain genetic disorders (e.g., trisomies 13, 18, and 21; Potter's syndrome [renal agenesis]; and myotonic dystrophy). Fetuses with neuromuscular disorders have a high rate of breech presentation, perhaps because they are less capable of movement within the uterus. Diagnosis is made by abdominal palpation (e.g., Leopold maneuvers) and vaginal examination and usually confirmed by ultrasound scan (Lanni & Seeds, 2007; Thorp, 2009).

During labor the descent of the fetus in a breech presentation may be slow because the breech is not as effective a dilating wedge as is the fetal head. There is risk of prolapse of the cord if the membranes rupture in early labor. The presence of meconium in amniotic fluid is not necessarily a sign of fetal distress because it results from pressure on the fetal abdominal wall as it traverses the birth canal. Assessment of FHR and pattern should

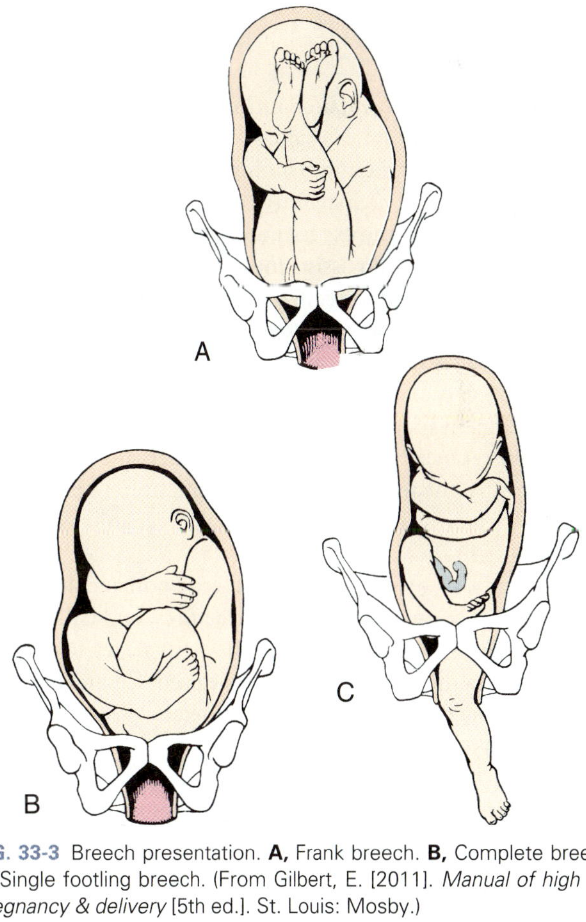

FIG. 33-3 Breech presentation. **A,** Frank breech. **B,** Complete breech. **C,** Single footling breech. (From Gilbert, E. [2011]. *Manual of high risk pregnancy & delivery* [5th ed.]. St. Louis: Mosby.)

be used to determine whether the passage of meconium is an expected finding associated with breech presentation or is an abnormal (nonreassuring) sign associated with fetal hypoxia. The heart tones of fetuses (FHTs) in a breech position are best heard at or above the umbilicus.

Vaginal birth is accomplished by mechanisms of labor that manipulate the buttocks and lower extremities as they emerge from the birth canal (Fig. 33-4). Risks associated with vaginal

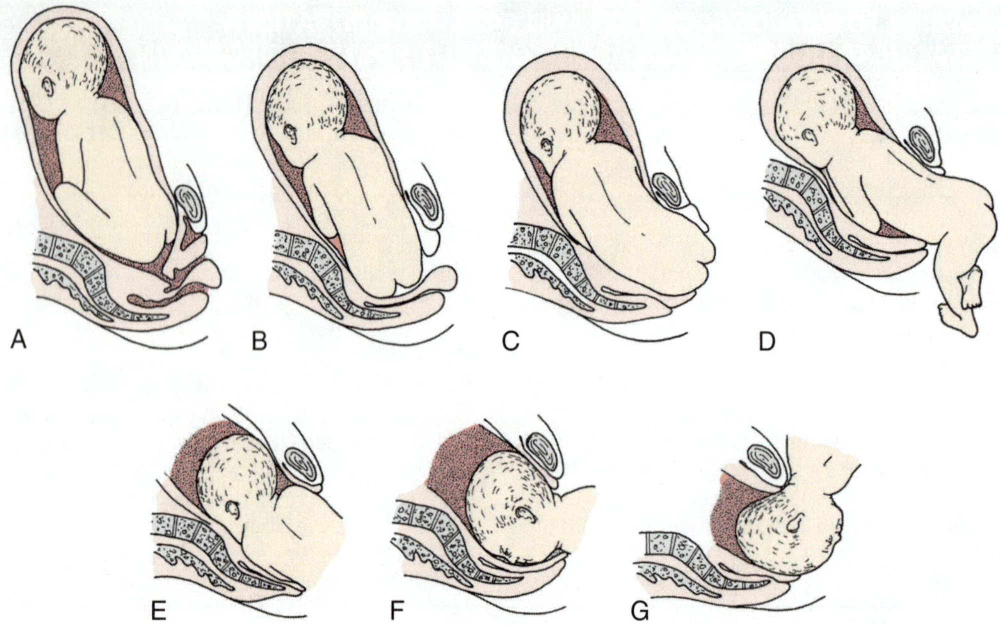

FIG. 33-4 Mechanism of labor in breech presentation. **A,** Breech before onset of labor. **B,** Engagement and internal rotation. **C,** Lateral flexion. **D,** External rotation or restitution. **E,** Internal rotation of shoulders and head. **F,** Face rotates to sacrum when occiput is anterior. **G,** Head is born by gradual flexion during elevation of fetal body.

birth from a breech presentation include prolapse of the umbilical cord (especially in single or double footling breech presentations) and trapping of the after-coming fetal head (especially with preterm infants). Safe vaginal birth from a breech presentation is largely dependent on the experience, judgment, and skill of the health care provider who assists the birth. Criteria for attempting a vaginal birth from a breech presentation are (Thorp, 2009):

- Frank or complete breech presentation
- Estimated fetal weight between 2000 and 3800 g
- Normal (gynecoid) maternal pelvis
- Flexed fetal head

External cephalic version (ECV) (see later discussion) may be tried to turn the fetus to a vertex presentation. If the attempt at ECV is unsuccessful, the woman usually gives birth by cesarean (Gilbert, 2011).

Face and brow presentations are uncommon and are associated with fetal anomalies, pelvic contractures, and CPD. Spontaneous vaginal birth is possible if the fetus flexes to a vertex presentation, although forceps often are used. Cesarean birth is indicated if the presentation persists, if fetal distress occurs, or if labor stops progressing.

Cesarean birth is usually necessary for a fetus in a transverse lie (i.e., shoulder) presentation, although ECV may be attempted after 36 to 37 weeks of gestation (Thorp, 2009).

Multifetal Pregnancy

Multifetal pregnancy is the gestation of twins, triplets, quadruplets, or more infants. Multiple gestations now account for more than 3% of all live births in the United States (Malone & D'Alton, 2009). The increasing number of twin gestations has been attributed to the use of fertility-enhancing medications and procedures and the older age of childbearing women. When compared with younger women, those age 35 years and older are naturally more likely to have a multifetal pregnancy. The rate of triplet and higher-order multiple pregnancies has been steadily declining since the all-time high rate of 193.5 per 100,000 in 1998. This decrease has been attributed to refinements in the treatments used for infertility (Cleary-Goldman, Chitkara, & Berkowitz, 2007; Malone & D'Alton; Martin et al., 2009).

Multiple births are associated with more complications (e.g., dysfunctional labor) than single births. The higher incidence of fetal and newborn complications and higher risk of perinatal mortality primarily stem from the birth of low birth weight infants resulting from preterm birth or IUGR (or both), in part related to placental dysfunction and twin-to-twin transfusion. Fetuses can experience distress and asphyxia during the birth process as a result of cord prolapse and the onset of placental separation with the birth of the first fetus. As a result, the risk for long-term problems such as cerebral palsy is higher among infants who were part of a multiple birth.

In addition, fetal complications such as congenital anomalies and abnormal presentations can result in dysfunctional labor and an increased incidence of cesarean birth. For example, in only 40% to 45% of all twin pregnancies do both fetuses present in the vertex position, the most favorable for vaginal birth. In 35% to 40% of the pregnancies, one twin may present in the vertex position and the other in a breech or transverse lie presentation (Malone & D'Alton, 2009).

The health status of the mother may be compromised by an increased risk for hypertension, anemia, and hemorrhage associated with uterine atony, placental abruption, and multiple or adherent placentas. Duration of the phases and stages of labor may vary from the duration experienced with singleton births.

Teamwork and planning are essential components of the management of childbirth in multiple pregnancies, especially those of higher-order multiples. The nurse plays a key role in coordinating the activities of many highly skilled health care professionals. Early detection and management of the maternal, fetal, and newborn complications associated with multiple births are essential to achieve a positive outcome for mother and babies. Maternal positioning and active support are used to enhance labor progress and placental perfusion. Stimulation of labor with oxytocin, epidural anesthesia, internal or external version, and forceps and vacuum assistance may be used to accomplish the vaginal birth of twins. Cesarean birth is almost always performed with higher-order multiple births. Each infant will have its own team of health care providers present at the birth. Emotional support that includes expression of feelings and full explanations of events as they occur and of the status of the mother and the fetuses and newborns is important to reduce the anxiety and stress the mother and her family experience.

Position of the Woman

The functional relationship among the uterine contractions, the fetus, and the mother's pelvis are altered by the maternal position. In addition, the position can provide a mechanical advantage or disadvantage to the mechanisms of labor by altering the effects of gravity and the body-part relationships that are important to the progress of labor. For example, the lateral position facilitates rotation from an occiput posterior position more effectively than the hands-and-knees position. Upright positions such as sitting and squatting for birth enhance fetal descent during bearing-down efforts, shorten the second stage of labor, reduce pain and perineal trauma, and decrease the need for forceps or vacuum assistance to facilitate vaginal birth (see Chapter 19) (Roberts & Hanson, 2007).

Discouraging maternal movement or restricting labor to the recumbent or lithotomy position may compromise progress. The incidence of dysfunctional labor in women confined to these positions is increased, resulting in a greater need for augmentation of labor or forceps-assisted, vacuum-assisted, or cesarean birth.

Psychologic Responses

Hormones and neurotransmitters released in response to stress (e.g., catecholamines) can cause dysfunctional labor. Sources of stress vary for each woman, but pain and the absence of a support person are two factors often related to dysfunctional labor. Confinement to bed and restriction of maternal movement can be a source of psychologic stress that compounds the physiologic stress caused by immobility in the unmedicated laboring woman. When anxiety is excessive, it can inhibit cervical dilation and result in prolonged labor and increased pain perception. Anxiety also causes increased levels of stress-related hormones (e.g., beta-endorphin, adrenocorticotropic hormone, cortisol, and epinephrine). These hormones act on the smooth muscles of the uterus. Increased levels can cause dysfunctional labor by reducing uterine contractility.

CARE MANAGEMENT

Risk assessment is a continuous process in the laboring woman. By reviewing the woman's past labor or labors and observing her physical and psychologic responses to the current labor, any factors that might contribute to dysfunctional labor should be identified. Nursing diagnoses, expected outcomes of care, and interventions are then established for each woman based on assessment findings. Many interventions for dysfunctional labor (e.g., ECV, cervical ripening, induction or augmentation of labor, and operative procedures [forceps- or vacuum-assisted birth, cesarean birth]) are implemented collaboratively with other members of the health care team. Commonly performed interventions are discussed in detail in the Obstetric Procedures section (see the Nursing Process box: Dysfunctional Labor).

When providing care for a woman who is experiencing labor or birth complications, all members of the health care team are responsible for complying with professional standards of care.

> **LEGAL TIP: Standard of Care—Labor and Birth Complications**
> - Document all assessment findings, interventions, and the woman's responses in the medical record according to unit protocols, procedures, and policies and professional standards.
> - Assess whether the woman (and her family, if appropriate) is fully informed about the procedures for which she is consenting.
> - Provide full explanations regarding what is happening and what needs to be done to help her and her baby.
> - Maintain safety in administering medications and treatments correctly.
> - Have telephone orders signed as soon as possible.
> - Provide care at the acceptable standard (e.g., according to unit protocols and professional standards).
> - If short staffing occurs in the unit and the nurse is assigned additional clients, the nurse should document that rejecting this additional assignment would have placed these clients in danger as a result of abandonment.
> - Continue maternal and fetal monitoring until birth according to the policies, procedures, and protocols of the birthing facility, even after a decision to carry out cesarean birth is made.

OBESITY

Excessive weight is an increasingly serious problem for children, adolescents, and adults living in affluent nations, including the United States, and pregnant women are no exception. The BMI is used to define obesity. Persons with a BMI of 30 or greater kg/m^2 are considered obese, whereas those with a BMI of 40 kg/m^2 or greater are classified as morbidly obese (Cunningham et al., 2010).

Obese women are at risk for several pregnancy complications, including venous thromboembolism and cesarean birth. In addition to having an increased risk for cesarean birth in general, obese women are also more likely to require emergency cesarean birth. As the woman's BMI increases, the risk of developing these complications also rises (Cunningham et al., 2010; Walters & Taylor, 2009, 2010).

CARE MANAGEMENT

Nursing care of obese women during labor and birth is challenging for a number of reasons. Sometimes standard furniture such as beds, chairs, and operating tables is simply not large enough to accommodate the woman's size. Extra-large furniture may not fit through a standard doorway, so room renovation may be necessary. Some hospitals have created rooms specifically designed to accommodate obese clients (Fig. 33-5). Continuous external FHR and contraction monitoring may be extremely difficult if not impossible to perform. Special equipment, such as extra-large blood pressure cuffs, is necessary to properly assess the woman's condition.

NURSING PROCESS

Dysfunctional Labor

ASSESSMENT

Women in labor are continuously assessed for signs that labor is progressing normally.

Past History

- Dysfunctional labor in a previous pregnancy

Physical

- Characteristics of uterine contractions (frequency, intensity, duration)
- Progress of cervical effacement and dilation
- Characteristics of FHR tracing (baseline rate, variability, presence of decelerations)
- Presentation, position, and station of fetus
- Status of amniotic membranes (intact or ruptured)
- Characteristics of maternal pelvis
- Maternal physical status including vital signs, elimination, energy level

Psychologic

- Anxiety

NURSING DIAGNOSES

Possible nursing diagnoses for women experiencing dysfunctional labor include:

***Risk for Injury (maternal or fetal)* related to:**

- interventions implemented for dysfunctional labor

***Powerlessness* related to:**

- loss of control

***Risk for Infection* related to:**

- premature rupture of membranes
- operative procedures

***Ineffective Individual Coping* related to:**

- inadequate support system
- exhaustion
- pain

EXPECTED OUTCOMES OF CARE

Expected outcomes include that the woman will:

- Be able to describe the causes and treatment of dysfunctional labor.
- Use measures recommended by the health care team to enhance the progress of labor and birth.
- Express relief of pain.
- Experience labor and birth with minimal or no complications, such as infection, injury, or hemorrhage.
- Give birth to a healthy infant who has experienced no fetal distress or birth injury.

PLAN OF CARE AND INTERVENTIONS

- Communicate pertinent assessment findings to the woman's primary health care provider immediately.
- Implement or assist with interventions as ordered or per protocol.
- Ensure that the woman and her significant other(s) receive an explanation regarding reason(s) for performing a particular intervention. (See the Obstetric Procedures section beginning on p. 799 for information regarding specific interventions.)
- Ensure that all questions are answered to the woman's (or support person or persons) satisfaction.
- Provide support and encouragement to the woman and her support persons during the labor and birth.

EVALUATION

The nurse can be reasonably assured that care was effective to the extent that the expected outcomes for care have been achieved.

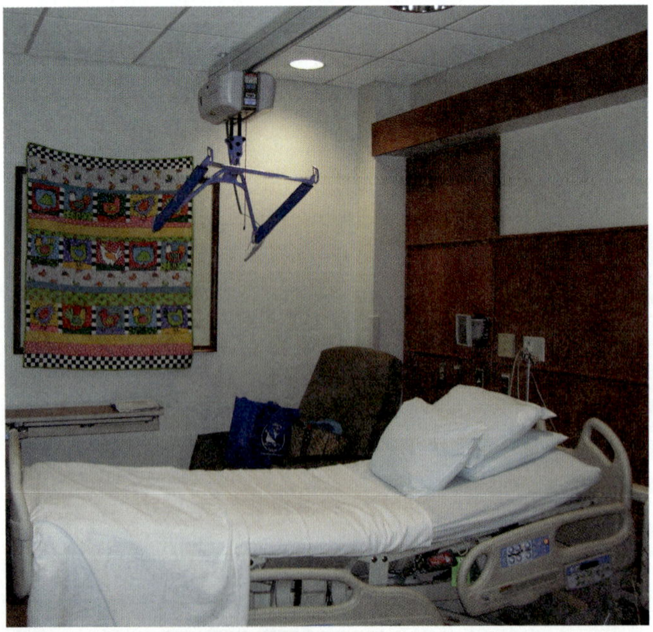

FIG. 33-5 Room specifically designed to accommodate obese pregnant clients. Note lift attached to ceiling for use in transferring women from the bed to chairs or stretchers. (Courtesy Dee Lowdermilk, Chapel Hill, NC.)

Even routine procedures will require more time and effort to accomplish when a woman is obese. This is extremely worrisome, given that obesity is a risk factor for emergency cesarean birth, when time is often of the essence. Establishing intravenous access, for example, may require multiple attempts, sometimes by multiple persons. Mobility is often a problem. Moving the woman from a labor room to the operating room and transferring her from a bed to the operating table may require the assistance of additional personnel or special equipment, especially if regional anesthesia is already in effect. If it is not, surgery may be further delayed by anesthetic complications, such as difficulty establishing an epidural or spinal block or accomplishing endotracheal intubation.

Postoperatively, obese women are at increased risk for blood clot formation. In the immediate recovery period, use of thromboembolic stockings (TED hose) and sequential compression device (SCD) boots help to decrease the chance for clot formation. Some women may also be given heparin prophylactically for clot prevention (Cunningham et al., 2010). Women should also be encouraged to get out of bed and begin ambulating as soon as possible.

Keeping the incision clean and dry to prevent wound infection and promote healing is another postoperative challenge.

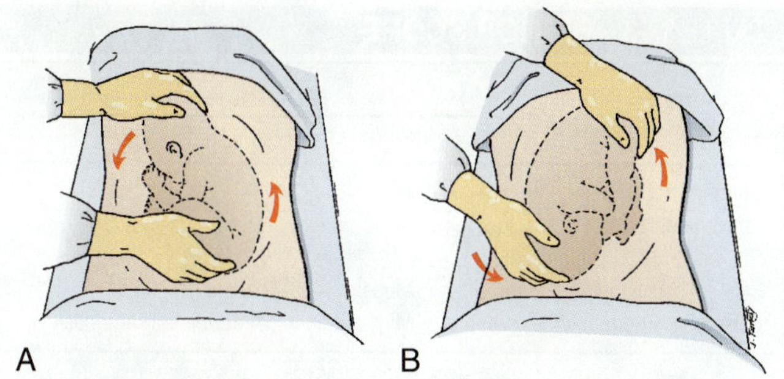

FIG. 33-6 External version of fetus from breech to vertex presentation. This must be achieved without force. **A,** Breech is pushed up out of pelvic inlet while head is pulled toward inlet. **B,** Head is pushed toward inlet while breech is pulled upward.

Many obese women have a *pannus* (large roll of abdominal fat) that overlies a lower abdominal transverse skin incision made just above the pubic area. The pannus causes the area to remain moist, which encourages infection development. Women should be taught to wash the incision with soap and water several times a day, drying the area well afterward. Sutures or staples used to close the skin incision are generally left in place longer than usual in order to avoid possible wound disruption when they are removed. Sometimes the skin and subcutaneous layers of the incision are left open to heal by secondary intention to avoid possible dehiscence. If this course of action is chosen, the woman and other family members must be taught to do dressing changes and wound care.

OBSTETRIC PROCEDURES

Version

Version is the turning of the fetus from one presentation to another. It may be performed externally or internally by the physician.

External Cephalic Version

External cephalic version (ECV) is used in an attempt to turn the fetus from a breech or shoulder presentation to a vertex presentation for birth. It may be attempted in a labor and birth setting after 37 weeks of gestation. ECV is accomplished by the exertion of gentle, constant pressure on the abdomen (Fig. 33-6). Before ECV is attempted, ultrasound scanning is done to determine the fetal position; locate the umbilical cord; rule out placenta previa; evaluate the adequacy of the maternal pelvis; and assess the amount of amniotic fluid, the gestational age, and the presence of any anomalies. An NST is performed to confirm fetal well-being, or the FHR and pattern are monitored for a period of time (i.e., 10 to 20 minutes). Informed consent is obtained. A tocolytic agent such as terbutaline often is given to relax the uterus and facilitate the maneuver. Contraindications to ECV include (Thorp, 2009):

- Uterine anomalies
- Third-trimester bleeding
- Multiple gestation
- Oligohydramnios
- Evidence of uteroplacental insufficiency
- A nuchal cord (identified by ultrasound)
- Previous cesarean birth or other significant uterine surgery
- Obvious CPD

ECV is most successful in a multiparous woman who has a normal amount of amniotic fluid and whose fetus is not yet engaged in the pelvis (Cunningham et al., 2010). If ECV is not successful, the ACOG recommends that the woman undergo planned cesarean birth (Thorp, 2009).

During an attempted ECV, the nurse continuously monitors the FHR and pattern, especially for bradycardia and variable decelerations; checks the maternal vital signs; and assesses the woman's level of comfort, because the procedure may cause discomfort. After the procedure is completed, the nurse continues to monitor maternal vital signs and uterine activity, and to assess for vaginal bleeding until the woman's condition is determined to be stable. FHR and pattern monitoring should continue for at least 1 hour. Women who are Rh negative should receive Rh immune globulin because the manipulation can cause fetomaternal bleeding (Lanni & Seeds, 2007; Thorp, 2009).

Internal Version

With internal version the fetus is turned by the physician, who inserts a hand into the uterus and changes the presentation to cephalic (head) or podalic (foot). Internal version is only rarely used, most often in twin gestations to deliver the second fetus. The safety of this procedure has not been documented; maternal and fetal injury is possible. Cesarean birth is the usual method for managing malpresentation in multifetal pregnancies. The nurse's role is to monitor the status of the fetus and to provide support to the woman.

Induction of Labor

Induction of labor is the chemical or mechanical initiation of uterine contractions before their spontaneous onset for the purpose of bringing about birth. Labor may be induced either electively or for indicated reasons. The rate of labor induction since 1990 has doubled to a rate of approximately 20% (Martin et al., 2009). It is likely that the rate of elective inductions is increasing more rapidly than the rate of indicated inductions. Additionally, there is concern that elective inductions may increase the risk of cesarean birth especially among primigravid women, and particularly those over the age of 35 (Martin et al.; Thorp, 2009; Wilson, 2007).

Induction of labor is indicated if continuing the pregnancy could be dangerous for either the woman or the fetus, and if no contraindications exist to artificial rupture of the membranes (amniotomy) or augmenting uterine contractions with oxytocin. Prior to labor induction, gestational age should be determined and any potential risks to the maternal-fetal unit evaluated. Women must be fully counseled regarding risks, benefits, and alternatives of labor stimulation methods as part of the process for informed consent (ACOG, 2009; Thorp, 2009). Box 33-8 lists indications and contraindications for labor induction.

An elective induction is one in which labor is initiated without a medical indication. Methods to ripen the cervix (e.g., application of prostaglandins) enhance the likelihood of successful induction and have therefore been a factor in the use of elective induction as an option for managing childbirth rather than waiting for labor to begin spontaneously. Many of these elective inductions are purely for the convenience of the woman or her primary health care provider. At times, however, labor may be electively induced to allay maternal fears and

BOX 33-8 INDICATIONS AND CONTRAINDICATIONS FOR LABOR INDUCTION

INDICATIONS
- Hypertensive complications of pregnancy: gestational hypertension, preeclampsia, eclampsia
- Fetal death
- Chorioamnionitis
- Maternal medical conditions: diabetes mellitus, renal disease, cardiopulmonary conditions, chronic hypertension, antiphospholipid syndrome
- Postterm pregnancy, especially when oligohydramnios is present
- Fetal compromise: intrauterine growth restriction, isoimmunization
- Premature rupture of membranes with established fetal maturity

CONTRAINDICATIONS
- Acute, severe fetal distress
- Shoulder presentation (transverse lie)
- Floating fetal presenting part
- Uncontrolled hemorrhage
- Umbilical cord prolapse
- Active genital herpes infection
- Placenta previa
- Previous uterine incision that prohibits a trial of labor

RELATIVE CONTRAINDICATIONS
- Grand multiparity (≥5 pregnancies that ended after 20 weeks of gestation)
- Multiple gestation
- Suspected cephalopelvic disproportion
- Breech presentations
- Inability to adequately monitor FHR or contractions (or both) throughout labor

Sources: Thorp, J. (2009). Clinical aspects of normal and abnormal labor. In R. Creasy, R. Resnik, J. Iams, C. Lockwood, & T. Moore (Eds.), *Creasy and Resnik's maternal-fetal medicine: Principles and practice* (6th ed.). Philadelphia: Saunders; American College of Obstetricians and Gynecologists (ACOG). (2009). *Induction of labor. ACOG Practice Bulletin No. 107.* Washington, DC: ACOG.

anxieties associated with prior perinatal losses or to ensure that experienced multispecialty personnel are available to handle anticipated maternal or neonatal complications immediately following birth (Battista & Wing, 2007; Moleti, 2009). The two major risks associated with elective labor induction at term are increased rates of cesarean birth and iatrogenic prematurity (Battista & Wing). In order to prevent iatrogenic prematurity, elective induction of labor should not be initiated until the woman reaches 39 completed weeks of gestation (ACOG, 2009; Cherouny, Federico, Haraden, Leavitt Gullo, & Resar, 2005).

Chemical, mechanical, physical, and alternative methods are used to ripen the cervix and induce labor. Intravenous oxytocin (Pitocin) and amniotomy are the most common methods used in the United States. Success rates for induction of labor are higher when the condition of the cervix is favorable, or inducible. Cervical ripeness is the most important predictor of successful induction. A rating system such as the **Bishop score** (Table 33-3) can be used to evaluate inducibility. For example, a score of 8 or more on this 13-point scale indicates that the cervix is soft, anterior, 50% or more effaced, and dilated 2 cm or more and that the presenting part is engaged. When the Bishop score totals 8 or more, induction of labor is usually successful (ACOG, 2009; Gilbert, 2011; Moleti, 2009). The Bishop score should be documented prior to the use of methods to ripen the cervix or induce labor.

TABLE 33-3 BISHOP SCORE

	SCORE			
	0	1	2	3
Dilation (cm)	0	1-2	3-4	≥5
Effacement (%)	0-30	40-50	60-70	≥80
Station (cm)	−3	−2	−1, 0	+1, +2
Cervical consistency	Firm	Medium	Soft	Soft
Cervical position	Posterior	Midposition	Anterior	Anterior

Cervical Ripening Methods

Chemical Agents. Preparations of prostaglandins E_1 (PGE_1) and E_2 (PGE_2) have been shown to be effective when used before induction to "ripen" (soften and thin) the cervix (see the Medication Guides for Prostaglandin E_1 and Prostaglandin E_2). In some cases, women spontaneously begin laboring after the administration of prostaglandin, thereby eliminating the need to administer oxytocin to induce labor. Additional advantages of prostaglandin use for cervical ripening include decreased oxytocin induction time and a decrease in the amount of oxytocin required for successful induction (Gilbert, 2011). PGE_1, although much less expensive and more effective than PGE_2 for inducing labor and birth, is associated with a higher risk for uterine tachysystole with abnormal (nonreassuring) fetal heart rate and pattern changes and passage of meconium into the aminotic fluid. Most of these adverse outcomes are associated with higher dose protocols (ACOG, 2009; Battista & Wing, 2007). Although the drug's manufacturer has acknowledged for several years that PGE_1 is effective for cervical ripening and labor induction, it has not yet been approved by the FDA for these uses (Thorp, 2009). PGE_2 in the form of a vaginal insert (dinoprostone [Cervidil]), although more expensive than PGE_1, has the major advantage of easy removal should adverse reactions, including uterine tachysystole, occur (Moleti, 2009).

Mechanical and Physical Methods. Mechanical dilators ripen the cervix by stimulating the release of endogenous prostaglandins. Balloon catheters (e.g., Foley catheter) can be inserted through the intracervical canal to ripen and dilate the cervix. The catheter balloon is inflated above the internal cervical os with 30 to 50 ml of sterile water. This process results in pressure and stretching of the lower uterine segment and the cervix, as well as the release of endogenous prostaglandins. It is especially helpful for women who cannot receive exogenous prostaglandin for cervical ripening. The balloon will fall out when cervical dilation reaches approximately 3 cm in about 8 to 12 hours after it is inserted. Evidence supports the insertion of a balloon catheter as a cervical ripening method especially since it is not associated with uterine tachysystole and fetal stress as are the prostaglandin methods (ACOG, 2009; Simpson, 2008).

Hydroscopic dilators (substances that absorb fluid from surrounding tissues and then enlarge) also can be used for cervical ripening. Laminaria tents (natural cervical dilators made from desiccated seaweed) and synthetic dilators containing

MEDICATION GUIDE

Prostaglandin E_1 (PGE_1): Misoprostol (Cytotec)

ACTION

PGE_1 ripens the cervix, making it softer and causing it to begin to dilate and efface it: stimulates uterine contractions.

INDICATIONS

- PGE_1 is used for preinduction cervical ripening (ripen cervix before oxytocin induction of labor when the Bishop score is 4 or less) and to induce labor or abortion (abortifacient agent); it has not yet been approved by the FDA for cervical ripening or labor induction (i.e., this is an off labeled use for obstetrics).
- Should not be used if the woman has a history of previous cesarean birth or other major uterine surgery.

DOSAGE AND ROUTE

- Misoprostol is available either as a 100- or a 200-mcg tablet. Therefore, tablets must be broken to prepare the correct dose. This preparation should take place in the pharmacy to ensure accurate doses.
- Recommended initial dose is 25 mcg. Insert intravaginally into the posterior vaginal fornix using the tips of index and middle fingers without the use of a lubricant. Repeat every 3 to 6 hours up to 6 doses in a 24-hour period or until an effective contraction pattern is established (three or more uterine contractions in 10 minutes), the cervix ripens (Bishop score of 8 or greater), or significant adverse effects occur.

ADVERSE EFFECTS

- Higher doses (e.g., 50 mcg every 6 hours) are more likely to result in adverse effects such as nausea and vomiting, diarrhea, fever, uterine tachysystole with or without an abnormal (nonreassuring) FHR and pattern, or fetal passage of meconium. The risk for adverse reactions is reduced with lower dosages and longer intervals between doses.

NURSING CONSIDERATIONS

- Explain the procedure to the woman and her family; ensure that an informed consent has been obtained as per agency policy.
- Assess the maternal-fetal unit, before each insertion and during treatment following agency protocol for frequency. Assess maternal vital signs and health status, FHR and pattern, and status of pregnancy, including indications for cervical ripening or induction of labor, signs of labor or impending labor, and the Bishop score. Recognize that an abnormal (nonreassuring) FHR and pattern; maternal fever, infection, vaginal bleeding, or hypersensitivity; and regular, progressive uterine contractions contraindicate the use of misoprostol.
- Use caution if the woman has a history of asthma, glaucoma, or renal, hepatic, or cardiovascular disorders.
- Have the woman void prior to insertion.
- Assist the woman to maintain a supine position with a lateral tilt or a side-lying position for 30 to 40 minutes after insertion.
- Prepare to swab the vagina to remove unabsorbed medication using a saline-soaked gauze wrapped around fingers or to administer terbutaline 0.25 mg subcutaneously if significant adverse effects occur.
- Initiate oxytocin for induction of labor no sooner than 4 hours after last dose of misoprostol was administered, following agency protocol, if ripening has occurred and labor has not begun.
- Document all assessment findings and administration procedures.

Sources: Moleti, C. (2009). Trends and controversies in labor induction. *MCN The American Journal of Maternal/Child Nursing, 34*(1), 40-47; Thorp, J. (2009). Clinical aspects of normal and abnormal labor. In R. Creasy, R. Resnik, J. Iams, C. Lockwood, & T. Moore (Eds.). *Creasy and Resnik's maternal-fetal medicine: Principles and practice* (6th ed.). Philadelphia: Saunders.

magnesium sulfate (Lamicel) are inserted into the endocervix without rupturing the membranes. As they absorb fluid, they expand and cause cervical dilation, and the release of endogenous prostaglandins. These dilators are left in place for 6 to 12 hours before being removed to assess cervical dilation. Fresh dilators are inserted if further cervical dilation is necessary. Synthetic dilators swell faster than natural dilators and become larger with less discomfort. When compared with prostaglandins, these mechanical methods achieved a lower rate of birth within 24 hours, but caused no change in the cesarean birth rate. Additionally, they were less likely to cause uterine tachysystole with or without changes in the fetal heart rate (ACOG, 2009; Thorp, 2009).

Hydroscopic dilators compare favorably with prostaglandins in terms of their effectiveness in ripening the cervix but are associated with increased discomfort at insertion and during expansion and with a higher incidence of postpartum maternal and newborn infections. They are a reliable alternative when prostaglandins are contraindicated or are unavailable. Nursing responsibilities for women who have dilators inserted include documenting the number of dilators and sponges inserted during the procedure, as well as the number removed, and assessment for urinary retention, rupture of membranes, uterine tenderness or pain, contractions, vaginal bleeding, infection, and fetal distress (Gilbert, 2011).

Amniotic membrane stripping or sweeping is a method of inducing labor through the release of prostaglandins and oxytocin. The procedure involves separation of the membrane from the wall of the cervix and lower uterine segment by inserting a finger into the internal cervical os and rotating it 360 degrees. Membrane stripping seems to work best when the woman is a primigravida at term with an unripe cervix and with the vertex well applied to the cervix. In some studies it has been associated with shorter pregnancies and a decreased likelihood of progressing past 42 weeks of gestation. The procedure is uncomfortable and increases the risk for infection, rupture of membranes, bleeding, and precipitous labor and birth (Simpson, 2008).

Physical methods such as sexual intercourse (prostaglandins in the semen and stimulation of contractions with orgasm), nipple stimulation (release of endogenous oxytocin from the pituitary gland), and walking (gravity applies pressure to the cervix, which stimulates the secretion of endogenous oxytocin) may be used by women to "self-induce" labor in an effort to "get it over with." Breast (nipple) stimulation has been shown to initiate or enhance labor, especially the latent phase of labor. Although orgasm does stimulate uterine contractions, there

MEDICATION GUIDE

Prostaglandin E_2 (PGE_2): Dinoprostone (Cervidil Insert; Prepidil Gel)

ACTION

PGE_2 ripens the cervix, making it softer and causing it to begin to dilate and efface; it stimulates uterine contractions. Dinoprostone is the only FDA-approved medication for cervical ripening or labor induction.

INDICATIONS

PGE_2 is used for preinduction cervical ripening (ripen cervix before oxytocin induction of labor when the Bishop score is 4 or less) and for inducement of labor or abortion (abortifacient agent). It is not recommended for use if the woman has a history of previous cesarean birth or other major uterine surgery.

DOSAGE AND ROUTE

Cervidil insert:

- Dosage is 10 mg of dinoprostone designed to be gradually released (approximately 0.3 mg/hr) over 12 hours. Insert is placed transvaginally into the posterior fornix of the vagina. The insert is removed after 12 hours or at the onset of active labor or earlier if tachysystole or abnormal FHR and patterns occur.

Prepidil gel:

- Dosage is 0.5 mg of dinoprostone in a 2.5-ml syringe. Gel is administered through a catheter attached to the syringe into the cervical canal just below the internal cervical os. Dose may be repeated every 6 hours as needed for cervical ripening up to a maximum cumulative dose of 1.5 mg (3 doses) in a 24-hour period.

ADVERSE EFFECTS

- Potential adverse effects include headache, nausea and vomiting, diarrhea, fever, hypotension, uterine tachysystole with or without an abnormal (nonreassuring) FHR and pattern, or fetal passage of meconium.

NURSING CONSIDERATIONS

- Explain the procedure to the woman and her family. Ensure that an informed consent has been obtained as per agency policy.
- Assess the maternal-fetal unit before each insertion and during treatment following agency protocol for frequency. Assess maternal vital signs and health status, FHR and pattern, and status of pregnancy, including indications for cervical ripening or induction of labor, signs of labor or impending labor, and the Bishop score. Recognize that an abnormal (nonreassuring) FHR and pattern; maternal fever, infection, vaginal bleeding, or hypersensitivity; and regular, progressive uterine contractions contraindicate the use of dinoprostone.
- Use caution if the woman has a history of asthma, glaucoma, or renal, hepatic, or cardiovascular disorders.
- Bring the gel to room temperature just before administration. Do not force the warming process by using a warm-water bath or other source of external heat such as microwave because heat may cause inactivation.
- Keep the insert frozen until just before insertion. No warming is needed.
- Have the woman void before insertion.
- Assist the woman to maintain a supine position with a lateral tilt or a side-lying position for at least 30 minutes after insertion of the gel or for 2 hours after placement of the insert.
- Allow the woman to ambulate after the recommended period of bed rest and observation.
- Prepare to pull the string to remove the insert and to administer terbutaline 0.25 mg subcutaneously if significant adverse effects occur. There is no effective way to remove the gel from the vagina if uterine tachysystole or abnormal (nonreassuring) FHR and patterns occur.
- Delay the initiation of oxytocin for induction of labor for 6 to 12 hours after the last instillation of the gel or for 30 to 60 minutes after removal of the insert, or follow agency protocol for induction if ripening has occurred but labor has not begun.
- Document all assessment findings and administration procedures.

Source: Moleti, C. (2009). Trends and controversies in labor induction. *MCN The American Journal of Maternal/Child Nursing, 34*(1), 40-47.

is inadequate evidence to support the belief that sexual intercourse enhances cervical ripening (Gilbert, 2011). Ambulation is an effective measure to augment labor (Moleti, 2009).

Alternative Methods. A variety of alternative methods have been used by women to stimulate cervical ripening and the onset of labor. For example, blue cohosh and castor oil can be used for their labor stimulation effects and black cohosh and evening primrose oil can ripen the cervix. Nurses must be knowledgeable about these preparations and ask about their use when assessing women during prenatal visits and on admission during labor. Women may accidentally take too much of the preparation or use it incorrectly. Also these preparations may potentiate the effect of pharmacologic methods to stimulate cervical ripening and uterine contractions, thereby increasing the potential for tachysystole and precipitous labor and birth (Gilbert, 2011; Moleti, 2009).

Acupuncture has been used effectively to induce labor and has been found, in several studies, to reduce the duration of labor, the use of oxytocin, and the rate of cesarean birth. Specific points have been identified to stimulate uterine contractions or to facilitate cervical dilation. More than one treatment may be required to establish labor (Gilbert, 2011; Moleti, 2009).

Amniotomy. Amniotomy (i.e., artificial rupture of membranes [AROM]) can be used to induce labor when the condition of the cervix is favorable (ripe) or to augment labor if progress begins to slow. Labor usually begins within 12 hours of the rupture. Amniotomy can decrease the duration of labor by up to 2 hours, even without oxytocin administration. However, if amniotomy does not stimulate labor, the resulting prolonged rupture may lead to intraamniotic infection. Variable FHR deceleration patterns can occur as a result of cord compression associated with umbilical cord prolapse or decreased aminotic fluid. Once an amniotomy is performed, the woman is committed to labor with an unknown outcome for how and when she will give birth. For this reason, amniotomy often is used in combination with oxytocin induction.

Before the procedure, the woman should be told what to expect. She also should be assured that the actual rupture of the membranes is painless for her and the fetus, although she may experience some discomfort when the Amnihook or other sharp instrument is inserted through the vagina and cervix (see the Procedure box: Assisting with Amniotomy). The presenting part of the fetus should be engaged and well applied to the cervix

PROCEDURE

Assisting with Amniotomy

PROCEDURE

- Explain to the woman what will be done.
- Assess fetal heart rate (FHR) and pattern before procedure begins to obtain a baseline reading.
- Place several underpads under the woman's buttocks to absorb the fluid.
- Position the woman on a padded bed pan, fracture pan, or rolled-up towel to elevate her hips.
- Assist the health care provider who is performing the procedure by providing sterile gloves and lubricant for the vaginal examination.
- Unwrap the sterile package containing an Amnihook or Allis clamp and pass the instrument to the primary health care provider, who inserts it alongside the fingers and then hooks and tears the membranes.
- Reassess the FHR and pattern.
- Assess the color, consistency, and odor of the fluid.
- Assess the woman's temperature every 2 hours or per protocol.
- Evaluate the woman for signs and symptoms of infection.

DOCUMENTATION

- Record the following:
  - Time of rupture
  - Color, odor, and consistency of the fluid
  - FHR and pattern before and after the procedure
  - Maternal status (how well procedure was tolerated)

prior to the procedure to prevent cord prolapse (Battista & Wing, 2007). The woman should also be free of active infection of the genital tract (e.g., herpes) and should be human immunodeficiency virus (HIV) negative. After rupture, the amniotic fluid is allowed to drain slowly. The color, odor, and consistency of the fluid are assessed (i.e., for the presence or absence of meconium or blood). The time of rupture is recorded.

! NURSNG ALERT

The FHR is assessed before and immediately after the amniotomy to detect any changes (e.g., transient tachycardia is common, but bradycardia and variable decelerations are not) that may indicate cord compression or prolapse.

The woman's temperature should be checked at least every 2 hours after rupture of membranes, more frequently if signs or symptoms of infection are noted. If her temperature is 38° C or higher, notify the primary health care provider. The nurse assesses for other signs and symptoms of infection, such as maternal chills, uterine tenderness on palpation, foul-smelling vaginal drainage, and fetal tachycardia. Comfort measures, such as frequently changing the woman's underpads and perineal cleansing, are implemented.

LEGAL TIP: Performing Amniotomy
Nurses should not perform amniotomy. This procedure should be done by the primary health care provider.

Oxytocin

Oxytocin is a hormone normally produced by the posterior pituitary gland. It stimulates uterine contractions and aids in milk let-down. Synthetic oxytocin (Pitocin) may be used either to induce labor or to augment a labor that is progressing slowly because of inadequate uterine contractions. Oxytocin is used in the majority of all births in the United States. It is also the drug most commonly associated with adverse events during childbirth. The most common errors involving oxytocin administration during labor are dose related (Clark, Simpson, Knox, & Garite, 2009; Mahlmeister, 2008; Simpson & Knox, 2009).

! SAFETY ALERT

Oxytocin was recently added to the list of high-alert medications designated by the Institute for Safe Medication Practices because it has the potential to cause significant harm when used inappropriately.

Oxytocin use can present hazards to the mother and fetus. Maternal hazards include placental abruption, uterine rupture, unnecessary cesarean birth due to abnormal (nonreassuring) FHR and patterns, postpartum hemorrhage, and infection. When placental perfusion is diminished by contractions that are too frequent or prolonged, the fetus can experience hypoxemia and acidemia, which eventually results in late decelerations and minimal or absent baseline variability. The goal of oxytocin use is to produce contractions of normal intensity, duration, and frequency while using the lowest dose of medication possible (Simpson & Knox, 2009).

The primary health care provider writes the order for the induction or augmentation of labor with oxytocin. The nurse implements the order by initiating the primary intravenous infusion and administering the oxytocin solution through a secondary line. The nurse's actions related to assessment and care of a woman whose labor is being induced are guided by hospital protocol and professional standards (see Fig. 33-7 and the Medication Guide: Oxytocin [Pitocin]).

The recommended protocol for administering oxytocin is to begin with a starting dose of 1 milliunit/min and to increase by 1 to 2 milliunits/min no more frequently than every 30 to 60 minutes (Simpson & Knox, 2009). This recommendation is based on research findings related to the pharmacokinetics of oxytocin. The uterus responds to oxytocin within 3 to 5 minutes of intravenous administration. The half-life of oxytocin (the time required to metabolize and eliminate half the dose) is approximately 10 to 12 minutes. Approximately 40 minutes is required to reach a steady state of oxytocin (the point in time when the rate of oxytocin administered intravenously equals the rate of oxytocin elimination) and for the full effect of a dosage increment to be reflected in more intense, frequent, and longer contractions (Mahlmeister, 2008) (see the Medication Guide: Oxytocin [Pitocin] and Fig. 33-7). Low-dose (physiologic) protocols such as the one described result in less uterine hyperstimulation, decreased fetal compromise, and significantly less use of oxytocin without affecting the duration of labor or cesarean birth rate (Battista & Wing, 2007; Gilbert, 2011).

MEDICATION GUIDE

Oxytocin (Pitocin)

ACTION

Oxytocin is a hormone produced in the posterior pituitary gland that stimulates uterine contractions and aids in milk let-down. Pitocin is a synthetic form of this hormone.

INDICATIONS

Oxytocin is used primarily for labor induction and augmentation.

DOSAGE AND ROUTE

- The intravenous solution containing oxytocin should be mixed in a standard concentration. Concentrations often used are 10 units in 1000 ml of fluid, 20 units in 1000 ml of fluid, or 30 units in 500 ml of fluid.
- Oxytocin is administered intravenously through a secondary line connected to the main line at the proximal port (connection closest to the intravenous insertion site). Oxytocin is always administered by pump.
- Begin oxytocin administration at 1 milliunit/min. Increase the rate by 1 to 2 milliunits/min, no more frequently than every 30 to 60 minutes based on the response of the maternal-fetal unit and the progress of labor.
- The goal of oxytocin administration is to produce acceptable uterine contractions as evidenced by:
  - Consistent achievement of 200 to 220 MVUs *or*
  - A consistent pattern of one contraction every 2 to 3 minutes, lasting 80 to 90 seconds, and strong to palpation

ADVERSE EFFECTS

- Possible maternal adverse effects include uterine tachysystole, placental abruption, uterine rupture, unnecessary cesarean birth caused by abnormal (nonreassuring) FHR and patterns, postpartum hemorrhage, and infection.
- Possible fetal adverse effects include hypoxemia and acidosis, eventually resulting in abnormal (nonreassuring) FHR and patterns.

NURSING CONSIDERATIONS

- Client and partner teaching and support:
  - Reasons for use of oxytocin (e.g., start or improve labor)
  - Effects to expect concerning the nature of contractions: the intensity of the contraction increases more rapidly, holds the peak longer, and ends more quickly; contractions will come regularly and more often
  - Monitoring to anticipate
- Continue to keep woman and her partner informed regarding progress.
- Remember that women vary greatly in their response to oxytocin; some require only very small amounts of medication to produce adequate contractions, while others need larger doses.
- Assessment:
  - Fetal status using electronic fetal monitoring; evaluate tracing every 15 minutes and with every change in dose during the first stage of labor and every 5 minutes during the active pushing phase of the second stage of labor.
  - Monitor the contraction pattern and uterine resting tone every 15 minutes and with every change in dose during the first stage of labor and every 5 minutes during the second stage of labor.
  - Monitor blood pressure, pulse, and respirations every 30 to 60 minutes and with every change in dose.
  - Assess intake and output; limit IV intake to 1000 ml in 8 hours; urine output should be 120 ml or more every 4 hours.
  - Perform vaginal examination as indicated.
  - Monitor for side effects, including nausea, vomiting, headache, hypotension.
  - Observe emotional responses of woman and her partner.
- Use a standard definition for uterine tachysystole that does not include an abnormal (nonreassuring) FHR and pattern or the woman's perception of pain (see the Emergency Box: Uterine Tachysystole with Oxytocin).
- The rate of oxytocin infusion should be continually titrated to the lowest dose that achieves acceptable labor progress. Usually the oxytocin dose can be decreased or discontinued after rupture of membranes and in the active phase of first stage labor.
- Documentation:
  - The time the oxytocin infusion is begun, and each time the infusion is increased, decreased, or discontinued
  - Assessment data as described above
  - Interventions for uterine tachysystole and abnormal (nonreassuring) FHR and patterns and the response to the interventions
  - Notification of the primary health care provider and that person's response

FHR, Fetal heart rate; *IV,* intravenous; *MVUs,* Montevideo units.

Sources: American College of Obstetricians and Gynecologists (ACOG). (2009). *Induction of labor. ACOG Practice Bulletin No. 107.* Washington, DC: ACOG; Clark, S., Simpson, K., Knox, G., & Garite, T. (2009). Oxytocin: New perspectives on an old drug. *American Journal of Obstetrics and Gynecology, 200*(1), 35,e1- e6; Mahlmeister, L. (2008). Best practices in perinatal care: Evidence-based management of oxytocin induction and augmentation of labor. *Journal of Perinatal and Neonatal Nursing, 22*(4), 259-263; Simpson, K. (2008). Labor and birth. In K. Simpson & P. Creehan (Eds.), *AWHONN's perinatal nursing* (3rd ed.). Philadephia: Lippincott Williams & Wilkins; Simpson, K., & Knox, G. (2009). Oxytocin as a high-alert medication: Implications for perinatal patient safety. *MCN The American Journal of Maternal/Child Nursing, 34*(1), 8-15.

High-dose protocols, in which the initial dose of oxytocin is larger and the dosage is increased more rapidly, have been found to result in shorter labors, less forceps-assisted births, and fewer cesarean births due to dystocia. However, high-dose protocols have been associated with more uterine hyperstimulation and more cesarean births related to fetal stress (Battista & Wing, 2007; Gilbert, 2011; Simpson & Knox, 2009). Some practitioners administer oxytocin in 10-minute pulsed infusions rather than as a continuous infusion. This method, which is more like endogenous secretion of oxytocin than the other approaches, is reported to be effective for labor induction but requires significantly less oxytocin use (Battista & Wing; Gilbert).

Nursing Considerations. An evidence-based written protocol for the preparation and administration of oxytocin should be established by the obstetric department (physicians, nurses) in each institution. Other safety measures recommended for use of this high-alert drug are using a standard concentration of oxytocin and a standard definition of uterine tachysystole that does not include an abnormal (nonreassuring) FHR or pattern or the woman's perception of pain. Additionally, standardized treatment of oxytocin-induced uterine tachysystole is recommended (Simpson & Knox, 2009) (see the Emergency box: Uterine Tachysystole with Oxytocin).

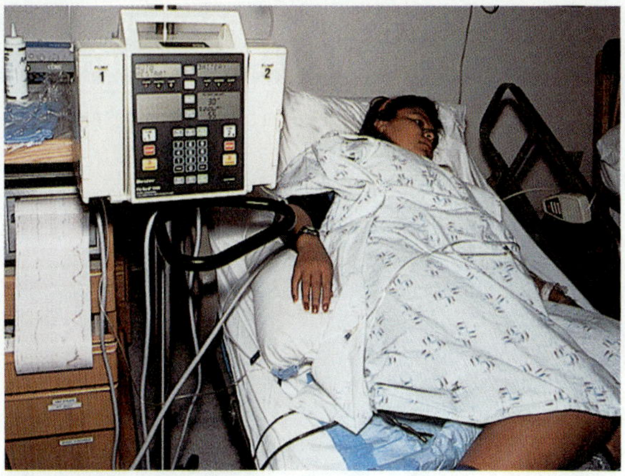

FIG. 33-7 Woman in side-lying position receiving oxytocin. (Courtesy Michael S. Clement, MD, Mesa, AZ.)

EMERGENCY

Uterine Tachysystole with Oxytocin

SIGNS

- More than five contractions in 10 minutes OR
- A series of single contractions lasting ≥2 minutes OR
- Contractions of normal duration occurring within 1 minute of each other

INTERVENTIONS (WITH NORMAL [REASSURING] FHR)

- Reposition or maintain woman in side-lying position (either side).
- Administer IV fluid bolus with 500 ml of lactated Ringer's solution.
- If uterine activity has not returned to normal after 10 minutes, decrease the oxytocin dose by at least half. If uterine activity has not returned to normal after another 10 minutes, discontinue the oxytocin infusion until fewer than five contractions occur in 10 minutes.

INTERVENTIONS (WTH ABNORMAL [NONREASSURING] FHR)

- Discontinue oxytocin infusion immediately.
- Reposition or maintain woman in side-lying position (either side).
- Administer IV fluid bolus with 500 ml of lactated Ringer's solution.
- Consider giving oxygen at 10 L/min if the above interventions do not resolve the abnormal (nonreassuring) FHR or pattern.
- If no response, consider giving 0.25 mg terbutaline subcutaneously according to unit protocol or standing orders.
- Notify primary health care provider of actions taken and maternal and fetal response.

RESUMPTION OF OXYTOCIN AFTER RESOLUTION OF TACHYSYSTOLE

- If the oxytocin infusion has been discontinued for less than 20 to 30 minutes, resume at no more than one half the rate that caused the tachysystole.
- If the oxytocin infusion has been discontinued for more than 30 to 40 minutes, resume at the initial starting dose.

Sources: Mahlmeister, L. (2008). Best practices in perinatal care: Evidence-based management of oxytocin induction and augmentation of labor. *Journal of Perinatal and Neonatal Nursing, 22*(4), 259-263; Simpson, K., & Knox, G. (2009). Oxytocin as a high-alert medication: Implications for perinatal patient safety. *MCN The American Journal of Maternal/Child Nursing, 34*(1), 8-15.

There has existed a need for standardizing the definition of excessive uterine contractions. The Eunice Kennedy Shriver National Institute of Child Health and Human Development, along with the ACOG and the Society for Maternal-Fetal Medicine, sponsored a workshop in April 2008 to review definitions, interpretation, and research recommendations for intrapartum fetal monitoring. Workshop participants also recommended standardizing definitions regarding uterine contractions for use in clinical practice. This group defined uterine tachysystole as more than five contractions in 10 minutes, averaged over a 30-minute window. The term *tachysystole* applies to both spontaneous and stimulated labor. Participants also recommended that use of the terms *hyperstimulation* and *hyperactivity* be abandoned because they are not defined (Macones, Hankins, Spong, Hauth, & Moore, 2008).

NURSING ALERT

If uterine tachysystole occurs, interventions are implemented immediately (see the Emergency Box: Uterine Tachysystole with Oxytocin). The primary health care provider is informed of the condition, the interventions initiated, and the maternal and fetal response.

Augmentation of Labor

Augmentation of labor is the stimulation of uterine contractions after labor has started spontaneously but progress is unsatisfactory. Augmentation is usually implemented for the management of hypotonic uterine dysfunction, resulting in a slowing of the labor process (protracted active phase). Common augmentation methods include oxytocin infusion and amniotomy. Noninvasive methods such as emptying the bladder, ambulation and position changes, relaxation measures, nourishment and hydration, and hydrotherapy should be attempted before initiating invasive interventions. The administration procedure and nursing assessment and care measures for augmenting labor with oxytocin are similar to those used for induction of labor with oxytocin (see the Medication Guide: Oxytocin [Pitocin]).

Some physicians advocate *active management of labor*, that is, augmentation of labor to establish efficient labor with the aggressive use of oxytocin so that the woman gives birth within 12 hours of admission to the labor unit. Advocates of active management believe that intervening early (as soon as a nulliparous labor is not progressing at least 1 cm/hr) with use of higher (pharmacologic) oxytocin doses administered at frequent increment intervals (e.g., a starting dose of 6 milliunits/min with increases of 6 milliunits/min every 15 minutes) shortens labor (Gilbert, 2011).

Additional components of the active management of labor include strict criteria to diagnose that the woman is indeed in active labor with 100% effacement, amniotomy within 1 hour of admission of a woman in labor if spontaneous rupture of the membranes has not occurred, and continuous presence of a personal nurse who provides one-on-one care for the woman while she is in labor. Many U.S. obstetricians emphasize using high-dose oxytocin protocols but do not implement all the other components of active management. At least one review of published studies on the effectiveness of active management of labor protocols concluded that the presence of a personal nurse who provides constant emotional and physical support is the only component associated with shorter labors and lower rates of cesarean birth (Clark et al., 2009; Gilbert, 2011).

The original active management of labor protocols were written for nulliparous women who began laboring spontaneously. However, active management of labor protocols have been implemented by some providers in the United States on women who were not appropriate candidates (Mahlmeister, 2008).

Operative Vaginal Birth

Operative vaginal births are accomplished with the assistance of forceps or vacuum extractor. Indications and prerequisites for the use of both instruments are similar. The decision to use forceps or vacuum is based on the experience and personal preference of the physician performing the procedure. There are several types of operative vaginal births, defined primarily by the station and position of the fetal head in relationship to the maternal pelvis (Table 33-4) (American Academy of Pediatrics [AAP] & ACOG, 2007). Forceps- and vacuum-assisted vaginal births have been declining. This decline has been attributed to the increasing rate of cesarean birth (Martin et al., 2009).

Forceps-Assisted Birth

A **forceps-assisted birth** is one in which an instrument with two curved blades is used to assist in the birth of the fetal head. The cephalic-like curve of the forceps commonly used is similar to the shape of the fetal head, with a pelvic curve to the blades conforming to the curve of the pelvic axis. The blades are joined by a pin, screw, or groove arrangement. These locks prevent the forceps from compressing the fetal skull (Fig. 33-8). There are several types of forceps-assisted births, defined primarily by the station and position of the fetal head in relationship to the maternal pelvis (see Table 33-4) (AAP & ACOG, 2007).

Maternal indications for forceps-assisted birth include a prolonged second stage of labor and the need to shorten the second stage of labor for maternal reasons (e.g., maternal exhaustion or maternal cardiopulmonary or cerebrovascular disease) (Nielsen, Galan, Kilpatrick, & Garrison, 2007). Fetal indications include birth of a fetus in distress or in certain abnormal presentations; arrest of rotation; or extraction of the head in a breech presentation. The use of forceps during childbirth has been decreasing, replaced by vacuum extraction or cesarean birth (Nielsen et al.; Thorp, 2009).

Certain conditions are required for a forceps-assisted birth to be successful. The woman's cervix must be fully dilated to prevent lacerations and hemorrhage. The bladder should be empty. The presenting part must be engaged—vertex presentation is desired. Membranes must be ruptured so that the position of the fetal head can be precisely determined and the forceps can firmly grasp the head during birth (Fig. 33-9). In addition, the size of the maternal pelvis must be assessed as adequate for the estimated fetal head circumference and weight.

Management. Both blades are positioned by the physician, and the handles are locked. Traction is usually applied during contractions. The mother may or may not be instructed to push during contractions, depending on physician preference. If a decrease in the fetal heart rate occurs, the forceps are removed and reapplied.

TABLE 33-4 DEFINITIONS FOR FORCEPS- AND VACUUM-ASSISTED BIRTHS

Outlet	Fetal scalp is visible on the perineum without manually separating the labia
Low	Fetal head is at least at the +2 station
Midpelvis	Fetal head is engaged (no higher than 0 station) but above the +2 station

Source: American Academy of Pediatrics (AAP) & American College of Obstetricians and Gynecologists (ACOG). (2007). *Guidelines for perinatal care* (6th ed.). Washington, DC: ACOG.

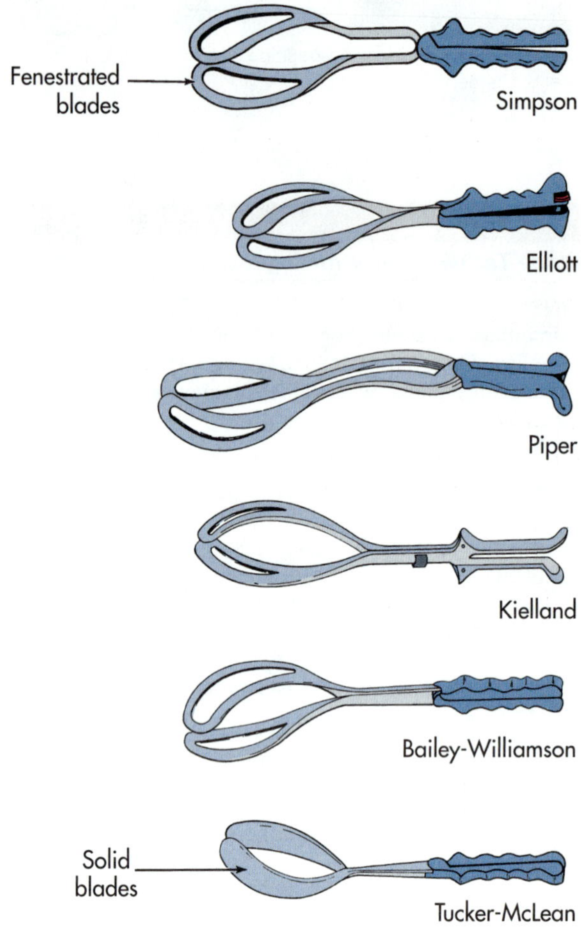

FIG. 33-8 Types of forceps. Piper forceps are used to assist delivery of the head in a breech birth.

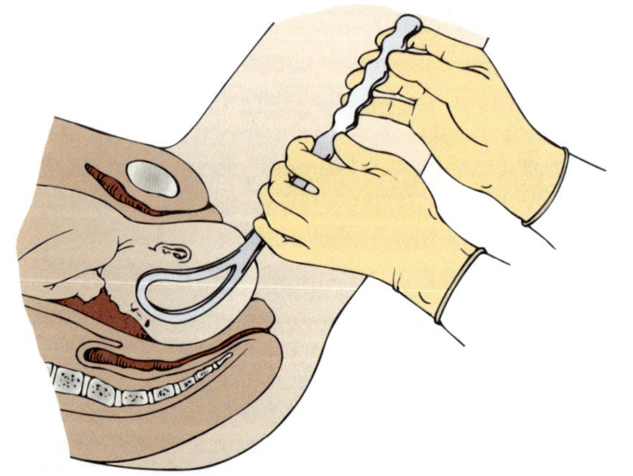

FIG. 33-9 Outlet forceps-assisted extraction of the head.

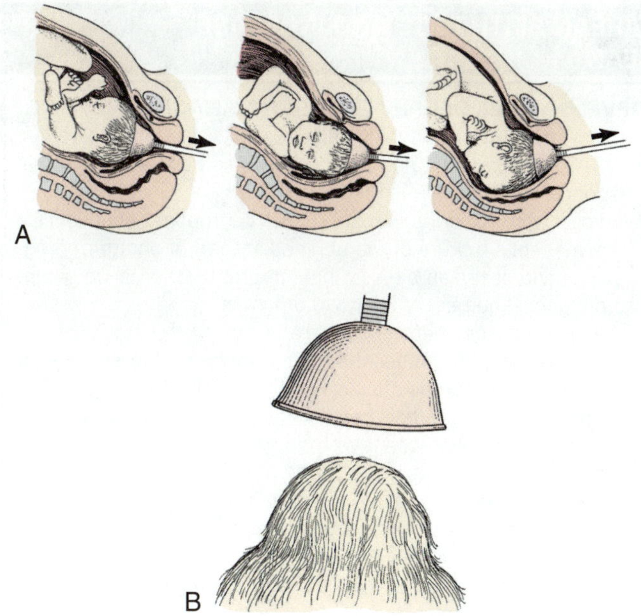

FIG. 33-10 Use of vacuum extraction to rotate fetal head and assist with descent. **A,** *Arrow* indicates direction of traction on the vacuum cup. **B,** Caput succedaneum formed by the vacuum cup.

! NURSING ALERT

Because compression of the cord between the fetal head and the forceps will cause a decrease in FHR, the FHR is assessed, reported, and recorded before and after application of the forceps.

Nursing Considerations. When a forceps-assisted birth is deemed necessary, the nurse obtains the type of forceps requested by the primary health care provider. The nurse may explain to the mother that the forceps blades fit the same way two tablespoons fit around an egg, with the blades placed in front of the baby's ears.

After birth the mother should be assessed for vaginal or cervical lacerations, urinary retention, and hematoma formation in the pelvic soft tissues, which may result from blood vessel damage. The infant should be assessed for bruising or abrasions at the site of the blade applications, facial palsy resulting from pressure of the blades on the facial nerve, and subdural hematoma. Newborn and postpartum caregivers should be told that a forceps-assisted birth was performed.

Vacuum-Assisted Birth

Vacuum-assisted birth, or vacuum extraction, is a birth method involving the attachment of a vacuum cup to the fetal head, using negative pressure to assist in the birth of the head (Fig. 33-10, *A*). It is generally not used to assist birth before 34 weeks of gestation. Indications for its use are the same as those for outlet forceps. Prerequisites for use include a completely dilated cervix, ruptured membranes, engaged head, vertex presentation, and no suspicion of CPD (Cunningham et al., 2010). There are several types of vacuum-assisted births, defined primarily by the station and position of the fetal head in relation to the maternal pelvis (see Table 33-4) (AAP & ACOG, 2007). Advantages of vacuum-assisted compared with forceps-assisted birth are the ease with which the vacuum can be placed and the need for less anesthesia. Also it is far easier to learn the skills necessary to safely use the vacuum than to gain a similar level of skill with forceps (Thorp, 2009).

BOX 33-9 ASSISTING WITH BIRTH BY VACUUM EXTRACTION

- Assess the fetal heart rate frequently during the procedure.
- Encourage the woman to push during contractions.
- If responsible for generating pressure for the vacuum, do not exceed the "green zone" indicated on the pump. Verify with the physician the amount of pressure to be generated.
- Document the number of pulls attempted, the maximum pressure used, and any pop-offs that occur.

Management. The vacuum cup is applied to the fetal head by the physician. There are basically two types of vacuum devices in use. One is a self-contained unit, which allows the physician to both position the cup on the baby's head and generate the desired amount of negative pressure to create a vacuum. When the other type of vacuum device is used, the physician applies the cup to the baby's head, after which the nurse connects the suction tubing attached to the cup to wall suction or a separate hand pump and generates the amount of pressure requested by the physician. With both devices, a caput develops inside the cup as the pressure is initiated (see Fig. 33-10, *B*). The woman is encouraged to push as traction is applied by the physician. The vacuum cup is released and removed after birth of the head. If vacuum extraction is not successful, a forceps-assisted or cesarean birth is usually performed.

Risks to the newborn include cephalhematoma, scalp lacerations, and subdural hematoma. Fetal complications can be reduced by strict adherence to the manufacturer's recommendations for method of application, amount of pressure to be generated, and duration of application. Maternal risks include perineal, vaginal, or cervical lacerations and soft-tissue hematomas.

Nursing Considerations. The nurse's role for the woman who has a vacuum-assisted birth is primarily one of support person and educator. The nurse can prepare the woman for birth and encourage her to remain active in the birth process by pushing during contractions. The fetal heart rate should be assessed frequently during the procedure. Documentation of the procedure in the medical record is important and is often the nurse's responsibility (Box 33-9). Neonatal caregivers should be told that the birth was vacuum assisted. After birth, the newborn must be observed for signs of trauma and infection at the application site and for cerebral irritation (e.g., poor sucking or listlessness). The newborn may also be at risk for hyperbilirubinemia and neonatal jaundice as bruising resolves. The parents may need to be reassured that the caput succedaneum usually disappears in 3 to 5 days (see Fig. 33-10, *B*) (Gilbert, 2011).

Cesarean Birth

Cesarean birth is the birth of a fetus through a transabdominal incision of the uterus. Whether cesarean birth is planned (scheduled) or unplanned, the loss of the experience of giving birth to a child in the traditional manner may have a negative effect on a woman's self-concept. An effort is therefore made to

BOX 33-10 SELECTED MEASURES TO REDUCE THE CESAREAN BIRTH RATE AND INCREASE THE RATE OF VAGINAL BIRTH AFTER CESAREAN

EDUCATE WOMEN REGARDING:
- Advantages and safety of the home environment for early or latent labor
- Indicators for hospital admission
- Management techniques to use during labor to enhance progress
- Nonpharmacologic measures to reduce pain and discomfort and enhance relaxation
- Safety and effectiveness of TOL and VBAC

ESTABLISH ADMISSION CRITERIA FOR WOMEN IN LABOR THAT:
- Distinguish clinical manifestations for false labor, latent (early) labor, and active labor.
- Conduct admission assessments in a separate admissions area.
- Send women in false or latent (early) labor home or keep them in the admissions area.
- Admit women in active labor to the labor and birth unit.

USE APPROPRIATE ASSESSMENT TECHNIQUES TO:
- Determine the status of the maternal-fetal unit.
- Establish an individualized rationale for initiating labor interventions such as epidural anesthesia, induction or augmentation, amniotomy, or cesarean birth.

INITIATE A DOULA PROGRAM THAT:
- Provides early, continuous one-to-one support for women in labor and for their partners

DEVELOP A PHILOSOPHY OF LABOR MANAGEMENT THAT:
- Supports admission during active labor
- Uses measures that promote, support, and encourage normal spontaneous labor
- Avoids automatic interventions such as routine induction for spontaneous rupture of membranes at term or postterm pregnancy and cesarean birth for breech presentation, twin gestation, genital herpes, or failure to progress
- Relies on assessment findings reflective of the status of the maternal-fetal unit rather than strict adherence to set ranges for the duration of the stages and phases of labor
- Uses intermittent rather than continuous electronic fetal monitoring of low risk pregnant women
- Focuses on measures that are known to enhance the progress of labor such as one-to-one support, ambulation, upright positions, maternal position changes, oral nutrition and hydration, and nonpharmacologic pain relief
- Uses nonpharmacologic measures in a manner that reduces their labor-inhibiting effects
- Establishes criteria for elective cesarean birth and TOL
- Encourages women who have had previous cesarean birth to participate in TOL to attempt a vaginal birth

TOL, Trial of labor; *VBAC,* vaginal birth after cesarean.

maintain the focus on the birth of the baby rather than on the operative procedure.

The purpose of cesarean birth is to preserve the life or health of the mother and her fetus. It may be the best choice for birth when evidence exists of maternal or fetal complications. Since the advent of modern surgical methods and care and the use of antibiotics, maternal and fetal morbidity and mortality have decreased. In addition, incisions are usually made into the lower uterine segment rather than in the muscular body of the uterus, thus promoting more effective healing. However, despite these advances, cesarean birth still poses threats to the health of the mother and infant.

The incidence of cesarean births has escalated to 32.3% of live births in 2008, the highest rate ever reported in the United States (Hamilton et al., 2010). Part of the reason for this rise is that a number of common risk factors for cesarean birth are increasing in frequency, especially in developed countries. These factors include fetal macrosomia, advanced maternal age, obesity, gestational diabetes, and multifetal pregnancy (Thorp, 2009). Malpractice concerns are another factor related to the elevated incidence, along with an increase in the number of cesareans done on maternal request, estimated to be 2.5% of all births in the United States (ACOG, 2007; Landon, 2007). An international estimate of the elective cesarean birth rate is much higher compared with the United States, between 4% and 18% (Collard, Diallo, Habinsky, Hentschell, & Vezeau, 2008, 2009).

As women age, the likelihood of their having a cesarean birth increases. The rationale for this increase may be related to biologic and medical factors, maternal and physician concerns, and the increased rate of multifetal pregnancies (Martin et al., 2009).

Approaches for managing labor and birth to reduce the rate of cesarean births while increasing the rate of VBAC are presented in Box 33-10. These approaches involve the combined efforts of health care professionals and pregnant women and their families. The type of nursing care given also may influence the rate of cesarean births. A labor management approach that uses one-to-one support and emphasizes ambulation, maternal position changes, relaxation measures, oral fluids and nutrition, hydrotherapy, and nonpharmacologic pain relief supports the physiologic progression of labor, reduces the incidence of dystocia, and increases the likelihood of a spontaneous vaginal birth (Albers, 2007; Hodnett, Gates, Hofmeyr, & Sakala, 2007). Several studies have found that the labor management approach that most consistently reduces cesarean birth rates is continuous, one-on-one, early-onset support of the laboring woman provided by another woman (e.g., doula, relative, friend, nurse, or nurse-midwife). The greatest reduction in risk for cesarean birth as well as a reduction in the use of epidural analgesia occurs when this woman is a doula, whose role is to spend all of her time providing physical and emotional support to the woman and providing emotional support and encouragement to the woman's partner (Berghella, Baxter, & Chauhan, 2008; Hodnett et al.; McGrath & Kennell, 2008).

Despite these efforts, the rate of cesarean birth is rising and the VBAC rate is decreasing. This decline may be due to reports of VBAC risks including rupture of the uterus, legal pressures, conservative practice guidelines, and debate regarding the relative benefits and risks of repeat cesarean birth versus vaginal birth. The declining trend in VBACs indicates that once a woman has a cesarean birth it is highly (92%) likely that her subsequent births will also be cesarean (Martin et al., 2009).

BOX 33-11 INDICATIONS FOR CESAREAN BIRTH

MATERNAL
- Specific cardiac disease (Marfan syndrome, unstable coronary artery disease)
- Specific respiratory disease (Guillain-Barré syndrome)
- Conditions associated with increased intracranial pressure
- Mechanical obstruction of the lower uterine segment (tumors, fibroids)
- Mechanical vulvar obstruction (condylomata)
- History of previous cesarean birth

FETAL
- Abnormal (nonreassuring) FHR or pattern
- Malpresentation (e.g., breech or transverse lie)
- Active maternal herpes lesions
- Maternal human immunodeficiency virus with a viral load of more than 1000 copies/ml
- Congenital anomalies

MATERNAL-FETAL
- Dysfunctional labor (cephalopelvic disproportion, "failure to progress" in labor)
- Placental abruption
- Placenta previa
- Elective cesarean birth

Sources: Duff, P., Sweet, R., & Edwards, R. (2009). Maternal and fetal infections. In R. Creasy, R. Resnik, J. Iams, C. Lockwood, & T. Moore (Eds.), *Creasy and Resnik's maternal-fetal medicine: Principles and practice* (6th ed.). Philadelphia: Saunders; Landon, M. (2007). Cesarean delivery. In S. Gabbe, J. Niebyl, & J. Simpson (Eds.), *Obstetrics: Normal and problem pregnancies* (5th ed.). Philadelphia: Churchill Livingstone; Thorp, J. (2009). Clinical aspects of normal and abnormal labor. In R. Creasy, R. Resnik, J. Iams, C. Lockwood, & T. Moore (Eds.), *Creasy and Resnik's maternal-fetal medicine: Principles and practice* (6th ed.). Philadelphia: Saunders.

Indications

Few absolute indications exist for cesarean birth. Today most are performed for conditions that might pose a threat to both the mother and the fetus if vaginal birth occurred, such as placenta previa or placental abruption (Landon, 2007). Box 33-11 lists common indications for cesarean birth.

Elective Cesarean Birth

Elective cesarean birth, sometimes referred to as cesarean on request or cesarean on demand, refers to a primary cesarean birth without medical or obstetric indication. Reasons given for elective cesarean birth include fear of the pain of childbirth and the mistaken belief that the surgery will prevent future problems with pelvic support, bladder and bowel incontinence, or sexual dysfunction. Although some nulliparous women may fear the pain of labor because of no firsthand experience, multiparous women may request a cesarean birth after a previous traumatic vaginal birth (Gardner, 2003). Other women desire an elective cesarean birth because of the convenience of planning a date, or having control and choice about when to give birth (Williams, 2005). At this time evidence is insufficient to recommend elective cesarean birth to prevent urinary or fecal incontinence later in life (Collard et al., 2008, 2009; Roberts & Mangan, 2009; Thorp, 2009).

Only limited data are available comparing cesarean births on request with planned vaginal births (ACOG, 2007). In a committee opinion (2007), the ACOG lists potential risks of cesarean birth on request that include a longer hospital stay for the woman, an increased risk of respiratory problems for the baby, and greater complications in subsequent pregnancies, including uterine rupture and placental implantation problems. The ACOG recommends that cesarean birth on request not be performed unless a gestational age of 39 weeks has been accurately determined. The ACOG does not recommend cesarean birth on request for women who desire additional children, because the risks for placenta previa, placenta accreta, and cesarean hysterectomy increase with each cesarean birth (ACOG, 2007). The Society of Obstetricians and Gynaecologists of Canada (SOGC) promotes natural childbirth. The organization does not promote elective cesarean birth but believes that the final decision as to the safest route of childbirth rests with the woman and her health care provider (SOGC, 2004).

CLINICAL REASONING

The Woman Seeking Elective Cesarean Birth

You are a nurse-midwife working at an active obstetric practice. Catherine, a primigravida at 20 weeks of gestation, arrives for her prenatal appointment. During the updating history she tells you that she is thinking about asking the obstetrician to schedule an elective cesarean birth once she reaches 38 weeks of gestation. She explains that she read an article in a magazine about how more women are choosing cesarean births to preserve their vaginas for satisfying sexual activity and to prevent problems with organs falling out and incontinence when they get older. Catherine adds that her friend had a scheduled cesarean when she had her first baby, and although there was pain after surgery, it was nothing like what her friend imagined labor pain would be like. Catherine asks the nurse-midwife if this is a good plan and one that would be safe for her and her baby because she and her partner want to have at least two more children over the next 5 years. She states, "I have always been very healthy and have not had any problems with my pregnancy so far—so a cesarean should be a breeze and I will know exactly when my baby will be born." What should the nurse discuss with Catherine to help her make an informed decision regarding how to manage her childbirth experience?

1. Evidence—Is there sufficient evidence regarding the benefits and risks of elective cesarean birth compared with a planned vaginal birth?
2. Assumptions—What assumptions can be made about the following issues related to childbirth?
   a. The effect of cesarean birth on plans for future pregnancies
   b. Ability of cesarean birth to preserve vaginal integrity and muscle support for pelvic organs
   c. Advantage of an approach that promotes normal birth for both the mother and her baby
3. If Catherine chooses this approach for her childbirth, what is the nursing priority in teaching her what she can anticipate with regard to her care before, during, and after her surgery as compared to what she could expect with a planned vaginal birth?
4. Does the evidence support your description of what to expect regarding each type of birth?
5. Are there alternative perspectives to your conclusion?

Spanish Guidelines—Cesarean Brith

Forced Cesarean Birth

A woman's refusal to undergo cesarean birth when indicated for fetal reasons is often described as a *maternal-fetal conflict.* Health care providers are ethically obliged to protect the well-being of both mother and fetus; a decision for one affects the other. If a woman refuses a cesarean birth that is recommended because of fetal jeopardy, health care providers must make every effort to find out why she is refusing and provide information that may persuade her to change her mind. If the woman continues to refuse surgery, then health care providers must decide if it is ethical to get a court order for the surgery. Every effort, however, should be made to avoid this legal step.

Surgical Techniques

The skin incision will either be vertical, extending from near the umbilicus to the mons pubis or transverse (Pfannenstiel) in the lower abdomen (Fig. 33-11). The transverse incision, sometimes referred to as the "bikini" incision, is performed more often. The type of skin incision is generally determined by the urgency of the surgery and the presence of any prior skin incisions (Landon, 2007). The type of skin incision does *not* necessarily indicate the type of uterine incision.

The two main types of uterine incision are the low transverse (Fig. 33-12, *A*) or vertical incision which may be either low or classic (see Fig. 33-12, *B* and *C*). Ideally the vertical incision is contained entirely within the lower uterine segment, but extension into the contractile portion of the uterus (e.g., a classic incision) is common (Landon, 2007). Indications for a vertical incision include an underdeveloped lower uterine segment, a transverse lie or preterm breech presentation, certain fetal anomalies such as massive hydrocephalus, and an anterior placenta previa (Landon). Because it is associated with a higher incidence of uterine rupture in subsequent pregnancies than is lower-segment cesarean birth, vaginal birth after a classic uterine incision is contraindicated.

The low transverse uterine incision is performed in more than 90% of cesarean births (see Fig. 33-12, *A*). Compared with the vertical incision, the transverse incision is preferred because it does not compromise the upper uterine segment, is easier to perform and repair, and is associated with less blood loss. It is also less likely to rupture in subsequent pregnancies (Landon, 2007).

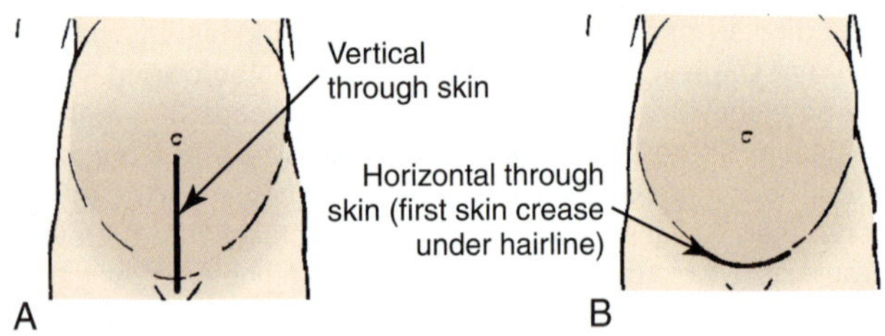

FIG. 33-11 Skin incisions for cesarean birth. **A,** Vertical. **B,** Horizontal (Pfannenstiel).

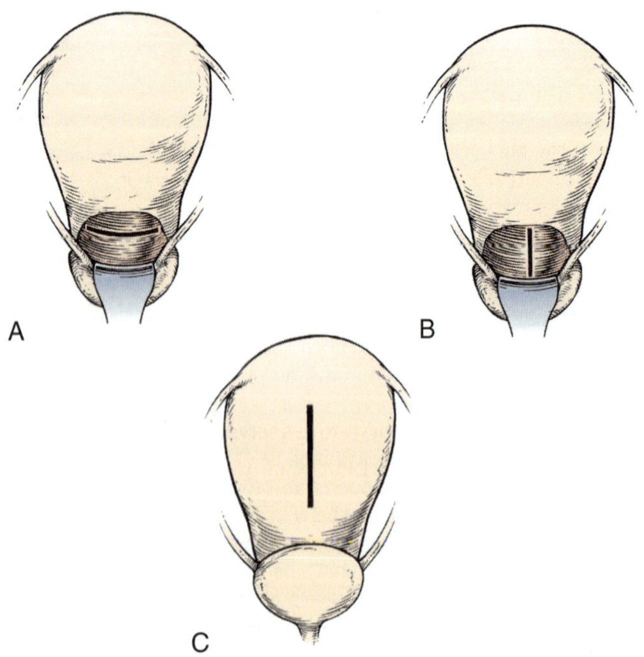

FIG. 33-12 Uterine incisions for cesarean birth. **A,** Low transverse incision. **B,** Low vertical incision. **C,** Classic incision, (From Gabbe, S., Niebyl, J., & Simpson, J. [2007]. *Obstetrics: Normal and problem pregnancies* [5th ed.]. Philadelphia: Churchill Livingstone.)

Complications and Risks

Possible maternal complications related to cesarean birth include aspiration, hemorrhage, atelectasis, endometritis, abdominal wound dehiscence or infection, urinary tract infection, injuries to the bladder or bowel, and complications related to anesthesia (Thorp, 2009). The fetus may be born prematurely if the gestational age has not been accurately determined. Fetal asphyxia can occur if the uterus and placenta are poorly perfused as a result of maternal hypotension caused by regional anesthesia (epidural or spinal) or maternal positioning. Fetal injuries (e.g., injuries caused by the scalpel) can also occur during the surgery. The newborn is more likely to require resuscitation efforts and develop respiratory complications (Roberts & Mangan, 2009; Thorp). In addition to these risks, the woman is at economic risk because the cost of cesarean birth is higher than that of vaginal birth, and a longer recovery period may require additional expenditures.

Anesthesia

Spinal, epidural, and general anesthetics are used for cesarean births. Epidural blocks are popular because women want to be awake for and aware of the birth experience. However, the choice of anesthetic depends on several factors. The mother's medical history or present condition, such as a spinal injury, hemorrhage, or coagulopathy, may rule out the use of regional anesthesia. Time is another factor, especially if there is an emergency and the life of the mother or infant is at stake. In an emergency, general anesthesia will most likely be used unless the woman already has an epidural block in effect. The woman herself is a factor. Either she may not know all the options or may have fears about having "a needle in her back" or about being awake and feeling pain. She needs to be fully informed about the risks and benefits of the different types of anesthesia so that she can participate in the decision whenever there is a choice.

Scheduled Cesarean Birth

Cesarean birth is scheduled or planned if labor and vaginal birth are contraindicated (e.g., complete placenta previa, active genital herpes, positive HIV status with a high viral load), if birth is necessary but labor is not inducible (e.g., hypertensive states that cause a poor intrauterine environment that threatens the fetus), or if this course of action has been chosen by the primary health care provider and the woman (e.g., a repeat cesarean birth).

Women who are scheduled for a cesarean birth have time to prepare for it psychologically. However, the psychologic responses of these women may differ. Those having a repeat cesarean birth may have disturbing memories of the conditions preceding the initial (primary) cesarean birth and of their experiences in the postoperative recovery period. They may be concerned about the added burdens of caring for the infant and perhaps other children while recovering from surgery. Others may feel glad that they have been relieved of the uncertainty about the date and time of the birth and are free of the pain of labor.

Unplanned Cesarean Birth

The psychosocial outcomes of unplanned or emergency cesarean birth are usually more pronounced and negative when compared with the outcomes associated with a scheduled or planned cesarean birth. Women and their families experience abrupt changes in their expectations for birth, postpartum care, and the care of the new baby at home. This may be an extremely traumatic experience for all.

The woman may approach the procedure tired and discouraged after an ineffective and difficult labor. Fear predominates as she worries about her own safety and well-being and that of her fetus. She may be dehydrated, with low glycogen reserves. Because preoperative procedures must be done rapidly, there is often little time for explanation of the procedures and the operation itself. Because maternal and family anxiety levels are high at this time, much of what is said may be forgotten or misunderstood. The woman may experience feelings of anger or guilt in the postpartum period. Fatigue is often noticeable in these women, and they need much supportive care.

After surgery, counseling strategies that have been implemented by nurses include providing women with opportunities to talk about their birth experience, express feelings about what happened, have their questions answered, address gaps in knowledge or understanding of events, connect the event with emotions and behavior, and talk about future pregnancies. More research is needed to determine how effective these strategies are for these women in influencing their views about the unplanned cesarean birth experience or on future pregnancies (Gamble & Creedy, 2004).

Prenatal Preparation

A discussion of cesarean birth should be included in all childbirth preparation classes. No woman can be guaranteed a vaginal birth, even if she is in good health and no indication of danger to the fetus exists before the onset of labor. Therefore, every woman needs to be aware of and prepared for the possibility of having a cesarean birth.

Childbirth educators should emphasize the similarities and differences between a cesarean and a vaginal birth. In support of the philosophy of family-centered birth, many hospitals have instituted policies that permit fathers and other partners and family members to share in these births as they do in vaginal births. Women who have undergone cesarean birth agree that the continued presence and support of their partners helped them respond more positively to the entire experience. In addition to preparing women for the possibility of cesarean birth, childbirth educators should empower them to believe in their ability to give birth vaginally and to seek care measures during labor that will enhance the progress of their labors and reduce their risk for cesarean birth.

Preoperative Care

Family-centered care is the goal for the woman who is to undergo cesarean birth and for her family. The preparation of the woman for cesarean birth is the same as that for other elective or emergency surgery. The primary health care provider discusses, with the woman and her family, the need for the cesarean birth and the prognosis for the mother and infant. A member of the anesthesia care team assesses the woman's cardiopulmonary status and describes the options for anesthesia. Women who are scheduled for an elective cesarean are often told to remain NPO (nothing by mouth) for at least 8 hours prior to the surgery (Roberts & Mangan, 2009). Informed consent is obtained for the procedure.

Blood tests are usually done a day or two before a planned cesarean birth or on admission to the labor and birth unit. Laboratory tests commonly ordered include a complete blood cell count and blood type and Rh status. Maternal vital signs and FHR and pattern are assessed according to hospital protocol until the operation begins. Intravenous fluids are started to maintain hydration and to provide an open line for the administration of blood or medications if needed. Other preoperative preparations include making sure that an informed consent form has been signed, inserting a retention (Foley) catheter to keep the bladder empty, and administering prescribed preoperative medications. In addition to medications given to prevent aspiration pneumonia, women may also receive prophylactic antibiotics to prevent postoperative infection. In the rare instance that an abdominal-mons shave or a clipping of pubic hair is ordered by the primary health care provider, it is performed in the operating room just prior to making the incision because shaving can result in injury of the integument thereby increasing the risk for infection. Often, TED hose and SCD boots will be placed on the woman's legs to prevent blood clot formation. Removal of contact lenses, dentures, nail polish, and jewelry may be optional, depending on hospital policies and the type of anesthesia used. If the woman wears glasses and is going to be awake, the nurse should make sure her glasses accompany her to the operating room so she can see her infant.

During the preoperative preparation, the support person is encouraged to remain with the woman as much as possible to provide continuing emotional support (if this action is culturally acceptable to the woman and support person). The nurse provides essential information about the preoperative procedures during this time. Although the nursing actions may be carried out quickly if a cesarean birth is unplanned, verbal communication, particularly explanations, is important. Silence can be frightening to the woman and her support person. The nurse's use of touch (if culturally appropriate) can communicate feelings of care and concern for the woman. The nurse can assess the woman's and her partner's perceptions about cesarean birth. As the woman expresses her feelings, the nurse may identify a potential for a disturbance in self-concept during the postpartum period that would need to be addressed. If there is time before the birth, the nurse can teach the woman about

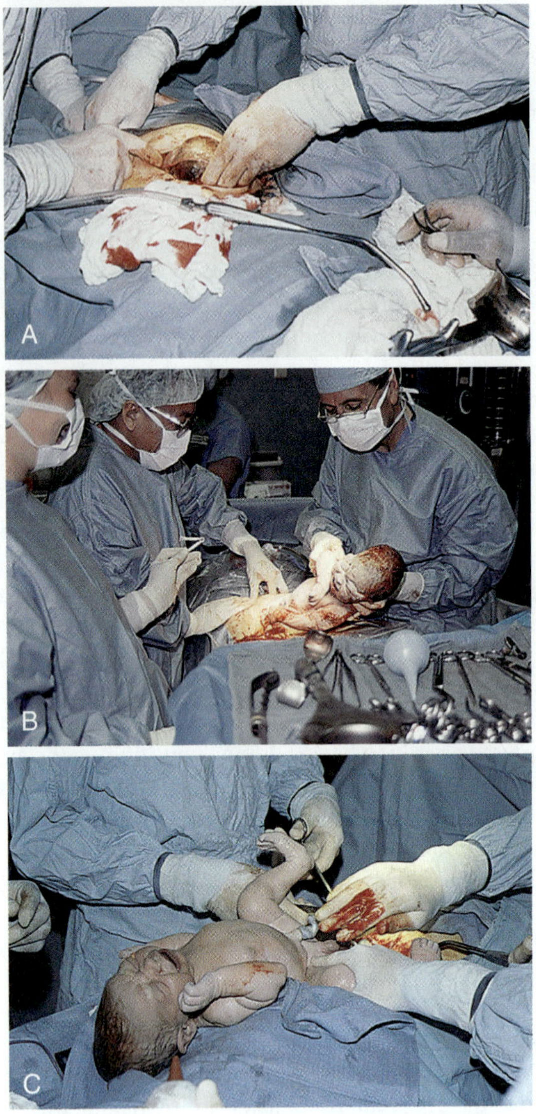

FIG. 33-13 Cesarean birth. **A,** "Bikini" incision has been made, the muscle layer is separated, the abdomen is entered, and the uterus has been exposed and incised; suctioning of amniotic fluid continues as head is brought up through the incision. Note small amount of bleeding. **B,** The neonate's birth through the uterine incision is nearly complete. **C,** A quick assessment is performed; note extreme molding of head resulting from cephalopelvic disproportion. (Courtesy Marjorie Pyle, RNC, Lifecircle, Costa Mesa, CA.)

postoperative expectations and about pain relief, turning, leg exercises, coughing, and deep-breathing measures.

Intraoperative Care

Cesarean births occur in operating rooms in the surgical suite or in the labor and birth unit. Staff members from the labor and birth unit may scrub and circulate during the surgery or these functions may be assumed by members of the hospital's surgery staff (Fig. 33-13). If possible, the partner, who is dressed appropriately for the operating room, accompanies the mother to the operating room and remains close to her for continued comfort and support. In unplanned cesarean birth, the nurse who cared for the woman during labor should be part of the nursing care team in the operating room if possible.

Video—Childbirth: Cesarean

The nurse who is circulating may assist with positioning the woman on the birth (operating) table. It is important to position her so that the uterus is displaced laterally to prevent compression of the inferior vena cava, which causes decreased placental perfusion. This is usually accomplished by placing a wedge under the hip or tilting the table to one side. The woman's legs should be strapped to the table to ensure proper positioning during the surgery. A retention (Foley) catheter is inserted into the bladder at this time if one is not already in place.

If the partner is not allowed or chooses not to be present, the nurse can stay in communication with him or her and give progress reports whenever possible. If the woman is awake during the birth, the nurse, anesthesia care provider, or both can tell her what is happening and provide support. She may be anxious about the sensations she is experiencing, such as the coldness of solutions used to cleanse the abdomen and pressure or pulling during the actual birth of the infant. She also may be apprehensive because of the bright lights or the presence of unfamiliar equipment and masked and gowned personnel in the room. Explanations can help to decrease the woman's anxiety.

A nurse from the labor and birth unit usually is present to provide care for the infant. In addition, a pediatrician or a nurse team skilled in neonatal resuscitation may also be present for the surgery because these infants are considered to be at risk until evidence of physiologic stability exists after the birth. A crib with resuscitation equipment is readied before surgery. Personnel who are responsible for care are expert not only in resuscitative techniques, but also in their ability to detect normal and abnormal infant responses (AAP & American Heart Association [AHA], 2006). After birth, if the infant's condition permits and the mother is awake, the baby can be placed skin-to-skin on the mother or can be given to the woman's partner to hold (Fig. 33-14). The infant whose condition is compromised is transported after initial stabilization to the nursery for observation and the implementation of appropriate interventions. In some institutions, the partner may accompany the infant; if not, personnel keep the family informed of the infant's progress and parent-infant contacts are initiated as soon as possible.

If family members cannot accompany the woman during surgery, they are directed to the surgical or obstetric waiting room. The physician then reports on the condition of the mother and infant to the family members after the birth is completed. Family members may be allowed to accompany the infant as she or he is transferred to the nursery, giving them an opportunity to see and admire the new baby.

LEGAL TIP: Disclosure of Client Information

Some mothers or fathers want the privilege of informing family and friends of the gender of the infant (if it was not known before birth) or other information about the birth. Before responding to requests for such information from people waiting outside the birthing area, the nurse should check to see if the mother has given consent for such information to be released and to whom.

Immediate Postoperative Care

Once surgery is completed, the mother is transferred to a post-anesthesia recovery area. After a cesarean birth, women have postoperative and postpartum needs that must be addressed. They are surgical clients as well as new mothers. Nursing assessments in this immediate postbirth period follow agency protocol and include degree of recovery from the effects of anesthesia,

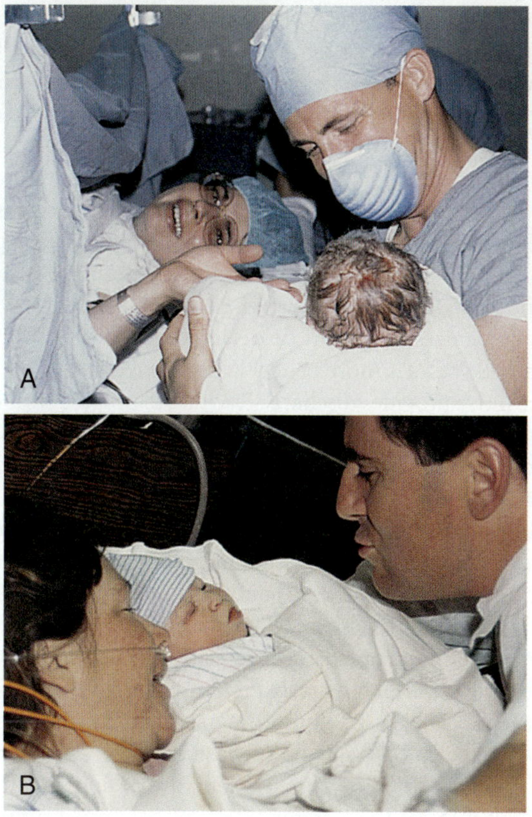

FIG. 33-14 **A,** Parents and their newborn. The physician manually removes the placenta, suctions the remaining amniotic fluid and blood from the uterine cavity, and closes the uterine incision, peritoneum, muscle layer, fatty tissue, and finally the skin, while the new family shares some time together. **B,** Parents become better acquainted with their newborn while mother rests after surgery. (Courtesy Marjorie Pyle, RNC, Lifecircle, Costa Mesa, CA.)

postoperative and postbirth status, and degree of pain. A patent airway is maintained, and the woman is positioned to prevent possible aspiration. Vital signs are taken every 15 minutes for 1 to 2 hours, or until stable. The condition of the incisional dressing and the fundus and the amount of lochia are assessed, as well as the intravenous intake and the urine output through the retention (Foley) catheter. Oxytocin usually is added to at least the first liter of the intravenous infusion to ensure that the fundus remains firmly contracted, thereby reducing blood loss (Roberts & Mangan, 2009). The woman is helped to turn and do coughing, deep-breathing, and leg exercises. Medications for pain relief should be administered before postoperative pain becomes severe.

If the baby is present, the mother and her partner are given some time alone with him or her to facilitate bonding and attachment. Breastfeeding can be initiated if the mother feels like trying. The woman is ready for discharge from the postanesthesia recovery area once her condition is stable and the effects of anesthesia have worn off (i.e., she is alert and oriented and able to feel and move her extremities).

Postoperative or Postpartum Care

The attitude of the nurse and other health care team members can influence the woman's perception of herself after a cesarean birth. The caregivers should stress that the woman is a new mother first and a surgical client second. This attitude helps the woman perceive herself as having the same problems and needs as other new mothers, while requiring supportive postoperative care.

The woman's physiologic concerns may be dominated by pain at the incision site and pain resulting from intestinal gas. For the first 24 hours following surgery, pain relief may be provided by epidural opioids, patient-controlled analgesia (PCA) or intravenous or intramuscular injections. The most commonly used analgesics include opioids (e.g., hydromorphone, morphine, nalbuphine) and NSAIDs (e.g., ketorolac [Toradol]). If opioids are used, an antiemetic (e.g., metoclopramide [Reglan]) is often administered either as needed by the woman or around the clock as long as the opioid is used. Palpation of the fundus with the possibility of massage should be performed after an analgesic is given to decrease pain (Roberts & Mangan, 2009). By 24 hours after surgery, women are generally changed to oral analgesics. Other comfort measures such as position changes, splinting of the incision with pillows, and relaxation and breathing techniques (e.g., those learned in childbirth classes) may be implemented (see the Teaching for Self-Management box: Postpartum Pain Relief After Cesarean Birth).

TEACHING FOR SELF-MANAGEMENT

Postpartum Pain Relief After Cesarean Birth

INCISIONAL

- Splint incision with a pillow when moving or coughing.
- Use relaxation techniques such as music, breathing, and dim lights.

GAS

- Walk as often as you can.
- Do not eat or drink gas-forming foods, carbonated beverages, or whole milk.
- Do not use straws for drinking fluids.
- Take antiflatulence medication if prescribed.
- Lie on your left side to expel gas.
- Rock in a rocking chair.

Women are often the best judges of what their bodies need and can tolerate, including the postoperative ingestion of foods and fluids. Some health care providers keep women NPO or allow only "sips and chips" (sips of clear fluids and teaspoons of crushed ice) until bowel sounds return. The diet is then advanced to full liquids. After women are passing flatus they can resume a regular diet (Gilbert, 2011). Because most women have an epidural or spinal anesthetic for surgery, most health care providers allow the early introduction of solid food if desired and tolerated. Women who eat early have been found to require less analgesia, and gastrointestinal problems do not occur (Abrams, Minassian, & Pickett, 2004). Intravenous fluids are usually continued until the woman is tolerating fluids orally. Ambulation and rocking in a rocking chair may relieve gas pains. Avoid gas-forming foods, ice chips, carbonated beverages, and using a straw to drink beverages to help limit gas formation, thereby minimizing the severity of gas pains (see the Teaching for Self-Management box: Postpartum Pain Relief After Cesarean Birth).

Nurses must be alert to a woman's physiologic needs, managing care to ensure adequate rest and pain relief. Mother-baby care (couplet care) for a cesarean birth mother may have to be modified according to her physical limitations as a surgical client.

Daily care includes perineal care, breast care, and routine hygienic care. The woman may shower after the original incisional dressing is removed, usually on the first postoperative day (if showering is acceptable according to the woman's cultural beliefs and practices). The indwelling (Foley) catheter usually is also removed on the first postpartum day. The woman is encouraged to be out of bed and ambulating several times each day as soon as the urinary catheter is removed. The nurse assesses the woman's vital signs, incision, fundus, and lochia according to hospital policies, procedures, or protocols. Breath sounds, bowel sounds, circulatory status of lower extremities, and urinary and bowel elimination patterns also are assessed. It is important to observe maternal emotional status and progress of attachment to her baby.

SAFETY ALERT

When getting out of bed, the woman should be taught to seek assistance initially especially when an intravenous line and catheter are still in place. Thereafter, when rising from a supine position, she should sit on the side of the bed first to determine if dizziness will occur, then stand at the bedside, and finally ambulate.

During the postpartum period, the nurse also can provide care that meets the psychologic and teaching needs of women who have had cesarean births. The nurse can explain postpartum procedures to help the woman participate in her recovery from surgery. The nurse can also help the woman plan care and visits from family and friends that will allow adequate rest periods. Providing information on and assistance with infant care can facilitate adjustment to her role as a mother. With adequate support, these women can benefit from mother-baby care to facilitate attachment and enhance involvement in newborn care. The woman is supported as she breastfeeds her baby by receiving individualized assistance to comfortably hold and position the baby at her breast. Use of the side-lying or football hold positions and supporting the newborn with pillows can enhance comfort and facilitate successful breastfeeding. The partner can be included in infant teaching sessions, and in explanations about the woman's recovery (Simpson, 2008).

SAFETY ALERT

When holding her baby or breastfeeding, a woman may become drowsy and even fall asleep because of the sedation that occurs with the use of analgesics. It is important that someone be with her during these times.

The couple also should be encouraged to express their feelings about the birth experience. Some parents are angry, frustrated, or disappointed that a vaginal birth was not possible. Some women express feelings of low self-esteem or a negative self-image. Others express relief and gratitude that the baby is healthy and safely born. It may be helpful for them to have the nurse who was present during the birth visit and help fill in "gaps" about the experience. Other psychologic and lifestyle concerns that have been reported include depression, feeling limited in activities, and changes in family interactions (Gamble & Creedy, 2004; Roberts & Mangan, 2009).

Discharge after cesarean birth is usually by the third postoperative day. The time is often determined by criteria established by the woman's insurance carrier or the federal government (e.g., diagnosis-related groups [DRGs]). The Newborn's and Mother's Health Protection Act of 1996 provides for a length of stay of up to 96 hours for cesarean births. These criteria may not coincide with the woman's physical or psychosocial readiness for discharge. Some states have added home care provisions for mothers who meet appropriate criteria for discharge and choose to leave sooner than the allowed length of stay. This policy recognizes that home care is less costly than hospital care and in most cases is more beneficial for recovery.

The nurse provides discharge teaching to prepare women for self-care and newborn care in a limited amount of time while still trying to ensure that the woman is comfortable and able to rest. The nurse must assess the woman's information needs and coordinate the health care team's efforts to meet them. Discharge teaching and planning should include information about nutrition; measures to relieve pain and discomfort; exercise and specific activity restrictions; time management that includes periods of uninterrupted rest and sleep; hygiene, breast, and incision care; timing for resumption of sexual activity and contraception; signs of complications (see the Teaching for Self-Management box: Signs of Postoperative Complications After Discharge Following Cesarean Birth); and infant care. The nurse assesses the woman's need for continued support or counseling to facilitate her emotional recovery from the birth. The woman's family and friends should be educated regarding her needs during the recovery process, and their assistance should be coordinated before discharge. Referral to support groups (e.g., www.birthrites.org) or to community agencies may be indicated to further promote the recovery process. A postdischarge program of telephone follow-up and home visits can facilitate the woman's full recovery after cesarean birth.

TEACHING FOR SELF-MANAGEMENT

Signs of Postoperative Complications After Discharge Following Cesarean Birth

Report the following signs to your health care provider:

- Temperature exceeding 38° C (100.4° F)
- Urination: dysuria, urgency, cloudy urine
- Lochia: heavier than a normal menstrual period, clots, odor
- Cesarean incision: redness, swelling, bruising, foul smelling discharge or bleeding, wound separation
- Severe, increasing abdominal pain

Trial of Labor

A **trial of labor (TOL)** is the observance of a woman and her fetus for a reasonable period (e.g., 4 to 6 hours) of spontaneous active labor to assess the safety of vaginal birth for the mother and infant. It may be initiated if the mother's pelvis is of questionable size or shape or if the fetus is in an abnormal presentation or position. By far the most common reason for a TOL is if the woman wishes to have a vaginal birth after a previous cesarean birth. A woman who has had a previous cesarean birth with a low transverse uterine incision may be a candidate for a TOL. Fetal sonography, maternal pelvimetry, or both may be done before a TOL to rule out CPD. During a TOL, the woman

BOX 33-12 SELECTION CRITERIA FOR VAGINAL BIRTH AFTER CESAREAN

- One previous low-transverse cesarean birth
- Clinically adequate pelvis
- No other uterine scars or history of previous rupture
- Physician immediately available throughout active labor who is capable of monitoring labor and performing an emergency cesarean birth if necessary
- Availability of anesthesia and personnel for emergency cesarean birth

Source: American College of Obstetricians and Gynecologists (ACOG). (2004). *Vaginal birth after a previous cesarean delivery. ACOG Practice Bulletin No. 54.* Washington, DC: ACOG.

is evaluated for active labor, including adequate contractions, engagement and descent of the presenting part, and effacement and dilation of the cervix.

The nurse assesses maternal vital signs and FHR and pattern and is alert for signs of potential complications. If complications develop, the nurse is responsible for initiating appropriate actions, including notifying the primary health care provider, and for evaluating and documenting the maternal and fetal responses to the interventions. Nurses must recognize that the woman and her partner are often anxious about her health and well-being and that of their baby. Supporting and encouraging the woman and her partner and providing information regarding progress can reduce stress and enhance the labor process and facilitate a successful outcome.

Vaginal Birth After Cesarean

Indications for primary cesarean birth, such as dysfunctional labor, breech presentation, or fetal distress, often are nonrecurring. Therefore, a woman who has had one cesarean birth with a low transverse incision may subsequently become pregnant, experience no contraindications to labor and vaginal birth during the pregnancy, and choose to attempt a VBAC. Box 33-12 lists selection criteria suggested by the ACOG for identifying candidates for VBAC. The overall success rate is approximately 70% to 80% (Landon, 2007). Benefits of VBAC include a shorter maternal hospital stay, less blood loss, fewer infections, and fewer thromboembolic events than with cesarean birth. Risks associated with VBAC include uterine rupture, hysterectomy, operative injury, and neonatal morbidity (ACOG, 2004).

Spontaneous labor with a ripe cervix is more likely to result in a successful VBAC than is labor that has been induced or augmented (ACOG, 2004). Induction or augmentation with oxytocin or prostaglandins increases the risk for uterine rupture, a major concern when a VBAC is attempted. If uterine stimulation is needed, oxytocin is the drug of choice because the risk for rupture is lower (Simpson, 2008). Women most likely to have a successful VBAC are those who are less than 35 years of age, whose fetus weighs less than 4000 g, and whose previous cesarean was performed for some reason other than failure of descent in second stage labor (Thorp, 2009).

Women are most often the primary decision makers with regard to choice of birth method. During the antepartal period, the woman should be given information about VBAC and encouraged to choose it as an alternative to repeat cesarean birth, as long as no contraindications exist. VBAC support groups (e.g., www.vbac.com) and prenatal classes can help prepare the woman psychologically for labor and vaginal birth. Women need to believe not only that their efforts during a TOL will be successful but also that they are fully capable of doing what is necessary to give birth vaginally. They must be given the opportunity to discuss their previous labor experience, including feelings of failure and loss of control, and to express concern they may have about how they will manage during their upcoming labor and birth. Not everyone is enthusiastic about TOL and VBAC. After being fully informed about the benefits and risks, more than 25% of potential candidates choose to have a repeat cesarean birth instead (Thorp, 2009).

If a woman chooses TOL, attention should be paid to her psychologic as well as physical needs during the TOL. Anxiety increases the release of catecholamines and can inhibit the release of oxytocin, thus delaying the progress of labor and possibly leading to a repeat cesarean birth. To alleviate such anxiety, the nurse can encourage the woman to use breathing and relaxation techniques and to change positions to promote labor progress. The woman's partner can be encouraged to provide comfort measures and emotional support. Collaboration among the woman in labor, her partner, the nurse, and other health care providers often results in a successful VBAC. If a TOL does not result in vaginal birth, the woman will need support and encouragement to express her feelings about having another cesarean birth. It is very important that this outcome not be labeled a failed VBAC.

Since 1996, VBAC rates have been decreasing, with the current rate being less than 10%. Both medical and nonmedical factors have contributed to this decline. In March 2010, the Eunice Kennedy Shriver National Institute of Child Health and Human Development and the NIH convened a consensus development conference to examine issues related to VBAC. The statement produced by the panel of experts affirmed that TOL is a reasonable option for many women who have had a previous cesarean birth (NIH, 2010a, 2010b).

The experts found, however, that many women who are appropriate candidates for TOL and VBAC do not have access to providers and health care facilities that are able and willing to offer this option. Two surveys of hospital administrators found that 30% of hospitals stopped offering VBAC because they could not meet all the prerequisites specified by ACOG (see Box 33-12). In addition, an ACOG member survey revealed that 30% of respondents stopped offering TOL and performing VBAC because of liability concerns. In order to remove some of the barriers to VBAC, the panel recommended that the VBAC guidelines published by professional associations be reevaluated, malpractice concerns be addressed, and additional research undertaken to better understand the medical and nonmedical factors that influence decision making for women who have had previous cesarean births (NIH, 2010a, 2010b).

POSTTERM PREGNANCY, LABOR, AND BIRTH

A **postterm pregnancy** (also sometimes referred to as a *postdate* or *prolonged pregnancy*) is one that extends beyond the end of week 42 of gestation, or 294 days from the first day of the last menstrual period (LMP). The incidence of postterm pregnancy is estimated to be between 4% and 14% (Resnik & Resnik, 2009). Many pregnancies are misdiagnosed as prolonged. The use of first-trimester ultrasound for pregnancy dating has confirmed that the first day of the LMP, traditionally used for pregnancy dating, is much less reliable as a predictor of true gestational age. Therefore, use of the LMP alone for pregnancy dating tends to greatly overestimate the number of postterm gestations (Divon, 2007; Resnik & Resnik).

The exact cause of true postterm pregnancy is still unknown. However, it is clear that the timing of labor is determined by complex interactions among the fetus, the placenta and membranes, the uterine myometrium, and the cervix. For example, congenital primary fetal adrenal hypoplasia and placental sulfatase deficiency cause low estrogen production. Low levels of estrogen may result in a decrease in prostaglandin precursors, thereby preventing normal cervical ripening, reducing the formation of oxytocin receptors in the myometrium, and delaying the onset of labor. Although postterm pregnancy is more common in primiparous women, a woman who experiences one postterm pregnancy is more likely to experience it again in subsequent pregnancies (Divon, 2007; Resnik & Resnik, 2009).

Clinical manifestations of postterm pregnancy include maternal weight loss (more than 3 lb/wk) and decreased uterine size (related to decreased amniotic fluid), meconium in the amniotic fluid, and advanced bone maturation of the fetal skeleton with an exceptionally hard fetal skull (Gilbert, 2011).

Maternal and Fetal Risks

Maternal risks are often related to dysfunctional labor, such as increased risk for perineal injury related to fetal macrosomia. Risk for hemorrhage and infection is higher. Interventions such as induction of labor with prostaglandins or oxytocin, forceps- or vacuum-assisted birth, and cesarean birth are more likely to be necessary. Each of these interventions, of course, carries its own set of risks. The woman also may experience fatigue, physical discomfort, and psychologic reactions such as depression, frustration, and feelings of inadequacy as she passes her estimated date of birth. Relationships with close friends and family members may become strained and the woman's negative feelings about herself may be projected as feelings of resentment toward the fetus (Gilbert, 2011).

Another complication associated with postterm pregnancy is abnormal fetal growth. Although the risk of having a small for gestational age infant is increased, only 10% to 20% of postterm fetuses are undernourished. Macrosomia (birth weight more than 4000 g) occurs far more often. Macrosomia occurs when the placenta continues to provide adequate nutrients to support fetal growth after 40 weeks of gestation. Macrosomic infants have an increased risk for birth injuries caused by difficult forceps-assisted births and shoulder dystocia (Resnik & Resnik, 2009).

Other fetal risks associated with postterm gestation are related to the intrauterine environment. After 43 to 44 weeks of gestation, the placenta begins to age. Enlarging areas of infarction and increased deposition of calcium and fibrin in its tissue decrease the placenta's reserve and may affect its ability to oxygenate the fetus. Decreased amniotic fluid (less than 400 ml), oligohydramnios, is the complication most frequently associated with postterm pregnancy. Because of the decreased amount of amniotic fluid, there is a potential for cord compression and resulting hypoxemia (Gilbert, 2011). Other potential complications include meconium-stained amniotic fluid, increased chance of meconium aspiration, and low Apgar scores. Oligohydramnios magnifies the effect of meconium staining. Having less than the normal amount of amniotic fluid available to dilute it makes the meconium thicker and stickier than it would otherwise be (Resnik & Resnik, 2009).

Postmaturity syndrome occurs in about 20% of neonates born following postterm pregnancies. Postmaturity syndrome is characterized by dry, cracked, peeling skin; long nails; meconium staining of skin, nails, and umbilical cord; and perhaps loss of subcutaneous fat and muscle mass (Gilbert, 2011).

CARE MANAGEMENT

The management of postterm pregnancy is still controversial. However, because perinatal morbidity and mortality increase greatly after 42 weeks of gestation, pregnancies are usually not allowed to continue after this time. In the United States, most physicians induce labor at 41 weeks of gestation. An alternative approach is to initiate twice-weekly fetal testing at 41 weeks of gestation. The testing generally consists of either a BPP or NST along with an assessment of amniotic fluid volume (see Chapter 26 for discussion of these tests). Evidence is insufficient to determine which of the two management approaches is better (Resnik & Resnik, 2009).

TEACHING FOR SELF-MANAGEMENT

Postterm Pregnancy

- Perform daily fetal movement counts.
- Assess for signs of labor.
- Call your primary health care provider if your membranes rupture or if you notice a decrease in or no fetal movement.
- Keep appointments for fetal assessment tests and cervical checks.
- Go to the hospital soon after labor begins.

During the postterm period, the woman is encouraged to assess fetal activity daily, assess for signs of labor, and keep appointments with her primary health care provider (see the Teaching for Self-Management box: Postterm Pregnancy). The woman and her family should be encouraged to express their feelings (e.g., frustration, anger, impatience, fear) about the prolonged pregnancy and helped to realize that these feelings are normal. At times the emotional and physical strain of a postterm pregnancy may seem overwhelming. Referral to a support group or another supportive resource may be needed.

During labor the fetus of a woman with a postterm pregnancy should be continuously monitored electronically for a more accurate assessment of the FHR and pattern. Inadequate fluid volume can lead to compression of the umbilical cord, which results in fetal hypoxia that is reflected in variable or prolonged deceleration patterns. If oligohydramnios is present, an amnioinfusion may be performed to restore amniotic fluid volume to maintain a cushioning of the cord. See Chapter 18 for additional information on amnioinfusion.

OBSTETRIC EMERGENCIES

Meconium-stained Amniotic Fluid

Meconium-stained amniotic fluid indicates that the fetus has passed meconium (first stool) before birth. Meconium-stained amniotic fluid is green. The consistency of the meconium fluid is often described as either thin (light) or thick (heavy), depending on the amount of meconium present. Three possible reasons for the passage of meconium are as follows: (1) it is a normal physiologic function that occurs with maturity (meconium passage being infrequent before weeks 23 or 24, with an increased incidence after 38 weeks) or with a breech presentation; (2) it is the result of hypoxia-induced peristalsis and sphincter relaxation; or (3) it may be a sequel to umbilical cord compression–induced vagal stimulation in mature fetuses.

The major risk associated with meconium-stained amniotic fluid is the development of meconium aspiration syndrome (MAS) in the newborn. MAS causes a severe form of aspiration pneumonia that occurs most often in term or postterm infants who have passed meconium in utero. MAS most likely results from a long-standing intrauterine process, rather than from aspiration immediately following birth as respirations are initiated (Rosenberg, 2007).

CARE MANAGEMENT

The presence of a team skilled in neonatal resuscitation is required at the birth of any infant with meconium-stained amniotic fluid. When meconium-stained amniotic fluid is present, the AAP and the AHA Neonatal Resuscitation Program no longer recommends routine suctioning of the newborn's mouth and nose on the perineum (after the head is out but before the rest of the baby is born) followed by endotracheal suctioning after birth. Instead, management of a newborn with meconium-stained amniotic fluid is based only on assessment of the baby's condition at birth. No clinical studies warrant basing tracheal suctioning guidelines simply on meconium consistency (AAP & AHA, 2006). See the Emergency box: Immediate Management of the Newborn with Meconium-Stained Amniotic Fluid for specific interventions.

EMERGENCY

Immediate Management of the Newborn with Meconium-Stained Amniotic Fluid

PRIOR TO BIRTH

- Assess the amniotic fluid for the presence of meconium after rupture of membranes.
- If the amniotic fluid is meconium stained, gather equipment and supplies before the birth that might be necessary for neonatal resuscitation.
- Have at least one person capable of performing endotracheal intubation on the baby present at the birth.

IMMEDIATELY AFTER BIRTH

- Assess the baby's respiratory efforts, heart rate, and muscle tone.
- Suction only the baby's mouth and nose, using either a bulb syringe or a 12- or 14-French suction catheter if the baby has:
    - Strong respiratory efforts
    - Good muscle tone
    - Heart rate >100 beats/min
- Suction below the vocal cords using an endotracheal tube to remove any meconium present before many spontaneous respirations have occurred or assisted ventilation has been initiated if the baby has:
    - Depressed respirations
    - Decreased muscle tone
    - Heart rate <100 beats/min

Source: American Academy of Pediatrics (AAP) & American Heart Association (AHA). (2006). *Textbook of neonatal resuscitation* (5th ed.). Elk Grove Village, IL: AAP; Dallas, TX: AHA.

! NURSING ALERT

Every birth should be attended by at least one person whose only responsibility is the baby and who is capable of initiating resuscitation. Either that person or someone else who is immediately available should have the skills required to perform a complete resuscitation, including endotracheal suctioning to remove meconium, if necessary.

Animation—Shoulder Dystocia

Shoulder Dystocia

Shoulder dystocia is an uncommon obstetric emergency that increases the risk for fetal and maternal morbidity and mortality during the attempt to accomplish birth vaginally. It is estimated that 0.6% to 1.4% of all vaginal births are complicated by shoulder dystocia (Cunningham et al., 2010). Shoulder dystocia is a condition in which the head is born, but the anterior shoulder cannot pass under the pubic arch. The incidence of shoulder dystocia has increased in recent years, perhaps because of larger birth weights or simply because more attention is now paid to documenting the condition (Cunningham et al.).

Fetopelvic disproportion related to excessive fetal size (more than 4000 g) or maternal pelvic abnormalities may be a cause of shoulder dystocia, although up to half of all cases of shoulder dystocia occur with smaller fetuses (Lanni & Seeds, 2007; Thorp, 2009). Other risk factors for shoulder dystocia include maternal diabetes (risk for macrosomia) and a history of shoulder dystocia with a previous birth. In half of all cases of shoulder dystocia, however, no risk factors are identified (Thorp). Shoulder dystocia cannot be accurately predicted or prevented (Cunningham et al., 2010). Signs that could indicate the presence of shoulder dystocia include slowing of the progress of the second stage of labor and formation of a caput succedaneum that increases in size. The nurse should observe for retraction of the fetal head against the perineum immediately following its emergence (turtle sign), an early sign of shoulder dystocia. External rotation does not occur (Jevitt, 2005; Thorp).

Fetal injuries are usually caused either by asphyxia related to the delay in completing the birth or to trauma from the maneuvers used to accomplish the birth. Complications related to trauma include brachial plexus and phrenic nerve injuries and fracture of the humerus or clavicle. The most serious complication is brachial plexus injury (Erb palsy), which occurs in 10% to 20% of infants born following shoulder dystocia. If brachial plexus injuries are recognized early and treated properly, 80% to 90% heal completely. Therefore, permanent neurologic injury is rare. The major maternal complications associated with shoulder dystocia are postpartum hemorrhage and rectal injuries (Thorp, 2009).

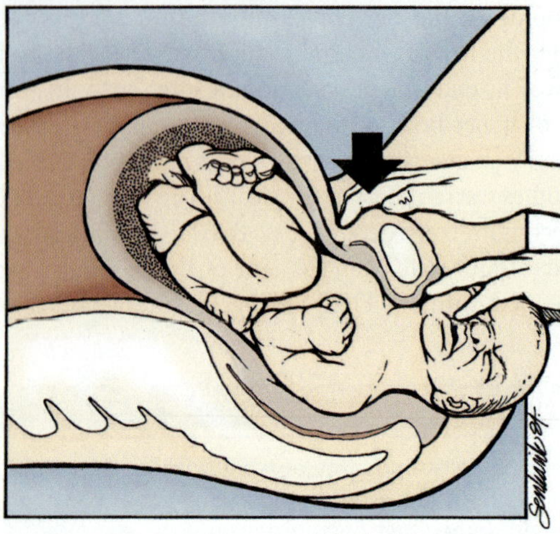

FIG. 33-15 Application of suprapubic pressure (From Gabbe, S., Niebyl, J., & Simpson, J. [2007]. *Obstetrics: Normal and problem pregnancies* [5th ed.]. Philadelphia: Churchill Livingstone).

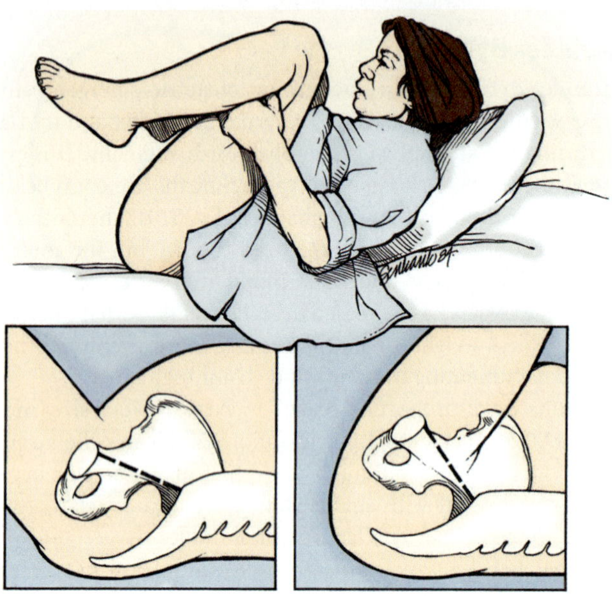

FIG. 33-16 McRoberts maneuver. (From Gabbe, S., Niebyl, J., & Simpson, J. [2007]. *Obstetrics: Normal and problem pregnancies* [5th ed.]. Philadelphia: Churchill Livingstone.)

CARE MANAGEMENT

Many maneuvers such as suprapubic pressure and maternal position changes have been suggested and tried to free the anterior shoulder, although no particular maneuver has been found to be most effective. Suprapubic pressure can be applied to the anterior shoulder (Fig. 33-15) in an attempt to push the shoulder under the symphysis pubis (Lanni & Seeds, 2007).

In the McRoberts maneuver (Fig. 33-16), the woman's legs are flexed apart, with her knees on her abdomen (Lanni & Seeds, 2007). This maneuver causes the sacrum to straighten, and the symphysis pubis to rotate toward the mother's head. The angle of pelvic inclination is decreased, which frees the shoulder. Suprapubic pressure can be applied at this time. The McRoberts maneuver is the preferred method when a woman is receiving epidural anesthesia.

Animation—Cord Prolapse

Having the woman move to a hands-and-knees position (the Gaskin maneuver), a squatting position, or lateral recumbent position also has been used to resolve cases of shoulder dystocia (Jevitt, 2005). However, the Gaskin maneuver requires that the woman be mobile, with no significant loss of motor function caused by regional anesthesia. Additionally, a wide and stable surface must be available (Lanni & Seeds, 2007).

Fundal pressure as a method of relieving shoulder dystocia should be avoided. Its use has been associated with neurologic complications (Gilbert, 2011).

When shoulder dystocia is diagnosed, the nurse should stay calm and immediately call for additional assistance (i.e., extra nurses, anesthesia care provider, and neonatal resuscitation team). The nurse then helps the woman assume the position or positions that may facilitate birth of the shoulders, assists the primary health care provider with these maneuvers and techniques during birth, and documents the maneuvers. The nurse also provides encouragement and support to reduce anxiety and fear.

Newborn assessment should include examination for fracture of the clavicle or humerus as well as brachial plexus injuries and asphyxia (Thorp, 2009). Maternal assessment should focus on early detection of hemorrhage and trauma to the vagina, perineum, and rectum.

Prolapsed Umbilical Cord

Prolapse of the umbilical cord occurs when the cord lies below the presenting part of the fetus. Umbilical cord prolapse may be occult (hidden, rather than visible) at any time during labor whether or not the membranes are ruptured (Fig. 33-17, *A* and *B*). It is most common to see frank (visible) prolapse directly after rupture of membranes, when gravity washes the cord in front of the presenting part (see Fig. 33-17, *C* and *D*). Contributing factors include a long cord (longer than 100 cm), malpresentation (breech or transverse lie), or an unengaged presenting part.

If the presenting part does not fit snugly into the lower uterine segment (e.g., as in hydramnios), when the membranes rupture, a sudden gush of amniotic fluid may cause the cord to be displaced downward. Similarly the cord may prolapse during amniotomy if the presenting part is high. A small fetus may not fit snugly into the lower uterine segment; as a result, cord prolapse is more likely to occur.

CARE MANAGEMENT

Prompt recognition of a prolapsed umbilical cord is important because fetal hypoxia resulting from prolonged cord compression (i.e., occlusion of blood flow to and from the fetus for more than 5 minutes) usually results in central nervous system damage or death of the fetus. Pressure on the cord may be relieved by the examiner putting a sterile gloved hand into the vagina and holding the presenting part off the umbilical cord (Fig. 33-18, *A* and *B*). The woman may also be assisted into a position such as a modified Sims (see Fig. 33-18, *C*), Trendelenburg, or knee-chest (see Fig. 33-18, *D*) position, in which gravity keeps the pressure of the presenting part off the cord. If the cervix is fully dilated, a forceps- or vacuum-assisted birth can be performed for the fetus in a cephalic presentation; otherwise, a cesarean birth is likely to be performed. Abnormal (nonreassuring) FHR and pattern (e.g., bradycardia, absent or minimal variability, and variable or prolonged decelerations), inadequate uterine relaxation, and bleeding also can occur as a result of a

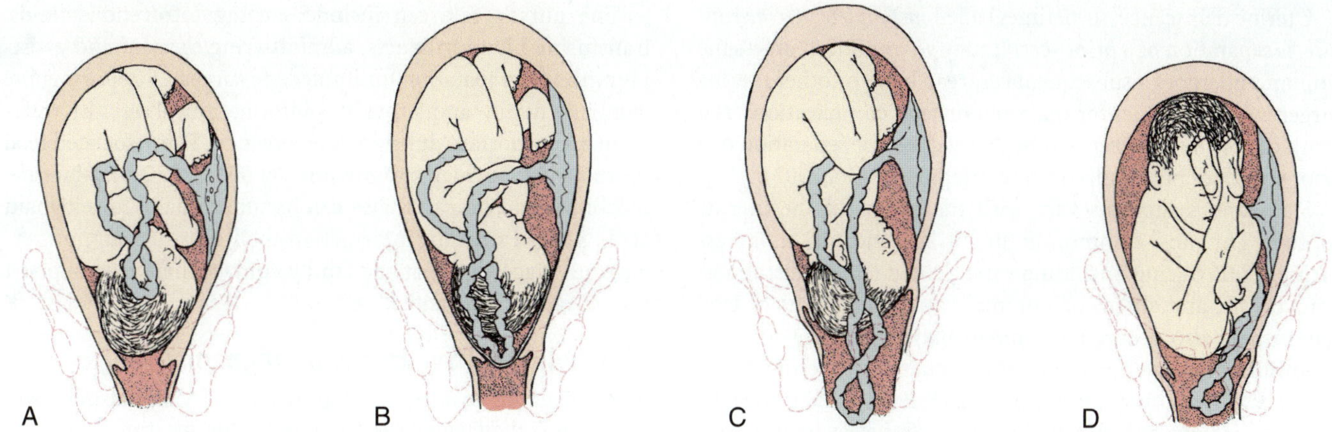

FIG. 33-17 Prolapse of umbilical cord. Note pressure of presenting part on umbilical cord, which endangers fetal circulation. **A,** Occult (hidden) prolapse of cord. **B,** Complete prolapse of cord. Note that membranes are intact. **C,** Cord presenting in front of the fetal head may be seen in vagina. **D,** Frank breech presentation with prolapsed cord.

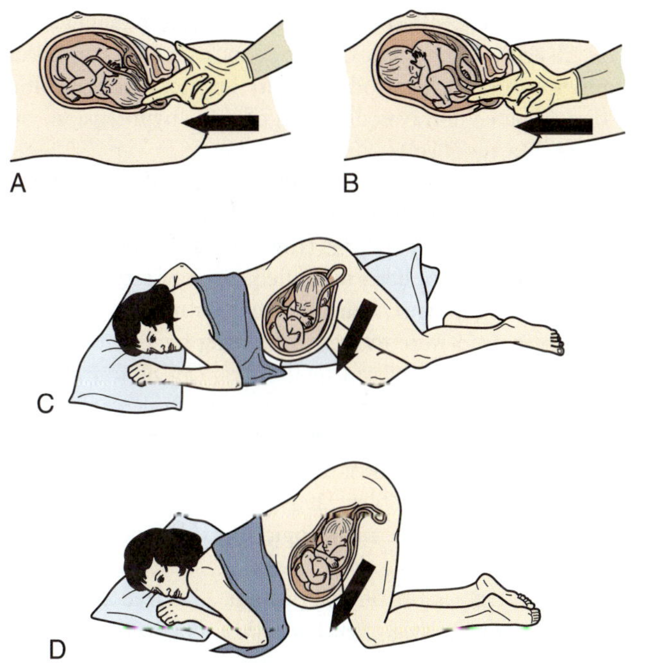

FIG. 33-18 *Arrows* indicate direction of pressure against presenting part to relieve compression of prolapsed umbilical cord. Pressure exerted by examiner's fingers in **A,** vertex presentation, and **B,** breech presentation. **C,** Gravity relieves pressure when woman is in modified Sims position with hips elevated as high as possible with pillows. **D,** Knee-chest position.

EMERGENCY

Prolapsed Umbilical Cord

SIGNS

- Variable or prolonged deceleration during uterine contractions
- Woman reports feeling the cord after membranes rupture.
- Cord is seen or felt in or protruding from the vagina.

INTERVENTIONS

- Call for assistance. Do not leave woman alone.
- Have someone notify the primary health care provider immediately.
- Glove the examining hand quickly and insert two fingers into the vagina to the cervix. With one finger on either side of the cord or both fingers to one side, exert upward pressure against the presenting part to relieve compression of the cord (see Fig. 33-18, *A* and *B*). Do not move your hand! Another person may place a rolled towel under the woman's right or left hip.
- Place woman into the extreme Trendelenburg or a modified Sims position (see Fig. 33-18, *C*), or a knee-chest position (see Fig. 33-18, *D*).
- If cord is protruding from vagina, wrap loosely in a sterile towel saturated with warm sterile normal saline solution. Do not attempt to replace cord into cervix.
- Administer oxygen to the woman by nonrebreather mask at 8 to 10 L/min until birth is accomplished.
- Start intravenous (IV) fluids or increase existing drip rate.
- Continue to monitor fetal heart rate (FHR) continuously, by internal fetal scalp electrode, if possible.
- Explain to woman and support person what is happening and the way it is being managed.
- Prepare for immediate vaginal birth if cervix is fully dilated, or cesarean birth if it is not.

prolapsed umbilical cord. Indications for immediate interventions are presented in the Emergency box: Prolapsed Umbilical Cord. Ongoing assessment of the woman and her fetus is critical to determine the effectiveness of each action taken. The woman and her family are often aware of the seriousness of the situation; therefore, the nurse must provide support by giving explanations for the interventions being implemented and their effect on the status of the fetus.

Rupture of the Uterus

Rupture of the uterus, in which there is complete nonsurgical disruption of all uterine layers, is a rare but very serious obstetric injury that occurs in 1 in 2000 births (Francois & Foley, 2007; Landon, 2007). During labor and birth the major risk factor for uterine rupture is a TOL for attempted VBAC. Other risk factors include labor induction, multiple prior cesarean births or other types of uterine surgery, multiparity, and trauma (Francois & Foley). The likelihood of uterine rupture depends on both the type and location of the previous uterine scar. Uterine rupture occurs most often with a previous classic incision (Landon).

Uterine dehiscence, sometimes called *incomplete uterine rupture,* is separation of a prior scar. It may go unnoticed unless the woman undergoes a subsequent cesarean birth or other uterine surgery. The potential for maternal or fetal complications as a result of uterine dehiscence is negligible because separation of a prior scar does not result in hemorrhage (Landon, 2007).

Signs and symptoms vary with the extent of the uterine rupture. The most common finding is an abnormal (nonreassuring) FHR tracing, including variable and late decelerations, bradycardia, and absent or minimal variability. A loss of fetal station may also occur. The woman may experience constant abdominal pain, uterine tenderness, a change in uterine shape, and cessation of contractions (Francois & Foley, 2007). She may also exhibit signs of hypovolemic shock caused by hemorrhage (i.e., hypotension, tachypnea, pallor, and cool, clammy skin). If the placenta separates, the FHR will be absent. Fetal parts may be palpable through the abdomen.

CARE MANAGEMENT

Prevention is the best treatment. Women who have had a classic cesarean birth are advised not to labor or attempt vaginal birth in subsequent pregnancies. Those at risk for uterine rupture are assessed closely during labor. Women whose labor is induced with oxytocin or prostaglandin (especially if their previous birth was cesarean) are monitored for signs of uterine tachysystole because this can precipitate uterine rupture. If tachysystole occurs, the oxytocin infusion is discontinued or decreased, and a tocolytic medication may be given to decrease the intensity of the uterine contractions (see the Emergency box: Uterine Tachysystole with Oxytocin). After giving birth, the woman is assessed for excessive bleeding, especially if the fundus is firm and signs of hemorrhagic shock are present.

If rupture occurs, management depends on the severity. A small rupture may be managed with a laparotomy and birth of the infant, repair of the laceration, and blood transfusions, if needed. Hysterectomy may be necessary if the rupture is large and difficult to close or if the woman is hemodynamically unstable (Francois & Foley, 2007).

The nurse's role can include starting intravenous fluids, transfusing blood products, administering oxygen, and assisting with the preparation for immediate surgery. Supporting the woman's family and providing information about the treatment are important during this emergency. The associated fetal mortality rate is high (approximately 50% to 70%). Maternal morbidity and mortality also can be substantial (Cunningham et al., 2010). Providing information about spiritual support services or suggesting that the family contact their own support system may be warranted.

Anaphylactoid Syndrome of Pregnancy

Anaphylactoid syndrome of pregnancy (ASP), also known as *amniotic fluid embolism,* is a rare but devastating complication of pregnancy characterized by the sudden, acute onset of hypoxia, hypotension, or cardiac arrest, and coagulopathy. ASP occurs during labor, during birth, or within 30 minutes after birth. This combination of sudden respiratory and cardiovascular collapse, along with coagulopathy, is similar to that observed in clients with anaphylactic or septic shock. In both conditions, a foreign substance is introduced into the circulation, resulting in disseminated intravascular coagulation, hypotension, and hypoxia (Martin & Foley, 2009).

In ASP the foreign substance that initiates the condition is presumed to be present in amniotic fluid that is introduced into the maternal circulation. However, the exact factor that initiates ASP has not been identified. In the past, particles of fetal debris (e.g., vernix, hair, skin cells, or meconium) found in amniotic fluid were thought to be responsible for initiating the syndrome; however, fetal debris can be found in the pulmonary circulation of most normal laboring women. Also fetal debris is identified in only 78% of women diagnosed with ASP. Although ASP is rare, the mortality rate is 61% or higher (Martin & Foley, 2009). About 50% of the neonates who survive have neurologic impairment (Schoening, 2006).

Maternal risk factors for ASP include advanced age, minority race, placenta previa, preeclampsia, and forceps-assisted or cesarean birth. Other factors commonly associated with the

EMERGENCY

Anaphylactoid Syndrome of Pregnancy

SIGNS

Respiratory Distress
- Restlessness
- Dyspnea
- Cyanosis
- Pulmonary edema
- Respiratory arrest

Circulatory Collapse
- Hypotension
- Tachycardia
- Shock
- Cardiac arrest

Hemorrhage
- Coagulation failure: bleeding from incisions, venipuncture sites, trauma (lacerations); petechiae, ecchymoses, purpura
- Uterine atony

INTERVENTIONS

Oxygenate
- Administer oxygen by nonrebreather face mask (8 to 10 L/min) or resuscitation bag delivering 100% oxygen.
- Prepare for intubation and mechanical ventilation.
- Initiate or assist with cardiopulmonary resuscitation. Tilt pregnant woman 30 degrees to side to displace uterus.

Maintain Cardiac Output and Replace Fluid Losses
- Position woman onto her side.
- Administer IV fluids.
- Administer blood products: packed cells, fresh-frozen plasma.
- Insert indwelling catheter, and measure hourly urine output.
- Correct coagulation failure
- Monitor fetal and maternal status.
- Prepare for emergency birth once woman's condition is stabilized.
- Provide emotional support to woman, her partner, and family.

development of ASP are rapid labor and meconium staining (Cunningham et al., 2010).

CARE MANAGEMENT

The immediate interventions for ASP are summarized in the Emergency Box: Anaphylactoid Syndrome of Pregnancy. Care must be instituted immediately. Cardiopulmonary resuscitation is often necessary. If cardiopulmonary arrest occurs, for optimal fetal survival, a perimortem cesarean birth should be accomplished within 4 minutes (Martin & Foley, 2009). The nurse's immediate responsibility is to assist with the resuscitation efforts.

If the woman survives, she is usually moved to a critical care unit. Additional interventions will likely include replacing blood and clotting factors and maintaining adequate hydration and blood pressure. The woman is usually placed on mechanical ventilation. Invasive hemodynamic monitoring may also be required (see Chapter 31) (Martin & Foley, 2009).

Support of the woman's partner and family is needed; they will be anxious and distressed. Brief explanations of what is happening are important during the emergency and can be reinforced after the immediate crisis is over. If the woman dies, emotional support and involvement of the perinatal loss support team or other resource for grief counseling is needed. Referral to grief and loss support groups would be appropriate (see Chapter 38). The nursing staff also may need help in coping with feelings and emotions that result from a maternal death.

KEY POINTS

- Preterm labor is uterine contractions with cervical change (e.g., effacement and dilation) that occurs between 20 weeks and 37 weeks of pregnancy; preterm birth is any birth that occurs before the completion of 37 weeks of pregnancy.
- The cause of preterm labor is unknown and is assumed to be multifactorial; therefore, it is not possible to predict with certainty which women will experience preterm labor and birth.
- Because the onset of preterm labor is often insidious and can be mistaken for normal discomforts of pregnancy, nurses should teach all pregnant women how to detect the early symptoms of preterm labor and to call their primary health care provider when symptoms occur.
- Bed rest, a commonly prescribed intervention for preterm labor, has many deleterious side effects and has never been shown to decrease preterm birth rates.
- The best reason to use tocolytic therapy is to achieve sufficient time to administer glucocorticoids in an effort to accelerate fetal lung maturity and reduce the severity of respiratory complications in infants born preterm. Additionally, time is allowed for transport of the woman prior to birth to a center equipped to care for preterm infants.
- If fetal or early neonatal death is expected, the parents and members of the health care team need to discuss the situation before the birth and decide on a management plan that is acceptable to everyone.
- Vigilance for signs of infection is an essential component of the care management for women with preterm PROM.
- Dysfunctional labor results from differences in the normal relations among any of the five factors affecting labor and is characterized by differences in the pattern of progress in labor.
- Obese women are at risk for several pregnancy complications, including venous thromboembolism and cesarean birth. Even routine procedures require more time and effort to accomplish when the client is obese.
- Uterine contractility is increased by the effects of oxytocin and prostaglandin and is decreased by tocolytic agents.
- Cervical ripening using chemical or mechanical measures can increase the success of labor induction.
- Expectant parents benefit from learning about operative obstetrics (e.g., forceps-assisted, vacuum-assisted, or cesarean birth) during the prenatal period.
- The basic purpose of cesarean birth is to preserve the life or health of the mother and her fetus.
- Unless contraindicated, vaginal birth is possible after a previous cesarean birth.
- Labor management that emphasizes one-to-one support of the laboring woman by another woman (e.g., doula, nurse, nurse-midwife) can reduce the rate of cesarean birth and increase the VBAC rate.
- A postterm pregnancy poses a risk to the mother and the fetus.
- Obstetric emergencies (e.g., meconium-stained amniotic fluid, shoulder dystocia, prolapsed cord, rupture of the uterus, and anaphylactoid syndrome of pregnancy) occur rarely but require immediate intervention to preserve the health or life of the mother and fetus or newborn.

Audio Chapter Summaries Access an audio summary of these Key Points on evolve

REFERENCES

Abrams., B., Minassian, D., & Pickett, K. (2004). Maternal nutrition. In R. Creasy, R. Resnik, J. Iams, C. Lockwood, & T. Moore (Eds.), *Creasy & Resnik's maternal-fetal medicine: Principles and practice* (5th ed.). Philadelphia: Saunders.

Albers, L. (2007). The evidence for physiologic management of the active phase of the first stage of labor. *Journal of Midwifery & Women's Health, 52*(3), 207–215.

American Academy of Pediatrics (AAP) & American College of Obstetricians and Gynecologists (ACOG). (2007). *Guidelines for perinatal care* (6th ed.). Washington, DC: ACOG.

American Academy of Pediatrics (AAP) & American Heart Association (AHA). (2006). *Textbook of neonatal resuscitation* (5th ed.). Elk Grove Village, IL: AAP; Dallas, TX: AHA.

American College of Obstetricians and Gynecologists. (ACOG). (2003). *Management of preterm labor*. ACOG Practice Bulletin No. 43. Washington, DC: ACOG.

American College of Obstetricians and Gynecologists (ACOG). (2004). *Vaginal birth after a previous cesarean delivery*. ACOG Practice Bulletin No. 54. Washington, DC: ACOG.

American College of Obstetricians and Gynecologists (ACOG). (2007). *Cesarean delivery on maternal request.* ACOG Committee Opinion no. 394. Washington, DC: ACOG.

American College of Obstetricians and Gynecologists (ACOG). (2009). *Induction of labor.* ACOG Practice Bulletin No. 107. Washington, DC: ACOG.

Battista, L., & Wing, D. (2007). Abnormal labor and induction of labor. In S. Gabbe, J. Niebyl, & J. Simpson (Eds.), *Obstetrics: Normal and problem pregnancies* (5th ed.). Philadelphia: Churchill Livingstone.

Berghella, V., Baxter, J., & Chauhan, S. (2008). Evidence-based labor and delivery management. *American Journal of Obstetrics & Gynecology, 199*(5), 445–454.

Bowers, N., Curran, C., Freda, M., Krening, C., Poole, J., Slocum, J., et al. (2008). High-risk pregnancy. In K. Simpson & P. Creehan (Eds.), *AWHONN's perinatal nursing* (3rd ed.). Philadelphia: Lippincott Williams & Wilkins.

Cesario, S. (2004). Reevaluation of Friedman's labor curve: A pilot study. *Journal of Obstetric, Gynecologic and Neonatal Nursing, 33*(6), 713–722.

Cherouny, P., Federico, F., Haraden, C., Leavitt Gullo, S., & Resar, R. (2005). *Idealized design of perinatal care. IHI Innovation series white paper.* Cambridge, MA: Institute for Healthcare Improvement. Available at www.IHI.org. Accessed August 9, 2010.

Clark, S., Simpson, K., Knox, G., & Garite, T. (2009). Oxytocin: New perspectives on an old drug. *American Journal of Obstetrics and Gynecology, 200*(1), 35.e1–e6.

Cleary-Goldman, J., Chitkara, U., & Berkowitz, R. (2007). Multiple gestations. In S. Gabbe, J. Niebyl, & J. Simpson (Eds.), *Obstetrics: Normal and problem pregnancies* (5th ed.). Philadelphia: Churchill Livingstone.

Collard, T., Diallo, H., Habinsky, A., Hentschell, C., & Vezeau, T. (2008/2009). Elective cesarean section: Why women choose it and what nurses need to know. *Nursing for Women's Health, 12*(6), 480–488.

Cunningham, F., Leveno, K., Bloom, S., Hauth, J., Rouse, D., & Spong, C. (2010). *Williams obstetrics* (23rd ed.). New York: McGraw-Hill.

Divon, M. (2007). Prolonged pregnancy. In S. Gabbe, J. Niebyl, & J. Simpson (Eds.), *Obstetrics: Normal and problem pregnancies* (5th ed.). Philadelphia: Churchill Livingstone.

Duff, P. (2007). Maternal and perinatal infection—bacterial. In S. Gabbe, J. Niebyl, & J. Simpson (Eds.), *Obstetrics: Normal and problem pregnancies* (5th ed.). Philadelphia: Churchill Livingstone.

Duff, P., Sweet, R., & Edwards, R. (2009). Maternal and fetal infections. In R. Creasy, R. Resnik, J. Iams, C. Lockwood, & T. Moore (Eds.), *Creasy and Resnik's Maternal-fetal medicine: Principles and practice* (6th ed.). Philadelphia: Saunders.

Francois, K., & Foley, M. (2007). Antepartum and postpartum hemorrhage. In S. Gabbe, J. Niebyl, & J. Simpson (Eds.), *Obstetrics: Normal and problem pregnancies* (5th ed.). Philadelphia: Churchill Livingstone.

Freda, M. (2006). It's time for preconception health! *MCN The American Journal of Maternal/Child Nursing, 31*(6), 346.

Friedman, E. (1989). Normal and dysfunctional labor. In W. Cohen, D. Ackers, & E. Friedman (Eds.), *Management of labor* (2nd ed.). Rockville, MD: Aspen.

Gamble, J., & Creedy, D. (2004). Content and processes of postpartum counseling after a distressing birth experience: A review. *Birth, 31*(3), 213–218.

Gardner, P. (2003). Previous traumatic birth: An impetus for requested cesarean birth. *Journal of Perinatal and Neonatal Education, 12*(1), 1–5.

Gennaro, S., Shults, J., & Garry, D. (2008). Stress and preterm labor and birth in black women. *Journal of Obstetric, Gynecologic and Neonatal Nursing, 37*(5), 538–545.

Gennaro, S., & Hennessy, M. (2003). Physiological and psychological stress: Impact on preterm birth. *Journal of Obstetric, Gynecologic and Neonatal Nursing, 32*(5), 669–675.

Gilbert, E. (2011). *Manual of high risk pregnancy & delivery* (5th ed.). St Louis: Mosby.

Grimes, D., & Nanda, K. (2006). Magnesium sulfate tocolysis: Time to quit. *Obstetrics and Gynecology, 108*(4), 986–989.

Hamilton, B., Martin, J., & Ventura, S. (2010). Birth: Preliminary data for 2008. *National Vital Statistics Reports, 58*(16), 1–18.

Hodnett, E., Gates, S., Hofmeyr, G., & Sakala, C. (2007). Continuous support for women during childbirth (Cochrane Review). *The Cochrane Database of Systematic Reviews, 2007,* 3, CD003766.

Iams, J., & Romero, R. (2007). Preterm birth. In S. Gabbe, J. Niebyl, & J. Simpson (Eds.), *Obstetrics: Normal and problem pregnancies* (5th ed.). Philadelphia: Churchill Livingstone.

Iams, J., Romero, R., & Creasy, R. (2009). Preterm labor and birth. In R. Creasy, R. Resnik, J. Iams, C. Lockwood, & T. Moore (Eds.), *Creasy and Resnik's maternal-fetal medicine: Principles and practice* (6th ed.). Philadelphia: Saunders.

Jevitt, C. (2005). Shoulder dystocia: Etiology, common risk factors, and management. *Journal of Midwifery & Women's Health, 50*(6), 485–497.

Landon, M. (2007). Cesarean delivery. In S. Gabbe, J. Niebyl, & J. Simpson (Eds.), *Obstetrics: Normal and problem pregnancies* (5th ed.). Philadelphia: Churchill Livingstone.

Lanni, S., & Seeds, J. (2007). Malpresentations. In S. Gabbe, J. Niebyl, & J. Simpson (Eds.), *Obstetrics: Normal and problem pregnancies* (5th ed.). Philadelphia: Churchill Livingstone.

Macones, G., Hankins, G., Spong, C., Hauth, J., & Moore, T. (2008). The 2008 National Institute of Child Health and Human Development Workshop Report on Electronic Fetal Monitoring: Update on Definitions, Interpretation, and Research Guidelines. *Journal of Obstetric, Gynecologic and Neonatal Nursing, 37*(5), 510–515.

Mahlmeister, L. (2008). Best practices in perinatal care: Evidence-based management of oxytocin induction and augmentation of labor. *Journal of Perinatal and Neonatal Nursing, 22*(4), 259–263.

Malone, F., & D'Alton, M. (2009). Multiple gestation: Clinical characteristics and management. In R. Creasy, R. Resnik, J. Iams, C. Lockwood, & T. Moore (Eds.), *Creasy and Resnik's maternal-fetal medicine: Principles and practice* (6th ed.). Philadelphia: Saunders.

Maloni, J., & Damato, E. (2004). Reducing the risk for preterm birth: Evidence and implications for neonatal nurses. *Advances in Neonatal Care, 4*(3), 166–174.

Maloni, J., & Park, S. (2005). Postpartum symptoms after antepartum bedrest. *Journal of Obstetric, Gynecologic and Neonatal Nursing, 34*(2), 163–171.

Martin, S., & Foley, M. (2009). Intensive care monitoring of the critically ill pregnant patient. In R. Creasy, R. Resnik, J. Iams, C. Lockwood, & T. Moore (Eds.), *Creasy and Resnik's maternal-fetal medicine: Principles and practice* (6th ed.). Philadelphia: Saunders.

Martin, J., Hamilton, B., Sutton, P., Ventura, S., Menacker, F., Kirmeyer, S., et al. (2009). Births: Final data for 2006. *National Vital Statistics Reports, 57*(7), 1–102.

McGrath, S., & Kennell, J. (2008). A randomized controlled trial of continuous labor support for middle-class couples: Effect on cesarean delivery rates. *Birth, 35*(2), 92–97.

Meis, P., & Society for Maternal-Fetal Medicine. (2005). 17 Hydroxyprogesterone for the prevention of preterm delivery. *Obstetrics & Gynecology, 105*(5 Pt 1), 1128–1135.

Mercer, B. (2007). Premature rupture of the membranes. In S. Gabbe, J. Niebyl, & J. Simpson (Eds.), *Obstetrics: Normal and problem pregnancies* (5th ed.). Philadelphia: Churchill Livingstone.

Mercer, B. (2009a). Assessment and induction of fetal pulmonary maturity. In R. Creasy, R. Resnik, J. Iams, C. Lockwood, & T. Moore (Eds.), *Creasy and Resnik's maternal-fetal medicine: Principles and practice* (6th ed.). Philadelphia: Saunders.

Mercer, B. (2009b). Premature rupture of the membranes. In R. Creasy, R. Resnik, J. Iams, C. Lockwood, & T. Moore (Eds.), *Creasy and Resnik's maternal-fetal medicine: Principles and practice* (6th ed.). Philadelphia: Saunders.

Moleti, C. (2009). Trends and controversies in labor induction. *MCN The American Journal of Maternal/Child Nursing, 34*(1), 40–47.

National Institutes of Health (NIH). (2010a). *Panel questions "VBAC bans," advocates expanded delivery options for women.* Available at www.nih.gov/news/health/mar2010/od 10. Accessed March 26, 2010.

National Institutes of Health (NIH). (2010b). *National institutes of health consensus development conference statement: NIH consensus development conference: Vaginal birth after cesarean: New insights.* Available at www.nih.gov/2010/images/vbac/vbac_statement.htm. Accessed March 26, 2010.

Nielsen, P., Galan, H., Kilpatrick, S., & Garrison, E. (2007). Operative vaginal delivery. In S. Gabbe, J. Niebyl, & J. Simpson (Eds.), *Obstetrics: Normal and problem pregnancies* (5th ed.). Philadelphia: Churchill Livingstone.

Resnik, J., & Resnik, R. (2009). Post-term pregnancy. In R. Creasy, R. Resnik, J. Iams, C. Lockwood, & T. Moore (Eds.), *Creasy & Resnik's maternal-fetal medicine: Principles and practice* (6th ed.). Philadelphia: Saunders.

Rideout, S. (2005). Tocolytics for pre-term labor: What nurses need to know. *AWHONN Lifelines, 9*(1), 56–61.

Ridley, R. (2007). Diagnosis and intervention for occiput posterior malposition. *Journal of Obstetric, Gynecologic and Neonatal Nursing, 36*(2), 135–143.

Roberts, J., & Hanson, L. (2007). Best practices in second stage labor care: Maternal bearing down and positioning. *Journal of Midwifery & Women's Health, 52*(3), 238–245.

Roberts, C., & Mangan, S. (2009). Special delivery: Know the risks of cesarean section. *OR Nurse 2009, 3*(2), 22–30.

Romero, R., & Lockwood, C. (2009). Pathogenesis of spontaneous preterm labor. In R. Creasy, R. Resnik, J. Iams, C. Lockwood, & T. Moore (Eds.), *Creasy and Resnik's maternal-fetal medicine: Principles and practice* (6th ed.). Philadelphia: Saunders.

Rosenberg, A. (2007). The neonate. In S. Gabbe, J. Niebyl, & J. Simpson (Eds.), *Obstetrics: Normal and problem pregnancies* (5th ed.). Philadelphia: Churchill Livingstone.

Schoening, A. (2006). Amniotic fluid embolism: Historical perspectives and new possibilities. *MCN The American Journal of Maternal/Child Nursing, 31*(2), 78–83.

Simpson, K. (2008). Labor and birth. In K. Simpson, & P. Creehan (Eds.), *AWHONN's perinatal nursing* (3rd ed.). Philadephia: Lippincott Williams & Wilkins.

Simpson, K., & Knox, G. (2009). Oxytocin as a high-alert medication: Implications for perinatal patient safety. *MCN The American Journal of Maternal/Child Nursing, 34*(1), 8–15.

Society of Obstetricians and Gynaecologists of Canada (SOGC). (2004). News. C-sections on demand—SOGC's position. *Birth, 31*(2), 154.

Stremler, R., Hodnett, E., Petryshen, P., Stevens, B., Weston, J., & Willan, A. (2005). Randomized controlled trial of hands-and-knees positioning for occipitoposterior position in labor. *Birth, 32*(4), 243–251.

Thorp, J. (2009). Clinical aspects of normal and abnormal labor. In R. Creasy, R. Resnik, J. Iams, C. Lockwood, & T. Moore (Eds.), *Creasy and Resnik's maternal-fetal medicine: Principles and practice* (6th ed.). Philadelphia: Saunders.

Walters, M., & Taylor, J. (2009/2010). Maternal obesity: Consequences and prevention strategies. *Nursing for Women's Health, 13*(6), 486–494.

Wener, M., & Lavigne, S. (2004). Can periodontal disease lead to premature delivery? *AWHONN Lifelines, 8*(5), 422–431.

Williams, D. (2005). The top 10 reasons elective cesarean section should be on the decline. *AWHONN Lifelines, 9*(1), 23–24.

Wilson, B. (2007). Assessing the effects of age, gestation, socioeconomic status, and ethnicity on labor inductions. *Journal of Nursing Scholarship, 39*(3), 208–213.

CHAPTER

34

Postpartum Complications

Deitra Leonard Lowdermilk

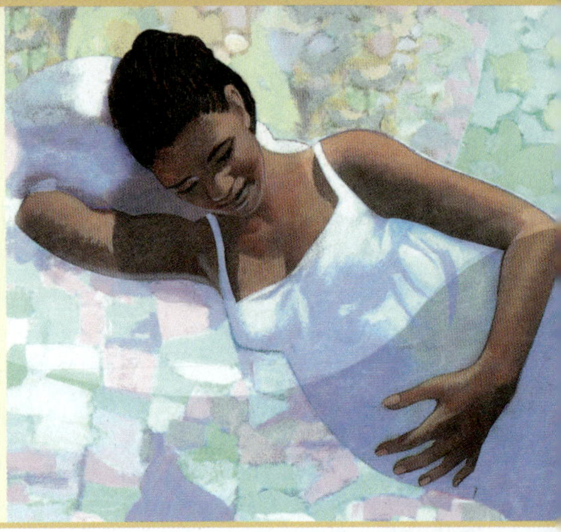

evolve WEBSITE

http://evolve.elsevier.com/Lowdermilk/MWHC/
Audio Glossary
Audio Key Points
NCLEX Review Questions
Nursing Care Plan
Postpartum Hemorrhage

LEARNING OBJECTIVES

- Identify the causes, signs and symptoms, and medical and nursing management of postpartum hemorrhage.
- Describe hemorrhagic shock as a complication of postpartum hemorrhage including management and hazards of therapy.
- Differentiate the causes of postpartum infection.
- Summarize assessment and care of women with postpartum infection.
- Describe thromboembolic disorders, including incidence, etiology, signs and symptoms, and management.
- Differentiate the role of the nurse in the hospital or birth center setting from the role of the home care nurse in assessing potential problems and managing care of women with postpartum physiologic complications.

Collaborative efforts of the health care team are needed to provide safe and effective care to the woman and family experiencing postpartum physiologic complications. This chapter focuses on hemorrhage and infection.

POSTPARTUM HEMORRHAGE

Definition and Incidence

Postpartum hemorrhage (PPH) continues to be a leading cause of maternal morbidity and mortality in the United States and worldwide (American College of Obstetricians and Gynecologists [ACOG], 2006; Johnson, Gregory, & Niebyl, 2007). It is a life-threatening event that can occur with little warning and is often unrecognized until the mother has profound symptoms. PPH has been traditionally defined as the loss of more than 500 ml of blood after vaginal birth and 1000 ml after cesarean birth (MacMullen, Dulski, & Meagher, 2005). A 10% change in hematocrit between admission for labor and postpartum or the need for erythrocyte transfusion also has been used to define PPH (Francois & Foley, 2007). However, defining PPH clinically is not a clear-cut undertaking. Diagnosis is often based on subjective observations, with blood loss often being underestimated by as much as 50% (Cunningham, Leveno, Bloom, Hauth, Rouse, & Spong, 2010).

Traditionally PPH has been classified as early or late with respect to the birth. Early, acute, or primary PPH occurs within 24 hours of the birth. Late or secondary PPH occurs more than 24 hours and up to 6 to 12 weeks postpartum (ACOG, 2006; Francois & Foley, 2007). Today's health care environment encourages shortened stays after birth, thereby increasing the potential for acute episodes of PPH to occur outside the traditional hospital or birth center setting.

Etiology and Risk Factors

Considering the problem of excessive bleeding with reference to the stages of labor is helpful. From birth of the infant until separation of the placenta, the character and quantity of blood passed can suggest excessive bleeding. For example, dark red blood is probably of venous origin, perhaps from varices or superficial lacerations of the birth canal. Bright red blood is arterial and can indicate deep lacerations of the cervix. Spurts of blood with clots can indicate partial placental separation. Failure of blood to clot or remain clotted indicates a pathologic condition or coagulopathy such as disseminated intravascular coagulation (see Chapter 28) (Francois & Foley, 2007).

Excessive bleeding may occur during the period from the separation of the placenta to its expulsion or removal. Commonly such excessive bleeding is the result of incomplete placental

CLINICAL REASONING

Postpartum Hemorrhage

Sara is a new staff RN on the mother-baby unit. One of her assigned clients (G4 P4) gave birth to a 9½-lb baby boy 4 hours ago after a long labor induced with oxytocin. The birth was vacuum assisted. She had a third-degree laceration that was repaired and a small cervical laceration that was not repaired. She has been having heavy lochia and her fundus has to be massaged frequently to firm it. Sara asks her nurse preceptor for advice about whether the woman is at risk for postpartum hemorrhage and if so what should be done.

1. Evidence—Is there sufficient evidence to draw conclusions about what advice the nurse preceptor should give?
2. Assumptions—Describe underlying assumptions about each of the following:
   a. Identifying risk factors for PPH
   b. Need for frequent assessments in the early postpartum period
   c. Use of oxytocic agents for prevention and management of PPH
3. What implications and priorities for nursing care can be made at this time?
4. Does the evidence objectively support your conclusion?
5. Are there alternative perspectives to your conclusion?

BOX 34-1 RISK FACTORS AND CAUSES OF POSTPARTUM HEMORRHAGE

Uterine atony
- Overdistended uterus
  - Large fetus
  - Multiple fetuses
  - Hydramnios
  - Distention with clots
- Anesthesia and analgesia
  - Conduction anesthesia
- Previous history of uterine atony
- High parity
- Prolonged labor, oxytocin-induced labor
- Trauma during labor and birth
  - Forceps-assisted birth
  - Vacuum-assisted birth
  - Cesarean birth
- Unrepaired lacerations of the birth canal
- Retained placental fragments
- Ruptured uterus
- Inversion of the uterus
- Placenta accreta, increta, percreta
- Coagulation disorders
- Placental abruption
- Placenta previa
- Manual removal of a retained placenta
- Magnesium sulfate administration during labor or the postpartum period
- Chorioamnionitis
- Uterine subinvolution

separation, undue manipulation of the fundus, or excessive traction on the cord. After the placenta has been expelled or removed, persistent or excessive blood loss usually is the result of atony of the uterus or prolapse of the uterus into the vagina. Late PPH can be the result of subinvolution of the uterus, endometritis, or retained placental fragments (Cunningham et al., 2010). Predisposing factors for PPH are listed in Box 34-1.

Uterine Atony

Uterine atony is marked hypotonia of the uterus. Normally, placental separation and expulsion are facilitated by contraction of the uterus, which also prevents hemorrhage from the placental site. The corpus is in essence a basket-weave of strong, interlacing smooth muscle bundles through which many large maternal blood vessels pass (see Fig. 4-3). If the uterus is flaccid after detachment of all or part of the placenta, brisk venous bleeding occurs, and normal coagulation of the open vasculature is impaired and continues until the uterine muscle is contracted.

Uterine atony is the leading cause of PPH, complicating approximately 1 in 20 births (Francois & Foley, 2007). It is associated with high parity, hydramnios, a macrosomic fetus, and multifetal gestation. In such conditions the uterus is "overstretched" and contracts poorly after the birth. Other causes of atony include traumatic birth, use of halogenated anesthesia (e.g., halothane) or magnesium sulfate, rapid or prolonged labor, chorioamnionitis, and use of oxytocin for labor induction or augmentation (Cunningham et al., 2010; Francois & Foley). PPH in a previous pregnancy is a predominant risk factor for recurrent PPH (Kominiarek & Kilpatrick, 2007).

Lacerations of the Genital Tract

Lacerations of the cervix, the vagina, and the perineum also are causes of PPH. Hemorrhage related to lacerations should be suspected if bleeding continues despite a firm, contracted uterine fundus. This bleeding can be a slow trickle, an oozing, or frank hemorrhage. Factors that influence the causes and incidence of obstetric lacerations of the lower genital tract include operative birth, precipitate birth, congenital abnormalities of the maternal soft parts, and contracted pelvis. Other possible causes of lacerations are size, abnormal presentation, and position of the fetus; relative size of the presenting part and the birth canal; previous scarring from infection, injury, or operation; and vulvar, perineal, and vaginal varicosities.

Extreme vascularity in the labial and periclitoral areas often results in profuse bleeding if laceration occurs. Hematomas also may be present.

Lacerations of the perineum are the most common of all injuries in the lower portion of the genital tract. These are classified as first, second, third, and fourth degree (see Chapter 19). An episiotomy may extend to become either a third- or fourth-degree laceration.

Prolonged pressure of the fetal head on the vaginal mucosa ultimately interferes with the circulation and may produce ischemic or pressure necrosis. The state of the tissues in combination with the type of birth may result in deep vaginal lacerations, with consequent predisposition to vaginal hematomas.

Pelvic hematomas may be vulvar, vaginal, or retroperitoneal in origin. Vulvar hematomas are the most common. Pain is the most common symptom, and most vulvar hematomas are visible. Vaginal hematomas occur more commonly in association with a forceps-assisted birth, an episiotomy, or primigravidity (Francois & Foley, 2007). During the postpartum period, if the woman reports a persistent perineal or rectal pain or a feeling of pressure in the vagina, a thorough examination is made. However, a retroperitoneal hematoma may cause minimal pain, and the initial symptoms may be signs of shock (Francois & Foley).

Cervical lacerations usually occur at the lateral angles of the external os. Most are shallow, and bleeding is minimal. More extensive lacerations may extend into the vaginal vault or into the lower uterine segment.

Retained Placenta

Nonadherent Retained Placenta

Nonadherent retained placenta may result from partial separation of a normal placenta, entrapment of the partially or completely separated placenta by an hourglass constriction ring of the uterus or mismanagement of the third stage of labor. Placental retention because of poor separation is common in very preterm births (20 to 24 weeks of gestation).

Management of nonadherent retained placenta is by manual separation and removal by the primary health care provider. Supplementary anesthesia is not usually needed for women who have had regional anesthesia for birth. For other women, administration of light nitrous oxide and oxygen inhalation anesthesia or intravenous (IV) thiopental facilitates uterine exploration and placental removal. After this removal, the woman is at continued risk for PPH and for infection.

Adherent Retained Placenta

Abnormal adherence of the placenta occurs for reasons unknown, but it is thought to result from zygotic implantation in an area of defective endometrium such that no zone of separation is present between the placenta and the decidua. Attempts to remove the placenta in the usual manner are unsuccessful, and laceration or perforation of the uterine wall may result, putting the woman at great risk for severe PPH and infection (Cunningham et al., 2010).

Unusual placental adherence may be partial or complete. The following degrees of attachment are recognized:

- *Placenta accreta*—slight penetration of myometrium by placental trophoblast
- *Placenta increta*—deep penetration of myometrium by placenta
- *Placenta percreta*—perforation of uterus by placenta

Bleeding with complete or total placenta accreta may not occur unless separation of the placenta is attempted. With more extensive involvement, bleeding will become profuse when removal of the placenta is attempted. Cesarean hysterectomy is indicated in approximately two thirds of women. If future fertility is desired, uterine conserving techniques may be attempted. Blood component replacement therapy is often necessary (Francois & Foley, 2007).

Inversion of the Uterus

Inversion of the uterus after birth is a potentially life-threatening but rare complication. The incidence of uterine inversion is approximately 1 in 2500 births (Francois & Foley, 2007), and the condition may recur with a subsequent birth. Uterine inversion may be partial or complete. Complete inversion of the uterus is obvious; a large, red, rounded mass (perhaps with the placenta attached) protrudes 20 to 30 cm outside the introitus. Incomplete inversion cannot be seen but must be felt; a smooth mass will be palpated through the dilated cervix. Contributing factors to uterine inversion include fundal implantation of the placenta, manual extraction of the placenta, short umbilical cord, uterine atony, leiomyomas, and abnormally adherent placental tissue (Francois & Foley). The primary presenting signs of uterine inversion are hemorrhage, shock, and pain in the absence of a palpable fundus abdominally.

Prevention—always the easiest, cheapest, and most effective therapy—is especially appropriate for uterine inversion. The umbilical cord should not be pulled on strongly unless the placenta has definitely separated.

Subinvolution of the Uterus

Late postpartum bleeding may occur as a result of **subinvolution** of the uterus. Recognized causes of subinvolution include retained placental fragments and pelvic infection.

Signs and symptoms include prolonged lochial discharge, irregular or excessive bleeding, and sometimes hemorrhage. A pelvic examination usually reveals a uterus that is larger than normal and that may be boggy.

CARE MANAGEMENT

Medical Management

Early recognition of PPH is critical to care management. The first step is to evaluate the contractility of the uterus. If the uterus is hypotonic, management is directed toward increasing contractility and minimizing blood loss.

Hypotonic Uterus. The initial management of excessive postpartum bleeding is firm massage of the uterine fundus (Hofmeyr, Abdel-Aleem, & Abdel-Aleem, 2008). Expression of any clots in the uterus, elimination of any bladder distention, and continuous IV infusion of 10 to 40 units of oxytocin added to 1000 ml of lactated Ringer's or normal saline solution also are primary interventions. If the uterus fails to respond to oxytocin, a 0.2-mg dose of ergonovine (Ergotrate) or methylergonovine (Methergine) may be given intramuscularly to produce sustained uterine contractions. However, administering a 0.25-mg dose of a derivative of prostaglandin $F_2\alpha$ (carboprost tromethamine [Carboprost; Hemabate]) intramuscularly is more common. It can also be given intramyometrially at cesarean birth or intraabdominally after vaginal birth (Francois & Foley, 2007). Prostaglandin E_2 (Dinoprostone) 20 mg vaginal or rectal suppository and rectal (800 to 1000 mcg) administration of misoprostol (Cytotec) also are used (ACOG, 2006) (see the Medication Guide for a comparison of drugs used to manage PPH). In addition to the medications used to contract the uterus, rapid administration of crystalloid solutions or blood or blood products or both will be needed to restore the woman's intravascular volume (Francois & Foley).

> **! NURSING ALERT**
>
> Use of ergonovine or methylergonovine is contraindicated in the presence of hypertension or cardiovascular disease. Prostaglandin $F_2\alpha$ should be used cautiously in women with cardiovascular disease or asthma (Francois & Foley, 2007).

MEDICATION GUIDE

Drugs Used to Manage Postpartum Hemorrhage

DRUG	ACTION	SIDE EFFECTS	CONTRAINDICATIONS	DOSAGE AND ROUTE	NURSING CONSIDERATIONS
Oxytocin (Pitocin)	Contraction of uterus; decreases bleeding	Infrequent: water intoxication, nausea and vomiting	None for PPH	10 to 40 units/L diluted in lactated Ringer's solution or normal saline at 125 to 200 milliunits/min IV; or 10 to 20 units IM	Continue to monitor vaginal bleeding and uterine tone
Methylergonovine (Methergine)*	Contraction of uterus	Hypertension, nausea, vomiting, headache	Hypertension, cardiac disease	0.2 mg IM every 2 to 4 hr up to five doses; may also be given intrauterine or orally	Check blood pressure before giving, and do not give if >140/90 mm Hg; continue monitoring vaginal bleeding and uterine tone
15-Methylprostaglandin $F_2\alpha$ (Prostin/15 m; Carboprost, Hemabate)	Contraction of uterus	Headache, nausea and vomiting, fever, tachycardia, hypertension, diarrhea	Avoid with asthma or hypertension	0.25 mg IM or intrauterine every 15 to 90 min up to eight doses	Continue to monitor vaginal bleeding and uterine tone
Dinoprostone (Prostin E_2)	Contraction of uterus	Headache, nausea and vomiting, fever, chills, diarrhea	Avoid with asthma or hypotension	20 mg vaginal or rectal suppository every 2 hr	Continue to monitor vaginal bleeding and uterine tone
Misoprostol (Cytotec)	Contraction of uterus	Headache, nausea and vomiting, diarrhea	History of allergy to prostaglandins	800 to 1000 mcg rectally once	Continue to monitor vaginal bleeding and uterine tone

IM, Intramuscularly; *IV,* intravenously; *PPH,* postpartum hemorrhage.
*Information about methylergonovine may also be used to describe ergonovine (Ergotrate).
Sources: American College of Obstetricians and Gynecologists (ACOG). (2006). *Postpartum hemorrhage.* ACOG Practice Bulletin No.76. Washington, DC: ACOG; Francois, K. & Foley, M. (2007). Antepartum and postpartum hemorrhage. In S. Gabbe, J. Niebyl, & J. Simpson (Eds.), *Obstetrics: Normal and problem pregnancies* (5th ed.). Philadelphia: Churchill Livingstone.

Oxygen can be given by nonrebreather face mask to enhance oxygen delivery to the cells. An indwelling urinary catheter is usually inserted to monitor urine output as a measure of intravascular volume. Laboratory studies usually include a complete blood count with platelet count, fibrinogen, fibrin split products, prothrombin time, and partial thromboplastin time. Blood type and antibody screen are done if not previously performed (Cunningham et al., 2010).

If bleeding persists, bimanual compression may be considered by the obstetrician or nurse-midwife. This procedure involves inserting a fist into the vagina and pressing the knuckles against the anterior side of the uterus, and then placing the other hand on the abdomen and massaging the posterior uterus with it. If the uterus still does not become firm, manual exploration of the uterine cavity for retained placental fragments is implemented. If the preceding procedures are ineffective, surgical management may be the only alternative. Surgical management options include vessel ligation (utero-ovarian, uterine, hypogastric), selective arterial embolization, and hysterectomy (Cunningham et al., 2010; Francois & Foley, 2007).

Bleeding with a Contracted Uterus. If the uterus is firmly contracted and bleeding continues, the source of bleeding still must be identified and treated. Assessment may include visual or manual inspection of the perineum, the vagina, the uterus, the cervix, or the rectum and laboratory studies (e.g., hemoglobin, hematocrit, coagulation studies, platelet count). Treatment depends on the source of the bleeding. Lacerations are usually sutured. Hematomas may be managed with observation, cold therapy, ligation of the bleeding vessel, or evacuation. Fluids and blood replacement may be needed (Francois & Foley, 2007).

Uterine Inversion. Uterine inversion is an emergency situation requiring immediate recognition, replacement of the uterus within the pelvic cavity, and correction of associated clinical conditions. Tocolytics (e.g., magnesium sulfate, terbutaline) or halogenated anesthetics may be given to relax the uterus before attempting replacement (Cunningham et al., 2010). Medical management of this condition includes repositioning the uterus, giving oxytocin after the uterus is repositioned, treating shock, and initiating broad-spectrum antibiotics (Cunningham et al.; Francois & Foley, 2007).

BOX 34-2 HERBAL REMEDIES FOR POSTPARTUM HEMORRHAGE*

HERB	ACTION
Witch hazel	Homeostatic
Lady's mantle	Homeostatic
Blue cohosh	Oxytocic
Cotton root bark	Oxytocic
Motherwort	Promotes uterine contraction; vasoconstrictive
Shepherd's purse	Promotes uterine contraction
Alfalfa leaf	Increases availability of vitamin K; increases hemoglobin; may promote uterine contraction
Nettle	Increases availability of vitamin K; increases hemoglobin; may promote uterine contraction
Raspberry leaf	Homeostatic; promotes uterine contraction
Yarrow	Homeostatic

*Usually used to promote uterine tone after the initial/emergency situation is controlled.

NOTE: Readers are advised to check the most current information about each specific herbal therapy to verify dose, methods of administration, side effects, and contraindications. Continued research is needed to determine efficacy of these herbal remedies.

Sources: Beal, M. (1998). Use of complementary and alternative therapies in reproductive medicine. *Journal of Nurse-Midwifery, 43*(3), 224-233; Born, D. & Barron, M. (2005). Herbal use in pregnancy: What nurses need to know. *MCN The American Journal of Maternal/Child Nursing, 30*(3), 201-208; Tiran, D. & Mack, S. (Eds.), (2000). *Complementary therapies for pregnancy and childbirth* (2nd ed.). Edinburgh: Baillière Tindall.

Subinvolution. Treatment of subinvolution depends on the cause. Ergonovine, 0.2 mg every 3 to 4 hours for 24 to 48 hours, and antibiotic therapy are the most common medications used (Cunningham et al., 2010). Dilation and curettage (D&C) may be needed to remove retained placental fragments or to debride the placental site.

Herbal Remedies

Herbal remedies have been used with some success to control PPH after the initial management and control of bleeding, particularly outside the United States. Some herbs have homeostatic actions, whereas others work as oxytocic agents to contract the uterus (Tiran & Mack, 2000). Box 34-2 lists herbs that have been used and their actions. However, published evidence of the safety and efficacy of herbal therapy is lacking. Evidence from well-controlled studies is needed before recommendations for practice can be made (Born & Barron, 2005).

Nursing Interventions

PPH may be sudden and even exsanguinating. The nurse must therefore be alert to the symptoms of hemorrhage and hypovolemic shock and be prepared to act quickly to minimize blood loss (Fig. 34-1 and Box 34-3). Immediate assessments, nursing

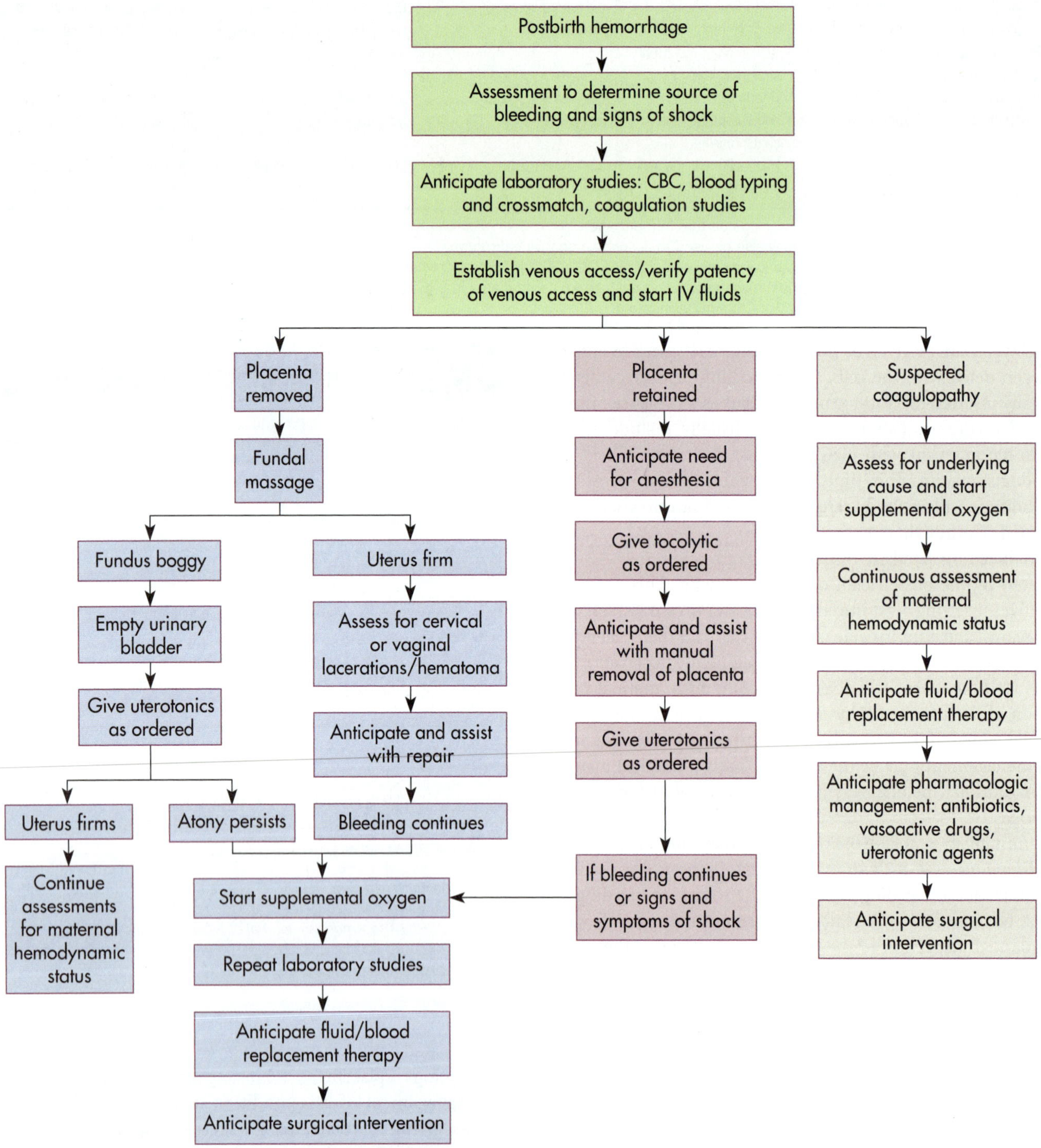

FIG. 34-1 Nursing assessments for postpartum bleeding. *CBC,* Complete blood count; *IV,* intravenous; *uterotonics,* medications to contract the uterus.

NURSING PROCESS

Postpartum Hemorrhage

ASSESSMENT

- Review the woman's history for factors that predispose to postpartum hemorrhage (PPH) (see Box 34-1).
- Assess the fundus to determine whether it is firmly contracted at or near the level of the umbilicus.
- Assess bleeding for color and amount.
- Inspect the perineum for signs of lacerations or hematomas.
- Assess vital signs every 15 minutes during the first 2 hours after birth to identify trends related to blood loss (e.g., tachycardia, tachypnea, decreasing blood pressure). However, vital signs may not be reliable indicators of shock immediately postpartum because of the physiologic adaptations of this period.
- Assess for bladder distention because a distended bladder can displace the uterus and prevent contraction.
- Assess the skin for warmth and dryness; nailbeds should be checked for color and promptness of capillary refill.
- Collect specimens or review reports of laboratory studies, specifically hemoglobin and hematocrit levels.

NURSING DIAGNOSES

Nursing diagnoses for women experiencing PPH include the following:

***Deficient Fluid Volume* related to:**
- excessive blood loss secondary to uterine atony, lacerations, or uterine inversion

***Risk for Imbalanced Fluid Volume* related to:**
- blood and fluid volume replacement therapy

***Risk for Infection* related to:**
- excessive blood loss or exposed placental attachment site
- multiple invasive procedures

***Risk for Injury* related to:**
- attempted manual removal of retained placenta
- administration of blood products
- operative procedures

***Fear or Anxiety* related to:**
- threat to self
- deficient knowledge regarding procedures and operative management

***Risk for Impaired Parenting* related to:**
- separation from infant secondary to treatment regimen

***Ineffective (Peripheral) Tissue Perfusion* related to:**
- excessive blood loss and shunting of blood to central circulation

EXPECTED OUTCOMES OF CARE

Expected outcomes of care for the woman experiencing PPH may include that the woman will:
- Maintain normal vital signs and laboratory values.
- Develop no complications related to excessive bleeding.
- Express an understanding of her condition, its management, and discharge instructions.
- Identify and use available support systems.

PLAN OF CARE AND INTERVENTIONS

Immediate nursing care of the woman with PPH includes:
- Assessments of vital signs, bleeding, and fundus
- Medication administration per protocol or orders
- Establishing or maintaining venous access
- Notifying the primary health care provider
- Providing explanations about interventions to woman and her family

(Care for specific problems that caused the bleeding and discharge teaching are discussed on pp. 826–830.)

EVALUATION

The nurse can be reasonably assured that care was effective to the extent that the expected outcomes were achieved.

BOX 34-3 NONINVASIVE ASSESSMENTS OF CARDIAC OUTPUT IN POSTPARTUM WOMEN WHO ARE BLEEDING

PALPATION OF PULSES (RATE, QUALITY, EQUALITY)
- Arterial

AUSCULTATION
- Heart sounds/murmurs
- Breath sounds

INSPECTION
- Skin color, temperature, turgor
- Level of consciousness
- Capillary refill
- Neck veins
- Mucous membranes

OBSERVATION
- Presence or absence of anxiety, apprehension, restlessness, disorientation

MEASUREMENT
- Blood pressure
- Pulse oximetry
- Urinary output

---

diagnoses, expected outcomes of care, and interventions are listed in the Nursing Process box.

The woman and her family will be anxious about her condition. The nurse can intervene by calmly providing explanations about interventions being performed and the need to act quickly.

After the bleeding has been controlled, the care of the woman with lacerations of the perineum is similar to that of women with episiotomies (analgesia as needed for pain and hot or cold applications as necessary). The need for increased roughage in the diet and increased intake of fluids is emphasized. Stool softeners may be used to assist the woman in reestablishing bowel habits without straining and putting stress on the suture lines.

! NURSING ALERT

To prevent injury to the suture line, a woman with third- or fourth-degree lacerations is not given rectal suppositories or enemas or digital rectal examinations.

The care of the woman who has experienced an inversion of the uterus focuses on immediate stabilization of hemodynamic status. This situation requires close observation of her response to treatment to prevent shock or fluid overload. If the uterus has been repositioned manually, care must be taken to avoid aggressive fundal massage.

Discharge instructions for the woman who has had PPH are similar to those for any postpartum woman. In addition, the woman should be told that she will probably feel fatigue, even exhaustion, and will need to limit her physical activities to conserve her strength. She may need instructions in increasing her dietary iron and protein intake and iron supplementation to rebuild lost red blood cell (RBC) volume. She may need assistance with infant care and household activities until she has regained strength. Some women have problems with delayed or insufficient lactation and postpartum depression (PPD). Referrals for home care follow-up or to community resources may be needed, such as Postpartum Support International at www.chss.iup.edu/postpartum (see the Nursing Care Plan).

HEMORRHAGIC (HYPOVOLEMIC) SHOCK

Hemorrhage may result in **hemorrhagic (hypovolemic) shock.** Shock is an emergency situation in which the perfusion of body organs may become severely compromised and death may occur. Physiologic compensatory mechanisms are activated

NURSING CARE PLAN

Postpartum Hemorrhage

NURSING DIAGNOSIS

Deficient fluid volume related to postpartum hemorrhage

Expected Outcome

Woman will demonstrate fluid balance as evidenced by stable vital signs, prompt capillary refill time, and balanced intake and output.

Nursing Interventions/*Rationales*

- Monitor vital signs, oxygen saturation, urine specific gravity, and capillary refill *to provide baseline data.*
- Measure and record amount and type of bleeding by weighing and counting saturated pads. If woman is at home, teach her to count pads and save any clots or tissue. If woman is admitted to hospital, save any clots and tissue for further examination *to estimate type and amount of blood loss for fluid replacement.*
- Provide quiet environment *to promote rest and decrease metabolic demands.*
- Give explanation of all procedures *to reduce anxiety.*
- Begin intravenous (IV) access with 18-gauge or larger catheter for infusion of isotonic solution as ordered *to provide fluid or blood replacement.*
- Administer medications as ordered, such as oxytocin, methylergonovine, or prostaglandin $F_2\alpha$, *to increase contractility of the uterus.*
- Insert indwelling urinary catheter *to provide the most accurate assessment of renal function and hypovolemia.*
- Prepare for surgical intervention as needed *to stop the source of bleeding.*

NURSING DIAGNOSIS

Ineffective tissue perfusion related to hypovolemia

Expected Outcomes

Woman will have stable vital signs, oxygen saturation, arterial blood gases, and adequate hematocrit and hemoglobin.

Nursing Interventions/*Rationales*

- Monitor vital signs, oxygen saturation, arterial blood gases, and hematocrit and hemoglobin *to assess for hypovolemic shock and decreased tissue perfusion.*
- Assess for any changes in level of consciousness *to assess for evidence of hypoxia.*
- Assess capillary refill, mucous membranes, and skin temperature *to note indicators of vasoconstriction.*
- Give supplementary oxygen as ordered *to provide additional oxygenation to tissues.*
- Suction as needed, and insert oral airway, *to maintain clear, open airway for oxygenation.*
- Monitor arterial blood gases *to provide information about acidosis or hypoxia.*
- Administer sodium bicarbonate if ordered *to reverse metabolic acidosis.*

NURSING DIAGNOSIS

Anxiety related to sudden change in health status

Expected Outcome

Woman will verbalize that anxious feelings are diminished.

Nursing Interventions/*Rationales*

- Using therapeutic communication, evaluate woman's understanding of events *to provide clarification of any misconceptions.*
- Provide calm, competent attitude and environment *to aid in decreasing anxiety.*
- Explain all procedures *to decrease anxiety about the unknown.*
- Allow woman to verbalize feelings *to permit clarification of information and promote trust.*
- Continue to assess vital signs or other clinical indicators of hypovolemic shock *to evaluate if psychologic response of anxiety intensifies physiologic indicators.*

NURSING DIAGNOSIS

Risk for infection related to blood loss and invasive procedures as a result of postpartum hemorrhage

Expected Outcomes

Woman will verbalize understanding of risk factors. Woman will demonstrate no signs of infection.

Nursing Interventions/*Rationales*

- Maintain Standard Precautions and use good handwashing technique when providing care *to prevent introduction of or spread of infection.*
- Teach woman to maintain good handwashing technique (particularly before handling her newborn) and to maintain scrupulous perineal care with frequent change and careful disposal of perineal pads *to avoid spread of microorganisms.*
- Monitor vital signs *to detect signs of systemic infection.*
- Monitor level of fatigue and lethargy, evidence of chills, loss of appetite, nausea and vomiting, and abdominal pain, *which indicate the extent of infection and serve as indicators of status of infection.*
- Monitor lochia for foul smell and profusion *as indicators of infection state.*
- Assist with collection of intrauterine cultures or other specimens for laboratory analysis *to identify specific causative organism.*
- Monitor laboratory values (i.e., white blood cell [WBC] count, cultures) *for indicators of type and status of infection.*
- Ensure adequate fluid and nutritional intake *to promote healthy recovery.*
- Administer and monitor broad-spectrum antibiotics as ordered *to prevent or treat infection.*
- Administer antipyretics as ordered and necessary *to reduce elevated temperature.*

Nursing Care Plan—Postpartum Hemorrhage

EMERGENCY

Hemorrhagic Shock

ASSESSMENTS	CHARACTERISTICS
Respirations	Rapid and shallow
Pulse	Rapid, weak, irregular
Blood pressure	Decreasing (late sign)
Skin	Cool, pale, clammy
Urinary output	Decreasing
Level of consciousness	Lethargy → coma
Mental status	Anxiety → coma
Central venous pressure	Decreased

INTERVENTION

- Summon assistance and equipment.
- Start intravenous infusion per standing orders.
- Ensure patent airway; administer oxygen.
- Continue to monitor status.

in response to hemorrhage. The adrenal glands release catecholamines, causing constriction of arterioles and venules in the skin, the lungs, the gastrointestinal tract, the liver, and the kidneys. The available blood flow is diverted to the brain and the heart and away from other organs, including the uterus. If shock is prolonged, the continued reduction in cellular oxygenation results in an accumulation of lactic acid and acidosis (from anaerobic glucose metabolism). Acidosis (reduced serum pH) causes arteriolar vasodilation; venule vasoconstriction persists. A circular pattern is established; that is, decreased perfusion, increased tissue anoxia and acidosis, edema formation, and pooling of blood further decrease the perfusion. Cellular death occurs. See the Emergency box for assessments and interventions for hemorrhagic shock.

Medical Management

Vigorous treatment is necessary to prevent adverse sequelae. Medical management of hypovolemic shock involves restoring circulating blood volume and treating the cause of the hemorrhage (e.g., lacerations, uterine atony, or inversion). To restore circulating blood volume, a rapid IV infusion of crystalloid solution is given at a rate of 3 ml infused for every 1 ml of estimated blood loss (e.g., 3000 ml infused for 1000 ml of blood loss). Packed RBCs are usually infused if the woman is still actively bleeding and no improvement in her condition is noted after the initial crystalloid infusion. Infusion of fresh-frozen plasma may be needed if clotting factors and platelet counts are below normal values (Cunningham et al., 2010; Francois & Foley, 2007).

Nursing Interventions

Hemorrhagic shock can occur rapidly, but the classic signs of shock may not appear until the postpartum woman has lost 30% to 40% of her blood volume. The nurse must continue to reassess the woman's condition, as evidenced by the degree of measurable and anticipated blood loss, and mobilize appropriate resources.

Most interventions are instituted to improve or monitor tissue perfusion. The nurse continues to monitor the woman's pulse and blood pressure. If invasive hemodynamic monitoring is ordered, the nurse may assist with the placement of the central venous pressure (CVP) or pulmonary artery (Swan-Ganz) catheter and monitor CVP, pulmonary artery pressure, or pulmonary artery wedge pressure as ordered (Gilbert, 2011) (see Chapter 31).

Additional assessments to be made include evaluating skin temperature, color, and turgor, as well as assessing the woman's mucous membranes. Breath sounds should be auscultated before fluid volume replacement, if possible, to provide a baseline for future assessment. Inspection for oozing at the sites of incisions or injections and assessment for the presence of petechiae or ecchymosis in areas not associated with surgery or trauma are critical in evaluating for disseminated intravascular coagulation (see Chapter 28).

Oxygen is administered, preferably by nonrebreather face mask, at 10 to 12 L/min to maintain oxygen saturation. Oxygen saturation should be monitored with a pulse oximeter, although measurements may not always be accurate in a woman with hypovolemia or decreased perfusion. Level of consciousness is assessed frequently and provides an additional indication of blood volume and oxygen saturation (Gilbert, 2011). In early stages of decreased blood flow the woman may report "seeing stars" or feeling dizzy or nauseated. She may become restless and orthopneic. As cerebral hypoxia increases, she may become confused and react slowly or not at all to stimuli. Some women complain of headaches (Curran, 2003). An improved sensorium is an indicator of improved perfusion.

Continuous electrocardiographic monitoring may be indicated for the woman who is hypotensive or tachycardic, continues to bleed profusely, or is in shock. A indwelling (Foley) catheter with a urometer is inserted to allow hourly assessment of urinary output. The most objective and least invasive assessment of adequate organ perfusion and oxygenation is urinary output of at least 30 ml/hr (Cunningham et al., 2010). Blood may be drawn and sent to the laboratory for studies that include hemoglobin and hematocrit levels, platelet count, and coagulation profile.

Fluid or Blood Replacement Therapy

Critical to successful management of the woman with a hemorrhagic complication is the establishment of venous access, preferably with a large-bore IV catheter. The establishment of two IV lines facilitates fluid resuscitation. Vigorous fluid resuscitation includes the administration of crystalloids (lactated Ringer's, normal saline solutions), colloids (albumin), blood, and blood components (Francois & Foley, 2007). Fluid resuscitation must be closely monitored because fluid overload may occur. Intravascular fluid overload occurs more frequently with colloid therapy than with other fluids. Transfusion reactions may follow the administration of blood or blood components, including cryoprecipitates. Even in an emergency, each unit should be checked per hospital protocol. Complications of fluid or blood replacement therapy include hemolytic reactions, febrile reactions, allergic reactions, circulatory overload, and air embolism.

LEGAL TIP: Standard of Care for Bleeding Emergencies

The standard of care for obstetric emergency situations such as PPH or hypovolemic shock is that provision should be made for the nurse to implement actions independently. Policies, procedures, standing orders or protocols, and clinical guidelines should be established by each health care facility in which births occur and should be agreed on by health care providers involved in the care of obstetric clients.

COAGULOPATHIES

When bleeding is continuous and no identifiable source is found, a coagulopathy may be the cause. The woman's coagulation status must be assessed quickly and continuously. The nurse can draw and send blood to the laboratory for studies. Abnormal results depend on the cause and can include increased prothrombin time, increased partial thromboplastin time, decreased platelets, decreased fibrinogen level, increased fibrin degradation products, and prolonged bleeding time. Causes of coagulopathies may be pregnancy complications such as idiopathic thrombocytopenic purpura or von Willebrand disease and disseminated intravascular coagulation.

Idiopathic Thrombocytopenic Purpura

Idiopathic or **immune thrombocytopenic purpura (ITP)** is an autoimmune disorder in which antiplatelet antibodies decrease the life span of the platelets. Thrombocytopenia, capillary fragility, and increased bleeding time are diagnostic findings. ITP may cause severe hemorrhage after cesarean birth or cervical or vaginal lacerations. The incidence of postpartum uterine bleeding and vaginal hematomas also is increased. Neonatal thrombocytopenia can result, but serious bleeding is unusual (Rosenberg, 2007).

Medical management focuses on control of platelet stability. If ITP was diagnosed during pregnancy, the woman likely was treated with corticosteroids or IV immunoglobulin. Platelet transfusions are usually given when bleeding is significant. A splenectomy may be needed if the ITP does not respond to medical management (Samuels, 2007).

von Willebrand Disease

von Willebrand disease (vWD), a type of hemophilia, is probably the most common of all hereditary bleeding disorders (Samuels, 2007). Although von Willebrand disease is rare, it is among the most common congenital clotting defects in U.S. women of childbearing age. It results from a deficiency or defect in a blood clotting protein called von Willebrand factor (vWF). There are as many as 20 variations of vWD disorders, most of which are inherited as autosomal dominant traits—types I and II are the most common (Cunningham et al., 2010). Symptoms include recurrent bleeding episodes such as nosebleeds or after tooth extraction, bruising easily, prolonged bleeding time (the most important test), factor VIII deficiency (mild to moderate), and bleeding from mucous membranes (Samuels). Although factor VIII increases during pregnancy, a risk for PPH still exists as levels of vWF begin to decrease (Cunningham et al.).

The woman may be at risk for bleeding for up to 4 weeks postpartum. The treatment of choice is administration of desmopressin, which promotes the release of vWF and factor VIII. It can be given nasally, intravenously, or orally. Transfusion therapy with plasma products that have been treated for viruses and contain factor VIII and vWF (e.g., Humate-P, Alphanate) also may be used (Lee & Abdul-Kadir, 2005; Samuels, 2007).

THROMBOEMBOLIC DISEASE

A thrombosis results from the formation of a blood clot or clots inside a blood vessel and is caused by inflammation **(thrombophlebitis)** or partial obstruction of the vessel. Three thromboembolic conditions are of concern in the postpartum period:

- *Superficial venous thrombosis:* involvement of the superficial saphenous venous system
- *Deep venous thrombosis:* involvement varies but can extend from the foot to the iliofemoral region
- *Pulmonary embolism:* complication of deep venous thrombosis occurring when part of a blood clot dislodges and is carried to the pulmonary artery, where it occludes the vessel and obstructs blood flow to the lungs

Incidence and Etiology

The incidence of thromboembolic disease in the postpartum period varies from approximately 1 in 1000 to 1 in 2000 women (Pettker & Lockwood, 2007). The incidence has declined in the past 20 years because early ambulation after childbirth has become the standard practice. The major causes of thromboembolic disease are venous stasis and hypercoagulation, both of which are present in pregnancy and continue into the postpartum period. Other risk factors include operative vaginal birth, cesarean birth, history of venous thrombosis or varicosities, obesity, maternal age older than 35 years, multiparity, infection, immobility, and smoking. Women with associated genetic risk factors are also at risk (Pettker & Lockwood).

Clinical Manifestations

Superficial venous thrombosis is the most frequent form of postpartum thrombophlebitis. It is characterized by pain and tenderness in the lower extremity. Physical examination may reveal warmth, redness, and an enlarged, hardened vein over the site of the thrombosis. Deep venous thrombosis is more common than superficial venous thrombosis during pregnancy than after the birth. It is characterized by unilateral leg pain, calf tenderness, and swelling (Fig. 34-2). Physical examination may reveal redness and warmth, but many women have few if any

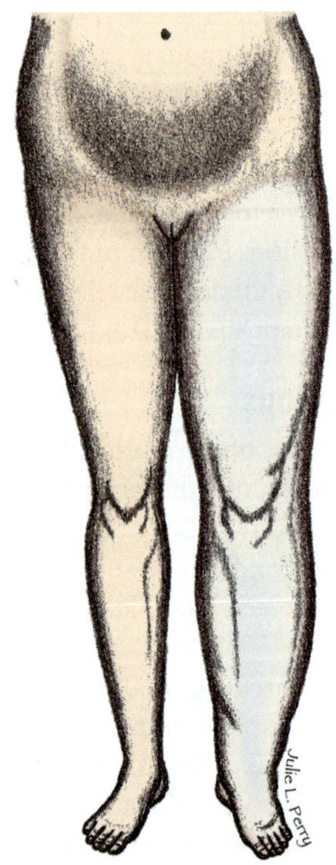

FIG. 34-2 Deep venous thrombophlebitis.

symptoms. A positive Homans sign may be present, but further evaluation is needed because the calf pain may be attributed to other causes, such as a strained muscle resulting from the birthing position (Pettker & Longwood, 2007). Acute pulmonary embolism is characterized by dyspnea and tachypnea (more than 20 breaths/min). Other signs and symptoms frequently seen include tachycardia (more than 100 beats/min), apprehension, cough, hemoptysis, elevated temperature, syncope, and pleuritic chest pain (Cunningham et al., 2010; Pettker & Lockwood).

Physical examination is not a sensitive diagnostic indicator for thrombosis. Venography is the most accurate method for diagnosing deep venous thrombosis; however, it is an invasive procedure that is associated with serious complications. Noninvasive diagnostic methods such as real-time and color Doppler ultrasound are commonly used. Cardiac auscultation may reveal murmurs with pulmonary embolism. Electrocardiograms are usually normal. Arterial oxygen pressure may be lower than normal (Katz, 2007a; Pettker & Lockwood, 2007).

Medical Management

Superficial venous thrombosis is treated with analgesia (nonsteroidal antiinflammatory agents), rest with elevation of the affected leg, and elastic stockings (Cunningham et al., 2010; Katz, 2007a). Local application of moist heat also may be used. Deep venous thrombosis is initially treated with anticoagulant (usually continuous IV heparin) therapy, bed rest with the affected leg elevated, and analgesia. After the symptoms have decreased, the woman may be fitted with elastic stockings to prevent venous congestion when she is allowed to ambulate. The woman is taught to put on the elastic stockings before getting out of bed. IV heparin therapy continues for 3 to 5 days or until symptoms resolve. Oral anticoagulant therapy (warfarin) is started during this time and will be continued for approximately 3 months. Continuous IV heparin therapy is used for pulmonary embolism until symptoms have resolved and is followed by subcutaneous heparin or oral anticoagulant therapy for up to 6 months (Pettker & Lockwood, 2007).

Nursing Interventions

In the hospital setting, nursing care of the woman with a thrombosis consists of continued assessments: inspecting and palpating the affected area; palpating peripheral pulses; checking for Homans sign; measuring and comparing leg circumferences; inspecting for signs of bleeding; monitoring for signs of pulmonary embolism including chest pain, coughing, dyspnea, and tachypnea; and assessing respiratory status for the presence of crackles. Laboratory reports are monitored for prothrombin or partial thromboplastin times. The woman and her family are assessed for their level of understanding about the diagnosis and their ability to cope during the unexpected extended period of recovery.

Interventions include explanations and education about the diagnosis and the treatment. The woman will need assistance with personal care as long as she is on bed rest; the family should be encouraged to participate in the care if that is what she and they wish. While the woman is on bed rest, she should be encouraged to change positions frequently but to avoid placing her knees in a sharply flexed position that could cause pooling of blood in the lower extremities. She also should be cautioned to avoid rubbing the affected area because this action could cause the clot to dislodge. Heparin and warfarin are administered as ordered, and the physician is notified if clotting times are outside the therapeutic level. If the woman is breastfeeding, she is assured that neither heparin nor warfarin is excreted in significant quantities in breast milk. If the infant has been discharged, the family is encouraged to bring the infant for feedings as permitted by hospital policy; the mother also can express milk to be sent home.

Pain can be managed with a variety of measures. Position changes, elevating the leg, and application of moist heat may decrease discomfort. Administration of analgesics or antiinflammatory medications may be necessary.

> **! NURSING ALERT**
>
> Medications containing aspirin are not given to women receiving anticoagulant therapy because aspirin inhibits synthesis of clotting factors and can lead to prolonged clotting time and increased risk of bleeding.

The woman is usually discharged home with oral anticoagulants and will need explanations about the treatment schedule and possible side effects. If subcutaneous injections are to be given, the woman and family are taught how to administer the medication and about site rotation. The woman and her family also should be given information about safe care practices to prevent bleeding and injury while she is receiving anticoagulant therapy, such as using a soft toothbrush and an electric razor. She also will need information about follow-up with her health care provider to monitor clotting times and to make sure the correct dose of anticoagulant therapy is maintained. The woman also should use a reliable method of contraception if taking warfarin because this medication is considered teratogenic (Gilbert, 2011). Oral contraceptives are contraindicated because of the increased risk for thrombosis (Cunningham et al., 2010).

POSTPARTUM INFECTIONS

Postpartum infection, or *puerperal infection,* is any clinical infection of the genital tract that occurs within 28 days after miscarriage, induced abortion, or childbirth. The definition used in the United States continues to be the presence of a fever of 38° C or more on 2 successive days of the first 10 postpartum days (not counting the first 24 hours after birth) (Katz, 2007b). Puerperal infection is probably the major cause of maternal morbidity and mortality throughout the world; endometritis is the most common cause. In the United States it occurs after approximately 2% of vaginal births and 10% to 15% of cesarean births (Katz, 2007b). Other common postpartum infections include wound infections, mastitis, urinary tract infections (UTIs), and respiratory tract infections.

The most common infecting organisms are the numerous streptococcal and anaerobic organisms. *Staphylococcus aureus,* gonococci, coliform bacteria, and clostridia are less common but serious pathogenic organisms that also cause puerperal infection. Postpartum infections are more common in women who have concurrent medical or immunosuppressive conditions or who had a cesarean or operative vaginal birth. Intrapartal factors such as prolonged rupture of membranes, prolonged labor, and internal maternal or fetal monitoring also increase

BOX 34-4 PREDISPOSING FACTORS FOR POSTPARTUM INFECTION

PRECONCEPTION OR ANTEPARTAL FACTORS
- History of previous venous thrombosis, urinary tract infection, mastitis, pneumonia
- Diabetes mellitus
- Alcoholism
- Drug abuse
- Immunosuppression
- Anemia
- Malnutrition

INTRAPARTAL FACTORS
- Cesarean birth
- Operative vaginal birth
- Prolonged rupture of membranes
- Chorioamnionitis
- Prolonged labor
- Bladder catheterization
- Internal fetal/uterine pressure monitoring
- Multiple vaginal examinations after rupture of membranes
- Epidural analgesia/anesthesia
- Retained placental fragments
- Postpartum hemorrhage
- Episiotomy or lacerations
- Hematomas

the risk of infection (Duff, 2007). Factors that predispose the woman to postpartum infection are listed in Box 34-4.

Endometritis

Endometritis is the most common postpartum infection. It usually begins as a localized infection at the placental site (Fig. 34-3) but can spread to involve the entire endometrium. Incidence is higher after cesarean birth than after vaginal birth. Assessment for signs of endometritis may reveal a fever (usually greater than 38° C); increased pulse; chills; anorexia; nausea; fatigue and lethargy; pelvic pain; uterine tenderness; or foul-smelling, profuse lochia (Duff, 2007). Leukocytosis and a markedly increased RBC sedimentation rate are typical laboratory findings of postpartum infections. Anemia also may be present. Blood cultures or intracervical or intrauterine bacterial cultures (aerobic and anaerobic) should reveal the offending pathogens within 36 to 48 hours.

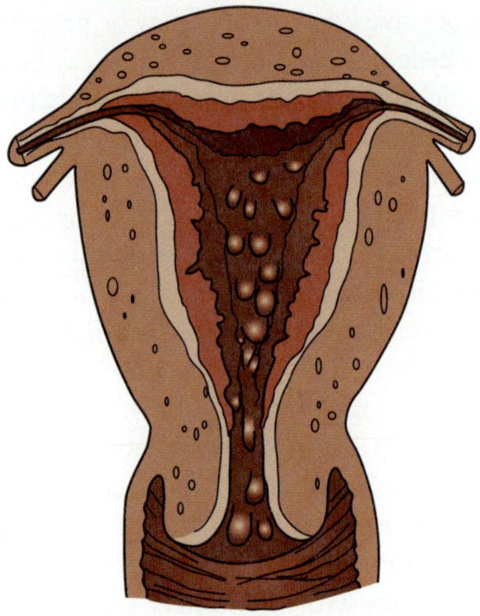

FIG. 34-3 Postpartum infection—endometritis.

Wound Infections

Wound infections also are common postpartum infections but often develop after the woman is at home. Sites of infection include the cesarean incision and the episiotomy or repaired laceration site. Predisposing factors are similar to those for endometritis (see Box 34-4). Signs of wound infection include erythema, edema, warmth, tenderness, seropurulent drainage, and wound separation. Fever and pain also may be present.

Urinary Tract Infections

UTIs occur in 2% to 4% of postpartum women. Risk factors include urinary catheterization, frequent pelvic examinations, epidural anesthesia, genital tract injury, history of UTI, and cesarean birth. Signs and symptoms include dysuria, frequency and urgency, low-grade fever, urinary retention, hematuria, and pyuria. Costovertebral angle (CVA) tenderness or flank pain may indicate upper UTI. Urinalysis results may reveal *Escherichia coli*, although other gram-negative aerobic bacilli also may cause UTIs.

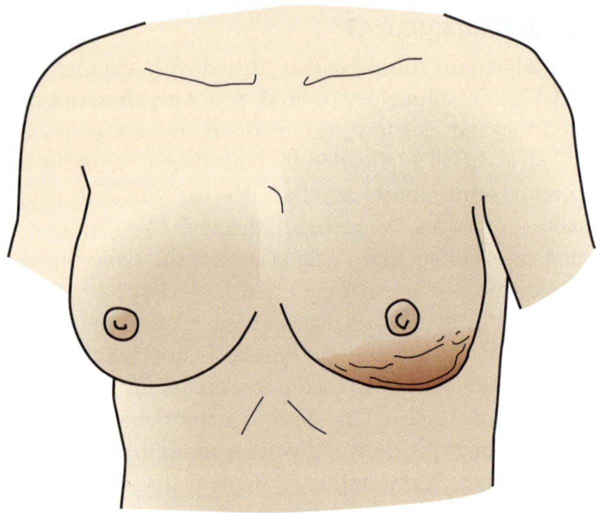

FIG. 34-4 Mastitis.

Mastitis

Mastitis affects approximately 1% to 10% of women soon after childbirth, most of whom are first-time mothers who are breastfeeding (Newton, 2007). Mastitis almost always is unilateral and develops well after the flow of milk has been established (Fig. 34-4). The infecting organism generally is the hemolytic *Staphylococcus aureus*. An infected nipple fissure usually is the initial lesion, but the ductal system is involved next. Inflammatory edema and engorgement of the breast soon obstruct the flow of milk in a lobe; regional, then generalized, mastitis follows. If treatment is not prompt, mastitis may progress to a breast abscess.

Symptoms rarely appear before the end of the first postpartum week and are more common in the second to fourth weeks. Chills, fever, malaise, and local breast tenderness are noted first. Pain, swelling, redness, and axillary adenopathy also may occur.

BOX 34-5 NURSING DIAGNOSES FOR WOMEN EXPERIENCING POSTPARTUM INFECTION

***Deficient Knowledge* related to:**
- Cause, management, course of infection
- Transmission and prevention of infection

***Impaired Tissue Integrity* related to:**
- Effects of infection process

***Acute Pain* related to:**
- Mastitis
- Puerperal infection
- Urinary tract infection

***Interrupted Family Processes* related to:**
- Unexpected complication to expected postpartum recovery
- Possible separation from newborn
- Interruption in process of realigning relationships after the addition of the new family member

***Risk for Impaired Parenting* related to:**
- Fear of spread of infection to newborn

CARE MANAGEMENT

Signs and symptoms associated with postpartum infection were discussed with each infection. Laboratory tests usually performed include a complete blood count, venous blood cultures, and uterine tissue cultures. Nursing diagnoses for women experiencing postpartum infection are listed in Box 34-5.

The most effective and least expensive treatment of postpartum infection is prevention. Good maternal perineal hygiene with thorough handwashing is emphasized. Strict adherence by all health care personnel to aseptic techniques during childbirth and the postpartum period is very important.

Management of endometritis consists of IV broad-spectrum antibiotic therapy (e.g., cephalosporins, penicillins, clindamycin, and gentamicin) and supportive care, including hydration, rest, and pain relief. Antibiotic therapy is usually discontinued 24 hours after the woman is asymptomatic (Duff, 2007).

Nursing measures including assessments of lochia, vital signs, and changes in the woman's condition continue during treatment. Comfort measures depend on the symptoms and can include cool compresses, warm blankets, perineal care, and sitz baths. Teaching should include side effects of therapy, prevention of spread of infection, signs and symptoms of worsening condition, and adherence to the treatment plan and the need for follow-up care. Women may need to be encouraged or assisted to maintain mother-infant interactions and breastfeeding (if allowed during treatment).

Treatment of wound infections may combine antibiotic therapy with wound debridement. Wounds may be opened and drained. Nursing care includes frequent wound and vital sign assessments and wound care. Comfort measures include sitz baths, warm compresses, and perineal care. Teaching includes good hygiene techniques (e.g., changing perineal pads front to back, handwashing before and after perineal care), self-care measures, and signs of worsening conditions to report to the health care provider. The woman is usually discharged to home for self-management or home nursing care after treatment is initiated in the inpatient setting.

Medical management for UTIs consists of antibiotic therapy, analgesia, and hydration. Postpartum women are usually treated on an outpatient basis; therefore, teaching should include instructions on how to monitor temperature, bladder function, and appearance of urine. The woman also should be taught about signs of potential complications and the importance of taking all antibiotics as prescribed. Other suggestions for prevention of UTIs include using proper perineal care, wiping from front to back after urinating or having a bowel movement, and increasing fluid intake.

Because mastitis rarely occurs before the postpartum woman who is breastfeeding is discharged, teaching should include warning signs of mastitis and counseling about the prevention of cracked nipples. Management includes support of breasts, local application of heat (or cold), adequate hydration, analgesics, and antibiotic therapy (e.g., dicloxacillin or flucloxacillin). Lactation can be maintained by emptying the breasts every 2 to 4 hours by breastfeeding, manual expression, or breast pump (Katz, 2007b) (see Chapter 25 for further information).

Postpartum women are usually discharged by 48 hours after birth, and often signs of infection may not be manifested until after the woman is at home. Nurses in birth centers and hospital settings must be able to identify women at risk for postpartum infection and provide anticipatory teaching and counseling before discharge. After discharge, telephone follow-up, hotlines, support groups, lactation counselors, home visits by nurses, and teaching materials (videos, written materials) can be used to decrease the risk of postpartum infections. Home care nurses must be able to recognize signs and symptoms of postpartum infection and provide the appropriate nursing care for women who need follow-up home care.

KEY POINTS

- Postpartum hemorrhage is the most common and most serious type of excessive obstetric blood loss.
- Hemorrhagic (hypovolemic) shock is an emergency situation in which the perfusion of body organs may become severely compromised, leading to significant risk of morbidity or death for the mother.
- The potential hazards of the therapeutic interventions may further compromise the woman with a hemorrhagic disorder.
- Clotting disorders are associated with many obstetric complications.
- The first symptom of postpartum infection is usually fever greater than 38° C on 2 consecutive days in the first 10 postpartum days (after the first 24 hours).
- Prevention is the most effective and inexpensive treatment of postpartum infection.

Audio Chapter Summaries Access an audio summary of these Key Points on evolve

REFERENCES

American College of Obstetricians and Gynecologists (ACOG). (2006). *Postpartum hemorrhage.* ACOG Practice Bulletin No. 76. Washington, DC: ACOG.

Born, D., & Barron, M. (2005). Herbal use in pregnancy: What nurses need to know. *MCN The American Journal of Maternal/Child Nursing, 30*(3), 201–208.

Cunningham, F., Leveno, K., Bloom, S., Hauth, J., Rouse, D., & Spong, C. (2010). *Williams obstetrics* (23rd ed.). New York: McGraw-Hill.

Curran, C. (2003). Intrapartum emergencies. *Journal of Obstetric, Gynecologic and Neonatal Nursing, 32*(6), 802–813.

Duff, P. (2007). Maternal and perinatal infection—bacterial. In S. Gabbe, J. Niebyl, & J. Simpson (Eds.), *Obstetrics: Normal and problem pregnancies* (5th ed.). Philadelphia: Churchill Livingstone.

Francois, K., & Foley, M. (2007). Antepartum and postpartum hemorrhage. In S. Gabbe, J. Niebyl, & J. Simpson (Eds.), *Obstetrics: Normal and problem pregnancies* (5th ed.). Philadelphia: Churchill Livingstone.

Gilbert, E. (2011). *Manual of high risk pregnancy & delivery* (5th ed.). St. Louis: Mosby.

Hofmeyr, G., Abdel-Aleem, H., & Abdel-Aleem, M. (2008). Uterine massage for preventing postpartum haemorrhage. *The Cochrane Database of Systematic Reviews, 2008,* 3, CD006431.

Johnson, T., Gregory, K., & Niebyl, J. (2007). Preconception and prenatal care: Part of the continuum. In S. Gabbe, J. Niebyl, & J. Simpson (Eds.), *Obstetrics: Normal and problem pregnancies* (5th ed.). Philadelphia: Churchill Livingstone.

Katz, V. (2007a). Postoperative counseling and management. In V. Katz, G. Lentz, R. Lobo, & D. Gershenson (Eds.), *Comprehensive gynecology* (5th ed.). Philadelphia: Mosby.

Katz, V. (2007b). Postpartum care. In S. Gabbe, J. Niebyl, & J. Simpson (Eds.), *Obstetrics: Normal and problem pregnancies* (5th ed.). Philadelphia: Churchill Livingstone.

Kominiarek, M., & Kilpatrick, S. (2007). Postpartum hemorrhage: A recurring pregnancy complication. *Seminars in Perinatology, 31*(3), 159–166.

Lee, C., & Abdul-Kadir, R. (2005). von Willebrand disease and women's health. *Seminars in Hematology, 42*(1), 42–48.

MacMullen, N., Dulski, L., & Meagher, B. (2005). Red alert: Perinatal hemorrhage. *MCN The American Journal of Maternal/Child Nursing, 30*(1), 46–51.

Newton, E. (2007). Breastfeeding. In S. Gabbe, J. Niebyl, & J. Simpson (Eds.), *Obstetrics: Normal and problem pregnancies* (5th ed.). Philadelphia: Churchill Livingstone.

Pettker, C., & Lockwood, C. (2007). Thromboembolic disorders. In S. Gabbe, J. Niebyl, & J. Simpson (Eds.), *Obstetrics: Normal and problem pregnancies* (5th ed.). Philadelphia: Churchill Livingstone.

Rosenberg, A. (2007). The neonate. In S. Gabbe, J. Niebyl, & J. Simpson (Eds.), *Obstetrics: Normal and problem pregnancies* (5th ed.). Philadelphia: Churchill Livingstone.

Samuels, P. (2007). Hematologic complications of pregnancy. In S. Gabbe, J. Niebyl, & J. Simpson (Eds.), *Obstetrics: Normal and problem pregnancies* (5th ed.). Philadelphia: Churchill Livingstone.

Tiran, D., & Mack, S. (Eds.), (2000). *Complementary therapies for pregnancy and childbirth* (2nd ed.). Edinburgh: Baillière Tindall.

CHAPTER

35

Acquired Problems of the Newborn

Debbie Fraser

evolve WEBSITE

http://evolve.elsevier.com/Lowdermilk/MWHC/

Audio Glossary
Audio Key Points
Critical Thinking Exercise
- Fetal Alcohol Syndrome

NCLEX Review Questions
Nursing Care Plans
- The Infant Experiencing Drug Withdrawal (Neonatal Abstinence Syndrome)
- The Infant of the Mother with Pregestational or Gestational Diabetes

LEARNING OBJECTIVES

- Summarize the care of the newborn with soft-tissue, skeletal, and nervous system injuries.
- Describe assessment and care of infants with birth trauma.
- Develop a plan of care for a neonate of a mother with diabetes.
- Describe in detail the assessment of a newborn with a suspected infection.
- Formulate nursing diagnoses for the infant and family for common bacterial and viral infections.
- Interpret the evidence available to guide the care of the infant at risk for group B streptococci (GBS) sepsis.
- Review implementation and evaluation of care of infants with infections; include their families.
- Analyze fetal and neonatal effects of maternal substance abuse during pregnancy.
- Describe concerns for fetal and neonatal well-being related to maternal use of caffeine and selective serotonin reuptake inhibitors during pregnancy.
- Describe the assessment and care of a newborn experiencing drug withdrawal (neonatal abstinence syndrome); include the infant's family.

This chapter deals with acquired problems of the newborn. *Acquired problems* refer to those conditions resulting from environmental factors rather than genetic circumstances. The focus is on birth trauma, the infant of a mother with diabetes, neonatal infections, effects of maternal substance abuse on the fetus and neonate, and effects of maternal use of caffeine and antidepressant medications during pregnancy.

BIRTH TRAUMA

Birth trauma or **birth injury** refers to physical injury sustained by a neonate during labor and birth. According to the Agency for Healthcare Research and Quality (AHRQ), the incidence of birth injuries in the United States is 1.84 per 1000 live births, excluding preterm and osteogenesis imperfecta births (AHRQ, 2008). Despite improvements in obstetric techniques; increased use of cesarean surgery for births that would be difficult vaginally; and decreased use of forceps, vacuum extraction, and version and extraction; birth injuries still are an important source of neonatal morbidity. Therefore, the clinician should consider the broad range of birth injuries in the differential diagnosis of neonatal clinical disorders (Mangurten, 2006).

The nurse's contribution to the welfare of the newborn begins with early observation and accurate recording. The prompt reporting of signs that indicate deviations from normal permits early initiation of appropriate therapy. In addition, nurses provide essential support and education to parents whose neonates experience birth injury.

In theory, some birth injuries are avoidable, especially with careful assessment of risk factors and appropriate planning for birth. The use of ultrasonography allows antepartum diagnosis of macrosomia, hydrocephalus, and unusual presentations. Elective cesarean birth can be chosen for some pregnancies to prevent significant birth injury. A small percentage of significant birth injuries are unavoidable despite skilled and competent obstetric care, as in especially difficult or prolonged labor or when the infant is in an abnormal presentation (Mangurten, 2006). Some injuries cannot be anticipated until the specific circumstances occur during birth. Emergency cesarean birth can provide last-minute salvage, but in these circumstances the injury may be truly unavoidable. The same injury can be caused in several ways. For example, a cephalhematoma can result from an obstetric technique such as forceps birth or vacuum extraction or from pressure of the fetal skull against the maternal pelvis.

Many injuries are minor and resolve readily in the neonatal period without treatment. Other traumas require some degree of intervention. A few are considered major trauma and serious enough to be fatal. Major trauma is often the result of instrumentation during birth (forceps or vacuum) and can occur concomitantly with other minor injuries. For example, a neonate who suffers a skull fracture is also likely to have a cephalhematoma (Cunningham, Leveno, Bloom, Hauth, Rouse, & Spong, 2010; Pressler, 2008).

Several factors predispose an infant to birth injuries. Maternal risk factors include age younger than 16 or older than 35, primigravida, uterine dysfunction that leads to prolonged or precipitate labor, preterm or postterm labor, and cephalopelvic disproportion. Oligohydramnios can increase the likelihood of birth trauma. Injury can result from dystocia caused by fetal macrosomia, multifetal gestation, abnormal or difficult presentation (not caused by maternal uterine or pelvic conditions), and congenital anomalies. Intrapartum events that can result in scalp injury include the use of internal monitoring of fetal heart rate (FHR) and collection of fetal scalp blood for acid-base assessment. Obstetric birth techniques can cause injury. Forceps- or vacuum-assisted birth, version and extraction, and cesarean birth are potential contributory factors. Often more than one factor is present, and multiple predisposing factors can be related to a single maternal condition (Mangurten, 2006; Pressler, 2008; Verklan & Lopez, 2011).

Birth injuries are usually classified according to their etiology (predisposing factors or mechanisms of injury) or anatomically. Table 35-1 is an example of anatomic classification of birth injuries.

TABLE 35-1 ANATOMIC CLASSIFICATION OF BIRTH INJURIES

SITE OF INJURY	TYPE OF INJURY
Scalp	Caput succedaneum Subgaleal hemorrhage Cephalhematoma
Skull	Linear fracture Depressed fracture Occipital osteodiastasis
Intracranial	Epidural hematoma Subdural hematoma (laceration of falx, tentorium, or superficial veins) Subarachnoid hemorrhage Cerebral contusion Cerebellar contusion Intracerebellar hematoma
Spinal cord (cervical)	Vertebral artery injury Intraspinal hemorrhage Spinal cord transection or injury
Plexus	Erb-Duchenne palsy Klumpke paralysis Total (mixed) brachial plexus injury Horner syndrome Diaphragmatic paralysis Lumbosacral plexus injury
Cranial and peripheral nerve	Radial nerve palsy Medial nerve palsy Sciatic nerve palsy Laryngeal nerve palsy Diaphragmatic paralysis Facial nerve palsy

Source: Verklan. M., & Lopez, S. (2011). *Neurologic disorders.* In S. Gardner, B. Carter, M. Enzman-Hines, & J. Hernandez (Eds.), *Merenstein & Gardner's handbook of neonatal intensive care* (7th ed.). St Louis: Mosby.

Soft-Tissue Injuries

Erythema, ecchymoses, petechiae, abrasions, lacerations, and edema of buttocks and extremities can be present. Localized discoloration can appear over presenting or dependent parts. Ecchymoses and edema can appear anywhere on the body and especially on the presenting body part from the application of forceps or vacuum cup. They also can result from manipulation of the infant's body during birth.

Bruises over the face can be the result of face presentation (Fig. 35-1). In a breech presentation, bruising and swelling can occur over the buttocks or genitalia (Fig. 35-2). The skin over the entire head can be ecchymotic and covered with petechiae caused by a tight nuchal cord. Petechiae, or pinpoint hemorrhagic areas, acquired during birth can extend over the upper portion of the trunk and face. These lesions are benign if they disappear within 2 days of birth and no new lesions appear. Ecchymoses and petechiae can be signs of a more serious disorder, such as thrombocytopenic purpura, if the hemorrhagic areas do not disappear spontaneously in 2 days. To differentiate hemorrhagic areas from skin rashes and discolorations such as mongolian spots, the nurse blanches the skin with two fingers. Because extravasated blood remains within the tissues, petechiae and ecchymoses do not blanch.

Forceps injury occurs at the site of application of the instrument. Forceps injury typically has a linear configuration across both sides of the face, outlining the placement of the forceps. The affected areas are kept clean to minimize the risk of secondary infection. These injuries usually resolve spontaneously within several days with no specific therapy.

Accidental lacerations can be inflicted with a scalpel during cesarean birth or with scissors during an episiotomy. These cuts can occur on any part of the body but most often are found on the scalp, buttocks, and thighs. Usually they are superficial, needing only to be kept clean. Butterfly adhesive strips will usually hold together the edges of more serious lacerations. Rarely are sutures needed.

Two of the most commonly occurring birth injuries are subconjunctival (scleral) and retinal hemorrhages. These injuries result from rupture of capillaries caused by increased *intracranial pressure (ICP)* during birth. They usually clear within 5 days after birth and present no problems; however, parents need reassurance about their presence.

Caput succedaneum and cephalhematoma are commonly seen in neonates, often as the result of pressure on the fetal head pushing through a dilated cervix. These are discussed in Chapter 23.

A more serious injury is **subgaleal hemorrhage,** which is bleeding into the subgaleal compartment (see Fig. 23-9, *C*).

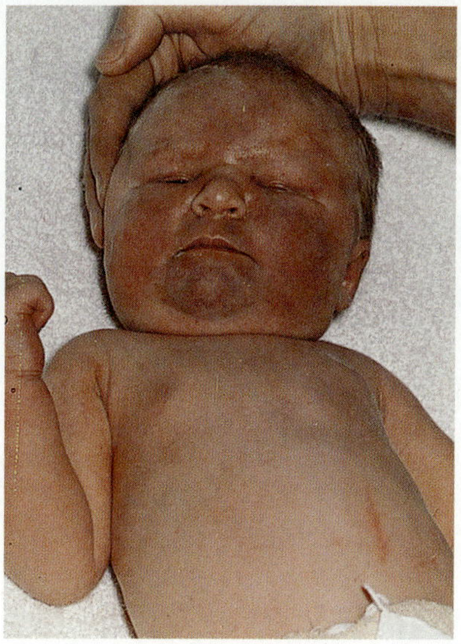

FIG. 35-1 Marked bruising on the entire face of an infant born vaginally after face presentation. Less severe ecchymoses were present on the extremities. Phototherapy was required for treatment of jaundice resulting from the breakdown of accumulated blood. (From O'Doherty, N. [1986]. *Neonatology: Micro atlas of the newborn.* Nutley, NJ: Hoffmann-La Roche.)

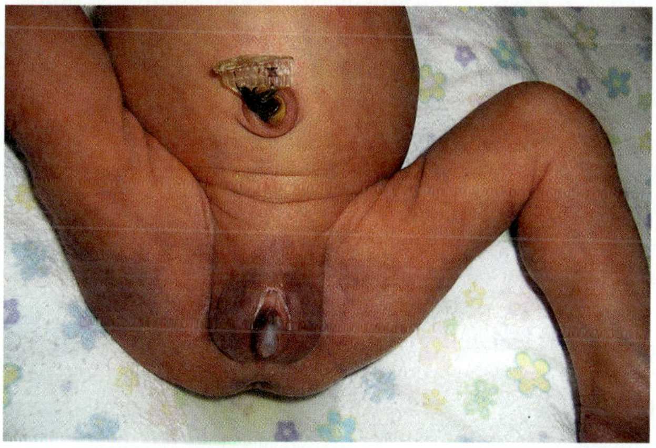

FIG. 35-2 Swelling of the genitals and bruising of the buttocks after a breech birth. Note the position of the infant's legs. (Courtesy Cheryl Briggs, RNC, Annapolis, MD.)

The subgaleal compartment is a potential space that contains loosely arranged connective tissue; it is located beneath the galea aponeurosis, the tendinous sheath that connects the frontal and occipital muscles and forms the inner surface of the scalp. The injury occurs as a result of forces that compress and then drag the head through the pelvic outlet (Verklan & Lopez, 2011). The bleeding extends beyond bone, often posteriorly into the neck, and continues after birth, with the potential for serious complications such as anemia, hypovolemic shock, or even death. Early detection of the hemorrhage is vital; serial head circumference measurements and inspection of the back of the neck for increasing edema and a firm mass are essential. A boggy scalp, pallor, tachycardia, and increasing head circumference can also be early signs of a subgaleal hemorrhage (Doumouchtsis & Arulkumaran, 2006). Computed tomography (CT) or magnetic resonance imaging (MRI) is useful in confirming the diagnosis. Replacement of lost blood and clotting factors is required in acute cases of hemorrhage. Another possible early sign of subgaleal hemorrhage is a forward and lateral

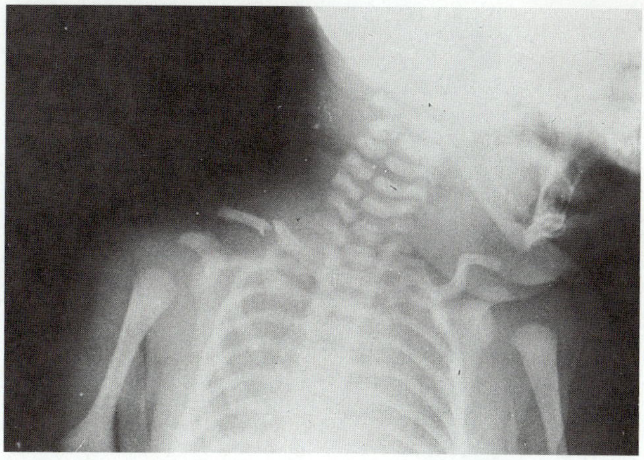

FIG. 35-3 Fractured clavicle after shoulder dystocia. (From O'Doherty, N. [1986]. *Neonatology: Micro atlas of the newborn.* Nutley, NJ: Hoffmann-La Roche.)

positioning of the infant's ears because the hematoma extends posteriorly. Monitoring the infant for changes in level of consciousness and a decrease in hematocrit is key to early recognition and management. An increase in serum bilirubin levels can be seen as a result of the breakdown of blood cells within the hematoma.

Skeletal Injuries

The newborn's immature, flexible skull can withstand a great degree of deformation (molding) before fracture results. Considerable force is required to fracture the newborn's skull. Two types of skull fractures typically are identified in the newborn: linear fractures and depressed fractures. The location of the fracture and involvement of underlying structures determine its significance. Linear fractures are most common in the parietal bones, require no treatment, and are usually of no clinical significance. Whenever a cephalhematoma or subarachnoid hemorrhage is present, a skull fracture should be suspected (Doumouchtsis & Arulkumaran, 2008).

The soft skull can become indented without laceration of either the skin or the dural membrane. These depressed fractures, or "ping-pong ball" indentations, can occur during difficult births from pressure of the head on the bony pelvis. They also can occur as a result of injudicious application of forceps. A CT scan is done to rule out bone fragments or underlying injury of the brain tissue. Management of depressed skull fractures is controversial; many resolve without intervention. Nonsurgical elevation of the indentation by using a manual breast pump or vacuum extractor has been reported. Surgery can be required in the presence of bone fragments or signs of increased ICP (Doumouchtsis & Arulkumaran, 2008).

The clavicle is the bone most often fractured during birth. Generally the break is in the middle third of the bone (Fig. 35-3). Dystocia, particularly shoulder impaction, is a risk factor for clavicular fracture. Other risk factors include vacuum-assisted birth and birth weight greater than 4000 g. Limited movement of the arm, crepitus over the bone, and the absence of the Moro reflex on the affected side are diagnostic. Except for use of gentle rather than vigorous handling, no accepted treatment for fractured clavicle exists, and the prognosis is good. A sign posted on the bassinet will alert care providers to the

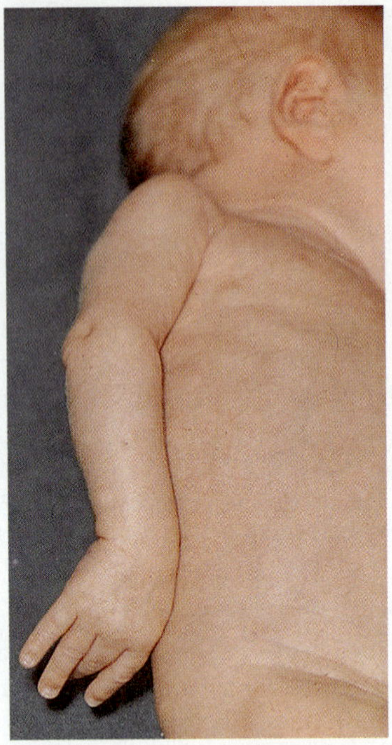

FIG. 35-4 Erb-Duchenne palsy in newborn infant. The Moro reflex was absent in right upper extremity. Recovery was complete. (From O'Doherty, N. [1986]. *Neonatology: Micro atlas of the newborn.* Nutley, NJ: Hoffmann-La Roche.)

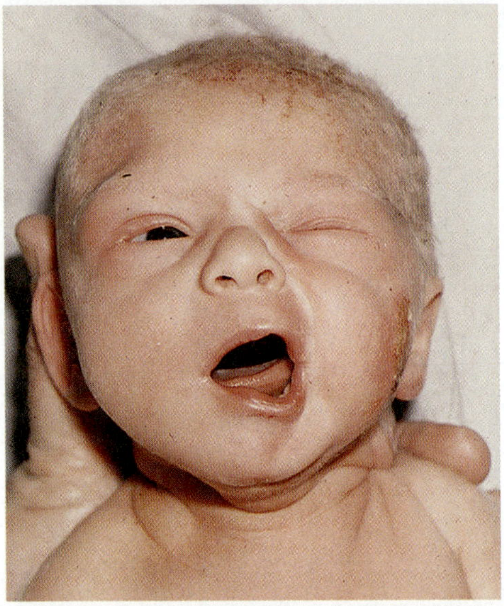

FIG. 35-5 Facial paralysis 15 minutes after forceps birth. Absence of movement on affected side is especially noticeable when infant cries. (From O'Doherty, N. [1986]. *Neonatology: Micro atlas of the newborn.* Nutley, NJ: Hoffmann-La Roche.)

need for careful handling. The figure-eight bandage appropriate for an older child should not be used for a newborn.

The humerus and femur can be fractured during a difficult birth. Fractures in newborns generally heal rapidly. Immobilization is accomplished with slings, splints, swaddling, and other devices.

The parents need support in handling these infants because they often are fearful of hurting them. Parents are encouraged to practice handling, changing, and feeding the affected neonate under the guidance of nursing staff prior to hospital discharge. This increases their confidence and knowledge and facilitates attachment. A plan for follow-up therapy is developed with the parents so that the times and arrangements for therapy are acceptable to them.

Peripheral Nervous System Injuries

Erb-Duchenne palsy (also called **Erb's palsy** or **brachial plexus injury**) is the most common type of paralysis associated with a difficult birth, occurring at rates of 0.5 to 2 per 1000 live births (Volpe, 2008) (Fig. 35-4). An increased risk of brachial plexus injury occurs with birth weight greater than 4000 g, shoulder dystocia, vaginal breech birth, forceps- or vacuum-assisted birth, maternal diabetes, and a prolonged second stage of labor. Injury to the upper plexus results from stretching or pulling the head away from the shoulder during the difficult birth. The arm hangs limply alongside the body. The shoulder and arm are adducted and internally rotated. The elbow is extended, and the forearm is pronated, with the wrist and fingers flexed; a grasp reflex can be present because finger and wrist movement remains normal (Adams-Chapman & Stoll, 2007).

Treatment is by intermittent immobilization across the upper abdomen, proper positioning, and range-of-motion (ROM) exercises. Gentle manipulation and ROM exercises are delayed until about the fifth day to prevent additional injury to the brachial plexus. Immobilization can be accomplished with a brace or splint or by pinning the infant's sleeve to his or her shirt.

Damage to the lower plexus or *Klumpke palsy* is less common. With lower arm paralysis the wrist and hand are flaccid, the grasp reflex is absent, and deep tendon reflexes are present; dependent edema and cyanosis can occur in the affected hand. Treatment consists of placing the hand in a neutral position, padding the fist, and gently exercising the wrist and fingers.

If edema or hemorrhage is responsible for the paralysis, the prognosis is good, and recovery can be expected in a few weeks. If laceration of the nerves has occurred and healing does not result in return of function within a few months, surgery can be indicated; however, return of function is variable. Full recovery is expected in 88% to 92% of infants (Volpe, 2008).

Facial paralysis (palsy) (Fig. 35-5) generally is caused by pressure on the facial nerve during birth. Risk factors include a prolonged second stage of labor and forceps-assisted birth. The face on the affected side is flattened and unresponsive to the grimace that accompanies crying or stimulation and the eye will remain open on the affected side. Moreover, the forehead will not wrinkle. Usually the infant's face appears distorted, especially when crying. Often the condition is transitory, resolving within hours or days of birth. Permanent paralysis is rare.

Treatment involves assistance with feeding, prevention of damage to the cornea of the open eye with the application of artificial tears or taping the eye closed, and supportive care of the parents. Feeding can be prolonged, with the milk flowing out the newborn's mouth around the nipple on the affected side. The parents will need understanding and sympathetic encouragement while learning how to feed and care for the infant, as well as how to hold and cuddle the baby.

Phrenic nerve injury almost always occurs as a component of brachial plexus injury rather than as an isolated problem. Injury is usually the result of traction on the neck and arm during birth. Injury to the phrenic nerve is usually unilateral, but can be bilateral, and results in diaphragmatic paralysis. Cyanosis and irregular thoracic respirations, with no abdominal movement on inspiration, are characteristic of paralysis of the diaphragm. Babies with diaphragmatic paralysis usually require mechanical ventilatory support, at least for the first few days after birth, and are at risk of developing pneumonia. In the presence of persistent respiratory distress, diaphragmatic pacing or surgical correction can be necessary.

Central Nervous System Injuries

All types of **intracranial hemorrhage (ICH)** occur in newborns. ICH as a result of birth trauma is more likely to occur in the term, large infant. Risk factors for ICH include primiparity, advanced maternal age, vacuum- or forceps-assisted birth, precipitous or prolonged second stage of labor, and increased fetal size (Limperopoulos, Robertson, Sullivan, Bassan, & du Plessis, 2009). In the newborn, more than one type of hemorrhage frequently occurs.

Subdural hemorrhage (hematoma), a collection of blood in the subdural space, most often is produced by the stretching and tearing of the large veins in the tentorium of the cerebellum, the dural membrane that separates the cerebrum from the cerebellum. When this type of bleeding occurs, the typical history includes a nulliparous mother, with the total labor and birth occurring in less than 2 or 3 hours; a difficult birth involving forceps application; or a large for gestational age (LGA) infant. Subdural hematoma occurs less frequently today because of improvements in obstetric care. However, it is especially serious because of its inaccessibility to aspiration by subdural tap (Askin & Wilson, 2007). Neonates with subdural hemorrhage usually present with apnea, unequal pupils, irritability, tense fontanel, seizures, and even coma (Doumouchtsis & Arulkamaran, 2008).

Subarachnoid hemorrhage, the most common type of ICH, occurs in term infants as a result of trauma and in preterm infants as a result of hypoxia. Small hemorrhages are the most common. Bleeding is of venous origin, and underlying contusion also can occur (Askin & Wilson, 2007).

The clinical presentation of hemorrhage in the term infant can vary considerably. In many infants signs are absent, and hemorrhaging is diagnosed only because of abnormal findings on lumbar puncture (e.g., red blood cells in the cerebrospinal fluid [CSF]). The initial clinical manifestations of neonatal subarachnoid hemorrhage can be the early onset of alternating depression and irritability, with refractory seizures or apnea. Occasionally the infant appears normal initially and then has seizures on the second or third day of life, followed by no apparent after effects.

In general, nursing care of an infant with ICH is supportive and includes monitoring of ventilatory and intravenous (IV) therapy, observation and management of seizures, and prevention of increased ICP. Minimal handling to promote rest and reduce stress should guide nursing care (Askin & Wilson, 2007).

Spinal cord injuries are usually the result of breech births, especially those difficult ones in which version and extraction were used. Brow and face presentations, dystocia, preterm birth, maternal nulliparity, and precipitate birth also have been identified as predisposing factors in these types of injuries. Stretching of the spinal cord, usually by forceful longitudinal traction on the trunk while the head is still firmly engaged in the pelvis, is the most common mechanism of injury. This injury is rarely seen today because cesarean birth is often used for breech presentation (Mangurten, 2006).

Clinical manifestations depend on the severity and location of the injury. High cervical cord injuries are more likely to cause stillbirths or rapid death of the neonate. Lower lesions cause an acute spinal cord syndrome. Common signs of spinal shock include flaccid extremities, diaphragmatic breathing, paralyzed abdominal movements, atonic anal sphincter, and distended bladder.

Therapy is supportive and usually unsatisfactory. Infants who survive present a therapeutic challenge that requires combined treatment from many health care providers: pediatrician, neurologist, neurosurgeon, urologist, orthopedist, nurse, physical therapist, and occupational therapist. Parents need to understand fully the implications of severe injury to the spinal cord and the overwhelming implications it presents for the family. (See the Nursing Process box: Birth Injury.)

INFANTS OF MOTHERS WITH DIABETES

No single physiologic or biochemical event can explain the diverse clinical manifestations seen in the infants of mothers with diabetes or infants of mothers with gestational diabetes. A better understanding of maternal and fetal metabolism, resulting in stricter control of maternal diabetes and improved obstetric and neonatal intensive care, has led to a decrease in the perinatal mortality rate in diabetic pregnancy. However, maternal diabetes continues to play a significant role in neonatal morbidity and mortality. Compared to nondiabetic pregnancies, infants born to mothers with diabetes are at an increased risk for complications such as congenital anomalies, macrosomia, birth trauma, perinatal asphyxia, stillbirth, preterm birth, respiratory distress syndrome (RDS), hypoglycemia, hypocalcemia, hypomagnesemia, cardiomyopathy, hyperbilirubinemia, and polycythemia. The degree of risk depends on the severity and duration of maternal disease. For example, women with vascular complications are more likely to have infants who are small for gestational age (SGA). All infants born to mothers with diabetes are at some risk for complications. The likelihood of these complications is reduced when maternal glucose levels are maintained within normal limits during the periconception period and during pregnancy (Cunningham, et al., 2010; Dudley, 2007; Jovanovic & Nakai, 2006).

Pathophysiology

The mechanisms responsible for the problems seen in infants of mothers with diabetes are not fully understood. In early pregnancy, fluctuations in blood glucose levels and episodes of ketoacidosis are believed to cause congenital anomalies. Later in pregnancy, when the mother's pancreas cannot release sufficient insulin to meet increased demands, maternal hyperglycemia results. Increased amounts of glucose cross the placenta and stimulate the fetal pancreas to release insulin. The combination of the increased supply of maternal glucose and other nutrients and increased fetal insulin results in excessive fetal growth called *macrosomia* (see later discussion).

Hyperinsulinemia accounts for many of the problems of the fetus or infant. In addition to fluctuating glucose levels,

NURSING PROCESS

Birth Injury

ASSESSMENT

- Maternal history including age, gravidity, parity, oligohydramnios, preterm or postterm labor, multifetal gestation, uterine dysfunction
- Intrapartum events: prolonged or precipitate labor, cephalopelvic disproportion, abnormal or difficult presentation, shoulder dystocia, use of internal fetal monitoring, collection of fetal scalp blood for acid-base measurement, forceps, vacuum extraction, version and extraction, cesarean birth
- Neonatal risk factors including prematurity, macrosomia, congenital anomalies
- Parental reactions, knowledge, and level of comfort in caring for infant with birth injury

NURSING DIAGNOSES

Possible nursing diagnoses include:

Infant

***Impaired Physical Mobility* related to:**
- brachial plexus injury

***Impaired Gas Exchange* related to:**
- diaphragmatic paralysis (partial or complete)

***Acute Pain* related to:**
- injury

***Injury* related to:**
- malpresentation, difficult birth, shoulder dystocia

Parents and Family

Anxiety* related to *Deficient Knowledge Regarding:
- injury and its cause
- management and therapy
- prognosis

***Grieving* related to:**
- possible sequelae of the birth injury

EXPECTED OUTCOMES OF CARE

Meeting the unique needs of the birth-injured newborn requires constant vigilance. Expected outcomes are established and priorities assigned. The overall outcomes for care of infants with birth trauma include:

- The newborn will have minimal or no sequelae of trauma.
- The infant will receive prompt and appropriate treatment.
- The parents will initiate and maintain a positive parent-infant relationship.
- The parents' and family's educational needs regarding the injury and its management will be met.

PLAN OF CARE AND INTERVENTIONS

Care of the infant with a birth injury is individualized based on the type of injury. See discussion on pp. 837–841.

EVALUATION

The nurse can determine that care has been effective if the outcomes for care have been achieved. That is, the injury receives prompt and appropriate therapy, the newborn has no or minimal sequelae of trauma, and the parents understand how to care for the infant.

maternal vascular involvement or superimposed maternal infection adversely affects the fetus. Normally, maternal blood has a more alkaline pH than does the carbon dioxide–rich fetal blood. This phenomenon encourages the exchange of oxygen and carbon dioxide across the placental membrane. When the maternal blood is more acidotic than the fetal blood, such as during ketoacidosis, little carbon dioxide or oxygen exchange occurs at the level of the placenta. The mortality rate for unborn babies resulting from an episode of maternal ketoacidosis may be as high as 50% or more (Lindsay, 2006).

Congenital Anomalies

The incidence of congenital anomalies among mothers with pregestational diabetes is more than three times that of pregnant women who do not have diabetes (Correa, Gilboa, Besser, Botto, Moore, & Hobbs, 2008). Elevated fasting blood glucose levels are correlated with an increased risk for anomalies in women with type 1 and type 2 diabetes (Jovanovic & Nakai, 2006). Gestational diabetes that is diagnosed in mid- to late pregnancy is usually not associated with an increased incidence of congenital anomalies. However, the risk of anomalies is increased in women with gestational diabetes with elevated fasting glucose or A_{1C} levels, especially during early pregnancy (Metzger, Buchanan, Coustan, de Leiva, Dunger, Hadden, et al., 2007). There is an increased incidence of congenital anomalies among women with gestational diabetes with prepregnancy obesity (Correa et al., 2008). In most defects associated with diabetic pregnancies, the structural abnormality occurs before the eighth week after conception. This reinforces the importance of control of blood glucose both before conception and in the early stages of pregnancy.

The most frequently occurring anomalies involve the cardiac, renal, musculoskeletal, and central nervous systems. The incidence of congenital heart lesions is three to five times higher than in the general population (Corrigan, Brazil, & McAuliffe, 2009). Coarctation of the aorta, transposition of the great vessels, and atrial or ventricular septal defects are the most common cardiac anomalies occurring in infants of mothers with diabetes. In the genitourinary system, renal agenesis (failure of the kidney to develop) and obstruction of the urinary tract have been associated with maternal diabetes. Central nervous system (CNS) anomalies include anencephaly, encephalocele, myelomeningocele, and hydrocephalus. The musculoskeletal system can be affected by *caudal regression syndrome* (*sacral agenesis*, with weakness or deformities of the lower extremities; malformation and fixation of the hip joints; and shortening or deformity of the femurs). Other defects noted in this population include gastrointestinal atresia and urinary tract malformations (see Chapter 36). Neonatal small left colon syndrome, also called lazy colon syndrome, occurs in up to 50% of infants born to mothers with diabetes (Thigpen, 2007). This syndrome is suspected when the infant fails to pass meconium and has abdominal distention and bile-stained vomitus. Contrast enemas show a greatly diminished caliber of the left colon from the splenic flexure to the anus. The syndrome is transient, with normal bowel function developing early in infancy.

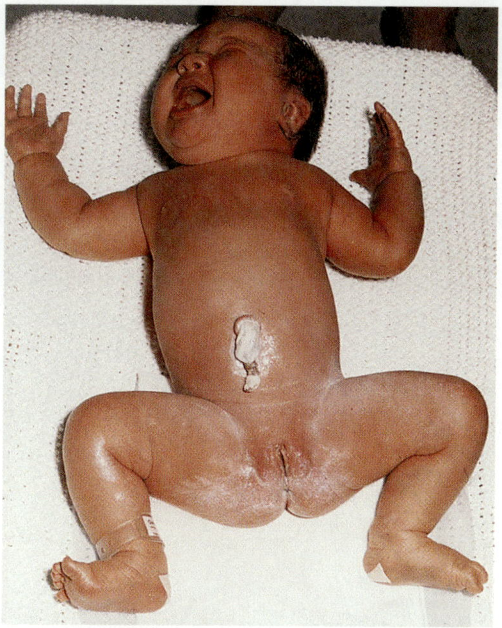

FIG. 35-6 Macrosomia. (From O'Doherty, N. [1986]. *Neonatology: Micro atlas of the newborn.* Nutley, NJ: Hoffmann-La Roche.)

Macrosomia

Despite improvements in the control of maternal blood glucose levels, the incidence of **macrosomia** is 50% in women with gestational diabetes and 40% in women with type 1 diabetes (Landon, Catalano, & Gabbe, 2007). At birth, the typical LGA infant has a round, cherubic ("tomato" or cushingoid) face, a chubby body, and a plethoric or flushed complexion (Fig. 35-6). The infant has enlarged internal organs (hepatosplenomegaly, splanchnomegaly, cardiomegaly) and increased body fat, especially around the shoulders. The placenta and umbilical cord are larger than average. Because insulin does not cross the blood-brain barrier, the brain is the only organ that is not enlarged. Infants of mothers with diabetes can be LGA but physiologically immature.

Insulin has been proposed as the primary growth hormone for intrauterine development. Maternal diabetes results in elevated maternal levels of amino acids and free fatty acids, along with hyperglycemia. As the nutrients cross the placenta, the fetal pancreas responds by producing insulin to match the fuel supply. The resulting accelerated protein synthesis, together with a deposition of excessive glycogen and fat stores, is responsible for the typical macrosomic infant. This is the infant most at risk for the neonatal complications of hypoglycemia, hypocalcemia, hyperviscosity, and hyperbilirubinemia. The excessive amounts of metabolic fuels presented to the fetus from the mother and the consequent fetal hyperinsulinism represent the basic pathologic mechanism in the diabetic pregnancy (Lindsay, 2006).

The excessive shoulder size in these infants often leads to dystocia, particularly because the head may be smaller in proportion to the shoulders than in a nonmacrosomic infant (Esakoff, Cheng, Sparks, & Caughey, 2009). Macrosomic infants, born vaginally or by cesarean after a trial of labor, can incur birth trauma such as clavicle fracture or Erb-Duchenne palsy. Despite increased vigilance in screening, and improvements in ultrasound techniques, the determination of macrosomia can be difficult to make.

Birth Trauma and Perinatal Hypoxia

Birth injury (resulting from macrosomia or method of birth) and perinatal hypoxia occur more often in infants of mothers with diabetes. Examples of birth trauma include cephalhematoma; paralysis of the facial nerve (cranial nerve VII) (see Fig. 35-5); fracture of the clavicle or humerus; brachial plexus paralysis, usually Erb-Duchenne palsy (right upper arm) (see Fig. 35-4); and phrenic nerve paralysis, invariably associated with diaphragmatic paralysis.

Respiratory Distress Syndrome

RDS in infants of mothers with diabetes is a much less common occurrence than in the past because of improved protocols to manage maternal glucose levels and enhanced antepartum fetal surveillance techniques to assess lung maturity. Among infants born to women with well-controlled diabetes who give birth at term, the risk of RDS is similar to that of the general population (Landon et al., 2007). RDS that occurs among infants of mothers with diabetes is more likely to be related to gestational age rather than to maternal diabetes (Cunningham et al., 2010). However, not all pregnant women with diabetes have well-controlled glucose levels. Maternal hyperglycemia can affect fetal lung maturity. In the fetus exposed to high levels of maternal glucose, synthesis of surfactant can be delayed because of the high fetal serum levels of insulin and/or glucose (Weindling, 2009). Fetal lung maturity, as evidenced by a lecithin/sphingomyelin (L/S) ratio of 2:1, is not reassuring if the mother has diabetes mellitus. For the infants of such mothers, an L/S ratio of 3:1 or more or the presence of **phosphatidylglycerol** (a component of surfactant) in the amniotic fluid is more indicative of adequate lung maturity.

Hypoglycemia

Hypoglycemia (blood glucose levels less than 40 mg/dl in term infants) affects many infants of mothers with diabetes. LGA and preterm infants have the highest risk. After constant exposure to high circulating levels of glucose, hyperplasia of the fetal pancreas occurs, resulting in hyperinsulinemia. Disruption of the fetal glucose supply occurs with the clamping of the umbilical cord, and the neonate's blood glucose level decreases rapidly in the presence of fetal hyperinsulinism. It can take several days for the newborn to regulate the secretion of insulin in response to a lower postnatal supply of glucose. Hypoglycemia is most common in the macrosomic infant, but the nurse should monitor blood glucose levels in all infants of mothers with known or suspected diabetes.

Asymptomatic or symptomatic hypoglycemia most frequently manifests within the first 1 to 6 hours after birth. Signs of hypoglycemia include jitteriness, apnea, tachypnea, and cyanosis. Many infants with hypoglycemia remain asymptomatic. Significant hypoglycemia can result in seizures. Hypoglycemia is worsened by the presence of hypothermia or respiratory distress.

Hypocalcemia and Hypomagnesemia

Hypocalcemia and hypomagnesemia have been reported to occur in as many as 50% of infants born to mothers with diabetes (Kalhan & Parimi, 2006). A number of these cases are related to hypoxia or prematurity; however, the overall incidence of hypocalcemia is higher than in nondiabetic women. Hypomagnesemia is believed to develop because of maternal renal losses that occur in diabetes. Hypocalcemia is associated with preterm birth, birth trauma, and perinatal asphyxia. Signs of hypocalcemia are similar to those of hypoglycemia, but they occur between 24 and 36 hours of age. Hypocalcemia should be considered if therapy for hypoglycemia is ineffective.

Cardiomyopathy

All infants of mothers with diabetes need careful observation for cardiomyopathy (disease affecting the structure and function of the heart) because an increased heart size is often found in these infants. Cardiomyopathy is more likely to occur in cases of poorly controlled maternal diabetes. Two types of cardiomyopathy can occur: hypertrophic and nonhypertrophic. Clinicians must be alert to identify the type of lesion correctly so that appropriate therapy is instituted. Both types of lesions are associated with respiratory symptoms and congestive heart failure.

Hypertrophic cardiomyopathy (HCM) is characterized by a hypercontractile and thickened myocardium. The ventricular walls are thickened, as is the septum, which in severe cases results in outflow tract obstructions. The mitral valve is poorly functioning. In nonhypertrophic cardiomyopathy (non-HCM), the myocardium is poorly contractile and overstretched. The ventricles are larger, and no outflow obstruction is found. Most infants are asymptomatic, but severe outflow obstruction can cause left ventricular heart failure.

Hyperbilirubinemia and Polycythemia

Infants of mothers with diabetes are at increased risk of developing hyperbilirubinemia. Many infants also are polycythemic. Polycythemia increases blood viscosity, thereby impairing circulation. In addition, this increased number of red blood cells to be hemolyzed increases the potential bilirubin load that the neonate must clear. The excessive red blood cells are produced in extramedullary foci (liver and spleen) in addition to the usual sites in bone marrow; therefore, liver function and bilirubin clearance can be adversely affected. Bruising associated with birth of a macrosomic infant will contribute further to high bilirubin levels.

Nursing Care

Nursing care depends on the neonate's particular problems. General care of the compromised infant is addressed in Chapter 37. If the maternal blood glucose level was well controlled throughout the pregnancy, the infant may require only monitoring. Because euglycemia (normal blood glucose levels) is not always possible, the nurse must promptly recognize and treat any consequences of maternal diabetes that arise. The most common problems experienced by infants of diabetic mothers that require intervention include birth trauma and perinatal asphyxia; RDS; difficult metabolic transition, including hypoglycemia and hypocalcemia; and congenital anomalies (see previous sections and the Nursing Care Plan: The Infant of the Mother with Pregestational or Gestational Diabetes).

TABLE 35-2 RISK FACTORS FOR NEONATAL SEPSIS

SOURCE	RISK FACTORS
Maternal	Low socioeconomic status
	Late or no prenatal care
	Poor nutrition
	Substance abuse
	Recently acquired sexually transmitted infection
	Untreated focal infection (urinary tract infection, vaginal, cervical)
	Systemic infection
	Fever
Intrapartum	Premature rupture of fetal membranes
	Maternal fever
	Chorioamnionitis
	Prolonged labor
	Premature labor
	Use of fetal scalp electrode
Neonatal	Multiple gestation
	Male
	Birth asphyxia
	Meconium aspiration
	Congenital anomalies of skin or mucous membranes
	Metabolic disorders (e.g., galactosemia)
	Absence of spleen
	Low birth weight
	Preterm birth
	Malnourishment
	Formula feeding
	Prolonged hospitalization
	Mechanical ventilation
	Umbilical artery catheterization or use of other vascular catheters

Source: Edwards, M. (2006). Postnatal bacterial infections. In R. Martin, A. Fanaroff, & M. Walsh (Eds.), *Fanaroff and Martin's neonatal-perinatal medicine: Diseases of the fetus and infant* (8th ed.). Philadelphia: Mosby.

NEONATAL INFECTIONS

Sepsis

Sepsis (presence of microorganisms or their toxins in blood or other tissues) continues to be one of the most significant causes of neonatal morbidity and mortality. The newborn infant is susceptible to infection. Maternal immunoglobulin M (IgM) does not cross the placenta. IgG levels in term infants are equal to maternal levels; however, in preterm infants the amount of IgG is directly proportional to gestational age (Stoll & Adams-Chapman, 2007). IgA and IgM require time to reach optimal levels after birth. Phagocytosis is less efficient. Serum complement levels are inadequate; serum complement (C1 through C6) is involved in immunologic reactions, some of which kill or lyse bacteria and enhance phagocytosis. Dysmaturity seen with intrauterine growth restriction (IUGR) and preterm and postdate birth further compromises the neonate's immune system.

Table 35-2 outlines risk factors for neonatal sepsis. Special precautions for preventing infection, as well as prompt recognition when it occurs, are necessary for optimal newborn care. Neonatal infections can be acquired in utero, during labor and birth, during resuscitation, and during the hospital stay.

Prenatal acquisition of infection occurs by organisms placentally transferred directly into the fetal circulatory system and transmitted from infected amniotic fluid, such as with herpes simplex virus (HSV), cytomegalovirus (CMV), and rubella. Microorganisms also can ascend from the vagina and pass

NURSING CARE PLAN

The Infant of the Mother with Pregestational or Gestational Diabetes

NURSING DIAGNOSIS

Risk for injury related to hypoglycemia, hypocalcemia, polycythemia, or hyperbilirubinemia secondary to maternal diabetes

Expected Outcome

Infant will exhibit blood glucose, serum calcium, hematocrit, and serum bilirubin levels that are within normal limits.

Nursing Interventions/*Rationales*

- Monitor blood glucose levels (<40 mg/dl indicative of hypoglycemia); serum calcium levels (<7 mg/dl indicative of hypocalcemia); and serum bilirubin levels (>15 mg/dl indicative of hyperbilirubinemia) *to assess and detect early onset to prevent complications.*
- Observe for signs of hypoglycemia (jitteriness, twitching, lethargy, apathy, convulsions, cyanosis, sweating, eye rolling, refusal to eat); hypocalcemia (jitteriness, apnea, high-pitched cry, abdominal distention); polycythemia (plethora); and hyperbilirubinemia (jaundice) *to assess and detect signs of onset to prevent complications.*
- Provide early feeding of infant, increased milk feedings/calcium supplements per physician order *to prevent or treat early hypocalcemia;* early and frequent feedings *to reduce hematocrit and enhance excretion of bilirubin in stool.*
- Administer intravenous glucose infusions per physician's order for infants with symptomatic hypoglycemia or those too ill to be fed orally safely *to treat hypoglycemia.*
- Reduce adverse environmental factors (e.g., excessive handling, cold stress) *that can predispose infant to hypoglycemia.*

NURSING DIAGNOSIS

Risk for impaired gas exchange related to lung immaturity or cardiomyopathy secondary to maternal diabetes

Expected Outcome

Infant will exhibit signs of adequate oxygenation (respiratory rate, rhythm, and amplitude, and blood gas levels within normal limits).

Nursing Interventions/*Rationales*

- Monitor infant's vital signs, oxygen saturation levels, blood gas levels per order, patency of airway *to evaluate pulmonary and circulatory status.*
- Avoid activities that can reduce body temperature and lead to cold stress, *which can induce respiratory distress.*
- Suction as needed *to keep airway patent and prevent aspiration.*
- Have resuscitation equipment and oxygen available *for prompt treatment of respiratory distress.*

NURSING DIAGNOSIS

Risk for ineffective thermoregulation related to physiologic immaturity; potential for infection related to immature immunologic defenses/environmental exposure. (See the Nursing Care Plan for the Normal Newborn in Chapter 24.)

NURSING DIAGNOSIS

Parental anxiety (risk for powerlessness, situational low self-esteem, ineffective coping) related to neonate's condition, management, and prognosis

Expected Outcome

Parents demonstrate understanding of prognosis and therapy for infant.

Nursing Interventions/*Rationales*

- Explain potential effects of maternal diabetic condition on newborn *to relieve fear of unknown and support ability to cope.*
- Encourage open communication (e.g., inform parents of ongoing condition, procedures, and treatment; answer questions; correct misperceptions; actively listen to parental concerns) *to provide support and help provide sense of control.*
- Encourage parents to interact with infant and to become involved in care routines *to foster emotional connection and to increase parental self-esteem.*

through the cervix. The membranes become infected and can rupture. Infection of the fetal skin and the respiratory or gastrointestinal tract can result.

During birth, contact with an infected birth canal can result in generalized or local infection. The upper airway and the gastrointestinal tract are the principal pathways for generalized infections. The conjunctiva and the oral cavity are the usual sites of local infection.

Postnatal infection is sometimes acquired during resuscitation or through the introduction of foreign objects such as indwelling catheters or endotracheal tubes. Nursery-associated infections may be transferred to the infant by the hands of the parents or health care personnel or spread from contaminated equipment. The umbilicus is a receptive site for cutaneous infection leading to sepsis (Edwards, 2006).

Neonatal bacterial infection is classified into two patterns according to the time of presentation. Early-onset or congenital sepsis usually manifests within 24 to 72 hours after birth, progresses more rapidly than later-onset infection, and has a mortality rate between 3% and 50% (Palazzi, Klein, & Baker, 2006). Early-onset infection is usually caused by microorganisms from the normal flora of the maternal vaginal tract, including group B streptococci, *Haemophilus influenzae, Listeria monocytogenes, Escherichia coli,* and *Streptococcus pneumoniae* (Venkatesh, Adams, & Weisman, 2011). It is associated with a history of obstetric complications, such as preterm labor, premature rupture of membranes, maternal fever during labor, and chorioamnionitis (Palazzi et al.).

Late-onset sepsis, occurring at approximately 7 to 30 days of age, can include maternally derived infection or health care–associated infection; the offending organisms are usually staphylococci, *Klebsiella* organisms, enterococci, *E. coli,* and *Pseudomonas,* or *Candida* species (Stoll & Adams-Chapman, 2007). Coagulase-negative staphylococci, considered to be primarily a contaminant in older children and adults, are commonly found to be the cause of septicemia in extremely low-birth-weight (ELBW) and very low-birth-weight (VLBW) infants. Additional infections of concern include methicillin-resistant *Staphylococcus aureus* (MRSA), vancomycin-resistant enterococci, and multidrug-resistant gram-negative pathogens (Stoll, 2007). Bacterial invasion can occur through sites such as the umbilical stump; the skin; mucous membranes of the eye, nose, pharynx, and ear; and internal systems such as the respiratory, nervous, urinary, and gastrointestinal (GI) systems.

Viral infections that are acquired perinatally can cause stillbirth, intrauterine infection, congenital malformations, and acute disease. These pathogens also can cause chronic infection, with subtle manifestations that can be recognized only after a prolonged period. It is important to recognize the manifestations of infections in the neonatal period to treat the acute infection and to prevent health care–associated infections in other infants, and to anticipate effects on the infant's subsequent growth and development.

Fungal infections are of great concern in the immunocompromised or premature infant. Occasionally fungal infections such as thrush are found in otherwise healthy term infants.

Septicemia refers to a generalized infection in the bloodstream. Pneumonia, the most common form of neonatal infection, is one of the leading causes of perinatal death and is caused by many of the same organisms that cause sepsis. Bacterial meningitis affects 1 in 2500 live-born infants (Edwards, 2006). Gastroenteritis is sporadic, depending on epidemic outbreaks. Local infections such as conjunctivitis and omphalitis occur frequently, but incidence rates are unavailable. Infection continues to be a significant factor in fetal and neonatal morbidity and mortality. Sequelae to septicemia include meningitis, disseminated intravascular coagulation (DIC), and septic shock.

Septic shock results from the toxins released into the bloodstream. The most common sign is a decrease in blood pressure, a vital sign often not assessed in the care of the neonate. The infant will often appear gray or mottled and can be noted to have cool extremities. Other signs are rapid, irregular respirations and pulse (similar to septicemia in general).

CARE MANAGEMENT

The development of systemic infection in the newborn can be influenced by maternal, peripartum, and neonatal risk factors. Onset within the first 48 hours of life is more often associated with prenatal or perinatal predisposing factors. Onset after 2 or 3 days more frequently reflects disease acquired at or

NURSING PROCESS

The Infant with Suspected Sepsis

ASSESSMENT

- History
  - Maternal history including illness during pregnancy; prenatal care; tests for infection (syphilis, chlamydia, hepatitis and HIV)
  - Group B streptococci screening result
  - Risk factors for infection including preterm labor, prolonged rupture of membranes, maternal fever or urinary tract infection, fetal tachycardia, evidence of chorioamnionitis, prolonged labor
  - Neonatal risk factors including prematurity, multiple gestation, birth asphyxia, need for invasive procedures, congenital anomalies of skin or mucous membranes
- Physical examination
  - Temperature, heart rate, respiratory rate, blood pressure
  - Tone and activity
  - Signs of respiratory distress
  - Abdominal distention
  - Skin rashes or lesions
- Laboratory tests
  - CBC (including a platelet and differential count)
  - Blood culture
  - Lumbar puncture
  - Chest x-ray
  - C-reactive protein (depending on institutional policy)
  - Urine for culture (depending on infant's age)

NURSING DIAGNOSES

Possible nursing diagnoses include:

Infant

Risk for Infection **related to:**
- maternal vaginal (or other) infection
- resuscitation or ventilation therapy
- presence of indwelling umbilical catheters, total parenteral nutrition (TPN), parenteral fluids
- intrauterine electronic fetal monitoring

Ineffective Thermoregulation **related to:**
- infection

Impaired Tissue Integrity **related to:**
- multiple supportive measures (e.g., biometric monitoring, TPN, inhalation therapy)

Acute Pain **related to:**
- multiple supportive measures

Parents and Family

Anxiety, Fear, or Grieving **related to:**
- uncertainty about infant's prognosis
- poor prognosis

Risk for Impaired Parenting **related to:**
- separation of parent and newborn
- feelings of inadequacy in caring for infant

EXPECTED OUTCOMES OF CARE

Expected outcomes for the newborn and parents are:

Newborn
- The newborn will remain free of sepsis.
- The newborn's early signs of sepsis will be recognized, and appropriate therapy will be instituted.
- If therapy is necessary, the newborn will have no harmful sequelae.

Parents
- Anxiety regarding infant's condition and prognosis will be relieved.
- Parents will interact with newborn and develop caregiving skills.
- Parental anxiety about care of the newborn will be relieved.

PLAN OF CARE AND INTERVENTIONS

- Parents and care providers will practice good hand hygiene.
- All equipment coming into contact with the newborn will be cleaned appropriately.
- National guidelines for space, visitation, and infection control practices will be followed.
- The newborn will receive prophylactic antibiotic eye ointment.
- A septic workup including the tests listed above will be done as soon as the risk for infection is recognized.
- Appropriate antibiotic and or antiviral treatment will be initiated promptly.

EVALUATION

Evaluation is based on the expected outcomes of care. The newborn remains free from infection or receives prompt and effective treatment if sepsis is present. The parents will interact with the newborn and their anxiety will be decreased or alleviated.

TABLE 35-3 SIGNS OF SEPSIS

SYSTEM	SIGNS
Respiratory	Apnea, bradycardia Tachypnea Grunting, nasal flaring Retractions Decreased oxygen saturation Acidosis
Cardiovascular	Decreased cardiac output Tachycardia Hypotension Decreased perfusion
Central nervous	Temperature instability Lethargy Hypotonia Irritability, seizures
Gastrointestinal	Feeding intolerance Abdominal distention Vomiting, diarrhea
Integumentary	Jaundice Pallor Petechiae
Metabolic	Hypoglycemia Hyperglycemia Metabolic acidosis
Hematologic	Thrombocytopenia Neutropenia

Source: Edwards, M. (2006). Postnatal bacterial infections. In R. Martin, A. Fanaroff, & M. Walsh (Eds.), *Fanaroff and Martin's neonatal-perinatal medicine: Diseases of the fetus and infant* (8th ed.). Philadelphia: Mosby.

subsequent to birth. (See the Nursing Process box: The Infant with Suspected Sepsis.)

The earliest clinical signs of neonatal sepsis are characterized by a lack of specificity. The nonspecific signs include lethargy, poor feeding, poor weight gain, and irritability. The nurse or parent can simply note that the infant is just not doing as well as before. Differential diagnosis can be difficult because signs of sepsis are similar to signs of noninfectious neonatal problems such as anemia or hypoglycemia. Additional clinical and laboratory information and appropriate cultures supplement the findings described. Table 35-3 outlines signs of sepsis.

Laboratory studies are important. Specimens for cultures include blood, CSF, and urine. Fluids such as urine and CSF can be evaluated by counterimmune electrophoresis or latex agglutination to help identify the bacteria. A complete blood cell (CBC) count with differential is performed to determine the presence of bacterial infection or increased or decreased white blood cell count (the latter is an ominous sign). The total neutrophil count, immature to total neutrophil (I/T) ratio, absolute neutrophil count, and C-reactive protein can be used to determine the presence of sepsis. Detection of viral deoxyribonucleic acid (DNA) or antibodies by polymerase chain reaction (PCR) amplification in fluids is also an important diagnostic tool (Edwards, 2006). Antepartum viral infection can be successfully treated with a number of antiviral medications to decrease viral replication and fetal transmission of disease; neonates can also be treated with antiviral medications such as acyclovir and ganciclovir. Treatment with antibiotics is initiated after blood cultures are obtained in neonates; in high risk infants with significant illness, antiviral or antibiotic treatment can begin once cultures are obtained. Once the pathogen is identified, antibiotic, antiviral, or antifungal therapy can be modified.

Preventive Measures

Virtually all controlled clinical trials have demonstrated that effective hand hygiene is responsible for the prevention of health care–associated infection in nursery units. Nursing is directly or indirectly responsible for minimizing or eliminating environmental sources of infectious agents in the nursery. Measures to be taken include implementing Standard Precautions, carefully and thoroughly cleaning the environment and equipment, frequently replacing used equipment (e.g., changing IV tubing per hospital protocol, cleaning resuscitation and ventilation equipment), and appropriately disposing of excrement and linens. Overcrowding must be avoided in nurseries. Guidelines for space, visitation, and general infection control in areas where newborns receive care have been established and published (American Academy of Pediatrics [AAP] & American College of Obstetricians and Gynecologists [ACOG], 2007).

Specific newborn care procedures are intended to prevent infection. These include the instillation of antibiotic ointment in newborns' eyes 1 to 2 hours after birth, bathing, and cord care (see Chapter 24).

Curative Measures

Breastfeeding or feeding the newborn breast milk from the mother is encouraged. Breast milk provides protective mechanisms (see Chapter 25). Colostrum contains immunoglobulin A (IgA), which offers protection against infection in the GI tract. Human milk contains iron-binding protein that exerts a bacteriostatic effect on *E. coli*. Human milk also contains macrophages and lymphocytes. The vulnerability of infants to common mucosal pathogens such as respiratory syncytial virus (RSV) can be reduced by passive transfer of maternal immunity in the colostrum and breast milk. Some evidence indicates that early enteral feedings with human milk (trophic or minimal enteral feedings) can be beneficial in establishing a natural barrier to infection in ELBW and VLBW infants (Anderson, Wood, Keller, & Hay, 2011).

Administering medications safely and correctly, taking precautions when performing treatments, and following isolation procedures are important interventions when a newborn has an infection. Monitoring the IV infusion rate and administering antibiotics are the nurse's responsibility. If the IV fluid the infant is receiving contains electrolytes, vitamins, or other medications, the nurse should check with the hospital pharmacy before adding antibiotics. The antibiotic (or other medication) can be deactivated or can form a precipitate when combined with other substances. To prevent this from occurring, a secondary line of the prescribed solution is attached with a three-way stopcock at the infusion site.

Care must be taken in suctioning secretions from any newborn's oropharynx or trachea; the secretions can be infected. Routine suctioning is not recommended and can further compromise the infant's immune status, as well as cause hypoxia and increase ICP. Isolation procedures are implemented as indicated according to hospital policy. Isolation protocols change rapidly, and the nurse is urged to participate in continuing education and in-service programs to remain up to date.

! NURSING ALERT

Artificial and long natural fingernails worn by nurses have been associated with serious neonatal infection and morbidity from organisms such as *Pseudomonas aeruginosa* and *Klebsiella* in the neonatal intensive care unit (NICU).

Transplacental Infections

The occurrence of certain maternal infections during early pregnancy is known to be associated with various congenital malformations and disorders. An acronym that is often used in clinical practice is TORCH, which stands for *t*oxoplasmosis, *o*ther (gonorrhea, hepatitis B, syphilis, varicella-zoster virus, parvovirus B19, and HIV), *r*ubella, *c*ytomegalovirus, and *h*erpes simplex virus) (Box 35-1). Additional organisms known to cause congenital infection include enteroviruses and parvovirus, leading some clinicians to suggest the need for a new more comprehensive acronym (Klein, Baker, Remington, & Wilson, 2006). With the advent of newer diagnostic methods, these viral infections can be diagnosed in utero and interventions planned based on the availability of intrauterine treatments.

Toxoplasmosis

Toxoplasmosis is a multisystem disease caused by the protozoan *Toxoplasma gondii* parasite, commonly found in cats, dogs, pigs, sheep, and cattle, with cats being the definitive host. In the United States risk factors for acquisition of toxoplasmosis include exposure to contaminated soil and consumption of raw or undercooked meats or seafood (oysters, clams, or mussels) (Jones, Dargelas, Roberts, Press, Remington, & Montoya, 2009). Changing cat litter is a known risk for toxoplasmosis. The risk of maternal-fetal transmission of acute infection is approximately 40% with the risk of transmission increasing as the pregnancy progresses. However, the earlier in pregnancy that fetal infection occurs, the greater the severity of congenital disease. Because many women are already seropositive for toxoplasmosis, the overall risk of a primary infection in pregnancy is quite low. The diagnosis of toxoplasmosis in the neonate is supported by elevated levels of cord blood serum IgM.

Most neonates infected with *T. gondii* in utero are asymptomatic at birth, although many will develop chorioretinitis and signs of CNS involvement such as learning disabilities (Cunningham et al., 2010). For some infected neonates, hydrocephalus is the only clinical sign of the disease (Remington, McLeod, Thulliez, & Desmonts, 2006). Up to 30% of infected infants are born with severe manifestations at birth. Clinical features ascribed to *T. gondii* infection include three key findings (classic triad) first described by Sabin (1942): hydrocephalus or microcephaly, chorioretinitis, and cerebral calcifications (Cunningham et al.). Severe toxoplasmosis is associated with preterm birth, growth restriction, microcephaly or hydrocephaly, microphthalmos, chorioretinitis, CNS calcification, thrombocytopenia, jaundice, and fever. Petechiae or a maculopapular rash also can be evident.

Infants with congenital toxoplasmosis are treated with pyrimethamine, combined with oral sulfadiazine; folic acid supplement is used to prevent anemia. Treatment should be continued for 1 year (AAP Committee on Infectious Diseases, 2009).

BOX 35-1 TRANSPLACENTAL (TORCH) INFECTIONS AFFECTING NEWBORNS

T Toxoplasmosis
O Other: gonorrhea, syphilis, varicella, hepatitis B virus (HBV), human immunodeficiency virus (HIV), parvovirus
R Rubella
C Cytomegalovirus (CMV) infections or cytomegalic inclusion disease (CMID)
H Herpes simplex virus (HSV) infection

Gonorrhea

The incidence of gonococcal infection in pregnant women ranges from 2.5% to 7.3%. Many women with gonorrhea often have a concurrent *Chlamydia trachomatis* infection (AAP Committee on Infectious Diseases, 2009). After rupture of membranes, ascending infection can result in orogastric contamination of the fetus. The organism can also invade mucosal surfaces such as the conjunctiva (ophthalmia neonatorum), the rectal mucosa, and the pharynx. Contamination can occur as the infant passes through the birth canal, or it may occur postnatally from an infected adult. Neonatal gonococcal arthritis, septicemia, meningitis, vaginitis, and scalp abscesses also can develop.

Eye prophylaxis (e.g., with 0.5% erythromycin ointment) is administered within the first hour after birth to prevent ophthalmia neonatorum (AAP & ACOG, 2007). Eye prophylaxis alone does not prevent systemic infection; therefore, infants with a gonococcal eye infection should receive one dose of ceftriaxone (Gowen, 2007). Infants with systemic gonococcal infection require hospitalization and 7 days of IV antibiotic therapy. Infants rarely die of overwhelming infection in the early neonatal period. With the prophylactic use of silver nitrate or antibiotics, the incidence of gonococcal conjunctivitis is less than 0.5% (Yudin & Gonik, 2006).

Syphilis

Congenital and neonatal syphilis have reemerged in recent years as significant health problems. Rates of congenital syphilis in the United States increased from 8.2 per 100,000 live births in 2005 to 10.1 per 100,000 live births in 2008 (Su, Berman, Davis, & Weinstock, 2010). It is estimated that for every 100 women diagnosed with primary or secondary disease, 2 to 5 infants will contract congenital syphilis. If syphilis during pregnancy is untreated, approximately 50% of neonates born to these women will have symptomatic congenital syphilis. Treatment failure can occur, particularly when treatment is given in the third trimester; therefore, infants born to women treated within 4 weeks of birth should be investigated for congenital syphilis (Woods, 2009). The following factors have been identified as placing the neonate at high risk for congenital syphilis: lack of or late prenatal care, maternal substance abuse, crack cocaine use in the mother or partner, multiple sexual partners, history of STI, poverty, homelessness, and HIV infection.

The fetus is usually infected in utero by transplacental infection, but infection of the amniotic fluid also can occur. The infant can also contract syphilis during contact with an active genital lesion at birth (Ingall, Sanchez, & Baker, 2006). The risk

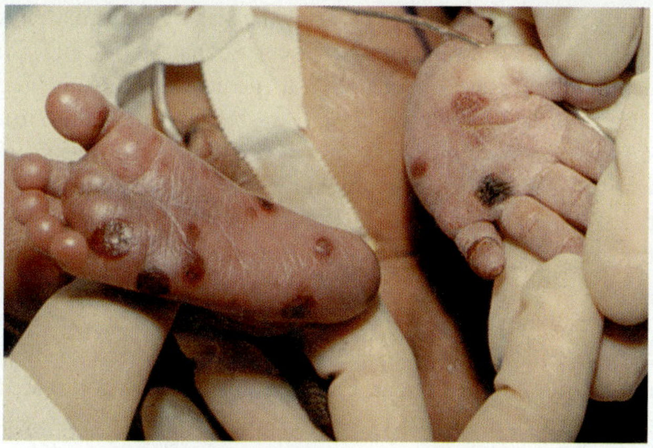

FIG. 35-7 Neonatal syphilis lesions on hands and feet. (Courtesy Mahesh Kotwal, MD, Phoenix, AZ.)

to the fetus and neonate varies according to the stage of maternal infection, with transmission during primary or secondary syphilis being more common. Untreated maternal disease results in stillbirth in 30% to 40% of cases. Prompt maternal treatment will eliminate most fetal infections; however, delayed treatment or a failure to obtain treatment can result in fetal effects that range from minor anomalies to preterm birth or fetal death. Damage to the fetus depends on when in gestation the infection occurred and the time that has elapsed before treatment. Congenital syphilis infection can be asymptomatic at birth in up to two thirds of infected infants. A portion of these infants will become symptomatic in the first 2 years of life, whereas others may take up to 20 years before displaying the effects of congenital infection (Woods, 2009).

Early congenital syphilis can result in prematurity, hydrops fetalis, and failure to thrive. Hepatosplenomegaly and jaundice are common. Hematologic findings include anemia, leukocytosis, and thrombocytopenia. Characteristic bony lesions occur in the long bones, the cranium, and the spine and include osteochondritis, osteomyelitis, and periostitis. Other findings include snuffles (copious clear mucous discharge from the nose), mucocutaneous lesions, edema, and a copper-colored maculopapular dermal rash first noticeable on the palms of the hands, the soles of the feet, and in the diaper area and around the mouth and the anus by the end of the first week of life in untreated infants (Fig. 35-7). *Condylomata* (elevated wartlike lesions) can be seen on mucous membranes, moist surfaces, or areas of the body affected by friction. Rough, cracked, mucocutaneous lesions of the lips heal to form circumoral radiating scars known as *rhagades*. Other involvement results in exfoliation (separation, flaking) of nails and loss of hair. Iritis and choroiditis are characteristic of infection of the eyes. The following can be noted: nephrotic syndrome secondary to renal infection; hepatitis with jaundice, lymphadenopathy, and inflammation of the pancreas, the testes, and the colon; and a pseudoparalysis of the extremities. In some infants, signs of congenital syphilis do not appear until late in the neonatal period. In these newborns, early signs such as poor feeding, slight hyperthermia, and snuffles can be nonspecific (Woods, 2009).

Medical Management. Treatment of the newborn should be carried out when the diagnosis of congenital syphilis is confirmed or suspected or when maternal treatment status is unknown or not well documented. The neonate should be treated when the mother was treated within 1 month of giving birth or does not respond to treatment, when medications other than penicillin were used for the mother, when the mother was treated appropriately but did not have sufficient serologic follow-up to assess response to treatment, and when inadequate neonatal follow-up is anticipated (Duff, Sweet, & Edwards, 2009).

The infant with symptomatic congenital syphilis should have a lumbar puncture, CBC, and long-bone radiography prior to treatment. If the results of these tests are normal, a single intramuscular dose of benzathine penicillin is recommended (Duff et al., 2009). If results are abnormal or there is concern about appropriate follow-up, a 10-day course of IV penicillin or intramuscular (IM) procaine penicillin can be given. If the mother was adequately treated before giving birth and serologic testing of the infant does not show syphilis, generally the infant is not treated with antibiotics. The infant is checked for antibody titer (received from the mother through the placenta) every 2 weeks for 3 months, at which time the test result should be negative. Some physicians recommend antibiotic therapy for asymptomatic or inconclusive cases.

Prognosis. In general, treatment of syphilis is more effective if it begins early rather than late in the course of the disease. However, a recurrence rate of 5% can be expected. Even adequate treatment of congenital syphilis after birth does not always prevent late (5 to 15 years after initial infection) complications. Potential complications include neurosyphilis, deafness, Hutchinson teeth (notched incisors), saber shins, joint involvement, saddle nose (depressed bridge), gummas (soft, gummy tumors) over the skin and other organs, interstitial keratitis (inflammation of the cornea), rhagades, frontal bossing, and mulberry molars (Woods, 2009).

Varicella-Zoster

The varicella-zoster virus, responsible for chickenpox and shingles, is a member of the herpes family. Approximately 90% of women in the childbearing years are immune; therefore the risk of infection in pregnancy is low: 5 per 10,000 pregnancies (Gershon, 2006).

Varicella transmission to the fetus can occur across the placenta when the disease is contracted in the first half of pregnancy, but this is relatively infrequent (about 2%). When transmission to the fetus does occur in the early part of pregnancy, the effects on the fetus include limb atrophy, neurologic abnormalities (hydrocephalus or microcephaly), and eye abnormalities (Gowen, 2007).

When maternal infection occurs in the last 3 weeks of pregnancy, 25% of infants born to these mothers will develop clinical varicella (Gershon, 2006). The severity of the infant's illness will increase greatly if maternal infection occurred within 5 days before or 2 days after birth (Tan & Koren, 2006). The mortality rate in severe illness is 30% (Gershon).

Seroimmune pregnant women exposed to active chickenpox can be given varicella-zoster immune globulin (VZIG), which does not reduce the incidence of infection but should decrease the effects of the virus on the fetus. The immunoglobulin must be given within 72 hours of exposure to be effective.

Infants born to mothers in whom chickenpox develops between 5 days before birth and 48 hours after should be given VZIG at birth because of the risk of severe disease (Tan & Koren, 2006). Acyclovir can be used to treat infants with generalized involvement and pneumonia (Myers, Seward, & LaRussa, 2007).

Term infants exposed to chickenpox after birth will have a mild or no infection if they are born to immune mothers. In those born to nonimmune mothers, chickenpox can develop, but the course is not usually severe. Experts are divided as to whether this group of infants should receive VZIG. Infants born before 28 weeks gestation are at risk regardless of their mother's status and probably benefit from VZIG if exposed to chickenpox (AAP Committee on Infectious Diseases, 2009).

Hepatitis B Virus

HBV infection during pregnancy is not associated with an increase in malformations, stillbirths, or IUGR; however, approximately 35% of infected fetuses will be born before term (Baley & Toltzis, 2006). The transmission rate of HBV to the newborn ranges from 70% to 90% when the mother is seropositive for both hepatitis B surface antigen (HBsAg) and hepatitis B e antigen (HBeAg) (AAP Committee on Infectious Diseases, 2009). Transmission occurs transplacentally, serum to serum, and by contact with contaminated urine, feces, saliva, semen, or vaginal secretions during birth. Infants are most frequently infected during birth or in the first few days of life. The rate of transmission is highest when the mother contracts the virus in the third trimester or early in the postpartum period (Bradley, 2006). These mothers will be positive for HBsAg. Transmission can occur through breast milk, but antigens also develop in formula-fed infants at the same or a higher rate, thus breastfeeding is not contraindicated. Diagnosis is made by viral culture of amniotic fluid, as well as the presence of HBsAg and IgM in the cord blood or infant's serum.

The majority of infants who become HBsAg positive are symptom free at birth, whereas some show evidence of acute hepatitis with changes in liver function. The mortality rate for full-blown hepatitis is 75%. Infants who become carriers are at high risk for chronic hepatitis, cirrhosis of the liver, or liver cancer even years later (Yudin & Gonik, 2006).

! NURSING ALERT

Infants whose mothers have antibodies for HBsAg or in whom hepatitis developed during pregnancy or the postpartum period should be treated with hepatitis B immunoglobulin (HBIG), 0.5 ml intramuscularly, as soon as possible after birth—within the first 12 hours of life. The hepatitis B vaccine also should be given at the same time but in a different site (AAP Committee on Infectious Diseases, 2009; Baley & Toltzis, 2006) (see Chapter 24).

Human Immunodeficiency Virus and Acquired Immunodeficiency Syndrome

Approximately 6000 pregnant women infected with HIV give birth each year in the United States. Due to the success of preventive strategies during pregnancy, the incidence of mother-to-child transmission has been reduced to approximately 1% to 2%. Universal HIV testing for all pregnant women allows for early identification and treatment of HIV-positive women during pregnancy, which decreases the risk of transmission to the fetus. Other strategies to prevent neonatal HIV infection include administration of antiviral medications during pregnancy and labor to women who are infected with the virus, administration of antiretrovirals to neonates for 6 weeks, and elective cesarean birth for women with HIV viral loads greater than 1000 copies per ml. In the United States, an additional strategy is the total avoidance of breastfeeding (AAP Committee on Pediatric AIDS, 2008).

Transmission of HIV from the mother to the fetus can occur transplacentally at various gestational ages. The risk of infection in an infant born to an HIV-positive mother (not treated) is approximately 12% to 40%. Transmission most often occurs during birth. Globally, approximately one third to one half of cases of mother-to-child transmission occur through breastfeeding (AAP Committee on Infectious Diseases, 2009).

Diagnosis of HIV infection in the neonate is complicated by the presence of maternal IgG antibodies that cross the placenta after 32 weeks of gestation. The most accurate test for newborns and infants younger than 18 months is the HIV-1 deoxyribonucleic acid (DNA) PCR assay, which is performed on neonatal blood, not cord blood (AAP Committee on Infectious Diseases, 2009). Follow-up testing for infants born to HIV-positive mothers is recommended at several intervals within the first year of life.

Typically the HIV-infected neonate is asymptomatic at birth. Early-onset illness (i.e., virus detected within 48 hours of birth) is attributed to prenatal infection. These infants develop opportunistic infections (*Candida* and *Pneumocystis jiroveci* pneumonia) and experience rapid progression of immunodeficiency that often results in death during the first 1 to 2 years of life.

The remainder of infants seroconvert over a period of months to years. By 1 year of life, the vast majority of perinatally infected infants show signs of infection. Some children infected at birth show no signs of disease 8 to 10 years later. The age of onset of symptoms predicts the length of survival.

The presenting signs and symptoms of HIV infection vary from severe immunodeficiency to nonspecific findings such as growth failure, parotitis, and recurrent or persistent upper respiratory tract infections. In the first year of life, lymphadenopathy and hepatosplenomegaly are common. The infant can have fever, chronic diarrhea, chronic dermatitis, interstitial pneumonitis, persistent thrush, and acquired immunodeficiency syndrome (AIDS)–defining opportunistic infections. Common secondary opportunistic infections include pneumonia, candidiasis, CMV, cryptosporidiosis, herpes simplex or herpes zoster, and disseminated varicella.

Although it is rare for an infant to be born with symptoms of HIV infection, all infants born to seropositive mothers should be presumed to be HIV positive until proven otherwise. Management begins by implementing Standard Precautions. Measures should also be taken to protect the infant from further exposure to maternal blood and body fluids. In the United States, breastfeeding is avoided completely if the mother is HIV positive. Regimens for the prevention of HIV transmission include antepartum, intrapartum, and neonatal treatment with highly active antiretroviral therapy (HAART).

The goal in the administration of antivirals is the suppression of the virus to undetectable concentrations; the available antiviral drugs do not, however, cure the child's disease. HIV diagnosis in the neonatal period combined with aggressive antibiotic treatment of opportunistic infections has the potential to prolong survival in children (AAP Committee on Infectious Diseases, 2009). Studies of HIV symptoms in children treated in the era of HAART show a significant decrease in the incidence of secondary opportunistic infections (Nesheim, Kapogiannis, Soe, Sullivan, Abrams, Farley, et al., 2007).

Counseling regarding the care of the mothers themselves, the family's care of the infant, and future pregnancies should be provided. The risk for transmission among members of the same household is minimal. Social services are required in these cases. If the parent chooses to keep the infant, home health care may be arranged. For more information and updated information, parents are referred to the National AIDS Hotline (1-800-342-AIDS).

In the United States, breastfeeding by the HIV-positive mother is contraindicated; however, in developing countries, the risks versus benefits in relation to number of infant deaths attributed to poor sanitary conditions and availability of an appropriate food supply for infants are considered. The World Health Organization and associated groups (2010) recommend that HIV-positive mothers who are taking antiretroviral medications should breastfeed for at least 12 months. For those who do not have access to ARV therapy, exclusive breastfeeding for 6 months is recommended. After 6 months, complementary foods are introduced and breastfeeding is continued until a safe, nutritional diet without breastmilk can be provided for the infant (WHO, UNICEF, UNFPA, UNAIDS, 2010).

The family must be counseled about vaccinations. All HIV-1–exposed infants should receive routine immunizations. There are specific guidelines for those with confirmed HIV infection (CDC, 2009a). It is usually safe to administer all inactivated vaccines to HIV-1–infected children. In the absence of severe immunosuppression, children with HIV-1 can receive varicella vaccine (CDC, 2009a).

Rubella Infection

Since the rubella vaccination program was begun in 1969, cases of congenital rubella infection have been reduced significantly; however, it is still seen occasionally in the newborn. Vaccination failures, lack of compliance, and the migration of nonimmunized persons result in periodic outbreaks of rubella, also known as German measles.

The risk of a congenitally infected infant varies with the gestational age of the fetus when maternal infection occurs. Abnormalities are most severe if the mother contracts the virus during the first trimester and rare if the disease occurs after that time (Cooper & Alford, 2006).

More than two thirds of infected infants show no apparent symptoms at birth, but sequelae can develop years later. Hearing loss, the most common result, appears to be progressive after birth. **Congenital rubella syndrome** includes cataracts or glaucoma, hearing loss, and cardiac defects (pulmonary artery stenosis, patent ductus arteriosus, or coarctation of the aorta). Multiple other abnormalities also are present, including IUGR, microphthalmia, hypotonia, hepatosplenomegaly, thrombocytopenic purpura, dermatoglyphic abnormalities, bony radiolucencies, microcephaly, and brain wave abnormalities. Severe infection can result in fetal death. Delayed effects of infection manifest as thyroid dysfunction, diabetes mellitus, growth hormone deficiency, myocarditis, and glaucoma (Baley & Toltzis, 2006).

SAFETY ALERT

The rubella virus has been cultured in infants for up to 18 months after birth. These infants are a serious source of infection to susceptible individuals, particularly women in the childbearing years. Extended pediatric isolation is mandatory until the noncontagious stage of rubella has been reached. The infant should be isolated until pharyngeal mucus and urine are free of virus (Best, 2007).

Cytomegalovirus Infection

CMV infection during pregnancy can result in miscarriage, stillbirth, or congenital or neonatal cytomegalic inclusion disease (CMID). It is the most common cause of congenital viral infections in humans, occurring in 40,000 newborns in the United States every year. Maternal-fetal transmission of CMV virus occurs in approximately one third of mothers with a primary CMV infection during pregnancy (Edwards, 2006).

The neonate with classic, full-blown CMID typically displays IUGR and has microcephaly, seizures, hypotonia, and lethargy. The neonate also has a rash, jaundice, and hepatosplenomegaly (Fig. 35-8). Anemia, thrombocytopenia, and hyperbilirubinemia are common (Malm & Engman, 2007). Intracranial, periventricular calcification often is noted on x-ray films. Mortality rates in symptomatic infants are 20% to 30%, with death resulting from hepatic failure, DIC, or secondary bacterial infection (Edwards, 2006). Congenital CMV can cause a variety of neurologic problems such as mental retardation, autism, learning disabilities, hearing loss, visual impairment, or blindness (Malm & Engman). Most (90%) affected infants are asymptomatic at birth (Kenneson & Cannon, 2007), although there is a 5% to 15% risk that they will develop later sequelae such as hearing loss and learning disabilities (Edwards). Hearing loss can be present at birth or may not be apparent until after the first year of life. The hearing loss is often progressive. Chorioretinitis,

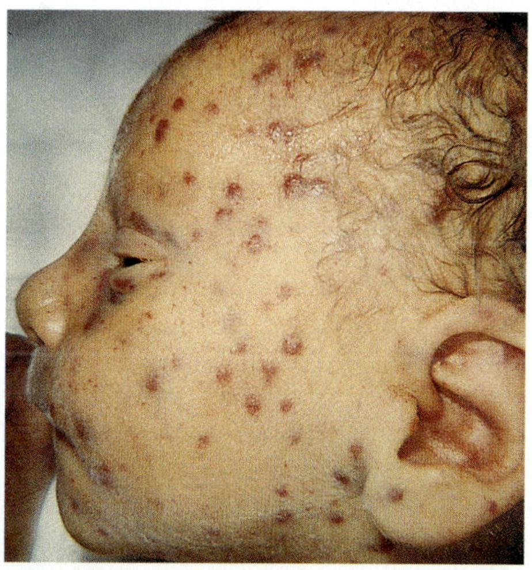

FIG. 35-8 Neonatal cytomegalovirus infection. Typical rash seen in a severely affected infant. (Courtesy David A. Clarke, Philadelphia, PA.)

microcephaly, mental retardation, and neuromuscular deficits can occur by 2 years of age. Some children are at risk for a defect in tooth enamel, resulting in severe caries (Edwards).

Elevated levels of cord blood IgM are suggestive of disease. The virus can be isolated from urine or saliva of the newborn. Differential diagnoses include other causes of jaundice, syphilis (positive Venereal Disease Research Laboratory [VDRL] findings), toxoplasmosis (positive Sabin-Feldman dye test result), hemolytic disease of the newborn (positive Coombs' test reaction), or coxsackievirus infection (positive culture).

CMV can be transmitted through breast milk while the mother has acute CMV infection. CMV infections acquired after birth are often asymptomatic and have no sequelae. Exceptions to this occur in preterm infants in whom postnatal acquisition of CMV can result in pneumonia, hepatitis, thrombocytopenia, and long-term neurologic sequelae.

Treatment of the infected newborn with ganciclovir is effective in decreasing neurologic sequelae, in particular sensorineural hearing loss. There is some evidence that administration of CMV-specific human immunoglobulin to the pregnant woman with primary CMV infection can help protect the fetus (Schleiss, 2008).

Herpes Simplex Virus

HSV infections among newborns are being diagnosed more frequently and are estimated to occur in as many as 1 in 3,000 to 1 in 20,000 births (AAP Committee on Infectious Diseases, 2009). The neonate can acquire the virus through transplacental infection, ascending infection by way of the birth canal, direct contamination during passage through an infected birth canal, or direct transmission from infected personnel or family (Malm, 2009).

Transplacental transmission of HSV infection to the neonate can occur during maternal infection; however, an ascending transcervical infection first involves the intact fetal membranes, causing chorioamnionitis. Transcervical infection can be accelerated by the use of internal fetal monitoring. The scalp electrodes break the fetal skin barrier and increase the risk of infection.

Congenital infection is rare and characterized by in utero destruction of normally formed organs. Affected infants are growth restricted and have skin lesions and scarring. They have severe psychomotor delays, with intracranial calcifications, microcephaly, hypertonicity, and seizures. They have eye involvement, including microphthalmos, cataracts, chorioretinitis, blindness, and retinal dysplasia. Some infants have patent ductus arteriosus, limb anomalies, and recurrent skin vesicles, with a short life expectancy.

HSV is most often transmitted from mother to neonate through viral shedding during passage through the birth canal. The risk of infection during vaginal birth in the presence of genital herpes has not been clearly delineated. It may be as high as 50% with active primary infection at term (Prober, 2008). Primary maternal infections after 32 weeks of gestation have a higher risk for the fetus and newborn than recurrent infections (Baley & Toltzis, 2006). If the mother is shedding HSV virus as a result of reactivated infection, the risk of transmission is only about 2% (AAP Committee on Infectious Diseases, 2009). This is possibly related to passive intrauterine immunity to herpes. Clinical and laboratory features associated with neonatal herpes include maternal primary HSV infection, vaginal birth, preterm birth, neonatal seizures, elevated liver enzymes, vesicular rash, and elevated CSF counts (Caviness, Demmler, & Selwyn, 2008). In approximately 70% of women whose infants have HSV infection, there are no symptoms or history of infection although serologic testing reveals evidence of herpesvirus (Baley & Toltzis, 2006).

Postnatal acquisition of the virus and spread within a nursery have been documented by DNA analysis. Parents have been implicated in neonatal infections. There also is concern regarding symptomatic and asymptomatic shedding among hospital personnel. Nursery personnel with cold sores should practice strict hand hygiene and wear a mask, but no evidence indicates that they should be removed from the nursery unless they have a herpetic whitlow (primary HSV infection of the terminal segment of a finger) (Baley & Toltzis, 2006).

Clinically, neonatal HSV infections are classified as disseminated infection (22%), CNS disease (34%), or localized infection of the skin, eye, or mouth (SEM) (40%) (Baley & Toltzis, 2006). Although the incubation period for HSV is 1 to 7 days, the onset of symptoms varies with the type of infection (Malm, 2009).

Disseminated infections are sepsis-like and can involve virtually every organ system, but primarily the liver, the adrenal glands, and the lungs are involved. By 5 to 11 days of age affected infants show signs of bacterial sepsis or shock. Death often results within 1 week of the onset of symptoms and is related to respiratory failure, pneumonitis, DIC with shock, and CNS complications (Baley & Toltzis, 2006; Malm, 2009).

In CNS disease, blood-borne seeding of the brain results in multiple lesions of cortical hemorrhagic necrosis. It also can occur alone or in association with oral, eye, or skin lesions. Brain involvement usually manifests in the second to fourth weeks of life. Skin lesions are apparent in 60% to 70% of the infants, and the CSF of less than 50% will reveal the virus. The presenting manifestations include lethargy, poor feeding, irritability, and local or generalized seizures. If untreated, the mortality rate in CNS disease approaches 50% with the vast majority of survivors experiencing severe sequelae such as microcephaly and blindness (Baley & Toltzis, 2006).

Localized HSV infections most often occur with skin findings or rarely with isolated oral cavity lesions (Fig. 35-9). Without treatment, CNS or disseminated disease develops in 70% of the infants with skin vesicles. Ocular involvement, which can occur alone, can be secondary to either HSV-1 or HSV-2. Ocular disease may not be discovered for months. Microphthalmos, cataracts, optic atrophy, and corneal scarring can result from chorioretinitis, keratitis, and retinal hemorrhage (Baley & Toltzis, 2006).

Gloves should be worn when caregivers are in contact with these infants. The neonate's eyes, oral cavity, and skin are inspected carefully for the presence of any lesions. Cultures are obtained from the mouth, the eyes, and any possible lesions. Circumcision, if performed, is delayed until the infant is ready to be discharged. The infant can be discharged with the mother if the infant's cultures are negative for the virus. As long as no suspicious lesions are present on the mother's breasts, breastfeeding is allowed. For the infant at risk, prophylactic topical eye

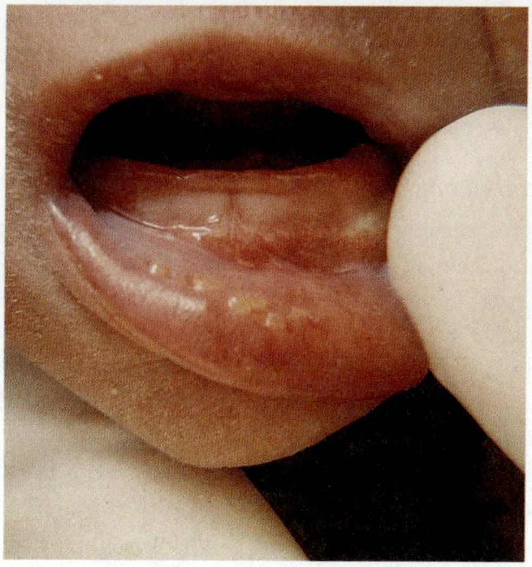

FIG. 35-9 Neonatal herpes simplex virus oral lesions. (Courtesy David A. Clarke, Philadelphia, PA.)

ointment (vidarabine) is administered for 5 days for prevention of keratoconjunctivitis. No current recommendations exist for prophylactic systemic therapy; each case should be considered individually. Blood, urine, and CSF specimens should be cultured when indicated clinically. If herpetic lesions first occur after 6 weeks of life, the risk of dissemination and severe illness is very low (Baley & Toltzis, 2006).

Therapy includes general supportive measures, as well as treatment with acyclovir. Duration of treatment is 21 days for infants with disseminated or CNS disease and 14 days for the skin-eye-mouth form of the disease (Malm, 2009). Continuing therapy is required in case of recurrence. When there is ocular involvement, ophthalmic ointment should be administered simultaneously (AAP Committee on Infectious Diseases, 2009).

Parvovirus B19

Parvovirus B19 is well known in older children as "fifth disease" or "slapped cheek illness" because of the characteristic facial appearance of the affected child. During pregnancy, infection can result in miscarriage, fetal anemia, hydrops fetalis, IUGR, and stillbirth. Vertical transmission of the parvovirus to the fetus occurs in about one third of maternal infections (de Jong, de Haan, Kroes, Beersma, Oepkes, Walther, et al., 2006) and the overall fetal loss rate after infection is about 5% to 10% (Tolfvenstam & Broliden, 2009).

The virus can be isolated from amniotic fluid, fetal blood, or tissues using DNA PCR assay. Viral load is not predictive of fetal morbidity and mortality (Cunningham et al., 2010).

There are no specific antiviral medications to treat parvovirus B19 infection and there is no vaccine. If a pregnant woman is confirmed with the infection, the fetus should be closely monitored for the development of fetal hydrops using serial ultrasound examinations (Tolfvenstam & Broliden, 2009). Protocols for intrauterine management have not been well developed, but intrauterine transfusion to treat anemia is the only currently accepted therapy (de Jong et al., 2006). There is insufficient evidence about the long-term effects of parvovirus (Cunningham et al., 2010).

Enterovirus

Enteroviruses include poliovirus, coxsackievirus, and echovirus. Nonpolio enteroviruses are among the most common viruses that infect humans. Enteroviral infections in the newborn account for about 10% of all reported cases of enterovirus infection in the United States (Khetsuriani, Lamonte-Fowlkes, Oberste, & Pallansch, 2006). Group B coxsackieviruses and echovirus 11 are the serotypes most commonly affecting neonates and can be transmitted transplacentally or through exposure to maternal blood or secretions during birth. The risk of transmission is increased with maternal enterovirus illness around the time of birth and a lack of maternal antibodies to the specific type of enterovirus. Antenatal transmission increases the risk of severe disease and death (Tebruegge & Curtis, 2009).

The onset of infection following perinatal transmission is usually within 1 to 2 weeks after birth. Usual presenting symptoms are fever, irritability, lethargy, and poor feeding; rash, respiratory symptoms and gastrointestinal symptoms also can occur. Clinical manifestations can be severe and include myocarditis, meningitis, respiratory distress, and hepatitis. Deaths are usually due to multiorgan involvement (Tebruegge & Curtis, 2009; Wikswo, Khetsuriani, Fowlkes, Zheng, Penaranda, Verma, et al., 2009).

Currently there is no vaccine or any treatment approved by the U.S. Food and Drug Administration (FDA) for nonpolio enteroviruses. Immunoglobulin is sometimes used to treat symptomatic infants. Pleconaril is under investigation as a treatment for enteroviral infection in neonates and infants (Tebruegge & Curtis, 2009).

Bacterial Infections

Group B Streptococci

GBS infection is a leading cause of neonatal morbidity and mortality in the United States (CDC, 2009d). The practice of giving prophylactic antibiotics to women in labor who are GBS positive has significantly reduced the incidence and severity of early-onset GBS infection in the newborn (Yudin & Gonik, 2006). In the United States, the incidence of early onset neonatal GBS infection is 0.4 per 1000 live births and the incidence of late-onset (after 7 days of age) infection is 0.3 per 1000 live births (CDC, 2009d).

Early-onset GBS infection in the neonate usually occurs in the first 7 days of life but most commonly manifests in the first 24 hours after birth. Risk factors for the development of early-onset GBS include low birth weight, preterm birth, rupture of membranes of more than 18 hours, maternal fever, previous GBS infant, maternal GBS bacteriuria, use of intrauterine fetal monitoring, maternal age less than 20 years, and Hispanic or African-American ethnicity. Early-onset disease usually results from vertical transmission from the birth canal and manifests as systemic infection or respiratory illness that mimics the symptoms of severe respiratory distress. The infant can rapidly develop pneumonia, shock, or meningitis. The mortality rate for early-onset infection is approximately 4%, with higher rates among preterm infants (AAP Committee on Infectious Diseases, 2009; Cunningham et al., 2010).

Late-onset GBS infections occur between 1 week and 3 months of age, with an average age at onset of 24 days. Infection can result from vertical transmission or from health care–associated infection or community exposure. Of infants with late-onset

GBS, 30% develop meningitis (Edwards, Nizet, & Baker, 2006). Mortality rates are less than for early-onset infection. Survivors often have neurologic damage (Cunningham et al., 2010).

For newborns with suspected GBS infection, the usual treatment is ampicillin in combination with an aminoglycoside. If GBS is identified as the cause of infection, penicillin G alone can be given (AAP Committee on Infectious Diseases, 2009).

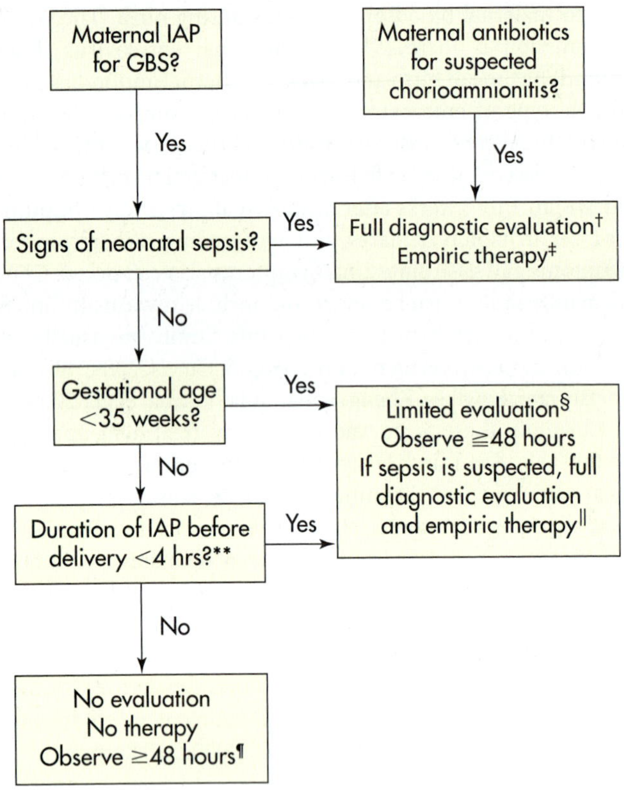

*If no maternal intrapartum prophylaxis for GBS was administered despite an indication being present, data are insufficient on which to recommend a single management strategy.
†Includes complete blood cell count and differential, blood culture, and chest radiograph if respiratory abnormalities are present. When signs of sepsis are present, a lumbar puncture, if feasible, should be performed.
‡Duration of therapy varies depending on results of blood culture, cerebrospinal fluid findings, if obtained, and the clinical course of the infant. If laboratory results and clinical course do not indicate bacterial infections, duration may be as short as 48 hours.
§CBC with differential and blood culture.
|| Applies only to penicillin, ampicillin, or cefazolin and assumes recommended dosing regimens.
¶A healthy-appearing infant who was ≥38 weeks of gestation at delivery and whose mother received ≥4 hours of intrapartum prophylaxis before delivery may be discharged home after 24 hours if other discharge criteria have been met and a person able to comply fully with instructions for home observation will be present. If any one of these conditions is not met, the infant should be observed in the hospital for at least 48 hours and until criteria for discharge are achieved.

FIG. 35-10 Sample algorithm for management of a newborn whose mother received intrapartum antimicrobial agents for prevention (IAP) of early-onset group B streptococcal disease or suspected chorioamnionitis. This algorithm is not an exclusive course of management. Variations that incorporate individual circumstances or institutional preferences may be appropriate. (From Schrag S., Gorwitz, R., Fultz-Butts, K., & Schuchat, A. [2002]. Prevention of perinatal group B streptococcal disease. Revised guideliness from CDC. *MMWR Morbidity and Mortality Weekly Report,* 51[RR11],1-22.)

Figure 35-10 provides a sample algorithm for the management of a neonate whose mother received intrapartum antibiotics for prevention (IAP) of group B streptococcal disease in the newborn or suspected chorioamnionitis.

Escherichia coli

E. coli is responsible for approximately 40% of cases of neonatal sepsis and 80% of cases of neonatal meningitis in the United States (AAP Committee on Infectious Diseases, 2009). It is found in the gastrointestinal tract soon after birth and makes up the bulk of human fecal flora. *E. coli* can cause a variety of neonatal infections, including omphalitis, diarrheal illness, pneumonia, peritonitis, urinary tract infections, and meningitis. Risk factors for the development of *E. coli* infections in the newborn include preterm birth, low birth weight, maternal infection, prolonged rupture of membranes, and septic or traumatic birth (AAP Committee on Infectious Diseases).

Neonates most often acquire *E. coli* from the maternal birth canal or rectum during birth, although it also can be hospital acquired through person-to-person transmission or from the hospital environment. Exposure to *E. coli* can result in no infection, infection without illness, gastroenteritis, or rarely, septicemia. Symptoms can appear within the first 24 hours after birth or several weeks later. Clinical signs of *E. coli* sepsis are relatively nonspecific and include fever, temperature instability, apnea, cyanosis, jaundice, hepatomegaly, lethargy or irritability, vomiting, abdominal distention, and diarrhea.

The usual treatment for *E. coli* infection in the newborn is ampicillin or an extended spectrum cephalosporin and an aminoglycoside. Treatment is continued for 1 to 14 days for bacteremia and 21 days for meningitis (AAP Committee on Infectious Diseases, 2009). Use of ampicillin in labor as prophylaxis against GBS disease has not been found to increase the risk of early-onset *E. coli* infection (Schrag, Hadler, Arnold, Martell-Cleary, Reingold, & Schuchat, 2006) but can result in more virulent *E. coli* disease resulting from ampicillin-resistant organisms (Bizzaro, Dembry, Baltimore, & Gallagher, 2008).

Staphylococcus aureus

Most staphylococcal infections in the newborn develop within the first few days after birth and involve the skin and soft tissue. Conjunctivitis, presenting with purulent eye discharge, is also a common manifestation of *S. aureus* infection. Skin lesions are typically small vesicles or pustules that are easily treated with topical antimicrobial agents. The skin lesions can appear as large fragile bullae containing clear or purulent fluid. These bullae rupture easily and leave moist, red, denuded areas of skin. A more severe bullous eruption due to staphylococcal infection is scalded skin syndrome characterized by widespread bullous lesions that easily rupture; fever and irritability are also present (Narendran & Hoath, 2006). *S. aureus* can cause serious problems such as abscesses, osteomyelitis, endocarditis, and septic arthritis. Breaks in the skin from IV catheters or scalp electrodes present an opportunity for the development of *S. aureus* abscesses. Colonization of the maternal genital tract with *S. aureus* is not uncommon although the potential for vertical transmission to the neonate is unclear (Andrews, Schelonka, Waites, Stamm, Cliver, & Moser, 2008). The major sources of colonization by *S. aureus* are the hands of medical and nursing personnel.

Although most strains of *S. aureus* are sensitive to semisynthetic penicillins, there are increasing concerns about methicillin-resistant strains (Gorwitz, 2008). MRSA has caused outbreaks of hospital-acquired infection in neonatal intensive care units and hospital nurseries (Fortunov, Hulten, Hammerman, Mason, & Kaplan, 2006).

Listeriosis

Listeriosis, caused by *Listeria monocytogenes,* is primarily a foodborne infection that can cause maternal and neonatal illness. Globally it is one of the three major causes of neonatal meningitis (Posfay-Barbe & Wald, 2009). The incidence of neonatal listeriosis in the United States is reported to be approximately 8.6 per 100,000 live births (CDC, 2009b). Although it is relatively uncommon and probably underdiagnosed, it occurs more frequently among pregnant women and those who are older or immunocompromised. Mother-to-child transmission occurs transplacentally, through ascending infection, or during birth. Prenatal infection causes chorioamnionitis or endometritis and should be suspected in cases of brown-stained amniotic fluid. It can also cause miscarriage, preterm birth, and stillbirth. Two forms of neonatal listeriosis are recognized: early onset and late onset. Signs of early-onset infection are present at birth or in the first 1 to 2 days. Manifestations of infection are sepsis-like symptoms, acute respiratory distress, pneumonia, and more rarely, meningitis or myocarditis. With severe infection the infant can have granulomatosis infantiseptum which is a widely disseminated granuloma, causing an erythematous rash with pale papules and abscesses in the liver, lungs, brain, kidneys, spleen, adrenal glands, and GI system (Posfay-Barbe & Wald, 2009). Late-onset listeriosis is more insidious and usually manifests as meningitis. Listeriosis in the newborn is treated with ampicillin and an aminoglycoside (AAP Committee on Infectious Diseases, 2009).

Chlamydia Trachomatis

Chlamydia trachomatis, the most common reportable sexually transmitted infection in the United States, causes neonatal conjunctivitis (25% to 50% of exposed infants) and pneumonia (5% to 20% of exposed infants). Neonatal infection is acquired by newborns in approximately half of all vaginal births by infected mothers and is known to occur in some infants born by cesarean with intact membranes (AAP Committee on Infectious Diseases, 2009). Chlamydial infection in pregnancy has also been suggested as a cause of early and late pregnancy loss, stillbirth, premature labor, and postpartum endometritis (Yudin & Gonik, 2006).

Neonatal chlamydial conjunctivitis (congestion and edema), with minimal discharge, develops within a few days to several weeks after birth and usually lasts 1 to 2 weeks. If untreated, it can progress to chronic follicular conjunctivitis with conjunctival scarring and corneal microgranulations.

Chlamydial pneumonia usually has a gradual onset, between 4 and 11 weeks of age, beginning with rhinorrhea and progressing to tachypnea and coughing (Yudin & Gonik, 2006). Signs may be quite subtle and often go unrecognized. It is speculated that pneumonia can occur as a result of movement of the organism from the conjunctiva into the lower respiratory tract; however, conjunctivitis is not a prerequisite to pneumonia.

Chlamydial conjunctivitis is treated with oral erythromycin or ethylsuccinate for 14 days. The recommended treatment for chlamydial pneumonia is oral azithromycin for 3 days or a 14-day regimen of erythromycin or ethylsuccinate. Erythromycin administration in infants younger than 6 weeks has been associated with an increased risk of infantile hypertrophic pyloric stenosis; therefore, parents should be educated regarding the symptoms of the condition (feeding intolerance, projectile vomiting, and abdominal distention) (AAP Committee on Infectious Diseases, 2009).

Fungal Infections

Candidiasis

Candida infections, formerly known as moniliasis, can occur in the newborn. *Candida albicans,* the organism usually responsible, can cause disease in any organ system. It is a yeastlike fungus (producing yeast cells and spores) that can be acquired during birth from a maternal vaginal infection; by person-to-person transmission; or from contaminated hands, bottles, nipples, or other articles. It usually is a benign disorder in the neonate, often confined to the oral and diaper regions (Wilson & da Cunha, 2007).

Candidal diaper dermatitis appears on the perianal area, inguinal folds, and lower portion of the abdomen. The affected area is intensely erythematous, with a sharply demarcated, scalloped edge, frequently with numerous satellite lesions that extend beyond the larger lesion. The source of the infection is through the GI tract. Treatment is an antifungal ointment, such as nystatin (Mycostatin) or miconazole 2% (Monistat), applied with each diaper change. The infant also can be given an oral antifungal preparation to eliminate any GI source of infection (Wilson & da Cunha, 2007).

Oral candidiasis (**thrush,** or mycotic stomatitis) is characterized by the appearance of white plaques on the oral mucosa, gums, and tongue. The white patches are easily differentiated from milk curds; the patches cannot be removed and tend to bleed when touched. In most cases, the infant does not seem to be in discomfort from the infection. A few infants seem to have some difficulty swallowing.

Infants who are sick, debilitated, or receiving antibiotic therapy are more susceptible to thrush. Those with cleft lip or palate, neoplasms, and hyperparathyroidism seem to be more vulnerable to mycotic infection.

The objectives of management are to eradicate the causative organism, to control exposure to *C. albicans,* and to improve the infant's resistance. Interventions include maintenance of scrupulous cleanliness to prevent reinfection (nursing personnel, parents, others). Careful hand hygiene is always essential. Clean surfaces should be provided for neonates. Proper cleanliness of the equipment and environment is essential. If the infant is breastfeeding, the mother also is treated with a topical antifungal preparation such as nystatin applied to the nipples.

For the infant, topical application of 1 ml nystatin over the surfaces of the oral cavity four times a day, or every 6 hours, is usually sufficient to prevent spread of the disease or prolongation of its course. Several other drugs can be used, including amphotericin B (Fungizone), clotrimazole (Lotrimin, Mycelex), fluconazole (Diflucan), or miconazole (Monistat, Micatin) given intravenously, orally, or topically. To prevent relapse, therapy should be continued for at least 2 days after the lesions disappear. Gentian violet solution can be used in addition to one of the antifungal drugs in chronic cases of oral thrush; however, the former does not treat GI candida and can irritate the oral mucosa.

Infants who are breastfed can acquire thrush from the mother. If the mother is colonized, treatment for mother and infant is recommended. Breastfeeding can continue even if the mother is receiving systemic antifungal medications.

COMMUNITY ACTIVITY

- Visit the March of Dimes website at www.marchofdimes.com. Go to the pregnancy and newborn link and click on complications. Select an infection or sexually transmitted disease. Review the client information about the disease and prevention strategies.
- Visit the Medline Plus website and research Neonatal Abstinence Syndrome. Review the client information about causes, symptoms, exams and tests (neonatal abstinence scoring system) and treatment.

SUBSTANCE ABUSE

Substance abuse during pregnancy is associated with significant fetal and neonatal risks. Other than alcohol and tobacco, cocaine and marijuana are the most commonly used substances by pregnant women. Maternal substance abuse is discussed in Chapter 32.

The adverse effects of exposure of the fetus to drugs are varied. They include transient behavioral changes such as alterations in fetal breathing movements or irreversible effects such as fetal death, IUGR, congenital anomalies, or mental retardation. Critical determinants of the effect of the drug on the fetus include the specific drug, the dosage, the route of administration, the genotype of the mother or fetus, and the timing of the drug exposure. Determining the specific effects of individual drugs on the fetus is made difficult by the common practice of polydrug use, errors or omissions in reporting drug use, and variations in the strength, purity, and types of additives found in street drugs. Maternal conditions such as poverty and malnutrition and comorbid conditions such as STIs further compound the difficulty in identifying the presence and consequences of intrauterine drug exposure. Figure 35-11 shows critical periods in human embryogenesis and the teratogenic effects of drugs. Table 35-4 summarizes the effects of commonly abused substances on the fetus and neonate.

Physiologic signs of withdrawal have been reported in neonates of mothers who use to excess such drugs as barbiturates, alcohol, opioids, or amphetamines. Prescription opioids such as oxycodone (Percodan, OxyContin) have been identified as increasingly popular drugs of abuse that can cause withdrawal symptoms in neonates. Serious withdrawal reactions can be seen in neonates whose mothers abuse psychoactive drugs. Withdrawal symptoms in the neonate are described as **neonatal abstinence syndrome.** This syndrome is characterized by symptoms of CNS irritability, respiratory distress, GI dysfunction, and autonomic dysfunction (Table 35-5). Withdrawal symptoms are more severe in newborns exposed to larger amounts of drugs for longer periods of time. The severity of withdrawal is also related to the timing of maternal drug use in relation to birth. Drug use close to the time of birth increases the severity of withdrawal, but delays the onset of symptoms (Fike, 2007).

Tobacco

According to the CDC (2009c), infants born to women who smoke are about 30% more likely to be preterm, weigh on average a half pound less, and have a threefold risk of sudden infant death syndrome (SIDS) as compared with infants born to nonsmokers. When other variables have been controlled, no clear association has been found between maternal smoking and congenital anomalies (Reed, Aranda, & Hales, 2006).

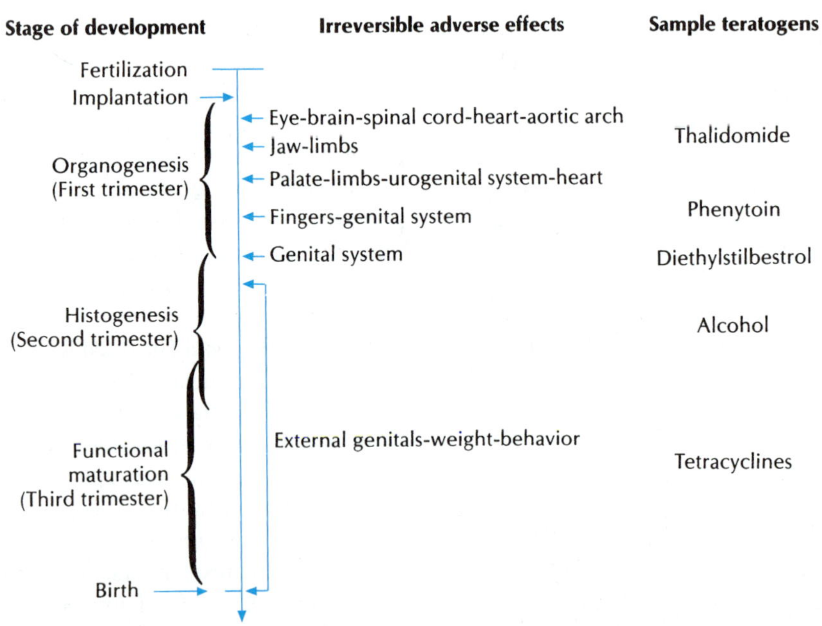

FIG. 35-11 Critical periods in human embryogenesis. (From Reed, M., Aranda, J., & Hales, B. [2006]. Developmental pharmacology. In R. Martin, A. Fanaroff, & M. Walsh (Eds.), *Fanaroff and Martin's neonatal-perinatal medicine: Diseases of the fetus and infant* [8th ed.]. St. Louis: Mosby.)

Nicotine and cotinine, the two pharmacologically active substances in tobacco, are found in higher concentrations in infants whose mothers smoke. These substances can be secreted in breast milk for up to 2 hours after the mother has smoked. Cigarette smoke contains more than 2000 compounds, including carbon monoxide, dioxin, cyanide, and cadmium. Long-term studies show residual effects beyond the neonatal period (Reed et al., 2006). Deficits in growth, in intellectual and emotional development, and in behavior have been documented (Shea & Steiner, 2008). These include poor auditory responsiveness, increased fine motor tremors, hypertonicity, and decreased verbal comprehension.

Increasing concern surrounds secondhand smoke and its potential effects on infants and children. Exposure to secondhand smoke increases the risk of ear infections, respiratory illnesses such as asthma and bronchitis, and SIDS (Best & Committee on Environmental Health, Committee on Native American Child Health, & Committee on Adolescence, 2009; Fleming & Blair, 2007). It is not clear whether the association between smoking and SIDS reflects in utero exposure or passive exposure postnatally, or both.

Smoking cessation during pregnancy greatly decreases the chance of fetal complications; therefore, women should be counseled regarding smoking cessation programs. Mothers and all others should refrain from smoking near the infant.

TABLE 35-4 SUMMARY OF NEONATAL EFFECTS OF COMMONLY ABUSED SUBSTANCES

SUBSTANCE	NEONATAL EFFECTS
Alcohol	Fetal alcohol syndrome (FAS): craniofacial anomalies, including short eyelid opening, flat midface, flat upper lip groove, thin upper lip; microcephaly; hyperactivity; developmental delays; attention deficits Alcohol-related birth defects (ARBDs): milder forms of FAS, cardiac anomalies, failure to thrive
Cocaine	Prematurity, small for gestational age, placental or cerebral infarctions, hyperactivity, difficult to console, hypersensitivity to noise and external stimuli, reduction in verbal reasoning
Heroin	Low birth weight, small for gestational age, neonatal abstinence syndrome (see Table 35-5)
Amphetamines	Small for gestational age, prematurity, poor weight gain, lethargy
Tobacco	Prematurity, low birth weight, increased risk for sudden infant death syndrome, increased risk for bronchitis, pneumonia, developmental delays

TABLE 35-5 SIGNS OF NEONATAL ABSTINENCE SYNDROME

SYSTEM	SIGNS
Respiratory	Irregular respirations, tachypnea, apnea, nasal flaring, chest retractions, intermittent cyanosis, rhinorrhea, nasal congestion
Neurologic	Irritability, tremors, shrill cry, incessant crying, hyperactivity, disturbed sleep pattern, seizures, hypertonicity, increased deep tendon reflexes, exaggerated Moro reflex
Autonomic dysfunction	Frequent yawning, frequent sneezing, tearing, excessive generalized sweating, mottling of skin, fever
Gastrointestinal	Abnormal feeding pattern, uncoordinated and ineffectual sucking and swallowing reflexes, incessant hunger, frantic sucking, refusal to feed, vomiting, regurgitation, diarrhea

Source: Fike, D. (2007). Substance-exposed newborn. In C. Kenner & J. Lott (Eds.), *Comprehensive neonatal care: An interdisciplinary approach* (4th ed.). St. Louis: Saunders.

Alcohol

Alcohol consumption during pregnancy is a growing concern. Alcohol ingestion during pregnancy is associated with both acute short- and long-term effects on the fetus and newborn, which are subsumed under the term *fetal alcohol spectrum disorders (FASDs)*. FASDs include specific conditions such as fetal alcohol syndrome (FAS), alcohol-related neurodevelopmental disorder (ARND), and alcohol-related birth defects (ARBD). FASDs are estimated to occur in as many as 9 to 10 of every 1000 births in the United States. However, the full extent of the problem is unknown and more prevalence studies are needed (Olson, Ohlemiller, O'Connor, Brown, Morris, Damus, & National Task Force on Fetal Alcohol Syndrome and Fetal Alcohol Effect, 2009).

The quantity of alcohol required to produce fetal effects is unclear, but it is known that infants born to heavy drinkers are at higher risk of congenital abnormalities than those born to moderate drinkers. Alcohol withdrawal can occur in neonates, particularly when maternal ingestion occurs near the time of birth. Signs and symptoms include jitteriness, increased tone and reflex responses, and irritability. Seizures are also common.

Fetal alcohol syndrome (FAS) is based on minimal criteria of signs in each of three categories: prenatal and postnatal growth restriction; CNS malfunctions, including mental retardation; and craniofacial features such as microcephaly, small eyes or short palpebral fissures, thin upper lip, flat midface, and an indistinct philtrum (Box 35-2). Neurologic problems in FAS children include some degree of IQ deficit, attention-deficit disorder, diminished fine motor skills, and poor speech. These children have been shown to lack inhibition, have no stranger anxiety, and lack appropriate judgment skills.

Infants exposed prenatally to alcohol who are affected but do not meet the criteria for FAS can be said to have **alcohol-related neurodevelopmental disorders (ARNDs)** or **alcohol-related birth defects (ARBDs)**. These disorders run the gamut from learning disabilities and behavioral problems to speech or language problems and hyperactivity. Often these problems are not detected until the child goes to school and learning problems become evident. Similar birth defects can be seen with other disorders, such as fetal hydantoin syndrome (from exposure to antiepileptic drugs); therefore, a careful history is needed.

Predictable abnormal patterns of fetal and neonatal morphogenesis are attributed to severe, chronic alcoholism in women who continue to drink heavily during pregnancy. The pattern of growth deficiency begun in prenatal life persists after birth, especially in the linear growth rate, rate of weight gain, and growth of head circumferences.

Ocular structural anomalies are common findings (Fig. 35-12). Limb anomalies and a variety of cardiocirculatory

Critical Thinking Exercise—Fetal Alcohol Syndrome

BOX 35-2 DIAGNOSTIC CRITERIA FOR FETAL ALCOHOL SYNDROME AND ALCOHOL-RELATED EFFECTS

1. Fetal alcohol syndrome (FAS) with confirmed maternal alcohol exposure*
   A. Confirmed maternal alcohol exposure
   B. Evidence of a characteristic pattern of facial anomalies that includes features such as short palpebral fissures and abnormalities in the premaxillary zone (e.g., flat upper lip, flattened philtrum, and flat midface)
   C. Evidence of growth restriction, as in at least one of the following:
   - Low birth weight for gestational age
   - Decelerating weight over time not due to nutrition
   - Disproportional low weight to height

   D. Evidence of central nervous system neurodevelopmental abnormalities, as in at least one of the following:
   - Decreased cranial size at birth
   - Structural brain abnormalities (e.g., microcephaly, partial or complete agenesis of the corpus callosum, cerebellar hypoplasia)
   - Neurologic hard or soft signs (as age appropriate), such as impaired fine motor skills, neurosensory hearing loss, poor tandem gait, poor eye-hand coordination
2. FAS without confirmed maternal alcohol exposure
   B, C, and D as above
3. Partial FAS with confirmed maternal alcohol exposure
   A. Confirmed maternal alcohol exposure
   B. Evidence of some components of the pattern of characteristic facial anomalies
   C or D as above *or*
   E. Evidence of a complex pattern of behavior or cognitive abnormalities that are inconsistent with developmental level and cannot be explained by familial background or environment alone, such as learning difficulties; deficits in school performance; poor impulse control; problems in social perception; deficits in higher level receptive and expressive language; poor capacity for abstraction or metacognition; specific deficits in mathematical skills; or problems in memory, attention, or judgment
4. Alcohol-related birth defects (ARBDs)†
   - Confirmed maternal alcohol exposure‡ and one or more congenital anomalies:

   Cardiac
   - Atrial septal defect
   - Aberrant great vessels
   - Ventricular septal defect
   - Tetralogy of Fallot

   Skeletal
   - Hypoplastic nails
   - Clinodactyly
   - Shortened fifth digits
   - Pectus excavatum and carinatum
   - Radioulnar synostosis
   - Klippel-Feil syndrome
   - Flexion contractures
   - Hemivertebrae
   - Camptodactyly
   - Scoliosis

   Renal
   - Aplastic, dysplastic, hypoplastic kidneys
   - Ureteral duplications
   - Hydronephrosis
   - Horseshoe kidneys

   Ocular
   - Strabismus
   - Retinal vascular anomalies
   - Refractive problems

   Auditory
   - Conductive hearing loss
   - Neurosensory heating loss

   Other
   - Virtually every malformation has been described in some infants with FAS. The etiologic specificity of most of these anomalies to alcohol teratogenesis remains uncertain.
5. Alcohol-related neurodevelopmental disorder (ARND)†
   - Confirmed maternal alcohol exposure‡ and D and/or E above

*A pattern of excessive intake characterized by substantial, regular intake or heavy episodic drinking. Evidence of this pattern may include frequent episodes of intoxication, development of tolerance or withdrawal, social problems related to drinking, legal problems related to drinking, engaging in physically hazardous behavior while drinking, or alcohol-related medical problems such as hepatic disease.

†In infants with both ARBD and ARND, both diagnoses should be rendered.

‡As further research is completed and as, or if, lower quantities or variable patterns of alcohol use are associated with ARBD or ARND, these patterns of alcohol use should be incorporated into the diagnostic criteria.

Sources: Committee to Study Fetal Alcohol Syndrome. (1996). Stratton, K., Howe, C., & Battaglia, F. (Eds.). *Fetal alcohol syndrome: Diagnosis, epidemiology, prevention, and treatment.* Washington, DC: National Academy Press; Bandstra, E., & Accornero, V. (2006). Infants of substance-abusing mothers. In R. Martin, A. Fanaroff, & M. Walsh (Eds.), *Fanaroff and Martin's neonatal-perinatal medicine: Diseases of the fetus and infant* (8th ed.). Philadelphia: Mosby.

anomalies, especially ventricular septal defects, pose problems for the child. Box 35-2 outlines physical findings in FAS. Mental retardation (IQ of 79 or less at age 7 years), hyperactivity, and fine motor dysfunction (poor hand-to-mouth coordination, weak grasp) add to the handicapping problems that maternal alcoholism can impose. Genital abnormalities are seen in daughters of alcohol-addicted mothers. Two thirds of newborns with FAS are girls; the cause of this altered fetal sex ratio is unknown. Severe and chronic alcoholism (ethanol toxicity), not maternal malnutrition, is responsible for the severity and consistency of postnatal performance problems (Bandstra & Accornero, 2006). High alcohol levels are lethal to the developing embryo. Lower levels cause brain and other malformations. Long-term prognosis (no studies are available) is discouraging even in an optimal psychosocial environment, when one considers the combination of growth failure and mental retardation.

Heroin

Heroin crosses the placenta and often results in IUGR in exposed infants, although the exact mechanisms of growth inhibition are not clear. There is an increased rate of stillbirths but not of congenital anomalies. Maternal heroin use increases the risk for meconium aspiration, increased neonatal death, microcephaly, neurobehavioral problems, and SIDS (Minozzi, Amato, Vecchi, & Davoli, 2008). If heroin users are placed on methadone maintenance treatment during pregnancy, perinatal outcomes are improved (Wisner, Sit, Reynolds, Altemus, Bogen, Sunder, et al., 2007).

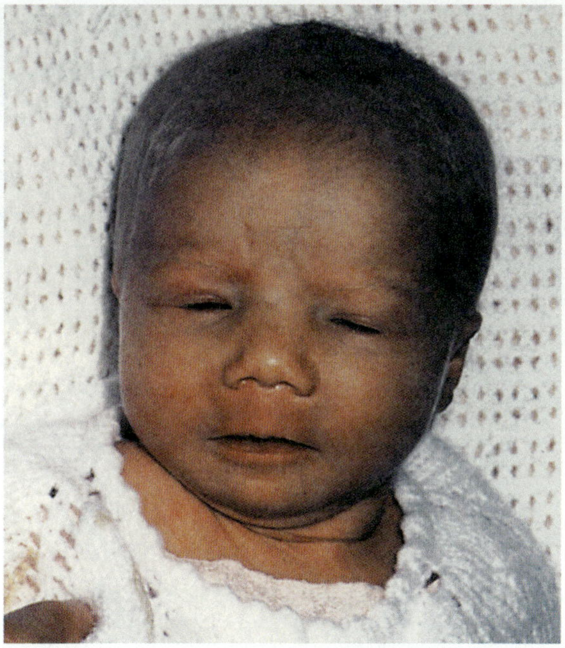

FIG. 35-12 Infant with fetal alcohol syndrome. (From Markiewicz, M., & Abrahamson, E. [1999]. *Diagnosis in color: Neonatology*. St. Louis: Mosby.)

Many of the medical complications attributed to heroin result from prematurity. Other risks include physical dependence in the fetus and the risk of exposure to infections, including hepatitis B and C viruses and HIV. Drug withdrawal in the mother is accompanied by fetal withdrawal, which can lead to fetal death. Maternal detoxification in the first trimester carries an increased risk of miscarriage. Detoxification in pregnancy is not recommended because of possible withdrawal-induced fetal distress. Methadone is often used in pregnancy to treat maternal drug cravings and prevent withdrawal.

Heroin withdrawal (neonatal abstinence syndrome) occurs in the majority of infants born to addicted mothers, usually within the first 12 to 48 hours of life. The signs depend on the length of maternal addiction, the amount of drug taken, and the time of injection before birth. The infant whose mother is taking methadone may not demonstrate signs of withdrawal until a week or so after birth. The symptoms of infants whose mothers used heroin or methadone are similar in nature. Initially the infant can be depressed. The withdrawal syndrome can manifest as a combination of any of the following signs. Most commonly, the infant is jittery and hyperactive. Usually the infant's cry is shrill and persistent. The infant can yawn or sneeze frequently. The tendon reflexes are increased, but the Moro reflex is decreased. The neonate can exhibit poor feeding and sucking, tachypnea, vomiting, diarrhea, hypothermia or hyperthermia, and sweating. In addition, an abnormal sleep cycle, with absence of quiet sleep and disturbance of active sleep, has been described in these infants (Bandstra & Accornero, 2006).

If withdrawal is not treated, vomiting, diarrhea, dehydration, apnea, and convulsions can develop. Death can follow. Therapy is individualized. Dehydration and electrolyte imbalance are prevented or treated. Usually one of the following drugs is ordered: phenobarbital, methadone, morphine syrup, or diazepam, singly or in combination.

NURSING ALERT

The use of naloxone (Narcan) is contraindicated in infants born to narcotic addicts because it may cause severe signs and symptoms of narcotic abstinence syndrome and seizures.

SAFETY ALERT

Methadone and morphine are high-alert medications, that is, they carry an increased risk of causing client injury or death if used incorrectly. Additional safety checks are put into place when these medications are administered to newborn infants (Institute for Safe Medication Practices, 2008).

Methadone

Methadone, a synthetic opiate, has been the therapy of choice for heroin addiction since 1965. Methadone crosses the placenta. An increasing number of infants have been born to methadone-maintained mothers, who seem to have better prenatal care and a somewhat better lifestyle than those taking heroin (Bandstra & Accornero, 2006).

Neonatal abstinence syndrome occurs in the majority of neonates born to women taking methadone. Neither the incidence or severity of symptoms has been correlated with methadone dose at delivery (Wisner et al., 2007). Methadone withdrawal resembles heroin withdrawal but tends to be more severe and prolonged. In addition, the incidence of seizures is higher. Seizures usually occur between days 7 and 10. Infants exhibit a disturbed sleep pattern similar to that seen in heroin withdrawal and have a higher birth weight than those in heroin withdrawal, usually appropriate for gestational age. No increased incidence of congenital anomalies is seen.

Late-onset withdrawal occurs at 2 to 4 weeks and can continue for weeks or months. A higher incidence of SIDS also has been reported in these infants (Bandstra & Accornero, 2006). This factor is important for perinatal nurses who coordinate follow-up care for the infant and education for the mother or other caregiver. Pediatric and community health nurses must know about the potential for withdrawal symptoms to occur.

Therapy for methadone withdrawal is similar to that for heroin withdrawal. Buprenorphine, a partial agonist–partial anatagonist synthetic opioid with a long duration of action, has gained acceptance and FDA licensing in the treatment of opioid addiction. Preliminary studies indicate that this drug has advantages over methadone in relation to neonatal outcomes such as severity of neonatal abstinence syndrome and length of hospital stay (Helmbrecht & Thiagarajah, 2008; Kakko, Heilig, & Sarman, 2008).

Methadone is not contraindicated during breastfeeding. Minimal amounts of methadone are transferred to the infant through breast milk. However, infants exposed to methadone are at greater risk for feeding problems (Wisner et al., 2007).

The long-term effects of methadone exposure are primarily related to neurodevelopmental outcomes. These neonates are at increased risk for developmental delays, poor fine motor coordination, lower intelligence, hyperactivity, learning and behavior disorders, and poor social adjustment. Researchers have noted that it is difficult to separate the effects of methadone from other factors in the environment that can influence neurobehavioral outcomes (Bandstra & Accornero, 2006; Helmbrecht & Thiagarajah, 2008).

Marijuana

Marijuana is the most common illicit drug used by pregnant women. Marijuana crosses the placenta, and its use during pregnancy can result in a shortened gestation and a higher incidence of IUGR. A review of studies examining the effects of marijuana during pregnancy found inconsistent results regarding the drug's effect on birth weight and gestational age (Schempf, 2007). No specific teratogenic effects have been identified. Some investigators have found a higher incidence of meconium staining of the amniotic fluid. Animal models suggest that marijuana smoking during pregnancy can increase carbon monoxide levels in the blood which reduces the amount of oxygen available to the fetus, but this has not been correlated with studies identifying short- or long-term effects on the fetus (Bandstra & Accornero, 2006).

Long-term effects of marijuana exposure can involve deficits in memory, attention, cognitive function, or motor skills (Wisner et al., 2007). Compounding the issue of the effects of marijuana is multidrug use, especially among adolescents, that combines the harmful effects of marijuana, tobacco, alcohol, and cocaine. Long-term follow-up studies on exposed infants are needed.

Cocaine

Cocaine crosses the placenta and is found in breast milk. Considerable controversy exists regarding the effects of cocaine on the fetus and neonate. There is a strong association between maternal cocaine use and both tobacco and marijuana use, which makes the determination of cocaine effects difficult. A large metaanalysis of 15,208 pregnancies did not find an association between illicit drug use and congenital anomalies (van Gelder, Reefhuis, Caton, Werler, Druschel, & Roeleveld, 2009). However, it is possible that habitual cocaine use in pregnancy has negative effects, many of which are too subtle to notice in the newborn and infancy periods. Cocaine is a recognized cause of placental abruption. Infants born to cocaine-abusing mothers show a high rate of perinatal morbidity, IUGR, low birth weight, and preterm birth (Box 35-3) (Bandstra & Accornero, 2006; Wisner et al., 2007).

Cocaine-dependent neonates do not experience a process of withdrawal as seen in narcotic-exposed infants but rather show neurotoxic effects of the drug. Signs of exposure have some of the same characteristics as those of heroin withdrawal but can be highly varied. There can be an increased risk for SIDS. The effects of prenatal exposure to cocaine on neonatal behavior have been studied extensively. Findings indicate that cocaine-exposed infants have limited ability to habituate to stimuli. As these children enter school, they demonstrate a reduced capacity for verbal reasoning and difficulties maintaining attention (Bandstra & Accornero, 2006).

BOX 35-3 FETAL AND NEONATAL EFFECTS OF MATERNAL COCAINE USE DURING PREGNANCY

PHYSICAL

- Preterm birth
- Decreased length
- Decreased head circumference
- Low birth weight
- Cerebral infraction
- Abnormal electroencephalogram (EEG)
- Seizures
- Atrial/ventricular arrhythmia
- Hypertension
- Decreased cardiac output
- Apnea
- Abnormal breathing pattern

BEHAVIORAL

- Irritability
- Tremors
- Abnormal sleep pattern
- Hypertonicity
- Increase In auditory startle response
- Disorganized behavior
- Lethargy
- Hyporeacitivity
- Poor interaction with caregivers

Sources: Weiner, S., & Finnegan, L. (2011). Drug withdrawal in the neonate. In S. Gardner, B. Carter, M. Enzman-Hines, & J. Hernandez (Eds), *Merenstein & Gardner's handbook of neonatal intensive care* (7th ed.). St Louis: Mosby; Pitts, K. (2010). Perinatal substance abuse. In M. Verklan & M. Walden (Eds.), *Core curriculum for neonatal intensive care nursing* (4th ed.), St. Louis: Saunders.

Methamphetamine

The fetal and neonatal effects associated with maternal use of methamphetamines in pregnancy are not well known. The limited data regarding the risk of congenital anomalies suggest little or no effect on organogenesis. A higher incidence of placental abruption, preterm birth, and IUGR is associated with methamphetamine use during pregnancy (Cunningham et al., 2010; Helmbrecht & Thiagarajah, 2008; Smith, LaGasse, Derauf, Grant, Shah, Arria, et al., 2006). Behavioral changes in infants exposed prenatally to methamphetamines include decreased arousal, increased stress, and alterations in movement (Smith et al., 2006).

Neonatal manifestations of methamphetamine withdrawal have not been clearly identified because of maternal polydrug use. After birth, infants can experience bradycardia or tachycardia that resolves as the drug is cleared from the infant's system. Lethargy can continue for several months, along with frequent infections and poor weight gain. Emotional disturbances and delays in gross and fine motor coordination can be seen during early childhood.

MDMA/Ecstasy

Increasing use of 3,4-methylenedioxymethamphetamine (MDMA), also known as "ecstasy," by adolescents and young adults of childbearing age heightens concerns related to fetal and neonatal effects of this substance. This illegal, synthetic psychoactive drug has hallucinogenic and stimulant properties. It alters the activity of neurotransmitters in the brain and causes increased heart rate and blood pressure. Animal studies have demonstrated that MDMA can be toxic to nerve cells containing serotonin, causing long-term damage. MDMA alters the body's temperature regulatory abilities and in high doses can cause a sharp increase in body temperature (hyperthermia) leading to liver, kidney, and cardiovascular system failure, and death (National Institute on Drug Abuse, 2009). This substance is transferred to the fetus through the placenta, but the effects on the developing fetus are not well substantiated in human studies. It is thought that maternal use of MDMA increases the risk of congenital anomalies in the fetus and that it can cause long-term problems with learning and memory. More research studies are needed to identify the effects of MDMA on the fetus and neonate (Fike, 2007).

Other Drugs of Concern

Caffeine

Caffeine is a mild CNS stimulant that is consumed on a regular basis by more than 85% of adults and children and 68% of pregnant women in the United States (Frary, Johnson, & Wang, 2005). Coffee is the primary source of caffeine for most Americans, although caffeine is also found in tea, chocolate, colas, energy drinks, guarana, and mate (a tea consumed primarily in South America).

The average half-life of caffeine ranges from about 3 to 7 hours with individual variation in metabolism related to genetic and environmental factors. During the second and third trimesters of pregnancy, caffeine metabolism is slowed due to hormonal influences. Caffeine readily crosses the placenta and is distributed to all fetal tissues. Because of immature liver function, fetuses metabolize caffeine very slowly.

Although caffeine has not been implicated as a teratogen in humans, there are concerns about caffeine consumption during pregnancy. The effects of caffeine seem to be dose dependent; that is, the risk increases with greater caffeine consumption. High maternal intake of caffeine (more than 200 to 300 mg/day) increases the risk of miscarriage and low birth weight (Higdon & Frei, 2006; Weng, Odouli, & Li, 2008).

The American Dietetic Association recommends that caffeine intake in pregnant women should not exceed 300 mg/day (Kaiser & Allen, 2008). The March of Dimes more conservatively recommends no more than 200 mg/day for women who are pregnant or are planning to become pregnant (March of Dimes, 2010).

Selective Serotonin Reuptake Inhibitors

Antidepressant medication is the mainstay treatment for maternal depression with selective serotonin reuptake inhibitors (SSRIs) being the first line of pharmacotherapy. Commonly prescribed SSRIs include citalopram, escitalopram, fluoxetine, fluvoxamine, paroxetine, and sertraline (Cunningham et al., 2010). The American College of Obstetricians and Gynecologists (2008) published guidelines for the use of psychiatric medications in women who are pregnant and breastfeeding. All medications that have been studied are known to cross the placenta and are transferred in breast milk. Their use should be determined by a risk/benefit analysis of the risks to the fetus/neonate with use of the medication weighed against risks of not treating the mother's psychiatric condition. Risks of nontreatment include noncompliance with prenatal care, poor nutrition, substance abuse, and interference with maternal-infant bonding (ACOG).

Based on current evidence, the ACOG (2008) has concluded that the absolute risk of any congenital abnormality associated with maternal SSRI use is small. However, certain medications carry greater risk than others. Because of the risk of cardiac defects associated with maternal paroxetine treatment, the ACOG (2008) warns that paroxetine use should be avoided during pregnancy and in women considering pregnancy. There have also been reports linking paroxetine use to other anomalies such as omphalocele, craniosynostosis, and anencephaly.

Fetal exposure to SSRIs predisposes the neonate to a behavioral syndrome resembling neonatal abstinence syndrome. Symptoms include irritability, agitation, tremors, nasal congestion, tachypnea, emesis, and diarrhea. This syndrome is usually mild and lasts for no longer than 2 days. In rare cases the syndrome is severe with seizures, hyperpyrexia, excessive weight loss, and respiratory problems (Cunningham et al., 2010). Persistent pulmonary hypertension in the newborn (PPHN) has been reported in infants who were exposed to maternal SSRIs after 20 weeks of gestation; the risk for PPHN was 6 to 12 per 1000 births (Chambers, Hernandez-Diaz, Van Marter, Werler, Louik, Jones, et al., 2006).

For parents who are concerned about maternal use of psychiatric medications and the fetal or neonatal effects, the nurse can direct them to the following websites: REPROTOX (www.reprotox.org) and TERIS (http://depts.washington.edu/terisweb) (ACOG, 2008).

CARE MANAGEMENT

The maternal history is the key to identification of newborns who are at risk because of maternal substance abuse or use of other drugs during pregnancy. Review of the prenatal record can reveal a medical and social history of drug use or abuse and any detoxification treatment that was used. There can also be other factors that contribute to neonatal outcomes and complications. For example, the woman who is addicted to narcotics or cocaine can have infections that compound the risk to the infant, including hepatitis, septicemia, and STIs, including AIDS (Bandstra & Accornero, 2006). In some cases there is no information in the prenatal record to suggest maternal substance abuse when the woman has, in fact, been using one or more substances during pregnancy.

The infant is assessed by means of the guidelines discussed in Chapter 24. The infant's gestational age and maturity are noted. The infant can have IUGR or be preterm with LBW. In utero exposure to some drugs results in observable malformations or dysmorphism (abnormality of shape). Neonatal behavior can arouse suspicion. Figure 35-13 provides an example of a scoring system for assessing withdrawal symptoms (neonatal abstinence syndrome). Because many women are multidrug users, the newborn initially may exhibit a confusing complex of signs. The nurse often is the first to observe the signs of drug withdrawal in the infant. The nurse's observations help the health care provider differentiate between signs of neonatal abstinence syndrome and other conditions, such as CNS disorder, sepsis, hypoglycemia, and electrolyte imbalance.

Urine or meconium screening can be used to identify substances abused by the mother. Urine screening is most commonly used, but its sensitivity is limited. Initially costly and of limited availability, tests of meconium collected on day 1 or 2 of life have been shown to be sensitive and reliable in detecting the

Signs	Score 0	1	2	3
Tremors (muscle activity of limbs)	Normal	Minimally ↑ when hungry or disturbed	Moderately or markedly ↑ when undisturbed, subside when fed or held snugly	Marked even when undisturbed, going on to seizure-like movements
Irritability (excessive crying)	None	Slightly ↑	Moderate to severe when disturbed or hungry	Marked even when undisturbed
Reflexes	Normal	Increased	Markedly increased	
Stools	Normal	Explosive, but normal frequency	Explosive, more than 8/day	
Muscle tone	Normal	Increased	Rigidity	
Skin abrasions	No	Redness of knees and elbows	Breaking of skin	
Respiratory rate/minute	<55	55 to 75	76 to 95	
Repetitive sneezing	No	Yes		
Repetitive yawning	No	Yes		
Vomiting	No	Yes		
Fever	No	Yes		

Scoring: Identification of newborn with narcotic withdrawal when score >17 (78% probability)

FIG. 35-13 Neonatal Abstinence Scoring System. (Source: Lipsitz, P. [1975]. A proposed narcotic withdrawal score for use with newborn infants: A pragmatic evaluation of its efficacy. *Clinical Pediatrics, 14*[6], 592-594.)

metabolites of several street drugs, including cocaine (López, Bermejo, Tabernero, Cabarcos, Alvarez, & Fernández, 2009).

Nursing Care

Planning for care of the infant born to a substance-abusing mother presents a challenge to the health care team. Parents are included in the planning for the newborn's care and for the care and support of the mother and her newborn at home. A multidisciplinary approach includes home health or community resource personnel (e.g., regulatory agencies such as child protective services).

Education and social support to prevent the abuse of drugs provide the ideal approach. However, given the scope of the drug abuse problem, total prevention is an unrealistic goal.

Nursing care of the drug-dependent neonate involves supportive therapy for fluid and electrolyte balance, nutrition, infection control, and respiratory care. Swaddling, holding, reducing stimuli, and feeding as necessary can be helpful in easing withdrawal (see the Nursing Care Plan: The Infant Experiencing Drug Withdrawal [Neonatal Abstinence Syndrome]). Specific suggestions for providing care to infants experiencing withdrawal are listed in Box 35-4.

Pharmacologic treatment is usually based on the severity of withdrawal symptoms, as determined by an assessment tool (see Fig. 35-13). When indicated, medications are given as ordered. Neonatal tincture of opium (0.4 mg/ml of morphine equivalent), phenobarbital, and, less commonly, paregoric may be used to control symptoms. Treatment may be needed for 2 weeks or more.

The issue of breastfeeding in this population is a difficult one. Although breast milk remains the optimal source of nutrition for these infants, care must be taken to avoid exposing the infant to additional drugs through the breast milk. According to the AAP Committee on Drugs (2001), nursing mothers should not ingest drugs of abuse including amphetamine, cocaine, heroin, marijuana, and phencyclidine because they are hazardous to the breastfeeding infant and to the mother.

NURSING CARE PLAN

The Infant Experiencing Drug Withdrawal (Neonatal Abstinence Syndrome)

NURSING DIAGNOSIS

Risk for injury related to hyperactivity, seizures secondary to passive narcotic addiction resulting from maternal substance abuse during pregnancy

Expected Outcome

Infant exhibits no signs of seizure activity.

Nursing Interventions/*Rationales*

- Administer phenobarbital, diazepam, or other medication per physician order *to decrease CNS irritability and control seizure activity.*
- Decrease environmental stimuli *that may trigger irritability and hyperactive behaviors.*
- Plan care activities carefully *to allow minimal stimulation.*
- Wrap infant snugly and hold tightly *to reduce self-stimulation behaviors and protect skin from abrasions.*
- If infant is cocaine addicted, position to avoid eye contact, swaddle infant, use vertical rocking techniques, and use a pacifier *to counter poor organizational response to stimuli and depressed interactive behaviors.*
- Monitor activity level, note the relation between activity level and external stimulation, and stop external stimulation *if it causes activity increase.*

NURSING DIAGNOSIS

Imbalanced nutrition: less than body requirements related to CNS irritability, poor suck reflex, vomiting, and diarrhea

Expected Outcome

Infant exhibits ingestion and retention of adequate nutrients and appropriate weight gain.

Nursing Interventions/*Rationales*

- Feed in frequent, small amounts, elevate head during and after feeding, and burp well *to diminish vomiting and aspiration.*
- Experiment with various nipples *to find one most effective in compensating for poor suck reflex.*
- Monitor weight daily and maintain strict intake and output *to evaluate success of feeding.*
- If intake is insufficient, feed by oral gavage per physician's order *to ensure ingestion of needed nutrients.*
- Have suction available as required *to reduce chances of aspiration.*

NURSING DIAGNOSIS

Risk for deficient fluid volume related to diarrhea and vomiting

Expected Outcome

Infant exhibits evidence of fluid homeostasis.

Nursing Interventions/*Rationales*

- Administer oral and parenteral fluids per physician order and regulate *to maintain fluid balance.*
- Monitor hydration status (skin turgor, weight, mucous membranes, fontanels, urine specific gravity, electrolytes) and intake and output *to evaluate for evidence of dehydration.*

NURSING DIAGNOSIS

Ineffective maternal coping, anxiety, powerlessness related to drug use, infant distress during withdrawal

Expected Outcomes

Woman will accept newborn's condition and participate in care activities, showing evidence of maternal-infant bonding process.

Nursing Interventions/*Rationales*

- Explain in a nonjudgmental way effects of maternal drug use on newborn and the withdrawal process *to provide understanding and reality concerning effects of drug use.*
- Encourage open communication (e.g., inform mother of ongoing condition, procedures, and treatment; answer questions; correct misperceptions; actively listen to her concerns) *to provide a sense of respect, provide support, and encourage a sense of control.*
- Encourage mother to interact with infant and to become involved in care routines *to foster emotional connection.*
- Explain how to do care procedures, how to avoid excess stimulation, and how to hold and rock infant *to enhance mother's care abilities and her sense of confidence and control.*
- If the mother is addicted to cocaine, explain infant's inability to interact, gaze aversion, arching back, and lack of response to cuddling *to enhance understanding of infant behaviors.*
- Make appropriate referrals to social agencies for treatment of maternal drug addiction, infant development programs, and other needed support services *to ensure adequate resources for care of self and infant.*

Nursing Care Plan—The Infant Experiencing Drug Withdrawal (Neonatal Abstinence Syndrome)

BOX 35-4 CARE OF THE INFANT EXPERIENCING WITHDRAWAL (NEONATAL ABSTINENCE SYNDROME)

- Place the infant in a side-lying position with the spine and legs flexed.
- Position the infant's hands in midline with the arms at the side.
- Carry the infant in a flexed position.
- When interacting with the infant, introduce one stimulus at a time when the infant is in a quiet, alert state.
- Watch for time-out or distress signals (gaze aversion, yawning, sneezing, hiccups, arching, mottled color).
- When the infant is distressed, swaddle in a flexed position and rock in a slow, rhythmic fashion.
- Put the infant in a sitting position with chin tucked down for feeding.

Drug dependence in the neonate is physiologic, not psychologic. Thus a predisposition to dependence later in life is not believed to be a factor. However, the psychosocial environment in which the infant is raised may create a tendency to addiction.

The mother requires considerable support. Her need for and her abuse of drugs can result in a decreased capacity to cope. The infant's withdrawal signs and decreased consolability stress her coping abilities even further. Family members also need support as they assist in caring for the infant. Home health care, treatment for addiction, and education are important considerations. Sensitive exploration of the woman's options for the care of her infant and herself and for future fertility management may help her see that she has choices. This approach helps communicate respect for the new mother as a person who can make responsible decisions.

CLINICAL REASONING

Narcotic Exposure in a Newborn

Annika is a female neonate born at 37 weeks of gestation to a G2 P1 mother, who, for the past 3 months, has been taking morphine for chronic pancreatitis. Following a spontaneous vaginal birth, Annika receives Apgar scores of 5 at 1 minute and 8 at 5 minutes. Annika is active and alert. In caring for this neonate and her mother you will need to determine a plan for monitoring Annika for signs of drug withdrawal.

1. Evidence—Is there sufficient evidence to draw conclusions about an appropriate plan for monitoring and treating Annika?
2. Assumptions—Describe underlying assumptions about each of the following issues:
   a. Symptoms of narcotic withdrawal
   b. Tools for assessing an infant with narcotic withdrawal
   c. Recommendations for managing an infant with narcotic withdrawal
3. What implications and priorities for nursing care can be drawn at this time?
4. Does the evidence objectively support your conclusion?
5. Are there alternative perspectives to your conclusion?

KEY POINTS

- A small percentage of significant birth injuries occur despite skilled and competent obstetric care.
- The same birth injury can be caused in several ways.
- The nurse's primary contribution to the welfare of the neonate begins with early observation, accurate recording, and prompt reporting of abnormal signs.
- Metabolic abnormalities of diabetes mellitus in pregnancy adversely affect embryonic and fetal development.
- Prepregnancy planning and good diabetic control, coupled with strict diabetic control during pregnancy, may prevent the embryonic, fetal, and neonatal conditions associated with pregnancies complicated by diabetes mellitus.
- Infection in the neonate can be acquired in utero, during birth, during resuscitation, and from within the nursery.
- The most common maternal infections during early pregnancy that are associated with various congenital malformations are caused by viruses.
- HIV transmission from mother to infant occurs transplacentally at various gestational ages, perinatally by maternal blood and secretions, and by breast milk.
- The nurse often is the first to observe signs of newborn drug withdrawal.
- Providing high-quality perinatal care to a varied population with multiple conditions is complicated by the special needs of high risk drug-dependent clients.
- Signs and symptoms of withdrawal in an infant vary in time of onset depending on the type and dose of drug involved.

Audio Chapter Summaries Access an audio summary of these Key Points on Evolve.

REFERENCES

Adams-Chapman, I., & Stoll, B. (2007). Nervous system disorders. In R. Kliegman, R. Behrman, H. Jenson, & B. Stanton (Eds.), *Nelson textbook of pediatrics* (18th ed.). Philadelphia: Saunders.

Agency for Healthcare Research and Quality (AHRQ), Center for Delivery Organization, and Markets. (2008). *National Healthcare Quality and disparities report, Table 10_4_1.1.* Available at. www.ahrq.gov/qual/qrdr08/10_patientsafety/T10_4_1-1.htm. Accessed July 27, 2010.

American Academy of Pediatrics (AAP) Committee on Drugs. (2001). The transfer of drugs and other chemicals into human milk. *Pediatrics, 108*(3), 776–789.

American Academy of Pediatrics (AAP) Committee on Pediatric AIDS. (2008). HIV testing and prophylaxis to prevent mother-to-child transmission in the United States. *Pediatrics, 122*(5), 1127–1134.

American Academy of Pediatrics (AAP) Committee on Infectious Diseases. (2009). *Red book: 2009 Report of the committee on infectious diseases* (28th ed.). Elk Grove Village, IL: American Academy of Pediatrics.

American Academy of Pediatrics (AAP) & American College of Obstetricians and Gynecologists (ACOG). (2007). *Guidelines for perinatal care* (6th ed.). Elk Grove Village, IL: The Academy.

American College of Obstetricians and Gynecologists (ACOG). (2008). Clinical management guidelines for obstetrician-gynecologists: Use of psychiatric medications during pregnancy and lactation. ACOG Practice Bulletin 92, 1–20, Washington, DC: ACOG.

Anderson, M., Wood, L., Keller, J., & Hay, W. (2011). Enteral nutrition. In S. Gardner, B. Carter, M. Enzman-Hines, & J. Hernandez (Eds.), *Merenstein & Gardner's handbook of neonatal intensive care* (7th ed.). St Louis: Mosby.

Andrews, W., Schelonka, R., Waites, K., Stamm, A., Cliver, S., & Moser, S. (2008). Genital tract methicillin-resistant *Staphylococcus aureus*: Risk of vertical transmission in pregnant women. *Obstetrical and Gynecological Survey, 63*(5), 284–286.

Askin, D., & Wilson, D. (2007). The high risk newborn and family. In M. Hockenberry & D. Wilson (Eds.), *Wong's nursing care of infants and children* (8th ed.). St. Louis: Mosby.

Association of Women's Health, Obstetric and Neonatal Nurses. (2007). *Evidence-based clinical practice guideline: Neonatal skin care* (2nd ed.). Washington, DC: The Association.

Baley, J., & Toltzis, P. (2006). Viral infections. In R. Martin, A. Fanaroff, & M. Walsh (Eds.), *Fanaroff and Martin's neonatal-perinatal medicine: Diseases of the fetus and infant* (8th ed.). Philadelphia: Mosby.

Bandstra, E., & Accornero, V. (2006). Infants of substance-abusing mothers. In R. Martin, A. Fanaroff, & M. Walsh (Eds.), *Fanaroff and Martin's neonatal-perinatal medicine: Diseases of the fetus and infant* (8th ed.). Philadelphia: Mosby.

Best, D. & Committee on Environmental Health, Committee on Native American Child Health, & Committee on Adolescence. (2009). Secondhand and prenatal tobacco smoke exposure. *Pediatrics, 124*(5), e1017–e1044.

Best, J. (2007). Rubella. *Seminars in Fetal and Neonatal Medicine, 12*(3), 182–192.

Bizzarro, M., Dembry, L., Baltimore, R., & Gallagher, P. (2008). Changing patterns in neonatal *Escherichia coli* sepsis and ampicillin resistance in the era of intrapartum antibiotic prophylaxis. *Pediatrics, 121*(4), 689–696.

Bradley, J. (2006). Hepatitis. In J. Remington, J. Klein, C. Baker, & C. Wilson (Eds.), *Infectious diseases of the fetus and newborn infant* (6th ed.). Philadelphia: Saunders.

Caviness, A., Demmler, G., & Selwyn, B. (2008). Clinical and laboratory features of neonatal herpes simplex infection: A case-control study, *Pediatric Infectious Disease Journal, 27*(5), 425–430.

Centers for Disease Control and Prevention (CDC). (2005). Guidelines for identifying and referring persons with fetal alcohol syndrome. *MMWR Morbidity and Mortality Weekly Report, Recommendations and Reports, 54*(RR-11), 1–15.

Centers for Disease Control and Prevention (CDC). (2009a). Guidelines for the prevention and treatment of opportunistic infections among HIV-exposed and HIV-infected children: Recommendations from the CDC, the National Institute of Health, the HIV Medicine Association of the Infections Diseases Society of America, the Pediatric Infectious Diseases Society, and the American Academy of Pediatrics. *MMWR Morbidity and Mortality Weekly Report, Recommendations and Reports, 58*(RR-11), 1–173.

Centers for Disease Control and Prevention (CDC). (2009b). Preliminary FoodNet data on the incidence of infection with pathogens transmitted commonly through food—10 states, 2008. *MMWR Morbidity and Mortality Weekly Report, Recommendations and Reports, 58*(13), 333–337.

Centers for Disease Control and Prevention (CDC). (2009c). *Tobacco use and pregnancy.* Available at www.cdc.gov/reproductivehealth/tobaccoUsePregnancy/index.htm. Accessed July 27, 2010.

Centers for Disease Control and Prevention. (2009d). Trends in perinatal group B streptococcal disease—United States, 2000-2006. *MMWR Morbidity and Mortality Weekly Report, Recommendations and Reports, 58*(5), 109–112.

Chambers, C., Hernandez-Diaz, S., Van Marter, L., Werler, M., Louik, C., Jones, K., et al. (2006). Selective serotonin-reuptake inhibitors and risk of persistent pulmonary hypertension of the newborn. *New England Journal of Medicine, 354*(6), 579–587.

Cooper, L., & Alford, C. (2006). Rubella. In J. Remington, J. Klein, C. Baker, & C. Wilson (Eds.), *Infectious diseases of the fetus and newborn infant* (6th ed.). Philadelphia: Saunders.

Correa, A., Gilboa, S., Besser, L., Botto, L., Moore, C., & Hobbs, C. (2008). Diabetes mellitus and birth defects. *American Journal of Obstetrics and Gynecology, 199*(3), 237, e1–e9.

Corrigan, N., Brazil, D., & McAuliffe, F. (2009). Fetal cardiac effects of maternal hyperglycemia during pregnancy. *Birth Defects Research Part A: Clinical and Molecular Teratology, 85*(6), 523–530.

Cunningham, F., Leveno, K., Bloom, S., Hauth, J., Rouse, D., & Spong, C. (2010). *Williams obstetrics* (23rd ed.). New York: McGraw-Hill.

de Jong, E., de Haan, T., Kroes, A., Beersma, M., Oepkes, D., Walther, F., et al. (2006). Parvovirus B19 infection in pregnancy. *Journal of Clinical Virology, 36*(1), 1–7.

Doumouchtsis, S., & Arulkumaran, S. (2006). Head injuries after instrumental vaginal deliveries. *Current Opinion in Obstetrics and Gynecology, 18*(2), 129–134.

Doumouchtsis, S., & Arulkumaran, S. (2008). Head trauma after instrumental births. *Clinics in Perinatology, 35*(1), 69–83.

Dudley, D. (2007). Diabetic-associated stillbirth: Incidence, pathophysiology and prevention. *Clinical Perinatology, 34*(4), 611–626.

Duff, P., Sweet, R., & Edwards, R. (2009). Maternal and fetal infections. In R. Creasy, R. Resnik, J. Iams, C. Lockwood, & T. Moore (Eds.), *Creasy & Resnik's maternal fetal medicine: Principles and practice* (6th ed.). Philadelphia: Saunders.

Edwards, M. (2006). Postnatal bacterial infections. In R. Martin, A. Fanaroff, & M. Walsh (Eds.), *Fanaroff and Martin's neonatal-perinatal medicine: Diseases of the fetus and infant* (8th ed.). Philadelphia: Mosby.

Edwards, M., Nizet, V., & Baker, C. (2006). Group B streptococcal infections. In J. Remington, J. Klein, C. Baker, & C. Wilson (Eds.), *Infectious diseases of the fetus and newborn infant* (6th ed.). Philadelphia: Saunders.

Esakoff, T., Cheng, Y., Sparks, T., & Caughey, A. (2009). The association between birthweight 4000 g or greater and perinatal outcomes in patients with and without gestational diabetes mellitus. *American Journal of Obstetrics and Gynecology, 200*(6), 672. e1–e4.

Fike, D. (2007). Substance-exposed newborn. In C. Kenner, & J. Lott (Eds.), *Comprehensive neonatal care: An interdisciplinary approach* (4th ed.). St. Louis: Saunders.

Fleming, P., & Blair, P. (2007). Sudden infant death syndrome and parental smoking. *Early Human Development, 83*(11), 721–725.

Fortunov, R., Hulten, K., Hammerman, W., Mason, E., & Kaplan, S. (2006). Community-acquired *Staphylococcus aureus* infections in term and near-term previously healthy neonates. *Pediatrics, 118*(3), 874–881.

Frary, C., Johnson, R., & Wang, M. (2005). Food sources and intakes of caffeine in the diets of persons in the United States. *Journal of the American Dietetic Association, 105*(1), 110–113.

Gershon, A. (2006). Chickenpox, measles and mumps. In J. Remington, J. Klein, C. Baker, & C. Wilson (Eds.), *Infectious diseases of the fetus and newborn infant* (6th ed.). Philadelphia: Saunders.

Gorwitz, R. (2008). A review of community-associated methicillin-resistant *Staphylococcus aureus* skin and soft tissue infections. *Pediatric Infectious Disease Journal, 27*(1), 1–7.

Gowen, C. (2007). Fetal and neonatal medicine. In R. Kliegman, H. Jenson, K. Marcdante, & R. Behrman (Eds.), *Nelson essentials of pediatrics* (5th ed.). Philadelphia: Saunders.

Helmbrecht, G., & Thiagarajah, S. (2008). Management of addiction disorders in pregnancy. *Journal of Addiction Medicine, 2*(1), 1–16.

Higdon, J., & Frei, B. (2006). Coffee and health: A review of recent human research. *Critical Reviews in Food Science and Nutrition, 46*(2), 101–123.

Ingall, D., Sanchez, P., & Baker, C. (2006). Syphilis. In J. Remington, J. Klein, C. Baker, & C. Wilson (Eds.), *Infectious diseases of the fetus and newborn infant* (6th ed.). Philadelphia: Saunders.

Institute for Safe Medication Practices. (2008). *ISMP's list of high-alert medications.* Available at www.ismp.org/Tools/highalertmedications.pdf. Accessed August 5, 2010.

Jones, J., Dargelas, V., Roberts, J., Press, C., Remington, J., & Montoya, J. (2009). Risk factors for *Toxoplasma gondii* infection in the United States. *Clinical Infectious Diseases, 49*(6), 878–884.

Jovanovic, L., & Nakai, Y. (2006). Successful pregnancy in women with type 1 diabetes: From preconception through postpartum care. *Endocrinology and Metabolic Clinics of North America, 35*(1), 79–97.

Kaiser, L., & Allen, L. (2008). Position of the American Dietetic Association: Nutrition and lifestyle for a healthy pregnancy outcome. *Journal of the American Dietetic Association, 108*(3), 553–561.

Kakko, J., Heilig, M., & Sarman, I. (2008). Buprenorphine and methadone treatment of opiate dependence during pregnancy: Comparison of fetal growth and neonatal outcomes in two consecutive case series. *Drug and Alcohol Dependence, 96*(1-2), 69–78.

Kalhan, S., & Parimi, P. (2006). Disorders of carbohydrate metabolism. In R. Martin, A. Fanaroff, & M. Walsh (Eds.), *Fanaroff and Martin's neonatal-perinatal medicine: Diseases of the fetus and infant* (8th ed.). Philadelphia: Mosby.

Kenneson, A., & Cannon, M. (2007). Review and meta-analysis of the epidemiology of congenital cytomegalovirus (CMV) infection. *Reviews of Medical Virology, 17*(4), 253–276.

Khetsuriani, N., Lamonte-Fowlkes, A., Oberste, M., & Pallansch, M. (2006). Enterovirus surveillance—United States, 1970-2005. *MMWR Morbidity and Mortality Weekly Report and Recommendations Surveillance Summaries, 55*(SS08), 1–20.

Klein, J., Baker, C., Remington, J., & Wilson, C. (2006). Current concepts of infections of the fetus and newborn infant. In J. Remington, J. Klein, C. Baker, & C. Wilson (Eds.), *Infectious diseases of the fetus and newborn infant* (6th ed.). Philadelphia: Saunders.

Landon, M., Catalano, P., & Gabbe, S. (2007). Diabetes mellitus complicating pregnancy. In S. Gabbe, J. Niebyl, & J. Simpson (Eds.), *Obstetrics: Normal and problem pregnancies* (5th ed.). Philadelphia: Churchill Livingstone.

Limperopoulos, C., Robertson, R., Sullivan, N., Bassan, H., & du Plessis, A. (2009). Cerebellar injury in term infants: Clinical characteristics, magnetic resonance imaging findings, and outcome. *Pediatric Neurology, 41*(1), 1–8.

Lindsay, C. (2006). Pregnancy complicated by diabetes mellitus. In R. Martin, A. Fanaroff, & M. Walsh (Eds.), *Fanaroff and Martin's neonatal-perinatal medicine: Diseases of the fetus and infant* (8th ed.). Philadelphia: Mosby.

López, P., Bermejo, A., Tabernero, M., Cabarcos, P., Alvarez, I., & Fernández, P. (2009). Cocaine and opiates use in pregnancy: Detection of drugs in neonatal meconium and urine. *Journal of Analytical Toxicology, 33*(7), 351–355.

Malm, G. (2009). Neonatal herpes simplex virus infection. *Seminars in Fetal and Neonatal Medicine, 14*(4), 204–208.

Malm, G., & Engman, M. (2007). Congenital cytomegalovirus infections. *Seminars in Fetal and Neonatal Medicine, 12*(3), 154–159.

Mangurten, H. (2006). Birth injuries. In R. Martin, A. Fanaroff, & M. Walsh (Eds.), *Fanaroff and Martin's neonatal-perinatal medicine: Diseases of the fetus and infant* (8th ed.). Philadelphia: Mosby.

March of Dimes. (2010). *Caffeine in pregnancy.* Available at www.marchofdimes.com/professionals/14332_1148.asp. Accessed January 8, 2010.

Metzger, B., Buchanan, T., Coustan, D., de Leiva, A., Dunger, D., Hadden, D., et al. (2007). Summary and recommendations of the fifth international workshop-conference on gestational diabetes mellitus. *Diabetes Care, 30*(Suppl. 2), S251–S260.

Minozzi, S., Amato, L., Vecchi, S., & Davoli, M. (2008). Maintenance agonist treatments for opiate dependent pregnant women. *The Cochrane Database of Systematic Reviews,* 2008, 2, CD006318.

Myers, M., Seward, J., & LaRussa, P. (2007). Varicella-zoster virus. In R. Kliegman, R. Behrman, H. Jenson, & B. Stanton (Eds.), *Nelson textbook of pediatrics* (18th ed.). Philadelphia: Saunders.

Narendran, V., & Hoath, S. (2006). The skin. In R. Martin, A. Fanaroff, & M. Walsh (Eds.), *Fanaroff and Martin's neonatal-perinatal medicine: Diseases of the fetus and infant* (8th ed.). Philadelphia: Mosby.

National Institute on Drug Abuse. (2009). *NIDA InfoFacts: MDMA (ecstasy).* Available at www.nida.nih.gov/infofacts/ecstasy.html. Accessed August 5, 2010.

Nesheim, S., Kapogiannis, B., Soe, M., Sullivan, K., Abrams, E., Farley, J., et al. (2007). Trends in opportunistic infections in the pre- and post-highly active antiretroviral therapy eras among HIV-infected children in the Perinatal AIDS Collaborative Transmission Study, 1986-2004. *Pediatrics, 120*(1), 100–109.

Olson, H., Ohlemiller, M., O'Connor, M., Brown, C., Morris, C., Damus, K., & National Task Force on Fetal Alcohol Syndrome and Fetal Alcohol Effect. (2009). *A call to action: Advancing essential services and research on fetal alcohol syndrome and fetal alcohol effect. — A report of the National Task Force on Fetal Alcohol Syndrome and Fetal Alcohol Effect.* Washington, DC: U.S. Department of Health and Human Services.

Palazzi, D., Klein, J., & Baker, C. (2006). Bacterial sepsis and meningitis. In J. Remington, J. Klein, C. Baker, & C. Wilson (Eds.), *Infectious diseases of the fetus and newborn infant* (6th ed.). Philadelphia: Saunders.

Posfay-Barbe, K., & Wald, E. (2009). Listeriosis. *Seminars in Fetal and Neonatal Medicine, 14*(4), 228–233.

Pressler, J. (2008). Classification of major newborn birth injuries. *Journal of Perinatal and Neonatal Nursing, 22*(1), 60–67.

Prober, C. (2008). Herpes simplex. In S. Long (Ed.), *Principles and practice of pediatric infectious diseases* (3rd ed.). Philadelphia: Churchill Livingstone.

Reed, M., Aranda, J., & Hales, B. (2006). Developmental pharmacology. In R. Martin, A. Fanaroff, & M. Walsh (Eds.), *Fanaroff and Martin's neonatal-perinatal medicine: Diseases of the fetus and infant* (8th ed.). Philadelphia: Mosby.

Remington, J., McLeod, R., Thulliez, P., & Desmonts, G. (2006). Toxoplasmosis. In J. Remington, J. Klein, C. Baker, & C. Wilson (Eds.), *Infectious diseases of the fetus and newborn infant.* Philadelphia: Saunders.

Sabin, A. (1942). Toxoplasmosis: A recently recognized disease of human beings. *Advances in Pediatrics, 1*(1), 1–56.

Schempf, A. (2007). Illicit drug use and neonatal outcomes: A critical review. *Obstetrical & Gynecological Survey, 62*(11), 749–757.

Schleiss, M. (2008). Congenital cytomegalovirus infection: Update on management strategies. *Current Treatment Options in Neurology, 10*(3), 186–192.

Schrag, S., Hadler, J., Arnold, K., Martell-Cleary, P., Reingold, A., & Schuchat, A. (2006). Risk factors for invasive, early-onset *Escherichia coli* infections in the era of widespread intrapartum antibiotic use. *Pediatrics, 118*(2), 570–576.

Shea, A., & Steiner, M. (2008). Cigarette smoking during pregnancy. *Nicotine and Tobacco Research, 10*(2), 267–278.

Smith, L., LaGasse, L., Derauf, C., Grant, P., Shah, R., Arria, A., et al. (2006). The infant development, environment, and lifestyle study: Effects of prenatal methamphetamine exposure, polydrug exposure, and poverty on intrauterine growth. *Pediatrics, 118*(3), 1149–1156.

Stoll, B. (2007). Infections in the neonatal infant. In R. Kliegman, R. Behrman, H. Jenson, & B. Stanton (Eds.), *Nelson textbook of pediatrics* (18th ed.). Philadelphia: Saunders.

Stoll, B., & Adams-Chapman, I. (2007). The high-risk infant. In R. Kliegman, R. Behrman, H. Jenson, & B. Stanton (Eds.), *Nelson textbook of pediatrics* (18th ed.). Philadelphia: Saunders.

Su, J., Berman, S., Davis, D., & Weinstock, H. (2010). Congenital syphilis—United States, 2003-2008. *MMWR, Morbidity and Mortality weekly Report, 59*(14), 413–417. Available at www.cdc.gov/mmwr/preview/mmwrhtml/mm5914a1.htm. Accessed August 5, 2010.

Tan, M., & Koren, G. (2006). Chickenpox in pregnancy: Revisited. *Reproductive Toxicology, 21*(4), 410–420.

Tebruegge, M., & Curtis, N. (2009). Enterovirus infections in neonates. *Seminars in Fetal and Neonatal Medicine, 14*(4), 222–227.

Thigpen, J. (2007). Gastrointestinal system. In C. Kenner, & J. Lott (Eds.), *Comprehensive neonatal nursing: An interdisciplinary approach* (4th ed.). St. Louis: Saunders.

Tolfvenstam, T., & Broliden, K. (2009). Parvovirus B19 infection. *Seminars in Fetal and Neonatal Medicine, 14*(4), 218–221.

van Gelder, M., Reefhuis, J., Caton, A., Werler, M., Druschel, C., & Roeleveld, N. (2009). Maternal periconceptional illicit drug use and the risk of congenital malformations. *Epidemiology, 20*(1), 60–66.

Venkatesh, M., Adams, K., & Weisman, L. (2011). Infection in the neonate. In S. Gardner, B. Carter, M. Enzman-Hines, & J. Hernandez (Eds.), *Merenstein & Gardner's handbook of neonatal intensive care* (7th ed.). St Louis: Mosby.

Verklan, M., & Lopez, S. (2011). Neurologic disorders. In S. Gardner, B. Carter, M. Enzman-Hines, & J. Hernandez (Eds.), *Merenstein & Gardner's handbook of neonatal intensive care* (7th ed.). St Louis: Mosby.

Volpe, J. (2008). *Neurology of the newborn* (5th ed.). Philadelphia: Saunders.

Weindling, A. (2009). Offspring of diabetic pregnancy: Short-term outcomes. *Seminars in Fetal and Neonatal Medicine, 14*(2), 111–118.

Weng, S., Odouli, R., & Li, D. (2008). Maternal caffeine consumption during pregnancy and the risk of miscarriage: A prospective cohort study. *American Journal of Obstetrics and Gynecology, 198*(3), 279, e1–e8.

Wikswo, M., Khetsuriani, N., Fowlkes, A., Zheng, X., Penaranda, S., Verma, N., et al. (2009). Increased activity of coxsackievirus B1 strains associated with severe disease among young infants in the United States, 2007-2008. *Clinical Infectious Diseases, 49*(5), e44–e51.

Wilson, D., & da Cunha, M. (2007). Health problems of the newborn. In M. Hockenberry, & D. Wilson (Eds.), *Wong's nursing care of infants and children* (8th ed.). St. Louis: Mosby.

Wisner, K., Sit, D., Reynolds, S., Altemus, M., Bogen, D., Sunder, K., et al. (2007). Psychiatric disorders. In S. Gabbe, J. Niebyl, & J. Simpson (Eds.), *Obstetrics: Normal and problem pregnancies* (5th ed.). Philadelphia: Churchill Livingstone.

Woods, C. (2009). Congenital syphilis. *Pediatric Infectious Disease Journal, 28*(6), 536–537.

WHO, UNICEF, UNFPA, & UNAIDS. (2010). *Guidelines on HIV and infant feeding.* Geneva: WHO. Available at http://whqlibdoc.who.int/publications/2010/9789241599535_eng.pdf. Accessed July 15, 2010.

Yudin, M., & Gonik, B. (2006). Perinatal infections. In R. Martin, A. Fanaroff, & M. Walsh (Eds.), *Fanaroff and Martin's neonatal-perinatal medicine: Diseases of the fetus and infant* (8th ed.). Philadelphia: Mosby.

CHAPTER

36

Hemolytic Disorders and Congenital Anomalies

M. Terese Verklan

evolve WEBSITE

http://evolve.elsevier.com/Lowdermilk/MWHC/

Audio Glossary

Audio Key Points

NCLEX Review Questions

Nursing Care Plan

The Infant with Hyperbilirubinemia

LEARNING OBJECTIVES

- Differentiate between physiologic and pathologic jaundice in the newborn.
- Develop a nursing plan of care for the prevention, identification, and management of the neonate with hyperbilirubinemia.
- Compare Rh and ABO incompatibility and the implications for neonatal outcomes.
- Explain nursing management to prevent the pathologic consequences of hyperbilirubinemia.
- Review prenatal diagnosis of neonatal disorders.
- Present assessment strategies during the postnatal period to aid in diagnosis of congenital disorders.
- Describe each congenital disorder presented in this chapter and identify the priority of nursing care for each.
- Describe preoperative and postoperative nursing care of the newborn.
- Develop a nursing care plan for parents of a newborn with a defect or disorder.

Many physiologic alterations occur in infants during the newborn period. The nurse must be alert to any deviations from normal, ranging from an obvious congenital anomaly, such as myelomeningocele, to a less obvious deviation such as a congenital heart defect that may not be symptomatic at birth. The nurse must possess the assessment skills necessary to detect any deviation from normal, as well as the knowledge base necessary to participate in the skilled care needed for affected infants. The nurse also must be cognizant of the special needs of the family with a child who is born with or acquires an abnormal condition.

The complications that affect newborns can stem from three basic problems: (1) problems relating to gestational age or intrauterine growth that does not follow normal patterns, such as a preterm birth; (2) acquired problems resulting from maternal or newborn physiologic factors, such as ABO incompatibility or respiratory distress; and (3) physical problems, such as congenital anomalies. This chapter focuses on acquired problems and congenital anomalies in the neonate.

HYPERBILIRUBINEMIA

Hyperbilirubinemia is a condition in which the total serum bilirubin level in the blood is increased. Values are abnormal based on gestational age, days of life, and the baby's general physical condition. Hyperbilirubinemia is characterized by a yellow discoloration of the skin, mucous membranes, sclera, and various organs. This discoloration is referred to as **jaundice,** or *icterus.* Jaundice is caused primarily by the accumulation in the skin of unconjugated bilirubin, a breakdown product of hemoglobin formed after its release from hemolyzed red blood cells (RBCs). Jaundice first appears in the infant's face and head and progresses downward toward the toes. It dissipates in the reverse order. Physiologic jaundice, discussed in Chapters 23 and 24, is the most common abnormal finding in newborns and is usually benign. The challenge in the care of neonates with hyperbilirubinemia is to distinguish physiologic jaundice from a serious clinical pathologic condition.

Physiologic Jaundice

Physiologic jaundice occurs in about 60% of healthy term newborns and almost all preterm infants (Watson, 2009). It typically arises more than 24 hours after birth. In both Caucasian and African-American infants, it is manifested by a progressive increase in the unconjugated bilirubin level in cord blood from 2 mg/dl to a mean peak of 5 to 6 mg/dl between 60 and 72 hours of age. In Asian and Native-American infants, the level may increase to 10 to 14 mg/dl between 72 and 120 hours of age. Resolution in Caucasian and African-American newborns is evidenced by a rapid decline in the unconjugated bilirubin level to 2 mg/dl by 5 days after birth; in Asian and Native-American infants, this takes 7 to 10 days.

Physiologic jaundice is more common in preterm infants in whom the serum bilirubin level typically reaches a mean peak of 10 to 12 mg/dl by the fifth or sixth day of life. It takes longer for the maximal concentration to be reached in preterm than in full-term infants because of the preterm infant's immature liver function and slower metabolic processes.

Pathologic Jaundice

Pathologic jaundice is the result of an increased level of total serum bilirubin that if left untreated can result in **acute bilirubin encephalopathy** or *kernicterus*. Although the terms are often used interchangeably, *acute bilirubin encephalopathy* describes the acute central nervous system manifestations seen in the first weeks after birth, whereas the term *kernicterus* is used to describe the chronic and permanent results of bilirubin toxicity (American Academy of Pediatrics [AAP] Subcommittee on Hyperbilirubinemia, 2004). Kernicterus, though rare, still occurs. Adherence to guidelines by the American Academy of Pediatrics (AAP Subcommittee on Hyperbilirubinemia) and a clinical position statement by the Association of Women's Health, Obstetric and Neonatal Nurses (AWHONN, 2005) should result in kernicterus becoming largely preventable. The following findings support a diagnosis of pathologic jaundice and, if encountered in an infant, warrant further investigation (Bradshaw, 2010; Watson, 2009):

- Serum bilirubin concentrations of greater than 4 mg/dl in cord blood
- Clinical jaundice evident within 24 hours of birth
- Total serum bilirubin levels increasing by more than 5 mg/dl in 24 hours or increasing at a rate of 0.5 mg/dl or more over a 4- to 8-hour period
- A serum bilirubin level in a term newborn that exceeds 15 mg/dl at any time or clinical jaundice lasting more than 10 days
- A serum bilirubin level in a preterm newborn that exceeds 10 mg/dl at any time
- Any case of visible jaundice that persists for more than 10 days of life in a term infant or 21 days in a preterm infant, unless the infant is receiving breast milk

AAP guidelines (2004) and the clinical position statement by AWHONN (2005) note the need for universal screening to identify elevated bilirubin level in newborns to facilitate the prevention of acute bilirubin encephalopathy and kernicterus. The use of hour-specific serum bilirubin levels to predict newborns at risk for rapidly rising levels is an official recommendation by the AAP Subcommittee on Hyperbilirubinemia (2004) for the monitoring of healthy neonates at 35 weeks of gestation or more before discharge from the hospital. Use of a nomogram helps determine which newborns might need further evaluation after discharge. In many institutions the nomogram is used to determine the infant's risk for development of hyperbilirubinemia requiring medical treatment or closer screening (see Fig. 24-8).

Risk factors recognized to place infants in the high risk category include gestational age less than 38 weeks, breastfeeding, previous sibling with significant jaundice, and jaundice appearing before discharge. It is recommended that healthy infants (35 weeks of gestation or greater) receive follow-up care and assessment of bilirubin within 3 days of discharge (if discharged at less than 24 hours) and a risk assessment with tools such as the hour-specific nomogram (see Box 36-1). Likewise, newborns discharged at 24 to 47.9 hours should receive follow-up evaluation within 4 days (96 hours), and those discharged between 48 and 72 hours should receive follow-up within 5 days (AAP Subcommittee on Hyperbilirubinemia, 2004). Other key elements of the recommendations of the AAP Subcommittee include promoting successful breastfeeding; recognizing that visual estimation of the degree of jaundice, particularly in darkly pigmented infants, can lead to errors; and providing parents with written and verbal information about newborn jaundice.

Many potential causes of pathologic hyperbilirubinemia are found in neonates (Box 36-2). The most common are hemolytic disorders of the newborn.

BOX 36-1 MONITORING FOR JAUNDICE AFTER EARLY DISCHARGE

If the infant is discharged from the hospital before 48 hours of age, the parents should receive written and verbal instructions regarding adequate hydration and assessment of the infant for the appearance of jaundice. Appropriate testing and follow-up of the infant should be available. A program of home phototherapy allows infants to receive treatment of uncomplicated hyperbilirubinemia after discharge from the hospital. For these infants, nurses provide monitoring of treatment and of serum bilirubin levels as outlined by hospital or agency policy.

Hemolytic Disease of the Newborn

Hemolytic diseases of the newborn occur most often if the blood groups of the mother and baby are different. The most common are ABO and Rh factor incompatibilities.

The four major blood groups in the ABO system are A, B, AB, and O. People with type A blood have A antigen; those with type B have B antigen; those with type AB have both A and B antigens; and those with type O have no antigens. In turn, people with type A blood have plasma antibodies to type B blood; those with type B blood have antibodies to type A blood; those with type AB blood have no antibodies; and those with type O blood have antibodies to types A and B blood. If a person is administered or exposed to an incompatible blood type, he or she will form antibodies against the antigen in that blood, with agglutination, or clumping, occurring as the antibodies in the plasma mix with the antigens of the different blood group.

The Rh factor, a genetically determined factor present on RBCs, can be a major source of incompatibility. Of the several forms of the Rh antigen, the D antigen is the most significant because it causes the most antibody production in a person who is Rh negative. A person who has the Rh factor is considered Rh positive; a person without it is considered Rh negative. For example, a mother who has A-negative blood has the A antigen, plasma antibodies to the B antigen, and no Rh factor on her RBCs.

Hemolytic disorders occur when maternal antibodies are present naturally or form in response to an antigen from the fetal blood crossing the placenta and entering the maternal circulation. The maternal antibodies of the immunoglobulin G

BOX 36-2 POTENTIAL CAUSES OF PATHOLOGIC HYPERBILIRUBINEMIA IN NEONATES

MATERNAL FACTORS
- Rh and ABO incompatibility
- Maternal infections
- Maternal diabetes
- Oxytocin administration during labor
- Maternal ingestion of sulfonamides, diazepam, or salicylates near time of birth

FETAL/NEWBORN FACTORS
- Prematurity
- Hepatic cell damage by infection or drugs
- Neonatal hyperthyroidism
- Polycythemia
- Intestinal obstruction such as meconium ileus
- Pyloric stenosis
- Biliary atresia
- Sequestered blood (e.g., from cephalhematomas, ecchymosis, or hemangiomas)
- Maternal blood swallowed by neonate

(IgG) class in turn cross the placenta, causing hemolysis of the fetal RBCs, resulting in hyperbilirubinemia and jaundice.

Rh Incompatibility

Rh incompatibility, or **isoimmunization,** occurs when an Rh-negative mother has an Rh-positive fetus who inherits the dominant Rh-positive gene from the father. If the mother is Rh negative and the father is Rh positive and homozygous for the Rh factor, all the offspring will be Rh positive. If the father is heterozygous for the factor, there is a 50% chance that each infant born of the union will be Rh positive and a 50% chance that each will be born Rh negative. An Rh-negative fetus is in no danger because it has the same Rh factor as the mother. An Rh-negative fetus with an Rh-positive mother also is in no danger. Only the Rh-positive fetus of an Rh-negative mother is at risk. From 10% to 15% of all Caucasian couples and about 5% of African-American couples have Rh incompatibility. It is rare in Asian couples due to the high incidence of ABO incompatibility, which is protective against Rh isoimmunization because of rapid destruction of the fetal RBCs which prevents Rh antigen exposure and maternal antibody production (Diehl-Jones & Askin, 2010). The incidence of Rh sensitization and resulting hemolytic disease of the newborn has decreased dramatically since the development of Rh_o(D) immunoglobulin in 1968. New treatment modalities, including early detection and fetal blood transfusions, have improved the outcome of affected fetuses.

The pathogenesis of Rh incompatibility is as follows. Hematopoiesis (the formation, production, and maintenance of blood cells) in the fetus is well established by the ninth week of gestation (Blackburn, 2007; Diehl-Jones & Askin, 2010). When fetal RBCs that contain the Rh antigen pass through the placenta into the maternal circulation absent the Rh antigen, the maternal immune system produces antibodies against the foreign fetal antigens. The process of antibody formation is called *maternal sensitization.* Sensitization can occur during pregnancy, birth, miscarriage or induced abortion, amniocentesis, external cephalic version, or trauma. Usually women become sensitized in their first pregnancy with an Rh-positive fetus but do not produce enough antibodies to cause lysis (destruction) of fetal blood cells. During subsequent pregnancies, antibodies form in response to repeated contact with the antigen from the fetal blood, and lysis of fetal RBCs results. The overall incidence of isoimmunization in Rh-negative mothers who are at risk is less than 10% and only 5% of mothers with isoimmunization have babies with hemolytic disease (Stoll, 2007). Multiple gestation, placental abruption, placenta previa, manual removal of the placenta, and cesarean birth increase the incidence of transplacental hemorrhage and the risk of isoimmunization.

Severe Rh incompatibility results in marked fetal hemolytic anemia because the fetal erythrocytes are destroyed by maternal Rh-positive antibodies. Although the placenta usually clears the bilirubin resulting from the RBC breakdown, in extreme cases fetal bilirubin levels increase. This results in fetal jaundice, also known as *icterus gravis.*

The fetus compensates for the anemia by producing large numbers of immature erythrocytes to replace those hemolyzed, thus the name for this condition: **erythroblastosis fetalis.** In **hydrops fetalis,** the most severe form of this disease, the fetus has marked anemia, cardiac decompensation, cardiomegaly, and hepatosplenomegaly. Hypoxia results from the severe anemia. In addition, because of the decreased intravascular oncotic pressure involved, fluid leaks out of the intravascular space. This results in generalized edema, as well as effusions into the peritoneal (ascites), pericardial, and pleural (hydrothorax) spaces. The placenta is often edematous, which, along with the edematous fetus, can cause the uterus to rupture.

Intrauterine or early neonatal death can occur as a result of hydrops fetalis, although intrauterine transfusions and early birth of the fetus can help to avert this. Intrauterine transfusion involves the infusion of Rh-negative, type O blood into the umbilical vein. The frequency of intrauterine transfusions varies according to institution and fetal hydropic status, but it can be as often as every 2 weeks until the fetus reaches pulmonary maturity at approximately 37 to 38 weeks of gestation. Studies of the use of intrauterine transfusions have demonstrated a high survival rate and low risk of disabilities in the surviving infant (Gruslin & Moore, 2006; Moise, 2010).

ABO Incompatibility

ABO incompatibility is the most common cause of hemolytic disease in the newborn, although the anemia that results is usually mild. ABO maternal blood group incompatibility occurs in approximately 20% of infants; however, only about 5% have clinical manifestations (Cunningham, Leveno, Bloom, Hauth, Rouse, & Spong, 2010). It occurs if the fetal blood type is A, B, or AB, and the maternal type is O. It occurs rarely in infants with type B blood born to mothers with type A blood. The incompatibility arises because naturally occurring anti-A and anti-B antibodies are transferred across the placenta to the fetus. Unlike the situation that pertains to Rh incompatibility, firstborn infants can be affected because mothers with type O blood already have anti-A and anti-B antibodies in their blood. Such a newborn can have a weakly positive direct Coombs' test (also referred to as a direct antiglobulin test [DAT]). The cord bilirubin level usually is less than 4 mg/dl, and any resulting hyperbilirubinemia usually can be treated with phototherapy. Exchange transfusions are required only occasionally. Although ABO incompatibility is a common cause of hyperbilirubinemia, it rarely precipitates significant anemia resulting from the hemolysis of RBCs.

Other Causes of Hemolytic Jaundice

It is not within the scope of this text to discuss the many potential causes of hemolytic jaundice in childhood. However, among African-Americans and persons of Mediterranean heritage there is a high incidence of glucose-6-phosphate dehydrogenase deficiency (G6PD) (Wilkins, 2010). Because it is a sex-linked disease, male offspring are affected more often than females. A deficiency of a red blood cell enzyme in combination with exposure to an oxidant stressor (such as sepsis) results in hemolysis and a decreased RBC life (Diehl-Jones & Askin, 2010). The increase in the destruction of RBCs overwhelms the immature neonatal liver's ability to conjugate the indirect bilirubin. Treatment is the same as for any newborn with rapidly rising serum bilirubin levels. Other metabolic and inherited conditions that increase hemolysis and can cause jaundice in the infant include galactosemia, Crigler-Najjar disease, and hypothyroidism (Blackburn, 2007).

Acute Bilirubin Encephalopathy

The goal of the care given the infant with hyperbilirubinemia is the prevention of **acute bilirubin encephalopathy,** which is caused by the deposition of bilirubin in the brain, especially within the basal ganglia, the cerebellum, and the hippocampus. Normally bilirubin does not cause harm because it is bound to albumin and carried to the liver to undergo conjugation. However, once albumin binding sites are saturated, the bilirubin circulates as unconjugated (indirect) bilirubin, which is highly lipid soluble and capable of crossing the blood-brain barrier. Circulation of unconjugated bilirubin can reach toxic levels and become deposited in the basal ganglia, resulting in the yellowish staining of the brain tissue and the necrosis of neurons.

Acute bilirubin encephalopathy, which can develop in newborns with no apparent signs of clinical jaundice, is directly related to the total serum bilirubin level, although these levels alone do not predict the risk of brain injury. In a term infant, a serum bilirubin level of 25 mg/dl is considered the upper limit, beyond which the risk for acute bilirubin encephalopathy increases. However, the condition can occur at much lower levels in premature infants or infants with other complications. In low birth weight preterm infants, a peak total serum bilirubin level as low as 6.5 mg/dl has been associated with the development of acute bilirubin encephalopathy (National Institute of Child Health and Human Development [NICHD], 1985; Watson, 2009).

Some of the perinatal events that increase the likelihood of acute bilirubin encephalopathy, even at these lower bilirubin levels, include hypoxia, asphyxia, acidosis, hypothermia, hypoglycemia, sepsis, treatment with certain medications, and hypoalbuminemia. In essence, any condition that interferes with the conjugation of bilirubin or competes for albumin-binding sites increases the risk that unconjugated bilirubin can pass through the blood-brain barrier and cause damage to the central nervous system.

Acute bilirubin encephalopathy is associated with acute and long-term signs of neurologic damage (AAP Subcommittee on Hyperbilirubinemia, 2004; Bradshaw, 2010; Volpe, 2008). The clinical manifestations typically appear between 2 and 6 days after birth and go through several phases as the disease progresses. During the first phase the newborn is hypotonic and lethargic and shows a poor suck and depressed or absent Moro reflex. These more subtle signs are followed by the appearance of a high-pitched cry, opisthotonos (severe muscle spasm that causes the back to arch acutely), spasticity, hyperreflexia, and fever. If allowed to progress to the third phase, the neonate will demonstrate a shrill cry, apnea, deep stupor to coma, seizures, and hearing and visual disturbances.

About half of the affected infants survive, although they often have permanent sequelae including extrapyramidal movement disorders (especially dystonia and athetosis), gaze abnormalities (especially an upward gaze), auditory disturbances (especially sensorineural hearing loss), intellectual deficits (rarely in the mentally retarded range), and enamel dysplasia of the deciduous teeth. Movement abnormalities and auditory disturbances are almost always present.

Kernicterus is the irreversible, chronic sequela of bilirubin toxicity (Bradshaw, 2010; Volpe, 2008; Watson, 2009). Over the first year of life a baby demonstrates the characteristic findings of hypotonia, active deep tendon reflexes, persistent tonic neck reflex, and difficulty meeting developmental milestones. Characteristics of a fully developed encephalopathy include the permanent sequelae identified above. Treatment for kernicterus is supportive.

CARE MANAGEMENT

It is important to determine the blood type and Rh factor of the pregnant woman prenatally. Early identification of the Rh-negative woman must occur, and care must be taken to prevent sensitization. The nurse must obtain a thorough history to assess for events that could have caused her to develop antibodies to the Rh factor. Such events include (1) previous pregnancy with an Rh-positive fetus; (2) transfusion with Rh-positive blood, which causes immediate sensitization; (3) miscarriage or induced abortion after 8 or more weeks of gestation; (4) amniocentesis performed for any reason; (5) premature separation of the placenta; and (6) trauma.

Because hematopoiesis is well developed in the fetus by the ninth week of gestation, a woman who has had a miscarriage or induced abortion after this time or has previously given birth to a child may have been inoculated with fetal blood at the time of placental separation. During amniocentesis, the needle can cause localized damage to the single layer of cells that separates the maternal and fetal circulation in the placenta, thereby allowing fetal RBCs to enter the maternal circulation.

If any of these events has occurred, the nurse checks the woman's record to determine whether she has received **Rh_o(D) immunoglobulin,** such as RhoGAM (WinGAM), which is a commercial preparation of passive antibodies against the Rh factor (see the Medication Guide, p. 499). This injection of anti-Rh antibodies destroys any fetal RBCs in the maternal circulation and blocks the maternal antibody production. RhoGAM is 90% effective in preventing sensitization. It is recommended

BOX 36-3 INDICATIONS FOR AMOUNT OF RH_0(D) IMMUNOGLOBULIN TO BE ADMINISTERED

50 mcg
- After chorionic villus sampling, ectopic pregnancy, miscarriage, or abortion before 13 weeks of gestation

300 mcg
- After any of the following events:
  - Miscarriage or induced abortion after 13 weeks of gestation
  - Percutaneous umbilical blood sampling
  - Amniocentesis
  - Placental abruption or placenta previa
  - Trauma
  - At 28 weeks of gestation
  - Within 72 hours of the preterm or term birth of an Rh-positive infant

MORE THAN 300 mcg
- After a large transplacental hemorrhage
- After a mismatched blood transfusion

that it be given to an Rh-negative mother at 28 weeks of gestation; within 72 hours after delivery; after an invasive procedure such as amniocentesis, chorionic villus sampling (CVS), or percutaneous umbilical blood sampling (PUBS); and any time there is a risk of fetal-maternal hemorrhage. It is also recommended after induced abortion and ectopic pregnancy (Box 36-3). (Diehl-Jones & Askin, 2010; Moise, 2010; Wong, DeSandre, Sibley, & Stevenson, 2006)

At the first prenatal visit of an Rh-negative woman with a fetus who may be Rh positive, an indirect **Coombs' test** should be done to determine whether she has antibodies to the Rh antigen. In this test the maternal blood serum is mixed with Rh-positive RBCs. If the Rh-positive RBCs agglutinate or clump, this indicates that maternal antibodies are present or that the mother has been sensitized. The dilution of the specimen of blood at which clumping occurs determines the titer, or level, of maternal antibodies. This titer indicates the degree of maternal sensitization. A level of 1:8 rarely results in fetal jeopardy. If the titer reaches 1:16, amniocentesis is performed to determine optical density (ΔOD) of amniotic fluid to estimate fetal hemolytic process (see Chapter 26). Rising bilirubin levels can indicate the need for an intrauterine transfusion. Genetic testing allows early identification of paternal zygosity at the RhD gene locus, thus allowing earlier detection of the potential for isoimmunization and precluding further maternal or fetal testing (Moise, 2010).

The indirect Coombs' test is repeated at 28 weeks. If the result remains negative, indicating that sensitization has not occurred, the woman is given an intramuscular injection of Rh_0(D) immunoglobulin. If the test result is positive, showing that sensitization has occurred, it is then repeated every 4 to 6 weeks to monitor the maternal antibody titer as just described.

Prevention of hyperbilirubinemia is the primary prenatal focus of care. The implementation of interventions focused on the care of the woman whose fetus is at risk for hyperbilirubinemia is essential to prevent problems in the newborn. Prenatal control of diabetes mellitus, prevention of maternal infection, avoidance of drugs such as diazepam and salicylates near the time of birth, and prevention of preterm birth reduce the risk.

The fetus and maternal antibody titers are monitored prenatally. Several methods are used to detect fetal anemia: amniocentesis to measure ΔOD 450, PUBS or cordocentesis, and middle cerebral artery peak systolic velocity (MCA-PSV). Although ultrasound-guided cordocentesis is the gold standard for detecting fetal anemia, MCA-PSV is being used increasingly as an accurate, noninvasive means to detect fetal anemia. This study is done using Doppler ultrasound (Moise, 2010).

If amniocentesis reveals that the ΔOD is high or the MCA-PSV is increased, cordocentesis is performed to assess fetal hematocrit. If the hematocrit is less than 30%, intrauterine transfusion is indicated (Moise, 2010). Intrauterine transfusion can be done every 1 to 2 weeks between 26 and 32 weeks. If the endangered fetus is at more than 32 weeks of gestation, a preterm birth may be indicated, usually by cesarean.

Postpartum interventions focus on preventing sensitization in the mother, if it has not occurred already, and treating any complications in the neonate resulting from the hemolysis of RBCs (see the Nursing Care Plan). The unsensitized Rh-negative mother whose baby is Rh positive should receive Rh_0(D) immunoglobulin within 72 hours of birth to prevent her from producing antibodies to the fetal blood cells that entered her bloodstream during the birth. One dose accommodates approximately 30 ml of fetal RBCs (Diehl-Jones & Askin, 2010).

At birth the neonate's cord blood is sent to the laboratory to determine the infant's blood type and Rh status. A direct Coombs' test is performed on this cord blood to determine whether there are maternal antibodies in the fetal blood. If antibodies are present, the titer, indicating the degree of maternal sensitization, is measured. If the titer is 1:64, an exchange transfusion is indicated. In addition, the prevention of or prompt therapy for perinatal asphyxia, acidosis, cold stress, sepsis, and hypoglycemia will decrease the newborn's risk for severe hemolytic disease and the susceptibility to kernicterus. Early feeding is initiated to stimulate stooling and thus facilitate the removal of bilirubin. See Chapter 24 for a discussion of phototherapy.

Exchange transfusions are needed infrequently because of the improved recognition of neonates at risk of hemolytic disease that can result from isoimmunization. Other factors must always be considered as well, particularly the clinical condition of the infant, because it is a procedure with potential complications. Guidelines for the initiation of exchange transfusion in relation to serum bilirubin levels in infants of more than 35 weeks of gestation can be found in the 2004 AAP Clinical Practice Guideline (AAP Subcommittee on Hyperbilirubinemia, 2004).

Exchange transfusion is accomplished by alternately removing a small amount of the infant's blood and replacing it with an equal amount of donor blood. Exchange transfusion replaces the RBCs that would otherwise be hemolyzed by circulating maternal antibodies, removes the antibodies responsible for hemolysis, and corrects the anemia caused by hemolysis of the infant's sensitized RBCs. It also reduces the serum bilirubin level in infants who have severe hyperbilirubinemia from any cause. If the infant has Rh incompatibility, type O Rh-negative blood is used for transfusion so the maternal antibodies still present in the infant do not hemolyze the transfused blood. Depending on the infant's size, maturity, and condition, amounts of 5 to 20 ml of the infant's blood are removed at one time and replaced

NURSING CARE PLAN

The Infant with Hyperbilirubinemia

NURSING DIAGNOSIS

Risk for injury related to hemolytic disease and treatment effects

Expected Outcomes

Bilirubin levels decrease with treatment; no evidence exists of harmful effects from phototherapy (e.g., no eye irritation, dehydration, temperature instability, or skin breakdown); and no complications occur from exchange transfusions.

Nursing Interventions/*Rationales*

- Initiate early feedings *to enhance excretion of bilirubin in stools.*
- Observe skin and mucous membranes for signs of jaundice, indicative of increasing bilirubin levels; monitor total serum bilirubin levels *to determine rate of increase and treatment response.*
- Note time of jaundice onset *to help distinguish physiologic from other causes of jaundice.*
- Observe for signs of hypoxia, hypothermia, hypoglycemia, and metabolic acidosis, *which occur as a result of hyperbilirubinemia and increase the risk of brain damage.*
- Initiate phototherapy per physician's order *to decrease bilirubin levels.*
- During phototherapy, shield infant's eyes *to prevent damage to corneas and retinas;* keep infant nude and change positions frequently *for maximal body surface exposure;* cleanse skin frequently *to prevent irritation;* maintain adequate fluid intake *to prevent dehydration;* monitor body temperature *to prevent hyperthermia.*
- Before exchange transfusion, keep infant on nothing-by-mouth (NPO) status (2 to 4 hours) *to prevent aspiration;* check donor blood for compatibility *to prevent transfusion reaction;* have resuscitation equipment (oxygen, Ambu bag, endotracheal tubes, laryngoscope) at bedside *in preparation for emergency action.*
- Assist physician with exchange transfusion procedure; track amounts of blood withdrawn and transfused *to maintain balanced blood volume;* maintain body temperature *to avoid hypothermia and cold stress;* monitor vital signs and observe *for signs of hypocalcemia, hypomagnesemia.*
- After transfusion, continue to monitor vital signs, signs of *hypocalcemia and hypomagnesemia; monitor for hypoglycemia;* check umbilical cord *for bleeding.*

NURSING DIAGNOSIS

Interrupted breastfeeding related to discharge of mother and continued hospitalization of infant

Expected Outcomes

Mother states desire to continue breastfeeding as much as possible and expresses and stores milk when she cannot come to the hospital to nurse the infant.

Nursing Interventions/*Rationales*

- Encourage the mother to come to the hospital to nurse infant as often as feasible for her *to maintain milk supply and encourage bonding.*
- Provide private and comfortable space for nursing that is available 24 hours per day *to support the mother in breastfeeding.*
- Instruct the mother in methods to express and store breast milk *to ensure a safe and adequate milk supply.*
- Provide written educational materials and audiovisual aids *to demonstrate proper techniques for expressing and storing milk and to allow the mother to learn at her own pace.*
- Recommend use of a breast pump and pump according to recommended guidelines (e.g., pump a minimum of five times a day; pump a minimum of 100 minutes a day; pump long enough to soften breasts) *to provide maximum stimulation for milk production.*
- Reassure the mother that infant's nutritional needs will be met through expressed milk or other methods *to allay anxiety.*
- Review the daily routine of the mother to advise her on ways to incorporate pumping into her daily schedule *to maintain her milk supply.*
- Provide information about breastfeeding support groups *to help the mother obtain emotional support from other breastfeeding mothers.*

NURSING DIAGNOSIS

Parental role conflict related to separation from hospitalized infant and interruptions of family life due to travel to hospital to see infant.

Expected Outcomes

Parents will share responsibilities for child care and home maintenance; parents will visit infant in hospital as often as feasible.

Nursing Interventions/*Rationales*

- Suggest to parents that they mutually establish a routine for child care for siblings and home maintenance *to enhance communication and provide necessary home activities.*
- Encourage parents to seek assistance and support from friends, relatives, and community groups such as their church *to meet their needs and ensure that a minimal level of appropriate functioning is maintained.*
- Encourage parents to travel to the hospital as often as is desirable and feasible *to promote breastfeeding and bonding with infant.*

NURSING DIAGNOSIS

Deficient knowledge related to administration of home phototherapy

Expected Outcome

Family demonstrates ability to provide home therapy.

Nursing Interventions/*Rationales*

- Explore family's willingness to try home phototherapy *to evaluate feasibility of home therapy option.*
- Explore family's understanding of jaundice and proposed therapy *to establish baseline for teaching.*
- Teach family with demonstration–return demonstration, allowing for several practice sessions, and supplement with written materials with pictorial representations *to ensure safe and optimal results.*
- Include the following in your instructions: placement of lamp or fiberoptic unit; proper eye care and patching; proper skin care; proper positioning under lamp; provision of increased fluid intake; monitoring of time under lamp; monitoring of temperature and skin, eyes, feeding patterns, stooling and voiding patterns; observation for complications *to ensure that the family understands and implements safe and effective use of phototherapy.*
- Stress importance of obtaining the prescribed bilirubin tests on schedule *as a way of tracking success of therapy.*
- Give parents a contact number if they have any questions while carrying out therapy *to offer ongoing support and increase parent comfort.*

with donor blood. The double volume or two-volume exchange replaces approximately 170 ml/kg of body weight, or 87% of the infant's total blood volume. The procedure requires approximately 1 hour. After the procedure, phototherapy is continued and the bilirubin levels are monitored every 4 hours (Martin & Cloherty, 2008; Watson, 2009; Wong et al., 2006).

The infant is monitored closely during and after the procedure, including the heart rate and rhythm, respirations, blood pressure, temperature, and perfusion. Preservatives in donor blood lower the infant's serum calcium and magnesium levels. It is not uncommon for calcium gluconate to be given during the exchange transfusion if symptoms of hypocalcemia become evident. Symptoms of hypocalcemia include jitteriness, irritability, convulsions, tachycardia, and electrocardiogram changes. The nurse monitors the neonate for hypoglycemia during the several hours after the exchange because the high glucose content of the preservatives can stimulate insulin secretion. These high risk neonates typically have dextrose support through an intravenous route (Martin & Cloherty, 2008; Watson, 2009).

Planning for rehabilitative measures is necessary if kernicterus occurs. The family will need the services of many community resources to care for the affected child. An interdisciplinary approach that includes social services must be taken.

CONGENITAL ANOMALIES

A **congenital anomaly** is a defect that is present at birth and can be caused by genetic or environmental factors, or both. It is defined as a physical, metabolic, anatomic, or behavioral deviation from the normal pattern of development (Moore & Persaud, 2007). Congenital defects are reported to occur in 2% to 3% of all live births (Bay, Steele, & Davis, 2007), but this number increases to approximately 6% by 5 years, when more anomalies are diagnosed. In addition, the incidence of congenital malformations in fetuses that are aborted is higher than that in infants who are born alive, thus adding to the overall incidence. Major congenital defects are the leading cause of death in infants younger than 1 year of age in the United States, accounting for 20.4% of infant deaths (Heron, Sutton, Xu, Ventura, Strobino, & Guyer, 2010). Although the incidences of other causes of neonatal mortality have decreased, the death rate associated with most congenital anomalies has essentially remained stable since 1932.

The desired and expected outcome of every wanted pregnancy is a normal, functioning infant with a good intellectual potential. Fulfillment of this hope depends on numerous hereditary and environmental factors. Probably all human characteristics have a genetic component, including those that produce symptoms or physical abnormalities that impair the fitness of the person. Some disorders or diseases occur through the influence of a single gene or the combined action of many genes inherited from the parents; others result from the action of the intrauterine environment. Many defects appear to occur as the result of multifactorial inheritance, the interaction of multiple genes with environmental factors that affect the embryonic development of the affected system. Examples of these include neural tube defects, congenital heart defects, developmental dysplasia of the hip, and cleft lip or palate. In about half of all cases of congenital anomalies, there is no identifiable cause. A chromosomal abnormality or gene alteration is responsible for approximately 40% of anomalies (Manning, 2009). Evidence indicates that maternal obesity is significantly linked to spina bifida, cardiac defects, diaphragmatic hernia, hypospadias, omphalocele, anorectal atresia, and limb reductions (Cunningham et al., 2010; Waller, Shaw, Rasmussen, Hobbs, Canfield, Siega-Riz, et al., 2007).

Ways of detecting and preventing some of the congenital anomalies are being improved continually, as are surgical techniques for the care of the fetus and newborn with certain anomalies. Promoting the availability of these services to populations at risk challenges community health care systems. An interdisciplinary team approach is vital for providing holistic care: the surgical treatment, rehabilitation, and education of the child, as well as psychosocial and financial assistance for the parents. Parental disappointment and disillusion add to the complexity of the nursing care needed for these infants.

The most common congenital anomalies that cause serious problems in the neonate are congenital heart disease, neural tube defects, cleft lip or palate, clubfoot, and developmental dysplasia of the hip. These are thought to result from the interaction of multiple genetic and environmental factors. Minor anomalies are less apparent but are important to identify because they can be a part of a characteristic pattern of malformations. That is, they can point to the presence of a more serious major anomaly and aid in its diagnosis. The presence of a minor anomaly indicates the need for further evaluation of the neonate for other anomalies. Minor malformations are more common in areas of the body that have variable features, such as the face and distal extremities. Some of the most common minor malformations include the lack of a helical fold of the pinna, low-set ears, alterations in hair pattern or texture, absent philtrum, or a hairy patch or birthmark over the vertebral column (Hudgins & Cassidy, 2006).

Cardiovascular System Anomalies

During fetal development, cell division and differentiation of the organs and tissues of a particular body system sometimes occur rapidly. During these critical periods particular body systems are more susceptible to environmental influences than they are later in gestation. For example, the critical period for the cardiovascular system is from week 3 of embryonic development to week 8, when many women are not aware that they are pregnant.

Congenital cardiac anomalies, with an overall prevalence of approximately 81 per 10,000 births, are the most common of all congenital malformations (Bernstein, 2007; Reller, Strickland, Riehle-Colarusso, Mahle, & Correa, 2009). Congenital heart defects (CHDs) are anatomic abnormalities in the heart that are present at birth, although they may not be diagnosed immediately. Congenital heart disease occurs more frequently in preterm infants. There is an increased likelihood of cardiac disease in neonates that are small for gestational age (SGA), as well as in those with congenital infections.

Ventricular septal defect, the most common type of heart defect with increased pulmonary blood flow (acyanotic lesion) has a prevalence of 27.5 per 10,000 births, and accounts for about 30% to 35% of all congenital heart defects. Tetralogy of Fallot has an incidence of 4.7 per 10,000 births, and is the most common cardiac defect with decreased pulmonary blood flow (cyanotic lesion) (Bernstein, 2007; Reller et al., 2009). Congenital heart defects are often associated with other extracardiac defects such as renal agenesis, omphalocele, tracheoesophageal fistula, and diaphragmatic hernias. Congenital heart disease is the leading cause of death in children with congenital defects (Bernstein, 2007).

The etiology of CHDs is multifactorial, chromosomal and/or genetic, and due to environmental teratogens (Sadowski, 2010). This is important information for parents because they often feel guilty thinking that they have done something to cause the defect. The etiology is also important when it comes to counseling the family regarding recurrence risks for future pregnancies. If the parent or a sibling is diagnosed with a CHD, the risk is increased 3- to 4-fold, and if two first-order relatives have a CHD, the recurrence risk is increased 10-fold (Park, 2008). Maternal factors that are known to be associated with a higher incidence of CHDs include the following (Hartas, Tsounias & Gupta-Malhotra, 2009):

- Rubella and cytomegalovirus
- Ingestion of folic acid antagonists, progesterone, estrogen, lithium, warfarin (Coumadin), or anticonvulsants such as phenytoin
- Use of the acne medication isotretinoin (Accutane)
- Alcohol intake
- Poor nutrition
- Radiation exposure
- Metabolic disorders such as diabetes mellitus and phenylketonuria
- Systemic lupus erythematosus
- Maternal age ≥40 years

Maternal smoking is associated with a greater risk of congenital heart disease. Infants born to women who are heavy smokers (≥25 cigarettes per day) have more than twice the risk of having a congenital septal defect (Malik, Cleves, Honein, Romitti, Botto, Yang, et al., 2008).

Maternal obesity can increase the risk of congenital heart anomalies. An above normal body mass index has been associated with an increased risk for all congenital heart defects, and specifically conotruncal defects, tetralogy of Fallot, total anomalous pulmonary venous return, hypoplastic left heart syndrome, right ventricular outflow tract defects, and septal defects (Gilboa, Correa, Botto, Rasmussen, Waller, Hobbs, et al., 2010).

Genetic factors are implicated in the pathogenesis of CHDs. It now appears that a much greater percentage of CHDs than believed to be true in the past can be attributed to single gene mutations. This recognition is based on animal models, studies of human familial patterns of inheritance, and the finding of cardiovascular defects as a part of syndromes exhibiting mendelian patterns of inheritance. An example of this is the identification of chromosome 22q11 deletions in infants with DiGeorge syndrome. This syndrome affects an estimated 1 in 4000 live births, making this one of the most frequent genetic disorders with congenital heart defects. The gene or genes located in the chromosomal region involved with DiGeorge syndrome appear to play a major role in the development of cardiovascular defects, particularly truncus arteriosus, absent pulmonary valve syndrome, tetralogy of Fallot, pulmonary atresia, and other abnormalities involving the aortic arch. Congenital heart disease is found in more than 50% of children with trisomy 21 (Down syndrome), 90% of neonates with trisomy 18 (Gilbert syndrome), and 40% of neonates with Turner syndrome (Bernstein, 2007).

TABLE 36-1 PHYSIOLOGIC CLASSIFICATION OF CARDIAC DEFECTS

CATEGORIES	EXAMPLES
Defects that result in increased pulmonary blood flow, often with congestive heart failure	Atrial and ventricular septal defects Patent ductus arteriosus
Defects that involve decreased pulmonary blood flow and typically result in cyanosis	Tetralogy of Fallot Tricuspid atresia
Defects that cause obstruction to blood flow out of the heart	Pulmonary stenosis; causes cyanosis Coarctation of the aorta; congestive heart failure, no cyanosis Subaortic stenosis; congestive heart failure, no cyanosis
Complex cardiac anomalies that involve a flow of mixed saturated and desaturated blood in the heart or great vessels	Transposition of the great vessels Total anomalous venous return

Although traditionally a CHD has been classified as either cyanotic or acyanotic, a classification that categorizes cardiac defects physiologically is now considered more descriptive. The first of the four categories in this classification includes defects that result in increased pulmonary blood flow. Examples of the CHDs in this category are defects that eventually manifest with congestive heart failure such as atrial and ventricular septal defects and patent ductus arteriosus. The second category includes defects that involve decreased pulmonary blood flow that produce cyanosis. The most common example of this type of defect is tetralogy of Fallot. The third category includes those defects that cause obstruction to blood flow out of the heart. Pulmonary stenosis is an example of an obstruction to the flow of blood out of the right side of the heart (ventricle) that causes cyanosis. Coarctation of the aorta and subaortic stenosis are examples of obstructions to the flow of blood out of the left side of the heart that can result in pulmonary venous congestion that leads to a left-sided congestive heart failure. The fourth category comprises those complex cardiac anomalies that involve blood flow composed of a mixed amount of oxygen saturated and oxygen desaturated blood in the heart or great vessels. These include such defects as transposition of the great vessels and total anomalous venous return (Table 36-1 and Fig. 36-1).

Severe CHDs often are evident immediately after birth, especially defects that cause cyanosis such as transposition of the great vessels. Infants with these anomalies are transferred directly to neonatal intensive care units, preferably those that are equipped to diagnose and medically/surgically treat these types of cardiac emergencies. Even though the structural or functional anomalies are always present at birth, the affected newborns can be asymptomatic because the defect is too small to interfere with sufficient blood flow to the lung for oxygenation or does not interfere with delivery of oxygenated blood to the tissues. With growth and maturation, the defect can become apparent as the infant or child is exposed to stresses such as growth demands or infection.

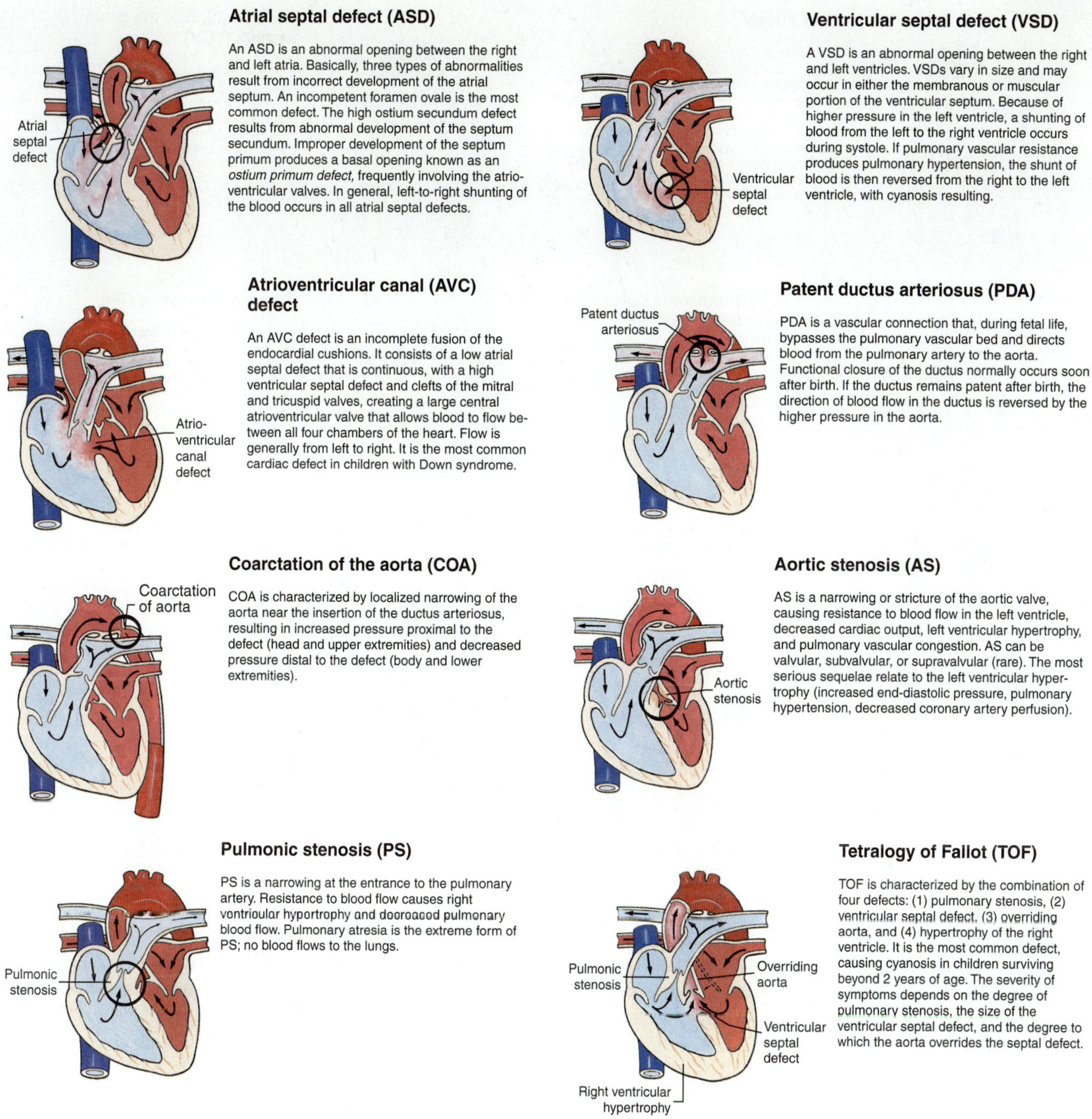

FIG. 36-1 Congenital heart abnormalities. (Modified from Hockenberry, M., & Wilson, D. [2011]. *Wong's nursing care of infants and children* [9th ed.]. St. Louis: Mosby.)

Continued

If symptoms are present at birth, they can be obvious with the first cry, which can be weak and muffled or loud and breathless. Affected newborns can exhibit cyanosis that is not relieved when given supplemental oxygen, with the cyanosis increasing whenever the child cries or is in the supine position. The bluish gray, dusky color of cyanotic infants can be mild, moderate, or severe. Other infants can be acyanotic and pale, with or without mottling on exertion, which includes crying, feeding, or stooling.

The affected newborn's activity level varies from restlessness to lethargy, and possibly unresponsiveness, except to pain. Persistent bradycardia (a resting heart rate of less than 80 beats/min) or tachycardia (a rate exceeding 160 beats/min) can be noted. The cardiac rhythm can be abnormal, and various murmurs may be heard. Signs of congestive heart failure and decreased tissue perfusion can also become evident (Hartas et al., 2009; Sadowski, 2010).

Because the cardiac and respiratory systems function together, cardiac disease can be manifested by respiratory signs and symptoms. The nurse assesses the respiratory rate while the newborn is in a resting state. Tachypnea, a respiratory rate greater than 60 breaths/min without dyspnea is typically a subtle clue that the baby possibly has a cardiac malformation. Increased respiratory depth or hyperpnea is often noted when the neonate has a cardiac lesion that is obstructing blood flow to the lung. Signs that can indicate the development of congestive heart failure are feeding difficulties and increasing respiratory distress, especially tachypnea such that the baby has to stop feeding to breathe.

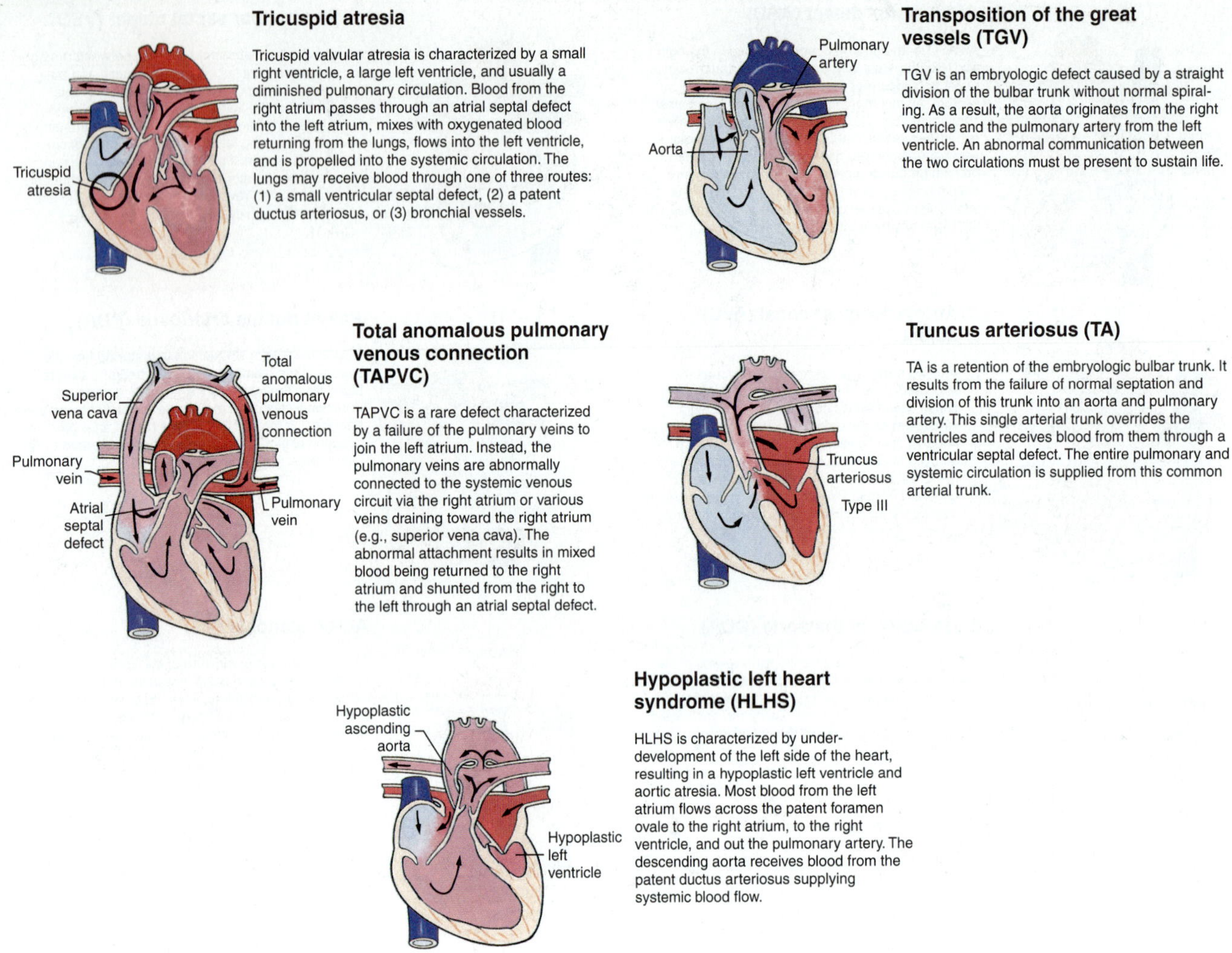

FIG. 36-1, cont'd Congenital heart anomalies.

A major role of the nurse is to assess infants for abnormal findings, which must be reported immediately. Newborns exhibiting these symptoms require prompt diagnosis and appropriate therapy in a neonatal or pediatric intensive care unit. Interventions include administering oxygen as ordered, administering cardiotonic and other medications such as diuretics that rid the body of accumulated fluid, decreasing the workload of the heart by maintaining a thermoneutral environment, feeding with the gavage method if necessary, and preventing crying if this precipitates cyanosis. Various diagnostic tests such as echocardiography and cardiac catheterization are performed to obtain specific information about the defect and the need for surgical intervention. Significant improvements in diagnosis, medical management, and surgical treatment of CHDs have caused the death rate to decrease significantly, with the result that more of these children are reaching adulthood (Hartas et al., 2009).

Central Nervous System Anomalies

Most congenital anomalies of the central nervous system (CNS) result from defects in the closure of the neural tube during fetal development. Although the cause of **neural tube defects (NTDs)** is unknown, they are thought to stem from the interaction of many genes that can be influenced by factors in the fetal environment. Environmental influences such as maternal treatment with anticonvulsants (e.g., valproic acid or carbamazepine), treatment with methotrexate (a chemotherapeutic medication), folic acid deficiency, and maternal diabetes have been implicated (Zupancic, 2008). Excessive maternal body heat exposure during the early first trimester, significant febrile illness, and lower socioeconomic status can increase the risk of an NTD (Sterk, 2010).

Maternal folic acid deficiency has a direct bearing on failure of the neural tube to close. Therefore, as a preventive measure, folic acid supplementation (0.4 mg/day) is recommended for women of childbearing age.

The incidence of NTD is about 1 per 1000 live births. However, the incidence varies according to race, geographic area, socioeconomic status, and ethnicity (Zupancic, 2008). Prevalence estimates for the two most common NTDs indicate that spina bifida occurs in approximately 18 of every 100,000 live births and anencephaly occurs in approximately 11 of every 100,000 live births (Mathews, 2008). Approximately 95% of all NTDs occur in families that have no history of NTDs. Primary NTDs have an increased recurrence rate in subsequent pregnancies although secondary NTDs do not. Primary NTDs are the result of failure of the anterior neuropore to close or a disruption of an already closed neural tube between 18 and 25 days of gestation (Moore & Persaud, 2007; Volpe, 2008). Myelomeningocele, encephalocele, and anencephaly are examples of primary NTDs. Secondary neural tube defects account for 5% of

NTDs. They are due to disruption in development of the lower sacral or coccygeal segments during secondary neurulation between 26 days and 8 weeks of gestation (Moore & Persaud; Volpe). Examples of secondary NTDs are meningocele, and sacral agenesis/dysgenesis.

Although an NTD is usually an isolated defect, it can occur with some chromosomal abnormalities and syndromes and with other defects such as cleft palate, ventricular septal defect, tracheoesophageal fistula, diaphragmatic hernia, imperforate anus, and renal anomalies. Some NTDs are diagnosed prenatally with fetal ultrasonography and the finding of elevated levels of alpha-fetoprotein in the amniotic fluid and maternal serum. Increased use of prenatal diagnostic techniques and termination of pregnancies have also had an effect on the overall incidence of birth of infants with NTDs.

Encephalocele and Anencephaly

Encephalocele and anencephaly are abnormalities resulting from failure of the anterior end of the neural tube to close. An **encephalocele** is a herniation of the brain and meninges through a skull defect. Treatment consists of surgical repair and shunting to relieve hydrocephalus, unless a major brain malformation is present. Most of these infants will have some degree of cognitive deficit. **Anencephaly** is the absence of both cerebral hemispheres and of the overlying skull. This condition is incompatible with life; many of the infants are stillborn or die within a few days of birth. Comfort measures are provided until the infant eventually dies of respiratory failure.

Spina Bifida

Spina bifida, the most common defect of the CNS, results from failure of the neural tube to close at some point. The two categories of spina bifida are spina bifida occulta and spina bifida manifesta. *Spina bifida occulta*, the milder form, is a malformation in which the posterior portion of the laminas fails to close, but the spinal cord or meninges do not herniate or protrude through the defect. Skin typically covers the opening in the spinal cord. There can also be a bulge under the skin where the ends of the spinal cord terminate in fatty tissue. Often a birthmark or a hairy patch is present above the defect.

Spina bifida manifesta occurs predominantly in the lumbar or lumbosacral regions and includes meningocele and myelomeningocele. A meningocele is a herniation of the meninges at the site of the defect in the vertebral column, and is typically covered by skin. The baby's neurologic function tends to be normal unless other abnormalities are present. A **myelomeningocele** is a herniation of the meninges and spinal cord at the site of the defect, with or without skin or vertebral covering (Fig. 36-2). The sac can tear easily, allowing cerebrospinal fluid (CSF) to leak out and providing an entry for infectious agents into the CNS. Because the nerves are involved, there are motor and sensory deficits below the lesion. Eighty percent of the lesions occur in the lumbar area and 95% of affected neonates will have hydrocephalus, typically due to an Arnold-Chiari malformation (Lynam & Verklan, 2010; Volpe, 2008). An Arnold-Chiari malformation results from the improper development and downward displacement of the hindbrain into the cervical spinal canal, which blocks the flow of CSF from communicating with the spinal column and results in the development of hydrocephalus. The long-term prognosis in an affected infant can be determined to a large extent at birth, with the degree of neurologic dysfunction related to the level of the lesion, as the level determines the nerves involved. Prenatal diagnosis makes possible a scheduled cesarean birth, allowing for more careful delivery of the infant's back to try to prevent rupture of the meningeal sac.

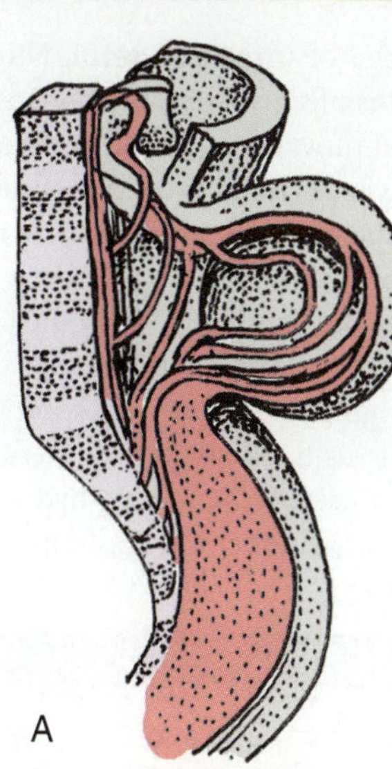

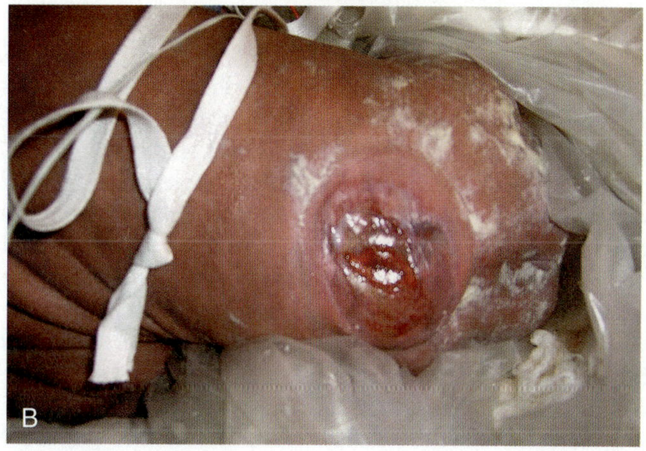

FIG. 36-2 **A,** Myelomeningocele. Note absence of vertebral arches. **B,** Myelomeningocele (spina bifida). (Courtesy Cheryl Briggs, RNC, Annapolis, MD.)

A major preoperative nursing intervention for a neonate with a myelomeningocele is to protect the protruding sac from injury, rupture, and resultant risk of CNS infection. Such infants should be positioned in a prone-kneeling position and the knees protected from skin breakdown. The sac should be covered with a sterile, moist, nonadherent dressing, and cared for using sterile technique. A drape should be placed over the buttocks below the lesion and secured using the drape's adhesive to keep the lesion free of meconium or stool. Neurosurgery and urology consultations should occur immediately after the neonate is admitted. A thorough physical examination will be done to evaluate the level of the injury, sensory involvement, sphincter control (anal wink), and measurement of the frontal-occipital circumference to assess for hydrocephalus (Lynam & Verklan, 2010; Volpe, 2008). Intake and output are recorded to document the number and character of the voidings and stools as well as the leakage of urine and stool. Nursing assessment includes observations of movement or absence of movement as well as the quality of movements of the lower extremities.

Nurses provide support and information to parents as they begin to learn to cope with an infant who has immediate needs for intensive care and who probably will have long-term needs as well. Based on the type and position of the lesion, along with the neonate's clinical condition, early surgical repair is advocated to preserve cognitive function, decrease the risk of sepsis, and improve prognosis for ambulation (Sterk, 2010). Surgical shunt procedures to prevent increasing hydrocephalus may be needed, such as a ventriculoperitoneal shunt.

! NURSING ALERT

Infants with myelomeningocele are at increased risk for developing latex sensitivity, so they must not come into direct or secondary contact with any products or equipment containing latex.

Maternal-fetal surgery to repair a fetal myelomeningocele is a promising new development in maternal-fetal intervention. The rationale for this intervention is based on direct and indirect evidence that some of the neural damage resulting from the myelomeningocele is acquired in the later part of gestation, caused by amniotic fluid exposure or trauma to the exposed neural elements. The improvement in hydrocephalus and the Arnold-Chiari II malformation can decrease the need for a ventriculoperitoneal shunt. There does not appear to be any improvement in neurologic function, including problems with continence. The term birth of an infant with myelomeningocele is a viable alternative to fetal repair. Numerous other significant issues have been addressed in the consideration of maternal-fetal surgery for this and other nonlethal anomalies (Hirose & Farmer, 2009).

Hydrocephalus

Hydrocephalus is a condition in which there is excess CSF in the ventricles of the brain due to overproduction (rare) or a decrease in reabsorption. The most common etiology for the neonate is excess ventricular CSF due to aqueductal flow obstruction. The obstruction prevents the CSF from leaving the head and flowing into the spinal column. Other etiologies include congenital viral infections, myelomeningocele with Arnold-Chiari malformation, and congenital masses or tumors (Lynam & Verklan, 2010; Volpe, 2008).

The neonate presents with an increasing frontal-occipital circumference because the head circumference is increasing at an abnormal rate as a result of the increase in CSF pressure (Fig. 36-3). The sutures are widened and the fontanels are full or bulging and tense. Classic signs of increasing intracranial pressure (vomiting, lethargy, and irritability) can be attributed to feeding intolerance. It is thought that "setting sun eyes," (eyes that are rotated downward) indicate permanent damage to the brain tissue. Serial head ultrasound is used to evaluate the evolving condition. Neurosurgery and genetics services are consulted to evaluate for the placement of a ventriculoperitoneal shunt versus placement of a reservoir and to assess for the presence of congenital anomalies (Lynam & Verklan, 2010; Volpe, 2008).

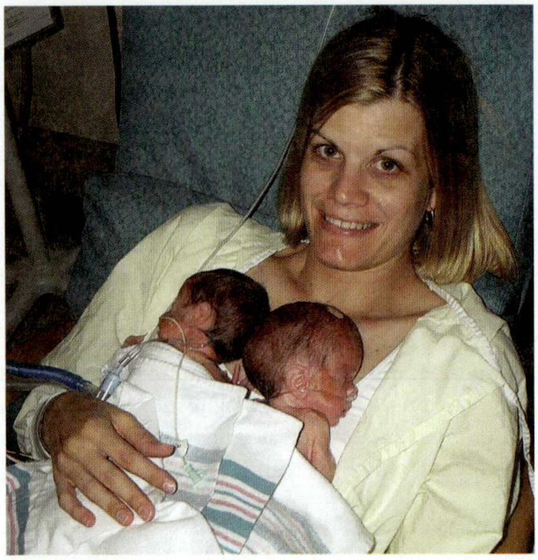

FIG. 36-3 Mother providing kangaroo care to preterm twins; the one on the right has hydrocephalus. The characteristic appearance is an enlarged head, thinning of the scalp, distended scalp veins, and a full fontanel. (Courtesy Cheryl Briggs, RNC, Annapolis, MD.)

The nurse provides support to the family by teaching and involving them in their baby's care as much as possible. Minimal stimulation protocols that promote the use of limited handling, dim lighting, and attention to the baby's cues will help keep the baby calm. The head needs to be positioned carefully, repositioned at least once every 4 hours, and attention given such that the head is not positioned on the shunt side postoperatively. Gel-filled pillows can provide some comfort for the neonate. The frontal-occipital circumference needs to be measured serially, and depending on the rate of increase, every 4 hours to every 24 hours. Neurologic assessments and observation for signs of increasing intracranial pressure should be done every 4 to 8 hours, depending on the baby's clinical condition.

The baby should be fed in a semi-reclining position with the head well-supported. The method, amount, and frequency of feeding depend on the infant's tolerance and energy level. The nurse should be alert to the possibility of emesis, a frequent occurrence in the presence of increased intracranial pressure, and should maintain aspiration precautions. Nonnutritive sucking, touching, and cuddling needs should be met.

In addition to serial intracranial ultrasonography, the diagnosis is also made using computed tomography and magnetic resonance imaging (MRI); antenatal diagnosis can be made by fetal ultrasonography. The surgical correction of hydrocephalus involves the placement of a shunt that goes from the ventricles of the brain usually to the peritoneum to allow the drainage of excess CSF. Damaged or destroyed brain tissue cannot be restored. The long-term prognosis in affected infants depends on the presence and extent of such tissue damage, along with the cause of the hydrocephalus, the presence of concurrent neurologic problems, and the long-term success of the shunt procedure.

Parent teaching regarding the shunt should be done both pre- and postoperatively. Providing handouts or if possible, seeing an infant with a shunt already in place can be helpful. Parents also need to be taught signs of a blocked shunt and signs of infection such as increasing intracranial pressure and changes in the baby's feeding patterns.

Microcephaly

Microcephaly refers to a head circumference that measures two or more standard deviations below the mean for age and sex (Lynam & Verklan, 2010). Brain growth is usually restricted and thus mental retardation is common. Maternal risk factors include congenital viral infections, chromosomal disorders, and malnutrition. Fetal and neonatal factors include inflammation, birth trauma, and sequelae of hypoxic-ischemic encephalopathy. If the result of an in utero insult, the baby is typically born with a small head and brain, which gives the forehead a backward sloping appearance. Diagnostic evaluations include a complete maternal history, evaluation of the events surrounding the birth, computed tomography (CT) or MRI to evaluate brain volume, and a neurologic assessment. Typically genetics and infectious disease consults are also obtained. Although neurologic deficits are not present at birth, developmental delays will become evident. The baby's outcome and prognosis depend on the severity of the microcephaly. Treatment for the infant is supportive. The parents will need support and education to help them learn to care for a child with cognitive impairment and developmental delays.

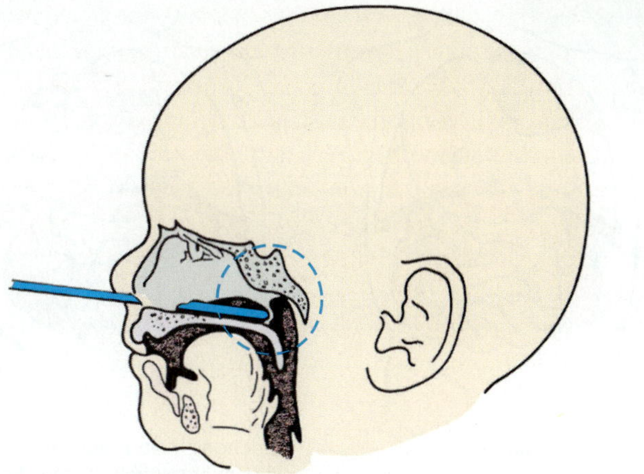

FIG. 36-4 Choanal atresia. Posterior nares are obstructed by membrane or bone either bilaterally or unilaterally. Infant becomes cyanotic at rest. With crying, newborn's color improves. Nasal discharge is present. Snorting respirations often are observed with increased respiratory effort. Newborn may be unable to breathe and eat at the same time. Diagnosis is made by noting inability to pass small feeding tube through one or both nares. (Used with permission of Ross Products Division, Abbott Laboratories, Inc., Columbus, OH 43216. From Clinical Education Aid #6, Copyright 1963, Ross Products Division, Abbott Laboratories, Inc.)

RESPIRATORY SYSTEM ANOMALIES

Screening for congenital anomalies of the respiratory system is necessary even in infants who are apparently normal at birth. Respiratory distress at birth or shortly thereafter can be the result of lung immaturity or anomalous development. Congenital laryngeal web and bilateral choanal atresia are readily apparent at birth. Respiratory distress caused by diaphragmatic hernia and tracheoesophageal fistula can appear immediately or be delayed, depending on the severity of the defect.

Laryngeal Web and Choanal Atresia

A laryngeal web, which is uncommon, results from the incomplete separation of the two sides of the larynx and is most often between the vocal cords. This is a surgical emergency such that perforation of the web using an endotracheal tube can be life saving. Choanal atresia (Fig. 36-4) is the most common congenital anomaly of the nose. The posterior nares can be blocked by a bony or soft-tissue obstruction. The obstruction can be unilateral or bilateral. The baby can display symptoms of respiratory distress and cyanosis or pallor that are relieved whenever the baby is crying. Inability to pass a suction catheter through the nose into the pharynx is highly suggestive of the diagnosis. Securing an oral airway into the posterior pharynx and maintaining the baby in the prone position will provide a patent airway and time to evaluate for the presence of other abnormalities. Definitive therapy involves creating a patency through the bony or soft tissue obstruction, and use of serial obturators to dilate the new airway passages (Pappas & Walker, 2010; Ringer & Hansen, 2008).

Congenital Diaphragmatic Hernia

Congenital diaphragmatic hernia (CDH) results from a defect in the formation of the diaphragm, allowing the abdominal organs to be displaced into the thoracic cavity. It occurs in approximately 1 in 3000 to 4000 live births and despite improvements in care management, the mortality rate remains high, at about 20% to 30% (Tsao & Lally, 2008). The etiology is unknown; however, it is not uncommon to find concomitant chromosomal anomalies, especially trisomies 12, 18, and 21, as well as abnormalities of the gastrointestinal, genitourinary, and central nervous systems. Intestinal malrotation is also associated with CDH. Approximately 80% of the hernias occur on the left side in the posterior diaphragm known as the foramen of Bochdalek (Holder, Klaassens, Tibboel, de Klein, Lee, & Scott, 2007; Ringer & Hansen, 2008). Poorer outcomes are associated with right-sided or bilateral defects (Brownlee, Howatson, Davis, & Sabharwal, 2009).

A small defect may not be detected on an early prenatal ultrasound. Fetuses with CDH tend to have polyhydramnios, which typically prompts the obstetrician to obtain an ultrasound. A major advantage of diagnosing CDH prenatally is that it allows the baby to be born in a tertiary hospital that is equipped to manage all the cardiorespiratory problems associated with the defect and to rapidly stabilize the neonate's precarious condition. Hernias can be repaired by fetal surgery in some research institutions; however, intrauterine surgical correction of CDH has met with poor neonatal outcomes in many cases. Severe defects can be managed with the baby being born by cesarean using the EXIT (EX-utero intrapartum treatment) procedure in which the neonate is transitioned immediately from placental support to extracorporeal membrane oxygenation (ECMO) (Ringer & Hansen, 2008).

Depending on the size of the defect and how much developed lung tissue is present, the baby may not be in any significant distress at birth. A small defect can distress the baby when feeding such that symptoms of respiratory distress (tachypnea, pallor, mottled, cyanosis) become evident. Babies with a large defect will have significant distress at birth because the viscera present in the thoracic cavity during embryonic life prevented the normal development of the lung (Fig. 36-5). Characteristic symptoms include respiratory distress, cyanosis, heart

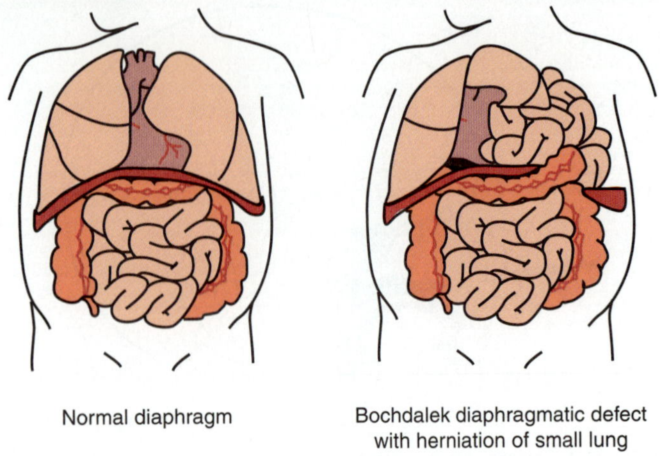

FIG. 36-5 **A**, Normal diaphragm separating the abdominal and thoracic cavities. **B**, Diaphragmatic hernia with a small lung and abdominal contents in the thoracic cavity. (From Erlich P., & Coran, A. [2007]. Diaphragmatic hernia. In R. Kliegman, R. Behrman, H. Jenson, & B. Stanton [Eds.], *Nelson textbook of pediatrics* [18th ed.]. Philadelphia: Saunders.)

sounds shifted to the right, and low blood pressure. There will be increasing distress as the bowels fill with air. The abdomen is scaphoid shaped and the chest appears barrel shaped due to the abdominal contents being in the chest. Diagnosis can be made on the basis of the x-ray finding of loops of intestine in the thoracic cavity and the absence of intestine in the abdominal cavity. The severity of the clinical picture is considered to be a neonatal emergency (Bradshaw, 2010; Ringer & Hansen, 2008).

Surgical repair is performed as soon as the infant is stable. Preoperative nursing interventions include participating in the stabilization of the infant's cardiopulmonary condition until surgical repair can be done. Inhaled nitrous oxide (NO) has been used in many centers with moderate success to treat the accompanying persistent pulmonary hypertension (Askin & Diehl-Jones, 2010). Gastric contents are aspirated and suction applied to decompress the gastrointestinal tract and prevent further cardiothoracic compromise. Oxygen therapy, mechanical ventilation, and the correction of acidosis are necessary in infants with large defects. Pulmonary hypertension can occur as a result of the lung hypoplasia. ECMO or high-frequency oscillatory ventilation can be used in infants with severe circulatory and respiratory complications (see Chapter 37) (Bradshaw, 2010; Migliazza, Bellan, Alberti, Auriemma, Burgio, Locatelli, & Colombo, 2007).

The prognosis depends largely on the degree of fetal pulmonary development and the success of surgical diaphragmatic closure, but the prognosis in severe cases is often poor. As a rule, finding the liver in the thorax is associated with the worst prognosis. Approximately 20% of infants with CDH die before they are able to have surgical repair. It is unclear whether the timing of the surgery or the condition of the infant at the time of repair is more important to improved outcomes (Bianco-Batlles, Mohamed, & Hammad, 2010). Overall survival rates have improved with the advent of inhaled NO, improved management of high-frequency ventilation, and ECMO. Of those who survive, some have chronic lung disease with long-term oxygen dependency, feeding difficulties, and gastroesophageal reflux (GER).

GASTROINTESTINAL SYSTEM ANOMALIES

Anomalies in the gastrointestinal (GI) system can occur anywhere along the GI tract, from the mouth to the anus. Some anomalies, such as cleft lip, omphalocele, and gastroschisis, are apparent at birth. Others, including cleft palate, esophageal atresia, pyloric stenosis, intestinal obstructions, and imperforate anus, become apparent as the infant is further assessed or becomes symptomatic.

Cleft Lip and Palate

Facial clefts are among the most common congenital anomalies. **Cleft lip** or **palate** is a congenital midline fissure, or opening, in the lip or palate resulting from failure of the primary palate to fuse (Fig. 36-6). One or both deformities can occur, and nasal deformity can be present. Multiple genetic and, to a lesser extent, environmental factors (e.g., maternal infection, maternal smoking, radiation exposure, alcohol ingestion, and treatment with medications such as corticosteroids, lithium, retinoids, and phenytoin) appear to be involved in their development. Approximately one third of cases of cleft lip or palate are associated with a major anomaly such as Pierre Robin syndrome (Manning, 2009).

Cleft lip with or without cleft palate occurs in approximately 10.48 per 10,000 live births. Cleft palate alone occurs in 6.39 per 10,000 live births (Centers for Disease Control and Prevention [CDC], 2006).

The defect can range from a simple notch in the lip to complete separation of the lip that extends to the floor of the nose. The treatment for a cleft lip is surgical repair, which usually is done between ages 6 and 12 weeks, if the infant is healthy and free of infection. Advances in surgical techniques have made it possible for some infants, particularly those with unilateral cleft lip, to have a near-normal appearance. The results of the repair depend on the severity of the defect, with more severe bilateral cleft lip requiring surgical repair done in stages (Thigpen, 2007).

Anomalies of the palate often occur in association with cleft lip. Cleft palate alone is more common in female infants and occurs more frequently as a constituent of certain syndromes. This defect can range from a cleft in the uvula to a complete cleft of the hard and soft palates that can be unilateral, bilateral, or midline. Feeding is difficult because the cleft lip renders the newborn unable to maintain a seal around a nipple; the cleft palate renders the infant unable to form a vacuum to maintain suction when feeding. In addition, the inability to suck and swallow normally allows milk to pool in the nasopharynx, which increases the likelihood of aspiration. Furthermore, as the infant attempts to suck, milk often comes out through the cleft and the nares. Although the degree of difficulty depends on the size of the cleft, feeding problems are greater in infants with a cleft palate than in those with a cleft lip. Breastfeeding can be successful in some infants, particularly if the infant has a cleft lip alone. Bottle feeding can be successful in some infants. There are special nipples, bottles, and appliances available to aid in feeding (Fig. 36-7). In general, parents of infants with these defects need education, support, and encouragement as they learn to feed their baby. This can help minimize anxiety and frustration while promoting competence and confidence in providing infant care. The type of surgical repair to close the

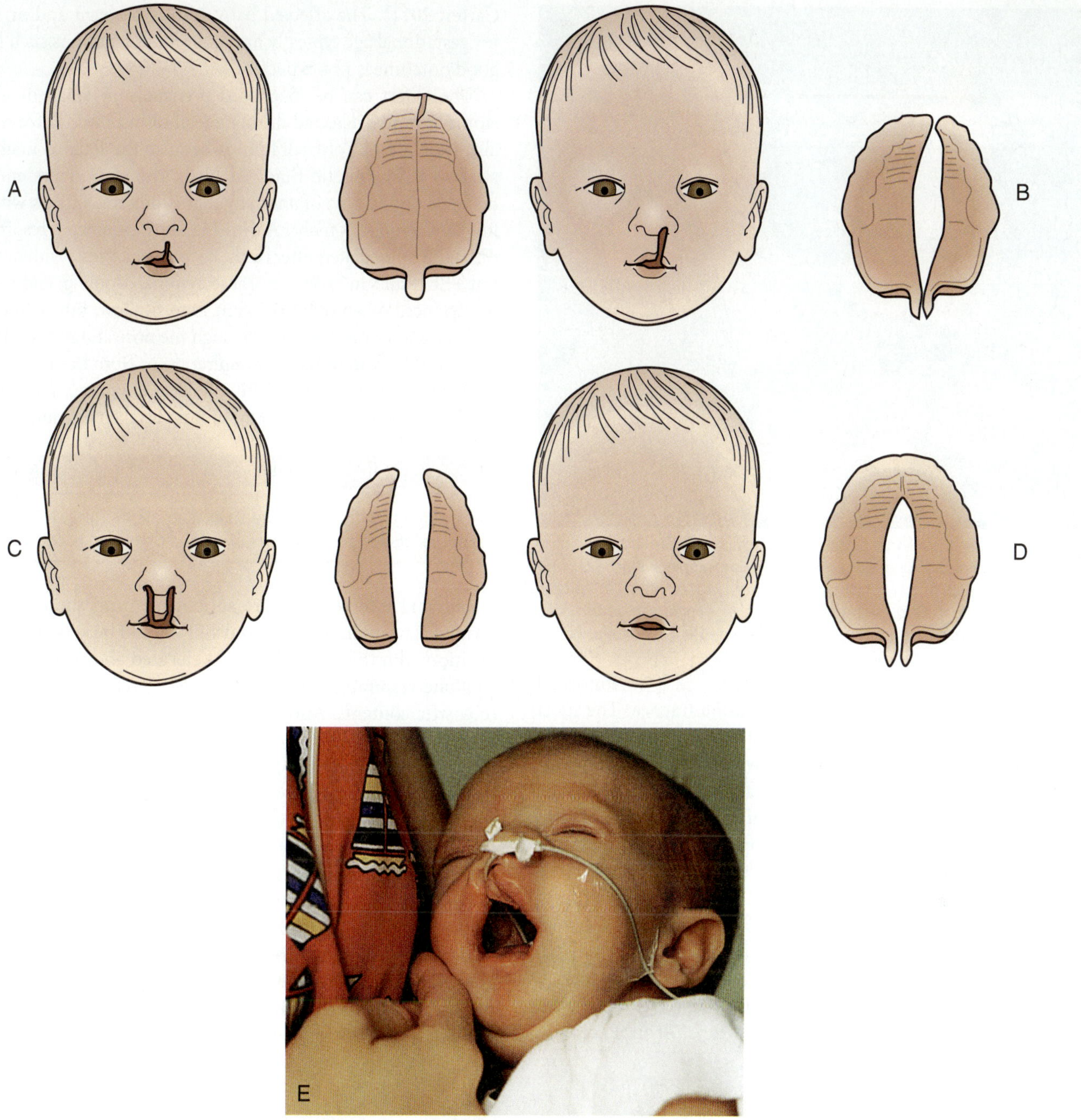

FIG. 36-6 Variations in clefts of lip and palate at birth. **A,** Notch in vermilion border. **B,** Unilateral cleft lip and cleft palate. **C,** Bilateral cleft lip and cleft palate. **D,** Cleft palate. **E,** Infant with complete unilateral cleft lip. Note the feeding tube. (**A-D,** From Hockenberry, M., & Wilson, D. [2011]. *Wong's nursing care of infants and children* [9th ed.]. St. Louis: Mosby. **E,** From Dickason, E., Silverman, B., & Kaplan, J. [1998]. *Maternal-infant nursing care* [3rd ed.]. St. Louis: Mosby.)

cleft palate is based on the degree of the cleft and, if severe, can necessitate repair done in stages. The cleft lip is usually repaired when the neonate reaches approximately 3600-4000 grams, and the palate is repaired at 1 to 2 years of age (Sterk, 2010). Early repair helps avert some of the speech problems that may occur in people with palate defects. Long-term care is often necessary for children with a cleft palate and involves the combined efforts of a health care team that includes acute care and community nurses; social workers; ear, nose, and throat and plastic surgeons; speech therapists; and orthodontists.

Parents of infants with a cleft lip or palate need much support, particularly in the case of a cleft lip, because this is both a cosmetic and functional defect. Recognizing that this may interfere with normal parent-infant bonding in the neonatal period, the nurse must assess for this and intervene appropriately.

Esophageal Atresia and Tracheoesophageal Fistula

Esophageal atresia (EA) and tracheoesophageal fistula (TEF), the most life-threatening anomalies of the esophagus, typically occur together, although they can occur singly. The prevalence of EA and TEF is approximately 2.37 per 10,000 live births (CDC, 2006). **Esophageal atresia** is a congenital anomaly in which the esophagus ends in a blind pouch, thus failing to form

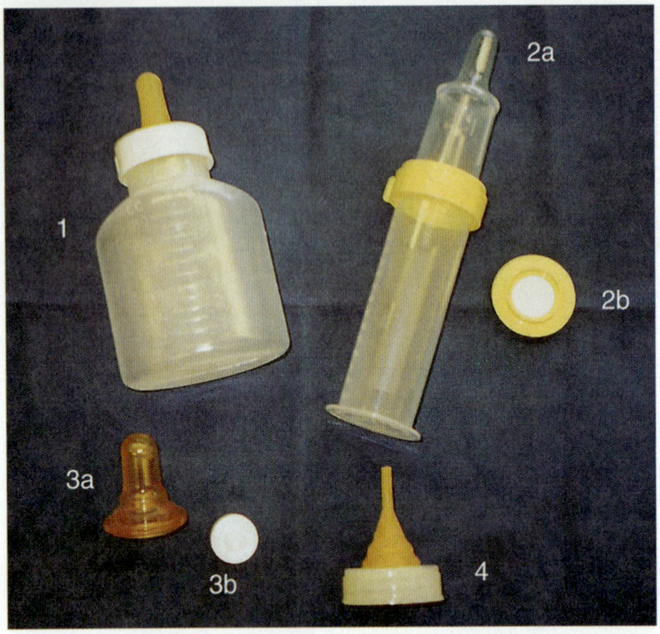

FIG. 36-7 Aids in feeding infants with cleft lip and palate *1*, Mead Johnson bottle and nipple for cleft palate. Cleft palate nipple system *(2a)* with valve *(2b)* to regulate flow. Haberman feeder *(3a)* with disk *(3b)* to control flow of milk. *4*, Ross cleft palate assembly. Nipple can be trimmed to accommodate palate size. (Courtesy Shannon Perry, Phoenix, AZ.)

a continuous passageway to the stomach. TEF is an abnormal connection between the esophagus and the trachea. The most common variant is the combination of a proximal EA, in which the esophagus ends in a blind pouch, with a distal TEF, in which the lower esophagus exits the stomach and is connected to the trachea by a fistula, rather than forming a continuous tube to the upper esophagus (Fig. 36-8). Variations of the anomalies are possible, depending on the presence or absence of a TEF, the site of the fistula, and the location and degree of the esophageal obstruction.

The presence of a midline defect such as EA or TEF is often accompanied by another significant embryonic defect such as a cardiac anomaly, cleft lip and/or palate, or vertebral, genitourinary, or abdominal wall defect (Lovvorn, Glenn, Pacetti, & Carter, 2011). The affected baby who is preterm and/or small for gestational age typically has other malformations such that a good outcome is not expected.

The defect can be diagnosed prenatally. A small or absent stomach can be detected during a fetal ultrasound. There is usually a history of polyhydramnios because the fetus is unable to swallow the amniotic fluid. At birth, the clinical presentation depends on the type of anomaly that is present. Infants with the life-threatening anomaly EA with TEF show significant respiratory difficulty immediately after birth. Esophageal atresia with or without TEF results in excessive oral secretions, drooling, and feeding intolerance. When fed, the infant may swallow, but then cough and gag and return the fluid through the nose and mouth. Respiratory distress can result from aspiration or from the acute gastric distention produced by the TEF. Choking, coughing, and cyanosis occur after even a small amount of fluid is taken by mouth.

! NURSING ALERT

Any infant with excessive oral secretions and respiratory distress should not be fed orally until a physician is consulted.

Nursing interventions are supportive until surgery is performed. The infant with EA and TEF should be kept in a supine position with the head of the bed elevated about 30 degrees to facilitate respiratory efforts and prevent reflux and aspiration of gastric contents. Antireflux and antacid medication may be given to minimize gastroesophageal reflux and prevent acid-induced pneumonitis. An orogastric tube (Replogle tube) is placed in the proximal esophageal pouch and attached to low continuous suction to remove secretions and decrease the possibility of aspiration (Lovvorn et al., 2011). The infant requires close observation and intervention to maintain a patent airway. Other supportive measures include thermoregulation, maintaining fluid and electrolyte balance intravenously as well as acid-base balance, and prevention of any further complications as a result of an associated defect. Surgical correction, done in one stage if possible, consists of ligating the fistula and anastomosing the two segments of the esophagus. The chances for

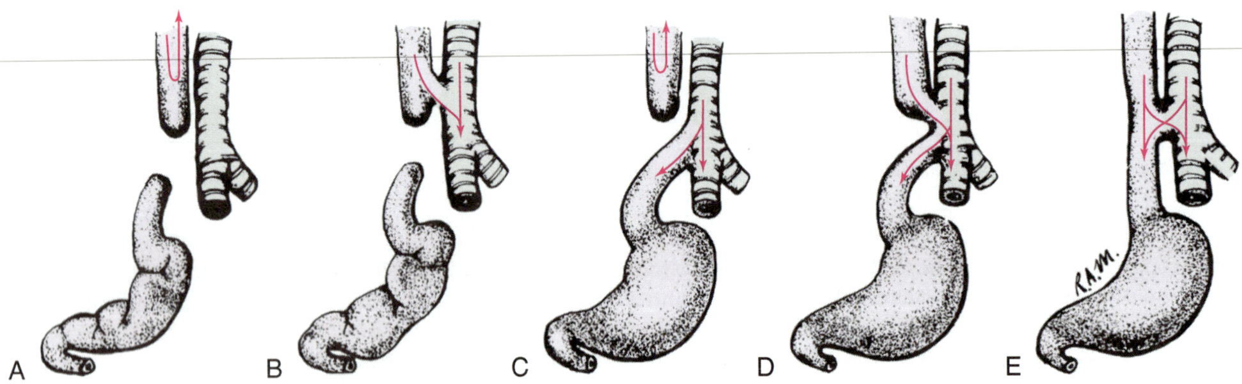

FIG. 36-8 Congenital atresia of esophagus and tracheoesophageal fistula. **A,** Upper and lower segments of esophagus end in blind sac, occurring in 5% to 8% of such infants. **B,** Upper segment of esophagus ends in atresia and connects to trachea by fistulous tract, occurring rarely. **C,** Upper segment of esophagus ends in blind pouch; lower segment connects with trachea by small fistulous tract, occurring in 80% to 95% of such infants. **D,** Both segments of esophagus connect by fistulous tracts to trachea, occurring in less than 1% of such infants. Infant may aspirate with first feeding. **E,** Esophagus is continuous but connects by fistulous tract to trachea; known as *H-type*. (From Hockenberry, M., & Wilson, D. [2011]. *Wong's nursing care of infants and children* [9th ed.]. St. Louis: Mosby.)

survival in those infants in a good risk category exceed 95% depending on the presence of associated defects and the infant's birth weight. Preterm infants with cardiac or chromosomal anomalies have the highest mortality rate. Many infants with EA and TEF will have postoperative issues related to feeding difficulties such as GER and esophageal strictures requiring periodic dilation (Bradshaw, 2010; Magnuson, Parry, & Chwals, 2006).

Omphalocele and Gastroschisis

Omphalocele and gastroschisis are two of the more common congenital defects of the abdominal wall. Omphalocele occurs in approximately 2 of every 10,000 live births, whereas the prevalence of gastroschisis is about 3.7 in 10,000 live births (CDC, 2006). An **omphalocele** is a covered defect of the umbilical ring into which varying amounts of the abdominal organs can herniate (Fig. 36-9, *A*). The peritoneal sac covering the defect can rupture during or after birth. Many of the infants born with an omphalocele are preterm and nearly 50% have an underlying chromosomal abnormality, usually trisomies 12, 18, or 21. Congenital heart defects are often associated with omphalocele (Lovvorn et al., 2011).

Gastroschisis is the herniation of the bowel through a defect in the abdominal wall to the right of the umbilical cord (see Fig. 36-9, *B*). No membrane covers the contents as it does with an omphalocele. Gastroschisis is 3 to 4 times more common than omphalocele and is not usually associated with other major congenital anomalies or syndromes. Intestinal atresia can occur with gastroschisis (Lovvorn et al., 2011).

The preoperative nursing care is similar for infants with either defect. Exposure of the viscera causes problems with thermoregulation and fluid and electrolyte balance. Immediately after birth, the neonate's torso should be placed in an impermeable, clear plastic bowel bag to decrease insensible water losses, maintain thermoregulation, and prevent contamination of the exposed viscera (Bradshaw, 2010). It is essential that the nurse assess the exposed viscera frequently to detect any changes in perfusion to the exposed abdominal contents. The baby should be placed in a side-lying position and the viscera supported with a blanket roll to prevent vascular compromise to a torqued intestine. Prior to surgery, the exposed viscera should be kept covered with sterile moistened saline gauze and plastic wrap. Gastric decompression with a Replogle tube (a special type of gastric tube) connected to low intermittent wall suction is also necessary to prevent aspiration pneumonia and to allow as much bowel as possible to be placed into the abdomen during surgery. Antibiotics, fluid and electrolyte replacement, and thermoregulation are needed for physiologic support (Lovvorn et al., 2011).

Surgery is usually performed soon after birth. If complete closure is impossible because of the small size of the defect and the large amount of viscera to be replaced, a Silastic silo or patch (Dow Corning, Midland, MI) is placed. This protects the contents as they are gradually placed back into the abdominal cavity and minimizes symptoms of respiratory distress as the increasing intraabdominal pressure pushes against the diaphragm. The defect is closed surgically after the exposed visceral contents have been reduced; this reduction process usually takes 7 to 10 days. The prognosis depends on the size of the defect and the presence of associated anomalies. It is generally expected that there will be complications related to intestinal dysfunction, such as feeding difficulties, dysmotility, or short-gut syndrome if a substantial amount of the intestine had to be removed.

Parental support is essential because the infant has an obvious disfiguring anomaly that can be shocking and repulsive in appearance. Depending on the size of the defect, the infant can also be critically ill before surgery. The nurse must be aware of the effect this may have on parental bonding and intervene appropriately as the parents cope with this crisis.

Gastrointestinal Obstruction

Congenital intestinal obstruction can occur anywhere in the GI tract and takes one of the following forms: atresia, which is a complete obliteration of the passage; partial obstruction, in which the symptoms can vary in severity and sometimes not be detected in the neonatal period; or malrotation of the intestine,

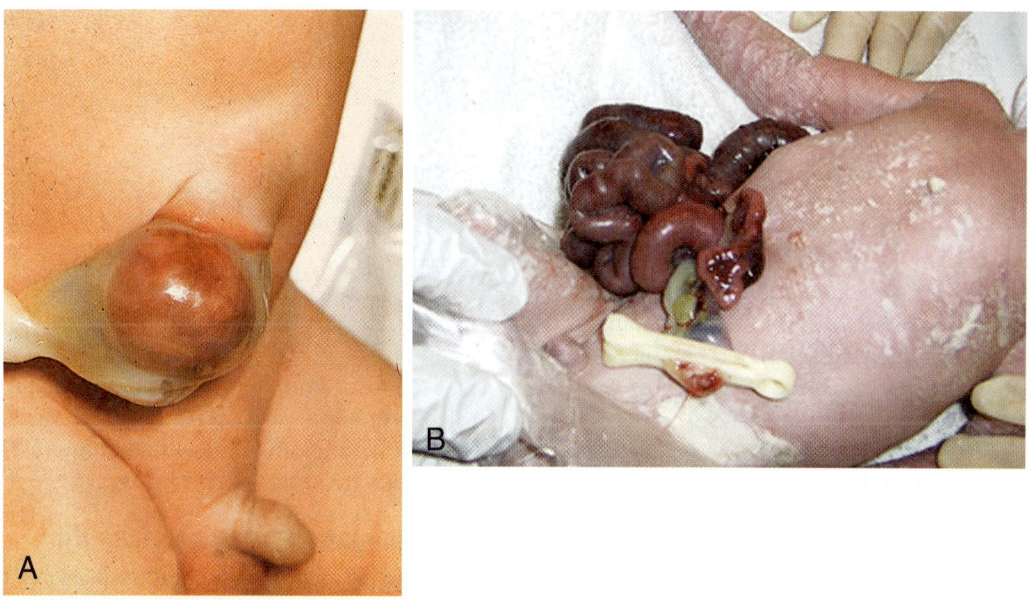

FIG. 36-9 **A,** Omphalocele. **B,** Gastroschisis of bowel and stomach. (**A,** From O'Doherty, N. [1986]. *Neonatology: Micro atlas of the newborn.* Nutley, NJ: Hoffmann-La Roche; **B,** courtesy Cheryl Briggs, RNC, Annapolis, MD.)

which leads to twisting of the intestine (volvulus) and obstruction. Esophageal atresia, discussed previously, is a type of GI obstruction. Duodenal atresia, midgut malrotation and volvulus, jejunoileal atresia, necrotizing enterocolitis, and meconium ileus are the most common causes of neonatal intestinal obstruction. Meconium ileus is an obstruction caused by impacted meconium; over 90% of infants who are born with meconium ileus have cystic fibrosis, a life-threatening chronic illness (Lowvorn et al., 2011).

Signs of neonatal intestinal obstruction occur early. It can be suspected in pregnant women with polyhydramnios. The neonate with an intestinal obstruction displays the following cardinal signs: bilious vomiting, abdominal distention, and failure to pass normal amounts of meconium in the first 24 hours. High intestinal obstruction is characterized by vomiting, even if the infant is not being fed orally. Distention usually indicates a low obstruction, with vomiting occurring later. Abdominal distention can elevate the diaphragm, which can cause respiratory difficulties.

Nursing care is aimed at supporting the infant until surgical intervention can be carried out to eliminate the obstruction. Oral feedings are withheld, an orogastric tube is placed to low intermittent wall suction, and intravenous therapy is initiated to provide needed fluid and electrolytes. In infants with an intestinal obstruction, surgery consists of resecting the obstructed area of bowel and anastomosing the nonaffected bowel, or creating an ostomy and allowing the bowel to rest. In recent years the survival rate for these infants has risen to 90% to 95% as a result of improved medical and nursing management, as well as a better understanding of the total problem.

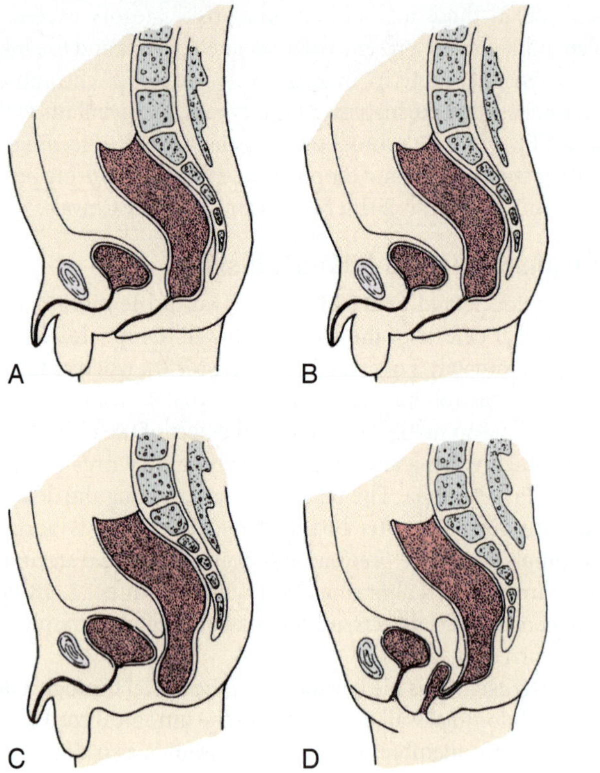

FIG. 36-10 Types of imperforate anus. Anal sphincter muscle may be present and intact. **A,** High lesion opening onto perineum through narrow fistulous tract. **B,** High lesion ending in fistulous tract to urinary tract. **C,** Low lesion in bowel passes through puborectal muscle. **D,** High lesion ending in fistulous tract to vagina.

Imperforate Anus

Imperforate anus is a term used to describe a wide range of congenital disorders involving the anus and rectum and genitourinary system (Fig. 36-10). These anomalies are relatively common, with an incidence of approximately 1 in 5000 live births (Bradshaw, 2010; Lovvorn et al., 2011). Occurring more in male than in female infants, they result from the failure of the urogenital sinus and cloaca to differentiate during weeks 7 and 8 of gestational life (Blackburn, 2007). Such infants have no anal opening, and commonly there is also a fistula from the rectum to the perineum or genitourinary system (Fig. 36-11). Types of anorectal malformations include the typical cloaca in females, which involves the vagina, colon, and urethra forming a single common passage in the perineum. Others include the low rectovaginal fistula (female) and rectourethral bulbar fistula (male). Imperforate anus can occur in isolation or in combination with other congenital defects such as esophageal atresia, duodenal atresia, renal anomalies, or vertebral anomalies. Extensive surgical repair is often required in stages for the more complex types of anorectal malformations. Infants with high imperforate anus typically have bowel incontinence even after surgical repair. In some cases the anomaly involves stenotic areas, or a thin translucent membrane can cover the anal opening. Treatment for such a membrane is anoplasty followed by daily dilation, which parents learn to do. The preoperative nursing care is similar to that described for other GI obstructions. Imperforate anus is often associated with other anomalies, with nearly half having additional genitourinary anomalies, which can complicate long-term care. Outcome is excellent with low imperforate anus (Bradshaw, 2010).

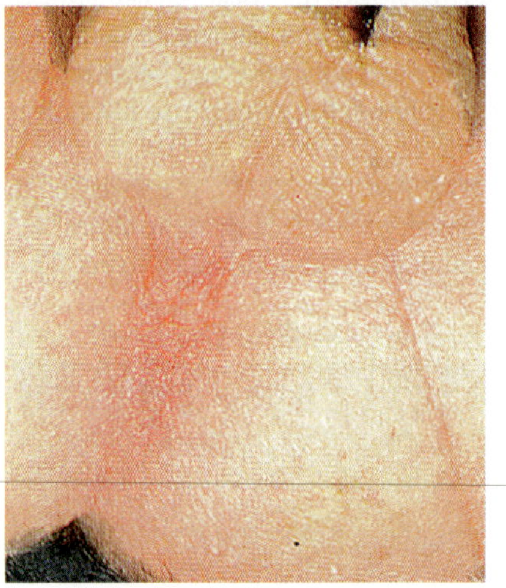

FIG. 36-11 Imperforate anus. (From Chessell, G., Jamieson, M., Morton, R., Petrie, J., & Towler, H. [1984]. *Diagnostic picture tests in clinical medicine* [vol. 2]. St. Louis: Mosby.)

MUSCULOSKELETAL SYSTEM ANOMALIES

The two most common musculoskeletal system anomalies seen in neonates are developmental dysplasia of the hip and congenital clubfoot. Both of these conditions must be detected and treated early for successful correction.

Developmental Dysplasia of the Hip

The broad term developmental dysplasia of the hip (DDH) describes a spectrum of disorders related to abnormal development of one or all of the components of the hip joint that

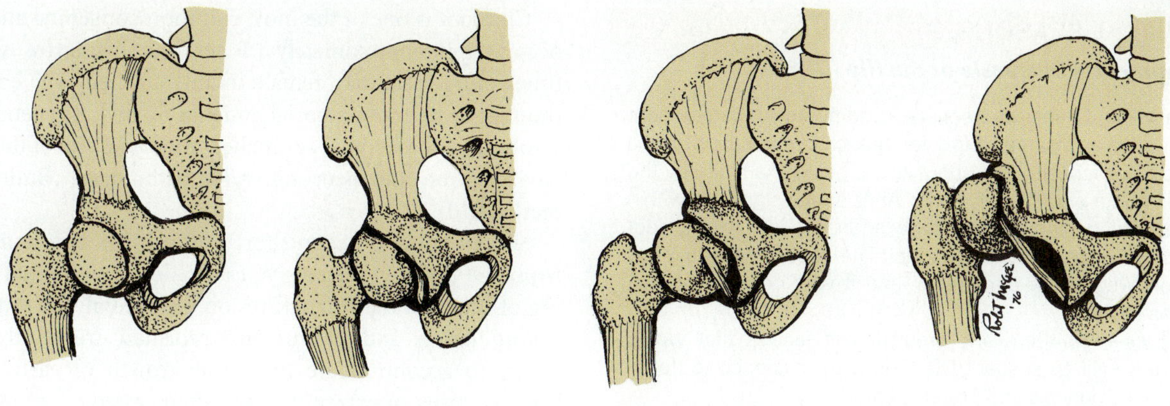

FIG. 36-12 Configuration and relationship of structures in developmental dysplasia of the hip.

can develop at any time during fetal life, infancy, or childhood. A change in terminology from congenital hip dysplasia (CHD) and congenital dislocation of the hip to DDH more properly reflects a variety of hip abnormalities in which there is a shallow acetabulum, subluxation, or dislocation.

The incidence of DDH in the United States is 1.5 per 1000 live births (Butler, 2007). The etiology is unknown, and believed to be multifactorial. Certain factors such as sex, birth order, family history, intrauterine position, birth type, joint laxity, and postnatal positioning are believed to affect the risk of DDH. Predisposing factors associated with DDH can be divided into three broad categories: (1) physiologic factors, which includes maternal hormone secretion and intrauterine positioning; (2) mechanical factors, which involves breech presentation, multiple fetus, oligohydramnios, and large infant size; other mechanical factors may include continued maintenance of the hips in adduction and extension that will in time cause a dislocation; and (3) genetic factors, which entail a higher incidence of DDH in siblings of affected infants, and an even greater incidence of recurrence if a sibling and one parent were affected.

Figure 36-12 illustrates the three degrees of DDH, which are described as follows:

- *Acetabular dysplasia (or preluxation)*—mildest form of DDH in which there is neither subluxation nor dislocation. There is a delay in acetabular development evidenced by osseous hypoplasia of the acetabular roof that is oblique and shallow, although the cartilaginous roof is comparatively intact. The femoral head remains in the acetabulum.
- *Subluxation*—accounts for the largest percentage of DDH. Subluxation implies incomplete dislocation of the hip and is sometimes regarded as an intermediate state in the development from primary dysplasia to complete dislocation. The femoral head remains in contact with the acetabulum, but a stretched capsule and ligamentum teres cause the head of the femur to be partially displaced. Pressure on the cartilaginous roof inhibits ossification and produces a flattened socket.
- *Dislocation*—The femoral head loses contact with the acetabulum and is displaced posteriorly and superiorly over the fibrocartilaginous rim. The ligamentum teres is elongated and taut. DDH is often not detected at the initial examination after birth; thus all infants should be carefully monitored for hip dysplasia at follow-up visits throughout the first year of life. In the newborn period dysplasia usually appears as hip joint laxity rather than as outright dislocation. Subluxation and the tendency to dislocate can be demonstrated by the Ortolani or Barlow tests. The Ortolani and Barlow tests are most reliable from birth to 2 or 3 months of age (see Fig. 23-11). Other signs of DDH are shortening of the limb on the affected side (Galeazzi sign, Allis sign), asymmetric thigh and gluteal folds, and broadening of the perineum (in bilateral dislocation).

! NURSING ALERT

The Ortolani and Barlow tests must be performed by an experienced clinician to prevent fracture or other damage to the hip.

Treatment is begun as soon as the condition is recognized because early intervention is more favorable to the restoration of normal bony architecture and function. The longer treatment is delayed, the more severe the deformity, the more difficult the treatment, and the less favorable the prognosis. The treatment varies with the age of the child and the extent of the dysplasia. The goal of treatment is to obtain and maintain a safe, congruent position of the hip joint to promote normal hip joint development and ambulation.

The hip joint is maintained by dynamic splinting in a safe position with the proximal femur centered in the acetabulum in an attitude of flexion and abduction. Of the numerous devices available, the Pavlik harness is the most widely used, and with time, motion, and gravity, the hip works into a more abducted, reduced position (www.pavlikharness.com). The harness is worn continuously until the hip is proved stable on clinical and radiographic examination, typically around 3 months. It has an 80% success rate for the treatment of classic DDH. If not effective, traction, casting, and even surgery can be necessary to stabilize the hip (Krasser, 2008).

! NURSING ALERT

The former practice of double- or triple-diapering for DDH is not recommended because it promotes hip extension, thus worsening proper hip development.

In addition to the major intervention of assessing and helping identify the disorder, another key nursing intervention is teaching the parents about the care of the infant as he/she

CLINICAL REASONING

Developmental Dysplasia of the Hip (DDH)

Anna, a 4.3-kg Caucasian neonate, is admitted to the newborn nursery after a cesarean birth for breech presentation. Anna appears to be a healthy newborn and is being examined by the pediatric nurse practitioner (PNP). Anna's vital signs are within the normal range and her physical examination is normal except for findings related to her left hip. The assessment findings were followed by an ultrasound, and it was determined that Anna has DDH.

1. Evidence—Are there any predisposing factors that would alert the PNP to suspect DDH? Is there evidence to determine her diagnosis and preferred treatment?
2. Assumptions—What assumptions can be made about the following items?
   a. Physical assessment techniques that will be done to assess for DDH
   b. The immediate plan of care for Anna after a diagnosis of DDH
   c. The ability for Anna's mother to breastfeed her daughter
   d. The effect of having an infant with a congenital disorder
   e. The trajectory of Anna's recovery
3. What implications and priorities for nursing care can be made at this time?
4. Does the evidence objectively support your conclusion?
5. Are there alternative perspectives to your conclusion?

will remain in the harness continuously during the treatment. Because the harness is worn during a time of maximal growth, it is necessary for the parents to adjust the infant's care to accommodate the infant's changing needs. The baby can develop a brachial plexus palsy due to increased tension of the shoulder harness if the harness is not modified according to the neonate's growth. Thorough and ongoing follow-up care is necessary, as is psychosocial support for the family (Butler, 2007).

Clubfoot

Congenital **clubfoot** is a deformity of the foot and ankle that includes forefoot adduction, midfoot supination, hindfoot varus, and ankle equinus. Deformities of the foot and ankle are described according to the position of the ankle and foot. The more common positions involve the following variations:

- *Talipes varus*—An inversion or a bending inward
- *Talipes valgus*—An eversion or bending outward
- *Talipes equinus*—Plantar flexion in which the toes are lower than the heel
- *Talipes calcaneus*—Dorsiflexion, in which the toes are higher than the heel

Most cases of clubfoot are a combination of these positions. The most frequently occurring type is the composite deformity *talipes equinovarus* (TEV). In this abnormality the foot appears C-shaped, pointing downward and inward; the ankle is inverted; and the Achilles tendon is shortened. The foot appears small, wide, and stiff, and the lower leg appears small because of hypoplasia of the calf muscles. Unless treated, further stiffening occurs, and bony changes will result. Unilateral clubfoot is somewhat more common than bilateral clubfoot and can occur as an isolated defect or in association with other disorders or syndromes, such as chromosomal aberrations, arthrogryposis (a generalized immobility of the joint), cerebral palsy, or spina bifida.

Clubfoot is one of the most common congenital anomalies, occurring in approximately 1.5 per 1000 live births, with two times more male than female infants affected. The etiology is thought to be multifactorial and can involve a genetic predisposition, chromosomal anomalies, abnormalities of the uterine environment, and neuromuscular pathologies (Butler, 2007; Sterk, 2010).

Serial casting is begun shortly after birth, before discharge from the nursery. Successive casts allow for gradual stretching of skin and tight structures on the medial side of the foot. Manipulation and casting are repeated frequently (every week) to accommodate the rapid growth of early infancy. The extremity or extremities are often casted or splinted until maximum correction is achieved, usually within 8 to 12 weeks. If needed, surgical correction is done before the infant begins to walk.

Because these infants are often placed in a cast before discharge, the nurse must teach parents necessary care, including how to protect the cast and assess the toes for neurovascular compromise. This is particularly important because of the potential for the infant to outgrow the cast. As is true with the birth of any child with an anomaly, the nurse should be supportive of the parents as they learn the ways to meet the infant's normal needs, as well as those brought about by the infant's physical problem.

Polydactyly

Occasionally an infant is born with extra digits on the hands or feet. In some instances, polydactyly is hereditary. If there is little or no bone involvement, the extra digit is tied with silk suture soon after birth. The finger or toe falls off within a few days, leaving a small scar. When there is bone involvement, surgical repair is indicated.

GENITOURINARY SYSTEM ANOMALIES

Anomalies involving the genitourinary system can be distressing to parents because they can be readily apparent and, in the case of some conditions, because of the concern about sexuality and reproductive functioning. These anomalies range from obvious anomalies of the external genitalia, such as hypospadias, to those involving internal organs that are not obvious but can cause damage to the urinary tract. An example of the latter is an obstruction in the urinary tract that can cause hydronephrosis, which is the abnormal collection of urine in the renal pelvis, that can eventually destroy the kidney.

Hypospadias and Epispadias

Hypospadias constitutes a range of penile anomalies associated with an abnormally located urinary meatus. The meatus can open below the glans penis or anywhere along the ventral surface of the penis, the scrotum, or the perineum. It is the most common anomaly of the penis, affecting approximately 88.7 in 100,000 male infants (Osterman, Martin, & Menacker, 2009). Hypospadias is classified according to the location of the meatus and the presence or absence of chordee, which is a ventral curvature of the penis (Figs. 36-13 and 36-14). The cause is unknown, although it is thought to be of multifactorial inheritance.

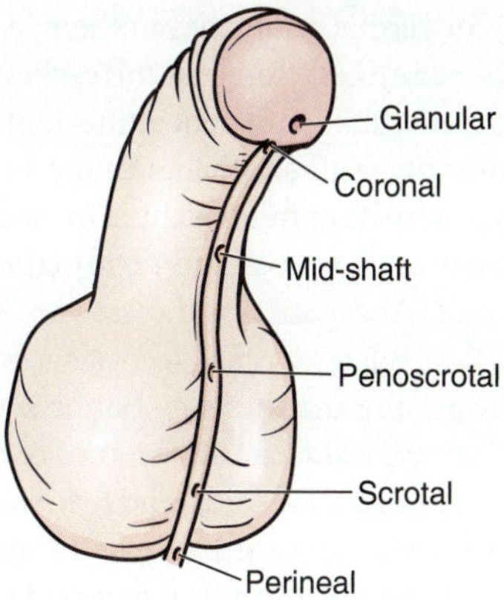

FIG. 36-13 Classification of hypospadias by position of the urethral meatus.

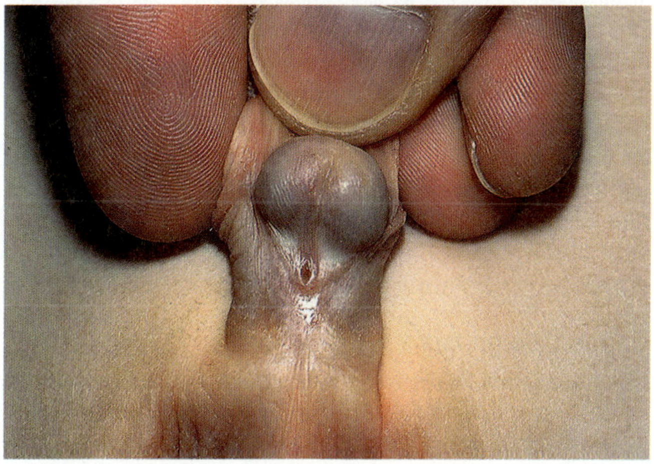

FIG. 36-14 Hypospadias. (Courtesy H. Gil Rushton, MD, Children's National Medical Center, Washington, DC.)

Mild cases of hypospadias are often repaired for cosmetic reasons and involve a single surgical procedure. In more severe cases, several surgeries are required to reconstruct the urethral opening and correct the chordee, thereby straightening the penis. The goals are to improve the appearance of the genitalia, make it possible for the child to urinate in a standing position, and have a sexually adequate organ. These infants are not circumcised because the foreskin can be needed during surgical repair. Repair is done early, between 6 and 12 months of age, so that the child's body image is not impaired (Botwinski, 2010).

Epispadias, a rare anomaly, results from failure of urethral canalization. About half of the affected infants are males who have a widened pubic symphysis and a broad spadelike penis with the urethral opening on the dorsal surface. In females there is a wide urethra and a bifid clitoris. Severity ranges from a mild anomaly to a severe one that is associated with exstrophy of the bladder. Surgical correction is necessary, and affected male infants should not be circumcised.

Exstrophy of the Bladder

The most common bladder anomaly is exstrophy (Fig. 36-15), which often occurs in conjunction with epispadias. It is rare, occurring in approximately 1 in 35,000 to 40,000 live births, and males are affected twice as often as females (Elder, 2007). It results from the abnormal development of the bladder, abdominal wall, and pubic symphysis that causes the bladder,

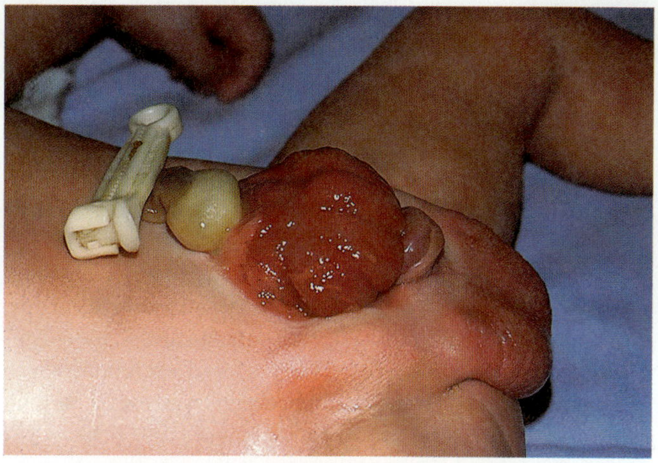

FIG. 36-15 Exstrophy of the bladder. (Courtesy H. Gil Rushton, MD, Children's National Medical Center, Washington, DC.)

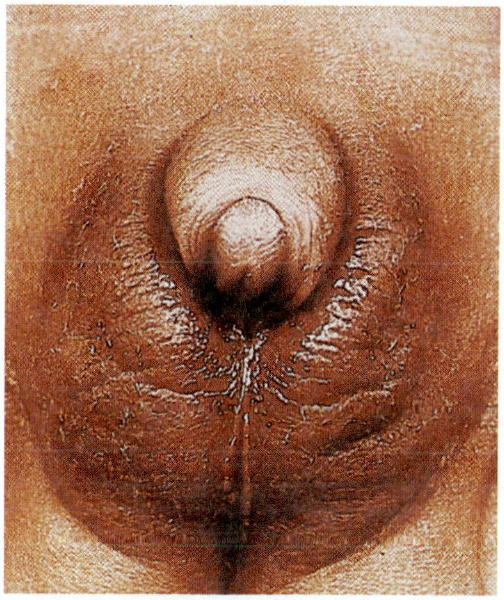

FIG. 36-16 Ambiguous external genitals (i.e., structure can be enlarged clitoral hood and clitoris or malformed penis). (Courtesy Edward S. Tank, MD, Division of Urology, Oregon Health Science University, Portland, OR.)

the urethra, and the ureteral orifices to be exposed. The bladder is visible in the suprapubic area as a red mass with numerous folds, with urine draining from it onto the infant's skin. Immediately after birth the exposed bladder should be covered with a sterile, nonadherent dressing to protect its delicate surface until closure can be performed. It is recommended that reconstructive surgery be started in the neonatal period, such that the bladder is closed within 48 hours. Parents will need detailed instruction along with support and encouragement as they deal with caring for an infant who has such an obvious defect. Repair is completed before school age, if possible, although some children never attain normal voiding patterns and later may be considered for surgery for urinary diversion.

Ambiguous Genitalia

The nurse is often the one to discover ambiguous genitalia in the newborn (Fig. 36-16) during a physical assessment. Erroneous or abnormal sexual differentiation can be a genetic aberration, such as congenital adrenal hypoplasia, which can be life threatening because it involves the deficiency of all adrenal cortical hormones. Other possible causes of sexual ambiguity include chromosomal abnormalities, defective sex hormone synthesis in male infants, and the placental transfer of masculinizing agents to female fetuses. Sex assignment should be based on data gathered from the following sources: maternal and family history, including the ingestion of steroids during pregnancy, and relatives with ambiguous genitalia or who died during the neonatal period; physical examination; chromosomal analysis (results are available in 2 to 3 days); endoscopy, ultrasonography, and radiographic contrast studies; biochemical tests, such as analysis of urinary steroid excretion, which helps detect several of the adrenal cortical syndromes; and, in some instances, laparotomy or gonad biopsy.

Assessment and management of a newborn with ambiguous genitalia requires urgency and sensitivity. Therapeutic intervention, including any counseling and surgery, should be started as soon as possible. Care is best managed by a multidisciplinary team consisting of the primary physician, pediatric endocrinologist, geneticist, surgeon, social worker, and nurses. An infant born with ambiguous genitalia should not receive a sex assignment until diagnostic testing provides enough information for a well-informed decision (Chi, Lee, & Neely, 2008).

An appropriate gender assignment should be based on the following: age at presentation, potential for mature sexual function, potential fertility, and the long-term psychologic and intellectual effect on the child and family. Parents need much support as they learn to deal with this very challenging situation.

CARE MANAGEMENT

Prenatal Diagnosis

Refined testing procedures are available to monitor fetal development. Prenatal diagnostic techniques such as amniocentesis, ultrasonography, alpha-fetoprotein measurements, chorionic villus sampling, PUBS, fetal nuchal translucency (FNT) screening, and gene probes contribute information to the database (see Chapter 26). Although they are a valuable adjunct to prenatal care, these tests cannot identify all congenital disorders. Furthermore, ethical issues surround such testing, and the nurse must be prepared to support the family's decision regarding these tests. If a disorder is detected and the family decides to proceed with the pregnancy, the advantage is that appropriate care can be made available for the infant immediately at birth.

The nurse reviews the maternal history and medical information in the prenatal record for risk factors associated with congenital disorders. These factors include various medical, surgical, and social conditions and their treatments (see Chapter 30); maternal infection (see Chapter 7); maternal endocrine and metabolic disorders (see Chapter 29); and infection and drug dependence in the newborn (see Chapter 35).

Perinatal Diagnosis

Many congenital anomalies require intervention soon after birth. By careful observations in the birth room or nursery, the nurse can identify most of these conditions. An excessive amount of amniotic fluid, **polyhydramnios,** is commonly associated with congenital anomalies in the newborn, and such infants should be examined closely at the earliest possible time.

Oligohydramnios, an insufficient amount of amniotic fluid, is associated primarily with anomalies of the urinary tract that prevent normal micturition in utero. It is most often associated with renal agenesis or dysplasia and obstructive lesions in the lower urinary tract. Anomalies of the ears are associated with renal abnormalities. Bilateral renal agenesis, resulting in oligohydramnios, commonly manifests as Potter syndrome, which is characterized by atypical facial appearance consisting of a flat nose, recessed chin, epicanthal folds, and low-set abnormal ears; limb abnormalities; pulmonary hypoplasia; and fetal growth restriction. These conditions can be diagnosed prenatally.

Postnatal Diagnosis

Apgar scoring and a brief assessment are completed for all neonates after birth. Any deviations from normal are reported to the primary health care provider immediately. A thorough assessment of all body systems follows to identify anomalies and determine the best management plan for the neonate and the family.

Some infants have multiple congenital anomalies. A recognized pattern of malformations is referred to as a *syndrome.* The most common is Down syndrome, affecting about 14 of every 10,000 births (CDC, 2006) (Fig. 36-17), with the diagnosis confirmed early in the neonatal period.

Genetic Diagnosis

Diagnostic procedures for the detection of genetic disorders are performed after birth at any time from the postnatal period through adulthood. Many tests exist for various disorders; only the most frequently used tests are discussed here.

Newborn Screening

The most widespread use of postnatal testing for genetic disease is the routine screening of newborns for inborn errors of metabolism such as phenylketonuria (PKU), galactosemia, hemoglobinopathy (sickle cell disease and thalassemias), and hypothyroidism; these are the minimum mandatory newborn screening tests in most states in the United States. Newborn screening testing in Canada varies by province.

An **inborn error of metabolism (IEM)** is the term applied to a large group of disorders caused by a metabolic defect that results from the absence of or change in a protein, usually an enzyme, and mediated by the action of a certain gene. These defects can involve any substrate produced from protein, carbohydrate, or fat metabolism. Inborn errors of metabolism are recessive disorders, so a person must receive a defective gene from each parent. The parents usually are unaffected because their normal dominant gene directs the synthesis of sufficient protein to meet their metabolic needs under normal circumstances.

With the advent of new biochemical techniques, it is possible to detect the abnormal gene responsible for causing an increasing number of these disorders early in the neonatal period so appropriate therapies to prevent further morbidity can be implemented. Deoxyribonucleic acid (DNA) sequencing along with mutational analysis, molecular diagnosis, and enzyme assays can be used to identify carriers, confirm the diagnosis, and play a role in genetic counseling with the family (Schiefelbein & Cheeseman, 2009; Sterk, 2010).

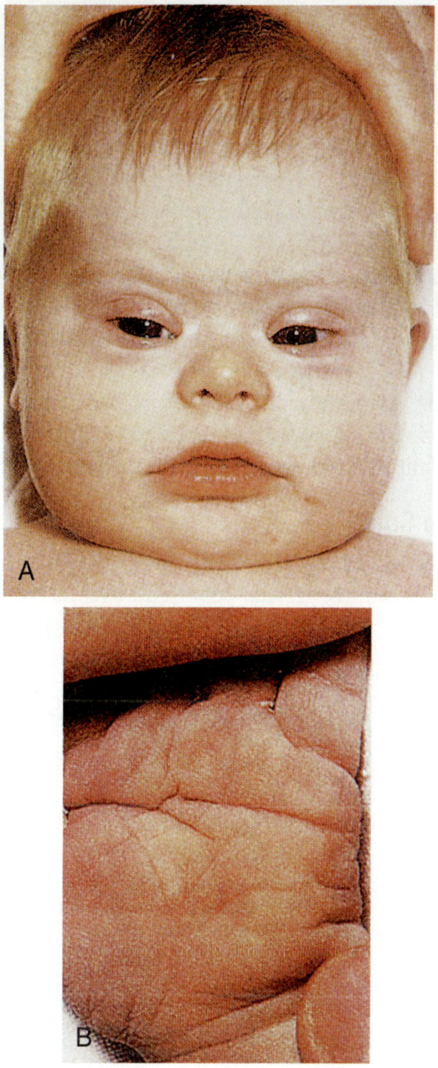

FIG. 36-17 **A,** Clinical features of Down syndrome. **B,** Simian crease. (From Zitelli, B., & Davis, H. [1997]. *Atlas of pediatric physical diagnosis* [3rd ed.]. St. Louis: Mosby.)

Phenylketonuria is an amino acid disorder that results from a deficiency of the enzyme phenylalanine dehydrogenase (see Chapter 3). This deficiency can cause elevated levels of phenylalanine that result in CNS damage. Severe effects of PKU are rare because of early recognition through newborn screening (Blackburn, 2007). The test for PKU is not reliable, however, until the newborn has ingested adequate amounts of breast milk or formula.

! NURSING ALERT

The nurse must document the initial ingestion of milk and perform the test for PKU at least 24 hours after that time.

If the infant has PKU, treatment includes a diet low in protein plus the addition of a special amino acid–containing formula that does not contain phenylalanine. Despite compliance with treatment, many affected children have some intellectual impairment. Successful management and outcome are largely dependent on early identification of the condition, modifying the diet, and compliance with the treatment regimen throughout the entire life (Sterk, 2010).

Galactosemia, caused by a deficiency of the enzyme galactose 1-phosphate uridyl transferase, results in the inability to convert galactose to glucose. Galactosemia can be detected by measuring the blood levels of galactose in the urine of newborns suspected of having the disease who have ingested formula containing galactose. Early symptoms are vomiting, weight loss, persistent jaundice, and CNS symptoms, including poor feeding, drowsiness, and seizures. *Escherichia coli* sepsis occurs in a large number of affected infants. If the disorder goes untreated, the galactose levels will continue to increase, and the affected infant will show failure to thrive, developmental delay, cataracts, jaundice, hepatomegaly, and cirrhosis of the liver, with death possibly occurring in the first month of life. Therapy consists of eliminating galactose from the diet and beginning a lactose-free diet. The condition precludes breastfeeding because lactose is present in breast milk (Sterk, 2010).

Congenital hypothyroidism results from a deficiency of thyroid hormones, and can be permanent (requires treatment for life) or transient (spontaneously resolves). All states in the United States routinely screen for hypothyroidism by measuring thyroxine (T_4) in a drop of blood obtained from a heelstick at 2 to 5 days of age. At this time the normally expected increase in T_4 is lacking in newborns with hypothyroidism. It is more often included as part of the newborn screen done in the first 24 to 48 hours or before discharge. Neonatal screening consists of an initial filter-paper blood-spot thyroxine (T_4) measurement followed by measurement of thyroid-stimulating hormone (TSH) in specimens with low T_4 values. Early screening can have false-positive results. Treatment is thyroid replacement. In the newborn, the results of thyroid function studies are elevated in comparison with values in older children; therefore, it is important to document the timing of the tests. In preterm and sick full-term infants, thyroid function levels are usually lower than in the healthy full-term infant. A repeat T_4 and TSH can be elevated after 30 weeks (corrected age) in newborns born before that time and after resolution of the acute illness in the sick full-term infant.

If the baby is untreated, symptoms usually appear after 6 weeks and include bradycardia; hypothermia; hypotension; hyporeflexia; abdominal distention; umbilical hernia; coarse, dry hair; thick, dry skin that feels cold; anemia; widely patent cranial sutures; and retarded bone age beginning at birth. The most disabling problem, however, is delayed development of the nervous system, leading to severe developmental delay. Once identified, treatment is started immediately using synthetic T_4 (L-thyroxine) as a thyroid replacement (Sterk, 2010).

Cytogenetic Studies

Abnormalities can occur in either the autosomes or the sex chromosomes. Chromosomal disorders often can be diagnosed on the basis of the clinical manifestations alone. However, an infant may have a clinical appearance that is only suggestive of a problem. Cytogenetic studies must be done to confirm or rule out a suspected diagnosis. Newer techniques in molecular cytogenetic analysis make possible a more precise identification of risk for having a fetus affected with a genetic defect such as phenylketonuria.

Disorders in the number or structure of chromosomes can be diagnosed by a *karyotype* (see Fig. 3-1). A karyotype is a photographic enlargement of the chromosomes arranged by their numbered pairs.

Abnormalities of the sex chromosomes make up about half of all the chromosomal abnormalities occurring in the newborn. The most common test for sex chromosome abnormalities is the buccal smear, using cells scraped from the mucosa inside the mouth. When prepared and stained, these show the number of inactive X chromosomes, also known as an *X-chromatin mass* or a *Barr body*. Each cell, whether male or female, has one genetically active X chromosome. Therefore, a normal female has one active X chromosome and one Barr body, which is on the inactive X chromosome. A normal male has no Barr bodies because he has only one genetically active X chromosome.

Dermatoglyphics

Dermatoglyphics is the study of the patterns formed by the ridges in the skin on the digits, palms, and soles. These patterns, formed early in development, are strongly correlated with the effects of chromosomes. The addition or deletion of genetic material produces alterations in the loops, swirls, and arches of the finger and toe prints, in the palm lines, and in the flexion creases on the palms of the hands and soles of the feet. Characteristic dermatoglyphic patterns have been noted for almost all the chromosomal abnormalities, including trisomies 13, 18, and 21.

An infant with Down syndrome (trisomy 21) can have a single palmar crease (Fig. 36-17), a single flexion crease of the fifth digit, and an open-field pattern on the ball of the foot (Matthews & Robin, 2011). The characteristic dermatoglyphic feature in a child with Turner syndrome is the large size of the dermal patterns on the fingers and toes. Certain fingerprint patterns also may be found in those people who have cardiac valvular problems later in life. Asymmetry of palmar ridges has been reported in congenital anomalies such as cleft lip and palate and congenital vertebral anomaly.

Newborn Care

A collaborative health team approach that includes specialists and community service representatives is needed in the care of infants with some disorders. Surgical intervention in

NURSING PROCESS

The Newborn with a Congenital Anomaly

ASSESSMENT

Newborn

The initial physical examination of the newborn (see Chapter 24) can reveal obvious congenital anomalies, although some anomalies are not evident until the infant is a few hours or days old. Ongoing assessment is important to identify the presence of anomalies.

Parents

The nurse assesses parental responses to a neonate with a congenital anomaly as well as their understanding of the anomaly and its implications for short- and long-term outcomes. It is also important to assess their willingness to participate in infant care. Family responses are also assessed.

NURSING DIAGNOSES

Nursing diagnoses for the newborn and the parents can include:

Newborn

Risk for Injury **related to:**
- presence of a congenital disorder

Risk for Infection **related to:**
- anomaly or its treatment

Impaired Gas Exchange **related to:**
- effects of congenital anomaly

Imbalanced Nutrition: Less than Body Requirements **related to:**
- effects of congenital anomaly

Delayed Growth and Development **related to:**
- inborn error of metabolism

Parents and Family

Grieving or Spiritual Distress **related to:**
- birth of a child with a defect

Compromised Family Coping **related to:**
- birth of a child with a defect

Deficient Knowledge **related to:**
- cause of the anomaly, its management, alternative courses of action, community resources, prognosis, and the care needed by the child after discharge

Anxiety **related to:**
- uncertainty regarding prognosis or ability to care for child

Risk for Impaired Parenting **related to:**
- birth of a child with a disorder or defect

EXPECTED OUTCOMES OF CARE

Expected outcomes can apply to the infant and to the parents and family. Expected outcomes for the infant include that he or she will:
- Maintain adequate physiologic functioning (airway, breathing, circulation).
- Remain free of infection.
- Receive adequate nutrition for growth.
- Grow and develop as normally as possible.

Expected outcomes for the parents and family include that they will:
- Demonstrate normal grief responses.
- Perceive the infant as a family member.
- Verbalize understanding of the anomaly, management, alternative courses of action, community resources, prognosis, and care needed after hospital discharge.
- Demonstrate ability to focus on new knowledge and skills needed to care for infant.
- Communicate feelings of anxiety.

PLAN OF CARE AND INTERVENTIONS

- Maintain a safe environment.
- Maintain Standard Precautions and use careful hand hygiene.
- Monitor for signs of infection.
- Maintain nutritional status.
- Provide support and information for parents.

Numerous other interventions are discussed in relation to specific anomalies.

EVALUATION

The nurse can be reasonably sure that care was effective to the extent that the expected outcomes for care have been achieved.

the neonatal period can be necessary for the infant requiring either immediate correction or a palliative procedure to relieve the symptoms of the anomaly until definitive correction can be done. There is a higher morbidity and mortality rate in neonates than in older children or adults undergoing similar procedures. However, despite these problems unique to neonates, advances in surgical techniques, anesthesia, and the nursing care given in intensive care nurseries have been responsible for decreasing the risk of surgery in neonates.

The health care team must be highly skilled to meet the needs of these high risk infants. In addition to stabilization of the infant's condition (oxygenation and perfusion of tissues), other preoperative interventions, such as orogastric tube placement for abdominal decompression, attention to thermoregulation and pain management, and the maintenance of fluid and electrolyte balance, are implemented to manage specific problems.

Parents and Family Support

While the infant is receiving optimal care, the parents have needs that must be met as they deal with the crisis of having an infant with an abnormal condition. The nurse carefully assesses their reactions, which are likely to be those typical of a grief response. Facilitating their understanding of the information given them about their infant's condition is a vital nursing intervention. A newly diagnosed disorder often implies the need for the implementation of a therapeutic regimen. For example, the disorder may be an inborn error of metabolism, such as PKU, which requires consistent and rigid adherence to a diet. The family may need help with securing the required formula and receiving counseling from the clinical dietitian. The nurse stresses the importance of maintaining the diet, keeping an adequate supply of special preparations, and avoiding the use of unauthorized substitutions.

Referral to appropriate agencies is another essential component of the follow-up management, and the nurse should make the parents aware of all possible sources of aid, including pertinent literature, parent groups, and national organizations. Many organizations and foundations, such as the Cystic Fibrosis Foundation and the Muscular Dystrophy Association, provide services and counseling for families of affected children. There are also numerous parent groups the family can join. There they can share experiences and receive mutual support in coping with problems similar to those of other group members. Nurses should be familiar with the services available in their community that provide assistance and education to families with these special problems.

A major nursing function is providing emotional support to the family during all aspects of the care of the infant born with a defect or disorder. The feelings stemming from the real or imagined threat posed by a congenital anomaly are as varied as the people being counseled. Responses may include apathy, denial, anger, hostility, fear, embarrassment, grief, and loss of self-esteem (see Chapter 38).

Parents benefit from seeing before-and-after pictures of other babies born with the same defect. Coupled with other verbal and nonverbal supportive care, this visual reassurance may be effective in allaying their concerns.

Families need much information, guidance, and support as they make decisions regarding the care of their infants. Once they have been given the facts and possible consequences and all the assistance they need in problem solving, the final decision regarding a course of action must be their own. It is then incumbent on health care providers to support the family's decision.

Nurses frequently encounter children with genetic diseases and families in which there is a risk that a disorder can be transmitted to or occur in an offspring. It is a responsibility of nurses to be alert to situations in which persons could benefit from a genetic evaluation and counseling, to be aware of the local genetic resources, to aid the family in finding services, and to offer support and care for children and families affected by genetic conditions. Local genetic clinics can be located through several sites, such as GeneTests (www.genetests.org), a publicly funded medical genetics information resource developed for physicians and other health care providers, which is available at no cost to all interested persons. Another resource is the National Society of Genetic Counselors (www.nsgc.org), which lists genetic counselors by states in the United States.

COMMUNITY ACTIVITY

- Visit the American Pregnancy Association website (www.americanpregnancy.org) and go to the birth defects and disorders link. Select a birth defect such as cleft lip and palate, congenital heart defects, or spina bifida. Review the information regarding neonatal effects, risk factors, diagnosis and resources. At the resources link, visit the website of the national organization. Locate a clinic that specializes in the care and treatment of the birth defect in your community.
- Visit the American Academy of Pediatrics website (www.aap.org). Go to the health topics link and search for jaundice. Review the questions and answers about jaundice for parents and the *management of hyperbilirubinemia in the newborn infant 35 or more weeks of gestation clinical practice guideline for health care providers.*

KEY POINTS

- Hyperbilirubinemia is caused by a variety of factors, including maternal-fetal Rh and ABO incompatibility.
- Erythroblastosis fetalis leads to anemia, edema, and the cytotoxic effects of unconjugated bilirubin.
- The injection of Rh_0(D) immunoglobulin in Rh-negative and Coombs' test–negative women provides passive immunity and minimizes the possibility of isoimmunization.
- Neonatal exchange transfusion with type O, Rh-negative RBCs serves to treat anemia and acidosis and to remove bilirubin, maternal antibodies, and fetal RBCs that are beginning to hemolyze.
- Major congenital defects are the leading cause of death in term neonates.
- The most common major congenital anomalies that cause serious problems in the neonate are congenital heart disease, neural tube defects, cleft lip or palate, and developmental dysplasia of the hip.
- Minor anomalies can be part of a characteristic pattern of malformations.
- Current technology permits the prenatal diagnosis of many congenital anomalies and disorders.
- The most widespread use of postnatal testing for genetic disease is the routine screening of newborns for inborn errors of metabolism.
- The curative and rehabilitative problems of an infant with a congenital disorder are often complex and require a multidisciplinary approach to care.
- Parents often need special instruction (e.g., meeting nutrition requirements, cast care, or home phototherapy) before they take a high risk infant home.
- The supportive care given to the parents of infants with an abnormal condition must begin at birth, or at the time of diagnosis and continue for years.

Audio Chapter Summaries Access an audio summary of these Key Points on Evolve

REFERENCES

American Academy of Pediatrics (AAP) Subcommittee on Hyperbilirubinemia. (2004). Management of hyperbilirubinemia in the newborn infant 35 or more weeks of gestation. *Pediatrics, 114*(1), 297–316.

Askin, D., & Diehl-Jones, W. (2010). Assisted ventilation. In M. Verklan & M. Walden (Eds.), *AWHONN core curriculum for neonatal intensive care nursing* (4th ed.). Philadelphia: Saunders.

Association of Women's Health, Obstetric and Neonatal Nurses (AWHONN). (2005). *Hyperbilirubinemia in the neonate: Risk assessment, screening, and management.* Washington, DC: AWHONN.

Bay, C., Steele, M., & Davis, H. (2007). Genetic disorders and dysmorphic conditions. In B. Zitelli & H. Davis (Eds.), *Atlas of pediatric physical diagnosis* (5th ed.). St. Louis: Mosby.

Bernstein, D. (2007). Congenital heart disease. In R. Kliegman, R. Behrman, H. Jenson, & B. Stanton (Eds.), *Nelson textbook of pediatrics* (18th ed.). Philadelphia: Saunders.

Bianco-Batlles, H., Mohamed, M., & Hammad, T. (2010). Mortality in infants with congenital diaphragmatic hernia: A study of the United States National Database. *Journal of Perinatology, 30*(8), 553–557.

Blackburn, S. (2007). *Maternal, fetal, and neonatal physiology: A clinical perspective* (3rd ed.). St. Louis: Saunders.

Botwinski, C. (2010). Renal and genitourinary disorders. In M. Verklan & M. Walden (Eds.), *AWHONN core curriculum for neonatal intensive care nursing* (4th ed.). Philadelphia: Saunders.

Bradshaw, W. (2010). Gastrointestinal disorders. In M. Verklan & M. Walden (Eds.), *AWHONN core curriculum for neonatal intensive care nursing* (4th ed.). Philadelphia: Saunders.

Brownlee, E., Howatson, A., Davis, C., & Sabharwal, A. (2009). The hidden mortality of congenital diaphragmatic hernia: A 20 year review. *Journal of Pediatric Surgery, 44*(2), 317–320.

Butler, J. (2007). Musculoskeletal system. In C. Kenner & J. Lott (Eds.), *Comprehensive neonatal care: An interdisciplinary approach* (4th ed.). St. Louis: Saunders.

Centers for Disease Control and Prevention (CDC). (2006). Improved national prevalence for 18 selected major birth defects—United States, 1999-2001. *MMWR Morbidity and Mortality Weekly Report, 54*(51, 52), 1301–1305.

Chi, C., Lee, H., & Neely, E. (2008). Ambiguous genitalia in the newborn. *NeoReviews, 9*(2), e78–e84.

Cunningham, F., Leveno, K., Bloom, S., Hauth, J., Rouse, D., & Spong, C. (2010). *Williams obstetrics* (23rd ed.). New York: McGraw-Hill.

Diehl-Jones, W., & Askin, D. (2010). Hematologic disorders. In M. Verklan & M. Walden (Eds.), *AWHONN core curriculum for neonatal intensive care nursing* (4th ed.). Philadelphia: Saunders.

Elder, J. (2007). Anomalies of the bladder. In R. Kliegman, R. Behrman, H. Jenson, & B. Stanton (Eds.), *Nelson textbook of pediatrics* (18th ed.). Philadelphia: Saunders.

Gilboa, S., Correa, A., Botto, L., Rasmussen, S., Waller, D., Hobbs, C., et al. (2010). Association between prepregnancy body mass index and congenital heart defects. *American Journal of Obstetrics and Gynecology, 202*(10), 51, e1–e10.

Gruslin, A., & Moore, T. (2006). Erythroblastosis fetalis. In R. Martin, A. Fanaroff, & M. Walsh (Eds.), *Fanaroff and Martin's neonatal-perinatal medicine: Diseases of the fetus and infant* (8th ed.). Philadelphia: Mosby.

Hartas, G., Tsounias, E., & Gupta-Malhotra, M. (2009). Approach to diagnosing congenital cardiac disorders. *Critical Care Nursing Clinics of North America, 21*(2), 27–36.

Heron, M., Sutton, P., Xu, J., Ventura, S., Strobino, D., & Guyer, B. (2010). Annual summary of vital statistics: 2007. *Pediatrics, 125*(1), 4–15.

Hirose, S., & Farmer, D. (2009). Fetal surgery for myelomeningocele. *Clinics in Perinatology, 36*(2), 431–438.

Holder, A., Klaassens, M., Tibboel, D., de Klein, A., Lee, B., & Scott, D. (2007). Genetic factors in congenital diaphragmatic hernia. *American Journal of Human Genetics, 80*(5), 825–845.

Hudgins, L., & Cassidy, S. (2006). Congenital anomalies. In R. Martin, A. Fanaroff, & M. Walsh (Eds.), *Fanaroff and Martin's neonatal-perinatal medicine: Diseases of the fetus and infant* (8th ed.). Philadelphia: Mosby.

Krasser, J. (2008). Orthopaedic problems. In J. Cloherty, E. Eichenwald, & A. Stark (Eds.), *Manual of neonatal care* (6th ed.). Philadelphia: Wolters Kluwer.

Lovvorn, H., Glenn, J., Pacetti, A., & Carter, B. (2011). Neonatal surgery. In S. Gardner, B. Carter, M. Enzman-Hines, & J. Hernandez (Eds.), *Merenstein & Gardner's handbook of neonatal intensive care* (7th ed.). St. Louis: Mosby.

Lynam, L., & Verklan, M. (2010). Neurologic disorders. In M. Verklan & M. Walden (Eds.), *Core curriculum for neonatal intensive care nursing* (4th ed.). Philadelphia: Saunders.

Magnuson, D., Parry, R., & Chwals, W. (2006). Selected abdominal gastrointestinal anomalies. In R. Martin, A. Fanaroff, & M. Walsh (Eds.), *Fanaroff and Martin's neonatal-perinatal medicine: Diseases of the fetus and infant* (8th ed.). Philadelphia: Mosby.

Malik, S., Cleves, M., Honein, M., Romitti, P., Botto, L., Yang, S., et al. (2008). Maternal smoking and congenital heart defects. *Pediatrics, 121*(4), e810–e816.

Manning, F. (2009). Imaging in the diagnosis of fetal anomalies. In R. Creasy, R. Resnik, J. Iams, C. Lockwood, & T. Moore (Eds.), *Creasy & Resnik's maternal-fetal medicine: Principles and practice* (6th ed.). Philadelphia: Saunders.

Martin, C., & Cloherty, J. (2008). Neonatal hyperbilirubinemia. In J. Cloherty, E. Eichenwald, & A. Stark (Eds.), *Manual of neonatal care* (6th ed.). Philadelphia: Wolters Kluwer.

Mathews, T. (2008). *Trends in spina bifida and anencephalus in the United States, 1991-2006.* Hyattsville, MD: U.S. Department of Health and Human Services, Centers for Disease Control and Prevention, National Center for Health Statistics. Available at http://www.cdc.gov/nchs/data/hestat/spine_anen/spine_anen.htm. Accessed August 6, 2010.

Matthews, A., & Robin, N. (2011). Genetic disorders, malformations, and inborn errors of metabolism. In S. Gardner, B. Carter, M. Enzman-Hines, & J. Hernandez (Eds.), *Merenstein & Gardner's handbook of neonatal intensive care* (7th ed.). St. Louis: Mosby.

Migliazza, L., Bellan, C., Alberti, D., Auriemma, A., Burgio, G., Locatelli, G., & Colombo, A. (2007). Retrospective study of 111 cases of congenital diaphragmatic hernia treated with early high-frequency oscillatory ventilation and presurgical stabilization. *Journal of Pediatric Surgery, 42*(9), 1526–1532.

Moise, K. (2010). Hemolytic disease of the fetus and newborn. In R. Creasy, R. Resnik, J. Iams, C. Lockwood, & T. Moore (Eds.), *Creasy & Resnik's maternal-fetal medicine: Principles and practice* (6th ed.). Philadelphia: Saunders.

Moore, K., & Persaud, T. (2007). Congenital anatomical anomalies or birth defects. In K. Moore & T. Persaud (Eds.), *The developing human: Clinically oriented embryology* (8th ed.). Philadelphia: Saunders.

National Institute of Child Health and Human Development. (1985). Randomized, controlled trial of phototherapy for neonatal hyperbilirubinemia: Executive summary. *Pediatrics, 75*(2), 385–386.

Osterman, M., Martin, J., & Menacker, F. (2009). Expanded health data from the new birth certificate, 2006. *National Vital Statistics Reports, 58*(5), 1–24.

Pappas, B., & Walker, B. (2010). Neonatal delivery room resuscitation. In M. Verklan & M. Walden (Eds.), *AWHONN core curriculum for neonatal intensive care nursing* (4th ed.). Philadelphia: Saunders.

Park, M. (2008). *Pediatric cardiology for practitioners* (5th ed.). St. Louis: Mosby.

Reller, M., Strickland, M., Riehle-Colarusso, T., Mahle, W., & Correa, A. (2009). Prevalence of congenital heart defects in metropolitan Atlanta, 1998-2005. *Obstetrical and Gynecological Survey, 64*(3), 156–157.

Ringer, S., & Hansen, A. (2008). Surgical emergencies in the newborn. In J. Cloherty, E. Eichenwald, & A. Stark (Eds.), *Manual of neonatal care* (6th ed.). Philadelphia: Wolters Kluwer.

Sadowski, S. (2010). Cardiovascular disorders. In M. Verklan & M. Walden (Eds.), *AWHONN core curriculum for neonatal intensive care nursing* (4th ed.). Philadelphia: Saunders.

Schiefelbein, J., & Cheeseman, S. (2009). Principles of genetics and their clinical application in the neonatal intensive care unit. *Critical Care Nursing Clinics of North America, 21*(1), 67–85.

Sterk, L. (2010). Congenital anomalies. In M. Verklan & M. Walden (Eds.), *AWHONN core curriculum for neonatal intensive care nursing* (4th ed.). Philadelphia: Saunders.

Stoll, B. (2007). Blood disorders. In R. Kliegman, R. Behrman, H. Jenson, & B. Stanton (Eds.), *Nelson textbook of pediatrics* (18th ed.). Philadelphia: Saunders.

Thigpen, J. (2007). Gastrointestinal system. In C. Kenner & J. Lott (Eds.), *Comprehensive neonatal care. An interdisciplinary approach* (4th ed.). St. Louis: Saunders.

Tsao, K., & Lally, K. (2008). The Congenital Diaphragmatic Hernia Study Group: A voluntary international registry. *Seminars in Pediatric Surgery, 17*(2), 90–97.

Volpe, J. (2008). *Neurology of the newborn* (5th ed.). Philadelphia: Saunders.

Waller, D., Shaw, G., Rasmussen, S., Hobbs, C., Canfield, M., Siega-Riz, A., et al. (2007). Prepregnancy obesity as a risk factor for structural birth defects. *Archives of Pediatric and Adolescent Medicine, 161*(8), 745–750.

Watson, R. (2009). Hyperbilirubinemia. *Critical Care Nursing Clinics of North America, 21*(1), 97–120.

Wilkins, I. (2010). Nonimmune hydrops. In R. Creasy, R. Resnik, J. Iams, C. Lockwood, & T. Moore (Eds.), *Creasy & Resnik's maternal-fetal medicine: Principles and practice* (6th ed.). Philadelphia: Saunders.

Wong, R., DeSandre, G., Sibley, E., & Stevenson, D. (2006). Neonatal jaundice and liver disease. In R. Martin, A. Fanaroff, & M. Walsh (Eds.), *Fanaroff and Martin's neonatal-perinatal medicine: Diseases of the fetus and infant* (8th ed.). Philadelphia: Mosby.

Zupancic, J. (2008). Neural tube defects. In J. Cloherty, E. Eichenwald, & A. Stark (Eds.), *Manual of neonatal care* (6th ed.). Philadelphia: Wolters Kluwer.

CHAPTER

37

Nursing Care of the High Risk Newborn

Carole Kenner and Susan Ellerbee

evolve WEBSITE

http://evolve.elsevier.com/Lowdermilk/MWHC/

Audio Glossary
Audio Key Points
Case Study — The Newborn at Risk
Critical Thinking Exercise
  Patent Ductus Arteriosus
NCLEX Review Questions
Nursing Care Plan
  The High Risk Preterm Newborn
Spanish Guidelines
  Intensive Care Nursery: Parent Teaching on First Visit
Video—Nursing Skills
  Performing Gavage Feeding

LEARNING OBJECTIVES

- Analyze differences in characteristics of preterm, late preterm, term, and postterm neonates.
- Discuss respiratory distress syndrome and the approach to treatment.
- Compare methods of oxygen therapy.
- Analyze the appropriate nursing interventions for nutritional care of the preterm infant.
- Discuss the pathophysiology of retinopathy of prematurity and bronchopulmonary dysplasia (BPD) and the risk factors that predispose preterm infants to these problems.
- Discuss pain assessment and management in the preterm infant.
- Describe the signs and symptoms of perinatal asphyxia.
- Analyze the pathophysiology of meconium aspiration syndrome and its clinical signs.
- Plan developmentally appropriate care for high risk infants.
- Discuss the needs of parents of high risk infants.
- Evaluate a neonatal transport plan.
- Explain appropriate responses and interventions the nurse can use in caring for families of preterm and high risk infants experiencing anticipatory grief or loss and grief in the neonatal period.
- Describe nursing care for late preterm infants admitted to mother-baby units.
- List specific discharge teaching needs for parents of late preterm infants admitted to mother-baby units.

Modern technology and expert nursing care have made important contributions to improving the health and overall survival of high risk infants. However, infants who are born considerably before term and survive are particularly susceptible to the development of problems related to their preterm birth. These problems are not limited to preterm infants. They can also occur in term and late preterm infants, although not so frequently, and include necrotizing enterocolitis, bronchopulmonary dysplasia (BPD), intraventricular and periventricular hemorrhage, and retinopathy of prematurity (ROP).

High risk infants are most often classified according to birth weight, gestational age, and predominant pathophysiologic problems (Box 37-1). Intrauterine growth rates differ among infants; factors such as heredity, placental insufficiency, and maternal disease influence intrauterine growth and birth weight. The classification system in the box encompasses birth weight and gestational age.

For the high risk infant, an accurate assessment of gestational age (see Chapter 24) is critical in helping the nurse identify the potential problems the newborn is likely to have. The response of the preterm, late preterm, or postterm infant to extrauterine life differs from that of the term infant. By understanding the physiologic basis of these differences, the nurse can assess these infants, determine the response of the preterm or postterm infant, and discern which problems are most likely to occur.

PRETERM INFANTS

The vast majority of high risk infants are those born at less than 37 weeks of gestation. This includes preterm and late preterm births. The preterm birth rate in the United States showed a

BOX 37-1 CLASSIFICATION OF HIGH RISK INFANTS

CLASSIFICATION ACCORDING TO SIZE

- *Low birth weight (LBW) infant:* an infant whose birth weight is less than 2500 g, regardless of gestational age
- *Very low birth weight (VLBW) infant:* an infant whose birth weight is less than 1500 g
- *Extremely low birth weight (ELBW) infant:* an infant whose birth weight is less than 1000 g
- *Appropriate for gestational age (AGA) infant:* an infant whose birth weight falls between the 10th and 90th percentiles on intrauterine growth curves
- *Small for date (SFD) or small for gestational age (SGA) infant:* an infant whose rate of intrauterine growth was restricted and whose birth weight falls below the 10th percentile on intrauterine growth curves
- *Large for gestational age (LGA) infant:* an infant whose birth weight falls above the 90th percentile on intrauterine growth charts
- *Intrauterine growth restriction (IUGR):* found in infants whose intrauterine growth is restricted (sometimes used as a more descriptive term for the SGA infant)
- *Symmetric IUGR:* growth restriction in which the weight, length, and head circumference are all affected
- *Asymmetric IUGR:* growth restriction in which the head circumference remains within normal parameters while the birth weight falls below the 10th percentile

CLASSIFICATION ACCORDING TO GESTATIONAL AGE

- *Premature (preterm) infant:* an infant born before completion of 37 weeks of gestation, regardless of birth weight
- *Late preterm infant:* an infant born between 34 0/7 and 36 6/7 weeks of gestation, regardless of birth weight
- *Full-term infant:* an infant born between the beginning of 38 weeks and the completion of 42 weeks of gestation, regardless of birth weight
- *Postmature (postterm) infant:* an infant born after 42 weeks of gestational age, regardless of birth weight

CLASSIFICATION ACCORDING TO MORTALITY

- *Live birth:* birth in which the neonate manifests any heartbeat, breathes, or displays voluntary movement, regardless of gestational age
- *Fetal death:* death of the fetus after 20 weeks of gestation and before birth, with absence of any signs of life after birth
- *Neonatal death:* death that occurs in the first 27 days of life; early neonatal death occurs in the first week of life and late neonatal death occurs at 7 to 27 days
- *Perinatal mortality:* total number of fetal and early neonatal deaths per 1000 live births

fairly steady increase from the early 1980s to 2006. Then, in 2006, the rate declined to 12.3% from 12.8%. The decrease occurred for all types of births, including cesareans, and induced and noninduced vaginal births (Martin, Osterman, & Sutton, 2010). What caused this decline and whether or not it will continue are subjects for ongoing research.

At times the nurse is able to anticipate problems, such as when a woman is admitted in preterm labor. At other times the birth of a high risk infant is unanticipated. In either case the personnel and equipment necessary for immediate care of the infant must be available.

Preterm infants are at risk because their organ systems are immature and they lack adequate reserves of bodily nutrients. The potential problems and care needs of the preterm infant weighing 2000 g differ from those of the term, postterm, or postmature infant of equal weight. If these infants have physiologic disorders and anomalies as well, they affect the infant's response to treatment. In general, the closer infants are to term from the standpoint of both gestational age and birth weight, the easier their adjustment to the external environment.

Preterm, low birth weight (LBW), and extremely low birth weight infants often require hospitalization beyond the typical 48 hours after birth. Their physiologic immaturity and associated problems can involve extensive use of technologic and pharmacologic interventions. The cost of the care required by preterm and LBW infants is estimated to be in the billions of dollars each year and continues to rise as the use of technology increases.

Varying opinions exist about the practical and ethical dimensions of resuscitation of **extremely low birth weight (ELBW)** infants (those infants whose birth weight is 1000 g or less). Ethical issues associated with resuscitation that nurses caring for such infants are confronted with include the following:

- Should resuscitation be attempted?
- Who should decide?
- Is the cost of resuscitation justified?
- Do the benefits of technology outweigh the burdens in relation to the quality of life?

All people involved (health care providers, nurses, parents, ethicists, clergy, attorneys) should participate in discussions addressing these controversial issues. Although there are no clear answers, such discussions help clarify the issues and promote more family-centered approaches to care. That care can involve sustaining life or providing care and support for a peaceful death. Nurses are key to the care of these infants and their families.

Late Preterm Infants

Infants born between 34 and 36 6/7 weeks of pregnancy are called "late preterm." The term, "late preterm," was developed by the National Institute of Child Health and Human Development (Raju, Higgins, Stark, & Lereno, 2006), replacing the previous terminology of *near-term*. By referring to these infants as late preterm, it conveys the concept that they are indeed premature with unique needs and potential problems associated with their early birth.

Late preterm infants are more likely than term infants to experience morbidity and mortality. They are at greater risk for complications such as respiratory distress, are more likely to require intensive and prolonged hospitalization, and to incur higher medical costs. They are more likely to die before 1 year of age and to suffer neurologic injury that results in long-term neurodevelopmental problems (Martin et al., 2010).

Common problems experienced by late preterm infants include thermoregulation, feeding difficulty, hyperbilirubinemia, hypoglycemia, infection, and respiratory problems. Care of the late preterm infant is discussed on pp. 922-923.

Physiologic Functions

Respiratory Function

The preterm infant is likely to have difficulty making the pulmonary transition from intrauterine to extrauterine life. Numerous problems can affect the respiratory systems of preterm infants and can include the following:

- Decreased number of functional alveoli
- Deficient surfactant levels
- Smaller lumen in the respiratory system
- Greater collapsibility or obstruction of respiratory passages
- Insufficient calcification of the bony thorax
- Weak or absent gag reflex
- Immature and friable capillaries in the lungs
- Greater distance between functional alveoli and the capillary bed

In combination, these deficits have the potential to severely hinder the preterm infant's respiratory efforts and can produce respiratory distress or apnea. Nurses must be alert to signs of respiratory distress or apnea and ready to intervene to promote adequate oxygenation.

Respiratory difficulty often follows a progressive pattern. Infants normally breathe between 30 and 60 breaths/min, relying significantly on their abdominal muscles to accomplish this. However, the respiratory rate can increase without a change in rhythm. Early signs of respiratory distress include flaring of the nares and an expiratory grunt. Depending on the cause, retractions can begin as subcostal, suprasternal, or clavicular retractions. If the infant shows increasing respiratory effort (e.g., seesaw breathing patterns, retractions, flaring of the nares, expiratory grunts, and/or apneic spells), this indicates deepening distress. A compromised infant's color progresses from pink to circumoral cyanosis and then to generalized cyanosis. Acrocyanosis deepens.

> **! NURSING ALERT**
>
> Acrocyanosis is a normal finding in the neonate, but central cyanosis indicates an underlying problem that requires further evaluation.

Periodic breathing is a respiratory pattern commonly seen in preterm infants. Such infants exhibit 5- to 10-second respiratory pauses followed by 10 to 15 seconds of compensatory rapid respirations. Such periodic breathing should not be confused with *apnea*, which is a 15- to 20-second cessation of respiration.

Cardiovascular Function

Evaluation of heart rate and rhythm, skin color, blood pressure, perfusion, pulses, oxygen saturation, and acid-base status provides information on the cardiovascular status. The nurse must be prepared to intervene if symptoms of hypovolemia or shock, or both, are found. These symptoms include hypotension, slow capillary refill (longer than 3 seconds), and continued respiratory distress despite the provision of oxygen and ventilation.

An accurate and timely blood pressure (BP) reading can assist in making an early diagnosis of cardiorespiratory disease and in monitoring the effects of fluid therapy. BP is monitored routinely in the sick neonate by internal or external means. Direct recording with arterial catheters is often used but carries the risks inherent in any procedure in which a catheter is introduced into an artery. An umbilical venous catheter can also be used to monitor the neonate's central venous pressure. Oscillometry (Dinamap) is a noninvasive, effective means for detecting alterations in systemic BP (hypotension or hypertension) and for identifying the need to implement appropriate therapy to maintain cardiovascular function.

Maintaining Body Temperature

Preterm infants are susceptible to temperature instability as a result of numerous factors. Because of their large body surface in relation to their weight, preterm infants are at high risk for heat loss. Other factors that place preterm infants at risk for temperature instability include the following:

- Minimal insulating subcutaneous fat
- Limited stores of brown fat (an internal source for the generation of heat present in normal term infants)
- Fragile capillaries
- Decreased or absent reflex control of skin capillaries (shiver response)
- Inadequate muscle mass activity (rendering the preterm infant unable to produce its own heat)
- Poor muscle tone, resulting in more body surface area being exposed to the cooling effects of the environment
- An immature temperature regulation center in the brain

The goal of thermoregulation is to create a **neutral thermal environment (NTE),** which is the environmental temperature at which oxygen consumption is minimal but adequate to maintain the body temperature (Bagwell, 2007). Armed with the knowledge of the four mechanisms of heat transfer (convection, conduction, radiation, and evaporation), the nurse can then create an environment for the preterm infant that prevents temperature instability (see Chapter 24). The infant is kept in a radiant warmer bed or in an incubator with control settings at a temperature to maintain the NTE. Because the preterm infant has few reserves (extra energy calories, minimal or no fat stores), cold sensitivity is a problem. This infant can easily lose heat and develop hypothermia. Physiologically the infant tries to conserve heat and burns more calories, and the metabolic system goes into overdrive, further stressing the already compromised neonate.

A critical nursing role is to prevent or minimize hypothermia and cold stress by recognizing the risk factors and using intervention strategies to prevent and treat such stress. Signs of cold stress are listed in Box 37-2.

The nurse should attempt to prevent hyperthermia. Given that overheating produces an increase in oxygen and calorie consumption, the infant is also jeopardized if he or she becomes hyperthermic. The preterm infant is not able to sweat and thus dissipate heat. Overheating can lead to apnea, tachycardia, and eventually bradycardia, as well as consumption of calories that the preterm infant cannot afford to expend (see Box 37-2).

BOX 37-2 SIGNS OF HYPOTHERMIA AND HYPERTHERMIA

HYPOTHERMIA
- Apnea
- Bradycardia
- Central cyanosis
- Coagulation defects (i.e., pulmonary hemorrhage)
- Hypoglycemia
- Hypotonia
- Hypoxia
- Feeding intolerance (abdominal distention, emesis, increased residuals)
- Increased metabolic rate
- Irritability
- Lethargy
- Metabolic acidosis
- Peripheral vasoconstriction (persistent pulmonary hypertension of the newborn)
- Poor weight gain (chronic hypothermia)
- Shivering (mature infants in presence of severe hypothermia)
- Weak cry or suck

HYPERTHERMIA
- Apnea
- Central nervous system depression
- Dehydration (increased insensible water loss)
- Flushed/red skin
- Hypernatremia
- Irritability
- Lethargy
- Poor feeding
- Seizures
- Sweating
- Tachycardia
- Tachypnea
- Warm to touch
- Weak or absent cry

Sources: Brand, M., & Boyd, H. (2010). Thermoregulation. In T. Verklan & M. Walden (Eds.), *AWHONN core curriculum for neonatal intensive care nursing* (4th ed.). Philadelphia: Saunders; Baumgart, S. (2008). Iatrogenic hyperthermia and hypothermia in the neonate. *Clinics in Perinatology, 35*(1), 183-197; Blackburn, S. (2007). *Maternal, fetal, and neonatal physiology: A clinical perspective* (3rd ed.). St. Louis: Saunders.

Central Nervous System Function

The preterm infant's central nervous system (CNS) is susceptible to injury as a result of the following problems:
- Birth trauma that includes damage to immature structures
- Bleeding from fragile capillaries
- An impaired coagulation process, including prolonged prothrombin time
- Recurrent hypoxic and hyperoxic episodes
- Predisposition to hypoglycemia
- Fluctuating systemic BP with concomitant variation in cerebral blood flow and pressure

In the preterm neonate, neurologic function is dependent on gestational age, associated illness factors, and predisposing factors such as intrauterine asphyxia, which can cause neurologic damage. Clinical signs of neurologic dysfunction can be subtle, nonspecific, or specific. Five categories of clinical manifestations should be thoroughly evaluated in the preterm infant: seizure activity, hyperirritability, CNS depression, elevated intracranial pressure (ICP), and abnormal movements such as decorticate posturing. Primary and tendon reflexes are generally present in preterm infants by 28 weeks of gestation; evaluation of these reflexes should be part of the neurologic examination.

Research evidence indicates that the developing nervous system has the ability to reorganize neural connection after injury, meaning that some injuries that would be permanent in adults are not so in infants. Certain neurologic signs appear to be predictive of later neurologic abnormalities. These signs include hypotonia, a decreased level of activity, weak cry for more than 24 hours, and an inability to coordinate suck and swallow. Ongoing assessment and documentation of these neurologic signs are needed for the purpose of discharge teaching and making follow-up recommendations, as well as for their predictive value.

Maintaining Adequate Nutrition

The goal of neonatal nutrition is to promote normal growth and development. However, the maintenance of adequate nutrition in the preterm infant is complicated by problems with intake and metabolism. The preterm infant has the following disadvantages with regard to intake: weak or absent suck, swallow, and gag reflexes; a small stomach capacity; and weak abdominal muscles. The preterm infant's metabolic functions are compromised by a limited store of nutrients, a decreased ability to digest proteins or absorb nutrients, and immature enzyme systems.

The nurse must continually assess the infant's ability to take in and digest nutrients. Some preterm infants require gavage or intravenous (IV) feedings instead of oral feedings. An area of research that holds promise for preterm infants is use of minimal enteral nutrition (MEN) that may be only 1 ml/hr (Anderson, Wood, Keller, & Hay, 2011; Mosqueda, Sapieqiene, Glynn, Wilson-Costello, & Weiss, 2008). These feedings stimulate the gastrointestinal (GI) system with minute amounts of breast milk or formula, usually given via gavage, so that when enteral feedings of greater volume can begin, the GI system is primed for nutrient absorption. They also may help to protect LBW infants from sepsis; however, more evidence is needed to support this relationship (Terrin, Passariello, Canani, Manguso, Paludetto, & Cascioli, 2009).

Maintaining Renal Function

The preterm infant's immature renal system is unable to (1) adequately excrete metabolites and drugs; (2) concentrate urine; or (3) maintain acid-base, fluid, or electrolyte balance. Therefore, intake and output, as well as specific gravity, must be assessed. Laboratory tests must be done to assess acid-base and electrolyte balance. Medication levels are monitored in preterm infants because certain medications can overwhelm the immature system's ability to excrete them.

Maintaining Hematologic Status

The preterm infant also is particularly predisposed to hematologic problems because of the following:
- Increased capillary fragility
- Increased tendency to bleed (prolonged prothrombin time and partial thromboplastin time)
- Slowed production of red blood cells resulting from rapid decrease in erythropoiesis after birth

- Loss of blood due to frequent blood sampling for laboratory tests
- Decreased red blood cell survival related to the relatively larger size of the red blood cell and its increased permeability to sodium and potassium

The nurse assesses such infants for any evidence of bleeding from puncture sites and the GI tract. Infants also are examined for signs of anemia (decreased hemoglobin and hematocrit levels, pale skin, increased apnea, lethargy, tachycardia, and poor weight gain). The amount of blood drawn for laboratory testing is closely monitored and recorded.

Resisting Infection

Preterm infants are at increased risk for infection because they have a shortage of stored maternal immunoglobulins, an impaired ability to make antibodies, and a compromised integumentary system (thin skin and fragile capillaries). Preterm infants exhibit various nonspecific signs and symptoms of infection (Box 37-3). Early identification and treatment of sepsis are essential (see Chapter 35). As with all aspects of care, strict attention to hand hygiene is the single most important measure to prevent health care–associated infections.

BOX 37-3 SIGNS AND SYMPTOMS OF INFECTION

Temperature instability
- Hypothermia
- Hyperthermia

Central nervous system changes
- Lethargy
- Irritability

Changes in color
- Cyanosis, pallor
- Jaundice

Cardiovascular instability
- Poor perfusion
- Hypotension
- Bradycardia/tachycardia

Respiratory distress
- Tachypnea
- Apnea
- Retractions, nasal flaring, grunting

Gastrointestinal problems
- Feeding intolerance
- Vomiting
- Diarrhea
- Glucose instability

Metabolic acidosis

Growth and Development Potential

Although it is impossible to predict with complete accuracy the growth and development potential of each preterm infant, some findings support an anticipated favorable outcome in the absence of ongoing medical problems that can affect growth, such as BPD, necrotizing enterocolitis, and CNS problems. The lower the birth weight, the greater the likelihood for negative outcomes.

The age of a preterm newborn is corrected by adding the gestational age and the postnatal age. For example, an infant born at 32 weeks of gestation 4 weeks ago would now be considered 36 weeks of age. The infant's corrected age at 6 months after the birth date is then 4 months, and the infant's responses are accordingly evaluated against the norm expected for a 4-month-old infant. The growth and development milestones (e.g., motor milestones, vocalization, growth) are corrected for gestational age until the child is approximately 2½ years old.

Certain measurable factors predict normal growth and development. The preterm infant experiences catch-up body growth during the first 2 years of life; this is most likely to occur when the infant has a normal birth length (Kliegman, 2006). The head is the first to experience catch-up growth, followed by a gain in weight and height. At the infant's discharge from the hospital, which usually occurs between 37 and 40 weeks of postconception age, the infant should exhibit the following characteristics:

- An ability to raise the head when prone and to hold the head parallel with the body when tested for the head-lag response
- An ability to cry with vigor when hungry
- An appropriate amount and pattern of weight gain according to a growth grid
- Neurologic responses appropriate for corrected age

At 39 to 40 weeks of corrected age, the infant should be able to focus on the examiner's or parent's face and to follow with his or her eyes.

Very low birth weight (VLBW) (<1500 g) survivors are at high risk for neurologic and/or cognitive disabilities in varying degrees of severity; these include cerebral palsy, borderline intelligence, and learning disabilities (Daily, Carter, & Carter, 2011). Ongoing research is focused on examining other factors including environmental ones that can cause adverse cognitive and neurodevelopmental outcomes for VLBW and ELBW babies by the time they reach infancy or school age.

CARE MANAGEMENT

The goal of care for the preterm infant is to provide an extrauterine environment that approximates the healthy intrauterine environment to promote normal growth and development. Physicians, nurses, nurse practitioners, infant developmental specialists, and respiratory therapists work together as a team to provide the intensive care needed.

The admission of a preterm newborn to the intensive care nursery usually represents an emergency situation. Immediately after admission, a rapid initial evaluation is done to determine the infant's need for lifesaving treatment. Resuscitation is started in the birthing unit, and the newborn's needs for warmth and oxygen are provided for during transfer to the nursery.

Nursing care is focused on the continuous assessment and analysis of the infant's physiologic status. Nurses fulfill many roles in providing the intensive and extended care that these infants require. In addition, they are the support persons and teachers during the first phase of the parents' adjustment to the birth of their preterm infant.

The nurse uses many technologic support systems to monitor the body responses and maintain the body functions of the infant. Technical skill must be combined with a gentle touch and concern about the traumatic effects of harsh lighting and the volume of machinery noise. Provision of individualized behavioral and environmental care has been shown to reduce infant stress, conserve energy, and promote better neurobehavioral outcomes (Gardner & Goldson, 2011). (See Nursing Process box on p. 899 and Nursing Care Plan on pp. 900-901.)

NURSING PROCESS

Late Preterm and Preterm Infant Care

ASSESSMENT

The late preterm or preterm infant must undergo an initial physical assessment for life-threatening problems. The stable infant may undergo a cursory gestational age assessment to identify risk factors.

NURSING DIAGNOSES

After assessment the nursing diagnoses for infants and their parents can include the following:

***Ineffective Breathing Pattern* related to:**

- decreased number of functional alveoli
- surfactant deficiency
- immature respiratory control
- increased pulmonary vascular resistance

***Ineffective Thermoregulation* related to:**

- immature CNS thermoregulatory control
- increased heat loss to environment and inability to produce heat
- greater body surface exposed to environment
- decreased brown fat reserves to produce body heat

***Risk for Infection* related to:**

- invasive procedures
- decreased immune response
- ineffective skin barrier

***Anxiety (parental)* related to:**

- lack of knowledge about infant's condition
- lack of knowledge regarding infant's prognosis (uncertain outcome)
- inability to perform expected caregiving activities
- neonatal intensive care unit environment noise and high-tech care

EXPECTED OUTCOMES OF CARE

Expected outcomes can apply both to the infant and to the parents. Expected outcomes are individualized and include that the infant will do the following:

- Maintain adequate physiologic functioning (airway, breathing, circulation).
- Receive adequate nutrition for growth.
- Maintain stable body temperature.
- Remain free of infection.
- Experience appropriate parent-infant interactions.

Expected outcomes for the parents include that they will do the following:

- Perceive the infant as a family member.
- Provide infant care confidently and competently.
- Experience pride and satisfaction in the care of the infant.
- Organize their time and energies to meet the love, attention, and care needs of the other members of the family, as well as their own needs.

PLAN OF CARE AND INTERVENTIONS

- Maintain neutral thermal environment.
- Maintain nutritional status using oral, gavage, or intravenous feeding as appropriate.
- Monitor amount of blood withdrawn for laboratory tests.
- Maintain Standard Precautions.
- Provide support and education for parents regarding infant's condition and care.

Numerous other nursing interventions are discussed in the text (see also Table 37-3).

EVALUATION

The nurse can be reasonably assured that care was effective to the extent that the expected outcomes for care have been achieved.

Physical Care

The environmental support measures for the preterm infant typically consist of the following equipment and procedures:

- An incubator or radiant warmer placed over the infant to control body temperature (NTE)
- Oxygen administration, depending on the infant's cardiopulmonary and circulatory status
- Electronic monitors as needed for the observation of respiratory and cardiac functions
- Assistive devices for positioning the infant in neutral flexion and with boundaries
- Clustering of care and minimization of stimulation according to infant cues

Various metabolic support measures that can be instituted consist of the following:

- Parenteral fluids to help support nutrition and maintain normal arterial blood gas (ABG) levels and acid-base balance
- IV access to facilitate the administration of antibiotic therapy if sepsis is a concern
- Blood work to monitor ABG levels, pH, blood glucose levels, electrolytes, and the status of blood cultures

Maintaining Body Temperature

The high risk infant is susceptible to heat loss and its complications. In addition, LBW infants can be unable to increase their metabolic rate because of impaired gas exchange, caloric intake restrictions, or poor thermoregulation. Transepidermal water loss is greater because of skin immaturity in very preterm infants (those at less than 28 weeks of gestation) and can contribute to temperature instability.

The preterm infant should be transferred from the birth room in a prewarmed incubator; ELBW infants can be placed in a polyethylene bag to decrease heat and water loss (Fig. 37-1). Skin-to-skin contact (kangaroo care) between the stable preterm infant and parent is a viable option for interaction because of the maintenance of appropriate body temperature by the infant (see pp. 910-911 for further discussion of kangaroo care).

High risk infants are cared for in the thermoneutral environment created by use of an external heat source. A probe to an external heat source supplied by a radiant warmer or a servo-controlled incubator is attached to the infant. The infant acts as a thermostat to regulate the amount of heat supplied by the external source. This idealized environment maintains an infant's normal body temperature between 36.5° and 37.2° C. Maintaining a thermoneutral condition in the youngest, most immature infants decreases the need for them to generate additional heat. The rationale is that this should increase physiologic stability and decrease oxygen consumption (Bosque & Haverman, 2009; Soll, 2008).

Care of the Hypothermic Infant. The hypothermic infant can appear pale and mottled; the skin is cool to touch, especially the extremities. Acrocyanosis and respiratory distress can occur as oxygen consumption increases in an effort to generate heat. As

NURSING CARE PLAN

The High Risk Preterm Newborn

NURSING DIAGNOSIS

Ineffective breathing pattern related to pulmonary and neuromuscular immaturity, decreased energy, fatigue

Expected Outcomes

Infant exhibits adequate oxygenation (i.e., arterial blood gases [ABGs] and acid-base within normal limits [WNL]; oxygen saturations 92% or greater; respiratory rate and pattern WNL; breath sounds clear; and absence of grunting, nasal flaring; minimal retractions, skin color WNL).

Nursing Interventions/*Rationales*

- Position neonate prone or supine, avoiding neck hyperextension *to promote optimum air exchange.* Use a side-lying position after feeding or in cases of excessive mucus production *to avoid aspiration.* Avoid Trendelenburg position *because it can cause increased intracranial pressure and reduce lung capacity.*
- Suction nasopharynx, trachea, and endotracheal tube as indicated *to remove mucus.* Avoid oversuctioning *because it can cause bronchospasm, bradycardia, and hypoxia and predispose neonate to intraventricular hemorrhage.*
- Administer oxygen and monitor neonatal response *to maintain oxygen saturation.*
- Maintain a neutral thermal environment *to conserve oxygen use.*
- Monitor arterial blood gases, acid-base balance, oxygen saturation, respiratory rate and pattern, breath sounds, and airway patency; observe for grunting, nasal flaring, retractions, and cyanosis *to detect signs of respiratory distress.*

NURSING DIAGNOSIS

Ineffective thermoregulation related to immature temperature regulation and minimal subcutaneous fat stores

Expected Outcome

Infant exhibits maintenance of stable body temperature within normal range for postconceptional age (36.5° to 37.2° C).

Nursing Interventions/*Rationales*

- Place neonate in a prewarmed radiant warmer *to maintain stable temperature.*
- Place temperature probe on neonatal abdomen *to control heat levels in radiant warmer.*
- Take axillary temperature periodically *to monitor temperature and cross-check functioning of warmer unit.*
- Avoid infant exposure to cool air and drafts, cold scales, cold stethoscopes, cold examination tables, and prolonged bathing *that predispose the infant to heat loss.*
- Monitor probe frequently *because detachment can cause overheating or warmer-induced hyperthermia.*
- Transfer infant to a servo-controlled open warmer bed or incubator *when temperature has stabilized.*

NURSING DIAGNOSIS

Risk for infection related to immature immune system

Expected Outcome

Infant exhibits no evidence of health care–associated infection.

Nursing Interventions/*Rationales*

- Institute scrupulous hand hygiene techniques before and after handling neonate, ensure all supplies and/or equipment are clean before use, and ensure strict aseptic technique with invasive procedures *to minimize exposure to infective organisms.*
- Prevent contact with persons who have communicable infections, and instruct parents in infection-control procedures *to minimize infection risk.*
- Administer prescribed antibiotics *to provide coverage for infection during sepsis workup.*
- Continuously monitor vital signs for stability *since instability, hypothermia, or prolonged temperature elevations serve as indicators for infection.*

NURSING DIAGNOSIS

Risk for imbalanced nutrition: less than body requirements related to inability to ingest nutrients secondary to immaturity

Expected Outcomes

Infant receives adequate amount of nutrients with sufficient caloric intake to maintain positive nitrogen balance; demonstrates steady weight gain.

Nursing Interventions/*Rationales*

- Administer parenteral fluid/total parenteral nutrition (TPN) as prescribed *to provide adequate nutrition and fluid intake.*
- Monitor for signs of intolerance to TPN, *which can interfere with effective replenishment of nutrients.*
- Periodically assess readiness to orally feed (i.e., strong suck, swallow, and gag reflexes) *to provide appropriate transition from TPN to oral feeding as soon as neonate is ready.*
- Advance volume and concentration of formula when orally feeding per unit protocol *to avoid overfeeding and feeding intolerance.*
- If mother desires to breastfeed when neonate is stable, demonstrate how to express milk *to establish and maintain lactation until infant can breastfeed.*

NURSING DIAGNOSIS

Risk for deficient fluid volume/excess fluid volume related to immature physiology

Expected Outcome

Infant exhibits evidence of fluid homeostasis.

Nursing Interventions/*Rationales*

- Administer parenteral fluids as prescribed and regulate carefully *to maintain fluid balance.* Avoid hypertonic fluids such as undiluted medications, and concentrated glucose *because they can cause excess solute load on immature kidneys.*
- Implement strategies (e.g., use of plastic covers and increase of ambient humidity) *that minimize insensible water loss.*
- Monitor hydration status (i.e., skin turgor, blood pressure, edema, weight, mucous membranes, fontanels, urine specific gravity, electrolytes) and intake and output *to evaluate for evidence of dehydration or overhydration.*

NURSING DIAGNOSIS

Risk for impaired skin integrity related to immature skin structure, immobility, or invasive procedures

Expected Outcome

Infant's skin remains intact, with no evidence of irritation or injury.

Nursing Interventions/*Rationales*

- Cleanse skin as needed with plain warm water and apply moisturizing agents to skin *to prevent dryness and reduce friction across skin surface.*
- When performing procedures: minimize use of tape and apply a skin barrier between tape and skin; use transparent elastic film for securing central and peripheral lines; use limb electrodes for monitoring or attach with hydrogel and rotate electrodes frequently; remove adhesives with soap and water rather than alcohol or acetone-based adhesive removers *to minimize skin damage.*

Nursing Care Plan—The High Risk Preterm Newborn

NURSING CARE PLAN

The High Risk Preterm Newborn—cont'd

- Monitor use of thermal devices such as warmers or heating pads carefully *to prevent burns.*
- Monitor skin closely for evidence of redness, rash, irritation, bruising, breakdown, ischemia, and infiltration *to detect and treat potential complications early.*

NURSING DIAGNOSIS

Risk for injury related to increased intracranial pressure (ICP) and intraventricular hemorrhage secondary to immature central nervous system

Expected Outcome

Infant will exhibit normal ICP with no evidence of intraventricular hemorrhage.

Nursing Interventions/*Rationales*

- Institute minimum stimulation protocol (i.e., minimal handling, clustering care techniques, avoidance of sudden head movements to one side, undisturbed sleep periods, light variations to simulate day and night, limiting personnel and equipment noise in environment) *to decrease stress responses, which can increase ICP.*
- Institute ordered pharmacologic and nonpharmacologic pain control methods *to manage pain and reduce physical stress.*
- Avoid hypertonic solutions and medications *because they increase cerebral blood flow.*
- Elevate head of bed 15 to 20 degrees *to decrease ICP.*
- Monitor vital signs *for evidence of ICP.*
- Recognize signs of overstimulation (i.e., flaccidity, yawning, irritability, crying, staring, active averting) *so stimulation can be stopped to allow rest.*

NURSING DIAGNOSIS

Impaired parenting related to separation and interruption of parent/infant attachment secondary to premature birth

Expected Outcomes

Parents establish contact with neonate; demonstrate competent parenting skills and willingness to care for neonate.

Nursing Interventions/*Rationales*

- Before parents' first visit to the NICU, prepare them by explaining what the neonate will look like, and what the equipment will look like and its function *to diminish fear and decrease sense of shock.*
- Keep parents informed about infant's condition (improvements and setbacks) and important aspects of infant's care; encourage and answer parental questions; actively listen to parents' concerns *to establish trust, open communication, and caring atmosphere to aid in coping.*
- Encourage parents to visit the NICU often; to name infant (if that is culturally appropriate); to touch, hold, or caress infant as physical condition permits; to be actively involved in infant's care; to bring personal items (i.e., clothing, stuffed animals, or pictures of family) *to allow for formation of emotional bond.*
- Reinforce parents' involvement and praise care endeavors *to increase self-confidence in their contribution.*
- Encourage parents to bring siblings to visit; explain to siblings what they are seeing; encourage siblings to draw pictures or write letters for infant and place in or near infant's crib *to promote family involvement, help ease sibling fears, and let them contribute to infant's care.*
- Refer parents to social services as needed *to ensure comprehensive care.*

NURSING DIAGNOSIS

Grieving related to perceived loss of premature infant

Expected Outcomes

Parents express feelings about the potential loss and seek support from staff, family, clergy, and other support systems.

Nursing Interventions/*Rationales*

- Encourage parents to express feelings about perceived loss of infant *to reinforce reality and help alleviate guilt.*
- Encourage parents to use family, friends, clergy, and other support persons *to enhance coping ability.*
- Plan time on each shift to sit and listen to parents *to demonstrate concern, empathy, and support.*
- Inform parents about support groups in the facility and the community *to encourage parents to use available resources.*

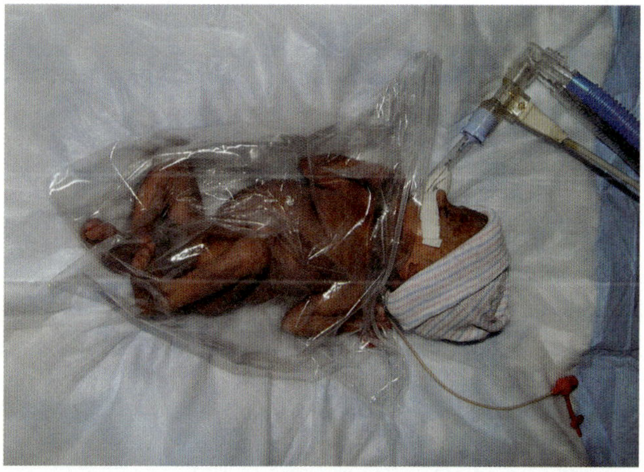

FIG. 37-1 Preterm infant in polyethylene bag to protect against heat loss. (Courtesy Cheryl Briggs, RNC, Annapolis, MD.)

hypothermia worsens, the infant can have apnea, bradycardia, and central cyanosis.

When an infant becomes hypothermic, rewarming should begin immediately by providing external heat. However, rapid changes in body temperature can cause apnea and acidosis. For the infant with mild hypothermia, slow rewarming is recommended. External heat sources should be slightly warmer than skin temperature and increased gradually until the infant's temperature is within the range of NTE. For the severely hypothermic infant (body temperature less than 35°C), more rapid rewarming is needed. Use of radiant heaters or heated water mattresses helps to prevent prolonged metabolic acidosis and hypoglycemia and reduces mortality (Brown & Landers, 2011).

Oxygen Therapy

Clinical criteria for identifying the need for oxygen administration include increased respiratory effort, respiratory distress with apnea, tachycardia, bradycardia, and central cyanosis with or without hypotonia. The need for oxygen should be substantiated by biochemical data (arterial oxygen pressure [Pao_2] of less than 60 mm Hg or an oxygen saturation of less than 92%). High risk infants often require saturations of more than 95% to maintain respiratory stability because their hemoglobin levels are frequently low. As the Pao_2 decreases, less oxygen is released from the hemoglobin, which increases the risk for cellular hypoxia.

Oxygen administered to an infant is warmed and humidified to prevent cold stress and drying of the respiratory mucosa. During the administration of oxygen, the concentration, volume, temperature, and humidity of the gas are carefully controlled. Delivery of oxygen for more than a few minutes requires the use of special equipment (hood, nasal cannula, positive-pressure mask, or endotracheal tube) because the concentration of free-flow oxygen cannot be monitored accurately. Free-flow oxygen into an incubator should not be used because the concentration fluctuates dramatically each time the doors or portholes are opened. The indiscriminate use of oxygen can be hazardous. Possible complications of oxygen therapy include ROP and BPD.

! NURSING ALERT

Administration of a therapeutic level of oxygen for a severely depressed infant can cause significant physiologic harm if given to an infant with mild respiratory disease.

Infants who need oxygen should have their respiratory status assessed accurately at least every hour. This includes a continuous pulse oximetry reading and at least one ABG measurement. There should also be hourly documentation of pulse oximetry readings as well as the amount of oxygen being administered and the mode of delivery (Gardner, Enzman-Hines, & Dickey, 2011). The interventions implemented are then determined on the basis of the findings yielded by the clinical assessment, including telemetry (pulse oximetry or $tcPo_2$ [skin oxygen tension] monitoring) and laboratory tests (Cifuentes & Carlo, 2007). The interventions ordered are those that can directly manage the underlying disease process and range from hood oxygen administration to ventilator therapy.

Hood Therapy. A hood can be used to administer oxygen to infants who do not require mechanical pressure support. The hood is a clear plastic cover that is sized to fit over the head and neck of the infant (Fig. 37-2, *A*). Inside the hood the infant receives the correct amount of oxygen. The nurse checks the oxygen level at least every hour because the concentration must be adjusted in response to the infant's condition. If the hood is removed for holding, feeding, or suctioning, an alternative source of oxygen must be provided (Gardner et al., 2011).

Nasal Cannula. Infants requiring low-flow amounts of oxygen can benefit from the use of a nasal cannula (see Fig. 37-2, *B*). These are of particular value for older infants who are recuperating but still require supplemental oxygen. They are the preferred method for home oxygen administration. Nasal cannulas permit the infant to receive an adequate, continuous flow of oxygen while allowing optimal vision, positioning, and parental holding. Infants also can breastfeed or bottle-feed while receiving oxygen by this method. Nasal cannulas come in

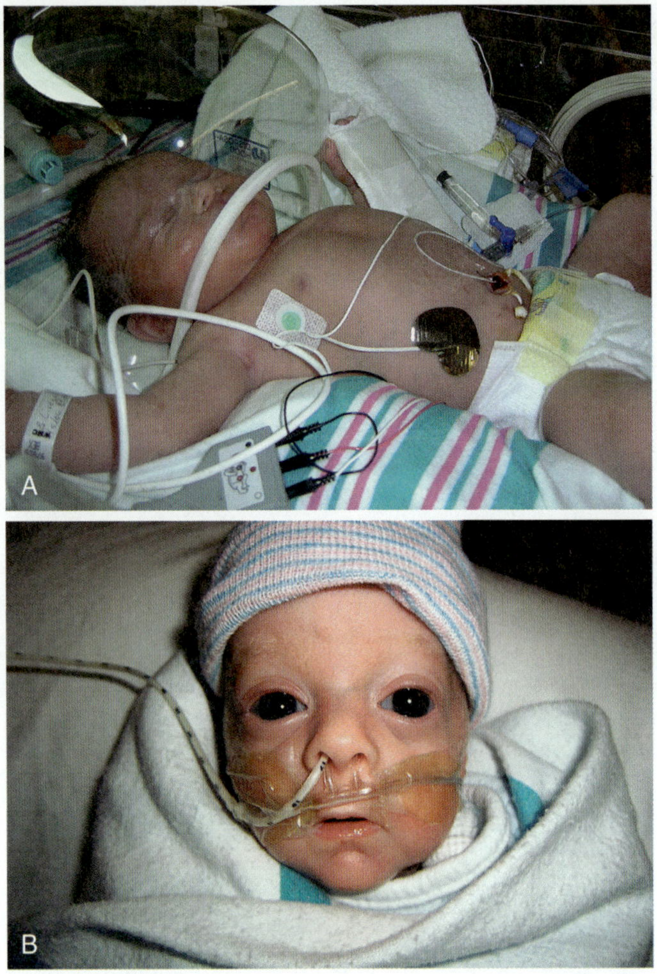

FIG. 37-2 **A**, Infant under hood. **B**, Infant with nasal cannula. (**A**, Courtesy Lauren and Brian LiVecchi, Raleigh, NC; **B**, courtesy Cheryl Briggs, RNC, Annapolis, MD.)

different sizes; proper fit is important. The nasal prongs must be inspected and cleaned frequently to make sure they are not partially obstructed by milk or secretions. Nasal cannulas allow easier feedings and psychosocial interactions.

Continuous Positive Airway Pressure Therapy. Infants who are unable to maintain an adequate Pao_2 despite the administration of oxygen by hood or nasal cannula may require the delivery of oxygen by using **continuous positive airway pressure (CPAP).** CPAP infuses oxygen or air under a preset pressure by means of nasal prongs, a face mask, or an endotracheal tube (Fig. 37-3). It is often achieved by sending the oxygen bubbling through water to the infant; this is referred to as bubble CPAP. Researchers are investigating whether the work of neonatal breathing is improved with bubble CPAP versus variable-flow devices (Polin, 2009). In either case, an orogastric tube should be used for decompression of the stomach during use of nasal prongs. CPAP increases the functional residual capacity, improves the diffusion time of pulmonary gases, including oxygen, and can decrease pulmonary shunting. If implemented early enough, CPAP may preclude the need for mechanical ventilation (Cifuentes & Carlo, 2007). CPAP can cause vascular shunting in the pulmonary beds, which can lead to persistent pulmonary hypertension and severe respiratory distress.

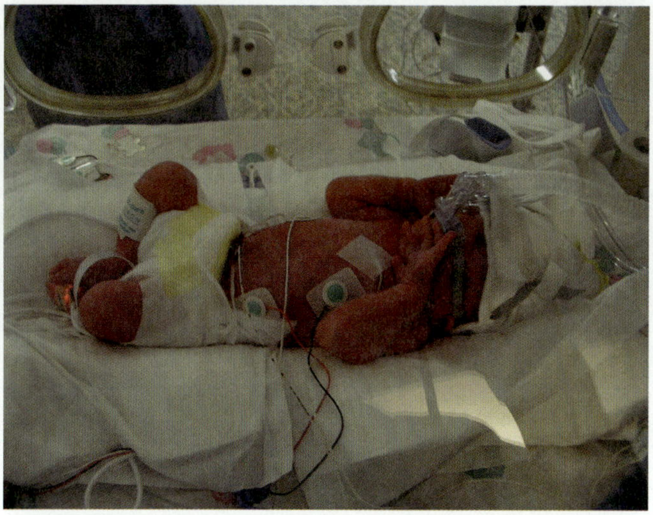

FIG. 37-3 Infant receiving ventilatory assistance with nasal continuous positive airway pressure (CPAP). (Courtesy Randi and Jacob Wills, Clayton, NC.)

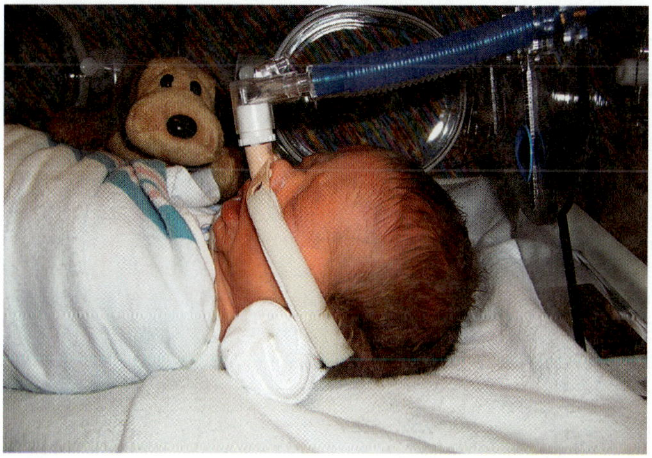

FIG. 37-4 Infant intubated and on ventilator. (Courtesy Cheryl Briggs, RNC, Annapolis, MD.)

Mechanical Ventilation. Mechanical ventilation must be implemented if other methods of therapy cannot correct abnormalities in oxygenation (Fig. 37-4). Its use is indicated whenever blood gas values reveal the existence of severe hypoxemia or severe hypercapnia. The condition of the infant who has apnea with bradycardia, ineffective respiratory effort, shock, asphyxia, infection, meconium aspiration syndrome, respiratory distress syndrome (RDS), or congenital defects that affect ventilation also can deteriorate and require intubation to reverse the process (Cifuentes & Carlo, 2007). Dexamethasone may be administered to prevent chronic lung disease in ventilator-dependent infants who are unlikely to survive without corticosteroids. It is not recommended for LBW infants (AAP & Canadian Paediatric Society, 2006).

The ventilator settings are determined by the infant's particular needs. The ventilator is set to provide a predetermined amount of oxygen to the infant during spontaneous respirations and mechanical ventilation in the absence of spontaneous respirations. Newer technologies in ventilation allow oxygen to be delivered at lower pressures and in assist modes, thereby preventing the overriding of the infant's spontaneous breathing and providing distending pressures within a physiologic range. Barotrauma and associated complications such as pneumothorax (accumulation of air in the pleural space) and pulmonary interstitial emphysema (PIE) (free air that accumulates in interstitial tissue) are decreased. See Table 37-1 for a description of the types of mechanical ventilation used in newborns.

Neonatal Resuscitation. In 2005 the American Heart Association published neonatal resuscitation guidelines (American Heart Association [AHA], 2005). A rapid assessment of infants can identify those who do not require resuscitation: those born at term gestation, with no evidence of meconium or infection in the amniotic fluid; those who are breathing or crying; and those with good muscle tone. If any of these characteristics is absent, the infant should receive the following actions in sequence: (1) initial steps in stabilization: provide warmth by placing the

TABLE 37-1 **COMMON METHODS FOR ASSISTED VENTILATION IN NEONATAL RESPIRATORY DISTRESS***

METHOD	DESCRIPTION	HOW PROVIDED
Continuous distending pressure—continuous positive airway pressure (CPAP)	Provides constant distending pressure to airway in spontaneously breathing infant	Nasal prongs or nasopharyngeal tubes Endotracheal tube Face mask Bubble CPAP uses water resistance
Intermittent mandatory ventilation (IMV)	Allows infant to breathe spontaneously at own rate but provides mechanical cycled respirations and pressure at regular preset intervals; infant may maintain asynchronous ventilation efforts, which diminishes effective gas exchange; uses positive end-expiratory pressure (PEEP)	Endotracheal tube
Synchronized intermittent mandatory ventilation (SIMV)	Mechanically delivered breaths are synchronized to the onset of spontaneous infant breaths; assist or control (A/C) mode facilitates full inspiratory synchrony; involves signal detection of onset of spontaneous respiration from abdominal movement, thoracic impedance, and airway pressure or flow changes; pressure support ventilation provides an inspiratory pressure assist when spontaneous breathing is detected to decrease infant's work of breathing	Patient-triggered infant ventilator with signal detector and A/C mode; endotracheal tube; SIMV, A/C, and pressure support are also referred to as patient-triggered ventilation
Volume guarantee ventilation	Delivers a predetermined volume of gas using an inspiratory pressure that varies according to the infant's lung compliance (often used in conjunction with SIMV)	Volume guarantee ventilator with flow sensor; endotracheal tube
High-frequency oscillation (HFO)	Application of high-frequency, low-volume, sine-wave flow oscillations to airway at rates between 480 and 1200 breaths/min	Variable-speed piston pump (or loudspeaker, fluidic oscillator); endotracheal tube
High-frequency jet ventilation (HFJV)	Uses a separate, parallel, low-compliant circuit and injector port to deliver small pulses or jets of fresh gas deep into airway at rates between 250 and 900 breaths/min	May be used alone or with low-rate IMV; endotracheal tube

baby under a radiant warmer, position the head in a position to open the airway, clear the airway with a bulb syringe or suction catheter, dry the baby, stimulate breathing, and reposition the baby; (2) ventilation; (3) chest compressions; and (4) administration of epinephrine or volume expansion or both. The decision to move from one category of action to the next is based on the assessment of respirations, heart rate, and color. Rapid decision making is imperative; 30 seconds are allotted for each step. The condition of the infant is reevaluated and the decision made whether to progress to the next step (Fig. 37-5).

Resuscitation of asphyxiated newborns with 21% oxygen rather than 100% oxygen shows promise. Proponents for room air resuscitation suggest that fewer complications are associated with oxidative stress and hyperoxemia when room air is administered. The 2005 American Heart Association resuscitation standards for neonatal resuscitation stress that resuscitation may begin with no supplemental oxygen (i.e., 21% or room air) but that if the infant's condition does not improve within 90 seconds, supplemental oxygen should be available for use. The stated goal is to minimize oxygen free radicals by preventing hyperoxia using supplemental oxygen at levels less than 100% (AHA, 2005). A review of several studies indicates that neonatal mortality is reduced by 30% to 40% when room air instead of 100% oxygen is used for neonatal resuscitation (Saugstad, 2007). Fluctuations in oxygen saturation are also deemed harmful. Experts recommend that oxygen saturations for ELBW infants be maintained between 85% and 93% but definitely not exceeding 95% (Saugstad).

! NURSING ALERT

Rates of retinopathy of prematurity and bronchopulmonary dysplasia are reduced in infants whose arterial oxygen saturation (SaO_2) is kept between 93% and 95%.

Surfactant Administration. Surfactant is a surface-active phospholipid secreted by the alveolar epithelium. Acting much the same as a detergent, this substance reduces the

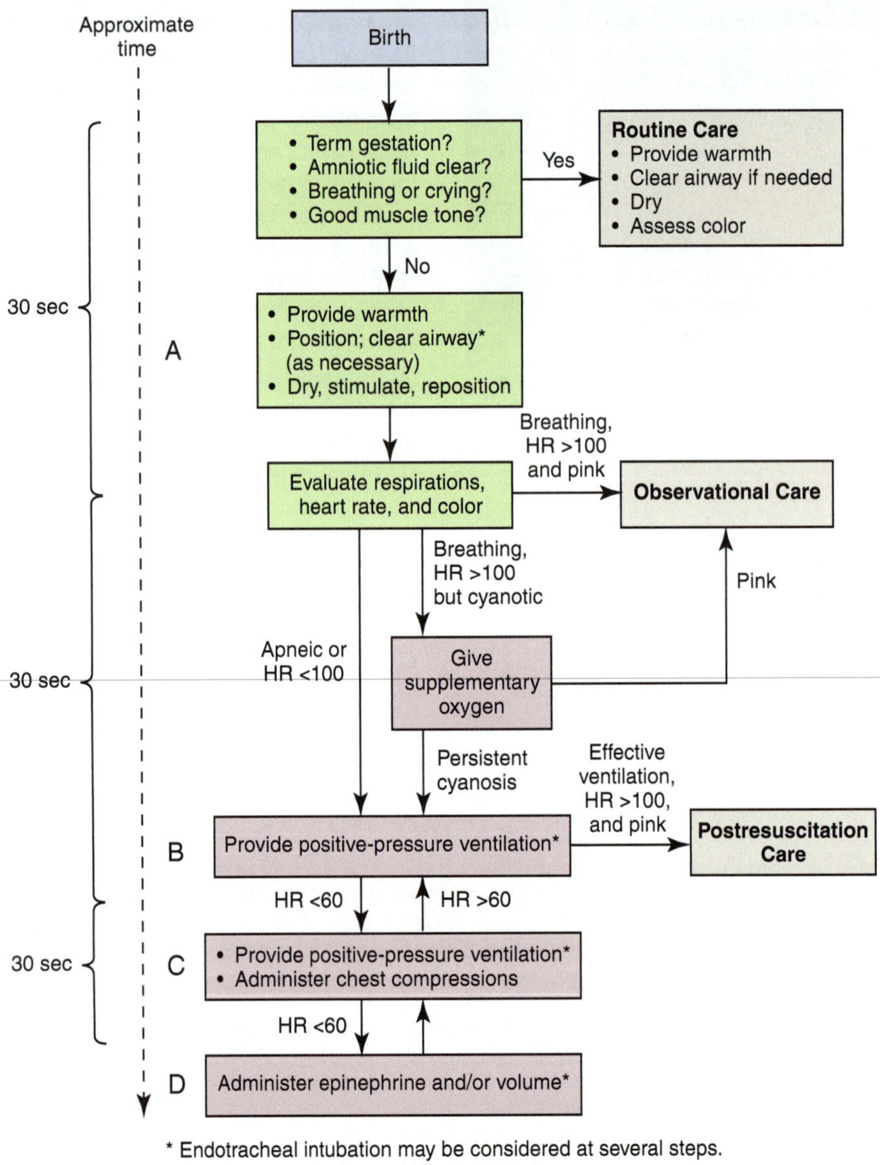

FIG. 37-5 Neonatal resuscitation flow algorithm. (From American Heart Association. [2005]. Neonatal resuscitation guidelines. *Circulation, 112*[24 Suppl], IV-188–IV-195.)

surface tension of fluids that line the alveoli and respiratory passages, resulting in uniform expansion and maintenance of lung expansion at low intraalveolar pressure. Before 34 weeks of gestation, most infants do not produce enough surfactant to survive extrauterine life. As a result, lung compliance is decreased, and not enough gas exchange occurs as the lungs become atelectatic and require greater pressures to expand.

Surfactant can be administered as an adjunct to oxygen and ventilation therapy. With administration of artificial surfactant, respiratory compliance is improved until the infant can generate enough surfactant on his or her own. Exogenous surfactant is either artificial or natural and is given in several doses through an endotracheal tube. The American Academy of Pediatrics (AAP) (Engle & AAP Committee on Fetus and Newborn, 2008) recommends the use of surfactant in infants with RDS as soon as possible after birth, especially ELBW infants and those not exposed to maternal antenatal steroids. The administration of antenatal steroids to the mother and surfactant replacement has decreased the incidence of RDS and concomitant morbidities. Use of artificial surfactant has been associated with a significantly reduced length of time on ventilators and oxygen therapy, and an increased survival rate in preterm infants. As with any drug therapy, the infant must be monitored for the occurrence of potential side effects such as a patent ductus arteriosus (PDA) and pulmonary hemorrhage (see the Medication Guide).

High-Frequency Ventilation. High frequency ventilation (HFV) is accomplished through the use of jet ventilators, oscillators, or high-frequency flow interrupters (Gardner et al., 2011). These methods provide smaller volumes of oxygen at a significantly more rapid rate (more than 300 breaths/min) than traditional mechanical ventilators. As a result, the intrathoracic pressure is decreased, and along with this, the risk of barotrauma.

Additional Therapies

Nitric Oxide Therapy. Inhaled nitric oxide (INO), delivered as a gas, causes potent and sustained pulmonary vasodilation in the pulmonary circulation. NO binds with hemoglobin in red blood cells and is inactivated after metabolism. INO is used in term and late preterm infants with conditions such as persistent pulmonary hypertension, meconium aspiration syndrome, pneumonia, sepsis, and congenital diaphragmatic hernia to decrease or reverse pulmonary hypertension, pulmonary vasoconstriction, acidosis, and hypoxemia. NO is a colorless, highly diffusible gas that can be administered through the ventilator circuit blended with oxygen. INO therapy can be used in conjunction with surfactant replacement therapy, high-frequency ventilation, or extracorporeal membrane oxygenation (ECMO). In the few studies conducted with human infants, positive results were seen: oxygen saturation improved, and no toxic effects from methemoglobin or increased levels of nitrogen oxide were documented. NO shows much promise in reducing adverse respiratory sequelae of being born prematurely. Its use has reduced the need for invasive technologies such as ECMO (Carlo, 2007; Gardner et al., 2011).

Extracorporeal Membrane Oxygenation (ECMO). ECMO is a very complex and costly treatment that is sometimes used to support life and allow treatment of intractable hypoxemia due to severe cardiac or respiratory failure. This therapy involves a modified heart-lung machine, although in ECMO the heart is not stopped, and blood does not entirely bypass the lungs. Blood is shunted from a catheter in the right atrium or right internal jugular vein by gravity to a servo-regulated roller pump, pumped through a membrane lung where it is oxygenated, and through a small heat exchanger where it is warmed,

MEDICATION GUIDE

Surfactant Replacement

DRUG/SOURCE

- Beractant* (Survanta) - Exogenous surfactant from bovine lung extract
- Poractant alpha* (Curosurf) – Modified porcine-derived minced lung extract
- Calfactant* (Infrasurf) – Natural surfactant extracted from calf lung lavage
- Lucinactant (Surfaxin): synthetic surfactant

ACTION

These medications provide exogenous surfactant to correct deficiency in lung immaturity.

INDICATIONS

Surfactants are used in the prevention and treatment of respiratory distress syndrome in premature infants. The drug should be administered to infants with RDS as soon as possible after intubation, regardless of gestational age or exposure to antenatal steroids. It should be given prophylactically to extremely preterm infants at high risk for RDS, especially if there was no exposure to antenatal steroids. Rescue surfactant may be given to infants with hypoxic respiratory failure that results from secondary surfactant deficiency; this includes meconium aspiration syndrome, sepsis or pneumonia, and pulmonary hemorrhage (Engle and the AAP Committee on Fetus and Newborn, 2008).

DOSAGE AND ROUTE

Dosage depends on the drug used. Administer via endotracheal tube.

ADVERSE REACTIONS

Adverse reactions are most often related to the dosage procedure and include oxygen desaturation, transient bradycardia, alterations in blood pressure, and drug reflux (Gardner, Enzman-Hines, & Dickey, 2011).

NURSING CONSIDERATIONS

Observe the infant's condition for changes. Diuresis can occur with improvement. Ventilator settings may need changing as the infant's ability to oxygenate increases.

*Bovine and porcine products can be objectionable to parents because of religious or cultural beliefs (Jewish, Islamic, or Hindu); prior to administering surfactant to infant, informed consent from parents is essential (Gardner et al., 2011).

Source: Engle, W., & American Academy of Pediatrics Committee on Fetus and Newborn. (2008). Surfactant replacement therapy for respiratory distress in the preterm and term neonate. *Pediatrics, 121*(2), 419-432; Gardner, S., Enzman-Hines, M., & Dickey, L. (2011). Respiratory diseases. In S. Gardner, B. Carter, M. Enzman-Hines, & J. Hernandez (Eds.). *Merenstein & Gardner's handbook of neonatal intensive care* (7th ed.). St. Louis: Mosby.

and then returned to the systemic circulation via a major artery such as the carotid artery to the aortic arch. ECMO provides oxygen to the circulation, allowing the lungs to "rest," and decreases pulmonary hypertension and hypoxemia in such conditions as persistent pulmonary hypertension of the newborn, congenital diaphragmatic hernia, sepsis, meconium aspiration, and severe pneumonia. ECMO is contraindicated for preterm infants younger than 34 weeks of gestation because of the anticoagulant therapy required in the pump and circuits, which can increase the potential for intraventricular hemorrhage in such infants (Carlo, 2007; Lund, 2010).

Partial Liquid Ventilation (PLV). For infants with severe RDS, the use of partial liquid ventilation (PLV) can improve outcomes. Perfluorocarbon liquid is instilled into the lungs during gaseous (mechanical) ventilation. PLV is beneficial to the surfactant deficient or immature lung because it reduces or eliminates surface tension, improves oxygenation through the re-creation of a fetal lung environment, and helps reexpand atelectatic areas. The safety and efficacy of PLV are being evaluated in the United States (Gardner et al., 2011).

Weaning from Respiratory Assistance. Respiratory assistance is weaned slowly as the infant's status improves. The infant is ready to be weaned from respiratory assistance once the ABG and oxygen saturation levels are maintained within normal limits. A spontaneous, adequate respiratory effort must be present, and the infant must show improved muscle tone during increased activity. Weaning is done in a stepwise and gradual manner. This can consist of the infant being extubated, placed on CPAP, and then weaned to oxygen by means of a hood or nasal cannula. Throughout the weaning process, the infant's oxygen levels are monitored by pulse oximetry, $TcPo_2$ monitoring, and blood gas levels.

The goal of weaning is the withdrawal of all oxygen support. However, some infants do not achieve this before discharge from the hospital and can require home oxygen therapy for several months. Throughout the weaning period the infant is assessed for signs and symptoms indicating poor tolerance of the process. These include an increased pulse, respiratory distress, or cyanosis, or a combination of these. If these occur, the amount of oxygen being delivered is increased, and weaning proceeds more slowly while further assessments are done. Underlying causes of intolerance of weaning may be BPD, a PDA, or CNS damage.

Nutritional Care

It is not always possible to provide enteral (by the GI route) nourishment to a high risk infant. Such infants are often too ill or weak to breastfeed or bottle feed because of respiratory distress or sepsis. Early enteral feeding of the asphyxiated neonate with a low Apgar score also is avoided to prevent bowel necrosis. In such cases, nutrition is provided parenterally. Those infants who require parenteral nutrition may have one or more of the following problems:

- Lack of a coordinated suck-and-swallow reflex
- Inability to suck because of a congenital anomaly
- Respiratory distress requiring aggressive ventilator support
- Asphyxiation with a potential for necrotizing enterocolitis

Type of Nourishment. The type, mode, and volume of feedings and the feeding schedule of the infant are determined on the basis of the findings yielded by assessment of the following variables:

- Initially, the birth weight, and then the current weight of the preterm infant
- Pattern of weight gain or loss (infants weighing less than 1500 g require more energy for growth and thermoregulation and may gain weight poorly with either breast- or bottle feedings)
- Presence or absence of suck-and-swallow reflex in all infants at less than 35 weeks of gestation
- Behavioral readiness to take oral feedings
- Physical condition, including presence or absence of bowel sounds, abdominal distention, or bloody stools, as well as presence and degree of respiratory distress or apneic episodes
- Residual from previous feeding, if being gavage fed
- Malformations (especially GI defects such as gastroschisis, omphalocele or esophageal atresia), including the need for a gastrostomy feeding tube
- Renal function, including urinary output and laboratory values (nitrogen balance, electrolyte balance, glucose level); preterm infants are especially susceptible to altered renal function

Human milk is the best source of nutrition for term and preterm infants. Even small preterm infants (28 to 36 weeks) are able to breastfeed if they have adequate sucking and swallowing reflexes and no other contraindications, such as respiratory complications or concurrent illness, are present. Preterm infants who are breastfed rather than bottle fed demonstrate fewer oxygen desaturations, absence of bradycardia, warmer-than-normal skin temperature, and improved coordination of breathing, sucking, and swallowing (Gardner & Lawrence, 2011). Mothers who wish to breastfeed their preterm infants are encouraged to pump their breasts until their infants are sufficiently stable to tolerate feeding at the breast. Appropriate guidelines for the storage of expressed mother's milk should be used to decrease the risk of milk contamination and destruction of its beneficial properties (Jones & Tully, 2006).

Commercially available preterm formulas are cow's milk–based and whey predominant, and have a higher concentration of protein, calcium, and phosphorus than term formulas to meet the unique needs of the preterm infant (AAP Committee on Nutrition, 2009). Most preterm formulas are either 22 or 24 cal/oz. Human milk with fortifier (protein, phosphorus, and calcium) is recommended for LBW preterm infants because it increases weight gain and improves bone mineralization better than nonfortified human milk (Gardner & Lawrence, 2011). Supplementation with iron, vitamin D, and multivitamins may be considered in exclusively breastfed LBW infants.

SAFETY ALERT

Contamination of powdered infant formula in hospitals by *Enterobacter sakazakii* has been associated with serious neonatal infections, necrotizing enterocolitis, and mortality. When possible, alternatives to powdered formula should be chosen; otherwise, the preparation of powdered formula for preterm infants should be carefully performed under strict aseptic technique, preferably in a pharmacy, and the formula properly refrigerated to prevent infection (AAP Committee on Nutrition, 2009). Continuous infusion of powdered formula should not exceed 4 hours.

Weight and Fluid Loss or Gain. The caloric, nutrient, and fluid requirements of high risk infants are greater than those of the term, normal newborn. Premature or dysmature (malnourished) newborns often have limited stores of nutrients and fluids. In addition, symptomatic or asymptomatic hypoglycemia, electrolyte imbalances, or other metabolic disturbances can develop in an infant whose nutritional intake is poor. Such hypoglycemia can cause serious damage to carbohydrate-dependent brain cells.

The infant's weight is measured and recorded daily, and the rate of weight loss or gain is calculated. Further depletion of weight and metabolic stores can occur as a result of one or a combination of the following factors:

- Birth asphyxia
- Increased respirations or respiratory effort
- PDA
- Hypothermic environment
- Insensible fluid loss caused by evaporation (with radiant heat or phototherapy)
- Vomiting, diarrhea, and dysfunctional absorption from the GI tract
- Growth demands (a preterm infant's growth rate approximates that of fetal growth during the last trimester and is at least two times faster than a term infant's growth rate after birth)
- Inability of the renal system to concentrate urine and maintain an adequate rate of urea excretion, as well as infant's inadequate response to antidiuretic hormone

The high risk newborn is predisposed to have weight and fluid losses because of the greater amount of fluid needed to meet the demands of the increased cellular metabolic processes (resulting from stress, repair, or growth). The body weight of preterm infants has a higher water content than that of their full-term counterparts (Hulzebos & Sauer, 2007). Most of this water is in the extracellular fluid compartment. Even with the early institution of fluid and nutrition intake, the preterm infant's weight and fluid losses seem exaggerated. Inadequate fluid intake, resulting from either delayed administration or insufficient volume, can further cause weight and fluid losses in the preterm infant.

Insensible water loss (IWL) is an evaporative loss that occurs largely through the skin (70%) and through the respiratory tract (30%). The basal IWL in a term infant is approximately 20 ml/kg/24 hr. It is significantly increased in preterm infants, and especially in ELBW infants with thin, gelatinous skin (Bell & Oh, 2005; Blackburn, 2007). The effects of radiant warmers, incubators, phototherapy, and other factors can increase the IWL. Humidifying the respiratory gases administered can prevent some of this loss.

During the first week of extrauterine life, the preterm infant can lose up to 15% of his or her birth weight. In contrast, a weight loss of up to only 7% to 10% is acceptable in a term, appropriate for gestational age (AGA) infant. After the initial week, a preterm infant's loss or gain during each 24-hour period should not exceed 2% of the previous day's weight. (To calculate a weight loss or gain, see Box 37-4.)

BOX 37-4 CALCULATION OF A WEIGHT LOSS OR GAIN

EXAMPLE 1

Day 1	1750 g (birth weight)	$\frac{70}{1750} = \frac{X\%}{100\%}$
Day 3	1680 g	$1750X = 7000$
	70 g loss	$1750X\overline{)7000.0}$ = 4.0
		X = 4.0% weight loss

EXAMPLE 2

Day 3	1680 g	$\frac{40}{1680} = \frac{X\%}{100\%}$
Day 4	1720 g	$1680X = 4000$
	40 g gain	$1680\overline{)4,000.00}$ = 2.38
		X = 2.4% weight gain

Increased stooling or voiding, increased evaporative losses, inadequate volume or incorrect fluid administration, and problems with malabsorption can cause weight loss. Implementation of interventions and frequent reassessment of the infant and the environment are necessary to correct the problems. Such interventions include adjusting the incubator temperature; "swamping" or providing high levels of humidity under a cover over the radiant warmer; monitoring and adjusting the volume and type of fluids being administered; assessing the urinary output, including the specific gravity; and assessing the blood glucose levels. Hyperglycemia results in urinary loss of glucose that can cause osmotic diuresis, which increases the risk of dehydration (Armentrout, 2010).

If the infant is gaining more than the expected amount of weight, this may be due to overfeeding or fluid retention. The nurse reports and records the findings and continues to assess the infant's fluid status, urinary output, and blood glucose levels. The interventions implemented are determined by the infant's specific disorder and nutritional needs.

Elimination Patterns. The infant's elimination patterns are assessed. This includes the frequency of urination, as well as the amount, color, pH, and specific gravity of the urine. The assessment of the infant's bowel movements includes the frequency of stooling and the character of the stool, as well as whether there is constipation, diarrhea, or loss of fats (steatorrhea). All of these findings are documented. The nurse may request guaiac tests to assess for blood in the stool, tests to detect stool-reducing substances, and a pH determination to assess for malabsorption. Infants with unexplained abdominal distention are assessed carefully to rule out the presence of hypomotility, obstructions of the GI tract, or necrotizing enterocolitis (NEC).

Oral Feeding. Nourishment by the oral route is preferred for the infant who has adequate strength and GI function. The best milk for an infant is from the mother. Breast milk can be fed by breast, bottle, cup, or spoon. Throughout the feeding the nurse assesses the newborn's tolerance of the procedure. Preterm infants can be put to breast for practice feeds and nonnutritive suckling as soon as medically stable. The nurse assists the mother by providing support and help as necessary when the infant breastfeeds. Referral to a lactation consultant is important.

The needs of the high risk infant must be considered when determining the type and frequency of the feedings. Many high risk infants cannot suck well enough to breastfeed or bottle feed

Video—Nursing Skills: Performing Newborn Gavage Feeding

until they have recovered from their initial illness or matured physically (corrected age more than 32 weeks of gestation). Mothers of high risk infants are encouraged to continue pumping breast milk, especially if theirs is a very premature infant who will not breastfeed for many weeks. Because of the significant breastfeeding attrition rates among these mothers, they need ongoing support and encouragement to continue pumping while their infant is not yet able to nurse. If no breast milk is available (from the mother or a milk bank), commercial formula is used. The calories, protein, and mineral content of commercial formulas vary. The type of nipple selected ("preemie," regular, orthodontic) depends on the infant's ability to suck from the specific type of nipple. The nurse also considers the energy the infant needs to expend in the process. However, the practice of delaying breastfeeding until the baby is able to effectively bottle-feed is not evidence based because studies continue to confirm that breastfeeding is less stressful than bottle feeding (Gardner & Lawrence, 2011).

Overfeeding of the preterm infant should be avoided because this can lead to abdominal distention, with apnea, vomiting, and possibly aspiration of the feeding. The nurse monitors the infant's abdominal girth when distention is obvious.

Gavage Feeding. Gavage feeding is a method of providing nourishment to the infant who is compromised by respiratory distress, the infant who is too immature to have a coordinated suck-and-swallow reflex, or the infant who is easily fatigued by sucking. In gavage feeding, breast milk or formula is given to the infant through a nasogastric or orogastric tube (Fig. 37-6). This spares the infant the work of sucking.

Gavage feeding can be done either with an intermittently placed tube providing a bolus feeding or continuously through an indwelling catheter. Infants who cannot tolerate large bolus feedings (those on ventilators for more than a week) are given continuous feedings. **Minimal enteral nutrition (MEN)** can be used to stimulate or prime the GI tract to achieve better absorption of nutrients when bolus or regular intermittent gavage feedings can be given (Blackburn, 2007).

Breast milk or formula can be supplied intermittently by using a syringe with gravity-controlled flow, or it can be given continuously by using an infusion pump. The type of fluid instilled is recorded with every syringe change. The volume of the continuous feedings is recorded hourly, and the residual gastric aspirate is measured every 2 to 4 hours. Aspirates of less than a one hour volume can be refed to the infant. For intermittent feedings, residuals of less than 50% of the previous feeding can be re-fed to the infant to prevent the loss of gastric electrolytes. Feeding is usually stopped if the residual is greater than 50% of the feeding or if residuals are increasing and is not resumed until the infant can be assessed for a possible feeding intolerance (Anderson, Wood, Keller, & Hay, 2011).

The orogastric route for gavage feedings is preferred because most infants are preferential nose breathers. Also when indwelling nasogastric tubes are used, there is a tendency toward nares necrosis; however, some infants do not tolerate oral tube placement. A small nasogastric feeding tube can be placed in older infants who would otherwise gag or vomit or in ones who are learning to suck. To insert the tube and give the feeding, the nurse should follow the sequence given in the Procedure box.

Gastrostomy Feedings. Gastrostomy feedings are used for infants with neurologic problems or certain congenital

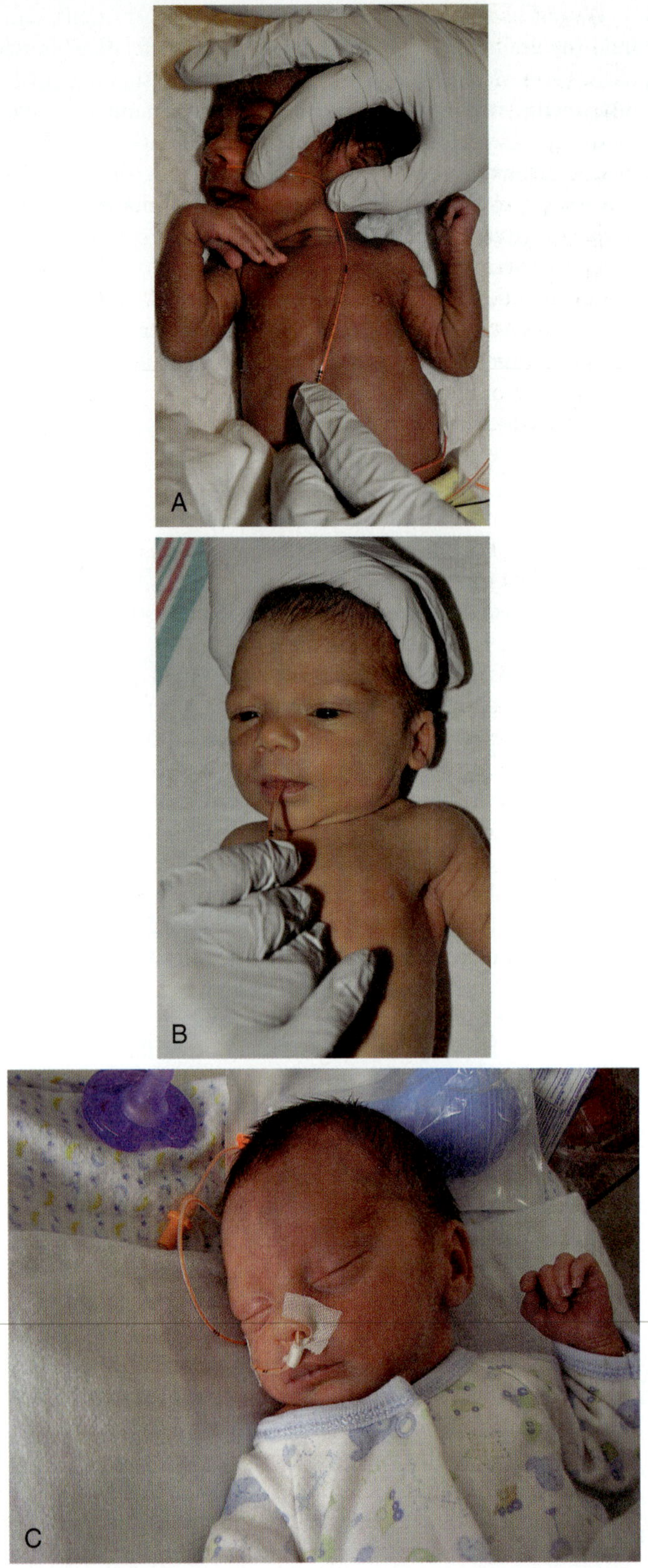

FIG. 37-6 Gavage feeding. **A,** Measurement of gavage feeding tube from tip of nose to earlobe and to midpoint between end of xiphoid process and umbilicus. Tape may be used to mark correct length on tube. For accurate measure, the infant should be facing up. **B,** Insertion of gavage tube using orogastric route. **C,** Indwelling gavage tube, nasogastric route. After feeding by orogastric or nasogastric tube, infant is propped on right side or placed prone (preterm infant) for 1 hour to facilitate emptying of stomach into small intestine. (**A** and **B,** Courtesy Cheryl Briggs, RNC, Annapolis, MD; **C,** courtesy Randi and Jacob Wills, Clayton, NC.)

PROCEDURE

Inserting a Gavage Feeding Tube

Equipment

- Infant feeding tube
  - For infants less than 1 kg, size 4-Fr tube
  - For infants more than 1 kg, size 5-Fr to 6-Fr
- Stethoscope
- Sterile water (lubricant)
- Syringe: 5 to 10 ml
- Tape, optional transparent dressing
- Gloves

1. Measure the length of the gavage tube from the tip of the nose to the earlobe to the midpoint between the xiphoid process and the umbilicus (see Fig. 37-6, *A*). Mark the tube with indelible ink or a piece of tape.
2. Lubricate the tip of the tube with sterile water and insert gently through the nose or mouth (see Fig. 37-6, *B*) until the predetermined mark is reached. Placement of the tube in the trachea will cause the infant to gag, cough, or become cyanotic.
3. Check correct placement of the tube by:
   a. Pulling back on the plunger to aspirate stomach contents. Lack of stomach aspirate or fluid is not necessarily evidence of improper placement. Aspiration of respiratory secretions may be mistaken for stomach contents; however, the pH of the stomach contents is much lower (more acidic) than the pH of respiratory secretions.
   b. Injecting a small amount of air (1-3 ml) into the tube while listening for gurgling by using a stethoscope placed over the stomach. Ensure that the tube is inserted to the mark; air entering the stomach may be heard even if the tube is positioned above the gastroesophageal (cardiac) sphincter.
   c. Abdominal or chest radiography. This is the only definitive way to verify tube placement.
4. Using tape or a transparent dressing, secure the tube in place and tape it to the cheek to prevent accidental dislodgment and incorrect positioning (see Fig. 37-6, *C*).
   a. Assess the infant's skin integrity before taping the tube.
   b. Edematous or very preterm infants should have a pectin barrier placed under the tape to prevent abrasions, or a hydrocolloid adhesive should be used to prevent epidermal stripping.
5. Tube placement *must* be assessed before each feeding.

Source: Anderson, M., Wood, L., Keller, J., & Hay, W. (2011). Enteral nutrition. In S. Gardner, B. Carter, M. Enzman-Hines, & J. Hernandez (Eds), *Merenstein & Gardner's handbook of neonatal intensive care* (7th ed.). St. Louis, Mosby.

malformations that require long-term gavage feedings (Ditzenberger, 2010). This involves the surgical placement of a tube through the skin of the abdomen into the stomach. The tube is then taped in an upright position to prevent trauma to the incision site. After the site heals, the nurse initiates small bolus feedings per the physician's orders. Feedings by gravity are done slowly over 20- to 30-minute periods. Special care must be taken to prevent rapid bolusing of the fluid because this can lead to abdominal distention, GI reflux into the esophagus, or respiratory compromise. Meticulous skin care at the tube insertion site is necessary to prevent skin breakdown or infections. In addition, intake and output are monitored scrupulously because these infants are prone to diarrhea until regular feedings are established.

Parenteral Nutrition. Supplemental parenteral fluids are indicated for infants who are unable to obtain sufficient fluids or calories by enteral feeding. Some of these infants are dependent on **total parenteral nutrition (TPN)** for extensive periods. The nurse assesses and documents the following in infants receiving parenteral fluids or TPN:

- Type and infusion rate of the solution
- Functional status of the infusion equipment, including the tubing and infusion pump
- Infusion site for possible complications (phlebitis, infiltration, dislodgment)
- Caloric intake
- Infant's responses to therapy

The physician or nurse practitioner orders TPN per the hospital protocol. These orders must specify the electrolytes and nutrients desired, as well as the volume and rate of infusion. The composition of calories, protein, and fats is calculated on an individual basis.

While caring for the infant receiving parenteral fluids or TPN, the nurse secures and protects the insertion site. Scrupulous hand hygiene is used before handling the TPN tubing or IV sites. Strict sterile technique is implemented for dressing changes (Ditzenberger, 2010). The nurse must observe the principles of neonatal skin care. The nurse also should inspect the infusion site for signs of infiltration and reposition the infant frequently to maintain body alignment and protect the site. Parents of infants need to be given explanations about TPN and the way in which the IV equipment and solutions affect their infant.

Advancing Infant Feedings. Feedings are advanced as assessment data and the infant's ability to tolerate the feedings warrant. Documentation of a preterm infant's sucking patterns also can be used to determine readiness to nipple feed. Feedings are advanced from passive (parenteral and gavage) to active (nipple and breastfeeding). At each step the nurse must carefully assess the infant's response to prevent overstressing the infant.

The infant receiving nutrition parenterally is gradually weaned off this type of nutrition. To do this the nourishment given by continuous or intermittent gavage feedings is increased while the parenteral fluids are decreased. Even the smallest infant is sometimes given MEN to stimulate the GI system to mature and to enhance caloric intake (Blackburn, 2007).

Feedings are advanced slowly and cautiously because if advanced too rapidly, the infant can develop vomiting (with an attendant risk of aspiration), diarrhea, abdominal distention, and apneic episodes. Rapid advancement also can cause fluid retention with cardiac compromise or a pronounced diuresis with hyponatremia.

If the infant needs additional calories, a commercial human milk fortifier can be added to the gavaged breast milk, or the number of calories per 30 ml of commercial formula can be increased. Soy and elemental formulas are used only for infants with very special dietary needs, such as allergies to cow's milk or chronic malabsorption. Calories in breast milk can be lost if the cream separates and adheres to the tubing during continuous infusion. This problem is decreased if microbore tubing is used for both continuous and intermittent gavage feedings.

The infant receiving gavage feedings progresses to bottle feeding or breast milk feedings. To do this the gavage feedings are decreased as the infant's ability to suckle breast milk or formula improves. Often during this transition, the infant is fed

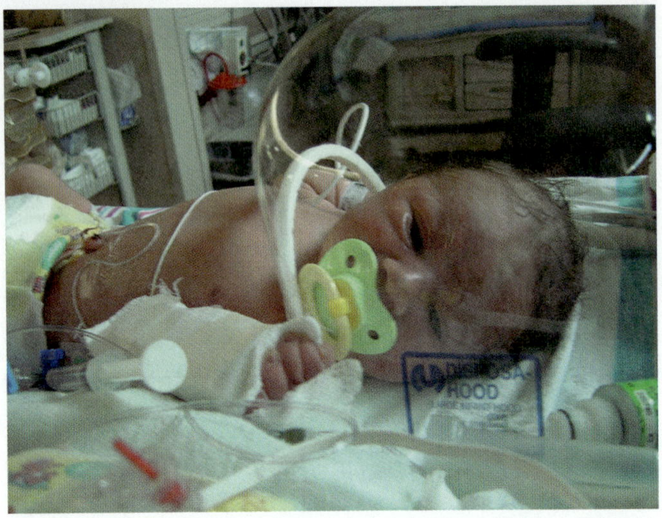

FIG. 37-7 Nonnutritive sucking. (Courtesy Lauren and Brian LiVecchi, Raleigh, NC.)

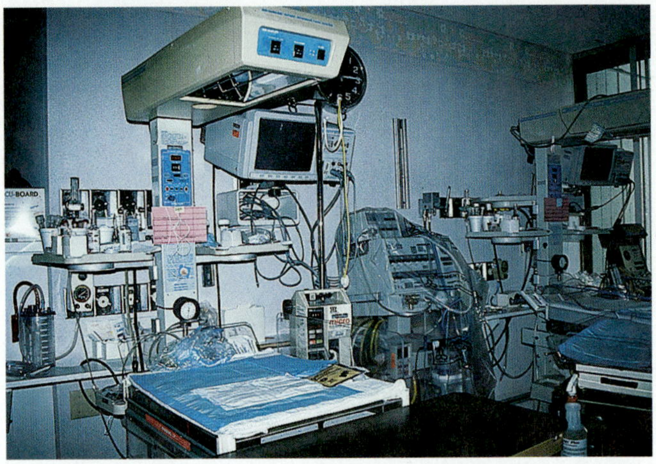

FIG. 37-8 Although necessary, neonatal intensive care unit equipment can contribute to significant environmental stimulation. Note bed, wall oxygen attachments, monitor, ventilator, incubator, and pumps, all of which have alarm systems. (Courtesy Marjorie Pyle, RNC, Lifecircle, Costa Mesa, CA.)

by both bottle or breast and gavage feeding to ensure the intake of both the prescribed volume of food and nutrients. However, when there is an indwelling tube, during breast or bottle feedings, some infants experience an increased respiratory effort, so nurses must watch for this. The parents need support during this transition because many families measure their parenting competence by how well they can feed their infant. For breastfed infants, it is important to weigh the infant before and after breastfeeding to determine the infant's intake (Hurst, 2007).

As the time of discharge nears, the appropriate method of feeding, as well as the assessments pertaining to the method (e.g., tolerance of feedings, status of gavage tube placement), are reviewed with the parents. The parents should be encouraged to interact with the infant by talking and making eye contact with the infant during the feeding. This is encouraged to stimulate the psychosocial development of the infant and to facilitate bonding and attachment.

Nonnutritive Sucking. If the gavage or the parenteral route nourishes the infant, **nonnutritive sucking** is encouraged for several reasons (Fig. 37-7). Allowing the infant to suck on a pacifier during gavage or between oral feedings can improve oxygenation. In addition, such nonnutritive sucking can lead to a decreased energy expenditure with less restlessness. It also promotes positive weight gain and better sucking skills (Harding, Law, & Pring, 2006).

Mothers of preterm infants should be encouraged to allow their infants to start sucking at the breast during kangaroo care (skin-to-skin). In some infants, the suck-and-swallow reflexes are coordinated as early as 32 weeks of gestation. If the neonate is unable to suck, the mother can place the infant near the nipple to encourage nuzzling or licking.

Infants with intrauterine growth restriction (IUGR) can have an age-appropriate sucking reflex but require thermoregulatory support, making it difficult to breastfeed. These infants also may benefit from nonnutritive sucking at the breast for short periods.

Skin Care

The skin of preterm infants is characteristically immature relative to that of full-term infants. Because of its increased sensitivity and fragility, the use of alkaline-based soap that might destroy the acid mantle of the skin is avoided. Vernix caseosa has benefits for the preterm infant's skin. Vernix acts as an epidermal barrier, decreases bacterial contamination of the skin through its antimicrobial peptides and proteins, and decreases transepidermal water loss (Lund, Kuller, Raines, Ecklund, Archambault, & O'Flaherty, 2007). Experts recommend that a validated skin assessment tool such as the Braden Q Scale or the Neonatal Skin Condition Score (NSCS) be used once daily to evaluate the high risk infant's skin condition so as to implement interventions aimed at minimizing skin breakdown (Curley, Razmus, Roberts, & Wypij, 2003; Lund & Osborne, 2004).

Environmental Concerns

Infants in NICUs also are exposed to high levels of auditory input from the various machine alarms, and this can have adverse effects (Fig. 37-8). In addition, continuous noise levels of 45 to 85 decibels (db) are common in NICUs. An incubator alone produces a constant noise level of 60 to 80 db, and each new piece of life-support equipment used adds another 20 db to the background noise. The infant's hearing may be damaged if it is exposed to a constant decibel level of 90 db or frequent decibel swings higher than 110 db. Cochlear damage has been recognized as a side effect of the NICU environment. Thus both conductive and sensorineural hearing losses have been identified in NICU graduates; these losses lead to long-term speech and language deficits (Haubrich, 2007; Krueger, Wall, Parker, & Nealis, 2005). Over time more emphasis has been placed on noise in the NICU and the adverse or long-term effects on neonates (White, 2007).

! NURSING ALERT

Routine hearing screening should be performed in all infants before discharge, with universal screening completed by no later than the third month of life.

Respiratory equipment or a phototherapy mask can alter the infant's vision, making it difficult for the infant to interact with caregivers and family members. The infant also may be unable to establish diurnal and nocturnal rhythms because of the continuous exposure to overhead lighting. In addition, sedation or pain medications affect the way in which the infant perceives the environment.

An additional concern in the care of infants is that some drugs used for infant therapy can potentiate environmental hazards. Diuretics (especially furosemide [Lasix]), antibiotics (gentamicin), and antimalarial agents can potentiate noise-induced hearing loss (Haubrich, 2007).

Research is ongoing to determine effects of light and noise on the preterm infant. Long-term problems are the focus of much research (Symington & Pinelli, 2006). Cycling of light and covering of incubators to reduce direct light hitting the retina are two areas of research. The retina of the immature infant has little protection from the nearly translucent eyelid, thus allowing light to almost continuously penetrate the retina unless it is artificially protected by dimming the lights or using incubator covers. Cycled lighting has been shown to have a positive effect on growth (White, 2007). Light and sound are adverse stimuli that add to an already stressed preterm infant. The result is stress cues, increased metabolic rate, increased oxygen and caloric use, and depression of the immune system. The nurse must monitor the macroenvironment and the microenvironment (unit and immediate environments) for sources of overstimulation. Providing a developmentally supportive environment can lead to decreased complications and length of stay. There are national recommendations for sound and light levels in the NICU.

Nurses can modify the environment to provide a developmentally supportive milieu. In that way the infant's neurobehavioral and physiologic needs can be better met, the infant's developing organization can be supported, and growth and development can be fostered (Symington & Pinelli, 2006).

Developmental Care

The goal of developmental care is to support each infant's efforts to become as well organized, competent, and stable as possible. Developmental care includes all care procedures and the physical and social aspects of care in the NICU (Als, Duffy, McAnulty, Rivkin, Vajapeyam, Mulkern, et al., 2004). The caregiver uses the infant's own behavior and physiologic functioning as the basis for planning care and providing interventions. Through caregiver observation, the infant's strengths, thresholds for disorganization, and vulnerable areas can be identified. The family is included in developmental care as the primary coregulators (Als et al.). Working together, the family and other caregivers provide opportunities to enhance the strengths of the family and the infant and to reduce the stress that is associated with the birth and care of high risk infants.

Reducing light and noise levels by instituting "quiet hours" at regularly scheduled times and positioning are just two of the ways in which nurses can support infants in their development. Sleep interruptions are minimized, and positioning and bundling the infant help promote self-regulation and prevent disorganization (Symington & Pinelli, 2006).

Positioning. The motor development of preterm infants permits less flexion than in term infants. Caregivers can provide a variety of positions for infants; side-lying and prone are preferred to supine (but only in the nursery) (Fig. 37-9). Body containment with use of blanket rolls, swaddling, holding the infant's arms in a crossed position, and secure holding provide boundaries. Use of facilitated tucking promotes self-regulation during feeding, procedures, and other stressful interventions. The prone position encourages flexion of the extremities; a sling or hip roll assists in maintaining flexion. Keeping the extremities close to the body helps calm the infant and decreases stimulation. Proper body alignment is necessary to prevent developmental problems that can affect the ability to walk as the child matures (Carrier, 2010).

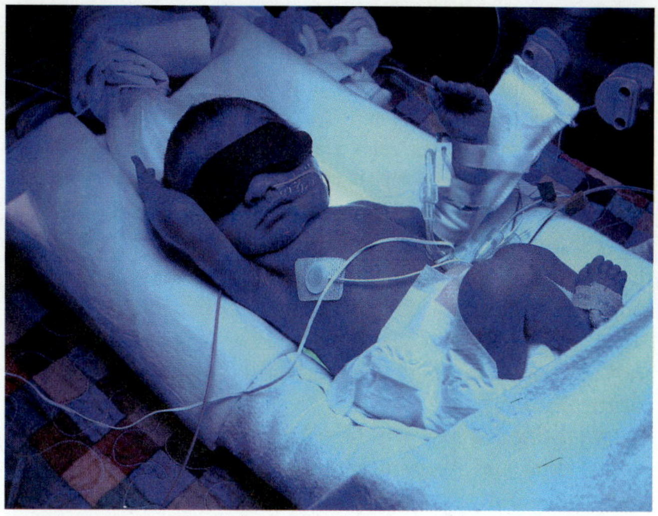

FIG. 37-9 Developmental care: positioning of preterm infant using containment while undergoing phototherapy. (Courtesy Randi and Jacob Wills, Clayton, NC.)

Reducing Inappropriate Stimuli. Staff can reduce unnecessary noise by closing doors or portholes on incubators quietly, placing only necessary objects gently on top of incubators, keeping radios at low volume, speaking quietly, and handling equipment noiselessly. Another source is internal noise created by mechanical sources such as CPAP. These noise sources must be considered when thinking about long-term effects on hearing. Earmuffs can be used during scans and transports (Mathur, Neil, McKinstry, & Inder, 2008).

Infants can be protected from light by dimming the lights during the night, placing a blanket over the incubator, or covering the infant's eyes with a mask. Sleep-wake cycles can be induced with such measures. Infants need periods in which there are no disruptions and sleep can occur. Clustering of care can promote longer uninterrupted periods of sleep (Carrier, 2010).

Infant Communication. Infants communicate their needs and ability to tolerate sensory stimulation through physiologic responses. The nurses and parents of high risk infants must therefore be alert to such cues. Although term infants may thrive on stimulation, this same stimulation in high risk infants can provoke physical symptoms of stress and anxiety (Symington & Pinelli, 2006).

Problems with noxious stimuli and barriers to normal contact can cause anxiety and tension. Clues to overstimulation include averting the gaze, hiccuping, gagging, or regurgitating food. Term infants exhibit a startle reflex, and preterm infants move all of their limbs in an uncoordinated fashion in response to noxious stimuli. An irregular respiratory rate or an increased heart rate can develop in severely distressed infants, and they may be unable to regain a calm state.

A relaxed infant state is indicated by stabilization of vital signs, closed eyes, and a relaxed posture. Nonintubated infants may make soothing verbal sounds when they are relaxed. Infants requiring artificial ventilation cannot cry audibly and often show their distress through posturing; they relax once their needs are met. As high risk infants heal and mature, they increasingly respond to stimuli in a self-regulated manner rather than with a dissociated response. Infants who do not show increased self-regulation should be evaluated for a neurologic problem.

Infant Stimulation. The Newborn Individualized Developmental Care and Assessment Program (NIDCAP, 2009) routinely integrates aspects of neurodevelopmental theory with caregivers' observations, environmental interventions, and parental support. Routine reassessment is built into the program's design. Developmental stimuli may consist of such simple measures as placing a waterbed mattress on the top of the infant's mattress, or kangaroo holding. The simplest calming technique is for the caregiver to use both hands to contain the infant's extremities close to the body. The care of the infant is organized to allow extended periods of undisturbed rest and sleep. Pain medications or sedatives should be administered consistently per the unit's protocol.

Infants acquire a sense of trust as they learn the feel, sound, and smell of their parents. High risk infants also must learn to trust their caregivers to obtain comfort. However, caregivers in the nursery also can inflict pain as part of the care they must give. For this reason it is important for parents and caregivers to use comforting interventions such as removing painful stimuli, stopping hunger, and changing wet or soiled clothing to foster trust. They can offer nonnutritive sucking or use oral sucrose for pain relief and topical creams before procedures to avoid pain. All of these techniques are part of developmental, supportive care (Carrier, 2010).

When the infant is ready for stimulation, the nurse has many options. Most infants can tolerate being held, even if only for short periods. Additional ways for the nurse or parents to stimulate infants include cuddling, rocking, singing, use of music therapy, and talking to the infant. These activities are beneficial and promote growth and weight gain as well as shorten the length of hospital stay. Stroking the infant's skin during medical therapy can provide tactile stimulation. The caregiver responds to the infant's cues by offering reassurance, providing nonnutritive sucking, stroking the infant's back, and talking to the infant. Infant massage is gaining evidence as a way to promote weight gain (Gardner & Goldson, 2011).

Mobiles and decals that can be changed frequently may be placed within the infant's visual range to stimulate the infant visually. Wind-up musical toys provide rhythmic distractions as long as they are not too loud. If the infant is receiving phototherapy, the protective eyepatches are removed periodically (e.g., during feeding) so that the infant can see the caregiver's face for short, comforting sessions.

Kangaroo Care. Although it must be individually adjusted, kangaroo care and short periods of gentle massage can help reduce stress in preterm infants (Fig. 37-10). The parent is bare-chested or may wear a loose-fitting, open-front top that has a modified marsupial-like pocket carrier for the infant. The undressed (except for diaper) infant is placed in a vertical position on the parent's bare chest, which permits direct eye contact, skin-to-skin sensations, and close proximity. Skin-to-skin contact can have a positive healing effect for the mother who had a high risk pregnancy. Additional benefits include early contact with mechanically ventilated infants, maintenance of neonatal thermal stability and oxygen saturation, increased feeding vigor and enhanced breastfeeding, maintenance of organized state, decreased pain perception during painful heelsticks, and minimal untoward effects of being held. The National Association of Neonatal Nurses developed a clinical practice guideline for kangaroo care for the stable healthy preterm infant ages 30 weeks or more of gestation (Ludington-Hoe, Morgan, & Abouelfettoh, 2008).

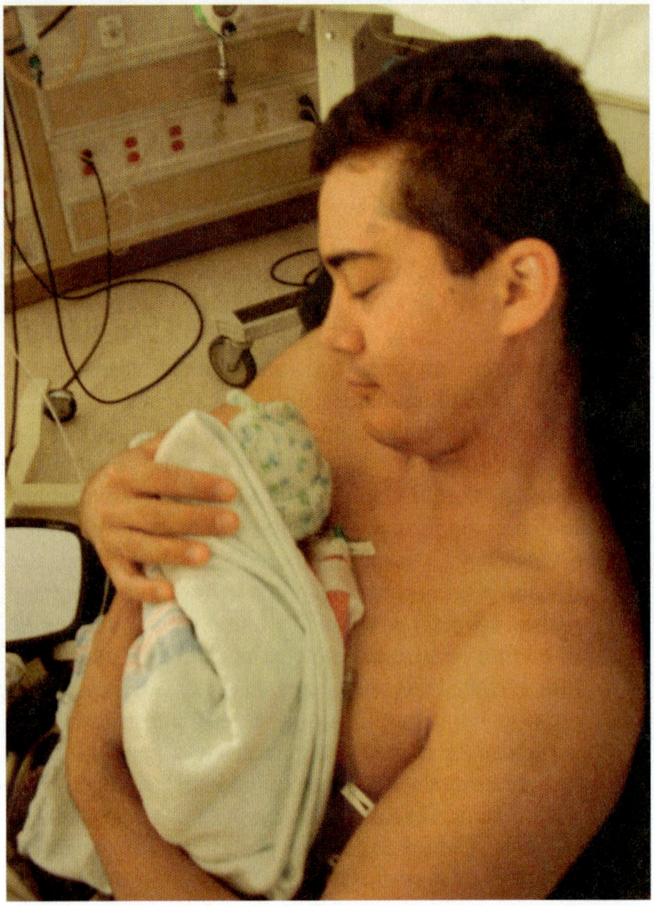

FIG. 37-10 Father holding infant in kangaroo care (Courtesy Randi and Jacob Wills, Clayton, NC.)

Parental Adaptation to Preterm Infant

Parents of premature infants often have difficulty in bonding and relating to their babies. The need to be empowered to recognize their competence and achieve competence is the basis of the Creating Opportunities for Parent Empowerment (COPE) program. This early educational-behavioral intervention model promotes more positive parent-infant interactions and enhanced ability to read and respond to infant cues (Melnyk, Feinstein, Alpert-Gillis, Fairbanks, Crean, Sinkin, et al., 2006; Siegel, Gardner, & Dickey, 2011).

Spanish Guidelines—Intensive Care Nursery: Parent Teaching on First Visit

Spanish Guidelines—Intensive Care Nursery: Parent Teaching on First Visit

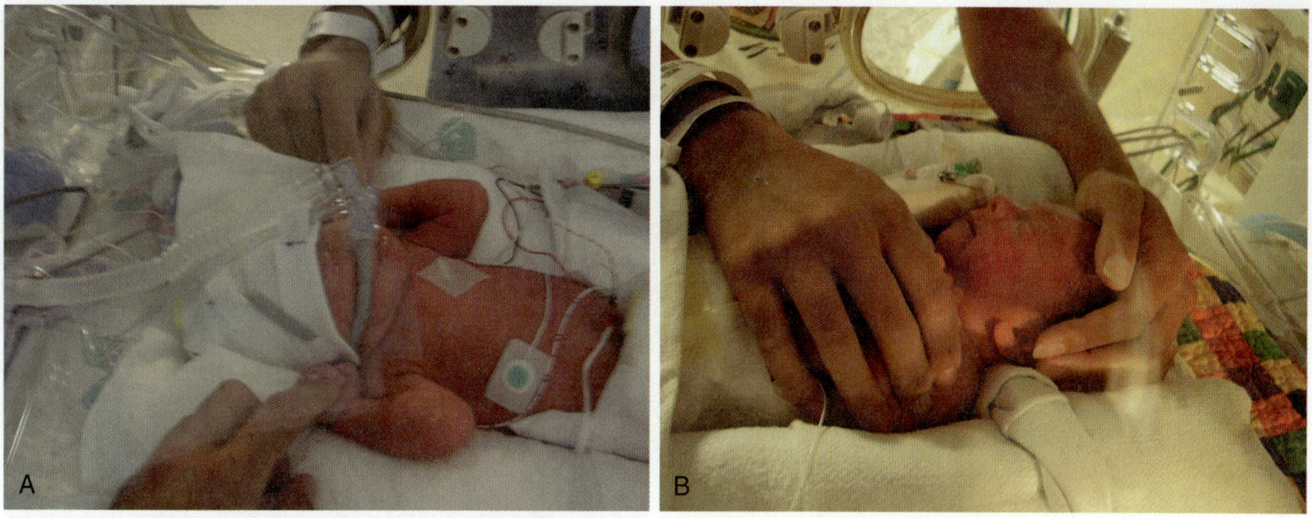

Fig. 37-11 **A**, Mother and father touch preterm infant. **B**, Mother caresses preterm infant. (Courtesy Randi and Jacob Wills, Clayton, NC.)

Parental Tasks. Parents of preterm infants must accomplish numerous psychologic tasks before effective relationships and parenting patterns can evolve. These tasks include the following:

- Experiencing **anticipatory grief** over the potential loss of an infant. The parent grieves in preparation for the infant's possible death, although the parent clings to the hope that the infant will survive. This process begins during labor and lasts until the infant dies or shows evidence of surviving. Anticipatory grief occurs when families have knowledge of an impending loss, such as when a baby is admitted to an NICU with problems or when a diagnosis of an anencephalic fetus is made with ultrasonography. The baby is still alive, but the prognosis is poor. Being able to anticipate the loss gives families an opportunity to plan, feel more in control of their situation, and say good-bye in a special way. However, some individuals or family members distance or detach themselves from the experience or from their loved ones as a way of protecting themselves from the pain of loss and grief. How a parent responds to this situation depends on religious, spiritual, and cultural beliefs. These must be considered when planning care. The nurse's role is to advocate for the family so that other health professionals realize that the family is grieving. Being fully present for these families and practicing active listening is important (see Chapter 38).
- The mother's acceptance of her failure to give birth to a healthy full-term infant. Grief and depression typify this phase, which persists until the infant is out of danger and is expected to survive.
- Resuming the process of relating to the infant. As the baby's condition begins to improve and the baby gains weight, is able to breastfeed or bottle-feed, and is weaned from the incubator or radiant warmer, the parent can begin the process of developing an attachment to the infant that was interrupted by the infant's critical condition at birth.
- Learning about the ways in which this baby differs in terms of his or her special needs and growth patterns, caregiving needs, and growth and development expectations.
- Adjusting the home environment to accommodate the needs of the new infant. Parents are encouraged to limit the number of visitors to minimize exposure of the infant to pathogens. The environmental temperature may have to be altered to optimize conditions for the infant.

Parental Responses. Physical contact with the infant is important to establish early bonding. If it is not possible for parents to hold the infant, they can touch and stroke the baby as they speak softly (Fig. 37-11). As the infant's condition improves, parents can hold the neonate and provide kangaroo care (see Fig. 37-10). They gradually begin to participate in infant activities, such as feeding, bathing, and changing. Parents go through numerous phases of adjustment as they learn to parent their infant. Nurses facilitate the transition to parenthood through their teaching and support of parental efforts.

Parental Support. The nurse as the support person and teacher is responsible for shaping the environment and making the caregiving responsive to the needs of the parents and infant. Nurses are instrumental in helping parents learn who their infant is and to recognize behavioral cues in his or her development and to use these cues in the care they provide (Aagaard & Hall, 2008; Carrier, 2010).

When a high risk birth is anticipated, the family can be given a tour of the NICU or shown a video to prepare them for the sights and activities of the unit. After an unanticipated preterm birth, the parents can be given a booklet, view a video, or have someone describe what they will see when they go to the unit to see their infant. As soon as possible, the parents should see and touch their infant so that they can begin to acknowledge the reality of the birth and the infant's true appearance and condition. They will need encouragement as they begin to accomplish the psychologic tasks imposed by the high risk birth. For the following reasons, a nurse or physician should be present during the parents' first visit to see the infant:

- To help them "see" the infant rather than focus on the equipment. The importance and purpose of the equipment that surrounds their infant should be explained to them.

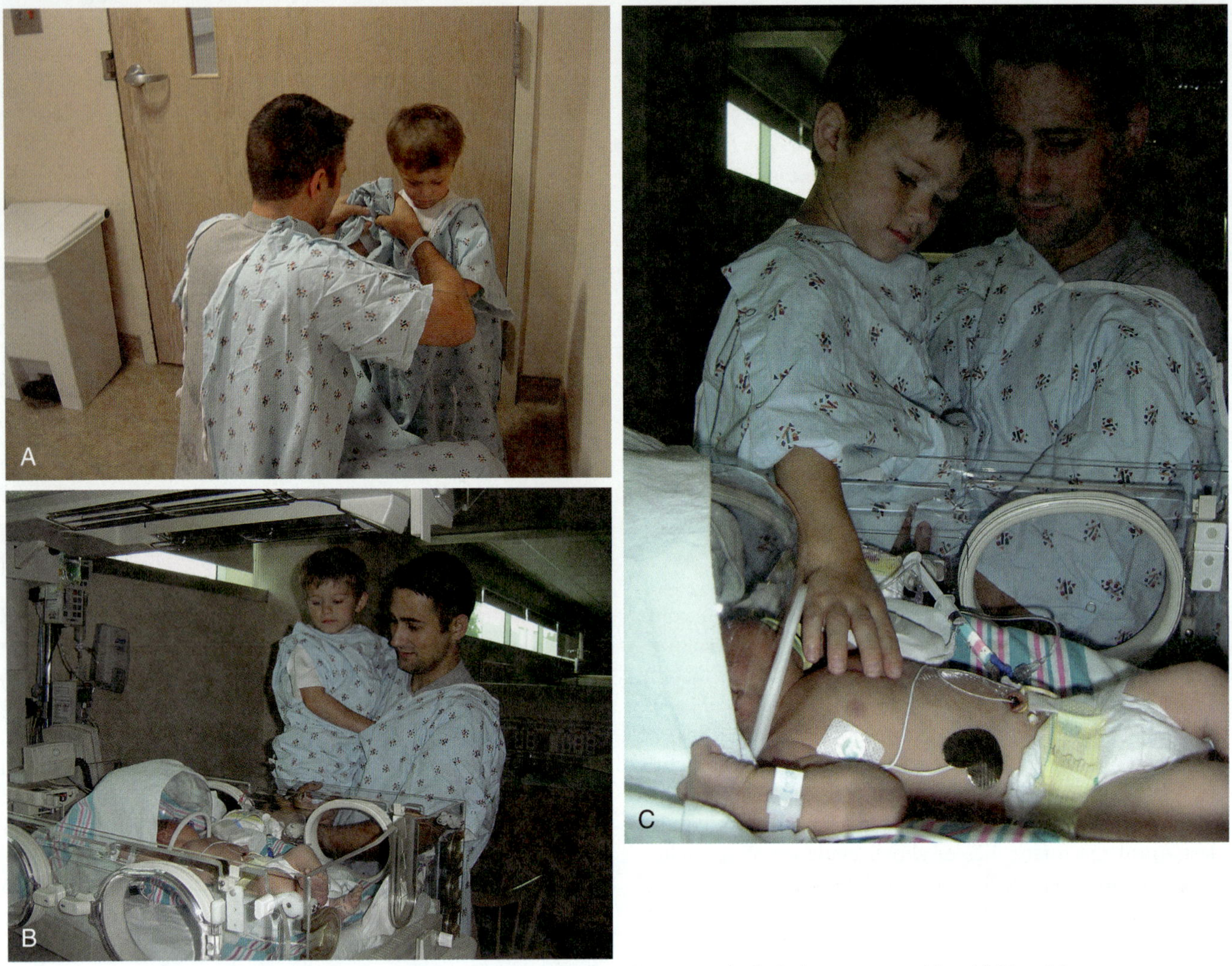

FIG. 37-12 Sibling visits newborn in the neonatal intensive care unit. **A,** Father prepares older child for visit. **B,** Sibling observes neonate at a safe distance. **C,** He reaches out to touch the infant. (Courtesy Lauren and Brian LiVecchi, Raleigh, NC.)

- To explain the characteristics normal for an infant of their baby's gestational age; in this way parents do not compare their child with a term, healthy infant.
- To encourage the parents to express their feelings about the pregnancy, labor, and birth and the experience of having a high risk infant
- To assess the parents' perceptions of the infant to determine the appropriate time for them to become actively involved in care

As soon as possible after the birth, the parents are given the opportunity to meet the infant in the en face position, to touch the infant, and to see his or her favorable characteristics. The premature or sick baby's appearance can be stressful to the parents. As soon as possible, depending primarily on her physical condition, the mother is encouraged to visit the nursery as desired and help with the infant's care. When the family cannot be present physically, staff members devise appropriate methods to keep them in almost constant touch with the newborn, such as with daily phone calls, notes written as if by the infant, or photographs of the infant.

The birth of a preterm or high risk infant affects the entire family. Nurses need to consider responses and reactions of grandparents and siblings as they provide individualized family-centered care for the infant and family. Grandparents often experience grief and sadness as they watch their own children experiencing the difficulties and challenges of having a preterm or high risk infant. They worry and are concerned about the well-being of their grandchild. Siblings also react to the birth of the preterm or high risk infant. If they are old enough to realize that the mother was supposed to be bringing home a new baby, they can be very confused when the baby must remain in the hospital. When possible it can be helpful to allow siblings to visit the new baby in the NICU environment so that they can see the infant (Fig. 37-12). Once the infant is brought home, some children are bewildered and angry at the seemingly disproportionate amount of parental time spent on the newborn. Nurses can facilitate visits by grandparents and siblings while the infant is hospitalized and can help parents anticipate possible reactions of siblings once the baby is discharged.

Some hospitals have support groups for the parents of infants in NICUs. These groups help parents experiencing anxiety and grief by encouraging them to share their feelings. Hospitals also often arrange to have an experienced NICU parent make contact with a new group member to provide additional support. The volunteer parents provide support by making hospital visits, phone calls, and home visits. Mothers in particular are prone to posttraumatic stress that can hinder their ability to interact with or care for their infant (Holditch-Davis, Bartlett, Blickman, & Miles, 2003). They need help in expressing their feelings and, when appropriate, referral for psychologic or family counseling.

Many NICUs use volunteers in varying capacities. After they have gone through the orientation program, volunteers can perform tasks such as holding the infants, stocking bedside cabinets, assembling parent packets, and, in some nurseries, feeding the infants.

Parental Maladaptation. The incidence of physical and emotional abuse is increased in infants who, because of preterm birth or high risk condition, are separated from their parents for a time after birth. Physical abuse includes varying degrees of poor nutrition, poor hygiene, and bodily harm. Emotional abuse ranges from subtle disinterest to outright dislike of the infant. Appropriate resources should be made available to assess the parent's feelings regarding the preterm infant's birth. In addition, proper guidance and counseling are made available, including posthospital discharge, to help families adjust to and care for the preterm infant. The ultimate goal is for the family to accept the infant and incorporate this new member into the existing family structure.

Parent Education

Some high risk infants can be discharged earlier than the expected time. The criteria showing an infant's readiness for early discharge are that the infant's physiologic condition is stable, the infant is receiving adequate nutrition, and the infant's body temperature is stable. The parents, or other caregivers, also need to exhibit physical, emotional, and educational readiness to assume responsibility for the care of the infant. Ideally, the home environment is adequate for meeting the needs of the infant. The parents also need to show that they know how to take the infant's temperature, know the signs and symptoms to report, and understand the dietary needs of the infant. Resources for parents and health care providers include http://prematurc-infant.com, www.vort.com/age/premature.html. www.neonatology.org, and www.familyvillage.wisc.edu.

Complications in High Risk Infants

Respiratory Distress Syndrome

Respiratory distress syndrome (RDS) refers to a lung disorder usually affecting preterm infants. Maternal and fetal conditions associated with a decreased incidence and severity of RDS include female gender, African-American race, maternal gestational hypertension, maternal drug abuse, maternal steroid therapy (betamethasone), chronic retroplacental abruption, prolonged rupture of membranes, and IUGR. The incidence and severity of RDS increase with a decrease in the gestational age. Perinatal asphyxia, hypovolemia, male gender, Caucasian race, maternal diabetes (types 1 and 2), second-born twin, familial predisposition, maternal hypotension, cesarean birth without labor, hydrops fetalis, and third-trimester bleeding are all factors that place an infant at increased risk for RDS. The incidence of RDS in infants weighing less than 1500 g is between 40% and 60% (Carlo, 2007; Cifuentes & Carlo, 2007).

RDS is caused by a lack of pulmonary surfactant, which leads to progressive atelectasis, loss of functional residual capacity, and a ventilation-perfusion imbalance with an uneven distribution of ventilation. This surfactant deficiency can be caused by insufficient surfactant production, abnormal composition and function, disruption of surfactant production, or a combination of these factors. The weak respiratory muscles and an overly compliant chest wall, common among preterm infants, further compromise the sequence of events that occurs. Lung capacity is further compromised by the presence of proteinaceous material and epithelial debris in the airways. The resulting decreased oxygenation, cyanosis, and metabolic or respiratory acidosis can cause the pulmonary vascular resistance (PVR) to be increased. This increased PVR can lead to right-to-left shunting and a reopening of the ductus arteriosus and foramen ovale (Fig. 37-13).

Clinical symptoms of RDS usually appear immediately after or within 6 hours of birth. Physical examination reveals crackles, poor air exchange, pallor, the use of accessory muscles (retractions) and, occasionally, apnea. Radiographic findings include a uniform reticulogranular appearance and air bronchograms (Rodriguez, Martin, & Fanaroff, 2006). The infant's clinical course typically is variable, usually with an increased oxygen requirement and increased respiratory effort as atelectasis, a loss of functional residual capacity, and ventilation-perfusion imbalance worsen.

RDS is a self-limiting disease that abates after 72 hours. This disappearance of respiratory signs coincides with the production of surfactant in the type 2 cells of the alveoli.

The treatment for RDS is supportive. Adequate ventilation and oxygenation must be established and maintained in an attempt to prevent ventilation-perfusion mismatch and atelectasis. Exogenous surfactant may be administered at birth or shortly after; this has the effect of altering the typical course of RDS. Positive-pressure ventilation, bubble CPAP, and oxygen therapy can be necessary during the respiratory illness. The prevention of complications associated with mechanical ventilation is critical. These complications include pulmonary interstitial emphysema, pneumothorax, pneumomediastinum, and pneumopericardium. The mortality and morbidity rates associated with RDS are attributed to the immature organ systems of the infant and the complications associated with the treatment of the disease (Rodriguez et al., 2006).

Acid-base balance is evaluated by monitoring the ABG values (Table 37-2). Frequent blood sampling requires arterial access either by umbilical artery catheterization or by a peripheral arterial line. Pulse oximetry and transcutaneous carbon dioxide and oxygen monitors document trends in ventilation and oxygenation. Capillary blood gas values indicate the pH and Pco_2 status in infants who are in more stable condition.

The maintenance of an NTE is critical to the care of infants with RDS. Infants with hypoxemia are unable to increase their metabolic rate when they experience cold stress (Rodriguez et al., 2006).

The clinical and radiographic presentation (radiodense lung fields and air bronchograms) of neonatal pneumonia can be similar to that of RDS. Fluid in the minor tissue also can be noted in infants with neonatal pneumonia. Therefore, sepsis evaluation, including blood culture and complete blood count (CBC) with differential, is done in infants with RDS to rule out

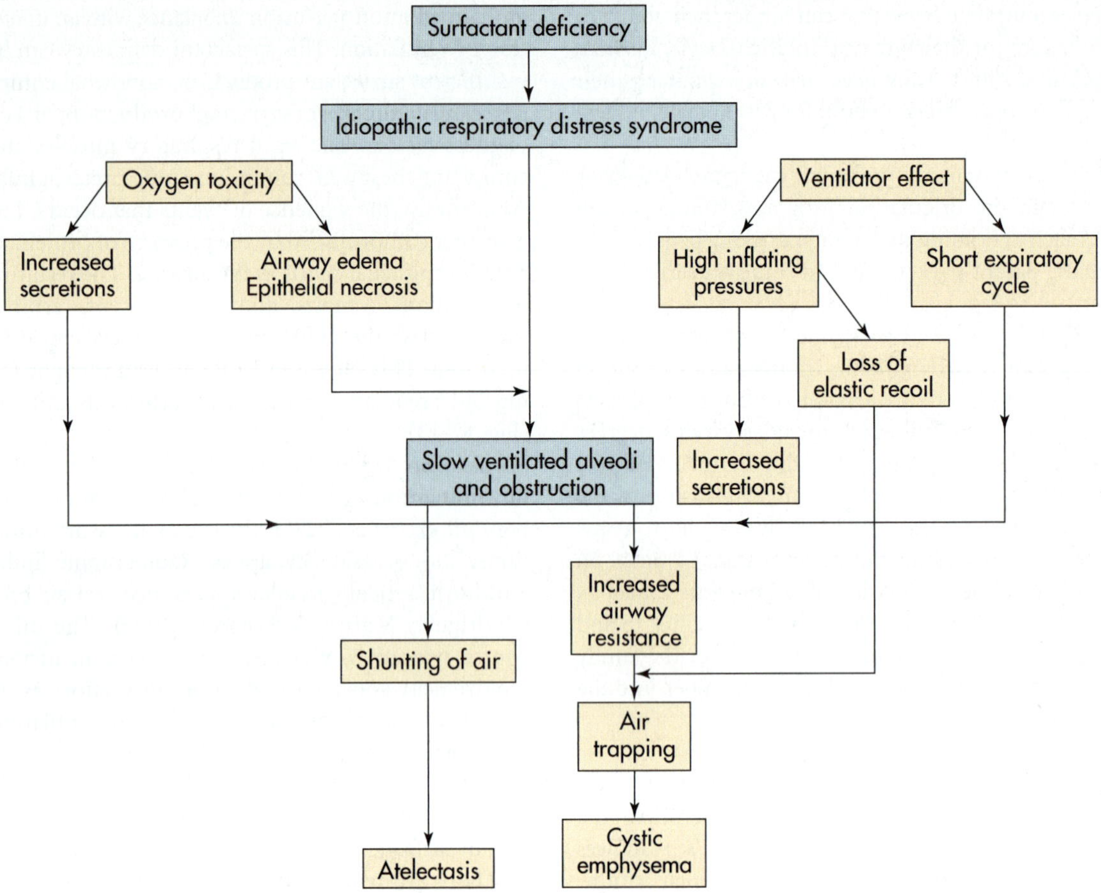

FIG. 37-13 Pathogenesis of respiratory distress syndrome (RDS). (Source: Gardner, S., Enzman-Hines, M., & Dickey, L. [2011]. Respiratory diseases. In S. Gardner, B. Carter, M. Enzman-Hines, & J. Hernandez [Eds.], *Merenstein and Gardner's handbook of neonatal intensive care* [7th ed.]. St. Louis: Mosby.)

TABLE 37-2 NORMAL ARTERIAL BLOOD GAS VALUES FOR NEONATES

VALUE	RANGE
pH	7.35-7.45
Arterial oxygen pressure (Pao_2)	60-80 mm Hg
Carbon dioxide pressure ($Paco_2$)	35-45 mm Hg
Bicarbonate (HCO^-_3)	18-26 mEq/L
Base excess	(−5) to (+5)
Oxygen saturation	92%-94%

Source: Wood, A. & Jones, D. (2011). Acid-base homeostasis and oxygenation. In S. Gardner, B. Carter, M. Enzman-Hines, & J. Hernandez (Eds.), *Merenstein & Gardner's handbook of neonatal intensive care* (7th ed.). St. Louis: Mosby.

neonatal pneumonia. Occasionally a lumbar puncture is done as part of the sepsis evaluation. Broad-spectrum antibiotics are begun while the results of cultures are awaited.

Fluid and nutrition must be maintained in the critically ill infant with RDS. Parenteral nutrition can be implemented to provide protein and fats to promote a positive nitrogen balance. Daily monitoring of the electrolyte values, urinary output, specific gravity, and weight help evaluate the infant's hydration status.

Frequent blood sampling can make blood transfusions necessary. The critically ill infant usually needs to have a venous hematocrit level of more than 40% to maintain adequate oxygen-carrying capacity.

! NURSING ALERT

Directed-donor blood may be requested by the family. This donor blood usually is obtained from a family member or close friend of the family who has the same blood type as the infant or a compatible blood type. It may be necessary to notify the infant's family of the potential need for blood transfusion on admission to allow for the processing of directed-donor blood.

Reassuring the family that stringent testing of all blood products is done can help alleviate some of their anxiety about the transmission of blood-borne pathogens such as human immunodeficiency virus (HIV) and hepatitis B. Because some religions prohibit the use of blood transfusions, it is critical to obtain a complete history from the family, including their religious preference. Alternative strategies for maintaining the infant's hematocrit may be used in these instances.

Complications Associated with Oxygen Therapy

Retinopathy of Prematurity. Retinopathy of prematurity (ROP) is a complex multicausal disorder that affects the developing retinal vessels of preterm infants. The normal retinal vessels begin to form in utero at approximately 16 weeks in response to an unknown stimulus. These vessels continue to develop until they reach maturity at approximately 42 to 43 weeks after conception. Once the retina is completely vascularized, the retinal vessels are not susceptible to ROP. The mechanism of injury in ROP is unclear. Oxygen tensions that are too high for the level of retinal maturity initially result in vasoconstriction. After oxygen therapy is discontinued, neovascularization occurs in the retina and vitreous, with capillary hemorrhages, fibrotic resolution, and possible retinal detachment. Scar tissue formation and consequent visual impairment can be mild or severe. The entire disease process in severe cases can take as long as several months to evolve. Examination by an ophthalmologist before discharge and a schedule for repeated examinations thereafter are recommended for the parents' guidance (Askin & Diehl-Jones, 2009b; Strodtbeck, 2007).

The key to the management of ROP is prevention of preterm birth and early detection. Blood oxygen levels in the preterm infant should be closely monitored and significant fluctuations avoided. Oxygen and ventilator settings should be adjusted to keep oxygen saturations within acceptable levels. Cryotherapy and laser photocoagulation are common treatments for ROP (Askin & Diehl-Jones, 2009b). Researchers are examining the effect of the NICU environment on the development of ROP in relation to light that shines directly through the very thin eyelid of very immature infants. Ambient lighting in the NICU is known to have an effect on the developing eye; although it may not directly cause ROP, it does contribute to other visual problems for the preterm infant. Another potential contributor to ROP is hyperglycemia, which apparently fosters vasoproliferation (Ertl, Gyarmati, Gaal, & Szabo, 2006). This factor needs much more study.

Bronchopulmonary Dysplasia. Bronchopulmonary dysplasia (BPD) is a chronic pulmonary iatrogenic condition caused by barotrauma from pressure ventilation and oxygen toxicity. The etiology of BPD is multifactorial and includes pulmonary immaturity, surfactant deficiency, lung injury and stretch, barotrauma, inflammation caused by oxygen exposure, fluid overload, ligation of a PDA, and a familial predisposition. With the advent of prenatal use of maternal steroids when preterm birth is expected coupled with use of exogenous surfactant in the neonate, most BPD or chronic lung disease (CLD) has been eliminated (Askin & Diehl-Jones, 2009a).

Clinical signs of BPD include tachypnea, retractions, nasal flaring, increased work of breathing, exercise intolerance (to handling and feeding), and tachycardia. Infants with BPD can have an increase in ventilatory requirements or are unable to be weaned from the ventilator. Auscultation of the lung fields in affected infants typically reveals crackles, decreased air movement, and occasionally expiratory wheezing. Hypoxia, hypercapnia, and respiratory acidosis are common (Askin, 2010).

The treatment for BPD includes oxygen therapy, nutrition, fluid restriction, and medications (diuretics, corticosteroids, bronchodilators). However, the key to the management of BPD is prevention of prematurity and RDS. Other therapies that can aid in prevention of BPD include antenatal steroids, prophylactic surfactant, avoidance of mechanical ventilation when possible, use of CPAP, gentle ventilation in the delivery room, and administration of vitamin A. Oxygen therapy may be continued in the home setting (Askin & Diehl-Jones, 2009a).

The prognosis for infants with BPD depends on the degree of pulmonary dysfunction and on the infant's overall health status. There is usually progressive normalization of pulmonary function, although abnormalities of small airways can persist. Mortality rates after hospital discharge are less than 10%; deaths are often due to complications such as respiratory infection (Askin, 2010).

Patent Ductus Arteriosus. The ductus arteriosus is a normal muscular contractile structure in the fetus connecting the left pulmonary artery and the dorsal aorta, diverting blood to the placenta for gas exchange. The duct constricts after birth as oxygenation, the levels of circulating prostaglandins, and the muscle mass increase. Other factors that promote ductal closure include catecholamines, low pH, bradykinin, and acetylcholine. When the fetal ductus arteriosus fails to close after birth, patent ductus arteriosus (PDA) occurs. During the first few days of life when a preterm or sick infant is under stress, the ductus arteriosus can reopen, leading to mottling and cyanosis. It can last only a few minutes until the stress is past, or it can remain open if the infant is quite unstable. The incidence of PDA in preterm infants is 20%, with an increasing incidence in VLBW infants and those with pulmonary disease (Carlo, Martin, & Fanaroff, 2006).

Critical Thinking Exercise—Patent Ductus Arteriosus

Although a small PDA can be asymptomatic, the clinical presentation in an infant with a significant PDA includes systolic murmur, active precordium, bounding peripheral pulses, tachycardia, tachypnea, crackles, and hepatomegaly. The systolic murmur is heard best at the second or third intercostal space at the upper left sternal border. An increased left ventricular stroke volume causes an active precordium.

Radiographic studies in infants with PDA typically show cardiac enlargement and pulmonary edema. ABG findings reveal hypercapnia and metabolic acidosis. Definitive diagnosis is through echocardiography, which can visualize a PDA and measure the amount of blood shunting across the PDA (Sadowski, 2010).

Medical management consists of ventilatory support, fluid restriction, and the administration of diuretics and indomethacin or ibuprofen (Ohlsson, Walia, & Shah, 2008; Sadowski, 2010). Ibuprofen and indomethacin inhibit prostaglandin synthesis and cause the PDA to constrict. There is some concern that indomethacin reduces blood flow to the brain, kidneys, and GI tract (Ohlsson et al.).

Ventilatory support is adjusted based on the ABG values. Fluid restriction and diuretic therapy are implemented to decrease cardiovascular volume overload. Surgical ligation is done when a PDA is clinically significant and medical management is ineffective.

Nursing management of the infant with PDA focuses on supportive care. The infant needs an NTE, adequate oxygenation, meticulous fluid balance, and parental support.

Germinal Matrix Hemorrhage–Intraventricular Hemorrhage. Germinal matrix hemorrhage–intraventricular hemorrhage (GMH-IVH) is one of the most common types of brain injury in neonates and is among the most severe from the standpoint of both short- and long-term outcomes. It is the most common type of intracranial hemorrhage, occurring almost exclusively in preterm infants. The risk of GMH-IVH increases with decreasing gestational age. The incidence of GMH-IVH is estimated to be 5% to 11%; it has shown a decline in recent years (de Vries, 2006). The decline in incidence is attributed to the prenatal use of corticosteroids and postnatal use of surfactant.

The germinal matrix is a loose network of cells abundantly supplied with tiny, fragile, thin-walled vessels. It lies beneath the lining of the lateral ventricles. This area is present and active until 34 to 35 weeks of gestation as a site for production of neurons and glial cells that gradually migrate to the cerebral cortex. The germinal matrix is especially vulnerable to alterations in cerebral blood flow related to blood pressure changes. Hemorrhage occurs when the tiny blood vessels rupture; the hemorrhage can extend into the lateral ventricles, then to the third and fourth ventricles, the subarachnoid space, and even into the white matter of the brain. Large clots can develop and create outflow obstruction from the ventricles (Volpe, 2008).

Infants who experience GMH-IVH are usually less than 34 weeks of gestation with a history of hypoxia, birth asphyxia, RDS, or other events causing impaired venous return or increased venous pressure. GMH-IVH is diagnosed in 50% of preterm infants within the first 24 hours and in 90% within the first 4 days. The hemorrhage progresses during the first few days of life in 20% to 40% of infants. Infants with GMH-IVH can be asymptomatic, develop symptoms gradually, or have an acute catastrophic presentation. Clinical signs suggestive of hemorrhage include decreasing hematocrit, full anterior fontanel, changes in activity level, and decreased muscle tone. With a catastrophic incident, the infant can develop stupor, coma, respiratory distress that progresses to apnea, decerebrate posturing, and seizures; there is a high mortality rate in these cases (Volpe, 2008).

Morbidity and mortality related to GMH-IVH are based on the severity of the hemorrhage and the associated problems. Small hemorrhages are usually associated with good outcomes and high survival rates. Infants with more severe hemorrhages, posthemorrhagic ventricular dilation, or periventricular leukomalacia have higher mortality rates and often long-term morbidity. Neurodevelopmental outcomes of GMH-IVH include hydrocephalus, cerebral palsy, developmental retardation, learning disorders, and sensory and attention problems (Volpe, 2008).

Care management begins with prevention of preterm birth, birth trauma, and hypoxic-ischemic injury. Antenatal steroids help to reduce the risk of GMH-IVH. Prompt and skilled resuscitation at birth minimizes hypoxia and ischemia. Nursing care focuses on recognition of factors that increase the risk of GMH-IVH, interventions to decrease the risk of bleeding, and supportive care to infants who have bleeding episodes. Ongoing assessment of vulnerable infants involves monitoring oxygenation and perfusion and avoiding or minimizing activities that increase cerebral blood flow. If GMH-IVH occurs, care is focused on maintaining oxygenation and perfusion, an NTE, and normoglycemia. The infant is positioned with the head in midline and the head of the bed elevated slightly to prevent or minimize fluctuations in intracranial blood pressure. Rapid infusions of fluids should be avoided. Blood pressure is monitored closely for fluctuations. The use of developmental interventions such as swaddling or containment during painful procedures can help promote greater physiologic stability (Blackburn & Ditzenberger, 2007).

Nursing support for parents includes assessment of their understanding and concerns related to the infant's condition. They need opportunities to discuss their feelings and ask questions about the infant's condition and care as well as the long-term prognosis. Nurses can demonstrate to parents how they can interact with the infant in a developmentally appropriate manner. Nurses can provide anticipatory guidance regarding ways the infant's needs and care will change as he or she matures. For many of these infants, a multidisciplinary approach to care is needed to address the neurodevelopmental sequelae of GMH-IVH and to plan for care after hospital discharge (Blackburn & Ditzenberger, 2007).

BOX 37-5 PROPOSED RISK FACTORS FOR NECROTIZING ENTEROCOLITIS

- Asphyxia
- Respiratory distress syndrome
- Umbilical artery catheter
- Exchange transfusion
- Early enteral feedings/hyperosmolar feedings
- Patent ductus arteriosus
- Congenital heart disease
- Polycythemia
- Anemia
- Shock
- Gastrointestinal infection

Necrotizing Enterocolitis. Necrotizing enterocolitis (NEC) is an acute inflammatory disease of the GI mucosa, commonly complicated by bowel necrosis and perforation. NEC occurs in up to 10% of all NICU admissions; 90% of cases are preterm infants (Caplan, 2006; Lambert, Christensen, Henry, Besner, Baer, Wiedmeier, et al., 2007). Reported mortality rates due to NEC range from 9% to 50% (Caplan). A national study showed rates of hospitalized neonates with NEC at about 16% and increasing to 20% among VLBW infants (Holman, Stoll, Curns, Yorita, Steiner, & Schonberger, 2006).

The exact etiology and pathophysiology of NEC are unclear, although many factors seem to contribute to its development (risk factors are listed in Box 37-5). Three primary conditions appear to be involved in the etiology of NEC. The first is intestinal ischemia that occurs as a result of asphyxia/hypoxia or events that cause a redistribution of blood flow away from the GI tract (e.g., hypotension, hypovolemia, severe stress). A second condition involved in the development of NEC seems to be bacterial colonization of the initially sterile GI tract with harmful organisms prior to the establishment of normal intestinal flora. *Klebsiella*, *Escherichia coli*, and *Clostridium* are common organisms involved in NEC. A third condition associated with the development of NEC is enteral feeding. The majority of infants with NEC had received some type of enteral feeding. It is thought that the feedings can provide a substrate for bacterial proliferation or that feedings can increase intestinal oxygen demand during absorption and results in tissue hypoxia. Breast milk seems to have a protective effect against the development of NEC—it is rare among infants who are exclusively fed breast milk. The use of probiotics shows promise in reducing the risk of NEC. Use of natural prophylactic probiotics such as *Bifidobacterium infantis* and *Streptococcus thermophilus* to enhance bowel flora appears to decrease the incidence of NEC (AlFaleh & Bassler, 2008; Barclay, Stenson, Simpson, Weaver, & Wilson, 2007). In addition, minimal enteral nutrition may help reduce the risk of NEC.

The onset of NEC in the term infant usually occurs between 1 and 3 days after birth, but can occur as late as 1 month. In the preterm infant, NEC usually occurs within the first 7 days, but can be delayed for up to 30 days. The signs of developing NEC are nonspecific, which is characteristic of many neonatal diseases. Some generalized signs include decreased activity, hypotonia, pallor, recurrent apnea and bradycardia, decreased oxygen saturation values, respiratory distress, metabolic acidosis, oliguria, hypotension, decreased perfusion, temperature instability, and cyanosis. GI symptoms include abdominal distention, increasing or bile-stained residual gastric aspirates, vomiting (bile or blood), grossly bloody stools, abdominal tenderness, and erythema of the abdominal wall (Bradshaw, 2010).

A diagnosis is confirmed by a radiographic examination that reveals bowel loop distention, pneumatosis intestinalis (air in the wall of the bowel), pneumoperitoneum, portal air, or a combination of these findings. The abnormal radiographic findings are caused by the bacterial colonization of the GI tract associated with NEC, resulting in ileus. Pneumatosis intestinalis, pneumoperitoneum, and portal air are caused by gas produced by the bacteria that invade the wall of the intestines and escape into the peritoneum and portal system when perforation occurs. The laboratory evaluation in such infants consists of a CBC with differential, coagulation studies, ABG analysis, measurement of serum electrolyte levels, and blood culture. The white blood cell count on the CBC can be either increased or decreased. The platelet count and coagulation study findings can be abnormal, showing thrombocytopenia and disseminated intravascular coagulation (DIC). Electrolyte levels can be abnormal, with leaking capillary beds and fluid shifts with the infection (Bradshaw, 2010; Caplan, 2006).

Management strategies are based on the degree of bowel involvement and the severity of the disease. The goal of treatment is to prevent progression of the NEC, intestinal perforation, and shock.

For the infant with suspected or confirmed NEC, oral or tube feedings are discontinued to rest the GI tract. An orogastric tube is placed and attached to low wall suction to provide gastric decompression. Parenteral therapy (often TPN) is begun. Because NEC is an infectious disease, control of the infection is imperative, with an emphasis on careful hand hygiene before and after infant contact. Antibiotic therapy may be instituted, and surgical resection is performed if perforation or clinical deterioration occurs. Therapy is usually prolonged, and recovery can be delayed by the formation of adhesions, the development of the complications associated with bowel resection, the occurrence of short-bowel syndrome (especially if the ileocecal valve is removed), or the development of intolerance to oral feedings. Some of these infants are candidates for intestinal transplants if they truly have short-bowel syndrome (Bradshaw, 2010; Caplan, 2006).

Families need education and support when faced with the crisis of having an infant with NEC. As part of the health care team, nurses can help parents understand the severity of the disease, treatment options, and care needed by the infant. When the disease is severe and the prognosis is poor, nurses are instrumental in supporting families with decision making and anticipatory grieving (Hughes, Baez, & McGrath, 2009).

Infant Pain Responses

The physiology of pain and pain assessment in the newborn are discussed in Chapter 24. This discussion focuses on pain assessment and management in the preterm infant.

Pain Assessment

Assessment of pain in the neonate is difficult because evaluation must be based on physiologic changes and behavioral observations. Pain is now considered the fifth vital sign, and its assessment is a requirement of The Joint Commission (TJC). A scale that examines multiple dimensions facilitates accurate assessment of neonatal pain (Spence, Gillies, Harrison, Johnston, & Nagy, 2005). Although behaviors such as vocalizations, facial expressions, body movements, and general state are common to all infants, they vary with different situations. Crying associated with pain is more intense and sustained. Facial expression is the most consistent and specific characteristic; scales are available for systematic evaluation of facial features, such as eye squeeze, brow bulge, and open mouth and taut tongue (Walden, 2007) (see Fig. 24-22). Most infants respond with increased body movements, but may be experiencing pain even when lying quietly with eyes closed. The preterm infant's response to pain may be behaviorally blunted or absent. An infant who receives a muscle-paralyzing agent such as vecuronium will be incapable of mounting a behavioral or visible pain response (Box 37-6), yet still feel pain.

! NURSING ALERT

When in doubt about the presence of pain in infants, the nurse should base the need for interventions on the following rule: Whatever is painful to an adult or child is painful to an infant unless proved otherwise. The nurse should anticipate pain and intervene promptly, without waiting for signs of pain to appear.

Several tools have been developed for the assessment of pain in the neonate. The CRIES assessment tool is discussed in Chapter 24 (see Table 24-4). Other instruments are the Pain Assessment Tool (PAT) (Hodgkinson, Bear, Thorn, & Van Blaricum, 1994); Scale for Use in Newborns (SUN) (Blauer & Gerstmann, 1998); Behavioral Pain Score (BPS) (Pokela, 1994); Distress Scale for Ventilated Newborn Infants (DSVNI) (Sparshott, 1995); Neonatal Infant Pain Scale (NIPS) (Lawrence, Alcock, McGrath, Kay, MacMurray, & Dulberg, 1993); and the Premature Infant Pain Profile (PIPP) (Stevens, Johnston, Petryshen, & Taddio, 1996). The PIPP is one of the most widely used scales for preterm infants because it considers behavioral, physiologic, and contextual indicators (Walden, 2007).

Memory of Pain

Preterm infants are subjected to a variety of repeated noxious stimuli, including multiple heelsticks, venipuncture, endotracheal intubation and suctioning, arterial sticks, chest tube placement, and lumbar puncture. The effects of pain caused by such procedures are not fully known, but researchers have begun to investigate potential consequences. From preliminary reports, it appears that a rewiring of the pain responses occurs

BOX 37-6 MANIFESTATIONS OF ACUTE PAIN IN THE NEONATE

PHYSIOLOGIC RESPONSES

Vital Signs
- Increased heart rate
- Increased blood pressure
- Rapid, shallow respirations

Oxygenation
- Decreased transcutaneous O_2 saturation ($tcPo_2$)
- Decreased arterial O_2 saturation (Sao_2)

Skin
- Pallor or flushing
- Diaphoresis
- Palmar sweating

Other Observations
- Increased muscle tone
- Dilated pupils
- Decreased vagal nerve tone
- Increased intracranial pressure
- Laboratory evidence of metabolic or endocrine changes
  - Hyperglycemia
  - Lowered pH
  - Elevated corticosteroids

BEHAVIORAL RESPONSES

Vocalizations: Observe Quality, Timing, and Duration
- Crying
- Whimpering
- Groaning

Facial Expression
- Grimacing
- Brow furrowed
- Chin quivering
- Eyes tightly closed
- Mouth open and squarish

Body Movements and Posture
- Limb withdrawal
- Thrashing
- Rigidity
- Flaccidity
- Fist clenching

Change in State
- Changes in sleep-wake cycles
- Changes in feeding behavior
- Changes in activity level
- Fussiness, irritability
- Listlessness

Modified from Hockenberry, M. (2007). *Wong's nursing care of infants and children* (8th ed.). St. Louis: Mosby.

in preterm infants who have been subjected to multiple painful treatments early in their lives. The nervous system networks of the preterm infant appear more dense and have more branches than those in the average infant, leading to the conclusion that the pain threshold and sensitivity in once preterm infants is heightened for life. There are also changes when the infant has undergone anesthesia (Anand, Johnston, Oberlander, Taddio, Lehr, & Walco, 2005; Aranda, Carlo, Hummel, Thomas, Lehr, & Anand, 2005).

Nurses' anecdotal reports suggest that infants show memory by exhibiting defensive behaviors when painful procedures are repeated. Nurses often describe infants who stiffen and withdraw when touched because human touch has repeatedly been associated with pain. Such infants often become hypervigilant and gaze intently at the hands rather than at the eyes of people who approach them.

These reports not only indicate that infants remember painful events but also show that continual exposure to pain affects development, especially in response to human contact.

Consequences of Untreated Pain in Infants

Despite research on the neonate's experience of pain, infant pain remains inadequately managed. This mismanagement is partially due to misconceptions regarding the effects of pain on the neonate, as well as a lack of knowledge of immediate and long-term consequences of untreated pain. Infants respond to noxious stimuli through physiologic indicators (increased heart rate and blood pressure, variability in heart rate and intracranial pressure, and decreases in arterial oxygen saturations and skin blood flow) and behavioral indicators (muscle rigidity, facial expression, crying, withdrawal, and sleeplessness). The physiologic and behavioral indicators, as well as a variety of neurophysiologic responses to noxious stimulation, are responsible for short- and long-term consequences of pain.

Pain Management

The International Evidence-Based Group for Neonatal Pain developed a Consensus Statement for the Prevention and Management of Pain in the Newborn (Anand & The International Evidence-Based Group for Neonatal Pain, 2001), which states that pain must be anticipated and prevented to avoid long-term consequences. Nonpharmacologic measures to alleviate pain include repositioning, swaddling, containment, cuddling, rocking, playing music, reducing environmental stimulation, providing tactile comfort measures and nonnutritive sucking, and using oral sucrose. However, nonpharmacologic measures may not be sufficient to decrease physiologic distress, even if behavioral responses such as crying are lessened. In preterm infants, additional stimulation such as stroking or environmental light or noise can *increase* physiologic distress (Walden, 2007). The effect of the NICU environment must be considered along with other forms of stimuli that can produce stress and pain.

Morphine is the most widely used opioid analgesic for pharmacologic management of neonatal pain, with fentanyl as an effective alternative. Continuous or bolus epidural or IV infusion of opioids provides effective and safe pain control. Other methods are epidural/intrathecal infusion, local and regional nerve blocks, and topical anesthetics, as well as general anesthesia for surgery (Walden, 2007).

Parents are universally concerned that their infants are feeling pain during procedures. Nurses need to address these concerns

EVIDENCE-BASED PRACTICE

Pat Gingrich

Non-Pharmacologic Pain Relief Measures for Newborns

ASK THE QUESTION

How can we decrease the pain and stress of painful procedures for newborns?

SEARCH FOR EVIDENCE

Search Strategies

Professional organization guidelines, meta-analyses, systematic reviews, randomized controlled trials, nonrandomized prospective studies and retrospective reviews since 2008.

Databases Searched

CINAHL, Cochrane, Medline, PUBMED, and the websites of the American Academy of Pediatrics and the National Guidelines Clearinghouse.

CRITICALLY ANALYZE THE DATA

Early pain experiences during the rapid brain growth of infancy can lead to the decrease in volume of the sensory areas of the brain and long-term changes in behavior. Preterm neonates are especially vulnerable to short-term stress from pain, leading to acidosis and respiratory distress. Newborns in intensive care units average a dozen or more painful procedures every day, most without sufficient pain relief. Pharmacologic pain relief measures may not be practical or advisable for fragile, low birth weight, or preterm infants. Non-pharmacologic pain relief measures offer some comfort and distraction, and may potentiate pharmacologic pain therapy.

Using sucrose is a well-known intervention for minor procedures. A Cochrane Database Systematic Review of 44 studies, totaling 3496 infants compared infants given sucrose to those given other care (water, pacifier, positioning or breastfeeding) during painful procedures. The use of sucrose decreased crying duration and the score for Premature Infant Pain Profile (PIPP) for heel stick. The reviewers concluded that sucrose use was safe and effective for single events, while cautioning that more research is needed for optimum doses and the safety of sucrose for very low birthweight babies (Stevens, Yamada, & Ohlsson, 2010).

A systematic review of 11 studies found evidence supporting the non-pharmacologic oral distraction measures of non-nutritive sucking (NNS), sucrose, breastfeeding, and breast milk. Effective tactile comfort measures included swaddling, holding, touching, positioning, and facilitative tucking (Yamada, Stinson, Lamba, Dickson, McGrath et al., 2008).

IMPLICATIONS FOR PRACTICE

Facilitated tucking is beneficial as a pain-relief measure for procedures such as suctioning or heel stick in preterm infants: one caretaker holds the baby's limbs in a flexed, midline position with two hands, while another administers the procedure. The tucking position should be held from three minutes prior to the procedure, to allow the infant to adapt to the stimuli, until 3 minutes post-procedure, to allow the infant time for recovery to baseline. While allowing ten minutes per procedure for two busy nurses might not be practical, holding the infant in the facilitated tuck position might be an excellent role for a family member or volunteer (Cignacco, Axelin, Stoffel, Sellam, Anand, & Engberg, 2010). A systematic review of 5 studies found that facilitated tucking resulted in more stable heart rate, increase in oxygen saturation, more normal sleep-wake state, and lower pain scores (Obeidat, Kahalaf, Callister, & Froelicher, 2009).

General principles for optimum pain management in the newborn involves knowing the additive or synergistic effects of pharmacologic and non-pharmacologic methods. Ideal timing for procedures would be during a state of quiet wakefulness, avoiding waking the infant from sleep. Try to allow two hours between painful stimuli. The nurse should keep the environment calm and relaxing, and place the infant on a warm sheet. Allow skin-to-skin contact to begin a few minutes before the procedure. Breastfeeding may be helpful for single procedures, but using this for frequent or routine procedures could interfere with the breastfeeding relationship. Assess pre-procedure pain as the fifth vital sign, and then monitor all vital signs until return to baseline post-procedure. For blood work, expert venipuncture is less painful and more effective for term or large babies than heel stick. For heel sticks, it is not advisable to warm or squeeze the heel, as it will not increase the uptake of blood, and may increase the pain. Distraction may include sensorial saturation, such as infant massage, sucrose administration via NNS and talking to the infant during the procedure (Lago, Garetti, Merazzi, Pieragostini, Ancora, Pirelli, et al., 2009).

References

Cignacco, E., Axelin, A., Stoffel, L., Sellam, G., Anand, K., & Engberg, S. (2010). Facilitated tucking as a non-pharmacological intervention for neonatal pain relief: Is it clinically feasible? *Acta Paediatrica*, July 6 epub.

Lago, P., Garetti, E., Merazzi, D., Pieragostini, L., Ancora, G., Pirelli, A., et al. (2009). Pain Study Group of the Italian Society of Neonatology. Guidelines for procedural pain in the newborn. *Acta Paediatrica, 98*(6), 932–939.

Obeidat, H., Kahalaf, I., Callister, L., & Froelicher, E. (2009). Use of facilitated tucking for nonpharmacological pain management in preterm infants: A systematic review. *Journal of Perinatal and Neonatal Nursing, 234*(4), 372–377.

Stevens, B., Yamada, J., & Ohlsson, A. (2010). Sucrose for analgesia in newborn infants undergoing painful procedures. *The Cochrane Database of Systematic Reviews, 2010*, 1, CD001069.

Yamada, J., Stinson, J., Lamba, J., Dickson, A., McGrath, P., et al. (2008). A review of systematic reviews on pain interventions in hospitalized infants. *Pain Research Management, 13*(5), 413–420.

and encourage the parents to speak with the health care professionals involved. Parents have the right to withhold consent for invasive procedures and are entitled to honest answers from those responsible for the infant's care. When appropriate, they also can help provide comfort measures for the infant. Kangaroo care is one parental intervention that comforts and calms the infant.

Parents want to know that nurses recognize pain in their infants and that the infants will be comfortable when they, the parents, are not present. They want to know that the nurse will advocate for comfort care for their baby. Although pain is considered a fifth vital sign, it cannot be assessed only at the time of vital signs. It must receive an ongoing evaluation of the pain level and the effectiveness of comfort measures used. This assessment is not lengthy but can be as simple as walking to the bedside and really looking at the infant's color, posture, movements, and breathing. Pain is a real phenomenon that is preventable in many instances. Pain management is a standard of care, and it is considered unethical not to prevent and effectively treat pain. Another growing area of neonatal nursing is end-of-life and palliative care. Most of this care centers on pain management. Palliative care is really comfort care that supports the needs of the preterm, sick neonate.

TABLE 37-3 **LATE PRETERM INFANT ASSESSMENT AND INTERVENTIONS**

RISK FACTORS	ASSESSMENT	INTERVENTIONS*
Respiratory distress (RD)	Assess for cardinal signs of RD (nasal flaring, grunting, tachypnea, central cyanosis, retractions), for presence of apnea especially during feedings, and for hypothermia, hypoglycemia.	Perform gestational age assessment; observe for signs of RD; monitor oxygenation by pulse oximetry; provide supplemental oxygen judiciously.
Thermal instability	Monitor axillary temperature every 30 min immediately after birth until stable; thereafter every 1-4 hr, depending on gestational age and ability to maintain thermal stability.	Provide skin-to-skin care immediately after birth for stable infant; implement measures to prevent excess heat loss (adjust environmental temperature, avoid drafts); bathe only after thermal stability has been maintained for 1 hr.
Hypoglycemia	Monitor for signs and symptoms of hypoglycemia; assess feeding ability (latch, nipple feeding); assess thermal stability, signs and symptoms of RD; monitor bedside glucose in infants with additional risk factors (mother with diabetes, prolonged labor, RD, poor feeding).	Initiate early feedings of human milk or formula; avoid dextrose water or water feedings; provide intravenous dextrose as necessary for hypoglycemia.
Jaundice	Observe for jaundice in first 24 hr; evaluate maternal-fetal history for additional risk factors that may cause increased hemolysis and circulating levels of unconjugated bilirubin (Rh, ABO, spherocytosis, bruising); assess feeding method, voiding, stooling patterns.	Monitor transcutaneous bilirubin, and note risk zone on hour-specific nomogram (see Fig. 24-8).
Feeding problems	Assess suck-swallow and breathing; assess for RD, hypoglycemia, thermal stability; assess latch-on, maternal comfort with feeding method; weight loss no more than 10% of birth weight.	Initiate early feedings—human milk or formula; ensure maternal knowledge of feeding method and signs of inadequate feeding (sleepiness, lethargy, color changes during feeding, apnea during feeding, decreased or absent urinary output).

*This list is not exhaustive of nursing interventions; additional interventions include those discussed under the care of the high risk infant in this chapter.
Source: Santa-Donato, A., Medoff-Cooper, B., Bakewell-Sachs, S., Askin, D., & Rosenberg, S. (2007). *Late preterm infant assessment guide.* Washington, DC: Association of Women's Health, Obstetric and Neonatal Nurses.

Late Preterm Infants

Late preterm infants are those born between 34 0/7 and 36 6/7 weeks of gestation (Raju et al., 2006). Because birth weights of late preterm infants often range from 2000 to 2500 g and they appear relatively mature in comparison to the smaller less mature infant, they are often cared for as if they are normal term infants. Risk factors for late preterm infants can easily be overlooked. Compared with term infants, late preterm infants are at increased risk for problems with thermoregulation, hypoglycemia, hyperbilirubinemia, feeding, sepsis, and respiratory function (Bakewell-Sachs, 2007; Darcy, 2009). Many of these healthy-appearing infants are admitted directly to postpartum units with their mothers or stay in the NICU only briefly (i.e., less than 24 hours). They are commonly discharged home at 2 to 3 days of age with their mothers. Discharge before 48 hours after birth is not recommended (Ramachandrappa & Jain, 2009).

Recognition of late preterm infants is essential to providing effective care. Initial physical assessment and assessment of gestational age are crucial to identifying these infants. Although the mother's estimated date of birth (EDB) can indicate a longer gestation, infant appearance, behaviors, and/or weight can indicate otherwise. The obstetric estimate of gestational age is usually reliable if it is based on a first-trimester ultrasound. However, if there is a discrepancy between the gestational age based on the obstetric estimate and newborn examination, it is better to rely on the estimate based on the newborn examination (Ramachandrappa & Jain, 2009).

The Association of Women's Health, Obstetric and Neonatal Nurses (AWHONN) published the *Late Preterm Infant Assessment Guide* (Santa-Donato, Medoff-Cooper, Bakewell-Sachs, Askin, & Rosenberg, 2007) for the education of perinatal nurses regarding the late preterm infant's risk factors and appropriate care and follow-up (Table 37-3).

Components of nursing care for late preterm infants and their parents are discussed in the following text. Frequent assessment is important. On mother-baby units, late preterm infants should be assessed more often than term infants—at least every 4 hours throughout their hospital stay. This includes vital signs and observation of a feeding.

Respiratory Distress. Late preterm infants are at increased risk for respiratory problems, including apnea. Close monitoring of respiratory status is essential and any changes are reported promptly to the primary health care provider. Car seat testing is indicated. Infants may go home on an apnea monitor. If possible, parents should attend an infant cardiopulmonary resuscitation (CPR) class or view a video about infant CPR. To help prevent respiratory infections the nurse should instruct the parents to limit the infant's contact with others outside the home. The nurse should review signs and symptoms of respiratory problems with the parents.

Thermoregulation. Late preterm infants have more difficulty with thermoregulation than term infants, and cold stress is a greater concern. They have less body fat than term infants, a higher ratio of surface area to body weight, decreased glycogen stores, and less mature mechanisms for increasing metabolism for heat. Stores of brown fat are smaller and quickly depleted. Cold stress can quickly lead to hypoglycemia. Nurses must closely monitor body temperature and teach parents to take the infant's temperature. Parents are encouraged to keep a record of this at home and to report high or low temperatures. It is important to remember that temperature instability is often an early sign of neonatal sepsis (Darcy, 2009).

Nutrition. Feedings should occur at least every 3 to 4 hours and according to infant feeding cues. Late preterm infants eat less than term neonates and have less energy reserves to do so. They can have difficulty coordinating sucking, swallowing, and breathing. Breastfeeding can be more problematic if the infant is sleepy and difficult to arouse for feedings. Late preterm infants are prone to early fatigue during feedings and fall asleep before consuming adequate volumes of milk. Nurses should observe at least one feeding every 8 hours. Early and extended skin-to-skin contact promotes breastfeeding. If supplementation is needed, expressed breast milk is the best option (Walker, 2008). To maximize the milk supply and milk transfer to the infant, mothers should use the electric breast pump after feedings while in the hospital and continue this process at home until the infant is able to successfully remove milk from the breasts and until the milk supply is well established. The mother-baby nurse or lactation consultant can provide instruction and assist breastfeeding mothers with using a breast pump. Mothers also need information regarding safe milk handling and storage guidelines (Jones & Tully, 2006). Parents should keep an intake and output record until their health care provider tells them otherwise and should share this record with the health care provider at each visit (Cleaveland, 2010; Walker, 2008).

Hypoglycemia. Late preterm infants are at risk for hypoglycemia. Hospital protocols may require routine monitoring of blood glucose until levels are stabilized and the infant is feeding adequately. Although the cut-off value for treatment remains uncertain (Garg & Devaskar, 2006), blood glucose values of less than 45 mg/dl, or symptoms of hypoglycemia, should be treated. Bedside monitoring of blood glucose levels at frequent intervals throughout the late preterm infant's hospital stay is recommended.

Hyperbilirubinemia. Neonatal hyperbilirubinemia is more common in late preterm infants because of immaturity of the liver, decreased gastric motility, and increased breakdown of red blood cells (RBCs) (Pappas & Walker, 2010). They are less able to conjugate and excrete bilirubin. Serum bilirubin levels tend to peak at 5 to 7 days and persist longer than in term infants. Hyperbilirubinemia is the most frequent reason for hospital readmission during the first week of life. Bilirubin levels are closely monitored before discharge and parents are instructed regarding signs of jaundice and when to notify the health care provider. Follow-up visits soon after hospital discharge are important for monitoring rising bilirubin levels (Darcy, 2010).

Infection. The immune systems of late preterm infants are immature; thus they are more likely to experience infections. Nurses should assess the infant for signs and symptoms of infection including temperature instability, lethargy, irritability, poor feeding, or vomiting. Before discharge, nurses provide education for the parents about the common signs and symptoms of infection.

> **CLINICAL REASONING**
>
> ***The Late Preterm Infant***
>
> A 2013-g (4-lb 7-oz) male infant is born at an estimated gestational age of 35 weeks. The parents are very excited about this birth because they have been trying to become pregnant for 6 years. The baby is placed on the mother's (Lucia's) abdomen after birth for skin-to-skin contact but does not breastfeed. The nurse assessing the baby notes that he has some mild grunting, nasal flaring, and intercostal retractions; he is taken to the transitional nursery for further evaluation and treatment. Jorge, the father, speaks little English but asks when they will be able to hold their son again. Lucia is crying and asks to have her baby brought back to her as soon as his condition is stable because she really wants to breastfeed him.
>
> 1. Evidence—Is evidence sufficient to draw conclusions about what to tell Lucia and Jorge about their infant son?
> 2. Assumptions—What assumptions can be made about the following?
>   a. The mother's and the father's reaction to their son's birth
>   b. The infant's expected progress
>   c. The possibility of Lucia breastfeeding the baby
> 3. What implications and priorities for nursing care can be drawn at this time?
> 4. Does the evidence objectively support your conclusion?
> 5. Are there alternative perspectives to your conclusion?

Postmature Infants

A pregnancy that is prolonged beyond 42 weeks is a postterm pregnancy, and the infant who is born is called postterm or *postmature.* Postmaturity can be associated with placental insufficiency, resulting in a fetus that has a wasted appearance (dysmaturity) at birth because of loss of subcutaneous fat and muscle mass. However, not all postmature infants will show signs of dysmaturity; some will continue to grow in utero and will be large at birth. Most postmature infants are oversized but otherwise normal, with advanced development and bone age. A postmature infant will have some, but not necessarily all, of the following physical characteristics:

- Generally a normal skull, but the reduced dimensions of the rest of the body in the presence of dysmaturity make the skull look inordinately large
- Dry, cracked (desquamating), parchment-like skin at birth
- Hard nails extending beyond the fingertips
- Profuse scalp hair
- Depleted subcutaneous fat layers, leaving the skin loose and giving the infant an "old person" appearance
- Long and thin body
- Absent vernix
- Often meconium staining (golden yellow to green) of skin, nails, and cord, indicative of a hypoxic episode in utero or a perinatal infection such as listeriosis
- Can have an alert, wide-eyed appearance symptomatic of chronic intrauterine hypoxia

The perinatal mortality rate is significantly higher in the postmature fetus and neonate. One reason for this is that during labor and birth the increased oxygen demands of the postmature fetus may not be met. Insufficient gas exchange in the postmature placenta also increases the likelihood of intrauterine hypoxia, which can result in the passage of meconium in utero, thereby increasing the risk for *meconium aspiration syndrome (MAS).*

Parents may be concerned about the appearance of the postmature infant. Nurses can help them understand reasons for the dry, peeling, skin and other characteristics of postmaturity. Initial bathing should be done with a mild soap. It can be helpful to moisturize the skin with a petrolatum-based ointment. Nurses need to be alert to common problems associated with postmaturity such as hypoglycemia and meconium aspiration (Lund & Kuller, 2007).

Meconium Aspiration Syndrome

Meconium staining of the amniotic fluid can be indicative of fetal distress, especially in a vertex presentation. It appears in 10% to 15% of all births (Dudell & Stoll, 2007). Many infants

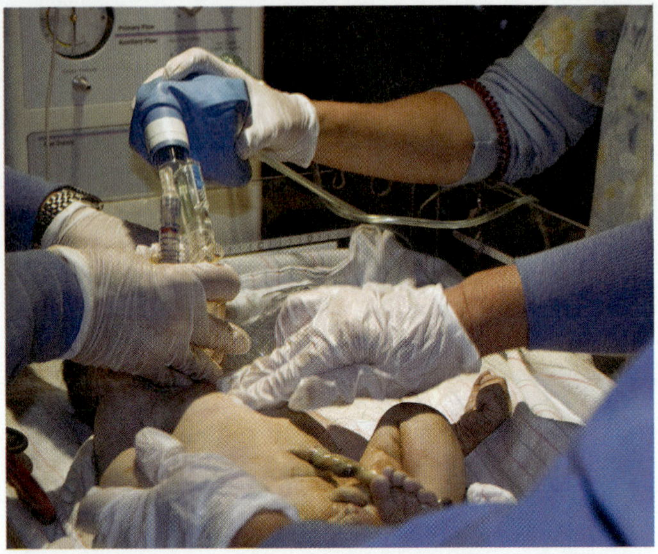

FIG. 37-14 Infant being resuscitated at birth. Meconium was present on the abdomen and umbilical cord. Infant was not breathing, and heart rate was 65 beats/min at birth. Respirations and heart rate were normal at 2 minutes. (Courtesy Shannon Perry, Phoenix, AZ.)

with meconium staining exhibit no signs of depression at birth; however, the presence of meconium in the amniotic fluid necessitates careful supervision of labor and close monitoring of fetal well-being. The presence of a team skilled in neonatal resuscitation is required at the birth of any infant with meconium-stained amniotic fluid (Fig. 37-14). The mouth and nares of the infant are not routinely suctioned on the perineum before the infant's first breath. However, for infants with meconium staining who are not vigorous, endotracheal suctioning should be performed immediately. Vigorous infants need no special handling (AHA, 2005; Velaphi & Vidyasagar, 2008).

If the infant is very depressed and the meconium is not removed from the airway at birth, it can migrate down to the terminal airways, causing mechanical obstruction leading to **meconium aspiration syndrome.** It also is possible that the fetus aspirated meconium in utero. Such meconium aspiration can cause a chemical pneumonitis. These infants can develop persistent pulmonary hypertension of the newborn, further complicating their management. Infants with MAS who receive surfactant can experience improved oxygenation, decreased severity of respiratory failure, and reduced need for ECMO (Engle & AAP Committee on Fetus and Newborn, 2008).

Persistent Pulmonary Hypertension of the Newborn

The term **persistent pulmonary hypertension of the newborn (PPHN)** is applied to the combined findings of pulmonary hypertension, right-to-left shunting, and a structurally normal heart. PPHN can occur either as a single entity or as the main component of MAS, congenital diaphragmatic hernia, RDS, hyperviscosity syndrome, or neonatal pneumonia or sepsis. PPHN also is called *persistent fetal circulation* (PFC) because the syndrome includes a reversion to fetal pathways for blood flow.

A brief review of the characteristics of fetal blood flow can help in visualizing the problems with PPHN (see Fig. 12-13). In utero, oxygen-rich blood leaves the placenta via the umbilical vein, goes through the ductus venosus, and enters the inferior vena cava. From there it empties into the right atrium and is mostly shunted across the foramen ovale to the left atrium, effectively bypassing the lungs. This blood enters the left ventricle, leaves via the aorta, and preferentially perfuses the carotid and coronary arteries. Thus the heart and brain receive the most oxygenated blood. Blood drains from the brain into the superior vena cava, reenters the right atrium, proceeds to the right ventricle, and exits via the main pulmonary artery. The lungs are a high-pressure circuit, needing only enough perfusion for growth and nutrition. The ductus arteriosus (connecting the main pulmonary artery and the aorta) is the path of least resistance for the blood leaving the right side of the fetal heart, shunting most of the cardiac output away from the lungs and toward the systemic system. This right-to-left shunting is the key to fetal circulation.

After birth, both the foramen ovale and the ductus arteriosus close in response to various biochemical processes, pressure changes within the heart, and dilation of the pulmonary vessels. This dilation allows virtually all of the cardiac output to enter the lungs, become oxygenated, and provide oxygen-rich blood to the tissues for normal metabolism. PPHN characteristically proceeds into a downward spiral of exacerbating hypoxia and pulmonary vasoconstriction. Prompt recognition and aggressive intervention are required to reverse this process (Cifuentes & Carlo, 2007).

The infant with PPHN is typically born at term or after term and has tachycardia and cyanosis. Management depends on the underlying cause of the persistent pulmonary hypertension. The use of ECMO has improved the chances of survival in these infants (see earlier discussion); however, it is considered a very invasive procedure. Use of NO as a pharmacologic intervention has increased, with great success. It acts as a vasodilator to decrease the pulmonary hypertension while increasing oxygenation (Konduri & Kim, 2009). This therapy is proving to work well either alone or with high-frequency ventilation. Another pharmacologic treatment is use of exogenous surfactant because some of these infants appear to be surfactant deficient. Use of environmental strategies such as decreasing adverse stimuli (excessive light and noise) to reduce stress is an area of ongoing research. This intervention is used in conjunction with other therapies.

Another mode of treatment for PPHN and other respiratory disorders of the newborn is high-frequency ventilation, a group of assisted ventilation methods that deliver small volumes of gas at high frequencies and limit the development of high airway pressure, thus reducing barotrauma. High-frequency ventilation decreases carbon dioxide while increasing oxygenation. It can be effectively used in conjunction with NO.

It is important to understand that PPHN is considered a cardiovascular and a respiratory problem. The lungs of these infants are healthy, but the hypertension of the cardiovascular system leads to their oxygenation problems.

Other Problems Related to Gestation

Small for Gestational Age and Intrauterine Growth Restriction

Infants who are small for gestational age (SGA; e.g., weight is below the 10th percentile expected at term) and infants who have IUGR (rate of growth does not meet expected growth pattern) are considered high risk. Among these infants perinatal mortality rates are 5 to 20 times greater than for normal term infants (Kliegman, 2006).

Various conditions can affect and impede growth in the developing fetus. Conditions occurring in the first trimester that affect all aspects of fetal growth (e.g., infections, teratogens, chromosomal abnormalities) or extrinsic conditions early in pregnancy result in symmetric IUGR (i.e., head circumference, length, and weight are all less than the 10th percentile). Conditions causing symmetric growth restriction result in an SGA infant, usually with a head circumference that is smaller than that of a term infant and reduced brain capacity. Growth restriction in later stages of pregnancy, as a result of maternal or placental factors, results in asymmetric growth restriction (with respect to gestational age, weight will be less than the 10th percentile, whereas length and head circumference will be greater than the 10th percentile). Infants with asymmetric IUGR have the potential for normal growth and development. There is relative sparing of head and brain growth while weight and somatic organ growth are more seriously altered (Furdon & Benjamin, 2010).

Several physical findings are characteristic of the SGA neonate (Furdon & Benjamin, 2010):

- Generally a normal skull, but the reduced dimensions of the rest of the body make the skull look inordinately large
- Reduced subcutaneous fat stores
- Loose and dry skin
- Diminished muscle mass, especially over buttocks and cheeks
- Sunken abdomen (scaphoid) as opposed to the well-rounded abdomen seen in normal infants
- Thin, yellowish, dry, and dull umbilical cord (normal cord is gray, glistening, round, and moist)
- Sparse scalp hair
- Wide skull sutures (inadequate bone growth)

Care of the SGA infant is based on the clinical problems present and is the same for preterm infants with similar problems. Gas exchange is supported by maintaining a clear airway and preventing cold stress. Hypoglycemia is treated with oral feedings (e.g., breast, formula) or IV dextrose as the infant's condition warrants. An external heat source (radiant warmer or incubator) is used until the infant is able to maintain an adequate body temperature. Nursing support of parents is the same as that given to parents of preterm infants.

Common problems that affect SGA (IUGR) infants are perinatal asphyxia, meconium aspiration, immunodeficiency, hypoglycemia, polycythemia, and temperature instability.

Perinatal Asphyxia. Commonly, IUGR infants have been exposed to chronic hypoxia for varying periods before labor and birth. Labor is a stressor to the normal fetus, but it is an even greater stressor for the growth-restricted fetus. The chronically hypoxic infant is severely compromised even by a normal labor and has difficulty compensating after birth. Appropriate management and resuscitation are essential for these depressed infants.

The birth of SGA babies with perinatal asphyxia can be associated with a maternal history of heavy cigarette smoking; preeclampsia; low socioeconomic status; multifetal gestation; gestational infections such as rubella, cytomegalovirus, and toxoplasmosis; advanced diabetes mellitus; and cardiac problems. The nursing staff must be alert to and prepared for possible perinatal asphyxia during the birth of an infant to a woman with such a history. Sequelae to perinatal asphyxia include MAS (see p. 924) and hypoglycemia.

Hypoglycemia. All high risk infants have an increased likelihood of developing hypoglycemia. Infants who experience physiologic stress can experience hypoglycemia as a result of a decreased glycogen supply, inadequate gluconeogenesis, or overutilization of glycogen stored during fetal and postnatal life. Preterm infants can also become hypoglycemic because of inadequate intake and increased metabolic demands as a result of illness factors. Evidence to support the concept that the preterm or high risk infant can tolerate lower levels of serum glucose any better than healthy term infants is insufficient (Blackburn, 2007) (see Chapter 23, p. 537, for discussion of hypoglycemia). The SGA infant, not unlike the preterm infant, is at increased risk for hypoglycemia as a result of decreased fetal stores and decreased rate of gluconeogenesis (McGowan, Rozance, Price-Douglas, & Hay, 2011).

Symptoms of hypoglycemia include poor feeding, hypothermia, and diaphoresis. CNS symptoms can include tremors and jitteriness, weak cry, lethargy, floppy posture, convulsions, or coma. Diagnosis is confirmed by blood glucose determinations performed by the laboratory, when suspected, or by unit visual methods with reagent strips such as Chemstrip-BG or Dextrostix (Kliegman, 2006). Blood glucose screening should be done on all high risk infants soon after birth and frequently during the first few hours until glucose levels stabilize.

Hyperglycemia. Hyperglycemia is defined as a blood glucose level greater than 125 mg/dl (whole blood) or a plasma glucose level of 145 to 150 mg/dl (Blackburn, 2007). This condition is seen primarily in ELBW and VLBW infants receiving parenteral nutrition with dextrose concentrations of 5% or higher. Hyperglycemia can be just as harmful to the preterm infant as hypoglycemia. Increased circulating levels of glucose can lead to osmotic changes, increased urine output, and fluid shifts in the already compromised CNS of the preterm infant. The net result of hyperglycemia can be cellular dehydration and intraventricular hemorrhage. Preterm infants undergoing stress such as surgical intervention can also become hyperglycemic with increased catecholamine release, which inhibits insulin release and glucose utilization (Blackburn). Therefore ELBW and VLBW infants should be monitored closely for both hypoglycemia and hyperglycemia during the acute phase of illness, while receiving parenteral nutrition, and perioperatively.

Polycythemia. Polycythemia or hyperviscosity of the blood is another common problem of the SGA infant. With polycythemia, there is an excess in circulating RBC mass. This condition is a result of fetal hypoxia and intrauterine stress that forces the body to produce more RBCs in an attempt to provide oxygen to the developing fetus. Polycythemia is associated with maternal preeclampsia, maternal smoking, maternal diabetes, and delayed cord clamping (Diehl-Jones & Askin, 2010). With hematocrit greater than 65% or venous hemoglobin greater than 22 g/dl, blood viscosity is increased. This can lead to compromised blood flow and reduced oxygenation of the body organs. Many infants with polycythemia are asymptomatic. Others present with plethora, cyanosis, CNS abnormalities (lethargy, jitteriness, seizures), respiratory distress, tachycardia, congestive heart failure, or hypoglycemia. Infants with polycythemia are at increased risk for hyperbilirubinemia. In some cases, a partial exchange transfusion to reduce the viscosity of the blood is necessary.

Heat Loss. SGA infants are particularly susceptible to temperature instability as a result of decreased brown fat deposits, decreased adipose tissue, large body surface exposure, and, in many instances, poor flexion, as well as decreased glycogen storage in major organs such as the liver and heart. Therefore, close attention must be given to maintain an NTE. Nursing considerations focus on maintenance of thermoneutrality to promote recovery from perinatal asphyxia because cold stress jeopardizes such recovery.

Large for Gestational Age Infants

The LGA infant is defined as an infant weighing 4000 g or more at birth. An infant is considered LGA despite gestation when the weight is more than the 90th percentile on growth charts or two standard deviations above the mean weight for gestational age. The LGA infant is at greater risk for morbidity than the SGA or preterm infant; such infants have an increased incidence of birth injuries, asphyxia, and congenital anomalies such as heart defects (Stoll & Adams-Chapman, 2007).

All pregnancies of longer than 42 weeks of gestation must be thoroughly evaluated. All large fetuses are monitored during a trial of labor, and preparation is made for a cesarean birth if abnormal fetal heart pattern or poor progress of labor occurs. LGA newborns can be preterm, term, or postterm; they may be infants of mothers with diabetes; or they can be postmature. Each of these problems carries special concerns. Regardless of coexisting potential problems, the LGA infant is at risk by virtue of size alone.

The nurse assesses the LGA infant for hypoglycemia and trauma resulting from vaginal or cesarean birth. Any specific birth injuries are identified and treated appropriately (see Chapter 35).

Discharge Planning

Discharge planning for the high risk newborn begins early in the hospitalization. Throughout the infant's hospitalization the nurse gathers information from the health care team members and the family. This information is used to determine the infant's and family's readiness for discharge. Discharge teaching for the high risk newborn family is extensive, requires time and planning, and cannot be adequately accomplished on the day of discharge. Information is provided about infant care, especially as it pertains to the particular infant's home care needs (e.g., supplemental oxygen, gastrostomy feedings, follow-up medical visits). Parents should be allowed to spend a night or two in a predischarge room providing care for the infant away from the NICU to become better acquainted with the necessary care and to have a time of transition in which questions can be answered regarding home care. Additional parent teaching should include bathing and skin care; requirements for meeting nutritional needs following discharge; safety in the home, including supine sleep position and prevention of infection (e.g., RSV); and medication administration.

Durable medical equipment and supplies required for the care of the infant in the home should be delivered to the home before the infant is discharged; parents and care providers should have ample opportunity and education in the use of the equipment. Parents of infants being discharged with special needs such as gavage or gastrostomy feedings, nasal cannula oxygen, tracheostomy, or colostomy should receive several days of thorough education in the procedure before discharge. Preterm infants have a high rate of emergency department visits and readmission to acute care centers; the family absolutely must have a health professional they can contact for questions regarding infant care and behavior once they are home. Parents should obtain an age-appropriate car seat before the discharge of their infant and demonstrate its use. Car seat safety is an essential aspect of discharge planning, and infants who were born at less than 37 weeks of gestation should have a period of observation in an appropriate car seat to monitor for possible apnea, bradycardia, and decreased Sao_2.

Before discharge all high risk or preterm infants should receive the appropriate immunizations, metabolic screening, hematologic assessment (bilirubin risk as appropriate), and evaluation of hearing. Successful discharge of high risk infants to their homes requires a multidisciplinary approach. Medical, nursing, social services, and other professionals (physical therapy, occupational therapy, developmental follow-up specialist) are crucial to the smooth transition of these infants and their families to the community and home. If the infant is transported back to the community hospital that referred either the mother before birth or the infant after birth, interfacility communication is essential to continuity of care.

Instruction in CPR is essential for parents of all infants but especially for those of infants at risk for life-threatening events. Infants considered at risk include those who are preterm, have apnea or bradycardia, or have a tendency to choke. Before taking their infant home, parents must be able to administer CPR. All parents should be encouraged to obtain instruction in CPR at their local Red Cross or other community agency, if it is not provided by the NICU.

Transport to and from a Regional Center

If a hospital is not equipped to care for a high risk mother and fetus or a high risk infant, transfer to a specialized perinatal or tertiary care center is arranged. Maternal transport ideally occurs with the fetus in utero because this has two distinct advantages: (1) the associated neonatal morbidity and mortality are decreased; and (2) infant-parent attachment is supported, thereby avoiding separation of the parents and infant. For a variety of reasons, however, it is not always possible to transport the mother before the birth. These reasons include imminent birth and unanticipated problems; therefore, physicians and nurses in level 1 and 2 facilities must have the skills and equipment necessary for making an accurate diagnosis and implementing emergency interventions to stabilize the infant's condition until transport can occur (Rojas, Shirley, & Rush, 2011). The goal of these interventions is to maintain the infant's condition within the normal physiologic range. Specific attention is given to the following areas:

- Vital signs
- Oxygen and ventilation
- Thermoregulation
- Acid-base balance
- Fluid and electrolyte levels
- Glucose level
- Developmental interventions

BOX 37-7 S.T.A.B.L.E. PROGRAM ON POST-RESUSCITATION AND POST-TRANSPORT STABILIZATION CARE OF SICK INFANTS

S – Sugar and safe care (safety, IV fluids, hypoglycemia, hyperglycemia, umbilical catheters)
T – Temperature (hypothermia)
A – Airway (respiratory distress, CPAP, mechanical ventilation, pneumothorax
B – Blood pressure (hypovolemic, cardiogenic, & septic shock)
L – Lab work (lab tests related to infection, sepsis)
E – Emotional support (for parents of infants in NICUs)

Source: The S.T.A.B.L.E. Program. (2010). *Program module objectives.* Available at www.stableprogram.org/stable/php. Accessed August 12, 2010.

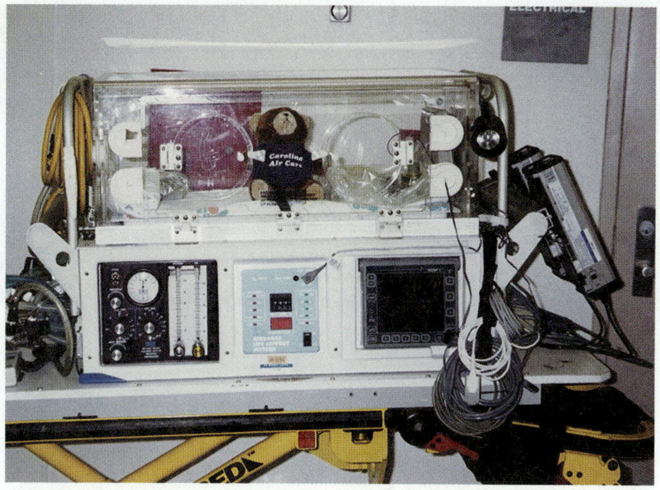

FIG. 37-15 Total life support system for transport of high risk newborns. (Courtesy UNC Hospitals, Carolina Air Care, Chapel Hill, NC.)

Transport teams can include physicians, nurse practitioners, nurses with expertise in neonatal intensive care, and respiratory therapists. The team must have expertise in resuscitation, stabilization, and provision of critical care during the transport, which can occur on the ground or in the air. In a neonatal transport, the team should provide information for the parents about the tertiary center. Transport teams can integrate an individual developmental plan of care into their caregiving efforts, thereby initiating multidisciplinary interventions early in the infant's life.

Health care professionals who are responsible for the early stabilization of newborns need specialized training to provide timely, efficient, and effective care. The S.T.A.B.L.E. training program (Box 37-7) is an evidence-based continuing education program that focuses on the postresuscitation and pretransport stabilization of sick neonates (Taylor & Price-Douglas, 2008). It has been endorsed by the March of Dimes and the American Academy of Pediatrics. Training includes an interactive didactic presentation and a posttest (www.stableprogram.org).

The birth of any high risk infant can cause profound parental stress. Parents can grieve the loss of the ideal infant. They are fearful of the possible eventual outcomes for the infant. They also must deal with the technologic world surrounding their infant, and amid all the equipment, it is sometimes difficult for them to perceive the infant and respond to his or her needs. Parents of high risk infants who have been transported to regional centers therefore need special support. As one way to deal with this problem, many intensive care units provide the family with a handbook or pictures of the tertiary care unit to help them understand what is going on around them. Parents should have the name and telephone number of a contact person at the regional center.

Infants are sometimes transferred back (back transport) to the referring facility; however, in most cases the infant is discharged home from the tertiary-care center. Preterm infants who require thermoregulation and gavage feedings may be cared for in community hospitals closer to home, which allows parents to visit their infant more easily and to work with their personal health care provider on the long-range outcomes for the infant. Specialized incubators make these trips possible (Fig. 37-15). However, parents may express mixed feelings about such return transports and may be reluctant to adapt to a different facility and group of caregivers. To minimize some of these concerns, giving the parents clear information about return transports during the initial discharge planning is important.

Anticipatory Grief

Families experience anticipatory grief when they are told of the impending death of their infant. Anticipatory grief prepares and protects parents who are facing a loss. Parents who have an infant with a debilitating disease (with or without a congenital deformity), but one that may not necessarily threaten the life of the child, also may experience anticipatory grief. An alteration in relationships, a change in lifestyle, and a very real threat to their hopes and dreams for the future may affect the day-to-day interaction of the family with their infant and the staff. Nurses can help facilitate the family's grieving process. If the nurse observes that a family member's daily interactions with the infant change, the nurse should assess the situation and request psychosocial support or intervention by a chaplain or social worker, if necessary.

Loss of an Infant

Parents who know their infant is going to die have a very difficult time. The parents need to direct their attention, energy, and caregiving activities toward the dying infant. However, some parents find it difficult to visit their infant even for short periods once a terminal diagnosis has been made. Grandparents also grieve but often are unsure how to comfort their own child (the infant's parent) during the period of impending death. Health care professionals can help by involving the family in the infant's care, providing privacy, answering questions, and preparing them for the inevitability of the death (see Chapter 38). There is a growing emphasis on hospice and palliative care for infants and their families.

The nursing staff also experiences grief. Many primary staff nurses find themselves grieving as if the infant were their own because they often have worked closely with the infant and family for weeks, or even months. Managers and other staff members must acknowledge this grief. Talking about the infant or attending the funeral can help the affected staff members resolve their feelings about the infant's death.

COMMUNITY ACTIVITY

- Visit the website of a hospital that offers neonatal intensive care in your community. How many beds does the unit have? What level of neonatal care is provided? Is the unit a major referral center for infants with complex medical or surgical problems? Are any special services available such as high frequency ventilation, or hypothermia for asphyxia? Does the unit participate in clinical research? What is the visitation policy for the parents and other family members? Are high-risk infants evaluated at an out-patient clinic for follow up after discharge? Contact the nurse manager and arrange a shadow experience at the clinic.
- Visit the website www.prematurity.org, which provides parental education, and support with a focus on special needs of premature infants. Review the information about the premature baby, premature child, and long term impacts. Research the availability of support groups for parents of premature infants in your community.

KEY POINTS

- Preterm infants are at risk for problems stemming from the immaturity of their organ systems.
- Nurses who work with preterm, late preterm, and other high risk infants observe them for respiratory distress and other early symptoms of physiologic disorders.
- The adaptation of parents to preterm, late preterm, or high risk infants differs from that of parents to normal term infants.
- Nurses can facilitate the development of a positive parent-child relationship.
- Nurses' skills in interpreting data, making decisions, and initiating therapy in newborn intensive care units are crucial to ensuring infants' survival.
- Pain management requires vigilant ongoing assessment, anticipation of painful events, and early interventions to prevent and diminish such a response.
- Nurses need to assess the macroenvironments and microenvironments of the infant and family to create a developmentally positive atmosphere.
- Developmental care is a philosophy that embraces family-centered care and awareness of the effect of environmental stimuli on the physical and psychologic well-being of the infant and family.
- Parents need special instruction (e.g., CPR, oxygen therapy, suctioning, developmental care) before they take home a high risk infant.
- SGA infants are considered at risk because of fetal growth restriction.
- The high incidence of fetal distress among postmature infants is related to the progressive placental insufficiency that can occur in a postterm pregnancy.
- Multidisciplinary health care teams including specially trained nurses transport high risk infants to and from special care units.
- Parents need assistance as they cope with anticipatory grief or loss and grief.

Audio Chapter Summaries Access an audio summary of these Key Points on Evolve

REFERENCES

Aagaard, H., & Hall, E. (2008). Mothers' experiences of having a preterm infant in the neonatal care unit: A meta-synthesis. *Journal of Pediatric Nursing, 23*(3), e26–e36.

AlFaleh, K., & Bassler, D. (2008). Probiotics for prevention of necrotizing enterocolitis in preterm infants. *The Cochrane Database of Systematic Reviews, 2008*, 1, CD005496.

Als, H., Duffy, F., McAnulty, G., Rivkin, M., Vajapeyam, S., Mulkern, R., et al. (2004). Early experience alters brain function and structure. *Pediatrics, 113*(4), 846–857.

American Academy of Pediatrics and Canadian Paediatric Society. (2006). Postnatal corticosteroids to treat or prevent chronic lung disease in preterm infants. *Pediatrics, 109*(2), 330–338.

American Academy of Pediatrics (AAP) Committee on Nutrition. (2009). *Pediatric nutrition handbook* (6th ed.). Elk Grove Village, IL: AAP.

American Heart Association (AHA). (2005). 2005 American Heart Association (AHA) guidelines for cardiopulmonary resuscitation (CPR) and emergency cardiovascular care (ECC) of pediatric and neonatal patients: Pediatric basic life support. *Circulation, 112*(Suppl. 24), 1–203.

Anand, K., & The International Evidence-based Group for Neonatal Pain. (2001). Consensus statement for the prevention and management of pain in the newborn. *Archives of Pediatric and Adolescent Medicine, 155*(2), 173–180.

Anand, K., Johnston, C., Oberlander, T., Taddio, A., Lehr, V., & Walco, G. (2005). Analgesia and local anesthesia during invasive procedures in the neonate. *Clinical Therapeutics, 27*(6), 844–876.

Aranda, J., Carlo, W., Hummel, P., Thomas, R., Lehr, V., & Anand, K. (2005). Analgesia and sedation during mechanical ventilation in neonates. *Clinical Therapeutics, 27*(6), 877–899.

Anderson, M., Wood, L., Keller, J., & Hay, W. (2011). Enteral nutrition. In S. Gardner, B. Carter, M. Enzman-Hines, & J. Hernandez (Eds.), *Merenstein & Gardner's handbook of neonatal intensive care* (7th ed.). St. Louis: Mosby.

Armentrout, D. (2010). Glucose management. In M. Verklan & M. Walden (Eds.), *AWHONN core curriculum for neonatal intensive care nursing* (4th ed.). St. Louis: Saunders.

Askin, D. (2010). Respiratory distress. In M. Verklan & M. Walden (Eds.), *AWHONN core curriculum for neonatal intensive care nursing* (4th ed.). St. Louis: Saunders.

Askin, D., & Diehl-Jones, W. (2009a). Pathogenesis and prevention of chronic lung disease in the neonate. *Critical Care Nursing Clinics of North America, 21*(1), 11–25.

Askin, D., & Diehl-Jones, W. (2009b). Retinopathy of prematurity. *Critical Care Nursing Clinics of North America, 21*(2), 213–233.

Bagwell, G. (2007). Resuscitation and stabilization of the newborn. In C. Kenner & J. Lott (Eds.), *Comprehensive neonatal care: A physiologic perspective* (4th ed.). St. Louis: Saunders.

Bakewell-Sachs, S. (2007). Near-term/late preterm infants. *Newborn & Infant Nursing Reviews, 7*(2), 67–71.

Barclay, A., Stenson, B., Simpson, J., Weaver, L., & Wilson, D. (2007). Probiotics for necrotizing enterocolitis: A systematic review. *Journal of Pediatric Gastroenterology and Nutrition, 45*(5), 569–576.

Bell, E., & Oh, W. (2005). Fluid and electrolyte management. In M. MacDonald, M. Seshia, & M. Mullett (Eds.), *Avery's neonatology: Pathophysiology and management of the newborn* (6th ed.). Philadelphia: Lippincott Williams & Wilkins.

Blackburn, S. (2007). *Maternal, fetal, and neonatal physiology: A clinical perspective* (3rd ed.). St. Louis: Saunders.

Blackburn, S., & Ditzenberger, G. (2007). Neurologic system. In C. Kenner & J. Lott (Eds.), *Comprehensive neonatal care: An interdisciplinary approach* (4th ed.). St. Louis: Saunders.

Blauer, T., & Gerstmann, D. (1998). A simultaneous comparison of three neonatal pain scales during common NICU procedures. *Clinical Journal of Pain, 14*(1), 39–47.

Bosque, E., & Haverman, C. (2009). Making babies real: Dressing infants in the NICU. *Neonatal Network, 28*(2), 85–92.

Bradshaw, W. (2010). Gastrointestinal disorders. In M. Verklan & M. Walden (Eds.), *AWHONN core curriculum for neonatal intensive care nursing* (4th ed.). St. Louis: Saunders.

Brown, V., & Landers, S. (2011). Heat balance. In S. Gardner, B. Carter, M. Enzman-Hines & J. Hernandez (Eds.), *Merenstein & Gardner's handbook of neonatal intensive care* (7th ed.). St. Louis: Mosby.

Caplan, M. (2006). Neonatal necrotizing enterocolitis. In R. Martin, A. Fanaroff & M. Walsh (Eds.), *Fanaroff and Martin's neonatal-perinatal medicine: Diseases of the fetus and infant* (8th ed.). Philadelphia: Mosby.

Carrier, C. (2010). Developmental support. In M. Verklan & M. Walden (Eds.), *AWHONN core curriculum for neonatal intensive care nursing* (4th ed.). St. Louis: Saunders.

Carlo, W. (2007). Respiratory system. In C. Kenner & J. Lott (Eds.), *Comprehensive neonatal care: A physiologic perspective* (4th ed.). St. Louis: Saunders.

Carlo, W., Martin, R., & Fanaroff, A. (2006). Assisted ventilation and complications of respiratory distress. In R. Martin, A. Fanaroff, & M. Walsh (Eds.), *Fanaroff and Martin's neonatal-perinatal medicine: Diseases of the fetus and infant* (8th ed.). Philadelphia: Mosby.

Cifuentes, J., & Carlo, W. (2007). Respiratory system. In C. Kenner & J. Lott (Eds.), *Comprehensive neonatal care: An interdisciplinary approach* (4th ed.). St. Louis: Saunders.

Cleaveland, K. (2010). Feeding challenges in the late preterm infant. *Neonatal Network, 29*(1), 37–41.

Curley, M., Razmus, I., Roberts, K., & Wypij, D. (2003). Predicting pressure ulcer risk in pediatric patients: The Braden Q scale. *Nursing Research, 52*(1), 22–33.

Daily, D., Carter, A., & Carter, B. (2011). Discharge planning and follow-up of the neonatal intensive care unit infant. In S. Gardner, B. Carter, M. Enzman-Hines, & J. Hernandez (Eds.), *Merenstein & Gardner's handbook of neonatal intensive care* (7th ed.). St. Louis: Mosby.

Darcy, A. (2009). Complications of the late preterm infant. *Journal of Perinatal and Neonatal Nursing, 23*(1), 78–86.

de Vries, L. (2006). Intracranial hemorrhage and vascular lesions. In R. Martin, A. Fanaroff, & M. Walsh (Eds.), *Fanaroff and Martin's neonatal-perinatal medicine: Diseases of the fetus and infant* (8th ed.). Philadelphia: Mosby.

Diehl-Jones, W., & Askin, D. (2010). Hematologic disorders. In M. Verklan & M. Walden (Eds.), *AWHONN core curriculum for neonatal intensive care nursing* (4th ed.). St. Louis: Saunders.

Ditzenberger, G. (2010). Nutritional management. In M. Verklan & M. Walden (Eds.), *AWHONN core curriculum for neonatal intensive care nursing* (4th ed.). St. Louis: Saunders.

Dudell, G., & Stoll, B. (2007). Respiratory tract disorders. In R. Kliegman, R. Behrman, H. Jenson, & B. Stanton (Eds.), *Nelson textbook of pediatrics* (18th ed.). Philadelphia: Saunders.

Engle, W., & American Academy of Pediatrics (AAP). Committee on Fetus and Newborn. (2008). Surfactant replacement therapy for respiratory distress in the preterm and term neonate. *Pediatrics, 121*(2), 419–432.

Ertl, T., Gyarmati, J., Gaal, V., & Szabo, I. (2006). Relationship between hyperglycemia and retinopathy of prematurity in very low birth weight infants. *Biology of the Neonate, 89*(1), 56–59.

Furdon, S., & Benjamin, K. (2010). Physical assessment. In M. Verklan & M. Walden (Eds.), *AWHONN core curriculum for neonatal intensive care nursing* (4th ed.). St. Louis: Saunders.

Gardner, S., Enzman-Hines, M., & Dickey, L. (2011). Respiratory diseases. In S. Gardner, B. Carter, M. Enzman-Hines & J. Hernandez (Eds.), *Merenstein & Gardner's handbook of neonatal intensive care* (7th ed.). St. Louis: Mosby.

Gardner, S., & Goldson, E. (2011). The neonate and the environment: Impact on development. In S. Gardner, B. Carter, M. Enzman-Hines & J. Hernandez (Eds.), *Merenstein & Gardner's handbook of neonatal intensive care* (7th ed.). St. Louis: Mosby.

Gardner, S., & Lawrence, R. (2011). Breastfeeding the neonate with special needs. In S. Gardner, B. Carter, M. Enzman-Hines, & J. Hernandez (Eds.), *Merenstein & Gardner's handbook of neonatal intensive care* (7th ed.). St. Louis: Mosby.

Garg, M., & Devaskar, S. (2006). Glucose metabolism in the late preterm infant. *Clinics in Perinatology, 33*(4), 853–870.

Harding, C., Law, J., & Pring, T. (2006). The use of non-nutritive sucking to promote functional sucking skills in premature infants: An exploratory trial. *Infant, 2*(6), 238–243.

Haubrich, K. (2007). Auditory system. In C. Kenner & J. Lott (Eds.), *Comprehensive neonatal care: A physiologic perspective* (4th ed.). St. Louis: Saunders.

Hodgkinson, K., Bear, M., Thorn, J., & Van Blaricum, S. (1994). Measuring pain in neonates: Evaluating an instrument and developing a common language. *Australian Journal of Advanced Nursing, 12*(1), 17–22.

Holditch-Davis, D., Bartlett, T., Blickman, A., & Miles, M. (2003). Posttraumatic stress symptoms in mothers of premature infants. *Journal of Obstetric, Gynecologic and Neonatal Nursing, 32*(2), 161–171.

Holman, R., Stoll, B., Curns, A., Yorita, K., Steiner, C., & Schonberger, L. (2006). Necrotising enterocolitis hospitalizations among neonates in the United States. *Paediatric and Perinatal Epidemiology, 20*(6), 498–506.

Hughes, B., Baez, L., & McGrath, J. (2009). Necrotizing enterocolitis: Past trends and current concerns. *Newborn and Infant Nursing Reviews, 9*(3), 156–162.

Hulzebos, C., & Sauer, P. (2007). Energy requirements. *Seminars in Fetal & Neonatal Medicine, 12*(1), 2–10.

Hurst, N. (2007). The 3 M's of breast-feeding the preterm infant. *Journal of Perinatal & Neonatal Nursing, 21*(3), 234–239.

Jones, F., & Tully, M. (2006). *Best practices for expressing, storing and handling human milk.* Raleigh, NC: Human Milk Banking Association of North America.

Kliegman, R. (2006). Intrauterine growth restriction. In R. Martin, A. Fanaroff, & M. Walsh (Eds.), *Fanaroff and Martin's neonatal-perinatal medicine: Diseases of the fetus and infant* (8th ed.). Philadelphia: Mosby.

Konduri, G., & Kim, U. (2009). Advances in the diagnosis and management of persistent pulmonary hypertension of the newborn. *Pediatric Clinics of North America, 56*(3), 579–600.

Krueger, C., Wall, S., Parker, L., & Nealis, R. (2005). Elevated sound levels within a busy NICU. *Neonatal Network, 24*(6), 33–37.

Lambert, D., Christensen, R., Henry, E., Besner, G., Baer, V., Wiedmeier, S., et al. (2007). Necrotizing enterocolitis in term neonates: Data from a multihospital health-care system. *Journal of Perinatology, 27*(7), 437–443.

Lawrence, J., Alcock, D., McGrath, P., Kay, J., MacMurray, S., & Dulberg, C. (1993). The development of a tool to assess neonatal pain. *Neonatal Network, 12*(6), 59–66.

Ludington-Hoe, S., Morgan, K., & Abouelfettoh, A. (2008). A clinical guideline for implementation of kangaroo care with premature infants of 30 or more weeks' postmenstrual age. *Advances in Neonatal Care, 8*(Suppl 3), S3–S23.

Lund, C. (2010). Extracorporeal membrane oxygenation. In M. Verklan & M. Walden (Eds.), *AWHONN core curriculum for neonatal intensive care nursing* (4th ed.). St. Louis: Saunders.

Lund, C., & Kuller (2007). Integumentary system. In C. Kenner & J. Lott (Eds.), *Comprehensive neonatal care: An interdisciplinary approach* (4th ed.). St. Louis: Saunders.

Lund, C., Kuller, J., Raines, D., Ecklund, S., Archambault, M., & O'Flaherty, P. (2007). *Neonatal skin care* (2nd ed.). Washington, DC: Association of Women's Health, Obstetric and Neonatal Nurses.

Lund, C., & Osborne, J. (2004). Validity and reliability of the neonatal skin condition score. *Journal of Obstetric, Gynecologic and Neonatal Nursing, 33*(3), 320–327.

McGowan, J., Rozance, P., Price-Douglas, W., & Hay, W. (2011). Glucose homeostasis. In S. Gardner, B. Carter, M. Enzman-Hines, & J. Hernandez (Eds.), *Merenstein & Gardner's handbook of neonatal intensive care* (7th ed.). St. Louis: Mosby.

Martin, J., Osterman, M., & Sutton, P. (2010). Are preterm births on the decline in the United States? Recent data from the National Vital Statistics System. *NCHS Data Brief, 39*. Hyattsville, MD: National Center for Health Statistics. Available at http://www.cdc.gov/nchs/data/databriefs/db24.htm. Accessed August 1, 2010.

Mathur, A., Neil, J., McKinstry, R., & Inder, T. (2008). Transport, monitoring, and successful brain MR imaging in unsedated neonates. *Pediatric Radiology, 38*(3), 260–264.

Melnyk, B., Feinstein, N., Alpert-Gillis, L., Fairbanks, E., Crean, H., Sinkin, R., et al. (2006). Reducing premature infants' length of stay and improving parents' mental health outcomes with the Creating Opportunities for Parent Empowerment (COPE) neonatal intensive care unit program: A randomized, controlled trial. *Pediatrics, 118*(5), e1414–e1427.

Mosqueda, E., Sapieqiene, L., Glynn, L., Wilson-Costello, D., & Weiss, M. (2008). The early use of minimal enteral nutrition in extremely low birth weight newborns. *Journal of Perinatology, 28*(4), 264–269.

NIDCAP. (2009). *NIDCAP federation international-newborn intensive and special care.* South Attleboro, MA. Available at www.nidcap.org/about.aspx. Accessed August 1, 2010.

Ohlsson, A., Walia, R., & Shah, S. (2008). Ibuprofen for the treatment of patent ductus arteriosus in preterm and/or low birth weight infants. *The Cochrane Database of Systematic Reviews, 2008*, 4, CD003481.

Pappas, B., & Walker, B. (2010). Care of the late preterm infant. In M. Verklan & M. Walden (Eds.), *AWHONN core curriculum for neonatal intensive care nursing* (4th ed.). St.Louis: Saunders.

Pokela, M. (1994). Pain relief can reduce hypoxemia in distressed neonates during routine treatment procedures. *Pediatrics, 93*(3), 379–383.

Polin, R. (2009). Bubble CPAP: A clash of science, culture, and religion. *Journal of Pediatrics, 154*(5), 633–634.

Raju, T., Higgins, R., Stark, A., & Lereno, K. (2006). Optimizing care and outcome for late-preterm (near term) infants: A summary of the workshop sponsored by the National Institute of Child Health and Human Development. *Pediatrics, 118*(3), 1207–1214.

Ramachandrappa, A., & Jain, L. (2009). Health issues of the late preterm infant. *Pediatric Clinics of North America, 56*(3), 565–577.

Rodriguez, R., Martin, R., & Fanaroff, A. (2006). Respiratory distress syndrome and its management. In R. Martin, A. Fanaroff, & M. Walsh (Eds.), *Fanaroff and Martin's neonatal-perinatal medicine: Diseases of the fetus and infant* (8th ed.). Philadelphia: Mosby.

Rojas, M., Shirley, K., & Rush, M. (2011). Perinatal transport. In S. Gardner, B. Carter, M. Enzman-Hines, & J. Hernandez (Eds.), *Merenstein & Gardner's handbook of neonatal intensive care* (7th ed.). St. Louis: Mosby.

Sadowski, S. (2010). Cardiovascular disorders. In M. Verklan & M. Walden (Eds.), *AWHONN core curriculum for neonatal intensive care nursing* (4th ed.). St. Louis: Saunders.

Santa-Donato, A., Medoff-Cooper, B., Bakewell-Sachs, S., Askin, D., & Rosenberg, S. (2007). *Late preterm infant assessment guide.* Washington, DC: Association of Women's Health, Obstetric and Neonatal Nurses.

Saugstad, O. (2007). Optimal oxygenation at birth and in the neonatal period. *Neonatology, 91*(4), 319–322.

Siegel, R., Gardner, S., & Dickey, L. (2011). Families in crisis: Theoretical and practical considerations. In S. Gardner, B. Carter, M. Enzman-Hines, & J. Hernandez (Eds.), *Merenstein & Gardner's handbook of neonatal intensive care* (7th ed.). St. Louis: Mosby.

Soll, R. (2008). Heat loss prevention in neonates. *Journal of Perinatology, 28*(Suppl. 1), S57–S57.

Sparshott, M. (1995). Assessing the behaviour of the newborn infant. *Paediatric Nursing, 7*(7), 14–16.

Spence, K., Gillies, D., Harrison, D., Johnston, L., & Nagy, S. (2005). A reliable pain assessment tool for clinical assessment in the neonatal intensive care unit. *Journal of Obstetric, Gynecologic and Neonatal Nursing, 34*(10), 80–86.

Stevens, B., Johnston, C., Petryshen, P., & Taddio, A. (1996). Premature Infant Pain Profile: Development and initial validation. *Clinical Journal of Pain, 12*(1), 13–22.

Stoll, B., & Adams-Chapman, I. (2007). The high-risk infant. In R. Kliegman, R. Behrman, H. Jenson, & B. Stanton (Eds.), *Nelson textbook of pediatrics* (18th ed.). Philadelphia: Saunders.

Strodtbeck, F. (2007). Ophthalmic system. In C. Kenner & J. Lott (Eds.), *Comprehensive neonatal care: An interdisciplinary approach* (4th ed.). St. Louis: Saunders.

Symington, A., & Pinelli, J. (2006). Developmental care for promoting development and preventing morbidity in preterm infants (review). *The Cochrane Database of Systematic Reviews, 2006*, 2, CD001814.

Taylor, R., & Price-Douglas, W. (2008). The S.T.A.B.L.E program: Postresuscitation/pretransport stabilization care of sick infants. *Journal of Perinatal and Neonatal Nursing, 22*(2), 159–165.

Terrin, G., Passariello, A., Canani, R., Manguso, F., Paludetto, R., & Cascioli, C. (2009). Minimal enteral feeding reduces the risk of sepsis in feed-intolerant very low birth weight newborns. *Acta Paediatrica, 98*(1), 31–35.

Tyson, J., & Kennedy, K. (2005). Minimal enteral nutrition for promoting feeding tolerance and preventing morbidity in parenterally fed infants. *The Cochrane Database of Systematic Reviews, 2005*, 3, CD000504.

Velaphi, S., & Vidyasagar, D. (2008). The pros and cons of suctioning at the perineum (intrapartum) and post-delivery with and without meconium. *Seminars in Fetal and Neonatal Medicine, 13*(6), 375–382.

Volpe, J. (2008). *Neurology of the newborn* (5th ed.). Philadelphia: Saunders.

Walden, M. (2007). Pain in the newborn and infant. In C. Kenner & J. Lott (Eds.), *Comprehensive neonatal care: A physiologic perspective* (4th ed.). St. Louis: Saunders.

Walker, M. (2008). Breastfeeding the late preterm infant. *Journal of Obstetric, Gynecologic and Neonatal Nursing, 37*(6), 692–701.

White, R. (2007). Recommended standards for the newborn ICU. *Journal of Perinatology, 27*(Suppl. 2), S4–S19.

CHAPTER

38

Perinatal Loss and Grief

Margaret Shandor Miles

evolve WEBSITE

http://evolve.elsevier.com/Lowdermilk/MWHC/
Audio Glossary
Audio Key Points
NCLEX Review Questions
Nursing Care Plan
Fetal Death: 24 Weeks of Gestation

LEARNING OBJECTIVES

- Describe the causes of perinatal loss.
- Describe the grieving process of parents who experience perinatal loss.
- Analyze the personal and societal issues that can complicate responses to perinatal loss.
- Formulate appropriate nursing diagnoses for parents experiencing perinatal loss.
- Identify specific nursing interventions to meet the special needs of parents and their families related to perinatal loss and grief.
- Differentiate among helpful and nonhelpful responses in caring for parents experiencing loss and grief.
- Discuss assessment and nursing interventions for parents experiencing complicated grief.

Becoming a parent is an important developmental milestone that most men and women in our society anticipate. Becoming a parent gives one social status, expands one's capacity for caring and for loving another, and adds immense responsibility to one's life. However, pregnancy and birth can also be associated with loss.

The focus of this chapter is to prepare the nurse to provide sensitive, supportive, and therapeutic interventions to parents experiencing perinatal loss in a variety of settings. An overview of the grief process is presented as a guide for assessing and understanding the responses of bereaved women, men, and their families. Guidelines for interventions are given and specific intervention approaches are discussed.

PERINATAL LOSS

During pregnancy parents plan for the birth, imagine what the birth will be like, and develop an image of the baby. The reality of childbirth can be inconsistent with the parents' hopes and dreams. In particular, the experience of preterm labor and birth or cesarean birth involves loss of the expected pregnancy and birth plans. Parents also may grieve over the sex or appearance of their child. For some parents, loss is associated with the birth of an infant who has a birth defect or chronic illness.

Although having children can be a strong desire and goal for women and men, not everyone is successful in achieving parenthood. For some couples, infertility can thwart their plans and desires for parenthood and cause intense feelings of grief (McGrath, Samra, Zukowsky, & Baker, 2010). When couples undergo infertility treatments, feelings of loss can intensify, especially when treatments fail and/or a pregnancy ends in an ectopic pregnancy loss or miscarriage. When infertility treatment is successful, loss and grief can confound the joy if selective reduction of multifetal pregnancy is done (Little, 2010).

Many women and their partners, whether infertile or not, experience **perinatal loss.** This includes ectopic pregnancy, fetal death, or miscarriage, all of which occur in the early months of pregnancy. These early pregnancy losses are often called "hidden" or "silent" because others in the women's network do not even know about the pregnancy and subsequent loss, or because family and friends do not feel comfortable bringing up the loss with the woman and her partner, resulting in acute grief and loneliness (Brier, 2008).

Women and their partners can suddenly be confronted with **stillbirth,** the birth of an infant who is not alive. Stillbirth is particularly devastating because it occurs suddenly and late in the pregnancy when expectant parents are preparing for the birth of a healthy infant (Cacciatore, 2010).

Couples also can face the death of an infant after birth who has serious health problems related to prematurity, severe congenital anomalies, genetic defects, or other complications. Some of these newborns survive only a few hours or die after days, weeks, or months in an intensive care unit, where complex highly technologic care and invasive treatments are used to try to save their lives. Many of these parents are confronted with making difficult end-of-life decisions about their baby (De Lisle-Porter & Podruchny, 2009). Another tragic loss for parents is death of an older infant from sudden infant death syndrome (SIDS).

Parents who face challenges in achieving and maintaining a pregnancy, learning about their infant's fatal or serious health problems, and coping with the loss of a fetus or death of an infant experience intense psychologic distress and grief. **Grief** involves the painful emotions and related behavioral and physical responses to a major loss. Grief can be particularly difficult with perinatal losses for a number of reasons. One is the societal belief that there are no barriers to getting pregnant, thus, perinatal losses are often hidden or private. Another is the expectation that once a woman is pregnant, the outcome will be a healthy live infant. As a result, our society tends to minimize or discount perinatal loss and lacks an understanding of the associated pain (Brier, 2008; Fretts, 2009).

Perinatal losses can be intensified for couples who delay pregnancy until the woman's career and the family's financial status are at the right point to take on the responsibilities of a child. Feelings of helplessness and loss of control can be very difficult when the couple experiences infertility or miscarriage. In many instances of perinatal loss, the lack of an identified cause for the loss can complicate grief. This is particularly difficult for women, who often feel personally responsible for infertility, miscarriage, and infant death. Some couples endure repeated losses, which can be devastating. Further, society allows too little time for mothers to grieve a perinatal loss and even less for men (O'Leary & Thorwick, 2006). Women and men who undergo perinatal losses often struggle with these issues alone and without the support they need because many perinatal losses are hidden or private.

Nurses have a powerful influence on how parents experience and cope with perinatal loss (Gold, 2007; Gold, Dalton, & Schwenk, 2007; Murphy & Merrell, 2009). Nurses encounter these parents in a variety of settings, including the antepartum, labor and birth, neonatal, postpartum, and gynecologic units of hospitals; and obstetric, gynecologic, and infertility outpatient clinics and general medical offices. In these settings nurses have opportunities to provide sensitive and caring interventions to parents. Parents have reported that their nurses were an important resource in helping them cope with their grief; parents tend to rate nurses as more supportive than physicians or other care providers (Gold, 2007).

Nurses in many inpatient settings have developed protocols that provide clear direction to all staff in how to help parents through this difficult process. In some units experienced nurses or social workers who are particularly comfortable in helping bereaved parents are designated as perinatal grief consultants. They are available to help parents and to help staff prepare for their roles with parents. In addition, many institutions now have follow-up programs involving telephone calls, home visits, and support groups that are effective in helping parents after discharge. These models for care of bereaved parents have evolved into more formalized perinatal hospice or palliative care programs in a variety of settings including prenatal diagnostic and genetic programs, maternity care clinics, and inpatient maternity and neonatal intensive care units (Breeze, Lees, Kumar, Missfelder-Lobos, & Murdoch, 2007; Leuthner & Jones, 2007; Murphy & Merrell, 2009; Rousch, Sullivan, Cooper, & McBride, 2007). It is important, then, that nurses are prepared to help parents deal with perinatal loss.

GRIEF RESPONSES

Grief or **bereavement** has been described as a cluster of painful responses experienced following a major loss or death. In a concept analysis of grief, Cowles and Rodgers (2000) identified attributes of grief: (a) grief is *dynamic* and involves an ever-changing complex of emotions, thoughts, and behaviors, (b) grief is *a process* that is enduring and has no time limit; (c) grief is *highly individualized* and manifested in many different ways from one person to the next; and (d) grief is *pervasive* in that it involves psychologic, social, physical, cognitive, behavioral, and affective responses and can affect every aspect of a person's life. Grief is experienced and expressed in an individualized manner and is particularly affected by the meaning of the loss to the person.

The model of grief presented here is based on years of clinical work by the author with bereaved parents and on the conceptualization of others regarding grief (Miles, 1984). It is hypothesized that parental grief responses occur in three overlapping phases (Box 38-1). There is an early period of acute distress and shock followed by a period of intense grief that includes emotional, cognitive, behavioral, and physical responses. Parents reach the phase of reorganization when they return to their usual level of functioning in society, although the pain associated with the death remains. There is general agreement that parental grief is a long-term process that can extend for months and years and that some aspects of their grief endure through life.

Acute Distress

The loss of a pregnancy or the death of an infant is an acute and distressing experience for mothers and fathers. The loss encompasses a loss of their identity as a mother or father and their many dreams related to parenthood (Arnold & Gemma, 2008). The immediate reaction to news of a perinatal loss or infant death encompasses a period of acute distress. Parents generally are in a state of shock and numbness. They can feel a sense of unreality, loss of innocence, and powerlessness as though they were in a bad dream or in a fog or trance-like state. Disbelief and denial can occur. Sadness, devastation, and depression as well as intense outbursts of emotion and crying are common. However, lack of affect, euphoria, and calmness can reflect numbness, denial, or a personal way of coping with stress.

Much of the literature and research on grief after perinatal loss and infant death has focused on the mother. Likewise, much of the attention during the time of a loss is on the mother; the father is expected to be her main support but is often not acknowledged as grieving, too. The response of fathers can be more variable than that of mothers and depends on the level

BOX 38-1 CONCEPTUAL MODEL OF PARENTAL GRIEF

PHASE OF ACUTE DISTRESS
- Shock
- Numbness
- Intense crying
- Depression

PHASE OF INTENSE GRIEF
- Loneliness, emptiness, yearning
- Guilt
- Anger, resentment, bitterness, irritability
- Fear and anxiety (especially about getting pregnant again)
- Disorganization
- Difficulties with cognitive processing
- Sadness and depression
- Physical symptoms

REORGANIZATION
- Search for meaning
- Reduction of distress
- Reentering normal life activities with more enthusiasm
- Can make plans, including decision about another pregnancy

Adapted from Miles, M. (1980). *The grief of parents...when a child dies.* Oak Brook, IL: Compassionate Friends; Miles, M. (1984). Helping adults mourn the death of a child. In H. Wass, & C. Corr (Eds.), *Childhood and death.* New York: Hemisphere.

of identification with the pregnancy. With early miscarriage or ectopic pregnancy, some fathers have not yet developed a strong investment in the wished-for child. However, many fathers are profoundly affected and do grieve deeply for a perinatal loss, yet their feelings are often ignored (O'Leary & Thorwick, 2006).

Fathers are distressed by the grief of the mother and often feel helpless as to how to help her with the intense pain (O'Leary & Thorwick, 2006). Some fathers appear stoic and unemotional to maintain the societal expectation that they are "strong" for the mother and other family members. It is important to realize that fathers can be experiencing deep pain beneath their calm and quiet appearance and need help in acknowledging these feelings. Because many fathers do not easily share feelings or ask for help, special efforts are needed to help them realize that they too have a right to receive support from others as they grieve.

During this time of acute distress parents face the first task of grief, accepting the reality of the loss. The pregnancy has ended or the baby has died, and their life has changed. Parents are often required to make many decisions, such as naming the infant and making funeral arrangements during this period when normal functioning is impeded and decisions are difficult to make. This can be especially painful and difficult for young couples who have limited or no previous experience with death. Grandparents are often called on to help make difficult decisions regarding funeral arrangements and/or disposition of the body because they have more life experience with taking care of these painful, yet required arrangements. However, some well-meaning grandparents and other family members try to take over all the decisions that must be made. It is critical for the nurse to remember that a very important role is always to be a client advocate and that the parents themselves should approve the final decisions.

Intense Grief

The phase of intense grief encompasses many difficult emotions as the parents work through their pain and adjust to life without the wished-for child. In the early months after the loss parents often experience feelings of loneliness, emptiness, and yearning. The mother may report that her arms ache to hold or nurse her baby and that she wakes to the sound of a baby crying. When her milk comes in, it is particularly poignant when there is no baby to breastfeed. Mothers and fathers can be preoccupied with thoughts about the wished-for child. Some women cope with these feelings by avoiding memories and by not talking about the baby, whereas others want to reminisce and discuss their loss over and over. Deciding what to do about the nursery and baby clothes is particularly difficult. Some women want the room taken down before they go home, whereas others want the room left intact until they have had time to grieve their loss. It is not unusual for a grandparent or other family member to want to rush home to take down the nursery with the thought that they would be sparing additional painful grief. In fact, their actions might only complicate the grief if parents were not involved in the decision. The bereaved parents, in their own time frame, must go through these types of experiences so that healing can take place.

During this phase of intense grief, guilt can emerge from the deep feelings of helplessness related to the inability to have somehow prevented the pregnancy loss or the death of the infant. Mothers are particularly vulnerable to feel guilt because of their sense of responsibility for the well-being of the fetus and baby. With many perinatal losses there is no clear cause of the event, leaving the woman to speculate about what she might have done or not done to cause the loss. Guilt can be intense if a mother thinks she is being punished for some unrelated event such as having had a prior induced abortion. Such self-blame is torture for mothers, and they need repeated emotional reassurance that they were not at fault. Guilt can occur when the mother or father begins enjoying life and experiencing happiness again despite the loss of the infant.

Other common responses during this phase of grief are anger, resentment, bitterness, or irritability. Anger is particularly poignant if the loss is perceived as senseless, and there is a need to blame others. Anger can be focused on the health care team who failed to save the pregnancy or infant. Some parents direct their anger toward God, who they blame for allowing the loss to occur. This can lead to a spiritual crisis. Anger also occurs toward family, friends, and peers when they do not provide the support bereaved parents need and want. Some parents focus their resentment on parents who do not appreciate their children or who neglect and abuse them. A sense of bitterness or generalized irritability, rather than frank anger, can be another response.

Fear and anxiety can occur during the grief process as a profound worry that something else bad might happen to another. Fear and anxiety are particularly poignant when the couple considers another pregnancy (DeBackere, Hill, & Kavanaugh, 2008). Some parents, especially mothers, are almost obsessed with the desire to become pregnant again; others struggle with whether they can cope with another potential loss.

Deep sadness and depression occur when the parent faces the full awareness of the reality of the loss. This often occurs several months after a perinatal loss and can continue for some time. Sadness and depression are often accompanied by disorganization and problems with cognitive processing. This leads to behavioral changes such as difficulty in getting things done, an inability to concentrate, restlessness, confused thought processes, difficulty in solving problems, and poor decision making. Disorganization and depression often cause difficulties in keeping up with work and family expectations. Additionally parents returning to work face issues such as handling well-meaning but painful comments or the silence of coworkers.

Physical symptoms of grief include fatigue, headaches, dizziness, or backaches. Parents are at risk for developing health problems, such as colds or hypertension. The grieving process makes it difficult for bereaved parents to sleep. Their appetites can be depressed or voracious. Lack of sleep and inadequate nutrition and fluids can complicate other grief responses.

Grief responses are very personal, ongoing, and difficult to endure. Some parents suppress or deny their feelings because of societal indifference toward pregnancy loss and infant death. Suppression of feelings may, on the surface, be more socially acceptable. However, denying the pain of grief can lead to eventual physical and emotional distress or illness. Many parents, especially mothers, want to tell their story over and over. This helps them actualize the loss and face their feelings. Sometimes parents begin to think they are the only individuals who have ever had such a rough time and that they are going crazy. Although bereaved parents have ups and downs for many months and even years after a child's death, few parents actually become mentally ill or commit suicide. Knowing that their feelings are normal and that others have felt the same is helpful. The grief process during this phase is often difficult for fathers (O'Leary & Thorwick, 2006). Some may continue to have difficulty sharing their feelings. A rift can occur if one parent, usually the mother, wants to talk about the loss and pain, and the other parent, often but not always the father, withdraws. Other signs of problems include reliance on alcohol and drugs, extramarital affairs, prolonged hours at work, and overinvolvement in activities outside the home as an escape.

Reorganization

From the time of the pregnancy loss or infant death, parents attempt to understand "why?" This leads to a long and intense search for meaning. At first the "why" is focused on the cause of death. Finding few good answers, parents focus next on "why me, why mine?" These questions lead some parents into an existential search about the meaning of life and death. "What does my loss mean to my life?" "What is life all about?" "What do I do with the rest of my life?" This search continues into the phase of reorganization and can lead to profound changes in the parents' views about the fragility of life.

Time helps to ease slowly the painful feelings of grief. Although some grief models focus on "letting go" as an important step in the grief process, bereaved parents often want to hold on to their relationship with their child (Davies, 2004). With perinatal loss, however, parents have few, if any, memories of their infant to provide a balance to their devastating loss, and this adds to their pain.

Over time the feelings become less painful. Reorganization occurs when the parent is better able to function at home and work, experiences a return of self-esteem and confidence, can cope with new challenges, and has placed the loss in perspective. Reorganization begins to peak sometime after the first year as parents begin to achieve the task of moving on with their lives. Enjoying the simple pleasures of life without feeling guilty, nurturing self and others, developing new interests, and reestablishing relationships are signs of moving on. For some women and families, another pregnancy and the birth of a subsequent child is an important step in moving on with their lives (Swanson, Connor, Jolley, Pettinato, & Wang, 2007). However, the term *recovery* is never used because the grief related to perinatal loss can continue in varying degrees for life.

Parents have shared that they will never forget the baby who has died, and they are not the same people as before the loss. The term *bittersweet grief* refers to the grief response that occurs with reminders of the loss. This typically happens at special anniversary dates related to the loss. Grief feelings also can be triggered during subsequent pregnancies and after birth (Côté-Arsenault & Marshall, 2000; DeBackere et al., 2008).

Resuming the sexual relationship is an important aspect of recovery, but it can be very complicated. Many parents are comforted with the belief that their babies were conceived in love, lived in love, and died in love. Their love and intimacy created this child, and parents can believe that they will never experience joy and closeness again. Once the doctor has given permission for resumption of sexual activities, parents can find it emotionally very difficult. Some couples have an increased need for sexual activity in an attempt for closeness and healing, whereas others have a decreased desire for sexual intimacy. It is important that parents are aware of some possible deep need from inside themselves to stop the emotional pain. Difficulties arise when the needs of the couple differ.

Sexuality also brings with it decisions about a future pregnancy. The decision to have another child involves intense and conflicting emotions (DeBackere et al., 2008). Parents want to be hopeful about having a normal healthy child but also have fears about having another loss. A deep fear of experiencing the pain of loss again can make the resumption of sexual activity difficult. These ambivalent feelings are normal, and couples will find themselves moving back and forth between the emotions of exhilaration and fear. The subsequent pregnancy after a loss is often filled with guarded emotions and great anxiety (Côté-Arsenault & Donato, 2007). The excitement that many others experience with a pregnancy is very different for previously bereaved parents (Côté-Arsenault, 2007). This distress can continue even after the birth of a healthy infant and affect maternal attachment to the new baby (Armstrong, 2007). Fathers also report anxiety about the outcome of the next pregnancy and increased their vigilance (Armstrong, 2007; O'Leary & Thorwick, 2006). Couples sometimes mark the progress of the pregnancy in terms of fetal development, waiting anxiously until the number of weeks of the previous loss have passed. The fear of repeated loss is especially high after a stillbirth.

FAMILY ASPECTS OF GRIEF

Grandparents and Siblings

It is extremely important for nurses taking care of grieving parents to keep in mind that they have an entire family to minister to, including especially grandparents and siblings.

Grandparents have hopes and dreams for a grandchild; these have been shattered. The grief of grandparents is often complicated by the fact that they are experiencing intense emotional pain by witnessing and feeling the immense grief of their own child. It is extremely difficult to watch their son or daughter experience unimaginable emotional trauma with very few ways to comfort and end their pain. As a result, the grief response can be complicated or delayed for grandparents. Some grandparents experience immense "survivor guilt" because they feel the death is out of order as they are alive and their grandchild has died.

The siblings of the expected infant also experience a profound loss. Most children have been prepared for having another child in the family once the pregnancy is confirmed. These children come in all ages and stages of development, and the nurse must consider this to understand how the child views the event and their loss experience. Given that young children are now often kept fully aware about a pregnancy and an expected brother or sister, they can have a great deal of difficulty understanding why there suddenly is no baby or the baby has not come home (Limbo & Kobler, 2009). A young child will respond to the reactions of his or her parents, picking up on the fact that they are behaving differently and are extremely sad. This can cause clinging, altered eating and sleeping patterns, or acting-out behaviors, yet it is a time when parents have limited patience for responding to and meeting the needs of the child. Older children have a more complete understanding of the loss. School-aged children can be frightened by the entire event, whereas teens can understand fully but feel awkward in responding.

Nurses can help to include siblings in grieving rituals to the extent the parents and the child feels comfortable. They may need to see the baby to actualize the loss. Nurses need to have a basic understanding about how children view death and grieve to reach out to siblings in an appropriate and sensitive manner. Nurses also need to help parents recognize and be sensitive to the grief of siblings, include them in family rituals, and keep the baby alive in the family memory. Nurses can direct parents to the website, "Children's Understanding of Death" (http://sidsnetwork.org/sibling/sibunderstanding.htm) for information about helping children cope with infant death.

CARE MANAGEMENT

Nursing care of mothers and fathers experiencing a perinatal loss begins the first time the parents are faced with the potential loss of their pregnancy or death of their infant. Supportive interventions are important when parents are anticipating loss, at the time of the loss, and after the parents have returned home (see the Nursing Process box).

In order to provide competent, compassionate, individualized care to grieving parents and their families, the nurse first conducts a thorough assessment. Several key areas to address include the following:

- The nature of the parental attachment with the pregnancy or infant, the meaning of the pregnancy and infant to the parent, and the related losses they are experiencing. Each pregnancy and birth has a special meaning to parents. Whether a woman has experienced a miscarriage or ectopic pregnancy, stillbirth, or death of an infant, it is important to gain some understanding of parents' perceptions of their unique loss. The meaning of the loss is determined by familial and cultural systems of the parents. Feelings about perinatal loss can range from feeling devastated to feeling relieved (Corbet-Owen & Kruger, 2001). Listening to parents tell their story and being sensitive to the language used to describe their experience can help nurses gain an understanding of the meaning of the loss. Open-ended questions are helpful: "Tell me about your labor and birth with Mia." Or, "When did you know you were miscarrying?" Mothers who have had a previous pregnancy loss may feel less attached, which can increase their feelings of guilt when a loss occurs.
- The circumstances surrounding the loss, including the level of preparation for the loss and the parents' level of understanding about the cause of the loss or death, and any related unresolved issues. While listening to the parents' stories, it is important to uncover any special experiences that may make their losses even more poignant. A history of infertility, repeated pregnancy losses, a previous stillbirth, or infant death can make this loss even more painful. In addition, other life circumstances such as illness of another family member, loss of a job, or other family stresses can increase the distress of parents. It also is helpful to know whether the mother and father perceived the loss to be totally unexpected, or whether they had some forewarning or preparation.
- The immediate response of the mother and father to the loss, whether their responses are complementary or problematic, and how their responses match with their past experiences, personalities, and behavioral and cultural backgrounds. An understanding of the usual responses to grief described earlier can be helpful in attempting to understand the unique grief responses of the mother and the father and other family members. As nurses work with families, they can uncover information about how the individual or family responded to a previous loss, or a personality or behavioral trait that may be involved in their responses to this grief. In particular, it is important to know about any history of infertility, previous pregnancy losses, or infant deaths and evaluate how that might affect parental responses. It also is important to be sensitive to different expectations during grief for men and women from different cultural groups (see section on cultural and spiritual needs of parents later in this chapter).
- The social support network of the parent (e.g., extended family, friends, coworkers, church) and the extent to which it has been activated. Support during a perinatal loss is important to most parents; however, it is important to assess the amount of support and the type of support that the parents desire. Some prefer to handle the tragedy alone for a time. Others want assistance in calling other family members, friends, and clergy to be with them and to help them with decisions.

Nursing care for grieving families should be comprehensive. It can be complex as the nurse considers the shock and numbness of the bereavement process and the varied grief responses of the parents and other family members during hospitalization. (See Nursing Care Plan on p. 947.)

NURSING PROCESS

Perinatal Grief

ASSESSMENT

- Attachment to the pregnancy or infant, meaning of the pregnancy and infant to the parent, and any related losses they are experiencing
- Circumstances surrounding the loss: preparation, understanding about the cause of the loss, and unresolved issues related to the loss
- Immediate responses to the loss
- Social support network

NURSING DIAGNOSES

Nursing diagnoses may involve issues experienced by the individual mother or father, or problems occurring within the couple or family because of the loss and subsequent grief. Possible nursing diagnoses include:

Anxiety **related to:**
- lack of experience regarding how to manage the loss
- worry about the partner
- concern over not achieving a pregnancy
- becoming pregnant again with risk of another loss

Ineffective Coping **related to:**
- inability to make decisions as a family
- difficulties in communication within the family
- conflicting coping patterns between mother and father

Powerlessness **related to:**
- infertility
- high risk pregnancy and birth
- unexpected cesarean birth
- inability to prevent the infant's death

Interrupted Family Processes **related to:**
- maternal depression leading to changes in role function
- inadequate communication of feelings between the grieving mother and father or partner
- lack of expected support from family
- behavioral and emotional reactions of siblings
- grief within the family system including grandparents and other relatives

Ineffective Sexuality Pattern (between the mother and father) **related to:**
- guilt and fear associated with sexuality
- loss of pleasure in sexual intercourse
- differences in sexual desires of each partner
- fear of getting pregnant again

Fatigue and Disturbed Sleep Pattern **related to:**
- inability to fall asleep because of grief
- waking in the night and thinking about the loss
- loss of sleep

Complicated Grieving **related to:**
- prolonged denial or avoidance of the loss
- intense guilt related to the loss
- continued anger about the loss
- serious depressive symptoms and despair
- loss of self-esteem
- intense grieving patterns that continue for more than a year
- social isolation due to grief
- feeling that life is meaningless

Situational Low Self-esteem **related to:**
- prolonged feelings of poor self-worth because of the loss
- feeling unworthy of having a child

Spiritual Distress **related to:**
- anger with God
- confusion about why prayers were not answered

EXPECTED OUTCOMES OF CARE

Expected outcomes are established and priorities assigned in parent-centered terms according to the mutual goals chosen by the parent(s) and the nurse. Expected outcomes are that the parents/family will:

- Actualize the loss.
- Feel supported by the nursing staff throughout their hospital stay and when visiting the clinic.
- Share experiences and verbalize feelings of grief as much as is culturally and personally appropriate.
- Understand the normal grief responses they and others in the family may experience at the time of and after the loss.
- Demonstrate increasing independence in participating in and making decisions that meet their needs and reflect their religious and cultural beliefs.
- Identify family, spiritual, health care, and community resources for support.
- Discuss problems or issues involving relationships with each other and family.
- Verbalize satisfaction with the care and support provided by their health care professionals.

PLAN OF CARE AND INTERVENTIONS

- Help the parents and other family members actualize the loss.
- Assist and support parents with decision making related to autopsy, organ donation, spiritual rituals, and disposition of the body.
- Help the bereaved parents acknowledge and express their feelings.
- Reassure and educate parents about the grief process and facilitate positive coping.
- Meet physical needs of the bereaved mother.
- Assist parents in communicating with, supporting, and getting support from family.
- Create memories for parents to take home.
- Communicate using a caring framework.
- Demonstrate concern and sensitivity about cultural and spiritual needs.
- Provide sensitive care after hospital discharge.

EVALUATION

The achievement of expected outcomes is determined when positive integration of the perinatal loss is expressed by the parents and family.

Checklists can be used to facilitate comprehensive care. Many hospitals use checklists for providing care, mobilizing members of the multidisciplinary health care team, communicating options the family has chosen, and keeping track of all the details in meeting the needs of bereaved parents (Figs. 38-1 and 38-2). Such checklists can be a permanent part of the chart. Documentation in the nursing notes of primary concerns, grief responses, health teaching, health care advice, and any referrals of the mother or other family members is essential to ensure consistency and continuity of care.

Interventions and support for parents from the nursing and medical staff after a perinatal loss or infant death are extremely important in their healing. Although parents often cannot recall details of their experiences at the time of death, they may recall

RTS Counselor ____________________ Date ____________________
Mother's name ____________________ Age ________ Due date ____________
Date of beginning of miscarriage ____________ Date of surgery ____________
# of Miscarriages ________ # of Children ________ Religion ____________________
Address ____________________ Occupation ____________________
Phone number ( ) ____________________ Marital status ____________________
Father's name ____________________ Age ________ Occupation ____________
Address ____________________ Phone number ( ) ____________________
Baby's name ____________________ Sex ____________________
Support people available ____________________ Children's names: ____________________
Problem areas ____________________ Physician ____________________
OK to send written material to home address ☐ Yes ☐ No

Date	Time	See Miscarriage Protocol RTS Manual	Comments	Initials
		Notify/Assign RTS counselor ☐ Yes ☐ No		
		Pastoral Care ☐ Yes ☐ No		
		Offered: ☐ Blessing ☐ Memorial Service ☐ Naming Ceremony ☐ Burial		
		Asked: "Would you like someone with you now?" ☐ Yes ☐ No		
		D&C/Surgical procedure discussed ☐ Yes ☐ No		
		Saw baby or tissue ☐ Mother ☐ Father		
		Touched and/or held baby ☐ Mother ☐ Father		
		If RH negative, RhoGAM given within 72 hrs ☐ Yes ☐ No		
		Patient's room flagged with door card ☐ Yes ☐ No		
		Photos taken: ☐ 35 mm ☐ Polaroid ☐ Given to parents ☐ On file		
		Footprints & handprints/weight & length: ☐ Given to parents ☐ On file		
		Grief process discussed ☐ Yes ☐ No		
		Incongruent grief discussed ☐ Yes ☐ No		
		Grief packet given ☐ Yes ☐ No		
		Info Brochure given to parents re: RTS PSG ☐ Yes ☐ No		
		Name/business card given ☐ Yes ☐ No		
		Regular OB/Midwife notified ____________ ☐ Memo ☐ Verbally		
		Childbirth Educator notified ____________ ☐ Yes ☐ No		
		Telephone number verified ☐ Yes ☐ No Optimal call time ________		
		Preg & Inf Loss Card sent to RTS Secretary ☐ Yes ☐ No		
		Given option to transfer from Maternity Unit ☐ Yes ☐ No		
		Genetic Studies ordered ☐ Yes ☐ No		
		Sex determination desired (tissue in NS only) ☐ Yes ☐ No		
		Would like another parent to call: ☐ Yes ☐ No ☐ Ask later		
		Parent contact: ____________________ Follow-up calls: eg. ☐ 1 wk, ☐ 3 wk, ☐ 4 mo, ☐ due date/anniv. date		

FIG. 38-1 Sample checklist for assisting parents experiencing miscarriage/ectopic pregnancy. (Used with permission of Bereavement Services. Copyright Lutheran Hospital—La Crosse, Inc., A Gundersen Lutheran Affiliate, La Crosse, WI.)

vividly minor events that were perceived as particularly painful or particularly helpful. However, care must be individualized for each parent and family. Parents whose infants were stillborn have noted that nurses were important in supporting them during periods of chaos, helping them meet and separate from the baby, and providing bereavement support (Saflund, Sjogren, & Wredling, 2004). Nurses also have an important role in helping parents who experience miscarriage, fetal death, or abortion related to a lethal fetal diagnosis (Breeze et al., 2007; Leuthner & Jones, 2007; Murphy & Merrell, 2009). Their grief can be overlooked because they are often treated as outpatients or have very brief hospital stays.

Furthermore, nurses should consider the cultural and spiritual beliefs and practices of individual parents and families. The interventions discussed later are general ideas about what may be helpful to parents.

Help the Mother, the Father, and Other Family Members Actualize the Loss

When a loss or death occurs, the nurse should be sure that parents have been honestly told about the situation by their physician or others on the health care team. It is important for their nurse to be with them during this time. With early pregnancy loss, it is recommended that the terminology "miscarriage" be used consistently (Cameron & Penney, 2005). With infant death, caregivers should use the words "dead" and "died," rather than "lost" or "gone," to assist the bereaved in accepting this reality. Parents need opportunities to tell their story about

Mother's discharge date: ______	Age ___ Gr ___ Para ___ L.C. ___ Due date ___
Mother's name: ______	Previous loss: ______
Address: ______	Date/Time delivered: ______
Phone number: ( ) ______	Date/Time death: ______
Father's name: ______	Baby's name: ______ Sex: ___
Address: ______	Children's name(s): ______ Age: ___
Phone number: ( ) ______	______ Age: ___
Optimal call time: ______	______ Age: ___
RTS Counselor: ______	Support people
Unit: ______ Ext ______	Attending MD &/or Pediatrician ______
Regular OB MD/Midwife: ______	Notify Peds Nurse Practitioner ______
Religion: ______	

Date	Time		Comments	Initials
		Notify/Assign RTS counselor ☐ Yes ☐ No		
		Pastoral Care notified ☐ Yes ☐ No		
		Funeral Home notified: ☐ Yes ☐ No Family Burial: ☐ Yes ☐ No		
		Saw baby when born and/or after delivery: ☐ Mother ☐ Father		
		Touched and/or held baby: ☐ Mother ☐ Father ☐ Siblings ☐ Grandparents ☐ Friends		
		Offered private time with their baby: ☐ Yes ☐ No		
		Baptism offered: (use seashell as vessel, give to parents) ☐ Yes ☐ No		
		Remembrance of Blessing offered: ☐ Yes ☐ No (can offer for any perinatal loss) ☐ Given to parents		
		Given option to transfer off Maternity Unit: ☐ Yes ☐ No		
		Patient's room flagged with door card ☐ Yes ☐ No		
		Autopsy: ☐ Yes ☐ No Genetic studies: ☐ Yes ☐ No Genetic Associate notified: ☐ Yes ☐ No		
		Regular Physician/Midwife notified of death: ☐ Yes ☐ No Memo sent to Physician/Midwife: ☐ Yes ☐ No		
		Section of Fetal monitor strip: ☐ Given to parents ☐ On file		
		ID Bands/Crib cards/Tape measure: ☐ Given to parents ☐ On file		
		Footprints/Handprints/Weight/Length recorded on "In Memory Of" sheet: ☐ Given to parents ☐ On file		
		Lock of hair offered: (ask permission) ☐ Yes ☐ No ☐ Given to parents ☐ On file		
		Mementos (clothing, hat, blanket, pacifier, crib cards, basin, baby ring, bear, thermometer, silk flower) ☐ Given to parents ☐ On file		
		Complimentary birth keepsake ☐ Given to parents ☐ On file		
		RTS Photos taken: (clothed, unclothed, w. props, family photo) 1) Polaroid - 3 or more ☐ Given to parents ☐ On file 2) 35 mm (6-12 pictures) ☐ Given to parents ☐ On file 3) Medical photos: ☐ Yes ☐ No		

FIG. 38-2 Sample checklist for assisting parents experiencing stillbirth or newborn death. (Used with permission of Bereavement Services. Copyright Lutheran Hospital—La Crosse, Inc., A Gundersen Lutheran Affiliate, La Crosse, WI.)

the events, experiences, and feelings surrounding the loss. This can help them come to terms with the reality of their loss. Listening to their pain and allowing time for them to absorb the information is important.

One way of actualizing the loss is to tell the parents the sex of the baby and give them the option of naming the fetus or to help them to name an infant who has died. Choosing a name helps make the baby a member of their family so that the baby can be remembered in a special way. Once the baby is named, the nurse should use the name when referring to the baby. Although naming can be helpful, it is important not to create the sense that the parents must name the "baby," especially in the case of an early pregnancy loss.

! NURSING ALERT

It is very important to be sensitive about naming. This is an individual decision that should never be imposed on parents. Beliefs and needs vary widely across individuals, cultures, and religions. Cultural taboos and rules in some religious faiths prohibit the naming of an infant who has died.

Date	Time		Comments	Initials
		Informed about postponing funeral until mother is able to attend: ☐ Yes ☐ No		
		Services/Funeral arrangements, options discussed: ☐ Self-transport ☐ Gravesite service ☐ Visitation ☐ Hospital chapel ☐ Cremation ☐ Funeral home ☐ Burial at foot or head of relative's grave ☐ Specific area for babies in cemetery ☐ Plan own service		
		Funeral arrangements made by: ☐ Mother ☐ Father Discussed: ☐ Seeing baby at funeral home ☐ Taking pictures there ☐ Providing outfit/toy for baby ☐ Dressing baby at funeral home		
		Grief information packet given to: ☐ Mother ☐ Father		
		Discussed grief process/incongruent grief with: ☐ Mother ☐ Father		
		Discussed grief conference: ☐ Yes ☐ No		
		RTS Parents Support Group brochure given to: ☐ Mother ☐ Father		
		RTS business card given to: ☐ Mother ☐ Father		
		Pregnancy & Infant Loss Card sent to RTS secretary: ☐ Yes ☐ No		
		Follow-up calls: 1 week: . . . . 3 weeks:. . . . . Due date:. . . . . 6-10 months: . . . . Anniversary date:.		
		Grief conference planned with parents: Date ________ Time ________ Place ______________ Letter of confirmation sent: ☐ Yes ☐ No		
		Parent Support Group, first meeting attended: Date: ________ Follow-up meetings attended: Dates ______________		
		Would like another parent to call: ☐ Yes ☐ No ☐ Ask later Parent contact: ______________		

FIG. 38-2, cont'd Sample checklist for assisting parents experiencing stillbirth or newborn death.

CLINICAL REASONING

The Bereaved Couple

One hour ago, Johanna gave birth to a stillborn female infant at 37 weeks of gestation. After an uneventful pregnancy, this was totally unexpected, and the obstetrician cannot identify any reason why this occurred. Her husband, Tyler, is at her side holding her hand as they both are crying softly. The baby was taken to the nursery after birth as they await the arrival of both sets of grandparents. As you enter the room to start your shift, you approach the couple quietly, place your hand on Johanna's arm and say, "I am very sorry." Johanna responds, "Why did this happen? I waited so long to have this baby. We wanted her so much. I did everything the doctor told me to do. My pregnancy was perfectly normal, and now my baby is dead. What did I do wrong?"

1. Evidence—Is there sufficient evidence to draw conclusions about meaning of the loss to Johanna and Tyler? About appropriate support for the couple as they experience the loss and grief of a stillborn infant?
2. Assumptions—What assumptions can be made about the following factors?
   a. The cause of the stillbirth
   b. The risk for complicated grief
   c. Seeing and holding the infant
3. What implications and priorities for nursing care can be drawn at this time?
4. Does the evidence objectively support your conclusion?
5. Are there alternative perspectives to your conclusion?

Research evidence supports the importance of parents' seeing or holding their fetus or infant (Gold et al., 2007). Most parents find this experience valuable and many indicate that they would have liked more time or more opportunities to do so. Seeing and holding the fetus or baby is important because it can help parents face the reality of the loss, reduces painful fantasies, and facilitates the grieving process. It should be noted, however, that while this is a beneficial experience for most parents, it can increase feelings of sadness about their loss and can even be traumatic for some individuals (Badenhorst & Hughes, 2007). Parents should be allowed to choose whether or not they want to see and/or hold their fetus or baby. They should never be made to feel they "should" see or hold their baby when this is something that they do not really want. Encouraging reluctant parents to hold or see their dead child by telling them that not seeing the child could make mourning more difficult is inappropriate. Obviously, this subject must be approached very carefully. The nurse might ask a question such as, "Some parents have found it helpful to see their baby. Would you like time to consider this?" is helpful because the need or willingness to see also may vary between the mother and father, it is extremely important to determine what each parent really wants. This should not be a decision made by one person or a decision made for the parents by grandparents or others. It is a good policy for the nurse to first tell them about this option and then give them time to think about it. Later the nurse can return and ask each parent individually what he or she decided.

In preparation for the visit with the baby, parents appreciate explanations about what to expect. Descriptions of the baby's appearance are important. For example, babies can have red, peeling skin resembling severe sunburn, dark discoloration similar to bruises, molding of the head that makes the head look soft and swollen, or birth defects. The nurse should make the baby look as normal as possible, and remember that parents see their baby with different eyes from health care professionals. Bathing the baby, applying lotion to the baby's skin, combing hair, placing identification bracelets on the arm and leg, dressing the baby in a diaper and special outfit, sprinkling powder in the baby's blanket, and wrapping the baby in a pretty blanket convey to the parents that their baby has been cared for in a special way. If the baby has been in the morgue, the nurse can place him or her underneath a warmer for 20 to 30 minutes and wrap the infant in a warm blanket before taking the infant to the parents. Cold cream rubbed over stiffened joints can help in positioning the baby. The use of powder and lotion stimulates the parents' senses and provides pleasant memories of their baby.

When bringing the baby to the parents, it is important to treat the baby as one would a live baby. Holding the baby close, touching a hand or cheek, using the baby's name, and talking with the parents about the special features of their child conveys that it is all right for them to do likewise. If a baby has a congenital anomaly, the nurse can help to desensitize the family by pointing out aspects of the baby that are normal. Nurses can help parents explore the baby's body as they desire. Parents often seek to identify family resemblance. A good question might be: "Who in your family does Michael resemble?"

Some families like to have the opportunity to bathe and dress their baby. Although the skin is fragile, parents can still apply lotion with cotton balls, sprinkle powder, tie ribbons, fasten the diaper, and place amulets, medallions, rosaries, or special toys or mementos in their baby's hands or alongside their baby. Volunteers in communities across the country make special burial clothes to give parents at this difficult time. Parents may want to perform other parenting activities, such as combing the hair, dressing the baby in a special outfit, wrapping the baby in a blanket, or placing the baby in a crib (Fig. 38-3).

Parents need to be offered time alone with their baby. They also need to know when the nurse will return and how to call if they should need anything. When possible, the family is placed in a private room with a rocking chair for the parents to sit in when holding their baby. This offers the mother and father special time together with their baby and with other family members (Fig. 38-4). Marking the door to the room with a special card helps remind the staff that this family has experienced a loss (Fig. 38-5).

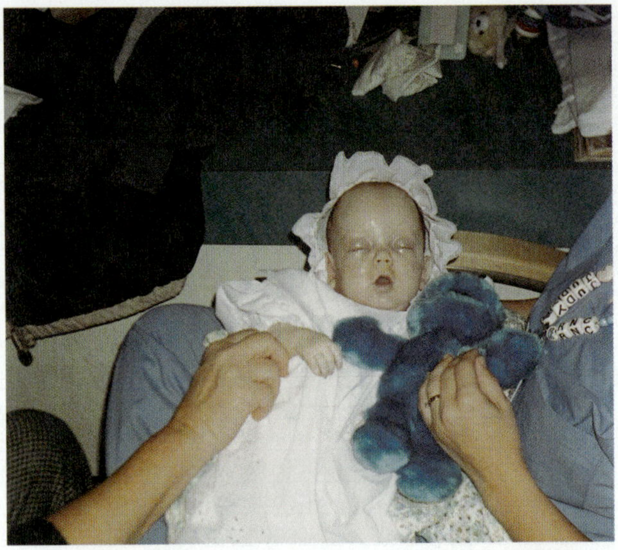

FIG. 38-3 Laura. (Courtesy Amy and Ken Turner, Cary, NC.)

It is difficult to predict how long and how often parents will need to spend time with their baby. These moments are the only ones they will have to parent their child while their child's physical presence is still with them. Some parents need only a few minutes; others need hours. It is extremely painful for some parents to say good-bye to their baby. They will tell the nurse when they are ready verbally and nonverbally. Nonverbal cues include when parents are no longer holding their child close to them or have placed the baby back in the crib. Grandparents should have the same opportunities to hold, rock, swaddle, and love their grandchildren so that their grief is started in a healthy way.

Help the Parents with Decision Making

At a time when they are experiencing the great distress of a perinatal loss, and especially if the loss was of an infant, parents have many decisions to make. Mothers, fathers, and extended families look to the medical and nursing staff for guidance in discerning what must be done immediately and what can wait and in understanding their options relative to each decision. Thus it is a primary responsibility of the nurse to help them and to advocate for them, because choices made during the time of their loss will influence their memories for a lifetime.

One decision might be related to conducting an autopsy. An autopsy can be very important in answering the question "why" if there is a chance that the cause of death can be determined. This information can be helpful in processing grief and perhaps preventing another loss. However, asking parents about an autopsy takes the utmost of sensitivity to personal, cultural, and religious views about an autopsy. (For a complete description of multicultural issues in requesting an autopsy, see Chichester [2007].) Some religions prohibit autopsy or limit the choice to times when it may help prevent another loss. Options for the type of autopsy, such as excluding the head, are available to parents. Note that the cost of an autopsy must be considered

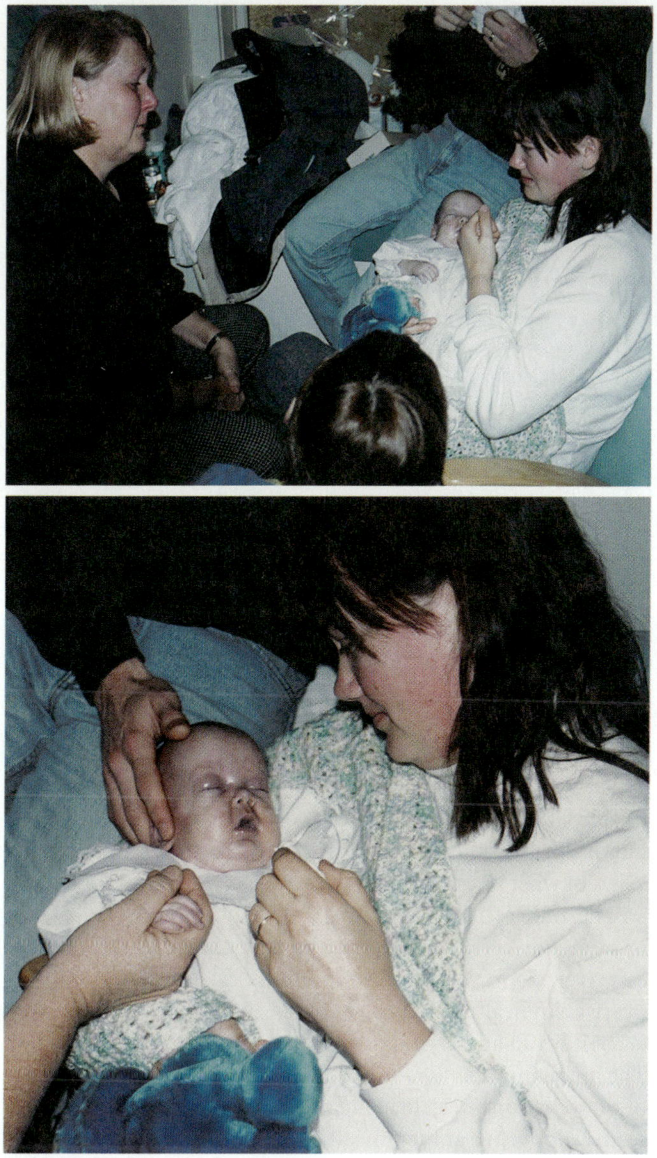

FIG. 38-4 Laura's family members say a special good-bye. (Courtesy Amy and Ken Turner, Cary, NC.)

because it is not covered by insurance and is expensive. Some parents feel that their baby has been through enough and prefer not to have further information about the cause of death. In any event, parents need time to make this decision. There is no need to rush them, unless there was evidence of contagious disease or maternal infection at the time of death.

Organ donation can be an aid to grieving and an opportunity for the family to see something positive associated with their experience. The federal Gift of Life Act and HCFA-3005-F, enacted in 1998, shifted the responsibility for determining organ donation potential from the hospital staff to the state's organ procurement organization (OPO). States and hospitals have clear procedures for how and when to call the OPO. Generally, if a death certificate is issued, a call must be made to the OPO. Once contacted, they will decide whether to talk to the family, and either an OPO representative or a designated requester will contact them. This allows requests to be made by trained personnel in a consistent and compassionate manner. The most common donation is of corneas; donation of corneas

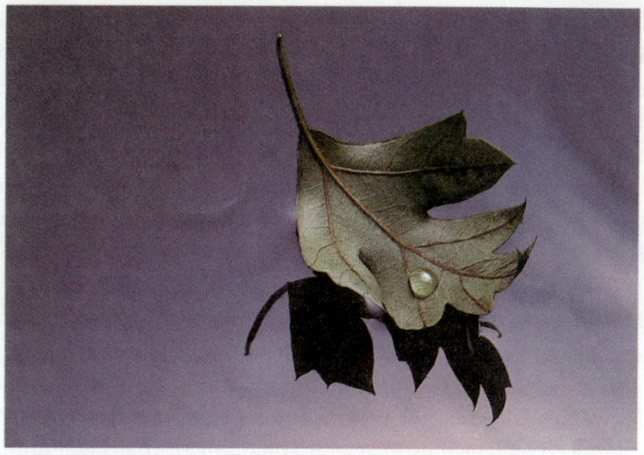

FIG. 38-5 Door card for room of mother who has had a perinatal loss. (Used with permission of Bereavement Services. Copyright Lutheran Hospital—La Crosse, Inc., A Gundersen Lutheran Affiliate, La Crosse, WI.)

from a baby can occur if the baby was born alive at 36 weeks of gestation or later.

Another important decision relates to spiritual rituals that can be helpful and important to parents. Support from the clergy should be offered to all parents. Parents may wish to have their own pastor, priest, rabbi, or spiritual leader contacted, or they may wish to see the hospital's chaplain. They may choose to do neither. Members of the clergy can offer the parents the opportunity for baptism when appropriate. Other rituals that can be important include a blessing, a naming ceremony, anointing, ritual of the sick, memorial service, or prayer.

One of the major decisions parents must make has to do with disposition of the body. Parents should be given information about the choices for the final disposition of their baby, regardless of gestational age. Nurses must be aware, however, of cultural and spiritual beliefs that can dictate the choices of parents, issues related to the cost of burial, alternatives to burial, and state laws related to burial. A baby younger than 20 weeks of gestation is considered a product of conception, whereas embryos, uterine tubes removed with an ectopic pregnancy, and tissue from a pregnancy obtained during a dilation and curettage are considered tissue. Many hospitals will make arrangements for the cremation of these infants or tissue. The nurse should know the hospital's policies and procedures and answer the parents' questions honestly. In most states if a fetus is at least 20 weeks and 1 day of gestational age or is born alive, it is the parents' responsibility to make the final arrangements for their baby, although some hospitals will offer free cremation. In this case, the family does not receive the ashes.

LEGAL TIP: Laws Regarding Live Birth

Laws in all states govern what constitutes a live birth. In most states a live birth is any products of conception expelled from a woman that show any signs of life. Signs of life are considered to be any muscle irritability, respiratory effort, or heart rate, regardless of gestational age. All nurses should be knowledgeable about their state laws regarding what constitutes a live birth and the forms that must be completed and filed in the case of fetal death, stillbirth, or newborn death.

Final disposition of all identifiable babies, regardless of gestational age, includes burial or cremation. Depending on the cemetery's policies, babies in caskets or the ashes from cremated babies can be buried in a special place designated for babies, at the foot of a deceased relative, in a separate plot, or in a mausoleum. Ashes also can be scattered in a designated area; many states have regulations regarding where ashes can be scattered. A local funeral director or a state's Vital Statistics Bureau should have information about the state's rules, codes, and regulations regarding live births, burial requirements, transportation of the deceased by parents, and cremation.

In making final arrangements for their baby, some parents want a special service. They can choose to have a service in the hospital chapel, visitation at a funeral home or their own home, a funeral service in a church, or a graveside service. Parents can make any of these services as special, personal, and memorable as they like. They can choose special music, poetry, or prose written by themselves or others.

If the family has decided on a funeral and burial, they still have decisions about which funeral home to call and where to bury the baby. Many couples live in an area distant from their family homes, and they may want to bury their child in their hometown or family cemetery. If the family desires cremation, they may want to have the option of obtaining the ashes. It is important to determine whether this will be done by the facility conducting the cremation.

Parents' hopes, dreams, self-esteem, and role expectations have been shattered with a perinatal loss; thus they have many needs. Unmet needs can form the basis of "if only" that may plague a mother or family for a lifetime and can be the foundation for the development of complicated bereavement. However, it is difficult for parents to know exactly what they can expect or what they need; thus the nurse as an advocate should lead by offering various options to meet specific needs. When a mother or family is able to verbalize needs, it is extremely important for the nurse to respond positively and to do everything to see that the request is met.

Families become unaware of time frames and do not care about the change of shifts or any needs the hospital system might have in "moving things along." When families are pushed or rushed into making decisions, in most cases, they make a decision in response to the health care system's needs, not their own. Actions such as naming the baby, seeing and holding the baby, disposition of the body, and funeral arrangements should never be rushed. In some cases, the mother is discharged home before these decisions are made. Then the family can think about them in the comfort of their home and contact the hospital in the following days to give their answers.

Help the Bereaved Parents Acknowledge and Express Their Feelings

One of the most important goals of the nurse is to validate the experience and feelings of the parents by encouraging them to tell their stories and listening with care (Corbet-Owen & Kruger, 2001). At the very least, the nurse should acknowledge the loss with a simple but sincere comment such as, "I'm sorry about the baby." Helping the parents to talk about their loss and the meaning it has for their lives and to share their emotional pain is the next step. Because nurses tend to be very focused on the physical and emotional needs of the mother, it is especially important to ask the father or partner directly about his or her views of what happened and the associated feelings of loss.

The nurse should listen patiently during the story of loss or grief; however, listening can be difficult and painful for the caregiver. The feelings and emotions of expressed grief can overwhelm health care professionals. Being with someone who is terribly sad and crying or sobbing can be extremely difficult. The initial impulse to reduce one's sense of helplessness is to say or do something to reduce their pain. Although such a response seems supportive at the time, it can stifle the further expression of emotion. Bereaved parents have identified many unhelpful responses made to them by well-meaning health care professionals, family, and friends. The nurse should resist the temptation to give advice or use clichés in offering support to the bereaved (Box 38-2). Nurses need to be comfortable with their own feelings of loss and grief to support and care for bereaved persons effectively. The nurse should have a presence of self, the willingness to be alongside, quietly supporting the bereaved in whatever expressions of feelings or emotions are appropriate for them. This presence leaves parents feeling that they were cared for. Leaning forward, nodding the head, and saying "Uh-huh" or "Tell me more" is often encouragement enough for the bereaved person to tell his or her story. Sitting through the silence can be therapeutic; silence gives the bereaved person an opportunity to collect thoughts and to process what he or she is sharing. Furthermore, careful assessment is important before using touch as a therapeutic technique. For some, touch is a meaningful expression of concern, but for others it is an invasion of privacy.

Bereaved parents have many questions surrounding the event of their loss that can leave them feeling guilty. This is particularly true for mothers. Such questions include "What did I do?" "What caused this to happen?" "What do you think I

BOX 38-2 WHAT TO SAY AND WHAT NOT TO SAY TO BEREAVED PARENTS

WHAT TO SAY

- "I'm sad for you."
- "How are you doing with all of this?"
- "This must be hard for you."
- "What can I do for you?"
- "I'm sorry."
- "I'm here, and I want to listen."

WHAT NOT TO SAY

- "God had a purpose for her."
- "Be thankful you have another child."
- "The living must go on."
- "I know how you feel."
- "It's God's will."
- "You have to keep on going for her sake."
- "You're young; you can have others."
- "We'll see you back here next year, and you'll be happier."
- "Now you have an angel in heaven."
- "This happened for the best."
- "Better for this to happen now, before you knew the baby."
- "There was something wrong with the baby anyway."

Used with permission of Bereavement Services. Copyright Lutheran Hospital—La Crosse, Inc., a Gundersen Lutheran Affiliate, La Crosse, WI.

should have, could have done?" Part of the grief process for bereaved parents is figuring out what happened, their role in the loss, why it happened to them, and why it happened to their baby. The nurse should recognize that the answers to these questions must be answered by the bereaved themselves; it is part of their healing. For example, a bereaved mother might ask, "Do you think that this was caused by painting the baby's room?" An appropriate response might be, "I understand you need to find an answer for why your baby died, but we really don't know why she died. What are some of the other things you have been thinking about?" Trying to give bereaved parents answers when there are no clear answers or trying to squelch their guilt feelings by telling them they should not feel guilty does not help them process their grief. In reality, many times there are no definite answers to the question of why this terrible thing has happened to them. However, factual information, such as data about the frequency of miscarriages in pregnant women or the fact that there usually is no clear cause of a stillbirth, can be helpful.

Feelings of anger, guilt, and sadness can occur immediately but often become more problematic in the early days and months after a loss. When a bereaved person expresses feelings of anger, it can be helpful to identify the feeling by simply saying, "You sound angry," or "You look angry." The nurse's willingness to sit down and listen to these feelings of anger can help the bereaved move past those surface feelings into the underlying feelings of powerlessness and helplessness in not being able to control the many aspects of the situation.

Normalize the Grief Process and Facilitate Positive Coping

While helping parents share their feelings of pain, it is critical to help them understand their grief responses and to feel they are not alone in these painful responses. Most parents are not prepared for the raw feelings that they experience or the fact that these painful, complex feelings and related behavioral reactions continue for many weeks or months. Thus reassuring them of the normality of their responses and preparing them for the length of their grief is important.

The nurse can help parents prepare for the emptiness, loneliness, and yearning; for the feelings of helplessness that can lead to anger, guilt, and fear; and for the cognitive processing problems, disorganization, difficulty making decisions; and sadness and depression that are part of the grief process. Many parents have reported feelings of fear that they were going crazy because of the many emotions and behavioral responses that leave them feeling totally out of control in the months after the loss.

It is essential for the nurse to reassure and educate bereaved parents about the grief process, including the physical, social, and emotional responses of individuals and families. Pamphlets about parental grief that are sensitive and brief can be very helpful (Geller, Psaros, & Kerns, 2006). Offering health teaching on the bereavement process alone is not enough, however. In the initial days after a loss, other strategies might include follow-up phone calls, referral to a perinatal grief support group, or providing a list of publications or websites intended for helping parents who have experienced a perinatal loss (Geller et al., 2006). Some important websites include www.compassionatefriends.org, www.resolve.org, www.mend.org, www.sidscenter.org, and www.natonalshareoffice.com. As with any referral, however, the nurse should first review the materials or the websites for accuracy and appropriateness.

To reduce relationship problems that can occur in grieving couples, nurses help them understand that they may respond and grieve in very different ways (Abboud & Liamputtong, 2005). Discongruent grieving can lead to serious marital problems and can be a risk factor for complicated bereavement. It is important to remind the couple of the importance of being understanding and patient with each other. A father may need encouragement to be able to share his grief with his wife, because of the desire to protect the woman from his pain or the need to appear strong.

Nurses can reinforce positive coping efforts and attempt to prevent negative coping (Abboud & Liamputtong, 2005). They can remind the parents of the importance of being patient and being good to themselves during the grief process. Additional suggestions are to encourage attempts to resume normal activities; reinforce and encourage positive ways to hold on to memories of the pregnancy or baby, while letting go; and help the parent to organize a plan for daily activities, if needed. In particular, nurses should discourage dependence on drugs and alcohol.

Meet the Physical Needs of the Postpartum Bereaved Mother

Coping with loss and grief after childbirth can be an overwhelming experience for the woman and her family. One particularly difficult aspect of the loss is hearing the sound of crying babies and witnessing the happiness of other families on the unit who have given birth to healthy infants. The mother should have the opportunity to decide if she wants to remain on the maternity unit or to move to another hospital unit. The nurse should help her to understand the positive and negative aspects of each choice. Postpartum care as well as grief support may not be as good on another hospital unit where the staff members are not experienced in postpartum and bereavement care.

The physical needs of a bereaved mother are the same as those of any woman who has given birth. The cruel reality for many bereaved mothers is that their milk comes in with no baby to nurse, their afterpains remind them of their emptiness, and gas pains feel as though a baby is still moving inside. The nurse should ensure that the mother receives appropriate medications and other interventions to reduce these physical symptoms. Adequate rest, diet, and fluids must be offered to replenish her physical strength.

Mothers need postpartum care instructions on discharge. They also need ideas about how to cope with problems with sleep such as decreasing food or fluids that contain caffeine, limiting alcohol and nicotine consumption, exercising regularly, and using strategies to promote rest such as taking a warm bath or drinking warm milk before bedtime, doing relaxation exercises, listening to restful music, or a having a massage.

Assist the Bereaved in Communicating with, Supporting, and Getting Support from Family

Providing sensitive care to bereaved parents means including their families in the grief process. Grandparents and siblings are particularly important when a perinatal loss has occurred. However, it is up to the parents to decide to what extent they want family involved in their grief process. If it is the parents' desire, nursing staff should allow children, grandparents, extended family members, and friends to be involved in the rituals surrounding the death, such as seeing and holding the baby. Such visits afford others the opportunity to become acquainted with the baby, to understand the parents' loss, to offer their support, and to say good-bye (see Fig. 38-4). This experience helps parents explain to their surviving children about their brother or sister and what death means, offers the children answers to their questions in a concrete manner, and helps the children in expressing their grief. Involving extended family and friends enables the parents to mobilize their social support system of people who will support the family not only at the time of loss but also in the future. Parents also need information about how grief affects a family. They may need help in understanding and coping with the potential differing responses of various family members. Frustrations can arise because of the insensitive or inadequate responses of other family members. Parents may need help in determining ways to let family members know how they feel and what they need.

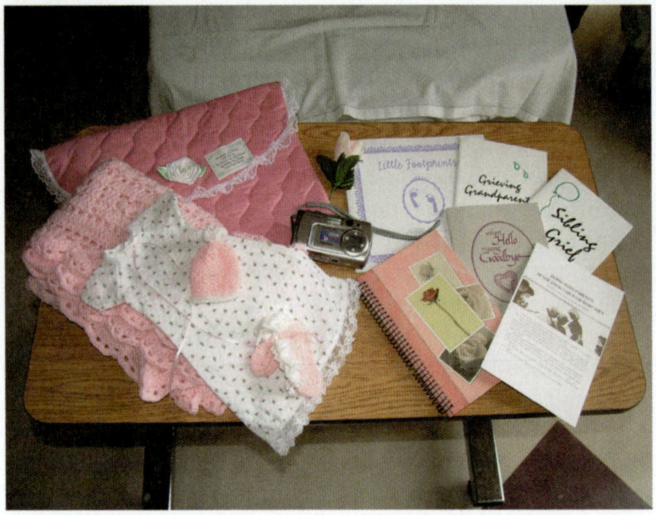

FIG. 38-6 A memory kit assembled at John C. Lincoln Hospital, Phoenix, AZ. Memory kits may include pictures of the infant, clothing, death certificate, footprints, identification bands, fetal monitor printout, and ultrasound picture. (Courtesy Julie Perry Nelson, Loveland, CO.)

Create Memories for Parents to Take Home

Parents may want tangible mementos of their baby to help them to actualize the loss. Some will bring in a previously purchased baby book. Special memory books, cards, and information on grief and mourning are available for purchase by parents or hospitals or clinics through national perinatal bereavement organizations (Fig. 38-6).

The nurse can provide information about the baby's weight, length, and head circumference to the family. Footprints and handprints can be taken and placed with the other information on a special card or in a memory or baby book. Sometimes it is difficult to obtain good handprints or footprints. Application of alcohol or acetone on the palms or soles can help the ink adhere to make the prints clearer, especially for small babies. When making prints, it is helpful to have a hard surface underneath the paper to be printed. The baby's heel or palm is placed down first, and the foot or hand is rolled forward, keeping the toes or fingers extended. If the print is not clear or well-defined, tracing around the baby's hands and feet can be done, although this distorts the actual size. A form of plaster of Paris can also be used to make an imprint of the baby's hand or foot.

Parents often appreciate articles that were in contact with or used in caring for the baby. This might include the tape measure used to measure the baby, baby lotions, combs or hairbrushes, clothing, hats, blankets, crib cards, and identification bands. The identification band helps the parents remember the size of the baby and personalizes the mementos. The nurse should ask parents if they wish to have these articles before giving them to the parents. A lock of hair can be another important keepsake. The nurse must ask the parents for permission before cutting a lock of hair, which can be removed from the nape of the neck, where it is not noticeable.

For some, pictures are the most important memento. Photographs are generally taken when it has been determined to be culturally acceptable to the family. It does not matter how tiny the baby is, what the baby looks like, or how long the baby has been dead. Pictures should include close-ups of the baby's face, hands, and feet and photos of the baby clothed and wrapped in a blanket as well as unclothed. If there are any congenital anomalies, close-ups of the anomalies also should be taken. Flowers, blocks, stuffed animals, or toys can be placed in the background to make the picture more special. Parents may want their pictures taken holding the baby. Keeping a camera nearby and taking pictures when parents are spending special time with their baby can provide special memories. Some parents have their own camera or video camera and appreciate having the nurse record them as they bathe, dress, hold, or diaper their baby.

Communicate Using a Caring Framework

Mothers, fathers, and extended families look to the nursing staff for support and understanding during the time of loss. One model for conceptualizing interventions was developed by Swanson based on her research with women experiencing perinatal loss (Swanson, Chen, Graham, Wojnar, & Petras, 2009). The framework identifies five components in a caring concept:

1. Knowing
2. Being with
3. Doing for
4. Enabling
5. Maintaining belief

Knowing implies that the nurse has taken the time to understand the perception of the loss and its meaning to the woman and her family. *Being with* involves how the nurse conveys acceptance of the various feelings and perceptions of each family member. *Doing for* refers to the activities performed by the nurse that provide physical care, comfort, and safety for the woman and her family. This can include offering pain medication or sitz baths, maintaining the patency of the intravenous line, performing postpartum checks, and giving back rubs. *Enabling* occurs when the nurse offers the woman and her family options for care. Offers of information, anticipatory guidance, choices for decision making, and support during hospitalization and after discharge help the family feel more in control of a situation in which they feel very much out of control. Enabling raises their self-esteem and allows them to feel more comfortable in asking for options according to their needs for memories and closure, rather than to the nurse's perception of their needs. *Maintaining belief* involves encouraging the woman and her family to believe in their own ability to pick up the pieces and begin to heal. The nurse spends time with the family, learns their inner strengths and coping abilities, and points out these inner resources to the family by saying, "I know this is a difficult time for you, but I have seen some of your inner strength and know that you will be able to make it through all of this."

Be Concerned About Cultural and Spiritual Needs of Parents

Given the growing diversity of the American culture, parents who experience perinatal loss can be from widely diverse cultural, ethnic, and spiritual groups. Many of the emotional responses and suggested interventions in this chapter are based on middle-class European-American views. Although there are likely no particular differences in the individual, intrapersonal experiences of grief based on culture, ethnicity, or religion, there are complex differences in the meaning of children and parenthood, the role of women and men, the beliefs and knowledge about modern medicine, views about death, mourning rituals and traditions, and behavioral expressions of grief. Thus the nurse must be sensitive to the responses and needs of parents from various cultural backgrounds and religious groups. To do this the nurse needs to be aware of his or her own values and beliefs and acknowledge the importance of understanding and accepting the values and beliefs of others who are different or even in conflict (Chichester, 2005). Furthermore, it is critical to understand that the individual and unique responses of a parent to a perinatal loss cannot be entirely predicted by their cultural or spiritual backgrounds. The nurse approaches each mother and father as an individual needing support during a profoundly difficult and distressing life experience.

It would be impossible to address all of the specific differences and needs of parents from diverse cultural and religious groups because of the complexity of this task and the lack of adequate research in this area of practice. Instead, some key concepts are presented and a few examples of areas of particular concern are given. For more detailed discussion of this topic, the reader is referred to an article by Melanie Chichester (2005).

The cultural meaning of children has a strong effect on the response of parents, extended family, and the community when an infant dies or is stillborn. For example, death of an infant or having a stillborn child shakes the foundation of a Jewish family and is surrounded by many cultural traditions, such as naming of the baby, burial, and mourning rituals (Shuzman, 2003). Likewise, in Hispanic families, children are deeply valued and there are many cultural differences associated with perinatal loss. Culture and religious beliefs often affect decision making surrounding stillbirth or death of an infant. Autopsies and cremation are not allowed by some religious groups, except under unusual circumstances (Chichester, 2007). Making a decision to end life-sustaining measures is more difficult for some groups. African-American parents can be less likely than Caucasians to make a decision to stop life-sustaining treatments in a mortally ill infant (Moseley, Church, Hempel, Yuan, Goold, & Freed, 2004). Photographs can conflict with beliefs of some cultures, such as among some Native Americans, Inuit, Amish, Hindus, and Muslims. Families from these cultures should be sensitively offered this opportunity but not pushed into having a photograph taken. In many cultures, decisions do not reside solely in the individual woman or couple but in the extended family. In Hispanic families, the concept of *la familia* is critical. Family decisions are usually made together and communicated through someone appointed by the family rather than the parents (Chichester, 2005). In Muslim families, the father typically makes the decisions.

Culture and religious beliefs also influence the customs following death. Many religious groups have rituals such as prayers, ritualistic washing and shrouding, or anointing with oil that are performed at the time of death. It is critical to ask parents about their needs as they relate to rituals at the time of and following death. For example, baptism is extremely important for Roman Catholics and some, but not all, Protestant groups. Baptism can be performed by a layperson, such as a nurse, in an emergency situation when a priest cannot be there in a timely fashion. The nurse should inquire about parental beliefs and preferences related to infant baptism. The nurse can offer to contact the hospital chaplain or the family's own clergy.

Expressions of grief vary across cultures from quiet and stoic to dramatic and hysterical responses. Muslims view death as a part of life and believe a baby's death is God's will. The Muslim mother may cry but loud wailing is not acceptable. The tearing of a garment, *keria*, may be done at the time of a death by Jewish parents. Hispanic parents and family members may be very demonstrative in their grief with loud wailing and weeping (Purnell & Paulanka, 2008). Some African-American women may use self-healing strategies that reflect inner processes, resources, and remedies (Van, 2001).

Provide Sensitive Care At and After Discharge

When leaving the hospital, mothers are often taken out in a wheelchair. This can be a devastating experience for the mother who has experienced a pregnancy loss. Leaving the hospital without a baby in her arms is a very empty and painful experience. It is especially difficult if others are seen leaving with babies; thus the discharge of mothers and fathers who have experienced a perinatal loss should be done with great sensitivity to their feelings. They should not be discharged at a time when other mothers with live babies are leaving. Giving the mother a special flower to carry in her arms can be a thoughtful gesture.

The grief of the mother and her family does not end with discharge; rather it really begins once they return home, attend the funeral, and start to live their lives without their baby. There are numerous models for providing follow-up care to parents after discharge and, although there is no solid evidence from sound clinical trials regarding the benefit of these programs, nonexperimental studies and clinical evaluations suggest these programs are helpful (Côté-Arsenault & Freije, 2004; Reilly-Smorawski, Armstrong, & Catlin, 2002). Programs include hospital-based bereavement teams who provide support during hospitalization and follow-up contacts.

Follow-up phone calls after a loss are helpful to some parents; however, it must be determined which parents do not want a follow-up call. The calls are made at predictably difficult times such as the first week at home, 1 month to 6 weeks later, 4 to 6 months after the loss, and at the anniversary of the death. Families who experienced a miscarriage, ectopic pregnancy, or death of a preterm baby can appreciate a phone call on the estimated date of birth. The calls provide an opportunity for parents to ask questions, share their feelings, seek advice, and receive information to help them in processing their grief.

A grief conference can be planned when parents return for an appointment with their physician or midwife, nurses, and other members of the health care team. At the conference, the loss or death of the infant is discussed in detail, parents are given information about the baby's autopsy report and genetic studies, and they have opportunities to ask the questions that have arisen since their baby's death. Parents appreciate the opportunity to review the events of hospitalization, go over the baby's and/or mother's chart with their primary health care provider, and talk with those who cared for them and their baby during hospitalization. This is an important time to help parents understand the cause of the loss, or to accept the fact that the cause will forever be unknown. This gives health care professionals the opportunity to assess how the family is coping with their loss and provide additional information and education on grief.

Some parents are very interested in finding a perinatal or parent grief support group. The opportunity to talk with others who have been through similar experiences, share memories of the pregnancy and the baby, and gain an understanding of the normality of the grief process have been generally found to be supportive (Côté-Arsenault & Freije, 2004). Over time, it is possibly the only place where bereaved parents can talk about the wished-for child and their grief. However, not all parents find such groups helpful.

When referring to a group, it is important to know something about the group and how it operates. For example, if a group has a religious base for their interventions, a nonreligious parent would not likely find the group to be helpful. If parents experiencing a perinatal loss are referred to a general parental grief group, they might feel overwhelmed with the grief of parents whose older children have died of cancer, suicide, or homicide. In addition, other parents can help to minimize the grief of parents following a perinatal loss. Thus the focus of the group needs to match the parents' needs.

Provide Postmortem Care

Preparation of the baby's body and transport to the morgue depend on the procedures and protocols developed by individual hospitals. The Joint Commission (www.jointcommission.org) requires that appropriate care is offered to the body after death. A sensitive and respectful approach for taking the fetus or infant to the morgue is the use of a "burial cradle," which makes the process more dignified for parents and the nursing staff. A burial cradle is a miniature coffin usually made of Styrofoam or wood (Fig. 38-7).

Postmortem care can be an emotional and sometimes difficult task for the nurse. However, nurses can find that providing postmortem care helps them in their own grief related to a perinatal loss. This is particularly true for neonatal intensive care nurses who have cared for an infant for several hours, days, or weeks.

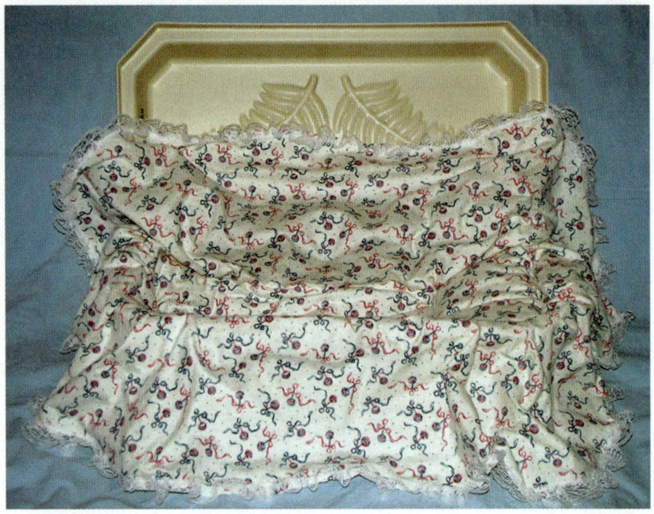

FIG. 38-7 Burial cradle. (Courtesy Shannon Perry, Phoenix, AZ.)

SPECIAL LOSSES

Prenatal Diagnoses with Negative Outcome

Early prenatal diagnostic tests such as ultrasonography, chorionic villus sampling, and amniocentesis can determine the well-being of the embryo or fetus. Reasons for prenatal testing include history of chromosomal abnormality in the family; three or more miscarriages; maternal age over 35 years; lack of fetal growth, movement, or heartbeat; and diabetes mellitus or other chronic illnesses. If the health care provider is certain that the baby has a serious genetic defect that will lead to death in utero or after birth (congenital anomalies incompatible with life or genetic disorders with severe mental retardation), the choice of interruption of a pregnancy via dilation and evacuation or induction of labor can be offered (Manning, 2009).

Foreknowledge of a prenatal diagnosis along with perception of the future low health status of the baby as well as multiple congenital problems intensify the grief response (Hunfeld, Tempels, Passchier, Hazebroek, & Tibboel, 1999). The decision to terminate a pregnancy is difficult and can pave the way for feelings such as guilt, despair, sadness, depression, and anger. The parent who decides to continue the pregnancy needs intensive support from the nursing staff. The time of labor and birth can be particularly difficult. The nurse should remember that parents can be grieving for not only the loss of the perfect child but also loss of expectations for their child's future. Thus nurses should assess how these parents feel about the experience, offer options for their memories as appropriate, and be a support person and good listener. Healing can take place when words can be given to feelings. Perinatal hospice care for parents experiencing prenatal diagnoses of lethal birth defects can be effective in helping families before and after their loss is actualized (Calhoun, Napolitano, Terry, Bussey, & Hoeldtke, 2003). Perinatal hospice does not have to be a formal program, although some do exist. It is the provision of care for families as they plan for the birth and probable death of their baby and involves support, information and resources. If the baby lives more than a few minutes or hours after birth, conventional hospice care may be incorporated into care management of the infant and family (Davis & Helzer, 2011).

NURSING CARE PLAN

Fetal Death at 24 Weeks

NURSING DIAGNOSIS

Risk for dysfunctional grieving related to fetal death, as evidenced by intense expressions of grief for prolonged period of time

Expected Outcome

Parents will identify appropriate ways to deal with grief.

Nursing Interventions/*Rationales*

- Prepare family for viewing infant by cleaning body and wrapping in clean blanket *to initiate and support the grieving process in a supportive setting.*
- Allow family quiet time to hold and view infant. Take pictures for family to keep *to provide reality of death and support the grieving process.*
- Provide a certificate for the family with vital statistics, along with identification bands, lock of hair (with parental permission), and footprints *to provide reality of situation and support the grieving process.*
- Provide spiritual support as needed to assist with religious services, such as baptism and memorial services, *to assist with religious practices.*
- Refer to appropriate community support groups *to facilitate grieving with group input and to share experiences.*

NURSING DIAGNOSIS

Situational low self-esteem related to fetal death as evidenced by mother's/family's intense feelings of guilt

Expected Outcomes

Mother/family will exhibit positive self-comments and adapt to death of fetus in a timely manner.

Nursing Interventions/*Rationales*

- Provide private time for expressions of feelings through therapeutic communication and active listening *to validate feelings.*
- Identify mother's/family's perception and feelings about fetal death *to correct any misconceptions and alleviate guilt.*
- Assist mother/family to identify positive coping mechanisms and support systems *to promote feelings of self-worth.*
- Refer to appropriate health professionals for further evaluation and counseling, such as social services, *to provide ongoing assistance as needed.*

NURSING DIAGNOSIS

Spiritual distress related to perinatal loss

Expected Outcome

Parents will verbalize a decrease in spiritual distress.

Nursing Interventions/*Rationales*

- Assess parent's spiritual preference *to reinforce parent's own beliefs.*
- Assist with spiritual rituals for parents and infant *to promote comfort for parents.*
- Provide opportunity for parents to express feelings about perinatal loss *to facilitate the grief process.*
- Assist parents in contacting the facility's chaplain or personal spiritual advisor *to provide spiritual support.*
- Attend memorial service/funeral if feasible *to provide support to parents and to help process grief of health care provider.*

NURSING DIAGNOSIS

Interrupted family processes related to inadequate communication of feelings between mother and father and other family members

Expected Outcome

Mother and father will discuss feelings involving relationship with each other and family members.

Nursing Interventions/*Rationales*

- Provide information to parents about how grief affects a family *to facilitate expression of grieving among family members.*
- Encourage mother and father to talk about their loss and its meaning to the family *to help the bereaved to acknowledge and express their feelings.*
- Include siblings and grandparents in discussions of the loss *to acknowledge feelings and grief of family members.*
- Offer follow-up contact (e.g., phone calls, grief conference) *to provide opportunity for parents to ask questions, share feelings, and to receive information to help them in processing their grief.*
- Refer family to perinatal or family support group if appropriate *to facilitate communication and sharing of the experience of loss with others who have had similar experiences.*

Loss of One in a Multiple Birth

The death of a twin or baby in a multifetal gestation during pregnancy, labor, birth, or after birth requires the mother and father (or partner) to parent and grieve at the same time. Such a death imposes a confusing and ambivalent induction into parenthood (Swanson, Kane, Pearsall-Jones, Swanson, & Croft, 2009). They can experience difficulty parenting their surviving child with all the joy and enthusiasm of new parents because their surviving child reminds them of what they have lost. Yet they can also have difficulty fully grieving their loss because their surviving child demands their attention. These parents can be at risk for altered parenting and complicated bereavement.

It is important to help the parents acknowledge the birth of all their babies. The nurse treats the parents as bereaved families, offering all the options previously discussed. With the parents' consent, photographs should be taken of the babies and parents should be offered the opportunity to hold their babies in their arms and have time to say good-bye to the baby who has died.

It is helpful to warn bereaved parents that well-meaning family members or friends may say, "Well, at least you have the other baby," implying that there should be no grief because they are lucky to have one at all. Parents need to be able to anticipate insensitivity to their loss and be empowered to say to those people, "That is not how I feel." By simply setting a boundary on what their feelings are, they are able to acknowledge the baby who died and then have an opportunity to share more about their feelings if they so choose.

Bereaved parents of multiples have special problems in coping with life without their anticipated "extra special" family, telling their surviving child about his or her twin, dealing with the possibility of that child's feelings of survivor guilt, and deciding on how to celebrate birthdays, death days, or special holidays, or anniversaries of the baby's death.

Adolescent Grief

Adolescent pregnancy accounts for many births in the United States. Each year, many adolescents experience perinatal loss, particularly as elective abortion or miscarriage. Adolescents grieve the loss of their babies through miscarriage, stillbirth, or newborn death and have significant emotional, social, and cognitive responses (Wheeler & Austin, 2001). These teens need emotional support from the nurses who care for them.

Often nurses and other health care professionals, as well as family members, believe that the adolescent's loss of her baby was for the best, so that the adolescent can move on with her life. Adolescent girls, then, may not receive the support they need from staff and family. In addition, adolescent girls often do not have the support from the father of the baby as compared with older women who have a perinatal loss; thus there is a great need to provide sensitive care to all adolescents who experience any type of perinatal loss.

The first step for the nurse in caring for a bereaved adolescent is to acknowledge the significance of giving birth, no matter what age the mother might be. Second, the nurse should make additional efforts to develop a trusting relationship in working with the adolescent. Third, the nurse should offer options for saying good-bye, and provide anticipatory guidance, support, and information to meet the adolescent at the point of her need. It can take longer for adolescents to process their grief because of their level of cognitive and emotional maturation. Being patient, saving mementos, and giving the adolescent information on how to contact the nurse are interventions that can help the adolescent accept the reality of the loss and process her grief.

COMPLICATED GRIEF

Although most parents cope adequately with the pain of their grief and return to some level of normal functioning, some have extremely intense grief reactions that last for a very long time; this response is **complicated grief.** It is also called complicated bereavement, prolonged grief, pathologic grief, or pathologic mourning (Zhang, El-Jawahri, & Prigerson, 2006). Complicated grief often results when there is sudden or traumatic loss, as occurs with stillbirth or termination of pregnancy due to lethal fetal anomalies (Cacciatore, 2010; Kersting, Kroker, Steinhard, Ludorff, Wesselman, Ohrmann, et al., 2007). Complicated grief differs from what is considered normal grief in its duration and the degree to which behavior and emotional state are affected (Badenhorst & Hughes, 2007). Risk factors for complicated grief include poor social support, history of mental health problems, and a more neurotic pre-loss personality (Badenhorst & Hughes, 2007). A study by Swanson and colleagues (2007) found that women who were still overwhelmed with grief at 1 year, had miscarried again, and/or were not pregnant, experienced six or more negative events in their lives and were distant from their partners.

Persons experiencing complicated grief seem to be in a state of chronic mourning. Evidence of complicated grief includes intense longing and yearning for the deceased, inability to trust others, excessive bitterness, difficulty moving on with one's life, feeling that life is empty or meaningless, hopelessness, loneliness, intense and continued guilt or anger, relentless depression or anxiety that interferes with role functioning, abuse of drugs (including prescription medications) or alcohol, severe relationship difficulties, high depressive symptomatology, low self-esteem, feelings of inadequacy, and suicidal thoughts or threats years after the loss has occurred (Swanson, 2000; Zhang et al., 2006).

Post traumatic stress disorder (PTSD) can occur following perinatal loss (Badenhorst & Hughes, 2007; Turton, Evans, & Hughes, 2009). Symptoms of posttraumatic stress include reliving the trauma, avoiding things and places that are reminders, panic attacks, physical symptoms such as chronic pain, feelings of mistrust, problems with relationships and daily activities, substance abuse, and depression.

Parents showing signs of complicated grief or posttraumatic stress should be referred for counseling. It is the responsibility of a qualified mental health professional to determine whether the parents are experiencing a normal, albeit intense grief response or whether they are also having a serious mental health problem such as depression. However, it is important when referring to a therapist or counselor that the referral is made to one who is experienced in grief counseling and knows how to help the bereaved; some therapists and counselors do not have an understanding of the special needs related to grief.

Making an appointment for counseling or therapy is a big step. The highest number of cancellations and "no shows" in a therapist's practice are intakes, or first visits; therefore, anything the nurse can do for a family or individual to help with that major hurdle is helpful. However, it also is important to remember that people can have symptoms but may not, for whatever reason, be ready to deal directly with these symptoms or may not have the energy to make the call. Enlisting a family member to encourage parents to seek such assistance can be helpful.

COMMUNITY ACTIVITY

- Visit the Healing Hearts Baby Loss Comfort website at www.babylosscomfort.com. Review the client information about the appropriate words to say, full term baby loss, and stillbirth and grief resources. Also, visit the websites of the National Stillbirth Society (www.stillnomore.org) and International Stillbirth Alliance (www.stillbirthalliance.org).
- Research the availability of a perinatal loss support group in your community. Visit the website of The Compassionate Friends (www.compassionatefriends.org), which provides support for families after the death of a child. Review the mission, vision statement, seven principles and credo of the organization. Locate a chapter of The Compassionate Friends in your area.

KEY POINTS

- Parental and infant attachment can begin before pregnancy with many hopes and dreams for the future.
- The gestational age of the baby influences neither the severity of the grief response nor the bereavement process.
- When a baby dies, all members of a family are affected, but no two family members grieve in the same way.
- When birth represents death, the role of the nurse is critical in caring for the woman and her family, regardless of the age of the woman or stage of gestation.
- An understanding of the grief process is fundamental in the implementation of the nursing process.
- Assessment of each family member's perception and experience of the loss is important.
- Culture and religion affect a family's response to and coping with perinatal death.
- Therapeutic communication and counseling techniques can help families identify their feelings, feel comfortable in expressing their grief, and understand their bereavement process.
- Follow-up after discharge can be an important component in providing care to families who have experienced a loss.
- Nurses need to be aware of their own feelings of grief and loss to provide a nonjudgmental environment of care and support for bereaved families.

Audio Chapter Summaries Access an audio summary of these Key Points on evolve

REFERENCES

Abboud, L., & Liamputtong, P. (2005). When pregnancy fails: Coping strategies, support networks and experiences with health care of ethnic women and their partners. *Journal of Reproductive and Infant Psychology, 23*(1), 3–18.

Armstrong, D. (2007). Perinatal loss and parental distress after the birth of a healthy infant. *Advances in Neonatal Care, 7*(4), 200–206.

Arnold, J., & Gemma, P. (2008). The continuing process of parental grief. *Death Studies, 32*(7), 658–673.

Badenhorst, W., & Hughes, P. (2007). Psychological aspects of perinatal loss. *Clinical Obstetrics and Gynaecology, 21*(2), 249–259.

Breeze, A., Lees, C., Kumar, A., Missfelder-Lobos, H., & Murdoch, E. (2007). Palliative care for prenatally diagnosed lethal fetal abnormality. *Archives of Disease in Childhood—Fetal & Neonatal Edition, 92*(1), 56–58.

Brier, N. (2008). Grief following miscarriage: A comprehensive review of the literature. *Journal of Women's Health, 17*(3), 451–464.

Cacciatore, J. (2010). Stillbirth: Patient-centered psychosocial care. *Clinical Obstetrics and Gynecology, 53*(3), 691–699.

Calhoun, B., Napolitano, P., Terry, M., Bussey, C., & Hoeldtke, N. (2003). Perinatal hospice: Comprehensive care for the family of the fetus with a lethal condition. *Journal of Reproductive Medicine, 48*(5), 343–348.

Cameron, M., & Penney, G. (2005). Terminology in early pregnancy loss: What women hear and what clinicians write. *Journal of Family Planning and Reproductive Health Care, 31*(4), 313–314.

Chichester, M. (2005). Multicultural issues in perinatal loss. *AWHONN Lifelines, 9*(4), 312–320.

Chichester, M. (2007). Requesting perinatal autopsy: Multicultural considerations. *MCN: The American Journal of Maternal/Child Nursing, 32*(2), 81–86.

Corbet-Owen, C., & Kruger, L. (2001). The health system and emotional care: Validating the many meanings of spontaneous pregnancy loss. *Family Systems of Health, 19*(4), 411–417.

Côté-Arsenault, D. (2007). Threat appraisal, coping, and emotions across pregnancy subsequent to perinatal loss. *Nursing Research, 56*(2), 108–116.

Côté-Arsenault, D., & Donato, K. (2007). Restrained expectations in late pregnancy following loss. *Journal of Obstetric, Gynecologic and Neonatal Nursing, 36*(6), 550–557.

Côté-Arsenault, D., & Freije, M. (2004). Support groups helping women through pregnancies after loss. *Western Journal of Nursing Research, 26*(6), 650–670.

Côté-Arsenault, D., & Marshall, R. (2000). One foot in-one foot out: Weathering the storm of pregnancy after perinatal loss. *Research in Nursing & Health, 23*(6), 473–485.

Cowles, K., & Rodgers, B. (2000). The concept of grief: An evolutionary perspective. In B. Rodgers & K. Knafl (Eds.), *Concept development in nursing: Foundations, techniques, and applications* (2nd ed.). Philadelphia: Saunders.

Davies, R. (2004). New understandings of parental grief: Literature review. *Journal of Advanced Nursing, 46*(5), 506–513.

Davis, D., & Helzer, S. (2011). Perinatal death and bereavement care. In E. Gilbert (Ed.), *Manual of high risk pregnancy and delivery* (5th ed.). St. Louis: Mosby.

DeBackere, K., Hill, P., & Kavanaugh, K. (2008). The parental experience of pregnancy after perinatal loss. *Journal of Obstetric, Gynecologic and Neonatal Nursing, 37*(5), 525–537.

De Lisle-Porter, M., & Podruchny, A. (2009). The dying neonate: Family-centered end-of-life care. *Neonatal Network, 28*(2), 75–83.

Fretts, R. (2009). The study of stillbirth. *American Journal of Obstetrics and Gynecology, 201*(5), 429–430.

Geller, P., Psaros, C., & Kerns, D. (2006). Web-based resources for health care providers and women following pregnancy loss. *Journal of Obstetric, Gynecologic and Neonatal Nursing, 35*(4), 523–532.

Gold, K. (2007). Navigating care after a baby dies: A systematic review of parent experiences with health providers. *Journal of Perinatology, 27*(4), 230–237.

Gold, K., Dalton, V., & Schwenk, T. (2007). Hospital care for parents after perinatal death. *Obstetrics and Gynecology, 109*(5), 1156–1166.

Hunfeld, J., Tempels, A., Passchier, J., Hazebroek, F., & Tibboel, D. (1999). Brief report: Parental burden and grief one year after the birth of a child with congenital anomaly. *Journal of Pediatric Psychology, 24*(6), 515–520.

Kersting, A., Kroker, K., Steinhard, J., Ludorff, K., Wesselman, U., Ohrmann, P., et al. (2007). Complicated grief after traumatic loss: A 14 month follow up study. *European Archives of Psychiatry and Clinical Neuroscience, 257*(8), 437–443.

Leuthner, S., & Jones, E. (2007). Fetal concerns program: A model for perinatal palliative care. *MCN The American Journal of Maternal/Child Nursing, 32*(5), 272–280.

Limbo, R., & Kobler, K. (2009). Will our baby be alive again? Supporting parents of young children when a baby dies. *Nursing for Women's Health, 13*(4), 302–311.

Little, C. (2010). Nursing considerations in the case of multifetal pregnancy reduction. *MCN: The American Journal of Maternal/Child Nursing, 35*(3), 166–171.

Manning, F. (2009). Imaging in the diagnosis of fetal anomalies. In R. Creasy, R. Resnik, J. Iams, C. Lockwood, & T. Moore (Eds.), *Creasy and Resnik's Maternal-Fetal Medicine* (6th ed.). Philadelphia: Saunders.

McGrath, J., Samra, H., Zukowsky, K., & Baker, B. (2010). Parenting after infertility: Issues for families and infants. *MCN: The American Journal of Maternal/Child Nursing, 35*(3), 156–164.

Miles, M. (1984). Helping adults mourn the death of a child. In H. Wass & C. Corr (Eds.), *Childhood and death.* New York: Hemisphere.

Moseley, K., Church, A., Hempel, B., Yuan, H., Goold, S., & Freed, G. (2004). End-of-life choices for African-American and white infants in a neonatal intensive-care unit: A pilot study. *Journal of the National Medical Association, 96*(7), 933–937.

Murphy, F., & Merrell, J. (2009). Negotiating the transition: Caring for women through the experience of early miscarriage. *Journal of Clinical Nursing, 18*(11), 1583–1591.

O'Leary, J., & Thorwick, C. (2006). Fathers' perspectives during pregnancy, postperinatal loss. *Journal of Obstetric, Gynecologic and Neonatal Nursing, 35*(1), 78–86.

Purnell, L., & Paulanka, B. (2008). *Transcultural health care: A culturally competent approach* (3rd ed.). Philadelphia: FA Davis.

Reilly-Smorawski, B., Armstrong, A., & Catlin, E. (2002). Bereavement support for couples following death of a baby: Program development and 14-year exit analysis. *Death Studies, 26*(1), 21–37.

Rousch, A., Sullivan, P., Cooper, R., & McBride, J. (2007). Perinatal hospice. *Newborn and Infant Nursing Reviews, 7*(4), 216–221.

Saflund, K., Sjogren, B., & Wredling, R. (2004). The role of caregivers after a stillbirth: Views and experiences of parents. *Birth, 31*(2), 132–137.

Shuzman, E. (2003). Facing stillbirth or neonatal death: Providing culturally appropriate care for Jewish families. *AWHONN Lifelines, 7*(6), 537–543.

Swanson, K. (2000). Predicting depressive symptoms after miscarriage: A path analysis based on the Lazarus paradigm. *Journal of Women's Health & Gender-Based Medicine, 9*(2), 191–206.

Swanson, K., Chen, H., Graham, J., Wojnar, D., & Petras, A. (2009). Resolution of depression and grief during the first year after miscarriage: A randomized controlled clinical trial of couples-focused interventions. *Journal of Women's Health, 18*(8), 1245–1257.

Swanson, K., Connor, S., Jolley, S., Pettinato, M., & Wang, T. (2007). Contexts and evolution of women's responses to miscarriage during the first year after loss. *Research in Nursing & Health, 30*(1), 2–16.

Swanson, P., Kane, R., Pearsall-Jones, J., Swanson, C., & Croft, M. (2009). How couples cope with the death of a twin or higher order multiple. *Twin Research and Human Genetics, 12*(4), 392–402.

Turton, P., Evans, C., & Hughes, P. (2009). Long-term psychosocial sequelae of stillbirth: Phase II of a nested case-control cohort study. *Archives of Women's Mental Health, 12*(1), 35–41.

Van, P. (2001). Breaking the silence of African American women: Healing after pregnancy loss. *Health Care for Women International, 22*(3), 229–243.

Wheeler, S., & Austin, J. (2001). The impact of early pregnancy loss on adolescents. *MCN: The American Journal of Maternal/Child Nursing, 26*(3), 154–159.

Zhang, B., El-Jawahri, A., & Prigerson, H. (2006). Update on bereavement research: Evidence-based guidelines for the diagnosis and treatment of complicated bereavement. *Journal of Palliative Medicine, 9*(5), 1188–1203.

A

abdominal Belonging or relating to the abdomen and its functions and disorders.

- **a. birth** Birth of a child through a surgical incision made into the abdominal wall and uterus; cesarean birth.
- **a. gestation** Implantation of a fertilized ovum outside the uterus but inside the peritoneal cavity.

abnormal (nonreassuring) fetal heart rate pattern Fetal heart rate pattern that indicates the fetus is not well oxygenated and requires intervention.

ABO incompatibility Hemolytic disease that occurs when the mother's blood type is O and the newborn's is A, B, or AB.

abortion Termination of pregnancy before the fetus is viable and capable of extrauterine existence, usually less than 20 weeks of gestation (or when the fetus weighs less than 500 g); miscarriage.

- **complete a.** Abortion in which fetus and all related tissue have been expelled from the uterus.
- **elective a.** Termination of pregnancy chosen by the woman that is not required for her physical safety.
- **habitual (recurrent) a.** Loss of three or more successive pregnancies for no known cause.
- **incomplete a.** Loss of pregnancy in which some but not all the products of conception have been expelled from the uterus.
- **induced a.** Purposeful interruption of a pregnancy before 20 weeks of gestation.
- **inevitable a.** Threatened loss of pregnancy that cannot be prevented or stopped and is imminent.
- **missed a.** Loss of pregnancy in which the products of conception remain in the uterus after the fetus dies.
- **septic a.** Loss of pregnancy in which there is an infection of the products of conception and the uterine endometrial lining, usually resulting from attempted termination of early pregnancy.
- **spontaneous a.** A pregnancy that ends as a result of natural causes before 20 weeks of gestation; preferred term is *miscarriage.* The 20-week marker is considered to be the point of viability, when a fetus may survive in an extrauterine environment.
- **therapeutic a.** Pregnancy that has been intentionally terminated for medical reasons.
- **threatened a.** Possible loss of a pregnancy; early symptoms are present (e.g., the cervix begins to dilate).

abruptio placentae Partial or complete premature separation of a normally implanted placenta from the uterus.

abstinence Refraining from sexual intercourse periodically or permanently.

acceleration Increase in FHR, usually seen as a reassuring sign.

accreta, placenta See *placenta accreta.*

acculturation Changes that occur within one group or among several groups when people from different cultures come in contact with one another.

acidosis Increase in hydrogen ion concentration resulting in a lowering of blood pH below 7.35.

acoustic stimulation test Antepartum test to elicit fetal heart rate response to sound; performed by applying sound source (laryngeal stimulator) to maternal abdomen over the fetal head.

acquaintance Process used by parents to get to know or become familiar with their new infant; an important step in *attachment.*

acrocyanosis Peripheral cyanosis; blue color of hands and feet in most infants at birth that may persist for 7 to 10 days.

active phase See *labor, active phase.*

acupressure Massage technique applied to specific points along certain energy pathways of the body called meridians. A form of treatment based in the theories of traditional Chinese medicine.

acupuncture A form of treatment using slender needles to stimulate points along energy pathways to correct, enhance, and rebalance the flow of body energy.

acute bilirubin encephalopathy Acute manifestations of bilirubin toxicity that occur during the first weeks after birth.

acute respiratory distress syndrome (ARDS) Set of symptoms including decreased compliance of lung tissue, pulmonary edema, and acute hypoxemia. The condition is similar to respiratory distress syndrome of the newborn.

adequate intakes (AIs) Recommended nutrient intakes estimated to meet the needs of almost all healthy people in the population. They are provided for nutrients or age-group categories where the available information is not sufficient to warrant establishing recommended dietary allowances.

adnexa Adjacent or accessory parts of a structure.

- **uterine a.** Ovaries and uterine (fallopian) tubes.

adjuvant chemotherapy Chemotherapy administered soon after surgical removal of the tumor.

AFI See *amniotic fluid index (AFI).*

AFP See *alpha-fetoprotein (AFP).*

afterbirth pains See *afterpains.*

afterload Ventricular wall tension during systole, or the resistance the blood meets as blood is ejected from the ventricles.

afterpains Painful uterine cramps that occur intermittently for approximately 2 or 3 days after birth and that result from contractile efforts of the uterus to return to its normal involuted condition. Also called *afterbirth pains.*

AGA Appropriate (growth) for gestational age.

AIs See *adequate intakes (AIs).*

alcohol-related birth defects (ARBDs) See alcohol-related neurodevelopmental disorders (ARNDs).

alcohol-related neurodevelopmental disorders (ARNDs) Infants exposed prenatally to alcohol who are affected but do not meet the criteria for fetal alcohol syndrome (FAS); these disorders run the gamut from learning disabilities and behavioral problems to speech or language problems and hyperactivity.

alkalosis Abnormal condition of body fluids characterized by a tendency toward an increased pH, such as from an excess of alkaline bicarbonate or a deficiency of acid.

allopathic, standard, or Western medicine Interchangeable terms used to describe the current U.S. health care system. With foundations in germ theory and reductionism, standard medical practice often focuses on one body system or disease complex. Treatments are often pharmaceutical or surgical and produce effects that are different from those of the disease complex.

alpha-fetoprotein (AFP) Fetal antigen; elevated levels in amniotic fluid are associated with neural tube defects.

alternative and complementary therapies Nontraditional approaches to health care and healing, often philosophically different from Western medicine. Often involve interventions that are said to induce healing from within the client or improve the internal environment so that the body, mind, or spirit can heal. Often referred to as "natural healing." *Alternative therapy* often refers to those modalities used in place of conventional (or other) health care. *Complementary therapy* refers to those modalities used in conjunction with conventional (or other) health care. Many therapies can be either alternative or complementary.

amenorrhea Absence or suppression of menstruation or menstrual flow.

amniocentesis Procedure in which a needle is inserted through the abdominal and uterine walls into the amniotic fluid; some fluid is withdrawn; used for assessment of fetal health and maturity.

amnioinfusion Infusion of room-temperature isotonic fluid (usually normal saline or lactated Ringer's solution) into the uterine cavity if the volume of amniotic fluid is low, in an attempt to increase the fluid around the umbilical cord and prevent compression during uterine contractions.

amnion Inner membrane of two fetal membranes that form the sac and contain the fetus and the fluid that surrounds it in utero.

amnionitis Inflammation of the amnion, occurring most frequently after early rupture of membranes.

amniotic Pertaining or relating to the amnion.

- **a. fluid** Fluid surrounding the fetus derived primarily from maternal serum and fetal urine.
- **a. fluid embolism** See *anaphylactoid syndrome of pregnancy (ASP).*
- **a. fluid index (AFI)** Estimation of amount of amniotic fluid by means of ultrasound to determine excess or decrease.
- **a. sac** Membrane "bag" that contains the fetus and fluid before birth.

amniotomy Artificial rupture of the fetal membranes (AROM), using a plastic AmniHook or surgical clamp.

analgesia Alleviation of the sensation of pain or the raising of the threshold for pain perception without loss of consciousness.

analgesic Any medication or agent that relieves pain.

- **opioid (narcotic) agonist** See *analgesic, opioid (narcotic) agonist.*
- **opioid (narcotic) agonist-antagonist** See *analgesic, opioid (narcotic) agonist-antagonist.*

opioid (narcotic) antagonist See *analgesic, opioid (narcotic) antagonist.*

anaphylactoid syndrome of pregnancy (ASP) Rare complication of pregnancy characterized by the sudden, acute onset of hypoxia, hypotension, or cardiac arrest and coagulopathy that can occur during labor or during birth or immediately after birth; also known as amniotic fluid embolism.

android pelvis Male type of pelvis; heart-shaped inlet.

anencephaly Congenital deformity characterized by the absence of both cerebral hemispheres (cerebrum and cerebellum) and the flat bones of the overlying skull.

anesthesia Encompasses analgesia, amnesia, relaxation, and reflex activity. Anesthesia abolishes pain perception by interrupting the nerve impulses to the brain. The loss of sensation may be partial or complete, sometimes with the loss of consciousness.

aneuploidy One of the two types of deviations from the correct number of chromosomes per cell, in which the numerical deviation is not an exact multiple of the haploid set. Having an abnormal number of chromosomes.

anovulatory Failure of the ovaries to produce, mature, or release eggs.

antenatal Occurring before or formed before birth (newborn).

a. glucocorticoids Medications administered to the mother for the purpose of accelerating fetal lung maturity when an increased risk exists for preterm birth between 24 and 34 weeks of gestation.

antepartal Before labor (maternal).

anthropoid pelvis Pelvis in which the anteroposterior diameter is equal to or greater than the transverse diameter; oval inlet.

anthropometric measurements Body measurements, such as height and weight.

antibody Specific protein substance made by the body that exerts restrictive or destructive action on specific antigens, such as bacteria, toxins, or Rh factor.

anticipatory grief See *grief, anticipatory.*

antigen Protein foreign to the body that causes the body to develop antibodies (e.g., bacteria, dust, Rh factor).

anxiety disorders Includes phobias, panic disorder, generalized anxiety disorder, obsessive-compulsive disorder, and post-traumatic stress disorder. Anxiety disorders are the most common mental disorder.

APF See *alpha-fetoprotein (AFP).*

Apgar score Numeric expression of the condition of a newborn obtained by rapid assessment at 1 and 5 minutes of age; developed by Dr. Virginia Apgar.

apnea Cessation of respirations for more than 15 seconds associated with generalized cyanosis.

ARBDs (alcohol-related birth defects) See *alcohol-related neurodevelopmental disorders (ARNDs).*

ARDS See *acute respiratory distress syndrome (ARDS).*

areola Pigmented ring of tissue surrounding the nipple.

secondary a. During the fifth month of pregnancy, a second faint ring of pigmentation seen around the original areola.

ARNDs See *alcohol-related neurodevelopmental disorders (ARNDs).*

AROM See *membranes, artificial rupture of (AROM).*

arterial pressure catheter A Teflon intravenous catheter, usually 20 gauge, that is placed in an artery and connected to a hemodynamic monitor by means of a pressure line to provide continuous measurements of the systolic, diastolic, and mean arterial blood pressures.

arteriolar vasospasm Diameter of arteriolar vessels diminishes, impeding blood flow to all organs and raising blood pressure.

ARTs See *assisted reproductive therapies (ARTs).*

Asherman's syndrome Intrauterine adhesions after inflammation and infection; one cause of impaired fertility.

ASP See *anaphylactoid syndrome of pregnancy (ASP).*

asphyxia Decreased oxygen with or without excess of carbon dioxide in the body.

perinatal a. Condition occurring in utero with the following biochemical changes: hypoxemia (lowering of Po_2), hypercapnia (increase in Pco_2), and respiratory and metabolic acidosis (reduction of blood pH).

aspiration pneumonia Inflammatory condition of the lungs and bronchi caused by the inhalation of vomitus containing acidic gastric contents.

assimilation Occurs when a cultural group loses its identity and becomes part of the dominant culture.

assisted reproductive therapies (ARTs) Treatments for infertility, including in vitro fertilization procedures, embryo adoption, embryo hosting, and therapeutic insemination.

asynclitism Oblique presentation of the fetal head at the superior strait of the pelvis; the pelvic planes and those of the fetal head are not parallel.

atony Absence of muscle tone. See also *uterine atony.*

atresia Absence of a normally present passageway.

biliary a. Absence of the bile duct.

choanal a. Complete obstruction of the posterior nares, which open into the nasopharynx, with membranous or bony tissue.

esophageal a. Congenital anomaly in which the esophagus ends in a blind pouch or narrows into a thin cord, thus failing to form a continuous passageway to the stomach.

attachment (1) The process by which a parent comes to love and accept a child and a child comes to love and accept a parent. (2) A specific and enduring affective tie to another person.

attitude Body posture or position.

fetal a. Relation of fetal parts to each other in the uterus (e.g., all parts flexed, all parts flexed except neck is extended).

general flexion a. Fetal posture in which the chin is flexed on the chest, the thighs are flexed on the abdomen, the legs are flexed at the knees, and the arms are crossed over the thorax.

augmentation of labor Stimulation of ineffective uterine contractions after labor has started spontaneously but is not progressing satisfactorily.

autoimmune disorders Body produces antibodies against itself, causing tissue damage.

autoimmunization Development of antibodies against constituents of one's own tissues (e.g., a man may develop antibodies against his own sperm).

autolysis "Self-digestive" process by which the uterus returns to a nonpregnant state after childbirth. The decrease in estrogen and progesterone levels after childbirth results in this destruction of excess hypertrophied uterine tissue.

autosomal dominant inheritance disorder Condition in which only one copy of a variant allele is needed for phenotypic expression.

autosomal inheritance Characteristics transmitted by genes on the autosomes, not the sex chromosomes.

autosomal recessive inheritance disorder Condition in which both genes of a pair are forms associated with the disorder to be expressed.

autosomes Any of the paired chromosomes other than the sex (X and Y) chromosomes.

azoospermia Absence of sperm in the semen.

B

baby blues See *postpartum blues.*

bag of waters Lay term for the sac containing amniotic fluid and fetus.

balanced translocation See *translocation, balanced.*

ballottement (1) Movability of a floating object, such as a fetus. (2) Diagnostic technique using palpation: a floating object, when tapped or pushed, moves away and then returns to touch the examiner's hand. (3) Passive movement of the unengaged fetus.

Bandl's ring Abnormally thickened ridge of uterine musculature between the upper and lower segments that occurs after a mechanically obstructed labor, with the lower segment thinning abnormally.

Bartholin cyst Most common benign lesion of the vulva; arises from obstruction of the Bartholin duct, which causes it to enlarge.

Bartholin glands Two small glands situated on either side of the vaginal orifice that secrete small amounts of mucus during coitus and that are homologous to the bulbourethral glands in the male.

basal body temperature Lowest body temperature of a healthy person taken immediately after awakening and before getting out of bed.

basalis, decidua See *decidua basalis.*

baseline fetal heart rate See *fetal heart rate (FHR), baseline.*

beaking See *cervical funneling.*

bearing-down effort "Secondary powers"; energy exerted by the woman during contractions to push out the baby.

Bell's palsy See *palsy, Bell's.*

bereavement The feelings of loss, pain, desolation, and sadness that occur after the death of a loved one.

bicornuate uterus Anomalous uterus that may be either a double or single organ with two horns.

bilateral tubal ligation (BTL) A method of female sterilization in which the uterine tubes are severed and ligated.

biliary atresia See *atresia, biliary.*

bilirubin Yellow or orange pigment that is a breakdown product of hemoglobin. It is carried by the blood to the liver, where it is chemically changed and excreted into the bile or is conjugated and excreted by the kidneys.

Billings method See *ovulation method.*

bimanual Performed with both hands.

b. palpation Examination of a woman's pelvic organs done by placement of one hand on the abdomen and one or two fingers of the other hand into the vagina.

biofeedback Technique that teaches the client to consciously control certain body functions usually thought of as unconscious (e.g., breathing, heart rate). Often involves electronic instrumentation that provides immediate visual and auditory feedback to assist the learning process.

biophysical profile (BPP) Noninvasive assessment of the fetus and its environment using ultrasonography and uterine fetal monitoring; includes fetal breathing movements, gross body movements, fetal tone, reactive fetal heart rate, and qualitative amniotic fluid volume.

biopsy Removal of a small piece of tissue for microscopic examination and diagnosis.

biorhythmicity Cyclic changes that occur with established regularity, such as sleeping and eating patterns.

biparietal diameter Largest transverse diameter of the fetal head; extends from one parietal bone to the other.

bipolar (or manic-depressive) disorder Mood disorder defined by the presence of one or more episodes of abnormally elevated energy leveles, cognition, and mood and one or more depressive episodes.

birth injury See *birth trauma.*

birth, late preterm See *preterm, late preterm birth.*

birth, preterm See *preterm birth.*

birth, very preterm See *preterm, very preterm birth.*

birth plan A tool by which parents can explore their childbirth options and choose those that are most important to them.

birth rate Number of live births per 1000 population per year. See also *fertility.*

birth trauma Physical injury sustained by a neonate during labor and birth. Also called *birth injury.*

Bishop score Rating system to evaluate inducibility of the cervix; a higher score increases the rate of successful induction of labor.

bittersweet grief See *grief, bittersweet.*

blastocyst Stage in the development of a mammalian embryo, occurring after the morula stage, that consists of an outer layer, or trophoblast, and a hollow sphere of cells enclosing a cavity.

blood pressure (BP) Pressure of the blood against the walls of the arteries.

bloody show Vaginal discharge that originates in the cervix and consists of blood and mucus; increases as cervix dilates during labor.

BMI See *body mass index (BMI).*

body mass index (BMI) Method of calculating appropriateness of weight for height (BMI = weight [kilograms]/height^2 [meters]).

BP See *blood pressure (BP).*

BPD See *bronchopulmonary dysplasia (BPD).*

BPP See *biophysical profile (BPP).*

brachial plexus injury See *Erb-Duchenne palsy.*

Bradley method Husband-coached childbirth using labor breathing techniques.

bradycardia Baseline FHR below 110 beats per minute.

Braxton Hicks sign Mild, intermittent, painless uterine contractions that occur during pregnancy. These contractions occur more frequently as pregnancy advances but do not represent true labor.

Brazelton assessment Method for assessing the interactional behavior of a newborn.

breakthrough bleeding Escape of blood occurring between menstrual periods; may be noted by women using chemical contraception (birth control pills).

breast self-examination (BSE) Self-palpation of breasts to detect for changes in breast tissue.

breech presentation Presentation in which buttocks or feet are nearest the cervical opening and are born first; occurs in approximately 3% of all births.

- **complete b.p.** Simultaneous presentation of buttocks, legs, and feet.
- **footling (incomplete) b.p.** Presentation of one or both feet.
- **frank b.p.** Presentation of buttocks, with hips flexed so that thighs are against abdomen.

bronchopulmonary dysplasia (BPD) Pulmonary condition affecting preterm infants who have experienced respiratory failure and have been oxygen dependent for more than 28 days.

brown fat Source of heat unique to neonates that is capable of greater thermogenic activity than ordinary fat. Deposits are found around the adrenals, kidneys, and neck, between the scapulas, and behind the sternum for several weeks after birth.

bruit, uterine See *uterine bruit.*

BSE See *breast self-examination (BSE).*

C

café-au-lait spot Patch of skin pigmentation.

calendar method See *rhythm method.*

cancer of the cervix See *cervical cancer.*

cancer of the ovaries See *ovarian cancer.*

cancer of the vulva See *vulvar carcinoma.*

Candida vaginitis Vaginal, fungal infection; formerly called *moniliasis.*

candidiasis Infection of the skin or mucous membrane by a yeastlike fungus, *Candida albicans*; see *thrush.*

capillary hydrostatic pressure Pressure in the arterial capillary system to promote the movement of fluid across the semipermeable membrane of the capillary wall from the vessel into the interstitial space. Measured as the *pulmonary capillary wedge pressure (PCWP).*

capsularis, decidua See *decidua capsularis.*

caput Occiput of fetal head appearing at the vaginal introitus preceding birth of the head.

- **c. succedaneum** Swelling of the tissue over the presenting part of the fetal head caused by pressure during labor.

carcinoma Malignant, often metastatic epithelial neoplasm; cancer.

carcinoma in situ (CIS) Diagnosed when the full thickness of epithelium is replaced with abnormal cells.

cardiac decompensation A condition of heart failure in which the heart is unable to maintain a sufficient cardiac output.

cardiac output (CO) Volume of blood ejected from the left ventricle in 1 minute, measured in liters per minute. Cardiac output is the product of stroke volume and heart rate (CO = HR × SV).

cardinal movements of labor The mechanism of labor in a vertex presentation; includes engagement, descent, flexion, internal rotation, extension, external rotation (restitution), and expulsion.

carpal tunnel syndrome Pressure on the median nerve at the point at which it goes through the carpal tunnel of the wrist. It causes soreness, tenderness, and weakness of the muscles of the thumb. Edema involving the peripheral nerves may result in carpal tunnel syndrome during the last trimester of pregnancy.

carrier Individual who carries a gene that does not exhibit itself in physical or chemical characteristics but that can be transmitted to children (e.g., a female carrying the trait for hemophilia, which is expressed in male offspring). Heterozygous individuals have only one variant allele and are unaffected clinically because their normal gene (wild-type allele) overshadows the variant allele. They are known as carriers of the recessive trait.

cephalhematoma NOTE: This is spelled *cephalohematoma* in some sources. Extravasation of blood from ruptured vessels between a skull bone and its external covering, the periosteum. Swelling is limited by the margins of the cranial bone affected (usually parietals).

cephalic Pertaining to the head.

- **c. presentation** Presentation of the fetal head.

cephalopelvic disproportion (CPD) Condition in which the infant's head is of such a shape, size, or position that it cannot pass through the mother's pelvis; can also be caused by maternal pelvic problems. Also called *fetopelvic disproportion (FPD).*

cerclage Use of nonabsorbable suture to keep a premature dilating cervix closed; released when pregnancy is at term to allow labor to begin.

certified midwife See *midwife, certified.*

cervical cancer The third most common reproductive cancer; begins as neoplastic changes in the cervical epithelium. Also called *cancer of the cervix.*

cervical cap Individually fitted contraceptive barrier for the cervix.

cervical conization Excision of a cone-shaped section of tissue from the endocervix.

cervical funneling Effacement of the internal cervical os. Also called *beaking.*

cervical intraepithelial neoplasia (CIN) Uncontrolled and progressive abnormal growth of cervical epithelial cells.

cervical mucus method See *ovulation method.*

cervical os "Mouth" or opening to the cervix.

cervical ripening Process of effecting physical softening and distensibility of the cervix in preparation for labor and birth.

cervix Lowest and narrow end of the uterus; the "neck." The cervix is situated between the external os and the body, or corpus, of the uterus, and its lower end extends into the vagina.

cesarean birth Birth of a fetus by an incision through the abdominal wall and uterus. See also *elective cesarean birth.*

Chadwick sign Violet bluish color of vaginal mucous membrane and cervix that is visible from about the fourth week of pregnancy; caused by increased vascularity.

chloasma Blotchy, brownish hyperpigmentation of the skin over the cheeks, nose, and forehead, especially in dark-complexioned pregnant women and some women taking oral contraceptives; also known as the *mask of pregnancy.*

choanal atresia See *atresia, choanal.*

cholecystitis Acute or chronic inflammation of the gallbladder.

cholelithiasis Presence of gallstones in the gallbladder.

choreoathetoid cerebral palsy Condition characterized by both choreiform (jerky, ticlike, twitching) and athetoid (slow, writhing) movements.

chorioamnionitis Bacterial infection of the amniotic cavity.

chorion Fetal membrane closest to the intrauterine wall that gives rise to the placenta and continues as the outer membrane surrounding the amnion.

chorionic villus Tiny vascular protrusions on the chorionic surface that project into the maternal blood sinuses of the uterus and that help form the placenta and secrete human chorionic gonadotropin.

chorionic villus sampling (CVS) Removal of fetal tissue from the placenta for genetic diagnostic studies.

chronic hypertension See *hypertension, chronic.*

chromosome Element within the cell nucleus carrying genes and composed of DNA and proteins. Threadlike package of genes and other DNA in the nucleus of a cell.

CIN See *cervical intraepithelial neoplasia (CIN).*

circumcision

- **female c.** Religious or cultural removal of a portion of the clitoris and labia; practiced in some Third World countries but illegal in the United States. Mutilating procedure that can cause problems in childbirth.
- **male c.** Excision of the prepuce (foreskin) of the penis, exposing the glans; may be done for religious or cultural reasons.

CIS See *carcinoma in situ (CIS).*

claiming process Process by which the parents identify their new baby in terms of likeness to other family members, differences, and uniqueness; the unique newcomer is thus incorporated into the family.

cleft lip Incomplete closure of the lip. Lay term used is harelip.

cleft palate Incomplete closure of the palate or roof of mouth; a congenital fissure.

climacteric The period of a woman's life when she is passing from a reproductive to a nonreproductive state, with regression of ovarian function. The cycle of endocrine, physical, and psychosocial changes that occurs during the termination of the reproductive years. Also called climacterium.

clinical benchmark Process used to compare one's own performance against the performance of the best in an area of service.

clitoris Female organ analogous to male penis; a small, ovoid body of erectile tissue situated at the anterior junction of the vulva.

clonus Hyperactive reflexes.

clubfoot Congenital deformity in which portions of the foot and ankle are twisted out of a normal position.

CNS Central nervous system.

CO See *cardiac output (CO).*

Cochrane Pregnancy and Childbirth Database Database of up-to-date systematic reviews and dissemination of views of randomized controlled trials of health care.

cohabiting-parent family Family form in which children live with two unmarried biologic parents or two adoptive parents.

coitus Penile-vaginal intercourse.

- **c. interruptus** Intercourse during which penis is withdrawn from vagina before ejaculation.

cold stress Excessive loss of heat that results in increased respirations and nonshivering thermogenesis to maintain core body temperature.

colloid osmotic pressure (COP) The gradient controlling whether fluid remains inside the capillary or moves into the interstitial space. Pressure in the arterial capillary system to prevent the movement of fluid across the semipermeable membrane of the capillary wall from the vessel into the interstitial space. The COP measures the "pulling" pressure of proteins in the plasma to retain fluid inside the vessel.

colostrum The creamy white to yellowish to orange premilk fluid that may be expressed from the nipples as early as 16 weeks of gestation; the fluid in the breast from pregnancy into the early postpartal period. It is more concentrated than mature milk and is extremely rich in immunoglobulins; it has higher concentrations of protein and minerals but less fat than mature milk; it is also rich in antibodies, which provide protection from many diseases; high in protein, which binds bilirubin; and laxative-acting, which speeds the elimination of meconium and helps loosen mucus.

colposcopy Examination of vagina and cervix with a colposcope (a stereoscopic binocular microscope that magnifies the view of the cervix) to identify neoplastic or other changes.

complete abortion See *abortion, complete.*

complete breech presentation See *breech presentation, complete.*

complicated bereavement See *grief, complicated.*

complicated grief See *grief, complicated.*

conception Union of the sperm and a single egg (ovum) resulting in fertilization; formation of the one-celled zygote, marks the beginning of a pregnancy.

conceptional age In fetal development the number of completed weeks since the moment of conception. Because the moment of conception is almost impossible to determine, conceptional age is estimated at 2 weeks less than gestational age.

conceptus Embryo or fetus, fetal membranes, amniotic fluid, and the fetal portion of the placenta.

condom Mechanical barrier worn on the penis for contraception or to protect against sexually transmitted infections (STIs); a "rubber."

condyloma acuminatum (plural condylomata acuminata) Wartlike growth on the skin usually seen near the anus or external genitals caused by human papillomavirus (HPV); genital warts. (Must be differentiated from condyloma latum seen in secondary syphilis.)

congenital Present or existing before birth as a result of either hereditary or prenatal environmental factors.

- **c. anomaly** A defect that is present at birth and can be caused by genetic or environmental factors, or both; defined as a physical, metabolic, anatomic, or behavioral deviation from the normal pattern of development.
- **c. diaphragmatic hernia** Malformation of diaphragm that allows displacement of the abdominal organs into the thoracic cavity.
- **c. rubella syndrome** Complex of problems, including hearing defects, cardiovascular abnormalities, and cataracts, caused by maternal rubella in the first trimester of pregnancy.

conization See *cervical conization.*

conjoined twins See *twins, conjoined.*

conjugate

- **diagonal c.** Radiographic measurement of distance from inferior border of symphysis pubis to sacral promontory; may be obtained by vaginal examination; 12.5 to 13 cm.
- **true c. (conjugata vera)** Radiographic measurement of distance from upper margin of symphysis pubis to sacral promontory; 1.5 to 2 cm less than diagonal conjugate.

conjunctivitis Inflammation of the mucous membrane that lines the eyelids and is reflected onto the eyeball.

conscious relaxation Technique used to release the mind and body from tension through conscious effort and practice.

consumptive coagulopathy See *disseminated intravascular coagulation (DIC).*

continuous positive airway pressure (CPAP) Method of infusing oxygen or air under a preset pressure by means of nasal prongs, a face mask, or an endotracheal tube.

contraception Intentional prevention of pregnancy (impregnation or conception) during sexual intercourse.

contractility Force and velocity of ventricular contractions when preload and afterload are held constant.

contraction ring See *Bandl's ring.*

contractions in labor Involuntary rhythmic tightening of the uterine muscle that act to expel the fetus and placenta from the uterus.

- **duration** Period from the beginning of the contraction to the end.
- **frequency** How often the contractions occur—the period from the beginning of one contraction to the beginning of the next.
- **intensity** Strength of the contraction at its peak.
- **interval** Period between uterine contractions, timed from the end of one contraction to the beginning of the next.
- **resting tone** The tension in the uterine muscle between contractions; relaxation of the uterus.
- **uterine c.** See *uterine contractions.*

contraction stress test (CST) Test to stimulate uterine contractions for the purpose of assessing fetal response; a healthy fetus does not react to contractions, whereas a compromised fetus demonstrates late decelerations in the fetal heart rate that are indicative of uteroplacental insufficiency.

Coombs' test Indirect: determination of Rh-positive antibodies in maternal blood. Direct: determination of maternal Rh-positive antibodies in fetal cord blood. A positive test result indicates the presence of antibodies or titer.

COP See *colloid osmotic pressure (COP).*

cordocentesis See *percutaneous umbilical blood sampling (PUBS).*

corpus luteum Yellow body. After rupture of the graafian follicle at ovulation, the follicle develops into a yellow structure that secretes progesterone and some estrogen in the second half of the menstrual cycle, atrophying about 3 days before sloughing of the endometrium in menstrual flow. If impregnation occurs, it continues to produce the hormones until the placenta can take over this function.

corpus luteum cysts Occur after ovulation and are possibly caused by an increased secretion of progesterone that results in an increase of fluid in the corpus luteum.

corrected age Taking into account the gestational age and the postnatal age of a preterm infant when determining expectations for development.

cotyledon One of the 15 to 28 visible segments of the placenta on the maternal surface, each made up of fetal vessels, chorionic villi, and an intervillous space.

counterpressure Pressure to sacral area of back during uterine contractions.

couplet care Care provided by one nurse, educated in both mother and infant care, who functions as the primary nurse for both mother and infant. Also called *mother-baby care* or *single-room maternity care.*

couvade syndrome The phenomenon of expectant fathers' experiencing pregnancy-like symptoms.

Couvelaire uterus See *uterus, Couvelaire.*

CPAP See *continuous positive airway pressure (CPAP).*

CPD See *cephalopelvic disproportion (CPD).*

cradle cap Common seborrheic dermatitis of infants consisting of thick, yellow, greasy scales on the scalp.

creatinine Substance found in blood and muscle; measurement of levels in maternal urine correlates with amount of fetal muscle mass and therefore fetal size.

crib death Unexpected and sudden death of an apparently normal and healthy infant that occurs during sleep and with no physical or autopsic evidence of disease. Also referred to as *sudden infant death syndrome (SIDS).*

cri du chat syndrome Rare congenital disorder recognized at birth by a kitten-like cry, which may prevail for weeks and then disappear. Other characteristics include low birth weight, microcephaly, "moon face," wide-set eyes, strabismus, and low-set misshapen ears. Infants are hypotonic; heart defects and mental and physical retardation are common. Also called *cat-cry syndrome.*

crowning Stage of birth when the top of the fetal head can be seen at the vaginal orifice as the widest part of the head distends the vulva.

cryosurgery Local freezing and removal of tissue without injury to adjacent tissue and with minimum blood loss, done with special equipment; uses a freezing technique that freezes abnormal cells, and when sloughing occurs, normal tissue is regenerated.

CSF Cerebrospinal fluid.

CST See *contraction stress test (CST).*

cul-de-sac of Douglas Pouch formed by a fold of the peritoneum dipping down between the anterior wall of the rectum and the posterior wall of the uterus; also called *Douglas's cul-de-sac, pouch of Douglas,* and *rectouterine pouch.*

culdocentesis Puncture of cul-de-sac of Douglas through the vagina for aspiration of fluid.

Cullen's sign Faint, irregularly formed hemorrhagic patches on the skin around the umbilicus. The discolored skin is blue-black and becomes greenish brown or yellow. Cullen's sign may appear 1 to 2 days after the onset of anorexia and the severe, poorly localized abdominal pains characteristic of acute pancreatitis. Cullen's sign is also present in massive upper gastrointestinal hemorrhage and ruptured ectopic pregnancy.

cultural competence Awareness, acceptance, and knowledge of cultural differences and adaptation of services to acknowledge and support the culture of the client.

cultural context Setting in which one considers the individual's and the family's beliefs and practices (culture).

cultural prescriptions Practices that are expected or acceptable; they tell women what to do.

cultural proscriptions Forbidden; taboo practices; they tell women what not to do.

curettage Scraping of the endometrium lining of the uterus with a curet to remove the contents of the uterus (as is done after an incomplete miscarriage or induced abortion) or to obtain specimens for diagnostic purposes. Also called *curet* or *curette.*

CVS See *chorionic villus sampling (CVS).*

cycle of violence Pattern of three phases: period of increasing tension, the abusive episode, and a period of contrition and kindness.

cystocele Bladder hernia: injury to the vesicovaginal fascia during labor and birth may allow herniation of the bladder into the vagina. Protrusion of the bladder downward into the vagina; develops when supporting structures in the vesicovaginal septum are injured.

D

D&C See *dilation and curettage (D&C).*

daily fetal movement count (DFMC) Maternal assessment of fetal activity; the number of fetal movements within a specific time are counted. Also called kick count.

DDH See *developmental dysplasia of the hip (DDH).*

death Cessation of life.

- **fetal d.** Intrauterine death; death of a fetus weighing 500 g or more and 20 weeks of gestation or more.
- **infant d.** Death during the first year of life.
- **maternal d.** Death of a woman as a result of a pregnancy or birth-related problem.
- **neonatal d.** Death of a newborn within the first 28 days after birth.
- **perinatal d.** Death of a fetus of 20 weeks of gestation or older or death of a neonate 28 days old or younger.

deceleration Slowing of fetal heart rate attributed to a parasympathetic response and described in relation to uterine contractions.

- **early d.** Onset corresponding to onset of uterine contraction, related to fetal head compression.
- **late d.** Onset after peak of contraction, continuing into interval after contraction; caused by uteroplacental insufficiency.
- **prolonged d.** Episode of slowing of fetal heart rate lasting longer than 2 minutes, but less than 10 minutes.
- **variable d.** Abrupt onset at any time unrelated to contraction; caused by cord compression.

decidua Mucous membrane, lining of uterus, or endometrium of pregnancy that is shed after giving birth.

- **d. basalis** The portion of the endometrium directly under the blastocyst, where the chorionic villi tap into the maternal blood vessels. Maternal aspect of the placenta made up of uterine blood vessels, endometrial stroma, and glands. It is shed in lochial discharge after delivery.
- **d. capsularis** That part of the decidual membranes surrounding the chorionic sac.
- **d. vera** Nonplacental decidual lining of the uterus.

decrement Decrease or stage of decline, as of a contraction.

deep tendon reflex (DTR) Reflex caused by stimulation of tendons, such as elbow, wrist, knee, triceps, and ankle jerk reflexes.

deletion Loss of chromosomal material and partial monosomy for the chromosome involved. The resulting clinical phenotype of either a terminal or an interstitial deletion depends on how much of the chromosome has been lost and the number and function of the genes contained in the missing segment.

- **interstitial d.** Deletion anywhere else in the chromosome except at the end.
- **microdeletion** Deletion too small to be detected by standard cytogenetic techniques.
- **terminal d.** Deletion at the end of a chromosome.

delivery (birth) Expulsion of the child with placenta and membranes by the mother or their extraction by the obstetric practitioner.

- **abdominal d.** See *abdominal birth.*

ΔOD_{450} (delta OD_{450}) Delta optical density (or absorbance) at 450 nm, obtained by spectral analysis of amniotic fluid. This prenatal test is used to measure the degree of hemolytic activity in the fetus and to evaluate fetal status in women sensitized to the Rh factor.

demand feeding Feeding a newborn every third hour or when the baby cries to be fed, whichever comes first.

deoxyribonucleic acid (DNA) Intracellular complex protein that carries genetic information, consisting of two purines (adenine and guanine) and two pyrimidines (thymine and cytosine).

dermoid cysts Germ cell tumors, usually occurring in childhood. These cysts contain substances such as hair, teeth, sebaceous secretions, and bones.

DES See *diethylstilbestrol (DES).*

desquamation Shedding of epithelial cells of the skin and mucous membranes.

developmental dysplasia of the hip (DDH) Abnormal development of the hip joint, resulting in instability of the hip causing one or both of the femoral heads to be displaced from the acetabulum (hip socket).

DFMC See *daily fetal movement count (DFMC).*

diabetes mellitus A group of metabolic diseases characterized by hyperglycemia resulting from defects in insulin secretion, insulin action, or both. Systemic disorder of carbohydrate, protein, and fat metabolism; caused by deficient insulin production or ineffective use of insulin at the cellular level.

diaphragmatic hernia See *congenital diaphragmatic hernia.*

diastasis recti abdominis Separation of the two rectus muscles along the median line of the abdominal wall. This is often seen in women with repeated childbirths or with a multiple gestation (e.g., triplets). In the newborn it is usually attributable to incomplete development.

Dick-Read method An approach to childbirth based on the premise that fear of pain produces muscular tension, producing pain and greater fear. The method includes teaching physiologic processes of labor, exercise to improve muscle tone, and techniques to assist in relaxation and prevent the fear-tension-pain mechanism.

dietary reference intakes (DRIs) Nutritional recommendations consisting of the recommended dietary allowances, adequate intakes, and tolerable upper intake levels, the upper limit of intake associated with low risk in almost all members of a population.

dilation of cervix Stretching of the external os from an opening a few millimeters in size to an opening large enough to allow the passage of the infant.

dilation and curettage (D&C) Vaginal procedure in which the cervical canal is stretched enough to admit passage of an instrument called a *curet* (or *curette*). The endometrium of the uterus is scraped with the curet to empty the uterine contents or to obtain tissue for examination.

displacement, uterine See *uterine displacement.*

disorganization A dimension of bereavement characterized by depression, anorexia, difficulty in concentration, and a generalized feeling of not feeling good about oneself physically and emotionally.

disparate twins See *twins, disparate.*

disseminated intravascular coagulation (DIC) Pathologic form of diffuse coagulation in which clotting that consumes large amounts of clotting factors, causing widespread external bleeding, internal bleeding, or both, and clotting; associated with abruptio placentae, eclampsia, intrauterine fetal demise, amniotic fluid embolism, and hemorrhage. Also called *consumptive coagulopathy.*

dizygotic Related to or proceeding from two zygotes (fertilized ova).

dizygotic twins See *twins, dizygotic.*

DNA See *deoxyribonucleic acid (DNA).*

dominant trait A trait or disorder expressed or phenotypically apparent when only one copy of an allele associated with the trait is present. Gene that is expressed whenever it is present in the heterozygous gene state (e.g., brown eyes are dominant over blue).

Doppler blood flow analysis Device for measuring blood flow noninvasively in the fetus and placenta to detect intrauterine growth restriction.

Douglas's cul-de-sac See *cul-de-sac of Douglas.*

doula A professional, experienced female labor attendant trained to provide labor support, including physical, emotional, and informational support to women and their partners during labor and birth.

Down syndrome (DS) Abnormality involving chromosome 21, that characteristically results in a typical picture of mental retardation and altered physical appearance. This condition was formerly called mongolism.

DRIs See *dietary reference intakes (DRIs).*

dry labor Lay term referring to labor in which amniotic fluid has already escaped. A "dry birth" does not exist. See *labor.*

DS See *Down syndrome (DS).*

dual diagnosis The coexistence of substance abuse and another psychiatric disorder.

DTR See *deep tendon reflex (DTR).*

DUB See *dysfunctional uterine bleeding (DUB).*

Dubowitz assessment Estimation of gestational age of a newborn based on criteria developed for that purpose.

ductus arteriosus In fetal circulation an anatomic shunt between the pulmonary artery and arch of the aorta. It is obliterated after birth by a rising Po_2 and a change in intravascular pressures in the presence of normal pulmonary function. It normally becomes a ligament after birth but in some instances remains patent; this is called *patent ductus arteriosus (PDA).*

ductus venosus In fetal circulation, a blood vessel carrying oxygenated blood between the umbilical vein and the inferior vena cava, bypassing the liver. It is obliterated and becomes a ligament after birth.

Duncan's mechanism Delivery of placenta with the maternal surface presenting, rather than the shiny fetal surface.

dysfunctional labor Long, difficult, or abnormal labor, caused by various conditions associated with the five factors affecting labor; also called *dystocia.*

dysfunctional uterine bleeding (DUB) Excessive uterine bleeding with no demonstrable organic cause, genital or extragenital; most frequently caused by anovulation. Subset of abnormal uterine bleeding.

dysmaturity See *intrauterine growth restriction (IUGR).*

dysmenorrhea Pain during or shortly before menstruation.

- **primary d.** Painful menstruation beginning 2 to 6 months after menarche, related to ovulation. Condition associated with abnormally increased uterine activity, due to myometrial contractions induced by prostaglandins in the second half of the menstrual cycle.
- **secondary d.** Acquired menstrual pain that develops later in life than primary dysmenorrhea, typically after age 25 years. This condition is associated with pelvic pathology, such as adenomyosis, endometriosis, pelvic inflammatory disease, endometrial polyps, or submucous or interstitial myomas (fibroids).

dyspareunia Painful sexual intercourse, for either sex.

dysplasia Any abnormal development of tissues or organs.

dystocia See *dysfunctional labor.*

E

ecchymosis Bruise; bleeding into tissue caused by direct trauma, serious infection, or bleeding diathesis.

eclampsia Onset of seizure activity or coma in a woman with preeclampsia, with no history of preexisting pathology, which can result in seizure activity. Severe complication of pregnancy of unknown cause and occurring more often in the primigravida; characterized by tonic and clonic convulsions, coma, high blood pressure, albuminuria, and oliguria occurring during pregnancy or shortly after birth.

ectoderm Outer layer of embryonic tissue giving rise to skin, nails, and hair.

ectopic Out of normal place.

- **e. pregnancy** Pregnancy in which the fertilized ovum is implanted outside of its normal place in the uterine cavity. Locations include the abdomen, uterine tubes, and ovaries.

ECV See *external cephalic version (ECV).*

EDB See *estimated date of birth (EDB).*

edema Generalized accumulation of interstitial fluid.

- **dependent e.** Edema of lower or most dependent parts of body where hydrostatic pressure is greater.
- **pitting e.** Edema that leaves a small depression or pit when pressure is applied to a swollen area.

effacement Thinning and shortening or obliteration of the cervix that occurs during late pregnancy or labor or both.

effleurage Gentle stroking used in massage.

EFM See *electronic fetal monitoring (EFM).*

Eisenmenger syndrome Pulmonary hypertension characterized by elevated pulmonary vascular resistance and right-to-left (or bidirectional) shunting in either atria or ventricles.

ejaculation Sudden expulsion of semen from the male urethra.

ELBW See *extremely low birth weight (ELBW).*

elective abortion See *abortion, elective.*

elective cesarean birth A primary cesarean birth without medical or obstetric indication; sometimes referred to as *cesarean on request* or *cesarean on demand.*

electronic fetal monitoring (EFM) Electronic surveillance of fetal heart rate by external and internal methods.

embolus Any undissolved matter (solid, liquid, or gaseous) that is carried by the blood to another part of the body and obstructs a blood vessel.

embryo Conceptus from the second or third week of development until about the eighth week after conception, when mineralization (ossification) of the skeleton begins. This period is characterized by cellular differentiation and predominantly hyperplastic growth.

emergency contraception Contraception that should be taken by a woman as soon as possible but within 120 hours of unprotected intercourse or birth control mishap to prevent unintended pregnancy.

emotional lability Rapid mood changes from irritability to anger or sadness to joy and cheerfulness; often seen in the first trimester of pregnancy.

encephalocele A herniation of the brain and meninges through a skull defect.

endocarditis Inflammation of the inner layer of the heart muscle (endocardium).

endocervical Pertaining to the interior of the canal of the cervix of the uterus.

endocrine glands Ductless glands that secrete hormones into the blood or lymph.

endometrial cancer Most common malignancy of the reproductive system; slow-growing tumor that usually develops in the fundus of the uterus and can spread directly to the myometrium and cervix, as well as to the reproductive organs.

endometriosis Characterized by the presence and growth of endometrial glands and stroma outside of the uterus. Tissue closely resembling endometrial tissue but located outside the uterus in the pelvic cavity. Symptoms may include pelvic pain or pressure, dysmenorrhea, dyspareunia, abnormal bleeding from the uterus or rectum, and sterility.

endometritis Postpartum uterine infection, often beginning at the site of the placental implantation.

endometrium Inner lining of the uterus that undergoes changes caused by hormones during the menstrual cycle and pregnancy; decidua.

endorphins Endogenous opioids secreted by the pituitary gland that act on the central and peripheral nervous systems to reduce pain.

energy healing A variety of techniques and disciplines that are said to augment, modulate, stimulate, or remedy certain deficiencies or blocks in the human energy system.

en face Face-to-face position in which the parent's and infant's faces are approximately 20 cm apart and on the same plane.

engagement In obstetrics, the entrance of the fetal presenting part into the superior pelvic strait and the beginning of the descent through the pelvic canal.

engorgement Distention or vascular congestion. In obstetrics, the process of swelling of the breast tissue brought about by an increase in blood and lymph supply to the breast as the body produces milk, which precedes true lactation. Occurring at about 72 to 96 hours after birth, it lasts about 48 hours and usually reaches a peak between the third and fifth postbirth days.

engrossment A parent's absorption, preoccupation, and interest in his or her infant; term typically used to describe the father's intense involvement with his newborn.

entrainment Phenomenon observed in the microanalysis of sound films in which the speaker moves several parts of the body and the listener responds to the sounds by moving in ways that are coordinated with the rhythm of the sounds. Infants have been observed to move in time to the rhythms of adult speech but not to random noises or disconnected words or vowels. Entrainment is believed to be an essential factor in the process of maternal-infant bonding.

epicanthus Fold of skin covering the inner canthus and caruncle that extends from the root of the nose to the median end of the eyebrow; characteristically found in certain races but may occur as a congenital anomaly.

epidural block Type of regional anesthesia produced by injection of a local anesthetic into the epidural (peridural) space.

epidural blood patch A patch formed by a few millimeters of the mother's blood occluding a tear or hole in the dura mater around the spinal cord.

episiotomy Surgical incision of the perineum at the end of the second stage of labor to enlarge the vaginal outlet, facilitate birth, and avoid laceration of the perineum.

episodic changes Changes from baseline patterns in the fetal heart rate that are not associated with uterine contractions.

epispadias Defect in which the urethral canal terminates on the dorsum of the penis or above the clitoris (rare).

Epstein's pearls Small white blebs found along the gum margins and at the junction of the soft and hard palates. They are a normal manifestation and are typically seen in the newborn. Similar to Bohn's nodules.

epulis Red raised nodule on the gums that bleeds easily; tumor-like benign lesion of the gingiva seen in pregnant women. Also called *gingival granuloma gravidarum.*

Erb-Duchenne palsy Paralysis caused by physical injury to the upper brachial plexus, occurring most often in childbirth from forcible traction during birth. The signs of Erb-Duchenne palsy include loss of sensation in the arm and paralysis and atrophy of the deltoid, the biceps, and the brachialis muscles. Also called *Erb's palsy* and *brachial plexus injury.*

Erb's palsy See *Erb-Duchenne palsy.*

ERT See *estrogen replacement therapy (ERT).*

erythema neonatorum See *erythema toxicum.*

erythema toxicum Innocuous pink papular neonatal rash of unknown cause, with superimposed vesicles appearing within 24 to 48 hours after birth and resolving spontaneously within a few days. Also called *erythema neonatorum, newborn rash,* or *flea bite dermatitis.*

erythroblastosis fetalis Hemolytic disease of the newborn usually caused by isoimmunization resulting from Rh incompatibility or ABO incompatibility.

esophageal atresia See *atresia, esophageal.*

estimated date of birth (EDB) Approximate date of birth. Usually determined by calculation using Nägele's rule; "due date."

estradiol An estrogen.

estriol Major metabolite of estrogen that increases during the second half of pregnancy with an intact fetoplacental unit (normal placenta, normal fetal liver and adrenals) and normal maternal renal function.

estrogen Female sex hormone produced by the ovaries and placenta.

estrogen replacement therapy (ERT) Exogenous estrogen given to women during and after menopause to prevent hot flashes, mood changes, osteoporosis, and genitourinary symptoms. Also called *estrogen therapy (ET).* See also *menopausal hormone therapy (MHT).*

ET (estrogen therapy) See *estrogen replacement therapy (ERT); menopausal hormone therapy (MHT).*

ethics Systematic inquiry into the principles of right and wrong conduct, of virtue and vice, and of good and evil as they relate to conduct.

ethnocentrism Belief in the rightness of one's culture's way of doing things.

euploid cell Cell with the correct or normal number of chromosomes within the cell.

eutocia Normal or natural labor or birth.

evidence-based practice Providing care based on evidence gained through research and clinical trials.

exchange transfusion Replacement of 75% to 85% of circulating blood by withdrawal of the recipient's blood and injection of a donor's blood in equal amounts, the purposes of which are to prevent an accumulation of bilirubin in the blood above a dangerous level, to prevent the accumulation of other byproducts of hemolysis in hemolytic disease, and to correct anemia and acidosis.

expulsive Having the tendency to drive out or expel.

- **e. contractions** Labor contractions that are characteristic of the second stage of labor.

extended family Family form that includes the nuclear family and other blood-related persons.

exenteration, pelvic See *pelvic exenteration.*

external cephalic version (ECV) Turning the fetus to a vertex position by exertion of pressure on the fetus externally through the maternal abdomen.

extracorporeal membrane oxygenation (ECMO) Oxygenation of blood external to body using cardiopulmonary bypass and a membrane oxygenator. Used primarily for newborns with refractory respiratory failure or meconium aspiration syndrome.

extrauterine Occurring outside the uterus.

- **e. pregnancy** Pregnancy in which the fertilized ovum implants itself outside the uterus.

extremely low birth weight (ELBW) A newborn birth weight 1000 g or less.

extrusion reflex Infant automatically extends tongue when it is stimulated.

F

facial paralysis Generally caused by pressure on the facial nerve during birth. Risk factors include a prolonged second stage of labor and forceps-assisted birth. Also called *facial palsy.*

facial palsy See *facial paralysis.*

facies Pertaining to the appearance or expression of the face; certain congenital syndromes typically cause a specific facial appearance.

FAD Fetal activity determination; also called *fetal activity test (FAT).*

failure to thrive Condition in which neonate's or infant's growth and development patterns are below the norms for age.

fallopian tubes Two canals or oviducts extending laterally from each side of the uterus through which the ovum travels, after ovulation, to the uterus; also called *uterine tubes.*

false labor Uterine contractions that do not result in cervical dilation, are irregular, are felt more in front, often do not last more than 20 seconds, and do not become longer or stronger.

false pelvis Part of the pelvis superior to a plane passing through the linea terminalis (brim or outlet).

family dynamics Process by which family members assume varying social roles.

family functions Activities carried out within families for the well-being of family members, including biologic, economic, educational, psychologic, and sociocultural aspects.

family stress theory Theory that explains how families react and adapt to stressors that they experience.

family systems theory Theory that conceptualizes the family as a unit and focuses on observing interactions among family members.

FAMs See *fertility awareness methods (FAMs).*

FAS See *fetal alcohol syndrome (FAS).*

feeding-readiness cues Infant responses that indicate optimal times to begin a feeding. The baby may make mouthing motions, suck a fist, or awaken and cry.

Ferguson reflex Reflex contractions of the uterus after stimulation of the cervix.

fern test The appearance of a fernlike pattern found on slides of certain fluids.

amniotic f.t. Test in which a drop of secretions from the vagina, placed on a slide, dries to form a fernlike pattern indicative of amniotic fluid and rupture of membranes.

ovulation f.t. Test in which cervical mucus, placed on a slide, dries in a branching pattern in the presence of high estrogen levels at the time of ovulation.

fertile period Period before and after ovulation during which the human ovum can be fertilized; usually 3 days before and 4 days after ovulation.

fertility Quality of being able to reproduce; also number of births per 1000 women ages 15 through 44 years. See also *birth rate.*

fertility awareness methods (FAMs) Methods of contraception, also known as periodic abstinence or natural family planning, that depend on identifying the beginning and end of the fertile period of the menstrual cycle. These methods provide contraception by relying on avoidance of intercourse during fertile periods.

fertility rate Births per 1000 women from 15 to 44 years of age.

fertilization Union of an ovum and a sperm.

fetal Pertaining or relating to the fetus.

f. alcohol effect (FAE) Lesser set of the same symptoms that make up fetal alcohol syndrome.

f. alcohol syndrome (FAS) Congenital abnormality or anomaly resulting from excessive maternal alcohol intake during pregnancy. It is characterized by typical craniofacial and limb defects, cardiovascular defects, intrauterine growth restriction, and developmental delay.

f. asphyxia See *asphyxia, fetal.*

f. attitude See *attitude, fetal.*

f. compromise Evidence such as a nonreassuring fetal heart rate pattern that indicates the fetus may be in jeopardy.

f. death See *death, fetal.*

f. lie Relation of the fetal spine to the maternal spine; that is, in vertical lie, maternal and fetal spines are parallel and the fetal head or breech presents; in transverse lie, fetal spine is perpendicular to the maternal spine and the fetal shoulder presents.

f. membrane See *membrane.*

f. presentation The part of the fetus that enters the pelvic inlet first.

f. heart rate (FHR) Beats per minute of the fetal heart. Normal range is 110 to 160 beats/min.

f. scalp spiral electrode Internal signal source for electronically monitoring the fetal heart rate.

f. sonogram See *ultrasound, fetal.*

f. tobacco syndrome Diagnostic term applicable to infants who fit the following criteria: mother who smoked more than five cigarettes a day during pregnancy and had no prenatal evidence of hypertension; infant has symmetric growth restriction, weighs less than 2500 g, and has no other cause of intrauterine growth restriction.

f. ultrasound See *ultrasound, fetal.*

fetopelvic disproportion (FPD) See *cephalopelvic disproportion (CPD).*

fetotoxic Poisonous or destructive to the fetus.

fetus Child in utero from approximately the eighth week after conception until birth.

FHR See *fetal heart rate (FHR).*

fibroadenoma Benign condition of the breast; discrete, usually solitary lumps less than 3 cm in diameter.

fibrocystic change Characterized by lumpiness, with or without tenderness, in both breasts. Fibrocystic breast condition involves the glandular breast tissue.

fibroid Fibrous, encapsulated connective tissue tumor, especially of the uterus.

fimbria Structure resembling a fringe, particularly the fringelike end of the uterine tube.

first stage of labor See *labor, first stage of labor.*

fissure Groove or open crack in tissue.

fistula Abnormal tubelike passage that forms between two normal cavities, possibly congenital or caused by trauma, abscesses, or inflammatory processes.

genital f. perforation between genital tract organs; most occur between the bladder and the genital tract (e.g., vesicovaginal); between the urethra and the vagina (urethrovaginal); and between the rectum or sigmoid colon and the vagina (rectovaginal).

flaccid Having relaxed, limp, or absent muscle tone.

flaring of nostrils Widening of nostrils (alae nasi) during inspiration in the presence of air hunger; sign of respiratory distress.

flea bite dermatitis See *erythema toxicum.*

flexion Opposite of extension. In obstetrics, resistance to the descent of the baby down the birth canal causes the head to flex, or bend, so that the chin approaches the chest. Thus the smallest diameter (suboccipitobregmatic) of the vertex presents.

general f. See *attitude, general flexion.*

follicle Small secretory cavity or sac.

graafian f. Mature, fully developed ovarian cyst containing the ripe ovum. The follicle secretes estrogens, and after ovulation the corpus luteum develops within the ruptured graafian follicle and secretes estrogen and progesterone.

follicle-stimulating hormone (FSH) Hormone produced by the anterior pituitary during the first half of the menstrual cycle. Stimulates development of the graafian follicle.

follicular cysts Develop most commonly in normal ovaries of young women as a result of the mature graafian follicle failing to rupture, or when an immature follicle does not resorb fluid after ovulation.

fontanel Broad area, or soft spot, consisting of a strong band of connective tissue contiguous with cranial bones and located at the junctions of the bones.

anterior f. Diamond-shaped area between the frontal and two parietal bones just above the baby's forehead at the junction of the coronal and sagittal sutures.

mastoid f. Posterolateral fontanel, usually not palpable.

posterior f. Small, triangular area between the occipital and parietal bones at the junction of the lambdoidal and sagittal sutures.

sagittal f. Soft area located in the sagittal suture, halfway between the anterior and posterior fontanels; may be palpated in normal newborns and in some neonates with Down syndrome.

sphenoid f. Anterolateral fontanel usually not palpable.

footling (incomplete) breech presentation See *breech presentation, footling.*

foramen ovale Septal opening between the atria of the fetal heart. The opening normally closes shortly after birth, but if it remains patent, surgical repair usually is necessary.

forceps Curved-bladed instruments used to protect head of fetus during birth and to apply traction to assist birth.

forceps-assisted birth Birth in which forceps are used to assist in delivery of the fetal head.

foreskin Prepuce, or loose fold of skin covering the glans penis.

fornix Any structure with an arched or vaultlike shape.

f. of the vagina Anterior and posterior spaces, formed by the protrusion of the cervix into the vagina, into which the upper vagina is divided.

fourth stage of labor See *labor, fourth stage of.*

fourth trimester Another term for the puerperium; the 3-month interval after the birth of the newborn that includes return of the reproductive organs to their nonpregnant state and psychologic adaptation to parenthood.

FPD (fetopelvic disproportion) See *cephalopelvic disproportion (CPD).*

frank breech presentation See *breech presentation, frank.*

fraternal twins Nonidentical twins that come from two separate fertilized ova.

free-standing birth center A center that provides prenatal, labor, birth, and postbirth care outside of a hospital setting.

frenulum Thin ridge of tissue in midline of undersurface of tongue extending from its base to varying distances from the tip of the tongue.

friability Easily broken. May refer to a fragile condition of the cervix, especially during pregnancy, that causes the cervix to bleed easily when touched.

Friedman's curve Labor curve; pattern of descent of presenting part and of dilation of cervix; partogram.

FSH See *follicle-stimulating hormone (FSH).*

fundus Dome-shaped upper portion of the uterus between the points of insertion of the uterine tubes.

funic souffle See *souffle, funic.*

funis Cordlike structure, especially the umbilical cord. See also *umbilical cord.*

G

galactorrhea Form of nipple discharge or lactation not associated with childbirth or breastfeeding; a bilaterally spontaneous, milky, sticky discharge. When associated with elevated prolactin levels, may be a symptom of a pituitary gland tumor.

galactosemia Inherited, autosomal recessive disorder of galactose metabolism, characterized by a deficiency of the enzyme galactose-1-phosphate uridyltransferase.

gamete Egg and sperm. Mature male or female germ cell; the mature sperm or ovum.

gamete intrafallopian transfer (GIFT) GIFT of ova and washed sperm into uterine tubes; requires women to have at least one normal uterine tube. Ovulation is induced as in *in vitro fertilization–embryo transfer (IVF-ET)*, and the oocytes are aspirated from follicles via laparoscopy. Semen is collected before laparoscopy, and sperm are capacitated by the same technique used for *IVF-ET*. The ova and sperm are then transferred to one uterine tube, permitting natural fertilization and cleavage.

gastroschisis Abdominal wall defect at base of umbilical stalk; herniation of the bowel through a defect in the abdominal wall to the right of the umbilical cord.

gastrostomy Surgical creation of an artificial opening into the stomach through the abdominal wall, performed to feed a client when oral feeding is not possible.

gate-control theory of pain Proposed in 1965 by Melzack and Wall, this theory explains the neurophysical mechanism underlying the perception of pain: the capacity of nerve pathways to transmit pain is reduced or completely blocked by using distraction techniques.

gavage Feeding by means of a tube passed through the nose or mouth to the stomach.

gene Basic physical unit of inheritance passed from parents to offspring; contains the information needed to specify traits.

general flexion See *attitude, general flexion.*

genetic Dependent on the genes. A genetic disorder may or may not be apparent at birth.

genetic counseling Process of determining the occurrence or risk of occurrence of a genetic disorder within a family and of providing appropriate information and advice about the courses of action that are available, whether care of a child already affected, prenatal diagnosis, termination of a pregnancy, sterilization, or artificial insemination is involved.

genetics Study of individual genes and their effect on relatively rare single gene disorders.

genital self-examination (GSE). See *vulvar self-examination (VSE).*

genitalia Organs of reproduction, especially the external genitals.

genogram Pictorial representation of family relationships and health history.

genome Entire set of genetic instructions found in each cell.

genomics Study of all the genes in the human genome together, including their interactions with each other, the environment, and the influence of other psychosocial factors and cultural factors.

genotype An individual's collection of genes. Hereditary combinations in an individual determining physical and chemical characteristics. Some genotypes are not expressed until later in life (e.g., Huntington's chorea); some hide recessive genes, which can be expressed in offspring; and others are expressed only under the proper environmental conditions (e.g., diabetes mellitus appearing under the stress of obesity or pregnancy).

gestation Period of intrauterine fetal development from conception through birth; the period of pregnancy.

gestational age In fetal development, the number of completed weeks counting from the first day of the last normal menstrual cycle.

gestational diabetes mellitus (GDM) Any degree of glucose intolerance with its onset or first recognition occurring during pregnancy.

gestational hypertension See *hypertension, gestational.*

gestational trophoblastic neoplasia (GTN) Persistent trophoblastic tissue that is presumed to be malignant.

GDM See *gestational diabetes mellitus (GDM).*

Ghb A_{1c} See *glycosylated hemoglobin (Ghb A_{1c}).*

GIFT See *gamete intrafallopian transfer (GIFT).*

gingival granuloma gravidarum See *epulis.*

gingivitis Inflammation of the gums characterized by redness, swelling, and tendency to bleed.

glans penis Smooth, round head of the penis, analogous to the female glans clitoris.

glomerulonephritis Noninfectious disease of the glomerulus of the kidney, characterized by proteinuria, hematuria, decreased urine production, and edema.

glucose tolerance test A test of the body's ability to use carbohydrates; used as a screening measure for gestational diabetes.

glycosuria Presence of glucose (a sugar) in the urine.

glycosylated hemoglobin (Ghb A_{1c}) Glycohemoglobin, a minor hemoglobin with glucose attached. Ghb A_{1c} concentration represents the average blood glucose level over the previous several weeks and is a measurement for glycemic control in diabetic therapy.

GnRH See *gonadotropin-releasing hormone (GnRH).*

gonad Gamete-producing gland or sex gland; the ovary or testis.

gonadotropic hormone Hormone that stimulates the gonads.

gonadotropin-releasing hormone (GnRH) Hormone released from hypothalamus that stimulates pituitary gland to produce follicle-stimulating hormone (FSH) and luteinizing hormone (LH).

Goodell sign Softening of the cervix, a probable sign of pregnancy, occurring during the second month.

graafian follicle (vesicle) See *follicle, graafian.*

gravida A woman who is pregnant.

gravidity Pregnancy.

grief A cluster of painful emotional and related behavioral and physical responses experienced following a major loss or death; also called *bereavement.*

- **anticipatory g.** Grief that predates the loss of a beloved object.
- **bittersweet g.** The resurgence of feelings and emotions that occur on remembering a loved one after the bereavement process has lessened.
- **complicated g.** Extremely intense grief reactions that last for a very long time; a state of chronic mourning. Also the persistent feelings of anger, guilt, loss, pain, and sadness over time that lead to feelings of hopelessness, helplessness, and diminishing self-worth that are signs and symptoms of clinical depression, which is different from the normal depression of bereavement. Also called *complicated bereavement, prolonged grief, pathologic grief,* or *pathologic mourning.*
- **g. responses** The physical, emotional, social, and cognitive responses to the death of a loved one.

grieving process A complex of somatic and psychologic symptoms associated with some extreme sorrow or loss, specifically the death of a loved one.

growth spurts Times of increased neonatal growth that usually occur at approximately 6 to 10 days, 6 weeks, 3 months, and 4 to 5 months. The increased caloric needs necessitate more frequent feedings to increase the amount of milk needed.

grunt, expiratory Sign of respiratory distress (hyaline membrane disease—see *respiratory distress syndrome [RDS]*—or advanced pneumonia) indicative of the body's attempt to hold air in the alveoli for better gaseous exchange.

GSE (genital self-examination) See *vulvar self-examination (VSE).*

GTN See *gestational trophoblastic neoplasia (GTN).*

guided imagery The use of imagination and thought processes in a purposeful way to change certain physiologic and emotional conditions.

gynecoid pelvis Pelvis in which the inlet is round instead of oval or blunt; typical female pelvis.

gynecology Study of the diseases of the female, especially of the genital, urinary, and rectal organs.

H

habitual (recurrent) abortion See *abortion, habitual.*

habituation An acquired tolerance from repeated exposure to a particular stimulus. Also called *negative adaptation*; a decline and eventual elimination of a conditioned response by repetition of the conditioned stimulus.

harlequin sign Rare color change of no pathologic significance occurring between the longitudinal halves of the neonate's body. When infant is placed on one side, the dependent half is noticeably pinker than the superior half.

hCG See *human chorionic gonadotropin (hCG).*

healing touch A combination of energetic healing techniques used by nurses and other health care professionals.

health promotion Motivation to increase well-being and actualize health potential.

Hegar sign Softening of the lower uterine segment that is classified as a probable sign of pregnancy and that may be present during the second and third months of pregnancy and is palpated during bimanual examination.

HELLP syndrome A laboratory diagnosis for a variant of severe preeclampsia that involves hepatic dysfunction, characterized by hemolysis (H), elevated liver enzymes (EL), and low platelet count (LP); it is not a separate illness.

hematocrit Volume of red blood cells per deciliter (dl) of circulating blood; packed cell volume (PCV).

hematoma Collection of blood in a tissue; a bruise or blood tumor.

hematopoiesis Production of blood cells; formation of blood.

hemoconcentration Increase in the number of red blood cells in proportion to the volume, resulting from either a decrease in plasma volume or increased erythropoiesis.

hemodilution An increase in fluid content of blood, resulting in diminution of the proportion of formed elements.

hemoglobin Component of red blood cells consisting of globin, a protein, and hematin, an organic iron compound.

- **h. electrophoresis** Test to diagnose sickle cell disease in newborns. Cord blood is used.

hemolytic disease of the newborn Breakdown of fetal red blood cells by maternal antibodies, usually from an Rh-negative mother.

hemorrhage, scleral See *subjunctival hemorrhage.*

hemorrhage, subconjunctival See *subconjunctival hemorrhage.*

hemorrhage, subgaleal See *subgaleal hemorrhage.*

hemorrhage, retinal See *retinal hemorrhage.*

hemorrhagic disease of newborn Bleeding disorder during first few days of life based on a deficiency of vitamin K.

hemorrhagic shock Clinical condition in which the peripheral blood flow is inadequate to return sufficient blood to the heart for normal function, particularly oxygen transport to the organs or tissue. Also called *hypovolemic shock.*

hereditary Pertaining to a trait or characteristic transmitted from parent to offspring by way of the genes; used synonymously with the term *genetic.*

hermaphrodite Person having genital and sexual characteristics of both sexes.

heterozygous Having two dissimilar genes at the same site, or locus, on paired chromosomes (e.g., at the site for eye color, one chromosome carrying the gene for brown, the other for blue).

high risk Increased possibility of suffering harm, damage, loss, or death. See also *risk factor.*

hirsutism Condition characterized by the excessive growth of hair.

HMD Hyaline membrane disease. See *respiratory distress syndrome (RDS).*

holism Philosophy that states that the whole is greater than the sum of its parts. In healing, refers to consideration and treatment of the whole client as a unified being. May include alternative and complementary modalities, but it is more a philosophical base than a modality in and of itself.

holistic medicine Health care treatment with techniques not commonly taught in U.S. medical schools or widely available in U.S. hospitals. May include a variety of disciplines involving diet, exercise, vitamin and nutritional supplements, bodywork, or alternative pharmacologic agents. Philosophy of medicine that encompasses holism.

holistic nursing Nursing practice that stems from the philosophy of holism, one that views the client as an integrated whole, and influenced by a variety of internal and external factors, including the biopsychosocial and spiritual dimensions of the person.

Homans sign Pain in the calf of the leg upon dorsiflexion of the foot with the leg extended; early sign of phlebothrombosis of the deep veins of the calf (deep vein thrombosis).

home birth Planned birth of the child at home, usually done under the supervision of a midwife.

homologous Similar in structure or origin but not necessarily in function.

homologous insemination Insemination in which the semen specimen is provided by the husband. The procedure is used primarily in cases of impotence or when the husband is incapable of sexual intercourse because of some physical disability.

homosexual family Family in which parents form a homosexual union (lesbian and gay), who may live together with or without children. Children may be the offspring of a previous heterosexual union, adopted, or conceived by one or both members of a homosexual couple through artificial insemination.

homozygous Having two similar genes at the same locus, or site, on paired chromosomes.

hormone Chemical substance produced in an organ or gland that is conveyed through the blood to another organ or part of the body, stimulating it to increased functional activity or secretion. See also specific hormones.

hormonal replacement therapy (HRT) Progestin and estrogen given for menopausal symptoms. Also called hormonal therapy (HT). See also *estrogen replacement therapy (ERT); menopausal hormone therapy (MHT).*

hot flash Transient, sudden sensation of warmth in neck, head, and chest experienced by some women during or after menopause, resulting from autonomic vasomotor disturbances that accompany changes in the neurohormonal activity of the ovaries, hypothalamus, and pituitary gland.

hot flush Visible red flush of skin and perspiration experienced by some women during or after menopause; see also *hot flash.*

HRT See *hormonal replacement therapy (HRT).*

HT (hormonal therapy) See *hormonal replacement therapy (HRT); menopausal hormone therapy (MHT).*

human chorionic gonadotropin (hCG) Hormone that is produced by chorionic villi; the biologic marker in pregnancy tests.

hyaline membrane disease (HMD) See *respiratory distress syndrome (RDS).*

hydatidiform mole A benign proliferative growth of the placental trophoblast in which the chorionic villi develop into edematous, cystic, avascular transparent vesicles that hang in a grapelike cluster. Gestational trophoblastic neoplasm usually resulting from fertilization of egg that has no nucleus or an inactivated nucleus. Also called *molar pregnancy.*

hydramnios Amniotic fluid in excess of 1.5 L; often indicative of fetal anomaly and frequently seen in poorly controlled, insulin-dependent diabetic pregnant women even if there is no coexisting fetal anomaly.

hydrocele Collection of fluid in a saclike cavity, especially in the sac that surrounds the testis, causing the scrotum to swell.

hydrocephalus Accumulation of cerebrospinal fluid (CSF) in the subdural or subarachnoid spaces; caused by overproduction (rare) of CSF or a decrease in reabsorption.

hydrops fetalis Most severe expression of fetal hemolytic disorder, a possible sequela to maternal Rh isoimmunization; infants exhibit gross edema (anasarca), cardiac decompensation, and profound pallor from anemia, and seldom survive.

hymen Membranous fold that normally partially covers the entrance to the vagina.

hyperbilirubinemia Condition in which the total unconjugated serum bilirubin concentration in the blood is elevated. Values are abnormal based on gestational age, days of life, and the baby's general physical condition. Hyperbilirubinemia is characterized by a yellow discoloration of the skin, mucous membranes, sclera, and various organs; caused by bilirubin levels that rise steadily over the first 3 to 4 days, peak around day 5, and decrease thereafter. See also *jaundice.*

hyperemesis gravidarum Abnormal condition of pregnancy characterized by vomiting excessive enough to cause weight loss, electrolyte imbalance, nutritional deficiencies, and ketonuria.

hyperesthesia Unusual sensibility to sensory stimuli, such as pain or touch.

hyperglycemia Excess glucose in the blood.

hyperinsulinemia Excess insulin in the blood.

hypermenorrhea See *menorrhagia.*

hyperplasia Increase in number of cells; formation of new tissue.

hyperreflexia Increased action of the reflexes.

hypertension Systolic blood pressure (BP) greater than 140 mm Hg or a diastolic BP greater than 90 mm Hg.

chronic h. Hypertension that is present before the pregnancy or develops before 20 weeks of gestation.

chronic h. with superimposed preeclampsia (1) In women with hypertension before 20 weeks of gestation: new-onset proteinuria (≥ 0.5 g protein in a 24-hour collection); (2) in women with both hypertension and proteinuria before 20 weeks of gestation: significant increase in hypertension, plus one of the following: new onset of symptoms; thrombocytopenia; or elevated liver enzymes.

gestational h. Onset of hypertension without proteinuria after week 20 of pregnancy.

hyperthermia Body temperature greater than 37.5° C.

hyperthyroidism Excessive functional activity of the thyroid gland.

hypertonic uterine dysfunction Uncoordinated, painful, frequent uterine contractions that do not cause dilation and effacement; primary dysfunctional labor.

hypertrophic cardiomyopathy Enlargement and loss of elasticity of the heart muscle, that is, the septum and the left ventricle, causing impaired filling during diastole resulting in decreased cardiac output.

hypertrophy Enlargement, or increase in size, of existing cells.

hyperventilation Rapid, shallow (or prolonged, deep) respirations resulting in respiratory alkalosis: a decrease in H^+ concentration and Pco_2 and an increase in the blood pH and the ratio of $NaHCO_3$ to H_2CO_3. Symptoms may include faintness, palpitations, and carpopedal (hands and feet) muscular spasms.

hypocalcemia Deficiency in calcium often seen in preterm infants, in infants of mothers with diabetes, or after long stressful labor in full-term infants.

hypofibrinogenemia Deficient level of a blood-clotting factor, fibrinogen, in the blood; in obstetrics, it occurs after complications of abruptio placentae or retention of a dead fetus.

hypogastric arteries Branches of the right and left iliac arteries carrying deoxygenated blood from the fetus through the umbilical cord, where they are known as umbilical arteries, to the placenta.

hypoglycemia Less than normal amount of glucose in the blood, usually caused by administration of too much insulin, excessive secretion of insulin by the islet cells of the pancreas, or dietary deficiency.

hypomenorrhea Scanty menstrual bleeding at normal intervals.

hypospadias Anomalous positioning of urinary meatus on undersurface of penis or close to or just inside the vagina.

hypothalamus Portion of the diencephalon of the brain forming the floor and part of the lateral wall of the third ventricle. It activates, controls, and integrates the peripheral autonomic nervous system, endocrine processes, and many somatic functions, such as body temperature, sleep, and appetite.

hypothermia Temperature that falls below normal range, that is, below 35º C, usually caused by exposure to cold.

hypothyroidism Deficiency of thyroid gland activity with underproduction of thyroxine.

congenital h. Results from a deficiency of thyroid hormones, and can be permanent (requires treatment for life) or transient (spontaneously resolves).

hypotonic uterine dysfunction Weak, ineffective uterine contractions usually occurring in the active phase of labor; often related to cephalopelvic disproportion or malposition of the fetus; secondary uterine inertia.

hypovolemic shock See *hemorrhagic shock.*

hypoxemia Reduction in arterial Po_2 resulting in metabolic acidosis by forcing anaerobic glycolysis, pulmonary vasoconstriction, and direct cellular damage.

hypoxia Insufficient availability of oxygen to meet the metabolic needs of body tissue.

hysterectomy Surgical removal of the entire uterus.

TAH-BSO Total abdominal hysterectomy and bilateral salpingo-oophorectomy; removal of uterus, both tubes, and both ovaries.

TVH Total vaginal hysterectomy.

hysterosalpingography Recording by x-rays of the uterus and uterine tubes after they are injected with radiopaque material.

hysterotomy Surgical incision into the uterus.

I

iatrogenic Caused by a health care provider's words, actions, or treatment.

ICP Intracranial pressure.

icterus See *jaundice.*

icterus neonatorum Jaundice in the newborn.

idiopathic peripartum cardiomyopathy A primary disease of the heart muscle with no apparent cause, occurring during the peripartum period.

idiopathic thrombocytopenic purpura (ITP) An autoimmune disorder in which antiplatelet antibodies decrease the life span of the platelets. Thrombocytopenia, capillary fragility, and increased bleeding time are diagnostic findings. Also called *immune thrombocytopenic purpura (ITP).*

IDM Infant of a mother with diabetes.

illness prevention Desire to avoid illness, detect it early, or maintain optimal functioning when illness is present.

immune thrombocytopenic purpura (ITP) See *idiopathic thrombocytopenic purpura (ITP).*

immunity

acquired i. Protection against microorganisms that develops in response to actual infection or transfer of antibody from an immune donor.

active i. Protection against specific microorganisms that develops in response to actual infection or vaccination.

natural i. Nonspecific protection against microorganisms. Natural immunity is the first line of defense and includes skin and phagocytic cells.

passive i. Protection against specific microorganisms that develops in response to the transfer of antibody or lymphocytes from an immune donor.

immunocompetent Ability of the immune system to respond appropriately to foreign antigens and to develop antigen-specific antibodies.

immunoglobin (Ig)

IgA Primary immunoglobulin in colostrum.

IgG Transplacentally acquired immunoglobulin that confers passive immunity to the fetus against the infections to which the mother is immune.

IgM Immunoglobulin neonate can manufacture soon after birth. Fetus produces it in the presence of amnionitis.

immunology The study of the components essential to the recognition and disposal of foreign (nonself or antigenic) material and maintenance of body defenses.

impaired fertility Inability to conceive or to carry fetus to live birth at a time a couple chooses to do so.

imperforate anus A term used to describe a wide range of congenital disorders involving the anus and rectum and genitourinary system.

implantation Embedding of the fertilized ovum in the uterine mucosa; nidation.

impotence Term designating a man's inability, partial or complete, to perform sexual intercourse or to achieve orgasm; erectile dysfunction.

inborn error of metabolism Hereditary deficiency of a specific enzyme needed for normal metabolism of specific chemicals (e.g., deficiency of phenylalanine hydroxylase results in phenylketonuria [PKU]; a deficiency of hexosaminidase results in Tay-Sachs disease).

incompetent cervix See *premature dilation of the cervix.*

incomplete abortion See *abortion, incomplete.*

increment Increase, or buildup, as of a contraction.

induced abortion See *abortion, induced.*

induction of labor Stimulation of uterine contractions before the spontaneous onset of labor.

inertia Sluggishness or inactivity; in obstetrics, refers to the absence or weakness of uterine contractions during labor.

inevitable abortion See *abortion, inevitable.*

infant Child who is under 1 year of age.

infective endocarditis Inflammation of the inner layer of the heart muscle (endocardium), caused by a bacterial infection.

infertility Decreased capacity to conceive. A serious medical concern that affects quality of life and is a problem for 10% to 15% of reproductive-age couples. The term *infertility* implies subfertility, a prolonged time to conceive, as opposed to *sterility,* which means inability to conceive.

informed consent Choice based on full comprehension of relevant information.

inhalation analgesia Reduction of pain by administration of anesthetic gas. Occasionally given during the second stage of labor. Consciousness is retained to allow the woman to follow instructions and to avoid the adverse effects of general anesthesia.

inlet Passage leading into a cavity.

pelvic i. Upper brim of the pelvic cavity.

insemination Introduction of semen into the vagina or uterus for impregnation.

therapeutic donor i. (TDI) Previously referred to as artificial insemination by donor; used when the male partner has no sperm or a very low sperm count (less than 20 million motile sperm per milliliter), the couple has a genetic defect, or the male partner has antisperm antibodies.

insensible water loss (IWL) Evaporative water loss that occurs mainly through the skin and respiratory tract.

insulin Hormone produced by the beta cells of the pancreatic islets of Langerhans; promotes glucose transport into the cells; aids in protein and lipid synthesis.

integrative health care Encompasses complementary and alternative therapies in combination with conventional Western modalities of treatment.

intermittent auscultation Involves listening to fetal heart sounds at periodic intervals to assess the *fetal heart rate (FHR).*

internal os Inside mouth or opening.

interstitial deletion See *deletion, interstitial.*

intertuberous diameter Distance between ischial tuberosities. Measured to determine dimension of pelvic outlet.

intervillous space Irregular space in the maternal portion of the placenta, filled with maternal blood and serving as the site of maternal-fetal gas, nutrient, and waste exchange.

intimate partner violence (IPV) The actual or threatened physical, sexual, psychologic, or emotional abuse by a spouse, ex-spouse, boyfriend, girlfriend, ex-boyfriend, ex-girlfriend, date, or cohabiting partner.

intoxication Development of a reversible substance-specific syndrome caused by the recent ingestion of or exposure to a substance. The symptoms of intoxication are attributable to the direct physiologic effects of the substance on the central nervous system.

intrapartum During labor and birth.

intrathecal Within the subarachnoid space.

intrauterine device (IUD) Small plastic or metal form placed in the uterus to prevent implantation of a fertilized ovum.

intrauterine growth restriction (IUGR) Fetal undergrowth of any cause, such as deficient nutrient supply or intrauterine infection, or associated with congenital malformation; birth weight below population 10th percentile corrected for gestational age.

intrauterine pressure catheter (IUPC) Catheter inserted into uterine cavity to assess uterine activity and pressure by electronic means.

intrauterine resuscitation Interventions initiated when abnormal (nonreassuring) fetal heart rate patterns are noted and are directed at improving intrauterine blood flow.

introitus Entrance into a canal or cavity such as the vagina.

intussusception Prolapse of one segment of bowel into the lumen of the adjacent segment.

in utero Within or inside the uterus.

in vitro fertilization (IVF) Fertilization in a culture dish or test tube.

in vitro fertilization–embryo transfer (IVF-ET) Ovarian stimulation using pharmacologic therapy results in multiple mature ova, which are collected at midcycle via intravaginal needle aspiration. The ova are fertilized with sperm in vitro (in a dish) for up to 6 days, then transferred to the uterus using ultrasound guidance.

inversion (1) Turning end for end, upside down, or inside out. (2) Deviation in which a portion of the chromosome has been rearranged in reverse order.

i. of the uterus Condition in which the uterus is turned inside out so that the fundus intrudes into the cervix or vagina, caused by a too vigorous removal of the placenta before it is detached by the natural process of labor.

involution (1) Rolling or turning inward. (2) Reduction in size of the uterus after birth and its return to its nonpregnant condition.

IPV See *intimate partner violence (IPV).*

isoflavones See *phytoestrogens.*

isoimmune hemolytic disease Breakdown (hemolysis) of fetal/neonatal Rh-positive red blood cells because of Rh antibodies formed by an Rh-negative mother who had been previously exposed to Rh-positive red blood cells.

isoimmunization Production of antibodies by one member of a species against something that is commonly found within that species (e.g., development of anti-Rh antibodies in an Rh-negative person; also called *Rh incompatibility*).

ITP See *idiopathic thrombocytopenic purpura (ITP).* Note: The acronym ITP is also known as *immune thrombocytopenic purpura.*

IUGR See *intrauterine growth restriction (IUGR).*

IUPC See *intrauterine pressure catheter (IUPC).*

IVF See *in vitro fertilization (IVF).*

IVF-ET See *in vitro fertilization and embryo transfer (IVF-ET).*

IWL See *insensible water loss (IWL).*

J

jaundice Yellow discoloration of the body tissues caused by the deposit of bile pigments (unconjugated bilirubin); also called *icterus.* See also *hyperbilirubinemia.*

breastfeeding-associated j. Also called *early-onset jaundice*; hyperbilirubinemia that occurs during the first 3 to 4 days of life; associated with insufficient breastfeeding and infrequent stooling.

breast milk j. Also called *late-onset jaundice*; hyperbilirubinemia that occurs between days 6 and 14 of life, usually in a healthy, breastfed infant; cause is unknown.

pathologic j. Jaundice usually first noticeable within 24 hours after birth; caused by some abnormal condition such as an Rh or ABO incompatibility and resulting in bilirubin toxicity (e.g., kernicterus); unconjugated hyperbilirubinemia that is either pathologic in origin or severe enough to warrant further evaluation and treatment. Also called *nonphysiologic jaundice.*

physiologic j. Yellow tinge to skin and mucous membranes in response to increased serum levels of unconjugated bilirubin; not usually apparent until after 24 hours; also called *neonatal jaundice, physiologic hyperbilirubinemia,* or *nonpathologic unconjugated hyperbilirubinemia.*

K

kangaroo care Skin-to-skin infant care, especially for preterm infants, which provides warmth to infant. Infant is placed naked or diapered against mother's or father's bare chest and is covered with parent's shirt or a warm blanket.

karyotype Pictorial analysis of the number, form, and size of an individual's chromosomes. Schematic arrangement of the chromosomes within a cell to demonstrate their numbers and morphology.

Kegel exercises Pelvic muscle exercises developed to strengthen the pubococcygeal muscles (supportive pelvic floor muscles) to control or reduce incontinent urine loss, and to provide support for the pelvic organs and control of the muscles surrounding the vagina and urethra. Also beneficial during pregnancy and postpartum.

kernicterus Bilirubin encephalopathy involving the deposit of unconjugated bilirubin in brain cells, resulting in death or impaired intellectual, perceptive, or motor function and adaptive behavior.

ketoacidosis The accumulation of ketone bodies in the blood as a consequence of hyperglycemia; leads to metabolic acidosis.

key informants Individuals in positions of leadership who can provide information about a situation.

Kleihauer-Betke test Laboratory test that detects the presence of fetal blood cells in the maternal circulation.

L

labia majora Two folds of skin containing fat and covered with hair that lie on either side of the vaginal opening and form each side of the vulva. (Singular, *labium majus.*)

labia minora Two thin folds of delicate, hairless skin inside the labia majora. (Singular, *labium minus.*)

labor Series of processes by which the fetus is expelled from the uterus; parturition; childbirth.

active phase Phase in first stage of labor from 4 to 7 cm in dilation.

augmentation of l. See *augmentation of labor.*

dry l. See *dry labor.*

dysfunctional l. See *dysfunctional labor.*

first stage of labor Begins with the onset of regular uterine contractions and ends with full cervical effacement and dilation; consists of three phases: the *latent phase* (through 3 cm of dilation), the *active phase* (4 to 7 cm of dilation), and the *transition phase* (8 to 10 cm of dilation).

fourth stage of labor Initial period of recovery from childbirth. It is usually considered to last for the first 1 to 2 hours after birth.

induction of l. See *induction of labor.*

latent phase Phase in first stage of labor from none to 3 cm in dilation.

precipitous l. See *precipitous labor.*

preterm l. See *preterm labor.*

second stage of labor The stage in which the infant is born. Begins with full cervical dilation (10 cm) and complete effacement (100%) and ends with the baby's birth.

third stage of labor Stage of labor from the birth of the baby to the expulsion of the placenta.

transition phase of labor Phase in first stage of labor from 8 to 10 cm in dilation.

labor, delivery, recovery (LDR) A single room where all steps of the birth process occur. Avoids having to move the woman to different rooms for each phase of the birth process. The woman is moved to a postpartum room after recovery.

labor, delivery, recovery, postpartum (LDRP) A single room where all steps of the birth process and hospitalization occur. The woman stays in the same room throughout her hospitalization.

laceration Irregular tear of wound tissue; in obstetrics, it usually refers to a tear in the perineum, vagina, or cervix caused by childbirth.

lactase Enzyme necessary for the digestion of lactose.

lactation Function of secreting milk or period during which milk is secreted.

l. consultant A health care professional who has specialized training in breastfeeding.

l. suppression Stopping the production of breast milk through the use of medication (rare) or nonpharmacologic interventions.

lactogen Medication or other substance that enhances the production and secretion of milk.

lactogenesis stage I Initial synthesis of milk components beginning at approximately 16 to 18 weeks of pregnancy; the breasts prepare for milk production by producing colostrum.

lactogenesis stage II Beginning of milk production 2 to 5 days postpartum.

lactose intolerance Inability to digest milk sugar (lactose) because of an inherited absence of the enzyme lactase in the small intestine.

lactosuria Presence of lactose in the urine during late pregnancy and during lactation. Must be differentiated from glycosuria.

Lamaze (psychoprophylaxis) method Method of preparation for childbirth developed in the 1950s by a French obstetrician, Fernand Lamaze, that gained popularity in the United States in the 1960s. It requires practice at home and coaching during labor and birth. The goals are to minimize fear and the perception of pain and to promote positive family relationships by using both mental and physical preparation.

Laminaria tent Cone of dried seaweed that swells as it absorbs moisture. Used to dilate the cervix nontraumatically in preparation for an induced abortion or in preparation for induction of labor.

lanugo Downy, fine hair characteristic of the fetus between 20 weeks of gestation and birth that is most noticeable over the shoulder, forehead, and cheeks but is found on nearly all parts of the body except the palms of the hands, soles of the feet, and the scalp.

laparoscopy Examination of the interior of the abdomen by insertion of a small telescope through the anterior abdominal wall.

large for gestational age (LGA) Exhibiting excessive growth for gestational age.

laser ablation Uses a laser mounted on a colposcope that allows precise direction of a beam of light (heat) to remove diseased tissue.

last menstrual period (LMP) Date of the first day of the last menstrual bleeding. In dating a pregnancy, the LMP is used to calculate the EDB.

latch (1) Placement of the infant's mouth over the nipple, areola, and breast, making a seal between the mouth and breast to create adequate suction for milk removal. (2) Attachment of the infant to the breast for feeding.

late preterm birth See *preterm, late birth.*

latent phase See *labor, latent phase.*

LBW See *low birth weight (LBW).*

LDR See *labor, delivery, recovery (LDR).*

LDRP See *labor, delivery, recovery, postpartum (LDRP).*

lecithin A phospholipid that decreases surface tension; surfactant.

lecithin/sphingomyelin ratio Ratio of lecithin to sphingomyelin in the amniotic fluid. It is used to assess maturity of the fetal lung.

LEEP See *loop electrosurgical excision procedure (LEEP).*

leiomyoma Slow-growing benign tumor arising from the muscle tissue of the uterus. Also known as fibroid tumor, fibroma, myoma, or fibromyoma.

Leopold maneuvers Four maneuvers for diagnosing the fetal position by external palpation of the mother's abdomen.

letdown or let-down reflex See *milk ejection reflex (MER).*

letting-go phase Interdependent phase after birth in which the mother and family move forward as a system with interacting members.

leukorrhea White or slightly gray mucoid discharge from the cervical canal or the vagina with a faint musty odor, which may be normal physiologically or caused by pathologic states of the vagina and endocervix (e.g., *Trichomonas vaginalis* infections).

LGA See *large for gestational age (LGA).*

LH See *luteinizing hormone (LH).*

libido Sexual drive.

lie Relationship existing between the long axis of the fetus and the long axis of the mother. In a longitudinal lie, the fetus is lying lengthwise or vertically, whereas in a transverse lie, the fetus is lying crosswise or horizontally in the uterus.

lightening Sensation of decreased abdominal distention produced by uterine descent into the pelvic cavity as the fetal presenting part settles into the pelvis. It usually occurs 2 weeks before the onset of labor in nulliparas.

linea nigra Pigmented line that appears on the middle of the abdomen and extends from the symphysis pubis toward the umbilicus, extending to the top of the fundus in the midline; seen in some women during the latter part of pregnancy.

linea terminalis Line dividing the upper (false) pelvis from the lower (true) pelvis.

lithotomy position Position in which the woman lies on her back with her knees flexed and with abducted thighs drawn up toward her chest.

live birth Birth in which the neonate, regardless of gestational age, manifests any heartbeat, breathes, or displays voluntary movement.

local infiltration anesthesia Process by which a substance such as a local anesthetic drug is deposited within the tissue to anesthetize a limited region.

local perineal infiltration anesthesia Process by which a local anesthetic medication is deposited within the tissue to anesthetize a limited region of the body.

lochia Uterine/vaginal discharge after childbirth (during the puerperium) consisting of blood, tissue, and mucus.

- **l. alba** Thin, yellowish to white, vaginal discharge that follows lochia serosa on about the tenth day after birth and that may last from 2 to 6 weeks postpartum; consists primarily of leukocytes and decidual cells but also contains epithelial cells, mucus, serum, and bacteria.
- **l. rubra** Red, distinctly blood-tinged vaginal flow that follows birth and lasts 2 to 4 days; consists mainly of blood and decidual and trophoblastic debris.
- **l. serosa** Serous, pinkish brown, watery vaginal discharge that follows lochia rubra until about the tenth day after birth; consists of old blood, serum, leukocytes, and tissue debris.

loop electrosurgical excision procedure (LEEP) This procedure uses a wire loop electrode that can excise and cauterize with minimal tissue damage; it is a standard treatment for cervical intraepithelial neoplasia in the United States.

low birth weight (LBW) A newborn birth weight less than 2500 g (5 lb, 8 oz).

low spinal (saddle) block anesthesia Type of regional anesthesia produced by injection of a local anesthetic solution into the cerebrospinal fluid intrathecal (subarachnoid) space in the spinal canal. See also *spinal anesthesia (block).*

L/S ratio See *lecithin/sphingomyelin ratio.*

lumpectomy Removal of the breast tumor and a small amount of surrounding healthy tissue to ensure there are clean margins. See also *mastectomy.*

lunar month Four weeks (28 days).

luteinizing hormone (LH) Hormone produced by the anterior pituitary that stimulates ovulation and the development of the corpus luteum.

luteotropin hormone (LTH) Lactogenic hormone; prolactin; an adenohypophyseal hormone.

lysozyme Enzyme with antiseptic qualities that destroys foreign organisms and that is found in blood cells of the granulocytic and monocytic series and is also normally present in saliva, sweat, tears, and breast milk.

M

maceration (1) Process of softening a solid by soaking it in a fluid. (2) Softening and breaking down of fetal skin from prolonged exposure to amniotic fluid as seen in a postterm infant. Also seen in a dead fetus.

macroglossia Hypertrophy of tongue or tongue large for oral cavity; seen in some preterm neonates and in neonates with Down syndrome.

macrophage Any phagocytic cell of the reticuloendothelial system, including Kupffer cells in the liver, splenocytes in the spleen, and histocytes in the loose connective tissue.

macrosomia Large body size as seen in neonates of mothers with diabetes or prediabetes defined in several different ways, including: a birth weight more than 4000 to 4500 g; birth weight greater than the 90th percentile; and estimates of neonatal adipose tissue.

magnetic resonance imaging (MRI) Noninvasive nuclear procedure for imaging tissues with high fat and water content; in obstetrics, uses include evaluation of fetal structures, placenta, and amniotic fluid volume.

malpractice Professional negligence that is the proximate cause of injury or harm to a client, resulting from a lack of professional knowledge, experience, or skill that can be expected in others in the profession or from a failure to exercise reasonable care or judgment in the application of professional knowledge, experience, or skill.

mammary duct ectasia An inflammation of the ducts behind the nipple.

mammary gland Compound gland of the female breast that is made up of lobes and lobules that secrete milk for nourishment of the young. Rudimentary mammary glands exist in the male.

mammography X-ray filming of the breast; examination technique used to screen for and evaluate breast lesions.

managed care System of guiding care to promote efficiency and cost-effectiveness.

MAP See *mean arterial pressure (MAP).*

Marfan syndrome An inherited disorder that is an autosomal dominant trait resulting in an abnormal condition characterized by elongation of the bones, causing significant musculoskeletal disturbances. Also usually associated with cardiovascular and eye abnormalities.

married-blended family Family formed as a result of divorce and remarriage, consisting of unrelated family members (stepparents, stepchildren, stepsiblings).

married-parent family Family form in which male and female partners are married and live with their children as an independent unit; parents can be biologic or adoptive.

MAS See *m. aspiration syndrome (MAS).*

mask of pregnancy See *chloasma.*

mastectomy Excision, or removal, of the mammary gland. See also *lumpectomy.*

- **modified radical m.** Removal of breast tissue, skin, and axillary nodes.
- **partial m.** Includes tylectomy, wide excision, and quadrantectomy or segmental mastectomy and involves removal of the tumor, which may be larger, along with a rim of healthy tissue around it, to ensure clear margins.

mastitis Infection in a breast, usually confined to a milk duct, characterized by influenza-like symptoms and redness and tenderness in the affected breast.

maternal adaptation Process that a woman goes through in adjusting to her version of the maternal role; includes three phases: taking in, taking hold, and letting go.

maternal mortality Death of a woman related to childbearing.

maturation (1) Process of attaining maximum development. (2) In biology, a process of cell division during which the number of chromosomes in the germ cells (sperm or ova) is reduced to one half the number (haploid) characteristic of the species.

maturational crisis Crisis that arises during normal growth and development, such as puberty.

McDonald sign Easy flexion of the fundus on the cervix.

mean arterial pressure (MAP) Average of systolic and diastolic blood pressures. An MAP of greater than 90 mm Hg in the second trimester is associated with an increase in the incidence of pregnancy-induced hypertension in the third trimester.

meatus Opening from an internal structure to the outside (e.g., urethral meatus).

mechanical ventilation Technique used to provide predetermined amount of oxygen; requires intubation.

mechanism of labor Movement of the fetus through the birth canal.

meconium First stools of infant: viscid, sticky; dark greenish brown, almost black; sterile; odorless.

m. aspiration syndrome (MAS) Function of fetal hypoxia: with hypoxia, the anal sphincter relaxes and meconium is released; reflex gasping movements draw meconium and other particulate matter in the amniotic fluid into the infant's bronchial tree, obstructing the airflow after birth.

m. ileus Lower intestinal obstruction by thick, putty-like, inspissated (dried) meconium that may be the result of deficiency of trypsin production in the newborn with cystic fibrosis.

m.-stained fluid In response to hypoxia, fetal intestinal activity increases and anal sphincter relaxes, resulting in the passage of meconium, which imparts a greenish coloration.

meditation Any activity that focuses the attention in the present moment and quiets and relaxes the mind and body in the process.

meiosis Process by which germ cells divide and decrease their chromosomal number by one half; produces gametes (eggs and sperm).

membrane(s) Thin, pliable layer of tissue that lines a cavity or tube, separates structures, or covers an organ or structure; in obstetrics, the amnion and chorion surrounding the fetus, which is also called the *fetal membrane*.

artificial rupture of m. (AROM) Rupture of membranes using a plastic AmniHook or surgical clamp. See also *amniotomy*.

premature rupture of m. (PROM) Rupture of amniotic sac and leakage of amniotic fluid beginning at least 1 hour before onset of labor at any gestational age.

preterm premature rupture of m. (PPROM) PROM that occurs before 37 weeks of gestation.

spontaneous rupture of m. (SROM) Rupture of membranes by natural means.

MEN See *minimal enteral nutrition (MEN)*.

menarche Onset, or beginning, of menstrual function; first menstruation.

meningocele A herniation of the meninges at the site of the defect in the vertebral column; typically covered by skin.

meningomyelocele Saclike protrusion of the spinal cord through a congenital defect in the vertebral column.

menopausal hormone therapy (MHT) Hormonal therapy for menopausal symptoms; either as *estrogen replacement therapy (ERT)* or *estrogen therapy (ET)*, in which a woman takes only estrogen, or *hormonal replacement therapy (HRT)* or *hormonal therapy (HT)*, in which she takes both estrogen and progestins.

menopause From the Latin mensis (month) and Greek pausis (to cease); refers only to the last menstrual period; unlike menarche, however, menopause can be dated with certainty only 1 year after menstruation ceases.

menorrhagia Excessive menstrual bleeding, in either duration or amount. Also known as hypermenorrhea.

menses (menstruation) (Latin plural of *mensis* "month.") Periodic uterine bleeding and vaginal discharge of bloody fluid from the nonpregnant uterus that occurs from the age of puberty to menopause, which begins approximately 14 days after ovulation.

menstruation See *menses (menstruation)*.

mentum Chin, a fetal reference point in designating position (e.g., "left mentoanterior" [LMA], meaning that the fetal chin is presenting in the left anterior quadrant of the maternal pelvis).

MER See *milk ejection reflex (MER)*.

mesoderm Embryonic middle layer of germ cells giving rise to all types of muscles, connective tissue, bone marrow, blood, lymphoid tissue, and urogenital system.

metastasis Spread of cancer from its original site to distant parts of the body. Results from seeding of cancer cells into the blood and lymph systems.

metrorrhagia Intermenstrual bleeding; refers to any episode of bleeding, whether spotting, menses, or hemorrhage, that occurs at a time other than the normal menses.

MHT See *menopausal hormone therapy (MHT)*.

microdeletion See *deletion, microdeletion*.

microcephaly Congenital anomaly characterized by abnormal smallness of the head in relation to the rest of the body and by underdevelopment of the brain, resulting in some degree of mental retardation.

midwife One who practices the art of helping and aiding a woman to give birth.

certified m. Midwife educated only in the discipline of midwifery (also known as direct-entry midwife).

certified nurse m. Registered nurse with advanced education in midwifery.

lay m. Midwife who learned skills through practice; has no formal education in midwifery.

milia Unopened sebaceous glands appearing as tiny, white, pinpoint papules on forehead, nose, cheeks, and chin of a neonate that disappear spontaneously in a few days or weeks.

milk ejection reflex (MER) Release of milk caused by the contraction of the myoepithelial cells within the milk glands in response to oxytocin; also called *letdown* or *let-down reflex*.

milk-leg Thrombophlebitis of femoral vein resulting in edema of leg and pain; may occur after difficult vaginal birth.

milk transfer Infant's removal of milk from the breast, which is dependent on correct latch and the efficiency of the baby's suck, as well as the mother's milk ejection reflex.

minimal enteral nutrition (MEN) Feeding small volumes of food to stimulate or prime the development of the immature gastrointestinal tract of the preterm infant, to achieve better absorption of nutrients when bolus or regular intermittent gavage feedings can be given. Also called *trophic feeding*.

miscarriage Spontaneous abortion; lay term usually referring to the loss of the fetus.

missed abortion See *abortion, missed*.

mitosis Process of somatic cell division in which a single cell divides, but both of the new cells have the same number of chromosomes as the first; body cells replicate to yield two cells with the same genetic makeup as the parent cell.

mitral valve prolapse (MVP) A disorder in which one or both of the cusp(s) of the mitral valve protrude backward into the left atrium during ventricular systole, resulting in incomplete closure of the valve. A midsystolic click or a late systolic murmur may be heard.

mitral valve stenosis Narrowing of the opening of the mitral valve caused by stiffening of valve leaflets, obstructing the blood flow from the atrium to the ventricle.

mittelschmerz Abdominal pain in the region of an ovary during ovulation that usually occurs midway through the menstrual cycle. Present in many women, mittelschmerz is useful for identifying ovulation, thus pinpointing the fertile period of the cycle.

molar pregancy See *hydatidiform mole*.

molding Overlapping of cranial bones or shaping of the fetal head to accommodate and conform to the bony and soft parts of the mother's birth canal during labor.

mongolian spot Bluish gray or dark nonelevated pigmented area usually found over the lower back and buttocks; present at birth in some infants, primarily nonwhite. The spot usually fades by school age.

mongolism See *Down syndrome (DS)*.

moniliasis See *candidiasis*.

monosomy Chromosomal aberration characterized by the absence of one chromosome from the normal diploid complement. Product of the union between a normal gamete and a gamete that is missing a chromosome.

monozygotic Originating or coming from a single fertilized ovum, such as identical twins.

monozygotic twins See *twins, monozygotic*.

mons veneris Pad of fatty tissue and coarse skin that overlies the symphysis pubis in the woman and that, after puberty, is covered with hair.

Montevideo units (MVUs) A method for evaluating the adequacy of uterine activity for achieving progress in labor. MVUs are calculated by subtracting the baseline uterine pressure from the peak contraction pressure for each contraction that occurs in a 10-minute window, and then adding together the pressures generated by each contraction that occurs during that period of time.

Montgomery glands Small, nodular prominences on the areolas around the nipples of the breasts that enlarge during pregnancy and lactation; hypertrophy of the sebaceous (oil) glands embedded in the primary areolae sebaceous glands. Also called *Montgomery tubercles* or *tubercules of Montgomery*.

mood disorders Disorders that have a disturbance in the prevailing emotional state as the dominant feature. Cause is unknown.

moratorium phase The second developmental task experienced by expectant fathers as identified by May. During this phase the expectant father adjusts to the reality of pregnancy.

morbidity (1) Condition of being diseased. (2) Number of cases of disease or of sick persons in relationship to a specific population; incidence.

morning sickness Nausea and vomiting that affect some women during the first few months of their pregnancy; may occur at any time of day.

Moro reflex Normal, generalized reflex in a young infant elicited by a sudden loud noise or by striking the table next to the child, resulting in flexion of the legs, an embracing posture of the arms, and usually a brief cry. Also called *startle reflex*.

mortality (1) Quality or state of being subject to death. (2) Number of deaths in relation to a specific population; incidence.

- **fetal m.** Number of fetal deaths per 1000 births (or per live births). See also *death, fetal.*
- **infant m.** Number of deaths per 1000 children 1 year of age or younger.
- **maternal m.** Number of maternal deaths per 100,000 births.
- **neonatal m.** (1) Number of neonatal deaths per 1000 births (or per live births). (2) Statistical rate of infant death during the first 28 days after live birth, expressed as the number of such deaths per 1000 live births in a specific geographic area or institution in a given period of time.
- **perinatal m.** Combined fetal and neonatal mortality. See also *death, perinatal.*

morula Developmental stage of the fertilized ovum in which there is a solid mass of cells resembling a mulberry.

mosaicism Condition, caused by nondisjunction, in which some somatic cells are normal, whereas others show chromosomal aberrations, either missing a chromosome or containing an extra chromosome.

mourning The process of finding the answers to the questions surrounding the loss, coping with grief responses, and determining how to live again.

MRI See *magnetic resonance imaging (MRI).*

multifactorial inheritance Inheritance of phenotypic characteristics resulting from two or more genes on different chromosomes acting together. See also *unifactorial inheritance.*

multifetal pregnancy Pregnancy in which there is more than one fetus in the uterus at the same time; multiple pregnancy.

multigravida A woman who has had two or more pregnancies.

multipara A woman who has completed two or more pregnancies to 20 or more weeks of gestation.

mutation Spontaneous and permanent change in the normal gene structure in a gene or chromosome in gametes that may be transmitted to offspring.

mutuality Component of parent-infant *attachment*; the infant's behaviors and characteristics elicit a corresponding set of parental behaviors and characteristics.

MVP See *mitral valve prolapse (MVP).*

MVUs See *Montevideo units (MVUs).*

mycotic stomatitis See *thrush.*

myelomeningocele External sac containing meninges, spinal fluid, and nerves that protrudes through defect in vertebral column.

myomectomy Removal of a tumor.

N

Nägele's rule Method for calculating the estimated date of birth (EDB) or "due date." Also called Naegele's rule.

narcotic antagonist A compound such as naloxone (Narcan) that promptly reverses the effects of narcotics such as meperidine (Demerol).

natal Relating or pertaining to birth.

navel Depression in the center of the abdomen, where the umbilical cord was attached to the fetus; umbilicus.

NEC See *necrotizing enterocolitis (NEC).*

necrotizing enterocolitis (NEC) Acute inflammatory bowel disorder that occurs primarily in preterm or low-birth-weight neonates. It is characterized by ischemic necrosis (death) of the gastrointestinal mucosa, which may lead to perforation and peritonitis; formula-fed infants are at higher risk for this disease.

negligence Commission of an act that a prudent person would not have done or the omission of a duty that a prudent person would have fulfilled, resulting in injury or harm to another person. In particular, in a malpractice suit a professional person is negligent if harm to a client results from such an act or such a failure to act, but it must be proved that other prudent persons of the same profession would ordinarily have acted differently under the same circumstances.

neonatal abstinence syndrome Signs and symptoms associated with drug withdrawal in the neonate.

neonatal mortality See *mortality, neonatal.*

neonatal narcosis Central nervous system depression in the newborn produced by an opioid or narcotic; may be exhibited by respiratory depression, hypertonia, lethargy, and delay in temperature regulation.

neonatology Branch of medicine that studies care of the neonate.

neoplasia Growth of new tissue; tumor that serves no physiologic function; may be benign or malignant.

neural tube Tube formed from fusion of the neural folds from which develop the brain and spinal cord.

- **n.t. defect (NTD)** Improper development of tube resulting in malformation of brain or spinal cord; see alpha-fetoprotein.

neurofibroma Benign, soft tumor.

neutral thermal environment (NTE) Environment that enables the neonate to maintain a body temperature of at least 36.5° C with minimum use of oxygen and energy.

nevus Natural blemish or mark; a congenital circumscribed deposit of pigmentation in the skin; mole.

- **n. flammeus** Port-wine stain; reddish, usually flat, discoloration of the face or neck. Because of its large size and color, it is considered a serious deformity.
- **n. vasculosus** Elevated lesion of immature capillaries and endothelial cells that regresses over a period of years. Also called a strawberry hemangioma.

newborn rash See *erythema toxicum.*

nidation Implantation of the fertilized ovum in the endometrium, or lining, of the uterus.

nipple confusion Difficulty experienced by some infants in mastering breastfeeding after having been given a pacifier or bottle. This problem appears to be more related to tactile sensation than flow of liquid.

nitrazine A pH indicator dye. Also called *phenaphthazine.*

nondirectiveness According to the principle of nondirectiveness, the individual who is providing genetic counseling respects the right of the individual or family being counseled to make autonomous decisions. Counselors using a nondirective approach avoid making recommendations and try to communicate genetics information in an unbiased manner.

nondisjunction Failure of two homologous chromosomes to separate during reduction division. One resulting cell contains both chromosomes, and the other contains none.

nonmaleficence The principle in bioethics directing us to act so as to avoid causing harm.

nonnutritive sucking Use of a pacifier by infants.

nonphysiologic jaundice See *jaundice, pathologic.*

nonshivering thermogenesis Infant's method of producing heat from brown fat by increasing metabolic rate.

nonstress test (NST) Evaluation of fetal response (fetal heart rate) to natural contractile uterine activity or to an increase in fetal activity.

no-parent family Family form in which children live independently in foster or kinship care, such as living with a grandparent.

normoglycemia Blood glucose level within normal limits; glycemic control.

nosocomial Pertaining to a hospital.

NST See *nonstress test (NST).*

NTD See *neural tube defect.*

NTE See *neutral thermal environment (NTE).*

nuchal cord Encircling of fetal neck by one or more loops of umbilical cord.

nuclear family Traditional family in which male and female partners and their children live as an independent unit, sharing roles, responsibilities, and economic resources.

nulligravida A woman who has never been pregnant.

nullipara A woman who has not completed a pregnancy with a fetus or fetuses who have reached 20 weeks of gestation.

nurse practitioner Registered nurse who has additional education to practice nursing in an expanded role.

O

observer style Characteristic style described by May that is displayed by expectant fathers who show a detached approach to involvement in their partner's pregnancy.

occipitobregmatic Pertaining to the occiput (the back part of the skull) and the bregma (junction of the coronal and sagittal sutures) or anterior fontanel.

occiput Back part of the head or skull.

occurrence risk Estimated risk given to a couple who has not yet had children, but are known to be at risk for having children with a genetic disease. See also *recurrence risk*.

OCT See *oxygen challenge test (OCT)*.

oligohydramnios Abnormally small amount or absence of amniotic fluid; often indicative of fetal urinary tract defect.

oligomenorrhea Infrequent menstrual periods characterized by intervals of 40 to 45 days or longer.

oliguria Urine output below 25 to 30 ml by the kidneys for 2 consecutive hours (in adults).

omphalitis Inflammation of the umbilical stump characterized by redness, edema, and purulent exudate in severe infections.

omphalocele Congenital defect resulting from failure of closure of the abdominal wall or muscles and leading to hernia of abdominal contents through the navel.

oocyte Primordial or incompletely developed ovum.

oogenesis Process of egg (ovum) formation; begins during fetal life in the female.

operculum Plug of mucus that fills the cervical canal during pregnancy; acts as a barrier against bacterial invasion.

ophthalmia neonatorum Infection in the neonate's eyes usually resulting from gonorrheal or other infection contracted when the fetus passes through the birth canal (vagina).

opisthotonos Tetanic spasm resulting in an arched, hyperextended position of the body.

oral glucose tolerance test Test for blood glucose after oral ingestion of a concentrated sugar solution.

orchitis Inflammation of one or both of the testes, characterized by swelling and pain, often caused by mumps, syphilis, or tuberculosis.

orifice Normal mouth, entrance, or opening, to any aperture.

os Mouth, or opening.

- **external o. (o. externum)** External opening of the cervical canal.
- **internal o. (o. internum)** Internal opening of the cervical canal.
- **o. uteri** Mouth, or opening, of the uterus.

ossification Mineralization of fetal bones.

osteoporosis Deossification of bone tissue resulting in structural weakness; generalized, metabolic disease characterized by decreased bone mass and increased incidence of bone fractures, especially after menopause.

outcomes-oriented care Measures effectiveness of care against benchmarks or standards.

outlet Opening by which something can leave.

- **pelvic o.** Lower aperture, or opening, of the true pelvis.

ovarian cancer The second most frequently occurring reproductive cancer, which causes more deaths than any other female genital tract cancer. Also called *cancer of the ovary*.

ovary One of two glands in the female situated on either side of the pelvic cavity that produces the female reproductive cell, the ovum, and two known hormones, estrogen and progesterone.

ovulation Periodic ripening and discharge of the ovum from the ovary, usually 14 days before the onset of menstrual flow; the release of a mature ovum from the ovary at intervals (usually monthly).

- **o. method** Control of fertility using evaluation of cervical mucus throughout the menstrual cycle; ovulation occurs just after the appearance of the peak mucus sign; Billings method.

ovum Female germ, or reproductive cell, produced by the ovary; egg.

oxygen toxicity Oxygen overdosage that results in pathologic tissue changes (e.g., retinopathy of prematurity, bronchopulmonary dysplasia).

oxytocics Drugs that stimulate uterine contractions, thus accelerating childbirth and preventing postbirth hemorrhage. They may be used to increase the let-down reflex during lactation.

oxytocin Hormone produced by the posterior pituitary that stimulates uterine contractions and the release of milk in the mammary gland (*let-down reflex*).

- **o. challenge test (OCT)** Evaluation of fetal response (*fetal heart rate*) to contractile activity of the uterus stimulated by exogenous oxytocin (Pitocin).

P

PAC See *pulmonary artery catheter (PAC)*.

$Paco_2$ Partial pressure of carbon dioxide in arterial blood.

palmar erythema Pinkish red, diffuse mottling or well-defined blotches seen over the palmar surfaces of the hands in about 60% of Caucasian women and 35% of African-American women during pregnancy; related primarily to increased estrogen levels.

palsy Permanent or temporary loss of sensation or ability to move and control movement; paralysis.

- **Bell's p.** Peripheral facial paralysis of the facial nerve (cranial nerve VII), causing the muscles of the unaffected side of the face to pull the face into a distorted position.
- **Erb's p.** See *Erb-Duchenne palsy*.
- **facial p.** See *facial paralysis*.

panic disorder Repeated, unprovoked episodes of intense fear, which develop without warning and are not related to any specific event.

Pao_2 Partial pressure of oxygen in arterial blood.

Pap (Papanicolaou) test Microscopic examination using scrapings from the cervix, endocervix, or other mucous membranes that will reveal, with a high degree of accuracy, the presence of premalignant or malignant cells.

PAP See *pulmonary artery pressure (PAP)*.

para Usually expressed as a number that refers to parity. See *parity*.

paracervical block Type of regional anesthesia produced by injection of a local anesthetic into the lower uterine segment just beneath the mucosa adjacent to the outer rim of the cervix (3 and 9 o'clock positions).

parental adjustment Process that a person goes through in adapting to the parental role; includes three stages: expectations, reality, and transition to mastery.

parity The number of pregnancies in which the fetus or fetuses have reached 20 weeks of gestation when they are born, not the number of fetuses (e.g., twins) born. Whether the fetus is born alive or is stillborn (fetus who shows no signs of life at birth) does not affect parity. See *para*.

parturient Woman giving birth.

parturition Process or act of giving birth.

patent Open.

- **p. ductus arteriosus (PDA)** Condition that occurs when the fetal *ductus arteriosus* fails to close after birth. Also see *ductus arteriosus*.

pathogen Substance or organism capable of producing disease.

pathologic jaundice See *jaundice, pathologic*.

pathologic mourning See *grief, complicated*.

pathological grief See *grief, complicated*.

Pco_2 Partial pressure of CO_2.

PCOS See *polycystic ovary syndrome (PCOS)*.

PCWP See *pulmonary capillary wedge pressure (PCWP)*.

PDA See *patent ductus arteriosus (PDA)*.

pelvic Pertaining or relating to the pelvis.

- **p. exenteration** A total exenteration involves removal of the perineum, the pelvic floor, the levator muscles, and all reproductive organs. Additionally, pelvic lymph nodes, rectum, sigmoid colon, urinary bladder, and distal ureters are removed, and a colostomy and ileal conduit are constructed.
- **p. inflammatory disease (PID)** Infectious process that most commonly involves the uterine (fallopian) tubes (salpingitis), uterus (endometritis), and more rarely, the ovaries and peritoneal surfaces. Usually secondary to sexually transmitted infections.
- **p. inlet** See *inlet, pelvic*.
- **p. outlet** See *outlet, pelvic*.
- **p. relaxation** Refers to the lengthening and weakening of the fascial supports of pelvic structures. Congenital or acquired weakness of the pelvic support structures.
- **p. tilt (rock)** Exercise used to help relieve low back discomfort during menstruation and pregnancy.

pelvimetry Measurement of dimensions and proportions of the pelvis to determine its capacity and ability to allow the passage of the fetus through the birth canal.

pelvis Bony structure formed by the sacrum, coccyx, innominate bones, and symphysis pubis and the ligaments that unite them.

- **android p.** See *android pelvis*.
- **anthropoid p.** See *anthropoid pelvis*.
- **gynecoid p.** See *gynecoid pelvis*.
- **platypelloid p.** See *platypelloid pelvis*.
- **true p.** Pelvis below the linea terminalis.

penis Male organ used for urination and copulation.

percutaneous umbilical blood sampling (PUBS) Procedure during which the fetal umbilical vessel is accessed for blood sampling or for transfusions. Also called *cordocentesis*.

perimenopause Period of transition of changing ovarian activity before menopause and through first few years of amenorrhea; precedes menopause and lasts about 4 years. During this time, ovarian function declines. Ova slowly diminish, and menstrual cycles may be anovulatory, resulting in irregular bleeding. The ovary stops producing estrogen, and eventually menses no longer occur.

perinatal Of or pertaining to the time and process of giving birth or being born.

perinatal loss Death of a fetus or infant through the twenty-eighth day after birth.

perinatal period Period extending from the twentieth or twenty-eighth week of gestation through the end of the twenty-eighth day after birth.

perinatologist Physician who specializes in fetal and neonatal care.

perineum A skin-covered muscular area that covers the pelvic structures. The perineum forms the base of the perineal body, a wedge-shaped mass that serves as an anchor for the muscles, fascia, and ligaments of the pelvis. Area between the vagina and rectum in the female and between the scrotum and rectum in the male.

periodic abstinence Contraceptive method in which a woman abstains from sexual intercourse during the fertile period of her menstrual cycle; also referred to as natural family planning (NFP) because no other form of birth control is used during this period.

periodic breathing Sporadic episodes of cessation of respirations for periods of 10 seconds or less not associated with cyanosis typically noted in preterm infants.

periodic changes Changes from baseline of the fetal heart rate that occur with uterine contractions.

periods of reactivity (newborn infant) First period (within 30 minutes after birth): brief cyanosis, flushing with crying; crackles, nasal flaring, grunting, retractions; heart sounds loud, forceful, irregular; alert; mucus; no bowel sounds; followed by period of sleep. Second period (4 to 8 hours after birth): swift color changes; irregular respiratory and heart rates; mucus with gagging; meconium passage; temperature stabilizing.

peripartum heart failure Inability of the heart to maintain an adequate cardiac output. Heart failure occurring during pregnancy.

periventricular Intraventricular hemorrhage, a common type of brain injury in preterm infants; prognosis depends on severity of hemorrhage.

persistent pulmonary hypertension of the newborn (PPHN) Combined findings of pulmonary hypertension, right-to-left shunting, and a structurally normal heart.

pessary Device placed inside the vagina to function as a supportive structure for the uterus.

petechiae Pinpoint hemorrhagic areas caused by numerous disease states involving infection and thrombocytopenia and occasionally found over the face and trunk of the newborn because of increased intravascular pressure in the capillaries during birth.

pH Hydrogen ion concentration.

phenotype An individual's observable traits. Refers to the observable expression of an individual's genotype, such as physical features, a biochemical or molecular trait, and even a psychologic trait. Expression of certain physical or chemical characteristics in an individual resulting from interaction between genotype and environmental factors.

phenylketonuria (PKU) Recessive hereditary disease that results in a defect in the metabolism of the amino acid phenylalanine caused by the lack of an enzyme, phenylalanine hydroxylase, that is necessary for the conversion of the amino acid phenylalanine into tyrosine. If PKU is not treated, brain damage may occur, causing severe mental retardation.

phimosis Tightness of the prepuce, or foreskin, of the penis.

phlebitis Inflammation of a vein with symptoms of pain and tenderness along the course of the vein, inflammatory swelling and acute edema below the obstruction, and discoloration of the skin because of injury or bruise to the vein, possibly occurring in acute or chronic infections or after procedures or childbirth.

phlebothrombosis Formation of a clot or thrombus in the vein; inflammation of the vein with secondary clotting.

phosphatidylglycerol A phospholipid, a component of pulmonary surfactant; its presence in amniotic fluid is considered a sign of fetal lung maturity when the pregnancy is complicated by maternal diabetes.

phototherapy Utilization of lights to reduce serum bilirubin levels by oxidation of bilirubin into water-soluble compounds that are then processed in the liver and excreted into bile and urine.

physiologic anemia A modest decrease in the hemoglobin concentration and hematocrit in pregnancy, caused by the relative excess of plasma.

physiologic jaundice See *jaundice, physiologic.*

phytoestrogens Plant compounds that have a weak estrogenic effect in the human body; used in the management of menopause as an alternative or complement to conventional hormone replacement therapy. Also known as isoflavones.

pica Unusual craving during pregnancy; the practice of consuming nonfood substances (e.g., clay, soil, and laundry starch) or excessive amounts of foodstuffs low in nutritional value (e.g., ice or freezer frost, baking powder or soda, and cornstarch), is often influenced by the woman's cultural background.

PID See *pelvic inflammatory disease (PID).*

pinch test Determines if nipples are everted or inverted by placing thumb and forefinger on areola and pressing inward. The nipple will stand erect or invert.

PKU See *phenylketonuria (PKU).*

placenta Latin, flat cake; afterbirth, specialized vascular disk-shaped organ for maternal-fetal gas and nutrient exchange. Normally it implants in the thick muscular wall of the upper uterine segment.

- **abruptio p.** See *abruptio placentae.*
- **battledore p.** Umbilical cord insertion into the margin of the placenta.
- **circumvallate p.** Placenta having a raised white ring at its edge.
- **p. accreta** Invasion of the uterine muscle by the placenta, thus making separation from the muscle difficult if not impossible.
- **p. increta** Deep penetration in myometrium by placenta.
- **p. percreta** Perforation of uterus by placenta.
- **p. previa** Placenta is implanted in the thin, lower uterine segment such that it completely or partially covers the cervix or is close enough to the cervix to cause bleeding when the cervix dilates or the lower uterine segment effaces. When transvaginal ultrasound is used, the placenta is classified as a complete placenta previa if it totally covers the internal cervical os. In a marginal placenta previa the edge of the placenta is seen on transvaginal ultrasound to be 2.5 cm or closer to the internal cervical os. When the exact relationship of the placenta to the internal cervical os has not been determined or in the case of apparent placenta previa in the second trimester, the term low-lying placenta is used.
- **p. retained** See *retained placenta.*
- **p. succenturiata** Accessory placenta.

placental Pertaining or relating to the placenta.

- **p. infarct** Localized, ischemic, hard area on the fetal or maternal side of the placenta.
- **p. souffle** See *souffle, placental.*

platypelloid pelvis Broad pelvis with a shortened anteroposterior diameter and a flattened, oval, transverse shape.

plethora Deep beefy-red coloration of a newborn caused by an increased number of blood cells (polycythemia) per volume of blood.

plugged milk ducts Milk ducts blocked by small curds of dried milk.

PMDD See *premenstrual dysphoric disorder (PMDD).*

PMS See *premenstrual syndrome (PMS).*

podalic Concerning or pertaining to the feet.

- **p. version** Shifting of the position of the fetus so as to bring the feet to the outlet during labor.

polycystic ovary syndrome (PCOS) Occurs when an endocrine imbalance results in high levels of estrogen, testosterone, and luteinizing hormone (LH) and decreased secretion of follicle stimulating hormone.

polycythemia Increased number of erythrocytes per volume of blood, which may be caused by large placental transfusion, fetus transfusion, or maternal-fetal transfusion, or it may be attributable to hypovolemia resulting from movement of fluid out of vascular into interstitial compartment.

polydactyly Excessive number of digits (fingers or toes).

polyhydramnios See *hydramnios.*

polyp Small tumor-like growth that projects from a mucous membrane surface.

- **uterine p.** Tumors that are on pedicles (stalks) arising from the uterine mucosa; may be endometrial or cervical in origin.

polyploidy One of the two types of deviations from the correct number of chromosomes per cell, in which the deviation is an exact multiple of the haploid number of chromosomes or one chromosome set (23 chromosomes).

polyuria Excessive secretion and discharge of urine by the kidneys.

position Relationship of an arbitrarily chosen fetal reference point, such as the occiput, sacrum, chin, or scapula on the presenting part of the fetus to its location in the front, back, or sides of the maternal pelvis.

positive signs of pregnancy Definite indication of pregnancy (e.g., hearing the fetal heartbeat, visualization and palpation of fetal movement by the examiner, sonographic examination).

postdate pregnancy See *postterm pregnancy.*

posterior Pertaining to the back.

- **p. fontanel** See *fontanel, posterior.*

postmature infant Infant born at or after the beginning of week 43 of gestation or later and exhibiting signs of dysmaturity.

postmenopause The time after menopause.

postnatal Happening or occurring after birth (newborn).

postpartum Happening or occurring after birth (mother).

p. blues A letdown feeling, accompanied by irritability and anxiety, which usually begins 2 to 3 days after giving birth and disappears within a week or two. Sometimes called the *baby blues.*

p. depression (PPD) Depression occurring within 6 months of childbirth, lasting longer than postpartum blues and characterized by a variety of symptoms that interfere with activities of daily living and care of the baby.

p. hemorrhage (PPH) Excessive bleeding after childbirth; traditionally defined as a loss of 500 ml or more after a vaginal birth and 1000 ml after a cesarean birth.

p. infection Any clinical infection of the genital canal that occurs within 28 days after miscarriage, induced abortion, or childbirth; in the United States, the presence of a fever of 38° C or more on 2 successive days of the first 10 postpartum days (not counting the first 24 hours after birth). Also called *puerperal infection.*

p. psychosis Symptoms begin as postpartum blues or depression but are characterized by a break with reality. Delusions, hallucinations, confusion, delirium, and panic can occur.

postterm pregnancy Pregnancy that extends beyond the end of week 42 of gestation. Also called *postdate pregnancy* or *prolonged pregnancy.*

posttraumatic stress disorder An anxiety disorder characterized by an acute emotional response to a traumatic event or situation such as sexual abuse.

PPD See *postpartum depression (PPD).*

PPH See *postpartum hemorrhage (PPH).*

PPHN See *persistent pulmonary hypertension of the newborn (PPHN).*

PPROM See *membrane(s), preterm premature rupture of (PPROM).*

precipitous labor Rapid or sudden labor of less than 3 hours beginning from onset of cervical changes to completed birth of neonate.

preconception care Care designed for health maintenance before pregnancy. Suggested components of preconception care are health promotion, risk assessment, and interventions.

preeclampsia A pregnancy-specific condition in which hypertension and proteinuria develop after 20 weeks of gestation or early in the puerperium in a previously normotensive woman; a vasospastic disease process characterized by increasing hypertension, proteinuria, and hemoconcentration.

pregestational diabetes Women who have either type 1 or type 2 diabetes before pregnancy, which may be complicated by vascular disease, retinopathy, nephropathy, or other diabetic sequelae. Almost all women with pregestational diabetes are insulin dependent during pregnancy.

pregnancy Period between conception through complete birth of the products of conception. The usual duration of pregnancy in the human is 280 days, 9 calendar months, or 10 lunar months.

abdominal p. See *abdominal gestation.*

ectopic p. See *ectopic pregnancy.*

extrauterine p. See *extrauterine pregnancy.*

predictive testing genetic testing used to clarify the genetic status of asymptomatic family members.

predispositional testing Testing for a gene mutation that indicates susceptibility for developing a condition; a positive result does not indicate a 100% risk of developing the condition.

preload The stretch of myocardial fiber at end-diastole. The ventricular end-diastole pressure and volume reflect this parameter.

premature dilation of the cervix Cervix that is unable to remain closed until a pregnancy reaches term because of a mechanical defect in the cervix resulting in dilation and effacement usually during the second or early third trimester of pregnancy.

premature infant Infant born before completing week 37 of gestation, irrespective of birth weight; preterm infant.

premature rupture of membranes (PROM) See *membrane(s), premature rupture of (PROM).*

premenstrual dysphoric disorder (PMDD) A more severe variant of premenstrual syndrome (PMS) in which 3% to 8% of women have marked irritability, dysphoria, mood lability, anxiety, fatigue, appetite changes, and a sense of feeling overwhelmed. The most common symptoms are those associated with mood disturbances.

premenstrual syndrome (PMS) Complex, poorly understood condition that includes one or more of a large number (more than 100) of physical and psychologic symptoms beginning in the luteal phase of the menstrual cycle, occurring to such a degree that lifestyle or work is affected, and followed by a symptom-free period.

premonitory Serving as an early symptom or warning.

prenatal Occurring or happening before birth.

prepartum Before birth; before giving birth.

prepuce Fold of skin, or foreskin, covering the glans penis of the male.

p. of the clitoris Fold of the labia minora that covers the glans clitoris.

presentation That part of the fetus that first enters the pelvis and lies over the inlet: may be head, face, breech, or shoulder.

breech p. See *breech presentation.*

cephalic p. See *cephalic presentation.*

presenting part That part of the fetus that lies closest to the internal os of the cervix.

pressure edema Edema of the lower extremities caused by pressure of the heavy pregnant uterus against the large veins; edema of fetal scalp after cephalic presentation (caput succedaneum).

presumptive signs of pregnancy Manifestations that are suggestive of pregnancy but are not absolutely positive. These include the cessation of menses, Chadwick's sign, morning sickness, and quickening.

presymptomatic testing Mutation analysis for a disorder in which symptoms are certain to appear if the individual lives long enough.

preterm

late p. birth Birth that occurs between 34 and 36 weeks of gestation.

p. birth Birth occurring before the completion of 37 weeks of gestation.

p. labor Uterine contractions causing cervical change that occur between 20 and 37 weeks of pregnancy.

p. pregnancy Pregnancy that has reached 20 weeks of gestation but ends before completion of 37 weeks of gestation.

p. premature rupture of membranes (PPROM) See *membrane(s), preterm premature rupture of (PPROM).* Also called *preterm PROM.*

very p. birth Birth that occurs before 32 weeks of gestation.

prevention Desire to avoid illness, detect it early, or maintain optimal functioning when illness is present.

previa, placenta See *placenta previa.*

primary dysmenorrhea See *dysmenorrhea, primary.*

primary survey The immediate response after trauma: the ABCs of resuscitation: establishment and maintenance of an airway, ensuring adequate breathing, and maintenance of an adequate circulatory volume.

primigravida A woman who is pregnant for the first time.

primipara A woman who has completed one pregnancy with a fetus or fetuses who have reached 20 weeks of gestation; woman who has carried a pregnancy to viability whether the child is dead or alive at the time of birth.

probable signs of pregnancy Manifestations or evidence that indicates that there is a definite likelihood of pregnancy. Among the probable signs are enlargement of abdomen, Goodell's sign, Hegar's sign, Braxton Hicks sign, and positive hormonal tests for pregnancy.

prodromal Serving as an early symptom or warning of the approach of a disease or condition (e.g., prodromal labor).

progesterone Hormone produced by the corpus luteum and placenta whose function is to prepare the endometrium of the uterus for implantation of the fertilized ovum, develop the mammary glands, and maintain the pregnancy.

prolactin A pituitary hormone that triggers milk production.

prolapse of the umbilical cord Umbilical cord lies below the presenting part of the fetus; may be frank (visible) or occult (hidden, rather than visible).

proliferative phase of menstrual cycle Preovulatory, follicular, or estrogen phase of the menstrual cycle.

prolonged grief See *grief, complicated.*

prolonged pregnancy See *postterm pregnancy.*

PROM See *membrane(s), premature rupture of (PROM).*

promontory of the sacrum Superior projecting portion of the sacrum at the junction of the sacrum and L5.

prophylactic (1) Pertaining to prevention or warding off disease or certain conditions. (2) Condom, or "rubber."

proscription Forbidden; taboo.

prostaglandin (PG) Substance present in many body tissues; has a role in many reproductive tract functions; used to induce abortions, cervical ripening for labor induction.

proteinuria Presence of protein in urine.

pruritus Itching.
pseudocyesis Condition in which the woman has all the usual signs of pregnancy, such as enlargement of the abdomen, cessation of menses, weight gain, and morning sickness, but is not pregnant; phantom or false pregnancy.
pseudopregnancy See *pseudocyesis.*
psychoprophylaxis Mental and physical education of the parents in preparation for childbirth, with the goal of minimizing fear and pain and promoting positive family relationships.
psychosis, postpartum See *postpartum psychosis.*
ptyalism Excessive salivation.
puberty Period in life in which the reproductive organs mature and one becomes functionally capable of reproduction; the entire transitional stage between childhood and sexual maturity.
pubic Pertaining to the pubis.
pubis Pubic bone forming the front of the pelvis.
PUBS See *percutaneous umbilical blood sampling (PUBS).*
pudendal nerve block Injection of a local anesthetic at the pudendal nerve root to produce numbness of the genital and perianal region.
puerperal infection See *postpartum infection.*
puerperium The interval between the birth of the newborn and the return of the reproductive organs to their normal nonpregnant state; also called the *fourth trimester of pregnancy* or the *postpartum period.* Period after the third stage of labor and lasting until involution of the uterus takes place, usually about 3 to 6 weeks.
pulmonary artery catheter (PAC) A flow-directed, balloon-tipped multilumen catheter made of polyvinyl chloride that is inserted into the pulmonary artery to provide continuous measurements of pulmonary artery pressure when the balloon is deflated and pulmonary capillary wedge pressures when the balloon is inflated. Sometimes called a *Swan-Ganz catheter*
pulmonary artery pressure (PAP) Systolic and diastolic pressures of blood in the pulmonary artery; reflects right afterload.
pulmonary capillary wedge pressure (PCWP) Pressure when the balloon of the *pulmonary artery catheter (PAC)* is inflated to obstruct right-sided pressures and to reflect left-sided pressures. Value is obtained during diastole, with the mitral valve open; it reflects left preload.
pulmonary vascular resistance (PVR) A measure for the tension required for the ejection of blood from the right ventricle into the circulation (afterload).
pulse oximetry Noninvasive method of monitoring oxygen levels by detecting the amount of light absorbed by oxygen-carrying hemoglobin.
PVR See *pulmonary vascular resistance (PVR).*
pyrosis A burning sensation in the epigastric and sternal region from stomach acid. Also called heartburn or "acid indigestion."

Q

quickening Maternal perception of fetal movement ("feeling life"); usually occurs between weeks 16 and 20 of gestation, but may be felt earlier by multiparous woman.

R

radical hysterectomy Involves removal of the uterus, the tubes, the ovaries, the upper third of the vagina, the entire uterosacral and uterovesical ligaments, and all of the parametrium on each side, along with pelvic node dissection encompassing the four major pelvic lymph node chains: ureteral, obturator, hypogastric, and iliac.
radioimmunoassay Pregnancy test that tests for the beta subunit of human chorionic gonadotropin using radioactively labeled markers.
rape Legal term that is defined differently by each state. Usually refers to forced sexual intercourse or penetration of the mouth, anus, or vagina by a body part or object without consent; it may or may not include the use of a weapon.
rape-trauma syndrome Characteristic symptoms seen in victims of rape and consisting of several phases; similar to posttraumatic stress syndrome.
RDAs See *recommended dietary allowances (RDAs).*
RDS See *respiratory distress syndrome (RDS).*
recessive trait A trait or disorder expressed or phenotypically, apparent only when two copies of the alleles associated with the trait are present. Genetically determined characteristic that is expressed only when present in the homozygotic state.
reciprocity Type of body movement or behavior that provides the observer with cues, such as the behavioral cues infants provide to parents and parents' responses to cues.
recommended dietary allowances (RDAs) Recommended nutrient intakes estimated to meet the needs of almost all (97% to 98%) of the healthy people in the population.
rectocele Herniation or protrusion of the anterior rectal wall through the relaxed or ruptured vaginal fascia and rectovaginal septum; it appears as a large bulge that may be seen through the relaxed introitus.
recurrence risk Estimated risk of a couple having a child with a specific genetic disease once they have produced one or more children with the same genetic disease.
referred pain Discomfort originating in a local area such as cervix, vagina, or perineal tissues but felt in the back, flanks, or thighs.
reflection Looking within for solutions and answers to certain dilemmas, using intuition and inner wisdom as guides for attainment of healing.
reflex Automatic response built into the nervous system that does not need the intervention of conscious thought (e.g., in the newborn, rooting, gagging, grasp).
reflex bradycardia Slowing of the heart in response to a particular stimulus.
refractory oliguria Oliguria not corrected with fluid challenge.
regional anesthesia Anesthesia of an area of the body by injection of a local anesthetic to block a group of sensory nerve fibers.
regurgitate Vomiting or spitting up of solids or fluids.
relaxation The absence or alleviation of mental, physical, and emotional tension through purposeful activities that quiet the mind and body.
reproductive tract infection Encompasses both sexually transmitted infections and other common genital tract infections.
residual urine Urine that remains in the bladder after urination.
respiratory distress syndrome (RDS) Condition resulting from decreased pulmonary gas exchange, leading to retention of carbon dioxide (increase in arterial Pco_2). Most common neonatal causes are prematurity, perinatal asphyxia, and maternal diabetes mellitus; hyaline membrane disease (HMD).
restitution In obstetrics, the turning of the fetal head to the left or right after it has completely emerged from the introitus as it assumes a normal alignment with the infant's shoulders.
resuscitation Restoration of consciousness or life in one who is apparently dead or whose respirations or cardiac function or both have ceased.
retained placenta Retention of all or part of the placenta in the uterus after birth.
retinal hemorrhage Injuries resulting from rupture of capillaries in the retina, caused by increased *intracranial pressure (ICP)* during birth.
retinopathy of prematurity (ROP) Associated with hyperoxemia, resulting in eye injury and blindness in premature infants.
retraction (1) Drawing in or sucking in of soft tissues of chest, indicative of an obstruction at any level of the respiratory tract from the oropharynx to the alveoli. (2) Retraction of uterine muscle fiber. After contracting, the muscle fiber does not return to its original length but remains slightly shortened, a unique attribute of uterine muscle that aids in preventing postbirth hemorrhage and results in involution.
retroflexion Bending backward.
- **r. of uterus** Condition in which the body of the uterus is bent backward at an angle with the cervix, the position of which usually remains unchanged.

retrolental fibroplasia (RLF) See *retinopathy of prematurity.*
retroversion Turning or a state of being turned back.
- **r. of uterus** Displacement of the uterus; the body of the uterus is tipped backward with the cervix pointing forward toward the symphysis pubis.

Rh factor Inherited antigen present on erythrocytes. The individual with the factor is known as positive for the factor.
Rh incompatibility See *isoimmunization.*
Rh immune globulin (RhIg) Solution of gamma globulin that contains Rh antibodies. Intramuscular administration of Rh immune globulin (trade name RhoGAM) prevents sensitization in Rh-negative women who have been exposed to Rh-positive red blood cells.
Rh_0(D) immunoglobulin A commercial preparation of passive antibodies against the Rh factor, such as RhoGAM (WinGAM).
rheumatic heart disease Permanent damage of the heart muscle and valves secondary to an autoimmune reaction in the heart tissue precipitated by rheumatic fever.
rhythm method Contraceptive method in which a woman abstains from sexual intercourse during the ovulatory phase of her menstrual cycle; calendar method.
ribonucleic acid (RNA) Element responsible for transferring genetic information within a cell; a template, or pattern.
ring of fire Burning sensation as vagina stretches and fetal head crowns.

risk factors Factors that cause a person or a group of people to be particularly vulnerable to an unwanted, unpleasant, or unhealthful event.

Ritgen maneuver Procedure used to control the birth of the head.

rooming-in unit Maternity unit designed so that the newborn's crib is at the mother's bedside or in a nursery adjacent to the mother's room.

rooting reflex Normal response of the newborn to move toward whatever touches the area around the mouth and to attempt to suck. This reflex usually disappears by 3 to 4 months of age.

ROP See *retinopathy of prematurity (ROP).*

rotation In obstetrics, the turning of the fetal head as it follows the curves of the birth canal downward.

rubella vaccine Live attenuated rubella virus given to clients who have not had rubella or who are serologically negative. Exposure to the rubella virus through vaccination causes the client to form antibodies, producing active immunity.

rugae Folds in the vaginal mucosa and scrotum.

S

Sao_2 monitoring Degree to which hemoglobin is saturated with oxygen, measured by a pulse oximeter. The normal Sao_2 range is 95% to 100%.

sac, amniotic See *amniotic sac.*

sacroiliac Of or pertaining to the sacrum and ilium.

sacrum Triangular bone composed of five united vertebrae and situated between L5 and the coccyx; forms the posterior boundary of the true pelvis.

safe passage Normal uneventful birth process for mother and child.

safe period The days in the menstrual cycle that are not designated as fertile days, that is, before and after ovulation.

sagittal suture Band of connective tissue separating the parietal bones, extending from the anterior to the posterior fontanel.

salpingo-oophorectomy Removal of a uterine tube and an ovary.

Schultze mechanism Delivery of the placenta with the fetal surfaces (shiny in appearance) presenting.

scrotum Pouch of skin containing the testes and parts of the spermatic cords.

second stage of labor See *labor, second stage of labor.*

secondary areola See *areola, secondary.*

secondary dysmenorrhea See *dysmenorrhea, secondary.*

secondary survey A complete physical assessment of all body systems after immediate resuscitation and stabilization after trauma to mother and fetus.

secretory phase of menstrual cycle Postovulatory, luteal, progestational, premenstrual phase of menstrual cycle; 14 days in length.

secundines Fetal membranes and placenta expelled after childbirth; afterbirth.

self-management Client provides care for self as part of plan of care.

semen Thick, white, viscid secretion discharged from the urethra of the male at orgasm; the transporting medium of the sperm.

semen analysis Basic test for male infertility; examination of semen specimen to determine liquefaction, volume, pH, sperm density, and normal morphology. Complete semen analysis includes the study of the effects of cervical mucus on sperm forward motility and survival, and evaluation of the sperm's ability to penetrate an ovum.

sensitization Development of antibodies to a specific antigen.

sensory behavior Responses of the five senses; indicate a readiness for social interaction.

sepsis Bacterial infections of the bloodstream.

septic abortion See *abortion, septic.*

septic shock Caused by the toxins released into the bloodstream in *septicemia.* The most common sign is a decrease in blood pressure, a vital sign often not assessed in the care of the neonate. The infant will often appear gray or mottled and can be noted to have cool extremities. Other signs are rapid, irregular respirations and pulse (similar to *septicemia* in general).

septicemia Generalized infection in the bloodstream.

sex chromosome Chromosome associated with determination of gender: the X (female) and Y (male) chromosomes. The normal female has two X chromosomes, and the normal male has one X and one Y chromosome.

sexual assault Intentional unwanted completed or attempted touching of the victim's genitals, anus, groin, or breasts, directly or through clothing as well as by voyeurism.

sexual decision making Selection of choices concerned with intimate and sexual behavior.

sexual history Past and present health conditions, lifestyle behaviors, knowledge, and attitudes related to sex and sexuality.

sexual response cycle The phases of physical changes that occur in response to sexual stimulation and sexual tension release. Divided into four phases: excitement phase, plateau phase, orgasmic phase, and resolution phase. The four phases occur progressively, with no sharp dividing line between any two phases. Specific body changes take place in sequence. The time, intensity, and duration for cyclic completion also vary for individuals and situations.

sexual violence Broad term that encompasses a wide range of sexual victimization including sexual harassment, sexual assault, and rape.

sexuality The part of life that has to do with being male or female.

sexually transmitted infections (STIs) Infections transmitted as a result of sexual activity with an infected individual; also called *sexually transmitted diseases (STDs).* Include more than 25 organisms that cause infections or infectious disease syndromes primarily transmitted by close, intimate contact.

SGA See *small for gestational age (SGA).*

shake test "Foam" test for lung maturity of fetus; more rapid than determination of lecithin/sphingomyelin ratio.

Sheehan syndrome Postpartum necrosis of the pituitary gland resulting from hypovolemic shock and disseminated intravascular coagulation.

shoulder dystocia Condition in which the head is born but the anterior shoulder cannot pass under the pubic arch to complete the birth of the entire fetus. See also *dysfunctional labor.*

sibling rivalry Jealousy and other negative behaviors exhibited by siblings in response to the addition of a new baby in the family.

sickle cell hemoglobinopathy Abnormal crescent-shaped red blood corpuscles in the blood.

SIL See *squamous intraepithelial lesion (SIL).*

Sims position Position in which the client lies on the left side with the right knee and thigh drawn upward toward the chest.

single-parent family Family form characterized by one parent (male or female) in the household. This may result from loss of spouse by death, divorce, separation, desertion, or birth of a child to a single woman.

single-room maternity care (SRMC) Variation of care sites where one nurse provides care to a mother and infant, that is, mother-baby units, labor-delivery-recovery-postpartum units (LDRPs).

singleton A single fetus.

situational crisis Crisis that arises suddenly in response to an external event or a conflict concerning a specific circumstance. The symptoms are transient, and the episode is usually brief.

sitz bath Application of moist heat to the perineum by sitting in a tub or basin filled with warm water.

SLE See *systemic lupus erythematosus (SLE).*

sleep-wake states Variations in the state of consciousness of infants.

small for gestational age (SGA) Inadequate growth for gestational age.

smegma Whitish secretion around labia minora and under foreskin of penis.

somatic cell Cell of the body of an individual that becomes differentiated and composes the tissues, organs, and parts of that individual. Diploid cell; not a gamete.

somatic pain Perineal discomfort resulting from stretching of perineal tissues.

sonogram See *ultrasonography.*

souffle Soft, blowing sound or murmur heard by auscultation.

- **funic s.** Soft, muffled, blowing sound produced by blood rushing through the umbilical vessels and synchronous with the fetal heart sounds.
- **placental s.** Soft, blowing murmur caused by the blood current in the placenta and synchronous with the maternal pulse.
- **uterine s.** Soft, blowing sound made by the blood in the arteries of the pregnant uterus and synchronous with the maternal pulse.

sperm Male sex cell. Also called *spermatozoon, spermatozoa.*

spermatogenesis Process by which mature spermatozoa are formed, during which the diploid chromosome number (46) is reduced by half (haploid, 23).

spermicide Chemical substance that kills sperm by reducing their surface tension, causing the cell wall to break down by a bactericidal effect or by creating a highly acidic environment. Also called *spermatocide.*

spina bifida The most common defect of the central nervous system (CNS); results from failure of the neural tube to close at some point.

- **s. b. manifesta** Occurs predominantly in the lumbar or lumbosacral regions and includes meningocele and myelomeningocele.
- **s. b. occulta** Congenital malformation of the spine in which the posterior portion of lami-

nas of the vertebrae fails to close but there is no herniation or protrusion of the spinal cord or meninges through the defect. The newborn may have a dimple in the skin or growth of hair over the malformed vertebrae.

spinal anesthesia (block) Regional anesthesia induced by injection of a local anesthetic agent into the subarachnoid space at the level of the third, fourth, or fifth lumbar interspace. See also *low spinal (saddle) block anesthesia.*

spinnbarkeit Formation of a stretchable thread of cervical mucus under estrogen influence at time of ovulation.

spiral electrode See *fetal scalp spiral electrode.*

spirituality The individual's connection to one's own values, purpose, and meaning of life. May encompass organized religion or belief in higher power or authority. Recognition of wisdom, imagination, spirit, intuition. A perception of the unity of nature and the interconnectedness of all beings. Inner strength.

splanchnic engorgement Excessive filling or pooling of blood within the visceral vasculature that occurs after the removal of pressure from the abdomen, such as birth of an infant, removal of an excess of urine from bladder, removal of large tumor.

spontaneous abortion See *abortion, spontaneous.*

spontaneous rupture of membranes (SROM) See *membrane(s), spontaneous rupture of (SROM).*

squamocolumnar junction Site in the endocervical canal where columnar epithelium and squamous epithelium meet, usually located just inside the cervical os; also called the *transformation zone*, the most common site for neoplastic changes; cells from this site are scraped for the Pap test.

squamous intraepithelial lesion (SIL) Term used to describe neoplastic changes of the cervix.

square window Angle of wrist between hypothenar prominence and forearm; one criterion for estimating gestational age of neonate.

SROM See *membrane(s), spontaneous rupture of (SROM).*

standard body weight An appropriate weight for height; a *body mass index (BMI)* within the normal range.

standard of care Level of practice that a reasonable, prudent nurse would provide.

state-related behavior Behavioral responses dependent on current state of infant.

station Relationship of the presenting fetal part to an imaginary line drawn between the ischial spines of the pelvis.

sterility (1) State of being free from living microorganisms. (2) Complete inability to reproduce offspring.

sterilization Surgical procedures intended to render a person infertile or unable to produce children.

stillbirth The birth of a baby after 20 weeks of gestation and 1 day or weighing 350 g (depending on the state code) that does not show any signs of life.

strawberry hemangioma See *nevus vasculosus.*

stress urinary incontinence (SUI) Loss of urine occurring with increased abdominal pressure (e.g., with coughing or sneezing).

stretch marks See *striae gravidarum.*

STIs See *sexually transmitted infections (STIs).*

striae gravidarum Shining, slightly depressed, reddish lines caused by stretching of the skin, often found on the abdomen, thighs, and breasts during pregnancy. These streaks turn to a fine pinkish white or silver tone in time in fair-skinned women and brownish in darker-skinned women. Also called *stretch marks.*

stroke volume Volume of blood ejected from the left ventricle during one cardiac cycle.

subconjunctival hemorrhage Injuries resulting from rupture of subconjunctival capillaries, caused by increased *intracranial pressure (ICP)* during birth.

subculture Group existing within a larger cultural system that retains its own characteristics.

subgaleal hemorrhage Bleeding into the subgaleal compartment, which is a potential space that contains loosely arranged connective tissue, located beneath the galea aponeurosis, the tendinous sheath that connects the frontal and occipital muscles and forms the inner surface of the scalp.

subinvolution Failure of a part (e.g., the uterus) to reduce to its normal size and condition after enlargement from functional activity (e.g., pregnancy).

suboccipitobregmatic diameter Smallest diameter of the fetal head—follows a line drawn from the middle of the anterior fontanel to the undersurface of the occipital bone.

substance abuse The continued use of substances despite related problems in physical, social, or interpersonal areas. Any use of alcohol or illicit drugs during pregnancy is considered abuse.

SUI See *stress urinary incontinence (SUI).*

supine hypotension Shock; fall in blood pressure caused by impaired venous return when gravid uterus presses on ascending vena cava, when woman is lying flat on her back; vena cava syndrome.

supply-meets-demand Physiologic basis for determining milk production. The volume of milk produced equals the amount of milk removed from the breast.

support systems Network from which people receive help in times of crisis.

surfactant Phosphoprotein necessary for normal respiratory function that prevents the alveolar collapse (atelectasis). See also *lecithin* and *L/S ratio.*

surgical menopause Occurs with hysterectomy and bilateral oophorectomy.

suture (1) Junction of the adjoining bones of the skull. (2) Procedure uniting parts by their being sewn together.

Svo_2 monitoring Percentage of saturation of hemoglobin with oxygen in mixed venous and arterial blood monitored with a fiberoptic pulmonary artery catheter that is connected to a bedside microprocessor. The Svo_2 reflects the balance between oxygen delivery and oxygen use.

Swan-Ganz catheter See *pulmonary artery catheter (PAC).*

symphysis pubis Fibrocartilaginous union of the bodies of the pubic bones in the midline.

synchrony Fit between an infant's cues and the parent's response.

syndactyly Malformation of digits, often seen as a fusion of two or more toes to form one structure.

systemic analgesia Analgesics administered either intramuscularly or intravenously that cross the blood-brain barrier and provide central analgesic effects.

systemic lupus erythematosus (SLE) A chronic inflammatory connective tissue disease affecting many systems, that is, the integumentary, renal, and nervous systems.

systemic vascular resistance (SVR) A measure of the tension required for the ejection of blood from the left ventricle into the circulation (afterload).

T

tachycardia Baseline fetal heart rate above 160 beats/min.

tachypnea Excessively rapid respiratory rate (e.g., in neonates, respiratory rate of 60 breaths/min or more).

tachysystole More than five uterine contractions in 10 minutes, averaged over a 30-minute window.

taking-hold phase Period after birth characterized by a woman becoming more independent and more interested in learning infant care skills; learning to be a competent mother is an important task.

taking-in phase Period after birth characterized by the woman's dependency; maternal needs are dominant, and talking about the birth is an important task.

talipes equinovarus Deformity in which the foot is extended and the person walks on the toes.

tandem nursing The practice of breastfeeding a newborn and an older child.

TDI See *insemination, therapeutic donor (TDI).*

telangiectasia Permanent dilation of groups of superficial capillaries and venules.

telangiectatic nevi Clusters of small, red, localized areas of capillary dilation frequently seen in neonates at the nape of the neck or lower occiput, upper eyelids, and nasal bridge that can be blanched with pressure of a finger. Also called stork bites.

telemedicine Use of communication technologies and electronic information to provide or support health care when participants are separated by distance.

telephonic nursing Services such as warm lines, nurse advice lines, and telephonic nursing assessments.

teratogenic agent Any drug, virus, or irradiation, the exposure to which can cause malformation of the fetus.

teratogens Nongenetic factors that cause malformations and disorders in utero.

teratoma Tumor composed of different kinds of tissue, none of which normally occurs together or at the site of the tumor.

term infant Live infant born between weeks 38 and 42 of completed gestation.

term pregnancy A pregnancy is considered to be at term if it advances to the completion of 37 weeks.

terminal deletion See *deletion, terminal.*

testis One of the glands contained in the male scrotum that produces the male reproductive cell, or sperm, and the male hormone, testosterone; testicle.

tetany, uterine Extremely prolonged uterine contractions.

tetraploid Cell that has four times the normal number of chromosomes (4N); example of a polyploidy.

thalassemia An anemia affecting Mediterranean and Southeast Asian populations in which there is an insufficient amount of globin produced to fill the red blood cells.

theca-lutein cysts Develop as a result of prolonged stimulation of the ovaries by human chorionic gonadotropin (hCG).

therapeutic abortion See *abortion, therapeutic.*

therapeutic donor insemination See *insemination, therapeutic donor.*

therapeutic rest Administration of analgesics to decrease pain and induce rest for management of *hypertonic uterine dysfunction.*

therapeutic touch A modern interpretation of the laying-on-of-hands for healing, as interpreted by Dolores Krieger, PhD, RN, and Dora Kunz, a noted healer. Originally taught within nursing programs.

thermal shift Drop and subsequent rise in basal body temperature around the time of ovulation.

thermistor probe Automatic sensor used to monitor skin temperature of infant under radiant warmer.

thermogenesis Creation or production of heat, especially in the body.

thermoregulation Control of temperature.

third stage of labor See *labor, third stage of labor.*

threatened abortion See *abortion, threatened.*

thrombocytopenia Abnormal hematologic condition in which the number of platelets is reduced, usually by destruction of erythroid tissue in bone marrow because of certain neoplastic diseases or an immune response to a drug.

thrombocytopenic purpura Hematologic disorder characterized by prolonged bleeding time, decreased number of platelets, increased cell fragility, and purpura, which result in hemorrhages into the skin, mucous membranes, organs, and other tissue.

thromboembolism Obstruction of a blood vessel by a clot that has become detached from its site of formation.

thrombophlebitis Inflammation of a vein with secondary clot formation.

thrombus Blood clot obstructing a blood vessel that remains at the place it was formed.

thrush Fungal infection of the mouth or throat that is characterized by the formation of white patches on a red, moist, inflamed mucous membrane and is caused by *Candida albicans.* Also called *mycotic stomatitis.*

toco- (toko-) Combining form that means childbirth or labor.

tocodynamometer See *tocotransducer.*

tocolysis Relaxation of the uterus. See also *tocolytic therapy.*

tocolytics Medications used to suppress uterine activity and relax the uterus in cases of preterm labor or tachysystole.

tocotransducer Electronic device for measuring uterine contractions. Also called a *tocodynamometer.*

TOL See *trial of labor (TOL).*

TORCH infections Collective name for toxoplasmosis, other infections (e.g., hepatitis), rubella virus, cytomegalovirus (CMV), and herpes simplex virus, a group of organisms capable of crossing the placenta; these infections can affect a pregnant woman and her fetus.

total parenteral nutrition (TPN) Administration of a nutritionally adequate hypertonic solution consisting of glucose, protein hydrolysates, minerals, and vitamins through an indwelling catheter into the superior vena cava.

toxicology screen Laboratory analysis of blood or urine to test for alcohol or drug content. Urine drug screening is the most common because it is noninvasive.

toxic shock syndrome A severe acute disease usually caused by *Staphylococcus aureus*; associated with high-absorbency tampon use during menstruation.

TPN See *total parenteral nutrition (TPN).*

tracheoesophageal fistula Congenital malformation in which there is an abnormal tubelike passage between the trachea and esophagus.

transformation zone See *squamocolumnar junction.*

transition—labor See *labor, transition phase.*

transition period—newborn Period from birth to 4 to 6 hours later; infant passes through period of reactivity, sleep, and second period of reactivity.

transition phase See *labor, transition phase.*

transition to parenthood Period of time from the preconception decision to conceive through the first months of having a child, during which parents define their parental roles and adjust to parenthood.

translocation Condition in which a chromosome breaks and there is an exchange of chromosomal material between two chromosomes; all or part of the broken chromosome is transferred to a different part of the same chromosome or to another chromosome.

balanced t. Translocation in which parts of the two chromosomes are exchanged equally. The individual is phenotypically normal because there is no extra chromosome material; it is just rearranged.

unbalanced t. Translocation in which part of a chromosome is transferred to a different chromosome; there is extra chromosomal material—extra of one chromosome but correct amount or deficient amount of other chromosome. The individual will be both genotypically and phenotypically abnormal.

trial of labor (TOL) Period of observation to determine if a laboring woman is likely to be successful in progressing to a vaginal birth.

***Trichomonas* vaginitis** Inflammation of the vagina caused by *Trichomonas vaginalis*, a parasitic protozoon, and characterized by persistent burning and itching of the vulvar tissue and a profuse, frothy, white discharge.

trimester One of three periods of about 3 months each into which pregnancy is divided.

triploid Cell that has three times the normal number of chromosomes (3N); example of a polyploidy.

trisomy Product of the union of a normal gamete with a gamete containing an extra chromosome. Condition whereby any given chromosome exists in triplicate instead of the normal duplicate pattern.

trophoblast Outer layer of cells of the developing blastodermic vesicle (blastocyst) that develops the trophoderm or feeding layer, which will establish the nutrient relationships with the uterine endometrium.

trophoblastic disease A condition in which trophoblastic cells covering the chorionic villi proliferate and undergo cystic changes, which may be malignant.

tubercles of Montgomery See *Montgomery glands.*

twins Two neonates from the same impregnation developed within the same uterus at the same time.

conjoined t. Twins who are physically united; Siamese twins.

disparate t. Twins who are different (e.g., in weight) and distinct from one another.

dizygotic t. Twins developed from two separate ova fertilized by two separate sperm at the same time; fraternal twins.

monozygotic t. Twins developed from a single fertilized ovum; identical twins.

U

UAE See *uterine artery embolization (UAE).*

UC See *uterine contraction (UC).*

UI See *urinary incontinence (UI).*

ultrasonography Use of high-frequency sound waves for a variety of obstetric diagnoses and for fetal surveillance.

fetal ultrasound Imaging technique using high-frequency sound waves to produce images of the fetus inside the uterus. Also called *sonogram.*

ultrasound transducer External signal source for monitoring fetal heart rate electronically.

umbilical cord Structure connecting the placenta and fetus and containing two arteries and one vein encased in a tissue called Wharton's jelly. The cord is ligated at birth and severed; the stump falls off in 4 to 10 days. Also called *funis.*

umbilical cord prolapse See *prolapse of the umbilical cord.*

umbilicus Navel, or depressed point in the middle of the abdomen that marks the attachment of the umbilical cord during fetal life.

unbalanced translocation See *translocation, unbalanced.*

unifactorial inheritance Inheritance of phenotypic characteristics controlled by a single gene. See also multifactorial inheritance.

UPI See *uteroplacental insufficiency (UPI).*

urethra Small tubular structure that drains urine from the bladder.

urinary frequency Need to void often or at close intervals.

urinary incontinence (UI) Disturbance in urinary control.

stress UI Due to sudden increases in intraabdominal pressure (such as that due to sneezing or coughing)

urge UI Caused by disorders of the bladder and urethra.

urinary meatus Opening, or mouth, of the urethra.

uterine Referring or pertaining to the uterus.

u. adnexa See *adnexa, uterine.*

u. artery embolization (UAE) Treatment during which polyvinyl alcohol (PVA) pellets are injected into selected blood vessels to block the blood supply to the fibroid and cause shrinkage and resolution of symptoms.

u. atony Relaxation of uterus; leads to postpartum hemorrhage. Failure of the uterine muscle to contract firmly.

u. contraction (UC) The primary power that acts involuntarily to expel the fetus and the placenta from the uterus.

u. displacement Variation of the normal placement of the uterus, which is normally held in anteversion by the round ligaments, with the cervix pulled backward and upward by the uterosacral ligaments.

u. inversion See *inversion of the uterus.*

u. ischemia Decreased blood supply to the uterus.

u. polyps See *polyps, uterine.*

u. prolapse Falling, sinking, or sliding of the uterus from its normal location in the body. The degree of prolapse can vary from mild to complete. In complete prolapse the cervix and body of the uterus protrude through the vagina, and the vagina is inverted.

u. souffle See *souffle, uterine.*

uteroplacental insufficiency (UPI) Decline in placental function—exchange of gases, nutrients, and wastes—leading to fetal hypoxia and acidosis; evidenced by late fetal heart rate decelerations in response to uterine contractions.

uterus Hollow muscular organ in the female designed for the implantation, containment, and nourishment of the fetus during its development and expulsion of fetus during labor and birth; also organ of menstruation.

Couvelaire u. Interstitial myometrial hemorrhage after premature separation (abruption) of placenta; if blood accumulates between the separated placenta and the uterine wall, it may produce a couvelaire uterus. The uterus appears purplish or bluish, rather than its usual "bubble gum pink" color; contractility is lost, causing boardlike rigidity of the uterus.

inversion of u. See *inversion of uterus.*

retroflexion of u. See *retroflexion of uterus.*

retroversion of u. See *retroversion of uterus.*

V

VBAC See *vaginal birth after cesarean (VBAC).*

vaccination Intentional injection of antigenic material given to stimulate antibody production in the recipient.

vacuum-assisted birth Birth involving attachment of vacuum cup to fetal head and using negative pressure to assist in birth of the fetus. Also called vacuum extraction.

vacuum curettage Uterine aspiration method of early abortion.

vacuum extraction See *vacuum-assisted birth.*

vagina Normally collapsed musculomembranous tube that forms the passageway between the uterus and the entrance to the vagina.

vaginal birth after cesarean (VBAC) Giving birth vaginally after having had a previous cesarean birth.

vaginismus Intense, painful spasm of the muscles surrounding the vagina.

Valsalva maneuver Any forced expiratory effort against a closed airway such as holding one's breath and tightening the abdominal muscles (e.g., pushing during the second stage of labor).

variability Normal irregularity of fetal cardiac rhythm; short term—beat-to-beat changes; long term—rhythmic changes (waves) from the baseline value.

varicocele Enlargement of veins of the spermatic cord.

varicosity (varicose veins) Swollen, distended, and twisted veins that may develop in almost any part of the body but are most commonly seen in the legs, caused by pregnancy, obesity, congenital defective venous valves, and occupations requiring much standing.

vasectomy Ligation or removal of a segment of the vas deferens, usually done bilaterally to produce sterility in the male.

VDRL test Abbreviation for Venereal Disease Research Laboratories test, a serologic flocculation test for syphilis.

vernix caseosa Protective gray-white fatty substance of cheesy consistency covering the fetal skin.

version Act of turning the fetus in the uterus to change the presenting part and facilitate birth.

external cephalic v. See *external cephalic version.*

podalic v. Shifting of the fetus's position so as to bring the feet to the outlet during birth.

vertex Crown or top of the head.

v. presentation Presentation in which the fetal head is nearest the cervical opening and is born first.

very low birth weight (VLBW) Refers to infant weighing 1500 g or less at birth.

vestibular schwannoma Tumor on the eighth cranial nerves, the hearing and balance nerves.

viable (viability) Capable (capability) of living outside the uterus; applied to a fetus that has reached a certain stage of development, usually 22 menstrual weeks (20 weeks of gestation); however, there are no clear limits of gestational age or weight.

vibroacoustic stimulation One of the methods of testing antepartum FHR response. Generally performed in conjunction with the NST and uses a combination of sound and vibration to stimulate the fetus. Also called the *fetal acoustic stimulation test.*

visceral pain Discomfort from cervical changes and uterine ischemia located over the lower portion of the abdomen and radiating to the lumbar area of the back and down the thighs.

VLBW See *very low birth weight (VLBW).*

von Willebrand disease (vWD) A type of hemophilia; probably the most common of all hereditary bleeding disorders.

VSE See *vulvar self-examination (VSE).*

vulva External genitalia of the female that consist of the labia majora, labia minora, clitoris, urinary meatus, and vaginal introitus.

vulvar carcinoma Cancer of the vulva.

vulvar self-examination (VSE) Systematic examination of the vulva by the woman.

vulvectomy Surgical removal of all or parts of the vulva.

complete v. Removal of the whole vulva, deep tissues, and the clitoris.

partial v. Removal of part of the vulva and deep tissues.

simple v. Removal of all of the vulva (external genital organs including the mons pubis, labia majora and minora, and possibly the clitoris). The clitoris usually can be saved if cancer is not present.

skinning v. Removal of the superficial vulvar skin; it is rarely performed.

vulvodynia Complex condition thought to be a chronic pain disorder of the vulvar area; this term is used if pain is present with no visible abnormality or no identified neurologic diagnosis.

vWD See *von Willebrand disease (vWD).*

W

walking survey Using one's senses while traveling through a community to obtain information about sociocultural characteristics and the environment, housing, transportation, and local community agencies.

warm line Telephone link between the new family and concerned caregivers or experienced parent volunteers; most often for support of newborn care and postpartum care after hospital discharge. A help line or consultation service, not a crisis intervention line.

weaning Process of changing from breastfeeding or bottle feeding to drinking from a cup.

Wharton's jelly White, gelatinous material surrounding the umbilical vessels within the cord.

witch's milk Secretion of a whitish fluid for about a week after birth from enlarged mammary tissue in the neonate, presumably resulting from maternal hormonal influences.

withdrawal (1) Physiologic or cognitive changes that occur after removal of the substance in the substance-dependent person; (2) removing penis from vagina before ejaculation (coitus interruptus).

womb See *uterus.*

X

X chromosome Sex chromosome in humans existing in duplicate in the normal female and singly in the normal male.

X linkage Genes located on the X chromosome.

X-linked dominant inheritance Mode of genetic inheritance by which a dominant gene is carried on the X chromosome.

X-linked recessive inheritance disorder Disorder for which the abnormal genes are carried on the X chromosome.

Y

Y chromosome Sex chromosome in the human male necessary for the development of the male gonads.

Z

ZIFT See *zygote intrafallopian transfer (ZIFT).*

zona pellucida Inner, thick membranous envelope of the ovum.

zygote Cell formed by the union of two reproductive cells or gametes; the fertilized ovum resulting from the union of a sperm and an ovum (egg).

zygote intrafallopian transfer (ZIFT) Similar to gamete intrafallopian transfer (GIFT) except that in ZIFT, after in vitro fertilization the ova are placed in the uterine tube during the zygote stage.

A

Abbreviations, 12, 13t
Abdomen
  distention of, 536
  newborn assessments, 556t–565t
  physical examination of, 84
  postpartum changes in, 481, 481f
  pregnancy-related changes in, 292, 293f–294f
  trauma examination, 753b
Abdominal discomfort, 304, 304f
Abdominal hysterectomy, 243f
Abdominal trauma
  blunt, 751
  penetrating, 751–752
Abduction of infants, 492
ABO incompatibility, 869–870
ABO system, 868
Abortion
  alternatives to, 192
  elective, 189. *See also* Induced abortion
  induced. *See* Induced abortion
  legalization of, 189
  spontaneous, 189, 670–675. *See also* Miscarriage; Perinatal loss
  therapeutic, 189
Abortus, 5b
Abruptio placentae
  classification of, 684
  clinical manifestations of, 681t, 684, 751b
  definition of, 683
  diagnosis of, 685
  etiology of, 683–684
  fetal outcomes of, 684–685
  incidence of, 683–684
  management of, 685
  maternal outcomes of, 684–685
  signs and symptoms of, 751b
  trauma as cause of, 751–752
Abused women
  documentation of abuse, 106, 107b
  health assessments, 79–81, 80f, 83b–84b
  history-taking, 339
  nursing interventions for, 105–109
  screenings, 79, 80f
Accelerated breast radiation, 225
Acceleration, of fetal heart rate, 416b, 423, 423b, 649–650
Acculturation, 21
Acetabular dysplasia, 885
Acid-base balance, 300, 915, 916t
Acinus, 64
Acquaintance, 508, 509f
Acquaintance rape, 109–110
Acrocyanosis, 530, 896b
Acroesthesia, 303
Acronyms, 12, 13t
Activated protein C resistance, 52–53
Activity restriction, for preterm labor, 784, 785b
Acupressure, 353f, 395–396, 395f
Acupuncture, 136, 395–396, 763, 802
Acute bilirubin encephalopathy, 538, 868, 870
Acute myelocytic leukemia, 264
Acute respiratory distress syndrome, 725–726
Adalat. *See* Nifedipine
Addiction, 74
Adenomatous polyposis coli gene, 55
Adolescent(s)
  in abusive relationships, 339
  adaptations to pregnancy, 335
  breasts in, 66t
  emotional level of, 73
  endometriosis in, 126
  father, 520
  health assessment in, 81
  health risks in, 73–74
  high-risk behaviors by, 32
  labia in, 66t
  mother, 519–520
  ovaries in, 66t
  reproductive system assessments in, 66t
  tasks for, 81
  uterus in, 66t
  vagina in, 66t
  as vulnerable population, 32
Adolescent pregnancy
  description of, 73–74
  grieving in, 947–948
  incidence of, 360
  intimate partner violence during, 103
  nursing care plan for, 361b
  nutritional needs during, 75, 319
  prenatal care, 360
  prevalence of, 9
  prevention of, 360
  substance abuse during, 767
Adoption, 208–209
Adrenal glands, 305
Advance directives, 82, 251b
Advil. *See* Ketoprofen
Aerobic exercise, 76
African-Americans
  childbearing beliefs, 26t–27t
  foods popular with, 326t–327t
  infant mortality rate in, 5–6
  intimate partner violence in, 102
  low-birth-weight infants, 5
  pain responses, 388b
  parenting beliefs, 26t–27t
  pica in, 318
Afterload, 740, 741f
Afterpains, 479
Aging, 82
Agranulocytosis, 706
Airway maintenance, 570–571
Airway obstruction
  in newborn, 599b
  in pregnant woman, 719
Alcohol use and abuse
  breast cancer risks, 215
  during breastfeeding, 626
  counseling about, 92
  description of, 75
  fetal effects of, 857–858, 857t
  maternal, 9, 351–352, 626, 638b, 761–762, 856f, 857–858, 858b
  during pregnancy, 351–352, 626, 638b, 761–762, 856f, 857–858, 858b
Alcohol use and abuse *(Continued)*
  sexual violence concerns, 110
  treatment for, 766
Alcoholics Anonymous, 766
Alcohol-related birth defects, 857, 858b
Alcohol-related neurodevelopmental disorders, 857, 858b
Aldomet. *See* Methyldopa
Aldosterone, 305
Alendronate sodium, 139, 140b
Alkalosis, 738
Alleles, 47
Allen's test, 744, 745b
Allodynia, 245
Alpha-fetoprotein, 641, 648–649, 699
Alternative therapies. *See* Complementary and alternative therapies
Ambiguous genitalia, 541, 887–888, 887f
Ambivalence, 331
Ambulation
  in labor, 452–453, 452f
  postpartum, 496
Ambulatory settings, 7
Amenorrhea, 120–121, 196
American Nurses Association *Health System Reform Agenda*, 1
Amniocentesis
  genetic testing uses of, 645–647
  indications for, 645–647, 871
  ultrasonography with, 642
Amnioinfusion, 429
Amnion, 274
Amniotic fluid
  analysis of, 646t
  assessment of, in first stage of labor, 448
  description of, 275–276
  fetal ingestion of, 281
  meconium-stained, 817, 817b
  volume of, 643
Amniotic fluid index, 643
Amniotic infection syndrome, 147
Amniotic membranes
  assessment of, in first stage of labor, 448
  stripping or sweeping of, for induction of labor, 801
Amniotomy, 802–803, 803b
Amphetamine, 763, 857t
Amylase, 535–536
Anal incontinence, 482
Analgesia and anesthesia, 397–408
  care management for, 408–412, 408b
  cesarean birth, 810
  circumcision, 587–588
  combined spinal-epidural, 406
  definitions, 398
  epidural. *See* Epidural anesthesia
  general, 407–408, 407f
  informed consent for, 408
  local, 400–401
  local perineal infiltration, 400–401
  maternal monitoring during, 412
  nerve block, 400–407
  nitrous oxide, 407
  nursing interventions for, 411b
Analgesia and anesthesia *(Continued)*
  opioid agonist analgesics, 398–399, 398b–399b
  opioid agonist-antagonist analgesics, 399–400, 399b
  opioid antagonists, 400, 400b
  patient-controlled
    description of, 248
    labor-related pain managed with, 398
  pudendal nerve block, 401, 401f
  regional, 411–412
  safety concerns, 412
  spinal. *See* Spinal anesthesia
  systemic, 398–400
Anaphylactoid syndrome of pregnancy, 820–821, 820b
Anaphylaxis, 410
Anaprox. *See* Naproxen sodium
Androgens, 205b
Android pelvis, 374, 376t
Anemia, 720–722
  definition of, 720
  folate deficiency, 721
  iron deficiency, 314, 720–721
  physiologic, 298
  in pregnancy, 720–722
  sickle cell, 721–722, 721b
Anencephaly, 876–877
Anesthesia. *See* Analgesia and anesthesia
Aneuploidy, 49
Angiomas, 301–302
Angiotensin-converting enzyme inhibitors, 716t
Anhydramnios, 429
Ankle clonus, 661, 661f
Ankyloglossia, 628
Anorexia nervosa, 75–76
Anovulation, 67, 131, 195–196, 481
Anovulatory bleeding, 121
Antabuse. *See* Disulfiram
Antenatal glucocorticoids, for fetal lung maturity, 790, 790b
Antepartum testing, 639, 639b
Anthropoid pelvis, 374, 376t
Anthropometric measurements, 321
Antibiotics, 572–573
Anticipatory grief, 913, 927
Anticipatory guidance, 88–93
Anticoagulant therapy, 714, 833
Anticonvulsant medications, 727–728
Antidepressant medications, 626, 758–759, 758t, 769–770, 776
Antihypertensive medications, 666, 666t
Antineoplastic drugs, 250
Antioxidants, 90
Antipsychotic medications, 760–761, 770t
Antiretroviral therapy, 158–159, 608
Antiviral medications
  genital herpes simplex virus managed with, 154
  human immunodeficiency virus treated with, 159
Anus, imperforate, 884, 884f
Anxiety
  grief and, 933
  pain-related, 388

Page numbers followed by "f" denote figures; "t," tables; "b," boxes.

Anxiety disorders
postpartum onset of, 775–776
during pregnancy, 759–761, 760t
Aortic stenosis, 712, 875f
Apgar score, 554–555, 554t, 555b
Apical pulse, 296, 531
Appendicitis, 304, 304f, 732
Appetite, 303, 482
Appropriate for gestational age, 569, 895b
Apresoline. *See* Hydralazine
Arachidonic acid, 610
Areola
pigmentation of, 64, 484
pregnancy-related changes in, 295–296
Areola-sparing mastectomy, 223
Arm recoil, 568
Arnold-Chiari malformation, 877
Aromatase inhibitors, 226
Aromatherapy, 396–397
Arousal, 69
Arterial blood gases, 738
Arterial pressure catheter, 744–745, 746f
Artificial sweeteners, 314, 315b
Asherman syndrome, 127, 197
Asian-Americans
childbearing beliefs, 26t–27t
parenting beliefs, 26t–27t
Asians, 103
Aspartame, 314
Assault, sexual. *See* Sexual assault
Assessments
community
data collection for, 29–30
definition of, 29–34
health data sources for, 29–30, 30f
family, 19, 22f
health. *See* Health assessment
home care, 36–37, 38f
newborn. *See* Newborn, assessment of
Assimilation, 21
Assisted reproductive therapies, 206–208
Association of Women's Health, Obstetric and Neonatal Nurses, 9, 10b
abortion and, 190
home care as defined by, 35
standards of practice, 11–12, 12b, 35
Asthma, 722, 723t, 723b
Asymptomatic bacteriuria, 730–731, 731b
Asynclitism, 381, 382f
Atenolol, 716t
Atrial fibrillation, 711
Atrial septal defect, 710, 875f
Atrioventricular canal defect, 875f
Attachment
behaviors associated with, 510, 510b
parental, 507–510, 508f, 508t
in prenatal period, 332
Attitude, fetal, 370, 372f
Atypical squamous cells, 253, 253b
Auditory brainstem response, 579, 579f
Auscultation, intermittent, 416–418, 418f, 418b
Autoimmune disorders, 728–729
Autopsy, 940–941
Autosomal dominant disorders, 52–53, 56
Autosomal recessive disorders, 53
Autosomes
abnormalities of, 48–51
definition of, 47
number of, 271
Axillary node dissection, 230b
Axillary temperature, 555
Azithromycin, 147

B

Babinski sign, 546t–549t
Baby Friendly Hospital Initiative, 609
Bacteremia, 792
Bacterial endocarditis, 711b
Bacterial vaginosis, 159–161, 160t
Balanced translocation, 51
Ballottement, 294, 295f, 330
Baptism, 945
Barbiturates, 397
Barlow test, 544, 544b, 885
Barotrauma, 903
Barr body, 890
Bartholin cysts, 244–245
Bartholin glands, 61, 61f
Basal body temperature, 69, 174, 174f, 198–200
Basal metabolic rate, 298–300
Basic care, 7
Bathing of newborn, 595–597, 596f, 596b–597b
Battered woman syndrome, 101t
Batterer, 98b
Battery, 95
Battledore placenta, 277, 685, 686f
Bearing down, 377, 464–466
Bed rest, 784, 784b–785b
Bell palsy, 728
Benzodiazepines
anxiety treated with, 759–760, 760t
pain management using, 397
postpartum use of, 775
Bereavement, 932, 942. *See also* Grief
Beta thalassemia, 722
Beta-adrenergic agents, 717
$Beta_2$-adrenergic agonists, 786, 787b–789b
Betamethasone, 790b
Bethesda system, 253, 253b
Biceps reflex, 660–661, 661f
Bicornuate uterus, 197f
Bile, 281
Bilirubin, 281, 575, 575f
Bimanual palpation, 86, 88f
Binge eating disorder, 76
Biochemical testing, 45
Biofeedback, 396
Bioidentical hormones, 136
Biologic marker methods, of contraception, 174–175, 176f
Biophysical profile, 643–644, 643t–644t, 682–683
Bioprosthetic heart valves, 713
Biopsy
breast, 220, 220f
cervical, 253
core needle, 220, 220f
endometrial, 201
sentinel node, 230, 261
Biorhythmicity, 512
Biotinidase deficiency, 578t
Biparietal diameter, 370, 372f–373f, 641
Birth. *See* Childbirth; Preterm birth
Birth ball, 453, 453f
Birth canal, 371
Birth centers, 365–366, 366f
Birth control, 169. *See also* Contraception; Contraceptives
Birth outcomes, 74
Birth plans, 365, 438, 438b
Birth rate, 5, 5b
Birth trauma, 574, 693, 837–841
anatomic classification of, 838t
avoidance of, 837–838
central nervous system, 841
clavicle fracture, 839–840, 839f, 843
definition of, 837
ecchymoses, 838, 839f
Erb's palsy, 817, 840, 840f
facial paralysis, 840, 840f
incidence of, 837
nursing process for, 842b
peripheral nervous system, 840–841, 840f
petechiae, 838
phrenic nerve injury, 840–841
predisposing factors, 838
retinal hemorrhage, 838
skeletal, 839–840, 839f
skull fractures, 839
soft-tissue injuries, 838–839, 839f
subarachnoid hemorrhage, 841
subconjunctival hemorrhage, 838
subdural hemorrhage, 841
subgaleal hemorrhage, 838–839
Birthing bed, 463f–464f, 464
Birthing chairs, 462–463
Birthing room, 465–467, 466f
Birthing stools, 463
Birthing table, 465, 465f
Bishop score, 800, 800t
Bisphenol A, 631b
Bisphosphonates, 139, 140b
Black cohosh, 136
Bladder. *See also* Genitourinary system
distention of, 493–494
exstrophy of, 887, 887f
postpartum changes in, 482, 493–494
Bladder infection, 731
Blastocyst, 273
Bleeding, 670–680
abruptio placentae
classification of, 684
clinical manifestations of, 681t, 684
definition of, 683
diagnosis of, 685
etiology of, 683–684
fetal outcomes of, 684–685
incidence of, 683–684
management of, 685
maternal outcomes of, 684–685
ectopic pregnancy. *See* Ectopic pregnancy
menstrual. *See* Menstrual bleeding
miscarriage as cause of. *See* Miscarriage
placenta previa, 680–683
clinical manifestations of, 680–681, 681t
diagnosis of, 682
etiology of, 680
fetal outcomes of, 681–682
home care for, 683
incidence of, 680
Bleeding *(Continued)*
management of, 682–683
maternal outcomes of, 681–682
nursing process for, 682b
types of, 681f
postpartum. *See* Postpartum hemorrhage
standard of care for, 831b
Blood. *See also* Hematologic system
composition of
postpartum changes, 483–484
pregnancy-related changes, 297–298
postpartal loss of, 493b
volume of
newborn, 532
postpartum changes, 483
pregnancy-related changes, 297–298, 737
Blood groups, 868
Blood pressure
labor-related changes, 383
measurement of, 297b
in newborn, 532
postpartum changes, 483t
pregnancy-related changes, 297
Blood replacement therapy, 831–832
Blood tests, 446–448
Blood types, 868
Blood urea nitrogen, 482
Bloody show, 437
Blunt trauma
abdominal, 751
thoracic, 751
Bochdalek diaphragmatic defect, 880f
Body language, 78
Body mass index, 75, 309, 319, 435
Body mechanics, 346–349, 348f
Body temperature
in newborn
assessment of, 555
discharge teaching about, 591
maintenance of, 571–572
phototherapy effects on, 585
postpartum changes, 483t
in preterm infant, 896, 899–901
Bonding, 507–510, 510b
Bone density testing, 133
Bone ossification, 283
Bony pelvis, 63, 63f, 372–374, 373f
Bowel elimination, 451–452
Bra, 350
Brachial plexus injury, 840
Brachioradial reflex, 661f
Brachytherapy, 225
Bradycardia, 422, 422t, 423f, 741
Braxton Hicks contractions, 279, 293, 354t–355t, 378
Brazelton Neonatal Behavioral Assessment Scale, 545, 545b
BRCA1/BRCA2
carriers of, 55
genetic testing for, 47
hereditary breast and ovarian cancer risks, 55, 214
Breakthrough bleeding, 128
Breast(s)
acinus of, 64
anatomy of, 64–65, 64f
distention of, 482
engorgement of, 495, 499, 625, 627–628, 627b, 628f
examination recommendations for, 89t

Breast(s) *(Continued)*
lactating, 611–613, 612f
lymphatic system of, 64
menstrual-related changes in, 64–65
physical examination of, 82, 83b–84b
postmenopausal changes in, 66t
postpartum changes in, 482
pregnancy-related changes in, 295–296
self-examination, 65, 65b–66b
stimulation of, for labor induction, 801–802
swelling of, in newborn, 541
vascular supply to, 64
Breast biopsy, 220, 220f
Breast cancer
alcohol consumption and, 215
biopsy evaluations, 220, 220f
chemoprevention of, 217
cigarette smoking and, 215
clinical manifestations of, 217–220
diagnosis of, 217–220, 220f, 228–232
dietary factors, 215
diethylstilbestrol and, 214
ductal carcinoma, 217
emotional support after diagnosis of, 228–232
etiologic factors, 214–215
family history of, 214
genetic risks, 216–217, 216b
hereditary, 54–55, 214
incidence of, 9, 214, 215f
inflammatory, 217
invasive, 217
lesion sites, 218f
lifestyle factors, 214
lymphatic spread of, 220–221, 221f
magnetic resonance imaging screenings, 220
mammography detection of, 9, 218–220, 218f
menopausal hormonal therapy and, 215
metastasis of, 217, 218t, 220–221, 221f
nursing care for, 228–233, 230b
nursing process for, 229b
obesity and, 215
pathophysiology of, 217
physical inactivity and, 215
during pregnancy, 263
prognosis for, 220–221
race and, 214, 215f
radiation treatment of, 225, 231–232
risk factors for, 214, 217, 217b
screening for, 218, 219b–220b
smoking and, 215
staging of, 218t
surgical treatment of, 221–223, 222f
axillary node dissection, 230b
discharge planning, 231
exercises after, 230, 231b
follow-up after, 230
lumpectomy, 221–222, 222f, 229–230, 263
lymph node dissection, 231b
mastectomy, 221–223, 222f
nursing care plan, 230b
partial mastectomy, 221–222, 222f
postoperative care, 228–231
Breast cancer *(Continued)*
preoperative care, 228
reconstruction after, 223–225, 224t–225t, 232b
sentinel node identification, 222
wound management, 229
treatment of
adjuvant systemic therapy, 225–228, 226b–227b, 231–232
chemotherapy, 225–228, 227b, 232
decision-making questions for, 221b
hormonal therapy, 226
radiation, 225, 231–232
surgical. *See* Breast cancer, surgical treatment of
Breast conditions
benign, 211–214
collaborative care for, 213–214
fibroadenomas, 212, 213t
fibrocystic changes, 211–212, 213t
intraductal papilloma, 213, 213t
lipoma, 213t
macromastia, 213
mammary duct ectasia, 213, 213t
micromastia, 213
nipple discharge, 212
macrocalcifications, 219–220
malignant. *See* Breast cancer
microcalcifications, 220
Breast implants, 215, 224t–225t
Breast milk
banking of, 625
cytomegalovirus transmission through, 852
description of, 610
expressing of, 622–623
frozen, 623
heating of, 623b
microwaving of, 623b
mood-stabilizing medications in, 775
nutrients in, 606, 610–611, 847
preterm infant feeding with, 906, 908
storage of, 622–623, 624b
uniqueness of, 613
Breast pumps, 622–623, 623f
Breast reconstruction, 223–225, 224t–225t, 232b
Breast self-examination, 65, 65b–66b
Breast shells, 346, 346f, 625, 626f
Breast surgery, 626
Breast-conserving surgery, 230b
Breastfeeding. *See also* Lactation
alcohol use during, 626
benefits of, 607, 608t
breast care during, 625
after breast surgery, 626
calcium intake during, 315–316
concerns during, 627–629
contraception and, 189, 626
contraindications, 608, 708
cultural influences on, 607, 609–610
definition of, 606
demand feeding, 616–617
duration of feedings, 617
effectiveness of, 617, 617b
by employed mothers, 623–624
food guide during, 313t
Breastfeeding *(Continued)*
frequency of feedings, 616–617
fussy baby, 619, 620b
Healthy People 2010 recommendations, 607
human immunodeficiency virus contraindications, 608, 851
ineffective, 620, 620b
insulin requirements during, 690, 700
jaundice related to, 538–539, 621
latch, 615–616, 616f
late preterm infants, 622
methadone use during, 859
mothers
concerns of, 627–629
follow-up, 629
maternal care during, 625–627
medication use by, 626–627, 774–775
monilial infections in, 628–629
reflexes in, 612f
substance abuse by, 767
multiple infants, 622, 622f
nipple soreness during, 628–629
nursing care plan for, 618b
nursing process for, 614b
obesity effects on, 324–325
oxytocin's role in, 612–613
pacifier use during, 618–619
phenylketonuria contraindications, 708
plugged milk ducts during, 629
positioning for, 614–615, 615f
during pregnancy, 626
preparation for, 345–346
preterm infants, 621–622, 906
promotion of, 499
psychotropic medication use during, 774–775
rates of, 607
recommendations for, 345, 607
removing infant from breast, 616f
resources for, 634b
selective serotonin reuptake inhibitor use during, 775
sexual stimulations during, 625
sleepy baby, 619, 620b
slow weight gain by newborn during, 620–621
smoking during, 626–627, 767
substance abuse during, 767, 862
supplemental feeding during, 617–619, 619b, 621f
support for, 607–609, 609b
thiazide diuretics effect on, 718
weaning, 624–625
weight loss during, 625
in workplace, 624
Breast-milk jaundice, 539, 621
Breathing. *See also* Respiratory system
modified-paced, 392–393, 393b
monitoring of, in second stage of labor, 464
paced techniques of, 392–393, 393b
patterned-paced, 393, 393b
periodic, 896
slow-paced, 392–393, 393b
techniques of, for labor-related pain, 392–393, 393b
Breech presentation, 370, 372f, 795–796, 795f, 838, 839f
Bronchopulmonary dysplasia, 917
Brow presentation, of fetus, 796
Brown fat, 534, 922
Bulb syringe, 570f, 570b
Bulimia nervosa, 76
Buprenorphine, 859
Burial cradle, 946, 946f
Burping, 631f
Butorphanol tartrate, 399, 399b
Butterfly needle, 580f

C

CA-125, 250
Café-au-lait spots, 52
Caffeine, 314, 314t, 627, 638b, 762, 861
CAGE questionnaire, 764b
Calan. *See* Verapamil
Calcitonin, 139
Calcium
for amenorrhea in female athlete triad patients, 121
daily intake of, 90, 121
deficiency of, 75
food sources of, 317b
osteoporosis prevention with, 133, 139
pregnancy intake of, 310t–311t, 315–316, 317b
Calendar-rhythm method, of contraception, 172
Cancer
breast. *See* Breast cancer
cervical. *See* Cervical cancer
colon. *See* Colon cancer
cultural influences on meaning of, 247b
endometrial. *See* Endometrial cancer
environmental factors, 54
gene mutations that cause, 54
genomics of, 54–55
metastasis of, 266
oncogenes and, 54
ovarian. *See* Ovarian cancer
during pregnancy, 264, 265–266
thyroid, 264
treatment of
chemotherapy. *See* Chemotherapy
fertility effects, 266
during pregnancy, 265–266
radiation. *See* Radiation therapy
tumor suppressor genes and, 54
uterine, 265
uterine tube, 262–263, 265
vaginal, 262, 265
vulvar, 260–266
Candida albicans, 161, 855
Candidiasis
newborn, 855–856
oral, 855
vulvovaginal, 160–161, 160t
Capacitation, 273
Capillary hydrostatic pressure, 738
Caput succedaneum, 542–543, 543f, 574, 838
Car seat, 594–595, 594b
Carbohydrates
dietary requirement, 610
infant requirements, 610
metabolism of, 537
Carboprost tromethamine, 674
Cardiac decompensation, 714, 714b, 718
Cardiac disease, 710, 710b

Cardiac output, 739–741
afterload, 740, 741f
definition of, 739, 748
description of, 298, 483, 719, 750
determinants of, 740–741, 740f
maternal position effects on, 739–740, 740t
noninvasive assessments of, 829b
normal, 748t
prepregnancy range of, 739, 750
thermodilution procedure for measuring, 746, 746b
Cardiogenic pulmonary edema, 749
Cardiomyopathy
hypertrophic, 844
in infants of mothers with diabetes mellitus, 844
peripartum, 713
Cardiopulmonary resuscitation
during labor, 821
of newborn, 597, 600b
parental teaching, 926
of pregnant woman, 719, 719b, 720f
Cardiopulmonary system, 739, 739f
Cardiovascular system. *See also* Heart
congenital anomalies of, 873–876, 874t, 875f. *See also* Congenital heart defects and disease
labor-related adaptations, 383
maternal disorders of, 709–719
aortic stenosis, 712
atrial septal defect, 710
bioprosthetic valves, 713
cardiac decompensation, 714, 714b, 718
care management for, 714–719
coarctation of the aorta, 710–711
Eisenmenger syndrome, 713
emergencies, 717b
heart transplantation, 714
incidence of, 709–710
infective endocarditis, 713
intrapartum management of, 716–718
ischemic heart disease, 712
Marfan syndrome, 712–713
mechanical prosthetic valves, 713
mitral valve prolapse, 711–712
mitral valve stenosis, 711
myocardial infarction, 712
nursing care plan for, 717b
nursing process for, 715b
patent ductus arteriosus, 710
peripartum cardiomyopathy, 713
postpartum management of, 718–719
primary pulmonary hypertension, 712
risk groups, 710b
tetralogy of Fallot, 711
valve replacement, 713
ventricular septal defect, 710
newborn adaptations, 530–532, 531t
postpartum changes, 483–484, 718–719
pregnancy-related adaptations, 296–298, 299t, 737, 738t, 750t
preterm infant, 896
Carpal tunnel syndrome, 303, 354t–355t
Carrier screening
cystic fibrosis, 45–46
description of, 45
Carriers, 53
Casein, 611
Cataflam. *See* Diclofenac
Catheter
arterial pressure, 744–745, 746f
intrauterine pressure, 793
nasopharyngeal, 570b
pulmonary artery. *See* Pulmonary artery catheter
Caudal regression syndrome, 842
Celecoxib (Celebrex), 122t
Census, 29
CenteringPregnancy, 336–337
Centers for Disease Control Standard Precautions, 40
Centers for Medicare & Medicaid Services, 4
Central nervous system
birth trauma to, 841
congenital anomalies of, 876–879, 877f
in preterm infant, 897
Central venous pressure lines, 747–748
Cephalhematoma, 542–543, 543f, 574, 838
Cephalic presentation, 370, 371f
Cephalopelvic disproportion, 794
Cerclage, cervical, 675, 676f
Certified midwives, 8
Certified nurse-midwives, 8, 364
Cervical cancer, 251–254
age of onset, 252
care management of, 254–260
chemotherapy for, 255, 260
clinical manifestations of, 252–254
complementary and alternative therapies for, 255b
cryosurgery for, 255–256
diagnosis of, 252–254, 263–264
etiology of, 251–252
FIGO classification of, 252t
human papillomavirus and, 252
incidence of, 251–252
invasive, 251–252, 264
laser ablation of, 256
loop electrosurgical excision procedure for, 253–254, 253f, 256, 256f
medical management of, 254–260
microinvasive, 251–252
Papanicolaou test for, 253, 263–264
pelvic exenteration for, 259–260, 260f
during pregnancy, 263–264
radiation therapy for, 254b, 256–259, 257f, 258b–259b
radical hysterectomy for, 255–256
recurrent, 259–260, 260f
surgical management of, 254–260
Cervical cap, 180–181, 180b
Cervical edema, 794
Cervical intraepithelial neoplasia, 251
Cervical mucus
functions of, 197
oral contraceptives effect on, 181
ovulation-detection method, 173–174, 173b
plug formation, 295, 295f
Cervical os, 62, 480
Cervical ripening
Bishop score for, 800, 800t
chemical agents for, 800
description of, 378
hydroscopic dilators for, 800–801
mechanical methods of, 800–802
methods of, 800–803
prostaglandin E_1 for, 800, 801b
Cervidil Insert. *See* Dinoprostone
Cervix
anatomy of, 62–63, 62f
assessment of, 81
biopsy of, 253
cerclage of, 675, 676f
colposcopy of, 253, 253f
dilation of
in labor, 377–378, 377f, 439t, 447f
recurrent premature, 675–676, 676f
effacement of, 376–377, 377f, 447f
funneling of, 675
incompetent, 675–676, 676f
lacerations of, 470, 826
length of, as preterm labor indicator, 781
postpartum changes in, 480
pregnancy-related changes in, 293–294, 295f
ripening of. *See* Cervical ripening
squamous epithelium of, 63
Cesarean birth, 807–814
accidental lacerations to neonate during, 838
anesthesia for, 810
complications of, 810, 833
definition of, 807–808
discharge after, 814, 814b
elective, 809–810, 809b
emergency, 837–838
epidural anesthesia for, 406. *See also* Epidural anesthesia
forced, 810
incidence of, 8, 808
incisions for, 810, 810f
indications for, 809, 809b
infection after, 833
intraoperative care for, 812, 812f
maternal reactions to, 811
pain management for, 398b
perimortem, 754
postoperative care for, 812–814, 813f, 813b
postpartum care, 813–814
in pregestational diabetes mellitus, 699
prenatal preparation of, 811
preoperative care for, 811–812
prevention of, 808b
purpose of, 808
risk factors for, 808
risks associated with, 810
scheduled, 810–811
spinal anesthesia for, 401, 402f
surgical techniques for, 810, 810f
unplanned, 811
vaginal birth after, 8, 364, 808, 808b, 815, 815b
Cesarean hysterectomy, 826
Chadwick sign, 295
Chain of custody, 114
Change, 766–767
Chemocautery, 206
Chemotherapy
breast cancer treated with, 225–228, 227b, 232
cervical cancer treated with, 255, 260
endometrial cancer treated with, 247, 247t
fetal effects of, 265
gynecologic cancers treated with, 247t
nursing care for, 248
during pregnancy, 264–265
side effects of, 232, 247t
vulvar cancer treated with, 261
Chest, 556t–565t, 753b
Chickenpox. *See* Varicella-zoster
Childbearing
beliefs and practices, cultural influences on, 24–27, 26t–27t, 27b
health promotion in, 28
Childbearing history, 338
Childbirth. *See also* Labor
abuse after, 107
birth plans, 365
cesarean. *See* Cesarean birth
complications of, 797b
cultural influences on, 439–441, 440b
education about, 363–367
emergencies during
anaphylactoid syndrome of pregnancy, 820–821, 820b
meconium-stained amniotic fluid, 817, 817b
shoulder dystocia, 817–818, 839f
umbilical cord prolapse, 818–819, 819f, 819b
uterine rupture, 819–820
emergency, 462b
environment for, 389
evidence-based practices, 455b
forceps-assisted, 806–807, 806f, 806t, 838
home, 366–367
hospital discharge after, 8
maternal death during, 755
perineal trauma, 470–471
positions for, 378, 379f, 430, 452–453, 452f–453f, 455b, 460–464, 461f, 463f
positive experience during, 433
preparation for
classes, 28, 392
maternal, 332–333
methods, 391
paternal, 334–335
preterm. *See* Preterm birth
primary health care providers for, 364–365, 365b
settings for, 365–367, 366f, 389
siblings during, 457
sociocultural context of, 502
Standard Precautions during, 442b
trauma to neonate during. *See* Birth trauma
trends in, 7–8
vacuum-assisted, 806t, 807, 807f, 807b, 838
vaginal. *See* Vaginal birth
vertex presentation, 466–467, 467f
Chinese culture, 326t–327t, 388b
Chlamydia, 146–147, 148t–149t, 162t, 855
Chlamydia trachomatis, 146, 848, 855
Chloasma, 301, 484

Choanal atresia, 879, 879f
Cholecystitis, 730
Cholelithiasis, 730
Cholesterol screening, 89t
Chorioamnionitis, 791–792, 855
Chorion, 274
Chorionic villi, 273–274, 277
Chorionic villus sampling, 647–648, 647f
Chromosomal abnormalities, 48–52
  aneuploidy, 49
  autosomal, 48–51
  incidence of, 48
  polyploidy, 49
  screening for, 344, 649
  sex chromosomes, 51–52
  structure-based, 51
  trisomy. *See* Down syndrome; Trisomy
Chromosomes, 47–48
  definition of, 45, 47
  haploid number of, 49
  homologous, 47, 271
  illustration of, 48f
  number of, 47
  S, 47–48, 283
  sex. *See* Sex chromosomes
  structural abnormalities of, 51
  X, 47–48, 283
  Y. *See* Y chromosome
Chronic hypertension, 656, 668
  definition of, 656
  with preeclampsia, 656
  pregestational diabetes mellitus and, 691
Chronosystem, 99, 100f
Circulatory system
  fetal, 279–280, 280f, 284t–286t, 532
  maternal, 739, 739f
Circumcision, 586–589
  benefits of, 586
  care management after, 588, 588b
  pain management for, 587–588
  positioning for, 587f
  prevalence of, 586
  reasons for, 586
  technique for, 587, 587f
Circumcision, female, 8–9, 73b
Claiming process, 508
Clarification, 78
Clavicle fracture, 544, 839–840, 839f
Clean-catch urine specimen, 343–344
Cleavage, 273
Cleft lip and palate, 880–881, 881f–882f
Client care standards, 736b
Climacteric, 69, 130
Clitoris, 61, 61f
Clomiphene citrate, 200, 205b
Clothing
  maternal, 350, 350f, 359
  newborn, 594, 594f
Clotting disorders, 685–686, 686b
Clubfoot, 544–545, 886
Coagulation
  in newborn, 539
  in pregnancy, 298, 299t
Coagulation factors, 281, 483, 577b
Coagulopathies, 832
Coarctation of the aorta
  maternal, 710–711
  newborn, 874, 875f
Cocaine, 763, 857t, 860b
Cochrane Pregnancy and Childbirth Database, 9–10
Coffee, 314, 314t
Cognitive restructuring, 331
Cognitive-behavioral therapy, 776
Cohabiting-parent family, 18–19
Coitus interruptus, 171
Cold stress, 534, 534f, 896, 897b, 922
Cold therapy, 396
Colic, 601
Colloid osmotic pressure, 657–658, 738
Colon cancer, 55
  adenomatous polyposis coli gene associated with, 55
  familial adenomatous polyposis, 54–55
  gene mutations associated with, 55
  hereditary nonpolyposis, 55, 246
  incidence of, 55
  in pregnancy, 264
  screening for, 89t
Colostrum, 482, 613, 626
Colporrhaphy, 238
Colposcopy, 253, 253f, 262
Combined estrogen-progestin contraceptives, 181–183
Combined spinal-epidural analgesia, 406
Comfort, 494–496
Commitment, psychiatric, 773b
Communication
  cultural considerations, 24, 79
  parent-infant, 511–512
  preterm infant, 911–912
  situation, background, assessment recommendation technique for, 13
  variations in, 79b
Community
  postpartum support resources, 505, 507b
  vulnerable populations in. *See* Vulnerable populations
  walking survey of, 30, 31b
Community assessment
  data collection for, 29–30
  definition of, 29–34
  health data sources for, 29–30, 30f
Community health
  indicators of, 29
  resources of, 29
Community health care
  access to, 29
  definition of, 7
  focus of, 18
  health departments, 29
Community-based health promotion, 28
  best practices for, 28
  preventive care levels in, 28
Complementary and alternative therapies. *See also* Herbal therapies
  cervical cancer treated with, 255b
  dysmenorrhea managed with, 123, 123t
  integrative health care use of, 3
  menopausal symptoms managed with, 136–137
  menstrual disorders managed with, 123, 123t
  pain management using, 390b
  during pregnancy, 351b
  types of, 3
Complementary feedings, 632–634
Complete blood count, 299t
Complete miscarriage, 671f, 672, 672t
Complicated grief, 948
Conception, 270–273
  cell division in, 270–271
  definition of, 270
  fertilization, 172, 273, 273f
  gametogenesis, 271–273, 271f–272f
  implantation, 273, 275f
  ovum. *See* Ovum
  sperm. *See* Sperm
Condom
  composition of, 177f, 181t
  failure rate for, 176
  female, 145, 176–177, 177f
  illustration of, 177f
  impediments to use of, 145–146
  natural skin, 176
  sexually transmitted infection prevention using, 145, 175
  technique for, 177b
  woman's suggestion for use of, 145–146
Conduction, 533
Condylomata acuminata, 849. *See also* Human papillomavirus
Condylomata lata, 152
Congenital adrenal hyperplasia, 578t, 816
Congenital anomalies, 873–879
  ambiguous genitalia, 887–888, 887f
  bladder exstrophy, 887, 887f
  cardiovascular system, 873–876
  care management of, 888–891
  central nervous system, 876–879, 877f
  cleft lip and palate, 880–881, 881f–882f
  cytogenetic studies for, 889–890
  definition of, 873
  epispadias, 886–887
  esophageal atresia, 881–883, 882f
  family support, 891
  gastrointestinal obstruction, 883–884
  gastrointestinal system, 880–884, 881f–884f
  gastroschisis, 883, 883f
  genetic diagnosis of, 888–889
  genitourinary system, 886–888, 887f
  hydrocephalus, 878
  hypospadias, 886–887, 887f
  imperforate anus, 884, 884f
  incidence of, 873
  microencephaly, 879
  musculoskeletal system, 884–886
  neural tube defects. *See* Neural tube defects
  nursing process for, 890–891, 890b
  omphalocele, 883, 883f
  parent support, 891
  perinatal diagnosis of, 888
  postnatal diagnosis of, 888
  prenatal diagnosis of, 888
  respiratory system, 879–880, 879f–880f
  tracheoesophageal atresia, 881–883, 882f
  types of, 873
Congenital diaphragmatic hernia, 879–880
Congenital heart defects and disease, 532
  classification of, 874, 874t
  coarctation of the aorta, 710–711, 874, 875f
  contraceptive counseling for women with, 718
  definition of, 873
  in Down syndrome, 49
  etiology of, 874
  genetic factors, 874
  illustration of, 875f
  maternal, 710–711
  risk factors for, 874
  signs and symptoms of, 875
  tetralogy of Fallot, 711, 873–874, 875f
  ventricular septal defect, 710, 873–874, 875f
Congenital hypothyroidism, 578t, 889
Congenital rubella syndrome, 851
Congenital syphilis, 848
Conization, 253–254, 253f
Conjoined twins, 286–287, 287f
Conjunctivitis, chlamydial, 855
Conscious relaxation, 349, 349b
Consent. *See* Informed consent
Constipation, 304, 325, 354t–355t
Consumers, 8–9
Continuous positive airway pressure, 902, 903f, 903t
Continuous subcutaneous insulin infusion, 697
Contraception, 169, 700
  barrier methods of, 175–181, 177f, 177b–179b
  basal body temperature method of, 174, 174f
  biologic marker methods of, 174–175, 176f
  breastfeeding and, 189, 626
  calendar-rhythm method of, 172
  in cancer survivors, 266
  cervical mucus ovulation-detection method of, 173–174, 173b
  coitus interruptus method of, 171
  definition of, 169
  discussions about, 170
  emergency, 170b, 184–185, 185t, 185b
  fertility awareness methods, 171–181, 172b
  future trends in, 189
  health promotion application to, 71, 72b
  hormonal methods of, 181–184
    combined estrogen-progestin contraceptives, 181–183
    progestin-only, 183–184
    transdermal system, 183, 183f
    vaginal contraceptive ring, 183, 183f
  informed consent for, 169, 170b
  lactational amenorrhea method of, 189
  Marquette Model of, 175
  multidisciplinary approach to, 169
  nursing care plan for, 171b
  nursing process for, 170b
  postpartum, 503
  Standard Days Method of, 172, 172f
  sterilization. *See* Sterilization
  symptoms-based methods of, 173–174
  symptothermal method of, 174, 175f
  TwoDay Method of, 173

Contraceptives
- barrier types of, 175–181, 177f, 177b–179b
- cervical cap, 180–181, 180b
- condom. *See* Condom
- counseling about, 171f
- diaphragm, 177–180, 177f, 178b–179b
- effectiveness of, 170, 171b
- failure of, 170
- intrauterine devices, 185–186, 185f, 186b
- oral. *See* Oral contraceptives
- progestin-only, 183–184, 729
- spermicides, 175–181, 176f
- sponge, 181

Contractility, 740–741
Contraction stress test, 651–652, 652f, 652b
Contractions. *See* Uterine contractions
Controlled emotions, 110–111
Convection, 533
Coombs' test, 649, 871
Cooper's ligaments, 64, 625
Coping
- facilitation of, 943
- intimate partner violence, 104
- mechanisms of, 339
- stress, 133

Cord. *See* Umbilical cord
Cordocentesis, 648
Core needle biopsy, 220, 220f
Coronary heart disease
- menopausal risks, 134
- risk factors for, 134

Corpus luteum, 67
Cortisol, 110
Cost containment, 4
Costovertebral angle, 834
Cough reflex, 570
Coumadin. *See* Warfarin
Counseling
- alcohol use, 92
- genetic. *See* Genetic counseling
- human immunodeficiency virus, 157, 157b
- nutritional, 88–90
- preconception, 70, 71b
- sexually transmitted infections, 146b

Counterpressure, 393
Couple. *See also* Father; Mother
- adolescent, 519b
- lesbian, 521
- parenthood adjustment, 516–519
- sexual intimacy by, 517

Couvade syndrome, 333
Couvelaire uterus, 684
Cow's milk
- description of, 610
- formulas using, 631

Crack cocaine, 763
Crawling reflex, 546t–549t
Cri du chat syndrome, 51
CRIES, 589, 590t, 919
Critically ill patients, 736–737
Crohn's disease, 730
Crossed extension reflex, 546t–549t
Crowning, 466
Crying, 551, 601, 601b, 919
Cryopreservation, 207b
Cryosurgery, 255–256
Cul-de-sac of Douglas, 61–62, 62f
Cultural beliefs, 21, 25–27, 26t–27t
Cultural competence, 21, 27–28, 79
Cultural knowledge, 21
Cultural prescriptions, 359
Cultural proscriptions, 359
Cultural relativism, 23–24
Cultural traditions, 21
Culture
- breastfeeding rates, 607, 609–610
- cancer meaning affected by, 247b
- childbearing beliefs and practices influenced by, 24–25, 27b
- childbirth affected by, 439–441, 440b
- communication affected by, 24
- diet affected by, 360
- family affected by, 18–19, 21–27
- family roles affected by, 25–27
- father's role affected by, 440
- food choices influenced by, 325–326, 326t–327t
- genetic testing affected by, 47
- health care affected by, 72
- infant feeding methods, 609–610
- infertility and, 198b
- intimate partner violence and, 101–103
- labor affected by, 439–441, 440b
- menopause perceptions affected by, 132
- nutrition affected by, 325–326, 326t–327t
- pain responses affected by, 388, 388b
- parenting affected by, 521–522
- perinatal loss responses, 945
- personal space affected by, 25
- postpartum period affected by, 502
- prenatal care affected by, 358–360
- time orientation affected by, 25

Cycled lighting, 911
Cyclic perimenstrual pain and discomfort, 121
Cyst(s)
- Bartholin, 244–245
- corpus luteum, 239, 265
- dermoid, 239
- follicular, 238
- ovarian, 238–240, 239f
- theca-lutein, 239

Cystic fibrosis, 45–46, 722–725
Cystitis, 731
Cystocele, 85, 235–236, 235f, 238, 238f
Cytogenetic testing, 45
Cytomegalovirus, 163t, 164, 164b, 851–852, 851f
Cytotec. *See* Misoprostol

D

Dactinomycin, 266
Daily fetal movement count, 640
Daily food plan, 325
Danazol (Danocrine), 126, 205b
Danger assessment tool, 103, 108f
Death. *See also* Perinatal loss
- fetal. *See* Fetal death
- maternal, 755
- newborn. *See* Newborn, death of

Decelerations, of fetal heart rate, 416b, 423–425, 424f–426f, 424b–426b
Decidua basalis, 273, 275f
Decidua capsularis, 273, 275f
Deep inferior epigastric perforator flap, 224t–225t
Deep tendon reflexes, 546t–549t, 660–661, 661f, 661t
Deep venous thrombosis, 832–833
Deletions, chromosomal, 51
Delusions, 769
Demand feeding, 616–617
Demerol. *See* Meperidine hydrochloride
Dental care, 346
Deoxyribonucleic acid. *See* DNA
Depo-Provera, 184, 184b
Depot medroxyprogesterone acetate, 184, 184b, 247
Depression
- medications for, 75, 758–759, 758t
- postpartum. *See* Postpartum depression

Dermatitis, 594
Dermatoglyphics, 890
Dermoid cysts, 239
Desquamation, 540
Development
- circulatory system, 279–280, 280f, 284t–286t
- critical periods in, 854f
- endocrine system, 282
- gastrointestinal system, 281, 284t–286t
- hepatic system, 281
- integumentary system, 283, 284t–286t
- milestones in, 284t–286t, 854f
- musculoskeletal system, 283, 284t–286t
- neurologic system, 282
- nongenetic factors that affect, 287
- preterm infant, 898
- renal system, 282, 284t–286t
- reproductive system, 283
- respiratory system, 281–282
- teratogen exposure during, 70, 274, 287, 349b

Developmental dysplasia of the hip, 543, 544f, 884–886, 885f
Dexamethasone, 790b
Diabetes mellitus, 688–690
- classification of, 689
- definition of, 689
- dietary modifications for, 325
- gestational, 689, 701–704, 842
- hyperglycemia, 689, 692t
- hypoglycemia, 692t, 693, 698b
- incidence of, 688–689
- infants of mothers with, 841–844
  - cardiomyopathy in, 844
  - congenital anomalies in, 842
  - hyperbilirubinemia in, 844
  - hyperinsulinemia in, 841–842
  - hypocalcemia in, 843–844
  - hypoglycemia in, 843
  - hypomagnesemia in, 843–844
  - macrosomia in, 843. *See also* Macrosomia
  - nursing care for, 844
  - nursing care plan for, 845b
  - pathophysiology of, 841–842
  - perinatal hypoxia in, 843
  - polycythemia in, 844
  - respiratory distress syndrome in, 843
- pathogenesis of, 689
- pregestational, 691–701
  - antepartum care of, 693–701
  - blood glucose
    - levels of, 695t
    - monitoring of, 697–699, 698b

Diabetes mellitus *(Continued)*
  - care management of, 693–701
  - cesarean birth in, 699
  - childbirth date determination, 699
  - definition of, 689
  - dietary management of, 695, 695b
  - exercise for, 695–696
  - fetal risks and complications, 693
  - fetal surveillance in, 699
  - hospitalization for, 699
  - insulin therapy for, 696–697, 696b, 697t
  - intrapartum care of, 699–700
  - intrauterine fetal demise risks, 692–693
  - maternal risks and complications, 691–693
  - mode of birth in, 699
  - nursing process for, 694b
  - oral contraceptives use in patients with, 700
  - postpartum care of, 700–701
  - preconception counseling, 691
  - resources for, 691b
  - urine testing in, 699
- resources for, 691b
- type 1, 689
- type 2, 689
- White's classification of, 689, 690t

Diabetic ketoacidosis, 692, 692t
Diaper dermatitis, 855
Diaper rash, 593–594
Diaphoresis, 482
Diaphragm (anatomy), 298
Diaphragm (contraceptive), 177–180, 177f, 178b–179b
Diastasis recti abdominis, 303, 303f, 481
Diastole, 739
Diclofenac, 122t
Diet. *See also* Nutrition
- breast cancer risks, 215
- cultural influences, 360
- diabetes mellitus managed with
  - gestational, 701
  - pregestational, 695, 695b
- dysmenorrhea managed with, 121
- hyperemesis gravidarum managed with, 706b
- phenylketonuria managed with, 707–708
- vegetarian, 326, 326t–327t

Diet history, 320–321, 322b
Dietary reference intakes, 308
Diethylstilbestrol
- breast cancer risks, 214
- cervical cancer risks, 252
- vaginal cancer risks, 262

DiGeorge syndrome, 874
Digestion, 535–536
Digoxin, 716t
Dilantin. *See* Phenytoin
Dilation and curettage, 673–675, 828
Dilation and evacuation, 191
Dilation of cervix
- in labor, 377–378, 377f, 439t, 447f
- recurrent premature, 675–676, 676f

Dilaudid. *See* Hydromorphone hydrochloride
Dinoprostone, 802b, 827b
Diphtheria, tetanus, acellular pertussis, 598t

Direct-entry midwives, 364
Disabilities, women with, 79
Discharge/discharge teaching
  cesarean birth, 814, 814b
  description of, 487–489, 488b–489b
  high risk newborns, 926–927
  postpartum. *See* Postpartum period, discharge
Disorganization phase, of rape-trauma syndrome, 110–111
Disseminated intravascular coagulation, 685–686
Distraction techniques, 391
Disulfiram, 762
Dizygotic twins, 286, 286f
DNA
  definition of, 47
  replication of, 270–271
DNA sequencing, 888
Documentation
  electronic fetal monitoring, 430, 431b
  home care, 38
  intimate partner violence, 106, 107b
  labor, 430–431, 431b, 467b
Domestic Abuse Intervention Project, 98, 99f
Domestic violence. *See* Intimate partner violence; Violence/violence against women
Dominant trait, 47–48
Dong quai, 136
Doppler blood flow analysis, 643
Dorsal penile nerve block, 587–588
Doulas, 8, 364–365, 456–457
"Dowager's hump," 133
Down syndrome
  advances in care for, 49–50
  characteristics of, 49, 49f, 889f
  congenital abnormalities and diseases associated with, 49
  dermatoglyphic patterns in, 890
  incidence of, 49
  life expectancy for, 49–50
  maternal age and, 49
  nursing care plan for, 50b
  screenings for
    maternal serum alpha-fetoprotein, 344
    multiple marker, 649
Dressings, 40
Drug testing, 762b, 861–862
Ductus arteriosus
  description of, 279–280, 531
  patent, 710, 875f, 917
Dysfunctional labor, 792–797. *See also* Dystocia
  abnormal patterns, 793–794, 793t
  care management of, 797
  definition of, 792
  hypertonic uterine dysfunction as cause of, 792
  hypotonic uterine dysfunction as cause of, 792–793
  maternal position and, 797
  nursing process for, 798b
  psychologic responses, 797
  risk factors for, 792
  secondary powers, 793, 793t
Dysfunctional uterine bleeding, 129–130, 130b
Dysmenorrhea, 121–123, 122t
Dyspareunia, 126, 132
Dystocia
  complications associated with, 794
  fetal causes of, 794–797
    anomalies, 794
    cephalopelvic disproportion, 794
    malposition, 794–795, 795b
    malpresentation, 795–796, 795f–796f
    multifetal pregnancy, 796–797
  pelvic, 794
  shoulder, 817–818, 818f
  soft-tissue, 794

E

Early decelerations, of fetal heart rate, 423, 424f, 424b
Ears. *See also* Hearing
  newborn assessments, 556t–565t
  physical examination of, 82, 83b–84b
Eating disorders
  anorexia nervosa, 75–76
  binge, 76
  bulimia nervosa, 76
  screening for, 76b
Ecchymoses, 574, 574f, 838, 839f
Eclampsia, 656, 667–668, 667b–668b
Ecological model, 99, 100f
Ecomap, 21, 23f
Ecstasy, 860–861
Ectoderm, 274, 274f
Ectopic pregnancy, 676–678
  abdominal, 677f
  classification of, 676–677
  clinical manifestations of, 677
  differential diagnosis of, 677–678
  etiology of, 676–677
  follow-up care, 678
  incidence of, 676–677
  medical management of, 677–678
  methotrexate for, 678b
  surgical management of, 678
Edema
  pitting, 660, 660f
  pulmonary, 738, 749
Edinburgh Postnatal Depression Scale, 770
Education
  childbirth, 363–367
  formula feeding, 629–630
  nutrition, 321–326, 345
  violence/violence against women, 93
Edward syndrome, 50–51
Effacement of cervix, 376–377, 377f, 447f
Effleurage, 393
Eisenmenger syndrome, 713
Elective abortion, 189
Elective cesarean birth, 809–810, 809b
Electroconvulsive therapy, 775
Electrolytes. *See also specific electrolyte*
  newborn, 535
  pregnancy-related changes, 301
Electronic fetal monitoring, 418
  antepartal assessment using, 649–652
    contraction stress test, 651–652, 652f, 652b
    indications for, 649, 649b
    nonstress test. *See* Nonstress test
  care management during, 425–428
  client teaching, 430, 430b
  description of, 415
Electronic fetal monitoring (*Continued*)
  disadvantages of, 428
  display for, 420, 420f
  documentation during, 430, 431b
  equipment for, 427b
  external, 419, 419t, 420f
  false-positive rates, 428
  family teaching, 430, 430b
  internal, 419, 419t, 420f
  maternal status after trauma, 750, 754
  nursing process for, 427b
  pattern recognition, 426–428
  purpose of, 418–419
  tracings, 426–428
  trauma assessments, 750, 754
Electronic medical record, 436f, 444f
Elimination. *See also* Voiding
  during labor, 450t, 451–452
  newborn, 592
  preterm infant, 907
Embryo
  development of, 274, 276f
  germ layers of, 274, 274f
  sex differentiation, 283
Emergency childbirth, 462b
Emergency contraception, 170b, 184–185, 185t, 185b
Emergency Medical Treatment and Active Labor Act, 435b
EMLA, 587–588
Emotional attachment, 332
Emotional lability, 331
Empathic responses, 78
Empty nest syndrome, 74
En face position, 517–518, 517f
Encephalocele, 877
Endocarditis
  bacterial, 711b
  infective, 713
  prophylaxis, 711b
Endocrine system
  fetal, 282
  labor-related changes in, 384
  physical examination of, 83b–84b
  postpartum changes, 481
  pregnancy-related changes in, 304–305
Endoderm, 274, 274f
Endometrial biopsy, 201
Endometrial cancer, 246–266
  assessment of, 246
  care management of, 246–248
  chemotherapy for, 247, 247t
  etiology of, 246
  evaluation of, 248
  FIGO classification of, 246, 246t
  hysterectomy for, 247, 249b
  incidence of, 246
  nursing diagnoses for, 246
  nursing management of, 247–248
  during pregnancy, 265
  psychologic care for patients with, 248
  treatment of, 247–248
Endometrial cycle, 67–68, 68f
Endometrial polyps, 240f
Endometriosis, 125–126
  nursing care plan for, 127b
  pain associated with, 123
  sites of, 126f
  treatment of, 126, 196b, 204–205
Endometritis, 197, 834–835, 834f
Endometrium
  anatomy of, 62
  lesions of, 125
Endorphins, 384, 388
Endothelial cell dysfunction, 657, 657f
Enema, 451–452, 498b
Engorgement of breasts, 495, 499, 625, 627–628, 627b, 628f
Enterobacter sakazakii, 906b
Enteroviruses, 853
Entrainment, 511–512
Environment
  cancer risks, 54
  hazards in, 78
  neutral thermal, 896, 915
  for newborn, 582–583
  preterm infants, 910–911, 910f
  risk prevention, 93
Enzyme-linked immunosorbent assay, 291
Epidermis, 283
Epidural anesthesia (block), 404–406
  advantages and disadvantages of, 405
  ambulation after, 496
  cesarean birth using, 810
  combined spinal-epidural, 406
  contraindications, 406
  hypotension secondary to, 405–406
  intrathecal opioids with, 406
  membrane levels for, 402f
  methods of, 405
  newborn effects, 407
  nursing interventions for, 411b
  obesity effects on, 404–405
  patient-controlled, 405
  popularity of, 404
  positioning for, 404
  side effects of, 405b
Epidural blood patch, 404, 404f
Epilepsy, 727–728, 727b
Episiotomy
  definition of, 470–471
  healing of, 480
  infection risks, 493
  interventions for, 492b
  local perineal infiltration anesthesia for, 400–401
  mediolateral, 470
  midline, 470
  types of, 471f
Epispadias, 886–887
Epithelial pearls, 541
Epstein's anomaly, 760
Epulis, 302
Erb's palsy, 817, 840, 840f
Ergonovine, 674, 826, 826b
Erythema toxicum, 540, 541f
Erythroblastosis fetalis, 869
Escherichia coli, 854
Esophageal atresia, 881–883, 882f
Estimated date of birth, 330, 922
Estimated date of delivery, 330
Estriol, 278
Estrogen
  functions of, 81
  glucose affected by, 690
  loss of, in older women, 81
  oral, 135t
  placental production of, 278
  postpartum deficiency of, 480–481
  transdermal, 135–136, 135t
Estrogen receptors, 221
Estrogen replacement therapy, 215. *See also* Menopausal hormonal therapy

Estrogen therapy. *See* Menopausal hormonal therapy
Estrogen-progestin
  combined estrogen-progestin contraceptives, 181–183
  oral, 135t
Ethical, legal, and social implications programs, 46
Ethical issues, 14
Ethnic diversity, 2
Ethnicity, 7–8
Ethnocentrism, 21
Euglycemia, 693, 844
Euploid cell, 48
European-Americans
  childbearing beliefs, 26t–27t
  parenting beliefs, 26t–27t
Evaporation, 533
Evidence-based practice
  Cochrane Pregnancy and Childbirth Database, 9–10
  definition of, 9–11
  Joanna Briggs Institute, 10–11
Evil eye, 511
Evista. *See* Raloxifene hydrochloride
Evoked otoacoustic emissions, 579, 579f
Exchange transfusions, 871
Excitement phase, of sexual response, 70t
Exercise. *See also* Physical activity
  amenorrhea associated with, 120–121
  description of, 76
  diabetes mellitus managed with
    gestational, 701
    pregestational, 695–696
  dysmenorrhea managed with, 121
  health benefits of, 90–91
  herpes simplex virus managed with, 154
  Kegel, 91, 91b, 138, 237, 345, 470, 481, 496, 498b
  in older women, 139
  osteoporosis prevention and, 139, 140f
  postpartum, 496, 497f
  posture, 140f
  in pregnancy, 319, 346, 347b, 348f, 359–360
  premenstrual syndrome managed with, 124
  uterine contractions occurring during, 696b
  weight-bearing, 139
Exosystem, 99, 100f
Expressed emotions, 110–111
Extended family, 18, 19f
External cephalic version, 796, 799f
External jugular vein, 742
Extracorporeal membrane oxygenation, 905–906, 924
Extremely low-birth-weight infant, 895, 895b
Extremities
  physical examination of, 84
  trauma examination, 753b
Extrusion reflex, 546t–549t
Eye contact, 511, 523
Eyes. *See also* Vision
  newborn
    assessment of, 556t–565t
    prophylaxis of, 572–573, 572f, 572b, 848
  physical examination of, 82, 83b–84b

F

Face presentation, of fetus, 796, 838, 839f
Facial paralysis, 840, 840f
Facies, 556t–565t
Facilitation, 78
Factor V Leiden, 52–53
Factor VIII deficiency, 832
Fad weight-loss programs, 75
Failure to rescue, 13
Fallopian tubes. *See* Uterine tubes
False labor, 434b
False pelvis, 63, 63f, 372
Familial adenomatous polyposis, 54–55
Family. *See also* Father; Grandparents; Mother; Parent(s); Siblings
  assessment of, 19, 22f
  challenges for, 17
  cohabiting-parent, 18–19
  community context of, 18–19
  cultural context of, 18–19, 21–27
  defining of, 18
  extended, 18, 19f
  functions of, 18, 501
  genogram of, 21, 23f
  graphic representation of, 21, 23f
  health care role of, 19
  homosexual, 19
  lesbian and gay, 19
  married-blended, 18
  married-parent, 18
  newborn relationships with, 475
  no-parent, 19
  nuclear, 18, 18f
  organization of, 18–19
  roles in, cultural influences on, 25–27
  single-parent, 19
  societal context of, 19
  structure of, 18–19, 501
Family health
  cultural factors related to, 21
  promotion of, 28
Family history
  definition of, 83b–84b
  importance of, in genetics, 45
  in prenatal care, 338
Family life cycle theory, 20t
Family nursing, 19
Family planning, 169, 503b–504b, 700
Family stress theory, 20t
Family support system, 338
Family systems theory, 20t, 28
Family theory, 19–21, 20t
Family-centered care, 8
Family-centered obstetric critical care, 754–755
Father. *See also* Couple; Family; Parent(s)
  adaptations to pregnancy by, 333–335
  adjustment to becoming, 515–516, 516f, 516t
  adolescent, 520
  attachment to child, 334
  cultural influences on role of, 440
  labor participation by, 439–440, 456, 465
  older than age 35, 520–521
  perinatal loss effects on, 932–933
  role as, 333
  support for, 456, 457b
Fatigue, postpartum, 495, 515
Fats, 610
Fat-soluble vitamins, 310t–311t, 317–318
Feeding. *See* Breastfeeding; Formula feeding
Female athlete triad, 121
Female condoms, 145, 176–177, 177f
Female genital mutilation, 8–9, 73b
Female infertility
  cervical factors, 197
  congenital causes of, 195
  diagnostic tests for, 198, 199t, 200b
  endometrial biopsy for, 201
  factors affecting, 195–197, 195b
  hormonal factors, 195–196
  hormone analysis, 200
  hysterosalpingography evaluations, 199t, 200–201, 201f
  hysteroscopy evaluations, 201
  laparoscopy evaluations, 199t, 201, 201f
  ovulatory factors, 195–196
  tubal/peritoneal factors, 196–197
  ultrasonography evaluations, 200, 200f
  uterine factors, 197
  vaginal factors, 197
Female reproductive system, 60–65. *See also specific anatomy*
  assessment of, 66t
  bony pelvis, 63, 63f
  breasts. *See* Breast(s)
  external structures of, 61, 61f
  internal structures of, 61–63, 62f
  in newborn, 541, 542f, 556t–565t
  structures of, 60–63, 61f
Female sterilization, 187–188, 187f, 188b
Femara. *See* Letrozole
Fentanyl citrate, 399, 399b, 406
Ferguson reflex, 377, 458, 464
Fern pattern, 437b
Ferritin, 720
Fertility
  awareness of, as contraception method, 171–181, 172b
  trends in, 5–6
Fertility control, 71–72
Fertility rate, 5b
Fertilization, 172, 273, 273f
Fetal alarm sign, 640
Fetal alcohol spectrum disorders, 351–352, 857
Fetal alcohol syndrome, 762, 856f, 857, 858b
Fetal attitude, 370, 372f
Fetal circulation, 382–383, 532, 924
Fetal death. *See also* Grief; Perinatal loss
  definition of, 895b
  nursing care plan for, 947b
  preterm birth as cause of, 790
Fetal fibronectin, 781, 783
Fetal heart rate
  abnormal patterns of, 416, 428, 428b, 459b
  accelerations of, 416b, 423, 423b, 649–650
  baseline, 416b, 421–422
  bradycardia, 422, 422t, 423f
  classification system for, 416b, 426
  decelerations of, 416b, 423–425, 424f–426f, 424b–426b
Fetal heart rate *(Continued)*
  description of, 280, 343, 343f, 382, 394–395
  electronic monitoring of. *See* Electronic fetal monitoring
  episodic changes in, 422–425
  first stage of labor assessments, 443
  intermittent auscultation of, 416–418, 418f, 418b
  internal monitoring of, 419, 420f
  monitoring of
    electronic. *See* Electronic fetal monitoring
    equipment for, 427b
    history of, 415
    intermittent auscultation, 416–418, 418f, 418b
    in second stage of labor, 465
    standards for, 428b
  patterns of, 416, 420–425, 428, 428b, 443, 465
  periodic changes in, 422–425
  point of maximal intensity of, 443, 445f
  tachycardia, 422, 422f, 422t
  trauma evaluations, 754
  variability of, 416b, 421–422, 421f
Fetal heart tones, 341, 343f, 445f, 795
Fetal hemoglobin, 280, 532
Fetal membranes, 274, 275f
Fetal ultrasound
  definition of, 45
  genetic testing uses of, 45
Fetal-maternal hemorrhage, 754
Fetomaternal hemorrhage, 645b
Fetoscope, 418f
Fetus
  abnormal growth of, 816
  alcohol abuse effects on, 856f, 857–858, 857t, 858b. *See also* Fetal alcohol syndrome
  amniotic fluid, 275–276. *See also* Amniotic fluid
  biophysical profile, 643–644, 643t–644t
  breech presentation of, 370, 372f, 795–796, 795f, 838, 839f
  caffeine effects on, 861
  chemotherapy effects on, 265
  circulatory system of, 279–280, 280f, 284t–286t
  cocaine effects on, 857t, 860, 860b
  death of. *See* Fetal death
  Doppler blood flow analysis of, 643
  echocardiography of, 699
  electronic monitoring of. *See* Electronic fetal monitoring
  endocrine system of, 282
  external cephalic version of, 796, 799f
  gastrointestinal system of, 281, 284t–286t
  growth of, 641–642
  head of
    description of, 369–370, 370f, 372f
    rotation of, 795b
  heart activity of, 641
  hematopoietic system of, 280–281, 870
  hemolytic disease of, 647
  hepatic system of, 281
  heroin effects on, 858–859
  hypoxemia in, 716

- Fetus *(Continued)*
  - immunoglobulin M production by, 539
  - immunologic system of, 283
  - insulin production by, 693
  - intrauterine development of, 276f
  - labor affected by. *See* Labor, fetal factors that affect
  - lie of, 370, 371f–372f, 796
  - liver of, 281
  - lungs of
    - description of, 279–280
    - maturity
      - assessment of, 647, 699
      - promotion of, 790, 790b
  - macrosomia in, 691, 794, 816, 841, 843f
  - magnetic resonance imaging uses, 645
  - malposition of, 794–795, 795b
  - malpresentation of, 795–796, 795f–796f
  - marijuana effects on, 860
  - maternal relationship with, 332
  - maternal substance abuse effects on, 856–861, 857t
  - maturation of, 279–283
  - methadone effects on, 859
  - methamphetamine effects on, 860
  - movements by, 294
  - musculoskeletal system of, 283, 284t–286t
  - neurologic system of, 282
  - occiput posterior position of, 794–795, 795b
  - pancreas of, 693
  - partial pressure of oxygen in, 531
  - paternal relationship with, 334
  - patient education about, 344
  - position of, 370–371, 373f
  - presentation of, 370, 371f, 462b, 795–796, 795f, 838, 839f
  - radiation therapy effects on, 265
  - renal system of, 282, 284t–286t
  - reproductive system of, 283
  - respiration by, 383
  - respiratory system of, 281–282
  - selective serotonin reuptake inhibitor effects on, 861
  - sensory awareness by, 282
  - sexually transmitted infection effects on, 162–164, 162t
  - shoulders of, 370
  - substance abuse effects on, 856–864, 857t, 863b
  - sucking motions by, 535
  - syphilis exposure, 848–849
  - trauma to, 749
  - ultrasonography indications, 641–644
  - version of, 796, 799, 799f
  - viability of, 279, 289
  - waste products from, 281
  - well-being assessments, 642–644, 644b, 699
- Fibroadenomas, 212, 213t
- Fibrocystic changes in breast, 211–212, 213t
- Fibroids, 129, 240–242
- Fine-needle aspiration, 212
- Fingernails, 283
- First heart sound, 531
- First trimester
  - abortion in, 190–191
  - chemotherapy contraindications in, 265
  - chromosomal abnormality screening in, 344
  - complications of, 342b
  - discomforts of, 354t–355t, 356b–357b
  - duration of, 330
  - miscarriage in. *See* Miscarriage
  - weight gain in, 311
- Fish, 313t, 314b
- FISH analysis, 51
- Fistula, genital, 237–238, 237f
- Flagyl. *See* Metronidazole
- Flap procedures, for breast reconstruction, 223, 224t–225t
- Flatulence, 354t–355t
- Fluid therapy, 831–832
- Fluids
  - in newborn, 535, 610
  - in pregnancy, 301, 310t–311t, 314
  - in preterm infants, 907
- Flunitrazepam, 110
- Fluoride, 317, 611
- Focusing techniques, for labor-related pain, 391–393, 392f
- Folate deficiency anemia, 721
- Folate/folic acid
  - deficiency of, 721
  - food sources of, 309b, 318, 721
  - supplementation of, 90, 307–308, 727, 876
- Follicle-stimulating hormone, 67
- Follicular cysts, 238
- Follitropins, 205b
- Fontanels, 283, 369–370, 370f, 381f, 556t–565t
- Food allergies, 321
- Food cravings, 318–319, 325–326, 354t–355t
- Food intake questionnaire, 322b
- Football hold, 615, 615f
- Foramen ovale, 279–280
- Forced cesarean birth, 810
- Forceps-assisted birth, 806–807, 806f, 806t, 838
- Forebrain, 282
- Foregut, 281
- Formula feeding, 629–634
  - bottles used in, 630–631, 631b
  - concerns regarding, 630
  - description of, 607–608
  - formulas
    - *Enterobacter sakazakii* contamination of, 906b
    - preparation of, 633b
    - types of, 631–632
  - nipples used in, 630–631
  - parent education about, 629–630
  - patterns of, 630
  - preterm infants, 906, 906b
  - readiness for, 630
  - self-management during, 633b
  - solid foods and, 632–634
  - technique used in, 630, 630f
  - weaning, 632
- Fornices, 61
- Fourchette, 61, 61f
- Fourth heart sound, 531
- Fractures
  - clavicle, 544, 839–840, 839f, 843
  - hip, 133
- Fractures *(Continued)*
  - osteoporosis-related, 133
  - skull, 839
- Fragile X syndrome, 54
- Fragile X-associated tremor/ataxia syndrome, 54
- Frank-Starling law, 740–741
- Freebasing, 763
- Frenulum, 61
- Friability, 293–294
- Full field digital mammography, 219
- Full-term infant, 895b
- Functional assessment
  - definition of, 83b–84b
  - in older women, 81
- Fundal pressure, 467, 818
- Fundus
  - description of, 474b
  - height measurements, 341–342, 342f
  - massage of, 493, 826
  - palpation of, 494f
  - postpartum descent of, 478
- Fungal infections, 855–856
- Furosemide, 716t
- Fussiness, 619, 620b

G

- Galactorrhea, 212
- Galactosemia, 578t, 889
- Galant reflex, 546t–549t
- Gallbladder, 304, 536, 730
- Gamete, 48
- Gamete intrafallopian transfer, 207–208, 207t, 208f
- Gametogenesis, 271–273, 271f–272f
- Gamma-aminobutyric acid, 97
- Ganciclovir, 852
- Gaskin maneuver, 818
- Gastrointestinal obstruction, 883–884
- Gastrointestinal stromal tumor, 54
- Gastrointestinal system. *See also specific anatomy*
  - congenital anomalies of, 880–884, 881f–884f
  - disorders of, 729–730
  - fetal, 281, 284t–286t
  - labor-related changes in, 384
  - in newborn, 535–536
  - postpartum changes, 482
  - pregnancy-related changes in, 303–304, 750t
- Gastroschisis, 883, 883f
- Gastrostomy feeding, 908–909
- Gate-control theory of pain, 388–389
- Gavage feeding, 908–910, 908f, 909b
- Gene therapy, 46
- General anesthesia, 407–408, 407f
- General flexion, 370, 371f
- Genes, 47–48
  - definition of, 43
  - function of, 47
  - human similarities in, 44
- Genetic counseling, 55–57
  - access to, 56
  - definition of, 55–56
  - emotional support during, 57
  - growth of, 55
  - nondirectiveness principle used in, 57
  - referral to, 56
  - risk estimations, 56–57
  - risk interpretation, 57
- Genetic Information Nondiscrimination Act, 216
- Genetic risk
  - estimation of, 56–57
  - interpretation of, 57
- Genetic testing
  - amniocentesis for, 645–647, 871
  - carrier screening, 45–46
  - commercially available, 45
  - congenital anomalies, 888–889
  - cultural influences, 47
  - decision to undergo, factors affecting, 47
  - direct-to-consumer, 43–44
  - ethical, legal, and social implications of, 46
  - fetal ultrasound for, 45
  - hereditary breast and ovarian cancer, 55
  - mandating of, 577–578
  - in mothers older than 35 years of age, 646b
  - perinatal loss secondary to, 946
  - population-based screening uses of, 45–46
  - predictive testing, 45
  - predispositional testing, 45
  - presymptomatic testing, 45
  - process of, 45
  - resources for, 604b
  - risks associated with, 46
  - single-gene disorders, 45
- Genetic transmission
  - description of, 47
  - inheritance patterns, 52–54
    - autosomal dominant, 52–53
    - autosomal recessive, 53
    - multifactorial, 52
    - unifactorial, 52–54
    - X-linked dominant, 53–54
    - X-linked recessive, 54
  - prevention methods, 57
- Genetics
  - advances in, 43
  - clinical, 47–54
  - competencies in, 44
  - definition of, 43
  - family history importance in, 45
  - future of, 57–58
  - nurse's role in, 57
  - nursing expertise in, 44
- Genital herpes simplex virus, 153–154, 153f, 162t–163t, 164
- Genital tract
  - infections of, 161b
  - lacerations of, 825–826
- Genital warts. *See* Human papillomavirus
- Genitals. *See also* Vagina
  - cleansing of, in newborn, 596b–597b
  - fistulas, 237–238, 237f
  - self-examination of, 65
- Genitourinary system. *See also* Bladder
  - congenital anomalies of, 886–888, 887f
  - physical examination of, 84
- Genogram, 21, 23f
- Genome, 43
- Genomics
  - cancer, 54–55
  - competencies in, 44
  - definition of, 43
  - nursing expertise in, 44
- Genotype, 45–48
- Germ layers, 274, 274f

Germinal matrix hemorrhage–intraventricular hemorrhage, 917–918
Gestational age
- appropriate for, 569, 895b
- assessment of, 342–343, 554b, 566–570
- estimation of, 567f–568f, 641
- large for, 895b, 926
- newborn behaviors affected by, 550
- small for, 569, 895b, 924–926
- ultrasonography assessments of, 641

Gestational diabetes mellitus, 689, 701–704, 703f, 703b, 842
Gestational hypertension, 655
- antihypertensive medications for, 666, 666t
- definition of, 655
- description of, 655t
- incidence of, 655
- persistence of, 667
- preeclampsia with. *See* Hypertensive disorders, preeclampsia

Gestational trophoblastic disease, 266, 266b, 678
Gingival hypertrophy, 302
Glabellar reflex, 546t–549t
Glans penis, 588
Glasgow Coma Scale, 752, 753b
Globoid-cell leukodystrophy, 53
Glomerular filtration rate, 300–301, 535
Gloves, 40, 166b, 852–853
Glucocorticoids, for fetal lung maturity, 790, 790b
Glucose
- blood
  - gestational diabetes mellitus, 702–704
  - medications for controlling, 702–704
  - pregestational diabetes mellitus, 695t, 697–699, 698b
- placental transport of, 690
- renal reabsorption of, 301

Glucose reflectance meter, 697
Glucose-6-phosphate dehydrogenase deficiency, 870
Glucosuria, 301
Glucuronyl transferase, 537
Gluteal skinfolds, 544
Glyburide, 702–704
Glycogen, 281
Glycosuria, 482
Glycosylated hemoglobin A_{1C}, 693
Gonadotropin-releasing hormone, 67
Gonadotropin-releasing hormone agonists
- endometriosis managed with, 126
- infertility treated with, 205b
- leiomyomas treated with, 241
- menorrhagia treated with, 129
- side effects of, 126
- uterine fibroids treated with, 241–242

Gonadotropin-releasing hormone antagonists, 205b
Gonorrhea
- description of, 147–149, 148t–149t, 162t, 848
- newborn exposure to, 848
- in pregnancy, 147, 162t, 848

Goodell sign, 293–294
Gowns, 166b
Graafian follicles, 67
Grandparents
- adaptations by, 331–332, 335–336, 336f, 525–526
- description of, 19
- grief responses by, 934–935
- grieving by, 927
- labor support by, 457
- role of, 525

Grasp reflex, 546t–549t, 556t–565t
Graves' disease, 706
Gravida, 289
Gravidity, 289–290
Grief, 932–934
- acute distress, 932–933
- adolescent pregnancy, 947–948
- anticipatory, 913, 927
- anxiety in, 933
- attributes of, 932
- complicated, 948
- conceptual model of, 933b
- definition of, 932
- family aspects of, 934–935
- grandparents, 934–935
- guilt during, 933
- intense, 933–934
- normalizing of, 943
- nursing process for, 936b
- physical symptoms of, 934
- reorganization, 934
- siblings, 934–935

Grief conference, 946
Group B streptococcus, 162, 344, 853–854
Guilt, 933
Gynecoid pelvis, 374, 376t
Gynecologic cancers. *See also specific cancer*
- chemotherapy for, 247t
- incidence of, 245
- nutritional management of problems caused by, 250b
- risk factors for, 77–78

Gynecologic disorders, 73, 77–78. *See also specific disorder*

H

Habituation, 551
Hair, 283
Hand hygiene, 166b, 582b
Hands-and-knees position, 452–453, 452f, 455b
Handwashing, 40
Head
- caput succedaneum, 542–543, 543f, 574, 838
- cephalhematoma, 542–543, 543f, 574, 838
- circumference of, 556t–565t, 565
- fetal
  - description of, 369–370, 370f, 372f
  - rotation of, 795b
- molding of, 542, 542f
- in newborn, 556t–565t
- physical examination of, 82, 83b–84b
- trauma examination, 753b

Headaches
- postdural puncture, 403–404, 404f
- postpartum, 484

Healing touch, 3f
Health assessment, 78–88
- abused women, 79–81, 80f
- adolescents, 81
- diagnostic procedures, 88
- disabilities, women with, 79
- hearing-impaired patients, 79
- interview, 78–79, 78f
- laboratory tests, 88
- midlife women, 81–82
- older women, 81–82
- physical examination. *See* Physical examination
- preeclampsia, 659–661
- spiritual wellness, 82, 82b
- visually impaired patients, 79

Health belief model, 20t
Health care
- barriers to, 4, 72–73, 336
- costs of, 4
- cultural influences on, 72
- culturally appropriate, 23b
- disparities in, 5, 31
- family's role in, 19
- financial barriers to, 72
- gender influences on, 72–73
- high-technology, 7
- level of, 7
- limited access to, 4
- reasons for seeking, 69–72
- safe practices for improving, 4, 4b
- sexual orientation effects on, 72–73

Health care delivery
- home care. *See* Home care
- networks for, 34

Health care systems
- medical errors, 4
- "never events" in, 4, 4b
- problems with, 3–5
- reforms in, 4, 72
- structure of, 3

Health departments, 29
Health disparities, 31
Health history, 82, 83b–84b, 321, 338
Health Insurance Portability and Accountability Act, 435
Health literacy, 5, 33
Health promotion
- anticipatory guidance for, 88–93
- contraception application of, 71, 72b
- exercise, 90–91
- health risk prevention, 93
- nutrition, 88–90
- sexual practices, 92
- stress management, 91–92
- substance use cessation, 92, 92b

Health protection, 93
Health Resources and Services Administration Health Disparities Collaboratives, 5
Health risk prevention, 93
Health screenings, 89t, 92. *See also* Screenings
Healthy aging, 82
Healthy People 2010
- breastfeeding goals, 607
- goals of, 2, 3b, 32

Hearing. *See also* Ears
- in newborn, 550
- screenings of, 89t, 578–579, 579f

Hearing impairment
- parents with, 523, 524b
- patients with, health assessment in, 79

Hearing loss, 851–852, 910
Heart. *See also* Cardiovascular system; Coronary heart disease
- congenital anomalies of. *See* Congenital heart defects and disease
- physical examination of, 82, 83b–84b
- pregnancy-related adaptations, 296, 296f
- ventricles of, 739

Heart rate
- as cardiac output determinant, 741
- fetal. *See* Fetal heart rate
- newborn, 531

Heart sounds, 531
Heart surgery, 716
Heart transplantation, 714
Heart valve replacement, 713
Heartburn, 304, 325, 354t–355t
Heat loss, 533, 926
Heat therapy, 396
Heelsticks, 579–580, 580f
Hegar sign, 293, 295f
HELLP syndrome, 658, 658b, 666–667
Hemabate. *See* Carboprost tromethamine
Hematocrit, 321, 483, 720
Hematologic system. *See also* Blood
- physical examination of, 83b–84b
- pregnancy-related changes in, 738, 750t
- in preterm infant, 897–898

Hematopoietic system
- fetal, 280–281
- newborn, 532–533

Hemodynamic monitoring, 739–749
- cardiac output. *See* Cardiac output
- central venous pressure lines for, 747–748
- circulation, 739, 739f
- data interpretation, 748–749, 748t
- invasive
  - arterial pressure catheter for, 744–745, 746f
  - data collection, 745–749
  - pressure lines, 745
  - pulmonary artery catheter for. *See* Pulmonary artery catheter
  - transesophageal echocardiography for, 741
  - venous access for, 742–743
- oxygenation, 746–747
- pulse oximetry, 746

Hemoglobin
- fetal, 280, 532
- postpartum changes, 483
- SC, 721
- SS, 721

Hemoglobin A_{1C}, glycosylated, 693
Hemolytic diseases of the newborn, 538, 868–869
Hemorrhage
- germinal matrix hemorrhage–intraventricular hemorrhage, 917–918
- intracranial, 841
- postpartum. *See* Postpartum hemorrhage
- postsurgical, 248
- retinal, 838
- subarachnoid, 841
- subconjunctival, 838
- subdural, 841
- subgaleal, 838–839

Hemorrhagic shock, 831b, 830–832
Hemorrhoids, 297, 298f, 480, 492b
Heparin, 716t
Hepatic system
  fetal, 281
  newborn, 536–539
Hepatitis A virus, 89t, 155
Hepatitis B virus, 155–156
  causes of, 155
  high-risk populations for, 155
  immunizations against, 89t, 146, 583, 583b, 598t
  management of, 155
  pregnancy exposure to, 163t, 850
  screening for, 155
Hepatitis B immune globulin, 584b, 598t
Hepatitis B surface antigen, 155, 850, 850b
Hepatitis C virus, 156
Herbal teas, 627
Herbal therapies. *See also* Complementary and alternative therapies
  history-taking, 338
  infertility managed with, 204
  menopausal symptoms managed with, 136, 136b
  menstrual disorders managed with, 123, 123t
  postpartum hemorrhage managed with, 827b, 828
  during pregnancy, 351, 351b
Herceptin. *See* Trastuzumab
Hereditary breast and ovarian cancer, 55
Hereditary nonpolyposis colon cancer, 55, 246
Hernia
  congenital diaphragmatic, 879–880
  hiatal, 303
  inguinal, 542
Heroin, 763–764, 857t, 858–859
Herpes simplex virus
  genital, 153–154, 153f, 162t–163t, 164
  newborn, 852–853, 853f
  transplacental transmission of, 852
Heterozygous, 47
Hiatal hernia, 303
High risk newborn
  anticipatory grief, 913, 927
  classification of, 894, 895b
  discharge planning for, 926–927
  hypoglycemia risks, 925
  late preterm infant as. *See* Late preterm infants
  parental stress, 927
  postmature infant as. *See* Postmature infants
  preterm infant as. *See* Preterm infants
  transport to and from a regional center, 926–927, 927f
High-frequency jet ventilation, 903t
High-frequency oscillation, 903t
High-frequency ventilation, 905
Highly active antiretroviral therapy, 850–851
High-risk pregnancy
  antepartal assessment using electronic fetal monitoring, 649–652
    contraction stress test, 651–652, 652f, 652b
    indications for, 649, 649b
    nonstress test. *See* Nonstress test
High-risk pregnancy *(Continued)*
  antepartum testing, 639, 639b
  assessment of, 637, 638b
  biochemical assessments, 645–649
    amniocentesis. *See* Amniocentesis
    chorionic villus sampling, 647–648, 647f
    Coombs' test, 649
    maternal serum alpha-fetoprotein, 648–649
    multiple marker screens, 649
    percutaneous umbilical blood sampling, 648, 648f
  biophysical assessments, 640–645
  biophysical profile, 643–644, 643t–644t
  biophysical risks, 637, 638b
  daily fetal movement count, 640
  definition of, 637
  increase in, 6–7
  magnetic resonance imaging for, 645
  nurse's role in assessment of, 652–653
  psychologic considerations, 639
  psychosocial risks, 637, 638b
  risk factors for, 6
  sociodemographic risks, 637, 638b
  ultrasonography of, 640–645, 640f–641f, 641t
High-technology care, 7
Hindbrain, 282
Hindgut, 281
Hip fractures, 133
Hirsutism, 239, 302
Hispanics. *See also* Mexican-Americans
  breastfeeding rates, 607
  childbearing beliefs, 26t–27t
  cultural characteristics of, 102
  intimate partner violence in, 102
  low-birth-weight infants in, 5
  pain responses, 388b
  parenting beliefs, 26t–27t
  preterm births in, 5, 780
History of present illness, 83b–84b
H1N1 pandemic, 724b
Hodgkin's disease, 264
Homan's sign, 832–833
Home birth, 366–367
Home care, 34–36
  assessments, 36–37, 38f
  client education in, 38
  client selection for, 35–36
  community focus on, 7
  definition of, 35
  documentation of, 38
  family education in, 38
  health services delivered in, 35
  high-technology, 36
  history of, 34
  nurse's preparations for, 36
  nursing considerations, 37–38
  nursing diagnoses, 36–37
  nursing practice guidelines, 35
  perinatal services, 35, 37b
  phototherapy, 35, 586
  placenta previa, 683
  plan of care, 36–37
  postpartum, 504–505
  postsurgery, 733b
  preterm labor, 784
  psychosocial assessment, 38b
Home care *(Continued)*
  referrals for, 35–36
  regulation of, 35
  safety considerations, 38–40
  technology applications for, 34–35
  visits, 35–36
  walk-through by nurse, 36–37
Home care agencies, 35
Home care nurse
  automobile safety, 39–40
  infection control, 40
  preparations for first home visit, 36
  safety issues for, 38–40
Homelessness, 33
Homeopathy, 136
Homocysteinuria, 578t
Homologous chromosomes, 47, 271
Homosexual family, 19
Homozygous, 47
Hood oxygen therapy, 902, 902f
Hormonal replacement therapy, 9, 141. *See also* Menopausal hormonal therapy
Hospitals
  discharge from, 8
  level of care in, 7
Hot flashes/flushes, 132, 136
Human chorionic gonadotropin
  ß-, 290, 677
  definition of, 290
  description of, 205b
  detection of, 290–291
  functions of, 278
  postpartum reductions in, 481
  pregnancy levels of, 278, 278f
  theca-lutein cysts caused by, 239
Human chorionic somatomammotropin, 278, 304–305
Human developmental ecology, 20t
Human Genome Project, 44–47
  advances made with, 57–58
  ethical, legal, and social implications, 46
  gene therapy, 46
  genetic testing from. *See* Genetic testing
  key findings of, 44
  pharmacogenomic testing, 46
Human immunodeficiency virus, 156–159
  antiretroviral therapy for, 158–159, 850–851
  breastfeeding contraindications, 608, 851
  in children, 11
  counseling associated with, 157, 157b
  diagnosis of, 850
  laboratory tests, 156
  management of, 157
  maternal, 157–159, 608
  newborn, 850–851
  pathophysiology of, 156
  in pregnancy, 157–159, 340b
  prevention of, 158b
  screening for, 156–157, 157b, 340b
  signs and symptoms of, 850
  transmission of, to infant, 850
Human milk. *See* Breast milk
Human Milk Banking Association of North America, 625
Human papillomavirus, 152–153
  cervical cancer and, 252
  description of, 89t
  incidence of, 152
  lesion sites for, 152, 152f
  in pregnancy, 152, 162t
  vaccinations against, 146
Human placental lactogen, 278, 304–305
Hydatidiform mole, 239, 266, 678–680
Hydralazine, 666t, 740
Hydramnios, 643, 691–692, 700
Hydrocele, 541
Hydrocephalus, 878
Hydromorphone hydrochloride, 398
Hydrops fetalis, 869
Hydroscopic dilators, 800–801
Hydrotherapy, 394–395, 394f
Hydroxychloroquine, 729
Hymen, 61, 61f
Hymenal tags, 84–85
Hyperbilirubinemia
  description of, 537, 538t, 575, 584–586, 621, 844
  hemolytic diseases of the newborn as cause of, 538, 868–869
  in late preterm infant, 923
  nursing care plan for, 872b
  pathologic jaundice, 538, 538t, 868, 869b
  physiologic jaundice, 537–538, 575, 867–868
  prevention of, 871
Hyperemesis gravidarum, 325, 353b, 704–706. *See also* Nausea and vomiting of pregnancy
Hyperglycemia, 689, 692t, 925
Hyperinsulinemia, 841–842
Hyperprolactinemia, 196
Hypertensive crisis, 774
Hypertensive disorders
  chronic hypertension, 656, 668
    definition of, 656
    with preeclampsia, 656
    pregestational diabetes mellitus and, 691
  classification of, 655–656, 655t
  eclampsia, 656, 667–668, 667b–668b
  gestational hypertension, 655
    antihypertensive medications for, 666, 666t
    definition of, 655
    description of, 655t
    incidence of, 655
    persistence of, 667
    preeclampsia with. *See* Hypertensive disorders, preeclampsia
  incidence of, 654
  morbidity and mortality associated with, 654–655
  preeclampsia, 656
    activity restriction for, 662, 663b
    assessment of, 662b
    care management of, 658–667
    causes of, 656–657
    chronic hypertension with, 656
    deep tendon reflexes testing, 660–661, 661f, 661t
    definition of, 656
    endothelial cell dysfunction associated with, 657, 657f
    etiology of, 656–657, 657f

Hypertensive disorders *(Continued)*
future risks, 667
gestational hypertension with
antihypertensive medications for, 666, 666t
dietary recommendations, 663b
intrapartum care for, 663–666
magnesium sulfate for, 664–666, 665b–666b
mild, 661–662
nursing care plan for, 664b
postpartum care for, 666–667
severe, 662–667
health assessment and screening, 659–661
HELLP syndrome, 658, 658b, 666–667
laboratory findings in, 656t
mild, 655t, 660b, 661–662
neurologic conditions associated with, 658
pathophysiology of, 657–658, 657f
physical examination of, 660–661
pitting edema tests, 660, 660f
prevention of, 658–659
proteinuria tests, 661
resources for, 656b
risk factors for, 656, 657b, 659b
severe, 655t, 662–667
signs of, 662b
Hyperthermia, 534, 896, 897b
Hyperthyroidism, 706–707, 707b
Hypertonic uterine dysfunction, 792
Hypertrophic cardiomyopathy, 844
Hyperventilation, 383, 387, 738
Hypervolemia, 483
Hypnosis, 396
Hypocalcemia, 576–577, 843–844
Hypochlorhydria, 729
Hypofibrinogenemia, 685
Hypoglycemia
description of, 534, 692t, 693, 698b
in high risk newborns, 925
in infants of mothers with diabetes mellitus, 843
in late preterm infant, 923
in newborn, 575–576
Hypogonadotropic amenorrhea, 120
Hypomagnesemia, 843–844
Hypomenorrhea, 127
Hypoplastic left heart syndrome, 875f
Hypospadias, 541, 886–887, 887f
Hypotension
epidural anesthesia-related, 405–406
interventions for, 428b
spinal anesthesia-related, 401, 403b
supine, 86, 279, 297, 341b, 349, 349f, 354t–355t, 383, 444f
Hypothalamic-pituitary cycle, 67, 68f
Hypothalamic-pituitary-axis system, 69
Hypothermia
in newborn, 571b
in preterm infant, 897b, 899–901, 901f
Hypothyroidism, 578t, 707, 889
Hypotonic uterine dysfunction, 792–793
Hypovolemia, 752
Hypovolemic shock, 494b, 830–832
Hypoxemia, 716
Hypoxia, fetal, 529
Hysterectomy
abdominal, 126, 243f, 247
definition of, 243
discharge planning and teaching, 244, 248
endometrial cancer treated with, 247, 249b
informed consent for, 243b
leiomyomas treated with, 243–244
pelvic examination after, 88
postoperative care for, 244, 244b, 248
preoperative care, 243–244, 243b
psychologic assessment before, 243
radical, 248, 255–256
self-management after, 244b
total abdominal, 126, 247
vaginal, 243, 243f
Hysterosalpingography, 197, 199t, 200–201, 201f
Hysteroscopy, 199t, 201

I

Ibandronate, 139
Ibuprofen, 122t
"Ice," 763
Icterus gravis, 869
Idiopathic thrombocytopenic purpura, 832
Illicit drugs, 75
Illness prevention
anticipatory guidance for, 88–93
definition of, 88
Imagery, 391–392
Immigrants, 32–33
Immune system
newborn, 539
postpartum changes, 484
Immunizations
newborn, 597, 598t
in pregnancy, 351
recommendations for, 89t
Immunoglobulin A, 539
Immunoglobulin G, 283, 539, 844
Immunoglobulin M, 155, 283, 539
Immunologic system, 283
Imperforate anus, 884, 884f
Implantation, 273, 275f
In vitro fertilization–embryo transfer, 206–207, 207t
Inborn errors of metabolism, 53
definition of, 888
phenylketonuria. *See* Phenylketonuria
screening for, 45, 578
Incapacitated rape, 110
Incarcerated women, 32
Incompetent cervix, 675–676, 676f
Incomplete miscarriage, 671f, 672t
Incontinence, urinary, 236–238
clinical manifestations of, 236–237
incidence of, 236
menopause-related, 132
nursing care for, 238
stress, 236
treatment of, 237–238
Inderal. *See* Propranolol
Indian culture, 326t–327t
Indicated preterm births, 780, 780b
Indirect Coombs' test, 871
Induced abortion, 188
alternatives to, 192
aspiration method of, 190–191
care management for, 190
complications after, 191b
decision to have, 190
definition of, 189
dilation and evacuation method, 191
first-trimester, 190–191
incidence of, 189
menstrual cycle resumption after, 191
methotrexate and misoprostol for, 191
mifepristone and misoprostol for, 191
nurses' rights and responsibilities related to, 190b
nursing considerations for, 192
nursing diagnoses for, 190b
prevalence of, 9
second-trimester, 191–192
Inevitable miscarriage, 671, 671f, 672t, 673
Infant. *See also* Newborn
abduction of, 492
body gestures by, 517f, 518
burping of, 631f
cocaine exposure effects on, 763, 857t, 860, 860b
cultural beliefs and practices, 590b
energy requirements, 610
feeding of
bottle, 617–619. *See also* Formula feeding
breastfeeding. *See* Breastfeeding
complementary, 632–634
cultural influences on, 609–610
formula feeding. *See* Formula feeding
methods of, 607–608
readiness cues by infant, 613, 630
solid foods, 632–634
supplemental, 617–619, 619b, 621f
health of, trends in, 17–18
large-for-gestational-age, 895b, 926
low-birth-weight. *See* Low-birth-weight infants
of mothers with diabetes. *See* Diabetes mellitus, infants of mothers with
nutrition for
breastfeeding. *See* Breastfeeding
carbohydrates, 610
fats, 610
fluids, 610
minerals, 611
nursing care plan, 618b
nutrients, 610–611
protein, 611
solid foods, 632–634
vitamins, 611
parent interactions with, 501, 510–511
adjustments in, 517–519
behavioral repertoires, 518–519
biorhythmicity, 512
communication, 511–512
cultural influences, 522
early contact, 510
entrainment, 511–512
Infant *(Continued)*
extended contact, 510–511
eye contact, 511
odor, 511
promotion of, 573–574, 589–591
reciprocity, 512
responsivity, 519
skin-to-skin contact, 510
social, 595–596
synchrony, 512
voice, 511
play in, 603t
postmature. *See* Postmature infants
preterm. *See* Preterm infants
safety of, 583, 583f, 592b
small-for-gestational-age, 569, 895b, 924–926
stimulation of, 601–603, 912
Infant mortality rate
definition of, 5b
international trends in, 6
in United States, 5–6
Infantile Krabbe's disease, 53
Infection. *See also specific infection*
in late preterm infant, 923
newborn. *See* Newborn, infections in
postpartum. *See* Postpartum period, infections
in preterm infants, 898
preterm labor risks, 781
signs and symptoms of, 898, 898b
vaginal. *See* Vaginal infections
Infection control
home care nurse, 40
measures for, 582–583
sexually transmitted infections, 165, 166b
Infective endocarditis, 713
Infertility, 71–72
age-related, 196
behaviors secondary to, 203, 203t
care management for, 197–209
causes of, 71
couples-specific assessments, 202
cultural considerations, 198b
diagnostic tests for, 198, 199t, 200b
factors associated with, 195–197
feelings associated with, 194
female
cervical factors, 197
congenital causes of, 195
diagnostic tests for, 198, 199t, 200b
endometrial biopsy for, 201
factors affecting, 195–197, 195b
hormonal factors, 195–196
hormone analysis, 200
hysterosalpingography evaluations, 199t, 200–201, 201f
hysteroscopy evaluations, 201
laparoscopy evaluations, 199t, 201, 201f
ovulatory factors, 195–196
tubal/peritoneal factors, 196–197
ultrasonography evaluations, 200, 200f
uterine factors, 197
vaginal factors, 197
grief responses for, 931
incidence of, 194
insurance coverage for, 198b

Infertility *(Continued)*
- interventions for, 202–209
  - adoption, 208–209
  - assisted reproductive therapies, 206–208
  - donor embryo, 207t, 208
  - gamete intrafallopian transfer, 207–208, 207t, 208f
  - herbal therapies, 204
  - intracytoplasmic sperm injection, 206–207, 207t
  - medications, 204–206, 205b
  - nonmedical, 204
  - nutrition, 204
  - ovarian stimulation therapy, 204
  - psychosocial, 202–204
  - surgical, 206
  - surrogate mothers, 208
  - therapeutic donor insemination, 207t, 208
  - in vitro fertilization–embryo transfer, 206–207, 207t
  - zygote intrafallopian transfer, 207t, 208
- male
  - factors affecting, 195b, 197
  - semen analysis for, 201–202, 201b
  - substance abuse as cause of, 197
  - ultrasonography evaluations, 202
- nursing care plan for, 202b
- nursing process for, 199b
- obesity and, 204
- ovulation detection, 198–200
- postcoital test for, 202
- prevalence of, 194
- prevention of, 72
- psychosocial effects of, 202–204
- religious considerations, 198b
- support systems, 203

Infibulation, 8–9
Inflammatory bowel disease, 730
Inflammatory breast cancer, 217
Influenza, 724b
Influenza immunization, 89t
Informed consent
- for contraception, 169, 170b
- for hysterectomy, 243b
- for sterilization, 188

Inguinal hernias, 542
Inguinal node dissection, 261
Inhibin A, 649
Insensible water loss, 907
Institute of Medicine
- ethnic disparity report by, 31
- medical errors, 4
- nursing competencies, 13, 14b
- racial disparity report by, 31

Insulin
- analogs, 696
- aspart, 697, 697t
- during breastfeeding, 690, 700
- continuous subcutaneous infusion of, 697
- glargine, 697, 697t
- lispro, 697, 697t
- postpartum needs, 700
- pregestational diabetes mellitus managed with, 696–697, 696b, 697t
- pregnancy needs for, 690f
- preparations of, 696–697, 697t
- self-administration of, 696b

Insulin pump, 697f
Insulin shock, 692t
Integrative health care, 3
Integumentary system. *See also* Skin
- development of, 283, 284t–286t
- disorders of, 726–727
- labor-related changes in, 383
- newborn, 539–541, 556t–565t
- postpartum changes, 484
- pregnancy-related changes in, 301–302, 301f, 302b, 726–727

Intense grief, 933–934
Intensive care unit, 736
Intermenstrual bleeding, 128–129, 129t
Intermittent auscultation, 416–418, 418f, 418b
Intermittent mandatory ventilation, 903t
Internal version, 799
International Lactation Consultant Association, 634b
International Society of Nurses in Genetics, 55
Internet, 29–30
Interpreter, 24–25, 24b, 441
Interstitial deletion, 51
Interview
- in first stage of labor, 437–438
- health assessment, 78–79, 78f
- prenatal, 337–339, 341

Intimate partner violence. *See also* Trauma
- in adolescents, 103
- in African-Americans, 102
- in Asians, 103
- assessment of, 104–105
- care management for, 103–105
- after childbirth, 107
- conceptual perspectives of, 97–99
- coping with, 104
- cultural considerations, 101–103
- danger assessment tool, 103, 108f
- definition of, 95
- documentation of, 106, 107b
- ecological model of, 99, 100f
- facts about, 102t
- feminist perspectives of, 98
- global incidence of, 101–102
- in Hispanics, 102
- historical perspective of, 96–97
- incidence of, 95–96
- mandatory reporting of, 104b
- medical costs associated with, 96
- myths about, 102t
- in Native Americans, 102–103
- nursing care plan for, 107b
- nursing interventions for, 105–109
- nursing process for, 106b
- during pregnancy, 103
- prevention of, 109
- psychologic perspectives of, 97–98, 98b
- reasons for seeking help, 103
- safety provisions, 106
- sociologic perspectives of, 98
- survivors of, 100–101
- theoretic perspectives of, 97–99
- women in, 100–103

Intracranial hemorrhage, 841
Intracytoplasmic sperm injection, 206–207, 207t
Intraductal papilloma, 213, 213t
Intrahepatic cholestasis, 304, 726–727
Intramural leiomyomas, 240, 241f
Intramuscular administration
- description of, 410–411
- in newborn, 583–584, 583b, 584f
- vastus lateralis, 584f

Intrauterine devices, 185–186, 185f, 186b
Intrauterine fetal demise, 692–693
Intrauterine growth restriction, 924–926
- asymmetric, 895b, 925
- definition of, 895b
- description of, 309, 341–342, 639b, 642, 681–682, 727, 780, 851–852
- symmetric, 895b, 925

Intrauterine pressure catheter, 793
Intravenous administration, 410
Invasive hemodynamic monitoring
- arterial pressure catheter for, 744–745, 746f
- data collection, 745–749
- pressure lines, 745
- pulmonary artery catheter for. *See* Pulmonary artery catheter
- transesophageal echocardiography for, 741
- venous access for, 742–743

Inversion of uterus, 826–827, 829
Inversions, 51
Involution of uterus, 478, 479f
Iron
- food sources of, 325b
- human milk levels of, 611
- pregnancy intake of, 310t–311t, 314–315, 325b
- supplementation of, 325, 325b, 707b

Iron deficiency anemia, 314, 720–721
Irritability, 551
Ischemic heart disease, 712
Islets of Langerhans, 282
Isoflavones, 136
Isoimmunization, 197
Isoptin. *See* Verapamil
Isotretinoin, 726b
Italian culture, 326t–327t

J

Japanese culture, 388b
Jarisch-Herxheimer reaction, 150b
Jaundice
- breastfeeding-associated, 538–539, 621
- definition of, 867
- early-onset, 621
- late-onset, 621
- monitoring for, after discharge, 868b
- newborn, 537–539
- pathologic, 538, 538t, 868, 869b
- phototherapy for, 574f
- physiologic, 537–538, 575, 867–868

Joanna Briggs Institute, 10–11

K

Kangaroo care, 878f, 912, 912f
Karyotype, 48, 48f, 890
Karyotyping, 645
Kegel exercises, 91, 91b, 138, 237, 345, 470, 481, 496, 498b
Kernicterus, 538, 868, 870
Ketoacidosis, 692, 692t
Ketones, 699
Ketoprofen, 122t
Ketorolac, 589
Key informants, 29
Kidneys. *See also* Renal system
- fetal, 282, 284t–286t
- newborn, 534–535
- pregnancy-related adaptations, 299t, 300–301, 750t
- pyelonephritis, 731

Klebsiella pneumoniae, 730
Kleihauer-Betke procedure, 648, 684
Klinefelter syndrome, 51–52
Klumpke palsy, 840
Knowledge, skills, and attitudes, 13
Krabbe's disease, infantile, 53

L

Labetalol hydrochloride, 666t
Labia majora
- anatomy of, 61, 61f
- postmenopausal changes in, 66t

Labia minora
- anatomy of, 61, 61f
- postmenopausal changes in, 66t

Labor. *See also* Childbirth
- abnormal patterns of, 793–794, 793t
- active management of, 805–806
- antibiotic prophylaxis during, 792
- augmentation of, 805–806
- bacterial endocarditis prophylaxis during, 711b
- cervical changes during, 376–377, 377f
- comfort during, 389
- complications of
  - chorioamnionitis, 791–792
  - description of, 448b
  - dystocia. *See* Dystocia; Labor, dysfunctional
  - premature rupture of the membranes. *See* Premature rupture of the membranes
  - standard of care for, 797b
- documentation during, 430–431, 431b
- dysfunctional, 792–797
  - abnormal patterns, 793–794, 793t
  - care management of, 797
  - definition of, 792
  - hypertonic uterine dysfunction as cause of, 792
  - hypotonic uterine dysfunction as cause of, 792–793
  - maternal position and, 797
  - nursing process for, 798b
  - psychologic responses, 797
  - risk factors for, 792
  - secondary powers, 793, 793t
- emergencies during, 459b
  - anaphylactoid syndrome of pregnancy, 820–821, 820b
  - meconium-stained amniotic fluid, 817, 817b
  - shoulder dystocia, 817–818, 818f, 839f
  - umbilical cord prolapse, 818–819, 819f, 819b
  - uterine rupture, 819–820
- emergency, 462b
- endocarditis prophylaxis during, 711b
- equipment for, 465, 465f
- evidence-based practices for, 448b

Labor (*Continued*)
  factors that affect, 369–378
    fetus. *See* Labor, fetal factors that affect
    passageway, 371–374, 373f–374f
    passenger, 369–371
    position, 378, 379f
    powers, 374–378
  false, 434b
  father's participation in, 439–440
  fetal adaptations to, 382–383
  fetal assessments during
    documentation of, 430–431, 431b
    monitoring. *See* Labor, fetal monitoring during
    pulse oximetry, 429
    scalp blood sampling, 429
    scalp stimulation, 428
    umbilical cord acid-base determinations, 428–429, 429t
    vibroacoustic stimulation, 428
  fetal factors that affect
    attitude, 370, 372f
    head, 369–370, 370f
    lie, 370, 371f–372f, 796
    position, 370–371, 373f
    presentation, 370, 371f
  fetal heart rate abnormalities during, 428b, 459b
  fetal monitoring during
    basis for, 415–416
    documentation of, 430–431, 431b
    electronic. *See* Electronic fetal monitoring
    intermittent auscultation, 416–418, 418f, 418b
    oxygen supply, 415–416
    techniques for, 416–420
  first stage of, 434, 468b–469b
    ambulation in, 452–453, 452f
    assessments, 434–448, 435f
      amniotic fluid, 448
      amniotic membranes, 448
      blood tests, 446–448
      culture, 439–441
      diagnostic tests, 446–448
      electronic medical record, 436f
      general systems, 442–443
      interview, 437–438
      laboratory tests, 446–448
      Leopold maneuvers, 443, 443b
      physical examination, 441–446
      prenatal data, 435–437
      psychosocial, 438, 439b
      respiratory status, 437
      stress, 438–439
      urine specimen analysis, 446
      uterine contractions, 443–445
      vaginal examination, 445–446, 445b, 447f
      vital signs, 443
    description of, 380
    doula's support during, 456–457
    elimination during, 450t, 451–452
    father's support during, 456
    fluid intake during, 450–451, 450t
    general hygiene during, 448–450, 450t
    grandparent's support during, 457

Labor (*Continued*)
    hands-and-knees position during, 452–453, 452f, 455b
    maternal progress in, 439t
    nurse's support during, 454–456
    nursing care, 448–457, 450t
    nursing care plan for, 449b
    nursing process for, 441b–442b
    nutrition in, 450t
    onset of, 434
    pain during, 386–387, 387f
    partner's support during, 456
    phases, 434
    positioning during, 452–453, 452f–453f, 455b, 461f, 463f
    stress effects on, 438–439
    supportive care during, 453–457
    touch during, 456
    urinary catheterization, 451
    voiding during, 451
  fourth stage of, 380, 472–475, 474b
  induction of, 799–805
    acupuncture for, 802
    amniotic membrane stripping or sweeping for, 801
    amniotomy for, 802–803, 803b
    breast stimulation for, 801–802
    cervical ripening for. *See* Cervical ripening
    contraindications, 800b
    definition of, 799
    elective, 799–800
    indications for, 799, 800b
    oxytocin for, 803–805, 804b
    sexual intercourse for, 801–802
  infection in, 459b
  instruments for, 465, 465f
  lateral position for, 455b
  lithotomy position in, 463f, 465
  maternal adaptations to, 383–384
  measurements in, 375t
  mechanisms of, 380–382
    descent, 381–382
    engagement, 381, 381f
    expulsion, 382
    extension, 382
    external rotation, 382
    flexion, 382
    internal rotation, 382
    restitution, 382
  medication administration methods in, 410–412
  non–English-speaking women in, 441
  onset of, 379–380
  physiologic adaptations to, 382–384
  positions for, 378, 379f, 430, 452–453, 452f–453f, 455b, 460–464, 461f, 463f
  postterm, 815–816
  precipitous, 794
  preterm. *See* Preterm labor
  process of, 378–382
  pushing in, 377–378
  second stage of, 457–458, 468b–469b
    active pushing phase, 458
    bearing-down efforts in, 464–465
    care management in, 458–471
    definition of, 457–458
    documentation during, 467b
    duration of, 457–458

Labor (*Continued*)
    father's support during, 465
    fetal heart rate in
      abnormalities of, 428b
      monitoring of, 465
    latent phase, 458
    maternal fear during, 464
    maternal progress in, 460t
    nursing process for, 461b
    pain during, 387, 387f
    perineal trauma, 470–471
    phases of, 380, 458
    positioning in, 378, 460–464, 461f, 463f
    prolonged, 393
    uterine contractions in, 460t
  siblings during, 457
  side-lying position for, 455b, 461f, 463–464
  signs preceding, 378–379, 380b
  squatting during, 460–462
  stages of, 380
  standing position for, 455b, 462–463
  supplies for, 465, 465f
  supportive care and measures during, 389b, 433, 453–457
  third stage of
    description of, 380, 468b–469b, 471–472
    duration of, 471
    nursing process for, 472b
    pain during, 387, 387f
    placental separation and expulsion, 471, 473f
  trial of, 814–815
  true, 434b
  upright position for, 455b, 460
  uterus
    activity of, 416t
    changes in, 376f
    contractions in. *See* Uterine contractions
  vaginal bleeding during, 459b
  version of fetus, 796, 799, 799f
Labor, delivery, and recovery, and postpartum rooms, 365, 366f, 434–435, 486
Lacerations
  accidental, during cesarean birth, 838
  cervical, 470, 826
  during cesarean birth, 575
  genital tract, 825–826
  interventions for, 492b
  perineal, 470, 493, 825, 829
  urethral, 470
  vaginal, 470
Lactated Ringer's solution, 411
Lactation. *See also* Breast milk; Breastfeeding
  anatomy of, 611–613
  breast anatomy in, 611–613, 612f
  calcium intake during, 315–316
  estimated energy requirement for, 496
  food guide during, 313t
  nutrition during, 319
  physiology of, 611–613
  psychotropic medication use during, 774–775
  resources for, 634b
  smoking during, 319
  suppression of, 499
  thiazide diuretics effect on, 718

Lactation room, 624, 624f
Lactational amenorrhea method, 189
Lactogenesis, 612–613, 612f, 700
Lacto-ovovegetarians, 326
Lactose intolerance, 315–316
Lacto-vegetarians, 326
Lamaze, 391, 391b, 454–455
Lanoxin. *See* Digoxin
Lanugo, 283, 540
Laparoscopy
  female infertility evaluations, 199t, 201, 201f
  supracervical hysterectomy, 243
  vaginal hysterectomy, 243
Large-for-gestational-age infant, 895b, 926
Laryngeal web, 879
Laser ablation, for cervical cancer, 256
Lasix. *See* Furosemide
Last menstrual period, 273–274, 291
Latch, 615–616, 616f
Late decelerations, of fetal heart rate, 423–424, 425f, 425b
Late preterm infants, 922–923
  breastfeeding of, 622
  definition of, 622, 895, 895b, 922
  description of, 569–570, 576b, 895–896
  hyperbilirubinemia in, 923
  hypoglycemia in, 923
  infection in, 923
  nursing process for, 899b
  nutrition for, 922–923
  prevalence of, 780
  problems associated with, 896
  recognition of, 922
  respiratory distress in, 922
  risks associated with, 922
  thermoregulation in, 922
Late-onset jaundice, 621
Latinos. *See* Hispanics
Lead, 318–319
Leading causes of death, 77b, 90b
Lecithin/sphingomyelin ratio, 647, 843
Leiomyomas, 240–244
  care management of, 241–244
  clinical manifestations of, 240–241
  definition of, 240
  diagnosis of, 240–241
  hysterectomy for, 243–244
  laser surgery for, 242
  medications for, 241–242
  myomectomy for, 242–243, 244b
  nursing process for, 241b
  soft-tissue dystocia caused by, 794
  surgical management of, 242–244
  types of, 241f
  uterine artery embolization for, 242, 242b
Leiomyomata, 129
Leopold maneuvers, 382, 443, 443b
Lesbian and gay family, 19
Lesbian couple, 521
Let-down reflex, 616, 767
Letrozole, 205b, 227b
Leukemia, 49, 264
Leukocytes, 532
Leukocytosis, 483, 532
Leukorrhea, 295, 354t–355t
Levonorgestrel, 185
Levonorgestrel/ethinyl estradiol, 182
Levothyroxine, 707
Lidocaine, 716t
Lie, of fetus, 370, 371f–372f, 796

- Life expectancy, 9, 32, 60
- Lifestyle modifications, for preterm labor, 784
- Ligaments, uterine, 61–62, 62f
- Lightening, 292, 378
- Linea nigra, 301, 301f, 484
- Linkage analysis, 45
- Lipase, 535–536
- Lipoma, 213t
- *Listeria monocytogenes*, 855
- Listeriosis, 321b, 855
- Literature search, 10b
- Lithium, 760
- Lithotomy position
  - during labor, 463f, 465
  - for pelvic examination, 80f, 84
  - during pregnancy, 86
  - supine hypotension concerns, 86
  - for women with disabilities, 80f
- Live birth, 895b, 941b
- Liver
  - fetal, 281
  - newborn, 536
  - pregnancy-related changes in, 304
- Local anesthetics, 400–401
- Local perineal infiltration anesthesia, 400–401
- Lochia, 474b, 479–480, 480t, 493
- Lochia alba, 479
- Lochia rubra, 479–480
- Lochia serosa, 479
- Loci, 47
- Loop electrosurgical excision procedure, 253–254, 253f, 256, 256f
- Lordosis, 302–303
- Loss. *See* Perinatal loss
- Low-birth-weight
  - definition of, 307, 780
  - preterm birth versus, 780
- Low-birth-weight infants
  - definition of, 5, 895b
  - extremely, 895, 895b
  - racial incidence of, 5
  - very, 895b
- Lumpectomy, 221–222, 222f, 229–230, 263
- Lungs. *See also* Breathing; Respiratory system
  - alveoli of, 529–530
  - fetal
    - description of, 279–280
    - maturity
      - assessment of, 647, 699
      - promotion of, 790, 790b
  - newborn, 529
  - physical examination of, 84
- Luteinizing hormone, 67, 174–175
- Lymph node dissection, 231b
- Lymphatic system
  - breast cancer metastasis through, 220–221, 221f
  - physical examination of, 82, 83b–84b
- Lyon hypothesis, 48

M

- Macromastia, 213
- Macrosomia, 691, 794, 816, 841, 843, 843f
- Macrosystem, 99, 100f
- Magnesium, 310t–311t, 316
- Magnesium sulfate
  - preeclampsia uses of, 664–666, 665b–666b
  - tocolytic uses of, 786, 787b–789b
- Magnet reflex, 546t–549t, 556t–565t
- Major depressive disorder, 768
- Male infertility
  - factors affecting, 195b, 197
  - semen analysis for, 201–202, 201b
  - substance abuse as cause of, 197
  - ultrasonography evaluations, 202
- Male reproductive system, 541, 542f, 556t–565t
- Male sterilization, 187f, 188–189
- Malignant melanoma, 264
- Malnutrition, 321, 323t
- Mammary duct ectasia, 213, 213t
- Mammary glands, 296. *See also* Breast(s)
- Mammography
  - breast cancer detection with, 218–220, 218f
  - computer-aided detection and diagnosis with, 219
  - full field digital, 219
  - recommendations for, 89t
- Mania, 769
- Maple syrup urine disease, 578t
- Marfan syndrome, 712–713
- Marijuana, 762, 860
- Marquette Model, of contraception, 175
- Married-blended family, 18
- Married-parent family, 18
- Mastectomy
  - breast reconstruction after, 223–225, 224t–225t, 232b
  - definition of, 222
  - modified radical, 222–223, 222f
  - nipple- and areola-sparing, 223
  - nipple-sparing, 223
  - partial, 221–222, 222f
  - pregnancy after, 263
  - prophylactic, 223
  - scar-sparing, 223
  - self-management after, 232b
  - skin-sparing, 223
  - total simple, 222, 222f
- Mastitis, 629, 834–835, 834f
- Masturbation, 358
- Maternal death, 755
- Maternal health, 17–18
- Maternal mortality
  - fetal deaths caused by, 351
  - pregnancy as cause of, 755
  - racial incidence of, 6
  - trauma as cause of, 749
  - trends in, 6
- Maternal mortality rate, 5b, 6
- Maternal phenylketonuria, 707–708
- Maternal role attainment, 514–515, 514t
- Maternal self-image, 501
- Maternal sensitivity, 514
- Maternal sensitization, 869
- Maternal serum alpha-fetoprotein, 344, 648–649, 699
- Maternity care, 8–9
- Maternity nursing
  - components of, 1
  - genetics involvement by, 44
  - milestones in, 2b
- McBurney's point, 304, 304f
- McGill Model of Nursing, 20t
- McRoberts maneuver, 818, 818f
- MDMA, 860–861
- Mean arterial pressure, 297
- Measles, mumps, rubella immunization, 89t
- Mechanical prosthetic valves, 713
- Mechanical ventilation, 903, 903f, 903t
- Meckel diverticulum, 281
- Meclofenamate, 122t
- Meconium, 281, 536, 536b, 861–862
- Meconium aspiration syndrome, 817, 923–924
- Meconium ileus, 281
- Meconium-stained amniotic fluid, 817, 817b
- Medical conditions, 77
- Medical errors
  - deaths caused by, 4
  - reduction in, 4
- Medical nutrition therapy, 325
- Medication history, 37–38
- Mediolateral episiotomy, 470
- Mefenamic acid, 122t
- Megestrol (Megace), 247
- Meiosis, 270–271, 273
- Melanoma, 264
- Melasma, 301
- "Melting pot," 21
- Menarche, 67
- Menopausal hormonal therapy, 134–137
  - breast cancer risks, 215
  - decision to use, 134
  - definition of, 134
  - guidelines for, 134–136, 135t
  - hormonal medications used in, 135t
  - side effects of, 134
- Menopause, 67–69, 130–141. *See also* Perimenopause
  - age of onset, 130
  - behavioral responses, 132–133
  - care management of, 137
  - coronary heart disease risks, 134
  - cultural influences on, 132
  - definition of, 69, 130
  - early, 196
  - hormonal changes associated with, 130
  - mood responses, 132–133
  - osteoporosis risks, 133–134, 133f
  - physiologic characteristics of, 131
  - sexual counseling, 137–141
  - symptom management in
    - bioidentical hormones for, 136
    - comfort measures, 137b
    - complementary and alternative therapies for, 136–137
    - hormonal therapy for. *See* Menopausal hormonal therapy
- Menorrhagia, 129
- Menotropins, 205b
- Menstrual bleeding
  - breakthrough, 128
  - cyclic alterations, 126–130
  - heavy, 128b
- Menstrual cycle
  - endometrial cycle, 67–68, 68f
  - hormones involved in, 119, 172
  - hypothalamic-pituitary cycle, 67, 68f
  - knowledge about, 120
  - length of, 67, 119
  - ovarian cycle, 67, 68f
  - physiology of, 119
  - variations in, 119
- Menstrual disorders, 72, 120–130
  - amenorrhea, 120–121, 196
  - cyclic bleeding alterations, 126–130
  - cyclic perimenstrual pain and discomfort, 121
  - dysfunctional uterine bleeding, 129–130, 130b
  - dysmenorrhea, 121–123, 122t
  - endometriosis, 125–126, 126f, 127b
  - herbal therapies for, 123, 123t
  - hypomenorrhea, 127
  - menorrhagia, 129
  - metrorrhagia, 127–129
  - nursing process for, 131b
  - oligomenorrhea, 127
  - premenstrual dysphoric disorder, 123–125, 123t
  - premenstrual syndrome, 123–125, 123t, 125b
  - types of, 72
- Menstruation, 67–69
  - back pain associated with, 387–388
  - breast changes during, 64–65
  - definition of, 67
  - postpartum resumption of, 481
- Mental health disorders
  - postpartum, 767–776
    - anxiety disorders, 775–776
    - depression. *See* Postpartum depression
    - mood disorders, 768–775
  - during pregnancy
    - anxiety disorders, 759–761, 760t
    - mood disorders, 757–759
    - prevalence of, 757
- Mental status examination, 83b–84b
- Menu planning, 325
- Meperidine hydrochloride, 398–399
- Mercury, 314b
- Mesoderm, 274, 274f
- Mesosystem, 99, 100f
- Metabolic acidemia, 429t
- Metabolic acidosis, 534
- Metformin, 204, 205b, 239
- Methadone, 763–764, 766, 859, 859b
- Methamphetamine, 763, 860
- Methergine. *See* Ergonovine
- Methotrexate
  - gestational trophoblastic disease treated with, 266
  - misoprostol and, for abortion, 191
- Methyldopa, 666t
- Methylergonovine (Methergine), 826, 826b, 827b
- 15-Methylprostaglandin $F_{2}\alpha$, 827b
- Metoclopramide, 397
- Metronidazole
  - candidiasis treated with, 160
  - trichomoniasis treated with, 162
- Metrorrhagia, 127–129
- Mexican-Americans. *See also* Hispanics
  - extended family in, 18
  - foods popular with, 326t–327t
  - pica in, 318–319
- Microdeletions, 51
- Microencephaly, 879
- Microinvasive carcinoma, 251–252
- Micromastia, 213
- Microsystem, 99, 100f
- Midbrain, 282
- Midcycle bleeding, 67
- Middle adults, 74

Middle cerebral artery peak systolic velocity, 871
Middle Eastern culture, 326t–327t, 388b
Midgut, 281
Midline episiotomy, 470
Midpelvis, 373
Midwives
  certified, 8
  direct-entry, 364
Mifepristone and misoprostol, for abortion, 191
Migrant women, 32–33
Milk, 315–316, 606. *See also* Breast milk; Cow's milk
Milk banking, 625
Milk ejection reflex, 612–613, 612f, 616
Milk stool, 536b
Millennium Development Goals, 2, 3b
Minimal enteral nutrition, 908
Minipill, 184
Minorities, 31–32. *See also specific minority group*
Mirtazapine, 758–759
Miscarriage, 670–675, 674b. *See also* Perinatal loss
  assessment of, 672t
  clinical manifestations of, 671–672
  dilation and curettage for, 673–675
  discharge teaching for, 675b
  etiology of, 670–671
  incidence of, 670–671
  initial care for, 672–675
  management of, 672–675
  medical management of, 673
  nursing process for, 673b
  parental support during, 937f
  resources for, 675b
  rupture of membranes as cause of, 671
  types of, 671, 671f
Misoprostol, 801b
  hypotonic uterus managed with, 826, 827b
  methotrexate and, for abortion, 191
  mifepristone and, for abortion, 191
Missed miscarriage, 671f, 672–673, 672t
Mitosis, 270
Mitral balloon valvuloplasty, 711
Mitral valve
  prolapse of, 711–712
  stenosis of, 711
Mittelschmerz, 69
Mittlestaining, 127–128
Mixed acidemia, 429t
Modified cow's milk, 610
Modified radical mastectomy, 222–223, 222f
Modified throne position, 412f
Modified-paced breathing, 392–393, 393b
Molar pregnancy, 239, 266, 678–680
Molding, 542, 542f
Molestation, 109
Molluscum contagiosum, 152
Mongolian spots, 540, 540f
Monilial infections, 628–629
Monoamine oxidase inhibitors, 758t, 774
Monosomy, 49, 51
Monozygotic twins, 286, 287f
Mons pubis, 61, 61f
Montevideo units, 416t, 419
Montgomery tubercles, 64, 64f, 295–296, 625
Mood disorders. *See also* Depression
  postpartum, 768–775
  during pregnancy, 757–759
Mood stabilizers, 760, 760t, 774–775
Morning sickness. *See* Nausea and vomiting of pregnancy
Moro reflex, 546t–549t, 839–840
Morphine, 406, 859b, 920
Mortality rate
  infant. *See* Infant mortality rate
  maternal, 5b, 6
  neonatal, 5–6, 5b
  perinatal. *See* Perinatal mortality rate
Morula, 273
Mosaicism, 51
Mother. *See also* Couple; Family; Parent(s)
  adolescent, 519–520
  death of, 755
  older than age 35, 74, 360–362, 520, 646b
  postpartum depression in. *See* Postpartum depression
  returning to employment, 623–624
  role attainment as, 514–515, 514t
  substance abuse by. *See* Substance abuse
Motivational interviewing, 767
Motor vehicle accidents, 749
Motrin. *See* Ibuprofen
Mouth
  newborn assessments, 556t–565t
  physical examination of, 82, 83b–84b
Multifactorial inheritance, 52
Multifetal pregnancy. *See also* Multiple births
  description of, 286–287, 286f–287f, 362–363
  dystocia caused by, 796–797
  perinatal loss in, 947
Multigravida, 289
Multipara, 289
Multiparous woman, 447f
Multiple births. *See also* Multifetal pregnancy
  breastfeeding, 622, 622f
  low-birth-weight infants secondary to, 5
  trend in, 5
Multiple marker screens, 649
Multiple sclerosis, 728
Mummy restraint, 580, 581f
Muñeco, 359
Musculoskeletal system. *See also* Fractures; Osteoporosis
  birth-related injuries to, 839–840, 839f
  fetal, 283, 284t–286t
  labor-related changes in, 383
  newborn, 542–545, 542f–544f, 839–840, 839f
  physical examination of, 83b–84b, 84
  postpartum changes, 484
  pregnancy-related changes in, 302–303, 302f, 750t
Music, 393–394
Mutation, 45
Mutuality, 507–508
Myasthenia gravis, 729
Myelomeningocele, 877, 877f
Myerson sign, 546t–549t
Myocardial infarction, 712
Myomas, 129
Myomectomy, 242–243, 244b
Myometrium, 62
MyPyramid, 322–323

N

Nägele's rule, 330, 330b
Nails, 302, 596b–597b
Nalbuphine hydrochloride (Nubain), 399, 399b
Naloxone hydrochloride (Narcan), 400, 400b, 859b
Naproxen sodium, 122t
Narcotics Anonymous, 766
Nasal cannula, 902, 902f
Nasopharyngeal catheter, 570b
National Association of Neonatal Nurses, 11–12
National Center for Complementary and Alternative Medicine, 3
National Center for Health Statistics, 29
National Comprehensive Cancer Network, 232b
National Friendly Access Program, 28
National Newborn Screening and Genetics Resource Center, 604b
National Quality Forum, 4, 4b
National Violence Against Women Survey, 95
National Violent Death Reporting System, 95–96
Native Americans
  childbearing beliefs, 26t–27t
  foods popular with, 326t–327t
  intimate partner violence in, 102–103
  pain responses, 388b
  parenting beliefs, 26t–27t
Natural family planning. *See* Fertility, awareness of
Natural skin condoms, 176
Nausea and vomiting of pregnancy. *See also* Hyperemesis gravidarum
  complementary and alternative therapies for, 353b
  management of, 325, 326b, 354t–355t
  onset of, 303
Neck
  hyperextension of, 752b
  newborn assessments, 556t–565t
  physical examination of, 82, 83b–84b
  trauma examination, 753b
Necrotizing enterocolitis, 918–919, 918b
Necrotizing osteochondritis, 579
Neisseria gonorrhoeae, 147, 150–151. *See also* Gonorrhea
Neonatal abstinence syndrome, 856, 857t, 859, 859f, 863b
Neonatal Infant Pain Scale, 589
Neonatal intensive care units, 910, 910f
Neonatal mortality rate, 5–6, 5b
Neonatal narcosis, 400
Neonatal resuscitation, 790, 903–904, 904f
Neonate. *See* Newborn
Neopresol. *See* Hydralazine
Nerve blocks, 400–407
Nervous system
  central. *See* Central nervous system
  embryologic development of, 282
Neural tube defects
  anencephaly, 876–877
  definition of, 307–308
  encephalocele, 877
  etiology of, 876
  folic acid supplementation to prevent, 307–308
  incidence of, 876–877
  maternal serum alpha-fetoprotein as screening tool for, 648, 699
  myelomeningocele, 877, 877f
  pregestational diabetes mellitus as risk factor for, 699
  prenatal diagnosis of, 877
  primary, 876–877
  secondary, 876–877
  spina bifida, 876–878, 877f
Neurofibromas, 52
Neurofibromatosis, 52
Neurologic system
  disorders of, 727–728
  fetal, 282
  labor-related changes in, 384
  physical examination of, 83b–84b, 84
  postpartum changes, 484
  pregnancy-related changes in, 303
Neuromuscular system, 545, 546t–549t
Neuropathic pain, 245
Neutral thermal environment, 896, 915
Nevi, 540, 541f
Nevus vasculosus, 540
New Ballard Score, 567, 569
New York Heart Association classification, of heart disease, 710
Newborn, 574–575. *See also* Infant
  abstinence syndrome in, 856, 857t
  acceptance of, 525b
  activities of daily living, 590–591, 598
  airway
    maintenance of, 570–571
    obstruction in, 599b
  assessment of
    gestational age, 566–570
    initial, 554–570, 554t
    neurologic, 565–566
    physical. *See* Newborn, physical assessment of
  bathing of, 595–597, 596f, 596b–597b
  behavioral characteristics of, 545–551
    factors influencing, 550
    gestational age effects, 550
    sleep-wake states, 549, 549f
  bilirubin in, 537–539, 537f
  birth injuries in. *See* Birth trauma
  birth weight of, 567–569
  blood pressure in, 532
  blood volume of, 532
  body temperature in
    assessment of, 555
    discharge teaching about, 591
    maintenance of, 571–572
    phototherapy effects on, 585
  body weight of, 556t–565t, 565
  brain growth in, 545
  breast tissue swelling in, 541
  breathing in

Newborn *(Continued)*
abnormalities, 570b
initiation of, 529–530
carbohydrate metabolism in, 537
cardiopulmonary resuscitation of, 597, 600b
cardiovascular system of
adaptations in, 530–532, 531t
congenital anomalies, 873–876, 874t, 875f
care of, 467
circumcision of. *See* Circumcision
coagulation in, 539
cocaine exposure effects on, 763, 857t, 860, 860b
cold stress effects, 534f, 896, 897b
congenital anomalies in, 873–879
ambiguous genitalia, 887–888, 887f
bladder exstrophy, 887, 887f
cardiovascular system, 873–876
care management of, 888–891
central nervous system, 876–879, 877f
cleft lip and palate, 880–881, 881f–882f
cytogenetic studies for, 889–890
definition of, 873
epispadias, 886–887
esophageal atresia, 881–883, 882f
family support, 891
gastrointestinal obstruction, 883–884
gastrointestinal system, 880–884, 881f–884f
gastroschisis, 883, 883f
genetic diagnosis of, 888–889
genitourinary system, 886–888, 887f
hydrocephalus, 878
hypospadias, 886–887, 887f
imperforate anus, 884, 884f
incidence of, 873
microencephaly, 879
musculoskeletal system, 884–886
neural tube defects. *See* Neural tube defects
nursing process for, 890–891, 890b
omphalocele, 883, 883f
parental support, 891
perinatal diagnosis of, 888
postnatal diagnosis of, 888
prenatal diagnosis of, 888
respiratory system, 879–880, 879f–880f
tracheoesophageal atresia, 881–883, 882f
types of, 873
consolability of, 551
crying by, 551, 601, 601b
cuddliness of, 551
day-night routines for, 599–601
death of. *See also* Perinatal loss
definition of, 895b
leading cause of, 6
preterm birth as cause of, 790
developmental dysplasia of the hips in, 543, 544f
developmental milestones for, 601–603, 602t, 603b
diagnostic tests, 577–582, 577b

Newborn *(Continued)*
diaper rash in, 593–594
digestion in, 535–536
discharge planning and teaching for, 591–603
body temperature, 591
clothing, 594, 594f
elimination, 592
follow-up care, 597
holding, 592–593, 593f
immunizations, 597, 598t
nail care, 596b–597b
nonnutritive sucking, 595
positioning, 592–593
rashes, 593–594
respirations, 591–592
umbilical cord care, 596–597, 596b–597b
drug dependence and withdrawal in, 863b, 864. *See also* Neonatal abstinence syndrome; Substance abuse
electrolyte balance in, 535
epidural anesthesia effects on, 407
erythema toxicum in, 540, 541f
extrauterine life transition, 528–529
eyes in
assessment of, 556t–565t
prophylaxis for, 572–573, 572f, 572b
family relationships, 475
feeding of
behaviors, 536
bottle, 617–619. *See also* Formula feeding
breastfeeding. *See* Breastfeeding
complementary, 632–634
cultural influences on, 609–610
discharge teaching about, 592
formula feeding. *See* Formula feeding
methods of, 607–608
readiness cues by infant, 613, 630
solid foods, 632–634
supplemental, 617–619, 619b, 621f
feet of, 544–545
female reproductive system in, 541, 542f, 556t–565t
first weeks with, 597–601
fluid balance in, 535
fractures in, 544, 839–840, 839f, 843
fussy, 619
gallbladder in, 536
gastrointestinal system in, 535–536
gestational age assessments, 566–570
glomerular filtration rate in, 535
habituation of, 551
hearing in, 550
heart rate in, 531
heart sounds in, 531
heat loss in, 533
hematopoietic system of, 532–533
hepatic system in, 536–539
high risk. *See* High risk newborn
holding of, 592–593, 593f
hyperbilirubinemia in, 537, 538t, 575, 584–586, 621, 844, 867–873, 869b
hyperthermia in, 534
hypoglycemia in, 575–576
hypothermia in, 571b

Newborn *(Continued)*
illness signs in, 603, 604b
immediate assessment of, 467
immune system in, 539
infections in, 844–846
bacterial, 853–856
candidiasis, 855–856
care management for, 846–861
chlamydia, 855
cytomegalovirus, 164, 851–852, 851f
enteroviruses, 853
Escherichia coli, 854
fungal, 855–856
gonorrhea, 848. *See also* Gonorrhea
group B streptococcus, 162, 853–854
hepatitis B virus, 850
herpes simplex virus, 154, 852–853, 853f
human immunodeficiency virus, 850–851
listeriosis, 855
parvovirus B19, 853
prevention against, 582–583
risks for, 539
rubella, 851
security of, 8
sepsis, 844–846, 844t, 846b, 847t
Staphylococcus aureus, 854–855
syphilis, 848–849, 849f
toxoplasmosis, 848
transplacental, 848–853
varicella-zoster virus, 849–850
initial assessment, 554–570, 554t
integumentary system in, 539–541, 556t–565t
interventions in, 570–574
intramuscular injections in, 583–584, 583b, 584f
iron storage in, 536
irritability of, 551
jaundice in. *See* Jaundice
kidneys in, 534–535
laboratory tests, 577–582, 577b
length of, 556t–565t
leukocytes in, 532
liver in, 536
lungs in, 529
male reproductive system in, 541, 542f, 556t–565t
Mongolian spots in, 540, 540f
of mothers with diabetes. *See* Diabetes mellitus, infants of mothers with
musculoskeletal system of
anatomy of, 542–545, 542f–544f
clubfoot, 886
congenital anomalies, 884–886
developmental dysplasia of the hip, 884–886, 885f
polydactyly, 886
myasthenia gravis in, 729
neurologic assessment in, 565–566
neuromuscular system in, 545, 546t–549t
nevi in, 540, 541f
nonnutritive sucking by, 595
nose breathing by, 530b
nursing care plan for, 566b
nursing process for, 569b
oxygen supply in, 571

Newborn *(Continued)*
pain management in, 588–589
parent interactions with, 501, 510–511
adjustments, 517–519
behavioral repertoires, 518–519
biorhythmicity, 512
communication, 511–512
cultural influences on, 522
early contact, 510
entrainment, 511–512
extended contact, 510–511
eye contact, 511
odor, 511
promotion of, 573–574, 589–591
reciprocity, 512
responsivity, 519
skin-to-skin contact, 510
social, 595–596
synchrony, 512
voice, 511
physical assessment of, 555b
abdomen, 556t–565t
anus, 556t–565t
baseline measurements, 565
body length, 565
body temperature, 555
chest, 556t–565t
chest circumference, 556t–565t
ears, 556t–565t
extremities, 556t–565t
eyes, 556t–565t
faces, 556t–565t
general appearance, 555
head circumference, 556t–565t, 565
initial, 555
mouth, 556t–565t
neck, 556t–565t
nose, 556t–565t
posture, 556t–565t
respiratory rate, 556t–565t, 565
vital signs, 555–565, 556t–565t
weight, 565
physiologic injuries in, 575–577
platelet count in, 533
play in, 603t
positioning of, 592–593
posture of, 556t–565t
protective environment for, 582–583
quieting of, 601, 601b
radiant warmer for, 465, 466f
rashes in, 593–594
reactivity periods, 529
red blood cells in, 532
reflexes in, 545, 546t–549t, 556t–565t
renal system in, 534–535
reproductive system in, 541–542, 556t–565t
respirations in, 591–592
respiratory distress in, 530
respiratory system in
adaptations, 529–530
congenital anomalies, 879–880
restraint of, 580, 581f, 582
safety of, 583, 583f, 592b
screenings in. *See also* Screenings
genetic, 577–578
hearing, 578–579, 578t, 579f
inborn errors of metabolism, 45
phenylketonuria, 45, 282, 578t
selective serotonin reuptake inhibitor effects on, 861

Newborn *(Continued)*
- sensory behaviors in, 550–551
- sensory stimulation in, 529–530
- sepsis in, 844–846, 844t, 846b, 847t
- sibling adaptation to, 523–525, 524f, 525b
- skeletal system in, 542–545, 542f–544f
- skin of, 556t–565t, 596b–597b
- sleep-wake states in, 549, 549f, 620b
- slow weight gain by, 620–621
- smell sense in, 550–551
- sodium reabsorption in, 535
- soft tissue injuries in, 574–575
- specimen collection, 579–582
  - heelstick, 579–580, 580f
  - urine, 580–582, 582f
  - venipuncture, 580, 580f–581f
- stimulation of, 601–603
- stomach of, 535
- stools in, 536, 536b, 556t–565t, 592, 617
- sweat glands in, 540
- taste sense in, 551
- teething in, 535
- temperament of, 551
- thermogenic system in, 533–534, 534f
- thermoregulation in, 533
- touch sense in, 551
- umbilical cord care in, 573, 574f
- vision in, 550
- voiding by, 534
- weight loss in, 528, 620
- white blood cell count in, 532

Newborns' and Mothers' Health Protection Act, 487–488
Nicotine, 74, 762, 857. *See also* Smoking
Nifedipine, 666t, 716t, 786–787, 787b–789b
Night eating syndrome, 76
Night sweats, 132
Nipple
- anatomy of, 64, 64f
- artificial, for formula feeding, 630–631
- carcinoma of, 217
- contraction test by stimulation of, 651–652
- discharge from, 212, 217–218
- inverted, 345–346, 346f, 625
- Paget's disease of, 217
- pigmentation of, 64, 301
- pinch test for, 345–346, 346f
- pregnancy-related changes in, 295–296, 301
- reconstruction of, 223–225
- soreness of, 495, 628–629
- tenderness of, 626

Nipple-erection reflex, 613
Nipple-sparing mastectomy, 223
Nitrazine, 437
Nitric oxide therapy, 905
Nitrous oxide analgesia, 407
Nondirectiveness, 57
Nondisjunction, 49, 51, 272f
Non–English-speaking women, 441
Nonnutritive sucking, 595, 910, 910f
Nonsteroidal anti-inflammatory drugs
- postoperative pain managed with, 248
- postpartum uses of, 495
- primary dysmenorrhea treated with, 122, 122t

Nonstress test, 649–651
- indications for, 649b, 799
- interpretation of, 650–651, 650f, 651b
- procedure for, 650
- vibroacoustic stimulation used in, 650–651, 651f

No-parent family, 19
Normodyne. *See* Labetalol hydrochloride
Nose
- newborn assessments, 556t–565t
- physical examination of, 82, 83b–84b

Nose breathing, 530b
Nuchal cord, 466–467, 540–541
Nuchal translucency, 642, 642f
Nuclear family, 18, 18f
Nulligravida, 289
Nullipara, 289
Nulliparous women
- pain perception in, 388
- partogram of, 447f

Nuprin. *See* Ketoprofen
Nurse
- cultural competence of, 21, 27–28
- genetics role of, 57
- home care. *See* Home care nurse

Nurse-client relationship, 344
Nurse-midwives
- certified, 8, 364
- childbirth using, 364
- safety of, 8b

Nursing, 9–11
Nursing Interventions Classification, 9, 10b
Nursing Outcomes Classification, 11, 11t
Nursing practice
- home care, 35
- standards of, 11–14, 12b

Nursing process
- birth trauma, 842b
- breast cancer, 229b
- breastfeeding, 614b
- contraception, 170b
- dysfunctional labor, 798b
- electronic fetal monitoring, 427b
- first stage of labor, 441b–442b
- grief, 936b
- infertility, 199b
- intimate partner violence, 106b
- late preterm infants, 899b
- leiomyomas, 241b
- menstrual disorders, 131b
- miscarriage, 673b
- neonatal sepsis, 846b
- newborn care, 569b
- pain management, 409b
- perimenopause, 138b
- postpartum depression, 772b
- postpartum hemorrhage, 829b
- preterm infants, 899b
- radiation therapy, 254b
- second stage of labor, 461b
- sepsis, 846b
- sexually transmitted infections, 165b
- substance abuse, 765b

Nutrition, 75–76. *See also* Diet
- adolescent pregnancy, 319
- assessment of, 321, 323t, 338
- client education regarding, 321–326
- counseling about, 88–90

Nutrition *(Continued)*
- cultural influences on, 325–326, 326t–327t
- deficiencies in, 75
- importance of, 75, 307
- infertility managed with, 204
- in labor, 450–451
- during lactation, 319
- late preterm infant, 922–923
- maternal education about, 345
- osteoporosis prevention through, 139
- postpartum, 323–325, 496
- preconception, 307–308
- preeclampsia and, 319
- during pregnancy, 308–318, 310t–311t
  - assessment of, 321
  - calcium, 310t–311t, 315–316, 317b
  - care management for, 320–326
  - client education, 321–326
  - energy, 308–313
  - fat-soluble vitamins, 310t–311t, 317–318
  - fiber, 310t–311t
  - fluids, 310t–311t, 314
  - fluoride, 317
  - folate, 310t–311t, 318
  - iodine, 310t–311t
  - iron, 310t–311t, 314–315
  - laboratory testing, 321
  - magnesium, 310t–311t, 316
  - maternal education about, 345
  - minerals, 310t–311t, 314–318
  - nursing care plan for, 324b
  - potassium, 317
  - protein, 310t–311t, 313–314
  - risk factors, 315b
  - sodium, 316–317
  - teaching about, 322–325
  - vitamin A, 310t–311t, 317–318
  - vitamin B_6, 310t–311t, 318
  - vitamin B_{12}, 310t–311t, 326
  - vitamin C, 310t–311t, 318
  - vitamin D, 310t–311t, 318
  - vitamin E, 310t–311t, 317
  - water, 310t–311t, 314
  - water-soluble vitamins, 310t–311t, 318
  - zinc, 310t–311t, 317
- preterm infants, 897, 906–927
- during radiation therapy, 257
- recommendations for, 139

Nutritional history, 338
Nystatin, 855–856

O

Obama, Barack, 4
Obesity, 75
- breast cancer risks, 215
- breastfeeding and, 324–325
- congenital heart anomaly risks, 874
- epidural anesthesia success affected by, 404–405
- fetal risks, 309
- health risks secondary to, 75
- high-risk pregnancies caused by, 6
- infertility risks, 204
- in pregnancy, 75, 312, 312b, 797–799, 798f
- prevalence of, 75

Obsessive-compulsive disorder, 759, 775
Obstetric critical care
- family-centered, 754–755
- hemodynamic monitoring. *See* Hemodynamic monitoring
- trauma. *See* Trauma

Obstetric history, 290, 290t
Obstetric intensive care unit, 735–737
Occupational history, 338–339
Occupational Safety and Health Administration, 40b
Occurrence risk, 56
Odor, 511
Office of Alternative Medicine, 3
Older women. *See also* Menopause
- estrogen loss in, 81
- health assessment in, 81–82
- health risks in, 74
- as vulnerable population, 32

Oligodactyly, 543
Oligohydramnios, 282, 429, 639b, 643, 816, 838, 888
Oligomenorrhea, 127
Oliguria, 748
Omphalocele, 883, 883f
Oncogenes, 54
Oncology Nursing Society, 44
Oogenesis, 271
Operculum, 295, 295f
Ophthalmia neonatorum, 147
Opiates, 763–764
Opioids
- agonists, 398–399, 398b–399b
- agonists-antagonists, 399–400, 399b
- antagonists, 400, 400b
- intrathecal, with epidural block, 406
- side effects of, 406

Opisthotonus, 870
Oral candidiasis, 855
Oral contraceptives
- advantages of, 181–182
- amenorrhea after discontinuation of, 196
- anticonvulsant medications effect on, 728
- combined estrogen-progestin, 181–183
- complications of, 183b
- contraindications, 182
- disadvantages of, 182
- discontinuation of, 182, 196
- drug interactions, 182, 182b
- dysmenorrhea managed with, 123
- endometrial cancer and, 246
- menstrual flow affected by, 127
- missed, 183f
- 91-day regimen, 182–183
- noncontraceptive benefits of, 181
- nursing considerations, 182
- polycystic ovary syndrome treated with, 239
- in pregestational diabetes mellitus patients, 700
- side effects of, 182

Oral glucose tolerance test, 701, 702b
Organ donation, 941
Orgasmic phase, of sexual response, 70t
Orthostatic hypotension, 787b
Ortolani maneuver, 544, 544b, 885
Oscillometry, 896
Osteoporosis
- bisphosphonates for, 139
- calcitonin for, 139
- calcium intake to prevent, 133, 139

Osteoporosis (Continued)
definition of, 133
exercise for, 139, 140f
fractures secondary to, 133
medications for, 139–141
nutritional recommendations for, 139
parathyroid hormone for, 141
perimenopause and, 133–134
prevention of, 139, 140b
skeletal changes associated with, 133f
Outcome and Assessment Information Set, 11
Outcomes-oriented care, 11
Ovarian cancer, 248–251
antineoplastic drugs for, 250
clinical manifestations of, 249–250
diagnosis of, 249–250
etiology of, 248–249
hereditary, 54–55
incidence of, 248–249
nursing considerations, 251
during pregnancy, 265
radiation therapy for, 251
recurrence of, 251
support for patient during, 251
symptom index for, 251
treatment of, 250–251
Ovarian cycle, 67, 68f
Ovarian cysts, 238–240, 239f
collaborative care for, 239
corpus luteum cysts, 239, 265
dermoid cysts, 239
follicular cysts, 238
polycystic ovarian syndrome, 239, 320–321
theca-lutein cysts, 239
Ovarian fibromas, 239–240
Ovarian stimulation therapy, 204
Ovaries
anatomy of, 62f, 63
postmenopausal changes in, 66t
Overweight, 75
Ovulation
basal body temperature before, 69, 198–200
definition of, 63
detection of, 198–200
estrogen levels after, 67
home predictor test kits for, 174–175, 176f, 198–200
postpartum resumption of, 503
progesterone levels after, 64
prostaglandins role in, 69
unpredictability of, 172
Ovulatory, 67
Ovum
description of, 272–273
fertilization of, 172, 273, 273f
illustration of, 273f
implantation of, 68
Oxygen supply, 571
Oxygen therapy, 901–905
assessments during, 902
complications of, 916–919
continuous positive airway pressure, 902, 903f, 903t
criteria for, 901–902
hood administration of, 902, 902f
mechanical ventilation, 903, 903f, 903t
nasal cannula for, 902, 902f
surfactant administration during, 904–905
weaning from, 906
Oxytocin
adverse reactions to, 804b
breastfeeding, 612–613
contraction test by stimulation of, 652
dosing of, 803, 804b
half-life of, 803
hazards associated with, 803
labor induction using, 803–805, 804b
lochia affected by, 479–480
nursing considerations for, 804–805
postpartum uses of
description of, 478–479
postpartum hemorrhage, 827b
production of, 304
uterine contractions, 613, 652
uterine tachysystole with, 805, 805b

P

Paced breathing techniques, 392–393, 393b
Pacifiers, 595, 595f, 618–619
Packed red blood cell volume, 720
Paget's disease of the nipple, 217
Pain, 364
behavioral signs of, 589
cesarean birth-related, 813b
circumcision-related, 587–588
emotional expressions of, 387
endometriosis, 123
gate-control theory of, 388–389
labor-related, 386–389
acupressure for, 395–396, 395f
acupuncture for, 395–396
analgesia and anesthesia for, 397–408
administration methods, 410–412
care management, 408–412, 408b
combined spinal-epidural, 406
definitions, 398
epidural. *See* Epidural anesthesia
general, 407–408, 407f
local, 400–401
maternal monitoring during, 412
nerve block, 400–407
nitrous oxide, 407
opioid agonist analgesics, 398–399, 398b–399b
opioid agonist-antagonist analgesics, 399–400, 399b
opioid antagonists, 400, 400b
pudendal nerve block, 401, 401f
regional, 411–412
safety concerns, 412
spinal. *See* Spinal anesthesia
systemic, 398–400
timing of, 408
anxiety associated with, 388
aromatherapy for, 396–397
biofeedback for, 396
breathing techniques for, 392–393, 393b
care management for, 408–412
cold therapy for, 396
comfort measures for, 389
complementary and alternative therapies for, 390b
counterpressure for, 393
Pain (Continued)
cultural influences on response to, 388, 388b
distraction techniques for, 391
effleurage for, 393
environmental influences on, 389
expression of, 387
focusing techniques for, 391–393, 392f
heat therapy for, 396
hypnosis for, 396
intradermal water block for, 397, 397f
music for, 393–394
neurologic origins of, 386–387
nonpharmacologic management of, 389–397, 408, 410b
nursing process for, 409b
pathways of, 401f
patient-controlled analgesia for, 398
perception of, 387
pharmacologic management of, 397–408, 398b
physiologic factors, 387–388
previous experience with, 388
relaxation techniques for, 391–393, 392f
response to, 387–389
sedatives for, 397
touch for, 396
transcutaneous electrical nerve stimulation for, 395, 395f
water therapy for, 394–395, 394f
menstruation-related. *See* Dysmenorrhea
in newborn, 588–589
nonpharmacologic management of, 389–397, 410b, 589
pelvic, 126
perception of, 387
pharmacologic management of, 397–408, 398b, 589
in preterm infant. *See* Preterm infant, pain in
referred, 386
somatic, 387
tolerance to, 387
Palmar grasp reflex, 546t–549t, 556t–565t
Pancreas. *See also* Insulin
embryologic development of, 282
fetal, 693
in pregnancy, 305
Panic attacks, 776
Pannus, 798–799
Papanicolaou test
cervical cancer detection using, 253, 263–264
description of, 86, 87b, 89t
pregnancy-related changes that affect, 293–294
Paradoxical respirations, 530
Paralytic ileus, 248
Parathyroid gland, 305
Parathyroid hormone, 141
Parent(s). *See also* Couple; Father; Mother
acquaintance, 508, 509f
anticipatory grief by, 913, 927
anticipatory guidance for, 598–599
attachment by, 507–510, 508f, 508t, 510b
Parent(s) (Continued)
bonding by, 507–510, 510b
claiming process by, 508
hearing-impaired, 523, 524b
infant interactions with, 501, 510–511
adjustments, 517–519
behavioral repertoires, 518–519
biorhythmicity, 512
communication, 511–512
cultural influences on, 522
early contact, 510
entrainment, 511–512
extended contact, 510–511
eye contact, 511
odor, 511
promotion of, 573–574, 589–591
reciprocity, 512
responsivity, 519
skin-to-skin contact, 510
social, 595–596
synchrony, 512
voice, 511
maternal role attainment, 514–515, 514t
perinatal loss. *See* Perinatal loss
preterm infant. *See* Preterm infant, parent
role of, after birth, 512–519
sensory-impaired, 522–523, 523b
tasks and responsibilities of, 512–514
visually impaired, 523, 523b
Parenteral nutrition, 909
Parenthood
care management in, 526
couple's adjustment to, 516–519
cultural influences, 521–522
paternal adjustment to, 515–516, 516f, 516t
personal aspirations affected by, 522
social support during, 521
socioeconomic influences, 522
transition to, 512, 513b, 515–516, 519–522, 526b
Parity, 289–290
Paroxetine, 758–759
Partial liquid ventilation, 906
Partial mastectomy, 221–222, 222f
Partial pressure of carbon dioxide, 300
Partial pressure of oxygen, 531, 746
Participant observation, 30
Partograms, 447f
Parvovirus B19, 853
Past health history, 83b–84b
Patau syndrome, 50–51
Patellar reflex, 660–661, 661f
Patent ductus arteriosus, 710, 875f, 917
Pathologic jaundice, 538, 538t, 868, 869b
Patient Protection and Affordable Care Act, 4
Patient-controlled analgesia
description of, 248
labor-related pain managed with, 398
Patient-controlled epidural anesthesia, 405
Patterned-paced breathing, 393, 393b
Pelvic canal, 373, 374f
Pelvic cavity, 373, 374f
Pelvic dystocia, 794

Pelvic examination, 84–86
in adolescents, 81
bimanual palpation, 86, 88f
external inspection, 84, 84f
external palpation, 84–85, 84f
after hysterectomy, 88
internal, 85–86
lithotomy position for, 80f, 84
in older women, 81
Papanicolaou test. *See* Papanicolaou test
during pregnancy, 86
prenatal, 339
procedure for, 86b
rectovaginal palpation, 86, 88f
specimen collection during, 86
vagina, 86
vulvodynia evaluations, 245
Pelvic exenteration, 259–260, 260f
Pelvic floor
anatomy of, 374
pregnancy-related changes in, 296f
Pelvic hematomas, 825–826
Pelvic inflammatory disease, 150–151, 151t
Pelvic inlet, 373, 382
Pelvic outlet, 373, 373f, 375t
Pelvic pain, 126
Pelvic relaxation, 235
Pelvic rocking, 348f
Pelvic support alterations, 234–238, 235f
Pelvic tilt, 348b
Pelvis
bony, 63, 63f, 372–374, 373f
fracture of, 751
gynecoid, 374, 376t
types of, 373, 376t
Penetrating abdominal trauma, 751–752
Penicillin, 150
Percutaneous arterial catheterization, 744
Percutaneous balloon mitral valvuloplasty, 711
Percutaneous umbilical blood sampling, 648, 648f
Periauricular papillomas, 540–541
Perimenopause. *See also* Menopause
age of onset, 130
behavioral responses, 132–133
bleeding changes during, 131
definition of, 130
description of, 69, 72
genital changes during, 131–132
health risks, 133–134, 133f
hot flashes or flushes during, 132, 136
mood responses, 132–133
night sweats associated with, 132
nursing process for, 138b
physical changes during, 131–133
vasomotor instability associated with, 132
Perimortem cesarean birth, 754
Perinatal asphyxia, 925
Perinatal care
continuum of, 34f
home-based, 35, 37b
regionalization of, 7
risk assessments, 7
Perinatal education, 363–367
Perinatal health, 29
Perinatal health nurse, 29
Perinatal hypoxia, 843
Perinatal loss, 931–932. *See also* Miscarriage; Stillbirth
actualizing of, 937–940
acute distress at, 932–933
adolescent pregnancy, 947–948
assessments, 935
autopsy decisions, 940–941
care management for, 935–946, 937f–939f
coping with, 932, 943
father's response to, 932–933
final disposition after, 941–942
funeral service, 942
grandparent responses to, 934–935
grief responses to. *See* Grief
multifetal pregnancy, 947
organ donation decisions, 941
parents
actualizing of loss to, 937–940
communication with, 943–945
coping by, 943
cultural needs of, 945
decision making by, 940–942
discharge of, 945–946
feelings of, 942–943
listening to, 942
memories for, 944, 944f
responses by, 932–933
spiritual needs of, 945
postmortem care, 946
sexuality after, 934
sibling responses to, 934–935
spiritual rites, 941
Perinatal mortality rate
collaborations to reduce, 7
definition of, 5b, 895b
in postmature infant, 923
Perinatal nursing
ethical issues in, 14
research in, 14
Perineal body, 61, 61f
Perineum. *See also* Episiotomy
anatomy of, 61, 61f
assessment of, 85
hygiene of, 345
lacerations to, 470, 493, 825, 829
postpartum changes in, 480–481
pregnancy-related changes in, 295
trauma to, 470–471
Periodic breathing, 896
Peripartum cardiomyopathy, 713
Peripheral vascular system, 82, 83b–84b
Peritoneum, 62
Persistent pulmonary hypertension of the newborn, 924
Personal hygiene, 345, 448–450
Personal protective equipment, 40, 166b
Personal space, 25
Pessaries, 238, 238f
Petechiae, 574, 838
Pharmacogenomics, 46
Phenergan. *See* Promethazine
Phenothiazines, 397
Phenotype, 45–48
Phenylalanine hydrolase, 707
Phenylketonuria
definition of, 53, 889
maternal, 707–708
newborn screening for, 45, 282, 578t
treatment of, 889
Phenytoin, 727
Phlebostatic axis, 742f
Phosphatidylglycerol, 843
Phototherapy, 35, 574f, 584–586, 911f
Phrenic nerve injury, 840–841
Physical activity. *See also* Exercise
description of, 90, 319
during pregnancy, 319, 346, 347b, 348f, 359–360
restrictions in, 662, 663b
Physical examination, 82–88
first stage of labor, 441–446
pelvic examination. *See* Pelvic examination
prenatal, 339, 341
preparation for, 82
recommendations, 89t
Physical fitness, 76
Physicians, 364
Physiologic anemia, 298
Physiologic edema, 301
Physiologic jaundice, 537–538, 575, 867–868
Physiologic retraction ring, 374, 376f
Phytoestrogens, 136
Pica, 318–319, 318f
Pitocin. *See* Oxytocin
Pitting edema, 660, 660f
Pituitary gland
hormones of, 481
in pregnancy, 304–305
Placenta, 277–279
abruption of. *See* Abruptio placentae
aging, 642
battledore, 277, 685, 686f
blood flow in, 293
drug passage across, 279
estrogen production by, 278
expulsion of, 471, 473f, 690
functions of, 277–279, 642
glucose transport across, 690
hormones produced by, 278, 481
infection passage across. *See* Transplacental infections
ischemia of, 657
maternal arterial blood, 279
metabolic functions of, 278–279
position of, 642
postpartum site of, 479
progesterone production by, 278, 278f
retained, 826
separation of, 471, 473f, 751, 824–825
structure of, 277–278, 277f
succenturiate, 685
ultrasonography evaluation of, 642
Placenta accreta, 826
Placenta increta, 826
Placenta percreta, 826
Placenta previa, 680–683
clinical manifestations of, 680–681, 681t
diagnosis of, 682
etiology of, 680
fetal outcomes of, 681–682
home care for, 683
incidence of, 680
management of, 682–683
maternal outcomes of, 681–682
nursing process for, 682b
types of, 681f
Placental growth factor, 659
Plan B, 184
Plantar grasp reflex, 546t–549t, 556t–565t
PlastiBell device, for circumcision, 587, 587f
Plateau phase, of sexual response, 70t
Platelet count, 533
Platypelloid pelvis, 374, 376t
Play, 603t
Plugged milk ducts, 629
Pneumonia, chlamydial, 855
Pneumothorax, 751
Point of maximal impulse, 296, 443, 531
Point-of-care testing, 7
Polycystic ovarian syndrome, 239, 320–321
Polycythemia, 532, 844, 925–926
Polydactyly, 543, 886
Polyhydramnios, 639, 643, 691–692, 888
Polyploidy, 49-50
Polyps
endometrial, 240f
uterine, 240, 240f
Popliteal angle, 568b
Population
aging of, 9
demographics of, 19
Population-based screening, 45–46
Port-wine stain, 540
Positions
for childbirth, 378, 379f, 430, 452–453, 452f–453f, 455b, 460–464, 461f, 463f
for physically disabled women, 79, 80f
Positive end-expiratory pressure, 725
Postanesthesia recovery, 473–474
Postcoital test, 202
Postdate, 289
Postdural puncture headache, 403–404, 404f
Postmature infants, 923–924
characteristics of, 923
definition of, 569, 923
meconium aspiration syndrome in, 923–924
perinatal mortality rate in, 923
persistent pulmonary hypertension of the newborn, 924
Postmenopausal women, 66t
Postmortem care, 946
Postpartum "blues," 515, 515b
Postpartum depression
assessment of, 773b
care management of, 770–775
community care for, 772–773
electroconvulsive therapy for, 775
etiology of, 768
irritability associated with, 769
medical management of, 769
nursing care for, 771–772, 771b
nursing process for, 772b
partner's reaction to, 772
prevention of, 771b
psychiatric hospitalization for, 773–774
with psychotic features, 769–770
psychotropic medications for, 774–775
referrals for, 772
risk factors for, 768, 768b
safety considerations, 773

Postpartum depression (Continued)
screening tools for, 770–771
selective serotonin reuptake inhibitors for, 861
without psychotic features, 768–769
Postpartum Depression Predictors Inventory, 770
Postpartum Depression Screening Scale, 770
Postpartum fatigue, 495, 515
Postpartum hemorrhage, 824–830
care management of, 826–830
definition of, 824
discharge instructions for, 830
etiology of, 824–825
genital tract lacerations, 825–826
inversion of uterus, 826–827, 829
retained placenta, 826
subinvolution of uterus, 826, 828
uterine atony, 825
herbal remedies for, 827b, 828
incidence of, 824
medical management of, 827b, 826–828
nursing assessments for, 828f
nursing care plan for, 830b
nursing interventions for, 828–830, 828f
nursing process for, 829b
risk factors for, 824–825, 825b
Postpartum period
abdominal changes in, 481, 481f
afterpains in, 479
ambulation in, 496
anal incontinence in, 482
bereavement, 943
bladder
changes in, 482
distention prevention, 493–494
blood components in, 483–484
bowel evacuation in, 482
bowel function in, 498
breastfeeding promotion, 499
breasts in, 482
cardiac output in, 483
cardiovascular system
description of, 483–484
disorders of, 718–719
cervix, 480
cesarean birth, 813–814
coagulation factors, 483
comfort in, 494–496
community resources, 505, 505b
complications in
coagulopathies, 832
hemorrhage. See Postpartum hemorrhage
idiopathic thrombocytopenic purpura, 832
infections. See Postpartum period, infections
thromboembolic disease, 832–833
von Willebrand disease, 832
complications of, 489t, 502–503
contraception in, 503
cultural diversity effects, 502
definition of, 478
depression in. See Postpartum depression
diabetes mellitus care in
gestational, 704
pregestational, 700–701
Postpartum period (Continued)
discharge
criteria for, 488–489, 488b
follow-up after, 504–505
infection presentation after, 835
law relating to, 487–488
legal considerations, 489b
planning for, 487–489
self-management, 502–503
teaching, 502–504
diuresis in, 482
endocrine system in, 481
excessive bleeding prevention in, 493–494
exercise in, 496, 497f
family planning in, 503b–504b
family structure and functioning in, 501
follow-up care, 504–505
gastrointestinal system in, 482
home visits, 504–505
immune system in, 484
infections, 833–835
care management of, 835
definition of, 833
endometritis, 834–835, 834f
mastitis, 834–835, 834f
nursing diagnoses for, 835b
predisposing factors, 834b
prevention of, 492–493, 835
urinary tract, 834–835
wound, 834–835
integumentary system in, 484
laboratory tests, 490
lactation suppression, 499
maternal cardiovascular disorders managed in, 718–719
maternal self-image in, 501
musculoskeletal system in, 484
neurologic system in, 484
nursing interventions in, 490–500
nursing process, 490b
nutrition in, 323–325, 498
parent-infant interactions, 501
pelvic muscular support, 481
perineum, 480–481
physical assessments, 489–490, 490b
preeclampsia with severe gestational hypertension, 666–667
pregestational diabetes mellitus care in, 700–701
prescribed medicines in, 503–504
psychologic complications of, 767–776
anxiety disorders, 775–776
depression. See Postpartum depression
mood disorders, 768–775
psychosocial needs, 500–502, 500b–501b
rest in, 494–496
Rh isoimmunization, 499–500, 499b–500b
rubella vaccination, 499, 499b
self-management, 502–503
sexual activity in, 503, 504b, 517
substance abuse management in, 767
support groups, 505
tetanus-diphtheria-acellular pertussis vaccination, 499
transfer from recovery area, 486–487
urethral changes, 482
Postpartum period (Continued)
urinary system in, 481–482
uterus
changes in, 478–480
contractions of, 478–479
tone, 493
vagina, 480–481
vaginal birth, 491b
varicella vaccination, 499, 499b
varicosities in, 484, 484f
vital signs in, 483, 483t
voiding in, 496–498
Postpartum psychosis, 769–770, 773
Postterm, 289, 569, 895b. See also Postmature infant
Postterm pregnancy, 815–816, 816b
Posttraumatic stress disorder, 759, 948
Posttraumatic stress syndrome
characteristics of, 101t
rape as cause of, 110
Posture
exercises for, 140f
newborn, 556t–565t
pregnancy-related changes in, 302–303, 346–349
Potassium, 317
Powers, 374–378
primary, 374–377
secondary, 377–378, 793, 793t
Prana, 396
Precipitous labor, 794
Preconception classes, 7
Preconception counseling and care, 70, 71b, 337, 691, 724–725
Predictive testing, 45
Predispositional testing, 45
Preeclampsia, 656
activity restriction for, 662, 663b
assessment of, 662b
care management of, 658–667
causes of, 656–657
chronic hypertension with, 656
deep tendon reflexes testing, 660–661, 661f, 661t
definition of, 656
description of, 316b
endothelial cell dysfunction associated with, 657, 657f
etiology of, 656–657, 657f
future risks, 667
gestational hypertension with
antihypertensive medications for, 666, 666t
dietary recommendations, 663b
intrapartum care for, 663–666
magnesium sulfate for, 664–666, 665b–666b
mild, 661–662
nursing care plan for, 664b
postpartum care for, 666–667
severe, 662–667
health assessment and screening, 659–661
HELLP syndrome, 658, 658b, 666–667
laboratory findings in, 656t
mild, 655t, 660b, 661–662
neurologic conditions associated with, 658
nutrition and, 319
pathophysiology of, 657–658, 657f
physical examination of, 660–661
pitting edema tests, 660, 660f
Preeclampsia (Continued)
prevention of, 658–659
proteinuria tests, 661
refractory oliguria caused by, 748
resources for, 656b
risk factors for, 656, 657b, 659b
severe, 655t, 662–667
signs of, 662b
Pregestational diabetes mellitus, 691–701
antepartum care of, 693–701
blood glucose
levels of, 695t
monitoring of, 697–699, 698b
care management of, 693–701
cesarean birth in, 699
childbirth date determination, 699
definition of, 689
dietary management of, 695, 695b
exercise for, 695–696
fetal risks and complications, 693
fetal surveillance in, 699
hospitalization for, 699
infant of mother with. See Diabetes mellitus, infants of mothers with
insulin therapy for, 696–697, 696b, 697t
intrapartum care of, 699–700
intrauterine fetal demise risks, 692–693
maternal risks and complications, 691–693
mode of birth in, 699
nursing process for, 694b
oral contraceptives use in patients with, 700
postpartum care of, 700–701
preconception counseling, 691
resources for, 691b
urine testing in, 699
Pregnancy. See also Childbirth; First trimester; Labor; Second trimester; Third trimester
abdomen changes in, 292, 293f–294f
abdominal discomfort in, 304, 304f
acceptance of, 331, 333
acid-base balance in, 300
adaptations to
grandparents, 331–332, 335–336
maternal, 289, 291–305, 330–336
paternal, 333–335
siblings, 335, 335b
adolescent. See Adolescent pregnancy
adrenal glands in, 305
alcohol use during. See Alcohol use and abuse, during pregnancy
anaphylactoid syndrome of, 820–821, 820b
anemia in, 720–722
anticoagulant therapy during, 714
appendicitis during, 732
appetite in, 303
asymptomatic bacteriuria in, 730–731, 731b
autoimmune disorders in, 728–729
basal metabolic rate in, 298–300
Bell palsy in, 728
bleeding in, 670–680
ectopic pregnancy. See Ectopic pregnancy
miscarriage as cause of. See Miscarriage

Pregnancy *(Continued)*
blood glucose levels in, 695t, 698
blood pressure during, 297, 297b
breast cancer during, 263
breast changes in, 295–296
breastfeeding during, 626
caffeine ingestion during, 314, 314t, 861
cancer during, 246, 263–266
cardiac output in, 298, 719
cardiopulmonary resuscitation during, 719, 719b, 720f
cardiovascular system
adaptations in, 296–298, 299t, 737, 738t, 750t
disorders of. *See* Cardiovascular system, maternal disorders of
cervical cancer during, 263–264
cervical changes in, 293–294, 295f
chemotherapy during, 264–265
chlamydia during, 162t
coagulation in, 298, 299t
cocaine use during, 763, 860, 860b
colloid osmotic pressure in, 738
colon cancer in, 264
complications of, 737b
critical illness during, 736–737
cultural beliefs and practices, 26t–27t
cystitis in, 731
cytomegalovirus exposure during, 163t, 164, 164b, 851
dermatologic disorders in, 302, 726–727
diagnosis of, 330, 330b. *See also* Pregnancy tests
discomforts of, 352–353, 356b–357b
ectopic. *See* Ectopic pregnancy
electrolyte balance in, 301
employment during, 349–350
endocrine system changes in, 304–305
endometrial cancer during, 265
energy needs during, 308–313
epilepsy in, 727–728, 727b
exercise during, 319, 346, 347b, 348f, 359–360
factors that affect, 308f
fluid balance in, 301
food guide during, 313t
gallbladder in, 304
gastrointestinal system
adaptations in, 303–304, 750t
disorders of, 729–730
gonococcal infections in, 147, 162t
grandparent adaptations to, 331–332, 335–336, 336f
group B streptococcus during, 162t
heart surgery during, 716
hematologic adaptations in, 738, 750t
herpes simplex virus during, 153–154, 162t–163t, 164
high-risk. *See* High-risk pregnancy
in homeless women, 33
human immunodeficiency virus in, 157–159, 340b
human papillomavirus in, 152, 162t
hypertensive disorders in. *See* Hypertensive disorders
indicators of, 292, 292t, 330
inflammatory bowel disease in, 730
insulin needs during, 690f

Pregnancy *(Continued)*
integumentary system
adaptations in, 301–302, 301f, 302b
disorders of, 726–727
intimate partner violence during, 95, 103
laboratory values during, 299t
length of, 273–274, 330
leukemia during, 264
liver in, 304
maternal adaptations to
acceptance, 331–332
childbirth preparations, 332–333
education about, 344
mother role, 331
relationship with fetus, 332
reordering of personal relationships, 331–332
systemic, 291–305, 302, 737, 749–750, 750t
maternal self-management in, 344–357
airline travel, 351
alcohol consumption, 351–352
body mechanics, 346–349, 348f
breastfeeding preparation, 345–346
cigarette smoking, 351–352, 352b
clothing, 350, 350f, 359
complementary and alternative therapies, 351b
dental care, 346
herbal preparations, 351, 351b
immunizations, 351
Kegel exercises, 91, 91b, 138, 237, 345, 470, 481, 496, 498b
nutrition, 345
personal hygiene, 345
physical activity, 346, 347b, 348f, 359–360
posture, 346–349, 348b
rest and relaxation, 349, 349f
travel, 350–351, 351f
urinary tract infections, 345
medical conditions during, 77
mental health disorders during
anxiety disorders, 759–761, 760t
mood disorders, 757–759
prevalence of, 757
metabolic changes associated with, 689–690
molar, 239, 266, 678–680
multifetal
description of, 286–287, 286f–287f, 362–363
dystocia caused by, 796–797
perinatal loss in, 947
multiple sclerosis in, 728
musculoskeletal system changes, 302–303, 302f, 750t
myasthenia gravis in, 729
nausea and vomiting of. *See also* Hyperemesis gravidarum
complementary and alternative therapies for, 353b
management of, 325, 326b, 354t–355t
onset of, 303
neurologic disorders in, 727–728
neurologic system changes, 303

Pregnancy *(Continued)*
nursing care during, 337b
nutrition during. *See* Nutrition, during pregnancy
obesity in, 75, 312, 312b, 797–799, 798f
ovarian cancer during, 265
pancreas in, 305
parathyroid gland in, 305
pelvic examination during, 86
physical activity during, 319, 346, 347b, 348f, 359–360
pituitary gland in, 304–305
postterm, 815–816, 816b
postural changes in, 302–303
preoperative care in, 732–733
psychosocial support in, 358
pulmonary capillary wedge pressure during, 744
pulmonary disorders in, 722–726
acute respiratory distress syndrome, 725–726
asthma, 722, 723t, 723b
cystic fibrosis, 722–725
influenza, 724b
pulmonary function in, 298, 300t
pyelonephritis in, 731
radiation therapy during, 265
rape as cause of, 759
renal system adaptations, 299t, 300–301, 750t
respiratory system adaptations, 298–300, 300t, 738, 750t
rubella exposure during, 163t, 164
sexual activity during, 332, 334, 353b, 357–358, 358f, 360
sexually transmitted infections in, 146b, 162–164, 162t
sibling adaptations to, 335, 335b
signs of, 292, 292t, 330
smoking during, 351–352, 352b, 761–762, 856–857, 857t
stomach changes in, 303–304
substance abuse during. *See* Substance abuse
surgery during, 732–733
syphilis during, 162t
systemic lupus erythematosus in, 728–729
thyroid cancer in, 264
thyroid gland in, 305
TORCH infections in, 162–164, 163t, 848
toxoplasmosis exposure during, 163–164, 163t, 848
trauma during. *See* Trauma, during pregnancy
urinary tract infections in, 730–732, 732b
uterine changes in, 292–294
vaginal changes in, 295
varicella-zoster exposure, 849
violence during, 78
vulva changes in, 295
weight gain in, 309–313, 309f, 311b, 312t, 320b
in women older than age 35, 74, 360–362
Pregnancy Risk Assessment Monitoring System, 761
Pregnancy tests, 290–291, 291f, 291b
Pregnancy-associated placental protein, 649
Preimplantation genetic diagnosis, 207

Preload, 740
Premature rupture of membranes, 675–676, 784, 791
Premenstrual dysphoric disorder, 123–125, 123t
Premenstrual syndrome, 123–125, 123t, 125b
Prenatal care
adolescent pregnancy, 360
barriers to, 336
benefits of, 7
collaborative care, 344–358
cultural influences, 358–360
description of, 73, 329
emotional response, 359
fetal assessments, 341–343
fetal heart tones, 341, 343f
fundal height, 341–342, 342f
gestational age, 342–343
health status, 343
goals of, 71b
laboratory tests, 340, 340t, 343–344
multidisciplinary approach to, 337
multifetal pregnancy, 362–363
multiparous women, 360–362
pelvic examination, 339
physical examination, 339, 341
prevalence of, 336
primiparous women, 362
purpose of, 336
racial and ethnic disparities in, 7–8
variations in, 358–363
visits
follow-up, 340–358
initial, 337–340
schedule of, 336
in women older than 35 years, 360–362
Prenatal interview, 337–339, 341
Prepidil Gel. *See* Dinoprostone
Prepuce, 61, 61f
Prescription drugs, 75
Presentation, fetal, 370, 371f–372f, 462b
Presymptomatic testing, 45
Preterm, 289, 569
Preterm birth
causes of, 780b, 781
definition of, 5, 779–780
fetal loss caused by, 790
HELLP syndrome as cause of, 658
incidence of, 894–895
indicated, 780, 780b
inevitable, 790
low birth weight versus, 780
neonatal loss caused by, 790
race and, 780
recurrent, 781
resources for, 784b
risk factors for, 780–781
sociodemographic factors associated with, 781
spontaneous, 780–781
very, 780
Preterm infants, 894–927
body temperature maintenance, 896, 899–901
breastfeeding of, 621–622, 906
cardiovascular function in, 896
care management of, 898
central nervous system function in, 897
cold stress in, 896, 897b
communication by, 911–912
complications in, 915–919

- Preterm infants *(Continued)*
  - bronchopulmonary dysplasia, 917
  - germinal matrix hemorrhage–intraventricular hemorrhage, 917–918
  - necrotizing enterocolitis, 918–919, 918b
  - patent ductus arteriosus, 917
  - respiratory distress syndrome, 915–916, 916f
  - retinopathy of prematurity, 916–917
- cycled lighting for, 911
- definition of, 895b
- development of
  - care to promote, 911–912
  - potential of, 898
- elimination patterns in, 907
- environmental concerns for, 910–911, 910f
- extracorporeal membrane oxygenation in, 905–906
- feeding of, 907–910, 908f
- fluid loss or gain in, 907
- formula feeding of, 906, 906b
- gastrostomy feeding of, 908–909
- gavage feeding of, 908–910, 908f, 909b
- growth and development potential of, 898
- hearing loss in, 910
- hematologic status in, 897–898
- hepatic problems in, 539
- hyperthermia in, 896, 897b
- hypothermia in, 897b, 899–901, 901f
- incidence of, 894–895
- infection resistance in, 898
- kangaroo care for, 912, 912f
- late, 922–923
  - breastfeeding of, 622
  - definition of, 622, 895b, 922
  - description of, 569–570, 576b
  - hyperbilirubinemia in, 923
  - hypoglycemia in, 923
  - infection in, 923
  - nursing process for, 899b
  - nutrition for, 922–923
  - prevalence of, 780
  - recognition of, 922
  - respiratory distress in, 922
  - risks associated with, 922
  - thermoregulation in, 922
- nitric oxide therapy in, 905
- nonnutritive sucking by, 910, 910f
- nursing care plan for, 900b–901b
- nursing process for, 899b
- nutritional care in, 897, 906–927
- oral feeding of, 907–908
- oxygen therapy in, 901–905
  - assessments during, 902
  - complications of, 916–919
  - continuous positive airway pressure, 902, 903f, 903t
  - criteria for, 901–902
  - hood administration of, 902, 902f
  - mechanical ventilation, 903, 903f, 903t
  - nasal cannula for, 902, 902f
  - surfactant administration during, 904–905
  - weaning from, 906

- Preterm infants *(Continued)*
  - pain in, 919–922
    - assessment of, 919
    - management of, 920–922, 921b
    - manifestations of, 919, 920b
    - memory of, 919–920
    - non-pharmacologic management of, 921b
    - untreated, 920
  - parenteral nutrition for, 909
  - parents
    - adaptation by, 912–915
    - education of, 915
    - maladaptation by, 915
    - responses by, 913, 913f
    - support for, 913–915
    - tasks for, 913–915
  - partial liquid ventilation in, 906
  - physical care for, 899–927
  - positions for, 911, 911f
  - renal function in, 897
  - respiratory function in, 896
  - risks for, 895
  - sibling responses to, 914, 914f
  - skin care of, 910
  - stimulation of, 912
  - stimuli reduction for, 911
  - surfactant administration in, 904–905, 905b
  - thermoregulation in, 896
  - total parenteral nutrition for, 909
  - weight loss or gain in, 907, 907b
- Preterm labor, 779–790
  - biochemical markers of, 781
  - care management of, 782–790
    - activity restriction, 784, 785b
    - bed rest, 784, 784b–785b, 785f
    - home care, 784
    - lifestyle modifications, 784
    - prevention, 782–783
  - causes of, 781
  - cervical length and, 781
  - client education about, 783
  - definition of, 779–780
  - diagnosis of, 783–784
  - early recognition of, 783–784
  - fetal fibronectin as indicator of, 781, 783
  - infection as risk for, 781
  - nursing care plan for, 782b
  - periodontal disease and, 781
  - recognition of, 357
  - risk factors for, 780–781, 780b
  - signs and symptoms of, 783b
  - tocolytic therapy for, 786–790, 786b–789b
  - uterine activity associated with
    - description of, 783b
    - suppression of, 786–790, 786b–789b
  - vaginal discharge associated with, 783b
- Preterm premature rupture of membranes, 780, 791, 791b
- Primary care providers
  - nurse-midwives as, 8
  - physicians as, 8
- Primary dysmenorrhea, 121–123
- Primary powers, 374–377
- Primary prevention, 28
- Primary pulmonary hypertension, 712
- Primigravida, 289

- Primipara, 289
- Procainamide (Pronestyl), 716t
- Procardia. *See* Nifedipine
- Professional publications, 29–30
- Progesterone
  - glucose affected by, 690
  - infertility treated with, 205b
  - placental production of, 278, 278f
  - postovulatory increases in, 64
  - postpartum decreases in, 481
  - pregnancy uses of, 304, 750
- Progesterone receptors, 221
- Progestin-only contraceptives, 183–184, 729
- Prolactin
  - anovulation caused by, 196
  - breastfeeding and, 612
  - pregnancy levels of, 304, 481
  - suckling-induced release of, 189
- Prolonged deceleration, of fetal heart rate, 423–424, 426f
- Promethazine, 397
- Prophylactic mastectomy, 223
- Propranolol, 716t
- Propylthiouracil, 706
- Prostaglandin(s)
  - definition of, 69
  - E_1, 800, 801b
  - E_2, 531, 826, 802b
  - $F_2\alpha$, 121
  - miscarriage managed with, 673
  - production of, 69
- Prostaglandin synthetase inhibitors, 787b–789b
- Prostin E_2. *See* Dinoprostone
- Protein
  - food sources of, 313, 313t, 314b
  - newborn requirements, 611
  - pregnancy intake of, 310t–311t, 313–314
- Proteinuria
  - description of, 301, 383
  - in preeclampsia, 661
- Proto-oncogenes, 54
- Pruritic urticarial papules and plaques of pregnancy, 726
- Pruritus, 726, 726f
- Pseudomenstruation, 283
- Psoriasis, 726
- Psychiatric commitment, 773b
- Psychological First Aid, 111–113
- Psychosis, 760
- Psychosocial assessment, 38b
- Psychotropic medications, 774–775
- Puberty, 67
- Pubic arch, 63, 63f
- Pudendal nerve block, 401, 401f
- Pull-to-sit reflex, 546t–549t
- Pulmonary artery catheter, 741–742
  - components of, 741, 742f
  - description of, 741
  - hemodynamic monitoring using, 741–745
  - insertion of, 743b
  - pressure readings with, 743–744
  - protocol for, 743b
  - troubleshooting of, 745b
  - venous access for, 742–743, 743b
  - waveforms, 743–744
- Pulmonary artery pressure, 741, 748, 748t
- Pulmonary capillary wedge pressure, 738, 744, 744b, 748, 748t

- Pulmonary disorders, 722–726
  - acute respiratory distress syndrome, 725–726
  - asthma, 722, 723t, 723b
  - cystic fibrosis, 722–725
  - influenza, 724b
- Pulmonary edema, 738, 749
- Pulmonary embolism, 832–833
- Pulmonary interstitial emphysema, 903
- Pulmonary surfactants, 281–282, 529–530
- Pulmonary vascular resistance, 740, 748t
- Pulmonic stenosis, 874, 875f
- Pulse, 483t
- Pulse oximetry, 429, 722, 746
- Purified protein derivative tuberculin test, 340
- Pyelonephritis, 731
- Pyrosis, 304, 321, 325, 354t–355t

Q

- Quality and Safety Education for Nurses, 13, 14b
- Quickening, 294
- Quinidine (Quinidex), 716t

R

- Race. *See also specific racial group*
  - birth rates based on, 5
  - breast cancer risks, 214, 215f
  - diversity in, 2
  - low-birth-weight infants based on, 5
  - maternal mortality rate based on, 6
  - prenatal care utilization based on, 7–8
  - preterm birth and, 780
- Radiation, of heat, 533
- Radiation therapy
  - breast cancer treated with, 225, 231–232
  - cervical cancer treated with, 254b, 256–259, 257f, 258b
  - complications of, 259
  - external, 257–258, 258b
  - fetal effects of, 265
  - internal, 258–259, 259b
  - intracavitary implant for, 257, 257f
  - nurse exposure to, 258
  - nursing process during, 254b
  - nutrition during, 257
  - ovarian cancer treated with, 251
  - during pregnancy, 265
  - vulvar cancer treated with, 261
- Radical hysterectomy
  - cervical cancer treated with, 255–256
  - ovarian cancer treated with, 248
- Radical vulvectomy, 261–262, 261f, 262b, 265
- Radioactive iodine, 706
- Radioimmunoassay tests, 290
- Radioreceptor assay, 291
- Raloxifene hydrochloride, 140–141, 217, 226, 227b
- Rape
  - acquaintance, 109–110
  - collaborative care for, 111–115
  - definition of, 109
  - discharge instructions, 115
  - emergency department protocol for, 112b
  - examination after, 113–114
  - history-taking after, 113

Rape (*Continued*)
- immediate care after, 114–115
- incapacitated, 110
- incidence of, 109
- laboratory tests, 113–114
- mental health consequences of, 110
- nursing diagnoses for, 114–115, 114b
- perpetrators of, 109–110
- physical examination after, 113–114
- pregnancy caused by, 759
- prevention classes, 115
- Psychological First Aid after, 111–113
- recovery after, 111
- statutory, 109
- stranger, 110

Rape-trauma syndrome, 101t, 110–111
Rashes, 593–594
Reactivity, 529
Recessive trait, 47–48
Reciprocal translocation, 51
Reciprocity, 512
Rectal suppositories, 498b
Rectocele, 85, 235–236, 235f, 238
Rectovaginal fistula, 237–238, 237f, 541
Rectovaginal palpation, 86, 88f
Rectum, 84
Rectus abdominis, 303, 303f
Recurrence risk, 56
Recurrent miscarriage, 672
Red blood cells, 532
Reflexes
- deep tendon, 546t–549t, 660–661, 661f, 661t
- newborn, 545, 546t–549t

Refugees, 32–33
Regional anesthesia, 411–412
Reglan. *See* Metoclopramide
Rehabilitation Act of 1973, 523
Relaxation
- conscious, 349, 349b
- labor-related pain managed with, 391–393, 392f
- during pregnancy, 349, 349f

Relaxin, 346–347
Religion
- description of, 82
- infertility and, 198b

Renal plasma flow, 300
Renal system. *See also* Kidneys
- pregnancy-related adaptations, 299t, 300–301, 750t
- preterm infants, 897

Repertoire of behaviors, 518–519
Reproductive system
- embryologic development of, 283
- female. *See* Female reproductive system
- male, 541, 542f, 556t–565t
- newborn, 541–542, 542f, 556t–565t
- pregnancy-related changes, 750t

Reproductive tract infection, 143
Research
- ethical guidelines for, 14
- perinatal nursing, 14
- women's health care, 14

Resolution phase, of sexual response, 70t
Respiratory acidemia, 429t
Respiratory alkalosis, 300
Respiratory distress, 530, 922
Respiratory distress syndrome, 843, 915–916, 916f
Respiratory rate, 556t–565t, 565
Respiratory syncytial virus, 847
Respiratory system. *See also* Breathing; Lung(s)
- congenital anomalies of, 879–880
- fetal, 281–282
- newborn adaptations, 529–530
- pregnancy-related adaptations in, 298–300, 300t, 738, 750t
- preterm infant, 896

Responsivity, 519
Rest and relaxation, 349, 349f, 491–496, 598–599
Resting tone, 445
Restraints, 580, 581f, 582
Resuscitation
- cardiopulmonary. *See* Cardiopulmonary resuscitation
- neonatal, 790, 903–904, 904f

Retained placenta, 826
Retinal hemorrhage, 838
Retinopathy of prematurity, 904b, 916–917
Retroplacental clot, 684
Review of systems, 83b–84b, 339
Rh factor, 868
Rh isoimmunization, 499–500, 499b–500b, 869
Rhagades, 849
Rheumatic heart disease, 711
Rh_o(D) immunoglobulin, 870–871, 871b
Right atrial pressure, 748, 748t
Right ventricle systolic pressure, 743
Risedronate sodium, 140b
Risk management, 12
Ritgen maneuver, 466, 467f
Ritodrine, 786
Robertsonian translocation, 51
Rooming-in, 510–511
Rooting reflex, 546t–549t, 613
Rubella
- newborn exposure to, 851, 851b
- pregnancy exposure to, 163t, 164
- vaccinations against, 499, 499b, 851

Rugae, 61
Rupture of membranes
- infection risks, 448
- miscarriage caused by, 671
- premature, 675–676, 784, 791
- preterm premature, 780, 791, 791b
- spontaneous, 437, 448
- tests for, 437b

Rural women, 33

S

Safety
- abused women, 106
- home care nurse, 38–40
- newborn, 583, 583f

Sao_2 monitoring, 746
Scalp stimulation, 428
Scarf sign, 568b
Scar-sparing mastectomy, 223
SCOFF questionnaire, 75–76
Screenings
- abuse-assessment, 79, 80f, 109
- bacterial vaginosis, 159–160
- bilirubin, 868
- breast cancer, 218, 219b–220b
- candidiasis, 161
- chlamydia, 146–147
- colon cancer, 89t
- eating disorders, 76b
- genital herpes simplex virus, 153–154
- gestational diabetes mellitus, 701, 703f
- gonorrhea, 147
- guidelines for, 89t
- hepatitis B virus, 155
- human immunodeficiency virus, 156–157, 157b
- human papillomavirus, 152
- maternal serum alpha-fetoprotein, 344, 648, 699
- multiple marker screens, 649
- pelvic inflammatory disease, 151
- phenylketonuria, 45, 282
- preeclampsia, 659–661
- recommendations, 89t, 92
- sickle cell, 340
- syphilis, 150
- trichomoniasis, 162
- triple-marker, 649
- triple-marker screens, 649

Seat belt, 351, 351f
Second heart sound, 531
Second trimester
- abortion in, 191–192
- complications of, 342b
- discomforts of, 354t–355t, 356b–357b
- duration of, 330

Secondary dysmenorrhea, 123
Secondary powers, 377–378, 793, 793t
Secondary prevention, 28
Secondhand smoke, 857
Sedatives, 397
Seizures
- eclamptic, 656, 667, 667b
- epileptic, 727

Selective serotonin reuptake inhibitors
- during breastfeeding, 775
- fetal effects of, 861
- postpartum depression treated with, 758t, 759
- premenstrual syndrome managed with, 124
- side effects of, 124

Self-examinations
- breast, 65, 65b–66b
- genital, 60–61
- vulvar, 85

Self-management, 8–9
Self-talk training, 776
Semen analysis, 201–202, 201b
Sensory behaviors, 550–551
Sentinel events, 12–13
Sentinel node
- biopsy of, 230, 261
- identification of, 222

Sepsis, in newborn, 844–846, 844t, 846b, 847t
Septic miscarriage, 672, 672t
Septic shock, 846
Septicemia, 846
Sequential compression device boots, 798
Serotonin/norepinephrine reuptake inhibitors, 758t
Sex chromosomes
- abnormalities of, 51–52, 890
- definition of, 47
- description of, 271

Sex differentiation, 283
Sexual abuse, 438
Sexual activity
- cultural influences, 360
- lubricating agents for, 138–139
- during menopause, 137–141
- after perinatal loss, 934
- postpartum, 503, 504b
- during pregnancy, 332, 334, 353b, 357–358, 358f, 360

Sexual assault. *See also* Rape
- collaborative care for, 111–115
- definition of, 109
- discharge instructions, 115
- emergency department protocol for, 112b
- examination after, 113–114
- forcible, 110
- history-taking after, 113
- immediate care after, 114–115
- incidence of, 109
- laboratory tests, 113–114
- mental health consequences of, 110
- physical examination after, 113–114
- prevention classes, 115
- Psychological First Aid after, 111–113

Sexual assault nurse examiners, 111
Sexual harassment, 109
Sexual history, 357
Sexual orientation, 72–73
Sexual practices, 77, 92
Sexual response, 69, 70t
Sexual violence, 109–115
- assault. *See* Sexual assault
- definition of, 109
- molestation, 109
- rape. *See* Rape
- reporting of, 110

Sexually transmitted infections
- care management of, 164–165
- chlamydia, 146–147, 148t–149t, 162t, 855
- condoms for prevention of, 145
- counseling for, 146b
- definition of, 143
- fetal effects of, 162–164, 162t
- genital herpes simplex virus, 153–154, 153f, 162t
- gonorrhea, 147–149, 148t–149t, 162t, 848
- human immunodeficiency virus. *See* Human immunodeficiency virus
- human papillomavirus. *See* Human papillomavirus
- incidence of, 143
- infection control for, 165, 166b
- nursing care plan for, 146b
- nursing process for, 165b
- pelvic inflammatory disease, 150–151, 151t
- in pregnancy, 146b, 162–164, 162t
- prevention of, 92, 143–146, 158b
- primary prevention of, 144
- psychosocial effects of, 164
- reporting of, 149b, 165, 165b
- risks for
  - description of, 77, 144, 144b
  - practices for reducing, 144–146, 145t
- self-management of, 164b
- sequelae of, 77
- Standard Precautions for, 166b
- syphilis, 149–150, 150f, 162t, 848–849
- types of, 144b
- vaccinations against, 146
- viral, 152–159
- viral hepatitis, 155–156

Sharps containers, 40
Shock
  hemorrhagic, 831b, 830–832
  hypovolemic, 494b, 830–832
  septic, 846
Shoulder dystocia, 817–818, 818f, 839f
Shoulder presentation, of fetus, 370, 372f
Sibling rivalry, 524
Siblings
  adaptations of
    to newborn, 523–525, 524f, 525b
    to pregnancy, 335, 335b
    to preterm infant, 914, 914f
  grief responses by, 934–935
  during labor and birth, 457
Sickle cell hemoglobinopathy, 721–722, 721b
Sickle cell screening, 340
Side-lying position, 455b, 461f, 463–464, 805f
Simian line, 540
Single-gene disorders, 45
Single-parent family, 19
Single-room maternity care, 574
Situation background assessment recommendation technique, 13
Sitz bath, 492b
Skene glands
  anatomy of, 61, 61f
  assessment of, 60
Skin. *See also* Integumentary system
  newborn, 556t–565t, 596b–597b
  physical examination of, 82, 83b–84b
  preterm infant, 910
Skin-sparing mastectomy, 223
Skin-to-skin contact, 533, 533f, 571b
Skull fractures, 839
Sleep-wake states, 549, 549f
Slow-paced breathing, 392–393, 393b
Small-for-gestational-age infant, 569, 895b, 924–926
Smell sense, 550–551
Smoking, 74–75. *See also* Nicotine
  breast cancer risks, 215
  breastfeeding affected by, 626–627, 767
  cessation of, 92, 92b, 352b, 765–766, 857
  effects of, 74
  high-risk pregnancy affected by, 638b
  during lactation, 319
  maternal, 351–352, 352b, 761, 856–857, 857t, 874
  during pregnancy, 351–352, 352b, 761, 856–857, 857t
  secondhand smoke, 857
Social history, 338–339
Social support, 521
Socioeconomic status, 74
Sodium
  excessive intake of, 317
  pregnancy intake of, 316–317
  reabsorption of, in newborn, 535
  restriction of, 316–317
Sodium nitroprusside, 716t, 740, 740b
Soft tissue
  birth injuries, 838–839, 839f
  dystocia, 794
Solid foods, 632–634
Somatic cells, 46
Somatic pain, 387
Soy-based formulas, 631
Specialty care, 7
Specimens, 579–582
  collection of, 40, 86
  heelstick, 579–580, 580f
  in home care settings, 40
  Papanicolaou test, 86, 87b, 89t
  pelvic examination, 86
  urine, 580–582, 582f
  venipuncture, 580, 580f–581f
Speculum examination
  in adolescents, 81
  insertion of speculum for, 85f
  in sexual assault victims, 114
Sperm, 273
  antibodies to, 197, 204
  capacitation of, 273
  ejaculation number of, 273
  illustration of, 273f
Spermatogenesis, 271
Spermicides, 145, 175–181, 176f
Sphingomyelin, 281
Spina bifida, 876–878, 877f
Spinal anesthesia, 401–404
  advantages and disadvantages of, 403
  cesarean birth uses of, 401, 402f
  combined spinal-epidural, 406
  headache caused by, 403–404, 404f
  hypotension caused by, 398, 403b
  membrane levels for, 402f
  monitoring during, 401–403
  nursing interventions for, 411b
  positioning for, 401, 403f
  side effects of, 405b
  voiding before and after, 411–412
Spinal cord, 282
Spinal shock, 841
Spinnbarkeit, 69
Spiritual wellness, 82, 82b
Sponge, contraceptive, 181
Sponge baths, 595, 596f
Spontaneous abortion, 189, 670–675
Spontaneous preterm births, 780–781
Spontaneous rupture of membranes, 437, 437b, 448
Squamocolumnar junction, 63
Squamous intraepithelial lesions, 251
Square window, 568b
St. John's wort, 775b
Stab wounds, 751
Stadol. *See* Butorphanol tartrate
Standard Days Method, of contraception, 172, 172f
Standard of care
  birth complications, 797b
  bleeding emergencies, 831b
  definition of, 12
  labor complications, 797b
Standard Precautions, 40, 166b, 442b
Standards of practice, 11–14, 12b, 35
Staphylococcus aureus, 854–855
Startle reflex, 546t–549t
Station, 371, 373f
Statutory rape, 109
Stepping reflex, 546t–549t
Sterilization, 186–189
  definition of, 186
  female, 187–188, 187f, 188b
  informed consent for, 188
  male, 187f, 188–189
  vasectomy, 187f, 188
Stethoscope, 418f
Stevia, 314
Stillbirth, 5b, 693, 931, 938f–939f. *See also* Perinatal loss
Stomach, 303–304, 535
Stools, 536, 536b, 556t–565t
"Stork bites," 540, 541f
Stranger rape, 110
Strawberry hemangioma, 540
Stress, 76
  coping with, 133
  management of, 91–92
  symptoms of, 76, 77b
Stress incontinence, 236
Stretch marks. *See* Striae gravidarum
Striae gravidarum, 301, 301f, 484
Stroke volume, 483, 739
Students Against Violence Everywhere, 109
Subarachnoid hemorrhage, 841
Subconjunctival hemorrhage, 574, 838
Subculture, 21
Subdural hemorrhage, 841
Subfertility, 194
Subgaleal hemorrhage, 838–839
Subinvolution of uterus, 478, 826, 828
Submucosal leiomyomas, 240, 241f
Suboccipitobregmatic diameter, 370, 373f
Subpubic angle, 373
Subpubic arch, 373, 374f
Subspecialty care, 7
Substance abuse, 761–767
  in adolescent pregnancy, 767
  alcohol, 75, 351–352, 626, 638b, 761–762. *See also* Alcohol use and abuse
  assessment of, 764–765, 765b
  barriers to treatment for, 761–762
  breastfeeding affected by, 767
  caffeine, 314, 314t, 627, 638b, 762, 861
  care management of, 764–767, 846–856, 861–864
  cessation of, 92
  cocaine, 763, 857t, 860, 860b
  collaborative care for, 765–767
  definition of, 761
  drug testing for, 762b
  drugs commonly abused, 762–764, 764b
  ecstasy, 860–861
  fetal effects of, 856–861, 857t
  heroin, 763–764, 858–859
  high-risk pregnancies caused by, 6
  illicit drugs, 75
  legal considerations for, 762
  male infertility secondary to, 197
  marijuana, 762, 860
  maternal, 9
  MDMA, 860–861
  methadone programs, 763–764, 766, 859, 859b
  methamphetamine, 763, 860
  nicotine, 762, 857
  nursing process for, 765b
  opiates, 763–764
  postpartum care, 767
  prescription drugs, 75
  prevalence of, 761
  risk factors for, 761
  screening for, 764, 764b
  smoking, 74–75, 92, 92b, 856–857, 857t
  treatment for, 761–762, 765–767
Succenturiate placenta, 685, 686f
Sucking reflex, 546t–549t
Suctioning, 570, 570f, 570b
Sudden infant death syndrome
  maternal smoking and, 856
  pacifiers for, 595, 595f, 618–619
  sleeping position to prevent, 592
Sufentanil citrate (Sufenta), 399, 406
Superficial inferior epigastric artery flap, 224t–225t
Superficial venous thrombosis, 832–833
Superior gluteal artery perforator flaps, 224t–225t
Supine hypotension, 86, 279, 297, 341b, 349, 349f, 354t–355t, 383, 444f
Supplemental feedings, 617–619, 619b, 621f
Suppositories, 498b
Suprapubic pressure, 818, 818f
Surfactants, 281–282, 529–530, 904–905, 905b, 915
Surgery
  breast, 626. *See also* Breast cancer, surgical treatment of
  breast-conserving, 230b
  cervical cancer treated with, 254–260
  heart, 716
  home care after, 733b
  during pregnancy, 732–733
  preoperative care, 732–733
Sutures, 369–370, 370f, 556t–565t
Svo_2 monitoring, 746–747
Swaddling, 589, 590f, 601
Swallowing reflex, 546t–549t
Sweat glands, 540
Symphysis pubis, 63, 63f
Symptothermal method, of contraception, 174, 175f
Synchronized intermittent mandatory ventilation, 903t
Synchrony, 512
Synclitism, 382f
Syncope, 354t–355t
Syndactyly, 543
Syphilis, 149–150, 150f, 162t, 848–849
Systemic lupus erythematosus, 728–729
Systemic vascular resistance, 738–739, 748, 748t
Systole, 739

T

Tachycardia, 422, 422f, 422t, 741
Tachypnea, 875
Talipes calcaneus, 886
Talipes equinovarus, 886
Talipes equinus, 886
Talipes valgus, 886
Talipes varus, 886
Tamoxifen, 217, 226, 226b
Tandem nursing, 626
Taste sense, 551
Tay-Sachs disease, 53
TeamSTEPPS, 13–14
Teamwork, 13, 146
Teenage birth rate, 5
Telangiectatic nevi, 540, 541f
Telehealth, 7, 35
Telemedicine, 35
Telephonic nursing, 34–35
Temperament, 551
Tenormin. *See* Atenolol

Tension headache, 303
Teratogens, 70, 274, 287, 349b
Terbutaline, 786, 787b–789b
Term, 289, 569
Terminal deletion, 51
Tertiary prevention, 28
Testosterone, 97
Tetanus-diphtheria immunization, 89t
Tetanus-diphtheria-acellular pertussis vaccination, 499
Tetralogy of Fallot
  maternal, 711
  newborn, 873–874, 875f
Tetraploid cell, 48–49
Thalassemia, 722
The Joint Commission
  medication abbreviations, acronyms, and symbols not to use, 12, 13t
  sentinel events, 12–13
  sexual assault, 111
Theca-lutein cysts, 239
Therapeutic abortion, 189
Therapeutic donor insemination, 207t, 208
Therapeutic rest, 792
Therapeutic touch, 396
Thermocautery, 206
Thermodilution procedure, 746, 746b
Thermometer, 555
Thermoregulation
  description of, 533
  in late preterm infant, 922
  in preterm infant, 896
Third heart sound, 531
Third trimester
  cardiac output in, 740b
  complications of, 342b
  discomforts of, 354t–355t, 356b–357b
  duration of, 330
Thoracic trauma, 751
Threatened miscarriage, 671, 671f, 672t
Throat, 82, 83b–84b
Thromboembolic disease, 832–833
Thromboembolic stockings, 798
Thrombophlebitis, 832, 832f
Thrush, 628, 855
Thyroid cancer, 264
Thyroid disorders, 706–707, 707b
Thyroid gland
  embryologic development of, 282
  in pregnancy, 305
Thyroid storm, 707b
Thyroxine, 282, 706, 889
Thyroxine-binding globulin, 305
Time orientation, 25
Tobacco. *See* Smoking
Tocolysis/tocolytic therapy, 429–430, 786–790, 786b–789b, 827
Tocotransducer, 419, 419t, 420f, 427b
Toenails, 283
Tongue extrusion reflex, 614
Tonic neck reflex, 546t–549t
Tonic-clonic seizures, 667, 667b
Toradol. *See* Ketorolac
TORCH infections, 162–164, 163t, 848
Total abdominal hysterectomy
  description of, 126
  endometrial cancer treated with, 247
Total anomalous pulmonary venous connection, 875f
Total parenteral nutrition, 909
Total simple mastectomy, 222, 222f
Touch, 396, 456, 511, 551
Toxic shock syndrome, 180–181, 180b
Toxoplasma gondii, 848
Toxoplasmosis, 163–164, 163t, 848
Tracheoesophageal atresia, 881–883, 882f
Trandate. *See* Labetalol hydrochloride
Transcultural nursing, 28
Transcutaneous bilirubinometry, 575
Transcutaneous electrical nerve stimulation, 395, 395f
Transdermal contraceptive system, 183, 183f
Transdermal estrogen, 135–136, 135t
Transepidermal water loss, 899
Transesophageal echocardiography, 741
Transformation zone, 251, 252f
Transient tachypnea of the newborn, 529–530
Transitional stool, 536b
Translocation, 51
Transplacental infections, 844–846
  cytomegalovirus, 851–852, 851f
  enteroviruses, 853
  gonorrhea, 848. *See also* Gonorrhea
  hepatitis B virus, 850
  herpes simplex virus, 852–853, 853f
  human immunodeficiency virus, 850–851
  parvovirus B19, 853
  prevention against, 582–583
  risks for, 539
  rubella, 851
  sepsis, 844–846, 844t, 846b, 847t
  syphilis, 848–849, 849f
  toxoplasmosis, 848
  varicella-zoster virus, 849–850
Transposition of the great vessels, 875f
Transvaginal ultrasonography, 200, 250, 640–641
Transverse rectus abdominis myocutaneous flap, 224t–225t
Trastuzumab, 46
Trauma. *See also* Intimate partner violence; Rape; Violence
  birth. *See* Birth trauma
  cortisol levels in response to, 110
  during labor. *See* Birth trauma
  during pregnancy, 749–754
    abruptio placentae secondary to, 751–752
    blunt abdominal, 751
    computed tomography evaluations, 752
    electronic fetal monitoring, 750, 754
    exploratory laparotomy for, 752–753
    factors that affect, 749
    fetal effects, 749–750
    fetal-maternal hemorrhage after, 754
    immediate stabilization of, 751–753
    mechanisms of, 751
    motor vehicle accidents, 749
    pelvic fracture, 751
    penetrating abdominal, 751–752
    perimortem cesarean birth in, 754
    physical examination of, 753b
    physiologic characteristics that affect, 749–750
Trauma *(Continued)*
    primary survey of, 752
    radiation exposure concerns, 754
    secondary survey of, 752–753, 753b
    thoracic trauma, 751
    ultrasound evaluations, 754
  rape-trauma syndrome, 101t, 110–111
  thoracic, 751
Travel, 350–351, 351f
Treponema pallidum, 149
Trial of labor, 814–815
Triceps reflex, 661f
Trichomonas vaginalis, 161
Trichomoniasis, 160t, 161–162
Tricuspid atresia, 875f
Tricyclic antidepressants, 759, 773b
Triiodothyronine, 706
Trimesters. *See* First trimester; Second trimester; Third trimester
Trinucleotide repeat expansion, 54
Triple-marker screens, 649
Triploid cell, 48–49
Trisomy
  causes of, 49, 271
  definition of, 49
  18, 50–51
  nondisjunction as cause of, 49, 51
  13, 50–51
  21. *See* Down syndrome
  XXY, 51–52
Trophoblast, 273, 275f
True labor, 434b
True pelvis, 63, 63f, 372, 374f
Truncus arteriosus, 875f
Trunk incurvation reflex, 546t–549t
Tumor ploidy, 221
Tumor suppressor genes, 54
Turner syndrome, 51
Twins, 286–287, 286f, 362, 622f
TwoDay Method, of contraception, 173
Type A blood, 868
Type ABO blood, 868
Type B blood, 868
Type O blood, 868

U

Ulcerative colitis, 730
Ultrasonography
  amniocentesis with, 642
  breast lump evaluations, 212
  fetal uses of, 641–644
  high-risk pregnancy, 640–645, 640f–641f, 641t
  infertility evaluations, 200, 200f, 202
  transvaginal, 200
Ultrasound transducer, 419, 419t, 427b
Umbilical artery velocity waveform, 643f
Umbilical cord
  acid-base determinations, 428–429, 429t
  anatomy of, 275f, 276–277
  care of, 573, 574f, 596–597, 596b–597b
  percutaneous umbilical blood sampling, 648, 648f
  prolapse of, 448b, 459b, 818–819, 819f, 819b
  separation of, 574f
  velamentous insertion of, 685, 686f
Unbalanced translocation, 51
Uninsured population, 4
United Nations Millennium Development Goals, 2, 3b
United States
  ethnic diversity in, 2
  health care systems in. *See* Health care systems
  infant mortality rate in, 5–6
  racial diversity in, 2
Urethra
  anatomy of, 61, 61f
  lacerations to, 470
  postpartum changes in, 482
Urethrocele, 85
Urethrovaginal fistula, 237, 237f
Urethrovesical angle, 236, 236f
Uric acid, 657
Urinary catheterization, 451
Urinary frequency, 300
Urinary incontinence, 236–238
  clinical manifestations of, 236–237
  incidence of, 236
  menopause-related, 132
  nursing care for, 238
  stress, 236
  treatment of, 237–238
Urinary system, 481–482
Urinary tract infections, 345, 692, 730–732, 732b, 834–835
Urinary tract trauma examination, 753b
Urine. *See also* Voiding
  components of, 482
  glucose testing, in pregestational diabetes mellitus, 699
Urine specimen
  labor assessments using, 446
  newborn, 580–582, 582f
Urobilinogen, 537, 537f
Ursodeoxycholic acid, 727
Uterine artery embolization, 129, 242, 242b
Uterine atony, 493, 825
Uterine contractions
  assessment of, 443–445, 446f
  back pain during, 795b
  blood pressure changes, 383
  Braxton Hicks, 279, 293, 354t–355t, 378
  characteristics of, 445, 445b
  definition of, 443
  discomfort associated with, 495
  electronic monitoring of, 445
  excessive, 805
  during exercise, 696b
  in first stage of labor, 445, 445b
  oxytocin's role in, 613, 652
  palpation of, 445
  pattern of, 445, 446f
  positioning during, 452–453, 452f–453f
  postpartum, 478–479
  resting tone, 445
  in second stage of labor, 460t
  suppression of, 786–790, 786b–789b
  terms used to describe, 374–376
  tocolysis effects on, 429–430
Uterine fibroids, 129, 240–242
Uterine tachysystole, 428b, 805, 805b
Uterine tone, 493
Uterine tubes
  adhesions on, 196–197
  anatomy of, 62f, 63

Uterine tubes *(Continued)*
cancer of, 262–263, 265
infertility and, 196–197
ligation of, 187f, 187b
occlusion of, 187, 187f
postmenopausal changes in, 66t
reconstruction of, 188
Uteroplacental insufficiency, 423–424, 425f, 637
Uterus
abnormalities of, 197f
anatomy of, 61–62, 62f, 374
bicornuate, 197f
bimanual palpation of, 86, 88f
blood flow in, 293
cancer of, 265
contracted, bleeding with, 827
couvelaire, 684
disorders of, 234–238
displacement of, 132, 234–235, 235f
distention of, 363
enlargement of, 292
functions of, 62
fundus of, 62, 62f
hypertonic dysfunction of, 792
hypotonic dysfunction of, 792–793, 826–827
infertility caused by abnormalities of, 197, 197f
inversion of, 826–827, 829
involution of, 478, 479f
ischemia of, 386
during labor, 376f, 416t
ligaments of, 61–62, 62f
physiologic retraction ring, 374, 376f
polyps of, 240, 240f
postmenopausal changes in, 66t
postpartum changes in, 478–480
pregnancy-related changes in, 292–294
prolapse of, 234–235, 235f, 237
retroversion of, 234–235
rupture of, 819–820
subinvolution of, 478, 826, 828
walls of, 62, 62f

V

Vacuum-assisted birth, 806t, 807, 807f, 807b, 838
Vagina. *See also* Labia majora; Labia minora
anatomy of, 61
cancer of, 262, 265
diaphragm insertion technique, 178b–179b
estrogen deficiency effects on, 131
hematomas of, 825–826
lacerations to, 470
menopausal changes in, 61
palpation of, 84–85
physical examination of, 86
postmenopausal changes in, 66t
postpartum changes in, 480–481
pregnancy-related changes in, 295
rectovaginal palpation, 86, 88f
secretions from, 61, 159, 295
trauma examination, 753b
Vaginal birth. *See also* Childbirth
in breech presentation, 795–796, 796f
forceps-assisted, 806–807, 806f, 806t, 838
infection after, 833
Vaginal birth *(Continued)*
operative, 806–814
postpartum care after, 491b
trauma during. *See* Birth trauma
vacuum-assisted, 806t, 807, 807f, 807b, 838
Vaginal birth after cesarean, 8, 364, 808, 808b, 815, 815b
Vaginal contraceptive ring, 183, 183f
Vaginal creams, 136
Vaginal disorders
collaborative care for, 237–238
cystocele, 85, 235–236, 235f, 238, 238f
genital fistulas, 237–238, 237f
rectocele, 85, 235–236, 235f, 238
Vaginal examination, for labor assessment, 445–446, 445b, 447f
Vaginal hysterectomy, 243, 243f
Vaginal infections, 159–162
bacterial vaginosis, 159–161, 160t
candidiasis, 160–161, 160t
group B streptococcus, 162, 344
infertility secondary to, 197
trichomoniasis, 160t, 161–162
wet smear tests for, 160t
Vaginal intraepithelial neoplasia, 262
Vaginal speculum, 85–86, 85f. *See also* Speculum examination
Vaginal wall, 85
Valproic acid, 728, 775
Valsalva maneuver, 383
Valve replacement, 713
Variable deceleration, of fetal heart rate, 424, 426f, 426b
Varicella-zoster
in newborn, 849–850
vaccination for, 499, 499b
Varicose veins, 354t–355t
Varicosities, 484, 484f
Vasa previa, 685
Vascular spiders, 301–302
Vasectomy, 187f, 188
Vasodilators, 740
Vasomotor instability, in perimenopausal period, 132
Vasopressors, 752
VBAC. *See* Vaginal birth after cesarean
Vegetarian diets, 326, 326t–327t
Velamentous insertion of umbilical cord, 685, 686f
Velocardiofacial syndrome, 51
Venipuncture, 580, 580f–581f
Venography, 833
Venous thromboembolism, 496
Ventricular septal defect
maternal, 710
newborn, 873–874, 875f
Verapamil, 716t
Vernix caseosa, 283, 539–540
Version, 796, 799, 799f
Vertex presentation, 466–467, 467f
Very low-birth-weight infant, 895b, 898
Very preterm birth, 780
Vesicovaginal fistula, 237, 237f
Vestibular schwannomas, 52
Vestibule, 61, 61f
Viability, 279, 289
Vibroacoustic stimulation, 428, 650–651, 651f
Violence/violence against women, 9, 78
care management for, 103–105
after childbirth, 107
Violence/violence against women *(Continued)*
coping with, 104
definition of, 95
documentation of, 106, 107b
education about, 93
forms of, 95
history-taking, 339
intimate partner violence. *See* Intimate partner violence
mandatory reporting of, 104b
nursing interventions for, 105–109
during pregnancy, 78
prevention of, 109
safety provisions, 106
screening for, 83b–84b
sexual. *See* Sexual violence
Viral hepatitis, 155–156
Vision. *See also* Eyes
in newborn, 550
screenings of, 89t
Visual impairment
parents with, 523, 523b
patients with, health assessment in, 79
Vital signs. *See also specific vital sign*
labor assessments, 443
newborn assessment, 555–565, 556t–565t
Vitamin A, 310t–311t, 317–318
Vitamin B_6, 310t–311t, 318
Vitamin B_{12}, 310t–311t, 326, 611
Vitamin C, 310t–311t, 318
Vitamin D
deficiency of, 133
description of, 90
food sources of, 139
newborn requirements, 611
pregnancy intake of, 310t–311t, 318
recommendations for, 139
Vitamin E, 136, 310t–311t, 317
Vitamin K, 539, 573, 573b, 583–584, 611, 727–728
Voice, 511
Voiding. *See also* Elimination
during labor, 451
newborn, 534
postpartum, 496–498
spinal anesthesia and, 411–412
Vomiting. *See* Nausea and vomiting of pregnancy
von Willebrand disease, 832
von Willebrand factor, 832
Vulnerable populations
adolescents. *See* Adolescent(s)
description of, 31–33
homeless, 33
incarcerated women, 32
low literacy, 33
migrants, 32–33
nursing implications of, 33–34
older women, 32. *See also* Older women
refugees, 32–33
rural women, 33
women, 31–33
Vulva
anatomy of, 61
cancer of, 260–266
hematomas of, 825–826
pregnancy-related changes in, 295
self-examination of, 85
Vulvar intraepithelial neoplasia, 260–261
Vulvectomy, 261–262, 261f, 262b, 265
Vulvodynia, 245
Vulvovaginitis, 159

W

Walking survey, 30, 31b
Warfarin, 716t
Warm lines, 34–35, 505
Water, 310t–311t, 314
Water aerobics, 139
Water therapy, 394–395, 394f
Weaning
breastfeeding, 624–625
formula feeding, 632
Weight gain
pregnancy, 309–313, 309f, 311b, 312t, 320b
preterm infants, 907, 907b
Weight loss
maternal, during breastfeeding, 625
newborn, 528–529, 620
preterm infants, 907, 907b
Weight-bearing exercises, 139
Well-woman care, 70–71
holistic approach to, 70–71
preconception health screenings, 70
Wharton's jelly, 277
Whey, 611
White blood cell count, 483, 532
"Witch's milk," 283, 541
Women
demographics of, 31
minority, 31–32
as vulnerable population, 31–33
Women's health
deficiencies in, 31
factors that affect, 9
Women's health care
ethical issues in, 14
research in, 14
Women's health nursing
focus of, 1
genetics involvement by, 44
Workplace hazards, 78
Wound infections, 834–835

X

X chromosome, 47–48, 283
X-chromatin, 890
X-inactivation, 48
X-linked dominant inheritance, 53–54
X-linked recessive disorders, 48, 54
Xylocaine. *See* Lidocaine

Y

Y chromosome
description of, 47
microdeletions in, 51
sex differentiation, 283
Yeast infections, 161, 628–629
Yellen clamp, for circumcision, 587, 587f
Yolk sac, 276
Young adults, 74
Yo-yo dieting, 75
Yutopar. *See* Ritodrine

Z

Zinc, 310t–311t, 317
Zoledronic acid, 139
Zona pellucida, 273, 274f
Zona reaction, 273
Zygote intrafallopian transfer, 207t, 208

FEATURES

CLINICAL REASONING

Abortion, 190
Admission of an Emergency Client to Labor and Delivery, 424
Assessment of Postpartum Bleeding, 480
Asymptomatic Bacteriuria, 731
The Bereaved Couple, 939
Breastfeeding: Engorgement and Nipple Soreness, 627
Breast Cancer Treatment Options, 221
Cardiovascular Disease—the Leading Cause of Death in Women, 90
Causes of Hyperglycemia in a Woman with Gestational Diabetes Mellitus (GDM), 704
Counseling About Genetic Risk, 57
Developmental Dysplasia of the Hip (DDH), 886
Encouraging Evidence-Based Birth Practices, 455
Family Planning and Contraceptive Use, 504
Fetal Assessment Using the Biophysical Profile, 645
Imbalanced Nutrition, 312
Infertility Counseling, 195
Informed Decision Making for Treatment of Leiomyoma, 240
Intimate Partner Violence, 96
The Late Preterm Infant, 923
Making Decisions Regarding Pain Management in Labor, 391
Narcotic Exposure in a Newborn, 864
Nausea in Pregnancy, 355
Nursing Care of the Critically Ill Pregnant Woman, 748
Postpartum Depression, 774
Postpartum Hemorrhage, 825
Pregnancy Testing, 291
Providing Culturally Appropriate Care, 23
Relief for Menstrual Discomfort, 122
Safety and Efficacy of Midwifery Care, 8
Second Stage Labor in a Woman with an Epidural, 380
Severe Complication of Preeclampsia, 658
STI Counseling in Pregnancy, 146
Third Trimester Vaginal Bleeding, 684
Transition to Parenthood for the Adolescent Couple, 519
Ultrasound Examination During Pregnancy, 283
Vaginal Bleeding on Depo-Provera, 184
The Woman Seeing Elective Cesarean Birth, 809

CULTURAL CONSIDERATIONS

Birth Practices in Different Cultures, 440
Breast Screening Practices, 219
Communication Variations, 79
Cultural Beliefs and Practices Related to Infant Care, 590
Female Genital Mutilation, 73
Fostering Bonding in Women of Varying Ethnic and Cultural Groups, 510
Meaning of Cancer, 247
Postpartum Period and Family Planning, 503
Questions to Ask to Elicit Cultural Expectations About Childbearing, 27
Some Cultural Beliefs About Pain, 388

EMERGENCY

Anaphylactoid Syndrome of Pregnancy, 820
Cardiopulmonary Resuscitation (CPR) for Infants, 600
Cardiopulmonary Resuscitation (CPR) for the Pregnant Woman, 719
Eclampsia, 667
Hemorrhagic Shock, 831
Hypovolemic Shock, 494
Immediate Management of the Newborn with Meconium-Stained Amniotic Fluid, 817
Interventions for Emergencies During Labor, 459
Maternal Hypotension with Decreased Placental Perfusion, 403
Prolapsed Umbilical Cord, 819
Relieving Airway Obstruction, 599
Supine Hypotension, 341
Uterine Tachysystole with Oxytocin, 805

EVIDENCE-BASED PRACTICE

The 2009 Influenza A (H1N1) Pandemic and Pregnancy, 724
An Ideal Solution: The Intrauterine Device, 186
Assessing for Postpartum Depression, 773
Benefits of Continuous Labor Support, 454
Cervical Cancer Treatment Options: Conventional and Complementary, 255
Complementary and Alternative Pain Management in Labor, 390
Education for Family Planning, 518
Endometriosis Treatments for Infertility, 196
Fetal Monitoring and the Machine That Goes "Beep", 417
Genetic Risk Assessment for Breast Cancer, 216
Heavy Menstrual Bleeding: Treatments to Improve Quality of Life, 128
How's My Baby Doing?, 644
Hypothermia Prevention and Skin-to-Skin Contact, 571
Interventions for Intimate Partner Violence, 105
Kegel, Kegel, Kegel!, 498
Non-Pharmacologic Pain Relief Measures for Newborns, 921
Perinatal Smoking Cessation, 352
The Precarious First Trimester, 674
Preeclampsia Risk Factors and Prevention, 659
Preterm Labor: Is Bed Rest (Especially in the Hospital) Really Best?, 785
Searching for and Evaluating the Evidence, 10
Stricter Glucose Tolerance Test in Pregnancy Will Mean Increased Diagnoses of Gestational Diabetes, 702
Supplemental Feeding, 619
Teaching Women Breast Self-Examination: Is It Worthwhile?, 66
Venus and Mars and HIV/STD Prevention Interventions, 158
What Else Should We Tell Our Pregnant Clients to Take, Besides Folic Acid?, 316

(Continued)

FEATURES—cont'd

MEDICATION GUIDE

Antenatal Glucocorticoid Therapy with Betamethasone or Dexamethasone, 790
Drugs Used to Manage Postpartum Hemorrhage, 827
Eye Prophylaxis: Erythromycin Ophthalmic Ointment, 0.5%, and Ophthalmic Ointment, 1%, 572
Hepatitis B Immune Globulin, 584
Hepatitis B Vaccine (Recombivax HB, Engerix-B), 583
Infertility Medications, 205
Letrozole (Femara), 227
Opioid Agonist Analgesics, 399
Opioid Agonist-Antagonist Analgesics, 399
Opioid Antagonist, 400
Oxytocin (Pitocin), 804
Prostaglandin E1 (PGE1): Misoprostol (Cytotec), 801
Prostaglandin E2 (PGE2): Dinoprostone (Cervidil Insert, Prepidil Gel), 802
Raloxifene Hydrochloride (Evista), 227
Rh Immune Globulin, RhoGAM, Gamulin Rh, HypRho-D, Rhophylac, 499
Surfactant Replacement, 905
Tamoxifen (Nolvadex), 226
Tocolytic Therapy for Preterm Labor, 787
Vitamin K: Phytonadine (AquaMEPHYTON, Konakion), 573

NURSING CARE PLAN

Adolescent Pregnancy, 361
Breastfeeding and Infant Nutrition, 618
Community and Home Care, 39
Discomforts of Pregnancy and Warning Signs, 356
Endometriosis, 127
The Family Living with a Child with Down Syndrome, 50
Fetal Death at 24 Weeks, 947
The High Risk Preterm Newborn, 900
Home Care Follow-up: Transition to Parenthood, 513
Hysterectomy for Endometrial Cancer, 249
Incorporating the Infant into the Family, 20
The Infant Experiencing Drug Withdrawal (Neonatal Abstinence Syndrome), 863
The Infant of the Mother with Pregestational or Gestational Diabetes, 845
The Infant with Hyperbilirubinemia, 872
Infertility, 202
Labor and Birth, 449
Nonpharmacologic Pain Management, 410
The Normal Newborn, 567
Nutrition During Pregnancy, 324
The Pregnant Woman with Gestational Diabetes, 703
The Pregnant Woman with Heart Disease, 717
Premenstrual Syndrome, 125
Preterm Labor, 782
Postpartum Care—Vaginal Birth, 491
Postpartum Depression (PPD), 771
Postpartum Hemorrhage, 830
Severe Preeclampsia, 664
Sexual Activity and Contraception, 171
The Woman Experiencing Intimate Partner Violence, 107
The Woman Having Breast Conserving Surgery and Axillary Node Dissection, 230

NURSING PROCESS

Asthma, 723
Breastfeeding Mother-Infant Pair, 614
Birth Injury, 842
Cardiac Disease, 715
Care of the Newborn and Family, 569
Contraception, 170
Dysfunctional Labor, 798
Electronic Fetal Heart Rate Monitoring, 427
Excessive Gestational Weight Gain, 320
First Stage of Labor, 441
The Infant with Suspected Sepsis, 846
Infertility, 199
Intimate Partner Violence, 106
Late Preterm and Preterm Infant Care, 899
Menstrual Disorders, 131
Mild Preeclampsia, 660
Miscarriage, 673
The Newborn with a Congenital Anomaly, 890
Nursing Care During Pregnancy, 337
Pain Management, 409
The Perimenopausal Woman, 138
Perinatal Grief, 936
Placenta Previa, 682
Postpartum Depression, 772
Postpartum Hemorrhage, 829
Postpartum Physical Concerns, 490
Postpartum Psychosocial Concerns, 501
Pregestational Diabetes, 694
Second Stage of Labor, 461
Substance Abuse, 765
Third Stage of Labor, 472
Transition to Parenthood, 526
The Woman with a Leiomyoma, 241
The Woman with a Sexually Transmitted Infection, 165
The Woman with Breast Cancer, 229
The Woman Having Radiation Therapy, 254

edition **10**

STUDY GUIDE

Maternity & Women's Health Care

Deitra Leonard Lowdermilk
RNC, PhD, FAAN

Shannon E. Perry
RN, PhD, FAAN

Kitty Cashion
RN, BC, MSN

Kathryn Rhodes Alden
RN, MSN, EdD, IBCLC

By

Karen A. Piotrowski, RNC, MSN
Associate Professor of Nursing
D'Youville College
Buffalo, New York

ELSEVIER
MOSBY

ELSEVIER
MOSBY

3251 Riverport Lane
Maryland Heights, MO 63043

STUDY GUIDE FOR MATERNITY & WOMEN'S HEALTH CARE, TENTH EDITION

ISBN: 978-0-323-07430-8

Notice

Knowledge and best practice in this field are constantly changing. As new research and experience broaden our knowledge, changes in practice, treatment and drug therapy may become necessary or appropriate. Readers are advised to check the most current information provided (i) on procedures featured or (ii) by the manufacturer of each product to be administered, to verify the recommended dose or formula, the method and duration of administration, and contraindications. It is the responsibility of the practitioner, relying on their own experience and knowledge of the patient, to make diagnoses, to determine dosages and the best treatment for each individual patient, and to take all appropriate safety precautions. To the fullest extent of the law, neither the Publisher nor the Authors assumes any liability for any injury and/or damage to persons or property arising out of or related to any use of the material contained in this book.

The Publisher

Executive Editor: Robin Carter
Managing Editor: Laurie K. Gower
Publishing Services Manager: Hemamalini Rajendrababu/Jeffrey Patterson
Project Manager: Deepthi Unni

Printed in the United States of America

Last digit is the print number: 9 8 7 6 5 4

INTRODUCTION

This *Study Guide* is designed to help students effectively use the textbook, *Maternity & Women's Health Care*, tenth edition. In addition to reviewing content of the text, this *Study Guide* encourages students to think critically in applying their knowledge.

Chapter Review Activities focus on recall and application of critical concepts and essential terminology. These activities are specifically designed to help you to identify the important content of the chapter and to test your level of knowledge and understanding after reading the chapter. Completion of each of the activities will provide you with an excellent resource to use when you are reviewing important content before course examinations. The knowledge that you attain by completing the activities will help you to develop the theoretical foundation that you will need to answer the critical thinking exercises that follow, to successfully pass course examinations and the NCLEX-RN© Examination, and to manage the care of your clients in the clinical setting. Answers or answer guidelines for the activities are provided in the Answer Key located at the end of this *Study Guide*.

Thinking Critically Exercises focus primarily on the application of critical chapter content. Typical client care situations are presented, and you are required to apply concepts found in the chapter to solve problems, to make decisions concerning care management, and to provide responses to a client's questions and concerns. These exercises may be completed by you on your own or with members of your study group. Completing the critical thinking exercises will help you prepare for clinical experiences, course examinations, and the NCLEX-RN Examination, all of which focus on problem solving and application of nursing knowledge. Guidelines for completing the exercises and specific chapter section, box, or table where the content for the answer is found are provided in the Answer Key located at the end of the *Study Guide*.

CONTENTS

UNIT ONE: INTRODUCTION TO MATERNITY & WOMEN'S HEALTH CARE

1. 21st Century Maternity and Women's Health Nursing, 1
2. Community Care: The Family and Culture, 7
3. Clinical Genetics, 17

UNIT TWO: WOMEN'S HEALTH

4. Assessment and Health Promotion, 23
5. Violence Against Women, 35
6. Reproductive System Concerns, 43
7. Sexually Transmitted and Other Infections, 53
8. Contraception and Abortion, 61
9. Infertility, 71
10. Problems of the Breast, 79
11. Structural Disorders and Neoplasms of the Reproductive System, 85

UNIT THREE: PREGNANCY

12. Conception and Fetal Development, 95
13. Anatomy and Physiology of Pregnancy, 101
14. Maternal and Fetal Nutrition, 109
15. Nursing Care of the Family During Pregnancy, 117

UNIT FOUR: CHILDBIRTH

16. Labor and Birth Processes, 131
17. Pain Management, 137
18. Fetal Assessment During Labor, 145
19. Nursing Care of the Family During Labor and Birth, 151

UNIT FIVE: POSTPARTUM

20. Postpartum Physiology, 163
21. Nursing Care of the Family During the Postpartum Period, 167
22. Transition to Parenthood, 177

UNIT SIX: THE NEWBORN

23. Physiologic and Behavioral Adaptations of the Newborn, 185
24. Nursing Care of the Newborn and Family, 193
25. Newborn Nutrition and Feeding, 205

UNIT SEVEN: COMPLICATIONS OF PREGNANCY

26. Assessment for Risk Factors in Pregnancy, 213
27. Hypertensive Disorders in Pregnancy, 221
28. Antepartum Hemorrhagic Disorders, 229
29. Endocrine and Metabolic Disorders in Pregnancy, 237
30. Medical-Surgical Problems in Pregnancy, 247
31. Obstetric Critical Care, 255
32. Mental Health Disorders and Substance Abuse in Pregnancy, 261
33. Labor and Birth Complications, 269
34. Postpartum Complications, 281

UNIT EIGHT: NEWBORN COMPLICATIONS
35. Acquired Problems of the Newborn, 287
36. Hemolytic Disorders and Congenital Anomalies, 297
37. Nursing Care of the High Risk Newborn, 305
38. Perinatal Loss and Grief, 315

Answer Key, 321

CHAPTER 1

21st Century Maternity and Women's Health Nursing

I. LEARNING KEY TERMS

MATCHING: Match the definition in Column I with the appropriate descriptive term from Column II.

COLUMN I

1. _______ Number of live births in 1 year per 1000 population.
2. _______ Embryo or fetus that is removed or expelled from the uterus at 20 weeks of gestation or less, weighs 500 g or less, or measures 25 cm or less.
3. _______ Number of maternal deaths from births and complications of pregnancy, childbirth, and the puerperium (the first 42 days after termination of the pregnancy) per 100,000 live births.
4. _______ An infant who at birth demonstrates no signs of life, such as breathing, heartbeat, or voluntary muscle movements.
5. _______ Number of stillbirths and number of neonatal deaths per 1000 live births.
6. _______ Number of births per 1000 women between the ages of 15 and 44 years (inclusive), calculated on a yearly basis.
7. _______ Infant whose weight at birth is less than 2500 g (5 lb, 8 oz).
8. _______ Number of deaths of infants less than 1 year of age per 1000 live births.
9. _______ Number of deaths of infants less than 28 days of age per 1000 live births.
10. _______ Infant born before 38 weeks of gestation.

COLUMN II

A. Fertility rate
B. Infant mortality rate
C. Birth rate
D. Maternal mortality rate
E. Neonatal mortality rate
F. Perinatal mortality rate
G. Low-birth-weight infant
H. Abortus
I. Stillbirth
J. Preterm infant

FILL IN THE BLANKS: Insert the term that corresponds to each of the following definitions or descriptions.

11. ______________________________ Specialty area of nursing practice that focuses on the care of childbearing women and their families through all stages of pregnancy and childbirth, as well as the first 4 weeks after birth.
12. ______________________________ Health care that focuses on the physical, psychologic, and social needs of women throughout their lives.
13. ______________________________ A set of goals that reflects the nation's agenda for improving health with the ultimate aims to increase the quality and years of healthy life and to eliminate health disparities.
14. ______________________________ A set of eight goals to be achieved by 2015 that respond to the world's main development challenges and adopted by 189 nations under the auspices of the United Nations.
15. ______________________________ Approach to health care that encompasses complementary and alternative therapies in combination with conventional Western modalities of treatment.
16. ______________________________ An umbrella term for the use of communication technologies and electronic information to provide or support health care when the participants are separated by distance.
17. ______________________________ Terms used to describe procedures in which part or all of the female external genitalia are removed for cultural or nontherapeutic reasons.
18. ______________________________ Trained and experienced female labor attendants who provide a continual one-on-one caring presence throughout the labor and birth process.

19. ______________________________ Term used to refer to a spectrum of abilities, ranging from reading an appointment slip to interpreting medication instructions.

20. ______________________________ Comprehensive standardized language that describes interventions performed by generalist or specialist nurses.

21. ______________________________ Health care that is based on information gained through research and clinical trials.

22. ______________________________ Approach to care that measures effectiveness of care against benchmarks or standards. It is a measure of the value of nursing using quality indicators and answers the question, "Did the client benefit or not benefit from the care provided?"

23. ______________________________ Guidelines for nursing practice that reflect current knowledge, represent levels of practice agreed on by leaders in the specialty, and can be used for clinical benchmarking.

24. ______________________________ Term used to refer to the level of practice that a reasonably prudent nurse would provide in the same or similar circumstances.

25. ______________________________ An evolving process that is used to identify risks, establish preventive practices, develop reporting mechanisms, and delineate procedures for managing lawsuits.

26. ______________________________ Term used by The Joint Commission to describe an unexpected occurrence involving death or serious physical or psychologic injury, or risk thereof.

27. ______________________________ Process used to evaluate the quality and quantity of nursing care by comparing the number of surgical clients who develop common complications who survive versus those who do not; in obstetrics, its aim is to evaluate the perinatal team's ability to decrease risk of adverse outcomes by measuring processes involved in common complications and emergencies.

28. ______________________________ Effort to provide nurses with the competencies to improve the quality and safety of the systems of health care in which they practice.

29. ______________________________ Technique that gives a specific framework for communication among health care providers. It is an easy to remember, useful, concrete mechanism for communicating important information that requires a clinician's immediate attention.

30. ______________________________ Approach developed by the Department of Defense's Patient Safety Program in collaboration with the Agency for Healthcare Research and Quality as a teamwork system for health professionals to provide higher quality, safer client care. It provides an evidence base to improve communication and teamwork skills.

II. REVIEWING KEY CONCEPTS

31. When assessing pregnant women, what factors would you recognize as having the potential to contribute to the rate of infant mortality in the United States?

32. The health care system in the United States faces many problems. DESCRIBE how the nurse can effect change in each of the following areas to improve the quality and effectiveness of health care available to Americans:
    - Structure

- Medical errors

- Cost

- Access

- Disparities

- Health literacy

33. The number of high risk pregnancies occurring in the United States is increasing. Briefly DISCUSS the factors that have been identified as contributing to this increase in incidence of high risk pregnancies.

34. IDENTIFY several factors and conditions that affect the health of women. For each factor and condition identified, DESCRIBE the effect it has had on women's health.

MULTIPLE CHOICE: Circle the correct option(s) and state the rationale for the option(s) chosen.

35. An integrative health care approach implies: (Circle all that apply.)
    A. The focus is on the whole person
    B. Conventional Western modalities of treatment are not included
    C. The beliefs, values, and desires of the client in terms of health and health care are respected
    D. Client autonomy is limited in terms of choosing alternative therapies
    E. The client's disease complex is considered when choosing treatment approaches

36. A nurse manager of a prenatal clinic should recognize that the most significant barrier encountered by pregnant women in accessing health care is:
    A. Lack of transportation to the clinic
    B. Child care responsibilities
    C. Inability to pay
    D. Deficient knowledge related to the benefits of prenatal care

37. Both worldwide and in the United States, the leading cause of maternal mortality is:
    A. Hemorrhage
    B. Infection
    C. Diabetes
    D. Gestational hypertension

38. Knowledge of trends in fertility and birth rates and infant mortality rates can guide nurses in targeting health care resources to those areas and clients in most need of intervention. Which statements accurately reflect current trends in the United States? (Circle all that apply.)
    A. Women between the ages 20 and 29 have the highest birth rate.
    B. Women in their 40s are less likely than younger women to give birth to twins.
    C. Births to unmarried women are more likely to result in a preterm birth or birth of a low-birth-weight infant.
    D. The infant mortality rate is a common indicator of the adequacy of prenatal care and the health of a nation as a whole.
    E. African-American women are two times more likely to die as a result of pregnancy than are non-Hispanic, white women.

39. After teaching a group of pregnant women about the hazards of smoking during pregnancy, a woman answers a question by listing the hazards. Which hazard, if included by the woman in her list, indicate the need for further teaching?
    A. Intrauterine growth restriction
    B. Congenital anomalies
    C. Low birth weight
    D. Premature labor and birth

40. Pregnant women who are obese are more likely to develop one or both of the two most frequently reported maternal risk factors. These factors include:
    A. Premature labor and infection
    B. Hemorrhage and gestational hypertension
    C. Infection and diabetes
    D. Diabetes and gestational hypertension

III. THINKING CRITICALLY

1. IMAGINE that you are the nursing director of an inner-city prenatal clinic that serves a large number of minority women, many of whom are younger than 20 years of age. DESCRIBE five nursing services you would provide for these women that would help reduce the potential for maternal and infant morbidity and mortality and low birth weight. Use the statistical data and risk behaviors presented in Chapter 1 to support the types of services you propose.

2. SUPPORT the accuracy of the following statement: An emphasis on high-technology medical care and lifesaving techniques will not reduce the rate of preterm and low-birth-weight infants in the United States.

3. PROPOSE three changes in health care and its delivery that you believe would improve the health status and well-being of mothers and their infants and reduce the rate of infant and maternal mortality. SUPPORT your answer by using the content presented in Chapter 1 and your own experiences with the health care system.

4. Many barriers interfere with a woman's participation in early and ongoing prenatal care. DESCRIBE incentives and services that you would offer to pregnant women to encourage their participation in prenatal care. State the rationale for your proposals. Your answer should reflect an understanding of the barriers.

5. At the prenatal clinic where you work, a change in health care focus is being implemented that will involve pregnant women and their families more completely in their care and promote self-management. What measures would you implement when caring for your clients that would support this change in focus?

6. Many clients who come to a prenatal clinic speak English as a second language and often have difficulty speaking fluently. EXPLAIN what measures nurses working in this clinic should use to ensure health literacy among their clients.

7. Medical errors are the leading cause of death in the United States. EXPLAIN the process that you will use as a student to prevent medical errors.

8. Imagine that you are the nurse manager of a postpartum unit that recently changed to a mother-baby form of care delivery. You now want to develop an evidence-based protocol that nurses on your unit will use to teach and guide breastfeeding women. Nurses on your unit are reluctant to participate in developing this protocol, stating, "The approach we use now when helping our breastfeeding moms works just fine—how can research make it better?" DESCRIBE the approach that you would use to convince these nurses that evidence-based practice enhances the quality and effectiveness of nursing care.

CHAPTER 2

Community Care: The Family and Culture

I. LEARNING KEY TERMS

MATCHING: Match the family described in Column I with the appropriate family category in Column II.

COLUMN I

1. ________ Miss M. lives with her 4-year-old adopted Korean daughter, Kim.
2. ________ Anne and Duane are married and live with their daughter, Susan, and Duane's mother, Ruth.
3. ________ Gloria and Andy are a married couple living with their new biologic baby girl, Annie, and their adopted son, Joseph.
4. ________ Tina and her brother Mark live with their grandmother, Irene, who is raising them.
5. ________ Carl and Allan are a gay couple living with Carl's daughter, Sally, and a son, Thomas, born through surrogacy whom they are raising together.
6. ________ The S. family consists of Jim; his second wife, Jane; and Jim's two daughters by a previous marriage.
7. ________ George and Denise, who are not married, live together with their daughter Rose.

COLUMN II

A. Cohabitating-parent family
B. Single-parent family
C. Homosexual family
D. Married-parent family
E. Extended family
F. Married (blended) family
G. No-parent family

MATCHING: Match the description in Column I with the appropriate cultural concept in Column II.

COLUMN I

8. ________ Mrs. M., a Mexican-American who just gave birth, tells the nurse not to include certain foods on her meal tray because her mother told her to avoid those foods while breastfeeding. The nurse tells her that she doesn't have to avoid any foods and should eat what is on the tray because it is good for her.
9. ________ Ms. P., an immigrant from Vietnam, has lived in the United States for 1 year. She tells you that although she enjoys the comfort of wearing blue jeans and sneakers for casual occasions, like shopping, she still wears traditional or "conservative" clothing for family gatherings.
10. ________ A Cambodian family immigrated to the United States and has been living in Denver for more than 5 years. The parents express concern about their children ages 10, 13, and 16, stating, "The children act so differently now. They are less respectful to us, want to eat only American food, and go to rock concerts. It's hard to believe they are our children."
11. ________ The Amish represent an important ethnic community in Lancaster, Pennsylvania.
12. ________ A nurse who is caring for a Native-American couple following the birth of their daughter arranges for them to take the placenta home for a ceremonial burial.

COLUMN II

A. Cultural relativism
B. Ethnocentrism
C. Assimilation
D. Subculture
E. Acculturation

FILL IN THE BLANKS: Insert the cultural concept that corresponds to each of the following definitions.

13. ______________________________ A unified set of values, attitudes, beliefs, and standards of behavior shared by a group of people.

14. ______________________________ A group existing within a larger cultural system that retains its own characteristics.

15. ______________________________ Recognizing that people from different cultural backgrounds comprehend the same objects and situations differently; that a culture determines a person's viewpoint.

16. ______________________________ Changes that occur within one group or among several groups when people from different cultures come into contact with one another and exchange and adopt each other's mannerisms, styles, and practices.

17. ______________________________ Process in which one cultural group loses its identity and becomes a part of the dominant culture.

18. ______________________________ A belief that one's cultural way of doing things is the right way, supporting the notion that "My group is the best."

19. ______________________________ Approach that involves respecting the differences in others including ethnicity, ethnoculture, and religious beliefs.

20. ______________________________ Type of time orientation that maintains a focus on achieving long-term goals; families or people who practice this time orientation are more likely to return for follow-up visits related to health care and to participate in primary prevention activities.

21. ______________________________ Type of time orientation of families or people who are more likely to strive to maintain tradition or the status quo and have little motivation for formulating future goals.

22. ______________________________ Type of time orientation of families or people who may have difficulty adhering to strict schedules and are often described as "living for the moment."

23. ______________________________ Cultural concept that reflects dimensions of personal comfort zones. Actions such as touching, placing the woman in proximity to others, taking away personal possessions, and making decisions for the woman can decrease personal security and heighten anxiety.

24. ______________________________ A unit of socialization and nurturing within a community that preserves and transmits culture.

25. ______________________________ Family structure in which male and female partners and their children live as an independent unit, sharing roles, responsibilities, and economic resources.

26. ______________________________ Family structure that includes the nuclear family and other people related by blood (kin) such as grandparents, aunts, uncles, and cousins.

27. ______________________________ Family structure in which children live with two unmarried biologic or adoptive parents.

28. ______________________________ Family category in which there is only one parent as head of the household; it is becoming an increasingly recognized structure in our society.

29. ______________________________ Family structure formed as a result of divorce and consisting of unrelated family members (stepparents, stepchildren, and stepsiblings) who join to create a new household.

30. ______________________________ Family structure in which gay or lesbian couples may live together with or without children.

31. ______________________________ Family structure in which children live independently in foster or kinship care such as living with a grandparent.

32. ______________________________ A family theory that views the family as a whole greater than the sum of its individual members and thus focuses on observing the interaction among family members rather than studying family members individually.

33. ______________________________ A family theory that focuses on the family as it moves through stages and relationships among family members as they progress through transitions.

34. ______________________________ A family theory concerned with the ways families react to stressful events; stress is studied within the internal and external contexts in which the family is living.

35. ______________________________ Family theory that involves a strength-based approach in clinical practice with families as opposed to a deficit approach.

36. ______________________________ Family theory with a focus on reducing cultural and environmental barriers that interfere with access to health care. Key elements include perceived susceptibility, perceived severity, perceived benefits, perceived barriers, cues to action, and confidence.

37. ______________________________ Family theory based on the belief that behavior is a function of the interaction of traits and abilities with the environment. Major concepts include ecosystem, niches, adaptive range, and ontogenetic development.

38. ______________________________ Term used for the family tree format of depicting relationships of family members over at least three generations; it provides valuable information about a family and its health.

39. ______________________________ Term used for a graphic portrayal of social relationships of the client and family including school, work, religious affiliations, and club memberships.

40. ______________________________ A community assessment technique that involves observing a community by traveling through it.

41. ______________________________ Groups within the community who are more likely to experience health status problems and negative health outcomes as a result of a variety of sociocultural, economic, and environmental risk factors.

42. ______________________________ Level of preventive care that involves health promotion and disease prevention activities to decrease the occurrence of illness and enhance general health and quality of life.

43. ______________________________ Level of preventive care that involves early detection of a disease and prompt treatment with the goal of curing the disease or slowing its progression and preventing subsequent disability; populations at risk for certain diseases are targeted.

44. ______________________________ Level of preventive care that focuses on rehabilitation of an individual who already has a disease back to as optimal a level of health as possible.

II. REVIEWING KEY CONCEPTS

45. DISCUSS why the nurse should take each of the following "products of culture" into consideration when providing care within a cultural context:

A. Communication

B. Personal space

C. Time orientation

D. Family roles

46. EXPLAIN the meaning of a CRASH course in cultural competency. Discuss how an international clinical placement applies the principles of CRASH in helping students/nurses to develop cultural competency.

47. STATE the rationale for the increasing emphasis on home- and community-based health care. How has this trend changed the demands placed on the community-based nurse?

48. Community health promotion requires the collaborative efforts of many individuals and groups within a community. CITE several programs that could be established to promote the health of a community's childbearing families.

49. EXPLAIN why each of the groups listed below has been identified as vulnerable populations of women:
   - Adolescent girls and older women
   - Racial and ethnic minorities
   - Incarcerated women
   - Refugees and migrant women
   - Homeless women

50. DESCRIBE the ways that nurses can provide care to perinatal clients using the telephone.

MULTIPLE CHOICE: Circle the correct option(s) and state the rationale for the option(s) chosen.

51. A family with open boundaries:
    A. Uses available support systems to meet its needs
    B. Is more prone to crisis, related to increased exposure to stressors
    C. Discourages family members from setting up channels
    D. Strives to maintain family stability by avoiding outside influences

52. Which nursing action is most likely to reduce a woman's anxiety and enhance her personal security as it relates to the concept of personal space needs?
    A. Touching the woman before and during procedures
    B. Providing explanations when performing tasks
    C. Ensuring that the woman has a talkative roommate to decrease loneliness
    D. Reducing the need for the woman to make decisions

53. A Native-American woman gave birth to a baby girl 12 hours ago. The nurse notes that the woman keeps her baby in the bassinet except for feeding and states that she will wait until she gets home to begin breastfeeding. The nurse recognizes that this behavior is most likely a reflection of:
    A. Embarrassment
    B. Delayed attachment
    C. Disappointment that the baby is a girl
    D. A belief that babies should not be fed colostrum

54. When caring for a pregnant woman who is Hispanic, the nurse should recognize that the woman may be guided by which cultural beliefs and practices during her pregnancy? (Circle all that apply.)
    A. Cool air currents can be dangerous during pregnancy.
    B. Prenatal care should begin very early in pregnancy.
    C. Milk should be avoided because it results in big babies and difficult births.
    D. Drinking chamomile tea should be avoided because it can cause preterm labor.
    E. The advice of both mothers and mothers-in-law should be followed during pregnancy.
    F. Pelvic examinations should not be performed by a male health care provider.

55. Regarding pregnancy and childbirth, European-American women are likely to believe that: (Circle all that apply.)
    A. The father of the baby should be actively involved in the labor and birth
    B. Pregnancy requires medical attention so prenatal care should begin early in pregnancy
    C. Birthing at home should be valued
    D. Pregnant women should participate in childbirth education
    E. The doctor is the head of the obstetric care team
    F. Mothers should not begin to breastfeed until milk comes in

56. A student nurse is planning to communicate with her postpartum client using an interpreter. Her instructor should provide further guidance if the student:
    A. Arranges for an older woman from the woman's country of origin to act as interpreter
    B. Stops periodically during the interaction to ask the interpreter how things are going
    C. Asks the woman questions while looking at the interpreter and speaking loudly so that the woman can hear the questions clearly
    D. Gathers culturally appropriate learning aids and reading materials to use during the interaction

57. Which health services represent the primary level of preventive care? (Circle all that apply.)
    A. Breast-self examination and testicular self-examination education programs
    B. Providing flu immunizations in pharmacies
    C. A safer-sex informational pamphlet provided to adolescents during a health education class
    D. Blood pressure and cholesterol screening at a health fair
    E. Instituting a wheelchair, cane, and walker exchange program for persons whose health insurance does not cover these items
    F. A car seat fitting fair at local auto dealerships

58. A student nurses' association is planning a health fair that will emphasize secondary level prevention activities. Which activities would their faculty adviser tell them to eliminate because it does not fit into their stated focus?
    A. Teaching participants how to check their radial pulse for rate and regularity
    B. Blood glucose monitoring
    C. Demonstration of relaxation measures to manage stress
    D. Breast models that participants can use to learn breast palpation techniques

59. When making a home visit, it is essential that the nurse use appropriate infection control measures. Of the measures listed below, which one is the most important?
    A. Including personal protective equipment in the home care bag
    B. Designating a dirty area with a trash bag to collect soiled equipment and supplies
    C. Wearing clean vinyl gloves for procedures that involve touching the client
    D. Performing hand hygiene using either soap and running water or a self-drying antiseptic solution

III. THINKING CRITICALLY

1. Nurses must avoid making stereotypical assumptions when caring for pregnant women from specific sociocultural or religious groups. EXPLAIN the process you would follow when providing culturally competent care that is reflective of a pregnant woman's unique values, beliefs, and behavioral patterns.

2. IMAGINE that you are a nurse working in a clinic that provides prenatal services to a multicultural community predominated by Hispanic-American, African-American, and Asian-American families. DESCRIBE how you would adapt care measures to reflect the cultural beliefs and practices of pregnant women and their families from each of the following cultural groups.
   A. Hispanic-American

   B. African-American

   C. Asian-American

3. Pamela is a 20-year-old Native-American. She is 3 months pregnant and has come to the prenatal clinic on the reservation where she lives for her first visit to obtain prenatal vitamins, which her friends at work told her are important.
   A. STATE the questions the nurse should ask to determine Pamela's cultural expectations about childbearing.

   B. DESCRIBE the communication approach you would consider when interviewing Pamela.

   C. IDENTIFY the Native-American beliefs and practices regarding childbearing that may influence Pamela's approach to her pregnancy and birth.

4. A nurse has been providing care to a Hispanic family. This family recently experienced the birth of twin girls at 38 weeks of gestation. It is the first birth experience for both parents and the first grandchildren for the extended family. Both newborns are healthy and living at home. DESCRIBE the cultural beliefs and practices that the family, as Hispanic, might use as guidelines to provide care to their newborn twin girls.

5. The nurse midwife at a prenatal clinic has been assigned to care for a Sunni refugee couple from Iraq who recently emigrated to the United States. The woman has just been diagnosed as 2 months pregnant. Neither she nor her husband speaks English. OUTLINE the process that this nurse should use when working with a translator to facilitate communication with this couple to enhance care management.

6. IMAGINE that you are a nurse who has just been hired to provide home health care. Before you begin seeing your clients, you realize that it would be helpful for you to become familiar with the neighborhood and resources in the community where your clients live.
   A. You decide to conduct a walking survey of this community. DESCRIBE how you would go about conducting this survey and gathering data.

   B. LIST the data you would see as essential to gather.

   C. DISCUSS how you would use the findings from your walking survey when providing health care to the clients you will be visiting.

7. Marie is a single parent of two young children ages 4 years and 1 year. She and her children have been homeless for 3 months since her husband abandoned her and she lost her job because she had no one to help her care for her children.
   A. DISCUSS the types of health problems for which Marie and her children are most vulnerable.

   B. Research indicates that approximately 20% of women who are homeless become pregnant. What factors related to being homeless could increase Marie's risk for becoming pregnant? If she did become pregnant, explain why it would be considered a high risk pregnancy.

   C. How would you, as a nurse, provide health care services to Marie and her children?

8. Consuelo is the wife of a migrant laborer. She and her husband, along with their two children, have been working on a California farm for 2 weeks. She has arrived at a health center established for migrant laborers. Consuelo states that she is 4 months pregnant. As the woman's health nurse practitioner assigned to care for Consuelo, what approaches would you use to ensure that she obtains quality health care that addresses her unique health risks as a migrant worker?

9. WRITE a series of questions that you would ask when making a postpartum follow-up call to a woman who gave birth 3 days ago.

10. Eileen gave birth to a son 36 hours ago. A home care nurse has been assigned to visit Eileen and her husband in their home to assess the progress of her recovery after birth, the health status of her newborn son, and the adaptation of family processes to the responsibilities of newborn care.
    A. OUTLINE the approach the nurse should take in preparing for this visit.

    B. DESCRIBE the nurse's actions during the visit using the care management process as a format.

    C. DISCUSS how the nurse should end the visit.

    D. IDENTIFY interventions the nurse should implement at the conclusion of the visit with Eileen and her husband.

E. SPECIFY how the nurse should protect her personal safety both outside and inside Eileen's home.

F. CITE the infection control measures the nurse should use when conducting the visit and providing care in Eileen's home.

11. Angela has recently been diagnosed with hyperemesis gravidarum and has been hospitalized to stabilize her fluid and electrolyte balance. The hospital-based nurse must evaluate Angela for referral to home care.
    A. STATE the criteria that this nurse should follow in order to determine Angela's readiness for discharge from hospital to home care.

    B. Angela has been discharged and will be receiving parenteral nutrition in her home. DISCUSS the additional information required related to high-technology home care.

    C. IDENTIFY specific home environment criteria that must be met to ensure the safety and effectiveness of Angela's treatment.

12. A nurse is seeking funding to start a home care agency designed to provide home visits to postpartum women and their families within 1 week of birth and follow-up visits as indicated. STATE the points the nurse should emphasize as a rationale for the importance of this health care service and the cost-effectiveness of funding such a service.

CHAPTER 3

Clinical Genetics

I. LEARNING KEY TERMS

MATCHING: Match the description in Column I with the appropriate genetic concept in Column II.

COLUMN I

1. _______ An individual's observable traits.
2. _______ Condition in which there is a mixture of cells, some with a normal number of chromosomes and others either missing a chromosome or containing an extra chromosome.
3. _______ Failure of chromosomes to separate.
4. _______ Basic physical units of inheritance that are passed from parents to offspring and contain the information needed to specify traits.
5. _______ An abnormality in chromosome number (the exact multiple of the haploid set is not present.)
6. _______ An individual's collection of genes.
7. _______ Union of a normal gamete and a gamete containing an extra chromosome, resulting in a cell with 47 chromosomes.
8. _______ A portion of the chromosome is rearranged in reverse order.
9. _______ X, Y
10. _______ A cell with the correct or normal number of chromosomes within it.
11. _______ Entire set of genetic instructions found in the nucleus of each human cell.
12. _______ Having two copies of the same allele for the same trait.
13. _______ Genes at corresponding loci on homologous chromosomes that code for different forms or variations of the same trait.
14. _______ Chromosomal material is exchanged between two chromosomes.
15. _______ Matched chromosomes, each having the same number and arrangement of genes.
16. _______ Loss of chromosomal material and partial monosomy for the chromosome involved.
17. _______ There are 22 pairs of these on each chromosome, one from each parent.
18. _______ Threadlike packages of genes and other DNA in a cell nucleus.
19. _______ Union of a normal gamete and a gamete missing a chromosome resulting in a cell with 45 chromosomes.
20. _______ A spontaneous and permanent change in normal gene structure.
21. _______ Pictoral analysis of the number, form, and size of an individual's chromosomes.
22. _______ Having two different alleles for a given trait.

COLUMN II

A. Genome
B. Chromosome
C. Homozygous
D. Gene
E. Sex chromosomes
F. Karyotype
G. Aneuploidy
H. Autosomes
I. Trisomy
J. Nondisjunction
K. Monosomy
L. Translocation
M. Mutation
N. Heterozygous
O. Alleles
P. Deletions
Q. Mosaicism
R. Euploid
S. Phenotype
T. Inversions
U. Genotype
V. Homologous

FILL IN THE BLANKS: Insert the term that corresponds to each of the following descriptions related to the study of genes and chromosomes.

23. ______________________________ The study of individual genes and their effect on relatively rare single-gene disorders.

24. ______________________________ The study of all the genes in the human genome together, including their interactions with each other, the environment, and the influence of other psychosocial and cultural factors.

25. ______________________________ Testing that involves the analysis of human DNA, RNA, chromosomes, or proteins to detect abnormalities related to an inherited condition.

26. ______________________________ Tests used to directly examine the DNA and RNA that make up a gene.

27. ______________________________ Tests that look at markers coinherited with a gene that causes a genetic condition.

28. ______________________________ Tests that examine the protein products of genes.

29. ______________________________ Tests that examine chromosomes.

30. ______________________________ Tests used to identify individuals who have a gene mutation for a genetic condition but do not show symptoms of the condition because it is a condition that is inherited in an autosomal recessive form.

31. ______________________________ Tests used to clarify the genetic status of asymptomatic family members. There are two specific types of these tests, namely ______________________________ tests (gene mutation is present and symptoms are certain to appear if the individual lives long enough) and ______________________________ tests (gene mutation is present but this positive result does not indicate that there is a 100% risk of developing the condition).

32. ______________________________ The use of genetic information to individualize drug therapy. A primary benefit is the potential to reduce adverse drug reactions.

33. ______________________________ Therapeutic approach that is based on the use of genetic information to correct inherited diseases.

FILL IN THE BLANKS: Insert the term that corresponds to each of the following descriptions related to patterns of genetic transmission.

34. ______________________________ Phenotypic characteristics resulting from two or more genes on different chromosomes acting together; it involves a combination of genetic and environmental factors.

35. ______________________________ Phenotypic characteristics controlled by a single gene; it is also known as single-gene inheritance.

36. ______________________________ Inherited disorder in which only one copy of a variant gene is needed for phenotypic expression.

37. ______________________________ Inherited disorder in which both genes of a pair are forms associated with the disorder to be expressed.

38. ______________________________ Disorder that follows the autosomal recessive pattern of inheritance; it occurs when a gene mutation reduces the efficiency of encoded enzymes to a level at which normal metabolism cannot occur.

39. ______________________________ Form of inheritance that mimics autosomal dominant inheritance, except that male-to-male transmission cannot occur unless the father has Klinefelter syndrome due to XY disomy.

40. ______________________________ Form of inheritance in which the abnormal gene is carried on the female chromosome; if the male receives the abnormal gene, the disorder will be expressed; a common example of this type of disorder is hemophilia.

II. REVIEWING KEY CONCEPTS

41. IDENTIFY five genetics-related activities that reflect the minimal amount of genetic and genomic competency expected of all nurses.

42. Couples referred for genetic counseling receive an estimation of risk for the genetic disorder of concern. EXPLAIN the difference between an estimate of occurrence risk and an estimation of recurrence risk.

43. Many nurses specialize in the area of genetic counseling. DISCUSS the major ethical, legal, and social implications (ELSI) associated with genetic testing that should guide the practice of these nurses.

MULTIPLE CHOICE: Circle the correct option(s) and state the rationale for the option(s) chosen.

44. Based on genetic testing of a newborn, a diagnosis of neurofibromatosis is made. The parents ask the nurse if this could happen to future children. Because this is an example of autosomal dominant inheritance, the nurse tells the parents:
    A. "For each pregnancy, there is a 50/50 chance the child will be affected by neurofibromatosis."
    B. "This will not happen again because the neurofibromatosis was caused by the harmful genetic effects of the infection you had during pregnancy."
    C. "For each pregnancy there is a 25% chance the child will be a carrier of the defective gene but unaffected by the disorder."
    D. "Because you already have had an affected child there is a decreased chance for this to happen in future pregnancies."

45. A female carries the gene for hemophilia on one of her X chromosomes. The father does not have hemophilia. Now that she is pregnant she asks the nurse how this might affect her baby. The nurse should tell her:
    A. A female baby has a 50% chance of also being a carrier.
    B. A male baby can be a carrier or have hemophilia.
    C. Female babies are never affected by this disorder.
    D. Hemophilia is always expressed if a male inherits the defective gene.

46. A pregnant woman carries a single gene for cystic fibrosis, an inborn error of metabolism. The father of her baby does not carry this gene. Which of the following is true regarding the genetic pattern of the inborn error of metabolism as it applies to this family?
    A. The pregnant woman has cystic fibrosis herself.
    B. There is a 50% chance her baby will have the disorder.
    C. There is a 25% chance her baby will be a carrier.
    D. There is no chance her baby will be affected by this disorder.

47. A woman has been diagnosed with factor V Leiden (FVL). The nurse caring for this woman would be alert for which of the following problems?
    A. Breast cancer
    B. Postpartum hemorrhage
    C. Deep vein thrombosis (DVT)
    D. Placenta previa

III. THINKING CRITICALLY

1. A nurse is providing genetic counseling to a pregnant woman and her partner. They are unsure about whether they should undergo genetic testing to determine if they are carriers of a genetic disorder. IDENTIFY the factors this nurse should keep in mind that can influence her clients' decision to have genetic testing or to refuse it.

2. SUPPORT THIS STATEMENT: All nurses must possess a basic understanding of and expertise in genetics to provide holistic family-centered care.

3. Angela has come for her first prenatal visit. IDENTIFY the questions the nurse should ask during the health history interview to determine if factors are present that would place Angela at risk for giving birth to a baby with an inheritable disorder.

4. Rachel and Joshua, who are Jewish, are newly married and planning for pregnancy. They express to the nurse their concern that Rachel has a history of Tay-Sachs disease in her family. Joshua has never investigated his family history.
   A. DESCRIBE the nurse's role in the process of assisting the couple to determine their genetic risk.

B. Both Rachel and Joshua are found to be carriers of the disorder. DISCUSS the estimation of risk and interpretation of risk as it applies to the couple for giving birth to a child who is normal, is a carrier, or is affected by the disorder.

C. OUTLINE the nurse's role in the education and emotional support of the couple now that a diagnosis and estimation of risk have been made.

CHAPTER 4

Assessment and Health Promotion

I. LEARNING KEY TERMS

FILL IN THE BLANKS: Insert the term that corresponds to each of the following descriptions related to the female reproductive system and breasts. Use the anatomic drawings (Figs. 4-1, 4-2, 4-4, and 4-6) in your textbook to visualize each of the structures as you are inserting the terms.

1. ______________________ Fatty pad that lies over the anterior surface of the symphysis pubis.
2. ______________________ Two rounded folds of fatty tissue covered with skin that extend downward and backward from the mons pubis; their purpose is to protect the inner vulvar structures.
3. ______________________ Two flat reddish folds composed of connective tissue and smooth muscle, which are supplied with nerve endings that are extremely sensitive.
4. ______________________ Hoodlike covering of the clitoris.
5. ______________________ Fold of tissue under the clitoris.
6. ______________________ Thin flat tissue formed by the joining of the labia minora; it is underneath the vaginal opening at the midline.
7. ______________________ Small structure underneath the prepuce composed of erectile tissue with numerous sensory nerve endings; it increases in size during sexual arousal.
8. ______________________ Almond-shaped area enclosed by the labia minora that contains openings to the urethra, Skene's glands, vagina, and Bartholin's glands.
9. ______________________ Bladder opening found between the clitoris and the vagina.
10. ______________________ Skin-covered muscular area between the fourchette and the anus that covers the pelvic structures.
11. ______________________ Fibromuscular collapsible tubular structure that extends from the vulva to the uterus and lies between the bladder and rectum. Its mucosal lining is arranged in transverse folds called ______________________. ______________________ and ______________________ glands secrete mucus that lubricates the vagina.
12. ______________________ Anterior, posterior, and lateral pockets that surround the cervix.
13. ______________________ Muscular pelvic organ located between the bladder and the rectum and just above the vagina. The ______________________ is a deep pouch, or recess, posterior to the cervix formed by the posterior ligament.
14. ______________________ Upper triangular portion of the uterus.
15. ______________________ Also known as the lower uterine segment, it is the short constricted portion that separates the corpus of the uterus from the cervix.
16. ______________________ Dome-shaped top of the uterus.
17. ______________________ Highly vascular lining of the uterus.
18. ______________________ Layer of the uterus composed of smooth muscles that extend in three different directions.
19. ______________________ Lower cylindric portion of the uterus composed of fibrous connective tissue and elastic tissue.

20. ______________________ Canal connecting the uterine cavity to the vagina. The opening between the uterus and this canal is the ______________________. The opening between the canal and the vagina is the ______________________.

21. ______________________ Location in the cervix where the squamous and columnar epithelia meet (the transformation zone); it is the most common site for neoplastic changes; cells from this site are scraped for the ______________________ test.

22. ______________________ Passageways between the ovaries and the uterus; they are attached at each side of the dome-shaped uterine fundus.

23. ______________________ Almond-shaped organs located on each side of the uterus; their two functions are ______________________ and the production of the hormones ______________________, ______________________, and ______________________.

24. ______________________ Structure that protects the bladder, uterus, and rectum; accommodates the growing fetus during pregnancy; and anchors support structures.

25. ______________________ The paired mammary glands.

26. ______________________ Segment of mammary tissue that extends into the axilla.

27. ______________________ Mammary papilla.

28. ______________________ Pigmented section of the breast that surrounds the nipple.

29. ______________________ Sebaceous glands that cause the areola to appear rough.

30. ______________________ Breast structures that are lined with epithelial cells that secrete colostrum and milk.

31. ______________________ Layer of tissue below the epithelium that contracts to expel milk from acini.

MATCHING: Match the descriptions related to the menstrual cycle in Column I with the appropriate term from Column II.

COLUMN I

32. ________ The first menstruation.

33. ________ Transitional stage between childhood and sexual maturity.

34. ________ Transitional phase during which ovarian function and hormone production decline.

35. ________ The last menstrual period dated with certainty once 1 year has passed after menstruation ceases.

36. ________ Period preceding the last menstrual period that lasts about 4 years; during this time ovarian function declines, ova diminish, more menstrual cycles become anovulatory, and irregular bleeding occurs.

37. ________ Periodic uterine bleeding that begins approximately 14 days after ovulation and lasting an average of 5 days.

38. ________ The cycle that involves cyclic changes in the lining of the uterus.

39. ________ Phase of the menstrual cycle during which the uterine lining grows rapidly and thickens from about the fifth day to the time of ovulation.

40. ________ Phase of the menstrual cycle during which the uterine lining becomes luxuriant with blood and glandular secretions suitable to protect and nurture a fertilized ovum.

COLUMN II

A. Menstruation
B. Hypothalamic-pituitary cycle
C. Gonadotropin-releasing hormone (GnRH)
D. Prostaglandins
E. Menarche
F. Luteinizing hormone
G. Graafian follicle
H. Spinnbarkeit
I. Secretory phase
J. Progesterone
K. Puberty
L. Ovarian cycle
M. Proliferative phase
N. Climacteric
O. Follicle-stimulating hormone

41. _______ Phase during which the blood supply to the functional uterine lining is blocked and necrosis develops; the functional layer separates from the basal layer, and menstrual bleeding begins.

42. _______ Cycle that involves secretion of hormones required to stimulate ovulation.

43. _______ Cycle that involves the changes in the ovary, leading to ovulation. It consists of two phases, namely, follicular and luteal.

44. _______ Structure that encloses the developing ovum; it ruptures at the time of ovulation, releasing the ovum.

45. _______ Hormone secreted by the hypothalamus when ovarian hormones are reduced to a low level. It stimulates the pituitary gland to secrete two critical hormones.

46. _______ Pituitary hormone that stimulates the development of follicles in the ovary.

47. _______ Pituitary hormone that stimulates the expulsion of the ovum from the graafian follicle and formation of the corpus luteum.

48. _______ Ovarian hormone that stimulates the thickening of the endometrium that occurs after menstruation and prior to ovulation; it is also responsible for changes in the cervix and cervical mucus.

49. _______ Stretchable quality of the cervical mucus at the time of ovulation.

50. _______ Ovarian hormone that is responsible for the changes in the endometrium that occur after ovulation to facilitate implantation should fertilization occur; it is also responsible for the rise in temperature that occurs after ovulation.

51. _______ Oxygenated fatty acids classified as hormones. They are thought to play an essential role in ovulation, transport of sperm, regression of the corpus luteum, and menstruation. By increasing the myometrial response to oxytocin, they also play a role in labor and dysmenorrhea.

P. Perimenopause
Q. Estrogen
R. Ischemic phase
S. Menopause
T. Endometrial cycle

II. REVIEWING KEY CONCEPTS

52. It is essential that guidelines for laboratory and diagnostic procedures be followed exactly to ensure the accuracy of the results obtained. OUTLINE the guidelines that should be followed when performing a Pap test in terms of each of the following:

A. Client preparation

B. Timing during examination when the specimen is obtained

C. Sites for specimen collection

D. Handling of specimens

E. Frequency of performance

53. During a clinical examination of a woman's breasts the nurse identifies a lump in one of the breasts. CITE the characteristics that the nurse should document regarding the palpated lump.

MULTIPLE CHOICE: Circle the correct option(s), and state the rationale for the option(s) chosen.

54. A 20-year-old woman tells the nurse that she performs breast self-examination (BSE) on a regular basis. The nurse evaluates the woman's understanding of BSE and ability to perform the technique correctly. Which actions by the woman indicate that she needs further instructions regarding BSE? (Circle all that apply.)
    A. Performs BSE every month on the first day of her menstrual cycle.
    B. Observes the size of her breasts, the direction of her nipples, and appearance of her skin including the presence of dimpling when looking at her breasts in the mirror.
    C. Lies down on her bed and puts a pillow under the shoulder of the breast she is going to palpate. Then she places the arm on that side under her head.
    D. Uses the tips of her four fingers to palpate her breast.
    E. Palpates her breast, using an overlapping circular pattern around her entire breast.
    F. Palpates her breasts again including up into her axilla while taking a shower.

55. When palpating the small breasts of a young slender woman, the nurse should:
    A. Wear clean gloves
    B. Lift hands when moving from one segment of the breast to another
    C. Use both hands
    D. Follow a systematic overlapping pattern

56. A nurse instructed a female client regarding vulvar self-examination (VSE). Which statement made by the client indicates that further instruction is needed?
   A. "I will perform this examination at least once a month, especially if I change sexual partners or am sexually active."
   B. "I will become familiar with how my genitalia look and feel so that I will be able to detect changes."
   C. "I will use the examination to determine when I should get medications at the pharmacy for infections."
   D. "I will wash my hands thoroughly before and after I examine myself."

57. A women's health nurse practitioner is going to perform a pelvic examination on a female client. Which nursing action would be least effective in enhancing the client's comfort and relaxation during the examination?
   A. Encourage the client to ask questions and express feelings and concerns before and after the examination.
   B. Ask the client questions as the examination is performed.
   C. Allow the client to keep her shoes and socks on when placing her feet in the stirrups.
   D. Instruct the client to place her hands over her diaphragm and take deep, slow breaths.

58. When assessing women it is important for a nurse to keep in mind the possibility that they are victims of violence. The nurse should:
   A. Use an abuse assessment screen during the assessment of every woman
   B. Recognize that abuse rarely occurs during pregnancy
   C. Assess a woman's legs and back as the most commonly injured areas
   D. Notify the police immediately if abuse is suspected

59. A 50-year-old woman asks the nurse practitioner about how often she should be assessed for the common health problems women of her age could experience. The nurse recommends:
   A. An endometrial biopsy every 3 to 4 years
   B. A fecal occult blood test annually
   C. A mammogram every other year
   D. Bone mineral density testing annually

60. Which statement is most accurate regarding persons who should participate in preconception counseling?
   A. All women and their partners as they make decisions about their reproductive future including becoming parents
   B. Women older than 40 years of age who wish to become pregnant
   C. Sexually active women who do not use birth control
   D. Women with chronic illnesses such as diabetes who are planning to get pregnant

61. To enhance the accuracy of the Pap test, the nurse should instruct the woman to:
   A. Schedule the test just prior to the onset of menses
   B. Stop taking birth control pills for 2 days before the test
   C. Avoid intercourse for 24 to 48 hours before the test
   D. Douche with a specially prepared antiseptic solution the night before the test

III. THINKING CRITICALLY

1. A nurse is teaching a group of young adult women about health promotion activities. As part of the discussion the nurse identifies preconception care as an important health promotion activity. One woman in the class asks, "I know you need to go for checkups once you are pregnant, but why would you need to see a doctor before you get pregnant? Isn't that a big waste of time and money?" EXPLAIN how the nurse should respond to this woman's question.

2. A group of nurse practitioners and midwives is establishing a women's health clinic in a large metropolitan area of New York. They will be serving a multiethnic population that consists of women ranging from adolescence to old age.
   A. Using an awareness that women most often initially seek health care for reproductive concerns, IDENTIFY the services the nurses at this new clinic should plan to offer.

   B. CITE the factors (barriers) that could interfere with the women in this community seeking health care at the clinic. Based on these barriers, DESCRIBE strategies these nurses could use to reduce the barriers to care and encourage the women to participate in the services offered at the clinic.

   C. Major goals of the nurses at this clinic are to promote the health of women in the community and prevent illness. DISCUSS the types of services the nurses should place a high priority on offering in order to achieve their goals. Include a rationale for each service proposed.

3. An inner-city women's health clinic serves a diverse population in terms of age, ethnic background, and health problems. DESCRIBE how the women's health nurse practitioner should adjust the approach for the following women with special needs. Each of the factors should influence a women's health nurse practitioner's approach when assessing the health of the women who come to the clinic for care.
   A. Adolescents

   B. Midlife and older women

C. Women with disabilities

D. Abused women

4. During a routine checkup for her annual Pap test, Julie, a 26-year-old, asks the nurse for advice regarding nutrition and exercise. Her body mass index (BMI) is 32, and she wants to "lose weight sensibly and keep it off." DISCUSS the advice the nurse should give to Julie.

5. Alice, a 30-year-old client, comes to the women's health clinic complaining of fatigue, insomnia, and feeling anxious. She works as a stockbroker for a major Wall Street brokerage firm. Alice states that although she enjoys the challenge of her job, she never can seem to find time for herself or to socialize with her friends. Alice tells the nurse practitioner that she has been drinking more and started to smoke again to help her to relax. She is glad that she has lost some weight, attributing this to her diminished appetite.
   A. STATE the physical and emotional signs of stress that the nurse should take note of when assessing Alice.

   B. DISCUSS how the nurse can help Alice cope with stress and its consequences in a healthy manner.

   C. Alice expresses interest in attempting to stop smoking. "I felt so much better when I stopped the first time. That was over 2 years ago and now here I am back at it again." DESCRIBE an approach the nurse could use to help Alice achieve a desired change in health behavior that is long lasting.

6. During a routine women's health checkup, a woman expresses concern to the nurse practitioner about the increase in violence against women. She states, "One of my friends was raped, and a colleague at work was beaten by her boyfriend." DISCUSS how the nurse practitioner should respond to this woman's concern, including measures she could use to protect herself from violence and injury.

7. IMAGINE that you are a nurse working at a clinic that provides health care to women. DESCRIBE how you would respond to each of the following concerns or questions of women who have come to the clinic for care.
   A. Serena, a 17-year-old, has just been scheduled for her first women's health checkup, which will include a pelvic examination and Pap test. She nervously asks if there is anything she needs to do to get ready for the examination.

   B. Andrea is trying to get pregnant. She wonders if there are signs she could observe in her body that would indicate that she is ovulating and therefore able to conceive a baby with her partner.

   C. When you are teaching a group of women of various ages about BSE, they ask you to describe the normal characteristics of the female breast and how these characteristics change as a woman gets older.

   D. Anne, 24 years old, asks the nurse about a recommended douche to use a couple of times a week to stay "nice and clean down there."

8. Julie, a 21-year-old client, has come to the women's health clinic for a women's health checkup. During the health history interview she becomes very anxious and states, "I have to tell you this is my first examination. I am very scared—my friends told me that it hurts a lot to have this examination." DESCRIBE how the nurse should respond in an effort to reduce Julie's anxiety.

9. As a nurse working in a women's health clinic, you have been assigned to interview Angie, a 25-year-old new client, to obtain her health history.
   A. LIST the components that should be emphasized in gathering Angie's history.

   B. WRITE a series of questions that you would ask to obtain data related to Angie's reproductive and sexual health and practices.

   C. DISCUSS the therapeutic techniques that you would use to facilitate communication. GIVE an example of each technique.

10. Self-examination of the breasts and vulva (genitalia) are important assessment techniques to teach a woman. OUTLINE the procedure that you would use to teach each technique to one of your clients. INCLUDE the teaching methodologies that you would use to enhance learning
    Breast self-examination

    Vulvar (genital) self-examination

11. Lu Chen is a 25-year-old exchange student from China who has been living in the United States for 3 months. This is the first time that she is away from home. She comes to the university women's health clinic for a checkup and to obtain birth control. DESCRIBE how the nurse assigned to Lu Chen would approach and communicate with her in a culturally sensitive manner.

12. Nurses working in women's health care must be aware of the growing problem of violence against women. All women should be screened when being assessed during health care for the possibility of abuse.
    A. DESCRIBE how you as a nurse would adjust the environment where the health history interview and physical examination will take place to elicit a woman's confidence and trust.

    B. IDENTIFY indicators of possible abuse that you would look for before the appointment and then during the health history interview and physical examination.

    C. STATE the questions you would ask to screen for abuse.

    D. DISCUSS the approach you would take if abuse is confirmed during the assessment.

13. When teaching a group of preadolescent girls about menstruation, one student asks the nurse, "What will happen to me when all of this stuff starts?" DESCRIBE what the nurse should tell the girls about the changes that they can expect and what is happening to their bodies during each of the following components of the menstrual cycle: Hypothalamic-pituitary cycle

Ovarian cycle

Endometrial cycle

14. As a student you may be assigned to assist a health care provider during the performance of a pelvic examination for one of your clients.
    A. DESCRIBE how you would:
       Prepare your client for the examination

       Support your client during the examination

       Assist your client after the examination

    B. DESCRIBE how you would assist the health care provider who is performing the examination.

15. Lara, a 16-year-old, has come to the women's health clinic where you are a women's health nurse practitioner. This is her first visit and she is accompanied by her mother. During the history Lara asks her mother to leave so she can have privacy. She expresses to you that her major concern is that she still has not had her first menstrual period and her breasts are not developing. You note that she is very thin. When you weigh her you discover that her BMI is 16. Despite this, Lara is concerned that she has gained a half a pound since her last weight at home, which she checks several times a week.
    A. DESCRIBE how you would address the nutritional problem that Lara is exhibiting.

    B. COMPARE AND CONTRAST each of the following eating disorders:
       Anorexia nervosa

       Bulimia nervosa

       Binge-eating disorder

CHAPTER 5

Violence Against Women

I. LEARNING KEY TERMS

FILL IN THE BLANKS: Insert the term that corresponds to the description related to violence against women.

1. ______________________ The most common form of violence against women. It refers to the actual or threatened physical, sexual, psychologic, or emotional abuse by a spouse, ex-spouse, boyfriend, girlfriend, ex-boyfriend, ex-girlfriend, date, or cohabitating partner.
2. ______________________ View of violence based on three phases in an IPV relationship. The first phase is a period of ______________________ leading to the second phase involving acute ______________________ followed by the third phase of calm and remorse called the ______________________ phase.
3. ______________________ A contemporary view of violence with the primary theme of male dominance and coercive control.
4. ______________________ View of violence based on the dynamic relationship between the individual and the environment. The ______________________ is the center of the model with her ______________________ as part of her immediate environment. At the next level or ______________________ are her children, family, friends, and the people and activities in her day-to-day life that are important to her. The ______________________ represents the community resources such as women's groups, violence prevention programs, and local resources. The ______________________ refers to organizations and formal agencies, health care systems, and providers such as nurses, the police, and the legal system. Finally, all of these are influenced by the ______________________, which includes the larger sociocultural beliefs, myths, and media. The ______________________ represents the influence of events over time.
5. ______________________ Broad term that encompasses a wide range of sexual victimization.
6. ______________________ Unwelcome degrading sexual remarks, jokes, contact, or behavior such as exhibitionism that makes the work or other environment uncomfortable or difficult.
7. ______________________ Intentional, unwanted, completed or attempted touching of the victim's genitals, anus, groin, or breasts, directly or through clothing as well as voyeurism. It also includes exhibitionism, exposing someone to pornography or images taken of the victim in a private context.
8. ______________________ Forced sexual intercourse or penetration of the mouth, anus, or vagina by a body part or object without consent; it may or may not include the use of a weapon.
9. ______________________ Penetration by a person who is 18 years or older of a person under the age of consent; specifics vary from state to state.
10. ______________________ Noncoital sexual activity between a child and adolescent or adult.
11. ______________________ Cluster of characteristic symptoms and related behaviors experienced by women in the weeks and months after they have been sexually assaulted. The three phases are ______________________, ______________________, and ______________________.
12. ______________________ A nurse educated in the specialty of forensic nursing and who is prepared to examine women who have been raped.

II. REVIEWING KEY CONCEPTS

13. Nurses caring for women should be alert for the presence of sociologic factors that have been associated with violence. IDENTIFY several of these factors that should be included as part of the assessment of women.

14. STATE how cultural beliefs and values can affect violence against women: its occurrence, how it is viewed, and the help sought by and provided to women who are abused. CITE examples from specific cultures.

15. Nurses working in women's health care should be aware of the characteristics typical of women who are abused and the persons who abuse them.
    A. CONTRAST the characteristics of women who are most likely to be in abusive relationships with the characteristics of women who are most likely to be in nonviolent relationships.

    B. CITE the characteristics of women who are most likely to seek assistance when they are abused.

    C. EXPLAIN why some women may not seek help when they are in an abusive relationship.

    D. CREATE a profile of persons most likely to become abusive partners.

16. A nurse is presenting a class related to IPV to a group of young college women. An expected outcome of this class is that *Women will describe the many forms that abuse can take*. DESCRIBE the information this nurse should present to the class to ensure that the outcome is achieved.

17. Clarise is a victim of IPV by her male partner. DESCRIBE how the nurse caring for Clarise could use the ABCDES tool to provide Clarise with the support she needs.

18. Nurses play an essential role in preventing the cycle of violence against women in our society. DESCRIBE several strategies school nurses can use to accomplish this goal.

19. Nurses working with victims of rape must realize that women are often reluctant to report the rape. INDICATE the factors that can deter women from reporting that they have been raped.

MULTIPLE CHOICE: Circle the correct option(s) and state the rationale for the option(s) chosen.

20. Men who are likely to abuse their female partner often exhibit which of the following characteristics? (Circle all that apply.)
    A. Low self-esteem
    B. Assertiveness
    C. Ability to express feelings verbally
    D. Intense interest in spending all of his time doing things with his partner
    E. Tolerance for frustration

21. A characteristic of women in abusive relationships is which of the following?
    A. Masochism
    B. Willingness to take a stand no matter what the cost
    C. Absence of typical feminine characteristics such as nurturing and compassion
    D. Tendency to isolate themselves from social relationships

22. A nurse caring for pregnant women needs to be aware that physical abuse during pregnancy can result in which of the following outcomes? (Circle all that apply.)
    A. Excessive weight gain
    B. Use of alcohol or tobacco as a means of coping
    C. Increased risk for giving birth to a low-birth-weight baby
    D. Postterm pregnancy
    E. Sexually transmitted infections (STIs)

23. Which of the following women is most likely to seek assistance when battered?
    A. A woman with a career
    B. A woman battered for the first time
    C. A woman who as a child saw her mother being abused by her father
    D. A woman who was abused as a child

24. A woman suspects that she has been raped by her date and that he put a "ruffie" (flunitrazepam [Rohypnol]) in the wine she was drinking. What signs would she describe to the SANE nurse to help to confirm that her suspicions are correct? (Circle all that apply.)
    A. Remembering what happened clearly
    B. Severe headache in the morning
    C. Feeling as if sex has occurred
    D. Feeling more intoxicated than usual with a similar amount of alcohol
    E. Feeling fuzzy or whoozy on awakening

III. THINKING CLEARLY

1. SUPPLY the facts to disprove each of the following myths concerning violence against women.
   A. IPV is primarily a problem of families who are at a low socioeconomic level and poorly educated.

   B. Violence affects only a small percentage of women in this country.

   C. Victims and perpetrators of IPV cannot change.

D. Battered women usually provoke their attack because they have a need to be beaten.

E. Being pregnant protects a woman from IPV.

2. OUTLINE an assessment format based on the ecological framework for IPV.

3. As a nurse working in a women's health clinic you must be alert to cues indicative of physical abuse.
   A. IDENTIFY the cues you would look for.

   B. Carol, a 24-year-old married client, comes to the clinic to confirm her belief that she is pregnant. During the assessment phase of the visit, you note cues that lead you to suspect that Carol is being abused by her husband. DISCUSS the approach you would take to confirm your suspicion that Carol is being abused.

   C. Carol admits to you that her husband beats her sometimes, and that "it has been increasing." Now she is afraid it will get worse because she "was not supposed to get pregnant." DISCUSS the nursing actions that you could take to help Carol.

D. LIST the possible reasons that Carol, now that she is pregnant, is experiencing an escalation of battering/abuse from her husband.

E. SPECIFY what you should avoid as you work with Carol.

F. EXPLAIN how you would determine the degree of danger Carol faces.

G. DISCUSS how Carol's pregnancy could be adversely affected by the violence she is experiencing.

H. DESCRIBE the behaviors Carol would most likely exhibit as an indication of her readiness to leave the abusive relationship.

I. IDENTIFY your legal responsibilities regarding confirmation that Carol is indeed being abused and reporting the abuse to authorities who can help Carol.

4. Marie has been raped. She is admitted to the emergency department for examination.
   A. EXPLAIN the advantage of having a SANE nurse care for Marie.

   B. DESCRIBE the nurse's responsibility in assessing Marie and in collecting and preserving the physical evidence of her rape.

   C. DISCUSS the nursing actions that should be used to meet the emotional needs of Marie at this time.

   D. OUTLINE how Marie's emotions and behaviors will be expressed and change as she progresses through the phases of the rape-trauma syndrome. IDENTIFY how a rape-trauma counselor should assess Marie during each phase.

   E. SPECIFY the interventions required prior to discharging Marie.

CHAPTER 6

Reproductive System Concerns

I. LEARNING KEY TERMS

FILL IN THE BLANKS: Insert the term that corresponds to each of the following descriptions related to menstrual disorders and experiences.

1. ______________________ Absence of menstrual flow. It is a clinical symptom of a variety of disorders but it is most commonly a result of pregnancy and is a classic sign of anorexia nervosa.
2. ______________________ Absence of menstrual flow related to a problem of the central hypothalamic-pituitary axis.
3. ______________________ Interrelatedness of disordered eating, amenorrhea, and altered bone mineral density.
4. ______________________ Collective term used to describe pain and discomfort associated with the menstrual cycle. The three main conditions included are ______________________, ______________________ and ______________________.
5. ______________________ Pain that occurs during or shortly before menstruation; it is one of the most common gynecologic problems for women in their childbearing years.
6. ______________________ Painful menstruation that occurs as a result of increased uterine activity due to myometrial contractions induced by excessive release of prostaglandins in the second half of the menstrual cycle.
7. ______________________ Acquired menstrual pain that typically develops after age 25 and is associated with pelvic pathology.
8. ______________________ A cluster of physical and psychologic symptoms beginning in the luteal phase of the menstrual cycle and followed by a symptom-free period.
9. ______________________ A more severe variant of premenstrual syndrome (PMS) with an emphasis on symptoms associated with mood disturbances such as marked irritability, dysphoria, mood lability, anxiety, and fatigue.
10. ______________________ Menstrual disorder characterized by the presence and growth of endometrial glands and stroma outside the uterus.
11. ______________________ Infrequent menstrual periods characterized by intervals of 40 to 45 days or longer.
12. ______________________ Scanty bleeding at normal intervals.
13. ______________________ or ______________________ Any episode of bleeding (e.g., spotting, menses, hemorrhage) that occurs at a time other than the normal menses.
14. ______________________ Small amount of bleeding or spotting that occurs at the time of ovulation (14 days before onset of the next menses); it is considered to be normal.
15. ______________________ Bleeding that occurs when the contraceptive pill does not maintain a sufficiently hypoplastic endometrium, resulting in shedding of the endometrium in small amounts at a time.
16. ______________________ or ______________________ Excessive menstrual bleeding, either in duration or amount.

17. ______________________________ Any form of uterine bleeding that is irregular in amount, duration, or timing and not related to regular menstrual bleeding.

18. ______________________________ Excessive uterine bleeding with no demonstrable organic cause, genital or extragenital; it is most frequently associated with anovulation.

19. ______________________________ First menstrual period.

20. ______________________________ Complete cessation of menses, said to have occurred when menstrual flow or spotting has ceased for 1 year.

21. ______________________________ or ______________________________ Period that encompasses the transition from normal ovulatory cycles to cessation of menses; it is marked by irregular menstrual cycles.

22. ______________________________ Cessation of the menstrual cycle that occurs as a result of hysterectomy and bilateral oophorectomy.

23. ______________________________ The period of time after menopause occurs.

24. ______________________________ Painful intercourse.

25. ______________________________ Visible red flush of the skin with perspiration.

26. ______________________________ Sudden warm sensation in neck, head, and chest.

27. ______________________________ Profuse perspiration and heat radiating from the body that disrupt sleep.

28. ______________________________ Generalized metabolic disease characterized by decreased bone mass and increased incidence of bone fractures.

29. ______________________________ or ______________________________ Substances found in certain plant foods (e.g., red clover, wild yams, dandelion greens, cherries) that are capable of interacting with estrogen receptors in the body.

II. REVIEWING KEY CONCEPTS

30. When caring for perimenopausal women it is important to not only recognize the expected changes associated with this period of transition but also to be able to explain to these women why these changes occur. IDENTIFY the manifestations and physiologic basis for each of the following expected changes:
    - Bleeding
    - Genital changes

- Vasomotor instability

- Mood and behavioral responses

MULTIPLE CHOICE: Circle the correct option(s) and state the rationale for the option(s) chosen.

31. Which woman is at greatest risk for developing hypogonadotropic amenorrhea?
    A. 48-year-old woman in Weight Watchers who lost 20 pounds over 6 months
    B. 14-year-old figure skater
    C. 18-year-old softball player
    D. 30-year-old (G3 P3003) breastfeeding woman

32. Pharmacologic preparations can be used to treat primary dysmenorrhea. Choose the preparation that is the least effective in relieving the symptoms of primary dysmenorrhea.
    A. Combined oral contraceptive (COC) pill
    B. Naproxen sodium (Anaprox)
    C. Acetaminophen (Tylenol)
    D. Ibuprofen (Motrin)

33. Women experiencing primary dysmenorrhea should be advised to avoid:
    A. Pretzels and potato chips
    B. Valerian
    C. Cranberry juice
    D. Whole-grain cereals

34. The nurse counseling a 30-year-old woman regarding effective measures to use to relieve symptoms associated with PMS could suggest that she: (Circle all that apply.)
    A. Decrease intake of fruits especially peaches and watermelon
    B. Take a bugleweed or evening primrose oil supplement
    C. Limit alcohol intake to less than 1 oz per day
    D. Reduce exercise during the luteal phase of the menstrual cycle when symptoms are at their peak
    E. Eat small, more frequent meals and snacks

35. A 28-year-old woman has been diagnosed with endometriosis. She has been placed on a course of treatment with danazol (Danocrine). The woman exhibits understanding of this treatment when she states: (Circle all that apply.)
    A. "Because this medication stops ovulation I do not need to use birth control."
    B. "I will experience more frequent and heavier menstrual periods when I take this medication."
    C. "I should follow a low-fat diet because this medication can increase the level of cholesterol in my blood."
    D. "I can experience a decrease in my breast size, oily skin, and hair growth on my face as a result of taking this medication."
    E. "I will need to spray this medication into my nose twice a day."
    F. "I may need to use a lubricant during intercourse to reduce discomfort."

36. A female client, age 26, describes scant bleeding between her menstrual periods. The nurse records this finding as:
    A. Metrorrhagia
    B. Oligomenorrhea
    C. Menorrhagia
    D. Hypomenorrhea

37. Dysfunctional uterine bleeding (DUB) is most likely to occur when women:
    A. Experience ovulatory cycles
    B. Weigh less than their expected body weight
    C. Experience signs of the onset of perimenopause
    D. Secrete high levels of prostaglandin

38. A 55-year-old woman tells the nurse that she has started to experience pain when she and her husband have intercourse. The nurse would record that this woman is experiencing:
    A. Dyspareunia
    B. Dysmenorrhea
    C. Dysuria
    D. Dyspnea

39. A 65-year-old woman is beginning treatment with alendronate sodium (Fosamax). Which statement by this woman indicates the need for further instructions?
    A. "I will take this medication first thing in the morning."
    B. "I will sit in a chair and read a book for about 30 minutes after I take this medication."
    C. "I will take this medication with a full glass of water."
    D. "I will eat my breakfast just before I take the medication."

40. Herbal preparations can be used as part of the treatment for a variety of menstrual disorders. Which herb is beneficial for a woman experiencing menorrhagia?
    A. Ginger
    B. Shepherd's purse
    C. Black cohosh root
    D. Black haw

III. THINKING CRITICALLY

1. Maria is a 16-year-old gymnast who has been training vigorously for a placement on the U.S. Olympic team. She has been experiencing amenorrhea, and the development of her secondary sexual characteristics has been limited. Maria expresses concern because her nonathletic friends have all been menstruating for at least 1 year and have well-developed breasts. After a health assessment, Maria was diagnosed with hypogonadotropic amenorrhea.
    A. STATE the risk factors for this disorder that Maria most likely exhibited during the assessment process.

    B. STATE one nursing diagnosis reflective of Maria's concern.

C. WRITE two expected outcomes for a plan of care for Maria.

D. OUTLINE a typical care management plan for Maria that addresses the issues associated with hypogonadotropic amenorrhea.

E. At Maria's all-female high school there is a large athletic department that emphasizes participation and excellence in a wide variety of sports. As the school nurse, you are concerned that there are other students like Maria who may be exhibiting signs of the female athlete triad. You have decided to institute an education program aimed at prevention and early detection of the triad.

1. Which sports should you emphasize with your program?

2. What measures should you include in your program as a means of prevention and early detection of the female athlete triad?

2. Mary, a 17-year-old who experienced menarche at age 16, comes to the women's health clinic for a routine checkup. She complains to the nurse that her last few periods have been very painful. "I have missed a few days of school because of it. What can I do to reduce the pain that I feel during my periods?" Physical examination and testing reveal normal structure and function of Mary's reproductive system. A medical diagnosis of primary dysmenorrhea is made.

A. WRITE several questions that the nurse should ask Mary to obtain a full description of her pain.

B. STATE the priority nursing diagnosis appropriate for Mary.

C. DESCRIBE what a nurse should tell Mary about the physiologic basis for her pain.

D. IDENTIFY several relief measures, including alternative therapies, for primary dysmenorrhea that a nurse could suggest to Mary.

3. Susan experiences physical and psychologic signs and symptoms associated with PMS during every ovulatory menstrual cycle.
   A. LIST the signs and symptoms most likely described by Susan that led to the diagnosis of PMS.

   B. IDENTIFY one nursing diagnosis that may be appropriate for Susan when she is experiencing the signs and symptoms of PMS.

   C. DESCRIBE the approach a nurse would use in helping Susan to deal with this menstrual disorder.

   D. STATE the symptoms that Susan would describe that could indicate she is also experiencing premenstrual dysphoric disorder (PMDD).

4. Lisa is 26 years old and has been diagnosed recently with endometriosis.
   A. LIST the signs and symptoms Lisa most likely exhibited to lead to this medical diagnosis.

   B. Lisa asks, "What is happening to my body as a result of this disease?" DESCRIBE the nurse's response.

   C. Lisa asks about her treatment options. "Are there medications I can take to make me feel better?" DESCRIBE the action/effect and potential side effects for each of the following pharmacologic approaches to treatment.
   Oral contraceptive pills

   Gonadotropin-releasing hormone agonists

   Androgenic synthetic steroids

   D. IDENTIFY support measures a nurse can suggest to assist Lisa to cope with the effects of endometriosis.

5. Jane, a 46-year-old slender white secretary, is at the beginning of the perimenopausal period. Her health history reveals a high intake of fast foods, coffee, and diet soft drinks especially Pepsi, along with a smoking habit of one pack per day. Jane states that her favorite leisure activities are reading, needlework, and playing Bingo two evenings a week. She expresses concern about the development of osteoporosis because her mother experienced the stress fractures and dowager's hump characteristic of this disorder. Jane requests information concerning what she can do to prevent this from happening to her.
   A. IDENTIFY the risk factors for osteoporosis present in this situation.

   B. DISCUSS the information you should give Jane regarding prevention measures that would reduce her risk for developing osteoporosis and its sequelae.

   C. LIST the signs Jane would exhibit if she begins to develop osteoporosis.

6. Heidi is a 50-year-old client experiencing the changes typical of perimenopause. Her BMI is 30. During a routine gynecologic checkup at the women's health clinic she tells her nurse practitioner that she is having a hard time coping with hot flashes, stress incontinence, and insomnia. Heidi also expresses concern about the vaginal dryness she is experiencing because it has resulted in discomfort and even pain when she and her husband have intercourse. She is also worried that her bones will get thin just like her mother's and grandmother's did. Heidi asks the nurse if there is anything she could suggest to reduce the discomfort associated with all these problems. She tells the nurse that several of her friends have been taking hormones and seem to be doing better, stating, "They told me that hormones cure everything from hot flashes to bad bones."
   A. DESCRIBE the relief measures the nurse practitioner should suggest to Heidi regarding:
      Hot flashes and flushes

      Insomnia

      Urogenital symptoms (e.g., vaginal dryness, stress incontinence, dyspareunia)

B. DISCUSS the approach the nurse practitioner should use to help Heidi decide about menopausal hormonal therapy (MHT).

C. Heidi decides to try MHT using a combined estrogen-progestin transdermal patch (CombiPatch). SPECIFY the instructions that Heidi should be given regarding this treatment to ensure its safety and effectiveness.

D. Heidi tells her nurse practitioner that she is very concerned about her potential for heart disease as a result of what is happening to her body with menopause. She asks the nurse why these changes occur and what she can do to promote her cardiac health.

E. Heidi is a computer expert and enjoys using the Internet to research a variety of topics and "chat" with persons who share her interests in quilting and mystery novels. DESCRIBE how the nurse could use Heidi's interest in and expertise with computers to direct her to appropriate websites that would provide her with reliable information and support during the perimenopausal period.

CHAPTER 7

Sexually Transmitted and Other Infections

I. LEARNING KEY TERMS

FILL IN THE BLANKS: Insert the term that corresponds to each of the following descriptions related to infections.

1. ______________________ Infections or infectious disease syndromes primarily transmitted by close intimate contact. The most common infections of this type in women are ______________________, ______________________, ______________________, ______________________, ______________________, and ______________________.
2. ______________________ Precautions used during sexual activity to prevent the transmission of pathogens.
3. ______________________ The physical barrier promoted for the prevention of sexual transmission of human immunodeficiency virus (HIV) and other sexually transmitted infections (STIs).
4. ______________________ Bacterial infection that is the most commonly reported STI in American women. This infection is often silent and is highly destructive to the female reproductive tract.
5. ______________________ The oldest communicable disease in the United States and second in terms of reported cases. Because it is a reportable communicable disease, health care providers are legally responsible for reporting all cases to health authorities.
6. ______________________ One of the earliest described STIs. It is caused by *Treponema pallidum,* a motile spirochete. ______________________ Primary lesion that appears 5 to 90 days after infection. ______________________ Broad, painless, pink-gray wartlike infectious lesion that may develop on the vulva, the perineum, or the anus.
7. ______________________ Infectious process that most commonly involves the uterine tubes, uterus, and more rarely ovaries and peritoneal surfaces.
8. ______________________ Infection, also called genital warts, that is the most common viral STI seen in ambulatory health care settings. ______________________ The visible lesions caused by infection with certain strains of this virus.
9. ______________________ A viral infection that is transmitted sexually and is widespread in the United States. It is characterized by painful, recurrent genital ulcers.
10. ______________________ Viral infection involving the liver acquired primarily through a fecal-oral route by ingestion of contaminated food—particularly milk, shellfish, or polluted water—or person-to-person contact.
11. ______________________ Viral infection involving the liver that is transmitted parenterally, perinatally, and through intimate contact. A vaccine is available to protect infants, children, and adults.
12. ______________________ Viral infection involving the liver that is the most common blood-borne infection in the United States. It is transmitted parenterally and through intimate contact. There is no vaccine available to provide protection against this infection.
13. ______________________ A retrovirus that is transmitted primarily through exchange of body fluids. Severe depression of the ______________________ system is associated with this infection and characterizes ______________________.

14. ______________________________ A normal vaginal flora that is present in 20% to 30% of healthy pregnant women. It has been associated with poor pregnancy outcomes and neonatal morbidity and mortality resulting from vertical transmission from the birth canal of the infected mother to the infant during birth.

15. ______________________________ Vaginal infection formerly called nonspecific vaginitis, *Haemophilus vaginitis,* or *Gardnerella*. It is the most common type of vaginitis today and is characterized by a profuse thin, whitish, gray, or milky discharge with a characteristic "fishy" odor.

16. ______________________________ A yeast infection that is the second most common type of vaginal infection in the United States. It is characterized by itching and a thick, white, lumpy discharge with a cottage cheese–like consistency.

17. ______________________________ A vaginal infection caused by an anaerobic one-celled protozoan with characteristic flagella. It is characterized by a copious yellowish green, frothy, mucopurulent, malodorous discharge.

18. ______________________________ A group of infections that can affect a pregnant woman and her fetus. The infecting organisms are capable of crossing the placenta and adversely affecting the development of the fetus.

19. ______________________________ A protozoal infection associated with the consumption of infested raw or undercooked meat and with poor handwashing after handling infected cat litter.

20. ______________________________ German or 3-day measles; the virus is transmitted by droplets.

21. ______________________________ Viral infection that may begin as a mononucleosis-like syndrome. It is primarily transmitted by close contact and has been isolated from semen, cervical and vaginal secretions, breast milk, placental tissue, urine, feces, and banked blood. It can lead to profound neurologic and sensory disorders if transmitted to the newborn.

22. ______________________________ Infection control measures that must be followed by health care providers when caring for all clients.

II. REVIEWING KEY CONCEPTS

MULTIPLE CHOICE: Circle the correct option(s) and state the rationale for the option(s) chosen.

23. Infections of the female midreproductive tract such as chlamydia are dangerous primarily because they:
    A. Are asymptomatic or silent
    B. Cause infertility
    C. Lead to pelvic inflammatory disease (PID)
    D. Are difficult to treat effectively

24. A finding associated with human papillomavirus (HPV) infection includes:
    A. White, curdlike adherent discharge
    B. Soft papillary swellings occurring singly or in clusters
    C. Vesicles progressing to pustules and then to ulcers
    D. Yellow to green frothy, malodorous discharge

25. A recommended medication effective in the treatment of vulvovaginal candidiasis is:
    A. Metronidazole
    B. Clotrimazole
    C. Benzathine penicillin
    D. Acyclovir

26. A woman is determined to be group B streptococci (GBS) positive at the onset of her labor. The nurse should prepare this woman for:
    A. Cesarean birth
    B. Isolation of her newborn after birth
    C. IV administration of penicillin G during labor
    D. Application of acyclovir to her labial lesions

27. When providing a woman who is recovering from primary herpes with information regarding the recurrence of herpes infection of the genital tract, the nurse tells her that: (Circle all that apply.)
    A. Fever and flulike symptoms occur only with primary infection
    B. Little can be done to control the recurrence of infection
    C. Transmission of the virus is possible only when lesions are open and draining
    D. Itching and tingling often occur prior to the appearance of vesicles
    E. Cleaning lesions twice a day with saline will help to prevent secondary infections
    F. Acyclovir therapy will cure herpes

28. A nurse is teaching a 20-year-old woman about risk-reduction measures. Which measure should the nurse emphasize as the most important?
    A. Using a female condom
    B. Knowing her partner
    C. Reducing the number of partners
    D. Getting the HPV vaccination

29. Cervical neoplasia has been linked to which of the following sexually transmitted infections?
    A. Herpes simplex virus (HSV)
    B. Human papillomavirus (HPV)
    C. Human immunodeficiency virus (HIV)
    D. Chlamydia

30. When assessing sexually active adults, the nurse must be alert for client behaviors that increase the risk for acquiring STIs. IDENTIFY two STI risk behaviors for each of the following categories:
    Sexual risk behaviors

    Drug-use related-risk behaviors

    Blood-related risk behaviors

31. Nurses who work on childbirth and postpartum units and in newborn nurseries must be guided by infection control principles when caring for their clients. DESCRIBE one implementation measure for each Standard Precautions category:
    - Hand hygiene
    - Use of personal protective equipment (PPE)
    - Respiratory hygiene and cough etiquette
    - Safe injection practices

32. OUTLINE the clinical manifestations and management guidelines for each common reproductive tract infection.
    - Chlamydia
    - Gonorrhea
    - Syphilis
    - Human papillomavirus
    - Genital herpes simplex virus
    - Bacterial vaginosis
    - Candidiasis
    - Trichomoniasis

33. STATE the infection represented by the group of infections known collectively as TORCH.

III. THINKING CRITICALLY

1. Terry, a 20-year-old, comes to a women's health clinic for her first visit.
   A. During the health history interview it is imperative that the nurse practitioner determine Terry's risk for contracting an STI, including HIV. DESCRIBE the approach you would take to determine this woman's risk for STIs.

   B. Terry asks the nurse about measures she can use to protect herself from STIs. CITE the major points that the nurse practitioner should emphasize when teaching Terry about prevention measures.

   C. Terry tells the nurse that she does not know if she could ever tell a partner that he must wear a condom. DESCRIBE the approach the nurse can take to enhance Terry's assertiveness and communication skills.

   D. Terry asks the nurse if it is too late for her to get the immunization for HPV. She states that she heard it prevents cervical cancer and therefore she would not need to bother getting a Pap smear every year. DISCUSS what the nurse should tell Terry.

2. Martha is 4 weeks pregnant. As part of her prenatal assessment it is discovered that she is HIV positive.
   A. STATE the modes of HIV transmission that could relate to Martha.

   B. LIST the clinical manifestations she most likely exhibited during her seroconversion to HIV positivity.

   C. OUTLINE the care management approach that nurses should use when caring for Martha during her pregnancy and after she gives birth.

   D. IDENTIFY the measures that can be used to reduce the risk of transmission of HIV from Martha to her baby.

3. Suzanne, a 20-year-old client, is admitted for suspected severe, acute PID.
   A. IDENTIFY the risk factors for PID that the nurse should be looking for in Suzanne's health history.

   B. A complete physical examination is performed to determine if the criteria for PID are met. SPECIFY the criteria that Suzanne's health care provider should be alert for during the examination.

C. Suzanne is hospitalized when the diagnosis of PID secondary to chlamydial infection is confirmed. IV antibiotics will be used as the primary medical treatment followed by oral antibiotics at the time of discharge. STATE three priority nursing diagnoses that are likely to be present during the acute stage of Suzanne's infection and treatment.

D. OUTLINE a nursing management plan for Suzanne.

E. LIST the recommendations for Suzanne's self-management during the recovery phase.

F. IDENTIFY the reproductive health risks that Suzanne may face as a result of the pelvic infection she experienced.

4. Laura has come to the women's health clinic on her campus because she has been informed that her boyfriend has been diagnosed with gonorrhea.
   A. STATE the essential areas of assessment the nurse should keep in mind when interviewing Laura during the health history and performing a physical examination.

   B. Diagnostic testing confirms that Laura has gonorrhea. Laura is very upset by the diagnosis, stating, "This is just awful—what kind of sex life can I have now?" CITE a nursing diagnosis that reflects Laura's concern.

C. OUTLINE a therapeutic plan that will assist Laura to take control of her self-management and prevent future infections.

5. Cheryl, a 27-year-old, is being treated for HPV. A primary diagnosis identified for Cheryl is acute pain related to lesions on the vulva and around the anus secondary to HPV infection. STATE the measures the nurse could suggest to Cheryl to reduce the pain from the condylomata and enhance their healing.

6. Mary, 20 years old, has just been diagnosed with a primary genital herpes simplex infection. In addition to the typical systemic symptoms, Mary exhibits multiple, painful genital lesions.
   A. Relief of pain and healing without the development of a secondary infection are two expected outcomes for care. IDENTIFY several measures that the nurse can suggest to Mary to help her achieve the expected outcomes of care.

   B. Mary asks the nurse if there is anything she can do so that this infection does not return and prevent transmission of the infection to her new partner. DISCUSS what the nurse should tell Mary about the recurrence of herpes infection and the influence of self-care measures.

7. Gloria tested positive for hepatitis B. DESCRIBE the measures that the nurse should teach Gloria in an effort to decrease the risk for transmission of the virus to other people in Gloria's life.

8. Sonya is concerned that she has been exposed to HIV and has come to the women's health clinic for testing.
   A. During the health history the nurse questions Sonya about behaviors that could have placed her at risk for HIV transmission. CITE the behaviors that the nurse would be looking for.

   B. EXPLAIN the testing procedure that will most likely be followed to determine Sonya's HIV status.

   C. OUTLINE the counseling protocol that should guide the nurse when caring for Sonya before and after the test.

   D. Sonya's test result is negative. DISCUSS the instructions the nurse should give Sonya regarding guidelines she should follow to reduce her risk for the transmission of HIV with future sexual partners.

CHAPTER

8

Contraception and Abortion

I. LEARNING KEY TERMS

FILL IN THE BLANKS: Insert the term that corresponds to each of the following descriptions regarding methods to prevent or plan pregnancy.

1. ______________________________ Term used for the intentional prevention of pregnancy during sexual intercourse.

2. ______________________________ Term used for the device and/or practice to decrease the risk of conceiving or bearing offspring.

3. ______________________________ Term that refers to the conscious decision on when to conceive, or to avoid pregnancy, throughout the reproductive years.

4. ______________________________ Percentage of contraceptive users expected to have an unplanned pregnancy during the first year, even when they use a method consistently and correctly.

5. ______________________________ Method that requires the male partner to withdraw his penis from the woman's vagina before he ejaculates.

6. ______________________________ Methods that depend on identifying the beginning and end of the fertile period of the menstrual cycle; they provide contraception by relying on avoidance of intercourse during fertile periods.

7. ______________________________ Method based on the number of days in each cycle, counting from the first day of menses. The fertile period is determined after accurately recording the lengths of menstrual cycles for at least 6 months.

8. ______________________________ Method based on monitoring and recording cervical secretions; each day the woman asks herself, (1) "Did I note secretions today?" and (2) "Did I note secretions yesterday?" If the answer to either is yes, she should avoid coitus or use a backup method of birth control. If the answer to both questions is no, her probability of getting pregnant is very low.

9. ______________________________ Method that requires the woman to recognize and interpret cyclic changes in the amount and consistency of cervical mucus that characterize her own unique pattern of changes.

10. ______________________________ Term used to refer to the stretchiness of cervical mucus.

11. ______________________________ Method based on variations in a healthy woman's lowest body temperature taken immediately after waking and before getting out of bed.

12. ______________________________ Term used to refer to the decrease and subsequent increase in temperature associated with ovulation.

13. ______________________________ Method that combines the basal body temperature (BBT) and cervical mucus methods with awareness of secondary cycle phase-related symptoms.

14. ______________________________ Methods based on detecting the sudden surge of luteinizing hormone (LH) that occurs approximately 12 to 24 hours before ovulation.

15. ______________________________ Chemical that destroys sperm. When inserted into the vagina it acts as a chemical barrier to sperm.

16. ______________________________ Thin, stretchable sheath that covers the penis or is inserted into the vagina.

17. ______________________________ Shallow, dome-shaped latex or silicone device with a flexible rim that covers the cervix resulting in a mechanical barrier to sperm.

18. ______________________________ A soft rubber or latex-free silicone dome with a firm but pliable brim that fits snugly around the base of the cervix close to the junction of the cervix and vaginal fornices.

19. ______________________ A small round polyurethane device that contains spermicide. It fits over the cervix and has a woven polyester loop to facilitate its removal.

20. ______________________ Form of oral contraceptive pill that provides a fixed dosage of estrogen and progesterone.

21. ______________________ Form of oral contraceptive pill that has varying amounts of progestin and sometimes the amount of estrogen within each cycle.

22. ______________________ Bleeding that occurs from 1 to 4 days after the last combined oral contraceptive is taken.

23. ______________________ Contraceptive form that delivers continuous levels of norelgestromin and ethinyl estradiol; a patch is applied to intact skin of the upper outer arm, the upper torso, the lower abdomen, or the buttocks on the same day once a week for 3 weeks followed by a week without the patch.

24. ______________________ Flexible device worn in the vagina to deliver continuous levels of etonorgestrel and ethinyl estradiol; the device is worn for 3 weeks, followed by a week without the device.

25. ______________________ Progestin only contraceptive pill.

26. ______________________ Progestin only IM injection providing contraception for approximately 3 months.

27. ______________________ Form of hormonal contraception in which a single flexible rod containing progestin is implanted subdermally, usually into the inner aspect of the upper arm.

28. ______________________ Small T-shaped device inserted into the uterine cavity. It is loaded with copper or levonorgestrel.

29. ______________________ Surgical procedures intended to render the person infertile. For the female the ______________________ are occluded. For the male, the ______________________ are occluded during a ______________________.

30. ______________________ Procedure used to restore tubal continuity (reanastomosis) after a sterilization procedure.

31. ______________________ Temporary method of birth control based on the surge of prolactin that occurs with breastfeeding.

32. ______________________ Purposeful interruption of a pregnancy before 20 weeks of gestation. If it is performed at the woman's request, it is termed an ______________________. If it is performed for reasons of maternal or fetal health or disease, it is termed a ______________________.

33. ______________________ Surgical method of performing an early induced abortion (less than 9 weeks of gestation); it is the most common abortion procedure used in the first trimester.

34. ______________________ Induced early abortion method using one of three drugs namely ______________________, ______________________, or ______________________.

35. ______________________ Surgical method used for a second-trimester abortion. It accounts for almost all procedures performed in the United States and results in more complications and greater costs than first-trimester abortions.

II. REVIEWING KEY CONCEPTS

MULTIPLE CHOICE: Circle the correct option(s) and state the rationale for the option(s) chosen.

36. A single young-adult woman received instructions from the nurse regarding the use of an oral contraceptive. The woman demonstrates a need for further instruction if she:
   A. Stops asking her sexual partners to use condoms with spermicide
   B. States her menstrual periods should be shorter with less blood loss
   C. Takes a pill every morning
   D. Uses a barrier method of birth control if she misses two or more pills

37. Oral contraception in the form of a combination of low-dose estrogen and progesterone:
   A. Reduces the pH of cervical mucus, thereby destroying sperm
   B. Protects against iron deficiency anemia by reducing menstrual blood loss
   C. Prevents the transmission of sexually transmitted diseases
   D. Is 90% effective in preventing pregnancy when used correctly

38. For some women the most distressing side effect of progestin-only contraception is:
   A. Irregular vaginal bleeding
   B. Headache
   C. Nervousness
   D. Nausea

39. A 36-year-old woman has chosen depot medroxyprogesterone acetate (DMPA, Depo-Provera) as the method of contraception most suitable for her lifestyle. Which statement made by the woman indicates a lack of understanding and a need for further instruction by the nurse?
   A. "I will need to receive another injection every 4 weeks."
   B. "I am going to watch my diet and exercise, because weight gain is common."
   C. "If I plan to continue with the Depo-Provera, I should have my bone density assessed."
   D. "This method will result in a smaller amount of thicker cervical mucus."

40. A woman with an intrauterine device (IUD) should confirm its placement by checking the IUD's string:
   A. After each menstrual period
   B. After intercourse
   C. At the time of ovulation
   D. During menstrual bleeding

41. When teaching women about the effective use of chemical barriers, the nurse should tell them to:
   A. Insert at least 2 hours prior to intercourse
   B. Use nonoxynol-9 (N-9) to inhibit the transmission of HIV
   C. Douche immediately after the last act of intercourse
   D. Reapply before each act of coitus

42. When using a cervical cap, the woman should be taught to:
   A. Apply spermicide only to the outside of the cap and around the rim
   B. Leave it in place for a minimum of 6 hours and maximum of 48 hours after the last act of coitus
   C. Continue to use the cap during menstrual periods
   D. Check the position of the cap and insert additional spermicide before each act of coitus.

43. Joyce has chosen the diaphragm as her method of contraception. Which action indicates that Joyce is using the diaphragm effectively? (Circle all that apply.)
   A. Joyce came to be refitted after healing was complete following the term vaginal birth of her son.
   B. Joyce applies a spermicide only to the rim of the diaphragm just before insertion.
   C. Joyce empties her bladder before inserting the diaphragm and after intercourse.
   D. Joyce applies more spermicide for each act of intercourse.
   E. Joyce removes the diaphragm within 1 hour of intercourse.
   F. Joyce always uses the diaphragm during her menstrual periods.

44. A woman must assess herself for signs that ovulation is occurring. Which signs are associated with ovulation? (Circle all that apply.)
    A. Increase in the level of LH in her urine 12 to 24 hours before ovulation
    B. Spinnbarkeit
    C. Drop in BBT during the luteal phase of her menstrual cycle
    D. Softened moist cervix which opens and rises in the vagina
    E. Decreased libido

45. A woman has had a ParaGard T380A IUD inserted. The nurse should recognize that the woman needs further teaching if she says: (Circle all that apply.)
    A. "This IUD remains effective for 10 years."
    B. "It is normal to experience an increase in bleeding and cramping within the first year after it has been inserted."
    C. "My IUD works by releasing progesterone."
    D. "I should avoid using NSAIDs like Motrin if I have cramping."
    E. "I must use risk prevention measures including condoms to prevent infections in my uterus."

46. A 40-year-old male has elected to have a vasectomy because he no longer wants to worry that a sexual partner will become pregnant. The nurse describes the procedure along with care requirements before and after the procedure. Which statement by the client indicates the need for further instruction? (Circle all that apply.)
    A. "I am glad I will not need to use a condom—I hate them!"
    B. "I will use ice packs for a few hours after I get home to reduce swelling and discomfort."
    C. "I will wear a scrotal support for a few days to reduce discomfort."
    D. "I will need to wait about 3 weeks before resuming sexual intercourse."
    E. "I should not expect to see a decrease in the amount of semen I ejaculate."

47. A nurse is working with a couple to help them choose a method of contraceptive that is right for them.
    A. LIST the factors that can influence the effectiveness of the contraceptive method they choose.

    B. Informed consent is a vital component when helping this couple to choose a contraceptive. STATE the elements of an informed consent that need to be met and documented as part of the decision-making process.

48. A woman is a little uncomfortable about checking her cervical mucus and asks the nurse what she could possibly find out about doing this assessment. STATE the useful purpose of self-evaluation of cervical mucus.

49. June's religious and cultural beliefs prohibit her from using any artificial method of birth control. She is interested in learning about fertility awareness methods (natural family planning) for contraception. FILL IN THE BLANKS in each of the following statements concerning this method.
   A. The two principal problems with fertility awareness methods are difficulty in determining the exact time of ______________________________ and difficulty in ______________________________ for several days before and after ovulation. Women with ______________________________ have the greatest risk for failure.
   B. Using the calendar method, June and her husband would abstain from day ______________________________ to day ______________________________ of her menstrual cycle because her shortest cycle was 23 days and her longest cycle was 33 days.
   C. Basal body temperature (BBT) will ______________________________ about ______________________________ degrees C at about the time of ovulation. After ovulation, because of increasing levels of ______________________________, the BBT will ______________________________ about ______________________________ degrees C. This change in BBT will last until ______________________________ days before menstruation.
   D. The ovulation method would require June to recognize and interpret the cyclic changes in the characteristics of her ______________________________ such as ______________________________ and ______________________________.
   E. The symptothermal method combines ______________________________ with ______________________________ methods in addition to awareness of secondary cycle phase-related symptoms.
   F. The home predictor test for ovulation detects the sudden surge of ______________________________ in the urine that occurs approximately ______________________________ hours before ovulation.

50. Alice and Bob use nonprescription chemical and mechanical contraceptive barriers. LABEL each of the following actions with "C" if correct or "I" if incorrect. INDICATE how the action should be changed for those actions labeled "I."
   A. ______________________________ When using a vaginal foam, Alice applies it just inside her vagina.
   B. ______________________________ Alice avoids using a spermicide with nonoxynol-9 as a lubricant if she and her husband plan to have anal intercourse.
   C. ______________________________ Alice reapplies the spermicide before each act of intercourse.
   D. ______________________________ Alice uses a female condom when her husband uses a condom during her fertile period because they want to have the added protection against getting pregnant.
   E. ______________________________ Bob applies a condom over his erect penis leaving an empty space at the tip.
   F. ______________________________ Bob often lubricates the outside of a latex condom with Vaseline, a petroleum-based lubricant.
   G. ______________________________ Alice and Bob will reuse the female condom if they have intercourse more than once because it is more expensive than the male condom.

III. THINKING CRITICALLY

1. A nurse working in a women's health clinic should be aware that toxic shock syndrome (TSS) is a possible complication for women who use a diaphragm or cervical cap as their method of contraception.
   A. CITE the prevention measures that the nurse should teach women to use to reduce their risk for TSS.

   B. IDENTIFY the clinical manifestations of TSS that the nurse should be alert for when assessing women who use diaphragms or cervical caps.

2. Kathy, an 18-year-old client, has come to Planned Parenthood for information on birth control methods and assistance with making her choice. She tells the nurse that she is planning to become sexually active with her boyfriend of 6 months and is worried about getting pregnant. She says, "I know I should know more about all of this but I just don't."
   A. STATE the nursing diagnosis that reflects Kathy's concern.

   B. OUTLINE the approach the nurse should use to help Kathy make an informed decision in choosing contraception that is right for her.

3. June plans to use combined oral contraceptive (COC) pills.
   A. DESCRIBE the mode of action for this type of contraception.

B. LIST the advantages of using COCs.

C. IDENTIFY the factors that, if present in June's health history, would constitute absolute or relative contraindications to the use of oral contraception with estrogen and progesterone.

D. When caring for June, the nurse must be alert for signs that she is experiencing adverse reactions related to the changing levels of estrogen and progestin. SPECIFY the estrogen and progesterone reactions the nurse should discuss with June.

E. Using the acronym ACHES, IDENTIFY the signs and symptoms that would require June to stop taking the pill and notify her health care provider.

A

C

H

E

S

F. SPECIFY the instructions the nurse should give June about taking the pill to ensure maximum effectiveness.

4. Beth has decided to try the cervical cap as her method of contraception.
   A. IDENTIFY factors that, if present in Beth's health history, would make her a poor candidate for this contraceptive method

   B. Following assessment, Beth is determined to be a good candidate for using the cervical cap. DESCRIBE the principles that the nurse should teach Beth to guide her in the safe and effective use of this method.

5. Anita has just had a ParaGard T380A copper IUD inserted. SPECIFY the instructions that the nurse should give Anita before she leaves the women's health clinic after the insertion.

6. Judy (6-4-0-2-4) and Allen, both age 36, are contemplating sterilization now that their family is complete. They are seeking counseling regarding this decision.
   A. DESCRIBE the approach a nurse should use in helping Judy and Allen make the right decision.

   B. The couple decide that Allen will have a vasectomy. DISCUSS the preoperative and postoperative care and instructions required by Allen.

7. Edna is 20 years old and unmarried. She is 8 weeks pregnant and is unsure about what to do. She comes to the women's health clinic and asks for the nurse's help in making her decision, stating, "I just cannot support a baby right now. I am alone and trying to finish my education. What can I do?"
   A. CITE the nursing diagnosis reflective of Edna's current dilemma.

   B. DESCRIBE the approach the nurse should take in helping Edna to make a decision that is right for her.

   C. Edna elects to have an abortion. A vacuum aspiration will be performed in the morning. Edna asks what will happen to her as part of the abortion procedure. DESCRIBE how the nurse should respond to Edna's question.

   D. IDENTIFY three nursing diagnoses related to Edna's decision and the procedure she is facing.

   E. DESCRIBE the nursing measures related to the physical care and emotional support that Edna will require as part of this procedure.

   F. OUTLINE the discharge instructions that Edna should receive.

8. A woman is 7 weeks pregnant and seeking an elective abortion. At this stage of gestation she would be a candidate for a medical abortion. CITE the three drugs that are used for this purpose in the United States and DESCRIBE how each drug works.

9. Marlee comes to the women's health clinic to report that she had unprotected intercourse the previous night. She is worried about getting pregnant because she is at midcycle and has already noticed signs of ovulation. Marlee tells the nurse that she hardly knows her partner and that her emotions just got the best of her. She is very anxious and asks the nurse what her options are.
   A. DESCRIBE the approach this nurse should use to assist Marlee with her concerns.

   B. After considering her options, Marlee elects to use Plan B. EXPLAIN what the nurse should tell Marlee about each of the following:
      - What Plan B entails

      - Timing of administration

      - Measures to decrease nausea and vomiting

   C. Prior to leaving, Marlee tells the nurse she is so glad that the Plan B regimen will mean that she will not have to worry about pregnancy. STATE how the nurse should respond.

CHAPTER 9

Infertility

I. LEARNING KEY TERMS

MATCHING: Match the description in Column I with the appropriate test in Column II.

COLUMN I

1. _______ Immunologic test to determine sperm and cervical mucus interaction.
2. _______ Basic test for male infertility.
3. _______ Test that uses fluid infused into the uterus via the cervix to help define the uterine cavity and the depth of the uterine lining via vaginal ultrasound.
4. _______ Examination of the lining of the uterus to assess its response to progesterone and to detect secretory changes and receptivity to implantation.
5. _______ Use of a flexible scope threaded through the cervix to directly view the uterine cavity.
6. _______ Test for adequacy of coital technique, cervical mucus, sperm, and degree of sperm penetration through cervical mucus.
7. _______ Examination of uterine cavity and tubes using radiopaque contrast material instilled through the cervix. It is often used to determine tubal patency and to release a blockage if present.
8. _______ Test used to visualize pelvic tissues and structures for a variety of reasons; it may be accomplished via a transabdominal or transvaginal approach.
9. _______ Visualization of pelvic structures intraperitoneally outside the uterus by inserting a small endoscope through an incision in the anterior abdominal wall.

COLUMN II

A. Laparoscopy
B. Postcoital test (PCT)
C. Ultrasonography
D. Timed endometrial biopsy
E. Hysterosalpingography
F. Sperm immobilization antibody reaction
G. Semen analysis
H. Sonohysterography
I. Hysteroscopy

FILL IN THE BLANKS: Insert the term that corresponds to each of the following descriptions related to alterations in fertility.

10. ______________________________ Term that refers to subfertility, a prolonged time to conceive.
11. ______________________________ Term that refers to an inability to conceive.
12. ______________________________ Collective term used to designate a variety of alternative measures to help infertile couples achieve the goal of a successful pregnancy and live birth.
13. ______________________________ A woman's eggs are collected from her ovaries, fertilized in the laboratory with sperm, and transferred into her uterus once normal embryo development has occurred.
14. ______________________________ Selection of one sperm cell that is injected directly into the egg to achieve fertilization.
15. ______________________________ Oocytes are retrieved from the ovary, placed into a catheter with sperm, and immediately transferred into the fimbriated end of the uterine tube, where fertilization takes place.
16. ______________________________ After in vitro fertilization the ova are placed in one uterine tube during the zygote stage.

17. ______________________________ Sperm from a person other than the male partner are used to inseminate the female partner.

18. ______________________________ Embryo(s) from one couple are transferred into the uterus of another woman who has contracted with the couple to carry the baby to term. This woman has no genetic investment in the child.

19. ______________________________ Process by which a woman is inseminated with the semen from the infertile woman's partner and then carries the fetus until birth.

20. ______________________________ The zona pellucida is penetrated chemically or manually to create an opening for the dividing embryo to hatch and to implant into the uterine wall.

21. ______________________________ A donated embryo is transferred to the uterus of an infertile woman at the appropriate time (normal or induced) of the menstrual cycle.

22. ______________________________ Form of early testing designed to eliminate embryos with serious genetic defects before implantation through one of the ARTs and to avoid future termination of pregnancy for genetic reasons.

23. ______________________________ Procedure used to freeze embryos for later implantation.

II. REVIEWING KEY CONCEPTS

MULTIPLE CHOICE: Circle the correct option(s) and state the rationale for the option(s) chosen.

24. A woman must assess herself for signs that ovulation is occurring. Which of the following is a sign associated with ovulation?
    A. Reduction in level of luteinizing hormone (LH) in the urine 12 to 24 hours prior to ovulation
    B. Spinnbarkeit
    C. Drop in basal body temperature (BBT) following ovulation
    D. Increase in amount and thickness of cervical mucus

25. A couple is to undergo a postcoital/timed intercourse test. The nurse should tell the couple which of the following about this test?
    A. Intercourse should occur daily for 3 days prior to the test.
    B. The test will be used to determine how sperm penetrate and survive in cervical mucus.
    C. The test will be scheduled for 2 days after menstruation ceases.
    D. The examination of cervical mucus must be performed within 30 minutes of intercourse.

26. Lifestyle and sexual practices can affect fertility. Which of the following practices could enhance a couple's ability to conceive?
    A. Use balanced nutrition and exercise to achieve a normal BMI.
    B. Abstain from alcohol.
    C. Avoid the use of lubricants during intercourse.
    D. Relax in a hot tub every day before going to bed.

27. A woman taking human menopausal gonadotropin for infertility should understand which of the following regarding this medication?
    A. She should take the medication orally, once a day after breakfast.
    B. The medication stimulates the pituitary gland to produce follicle-stimulating hormone (FSH) and luteinizing hormone (LH).
    C. She must report for ultrasound testing as scheduled to monitor follicular development.
    D. Clomiphene citrate should be taken daily, along with human chorionic gonadotropin, until ovulation occurs.

28. An infertile woman may be given nafarelin acetate (Synarel) in order to achieve which of the following therapeutic outcomes?
    A. Stimulation of her pituitary gland
    B. Shrinkage of endometrial implants
    C. Induction of ovulation
    D. Relaxation prior to intercourse

29. When caring for a woman scheduled for a hysterosalpingogram, the nurse should do which of the following?
    A. Ensure that the woman is in the secretory phase of her menstrual cycle.
    B. Explain to the woman that the procedure will allow her to conceive.
    C. Report any uterine cramping immediately because it may indicate that her uterus was perforated during the procedure.
    D. Change the woman's position if she complains of shoulder pain following the procedure.

30. STATE the type of infertility problem each of the following medications is designed to treat and explain the mechanism of action. (NOTE: You may want to consult the *Physicians' Desk Reference* (PDR) or a nurse's drug manual for more in-depth information on each of these medications.)
    clomiphene citrate

    follitropins (purified FSH)

    GnRh antagonists (ganirelix acetate)

    progesterone

    GnRh agonists (nafarelin acetate, leuprolide acetate)

Androgens (danazol)

menotropins (human menopausal gonadotropin)

human chorionic gonadotropin (hCG)

metformin

letrozole

III. THINKING CRITICALLY

1. Mary and Jim have come for their first visit to the fertility clinic. The nurse needs to instruct them about the interrelated structures, functions, and processes essential for conception, emphasizing that they are a biologic unit of reproduction.
   A. PREPARE a lesson plan that explains each component required for normal fertility. INCORPORATE anatomic illustrations to clarify descriptions.

   B. SUPPORT the following statement: Assessment of infertility must involve both partners.

2. Mark and his wife, Mary, are undergoing testing for impaired fertility.
   A. DESCRIBE the nursing support measures that should be used when working with this couple.

   B. LIST the components of the assessment for both Mary and Mark.
      Assessment for the woman

      Assessment for the man

   C. Mark must provide a specimen of semen for analysis. DESCRIBE the procedure he should follow to ensure accuracy of the test.

   D. STATE the semen characteristics that will be assessed.

   E. A postcoital test (PCT) is part of the diagnostic process for Mary and Mark. DESCRIBE the instructions you would give them to maximize the effectiveness and accuracy of the test.

F. During the assessment process Mark admits that he smokes a pack of cigarettes every 1 or 2 days and drinks at least two beers each weekday and a few more on the weekend. He tells the nurse that he does this as a way of relieving the stress from his job. DISCUSS how the nurse should respond to these lifestyle issues.

3. ARTs are being developed and perfected, creating a variety of ethical, legal, financial, and psychosocial concerns. DISCUSS the issues and concerns engendered by these alternative technologies.

4. Suzanne has been scheduled for a diagnostic laparoscopy to determine the basis of her infertility.
   A. INDICATE when during the menstrual cycle this test should be performed.

   B. SPECIFY the measures required to prepare Suzanne for this procedure.

   C. Suzanne asks the nurse why the test is needed and what will be done during the test. DESCRIBE the nurse's response.

   D. SPECIFY the postprocedural care measures required, including the discharge instructions that Suzanne should receive.

5. Sara and Ben have been trying to conceive for 3 years. They have come to an infertility clinic to find out what is wrong. They are distraught because they have been trying so long to get pregnant. They tell the nurse that they just cannot believe what is happening to them. "None of our friends and no one in our family is having a problem—what's wrong with us?" A diagnosis of infertility is made, necessitating that Sara and Ben make decisions about treatments, use of alternative birth technologies, and adoption.
   A. IDENTIFY the responses that Sara and Ben might exhibit related to the diagnosis of infertility. DESCRIBE one nursing action for each of the responses you have identified.

   B. DISCUSS how the nurse should guide this couple through the decision-making process that is required to determine a course of action that is right for both of them.

   C. The nurse is aware that Sara and Ben as a devout Jewish couple may be influenced by cultural and religious beliefs and practices as they make decisions regarding assessment and treatment for infertility. EXPLAIN the approach the nurse should take to identify and then incorporate these beliefs and practices in planning care with the couple.

CHAPTER 10

Problems of the Breast

I. LEARNING KEY TERMS

MATCHING: Match the description in Column I with the appropriate breast disorder in Column II.

COLUMN I

1. _______ Most common benign breast problem characterized by lumpiness with or without tenderness in both breasts.
2. _______ Fatty unilateral breast tumor that is soft, round, nontender, and mobile with discrete borders.
3. _______ Breast hyperplasia characterized by very large, heavy breasts.
4. _______ Unilateral, discrete, small, usually nontender lump; it is unresponsive to dietary changes or hormone therapy.
5. _______ Spontaneous, bilateral, milky, sticky breast discharge unrelated to malignancy.
6. _______ Very small breasts.
7. _______ Inflammation of the ducts behind the nipples resulting in a thick, sticky, white, or colored discharge. Burning pain, itching, or a palpable mass behind the nipple may be experienced.
8. _______ Small, nonpalpable benign lesions in the terminal nipple ducts most often occurring in women 30 to 50 years of age; it is characterized by a serous, serosanguineous, or bloody nipple discharge.

COLUMN II

A. Fibroadenoma
B. Fibrocystic changes
C. Intraductal papilloma
D. Mammary duct ectasia
E. Lipoma
F. Galactorrhea
G. Macromastia
H. Micromastia

II. REVIEWING KEY CONCEPTS

9. DEFINE each of the following treatment approaches used in the care of women with breast cancer, and briefly describe the rationale for their selection.
   A. Chemoprevention

   B. Lumpectomy

C. Mastectomy (partial, modified radical, total [simple], preventive/prophylactic)

D. Breast reconstruction (Timing: simultaneous, staged, delayed; Types: implants, flap procedures)

E. Radiation

F. Adjuvant systemic therapy (adjuvant chemotherapy; hormonal therapy); chemotherapy

MULTIPLE CHOICE: Circle the correct option(s) and state the rationale for the option(s) chosen.

10. When teaching a group of women about breast cancer, the nurse should emphasize: (Circle all that apply.)
    A. The incidence of breast cancer is highest among African-American women
    B. One in eight American women will develop breast cancer in her lifetime
    C. The mortality rate from breast cancer has been declining since 1990
    D. Breast cancer is most prevalent among women in their 30s and 40s
    E. Most women diagnosed with breast cancer have a family history of the disease

11. The physician of a 46-year-old premenopausal woman with breast cancer has prescribed tamoxifen (Nolvadex) beginning in the postoperative period following a lumpectomy. What should the nurse teach this woman regarding tamoxifen?
    A. It will help to relieve postoperative discomfort.
    B. She will take 100 mg of tamoxifen four times a day.
    C. Tamoxifen works by blocking the action of progesterone on breast tissue.
    D. She may experience hot flashes and menstrual irregularities when taking tamoxifen.

12. When providing discharge instructions to a woman who had a modified right radical mastectomy, the nurse should emphasize the importance of:
    A. Reporting any tingling or numbness in her incisional site or right arm immediately
    B. Telling health care providers not to take a blood pressure or draw blood from her right arm
    C. Learning how to use her left arm to write and accomplish the activities of daily living, such as brushing her hair
    D. Avoiding the use of any deodorant in her right axillary area.

13. A 26-year-old woman has just been diagnosed with fibrocystic changes in her breasts. Which nursing diagnosis is appropriate for this woman?
    A. Acute pain related to cyclic enlargement of breast cysts
    B. Risk for infection related to altered integrity of the areola associated with accumulation of a thick sticky discharge from both nipples
    C. Anxiety related to anticipated surgery to remove the cysts in her breasts
    D. Fear related to high risk for breast cancer

14. When assessing a woman with a diagnosis of fibroadenoma, the nurse would expect to find:
    A. Bilateral tender lumps behind the nipple
    B. Milky discharge from one or both nipples
    C. Soft and nonmovable lumps
    D. Firm, well-delineated, movable lump in one breast

15. The doctor has prescribed raloxifene hydrochloride for a 58-year-old postmenopausal woman. Which statements indicate that the woman understands the nurse's instructions regarding this medication? (Circle all that apply.)
    A. "I should stop taking my calcium supplement when I am taking this medication."
    B. "This drug can reduce my risk for breast cancer."
    C. "I must take this medication on an empty stomach once a week."
    D. "I will report to my doctor if I notice swelling in my hands and feet."
    E. "I may start experiencing hot flashes again when taking this medication."

III. THINKING CRITICALLY

1. Breast cancer is a major health problem facing women in the United States. IMAGINE that you are a nurse who has been invited to discuss the issue of breast cancer with a group of women.
    A. OUTLINE the information that you would give these women about the risk factors associated with breast cancer.

    B. The ages of the women in your class range from 26 to 65 years. SPECIFY the breast screening examinations you would recommend for women across the life span. INDICATE the frequency at which each examination should be performed, according to the American Cancer Society.

    C. DISCUSS several factors that could inhibit these women from participating in the breast screening examinations you identified. SUGGEST several strategies that can be used to overcome these inhibiting factors.

D. One of the women asks you to discuss the signs that would be associated with breast cancer. DISCUSS the clinical manifestations that are strongly suggestive of breast cancer.

E. Another woman asks you what would happen if she finds a lump in her breast. SPECIFY the diagnostic tests she could anticipate.

F. Finally, a woman asks whether breast cancer is hereditary, as she had heard. She further states that she must not have the gene for breast cancer because no one in her family that she knows of has or has had breast cancer.

2. Jane's mother died from breast cancer at the age of 36. Now at 30 years of age, Jane is concerned about her chances of developing breast cancer herself. She asks you about tests available to detect the gene for breast cancer and wonders if she should have a test performed. She doesn't want to take it if it's not necessary because it is so expensive. Further, she is worried that if her test is positive she will lose her health insurance coverage. DISCUSS your response to Jane's concerns.

3. Mary Anne, a 24-year-old, comes to the women's health clinic complaining that her breasts feel lumpy.
   A. OUTLINE the assessment process that should be used to determine the basis for Mary Anne's complaint.

   B. A diagnosis of fibrocystic breast changes is made. DESCRIBE the clinical manifestations Mary Anne most likely exhibited to support this diagnosis.

C. STATE one nursing diagnosis that the nurse would identify as a priority when preparing a plan of care for Mary Anne.

D. IDENTIFY measures the nurse could suggest to Mary Anne for lessening the symptoms she experiences related to fibrocystic changes.

E. Mary Anne expresses fear that she is now at very high risk for breast cancer. DESCRIBE how the nurse should respond to Mary Anne's expressed fear.

4. Molly, 50 years old, found a lump in her left breast during a breast self-examination. She comes to the women's health clinic for help.
   A. DESCRIBE the diagnostic protocol that should be followed to determine the basis for the lump Molly found in her breast.

   B. Molly's lump is diagnosed as cancerous. DESCRIBE the emotional effect that this diagnosis and the treatment is likely to have on Molly and her family.

   C. Molly elects to have a modified radical mastectomy based on the information provided by her oncologist regarding her cancer and in consultation with her husband. IDENTIFY two priority nursing diagnoses and OUTLINE the nursing care management for each of the following phases of Molly's treatment.
   Preoperative phase

   Immediate postoperative phase

D. Molly will be discharged within 48 hours after her surgery. DESCRIBE the instructions that the nurse should give Molly to prepare her for self-care at home.

E. DISCUSS support measures the nurse should use to address the concerns that Molly and her husband will most likely experience and express.

5. Susan has been diagnosed with breast cancer. Her initial treatment included a lumpectomy. In addition, Susan's physician has prescribed adjuvant hormonal therapy using tamoxifen. EXPLAIN to Susan and her family what this medication is and how it works. USE a drug manual to obtain information regarding administration, dosage, and side effects that you will incorporate into a teaching plan to ensure that Susan takes the medication effectively and safely.

6. Annie is a 36-year-old client about to begin chemotherapy for treatment of breast cancer.
   A. OUTLINE a teaching plan the nurse would use to prepare Annie and her family for what to expect regarding this treatment method.

   B. IDENTIFY two priority nursing diagnoses the nurse should address when developing a plan of care for Annie during her treatment. DESCRIBE two nursing interventions for each nursing diagnosis identified, including the use of alternative therapies.

CHAPTER 11

Structural Disorders and Neoplasms of the Reproductive System

I. LEARNING KEY TERMS

MATCHING: Match the description in Column I with the appropriate disorder in Column II.

COLUMN I

1. _______ The most common malignancy of the female reproductive system usually seen in women between the ages of 50 and 65 years.
2. _______ Herniation of the anterior rectal wall through the relaxed or ruptured vaginal fascia and rectovaginal septum.
3. _______ Development of multiple follicular cysts that occurs when an endocrine imbalance results in high levels of estrogen, testosterone, and luteinizing hormone and decreased secretion of follicle-stimulating hormone.
4. _______ Spectrum of disorders that includes hydatidiform mole, invasive mole, and choriocarcinoma.
5. _______ Tumors that are on pedicles usually originating from the mucosa of the cervix or endometrium.
6. _______ Perforations between genital tract organs, with most occurring between the bladder and the vagina.
7. _______ Germ cell tumors, usually occurring in childhood; they contain substances such as hair, teeth, sebaceous secretions, and bones.
8. _______ Protrusion of the bladder downward into the vagina that develops when supporting structures in the vesicovaginal septum are injured.
9. _______ Slow-growing benign tumors arising in uterine muscle tissue; their growth is influenced by ovarian hormones.
10. _______ Spread of cancer from its original site.
11. _______ Vulvar pain syndrome or vulvovestibulitis; chronic pain disorder of the vulvar area.
12. _______ The most common benign lesion of the vulva.
13. _______ Form of cancer that is strongly linked to the human papillomavirus (types 16 and 18).
14. _______ Reproductive cancer with a high mortality rate as a result of being frequently diagnosed in an advanced stage.
15. _______ Downward displacement of the uterus as a result of pelvic relaxation.

COLUMN II

A. Cystocele
B. Leiomyomas (fibroid tumors)
C. Endometrial cancer
D. Cervical cancer
E. Ovarian cancer
F. Rectocele
G. Polyps
H. Genital fistulas
I. Bartholin cyst
J. Gestational trophoblastic disease (GTD)
K. Uterine prolapse
L. Polycystic ovary syndrome (PCOS)
M. Dermoid cysts
N. Vulvodynia
O. Metastasis

FILL IN THE BLANKS: Insert the treatment that corresponds to each of the following descriptions.

16. ______________________________ Device used to support the uterus and hold it in the correct position.

17. ______________________________ Surgery used to repair a cystocele.

18. ______________________________ Surgery used to repair a rectocele.

19. ______________________________ Surgical removal of a leiomyoma (fibroid).

20. ______________________________ Injection of polyvinyl alcohol (PVA) pellets into selected blood vessels to block the blood supply to a leiomyoma (fibroid) in order to cause shrinkage and resolution of symptoms.

21. ______________________________ Use of electrocauterization to destroy small fibroids through a laparoscopic (abdominal) or hysteroscopic (vaginal) approach.

22. ______________________________ Vaporization of tissue inside the uterus.

23. ______________________________ Surgical removal of the entire uterus.

24. ______________________________ Surgical removal of both ovaries and both uterine tubes.

25. ______________________________ Examination of the cervix using a stereoscopic binocular microscope that magnifies the view of the cervix.

26. ______________________________ Removal of a wedge of tissue from the exocervix and endocervix to establish a diagnosis or effect a cure.

27. ______________________________ Treatment that involves destroying abnormal cells by freezing them. Cells slough off and are replaced with the regeneration of normal tissue.

28. ______________________________ Treatment for cervical intraepithelial neoplasia that involves use of a wire loop electrode that can excise and cauterize with minimal tissue damage.

29. ______________________________ Surgical procedure involving the removal of the uterus, tubes, ovaries, and the upper third of the vagina along with certain pelvic ligaments and lymph nodes and a portion of the parametrium while preserving the bladder, rectum, and ureters.

30. ______________________________ Surgical removal of the perineum, pelvic floor, levator muscles, all reproductive organs, pelvic lymph nodes, rectum, sigmoid colon, urinary bladder, and distal ureters. A colostomy and ileal conduit are constructed.

31. ______________________________ Surgical removal of part or all of the vulva (mons pubis, labia majora and minora, and, possibly, the clitoris).

32. ______________________________ Surgical removal of entire vulva, deep tissues, and the clitoris.

II. REVIEWING KEY CONCEPTS

33. EXPLAIN why ovarian cancer is called the silent disease.

MULTIPLE CHOICE: Circle the correct option(s), and state the rationale for the option(s) chosen.

34. A 60-year-old woman has been diagnosed with a mild prolapse of her uterus. The nurse practitioner could suggest that this woman: (Circle all that apply.)
   A. Assume a knee-chest position for a few minutes several times a day
   B. Use a specially fitted pessary to support her uterus and hold it in the correct position
   C. Begin progestin-only hormone replacement therapy
   D. See a surgeon to discuss the possibility of having an anterior repair (colporrhaphy) performed
   E. Perform Kegel exercises several times each day

35. A 35-year-old woman has recently been diagnosed with two leiomyomas in the body of her uterus. This woman can expect to experience which clinical manifestations? (Circle all that apply.)
    A. Shrinkage of tumors if she becomes pregnant
    B. Diarrhea
    C. Dysmenorrhea
    D. Acute abdominal pain
    E. Abnormal uterine bleeding

36. Which measure is the *least* effective in relieving the stress urinary incontinence experienced by a 60-year-old woman with pelvic relaxation?
    A. Performing Kegel exercises
    B. Reducing her intake of oral fluids to 1 L or less per day
    C. Emptying her bladder on a regular basis every 2 hours
    D. Participating in a smoking cessation program to relieve her smoker's cough

37. A 38-year-old premenopausal woman has had a total abdominal hysterectomy (TAH) performed as a result of fibroid tumors that have been increasing in size and causing menorrhagia. Postoperative care for this woman would include instructions regarding:
    A. Taking hormone replacement therapy (HRT), which will begin prior to discharge
    B. Avoiding vigorous exercise and heavy lifting for at least 6 weeks
    C. Performing a Betadine douche daily for the first week postoperatively
    D. Turning, coughing, and deep breathing every 4 hours for the first 24 hours

38. A woman has been diagnosed with carcinoma in situ (CIS) of the cervix. The nurse should prepare this woman for which treatment measure?
    A. Uterine artery embolization (UAE)
    B. Radical hysterectomy
    C. Cervical conization with follow-up Pap tests and colposcopy
    D. Intracavitary and external radiation therapy

III. THINKING CRITICALLY

1. When caring for women across the life span, it is critical that the nurse be alert for risk factors associated with the three most common types of reproductive system cancer.
    A. IDENTIFY the risk factors that increase a woman's vulnerability to the following:
       Endometrial cancer

       Ovarian cancer

       Cervical cancer

B. DESCRIBE how you as a nurse would use this information when providing health care to women.

2. Denise (6-5-0-1-5), a 60-year-old postmenopausal client, has been diagnosed with a moderate uterine prolapse along with cystocele and rectocele.
   A. DESCRIBE the clinical manifestations Denise most likely exhibited to lead to this diagnosis.

   B. IDENTIFY two priority nursing diagnoses related to the signs and symptoms Denise is most likely experiencing. WRITE one expected outcome for each of the nursing diagnoses identified.

   C. OUTLINE the care management approach recommended for Denise's health problem.

   D. Denise will use a pessary during the day until a surgical repair can be accomplished.
      1. IDENTIFY one nursing diagnosis associated with pessary use.

      2. SPECIFY the instructions the nurse should give to Denise regarding the use and care of a pessary.

E. Denise has a vaginal hysterectomy and an anterior and posterior colporrhaphy. OUTLINE the postoperative care Denise will require in order to heal without complications.

3. Marie, age 40, has been diagnosed with two leiomyomas (fibroid tumors).
   A. DESCRIBE the clinical manifestations most likely exhibited by Marie.

   B. COMPARE the commonly used therapeutic approaches for fibroid tumors. INCLUDE in your answer the criteria that Marie's gynecologist will consider when making a recommendation for treatment.

   C. After consultation with her gynecologist, Marie chooses uterine artery embolization as her treatment. OUTLINE a plan of care for Marie during her preoperative and postoperative periods.

4. Louise, age 60, has been diagnosed with endometrial cancer. Because of the early stage of the carcinoma, a total abdominal hysterectomy and bilateral salpingo-oophorectomy is the form of treatment chosen.
   A. IDENTIFY one nursing diagnosis relevant for the preoperative period and one nursing diagnosis relevant for the postoperative period. STATE an expected outcome for each nursing diagnosis identified.

   B. OUTLINE the nursing care and support required for each of the following stages in Louise's treatment.
      Preoperative stage

Postoperative stage

C. SPECIFY the instructions that Louise should receive in preparation for discharge about caring for herself once at home.

D. DISCUSS how Louise's cultural beliefs could affect her responses to her diagnosis of cancer and the need to have her reproductive organs removed.

E. IDENTIFY one nursing diagnosis associated with Louise's likely emotional response to her diagnosis and treatment.

F. DISCUSS the support measures the nurse could use to meet Louise's emotional and psychosocial needs as she recovers.

5. Laura has been diagnosed with invasive carcinoma of the cervix and is about to begin a course of radiation therapy.
   A. IDENTIFY two priority nursing diagnoses associated with the course of treatment that Laura is about to undergo. WRITE one expected outcome for each nursing diagnosis identified.

B. USE the following outline to summarize the care and support Laura will require at each stage of her treatment regimen.

External radiation

- Pretreatment care

- Care during treatment

- Posttreatment care and instructions

Internal radiation

- Pretreatment care

- Care during treatment

- Posttreatment care and instructions

C. DESCRIBE the self-protection measures the nurse should use when caring for a woman receiving internal radiation therapy.

6. Pat is recovering from a radical vulvectomy that was performed to treat invasive vulvar cancer.
   A. IDENTIFY three nursing measures related to the expected outcome: Pat will heal without the development of infection.

   B. IDENTIFY three nursing measures related to the expected outcome: Pat will maintain appropriate sexual functioning.

   C. DISCUSS the discharge instructions Pat should receive.

7. DISCUSS the issues and emotions that can confront a pregnant woman, her family, and her health care providers when the woman is diagnosed with cancer.

8. Angela has been diagnosed with advanced ovarian cancer. Metastasis has occurred, and as a result she will be starting another course of chemotherapy.
   A. OUTLINE the measures you would recommend to relieve the following anticipated problems associated with chemotherapy.
      Altered taste and anorexia

Nausea and vomiting

Stomatitis

Constipation

Diarrhea

B. DESCRIBE the approach you would use to support Angela and her family as they cope with the effects of the chemotherapy and the diagnosis of advanced cancer.

CHAPTER 12

Conception and Fetal Development

I. LEARNING KEY TERMS

FILL IN THE BLANKS: Insert the term that corresponds to each of the following descriptions related to conception and fetal development.

1. ______________________ Union of a single egg and sperm. It marks the beginning of a pregnancy.
2. ______________________ Male and female germ cell. The male germ cell is a ______________________ and the female germ cell is an ______________________.
3. ______________________ The process by which body (somatic) cells replicate to yield two cells, each with the same genetic makeup as the parent cell.
4. ______________________ The process by which germ cells divide and decrease their chromosome number by half.
5. ______________________ A cell with 23 single chromosomes.
6. ______________________ A cell with 46 chromosomes or 23 pairs.
7. ______________________ Process whereby gametes are formed and mature. For the male the process is called ______________________, and for the female the process is called ______________________.
8. ______________________ Process of successful penetration of the membrane surrounding the ovum by a sperm.
9. ______________________ The first cell of the new individual.
10. ______________________ The 16-cell solid ball of cells that develops within 3 days of fertilization.
11. ______________________ Term used to refer to the solid cell ball when a cavity becomes recognizable within it. The outer layer of cells surrounding this cavity is called the ______________________.
12. ______________________ Attachment process whereby the blastocyst burrows into the endometrium at 6 to 10 days after conception.
13. ______________________ Finger-like projections develop out of the trophoblast and extend into the blood-filled spaces of the endometrium.
14. ______________________ Term used to refer to the endometrium during pregnancy.
15. ______________________ Term used to refer to the developing baby from day 15 until about 8 weeks from conception.
16. ______________________ The term used to refer to the developing baby from 9 weeks of gestation to the end of pregnancy.
17. ______________________ Membranes that surround the developing baby and the fluid. The ______________________ is the outer layer of these membranes and the ______________________ is the inner layer.

18. ______________________________ Fluid that surrounds the developing baby in utero. ______________________________ refers to a decreased amount of the fluid (<300 ml). ______________________________ refers to an excessive amount of the fluid (>2 L).

19. ______________________________ Structure that connects the developing baby to the placenta. It contains three vessels, namely, two ______________________________ and one ______________________________. ______________________________ is the connective tissue that prevents compression of the blood vessels to ensure continued nourishment of the developing baby. When it is wrapped around the fetal neck, it is called a ______________________________.

20. ______________________________ Structure composed of 15 to 20 lobes/areas called cotyledons; it serves as a means of metabolic exchange and produces several hormones including ______________________________, which is the hormone that is the basis of pregnancy tests.

21. ______________________________ Capability of fetus to survive outside the uterus.

22. ______________________________ Special circulatory pathway that allows fetal blood to bypass the lungs.

23. ______________________________ Shunt that allows most of fetal blood to bypass the liver and pass into the inferior vena cava.

24. ______________________________ Opening between the atria of the fetal heart.

25. ______________________________ Formation of blood.

26. ______________________________ Surface-active phospholipid that needs to be present in fetal/newborn lungs to facilitate breathing after birth. The ______________________________ ratio can be performed using amniotic fluid to determine fetal lung maturity.

27. ______________________________ Maternal perception of fetal movement that occurs sometime between 16 and 20 weeks of gestation.

28. ______________________________ Dark green to black tarry substance that contains fetal waste products and accumulates in the fetal intestines.

29. ______________________________ Twins that are formed from two zygotes. They are also called ______________________________ twins.

30. ______________________________ Twins that are formed from one fertilized ovum that then divides. They are also called ______________________________ twins.

31. ______________________________ Environmental substances or exposures that cause abnormal fetal development.

II. REVIEWING KEY CONCEPTS

32. Each of the following structures plays a critical role in fetal growth and development. DESCRIBE the functions of these structures.
    - Yolk sac

- Amniotic membranes and fluid

- Umbilical cord

- Placenta

33. NAME the three primary germ layers and identify the tissues or organs that develop from each layer.

MULTIPLE CHOICE: Circle the correct option(s), and state the rationale for the option(s) chosen.

34. When teaching a class of pregnant women about fetal development, the nurse would include which statements? (Circle all that apply.)
    A. The sex of your baby is determined by the 9th week of pregnancy.
    B. Your baby will be able to suck and hiccup while in your uterus.
    C. The baby's heart begins to pump blood during the 10th week of pregnancy.
    D. The baby's heart beat will be audible using a special ultrasound stethoscope beginning at the 18th week of pregnancy.
    E. You should be able to feel your baby move by week 16 to 20 of pregnancy.
    F. By the 24th week of your pregnancy you will notice your baby responding to sounds in the environment including music and your voice.

35. The results of an amniocentesis show that the pregnant woman's L/S ratio is 2:1. This result indicates that:
    A. The woman is in her second trimester of pregnancy
    B. The newborn should be able to maintain effective respiration after birth
    C. The fetus has most likely developed a renal problem
    D. An open neural tube defect is present

36. If a pregnant woman's intake of iron is sufficient, her newborn will have enough iron stored in its liver to last approximately how many months after birth?
    A. 1 month
    B. 3 months
    C. 5 months
    D. 9 months

37. When caring for pregnant women, the nurse would recognize that a woman with which disorder has the greatest risk for giving birth to a macrosomic newborn?
    A. Diabetes
    B. Anemia
    C. Hyperthyroidism
    D. Hypertension

III. THINKING CRITICALLY

1. IMAGINE that you are a nurse-midwife working in partnership with an obstetrician. FORMULATE a response to each of the following concerns or questions directed to you from some of your prenatal clients.
    A. June (2 months pregnant), Mary (5 months pregnant), and Alice (7 months pregnant) each ask for a description of their fetus at the present time.

       June

       Mary

       Alice

    B. Jessica states that a friend told her that babies born after about 35 weeks have a better chance to survive because they can breathe more easily. She asks if this is truc.

    C. Beth, who is 1 month pregnant, states that she heard that women who are pregnant experience quickening. She wants to know what that could mean and if it hurts.

D. Susan, who is 6 months pregnant, states that she read in a magazine that a fetus can actually hear and see. She feels that this is totally unbelievable!

E. Alexa is 2 months pregnant. She asks how the sex of her baby is determined and if a sonogram could tell if she is having a boy or a girl.

F. Karen is pregnant for the first time. She reveals that she has a history of twins in her family. She wants to know what causes twin pregnancies to occur and what the difference is between identical and fraternal twins.

G. Louise is beginning her second trimester. She tells the nurse that a friend who just had a baby told her that her position and activity can affect how her baby grows and develops. Louise asks if this is true.

CHAPTER 13

Anatomy and Physiology of Pregnancy

I. LEARNING KEY TERMS

MATCHING: Match the assessment finding in Column I with the appropriate descriptive term in Column II.

COLUMN I

1. _______ Menstrual bleeding no longer occurs.
2. _______ Fundal height decreased, fetal head in pelvic inlet.
3. _______ Cervix and vagina violet bluish.
4. _______ Swelling of ankles and feet at the end of the day.
5. _______ Cervical tip softened.
6. _______ Lower uterine segment is soft and compressible.
7. _______ Fetal head rebounds with gentle, upward tapping through the vagina.
8. _______ White or slightly gray mucoid vaginal discharge with faint, musty odor.
9. _______ Enlarged sebaceous glands in areola on both breasts.
10. _______ Plug of mucus fills endocervical canal.
11. _______ Pink stretch marks or depressed streaks on breasts and abdomen.
12. _______ Thick creamy yellowish fluid expressed from nipples.
13. _______ Cheeks, nose, and forehead blotchy, brownish hyperpigmentation.
14. _______ Pigmented line extending up abdominal midline.
15. _______ Red raised nodule on gums; bleeds after brushing teeth.
16. _______ Heartburn experienced after supper.
17. _______ Lumbosacral curve accentuated.
18. _______ Paresthesia and pain in right hand radiating to elbow.
19. _______ Spotting following cervical palpation or intercourse.
20. _______ Hematocrit decreased to 36% and hemoglobin to 11 g/dl.
21. _______ Vascular spiders on neck and thorax.
22. _______ Palms pinkish red, mottled.
23. _______ Abdominal wall muscles separated.
24. _______ Varicosities around the anus.

COLUMN II

A. Colostrum
B. Operculum
C. Amenorrhea
D. Angiomas
E. Pyrosis
F. Friability
G. Striae gravidarum
H. Physiologic anemia
I. Linea nigra
J. Ballottement
K. Chadwick sign
L. Diastasis recti abdominis
M. Lordosis
N. Leukorrhea
O. Chloasma (mask of pregnancy; facial melasma)
P. Lightening
Q. Hemorrhoids
R. Palmar erythema
S. Goodell sign
T. Physiologic/dependent edema
U. Hegar sign
V. Montgomery tubercles
W. Carpal tunnel syndrome
X. Epulis (gingival granuloma gravidarum)

FILL IN THE BLANKS: Insert the term that corresponds to each of the following descriptions related to pregnancy.

25. ______________________ Pregnancy.
26. ______________________ The number of pregnancies in which the fetus or fetuses have reached 20 weeks when they are born, not the number of fetuses (e.g., twins) born. The numeric designation is not affected by whether the fetus is born alive or is stillborn (i.e., showing no signs of life at birth).
27. ______________________ A woman who is pregnant.
28. ______________________ A woman who has never been pregnant.
29. ______________________ A woman who has not completed a pregnancy with a fetus or fetuses who have reached 20 weeks of gestation.
30. ______________________ A woman who is pregnant for the first time.
31. ______________________ A woman who has completed one pregnancy with a fetus or fetuses who have reached 20 weeks of gestation.
32. ______________________ A woman who has had two or more pregnancies.
33. ______________________ A woman who has completed two or more pregnancies to 20 weeks of gestation.
34. ______________________ Capacity to live outside the uterus at about 22 to 24 weeks of gestation and weighing at least 500 g.
35. ______________________ Designation given to a pregnancy that has reached 20 weeks of gestation but ends before completion of 37 weeks of gestation.
36. ______________________ Designation given to a pregnancy from the completion of 37 weeks of gestation to the end of week 42 of gestation.
37. ______________________ Designation given to a pregnancy that goes beyond 42 weeks of gestation.
38. ______________________ Presence of this biochemical marker in maternal urine or serum results in a positive pregnancy test result.
39. ______________________ Pregnancy-related changes felt by a woman.
40. ______________________ Pregnancy-related changes that can be observed by an examiner.
41. ______________________ Signs that can be attributed only to the presence of a fetus.
42. ______________________ Uterine contractions that can be felt through the abdominal wall soon after the fourth month of pregnancy.
43. ______________________ A rushing or blowing sound of maternal blood flow through the uterine arteries to the placenta that is synchronous with the maternal pulse.
44. ______________________ Sound of fetal blood coursing through the umbilical cord; it is synchronous with the fetal heart rate.
45. ______________________ Fetal movements first felt by the pregnant woman at 16 to 18 weeks of gestation.
46. ______________________ Change in blood pressure as a result of compression of abdominal blood vessels and decrease in cardiac output when a woman lies down on her back.
47. ______________________ Itching of the skin that occurs during pregnancy.
48. ______________________ Nonfood cravings for substances such as ice, clay, and laundry starch.
49. ______________________ Excessive salivation

II. REVIEWING KEY CONCEPTS

50. DESCRIBE the obstetric history for each of the following women, using both the 2-digit and 5-digit systems.
    A. Nancy is pregnant. Her first pregnancy resulted in a stillbirth at 36 weeks of gestation, and her second pregnancy resulted in the birth of her daughter at 42 weeks of gestation.

    B. Marsha is 6 weeks pregnant. Her previous pregnancies resulted in the live birth of a daughter at 40 weeks of gestation, the live birth of a son at 38 weeks of gestation, and a spontaneous abortion at 10 weeks of gestation.

    C. Linda is experiencing her fourth pregnancy. Her first pregnancy ended in a spontaneous abortion at 12 weeks, the second resulted in the live birth of twin boys at 32 weeks, and the third resulted in the live birth of a daughter at 39 weeks.

51. When assessing a pregnant woman a nurse should keep in mind that baseline vital sign values will change as she progresses through her pregnancy. DESCRIBE how each of the following change as pregnancy progresses.
    - Blood pressure

    - Heart rate and patterns

    - Respiratory rate and patterns

- Body temperature

52. CALCULATE the mean arterial pressure (MAP) for each of the following BP readings.
    - 120/76
    - 114/64
    - 110/80
    - 150/90

53. SPECIFY the value changes that occur in the following laboratory tests. STATE the rationale for these changes in terms of the expected physiologic adaptations to pregnancy.
    - CBC: hematocrit, hemoglobin, white blood cell count, platelets

- Clotting activity

- Acid-base balance

- Urinalysis

54. DISCUSS how and why the levels of each of the following substances changes during pregnancy.
    - Parathyroid hormone

    - Insulin

    - Estrogen

    - Progesterone

- Thyroid hormones

- Human chorionic gonadotropin (hCG)

MULTIPLE CHOICE: Circle the correct option(s), and state the rationale for the option(s) chosen.

55. When assessing pregnant women during routine prenatal checkups, which findings would be categorized as probable signs of pregnancy? (Circle all that apply.)
    A. Human chorionic gonadotropin in the urine
    B. Breast tenderness
    C. Morning sickness
    D. Fetal heart sounds
    E. Ballottement
    F. Hegar sign

56. A pregnant woman with four children reports the following obstetric history: a stillbirth at 32 weeks of gestation, triplets (2 sons and a daughter) born via cesarean section at 30 weeks of gestation, a spontaneous abortion at 8 weeks of gestation, and a daughter born vaginally at 39 weeks of gestation. What accurately expresses this woman's current obstetric history, using the 5-digit system?
    A. 5-1-4-1-4
    B. 4-1-3-1-4
    C. 5-2-2-0-3
    D. 5-1-2-1-4

57. An essential component of prenatal health assessment of pregnant women is the determination of vital signs. An expected change in vital sign findings as a result of pregnancy is:
    A. Increase in systolic BP by 30 mm Hg or more after assuming a supine position
    B. Increase in diastolic BP by 5 to 10 mm Hg beginning in the first trimester
    C. Increased awareness of the need to breathe as pregnancy progresses
    D. Gradual decrease in baseline pulse rate of approximately 20 beats/min

58. A woman exhibits understanding of instructions for performing a home pregnancy test to maximize accuracy if she:
    A. Uses urine collected at the end of the day, just before going to bed
    B. Avoids using Tylenol or aspirin for a headache for about 1 week prior to performing the test
    C. Performs the test on the day after she misses her first menstrual period
    D. Records the day of her last menstrual period and her usual cycle length

59. During an examination of a pregnant woman, the nurse notes that the woman's cervix is soft on its tip. The nurse documents this finding as:
    A. Friability
    B. Goodell sign
    C. Chadwick sign
    D. Hegar sign

III. THINKING CRITICALLY

1. DESCRIBE how a nurse should respond to each of the following client concerns and questions.
   A. Tina is 16 weeks pregnant. She calls the prenatal clinic to report that she noticed slight painless spotting this morning. She reveals that she did have intercourse with her partner the night before.

   B. Lisa suspects she is pregnant because her menstrual period is already 3 weeks late. She asks her friend, who is a nurse, how to use the pregnancy test that she just bought so that she can obtain the best results.

   C. Joan is 3 months pregnant. She tells the nurse that she is worried because a friend told her that vaginal and bladder infections are more common during pregnancy. She wants to know if this could be true and, if so, why.

   D. Tammy, who is 20 weeks pregnant, tells the nurse that she has noted some "problems" with her breasts: There are "little pimples" near her nipples, and her breasts feel "lumpy and bumpy" and "leak a little" when she performs a breast self-examination (BSE).

   E. Tamara is concerned because she read in a book about pregnancy that a pregnant woman's position could affect her circulation, especially to the baby. She asks what positions are good for her circulation now that she is pregnant.

   F. Beth, a pregnant client, calls to tell the nurse that she had a nosebleed this morning and has noticed occasional feelings of fullness in her ears. She asks if these are anything to worry about.

G. Karen is 7 months pregnant and works as a secretary full time. She asks the nurse if she should take a "water pill" that a friend gave her, because she has noticed that her ankles "swell up" at the end of the day.

H. Jan is in her third trimester of pregnancy. She tells the nurse that her posture seems to have changed and that she occasionally experiences low back pain.

I. Monica, who is 36 weeks pregnant with her first baby, calls the clinic stating that she knows the baby is coming because she felt some uterine contractions before getting out of bed in the morning. Monica confirms that they seem to have decreased in intensity and frequency since she has gotten out of bed and walked around.

J. Nina is a primigravida who is at 32 weeks of gestation. When she comes for a prenatal visit, she reports that she has been experiencing occasional periods of shortness of breath during the day and sometimes has to use an extra pillow to sleep comfortably. Nina expresses concern that she is developing a breathing problem.

K. Shade, a primigravida, is at 26 weeks of gestation. She has recently begun to experience difficulty moving her bowels. Shade reports that she has a bowel movement every 2 days or so now instead of daily and that her stool is firmer and a little harder to pass.

2. Accurate BP readings are critical if significant changes in the cardiovascular system are to be detected as a woman adapts to pregnancy during the prenatal period. WRITE a protocol for BP assessment that can be used by nurses working in a prenatal clinic to ensure accuracy of the results obtained during BP assessment.

CHAPTER 14

Maternal and Fetal Nutrition

I. LEARNING KEY TERMS

FILL IN THE BLANKS: Insert the term that corresponds to each of the following descriptions.

1. ______________________ Birth weight of 2500 g or less.
2. ______________________ The best way to ensure that adequate nutrients are available for the developing fetus.
3. ______________________ Nutrient, the adequate intake of which is important for decreasing risk for ______________________ or failures in the closure of the neural tube. An intake of ______________________ daily is recommended for all women capable of becoming pregnant.
4. ______________________ Recommendations for daily nutritional intakes that meet the needs of almost all healthy members of the population.
5. ______________________ Method used to evaluate the appropriateness of weight for height. If the calculated value is less than 18.5 the person is considered to be ______________________. If the calculated value is between 18.5 and 24.9 the person is considered to be ______________________. If the calculated value is between 25 and 29.9 the person is considered to be ______________________ and if the calculated value is 30 or greater the person is considered to be ______________________.
6. ______________________ Presence of ketones in the urine as a result of catabolism of fat stores; it has been found to correlate with the occurrence of ______________________.
7. ______________________ Normal adaptation that occurs during pregnancy when the plasma volume increases more rapidly than RBC mass.
8. ______________________ Inability to digest milk sugar because of the absence of the lactase enzyme in the small intestine.
9. ______________________ The practice of consuming nonfood substances such as ______________________, ______________________, and ______________________ or excessive amounts of food stuffs low in nutritional value such as ______________________, ______________________, ______________________, and ______________________.
10. ______________________ Urge to consume specific types of foods such as ice cream, pickles, and pizza during pregnancy.
11. ______________________ Infection that can occur as a result of consuming unpasteurized milk or products made with unpasteurized milk; it increases the risk for miscarriage, premature birth, and stillbirth.
12. ______________________ Body measurements such as height and weight.
13. ______________________ Guide that can be used to make daily food choices during pregnancy and lactation, just as during other stages of the life cycle.
14. ______________________ A discomfort most commonly experienced in the first trimester of pregnancy; it usually causes only mild to moderate nutritional problems but may be a source of substantial discomfort.

15. ______________________________ Severe and persistent vomiting during pregnancy causing weight loss, dehydration, and electrolyte abnormalities.

16. ______________________________ Discomfort of pregnancy characterized by infrequent and difficult passage of hard, dry stool.

17. ______________________________ Discomfort of pregnancy that is usually caused by reflux of gastric contents into the esophagus.

II. REVIEWING KEY CONCEPTS

18. INDICATE the importance of each of the following nutrients for healthy maternal adaptation to pregnancy and optimum fetal growth and development. Indicate three food/fluid sources for each of the nutrients.

NUTRIENT	IMPORTANCE FOR PREGNANCY	MAJOR FOOD SOURCES
PROTEIN		
IRON		
CALCIUM		
SODIUM		
FAT-SOLUBLE VITAMINS		
WATER-SOLUBLE VITAMINS		

19. When assessing pregnant women, it is critical that nurses be alert for factors that could place women at nutritional risk so that early intervention can be implemented. NAME five such indicators or risk factors of which the nurse should be aware. CITE three strategies a nurse could use in an attempt to reduce nutritional risk for pregnant women based on the risks named.

20. CITE the pregnancy-related risks associated with the following nutritional problems.
    A. Underweight women

B. Inappropriate weight gain during pregnancy (inadequate; excessive)

C. Obese women

21. At her first prenatal visit, Marie, a 20-year-old primigravida, reports that she has been a strict vegetarian for the past 3 years. IDENTIFY two major guidelines that the nurse should follow when planning menus with Marie.

22. Evaluation of nutritional status is an essential part of a thorough physical assessment of pregnant women. CITE four signs of good nutrition and four signs of inadequate nutrition that the nurse should observe for during the assessment of a pregnant woman.

23. CALCULATE the BMI for each of the following women, then determine the recommended weight gain and pattern for each based on her BMI.

WOMAN	BMI	WEIGHT GAIN (TOTAL; PATTERN)
A. June: 1.60 m, 55 kg		
B. Alice: 1.65 m, 82 kg		
C. Ann: 1.70 m, 50 kg		

MULTIPLE CHOICE QUESTIONS: Circle the correct option(s) and state the rationale for the option(s) chosen.

24. A nurse teaching a pregnant woman about the importance of iron in her diet would tell her to consume which foods as good sources of iron? (Circle all that apply.)
    A. Whole grain breads and cereals
    B. Oranges
    C. Salmon
    D. Raisins
    E. Spinach
    F. Tomatoes

25. A 30-year-old pregnant woman with a BMI of 28 asks the nurse about recommendations for diet and weight gain during pregnancy. What should the nurse tell this woman?
    A. Counsel her to begin a lifestyle change for weight reduction
    B. Recommend a total weight gain goal of 4 kg during pregnancy
    C. Set a weight gain goal of 0.3 kg per week during the second and third trimesters
    D. Limit her third-trimester calorie increase to no more than 600 kcal more than prepregnant needs

26. A 25-year-old pregnant woman is at 10 weeks of gestation. Her BMI is calculated to be 24. Regarding weight gain during pregnancy, the nurse should recommend:
    A. A total weight gain of 18 kg
    B. First-trimester weight gain of 1 to 2 kg
    C. Weight gain of 0.4 kg each week for 40 weeks
    D. Weight gain of 3 kg per month during the second and third trimesters

27. A pregnant woman at 6 weeks of gestation tells her nurse-midwife that she has been experiencing nausea with occasional vomiting every day. As an effective relief measure, the nurse should recommend:
    A. Eating starchy foods such as buttered popcorn or peanut butter with crackers in the morning before getting out of bed
    B. Avoiding eating before going to bed at night
    C. Altering eating patterns to small meals every 2 to 3 hours
    D. Skipping a meal if nausea is experienced

28. A woman demonstrates an understanding of the importance of increasing her intake of foods that are good sources of folic acid (50 mcg or more) when she includes which foods in her diet? (Circle all that apply.)
    A. Baked haddock
    B. Lentil soup
    C. Scrambled eggs
    D. Fruit salad of papaya and oranges
    E. Steamed asparagus
    F. Corn on the cob

29. A nurse taught a pregnant woman about the importance of iron and taking her iron supplement daily. Which statement by the woman indicates the need for further instruction?
    A. "I take my iron supplement at bedtime with a cup of tea."
    B. "I include a lot of citrus fruit and tomatoes in my diet."
    C. "My stools can turn black or dark green."
    D. "I need to keep track of my bowel movements because taking iron can lead to constipation."

30. A 30-year-old woman at 16 weeks of gestation comes for a routine prenatal visit. Her 24-hour dietary recall is evaluated by the nurse. Which entry indicates that this woman needs further instructions regarding nutrient needs during pregnancy?
    A. Eight ounces total from the meat, poultry, fish, dry beans, eggs, and nuts group
    B. Three cups of vegetables and two cups of fruit
    C. Seven ounces of grains including whole grain bread and bran cereal
    D. Three cups from the milk, yogurt, and cheese group

III. THINKING CRITICALLY

1. Nutrition and weight gain are important areas of consideration for nurses who care for pregnant women. In addition, weight gain is often a source of stress and body image alteration for the pregnant woman. DISCUSS the approach you would use in each of the following situations.
   A. Kelly (150 cm and 55 kg) complains to you that her physician recommended a weight gain of approximately 30 pounds (14 kg) during her pregnancy. She states, "Babies only weigh about 7 pounds when they are born. Why do I have to gain much more than that?"

   B. Kate (160 cm and 68 kg) has just found out that she is pregnant. She states, "I am so glad to be pregnant. I love to eat, and now I can start eating for two. It will be great not to have to watch the scale or what I eat."

   C. June tells you that she does not have to worry about her nutrient intake during her pregnancy. "I take plenty of vitamins—everything from A to Z."

   D. Mary, a primigravida beginning her second month of pregnancy, asks you why she needs to increase her intake of so many nutrients during pregnancy and state, "I work every weekday and rely on fast foods to get through the week, though I try to eat better over the weekends."

   E. Sara (BMI = 28.7) is 1 month pregnant. She asks you for dietary guidance, including a weight reduction diet because she does not want to gain too much weight with this pregnancy.

F. Beth is 2 months pregnant. She states, "I have cut down on my water intake. I do get a little thirsty, but it's worth it because I don't have to urinate so often."

G. Hedy is 2 months pregnant and has come for her second prenatal visit. During a discussion about nutritional needs during pregnancy she states, "I know I will never get enough calcium because I get sick when I drink milk."

H. Lara is 36 weeks pregnant. She states that she would like to breastfeed her baby but is concerned about getting back into shape and losing weight after the baby is born. "My friends told me that I will lose weight more slowly since I will not be able to start on a weight reduction diet as long as I am breastfeeding."

I. Jean intends to breastfeed her infant until she returns to work in 6 months. She asks you what guidelines she should follow so that she makes good breast milk for her baby.

2. Yvonne's hemoglobin is 13 g/dl and her hematocrit is 37% at the onset of her pregnancy. She asks the nurse if she will have to take iron during her pregnancy if she tries to follow a good diet. "My friend took iron when she was pregnant and it made her sick to her stomach." DISCUSS the appropriate response by the nurse.

3. IDENTIFY three nursing measures appropriate for each of the following nursing diagnoses:
   A. Imbalanced nutrition: less than body requirements related to inadequate intake associated with moderate nausea and vomiting (morning sickness) associated with pregnancy.

   B. Constipation related to decreased intestinal motility associated with increased progesterone levels during pregnancy.

   C. Acute pain related to reflux of gastric contents into the esophagus following dinner.

4. Gloria is an 18-year-old Native-American (165 cm and 45 kg) who has just been diagnosed as 8 weeks pregnant. In her discussions with you at her first prenatal visit, she expresses a lack of knowledge regarding the nutritional requirements of pregnancy and an interest in learning about what to eat because she wants to have a healthy baby.
   A. OUTLINE the approach that you would use to help Gloria learn about and meet the nutritional requirements of her pregnancy.

   B. Plan a 1-day menu that incorporates Gloria's nutritional needs and reflects the traditions of her culture.

CHAPTER 15

Nursing Care of the Family During Pregnancy

I. LEARNING KEY TERMS

FILL IN THE BLANKS: Insert the term that corresponds to each of the following descriptions.

1. ______________________ Indicators of pregnancy that can be caused by conditions other than gestation and are not reliable for diagnosis; they include subjective symptoms and objective signs.
2. ______________________ Indicators of pregnancy that are detected by an examiner and are mainly related to physical changes in the uterus; they strongly suggest pregnancy but are not conclusive.
3. ______________________ Indicators of pregnancy that are directly attributed to the fetus.
4. ______________________ Method used to determine the expected date of birth by subtracting ______________________ from and adding ______________________ and ______________________ (if appropriate) to the first day of the last menstrual period.
5. ______________________ One of three periods of pregnancy, each of which is approximately 3 months in length.
6. ______________________ Change in blood pressure that can occur when a pregnant woman lies on her back and the ______________________ and the ______________________ are compressed by abdominal contents, including the uterus.
7. ______________________ Uterine measurement that is performed beginning in the second trimester as one indicator of the progress of fetal growth.
8. ______________________ Test used to determine whether the nipple is everted or inverted; achieved by placing thumb and forefinger on the areola and gently pressing inward.
9. ______________________, ______________________, ______________________, ______________________, and ______________________ Tasks that are accomplished by parents as they adapt to the changes of pregnancy and impending parenthood.
10. ______________________ Rapid unpredictable changes in mood related to profound hormonal changes and concerns about finances and changed lifestyle.
11. ______________________ Emotional state of having conflicting feelings about a pregnancy simultaneously.
12. As a pregnant woman establishes a relationship with her fetus and emotional attachment begins, she progresses through three phases. In phase one she accepts the ______________________ and needs to be able to state ______________________. In phase two the woman accepts the ______________________. She can now say ______________________. Finally, in phase three the woman prepares realistically for the ______________________ and ______________________. She expresses the thought ______________________.
13. ______________________ Phenomenon of an expectant father's experiencing pregnancy-like symptoms such as nausea, weight gain, and other physical symptoms.

14. ______________________ The first period of paternal adaptation, during which the father accepts the ______________________. During the second or ______________________ phase, the father adjusts to the reality of the pregnancy. The developmental task is to ______________________. The father becomes actively involved in the pregnancy and the relationship with his child during the third or ______________________ phase. The developmental task is to negotiate with his partner the role he is to play in ______________________ and to prepare for ______________________.

15. ______________________ Cultural practices that tell a woman what to do during pregnancy.

16. ______________________ Cultural practices that tell a woman what not to do during pregnancy; they establish ______________________.

17. ______________________ Screening test done between 16 to 18 weeks of gestation; elevated levels are associated with neural tube defects and multiple gestations; low levels are associated with Down syndrome.

18. ______________________ Blood test performed at 16 to 18 weeks of gestation to screen for Down syndrome by measuring maternal serum levels of ______________________, ______________________, and ______________________.

19. ______________________ Woman professionally trained to provide physical, emotional, and informational support to women and their partners during labor and birth.

20. ______________________ Tool that can be used by parents to explore their childbirth options and choose those that are most important to them; it serves as a tentative guide because the realities of what is feasible may change as the actual labor and birth progress.

II. REVIEWING KEY CONCEPTS

21. CALCULATE the expected date of birth (EDB) for each of the following pregnant women using Nägele's rule.
   A. Diane's last menses began on May 5, 2010, and the last day occurred on May 10, 2010.

   B. Sara had intercourse on February 21, 2011. She has not had a menstrual period since the one that began on January 14, 2011, and ended 5 days later.

   C. Beth's last menstrual period began on September 4, 2010, and ended on September 10, 2010. Beth noted that her basal body temperature (BBT) rose on the morning of September 28, 2010.

22. Cultural beliefs and practices are important influencing factors during the prenatal period.
    A. DESCRIBE how cultural beliefs can affect a woman's participation in prenatal care as it is defined by the Western Biomedical Model of Care.

    B. IDENTIFY one prescription and one proscription for each of the following areas. EXPLAIN how these beliefs can affect prenatal health care and practices.
    - Emotional response

    - Clothing

    - Physical activity and rest

    - Sexual activity

    - Diet

23. OUTLINE the assessment measures that should be used and the data that should be collected during each component of the initial prenatal visit and the follow-up prenatal visits.

INITIAL PRENATAL VISIT

Health History Interview

Physical Examination

Laboratory and Diagnostic Testing

FOLLOW-UP PRENATAL VISITS

Updating History Interview

Physical Examination

Fetal Assessment

Laboratory and Diagnostic Testing

24. Marie asks the nurse what can be done during a prenatal visit to make sure that her baby is healthy and doing well. IDENTIFY and DESCRIBE what the nurse could tell Marie about the components of fetal assessment that will determine her baby's health status.

25. Nurses responsible for the care management of pregnant women must be alert for warning signs of complications that women could develop as pregnancy progresses from trimester to trimester.
    A. LIST the signs of potential complications (warning signs) for each trimester of pregnancy. INDICATE possible cause(s) for each sign listed.

    B. DESCRIBE the approach a nurse should take when discussing potential complications with a pregnant woman and her family.

26. Nurses working in a prenatal clinic become concerned that the fundal height measurement technique they each used varied and resulted in variations in findings. They decide to create a protocol for fundal measurement that will facilitate accuracy. DISCUSS what they should include in the protocol that they create.

27. IDENTIFY four factors that a nurse should use to estimate the gestational age of a fetus.

28. Prevention of injury is an important goal for nurses as they teach pregnant women about how to care for themselves during pregnancy.
    A. DESCRIBE three principles of body mechanics that a pregnant woman should be taught to prevent injury.

B. IDENTIFY five safety guidelines that the nurse should include in a pamphlet titled "Safety During Pregnancy" that will be distributed to pregnant women during a prenatal visit.

29. During the third trimester, parents often make a decision concerning the method they will use to feed their newborn. LIST the contraindications for breastfeeding.

MULTIPLE CHOICE: Circle the correct option(s) and state the rationale for the option(s) chosen.

30. A nurse is assessing a pregnant woman during a prenatal visit. Several presumptive indicators of pregnancy are documented. Presumptive indicators include: (Circle all that apply.)
A. Nausea and vomiting
B. Quickening
C. Hegar sign
D. Palpation of fetal movement by the nurse
E. Amenorrhea
F. Positive pregnancy test

31. A woman's last menstrual period (LMP) began on November 9, 2010, and it ended on November 14, 2010. Using Nägele's rule, the estimated date of birth is:
A. July 2, 2011
B. July 7, 2011
C. August 16, 2011
D. August 21, 2011

32. A woman at 30 weeks of gestation assumes a supine position for a fundal measurement and Leopold maneuvers. She begins to complain about feeling dizzy and nauseated. Her skin feels damp and cool. The nurse's first action is to:
A. Assess the woman's blood pressure and pulse
B. Provide the woman with an emesis basin
C. Elevate the woman's legs 20 degrees from her hips
D. Turn the woman onto her side

33. During an early-bird prenatal class, a nurse teaches a group of newly diagnosed pregnant women about their emotional reactions during pregnancy. What topics should the nurse discuss with the women? (Circle all that apply.)
A. Sexual desire (libido) usually increases during the second trimester of pregnancy.
B. A referral for counseling should be sought if a woman experiences conflicting feelings about her pregnancy in the first trimester.
C. Rapid, unpredictable mood swings reflect gestational bipolar disorder.
D. A quiet period of introspection is often experienced around the time a woman feels her baby move for the first time.
E. A woman's own mother is usually her greatest source of emotional support during pregnancy.
F. Attachment to her baby begins late in the third trimester, when she begins attending childbirth preparation classes and realizes the baby will arrive soon.

34. The nurse evaluates a pregnant woman's knowledge about prevention of urinary tract infections at the prenatal visit following a class on infection prevention that the woman attended. The nurse recognizes that the woman needs further instruction when she tells the nurse about which measures that she now uses to prevent urinary tract infections? (Circle all that apply.)
    A. "I drink about one quart of fluid a day."
    B. "I have stopped using bubble baths and bath oils."
    C. "I have started wearing panty hose and underpants with a cotton crotch."
    D. "I have yogurt for lunch or as a bedtime snack every other day."
    E. "I only have intercourse with my husband once a week now because it could lead to bladder infections."
    F. "If I drink cranberry juice at least twice a day I will not get an infection."

35. Doulas are becoming important members of a laboring woman's health care team. Which activity should be expected as part of the doula's responsibilities?
    A. Monitoring hydration of the laboring woman, including adjusting IV flow rates
    B. Interpreting electronic fetal monitoring tracings to determine the well-being of the maternal-fetal unit
    C. Eliminating the need for the husband/partner to be present during labor and birth
    D. Providing continuous support throughout labor and birth, including explanations of labor progress

III. THINKING CRITICALLY

1. A health history interview of the pregnant woman by the nurse is included as part of the initial prenatal visit.
    A. STATE the purpose of the health history interview.

    B. WRITE two questions for each component that is included in the initial health history interview. Questions should be clear, concise, and understandable. Most of the questions should be open ended to elicit the most complete response from the client.

    C. WRITE four questions that should be included when doing an updating health history interview during follow-up visits.

2. IMAGINE that you are a nurse working in a prenatal clinic. You have been assigned to be the primary nurse for Martha, an 18-year-old, who has come to the clinic for confirmation of pregnancy. She tells you that she knows she is pregnant because she has already missed three periods, and a home pregnancy test that she did last week was positive. Martha states that she has had very little contact with the health care system, and the only reason she came today is because her boyfriend insisted that she "make sure" she is really pregnant. DESCRIBE the approach that you would take regarding data collection and nursing intervention that is appropriate for this woman.

3. Terry is a primigravida in her first trimester of pregnancy. She is accompanied by her husband, Tim, to her second prenatal visit. ANSWER each of the following questions asked by Terry and Tim:
   A. "At the last visit I was told that my baby's estimated date of birth is December 25, 2010! Can I really count on my baby being born on Christmas Day?"

   B. "Before I became pregnant, my friend told me I should be doing Kegel exercises. I was too embarrassed to ask her about them. What are they, and is it safe for me to do them while I am pregnant?"

   C. "What effect will pregnancy have on our sex life? We are willing to abstain during pregnancy if we must to keep our baby safe."

   D. "This morning sickness I am experiencing is driving me crazy. I become nauseated in the morning and again late in the afternoon. Occasionally I vomit or have the dry heaves. Will this last for my entire pregnancy? Is there anything I can do to feel better?"

4. Tara is 2 months pregnant. She tells the nurse at the prenatal clinic that she is used to being active and that she exercises every day. Now that she is pregnant she wonders if she should shorten or stop her exercise routine. DISCUSS the nurse's response to Tara.

5. WRITE one nursing diagnosis for each of the following situations. STATE one expected outcome, and LIST appropriate nursing measures for the nursing diagnosis you identified.
   A. Beth is 6 weeks pregnant. During the health history interview she tells you that she has limited her intake of fluids and tries to hold her urine as long as she can because "I just hate having to go to the bathroom so frequently."

Nursing Diagnosis	Expected Outcome	Nursing Measures

   B. Doris, who is 23 weeks pregnant, tells you that she is beginning to experience more frequent lower back pain. You note that when she walked into the examining room, her posture exhibited a moderate degree of lordosis and neck flexion. She was wearing shoes with 2-inch-high narrow heels.

Nursing Diagnosis	Expected Outcome	Nursing Measures

   C. Lisa, a primigravida at 32 weeks of gestation, comes for a prenatal visit accompanied by her partner, the father of the baby. They both express anxiety about the impending birth of the baby and how they will handle the experience of labor. Lisa is especially concerned about how she will survive the pain, and her partner is primarily concerned about how he will help Lisa cope with labor and make sure she and the baby are safe.

Nursing Diagnosis	Expected Outcome	Nursing Measures

6. Jane is a primigravida in her second trimester of pregnancy. ANSWER each of the following questions asked by Jane during a prenatal visit.
   A. "Why do you measure my abdomen every time I come in for a checkup?"

   B. "How can you tell if my baby is doing okay?"

   C. "I am going to start changing the way that I dress now that I am beginning to show. Do you have any suggestions I could follow, especially because I have a limited amount of money to spend?"

   D. "What can I do about gas and constipation? I never had much of a problem before I was pregnant."

   E. "Since yesterday I have started to feel itchy all over. Do you think I am coming down with some sort of infection?"

   F. "I will be flying out to Chicago to visit my father in 1 month. Is airline travel safe for me when I am 5 months pregnant?"

7. While a nurse is measuring a pregnant woman's fundus, the woman becomes pale and diaphoretic. The woman, who is at 23 weeks of gestation, states that she feels dizzy and lightheaded.
   A. STATE the most likely explanation for the assessment findings exhibited by this woman.

   B. DESCRIBE the nurse's immediate action.

8. Kelly is a primigravida in her third trimester of pregnancy. ANSWER each of the following questions asked by Kelly during a prenatal visit.
   A. "My husband and I have decided to breastfeed our baby, but friends told me it is very difficult if my nipples do not come out. Is there any way I can tell now if my nipples are okay for breastfeeding?"

   B. "My ankles are swollen by the time I get home from work late in the afternoon (Kelly teaches second grade). I have been trying to drink about 3 liters of fluid every day. Should I reduce the amount of liquid I am drinking or ask my doctor for a water pill?"

   C. "I woke up last night with a terrible cramp in my leg. It finally went away, but my husband and I just did not know what to do. What if this happens again tonight?"

9. Tanisha, a pregnant woman at 26 weeks of gestation, and her husband, George, tell the nurse at a prenatal visit that their friends who live in another state just had a baby 2 months ago and employed a doula to help them during childbirth. Their friends recommended that they do the same because the doula was wonderful. Tanisha and George are unsure whether they should spend the extra money, asking the nurse exactly what these doulas do and where they could find one.
   A. DESCRIBE what the nurse should tell this couple about the role of the doula during labor and birth including how it could be of benefit to them.

   B. STATE what the nurse should tell this couple about how to find a doula and the importance of interviewing her before they make a commitment to ensure that she is a good "fit" for them.

10. Carol is 4 months pregnant and is beginning to "show." She asks the nurse what she should expect as a reaction from her 13-year-old daughter and 3-year-old son. DESCRIBE the response the nurse would make.

11. Your neighbor, Jane Smith, is in her second month of pregnancy. Knowing that you are a nurse, her husband, Tom, confides in you that he just "cannot figure Jane out. One minute she is happy, and the next minute she is crying for no reason at all! I do not know how I will be able to cope with this for 7 more months."
    A. WRITE a nursing diagnosis and expected outcome that reflects Tom's concern.

    B. DISCUSS how you would respond to his concern.

12. Jim's partner, Mary, is 5 months pregnant. He tells you that sometimes he feels "left out" of Mary's pregnancy and asks you if he is important to Mary as her partner and the father of the baby. SPECIFY how you would answer his question.

13. Jennifer (2-1-0-0-1) and her husband, Dan, are beginning their third trimester of a low risk pregnancy. As you work with them on their birth plan, they tell you that they are having trouble making a decision about their choice of a birth setting. They experienced a delivery room birth with their first child. Jennifer states, "My first pregnancy was perfectly normal just like this one, but the birth was disappointing, so medically focused with monitors, IVs, and staying in bed." They ask you for your advice about the different birth settings they have heard and read about, namely labor, delivery, recovery, and postpartum (LDRP) rooms at their local hospital, the birthing center a few miles from their home, and even their own home. DESCRIBE the approach you would take to guide Jennifer and Dan in their decision making regarding a birth setting.

14. Tony and Andrea are considering the possibility of giving birth to their second baby at home. They have been receiving prenatal care from a certified nurse-midwife who has experience with home birth. Their 5-year-old son and both sets of grandparents want to be present for the birth.
    A. DISCUSS the decision-making process that Tony and Andrea should follow to ensure that they make an informed decision that is right for them and their family.

    B. Tony and Andrea decide that home birth is an ideal choice for them. OUTLINE the preparation measures you would recommend to Tony and Andrea to ensure a safe and positive experience for everyone.

CHAPTER 16

Labor and Birth Processes

I. REVIEWING KEY TERMS

FILL IN THE BLANKS: Insert the term that corresponds to each of the following descriptions.

1. ______________, ______________, ______________, ______________, and ______________. The five factors (5 Ps) affecting the process of labor and birth.
2. ______________ Membranous-filled spaces that are located where the sutures in the fetal/neonatal skull intersect.
3. ______________ Overlapping of the bones of the fetal skull that occurs during childbirth, thereby temporarily changing its shape and facilitating the skull's passage through the birth canal.
4. ______________ Part of the fetus that enters the pelvic inlet first and leads through the birth canal during labor. The three main types are ______________ (head first), ______________ (buttocks first), and ______________.
5. ______________ Part of the fetal body that is first felt by the examining finger during a vaginal examination. The four types are ______________, ______________, ______________, and ______________.
6. ______________ Presentation that occurs when the fetal head is fully flexed, making the fetal occiput the part first felt by the examining finger.
7. ______________ Relationship of the fetal spine (long axis) to the maternal spine (long axis). ______________ Term used when the spines are parallel. ______________ Term used when the spines are perpendicular (at right angles).
8. ______________ Relationship of the fetal body parts to one another. ______________ The most common type of relationship.
9. ______________ Largest transverse diameter of the fetal skull.
10. ______________ Smallest anteroposterior diameter of the fetal skull to enter the maternal pelvis when the fetal head is in complete flexion.
11. ______________ Relationship of the fetal presenting part (occiput, mentum, sacrum, scapula) to the four quadrants of the maternal pelvis.
12. ______________ This is said to have occurred when the largest transverse diameter of the presenting part has passed through the pelvic inlet and into the true pelvis, reaching the level of the ischial spines.
13. ______________ Relationship of the fetal presenting part to an imaginary line drawn between the ischial spines. It is measured in ______________ above or below the ischial spines, thereby serving as a method of determining the progress of fetal ______________.
14. ______________ Process of shortening and thinning of the cervix during the first stage of labor. Progress is expressed in percentages from 0% to 100%.

15. ______________________ Enlargement and widening of the cervical opening (os) and the cervical canal that occurs during labor. Progress is expressed in centimeters from less than 1 cm to 10 cm when complete.

16. ______________________ Descent of the fetal presenting part into the true pelvis approximately 2 weeks before term in the primigravida and in the multiparous woman once true labor is in progress.

17. ______________________ Primary powers of labor. They are responsible for ______________________ and ______________________.

18. ______________________ Secondary powers of labor accomplished when the woman bears down or pushes.

19. ______________________ Brownish or blood-tinged cervical mucoid discharge representing the passage of the mucous plug as the cervix ripens in preparation for labor.

20. ______________________ Term used to refer to the movements of the fetus in a vertex presentation as it turns and adjusts its head to facilitate passage through the maternal birth canal. These seven movements are ______________________, ______________________, ______________________, ______________________, ______________________, ______________________, and ______________________.

21. ______________________ Term used to refer to the maternal urge to bear down, which occurs when the fetal presenting part reaches the perineal floor stimulating stretch receptors and causing release of oxytocin.

22. ______________________ Pushing method characterized by a closed glottis with prolonged breath holding and bearing down.

23. The first stage of labor begins with the onset of ______________________ and ends with full ______________________. It is divided into three phases, namely, ______________________, ______________________, and ______________________.

24. The second stage of labor lasts from the time the ______________________ to the ______________________.

25. The third stage of labor lasts from the ______________________ until the ______________________.

26. The fourth stage of labor is the period of ______________________ when homeostasis is reestablished.

27. ______________________, ______________________, ______________________, and ______________________. Four factors that affect fetal circulation during labor.

II. REVIEWING KEY CONCEPTS

28. LABEL the following illustrations of the fetal skull and the maternal pelvis with the appropriate landmarks and diameters.

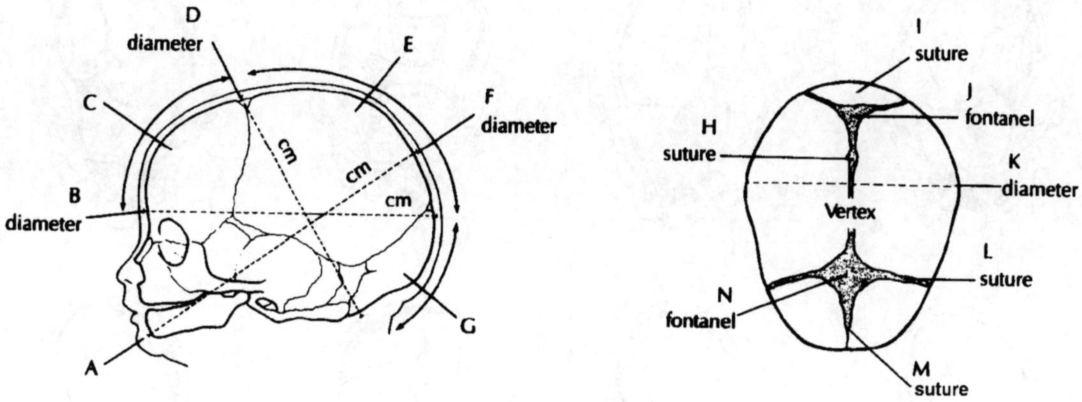

A **Fetal Skull**

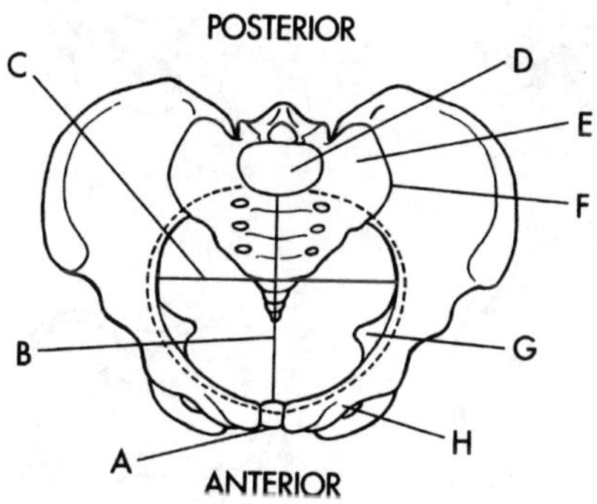

Pelvic Brim from Above

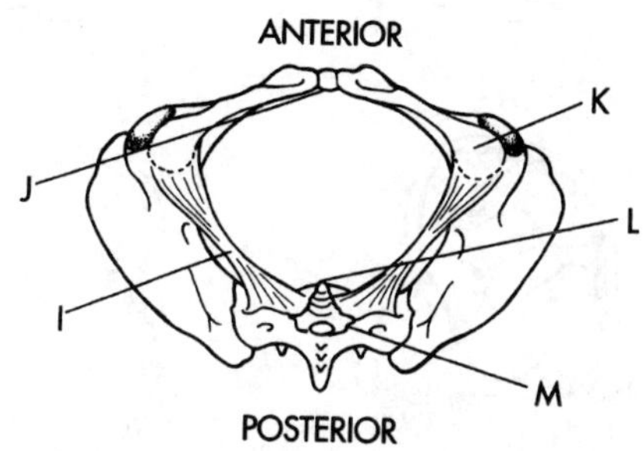

Pelvic Outlet from Above

B **Maternal Pelvis**

29. INDICATE the presentation, presenting part, position, lie, and attitude of the fetus for each of the following illustrations.

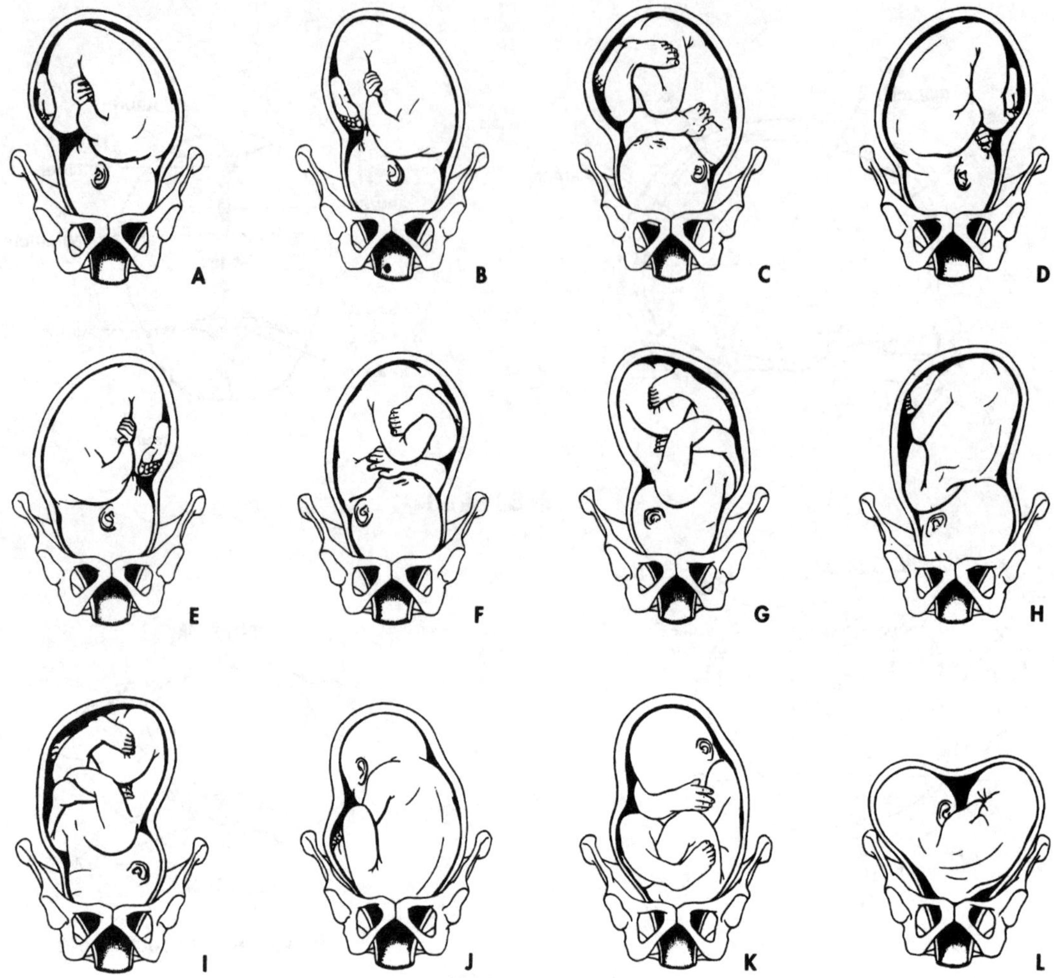

MULTIPLE CHOICE: Circle the correct option(s), and state the rationale for the option(s) chosen.

30. A vaginal examination during labor reveals the following information: LOA, –1, 75%, 3 cm. An accurate interpretation of these data includes: (Circle all that apply.)
   A. Attitude: flexed
   B. Station: 3 cm below the ischial spines
   C. Presentation: cephalic
   D. Lie: longitudinal
   E. Effacement: 75% complete
   F. Dilation: 9 cm more to reach full dilation

31. Changes occur as a woman progresses through labor. What maternal adaptations are expected during labor? (Circle all that apply.)
   A. Increase in both systolic and diastolic blood pressure during uterine contractions in the first stage of labor
   B. Decrease in white blood cell count
   C. Slight increase in baseline pulse and respiratory rates
   D. Decrease in gastric motility leading to nausea and vomiting, especially during the transition phase.
   E. Proteinuria 2+
   F. Hyperglycemia

32. When instructing a group of primigravid women about the onset of labor, the nurse tells them to be alert for:
    A. Urinary retention
    B. Weight gain of 2 kg
    C. Quickening
    D. Energy surge

III. THINKING CRITICALLY

1. During a prenatal class you are going to teach the women and their partners about the process of labor and how it progresses. You decide that the best approach is to use models and illustrations representing the 5 Ps of labor and the cardinal movements to describe the labor process.
   A. OUTLINE what you will present related to the 5 Ps. IDENTIFY the visual aids you will use.

   B. OUTLINE what you will present related to the cardinal movements. IDENTIFY the visual aids you will use.

2. As part of their care of the laboring woman, nurses perform vaginal examinations and interpret the results. STATE the meaning of each of the following vaginal examination findings.

EXAM I	EXAM II	EXAM III	EXAM IV
ROP	RMA	LST	OA
−1	0	+1	+3
50%	25%	75%	100%
3 cm	2 cm	6 cm	10 cm

3. Brooke is a primigravida. During a prenatal visit at 34 weeks of gestation, she asks you the following questions regarding her approaching labor. DESCRIBE how you would respond.
   A. "What gets labor to start?"

   B. "Are there things I should watch for that would tell me my labor is getting closer to starting?"

   C. "How long can I expect my labor to last once it gets started?"

   D. "My friend just had a baby, and she told me the nurses kept helping her to change her position, to get in and out of bed, and to walk! Isn't that dangerous for the baby and painful for the mom?"

CHAPTER 17

Pain Management

LEARNING KEY TERMS

MATCHING: Match the description in Column I with the appropriate pharmacologic method for pain management during childbirth in Column II.

COLUMN I

1. _______ Abolition of pain perception by interrupting nerve impulses to the brain. Loss of sensation (partial or complete) and sometimes loss of consciousness occurs.
2. _______ Method used to repair a tear or hole in the dura mater around the spinal cord as a result of spinal anesthesia; the goal is to prevent or treat postdural puncture headaches (PDPHs).
3. _______ Single-injection, subarachnoid anesthesia useful for pain control during vaginal or cesarean birth but not for labor.
4. _______ Systemic analgesic such as nalbuphine and butorphanol that relieves pain without causing significant maternal or neonatal respiratory depression and less likely to cause nausea and vomiting.
5. _______ Provides rapid perineal anesthesia for performing and repairing an episiotomy or lacerations.
6. _______ Anesthetic gas mixed with oxygen, which is inhaled beginning 30 seconds before the onset of a contraction to reduce but not eliminate pain during the first and second stages of labor.
7. _______ Injection of an opioid agonist analgesic into the spinal fluid to relieve pain associated with labor and following cesarean birth.
8. _______ Class of drug used to decrease anxiety, increase sedation, and reduce nausea and vomiting but which may impair the analgesic efficacy of opioids.
9. _______ Drug that promptly reverses the effects of opioids, including maternal and neonatal CNS depression especially respiratory depression.
10. _______ Systemic analgesic such as meperidine or fentanyl that relieves pain and creates a feeling of well-being, but can result in respiratory depression, nausea, and vomiting.
11. _______ Alleviation of pain sensation or raising of the pain threshold without loss of consciousness.
12. _______ Relief from pain of uterine contractions and birth by injecting a local anesthetic agent and/or an opioid agonist analgesic into the peridural space.
13. _______ Relief from pain in the lower vagina, vulva, and perineum, making it useful if an episiotomy is to be performed or forceps- or vacuum-assistance is required to facilitate birth.

COLUMN II

A. Opioid agonist-antagonist analgesic
B. Anesthesia
C. Analgesia
D. Phenothiazine
E. Epidural analgesia/anesthesia (block)
F. Autologous epidural blood patch
G. Local perineal infiltration anesthesia
H. Spinal anesthesia (block)
I. Opioid antagonist
J. Nitrous oxide
K. Pudendal nerve block
L. Opioid agonist analgesic
M. Intrathecal analgesia

FILL IN THE BLANKS: Insert the term that corresponds to each of the following descriptions.

14. ______________________________ Type of pain that predominates during the first stage of labor and is located over the lower abdomen; it results from cervical changes, distention of the lower uterine segment, and uterine ischemia.

15. ______________________________ Type of pain that predominates during the second stage of labor; it results from stretching and distention of perineal tissues and the pelvic floor to allow passage of the fetus, from distention and traction on the peritoneal and uterocervical supports during contractions, and from lacerations of soft tissues.

16. ______________________________ Type of pain felt in areas of the body other than the area of pain origin. During labor and birth, pain originating in the uterus radiates to the abdominal wall, lumbosacral area of the back, iliac crests, gluteal area, and down the thighs.

17. ______________________________ Theory of pain based on the principle that certain nerve cell groupings within the spinal cord, brainstem, and cerebral cortex have the ability to modulate the pain impulse through a blocking mechanism. According to this theory, pain sensations travel along sensory nerve pathways to the brain, but only a limited number of sensations or messages can travel through these nerve pathways at one time.

18. ______________________________ Endogenous opioids secreted by the pituitary gland that act on the central and peripheral nervous systems to reduce pain.

19. ______________________________ Paced breathing technique during which the woman breathes at approximately half her normal rate. It is usually the first technique used in early labor when the woman can no longer talk or walk her way through a contraction.

20. ______________________________ Paced breathing technique during which the woman breathes at an accelerated rate which should not exceed twice her resting respiratory rate.

21. ______________________________ Full breath taken at the beginning of a contraction to greet it and end of each contraction to blow it away.

22. ______________________________ Paced breathing technique that combines breaths and puffs in a ratio (e.g., 3:1 or 4:1) as a means to enhance concentration during the transition phase of the first stage of labor.

23. ______________________________ Rapid, deep breathing that can be an undesirable outcome of the more rapid and more shallow types of paced breathing techniques; it can result in ______________________________.

24. ______________________________ Light stroking of the abdomen or other body part in rhythm with breathing during contractions.

25. ______________________________ Steady pressure applied against the laboring woman's sacrum by the nurse or coach using the fist or heel of the hand or a firm object (e.g., tennis ball); it is especially helpful during back labor.

26. ______________________________ Nonpharmacologic comfort measure that uses the buoyancy of the warm water to provide support for tense muscles, relief from discomfort, and general body relaxation.

27. ______________________________ Nonpharmacologic pain control technique that involves placing two pairs of electrodes on either side of the woman's thoracic and sacral spine to provide continuous low-intensity electrical impulses or stimuli that can be increased during a contraction.

28. ______________________________ Nonpharmacologic pain control technique that is based on the application of pressure, heat, or cold on specific body points called tsubos.

29. ______________________________ Insertion of fine needles into specific areas of the body to restore the flow of qi (energy) and to decrease pain.

30. ______________________________ Technique that uses the concept of energy fields within the body called prana that are thought to be deficient in some people who are in pain. It involves the laying-on-of hands by a specially trained person to redirect energy fields associated with pain.

31. ______________________________ Form of deep relaxation, similar to daydreaming or meditation; the person enters a state of focused concentration and the subconscious mind can be more easily accessed.

32. ______________________________ Nonpharmacologic pain control technique based on the premise that a person can recognize his or her body's physical signals and use mental processes to change or control certain internal physiologic events.

33. ______________________ Use of essential oils from plants, flowers, herbs, and trees to promote health and well-being, enhance relaxation, and treat illnesses.

34. ______________________ Injection of small amounts of sterile water using a fine needle into four locations on the lower back to relieve low back pain.

35. ______________________ State of CNS depression in the newborn produced by an opioid.

II. REVIEWING KEY CONCEPTS

36. EXPLAIN the theoretic basis for using such techniques as massage, stroking, music, and imagery to reduce the sensation of pain during childbirth.

37. Nurses working on childbirth units must be knowledgeable regarding the use of a variety of nerve block analgesia and anesthesia methods to ensure that they manage them in a safe and effective manner. COMPLETE the following table by listing the effects, criteria/timing for use, and care management for each of the analgesic/anesthetic methods.

METHOD	EFFECTS	CRITERIA/TIMING	CARE MANAGEMENT
Local perineal infiltration anesthesia			
Pudendal nerve block			
Spinal anesthesia (block)			
Epidural anesthesia or analgesia (block)			
Combined spinal-epidural analgesia			
Epidural and intrathecal opioids			

MULTIPLE CHOICE: Circle the correct option(s), and state the rationale for the option(s) chosen.

38. In her birth plan, a woman requests that she be allowed to use the new whirlpool bath during labor. When implementing this woman's request, the nurse should:
    A. Assist the woman to maintain a reclining position when in the tub
    B. Tell the woman she will need to leave the tub as soon as her membranes rupture
    C. Begin hydrotherapy when the woman is in active labor
    D. Limit her to no longer than 1 hour in the tub

39. A variety of medications may be administered to women during labor. Which medication is used primarily to reduce anxiety and relieve nausea?
 A. naloxone (Narcan)
 B. hydroxyzine (Vistaril)
 C. butorphanol tartrate (Stadol)
 D. fentanyl citrate (Sublimaze)

40. The physician has ordered nalbuphine hydrochloride (Nubain) 10 mg IV every 3 to 4 hours as needed for pain associated with labor. In fulfilling this order, the nurse knows that:
 A. This medication is a potent opioid agonist analgesic
 B. The dosage of the analgesic is too high for IV administration, necessitating a new order
 C. This is the analgesic of choice if the laboring woman is opioid dependent
 D. This analgesic is unlikely to cause significant maternal or fetal/neonatal respiratory depression

41. Following administration of fentanyl (Sublimaze) IV for pain associated with uterine contractions, a woman's labor progresses more rapidly than expected. The physician orders that a stat dose of naloxone (Narcan) 1 mg IV be administered to the woman to reverse respiratory depression in the newborn after its birth. In fulfilling this order, the nurse knows that:
 A. Question the route because this medication should be administered orally
 B. Recognize that the dose is too low
 C. Assess the woman's level of pain because it will return abruptly
 D. Observe the maternal pulse for bradycardia

42. An anesthesiologist is preparing to begin a continuous epidural block using a combination local anesthetic and opioid analgesic as a pain relief measure for a laboring woman. Nursing measures related to this type of nerve block include: (Circle all that apply.)
 A. Assist the woman into a modified Sims position or upright position with back curved for administration of the block
 B. Alternate her position from side to side every hour
 C. Assess the woman for headaches because they commonly occur in the postpartum period if an epidural is used for labor
 D. Assist the woman to urinate at least every 2 hours during labor to prevent bladder distention
 E. Prepare the woman for use of forceps- or vacuum-assisted birth because she will be unable to bear down
 F. Assess blood pressure frequently because severe hypotension can occur

43. Administering an opioid antagonist to a woman who is opioid dependent will result in the opioid abstinence syndrome. The nurse would recognize which clinical manifestations as evidence that this syndrome is occurring? (Circle all that apply.)
 A. Yawning
 B. Coughing
 C. Piloerection
 D. Anorexia
 E. Dry skin, eyes, and nose
 F. Miosis

44. After induction of a spinal block in preparation for an elective cesarean birth, a woman's blood pressure decreases from 124/76 to 96/60. The nurse's initial action is to:
 A. Administer a vasopressor intravenously to raise the blood pressure
 B. Change the woman's position from supine to lateral
 C. Begin to administer oxygen by mask at 10 to 12 L/min
 D. Notify the woman's health care provider

III. THINKING CRITICALLY

1. You are caring for Latisha, a primigravida in active labor, and her partner. Her primary nursing diagnosis at this time is acute pain related to the processes involved in labor and birth. IDENTIFY the factors that you feel could influence this nursing diagnosis, and DESCRIBE how these factors influence Latisha's pain experience.

2. Martina is a primigravida in labor. She tells her nurse that she needs something for pain "NOW!"
   A. DESCRIBE the approach that Martina's nurse should use in responding to her request.

   B. The nurse prepares to administer meperidine hydrochloride (Demerol) 25 mg IV as ordered by Martina's primary health care provider. The nurse knows that this medication will not only affect Martina but also will cross her placenta and affect the fetus.
      1. IDENTIFY the maternal reactions to this medication for which the nurse must be alert when assessing Martina after the meperidine is administered.

      2. LIST three factors that influence the effect systemic analgesics have on the fetus/newborn.

      3. IDENTIFY the fetal/newborn effects that can occur after administration of meperidine.

3. A woman in labor asks the nurse why the pain medication she is getting is put into her IV tubing instead of into her buttocks like the last time she was in labor. EXPLAIN what the nurse should tell this woman about why the IV route is preferred to the IM route for the administration of systemic analgesics during labor.

4. A nurse working with a group of expectant fathers is asked if there really is "a physical reason for all the pain women say they feel when they are in labor." DESCRIBE the response that this nurse should give.

5. Nurses working on childbirth units must be sensitive to their clients' pain experiences.
   A. DESCRIBE how women experience pain during childbirth and how they will express it. CREATE a pain assessment guide that you can use in the clinical setting when caring for clients in pain, including women in labor.

   B. DESCRIBE specific measures nurses can use to alter the laboring woman's perception of pain.

6. On admission to the labor unit in the latent phase of labor, Kimberly (2-0-0-1-0) and her husband Maurice tell you that they are so glad they took Lamaze classes and did so much reading about childbirth. "We will not need any medication now that we know what to do. But most importantly, our baby will be safe!" DESCRIBE how you would respond if you were their primary nurse for childbirth.

7. IMAGINE you are the nurse manager of a labor and birth unit. Major renovations are being planned for your unit, and your input is required. You and your staff nurses believe that water therapy including the use of showers and whirlpool baths is a beneficial nonpharmacologic method to relieve pain and discomfort and to enhance the progress of labor. DISCUSS the rationale you would use to convince planners that installation of a shower and a whirlpool bath into each birthing room is cost-effective.

8. Tara has been in labor for 4 hours. Her blood pressure had been stable, averaging 130/80 when assessed between contractions, and the FHR pattern consistently exhibited criteria of a reassuring pattern. An epidural block was initiated. Shortly afterward during assessment of maternal vital signs and FHR, Tara's blood pressure decreased to 102/60 and the FHR pattern began to exhibit a decrease in rate and variability.
   A. STATE what Tara is experiencing. SUPPORT your answer, and EXPLAIN the physiologic basis for what is happening to Tara.

   B. WRITE a nursing diagnosis that reflects this occurrence.

   C. LIST the immediate nursing actions.

9. Moira, a primigravida, has elected to receive a continuous epidural block as her pharmacologic method of choice during childbirth.
   A. IDENTIFY the assessment procedures that should be used to determine Moira's readiness for the initiation of the epidural block.

B. DESCRIBE the preparation methods that should be implemented.

C. DESCRIBE two positions you could help Moira assume for the induction of the epidural block.

D. OUTLINE the nursing care management interventions recommended while Moira s receiving the epidural block to ensure her well-being and that of her fetus.

CHAPTER 18

Fetal Assessment During Labor

I. LEARNING KEY TERMS

MATCHING: Match the definition in Column I with the appropriate term related to FHR pattern from Column II.

COLUMN I

1. _______ Average FHR range of 110 to 160 beats/min at term as assessed during a 10-minute segment that excludes periodic or episodic changes and periods of marked variability.
2. _______ Persistent (10 minutes or longer) baseline FHR below 110 beats/min.
3. _______ Visually apparent decrease in the FHR of 15 beats/min or more below the baseline, that lasts more than 2 minutes but less than 10 minutes.
4. _______ Changes from baseline patterns in FHR that occur with uterine contractions.
5. _______ Persistent (10 minutes or longer) baseline FHR greater than 160 beats/min.
6. _______ Expected irregular fluctuations in the baseline FHR of 2 cycles per minute or greater as a result of the interaction of the sympathetic and parasympathetic nervous systems.
7. _______ Visually apparent gradual FHR decrease starting with the onset of a contraction in response to fetal head compression.
8. _______ Visually apparent gradual FHR decrease after the start of a uterine contraction in response to uteroplacental insufficiency; the lowest point occurs after the peak of the contraction and baseline rate is not usually regained until the uterine contraction is over.
9. _______ Visually abrupt FHR decrease any time during a contraction in response to umbilical cord compression.
10. _______ Visually apparent abrupt increase in the FHR of at least 15 beats/min or greater above the baseline rate that lasts 15 seconds or more with return to baseline less than 2 minutes from the beginning of the increase.
11. _______ Changes in FHR from baseline that are not associated with uterine contractions.

COLUMN II

A. Acceleration
B. Early deceleration
C. Variability
D. Late deceleration
E. Variable deceleration
F. Tachycardia
G. Prolonged deceleration
H. Bradycardia
I. Baseline FHR
J. Periodic changes
K. Episodic changes

FILL IN THE BLANKS: Insert the term that corresponds to each of the following descriptions related to fetal assessment.

12. ______________________ Deficiency of oxygen in the arterial blood.
13. ______________________ Inadequate supply of oxygen at the cellular level.
14. ______________________ Method of listening to fetal heart sounds at periodic intervals to assess the FHR using a Leff scope, DeLee-Hillis fetoscope, or an ultrasound device.

15. ______________________________ External monitoring instrument that works by reflecting high-frequency sound waves off the fetal heart and valves to assess and record the FHR pattern. It is placed over the area of ______________________________ after conductive gel is applied to its surface.

16. ______________________________ External monitoring instrument that measures uterine activity (e.g., frequency, regularity, and approximate duration of uterine contractions) transabdominally. It is placed over the ______________________________.

17. ______________________________ Internal monitoring instrument that is attached to the fetal presenting part to assess FHR pattern.

18. ______________________________ Internal monitoring instrument that is solid or fluid filled; it is inserted into the intrauterine cavity to measure uterine activity (e.g., frequency, duration, and intensity of uterine contractions).

19. ______________________________ Method of assessment that monitors fetal oxygen saturation levels.

20. ______________________________ Method used to obtain fetal blood in order to assess the pH of the blood.

21. ______________________________ Instillation of room-temperature isotonic fluid (e.g., normal saline or lactated Ringer's) into the uterine cavity if the volume of amniotic fluid is low to relieve intermittent cord compression that results in variable decelerations and transient fetal hypoxemia.

22. ______________________________ An abnormally small amount of amniotic fluid.

23. ______________________________ Absence of amniotic fluid.

24. ______________________________ Relaxation of the uterus that can be achieved through the administration of drugs that inhibit uterine contractions. The most commonly used for this purpose is ______________________________.

25. ______________________________ Assessment method used immediately after birth as an adjunct to the Apgar score; it measures pH, Po_2, and Pco_2 of the newborn's blood and reflects the acid-base status of the newborn at birth.

26. ______________________________ Group of interventions initiated when an abnormal (nonreassuring) FHR pattern is noted to improve uteroplacental perfusion and increase maternal oxygenation and cardiac output. Basic corrective measures include ______________________________, ______________________________, and ______________________________.

II. REVIEWING KEY CONCEPTS

27. It is critical that a nurse working on a labor unit be knowledgeable concerning factors associated with a reduction in fetal oxygen supply, characteristics of normal (reassuring) and abnormal (nonreassuring) FHR patterns, and the characteristics of normal uterine activity.
    A. DESCRIBE the factors associated with a reduction in fetal oxygen supply.

    B. STATE the characteristics of normal (reassuring) FHR patterns.

C. STATE the characteristics of abnormal (nonreassuring) FHR patterns.

D. STATE the characteristics of normal uterine activity during labor.

E. STATE the meaning and criteria for each of the following categories of FHR tracings:
- Category I

- Category II

- Category III

FILL IN THE BLANKS: In general, the recommended frequency of FHR assessment depends on the risk status of the mother and the stage of labor. Insert the appropriate time for each of the following assessment recommendations:

28. Low risk client (risk factors are absent during labor): Auscultate FHR or assess tracing every ______________________ in the first stage of labor and every ______________________ in the second stage of labor.
29. High risk client (risk factors are present during labor): Auscultate FHR or assess tracing every ______________________ in the first stage of labor and every ______________________ in the second stage of labor.

30. The five essential components of the FHR tracing that must be evaluated at the recommended frequency for the maternal risk status are ______________________, ______________________, ______________________, ______________________, and ______________________.

31. STATE the legal responsibilities related to fetal monitoring for nurses who care for women during childbirth.

MULTIPLE CHOICE: Circle the correct option(s) and state the rationale for the option(s) chosen.

32. A laboring woman's uterine contractions are being internally monitored. When evaluating the monitor tracing, which finding is a source of concern and requires further assessment?
    A. Frequency every 2½ to 3 minutes
    B. Duration of 80 to 85 seconds
    C. Intensity during a uterine contraction of 85 to 90 mm Hg
    D. Average resting pressure of 20 to 25 mm Hg

33. External electronic fetal monitoring will be used for a woman just admitted to the labor unit in active labor. Guidelines the nurse should follow when implementing this form of monitoring are to: (Circle all that apply.)
    A. Use Leopold maneuvers to determine correct placement of the tocotransducer
    B. Assist the woman to maintain a dorsal recumbent position to ensure accurate monitor tracings that can be easily evaluated
    C. Apply contact gel to the ultrasound transducer prior to application over the point of maximum intensity
    D. Reposition the tocotransducer when the fetus changes its position
    E. Caution the woman to avoid effleurage when the transducers are in place
    F. Palpate the fundus periodically to estimate the intensity of the uterine contractions

34. A nurse caring for women in labor should be aware of signs characterizing normal (reassuring) and abnormal (nonreassuring) FHR patterns. What would be characteristic of abnormal patterns?
    A. Moderate baseline variability
    B. Average baseline FHR of 100 beats/min
    C. Acceleration of the FHR with movement
    D. Late deceleration patterns approximately every three or four contractions
    E. FHR of 170 beats/min between contractions
    F. Early deceleration patterns when the cervix dilated to 7 cm

35. A laboring woman's temperature is elevated as a result of an upper respiratory infection. The FHR pattern that reflects maternal fever is:
    A. Diminished variability
    B. Variable decelerations
    C. Tachycardia
    D. Early decelerations

36. A nulliparous woman is in the active phase of labor and her cervix has progressed to 6 cm dilation. The nurse caring for this woman evaluates the external monitor tracing and notes the following: decrease in FHR shortly after onset of several uterine contractions returning to baseline rate by the end of the contraction; shape is uniform. Based on these findings, the nurse should:
    A. Change the woman's position to her left side
    B. Document the finding on the woman's chart
    C. Notify the physician
    D. Perform a vaginal examination to check for cord prolapse

37. When evaluating the external fetal monitor tracing of a woman whose labor is being induced, the nurse identifies signs of persistent late deceleration patterns and begins intrauterine resuscitation interventions. What indicates that the appropriate interventions were implemented in the recommended order of priority?
    1. Increase rate of maintenance IV solution.
    2. Palpate uterus for tachysystole.
    3. Discontinue oxytocin (Pitocin) infusion.
    4. Change maternal position to a lateral position, then elevate her legs if woman is hypotensive.
    5. Administer oxygen at 8 to 10L/min by nonrebreather face mask.
       A. 2, 1, 5, 4, 3
       B. 4, 1, 2, 3, 5
       C. 5, 3, 4, 1, 2
       D. 4, 5, 1, 2, 3

III. THINKING CRITICALLY

1. Nurses working on a childbirth unit at a small rural hospital primarily use intermittent auscultation with an ultrasound fetoscope to assess fetal health and well-being during the labors of low risk women.
   A. STATE the advantages and disadvantages of intermittent auscultation as a method of fetal assessment during childbirth.

   B. CREATE a protocol that these nurses could follow when monitoring the fetus using the intermittent auscultation method.

2. A nurse caring for a laboring woman in active labor notes an abnormal (nonreassuring) FHR pattern when evaluating the monitor tracing. DESCRIBE the action the nurse should take based on this finding.

3. Darlene, a primigravida in active labor, has just been admitted to the labor unit. She becomes very anxious when external electronic monitoring equipment is set up. She tells the nurse that her father had a heart attack 2 months ago. "He was so sick they had to put him on a monitor, too. Does this mean that my baby has a heart problem just like my father?"
   A. DESCRIBE the response this nurse should make to address Darlene's expressed concern.

B. OUTLINE the care measures that this nurse should implement to ensure that the EFM is used in an effective manner to provide accurate data and to ensure that Darlene remains comfortable during this assessment technique.

4. Terry is a primigravida at 43 weeks of gestation. Her labor is being stimulated with oxytocin administered IV. Her contractions have been increasing in intensity with a frequency of every 2 to 2½ minutes and a duration of 80 to 85 seconds. She is currently in a supine position with a 30-degree elevation of her head. On observation of the monitor tracing, you note that during the last two contractions the FHR decreased after the contraction peaked and did not return to baseline until about 10 seconds into the rest period. A slight decrease in variability and baseline rate was observed.
   A. IDENTIFY the pattern described and the possible factors responsible for it.

   B. DESCRIBE the actions you would take. State the rationale for each action.

5. Taisha is a multiparous client in active labor. Her membranes rupture and the nurse caring for her immediately evaluates the EFM tracing.
   A. What type of periodic FHR pattern would the nurse be alert for when evaluating the tracing? EXPLAIN the rationale for your answer.

   B. STATE the actions the nurse should take in order of priority if the pattern is noted.

CHAPTER 19

Nursing Care of the Family During Labor and Birth

I. LEARNING KEY TERMS

FILL IN THE BLANKS: Insert the term that corresponds to each of the following descriptions related to the process of labor.

1. The first stage of labor begins with the onset of ______________ and ends with complete cervical ______________ and ______________. A blood- tinged mucous discharge (bloody show) from the vagina usually indicates the passage of the ______________.
2. During the latent phase of the first stage of labor the cervix dilates up to ______________ cm in approximately ______________ to ______________ hours. Cervical dilation progresses from ______________ to ______________ cm in about ______________ to ______________ hours during the active phase of the first stage of labor. The duration of the transition phase is approximately ______________ to ______________ minutes and the cervix dilates from ______________ to ______________ cm.
3. The second stage of labor is the stage in which the ______________. It begins with full cervical ______________ and complete ______________ It ends with the ______________. This stage is divided into the ______________ phase, a period of rest and calm (laboring down) and the phase of ______________ (descent). The only certain objective sign that the second stage has begun is the inability to feel the ______________ during a vaginal examination.
4. The third stage of labor lasts from the ______________ until the ______________ Detachment of the placenta from the wall of the uterus or separation is indicated by a firmly contracting ______________, change in the shape of the uterus from ______________ to ______________, a sudden ______________ from the introitus, apparent ______________, and the finding of ______________ or of ______________ at the introitus.
5. The fourth stage of labor is considered to be the first ______________ after birth. During this stage the mother and newborn recover from the physical process of childbirth and get to know each other.
6. ______________ Federal regulation enacted to ensure that pregnant women obtain the care they require during emergencies and when in labor.
7. ______________ Graphic chart on which cervical dilation and station are plotted to assist in early identification of deviations from expected labor patterns.

8. ______________________________ Trained experienced female labor attendant who provides a continuous one-on-one caring presence throughout the labor and birth of the woman she is attending.

9. ______________________________ Traditional labor position in which the woman lies on her back with her legs raised in stirrups.

MATCHING: Match the description in Column I with the appropriate term from Column II.

COLUMN I

10. ________ Appearance of fetal intestinal contents in the amniotic fluid, giving it a greenish color.
11. ________ Prolonged breath holding while bearing down (closed glottis pushing).
12. ________ Burning sensation of acute pain as vagina stretches and crowning occurs.
13. ________ Artificial rupture of membranes (AROM, ARM).
14. ________ Occurs when widest part of the head (biparietal diameter) distends the vulva just before birth.
15. ________ Incision into perineum to enlarge the vaginal outlet.
16. ________ Test to determine if membranes have ruptured by assessing pH of the fluid.
17. ________ Technique used to control birth of fetal head and protect perineal musculature.
18. ________ Method of breathing during bearing-down efforts characterized by a strong expiratory grunt or groan.
19. ________ Expulsion of placenta with fetal side emerging first.
20. ________ Cord encircles the fetal neck.
21. ________ Method used to palpate fetus through abdomen.
22. ________ Occurs when pressure of presenting part against pelvic floor stretch receptors results in a woman's perception of an urge to bear down.
23. ________ Frondlike crystalline pattern created by amniotic fluid when it is placed on a glass slide.
24. ________ Classification of medication that stimulates the uterus to contract (a uterotonic).
25. ________ Expulsion of placenta with maternal surface emerging first.
26. ________ Application of a gentle yet steady force with hands pressed against the uterus.
27. ________ Protrusion of umbilical cord in advance of the presenting part.

COLUMN II

A. Ritgen maneuver
B. Episiotomy
C. Oxytocic
D. Ferguson reflex
E. Shultz mechanism
F. Valsalva maneuver
G. Ring of fire
H. Crowning
I. Duncan mechanism
J. Amniotomy
K. Nuchal cord
L. Prolapse of umbilical cord
M. Nitrazine test
N. Leopold maneuvers
O. Ferning
P. Meconium staining
Q. Open-glottis pushing
R. Fundal pressure

FILL IN THE BLANKS: Insert the term that corresponds to each of the following descriptions related to the characteristics of the powers of labor (view Fig. 19-7 as you work on inserting the terms).

28. ______________________________ The primary powers of labor that act involuntarily to expel the fetus and the placenta from the uterus.

29. ______________________________ "Building up" of a contraction from its onset.

30. ______________________________ The peak of a contraction with an intrauterine pressure less than 80 mm Hg.

31. ______________________________ "Letting down" of a contraction.

32. ______________________________ How often uterine contractions occur; the time that elapses from the beginning of one contraction to the beginning of the next contraction.

33. ______________________________ The strength of a contraction at its peak.

34. ______________________________ The time that elapses between the onset and the end of a contraction.

35. ______________________________ The tension of the uterine muscle between contractions.

36. ______________________________ Period of rest between contractions.

37. ______________________________ An involuntary urge to push in response to the Ferguson reflex.

II. REVIEWING KEY CONCEPTS

38. When caring for women in labor a nurse should periodically palpate the uterus during and between contractions. DESCRIBE how the nurse should assess frequency, duration, intensity, and relaxation using palpation.

39. Laura (3-1-1-0-1) has just been admitted in the latent phase of the first stage of labor. As part of the admission procedure, you review her prenatal record and interview her regarding what she has observed regarding her labor and discuss her current health status.

    A. LIST the essential data you would need to obtain from her prenatal record to plan appropriate care for Laura.

    B. IDENTIFY the information required regarding the status of Laura's labor.

    C. STATE the information required regarding Laura's current health status.

40. A nurse caring for a laboring woman needs to be alert for signs indicative of obstetric emergencies during labor. STATE the signs reflecting each of the following emergencies and EXPLAIN what the nurse should do if a laboring woman exhibits signs that the emergency is occurring.

    Abnormal (nonreassuring) fetal heart rate and pattern

    Inadequate uterine relaxation

Vaginal bleeding

Infection

Prolapse of the cord

41. IDENTIFY two advantages for each of the following labor positions.
    Semirecumbent

    Upright

    Lateral

    Hands and knees

42. OUTLINE the critical factors to be included in the physical assessment of the maternal-fetal unit during labor.

43. INDICATE the laboratory and diagnostic tests that are recommended during labor. State the purpose for each.

44. IDENTIFY the factors that can influence the duration of the second stage of labor.

45. DESCRIBE the maternal positions recommended to enhance the effectiveness of a woman's bearing-down efforts during the second stage of labor. STATE the basis for each position's effectiveness in facilitating the descent and birth of the fetus.

46. EXPLAIN why the nurse should encourage a woman planning to breastfeed to begin breastfeeding during the fourth stage of labor.

MULTIPLE CHOICE: Circle the correct option(s) and state the rationale for the option(s) chosen.

47. Following spontaneous rupture of the membranes, a variable deceleration pattern appears on the monitor tracing and the umbilical cord is observed to be protruding slightly below the vaginal introitus. It is essential that the nurse caring for this woman perform which of the following measures to prevent fetal hypoxia: (Circle all that apply.)
    A. Elevate the woman's legs
    B. Call someone to notify the woman's primary health care provider
    C. Insert fingers into the vagina and push up against the presenting part
    D. Administer oxygen at 8 to 10L/min via a face mask
    E. Place the woman in a modified Sims position
    F. Wrap the cord with a compress saturated in cool tap water

48. A primigravida calls the hospital and tells a nurse on the labor unit that she knows that she is in labor. The nurse's initial response is:
A. "Tell me why you know that you are in labor."
B. "How far do you live from the hospital?"
C. "When is your expected date of birth?"
D. "Have your membranes ruptured?"

49. A woman's amniotic membranes have apparently ruptured. The nurse assesses the fluid to determine its characteristics and confirm membrane rupture. An expected assessment finding of membrane rupture is:
A. pH 5.5
B. Absence of ferning
C. Pale straw-colored fluid with white flecks
D. Strong odor

50. When admitting a primigravida to the labor unit, the nurse observes for signs that indicate that the woman is in true labor and should be admitted. The nurse recognizes which of the followinge signs as indicative of true labor: (Circle all that apply.)
A. Woman reports that her contractions seem stronger since she walked from the car to her room on the labor unit
B. Cervix feels soft and is 50% effaced
C. Woman perceives pain to be in her back or abdomen above the level of the navel
D. Fetus is engaged in the pelvis at zero station
E. Cervix is in the posterior position
F. Woman continues to feel her contractions intensify following a back rub and with use of effleurage

51. A vaginal examination is performed on a multiparous woman who is in labor. The results of the examination were documented as 4 cm, 75%, +2, LOT. An accurate interpretation of these data is that:
A. Woman is in the latent phase of the first stage of labor
B. Station is 2 cm above the ischial spines
C. Presentation is cephalic
D. Lie is transverse

52. A physical care measure for a laboring woman that has been identified as unlikely to be beneficial and may even be harmful is:
A. Allowing the laboring woman to drink fluids and eat light solids as tolerated
B. Administering a Fleet enema at admission
C. Ambulating periodically throughout labor as tolerated
D. Using a whirlpool bath once active labor is established

III. THINKING CRITICALLY

1. Alice, a primigravida, calls the labor unit. She tells the nurse that she thinks she is in labor. "I have had some pains for about 2 hours. Should my husband bring me to the hospital now?"
A. DESCRIBE how the nurse should approach this situation.

B. WRITE several questions the nurse could use to elicit the appropriate information required to determine the course of action required.

C. Based on the data collected during the telephone interview, the nurse determines that Alice is in very early labor. Because she lives fairly close to the hospital, she is instructed to stay home until her labor progresses. OUTLINE the instructions and recommendations for care Alice and her husband should be given.

2. ANALYZE the assessment findings documented for each of the following women.

Denise (2-0-0-1-0)	Teresa (4-3-0-0-3)	Danielle (2-1-0-0-1)
5 cm	9 cm	2 cm
moderate	very strong	mild
q4 min	q2-3 min	q6-8 min
40-55 sec	65-75 sec	30-35 sec
0	+2	–1

A. IDENTIFY the phase of labor being experienced by each woman.

B. DESCRIBE the behavior and appearance you would expect to be exhibited by each woman.

C. SPECIFY the physical care and emotional support measures you would implement if you were caring for each of these women.

D. Denise's husband, Sam, is her major support person during labor. The nurse observes that he is beginning to appear fatigued and "stressed" after being with Denise since her admission 5 hours ago. DESCRIBE the actions this nurse can take to support Sam and his efforts to care for Denise.

3. DESCRIBE the procedure that should be followed before auscultating the FHR or applying an ultrasound transducer to the abdomen of a laboring woman. EXPLAIN the rationale for using this procedure.

4. Tonya, a client in active labor, begins to cry during a vaginal examination to assess her status. "Why not watch the monitor to see how I am progressing instead of doing these vaginal exams? They really hurt and they are embarrassing!"
   A. DESCRIBE the response the nurse should make to Tonya's concern.

   B. DISCUSS the measures the nurse could use to meet Tonya's safety and comfort needs during a vaginal examination.

5. Tasha is dilated 6 cm. Her coach comes to tell you that her "water just broke with a gush!" IDENTIFY each action you would take in this situation, in order of priority. STATE the rationale for the actions you have identified.

6. Sara, a 17-year-old primigravida, is admitted in the latent phase of labor. Her boyfriend, Dan, is with her as her only support. They appear committed to each other. During the admission interview Sara tells you that they did not go to any classes because she was embarrassed about not being married. Both Sara and Dan appear very nervous, and assessment indicates they know little about what is happening, what to expect, and how to work together with the process of labor. IDENTIFY the nursing diagnosis reflected in these data. STATE one expected outcome and LIST nursing measures appropriate for the diagnosis you identified.

Nursing Diagnosis	Expected Outcome	Nursing Measures

7. Identifying a laboring couple's cultural and religious beliefs and practices regarding childbirth is a critical factor in providing culturally sensitive care that enhances the couple's sense of control and eventual satisfaction with their childbirth experience.
   A. LIST the questions you would ask when assessing a couple's cultural and religious preferences for childbirth.

   B. DISCUSS the importance of considering the couple's cultural and religious preferences when planning and implementing care.

8. Cori (4-3-0-0-3) is in latent labor. She and her husband are being oriented to the birthing room. Their last birth occurred in a delivery room 10 years ago. Both she and her husband are amazed by the birthing room and the birthing bed that will allow her to give birth in an upright position. They are also informed that changes in bearing-down efforts now allow a woman to follow her own body feelings and even to vocalize with pushing. Both Cori and her husband state that with every other birth they put her legs in stirrups, she held her breath for as long as she could, and pushed quietly. "Everything turned out okay, so why should we change?" DESCRIBE the response the primary nurse caring for this couple should make to their concerns.

9. A nurse living in a rural area is called to her neighbor's home to assist his wife who is in labor. "Everything is happening so fast. She says she is ready to deliver!"
   A. IDENTIFY the measures the nurse can use to reassure and comfort the woman.

   B. Shortly after the nurse arrives, crowning begins. STATE what the nurse should do.

   C. DESCRIBE the action the nurse should take after the birth of the head.

   D. LIST the measures the nurse should use to prevent excessive neonatal heat loss after its birth.

   E. IDENTIFY the infection control measures that should be implemented during a home birth.

   F. SPECIFY the measures the nurse should use to prevent excessive maternal blood loss or hemorrhage until the ambulance arrives.

   G. OUTLINE the information the nurse should document regarding the childbirth.

10. Beth is in the descent phase of the second stage of labor. She is actively pushing/bearing down to facilitate birth. INDICATE the criteria a nurse would use to evaluate the correctness of Beth's technique.

11. IMAGINE that you are participating in a panel discussion on childbirth practices. Your topic is "Episiotomy—is it needed to ensure the safety and well-being of the laboring woman and her fetus?" OUTLINE the information you would include in your presentation.

12. Imagine that you are a staff nurse on a childbirth unit. Your hospital is instituting a change in policy that would allow the participation of children in the labor and birth process of their mother. You are asked to be a part of the committee that will formulate the guidelines regarding sibling participation during childbirth. DISCUSS the suggestions you would make to help ensure a positive outcome for parents, children, and health care providers.

13. Annie is a primipara in the fourth stage of labor following a long and difficult childbirth process.
    A. IDENTIFY the essential nursing assessment and care measures required to insure Annie's safety and recovery during this stage of her labor.

    B. As she performs the first assessment, the nurse notes that Annie seems disinterested in her baby. She looks him over quickly and then asks the nurse to take him back to the nursery. IDENTIFY the factors that could be accounting for Annie's behavior.

    C. DISCUSS the nursing measures you would use to encourage future maternal-newborn interactions and facilitate the attachment process.

14. Felisha is a primipara who gave birth to a baby girl 15 minutes ago. Her baby is very alert and interacting well with both parents. The nurse encourages her to attempt to breastfeed her baby, but Felisha asks why she needs to breastfeed now because she feels a little tired and is unsure about what to do. DESCRIBE the approach this nurse should take to assist Felisha to breastfeed comfortably. INCLUDE a response to her question about why breastfeeding her newborn during the fourth stage of labor is beneficial to her and her baby.

CHAPTER 20

Postpartum Physiology

I. LEARNING KEY TERMS

FILL IN THE BLANKS: Insert the term that corresponds to each of the following descriptions.

1. ______________________________ Profuse sweating that occurs after birth, especially at night, to rid the body of fluid retained during pregnancy.
2. ______________________________ Uncomfortable uterine cramping that occurs during the early postpartum period as a result of periodic relaxation and vigorous contractions.
3. ______________________________ The lactogenic hormone secreted by the pituitary gland of lactating women.

   ______________________________ is another pituitary hormone that is responsible for uterine contraction and the let-down reflex.
4. ______________________________ Surgical incision of the perineum to facilitate birth.
5. ______________________________ Failure of the uterine muscle to contract firmly. It is the most frequent cause of excessive postpartum bleeding.
6. ______________________________ An anal varicosity.
7. ______________________________ Return of the uterus to a nonpregnant state.
8. ______________________________ The self-destruction of excess hypertrophied uterine tissue as a result of the decrease in estrogen and progesterone level following birth.
9. ______________________________; ______________________________ Terms used interchangeably with *postpartum* to refer to the period of recovery after childbirth that lasts approximately 6 weeks, although the time can vary from woman to woman.
10. ______________________________ Separation of the abdominal wall muscles related to the effect of the enlargement of the uterus on the abdominal musculature.
11. ______________________________ Post-childbirth uterine discharge or flow.
12. ______________________________ The bright red bloody uterine discharge that occurs for the first few days following birth; it consists primarily of blood and decidual tissue and trophoblastic debris and may contain small clots.
13. ______________________________ The pink to brownish uterine discharge that begins about 3 to 4 days after birth; it consists of old blood, serum, leukocytes, and tissue debris and continues for 10 to 14 days.
14. ______________________________ The yellowish white flow that begins about 10 days after birth and continues for 2 to 6 weeks; it consists of leukocytes, decidua, epithelial cells, mucous, serum, and bacteria.
15. ______________________________ Term used to describe distended, firm, tender, and warm breasts during the postpartum period.
16. ______________________________ Failure of the uterus to return to a nonpregnant state. The most common causes for this failure are retained ______________________________ and ______________________________.
17. ______________________________ Medication usually administered IV or IM immediately after expulsion of the placenta to ensure that the uterus remains firm and well contracted.
18. ______________________________ Discomfort or pain with intercourse.

19. ______________________ Exercises that help strengthen perineal muscles and encourage healing.

20. ______________________ Yellowish fluid produced in the breasts before lactation.

21. ______________________ Increased production of urine that occurs in the postpartum period to rid the body of excess tissue fluid retained during pregnancy.

22. ______________________ Lengthening and weakening of the fascial supports of pelvic structures, which include the uterus, vagina, urethra, bladder, and rectum.

II. REVIEWING KEY CONCEPTS

23. When caring for a woman following vaginal birth, it is of critical importance for the nurse to assess the woman's bladder for distention.
    A. EXPLAIN why bladder distention is more likely to occur during the immediate postpartum period.

    B. IDENTIFY the problems that can occur if the bladder is allowed to become distended.

24. CITE the factors that can interfere with bowel elimination in the postpartum period.

25. EXPLAIN why hypovolemic shock is less likely to occur in the postpartum woman experiencing a normal or average blood loss.

26. INDICATE the factors that place a postpartum woman at increased risk for the development of thrombophlebitis.

27. COMPARE AND CONTRAST the characteristics of lochial bleeding and nonlochial bleeding.

MULTIPLE CHOICE: Circle the correct option(s) and state the rationale for the option(s) chosen.

28. A nurse has assessed a woman who gave birth vaginally 12 hours ago. Which finding would require further assessment?
    A. Bright to dark red uterine discharge
    B. Midline episiotomy—approximated, moderate edema, slight erythema, absence of ecchymosis
    C. Protrusion of abdomen with sight separation of abdominal wall muscles
    D. Fundus firm at 1 cm above the umbilicus and to the right of midline

29. A woman, 24 hours after giving birth, complains to the nurse that her sleep was interrupted the night before because of sweating and the need to have her gown and bed linen changed. The nurse's first action is to:
    A. assess this woman for signs of infection
    B. explain to the woman that the sweating represents her body's attempt to eliminate the fluid that was accumulated during pregnancy
    C. notify her physician of the finding
    D. document the finding as postpartum diaphoresis

30. Which woman at 24 hours following birth is least likely to experience afterpains?
    A. Primipara who is breastfeeding her twins that were born at 38 weeks of gestation
    B. Multipara who is breastfeeding her 10-pound full-term baby girl
    C. Multipara who is bottle feeding her 8-pound baby boy
    D. Primipara who is bottle feeding her 7-pound baby girl

III. THINKING CRITICALLY

1. DESCRIBE how you would respond to each of the following typical questions/concerns of postpartum women.
   A. Mary is a primipara who is breastfeeding. "Why am I experiencing so many painful cramps in my uterus? I thought this happens only in women who have had babies before."

   B. Susan is being discharged after giving birth 20 hours ago. "For how many days should I be able to palpate my uterus to make sure it is firm?"

   C. June is a primipara. "My friend, who had a baby last year, said she had a flow for 6 weeks. Isn't that a long time to bleed after having a baby?"

D. Jean is 24 hours postpartum. "I cannot believe it—I look as if I am still pregnant! How can this be?"

E. Marion is 1 day postpartum. "It seems like I am urinating all the time—do you think that I have a bladder infection?"

F. Joan is a primipara who is breastfeeding her baby. "My friend told me that I cannot get pregnant as long as I continue to breastfeed. This is great because I do not like to use birth control."

G. Alice, a multipara, is concerned. She states, "My doctor is not going to give me a drug to dry up my breasts like I had with my first baby. How will my breasts ever get back to normal now?"

H. Andrea, a primipara, is 1 day postpartum. While breastfeeding her baby she confides to the nurse that she does not know how long she will continue to breastfeed. "My husband and I have always had a satisfying sex life, but my friend told me that as long as I breastfeed, intercourse is painful."

CHAPTER 21

Nursing Care of the Family During the Postpartum Period

I. LEARNING KEY TERMS

FILL IN THE BLANKS: Insert the term that corresponds to each of the following descriptions regarding the postpartum period.

1. ______________________ Nursing care management approach in which one nurse cares for both the mother and her infant. It is also called ______________________.
2. ______________________ Term used for the decreasing length of hospital stays of mothers and their babies after low risk births. Other terms used are ______________________ and ______________________.
3. ______________________ Classification of medications that stimulate contraction of the uterine smooth muscle.
4. ______________________ Failure of the uterine muscle to contract firmly. It is the most frequent cause for excessive bleeding following childbirth.
5. ______________________ Perineal treatment that involves sitting in warm water for approximately 20 minutes to soothe and cleanse the site and to increase blood flow, thereby enhancing healing.
6. ______________________ Menstrual-like cramps experienced by many women as the uterus contracts after childbirth.
7. ______________________ Dilation of the blood vessels supplying the intestines as a result of the rapid decease in intraabdominal pressure after birth. It causes blood to pool in the viscera and thereby contributes to a drop in blood pressure called ______________________ when the woman who has recently given birth sits or stands, first ambulates, or takes a warm shower.
8. ______________________ Complaint of pain in calf muscles when the foot is sharply dorsiflexed; it could signal the presence of a deep vein thrombosis (DVT).
9. ______________________ Exercises that can assist women to regain muscle tone that is often lost when pelvic tissues are stretched and torn during pregnancy and birth.
10. ______________________ Swelling of breast tissue caused by increased blood and lymph supply to the breasts as the body begins the process of lactation; it occurs about 72 to 96 hours after birth.
11. ______________________ Vaccine that can be given to postpartum women whose antibody titer is less than 1:8 or whose EIA level is less than 0.8. It is used to prevent nonimmune women from contracting this TORCH infection during a subsequent pregnancy.
12. ______________________ Blood product that is administered to Rh-negative, antibody (Coombs')-negative women who give birth to Rh-positive newborns. It is administered at 28 weeks of gestation and again within 72 hours after birth.
13. ______________________ Telephone-based postpartum consultation service that can provide information and support; it is not a crisis intervention line to be used for emergencies.

II. REVIEWING KEY CONCEPTS

14. A postpartum woman at 6 hours after a vaginal birth is having difficulty voiding. LIST the measures that you would try to help this woman void spontaneously.

15. IDENTIFY the measures the nurse should teach a postpartum woman in an effort to prevent the development of thrombophlebitis.

16. STATE the two most important interventions that can be used to prevent excessive postpartum bleeding in the early postpartum period. Indicate the rationale for the effectiveness of each intervention you identified.

17. A nurse is planning a home visit to a woman who gave birth 5 days ago. What signs, if exhibited by the woman, indicate the potential for postpartum psychosocial complications?

MULTIPLE CHOICE: Circle the correct option(s) and state the rationale for the option(s) chosen.

18. A nurse is prepared to assess a postpartum woman's fundus. To facilitate the accuracy and comfort of the examination, the nurse should tell the woman to:
    A. Elevate the head of her bed
    B. Place her hands under her head
    C. Flex her knees
    D. Lie flat with legs extended and toes pointed

19. The expected outcome for care when methylergonovine (Methergine), an oxytocic, is administered to a postpartum woman is that the woman will:
    A. Demonstrate expected lochial characteristics
    B. Achieve relief of pain associated with uterine cramping
    C. Remain free from infection
    D. Void spontaneously within 4 hours of birth

20. A nurse is preparing to administer RhoGAM to a postpartum woman. Before implementing this care measure the nurse should:
    A. Ensure that medication is given at least 24 hours after the birth
    B. Verify that the indirect and direct Coombs' test results are negative
    C. Make sure that the newborn is Rh negative
    D. Cancel the administration of the RhoGAM if it was given to the woman during her pregnancy

21. When teaching a postpartum woman with an episiotomy about using a sitz bath, the nurse should emphasize:
    A. Using sterile equipment
    B. Filling the sitz bath basin with hot water (at least 42° C)
    C. Taking a sitz bath once a day for 10 minutes
    D. Squeezing her buttocks together before sitting down, then relaxing them

22. Before discharge at 2 days postpartum, the nurse evaluates a woman's level of knowledge regarding the care of her episiotomy. Which statements made by the woman indicate the need for further instruction before she goes home? (Circle all that apply.)
    A. "I will wash my stitches at least once a day with mild soap and warm water."
    B. "I will change my pad every time I go to the bathroom—at least four times each day."
    C. "I will continue to apply ice packs to my perineum to reduce swelling."
    D. "I will use my squeeze bottle filled with warm water to cleanse my stitches after I urinate."
    E. "I will wear a pair of clean, disposable gloves when I wash my stitches and change my pad just like the nurses did."
    F "I will apply the anesthetic cream to my stitches at least six times per day."

23. When assessing postpartum women during the first 24 hours after birth the nurse must be alert for signs which could indicate the development of postpartum physiologic complications. Which signs are of concern to the nurse? (Circle all that apply.)
    A. Temperature—38° C
    B. Fundus—midline, boggy
    C. Lochia—three quarters of pad saturated in 3 hours
    D. Positive Homans sign in right leg
    E. Anorexia
    F. Voids approximately 150 to 200 ml of urine for each of the first 3 voidings after birth

III. THINKING CRITICALLY

1. Marie just gave birth to her second child. She plans to bottle-feed her baby just like she did for her first child who was born 12 years ago. She asks the nurse what medication her doctor ordered to "dry up her milk." DESCRIBE how the nurse should respond to Marie's question and assist her with the process of lactation suppression.

2. Tara is breastfeeding at 12 hours postpartum. She requests medication for pain. DESCRIBE the approach that you would take when fulfilling Tara's request.

3. When caring for a woman who gave birth 4 hours earlier, the nurse notes an excessive rubra flow and early signs of hypovolemic shock.
   A. STATE the criteria that the nurse should have used to determine that the flow is rubra and excessive and that the early signs of hypovolemic shock are being exhibited.

   B. IDENTIFY the nurse's priority action in response to these assessment findings.

   C. IDENTIFY additional interventions that a nurse may need to implement to ensure this woman's safety and to prevent the development of further complications.

4. Carrie is a postpartum client awaiting discharge. Because her rubella titer indicates that she is not immune, a rubella vaccination has been ordered before discharge. STATE what you would tell Carrie with regard to this vaccination.

5. A physician has written the following order for a postpartum woman: "Administer RhoGAM [Rh immunoglobulin] if indicated." DESCRIBE the actions the nurse should take in fulfilling this order.

6. Susan, a postpartum breastfeeding client, confides to the nurse, "My partner and I have always had a very satisfying sex life even when I was pregnant. My sister told me that this will definitely change now that I have had a baby." DESCRIBE what the nurse should tell Susan regarding sexual changes and activity after birth.

7. IDENTIFY the priority nursing diagnosis as well as one expected outcome and appropriate nursing management for each of the following situations.
   A. Tina is 2 days postpartum. During a home visit the nurse notes that Tina's episiotomy is edematous, slightly reddened, with approximated wound edges and no drainage. A distinct odor is noted and there is a buildup of secretions and the HurriCaine gel Tina uses for discomfort. During the interview Tina reveals that she is afraid to wash the area. "I rinse with a little water in my peribottle in the morning and again at night. I also apply plenty of my gel."

Nursing Diagnosis	Expected Outcome	Nursing Management

   B. Erin, who gave birth 3 days ago, has not had a bowel movement since a day or two before labor. She tells the visiting nurse during the interview that she has been avoiding "fiber" foods for fear that the baby will get diarrhea. Her activity level is low. "My family is taking good care of me. I do not have to lift a finger! Besides I would prefer to wait until my episiotomy is less sore before trying to have a bowel movement."

Nursing Diagnosis	Expected Outcome	Nursing Management

   C. Mary gave birth 24 hours ago. She complains of perineal discomfort. "My hemorrhoids and stitches are killing me, but I do not want to take any medication because it will get into my breast milk and hurt my baby."

Nursing Diagnosis	Expected Outcome	Nursing Management

8. Dawn gave birth 8 hours ago. On palpation, her fundus was found to be two fingerbreadths above the umbilicus and deviated to the right of midline. It was also assessed to be less firm than previously noted.
   A. STATE the most likely basis for these findings.

   B. DESCRIBE the action that the nurse should take based on these assessment findings.

9. Jill gave birth 3 hours ago. During labor epidural anesthesia was used for pain relief. Jill's primary health care provider has written the following order: "Out of bed and ambulating when able." DISCUSS the approach the nurse should take in safely fulfilling this order.

10. Taisha and her husband Raushaun are expecting their first baby. They have been given the option by their nurse-midwife of early postpartum discharge but are unsure of what to do.
    A. DESCRIBE the approach the nurse-midwife could take to help this couple make a decision that is right for them.

    B. Taisha and Raushaun decide to take the option of early discharge within 12 hours of birth. DESCRIBE the nurse's legal responsibility as she prepares this couple for discharge following the birth of their daughter.

    C. LIST the criteria for discharge that Taisha and her newborn must meet before discharge from the hospital to home.
    Maternal criteria

Newborn criteria

General criteria

D. OUTLINE the essential content that must be taught before discharge. A home visit by a nurse is planned for Taisha's third postpartum day.

11. Cultural beliefs and practices must be considered when planning and implementing care in the postpartum period.
    A. DISCUSS the importance of using a culturally sensitive approach when providing care to postpartum women and their families.

    B. Kim, a Korean-American, has just given birth. Assessment reveals that she and her family are guided by beliefs and practices based on a balance of heat and cold. DESCRIBE how the nurse would adjust typical postpartum care in order to respect and accommodate Kim's cultural beliefs and practices.

    C. A Muslim woman has been admitted to the postpartum unit following the birth of her second son. DESCRIBE the approach you would use in managing this woman's care in a culturally sensitive manner.

12. Tamara delivered vaginally 8 hours ago. She has a midline episiotomy.
    A. DESCRIBE the position that Tamara should assume in order to facilitate palpation of her fundus.

    B. IDENTIFY the characteristics of Tamara's fundus that should be assessed.

    C. DESCRIBE the position Tamara should assume in order to facilitate the examination of her episiotomy.

    D. IDENTIFY the characteristics that should be assessed to determine progress of healing and adequacy of Tamara's perineal self-care measures.

    E. STATE the characteristics of Tamara's uterine flow that should be assessed.

13. IMAGINE that you are the nurse who cared for a woman during her labor and birth and her recovery during the fourth stage of labor. OUTLINE the information that you would report to the mother-baby nurse when you transfer the new mother and her baby to her room on the postpartum unit.

14. Infection control measures should guide the practice of nurses working on a postpartum unit.
    A. DISCUSS the measures designed to prevent transmission of infection from person to person.

    B. DISCUSS measures a postpartum woman should be taught to reduce her risk of infection.

CHAPTER 22

Transition to Parenthood

I. LEARNING KEY TERMS

FILL IN THE BLANKS: Insert the appropriate term for each of the following descriptions regarding parent-infant interaction and parenting.

1. ______________________ Process by which a parent comes to love and accept a child and a child comes to love and accept a parent. The term ______________________ is often used to refer to this process.
2. ______________________ Process that occurs as parents interact with their newborn and maintain close proximity as they identify the infant as an individual and claim him or her as a member of the family.
3. ______________________ Infant behaviors and characteristics call forth a corresponding set of parental behaviors and characteristics.
4. ______________________ Infant behaviors such as crying, smiling, and cooing that initiate the contact and bring the caregiver to the child.
5. ______________________ Infant behaviors such as rooting, grasping, and postural adjustments that maintain the contact.
6. ______________________ Process in which parents identify the new baby, first in terms of likeness to other family members, then in terms of differences, and finally in terms of uniqueness.
7. ______________________ Position used for mutual gazing in which the parent's face and the infant's face are approximately 20 cm (8 inches) apart and are on the same plane.
8. ______________________ Newborns move in time with the structure of adult speech by waving their arms, lifting their heads, and kicking their legs, seemingly "dancing in tune" to a parent's voice.
9. ______________________ Personal biorhythm developed by the infant; parents facilitate this process by giving consistent loving care and using their infant's alert state to develop responsive behavior and thereby increase social interaction and opportunities for learning.
10. ______________________ Type of body movement or behavior that provides the observer with cues. The observer or receiver interprets those cues and responds to them.
11. ______________________ The "fit" between the infant's cues and the parents' response.
12. ______________________ Period from the decision to conceive through the first months of having a child.
13. ______________________ Phase of maternal adjustment that occurs during the first 24 hours (range of 1 to 2 days) when the woman focuses on herself and meeting basic needs with a reliance on others for comfort, rest, closeness, and nourishment. She is often talkative and desires to discuss her childbirth experience.
14. ______________________ Phase of maternal adjustment that begins on the second or third day postpartum and lasts for about 10 days to several weeks during which the woman focuses on caring for her baby and becoming competent as a mother; she is eager to learn and to practice and may experience baby blues.
15. ______________________ Phase of maternal adjustment during which the woman reasserts her relationship with her partner and resumes sexual intimacy.
16. ______________________ Process of transformation and growth of the mother identity during which the woman learns new skills and increases her confidence in herself as she meets new challenges in caring for her child(ren).

17. ______________________ The quality of a mother's sensitive behaviors that are based on her awareness, perception, and responsiveness to infant cues and behaviors.

18. ______________________ Social process in maternal transition during which the woman makes a commitment to being a mother, actively cares for her child, and experiences his or her presence.

19. ______________________ Social process in maternal transition during which the woman learns how to mother and adapt to a changed relationship with her partner, family, and friends; she examines herself in relation to the past and present and comes to view herself as a mother.

20. ______________________ Period surrounding the first day or two of birth, characterized by heightened joy and feelings of well-being. ______________________ Period following birth that is characterized by emotional lability, depression, a let-down feeling, restlessness, fatigue, insomnia, anxiety, sadness, and anger. Lability peaks around the fifth day postpartum and subsides by the tenth day.

21. ______________________ Father's absorption, preoccupation, and interest in his infant.

II. REVIEWING KEY CONCEPTS

22. Attachment of the newborn to parents and family is critical for optimum growth and development.
    A. LIST conditions that must be present for the parent-newborn attachment process to begin favorably.

    B. DISCUSS how nurses should assess the progress of attachment between parents and their new baby.

    C. IDENTIFY what nurses can do to facilitate the process of attachment in the immediate postbirth period.

23. DESCRIBE three parental tasks and responsibilities that are part of parental adjustment to a new baby.

24. DISCUSS how each of the following forms of parent-infant contact can facilitate attachment and promote the family as a focus of care.
    A. Early contact

    B. Extended contact

25. DESCRIBE how a mother's touching of her newborn progresses during the immediate postbirth period.

26. DESCRIBE how each of the following factors influences the manner in which parents respond to the birth of their child. STATE two nursing implications/actions related to each factor.
    Adolescent parents

    Parental age older than 35

    Social support

    Culture

    Lesbian couple

Socioeconomic conditions

Personal aspirations

Sensory impairment

27. COMPARE AND CONTRAST Ruben's *Maternal Role Attainment Model of Maternal Adjustment After Birth* with Mercer's *Becoming a Mother* Model.

MULTIPLE CHOICE: Circle the correct option(s) and state the rationale for the option(s) chosen.

28. During the final phase of the claiming process of a newborn, a mother might say:
    A. "She has her grandfather's nose."
    B. "His ears lie nice and flat against his head, not like mine and his sister's, which stick out."
    C. "She gave me nothing but trouble during pregnancy, and now she is so stubborn she won't wake up to breastfeed."
    D. "He has such a sweet disposition and pleasant expression. I have never seen a baby quite like him before."

29. Which nursing action is least effective in facilitating parent attachment to their new infant?
    A. Referring the couple to a lactation consultant to ensure continuing success with breastfeeding
    B. Keeping the baby in the nursery as much as possible for the first 24 hours after birth so the mother can rest
    C. Extending visiting hours for the woman's partner or significant other as they desire
    D. Providing guidance and support as the parents care for their baby's nutrition and hygiene needs

30. Which behavior illustrates engrossment?
    A. A father is sitting in a rocking chair, holding his new baby boy, touching his toes, and making eye contact.
    B. A mother tells her friends that her baby's eyes and nose are just like hers.
    C. A mother picks up and cuddles her baby girl when she begins to cry.
    D. A grandmother gazes into her new grandson's face, which she holds about 8 inches away from her own; she and the baby make eye-to-eye contact.

31. A woman expresses a need to review her labor and birth experience with the nurse who cared for her while in labor. This behavior is most characteristic of which phase of maternal postpartum adjustment?
    A. Taking-hold (dependent-independent phase)
    B. Taking-in (dependent phase)
    C. Letting-go (interdependent)
    D. Postpartum blues (baby blues)

32. Before discharge, a postpartum woman and her partner ask the nurse about the baby blues. "Our friend said she felt so let down after she had her baby, and we have heard that some women actually become very depressed. Is there anything we can do to prevent this from happening to us or at least to cope with the blues if they occur?" The nurse could tell this couple:
    A. "Postpartum blues usually happen in pregnancies that are high risk or unplanned, so there is no need for you to worry."
    B. "Try to become skillful in breastfeeding and caring for your baby as quickly as you can."
    C. "Get as much rest as you can and sleep when the baby sleeps, because fatigue can precipitate the blues or make them worse."
    D. "I will call your doctor before you leave to get you a prescription for an antidepressant to prevent the blues from happening."

III. THINKING CRITICALLY

1. Jane and Andrew are parents of a newborn girl. DESCRIBE what you would teach them regarding the communication process as it relates to their newborn.
   A. Techniques they can use to communicate effectively with their newborn.

   B. The manner in which the baby is able to communicate with them.

2. Allison had a difficult labor that resulted in an emergency cesarean birth under general anesthesia. She did not see her baby until 12 hours after her birth. Allison tells the nurse who brings the baby to her room, "I am so disappointed. I had planned to breastfeed my baby and hold her close, skin to skin, right after her birth just like all the books say. I know that this is so important for our relationship." DESCRIBE how the nurse should respond to Allison's concern.

3. Angela is the mother of a 1-day-old boy and a 3-year-old girl. As you prepare Angela for discharge, she states, "My little girl just saw her brother. She says she loves him and cannot wait for him to come home. I am so glad that I do not have to worry about any of that sibling rivalry business!" INDICATE how you would respond to Angela's comments.

4. Sara and Ben have just experienced the birth of their first baby. They are very happy with their baby boy but appear very unsure of themselves and are obviously anxious about how to tell what their baby needs. Sara is trying very hard to breastfeed and is having some success but not as much as she had hoped. Both parents express self-doubt about their ability to succeed at the "most important role in our lives."
   A. STATE the nursing diagnosis that is most appropriate for this couple.

   B. DESCRIBE what the nurse caring for this family can do to facilitate the attachment process.

5. Mary and Jim are the parents of three sons. They very much wanted to have a girl this time, but after a long and difficult birth they had another son who weighed 10 pounds. His appearance reflects the difficult birth process: occipital molding, caput succedaneum, and forceps marks on each cheek. Mary and Jim express their disappointment not only in the appearance of their son but also in the fact that they had another boy. "This was supposed to be our last child—now we just do not know what we will do." DISCUSS how you would facilitate Mary and Jim's attachment to their son and reconcile their fantasy ("dream") child with the reality of their actual child.

6. Dawn and Matthew have just given birth to their first baby. This is the first grandchild for both sets of grandparents. The grandmothers approach the nurse to ask how they can help the new family, stating, "We want to help Dawn and Matthew but at the same time not interfere with what they want to do." DISCUSS the role of the nurse in helping these grandparents recognize their importance to the new family and develop a mutually satisfying relationship with Dawn, Matthew, and the new baby.

7. Jane is 2 days postpartum. When the nurse makes a home visit, Jane is found crying. Jane states, "I have such a let-down feeling. I cannot understand why I feel this way when I should be so happy about the healthy outcome for myself and my baby." Jane's husband confirms her behavior and expresses confusion as well, stating, "I wish I knew what to do to help her." Identify the priority nursing diagnosis and one expected outcome for this situation. DESCRIBE the recommended nursing management for the nursing diagnosis you have identified.

Nursing Diagnosis	Expected Outcome	Care Management

8. Ali has just become a father with the birth of his first child, a baby boy.
   A. DESCRIBE the process Ali will follow as he adjusts to fatherhood.

   B. IDENTIFY several measures the nurse caring for Ali's wife and baby boy can use to facilitate his adjustment to fatherhood and attachment to his baby.

CHAPTER 23

Physiologic and Behavioral Adaptations of the Newborn

I. LEARNING KEY TERMS

FILL IN THE BLANKS: Insert the term that corresponds to each of the following descriptions related to newborn characteristics and care.

1. ______________________ Protein manufactured in type II cells of the lungs that reduces surface tension, thereby decreasing the pressure required to keep alveoli open with inspiration and preventing total alveolar collapse on exhalation; alveolar stability is maintained.

2. ______________________ Maintenance of balance between heat loss and heat production.

3. ______________________ Generation of heat.

4. ______________________ Heat production process unique to the newborn accomplished primarily by brown fat and secondarily by increased metabolic activity in the brain, heart, and liver.

5. ______________________ Environment in which heat balance for the newborn is maintained; it is at the temperature that allows the newborn to maintain a normal body temperature to minimize oxygen and glucose consumption.

6. ______________________ Flow of heat from the body surface to cooler ambient air. Two measures to reduce heat loss by this method are to keep the ambient air at 24° C and wrap the infant who is in an open bassinet.

7. ______________________ Loss of heat from the body surface to a cooler, solid surface not in direct contact but in relative proximity. To prevent this type of heat loss, cribs and examining tables are placed away from outside windows and care is taken to avoid direct air drafts.

8. ______________________ Loss of heat that occurs when a liquid is converted to vapor; in the newborn heat loss occurs when moisture from the skin is vaporized. This heat loss can be intensified by failure to dry the newborn directly after birth or by drying the newborn too slowly after a bath.

9. ______________________ Loss of heat from the body surface to cooler surfaces in direct contact. When admitted to the nursery, the newborn is placed in a warmed crib to minimize heat loss. Placing a protective cover on the scale when weighing the newborn will also minimize heat lost by this method.

10. ______________________ High body temperature (>37.5° C) that develops more rapidly in the newborn than in the adult. The newborn has a decreased ability to increase evaporative skin water losses because sweat glands do not function sufficiently to allow the newborn to sweat; serious overheating can cause cerebral damage from dehydration or heat stroke and death.

11. ______________________ Pinkish, easily blanched areas on the upper eyelids, nose, upper lip, back of head, and nape of neck. They are also known as stork bites.

12. ______________________ Overlapping of cranial bones to facilitate passage of the fetal head through the maternal pelvis during the process of labor and birth.

13. ______________________ Generalized, easily identifiable edematous area of the scalp usually over the occiput.

14. ______________________ Collection of blood between skull bone and its periosteum as a result of pressure during birth; it does not cross a suture line.

15. ______________________ Bluish black pigmented areas usually found on back and buttocks.

16. ______________________ Bluish discoloration of the hands and feet, especially when chilled; it is a normal finding in the first 24 hours after birth related to vasomotor instability, capillary stasis, and a high hemoglobin level.

17. ______________________________ White cheeselike substance that coats and protects the fetus's skin while in utero.

18. ______________________________ White facial pimples caused by distended sebaceous glands.

19. ______________________________ Yellowish skin discoloration caused by increased levels of serum bilirubin (hyperbilirubinemia).

20. ______________________________ Nonpathologic unconjugated hyperbilirubinemia that occurs in approximately 60% of term newborns and 80% of preterm newborns.

21. ______________________________ Acute manifestations of bilirubin toxicity that occur during the first weeks after birth; these can include lethargy, hypotonia, irritability, seizures, coma, and death.

22. ______________________________ Irreversible, long-term consequences of bilirubin toxicity such as hypotonia, delayed motor skills, hearing loss, cerebral palsy, and gaze abnormalities.

23. ______________________________ Hyperbilirubinemia that can be manifested by breastfed newborns. Early onset, which begins in the first 2 to 4 days of age, is associated with ineffective breastfeeding. The etiology of the late-onset form, which can begin at age 4 or 5 days and persist for up to 12 weeks, is uncertain but could be related to factors found naturally in breast milk.

24. ______________________________ Thick, dark green-black stool formed during fetal life and usually passed within 24 hours of birth.

25. ______________________________ Sudden, transient newborn rash characterized by erythematous macules, papules, and small vesicles.

26. ______________________________ Condition in which the urethral opening is located in an abnormal position, on or adjacent to the glans instead of at the normal position on the tip of the penis.

27. ______________________________ Accumulation of fluid in the scrotum, around the testes.

28. ______________________________ Small whitish areas found on the gum margins and at the juncture of the hard and soft palates.

29. ______________________________ Membranous area formed where skull bones join.

30. ______________________________ Soft, downy hair on face, shoulders, and back.

31. ______________________________ Bruise.

32. ______________________________ Peeling of the skin that occurs in the term infant a few days after birth; if present at birth it may be an indication of postmaturity.

33. ______________________________ Flat red to purple birth mark composed of a plexus of newly formed capillaries in the papillary layer of the corium; it varies in size, shape, and location, but is usually found on the neck and face. It does not blanch under pressure or disappear.

34. ______________________________ Birth mark consisting of dilated, newly formed capillaries occupying the entire dermal and subdermal layers with associated connective tissue hypertrophy; it is typically a raised, sharply demarcated bright or dark red, rough-surfaced swelling that may proliferate and become more vascular as the infant grows; usually is found as a single lesion on the head.

35. ______________________________ Slightly blood-tinged mucoid vaginal discharge associated with an estrogen decrease after birth.

36. ______________________________ Foreskin.

37. ______________________________ White cheesy substance commonly found under the foreskin.

38. ______________________________ Small, white, firm cysts seen at the tip of the foreskin.

39. ______________________________ Missing digits.

40. ______________________________ Extra digits, fingers or toes.

41. ______________________________ Fused fingers or toes.

FILL IN THE BLANKS: Insert the term that corresponds to each of the following descriptions related to newborn behavioral adaptations and characteristics.

42. ______________ Variations in the state of consciousness of newborn infants.

43. ______________ and ______________ The two sleep states. The newborn sleeps about ______________ hours a day, with periods of wakefulness gradually ______________.

44. ______________, ______________, ______________, and ______________ The four wake states.

45. ______________ The optimum state of arousal in which the infant can be observed smiling, responding to voices, watching faces, vocalizing, and moving in synchrony with speech.

46. ______________ Ability of the newborn to respond to internal and external environmental factors by controlling sensory input and regulating the sleep-wake states, thereby making smooth transitions between states.

47. ______________ Protective mechanism that allows the infant to become accustomed to environmental stimuli. It is a psychologic and physiologic phenomenon in which the response to a constant or repetitive stimulus is decreased.

48. ______________ Quality of alert states and ability to attend to visual and auditory stimuli while alert.

49. ______________ Individual variations in a newborn's primary reaction pattern.

MATCHING: Match the description in Column I with the appropriate newborn reflex from Column II.

COLUMN I

50. ______ Place infant in a supine position and apply pressure to feet with fingers when the lower limbs are semi-flexed—legs extend against examiner's pressure.

51. ______ Place infant supine on flat surface and make a loud abrupt noise—symmetric abduction and extension of arms, fingers fan out, thumb and forefinger form a C; arms are then adducted into an embracing motion and return to relaxed flexion and movement.

52. ______ Place finger in palm of hand or at base of toes—infant's fingers curl around examiner's finger, toes curl downward.

53. ______ Place infant prone on flat surface, run finger down side of back first on one side then down the other 4 to 5 cm lateral to spine—body flexes and pelvis swings toward stimulated side.

54. ______ Tap over forehead, bridge of nose, or maxilla when eyes are open—blinks for first four or five taps.

55. ______ Use finger to stroke sole of foot beginning at heel, upward along lateral aspect of sole, then across ball of foot—all toes hyperextend, with dorsiflexion of big toe.

56. ______ Anal sphincter responds to touch by opening and closing.

57. ______ Testes retract when infant is chilled.

58. ______ Touch infant's lip, cheek, or corner of mouth with nipple—turns head toward stimulus, opens mouth, takes hold, and sucks.

59. ______ Place sleepy infant in a supine position, turn head quickly to one side—arm and leg extend on side to which head is turned while opposite arm and leg flex.

60. ______ Hold infant vertically, allowing one foot to touch table surface—infant alternates flexion and extension of its feet.

61. ______ Touch or depress tip of tongue—tongue is forced outward.

62. ______ Place infant in a supine position, then extend one leg, press knee downward, and stimulate bottom of foot—opposite leg flexes, adducts, and then extends.

COLUMN II

A. Rooting
B. Grasp
C. Extrusion
D. Glabellar (Myerson sign)
E. Tonic neck (fencing)
F. Moro
G. Stepping (walking)
H. Wink reflex
I. Babinski
J. Truncal incurvation (Galant)
K. Magnet
L. Cremasteric
M. Crossed extension

II. REVIEWING KEY CONCEPTS

63. The most critical adjustment that a newborn must make at birth is the establishment of respirations. LIST the factors that are responsible for the initiation of breathing after birth.

64. During the first 6 to 8 hours after birth, newborns experience a transitional period characterized by three phases of instability. INDICATE the timing/duration and typical behaviors for each phase of this transitional period.
    FIRST PERIOD OF REACTIVITY

    PERIOD OF DECREASED RESPONSIVENESS

    SECOND PERIOD OF REACTIVITY

65. EXPLAIN how each of the following factors influence newborn behavior:
    - Gestational age

    - Time

• Stimuli

• Medication

MULTIPLE CHOICE: Circle the correct option(s) and state the rationale for the option(s) chosen.

66. A newborn, at 5 hours old, wakes from a sound sleep and becomes very active and begins to cry. Which signs if exhibited by this newborn indicate expected adaptation to extrauterine life? (Circle all that apply.)
    A. Increased mucus production
    B. Passage of meconium
    C. Heart rate of 160 beats/min
    D. Respiratory rate of 24 breaths/min and irregular
    E. Fine crackles on auscultation
    F. Expiratory grunting with nasal flaring

67. When assessing a newborn boy at 12 hours of age, the nurse notes a rash on his abdomen and thighs. The rash appears as irregular reddish blotches with scattered papules. The nurse:
    A. Documents the finding as erythema toxicum
    B. Isolates the newborn and his mother until infection is ruled out
    C. Applies an antiseptic ointment to each lesion
    D. Requests nonallergenic linen from the laundry

68. A breastfed full-term newborn girl is 12 hours old and is being prepared for early discharge. If present, which assessment findings could delay discharge? (Circle all that apply.)
    A. Dark green-black stool, thick consistency
    B. Yellowish tinge in sclera and on face
    C. Swollen breasts with a scant amount of thin discharge
    D. Blood-tinged mucoid vaginal discharge
    E. Blood glucose level of 35 mg/dl
    F. Acrocyanosis

69. As part of a thorough assessment of a newborn the pediatric nurse practitioner (PNP) should check for hip dislocation and dysplasia. Which technique does the PNP use?
    A. Check for syndactyly bilaterally
    B. Stepping or walking reflex
    C. Magnet reflex
    D. Ortolani maneuver

70. When assessing a newborn after birth, the nurse notes flat, irregular, pinkish marks on the bridge of the nose, nape of neck, and over the eyelids. The areas blanch when pressed with a finger. The nurse documents this finding as:
    A. Milia
    B. Nevus vasculosus
    C. Telangiectatic nevi
    D. Nevus flammeus

III. THINKING CRITICALLY

1. When caring for newborns especially during the transition period following birth, the nurse recognizes that newborns are at increased risk for cold stress.
   A. EXPLAIN the basis for this risk

   B. STATE the dangers that cold stress poses for the newborn.

   C. IDENTIFY one nursing diagnosis and one expected outcome related to this danger.

   D. DESCRIBE care measures the nurse should implement to prevent cold stress from occurring.

2. After a long and difficult labor, baby boy James was born with a caput succedaneum, significant molding over the occipital area, and a small cephalhematoma over the right parietal bone. Low forceps were used for the birth, resulting in ecchymotic areas on both cheeks. James's parents tell the nurse that they are very concerned that James may have experienced brain damage. DESCRIBE what the nurse should tell the parents about these assessment findings.

3. Mary and Jim are concerned that their baby boy, born 2 days ago via a cesarean birth, appears to look a little "yellow," especially his eyes. They ask the nurse if there is some thing wrong with their baby's liver. After examination of the baby, a diagnosis of physiologic jaundice is made.
   A. LIST the criteria used to make this diagnosis.

   B. EXPLAIN to Mary and Jim what caused their baby to appear yellow.

4. Susan and Allen are first-time parents of a baby girl. They ask the nurse about their baby's ability to see and hear things around her and to interact with them.
   A. SPECIFY what the nurse should tell these parents about the sensory capabilities of their healthy full-term newborn.

   B. NAME four stimuli Susan and Allen could provide for their baby that would help foster her development.

   C. DESCRIBE what the nurse should tell the parents about the best time to interact with their newborn.

5. Tonya and Sam, an African-American couple, express concern that their new baby girl has several bruises on her back and buttocks. They ask if their baby was injured during birth or in the nursery. DESCRIBE the appropriate response of the nurse to this couple's concern.

CHAPTER 24

Nursing Care of the Newborn and Family

I. LEARNING KEY TERMS

FILL IN THE BLANKS: Insert the term that corresponds to each of the following descriptions of newborns and their care.

1. ______________________ Tool used to rapidly assess the newborn's transition to extrauterine existence at 1 and 5 minutes after birth; it is based on five signs that indicate his or her physiologic state, namely: ______________________, ______________________, ______________________, ______________________, and ______________________.
2. ______________________ Device used to suction mucus and secretions from the newborn's mouth and nose immediately after birth and when needed.
3. ______________________ Automatic sensor usually placed on the upper quadrant of the abdomen immediately below the right or left costal margin; it is attached to the radiant warmer and monitors the newborn's skin temperature.
4. ______________________ Instillation of antibiotic ointment into the eyes of a newborn after birth.
5. ______________________ Inflammation of the newborn's eyes from gonorrheal or chlamydial infection contracted by the newborn during passage through the mother's birth canal. ______________________ or ______________________ ointment is usually instilled into the newborn's eyes within 1 to 2 hours after birth to prevent this infection.
6. ______________________ Medication administered intramuscularly to the newborn to prevent neonatal hemorrhagic disease; it is administered in a dose of 0.5 to 1 mg using a 25-gauge, 5/8- to 7/8-inch inch needle.
7. ______________________ Scale used to assess and estimate a newborn's gestational age at birth; the initial assessment should be performed within the first 48 hours of life to ensure accuracy and assesses physical and neurologic maturity.
8. ______________________ Term used to describe an infant whose birth weight falls between the 10th and 90th percentiles as a result of growing at a normal rate during fetal life regardless of length of gestation.
9. ______________________ Term used to describe an infant whose birth weight falls above the 90th percentile as a result of growing at an accelerated rate during fetal life regardless of length of gestation.
10. ______________________ Term used to describe an infant whose birth weight falls below the 10th percentile as a result of growing at a restricted rate during fetal life regardless of length of gestation.
11. ______________________ Infant born before the completion of 37 weeks of gestation, regardless of birth weight.
12. ______________________ Infant born at 34 to 36 weeks of gestation; this infant has risk factors due to his or her physiologic immaturity that require close attention by nurses.
13. ______________________ Infant born between the beginning of week 38 and the end of week 42 of gestation.
14. ______________________ Infant born after the completion of 42 weeks of gestation.
15. ______________________ Infant born after the completion of 42 weeks of gestation and showing the effects of progressive placental insufficiency.

16. ______________________________ Pinpoint hemorrhagic areas acquired during birth that may extend over the upper trunk and face; they are benign if they disappear within 2 to 3 days of birth and no new lesions appear.

17. ______________________________ One of the products derived from the hemoglobin released with the breakdown of red blood cells and the myoglobin in muscle cells; its accumulation in the blood results in a yellowish discoloration of the skin, sclera, and oral mucous membranes.

18. ______________________________ Yellowish discoloration of the integument and sclera that first appears after the first 24 hours of life and disappears by the end of the seventh day of life.

19. ______________________________ Test performed to distinguish cutaneous jaundice of the skin from normal skin color. It is performed by applying pressure with a finger over a bony area such as the nose, forehead, or sternum for several seconds to empty all capillaries in the spot. The area will appear yellow when the finger is removed if jaundice is present.

20. ______________________________ Device used for noninvasive monitoring of bilirubin via cutaneous reflectance measurements; it allows for repetitive estimation of bilirubin and works well on both dark- and light-skinned newborns.

21. ______________________________ Infection characterized by white plaques on cheeks or tongue that bleed if touched.

22. ______________________________ Blood glucose concentration less than adequate to support neurologic, organ, and tissue function during the early newborn period; the precise level at which this occurs in every neonate is not known though intervention is usually required if the blood glucose level falls below 40 mg/dl.

23. ______________________________ Serum calcium level less than 7.8 to 8 mg/dl in the term infant and less than 7 mg/dl in the preterm infant.

24. ______________________________ Newborn respiratory rate of less than 25 breaths/min.

25. ______________________________ Newborn respiratory rate of greater than 60 breaths/min.

26. ______________________________ The most important single measure in the prevention of neonatal infection.

27. ______________________________ Use of light to treat hyperbilirubinemia.

28. ______________________________ Surgical procedure that involves removing the prepuce (foreskin) of the glans penis.

29. ______________________________ Postoperative pain scale for newborns. A score is determined by evaluating five signs, namely ______________________________, ______________________________, ______________________________, ______________________________, and ______________________________.

II. REVIEWING KEY CONCEPTS

Neonatal nurses are responsible for the assessment of the physiologic integrity of newborns. As part of this responsibility, the nurse must be aware of the significance of data collected. LABEL each of the following assessment findings, if present, in a group of three full-term 12-hour-old newborns who are all in the quiet alert state, as "N" (reflective of normal adaptation or acceptable variation to extrauterine life) or "P" (reflective of potential problems with adaptation to extrauterine life).

______________ 30. Crackles on auscultation of the lungs

______________ 31. Respirations: 36 breaths/min, irregular, shallow

______________ 32. Episodic apnea lasting 5 to 10 seconds

______________ 33. Nasal flaring and sternal retractions

______________ 34. Slight bluish discoloration of hands and feet

______________ 35. Blood pressure 86/44

______________ 36. Apical heart rate: 126 beats/min with murmurs

______________ 37. Temperature 36° C.

______________ 38. Pink-tinged stains on diaper with first two voidings

_____________ 39. Two small white cysts at gum margins and on palate

_____________ 40. Boggy, edematous swelling over occiput

_____________ 41. Overlapping of parietal bones

_____________ 42. White pimple-like spots on nose and chin

_____________ 43. Jaundice on face

_____________ 44. Regurgitation of small amount of milk following first two feedings

_____________ 45. Liver palpated at 1 cm below right costal margin

_____________ 46. Absence of bowel elimination since birth

_____________ 47. Spine straight with dimple and small tuft of hair at the base

_____________ 48. Adhesion of prepuce—unable to fully retract foreskin

_____________ 49. Edema of labia majora

_____________ 50. Flaring of toes and hyperextension of big toe when sole is stroked upward

_____________ 51. Hematocrit 36% and hemoglobin 12 g/dl

_____________ 52. White blood cell count (WBC) 20,000/mm^3

_____________ 53. Blood glucose 45 mg/dl

54. OUTLINE the specific measures nurses should use when caring for newborns to ensure a safe and protective environment.

55. When assessing newborns, nurses should be alert for evidence of physical injuries sustained by the newborn during the labor and birth process.
    A. IDENTIFY the factors that can lead to soft tissue injuries in the newborn.

B. When assessing a newborn after a difficult birth, what soft tissue injuries would the nurse look for?

56. Preparing parents for the discharge of their newborn requires informing them about the essential aspects of newborn care. IDENTIFY three points that you would emphasize when teaching parents about each of the following aspects of newborn characteristics and care. Include teaching methodologies you would use.
   A. Vital signs: temperature and respirations

   B. Elimination: urinary and bowel

   C. Positioning and holding

   D. Safety

   E. Hygiene: bathing, cord care, and skin care

57. A nurse is measuring a full-term newborn boy 1 hour after his birth. SPECIFY the guidelines this nurse should follow to ensure accuracy of the findings and safety of the newborn when measuring him. INDICATE the expected range for the term newborn.
    Weight

    Head circumference

    Chest circumference

    Abdominal circumference

    Length

58. Nurses caring for newborns are often required to collect blood and urine specimens for laboratory testing. OUTLINE the guidelines nurses should use for each of the following specimen collection techniques.
    Heelstick

Venipuncture

Collection bag for specimen collection

59. Maintaining a patent airway and supporting respirations to ensure an adequate oxygen supply in the newborn are essential focuses of nursing care management of the newborn, especially in the early postbirth period.
   A. STATE the four conditions that are essential for maintaining an adequate oxygen supply in the newborn.

   B. LIST four signs that the nurse who is assessing a newborn would recognize as indicative of abnormal breathing.

   C. DESCRIBE three methods of relieving airway obstruction in an infant.

MULTIPLE CHOICE: Circle the correct option(s) and state the rationale for the option(s) chosen.

60. A newborn male is estimated to be at 40 weeks of gestation following an assessment using the New Ballard Scale. Ballard Scale findings consistent with this newborn's full-term status are: (Circle all that apply.)
   A. Apical pulse rate of 120 beats/min, regular, and strong
   B. Popliteal angle of 160°
   C. Weight of 3200 g, placing him at the 50th percentile
   D. Thinning of lanugo with some bald areas
   E. Testes descended into the scrotum
   F. Elbow does not pass midline when arm is pulled across the chest

61. The nurse evaluates the laboratory test results of a newborn who is 4 hours old. Which results require notifying the pediatrician? (Circle all that apply.)
    A. Hemoglobin 20 g/dl
    B. Hematocrit 54%
    C. Glucose 34 mg/dl
    D. Total serum bilirubin in peripheral blood 9 mg/dl
    E. White blood cell count 24,000/mm^3
    F. Calcium 8 mg/dl

62. A newborn male has been designated as large for gestational age. His mother was diagnosed with gestational diabetes late in her pregnancy. The nurse should be alert for signs of hypoglycemia. Which assessment findings are consistent with a diagnosis of hypoglycemia?
    A. High-pitched cry
    B. Jitteriness
    C. Hyperthermia
    D. Laryngospasm

63. A radiant warmer will be used to help a newborn girl to stabilize her temperature. The nurse implementing this care measure should:
    A. Undress and dry the infant before placing her under the warmer.
    B. Set the control panel between 35° and 38° C
    C. Place the thermistor probe on her abdomen just below her umbilical cord
    D. Assess her rectal temperature every hour until her temperature stabilizes

64. A newborn male has been scheduled for a circumcision. Essential nursing care measures following this surgical procedure include:
    A. Administering oral acetaminophen every 6 hours for a maximum of 20 mg/kg in 24 hours
    B. Applying petroleum jelly or A&D ointment to the site with every diaper change until the site is healed
    C. Checking the penis for bleeding every 15 minutes for the first 4 hours
    D. Teaching the parents to remove the yellowish exudate that forms over the glans using a diaper wipe

65. A physician has ordered that a newborn receive a hepatitis B vaccination prior to discharge. In fulfilling this order the nurse should: (Circle all that apply.)
    A. Confirm that the mother is hepatitis B positive before the injection is given
    B. Obtain parental consent prior to administering the vaccination
    C. Inform the parents that the next vaccine in the series needs to be given at 1 month
    D. Administer the injection into the vastus lateralis muscle
    E. Use a 1-inch 23-gauge needle
    F. Insert the needle at a 45-degree angle

66. A nurse is preparing to administer erythromycin ophthalmic ointment 0.5% to a newborn after birth. Which nursing actions are appropriate? (Circle all that apply.)
    A. Administer the ointment within 30 minutes of the birth.
    B. Wear gloves.
    C. Cleanse the eyes if secretions are present.
    D. Squeeze an ointment ribbon of 3 cm into the lower conjunctival sac.
    E. Wipe away excess ointment after 1 minute.
    F. Apply the ointment from the inner to outer canthus.

III. THINKING CRITICALLY

1. Apgar scoring is a method of newborn assessment used in the immediate postbirth period, at 1 and 5 minutes. Indicate the Apgar score for each of the following newborns.
   a. Baby boy Smith at 1 minute after birth:
      Heart rate—160 beats/min
      Respiratory effort—good, crying vigorously
      Muscle tone—active movement, well flexed
      Reflex irritability—cries with stimulus to soles of feet
      Color—body pink, feet and hands cyanotic
      Score: ____________________
      Interpretation:

   b. Baby girl Doe at 5 minutes after birth:
      Heart rate—102 beats/min
      Respiratory effort—slow, irregular with weak cry
      Muscle tone—some flexion of extremities
      Reflex irritability—grimace with stimulus to soles of feet
      Color—pale
      Score: ____________________
      Interpretation:

2. Baby girl June was just born.
   A. OUTLINE the protocol that the nurse should follow when assessing June's physical status during the first 2 hours after her birth.

   B. STATE the nurse's legal responsibility regarding identification of June and her mother after birth.

   C. IDENTIFY the priority nursing diagnosis for the first 2 hours after birth.

   D. CITE the priority nursing care measures that the nurse must implement to ensure June's well-being and safety during the first 2 hours after birth.

E. DESCRIBE the emotional and physiologic benefits of early contact between the mother and her newborn.

3. Baby boy Tim is 24 hours old. The nurse is preparing to perform a physical examination of this newborn before his discharge.
   A. LIST the actions the nurse should take in order to ensure safety and accuracy. Include the rationale for the actions identified.

   B. IDENTIFY the major points that should be assessed as part of this physical examination.

   C. SUPPORT the premise that Tim's parents should be present during this examination.

4. Baby girl Susan has an accumulation of mucus in her nasal passages and mouth, making breathing difficult.
   A. STATE the nursing diagnosis represented by the assessment findings.

   B. LIST the steps that the nurse should follow when clearing Susan's airway using a bulb syringe.

C. If mucus accumulation continues and breathing is compromised, use of a nasopharyngeal catheter with mechanical suction may be required. LIST the guidelines a nurse should follow when using this method to clear the newborn's airway.

5. Susan and James are taking their newly circumcised (6 hours postprocedure) baby home. This is their first baby and they express anxiety concerning care of both the circumcision and the umbilical cord.
   A. STATE one nursing diagnosis related to this situation.

   B. STATE one expected outcome related to the nursing diagnosis identified.

   C. SPECIFY the instructions that the nurse should give to Susan and James regarding assessment of both sites and the care measures required to facilitate healing.

6. Andrew and Marion are parents of a newborn, 30 hours old, who has developed hyperbilirubinemia. They are very concerned about the color of their baby and the need to put the baby under special lights. "A relative was yellow just like our baby and later died of liver cancer!"
   A. DESCRIBE how the nurse should respond to Andrew and Marion's concern.

   B. DESCRIBE the blanch test as a method of assessment for jaundice.

C. IDENTIFY the expected assessment findings and physiologic effects related to hyperbilirubinemia.

D. LIST the precautions and care measures required by the newborn undergoing phototherapy in order to prevent injury to the newborn yet maintain the effectiveness of the treatment. STATE the rationale for each action identified.

7. A newborn is scheduled for a circumcision. The nurse caring for this newborn is aware that he will experience pain as a result of this procedure.

A. DESCRIBE the most common newborn behavioral responses to pain.

B. INDICATE how a newborn's vital signs and integument will change when he or she experiences pain.

C. EXPLAIN how the CRIES assessment can be used to monitor a newborn's pain during circumcision.

D. OUTLINE the nonpharmacologic and the pharmacologic measures the nurse could use or suggest be used to minimize the pain experience and its effects and maximize the newborn's ability to cope with the pain and recover.

8. You are caring for a newborn girl born vaginally 30 minutes ago. As part of your care of this newborn, you are required to administer two medications as listed below. STATE the purpose for each of the medications and the guidelines you would follow to ensure their safe and effective administration.
   A. Erythromycin ophthalmic ointment 0.5%

   B. Vitamin K (AquaMEPHYTON) 0.5 mg IM

9. Mary and Jim are concerned because their breastfed baby boy, who weighed 8 lb 6 oz at birth, now, at 2 days of age, "weighs only 7 lb 14 oz." They wonder if Mary should stop breastfeeding as a result of this continuing weight loss. Mary states, "Maybe my breast milk is just not good enough to help my baby grow." DESCRIBE how you would respond to their concern.

CHAPTER 25

Newborn Nutrition and Feeding

I. LEARNING KEY TERMS

FILL IN THE BLANKS: Insert the term that corresponds to the following descriptions of breast structures and the breastfeeding process.

1. ______________________________ Structures in the breast that are composed of alveoli, milk ductules, and myoepithelial cells. There are approximately 15 to 20 of these structures in each female breast.
2. ______________________________ Milk-producing cells.
3. ______________________________ Breast structures that transport milk from the milk-producing cells to the nipple; they form a complex intertwining network.
4. ______________________________ Cells that surround the alveoli; these cells contract in response to oxytocin, resulting in the milk ejection reflex or let-down.
5. ______________________________ Rounded, pigmented section of tissue surrounding the nipple.
6. ______________________________ The process of milk production.
7. ______________________________ The lactogenic hormone secreted by the anterior pituitary gland in response to the infant's suck and emptying of the breast.
8. ______________________________ Posterior pituitary hormone that triggers the let-down reflex.
9. ______________________________ Reflex response of the nipple when the infant cries, suckles, or rubs against the breast; this response propels milk through the milk ducts to the nipple pores.
10. ______________________________ Nipple type that becomes hard, erect, and protrudes on stimulation, thereby facilitating latch. ______________________________ Nipple type that remains flat and soft and does not protrude even when stimulated.
11. ______________________________ Plastic device that can be placed over the nipple and areola to keep clothing off the nipple and put pressure around its base to promote protrusion of the nipple.
12. ______________________________ Very concentrated, high-protein, antibody-rich substance present in the breasts before the formation of milk.
13. ______________________________ Difficulty in knowing how to latch on to the breast after having taken a bottle or artificial nipple (pacifier).
14. ______________________________ Newborn behaviors that indicate hunger and a desire to eat such as hand-to-mouth movements, rooting, and mouth and tongue movements.
15. ______________________________ or ______________________________ Reflex triggered by the contraction of myoepithelial cells as a result of oxytocin stimulation. Colostrum, and later milk, is transported to the nipple.
16. ______________________________ Reflex stimulated when a hungry baby's lower lip is touched. The baby opens its mouth and begins to suck.
17. ______________________________ Placement of the infant's mouth over the nipple, areola, and breast, making a seal between the mouth and the breast to create adequate suction for milk removal.
18. ______________________________ Breast response that occurs around the third to fifth day, when the "milk comes in" and blood supply to the breasts increases. The breasts become tender, swollen, hot and hard, and even shiny and red.

19. ______________________________ Breastfeeding position in which the mother holds the baby's head and shoulders in her hand with the baby's back and body tucked under her arm.

20. ______________________________ Breastfeeding position in which the baby's head is positioned in the crook of the mother's arm and the mother and baby are "tummy to tummy."

21. ______________________________ Health care professional who specializes in breastfeeding and may be available to assist a new mother with breastfeeding while in the hospital or after discharge.

22. ______________________________ Infection of the breast manifested by a swollen, tender breast and sudden onset of flulike symptoms.

23. ______________________________ Oral infection caused by a fungus or yeast.

24. ______________________________ Short or tight frenulum, which interferes with extrusion and effective sucking.

25. ______________________________ Process whereby the infant is gradually introduced to drinking from a cup and eating solid food while breastfeeding and bottle feeding is reduced by gradually decreasing the number of feedings.

26. ______________________________ Milk that is initially released with breastfeeding; it is bluish white, is composed of part skim milk and part whole milk, and provides primarily lactose, protein, and water-soluble vitamins.

27. ______________________________ Milk that is let down 10 to 20 minutes into the feeding; often called the cream, it is denser in calories from fat necessary for optimal growth and contentment between feedings.

28. ______________________________ Foods or liquids given to the infant in addition to breast milk or formula.

II. REVIEWING KEY CONCEPTS

29. A nurse has been asked to participate in a women's health seminar for women of childbearing age in the community. Her topic is "Breastfeeding: The Goals for Healthy People 2010/2020 and Beyond." OUTLINE the points that this nurse should emphasize to help women appreciate the benefits of breastfeeding and seriously consider breastfeeding when they have a baby.

30. It is important that a breastfeeding woman alter the position she uses for breastfeeding as one means of preserving nipple and areolar integrity. DESCRIBE four positions the nurse should demonstrate to a woman who is breastfeeding her newborn.

31. Infants exhibit feeding cues as they recognize and express their hunger.
    A. IDENTIFY feeding cues of the infant.

    B. STATE why the new mother should be guided by these cues when determining the timing of feeding sessions.

32. A proper latch is essential for effective breastfeeding and preservation of nipple and areolar tissue integrity.
    A. INDICATE the steps the nurse should teach a breastfeeding woman to follow to ensure a proper latch

    B. When observing a woman breastfeeding, it is essential that the nurse determine the effectiveness of the latch. STATE the signs a nurse should look for that would indicate a proper latch

    C. DESCRIBE the way a woman should remove her baby from her breast after feeding is completed.

MULTIPLE CHOICE: Circle the correct option(s) and state the rationale for the option(s) chosen.

33. During a home visit, the mother of a 1-week-old infant son tells the nurse that she is very concerned about whether her baby is getting enough breast milk. The nurse should tell this mother that at 1 week of age a well-nourished newborn should exhibit:
    A. Weight gain sufficient to reach his birth weight
    B. A minimum of three bowel movements each day of soft yellow seedy stools
    C. Approximately 10 to 12 wet diapers each day
    D. Breastfeeding at a frequency of every 4 hours or about 6 times each day

34. A woman is trying to calm her fussy baby daughter in preparation for feeding. She exhibits a need for further instruction if she:
    A. Removes all clothing from infant except the diaper
    B. Dims lights in the room and turns off the television
    C. Gently rocks the baby and talks to her in a low voice
    D. Allows the baby to suck on her finger

35. The nurse should teach breastfeeding mothers about breast care measures to preserve the integrity of the nipples and areola. What should the nurse include in these instructions?
    A. Cleanse nipples and areola twice a day with mild soap and water.
    B. Apply vitamin E cream to nipples and areola at least four times each day before a feeding.
    C. Insert plastic-lined pads into the bra to absorb leakage and protect clothing.
    D. Apply modified lanolin to both dry and sore nipples.

36. A breastfeeding woman asks the nurse about a reliable and safe method of birth control she should use during the postpartum period. The best recommendation for a safe, yet effective method during the first 6 weeks after birth is:
    A. Combination oral contraceptive that she used before she was pregnant
    B. Barrier method using a combination of a condom and spermicide foam
    C. Resume using the diaphragm she used prior to getting pregnant
    D. Complete breastfeeding—baby only receives breast milk for nourishment

37. A woman has determined that bottle feeding is the best feeding method for her. Instructions the woman should receive regarding this feeding method include:
    A. Check nipple before feeding to ensure that it allows passage of formula in a slow stream
    B. Sterilize water by boiling, then cool and mix with formula powder or concentrate
    C. Expect a 2-week-old newborn to drink approximately 90 to150 ml of formula at each feeding
    D. Microwave refrigerated formula for about 2 minutes before feeding the newborn

38. At a home visit 1 week after birth, a nurse is evaluating a woman's breastfeeding technique. Which actions indicate that the woman needs further instruction regarding breastfeeding to ensure success? (Circle all that apply.)
    A. Waits to feed her baby until he wakes up and begins to cry
    B. Massages a small amount of breast milk into her nipple and areola before and after each feeding
    C. Squeezes her nipple and areola between her thumb and forefinger then inserts her nipple into the baby's mouth
    D. Positions her baby supporting back and shoulders securely and then brings her breast toward the baby putting the nipple in the baby's mouth
    E. Inserts her finger into the corner of her baby's mouth between the gums before removing the baby from the breast
    F. Feeds her baby approximately 20 minutes on each breast

39. A new breastfeeding mother asks the nurse how to prevent nipple soreness. The nurse tells this woman that the key to preventing sore nipples is:
    A. Limiting the length of breastfeeding to no more that 10 minutes on each breast until the milk comes in
    B. Apply lanolin to each nipple and areola after each feeding
    C. Correct latch and removal from the breast
    D. Using breast shells to protect the nipples and areola between feeding

III. THINKING CRITICALLY

1. Tonya is bottle feeding her baby. She expresses concern to the nurse at the well-baby clinic about heart disease and cholesterol levels as they relate to her 2-month-old baby. She tells the nurse that her family has a history of cardiac disease and hypertension and she has already changed her diet and wants to do the same for her baby. Tonya asks, "When should I start giving my baby skim milk instead of the prepared formula that I am using, which seems to contain quite a bit of fat?" DISCUSS how the nurse should respond to Tonya's question.

2. Elise and her husband, Mark, are experiencing their first pregnancy. During one of their prenatal visits they tell the nurse that they are as yet unsure about the method they want to use for feeding their baby. "Everyone has an opinion—some say breastfeeding is best, yet others tell us that bottle feeding is more convenient, especially because the father can help. What should we do?"
   A. IDENTIFY one nursing diagnosis and one expected outcome appropriate for this situation.

   B. DISCUSS why it is important for the pregnant couple to make this decision together.

   C. INDICATE why is it preferable to make this decision during the prenatal period rather than waiting until the baby is born.

   D. DESCRIBE how the nurse could use the decision-making process to assist Elise and Mark to choose the method that is best for them.

3. Mary, as a first-time breastfeeding mother, has many questions. DESCRIBE how you would respond to the following questions and comments.
   A. "I am so afraid that I will not make enough milk for my baby. My breasts are not as large as some of my friends who breastfeed."

   B. "Everyone keeps talking about this let-down that is supposed to happen. What is it and how will I know I have it?"

C. "How can I possibly know if breastfeeding is going well and my baby is getting enough if I cannot tell how many ounces he gets with each feeding?"

D. "It is only the first day that I am breastfeeding and my nipples already feel sore. What can I do to relieve this soreness and prevent it from getting worse?"

E. "My friends all told me to watch out for the fourth day and engorgement. What can I do to keep it from being too bad and to take care of myself when it occurs?"

F. "Every time I breastfeed, I get cramps and my flow seems to get heavier. Is there something wrong with me?"

G. "I am so glad I do not have to worry about getting pregnant again as long as I am breastfeeding. I hate using birth control and my friend told me I do not have to as long as I am breastfeeding."

H. "What should I do when I am ready to stop breastfeeding my baby?"

4. Susan is 2 days old. She last fed 5 hours ago. Her mother tells the nurse that Susan is so sleepy that she just does not have the heart to wake her.
   A. IDENTIFY one nursing diagnosis and one expected outcome appropriate for this newborn.

   B. DISCUSS the approach the nurse should take with regard to this situation.

5. Alice has decided that for personal and professional reasons, bottle feeding with a commercially prepared formula is the feeding method that is best for her. She tells the nurse that she hopes she made a good decision for her baby. "I hope she will be well nourished and feel that I love her even though I am bottle feeding."
   A. DESCRIBE how the nurse should respond to Alice's concern.

   B. STATE three guidelines for bottle-feeding technique that the nurse should teach Alice to ensure the safety and health of her baby.

6. Prior to discharge, a nurse is evaluating a woman's ability to breastfeed and her newborn's response to breastfeeding.
   A. IDENTIFY the factors that the nurse should assess before and during breastfeeding to ensure that the mother and newborn are ready to breastfeed at home.

   B. After determining that breastfeeding is progressing well the woman is discharged. One week later the nurse calls the woman to discuss breastfeeding. WRITE several questions this nurse should ask to determine if breastfeeding is continuing to progress normally.

CHAPTER 26

Assessment for Risk Factors in Pregnancy

I. LEARNING KEY TERMS

FILL-IN-THE-BLANKS: Insert the term that corresponds to each of the following descriptions.

1. ______________________________ A pregnancy in which the life or health of the mother or her fetus is jeopardized by a disorder coincidental with or unique to pregnancy.
2. ______________________________ Assessment of fetal activity by the mother; it is a simple yet valuable method for monitoring the condition of the fetus. The ______________________________ refers to the cessation of fetal movements entirely for 12 hours.
3. ______________________________ Diagnostic test that involves the use of sound having a frequency higher than that detectable by humans to examine structures inside the body. During pregnancy it can be done by using either the ______________________________ or ______________________________ approach.
4. ______________________________ Decreased or deficient amount of amniotic fluid.
5. ______________________________ Increased or excessive amount of amniotic fluid
6. ______________________________ Noninvasive study of blood flow in the fetus and placenta.
7. ______________________________ Noninvasive dynamic assessment of the fetus and its environment that is based on acute and chronic markers of fetal disease. It uses both real-time ______________________________ and external ______________________________. This test includes assessment of five variables, namely ______________________________, ______________________________, ______________________________, ______________________________, and ______________________________.
8. ______________________________ Noninvasive radiologic technique used for obstetric and gynecologic diagnosis by providing excellent pictures of soft tissue without the use of ionizing radiation.
9. ______________________________ Prenatal diagnostic test performed to obtain amniotic fluid to examine the fetal cells it contains.
10. ______________________________ Prenatal diagnostic test that provides direct access to the fetal circulation during the second and third trimesters.
11. ______________________________ Procedure that involves the removal of a small tissue specimen from the fetal portion of the placenta. Because this tissue originates from the zygote, it reflects the genetic makeup of the fetus; it is performed between 10 and 12 weeks of gestation.
12. ______________________________ Test used as a screening tool for neural tube defects in pregnancy. The test is ideally performed between ______________________________ and ______________________________ weeks of gestation.
13. ______________________________ Test used to screen for Down syndrome. It is performed between ______________________________ and ______________________________ weeks of gestation. The levels of three markers, namely ______________________________, ______________________________, and

________________, in combination with maternal ________________ are used to determine risk. The ________________ test adds an additional marker called inhibin A to increase the accuracy of screening for Down syndrome in women more than 35 years of age.

14. ________________ Screening test for Rh incompatibility by examining the serum of Rh-negative women for Rh antibodies.

15. ________________ Test based on the fact that the heart rate of a healthy awake fetus with an intact central nervous system usually accelerates in response to its own movement.

16. ________________ Test used to determine fetal response to sound; the expected response is acceleration of the fetal heart rate.

17. ________________ Test used to identify the jeopardized fetus who is stable at rest but shows evidence of compromise when exposed to the stress of uterine contractions. If the resultant hypoxia of the fetus is sufficient, a deceleration of the FHR will result. Two methods used for this test are the ________________ ________________ test and the ________________ test.

18. ________________ Goal of antepartal assessment during the first and second trimesters.

19. ________________ and ________________ Two major goals of antepartal assessment during the third trimester.

II. REVIEWING KEY CONCEPTS

20. EXPLAIN how risk factors in each of the following categories could place the maternal-fetal unit in jeopardy. Identify several strategies that a nurse could use to eliminate or reduce the risk.
Biophysical factors:

Psychosocial factors:

Sociodemographic factors:

Environmental factors:

21. DISCUSS the role of the nurse when caring for high risk pregnant women who are required to undergo antepartal assessment testing to determine fetal well-being.

22. STATE two risk factors for each of the following pregnancy-related problems:
Polyhydramnios

Intrauterine growth restriction

Oligohydramnios

Chromosomal abnormalities

MULTIPLE CHOICE: Circle the correct option(s) and state the rationale for the option(s) chosen.

23. A 34-year-old woman at 36 weeks of gestation has been scheduled for a biophysical profile. She asks the nurse why the test needs to be performed. The nurse tells her that the test is performed because it:
    A. Determines how well her baby will breathe after it is born
    B. Evaluates the response of her baby's heart to uterine contractions
    C. Measures her baby's head and length
    D. Observes her baby's activities in utero to ensure that her baby is getting enough oxygen

24. As part of preparing a 24-year-old woman at 42 weeks of gestation for a nonstress test, the nurse should:
    A. Tell the woman to fast for 8 hours before the test
    B. Explain that the test will evaluate how well her baby is moving inside her uterus
    C. Show her how to indicate when her baby moves
    D. Attach a spiral electrode to the presenting part to determine FHR patterns

25. A 40-year-old woman at 18 weeks of gestation is having a triple marker test performed. She is obese, and her health history reveals that she is Rh negative. The primary purpose of this test is to screen for:
   A. Spina bifida
   B. Down syndrome
   C. Gestational diabetes
   D. Rh antibodies

26. During a contraction stress test, four contractions lasting 45 to 55 seconds were recorded in a 10-minute period. A late deceleration was noted during the third contraction. The nurse conducting the test documents the result as:
   A. Negative
   B. Positive
   C. Equivocal-suspicious
   D. Unsatisfactory

27. A pregnant woman is scheduled for a transvaginal ultrasound test to establish gestational age. In preparing this woman for the test the nurse should:
   A. Place the woman in a supine position with her hips elevated on a folded pillow
   B. Instruct her to come for the test with a full bladder
   C. Administer an analgesic 30 minutes before the test
   D. Lubricate the vaginal probe with transmission gel

28. A pregnant woman at 42 weeks of gestation is undergoing a nonstress test. During the test an evaluation of the monitor tracing indicated that two accelerations of the fetal heart rate occurred within a 20-minute period. The first acceleration of 18 beats/min lasted 20 seconds and the second acceleration of 20 beats/min lasted 16 seconds. The nurse conducting the test records the test result as:
   A. Reactive
   B. Positive
   C. Nonreactive
   D. Equivocal hyperstimulatory

III. THINKING CRITICALLY

1. Annie is a primigravida who is at 10 weeks of gestation. Her prenatal history reveals that she was treated for pelvic inflammatory disease 2 years ago. She describes irregular menstrual cycles and is therefore unsure about the first day of her last menstrual period. Annie is scheduled for a transvaginal ultrasound.
   A. CITE the likely reasons for the performance of this test.

   B. DESCRIBE how the nurse should prepare Annie for this test.

2. Latisha, pregnant at 20 weeks of gestation, is scheduled for a series of transabdominal ultrasounds to monitor the growth of her fetus. DESCRIBE the nursing role as it applies to Latisha and transabdominal ultrasound examinations.

3. Mary is at 42 weeks of gestation. Her physician has ordered a biophysical profile (BPP). She is very upset and tells the nurse, "All my doctor told me is that this test will see if my baby is okay. I do not know what is going to happen and if it will be painful to me or possibly harmful for my baby."
   A. STATE a nursing diagnosis that reflects this situation.

   B. DESCRIBE how the nurse should respond to Mary's concerns.

   C. Mary receives a score of 8 for the BPP. LIST the factors that were evaluated to obtain this score and specify the meaning of Mary's test result of 8.

4. Jan, age 42, is 18 weeks pregnant. Because of her age Jan's fetus is at risk for genetic anomalies. Jan's blood type is A negative and her partner's, the father of her baby, is B positive. Her primary health care provider has suggested an amniocentesis. DESCRIBE the nurse's role in terms of each of the following:
   A. Preparing Jan for the amniocentesis.

   B. Supporting Jan during the procedure.

   C. Providing Jan with postprocedure care and instructions.

5. Susan, who has diabetes and is in week 36 of pregnancy, has been scheduled for a nonstress test.
   A. DISCUSS what you would tell Susan about the purpose of this test and what will be learned about her baby's well-being.

   B. DESCRIBE how you would prepare Susan for this test.

   C. DISCUSS how you would conduct the test.

   D. INDICATE the criteria you would use to determine if the result of the test was:
   Reactive

   Nonreactive

6. Beth is scheduled for a contraction stress test following a nonreactive result on a nonstress test. Nipple stimulation will be used to induce the required contraction pattern.
   A. DISCUSS what you would tell Beth about the purpose of this test and what will be learned about the well-being of her fetus.

   B. DESCRIBE how you would prepare Beth for the test.

C. INDICATE how you would conduct the test.

D. STATE how you would conduct the test differently if exogenous oxytocin (Pitocin) is used instead of nipple stimulation.

E. INDICATE the criteria you would use to determine if the result of the test is:
Negative

Positive

Equivocal suspicious

Equivocal hyperstimulatory

Unsatisfactory

CHAPTER 27

Hypertensive Disorders in Pregnancy

I. LEARNING KEY TERMS

MATCHING: Match the client description in Column I with the appropriate diagnosis from Column II.

COLUMN I

1. _______ During a prenatal visit at 30 weeks of gestation, Angela's blood pressure was 156/98 and has ranged between 142/92 to 150/90 since the 28th week of her pregnancy; her urinalysis indicated a protein level of 2+ using a dipstick; biceps and patellar reflexes are 2+.
2. _______ At 37 weeks of gestation, Mary's BP rose from a prepregnant baseline of 118/66 to 142/88. No other problematic signs and symptoms including proteinuria were noted.
3. _______ Susan, a 34-year-old pregnant client, has had a consistently high BP ranging from 148/92 to 160/98 since she was 28 years old. Her weight gain has followed normal patterns, and urinalysis remains normal as well.
4. _______ At 32 weeks of gestation, Maria, with hypertension since 28 weeks, hyperactive DTRs with clonus, and proteinuria of 4+, has a convulsion.
5. _______ Shawna is a primigravida at 28 weeks of gestation. Her BP has risen to 160/110 and higher. Proteinuria is at 3+. She has been complaining of a headache and states she needs to wear sunglasses even indoors because light hurts her eyes.
6. _______ Dawn has been hypertensive since her 24th week of pregnancy. Urinalysis indicates a protein content of 3+. Further testing reveals a platelet count of 95,000 and elevated AST and ALT levels; she has begun to experience nausea with some vomiting and epigastric pain.

COLUMN II

A. Eclampsia
B. Chronic hypertension
C. Gestational hypertension
D. HELLP syndrome
E. Preeclampsia (mild)
F. Preeclampsia (severe)

FILL IN THE BLANKS: Insert the term that corresponds to each of the following descriptions of hypertensive disorders during pregnancy.

7. ____________________ Onset of hypertension without proteinuria after the 20th week of pregnancy; it is the most common cause of hypertension during pregnancy and usually develops at or after 37 weeks of gestation.
8. ____________________ Hypertension that is present before pregnancy or that is diagnosed before the 20th week of pregnancy.
9. ____________________ Pregnancy-specific condition in which hypertension and proteinuria develop after 20 weeks of gestation in a previously normotensive woman.
10. ____________________ A systolic blood pressure greater than 140 mm Hg or a diastolic blood pressure greater than 90 mm Hg. The elevated values must be present on ____________________ separate occasions at least ____________________ hours apart but within a maximum of a ____________________ -week period.
11. ____________________ A protein concentration at or above 30 mg/dl (greater than 1+ on dipstick measurement) in at least two random urine samples collected at least 6 hours apart.

12. ______________________ Accumulation of fluid in the tissues of the lowest or most dependent parts of the body, where hydrostatic pressure is the greatest. For ambulating women it is first evident in ______________________, and if the pregnant woman is confined to bed, it occurs in the ______________________ region.

13. ______________________ Onset of seizure activity or coma in the woman diagnosed with preeclampsia, with no history of preexisting pathology that can result in seizure activity.

14. ______________________ A laboratory diagnosis for a variant of severe preeclampsia that involves hepatic dysfunction; it is characterized by ______________________, elevated ______________________, and low ______________________.

15. ______________________ Activity in blood vessels that diminishes their diameter, thereby impeding blood flow to all organs and raising blood pressure.

II. REVIEWING KEY CONCEPTS

16. DESCRIBE the assessment technique used to determine if the following findings are present in women with preeclampsia. (Note: You may wish to review this information in a physical assessment textbook for a complete explanation of each technique.)

Hyperreflexia

Ankle clonus

Proteinuria

Pitting edema

MULTIPLE CHOICE: Circle the correct option(s) and state the rationale for the option(s) chosen.

17. When measuring the blood pressure to ensure consistency and to facilitate early detection of blood pressure changes consistent with preeclampsia, the nurse should:
    A. Place the woman in a sitting position with feet flat on the floor
    B. Allow the woman to rest for 10 minutes after positioning before measuring her blood pressure
    C. Record Korotkoff phase IV (muffled sound) as the diastolic pressure
    D. Use a proper sized cuff that covers at least 50% of her upper arm

18. When caring for a woman with mild preeclampsia, it is critical that during assessment the nurse be alert for signs of progress to severe preeclampsia. Progress to severe preeclampsia is indicated by this assessment finding:
    A. Proteinuria greater than 2+, in two specimens collected 6 hours apart
    B. Platelet count of 180,00/mm^3
    C. Positive ankle clonus response
    D. Blood pressure of 154/94 and 156/100, 6 hours apart

19. A woman's preeclampsia has advanced to the severe stage. She is admitted to the hospital and her primary health care provider has ordered an infusion of magnesium sulfate be started. In implementing this order, the nurse should: (Circle all that apply.)
    A. Prepare a solution of 20 g of magnesium sulfate in 100 ml of 5% glucose in water
    B. Monitor maternal vital signs, FHR patterns, and uterine contractions every hour
    C. Expect the maintenance dose to be approximately 2 g/hr
    D. Administer a loading dose of 4 to 6 g over 15 to 30 minutes
    E. Prepare to administer hydralazine (Apresoline) if signs of magnesium toxicity occur
    F. Report a respiratory rate of 12 breaths or less per minute to the primary health care provider immediately

20. The primary expected outcome for nursing care associated with the administration of magnesium sulfate would be met if which assessment finding is present? The woman:
    A. Exhibits a decrease in both systolic and diastolic blood pressure
    B. Experiences no seizures
    C. States that she feels more relaxed and calm
    D. Urinates more frequently resulting in a decrease in pathologic edema

21. A woman has been diagnosed with mild preeclampsia and will be treated at home. In teaching this woman about her treatment regimen for mild preeclampsia, the nurse should tell her to: (Circle all that apply.)
    A. Follow a low-salt diet
    B. Use a dipstick to check her urine for protein
    C. Maintain a fluid intake of six to eight 8-ounce glasses of water each day
    D. Increase the roughage in her diet
    E. Perform gentle range of motion exercises of her upper and lower extremities
    F. Ask her friends to avoid visiting or calling her because she needs to rest.

22. A woman with severe preeclampsia is receiving nifedipine (Procardia). She asks the nurse what this medication is for. The nurse should tell her that nifedipine is used to:
    A. Prevent seizures
    B. Relieve the headaches she is starting to have
    C. Decrease her blood pressure
    D. Reduce the edema in her hands and legs

23. A woman with preeclampsia gave birth by cesarean section 1 hour ago. She is still receiving a magnesium sulfate infusion at 1 g/hr. A major concern regarding the administration of magnesium sulfate at this time is:
    A. Increased risk for seizures
    B. Central nervous system depression
    C. Hypotension
    D. Diuresis

24. Following vaginal birth 2 hours ago a woman with preeclampsia is experiencing a heavy flow as a result of a boggy uterus. It is determined that she will require medication to reduce the amount of blood loss. Which medication would the nurse anticipate administering?
   A. Methylergonovine (Methergine)
   B. Calcium gluconate
   C. Oxytocin (Pitocin)
   D. Labetalol (Normodyne)

25. A woman, at 35 weeks of gestation with preeclampsia, has a seizure. Immediately after the seizure, the nurse's priority action is to:
   A. Evaluate FHR and pattern for signs of decreasing variability, late decelerations, or bradycardia
   B. Assess status of the maternal airway, respiratory effort, and pulse
   C. Determine if membranes have ruptured and if the amniotic fluid contains meconium
   D. Prepare to increase the amount of magnesium sulfate being infused from 1 g/hr to 2 g/hr

III. THINKING CRITICALLY

1. Hypertension during pregnancy can result in serious health problems for the woman and her fetus. As a result, nurses working with pregnant women need to be consistent in the technique they use to monitor blood pressure changes. DEVELOP a protocol nurses could follow to ensure the accuracy of blood pressure measurement during pregnancy.

2. Preeclampsia is a serious complication of pregnancy. CREATE a profile of two women who, when pregnant, are at risk for preeclampsia (use different risk factors for each profile that you create). EXPLAIN how nurses working with these women could identify the risks these women present.

3. Amber, a primigravida at 30 weeks of gestation, is diagnosed with mild preeclampsia. The nurse caring for Amber recognizes that preeclampsia and eclampsia can affect both maternal and fetal well-being.
   A. DESCRIBE how preeclampsia and eclampsia can adversely affect the health and well-being of Amber's fetus.

   B. Amber is concerned about her diagnosis, stating, "I know this can have an effect on my baby, so I will do whatever necessary to keep both of us safe. But how will you and I know my baby is doing okay?" INDICATE the fetal surveillance measures recommended for women experiencing preeclampsia that the nurse should discuss with Amber.

4. Jean (2-1-0-0-1) is at 30 weeks of gestation and has been diagnosed with mild preeclampsia. The treatment plan includes home care with limited activity consisting of bed rest with bathroom privileges and out of bed twice a day for meals, appropriate nutrition, and stress reduction. She and her husband are very anxious about the diagnosis and are also concerned about how they will manage the care of their active 3-year-old daughter, Anne.

   A. INDICATE the clinical manifestations that indicate this diagnosis.

   B. LIST three priority nursing diagnoses for Jean and her family.

   C. DESCRIBE how you would help this couple organize their home care routine.

   D. SPECIFY what you would teach them with regard to assessment of Jean's status in terms of each of the following:

   Blood pressure

   Weight

   Protein in urine

Fetal well-being

Signs of a worsening condition

E. DESCRIBE the instructions you would give Jean regarding her nutrient and fluid intake.

F. DISCUSS the measures Jean can use to cope with the boredom and alteration in circulation and muscle tone that accompany activity restrictions including bed rest.

G. Limited activity can lead to a nursing diagnosis of risk for constipation related to changes in bowel function associated with pregnancy and limited activity. CITE two measures that Jean can use to enhance bowel elimination and prevent constipation.

5. Ellen, pregnant at 37 weeks of gestation, is admitted to the hospital with a diagnosis of severe preeclampsia.
   A. INDICATE the signs and symptoms that indicate this diagnosis.

   B. LIST three priority nursing diagnoses for Ellen.

C. SPECIFY the measures that should be taken to protect Ellen and her fetus from injury.

D. Ellen's physician orders magnesium sulfate to be infused at 4 g in 20 minutes as a loading dose, then a maintenance intravenous infusion of 2 g/hr.

1. CREATE a protocol that will be a guide nurses can follow when administering the magnesium sulfate infusion.

2. WRITE one nursing diagnosis related to the treatment with magnesium sulfate.

3. EXPLAIN the expected therapeutic effect of magnesium sulfate to Ellen and her family.

4. LIST the maternal-fetal assessments that should be accomplished on a regular basis during the infusion of magnesium sulfate.

5. IDENTIFY the progressive signs of magnesium sulfate toxicity.

6. STATE the interventions that must be instituted immediately if magnesium sulfate toxicity occurs.

E. Despite all prevention efforts, Ellen has a convulsion.
   1. SPECIFY the nursing measures that should be implemented at the onset of the convulsion and immediately afterward.

   2. LIST the problems that can occur as a result of the convulsion that Ellen experienced.

F. Ellen successfully gave birth vaginally despite her high risk status. DESCRIBE Ellen's care management during the first 48 hours of her postpartum recovery period.

CHAPTER 28

Antepartum Hemorrhagic Disorders

I. LEARNING KEY TERMS

FILL IN THE BLANKS: Insert the appropriate term for each description of antepartal bleeding.

1. ______________________, ______________________, ______________________, and ______________________ The common bleeding disorders of early pregnancy.
2. ______________________ and ______________________ The common bleeding disorders of late pregnancy.
3. ______________________ Pregnancy that ends as a result of natural causes before 20 weeks of gestation, the point of viability when the fetus may survive outside the uterus. The five types are ______________________, ______________________, ______________________, ______________________ and ______________________.
4. ______________________ Term used to refer to three or more spontaneous pregnancy losses prior to 20 weeks of gestation.
5. ______________________ Placental hormone used in the diagnosis of pregnancy and pregnancy loss.
6. ______________________ Surgical procedure in which the cervix is widened and an instrument is inserted to scrape the uterine walls and remove uterine contents.
7. ______________________ A cause of late miscarriage; it is traditionally defined as passive and painless dilation of the cervix during the second trimester.
8. ______________________ Procedure in which a suture is placed around the cervix beneath the mucosa to constrict the internal os of the cervix.
9. ______________________ Pregnancy in which the fertilized ovum is implanted outside the uterine cavity, usually in the ampulla or largest part of the uterine tube.
10. ______________________ An ecchymotic blueness around the umbilicus indicating hematoperitoneum; it may develop in an undiagnosed intraabdominal ectopic pregnancy.
11. ______________________ A gestational trophoblastic disease (GTD); it is a benign proliferative growth of the placental trophoblast.
12. ______________________ A group of pregnancy-related trophoblastic proliferative disorders without a viable fetus.
13. ______________________ Term used to refer to the result of fertilization of an egg with a lost or inactivated nucleus; it resembles a bunch of white grapes; there is an increased risk for persistent GTD.
14. ______________________ Term used to refer to the result of two sperm fertilizing an apparently normal ovum; embryonic or fetal parts and an amniotic sac are often present in the uterus.
15. ______________________ One of the GTD diseases; it is now considered to be the most successfully treated gynecologic cancer.
16. ______________________ Implantation of the placenta in the lower uterine segment such that it completely or partially covers the cervix or is close enough to the cervix to cause bleeding when dilation or effacement occurs.

17. ______________________________ Detachment of part or all of a normally implanted placenta from the uterus.

18. ______________________________ Disorder of the uterus in which blood accumulates between a separating placenta and the uterine wall; the uterus appears purple or blue, it is ecchymotic, and contractility is lost.

19. ______________________________ Placental anomaly wherein the cord vessels begin to branch at the membranes and then course into the placenta.

20. ______________________________ Marginal insertion of the cord into the placenta.

21. ______________________________ Placenta is divided into two or more separate lobes.

22. ______________________________ Pathologic form of clotting that is diffuse and consumes large amounts of clotting factors, causing widespread external bleeding, internal bleeding, or both, and clotting.

II. REVIEWING KEY CONCEPTS

23. Disseminated intravascular coagulation (DIC) is an acute, life-threatening disorder that can occur during pregnancy.
    A. IDENTIFY the obstetric risk factors for the development of DIC. EXPLAIN how these risk factors can lead to DIC.

    B. DESCRIBE the pathophysiology that leads to DIC.

    C. INDICATE the clinical manifestations of DIC that would be noted during physical examination and with laboratory testing.

    D. DESCRIBE four priority nursing measures that should be used when caring for a woman experiencing DIC.

24. DESCRIBE the effect that bleeding during pregnancy can have on maternal and fetal well-being.

MULTIPLE CHOICE: Circle the correct option(s), and state the rationale for the option(s) chosen.

25. A primigravida at 10 weeks of gestation reports mild uterine cramping and slight vaginal spotting without passage of tissue. When she is examined, no cervical dilation is noted. The nurse caring for this woman should:
    A. Anticipate that the woman will be sent home with instructions to limit her activity and to avoid stress or orgasm
    B. Prepare the woman for a dilation and curettage
    C. Notify a grief counselor to assist the woman with the imminent loss of her fetus
    D. Tell the woman that the doctor will most likely perform a cerclage to help her maintain her pregnancy

26. A woman is admitted through the emergency department with a medical diagnosis of ruptured ectopic pregnancy. The primary nursing diagnosis at this time is:
    A. Acute pain related to irritation of the peritoneum with blood
    B. Risk for infection related to tissue trauma
    C. Deficient fluid volume related to blood loss associated with rupture of the uterine tube
    D. Anticipatory grieving related to unexpected pregnancy outcome

27. A woman diagnosed with an ectopic pregnancy is to receive methotrexate. The nurse should explain to the woman that: (Circle all that apply.)
    A. Methotrexate is an analgesic that will relieve the dull abdominal pain she is experiencing
    B. She should avoid alcohol until her primary care provider tells her the treatment is complete
    C. She will receive the medication intramuscularly
    D. She must stop taking folic acid supplements as long as she is on methotrexate.
    E. Her partner should use a condom during intercourse
    F. She must return for a measurement of her progesterone level to determine if a second dose of methotrexate is required.

28. A pregnant woman at 32 weeks of gestation comes to the emergency department because she has begun to experience bright red vaginal bleeding. She reports that she has no pain. The admission nurse suspects that the woman is experiencing:
    A. Abruptio placentae
    B. Disseminated intravascular coagulation
    C. Placenta previa
    D. Preterm labor

29. A pregnant woman at 38 weeks of gestation diagnosed with marginal placenta previa has just given birth to a healthy newborn male. The nurse recognizes that the immediate focus for the care of this woman is:
    A. Preventing hemorrhage
    B. Relieving acute pain
    C. Preventing infection
    D. Fostering attachment of the woman with her new son

III. THINKING CRITICALLY

1. Andrea is admitted to the hospital, where a diagnosis of acute ruptured ectopic pregnancy in her fallopian tube is made.
    A. STATE the risk factors associated with ectopic pregnancy.

B. DESCRIBE the findings that were most likely experienced and exhibited by Andrea as her ectopic pregnancy progressed and then ruptured.

C. IDENTIFY the other health care problems that share the same or similar clinical manifestations as ectopic pregnancy.

D. STATE the major care management problem at this time. SUPPORT your answer.

E. IDENTIFY two priority nursing diagnoses appropriate for Andrea.

F. OUTLINE the nursing measures Andrea will require during the preoperative and postoperative period.

2. Janet is 10 weeks pregnant. She comes to the clinic and states that she has been experiencing slight bleeding with mild cramping for about 4 hours. No tissue has been passed, and pelvic examination reveals that the cervical os is closed.
   A. INDICATE the most likely basis for Janet's signs and symptoms.

   B. OUTLINE the expected care management of Janet's problem.

3. Denise, a primigravida, calls the clinic. She is crying while she tells the nurse that she has noted "a lot of bleeding" and that she is sure she is losing her baby.
   A. WRITE several questions the nurse should ask Denise in order to obtain a more definitive picture of the bleeding she is experiencing.

   B. Denise is admitted to the hospital for further evaluation. A medical diagnosis of incomplete miscarriage is made. DESCRIBE the assessment findings that indicate the diagnosis of incomplete miscarriage.

   C. STATE the nursing diagnosis that takes priority at this time.

   D. OUTLINE the nursing measures that are appropriate for the priority nursing diagnosis you identified and for the expected medical management of Denise's health problem.

   E. SPECIFY the instructions that Denise should receive prior to her discharge from the hospital.

   F. LIST the nursing measures appropriate for a nursing diagnosis of anticipatory grieving related to unexpected outcome of pregnancy.

4. Marsha (5-0-1-4-0) is pregnant, at 12 weeks of gestation. She has a history of early and recurring pregnancy loss. In an attempt to maintain the current pregnancy to term, a prophylactic cerclage has been performed. OUTLINE the discharge care and instructions the nurse should give Marsha to ensure her safe recovery at home.

5. Mary has been diagnosed with hydatidiform mole (complete).
   A. IDENTIFY the typical signs and symptoms Mary most likely exhibits to establish this diagnosis.

   B. SPECIFY the posttreatment care and instructions that the nurse should include in a follow-up management plan with Mary and her family.

6. Two pregnant women are admitted to the labor unit with vaginal bleeding. Sara is at 29 weeks of gestation and is diagnosed with marginal placenta previa. Jane is at 34 weeks of gestation and is diagnosed with a moderate (grade II) premature separation of the placenta (abruptio placentae).
   A. COMPARE the clinical picture each of these women is likely to exhibit during assessment.

   B. IDENTIFY two priority nursing diagnoses for both Sara and Jane.

C. CONTRAST the care management approach required by each of the women as it relates to her diagnosis and the typical medical management.

D. INDICATE the considerations that must be given top priority following birth for each of these women.

CHAPTER 29

Endocrine and Metabolic Disorders in Pregnancy

I. LEARNING KEY TERMS

1. EXPLAIN the interrelationship of each of the following clinical manifestations associated with diabetes mellitus.
   Hyperglycemia

   Polyuria

   Glycosuria

   Polydipsia

   Ketoacidosis and acetonuria

   Weight loss

   Polyphagia

FILL IN THE BLANKS: Insert the term that corresponds to each of the following descriptions.

2. ______________________ Group of metabolic diseases characterized by hyperglycemia resulting from defects in insulin secretion, insulin action, or both.

3. ______________________ Excretion of large volumes of urine.

4. ______________________ Excessive thirst.

5. ______________________ Eating excessive amounts of food.

6. ______________________ Results when unusable glucose is excreted.

7. ______________________ Metabolic disease that occurs when pancreatic islet beta cells are destroyed, resulting in an absolute insulin deficiency; an autoimmune process may be involved in its etiology.

8. ______________________ Metabolic disease resulting in insulin resistance and relative rather than absolute insulin deficiency.

9. ______________________ Label given to type 1 or type 2 diabetes that existed before pregnancy.

10. ______________________ Any degree of glucose intolerance with onset or first recognition occurring during pregnancy.

11. ______________________ Key to optimal outcome of a diabetic pregnancy before conception and throughout pregnancy.

12. ______________________ Excessive amount of amniotic fluid.

13. ______________________ Less than the normal amount of glucose in the blood

14. ______________________ Excess glucose in the blood

15. ______________________ Accumulation of ketones in the blood resulting from hyperglycemia and leading to metabolic acidosis; it occurs most often during the second and third trimesters when the diabetogenic effect of pregnancy is the greatest.

16. ______________________ Normal blood glucose level with preprandial range of ______________________ and 1-hour postprandial range no higher than ______________________.

17. ______________________ Result of excessive fetal growth in utero; newborn weighs more than 4000 to 4500 g at birth or is above the 90th percentile.

18. ______________________ Blood test that evaluates glycemic control over the previous 4 to 6 weeks.

19. ______________________ Measurement of blood glucose levels prior to eating. Acceptable results for this test range from ______________________ to ______________________ during pregnancy.

20. ______________________ Measurement of blood glucose levels 1 to 2 hours after eating; acceptable results for 1 hour after meals range from ______________________ to ______________________.

21. ______________________ Substance in amniotic fluid that is a better predictor of fetal lung maturity than is the L/S ratio in pregnancies complicated by diabetes.

22. ______________________ Excessive vomiting during pregnancy resulting in a weight loss of at least 5% of prepregnancy weight and is accompanied by dehydration, electrolyte imbalance, ketosis, and acetonuria.

II. REVIEWING KEY CONCEPTS

23. Women with diabetes mellitus are attending a preconception care class regarding the risks of pregnancy for mother and fetus and how to prevent or minimize the complications that can result. DISCUSS the major maternal and fetal/neonatal risks and complications associated with diabetic pregnancies (pregestational and gestational) that should be included in this class. SUGGEST several measures a nurse could include in the class to reduce the risk for these complications.

24. Rosario, a woman with type 1 diabetes, has just discovered that she is pregnant. She is concerned that pregnancy will affect her diabetes and her diabetes will affect her pregnancy and baby. EXPLAIN to Rosario the metabolic changes that occur during pregnancy and indicate how these changes will affect her care management during the first trimester, the second and third trimesters, and the postpartum period of her pregnancy.

25. DISCUSS how each of the following types of insulin are used during pregnancy to achieve and maintain euglycemia. Give an example of each type of insulin.
    A. Rapid acting

    B. Short acting

    C. Intermediate acting

    D. Long acting

26. Magda, a 28-year-old Hispanic-American, is pregnant for the first time. Her BMI is 29. She asks you why she needs to have a glucose test done at 24 weeks into her pregnancy because she does not have diabetes like her mother does.
    A. EXPLAIN to Magda the current recommendations for screening for and diagnosing of gestational diabetes mellitus. Include in your explanation the risk factors Magda presents that make screening especially important and what the glucola screening involves.

    B. The results of Magda's test is 145 mg/dl. What would you anticipate as the next step?

    C. STATE the results that confirm a diagnosis of gestational diabetes.

27. You are part of a health care team caring for two pregnant women. One is Anna, who is hypothyroid, and the other is Tanisha, who is hyperthyroid. DESCRIBE how their pregnancies will be affected by their thyroid disorder and compare the management approach you anticipate.

MULTIPLE CHOICE: Circle the correct option(s) and state the rationale for the option(s) chosen.

28. A pregestational diabetic woman at 20 weeks of gestation exhibits the following: thirst, nausea and vomiting, abdominal pain, drowsiness, and increased urination. Her skin is flushed and dry, and her breathing is rapid, with a fruity odor. A priority nursing action when caring for this woman is to:
    A. Provide the woman with a simple carbohydrate immediately
    B. Request an order for an antiemetic
    C. Assist the woman into a lateral position to rest
    D. Administer insulin according to the woman's blood glucose level

29. During her pregnancy a woman with pregestational diabetes has been monitoring her blood glucose level several times a day. Which level requires further assessment?
    A. 85 mg/dl—15 minutes prior to breakfast
    B. 90 mg/dl—prior to lunch
    C. 140 mg/dl—2 hours after lunch
    D. 135 mg/dl—1 hour after supper

30. Specific guidelines should be followed when planning a diet with a pregestational diabetic woman (BMI 24) to ensure a euglycemic state. Which dietary practices does the woman need to modify? (Circle all that apply.)
    A. Follows a diet that reflects 45 kcal per kg daily based on her preconception BMI
    B. Eats three meals a day along with a midmorning, a midafternoon, and a bedtime snack
    C. Drinks a cup of tea and a piece of dry toast as her bedtime snack
    D. Divides her daily carbohydrate intake at 50% simple carbohydrates and 50% complex carbohydrates
    E. Maintains a fat intake of approximately 25% of the total daily kcal recommendation
    F. Monitors the appropriateness of her nutritional intake by checking her blood glucose levels before and after meals

31. An obese pregnant woman with gestational diabetes is learning self-injection of insulin. While evaluating the woman's technique for self-injection, the nurse evaluates that the woman understands the instructions when she: (Circle all that apply.)
    A. Washes her hands and puts on a pair of clean gloves
    B. Gently rotates the NPH insulin vial to fully mix the insulin
    C. Draws the NPH insulin into her syringe first when mixing it with regular insulin
    D. Spreads her skin taut and punctures the skin at a 90-degree angle
    E. Cleanses the injection site vigorously with an alcohol swab
    F. Covers the injection site with a sterile gauze as she removes the needle then applies gentle pressure

32. A woman has just been admitted with a diagnosis of hyperemesis gravidarum. She has been unable to retain any oral intake and as a result has lost weight and is exhibiting signs of dehydration with electrolyte imbalance and acetonuria. The nurse anticipates that the care management of this woman will include:
    A. Administering vitamin K to control nausea and vomiting
    B. Separating liquids from solids, alternating them every 2 to 3 hours
    C. Avoiding oral hygiene until the woman is able to tolerate oral fluids
    D. Providing three daily meals of bland foods with warm fluids once the woman is able to tolerate oral intake

III. THINKING CRITICALLY

1. Mary is a 24-year-old diabetic client. When Mary informed her gynecologist that she and her husband were trying to get pregnant, she was referred to an endocrinologist for preconception counseling. Mary tells the nurse that she just cannot understand why this is necessary. She says, "I have had diabetes since I was 12 years old, and I have not had many problems. All I want to do is get pregnant!" DISCUSS how the nurse should respond to Mary's comments.

2. Luann is a 25-year-old nulliparous client in her first trimester of pregnancy (sixth week of gestation). She has had type 1 diabetes since she was 15 years old. Recently she has been experiencing some nausea and is eating less as a result. She took her usual dose of lispro (Humalog) and NPH (Humulin N) insulin prior to eating a very light breakfast of tea and a piece of toast. Just before her midmorning snack at work, she began to experience nervousness and weakness. She felt dizzy and became diaphoretic and pale.
    A. IDENTIFY the problem that Luann is experiencing. INDICATE the basis for her symptoms.

    B. DESCRIBE the action that Luann should take.

C. LIST several "glucose boosters" that Luann should have on hand should this problem occur again.

D. STATE what Luann should do after she takes the action described in B.

3. Judy's pregnancy has just been confirmed. She also has type 1 diabetes.
   A. As a result of her high risk status, a variety of additional assessment measures are emphasized during her prenatal period to evaluate the status of her fetus. IDENTIFY these additional assessment measures and their relevance in a diabetic pregnancy.

   B. DISCUSS the stressors that might confront Judy and her family as a result of her status as a diabetic woman who is pregnant.

   C. WRITE two nursing diagnoses that reflect Judy's health status.

   D. INDICATE the activity and exercise recommendations that Judy should be given.

E. OUTLINE the required nursing interventions and health teaching for the following major care components at each stage of Judy's pregnancy.
- Diet

- Blood glucose monitoring

- Insulin therapy

F. After birth, Judy, who will be bottle feeding, asks the nurse about birth control. DISCUSS the birth control options that would be best for Judy and her partner.

4. Elena (2-1-0-0-1) is a 32-year-old Hispanic-American in week 28 of her pregnancy. Her BMI is 30. Her mother, who is 59, was recently diagnosed with type 2 diabetes. Elena's first pregnancy resulted in the birth of a 10-pound 6-ounce daughter who is now 2 years old. A 1-hour, 50 g oral glucose tolerance test last week revealed a glucose level of 152 mg/dl. A 3-hour oral glucose tolerance test was done yesterday, with the following results: fasting—110 mg/dl, 1 hour—192 mg/dl, 2 hours—166 mg/dl, 3 hours—142 mg/dl.
   A. IDENTIFY the complication of pregnancy Elena is exhibiting. STATE the rationale for your answer.

   B. LIST the risk factors for this health problem that are present in Elena's assessment data.

C. DESCRIBE the pathophysiology involved in creating Elena's problem.

D. OUTLINE the ongoing assessment measures necessitated by Elena's health problem.

E. STATE two nursing diagnoses for Elena and her fetus.

F. STATE the dietary changes Elena will have to make to maintain glycemic control during the rest of her pregnancy.

G. Based on blood glucose levels, it was determined that despite Elena's adherence to the prescribed diet, she will need to take insulin. When told, Elena becomes very upset, stating that she is sure she will not be able to give herself shots. DESCRIBE how the nurse should approach this situation.

H. Before discharge after the full-term vaginal birth of her second daughter who was determined to be appropriate for gestational age (AGA), Elena asks the nurse if the health problem she experienced during this pregnancy will continue now that she has had her baby. She also wonders if it will happen with her next pregnancy, because she wants to get pregnant again soon so she can "try for a son." DISCUSS the response the nurse should give to address Elena's concerns.

5. Marie, a 19-year-old obese primigravida, is diagnosed with hyperemesis gravidarum at 14 weeks of gestation. She is unmarried and lives at home with her parents. The father of Marie's baby recently told her that he wants nothing to do with her or the baby. Marie is in the second semester of her sophomore year in college and is worried about how having a baby will affect her goals of obtaining a college degree and pursuing a career as a teacher. She states that she cannot bear the thought of having an abortion or giving her baby up for adoption. Her parents are upset about the pregnancy but are willing to help her as much as they can, emphasizing that as the baby's mother, she will be its major caregiver. Marie is admitted to the high risk antepartal unit.
   A. IDENTIFY the etiologic factors that may have contributed to Marie's current health problem.

   B. LIST the physiologic and psychologic factors that the nurse should be alert for when assessing Marie on her admission.

   C. STATE two nursing diagnoses related to Marie's current health status.

   D. OUTLINE the nursing care measures appropriate for Marie while she is hospitalized.

   E. Once stabilized, Marie is discharged to home care. She is able to tolerate oral food and fluid intake. EXPLAIN the important care measures that the nurse should discuss with Marie and her family before she goes home.

CHAPTER 30

Medical-Surgical Problems in Pregnancy

I. LEARNING KEY TERMS

FILL IN THE BLANKS: Insert the term that corresponds to each of the following descriptions.

1. ______________________ Inability of the heart to maintain a sufficient cardiac output.
2. ______________________ Classification system for cardiovascular disorders developed by the New York Heart Association. Class I implies: ______________________. Class II implies: ______________________. Class III implies: ______________________. Class IV implies: ______________________.
3. ______________________ Type of congenital heart defect that results in an abnormal opening between the atria.
4. ______________________ Type of congenital heart defect that results in an abnormal opening between the right and left ventricles.
5. ______________________ Type of congenital heart defect that involves failure of the ductus arteriosus to close; it results in a right-to-left shunt.
6. ______________________ Type of congenital heart defect that results in a localized narrowing of the aorta near the insertion of the ductus; it is an acyanotic heart lesion.
7. ______________________ Type of congenital heart defect that results in an abnormal opening between the ventricles, pulmonary stenosis, overriding aorta, and right ventricular hypertrophy; it is a cyanotic heart lesion.
8. ______________________ Narrowing of the opening of the aortic valve leading to an obstruction to left ventricular ejection.
9. ______________________ Acute ischemic event involving the heart.
10. ______________________ Development of congestive heart failure in the last month of pregnancy or within the first 5 months postpartum; there is lack of another cause for heart failure and absence of heart disease prior to the last month of pregnancy.
11. ______________________ Narrowing of the opening of the valve between the left atrium and the left ventricle of the heart by stiffening of the valve leaflets, which obstructs blood flow from the atrium to the ventricles. It is the characteristic lesion resulting from rheumatic heart disease.
12. ______________________ Inflammation of the innermost lining of the heart caused by invasion of microorganisms.
13. ______________________ Right-to-left or bidirectional shunting at either the atrial or ventricular level, combined with elevated pulmonary vascular resistance.
14. ______________________ Common, usually benign cardiac condition that involves the protrusion of the leaflets of the mitral valve back into the left atrium during ventricular systole, allowing some backflow of blood.
15. ______________________ Autosomal dominant genetic disorder characterized by generalized weakness of the connective tissue, resulting in joint deformities, ocular lens dislocation, and weakness of the aortic wall and root.

16. ______________________________ Disorder characterized by constriction of the arteriolar vessels in the lungs, leading to an increase in the pulmonary artery pressure.

17. ______________________________ Reduction of the oxygen-carrying capacity of the blood primarily caused by an iron deficiency; the heart attempts to compensate by increasing the cardiac output; hemoglobin is less than 11 g/dl in the first and third trimesters and 10.5 g/dl in the second trimester.

18. ______________________________ Deficiency that, if present during conception and early pregnancy, is associated with an increased incidence of neural tube defects, cleft lip, and cleft palate.

19. ______________________________ Disease caused by the presence of abnormal hemoglobin in the blood. It is a recessive, hereditary, familial hemolytic anemia that affects those of African-American and Mediterranean ancestry.

20. ______________________________ Anemia in which an insufficient amount of hemoglobin is produced to fill red blood cells.

21. ______________________________ Chronic inflammatory disorder involving the tracheobronchial airways with increased airway responsiveness to a variety of stimuli; it is characterized by exacerbations and remissions.

22. ______________________________ Respiratory disorder in which the lungs are unable to maintain levels of oxygen and carbon dioxide within normal limits; it is also know as shock lung.

23. ______________________________Autosomal recessive genetic disorder in which exocrine glands produce excessive viscous secretions, which causes problems with both respiratory and digestive functions.

24. ______________________________ Generalized itching during pregnancy without the presence of a rash; it is often limited to the abdomen and is usually caused by skin distention and development of striae.

25. ______________________________ Common pregnancy-specific cause of pruritus in pregnancy; it is also termed polymorphic eruption of pregnancy and is most common in primigravidas during the third trimester.

26. ______________________________ Disorder of the brain that causes recurrent seizures; it is the most common major neurologic disorder accompanying pregnancy.

27. ______________________________Patchy demyelinization of the spinal cord and the CNS; it may be a viral disorder.

28. ______________________________ Chronic, multisystemic inflammatory disease that affects the skin, joints, kidneys, lungs, nervous system, liver, and other body organs; it is the most common serious autoimmune disease affecting women of reproductive age.

29. ______________________________ Autoimmune motor (muscle) end-plate disorder that involves acetylcholine use and affects the motor function at the myoneural junction; it results in muscle weakness, particularly of the eyes, face, tongue, neck, limbs, and respiratory muscles.

30. ______________________________ Presence of gallstones in the gallbladder.

31. ______________________________ Inflammation of the gallbladder.

32. ______________________________ Disorder of the intestine including ulcerative colitis and Crohn's disease.

33. ______________________________ Most common medical complication of pregnancy, occurring in approximately 20% of all pregnancies and is responsible for 10% of all hospitalizations during pregnancy.

34. ______________________________ Most common nongynecologic condition necessitating abdominal surgery during pregnancy.

35. ______________________________ Acute idiopathic facial paralysis.

II. REVIEWING KEY CONCEPTS

36. Sara, who has been diagnosed with mitral valve stenosis class II heart disease, is considering pregnancy. She and her husband ask the nurse during a preconception care visit to explain the potential risks that Sara and their potential fetus face as a result of her cardiac status. DESCRIBE how the nurse should approach the question Sara and her husband have. Include the maternal and fetal complications that are more common among pregnant women who have cardiac problems in your answer.

37. EXPLAIN the modifications that should be made in the protocol used for cardiopulmonary resuscitation (CPR) and the abdominal thrust maneuver when a woman is pregnant.

MULTIPLE CHOICE: Circle the correct option(s), and state the rationale for the option(s) chosen.

38. When assessing a pregnant woman at 28 weeks of gestation who is diagnosed with mitral valve stenosis, it is important that the nurse be alert for signs and symptoms indicating cardiac decompensation. Signs and symptoms of cardiac decompensation include: (Circle all that apply.)
    A. Dry, hacking cough
    B. Orthopnea
    C. Wheezing with inspiration and expiration
    D. Rapid pulse that is irregular and weak
    E. Woman reports that shoes and rings are tight
    F. Supine hypotension

39. A woman at 30 weeks of gestation with a class II cardiac disorder calls her primary health care provider's office and speaks to the nurse practitioner. She tells the nurse that she has been experiencing a frequent moist cough for the past few days. In addition, she has been feeling more tired and is having difficulty completing her routine activities as a result of some difficulty with breathing. The nurse's best response is:
    A. "Have someone bring you to the office so we can assess your cardiac status."
    B. "Try to get more rest during the day, because this is a difficult time for your heart."
    C. "Take an extra diuretic tonight before you go to bed, because you may be developing some fluid in your lungs."
    D. "Ask your family to come over and do your housework for the next few days so you can rest."

40. A pregnant woman with a valvular disorder of her heart requires medication to prevent clot formation. In preparing the woman for this treatment measure, the nurse expects to teach the woman about self-administration of:
    A. Furosemide (Lasix)
    B. Propranolol (Inderal)
    C. Heparin
    D. Warfarin (Coumadin)

41. At a previous antepartal visit, the nurse taught a pregnant woman diagnosed with a class II cardiac disorder about measures to use to lower her risk for cardiac decompensation. This woman indicates a need for further instruction if she:
    A. Increases roughage in her diet
    B. Remains on bed rest, getting out of bed only to go to the bathroom
    C. Sleeps 10 hours every night and rests after meals
    D. States she will call the nurse immediately if she experiences any pain or swelling in her legs

42. A pregnant woman has been diagnosed with cholelithiasis. An important component of her treatment regimen is dietary modification. The nurse helps this woman plan a diet that:
    A. Reduces dietary fat to approximately 60 g per day
    B. Limits protein to 30% of total calories
    C. Chooses foods that ensure that most calories come from carbohydrates
    D. Avoids putting spices in foods

III. THINKING CRITICALLY

1. Serena, a 30-year-old pregnant client at 24 weeks of gestation, begins to complain of pain in her lower abdomen, nausea with some vomiting, and anorexia. Her husband brings her to the emergency department.
    A. IDENTIFY the factors that will make it difficult for the doctor to diagnose the condition causing Serena's clinical manifestations.

    B. Serena is diagnosed with appendicitis. EXPLAIN why it is vital that surgical treatment occur prior to rupture of the appendix.

    C. CITE the major fears Serena and her husband will have about the impending surgery.

    D. OUTLINE the preoperative and postoperative care Serena will require.

    E. Serena's surgery was successful, and she is discharged to home. IDENTIFY the nursing considerations and topics for teaching related to the discharge planning process for Serena as a pregnant woman who is recovering from surgery.

2. Linda, age 26, had rheumatic fever as a child and subsequently developed mitral valve stenosis. She is 6 weeks pregnant. She is classified as class II according to the New York Heart Association functional classification of organic heart disease. This is the first pregnancy for Linda and her husband, Sam.
   A. IDENTIFY two nursing diagnoses appropriate for Linda related to her cardiac status and her anticipated care management. STATE an expected outcome for each nursing diagnosis identified.

   B. DISCUSS a recommended therapeutic plan for Linda that will reduce her risk for cardiac decompensation in terms of each of the following:
      - Rest/sleep/activity patterns

      - Prevention of infection

      - Nutrition

      - Bowel elimination

   C. IDENTIFY several physiologic and psychosocial factors that could increase the stress placed on Linda's heart during her pregnancy.
      - Physiologic factors

- Psychosocial factors

D. LIST the subjective symptoms that the nurse should teach Linda and her family to look for as indicators of possible cardiac decompensation.

E. LIST the objective signs that indicate that Linda is experiencing signs of cardiac decompensation and heart failure.

F. Linda is admitted to the labor unit. Her cardiac condition is still classified as class II. OUTLINE the nursing measures designed to assess Linda and promote optimum cardiac function during labor and birth.

G. Linda should be observed carefully during the postpartum period because cardiac risk continues. INDICATE the physiologic events after birth that place Linda at risk for cardiac decompensation.

H. IDENTIFY two nursing diagnoses appropriate for the first 24 to 48 hours of Linda's postpartum period.

I. DISCUSS the measures the nurse can use to reduce the stress placed on Linda's heart during the postpartum period.

J. Linda indicates that she wishes to breastfeed her infant. DESCRIBE the nurse's response.

K. IDENTIFY the important factors to be considered when preparing Linda's discharge plan.

3. Allison is a pregnant woman with a cardiac disorder. As part of her medical regimen, her primary health care provider substituted subcutaneous heparin for the oral warfarin sodium (Coumadin) she had been taking before pregnancy.
   A. Allison states, "I cannot give myself a shot! Why can't I just take the medication orally?" DISCUSS how you would respond as to the purpose of heparin and why it must be used instead of the Coumadin she is used to taking.

   B. INDICATE the information that the nurse should give Allison to ensure safe use of the heparin.

4. Jean is a primigravida at 4 weeks of gestation. She has been an epileptic for several years, and her seizures have been controlled with phenytoin (Dilantin). Jean expresses concern regarding how her medication use will affect her pregnancy and her baby. She wants to stop taking the Dilantin. DESCRIBE the approach you would take in addressing Jean's concern and the course of action she is contemplating.

CHAPTER 31

Obstetric Critical Care

I. LEARNING KEY TERMS

FILL IN THE BLANKS: Insert the term that corresponds to each of the following descriptions.

1. ______________________ Gradient controlling whether fluid remains inside the capillary or moves into the interstitial space. The force to keep fluid inside the vessel is the pulling pressure of the colloids or proteins present in the plasma.
2. ______________________ The force exerted to push fluids through the membrane; it is measured as the ______________________.
3. Normal arterial blood gas values for pregnancy reflect a chronic state of compensated ______________________.
4. ______________________ Hematologic change in pregnancy that increases the risk for thrombus formation whenever hemoconcentration develops, as occurs with severe preeclampsia or dehydration.
5. ______________________ Measure of the tension required for the ejection of blood into the circulation (afterload).
6. ______________________ Period of the cardiac cycle when both ventricles are relaxed and filling.
7. ______________________ Period of the cardiac cycle when both ventricles contract.
8. ______________________ Volume of blood ejected from the left ventricle in 1 minute; it is measured in liters per minute.
9. ______________________ Volume of blood ejected from the left ventricle during one cardiac cycle; it is a result of three factors, namely ______________________, ______________________ and ______________________.
10. ______________________, ______________________, ______________________, and ______________________ The four major determinants of cardiac output.
11. ______________________ Volume of blood in the ventricles at the end of diastole; it is determined by intraventricular pressure and volume.
12. ______________________ Ventricular wall tension during systole, or the resistance the blood meets as it is ejected from the ventricles.
13. ______________________ Inotropic state of the heart.
14. ______________________ Method that provides continuous measurements of preload, afterload, myocardial contractility, and heart rate in the critically ill pregnant woman so that therapeutic manipulation may be made quickly at the bedside in response to changes in client status. A ______________________ or ______________________ is used to gather these measurements.
15. ______________________ Catheter that provides measurements of systolic, diastolic, and mean arterial pressures and provides access for arterial blood gas sampling and analysis.

16. ______________________________ Test performed prior to radial artery puncture to validate adequate collateral circulation into the hand by demonstrating a patent ulnar artery.

17. ______________________________ Method used to evaluate the saturation of hemoglobin with oxygen (Sao_2).

18. ______________________________ Method used to evaluate the percentage of saturation of hemoglobin with oxygen in mixed venous and arterial blood; it involves the insertion of a fiberoptic PAC.

19. ______________________________ Urine output of less than 20 to 30 ml for 2 consecutive hours.

20. ______________________________ The leading nonobstetric cause of maternal mortality.

II. REVIEWING KEY CONCEPTS

21. Obstetric intensive care units are becoming more common as options for obstetric critical care.
    A. EXPLAIN the rationale for the health care option of the obstetric intensive care unit.

    B. CITE several indicators for use of obstetric critical care.

22. EXPLAIN the factors present during labor and the postpartum period that are responsible for altering the cardiac output. INDICATE how cardiac output is altered.
    - Labor

    - Postpartum period

23. Oxygen delivery to and use by peripheral tissues must be adequate; therefore, its assessment is an essential aspect of the care of a critically ill pregnant woman. DESCRIBE each of the following techniques that monitor oxygenation. INDICATE expected values as part of your description.
    A. Arterial blood gas determinations

B. Pulse oximetry

C. Svo_2 monitoring

MULTIPLE CHOICE: Circle the correct option(s), and state the rationale for the option(s) chosen.

24. A nurse caring for a pregnant woman evaluates the woman's most recent arterial blood gas (ABG) values. Which arterial blood gas value falls within the expected range for a pregnant woman?
    A. pH: 7.30
    B. Po_2: 105 mm Hg
    C. Pco_2: 50 mm Hg
    D. Bicarbonate: 16 mEq/L

25. A pulmonary artery catheter will be one of the monitoring techniques used during the care of a critically ill pregnant woman. As part of the protocol for a pulmonary artery catheter insertion and care, the nurse will: (Circle all that apply.)
    A. Assist the woman into a supine position, with the head of the bed elevated slightly to facilitate catheter insertion
    B. Ensure that a signed informed consent is attached to the woman's chart
    C. Perform catheter site care once per shift or daily according to unit infection control policy
    D. Keep hydralazine on hand in case an arrhythmia develops
    E. Apply pressure to the catheter site for 10 minutes following the catheter's removal.
    F. Document the woman's response to the insertion procedure.

26. A nurse is performing a full assessment of a pregnant trauma victim just admitted to the emergency department. As part of the assessment, the nurse determines the woman's Glasgow Coma Scale score. Which data should the nurse use in calculating this score? (Circle all that apply.)
    A. Eyes opened to verbal command
    B. Blood pressure 110/60
    C. Pupils constricted equally to light
    D. Able to indicate location of pain
    E. Apical pulse 98 beats/min, regular, moderate strength
    F. Communication clear but is unsure where she is and what happened to her

27. When positioning a critically ill pregnant woman, which position should the nurse use to provide optimal cardiac output?
    A. Supine position
    B. Prone position
    C. Fowler position
    D. Right or left lateral position

28. The most common risk associated with an intraarterial line is:
    A. Hemorrhage
    B. Thrombus formation
    C. Embolization
    D. Infection

29. A critically ill pregnant woman is to have an arterial pressure catheter inserted to monitor her systolic, diastolic, and mean arterial pressures. Before insertion the nurse performs an Allen test and reports the results to the physician who will be inserting the catheter. When performing this test, the nurse should:
    A. Perform the test on the woman's dominant hand
    B. Occlude the ulnar and radial arteries simultaneously while raising the hand
    C. Instruct the woman to keep her fist tightly clenched during the test
    D. Release pressure on both arteries at the same time, noting the time for capillary refill

III. THINKING CRITICALLY

1. Annie is in her 28th week of pregnancy. She was in an automobile accident and as a result was admitted to an obstetric intensive care unit for observation and treatment of severe injuries.
    A. Annie's physician orders arterial blood gases and the insertion of an arterial pressure catheter into the radial artery to evaluate her cardiopulmonary status. DESCRIBE the protocol that should be followed before obtaining the arterial blood sample and inserting the arterial pressure catheter.

    B. STATE the two major purposes for inserting an arterial pressure catheter.

    C. EXPLAIN why the nurse caring for Annie should assess her blood pressure periodically using a sphygmomanometer.

    D. Annie's blood gas values are: pH 7.43, Po_2 106, Pco_2 30, and Hco_3 22. ANALYZE these values to determine if each is within the normal range for a pregnant woman.

    E. The Glasgow Coma Scale is used to help determine Annie's neurologic integrity and the extent of any head injury Annie may have sustained during the automobile accident. IDENTIFY the three major assessment categories of the scale, and GIVE one example of how you would evaluate each.

F. SPECIFY the positions you would use to enhance Annie's cardiac output. SUPPORT your answer.

G. DESCRIBE how the nurse can provide supportive care to Annie and her family.

2. Trauma continues to be a common complication during pregnancy that may require obstetric critical care.
   A. DISCUSS the significance of this complication using statistical data to describe the scope of the problem in terms of incidence, timing during pregnancy, and forms of trauma.

   B. INDICATE the effects trauma can have on pregnancy.

   C. EXPLAIN how each of the following physiologic and anatomic adaptations to pregnancy can affect the type and extent of injuries a woman could experience as a result of trauma.
      - Location of bladder and uterus
      - Elevation of progesterone levels
      - Changes in hemodynamic (cardiopulmonary) function

D. DESCRIBE the potential efect of trauma on the fetus.

E. SPECIFY the potential effects of each of the following mechanisms of trauma.

- Blunt abdominal trauma

- Penetrating abdominal trauma

- Thoracic trauma

F. Priorities of care for a pregnant woman following trauma must be to ______________________ and ______________________ first and then consider ______________________. This method of approach in care management is important because ______________________ survival is dependent on ______________________ survival.

G. OUTLINE the major components of the primary and secondary survey of a pregnant woman who has experienced trauma.

1. Primary survey

2. Secondary survey

CHAPTER 32

Mental Health Disorders and Substance Abuse in Pregnancy

I. LEARNING KEY TERMS

FILL IN THE BLANKS: Insert the term that corresponds to each of the following descriptions.

1. ______________________________ Group of mental health disorders that have as their dominant feature a disturbance in the prevailing emotional state.
2. ______________________________ The most common group of mental health disorders.
3. ______________________________ Anxiety disorder that is characterized by irrational fears that lead a person to avoid common objects, events, or situations.
4. ______________________________ Anxiety disorder that is characterized by repeated, unprovoked episodes of intense fear that develop without warning and are not related to any specific event.
5. ______________________________ Anxiety disorder characterized by constant worry unrelated to any event.
6. ______________________________ Anxiety disorder characterized by recurrent, persistent, and intrusive thoughts that cause anxiety which a person tries to control by performing repetitive behaviors.
7. ______________________________ Anxiety disorder that can be precipitated by highly stressful events such as sexual assault and military combat.
8. ______________________________ Postpartum mood disorder characterized by an intense and pervasive sadness with severe and labile mood swings. The woman experiences feelings of intense fear, anxiety, irritability, and despondency that persists past the baby's first few weeks of life.
9. ______________________________ Syndrome most often characterized by depression, delusions, hallucinations, elements of delirium or disorientation, extreme deficits in judgment, and thoughts by the mother of harming either the infant, herself, or both.
10. ______________________________ Mood disorder preceded or accompanied by manic episodes and characterized by elevated, expansive, or irritable moods that often alternate with periods of depression.
11. ______________________________ Discrete periods in which there is a sudden onset of intense apprehension, fearfulness, or terror.

II. REVIEWING KEY CONCEPTS

12. Before major depression can be diagnosed, the client must experience at least five specific signs and symptoms nearly every day. DESCRIBE the signs and symptoms used to diagnose major depression.

13. EXPLAIN why diagnostic assessment of pregnant women for depression is difficult. STATE the cues for which the nurse could look in an effort to facilitate diagnosis of depression.

14. It is essential to screen pregnant women for substance abuse early in pregnancy.
    A. STATE the purpose for the CAGE questionnaire and the 4 Ps Plus screening tool.

    B. COMPARE each tool and explain which tool is more suited to pregnancy.

    C. INDICATE the question represented by each letter:
    C
    A
    G
    E

    D. STATE the meaning of each of the 4 Ps on the 4 Ps Plus screening tool.

15. SPECIFY the harmful effects that use of each of the following substances can have on the pregnant woman and her fetus/newborn.
    - Nicotine

    - Caffeine

- Alcohol

- Marijuana

- Cocaine

- Methamphetamine

- Opiates

MULTIPLE CHOICE: Circle the correct option(s) and state the rationale for the option(s) chosen.

16. Nurses caring for postpartum women experiencing depression need to be aware of the safety of administering antidepressants. Which antidepressant should be avoided by women who wish to continue breastfeeding?
    A. Desipramine (Norpramin)
    B. Sertraline (Zoloft)
    C. Doxepin (Sinequan)
    D. Paroxetine (Paxil)

17. Which measure is least effective in helping a woman prevent postpartum depression?
    A. Share feelings and emotions with family members and her partner.
    B. Recognize that emotional problems after having a baby are not unusual.
    C. Care for the baby by herself to increase her level of self-confidence and self-esteem.
    D. Ask friends or family members to take care of the baby while she sleeps or has a date with her partner.

18. A pregnant woman being treated for major depression arrives for her first prenatal visit. During the health history interview she shows the nurse the cough medicine that she just bought for a cold. The nurse notes that the cough medicine contains dextromethorphan. The nurse is concerned if the woman reports taking which medication for her depression?
    A. Citalopram (Celexa)
    B. Desipramine (Norpramin)
    C. Doxepine (Sinequan)
    D. Amoxapine (Asendin)

19. A priority question to ask a woman experiencing postpartum depression is:
    A. Have you thought about hurting yourself?
    B. Does it seem like your mind is filled with cobwebs?
    C. Have you been feeling insecure, fragile, or vulnerable?
    D. Does the responsibility of motherhood seem overwhelming?

20. The nurse should recognize that a complication of pregnancy associated with the intravenous use of cocaine is:
    A. Prolonged, difficult labor
    B. Premature separation of the placenta
    C. Increased risk for vaginal and urinary tract infections
    D. Premature rupture of membranes

21. When conducting a health history interview during a pregnant woman's first prenatal visit, the nurse must determine if the woman is substance dependent. The nurse's first question should relate to the woman's use of:
    A. Alcohol
    B. Caffeine
    C. Cocaine
    D. Over-the-counter and prescription medications

III. THINKING CRITICALLY

1. CREATE two profiles of women who, based on the risk factors they exhibit, are at increased risk for postpartum depression. USE different risk factors for each profile.

2. A common nursing diagnosis for a woman with postpartum depression who is hospitalized is the following: risk for impaired parenting related to limited ability of the mother to interact with and care for her infant, secondary to postpartum depression. IDENTIFY the nursing measures appropriate for this nursing diagnosis.

3. IMAGINE that you are a nurse working on a postpartum mother-baby unit. You have been asked to develop a teaching plan regarding postpartum depression that will be incorporated into the standard postpartum discharge instructions presented to postpartum women and their families.
    A. OUTLINE the teaching plan that you would develop regarding postpartum depression—its identification, prevention, and treatment.

B. CREATE a handout regarding the most critical points covered in your teaching plan that new parents can take home and use as a reference.

4. Julia is a 20-year-old primigravida at 16 weeks of gestation. When you assess her during her first prenatal visit, you suspect that she may be using cocaine.
   A. LIST several clinical manifestations that would lead the nurse to suspect that Julia is using cocaine.

   B. DESCRIBE the effect that cocaine use can have on Julia's pregnancy and on her fetus.

   C. EXPLAIN how the nurse should seek confirmation that Julia is indeed using cocaine.

   D. Julia confirms that she is using cocaine sometimes and that she can quit on her own, stating, " I know what can happen if you are pregnant and go to a treatment program. My friend went to one, and she was put in jail—and they ended up taking her baby away." DISCUSS the legal implications of cocaine use during pregnancy and the barriers women face in seeking and accepting treatment for their addiction.

   E. EXPLAIN how you can use the process of change, including the importance of readiness to make a change, in helping Julia.

F. EXPLAIN the considerations that should guide the nurse when planning care and setting expected outcomes for Julia as a pregnant woman who abuses illicit drugs.

G. INDICATE the nursing measures appropriate for Julia who is addicted to cocaine during pregnancy, childbirth, and the postpartum period.

5. Mary, a 23-year-old primipara beginning her second week postpartum, is bottle feeding her baby. Two months ago she and her husband, Tom, moved from Buffalo, where they had lived all their lives, to Los Angeles to take advantage of a career opportunity for Tom. They live in a community with many other young couples who are also starting families but have not had time to make friends with any of them. Last month they joined the Catholic church near their home so their baby can be baptized when the time comes. Tom tries to help Mary with the baby, but he has to spend long hours at work to establish his position. Mary's prenatal record reveals that she often exhibited anxiety about her well-being and that of her baby. During a home visit by a nurse as part of an early discharge program, Mary tells the nurse that she always wants to sleep and just cannot seem to get enough rest. Mary is very concerned that she is not being a good mother and states, "Sometimes I just do not know what to do to care for my baby the right way. I feel so bad that I am not breastfeeding my baby but I just could not handle it because I heard how hard it is to do successfully. It seems that Tom enjoys spending what little time he has at home with the baby and not with me. I even find myself yelling at him for the silliest things." The nurse recognizes that Mary is exhibiting behaviors strongly suggestive of postpartum depression.

   A. INDICATE the signs and symptoms that Mary exhibited that led the nurse to suspect postpartum depression.

   B. SPECIFY the predisposing factors for postpartum depression that are present in Mary's situation.

   C. WRITE several questions that the nurse could ask Mary to determine the depth of the postpartum depression that she is experiencing.

D. WRITE one nursing diagnosis that is reflective of Mary and Tom's current situation.

E. DESCRIBE the measures the nurse could use to help Mary and Tom cope with postpartum depression.

6. IMAGINE that you are an advanced practice nurse who specializes in the treatment of men and women who are alcohol and drug dependent. You have been hired to establish a treatment program specifically designed for pregnant women. OUTLINE the approach you would take to ensure that the program you establish takes into consideration the unique characteristics of women who abuse alcohol and drugs.

CHAPTER

33

Labor and Birth Complications

I. LEARNING KEY TERMS

FILL IN THE BLANKS: Insert the term that corresponds to each of the following descriptions.

1. ______________________ Cervical changes and uterine contractions occurring between 20 and 37 weeks of pregnancy.
2. ______________________ Any birth that occurs before the completion of 37 weeks of pregnancy.
3. ______________________ Birth that occurs between 34 and 36 weeks of gestation.
4. ______________________ Birth that occurs before 32 weeks of gestation; the great majority of deaths and most serious morbidity occur to infants born at this time.
5. ______________________ Weight at the time of birth of 2500 g or less.
6. ______________________ Condition of inadequate fetal growth not necessarily correlated with the initiation of labor.
7. ______________________ Glycoprotein found in plasma and produced during fetal life; its reappearance in the cervical mucus between 24 and 34 weeks of gestation could predict preterm labor.
8. ______________________ Rupture of the amniotic sac and leakage of amniotic fluid beginning at least 1 hour before the onset of labor at any gestational age.
9. ______________________ Rupture of the amniotic sac and leakage of fluid before the completion of 37 weeks of gestation with infection often preceding this rupture, but the etiology remains unknown.
10. ______________________ An infection of the amniotic cavity that is potentially life-threatening for the fetus and the woman.
11. ______________________ Long, difficult, or abnormal labor caused by various conditions associated with the five factors affecting labor.
12. ______________________ Abnormal uterine contractions that prevent the normal progress of cervical dilation and effacement (primary powers) or descent (secondary powers).
13. ______________________ or ______________________ Abnormal uterine activity often experienced by an anxious first-time mother who is having painful and frequent contractions that are ineffective in causing cervical dilation and effacement to progress.
14. ______________________ or ______________________ Abnormal uterine activity that usually occurs when a woman initially makes normal progress into the active phase of labor but then uterine contractions become weak and inefficient or stop altogether.
15. ______________________ Abnormal labor caused by contractures of the pelvic diameters that reduce the capacity of the bony pelvis, including the inlet, midpelvis, outlet, or any combination of these planes.
16. ______________________ Abnormal labor caused by obstruction of the birth passage by an anatomic abnormality other than that involving the bony pelvis; the obstruction may result from placenta previa, leiomyomas (uterine fibroid tumors), ovarian tumors, or a full bladder or rectum.
17. ______________________ Abnormal labor caused by fetal anomalies, excessive fetal size, malpresentation, malposition, or multifetal pregnancy.
18. ______________________ Excessive fetal size.

19. ______________________ or ______________________ Abnormal labor caused by excessive fetal size in relation to the size of the maternal pelvis.

20. ______________________ The most common fetal malposition.

21. ______________________ The most common form of malpresentation.

22. ______________________ Gestation of twins, triplets, quadruplets, or more.

23. ______________________ Labor pattern defined as a latent phase that exceeds 20 hours in nulliparas and exceeds 14 hours in multiparas.

24. ______________________ Labor pattern defined as an active phase during which cervical dilation occurs at a rate of less than 1.2 cm/hr in nulliparas and less than 1.5 cm/hr in multiparas.

25. ______________________ Labor pattern defined as no progress in dilation for 2 hours or more in both nulliparas and multiparas.

26. ______________________ Labor pattern during which fetal progress through the birth canal occurs at a rate of less than 1 cm/hr in nulliparas and less than 2 cm/hr in multiparas.

27. ______________________ Labor pattern defined as no change in fetal progress through the birth canal during the deceleration phase and second stage of labor.

28. ______________________ Labor pattern that lasts less than 3 hours from the onset of contractions to the time of birth often resulting from hypertonic uterine contractions that are tetanic in intensity. For nulliparas, dilation is greater than 5 cm in 1 hour and for multiparas, dilation is 10 cm in 1 hour.

29. ______________________ Attempt to turn the fetus from a breech or shoulder presentation to a vertex presentation for birth by exerting gentle, constant pressure on the abdomen.

30. ______________________ Observance of a woman and her fetus for a reasonable period of spontaneous active labor (e.g., 4 to 6 hours) to assess the safety of a vaginal birth for both.

31. ______________________ Chemical or mechanical initiation of uterine contractions before their spontaneous onset for the purpose of bringing about the birth.

32. ______________________ Rating system used to evaluate the inducibility of the cervix. The five characteristics assessed are ______________________, ______________________, ______________________, ______________________, and ______________________.

33. ______________________ Artificial rupture of the membranes often used to induce labor when the cervix is ripe or to augment labor if the progress begins to slow.

34. ______________________ Stimulation of uterine contractions after labor has started spontaneously but progress is unsatisfactory. Common methods include ______________________ infusion and ______________________.

35. ______________________ More than five uterine contractions in 10 minutes averaged over a 30-minute window.

36. ______________________ Birth method in which an instrument with two curved blades is used to assist the birth of the fetal head.

37. ______________________ or ______________________ Birth method involving the attachment of a vacuum cup to the fetal head using negative pressure.

38. ______________________ Birth of the fetus through a transabdominal incision of the uterus.

39. ______________________ or ______________________ Pregnancy that extends beyond the end of week 42 of gestation. ______________________ Syndrome characterized by dry, cracked, peeling skin; long nails; meconium staining of skin, nails, and umbilical cord; and perhaps loss of subcutaneous fat and muscle mass.

40. ______________________ Uncommon obstetric emergency in which the head of the fetus is born but the anterior shoulder cannot pass under the pubic arch. Two major causes are ______________________ or maternal ______________________.

41. ______________________ Obstetric emergency in which the umbilical cord lies below the presenting part of the fetus; it may be occult (hidden) or more commonly frank (visible).

42. ______________________ Nonsurgical disruption of all uterine layers; it is a rare but very serious obstetric injury occurring during labor and birth. The major risk factor for its occurrence is ______________________.

43. ______________________ or ______________________ Obstetric emergency in which amniotic fluid enters the maternal circulation triggering a rapid, complex series of pathophysiologic events leading to DIC, hypotension, and hypoxia.

II. REVIEWING KEY CONCEPTS

44. When caring for pregnant women, what factors would alert the nurse to the woman's increased risk for spontaneous preterm labor and birth?

45. EXPLAIN why bed rest may be more harmful than helpful as a component of preterm labor care management.

MATCHING: Match the description of medications used as part of the management of preterm labor in Column I with the appropriate medication listed in Column II.

COLUMN I

46. ________ Beta$_2$-adrenergic receptor agonist, often administered intravenously, is the only drug approved by the FDA for the purpose of suppressing uterine contractions.

47. ________ An antenatal glucocorticoid used to accelerate fetal lung maturity when there is risk for preterm birth.

48. ________ Beta$_2$-adrenergic receptor agonist often administered subcutaneously using a syringe or pump; it inhibits uterine activity and causes bronchodilation.

49. ________ A calcium channel blocker that relaxes smooth muscles including those of the contracting uterus; maternal hypotension is a major concern.

50. ________ Classification of medications given to arrest labor after uterine contractions and cervical change have occurred.

51. ________ A central nervous system (CNS) depressant used during preterm labor for its ability to relax smooth muscles including the uterus; it is administered intravenously.

52. ________ A prostaglandin synthesis inhibitor that relaxes uterine smooth muscle; it is administered orally or rectally.

COLUMN II

A. tocolytic
B. betamethasone
C. ritodrine (Yutopar)
D. terbutaline (Brethine)
E. magnesium sulfate
F. nifedipine (Procardia)
G. indomethacin (Indocin)

MATCHING: Match the description of medications used during the process of stimulating uterine contractions and cervical ripening in Column I with the medication listed in Column II.

COLUMN I

53. _______ Tocolytic medication administered subcutaneously to suppress uterine tachysystole.

54. _______ Classification of medications that can be used to ripen the cervix, stimulate uterine contractions, or both.

55. _______ Cervical ripening agent in the form of a vaginal insert that is placed in the posterior fornix of the vagina.

56. _______ Cervical ripening agent in the form of a gel that is inserted into the cervical canal just below the internal os.

57. _______ Pituitary hormone used to stimulate uterine contractions in the augmentation or induction of labor.

58. _______ Natural cervical dilator made from desiccated seaweed.

59. _______ Synthetic dilator containing magnesium sulfate.

60. _______ Cervical ripening agent, used in the form of a tablet, that is most commonly inserted intravaginally into the posterior fornix.

COLUMN II

A. oxytocin (Pitocin)
B. misoprostol (Cytotec)
C. dinoprostone (Cervidil)
D. dinoprostone (Prepidil)
E. terbutaline (Brethine)
F. prostaglandin
G. laminaria tent
H. lamicel

61. DESCRIBE how each of the five factors of labor can cause labor to be long, difficult, or abnormal. Explain how these factors interrelate.

62. EXPLAIN the treatment approach of therapeutic rest.

63. Angela (1-0-0-0-0) is experiencing hypertonic uterine dysfunction and Helena (3-1-0-1-1) is experiencing hypotonic uterine dysfunction. COMPARE AND CONTRAST each woman's labor in terms of causes/precipitating factors, maternal-fetal effects, change in pattern of progress, and care management.

A. Angela: hypertonic uterine dysfunction

B. Helena: hypotonic uterine dysfunction

64. IDENTIFY four indications for oxytocin induction and four contraindications to the use of oxytocin to stimulate the onset of labor.

Indications

Contraindications

MULTIPLE CHOICE: Circle the correct option(s) and state the rationale for the option(s) chosen.

65. When assessing a pregnant woman, the nurse is alert for factors associated with preterm labor. Which factors if exhibited by this woman increases her risk for spontaneous preterm labor and birth? (Circle all that apply.)
   A. Caucasian race
   B. Obstetric history: 3-0-2-0-1
   C. History of bleeding at 20 weeks
   D. Currently being treated for second bladder infection in 2 months
   E. Employed as a nurse in a trauma ICU
   F. BMI of 22 and height of 158 cm

66. Bed rest for prevention of preterm birth can result in: (Circle all that apply.)
   A. Bone demineralization with calcium loss
   B. Weight gain
   C. Fatigue
   D. Dysphoria and guilt
   E. Increase in cardiac output
   F. Emotional lability

67. A woman's labor is being suppressed using IV magnesium sulfate. Which measure should be implemented during the infusion?
   A. Limit intravenous fluid intake to 125 ml/hr.
   B. Discontinue infusion if maternal respirations are less than 14 breaths/min.
   C. Ensure that indomethacin is available should toxicity occur.
   D. Assist woman to maintain a comfortable semirecumbent position.

68. A physician has ordered that dinoprostone (Cervidil) be administered to ripen a pregnant woman's cervix in preparation for an induced labor. In fulfilling this order, the nurse should:
   A. Insert the dinoprostone into the cervical canal just below the internal os
   B. Tell the woman to remain in bed for at least 15 minutes
   C. Observe the woman for signs of uterine tachysystole
   D. Remove the dinoprostone as soon as the woman begins to experience uterine contractions

69. A nulliparous woman experiencing a postterm pregnancy is admitted for labor induction. Assessment reveals a Bishop score of 9. The nurse should:
   A. Call the woman's primary health care provider to order a cervical ripening agent
   B. Mix 20 units of oxytocin (Pitocin) in 500 ml of 5% glucose in water
   C. Piggyback the oxytocin solution into the port nearest the drip chamber of the primary IV tubing
   D. Begin the infusion at a rate between 1 milliunits/min as determined by the induction protocol

70. A woman's labor is being induced. The nurse assesses the woman's status and that of her fetus and the labor process just before an infusion increment of 2 milliunits/min. The nurse discontinues the infusion and notifies the woman's primary health care provider if during this assessment she notes:
   A. Frequency of uterine contractions: every 1½ minutes
   B. Variability of FHR: present
   C. Deceleration patterns: early decelerations noted with several contractions
   D. Intensity of uterine contractions at their peaks: 80 to 85 mm Hg

71. A laboring woman's vaginal examination reveals the following: 3 cm, 50%, LSA, 0. The nurse caring for this woman should:
   A. Place the ultrasound transducer in the left lower quadrant of the woman's abdomen
   B. Recognize that passage of meconium would be a definitive sign of fetal distress
   C. Expect the progress of fetal descent to be slower than usual
   D. Assist the woman into a knee-chest position for each contraction

72. A nurse is caring for a pregnant woman at 30 weeks of gestation in preterm labor. The woman's physician orders betamethasone 12 mg IM for two doses with the first dose to begin at 11 AM. In implementing this order the nurse should:
   A. Consult the physician because the dose is too high
   B. Explain to the woman that this medications will reduce her heart rate and help her to breathe easier
   C. Assess the woman for tachycardia and hypotension
   D. Schedule the second dose for 11 AM the next day

73. A nurse caring for a pregnant woman suspected of being in preterm labor recognizes this sign as diagnostic of preterm labor.
   A. Cervical dilation of at least 2 cm
   B. Uterine contractions occurring every 15 minutes
   C. Spontaneous rupture of the membranes
   D. Presence of fetal fibronectin in cervical secretions

74. A woman at 27 weeks of gestation experiences some mild uterine cramping. Which actions should she take? (Circle all that apply.)
   A. Empty her bladder
   B. Call her nurse midwife immediately
   C. Relax in a chair
   D. Drink two to three glasses of water or juice
   E. Palpate her uterus for 1 hour
   F. Resume the activity she was doing if the cramping subsides

75. A woman is in active labor. On spontaneous rupture of her membranes, the nurse caring for this woman notices variable deceleration patterns during evaluation of the monitor tracing. When preparing to perform a vaginal examination, the nurse observes a small section of the umbilical cord protruding from the vagina. What should the nurse do next?
   A. Increase the IV drip rate.
   B. Administer oxygen to the woman via mask at 8 to 10 L/min.
   C. Place a sterile gloved hand into the vagina and hold the presenting part off the cord while calling for assistance.
   D. Wrap the cord loosely with a sterile towel saturated with warm normal saline.

III. THINKING CRITICALLY

1. IMAGINE that you are a nurse-midwife working at an inner-city women's health clinic. You are concerned about the rate of preterm labor and birth among the pregnant women who come to your clinic for care. OUTLINE a preterm labor and birth prevention program that you would implement at your clinic to reduce the rate of preterm labors and birth.

2. Sara, a primiparous client (2-0-1-0-1) at 22 weeks of gestation, comes to the clinic for her scheduled prenatal visit. She is anxious because her last labor began at 26 weeks and she is worried that this will happen again. "I had no warning the last time. Is there anything I can do this time to have my baby later or at least know that labor is starting so I can let you know?"
   A. IDENTIFY the signs of preterm labor that the nurse-midwife should teach Sara.

   B. EXPLAIN how the nurse-midwife could help Sara implement a plan to reduce her risk for preterm labor.

   C. Three weeks later Sara calls the clinic and tells her nurse-midwife that she has been having uterine contractions about every 8 minutes or so for the last hour. She is admitted for possible tocolytic therapy. SPECIFY the criteria that Sara must meet before tocolysis can be safely initiated.

   D. Sara is started on a tocolysis regimen that involves IV administration of magnesium sulfate. OUTLINE the nursing care measures that must be implemented during the infusion to ensure the safety of Sara and her fetus.

E. The nurse is preparing to give Sara a dose of betamethasone 12 mg as ordered by the physician.
   1. STATE the purpose of this medication.

   2. EXPLAIN the protocol that the nurse should follow in fulfilling this order.

3. Debra has been experiencing signs of preterm labor. After a period of hospitalization, her labor was successfully suppressed and she was discharged to be cared for at home. Debra is receiving nifedipine (Procardia) 30 mg every 12 hours for 48 hours. She will palpate her uterine activity daily. Debra must also remain on bed rest most of the day with time up to use the bathroom and for meals.
   A. OUTLINE what the nurse should teach Debra regarding the self-administration of nifedipine.

   B. IDENTIFY the side effects of nifedipine that the nurse should teach Debra before discharge.

   C. DESCRIBE the instructions that Debra should be given regarding palpating her uterus for contractions.

   D. Debra has two children who are 5 and 8 years old. SPECIFY the suggestions you would give to help Debra and her children cope with the bed rest requirement ordered by Debra's primary health care provider.

4. Denise, a primigravida has reached the second stage of her labor with her fetus at zero station and positioned LOP. She is experiencing intense low back pain. Denise did not attend any childbirth classes and is having difficulty pushing effectively. Epidural analgesia is being used for pain control.
   A. IDENTIFY the factors that can have a negative effect on the secondary powers of labor (bearing-down efforts). Indicate those factors most likely implicated in Denise's situation.

   B. DESCRIBE how you would help Denise use her expulsive forces to facilitate the descent and birth of her baby.

   C. SPECIFY the positions that would be recommended based on the position of the presenting part of Denise's fetus.

5. Anne, a primigravida attended Lamaze classes with her husband, Mark. They were looking forward to working together during the labor and birth of their baby. Because of fetal distress, an emergency low-segment cesarean section with a transverse incision was performed after 18 hours of labor. Even though Anne and her son are in stable condition and she is glad that "everything turned out okay" for her son, she expresses a sense of failure, stating, "I could not manage to give birth to my son in the normal way and now I never will!"
   A. LIST the preoperative nursing measures that should have been implemented to prepare Anne physically and emotionally for the unexpected cesarean birth.

   B. SPECIFY the assessment measures that are critical when Anne is recovering following birth.

   C. STATE the postoperative nursing care measures that Anne requires.

D. Identify the nursing diagnosis reflected in Anne's statement, "I could not manage to give birth to my baby in the normal way and now I never will." SPECIFY the support measures the nurse could use to put her cesarean birth into perspective.

6. A vaginal examination reveals that Marie's fetus is RSA. SPECIFY the considerations that the nurse should keep in mind when providing care for Marie.

7. Angela (2-0-0-1-0) is at 42 weeks of gestation and has been admitted for induction of her labor.
   A. Assessment of Angela at admission included determination of her Bishop score. STATE the purpose of the Bishop score and identify the factors that are evaluated.

   B. Angela's score was 5. INTERPRET this result in terms of the planned induction of her labor.

   C. Angela's primary health care provider ordered that dinoprostone (Cervidil) be inserted. STATE the purpose of the dinoprostone, method of application, and its potential side effects.

   D. Before induction of her labor, Angela's primary health provider performs an amniotomy.
      1. STATE the rationale for performing an amniotomy at this time.

2. SPECIFY the nursing responsibilities before, during, and after this procedure.

E. Indicate which of the following actions reflect appropriate collaborative care (A) for Angela during the induction of her labor with IV oxytocin. If the action is not appropriate (NA), state what the correct action would be.

1. _______ Assist Angela into a lateral or upright position.
2. _______ Apply an external electronic fetal monitor and obtain a baseline strip of FHR and pattern.
3. _______ Explain to Angela what to expect and techniques used.
4. _______ Add 20 units of oxytocin (Pitocin) into 500 ml of an isotonic electrolyte solution.
5. _______ Piggyback the oxytocin solution into the port nearest the IV insertion site of the primary IV.
6. _______ Begin infusion at 4 milliunits/min.
7. _______ Increase oxytocin by 1 to 2 milliunits/min at 5- to 10-minute intervals after the initial dose until the desired pattern of contractions is achieved.
8. _______ Stop increasing the dosage and maintain level of oxytocin when active labor is established, contractions occur every 2 to 3 minutes, last 80 to 90 seconds, and are estimated to be strong using palpation.
9. _______ Monitor maternal blood pressure and pulse every 15 minutes and after every increment.
10. _______ Monitor FHR pattern and uterine activity every 15 minutes and before and after every increment.
11. _______ Limit IV intake to 1500 ml/8 hours.

F. STATE the reportable conditions associated with oxytocin (Pitocin) induction for which the nurse must be alert when managing Angela's labor.

G. The nurse notes a pattern of excessive uterine activity when evaluating Angela's monitor tracing. LIST the actions the nurse should take in order of priority.

8. Lora is a 37-year-old nulliparous client beginning her 42nd week of pregnancy. She and her primary health care provider have decided on a conservative "watchful waiting" approach because both she and her fetus are not experiencing distress.
   A. In helping Lora make this decision, the risks she and her fetus face as a result of a postterm pregnancy were explained. IDENTIFY the risks that Lora should have considered in making her decision.

   B. STATE the clinical manifestations that Lora is likely to experience as her pregnancy continues.

   C. OUTLINE the typical care management measures that should be implemented to ensure the safety of Lora and her fetus.

   D. SPECIFY the instructions that the nurse should give to Lora regarding her self-care as she awaits the onset of labor.

CHAPTER 34

Postpartum Complications

I. LEARNING KEY TERMS

FILL IN THE BLANKS: Insert the term that corresponds to each of the following descriptions of postpartum complications.

1. ______________________ Loss of more than 500 ml of blood after vaginal birth or 1000 ml of blood after cesarean birth. Additional criteria that may be used are a 10% change in hematocrit between admission for labor and postpartum or the need for erythrocyte transfusion. It can be classified as ______________________ if it occurs within the first 24 hours after birth or ______________________ if it occurs more than 24 hours after birth and up to 6 weeks postpartum.
2. ______________________ Marked hypotonia of the uterus. It is the leading cause of PPH complicating approximately 1 in 20 births.
3. ______________________ Most common of all injuries in the low portion of the genital tract; they are classified as first, second, third, and fourth degree.
4. ______________________ Accumulation of blood in the connective tissue as a result of blood vessel damage. ______________________ are the most common type following birth.
5. ______________________ Term used to refer to slight penetration of the myometrium by placental trophoblast.
6. ______________________ Term used to refer to deep penetration of the myometrium by the placenta.
7. ______________________ Term used to refer to perforation of the uterus by the placenta.
8. ______________________ Turning of the uterus inside out after birth; it may be partial or complete.
9. ______________________ Delayed return of the enlarged uterus to normal size and function following birth. Recognized causes of this delay include ______________________ and ______________________.
10. ______________________ Emergency situation in which profuse blood loss can result in severely compromised perfusion of body organs. Death may occur.
11. ______________________ Disorder in which coagulation is compromised, resulting in continuous bleeding.
12. ______________________ Abnormally low platelet level.
13. ______________________ Autoimmune disorder in which antiplatelet antibodies decrease the life span of the platelets.
14. ______________________ Type of hemophilia; it is probably the most common of all hereditary bleeding disorders.
15. ______________________ Formation of a blood clot or clots inside a blood vessel.
16. ______________________ Formation of a clot in a blood vessel as result of inflammation.

17. ______________________________ Thromboembolic condition that involves the superficial saphenous venous system.

18. ______________________________ Thromboembolic condition in which involvement varies. It can extend from the foot to the iliofemoral region.

19. ______________________________ Complication of DVT that occurs when part of a blood clot dislodges and is carried to the pulmonary artery, where it occludes the vessel and obstructs blood flow to the lungs.

20. ______________________________ Any clinical infection of the genital canal that occurs within 28 days after miscarriage, induced abortion, or childbirth.

21. ______________________________ Infection located in the lining of the uterus; it is the most common cause of postpartum infection; it usually begins as a localized infection at the placental site but can spread to involve the entire lining.

22. ______________________________ Infection of the breast soon after childbirth affecting approximately 1% to 10% of women, most of whom are primiparous breastfeeding women.

II. REVIEWING KEY CONCEPTS

23. STATE the twofold focus of medical management of hemorrhagic shock.

24. STATE the standard of care for bleeding emergencies.

MULTIPLE CHOICE: Circle the correct option(s), and state the rationale for the option(s) chosen.

25. Methylergonovine (Methergine) 0.2 mg is ordered for a woman who gave birth vaginally 1 hour ago; it is to be administered intramuscularly to treat a profuse lochial flow with clots. Her fundus is boggy and does not respond well to massage. She is still being treated for preeclampsia with IV magnesium sulfate at 1 g/hr. Her blood pressure, measured 5 minutes ago, was 155/98 mm Hg. In fulfilling this order, the nurse should:
    A. Measure the woman's blood pressure again 5 minutes after administering the medication
    B. Question the order, based on the woman's hypertensive status
    C. Administer the methylergonovine because it is the best choice to counteract the possible uterine relaxation effects of the magnesium sulfate infusion the woman is receiving.
    D. Tell the woman that the medication will lead to uterine cramping

26. A postpartum woman in the fourth stage of labor received 15-methylprostaglandin $F_{2\alpha}$ (Hemabate) 0.25 mg intramuscularly. The expected outcome of care for the administration of this medication is:
    A. Relief from the pain of uterine cramping
    B. Prevention of intrauterine infection
    C. Reduction in the blood's ability to clot
    D. Limitation of excessive blood loss that is occurring after birth

27. The nurse responsible for the care of postpartum women recognizes that the first sign of puerperal infection most likely is:
    A. Temperature elevation of 38° C or higher after the first 24 hours following birth
    B. Increased white blood cell count
    C. Foul-smelling profuse lochia
    D. Bradycardia

28. A breastfeeding woman's cesarean birth occurred 2 days ago. Investigation of the pain, tenderness, and swelling in her left leg led to a medical diagnosis of deep vein thrombosis (DVT). Care management for this woman during the acute stage of the DVT involves: (Circle all that apply.)
    A. Explaining that she will need to stop breastfeeding until anticoagulation therapy is completed
    B. Administering warfarin (Coumadin) orally
    C. Placing the woman on bed rest with her left leg elevated
    D. Fitting the woman with an elastic stocking so that she can exercise her legs
    E. Telling her to avoid changing her position for the first 24 hours
    F. Administering heparin intravenously for 3 to 5 days

III. THINKING CRITICALLY

1. Andrea is a multiparous woman (6-5-1-0-7) who gave birth to full-term twins vaginally 1 hour ago. Oxytocin (Pitocin) was used to augment her labor when hypotonic uterine contractions protracted the active stage of her labor. Special forceps were used to assist the birth of the second twin. Currently her vital signs are stable; her fundus is at the umbilicus, midline and firm; and her lochial flow is moderate to heavy without clots.
    A. Early postpartum hemorrhage is a major concern. STATE the factors that have increased Andrea's risk for hemorrhage at this time.

    B. IDENTIFY the priority nursing diagnosis at this time.

    C. During the second hour after birth, the nurse notes that Andrea's perineal pad became saturated in 15 minutes and that a large amount of blood had accumulated on the bed under her buttocks. DESCRIBE the nurse's initial response to this finding. STATE the rationale for the action you described.

    D. The nurse prepares to administer 10 units of oxytocin intravenously as ordered by Andrea's physician. EXPLAIN the guidelines the nurse should follow in fulfilling this order.

E. During the assessment of Andrea, the nurse must be alert for signs of developing hemorrhagic shock. CITE the signs the nurse would be watching for.

F. DESCRIBE the measures that the nurse should use to care for Andrea's physiologic needs, and support her and her family and attempt to reduce their anxiety.

2. Nurses working on a postpartum unit must be constantly alert for signs and symptoms of puerperal infection in their clients. You have been assigned to present a nursing inservice presentation titled, "Postpartum Uterine Infection—An Update." PREPARE a teaching plan that includes each of the following components.
   A. Factors that can increase a postpartum woman's risk for puerperal infection.

   B. Infection prevention measures that nurses should be using when caring for postpartum women.

   C. Typical clinical manifestations of endometritis for which nurses should be alert when assessing postpartum women.

   D. Two nursing diagnoses that are appropriate for women diagnosed with endometritis.

E. Critical nursing measures that are essential in care management related to puerperal infection using the nursing diagnoses as an organizing framework.

3. Sara, a primiparous breastfeeding mother at 2 weeks postpartum, calls her nurse-midwife to tell her that her right breast is painful and that she is "not feeling well."
   A. EXPLAIN the assessment findings the nurse-midwife would be alert for to determine whether Sara is experiencing mastitis.

   B. A medical diagnosis of mastitis of Sara's right breast is made. STATE two nursing diagnoses appropriate for this situation.

   C. DESCRIBE the treatment measures and health teaching that Sara, who wishes to continue to breastfeed, needs regarding her infection and breastfeeding.

   D. IDENTIFY several behaviors that Sara should learn to prevent recurrence of mastitis.

4. Susan is a 36-year-old obese multiparous client (4-3-0-1-3) who experienced a cesarean birth 2 days ago. She has no previous history of pregnancy-related complications. When asked, she admits to smoking but has been trying to cut down from her usual half pack every 1 to 2 days. A major complication of the postpartum period for Susan is the development of thromboembolic disease.
   A. STATE the risk factors for this complication that Susan presents.

B. When assessing Susan on the afternoon of her second postpartum day, the nurse notes signs indicative of deep vein thrombosis (DVT). LIST the signs the nurse most likely observed.

C. A medical diagnosis of DVT is confirmed. STATE one nursing diagnosis appropriate for this situation.

D. OUTLINE the expected care management for Susan during the acute phase of the DVT.

E. On discharge, Susan will be taking warfarin for at least 3 months. SPECIFY the discharge instructions that Susan and her family should receive.

CHAPTER 35

Acquired Problems of the Newborn

I. LEARNING KEY TERMS

FILL IN THE BLANKS: Insert the term that corresponds to each of the following descriptions.

1. ______________________ Physical injury sustained by a neonate during labor and birth.
2. ______________________ Rupture of the capillaries within the eye caused by increased intracranial pressure during birth. They usually clear within 5 days after birth and present no problems.
3. ______________________ Bruises; may appear on the face as the result of a face presentation, or on the buttocks and genitalia with a breech presentation.
4. ______________________ Pinpoint hemorrhagic areas.
5. ______________________ The bone most frequently fractured during birth.
6. ______________________ or ______________________ Brachial paralysis of the upper portion of the arm; it is the most common type of paralysis associated with a difficult birth.
7. ______________________ Failure of the kidney to develop.
8. ______________________ Sacral agenesis with weakness or deformities of the lower extremities, malformation and fixation of the hip joints, and shortening or deformity of the femurs.
9. ______________________ Excessive fetal growth resulting in a large for gestational age (LGA) newborn; often associated with women who have pregestational or gestational diabetes.
10. ______________________ Component of surfactant; it is more indicative of adequate fetal lung maturity when present in amniotic fluid of women with diabetes.
11. ______________________ Blood glucose levels less than 40 mg/dl in term infants.
12. ______________________ Disease affecting the structure and function of the heart.
13. ______________________ Increased number of red blood cells; results in increased viscosity of the blood. ______________________ Results when the excessive red blood cells are hemolyzed.
14. ______________________ Presence of microorganisms or their toxins in blood or other tissues; it is one of the most significant causes of neonatal morbidity and mortality.
15. ______________________ Generalized infection in the bloodstream.
16. ______________________ Disorder that results from toxins released into the bloodstream by microorganisms. The most common sign is hypotension. The infant will appear gray or mottled and will have cool extremities.
17. ______________________ Administration of an antibiotic ointment (e.g., erythromycin) into the eyes of the newborn within 1 hour of birth to prevent ophthalmia neonatorum.
18. ______________________ Elevated wartlike lesions characteristic of congenital syphilis.
19. ______________________ Copious clear mucous discharge from the nose characteristic of congenital syphilis.
20. ______________________ Combination drug treatment used during antepartum, intrapartum, and neonatal periods that has almost completely eliminated mother-to-child HIV transmission in developed countries.

21. ______________________ Infections caused by an organism that usually does not cause illness; it is an outcome of HIV infection related to the suppression of immunologic activity. These infections include candidiasis and *Pneumocystis jiroveci* pneumonia (PCP).

22. ______________________ Infection know as fifth disease or "slapped cheek illness" in older children.

23. ______________________ Microorganism that is a leading cause of neonatal morbidity and mortality in the United States. Women who are positive for this microorganism are given prophylactic antibiotics when in labor.

24. ______________________ Primarily a food-borne infection causing maternal and neonatal illness; it is one of the three major causes of neonatal meningitis globally.

25. ______________________ Oral candidiasis; it is characterized by adherent white plaques on the oral mucosa, gums, and tongue.

26. ______________________ Acute and long-term outcome of alcohol ingestion during pregnancy; it is characterized by prenatal and postnatal growth restriction, CNS malfunctions (e.g., mental retardation), and distinctive craniofacial features (e.g., microcephaly, small eyes).

27. ______________________ Term given to the group of signs and symptoms associated with drug withdrawal in the neonate.

II. REVIEWING KEY CONCEPTS

28. IDENTIFY the most common congenital anomalies experienced by infants with diabetic mothers in terms of each of the following:

Cardiac

Central nervous system

Musculoskeletal

Renal

29. STATE the infections(s) represented by each letter in the acronym TORCH.

T

O

R

C

H

30. Sepsis is one of the most significant causes of neonatal morbidity and mortality.

A. INDICATE the primary modes of infection transmission for each of the periods listed below.

- Prenatal

- Perinatal

- Postnatal

B. IDENTIFY the major risk factors that, if present, should alert the nurse to an increased potential for infection in the neonate.

C. LIST the signs a neonate might exhibit that would indicate that sepsis is present.

D. DESCRIBE two effective nursing measures for each of the following categories.
- Preventive measures

- Curative measures

MULTIPLE CHOICE: Circle the correct option(s), and state the rationale for the option(s) chosen.

31. When assessing a newborn after birth, the nurse notes the following: limited movement of left arm with crepitus at the shoulder and absence of Moro reflex on left side. The nurse suspects:
    A. Brachial plexus injury
    B. Fracture of the clavicle
    C. Phrenic nerve injury
    D. Intracranial hemorrhage on the right side of the brain

32. A nurse is caring for a male newborn whose mother had gestational diabetes during pregnancy. His estimated gestational age is 41 weeks, and his weight indicates that he is macrosomic. When assessing this newborn, the nurse should be alert for which findings associated with macrosomia? (Circle all that apply.)
    A. Fracture of the femur
    B. Hypocalcemia
    C. Blood glucose level of 38 mg/dl
    D. Signs of a congenital heart defect
    E. Pale complexion
    F. Round "cherubic" face

33. A woman who developed hepatitis B during pregnancy gives birth vaginally to a healthy baby boy. Her baby is receiving hepatitis B immunoglobulin (HBIg) 0.5 mg IM 2 hours after birth. When should he receive his first dose of the hepatitis B vaccine?
    A. At the same time as the HBIg but in a different site
    B. One month after birth
    C. Six months after birth
    D. One year after birth

34. A woman was discovered to be HIV positive as part of routine screening during pregnancy. She was immediately treated with HAART. She just gave birth to a baby girl. Care management of this newborn includes:
    A. Encouraging the mother to breastfeed to protect her infant from infection
    B. Teaching the mother about the importance of taking her infant for routine immunizations
    C. Isolating the newborn in a special nursery
    D. Initiating HAART treatment as soon as the newborn is diagnosed as HIV positive

35. A woman in labor admits that she used heroin during her pregnancy. After the birth of her baby boy, the nurse caring for him must be alert for which signs that indicate neonatal abstinence syndrome? (Circle all that apply.)
    A. Sleepiness
    B. Poor feeding
    C. Bradypnea
    D. Hyperthermia or hypothermia
    E. Diarrhea
    F. Frequent yawning

III. THINKING CRITICALLY

1. Birth trauma, although decreasing in incidence, is still an important source of neonatal morbidity. Nurses caring for women in labor should be aware of the factors that predispose infants to injury during the process of birth.
    A. IDENTIFY the factors that increase fetal vulnerability to injury and trauma at birth.

    B. DESCRIBE an approach to labor and birth care that can reduce the incidence of birth injuries.

C. Baby boy Timothy's right clavicle was fractured during birth as a result of shoulder dystocia. DESCRIBE the signs Timothy most likely exhibited that alerted the nurse that his clavicle was fractured.

D. EXPLAIN to Timothy's parents the most likely care approach related to his fracture.

2. Baby boy Robert, weighing 11 lb 4 oz, was born 1 hour ago. His mother, a primipara, had gestational diabetes mellitus.

A. Robert's mother is thrilled at his size stating, "He looks so healthy and well nourished, not like the skinny babies in the nursery." EXPLAIN what the nurse caring for Robert should tell his parents about the reason for his large size.

B. DESCRIBE the typical characteristics exhibited by a macrosomic infant such as Robert.

C. Robert, as a macrosomic infant, is most at risk for the complications of ________________,

________________, ________________, and ________________.

D. DESCRIBE the physiologic basis for and the warning signs of each of the potential complications for which the nurse should be aware when assessing Robert during the first 24 hours after his birth.

3. Baby girl Susan was born 2 hours ago. Her mother tested positive for HBsAg antibodies as a result of infection with hepatitis B virus (HBV).
   A. DESCRIBE the protocol that should be followed in providing care for Susan.

   B. Susan's mother asks the nurse if she can breastfeed her baby daughter. DISCUSS the nurse's response to the mother's question.

4. Baby boy Andrew is a full-term newborn who was just now born by spontaneous vaginal delivery. Genital herpes recurred in his mother, and her membranes ruptured before the onset of labor.
   A. IDENTIFY the four modes of transmission for HSV to the newborn. INDICATE the mode most likely to have transmitted the infection to Andrew.

   B. LIST the clinical signs Andrew would exhibit as evidence of a disseminated infection, CNS involvement, and localized HSV infection.

   C. DESCRIBE the recommended nursing measures related to each of the following:
   Management after birth, prior to discharge

   Vidarabine eye ointment

5. Baby girl Mary is 1 day old. Her mother is HIV positive but received no treatment during pregnancy.
   A. DISCUSS Mary's potential for HIV infection.

   B. IDENTIFY four strategies that can be used to prevent the transmission of HIV to newborns.

   C. OUTLINE the protocol that most likely will be followed to determine if Mary is HIV positive.

   D. NAME the opportunistic infections, if contracted by Mary, that would strongly suggest that she is infected with HIV.

   E. DESCRIBE the care measures recommended for Mary.

   F. Mary's mother wishes to breastfeed Mary because she has read that it can prevent infection. DISCUSS the nurse's response to this mother's question.

6. Thomas, a healthy 2-day-old newborn, has developed thrush.
   A. DESCRIBE the signs most likely exhibited by Thomas that led to this diagnosis.

B. NAME the modes of transmission for this infection.

C. DISCUSS the care management required by Thomas as a result of his yeastlike fungal infection.

7. Jane, a newborn, has been diagnosed with fetal alcohol syndrome (FAS) as a result of moderate to sometimes heavy binge drinking by her mother throughout pregnancy.
   A. DESCRIBE the characteristics Jane most likely exhibited to establish the diagnosis of FAS.

   B. STATE three long-term effects Jane could experience as she gets older.

   C. DESCRIBE two nursing measures that could be effective in promoting Jane's growth and development.

8. Maternal substance abuse can be harmful to fetal and newborn health status, as well as to growth and development. Susan has just been born. Her mother used cocaine during pregnancy.
   A. IDENTIFY the effects Susan may exhibit as a result of exposure to cocaine while in utero.

   B. OUTLINE the care measures appropriate for both Susan and her mother during hospitalization and after discharge.

9. Tony is a 2-hour-old newborn. It is suspected that his mother abused drugs during pregnancy.
   A. LIST the signs associated with neonatal abstinence syndrome that the nurse should observe for when assessing Tony.

   B. Tony begins to exhibit signs that confirm that his mother used heroin during pregnancy. CITE two nursing diagnoses that would be appropriate for Tony.

   C. OUTLINE the care management that Tony and his mother will require as Tony progresses through withdrawal.

CHAPTER 36

Hemolytic Disorders and Congenital Anomalies

I. LEARNING KEY TERMS

FILL IN THE BLANKS: Insert the hematologic disorder or congenital anomaly represented by each of the following descriptions.

1. ______________________ Condition in which the total serum bilirubin level in the blood is increased.
2. ______________________ Yellow discoloration of the skin, mucous membranes, sclera, and various organs associated with elevated bilirubin levels in the blood. It is termed ______________________ when it occurs more than 24 hours after birth, and ______________________ if it is evident beginning in the first 24 hours after birth.
3. ______________________ Condition that occurs when an Rh-negative mother has an Rh-positive fetus who inherits the dominant Rh-positive gene from the father.
4. ______________________ Term used to refer to an Rh-negative mother's formation of antibodies capable of destroying the red blood cells of an Rh-positive fetus; this occurs with exposure of the mother to Rh-positive blood during pregnancy, birth, abortion, amniocentesis or trauma.
5. ______________________ Complication of Rh incompatibility in which erythrocytes are destroyed by maternal Rh-positive antibodies; this can result in an increase in fetal bilirubin levels.
6. ______________________ Complication of Rh incompatibility that results in fetal compensation for red blood cell destruction by producing large numbers of immature erythrocytes to replace those that are hemolyzed.
7. ______________________ The most severe form of Rh incompatibility; it is characterized by marked anemia, cardiac decompensation, cardiomegaly, hepatosplenomegaly, hypoxia, and fluid leakage into the intravascular space, resulting in generalized edema and fluid effusion into the peritoneal, pericardial, and pleural spaces.
8. ______________________ Disorder caused by deposition of bilirubin in the brain, resulting in acute central nervous system manifestations during the first weeks after birth.
9. ______________________ Term used to refer to the chronic and permanent results of bilirubin toxicity.
10. ______________________ Maternal blood test, used to determine whether the mother has antibodies to the Rh antigen.
11. ______________________ Test performed on cord blood to determine whether there are maternal antibodies in the fetal blood.
12. ______________________ Defect present at birth that is caused by genetic or environmental factors, or both.
13. ______________________ A group of disorders that results from the absence of or change in a protein, usually an enzyme, and mediated by the action of a certain gene (autosomal recessive inheritance). Examples include phenylketonuria and galactosemia.
14. ______________________ A small head circumference restricting brain growth and leading to mental retardation.
15. ______________________ Urinary meatus opens below the glans penis or anywhere along the ventral surface of the penis, scrotum, or peritoneum.

16. ______________________________ Urinary meatus opens on the dorsal surface of the penis.

17. ______________________________ Abnormal development of the bladder, abdominal wall, and pubic symphysis that causes the bladder, urethra, and ureteral orifices to be exposed.

18. ______________________________ Excess cerebrospinal fluid (CSF) in the ventricles of the brain as a result of overproduction, decrease in reabsorption, or an aqueductal flow obstruction of CSF; it is characterized by a bulging anterior fontanel, an abnormal increase in the circumference of the head, and an increasing CSF pressure.

19. ______________________________ Term used to refer to the group of anatomic abnormalities of the heart that are present at birth and are the most common of all congenital malformations; ventricular septal defects and tetralogy of Fallot are two common forms of this type of congenital disorder.

20. ______________________________ The most common form of clubfoot. The foot points downward and inward, the ankle is inverted, and the Achilles tendon is shortened, all making the foot appear C shaped.

21. ______________________________ The most common congenital anomaly of the nose consisting of a unilateral or bilateral bony or soft tissue septum obstructing the posterior nares.

22. ______________________________ The most common defect of the CNS resulting from failure of the neural tube to close at some point.

23. ______________________________ Type of neural tube defect in which the posterior portion of the laminas fail to close but the spinal cord or meninges do not herniate or protrude through the defect; often a birthmark or hairy patch is present above the defect.

24. ______________________________ Type of neural tube defect in which an external sac containing the meninges and cerebrospinal fluid protrudes through a defect in the vertebral column.

25. ______________________________ Covered (with a peritoneal sac) defect of the umbilical ring into which varying amounts of the abdominal organs may herniate.

26. ______________________________ Herniation of the bowel through a defect in the abdominal wall to the right of the umbilical cord. No membrane covers the intestines.

27. ______________________________ Congenital anomaly in which the passageway from the mouth to the stomach ends in a blind pouch failing to form a continuous passageway to the stomach.

28. ______________________________ Congenital anomaly characterized by an abnormal connection between the esophagus and the trachea.

29. ______________________________ Term used to describe absence of an anal opening; commonly it is accompanied by a fistula from the rectum to the perineum or to the genitourinary system.

30. ______________________________ Term used to describe a spectrum of disorders related to the abnormal development of one or all of the components of the hip joint that may develop at any time during fetal life, infancy, or childhood.

31. ______________________________ Herniation of the brain and meninges through a skull defect.

32. ______________________________ Congenital disorder characterized by the absence of both cerebral hemispheres and the overlying skull. It is incompatible with life.

33. ______________________________ Disorder characterized by displacement of the abdominal organs into the thoracic cavity through a defect in the formation of the diaphragm.

34. ______________________________ Type of neural tube defect in which an external sac containing the meninges, cerebrospinal fluid, and nerves protrudes through a defect in the vertebral column.

35. ______________________________ Commonly occurring congenital midline fissure, or opening, in the lip or palate resulting from failure of the primary palate to fuse; one or both deformities may occur, and nasal deformity may also be present.

36. ______________________________ Erroneous or abnormal sexual differentiation.

37. ______________________________ An excessive amount of amniotic fluid.

38. ______________________________ An insufficient amount of amniotic fluid.

39. ______________________________ Studies of chromosomes done to confirm or rule out a suspected chromosomal disorder.

40. ______________________________ Study of the patterns formed by the ridges in the skin on the digits, palms, and soles; they are strongly correlated with the effects of chromosomes.

II. REVIEWING KEY CONCEPTS

41. EXPLAIN the pathogenesis of ABO incompatibility.

42. Congenital anomalies affect the health and well-being of infants.
    A. SPECIFY the assessment techniques and considerations that guide prenatal diagnosis of congenital anomalies.

    B. EXPLAIN why observation of the amount of amniotic fluid can be helpful in the perinatal diagnosis of certain congenital anomalies.

    C. INDICATE how each of the following types of postnatal tests can be used to diagnose an infant with a congenital anomaly.
    - Newborn screening

    - Cytogenetic studies

    - Dermatoglyphics

43. Congenital heart defects (CHDs) are a major cause of death in the first year of life.
    A. LIST several maternal factors associated with a higher incidence of CHDs.

    B. IDENTIFY the four physiologic classifications of CHDs, and GIVE one example for each classification.

    C. Nurses caring for newborns after birth need to include assessment for CHDs as part of a thorough and ongoing assessment of their health status. DESCRIBE the signs that may be exhibited at birth by an infant with a CHD.

MULTIPLE CHOICE: Circle the correct option(s), and state the rationale for the option(s) chosen.

44. A nurse is caring for a full-term newborn who is Rh positive. His mother (3-2-0-1-2), who is Rh negative, was never treated to prevent sensitization with her previous pregnancies. When assessing the newborn, the nurse must be alert for signs indicative of pathologic jaundice. Which sign alerts the nurse to this disorder?
    A. Jaundice in face including sclera beginning at 36 hours after birth
    B. Serum bilirubin level on the second day of life of 16 mg/dl
    C. Serum bilirubin concentration of 2 mg/dl in cord blood
    D. Total serum bilirubin level increase of 3 mg/dl in 24 hours

45. An Rh-negative woman (2-2-0-0-2) just gave birth to an Rh-positive baby boy. The direct and indirect Coombs' test results are negative. Based on these data, the nurse anticipates to:
    A. Prepare to administer RhoGAM to the newborn within 24 hours of his birth
    B. Observe the newborn closely for signs of pathologic jaundice
    C. Tell the woman that she will not need to receive RhoGAM after this birth because both Coombs' test results are negative
    D. Administer Rh_0(D) immunoglobulin (RhoGAM) intramuscularly to the woman within 72 hours of her baby's birth

46. A newborn female has been diagnosed with myelomeningocele. An important nursing measure to protect the newborn from injury and further complications during the preoperative period is:
    A. Maintain the newborn in a lateral position
    B. Measure the frontal-occipital circumference to assess for hydrocephalus
    C. Cover the sac with Vaseline gauze to protect it from drying out
    D. Change the diaper frequently to prevent contamination of the sac with meconium

III. THINKING CRITICALLY

1. Pathologic jaundice is a serious health problem with the potential for severe complications that can permanently affect the life and health of the infant.
   A. CONTRAST physiologic and pathologic jaundice in terms of time of onset, time of resolution, and expected serum levels of unconjugated bilirubin.

   B. EXPLAIN the underlying physiologic process that leads to hyperbilirubinemia in the newborn.

   C. LIST the potential causes for pathologic jaundice.

   D. IDENTIFY the measures found to be effective in preventing hyperbilirubinemia.

2. Angela, who is Rh negative, had a spontaneous abortion at 13 weeks of gestation, which resulted in what she said was just a heavier than usual menstrual period. Six months later she became pregnant again.
   A. DESCRIBE the physiologic basis for Rh incompatibility and the occurrence of sensitization.

   B. An indirect Coombs' test is positive. STATE the meaning of this finding.

C. INDICATE if Angela is or is not a candidate for RhoGAM. SUPPORT your answer.

D. DESCRIBE RhoGAM (Rh immunoglobulin) and its use.

E. Angela's fetus is at risk for erythroblastosis fetalis and hydrops fetalis. EXPLAIN each of these conditions—what they are and the implications of their occurrence for the health status of Angela's baby.

- Erythroblastosis fetalis

- Hydrops fetalis

F. DESCRIBE the treatment approaches that can be used to prevent intrauterine fetal death and early neonatal death for Angela's baby.

3. Baby girl Jennifer was born with spina bifida cystica, myelomeningocele. DESCRIBE the measures the nurse should use to manage Jennifer's care and help her parents cope with this congenital anomaly.

4. Baby boy Thomas was just born. He is exhibiting signs that the nurse-midwife and the neonatologist believe are consistent with a diaphragmatic hernia.
   A. IDENTIFY the clinical manifestations that Thomas most likely exhibited to cause his health care providers to suspect diaphragmatic hernia.

   B. STATE the priority nursing diagnosis for Thomas.

   C. OUTLINE the essential care measures during the immediate postbirth period.

5. Baby girl Denise was born with a cleft lip and palate.
   A. STATE three nursing diagnoses faced by Denise and her parents. DISCUSS the rationale for each nursing diagnosis stated.

   B. OUTLINE several nursing measures that will need to be implemented to ensure Denise's well-being until surgical repair can be accomplished.

CHAPTER

37

Nursing Care of the High Risk Newborn

I. LEARNING KEY TERMS

FILL IN THE BLANKS: Insert the term that corresponds to each of the following descriptions related to gestational age and intrauterine growth.

1. ______________________ Infant whose birth weight is less than 2500 g, regardless of gestational age.
2. ______________________ Infant whose birth weight is less than 1500 g.
3. ______________________ Infant whose birth weight is less than 1000 g.
4. ______________________ or ______________________ Infant born before completion of 37 weeks of gestation, regardless of birth weight. These infants are at risk because their organ systems are immature and they lack adequate physiologic reserves to function in an extrauterine environment.
5. ______________________ Infant born between 34 6/7 and 36 6/7 weeks of gestation regardless of birth weight; by nature of their limited gestation, these infants remain at risk for problems related to thermoregulation, hypoglycemia, hyperbilirubinemia, sepsis, and respiratory function.
6. ______________________ Infant born between the beginning of 38 weeks and the completion of 42 weeks of gestation, regardless of birth weight.
7. ______________________ or ______________________ An infant born after 42 weeks of gestational age, regardless of birth weight.
8. ______________________ Infant whose birth weight falls above the 90th percentile on intrauterine growth curves.
9. ______________________ Infant whose birth weight falls between the 10th and the 90th percentiles on intrauterine growth curves.
10. ______________________ Infant whose rate of intrauterine growth was restricted and whose birth weight falls below the 10th percentile on intrauterine growth curves.
11. ______________________ Rate of fetal growth that does not meet expected growth patterns.
12. ______________________ Type of inhibited fetal growth in which the weight, length, and head circumference are all affected.
13. ______________________ Type of inhibited fetal growth in which the head circumference remains within normal parameters and the birth weight falls below the 10th percentile.
14. ______________________ Birth in which the neonate manifests any heartbeat, breathes, or displays voluntary movement, regardless of gestational age.
15. ______________________ Death of a fetus after 20 weeks of gestation and before delivery, with absence of any signs of life after birth.
16. ______________________ Death that occurs in the first 27 days of life; it is described as early if it occurs in the first week of life and late if it occurs at 7 to 27 days.
17. ______________________ Total number of fetal and early neonatal deaths per 1000 live births.
18. ______________________ Respiratory pattern commonly seen in preterm infants; such infants exhibit 5- to 10-second respiratory pauses followed by 10 to 15 seconds of compensatory rapid respirations.

19. ______________________________ Cessation of respirations for 15 to 20 seconds or more.

20. ______________________________ Noninvasive, effective means for detecting alterations in systemic blood pressure (hypotension or hypertension) and for identifying the need to implement appropriate therapy to maintain cardiovascular function.

21. ______________________________ The environmental temperature at which oxygen consumption is minimal but adequate to maintain the body temperature.

22. ______________________________ Surface-active phospholipid secreted by the alveolar epithelium; it reduces the surface tension of fluids that line the alveoli and respiratory passages, resulting in uniform expansion and maintenance of lung expansion at low intraalveolar pressure.

23. ______________________________ Evaporative loss that occurs largely through the skin and respiratory tract; it is increased in preterm infants.

24. ______________________________ Method of providing breast milk or formula through a nasogastric tube or orogastric tube; feeding can be accomplished either with a tube inserted at each feeding (bolus) or continuously through an indwelling catheter.

25. ______________________________ Method of feeding that involves the surgical placement of a tube through the skin of the abdomen into the stomach.

26. ______________________________ Sucking on a pacifier during tube or parenteral feeding or between oral feedings to improve oxygenation and facilitate earlier transition to nipple feeding; this type of sucking may lead to decreased energy expenditure with less restlessness and to positive weight gain and better sucking skills.

27. ______________________________ Method that can be used to provide maternal or paternal skin-to-skin contact with their newborn and to reduce stress in the infant.

28. ______________________________ Hyperviscosity of the blood related to an excess in circulating red blood cell mass.

II. REVIEWING KEY CONCEPTS

29. The preterm infant is vulnerable to a number of complications related to immaturity of physiologic functions. IDENTIFY the potential problems and their physiologic basis for each of the areas listed below.
    - Respiratory function
    - Cardiovascular function
    - Maintaining body temperature

- Central nervous system function

- Maintaining adequate nutrition

- Maintaining renal function

- Maintaining hematologic status

- Resisting infection

MATCHING: Match the description in Column I with the appropriate complication associated with the high risk newborn in Column II.

COLUMN I

30. _______ Complex, multicausal disorder that affects the developing blood vessels in the eyes; it is often associated with oxygen tensions that are too high for the level of retinal maturity initially resulting in vasoconstriction and continuing problems after the oxygen is discontinued. Scar tissue formation and consequent visual impairment may be mild or severe.
31. _______ Acute inflammatory disease of the gastrointestinal mucosa commonly complicated by perforation; intestinal ischemia, colonization by pathogenic bacteria, and enteral feeding all play an important role in its development.
32. _______ Occurs when the fetal shunt between the left pulmonary artery and the dorsal aorta fails to constrict after birth or reopens after constriction has occurred.

COLUMN II

A. Bronchopulmonary dysplasia (BPD)
B. Retinopathy of prematurity (ROP)
C. Patent ductus arteriosus (PDA)

33. _______ Chronic lung disease with a multifactorial etiology that includes pulmonary immaturity, surfactant deficiency, lung injury and stretch, barotrauma, inflammation caused by oxygen exposure, fluid overload, ligation of a PDA, and familial predisposition. Incidence has decreased with prenatal use of maternal steroids when preterm birth is expected coupled with the use of exogenous surfactant.

34. _______ Lung disorder caused by a lack of pulmonary surfactant, which leads to progressive atelectasis, loss of functional residual capacity, and ventilation-perfusion imbalance with an uneven distribution of ventilation; it usually affects preterm infants and a small percentage of term and late preterm infants.

35. _______ Combined findings of pulmonary hypertension, right-to-left shunting, and a structurally normal heart; it is also called persistent fetal circulation because the syndrome includes reversion to fetal pathways for blood flow.

36. _______ One of the most common types of brain injury encountered in the neonatal period and among the most severe in both short- and long-term outcomes; incidence is decreasing related to prenatal use of corticosteroids and postnatal use of surfactant

D. Persistent pulmonary hypertension of the newborn (PPHN)
E. Germinal matrix hemorrhage–intraventricular hemorrhage (GMH-IVH)
F. Necrotizing enterocolitis (NEC)
G. Respiratory distress syndrome (RDS)

37. Joshua was born at 35 weeks of gestation and James was born at 43 weeks of gestation. COMPARE the care management needs of Joshua and James based on needs and risks associated with their gestational age.

MULTIPLE CHOICE: Circle the correct option(s) and state the rationale for the option(s) chosen.

38. Preterm infants are at increased risk for developing respiratory distress. The nurse should assess for signs that would indicate that the newborn is having difficulty breathing. Signs of respiratory distress are: (Circle all that apply.)
A. Use of abdominal muscles to breathe
B. Expiratory grunting
C. Periodic breathing pattern
D. Suprasternal retraction
E. Nasal flaring
F. Acrocyanosis

39. When caring for a preterm infant at 30 weeks of gestation, the nurse should recognize that the newborn's primary nursing diagnosis is:
A. Risk for infection related to decreased immune response
B. Ineffective breathing pattern related to surfactant deficiency and weak respiratory muscle effort
C. Ineffective thermoregulation related to immature thermoregulation center
D. Imbalanced nutrition: less than body requirements related to ineffective suck and swallow

40. A nurse is preparing to insert a gavage tube and feed a preterm newborn. As part of the protocol for this procedure the nurse should: (Circle all that apply.)
A. Determine the length of tubing to be inserted by measuring from tip of nose to lobe of ear to midpoint between xiphoid process and umbilicus
B. Coat the tube with sterile water to ease passage
C. Insert the tube through the nose as the preferred route for most infants
D. Check placement of the tube by injecting 2 to 3 ml of sterile water into the tube and listening for gurgling with a stethoscope
E. Assess residual gastric aspirate every 4 hours
F. Provide nonnutritive sucking during gavage feedings

41. Evaluating blood gas values provides essential information about the effectiveness of the preterm newborn's respiratory effort and oxygen administration measures. Which arterial blood gas values indicate adequate gas exchange? (Circle all that apply.)
   A. pH 7.40
   B. Pao_2 75 mm Hg
   C. $Paco_2$ 48 mm Hg
   D. HCO_3 14 mEq/L
   E. Base excess –6
   F. Oxygen saturation 93%

42. Preterm newborns are at increased risk for infection. The most important measure to prevent iatrogenic infections in the preterm newborn is to:
   A. Monitor vital signs for instability
   B. Teach parents infection control measures
   C. Cleanse the newborn's skin with plain warm water
   D. Perform hand hygiene

43. Preterm infants are at risk for cold stress. Which signs should alert the nurse that the preterm infant he or she is caring for may be hypothermic? (Circle all that apply.)
   A. Acrocyanosis
   B. Emesis
   C. Irritability
   D. Periodic breathing pattern
   E. Bradycardia
   F. Abdominal distention

III. THINKING CRITICALLY

1. Baby girl Jane was born 12 hours ago at 28 weeks of gestation. Oxygen therapy is a vital component of her care because she has been experiencing respiratory distress since birth.
   A. IDENTIFY the criteria that were used to determine that baby Jane needed supplemental oxygen.

   B. CREATE a set of general guidelines that reflects the recommended principles for safe and effective administration of oxygen to a compromised newborn.

   C. Baby girl Jane's respiratory status is improving and her health care providers are preparing to begin the process of weaning her from the oxygen. DESCRIBE signs that indicate that Jane is ready to be weaned from oxygen therapy.

D. OUTLINE the guidelines that should be followed when weaning Jane from oxygen therapy.

2. Anne, a 3 lb, 12 oz (1705 g) preterm newborn at 32 weeks of gestation, is admitted to the neonatal intensive care unit (NICU) after her birth for observation and supportive care. Anne's nutritional needs are a critical concern in her care. Oral feedings of maternal colostrum and breast milk are attempted first.
   A. STATE the assessment data that the nurse should document after each of Anne's feedings to indicate feeding method effectiveness.

   B. The nurse determines that Anne's suck is weak and she becomes too fatigued during oral feedings to obtain sufficient nutrients and fluid. The nurse confers with the neonatologist and a decision is made to provide intermittent gavage feedings with occasional oral feedings. DESCRIBE the guidelines the nurse should follow when inserting the gavage tube.

   C. STATE the priority nursing diagnosis for Anne.

   D. DISCUSS the principles the nurse should follow before, during, and after a gavage feeding to ensure safety and maximum effectiveness.

   E. OUTLINE the protocol that should be followed when advancing Anne back to full oral feeding.

3. The NICU is a stressful environment for preterm infants and their families.
   A. IDENTIFY the common sources of stress facing infants and their families in an intensive care environment.
      Infant stressors

      Family stressors

   B. Nurses working in the NICU and parents must be aware of infant behavioral cues and adjust stimuli accordingly. LIST infant behavioral cues that indicate readiness for interaction and stimulation and behavioral cues that signal a need for a time-out.
      Approach behaviors (cues to a relaxed state)

      Avoidance behaviors (cues to overstimulation)

   C. IDENTIFY specific measures that can be used to protect infants from overstimulation and yet provide appropriate stimulation to meet the developmental and emotional needs of infants.

   D. SPECIFY the guidelines that should be followed regarding infant positioning.

4. Marion is beginning her 43rd week of pregnancy.
   A. SUPPORT THIS STATEMENT: Perinatal mortality is significantly higher in the postmature fetus and neonate.

   B. STATE the assessment findings that are typical of a postmature infant.

   C. DISCUSS the two major complications that can be experienced by a postmature infant.

5. Janet, a pregnant client at term, is in labor. On the basis of serial ultrasound findings, her fetus is estimated to be smaller than it should be as a consequence of Janet's heavy smoking during pregnancy and her high risk status related to preeclampsia.
   A. IDENTIFY three major complications facing Janet's baby during labor, birth, and the postpartum period.

   B. DESCRIBE the physiologic basis for each potential complication and the signs and symptoms indicative of its presence.

6. Marion is at 24 weeks of gestation and is in preterm labor. Her primary health care provider determines that preterm birth is inevitable and has elected to transport Marion to a tertiary center before she gives birth, to maximize the survival potential of her unborn infant.
   A. EXPLAIN the advantages of transport before birth.

   B. Marion gives birth before she can be transported. Her baby will be transported to the tertiary center once stable. INDICATE the needs of this preterm baby that must be stabilized before transport.

C. IDENTIFY the measures that the nurse should use to support Marion and her family as her newborn is transported to the tertiary center.

7. Anita and Juan are the parents of a 2-day-old preterm newborn boy. Their baby, who is 27 weeks gestation and weighs 1 kg, is in the NICU and will be in the hospital for several weeks or longer. The nurse caring for this baby recognizes that he must also provide supportive care for Anita and Juan.
   A. As parents of a preterm infant, Anita and Juan must accomplish several tasks as they develop a relationship with their baby boy and prepare to care for him. IDENTIFY these tasks and a nursing care measure that can be used to help Anita and Juan successfully accomplish the task.

   B. STATE the behaviors the nurse should assess as he observes Anita and Juan with their baby. CATEGORIZE these behaviors in terms of behaviors that indicate effective coping and those that indicate ineffective coping and maladaptation.

8. IMAGINE that you are a nurse working in a NICU caring for an infant at 26 weeks of gestation born 2 hours ago. He is exhibiting signs of increasing dyspnea. The neonatologist orders that surfactant be administered. The baby's parents become very upset and tell you, "Our baby is already having a hard time breathing. What can this surfactant stuff do except make it worse for him?"
   A. DESCRIBE what you would tell these parents regarding the purpose of exogenous surfactant administration to the preterm newborn.

   B. EXPLAIN how you would inform the parents about how the surfactant is administered.

9. The nurse manager of a NICU attended a national nursing conference on NICU innovations in care. She was very impressed by the presentation on kangaroo care and decides to institute it at the NICU she manages. DESCRIBE the approach that she should take to inform her nurses about the change she wishes to make and encourage their full participation in its implementation.

10. IMAGINE that you are a nurse working in a NICU. You have been assigned to care for Tim, a 1-day-old infant born at 30 weeks of gestation. As you begin his care you take note of all the lines and tubes attached to him and realize that you must consider the pain Tim is experiencing as part of your plan of care.
    A. EXPLAIN how you would distinguish common newborn responses from those that could indicate that Tim is experiencing discomfort and pain.

    B. Reports indicate that newborns have memory of the pain they experience. DESCRIBE behaviors that you would look for that could indicate that Tim is forming a memory of painful experiences.

    C. DESCRIBE what could happen to Tim if you neglected to recognize his pain experience and incorporate pain relief measures into your plan of care.

    D. DISCUSS how you would use each of the following strategies to manage the pain Tim is experiencing:
    - Nonpharmacologic measures

    - Pharmacologic measures

CHAPTER 38

Perinatal Loss and Grief

I. LEARNING KEY TERMS

FILL-IN-THE-BLANKS: Insert the term that corresponds to each of the following descriptions related to perinatal loss and grief.

1. ______________________ or ______________________ A cluster of painful responses experienced following a major loss or death.
2. ______________________ The immediate reaction to news of perinatal loss or infant death; it is characterized by a state of shock and numbness, a sense of unreality, powerlessness, disbelief, and denial.
3. ______________________ Phase of the grief response that encompasses many difficult emotions as the parents work through their pain and adjust to life without the wished-for child; it is characterized by feelings of loneliness, emptiness, and yearning that occur in the early months after the loss.
4. ______________________ Phase of the grief response characterized by behavioral changes such as difficulty in getting things done, an inability to concentrate, restlessness, confused thought processes, difficulty solving problems, and poor decision making often occurring for several months after the loss.
5. ______________________ Phase of the grief response that occurs when parents are better able to function at home and at work, experience a return of self-esteem and confidence, can cope with new challenges, and have placed the loss in perspective. It peaks sometime after the first year as parents begin to achieve the task of moving on with their lives and enjoying simple pleasures of life without feeling guilty.
6. ______________________ The grief response that occurs with reminders of the loss; it typically happens at special anniversary dates related to the loss and during subsequent pregnancies and after birth.
7. ______________________ Model developed by Swanson that conceptualizes intervention with women and families experiencing perinatal loss. It involves five components, namely ______________________, ______________________, ______________________, ______________________, and ______________________.
8. ______________________ Extremely intense grief reaction that lasts for a very long time.

II. REVIEWING KEY CONCEPTS

9. Mary, a pregnant client at 24 weeks of gestation, has been admitted to the labor unit following a prenatal visit at her health care provider's office. Fetal death is suspected and eventually confirmed. IDENTIFY the phase of grief response represented by each of the comments made by Mary as she reacts to her loss. DESCRIBE each phase in terms of expected duration, behaviors typically exhibited, and emotions experienced.
   A. "The doctor says he cannot find my baby's heartbeat or feel my baby move. He thinks my baby has died. I know you will hear my baby's heartbeat because you have a monitor here. My baby is okay—I just know it!"

B. "I know this never would have happened if I had quit my job as a legal secretary. My mom told me that pregnant women should take it easy. If I had listened I would have my baby in my arms right now!"

C. "Since my baby died I just cannot seem to concentrate on even the simplest things at home and at work. I always seem to feel tired and out of sorts."

D. "It is going to be hard. I will always remember my little baby boy and the day he was supposed to be born. But I know that my husband and I have to go on with our lives."

10. EXPLAIN how a father's grief response may differ from that of his partner, the mother.

11. EXPLAIN how you would use each of the five components of the Caring Framework to support grieving parents and families.

12. DESCRIBE how you, as a nurse, would help parents and other family members actualize the loss of their newborn.

13. Nurses working with families experiencing loss must be able to distinguish normal grieving behaviors from those that indicate complicated grief (bereavement).
    A. IDENTIFY those behaviors that characterize complicated grief (bereavement).

    B. DESCRIBE the approach a nurse should take if signs of complicated grief (bereavement) are noted.

MULTIPLE CHOICE: Circle the correct option(s), and state the rationale for the option(s) chosen.

14. A woman gave birth to twin girls, one of whom was stillborn. Which nursing action would be *least* helpful in supporting the woman as she copes with her loss?
    A. Remind her that she should be happy that one daughter survived and is healthy.
    B. Assist the woman to take pictures of both babies.
    C. Encourage the woman to hold the deceased twin in her arms to say good-bye.
    D. Offer her the opportunity for counseling to help her with her grief and that of her surviving twin as she gets older.

15. During the acute distress phase of the grief response parents are most likely to experience:
    A. Fear and anxiety about future pregnancies
    B. Difficulty with cognitive processing
    C. Search for meaning
    D. Shock and numbness

16. A 17-year-old woman experiences a miscarriage at 12 weeks of gestation. When she is informed about the miscarriage she begins to cry, stating that she was upset about her pregnancy at first, and now she is being punished for not wanting her baby. The nurse's best response is:
    A. "You are still so young, you probably were not ready for a baby right now."
    B. "This must be so hard for you. I am here if you want to talk."
    C. "At least this happened early in your pregnancy before you felt your baby move."
    D. "God must have a good reason for letting this happen."

III. THINKING CRITICALLY

1. Jane (2-1-0-0-1) is a 21-year-old admitted with vaginal bleeding at 13 weeks of gestation. She experiences a miscarriage. Jane is accompanied by her husband, Tom. Her 5-year-old daughter is at home with Jane's mother.
    A. DESCRIBE the approach you would take to develop a plan of individualized support measures for Jane as she and her family cope with their loss.

B. CITE questions and observations you would use to gather the information required to create an individualized plan of care.

C. FORMULATE three nursing diagnoses appropriate for Jane and her family.

D. IDENTIFY the therapeutic communication techniques you should use to help Jane and Tom acknowledge and express their feelings and emotions about their loss.

E. At discharge Jane is crying. She tells you, "I know it must have been something I did wrong this time, since my first pregnancy was okay. We wanted to give our daughter a baby brother or sister." INDICATE whether the following responses would be therapeutic (T) or nontherapeutic (N). SPECIFY how you would change the responses determined to be nontherapeutic.

_______ 1. "You are still young. As soon as your body heals, you will be able to try to have another baby."

_______ 2. "What can I do that would help you and Tom cope with what happened?"

_______ 3. "Do not worry. I am sure you did everything you could to have a healthy pregnancy."

_______ 4. "It was probably for the best. Fetal loss at this time is usually the result of defective development."

_______ 5. "You sound like you are blaming yourself for what happened. Let's talk about it."

_______ 6. "This must be difficult for you and your family."

_______ 7. "If it had to happen, it is best that it happened this early in the pregnancy before you and your family became attached to the fetus."

_______ 8. "You really should concentrate on your little daughter rather than thinking so much about the baby you lost."

_______ 9. "I feel sad about the loss that you and Tom are experiencing."

_______ 10. "Would you and Tom like to speak to our hospital's chaplain before you are discharged?"

2. Angela gave birth vaginally to a stillborn fetus at 38 weeks of gestation. In addition to emotional support, her physical needs must be recognized and met. IDENTIFY these physical needs and how you would meet them.

3. Anita gave birth to a baby boy who died shortly thereafter as a result of multiple congenital anomalies, including anencephaly. She and her husband, Bill, are provided with the opportunity to see their baby.
   A. DISCUSS how the nurse can help Anita and Bill make a decision that is right for them about seeing their baby.

   B. Anita and Bill decide to see their baby. SPECIFY the measures the nurse can use to make the time Anita and Bill spend with their baby as easy as possible and to provide them with an experience that will facilitate the grieving process.

4. Tara is at 16 weeks of gestation. A sonogram reveals that her fetus has anencephaly. Her primary health care provider recommends a therapeutic abortion. DISCUSS the role of the nurse in supporting Tara as she makes her decision about the abortion and copes with her grief.

Answer Key

CHAPTER 1: 21ST CENTURY MATERNITY AND WOMEN'S HEALTH NURSING

I. Learning Key Terms

1. C, 2. H, 3. D, 4. I, 5. F, 6. A, 7. G, 8. B, 9. E, 10. J
11. Maternity nursing
12. Women's health care
13. *Healthy People 2010, 2020*
14. Millennium Developmental Goals (MDGs)
15. Integrative health care
16. Telehealth
17. Female genital mutilation, infibulation, circumcision
18. Doula
19. Health literacy
20. Nursing Interventions Classification (NIC)
21. Evidence-based practice
22. Outcomes-oriented care
23. Standards of practice
24. Standard of care
25. Risk management
26. Sentinel event
27. Failure to rescue
28. QSEN
29. SBAR
30. Team STEPPS

II. Reviewing Key Concepts

31. Factors contributing to infant mortality: see Infant Mortality section, which identifies several physical and psychosocial factors.
32. Problems of the U.S. health care system: see sections related to each of the problems listed to help you with your answer.
33. See Increase in High Risk Pregnancies section for a discussion of the physical as well as psychosocial factors that have led to the increase in incidence.
34. Factors/conditions affecting health of women: see Health of Women section; discuss such factors as race, violence, aging, adolescent pregnancy, cancer, poverty, access to health care.
35. Choices A, C, and E are correct; conventional Western modalities are included and client autonomy and decision making are encouraged.
36. Choice C is correct; although the other options are important, inability to pay, which relates to inadequate or no health care insurance, is the most significant barrier.
37. Choice D is correct.
38. Choices A, C, and D are correct; women in their 40s are more likely to give birth to twins; African-American women have a maternal mortality rate that is three times higher than Caucasian women.
39. Choice B is correct; smoking is not associated with anomalies; because smoking adversely affects circulation and thus placental perfusion, A, C, and D are all possible complications of smoking.
40. Choice D is correct; both diabetes and gestational hypertension are associated with obesity.

III. Thinking Critically

1. Nursing director of inner-city prenatal clinic; answer should incorporate application of each of the following:
   - Biostatistics and contributing factors
   - Factors associated with high risk pregnancy and measures to reduce them
   - Benefits of prenatal care; effect of and reasons for inadequate prenatal care
   - Importance of self-management and consumer involvement; devise ways to enhance health literacy and to encourage participation in prenatal care by overcoming barriers
2. High technology will not reduce rate of preterm birth and LBW infants: discuss the following topics when formulating an answer:
   - Factors associated with LBW and IMR
   - Factors that escalate rate of high risk pregnancy
   - High-tech care: what it can and cannot do; answer should reflect factors associated with IMR, the high cost of care management for high risk pregnancies and compromised infants as compared with the cost and effectiveness of early, ongoing, comprehensive prenatal care.
3. Three proposed changes with rationales: changes proposed should reflect efforts toward improving access to care, using evidence-based approaches and standards to guide care, and creating health care services that address the factors associated with poor pregnancy outcomes and medical errors.
4. Barriers to prenatal care: see Limited Access to Care section; address solutions to such barriers as inability to pay, lack of transportation, dependent child care, minority status, cultural beliefs, young maternal age, and single status. Be creative and innovative in the approaches that you propose.
5. Involving consumers and promoting self-management: Care measures proposed should include health teaching; self-assessment measures; guiding decision making by providing information regarding the pros and cons of care choices available; communication and counseling techniques should be included; substance abuse counseling; referral to support groups.
6. Facilitating health literacy: see Health Literacy section; include therapeutic communication

techniques, culturally sensitive approaches, and preparation of bilingual written materials in answer.

7. Process to use to prevent medical errors: see Reducing Medical Errors section and access the Patient Fact Sheet identified when formulating your answer.
8. Value of evidence-based practice: see Evidence-Based Practice, Cochrane Pregnancy and Childbirth Database, and Joanna Briggs Institute sections for ideas for answer.

CHAPTER 2: COMMUNITY CARE: THE FAMILY AND CULTURE

I. Learning Key Terms

1. B, 2. E, 3. D, 4. G, 5. C, 6. F, 7. A, 8. B, 9. E, 10. C, 11. D, 12. A
13. Culture
14. Subculture
15. Cultural relativism
16. Acculturation
17. Assimilation
18. Ethnocentrism
19. Cultural competence
20. Future-orientation
21. Past-orientation
22. Present-orientation
23. Personal space
24. Family
25. Nuclear
26. Extended
27. Cohabitating parent
28. Single parent
29. Married blended
30. Homosexual
31. No parent family
32. Family systems theory
33. Family life cycle theory
34. Family stress theory
35. McGill model of nursing
36. Health belief model
37. Human developmental ecology
38. Genogram
39. Ecomap
40. Walking survey
41. Vulnerable populations
42. Primary prevention
43. Secondary prevention
44. Tertiary prevention

II. Reviewing Key Concepts

45. Discuss purpose of incorporating products of culture when providing care: see Childbearing Beliefs and Practices section for a discussion of communication, personal space, time orientation, and family roles including how the nurse should consider each area when communicating with and caring for clients in a culturally sensitive manner.
46. Culturally Competent practice: see Developing Cultural Competency section which identifies the components of this approach.
47. Rationale for increasing emphasis on home- and community-based health care: see Home Care in the Community and Guidelines for Nursing Practice to formulate your answer. Consider changes in length of hospital stays, portability of technology, influence of insurance reimbursement, and the need to reduce health care costs in your answer; describe the need for nurses to broaden their scope of practice.
48. Community-based health promotion activities for childbearing families: see Community Health Promotion and Levels of Preventive Care sections to formulate an answer.
49. Cite problems faced by several vulnerable populations: see separate sections for each of the identified vulnerable populations listed to formulate an answer.
50. Ways nurses can use of the telephone to provide health services: see Communication and Technology Applications section; include warm lines, advice lines, and telephonic nursing assessment, consultation, and education.
51. Choice A is correct; choices B, C, and D reflect the characteristics of families with closed boundaries; they are more prone to crises because they have a narrow network to help them in times of stress.
52. Choice B is correct; providing explanations, especially when performing tasks that require close contact, can help avoid misunderstandings; touching the client, putting the client in proximity to others, and taking away the right to make decisions can be interpreted by clients in some cultures as invading their personal space.
53. Choice D is correct; choices A, B, and C are incorrect interpretations based on the woman's culture and customs; Native Americans may use cradle boards and avoid handling their newborn often; they should not be fed colostrum.
54. Choices A, C, E, and F are correct; prenatal care should begin late in pregnancy, chamomile tea is thought to ensure effective labor.
55. Choices A, B, D, and E are correct; birthing in an institutional setting is valued and breastfeeding should start as soon as possible after birth.
56. Choice C is correct; the student should be looking at the woman while speaking and asking questions through the interpreter; a normal tone of voice should be used
57. Choices B, C, and F are correct; A and D are secondary levels of prevention, and E is a tertiary level of prevention
58. Choice C is correct because it represents the primary level of prevention.
59. Choice D is correct; although A and B are appropriate they are not the most important; gloves are not needed unless the possibility of contacting body substances is present.

III. Thinking Critically

1. Process for providing culturally competent care: see The Family in a Cultural Context section and Box 2-2; incorporate the components of culturally competent care in answer; use questions in Cultural Considerations box to assess a client's cultural beliefs.
2. Imagine that you are a nurse working in a multicultural prenatal clinic: use Table 2-2 to formulate your answer; consider components of communication, personal space, time orientation, family roles; identify the degree to which each woman/family adheres to their cultures, beliefs, and practices; do not stereotype.
3. Pamela, a Native-American pregnant woman.
   A. Questions to ask: see questions listed in the Cultural Considerations box.
   B. Communication approach to use: see Childbearing Beliefs and Practices section; include concepts of communication patterns, space, time, and family roles when formulating your answer.
   C. Identify Native-American beliefs and practices: see Table 2-2 to formulate your answer; remember to determine her individual beliefs and practices to avoid stereotyping.
4. Hispanic family—recent birth of twin girls: describe cultural beliefs and practices: Table 2-2 outlines newborn care guidelines for several ethnic groups, including those Hispanic families are likely to follow.
5. Sunni refugee couple from Iraq seeking prenatal care (see Communication: Use of an Interpreter section and Box 2-1).
   - Consider the process of working with a translator; show respect for this couple by addressing questions and comments to them and not to the translator; recognize that the husband may wish to be present and a female interpreter would be required.
   - Box 2-1 outlines the preparation measures, interaction during the interview, and consultation with translator before, during, and after the interview—learn about the culture and prepare questions.
   - Consider the stressors faced by refugees/immigrants and the health care needs they present.
   - Research Iraq and become familiar with Sunni cultural/religious beliefs and practices and the current political and religious turmoil that led this couple to come to the United States.
6. Home care nurse must become familiar with neighborhoods and their resources (see Data Collection and Sources of Community Health Data section).
   A. Walking survey: a walking survey involves use of observation skills during a trip through a community.
   B. Components of a Community Walk-Through are outlined in Box 2-3.
   C. Use of findings: discusses each of the survey's components; describe how each of these components can reflect a community's strengths and problems; strengths can be used to provide clients with needed support; nurse can mobilize community leaders to solve identified problems; try using the survey to assess your community and the community in which your college is located.
7. Marie, a single parent of two children, is homeless (see Homeless Women and Implications for Nursing sections).
   A. Basis for health problems to which she and her children are most vulnerable: lack of preventive care and resources, limited to no access to primary care resulting in the use of emergency departments for health care
   B. Marie's vulnerability for pregnancy: victimization, economic survival, lack of access to health care and birth control measures, need for closeness and intimacy, doubt fertility
   C. Principles to guide nurse when providing care: treat with respect and dignity, case management to coordinate care to meet multiple needs, flexible appointment times providing service when they come in, make each interaction count, be purposeful, keep her empowered, help her reconnect with her support system if possible and appropriate
8. Consuelo, pregnant wife of a migrant worker and mother of two (see Refugee and Migrant Women section).
   - Begin by confirming that she is pregnant.
   - Consider pregnancy risks she faces; evaluate exposure to teratogens.
   - Concerns to address include limited access to and use of contraceptives, increased rate of STIs, poor nutrition.
   - Lack of trust and fear of deportation may be barriers to seeking and continuing with prenatal care.
9. List questions for a postpartum follow-up telephone call: see Communication and Technology Applications section; include questions guided by expected postpartum physical and emotional changes; ask her how she is feeling and managing, condition of her newborn (eating, sleeping, eliminating), response of other family members to newborn, sources of happiness and stress, adequacy of help and support being received and need for additional support or referrals.
10. Home visit to a postpartum woman at 36 hours after birth: see Boxes 2-4 and 2-5, and Care Management, Preparing for a Home Visit section to answer each component of this exercise, including the approach you would take to prepare, your actions during the visit, safety precautions and

infection control measures you would follow, how you would end the visit, and the interventions you would follow after the visit, including documentation of assessments, actions, and responses.

11. Angela, a pregnant woman with hyperemesis gravidarum: see Home Care in the Community—Perinatal Services and Client Selection and Referral sections for A and B and Care Management for C.
    A. Criteria for discharge readiness: include criteria related to Angela's health status and that of her fetus, availability of qualified home care professionals, family resources, and cost effectiveness of discharging her to home care.
    B. Information needed to institute high-tech care in the home: medical diagnosis and prognosis, treatment required, medication history, drug dosing information, and type of infusion access device that will be used.
    C. Home environment criteria: safe place to store medications and infusion supplies; do a walk-through inspection to determine temperature of the home, general cleanliness, adequacy of area to prepare and administer prescribed treatment.
12. Importance and cost-effectiveness of home health care services for postpartum women and their families: see Perinatal Services section; include the following in your answer:
    - Ability to observe firsthand, the home environment and family dynamics; natural; adequacy of resources; safety.
    - Teaching can be tailored to the woman, her family, and her home.
    - Services are less expensive than hospital.
    - Prevention, early detection, and treatment measures can be offered.
    - Services may lead to long-term positive effects on parenting and child health.
    - Use research findings and recommendations of professional organizations to validate proposal.
    - Investigate insurance reimbursement for home care.

CHAPTER 3: CLINICAL GENETICS

I. Learning Key Terms

1. S, 2. Q, 3. J, 4. D, 5. G, 6. U, 7. I, 8. T, 9. E, 10. R, 11. A, 12. C, 13. O, 14. L, 15. V, 16. P, 17. H, 18. B, 19. K, 20. M, 21. F, 22. N
23. Genetics
24. Genomics
25. Genetic testing
26. Direct (molecular) testing
27. Linkage analysis
28. Biochemical testing
29. Cytogenic testing
30. Carrier screening tests
31. Predictive testing; presymptomatic; predispositional
32. Pharmacogenomic testing
33. Gene therapy
34. Multifactorial
35. Unifactorial
36. Autosomal dominance
37. Autosomal recessive
38. Inborn error of metabolism
39. X-linked dominant
40. X-linked recessive

II. Reviewing Key Concepts

41. Identify five main genetics-related nursing activities: see Nursing Expertise in Genetics and Genomics section.
42. Explain difference between occurrence and recurrence risk: see Genetic Counseling—Estimation of Risk section.
43. Ethical issues related to Human Genome Project: see Human Genome Project—Ethical, Legal, and Social Implications section—consider effect of being able to determine vulnerability to certain disorders and the effect this can have on an individual physically, socially, economically, and emotionally; consider possibility of altered relationships engendered by the information and the potential for discrimination/stigmatization.
44. A is correct; autosomal dominant inheritance is unrelated to exposure to teratogens; each pregnancy has the same potential for expression of the disorder; there is no reduction if one child is already affected; if the gene is inherited, the disorder is always expressed.
45. D is correct; there is a 25% chance females will be carriers; if males inherit the X-chromosome with the defective gene, the disorder will be expressed and they can transmit the gene to female offspring; females are affected if they receive the defective gene from both parents.
46. D is correct; cystic fibrosis, as an inborn error of metabolism, follows an autosomal recessive pattern of inheritance; two defective genes (one from each parent) are required for the disorder to be expressed; she does not have the disorder and the father does not have the defective gene; therefore, none of their children will have the disorder, but there will be a 50% chance they will be carriers of the defective gene.
47. C is correct; factor V Leiden (FVL) affects the body's clotting mechanism by increasing the woman's risk for deep vein thrombosis (DVT) and pulmonary embolism (PE).

III. Thinking Critically

1. Factors influencing decision regarding genetic testing: see Factors Influencing the Decision to Undergo Genetic Testing section. Factors can include family pressures, responsibility to others, access to testing, cultural/ethical beliefs.

2. Support of statement that nurses should have basic understanding of genetics: see Nursing Expertise in Genetics and Genomics section. Answer should reflect the rapid advance in genetic-based treatment and the ability to diagnose genetic disorders; emphasize the nurse's role as teacher and advocate.
3. Questions to determine if risk factors for inheritable disorders are present: ask questions that would elicit information regarding health status of family members, abnormal reproductive outcomes, history of maternal disorders, drug exposures, and illnesses, advanced maternal and paternal age, and ethnic origin.
4. Couple facing a genetic disorder.
   A. Nurse's role in determining genetic risk: Tay-Sachs is an autosomal recessive disorder that follows a unifactorial pattern of inheritance; Joshua needs to be tested because he must also be a carrier, which would produce a child with the disorder; emphasize the nurse's role in terms of emotional support, facilitation of the decision-making process, and interpretation of diagnostic test results and how they can influence future childbearing decisions. Consider factors that can influence the decision to participate or not participate in testing.
   B. Inheritance possibility when both parents carry the defective recessive gene: there is a 25% chance child will be normal, a 25% chance that child will express the disorder, and a 50% chance that child will be a carrier; this pattern is the same for every pregnancy; there is no reduction in risk from one pregnancy to another.
   C. Education and emotional support: discuss the nature of this disorder, extent of risk, and consequences if the child inherits the disorder; discuss options available including amniocentesis, continuing or not continuing the pregnancy if the child is affected; discuss use of reproductive technology or adoption; be sensitive to cultural and religious beliefs; encourage expression of feelings; refer for further counseling or support groups as appropriate.

CHAPTER 4: ASSESSMENT AND HEALTH PROMOTION

I. Learning Key Terms

1. Mons pubis
2. Labia majora
3. Labia minora
4. Prepuce
5. Frenulum
6. Fourchette
7. Clitoris
8. Vestibule
9. Urethra (urinary meatus)
10. Perineum
11. Vagina, rugae, Skene's, Bartholin's
12. Fornices
13. Uterus, cul-de-sac of Douglas
14. Corpus
15. Isthmus
16. Fundus
17. Endometrium
18. Myometrium
19. Cervix
20. Endocervical canal, internal os, external os
21. Squamocolumnar junction; Papanicolaou (Pap)
22. Uterine (fallopian) tubes
23. Ovaries, ovulation, estrogen, progesterone, androgen
24. Bony pelvis
25. Breasts
26. Tail of Spence
27. Nipple
28. Areola
29. Montgomery glands (tubercles)
30. Acini
31. Myoepithelium
32. E, 33. K, 34. N, 35. S, 36. P, 37. A, 38. T, 39. M, 40. I, 41. R, 42. B, 43. L, 44. G, 45. C, 46. O, 47. F, 48. Q, 49. H, 50. J, 51. D

II. Reviewing Key Concepts

52. Guidelines for performing a Pap smear: guidelines for each component of the procedure are outlined in the Procedure box—Papanicolaou Test.
53. Characteristics of a palpated lump: location, size, mobility, consistency, tenderness, type of borders.
54. Choices A and D are correct; a woman should perform BSE every month at the end of menstruation when the breasts are the least tender; she should use the finger pads of her three middle fingers for palpation.
55. Choice D is correct; clean gloves are required only if open lesions are present and when compressing the nipple if discharge is anticipated; fingers should not be lifted; two hands are used for women with large, pendulous breasts.
56. Choice C is correct; self-examination should not be used for self-diagnosis but rather to detect early changes, which would call for the guidance of a health care provider.
57. Choice B is correct; do not ask questions during the examination because it may distract the client, interfering with relaxation measures she may be using; offer explanations only as needed during the examination.
58. Choice A is correct; all women should be screened because abuse can happen to any woman; abuse often escalates during pregnancy; the most commonly injured sites are head, neck, chest, abdomen, breasts, and upper extremities. If abuse is suspected, the nurse needs to assess further to encourage disclosure and then assist the woman

to take action and formulate a plan. Nurses should follow the laws of their state with regard to reporting instances of abuse.

59. Choice B is correct; bone mineral density testing should be initiated at 65 years of age or older unless risk factors are present; endometrial biopsies are not recommended on a routine basis for most women but women at risk for endometrial cancer should have one done at menopause; mammograms should be done annually for women 50 years of age and older.
60. Choice A is correct; all women—not just specific groups—should participate in preconception care approximately 1 year before planning to get pregnant.
61. Choice C is correct; women should not use vaginal medications or douche for 24 hours before the test; OCPs can continue; the best time for the test is midcycle.

III. Thinking Critically

1. Importance of preconception care: see Preconception Counseling and Care section and Box 4-1; this nurse should:
   - Define preconception counseling and what it entails, and stress the importance of both partners' participation.
   - Identify the effect that a woman's health status and lifestyle habits have on the developing fetus during the first trimester.
   - Describe how preconception counseling can assist a couple to choose the best time to begin a pregnancy.
2. Establishing a woman's health clinic.
   A. Services to be offered: see the Reasons for Entering the Health Care System section, in which several services are discussed, including those related to: pregnancy, health promotion and screening, fertility, sexuality, menstruation, and menopause.
   B. Barriers: see the Barriers to Seeking Health Care section. Discuss financial, cultural, and gender issues as barriers; use barriers to create strategies, including advocating for universal health insurance, providing culturally sensitive services; improving access, including transportation and child care provisions and longer hours open; innovative incentives.
   C. Services to meet goal of health promotion and prevention: see Box 4-6 and Table 4-3.
      - Consider common risk factors for health problems, leading causes of death among women, and behaviors that increase risk for health problems
      - Create programs that address age-specific issues; for example, puberty, teen pregnancies, menopause.
      - Address the appropriate focus areas for women in *Healthy People 2010/2020.*
      - Follow recommended health screening guidelines in Table 4-3.
3. State how age, disabilities, and abuse can influence health assessment of women: see specific sections for each factor in the health assessment.
4. Woman requesting advice regarding diet and exercise to lose weight: see Nutrition, Obesity, and Exercise sections.
   - BMI falls in the obese range.
   - Review risks for health disorders that are associated with being overweight.
   - Start with 24-hour to 3-day nutritional recall; based on analysis of woman's current nutritional habits, suggest use of the new food pyramid, emphasize complex carbohydrates and foods high in iron and calcium; recommend reduced fat intake; ensure adequate fluid intake, avoiding those high in sugar, alcohol, or caffeine; use weight changes and activity patterns to determine adequacy of caloric intake.
   - Aerobic exercise: discuss weight-bearing vs. non–weight-bearing exercises as well as frequency and duration of exercise sessions for maximum benefit; associate exercise with weight loss and the maintenance of appropriate weight.
5. Woman experiencing stress.
   A. Physical and emotional signs of stress: see Stress section and Box 4-5 for a listing of typical physical, behavioral, and psychologic signs of stress.
   B. Stress management: see Stress Management section.
      - Help Alice formulate her goals in life and set priorities; work on time management to allow for relaxation time.
      - Discuss her interests, hobbies to be incorporated into a stress management program designed for her; develop alternatives to alcohol and smoking for relaxation, such as biofeedback, guided imagery, yoga.
      - Refer to support group for stress management.
      - Suggest literature and Internet sites that may be beneficial.
   C. Smoking cessation: see Substance Use Cessation section and Box 4-9.
      - Use the Five A's formula.
      - Have Alice describe her smoking.
      - Discuss how she stopped before.
      - Suggest a variety of strategies for stopping smoking; encourage her to make a decision on a method that is right for her.
6. Woman's concern regarding violence against women: see Violence Against Women, abused women, and Health Protection sections.
   - Discuss woman's current circumstances and what she does now to protect herself.
   - Discuss how she changed her behavior based on the experiences of her friends; how she helped or

did not help her friends; her evaluation of how the legal and health care system met the needs of her friends; discuss what could have and should have been done to help her friends.
- Discuss protective and legal services, including hotlines, emergency centers; facilitate access to services to promote assertiveness, self-defense techniques, self-help groups.

7. Nurses' responses to concerns and questions of women.
   A. How to get ready for first gynecologic examination: explain what will occur and each guideline to follow for preparation and why each is important for the accuracy of the test.
   B. Signs indicating ovulation: see Ovarian Cycle and other Cyclic Changes sections, in which signs of ovulation are described.
   C. Breast characteristics across the life span: see Table 4-1, which outlines characteristics of breasts of adolescent, adult, and postmenopausal women.
   D. Douching: see Internal Structures section; describe how vaginal secretions protect reproductive tract and how douching could alter this function and also injure the mucosa, thereby increasing the risk for infection; describe how she should cleanse her genitalia.
8. Woman anxious about first gynecologic examination: see Pelvic Examination section and Procedure box—Assisting with Pelvic Examination. Discuss.
   - Teach her about the examination.
   - Encourage her to ask questions and to verbalize concerns.
   - Describe simple relaxation measures.
   - Ensure privacy and be sensitive to modesty.
9. Health history of a new client at a women's health clinic.
   A. Components: see History section and Box 4-8 for a list and description of components.
   B. Writing questions: use components of health history as a guide; write questions that are open ended, clear, concise; address only one issue; progress from general to specific.
   C. Therapeutic communication techniques with examples: see Interview, Cultural Considerations, Communication Variations, and Women with Special Needs sections and Cultural Considerations box for a description of communication techniques to use.
      - How to be sensitive and nonjudgmental in your approach; use a relaxed, confident, professional manner.
      - Consider the culture of the client and any special needs, including those related to sensory deficit.
      - Adjust the environment and provide privacy.
      - Ensure confidentiality.
10. Teaching self-examination techniques: each teaching plan should include cognitive, psychomotor, and affective teaching-learning techniques; describe a variety of methodologies, including discussion, exploration of feelings, provision of literature; demonstrate and have client redemonstrate using practice models and then the clients themselves as appropriate.
    Breast self-examination: see Teaching for Self-Management box—BSE and Evidence-Based Practice box—Teaching Women Breast Self-Examination.
    Vulvar (genital) Self-Examination: see Vulvar Self-Examination section.
11. Culturally sensitive approach to women's health care: review the Cultural Competence section in Chapter 2 and Cultural Considerations section and box of this chapter; use the 4 Cs of cultural competence to determine how to:
    - Approach the woman in a respectful and calm manner.
    - Consider modifications in the examination to maintain the woman's modesty.
    - Incorporate communication variations such as conversational style, pacing, spacing, eye contact, touch, time orientation.
    - Take time to learn about the woman's cultural beliefs and practices regarding well-woman assessment and care.
12. Screening for abuse when providing well-woman care.
    A. Adjusting the environment: provide for comfort and privacy; assess the woman alone, without her partner or adult children present.
    B. Abuse indicators: see the Abused Women section for identification of several indicators of possible abuse and areas of the body most commonly injured including during pregnancy; specific somatic complaints; and inadvisable behaviors, including a pattern of canceling health care appointments.
    C. Questions to ask: see Figure 4-10, which lists questions that all women should be asked in a very direct manner.
    D. Use the following approach if abuse is confirmed:
       - Acknowledge the abuse, and affirm that it is unacceptable and common; tell her that you are concerned, and that she does not deserve it.
       - Communicate that it can recur; cite the cycle of violence (see Chapter 5); tell her that help is available; empower her to use this help.
       - Help her to formulate an escape plan.
13. Describe events in each cycle composing the menstrual cycle: see Hypothalamic-Pituitary Cycle, Ovarian Cycle, and Endometrial Cycle subsections of the Menstrual Cycle for a full description of the events and changes characteristic of each cycle; include teaching methodologies you would use to enhance the effectiveness of presentation. Encourage the young women to discuss their concerns regarding these changes.

14. Assisting with a pelvic examination: see Procedure boxes—Assisting with Pelvic Examination and Papanicolaou Smear and Pelvic Examination sections to formulate your answer; information is included regarding client preparation and assisting the health care provider.
15. Adolescent client at women's health clinic who exhibits signs of a possible eating disorder. Based on her BMI of 16 this woman is underweight (Nutritional Deficiencies section).
    A. Use the SCOFF questions (Box 4-4) to screen for an eating disorder and what it could be; complete a nutritional assessment including what she eats, how much she eats, when, and where; discuss her exercise patterns; ask her about how she should look and how much she should weigh; discuss the connection between her BMI and nutritional patterns and her lack of menses and breast development.
    B. See sections for each of the eating disorders listed and compare them.

CHAPTER 5: VIOLENCE AGAINST WOMEN

I. Learning Key Terms

1. Intimate partner violence (IPV)
2. Cycle of violence model, increasing tension, battery, "honeymoon"
3. Feminist perspective
4. Ecological model, individual woman, intimate partner relationship, microsystem, mesosystem, exosystem, macrosystem, chronosystem
5. Sexual violence
6. Sexual harassment
7. Sexual assault
8. Rape
9. Statutory rape
10. Molestation
11. Rape-trauma syndrome; acute (disorganization), outward adjustment, long-term process (reorganization)
12. Sexual assault nurse examiner (SANE)

II. Reviewing Key Concepts

13. Sociologic factors associated with violence: see Sociologic Perspective section for several significant factors.
14. Cultural influence on violence against women: see Cultural Considerations section. Answer should reflect:
    - Factors true for all cultures, such as role and expected behavior of men and women, importance of family, and roles within the family, to whom you go when experiencing problems; approach to health care; definition of what violence and abuse means; effect of environmental stressors; and availability of resources
    - Examples from a variety of cultures given for each factor (see separate sections)
15. Characteristics of women in abusive relationships and men who are abusers.
    A. Characteristics of women in abusive relationships contrasted with those who are not: see Women Experiencing IPV section for the identification of several characteristics for women in violent and nonviolent relationships.
    B. Characteristics of women who seek help (see Care Management section): beaten severely and frequently, never experienced or witnessed abuse in their own families, have alternatives in terms of jobs or careers.
    C. Barriers to seeking help (see Care Management section): avoid stigma and involvement of police, fear they will not be believed or of reprisal from abuser.
    D. Characteristics of persons who are likely to abuse: see Box 5-1 for a list of many characteristics of a potential male batterer.
16. Forms of abuse: forms of abuse are illustrated in Figure 5-1.
17. The use of the ABCDEs tool when caring for an abused woman: see Plan of Care and Interventions section for a full description of this tool and how it is used.
18. Strategies to prevent cycle of violence: see Prevention section of Nursing Interventions, which describes many prevention strategies across the life span.
19. Factors that deter women from reporting rape: see Sexual Violence section, which discusses several deterrents to reporting rape.
20. Choices A and D are correct; characteristics of a potential batterer include deficits in assertiveness, low tolerance for frustration, inadequate verbal skills especially with regard to expressing feelings, and an unusual amount of jealousy leading to often expecting his partner to spend all of her time with him (see Box 5-1).
21. Choice D is correct; battered women are often isolated as a result of fear, the stigma society places on them because of the false belief that they must enjoy being abused, and restrictions on their activities by their partner; typical feminine characteristics are more apparent in women in abusive relationships whereas assertiveness, independence, and willingness to take a stand are more characteristic of women who are in nonviolent relationships.
22. Choices B, C, and E are correct; anxiety and depression can lead to use of alcohol, tobacco, and drugs as a means of coping; inadequate diet results in low maternal weight gain increasing the risk for anemia and giving birth to an LBW newborn; the rate of preterm birth and LBW is increased; abused women are more likely to experience sexually transmitted infections, pelvic pain, and bleeding.
23. Choice A is correct; women who experience repeated and severe abuse, have never witnessed or

experienced abuse in their own families, and have alternatives such as a job or career are more likely to seek assistance.

24. Choices C, D, and E are correct; there is no recall after taking a drink laced with the drug; severe headache is not characteristic of having been drugged but feeling fuzzy when waking up is characteristic.

III. Thinking Critically

1. Disproving myths regarding violence against women: use the Introduction section for statistical information regarding the incidence and demographics of violence against women, Table 5-2, Perspectives on Violence, and IPV sections to disprove myths A, B, C, and D; use IPV During Pregnancy section to disprove myth E; in addition to your textbook, you can use the Internet to gather information to dispel the myths.
2. Ecological framework (see Conceptual and Theoretical Perspectives section and Fig. 5-2) to create your outline.
3. Cues indicative of physical abuse.
   A. Identify cues: see IPV During Pregnancy and Care Management sections and Nursing Process box for IPV
      - Typical injuries
      - Psychosocial findings
      - Behaviors related to health care
   B. Suspicion that pregnant woman is being abused: see Care Management and IPV During Pregnancy sections.
      - Use appropriate communication techniques including direct questions (see Fig. 5-3).
      - Perform interview and examination in a private setting; female health care provider might be helpful.
      - If injuries are noted, tell her that these are common in women who are abused; tell her she is not responsible for another person's abusive behavior.
      - Consider legal implications.
   C. Abuse is confirmed: see Nursing Interventions section; describe how you would use the ABCDES of caring as a framework for helping Carol.
   D. Why pregnancy leads to violence: see IPV During Pregnancy section; discuss such factors as stress of pregnancy, jealousy of fetus, anger, attempt to end the pregnancy.
   E. Approach to avoid: avoid being judgmental, such as evaluating Carol's actions and responses to violence in terms of how the nurse would act in the same situation or to rush her; Carol needs to be helped at her own pace, but formulating an escape plan is critical.
   F. Use Figure 5-3 to evaluate the degree of danger.
   G. Adverse effects of violence on pregnancy: many adverse effects are identified in IPV During Pregnancy section.
   H. Indicators for readiness to leave abusive relationship: see Nursing Interventions section
      - Exhibits capability to plan for and invest in herself
      - Recognizes that abuse is part of a continuing pattern
      - Expresses desire to leave; needs to leave when no abuse is occurring with reassurance of available economic and social support to make it on her own
   I. Legal responsibilities of the nurse (see Legal Tip—Mandatory Reporting of Domestic Violence).
      - Full documentation of the abuse should be done (see Box 5-2 for guidelines to follow).
      - Know your state's requirement regarding the reporting of abuse/battering.
4. For a woman who has been raped, see Sexual Violence section.
   A. Sexual assault nurse examiner: see Collaborative Care section; this nurse is fully prepared to care for rape victims and collect essential evidence.
   B. Nurse's responsibility to assess and to collect and preserve evidence of the rape: see The Sexual Examination section, Legal Tips—(Collection of Evidence and Documentation) and Box 5-3 for adult sexual assault protocol to follow; be sure that answer includes data that must be collected, how to care for evidence, and legal requirements.
   C. Nurse's actions to meet emotional needs: emotional support measures can be found throughout the Collaborative Care section including the section on psychologic first aid; consider how you would help her before, during, and after the examination as well as the importance of follow-up care after discharge.
   D. Phases of rape-trauma syndrome: behaviors and emotions and counselor support required: see Rape Trauma section for sections related to each phase.
   E. Discharge interventions: see Discharge and After Discharge sections; describe each of the following in your answer: medications, instructions, resources, getting home, follow-up.

CHAPTER 6: REPRODUCTIVE SYSTEM CONCERNS

I. Learning Key Terms

1. Amenorrhea
2. Hypogonadotropic amenorrhea
3. Female athlete triad
4. Cyclic perimenstrual pain and discomfort (CPPD), dysmenorrhea, premenstrual syndrome (PMS), premenstrual dysphoric disorder (PDD)
5. Dysmenorrhea
6. Primary dysmenorrhea
7. Secondary dysmenorrhea
8. Premenstrual syndrome (PMS)
9. Premenstrual dysphoric disorder (PDD)

10. Endometriosis
11. Oligomenorrhea
12. Hypomenorrhea
13. Metrorrhagia, intermenstrual bleeding
14. Mittlestaining
15. Breakthrough bleeding
16. Menorrhagia, hypermenorrhea
17. Abnormal uterine bleeding (AUB)
18. Dysfunctional uterine bleeding (DUB)
19. Menarche
20. Menopause
21. Perimenopause, climacteric
22. Surgical menopause
23. Postmenopause
24. Dyspareunia
25. Hot flush
26. Hot flash
27. Night sweats
28. Osteoporosis
29. Phytoestrogens, isoflavones

II. Reviewing Key Concepts

30. Describe changes associated with perimenopause: use separate section for each expected change in the Menopause section to complete this activity.
31. Choice B is correct; the 14-year-old reflects several of the risk factors associated with this menstrual disorder, namely participating in a sport that is stressful, subjectively scored, requires contour revealing clothing, and success is favored by a prepubertal body shape.
32. Choice C is correct; A, B, and D all interfere with prostaglandin synthesis, whereas acetaminophen has no antiprostaglandin properties; prostaglandins are a recognized factor in the etiology of primary dysmenorrhea.
33. Choice A is correct; decreasing the ingestion of salty foods and refined sugars 7 to 10 days before menses decreases fluid retention; asparagus and cranberry juice have a natural diuretic effect that can reduce edema and related discomforts; valerian is a herb that reduces menstrual cramping.
34. Choices B, C, and E are correct; alcohol as well as tobacco and caffeine can worsen symptoms, whereas exercise especially during the luteal phase relieves symptoms, as can fruits, especially peaches and watermelon and whole grains; sodium intake should be less than 3 g daily; bugleweed and evening primrose oil can reduce breast discomfort.
35. Choices C, D, and F are correct; women taking danazol often experience reversible masculinizing changes; it is taken orally for a 3- to 4-month period; ovulation may not be fully suppressed; therefore, birth control is essential because the medication is teratogenic; amenorrhea, not increased bleeding, occurs.
36. Choice A is correct; oligomenorrhea—infrequent menses; menorrhagia—excessive bleeding during menses; hypomenorrhea—scanty bleeding at normal intervals.
37. Choice C is correct; DUB is most commonly associated with anovulatory cycles in women at the extremes of their reproductive years (puberty, perimenopause); it can also occur when women secrete low levels of progesterone; it is associated with obesity; increased prostaglandins is associated with dysmenorrheal.
38. Choice A is correct; dysmenorrhea is painful menstruation; dysuria is painful urination; dyspnea is difficulty breathing.
39. Choice D is correct; alendronate sodium (Fosamax) should be taken on an empty stomach with a glass of water to enhance absorption; remaining upright will help decrease GI symptoms.
40. Choice B is correct; see Table 6-2 for an explanation of each herb.

III. Thinking Critically

1. Woman with hypogonadotropic amenorrhea (see Hypogonadotropic Amenorrhea section).
   A. Risk factors exhibited: athletic competition subjectively scored, endurance sport favoring low body weight, inappropriate body composition, nutritional deficits related to need to maintain body size, stress and vigorous exercise, need to wear body-revealing clothing, prepubertal body shape or weight categories favor success or ability to participate.
   B. Nursing diagnosis: disturbed body image related to delayed onset of menstruation and development of secondary sexual characteristics; anxiety can also be a nursing diagnosis.
   C. Expected outcomes: Maria will:
      - Verbalize understanding regarding basis for delayed onset of pubertal changes
      - Participate in a therapeutic regimen that will favor age-appropriate physical development
   D. Care management: see Management section for several nursing interventions.
   E. See Hypogonadotropic Amenorrhea for a list of sports of concern and the rationale for the concern; measures should include education, one-on-one counseling, screening in terms of BMI and nutrition; involve coaches and families in the program.
2. Woman with primary dysmenorrhea (see Primary Dysmenorrhea section).
   A. Questions regarding pain should gather data related to timing of the pain, its characteristics, severity, relief measures she has tried and their level of effectiveness; what makes the pain worse or better, woman's knowledge level regarding reason for the pain; effect of pain on daily activities and relationships.
   B. Nursing diagnoses: consider the areas of acute pain and ineffective role performance as the focus for nursing management of this woman's primary dysmenorrhea; use assessment data to determine which nursing diagnosis will take precedence.

C. Physiologic basis of pain: dysmenorrhea is a physiologic rather than pathologic process associated with ovulatory cycles and the secretion of estrogen and progesterone leading to the release of prostaglandins which cause the uterus to contract and vasospasm to occur resulting in uterine ischemia and pain.

D. Relief measures: see Management section and Tables 6-1 and 6-2 for several measures; be sure to discuss basis of the problem, how each measure suggested works to provide relief, and how/when they should be used; assist woman to choose measures that are best for her.

3. Woman experiencing PMS (see PMS and PMDD section).
   A. Signs and symptoms of PMS (see PMS section for a full description of signs and symptoms): include physical and psychologic signs and symptoms; clinical manifestations are usually related to effects of fluid retention, behavioral and emotional changes, cravings, headache, fatigue/energy level, and backache.
   B. Nursing diagnosis: nursing diagnoses could include acute pain, activity intolerance, disturbed sleep pattern, ineffective role performance; use assessment findings to determine those that apply to a particular client, including those that are priority.
   C. Nursing approach: see Management section, Tables 6-1 and 6-2, and Nursing Care Plan for several pharmacologic and nonpharmacologic measures; include how you would work with the woman to explain the basis of PMS and to choose the measures to include in an individualized plan of care.
   D. See PMS and PMDD section for a full description of this disorder.
4. Woman with endometriosis (see Endometriosis section).
   A. Clinical manifestations: dysmenorrhea (secondary), pelvic pain and heaviness, thigh pain, diarrhea, constipation, painful defecation, dyspareunia, abnormal bleeding, and infertility.
   B. Pathophysiology of the disorder: growth of endometrial tissue outside uterus, mainly in the pelvis; implants respond to cyclic changes in hormones; bleeding of implants leads to inflammatory response, formation of scar tissue/adhesions, fibrosis, anemia; impaired fertility can occur.
   C. Pharmacologic management: each medication is discussed in the Management section.
   D. Support measures: see Management section and Nursing Care Plan for several measures such as educate regarding disease process; discuss treatment options; refer to support groups and counseling as appropriate, work with couple together and separately to allow for expression of feelings and concerns; review options for pregnancy since infertility can be an outcome.
5. Woman at risk for osteoporosis (see Osteoporosis section).
   A. Risk factors exhibited: Caucasian, age, slender/thin, family history of osteoporosis, smokes, sedentary lifestyle, dietary risks related to inadequate calcium coupled with excess intake of fast food, caffeine, and soft drinks
   B. Prevention measures (see Box 6-2): specifically address risk factors presented by the woman, in this case including nutrition, smoking, exercise and activity patterns; encourage bone density testing.
   C. Signs of osteoporosis: see Figure 6-2; decrease in height, back pain especially lower back, dowager's hump (kyphosis), fractures
6. Woman experiencing perimenopausal changes (see Menopause section)
   A. Relief measures (see specific subsection for each change, Teaching for Self-Management box—Comfort Measures, Box 6-2, Table 6-4, and Alternative Therapies, Sexual Counseling, and Midlife Support Groups sections): discuss each change, why it occurs, and several relief options; encourage the woman and her partner to be involved in the process of coping with the changes of the perimenopause period and the decisions that have to be made.
   B. Decision making regarding MHT (see Menopausal Hormonal Therapy section, Box 6-2, and Table 6-4): answer should include benefits, risks, side effects, preparations and administration, duration of treatment, and alternatives.
   C. Instructions for use of transdermal patch: see Treatment Guidelines section: apply to trunk and upper arms, not on breasts; check site for irritation, alternate sites, apply at recommended frequency to hairless, clean, dry, intact site; emphasize importance of regular and ongoing health care to monitor effects of hormone use.
   D. Heart disease concerns: see Coronary Heart Disease section and sections related to nutrition and exercise for the information to tell this client why there is risk for heart disease and what she can do about it; with a BMI indicating obesity, weight loss will decrease not only the risk for heart disease but also hypertension and type 2 diabetes.
   E. Use of Internet: provide Heidi with a list of appropriate sites with which to start; give her guidelines regarding how to find sites and how to evaluate sites she finds including sponsor, currency, accuracy; caution her to seek advice of health care provider before beginning a recommended treatment or to seek information if she has questions.

CHAPTER 7: SEXUALLY TRANSMITTED AND OTHER INFECTIONS

I. Learning Key Terms

1. Sexually transmitted infections (STIs) or sexually transmitted diseases (STDs), chlamydia, HPV, gonorrhea, HSV-2, syphilis, HIV

2. Risk-reduction measures
3. Condom (male, female)
4. Chlamydia
5. Gonorrhea
6. Syphilis, chancre, condylomata lata
7. Pelvic inflammatory disease (PID)
8. Human papillomavirus (HPV), condylomata acuminata
9. Genital herpes simplex virus (HSV)
10. Hepatitis A virus (HAV)
11. Hepatitis B virus (HBV)
12. Hepatitis C virus (HCV)
13. Human immunodeficiency virus (HIV), immunologic, acquired immunodeficiency syndrome (AIDS)
14. Group B streptococci (GBS)
15. Bacterial vaginosis (BV)
16. Candidiasis (vulvocandidiasis)
17. Trichomoniasis
18. TORCH
19. Toxoplasmosis
20. Rubella
21. Cytomegalovirus (CMV)
22. Standard Precautions

II. Reviewing Key Concepts

23. Choice A is correct; because these infections are often asymptomatic, they can go undetected and untreated, causing more severe damage, including ascent of the pathogen into uterus and pelvis resulting in PID and infertility; many effective treatment measures are available, including treatment for chlamydia.
24. Choice B is correct; A is indicative of candidiasis; C is indicative of genital HSV; D is indicative of trichomoniasis.
25. Choice B is correct; metronidazole is used to treat bacterial vaginosis and trichomoniasis; benzathine penicillin is used to treat syphilis; acyclovir is used to treat genital herpes.
26. Choice C is correct; cesarean section or isolation is not required; there are no lesions with this bacterial infection; antiviral medication is not appropriate.
27. Choices A, D, and E are correct; recurrent infections commonly involve only local symptoms that are less severe; stress reduction, healthy lifestyle practices, cleansing lesions, and acyclovir can reduce recurrence rate and prevent secondary infection; viral shedding can occur before lesions appear during the prodromal stage; acyclovir cannot cure herpes but can keep it in control.
28. Choice B is correct; although A, C, and D are measures that should be followed, knowing her partner including his sexual history and presence of any manifestations of infection is essential.
29. Choice B is correct; several HPV serotypes are thought to have oncogenic potential and are therefore the primary cause of cervical cancer.
30. Common risk factors for STIs: Box 7-2 cites many common risk behaviors according to sexual, drug use-related, and blood-related risks.
31. Infection control principles and practices: see Box 7-3 for a full explanation of Standard Precautions.
32. Outline of common reproductive infections: see each infection's section for information related to typical clinical manifestations and management guidelines.
33. Meaning of TORCH: see TORCH Infections section and Table 7-7 for the infections represented by each letter.

III. Thinking Critically

1. Woman attending first visit at a women's health clinic.
   A. Determining risk for STIs: see Box 7-2 to determine areas of risk; discuss the development of a therapeutic relationship including use of therapeutic communication techniques in order to facilitate trust and full disclosure; consider importance of vulvar self-examination for early detection.
   B. Major points to emphasize for STI prevention: see Prevention and Risk Reduction Measures sections and Table 7-1.
      - Know partner.
      - Avoid many partners or partners who have had many previous partners.
      - Insist on barrier method; be prepared.
      - Do not make decisions based on appearances and unfounded assumptions.
      - Carefully examine partner.
      - Know low risk sexual practices and those that are unsafe or risky.
   C. Measures to help client develop assertiveness and communication skills related to safer sexual practices.
      - Begin by stressing the seriousness of the infections and the risk for transmission she faces by not using prevention measures; emphasize importance of discussing prevention measures including condom use with partner at a time removed from sexual activity.
      - Role-play using possible partner responses for woman to react to; rehearse how she will handle various situations so she can sort out her feelings and fears ahead of time.
      - Reassure her that her reluctance is not unusual.
   D. HPV vaccine (see Risk Reduction Measures section and HPV section); emphasize that although still within the age range of 13 to 26 to receive a catch-up vaccine, it is less effective when given after the woman is sexually active; it is also not effect for all forms of HPV, so regular Pap smears are still very important.
2. Pregnant woman diagnosed as HIV positive at 4 weeks of gestation.
   A. Heterosexual transmission of HIV to women: see HIV section; consider exchange of body fluids (semen, blood, vaginal secretions); IV drug use by herself or her partner; history of multiple STIs

B. Clinical manifestations during seroconversion: viremic, influenza-type responses along with abnormal CBC results

C. Management: see Management section for a discussion of measures for nonpregnant and pregnant women, including education regarding transmission prevention, infection control measures to maintain resistance to infection, contraceptive methods, and signs of disease progress; use a multidisciplinary care approach with a holistic focus; prescribe prophylactic medication, and make referrals as needed.

D. Measures to reduce transmission to baby: see HIV—Counseling for HIV testing and HIV and Pregnancy sections; discuss several measures including use of HAART, scheduled cesarean at 38 weeks, avoiding breastfeeding, and lifestyle changes.

3. Woman with severe PID (see Pelvic Inflammatory Disease section).

A. Risk factors: several factors are listed, including those related to menstrual history, age, contraceptive method used, recent reproductive tract problem or procedure, sexual behavior, and genital hygiene including douching.

B. Diagnostic criteria: include such findings as oral temperature of 38.3° C or higher, discharge, elevated erythrocyte sedimentation rate, bilateral adnexal tenderness, cervical motion tenderness, elevated C-reactive protein, lower abdominal tenderness.

C. Nursing diagnoses during acute phase: nursing diagnoses will most likely include acute pain, anxiety (effect on sexuality and future fertility), impaired physical mobility, constipation/diarrhea, and impaired urinary elimination.

D. Management guidelines: see Management section; management outline should include measures for each of the following areas:

- Position and activity/rest
- Comfort measures; nutrition and fluid balance
- Emotional support measures
- Health education: for now and with discharge

E. Self-management during recovery phase: see Management section and Teaching for Self-Management boxes—Sexually Transmitted Infections and Prevention of Genital Tract Infections for several suggestions and prevention of genital tract infection for the future; emphasize activity restrictions, importance of rest, good nutrition, taking medications completely, and follow-up.

F. Reproductive risks: tubal obstructions and adhesions leading to ectopic pregnancy or infertility, chronic pelvic pain, dyspareunia, abscesses.

4. Woman diagnosed with gonorrhea.

A. Essential assessment areas during health history: Box 7-2 outlines points to emphasize during assessment; be sure to discuss with her measures she has been using to reduce the risk of STIs; determine why she may or may not be using these measures.

B. Nursing diagnosis: anxiety related to potential effect of STI on future sexual function *or* ineffective sexuality pattern related to recent diagnosis of STI is indicated.

C. Management

- Educate about STIs.
- Discuss self-care measures: see Teaching for Self-Management boxes—Sexually Transmitted Infections and Prevention of Genital Tract Infections.
- Discuss risk-reduction practices (Table 7-1) and practice assertiveness with partners.
- Review Genital Self-Examination (see technique Chapter 4).

5. Reducing pain of condylomata associated with HPV infection: see HPV—Management section for several suggestions related to cleansing, reducing moisture, what to wear, measures to enhance healing.

6. Woman diagnosed with herpes simplex virus 2 (see HSV—management section).

A. Measures to relieve pain and prevent secondary infection: see HSV—Management section for several measures to include in the answer.

- Correct use of antiviral medications (Table 7-2)
- Care of lesions
- Use of alternative treatments
- What to wear
- Comfort measures including use of analgesics
- Diet and lifestyle to enhance healing.

B. Preventing/reducing recurrence.

- Educate regarding HSV.
- Keep diary.
- Educate regarding stress-reduction measures and how to prevent transmission.

7. Measures to prevent transmission of hepatitis B virus (see HBV—Management section): use immunoprophylaxis for household members and sexual contacts, maintain high levels of personal hygiene, carefully dispose of items contaminated with blood or body fluids including saliva, use risk-reduction practices (Table 7-1).

8. Woman concerned about exposure to HIV (see HIV section).

A. Risky behaviors (see Box 7-2 and Table 7-1): exposure to contaminated body fluids, including semen and blood; discuss sexual practices and partners as well as possible IV drug use.

B. Testing procedure: see Screening and Diagnosis section, and Legal Tip: HIV Testing box for full description of types of tests and testing protocol, counseling required, and legal implications; nurse should witness an informed consent, tell the woman how long it will take for the results to be available, consider ethical issues of confidentiality and privacy, and use a nonjudgmental, empathic approach.

C. Counseling protocol: counseling should occur before and after testing, by the same person, in a private area with no interruptions; all assessments, actions, and responses should be documented; describe pretest and posttest counseling and teaching.
D. Instructions following a negative test result: use Sonya's risky behaviors as a basis for discussing prevention measures, including risk reduction practices; discuss effect HIV could have on Sonya's health and on the health of her fetus when she is pregnant.

CHAPTER 8: CONTRACEPTION AND ABORTION

I. Learning Key Terms

1. Contraception
2. Birth control
3. Family planning
4. Contraceptive failure rate
5. Coitus interruptus
6. Fertility awareness methods, natural family planning (NFP), periodic abstinence
7. Calendar rhythm method
8. Two-day method
9. Ovulation method
10. Spinnbarkeit
11. Basal body temperature (BBT) method
12. Thermal shift
13. Symptothermal
14. Biologic marker methods
15. Spermicide
16. Condom
17. Diaphragm
18. Cervical cap
19. Contraceptive sponge
20. Monophasic pill
21. Multiphasic pill (biphasic, triphasic)
22. Withdrawal bleeding
23. Transdermal contraceptive system
24. Vaginal contraceptive ring
25. Minipill
26. Depo-Provera (DMPA, depot medroxyprogesterone acetate)
27. Implanon
28. Intrauterine device (IUD)
29. Sterilization, oviducts (uterine fallopian tubes), sperm ducts (vas deferens), vasectomy
30. Tubal reconstruction
31. Lactation amenorrhea method (LAM)
32. Induced abortion, elective abortion, therapeutic abortion
33. Aspiration (vacuum or suction curettage)
34. Medical abortion; methotrexate, misoprostol, mifepristone
35. Dilation and evacuation

II. Reviewing Key Concepts

36. Choice A is correct; oral contraception provides no protection from STIs; therefore, a condom and spermicide are still recommended to prevent transmission; B, C, and D reflect appropriate actions and recognition of the effects of OCPs.
37. Choice B is correct; cervical mucus is thickened, thereby inhibiting sperm penetration; ovulation and the development of the endometrium are also inhibited; there is no protection from STIs; the overall effectiveness rate is nearly 100% if used correctly.
38. Choice A is correct; women often complain of the irregular bleeding that occurs with progestin-only contraceptives.
39. Choice A is correct; the injection is repeated every 11 to 13 weeks; B, C, and D are accurate.
40. Choice A is correct; the string should be checked after menses; a missing string or one that becomes longer or shorter should be checked by a health care professional.
41. Choice D is correct; maximum spermicide effectiveness lasts no longer than 1 hour; foams and jellies/creams have a nearly instant effect, whereas tablets and suppositories require 10 to 30 minutes to dissolve, and film takes about 5 minutes; douching or rinsing should not occur for at least 6 hours after the last act of coitus; frequent use of N-9 especially for anal intercourse may disrupt mucosa, increasing rather than decreasing the risk of HIV transmission.
42. Choice B is correct; spermicide should be applied inside the cap but not around the rim because a seal will not form to keep the cap in place; use during menses increases the risk for toxic shock syndrome; checking the cap's position is all that is required before each subsequent act of coitus.
43. Choices A, C, and D are correct; spermicide should be spread on both surfaces of the diaphragm; it should not be removed for at least 6 hours nor should it be used during menses because of the risk for TSS.
44. Choices A, B, and D are correct; BBT rises during the luteal phase and libido increases.
45. Choices C and D are correct; there is no hormone in this IUD; copper serves as a spermicide and it inflames the endometrium, preventing fertilization; NSAIDs are recommended to decrease cramping,
46. Choices A and D are correct; condoms are still needed to reduce risk for STIs and to prevent pregnancy until two consecutive sperm counts are at zero; he may become sexually active when desired but needs to use a condom since sperm may still be in the ejaculate.
47. Couple making decision regarding contraceptive method to use,
    A. Factors influencing effectiveness: see full list in Box 8-1.

B. Informed consent: see Legal Tip—Informed Consent in Care Management section; use BRAIDED format.

48. Purpose for self-assessment of cervical mucus: see Ovulation Method section and Teaching for Self-Management box—Cervical Mucous Characteristics for a description of the rationale for checking cervical mucus.
49. Fertility awareness (natural family planning) methods for contraception
    A. ovulation, exercising restraint, irregular menstrual cycles
    B. 5, 22
    C. decrease, 0.5°, progesterone, increase, 0.2° to 0.5°, 2 to 4
    D. cervical mucus, amount, consistency
    E. basal body temperature (BBT), cervical mucus
    F. luteinizing hormone (LH), 12 to 24
50. Use of nonprescription barrier methods.
    A. I
    B. C
    C. C
    D. I
    E. C
    F. I
    G. I

III. Thinking Critically

1. Toxic shock syndrome: see Diaphragms section
    A. Prevention measures when using diaphragm/cervical cap: removal 6 to 8 hours after intercourse as recommended; avoid use during menses; awareness of danger signs of TSS.
    B. Clinical manifestations: see Nursing Alert for several signs.
2. Woman seeking assistance with making choice regarding birth control method (see Nursing Process box for contraception and Nursing Care Plan for sexual activity and contraception).
    A. Nursing diagnosis: deficient knowledge related to methods of contraception *or* anxiety related to lack of knowledge regarding contraception.
    B. Approach for nurse to use to assist with decision making; include the following areas in answer:
        - Assess level of knowledge and health status.
        - Describe methods; determine preferences for or objections to.
        - Determine level of contraceptive involvement desired.
3. Woman choosing to use combination estrogen-progestin oral contraceptive (see Hormonal Methods section).
    A. Mode of action; see Oral Contraceptive section for a description of how method works.
    B. Advantages: see Advantages section for several benefits of COCs.
    C. Contraindications: see Disadvantages and Side Effects section, which lists several reasons for not using COCs.
    D. Specify side effects related to changing levels of estrogen and progesterone (see Disadvantages and Side Effects section).
    E. Signs and symptoms requiring woman to stop taking the OCP and notifying her health care provider: see Signs of Potential Complications box—Oral Contraceptives for full explanation of ACHES.
    F. Instructions for the client: Include a description of each of the following in your answer: directions on package, importance if using own pills and taking at same time every day, side effects/adverse reactions, interactions with other medications, need for STI protection, backup method, what to do when missing a pill(s).
4. Woman using a cervical cap (see Cervical Cap section and Teaching for Self-Management box—Insertion and Removal of Cervical Cap).
    A. Factors making client a poor candidate for using cap: several factors are identified in this section.
    B. Client instructions for safe and effective use; include a discussion of each of the following:
        - Know when and how to insert and remove, check placement, and use spermicide.
        - Avoid using during menses or for at least 6 weeks postpartum.
        - Check fit annually and after gynecologic surgery, birth, major weight changes.
5. Instructions following IUD insertion (see IUD section).
    - See Signs of Potential Complications box—IUDs, which defines the acronym PAINS to identify signs of problems.
    - Teach how and when to check string.
    - Stress importance of appropriate genital hygiene and risk reduction measures.
    - Inform when IUD needs to be replaced.
6. Couple contemplating sterilization (see Sterilization section).
    A. Decision-making approach: nurse acts as facilitator to help couple explore the pros and cons of sterilization itself and the options available for male and female
    B. Preoperative and postoperative care measures and instructions for vasectomy; fully discuss each of these areas in your answer.
        - Preoperative: health assessment; witness an informed consent.
        - Postoperative: prevention and early detection of bleeding and infection; self-management measures.
        - Caution that sterility is not immediate and what to do.
        - STI protection.
7. Woman contemplating elective abortion (see Induced Abortion section and Box 8-4).

A. Nursing diagnosis: decisional conflict related to unplanned pregnancy and need to complete education.
B. Describe approach: use therapeutic communication techniques to establish trusting relationship; discuss alternatives available to her and the consequences of each; nurse facilitates decision-making process, and the client makes the decision; make appropriate referrals to help her with the decision.
C. Procedure for vacuum aspiration: see Aspiration section for full description of procedures.
D. Nursing diagnoses: consider fear/anxiety, anticipatory grieving, risk for deficient fluid volume (blood loss), risk for infection, acute pain.
E. Nursing measures for care and support: answer should reflect assessment and physical care and emotional support.
F. Discharge instructions: answer should include observation for signs of complications (see Safety Alert) infection prevention, observation for signs of complications; activity restrictions, resumption of sexual relations, use of birth control and risk reduction measures; follow-up appointment and importance of stress reduction.

8. Drugs used for medical abortions—how they work; see Medical Abortion section. Describe methotrexate, misoprostol (Cytotec), and mifepristone.
9. Woman seeking assistance following unprotected intercourse (see Emergency Contraception section).
   A. Nursing approach.
      - Explore possibility of pregnancy and options related to continuing pregnancy if it occurs (keeping baby, adoption).
      - Explore options for emergency contraception to prevent pregnancy: methods available, how each works, timing, side effects, how administered.
      - Emphasize importance of follow-up to check for effectiveness of method used and occurrence of infection.
      - Discuss methods of contraception and safer sex measures to prevent recurrence of this situation.
   B. Using Plan B (see Emergency Contraception section Nursing Alert, and Table 8-2) for the information to complete this exercise.
   C. Nurse must emphasize that while risk for pregnancy is reduced by 89%; pregnancy is still possible; therefore, follow-up is essential. In addition, infection is also still possible.

CHAPTER 9: INFERTILITY

I. Learning Key Terms

1. F, 2. G, 3. H, 4. D, 5. I, 6. B, 7. E, 8. C, 9. A
10. Infertility
11. Sterility
12. Assisted reproductive therapies (ARTs)
13. In vitro fertilization and embryo transfer (IVF & ET)
14. Intracytoplasmic sperm injection
15. Gamete intrafallopian transfer (GIFT)
16. Zygote intrafallopian transfer (ZIFT)
17. Therapeutic donor insemination
18. Gestational carrier (embryo host)
19. Surrogate motherhood
20. Assisted hatching
21. Donor embryo (embryo adoption)
22. Preimplantation genetic diagnosis (PGD)
23. Cryopreservation of human embryos

II. Reviewing Key Concepts

24. Choice B is correct; spinnbarkeit refers to stretchiness of cervical mucus at ovulation to facilitate passage of sperm; there is an LH surge prior to ovulation; BBT rises in response to increased progesterone after ovulation; cervical mucus becomes thinner and more abundant with ovulation.
25. Choice B is correct; the couple should abstain from intercourse for 2 to 4 days before expected ovulation; the test is scheduled for the expected time of ovulation; the woman should be examined within several hours after ejaculation of semen into vagina.
26. Choice A is correct; both male and female obesity can adversely affect fertility; water-soluble lubricants can be safely used; daily hot tubs or saunas may increase scrotal temperature enough to interfere with spermatogenesis; although excessive alcohol use can cause erectile dysfunction, abstention from alcohol is not necessary.
27. Choice C is correct; this medication provides LH and FSH, causing a powerful ovulation stimulation that can result in multiple pregnancy; therefore, regular ovarian ultrasound and monitoring of estradiol levels are required to prevent hyperstimulation. It is administered intramuscularly and is used when clomiphene fails to induce ovulation; it is followed by administration of hCG.
28. Choice B is correct; nafarelin is used to create a pseudomenopause when a woman has endometriosis to cause the implants to atrophy and shrink, thereby increasing the chance that a woman will be fertile after treatment.
29. Choice D is correct; with passage of radiopaque dye, this test could straighten or unblock the uterine tube if that is the cause of the infertility—it is not a guarantee she will conceive; it is performed 4 to 5 days after menstruation (proliferative phase); uterine cramping and referred pain to the shoulder are expected findings and are treated with mild analgesics and position changes.
30. Medications used in the treatment of infertility: use Medication Guide—Infertility Medications and Medical section to describe the mode of action and purpose for each medication listed.

II. Thinking Critically

1. Couple receiving care for infertility: see Factors Associated with Infertility section, Nursing Process box—Infertility, and Nursing Care Plan Infertility, and Boxes 9-1 and 9-2.
   A. Identify/describe components for normal fertility: components required for conception and pregnancy are identified and described in this section.
   B. Support statement that assessment for infertility must involve both partners: Box 9-5 identifies findings favorable for fertility indicating male and female factors; cite statistics related to male and female factors associated with infertility.
2. Couple undergoing testing for infertility.
   A. Nursing support measures: see Psychosocial section of Interventions and Box 9-2; Nurses must feel comfortable with their own sexuality and recognize common responses to infertility; help couple to:
      - Express feelings and openly discuss sexuality issues
      - Grieve the loss of fertility and inability to have biologic children if that is the outcome
      - Refer to support groups and adoption agencies as appropriate
   B. Female and male assessment components: see appropriate text sections and Boxes 9-1 and 9-2 and Table 9-1 for a full explanation of the components for each assessment.
   C. Procedure for semen analysis: see Semen Analysis section for essential guidelines to Ensure test result accuracy.
   D. Semen characteristics evaluated: see Box 9-6 for a full list of characteristics in terms of liqucfaction, volume, pH, density, and morphology.
   E. Postcoital (PCT) test instructions: see Assessment of Couple—Postcoital Test section for a review of instructions that must be followed to ensure test result accuracy.
   F. Effect of male smoking and alcohol use on fertility: see Male Infertility section and Box 9-2. Depending on number of cigarettes smoked each day, smoking can result in abnormal sperm, decreased number of sperm, and chromosomal damage; include in your answer the potential effect of secondhand smoke on the smoker's partner and on the fetus, should pregnancy occur. In addition to sperm/genetic damage, alcohol use can result in erectile dysfunction depending on the amount of alcohol used.
3. Concerns engendered by assisted reproductive technologies: see Assisted Reproductive Therapies section and Boxes 9-3, 9-4, and 9-7. In your answer, discuss who should pay; who are the biologic parents; marital status; ownership of ovum, sperm, embryos; seeking the "perfect" child; risk for multiple gestation; reduction abortions.
4. Woman scheduled for a diagnostic laparoscopy: see Laparoscopy section, Figure 9-4, and Table 9-1.
   A. Timing: early in menstrual cycle to avoid disturbing a possible fertilized ovum.
   B. Preprocedure care measures: NPO depending on anesthesia used: for 8 hours, void before procedure, bowel preparation may be required.
   C. Purpose and process of the procedure—describe each of the following: diagnostic and therapeutic purposes and process (what will happen).
   D. Postprocedure care measures: discuss assessment of status; physical care and emotional support measures; timing of discharge criteria, discharge instructions, prevention of complications.
5. Couple experiencing problems with fertility.
   A. Typical responses and nursing actions: see Table 9-2 for description of reactions and several recommended nursing actions.
   B. Guiding the decision-making process: see Box 9-7.
      - Discuss meaning of fertility and having biologic children for this couple and for their family.
      - Fully inform couple of diagnostic tests and treatment options so that informed decision can be made.
      - Review financial considerations, including what insurance will cover (see Box 9-4).
      - Encourage couple to define what they are willing to endure physically, emotionally, and financially to have a biologic child; discuss alternatives to biologic children.
      - Refer to support groups.
   C. Religious and cultural beliefs and practices that can influence decision making regarding treatment of infertility (see Box 9-3).

CHAPTER 10: PROBLEMS OF THE BREAST

I. Learning Key Terms

1. B, 2. E, 3. G, 4. A, 5. F, 6. H, 7. D, 8. C

II. Reviewing Key Concepts

9. Definitions of treatment approaches: see Surgery, Breast Reconstruction, Radiation, and Adjuvant Treatment sections and Table 10-4 for a full description of each treatment approach.
10. Choices B and C are correct; breast cancer is more common among Caucasian women but the mortality rate is higher for African-American women; it is most prevalent among women 55 years of age, and 70% to 80% of women with breast cancer do not have a family history.
11. Choice D is correct; tamoxifen reduces growth and inhibits recurrence of estrogen-sensitive breast cancer; usual dose is 20 to 40 mg, po, once or twice a day depending on dosage; because it is an antiestrogen medication, signs of estrogen deficit

such as hot flashes and menstrual irregularities can occur.

12. Choice B is correct; the right arm should be used as much as possible to maintain mobility and prevent lymphedema; tingling and numbness are expected findings for as long as a few months after surgery; deodorant may be used, but not a strong one.
13. Choice A is correct; acute pain is a common finding; it usually begins a week before the onset of menses; leakage from nipples is not associated with this disorder; surgery is unlikely; cancer risk is not high because fibrocystic changes are part of the normal involutional patterns of the breast.
14. Choice D is correct; fibroadenomas are generally small, unilateral, firm, nontender, movable lumps; borders are discrete and well defined; discharge is not associated with this breast disorder.
15. Choices B, D, and E are correct; the woman should continue to take her calcium supplement because the medication will also treat her osteoporosis; the medication is taken daily with or without food.

III. Thinking Critically

1. Educating women about breast cancer: see Malignant Conditions of the Breast section.
   A. Information regarding risk factors: see Etiologic factors section and Box 10-1 to determine risk factors to teach women; identify factors, degree of risk they represent alone and in combination; include research findings; discuss how risk factors can influence health care including suggestions for assessment methods and frequency, lifestyle changes, and prevention methods for very high risk women.
   B. Breast screening recommendations: see Table 10-3 and Box 10-2 for recommendations for women ages 20 to 39 and 40 and older.
   C. Factors inhibiting women from participating in breast screening and strategies to encourage compliance: see Clinical Manifestations and Diagnosis section and Cultural Considerations box—Breast Screening Practices.
      - Inhibiting factors: culture, lack of knowledge and time, fear, finances and insurance coverage, age, culture, and access.
      - Strategies: reminder postcards, buddy system, insurance coverage, teaching days and programs for women and health care providers, advertisements in the media, mobile clinics to bring health screening to neighborhoods, flexible clinic hours, free screening and walk-in self referrals; present several and get their feedback; encourage them to offer other suggestions.

   D. Manifestations suggestive of breast cancer: see Clinical Manifestations and Diagnosis section for a full explanation of the manifestations.
   E. Diagnostic tests if a lump is found: describe each test and its importance in the diagnostic process—mammography, ultrasound, MRI, biopsy of tumor tissue or fluid.
   F. Genetic basis for breast cancer: see Etiologic Factors section; discuss pros and cons for genetic testing and the risks for genetically transmitted breast cancer.
2. Woman's concern regarding the genetic risk for breast cancer: see Malignant Conditions of the Breast—Etiologic Factors section.
   - Tell her most cancers are not related to genetic factors; 70% to 80% of women with breast cancer do not have a family history.
   - Obtain a full family history regarding breast and other cancers focusing on other family members diagnosed with breast cancer.
   - Discuss BRCA testing and its meaning; discuss the Genetic Information Nondiscrimination Act (GINA).
   - Help her explore what she would do if results are positive.
   - Encourage BSE and clinical breast examination.
3. Woman with fibrocystic breast change; see Fibrocystic Changes section.
   A. Assessment process to diagnose fibrocystic change: include a description of each component.
      - History, physical assessment, clinical breast examination
      - Diagnostic testing: ultrasonography; fluid aspirated if necessary; fine-needle aspiration

   B. Clinical manifestations: describe the bilateral changes that occur in size and tenderness with the menstrual cycle.
   C. Nursing diagnosis: based on assessment findings and time in menstrual cycle; can include acute pain, anxiety.
   D. Relief measures: try several approaches to find the combination that works the best—keep a diary; include such measures as analgesics, support, dietary changes, vitamin E, diuretics.
   E. Risk for cancer: very low and depends on type of cellular change; risk is primarily related to atypical hyperplasia.
4. Woman with lump in left breast (see Malignant Conditions of the Breast; Nursing Process Box, and Nursing Care Plan).
   A. Diagnostic protocol: describe each component. (see Clinical Manifestations and Diagnosis section).
      - History and physical examination including clinical breast examination; document characteristics of the lump and associated findings
      - Mammography, ultrasound, biopsy, MRI
      - Laboratory testing

   B. Emotional effect of cancer diagnosis (see Care Management—Emotional Support after Diagnosis section): answer should include description of emotional reactions, such as:

- Shock, denial, fear
- Disruption caused by diagnosis: role changes, finances, body image, sexual function
- Review decision-making questions she and her family should ask; see Box 10-3.

C. Nursing diagnoses and care management
- Preoperative period
  - Nursing diagnoses; see Preoperative Care section; could include fear/anxiety, anticipatory grieving; risk for ineffective family and individual coping are likely to be priority diagnoses.
  - Preoperative teaching and typical surgical care measures; Reach for Recovery volunteer may be asked to come and speak to the woman and her family.
- Immediate postoperative period; see Immediate Postoperative Care section and Nursing Care Plan.
  - Nursing diagnoses would include acute pain, risk for infection, impaired skin integrity, risk for deficient fluid volume.
  - Typical postoperative care along with elevation of arm; avoid using arm for BP, IV, blood draws, and medications; follow protocol for movement and use of affected arm; check for bleeding; assist with position changes; leg exercises; and coughing and deep breathing.
- Emotional support throughout

D. Preparing Molly for self-management at home: see Box 10-5 and Teaching for Self-Management box—After a Mastectomy; instructions should address pain control; signs of expected changes and complications; infection prevention; wound, dressing, and drainage care; BSE; arm exercises and use of arm for activities of daily living; time for follow-up appointment.

E. Support measures.
- Help woman and partner deal with change in appearance and treatment regimen.
- Refer to community resources and support groups.
- Discuss follow-up treatments and the process of reconstruction; use of prostheses; provide emotional support with first view of incision.

5. Tamoxifen therapy (see Adjuvant Therapy section and the Medication Guide for Tamoxifen).
   - Oral antiestrogen medication; be prepared for menopause-like symptoms such as hot flashes.
   - Plan should include action/purpose, dosage, and how to take effectively; adverse reactions to watch for and what to do if they occur.
6. Woman with breast cancer beginning chemotherapy: see Chemotherapy and Teaching Needs for the Client and Family Undergoing Adjuvant Therapies sections.

   A. Teaching plan.
   - Name of medication, route of administration, treatment schedule, timing, length of time for administration
   - Payment—insurance coverage
   - Side effects and how to manage them including use of alternative therapies
   - Teratogenic potential
   - Required follow-up care
   - Expected effect of treatment on her daily life; adjustments that will need to be made

   B. Nursing diagnoses: use assessment findings to determine which diagnosis would apply and their priority for this client.
   - Imbalanced nutrition: less than body requirements
   - Risk for infection
   - Disturbed body image
   - Interrupted family processes
   - Ineffective role performance
   - Fear/anxiety

   Nursing Interventions: see Nursing Process box and Nursing Considerations section.

CHAPTER 11: STRUCTURAL DISORDERS AND NEOPLASMS OF THE REPRODUCTIVE SYSTEM

I. Learning Key Terms

1. C, 2. F, 3. L, 4. J, 5. G, 6. H, 7. M, 8. A, 9. B, 10. O, 11, N, 12. I, 13. D, 14. E, 15. K
16. Pessary
17. Anterior repair (colporrhaphy)
18. Posterior repair (colporrhaphy)
19. Myomectomy
20. Uterine artery embolization (UAE)
21. Laser surgery
22. Hysteroscopic uterine ablation
23. Hysterectomy
24. Bilateral salpingo-oophorectomy (BSO)
25. Colposcopy
26. Conization
27. Cryosurgery
28. Loop electrosurgical excision procedure (LEEP)
29. Radical hysterectomy
30. Total pelvic exenteration
31. Simple vulvectomy
32. Radical vulvectomy

II. Reviewing Key Concepts

33. Ovarian cancer, a "silent" cancer: see Cancer of Ovary—Incidence and Etiology and Clinical Manifestations and Diagnosis sections for full explanation.
34. Choices B and E are correct; a knee-chest position is appropriate for a retroverted uterus; anterior colporrhaphy is performed to repair a cystocele; vaginal or abdominal hysterectomy would be performed if needed; estrogen may be used to improve tissue tone.

35. Choices C and E are correct; fibroids are dependent on estrogen for growth; therefore, they will increase in size during pregnancy and shrink with menopause; abnormal uterine bleeding is the most common clinical manifestation and can lead to anemia if severe; constipation, low dull abdominal pain and pressure, dysmenorrhea, and backache are other common signs and symptoms as the tumors enlarge.
36. Choice B is correct; reducing fluid intake can be dangerous because fluids are required to prevent urinary tract infection; A, C, and D are all effective in reducing urinary incontinence.
37. Choice B is correct; only the uterus was removed; therefore, HRT will not be needed; turning, coughing, and deep breathing should be performed at least every 2 hours for the first 24 hours; no douching is required and should be avoided.
38. Choice C is correct; CIS is noninvasive and therefore cervical conization with follow-up is the appropriate treatment choice; the LEEP procedure can be used for the conization; UAE is used in the treatment of fibroid tumors and radiation for invasive forms of cancer.

III. Thinking Critically

1. Reproductive tract cancers.
   A. Risk factors: see Incidence and Etiology section for each of the cancers listed for identification of risk factors.
   B. Use of risk factors: encourage early detection; teaching measures such as more frequent, earlier examination for those at high risk; use the risk factors to identify specific measures for each type of cancer (e.g., infection prevention measures for cervical cancer).
2. Woman diagnosed with moderate uterine prolapse along with cystocele and rectocele; see Uterine Displacement and Prolapse, Cystocele and Rectocele, and Collaborative Care sections.
   A. Clinical manifestations: see Clinical Manifestations section; several manifestations are described for each disorder.
   B. Two priority nursing diagnoses with expected outcomes.
      - Constipation related to altered position of uterus, rectum, and bladder; woman will experience regular, soft-formed bowel elimination.
      - Ineffective sexuality patterns related to vaginal change associated with uterine prolapse, cystocele, and rectocele; woman will openly discuss measures to enhance sexual function.
   C. Management of uterine prolapse, cystocele and rectocele: see Collaborative Care section; answer should include use of Kegel exercises, diet changes, stool softeners, mild laxatives, pessary.
   D. Using a pessary.
      1. Nursing diagnosis—risk for infection related to insertion of pessary.
      2. Instructions for use—tailor instructions for the type that is used; include how to insert and remove, how to care for and cleanse, genital hygiene measures, signs indicative of infection.
   E. Postoperative care following vaginal hysterectomy and colporrhaphy (see Postoperative Care section, Box 11-3, and Teaching for Self-Management box—Care After Myomectomy or Hysterectomy); discuss each of the following measures:
      - Ensure cleanliness; prevention of postoperative complications.
      - Keep bowel and bladder empty; discuss activity and rest requirements.
      - Check for pain, bleeding, infection.
3. Woman with fibroids (see Benign Neoplasms—Leiomyomas section and Nursing Process Box—Woman with a Leiomyoma).
   A. Clinical manifestations: see Clinical Manifestations and Diagnosis section for several manifestations.
   B. Compare treatment approaches and factors considered for choice (see Medical Management and Surgical Management sections); discuss medications such as GnRH agonists such as leuprolide (Lupron) to shrink the tumor and medications to treat symptoms, uterine artery embolization, myomectomy, laser surgery, electrocautery, hysterectomy.
   C. Care management after UAE: see UAE section and Teaching for Self-Management box—Care After UAE for several measures that should be implemented.
4. Woman with endometrial cancer.
   A. Nursing diagnosis for preoperative and postoperative periods: see Cancer of the Endometrium Section and Nursing Care Plan.
      - Preoperative: fear related to diagnosis of uterine cancer and anticipated surgery; woman will openly discuss fears and concerns with health care provider and family.
      - Postoperative: acute pain, risk for deficient fluid volume, risk for infection; eventually disturbed body image, ineffective sexuality patterns; an expected outcome for pain would be woman will experience reduction in pain when relief measures are implemented.
   B. Nursing care and support.
      - Preoperative; see Preoperative Care section and Box 11-2: preoperative teaching, typical physical measures for major abdominal surgery; consider issue of informed consent; see Box 11-1.
      - Postoperative: see Postoperative Care section and Box 11-3; measures included in

plan should be assessment of physical and emotional status, fluid intake, measures to prevent postoperative complications, wound care, perineal care, pain relief and comfort measures, recommend position changes.

C. Discharge instructions: see Discharge Planning and Teaching section and Teaching for Self-Management box—Woman Who Has Had a Myomectomy or Hysterectomy for a full explanation of teaching topics.

D. Cultural issues (see Cultural Considerations box—Meaning of Cancer): body image, meaning of uterus and fertility in her culture; meaning of death; responses to pain.

E. Nursing diagnosis related to diagnosis and treatment: Anxiety *or* disturbed body image related to effects of surgery and possibility of ongoing treatment for cancer; also consider ineffective sexuality patterns that could interfere with her emotional health and recovery.

F. Support measures during recovery.
   - Provide time to discuss fears, and feelings regarding self as woman and sexuality; ask questions.
   - Involve significant others.
   - Teach about effects of surgery and other treatment measures that may be used; discuss the use of alternative therapies.
   - Refer to support groups.

5. Woman with invasive cancer of the cervix: see Cancer of Cervix section.
   A. Nursing diagnoses with expected outcomes (see Nursing Process box—Woman Having Radiation Therapy).
      - Fear related to concerns about cancer and effects of radiation treatments; woman will openly express fears regarding diagnosis and treatment with health care provider and family.
      - Impaired skin integrity related to effects of radiation on tissue; will use appropriate measures to reduce skin breakdown and enhance healing; see Box 11-4 related to the importance of nutrition.
   B. Outline of the care and support required for external radiation and internal radiation; see sections for each type of radiation therapy and the Teaching for Self-Management boxes related to radiation therapy and Box 11-4 for points to highlight when completing the outline; be sure to include emotional support measures along with the physical care measures.
   C. Self-protection measures: see Internal Therapy section and Safety Alert for precautions to follow; emphasize wearing of film badge, use of careful isolation techniques, and planning nursing care to reduce exposure; distance, time, and shielding are three ways to control exposure.

6. Woman recovering from a radical vulvectomy (see Cancer of the Vulva section).
   A and B. Nursing measures to prevent infection and maintain sexual functioning: see Nursing Management section of Cancer of the Vulva for a full list of nursing care measures for each expected outcome of care.
   C. Discharge instructions: see Teaching for Self-Management box—Care After Radical Vulvectomy to determine critical discharge instructions that should be given to this woman to enhance healing and prevent complications.

7. Cancer during pregnancy (see Cancer Therapy and Pregnancy section); answer should include:
   - Issues and emotions regarding the mother, fetus, and impact of treatment
   - Potential for pregnancy termination
   - Review of options for treatment with their potential effect on the maternal-fetal unit
   - Ethical considerations for treatment and its effect on fetal well-being—a critical component of decision making

8. Woman receiving chemotherapy for treatment of advanced ovarian cancer: see Cancer of Ovary—Therapeutic Management and Nursing Implications.
   A. Measures to relieve selected chemotherapy-related problems: see Table 11-2 and Box 11-4; be sure to include an explanation of why the problems occur and why suggested relief measures are safe and effective.
   B. Support measure: see Nursing Implications section and Legal Tip—Advance Directives; consider discussion of such issues as stages of grief, advance directives, services of hospice, Internet resources, and alternative and complementary therapies.

CHAPTER 12: CONCEPTION AND FETAL DEVELOPMENT

I. Learning Key Terms

1. Conception
2. Gametes, sperm, ovum (egg)
3. Mitosis
4. Meiosis
5. Haploid
6. Diploid
7. Gametogenesis, spermatogenesis, oogenesis
8. Fertilization
9. Zygote
10. Morula
11. Blastocyst, trophoblast
12. Implantation
13. Chorionic villi
14. Decidua
15. Embryo
16. Fetus
17. Amniotic membranes, chorion, amnion
18. Amniotic fluid, oligohydramnios, hydramnios
19. Umbilical cord, arteries, vein, Wharton's jelly, nuchal cord
20. Placenta, human chorionic gonadotropin (hCG)

21. Viability
22. Ductus arteriosus
23. Ductus venosus
24. Foramen ovale
25. Hematopoiesis
26. Surfactants, lecithin-sphingomyelin (L/S)
27. Quickening
28. Meconium
29. Dizygotic, fraternal
30. Monozygotic, identical
31. Teratogens

II. Reviewing Key Concepts

32. Describe the functions of yolk sac, amniotic fluid and membranes, umbilical cord, placenta: see individual sections for each of these structures in the Development of the Embryo.
33. Name the primary germ layers and identify tissues and organs developed from each layer: see Primary Germ Layers section to complete this activity.
34. Choices B, E, and F are correct; feeling of movement is called quickening; the sex of a baby is determined at conception; the heart begins to pump blood by the third week, and a beat can be heard with ultrasound by the eighth week of gestation.
35. Choice B is correct; the L/S ratio is a test to determine the presence of the surfactants lecithin and sphingomyelin; it becomes 2:1 indicating lung maturity at approximately 35 weeks of gestation; an elevated alpha-fetoprotein level is an indicator for an open neural tube defect; renal disorders usually are indicated by a decreased amount of amniotic fluid.
36. Choice C is correct; the healthy newborn of a well-nourished mother will not need iron sources until about 5monhts of age; iron-fortified cereal is usually introduced at this time.
37. Choice A is correct; if a woman's diabetes is uncontrolled, maternal hyperglycemia will produce fetal hyperglycemia and stimulate hyperinsulinemia, resulting in increased fetal growth (macrosomia or large for gestational age); lung maturation is inhibited and neonatal hypoglycemia can occur; strict control of maternal glucose levels before and during pregnancy will reduce the risk.

III. Thinking Critically

1. A. Progress of development at 2 months, 5 months, and 7 months: see Table 12-1 to formulate your answer; use of illustrations and life-size models will facilitate learning.
   B. Survival after 35 weeks of gestation: discuss how the respiratory system develops including the critical factor surfactant production; describe how surfactant helps the newborn to breathe.
   C. Quickening: explain that this is the woman's perception of fetal movement that occurs at about 16 to 20 weeks of gestation; describe how the fetus moves; it will not hurt but can be uncomfortable and interfere with sleep toward the end of pregnancy; fetus will develop its own sleep-wake cycle.
   D. Fetal-sensory perception: discuss sensory capability of the fetus using the Sensory Awareness section of Fetal Maturation; fetus can hear sounds such as parents' voices and respond to light touch; encourage Susan to interact with her fetus.
   E. Sex determination: discuss function of X and Y chromosomes; sex of her fetus will become recognizable around 12 weeks of gestation.
   F. Multifetal Pregnancy—twins: see section for each type of twinning in your answer; discuss monozygotic (identical) and dizygotic (fraternal) twinning and how each occurs; emphasize that fraternal twinning tends to occur in families.
   G. Influence of activity and position on fetal growth and development (see Placental section Functions): discuss differences in circulation through placenta in various positions including supine, lateral, sitting, and standing; discuss the effect of excessive exercise on placental circulation; emphasize that efficient circulation through the placenta is important to ensure an adequate supply of oxygen and nutrients for growth and development.

CHAPTER 13: ANATOMY AND PHYSIOLOGY OF PREGNANCY

I. Learning Key Terms

1. C, 2. P, 3. K, 4. T, 5. S, 6. U, 7. J, 8. N, 9. V, 10. B, 11. G, 12. A, 13. O, 14. I, 15. X, 16. E, 17. M, 18. W, 19. F, 20. H, 21. D, 22. R, 23. L, 24, Q
25. Gravidity
26. Parity
27. Gravida
28. Nulligravida
29. Nullipara
30. Primigravida
31. Primipara
32. Multigravida
33. Multipara
34. Viability
35. Preterm
36. Term
37. Postdate, postterm
38. Human chorionic gonadotropin (hCG)
39. Presumptive changes
40. Probable changes
41. Positive signs
42. Braxton Hicks sign
43. Uterine souffle
44. Funic souffle
45. Quickening
46. Supine hypotensive syndrome
47. Pruritus gravidarum
48. Pica
49. Ptyalism

II. Reviewing Key Concepts

50. Obstetric history using 2-digit and 5-digit systems: Nancy (3-2; 3-1-1-0-1); Marsha (4-2; 4-2-0-1-2); Linda (4-2; 4-1-1-1-3) see Gravidity and Parity section and Table 13-1.
51. Changes in vital signs as pregnancy progresses.
    - Blood pressure and heart-rate patterns—see Table 13-4 and Cardiovascular System section; blood pressure decreases and returns to prepregnant levels by term—it is affected by several factors including maternal position and level of anxiety; pulse increases by 10 to 15 beats/min; murmurs and palpitations can occur.
    - Respiratory patterns—see Table 13-5 and Respiratory System section; breathing becomes more thoracic in nature and volume is deeper with a slight increase in rate; some shortness of breath may be experienced in the second trimester as the diaphragm is pushed up by the enlarging uterus; continues until lightening occurs.
    - Temperature—baseline temperature rises slightly as a result of the increase in BMR and the progesterone effect; women may complain of heat intolerance.
52. Mean arterial pressure (MAP) calculation: see Box 13-2 use the following formula:

$$\frac{\text{systolic} + 2(\text{diastolic})}{3}$$

    Answers are: 91, 81, 90, 110
53. Specify value changes for selected laboratory tests during pregnancy.
    - CBC: see Tables 13-3 and 13-4 and Blood Volume and Composition section.
    - Clotting activity: see Circulation and Coagulation times section and Table 13-3.
    - Acid-base balance: see Acid-Base section and Table 13-3.
    - Urinalysis: see Fluid and Electrolyte Balance section and Table 13-3.
54. Changes in endocrine function and secretions of hormones: see Endocrine System section for a description of each hormone and how and why hormonal levels change with pregnancy.
55. Choices A, E, and F are correct; hCG indicates a positive pregnancy test and is a probable sign along with ballottement and Hegar sign; breast tenderness and morning sickness are presumptive signs; fetal heart sounds are a positive sign of pregnancy.
56. Choice D is correct; gravida (total number of pregnancies including the present one is 5); para (term birth of daughter at 39 weeks = 1; stillbirth at 32 weeks and triplets at 30 weeks = 2; spontaneous abortion at 8 weeks = 1; total number of living children = 4).
57. Choice C is correct; although little change occurs in respiratory rate, breathing becomes more thoracic in nature with the upward displacement of the diaphragm; women normally experience a greater awareness of breathing at rest and may even complain of dyspnea as pregnancy progresses; supine hypotension syndrome occurs as a result of vena cava and aorta compression by the uterus when the woman is in a supine position; baseline pulse rate increases by 10 to 15 beats/min; systolic and diastolic pressure decreases beginning in the second trimester. returning to prepregnant levels in the third trimester.
58. Choice D is correct; recording cycle information assists with accuracy of diagnosis; C reflects the most common error of performing this test too soon, she will need to repeat the test in 1 week if the result is negative; first-voided morning specimens should be used because they are the most concentrated and are apt to have the largest amount of hCG; anticonvulsants, tranquilizers, diuretics, and promethazine can result in inaccurate results.
59. Choice B is correct; friability refers to cervical fragility resulting in slight bleeding when scraped or touched; Chadwick sign refers to a deep bluish cervix and vagina as a result of increased circulation; Hegar sign refers to softening and compressibility of the lower uterine segment.

III. Thinking Critically

1. Responses to client concerns and questions.
    A. Spotting after intercourse: discuss cervical and vaginal friability and increased vascularity; makes the vagina and cervix softer and more delicate, so spotting after intercourse is expected; caution that any bleeding should be reported so it can be evaluated.
    B. Use of home pregnancy test: see Teaching for Self Management box—Home Pregnancy Testing; emphasize the importance of following directions because each brand of test is slightly different; use first-voided morning specimen for the most concentrated urine, and notify health care provider regardless of the test result.
    C. Bladder and vaginal infections: discuss effect of increased vaginal secretions and of changes in urinary elimination including stasis of urine that contains nutrients and has a higher pH; review prevention measures at this time.
    D. Breast changes with pregnancy: discuss changes in beasts, such as enlargement of Montgomery's glands and development of lactation structures resulting in larger breasts that are tender during the first trimester; changes in consistency and presence of lumpiness during BSE and leakage of fluid; changes are bilateral.
    E. Effects of pregnant woman's position: discuss supine hypotensive syndrome and importance of the lateral position when at rest.
    F. Nosebleeds: discuss effect of estrogen-stimulated increase in upper airway vascularity.
    G. Ankle edema: explain effect of the enlarging uterus and the dependent position of her legs

on circulation; discuss measures to reduce edema; caution her to never take someone else's medications or to self-medicate herself.

H. Posture and low back pain: explain why lordosis occurs and what she can do to relieve low back pain.

I. Braxton Hicks: the woman is describing false labor contractions because they diminish with activity; these contractions facilitate blood flow and promote oxygen delivery to the fetus; compare these contractions with true labor contractions.

J. Shortness of breath: explain that what she is experiencing is a result of increased sensitivity of her respiratory center to carbon dioxide, compensation for a mild respiratory alkalosis, and the elevation of her diaphragm by the enlarging uterus; assess the woman for signs of pulmonary edema to be sure the shortness of breath is physiologic rather than pathologic.

K. Changes in bowel function: explain changes in elimination patterns, why they occur, and what she can safely do to prevent constipation and enhance bowel elimination.

2. Blood pressure protocol: see Blood Pressure section and Box 13-1 consider the effects of maternal age, activity and stress level, health status, arm, and position; protocol should emphasize consistency in arm and position used, size of cuff, time provided for relaxation prior to measurement; repeat if finding is inconsistent with woman's baseline or is abnormal.

CHAPTER 14: MATERNAL AND FETAL NUTRITION

I. Learning Key Terms

1. Low birth weight (LBW)
2. Healthful diet before conception
3. Folate (folic acid); neural tube defects; 0.4 mg (400 mcg)
4. Dietary Reference Intakes (DRIs)
5. Body Mass Index (BMI); underweight; normal weight; overweight; obese
6. Ketonuria; preterm labor
7. Physiologic anemia
8. Lactose intolerance
9. Pica, clay, dirt, laundry starch, ice, baking powder, baking soda, cornstarch
10. Food cravings
11. Listeriosis
12. Anthropometric measurements
13. MyPyramid
14. Morning sickness (nausea and vomiting of pregnancy)
15. Hyperemesis gravidarum
16. Constipation
17. Pyrosis (heartburn)

II. Reviewing Key Concepts

18. Indicate nutrient requirements during pregnancy and food/fluid sources for each: see separate sections for each nutrient in Nutrient Needs During Pregnancy section and Table 14-1 to complete the table.
19. Indicators of nutritional risk: see Box 14-4 to identify the five risk indicators; consider the woman's lifestyle, age, culture, socioeconomic status when developing risk-reduction strategies.
20. Cite pregnancy-related risks associated with nutritional problems: see Weight Gain. Pattern Weight Gain, Hazards of Restricting Adequate Weight Gain, and Excessive Weight Gain sections, Nursing Process box—Excessive Gestational Weight Gain, and Box 14-2 to complete this activity.
21. Guidelines for strict vegetarians during pregnancy: see Vegetarian Diets section.
    - These diets tend to be low in vitamins B_{12} and B_6, iron, calcium, zinc, and perhaps calories; supplements may be needed.
    - Food needs to be combined to ensure that all essential amino acids are provided.
22. Signs of good and inadequate nutrition: see Table 14-5 for several signs of good and inadequate nutrition.
23. Determining recommended pregnancy weight gain pattern: see Weight Gain and Pattern of Weight Gain sections of Energy Needs and Box 14-2 to determine weight gain patterns based on each woman's BMI; keep in mind that each woman should gain 1 to 2 kg in the first trimester; weight gain per week is recommended for the second and third trimesters.
    a. June: BMI 21 (normal weight); total 11.5-16 kg; 0.4 kg/week
    b. Alice: BMI 30 (obese); total 5-9 kg; 0.2 kg/week
    c. Ann: BMI 17 (underweight); total 12.5 to 18 kg; 0.5 kg/week
24. Choices A, D, and E are correct; oranges and tomatoes contain vitamin C, which enhances iron absorption.
25. Choice C is correct; BMI indicates that this woman is overweight; she should not consider a weight loss regimen until healing is complete in the postpartum period; she should gain 7 to 11.5 kg; increase in calories should reflect energy expenditure of the pregnancy during the third trimester, which would be approximately 452 kcal.
26. Choice B is correct; BMI indicates woman is at a normal weight; total gain should be 11.5 to 16 kg representing a gain of 0.4 kg/week and 1.6 kg/month during the second and third trimesters.
27. Choice C is correct; small, frequent meals are better tolerated than large meals that distend the stomach; hunger can worsen nausea; therefore, meals should not be skipped; dry, starchy foods should be eaten in the morning and at other times

during the day when nausea occurs; fried, fatty, and spicy foods should be avoided; a bedtime snack is recommended.

28. Choices B, D, and E are correct; legumes are a good source for folic acid along with whole grains and fortified cereals, oranges, papaya, asparagus, liver, and green leafy vegetables; choices A, C, and F are not good sources of folic acid though they do supply other important nutrients for pregnancy (see Box 14-1).
29. Choice A is correct; iron should not be taken at the same time as tea because tea decreases the absorption of iron as does bran, coffee, milk, egg yolks, and oxalates in spinach and Swiss chard; vitamin C–containing foods such as citrus fruit and tomatoes enhance absorption of iron.
30. Choice A is correct; up to 5.5-6.5 oz total are suggested for meat, poultry, fish, dry beans, eggs, and nut group during pregnancy; choices B, C, and D are all appropriate for pregnancy (see Table 14-3).

III. Thinking Critically

1. Nutrition and weight gain concerns during pregnancy.
   A. Concern regarding amount of recommended weight gain during pregnancy.
      - Identify components of maternal weight gain (see Table 14-2); use Figure 14-2 to illustrate how the weight gain is distributed over weeks of gestation.
      - Discuss effect of maternal weight gain on fetal growth and development; association between inadequate maternal weight gain and low birth weight and infant morbidity and mortality.
      - Discuss weight gain total and pattern recommended for a woman with a BMI of 24 (normal weight); discuss appropriate measures for weight loss after birth.

   B. Eating for two during pregnancy.
      - Place emphasis on quality of food that meets nutritional requirements, not on the quantity of food.
      - Discuss expected weight gain total and pattern for a woman with overweight BMI of 27.
      - Excessive weight gain during pregnancy may be difficult to lose after pregnancy and could lead to chronic obesity; excessive fetal size and childbirth problems could also result.

   C. Vitamin supplementation during pregnancy: determine what and how much she takes; compare to recommendations for pregnancy; discuss potential problems with toxicity, especially with overuse of fat-soluble vitamins.

   D. Factors that increase nutritional needs during pregnancy: growth and development of uterine-placental-fetal unit, expansion of maternal blood volume and RBCs, mammary changes, increased BMR.

   E. Weight reduction diets during pregnancy.
      - BMI indicates overweight status; a gain of 7 to 11.5 kg during pregnancy is recommended.
      - Discuss hazards of inadequate caloric intake during pregnancy in terms of growth and development of fetus and pregnancy-related structures; effect of ketoacidosis.
      - Discuss quality foods and development of good nutritional habits to be used during the postpartum period as part of a sensible weight loss program.
      - Discuss importance of exercise and activity during pregnancy.

   F. Reduction of water intake: discuss importance of fluid to meet demands of pregnancy-related changes, regulate temperature, prevent constipation and UTIs; consider possible association between dehydration and preterm labor and oligohydramnios.

   G. Lactose intolerance: discuss basis for problem; reduce lactose intake by using lactose-free products, nondairy sources of calcium and calcium supplements; take lactase supplements; see Calcium section and Box 14-6, Calcium Sources for Women Who Do Not Drink Milk.

   H. Weight loss lactation: discuss weight loss patterns with lactation; emphasize that pregnancy fat stores are used during lactation with a resultant weight loss; inform her of increased need for nutrients, calories, and fluids, which are used up with lactogenesis.

   I. Nutrition guidelines for lactation: adequate calcium intake, a balanced intake of nutrients (about 330 kcal above nonpregnant intake) or at least 1800 kcal/day, adequate fluid intake (should not experience thirst), and avoid tobacco, alcohol, and excessive caffeine.

2. Taking iron supplements effectively: see Iron section of Nutrient Needs, Teaching for Self-Management box—Iron Supplementation, and Table 14-1 for iron sources.
   - Discuss importance of iron.
   - Emphasize importance of vitamin C for iron absorption; discuss food sources high in iron and vitamin C.
   - Discuss ways to take iron supplements to enhance absorption and minimize side effects including GI upset and constipation.

3. Nursing measures appropriate for each nursing diagnosis: see appropriate section for each nutrition-related discomfort in Coping with Nutritional-Related Discomforts of Pregnancy section.
   A. Imbalanced nutrition: less than body requirements related to inadequate intake associated with nausea and vomiting: see Nausea and Vomiting section and Box 14-8 for several relief measures.

   B. Constipation related to decreased intestinal motility associated with effects of increased progesterone and enlarging uterus: see Constipation section; include adequate fluid and roughage/fiber intake, exercise and activity, regular time for elimination.

C. Acute Pain related to reflux of gastric contents into esophagus associated with progesterone effect on gastric motility: see Pyrosis section; small frequent meals, drink fluids between not with meals, avoid spicy foods, remain upright after eating.

4. Native-American woman—nutritional needs.
   A. Counseling approach.
      - Assess her current nutritional status and habits; obtain a diet history.
      - Analyze current patterns as a basis for menu planning.
      - Discuss weight gain pattern for an underweight woman.
      - Use a variety of teaching methods; keep woman actively involved.
      - Emphasize importance of good nutrition for herself and her newborn.
   B. Menu plan: use Table 14-6 for Native-American foods and Table 14-3 for servings of required nutrients for a 1-day menu; distribute throughout day—meals/snacks.

CHAPTER 15: NURSING CARE OF THE FAMILY DURING PREGNANCY

I. Learning Key Terms

1. Presumptive
2. Probable
3. Positive
4. Nägele's Rule, 3 months, 7 days, 1 year
5. Trimester
6. Supine hypotension, vena cava, aorta
7. Fundal height
8. Pinch
9. Accepting the pregnancy, identifying with role of parent, reordering personal relationships, establishing relationship with the fetus, preparing for childbirth
10. Emotional lability (mood swings/changes)
11. Ambivalence
12. Biologic fact of pregnancy, "I am pregnant," growing fetus as distinct from herself, "I am going to have a baby," birth, parenting of the child, "I am going to be a mother"
13. Couvade syndrome
14. Announcement phase, biologic fact of pregnancy, moratorium, accept the pregnancy, focusing, labor, parenthood
15. Prescriptions
16. Proscriptions, taboos
17. Maternal serum alpha-fetoprotein (MSAFP)
18. Triple screen (multiple marker), alpha-fetoprotein, human chorionic gonadotropin, unconjugated estriol
19. Doula
20. Birth plan

II. Reviewing Key Concepts

21. Calculate expected date of birth: use Nägele's rule: subtract 3 months and add 7 days, and 1 year (if appropriate) to the first day of the last menstrual period.
    A. February 12, 2011
    B. October 21, 2011
    C. June 11, 2011
22. Cultural beliefs and practices: see Variations in Prenatal Care—Cultural Influences section.
    A. Describe how cultural beliefs affect participation in prenatal care. Consider the following factors: beliefs regarding pregnancy and health care during pregnancy, finances, and transportation, communication difficulties, concern regarding modesty.
    B. Prescriptions and proscriptions: see specific sections for emotional response, clothing, physical activity and rest, sexual activity, diet.
23. Complete outline regarding components of initial and follow-up visits; see Initial Visit and Follow-up Visits sections to complete the outline.
24. Components of fetal assessment: see Follow-up Visits section, which describes several assessment measures of the mother and of the fetus directly; include what a mother can do to assess her fetus, such as daily fetal movement counts beginning at approximately 27 weeks of gestation.
25. Warning signs of potential complications during pregnancy.
    A. List signs of complications: see Signs of Potential Complications box, which lists signs according to the first, second, and third trimesters.
    B. Nursing approach when discussing signs of complications with pregnant woman and her family: see Recognizing Potential Complications section.
       - Discuss the signs, possible causes, when and to whom to report.
       - Present the signs verbally and in written form.
       - Provide time to answer questions and discuss concerns; make follow-up phone calls.
       - Gather full information of signs that are reported; use information as a basis for action.
       - Document all assessments, actions, and responses, including the date(s) that information regarding these signs was given, the methodology used, and the woman's reaction to the information.
26. Creating a protocol for fundal measurement: see Measurement of Fundal Height section and Figure 15-7; consider woman's position, type of measuring device used, measurement method, and conditions of the examination, such as an empty bladder and relaxed or contracted uterus. Document any variations from the protocol when recording a measurement.

27. Factors used to estimate gestational age: see Fetal Assessment—Gestational Age section for a discussion of these factors.
28. Prevention of injury.
    A. Principles of body mechanics: see Figure 15-12, and Teaching for Self-Management box—Posture and Body Mechanics.
    B. Safety guidelines: see Teaching for Self-Management box—Safety During Pregnancy and the prevention measures identified in Education for Self-Management section.
29. Contraindications for breastfeeding: see Preparation for Breastfeeding section which identifies several reasons why breastfeeding would not be recommended.
30. Choices A, B, and E are correct; C and F are probable signs, and F is a positive sign, diagnostic of pregnancy.
31. Choice C is correct; use Nägele's rule by subtracting 3 months and adding 7 days and 1 year (if appropriate) to the first day of the last menstrual period, which in this case is November 9, 2010.
32. Choice D is correct; supine hypotension related to compression of aorta and vena cava is being experienced; the first action is to remove the cause of the problem by turning the woman onto her side; this should alleviate the symptoms being experienced, including nausea; assessment of vital signs can occur after the woman's position is changed.
33. Choices A and D are correct; during this normal quiet period a woman focuses on her fantasy child as the attachment process is occurring; sexual desire is decreased during the first and third trimesters and increased in the second; ambivalence and mood swings are common responses when preparing for a new role and reacting to hormonal changes; safe passage and birth preparation is a primary concern during the third trimester; a woman's partner is usually the most important person.
34. Choices A, E, and F are correct; intake of at least 2 to 3 L per day is recommended; she does not have to reduce having intercourse but rather to void before and after intercourse and then drink a large glass of water; the effectiveness of cranberry juice has not be proven; additional methods of preventing UTIs include frequent, regular urination; good genital hygiene; and avoiding wearing tight-fitting jeans for long periods.
35. Choice D is correct; continuous support is critical and involves praise, encouragement, reassurance, comfort measures, physical contact, as well as explanations; the doula does not get involved in clinical tasks; he or she is not a substitute for the father but rather encourages his participation as a partner in supporting the laboring woman.

III. Thinking Critically

1. Health history interview: see Initial Visit and Follow-up Visits sections.
    A. Purpose of the health history interview.
        - Establish therapeutic relationship.
        - Planned time for purposeful communication to gather baseline data related to the woman's subjective appraisal of her health status and to gather objective information based on observation of the woman's affect, posture, body language, skin color, and other physical and emotional signs.
        - Update information and compare with baseline information during follow-up interviews.
    B. Write two questions for each component of initial health history interview: be sure questions reflect principles of effective questioning; consider the need to ask follow-up questions to clarify and gather further information when a problem is identified.
    C. Write four questions for the follow-up health history interviews: focus on updating baseline information and asking questions related to anticipated events and expected changes for the woman's gestational age at the time of the visit.
2. Care of woman at initial visit who is anxious and unsure about prenatal care: answer should emphasize:
    - Establishing a therapeutic, trusting relationship so woman will feel comfortable continuing with prenatal care.
    - Teaching the woman about the importance of prenatal care for her health and that of her baby; determine if barriers are present that may limit participation in prenatal care.
    - Involving her boyfriend in the care process so he will encourage her participation in prenatal care; consider that the father of the baby is often considered to be the most significant person.
    - Following guidelines for health history interview, physical examination, and laboratory testing; ensure privacy and comfort during the examination and teach her about how her body is changing and will continue to change with pregnancy.
    - Evaluating the desire for this pregnancy and the need for community agency support.
3. Couple during first trimester—concerns and questions.
    A. Accuracy of EDB: reliability depends on the accuracy of date used and the regularity of her menstrual cycles; most women give birth within 1 week before and 1 week after the expected date of birth.
    B. Kegel exercises: use pelvic muscle exercises to maintain muscle tone and ability to support pelvic organs; see Kegel Exercises section of Education for Self-Care (see Chapter 5: Teaching for Self-Management box—Kegel Exercises).
    C. Effect of pregnancy on sexuality: see Sexual Counseling section and Teaching for Self-Management box—Sexuality in Pregnancy

and Figure 15-19; emphasize that intercourse is safe as long as pregnancy is progressing normally and it is comfortable for the woman; sexual expression should be in tune with the woman's changing needs and emotions; inform that spotting can normally occur related to the fragility of the vaginal mucosa and cervix and that changes in positions and activities may be helpful as pregnancy progresses.

D. Morning sickness: see Table 15-2 (first trimester section) and Box 15-6; fully assess what she is experiencing, then discuss why it happens, how long it will likely last, and relief measures that are safe and effective including complementary and alternative approaches (also see Nutritional Discomforts section of Chapter 14).

4. Physical activity and exercise in pregnancy: see Physical Activity section of Education for Self-Management and Teaching for Self-Management box—Exercise Tips for Pregnant Women; assess her usual pattern of exercise and activity and consider their safety during pregnancy; discuss precautions and guidelines for safe, effective exercise; emphasize that moderate physical activity benefits her and her baby and will prepare her for the work of labor and birth; caution her to take note of the effects of exercise in terms of temperature, heart rate, and feeling of well-being.

5. Nursing diagnoses; expected outcomes and nursing measures for women in various situations during pregnancy.

   A. Risk for urinary tract infection related to lack of knowledge regarding changes of the renal system during pregnancy.
      - Woman will drink at least 2 to 3 L of fluids per day; will empty bladder at first urge.
      - Explain changes that occur in the renal system during pregnancy; increase fluid intake, use acid-ash–forming fluids, void frequently including before going to bed to keep bladder empty, void before and after intercourse then drink a full glass of water, perform good perineal hygiene and wear appropriate clothing, use lateral position to enhance renal perfusion and urine formation.

   B. Acute pain in lower back related to neuromuscular changes associated with pregnancy at 23 weeks of gestation.
      - Woman will experience lessening of lower back pain following implementation of suggested relief measures.
      - Explain basis for lower back pain and relief measures including back massage, pelvic rock, and posture changes (see Teaching for Self-Management—Posture and Body Mechanics, Table 15-2 and Fig. 15-11); encourage woman to change her footwear for better stability and safety.

   C. Anxiety related to lack of knowledge concerning the process of labor and birth and appropriate measures to cope with the pain and discomfort.
      - Couple will enroll in a childbirth education program in the seventh month of pregnancy.
      - Explain the childbirth process and describe the many nonpharmacologic and pharmacologic measures to relieve pain; discuss role of coach and possibility of hiring a doula; make a referral to a childbirth education program and assist with the preparation of a birth plan; discuss childbirth options and prebirth preparations (see Childbirth and Perinatal Education section).

6. Woman in the second trimester—questions and concerns.

   A. Purpose of fundal height measurement: indirect assessment of how her fetus is growing.
   B. Determining fetal health status: discuss FHR (let her listen) and fetal movement assessments (tell her how).
   C. Clothing choices during pregnancy: consider safety and comfort in terms of low-heeled shoe and nonrestrictive clothing.
   D. Gas and constipation: see Table 15-2 (second trimester section); assess problem and lifestyle factors that may be contributing to the problem; determine what she has tried so far; discuss why it occurs and appropriate relief measures (fluids, roughage, activity).
   E. Itchiness: if the woman is experiencing noninflammatory pruritus, use Table 15-2 (second trimester section) for basis of discomfort and relief measures; be sure to rule out rashes related to infection or allergic reactions.
   F. Travel during pregnancy: see Travel section of Education for Self-Management; tell her that she may travel if her pregnancy is progressing normally; emphasize importance of staying hydrated, wearing seat belt and shoulder harness, doing breathing and lower extremities exercises, ambulating every hour for 15 minutes, and voiding every 2 hours.

7. Woman experiencing supine hypotension syndrome: see Emergency box—Supine Hypotension.

   A. Explanation of assessment findings: supine hypotension.
   B. Immediate action: turn her onto her side and maintain the position until vital signs stabilize and signs and symptoms diminish; place wedge to maintain a lateral tilt, then continue the assessment; when completed, help her to rise slowly to an upright position—observe for signs of postural hypotension.

8. Woman during third trimester—questions and concerns

   A. Nipple condition for breastfeeding: see Preparation for Breastfeeding section and

Figures 15-9 and 15-10 for several measures she can use and what to avoid.

B. Ankle edema: see Table 15-2 (third trimester section); discuss basis of the edema and encourage use of lower extremities exercises and elevation of legs periodically during the day (Fig. 15-15); emphasize importance of fluid intake and sleeping in a lateral position (Fig. 15-13) to enhance kidney function, increasing the amount of excess fluid mobilized and excreted in urine.

C. Leg cramps: see Table 15-2 (third-trimester section) and Figure 15-16; discuss basis of leg cramps, then demonstrate relief measures such as pressing weight onto foot when standing or dorsiflexing the foot while lying in bed; avoid pointing the toes; ensure adequate intake of calcium.

9. Choosing a doula (see Doulas section in Perinatal Care Choices and Box 15-7 to formulate your answer). Include relevant Internet sites to recommend to the couple.

   A. Role of doula: describe what a doula does; cite research that illustrates the benefits of using a doula for labor support; emphasize that the doula's role is to provide physical, emotional, and informational care and that his or her role does not involve the performance of clinical tasks.

   B. Finding a doula: community contacts, other health care professions especially those involved in childbirth care or education, organizations such as DONA, persons who have used a doula; emphasize the importance of starting early so that there is time to make the right choice; discuss questions to ask during an interview with a prospective doula and put these questions in writing so that the woman will have them to refer to during the interview.

10. Sibling reactions to mother's pregnancy: see Sibling Adaptation section of Preparing for Childbirth and Box 15-2, which provides tips for sibling preparation; emphasize importance of considering each child's developmental level; prepare children for prenatal events, time during hospitalization, and the homecoming of the new baby; refer to sibling classes and encourage sibling visitation after birth; suggest books, DVDs, and Internet sites that parents could use to prepare their children for birth.

11. Expectant father concerned about wife's mood swings.

    A. Nursing diagnoses: deficient knowledge regarding pregnant spouse's mood changes related to lack of experience with pregnancy; Tom will explain basis for wife's mood swings and strategies that he can use to cope with these changes and support his spouse.

    B. Nurse's response: see Maternal Adaptation section and Table 15-2 (first-trimester section); discuss the basis for the mood swings and experiences during the first trimester including ambivalence; identify measures he can use to support her.

12. Woman experiencing introspection: see Reordering Personal Relationships section; explain that she is concentrating on having a baby and forming a relationship with the fetus; emphasize her partner's important role as a caregiver and nurturer.

13. Birth plan development and deciding on a birth setting: see Birth Plan section.
    - Purpose of birth plan: means of open communication about the childbirth process between the woman and her partner and with the health care providers in an effort to have a childbirth experience that meets their expectations and wishes as closely as possible; it is a tool that couples can use to stay in control and in this case to experience a more satisfying childbirth.
    - Guidelines for formation of birth plan: begin discussion early in pregnancy so that full consideration can be given to each option; identify components that should be included in the plan; facilitate decision making concerning the options available; recognize risk status implications for care options.
    - Topics for discussion/decision making: partner's role during childbirth and who will be present; setting for the birth; labor management measures including pain control, comfort measures, positions, events at the birth, newborn, and postpartum care (e.g., celebratory activities, breastfeeding, mother-baby care).
    - Birth setting choice is an essential component of a birth plan.
      - Descriptions of each option, along with the criteria for use and the advantages and disadvantages.
      - Onsite visits and interaction with health care providers responsible for care at each site should be encouraged.
      - Speak to couples who gave birth in these settings to get their impressions.
      - Emphasize that the decision is theirs and that they should choose what is comfortable for them; a decision should be made on the basis of a full understanding of each option.

14. Home birth (see Home Birth section).

    A. Discuss decision-making process.
       - Fully review advantages and disadvantages of home birth so that an informed decision can be made and appropriate arrangements can be devised to enhance the advantages and offset the disadvantages.
       - Speak to couples who have experienced a home birth.

    B. Preparation measures.
       - Preparation of home, including obtaining supplies and equipment, arranging for medical backup and transportation in the

event of an emergency; measures to increase safety should be emphasized.
- Choosing and preparing the persons who will be attending, including children and grandparents.

CHAPTER 16: LABOR AND BIRTH PROCESSES

I. Learning Key Terms

1. Passenger (fetus and placenta), passageway, powers, position of the mother, psychologic response
2. Fontanels
3. Molding
4. Presentation, cephalic, breech, shoulder
5. Presenting part, occiput, chin (mentum), sacrum, scapula
6. Vertex presentation
7. Fetal lie, longitudinal lie, transverse lie
8. Attitude, general flexion
9. Biparietal diameter
10. Suboccipitobregmatic diameter
11. Fetal position
12. Engagement
13. Station, centimeters, descent
14. Effacement
15. Dilation
16. Lightening ("dropping")
17. Involuntary uterine contractions, effacement, dilation
18. Voluntary bearing-down efforts (abdominal muscle contraction)
19. Bloody show
20. Cardinal movements of labor (mechanism of labor), engagement, descent, flexion, internal rotation, extension, external rotation (restitution), expulsion
21. Ferguson reflex
22. Valsalva maneuver
23. Regular uterine contractions, dilation of cervix, latent, active, transition
24. Cervix is fully dilated, birth of the fetus
25. Birth of the fetus, placenta is delivered
26. Recovery following birth
27. Maternal position, maternal blood pressure, uterine contractions, umbilical cord blood flow

II. Reviewing Key Concepts

28. Label illustrations.
    Fetal skull: A. mentum (chin); B. occipitofrontal diameter; C. frontal bone (sinciput); D. suboccipitobregmatic diameter; E. parietal bone (vertex); F. occipitomental diameter; G. occiput; H. sagittal suture; I. lambdoid suture; J. posterior fontanel; K. biparietal diameter; L. coronal suture; M. frontal suture; N. anterior fontanel (bregma)
    Maternal pelvis: A. symphysis pubis; B. anteroposterior diameter of inlet; C. transverse diameter of the inlet; D. sacral promontory; E. sacrum; F. sacroiliac joint; G. ischial spine; H. pubic bone; I. sacrotuberous ligament; J. pubic arch; K. ischial tuberosity; L. coccyx; M. sacroiliac joint
29. Indicate presentation, presenting part, position, lie, and attitude represented by each illustration.
    A. Cephalic (vertex), occiput, LOA, longitudinal, flexion
    B. Cephalic (vertex), occiput, LOT, longitudinal, flexion
    C. Cephalic (vertex), occiput, LOP, longitudinal, flexion
    D. Cephalic (vertex), occiput, ROA, longitudinal, flexion
    E. Cephalic (vertex), occiput, ROT, longitudinal, flexion
    F. Cephalic (vertex), occiput, ROP, longitudinal, flexion
    G. Cephalic (face), mentum, LMA, longitudinal, extension
    H. Cephalic (face), mentum, RMP, longitudinal, extension
    I. Cephalic (face), mentum, RMA, longitudinal, extension
    J. Breech, sacrum, LSA, longitudinal, flexion
    K. Breech, sacrum, LSP, longitudinal, flexion
    L. Shoulder, scapula, ScA, transverse, flexion
30. Choices A, C, D, and E are correct; the presenting part is 1 cm above the ischial spines as indicated by the "–1"; attitude is flexion of head and neck as indicated by the occiput ("O") as the presenting part; the lie is longitudinal as indicated by the cephalic presentation; effacement of the cervix is 75% complete and it is 3 cm dilated requiring 7 more cm for full dilation to 10 cm.
31. Choices C and D are correct; systolic blood pressure increases with uterine contractions in the first stage while both systolic and diastolic blood pressure increase during a contraction and remain slightly elevated between contractions in the second stage; white blood cell count increases, gastric motility decreases and can lead to nausea and vomiting especially during the transition phase of the first stage of labor, a decrease in blood glucose and proteinuria of 1+ can be expected (see Box 16-2).
32. Choice D is correct; quickening refers to the woman's first perception of fetal movement at 16 to 20 weeks of gestation; lightening accompanied by urinary frequency and weight loss of 0.5 to 1 kg occur to signal that the onset of labor is near; backache, stronger Braxton Hicks and bloody show are also noted.

III. Thinking Critically

1. Teaching a class on the process of labor.
   A. Describe five factors and how they affect the process of childbirth: see separate sections for four of the factors in Factors of Labor section and Chapter 17 for the fifth factor; consider the factors of passenger, passage, powers, position of mother,

psychologic response of mother; be sure to identify the visual aids you would use to facilitate learning.

B. Explain how the cardinal movements of labor facilitate birth: see Mechanism of Labor section in Process of Labor; describe engagement and descent, flexion, internal rotation, extension, external rotation and restitution, expulsion.

2. Analysis of vaginal examinations.
   - Exam I: ROP (right occiput posterior, cephalic [vertex] presentation, longitudinal lie, flexed attitude), –1 (station at one centimeter above the ischial spines), 50% effaced, 3 cm dilated.
   - Exam II: RMA (right mentum anterior, cephalic [face] presentation, longitudinal lie, extended attitude), 0 (station at the ischial spines, engaged), 25% effaced, 2 cm dilated.
   - Exam III: LST (left sacrum transverse, breech presentation, longitudinal lie, flexed attitude), +1 (station at one centimeter below the ischial spines), 75% effaced, 6 cm dilated.
   - Exam IV: OA (occiput anterior, cephalic [vertex] presentation, longitudinal lie, flexed attitude), +3 (station at 3 centimeters below the ischial spines near or on the perineum), 100% effaced, 10 cm (fully dilated).
3. Woman with questions and concerns about process of labor.
   A. Onset of labor: see Onset of Labor section; explain in simple terms the interaction of maternal and fetal hormones, uterine distention, placental aging, increase in prostaglandin level, increase in estrogen level, and decrease in progesterone.
   B. Signs of preceding labor: see Signs Preceding Labor section and Box 16-1 for a discussion of all of the signs that occur prior to the onset of labor; keep in mind that she is a primigravida.
   C. Duration of labor: see Stages of Labor section for approximate times for each stage; give woman ranges rather than absolute numbers especially because this is her first labor; discuss her role in facilitating the progress of labor.
   D. Position changes during labor; see Position of Laboring Woman section and Figure 16-12; answer should include each of the following:
      - Emphasize that the position of the woman is one of the 5 Ps of labor.
      - Discuss each position and describe its effect.
      - Demonstrate each position and have her practice each of them with her partner.
      - Emphasize the beneficial effects of ambulation and changing positions on fetus, circulation, comfort, and progress.

CHAPTER 17: PAIN MANAGEMENT

I. Learning Key Terms

1. B, 2. F, 3. H, 4. A, 5. G, 6. J, 7. M, 8. D, 9. I, 10. L, 11. C, 12. E, 13. K
14. Visceral pain
15. Somatic pain
16. Referred pain
17. Gate control
18. Endorphins
19. Slow-paced breathing
20. Modified-paced breathing
21. Deep cleansing breath
22. Patterned-paced (pant-blow) breathing
23. Hyperventilation; respiratory alkalosis
24. Effleurage
25. Counterpressure
26. Water therapy (hydrotherapy)
27. Transcutaneous electrical nerve stimulation (TENS)
28. Acupressure
29. Acupuncture
30. Therapeutic touch
31. Hypnosis
32. Biofeedback
33. Aromatherapy
34. Intradermal water block
35. Neonatal narcosis

II. Reviewing Key Concepts

36. Theoretic basis for effectiveness of massage, stroking, music, and imagery in reducing sensation of pain: discuss the gate-control theory of pain; see Childbirth Preparation and Nonpharmacologic Management of Pain and Gate-Control Theory of Pain sections; each of the methods listed are examples of gate-control technique.
37. Complete table related to nerve block analgesic and anesthetic methods: see appropriate sections in Pharmacologic Management of Pain for each method cited in the table.
38. Choice C is correct; beginning in active labor reduces the risk that labor will slow down; there is no limit to the time a woman can stay in the tub; woman can and should change her position while in the bath, using lateral and hand-and-knees when indicated; there is no evidence indicating an increased risk for infection when membranes are ruptured; however, tubs must be carefully cleansed; contractions may slow if bath is begun in the latent phase.
39. Choice B is correct; naloxone hydrochloride (Narcan) is an opioid antagonist; butorphanol tartrate (Stadol) is an opioid agonist–antagonist analgesic; fentanyl citrate (Sublimaze) is an opioid agonist analgesic.
40. Choice D is correct; nalbuphine hydrochloride (Nubain) is an opioid agonist-antagonist analgesic; a 10-mg dose is appropriate for IV administration; the antagonist component of this medication could precipitate withdrawal symptoms if the woman is opioid dependent.

41. Choice C is correct; as an opioid antagonistic it will reverse the effects of the opioid agonist analgesic administered for pain; maternal adverse reactions include hypotension/hypertension, tachycardia, hyperventilation, nausea, and vomiting; Narcan is administered intravenously at a dose of 0.4 to 2 mg depending on the amount of opioid agonist analgesic given and the degree of CNS depression; it may be repeated at 2- to 3-minute intervals if needed for adequate reversal; Narcan is only given parenterally.
42. Choices A, B, D, and F are correct; position with a curved back separates the vertebrae and facilitates administration of the anesthetic; alternating lateral positions after administration will prevent supine hypotension; she should be encouraged to empty her bladder every 2 hours; because the dura is not punctured, there is no leakage of cerebrospinal fluid, making spinal headache rare; the dosage can be adjusted to allow her to push during the second stage of labor.
43. Choices A, C, and D are correct; sneezing, rhinorrhea, sweating, lacrimation, and mydriasis also occur (see Signs of Potential Complications—Maternal Opioid Abstinence Syndrome box).
44. Choice B is correct; changing the woman to a lateral position will enhance cardiac output and raise her BP; because compression of the abdominal aorta and vena cava is removed, the other actions will follow (see Emergency box—Maternal Hypotension with Decreased Placental Perfusion).

III. Thinking Critically

1. Factors influencing nursing diagnosis of acute pain: see Factors Influencing Pain Response section for a discussion of many factors such as endorphin level, anxiety and fear, culture, previous experience, knowledge and expectations, childbirth preparation, available support and comfort, physical condition of the woman at the onset of labor, history of substance abuse or sexual abuse, environmental factors.
2. Systemic analgesic administration to a woman in labor: see Systemic Analgesics section of Pharmacologic Pain Management, Opioid Agonist Analgesics Medication Guide, and Nursing Process box—Pain Management.
   A. Approach nurse should follow in pain relief; consider importance of a full assessment of this woman regarding her pain and what this assessment should include.
   B. Administering meperidine.
      1. Maternal reactions: discuss effect on pain and relaxation as well as on her vital signs including breathing and blood pressure.
      2. Factors influencing effect of systemic analgesics on fetus: maternal dosage, characteristics of the specific drug, route, time when administered during labor.
      3. Fetal/newborn effects: describe CNS depression as a result of the direct effect of the drug when it crosses the placenta and/or the indirect effect of the mother resulting in respiratory depression, decreased alertness, and delayed sucking after birth.
3. IV administration of systemic analgesics as the preferred route; see Administration of Medication section for an explanation of the rationale; include in answer that IV administration results in a faster, more predictable onset of action; a higher level of analgesia occurs at a lower dosage.
4. Explaining basis of childbirth pain to expectant fathers: see Neurologic Origins of Pain section and Box 17-1; describe why pain occurs and its very real basis; discuss visceral, somatic, and referred pain, how women experience the pain, and factors that influence the experience; identify measures they can use to help their partners reduce and cope with the pain.
5. Nurse sensitivity to client's pain experience.
   A. Experience and expression of pain in labor: see Expression of Pain and Factors influencing the Pain Response section; discuss physiologic effects, sensory responses, emotional responses, and affective expressions.
   B. Measures to alter perception of pain: see Perception of Pain and Nonpharmacologic Pain Management sections; consider the specific factors influencing each woman's response when determining measures to use.
6. Working with couple with unrealistic, inaccurate views regarding pain and pain relief during labor.
   - Inform couple regarding the basis of pain and its potentially adverse effects on the maternal-fetal unit and the progress of labor.
   - Discuss a variety of nonpharmacologic and pharmacologic measures that are safe and effective to use during labor and which can have beneficial effects on the maternal-fetal unit and can enhance the progress of labor.
   - Emphasize that the mother and fetus will be thoroughly assessed before, during, and after use of any measure to ensure safety.
7. Benefits of water therapy: see Water Therapy (Hydrotherapy) section.
   - Describe the beneficial effects of water therapy and how it can facilitate the labor process, create a more positive experience with fewer complications, including cesarean birth; use research findings to substantiate these claims.
   - Describe the successful experiences of other agencies that have implemented water therapy; state how it has affected the number of births.
   - Use favorable reports of women who have used water therapy; consider how this could affect other women preparing for childbirth.
   - Prepare a cost-benefit analysis.
8. Occurrence of hypotension after administration of epidural block during labor: see Emergency

box—Maternal Hypotension with Decreased Placental Perfusion.

A. What is being experienced by this woman: maternal hypotension related to effect of epidural anesthesia/analgesia (block); fully describe why this happens and its effect on the maternal-fetal unit.
B. Nursing diagnosis: ineffective tissue perfusion to placenta related to maternal hypotension associated with epidural block anesthesia.
C. Immediate nursing actions: in answer, take a data, action, response approach; discuss measures used to enhance perfusion and ensure oxygenation, then determine response to actions taken; consider when to notify primary health care provider.

9. Woman receiving an epidural block: see Epidural Analgesia/Anesthesia [Block] section of Pharmacologic Management of Discomfort and the Care Management sections; Nursing Process box related to Pain Management, and Boxes 17-5 and 17-6.
   A. Assessment prior to induction of block: describe how you would determine status of maternal-fetal unit, progress of labor in terms of phase and contraindications to use.
   B. Preparation measures: answer should reflect actions related to explanation of procedures used, informed consent, hydration, bladder condition.
   C. Positions for induction: lateral (modified Sims with back curved forward) or sitting with back curved forward to separate vertebrae; assist her with assuming and maintaining the position without movement during the induction; it is important to avoid severe spinal flexion.
   D. Nursing management during the epidural block; include in the outline: assessment of the response, maintenance of fluid balance, assistance with elimination and positioning, prevention of complications.

CHAPTER 18: FETAL ASSESSMENT DURING LABOR

I. Learning Key Terms

1. I, 2. H, 3. G, 4. J, 5. F, 6. C, 7. B, 8. D, 9. E, 10. A, 11. K
12. Hypoxemia
13. Hypoxia
14. Intermittent auscultation
15. Ultrasound transducer, maximal intensity of FHR
16. Tocotransducer (tocodynamometer), fundus
17. Spiral electrode
18. Intrauterine pressure catheter (IUPC)
19. Fetal pulse oximetry
20. Fetal scalp blood sampling
21. Amnioinfusion
22. Oligohydramnios
23. Anhydramnios
24. Tocolysis, terbutaline (Brethine)
25. Umbilical cord acid-base determination
26. Intrauterine resuscitation; supplemental oxygen, maternal position change, increasing IV infusion rate

II. Reviewing Key Concepts

27. Factors that affect fetal oxygen supply and characteristics of FHR and uterine activity.
    A. Factors that can reduce fetal oxygen supply: see Fetal Response section for a discussion of these factors.
    B. Characteristics of (normal) reassuring FHR patterns: see Fetal Response section and Box 18-1.
    C. Characteristics of abnormal (nonreassuring) FHR patterns: see Fetal Response section and Box 18-1.
    D. Characteristics of normal and abnormal uterine activity: see Table 18-1.
    E. Meaning and criteria for categories I, II, and III: see Categorizing FHR Tracings section and Box 18-1.
28. 30 minutes, 15 minutes
29. 15 minutes, 5 minutes
30. Baseline rate, baseline variability, accelerations, decelerations, changes or trends over time
31. Legal responsibilities related to fetal monitoring during childbirth: see Nurse Alert in Intermittent Auscultation section and Legal Tip—Fetal Monitoring Standards; evaluate FHR pattern at frequency that reflects professional standards, agency policy, and condition of maternal-fetal unit; consider the correct interpretation of FHR pattern as normal (reassuring) or abnormal (nonreassuring); take appropriate action; evaluate response to actions taken; notify primary health care provider in a timely fashion; know the chain of command if a dispute about interpretation occurs; document assessment findings, actions, and responses.
32. Choice D is correct; the average resting tone during labor should be 10 mm Hg; A, B, and C are all findings within the expected ranges.
33. Choices C and F are correct; Leopold maneuvers are used to locate the PMI for correct placement of the ultrasound transducer; the tocotransducer is always placed over the fundus; the ultrasound transducer's position needs to change with fetal movement; the tocotransducer cannot assess intensity of contractions; therefore, periodic palpation is an essential assessment measure.
34. Choices B, D, and E are correct; the baseline rate should be 110 to 160 beats/min; accelerations should occur with fetal movement; no late deceleration pattern of any magnitude is normal (reassuring), especially if it is repetitive or uncorrectable; early deceleration patterns are expected findings when head compression occurs.

35. Choice C is correct; the FHR increases as the maternal core body temperature elevates; therefore, tachycardia is the pattern exhibited; it is often a clue of intrauterine infection because maternal fever is often the first sign; diminished variability reflects hypoxia, variable decelerations are characteristic of cord compression, and early decelerations are characteristic of head compression.
36. Choice B is correct; the pattern described is an early deceleration pattern, which is considered to be benign, requiring no action other than documentation of the finding; changing a woman's position and notifying the physician would be appropriate if abnormal (nonreassuring) signs such as late or variable decelerations were occurring; prolapse of cord is associated with variable decelerations as a result of cord compression.
37. Choice B is correct; see Box 18-5 for the rationale.

III. Thinking Critically

1. Intermittent auscultation to assess fetal status during labor: see Intermittent Auscultation section and Figure 18-1.
   A. State advantages and disadvantages.
      - Advantages: high-touch/low-tech approach, natural method facilitating activity, comfortable, noninvasive.
      - Disadvantages: inconvenient and time consuming, increased anxiety if nurse has difficulty locating PMI, less information about FHR pattern is obtained, less accurate.

   B. Protocol to follow: cite the six specific guidelines that should be used (see Box 18-2).
2. Nonreassuring pattern noted on evaluation of a monitor tracing: see Nursing Management of Abnormal Patterns section; evaluate the tracing according to the five essential components and implement intrauterine resuscitation measures as appropriate; actions that most often involve repositioning the mother, administering oxygen, altering rate of IV, discontinuing oxytocin (Pitocin), assessing for possible causes, notifying primary health care provider, and preparing for emergency treatment.
3. Woman concerned about use of external monitoring to assess her fetus and labor.
   A. Client/family teaching when electronic fetal monitoring is used: see Box 18-9 and Client and Family Teaching section.
      - Discuss how fetus responds to labor and how the monitor will assess these responses.
      - Explain the advantages of monitoring.
      - Show her a monitor strip and explain what it reveals; tell her how to use the strip to help her with breathing techniques.

   B. Nursing care measures for woman being monitored externally: see Client and Family Teaching section Nursing Process box—Electronic Fetal Heart Rate monitoring and Box 18-9 for a detailed outline related to assessing tracings and maternal responses, palpation of contractions, and caring for woman in terms of comfort, changing position, transducer placement and site care, and keeping her and her family informed about fetal and maternal status and progress of labor.
4. Woman whose labor is being induced and monitored externally.
   A. Pattern described and causative factors: late deceleration patterns as a result of uteroplacental insufficiency associated with intense uterine contractions, supine position (supine hypotension), and placental aging related to postterm gestation of 43 weeks (see Figs. 18-5, 18-8, and 18-11).
   B. Nursing interventions: see Nursing Management of Abnormal Pattern and Table 18-3 and Boxes 18-5 and 18-8; discontinue oxytocin to stop stimulation of contractions but continue primary infusion; change to lateral position and elevate legs to enhance uteroplacental perfusion; administer oxygen via mask to increase oxygen availability to fetus; assess response to actions and notify primary health care provider; see Documentation section for guidelines related to recording findings organized around data, action, and response.
5. Evaluation of monitor tracing following rupture of membranes.
   A. Nurse should be alert for variable deceleration pattern (see Variable Deceleration section and Fig. 18-12).
   B. Action to take if variable decelerations occur: see Boxes 18-5 and 18-6.

CHAPTER 19: NURSING CARE OF THE FAMILY DURING LABOR AND BIRTH

I. Learning Key Terms

1. Regular uterine contractions, effacement, dilation, mucous plug
2. 3, 6, 8, 4, 7, 3, 6, 20, 40, 8, 10
3. Infant is born, cervical dilation, effacement, baby's birth, latent, active pushing, cervix
4. Birth of the baby, placenta is expelled, fundus, discoid, globular ovoid, gush of dark blood, lengthening of umbilical cord, vaginal fullness, fetal membranes
5. 1-2 hours
6. Emergency Medical Treatment and Active Labor Act (EMTALA)
7. Partogram
8. Doula
9. Lithotomy

10. P	11. F	12. G	13. J	14. H	15. B
16. M	17. A	18. Q	19. E	20. K	21. N
22. D	23. O	24. C	25. I	26. R	27. L

28. Uterine contractions
29. Increment
30. Acme
31. Decrement

32. Frequency
33. Intensity
34. Duration
35. Resting tone
36. Interval
37. Bearing-down effort

II. Reviewing Key Concepts

38. Assessing uterine contractions using palpation (see Assessment of Uterine Contractions section); place hand on fundus to time several contractions to establish a pattern of frequency and duration; palpate entire uterus periodically to note differences in tone; use comparisons of tip of nose, chin, and forehead to gauge intensity and tone during the peak of a contraction and during the period of rest.
39. Admission of woman in labor (see Assessment section of Care Management, First Stage of Labor and Nursing Process box—First Stage of Labor).
    A. Information from prenatal record: see Prenatal Data section; include such information as age, weight gain, health status and medical problems during pregnancy, past and present obstetric history (gravida, para), including outcomes and problems encountered, laboratory and diagnostic test results, EDB, baseline data from pregnancy, including vital signs and FHR.
    B. Information regarding status of labor: see Teaching for Self-Management box—How to Distinguish True Labor from False Labor; factors distinguishing false from true labor, uterine contractions (onset, characteristics), show, status of membranes, fetal movement, discomfort (location, characteristics), any other signs of the onset of labor experienced.
    C. Information regarding current health status: health problems, respiratory status, allergies, character and time of last oral intake, emotional status.
40. Signs indicative of obstetric emergencies: see Emergency box—Interventions for Emergencies that lists signs of emergencies such as abnormal (nonreassuring) FHR and pattern, inadequate uterine relaxation, vaginal bleeding, infection, and cord prolapse.
41. Labor positions and their advantages: see Box 19-5 and Ambulation and Positioning section of Nursing Care—First Stage of Labor.
42. Critical maternal-fetal factors to assess during labor: see appropriate sections that discuss general systems assessment, vital signs, Leopold maneuvers, assessment of FHR and pattern, assessment of uterine contractions, vaginal examination, and tests for ruptured membranes; see Table 19-1, Box 19-2, and Nursing Process box—First Stage of Labor.
    - Maternal factors: vital signs, uterine activity, cervical changes, show/bleeding/amniotic fluid, behavior, appearance, mood, energy level, bearing-down effort, use of childbirth preparation methods.
    - Fetal factors: FHR pattern, activity level, progress in cardinal movements of labor, passage of meconium.
43. Laboratory and diagnostic tests during labor: see Laboratory and Diagnostic Tests section of Assessment, First Stage of Labor, CBC, blood type and Rh factor, analysis of urine, dipstick for protein, glucose, acetone, Nitrazine and ferning tests for amniotic fluid; additional tests such as HIV or drug screening, vaginal cultures may be done depending on state laws and maternal condition.
44. Factors influencing duration of second stage of labor: use of regional anesthesia such as epidural block, quality of bearing-down efforts and positions used, parity, size, presentation, and position of fetus, maternal pelvic adequacy, maternal physical status, including energy level, support measures provided.
45. Second stage positions: see Maternal Position section; see Figures 19-15, 19-16, and 19-17; describe squatting, side-lying, semirecumbent, standing, hands-and-knees.
46. Encouraging breastfeeding during the fourth stage of labor stimulates the production of oxytocin to contract the uterus and decrease blood loss; takes advantage of newborn's alert state to interact with the newborn, facilitate the process of attachment, and enhance the success of breastfeeding because the newborn is ready to feed and success is likely; colostrum stimulates peristalsis, thereby facilitating excretion of bilirubin in meconium; be sure to provide support, privacy, and positive reinforcement; keep breastfeeding period short related to maternal fatigue.
47. Choices B, C, D, and E are correct; goal is to remove pressure from the cord and keep it intact and functioning; raising a woman's legs will not do this but a knee-chest position would; cord should be wrapped in a sterile compress moistened with warm sterile normal saline.
48. Choice A is correct; although choices B, C, and D are all important questions, the first question should gather information regarding whether or not the woman is in labor.
49. Choice C is correct; pH of amniotic fluid is alkaline at 6.5 or higher, ferning is noted when examining fluid with a microscope, and the fluid is relatively odorless; a strong odor is strongly suggestive of infection; white flecks indicate vernix caseosa.
50. Choices A, B, D, and F are correct; pain of true labor is usually felt in the lower back radiating to the lower portion of the abdomen; cervix should be moving toward an anterior position.
51. Choice C is correct; O or occiput indicates a vertex presentation with the neck fully flexed and the occiput in the transverse section (T) of the woman's pelvis; the station is 2 cm below the ischial spines

(+2); the woman is in the active phase of labor as indicated by 4 cm of dilation; the lie is longitudinal because the head (cephalic/vertex) is presenting.

52. Choice B is correct; research has indicated that enemas are not needed during labor; according to research findings A, C, and D have all been found to be beneficial and safe during pregnancy.

III. Thinking Critically

1. Woman thinking she is in labor calls nurse (see Teaching for Self-Management box—How to Distinguish True Labor from False Labor).
   A. Nursing approach: determine the status of her labor, asking her to describe what she is experiencing and comparing her description to the characteristics of true and false labor.
   B. Write questions: questions should be clear, concise, open ended, and directed toward distinguishing her labor status and determining the basis for action.
   C. Instructions for home care of woman in latent labor: discuss comfort measures, distracting activities, measures to reduce anxiety, and measures to enhance the labor process; inform regarding assessment measures to determine progress and identify signs of problems, when and whom to call, and when to come to the hospital; the nurse should notify the woman's primary health care provider to confirm plan for woman to stay home until labor progresses; follow-up calls should be made to check on progress.
2. Women in first stage of labor at various phases.
   A. Identify phase of labor: see Table 19-1 to determine phase; Denise (active); Teresa (transition); Danielle (latent).
   B. Describe behavior and appearance: see Table 19-1 for descriptions; consider the phase of the woman's labor when formulating your answer.
   C. Specify physical care and emotional support required: see Nursing Process box for First Stage of Labor for care measures required by each woman according to her phase of labor.
   D. Support of husband who is fatigued and "stressed"; see Nursing Care section—Supportive Care During Labor and Birth, Box 19-6, and Support of the Father or Partner section in Second Stage of Labor for several measures the nurse can use to help the support person of the laboring woman.
3. Procedure for locating point of maximum intensity (PMI) before auscultation of FHR or application of ultrasound transducer: realize that presentation and position affect location of PMI (see Procedure box—Leopold Maneuvers and Fig.19-6) and that Leopold maneuvers will facilitate location of this point; the PMI will change as the fetus progresses through the birth canal.
4. Woman experiencing difficulty with vaginal examinations during labor (see Vaginal Examination section of Physical Examination First Stage of Labor and Procedure box for Vaginal Examination of Laboring Woman).
   A. Nurse's response to concern: explain purpose of the examination and the information that will be obtained during each examination in terms of the progress of labor and the status of the fetus; compare findings obtained from a vaginal examination with information on the monitor tracing.
   B. Measures to enhance comfort and safety: deep breathing and gentleness during the examination; limit frequency and explain why each examination is needed, what you are doing, and the results you are obtaining; acknowledge her feelings and ensure her privacy; use infection control measures such as perineal care before, sterile gloves and lubricant to perform; never perform the examination when active bleeding is present.
5. Actions and rationale when membranes rupture: immediate assessment of the FHR and pattern (prolapse of the cord could have occurred, compressing the cord and leading to hypoxia and variable deceleration patterns); vaginal examination (status of cervix, check for cord prolapse); assess fluid, document findings, and notify primary health care provider; cleanse perineum as soon as possible once status of fetus, mother, and labor is determined; strict infection control measures are critical after rupture because risk for infection increases.
6. Sara, a 17-year-old primigravida in the latent phase of labor.
   - Nursing diagnosis: anxiety related to lack of knowledge and experience regarding the process of childbirth.
   - Expected outcome: couple will cooperate with measures to enhance progress of labor as their anxiety level decreases.
   - Nursing measures: provide full, simple explanations about each aspect of labor and care measures required as they occur; demonstrate and assist with simple breathing and relaxation techniques; make use of phases of labor to tailor health teaching (doing more during latent phase and less as labor progresses); model coaching and comfort measures father can perform.
7. Cultural and religious beliefs and practices during labor:
   A. Questions to determine cultural and religious preferences: Cultural Factors and Culture and Father Participation sections and Cultural Considerations box; use questions to determine support persons, gender of caregivers, acceptable comfort measures, oral intake, positions to use.
   B. Importance of determining cultural preferences: see Cultural Considerations box; consider

preferences so couple can act in ways that are comfortable to enhance the progress of labor and their view of health care providers; such an approach demonstrates respect, concern, and caring and provides the couple with positive memories of their childbirth experience that will be helpful should they experience childbirth again.

8. Couple surprised by changes in approaches to facilitate the labor process.
   - Discuss advantages of new approaches: internal locus of control (listening to her own body); maternal positions that enhance circulation to the placenta and apply the principle of gravity to facilitate and even shorten labor; new bearing-down efforts are safer (better oxygenation for fetus) and more effective (less tiring while applying effective force to facilitate descent).
   - Use illustrations, model, and DVD to help couple learn techniques.
   - Demonstrate positions; help them to try.
9. Home birth (see Mechanism of Birth Vertex Presentation, Immediate Assessment and Care of Newborn, and Fourth Stage sections, Boxes 19-7 [Guidelines for Assistance at the Emergency Birth of a Fetus in the Vertex Presentation], 19-8, and 19-9, and Nursing Process boxes for each stage of labor).
   A. Measures to reassure and comfort: use eye contact; assume a relaxed, calm, and confident manner; explain what is happening and what you are going to be doing to help her give birth; inform her and her husband about what they will need to do.
   B. Crowning (guideline 6): break membranes, tell her to pant or blow to reduce force, use Ritgen maneuver to control delivery of the head without trauma to fetus or to maternal soft tissues.
   C. Actions after appearance of head (guideline 7): check for cord around neck, support head during external rotation and restitution, and ease shoulders out one at a time with anterior first, then posterior.
   D. Prevention of neonatal heat loss (guidelines 11 and 12). dry baby, wrap up with mother, cover head.
   E. Infection control (Box 19-3): use Standard Precautions during childbirth adapting to the home setting; use handwashing, clean materials, wear gloves if available.
   F. Prevention of bleeding (guideline 17): breastfeed, assess fundus and massage prn, expel clots if present once fundus is firm, assess bladder and encourage voiding, allow placenta to separate naturally.
   G. Documentation (guideline 20, items a-i): include date, time, assessment of mother and newborn, family present, events, blood loss, Apgar.
10. Criteria of effective pushing: see Maternal Position and Bearing-Down Efforts sections of Second Stage of Labor; cleansing breaths to begin and end each contraction; open-glottis pushing with no breath holds longer than 6 to 8 seconds; frequent catch breaths; strong expiratory grunt; upright or lateral position.
11. Is an episiotomy needed? See Perineal Trauma related to Childbirth section; compare episiotomies with spontaneous lacerations in terms of tissue affected, long-term sequelae, healing process, discomfort; compare reasons given for performing an episiotomy with what research findings demonstrate to be true.
12. Siblings at childbirth: include research findings regarding effect of sibling participation on family and on the sibling; consider the developmental readiness of the child and use developmental principles to prepare him or her for the experience; offer family and sibling classes to prepare them for participation in the birth process; evaluate parental comfort with this option; arrange for a support person to remain with the child during the entire childbirth process.
13. Primipara during the fourth stage of labor (see Fourth Stage of Labor and Family, Newborn Relationships sections, Nursing Process box—Third Stage of Labor).
   A. Essential nursing assessment and care measures during the fourth stage of labor: see Box 19-9 and Fourth Stage of Labor section.
   B. Factors accounting for disinterest in newborn: exhaustion, discomfort, cultural beliefs, disappointment, difficult labor and birth, taking-in stage of recovery.
   C. Nursing measures to encourage maternal-newborn interaction: continue to assess response to newborn, provide time for close contact with newborn when she is more comfortable and rested, help her meet her needs during the taking-in stage in terms of comfort, rest, and desire to review what happened during the process of labor and birth.
14. Breastfeeding in the fourth stage of labor: recognize that the reluctance is related to lack of experience, knowledge, and fatigue. Take these factors into consideration when formulating answer, which should include measures to ensure privacy, to support and encourage her attempt; take note of signs of fatigue and keep the session short, praise her attempt, and explain benefits of breastfeeding at this time for her and for her baby.

CHAPTER 20: POSTPARTUM PHYSIOLOGY

I. Learning Key Terms

1. Postpartal diaphoresis
2. Afterpains
3. Prolactin, oxytocin
4. Episiotomy

5. Atony
6. Hemorrhoid
7. Involution
8. Autolysis
9. Puerperium; fourth trimester
10. Diastasis recti abdominis
11. Lochia
12. Lochia rubra
13. Lochia serosa
14. Lochia alba
15. Engorgement
16. Subinvolution; retained placental fragments; infection
17. Exogenous oxytocin (Pitocin)
18. Dyspareunia
19. Kegel exercises
20. Colostrum
21. Postpartal diuresis
22. Pelvic relaxation

II. Reviewing Key Concepts

23. Assessing the bladder for distention: see Urethra and Bladder section of Urinary System.
    A. Risk for bladder distention: birth-induced trauma to urethra and bladder; edematous urethra; increased bladder capacity and diuresis; diminished sensation of bladder fullness related to use of conduction anesthesia; pelvic soreness, lacerations, and episiotomy
    B. Implications of bladder distention.
       - Bladder pushes uterus up and to side, inhibiting uterine contraction, which leads to excessive bleeding.
       - Distention can lead to stasis of urine, increasing risk for UTI.
24. Factors interfering with bowel elimination: see Bowel Evacuation section of Gastrointestinal System; decreased muscle tone, effect of progesterone on peristalsis, prelabor diarrhea, limited oral intake and dehydration from labor, anticipated discomfort related to hemorrhoids and perineal trauma lead to resisting the urge to defecate.
25. Hypovolemic shock is less likely: see Blood Volume section of Cardiovascular System; pregnancy-induced hypervolemia allows most women to tolerate a considerable blood loss; size of maternal vascular bed decreases with expulsion of placenta, loss of stimulus for vasodilation, and extravascular water stores of pregnancy is mobilized back into vascular system for excretion.
26. Risk for thrombophlebitis: see Coagulation Factors section of Blood Components; increase in clotting factors and fibrinogen levels during pregnancy continues into the postpartum period; hypercoagulable state combined with vessel damage during childbirth and decreased activity level of the postpartum period increase risk for thrombus formation.
27. Compare and contrast lochial and nonlochial bleeding: see Table 20-1 for the information to complete your answer.
28. Choice D is correct; fundus should be at midline; deviation from midline could indicate a full bladder; bright to dark red uterine discharge refers to lochia rubra; edema and erythema are common shortly after repair of a wound; decreased abdominal muscle tone and enlarged uterus result in abdominal protrusion; separation of the abdominal muscle walls, diastasis recti abdominis, is common during pregnancy and the postpartum period.
29. Choice B is correct; the woman is describing the normal finding of postpartum diaphoresis, which is the body's attempt to excrete fluid retained during pregnancy; documentation is important but not the first nursing action; infection assessment and physician notification are not needed at this time.
30. Choice D is correct; afterpains are most likely to occur in the following circumstances: multiparity, overdistention of the uterus (macrosomia, multifetal pregnancy), breastfeeding (endogenous oxytocin secretion), and administration of an oxytocic.

III. Thinking Critically

1. Postpartum women express questions and concerns.
   A. Afterpains: breastfeeding with newborn sucking causes the posterior pituitary to secrete oxytocin, stimulating the let-down reflex; uterine contractions are also stimulated, leading to afterpains, which will occur for the first few days postpartum.
   B. Length of time fundus can be palpated: see Involution Process section of Uterus and Figure 20-1; progress of uterine descent in the abdomen is described; within 2 weeks of childbirth, the uterus is again located within the pelvis.
   C. Stages and duration of lochia: see Lochia section of Uterus; discuss characteristics of rubra, serosa, and alba lochia in terms of color, consistency, amount, odor, and duration; explain that the contents of the flow including the amount of blood change as progress is made from stage to stage.
   D. Protruding abdomen: see Abdomen section; enlarged uterus along with stretched abdominal muscles with diminished tone creates a still-pregnant appearance for the first few weeks after birth; by 6 weeks the abdominal wall will return to approximately its prepregnant state; skin will regain most of its elasticity and striae will fade but remain; discuss exercise and a sensible weight loss program to facilitate the return of tone and diminish protrusion.
   E. Diuresis: see Postpartal Diuresis section of Urinary System; discuss normalcy of these processes designed to rid the body of fluid retained during pregnancy; be sure to ask questions related to characteristics of

the urination including amount, frequency, appearance of urine, experience of pain such as burning to rule out urinary tract infection or urinary retention with voiding of overload in frequent, small amounts.

F. Breastfeeding as a reliable contraceptive method: see Pituitary Hormones and Ovarian Function section; emphasize that breastfeeding is not a reliable method because return of ovulation is unpredictable and may precede menstruation; discuss appropriate contraceptive methods for a breastfeeding woman, taking care to avoid hormonal-based methods until lactation is well established.

G. Lactation suppression in bottle-feeding woman: see Nonbreastfeeding Mothers section of Breast; congestion of veins and lymphatics along with some filling of milk begins to occur when estrogen and progesterone levels fall with expulsion of the placenta; because milk is not removed, the cycle shuts down and the milk is absorbed into the circulatory system; she will need to support her breasts with a snug bra/binder and avoid applying warmth on her breasts and expressing any of the milk or stimulating her nipples; ice pack application and analgesics can be used for discomfort.

H. Sexuality during the postpartum period of breastfeeding women: see Vagina and Perineum section of Reproductive System and Associated Structures; discuss role of prolactin in suppressing estrogen secretion, thereby inhibiting vaginal lubrication and resulting in vaginal dryness and dyspareunia, which will persist until ovulation resumes; use of water-soluble lubricant or a spermicide used with a condom for birth control can reduce discomfort.

CHAPTER 21: NURSING CARE OF THE FAMILY DURING THE POSTPARTUM PERIOD

I. Learning Key Terms

1. Couplet care; mother-baby care (single-room maternity care)
2. Early postpartum discharge, shortened hospital stay, 1-day maternity stay
3. Oxytocic
4. Uterine atony
5. Sitz bath
6. Afterpains (postbirth pains)
7. Splanchnic engorgement, orthostatic hypotension
8. Homans sign
9. Kegel
10. Engorgement
11. Rubella
12. RhoGAM (Rh immunoglobulin)
13. Warm line

II. Reviewing Key Concepts

14. Measures to assist with voiding: see Prevention of Bladder Distention section; help her assume an upright position on bedpan or in bathroom, listen to running water, put hands in warm water, pour water over vulva with peribottle, stand in a shower, or sit in a sitz bath, provide analgesics.
15. Measures to prevent thrombophlebitis: see Ambulation section; exercise legs with active ROM of knees, ankles, feet, and toes; early ambulation; wear support hose (if varicosities are present); keep well hydrated.
16. Two interventions to prevent postpartum hemorrhage in early postpartum period: see Prevention of Excessive Bleeding section.
    - Maintain uterine tone: massage fundus if boggy, expel clots when fundus is firm, administer oxytocic medications, breastfeed or stimulate nipples.
    - Prevent bladder distention.
17. Signs of potential psychosocial complications during postpartum period: see Signs of Potential Complications—Postpartum Psychosocial Concerns box to formulate your answer.
18. Choice C is correct; the woman should be assisted into a supine position with head and shoulders on a pillow, arms at sides, and knees flexed; this facilitates relaxation of abdominal muscles and allows deep palpation.
19. Choice A is correct; Methergine as an oxytocic contracts the uterus, thereby preventing excessive blood loss; lochia will therefore reflect expected characteristics; this medication can cause uterine contractions that are severe enough to require an analgesic.
20. Choice B is correct; a direct and indirect Coombs' must be negative, indicating that antibodies have not been formed, before RhoGAM can be given; it must be given within 72 hours of birth; the newborn needs to be Rh positive; it is often given in the third trimester and then again after birth.
21. Choice D is correct; squeezing the buttocks together before sitting down will reduce pulling on any perineal repairs; this is a medical aseptic procedure; therefore, clean not sterile equipment is used; the water should be warm at 38° to 40.6° C; it is used at least twice a day for 20 minutes each time.
22. Choices C, E, and F are correct; ice packs are used during the first 2 hours after birth to decrease edema; topical medications should be used sparingly only three or four times per day; gloves are not needed but she should wash her hands before and after perineal care.
23. Choices B, D, and E are correct; temperature of 38° C during the first 24 hours may be related to deficient fluid and is therefore not a concern; fundus should be midline but firm not boggy; saturation of the pad in 15 minutes or less would be a concern; a positive Homans sign could indicate

DVT; usually women have a good appetite and eat well after birth; each voiding should be at least 100 to 150 ml.

III. Thinking Critically

1. Measures for bottle-feeding mother to suppress lactation and relieve discomfort of engorgement: see Lactation Suppression section; wear supportive bra or a breast binder continuously for at least the first 72 hours postpartum, avoid stimulating breasts (no warm water during shower, no infant sucking, no pumping or removal of milk), apply ice packs intermittently to relieve soreness and use cabbage leaves, mild analgesics.
2. Pain relief for a postpartum breastfeeding mother: see Promotion of Comfort, Rest, Ambulations, and Exercise section; assess characteristics of pain (severity, location, relief measures already tried and effectiveness); use a combination of pharmacologic and nonpharmacologic measures as indicated by the nature of the pain being experienced; if breastfeeding, administer a systemic analgesic just after a feeding session; make sure medication is not contraindicated for breastfeeding women.
3. Woman exhibiting signs of hemorrhage and shock (see Prevention of Excessive Bleeding section and Emergency box—Hypovolemic Shock).
   A. Criteria to determine if flow is excessive: note length of time pad was worn and the degree to which it was saturated with blood; check the bed to determine if lochia has pooled under buttocks; pad saturation in 15 minutes or less indicates a profuse flow.
   B. Priority action: assess fundus and massage if boggy; once firm, express clots, check bladder for distention and assist to empty, and administer oxytocics if ordered; take note of vital sign findings and changes in behavior; notify the primary health care provider to discuss assessment findings, actions taken, and responses.
   C. Additional interventions: see list of measures identified in Emergency box—Hypovolemic Shock.
4. Administering rubella vaccine to a postpartum woman: see Health Promotion for Planning Future Pregnancies and Children section; recheck titer results and order; determine if woman or any household members are immunocompromised; check allergies (duck eggs); inform her of side effects and emphasize that she must not become pregnant for at least 1 month after the immunization.
5. Administering RhoGAM to a postpartum woman: see Health Promotion for Planning Future Pregnancies and Children section and Medication Guide; check woman's and newborn's Rh status and Coombs' test results; obtain RhoGAM and check all identification data; administer intramuscularly; woman must be Rh negative and indirect Coombs' negative; newborn must be Rh positive and direct Coombs' negative; ensure that it is administered within 72 hours after birth; provide woman with documentation that she received RhoGAM.
6. Sexual changes after pregnancy and childbirth: see Sexual Activity and Contraception section and Teaching for Self-Management box—Resumption of Sexual Activity; identify changes that may occur; discuss physical and emotional readiness of the woman; stress importance of open communication; discuss how to prevent discomfort in terms of position and lubrication; emphasize the importance of birth control because return of ovulation cannot be predicted with accuracy.
7. Postpartum women—nursing diagnoses, expected outcomes, and nursing management.
   A. Nursing diagnosis: risk for infection of episiotomy related to ineffective perineal hygiene measures.
      Expected outcome: episiotomy will heal without infection.
      Nursing management: see Prevention of Infection section and Box 21-2 for full identification of measures to enhance healing and prevent infection.
   B. Nursing diagnosis: constipation related to inactivity and lack of knowledge regarding bowel elimination patterns after childbirth.
      Expected outcome: woman will have soft formed bowel movement.
      Nursing management: see Promotion of Normal Bladder and Bowel Patterns section; determine usual elimination patterns and measures used to enhance elimination; encourage activity, roughage, fluids; obtain order for mild combination stool softener-laxative.
   C. Nursing diagnosis: acute pain related to episiotomy and hemorrhoids.
      Expected outcome: woman will experience a reduction in pain following implementation of suggested relief measures.
      Nursing management: see Promotion of Comfort, Rest, Ambulation, and Exercise section, Nursing Care Plan, and Box 21-2; emphasize nonpharmacologic relief measures such as perineal care, sitz bath, topicals, side-lying position, Kegel exercises, measures to enhance bowel and bladder elimination; use pharmacologic measures if local measures are ineffective or pain is severe.
8. Fundus above umbilicus and to the right of midline.
   A. Most likely basis for finding: bladder distention; confirm by palpating the bladder and asking the woman to describe the last time she voided.
   B. Nursing action: assist woman to empty bladder; measure amount voided and assess characteristics of the urine; palpate bladder and fundus again to determine response;

catheterization may be required if she is unable to empty her bladder fully because a distended bladder can lead to uterine atony with excessive bleeding and UTIs.

9. Resumption of physical activity after giving birth: see Promotion of Comfort, Rest, Ambulation, and Exercise section.
   - Assess postanesthesia recovery and physical stability, including return of strength, mobility, and sensation in lower extremities.
   - Assist and supervise first few times out of bed because orthostatic hypotension can cause her to be dizzy and fall.
   - Show her where the call light is and what to do if she is alone and begins to feel dizzy or lightheaded.
10. Early discharge option.
    A. Decision making regarding early discharge: discuss the advantages and disadvantages of early discharge; the nurse should discuss these with the couple in terms of their own situation; explore the reasons why they are contemplating early discharge and the determine the quality of support they will have after discharge.
    B. Nurse's legal responsibility: assess woman, newborn, and family to confirm that criteria for discharge are fully met; notify primary health care provider if criteria are not met; document all assessment findings, actions, and responses.
    C. Criteria for discharge—maternal, newborn, general; see Box 21-1.
    D. Outline essential content that must be taught before discharge: see Discharge Teaching section; include information regarding self- and newborn care, signs of complications, prescribed medications; arrange for first postpartum checkup and for a follow-up telephone call or home visit usually within 1 to 2 days after discharge.
11. Cultural beliefs and practices (see Effect of Cultural Diversity section).
    A. Importance of using a culturally sensitive approach: recognition of cultural beliefs and practices is essential to meet her individual needs; such an approach demonstrates respect, caring, and concern and helps to foster trust and cooperation with creating a plan of care.
    B. Korean-American woman—heat and cold balance: ask woman about the substances and practices that she identifies to be hot and cold, then intervene appropriately; realize the self-management may not be a priority and that she may seek guidance from older women in her family or community; see Cultural Considerations box—Postpartum Period and Family Planning.
    C. Muslim woman in postpartum period: see Cultural Considerations box—Postpartum Period and Family Planning; emphasize diet modification and modesty.
12. Performing a postpartum assessment 8 hours after vaginal birth (see content of this chapter related to assessment and the content related to the fourth stage of labor in Chapter 19).
    A. Position for fundal palpation: supine, head and shoulder on pillow, arms at sides, knees slightly flexed.
    B. Fundal characteristics to assess: consistency (firm or boggy), height (above, at, below umbilicus), location (midline or deviated to the right or left).
    C. Position for assessment of perineum: lateral or modified Sims position with upper leg flexed on hip; wear gloves for this portion of the assessment, which will involve contact with body fluids including blood (Standard Precautions).
    D. Episiotomy characteristics to assess: REEDA (redness, edema, ecchymosis, drainage, approximation); presence of hematoma; adequacy of hygiene, including cleanliness, presence of odor, method used to cleanse perineum and to apply topical preparations
    E. Characteristics of lochia to assess: stage, amount, odor, clots.
13. Recovery room nurse report: see Transfer from Recovery Area section and Table 21-1 for a discussion of essential information that should be reported regarding the woman, the baby, and the significant events and findings from her prenatal and childbirth periods.
14. Using infection control measures (see Prevention of Infection section).
    A. Measures to prevent transmission of infection from person to person: clean environment, handwashing, use of Standard Precautions, proper care and use of equipment.
    B. Infection prevention measures to teach the woman: avoid walking barefoot, handwashing, hygiene measures (general, breast, perineal), prevention of bladder infection, measures to enhance resistance to infection, including nutrition and rest.

CHAPTER 22: TRANSITION TO PARENTHOOD

I. Learning Key Terms

1. Attachment, bonding
2. Acquaintance
3. Mutuality
4. Signaling behaviors
5. Executive behaviors
6. Claiming
7. En face (face to face)
8. Entrainment
9. Biorhythmicity
10. Reciprocity
11. Synchrony

12. Transition to parenthood
13. Dependent (taking-in)
14. Dependent-independent (taking-hold)
15. Interdependent (letting-go)
16. Becoming a mother
17. Maternal sensitivity
18. Engagement
19. Experiencing herself as a mother
20. "Pink" period, "blue" period
21. Engrossment

II. Reviewing Key Concepts

22. Attachment of newborn to parents and parents to newborn (see Parental Attachment, Bonding, and Acquaintance section).
    A. Conditions that facilitate attachment: emotionally and physically healthy parents, competent in communication and caregiving; parent and newborn fit in terms of state, temperament, and gender; parental proximity to infant and time for interaction; adequate social support system; positive feedback and mutually satisfying interaction with newborn; health status of newborn.
    B. Assessment of process of attachment: see Assessment of Attachment Behaviors section and Box 22-1, for specific behaviors indicating the quality of the attachment that is developing; it is critical that nurses provide opportunities for parent-infant contact and to be present during these contacts to observe the interaction.
    C. Facilitation of attachment process: see Tables 22-1, 22-2, and 22-3 for several measures nurses can use to help parents and newborns interact with each other and become attached; consider the conditions for attachment that you identified in ***A*** above to develop creative nursing approaches.
23. Parental tasks: see Parental Tasks and Responsibilities section for a description of each of the tasks of reconciling actual child with fantasy child, becoming adept in infant care, and establishing a place for the newborn within the family group.
24. Parent-infant contact: see specific sections for each form of contact in Parent-Infant Contact.
    A. Early contact: important to provide time for parents to see, touch, and hold their newborn as soon as possible after birth; stress that attachment is an ongoing process; interference with this early contact because of maternal and/or newborn problems should not have a long-term effect as long at it is balanced by opportunities for close contact as soon as possible after birth as appropriate for maternal and/or newborn condition.
    B. Extended contact: family-centered care, mother-baby care, and use of LDRP/LDR rooms to facilitate this type of contact.
25. Progress of a mother's touch as she becomes acquainted with her newborn: see Touch section for a description of touch as it progresses from an exploration with fingertips gentle stroking, patting, and rubbing.
26. Factors influencing parental responses to the birth of their child: see section for each factor in the Diversity in Transition to Parenthood and Parental Sensory Impairment sections and Box 22-2.
27. Compare and contrast two theories of maternal adjustment after birth: Mercer's theory (see Becoming a Mother section) and Rubin's theory (see Table 22-4); in your comparison, you should include a description of the stages proposed by Rubin and Mercer along with the behaviors of women and the tasks they must accomplish.
28. Choice D is correct; choice A reflects the first phase of identifying likenesses; choice B reflects the second phase of identifying differences; choice C reflects a negative reaction of claiming the infant in terms of pain and discomfort; choice D reflects the third or final stage of identifying uniqueness.
29. Choice B is correct; early close contact is recommended to initiate and enhance the attachment process.
30. Choice A is correct; engrossment refers to a father's absorption, preoccupation, and interest in his infant; choice B represents the claiming process phase I identifying likeness; choice C represents reciprocity; choice D represents en face or face-to-face position with mutual gazing.
31. Choice B is correct; taking-in is the first 1 to 2 days of recovery following birth; other behaviors exhibited include reliance on others to help her meet needs, being excited, and talkative.
32. Choice C is correct; approximately 50% to 80% of women experience postpartum blues; new parents should be reassured that their skills as parents develop gradually and they should seek help to develop these skills; postpartum blues that are self-limiting and short lived do not require psychotropic medications; support and care of the postpartum woman and her newborn by her partner and family is the most effective prevention and coping strategy; feelings of fatigue from childbirth and meeting demands of newborn can accentuate feelings of depression.

III. Thinking Critically

1. Teaching parents communication skills with their newborns (see Communication between Parent and Infant section).
    A. Communication techniques: discuss touch, eye contact, voice, and odor; demonstrate techniques, have parents try, and point out newborn response in terms of quieting, alerting, making eye contact, gazing; help parents interpret cues.
    B. Newborn's communication: point out infant responses; discuss processes of entrainment,

biorhythmicity, reciprocity, synchrony, and repertoire of behaviors.

2. Woman following emergency cesarean birth: disappointment with lack of immediate bonding time with newborn.
   - Discuss concepts of early and extended contact.
   - Emphasize that the parent-infant attachment process is ongoing—her emotional bond with her baby will not be weaker.
   - Help her meet her own physical and emotional needs so that she develops readiness to meet her newborn's needs.
   - Help her get to know her baby, interact with and care for him; point out newborn characteristics, including how the baby is responding to her efforts.
   - Show her how to communicate with her newborn and how her newborn communicates with her.
   - Arrange for follow-up after discharge to assess how attachment is progressing.
3. Sibling adjustment to newborn: see Sibling Adaptation section and Box 22-4, which identify strategies parents can use to help their other children accept a new baby; caution her that adjustment takes time and is strongly related to the developmental level and experiences of the sibling(s); give mother suggestions regarding what she can do now and what she did previously.
4. Parents unsure and anxious about caring for their newborn (see Nursing Care Plan, Home Care Follow-up, Transition to Parenthood and Parental Role after Birth sections, and Nursing Process box—Transition to Parenthood).
   A. Nursing diagnosis: risk for impaired parent-infant attachment related to lack of knowledge and feeling of incompetence regarding infant care.
   B. Nursing measures to facilitate attachment can include the following:
      - Perform newborn assessment with parents present, pointing out newborn characteristics and encouraging parents to participate and ask questions.
      - Demonstrate newborn care measures and provide time for parents to practice and obtain feedback.
      - Provide extended contact time with newborn, such as longer visiting hours and rooming-in, until discharge.
      - Make referral for follow-up with telephone contacts and home visits; refer to parenting classes and support groups, lactation consultant and La Leche.
      - Recommend books, magazines, DVDs, and interactive Internet sites that discuss newborns and their care.
5. Parental disappointment with newborn's gender and appearance: see Parental Tasks and Responsibilities section; foster attachment, acquaintance, and claiming; help parents get acquainted with the infant and to reconcile the real child with the fantasy child; discuss the basis of molding, caput succedaneum, and forceps marks and how they will be resolved; be alert for problems with attachment and care so follow-up can be arranged.
6. Grandparent adjustment: see Grandparent Adaptation section; observe interaction between grandparents and parents, taking note of signs of effective interaction and conflict; involve grandparents in teaching sessions as appropriate for this family; spend time with grandparents to help them be supportive without "taking over" or being critical; help the new parents recognize the unique role grandparents can play as parenting role models, nurturers, and providers of respite care.
7. Woman experiencing postpartum blues.
   - Nursing diagnosis: ineffective maternal coping related to hormonal changes and increased responsibilities following birth.
   - Expected outcome: woman will report feeling more contented with her role as mother following the use of recommended coping strategies.
   - Care management: see Postpartum Blues section and Teaching for Self-Management box—Coping with Postpartum Blues to identify behaviors that should be assessed in order to determine the level of blues she is experiencing; involve both Jane and her husband in the teaching session and in the development of a plan for coping with the blues; this must occur early to prevent development of postpartum depression.
8. Discussion of paternal adjustment: see Becoming a Father section and Table 22-5 to discuss the transition process to fatherhood and nursing measures that provide the father with support, teaching, demonstrations, practice, and interaction time with the newborn.

CHAPTER 23: PHYSIOLOGIC AND BEHAVIORAL ADAPTATIONS OF THE NEWBORN

I. Learning Key Terms

1. Surfactant
2. Thermoregulation
3. Thermogenesis
4. Nonshivering thermogenesis
5. Neutral thermal environment
6. Convection
7. Radiation
8. Evaporation
9. Conduction
10. Hyperthermia
11. Telangiectatic nevi
12. Molding
13. Caput succedaneum
14. Cephalhematoma
15. Mongolian spots
16. Acrocyanosis

17. Vernix caseosa
18. Milia
19. Jaundice
20. Physiologic jaundice
21. Acute bilirubin encephalopathy
22. Kernicterus
23. Breast milk jaundice
24. Meconium
25. Erythema toxicum (erythema neonatorum; flea bite dermatitis)
26. Hypospadias
27. Hydrocele
28. Epstein pearls
29. Fontanel
30. Lanugo
31. Ecchymosis
32. Desquamation
33. Port-wine stain (nevus flammeus)
34. Strawberry hemangioma
35. Pseudomenstruation
36. Prepuce
37. Smegma
38. Epithelial pearls
39. Oligodactyly
40. Polydactyly
41. Syndactyly
42. Sleep-wake states
43. Deep, light, 17, increasing
44. Drowsy, quiet-alert, active alert, crying
45. Quiet-alert
46. State modulation
47. Habituation
48. Orientation
49. Temperament
50. K, 51. F, 52. B, 53. J, 54. D, 55. I, 56. H, 57. L, 58. A, 59. E, 60. G, 61. C, 62. M

II. Reviewing Key Concepts

63. Factors initiating breathing after birth: see Respiratory System section for a description of how a newborn begins to breathe, including effect of pressure changes, chilling, noise, light, and other sensations associated with birth and chemoreceptor activation of respiratory center.
64. Describe phases of newborn transition period to extrauterine life: see Transition to Extrauterine Life section for identification of each phase and description of timing/duration and typical newborn behaviors for each phase.
65. Factors affecting newborn behavior: see sections related to each factor to formulate your answer.
66. Choices A, B, and C are correct; the newborn at 5 hours old is in the second period of reactivity, during which tachycardia, tachypnea, increased muscle tone, skin color changes, increased mucus production, and passage of meconium are normal findings; respiratory rate should range between 30 and 60 breaths/min; expiratory grunting and nasal flaring are signs of respiratory distress; crackles commonly present in the first period of reactivity immediately following birth should be absent during the second period representing the absorption of lung fluid into the circulatory system.
67. Choice A is correct; the rash described is erythema toxicum; it is an inflammatory response that has no clinical significance and requires no treatment because it will disappear spontaneously.
68. Choices B and E are correct; physiologic jaundice does not appear until 24 hours after birth; further investigation would be needed if it appears during the first 24 hours, because this is consistent with pathologic jaundice; glucose levels should range between 50 to 60 mg/dl and should not be lower than 40 mg/dl; acrocyanosis is normal for 7 to 10 days after birth.
69. Choice D is correct; choices B and C are common newborn reflexes used to assess integrity of neuromuscular system; syndactyly refers to webbing of the fingers.
70. Choice C is correct; telangiectatic nevi are known as stork bite marks and can appear on the eyelids; milia are plugged sebaceous glands and appear like white pimples; nevus vasculosus or a strawberry mark is a raised, sharply demarcated, bright or dark red swelling; nevus flammeus is a port-wine, flat red to purple lesion that does not blanch with pressure.

III. Thinking Critically

1. Newborn—risk for cold stress (see Thermogenic System section).
   A. Basis for cold stress: see Thermogenesis section to formulate answer including newborn's ability to generate and conserve heat.
   B. Dangers of cold stress (see Fig. 23-2): metabolic and physiologic problems related to increased oxygen need and consumption; oxygen and energy diverted from brain cell and cardiac function and growth to thermogenesis; vasoconstriction results in respiratory distress, reopening of the ductus arteriosus, acidosis, and increasing the level of bilirubin; hypoglycemia can occur as a result of increased glucose utilization.
   C. Nursing diagnosis: risk for imbalanced body temperature— hypothermia related to immature thermoregulation associated with newborn status; Expected outcome: newborn's temperature will stabilize between 36.5° and 37.2° C within 8 to 10 hours of birth.
   D. Measures to stabilize newborn temperature and prevent cold stress: implement measures that reflect application of heat loss mechanisms of convection, radiation, evaporation, and conduction.
      - Dry infant and cover with warmed blankets or wrap with mother.
      - Cover head and feet; double wrap.

- Use radiant warmer to stabilize temperature, assess newborn, and perform procedures.
- Adjust environment in terms of temperature and drafts (nursery and mother's room).
- Place bassinet away from drafts and outside windows.
- Maintain adequate nutrition (caloric intake).

2. Parental concern regarding head variations: see Integumentary System and Skeletal System sections; discuss each finding in terms of cause, significance for the newborn's health status and adjustment, and how/when it will be resolved; refer to Figures 23-8 and 23-9 to facilitate parental understanding; perform a thorough newborn assessment with parents present to reassure the parents.
3. Physiologic jaundice (see Conjugation of Bilirubin and Newborn Jaundice section).
   A. Criteria for diagnosis: see Physiologic section for a full explanation of clinical manifestations.
   B. Explanation to parents: discuss why the jaundice occurs and its common occurrence among healthy newborns; emphasize how frequent feeding with associated bowel movements will be helpful in treating the jaundice by increasing the loss of bilirubin in the stool.
4. Parental interest in newborn's sensory capabilities (see Sensory Behaviors section).
   A. What nurse should tell parents: discuss and demonstrate newborn's capability regarding vision, hearing, touch, taste, and smell.
   B. Stimuli parents can provide to facilitate newborn development: face-to-face/eye-to-eye contact, objects (bright or black-and-white changing, complex patterns), sound (talking to infant, music, heartbeat simulator), touch (infant massage, cuddling).
   C. Tell parents that the best time to interact with their newborn is during the quiet-alert state; describe what this state is and how they will know she is in it.
5. Parental concern regarding "bruises" on newborn's back and buttocks: discuss the characteristics and cause of Mongolian spots (see Mongolian Spots section of Integumentary System section and Fig. 23-4).

CHAPTER 24: NURSING CARE OF THE NEWBORN AND FAMILY

I. Learning Key Terms

1. Apgar score, heart rate, respiratory rate, muscle tone, reflex irritability, color
2. Bulb syringe
3. Thermistor probe
4. Eye prophylaxis
5. Ophthalmia neonatorum, erythromycin, tetracycline
6. Vitamin K
7. New Ballard Scale
8. Appropriate for gestational age (AGA)
9. Large for gestational age (LGA)
10. Small for gestational age (SGA)
11. Preterm
12. Late preterm
13. Term
14. Postterm
15. Postmature
16. Petechiae
17. Bilirubin
18. Physiologic jaundice
19. Blanch test
20. Transcutaneous bilirubinometry (TcB)
21. Thrush
22. Hypoglycemia
23. Hypocalcemia
24. Bradypnea
25. Tachypnea
26. Handwashing (hand hygiene)
27. Phototherapy
28. Circumcision
29. CRIES: crying, requires oxygen for saturation of 95%, increased vital signs, expression, sleepless

II. Reviewing Key Concepts

30. P, 31. N, 32. N, 33. P, 34. N, 35. N, 36. N, 37. P, 38. N, 39. N, 40. N, 41. N, 42. N,43. P, 44. N, 45. N, 46. N, 47. P, 48. N, 49. N, 50. N, 51. P, 52. N, 53. N
54. Creation of a protective environment in terms of infection control and safety: see Protective Environment section to formulate answer that includes discussion of each of the following:
    A. Environmental modifications
    B. Infection control measures
    C. Safety in terms of security precautions and identification measures
55. Birth trauma.
    A. Factors leading to soft tissue injuries: see Birth Injuries section to identify several factors.
    B. Soft-tissue injuries that can occur after a difficult birth: see Soft Tissue Injuries section for a description of several injuries that can occur.
56. Health teaching in preparation for discharge: see Box 24-9 and specific sections for teaching topics identified in Discharge Planning and Teaching section; be sure to include methodologies that reflect cognitive, psychomotor, and affective learning.
57. Guidelines for weighing and measuring newborn: see Table 24-2 and Baseline Measurements of Physical Growth section for guidelines to follow and expected findings; wear gloves if performed before first bath.
    A. Weight: balance scale, cover scale with clean scale paper, place undressed infant on scale, keep hand hovering over infant, never turn

away; weigh at the same time of day when hospitalized.

B. Head circumference: measure the widest part of head just above ears and eyebrows; repeat if molding is present at birth.
C. Chest circumference: measure across nipple line.
D. Abdominal circumference: measure just above the level of umbilicus.
E. Length: measure from crown to rump, then rump to heels.

58. Specimen collection guidelines: see Collection of Specimens section and Figures 24-10, 24-11, and 24-14 for procedure to follow for heelstick, venipuncture, and urine collection bag; include a description of restraint methods that should be used (see Figs. 24-12 and 24-13).
59. Maintaining a patent airway and supporting respirations (see Airway Maintenance section).
    A. Four conditions essential for maintaining an adequate oxygen supply: clear, patent airway; adequate respiratory effort; functioning cardiopulmonary system; adequate thermoregulation.
    B. Signs of respiratory distress: see Signs of Potential Complications box—Abnormal Newborn Breathing for a list of the signs to observe for; consider how respiratory signs change from the first period of reactivity to second period of reactivity.
    C. Three methods of relieving airway obstruction: see Airway Maintenance and Maintaining an Adequate Oxygen Supply sections, Procedure boxes for Suctioning with Bulb Syringe and Nasopharyngeal Catheter, and Figure 24-2; reposition infant, use a bulb syringe or mechanical suction; take note of effectiveness of the methods used.
60. Choices D, E, and F are correct; thinning of lanugo with bald spots, absence of scarf sign, and descended testes are assessed and the New Ballard Scale and are consistent with full-term status; pulse and weight are not part of the Ballard scale; the popliteal angle for a full-term newborn is 100 degrees or less.
61. Choices C and D are correct; glucose should be 45 to 65 mg/dl; total serum bilirubin in peripheral blood should be 6 mg/dl or less in the first 24 hours after birth; A, B, E, and F all fall within the expected range (see Box 24-6).
62. Choice B is correct; signs of hypoglycemia include apnea, jitteriness, respiratory distress, poor feeding, lethargy, hypotonia, hypothermia, and seizures; laryngospasm and a high-pitched cry are signs of hypocalcemia.
63. Choice A is correct; the control panel should be set between 36° and 37° C; the probe should be placed in one of the upper quadrants of the abdomen below the intercostal margin, never over a rib; axillary, not rectal, temperatures should be taken.
64. Choice B is correct; acetaminophen should be given every 4 hours for a maximum of 5 doses in 24 hours at 75 mg/kg/day; the site should be checked every 15 to 30 minutes for the first hour then every hour for 4 to 6 hours; diaper wipes should not be used on the site because they contain alcohol, which delays healing and causes discomfort; the yellow exudate is a protective film that forms in 24 hours and should not be removed.
65. Choices B, C, and D are correct; mother does not have to be hepatitis B positive for the vaccine to be given to her newborn; use a 5/8-inch 25-gauge needle and insert it at a 90-degree angle.
66. Choices B, C, E, and F are correct; administer within 1 to 2 hours and squeeze a 1- to 2-cm ribbon of ointment into the lower conjunctival sac.

II. Thinking Critically

1. Apgar scoring: see Table 24-1 and Initial Assessment and Apgar Scoring section
   A. Baby boy Smith: heart rate: 160 (2); respiratory effort: good, crying (2); muscle tone: flexion, active movement (2); reflex irritability: cry with stimulus (2); color: acrocyanosis (1); score is 9; interpretation: score of 7 to 10 indicates that the infant is not having difficulty adjusting to extrauterine life
   B. Baby girl Doe: heart rate: 102 (2); respiratory effort: slow, irregular, weak cry (1); muscle tone: some flexion (1); reflex irritability: grimace with stimulus (1); color: pale (0); score is 5; interpretation: score of 4 to 6 indicates moderate difficulty adjusting to extrauterine life.
2. Assessment of newborn girl:
   A. Protocol for assessment during first 2 hours: see Table 24-1 (Apgar score) and Box 24-2 (Initial Physical Assessment by Body System), Initial Assessment and Apgar Scoring section to prepare your outline.
   B. Nurse's responsibility for newborn identification at birth: see Protective Environment—Safety Factors section; complete the identification process before mother and newborn are separated; attach matching ID bands to both (father also in some cases) immediately after birth; take newborn's footprint and mother's fingerprint(s) and place on appropriate form.
   C. Priority nursing diagnosis for the first 24 hours: consider nursing diagnoses related to breathing and to thermoregulation (see Nursing Process box).
   D. Priority nursing care measures—discuss each of the following areas:
      - Stabilization of respiration and airway patency
      - Maintenance of body temperature
      - Immediate interventions in terms of identification, prophylactic medications, promotion of parent-infant interaction

E. Benefits of early contact between mother and newborn are described in the Promoting Parent-Infant Interaction section.

3. Performing a physical examination of newborn before discharge.
   A. Actions to ensure safety and accuracy: well-lighted, warm, and draft-free environment; undress as needed; place on firm surface with constant supervision; progress in a systematic manner from cleanest to dirtiest area; see Box 24-4: Performing a Physical Examination of the Newborn.
   B. Major areas assessed (see Table 24-2 and Chapter 23 for Assessment of Newborn Reflexes): areas to include general appearance and posture; vital signs and weight; integument; head and neck; abdomen and back; genitalia and anus; elimination patterns; extremities; neurologic system, including reflexes; behavioral characteristics.
   C. Rationale for presence of parents: chance to observe parent-infant interactions and to identify and meet learning needs; foster active involvement in assessment and care of their newborn; encourage discussion of concerns and asking of questions; chance to explain and demonstrate newborn characteristics and capabilities.
4. Newborn with mucus in airway (see Airway Maintenance and Maintaining an Adequate Oxygen Supply sections and Procedure Boxes for Suctioning with a Bulb Syringe, Nasopharyngeal Catheter with a Mechanical Suction Apparatus).
   A. Nursing diagnosis: impaired gas exchange related to upper airway obstruction with mucus.
   B. Steps using bulb syringe: suction mouth first, then nose; compress bulb before insertion; insert tip along side of mouth not over tongue, which could stimulate the gag reflex and sucking; release compression slowly; continue until breathing sounds clear; teach parents how to use bulb syringe.
   C. Guidelines for use of mechanical suction: suction for 5 seconds or less per insertion; use <80 mm Hg setting; lubricate catheter with sterile water; insert along base of tongue or horizontally through nose into nares; repeat until breathing/cry sounds clear.
5. Care of circumcision and umbilical cord sites.
   A. Nursing diagnosis: risk for infection related to removal of foreskin and healing umbilical cord site.
   B. Expected outcome: cord and circumcision site will heal without infection.
   C. Teaching about care: see Boxes 24-7 and 24-9 and Umbilical Cord Care and Circumcision section emphasize importance of assessing sites for infection and progress of healing; discuss measures to keep areas clean and dry and to enhance comfort; teach parents how to assess circumcision site for bleeding and what to do if it occurs, and emphasize importance of assessing urination and what to do if the newborn has difficulty voiding; demonstrate skills and assist parents to redemonstrate.
6. Newborn with hyperbilirubinemia (see Therapy for Hyperbilirubinemia section, Physiologic Problems section).
   A. Responding to parental concerns: tell parents in simple terms that their newborn is exhibiting physiologic jaundice, explaining why it occurs, what effect it will have on their newborn's health, and how it will be resolved; emphasize that their newborn's form of jaundice is a common and naturally occurring physiologic process as the newborn adjusts to extrauterine life.
   B. Blanch test: apply pressure with finger over a bony area (nose, forehead, sternum) for several seconds to empty capillaries at the spot; if jaundice is present, the blanched area will appear yellow before the capillaries fill.
   C. Expected findings of physiologic hyperbilirubinemia: jaundice (cephalocaudal, proximodistal progression), watery greenish stools, sleepiness, alteration in bilirubin levels that follows a specific pattern and degree of elevation (see Chapter 23).
   D. Precautions and care measures during phototherapy: increase fluids and feed at least every 3 hours; cover eyes, removing periodically to assess condition and allow for interaction with parents; monitor temperature for increases or decreases; cleanse stools promptly; do not put lotions on skin; place undressed under lights and change position every 2 hours to expose as much skin to the lights as possible; remove from under lights for feeding, cuddling, and interaction with parents.
7. Newborn scheduled for a circumcision—pain concerns (see Neonatal Pain and Circumcision—Procedural Pain Management sections, Table 24-4, Box 24-7 and Figs. 24-22 and 24-23).
   A. Common behavioral responses to pain: see Behavioral Responses section for several examples.
   B. Changes in vital signs and integument: see Assesment of Neonatal Pain section and Table 24-4 for several examples.
   C. CRIES tool (see Table 24-4).
   D. Nonpharmacologic and pharmacologic relief measures: see Management of Neonatal Pain section.
      - Nonpharmacologic: swaddle, nonnutritive sucking, take to parent, distract, apply Vaseline ointment, change diaper promptly, avoid pressure on site when holding or positioning.
      - Pharmacologic: local anesthesia, topical preparations, nonopioid systemic analgesics.

8. Administration of medications to newborns after birth: see Medication Guide for each of the medications to develop the guidelines to ensure safe and effective administration of erythromycin ophthalmic ointment 5% and vitamin K 0.5 mg IM.
9. Parental concern about weight loss: see Baseline Measurements of Physical Growth section and Table 24-2; determine percentage of weight loss, making sure it does not exceed 10%; explain that their newborn's weight loss of 6% is within the expected range for weight loss after birth; discuss the cause of the loss and feeding measures, and inform them that the birth weight should be regained within 2 weeks.

CHAPTER 25: NEWBORN NUTRITION AND FEEDING

I. Learning Key Terms

1. Lobes
2. Alveoli
3. Milk ducts
4. Myoepithelial cells
5. Areola
6. Lactation (lactogenesis)
7. Prolactin
8. Oxytocin
9. Nipple erection reflex
10. Everted, inverted
11. Breast shell
12. Colostrum
13. Nipple confusion
14. Feeding readiness cues
15. Let-down; milk ejection
16. Rooting reflex
17. Latch
18. Engorgement
19. Football (clutch) hold
20. Cradle (traditional) hold
21. Lactation consultant
22. Mastitis
23. Thrush
24. Tongue-tie
25. Weaning
26. Foremilk
27. Hindmilk (cream)
28. Complementary feeding

II. Reviewing Key Concepts

29. Teaching group of women about breastfeeding: see Benefits of Breastfeeding section and Table 25-1; emphasize the importance and benefits of breastfeeding for infants, mothers, and family/society.
30. Breastfeeding positions: see Positioning section and Figure 25-5; describe the positions of football hold, cradle (traditional), modified cradle (across the lap), and side-lying; included in the demonstration should be an explanation of the rationale for alternating positions.
31. Feeding readiness cues: see Care Management section.
    A. Cues: hand-to-mouth or hand-to-hand movements, sucking motions, strong rooting reflex, mouthing, tongue movements; crying is a late sign.
    B. Rationale for feeding according to these cues: if cues are missed, baby may cry vigorously, become distraught, shut down, or withdraw into a deep sleep; these behaviors will make feeding more difficult or impossible; feeding when the infant exhibits readiness enhances the chance of success.
32. Proper latch (see Latch section).
    A. Steps to ensure proper latch: apply colostrum/milk to areola/nipple (lubricate and entice), support the breast (see Fig. 25-6), hold baby close and tickle baby's lower lip with the breast nipple to stimulate the rooting reflex—mouth opening and extrusion of tongue occurs; pull baby onto nipple and areola; bring infant to the breast.
    B. Signs of proper latch: see Figure 25-6; nose, cheeks, and chin touch the breast, firm, tugging sensation on the nipple but no pinching or pain; baby's cheeks are rounded and jaw glides smoothly with sucking; swallow is audible.
    C. Removal of baby from breast: see Figure 25-7; break suction by inserting finger in the side of baby's mouth between gums and leaving the finger in until nipple is completely out of the baby's mouth.
33. Choice B is correct; soft, yellow seedy stools are very characteristic of the stools of breastfed babies; birth weight is regained in 10 to 14 days; six to eight wet diapers are expected at this time; should be fed every 2 to 3 hours for at total of 8 to 10 times per day.
34. Choice A is correct; swaddling is recommended; choices B, C, and D are all appropriate actions to calm a fussy baby.
35. Choice D is correct; no soap should be used because it could dry the areola and nipple and increase the risk for irritation; vitamin E should not be used especially before a feeding because it is a fat-soluble vitamin that the infant could ingest when breastfeeding; lanolin or colostrum/milk are the preferred substances to be applied to the area; plastic liners can trap moisture and lead to sore nipples.
36. Choice B is correct; a combination hormonal contraceptive could decrease the milk supply if given before lactation is well established during the first 6 weeks after birth; after 6 weeks a progestin-only contraceptive could be used because it is the least likely hormonal contraceptive to affect lactation; even complete breastfeeding is not considered to be a reliable method because ovulation can occur unexpectedly even before

the first menstrual period; diaphragm used before pregnancy would have to be checked after healing has occurred and lochia has ceased to see if it fits properly before the woman uses it again.

37. Choice C is correct; nipple should allow only the passage of a slow drip; tap water can be used unless the water supply is unsafe or if otherwise instructed; formula should never be heated in the microwave because it could be overheated or unevenly heated.
38. Choices A, C, and D are correct; bring baby to breast not breast to baby; feeding should occur when baby begins to exhibit feeding readiness cues; breast should be supported with thumb on top and four fingers under back edge of areola and gently compress.
39. Choice C is correct; limiting length of feeding does not protect the nipples and areola; B and D are correct actions but not the most important.

III. Thinking Critically

1. Bottle-feeding mother wishes to give her newborn skim milk to prevent cardiac problems: see Fat section of Nutrient Needs; emphasize the importance of fat in the newborn's diet for energy and supplying essential fatty acids for growth and tissue maintenance, cell membranes, and hormone production; at least 15% of calories must come from fat; skim and low-fat milk lack essential fatty acids; whole milk should not be given until after the first year of life
2. Infant feeding method decision making during prenatal period (see Choosing an Infant Feeding Method section).
   A. Nursing diagnosis: decisional conflict regarding feeding method for their newborn related to lack of knowledge and experience with newborn feeding methods.
   Expected outcome: couple will choose the feeding method for their newborn that is most comfortable for them.
   B. Rationale for couple making the decision together: both should learn about the pros and cons of feeding methods with an emphasis on the benefits of breastfeeding and how the partner can help with the method.
   C. Making decision prenatally: the prenatal period is a less stressful time, allowing for full consideration of options, how feeding methods would be incorporated into life activities (such as work outside the home), and learning about breastfeeding by attending a prenatal breastfeeding class and reading.
   D. How the nurse can facilitate decision-making process: provide information about feeding methods in a nonjudgmental manner while still emphasizing the importance of breastfeeding as the preferred method, dispel myths, address personal concerns of the couple, and make needed referrals to WIC, lactation consultant, breastfeeding classes, and La Leche League.
3. Breastfeeding mother's questions and concerns.
   A. Breast size: discuss development of lactation structures during pregnancy; emphasize the importance of this development and not the breast size for successful lactation.
   B. Let-down reflex: explain what it is and why it happens (including physical and emotional triggers); emphasize its importance in providing the infant with hindmilk.
   C. Signs that breastfeeding is going well: see Indicators of Effective Breastfeeding section and Box 25-2, which identify maternal and newborn indicators of effective breastfeeding; put the indicators in writing and go over each one; provide contact person if mother is concerned.
   D. Nipple soreness: see Sore Nipples section; discuss and demonstrate measures to prevent and to treat sore nipples, including, most important, good breastfeeding techniques such as latch, removal, and alternating starting breast and positions; discuss breast care measures such as air-drying nipples, avoiding soap, and applying colostrum/milk or purified lanolin after feeding, using breast shells.
   E. Engorgement: see Engorgement section; begin by describing engorgement, what it is and why it occurs and when; prevention of excessive engorgement includes frequency of feeding every 2 to 3 hours on each breast (use pumping to soften second breast if needed); relief measures include warm shower and massage before feeding, ice between feedings, supportive bra; emphasize the temporary, self-limiting nature of engorgement, analgesics such as ibuprofen or acetaminophen.
   F. Afterpains and increased flow: explain that oxytocin is released as a result of infant sucking; this triggers the let-down reflex and stimulates the uterus to contract, causing afterpains for the first 3 to 5 days after birth; oxytocin also reduces excessive bleeding, though the contractions can cause flow already in the uterus to be expelled, giving the impression of an increased flow.
   G. Breastfeeding as a birth control method: see Breastfeeding and Contraception section; emphasize that breastfeeding is not an effective contraceptive method; although ovulation may be delayed, its return cannot be predicted with accuracy and may occur before the first menstrual period; discuss contraceptive methods that are safe to use with breastfeeding and resuming sexual intercourse during the postpartum period.
   H. Weaning: see Weaning section; emphasize that weaning needs to be a gradual process, eliminating one feeding at a time, beginning with the one the baby is most likely to sleep

through; discuss the use of bottles and cups; use of formula, cow's milk, and/or solids depends on the age of infant at the time of weaning.

4. Infrequent feeding of sleeping baby (see Frequency and Duration of Feeding and Sleepy Baby sections, Nursing Care Plan and Nursing Process boxes and Box 25-3).
   A. Nursing diagnosis: imbalanced nutrition: less than body requirements related to infrequent feeding of newborn.
   Expected outcome: mother will awaken infant every 2 to 3 hours during the day and every 4 hours at night to feed the infant, achieving approximately 8 to 12 feedings per day.
   B. Nursing approach: discuss feeding readiness cues to facilitate proper timing of feedings; discuss techniques to wake sleeping baby and signs indicating adequate intake; discuss potential problems associated with feedings that are too infrequent.
5. Bottle-feeding mother (see Formula Feeding section and Teaching for Self-Management box—Formula Preparation and Feeding).
   A. Nurse's response to mother's concern: discuss how the mother can facilitate close contact and socialization with the infant during feeding: sitting comfortably, touching, singing, and talking quietly to newborn to make feeding a pleasant time for both; reassure that properly prepared formulas will fully meet her newborn's need for nutrients and fluid.
   B. Guidelines for bottle feeding: discuss how to choose a formula type; amount and frequency of feedings; how to prepare formula (follow directions for dilution exactly), warming formula correctly, discarding leftover formula, and bottle and nipple cleansing; principles of the feeding process, including semi-upright position, not propping bottles, fluid filling the nipple to limit air consumption, cues of feeding readiness and satiety, and burping.
6. Assessment of breastfeeding mother and infant to ensure that mother and infant are ready for discharge
   A. Factors to assess: see Care Management and Boxes 25-2 and 25-5 to determine what to assess; it is essential to assess maternal feeding technique, level of knowledge, and confidence as well as newborn responses and physical status.
   B. Assessment 1 week after discharge: formulate questions that address the factors that you identified in **A** above; in addition ask questions about such areas as frequency and duration of feedings, breastfeeding techniques used, how she feels about breastfeeding and how well she feels she is doing, family support for breastfeeding; her ability to rest; nutrient and fluid intake.

CHAPTER 26: ASSESSMENT FOR RISK FACTORS IN PREGNANCY

I. Learning Key Terms

1. High risk pregnancy
2. Daily fetal movement count (DFMC), fetal alarm signal
3. Ultrasonography, transvaginal, transabdominal
4. Oligohydramnios
5. Polyhydramnios (hydramnios)
6. Doppler blood flow analysis
7. Biophysical profile (BPP), ultrasound, electronic fetal monitoring, fetal breathing movements, fetal body movements, fetal tone, nonstress test (fetal heart rate reactivity), amniotic fluid volume
8. Magnetic resonance imaging (MRI)
9. Amniocentesis
10. Percutaneous umbilical blood sampling (PUBS)
11. Chorionic villus sampling (CVS)
12. Maternal serum alpha-fetoprotein (MSAFP), 16, 18
13. Triple-marker; 16, 18; MSAFP; unconjugated estriol; hCG; age; quad screen
14. Indirect Coombs'
15. Nonstress test
16. Vibroacoustic stimulation test (fetal acoustic stimulation test)
17. Contraction stress test, nipple-stimulated contraction stress, oxytocin-stimulated contraction stress
18. Diagnosis of fetal anomalies
19. Determine if the intrauterine environment continues to be supportive of the fetus, determine timing of childbirth for women at risk for uteroplacental insufficiency (UPI)

II. Reviewing Key Concepts

20. Factors placing a pregnant woman and her fetus/newborn at risk and identification of strategies to eliminate or reduce the risk: see Box 26-1, which describes several risk factors in each category listed.
21. Role of nurse when caring for high risk pregnant women undergoing antepartal testing: see Nurse's Role in Assessment of the High Risk Pregnancy section; answer should emphasize education, support measures as well as assisting with or performing the test and follow-up care.
22. Risk factors for pregnancy-related problems: see Box 26-2, which lists risk factors for each pregnancy-related problem identified.
23. Choice D is correct; an amniocentesis with analysis of amniotic fluid for the L/S ratio and presence of phosphatidylglycerol (Pg) is used to determine pulmonary maturity; choice B refers to a contraction stress test; choice C refers to serial measurements of fetal growth using ultrasound.
24. Choice C is correct; food/fluid is not restricted before the test to stimulate fetal movement; the test will evaluate the response of the FHR to fetal

movement—acceleration is expected; external not internal monitoring is used.

25. Choice B is correct; the triple-marker test is used to screen the older pregnant woman for the possibility that her fetus has Down syndrome; serum levels of AFP, unconjugated estriol, and hCG are measured; maternal serum alpha-fetoprotein alone is the screening test for open neural tube defects such as spina bifida; a 1-hour, 50-g glucose test is used to screen for gestational diabetes; amniocentesis and Coombs' testing are be used to check for Rh antibodies and sensitization.
26. Choice C is correct; an equivocal suspicious result is recorded when late decelerations occur with less than 50% of the contractions; see Box 26-8 for a full explanation of the results.
27. Choice A is correct; a supine position with hips elevated enhances the view of the uterus; a lithotomy position may also be used; a full bladder is not required for the vaginal ultrasound but is needed for most abdominal ultrasounds; during the test the woman may experience some pressure but medication for pain relief before the test is not required; contact gel is used with the abdominal ultrasound; water-soluble lubricant may be used to ease insertion of the vaginal probe.
28. Choice A is correct; B and D are types of results for the contraction stress test; see Boxes 26-7 and 26-8 for a full explanation of results for both the NST and the CST.

III. Thinking Critically

1. Woman scheduled for transvaginal ultrasound (see Ultrasonography section).
   A. Cite reasons for test for this woman: to determine location of gestational sac because PID could have resulted in narrowing of fallopian tube, thereby increasing risk for ectopic pregnancy; in addition, a determination of gestational age and estimation of date of birth would be done related to irregular cycles and unknown date of LMP.
   B. Preparation for the test: explain purpose of test, how it will be performed, and how it will feel; assist her into a lithotomy position or supine position with hips elevated on a pillow; point out structures on monitor as test is performed.
2. Nurse's role in transabdominal ultrasound for monitoring fetal growth: see Ultrasonography section; instruct woman to come for test with full bladder if appropriate; explain purpose of test and method of examination; assist her into a supine position with head and shoulders elevated on pillow and hip slightly tipped to right or left side; observe for supine hypotension during test and orthostatic hypotension when rising to upright position after test; indicate how the fetus is being measured and point out fetus and its movements if the woman wishes to know.
3. Woman having biophysical profile (see Biophysical Profile section and Tables 26-2 and 26-3 for identification of variables tested; scoring).
   A. Nursing diagnosis: anxiety related to unexpected need to undergo a biophysical profile.
   B. Nurse's response to woman's concern about the test: describe how the test will be performed using real-time ultrasound and external electronic fetal monitoring; explain that the purpose of the test is to view the fetus within its environment, to determine the amount of amniotic fluid, and assess the FHR response to fetal activity.
   C. Meaning of score obtained: a score of 8 to 10 is a normal result.
4. Amniocentesis (see Amniocentesis section and Nurse's Role in the Assessment of the High Risk Pregnancy section).
   A. Preparing woman: explain procedure, witness informed consent, assess maternal vital signs and health status and FHR before the test; ensure that ultrasound is performed to locate placenta and fetus before the test.
   B. Supporting woman during the procedure: explain what is happening and what she will be feeling; help her relax; encourage her to ask questions and voice concerns and feelings; assess her reactions.
   C. Postprocedure care and instructions: monitor maternal vital signs and status and FHR; tell her when test results should be available and whom to call; administer RhoGAM because she is Rh negative; teach her to assess herself for signs of infection, bleeding, rupture of membranes, and uterine contractions; make a follow-up phone call to check her status.
5. Nonstress test (see Nonstress Test section and Boxes 26-6 and 26-7).
   A. Tell woman about purpose of test: test measures response of FHR to fetal activity to determine adequacy of placental perfusion and fetal oxygenation.
   B. Preparation of woman for test: tell her that she can eat before and during the test; schedule test at a time of day that fetus is usually active; assist woman into a reclining chair or semi-Fowler position with a left or right tilt.
   C. Indicate how test is conducted: attach tocotransducer over the fundus and ultrasound transducer at site of PMI; instruct woman to indicate when fetus moves; assess change, if any, in FHR following the movement.
   D. Analyze the results: see Box 26-7 and Figs. 26-10 and 26-11 for the criteria to determine the test result and to document it as reactive: good variability and normal baseline with accelerations following fetal movement that meet criteria for a reactive result; as nonreactive—no accelerations with movement or the accelerations that do occur do not meet the criteria and limited variability.

6. Contraction stress test (see Contraction Stress Test section and Box 26-8).
   A. Tell woman about purpose of test: the test is a way of determining how her fetus will react to the stress of uterine contractions as they would occur during labor; uterine contractions decrease perfusion through placenta leading to fetal hypoxia; late decelerations during this test could be interpreted as an early warning of fetal compromise.
   B. Preparation: assess woman's vital signs, general health status, and contraindications for the test; attach external electronic fetal monitor and assess FHR and uterine activity; assist woman into a lateral, semi-Fowler, or seated position; determine if an informed consent is required since contractions will be stimulated
   C. Indicate how the test is performed: see Nipple-Stimulation Contraction Stress Test section; stimulate nipple(s) according to protocol until three contractions of good quality occur in a 10-minute period; make sure that contractions subside after the test and assess maternal and fetal responses.
   D. Use of oxytocin to stimulate contractions: see Oxytocin-Stimulated Contraction Stress Test section; administer oxytocin (Pitocin) intravenously (similar to induction of labor but with lower dosages) according to protocol, increasing rate until uterine contractions meet criteria indicated for a nipple-stimulated CST; monitor woman, fetus, and contractions during the test and afterward until contractions subside.
   E. Analyze the results: see Box 26-8 and Fig. 26-13 for criteria used to interpret the test results and to document it as negative, positive, equivocal-suspicious, equivocal-hyperstimulatory, and unsatisfactory.

CHAPTER 27: HYPERTENSIVE DISORDERS IN PREGNANCY

I. Learning Key Terms

1. E, 2. C, 3. B, 4. A, 5. F, 6. D
7. Gestational hypertension
8. Chronic hypertension
9. Preeclampsia
10. Hypertension, 2, 4 to 6, 1
11. Proteinuria,
12. Dependent edema, ankles, sacrum
13. Eclampsia
14. HELLP syndrome, hemolysis, liver enzymes, platelets
15. Arteriolar vasospasm

II. Reviewing Key Concepts

16. Assessment techniques to determine findings associated with preeclampsia: see Care Management—Physical Examination section and use a physical assessment textbook to further explain each assessment technique.
    - Hyperreflexia and ankle clonus: see Table 27-4, which grades DTR responses and Figure 27-4 for illustrations depicting performance of DTRs and ankle clonus.
    - Proteinuria: describe dipstick and 24-hour urine collection methods to determine level of protein in urine.
    - Pitting edema: see Figure 27-3, which illustrates assessment of pitting edema and classifications.
17. Choice A is correct; the woman should rest for at least 5 minutes after assuming her position, and the cuff should cover 80% of the upper arm or be 1.5 times the length of the upper arm; either Korotkoff V alone or with IV should be used when recording the diastolic pressure.
18. Choice C is correct; with severe preeclampsia the DTRs should be ≥3+ with positive ankle clonus, the BP should be >160/110, with a platelet count of <100,000/mm3, which reflects thrombocytopenia; proteinuria should be 3+ or greater.
19. Choices C, D, and F are correct; a respiratory rate of 12 breaths/min indicates CNS depression caused by the magnesium sulfate; the solution should be 40 g in 1000 ml of Ringer's lactate; assessment should occur every 15 to 30 minutes, and the maintenance dose should be 2 g/hr; calcium gluconate is the antidote for magnesium sulfate toxicity while hydralazine (apresoline) is used to lower blood pressure.
20. Choice B is correct; magnesium sulfate acts as a CNS depressant and is given to prevent seizures.
21. Choices B, C, D, and E are correct; a clean-catch midstream urine specimen should be used to assess urine for protein using a dipstick; fluid intake should be 6 to 8 glasses a day along with roughage to prevent constipation; gentle exercise improves circulation and helps preserve muscle tone and a sense of well-being; no sodium restriction is required except for limiting excessively salty foods; diversional activities including contact with friends will decrease boredom and stress.
22. Choice C is correct; nifedipine (Procardia) is a calcium channel blocker used to decrease blood pressure.
23. Choice B is correct; magnesium sulfate is a CNS depressant that potentiates the action of other CNS depressants such as opioid analgesics; it reduces the risk for seizures but is unlikely to cause hypotension; diuresis is a common expected finding in the postpartum period.
24. Choice C is correct; Oxytocin (Pitocin) as an oxytocic medication is safe and effective to use to contract the uterus and reduce blood loss because it will not increase blood pressure as can methylergonovine (Methergine) another oxytocic medication; calcium gluconate is the antidote used for magnesium sulfate toxicity; labetalol (Normodyne) is an antihypertensive medication.

25. Choice B is correct; although A, C, and D are all appropriate actions they are not the first priority; remember the ABCs—airway, breathing, circulation—when considering the priority action.

III. Thinking Critically

1. Protocol to ensure accurate blood pressure measurement: see Box 13-1; emphasize consistency in position of woman and her arm, the arm used, size of cuff, and provision of a rest period prior to the measurement; consider teaching these principles to the pregnant woman and her family.
2. Profile of two women at risk for preeclampsia: see Preeclampsia section and Box 27-1 for information on risk factors to use when creating the profiles; be sure to use different risk factors for each profile created.
3. Preeclampsia and eclampsia: effect on fetal well-being.
   A. Describe effect: see Morbidity and Mortality and Pathophysiology sections and Figures 27-1, and 27-2; many major effects on fetal health are described.
   B. Fetal surveillance measures: see Mild Gestational Hypertension and Mild Preeclampsia—Maternal and Fetal Assessment section for the surveillance measures that are commonly used; emphasize to woman the importance of ongoing prenatal care.
4. Woman with mild preeclampsia: home care.
   A. Clinical manifestations: see Table 27-2, which differentiates between mild and severe preeclampsia in terms of maternal and fetal effects; Table 27-3 lists the changes in laboratory values.
   B. Three priority nursing diagnoses (see Nursing Process box): nursing diagnoses should consider physiologic effects of preeclampsia such as ineffective tissue perfusion—placenta, risk for injury to mother or fetus; psychosocial effects: anxiety, ineffective individual/ family coping, powerlessness, ineffective role performance, interrupted family processes; assessment findings should guide the choice and priority of nursing diagnoses, especially with regard to those that apply to psychosocial effects.
   C. Organization of home care: see Mild Gestational Hypertension and Mild Preeclampsia section and Nursing Process box; help couple mobilize their support system, make referrals to home care if needed, discuss frequency of prenatal visits and antepartal testing.
   D. Teaching regarding assessment of status and signs of a worsening condition: see Table 27-2 and Teaching for Self- Management box—Assessing and Reporting Clinical Signs of Preeclampsia; discuss signs and put them in writing so couple can refer to them at home; have woman keep a daily diary of her findings, feelings, and concerns; teach woman and family to take BP, weigh accurately, assess urine, determine daily fetal movement counts, and whom to call if problems or concerns arise.
   E. Instructions about nutrition and fluid intake: see Diet section and Teaching for Self-Management box—Diet for Preeclampsia for several food and fluid recommendations.
   F. Coping with bed rest: see Activity Restrictions section, Teaching for Self-Management box—Coping with Activity Restrictions and Nursing Process boxes; explain rationale for bed rest and activity restrictions; clarify what this restriction means; discuss importance of lateral position when in bed, gentle ROM exercises, relaxation exercises, and nonstressful, calming diversional activities.
   G. Risk for constipation: see Teaching for Self-Management boxes—Nutrition and Coping with Activity Restriction; discuss roughage, fluid, and activity.
5. Woman with severe preeclampsia—hospital care (see Severe Gestational Hypertension and Severe Preeclampsia section).
   A. Signs and symptoms: see Table 27-2, which differentiates between mild and severe preeclampsia in terms of maternal and fetal effects; Table 27-3 lists changes in laboratory values.
   B. Three priority nursing diagnoses (see Nursing Process boxes): impaired tissue perfusion, risk for impaired gas exchange, and injury take priority as the physiologic nursing diagnoses because her condition is worsening and the safety of the maternal-fetal unit is jeopardized; anxiety or fear is the priority psychosocial nursing diagnosis.
   C. Measures to protect mother and fetus: see Box 27-2, which lists precautionary measures in erms of environmental modifications, seizure precautions, and readiness of emergency medications and equipment.
   D. Administration of magnesium sulfate: see Box 27-3 and Magnesium Sulfate section.
      (1) Create a protocol: list the guidelines for preparing and administering the medication solution safely including dosage, IV solution, and infusion rate; identify essential assessment measures that must be completed and documented before and during the infusion.
      (2) Nursing diagnosis: risk for ineffective breathing pattern related to the CNS depressant effects of magnesium sulfate infusion.
      (3) Explain expected therapeutic effect: discuss that this medication is used for its CNS depressant effects to prevent convulsions; describe how it will be given, how she will

feel, and what will be done while she is receiving the infusion.
(4) Maternal-fetal assessments: VS, FHR pattern, intake and output, urine for protein, DTRs and ankle clonus, signs of improvement or worsening condition including signs of an imminent seizure.
(5) Signs of magnesium sulfate toxicity: hyporeflexia, respiratory depression, oliguria, diminished LOC.
(6) Immediate action: discontinue the magnesium sulfate infusion, administer calcium gluconate slowly, IV push according to protocol.

E. Seizure occurs: see Eclampsia section and Emergency box—Eclampsia.
(1) Emergency measures at onset of convulsion and immediately following.
- Emphasize importance of maintaining a patent airway, preventing injury, and calling for help.
- Observe effect of seizure on mother and fetus.
- Document the event and care measures implemented during and after seizure.
- Provide comfort and reassurance after the convulsion; orient to what happened; never leave alone because another seizure could occur or signs of complications can begin; inform family.

(2) List problems that can occur: rupture of membranes, preterm labor and birth, altered LOC, abruptio placentae, fetal distress.

F. Postpartum period recovering from eclampsia (see Postpartum Care section); discuss each of the following components of care:
- Comprehensive assessment with emphasis on signs of hemorrhage, impending seizures, and status of preeclampsia
- Precautionary measures
- Medications that may be given
- Emotional and psychosocial support for woman and her family; parent-infant interaction
- Information to give to woman and family

CHAPTER 28: ANTEPARTUM HEMORRHAGIC DISORDERS

I. Learning Key Terms

1. Miscarriage (spontaneous abortion), premature dilation of the cervix, ectopic pregnancy, hydatidiform mole (molar pregnancy)
2. Placenta previa, premature separation of the placenta (abruptio placentae or placental abruption)
3. Spontaneous (abortion) miscarriage, threatened, inevitable, incomplete, complete, missed
4. Recurrent (habitual) miscarriage
5. Human chorionic gonadotropin (hCG)
6. Dilation and curettage (D&C)
7. Recurrent premature dilation of the cervix (incompetent cervix)
8. Cerclage
9. Ectopic (tubal) pregnancy
10. Cullen sign
11. Hydatidiform mole (molar pregnancy)
12. Gestational trophoblastic disease (GTD)
13. Complete hydatidiform mole
14. Partial hydatidiform mole
15. Gestational trophoblastic neoplasia (GTN)
16. Placenta previa
17. Premature separation of the placenta (abruptio placentae)
18. Couvelaire uterus
19. Velamentous insertion of the cord (vasa previa)
20. Battledore placenta
21. Succenturiate placenta
22. Disseminated intravascular coagulation (DIC) or consumptive coagulopathy

II. Reviewing Key Concepts

23. DIC in pregnancy (see Clotting Disorders in Pregnancy—Disseminated Intravascular Coagulation section).
    A. Obstetric risk factors for DIC: abruptio placentae, retained dead fetus, anaphylactoid syndrome, severe preeclampsia, HELLP syndrome, and gram-negative sepsis.
    B. Pathophysiology of DIC: see Disseminated Intravascular Coagulation section for an explanation of what goes wrong with clotting and why.
    C. Clinical manifestations: see Box 28-2 for a list of manifestations.
    D. Priority nursing care measures: see Management section; discuss thorough assessment, treatment of underlying cause, positioning, administration of blood/blood products and oxygen as ordered, education and emotional support of woman and family; closely monitor renal function including urinary output.
24. Effect of bleeding: see chapter introductory section for a discussion of the harmful effects of blood loss for the mother and fetus.
25. Choice A is correct; the woman is experiencing a threatened miscarriage; therefore, expectant management is attempted first though there are no research-proven therapies; B and C reflect management of an inevitable and complete or incomplete abortion; cerclage or suturing of the cervix is done for recurrent spontaneous miscarriage associated with premature dilation of the (incompetent) cervix.
26. Choice C is correct; A, B, and D are appropriate nursing diagnoses, but deficient fluid volume is the most immediate concern, placing the woman's well-being at greatest risk.
27. Choices B, C, and D are correct; methotrexate destroys rapidly dividing cells, in this case the fetus and placenta, to avoid rupture of tube and need for surgery; vitamins (folic acid) and alcohol increase

the risk for side effects with this medication; the woman should not put anything into her vagina; she needs to return periodically to check her hCG level.

28. Choice C is correct; the clinical manifestations of placenta previa are described; dark red bleeding with pain is characteristic of abruptio placentae; massive bleeding from many sites is associated with DIC; bleeding is not an expected sign of preterm labor.
29. Choice A is correct; hemorrhage is a major potential postpartum complication because the implantation site of the placenta is in the lower uterine segment, which has a limited capacity to contract after birth; infection is another major complication, but it is not the immediate focus of care; B and D are also important, but not to the same degree as hemorrhage, which is life threatening.

III. Thinking Critically

1. Woman with ruptured ectopic pregnancy: see Ectopic Pregnancy section.
   A. Risk factors: see Incidence and Etiology section for several risk factors.
   B. Assessment of findings: see Clinical Manifestations section; discuss findings beginning with signs of an unruptured tubal pregnancy, which are subtle and often missed; signs of rupture are more acute and may be mistaken for other acute abdominal conditions.
   C. Differential diagnosis (other health care problems): see Tubal Pregnancy Management section; miscarriage, appendicitis, salpingitis, ruptured ovarian cyst.
   D. Major care management problem: hemorrhage; much of the blood accumulates in the abdominal cavity.
   E. Two priority nursing diagnoses: deficient fluid volume and acute pain as well as fear/anxiety and anticipatory grief
   F. Nursing measures for the preoperative and postoperative periods: see Initial Care and Follow-up Care sections; assessment, general preoperative and postoperative care measures, fluid replacement, major emphasis on emotional support to facilitate grieving, discussion of effect of rupture on future pregnancies, referral for counseling as appropriate, prepare for discharge with instructions for postoperative self-care including self-assessment for complications such as infection, measures to enhance healing, importance of follow-up appointment to assess progress of physical and emotional recovery.
2. Woman with signs of miscarriage: see Table 28-1.
   A. Basis for signs and symptoms: signs indicate the woman is experiencing a threatened miscarriage.
   B. Expected care management: bed rest, sedation, avoidance of stress and orgasm; follow progress with hCG and progesterone levels and ultrasound to assess integrity of gestational sac; watch for signs of progress to inevitable abortion; caution her to save peripads and tissue passed.
3. Woman with signs of miscarriage: see Table 28-1, Nursing Process box—Miscarriage, Teaching for Self-Management box—Discharge Teaching for the Woman After Early Miscarriage.
   A. Questions: determine what she means by a lot of bleeding and if she is experiencing any other signs and symptoms related to miscarriage such as pain and cramping; determine the gestational age of her pregnancy and if there is anyone to bring her to the hospital for evaluation.
   B. Assessment findings indicative of an incomplete miscarriage: heavy, profuse bleeding, severe cramping, passage of tissue, cervix is dilated with tissue present.
   C. Priority nursing diagnosis at this time: deficient fluid volume related to blood loss secondary to incomplete abortion.
   D. Outline nursing measures: prepare woman for the prompt termination of her pregnancy—assess before and after procedure (e.g., dilation and curettage), explain what will occur, provide emotional support, refer for counseling if needed, prepare for discharge, and arrange for follow-up to assess physical and emotional status; include immediate and postprocedure care.
   E. Discharge instructions: see Home Care section and Teaching for Self-Management box—Discharge Teaching for the Woman After Early Miscarriage; advise regarding signs and symptoms of complications (bleeding, infection), what to expect regarding progress of healing (pain, discharge), measures to prevent complications (hygiene, nutrition, rest); advise her to allow for physical and emotional healing before considering another pregnancy.
   F. Nursing measures for anticipatory grieving: see Follow-up Care at Home section and Teaching for Self-Management box—Discharge Teaching for the Woman After Early Miscarriage; acknowledge her loss and provide time for her to express her feelings; inform her about how she may feel (mood swings, depression); refer her for grief counseling, support groups, clergy; make follow-up phone calls (see Chapter 38).
4. Care of woman following cerclage: see Premature Dilation of the Cervix section. Answer should include the following care measures:
   - Assessment for uterine contractions, rupture of membranes, infection
   - Explanation of activity restrictions, warning signs including those that require immediate transfer to the hospital, and treatments including medications
   - Discussion of her feelings regarding the pregnancy and her understanding of her health problem and its treatment

- Identification and involvement of support system as appropriate

5. Woman with complete hydatidiform mole: see Hydatidiform Mole section.
   A. Typical signs and symptoms: see Clinical Manifestations section for a description of assessment findings.
   B. Posttreatment instructions: see Management and Follow-up Care sections; frequent physical and pelvic examinations, regular measurement of serum hCG levels following protocol for frequency; emphasize importance of follow-up assessments and strict birth control (avoid use of IUD) to prevent pregnancy until hCG levels have been normal for a specified period of time; provide time to discuss knowledge of disorder, treatment, and follow-up and to express feelings; referral to support group may be helpful.
6. Comparison of a woman with marginal placenta previa to a woman with abruptio placentae, grade II
   A. Comparison of findings: see Placenta Previa and Abruptio Placentae sections and Table 28-2 to compare findings for each disorder in terms of characteristics of bleeding, uterine tone, pain and tenderness, and ultrasound findings regarding location of placenta and fetal presentation/position, hypertension associations, and fetal effects.
   B. Priority nursing diagnoses: consider diagnoses related to major physical problems such as deficient fluid volume related to blood loss, ineffective tissue perfusion (placenta), and risk for fetal injury; pain would be another major nursing diagnosis as the placenta continues to separate; major psychosocial nursing diagnoses could include fear/anxiety, interrupted family processes, and anticipatory grieving.
   C. Comparison of care management approaches: consider home care versus hospital care for woman with placenta previa; hospital care is the safest approach for woman experiencing abruptio placentae; discuss active versus expectant management for each disorder.
   D. Postpartum considerations: potential complications should be the basis for the special postpartum care requirements; describe each major complication and the basis for its occurrence: hemorrhage and infection are the major physiologic complications that need to be addressed; emotional and psychosocial support are important related to the high risk nature of the pregnancy, especially if fetal loss, maternal loss, or both was the outcome.

CHAPTER 29: ENDOCRINE AND METABOLIC DISORDERS IN PREGNANCY

I. Learning Key Terms

1. Interrelationship of the clinical manifestations of diabetes mellitus: see Pathogenesis section of Diabetes Mellitus for a full description of each of the clinical manifestations listed in terms of cause and interrelationship with one another.
2. Diabetes mellitus
3. Polyuria
4. Polydipsia
5. Polyphagia
6. Glycosuria
7. Type 1 diabetes mellitus
8. Type 2 diabetes mellitus
9. Pregestational
10. Gestational
11. Glycemic control
12. Hydramnios (polyhydramnios)
13. Hypoglycemia
14. Hyperglycemia
15. Diabetic ketoacidosis (DKA)
16. Euglycemia, 65 to 95 mg/dl, 130 to140 mg/dl
17. Macrosomia
18. Glycosylated hemoglobin (hemoglobin A_{1c})
19. Fasting blood glucose, 65 mg/dl, 95 mg/dl
20. Postprandial blood glucose, 130 mg/dl, 140 mg/dl
21. Phosphatidylglycerol
22. Hyperemesis gravidarum

II. Reviewing Key Concepts

23. Maternal and fetal/neonatal risks and complications related to pregestational diabetes: see Pregestational Diabetes Mellitus—Maternal Risks/Complications, and Fetal Risks and Gestational Diabetes—Maternal-Fetal Risks sections for a list with explanations of the risks/complications; describe why these risks/complications are more likely to occur in women with diabetes; explain to the woman what they can do to reduce the risk by regular health care, maintaining euglycemia and a normal BMI, exercising, reducing stress etc.
24. Explain metabolic changes in pregnancy and effect on diabetes management: see Metabolic Changes Associated with Pregnancy section of Diabetes Mellitus for a description related to changes associated with pregnancy and the postpartum period; include how the need for insulin changes from trimester to trimester.
25. Types of insulin and how they work: see Insulin Therapy section and Table 29-4 for a discussion of each type of insulin with examples; you may also wish to use a nursing drug manual for further information on the types of insulin.
26. Recommendations for screening for and diagnosing gestational diabetes: see Screening for Gestational Diabetes Mellitus section for current guidelines related to screening and criteria for diagnosis.
    A. Explain to woman the risk factors she presents for GDM—discuss what it is and why screening is important for her and her baby.
    B. Result of 130 to 140 mg/dl is a positive screen requiring further testing by an oral glucose tolerance test (OGTT); explain to the woman what this means and how to prepare for the diagnostic test.

C. Diagnosis is made if two or more of the values are met or exceeded.

27. State effect of thyroid disorders on reproduction and pregnancy: see Thyroid Disorders section for a full description of hyperthyroidism and hypothyroidism; consider effects of these disorders on reproductive development, sexuality, fertility in terms of ability to conceive and to sustain a pregnancy to viability, potential fetal/newborn complications related to maternal treatment of her thyroid disorder.
28. Choice D is correct; the woman is exhibiting signs of DKA; insulin is the required treatment, with the dosage dependent on blood glucose level; IV fluids may also be required; A is the treatment for hypoglycemia; B and C, although they may increase the woman's comfort, are not the priority.
29. Choice C is correct; a 2-hour postprandial blood glucose should be less than 120 mg/dl; A, B, and D all fall within the expected normal ranges for premeal and postmeal levels (see Table 29-3).
30. Choices A, C, and D are correct; based on a normal BMI (19.8 to 26) calories should be 30 to 40 kcal/kg each day; the bedtime snack needs to be substantial to prevent starvation ketoacidosis; simple carbohydrates should be avoided.
31. Choices B, D, and F are correct; washing hands is important, but gloves are not necessary for self-injection; vial should be gently rotated, not shaken; regular insulin should be drawn into the syringe first; because she is obese, a 90-degree angle with skin taut is recommended; gentle rather than vigorous cleansing of the skin with alcohol is required.
32. Choice B is correct; oral hygiene is important when NPO and after vomiting episodes to maintain the integrity of oral mucosa and teeth; taking fluids between (not with) meals reduces nausea, thereby increasing tolerance for oral nutrition; vitamin B_6 (pyridoxine) is one of the first-line antiemetic drugs used.

III. Thinking Critically

1. Preconception counseling for a woman with diabetes mellitus: see Preconception Counseling section. In your answer:
   - Discuss purpose in terms of planning pregnancy for the optimum time when glucose control is established within normal ranges and why this is important.
   - Discuss how her diabetes management will need to be altered during pregnancy; include her husband, because his health is important, as is his support during pregnancy.
2. Pregnant woman with pregestational diabetes experiencing hypoglycemia (see Tables 29-2 and 29-4, Teaching for Self-Management box—Treatment for Hypoglycemia, and Metabolic Changes Associated with Pregnancy and Pregestational Diabetes Mellitus sections).
   A. Problem: signs and symptoms suggest hypoglycemia resulting from insufficient caloric intake with no adjustment in insulin dosage.
   B. Action: see Table 29-2 and Teaching for Self-Management box for a discussion of the action to take in sequence.
   C. Glucose boosters: see Teaching for Self-Management box for a list of substances that provide 15 g of simple carbohydrate.
   D. Follow-up actions: after ingesting the simple carbohydrate, the woman should wait 15 minutes, then check her blood glucose level again; based on the finding further action may need to be taken; be sure to discuss with the woman how to reduce the risk that the problem will recur (see Teaching for Self-Management box—Treatment for Hypoglycemia).
3. Woman with pregestational diabetes: care management.
   A. Additional antepartal fetal assessments: see Fetal Surveillance section, which describes several tests.
   B. Stressors facing woman and family: alteration in daily living, including usual diabetes management, need for additional antepartal testing and prenatal visits, financial implications.
   C. Nursing diagnoses (see Nursing Process box—Pregestational Diabetes): consider both physiologic and psychosocial concerns; consider areas of deficient knowledge, anxiety/fear, ineffective coping, risk for maternal or fetal injury, imbalanced nutrition.
   D. Activity/exercise recommendations: see Exercise section; recommend exercises according to her diabetic status; discuss when she should exercise, and emphasize the importance of checking blood glucose level, adjusting caloric intake and insulin administration accordingly.
   E. Complete outline related to care management during antepartum, intrapartum, and postpartum periods: see specific sections for diet, glucose monitoring, and insulin and the Teaching for Self-Management boxes, Tables 29-3 and 29-4, and Nursing Process box for information regarding interventions and health teaching.
   F. Birth control recommendations: see Postpartum section; discuss risks and benefits of a variety of methods, including their effect on glucose levels and infection; stress importance of delaying intercourse until healing is complete to prevent infection; discuss effect of another pregnancy and its timing.
4. Hispanic woman with gestational diabetes: see Gestational Diabetes section.
   A. Complication of pregnancy exhibited with validating findings: gestational diabetes; 50-g glucose test result 152 mg/dl (135 to 145 mg/dl or greater) represents a positive screen; 3-hour glucose test reveals three values

exceeding the normal range (fasting, 1-hour result, and 2-hour result—see Fig. 29-4).

B. Risk factors exhibited: older than 25 years of age, Hispanic, BMI indicates obesity, woman's mother has type 2 diabetes, previous birth of baby >4500 g (9.9 lb).

C. Pathophysiology of gestational diabetes: see Metabolic Changes associated with Pregnancy and Gestational Diabetes sections for a description of the pathophysiology involved.

D. Ongoing assessment: see Care Management—Antepartum section; emphasize importance of monitoring blood glucose levels at recommended times, antepartal fetal surveillance measures, and increased frequency of prenatal visits.

E. Nursing diagnoses.
   - Anxiety related to diagnosis of ineffective glucose metabolism during pregnancy associated with gestational diabetes
   - Risk for fetal injury related to excessive intrauterine growth associated with uncontrolled gestational diabetes

F. Dietary changes: see Diet section, which provides guidelines to follow in terms of nutrient proportion and meal distribution.

G. Administration of insulin: see Medications for Controlling Blood Glucose Levels section and Teaching for Self-Management box—Self-Administration of Insulin for the information required to respond to the woman's concern and what to teach her; commend her for her positive efforts to follow the prescribed diet and provide her with the emotional support she will need to perform the skill of administering insulin safely and effectively; enlist family support if needed; incorporate teaching methodologies that represent cognitive, psychomotor, and affective learning.

H. Implications of gestational diabetes mellitus: see Postpartum section for a description of recovery of glucose control and implications for her future related to the development of diabetes for herself and her children; discuss what the woman can do to reduce her risk for future glucose metabolism problems including diet modification, exercise, and weight loss.

5. Woman with hyperemesis gravidarum: see Hyperemesis Gravidarum section.

   A. Predisposing/etiologic factors: see Hyperemesis Gravidarum Etiology section, which identifies several physiologic and psychologic factors, including the factors present in this situation: nullipara, obesity, ambivalence about pregnancy, lifestyle alterations; additional factors include multifetal pregnancy, molar pregnancy, body change concerns, history of migraines.

   B. Assessment of physiologic and psychosocial factors upon admission (see Care Management—Assessment Section).
      - Physiologic: full description of nausea and vomiting, presence of other GI symptoms, relief measures used, weight including changes, vital signs, signs of fluid, electrolyte, and acid-base imbalances, urine check for ketones (ketonuria) and specific gravity, CBC, serum electrolytes, liver enzymes, bilirubin levels.
      - Psychosocial: discuss concerns regarding self and pregnancy; assess support system.

   C. Priority nursing diagnoses: deficient fluid volume, risk for fetal and maternal injury, anxiety, powerlessness, ineffective individual or family coping; woman's condition and circumstances will determine the priority with physiologic diagnoses taking precedence in the acute phase

   D. Care measures during hospitalization.
      - Restore fluid and electrolyte balance with IV administration of fluids, electrolytes, and nutrients.
      - Restore ability to tolerate oral nutrition: gradual progression from NPO to full diet.
      - Monitor progress to determine effectiveness of therapeutic regimen, readiness for discharge, and need for continuing treatment with home care.
      - Provide psychosocial support for woman and her family; make referrals as appropriate; offer comfort measures including oral care and provide a calm, restful environment free of odors.
      - Teach woman and family about the disorder, how it is treated, its effect on pregnancy and fetus.

   E. Home care:
      - Discuss follow-up care requirements, types of foods to eat, and ways to eat (similar to recommendations for morning sickness); see Teaching for Self-Management—Diet for Hyperemesis.
      - Include family in plan of care, especially with regard to meal preparation and support and encouragement of the woman.
      - Teach woman how to assess herself in terms of weight, urine for ketones, signs of developing problems that should be reported including weight loss, return of nausea and vomiting, pain, dehydration.

CHAPTER 30: MEDICAL-SURGICAL PROBLEMS IN PREGNANCY

I. Learning Key Terms

1. Cardiac decompensation
2. Functional classification of organic heart disease, asymptomatic without limitation of physical activity, symptomatic with slight limitation of activity, symptomatic with marked limitation of

activity, symptomatic with inability to carry on any physical activity without discomfort
3. Atrial septal defect (ASD)
4. Ventricular septal defect (VSD)
5. Patent ductus arteriosus (PDA)
6. Coarctation of the aorta
7. Tetralogy of Fallot
8. Aortic stenosis
9. Myocardial infarction (MI)
10. Peripartum cardiomyopathy
11. Mitral valve stenosis
12. Infective endocarditis
13. Eisenmenger syndrome
14. Mitral valve prolapse
15. Marfan syndrome
16. Primary pulmonary hypertension
17. Anemia
18. Folic acid deficiency
19. Sickle cell hemoglobinopathy
20. Thalassemia
21. Asthma
22. Acute respiratory distress syndrome (ARDS)
23. Cystic fibrosis
24. Pruritus gravidarum
25. Pruritic urticarial papules and plaques of pregnancy (PUPPS)
26. Epilepsy
27. Multiple sclerosis (MS)
28. Systemic lupus erythematosus (SLE)
29. Myasthenia gravis (MG)
30. Cholelithiasis
31. Cholecystitis
32. Inflammatory bowel disease
33. Urinary tract infection (UTI)
34. Appendicitis
35. Bell's palsy

II. Reviewing Key Concepts

36. Maternal and fetal complications related to maternal cardiovascular problems: see Cardiovascular Disorders section and Box 30-1; increased risk for miscarriage, preterm labor and birth, IUGR, maternal mortality, and stillbirth; help the couple to recognize that MVS represents a low risk but that could change as pregnancy progresses; emphasize the importance of regular health care and lifestyle practices that include diet, rest/exercise balance, and stress reduction including infection prevention.
37. Modifications in CPR and abdominal thrust maneuver when a woman is pregnant: see Cardiopulmonary Resuscitation of the Pregnant Woman section, Emergency box—Cardiopulmonary Resuscitation for the Pregnant Woman, and Figure 30-1, which cover the recommended modifications, based on anatomic changes that occur during pregnancy, for safe and effective CPR and the abdominal thrust maneuver.
38. Choices B, D, and E are correct; other signs of cardiac decompensation include moist, frequent cough, and crackles at bases of lungs; supine hypotension is a common finding during pregnancy related to compression of vena cava and aorta, not cardiac decompensation; wheezing is characteristic of narrowed air passages and not fluid in the lungs as would occur with pulmonary edema associated with cardiac decompensation.
39. Choice A is correct; this woman is exhibiting signs of cardiac decompensation; further information regarding her cardiac status is required to determine what further action would be needed.
40. Choice C is correct; furosemide (Lasix) is a diuretic; propranolol (Inderol) is used to manage hypertension and cardiac dysrhythmias; heparin is a large-molecule anticoagulant that does not cross the placenta or cause teratogenic effects as does warfarin (Coumadin) which does cross the placenta potentially causing teratogenic effects.
41. Choice B is correct; bed rest is not required for a woman with a class II designation; she will need to avoid heavy exertion and stop activities that cause fatigue and dyspnea; actions in A, C, and D are all appropriate and recommended for class II.
42. Choice C is correct; fat should be reduced to 40 to 50 g; protein should be limited to 10% to 12% of total calories; fatty/fried foods should be avoided.

III. Thinking Critically

1. Pregnant women requiring abdominal surgery.
   A. Factors that complicate diagnosis and treatment for abdominal problems: see Surgery During Pregnancy section for several reasons why diagnosis is more difficult including displacement of abdominal organs and changes in clinical manifestations; treatment is more complicated as a result of the cardiovascular and respiratory changes associated with pregnancy and presence of an enlarged uterus and fetus.
   B. Importance of treating appendicitis before rupture: see Appendicitis section for goal of early diagnosis and prompt treatment; consider maternal and fetal effects of late diagnosis, after rupture including the need to use medications and the potential for preterm labor and fetal loss.
   C. Fears often expressed by women undergoing surgery and her family: fear of losing baby, the effects of the procedure and medications on fetal well-being and the course of the pregnancy; women and family members should be encouraged to express their fears, concerns, and questions.
   D. Outline pre- and postoperative care requirements: see Management—Hospital section; outline should include assessment and care measures.
   E. Discharge planning: see Home Care section and Box 30-3; teach woman and family about what to watch for, care of incision site, activity and rest considerations, and nutrition guidelines for healing and recovery; include assessing for changes in fetal status and for signs of preterm labor.

2. Pregnant woman with mitral valve stenosis—class II; see Cardiovascular Disorders section.
   A. Two nursing diagnoses (see Nursing Process box—Cardiac Disease and Nursing Care Plan—The Pregnant Woman with Heart Disease): several nursing diagnoses and expected outcomes of care are listed in the Assessment and Nursing Diagnoses section. Use assessment findings to determine the priority for a specific pregnant woman.
      - Fear/anxiety would be a top priority psychosocial nursing diagnosis for this woman because it is her first pregnancy and she does not really know what to expect; expected outcome: the woman/couple will openly express concerns and seek information as needed.
      - Physiologically, activity intolerance, risk for ineffective tissue perfusion, and decreased cardiac output would be priorities as pregnancy advances and the cardiac workload increases; expected outcome: woman will follow recommended therapeutic regimen to reduce stress on her heart.
   B. Recommended therapeutic plan for a pregnant woman designated as class II: see Care Management—Antepartum section and Nursing Process box focusing on specific guidelines for class II and descriptions of recommended care measures for each area; fully discuss measures for each area in answer including a rationale for use and effectiveness.
      - Rest/sleep/activity patterns: activities to avoid and importance of rest (include rest recommendations).
      - Prevention of infection: infection is a major stressor that can increase risk for decompensation.
      - Nutrition: nutrients to include in a well-balanced diet; avoid weight gain that exceeds the recommended range for her BMI.
      - Bowel elimination: prevent constipation.
   C. Factors increasing stress.
      - Physiologic stress: anemia, infection, edema, constipation
      - Psychosocial stress: depression, anxiety and fear, financial concerns, anger, impaired social interactions, feelings of inadequacy, cultural expectations, inadequate support system
   D. Subjective symptoms of cardiac decompensation: see Signs of Complications box—Cardiac Decompensation.
   E. Objective signs of cardiac decompensation: see Signs of Complications box—Cardiac Decompensation.
   F. Care during labor: see Intrapartum section, which identifies specific measures for each area.
      - Comprehensive assessment for decompensation along with routine assessments related to labor and birth.
      - Decrease fear and anxiety with support measures and creating a calm environment.
      - Provide pain relief using pharmacologic and nonpharmacologic measures.
      - Vaginal birth is the best approach; include recommendations for measures to enhance labor process, positioning, breathing exercises, pushing techniques.
      - Prevent postpartum bleeding; medications to use.
   G. Risk for postpartum cardiac decompensation: see Postpartum—nursing Alert for a discussion of the basis of cardiac decompensation in first 24 to 48 hours after birth.
   H. Nursing diagnoses for early postpartum period.
      - Risk for excess fluid volume related to extravascular fluid shifts following birth would be the top priority physiologic nursing diagnosis.
      - Ineffective breastfeeding, risk for impaired mother-infant attachment, *or* situational low self-esteem can be priority psychosocial nursing diagnoses related to the woman's need for activity reduction and limited ability to care for newborn on her own.
   I. Stress reduction during postpartum period: see Postpartum section; encourage rest in a lateral position; assist with ADLs and progressive ambulation; provide for pain relief and comfort; emphasize measures to prevent infection and constipation; assist with newborn care while keeping newborn nearby so she can see and touch her baby.
   J. Breastfeeding: breastfeeding is allowed, but the woman will need extra support and rest because of the increased energy demands associated with lactation; medications used for the mother must be evaluated for their effect on the newborn.
   K. Discharge plan—emphasize the following:
      - Follow-up with health care providers for assessment of postpartum recovery and cardiac status.
      - Contraception, future pregnancy, and sexuality issues.
      - Assistance with infant, self, and home care; make referrals as needed.
      - Importance of balancing rest and activity.
      - Instruct regarding the healing process, how to assess progress, and prevent complications.
3. Pregnant woman with cardiac disorder needs to take heparin (see Antepartum section and Table 30-1).
   A. Explain why heparin instead of warfarin (Coumadin) will be used: discuss importance of taking an anticoagulant to prevent thrombus formation; inform that warfarin will cross the placenta and could cause congenital anomalies and fetal hemorrhage; heparin does not cross the placenta.
   B. Information to ensure safe use of heparin.

- Safe administration; teach subcutaneous injection technique to Allison and family.
- Stress importance of routine blood tests to assess clotting ability.
- Discuss alternative sources for folic acid.
- Review side effects including unusual bleeding and bruising and measures to prevent injury (use soft toothbrush, no razors to shave).

4. Pregnant woman with epilepsy: see Epilepsy section; inform her that effects of pregnancy on epilepsy are unpredictable; convulsions may injure her or her fetus and lead to miscarriage, preterm labor, or separation of the placenta; medications, which will be given in the lowest therapeutic dose, must be taken to prevent convulsions; folic acid supplementation is important because anticonvulsants deplete folic acid stores, increasing the risk for neural tube defects.

CHAPTER 31: OBSTETRIC CRITICAL CARE

I. Learning Key Terms

1. Colloid osmotic pressure (COP)
2. Capillary hydrostatic pressure, pulmonary capillary wedge pressure (PCWP)
3. Respiratory alkalosis
4. Hypercoagulable state
5. Systemic vascular resistance (SVR)
6. Diastole
7. Systole
8. Cardiac output
9. Stroke volume, preload, afterload, contractility
10. Heart rate, preload, afterload, contractility
11. Preload
12. Afterload
13. Contractility
14. Invasive hemodynamic monitoring; pulmonary artery catheter (PAC), Swan-Ganz catheter
15. Arterial pressure catheter
16. Allen test
17. Pulse oximetry (Sao_2 monitoring)
18. Svo_2 monitoring
19. Oliguria
20. Trauma

II. Reviewing Key Concepts

21. Increasing use of obstetric intensive care units
    A. Rationale for obstetric critical care units: see Obstetric Intensive Care Unit and Equipment and Expertise sections for a description of this form of care delivery and the rationale for its use; discuss that these units address the unique needs of the pregnant woman; these needs will be met by health care providers who have expertise in the physical and hemodynamic differences during pregnancy; there are also increasing numbers of women who require this type of specialized care.
    B. Indications for use: see Indications for Obstetric Critical Care section and Box 31-1 for several reasons when this form of care would be used.
22. Factors responsible for altering cardiac output during labor and the postpartum periods: see Hemodynamic Monitoring—Cardiac Output section for a description of changes and why they occur in labor and after birth.
23. Techniques used to monitor oxygenation: see specific section in Hemodynamic Monitoring—Oxygenation.
    A. Arterial blood gas analysis: reflects dissolved oxygen in plasma, which is 1% to 2% of total oxygen content; requires arterial puncture or an arterial catheter; see Table 13-3 p 299 for normal nonpregnant and pregnant ABG values.
    B. Pulse oximeter: measures oxygen bound to hemoglobin and available for cellular use; the oxygen saturation of hemoglobin represents 98% to 99% of total oxygen content; values for pregnancy range from 97% to 100%.
    C. Svo_2 monitoring: reflects balance between oxygen delivery and oxygen use; requires insertion of a fiberoptic PAC that is connected to a bedside microprocessor for a continuous Svo_2 value; normal value is 60% to 80%.
24. Choice B is the correct answer; pH ranges from 7.40 to 7.45; Po_2 during pregnancy ranges from 104 to 108 mm Hg; Pco_2 during pregnancy ranges from 27 to 32 mm Hg; bicarbonate during pregnancy ranges from 18 to 31 mEq/L (see Table 13-3 p 299).
25. Choices B, C, and F are correct; woman should be assisted into a slight Trendelenburg position with hip wedge; lidocaine hydrochloride should be on hand for arrhythmias; pressure is applied for 5 minutes on catheter removal (see Box 31-2).
26. Choices A, D, and F are correct; see Box 31-6 for the Glasgow Coma Scale.
27. Choice D is correct; although the knee-chest position provides the best cardiac output, it is not an appropriate position for a critically ill pregnant woman; lateral positions provide the next best cardiac output; sitting and supine are the least effective positions in terms of cardiac output (see Table 31-3).
28. Choice D is correct, hemorrhage, thrombus formation and embolization are also risks; they are less common than infection and more severe.
29. Choice B is correct; test the nondominant hand; tell client to clench and unclench fist to facilitate venous drainage; only release pressure on the ulnar artery—capillary refill should occur in 5 seconds or less (see Box 31-4).

III. Thinking Critically

1. Pregnant woman in obstetric critical care unit as a result of trauma.
    A. Insertion of an arterial pressure catheter: see Arterial Pressure Catheter section of Hemodynamic Monitoring and Box 31-4 (Allen

test); perform Allen test on nondominant hand to assess quality of circulation from ulnar artery in case of damage during puncture of radial artery; explain procedure to woman; comfort and support her during the procedure because stress and restlessness alter arterial blood gases and increase risk for arterial damage; ensure signed consent is on the chart.

B and C: Purposes for an arterial pressure catheter and periodic cuff pressure reading: see Arterial Pressure Catheter section for a discussion of both methods of arterial pressure assessment; the arterial pressure catheter is inserted when frequent and accurate BP measurements are needed as well as ABG determinations

D. Blood gas analysis: see Table 13-3 p 299; values fall within the normal range for a pregnant woman.

E. Glasgow Coma Scale: see Box 31-6 for a description of this scale.

F. Positions to enhance cardiac output in a pregnant woman: see Table 31-3 and Cardiac Output-Positional Changes section to determine cardiac output in a variety of positions; note that the lateral positions support an appropriate cardiac output.

G. Supportive care measures for woman and family: see Family-Centered Maternity Care section; consider components of open visitation, parent-infant interaction and attachment, sibling and family visitation, information giving, and grief support.

2. Trauma during pregnancy: see Trauma During Pregnancy section.
   A. Significance of problem: see Significance section; use statistics to describe the problem of trauma in terms of incidence in general and then for specific causes of trauma.
   B. Effects of trauma: see Significance section for the major effects of fetal and maternal trauma and the influencing factors that determine the severity of the effect.
   C. Maternal physiologic and anatomic adaptations that affect type and extent of trauma: see Maternal Physiologic Characteristics section and Table 31-6 for a discussion of influence of bladder and uterine location, progesterone levels, and hemodynamic changes coupled with maternal position.
   D. Effect of trauma on fetus: fetal injury (skull fracture, intracranial hemorrhage, prematurity); death related to maternal death or abruptio placentae, altered oxygenation, PROM, fetomaternal transfusion.
   E. Potential effects of mechanisms of trauma: see specific section for each mechanism in Mechanisms of Trauma section for a full description.
   F. Resuscitate the woman, stabilize her condition, fetal needs, fetal, maternal.
   G. Outline primary and secondary surveys: see Primary Survey and Secondary Survey sections to highlight the important components of each.

CHAPTER 32: MENTAL HEALTH DISORDERS AND SUBSTANCE ABUSE IN PREGNANCY

I. Learning Key Terms

1. Mood disorders
2. Anxiety disorders
3. Phobia
4. Panic disorder
5. Generalized anxiety disorder (GAD)
6. Obsessive-compulsive disorder (OCD)
7. Posttraumatic stress disorder (PTSD)
8. Postpartum depression without psychotic features
9. Postpartum depression with psychotic features (postpartum psychosis)
10. Bipolar disorder
11. Panic attacks

II. Reviewing Key Concepts

12. Diagnostic criteria for diagnosis of major depression: see Mood Disorders section, which lists several criteria, at least five of which must be present nearly every day.
13. Difficulty of diagnosing depression during pregnancy: see Nursing Alert— Mood Disorders During Pregnancy, which explains the difficulty and provides several diagnostic cues.
14. Screening for substance abuse: see Substance Abuse during Pregnancy—Care Management section and Boxes 32-1 and 32-2.
    A and B. Purpose for and comparison of assessment tools: CAGE questionnaire to screen for alcohol use and 4 Ps Plus screen for alcohol and other substances.
    C. Questions represented by each letter: CAGE (Box 32-1).
    D. Meaning of each P (Box 32-2).
15. Maternal and fetal/newborn effects of a variety of substances: see specific section for each substance to gather the information needed to complete your answer.
16. Choice C is correct; doxepin (Sinequan) (L5—high lactation risk category) is not used because it can lead to neonatal respiratory depression; A, B, and D are antidepressants that are classified as L2, which is a low lactation risk category and therefore considered safe for breastfeeding women (see Table 32-1).
17. Choice C is correct; the woman needs to avoid being a superwoman and placing unrealistic expectations on herself; sharing feelings, rest, and some time away from the baby are all adaptive coping mechanisms.
18. Choice A is correct; citalopram (Celexa) as an SSRI if taken along with dextromethorphan increases the risk for serotonin syndrome.
19. Choice A is correct; although the other questions are all appropriate, the potential for harming herself or her baby represents the most serious and very real concern.

20. Choice B is correct; acute onset of labor with long hard uterine contractions and precipitous birth are characteristic of cocaine use; premature rupture of the membranes is associated with heroin use in pregnancy; IV use increases the risk for blood-borne infections.
21. Choice D is correct; the nurse should follow a sequence that establishes trust by starting with questions about substances that are least problematic for the woman and her fetus and are therefore the easiest to answer and to progress to questions about substances that are more problematic and therefore more difficult to answer; questions about caffeine, then alcohol and tobacco, and lastly illicit drugs such as cocaine should be asked.

III. Thinking Critically

1. Profiles of women at risk for postpartum depression: see Postpartum Psychologic Complications—Etiology and Risk Factors sections and Box 32-3 for the risk factors you will need to develop your profiles; be sure to use different risk factors for each profile.
2. Nursing diagnosis— risk for impaired parenting: see Psychiatric Hospitalization section, which discusses measures to facilitate maternal-infant attachment.
3. Discharge teaching plan related to postpartum depression: see Postpartum Psychologic Complications section, Box 32-3, and Teaching for Self-Management box—Activities to Prevent Postpartum Depression; outline should cover such topics as what postpartum depression is, why it can occur, risks for its occurrence, and signs to look for; woman and her family should be part of the teaching; handout should include the highlights of the teaching plan content along with who to contact, community agencies/supports, and Internet sites.
4. Woman suspected of cocaine use during pregnancy; see Cocaine and Methamphetamine section and Nursing Process box—Substance Abuse.
   A. Cite clinical manifestations associated with cocaine use: women on cocaine often appear euphoric, energetic, self-confident, sociable; psychotic symptoms as well as agitation and impaired judgment may be exhibited; vital signs may be altered and nasal changes can occur.
   B. Impact of use: discuss effect on woman and her fetus with special emphasis on increased risk for infections including blood-borne and circulatory changes.
   C. Assessment approach by the nurse (see Care Management—Screening); approach should be nonjudgmental ensuring privacy and confidentiality; begin by asking questions about the use of over-the-counter drugs and prescription drugs.
   D. Legal implications and barriers: see Barriers to Treatment and Legal Considerations sections and Legal Tip—Drug Testing During Pregnancy; answer should include the legal responsibilities of a nurse, the barriers facing the woman, and—very important—how you would try to break down these barriers so that this woman would be more receptive to entering a treatment program.
   E. Process of change and readiness for change: see Care Management—Substance Abuse During Pregnancy section.
      - See pregnancy as a window of opportunity for motivation to change.
      - Identify the steps a nurse should follow to identify women who are ready for change and the degree of readiness and supportive nursing interventions to facilitate change.
      - Identify problem with abuse and readiness for change (Prochaska-DiClemente model).
      - Use supportive interventions and motivational interviewing.
   F. Considerations when planning care.
      - Consider the characteristics of substance abusers, including depression related to negative life experiences (e.g., violence); substance abuse may serve as a means of relieving loneliness and emptiness; abusers may have grown up in an environment where abuse is common and have had little opportunity to learn sober living skills.
      - These characteristics can make change and recovery very difficult and interfere with their ability to be caring and nurturing parents; follow-up care is critical for safety of mother and the newborn.
      - Determine readiness for change and use measures that will facilitate change, including the window of opportunity for change that pregnancy presents.
   G. Nursing measures.
      - Assist with decreasing then stopping substance abuse; educate about effects of substances on pregnancy and fetus; be clear and confront if necessary; make referrals for treatment and to help woman deal with negative life experiences that may be contributing to the abuse of substances as a coping mechanism; assess progress and perform toxicology screens as indicated.
      - Recognize that ability to cope with childbirth may be limited; plan for toxicology screens of newborn.
      - Assess progress of maternal-newborn attachment and mother's level of knowledge and skill regarding newborn care; plan for discharge with the safety of the newborn of utmost importance; make arrangements for home visit follow-up and referral to services that will help mother to care for her baby and continue treatment; notify child protective services if indicated.

5. Woman with postpartum depression (see Postpartum Psychologic Complications section).
   A. Signs and symptoms indicative of postpartum depression: fatigue, concerned about being a good mother but has a low level of self-esteem and self-confidence regarding her effectiveness, expressed jealousy of her husband's seemingly greater enjoyment when spending time with baby than with her, and angry outbursts directed against husband (see Box 32-3).
   B. Predisposing factors: prenatal anxiety, meager social support and stressful life events (recent relocation, husband busy with new job, no friends locally), bottle feeding, mother unemployed and inexperienced with newborn care, 23 years of age.
   C. Questions: see Postpartum Psychologic complications—Care Management section and Box 32-3 to formulate questions related to risk factors for postpartum depression and also questions related to common manifestations; be sure to directly ask Mary about contemplating harm to self or baby; use open-ended questions that encourage full expression of feelings and thoughts.
   D. Nursing diagnoses: several nursing diagnoses are listed in the Nursing Process box and the Nursing Care Plan; at this point, fatigue, situational low self-esteem, ineffective individual coping, risk for impaired parenting seems to be paramount, but risk for violence toward self and infant is a critical ongoing nursing diagnosis, especially if postpartum depression is not identified and treated early.
   E. Measures to cope with postpartum depression: see Care Management—Nursing Care in the Home and Community section; include husband in discussions and planning, consider relationship with partner and suggest changes and resources they could seek out from their church and childrearing couples in their community; emphasize safety measures for mother or newborn; referral for psychiatric care with possible use of psychotropic/antidepressant medications if postpartum depression is determined to be moderate to severe; frequent follow-up to check progress is critical.
6. Principles to follow for providing care to women who abuse alcohol or drugs: see Substance Abuse during Pregnancy—Collaborative Care section for description of principles to follow; emphasize:
   - Family focus
   - Empowerment building
   - A community-based multidisciplinary approach with multiplicity of services; comprehensive, coordinated, holistic treatment
   - Continuum of care with consistent caregiver that allows for development of a trusting nonjudgmental relationship with health care provider and a mostly female staff

CHAPTER 33: LABOR AND BIRTH COMPLICATIONS

I. Learning Key Terms

1. Preterm labor
2. Preterm birth
3. Late preterm birth
4. Very preterm birth
5. Low birth weight (LBW)
6. Intrauterine growth restriction (IUGR)
7. Fetal fibronectins
8. Premature rupture of membranes (PROM)
9. Preterm premature rupture of membranes (PPROM)
10. Chorioamnionitis
11. Dystocia
12. Dysfunctional labor
13. Hypertonic uterine dysfunction, primary dysfunctional labor
14. Hypotonic uterine dysfunction, secondary uterine inertia
15. Pelvic dystocia
16. Soft tissue dystocia
17. Fetal dystocia
18. Macrosomia
19. Cephalopelvic disproportion (CPD), fetopelvic disproportion (FPD)
20. Occipitoposterior
21. Breech
22. Multifetal pregnancy
23. Prolonged latent phase
24. Protracted active phase
25. Secondary arrest
26. Protracted descent
27. Arrest of descent
28. Precipitous labor
29. External cephalic version (ECV)
30. Trial of labor
31. Induction of labor
32. Bishop score, dilation (cm), effacement (%), station (cm), cervical consistency, cervical position
33. Amniotomy
34. Augmentation of labor, oxytocin, amniotomy
35. Uterine tachysystole
36. Forceps-assisted birth
37. Vacuum-assisted birth; vacuum extraction
38. Cesarean birth
39. Postterm, postdate, dysmaturity syndrome
40. Shoulder dystocia, fetopelvic disproportion related to excessive fetal size (macrosomia), pelvic abnormalities
41. Prolapse of umbilical cord
42. Rupture of the uterus, trial of labor for attempted vaginal birth after cesarean (VBAC)
43. Amniotic fluid embolism (AFE); anaphylactoid syndrome of pregnancy

II. Reviewing Key Concepts

44. Identify factors associated with risk for spontaneous preterm labor and birth: use Box 33-1 and Predicting

Spontaneous Preterm Labor and Birth section to complete this activity.

45. Bed rest more harmful than helpful: see Activity Restriction section and Box 33-4.
    - Discuss the adverse effects of bed rest in terms of maternal physical and psychosocial effects and the effects on the woman's support system.
    - Cite the fact that there is no research evidence to support the effectiveness of bed rest in preventing preterm birth or decreasing preterm birth rates.
46. C 47. B 48. D 49. F 50. A 51. E 52. G
53. E 54. F 55. C 56. D 57. A 58. G 59. H 60. B
61. Five factors that cause dystocia: see Dystocia section and specific sections for each factor.
    - Powers: dysfunctional labor (ineffective uterine contractions or bearing-down efforts)
    - Passage: altered pelvic diameters/shape; soft tissue abnormality
    - Passenger: malpresentation or malposition, anomalies, size, number
    - Psychologic response of mother: past experiences, preparation, culture, support system, stress and anxiety level
    - Position of mother: ability and willingness to assume positions that facilitate uteroplacental perfusion and fetal descent
62. Therapeutic rest: see Hypertonic Uterine Dysfunction section.
    - Purpose: help woman experiencing hypertonic uterine dysfunction to rest/sleep so active labor can begin usually after a 4- to 6-hour rest period.
    - What: use of shower or warm bath for relaxation, comfort measures, administration of analgesics to inhibit contractions, reduce pain, and encourage rest/sleep and relaxation.
63. Compare and contrast hypertonic uterine dysfunction and hypotonic uterine dysfunction: see Dysfunctional Labor section, Nursing Process Box—Dystocia, and Table 33-1 for information related to each dysfunctional labor pattern in terms of causes/precipitating factors, maternal fetal effects, changes in labor progress, and care management.
64. Indications and contraindications for oxytocin induction of labor: see Box 33-8, where several indicators and contraindications for induction are listed.
65. Choices B, C, D, and E are correct; women who are underweight or overweight/obese, have high stress jobs, are members of the non-Hispanic black race, or have a history of preterm birth, multiple abortions, infections of the genitourinary tract, including UTIs and reproductive tract such as bacterial vaginosis, and bleeding in the second trimester are at increased risk for preterm labor and birth.
66. Choices A, C, D, and F are correct; weight loss, not gain, occurs and cardiac output is decreased.
67. Choice A is correct; magnesium sulfate is a CNS depressant; woman should alternate lateral positions to decrease pressure on cervix, which could stimulate uterine contractions; calcium gluconate would be used if toxicity occurs; infusion should be discontinued if respiratory rate is less than 12.
68. Choice C is correct; it is inserted into the posterior vaginal fornix; the woman should remain in bed for 2 hours; caution should be used if the woman has asthma; therefore, ensure that physician is aware; the insert is removed for severe side effects such as uterine tachysystole; dinoprostone (Cervidil) often stimulates contractions and may even induce the onset of labor, eliminating or reducing the need for oxytocin (Pitocin); it should be removed after 12 hours or with onset of active labor.
69. Choice D is correct; a Bishop score of 9 indicates that the cervix is already sufficiently ripe for successful induction; it is currently recommended that 30 units of oxytocin (Pitocin) be mixed in 500 ml of an electrolyte solution such as Ringer's lactate; the oxytocin solution is piggybacked at the proximal port (port nearest the insertion site).
70. Choice A is correct; uterine contractions should not occur more frequently than 5 uterine contractions in 10 minutes to allow for an adequate rest period between contractions; choices B, C, and D are all expected findings within the normal range.
71. Choice C is correct; the presentation of this fetus is breech; the soft buttocks are a less efficient dilating wedge than the fetal head; therefore, labor may be slower; the ultrasound transducer should be placed to the left of the umbilicus at a level at or above it; passage of meconium is an expected finding as a result of pressure on the abdomen during descent; knee-chest position would be used for occipitoposterior positions.
72. Choice D is correct; the dosage is correct at 12 mg × 2 doses; this medication will stimulate her baby's lungs to produce surfactant and help him or her to breathe more easily should birth occur; dosages should be spaced 24 hours apart; therefore, the next dose should be given at 11 AM the next day; tachycardia and hypotension are not effects of this medication.
73. Choice A is correct; the definitive sign of preterm labor is significant change in the cervix; while uterine contractions do occur they must occur at a frequency of more than six uterine contractions per hour and cause significant changes in the cervix; the pregnancy must be at 20 to 37 weeks of gestation.
74. Choices A, D, and E are correct; See Teaching for Self-Management box—What to Do if Symptoms of Preterm Labor Occur.
75. Choice C is correct; although A, B, and D are appropriate actions along with changes in her position, removing pressure from the cord to preserve perfusion is the priority. (see Emergency box—Prolapsed Umbilical Cord).

III. Thinking Critically

1. Preterm labor and birth prevention program: see Predicting Spontaneous Preterm Labor and Birth and Prevention and Early Recognition and Diagnosis sections.

- Why: preterm birth is a major factor contributing to perinatal morbidity and mortality; early detection is critical for successful tocolysis and antenatal glucocorticoid therapy.
- Many risk factors for preterm labor have been identified (Boxes 33-1 and 33-2), but risk scoring systems miss many women who go into preterm labor.
- All women should be taught signs of preterm labor and measures to prevent based on risk factors identified that can be manipulated by changes in lifestyle behaviors (see Box 33-3).

2. Woman with a history of preterm labor and birth.
   A. Identify signs of preterm labor: see Box 33-3 as a guide for teaching Sara about preterm labor; see if Sara can retrospectively remember experiencing these vague signs with her first pregnancy.
   B. Implementation of plan to prevent preterm labor.
      - Evaluate Sara's lifestyle for risky behaviors and health history for risk factors for preterm labor.
      - Discuss how certain factors identified could be changed to reduce her risk, especially related to lifestyle (see Lifestyle Modifications section).
      - Consider modification of sexual activity, stress level, activity (work, home), and hygiene (prevent genitourinary [GU] tract infections).
   C. Criteria for use of tocolysis: assess Sara to make sure that she is indeed in labor and that she does not exhibit contraindications to tocolysis (see Suppression of Uterine Activity section and Box 33-5).
   D. Nursing measures during magnesium sulfate infusion to suppress preterm labor: see Box 33-6, Suppression of Uterine Activity section, and Medication Guide, Tocolytic Therapy for Preterm Labor.
      - Assess for labor progress and maternal-fetal responses to magnesium sulfate.
      - Monitor and regulate infusion following protocol for increments in dosage of magnesium sulfate.
      - Measure intake and output.
      - Provide support and encouragement.
      - Maintain bed rest in lateral position.
   E. Administration of betamethasone: see Promotion of Fetal Lung Maturity section.
      1. Purpose: stimulation of fetal surfactant production.
      2. Protocol: see Medication Guide, Antenatal Glucocorticoid Therapy; assess Sara for signs of infection and pulmonary edema, explain action and indications for use, administer IM deep into gluteal muscle, 12 mg, twice, 24 hours apart, observe for adverse effects.
3. Woman experiencing preterm labor discharged to home care (see Suppression of Uterine Activity and Home Care sections and Nursing Care Plan).
   A. Teach her how to take the medication, how the medication works, and the side effects of nifedipine (Procardia) to watch for and whom to call if they should appear; teach her how to assess her vital signs, especially how to assess her blood pressure.
   B. Side effects of nifedipine: see Medication Guide, Tocolytic Therapy for Preterm Labor, which lists signs that should be taught to the client.
   C. Instructions regarding palpating uterine activity: discuss how often to monitor (once or twice a day while lying on side); teach her how to palpate abdomen for uterine contractions: palpate over fundus where uterine contractions are most intense to determine characteristics and then palpate over entire uterus to determine generalized tone; tell her what activity could indicate preterm labor and who to call.
   D. Coping with bed rest/activity restriction: see Home Care section, Teaching for Self-Management box—Suggested Activities for Children of Women on Activity Restriction, and Figure 33-2; identify the members of her support system and include them in discussions of how bed rest/activity limitations will be managed and how they can help; make referrals to home care agencies if needed.
4. Woman with occipitoposterior position and difficulty bearing down (see Dystocia—Fetal Causes—Malposition section and Box 33-7).
   A. Identifying factors that have a negative effect on bearing-down efforts: amount of analgesia/anesthesia used, exhaustion, maternal position, lack of knowledge about how to push effectively, lack of sleep, inadequate food and fluid intake.
   B. Measures to facilitate bearing-down efforts: coach her in BDE, help her into an appropriate position, apply counterpressure to sacrum, demonstrate open-glottis pushing and coach her efforts with every contraction, help her to begin pushing when Ferguson reflex is perceived; reduce epidural medication to a minimum effective dose.
   C. Recommended positions: hand-and-knees or lateral position on the same side as the fetal back when the fetus is in an occipitoposterior position can be very effective in facilitating internal rotation and reducing back pain (see Box 33-7 for many additional techniques).
5. Emergency cesarean birth (see Cesarean Birth section).
   A. Preoperative measures (see Preoperative Care section): implement typical preoperative care measures as for any major surgery in a calm

and professional manner, explaining the purpose of each measure that must be performed; use a family-centered approach; discuss what will happen; witness an informed consent; assess fetal-maternal unit, insert Foley catheter, start or maintain IV infusion, provide emotional support.

B. Immediate postoperative measures: see Immediate Postoperative Care section; assess for signs of hemorrhage, pain level, respiratory effort, renal function, circulatory status to extremities, signs of postanesthesia recovery, emotional status, and attachment/reaction to newborn.

C. Ongoing postoperative care measures: see Postoperative or Postpartum Care section, Teaching for Self-Management boxes: Postpartum Pain Relief After Cesarean Birth, and Signs of Postoperative Complications After Discharge Following Cesarean Birth; measures include assessment of recovery, pain relief, coughing and deep breathing, leg exercises and assistance with ambulation, nutrition and fluid intake (oral, IV); provide opportunities for interaction with and care of newborn, assisting her as needed; provide emotional support to help her deal with her disappointment and feelings of failure; help her and her family prepare for discharge making referrals as needed.

D. Nursing diagnosis: situational low self-esteem related to inability to reach goal of a vaginal birth secondary to occurrence of fetal distress.
- Discuss and review why Anne needed a cesarean birth, how she performed during labor, and that she had no control over the fetal distress.
- Discuss vaginal birth after cesarean (VBAC) and likelihood of it being an option because the reason for her primary cesarean (fetal distress) may not occur again; discuss trial of labor next time to determine her ability to proceed to vaginal birth.
- Use follow-up phone calls to assess progress in accepting cesarean birth.

6. Fetal position/presentation—RSA: see Dystocia—Malpresentation section; right sacrum anterior (RSA) indicates a breech presentation; consider that descent may be slower, meconium is often expelled, increasing danger of meconium aspiration, and risk for cord prolapse is increased; depending on progress of labor and maternal characteristics, cesarean or vaginal birth may occur or external cephalic version (ECV) may be attempted.

7. Induction of labor (see Induction of Labor section and Box 33-8).

A. Bishop score: see Table 33-3 for factors assessed to determine degree of cervical ripening in preparation for labor process; it is used to determine if a cervical ripening method will need to be used to increase the chances of a successful labor induction.

B. Score of 5 for a nulliparous woman: her score should be greater than 9 to ensure a successful induction; a score of 5 indicates a cervix that is not fully ripe; therefore, cervical ripening will be needed before induction to enhance its success.

C. Administration of dinoprostone (Cervidil): see Cervical Ripening Methods section and Medication Guide Prostaglandin E_2 for guidelines for use and adverse reactions; consider how and where it is inserted, protocol to follow after the insertion, and adverse reactions and what to do if they occur.

D. Amniotomy: see Amniotomy section and Procedure box—Assisting with Amniotomy; explain what will happen, how it will feel, and why it is being done; assess maternal-fetal unit before and after the procedure; document findings; support woman during procedure telling her what is happening; document procedure and outcomes/reactions appropriately.

E. Induction protocol (see Medication Guide—Oxytocin [Pitocin]).
1. A 2. A 3. A 4. NA 5. A
6. NA 7. NA 8. A 9. NA 10. A
11. NA

F. Major side effects of oxytocin (Pitocin) induction: tachysystole, uterine rupture, nonreassuring FHR patterns, abruptio placentae.

G. Actions if uterine tachysystole occurs: see Emergency box—Uterine Tachysystole with Oxytocin, which lists signs related to uterine contractions and abnormal (nonreassuring) FHR patterns as well as immediate interventions such as discontinuing the induction, maintaining the primary infusion of fluid, turning the woman onto her side, administering oxygen via face mask, monitoring response of maternal-fetal unit to actions, notifying primary health care provider, and preparing for possible administration of terbutaline to suppress contractions.

8. Postterm pregnancy (see Postterm Pregnancy, Labor, and Birth section).

A. Maternal-fetal risks related to postterm pregnancy: see Maternal-Fetal Risks section; maternal risk relates to excessive size of fetus and hardness of fetal skull, which increases risk for dystocia; fetal risk relates to postmaturity syndrome as the placenta ages and a stressful prolonged labor and birth process, including increased risk for birth injury and neonatal hypoglycemia; macrosomia can result in shoulder dystocia and maternal/fetal birth injury.

B. Clinical manifestations: maternal weight loss, decrease in uterine size, meconium in amniotic fluid, advanced fetal bone maturation including the skull.

C. Care measures to ensure safety of maternal-fetal unit: see Care Management section.
   - Continue prenatal care with more frequent visits.
   - Antepartal assessments, including daily fetal movement counts, NST, amniotic fluid volume assessments, BPP, CST, Doppler blood flow measurements, cervical checks for ripening.
   - Emotional support.
   - Prepare for cervical ripening, induction of labor, monitoring for late and variable deceleration patterns, amnioinfusion, forceps- or vacuum-assisted or cesarean birth.

D. Instructions for self-care at home: see Teaching for Self-Management box—Postterm Pregnancy.
   - Make sure Lora knows how to assess fetal movements and signs of labor.
   - Emphasize importance of keeping all appointments for prenatal care and antepartal assessments.
   - Identify whom to call with concerns, questions, and reports of changing status such as onset of labor or change in fetal movement pattern.

CHAPTER 34: POSTPARTUM COMPLICATIONS

I. Learning Key Terms

1. Postpartum hemorrhage (PPH), early (acute, primary), late (secondary)
2. Uterine atony
3. Perineal lacerations
4. Hematoma, vulva hematomas
5. Placenta accreta
6. Placenta increta
7. Placenta percreta
8. Inversion of the uterus
9. Subinvolution, retained placental fragments, pelvic infection
10. Hemorrhagic (hypovolemic) shock
11. Coagulopathy
12. Thrombocytopenia
13. Idiopathic (immune) thrombocytopenic purpura (ITP)
14. von Willebrand disease
15. Thrombosis
16. Thrombophlebitis
17. Superficial venous thrombosis
18. Deep venous thrombosis
19. Pulmonary embolism
20. Postpartum (puerperal) infection
21. Endometritis
22. Mastitis

II. Reviewing Key Concepts

23. Twofold focus of management of hemorrhagic shock: see Hemorrhagic (Hypovolemic) Shock—Medical Management section; restore circulating blood volume and perfusion and treat the cause of the hemorrhage.
24. Standard of care for bleeding emergencies: see Hemorrhagic (Hypovolemic) Shock—Legal Tip section for a description of the standard of care that focuses on provisions made for the nurse to implement actions independently and establishment of policies, procedures, standing orders or protocols, and clinical guidelines; the nurse should never leave the client alone.
25. Choice B is correct; although BP should be taken before and after administration of Methylergonovine (Methergine), the woman's hypertensive status would be a contraindicating factor for its use, especially if administered parenterally—therefore, the order should be questioned; a more appropriate choice would be oxytocin (Pitocin); Methergine should not be given if the BP is greater than 140/90.
26. Choice D is correct; 15-methylprostaglandin F_{2a} (Hemabate) is a powerful prostaglandin that is given to treat excessive uterine blood loss or hemorrhage related to uterine atony; it has no action related to pain, infection, or clotting.
27. Choice A is correct; puerperal infections are infections of the genital tract after birth; pulse will increase, not decrease, in response to fever; B and C will also occur but are not the first signs exhibited.
28. Choices C and F are correct; heparin and warfarin are safe for use by breastfeeding women; heparin, usually administered intravenously for the first 3 to 5 days, is the anticoagulant of choice during the acute stage of DVT; after acute phase, warfarin (Coumadin) is begun orally; woman should be fitted for elastic stockings after the acute stage is past when edema subsides; the woman should be encouraged to change her position when on bed rest.

III. Thinking Critically

1. Postpartum woman at risk for postpartum hemorrhage: see PPH section.
   A. Risk factors for early postpartum hemorrhage: see Etiology and Risk Factors and Uterine Atony sections and Box 34-1; discuss increased likelihood for uterine atony as a result of parity (6-5-1-0-7), vaginal full-term twin birth 1 hour ago, hypotonic uterine dysfunction treated with oxytocin (Pitocin), use of forceps for birth, increased manipulation with birth of twins; increased size and stretch of uterus with a multiple gestation.
   B. Nursing diagnosis (see Nursing Process Box and Nursing Care Plan for Postpartum Hemorrhage): risk for deficient fluid volume related to moderate to heavy blood loss associated with vaginal birth of twins.
   C. Nurse's response to excessive blood loss in 15 minutes: see Medical Management and Nursing Interventions sections; most common cause of the excessive blood loss 1 hour after birth would

be uterine atony, especially because woman exhibits several risk factors; discuss each of the following with rationale for action.
- Assess fundus; massage as the priority action.
- Express clots.
- Check bladder for distension and perineum for swelling; ask woman about experiencing perineal pressure.

D. Guidelines for administering oxytocin (Pitocin) IV: use Medication Guide—Drugs Used to Manage Postpartum Hemorrhage in explaining guidelines for administration in terms of dose/route, side effects, nursing management, including assessment and maternal support.

E. Signs of developing hemorrhagic (hypovolemic) shock: see Hemorrhagic (Hypovolemic) Shock section and Emergency box—Hemorrhagic Shock, which identifies the priority assessment a nurse should perform and the findings that would indicate progress from hemorrhage to shock; assessment includes VS, skin, urinary output, level of consciousness, and mental status; assessment should be frequent and findings compared to one another to note change.

F. Nursing measures to support the woman and family: see Nursing Interventions section, Nursing Process box, and Nursing Care Plan for Postpartum Hemorrhage.
- Explain progress.
- Discuss physiologic care; consider approach to take and organization of care.
- Comfort and support measures.
- Opportunities for interaction with newborn.

2. Puerperal infection: see Postpartum Infection section.
   A. Risk factors: see Box 34-4; consider preconception, antepartal, and intrapartal factors.
   B. Infection prevention measures: see Care Management section; emphasize measures to maintain resistance to infection. (nutrition, rest, hygiene); use of Standard Precautions including handwashing, proper use of gloves, and care of equipment; teach woman about prevention measures including genital hygiene and safer sex practices.
   C. Typical signs of endometritis: see Endometritis section for a description of typical clinical manifestations to guide assessment.
   D. Nursing diagnoses (see Box 34-5): acute pain related to effects of infection in uterine tissue; interrupted family process *or* anxiety *or* ineffective individual or family coping related to unexpected postpartum complication (use assessment findings to determine priority psychosocial nursing diagnoses).
   E. Nursing measures: see Care Management section, which discusses many nursing interventions for each nursing diagnosis identified.
3. Woman with mastitis: see Mastitis section.
   A. Assessment findings associated with mastitis: see Mastitis for typical signs this woman would exhibit.
   B. Nursing diagnoses: acute pain related to inflammation of right breast associated with mastitis; ineffective breastfeeding *or* anxiety related to interruption of breastfeeding while taking antibiotics or related to concerns regarding transmission of infection to newborn.
   C. Treatment measures; see Care Management section for several measures, including medications used including antibiotic therapy, local applications to enhance comfort, breast support, adequate hydration and nutrition, and pumping of breasts to maintain lactation if breastfeeding is prohibited because of medications being used for treatment.
   D. Measures to prevent recurrence of mastitis: see Care Management section; focus on good breastfeeding techniques, breast care to maintain integrity of areolae and nipples, early detection and treatment of cracks, and cleanliness including strict hand hygiene measures.
4. Woman with deep vein thrombosis: see Thromboembolic Disease section.
   A. Risk factors: see Incidence and Etiology section; in addition to venous stasis and hypercoagulability of pregnancy continuing into the postpartum period, other risk factors for this woman would be cesarean birth, obesity, age over 35 years, multiparity, and smoking.
   B. Signs and symptoms indicative of DVT: see Clinical Manifestations section for a description of typical clinical manifestations.
   C. Nursing diagnosis: anxiety related to unexpected development of a postpartum complication.
   D. Expected care management: see Medical Management and Nursing Interventions sections; discuss what should be included in each of the following sections of your outline: assessment, anticoagulant therapy, activity level, pain management, leg support, reassurance that breastfeeding is safe, emotional support, assistance with care of self and newborn.
   E. Discharge instructions.
      - How to assess leg and assess for signs of unusual bleeding; proper use of elastic/support stockings.
      - How to take anticoagulant safely and importance of follow-up to assess progress.
      - Practices to prevent bleeding while taking an anticoagulant and importance of avoiding pregnancy because warfarin is teratogenic.

CHAPTER 35: ACQUIRED PROBLEMS OF THE NEWBORN

I. Learning Key Terms

1. Birth trauma (birth injury)
2. Subconjunctival (scleral and retinal) hemorrhages
3. Ecchymoses
4. Petechiae
5. Clavicle

6. Erb-Duchenne palsy, brachial plexus injury
7. Renal agenesis
8. Caudal regression syndrome
9. Macrosomia
10. Phosphatidylglycerol
11. Hypoglycemia
12. Cardiomyopathy
13. Polycythemia, hyperbilirubinemia
14. Sepsis
15. Septicemia
16. Septic shock
17. Eye prophylaxis
18. Condylomata
19. Snuffles
20. Highly active antiretroviral therapy (HAART)
21. Opportunistic infection
22. Parvovirus B19
23. Group B streptococci
24. Listeriosis
25. Thrush
26. Fetal alcohol syndrome (FAS)
27. Neonatal abstinence syndrome

II. Reviewing Key Concepts

28. Common congenital anomalies experienced by infants of women with diabetes: see Infants of Diabetic Mothers—Congenital Anomalies section for the identification of anomalies in each category.
29. Infections represented by TORCH: see Transplacental Infections section and Box 35-1 for infections represented by each letter.
30. Sepsis: see Neonatal Infections section.
    A. Modes of transmission of infection: see Sepsis and Care Management sections for a review of prenatal, perinatal, and postnatal transmission modes.
    B. Risk factors: see Care Management section and Table 35-2, which lists risk factors according to maternal, intrapartum, and neonatal sources.
    C. Signs of sepsis exhibited by neonate: see Table 35-3 and Care Management section for a list of signs according to body systems.
    D. Effective nursing measures: see appropriate sections for Preventive Measures and Curative Measures in the Care Management section.
31. Choice B is correct; findings are consistent with a bone fracture, in this case the clavicle.
32. Choices B, C, and F are correct; macrosomic infants are at increased risk for hypoglycemia (e.g., a blood glucose level of 38 mg/dl would be considered hypoglycemia); hypocalcemia is also common; fracture and trauma are more common in the upper body such as the humerus and clavicle; the newborn of a pregestational diabetic mother is more likely to experience congenital anomalies such as heart defects; there is no increased risk over the general population with gestational diabetes; the complexion is characteristically plethoric or flushed.
33. Choice A is correct; the second dose is given at one month and the third at 6 months.
34. Choice B is correct; isolation is not required and breastfeeding is contraindicated because of the potential for viral transmission; the nurse should be using Standard Precautions as would be used with all clients; HAART is used to prevent transmission of HIV—the chance of this newborn becoming HIV positive is very low because the mother was treated during pregnancy.
35. Choices B, D, E, and F are correct; signs of abstinence syndrome also include little sleep, tachypnea, jitteriness, hyperactivity, shrill cry, vomiting.

III. Thinking Critically

1. Birth Trauma: see Birth Trauma section.
    A. Risk factors for trauma: see Birth Trauma section for a discussion of maternal and fetal factors and intrapartum techniques that predispose a newborn to birth injury.
    B. Approach to reduce birth injuries; consider an approach that facilitates labor progress including maternal movement, comfort measures, and support.
    C. Signs of fractured clavicle: see Skeletal Injuries section; signs include limited motion of arm and absence of Moro reflex on affected side, crepitus over the bone.
    D. Treatment: there is no accepted standard treatment; care is limited to gently handling and supporting shoulder when changing clothes and moving and proper alignment; alert caregivers and parents regarding need for special handling; support and reassure parents.
2. Macrosomic infant: see Neonatal Complications—Macrosomia section.
    A. Pathophysiologic basis for macrosomia: discuss the effect of fetal insulin secretion in response to maternal blood glucose levels during pregnancy; discuss the rationale for frequent monitoring of the baby's blood glucose levels until stabilized after birth; it also is important to discuss the importance of good nutrition patterns, exercise habits, and maintaining a normal BMI for herself and the rest of her family including her new baby. She is at risk for type 2 diabetes as are her children.
    B. Characteristics: see Macrosomia section and Fig. 35-6, which describes several characteristics that can be noted with assessment of the newborn.
    C. Hypoglycemia, hypocalcemia, polycythemia/hyperviscosity, hyperbilirubinemia
    D. Warning signs of potential complications: see section for each complication identified in answer for **C**.
3. Newborn whose mother is hepatitis B positive: see Hepatitis B virus section.
    A. Protocol for newborn care: discuss use of hepatitis B immunoglobulin and hepatitis B vaccine, including when and how to administer.
    B. Safety of breastfeeding: it is safe to breastfeed after the infant has been cleansed and the

vaccine and immunoglobulin have been administered.

4. Newborn whose mother has active herpes at the time of birth: see Herpes Simplex Virus section.
   A. Four modes of transmission: transplacental, ascending by way of birth canal, direct contamination during passage through birth canal (mode for this baby), and direct transmission to the newborn by an infected person.
   B. Clinical signs of active infection in the newborn: see HSV section for signs of infection in each category.
   C. Recommended nursing measures related to: see Care Management section.
      - Management after birth, prior to discharge: discuss assessment measures including inspection of eyes, oral cavity, and skin for lesions, infection control measures including use of gloves when appropriate, specimen collection for culture with evaluation of results as criteria for discharge, and appropriateness of breastfeeding.
      - Vidarabine therapy: discuss how and why it is used and for how long.
5. Newborn whose mother is HIV positive: see HIV/AIDS section.
   A. Potential for newborn infection: there is a 12% to 40% risk for transmission of the mother was not treated during pregnancy; the risk is reduced to 1% to 2% if she was treated.
   B. Strategies to prevent transmission: universal HIV testing, HAART treatment during pregnancy, labor, and to the newborn for 6 weeks, elective cesarean section, and avoiding breastfeeding.
   C. Testing protocol: discuss tests used and time performed as well as factors that can influence test accuracy.
   D. Opportunistic infections: common infections can include *Pneumocystis jiroveci* pneumonia, candidiasis, CMV infection, cryptosporidiosis, herpes simplex or herpes zoster, disseminated varicella.
   E. Care measures: discuss use of Standard Precautions, cleansing of skin, antimicrobial and immunization administration—also counseling, referrals, and follow-up care.
   F. Breastfeeding safety: because breast milk can contain the virus, the newborn should not be breastfed; teach mother how to bottle feed and demonstrate how she can have close contact with her newborn during feeding; discuss risk breastfeeding poses citing statistics; inform the mother about the safe use of immunizations for her newborn.
6. Infant with thrush: see Fungal Infection—Candidiasis section.
   A. Signs: white adherent patches on mucosa, gums, and tongue that bleed when touched.
   B. Modes of transmission: maternal vaginal infection during birth, person-to-person contact, contaminated hands, bottles, nipples, or other articles.
   C. Management: discuss assessment of mother for signs of fungal infection, use of standard precautions/infection control measures, cleanliness, measures to improve resistance to infection, and procedure for administration of an antifungal preparation, discuss treatment of infant (mouth) and mother (e.g., breasts) together.
7. Newborn with fetal alcohol syndrome—FAS: see Substance Abuse—Alcohol section.
   A. Typical characteristics: see Box 35-2 and Figure 35-12 for a full description of the newborn diagnosed with FAS.
   B. Long-term effects: several are described in the Alcohol section, including those related to learning behaviors and fine motor dysfunction; also increased incidence of congenital anomalies.
   C. Nursing measures: see Alcohol and Care Management sections for several ideas; involve parents in care of newborn, encouraging attachment; teach parents what to expect about their child's behavior; help the parents to create a warm and caring home environment that enhances development; make appropriate referrals to community services for the newborn as well as treatment program for the mother to help her with her alcohol abuse problem (father may also need assistance).
8. Effect of maternal abuse of cocaine on the newborn: see Substance Abuse section.
   A. Effect of cocaine exposure: see Box 35-3 for list of neonatal effects in terms of physical and behavioral assessment findings.
   B. Care of newborn and mother: see Cocaine and Care Management section for a discussion of supportive care for the newborn and counseling for the mother; ensure she is able to care for her newborn independently, making referrals as needed.
9. Newborn of mother suspected of abusing drugs during pregnancy (see Heroin and Care Management sections Nursing Care Plan for Infant Experiencing Withdrawal), and Fig. 35-13.
   A. Signs of neonatal abstinence syndrome: see Table 35-5 for a list of signs in terms of respiratory, neurologic, gastrointestinal function, and autonomic dysfunction
   B. Nursing diagnoses: deficient fluid volume related to inadequate fluid intake and increased fluid loss associated with heroin withdrawal; disorganized infant behavior *or* disturbed sleep pattern related to withdrawal from heroin; risk for infection related to risky maternal behaviors associated with drug abuse.

C. Care management: encourage parent participation in care of newborn providing education and social support as needed; maintain nutrition, fluid, and electrolyte balance with careful management of feeding; infection control and respiratory care; swaddling and holding; stimuli reduction; pharmacologic treatment as appropriate; discharge planning and referral.

CHAPTER 36: HEMOLYTIC DISORDERS AND CONGENITAL ANOMALIES

I. Learning Key Terms

1. Hyperbilirubinemia
2. Jaundice (icterus), physiologic, pathologic
3. Rh incompatibility (isoimmunization)
4. Maternal sensitization
5. Fetal hemolytic anemia
6. Erythroblastosis fetalis
7. Hydrops fetalis
8. Acute bilirubin encephalopathy
9. Kernicterus
10. Indirect Coombs' test
11. Direct Coombs' test
12. Congenital
13. Inborn errors of metabolism
14. Microcephaly
15. Hypospadias
16. Epispadias
17. Exstrophy of the bladder
18. Hydrocephalus
19. Congenital heart defects
20. Talipes equinovarus
21. Choanal atresia
22. Spina bifida
23. Spinal bifida occulta
24. Meningocele (spina bifida manifesta)
25. Omphalocele
26. Gastroschisis
27. Esophageal atresia
28. Tracheoesophageal fistula
29. Imperforate anus
30. Developmental dysplasia of the hip (DDH)
31. Encephalocele
32. Anencephaly
33. Congenital diaphragmatic hernia
34. Myelomeningocele (spina bifida manifesta)
35. Cleft lip or palate
36. Ambiguous genitalia
37. Hydramnios (polyhydramnios)
38. Oligohydramnios
39. Cytogenic studies
40. Dermatoglyphics

II. Reviewing Key Concepts

41. Physiologic basis for ABO incompatibility: see Hemolytic Disease of the Newborn—ABO Incompatibility section for an explanation of the pathophysiology.
42. Congenital anomalies.
    A. Assessment techniques/considerations guiding prenatal diagnosis: see Care Management—Prenatal Diagnosis section for an overview of techniques that are commonly used for diagnosis during the prenatal period.
    B. Observations of amount of amniotic fluid: see Care Management—Perinatal Diagnosis section; hydramnios (polyhydramnios) and oligohydramnios are associated with congenital anomalies; a thorough assessment of newborn is indicated if either amniotic fluid abnormality is found to be present.
    C. Specific types of postnatal tests for diagnosis of congenital anomalies: see specific sections for each type of test in Postnatal Diagnosis section.
    - Newborn screening: testing for inborn errors of metabolism.
    - Cytogenetic studies: chromosomal examination to confirm suggestive but not diagnostic clinical appearance.
    - Dermatoglyphics: study of the pattern of ridges in the skin of the hands, digits, and feet.
43. Congenital heart defects: see Cardiovascular System Anomalies section.
    A. Maternal factors associated with higher risk: several factors are discussed in this section including rubella, alcohol intake, certain medications, tobacco use, and maternal age.
    B. Four physiologic classifications; include one example of each: see Table 36-1 for the list of classifications with some examples of each.
    C. Signs that could indicate CHD: discuss characteristics of cry, color of skin (e.g., cyanosis and when it occurs), activity level (e.g., restless, lethargic, responsiveness) and effect of activity such as crying, feeding, and stooling on color and breathing, VS, respiratory status.
44. Choice B is correct; at 16 mg/dl the serum bilirubin exceeds the 15 mg/dl limit on the second day of life; other signs of pathologic hyperbilirubinemia include serum bilirubin concentration in cord blood >4 mg/dl, increase of >5 mg/dl in 24 hours, and appearance of jaundice within the first 24 hours after birth.
45. Choice D is correct; RhoGAM should be administered intramuscularly to the mother within 72 hours of birth; pathologic jaundice is unlikely because Coombs' test results indicate that antibodies have not been formed to destroy the newborn's RBCs; RhoGAM is given to prevent formation of antibodies; it would not be given if antibodies have already been formed as indicated by positive Coombs' test results.
46. Choice B is correct; kneeling or prone position prevents pressure on the sac that could cause damage; sterile, moist nonadherent dressings are used to protect the cord; a drape should be placed over the buttocks below the lesion—diapers are not used.

III. Thinking Critically

1. Pathologic jaundice (see Hyperbilirubinemia section).
   A. Contrast pathologic and physiologic jaundice: see Physiologic and Pathologic sections for information regarding onset, resolution, and serum bilirubin levels to complete the comparison.
   B. Physiologic process that leads to hyperbilirubinemia: see Hyperbilirubinemia section; discuss the effect of RBC destruction including the number of RBCs and the speed at which they are destroyed.
   C. Potential causes for pathologic jaundice: see Pathologic Jaundice section and Box 36-2 for a list of maternal causes and fetal/newborn causes.
   D. Effective prevention measures: see Hyperbilirubinemia—Care Management section; measures are described; fully discuss.
      - Identification of mother and newborn at risk and institute appropriate measures; determine maternal blood type and RH factor early in pregnancy.
      - Prevention of and prompt therapy for asphyxia, acidosis, sepsis, cold stress, hypoglycemia.
      - Administration of RhoGAM promptly; take note of any potential for sensitization during pregnancy if the woman is Rh negative (e.g., postamniocentesis).
      - Promotion of early feeding to stimulate stooling and thereby removal of bilirubin.
2. Pregnant woman who is Rh negative (see Hyperbilirubinemia section).
   A. Physiologic basis: see Rh Incompatibility section; if an Rh-negative mother's blood comes into contact with the blood of her Rh-positive fetus, she will form antibodies against Rh-positive blood that can then be transferred via the placenta to the fetus; if a fetus is Rh positive, the presence of these antibodies in its bloodstream will result in destruction of its RBCs (hemolysis).
   B. Meaning of a positive indirect Coombs' test: indicates that the woman has formed antibodies, probably as a result of her miscarriage and not receiving RhoGAM to prevent antibody formation.
   C. Candidate to receive RhoGAM: woman is not a candidate because RhoGAM cannot be given once antibodies or sensitization has occurred.
   D. RhoGAM purpose and use: prevents sensitization by injecting passive antibodies against the Rh factor that will destroy any fetal RBCs that may have entered maternal circulation before the maternal immune system is activated; Rh-negative mothers who are indirect Coombs' negative should receive RhoGAM after an abortion, after specific invasive tests such as CVS and amniocentesis, during the third trimester, and within 72 hours after the birth of an Rh-positive, direct Coombs'-negative newborn.
   E. Newborn complications: see Rh Incompatibility section, in which both erythroblastosis fetalis and hydrops fetalis are described.
   F. Prevention of perinatal mortality: regular pregnancy testing to check bilirubin levels, anemia, and antibody titers; intrauterine transfusions and early birth if the Rh antibody titer rises to dangerous levels and bilirubin is increasing'
3. Care management of newborn born with myelomeningocele: see CNS Anomalies—Spina Bifida section.
   - Preoperative and postoperative measures, including how to position newborn to protect the site, assessment of neurologic function, prevent trauma, rupture, and infection of the site, site care.
   - Parental support, including facilitate attachment process, provide information and emotional care, prepare for surgical interventions, make referrals for long-term care for parents and child to help them adjust to and cope with the effects of the congenital anomaly.
4. Newborn with a diaphragmatic hernia: see Respiratory System Anomalies—Congenital Diaphragmatic Hernia section.
   A. Clinical manifestations exhibited are influenced by the degree of the defect : respiratory distress which worsens as intestine fills with air, diminished breath sounds, cyanosis, heart sounds in the right chest, low blood pressure, barrel-shaped chest with flat/scaphoid abdomen, bowel in the chest.
   B. Nursing diagnosis: impaired gas exchange related to inability to fully expand lungs associated with diaphragmatic hernia.
   C. Care measures in immediate postbirth period.
      - Position: head and chest elevated, affected side down to allow normal lung to fully expand.
      - Aspirate gastric contents to decompress gastrointestinal tract.
      - Oxygen therapy, mechanical ventilation, and correction of acidosis.
5. Newborn with cleft lip and palate: see Gastrointestinal System Anomalies—Cleft Lip and Palate section.
   A. Nursing diagnoses: imbalanced nutrition: less than body requirements, risk for ineffective airway clearance, risk for impaired parent-infant attachment; all of these are related to defective and incomplete development of the lip and palate.
   B. Nursing measures.
      - Maintain airway patency while ensuring adequate hydration and nutrition using devices that prevent passage of milk into airway.

- Support and facilitate parental attachment to infant and skill with feeding; prepare parents for discharge.
- Explain the condition, how it occurs, what it entails, and how and when it will be repaired.
- Refer to support group.

CHAPTER 37: NURSING CARE OF THE HIGH RISK NEWBORN

I. Learning Key Terms

1. Low-birth-weight (LBW)
2. Very low-birth weight (VLBW)
3. Extremely low-birth-weight (ELBW)
4. Premature, preterm
5. Late preterm
6. Full term
7. Postmature, postterm
8. Large for gestational age (LGA)
9. Appropriate for gestational age (AGA)
10. Small for date (SFD) or small for gestational age (SGA)
11. Intrauterine growth restriction (IUGR)
12. Symmetric IUGR
13. Asymmetric IUGR
14. Live birth
15. Fetal death
16. Neonatal death
17. Perinatal mortality
18. Periodic breathing
19. Apnea
20. Oscillometry (Dinamap)
21. Neutral thermal environment
22. Surfactant
23. Insensible water loss (IWL)
24. Gavage feeding
25. Gastrostomy tube feeding
26. Nonnutritive sucking
27. Kangaroo care
28. Polycythemia

II. Reviewing Key Concepts

29. Identify physiologic problems of the preterm newborn: physiologic functions and potential problems are discussed in specific sections of Preterm Infant—Physiologic Function section.
30. B 31.F 32. C 33. A 34. G 35. D 36. E
37. Comparing needs of late preterm and full-term newborns: see Late Preterm Infants and Postmature Infants sections and Table 37-3 to complete your comparison.
38. Choices B, D, and E are correct; retractions, nasal flaring, and expiratory grunting reflect increased effort and work to breathe; choices A, C, and F are all expected findings consistent with efficient respiratory effort in the preterm newborn.
39. Choice B is correct; although choices A, C, and D are appropriate and important, respiration with adequate gas exchange takes precedence, especially because adequate surfactant is not produced before 32 weeks of gestation.
40. Choices A, B, E, and F are correct; air, not sterile water, is used to check placement before feeding; because newborns are nose breathers, the mouth is the preferred route for insertion unless the infant is unable to tolerate. (see Procedure box—Inserting a Gavage Feeding Tube and Fig. 37-6).
41. Choices A, B, and F are correct; see Table 37-2 for normal arterial gas values for neonates.
42. Choice D is correct; monitoring vital signs is an assessment measure; cleansing the skin and teaching parents are important but not the single most important action; hand hygiene practiced by everyone in contact with the preternm newborn is critical.
43. Choices B, C, E, and F are correct; acrocyanosis and periodic breathing patterns are expected findings but central cyanosis and apnea reflect hypothermia.

III. Thinking Critically

1. Oxygen therapy for the newborn experiencing respiratory distress: see Respiratory Function and Oxygen Therapy sections.
   A. Criteria to determine need for oxygen include increased effort to breathe, respiratory distress with apnea, tachycardia or bradycardia, central cyanosis, Pao_2 less than 60 mm Hg, oxygen saturation less than 92%.
   B. Guidelines for safe and effective administration of oxygen: observe respiratory status every hour with continuous pulse oximetry and arterial blood gas measurement as warranted, vital signs, controlled oxygen concentration, volume, temperature and humidity; oxygen should be warm and humidified.
   C. Signs of readiness: see Weaning from Respiratory Assistance section to formulate your answer; include signs of respiratory distress are no longer exhibited, ABGs and oxygen saturation are maintained within normal limits, newborn displays spontaneous adequate respiratory effort without difficulty and exhibits good color and improved muscle tone during increased activity.
   D. Guidelines: approach carefully, proceeding in a stepwise manner from one method to another with close observation for signs of good or poor tolerance of the change; reassure and keep parents informed throughout the process of weaning, pointing out signs that their newborn is breathing effectively and is well oxygenated.
2. Meeting nutritional needs of a preterm infant (see Nutritional Care and Gavage Feeding sections).
   A. Assessment to determine effectiveness of feeding method: observe for ability to suck and swallow and the coordination of each; signs of respiratory distress during the feeding; length of time for the feeding and the amount

ingested; presence of regurgitation, vomiting, or abdominal distention after feeding; daily weight gains and losses and elimination patterns.

B. Guidelines to follow when inserting a gavage tube: see Gavage Feeding section, Procedure box—Inserting a Gavage Feeding Tube, and Figure 37-6; emphasize tubing choice and measurement of length, insertion without trauma and securing to maintain placement, checking placement.

C. Nursing diagnosis: imbalanced nutrition: less than body requirements related to weak suck associated with premature status.

D. Principles to follow before, during, and after a gavage feeding:
   - Assess nutritional status (e.g., weight, elimination patterns, abdominal circumference) and tolerance of feedings (volume of residual gastric aspirate); check skin at site where tubing is secured.
   - Initiate measures to prevent aspiration with proper tube insertion, removal, and position check techniques.
   - Instill breast milk or formula at rate prescribed: assist mother to pump breasts.
   - Cuddle, swaddle infant during feedings; involve parents; use nonnutritive sucking: see Figure 37-7.
   - Document assessment findings and specifics of the procedure including newborn tolerance.

E. Advancing to oral feeding: see Advancing Infant Feedings section; proceed cautiously, checking for GI, nutritional, fluid, and electrolyte signs of tolerance or intolerance for advancement; decrease gavage feedings as ability to suck improves.

3. NICU environment: see Environmental Concerns section, Nursing Care Plan—High Risk Preterm Newborn, and Fig. 37-8.

   A. Common stressors
   - Infant stressors: continuous exposure to light and noise; administration of sedatives and pain medications; invasive procedures and medications required for treatment.
   - Family stressors: size and compromised and often fluctuating health status of their newborn; difficulty interacting with newborn and making eye contact; increased learning needs regarding status of newborn and care needs; concern regarding potential disabilities.

   B. Identify approach and avoidance newborn behaviors: see Developmental Care section for a description of these behaviors.

   C. Measures to provide a balance of stimuli for the newborn: see Developmental Care—Infant Communication section for many ideas, including waterbeds, kangaroo care, bundling, coordinated plan of care to provide for period of interrupted rest and sleep, use pain medications and sedatives as needed, provide diurnal light patterns, decrease noise level; use stroking, talking, mobiles, decals, music, and windup toys for stimulation.

   D. Guidelines for infant positioning: see Positioning section and Fig. 37-9; change position frequently, observing effect of position change on breathing and oxygenation and preventing aspiration; consider boundaries, body alignment, sense of security and comfort when positioning; teach parents; use facilitated tucking and blanket swaddling.

4. Postterm pregnancy: see Postmature Infant section.

   A. Rationale for increased mortality: increased oxygen demands are not met especially during labor and birth when contractions combine with an aging placenta to diminish perfusion and increase the likelihood for impaired gas exchange, leading to hypoxia and passage of meconium into amniotic fluid; risk for aspiration of meconium into lungs.

   B. Typical assessment findings among others include thin, emaciated appearance (dysmature) due to loss of subcutaneous fat and muscle mass; peeling of skin; meconium staining on fingernails; long hair and nails; absence of vernix.

   C. Two major complications: meconium aspiration syndrome and persistent pulmonary hypertension of the newborn (PPHN); see separate section that describes each complication.

5. Birth of a small for gestational age newborn (see Small for Gestational Age and Intrauterine Growth Restriction sections).

   A. Major complications: perinatal asphyxia with possible passage of meconium and aspiration, hypoglycemia and hyperglycemia, polycythemia, heat loss (cold stress).

   B. Physiologic basis for each identified complication: see separate section for each complication.

6. Transport to a tertiary center (see Transport to and from a Regional Center section, Box 37-7, and Fig. 37-15)

   A. Advantages of transport before birth.
   - Associated neonatal morbidity and mortality are decreased.
   - Infant-parent attachment is supported because separation is avoided.

   B. Stabilization of needs before transport: VS, oxygenation and ventilation, thermoregulation, acid-base balance, fluid/electrolyte status, glucose levels, and developmental interventions.

   C. Support measures for family: provide information about center (location, visiting hours, phone number, caregivers' names, rules), one parent accompany infant, see infant before transport, get status updates.

7. Parents of a preterm newborn (see Parental Adaptation to Preterm Infant and Parental Support sections and Nursing Care Plan—High Risk Preterm Newborn).

A. Identify parental tasks and nursing measures to help parents: measures should include ideas regarding helping parents get to know their newborn, informing of status, educating regarding care needs, providing emotional support and help with the grieving process, making referrals to parents groups and home care agencies, mobilizing family support system
B. Assessment of attachment progress and coping ability of parents: see Parental Responses and Parental Maladaptation sections and attachment content in Chapter 22 to formulate your answer; include progress of touch, eagerness to help with care, asking questions and demonstrating interest in status, visiting practices, and bringing items from home to identify the newborn as their own and part of a family.

8. Surfactant administration to preterm infant born at 26 weeks of gestation: see Oxygen Therapy—Surfactant section, and Medication Guide—Surfactant Replacement.
   A. Purpose of exogenous surfactant administration; preterm infant born before 34 weeks of gestation will be unable to produce enough surfactant to survive extrauterine life; exogenous surfactant will facilitate alveoli expansion and stability, easing respirations, and enhancing gas exchange until the newborn can produce sufficient quantities on its own; it is administered in several doses via an endotracheal tube directly into the lungs.
   B. Informing and reassuring parents; show parents how their baby is having difficulty breathing; discuss surfactant—what it does, how it can help their baby by preventing complications and increasing their baby's chances of survival, and why their baby does not have enough, thereby causing difficulty breathing; show them how it will be administered, including how their baby's comfort needs will be met and then, after administration, point out how it is helping their baby to breathe.
9. Kangaroo care: see Kangaroo Care section and Figure 37-10; explain what it is and why it is used; show pictures/film; report testimony of effectiveness from parents and nurses who have used kangaroo care; involve nurses and parents who had/have children in the NICU in creating the protocol that will be used to implement this form of care.
10. Pain of a newborn in NICU: see Infant Pain Responses section and Chapter 24 including Table 24-4.
    A. Explain how the newborn expresses pain: see Pain Assessment section and Box 37-6 for a list of behavioral responses in several categories; describe behaviors such as crying, body movements, and facial expressions and how they differ when infant is in pain when compared with common newborn responses.
    B. Evidence of infant pain memory: see Memory of Pain section for defensive-type behaviors that an infant might exhibit when painful procedures are repeated.
    C. Consequences of untreated pain: see Consequences of Untreated Pain in Infants section, which discusses physiologic and behavioral responses when pain is not relieved and how these responses can interfere with growth and development and positive adaptations to extrauterine life.
    D. Management strategies: see Pain Management section and Chapter 24; several measures are discussed for each type of relief measures; consider involvement of family in pain relief and tell them what you are doing to keep baby comfortable; show them how their baby is indicating that relief measures are working.

CHAPTER 38: PERINATAL LOSS AND GRIEF

I. Learning Key Terms

1. Grief, bereavement
2. Acute distress
3. Intense grief
4. Disorganization
5. Reorganization
6. Bittersweet grief
7. Caring framework, knowing, being with, doing for, enabling, maintaining belief
8. Complicated grief (Bereavement)

II. Reviewing Key Concepts

9. Pregnant woman at 24 weeks of gestation with suspected fetal death: see separate sections for a description of each phase and Box 38-1
   A. Acute distress
   B. Intense grief
   C. Disorganization
   D. Reorganization
10. Father's grief responses: see Acute Distress section; discuss each of the following:
    - Distressed by maternal grief
    - May be less able to share deep intense grief; special efforts are required to give them the support they may need
    - Experience a variable response depending on the degree to which he identified with the pregnancy
11. Use of the five components of the caring framework developed by Swanson to support grieving parents: see Communicate Using a Caring Framework section for a description of each component. Explain how you would use each of the following to help parents:
    - Knowing
    - Being with
    - Doing for
    - Enabling
    - Maintaining belief

12. Actualizing the loss: see Help the Mother, Father, and Other Family Members Actualize the Loss and Create Memories for Parents to Take Home sections; tangible memories of the baby can help parents actualize (make it a reality) the loss; help them participate in the options that are most appealing and comfortable for them; use baby's name and words such as dead and died; help parents tell their story; many other ideas are presented in these sections.
13. Complicated grief (bereavement): see Complicated grief (Bereavement) section.
    A. Characteristic behaviors: several behaviors are described in this section.
    B. Nursing approach: refer for counseling to a therapist or counselor who is experienced in grief counseling; be persistent in getting individual or family into counseling, especially to the first visit, enlisting other family members to help.
14. Choice A is correct; telling her to be happy that one twin survived may be interpreted that she should not grieve the loss of the daughter who died—the loss must be acknowledged and the tasks for mourners accomplished; B, C, and D are all appropriate responses by the nurse with B and C helpful in actualizing the loss.
15. Choice D is correct; A and B represent the intense grief phase and C represents the reorganization phase.
16. Choice B is correct; see Box 38-2; note that A, C, and D are in the category of what not to say, whereas B represents a response that acknowledges the difficulty of the loss and offers an opportunity for expression of feelings.

III. Thinking Critically

1. Family experiencing miscarriage at 13 weeks of gestation.
    A. Approach to individualize support measures: see Care Management section.
        - Begin with assessment to determine best approach to take for this couple.
        - Determine nature of the parental attachment with the pregnancy and the meaning of the pregnancy and birth to the parents.
        - Circumstances surrounding the loss—listen to their story.
        - The immediate response of each parent to the loss—do they match?
        - Persons comprising their social network and how can they support them; do the parents want their support?
    B. Cite questions and observations to gather information required to create an individualized plan of care: use each of the areas identified in **A** to formulate questions and organize observations.
    C. Nursing diagnoses: see Nursing Process box—Perinatal Grief; consider assessment findings to determine nursing diagnoses and their priority for a specific family.
        - Nursing diagnoses associated with emotional effects of grief: situational low self-esteem, spiritual distress, anxiety, ineffective individual coping
        - Nursing diagnoses associated with effect on family including other child and grandparents: interrupted family processes, ineffective family coping
        - Nursing diagnoses related to the physical effects of the grief process: fatigue, disturbed sleep pattern, imbalanced nutrition
    D. Therapeutic communication techniques to help couple express feelings and emotions: see Communicate Using a Caring Framework and Help the Bereaved Parents Acknowledge and Express Their Feelings sections and Box 38-2; examples of therapeutic communication techniques include encouraging expression of feelings by leaning forward, nodding, reflection, saying "tell me more"; observe nonverbal cues; use touch as appropriate; listen patiently and use silence while couple tell their story; avoid giving advice or using clichés, reassure regarding normalcy of emotions.
    E. Analysis of nurse responses: N, T, N, N, T, T, N, N, T, T
2. Physical needs of postpartum woman following stillbirth: see Meet the Physical Needs of the Postpartum Bereaved Mother section.
    - Provide option of staying on maternity unit or transferring to another—discuss the advantages and disadvantages of each option.
    - Provide option for room assignment (away from nursery).
    - Assist with breast care (milk coming in is a reminder of the loss).
    - Emphasize the importance of analgesics and comfort measures to help with rest and sleep.
    - Encourage adequate nutrition, fluids, balance of activity and rest to enhance strength and healing.
3. Birth of baby who died with anencephaly.
    A. Making the decision to see the baby: see Help Mother and Father and Other Family Members to Actualize the Loss, Create Memories for Parents to Take Home; and Help the Parents with Decision Making sections.
        - Tell them about the option to see the baby; consider that each parent may have different feelings.
        - Give them time to think about the option so they can choose what is best for them.
        - Come back and ask them their decision; if they are unsure or say no, ask again before discharge.
    B. Measures to help the couple when they see their baby.

- Explain to parents how the baby will look so they know what to expect.
- Prepare baby making it look as normal as possible—bathe, use powder, comb hair, put on ID bracelet, dress, wrap in a pretty blanket (get help from a funeral director if needed); give parents the opportunity to provide care because they may want to help bathe and dress the baby and leave mementos.
- Treat baby as one would a live baby when bringing baby to parents—use name, touch cheek, talk about baby's features emphasizing those that are normal, or resemble family members including themselves.
- Provide time alone with baby and adjust length of time with the baby to meet their needs—observe for cues that tell you they need more time or that they are done.
- Determine what else they would need to make a memory—footprint, photograph, lock of hair, etc.

4. Role of the nurse in supporting a pregnant woman at 16 weeks who is told her baby has anencephaly: see Prenatal Diagnosis with Negative Outcome and Be Concerned About Cultural and Spiritual Needs of Parents sections.
   - Fully explain anencephaly, and discuss her options.
   - Be a good listener encouraging her to express how she feels about the experience, including cultural and religious beliefs and values that will guide the option that she will choose.
   - Respect her decision and provide her with follow-up support including referral to a perinatal hospice program if she decides to continue the pregnancy or after elective abortion if that is her choice; if elective abortion is her choice, determine if she wishes to see the fetus.